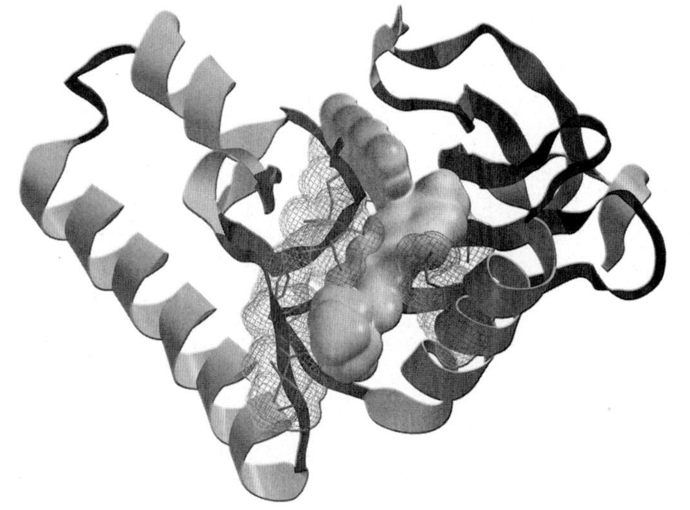

FOYE'S Principles of Medicinal Chemistry

SIXTH EDITION

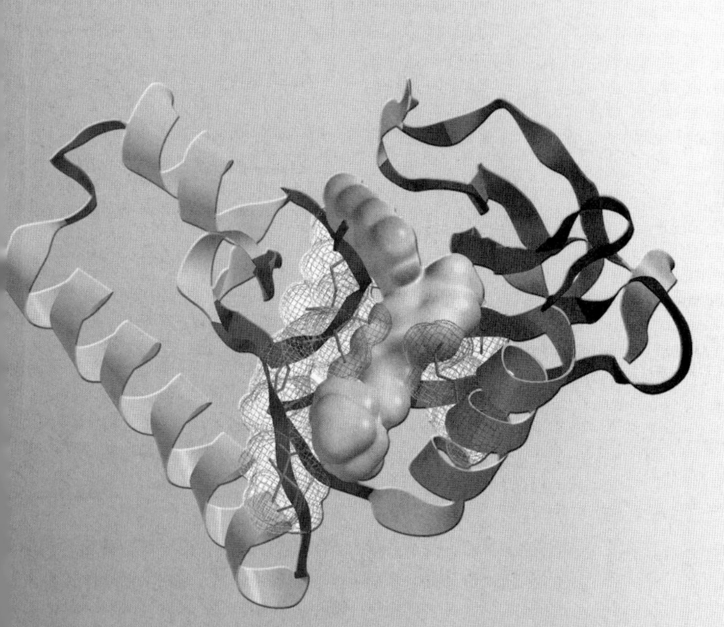

FOYE'S Principles of Medicinal Chemistry

SIXTH EDITION

Edited By

THOMAS L. LEMKE, PHD

Professor Emeritus
College of Pharmacy
University of Houston
Houston, Texas

DAVID A. WILLIAMS, PHD

Professor Emeritus of Chemistry
Massachusetts College of Pharmacy and Health Sciences
Boston, Massachusetts

Assistant Editors

VICTORIA F. ROCHE, PHD

Senior Associate Dean
School of Pharmacy and Health Professions
Creighton University
Omaha, Nebraska

S. WILLIAM ZITO, PHD

Professor of Pharmaceutical Sciences
College of Pharmacy and Allied Health Professions
St. John's University
Jamaica, New York

Wolters Kluwer Health | Lippincott Williams & Wilkins

Philadelphia • Baltimore • New York • London
Buenos Aires • Hong Kong • Sydney • Tokyo

Acquisitions Editor: David Troy
Managing Editor: Meredith Brittain
Marketing Manager: Christen Murphy
Production Editor: Hearthside Publishing Services
Designer: Sunflower Publishing Services
Graphic Artist: Nicole Williams
Compositor: Aptara

Cover image courtesy of Wavefunction, Inc. The ribbon display (green and red) is tyrosine kinase. The "active site" for tyrosine kinase is shown as tube display with a mesh-style electrostatic potential map (a charge distribution map), with the drug imatinib shown in the "active site" with a solid-color style electrostatic potential map (where the colors toward red depict negative potential; colors toward blue depict positive potentials; and colors such as yellow, orange, green, and violet depict intermediate values). Imatinib (a 2-phenyl amino pyrimidine derivative, a.k.a. CGP57148B, STI571 or Gleevec®) is a selective inhibitor of several tyrosine kinases that binds to the ATP-binding pocket of tyrosine kinase and blocks the activities of Abl, c-kit, and PDGFR. It is used for treating chronic myelogenous leukemia (CML), gastrointestinal stromal tumors (GISTs), and a number of other malignancies.

Sixth Edition

Copyright © 2008, 2002, 1995, 1989, 1981, 1974
Lippincott Williams & Wilkins, a Wolters Kluwer business.

351 West Camden Street
Baltimore, MD 21201

530 Walnut Street
Philadelphia, PA 19106

Printed in the USA

All rights reserved. This book is protected by copyright. No part of this book may be reproduced or transmitted in any form or by any means, including as photocopies or scanned-in or other electronic copies, or utilized by any information storage and retrieval system without written permission from the copyright owner, except for brief quotations embodied in critical articles and reviews. Materials appearing in this book prepared by individuals as part of their official duties as U.S. government employees are not covered by the above-mentioned copyright. To request permission, please contact Lippincott Williams & Wilkins at 530 Walnut Street, Philadelphia, PA 19106, via email at permissions@lww.com, or via website at lww.com (products and services).

9 8 7 6 5 4

Library of Congress Cataloging-in-Publication Data

Foye's principles of medicinal chemistry / edited by Thomas L. Lemke . . . [et al.]. — 6th ed.
p. ; cm.
Includes bibliographical references and index.
ISBN 978-0-7817-6879-5
1. Pharmaceutical chemistry. I. Foye, William O. II. Lemke, Thomas L.
III. Title: Principles of medicinal chemistry.
[DNLM: 1. Chemistry, Pharmaceutical. QV 744 F7962 2008]
RS403.P75 2008
616.07′56—dc22

2007026228

DISCLAIMER

Care has been taken to confirm the accuracy of the information present and to describe generally accepted practices. However, the authors, editors, and publisher are not responsible for errors or omissions or for any consequences from application of the information in this book and make no warranty, expressed or implied, with respect to the currency, completeness, or accuracy of the contents of the publication. Application of this information in a particular situation remains the professional responsibility of the practitioner; the clinical treatments described and recommended may not be considered absolute and universal recommendations.

The authors, editors, and publisher have exerted every effort to ensure that drug selection and dosage set forth in this text are in accordance with the current recommendations and practice at the time of publication. However, in view of ongoing research, changes in government regulations, and the constant flow of information relating to drug therapy and drug reactions, the reader is urged to check the package insert for each drug for any change in indications and dosage and for added warnings and precautions. This is particularly important when the recommended agent is a new or infrequently employed drug.

Some drugs and medical devices presented in this publication have Food and Drug Administration (FDA) clearance for limited use in restricted research settings. It is the responsibility of the health care provider to ascertain the FDA status of each drug or device planned for use in their clinical practice.

To purchase additional copies of this book, call our customer service department at **(800) 638-3030** or fax orders to **(301) 223-2320**. International customers should call **(301) 223-2300**.

Visit Lippincott Williams & Wilkins on the Internet: http://www.lww.com. Lippincott Williams & Wilkins customer service representatives are available from 8:30 am to 6:00 pm, EST.

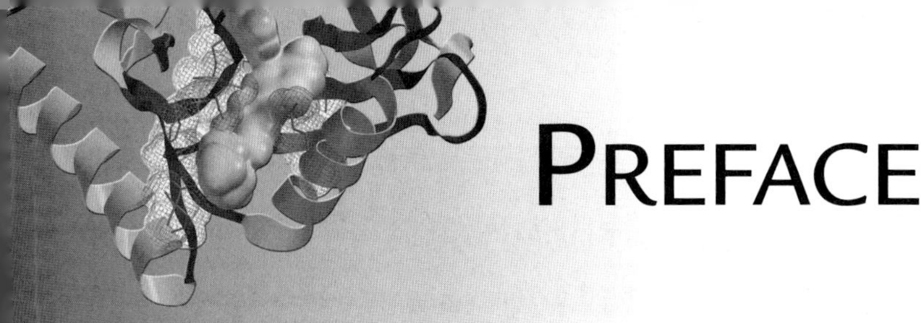

PREFACE

As defined by IUPAC, medicinal chemistry is a chemistry-based discipline, involving aspects of biological, medical and pharmaceutical sciences. It is concerned with the invention, discovery, design, identification and preparation of biologically active compounds, the study of their metabolism, the interpretation of their mode of action at the molecular level and the construction of structure-activity relationships (SAR), the relationship between chemical structure and pharmacological activity for a series of compounds.

As we look back 33 years to the first edition of *Foye's Principles of Medicinal Chemistry* and nearly 60 years to the first edition of Wilson and Gisvold's textbook, *Organic Chemistry in Pharmacy* (later renamed *Textbook of Organic Medicinal and Pharmaceutical Chemistry*), we can examine how the teaching of medicinal chemistry has evolved over the last half of the 20th century. Fifty years ago the approach to teaching drug classification was based on chemical functional groups; in the 1970s it was the relationship between chemical structure and pharmacological activity for a series of compounds, and today it is the integration of these principles with pharmacology and therapeutics into a single multi-semester course called pharmacodynamics, pharmacotherapeutics, or another similar name. Drug discovery and development maintains its role in traditional drug therapy, but its application to pharmacogenomics may well become the treatment modality of the future. The scope of knowledge in organic chemistry, biochemistry, pharmacology, and therapeutics allows students to make generalizations connecting the physicochemical properties of small organic molecules and peptides to the receptor and biochemical properties of living systems. As a consequence, these generalizations, validated by repetitive examples, emerge in time as principles of drug discovery and drug mechanisms, principles that describe the structural relationships between diverse organic molecules and the biomolecular functions that predict their mechanisms toward controlling diseases.

Medicinal chemistry is central to modern drug discovery and development. For most of the 20th century, the majority of drugs were discovered either by identifying the active ingredient in traditional natural remedies, by rational drug design, or by serendipity. Medicinal chemistry has advanced during the past several decades from not only synthesizing new compounds but to understanding the molecular basis of a disease and its control, identifying biomolecular targets implicated as disease-causing, and ultimately inventing specific compounds (called "hits") that block the biomolecules from progressing to an illness or stop the disease in its tracks. Medicinal chemists use structure-activity relationships to improve the "hits" into "lead candidates" by optimizing their selectivity against the target and reducing their activity against nontargets, and ADME (pharmacokinetics) to understand how the body causes drug clearance, what's involved in drug distribution, and the nature of the molecules that control those factors.

We are both medicinal chemists, and our approaches to editing this sixth edition of *Foye's Principles of Medicinal Chemistry* are influenced by our respective academic backgrounds. We believe that our collaboration on this textbook represents a melding of our perspectives that will provide new dimensions of appreciation and understanding for all students. In editing this multi-authored book we have tried to ensure a more-or-less consistent style in the organization of the respective chapters.

ORGANIZATIONAL PHILOSOPHY

The organizational approach we take in this textbook builds from the principles of drug discovery, physicochemical properties of drug molecules, and ADMET (absorption-distribution-metabolism-excretion-toxicity) to their integration into therapeutic substances. Our challenge has been to provide a comprehensive description of drug discovery and pharmacodynamic agents in an introductory textbook. To address the increasing emphasis in U.S. pharmacy schools to integrating medicinal chemistry with pharmacology and clinical pharmacy and the creation of one-semester principle courses, we organized the book into four parts: Part I: Principles of Drug Discovery; Part II: Drug Receptors Affecting Neurotransmission and Enzymes as Catalytic Receptors; Part III: Pharmacodynamic Agents (with further subdivision into drugs affecting different systems of the body); and Part IV: Disease State Management. Parts I and II are designed for the one-semester course in principles of drug discovery and Parts II through IV for an integrated course or courses in pharmacodynamics/pharmacotherapeutics.

WHAT IS NEW IN THIS EDITION

The pharmacist sits at the interphase between the healthcare system and the patient. The pharmacist has the responsibility for improving the quality of life of the patient by assuring the appropriate use of pharmaceuticals. To do this appropriately, the pharmacist must bring together the basic sciences of chemistry, biology, biopharmaceutics and pharmacology with the clinical sciences. In an attempt to relate the importance of medicinal chemistry to the clinical sciences, each of the chapters in Part III, Pharmacodynamic Agents, and Part IV, Disease State Management, includes the following:

- **A clinical significance section:** Near the beginning of the chapter, a prominent scientist has provided a statement of the clinical significance of medicinal chemistry to the particular subject matter.
- **A case study:** Each of these chapters ends with a case study (see the "Introduction to Medicinal Case Studies" section of this preface).

In addition, the reader will find at the beginning of most chapters a list of drugs (presented by generic or chemical names) discussed in that chapter.

Several new chapters appear in the sixth edition, including Chapter 15, Amino Acid Neurotransmitters in the Central Nervous System; Chapter 17, Phosphodiesterase Inhibitors; Chapter 21, Antidepressants; and Chapter 44, Asthma and Chronic Obstructive Pulmonary Disease. In addition, previously included material has been updated and reorganized into Chapter 45, Men's Health, and Chapter 46, Women's Health.

Lastly, color plates have been added to this edition to help the reader visualize drug-receptor interactions. Such interactions cannot easily be appreciated by word descriptions and are difficult to see in black-and-white figures. The editors hope that the beauty and complexity of drug-receptor interactions will excite the imagination of the reader.

STUDENT AND INSTRUCTOR RESOURCES

Student Resources

A Student Resource Center at http://thePoint.lww.com/lemke6e includes the following materials:

- Interactive practice quizzes
- Additional case studies and answers
- Answers to the problems in Chapter 2
- A Drug Update section with short monographs of new drugs (complete with references) that have appeared on the market since publication of the latest edition of this book
- An Image Bank that contains the figures and tables from the textbook

Instructor Resources

We understand the demand on an instructor's time, so to help make your job easier, you will have access to Instructor Resources upon adoption of *Foye's Principles of Medicinal Chemistry, 6th edition.* An Instructor's Resource Center at http://thePoint.lww.com/lemke6e includes the following:

- Answers to the case studies that appear in the book
- The resources listed in the student resources section, above

ACKNOWLEDGMENTS

We are indebted to our knowledgeable contributors, for without them this book would not exist; to Vickie Roche and Sandy Zito for creating the case studies; to our respective Deans, Department Chairs, and senior administrators for allowing us the time and facilities to complete this book; to Stephen Kerr, who reviewed Ch. 21; to Brian L. LaRowe and Vicki Nussbaum, for reviewing the case studies; and to colleagues at various institutions who carefully reviewed portions of the chapter manuscripts for accuracy and wrote the clinical significance sections.

We gratefully acknowledge many other people who assisted and encouraged us in writing and editing this sixth edition. These include the managing editor Meredith Brittan for her tactfulness in keeping us on schedule, Matt Hauber who has been a part of the publication team for the last several editions, and the other editorial staff members at LWW. We owe a very special ***thank you*** to our devoted wives for their understanding and sacrifices over the past several years.

With the publication of this sixth edition of this book, we celebrate and commemorate the contributions of William O. Foye, whose vision founded this textbook. We also commemorate the contributions of Charles Wilson and Ole Gisvold, who founded the first textbook in pharmaceutical and medicinal chemistry and introduced many of us to the world of medicinal chemistry, and the contributions of research mentors who influenced our teachings in medicinal chemistry, William O. Foye, Edward Smissman, and Philip S. Portoghese.

Thomas L. Lemke PhD
Professor Emeritus
College of Pharmacy
University of Houston
Houston, Texas

David A. Williams PhD
Professor Emeritus of Chemistry
Massachusetts College of Pharmacy and Health Sciences
Boston, Massachusetts

INTRODUCTION TO MEDICINAL CHEMISTRY CASE STUDIES

We are pleased to share our newest medicinal chemistry case studies with student and faculty users of *Foye's Principles of Medicinal Chemistry, 6th edition.* One case study is provided at the end of most chapters. This preface is written to explain their scope and purpose, and help those who are unfamiliar with our technique of illustrating the therapeutic relevance of chemistry get the most out of the exercise.

Like the more familiar therapeutic case studies, medicinal chemistry case studies are clinical scenarios that present a patient in need of a pharmacist's expert intervention. The learner, in the role of the pharmacist, evaluates the patient's clinical and personal situation and makes a drug product selection from a limited number of therapeutic choices. However, in a medicinal chemistry case study, only the structures of the potential therapeutic candidates are given. To make their professional recommendation, students must conduct a thorough analysis of key *structure activity relationships (SAR)* in order to predict such things as relative potency, receptor selectivity, duration of action and potential for adverse reactions, and then apply the knowledge gained to meet the patient's therapeutic needs.

The therapeutic choices we offer in each case have been carefully selected to allow students to thoroughly review the therapeutically relevant chemistry of the classes of drugs used to treat a particular disease. By working thoughtfully and scientifically through the cases, students will not only master chemical concepts and principles and reinforce basic SAR, but also learn how to actively use their unique knowledge of drug chemistry when thinking critically about patient care. This skill will be invaluable to you when, as a practitioner, you are faced with a full gamut of therapeutic options to analyze in order to ensure the best therapeutic outcomes for your patients.

In short, here's what we hope you will gain by working our cases.

- Mastery of the important concepts needed to be successful in the medicinal chemistry component of your pharmacy curriculum;
- An understanding of the relevance of drug chemistry to pharmacological action and therapeutic utility, and the ability to discriminate between therapeutic options based on that understanding;
- An enhanced ability to think critically and scientifically about drug use decisions;
- A commitment to caring about the impact of your professional decisions on your patients' quality of life;
- An appreciation of your unique role as the chemist of the health care team.

We hope you find these case studies both challenging and enjoyable, and encourage you to use them as a springboard to more in-depth discussions with your faculty about the role of chemistry in rational therapeutic decision-making.

Victoria F. Roche, PhD
Senior Associate Dean
School of Pharmacy and Health Professions
Creighton University
Omaha, Nebraska

S. William Zito, PhD
Professor of Pharmaceutical Sciences
College of Pharmacy and Allied Health Professions
St. John's University
Jamaica, New York

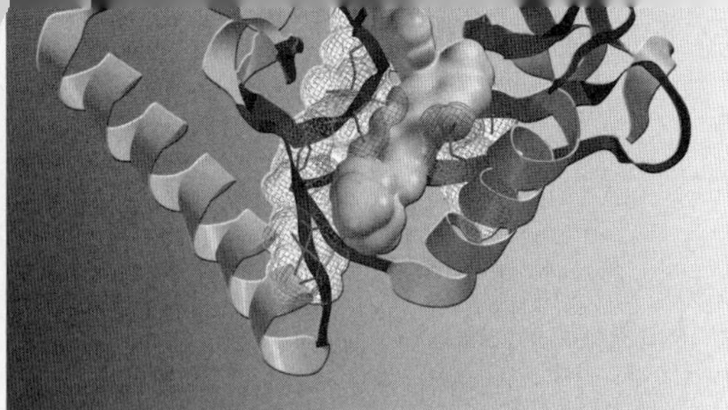

CONTRIBUTORS

Ali Banijamali, PhD
Research Fellow
Chemtura Corporation
Middlebury, CT

Raymond Booth, PhD
Associate Professor
University of Florida
Gainesville, FL

Ronald Borne, PhD
Professor Emeritus
University of Mississippi
Oxford, MS

Robert W. Brueggemeier, PhD
Dean, College of Pharmacy
Professor, Division of Medicinal Chemistry and Pharmacognosy
Ohio State University College of Pharmacy
Columbus, OH

Bruce Currie, PhD
Professor of Medicinal Chemistry
Chair, Department of Pharmaceutical Sciences
School of Pharmacy
Loma Linda University
Loma Linda, CA

Kevin Dalby, PhD
Associate Professor
Division of Medicinal Chemistry
The University of Texas at Austin
Austin, TX

James T. Dalton, PhD
Kimberly Professor
Division of Pharmaceutics
Ohio State University College of Pharmacy
Columbus, OH

Malgorzata Dukat-Glennon, PhD
Associate Professor
School of Pharmacy
Virginia Commonwealth University
Richmond, VA

E. Kim Fifer, PhD
Professor
University of Arkansas for Medical Sciences
Little Rock, AR

David Fries, PhD
Professor
University of the Pacific
Stockton, CA

Elmer Gentry, PhD
Associate Professor
Midwestern University
Glendale, AZ

Richard Glennon, PhD
Professor and Chair
Virginia Commonwealth University
Richmond, VA

Robert Griffith, PhD
Associate Professor
West Virginia University
Morgantown, WV

Marc Harrold, BS, PhD
Professor
Duquesne University
Pittsburgh, PA

Sunil Jambhekar, BPharm., PhD
Professor
LECOM–Bradenton
School of Pharmacy
Bradenton, FL

David A. Johnson, PhD
Associate Professor
Mylan School of Pharmacy
Duquesne University
Pittsburgh, PA

Stephen Kerr, BSc, PhD
Assistant Professor
Massachusetts College of Pharmacy and Health Sciences
Boston, MA

A. Douglas Kinghorn, PhD, DSc
Jack Beal Professor and Chair
Division of Medicinal Chemistry & Pharmacognosy
Ohio State University College of Pharmacy
Columbus, OH

James Knittel, PhD
Associate Professor
University of Cincinnati
Cincinnati, OH

John L. Krstenansky, PhD
Associate Professor
Loma Linda University
Loma Linda, CA

Barbara LeDuc, PhD
Associate Professor
Massachusetts College of Pharmacy and Health Sciences
Boston, MA

Thomas L. Lemke, PhD
Professor Emeritus
University of Houston
Houston, TX

Mark Levi, PhD
Research Instructor
University of Arkansas for Medical Sciences
Little Rock, AR

Matthias Lu, PhD
Professor
College of Pharmacy
University of Illinois at Chicago
Chicago, IL

Timothy Maher, PhD
Professor
Massachusetts College of Pharmacy and Health Sciences
Boston, MA

Ahmed Mehanna, PhD
Professor
Massachusetts College of Pharmacy and Health Sciences
Boston, MA

Duane Miller, PhD
Professor, Chair and Associate Dean
University of Tennessee
Memphis, TN

Lester Mitscher, BS, PhD
University Distinguished Professor
Kansas University
Lawrence, KS

Michael Mokotoff, PhD
Professor Emeritus
University of Pittsburgh
Pittsburgh, PA

Wendel Nelson, PhD
Professor
University of Washington
Seattle, WA

John Neumeyer, PhD
Matthews Distinguished Professor (Emeritus)
Harvard Medical School
Belmont, MA

Douglas Pisano, PhD
Professor and Associate Provost of Pharmacy Education
Massachusetts College of Pharmacy and Health Sciences
Boston, MA

Gary Rankin, PhD
Professor and Chair
Marshall University
Huntington, WV

Ronald Reid, BSP, PhD
Professor
University of British Columbia
Vancouver, British Columbia

Victoria F. Roche, PhD
Senior Associate Dean
School of Pharmacy and Health Professions
Creighton University
Omaha, NE

Robert Sindelar, BA, MS, PhD
Professor and Dean
University of British Columbia
Vancouver, British Columbia

William Soine, PhD
Professor Emeritus
Virginia Commonwealth University
Richmond, VA

Marilyn Speedie, PhD
Dean and Professor
University of Minnesota
St. Paul, MN

David Triggle, PhD
Professor
University at Buffalo
The State University of New York
Buffalo, NY

David A. Williams, PhD
Professor Emeritus of Chemistry
Massachusetts College of Pharmacy and Health Sciences
Boston, MA

Norman Wilson, BSc, PhD, CChem, FRSC
University of Edinburgh
Edinburgh, Scotland

Patrick M. Woster, BS, PhD
Professor
Wayne State University
Detroit, MI

Xiang-Qun (Sean) Xie, Ph.D., MBA
Professor
Drug Discovery Institute
University of Pittsburgh
Pittsburgh, PA

Robin Zavod, BS, MS, PhD
Associate Professor
Midwestern University
Downers Grove, IL

S. William Zito, PhD
Professor of Pharmaceutical Sciences
College of Pharmacy and Allied Health Professions
St. John's University
Jamaica, NY

WRITERS OF "CLINICAL SIGNIFICANCE" SECTIONS

Kimberly Birtcher, PharmD
Clinical Assistant Professor
Department of Clinical Sciences and Administration
College of Pharmacy
University of Houston
Houston, TX

Heidi H. Bragg, RPh
Clinical Assistant Professor
Department of Clinical Sciences and Administration
College of Pharmacy
University of Houston
Houston, TX

Elizabeth Coyle, PharmD
Clinical Assistant Professor
Department of Clinical Sciences and Administration
College of Pharmacy
University of Houston
Houston, TX

Joseph V. Etzel, PharmD
Assistant Dean of Student Affairs
Associate Clinical Professor of Pharmacy
College of Pharmacy and Allied Health Professions
St. John's University
Jamaica, NY

Laura Gerard, PharmD, BCPS
Clinical Assistant Professor
Department of Clinical Sciences and Administration
College of Pharmacy
University of Houston
Houston, TX

Michael Gonyeau, PharmD
Associate Clinical Specialist
Department of Pharmacy Practice
Bouvé College of Health Sciences
Northeastern University
Boston, MA

Catherine L. Hatfield, PharmD
Clinical Assistant Professor
Department of Clinical Sciences and Administration
College of Pharmacy
University of Houston
Houston, TX

David Hayes, PharmD
Clinical Assistant Professor
Department of Clinical Sciences and Administration
College of Pharmacy
University of Houston
Houston, TX

Jill T. Johnson, PharmD, BCPS
Associate Professor
Department of Pharmacy Practice
College of Pharmacy
University of Arkansas for Medical Sciences
Little Rock, AR

Matthias Lu, PhD
Professor
College of Pharmacy
University of Illinois at Chicago
Chicago, IL

Dalia R. Mack, PharmD
Assistant Clinical Specialist
Department of Pharmacy Practice
Bouvé College of Health Sciences
Northeastern University
Boston, MA

Kathryn Neill, PharmD
Assistant Professor
Critical Care Specialist
Department of Pharmacy Practice
College of Pharmacy
University of Arkansas for Medical Sciences
Little Rock, AR

Edith A. Nutescu, PharmD
Clinical Associate Professor
Director, Antithrombosis Center
College of Pharmacy
The University of Illinois at Chicago
Chicago, IL

Kelly Nystrom, PharmD, BCOP
Assistant Professor
Pharmacy Practice Department
School of Pharmacy and Health Professions
Creighton University
Omaha, NE

Nancy Ordonez, PharmD
Clinical Assistant Professor
College of Pharmacy
University of Houston
Houston, TX

Nathan A. Painter, PharmD
Assistant Professor of Pharmacy Practice
School of Pharmacy
Loma Linda University
Loma Linda, CA

Thomas L. Rihn, PharmD
Senior Vice President and Chief Clinical Officer
University Pharmacotherapy Associates and Associate Professor of Clinical Pharmacy
School of Pharmacy
Duquesne University
Pittsburgh, PA

Jeffrey T. Sherer, PharmD, MPH, BCPS, CGP
Clinical Assistant Professor
College of Pharmacy
University of Houston
Houston, TX

Douglas Slain, PharmD, BCPS
Associate Professor
College of Pharmacy
West Virginia University
Morgantown, WV

Christian Teter, PharmD
Assistant Professor
Department of Pharmacy Practice
Bouvé College of Health Sciences
Northeastern University
Boston, MA

Mark D. Watanabe, PharmD, PhD, BCPP
Assistant Clinical Specialist
Department of Pharmacy Practice
Bouvé College of Health Sciences
Northeastern University
Boston, MA

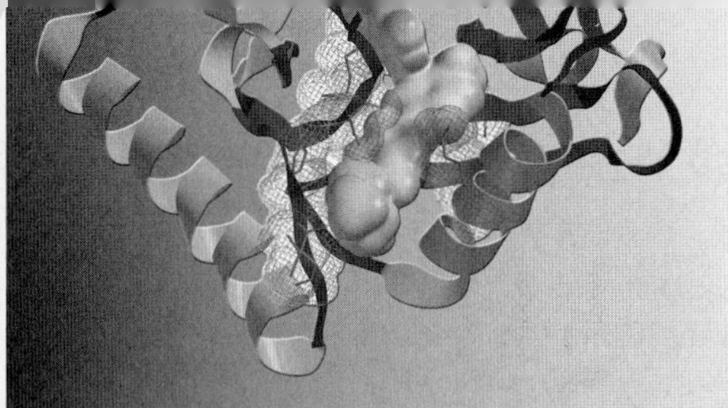

Reviewers

Stelvio Bandiera, PhD
Professor, Faculty of Pharmaceutical Sciences
The University of British Columbia
Vancouver, British Columbia

Jesse Blankenship
Johns Hopkins University
Baltimore, Maryland

Michael R. Borenstein, PhD
Chairman
Temple University
Philadelphia, Pennsylvania

Jack DeRuiter, PhD
Associate Professor
Auburn University
Auburn, Alabama

Philip G. Kerr, PhD
School of Biomedical Sciences
Charles Sturt University
Wagga Wagga, NSW, Australia

Brian L. LaRowe, MSc, RPh
Senior Clinical Pharmacist, Clinical Instructor
University of Wisconsin Hospital/Clinics, University of Wisconsin School of Pharmacy
Madison, Wisconsin

Vicki Nussbaum, PharmD, BCOP
Clinical Pharmacist
University of Wisconsin-Madison
Madison, Wisconsin

Amjad Qandil, PhD
Faculty of Pharmacy
Jordan University of Science and Technology
Jordan

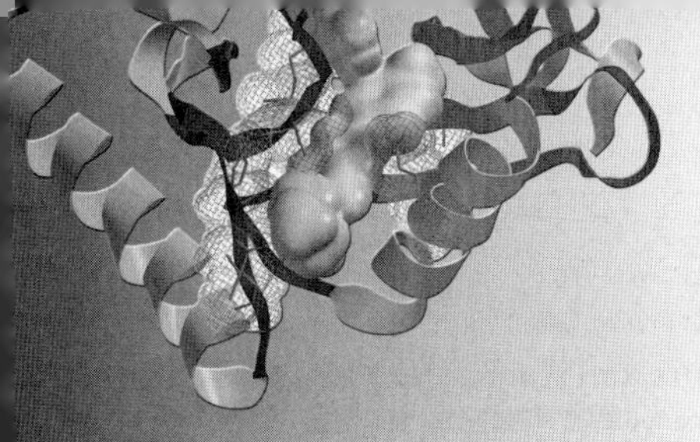

Contents

Historical Perspective of Medicinal Chemistry

JOHN L. NEUMEYER

"The unprecedented increase in human life expectancy, which has almost doubled in a hundred years, is mainly due to drugs and to those who discovered them." (1)

HISTORY AND EVOLUTION OF MEDICINAL CHEMISTRY

Just as in all fields of science, the history of medicinal chemistry is comprised of the ideas, knowledge, and available tools that have advanced contemporary knowledge. The spectacular advances in medicinal chemistry over the years are no exception. Burger (1) stated that "the great advances of medicinal chemistry have been achieved by two types of investigators: those with the genius of prophetic logic, who have opened a new field by interpreting correctly a few well-placed experiments, whether they pertained to the design or the mechanism of action of drugs; and those who have varied patiently the chemical structures of physiologically active compounds until a useful drug could be evolved as a tool in medicine."

To place the development of medicinal chemical research into its proper perspective, one needs to examine the evolution of the ideas and concepts that have led to our present knowledge.

Drugs of Antiquity

The oldest records of the use of therapeutic plants and minerals are derived from the ancient civilizations of the Chinese, the Hindus, the Mayans of Central America, and the Mediterranean peoples of antiquity. The Emperor Shen Nung (2735 BC) compiled what may be called a pharmacopeia, including *ch'ang shang*, an antimalarial alkaloid, and *ma huang*, from which ephedrine was isolated. Chaulmoogra fruit was known to the indigenous American Indians, and the ipecacuanha root containing emetine was used in Brazil for the treatment of dysentery and diarrhea and is still used for the treatment of amebiasis. The early explorers found that the South American Indians also chewed cocoa leaves (containing cocaine) and used mushrooms (containing tryptamine) as hallucinogens. In ancient Greek apothecary shops could be found herbs such as opium, squill, hyoscyamus, and viper toxin and such metallic drugs as copper and zinc ores, iron sulfate, and cadmium oxide.

The Middle Ages

The basic studies of chemistry and physics shifted from the Greco-Roman to the Arabian alchemists between the thirteenth and sixteenth centuries. Paracelsus (1493–1541) glorified antimony and its salts in elixirs as cure-alls in the belief that chemicals could cure disease.

The Nineteenth Century Age of Innovation and Chemistry

The nineteenth century saw a great expansion in the knowledge of chemistry, which greatly extended the herbal pharmacopeia that had previously been established. Building on the work of Lavoisier, chemists throughout Europe refined and extended the techniques of chemical analysis. The synthesis of acetic acid by Kolbe in 1845 and of methane by Berthelot in 1856 set the stage for organic chemistry. Pharmacognosy, the science that deals with medicinal products of plant, animal, or mineral origin in their crude state, was replaced by physiological chemistry. The emphasis was shifted from finding new medicaments from the vast world of plants to finding the active ingredients that accounted for their pharmacologic properties. The isolation of morphine by Sertürner in 1803, of emetine from ipecacuanha by Pelletier in 1816, and his purification of caffeine, quinine, and colchicine in 1820 all contributed to the increased use of "pure" substances as therapeutic agents. The nineteenth century also contributed to the use of digitalis by William Withering, the English physician and botanist, for the treatment of dropsy. Niemann isolated cocaine in 1860 and the active ingredient, physostigmine, from the calabar bean in 1864. As a result of these discoveries and the progress made in organic chemistry, the pharmaceutical industry came into being at the end of the nineteenth century.

The Twentieth Century and the Pharmaceutical Industry

Diseases of protozoal and spirochetal origin responded to synthetic chemotherapeutic agents. Interest in synthetic chemicals that could inhibit the rapid reproduction of pathogenic bacteria and enable the host organism to cope with invasive bacteria was dramatically increased when Domagk reported that the red dyestuff 2,4-diaminoazobenzene-4′-sulfonamide (Prontosil) dramatically cured dangerous, systemic Gram-positive bacterial infections in man and animals. The observation by Woods and Fildes in 1940 that the bacteriostatic action of sulfonamide-like drugs was antagonized by *p*-aminobenzoic acid was one of the early examples in which a balance of stimulatory and inhibitory properties depends on the structural analogies of chemicals.

Together with the discovery of penicillin by Fleming in 1929 and its subsequent examination by Florey and Chain in 1941, this led to a water soluble powder of much higher antibacterial potency and lower toxicity than those of previously known synthetic chemotherapeutic agents. With the discovery of a variety of highly potent anti-infective agents, a significant change was introduced into medical practice.

DEVELOPMENTS LEADING TO VARIOUS MEDICINAL CLASSES

Psychopharmacologic Agents and the Era of Brain Research

Psychiatrists have been using agents that are active in the central nervous system for hundreds of years. Stimulants and depressants were used to modify the mood and mental states of psychiatric patients. Amphetamine, sedatives, and hypnotics were used to stimulate or depress the mental states of patients. The synthesis of chlorpromazine by Charpentier ultimately caused a revolution in the treatment of schizophrenia, but who really discovered chlorpromazine? Charpentier, who first synthesized the molecule in 1950 at Rhone-Poulenc's research laboratory; Simon Courvoisier, who reported distinctive effects on animal behavior; Henri Laborit, a French military surgeon who first noticed distinctive psychotropic effects in man; or Pierre Deniker and Jean Delay, French psychiatrists who clearly outlined what has now become its accepted use in psychiatry and without whose endorsement and prestige Rhone-Poulenc might never have developed it further as an antipsychotic. Because of the bitter disputes over the discovery of chlorpromazine, no Nobel Prize was ever awarded for what has been the single most important breakthrough in psychiatric treatment.

The discovery of the antidepressant effects of the antitubercular drug iproniazid led to the first-generation tricyclic antidepressant imipramine in 1957 and the monoamine oxidase inhibitor phenelzine. These were followed by present-day selective serotonin reuptake inhibitors, such as fluoxetine (Prozac). The antianxiety agents in the benzodiazepine class are examples of the serendipitous discovery of new drugs based on random screening of chemicals synthesized in the laboratory. The discovery of these drugs also was based on observations made by pharmacologists who recognized significant animal signs during general biologic screening of random chemicals. In 1946, F.M. Berger and, in 1957, L.O. Randall, working at Hoffmann LaRoche Laboratories, independently observed unusual and characteristic paralysis and relaxation of voluntary muscles in laboratory animals for different series of compounds. At this point, the treatment of ambulatory, anxious patients with meprobamate and of psychotic patients with one of the aminoalkylphenothiazine drugs was possible. There was a need for drugs of greater selectivity in the treatment of anxiety because of the side effects often encountered with phenothiazines. Leo Sternback, a chemist working in the research laboratory of Hoffman-LaRoche in New Jersey, decided to reinvestigate a relatively unexplored class of compounds that he had studied in the 1930s, when he was a postdoctoral fellow at the University of Cracow in Poland. He synthesized approximately 40 compounds in this series, all of which were disappointing in pharmacologic tests, after which the project was abandoned. In 1957, during a cleanup of the laboratory, one compound synthesized 2 years earlier had crystallized and was submitted for testing to L.O. Randall, a pharmacologist. Shortly thereafter, Randall reported that this compound was hypnotic and sedative and had antistrychnine effects similar to those of meprobamate. The compound was named chlordiazepoxide and marketed as Librium in 1960, just 3 years after the first pharmacologic observations by Randall. Structural modifications of benzodiazepine derivatives were undertaken, and a compound 5- to 10-fold more potent than chlordiazepoxide was synthesized in 1959 and marketed as diazepam (Valium) in 1963. The synthesis of many other experimental analogues soon followed, and by 1983, approximately 35 benzodiazepine drugs were available for therapy (see Chapter 22). Benzodiazepines are used in the pharmacotherapy of anxiety and related emotional disorders and in the treatment of sleep disorders, status epilepticus, and other convulsive states. They are used as centrally acting muscle relaxants, for premedication, and as inducing agents in anesthesiology.

Endocrine Therapy and Steroids

The first pure hormone to be isolated from an endocrine gland was epinephrine, which led to further molecular modifications in the area of sympathomimetic amines. Subsequently, norepinephrine was identified from sympathetic nerves. The development of chromatographic techniques allowed the isolation and characterization of a multitude of hormones from a single gland. In 1914, biochemist Edward Kendall isolated thyroxine (T_4) from the thyroid gland. He subsequently won the Nobel Prize in Physiology or Medicine in 1950 for his discovery of the activity of cortisone. Two of the hormones of the thyroid gland, T_4 and liothyronine (T_3,3,5,3′-triiodo-thyronine) have similar effects in the body, regulating metabolism, whereas the two hormones from the posterior pituitary gland, vasopressin, which exerts pressor and antidiuretic activity, and oxytocin, which stimulates lactation and uterine motility, differ considerably both in their chemical structure and physiological activity (Fig. I.1).

Less than 50 years after the discovery of oxytocin in 1904 by Sir Henry Dale, who found that an extract from the human pituitary gland contracted the uterus of a pregnant cat, the biochemist du Vigneud synthesized the cyclic peptide hormone. His work resulted in the Nobel Prize in Chemistry in 1955.

A major achievement in drug discovery and development was the discovery of insulin in 1921 from animal sources. Frederick G. Bunting and Charles H. Best, working in the laboratory of John J.R. McLeod at the University of Toronto, isolated the polypeptide hormone and began testing it in dogs. By 1922, researchers, with the

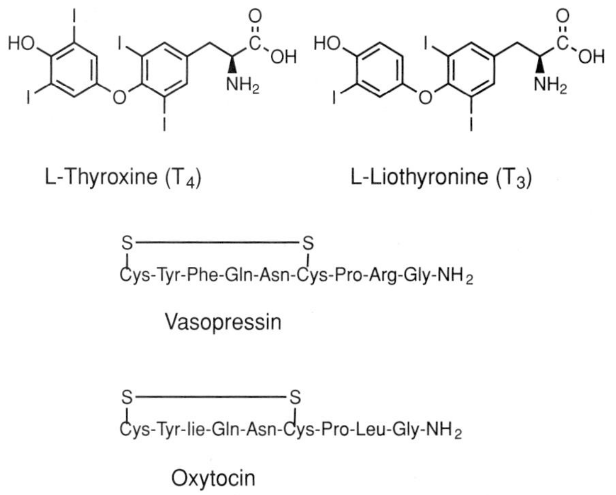

L-Thyroxine (T_4) L-Liothyronine (T_3)

Cys-Tyr-Phe-Gln-Asn-Cys-Pro-Arg-Gly-NH_2

Vasopressin

Cys-Tyr-Iie-Gln-Asn-Cys-Pro-Leu-Gly-NH_2

Oxytocin

Fig. I.1. Hormones from the endocrine glands.

help of James B. Collip and the pharmaceutical industry, were able to purify and produce animal-based insulin in large quantities. Insulin soon became a major product for Eli Lilly & Co. and Novo Nordisk, a Danish pharmaceutical company. In 1923, McLeod and Bunting were awarded the Nobel Prize in Medicine or Physiology, and after much controversy, they shared the prize with Collip and Best. For the next 60 years, cattle and pigs were the major sources of insulin. With the development of genetic engineering in the 1970s, new opportunities arose for making synthetic insulin that is chemically identical to human insulin. In 1978, the biotech company Genentech and the City of Hope National Medical Center produced human insulin in the laboratory using recombinant DNA technology. By 1982, Lilly's Humulin became the first genetically engineered drug to be approved by the U.S. Food and Drug Administration (FDA). At about the same time, Novo Nordisk began selling the first semisynthetic human insulin made by enzymatically converting porcine insulin. Novo Nordisk also was using recombinant technology to produce insulin. Recombinant insulin was a significant milestone in the development of genetically engineered drugs, and it combined the technologies of the biotech companies with the know-how and resources of the major pharmaceutical industries. Inhaled insulin was approved by the FDA in 2006. Many drugs are now available (see Chapter 32) to treat the more common type 2 diabetes, in which natural insulin production in the human needs to be increased. Insulin had been the only treatment for type 1 diabetes until 2005, when the FDA approved Amylin Pharmaceuticals' Symlin to control blood sugar levels in combination with the polypeptide hormone. The isolation and purification of several polypeptide hormones of the anterior pituitary and hypothalamic-releasing hormones now makes it possible to produce synthetic peptide agonists and antagonists that have important diagnostic and therapeutic applications.

Extensive and remarkable advances in the endocrine field have been made through an understanding, development, and utilization of steroid hormones. The isolation and characterization of minute amounts of the active principles of the sex glands and from the adrenal cortex eventually led to their total synthesis. The various male and female sex hormones are used in the treatment of a variety of disorders associated with sexual development and the sexual cycles of males and females as well as in the selective therapy of malignant tumors of the breast and prostate gland. Synthetic modifications of the structure of the male and female hormones have furnished improved hormonal compounds, such as the anabolic agents (see Chapter 45). Since early days, women have ingested every manner of substance as birth control agents. In the early 1930s, Russell Marker found that for hundreds of years, Mexican women had been eating wild yams of the *Dioscorea* genus for contraception, apparently successfully. Marker determined that diosgenin is abundant in yams and has a structure similar to that of progesterone. Marker was able to convert diosgenin into progesterone, a substance known to stop ovulation in rabbits. Progesterone, however, is destroyed by the digestive system when ingested. In 1950, Carl Djerassi, a chemist working at the Syntex Laboratories in Mexico City, synthesized norethindrone, the first orally active contraceptive steroid, by a subtle modification of the structure of progesterone. Gregory Pincus, a biologist working at the Worcester Foundation for Experimental Biology in Massachusetts studied Djerassi's new steroid together with its double-bond isomer norethynodrel (Fig. I.2).

By 1956, clinical studies led by John Rock, a gynecologist, showed that progesterone, in combination with norethindrone, was an effective oral contraceptive. G.D. Searle was the first on the market with Enovid, a combination of mestranol and norethynodrel. In 2005. approximately 11 million American women, and approximately 100 million women worldwide, were using oral contraceptive pills. In 1993, the British weekly *The Economist* considered the pill to be one of the seven wonders of the

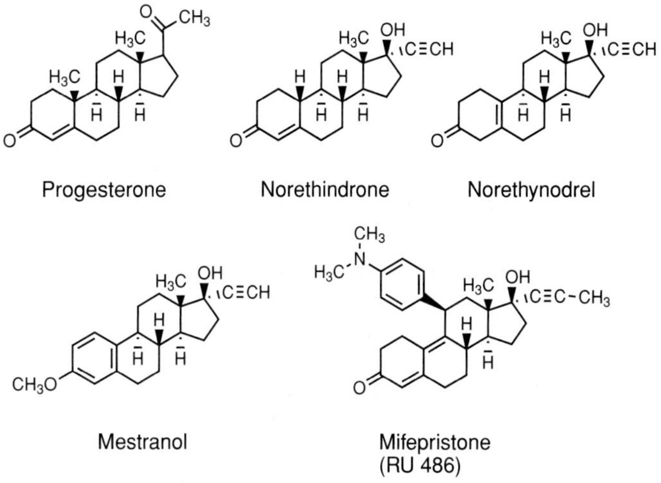

Progesterone Norethindrone Norethynodrel

Mestranol Mifepristone (RU 486)

Fig. I.2. Steroidal agents.

modern world, bringing about major changes in the economic and social structure for women throughout the world.

In the early 1930s, chemists recognized the similarity of a large number of natural products, including the cortical steroids, such as hydrocortisone. The medicinal value of Kendall's Compound F and Reichstein's Compound M was quickly recognized. The 1950 Nobel Prize in Physiology or Medicine was awarded to Philip S. Hench, Edward C. Kendall, and Tadeus Reichstein "for their discovery relating to the hormones of the adrenal cortex, their structure and biological effects" (2).

An interesting development in the study of glucocorticoids led to the synthesis in 1980 of the "abortion pill," RU-486, by Etienne-Emile Beaulieu, a consultant to the French pharmaceutical company Rousel-Uclaf. Researchers at that time were investigating glucocorticoid antagonists for the treatment of breast cancer, glaucoma, and Cushing's syndrome. In screening RU-486, researchers at Rousel-Uclaf found that it had both antiglucocorticoid activity as well as high affinity for progesterone receptors, where it could be used for fertility control. Also known as mifepristone (Mifeprex), RU-486 entered the French market in 1988. but sales were suspended by Rousel-Uclaf when antiabortion groups threatened to boycott the company. In 1994, the company donated the U.S. rights to the New York City–based Population Council, a nonprofit reproductive and population control research institution. Mifepristone is now administered in doctors' offices as a tablet in combination with misoprostol, a prostaglandin that causes uterine contractions to help expel the embryo. The combination of mifepristone and misoprostol is more than 90% effective. Plan B, also known as the "morning-after pill," has been referred to as an emergency contraceptive. It contains norgestrel, the same progestin that is in the pill. It should be taken within 3 days of unprotected sex and can reduce the risk of pregnancy by 89%.

Anesthetics and Analgesics

The first use of synthetic organic chemicals for the modulation of life processes occurred when nitrous oxide, ether, and chloroform were introduced in anesthesia during the 1840s. Horace Wells, a dentist in Hartford, Connecticut, administered nitrous oxide during a tooth extraction, and Crawford Long, a Georgia physician, employed ether as an anesthetic for excising a growth on a patient's neck. It was William Morton, a 27-year-old dentist, however, who gave the first successful public demonstration of surgical anesthesia on October 16, 1846, at the surgical amphitheater that is now called the Ether Dome at Massachusetts General Hospital. Morton attempted to patent his discovery but was unsuccessful, and he died penniless in 1868. Chloroform also was used as an anesthetic at St. Bartholomew's Hospital in London. In Paris, Pierre Fluorens tested both chloroform and ethyl chloride as anesthetics in animals.

The potent analgesic and euphoric properties of the extract of the opium poppy have been known for thousands of years. In the sixteenth century, the Swiss physician and alchemist Paracelsus (1493–1541) popularized the use of opium in Europe. At that time, an alcoholic solution of opium, known as laudanum, was the method of administration. Morphine was first isolated in pure crystalline form from opium in 1805 by the German apothecary Friedrich W. Sertürner, who named the compound "morphium," after Morpheus, the Greek god of dreams. It took another 120 years before the structure of morphine was elucidated by Sir Robert Robinson at the University of Oxford. The chemistry of morphine and the other opium alkaloids obtained from *Papaver somniferum* have fascinated and occupied chemists for more than 200 years, resulting in many synthetic analgesics that are available today (see Chapter 24). (-)-Morphine was first synthesized by Marshall Gates at the University of Rochester in 1952. Although a number of highly effective, stereoselective synthetic pathways have been developed, it is unlikely that a commercial process can compete with its isolation from the poppy. Diacetylmorphine, known as heroin, is highly addictive and induces tolerance. The illicit worldwide production of opium now exceeds the pharmaceutical production by almost 10-fold. In the United States, some 800,000 people are chemically addicted to heroin, and a growing number are becoming addicted to oxycontin, a synthetic opiate also known as oxycodone. Another synthetic opiate, methadone, blocks the opiate receptors in the brain, curbing the craving for heroin or morphine. A series of studies in the 1960s at Rockefeller University by Vincent Dole and his wife, Marie Nyswander, found that methadone also could be a viable maintenance treatment to keep addicts from heroin. It is estimated that approximately 250,000 addicts are taking methadone in the United States. Unfortunately, it has not been widely recognized in the United States that opiate addiction is a medical condition for which there is no known cure. More than 80% of U.S. heroin addicts lack access to methadone treatment facilities, primarily because of the strong stigma against drug users and the medical distribution of methadone.

Only within the last 25 years have scientists begun to understand the effects of opioid analgesics at the molecular level. In 1954, Beckett and Casey at the University of London proposed that opiate effects were receptor mediated, but it was not until the early 1970s that the stereospecific binding of opiates to specific receptors was demonstrated. The characterization and classification of three different types of opioid receptors (μ, κ, and δ) by W.R. Martin formed the basis of our current understanding of opioid pharmacology. The demonstration of stereospecific binding of radiolabeled ligands to opioid receptors led to the development of radioreceptor-binding assays for each of the opioid receptor types, a technique that has been of major importance in the identification of selective opioids as well as many other receptors. In 1973, Avram Goldstein, Solomon Snyder, Ernst Simon, and Lars Terenius independently described saturable, stereospecific binding sites for opiate drugs in the mammalian nervous system. Shortly thereafter, John Hughes and Hans Kosterlitz, working at the University of Aberdeen in Scotland, described the isolation from pig brains of two pentapeptides that exhibited morphine-like actions on the guinea pig ileum. At about the same time, Goldstein reported the presence of peptide-like substances in the pituitary gland that showed opiate-like activity. Subsequent research revealed three distinct families of opiate peptides: the enkephalins, the endorphins, and the dynorphins.

Hypnotics and Anticonvulsants

Since antiquity, alcoholic beverages and potions containing laudanum, an alcoholic extract of opium, and various other plant products have been used to induce sleep. Bromides were used in the middle of the nineteenth century as a sedative-hypnotic, as was chloral hydrate, paraldehyde, urethane, and sulfenal. Von Mering, on the assumption that a structure having a carbon atom carrying two ethyl groups would have hypnotic properties, investigated diethyl acetyl urea, which proved to be a potent hypnotic. Further investigations led to 5,5-diethylbarbituric acid, a compound synthesized 20 years earlier, in 1864, by Adolph von Beyer. Phenobarbital was synthesized by the Bayer Pharmaceutical Company and introduced to the market under the name Luminol (Fig. I.3). The compound was effective as a hypnotic, but it also exhibited anticonvulsant properties. The success of phenobarbital led to the testing of more than 2,500 barbiturates, of which approximately 50 were used clinically, many of which are still in clinical use. Modification of the barbituric acid molecule also led to the development of the hydantoins. Phenytoin, also known as diphenylhydantoin or Dilantin, was first synthesized in 1908, but its anticonvulsant properties were not discovered until 1938. Because phenytoin was not a sedative at ordinary doses, it established that antiseizure drugs need not induce drowsiness and encouraged the search for drugs with selective antiseizure action (Fig. I.3).

Phenobarbital Phenytoin

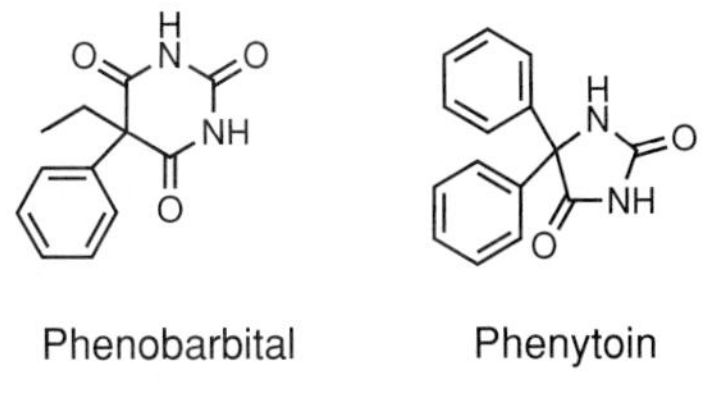

Fig. I.3. Examples of early an early hypnotic and anticonvulsant.

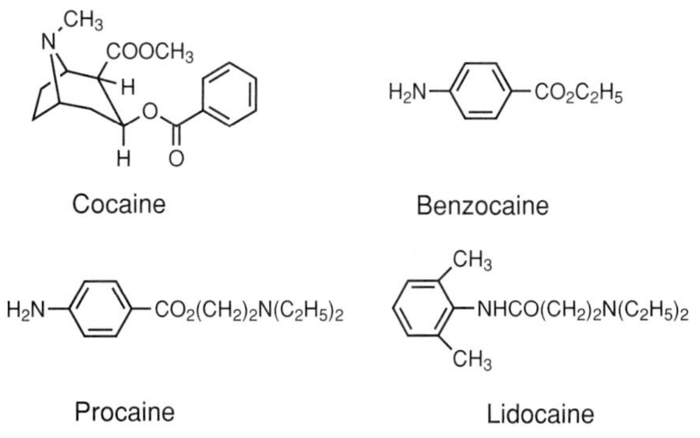

Local Anesthetics

The local anesthetics can be traced back to the naturally occurring alkaloid cocaine isolated from *Erythroxylon coca*. A Viennese ophthalmologist, Carl Koller, had experimented with several hypnotics and analgesics for use as a local anesthetic in the eye. His friend, Sigmund Freud, suggested that they attempt to establish how the South American Indians allayed fatigue by chewing leaves of the coca bush. Cocaine had been isolated from the plant by the chemist Albert Niemann at Gothenburg University, Sweden, in 1860. Koller found that cocaine numbed the tongue; thus, he discovered a local anesthetic. He quickly realized that cocaine was an effective, nonirritating anesthetic for the eye, leading to the widespread use of cocaine in both Europe and the United States. Richard Willstatter in Munich determined the structure of both cocaine and atropine in 1898 and succeeded in synthesizing cocaine 3 years later. Although today cocaine is of greater historic than medicinal importance and is widely abused, few developments in the chemistry of local anesthetics can disclaim a structural relationship to cocaine (Fig. I.4). Benzocaine, procaine, tetracaine, and lidocaine can all be considered structural analogues of cocaine, a classic example of how structural modification of a natural product can lead to useful therapeutic agents.

Cocaine Benzocaine

Procaine Lidocaine

Fig. I.4. Synthetic local anesthetics development based on the structure of cocaine.

Drugs Affecting Renal and Cardiovascular Function

Included in the category are the diuretics, vasopressin, rennin and angiotensin drugs used in the treatment of myocardial ischemia, pharmacotherapy of congestive heart failure, antiarrythmic drugs, and drugs used in therapy for hypercholesterolemia. Use of the cardiac drug digoxin dates back to the folk-remedy foxglove, attributed to William Withering, who in 1775 discovered that the foxglove plant, *Digitalis purpurea,* was beneficial to those suffering from abnormal fluid buildup. The active principles of digitalis were isolated in 1841 by E. Humolle and T. Quevenne in Paris. These active principles consisted mainly of digitoxin. The other glycosides of digitalis were subsequently isolated in 1869 by Nativelle and in 1875 by Schmiedberg. The correct structure of digitoxin was established more than 50 years later by Adolf Windaus at Gothenburg University. In 1929, Sydney Smith at Burroughs Welcome isolated and separated a new glycoside from *Digitalis purpurea,* known as digoxin. This is now the most widely used cardiac glycoside.

Today, dried foxglove leaves are processed to yield digoxin, much like the procedure used by Withering. It takes approximately 1,000 kg of dried foxglove leaves to make 1 kg of pure digoxin.

The group of drugs used in the therapy for hypercholesterolemia has received the greatest success and financial reward for the pharmaceutical industry during the last decade. Cholesterol-lowering drugs, known as statins, are one of the cornerstones in the prevention of both primary and secondary heart diseases. Drugs such as Merck's lovastatin (Mevacor) and Pfizer's Lipitor are a huge success. In 2004, Lipitor was the world's top-selling drug, with sales of more than $10 billion. As a class, cholesterol- and triglyceride-lowering drugs were the world's top category, with sales exceeding $30 billion.

The discovery of the statins can be credited to Akira Endo, a research scientist at Sankyo Pharmaceuticals in Japan (3). Endo's 1973 discovery of the first anticholesterol statin has almost been relegated to obscurity. The story of his research and the discovery of lovastatin are not typical but often escape attention. When Endo joined Sankyo after his university studies to investigate food ingredients, he searched for a fungus that produced an enzyme to make fruit juice less pulpy. The search was a success, and Endo's next assignment was to find an enzyme that would block the production of cholesterol, known as HMG-CoA reductase. With Endo's interest and background, he searched for fungi that would block this enzyme. After testing 6,000 fungal broths, he found such a fungus in 1973. A substance made by a mold, *Penicillium citrinum*, produced a potent inhibitor of the enzyme that helps the body to make cholesterol, and it was named compactin. The substance did not work in rats, but it did work in hens and dogs. Endo's bosses were unenthusiastic about his discovery and discouraged further research with this compound. With the collaboration of Akira Yamamoto, a physician treating patients with extremely high cholesterol because of a genetic defect, Endo prepared samples of his drug and had it administered to an 18-year-old woman by Yamamoto. Further testing in nine patients led to an average lowering of cholesterol of 27%.

In 1978, using a different fungus, Merck discovered a substance that was nearly identical to Endo's; this one was named lovastatin. Merck held the U.S. rights and, in 1987, started marketing it in the United States as Mevacor, the first FDA-approved statin. Sankyo eventually gave up compactin and pursued another statin, which they licensed to Bristol-Myers Squibb, and it was sold as Pravachol.

In 1985, Michael S. Brown and Joseph Goldstein won the Nobel Prize in Physiology or Medicine for their work in cholesterol metabolism. It was only in January of 2006 that Endo received the Japan Prize, considered by many to be equivalent to the Nobel Prize. There is no doubt that millions of people whose lives have been—and will be—extended through statin therapy owe their longevity to Akira Endo.

Anticancer Agents

Sulfur mustard gas was used as an offensive weapon by the Germans during World War I, and the related nitrogen mustards were manufactured by both sides in World War II. Later, investigations showed that the toxic gasses had destroyed the blood's white cells, which subsequently led to the discovery of drugs used in leukemia therapy. These compounds, although effective antitumor agents, were very toxic. 6-Mercaptopurine was really the first effective leukemia drug and was developed by George Hitchings and his technician, Gertrude Elion, who, working together at Burroughs Welcome Research Laboratories, shared the Nobel Prize in 1988 (Fig. I.5). By a process now termed "rational drug design," Hitchings hypothesized that it might be possible to use antagonists to stop bacterial or tumor cell growth by interfering with nucleic acid biosynthesis in a way similar to how sulfonamides blocked cell growth.

Unlike many cancer drugs available today, cisplatin is an inorganic molecule with a simple structure (Fig. I.5). Cisplatin interferes with the growth of cancer cells by binding to DNA and interfering with the cells' repair mechanism, eventually causing cell death. It is used to treat many types of cancer, but primarily testicular, ovarian, bladder, lung, and stomach cancers. Cisplatin is now the gold standard against which new medicines are compared. It was first synthesized in 1845, and its structure was elucidated by Alfred Werner in 1893. It was not until the early 1960s, however, when Barnett Rosenberg, a professor of biophysics and chemistry at Michigan State University, observed the compound's effect in cell division, which prompted him to test cisplatin against tumors in mice. The compound was found to be effective and entered clinical trials in 1971. There is an important lesson to be learned from Rosenberg's development of cisplatin. As a biophysicist and chemist, Rosenberg realized that when he was confronted with interesting results for which he could not find explanations, he needed to enlist the help and expertise of researchers in microbiology, inorganic chemistry, molec-

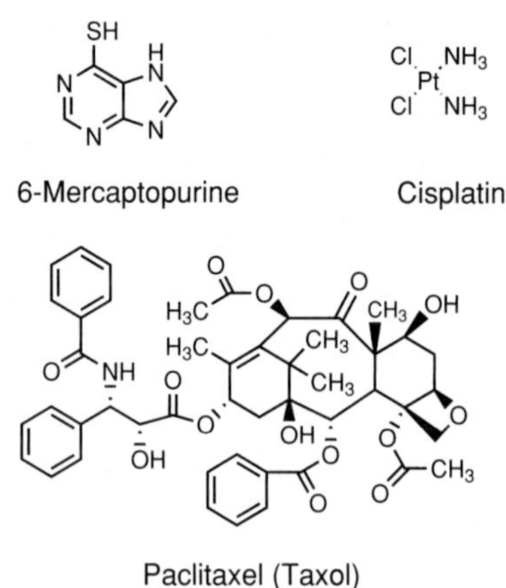

Fig. I.5. Anticancer drugs.

ular biology, biochemistry, biophysics, physiology, and pharmacology. Such a multidisciplinary approach is the key to the discovery of modern medicines today. Although cisplatin is still an effective drug, researchers have found second-generation compounds, such as carboplatin, which has less toxicity and fewer side effects.

The third compound in this class of anticancer agents is Taxol, which was discovered in 1963 by Monroe E. Wall and Masukh C. Wani at Research Triangle Park in North Carolina (Fig. I.5). Taxol was isolated from extracts of the bark of the Pacific yew tree, *Taxus brevifolia.* The extracts showed potent anticancer activity. By 1967, Wall and his coworkers had isolated the active ingredients, and in 1971, they had established the structure of the compound. Susan Horwitz, working at the Albert Einstein College of Medicine in New York, studied the mechanism of how Taxol kills cancer cells. She discovered that Taxol works by stimulating the growth of microtubules and by stabilizing the cell structures so that the killer cells are unable to divide and multiply. It was not until 1993, however, that Taxol, generically called paclitaxel, was brought to the market by Bristol-Myers Squibb, but it soon became an effective drug for treating ovarian, breast, and certain forms of lung cancers. The product became a huge commercial success, with annual sales of approximately $1.6 billion in 2000.

Old Drugs as Targets for New Drugs

> Cannabis is used throughout the world for diverse purposes and has a long history characterized by usefulness, euphoria or evil, depending on one's point of view. To the agriculturist cannabis is a fiber crop; to the physician of a century ago it was a valuable medicine; to the physician of today it is an enigma; to the user, a euphoriant; to the police, a menace; to the trafficker, a source of profitable danger; to the convict or parolee and his family, a source of sorrow (4).

The plant *Cannabis sativa,* the source of marijuana, has a long history in folk medicine, where it has been used for such ills as menstrual pain and the muscle spasms that affect multiple sclerosis sufferers. As in so many other areas of drug research, progress was achieved through the understanding of the pharmacology and biogenesis of a naturally occurring drug only when the chemistry had been well established and researchers had at their disposal pure compounds of known composition and stereochemistry. Cannabis is no exception in this respect, with the last 50 years producing the necessary know-how in the chemistry of the cannabis constituents so that chemists could devise practical and novel synthetic schemes to provide the pharmacologists with pure substances. The isolation and determination of the structure of tetrahydrocannabinol (Δ^9-THC), the principal active ingredient, was determined in 1964 by Rafael Mechoulam at Hebrew University in Israel. Although cannabis and some of its structural analogs have been—and are still—used in medicine, during the last few years research has focused on the endocannabinoids and their receptors as targets for drug development. It was shown that Δ^9-THC exerts its effects by binding to receptors that are targets of naturally occurring molecules, termed endocannabinoids, that have been involved in controlling learning, memory, appetite, metabolism, blood pressure, emotions such as fear and anxiety, inflammation, bone growth, and cancer. It is no surprise then that drug researchers are focusing on developing compounds that either act as agonists or antagonists of the endocannabinoids. In 1990, Lisa Matsuda and Tom Bonner at the National Institutes of Health cloned a Δ^9-THC receptor, now called CB_1, from a rat brain. Shortly thereafter, Mechoulam's group identified the first of these endogenous cannabinoids, called anandamide, and a few years later identified 2-arachidonylgyclerol. In 1993, the second cannabinoid receptor, CB_2, was cloned by Muna Abu-Shaar at the Medical Research Council in Cambridge, United Kingdom. The drug rimonabant, an endocannabinoid antagonist under development by the French pharmaceutical company Sanofi-Aventis, is the drug closest to clinical development. The drug binds to CB_1, but not CB_2, receptors and promotes weight loss. Efforts to develop other endocannabinoids as therapeutic agents are in full swing at many laboratories and include preclinical testing for epilepsy, pain, anxiety, and diarrhea. Thus, a new series of drugs may soon be on the market that are not centered on marijuana itself but, rather, are inspired by its active ingredient, Δ^9-THC, mimicking the endogenous substances acting in the brain or the periphery.

MOLECULAR IMAGING

Clinicians now have at their disposal a variety of diagnostic tools to help obtain information about the pathophysiological status of internal organs. The most widely used methods for noninvasive imaging are scintigraphy, radiography (x-ray and computed tomography), ultrasonography, positron-emission tomography (PET), single-photon emission computed tomography (SPECT), and magnetic resonance imaging (MRI). Chemists continue to make important contributions to the preparation of radiopharmaceuticals and contrast agents. These optical, nuclear, and magnetic methods are increasingly empowered by new types of imaging agents. These modalities are now routinely being used to judge the effectiveness of new and old drugs to treat disease and to monitor the response to therapies.

The expanded use of the cyclotron in the late 1930s and of the nuclear reactor in the early 1940s made available a variety of radionuclides for potential applications in medicine. The field of nuclear medicine was founded with reactor-produced radioiodine for the diagnosis of thyroid dysfunction. Soon, other radioactive tracers, such as ^{18}F, ^{123}I, ^{131}I, ^{99m}Tc, and ^{11}C, became available. Together with more sensitive radiation detection instruments and cameras, this made it possible to study many organs of the body, such as the liver, kidney, lung, and brain. The diagnostic value of these noninvasive techniques served to establish nuclear medicine and radiopharmaceutical chemistry as distinct specialties. A radiopharmaceutical is defined as any pharmaceutical that contains a radionuclide (5).

Historically, radioiodine has a special place in nuclear medicine. In 1938, Hertz, Roberts, and Evans first demonstrated the uptake of ^{128}I by the thyroid gland. With a longer half life (8 days), ^{131}I later became available and is now widely used. Although iodine has 24 known isotopes, ^{123}I, ^{131}I, and ^{125}I are the only ones currently used in medicine. At present, the most widely used PET radiopharmaceutical is the glucose analogue ^{18}F-FDG (2-fluoro-2-deoxy-D-glucose; half-life = 1.8 hours); it is routinely employed for functional studies of brain, heart, and tumor growth. The process is derived from the earlier animal studies quantifying regional glucose metabolism with [^{14}C]-2-dexoyglucose, which passes through the blood-brain barrier by the same carrier-facilitated transport system used for glucose. With the advancement in highly selective PET and SPECT ligands, the potential of the noninvasive imaging procedures will achieve wider application both in pharmacologic research and in the diagnosis of central nervous system disorders.

THE NEXT WAVE IN DRUG DISCOVERY

Genomics

Gleevec (imatinib) was discovered through the combined use of high-throughput screening and medicinal chemistry that resulted in the successful treatment of chronic myeloid leukemia. By molecular modifications, improved activity against the platelet-derived growth factor receptor (PDGFR) and tyrosine kinase as well as the loss of serine/threonine kinase inhibition were obtained. As a result of the success of Gleevec, scientists are modifying their drug discovery and development strategies to consider the patient's genes, without abandoning the more traditional drugs. It has been known for many years that genetics plays an important role in an individual's well-being. Attention is now being paid to manipulating the proteins that are produced in response to malfunctioning genes by inhibiting the out-of-control tyrosine kinase enzymes in the body that play such an important role in cell signaling events in growth and cell division. Using the knowledge obtained from the Human Genome Project, scientists with a knowledge of the sequencing of DNA and genes of various species have shown that some cancers are caused by genetic errors that direct the biosynthesis of dysfunctional proteins. Because proteins carry out the instructions from the genes located on the DNA, dysfunctional proteins, such as the kinases, deliver the wrong message to the cells, making them cancerous. The emphasis is now on inhibiting the proteins to slow the progression of the cancerous growth.

An emphasis in the pharmaceutical industry as well as in academia is to develop drug formulations that guarantee therapies will reach specific targets in the body. Vaccines based on a proprietary plasmid DNA that will activate skeletal muscles to manufacture desired proteins and antigens are being developed. Plasmid DNA vaccine technology represents a fundamentally new means of treatment that is of great importance for the future of drug targeting. Currently, the number of products coming out of biotechnology companies is increasing. Biotechnology drug discovery and drug development tools are used to create the more traditional small molecules. The promise of pharmacogenetics lies in the potential to identify sources of interindividual variability in drug responses that affect drug delivery and safety. Recent success stories in oncology demonstrate that the field of pharmacogenetics has progressed substantially. The knowledge created through pharmacogenetic trials can contribute to the development of patient-specific medicines as well as to improved decision making along the research and development value chain (6).

Combinatorial Chemistry and High-Throughput Screening

No discussion of the history and evolution of medicinal chemistry would be complete without briefly mentioning combinatorial chemistry and high-throughput screening. Combinatorial chemistry is one of the new technologies developed by academics and researchers in the pharmaceutical and biotechnology industries to reduce the time and cost associated with producing effective, marketable, and competitive new drugs. Chemists use combinatorial chemistry to create large populations of molecules that can be screened efficiently, generally using high-throughput screening. Thus, instead of synthesizing a single compound, combinatorial chemistry exploits automation and miniaturization to synthesize large libraries of compounds. Combinatorial organic synthesis is not random but, rather, systematic and repetitive, using sets of chemical "building blocks" to form a diverse set of molecular entities.

Random screening has been a source of new drugs for several decades. Many of the drugs currently on the market were developed from leads identified through screening of natural products or compounds synthesized in the laboratory. In the late 1970s and 1980s, however, screening fell out of favor in the industry. Using traditional methods, the number of novel selective leads that were generated did not make this approach cost-effective. The last 25 years have seen an enormous advance in our understanding of critical cellular processes, leading to a more rationally designed approach in drug discovery. The availability of cloned genes for use in high-throughput screening to identify new molecules has led to a reexamination of the screening process. Targets now are often recombinant proteins (i.e., receptors) produced from cloned genes that are heterologously expressed in a number of ways. Combinatorial libraries complement the enormous numbers of synthetic libraries available from new and old synthetic programs. The development and use of robotics and automation have made it possible to screen large numbers of compounds in a short period of time. It also should be emphasized that computerized data systems and analysis of the data have facilitated the handling of the information being generated, leading to the identification of new leads.

SUMMARY

It is fair to say that more than 50% of the drugs in use today had their origin in a plant, animal, or mineral that had been used as cures for alleviating diseases occurring in humans. Examples of a number of discoveries of important drugs in use today are recounted as "case studies" in the drug discovery process and are described in more detail in the following chapters. The discoveries briefly described are, in large measure, a result of the increased sophistication brought to bear in the isolation, identification, structure determination, and synthesis of the active ingredients of the drugs used empirically hundreds of years ago.

The emergence of the pharmaceutical industry took place in conjunction with the advances in organic/ medicinal/pharmaceutical chemistry, pharmacology, bacteriology, biochemistry, and medicine as distinct fields of science in the late nineteenth century. Current research efforts are now focused not only on discovering new, biologically active compounds using ever increasingly sophisticated technology but also on gaining a better understanding of how and where drugs exert their effects at the molecular level. One should not underestimate, however, that the discoveries in the twentieth and twenty-first centuries, and before, represent an amazing amount of insight, determination, and luck by researchers in chemistry, pharmacology, biology, and medicine. We owe gratitude and admiration to those earlier scientists who had the imagination and inspiration to develop drugs to cure so many illnesses.

References

1. Burger A. The practice of medicinal chemistry. Burger A, eds. Medicinal Chemistry, New York. New York: Wiley, 1970: 4–9.
2. Daemmrich A, Bowden ME. A rising drug industry. Chem & Eng News. Am Chem Soc, 2005; 83(25): 28–42.
3. Landers P. Stalking cholesterol: How one scientist intrigued by molds found first statin; feat of Japan's Dr. Endo led to heart-care revolution but brought him nothing; nature as a drug laboratory. The Wall Street Journal. (Eastern edition), Jan. 9, 2006: A.1.
4. Miloriya TH. Marijuana in medicine: past, present and future. California Medicine 1969;110(1):34–40.
5. Counsel RE, Weichert JP. Agents for organ imaging. In: Foye WO, Lemke TL, Williams DA, eds. Principles of Medicinal Chemistry. 4th ed. Baltimore: Williams & Wilkins, 1995; Chap 43:927–947.
6. Mullin R. The next wave of biopharmaceuticals. Chem & Eng News. Am Chem Soc, 2005;83(35):16–19.

Suggested Readings

Djerassi C. The Politics of Contraception. New York: Norton, 1970.

Healy D. The Antidepressant Era. Cambridge, MA: Harvard University Press, 1998.

Marx J. Drugs Inspired by a Drug. Sci. 2006; 311:322–325.

Meyer P. Discovering new drugs: The legacy of the past, present approaches, and hopes for the future. In: Wermuth G, ed. The Practice of Medicinal Chemistry. London: Academic Press, 1996:11–24.

Podolsky ML. Cures Out of Chaos. Williston, VT: Harwood Academic, 1997.

Sheehan JC. The Enchanted Ring—The Untold Story of Penicillin. Cambridge, MA: MIT Press, 1982.

PART I

PRINCIPLES OF DRUG DISCOVERY

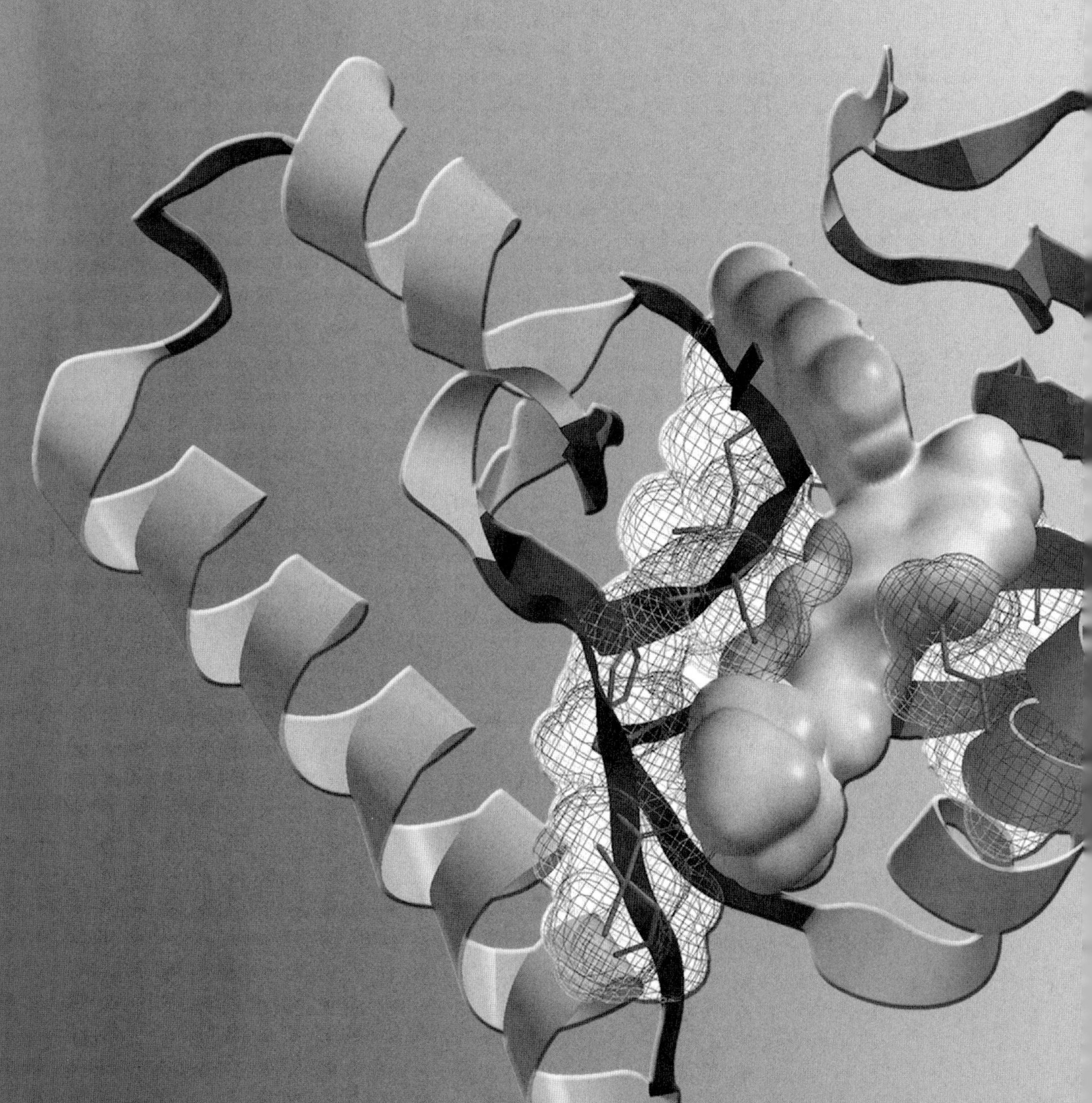

1. *Drug Discovery from Natural Products*

A. Douglas Kinghorn

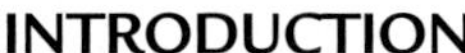

INTRODUCTION

"Pharmacognosy" is one of the oldest established pharmaceutical sciences, and the term has been used for nearly two centuries. Initially, this term referred to the investigation of medicinal substances of plant, animal, or mineral origin in their crude or unprepared state, used in the form of teas, tinctures, poultices, and other types of formulation (1–4). By the middle of the twentieth century, however, the chemical components of such crude drugs began to be studied in more detail. Today, the subject of pharmacognosy is highly interdisciplinary, and it incorporates aspects of analytical chemistry, biochemistry, biosynthesis, biotechnology, ecology, ethnobotany, microbiology, molecular biology, organic chemistry, and taxonomy, among others (5). The term "pharmacognosy" is defined on the Web site of the American Society of Pharmacognosy (http://www.phcog.org) as "the study of the physical, chemical, biochemical, and biological properties of drugs, drug substances, or potential drugs or drug substances of natural origin, as well as the search for new drugs from natural sources."

There seems little doubt that humans have used natural drugs since before the advent of written history. In addition to their use as drugs, the constituents of plants have afforded poisons for darts and arrows used in hunting and euphoriants with psychoactive properties used in rituals. The actual documentation of drugs derived from natural products in the Western world appears to date back as far to the Sumerians and Akkadians in the third century BC as well as to the Egyptian *Ebers Papyrus* (approximately 1,600 BC). Other important contributions on the uses of drugs of natural origin were documented by Dioscorides (*De Materia Medica*) and Pliny the Elder in the first century AD and by Galen in the second century. Written records also exist from about the same time period regarding plants used in both Chinese traditional medicine and Ayurvedic medicine. Then, beginning approximately 500 years ago, information concerning medicinal plants began to be documented in herbals. In turn, the laboratory study of natural product drugs commenced approximately 200 years ago, with the purification of morphine from opium. This corresponds with the beginnings of organic chemistry as a scientific discipline. Additional drugs isolated from plant sources in the nineteenth century included atropine, caffeine, cocaine, nicotine, quinine, and strychnine, and in the twentieth century, digoxin, reserpine, paclitaxel, vincristine, and chemical precursors of the steroid hormones. Even as we enter the twenty-first century, approximately three-quarters of the world's population is reliant on primary health care from systems of traditional medicine, including the use of herbs. In recent years, a more profound understanding has emerged of the chemical and biological aspects of plants used in the traditional medicine of countries such as the People's Republic of China, India, Indonesia, and Japan, in addition to the medicinal plants used in Latin America and Africa. Many important scientific observations germane to natural product drug discovery have been made as a result (1–4).

By the mid-twentieth century, therapeutically useful alkaloids had been purified and derivatized from the ergot fungus, as uterotonic and sympatholytic agents. Then, the penicillins were isolated, along with further major structural classes of effective and potent antibacterials from terrestrial microbes, and these and later antibiotics revolutionized the treatment of infectious diseases. Of the types of organisms producing natural products, terrestrial microorganisms have been found to afford the largest number of compounds currently used as drugs for a wide range of human diseases, and these include antimicrobial agents, the "statin" cholesterol-lowering agents, immunosuppressive agents, and several anticancer agents (1–4).

At the beginning of the twenty-first century, there is much interest in the discovery and development of drugs from marine animals and plants. To date, however, marine organisms have had a relatively brief history as sources of drugs. Although the oceans occupy 70% of the surface of the earth, an intense effort to investigate the chemical structures and biological activities of marine fauna and flora has only been ongoing for approximately 30 years. Two established drugs based on marine-derived nucleoside model compounds are the antileukemic agent cytosine arabinoside and the antiviral agent, adenine arabinoside (6).

The term "natural product" generally is taken to mean a compound that has no known primary biochemical role in the producing organism. Such small-molecular-weight organic molecules also may be referred to as "secondary metabolites," and they are biosynthesized by the producing organism in a biologically active chiral form to increase the chances of survival, such as by repelling predators or, in the case of terrestrial plants, serving as insect pollination attractants (1–4). There have been a number of studies to investigate the physicochemical parameters of natural products in recent years, and it has been concluded that "libraries," or collections of these substances, tend to afford a higher degree of "drug-likeness" when compared to compounds in either synthetic or combinatorial "libraries" (7,8). This characteristic might well be expected, because natural products are produced by living systems, where they are subject to transport and diffusion at the cellular level. Small-molecule natural products are capable of modulating protein–protein interactions and, thus, can affect cellular processes that may be modified in disease states. When compared to synthetic compounds, natural products tend to have more protonated amine and free hydroxy functionalities and more single bonds, with a greater number of fused rings containing more chiral centers. Natural products also differ from synthetic products in the average number of halogen, nitrogen, oxygen, and sulfur atoms, in addition to their steric complexity (9). It is considered that natural products and synthetic compounds occupy different regions of "chemical space"; hence, they each tend to contribute to the overall chemical diversity required in a drug discovery program (7,8). Fewer than 20% of the ring systems produced among natural products are represented in currently used drugs (8). Naturally occurring substances may serve either as drugs in their native or unmodified form or as "lead" compounds (prototype bioactive molecules) for subsequent semisynthetic or totally synthetic modification—for example, to improve biological efficacy or to enhance solubility (7–10).

In the present era of efficient drug design by chemical synthesis aided by computational and combinatorial techniques, and with other new drugs obtained increasingly through biotechnological processes, it might be expected that traditional natural products no longer have any significant role to play in this regard. Indeed, during the past decade, emphasis on the screening of natural products for new drugs by pharmaceutical companies has decreased, with greater reliance being placed on screening large "libraries" or collections of synthetic compounds (7,8,10). In a landmark review article, however, Newman et al. (11) from the U.S. National Cancer Institute pointed out that from 1982 to 2002, approximately 28% of the new chemical entities in Western medicine were either natural products per se or derived from natural products. Thus, of 1,031 new chemical entities over this 22-year period, 5% were unmodified natural products, and 23% were semisynthetic agents based on natural product lead compounds. An additional 14% of the synthetic compounds were designed based on knowledge of a natural product "pharmacophore" (the region of the molecule containing the essential organic functional groups that directly interact with the receptor active site and, therefore, confers, the biologic activity of interest). Furthermore, in the thirteenth revision of the *World Health Organization Model List of Essential Medicines*, of approximately 300 drugs considered necessary for the practice of medicine, approximately 210 are small-molecular agents. Of these, more than 40 are unmodified natural products, 25 are semisynthetic drugs based on natural product prototypes, and more than 70 are either synthetic drugs based on natural product prototype molecules or synthetic mimics of natural products (12). The launch of new natural product drugs in the United States, Europe, and Japan has continued in the early years of the present decade of this new century, and such compounds introduced to the market recently have been reviewed by Butler (13).

Thus, the secondary metabolites of organisms generally are recognized to afford a source of small-organic molecules of outstanding chemical diversity that are highly relevant to the contemporary drug discovery process. Potent and selective leads are obtained from increasingly exotic organisms as collection efforts venture into increasingly inhospitable locales throughout the world, such as deep caves in terrestrial areas and thermal vents on the ocean floor. On occasion, a natural product lead compound may help to elucidate a new mechanism of interaction with a biological target for a disease state under investigation. Natural products may serve to provide molecular inspiration in certain therapeutic areas for which there are only a limited number of synthetic lead compounds. A widespread perception remains, however, that the resupply of the source organism of a secondary metabolite of interest may prove to be problematic and, consequently, will hinder the timely, more detailed biological evaluation of a compound that is available initially only in milligram quantities. In addition, natural product extracts have been regarded by some as being incompatible with the modern rapid screening techniques and the successful market development of a natural product-derived drug as being too time-consuming (7,8,13). A further consideration of the factors involved in the discovery of drugs from natural products will be presented in the next section. This will be followed by examples of natural products currently used in various therapeutic categories as well as a few selected representatives with future clinical potential.

NATURAL PRODUCTS AND DRUG DISCOVERY

Collection of Source Organisms

There are at least five recognized approaches to the choice of plants and other organisms for the laboratory investigation of their biological components: random screening; selection of specific taxonomic groups, such as families or genera; a chemotaxonomic approach in which restricted classes of secondary metabolites, such as alkaloids, are sought; an information-managed approach, which involves the target collection of species selected by database surveillance; and selection by an ethnomedical approach (e.g., by investigating remedies used in traditional medicine by "shamans" or medicine men or women) (14). In fact, if plant-derived natural products are taken specifically, it has been estimated that of 122 drugs of this type used worldwide from a total of 94 species, 72% can be traced to the original ethnobotanical uses that have been documented for their plant of origin (14). The need for increased research concerning natural product discovery involving ethnobotany should be regarded as urgent because of the accelerating loss in developing countries of indigenous cultures and languages, inclusive of knowledge of traditional medical practice (15). It is common, however, for a given medicinal plant to be used ethnomedically in more than one disease context, which sometimes may obscure its therapeutic utility for a specific disease condition. Another manner in which drugs have been developed from terrestrial plants and fungi is through following up on observations of the causes of livestock poisoning, leading to new drugs and molecular tools for biomedical investigation (16). When the origin of plants with demonstrated inhibitory effects in experimental tumor systems was considered at the U.S. National Cancer Institute, medicinal or poisonous plants with uses as either anthelmintics or arrow and homicidal poisons were three- to fourfold more likely to be active in this regard than species screened at random (17).

Some shallow-water marine specimens may be collected simply by wading or snorkeling down to 20 feet below the water surface, but scuba diving permits the collection of organisms to depths of 120 feet. Deep-water collections of marine animals and plants have been made by dredging and trawling and through the use of manned and unmanned submersible vessels. Collection strategies for specimens from the ocean must take into account marine macroorganism-microorganism associations that may be involved in the biosynthesis of a particular secondary metabolite of interest (18). Thus, there seems to be a complex interplay between many marine host invertebrate animals and symbiotic microbes that inhabit them, and several bioactive compounds previously thought to be of animal origin may be produced by their associated microorganisms instead (19).

The process of collecting or surveying a large set of flora (or fauna) for the purpose of biological evaluation and isolation of lead compounds is called "biodiversity prospecting" (20). Many natural product collection programs are focused on tropical rain forests to take advantage of the inherent biological diversity (or "biodiversity") evident there, with the hope of harnessing as broad a profile of chemical classes as possible among the secondary metabolites produced by the species to be obtained. To exemplify this, there may be more tree species in a relatively small area of a tropical rainforest than in the whole of the temperate regions of North America. A generally accepted explanation for the high biodiversity of secondary metabolites in humid forests in the tropics is that these molecules are biosynthesized (a process of chemical synthesis by the host organism) for ecological roles in response to a continuous growing season under elevated temperatures, high humidity, and great competition resulting from the high species density present. Maximal biodiversity in the marine environment is found on the fringes of the ocean or sea bordering land, where intense competition for attachment space exists among sessile (nonmoving) organisms, such as algae, corals, sponges, and some other invertebrate animals space (21).

Great concern should be expressed about the continuing erosion of tropical rain forest species, which is accelerating as the twenty-first century begins (22). Approximately 25 "hot spots" of especially high biodiversity have been proposed that represent 44% of all vascular plant species and 35% of all species of vertebrates in approximately 1.4% of the earth's surface (23). At present, many of the endemic (or native) species to these biodiversity "hot spot" areas have been reported to be undergoing massive habitat loss and are threatened with extinction, especially in tropical regions (22,23).

Following the United Nations Convention on Biological Diversity, which was passed in Rio de Janeiro in 1992, biological or genetic materials are owned by the country of origin (20). A major present-day component of being able to gain access to the genetic resources of a given country for the purposes of drug discovery and other scientific study is the formulation of a Memorandum of Agreement, which itemizes access, previous informed consent (involving human subjects in cases where ethnomedical knowledge is divulged), intellectual property related to drug discovery, and equitable sharing of the financial benefits that may accrue from the project, such as patent royalties and licensing fees (20). When access to marine organisms is desired, the United National Convention on the Law of the Sea must be considered as well (24).

Once a formal "benefit sharing" agreement is on hand, the organism collection process can begin. Usually, 0.3 to 1 kg of each dried plant sample and approximately 1 kg wet weight of a marine organism are initially collected for preliminary screening studies (25). In the case of a large plant (tree or shrub), it is typical to collect up to four different organs or plant parts, because the secondary metabolite composition may vary considerably between the leaves, where photosynthesis occurs, and the storage or translocation organs, such as the roots and bark. Increasing evidence suggests that considerable variation in the profile of secondary metabolites occurs in the same plant organ when collected from different habitats, depending on local environmental conditions; thus, it may be worth reinvestigating even well-studied species in drug discovery projects (26). Taxa that are endemic to a particular country or region generally are of higher priority than pandemic weeds. It is very important not to remove all quantities of a desired species at the site of collection to conserve the native germplasm encountered. Also, rare or endangered species should not be collected; a listing of the latter is maintained, for example, by the *Red List of Threatened Species* of the International Union for Conservation of Nature and Natural Resources (http://www.redlist.org), covering terrestrial, marine, and freshwater organisms.

A crucial aspect of the organism collection process is to deposit voucher specimens representative of the species collected in a central repository, such as an herbarium or a museum, so that this material can be accessed by other scientists. It is advisable to deposit specimens in more than one repository, including regional and national institutions of the country in which the organisms were collected. Collaboration with general and specialist taxonomists is very important, because without an accurate identification of a source organism, the value of subsequent isolation, structure elucidation, and biological evaluation studies will be greatly reduced.

Organisms for natural product drug discovery work may be classified into the Kingdoms Eubacteria (bacteria, cyanobacteria [or "blue-green algae"]), Archaea (halobacterians, methanogens), Protoctista (e.g., protozoa, diatoms, "algae" [including red algae, green algae]), Plantae (land plants [including mosses and liverworts, ferns, and seed plants]), Fungi (e.g., molds, yeasts, mushrooms), and Animalia (mesozoa [wormlike invertebrate marine parasites], sponges, jellyfish, corals, flatworms, roundworms, sea urchins, mollusks [snails, squid], segmented worms, arthropods [crabs, spiders, insects], fish, amphibians, birds, mammals) (20). Of these, the largest numbers of organisms are found for arthropods, inclusive of insects (~950,000 species), with only a relatively small proportion (5%) of the estimated 1.5 million fungi in the world having been identified. At present, with 300,000 to 500,000 known species, plants are the second-largest group of classified organisms, representing approximately 15% of our biodiversity. Of the 28 major animal phyla, 26 are found in the sea, with eight of these exclusively so. More than 200,000 species of invertebrate animals and algal species have been found in the sea (5,18,20). During the last decade, a high proportion of the new natural product molecules was isolated from fungal sources (27). An area of investigation with great potential for expansion in the future will be microbes, particularly actinomycetes and cyanobacteria of marine origin, especially if techniques can be developed for their isolation and culturing in the laboratory (28). Along the same lines, endophytes (microorganisms that reside in the tissue of living plants) have been found to produce an array of biologically interesting new compounds and are worthy of more intensive investigation (29). Interestingly, in a survey regarding the origin of 30,000 structurally assigned lead compounds of natural origin, these compounds were derived from animals (13%), bacteria (33%), fungi (26%), and plants (27%) (9). A basic premise inherent in natural product drug discovery work is that the greater the degree of phylogenetic (taxonomic) diversity of the organisms sampled, the greater the resultant chemical diversity. Therefore, whereas natural product researchers tend to specialize in the types of organism on which they work, it is reasonable to envisage that the future investigation of all the major groups mentioned above will provide dividends in terms of affording new prototype biologically active compounds of use in drug discovery.

Preparation of Initial Extracts and Preliminary Biological Screening

Different laboratories tend to adopt different procedures for initial extraction of the source organisms being investigated, but typically, terrestrial plants undergo extraction initially with a polar solvent, such as methanol or ethanol, then this extract is subjected to a defatting (lipid-removing) partition with a nonpolar solvent, such as hexane or petroleum ether. Finally, the residue is partitioned between a semipolar organic solvent, such as chloroform or dichloromethane, and a polar aqueous solvent (26). Marine and aquatic organisms are commonly extracted fresh into methanol or a mixture of methanol and dichloromethane (25). A peculiarity of working on plant extracts is the need to remove a class of compounds known as "vegetable tannins" or "plant polyphenols" before subsequent biological evaluation, because these compounds act as interfering substances in enzyme inhibition assays as a result of precipitating proteins in a nonspecific manner. Several methods to remove plant polyphenols have been proposed, such as passage over polyvinylpyrrolidone and polyamide, on which they are retained. Alternatively, partial removal of these interfering substances may be effected by washing the final semipolar organic layer with an aqueous sodium chloride solution (25). It should be noted, however, that active interest remains in pursuing purified and structurally characterized vegetable tannins for their potential medicinal value (30,31). Caution also needs to be expressed in regard to common saturated and unsaturated fatty acids that might be present in natural product extracts, because these may interfere with various enzyme-inhibition and receptor-binding assays (32). Fatty acids and other lipids may largely be removed from more polar natural product extracts using the defatting solvent partition stage mentioned above.

Drug discovery from organisms is a "biology-driven" process, and as such, biological activity evaluation is at the heart of the drug discovery process from crude extracts prepared from organisms. So-called "high-throughput" screening (HTS) assays have become widely used for affording new leads. In this process, large numbers of crude extracts from organisms can be simultaneously evaluated in a cell- or noncell-based format, usually utilizing multiwell microtiter plates (33). Cell-based in vitro bioassays allow a considerable degree of biological relevance, and manipulation may take place so that a selected cell line may involve a genetically altered organism (34) or incorporate a reporter gene (20,33). In noncellular (cell-free) assays, natural product extracts and their purified constituents may be investigated for their effects on enzyme activity (30,32) or receptor binding (35). Other homogenous and separation-based assays that are suitable for the screening of natural products have been reviewed (36). For maximum efficiency and speed, HTS may be automated through the use of robotics and may be rendered a more effective process through miniaturization.

Methods for Compound Structure Elucidation and Identification

Bioassay-directed fractionation is the process of isolating pure active constituents from some type of biomass (e.g., plants, microbes, marine invertebrates) using a decision tree that is dictated solely by bioactivity. A variety of chromatographic separation techniques are available for these purposes, including those based on adsorption on sorbents, such as silica gel, alumina, Sephadex, and more specialized solid phases, and methods involving partition chromatography inclusive of countercurrent chromatography. Recent improvements have been made in column technology, automation of high-performance liquid chromatography (HPLC; a technique often used for final compound purification), and compatibility with HTS methodology (13). Routine structure elucidation is performed using combinations of spectroscopic procedures, with particular emphasis on one- and two-dimensional ^{1}H- and ^{13}C-nuclear magnetic resonance (NMR) spectroscopy and mass spectrometry (MS). Considerable progress has been made in the development of cryogenic and microcoil NMR probe technology for the determination of structures in submilligram amounts of natural products (8). In addition, the automated processing of spectroscopic data for the structure elucidation of natural products is a practical proposition (37). Another significant advance is the use of "hyphenated" analytical techniques for rapid determination of the structure of natural products without the need for a separate isolation step, such as liquid chromatography-NMR (LC-NMR) and LC-NMR-MS (8,13). The inclusion of an on-line solid-phase extraction (SPE) cartridge is advantageous in the identification of natural product molecules in crude extracts using LC-NMR (38).

"Dereplication" is a process of determining whether an observed biological effect of an extract or specimen is caused by a known substance. This is applied during natural product drug discovery programs in an attempt to avoid the reisolation of compounds of previously determined structure. A step like this is essential to prioritize the resources available to a research program so that the costly stage of bioassay-directed fractionation on a promising lead crude extract can be devoted to the discovery of biologically active agents representing new chemotypes (39). This has been particularly necessary for many years in studies on anti-infective agents from actinomycetes and bacteria, and it is applied routinely to extracts from higher plants and marine invertebrates. Methods for dereplication must be sensitive, rapid, and reproducible, and the chemical methods employed generally contain a mass spectrometric component (39). For example, the eluant (effluent) from an HPLC separation of crude natural product extracts may be split into two portions so that the major part is plated out into a microtiter plate, with the wells then evaluated in an in vitro bioassay of interest. The fractions from the minor portion of the column eluant are introduced into a mass spectrometer, and the molecular weights of compounds in active fractions can be determined. This information may then be introduced into an appropriate natural product database, and tentative identities of the active compounds in the active wells can be determined (26,39).

"Metabolomics" is a recently developed approach in which the entire or "global" profile of secondary metabolites in a system (cell, tissue, or organism) is catalogued under a given set of conditions. Secondary metabolites may be investigated by a detection step, such as MS, after a separation step, such as gas chromatography, HPLC, or capillary electrophoresis (40). This type of technology has particular utility in systematic biology, genomics research, and biotechnology, and it should have value in future natural product drug discovery (40,41).

Compound Development

A major challenge in the overall natural product drug discovery process is to obtain larger amounts of a biologically active compound of interest for additional laboratory investigation and potential preclinical development. One strategy that can be adopted when a plant-derived, active compound is of interest is to recollect the species of origin. To maximize the likelihood that the recollected sample will contain the bioactive compound of previous interest, the plant recollection should be carried out in the same location as the initial collection, on the same plant part, and during the same time of the year (26). Some success has been achieved with the production of terrestrial plant and marine cyanobacterial secondary metabolites via plant tissue culture and aquaculture, respectively. For microbes of terrestrial origin, compound scale up often can be carried out through cultivation and large-scale fermentation.

Evaluation of crude extracts of organisms is not routinely carried out in animal models because of limitations of either test material or other project resources, but it is of great value to test in vitro-active natural products in a pertinent in vivo method to obtain a preliminary indication regarding the worthiness of a lead compound for preclinical development. A number of "secondary discriminator" bioassays also provide an assessment of whether a given in vitro-active compound is likely to be active in vivo, and these require quite small amounts of test material. For example, the in vivo hollow-fiber assay was developed at the U.S. National Cancer Institute for the preliminary evaluation of potential anticancer agents, and it uses confluent cells of a tumor model of interest deposited in polyvinylidene fluoride fibers that are implanted in nude mice (26,42). It also is important for pure bioactive compounds to be evaluated mechanistically for their effects on a particular biological target, such as on a given stage of the life cycle of a pathogenic organism or on a cancer cell. Needless to say, a pure natural product of novel structure with in vitro and in vivo activity against a particular biological target relevant to human disease acting through a previously unknown mechanism of action is of great value in the drug discovery process.

Once a bioactive natural product lead is obtained in gram quantities, it is treated in the same manner as a synthetic drug lead and, thus, subjected to pharmaceutical development leading to preclinical and clinical trials. This includes lead optimization via medicinal chemistry, combinatorial chemistry, computational chemistry, as well as formulation, pharmacokinetics, and drug metabolism studies, as described elsewhere in this volume. Often, a lead natural product is obtained from its organism of origin along with several naturally occurring structural analogues, permitting a preliminary study of the structure-activity relationship to be conducted. This information may be supplemented with data obtained by microbial biotransformation or the production of semisynthetic analogues to allow researchers to glean some initial information about the pharmacophoric site(s) of the naturally occurring molecule (7,8,10).

"Combinatorial biosynthesis" is a contemporary approach with the ability not only to produce new natural product analogues but also to afford new drug candidates per se. This methodology involves the engineering of biosynthetic gene clusters in microorganisms. For example, the modification of bacterial polyketide synthases has led to the production of some 200 new polyketides that do not occur naturally (43).

SELECTED EXAMPLES OF NATURAL PRODUCT-DERIVED DRUGS

In this section, examples are provided of both naturally occurring substances and synthetically modified compounds based on natural products with drug use. Many of the examples shown reflect considerable structural complexity, and the compounds introduced to the market have been obtained from organisms of very wide diversity. More detailed treatises with many more examples of natural product drugs also may be found (1–4). Several recent reviews have summarized newly introduced natural product drugs introduced to the market in recent years as well as substances on which clinical trials are being conducted (6,13,44,45).

Drugs for Cardiovascular and Metabolic Diseases

A very close relationship exists between natural product drugs and the treatment of cardiovascular and metabolic diseases. The powdered leaves of *Digitalis purpurea* have been used in Western medicine for more than 200 years, with the major active constituent being the cardiac (steroidal) glycoside digitoxin, which is still used for the treatment of congestive heart failure and atrial fibrillation. A more widely used drug today is digoxin, a constituent of *Digitalis lanata*, which has a rapid action and is more rapidly eliminated from the body than digitoxin. Deslanoside (deacetyllanatoside C) is a hydrolysis product of the *D. lanata* constituent lanatoside C and is used for rapid digitalization (1–4). The "statin" drugs used for lowering blood cholesterol levels are based on the lead compound mevastatin (formerly known as compactin), produced by cultures of *Penicillium citrinum*, and were discovered using a 3-hydroxy-3-methylglutaryl–coenzyme A reductase assay. Because hypercholesterolemia is regarded as one of the major risk factors for coronary heart disease, several semisynthetic and synthetic compounds modeled on the mevastatin structure (inclusive of the dihydroxycarboxylic acid side chain), including atorvastatin, fluvastatin, pravastatin, and simvastatin, now have extremely wide therapeutic use. Lovastatin is a natural product drug of this type, isolated from *Penicillium brevecompactum* and other organisms (2). There also is a history of the successful production of cardiovascular agents from a terrestrial vertebrate—namely, the angiotensin-converting enzyme inhibitors, captopril and enalapril, which were derived from teprotide, a nonapeptide isolated from the pit viper, *Bothrops jararaca* (44).

D-Phe-L-Pro-L-Arg-L-Pro-Gly-Gly-Gly-Gly-L-Asn-Gly-L-Asp-L-Phe-L-Glu-L-Glu-L-Ile-L-Pro-L-Glu-L-Glu-L-Tyr-L-Leu

Bivalirudin

L-His-Gly-L-Glu-Gly-L-Thr-L-Phe-L-Thr-L-Ser-L-Asp-L-Leu-L-Ser-L-Lys-L-Gln-L-Met-L-Glu-L-Glu-L-Glu-L-Ala-L-Val-L-Arg-L-Leu-L-Phe-L-Ile-L-Glu-L-Trp-L-Leu-L-Lys-L-Asn-Gly-Gly-L-Pro-L-Ser-L-Ser-Gly-L-Ala-L-Pro-L-Pro-L-Pro-L-Ser-NH_2

Exenatide

Two more new drugs derived from a vertebrate and an invertebrate source, respectively, are bivalirudin and exenatide. Bivalirudin is a specific and reversible direct thrombin inhibitor that is administered by injection and is used to reduce the incidence of blood clotting in patients undergoing coronary angioplasty. This compound is a synthetic, 20-amino-acid peptide modeled on hirudin, a substance in the saliva of the leech, *Haementeria officinalis* (46,47). Exenatide is a synthetic version of a 39-amino-acid peptide (exenatid-4) produced in the salivary secretions of a lizard native to the southwestern United States and northern Mexico called the Gila monster, *Heloderma suspectum*, and it acts in the same manner as glucagon-like peptide-1 (GLP-1), a naturally occurring hormone. This drug also is administered by injection, and it enables improved glycemic control in patients with type 2 diabetes (44,48).

Central Nervous System Drugs

A comprehensive review has appeared regarding natural products (mostly of experimental value) that affect the central nervous system, inclusive of analgesics, antipsychotics, anti-Alzheimer's disease agents, antitussives, anxiolytics, and muscle relaxants, among other categories (49). The authors point out in this review that apart from the extensive past literature concerning plants and their constituents as hallucinogenic agents, this area of research on natural products is not well developed but is likely to be very productive in the future.

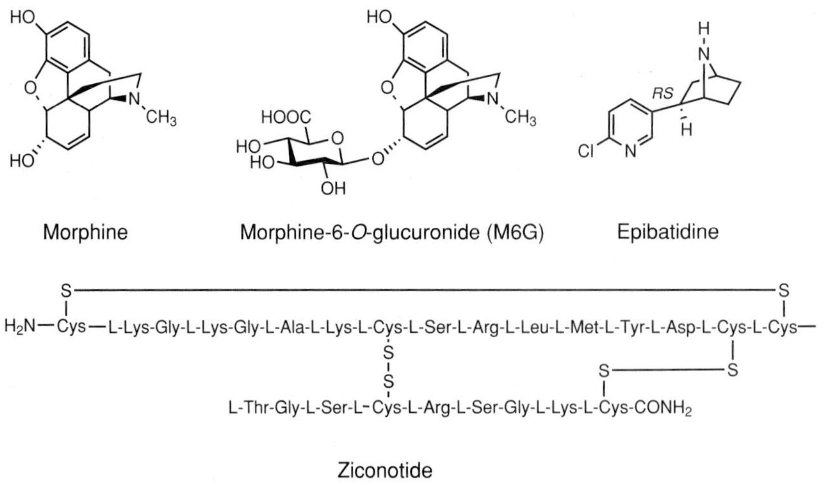

Morphine Morphine-6-*O*-glucuronide (M6G) Epibatidine

Ziconotide

Fig. 1.1. Analgesic compounds of natural origin or derived from naturally occurring analgesics.

The morphinan isoquinoline alkaloid, (-)-morphine, is the most abundant and important constituent of the dried latex (milky exudate) of *Papaver somniferum* (opium poppy), and the prototype of the opioid analgesics, being selective for μ opioid receptors (Fig. 1.1). This compound may be considered to be the paramount natural product lead compound, with many thousands of derivatives synthesized in an attempt to obtain derivatives with strong analgesic potency but without any addictive tendencies (1–4). One derivative now in late clinical trials as a pain treatment is morphine-6-glucuronide (M6G) (Fig. 1.1), the major active metabolite of morphine, with fewer side effects than the parent compound (44,50). The pyridine alkaloid epibatidine (Fig. 1.1), isolated from a dendrobatid frog, *Epipedobates tricolor*, found in Ecuador, activates nicotinic receptors and has an analgesic activity 200-fold more potent than that of morphine. The drug potential of epibatidine is limited by its concomitant toxicity, but it is an important lead compound for the development of future new analgesic agents with less addictive liability than the opiate analgesics (51). A nonopioid analgesic, ziconotide, which is prescribed for the amelioration of chronic pain, has been introduced to the market recently (Fig. 1.1). This drug is a synthetic version of the peptide ω-conotoxin MVIIA. The conotoxin class is produced by the cone snail, *Conus magus*, and these compounds are peptides with 24- to 27-amino-acid residues. Ziconotide selectively binds to N-type voltage-sensitive neuronal channels, causing a blockage of neurotransmission and a potent analgesic effect (44,52). This is one of the first examples of a new natural product drug from a marine source.

(-)-Δ^9-*trans*-Tetrahydrocannabinol (THC) is the major psychoactive (euphoriant) constituent of marijuana, *Cannabis sativa.* The synthetic form of THC (dronabinol) was approved approximately 20 years ago to treat nausea and vomiting associated with cancer chemotherapy, and it has been used for a lesser amount of time to treat appetite loss in patients with HIV/AIDS (44). More recently, an approximately 1:1 mixture of THC and the structurally related marijuana constituent cannabidiol has been approved in Canada for the alleviation of neuropathic pain and spasticity for patients with multiple sclerosis and is administered in low doses as a buccal spray (53). Considerable interest exists in using cannabinoid derivatives based on THC for medicinal purposes, but it is necessary to minimize the central nervous system effects of these compounds.

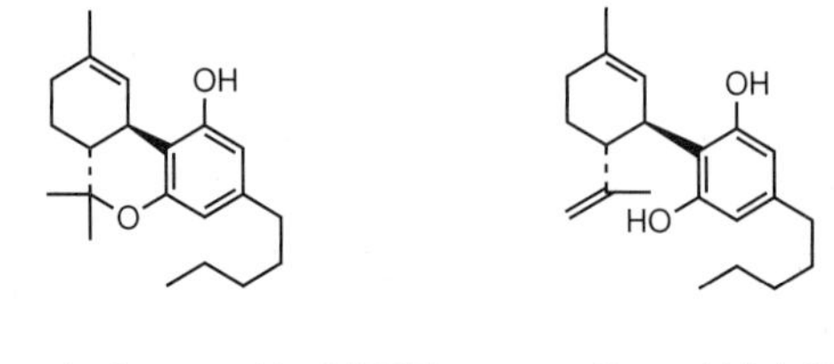

Tetrahydrocannabinol (THC) Cannabidiol (CBD)

Another important natural product lead compound is the tropane alkaloid ester atropine [(±)-hyoscyamine], from the plant *Atropa belladonna* (deadly nightshade) Atropine has served as a prototype molecule for several anticholinergic and antispasmodic drugs. One recently introduced example of an anticholinergic compound modeled on atropine is tiotropium bromide, which is used for the maintenance treatment of bronchospasm associated with chronic obstructive pulmonary disease (54).

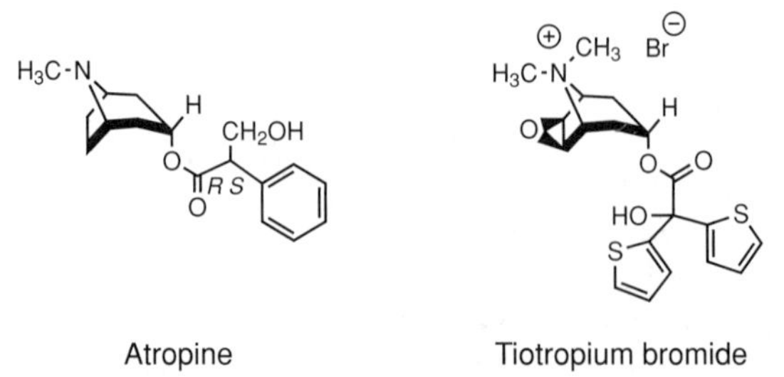

Atropine Tiotropium bromide

In the category of anti-Alzheimer's disease agents, galanthamine hydrobromide is a selective acetylcholinesterase inhibitor that slows neurological degeneration by inhibiting this enzyme and by interacting with the nicotinic receptor (55). Galanthamine (also known as "galantamine") is classified as an Amaryllidaceae alkaloid and has been obtained from several species in this family. Because commercial synthesis is not yet economic, it is obtained from the bulbs of *Leucojum aestivum* (snowflake) and *Galanthus* spp. (snowdrops) (1–4). Some evidence indicates an ethnomedical basis for the current use of galanthamine (56).

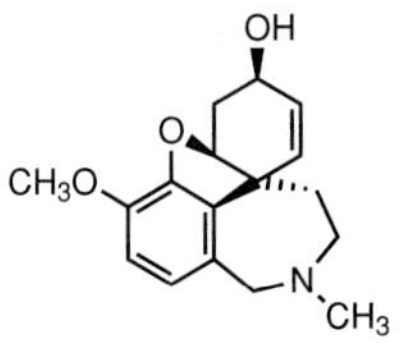

Galanthamine

Anti-infective Agents

Since the introduction of penicillin G (benzylpenicillin) to chemotherapy as an antibacterial agent in the 1940s, natural products have been the most important subcategory of anti-infective agents. As well as the discovery of additional penicillins more resistant to acid hydrolysis and to the β-lactamase enzyme, other classes of antibacterials that have been developed from natural product sources are the aminoglycosides, cephalosporins, glycopeptides, macrolides, rifamycins, and tetracyclines. Antifungals, such as griseofulvin and the polyenes, and the avermectins, such as the antiparasitic drug ivermectin, also are of microbial origin (1–4). Of the approximately 90 drugs in this category that were introduced in Western countries (inclusive of Japan) from 1981 to 2002, almost 80% can be related to a microbial origin (11). In spite of this, relatively few major pharmaceutical companies are currently working on the discovery of new anti-infective agents from natural sources, both because of possible bacterial resistance against new agents and because of concerns in regard to regulation (44). Higher plants also have afforded important anti-infective agents, perhaps most significantly the quinoline alkaloid quinine, obtained from the bark of several *Cinchona* spp. found in South America, including *C. ledgeriana* and *C. succirubra*. Quinine continues to be used for the treatment of multidrug-resistant malaria and was the template molecule for the synthetic antimalarials chloroquine, primaquine, and mefloquine (1–4).

The following examples, shown in Figure 1.2, have been chosen to represent an array of different structural types of antibacterial agents recently introduced into therapy (44). Biapenem is a carbapenem (a group of β-lactam antibiotics in which the sulfur atom in the thiazolidine ring is replaced by a carbon atom) and is based on thienamycin, isolated from *Streptomyces cattleya*. It is a broad-spectrum antibacterial and is more stable to hydrolysis by human renal dihydropeptidase-1 (DHP-1) than other antibiotics in its structural class (57). Tigecycline is a member of the glycylcycline class of tetracycline antibacterials and is the 9-*tert*-butylglycylamido derivative of minocycline, a semisynthetic derivative of chlortetracycline from *Streptomyces aureofaciens*. This is a broad-spectrum antibiotic, with activity against methicillin-resistant *Staphylococcus aureus* (58,59). Daptomycin is the prototype member of the cyclic lipopeptide class of antibiotics,

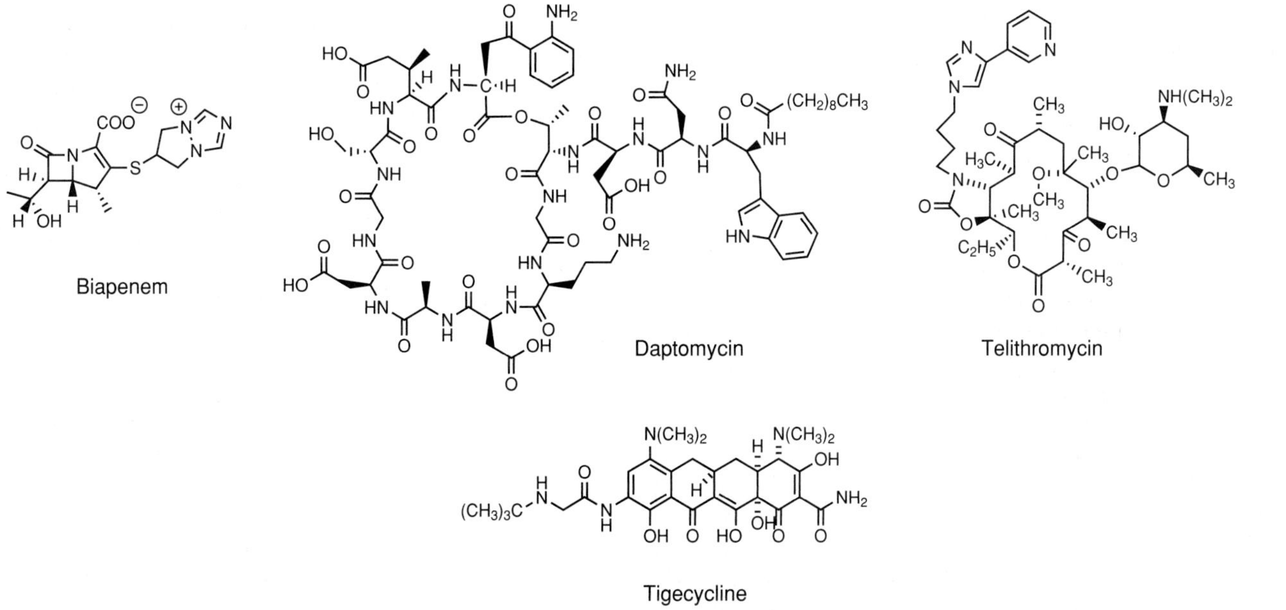

Biapenem

Daptomycin

Telithromycin

Tigecycline

Fig. 1.2. Natural occurring anti-infective agents.

and although isolated initially from *Streptomyces roseosporus*, it is now produced by semisynthesis. This compound binds to bacterial cell membranes, disrupting the membrane potential, and blocks the synthesis of DNA, RNA, and proteins. Daptomycin is bactericidal against Gram-positive organisms (inclusive of vancomycin-resistant *Enterococcus faecalis* and *E. faecium*) and is approved for the treatment of complicated skin and dermal infections (60,61). Telithromycin is a semisynthetic derivative of the 14-membered macrolide erythromycin A, from *Saccharopolyspora erythraea*, and is a macrolide of the ketolide class that lacks a cladinose sugar but has an extended alkyl–aryl unit attached to a cyclic carbamate unit. It binds to domains II and V of the 23S rRNA unit of the bacterial 50S ribosomal unit, leading to inhibition of the ribosome assembly and protein synthesis. This macrolide antibiotic is used to treat bacteria that infect the lungs and sinuses, including community-acquired pneumonia caused by *Streptomyces pneumoniae* (62,63).

Natural products have been a fruitful source of antifungal agents in the past, with the echinocandins being a recently introduced group of lipopeptides (44). Of these, three compounds are now approved drugs, including the acetate of caspofungin, which is a semisynthetic derivative of pneumocandin B_0, a fermentation product of *Glarea lozoyensis*. Caspofungin inhibits the synthesis of the fungal cell wall β(1,3)-D-glucan by noncompetitive inhibition of the enzyme β(1,3)-D-glucan synthase, producing both a fungistatic and a fungicidal effect (64). The compound is administered by slow intravenous infusion and is useful for treating infections by *Candida* and *Aspergillus* spp. (65).

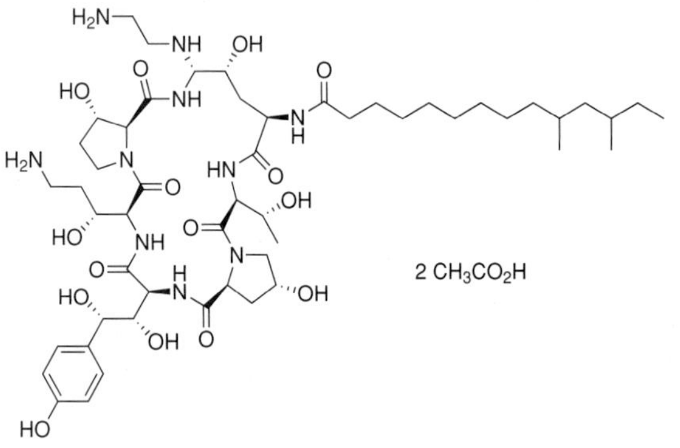

$2\ CH_3CO_2H$

Caspofungin

Malaria remains a parasitic scourge that is still increasing in incidence. In 1972, the active principle from *Artemisia annua*, a plant used for centuries in Chinese traditional medicine to treat fevers and malaria, was established as a novel antimalarial chemotype. This compound, artemisinin ("qinghaosu" in Chinese), is a sesquiterpene lactone with an endoperoxide group that is essential for activity, and it reacts with the iron in heme in the malarial parasite, *Plasmodium falciparum* (Fig. 1.3). Because this compound is poorly soluble in water, a number of derivatives have been produced with improved formulation, including arteether and artemether. Animal

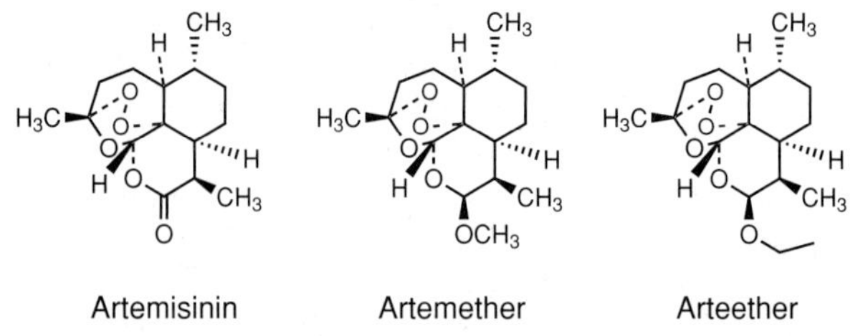

Artemisinin Artemether Arteether

Fig. 1.3. Artemisinin and two derivatives used for the treatment of malaria.

experiments have suggested that artemisinin derivatives are neurotoxic, but this may not be the case in patients with malaria (1–4). Artemisinin-based combination treatments, such as coartemether (artemether and lumefantrine), are now widely used for treating drug-resistant falciparum malaria (66). Coartemether also is known as Artemisinin Combination Therapy and is registered in approximately 75 countries. A second ether derivative of artemisinin, arteether, also has been developed and is registered in the Netherlands (67).

Anticancer Agents

For several decades, natural products have served as a very useful group of structurally diverse cancer chemotherapeutic agents, and many of our most important anticancer agents are of microbial or plant origin. Thus, the antitumor antibiotics include the anthracyclines (daunorubicin, doxorubicin, epirubicin, idarubucin, and valrubucin), bleomycin, dactinomycin (actinomycin D), mitomycin C, and mitoxantrone. Four main classes of plant-derived antitumor agents are used—namely, the vinca (*Catharanthus* spp.) bisindole alkaloids (vinblastine, vincristine, and vinorelbine), the semisynthetic epipodophyllotoxin derivatives (etoposide, teniposide, and etoposide phosphate), the taxanes (paclitaxel and docetaxel), and the camptothecin analogues (irinotecan and topotecan) (Fig. 1.4).

The parent compounds, paclitaxel (originally called "taxol") and camptothecin, were both discovered in the laboratory of the late Monroe E. Wall and Mansukh Wani at Research Triangle Institute in North Carolina (Fig. 1.4). Like some other natural product drugs, several years elapsed between the initial discovery of these substances and their ultimate clinical approval in either a chemically unmodified or modified form (68). One of the factors that served to delay the introduction of paclitaxel to the market was the need for the large-scale acquisition of this compound from a source other than from the bark of its original plant of origin, the Pacific yew, *Taxus brevifolia*, because this would involve destroying the slow-growing tree. Paclitaxel and its semisynthetic analogue docetaxel may be produced by partial synthesis. To enable this, the diterpenoid "building block," 10-deacetylbaccatin III, is used as a starting material. This material can be isolated from the needles of the ornamental yew, *Taxus baccata*, a renewable botanical resource that can be cultivated in greenhouses (68). More recently, the plant tissue culture of *Taxus Chinensis* has become available for the commercial production of

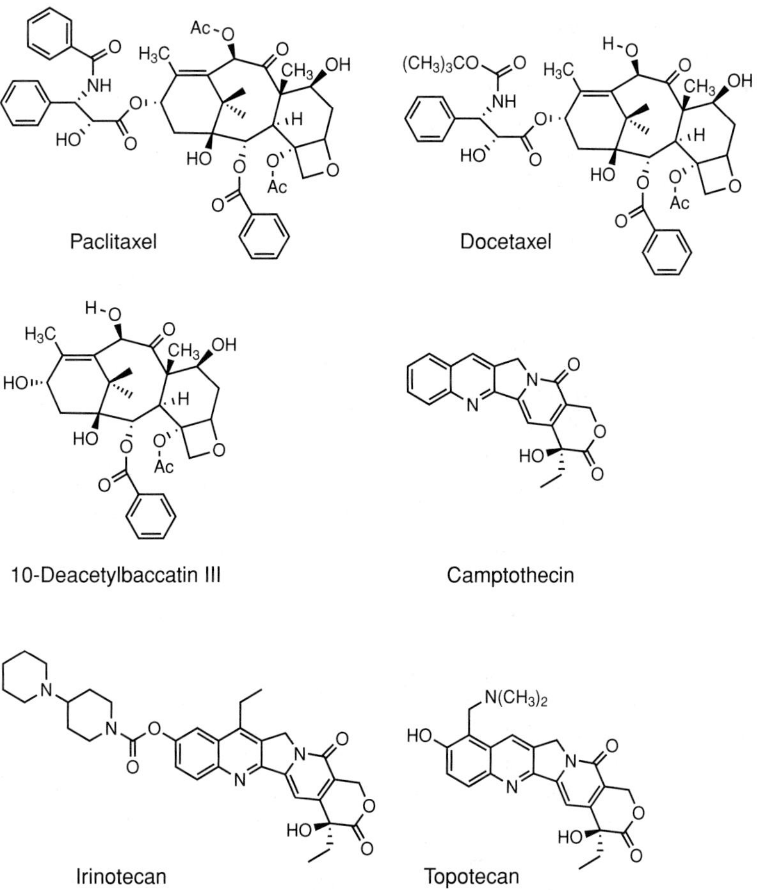

Fig. 1.4. Lead anticancer compounds paclitaxel, camptothecin, and their respective derivatives.

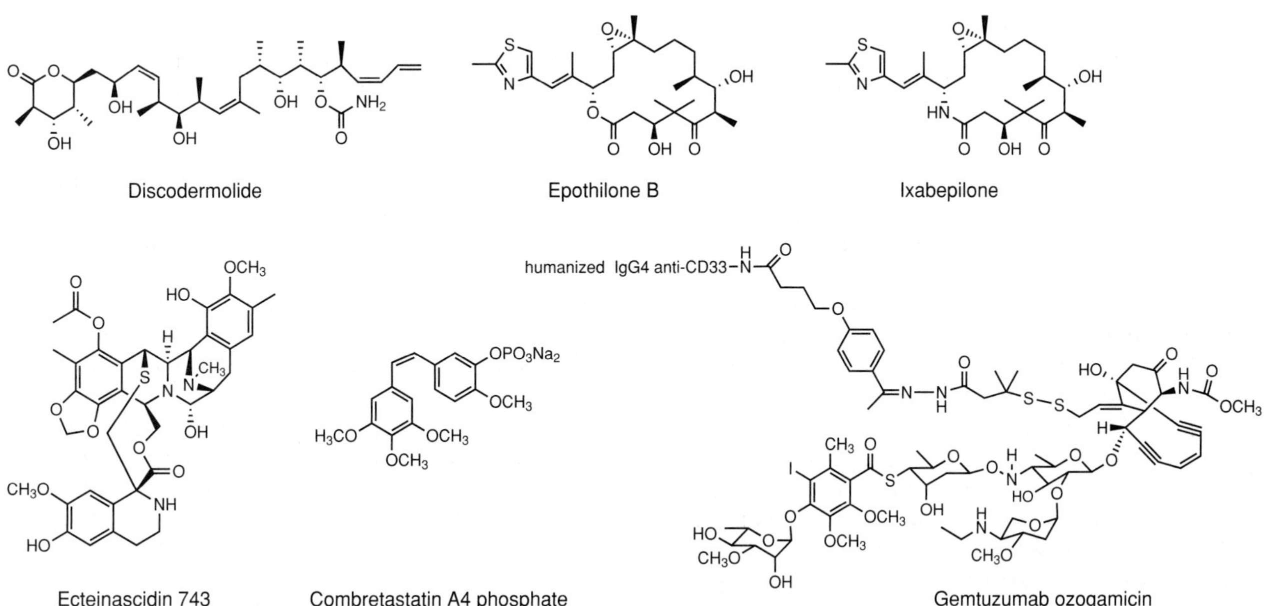

Fig. 1.5. Potential cancer chemotherapeutic agents from marine, bacterial, plant, and fungal origin.

paclitaxel. The initial source plant of camptothecin, *Camptotheca acuminata*, is a rare species found in southern regions of the People's Republic of China. Today, camptothecin is produced commercially not only from cultivated *C. acuminata* trees in mainland China but also from the roots of *Nothapodytes nimmoniana* (formerly known as both *N. foetida* and *Mappia foetida*), which is found in the southern regions of the Indian subcontinent (69). Interestingly, these two antineoplastic agents are particularly important both because of the clinical effectiveness of their derivatives as cancer chemotherapeutic agents and because they are prominent lead compounds for synthetic optimization. Numerous taxanes and camptothecin derivatives are now in clinical trials (43,44). Endophytic fungi also have been reported to produce paclitaxel (29) and camptothecin (70), so in the future, it may be possible to produce these important compounds by fungal fermentation rather than by cultivation. Paclitaxel and camptothecin were each found to exhibit a unique mechanism of action for the inhibition of cancer cell growth: Paclitaxel promotes the polymerization of tubulin and the stabilization of microtubules, whereas camptothecin was the first inhibitor of the enzyme DNA topoisomerase I (68).

A large number of other new natural products of diverse origin have great potential for future therapeutic use as anticancer agents. Several other natural product molecules or their derivatives have been shown to have a action similar to that of paclitaxel against tubulin and are now either in clinical trials or preclinical development; these include dictyostatin-1, eleutherobin, laulimalide, and sarcodictyin, all of which are marine origin (6,43,44,71). Also included in this group is discodermolide, a polyketide lactone from the marine sponge, *Discodermia dissoluta*, which has now been synthesized (71,72), and several epothilones from the terrestrial myxobacterium *Sorangium cellulosum*, of which epothilone B and its semisynthetic derivative ixabepilone are representative (Fig. 1.5) (70,73). Two further examples of promising new anticancer agents are combretastatin A4 phosphate, a water-soluble prodrug of combretastatin A4 from the South African plant, *Combretum caffrum*, and ecteinascidin 743 (ET-743; trabectedin), biosynthesized from the marine tunicate, *Ecteinascidia turbinata*, but now produced by partial synthesis from a microbial metabolite (Fig. 1.5). Combretastatin A4 phosphate binds to tubulin and also affects tumor blood flow, and it is being evaluated along with other cytotoxic agents and radiotherapy (70,74). ET-743 binds to the minor groove of DNA, blocks cells in the G_2/M phase, and is being evaluated in patients with soft-tissue sarcoma (70,75). An example of a natural product derivative that has been recently introduced into cancer chemotherapy is gemtuzumab ozogamicin (Fig. 1.5). This is a conjugated molecule in which the highly active enediyne DNA-damaging agent component, calichaemicin γ1, produced by *Micromonospora echinospora*, is linked to a monoclonal antibody that binds specifically to the CD33 cell-surface antigen of acute myeloid leukemic cells, where the enediyne is released (8,76).

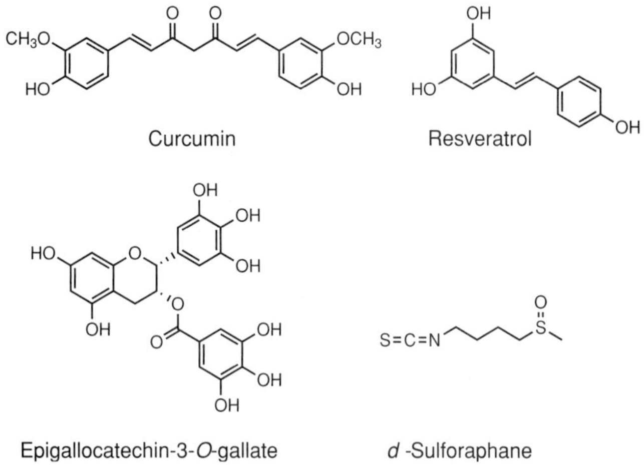

Curcumin

Resveratrol

Epigallocatechin-3-*O*-gallate

d-Sulforaphane

Fig. 1.6. Naturally occurring cancer chemopreventive agents.

Cancer chemoprevention is regarded as the use of synthetic or natural agents to inhibit, delay, or reverse the process of carcinogenesis through intervention before the appearance of invasive disease. This new approach toward the management of cancer has involved gaining a better understanding of the mechanism of action by cancer chemopreventive agents (77). Among the natural products that have been studied for this purpose, there has been a renewed interest in the effects of the phytochemical components of the diet, and some of these compounds have been found to block cancer initiation ("blocking agents") or to reverse tumor promotion and/or progression ("suppressing agents") (77). Members of many different structural types of plant secondary metabolites have been linked to potential cancer chemopreventive activity (78). Recently, approximately 35 foods of plant origin have been found to produce cancer chemopreventive agents, such as curcumin from turmeric, epigallocatechin 3-*O*-gallate from green tea, *trans*-resveratrol from grapes and certain red wines, and *d*-sulforaphane from broccoli (Fig. 1.6) (79).

Immunomodulators

The fungal-derived cyclic peptide cyclosporine (cyclosporin A) was found some years ago to be an immunosuppressive agent in organ and tissue transplant surgery. Another compound with this same type of use and that also acts by the inhibition of T-cell activation is the macrolide tacrolimus (FK-506), from *Streptomyces tsukubaensis* (2).

Two further natural product–derived immunosuppressants have been introduced recently, mycophenolate sodium and everolimus (Fig. 1.7) (44). The active principle of both mycophenolate sodium and an earlier introduced form, mycophenolate mofetil (a morpholinoethyl derivative), is mycophenolic acid, obtained from several *Penicillium* spp. This compound is a reversible inhibitor of inosine monophosphate dehydrogenase, which is involved in guanosine nucleotide synthesis (80).

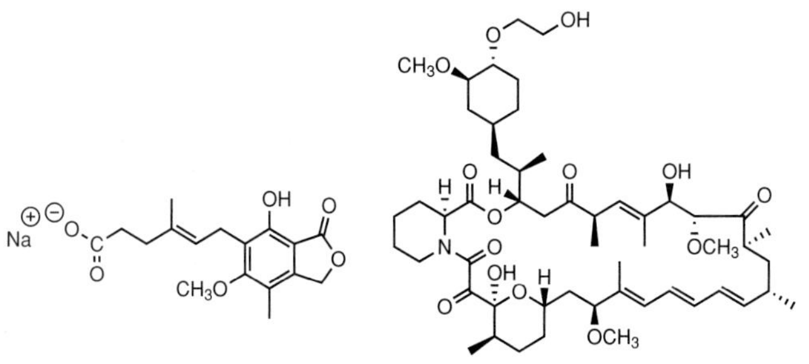

Fig. 1.7. Naturally occurring immunosuppressants.

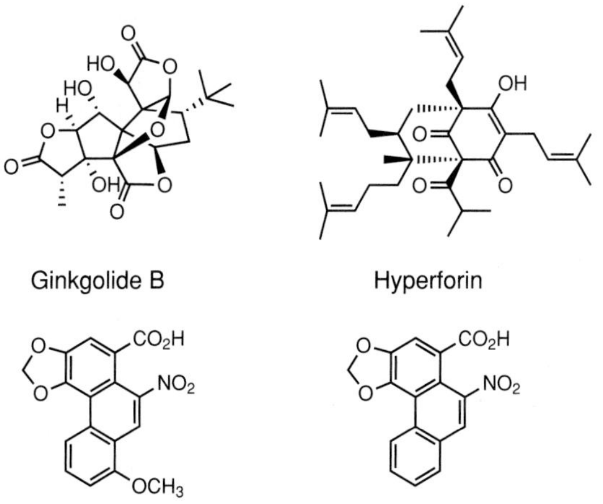

Fig. 1.8. Chemicals found in various botanical dietary supplements.

Everolimus is an orally active, semisynthetic 40-*O*-(2-hydroxyethyl) derivative of rapamycin (also known as sirolimus) and was originally obtained from *Streptomyces hygroscopicus*. Everolimus is a proliferation inhibitor that blocks growth factor-mediated signal transduction and prevents organ rejection through a different mechanism than mycophenolate mofetil (81).

BOTANICAL DIETARY SUPPLEMENTS

The use of phytomedicines (herbal remedies) as prescription products has been well established in Germany and several other countries of Western Europe for approximately 25 years. Approximately 80% of physicians in Germany prescribe phytomedicines through the orthodox health care system. During the last decade, there has been a large influx of botanical products into community pharmacy practice and health food stores in the United States as a result of the Dietary Supplement Health and Education Act in 1994. Such products are regulated by the U.S. Food and Drug Administration as foods rather than drugs, and they must adhere to requirements in regard to product labeling and acceptable health claims (82). Currently, among the most popular botanical products used in the United States are those containing black cohosh, cranberry, echinacea, evening primrose, garlic, ginkgo, ginger, ginseng, green tea, milk thistle, saw palmetto, soy, St. John's wort, and valerian. These are purchased as either the crude powdered form in compressed tablets or capsules or as galenical preparations, such as extracts or tinctures, and they frequently are ingested in the form of a tea (82). In addition to the United States, a parallel increased interest in herbal remedies has occurred in Europe, Canada, and Australia, in part because of an overall greater awareness of complementary and alternative medicine. Many clinical trials focusing on these products have been conducted in Europe, and some are occurring in the United States under the sponsorship of the National Institutes of Health.

The recent widespread introduction of a large number of botanical dietary supplements has opened a new door in terms of research inquiry for natural product scientists in the United States. Not all of these products, however, have a well-documented efficacy (82). Three important needs in the scientific investigation of herbal remedies are the characterization of active principles (when these are not known), the development of rigorous and validated analytical methods for quality-control procedures, and the determination of potential toxicity and interactions with prescription medications (83). Unlike compounds approved as single-chemical drugs, it is accepted that combinations of plant secondary metabolites may be responsible for the physiological effects of herbal medicines. For example, both the terpene lactone (e.g., ginkgolide B) (Fig. 1.8) and flavonoid glycoside constituents of *Ginkgo biloba* leaves are regarded as being necessary for mediation of the symptoms of peripheral vascular disease, for which this phytomedicine is used in Europe (82). Moreover, an acetone-soluble extract of *G. biloba* containing standardized amounts of flavone glycosides (24%) and terpene lactones (6%) has been used in many clinical trials on this herb (82). If the "active principles" of an herbal remedy are known or can be discovered, these substances can act as reference standards, and their specified concentration levels can be quantified in chemical quality-control procedures, which are predominantly performed by HPLC. A number of official monographs for the standardization of botanical dietary supplements have been developed over the last decade in the United States (84). Other scientific challenges regarding herbal remedies are to establish more completely their dissolution, bioavailability, and shelf life. These products should be free of adulteration (the deliberate addition of nonauthentic plant material or of biologically active or inactive compounds); free of other additives, such as herbicides, pesticides, heavy metals, and solvent residues; and free of microbial and biological contaminants (82–84).

Unfortunately, many herbal remedies may pose toxicity risks or be involved in harmful drug interactions. A drastic example of toxicity caused by a herbal product involves the Chinese medicinal plant *Aristolochia fangchi*, which was substituted in error for another Chinese plant in a weight-reducing regimen taken by a number of women in Belgium approximately 15 years ago. Several years later, this product was linked to the generation of severe renal disease, characterized as interstitial fibrosis with atrophy of the tubules, as well as the development of tumors. These toxic symptoms, also known as "Chinese herb nephropathy," were attributed to the presence of the phenanthrene derivatives, aristolochic acids I and II (Fig. 1.8), produced by *A. fangchi*, which have been found experimentally to intercalate with DNA (85). The presence of high levels of the phloroglucinol derivative hyperforin (Fig. 1.8) in St. John's wort, *Hypericum perforatum*, products has been found to induce cytochrome P450 enzymes (particularly CYP34A), leading to decreased plasma concentrations of prescription drugs that are coadministered, such as alprazolam, cyclosporine, digoxin, indinavir, irinotecan, simvastatin, and warfarin, as well as oral contraceptives (86).

FUTURE PROSPECTS

The beginning years of the twenty-first century seem opportune for renewed efforts to be made in regard to the discovery of new secondary-metabolite, prototype biologically active compounds from animals, fungi, microorganisms, and plants of both terrestrial and marine origin. Although many pharmaceutical companies have reduced their investment in natural product research in favor of screening libraries of synthetic compounds and combinatorial chemistry, this has coincided with disappointing numbers of single-chemical entities being introduced as new drugs in recent years (8,11,13). Fortunately, many smaller "biotech" companies have actively taken up the challenge of contemporary natural product drug discovery from organisms (87). There continues to be a steady stream of new natural product-derived drugs introduced for the treatment of many common human diseases (e.g., cancer, cardiovascular diseases, neurological conditions) (13,43). There is ample potential, however, for much greater utilization of natural product-derived compounds in the treatment or prophylaxis of such major worldwide scourges as HIV/AIDS, tuberculosis, hepatitis C, and tropical diseases (inclusive of lymphatic filariasis, leishmaniasis, and schistosomiasis). The search for such agents should be enhanced by the availability of extensive libraries of taxonomically authenticated crude extracts of terrestrial and marine origin as well as pure secondary metabolites from microorganisms, plants, and animals. In addition, this will be facilitated by recently developed techniques, such as biocatalysis, combinatorial biosynthesis, combinatorial and computational chemistry, metabolic engineering, and tissue culture. The high "drug-like" quality of natural product molecules stands as a constant, and it only remains for natural product chemists and biologists to investigate these substances in the most technically ingenious and expedient ways.

It should not be thought that, after approximately 200 years of investigation, the prospects of finding new drugs of natural origin are nearing exhaustion; much hope for success remains in this type of endeavor. For example, if one considers plants, less than 20% have been evaluated chemically or biologically. Moreover, of approximately 21,000 alkaloids, which are mainly of plant origin, about 75% have never been subjected to testing in a bioassay (87). The urgency of performing this type of work cannot be understated in view of the increasing erosion of natural resources that will accelerate as the twenty-first century progresses.

References

1. Evans WC. Trease and Evans' Pharmacognosy. 15th Ed. New York: WB Saunders, 2002.
2. Dewick PM. Medicinal Natural Products: A Biosynthetic Approach. 2nd Ed. New York: John Wiley & Sons, 2002.
3. Samuelsson G. Drugs of Natural Origin. A Textbook of Pharmacognosy. 5th Rev. Ed. Stockholm: Swedish Pharmaceutical Press, 2004.
4. Heinrich M, Barnes J, Gibbons S, et al. Fundamentals of Pharmacognosy and Phytotherapy. Edinburgh: Churchill Livingstone, 2004.
5. Kinghorn AD. Pharmacognosy in the 21st century. J Pharm Pharmacol 2001;53:135–148.
6. Newman DJ, Cragg GM. Marine natural products and related compounds in clinical and advanced clinical trials. J Nat Prod 2004;67:1216–1238.
7. Clardy J, Walsh C. Lessons from natural molecules. Nature 2004;432: 829–837.
8. Koehn FE, Carter GT. The evolving role of natural products in drug discovery. Nat Rev Drug Discov 2005;4:206–220.
9. Henkel T, Brunne RM, Muller H, et al. Statistical investigation into the structural complementarity of natural products and synthetic compounds. Angew Chem Int Ed Eng 1999;38:643–647.
10. Paterson I, Anderson EA. The renaissance of natural products as drug candidates. Science 2005;310:451–453.
11. Newman DJ, Cragg GM, Snader KM. Natural products as sources of new drugs over the period 1981–2002. J Nat Prod 2003;66:1022–1037.
12. Jones WP, Chin YW, Kinghorn AD. The role of pharmacognosy in modern medicine and pharmacy. Curr Drug Targets 2006;7:247–264.
13. Butler MS. The role of natural product chemistry in drug discovery. J Nat Prod 2004;67:2141–2153.
14. Fabricant DS, Farnsworth NR. The value of plants used in traditional medicine for drug discovery. Environ Health Perspect 2001;109:69–75.
15. Lewis WH. Pharmaceutical discoveries based on ethnomedicinal plants: 1985 to 2000 and beyond. Econ Bot 2003;57:126–134.
16. James LF, Panter KE, Gaffield W, et al. Biomedical applications of poisonous plant research. J Agric Food Chem 2004;52:3211–3230.
17. Spjut RW. Relationships between folklore and antitumor activity: an historical review. Sida 2005;21:2205–2241.
18. McConnell OJ, Longley RE, Koehn FE. The discovery of marine natural products with therapeutic potential. In: Gullo VP, ed. The Discovery of Natural Products with Therapeutic Potential. Boston: Butterworth-Heinemann, 1993:109–174.
19. Piel J. Metabolites from symbiotic bacteria. Nat Prod Rep 2004;21: 519–538.
20. Tan GT, Gyllenhaal C, Soejarto DD. Biodiversity as a source of anticancer agents. Curr Drug Targets 2006;7:265–277.
21. Simmons TL, Andrianosolo E, McPhail K, et al. Marine natural products as anticancer drugs. Mol Cancer Ther 2005;4:335–342.
22. Pitman NCA, Jørgensen PM. Estimating the size of the world's threatened flora. Science 2002;298:989.
23. Myers N, Mittermeier RA, Mittermeier CG, et al. Biodiversity hotspots for conservation priorities. Nature 2000;403;853–858.
24. Farrier D, Tucker L. Access to marine bioresources: hitching the conservation car to the bioprospecting horse. Ocean Dev Int Law 2001;32: 213–239.
25. Hallock YF, Cragg GM. National Cooperative Drug Discovery Groups (NCDDGs): a successful model for public private partnerships in cancer drug discovery. Pharm Biol 2003;41(Suppl):78–91.
26. Kinghorn AD, Farnsworth NR, Soejarto DD, et al. Novel strategies for the discovery of plant-derived anticancer agents. Pharm Biol 2003;41(Suppl): 53–67.
27. Berdy J. Bioactive microbial metabolites: a personal view. J Antibiot 2005; 58:1–26.
28. Fenical W, Jensen PR, Kauffman C, et al. New anticancer agents from cultured and collected marine organisms. Pharm Biol 2003;41(Suppl):6–14.
29. Strobel G, Daisy B, Castillo U, et al. Natural products from endophytic microorganisms. J Nat Prod 2004;67:257–268.

30. Nonaka G-I, Nishioka E, Nishizawa M, et al. Anti-AIDS agents. 2. Inhibitory effects of tannins on HIV reverse transcriptase and HIV replication in H9 lymphocyte cells. J Nat Prod 1990;53:587–595.
31. Okuda T. Systematics and health effects of chemically distinct tannins in medicinal plants. Phytochemistry 2005;66:2012–2031.
32. Balunas MJ, Su B, Landini S, et al. Interference by naturally occurring fatty acids in a noncellular enzyme-based aromatase bioassay. J Nat Prod 2006;69: 700–703.
33. Silverman L, Campbell R, Broach JR. New assay technologies for high-throughput screening. Curr Opin Chem Biol 1998;2:397–403.
34. Jacob MR, Walker LA. Natural products and antifungal drug discovery. In: Ernst EJ, Rogers P, eds. Methods in Molecular Medicine, vol 118: Antifungal Agents: Methods and Protocols. Totowa, NJ: Humana Press, 2005:83–109.
35. Mora FD, Jones DK, Desai PV, et al. Bioassay for the identification of natural product-based activators of peroxisome proliferator-activated receptor-γ (PPARγ): the marine sponge metabolite psammaplin A activates PPARγ and induces apoptosis in human breast cancer cells. J Nat Prod 2006;69: 547–552.
36. Walters WP, Namchuk M. Designing screens: how to make your hits a hit. Nat Rev Drug Discov 2003;2:259–266.
37. Steinbeck C. Recent developments in automated structure elucidation of natural products. Nat Prod Rep 2004;21:512–518.
38. Clarkson C, Stærk D, Hansen SH, et al. Hyphenation of solid-phase extraction with liquid chromatography and nuclear magnetic resonance: application of HPLC-DAD-SPE-NMR to identification of constituents of *Kanahia laniflora*. Anal Chem 2005;77:3547–3553.
39. Dinan L. Dereplication and partial identification of compounds. In: Sarker SD, Latif Z, Gray AI, eds. Methods in Biotechnology, vol. 20: Natural Products Isolation. 2nd Ed. Totowa, NJ: Humana Press, 2005:297–321.
40. Sumner LW, Mendes P, Dixon RA. Plant metabolomics: large-scale phytochemistry in the functional genomics era. Phytochemistry 2003;62:817–836.
41. Rochfort S. Metabolomics revisited: a new "omics" platform technology for systems biology and implications for natural products research. J Nat Prod 2005;68:1813–1820.
42. Hollingshead MG, Alley MC, Camalier RF, et al. In vivo cultivation of tumor cells in hollow fibers. Life Sci 1995;25:131–141.
43. Weissman KJ, Leadlay PF. Combinatorial biosynthesis of reduced polyketides. Nat Rev Microbiol 2005;3:925–936.
44. Butler MS. Natural products to drugs: natural product derived compounds in clinical trials. Nat Prod Rep 2005;22:162–195.
45. Cragg GM, Newman DJ. A tale of two tumor targets: topoisomerase I and tubulin. The Wall and Wani contribution to cancer chemotherapy. J Nat Prod 2004;67:232–244.
46. Ledizet M, Harrison LM, Koski RA, et al. Discovery and preclinical development of antithrombotics from hematophagous invertebrates. Curr Med Chem Cardiovasc Hematol Agents 2005;3:1–10.
47. Moen MD, Keating GM, Wellington K. Bivalirudin. A review of its use in patients undergoing percutaneous coronary intervention. Drugs 2005;65:1869–1891.
48. Buse JB, Henry RR, Han J, et al. Effects of exenatide (exendin-4) on glycemic control over 30 weeks in sulfonylurea-treated patients with type-2 diabetes. Diabetes Care 2004;27:2628–2635.
49. Clement JA, Yoder BJ, Kingston DGI. Natural products as a source of CNS-active agents. Mini-Rev Org Chem 2004;1:183–208.
50. Lotsch J, Geisslinger G. Morphine-6-glucuronide: an analgesic of the future? Clin Pharmacokinet 2001;40:485–499.
51. Daly JW, Spande TF, Garraffo HM. Alkaloids from amphibian skin: a tabulation of over 800 compounds. J Nat Prod 2005;68:1556–1575.
52. Miljanich GP. Ziconotide: neuronal calcium channel blocker for treating severe chronic pain. Curr Med Chem 2004;11:3029–3040.
53. Burns TL, Ineck JR. Cannabinoid analgesia as a potential new therapeutic option in the treatment of chronic pain. Ann Pharmacother 2006;40:251–260.
54. Mundy C, Kirkpatrick P. Fresh from the pipeline. Tiotropium bromide. Nat Rev Drug Disc 2004;3:643–644.
55. Suh WH, Suslick KS, Suh Y-H. Therapeutic agents for Alzheimer's disease. Curr Med Chem Central Nervous System Agents 2005;5:259–269.
56. Heinrich M, Teoh HL. Galanthamine from snowdrop—the development of a modern drug against Alzheimer's disease from local Caucasian knowledge. J Ethnopharmacol 2004;92:147–162.
57. Perry CM, Ibbotson T. Biapenem. Drugs 2002;62:2221–2234.
58. Milatovic D, Schmitz F-J, Verhoef J, et al. Activities of the glycylcycline tigecycline (GAR-936) against 1,924 recent European clinical bacterial isolates. Antimicrob Agents Chemother 2003;47:400–404.
59. Zhanel GG, Karlowsky JA, Rubenstein E, et al. Tigecycline: a novel glycylcycline antibiotic. Exp Rev Anti-infect Ther 2006;4:9–25.
60. Baltz RH, Maio V, Wrigley SK. Natural products to drugs: daptomycin and related lipopeptide antibiotics. Nat Prod Rep 2005;22:717–741.
61. Adler JD. Daptomycin, a new drug class for the treatment of Gram-positive infections. Drugs of Today 2005;41:81–90.
62. Berisio R, Harms J, Schleunzen F, et al. Structural insight into the antibiotic action of telithromycin against resistant mutants. J Bacteriol 2003;185: 4276–4279.
63. Speirs KM, Zervos MJ. Telithromycin. Exp Rev Anti-infect Ther 2004;2: 685–693.
64. Letscher-Bru V, Herbrecht R. Caspofungin: the first representative of a new antifungal class. J Antimicrob Chemother 2003;51:513–521.
65. McCormack PL, Perry CM. Caspofungin: a review of its use in the treatment of fungal infections. Drugs 2005;65:2049–2068.
66. Wernsdorfer WH. Coartemether (artemether and lumefantrine): an oral antimalarial drug. Expert Rev Anti-infect Ther 2004;2:181–196.
67. Yeates RA. Artemotil (Artecef). Curr Opin Invest Drugs 2002;3:545–549.
68. Oberlies NH, Kroll DJ. Camptothecin and taxol: historic achievements in natural products research. J Nat Prod 2004;67:129–135.
69. Padmanabha BV, Chandrashekar M, Ramesha BT, et al. Patterns of accumulation of camptothecin, an anticancer alkaloid, in *Nothapodytes nimmoniana* Graham, in the Western Ghats, India: implications for identifying high-yielding sources of the alkaloid. Curr Sci 2006;90:95–100.
70. Puri SC, Verma V, Amna T, et al. An endophytic fungus from *Nothapodytes foetida* that produces camptothecin. J Nat Prod 2005;68:1717–1719.
71. Cragg GM, Kingston DGI, Newman DJ, eds. Anticancer Agents from Natural Products. Boca Raton, FL: Taylor & Francis/CRC Press, 2005.
72. Mickel SJ. Toward a commercial synthesis of (+)-discodermolide. Curr Opin Drug Discov Dev 2004;7:869–881.
73. Zhuang SH, Agrawal M, Edgerly M, et al. A Phase I clinical trial of ixabepilone (BMS-247550), an epothilone B analog, administered intravenously on a daily schedule for 3 days. Cancer 2005;103:1932–1938.
74. Cooney MM, Ortiz J, Bukowski RM, et al. Novel vascular targeting/disrupting agents: combretastatin A4 phosphate and related compounds. Curr Oncol Rep 2005;7:90–95.
75. Fayette J, Coquard IR, Alberti L, et al. ET-743: a novel agent with activity in soft-tissue sarcomas. Oncologist 2005;10:827–832.
76. Fenton C, Perry CM. Gemtuzumab ozogamicin: a review of its use in acute myeloid leukemia. Drugs 2005;65:2405–2427.
77. Kelloff GJ, Hawk ET, Sigman CC, eds. Cancer Chemoprevention, vol. 1: Promising Cancer Chemopreventive Agents. Totowa, NJ: Humana Press, 2004.
78. Kinghorn AD, Su B-N, Jang DS, et al. Natural inhibitors of carcinogenesis. Planta Med 2004;70:691–705.
79. Surh Y-J. Cancer chemoprevention with dietary phytochemicals. Nat Rev Cancer 2003;3;768–780.
80. Curran MP, Keating GM. Mycophenylate delayed release: prevention of renal transplant rejection. Drugs 2005;65:799–805.
81. Chapman TM, Perry CM. Everolimus. Drugs 2004;64:861–872.
82. Robbers JC, Tyler VE. Tyler's Herbs of Choice. The Therapeutic Use of Phytomedicinals. New York: The Haworth Herbal Press, 1999.
83. Cardellina JH. Challenges and opportunities confronting the botanical dietary supplement industry. J Nat Prod 2001;65:1073–1081.
84. Schiff PL Jr, Srinivasan VS, Giancaspro GI, et al. The development of USP botanical dietary supplement monographs, 1995–2005. J Nat Prod 2006;69: 464–472.
85. IARC Monographs on the Evaluation of Carcinogenic Risks to Humans, vol. 82: Some Traditional Herbal Medicines, Some Mycotoxins, Naphthalene, and Styrene. Lyon: IARC Press, 2002.
86. Madabushi R, Frank B, Drewelow B, et al. Hyperforin in St. John's wort drug interactions. Eur J Clin Pharmacol 2006;62:225–233.
87. Cordell GA, Colvard MA. Some thoughts on the future of ethnopharmacology. J Ethnopharmacol 2005;100:5–14.

2. *Drug Design and Relationship of Functional Groups to Pharmacologic Activity*

JAMES J. KNITTEL AND ROBIN M. ZAVOD

Medicinal chemistry is the discipline concerned with determining the influence of chemical structure on biological activity. As such, it is necessary for the medicinal chemist to understand not only the mechanism by which a drug exerts its effect but also the physicochemical properties of the molecule. The term "physicochemical properties" refers to the influence of the organic functional groups within a molecule on its acid-base properties, water solubility, partition coefficient, crystal structure, stereochemistry, and so on. All these properties influence the absorption, distribution, metabolism excretion, and toxicity of the molecule. To design better medicinal agents, the medicinal chemist needs to understand the relative contributions that each functional group makes to the overall physicochemical properties of the molecule. Studies of this type involve modification of the molecule in a systematic fashion and determination of how these changes affect biological activity. Such studies are referred to as studies of structure–activity relationships (SARs)—that is, what structural features of the molecule contributes to, or takes away from, the desired biological activity of the molecule of interest.

Because of the fundamental nature of the subject matter, this chapter includes numerous case studies throughout (as boxes) as well as at the end. In addition, a list of study questions at the end of—and unique to—this chapter provides further self-study material regarding the subject of drug design.

INTRODUCTION

Chemical compounds, usually derived from plants and other natural sources, have been used by humans for thousands of years to alleviate pain, diarrhea, infection, and various other maladies. Until the nineteenth century, these "remedies" were primarily crude preparations of plant material of unknown constitution. The revolution in synthetic organic chemistry during the nineteenth century produced a concerted effort toward identification of the structures of the active constituents of these naturally derived medicinals and synthesis of what were hoped to be more efficacious agents. By determining the molecular structures of the active components of these complex mixtures, it was thought that a better understanding of how these components worked could be elucidated.

Relationship Between Molecular Structure and Biological Activity

Early studies of the relationship between chemical structure and biological activity were conducted by Crum-Brown and Fraser (1) in 1869. They showed that many compounds containing tertiary amine groups became muscle relaxants when converted to quaternary ammonium compounds. Compounds with widely differing pharmacologic properties, such as strychnine (a convulsant), morphine (an analgesic), nicotine (deterrent, insecticide), and atropine (anticholinergic), could be converted to muscle relaxants with properties similar to those of tubocurarine when methylated (Fig. 2.1). Crum-Brown and Fraser therefore concluded that muscle-relaxant activity required a quaternary ammonium group

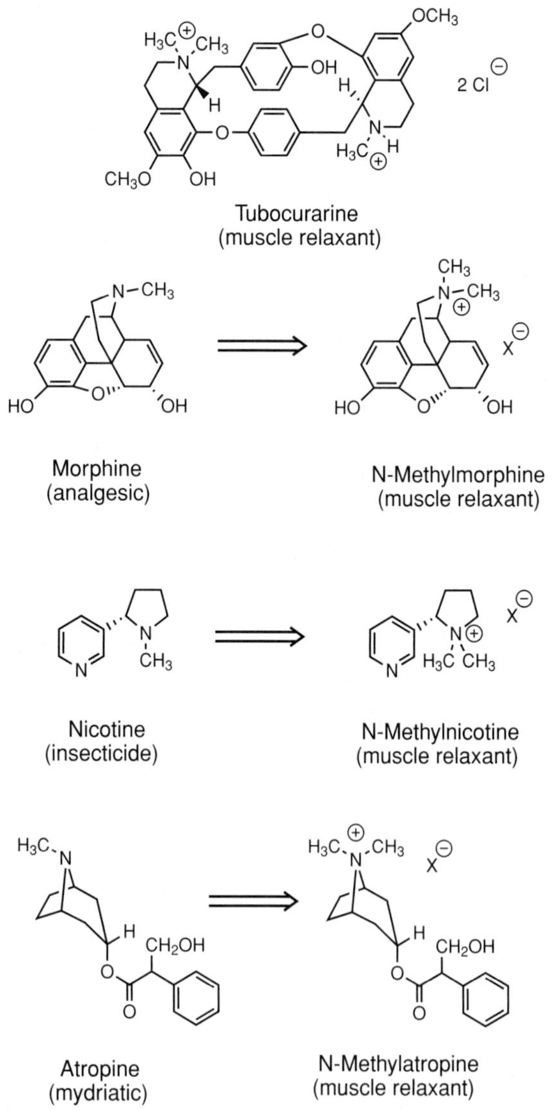

Tubocurarine
(muscle relaxant)

Morphine
(analgesic)

N-Methylmorphine
(muscle relaxant)

Nicotine
(insecticide)

N-Methylnicotine
(muscle relaxant)

Atropine
(mydriatic)

N-Methylatropine
(muscle relaxant)

Fig. 2.1. Effects of methylation on biological activity.

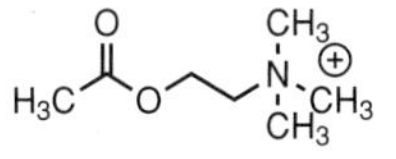

Fig. 2.2. Acetylcholine, a neurotransmitter.

within the chemical structure. This initial hypothesis was later disproven by the discovery of the natural neurotransmitter and activator of muscle contraction, acetylcholine (Fig. 2.2). Even though Crum-Brown and Fraser's initial hypothesis concerning chemical structure and muscle relaxation was incorrect, it demonstrated the concept that molecular structure influences the biological activity of chemical compounds.

With the discovery by Crum-Brown and Fraser that quaternary ammonium groups could produce compounds with muscle-relaxant properties, scientists began looking for other organic functional groups that would produce specific biological responses. The thinking during this time was that specific chemical groups, or nuclei (rings), were responsible for specific biological effects. This lead to the postulate, which took some time to disprove, that "one chemical group gives one biological action" (2). Even after the discovery of acetylcholine by Loewi and Navrati (3), which effectively dispensed with Crum-Brown and Fraser's concept of all quaternary ammonium compounds being muscle relaxants, this was still considered to be dogma and took a long time to replace.

Selectivity of Drug Action and Drug Receptors

Although the structures of many drugs or xenobiotics, or at least the composition of functional groups, were known at the start of the twentieth century, how these compounds exerted their effects was still a mystery. Utilizing his observations regarding the staining behavior of microorganisms, Ehrlich (4) developed the concept of drug receptors. He postulated that certain "side chains" on the surfaces of cells were "complementary" to the dyes (or drug), thereby allowing the two substances to combine. In the case of antimicrobial compounds, this combining of the chemical to the "side chains" produced a toxic effect. This concept effectively was the first description of what later became known as the receptor hypothesis for explaining the biological action of chemical compounds. Ehrlich also discussed selectivity of drug action via the concept of a "magic bullet" for compounds that would eradicate disease states without producing undue harm to the organism being treated (i.e., the patient). This concept was later modified by Albert (5) and generally is referred to as "selective toxicity." Utilizing this concept, Ehrlich developed organic arsenicals that were toxic to trypanosomes as a result of their irreversible reaction with mercapto groups (-SH) on vital proteins within the organism. The formation of As-S bonds resulted in death to the target organism. It was soon learned, however, that these compounds were toxic not only to the target organism but also to the host once certain blood levels of arsenic were achieved.

The "paradox" that resulted after the discovery of acetylcholine—how one chemical group can produce two different biological effects (i.e., muscle relaxation and muscle contraction)—was explained by Ing (6) using the actions of acetylcholine and tubocurarine as his examples. Ing hypothesized that both acetylcholine and tubocurarine act at the same receptor, but that one molecule fits to the receptor in a more complementary manner and "activates" it, causing muscle contraction. (Ing did not elaborate just how this activation occurred.) The blocking effect of the larger molecule, tubocurarine, could be explained by its occupation of part of the receptor, thereby preventing acetylcholine, the smaller molecule, from interacting with the receptor. With both molecules, the quaternary ammonium functional group is a common structural feature and interacts with the same region of the receptor. If one closely examines the structures of other compounds with opposing effects on the same pharmacologic system, this appears to be a common theme: Molecules that block the effects of natural neurotransmitters (antagonists) generally are larger in size than the native compound. Both agonists and antagonists share common structural features, however, thus providing support to the concept that the structure of a molecule, its composition and arrangement of chemical functional groups, determines the type of pharmacologic effect that it possesses (i.e., SAR). Thus, compounds that are muscle relaxants acting via the cholinergic nervous system will possess a quaternary ammonium or protonated tertiary ammonium group and will be larger than acetylcholine.

Structure–activity relationships are the underlying principle of medicinal chemistry. Similar molecules exert similar biological actions in a qualitative sense. A corollary to this is that structural elements (functional groups) within a molecule most often contribute in an additive manner to the physicochemical properties of a molecule and, therefore, to its biological action. One need only peruse the structures of drug molecules in a particular pharmacologic class to become convinced of this (e.g., histamine H_1 antagonists, histamine H_2 antagonists, and β-adrenergic antagonists). The objective of medicinal chemists in their quest for better medicinal agents (drugs) is to discover what functional groups within a specific structure are important for its pharmacologic activity and how can these groups be modified to produce more potent, selective, and safer compounds.

An example of how different functional groups can yield compounds with similar physicochemical properties is shown with sulfanilamide antibiotics. In Figure 2.3, the structures of sulfanilamide and *p*-aminobenzoic acid (PABA) are shown. In 1940, Woods (7) demonstrated that PABA was capable of reversing the antibacterial action of sulfanilamide (and other sulfonamides antibacterials) and that both PABA and sulfanilamide had similar steric and electronic properties. Both compounds contain acidic functional groups, with PABA containing an aromatic carboxylic acid and sulfanilamide an aromatic sulfonamide. When ionized at physiological pH,

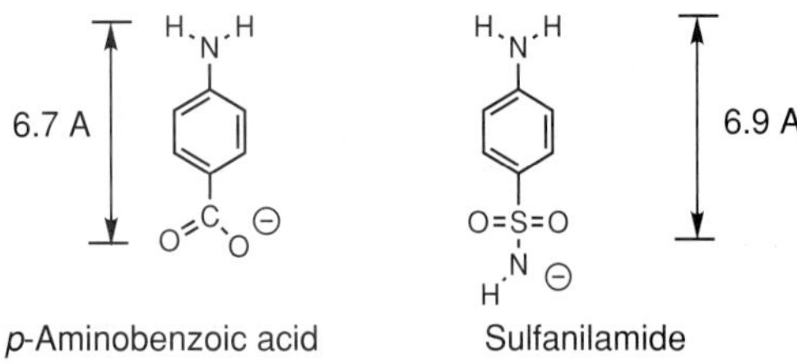

Fig. 2.3. Ionized forms of *p*-aminobenzoic acid (PABA) and sulfanilamide, with comparison of the distance between amine and ionized acids of each compound. Note how closely sulfanilamide resembles PABA.

both compounds have a similar electronic configuration, and the distance between the ionized acid and the weakly basic amino group also is very similar. It should therefore be no surprise that sulfanilamide acts as an antagonist to PABA metabolism in bacteria.

PHYSICOCHEMICAL PROPERTIES OF DRUGS

Acid-Base Properties

The human body is 70 to 75% water, which amounts to approximately 51 to 55 L of water for a 160-lb (73-kg) individual. For an average drug molecule with a molecular weight of 200 g/mol and a dose of 20 mg, this leads to a solution concentration of approximately 2×10^{-6} M. When considering the solution behavior of a drug within the body, we therefore are dealing with a dilute solution, for which the Brönsted-Lowry (8) acid-base theory is most appropriate for explaining and predicting acid-base behavior. This is a very important concept in medicinal chemistry, because the acid-base properties of drug molecules directly affect absorption, excretion, and compatibility with other drugs in solution. According to the Brönsted-Lowry Theory, an "acid" is any substance capable of yielding a proton (H^+), and a "base" is any substance capable of accepting a proton. When an acid gives up a proton to a base, it is converted to its "conjugate base." Similarly, when a base accepts, a proton it is converted to its "conjugate acid" (Eqs. 2.1 and 2.2):

Eq. 2.1 $CH_3COOH + H_2O \rightleftharpoons CH_3COO^{\ominus} + H_3O^{\oplus}$

Acid	Base	Conjugate	Conjugate
(acetic acid)	(water)	base	acid
		(acetate)	(hydronium)

Eq. 2.2 $CH_3NH_2 + H_2O \rightleftharpoons CH_3NH_3^{\oplus} + {}^{\ominus}OH$

Base	Acid	Conjugate	Conjugate
(methylamine)	(water)	acid	base
		(methylammonium)	(hydroxide)

Note that when an acid loses its proton, it is left with an extra pair of electrons that are no longer neutralized by the proton. This is the "ionized" form of the acid and is now more water soluble because of the charge. Because the acid has lost its proton, it also often is referred to as having undergone "dissociation." Many different organic functional groups behave as acids, and these are listed in Table 2.1. It is important that the student learn to recognize these functional groups and their relative acid strengths. This will help the student to predict absorption, distribution, excretion, and potential incompatibilities between drugs.

When a base is converted to its conjugate acid, it too becomes ionized. In this instance, however, it becomes positively charged because of the presence of the extra proton. Most basic drugs usually are derived from primary, secondary, and tertiary amines or imino amines, such as guanidines and amidines. Other organic functional groups that act as bases are shown in Table 2.2. Again, the student should become familiar with these functional groups and be able to readily recognize them by name and relative strengths.

Organic functional groups that cannot give up or accept a proton are considered to be "neutral" (or "nonelectrolytes") with respect to their acid-base properties. Common functional groups of this type are shown in Table 2.3. In the case of quaternary ammonium compounds, the molecule is not electrically neutral, even though it is neither acidic nor basic. Additional reading on the acid-base behavior of the functional groups listed in Tables 2.1 through 2.3 can be found in Gennaro (9) and Lemke (10). Further review of organic functional groups and their acid-base properties can be found at http://www-home.cr.duq.edu/~harrold/.

A molecule may contain multiple functional groups and, therefore, possess both acidic and basic properties. For example, ciprofloxacin (Fig. 2.4), a fluoroquinolone antibiotic, contains a secondary alkylamine, two tertiary arylamines (aniline-like amines), and a carboxylic acid. The two arylamines are weakly basic and, therefore, do not contribute significantly to the acid-base properties of ciprofloxacin. Depending on the pH of the solution (or tissue), this molecule will either accept a proton (secondary alkylamine), yield a proton (carboxylic acid), or both. Thus, it is amphoteric (both acidic and basic) in its properties. Figure 2.5 shows the acid-base behavior of ciprofloxacin at two different locations of the gastrointestinal tract. Note that at a given pH (e.g., pH 1.0–3.5), only one of the functional groups (the alkylamine) is ionized. To be able to make this prediction, one has to understand the relative acid-base strength of acids and bases. Thus, one needs to know which acid or base within a molecule containing multiple functional groups is the strongest and which acid or base is the weakest. The concept of pK_a not only indicates the relative acid-base strength of organic functional groups but also allows one to calculate, for a given pH, exactly how much of the molecule is in the ionized and un-ionized form, which therefore allows prediction of relative water solubility, absorption, and excretion for a given compound.

Table 2.1. Common Acidic Organic Functional Groups and Their Ionized (Conjugate Base) Forms

Acids (pKa)			Conjugate Base
Phenol (9-11)	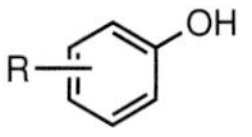	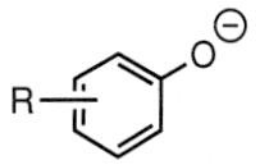	Phenolate
Sulfonamide (9-10)	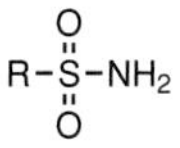 $R-SO_2-NH_2$	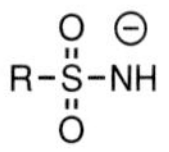 $R-SO_2-NH^{\ominus}$	Sulfonamidate
Imide (9-10)	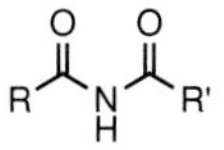	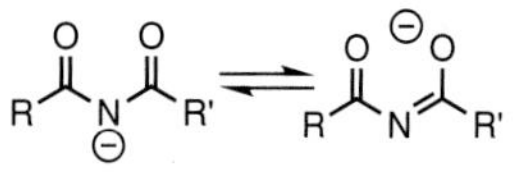	Imidate
Alkylthiol (10-11)	R-SH	$R-S^{\ominus}$	Thiolate
Thiophenol (9-10)	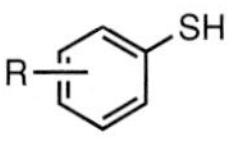	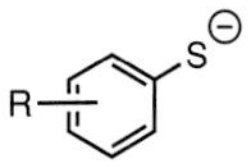	Thiophenolate
N-Arylsulfonamide (6-7)	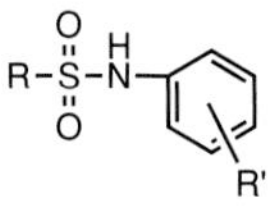	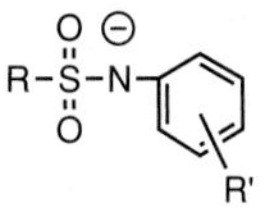	N-Arylsulfonamidate
Sulfonimide (5-6)	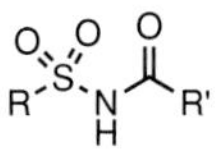	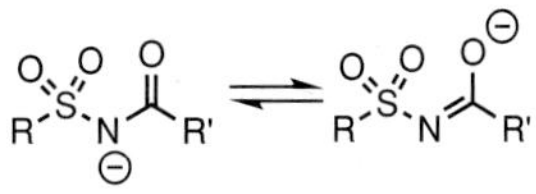	Sulfonimidate
Alkylcarboxylic acid (5-6)	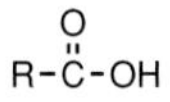 R-C(=O)-OH	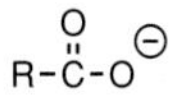 $R-C(=O)-O^{\ominus}$	Alkylcarboxylate
Arylcarboxylic acid (4-5)	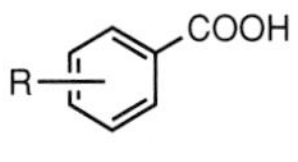	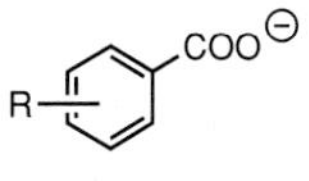	Arylcarboxylate
Sulfonic acid (0-1)	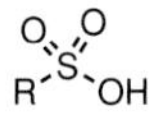 $R-SO_2-OH$	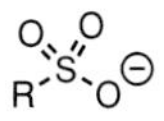 $R-SO_2-O^{\ominus}$	Sulfonate

Acid strength usually increases as one moves down the table.

Relative Acid Strength (pK_a)

Strong acids and bases completely dissociate or accept a proton in aqueous solution to produce their respective conjugate bases and acids. For example, mineral acids, such as HCl, or bases, such as NaOH, undergo 100% dissociation in water, with the equilibrium shifted completely to the right side, as shown in Equations 2.3 and 2.4:

Eq. 2.3 $$HCl + H_2O \rightleftharpoons Cl^{\ominus} + H_3O^{\oplus}$$

Eq. 2.4 $$NaOH + H_2O \rightleftharpoons Na^{\oplus} + OH^{\ominus} + H_2O$$

Acids and bases of intermediate or weak strength, however, incompletely dissociate or accept a proton, and the equilibrium lies somewhere in between. The equilibrium is such that all possible species may exist. Note that in Equations 2.3 and 2.4, water is acting as a base in one instance and as an acid in the other. Water is amphoteric—that is, it may act as an acid or a base, depending on the conditions. Because we are always dealing with a dilute aqueous solution, the strongest base that can be present is OH^-, and the strongest acid is H_3O^+. This is known as the "leveling effect" of water. Thus, some organic functional groups that are considered to be acids or bases with respect to their chemical reactivity do not behave as such under physiological conditions in aqueous solution. For example, alkyl alcohols, such as ethyl alcohol, are not sufficiently acidic to undergo ionization to a significant extent in aqueous solution. Water is not sufficiently basic to remove the proton from the alcohol to form the ethoxide ion (Eq. 2.5). Therefore, under physiological conditions, alcohols may be considered to be neutral with respect to acid-base properties:

Eq. 2.5 $$CH_3CH_2OH + H_2O \rightleftharpoons CH_3CH_2O^- + H_3O^{\oplus}$$

Table 2.2. Common Basic Organic Functional Groups and Their Ionized (Conjugate Acid) Forms

Base (pKa)			Conjugate Acid
Arylamine (9-11)	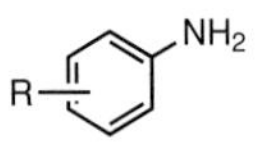 $R-C_6H_4-NH_2$	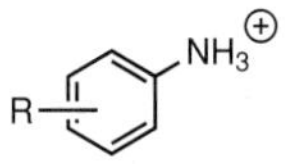 $R-C_6H_4-NH_3^{\oplus}$	Arylammonium
Aromatic amine (5-6)	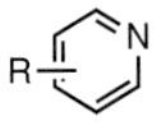 R-pyridine (N)	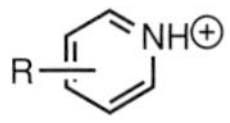 R-pyridinium (NH⊕)	Aromatic ammonium
Imine (3-4)	R-CH=NH	R-CH=NH⊕	Iminium
Alkylamines (2^0 - 10-11) (1^0 - 9-10)	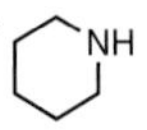 piperidine (NH); $R-NH_2$	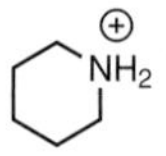 piperidinium ($NH_2^{\oplus}$); $R-NH_3^{\oplus}$	Alkylammonium
Amidine (10-11)	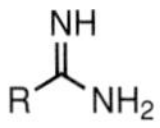 $R-C(=NH)NH_2$	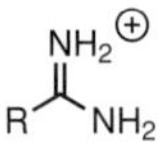 $R-C(=NH_2^{\oplus})NH_2$	Amidinium
Guanidine (12-13)	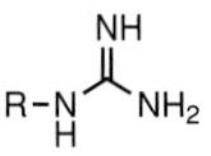 $R-NH-C(=NH)NH_2$	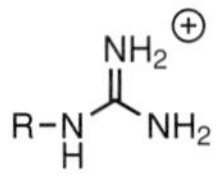 $R-NH-C(=NH_2^{\oplus})NH_2$	Guanidinium

Predicting the Degree of Ionization of a Molecule

From general principles, it is possible to predict if a molecule is going to be ionized or un-ionized at a given pH simply by knowing if the functional groups on the molecule are acidic or basic. To be able to quantitatively predict the degree of ionization of a molecule, however, one must know the pK_a values of the acidic and basic functional groups that are present and the pH of the environment to which the compound will be exposed. The Henderson-Hasselbalch equation (Eq. 2.6) can be used to calculate the percentage ionization of a compound at a given pH (this equation was used to calculate the major forms of ciprofloxacin in Fig. 2.5):

Eq. 2.6
$$pK_a = pH + \log \frac{[\text{acid form}]}{[\text{base form}]}$$

The key to understanding the use of the Henderson-Hasselbalch equation for calculating percentage ionization is to realize that this equation relates a constant, pK_a, to the ratio of acidic form to the basic form of the drug. Because pK_a is a constant for any given molecule, the ratio of acid to base will determine the pH of the solution. Conversely, a given pH determines the ratio of acid to base. A sample calculation is shown in Figure 2.6 for the sedative hypnotic amobarbital.

When dealing with a base, the student must recognize that the conjugate acid is the ionized form of the drug. Thus, as one should expect, a base behaves in a manner opposite to that of an acid. Figure 2.7 shows the calculated percentage ionization for the decongestant phenylpropanolamine. It is very important to recognize that for a base, the pK_a refers to the conjugate acid or ionized

Table 2.3. Common Organic Functional Groups That Are Considered Neutral Under Physiologic Conditions

$R-CH_2-OH$ Alkyl alcohol	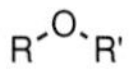 R-O-R' Ether	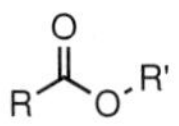 R-C(=O)-O-R' Ester	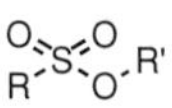 $R-SO_2-O-R'$ Sulfonic acid ester
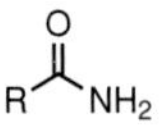 $R-C(=O)-NH_2$ Amide	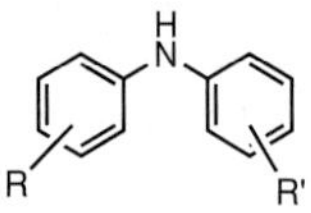 R-Ar-NH-Ar-R' Diarylamine	R-C≡N Nitrile	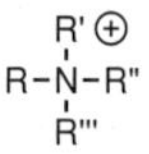 R-N⊕(R')(R'')-R''' Quaternary ammonium
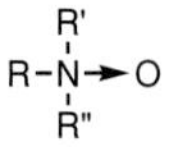 R-N(R')(R'')→O Amine oxide	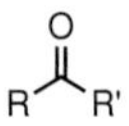 R-C(=O)-R' Ketone & Aldehyde	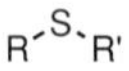 R-S-R' Thioether	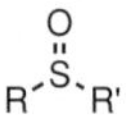 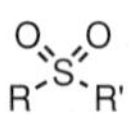 R-S(=O)-R' Sulfoxide; $R-SO_2-R'$ Sulfone

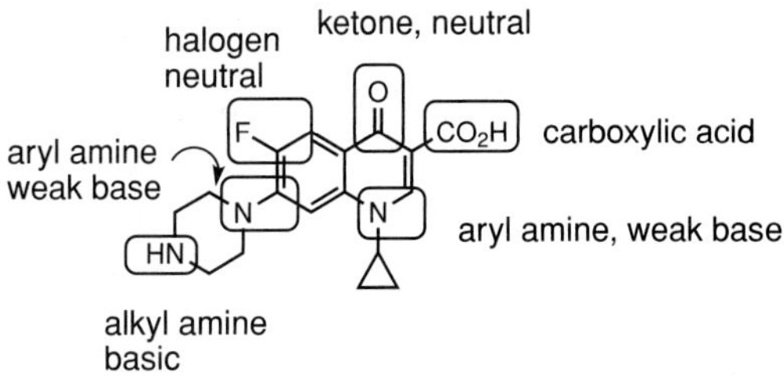

Fig. 2.4. Chemical structure of ciprofloxacin showing the various organic functional groups.

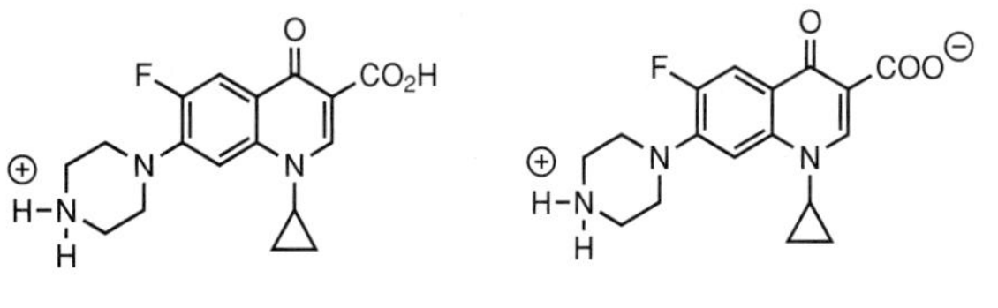

Stomach (pH 1.0 - 3.5)

Colon (pH 5.6-7)

Fig. 2.5. Predominate forms of ciprofloxacin at two different locations within the gastrointestinal tract.

form of the compound. To thoroughly comprehend this relationship, the student should calculate the percentage ionization of an acid and a base at different pH values.

Water Solubility of Drugs

The solubility of a drug molecule in water greatly affects the routes of administration that are available as well as its absorption, distribution, and elimination. Two key concepts to keep in mind when considering the water (or fat) solubility of a molecule are the hydrogen bond–forming potential of the functional groups in the molecule and the ionization of functional groups.

Hydrogen Bonds

Each functional group capable of donating or accepting a hydrogen bond will contribute to the overall water solubility of the compound and increase the hydrophilic (water-loving) nature of the molecule. Conversely, func-

Absorption/Acid-Base Case

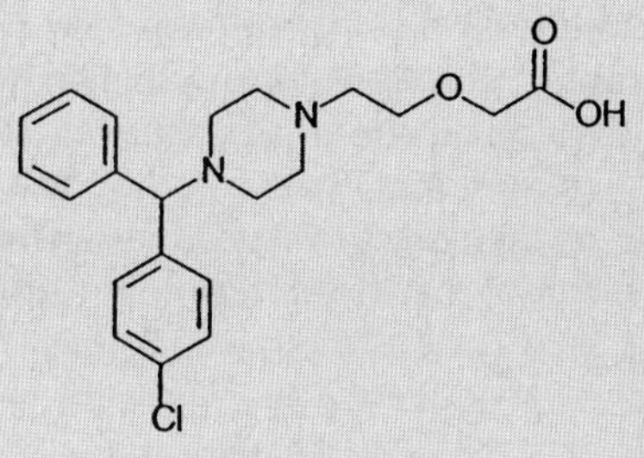

Cetirizine (Zyrtec)

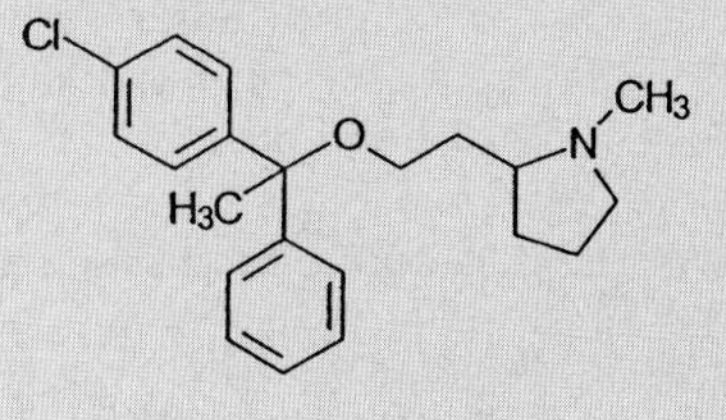

Clemastine (Tavist)

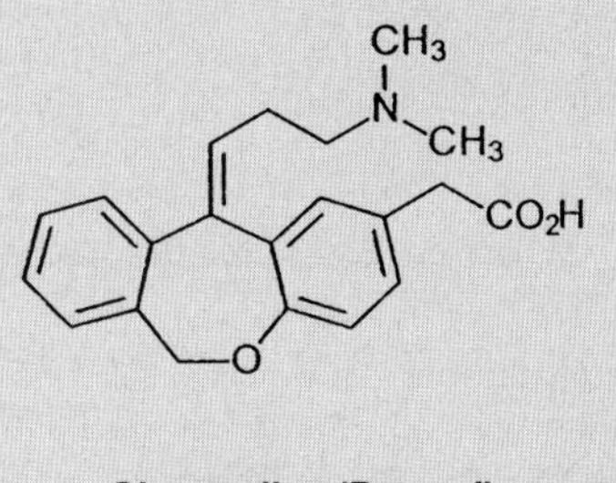

Olopatadine (Patanol)

A long-distance truck driver comes into the pharmacy complaining of seasonal allergies. He asks you to recommend an agent that will act as an antihistamine but that will not cause drowsiness. He regularly takes TUMS for indigestion because of the bad food that he eats while on the road.

1. Identify the functional groups present in Zyrtec and Tavist, and evaluate the effect of each functional group on the ability of the drug to cross lipophilic membranes (e.g., blood-brain barrier). Based on your assessment of each agent's ability to cross the blood-brain barrier (and, therefore, potentially cause drowsiness), provide a rationale for whether the truck driver should be taking Zyrtec or Tavist.
2. Patanol is sold as an aqueous solution of the hydrochloride salt. Modify the structure above to show the appropriate salt form of this agent. This agent is applied to the eye to relieve itching associated with allergies. Describe why this agent is soluble in water and what properties make it able to be absorbed into the membranes that surround the eye.
3. Consider the structural features of Zyrtec and Tavist. In which compartment (stomach [pH 1] or intestine [pH 6–7]) will each of these two drugs be best absorbed?
4. TUMS neutralizes stomach acid to pH 3.5. Based on your answer to question 3, determine whether the truck driver will get the full antihistaminergic effect if he takes his antihistamine at the same time that he takes his TUMS. Provide a rationale for your answer.

Acid-Base Chemistry/Compatibility Cases

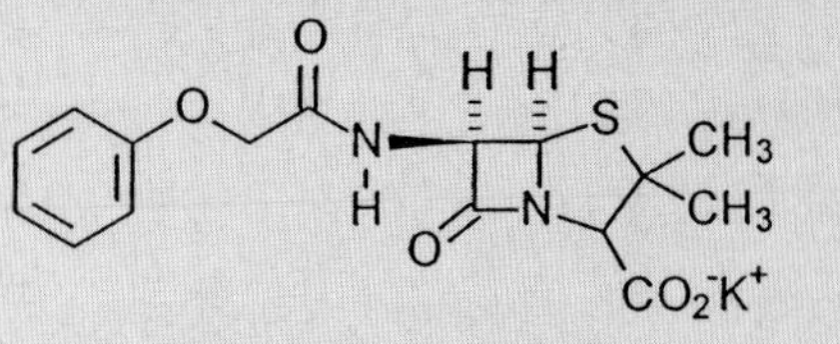

Penicillin V Potassium

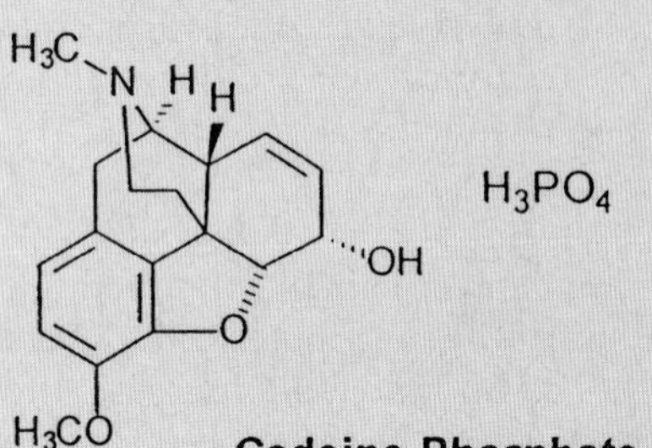

Codeine Phosphate

The IV technician in the hospital pharmacy gets an order for a patient that includes the two drugs drawn below. She is unsure if she can mix the two drugs together in the same IV bag and is not certain how water soluble the agents are.

1. Penicillin V potassium is drawn in its salt form, whereas codeine phosphate is not. Modify the structure above to show the salt form of codeine phosphate. Determine the acid-base character of the functional groups in the two molecules drawn above as well as the salt form of codeine phosphate.
2. As originally drawn above, which of these two agents is more water soluble? Provide a rationale for your selection that includes appropriate structural properties. Is the salt form of codeine phosphate more or less water soluble than the free base form of the drug? Provide a rationale for your answer based on the structural properties of the salt form of codeine phosphate.
3. What is the chemical consequence of mixing aqueous solutions of each drug in the same IV bag? Provide a rationale that includes an acid-base assessment.

tional groups that cannot form hydrogen bonds will not enhance hydrophilicity and will actually contribute to the hydrophobicity (water-hating) nature of the molecule. Hydrogen bonds are a special case of what generally are referred to as dipole–dipole bonds. Dipoles result from unequal sharing of electrons between atoms within a covalent bond. This unequal sharing of electrons results when two atoms involved in a covalent bond have significantly different electronegativities. As a result, partial ionic character develops between the two atoms, producing a permanent dipole—that is, one end of the covalent bond has higher electron density than the other. When two molecules containing dipoles approach one another, they align such that the negative end of one dipole is electrostatically attracted to the positive end of the other. When the positive end of the dipole is a hydrogen atom,

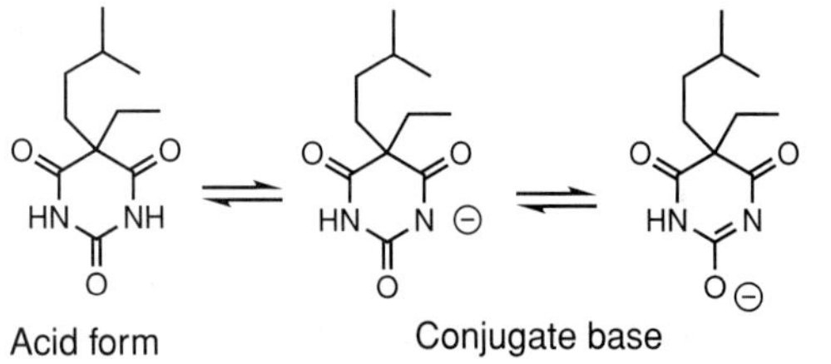

Acid form
pK_a 8.0

Conjugate base

Question: At a pH of 7.4, what is the percent ionization of amobarbital?

Answer:

$$8.0 = 7.4 + \log \frac{[\text{acid}]}{[\text{base}]}$$

$$0.6 = \log \frac{[\text{acid}]}{[\text{base}]}$$

$$10^{0.6} = \frac{[\text{acid}]}{[\text{base}]} = \frac{3.98}{1}$$

$$\%\ \text{acid form} = \frac{3.98 \times 100}{4.98} = 79.9\%$$

Fig. 2.6. Calculation of percentage ionization of amobarbital. Calculation indicates that 80% of the molecules are in the acid (or protonated) form, leaving 20% in the conjugate base (ionized) form.

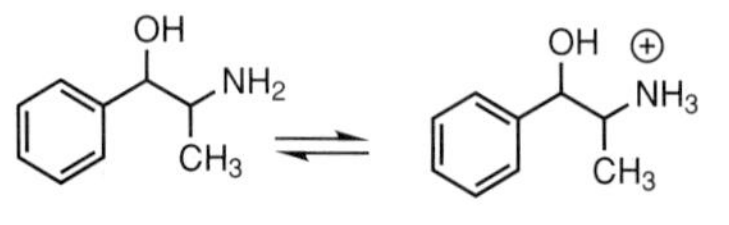

Base form

Conjugate acid form
pK_a 9.4

Question: What is the % ionization of phenylpropanolamine at pH 7.4?

Answer:

$$9.4 = 7.4 + \log \frac{[\text{acid}]}{[\text{base}]}$$

$$2.0 = \log \frac{[\text{acid}]}{[\text{base}]}$$

$$10^{2} = \frac{[\text{acid}]}{[\text{base}]} = \frac{100}{1}$$

$$\%\ \text{ionization} = \frac{100 \times 100}{101} = 99\%$$

Fig. 2.7. Calculation of percentage ionization of phenylpropanolamine. Calculation indicates that 99% of the molecules are in the acid form, which is the same as the percentage ionization.

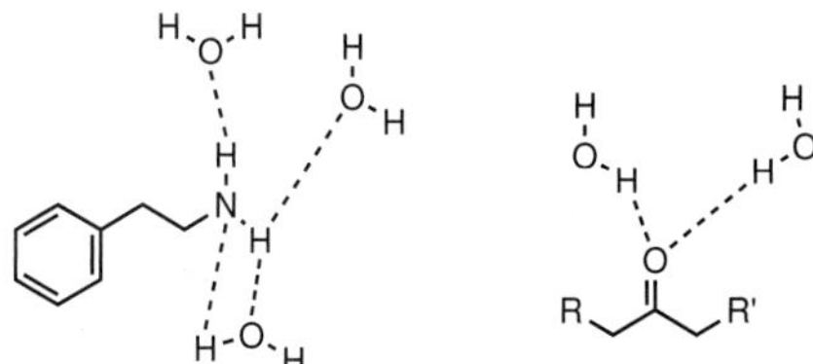

Fig. 2.8. Examples of hydrogen-bonding between water and hypothetical drug molecules.

this interaction is referred to as a "hydrogen bond" (or H-bond). Thus, for a hydrogen bond to occur, at least one dipole must contain an electropositive hydrogen. The hydrogen atom must be involved in a covalent bond with an electronegative atom, such as oxygen (O), nitrogen (N), sulfur (S) or selenium (Se). Of these four elements, only oxygen and nitrogen contribute significantly to the dipole, and we will therefore concern ourselves only with the hydrogen-bonding capability of OH and NH groups. (This is only in reference to functional groups that "donate" hydrogen bonds.)

Even though the energy involved for each hydrogen bond is small (1–10 kcal/mol/bond), it is the additive nature of multiple hydrogen bonds that contributes to water solubility. We will see in Chapter 4 that this same bonding interaction also is important in drug–receptor interactions. Figure 2.8 shows several possible hydrogen bond types that may occur with different organic functional groups and water. As a general rule, the more hydrogen bonds that are possible, the greater the water solubility of the molecule. Table 2.4 lists several common organic functional groups and the number of potential hydrogen bonds for each. Note that this table does not take into account the possibility of intramolecular hydrogen bonds that could form. Each intramolecular hydrogen bond decreases water solubility (and increases lipid solubility), because one less interaction with solvent occurs.

Table 2.4. Common Organic Functional Groups and Their Hydrogen-Bonding Potential

Functional Groups	Number of Potential H-bonds
R-OH	3
R-C(=O)-R'	2
R-NH₂	3
R-NH-R'	2
R-N(R')-R"	1
R-C(=O)-O-R'	2

Absorption/Binding Interactions Case

A 24-year-old man comes into the pharmacy and asks you to recommend a treatment for the itching and burning he has recently noticed on both feet. He indicates that he would prefer a cream rather than a spray or a powder. Your recommendation to this patient is to use Lamisil®, a very effective topical antifungal agent that is sold over-the-counter.

Terbinafine (Lamisil)

1. Identify the structural characteristics and the corresponding properties that make terbinafine an agent that can be utilized topically.
2. The biological target of drug action for terbinafine is squalene epoxidase. Consider each of the structural features of this antifungal agent, and describe the type of interactions that the drug will have with the target for drug action. Which amino acids are likely to be present in the active site of this enzyme?

Ionization

In addition to the hydrogen-bonding capability of a molecule, another type of bonding interaction plays an important role in determining water solubility: ion–dipole interaction. This type of interaction comes into play when one deals with organic salts. Ion–dipole interactions develop between either a cation or anion and a formal dipole, such as water. A cation, having a deficiency in electron density, will be attracted to regions of high electron density. When dealing with water, this would be the two lone pairs of electrons associated with the oxygen atom. An anion will associate with regions of low electron density or the positive end of the dipole. In the case of water as solvent, this would be the hydrogen atoms (Fig. 2.9).

Fig. 2.9. Examples of ion–dipole interactions.

Not all organic salts are necessarily very water soluble. To associate with enough water molecules to become soluble, the salt must be highly dissociable; in other words, the cation and anion must be able to separate and interact with water molecules. Highly dissociable salts are those formed from strong acids with strong bases (e.g., sodium chloride), weak acids with strong bases (e.g., sodium phenobarbital), or strong acids with weak bases (e.g., atropine sulfate). Examples of strong acids (strong acids are 100% ionized in water [i.e., no ionization constants or pK_a values of <1]) include the hydrohalic acids (hydrochloric, hydrobromic, and hydrofluoric), sulfuric, nitric, and perchloric acid. All other acids are partially ionized with pK_a values from 1–14 and are therefore considered to be moderate or weak acids, such as phosphoric, tartaric and acetic acids. Sodium hydroxide, potassium hydroxide, and calcium hydroxide are strong bases, because they are 100% ionized, whereas the other bases, such as amines, are moderate or weak bases. The magnitude of the pK_a values is a measure of acid or base strength. Thus, the salt of a carboxylic acid and of an alkylamine is a salt of a weak acid and weak base, respectively, and therefore does not dissociate appreciably and may or may not be very water soluble, depending on their molecular weights: Low-molecular-weight salts generally are water soluble, and high-molecular-weight salts are water insoluble. Some examples of common organic salts used in pharmaceutical preparations are provided in Figure 2.10.

When dealing with the water solubility of ionized molecules, one also must consider the possibility of intramolecular ionic interactions. Compounds with ionizable functional groups that produce opposite charges have the potential to interact with each other rather than with water molecules. When this occurs, such compounds often become very insoluble in water. A classic example is the amino acid tyrosine (Fig. 2.11). Tyrosine contains three very polar functional groups, with two of these groups (the alkylamine and carboxylic acid) capable of being ionized, depending on the pH of the solution. The phenolic hydroxyl also is ionizable (pK_a 9–10), but it does not contribute much to the ionization of tyrosine under the conditions most often encountered in pharmaceutical formulations or physiologic conditions (<1% at pH 7). Because of the presence of three very polar functional groups (two of them being ionizable), one would therefore expect tyrosine to be very soluble in water, yet its solubility is only 0.45 g/1,000 mL. Because the basic alkylamine (pK_a 9.1 for the conjugate acid) and the carboxylic acid (pK_a 2.2) can react with one another to form a zwitterionic molecule, the two charged groups are sufficiently close to allow a strong ion–ion interaction to form, thereby keeping each of these groups from forming ion–dipole interactions with the surrounding water molecules. The lack of interaction of the ions with the water dipoles results in a molecule that is very insoluble (Fig. 2.12). Not all zwitterions or multiply charged molecules show this behavior; only those containing ionized functional groups that are close enough to interact to form an ion–ion interaction will be poorly soluble. Generally, the greater the separation between charges, the more highly water soluble one would expect the molecule will be. This is only true, however, to up to a certain number of carbon atoms. This will be discussed in more detail below.

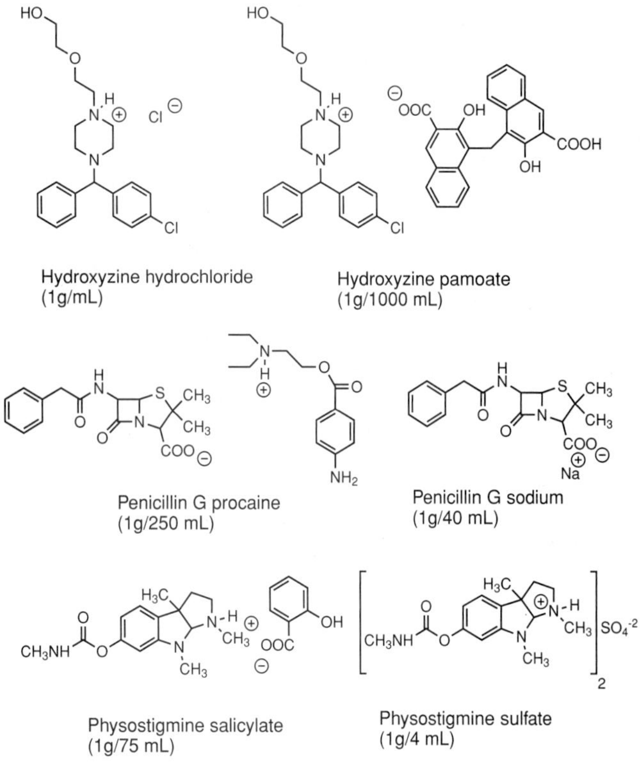

Hydroxyzine hydrochloride (1g/mL)

Hydroxyzine pamoate (1g/1000 mL)

Penicillin G procaine (1g/250 mL)

Penicillin G sodium (1g/40 mL)

Physostigmine salicylate (1g/75 mL)

Physostigmine sulfate (1g/4 mL)

Fig. 2.10. Water solubilities of different salt forms of selective drugs.

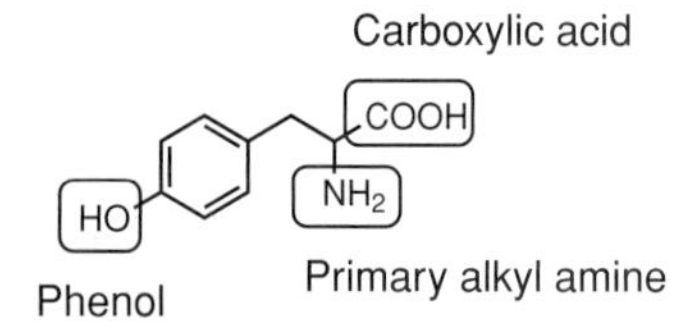

Carboxylic acid

Phenol

Primary alkyl amine

Fig. 2.11. Organic functional groups in tyrosine (see text for pK_a values).

Predicting Water Solubility: Empiric Approach

Lemke (10) has developed an empiric approach to predicting the water solubility of molecules based on the carbon-solubilizing potential of several organic functional groups. If the solubilizing potential of the functional groups exceeds the total number of carbon atoms present, then the molecule is considered to be water

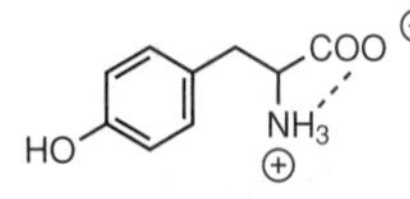

Fig. 2.12. Zwitterionic form of tyrosine showing ion–ion bond.

Binding Interactions

Each of these drug molecules interacts with a different biological target and elicits a unique pharmacologic response. For each of the three molecules, list the types of binding interactions that are possible with a target for drug action. For each type of binding interaction, provide one example of an amino acid that could participate in that interaction.

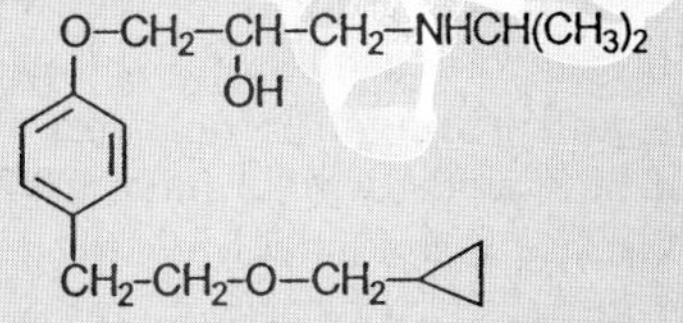

Betaxolol (Betoptic)

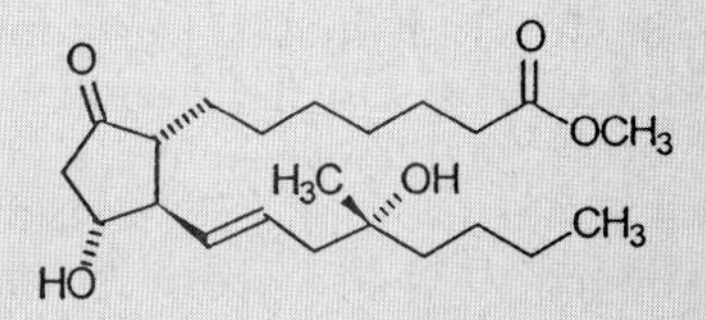

Misoprostol (Cytotec)

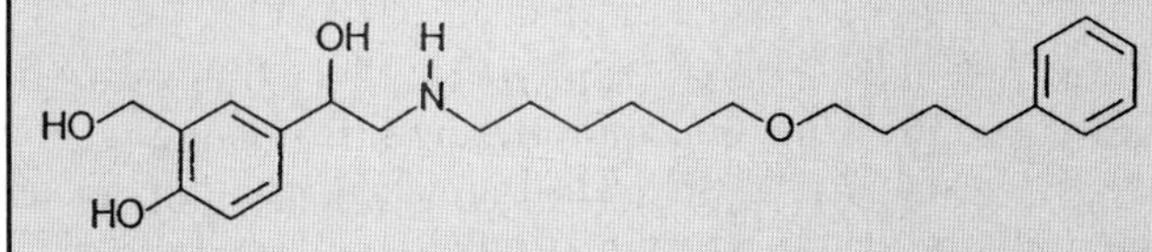

Salmeterol (Serevent)

Example: Binding Interaction: Van der Waals
Amino Acid: leucine

soluble. Otherwise, it is considered to be water insoluble. Functional groups that can interact either through intramolecular hydrogen or ion–ion interactions will decrease the solubilizing potential of each group. It is difficult to quantitate how much such interactions will take away from water solubility, but recognizing these interactions will allow one to explain anomalous results.

Table 2.5 shows the water-solubilizing potential for several organic functional groups that are common to many drugs. Because most drug molecules contain more than one functional group (i.e., are polyfunctional), the second column in the table will be used most often. A couple of examples for predicting water solubility will be used to demonstrate Lemke's method. Anileridine (Fig. 2.13) is a narcotic analgesic containing three organic functional groups that contribute to water solubility: an aromatic amine (very weak base), a tertiary alkylamine (weak base), and an ester (neutral). There are a total of 21 carbon atoms in the molecule, with a solubilizing potential from

Water/Lipid Solubility Case

When you look at any drug molecule, there are a number of functional groups present that contribute to the properties of that drug molecule. Identify the types of functional groups in each molecule and to which physical properties (water/lipid solubility) each contributes.

1. Structural Feature Physical Property

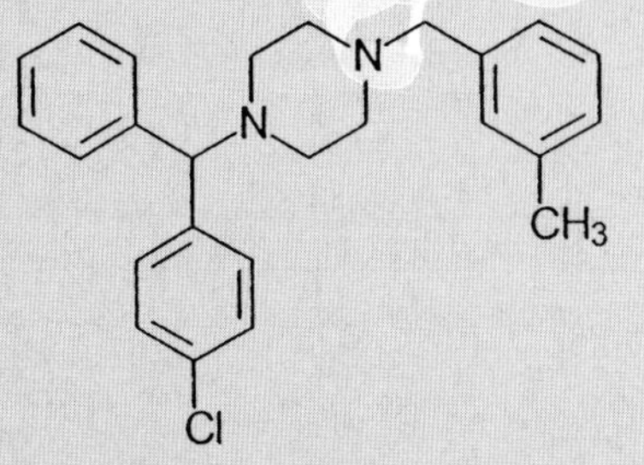

Meclizine (Antivert)

2. Structural Feature Physical Property

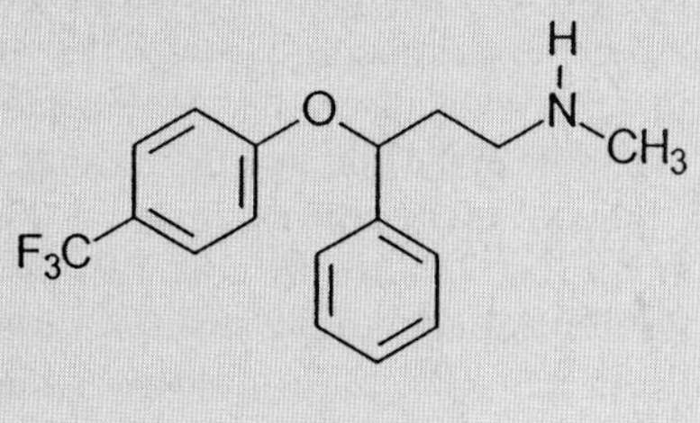

Fluoxetine (Prozac)

3. Structural Feature Physical Property

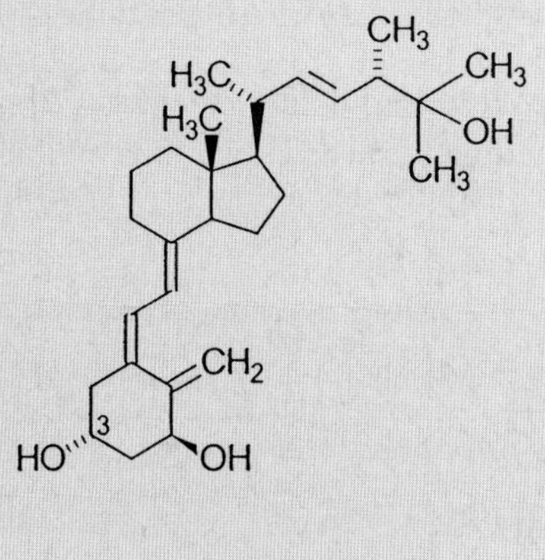

1, 25-dihydroxy Vit D_2

Table 2.5. Water-solubilizing Potential of Organic Functional Groups in a Mono- or Polyfunctional Molecule

Functional Group	Monofunction Molecule	Polyfunctional Molecule
Alcohol	5 to 6 carbons	3 to 4 carbons
Phenol	6 to 7 carbons	3 to 4 carbons
Ether	4 to 5 carbons	2 carbons
Aldehyde	4 to 5 carbons	2 carbons
Ketone	5 to 6 carbons	2 carbons
Amine	6 to 7 carbons	3 carbons
Carboxylic acid	5 to 6 carbons	3 carbons
Ester	6 carbons	3 carbons
Amide	6 carbons	2 to 3 carbons
Urea, carbonate, carbamate		2 carbons

Water solubility is defined as greater than 1% solubility (9).

the three functional groups of nine carbon atoms. Because the solubilizing potential of the functional groups is less than the total number of carbons that are present, the prediction would be that anileridine is insoluble in water. This is, indeed, the case: Its solubility is reported in the U.S. Pharmacopeia (USP) as 1 g/10,000 mL, or 0.01%. When the hydrochloride salt of anileridine is considered, however, not only do the three functional groups contribute a solubilizing potential of nine carbon atoms, the positive charge of the alkylammonium also contributes to its solubility. Lemke (10) estimates that each charge on a molecule (cationic or anionic) contributes a solubilizing potential of 20 to 30 carbon atoms. Thus, the solubilizing potential for these groups in anileridine hydrochloride is 29 to 39 carbon atoms, which is more than the total number of carbon atoms in the molecule. The compound should therefore be soluble in water, and it is (to the extent of 0.2 g/ml, or 20%). Problem 6 at the end of this chapter provides more opportunity to utilize this approach to predict water solubility for several compounds. Solubility data for these compounds can be found in the USP. The student should be able to rationalize any discrepancies between their results and the USP data.

Predicting Water Solubility: Analytical Approach

Another method for predicting water solubility involves calculating an approximate logP, or log of the partition coefficient for a molecule. This approach is based on an approximation method developed by Cates (11) and discussed in Lemke (10). In this approach, one sums the hydrophobic or hydrophilic properties of each functional group present in the molecule. Before we can calculate logP values, we must first digress to a brief explanation of the concept of partition coefficient.

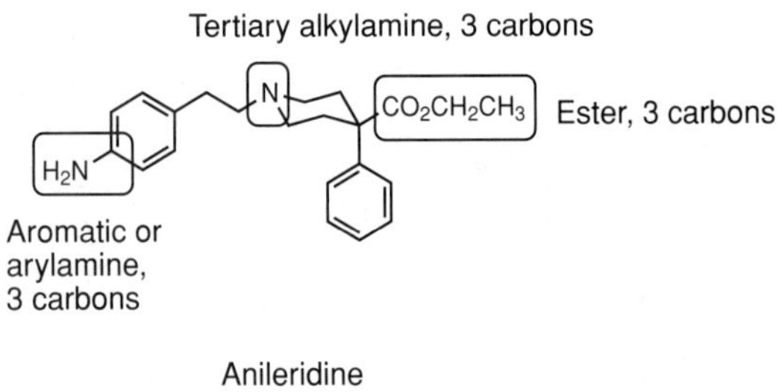

Tertiary alkylamine, 3 carbons

$CO_2CH_2CH_3$ Ester, 3 carbons

H_2N

Aromatic or arylamine, 3 carbons

Anileridine

Fig. 2.13. Identification of functional groups in anileridine.

In its simplest form, the partition coefficient, P, refers to the ratio of the concentrations of drug in octanol to that in water. Octanol is used to mimic the amphiphilic nature of lipid, because it has a polar head group (primary alcohol) and a long hydrocarbon chain, or tail, such as that of fatty acids, which make up part of a lipid membrane. Because P is logarithmically related to free energy (12), it generally is expressed as logP and, therefore, is the sum of the hydrophobic and hydrophilic characteristics of the organic functional groups making up the structure of the molecule. Thus, logP is a measure of the solubility characteristics of the entire molecule. Because each organic functional group contained within the molecule contributes to the overall hydrophobic/hydrophilic nature of the molecule, a hydrophobic/hydrophilic value (the hydrophobic substituent constant, π) can be assigned to each organic functional group. Equation 2.7 defines this relationship:

Eq. 2.7 $$\text{LogP} = \Sigma\pi \text{ (fragments)}$$

When calculating logP from hydrophobic substituent constants, the sum is usually referred to as logP_{calc} or ClogP or MaclogP (16) to distinguish it from an experimentally determined value (logP_{meas}). Over the years, extensive tables of π values have been compiled for organic functional groups and molecular fragments (12–15). Table 2.6 is a highly abbreviated summary of π values from Lemke (10), based largely on the manuscript by Cates (11). Using the values in this table, it is possible to obtain a fairly reasonable estimate for the water solubility of many organic compounds (shown as logP).

As an example, we will once again use the narcotic analgesic anileridine to demonstrate the calculation of logP. This compound has a total of 22 carbon atoms, some aliphatic and some aromatic. We need to separate these, because aromatic carbon atoms, because of delocalized π orbitals for the sp^2 hybridized atoms, are more polar than aliphatic carbons. The compound also contains one tertiary alkylamine, one aryl amine, and one ester. Note that when dealing with esters and amides, the oxygen, nitrogen, and ester/amide carbon are counted in this π value. The remaining aliphatic carbons are then counted. Figure 2.14 summarizes the logP calculation for anileridine. The calculation gives a ClogP value for anileridine of +4.8. Water solubility as defined by the USP is solubility of greater than 3.3%, which equates to an approximate logP of +0.5. Values less than +0.5 are therefore considered to be water soluble, and those greater than +0.5 are considered to be water insoluble. According to our calculation, anileridine would be predicted to be insoluble in water.

Binding Interactions/Solubility Case

JK presents a prescription for her 6-month-old daughter for Donatussin Drops. She wants to know if this medication will have an effect on her daughter's alertness.

Components of Donatussin:

Phenylephrine (decongestant)
Chlorpheniramine (antihistamine)
Guaifenesin (expectorant)

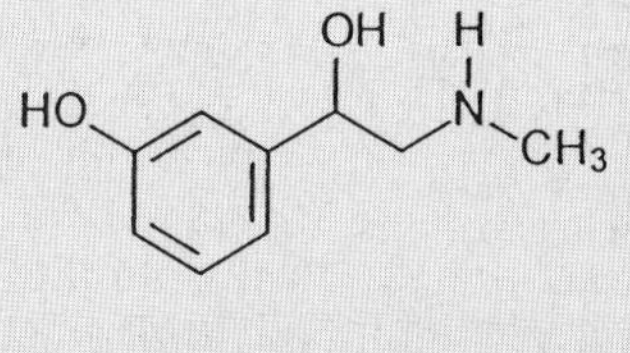

Phenylephrine

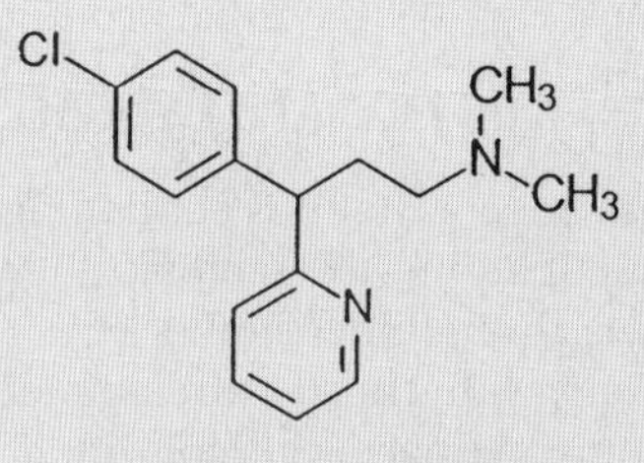

Chlorpheniramine

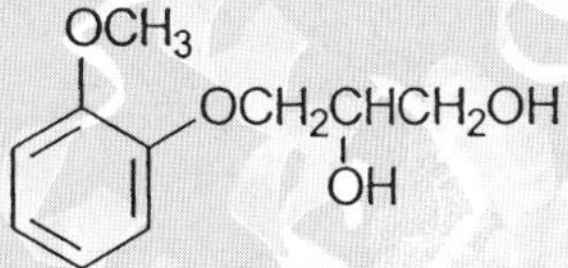

Guaifenesin

1. Identify the structural features/functional groups of phenylephrine and guaifenesin that contribute to improved water solubility (medication given as drops). List the type(s) of interactions that these groups have with water, and draw an example of these interactions (with appropriate labels) below.
2. Evaluate each of the three molecules, and determine if each molecule contains any functional groups that will allow the drug to cross the blood-brain barrier and have an effect on this child's alertness (create a list of relevant functional groups for each molecule). Based on your evaluation, which agent is likely to have the most significant effect? Identify what property is necessary for these agents to cross this biological membrane.
3. Identify the binding interactions that chlorpheniramine and guaifenesin could have with their respective targets for drug action. Be sure to identify which functional groups will participate in each of these binding interactions.

This calculation agrees with the more empiric procedure discussed earlier.

Other sample calculations are shown in Figure 2.15, and several problems are provided at the end of this chapter. In Figure 2.15, MlogP values (when available) and ClogP values obtained from the ClogP 4.0 program MaclogP (16) are included for comparison purposes. Even though the π values from Table 2.6 are not as extensive as those in the computer program, there is good general agreement with most of these compounds regarding their solubility (or insolubility) in water. In addition, other programs besides ClogP are available to predict logP values; some of these programs are available on the Internet. One must keep in mind that because of the assumptions made in these programs, they may not produce results in total agreement with measured values or other prediction programs. At this time, it generally is agreed that the ClogP values calculated from ClogP 4.0 (16) are the most accurate. Other programs for calculating logP values

Table 2.6. Hydrophilic-lipophilic Values (π V) for Organic Fragments (10)

Fragments	π Value
C (aliphatic)	+0.5
Phenyl	+2.0
Cl	+0.5
O_2NO (nitrate ester)	+0.2
IMHB (intramolecular hydrogen bond)	+0.65
S	0.0
O=C–O (carboxyl)	−0.7
O=C–N (amide, imide)	−0.7
O (hydroxyl, phenol, ether)	−1.0
N (amine)	−1.0
O_2N (aliphatic)	−0.85
O_2N (aromatic)	−0.28

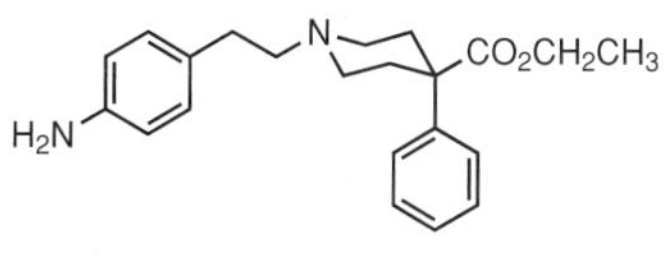

Fragments	π
2 amines	-2.0
9 aliphatic carbons	+3.5
2 phenyl rings	+4.0
1 ester (O=C–O)	-0.7
logP	+4.8

Fig. 2.14. Calculation of logP for anileridine.

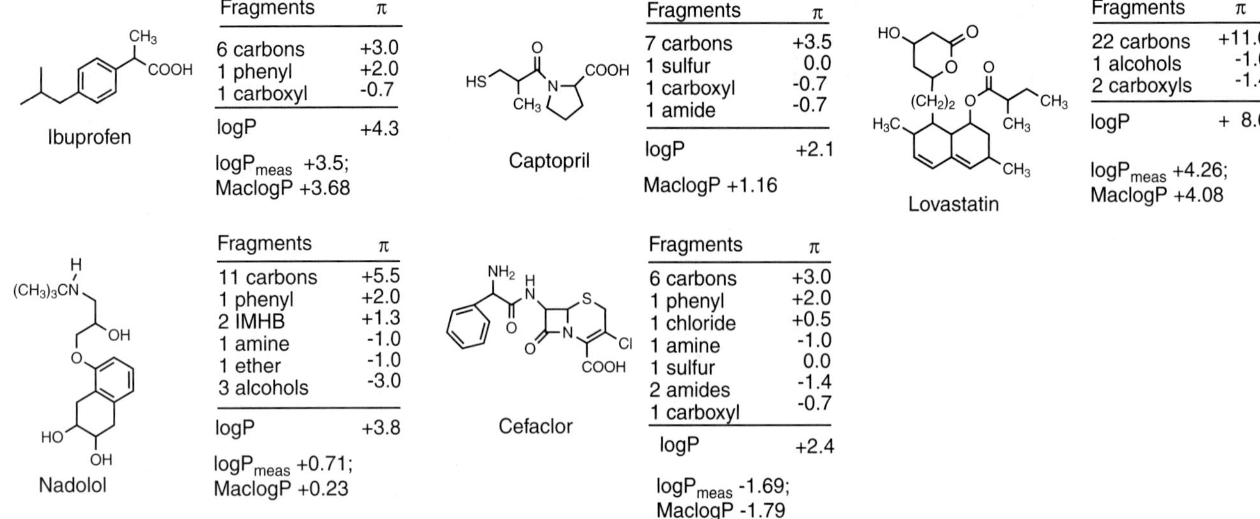

Fig. 2.15. LogP calculations for selected compounds.

such as Molinspiration (17) and Interactive Analysis (18), use different methods and assumptions and, therefore, do not always agree with ClogP predictions or experimentally determined values. This is not to say the latter two programs do not give accurate results. Often, one or all of the programs will agree with measured values, and with other molecules, none of the programs agree, especially as the number of hydrogen-bond acceptors and hydrogen-bond donor group increase.

Predicting the percentage ionization or water solubility of a molecule should not be viewed as an exercise in arithmetic but also as a way to understand the solution behavior of molecules, especially when dealing with admixtures and differences among molecules in their pharmacokinetics. The ionization state of a molecule influences its water solubility as well as its ability to traverse membranes and, therefore, its ability to be absorbed. Serum protein binding (and, therefore, the amount of free drug available for receptor binding) also is greatly influenced by the ionization state and the hydrophilic/hydrophobic nature of the molecule.

> **Questions We Can Now Answer about Any Drug Molecule**
>
> Based on your knowledge of acid-base chemistry, from where will this drug primarily be absorbed?
> What is the solubility of the drug in the stomach, plasma, or an aqueous IV?
> What are the possible interactions that the drug could have with its respective target for drug action?
> What is the compatibility of the drug if mixed with other drugs?
> How should this drug be delivered? Is it stable in stomach acid?

STEREOCHEMISTRY AND DRUG ACTION

Stereoisomers are compounds containing the same number and kinds of atoms, the same arrangement of bonds, but different three-dimensional structures; in other words, they only differ in the three-dimensional arrangements of atoms in space. Stereoisomers are subdivided into two types, enantiomers and diastereoisomers. Enantiomers are compounds for which the three-dimensional arrangement of atoms is such that they are nonsuperimposable mirror images. Diastereoisomers are all stereoisomeric compounds that are not enantiomers. Thus, the term "diastereoisomer" includes compounds containing double bonds (geometric isomers) as well as ring systems. Unlike enantiomers, diastereoisomers exhibit different physicochemical properties, including, but not limited to, melting point, boiling point, solubility, and chromato-

> **Learning the Lingo: Drug Molecule Evaluation**
>
> *Analysis of Individual Functional Groups:*
> Name of functional group
> Shape of functional group
> Hydrophobic vs. hydrophilic character
> Polar vs. nonpolar character
> Acidic vs. basic (pK_a) character
> Binding interactions
> Chemical/enzymatic stability
>
> *Analysis of the Whole Drug Molecule:*
> Looking for functional group balance: water solubility and absorption
> Ionization issues: effect on solubility and absorption
> Drug combinations: acid-base interactions
> Drug interactions with biological target: good fit or not?
> Stability and bioavailability: route of administration

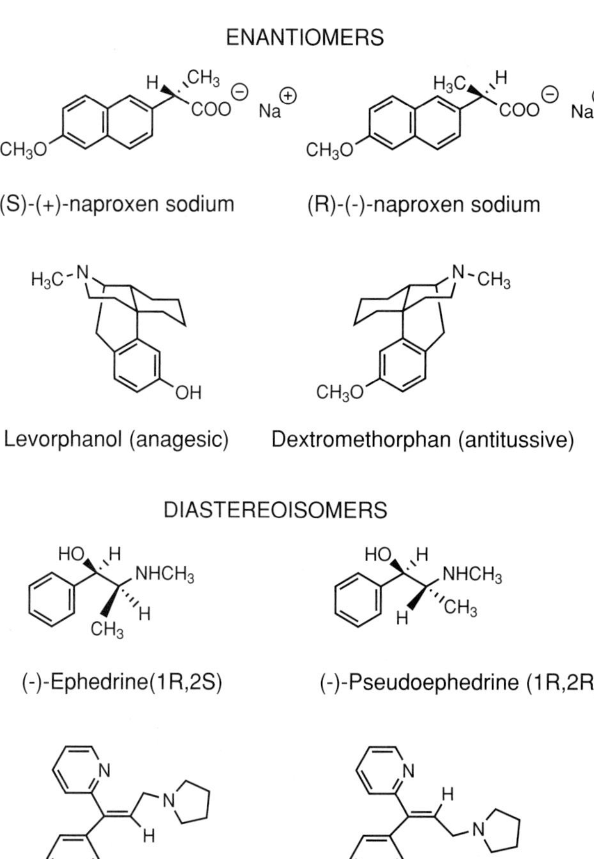

Fig. 2.16. Examples of stereoisomers.

graphic behavior. These differences in physicochemical properties allow the separation of diastereoisomers from mixtures utilizing standard chemical separation techniques, such as column chromatography or crystallization. Enantiomers cannot be separated using such techniques unless a chiral environment is provided or they are converted to diastereoisomers (e.g., salt formation with another enantiomer). Examples of enantiomers and diastereoisomers are provided in Figure 2.16.

The physicochemical properties of a drug molecule are dependent not only on what functional groups are present in the molecule but also on the spatial arrangement of these groups. This becomes an especially important factor when a molecule is subjected to an asymmetric environment, such as the human body. Because proteins and other biological macromolecules are asymmetric in nature, how a particular drug molecule interacts with these macromolecules is determined by the three-dimensional orientation of the organic functional groups that are present. If crucial functional groups are not occupying the proper spatial region surrounding the molecule, then productive bonding interactions with the biological macromolecule (or receptor) will not be possible, potentially negating the desired pharmacologic effect. If, however, these functional groups are in the proper three-dimensional orientation, the drug can produce a very strong interaction with its receptor. It therefore is very important for the medicinal chemist developing a new molecular entity for therapeutic use to understand not only what functional groups are responsible for the drug's activity but also what three-dimensional orientation of these groups is needed.

Approximately one in every four drugs currently on the market can be considered to be an isomeric mixture, yet for many of these compounds, the biological activity may reside in only one isomer (or at least predominate in one isomer). The majority of these isomeric mixtures are what are referred to as "racemic mixtures" (or "racemates"). These are compounds, usually synthetic, that contain equal amounts of both possible enantiomers, or optical isomers. Enantiomers also are referred to as chiral compounds, antipodes, or enantiomorphs. When introduced into an asymmetric, or chiral, environment, such as the human body, enantiomers will display different physicochemical properties, producing significant differences in their pharmacokinetic and pharmacodynamic behavior. Such differences can result in adverse side effects or toxicity, because one or more of the isomers may exhibit significant differences in absorption (especially active transport), serum protein binding, and metabolism. With the latter, one isomer may be converted into a toxic substance or may influence the metabolism of another drug. To discuss further the influence of stereochemistry on drug action, some of the basic concepts of stereochemistry need to be reviewed.

Stereochemical Definitions

Designation of Absolute Configuration

At first, enantiomers were distinguished by their ability to rotate the plane of polarized light. Isomers rotating light to the right, or in a clockwise direction, were designated as dextrorotatory, and this was indicated by a (+)-sign before the chemical name (e.g. (+)-amphetamine or dextroamphetamine). The opposite designation, levorotatory or (−)-, was given to compounds that rotated the plane of polarized light to the left, or in a counterclockwise direction. The letters d- and ℓ- were formerly used to indicate (+)- and (−)-, respectively. A racemate (racemic mixture)—that is, a 1:1 mixture of enantiomers—is indicated by a (±)- before the compound name. The student should be aware that this method of nomenclature is based on a physical property of the molecule and does not provide any information concerning the absolute configuration or three-dimensional arrangement of atoms around the chiral center. Because rotation of the plane of polarized light is a physical property, both the magnitude and direction of rotation can vary, depending on the conditions. Thus, temperature, solvent, and concentration of the substance are three factors that need to be considered when reporting optical rotations. A good example of this is the antibiotic chloramphenicol. There are two chiral centers in this molecule, resulting in four possible stereoisomers. The isomer shown here is dextrorotatory when its optical rotation is measured in ethanol but levorotatory when measured in ethyl acetate. Obviously, the simple measurement of a physical property, such as rotation of the plane of polarized light, is not sufficient for assignment of the absolute configuration of a molecule.

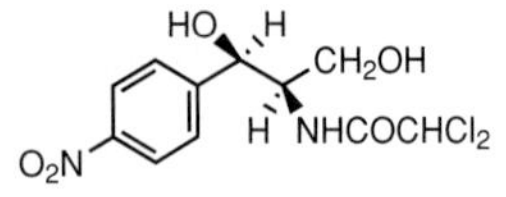

Chloramphenicol

In the late nineteenth century, Fisher and Rosanoff developed a system of nomenclature based on the structure of glyceraldehyde (Fig. 2.17). Because at this time no methods were known for determining the absolute three-dimensional arrangement of atoms in space, the two isomers of glyceraldehyde were arbitrarily assigned the designation of D-(+)- and L-(−). It was not until the 1950s that the absolute configurations were determined, and it was found that Fisher had fortuitously guessed correctly. Assignments of configuration to other molecules were done based on their relationship to D- or L-glyceraldehyde via synthesis or chemical degradation, irrespective of the observed direction of rotation of the plane of polarized light. Thus, via chemical degradation, it was possible to determine that (+)-glucose, (−)-2–deoxyribose, and (−)-fructose had the same terminal configuration as D-(+)-glyceraldehyde and, therefore, were given the D-absolute configuration. Amino acids were assigned based on their relationship to D-(+)- and L-(−)-serine (Fig. 2.17). Unfortunately, this system becomes very cumbersome with molecules containing more than one chiral center.

In 1956, a new system of nomenclature was introduced by Cahn et al. (19) and has since become known as the Sequence Rule or CIP system. With this system, atoms attached to a chiral center are ranked according to their atomic number. Highest priority is given to the atom with the highest atomic number, and subsequent atoms are ranked accordingly, from highest to lowest. When a decision cannot be made regarding priority—for example, two atoms with the same atomic number attached to the chiral center—the process continues to the next atom until a decision can be made. The molecule is then viewed from the side opposite the lowest-priority atom, and the priority sequence from highest to lowest is determined. If the sequence is to the right, or clockwise, the chiral center is designated as the (R)-absolute configuration. The designation is (S) when the priority sequence is to the left, or counterclockwise. An example of this is seen in the neurotransmitter norepinephrine.

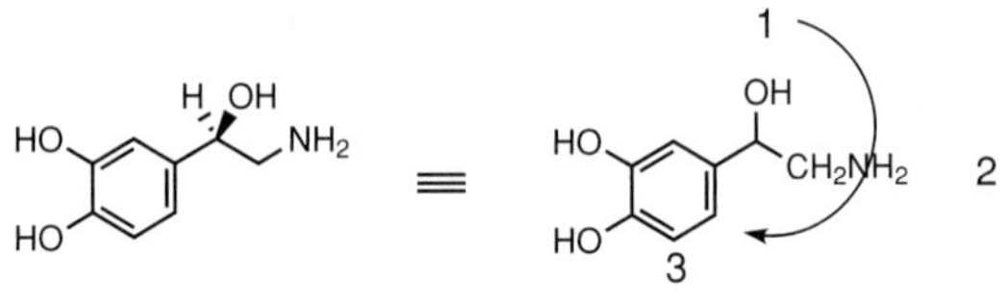

Norepinephrine

R

Degradation studies demonstrated that (−)-norepinephrine is related to D-(−)-mandelic acid; therefore, it was given the D-designation using the Fisher system. With the CIP system, norepinephrine is assigned the (R)-absolute configuration.

The student should note that the CIP system of nomenclature uses a set of arbitrary rules and, therefore, should be viewed as a system that keeps track of absolute configuration only. In many instances, two molecules may have different absolute configurations as designated by the CIP system but the same relative orientation of the functional groups relevant for biological activity. A case in point is the absolute configuration of the nonselective β-adrenergic antagonist propranolol as compared to norepinephrine. Because of the ether oxygen, the priority sequence of the functional groups about the chiral center results in the assignment of the (S)-absolute configuration for the more active enantiomer of propranolol. Close inspection of both (R)-norepinephrine and (S)-propranolol, however, shows that the hydroxy group, basic amine, and aromatic rings of both compounds occupy the same regions in three-dimensional space.

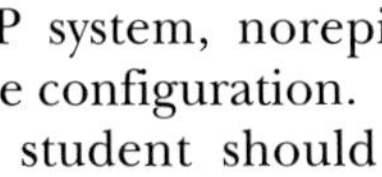

(R)-Norepinephrine 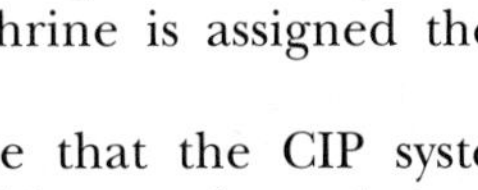 (S)-Propranolol

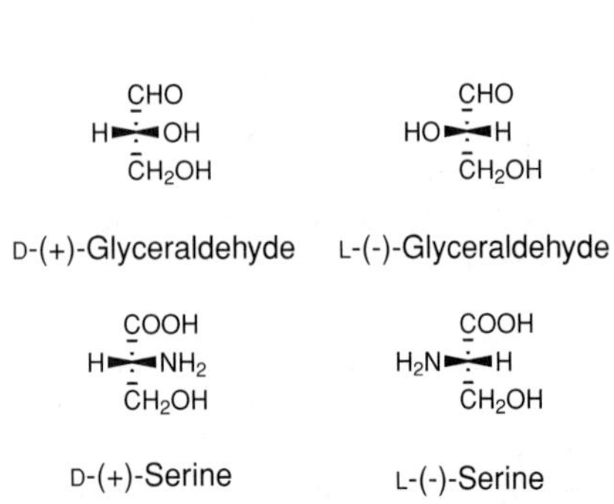

D-(+)-Glyceraldehyde L-(-)-Glyceraldehyde

D-(+)-Serine L-(-)-Serine

Fig. 2.17. Relationship of optical isomers of serine to D- and L-glyceraldehyde.

Stereochemistry and Biological Activity

Easson-Stedman Hypothesis

In 1886, Piutti (20) reported different physiologic actions for the enantiomers of asparagine, with (+)-asparagine having a sweet taste and (−)-asparagine a bland one. This was one of the earliest observations that enantiomers can exhibit differences in biological action.

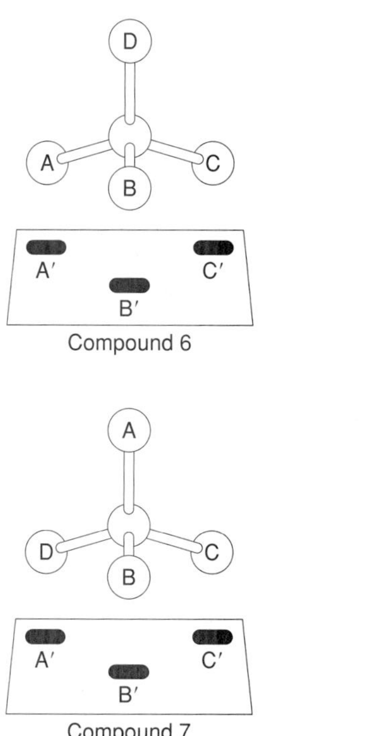

Fig. 2.18. Optical isomers. Only in compound 6 do the functional groups A, B, and C align with the corresponding sites of binding on the asymmetric surface.

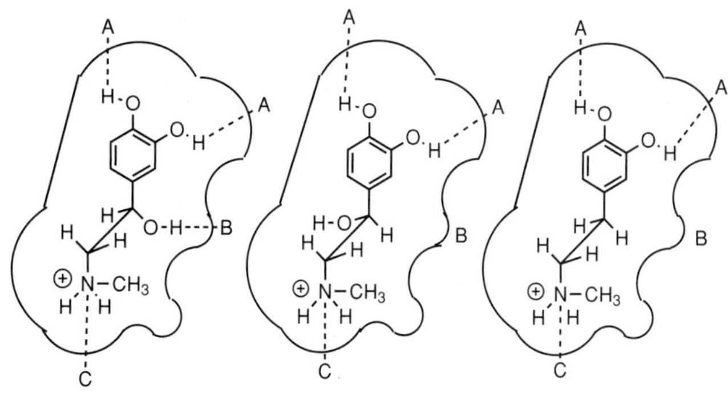

Fig. 2.19. Drug receptor interaction of (R)-(−)-epinephrine, (S)-(+)-epinephrine, and N-methyldopamine.

In 1933, Easson and Stedman (21) reasoned that differences in biological activity between enantiomers resulted from selective reactivity of one enantiomer with its receptor. They postulated that such interactions require a minimum of a three-point fit to the receptor. This is demonstrated in Figure 2.18 for two hypothetical enantiomers. In Figure 2.18, the letters A, B, and C represent hypothetical functional groups that can interact with complementary sites on the hypothetical receptor surface, represented by A′, B′, and C′. Only one enantiomer is capable of attaining the correct orientation to enable all three functional groups to fit their respective sites on the receptor surface. The lack of achieving the same interactions by the other enantiomer explains its reduced biological activity, because it is unable to properly fit into the receptor and, therefore, cannot "trigger" the appropriate change in the receptor conformation. The Easson-Stedman Hypothesis states that the more potent enantiomer must be involved in a minimum of three intermolecular interactions with the receptor surface and that the less potent enantiomer only interacts with two sites. This can be illustrated by looking at the differences in vasopressor activity of (R)-(−)-epinephrine, (S)-(+)-epinephrine and the achiral N-methyldopamine (Fig. 2.19). With (R)-(−)-epinephrine, the three points of interaction with the receptor site are the substituted aromatic ring, β-hydroxyl group, and the protonated secondary ammonium group. All three functional groups interact with their complementary binding sites on the receptor surface, producing the necessary interactions that stimulate the receptor. With (S)-(+)-epinephrine, only two interactions are possible (the protonated secondary ammonium and the substituted aromatic ring). The β-hydroxyl group occupies the wrong region of space and, therefore, cannot interact properly with the receptor. N-methyldopamine can achieve the same interactions with the receptor as (S)-(+)-epinephrine; therefore, it is not surprising that its vasopressor response is the same as that of (S)-(+)-epinephrine and less than that of (R)-(−)-epinephrine.

Not all stereoselectivity seen with enantiomers can be attributed to differences in reactivity at the receptor site. Differences in biological activity also can result from differences in the ability of each enantiomer to reach the receptor site. Because the biological system encountered by the drug is asymmetric, each enantiomer may experience selective penetration of membranes, metabolism, and absorption at sites of loss (e.g., adipose tissue) or excretion. Figure 2.20 shows the selective phases that enantiomers may encounter before reaching the receptor. Not all of these processes may be encountered by a particular enantiomer, but such processes may provide enough of an influence to cause one enantiomer to produce a significantly better pharmacologic effect than the other. Conversely, such processes also may contribute to untoward effects of a particular enantiomer. The student

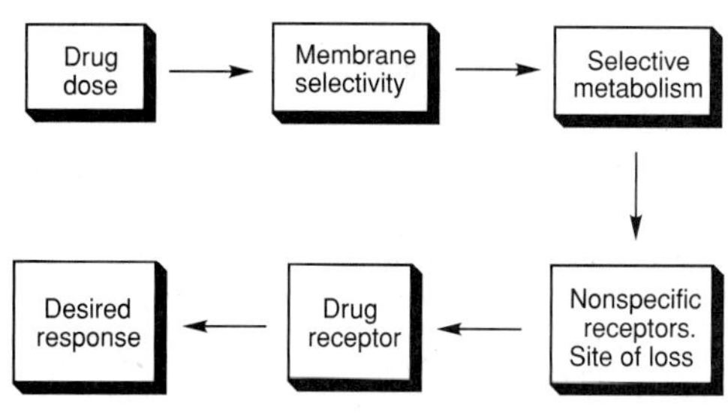

Fig. 2.20. Selective phases to which optical isomers may be subjected before biological response.

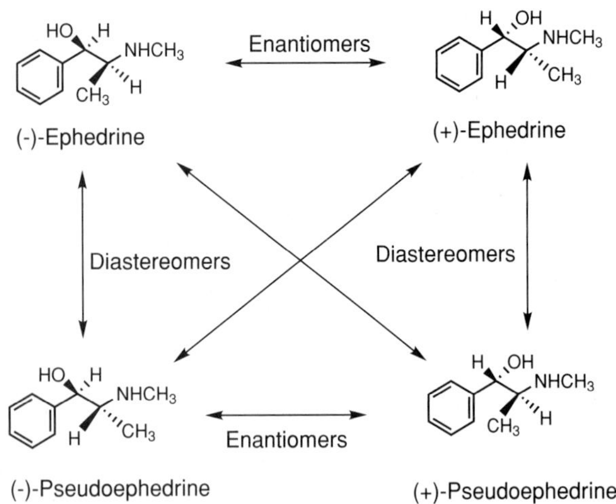

Fig. 2.21. Relationship between the diastereomers of ephedrine and pseudoephedrine.

must continually keep in mind that not all pharmacologic effects of a drug are necessarily beneficial to the patient, and differences in pharmacologic action among stereoisomers provide excellent examples of this concept.

Diastereomers

As mentioned earlier, diastereoisomers are compounds that are nonsuperimposable, nonmirror-image isomers. Such compounds can result from the presence of more than one chiral center in the molecule, double bonds, or ring systems. These isomers have different physicochemical properties; thus, differences in biological activity between such isomers often can be attributed to these properties.

Compounds containing more than one chiral center probably are the most common type of diastereoisomer used as drugs. The classic example of compounds of this type is the diastereoisomers ephedrine and pseudoephedrine (Fig. 2.21). When a molecule contains two chiral centers, there can be as many as four possible stereoisomers consisting of two sets of enantiomeric pairs. For each enantiomeric pair, there is inversion of both chiral centers, whereas the difference between diastereomers is inversion of only one chiral center (Problem 9 at the end of this chapter helps to illustrate this point).

Figure 2.22 shows several examples of other compounds that contain two or more chiral centers and, therefore, are diastereoisomeric (see Problem 10 at the end of this chapter).

Restricted bond rotation caused by carbon–carbon double bonds (alkenes or olefins) and similar systems, such as imines (C═N), can produce stereoisomers. These also are referred to as geometric isomers, although they more properly are classified as diastereoisomers. In compounds of this type, substituents can be oriented on

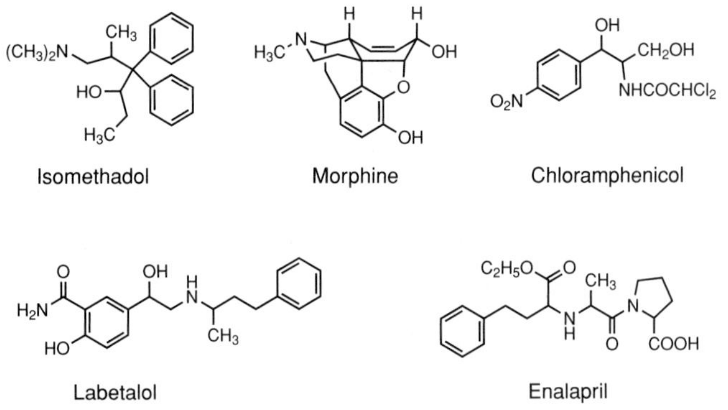

Isomethadol   Morphine   Chloramphenicol

Labetalol   Enalapril

Fig. 2.22. Examples of chiral drugs with two or more asymmetric centers.

the same side or on opposite sides of the double bond. The alkene 2-butene is a simple example of this.

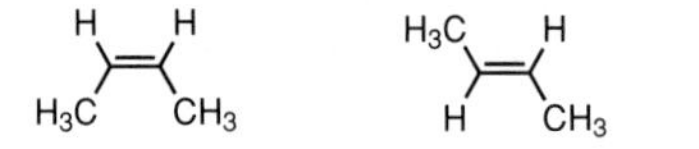

cis or Z isomer   trans or E isomer

With 2-butene, it is readily apparent that the methyl groups may be on the same side or on opposite sides of the double bond. When they are on the same side, the molecule is defined as the *cis*- or *Z*-isomer (from the German *zusammen,* meaning "together"); when they are on opposite sides, the designation is *trans*- or *E*- (from the German *entgegen,* meaning "opposite"). With simple compounds, such as 2-butene, it is easy to determine which groups in the molecule are *cis* or *trans* to one another. This becomes more difficult to determine, however, with more complex structures, in which it is less obvious which substituents should be referred to when naming the compound. In 1968, Blackwood et al. (22) proposed a system for the assignment of "absolute" configuration with respect to double bonds. Using the CIP sequence rules, each of the two substituents attached to the carbon atoms comprising the double bond are assigned a priority of 1 or 2, depending on the atomic number of the atom attached to the double bond. When two substituents of higher priority are on the same side of the double bond, this isomer is given the designation of *cis* or *Z*. When the substituents are on opposite sides, the designation is *trans* or *E*. The histamine H_1-receptor antagonist triprolidine (Fig. 2.23) is a good example for

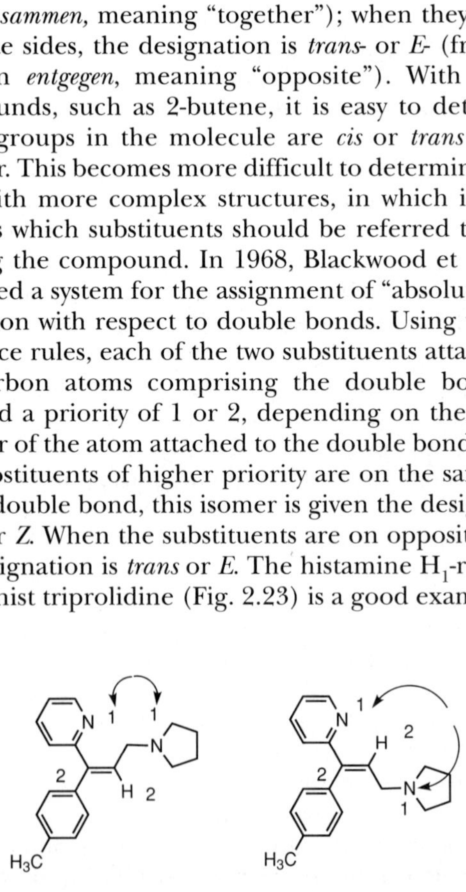

Fig. 2.23. Geometric isomers of triprolidine.

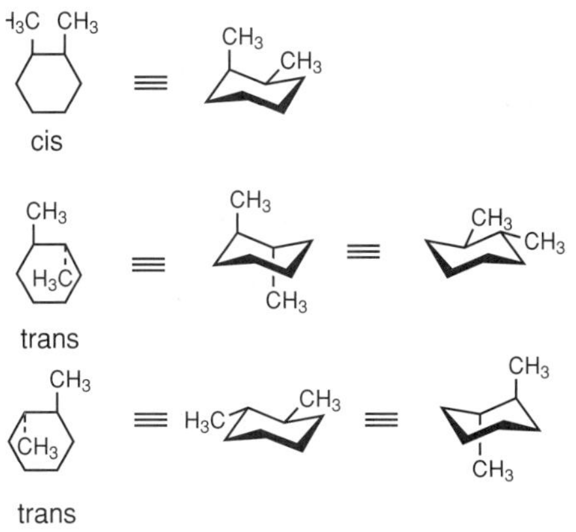

Fig. 2.24. Diastereomers of 1,2-dimethylcyclohexane.

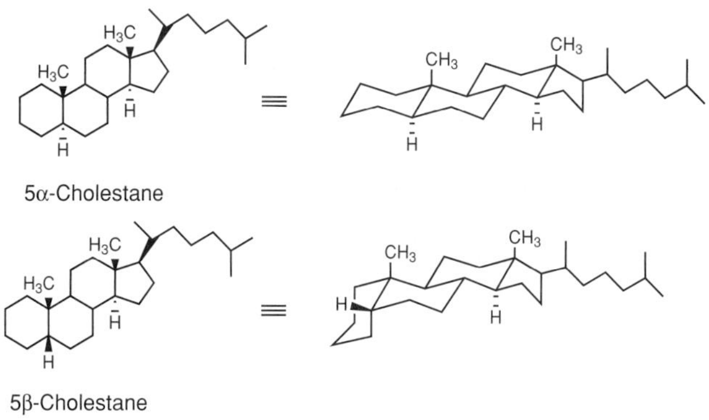

Fig. 2.25. The 5α and 5β conformations of the steroid nucleus cholestane.

demonstrating how this nomenclature system works. The *E*-isomer of triprolidine is more active both in vitro and in vivo, indicating that the distance between the pyridine and pyrrolidine rings is critical for binding to the receptor.

Diastereoisomers (as well as enantiomers) also can be found in cyclic compounds. For example, the cyclic alkane 1,2-dimethylcyclohexane can exist as *cis/trans*-diastereoisomers, and the *trans* isomer also can exist as an enantiomeric pair. In Figure 2.24, each of the *trans*-enantiomorphs are depicted in the two possible chair conformations for the cyclohexane ring. Cyclohexane rings can exhibit significant conformational freedom that allows for the possibility of conformational isomers. Isomers of this type will be discussed in the next section. When two or more rings share a common bond (e.g., decalin), rotation around the bonds is even more restricted, preventing ring "flipping" (through conformational rigidity) from occurring, thereby producing diastereoisomers and enantiomers.

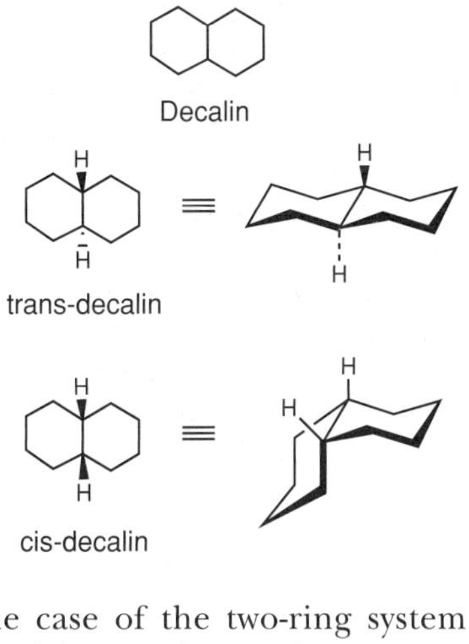

In the case of the two-ring system of decalin, the rings can join together at the common bond in either the *trans* or *cis* configuration as shown. Steroids, a class of medicinally important compounds consisting of four fused rings (three cyclohexanes and one cyclopentane), exhibit significantly different biological activity when the first two cyclohexane rings are fused into different configurations, referred to as the 5α- or 5β-isomers (Fig. 2.25). The β-designation indicates that the substituent in the 5-position is below the "plane" of the ring system; the β-designation refers to the substituent being above this plane. What appears to be a very minor change in orientation for the substituent results in a very drastic change in the three-dimensional shape of the molecule and in its biological activity. Figure 2.25 shows the diastereoisomers 5α-cholestane and 5β-cholestane as examples. The chemistry and pharmacology of steroids will be discussed in more detail in Chapters 32 (Adrenocorticoids), 45 (Estrogens and Progestins), and 46 (Androgens).

Conformational Isomerism

With conformational isomerism, we are dealing with a dynamic process—that is, isomerization takes place via rotation about one or more single bonds. Such bond rotation results in nonidentical spatial arrangement of atoms in a molecule. Changes in spatial orientation of atoms because of bond rotation results in different conformations (or rotamers), whereas conversion of one enantiomer into another (or diastereoisomer) requires the breaking of bonds, which has a much higher energy requirement than rotation around a single bond. The neurotransmitter acetylcholine can be used to demonstrate the concept of conformational isomers.

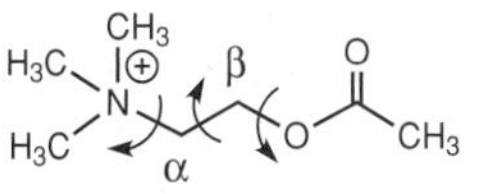

Acetylcholine

Each single bond within the acetylcholine molecule is capable of undergoing rotation, and at room temperature, such rotations readily occur. Even though rotation around single bonds was shown by Kemp and Pitzer (23) in 1936 not to be free but, rather, to have an energy

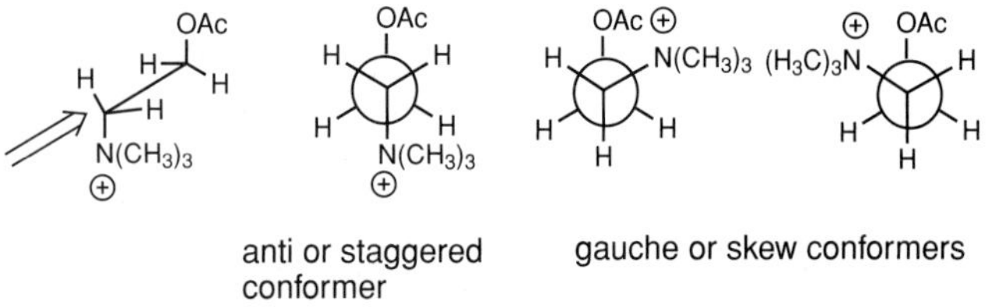

OAc H H H H H N(CH3)3 ⊕

anti or staggered conformer

gauche or skew conformers

Fig. 2.26. Anti and gauche conformations of acetylcholine.

barrier, this barrier is sufficiently low that at room temperature, acetylcholine exists in many interconvertible conformations (see Chapter 12). Close observation reveals that rotation around the central Cα–Cβ bond produces the greatest spatial rearrangement of atoms compared to rotation around any other bond within the molecule. In fact, several rotatable bonds in acetylcholine produce redundant structures, because all of the atoms attached to one end of some bonds are identical, resulting in no change in spatial arrangement of atoms (e.g., methyl groups). When viewed along the Cα–Cβ bond, acetylcholine can be depicted in the sawhorse or Newman projections, as shown in Figure 2.26. When the ester and trimethylammonium group are 180° apart, the molecule is said to be in the anti, or staggered, conformation (or conformer or rotamer). This conformation allows maximum separation of the functional groups and, therefore, considered to be the most stable conformation energetically. Other conformations possibly are more stable if factors other than steric interactions come into play (e.g., intramolecular hydrogen bonds). Rotation of one end of the Cα–Cβ bond by 120° or 240° results in the two gauche, or skew, conformations shown in Figure 2.26. These are considered to be less stable than the anticonformer, although some studies suggest that an electrostatic attraction between the electron-poor trimethylammonium and electron-rich ester oxygen stabilizes this conformation. Rotation by 60°, 180°, and 240° produce conformations in which all of the atoms overlap, or what are referred to as eclipsed conformations. These are the least stable conformers.

An interesting observation can be made with the two gauche conformers shown in Figure 2.26. These conformers are not distinct molecules, and they only exist for a transient period of time at room temperature. If these could be "frozen" into the conformations shown, however, they would be nonsuperimposable mirror images or enantiomers. Thus, a compound that is achiral, such as acetylcholine, can exhibit prochirality if certain conformational isomers can be formed. It is quite possible that such a situation could exist when acetylcholine binds to one of its receptors. Studies have suggested that the gauche conformation is the form that binds to the nicotinic receptor. whereas the anti form, which is achiral, binds to the muscarinic receptor.

DRUG DESIGN: DISCOVERY AND STRUCTURAL MODIFICATION OF LEAD COMPOUNDS

Natural Product Screening

Perhaps the most difficult aspect of drug discovery for the medicinal chemist is that of lead discovery. Until the late nineteenth century, the development of new chemical entities for medicinal purposes was achieved primarily through the use of natural products, generally derived from plant sources (see Chapter 1). As the colonial powers of Europe discovered new lands in the Western Hemisphere and colonized Asia, the Europeans learned from the indigenous peoples of the newly discovered lands of remedies for many ailments derived from herbs. Salicylic acid was isolated from the bark of willow trees after learning that Native Americans brewed the bark to treat inflammatory ailments. Further development of this lead compound by the Bayer Corporation of Germany resulted in acetylsalicylic acid, or aspirin, the first nonsteroidal anti-inflammatory agent. South American natives used a tea obtained by brewing Cinchona bark to treat chills and fever. Further study in Europe led to the isolation of quinine and quinidine, which subsequently were used to treat malaria and cardiac arrhythmias, respectively. Following leads such as these, chemists of the late nineteenth and early twentieth centuries began to seek new medicinals from plant sources and to assay them for many types of pharmacologic actions. This approach to drug discovery often is referred to as "natural product screening." With this approach, compounds were isolated from natural sources based on information obtained from indigenous peoples in many parts of the world. Until the mid-1970s, this was one of the major approaches to obtaining new chemical entities as leads for new drugs. Unfortunately, this approach declined in favor of what were then considered to be more rational approaches to drug design developed during that period (see below). Recently, however, because heightened awareness of the fragility of ecosystems, especially the rainforests, there has been a resurgence of screening products from plants before they become extinct. A new field of pharmacology, called "ethnopharmacology," has emerged as a result. Ethnopharmacology is the term used for the discipline of identifying potential natural product sources with medicinal products based on native lore.

Compounds isolated from natural sources usually are tested in bioassays for the ailment that the plant material has been described to treat. Sometimes, this may require several bioassays, because the plant has been reported to be effective against several ailments. Often, the treatment of different ailments requires different methods of preparation (e.g., brewing, chewing, or direct application to wounds) or different parts of the same plant (e.g., roots, stem, leaves, flowers, or sap). Each method of administration or part of the plant may involve one or more different chemical compounds to produce the desired outcome. One can readily see that isolation of active constituents from plants that may be useful as medicinals is not a simple process. A number of variables may influence the amount of active compound or compounds and, ultimately, the pharmacologic activity of the extract.

Drug Discovery via Random Screening of Synthetic Organic Compounds

This approach to discovering new chemical structures for a particular biological action began in the 1930s, after the discovery of the sulfonamide class of antibacterials. Thousands of compounds and their synthetic intermediates were assayed in search of new structures that possessed antibacterial activity. All compounds available to the investigator (natural products, synthetic compounds), regardless of structure, were tested in the assays available at the time. This approach also was applied in the 1960s and 1970s in an effort to find agents that were effective against cancer. Some groups did not limit themselves to a particular biological activity but, rather, tested compounds in a wide variety of assays. This approach was a precursor to what is now referred to as high-throughput screening assays, which involve the bioassay of thousands of compounds in hundreds to thousands of bioassays simultaneously. This only became possible with the advent of computer-controlled robotic systems for the assays and combinatorial chemistry techniques. These will be discussed further below.

What is crucial for random screening to be successful is a good bioassay system for the pharmacologic action of interest. Unfortunately, this means of lead discovery is very inefficient, because no rational approach is taken to what compounds are to be tested to find new lead structures. Random screening eventually gave way to dedicated screening and rational design techniques.

Drug Discovery via Targeted Dedicated Screening and Rational Drug Design

This approach is more or less random in nature and involves greater knowledge of the therapeutic targets and some actual design based on physicochemical properties. Testing usually is done with one or two models (e.g., specific receptor systems or enzymes) based on the therapeutic target. The design aspect often involves molecular modeling and the use of quantitative SARs to better define the physicochemical properties that are crucial for biological activity. The drawback of these approaches is that they are better for developing a lead compound than for discovering a lead compound.

Drug Discovery via Drug Metabolism Studies

New compounds have been "discovered" by investigating the metabolism of compounds that already are clinical candidates or, in rare instances, are already on the market. Metabolites of known compounds are isolated and then assayed for biological effects either on the same

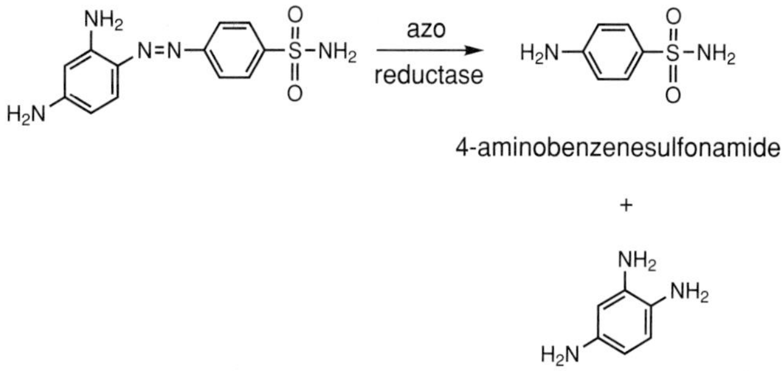

Fig. 2.27. Metabolic conversion of prontosil to 4-aminobenzenesulfonamide.

target system or with a broader screen of several other target systems. The latter will be more useful if the metabolite being studied is a chemical structure that has been radically altered from the parent molecule through some unusual rearrangement reaction. More often, the metabolite is not radically different from the parent molecule and, therefore, would be expected to have similar pharmacologic effects. The advantage is that a metabolite may possess better pharmacokinetic properties, such as a longer duration of action, better absorption orally, or less toxicity with fewer side effects (e.g., terfenadine and its antihistaminic metabolite, fexofenadine). The sulfonamide antibacterial agents were discovered in this way. The azo dye Prontosil was found to have only antibacterial action in vivo, but it was soon discovered that this compound required metabolic reduction of the diazo group to produce 4-aminobenzene sulfonamide (Fig. 2.27). The sulfonamide mimics the physicochemical properties of PABA, a crucial component in microbial metabolism. This results in the sulfonamide acting as a competitive inhibitor of the enzyme that uses PABA as a substrate.

Drug Discovery from the Observation of Side Effects

An astute clinician or pharmacologist may detect a side effect in a patient or animal model that could lead, on further development, to a new therapeutic use for a particular chemical structure. Further development may even lead to an entirely new chemical class. Discovery of new lead compounds via exploitation of side-effect profiles of existing agents has occurred several times and will be discussed below.

One of the more interesting cases of drug development is that of the phenothiazine antipsychotics (see Chapter 22). These compounds can be traced back to the first histamine H_1-receptor antagonists developed in the 1930s. In 1937, Bovet (24) was the first to recognize that it should be possible to antagonize the effects of histamine and, thereby, treat allergic reactions. He tested compounds that were known to act on the autonomic nervous system and, eventually, discovered that benzodioxanes (Fig. 2.28) were capable of significant antagonism

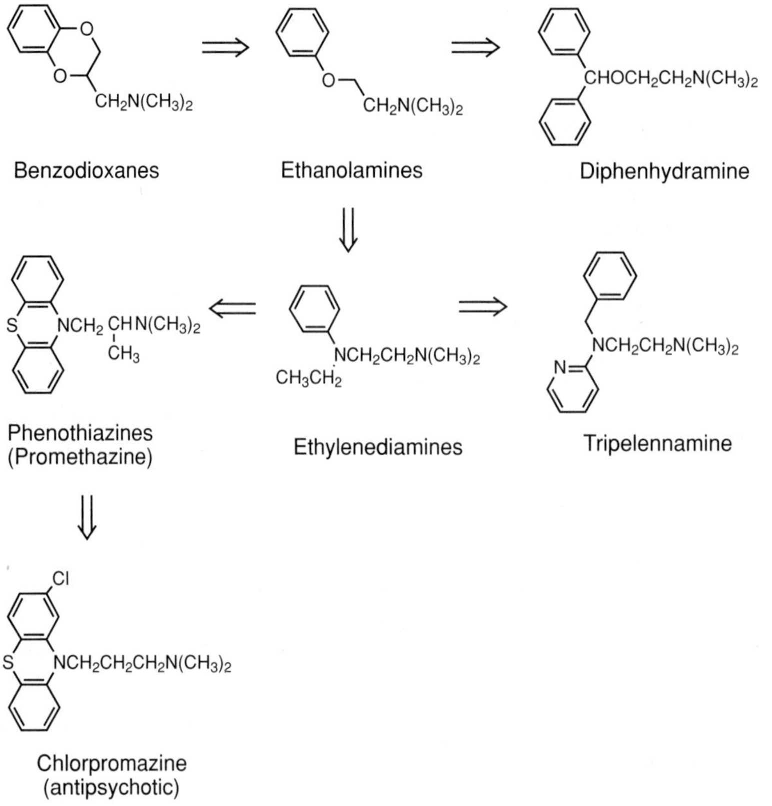

Benzodioxanes ⟹ Ethanolamines ⟹ Diphenhydramine

Ethanolamines ⟹ Ethylenediamines

Phenothiazines (Promethazine) ⟸ Ethylenediamines ⟹ Tripelennamine

Phenothiazines (Promethazine) ⟹ Chlorpromazine (antipsychotic)

Fig. 2.28. Development of phenothiazine-type antipsychotic drugs.

of the effects of histamine. During an attempt to improve the antihistaminic action of the benzodioxanes, it was discovered that ethanolamines also provided significant antihistaminic activity. Further development of this class ended up generating two different classes of antihistamines. One approach led to the development of the diphenhydramine class of antihistamines and is represented by the first clinically useful H_1-receptor antagonist developed in the United States, diphenhydramine (Fig. 2.28). The other approach led to the ethylenediamine class, represented by tripelennamine (Fig. 2.28) (see Chapter 37).

Incorporation of the aromatic rings of the ethylenediamines into the tricyclic phenothiazine structure produced compounds (e.g., promethazine) with good antihistaminic action and relatively strong sedative properties (see Chapter 37). At first, these compounds were found to be useful as antihistamines, but their very strong sedative properties also lead to their use as potentiating agents for anesthesia (25). Further development to increase the sedative properties of the phenothiazines resulted in the development of chlorpromazine in 1950 (26).

Chlorpromazine was found to produce a tendency for sleep, but unlike the previous phenothiazines, it also produced a disinterest in patients regarding their surroundings and, with patients suffering psychiatric disorders, an ameliorative effect on the psychosis as well as a relief of anxiety and agitation. These observations suggested that chlorpromazine had potential for the treatment of psychiatric disorders. Thus, what started out as an attempt to improve antihistaminic activity ultimately resulted in an entirely new class of chemical entity useful in an unrelated disorder (27).

Another example of how new chemical entities can be derived from compounds with unrelated biological effects is that of the development of the potassium channel agonist diazoxide (Fig. 2.29). This compound was developed as a result of the observation that the thiazide diuretics, such as chlorothiazide, not only had a diuretic component, because of inhibition of sodium absorption in the distal convoluted tubule, but also a direct effect on the renal vasculature. Structural modification to enhance this direct effect led to the development of diazoxide and related potassium channel agonists for the treatment of hypertension (see Chapter 29).

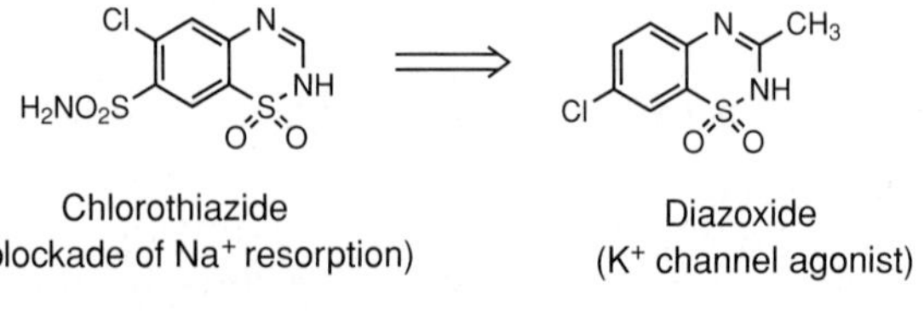

Chlorothiazide (blockade of Na^+ resorption) ⟹ Diazoxide (K^+ channel agonist)

Fig. 2.29. Structural similarity of chlorothiazide (a diuretic), and diazoxide (an antihypertensive that acts via opening of K^+ channels).

REFINEMENT OF THE LEAD STRUCTURE

Determination of the Pharmacophore

Once a lead compound has been discovered for a particular therapeutic use, the next step is to determine the pharmacophore for this compound. The pharmacophore of a drug molecule is that portion of the molecule containing the essential organic functional groups that directly interact with the receptor active site and, therefore, confers on the molecule the biological activity of interest. Because drug–receptor interactions can be very specific, the pharmacophore may constitute a small portion of the molecule. It has been found on several occasions that what seem to be very complex molecules can be reduced to simpler structures with retention of the desired biological action. An example of this is the narcotic analgesic morphine, which is a tetracyclic compound with five chiral centers. Not only would simplification of the structure possibly provide molecules with fewer side effects, a reduction in the number of chiral centers would greatly simplify the synthesis of morphine derivatives and, thereby, decrease cost. Figure 2.30 shows how the morphine structure has been simplified in the search for compounds with fewer deleterious side effects, such as respiratory depression and addiction potential. Within each class are analogues that are less potent, equipotent, and many times more potent than morphine. It can be readily seen from the figure that the pharmacophore of morphine must consist of a tertiary alkylamine that is at least four atoms away from an aromatic ring. A more detailed discussion of the chemistry and pharmacology of morphine can be found in Chapter 24.

4,5α-Epoxymorphinans

Morphinans

Benzomorphans

4-Phenylpiperidines

Methadones

Fig. 2.30. Morphine pharmacophore and its relationship to analgesic derivatives.

Alterations in Alkyl Chains: Chain Length, Branching, and Rings

Alterations in alkyl chains, such as increasing or decreasing chain length (homologation), branching, and changing ring size, can have profound effects on the potency and pharmacologic activity of the molecule. Simply changing the length of an alkyl chain by one CH_2 unit or branching the chain will alter the lipophilic character of the molecule and, therefore, its properties of absorption, distribution, and excretion. If the alkyl chain is directly involved in the receptor interaction, then chain length and branching can alter the binding characteristics. Molecules that are conformationally flexible may become less flexible if branching is introduced at a key position of an alkyl chain. Changes in conformation will affect the spatial relationship of functional groups in the molecule, thereby influencing receptor binding. Changes as small as one CH_2 unit may seem trivial at first, but in many instances, such small changes are important aspects in the design of analogues.

An example in which simply increasing hydrocarbon chain length has significant effects not only on potency but also on the agonistic or antagonistic action of a molecule is provided by a series of N-alkyl morphine analogues (Fig. 2.31). In this series, going from R=CH_3 (morphine) to R=$CH_2CH_2CH_3$ (N-propylnormorphine) produces a pronounced decrease in agonist activity and an increase in antagonist activity. When R=$CH_2CH_2CH_2CH_3$ (N-butylnormorphine), the compound is totally devoid of agonist or antagonist activity (i.e., the compound is inactive), but further increases in chain length (R=$CH_2CH_2CH_2CH_2CH_3$ and R=$CH_2CH_2CH_2CH_2CH_2CH_3$) produce compounds with increasing potency as agonists. When R is β-phenylethyl, the compound is a full agonist, with a potency approximately 14-fold that of morphine (28,29).

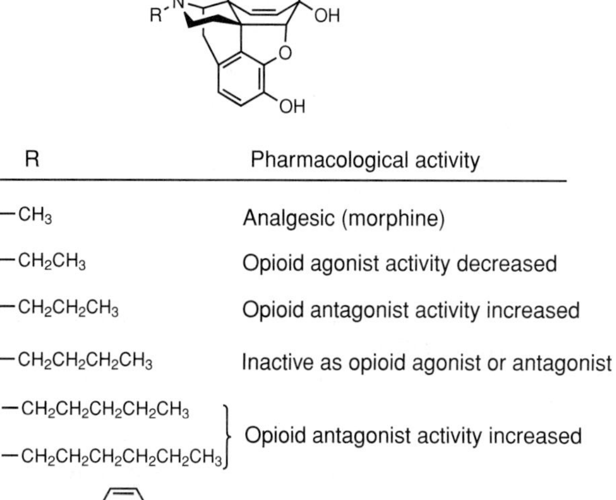

R	Pharmacological activity
$-CH_3$	Analgesic (morphine)
$-CH_2CH_3$	Opioid agonist activity decreased
$-CH_2CH_2CH_3$	Opioid antagonist activity increased
$-CH_2CH_2CH_2CH_3$	Inactive as opioid agonist or antagonist
$-CH_2CH_2CH_2CH_2CH_3$	Opioid antagonist activity increased
$-CH_2CH_2CH_2CH_2CH_2CH_3$	Opioid antagonist activity increased
$-CH_2CH_2$-phenyl	14X potency of morphine

Fig. 2.31. Effect of alkyl chain length on activity of morphine.

Branching of alkyl chains also can produce drastic changes in potency and pharmacologic activity. If the mechanism of action is closely related to the lipophilicity of the molecule, then branching of a hydrocarbon chain will result in a less lipophilic compound and significantly altered biological effect. This decrease in lipophilicity as the result of hydrocarbon chain branching results from the chain becoming more compact and, therefore, produces less disruption of the hydrogen-bonding network of water. If the hydrocarbon chain is directly involved in receptor interactions, then branching can produce major changes in pharmacologic activity. For example, consider the phenothiazines promethazine and promazine:

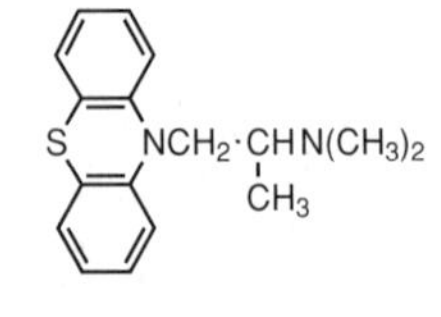

Promethazine 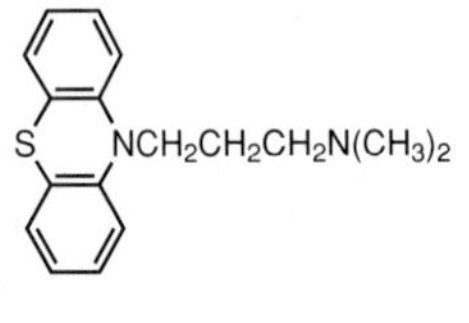 Promazine

The primary pharmacologic activity of promethazine is that of an antihistamine, whereas promazine is an antipsychotic. The only difference between the two is the alkylamine side chain. In the case of promethazine, it contains a isopropylamine side chain, whereas promazine has a *n*-propylamine. In this case, the small change of one carbon atom from a branched to a linear hydrocarbon radically alters the pharmacologic activity.

Position isomers of substituents on aromatic rings also may possess different pharmacologic properties. Substituents on aromatic rings can alter the electron distribution throughout the ring, which in turn can affect how the ring interacts with the receptor. Ring substituents also may influence the conformation of a flexible molecule, especially if they are located ortho to flexible side chains and can participate in steric or electronic intramolecular interactions (e.g., hydrogen, ion–dipole, or ion–ion bonds). Ring substituents influence the conformations of adjacent substituents via steric interactions and may significantly affect receptor interactions. Aromatic methoxy groups ortho to two other substituents take on a conformation perpendicular to the plane of the aromatic ring in hallucinogenic phenylalkylamines (Fig. 2.32) and can explain the lack of hallucinogenic activity in these compounds (30).

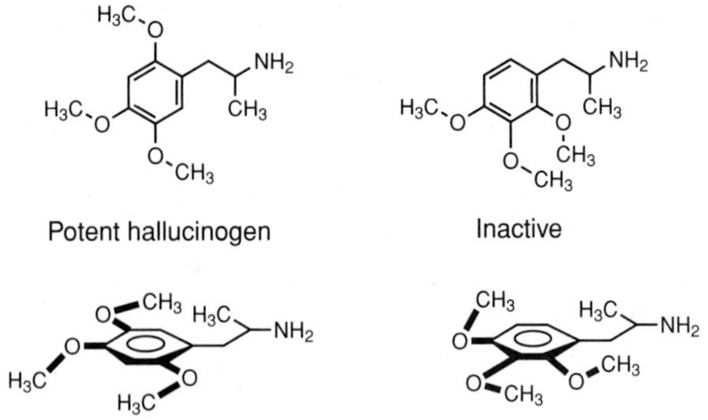

Potent hallucinogen Inactive

Fig. 2.32. Effect of positional isomers on structural conformation and biological activity.

FUNCTIONAL GROUP MODIFICATION: ISOSTERISM AND BIOISOSTERISM

Isosterism

When a lead compound is first discovered for a particular disease state, it often lacks the required potency and pharmacokinetic properties suitable for making it a viable clinical candidate. These may include undesirable side effects, physicochemical properties, other factors that affect oral bioavailability (see Chapter 9), and adverse metabolic or excretion properties. These undesirable properties could be the result of specific functional groups in the molecule. The medicinal chemist therefore must modify the compound to reduce or eliminate these undesirable features without losing the desired biological activity. Replacement or modification of functional groups with other groups having similar properties is known as "isosteric replacement," or "bioisosteric replacement."

In 1919, Langmuir (31,32) first developed the concept of chemical isosterism to describe the similarities in physical properties among atoms, functional groups, radicals, and molecules. The similarities among atoms described by Langmuir primarily resulted from the fact that these atoms contained the same number of valence electrons and came from the same columns within the periodic table. This concept was limited to elements in adjacent rows and columns, inorganic molecules, ions, and small organic molecules, such as diazomethane and ketene. Table 2.7 shows a comparison of the physical properties of N_2O and CO_2 to illustrate Langmuir's concept.

To account for similarities between groups with the same number of valence electrons but different numbers of atoms, Grimm (33) developed his hydride displacement law. This is not a "law" in the strict sense but, rather, more an illustration of similar physical properties among closely related functional groups. Table 2.8 presents an example of hydride displacement. Descending diagonally from left to right in the table, hydrogen atoms are progressively added to maintain the same number of

Table 2.7. Comparison of Physical Properties of N_2O and CO_2

Property	N_2O	CO_2
Viscosity at 20°C	148×10^{-6}	148×10^{-6}
Density of liquid at 10°C	0.856	0.858
Refractive index of liquid, D line 16°C	1.193	1.190
Dielectric constant of liquid at 0°C	1.593	1.582
Solubility in alcohol at 15°C	3.250	3.130

Table 2.8. Grimm's Hydride Displacement "Law"

C	N	O	F	Ne
	CH	NH	OH	FH
		CH_2	NH_2	OH_2
			CH_3	NH_3

valence electrons for each group of atoms within a column. Within each column, the groups are considered to be "pseudoatoms" with respect to one another. Thus, NH_2 is considered to be isosteric to OH, and so on. This early view of isosterism did not consider the actual location, motion, and resonance of electrons within the orbitals of these functional group replacements. Careful observation of this table reveals that some groups do share similar physicochemical properties, but others have very different properties, despite having the same number of valence electrons. For example, OH and NH_2 share similar hydrogen-bonding properties and, therefore, should be interchangeable if that is the only criterion necessary. The NH_2 group is basic, however, whereas the OH is neutral. Hence, at physiological pH, the NH_2 group would be in its protonated, or conjugate acid, form and give the molecule a positive charge. If OH is being substituted by NH_2, the additional positive charge could have a significant effect on the overall physicochemical properties of the molecule in which it is being introduced. The difference in physicochemical properties of the CH_3 group relative to the OH and NH_2 groups is even greater. In addition to basicity and acidity, this "law" fails to take into account other important physicochemical parameters, such as electronegativity, polarizability, bond angles, size, shape of molecular orbitals, electron density, and partition coefficients, all of which contribute significantly to the overall physicochemical properties of a molecule.

Instead of considering only partial structures, Hinsberg (34) applied the concept of isosterism to entire molecules. He developed the concept of "ring equivalents"—that is, groups that can be exchanged for one another in aromatic ring systems without drastic changes in physicochemical properties relative to the parent structure. Benzene, thiophene, and pyridine illustrate this concept (Fig. 2.33). A –CH=CH- group in benzene is replaced by the divalent sulfur, -S-, in thiophene, and a –CH= is replaced by the trivalent –N= to give pyridine. The physical properties of benzene and thiophene

Tripelennamine Methaphenilene

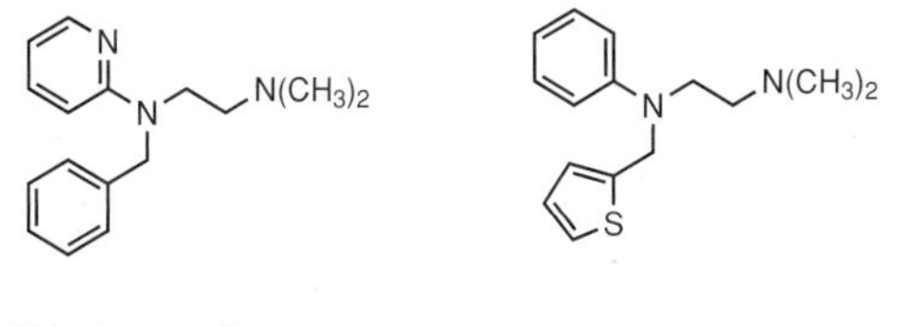

Fig. 2.33. Isosteric substitution of thiophene for benzene and benzene for pyridine.

are very similar. For example, the boiling point of benzene is 81.1°C, and that of thiophene is 84.4°C (at 760 mm Hg). Pyridine, however, deviates, with a boiling point of 115 to 116°C. Hinsberg therefore concluded that divalent sulfur (-S- or thioether) must resemble –C=C- in shape, and these groups were considered to be isosteric. Note that hydrogen atoms are ignored in this comparison. Today, this isosteric relationship is seen in many drugs (e.g., H_1-receptor antagonists) (Fig. 2.33).

Bioisosterism

It is difficult to relate biological properties to physicochemical properties of individual atoms, functional groups, or entire molecules, because many physicochemical parameters are involved simultaneously and, therefore, are difficult to quantitate. Simple relationships as described above often do not hold up across the many types of biological systems seen with medicinal agents. That is, what may work as an isosteric replacement in one biological system (or a given drug receptor, enzyme, etc.) may not work in another system. Because of this, it was necessary to introduce the term "bioisosterism" to describe functional groups related in structure and having similar biological effects. Friedman (35) introduced the term bioisosterism and defined it as follows: "Bioisosteres are (functional) groups or molecules that have chemical and physical similarities producing broadly similar biological properties." Recently, Burger (36) expanded this definition to take into account biochemical views of biological activity: "Bioisosteres are compounds or groups that possess near equal molecular shapes and volumes, approximately the same distribution of electrons, and which exhibit similar physical properties such as hydrophobicity. Bioisosteric compounds affect the same biochemically associated systems as agonist or antagonists and thereby produce biological properties that are related to each other." The key point is that the same pharmacologic target is influenced by bioisoteres as agonists or antagonists. What may work as a bioisosteric group in one biological system may not have similar effects on another.

Classical and Nonclassical Bioisosteres

Bioisosteric groups can be subdivided into two categories: classical and nonclassical bioisosteres. Functional groups that satisfy the original conditions of Langmuir and Grimm are referred to as classical bioisosteres. Nonclassical bioisosteres do not obey steric and electronic definitions of classical bioisoteres and do not necessarily have the same number of atoms as the substituent they replace. A wider set of compounds and functional groups are encompassed by nonclassical bioisoteres that produce, at the molecular level, qualitatively similar agonistic or antagonistic responses. In animals, many hormones, neurotransmitters, and so on with very similar structures and biological actions can be classified as bioisosteres. An example would be the insulins isolated from various mammalian species. Even though these insulins may differ by several amino acid residues, they

Table 2.9. Classical Bioisosteres (Groups Within the Row Can Replace Each Other)

Monovalent bioisosteres

F, H
OH, NH
F, OH, NH or CH_3 for H
SH, OH
Cl, Br, CF_3

Divalent bioisosteres:

—C=S, —C=O, —C=NH, —C=C—

Trivalent atoms or groups:

—CH=, —N=
—P=, —As=

Tetrasubstituted atoms:

$-\overset{|}{\underset{|}{N}}{}^{\oplus}-$ $-\overset{|}{\underset{|}{C}}-$ $-\overset{|}{\underset{|}{P}}{}^{\oplus}-$ $-\overset{|}{\underset{|}{As}}{}^{\oplus}-$

Ring equivalents:

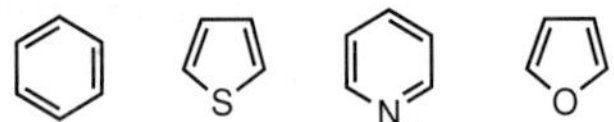

still produce the same biological effects. (If this did not occur, the use of insulin to treat diabetes would have had to wait another 60 years for recombinant DNA technology to allow production of human insulin.)

What may be a successful bioisosteric replacement for a given molecule interacting with a particular receptor quite often has no effect or abolishes biological activity in another. Thus, the use of bioisosteric replacement (classical or nonclassical) in drug design is highly dependent on the biological system being investigated. No hard-and-fast rules exist to determine what bioisosteric replacement is going to work with a given molecule, although as the following tables and examples demonstrate, some generalizations are possible. The medicinal chemist, however, must still rely on experience and intuition to decide the best approach to use when applying this strategy.

Each category of bioisostere can be further subdivided as shown below, and examples are provided in Table 2.9:

I. Classical bioisosteres
  A. Monovalent atoms and groups
  B. Divalent atoms and groups
  C. Trivalent atoms and groups
  D. Tetrasubstituted atoms
  E. Ring equivalents
II. Nonclassical bioisoteres
  A. Exchangeable groups
  B. Rings versus noncyclic structure

Classical Bioisosteres

Substitution of hydrogen by fluorine is one of the most common monovalent isosteric replacements. Sterically, hydrogen and fluorine are quite similar, with their van der Waal's radii being 1.2 and 1.35 Å, respectively. Because fluorine is the most electronegative element in the periodic table, any differences in biological activity resulting from replacement of hydrogen with fluorine can be attributed to this property.

R =	Cl	Br	CF_3
σ	+0.23	+0.23	+0.54
π	+0.71	+0.86	+0.88
E_s	-0.97	-1.16	-2.40

Fig. 2.34. Isosteric replacement of chlorine in thiazide diuretics. Comparison of physicochemical properties of the substituents.

A classic example of hydrogen replacement by fluorine is development of the antineoplastic agent 5-fluorouracil from uracil. Another example is shown in Figure 2.34, in which the chlorine of chlorothiazide has been replaced with bromine or a trifluoromethyl group. For each of the substitutions, the electronic (σ, where σ^+ is electron withdrawing and σ^- is electron donating) and hydrophobic (π) properties of each group are maintained relatively constant, but the size of each group varies significantly, as indicated by the Taft steric parameter (E_s).

Figure 2.35 shows an example of classical isosteric substitution of an amino group for a hydroxyl group in folic acid. The amino group is capable of mimicking the tautomeric forms of folic acid and providing the appropriate hydrogen bonds to the enzyme active site.

A tetravalent bioisosteric replacement study was done by Grisar et al. (37) with a series of α-tocopherol analogues (Fig. 2.36). α-Tocopherol has been shown to scavenge

Folic acid X = OH
Aminopterin X = NH_2

Fig. 2.35. Isosteric replacement of OH by NH_2 in folic acid and possible tautomers of folic acid and aminopterin.

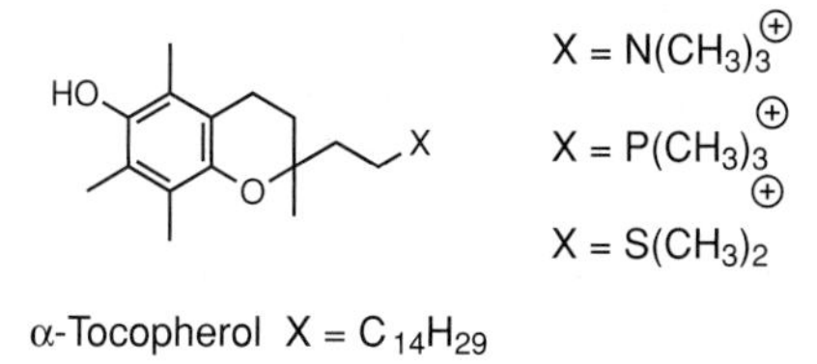

Fig. 2.36. Tetravalent bioisosteres of α-tocopherol.

lipoperoxyl and superoxide radicals and to accumulate in heart tissue. This is thought to be part of its mechanism of action for reducing cardiac damage resulting from myocardial infarction. All of the bioisosteric analogues were found to produce similar biological activity.

Nonclassical Bioisoteres

As mentioned earlier, nonclassical bioisosteres are replacements of functional groups not defined by classical definitions. Some of these groups, however, mimic spatial arrangements, electronic properties, or some other physicochemical property of the molecule or functional group critical for biological activity. One example is the use of a double bond to position essential functional groups into a particular spatial configuration critical for activity. This is shown in Figure 2.37 with the naturally occurring hormone estradiol and the synthetic analogue diethylstilbestrol. The *trans* isomer of diethylstilbestrol has approximately the same potency as estradiol, whereas the *cis* isomer is only one-fourteenth as active. In the *trans* configuration, the phenolic hydroxy groups mimic the correct orientation of the phenol and alcohol in estradiol (38,39). This is not possible with the *cis* isomer, and more flexible analogues (Fig. 2.37) have little or no activity (40,41).

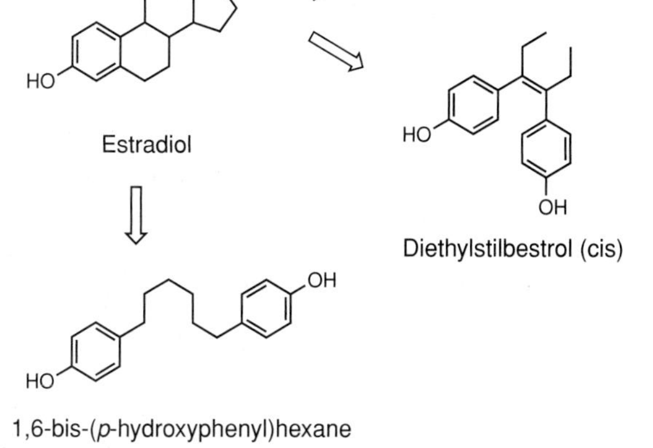

Fig. 2.37. Noncyclic analogs of estradiol.

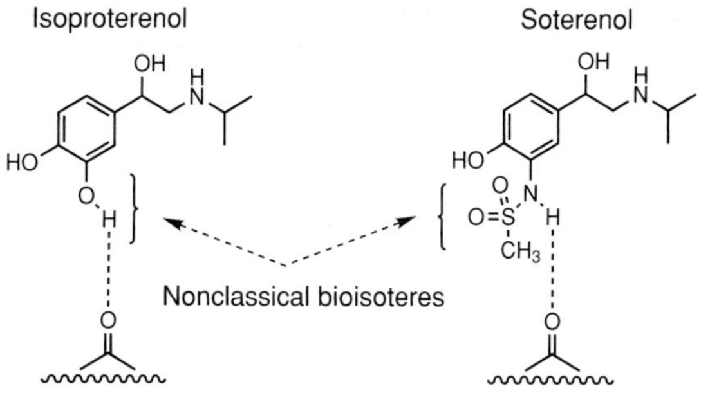

Fig. 2.38. Bioisosteric replacement of m-OH of isoproterenol with a sulfonamido group and similar hydrogen-bonding capacity to a possible drug receptor.

Another example of a nonclassical replacement is that of a sulfonamide group for a phenol in catecholamines (Fig. 2.38). With this example, steric factors appear to have less influence on receptor binding than acidity and hydrogen-bonding potential of the functional group on the aromatic ring. Both the phenolic hydroxyl of isoproterenol and the acidic proton of the arylsulfonamide have nearly the same pK_a (~10) (42). Both groups are weakly acidic and capable of losing a proton and interacting with the receptor as anions or participating as hydrogen-bond donors at the receptor, as shown in Figure 2.38. Because the replacement is not susceptible to metabolism by catechol O-methyltransferase, it also has the added advantages of increasing the duration of action and making the compound orally active. Other examples of successful bioisosteric replacements are shown in Table 2.10, and a more detailed description of the role of bioisosterism can be found in the review by Patani and LaVoie (43).

SUMMARY

Medicinal chemistry involves the discovery of new chemical entities for the treatment of disease and the systematic study of the SARs of these compounds. Such studies provide the basis for development of better medicinal agents from lead compounds found via random screening, systematic screening, and rational design. The role of the medicinal chemist is to increase the potency and duration of action of newly discovered compounds and to decrease adverse side effects. Without a thorough understanding of the physicochemical properties of the organic functional groups that comprise any given structure, this task would be impossible.

For the pharmacist, it is also important to understand the physicochemical properties of the medicinal agents that he or she is dispensing. Such knowledge will help the practicing pharmacist not only to better understand the clinical properties of these compounds but also to anticipate the properties of new agents that appear on the

Table 2.10. Nonclassical Bioisosteric Replacements

Compounds	Bioisosteric Replacement	References
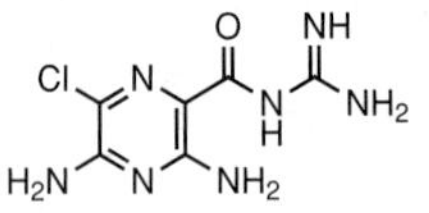	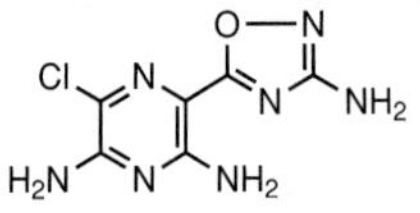	40
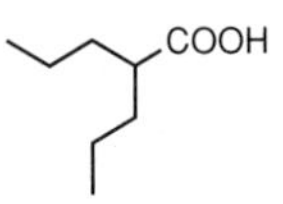	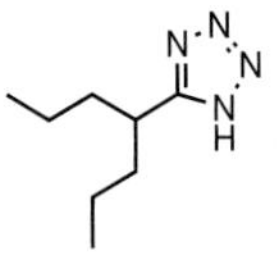	41
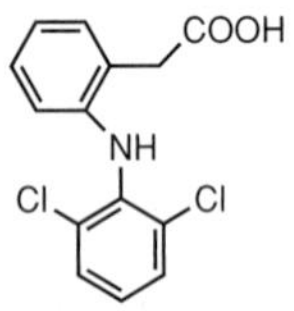	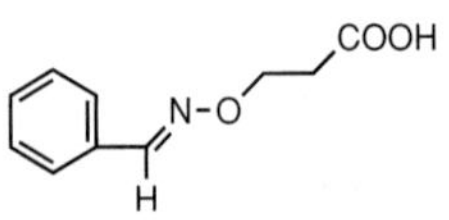	42
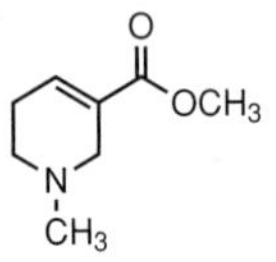	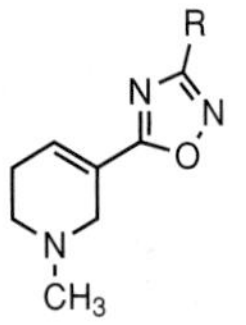	43
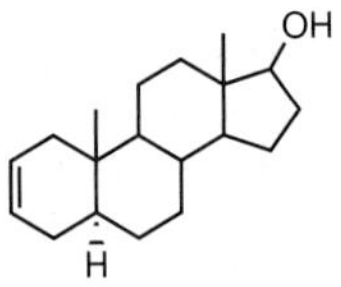	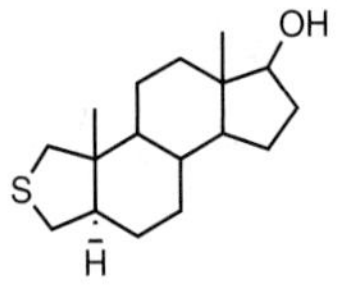	44
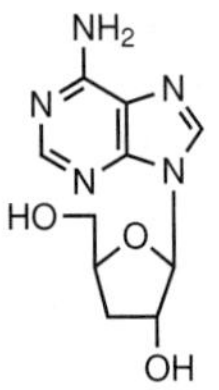	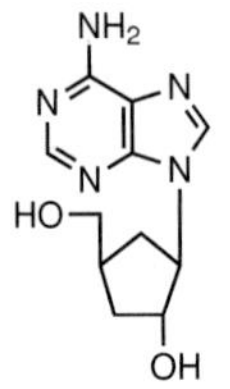	45
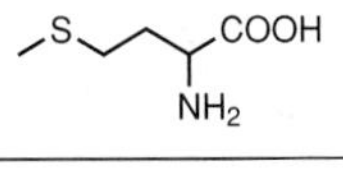	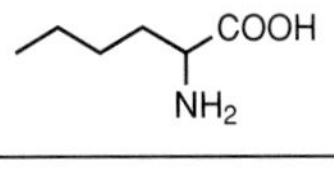	46

market. An understanding of the chemical properties of the molecule will allow the pharmacist to anticipate formulation problems (especially IV admixtures) as well as potential adverse interactions with other drugs as the result of serum protein binding and metabolism.

PROBLEMS

The following problems are provided for additional study:

1. Calculate the percentage ionization of amobarbital at pH 2.0, 5.5, and 8.0. What trend is seen?
2. Calculate the percentage ionization of phenylpropanolamine at pH 2.0, 5.5, and 8.0. Compare these results with those obtained in Problem 1.
3. Calculate the percentage ionization of sulfacetamide in the stomach, duodenum, and ileum. Draw the structure of the predominate form of the drug in each tissue.
4. Referring to Figure 2.15, redraw each compound in its ionized form.
5. For the organic functional groups listed in Table 2.4, name each functional group, and redraw them, showing all potential hydrogen bonds with water.
6. Using the empiric method of Lemke, predict the water solubility for each of the following molecules (*Note:* Water solubility is defined as >1% solubility):

Aspirin	Carphenazine maleate
Chlordiazepoxide	Codeine
Codeine phosphate	Cyproheptadine hydrochloride
Haloperidol	Phenytoin

7. Calculate the logP value for each of the following:

Aspirin	Carphenazine
Codeine	Cyproheptadine
Haloperidol	Chlordiazepoxide
Phenytoin	

8. Using the Merck Index, find the chemical structures for the following empirical formulae. List as many physicochemical properties as possible for each compound, and compare them within each group of isomers:

$$C_4H_{10}O_2 \quad C_5H_8O$$
$$C_5H_{11}O_2 \quad C_7H_7NO_2 \quad C_8H_8O_2$$
$$C_{12}H_{17}NO_3$$
$$C_{20}H_{30}O_2$$

9. Using the Cahn-Ingold-Prelog rules, assign the absolute configuration to each chiral center of ephedrine and pseudoephedrine (Fig. 2.21).
10. For the compounds shown in Figure 2.22, indicate, using an *, where the chiral centers are in each molecule.
11. Draw each possible stereoisomer for chloramphenicol and enalapril. Assign the absolute sterechemistry to each chiral center.
12. I. Draw the Newman projection along the CH_3-N bond of acetylcholine in the staggered conformation. Rotate the bond 120° and 240°. Are these rotameters conformational isomers? Explain why or why not.
    II. Repeat the above exercise with the N1–C2 bond of acetylcholine.
13. Draw the three most stable rotameters of norepinephrine. Of these rotameters, is there the possibility of an intramolecular interaction that would stabilize what normally would be considered an unstable rotameter? Explain.

References

1. Crum-Brown A, Fraser TR. On the connection between chemical constitution and physiological action. Part 1: on the physiological action of the ammonium bases derived from Strychia, Brucia, Thebia, Codeia, Morphia, and Nicotia. Trans R Soc Edinburgh 1869;25:257–274.

2. Ariëns EJ. A General Introduction to the Field of Drug Discovery. In: Ariëns EJ, ed. Drug Design. New York: Academic Press, 1971;1:689–696.
3. Loewi O, Navrati E. Über humorale Übertragbarkeit der Herznervenwirkung XI Mitteilung. Über den Mechanismus der Vaguswirkung von Physostigmin und Ergotamine. Plugers Arch Ges Physiol Menshen Tiere 1926;214:689–696.
4. Ehrlich P. On immunity with special reference to cell life. In: Himmelweit F, ed. Collected Papers of Paul Ehrlich. London: Pergamon, 1957, pp. 178–195.
5. Albert A. The long search for valid structure–action relationships in drugs. J Med Chem 1982;25:1–5.
6. Ing HR. The curariform action of onium salts. Physiol Rev 1936;16:527–544.
7. Woods DD. The relation of *p*-aminobenzoic acid to the mechanism of the action of sulfanilamide. Br J Exp Pathol 1940;21:74–90.
8. Kauffman GB. The Brönsted-Lowry acid-base concept. J Chem Ed 1988;85: 28–31.
9. Gennaro AR. Organic pharmaceutical chemistry. In: Gennaro AR, ed. Remington's Pharmaceutical Sciences. 21st ed. Easton, PA: Mack Publishing, 2006:386–409.
10. Lemke TL. Review of Organic Functional Groups: Introduction to Medicinal Organic Chemistry. 4th ed. Philadelphia: Lippincott Williams & Wilkins, 2003.
11. Cates LA. Calculation of drug solubilities by pharmacy students. Am J Pharm Ed 1981;45:11–13.
12. Fujita T. The extrathermodynamic approach to drug design. In: Hansch C, ed. Comprehensive Medicinal Chemistry. New York: Pergamon Press, 1990;4: 497–560.
13. Tute MS. Principles and practice of Hansch analysis: a guide to structure–activity correlation for the medicinal chemist. In: Harper NJ, Simons AB, eds. Advances in Drug Research. London: Academic Press, 1971;6:1–77.
14. Hansch C, Leo A. Substituent Constants for Correlation Analysis in Chemistry and Biology. New York: John Wiley, 1979.
15. Hansch C, Leo A. Exploring QSAR: Hydrophobic, Electronic, and Steric Constants. Washington, D.C.: American Chemical Society, 1995.
16. ClogP 4.0®. BioByte Corp., Claremont, CA.
17. Molinspiration Chemoinformatics. http://www.molinspiration.com, last accessed March 6, 2007.
18. Interactive Analysis. http://www.logP.com, last accessed March 6, 2007.
19. Cahn RS, Ingold CK, Prelog V. The specification of asymmetric configuration in organic chemistry. Experientia 1956;12:81–94.
20. Piutti A. Su rune nouvelle espec d'asparagine. Compt Red 1886;103:134–138.
21. Easson LH, Stedman E. Studies on the relationship between chemical constitution and physiological action. V. Molecular dissymmetry and physiological activity. Biochem J 1933;27:1257–1266.
22. Blackwood JE, Gladys CL, Loening KL, et al. Unambiguous specification of stereoisomerism about a double bond. J Am Chem Soc 1968;90:509–510.
23. Kemp JD, Pitzer KS. Hindered rotation of the methyl groups in ethane. J Chem Phys 1936;4:749.
24. Bovet D, Staub A. Action Protectice des Ethers Phenoliques au cours de L'intoxication Histaminique. C R Soc Biol (Paris) 1937;124:547–549.
25. Laborit H, Huguenard P, Alluaume R. Un nouveau stabilisateur vegetatif, le 4560 RP. Presse Med 1952;60:206–208.
26. Charpentier P, Gaillot P, Jacob R, et al. Recherches sur les Dimethylaminopropyl N-phenothiazines. C R Acad Sci (Paris) 1952;325:59–60.
27. Delay J, Deniker P, Hurl JM. Utilisation en Thirapeutique Psychiatrique d'une Phenothiazine d'action Centrale elective. Ann Med Psychol (Paris) 1952;110:112–117.
28. McCawley EL, Hart ER, Marsh DF. The preparation of N-allylnormorphine. J Am Chem Soc 1941;63:314.
29. Clark RL, Pessolano AA, Weijlard J, et al. N-substituted epoxymorphinans. J Am Chem Soc 1953;75:4964–4967.
30. Knittel JJ, Makriyannis A. Studies on phenethylamine hallucinogens. 2. Conformations of arylmethoxyl groups using ^{13}C NMR. J Med Chem 1981;24: 906–909.
31. Langmuir I. The arrangement of electrons in atoms and molecules. J Am Chem Soc 1919;41:868–934.
32. Langmuir I. Isomorphism, isosterism, and covalence. J Am Chem Soc 1919;41:1543–1559.
33. Grimm HG. Über Ban und Grösse der Nichtmetallhydride. Z Elekrochemie. 1925;31:474–480.
34. Hinsberg O. The sulfur atom. J Prakt Chem 1916;93:302–311.
35. Friedman HL. Influence of Isosteric Replacements upon Biological Activity. In: Symposium on Chemical–Biological Correlation. Publication 206. Washington, D.C.: Natl. Acad. Sci., 1951:206:295–358.
36. Burger A. Isosterism and bioisosterism in drug design. Prog Drug Res 1991;37:288–371.
37. Grisar JM, Marciniak G, Bolkenius FN, et al. Cardioselective ammonium, phosphonium, and sulfonium analogues of α-tocopherol and ascorbic acid that inhibit in vitro and ex vivo lipid peroxidation and scavenge superoxide radicals. J Med Chem 1995;38:2880–2886.
38. Dodds EC, Goldberg L, Lawson W, et al. Estrogenic activity of certain synthetic compounds. Nature 1938;141:247–248.
39. Walton E, Brownlee G. Isomers of stilbestrol and its esters. Nature 1943;151;305–306.
40. Blanchard EW, Stuart AH, Tallman RC. Studies on a new series of synthetic estrogenic substances. Endocrinology 1943;32:307–309.
41. Baker BR. Some analogues of hexestrol. J Am Chem Soc 1943;65:1572–1579.
42. Larsen AA, Gould WA, Roth HR, et al. Sulfonanilides. II. Analogues of catecholamines. J Med Chem 1967;10:462–472.
43. Patani GA, LaVoie EJ. Bioisosterism: a rational approach in drug design. Chem Rev 1996;96:3147–3176.

3. *Molecular Modeling and In Silico Drug Design*

XIANG-QUN (SEAN) XIE

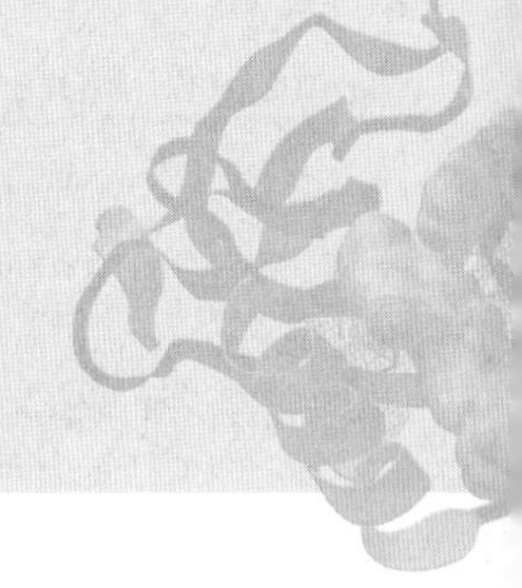

INTRODUCTION

Molecular modeling allows scientists to use computers to visualize molecules, to discover new lead compounds for drugs, or to refine existing drugs in silico. It enables computational chemists to rigorously study molecular behavior in ways that are not possible in the laboratory. "Molecular modeling" is a term for which the definition has evolved along with the capabilities of computer hardware and algorithms. The term referred to software capable of displaying and manipulating simple structures of molecules. As computers became faster and algorithms more accurate, the term grew to include algorithms for calculating the structures of small molecules, such as the pioneering work of Hendrickson (1). Modern molecular modeling software is used to study small molecules, proteins, lipids, DNA, and nonbiological work. One goal of molecular modeling is to develop a sufficiently accurate model of the system so that the physical experiments may not be necessary.

As we learn about physical chemistry, we extend that understanding to new systems of interest, but the transition from simple molecules to more complicated systems is limited by our human abilities. We can imagine a butane molecule and imagine both how and why different conformers are preferred. When we tackle pentane or combinations of functional groups, however, it becomes difficult to simultaneously consider the relative effects of electrostatics, steric interactions, and bulk properties, such as solubilities. Fortunately, we can construct models in software that allow us to properly treat all of these interactions. The scientific field of molecular modeling or, more generally, computational chemistry is the practice of simulation of molecular systems with sufficient detail to address a question of interest.

Furthermore, computational chemistry has advanced from the classical quantum mechanical ab initio calculations to semiempirical molecular orbital calculations and molecular mechanics empirical force fields. The tremendous development of the new generation of simulation techniques (e.g., molecular dynamics, Monte Carlo, docking, and virtual screening) and advanced computer hardware provides high computing power and various molecular modeling or computational chemistry approaches. Actually, the term "molecular modeling" has expanded over the last decades from a tool to visualize three-dimensional (3D) molecular structures (Fig. 3.1) and to simulate, predict, and analyze the properties and behaviors of molecules on an atomic level to a data-mining and *in silico* drug design platform to organize many compounds and their properties into databases and to perform virtual drug screening via 3D database searches for novel drug compounds.

The diverse molecular modeling packages have converged to offer a core of similar capabilities for manipulating molecules. They differ in their user interfaces and level of sophistication. Several newly emerged programs have specialized functions for fields such as virtual drug screening, virtual combinatorial chemistry, de novo drug design, chemical synthesis pathway prediction, and toxicology (absorption, distribution, metabolism, and excretion [ADME]) prediction as reviewed in literature (2–10). Various computer molecular modeling software programs are available for computational chemistry (described later); however, several pitfalls are associated with computational chemistry. Software packages are marketed to simplify our work by providing extensive default choices, which simplifies a calculation. The default parameters sometimes are incapable of providing a meaningful result. It is the user's responsibility to determine the appropriate methods and parameters for the quality of the result needed. A second pitfall is overinterpreting of the results while ignoring the experimental data. Little effort is made in most packages to provide error analysis and data integrity tests. A good application of computational chemistry techniques ensures that a level of accuracy appropriate to the question is used and balances the amount of computer time necessary with the importance of the result. An appreciation of molecular modeling and its pitfalls requires an understanding of the fundamentals presented in this chapter.

In this chapter, we shall discuss the basis and common applications of molecular modeling methods so that readers may appreciate its usefulness and be wary of its shortcomings. The cost for an improved understanding of what computational chemistry techniques can accomplish is an investment of time to understand the mathematical basis for representing atoms and molecules in software. Once the reader is equipped with a basic appreciation of the molecular model, the different methods and applications available to the practitioner make more sense. A brief review of the physical principles is provided to help medicinal chemists to recall the mathematical basis underlying the subsequent computational techniques. The techniques described in this chapter include molecular mechanics, molecular dynamics simulations, Monte Carlo techniques, ligand docking, and virtual screening methods. This chapter also covers the modern computer-aided drug design approaches, including ligand-based design and receptor-based design, along with the practical aspects of these techniques and applications.

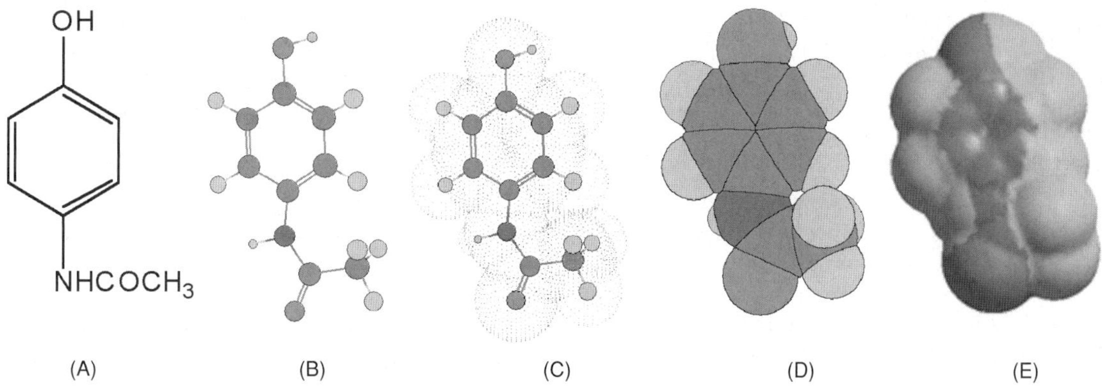

Fig. 3.1. Visualization of a drug molecule N-(4-hydroxy-phenyl)-acetamide (Tylenol or acetaminophen) computerized with different levels of graphic representations. (A) Molecular structure of the drug Tylenol. (B) Ball-stick model showing atomic positions and types. (C) Ball-stick model with van der Waals dot surfaces. (D) Space-filled model showing van der Walls radii of the oxygen, nitrogen, and carbon atoms. (E) Solvent accessible surface model (solid) (solvent radius, 1.4Å). (See color plate.)

COMPUTATIONAL CHEMISTRY APPROACHES

Molecular modeling or, more generally, computational chemistry is the scientific field of simulation of molecular systems. An effective simulation must include enough of the underlying physical and quantum chemistry to capture the behavior of the system of interest. This chapter, however, tends to focus on computational chemistry techniques and applications to meet its objectives.

Basically, computational methods can be thermodynamically rigorous by considering the components of the free energy of the system ($\Delta G = \Delta H - T\Delta S$). Once it can be estimated, the free energy of a system can be used to assess many interesting aspects of the system. In drug design, the free energy may be used to assess whether a modification to a drug increases or decreases target binding. In developing formulations, it can be used to estimate the relative stability of different compounds. In synthesis, it may be used to determine if the system is at equilibrium or how fast and to what extent it is likely to undergo a reaction. The central, descriptive role of the free energy, ΔG, makes it a worthwhile target for computational methods. In addition, the enthalpy (ΔH) of a system may be estimated as the energy required for assembling the constituents into a particular configuration. Consequently, the energy of the system is a function of the type and number of atoms and their positions. Molecular modeling software is designed to calculate this efficiently. To date, four levels of theory have matured and found widespread use in molecular modeling: ab initio, density functionals, semiempirical methods, and empirical force fields. For example, the configurational energy of the butane molecule in Figure 3.2 (black line) could be calculated by each of these methods. The first three are quantum mechanical methods and are based on different solutions to Schrödinger equation. Empirical force fields are an example of molecular mechanics approaches and are based on simple functions that are fit to experimental data. These implicitly include quantum effects and, consequently, are much faster to compute.

An understanding of the different levels of theory is important in the design of a computational study. In general, the more detailed the description (i.e., a higher level of theory), the more accurate and generally useful the results. On the other hand, the more detailed the description, the longer the calculation takes. For example, quantum mechanical methods offer some of the most detailed and robust expressions for the energy. They are lengthy calculations for small systems (10–100 atoms) and intractable for larger ones. Empirical force fields were developed to capture much of the behavior of systems but are much faster. A typical empirical force field calculation can be 10^4-fold faster than a quantum mechanical model. Because the available computing resources place a practical limit on our studies, it is appropriate to match the level of theory to the question. To be effective, the level of theory must contain terms necessary to reproduce the effect under study. For example, to study electron rearrangement, it must contain explicit terms for electrons. Although this seems obvious, molecular modeling software packages often make it easy for the casual user to use the wrong tool, which can result

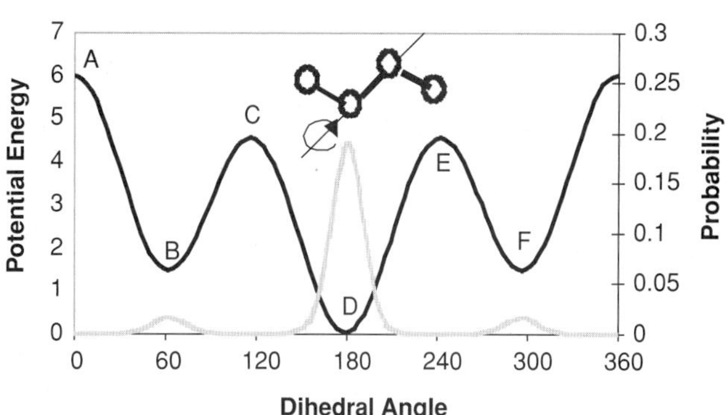

Fig. 3.2. Potential energy surface of a dihedral angle in butane.

in misleading findings. Therefore, each of the four levels of theory will be covered later.

Molecular Behavior: Computing the Energy of a Model system

The energy of a set of molecules plays a central role in computational chemistry, so it figures prominently in this chapter. If an algorithm can estimate the energy of the system, then many important properties may be derived from it. In an ideal world with infinitely fast computers, the energy would be computed from first principles (ab initio) using our most precise level of quantum theory. On today's computers, however, this level of theory could take days or months to calculate—even for a simple system. So, in practice, various approximations must be introduced that reduce the calculation time while adding an acceptably small effect on the result. As long as we are aware of the approximations and the errors they introduce, we are free to take this more expedient route. When designing a study, a computational chemist must carefully select the appropriate level of theory to derive meaningful results in a reasonable amount of time.

Four levels of theory (or accuracy) will be introduced in later sections to compute the energy of a system, ranging from empirical force fields to quantum chemistry. Fortunately, all of these methods are used to quantify the physicochemistry concepts with which we have become familiar. For example, consider the familiar conformations of butane. The central dihedral angle of butane and its associated energy are shown in Figure 3.2. The *trans* conformation (D in Fig. 3.2) is the lowest energy, because it reduces the steric interaction between the terminal methyl groups. For any given rotation about this central angle, the associated energy may be computed using any of the four levels of theory introduced in the next section.

Small molecules are comprised of bonded atoms and, typically, adopt the most favorable conformation. This one-dimensional potential energy surface (Fig. 3.2, black line) represents the excess conformational energy for the dihedral angle formed by the four carbons in butane, for example. Butane has the *trans* (180°) configuration (D in Fig. 3.2) as its favorable, low-energy state. The *cis* (0°) position (A in Fig. 3.2) is the relative maximum. The gauche (60° and 300°) positions (B and F, respectively, in Fig. 3.2) are local minima. The probability of a given state also is shown in Fig. 3.2 (gray line).

Prediction of a molecule's behavior demands that we consider more than the energy of a single configuration. For example, if we wish to predict what conformation a butane molecule is most likely to adopt, we must consider the energy of its current state as well as the energy of the states it might adopt. If we only compute the energy of the butane molecule in its gauche conformation (B or F in Fig. 3.2), we would not observe that it would be more stable in the *trans* conformation. We can use the energy profile for butane in Figure 3.2 to determine how likely a given conformation is populated (gray line in Fig. 3.2). Similarly, if we are interested in how a drug binds to its target, we should consider all of the binding sites—not just one. To increase the utility of the study, we should consider the energy of the nearly infinite number of states it could adopt. Several methods, including molecular mechanics, molecular dynamics, and Monte Carlo methods, will be introduced later to address the possible states.

Quantum Mechanics: Energies Derived from Theory

Generally, molecular modeling methods can be categorized as molecular mechanics and quantum mechanics (molecular orbital) methods. Quantum mechanics is basically molecular orbital calculation and offers the most detailed description of a molecule's chemical behavior. An example of molecular orbitals of HOMO and LUMO calculation is illustrated in Figure 3.3. The surface type of HOMO is the highest-occupied molecular orbitals, and LUMO represent the lowest-unoccupied molecular orbitals. The shapes and symmetries of HOMO and LUMO are crucial in predicting the reactivity of a species and the stereochemical and regiochemical outcome of a chemical reaction. Several molecular properties (Table 3.1) are only accessible with these methods, because they explicitly require a description of the molecule's electronic structure. It is important to understand their foundation as well as their relative accuracy and generality.

Quantum mechanics is based on the extended Schrödinger equation to describe the motion of the nucleus and electrons on the potential energy surface:

Eq. 3.1 $$H\Psi = E\Psi = (U + K)\,\Psi$$

where H is the Hamiltonian for the system, Ψ (pronounced "p-sigh") is the wavefunction, and E is the energy. Simply put, the Hamiltonian is an "operator," a mathematical construct that operates on the molecular orbital, Ψ, to determine the energy. The total energy E

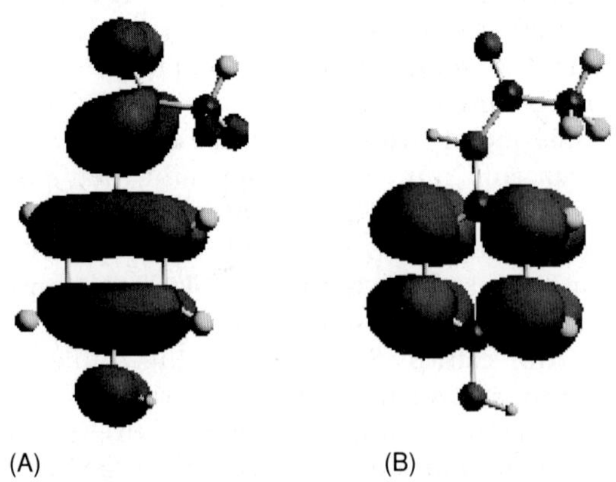

Fig. 3.3. Graphic visualization of molecular orbital surface HOMO/LUMO calculation for the drug molecule acetaminophen. (See color plate.)

Table 3.1. Summary of Molecular Modeling Methodologies and Their Capabilities

		Quantum mechanical Calculations		
	Empirical Force Fields Calculations	Ab initio	Density Functional Theory	Semiempirical
Basic principle	Hamiltonian equation		Schrödinger's equation	
Level of computing	Atoms		Electrons, nuclei orbital	
Parameterization	By atom type and charge	None		
Geometry optimization	Yes	Yes	Yes	Yes
Molecular dynamics	Yes	No	No	Limited
Vibration spectra	Yes	Yes	Yes	Yes
Heat formation ΔH (enthalpy)	Relative	Yes	Yes	Yes
Binding energy ΔG (free energy)	Yes	No	Yes (but not accurate)	Yes
Electrostatics	Yes	Yes	Yes	Yes
Hydrophobicity and lipophilicity	Yes	No	No	No
Proton and electron affinity	No	Yes	Yes	Yes
Tractable number of atoms	<50,000	<50	<200	<200
Tractable number of compounds	1	1	1	1
Relative CPU time/iteration	104	108	106	106
Disk space requirements	5–5,000 MB	5–2,000 MB	5–1,000 MB	5–10 MB
Memory requirements (RAM)	5–100 MB	5–1,000 MB	5–100 MB	5–100 MB
Popular programs	AMBER CHARMM CVFF	GAUSSIAN GAMESS-US GAMESS-UK JAGUAR	DFT++ GAUSSIAN GAMESS-US GAMESS-UK JAGUAR	AMPAC MOPAC

contains the potential energy (U) energy and kinetic energy (K) components. The wavefunction Ψ describes the distribution of the electrons around the molecule (e.g., *s*, *p*, *d*, *f*, . . . orbitals and their complex shape). Hamiltonian H is shorthand notation for operations necessary to add up the total energy of the system. So, quantum mechanical methods are the most rigorous methods in use for describing the energy, and they include quantum effects explicitly. Typically, three quantum mechanical calculations are used for molecular modeling: ab initio, density functionals, and semiempirical methods.

Ab Initio Methods

Ab initio methods (11), derived "from the beginning" premises of quantum theory, is one of the quantum mechanical calculations based on the Hartree-Fock self-consistent field theory with one-electron molecular orbital. This method that uses no experimental data is based on variation theory to seek the nuclear geometry of the molecule or hydrogen-bonded complex with lowest energy.

Hartree and Fock simplified calculations by combining the electrons into an averaged field. This allowed the Hamiltonian to be calculated for each electron independently using a new term for its interaction with the overall electron cloud. So, low-energy conformations, especially for global conformation searches, require very large amounts of computer time, both because atomic Cartesian coordinates are allowed to vary and because the nuclear configuration of minimum energy is sought. This involves a global search in $3(N - 1)$ dimensions, where N is the number of atoms in the molecule or assemblage of molecules. Basically, the ab initio method is initially introduced only as satisfactory for modeling small molecules (11), whereas more computational work has been reported using ab initio method as the high computing horsepower and capability lately become available. Many properties of molecules may be determined following a successful determination of the molecular orbitals and their occupancy, such as dipole moments, magnetic susceptibility, chemical shielding, spin–spin coupling constants, and electron affinities. Several versions of ab initio methods are available. Commercial software packages tend to have more sophisticated user interfaces, such as Gaussian series (12). It requires no a priori assumptions about the structure and only needs the atomic positions. Unlike experimental methods of structural analysis, no basis exists for estimating the error associated with a particular calculation; however, calculations are performed at successively more accurate levels, each of which requires more computer time. In addition, academic versions at low cost and with a variety of methods under development are available, including GAMESS (13,14) (http://www.msg.ameslab.gov/GAMESS) and GAMESS-UK (15) (http://www.cfs.dl.ac.uk/gamess-uk/).

Density Functional Theory

Basically, density functional theory (DFT) is similar to the ab initio method, but it is not based on a wavefunction. Instead, the energy is computed as a functional of the electron density (16). The DFT methods were developed that are much faster than Gaussian-style programs. Currently, many functional approximations are in use. The most common implementation of DFT is through the Kohn-Sham method (sometimes called the Kohn-Sham theory) (17). Within the framework of Kohn-Sham DFT, the many-body complex of interacting electrons in a static external potential is reduced to a tractable problem of noninteracting electrons moving in an effective potential. The effective potential includes the external potential and the effects of the Coulomb interactions between the electrons (e.g., the exchange and correlation interactions). DFT was not considered to be accurate enough, however, for calculations in quantum chemistry until the 1990s, when the approximations used in the DFT theory were greatly refined to better model the exchange and correlation interactions. DFT is now a leading method for calculations of electronic structure. Nevertheless, despite the improvements in DFT, difficulties remain in using DFT to properly describe intermolecular interactions, especially van der Waals forces (dispersion).

Density functional theory is a successful approach for the description of ground-state properties of metals, semiconductors, and insulators. It also has become an attractive method to calculate complex materials, such as proteins and carbon nanotubes. For example, DFT calculation has been used to compute anion-binding properties of 2,6-diamidopyridine dipyrromethane hybrid macrocycles (18), to predict drug resistance of HIV-1 reverse transcriptase to nevirapine through point mutations (19), and to analyze the β_2-adrenergic G protein–coupled receptor (20). A free DFT software program also is available (http://dft.physics.cornell.edu/). The detailed techniques and potential applications of DFT as well as drug design were described in a recent review (21).

Semiempirical Molecular Orbital Methods

Semiempirical calculations are based on the same or related quantum mechanical principles above but make approximations or assumptions for the majority of the electron–electron interactions to simplify the computations or to include some empirical parameters based on experimental data (22). Three types of semiempirical methods, which differ in their approach to approximation, have been used extensively for conformational calculations on medium-size biological molecules, including the CNDO (complete neglect of differential overlap) (23), MNDO (Modified Neglect of Differential Overlap; a part of the MOPAC program) (24), and PCILO (Perturbation Configuration Integration Using Localized Orbital) (25). Both CNDO and MNDO simplify the computations by neglecting (or partially neglecting) the differentials in the energy calculations for the valence electrons, and both treat the inner-shell electron as a core that screens the nuclear charge. In PCILO calculations, the molecular orbitals are not expanded in the usual LCAO (linear combination of atomic orbitals) form but, rather, in pairwise hybrids. It uses perturbation theory rather than variation theory to obtain the wavefunctions and to calculate the energy. The PCILO method is too computationally intensive for macromolecules. The global searching problem can be severe for even small molecules with a significant number of variable torsion angles.

The MOPAC program (Molecular Orbital PACkag) (26) is one of the popular quantum mechanical semiempirical methods. The AM1 (Austin Model 1), developed by Michael Dewar (26), is a generalization of the modified neglect of differential diatomic overlap (MNDO) approximation. Often, AM1 is implemented in the MOPAC, and MOPAC(AM1) has been widely used to minimize molecular conformations, to calculate electronic configuration, and to predict such properties as electron distribution and partial charges. The semiempirical methods are dramatically (100- to 1,000-fold) faster and are suitable for many applications. The results of AM1 calculations often are used as the starting points for parameterizations (e.g., atomic charges) of force fields in molecular dynamics simulations (27,28) and CoMFA quantitative structure–activity relationship (QSAR) modeling studies (29).

Molecular Mechanics: Energies Approximated from Experimental Data

Molecular mechanics is based on simple empirical approximations of atomic and molecular interactions. The Hamiltonian in molecular mechanics classically describes the energy of the whole system as the sum of the inter- and intramolecular interactions. Simply put, the energy of a molecular system is evaluated two atoms at a time, without quantum mechanics. The generic molecular mechanics potential energy function is given in Figure 3.4 and further breaks down the pairwise interactions into bonded interactions (or internal coordinates) and nonbonded interactions. Atoms that are connected via one to three bonds are treated with internal coordinates. The nonbonded terms include an electrostatic and van der Waals component. This type of potential energy function sometimes is referred to as an empirical force field, because the energetic terms have simple forms and parameters that are derived from experimental data and ab initio calculations.

It is on this expression that the whole field of molecular mechanics, conformational calculations, and molecular dynamics simulations rest. A "force field" therefore just includes an analytical energy function and its associated set of numerical parameters. In other words, the force field is an empirical fit to the potential energy of a molecular system. It defines the coordinates to be used

$$E = \sum_{Bond}\frac{1}{2}k_r\left(rb - br_0\right)^2 + \sum_{Angle}\frac{1}{2}k_\theta\left(\theta - \theta_0\right)^2 + \sum_{Dihedral}\frac{1}{2}k_\phi[1+\cos(n\phi+\delta)] + \sum_{Coulomb}\frac{q_i q_j}{\varepsilon r_{ij}} + \sum_{vdw}\varepsilon\left[\frac{A_{ij}}{r_{ij}^{12}} - \frac{B_{ij}}{r_{ij}^{6}}\right]$$

Fig. 3.4 A generic empirical force field equation.

(the bond lengths, b, and angles, θ, ϕ); the functional mathematical forms ranging from simple quadratic to Morse functions, Fourier expansions, Leonard-Jones potentials, and so on; and the parameters adjusted in the empirical fit of the potential energy surface. Simply said, the force field is the description of the potential energy of a molecule as a function of its position (or coordinates) of all the atoms, as described below.

Bonded Interactions

The bonded interactions or internal coordinates (short-range energy terms) are used to better approximate the interaction of adjacent atoms. The bond, angle, and dihedral terms are used to treat atoms that are separated by one, two, and three bonds. To better illustrate the bonded energy terms, we can consider that the calculation of internal energies in molecular mechanics is simply based on the Newtonian laws of classical mechanics (30–32). Molecules are treated as if they consist of an assembly of soft rubber balls (or atoms) and springs (or bonds), as shown below. Each ball (or atom) is the junction point between springs (or chemical bonds), which have, at their equilibrium state, bond length (b_0), bond angle (θ_0) and torsion angle (ϕ_0), with appropriate values of stretching (k_b), bending (k_θ) and twisting (k_ϕ) force constants, respectively (Fig. 3.5).

Principally, for small deviations from the equilibrium values, Hooke's Law is applied:

Eq. 3.2 $$f = kx$$

where the force, f, on the spring (or bond) needed to stretch an ideal spring is proportional to its elongation x, and where k is the force constant or spring constant of the spring. The extension of Hooke's Law to a molecular system is illustrated in Figure 3.5 with respect to bond stretching, bond angle bending, and torsion angle. Hooke's Law can approximate the bond vibration:

Eq. 3.3

$$E_{\text{Bond Vibration}} = \frac{1}{2}k_b(b-b_0)^2 + \frac{1}{2}k_0(\theta-\theta_0)^2 + \frac{1}{2}k_\phi(1-\cos(n\phi + \delta))$$

where k_b, k_Θ, and k_ϕ are the bond and angle force constants. These three parameters are specific to the type atoms and the bond order (e.g., —C—C—, —C=C—, and —C—N). The values for the parameters are derived from x-ray crystallographic structures and infrared spectra. The squared term in Hooke's Law results in both compression (negative displacement) and expansion (positive displacement) of the bond from its equilibrium value increasing the energy.

The "bond term" is symmetric about the equilibrium bond length, and we know this is an approximation. It actually takes more energy to compress the bond than to stretch it. If necessary, we can use a Morse function that takes more time to compute but does a better job. In general, as long as the bond length is not too far from the equilibrium, the approximation is a good one (Fig. 3.5):

Eq. 3.4 $$E_{\text{bond}} = \frac{1}{2}k_b(b-b_0)^2$$

The "angle term" uses a similar term to increase the energy when the bond angle bends or deviates from its equilibrium value (Fig. 3.5):

Eq. 3.5 $$E_{\text{angle}} = \frac{1}{2}k_\theta(\theta - \theta_0)$$

The energy of the dihedral angles must be periodic, because, for example, dihedral angles across single bonds are free to rotate. This term's potential energy surface is the same as the butane central dihedral angle (Fig. 3.2) and is treated as a sum of cosine terms (Fig. 3.6):

Eq. 3.6 $$E_{\text{dihedral}} = k_\phi(1 + \cos(n\phi + \delta))$$

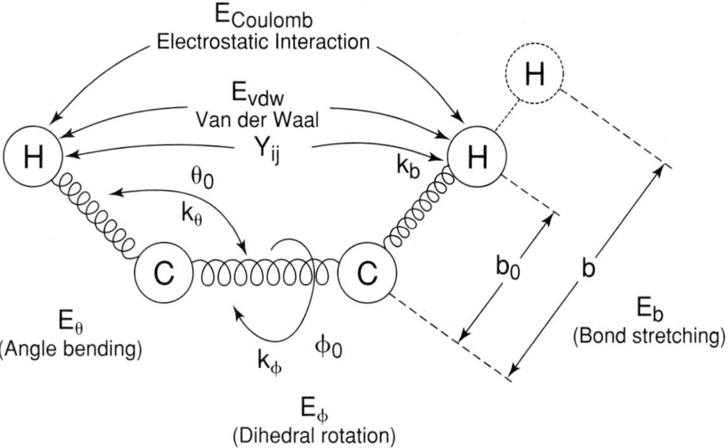

Fig. 3.5. Graphic representation of the bonded and nonbonded interactions and the corresponding energy terms.

where k_ϕ is the dihedral force constant, n determines the periodicity of the term, and δ adjusts phase for each term. The parameters for this term are adjusted to reproduce infrared and crystallographic data.

Nonbonded Interactions

The nonbonded interactions (long-range energy terms; i.e., the electrostatic and van der Waals terms) are applied to nearly all pairs of atoms. They are not computed for pairs of atoms treated by the internal coordinates, because the bond, angle, and dihedral terms provide a better approximation of their interaction. The nonbonded terms usually are smaller in magnitude individually, but they can have a dominant effect because of the large number. The number of atom pairs is $N(N-1)/2$, where N is the number of atoms in the system. A typical model of a protein (without solvent) might have 5,000 atoms, with 25,000,000 atom-pair interactions and 15,000 internal coordinate terms to calculate. It is no surprise that the nonbonded interactions usually take more than 90% of the computer time for a simulation. Several methods exist for reducing the number of interactions that need to be calculated, but each introduces artifacts. Recently, the Ewalds method has gained general acceptance as a way to include all interactions within an acceptable amount of computation (33) using some mathematical cleverness and periodic boundary conditions. The nonbonded terms usually include electrostatic interactions and van der Waals interaction, which are almost the same for all force field programs and are expressed as coulombic interactions as well as Lennard-Jones type potentials, respectively. All of them are a function of the distance between atom pairs, r_{ij} (nonbond cutoff distances) (Fig. 3.5).

Electrostatic interactions between atoms (e.g., atoms i and j), either within a molecule or between adjacent molecules, are calculated using Coulomb's Law by means of an atomic point-charge model. Each atom is assigned a charge to represent both formal and partial charges that arise because of unequal sharing of electrons. The partial charges frequently are derived from quantum mechanical calculations that are described in the previous section. Although the form of Coulomb's Law is simple, it captures the underlying physics. The magnitude of the interaction is proportional to the atoms' charges (q_i and q_j) and inversely proportional to their separation (r_{ij}) and the dielectric constant (ε):

Eq. 3.7
$$E_{\text{Coulomb}} = \frac{q_i q_j}{\varepsilon r_{ij}}$$

The dielectric constant ε is a bulk property of the environment of a system. The dielectric of a vacuum is one, which implies that no polarization of the environment exists. If a solvent, such as water or methanol, is explicitly included in the system, then a dielectric of one is used, because the orientation of the solvent molecules will polarize in the presence of the electric field. If water is the solvent, it is possible to use continuum models and, thus, reduce the amount of computation required. This does add artifacts to the simulation. These artifacts are fairly well characterized, however, and the computation time is dramatically reduced. In some case, two different dielectric constants were used to mimic the different biological environments. For example, in a membrane protein structural modeling, the dielectric constant was set to a value of five for simulating the hydrophobic transmembrane environment and the dielectric constant to 80 for mimicking the hydrophilic loop environment in the two phases of computer simulations (34).

Van der Waal term describes a more complex interaction between nonbonded atoms. Atoms (e.g., atoms i and j) are attracted to each other by weak dispersion forces (also called London forces) linked to small oscillating dipoles created by electron cloud fluctuation. Atoms also are repelled by each other because of the Pauli exclusion principle, which states that no two electrons may share the same quantum numbers. The van der Waals interaction between two atoms (e.g., atoms i and j) arises from a balance between repulsive and attractive forces. At a large distance, a net attraction or dispersion force exists between all (even neutral) atoms because of the concerted oscillation of their electrons, and the forces become stronger linearly as $1/r$ to the sixth power increases. At close range, however, the electrons and nuclei strongly repel each other, and the forces of repulsion become more repulsive linearly as $1/r$ to the 12th power increases. The attractive interaction usually is longer range than the repulsion, but as the distance become short, the repulsive interaction becomes dominant. This gives rise to a minimum in the energy. Positioning of the atoms at the optimal distances stabilizes the system. Both the value of energy at the minimum (E^*) and the optimal separation of atoms (r^*, or the sum of Van der Waals radii of the atoms) depend on chemical type of these atoms. The van der Waals interaction most often is modeled using the Lennard-Jones 6-12 potential, which expresses the interaction energy using the atom-type dependent constants A_{ij} and B_{ij}. Experimental data for the energy of interaction can be fit with a Lennard-Jones, or 6-12, function:

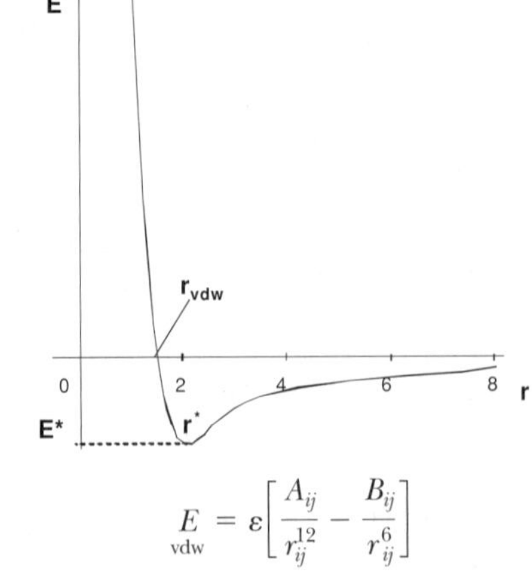

Eq. 3.8
$$E_{\text{vdw}} = \varepsilon\left[\frac{A_{ij}}{r_{ij}^{12}} - \frac{B_{ij}}{r_{ij}^{6}}\right]$$

where r_{ij} is the distance between the atoms (i and j), The constant A_{ij} and B_{ij} values may be determined by a variety of experimental methods, such as nonbonding distances in crystals and gas-phase scattering measurements.

Force fields

The above internal coordinates and nonbonded interaction terms comprise the force field equations in molecular mechanics to calculate the potential energy of a molecular system. The basic form of empirical force fields has been varied as part of efforts to improve their treatment of various biological systems. Extensive work has been done on the systematic improvement of the both the form and the parameters used (35). However, this consensus form is common to AMBER (36), CHARMM (37), and CVFF (38), three popular classical empirical force fields.

AMBER (ASSISTED MODEL BUILDING AND ENERGY REFINEMENT). The AMBER force field was developed by Peter Kollman and coworkers (39) at the University of California, San Francisco. In addition to the common terms of generic force fields, AMBER has a hydrogen-bond energy term that augments the electrostatic description of the hydrogen bond and estimates the relative contribution of energy from hydrogen-bonding. AMBER defines the atomic partial charges by using a charge-fitting scheme that replicates the electrostatic potential at a distance out from the nucleus, with only the atom centers having charge. An extended version of AMBER (40) has been parameterized and widely used for proteins and DNA. AMBER also is the name for the molecular dynamics simulation package that implements these force fields. Further development of both the force fields and software is now coordinated by David A. Case at the Scripps Research Institute.

CHARMM (CHEMISTRY AT HARVARD MACROMOLECULAR MECHANICS). The CHARMM force field, originally developed at Harvard, has been widely used for both small molecules and macromolecules (37). This force field has two additional energy terms, including the improper term that accounts for the out-of-plane bending with the out of plan angle ($\omega - \omega_0$) and the force constant (k_ω) as well as the cross-term (Urey-Bradley component) that accounts for angle bending using 1,3-nonbonded interactions with the respective force constant (k_u) and the distance (U) between the 1,3-atoms in the harmonic potential. In addition, CHARMM uses different protocols to develop the partial atomic charges by beginning with the Mullikin charges and then strategically places a water molecule near any polar group. The extended CHARMM development project involves a network of developers in the United States and elsewhere working with Martin Karplus and his group at Harvard to develop and maintain the CHARMM program.

CVFF (CONSISTENT VALENCE FORCE FIELD). The CVFF is the original force field provided with the Discover program (41) and is a generalized valence force field (42). Valence charge and atom-type parameters are provided for amino acids, water, and a variety of other functional groups. The force field expression consists of additional energy terms (i.e., the cross-terms that account for interactions between the four internal coordinates). The cross-terms represent the coupling between the adjacent bond–bond, the angle–angle term, the bond–angle term, the valence angle–torsion angle, and improper torsions. Such cross-terms are important for accurately reproducing experimental properties (e.g., vibrational frequencies) but can cause problems during the initial refinement of strongly distorted structures (derivatives > 100 kcal/mol/Å). So, both cross-terms and the Morse potential should be used only with the reasonably optimized structures.

OTHER FORCE FIELDS. In addition to the classical force fields above, many other force fields have been developed for small drug molecules or macromolecules. The MM2, MM3, and MM4 force fields were developed by Norman L. Allinger for a broad range of chemicals, and CFF is a family of force fields adapted to a broad variety of organic compounds, polymers, metals, and so on. The MMFF force field was developed at Merck for a broad range of chemicals. ReaxFF is a reactive force field, developed by William Goddard and coworkers, is fast, transferable, and the computational method of choice for atomistic-scale dynamics simulations of chemical reactions.

These programs are organized quite differently. The most popular commercial packages offer mature, sophisticated user interfaces, with easier point-and-click interfaces for many functions. The academic versions typically offer more advanced features and methods that are still under development. Their user interfaces are improving but lack robust point-and-click interfaces. Each offers advantages and disadvantages that must be considered before selecting one program and spending the time to learn it.

The advantages of empirical force field methods lie in their ability to treat thousands of atoms and their direct connection with statistical thermodynamics. Many biological systems, such as enzymes, proteins, and DNA and their complexes, are within the range of molecular mechanics. Scoring functions and simulations based on empirical force fields have successfully analyzed binding modes, folding mechanisms, and allosteric effects. The simulations may be analyzed with statistical thermodynamics methods to estimate the free energy of binding or folding. Trajectories of atoms may be used to derive diffusion constants or to compare with nuclear magnetic resonance (NMR) estimates of atomic motion. The flexibility of empirical force field methods must be balanced with the time required to develop parameters for a new system. Proteins, nucleotides, and carbohydrates parameter sets continue to evolve but have been useful for more than 10 years. Novel lead compounds often will require parameterization to achieve meaningful results.

Molecular Mechanics Energy Minimization

Molecular mechanics is an approach of energy minimization that finds stable, low-energy conformations by changing the geometry of a structure or identifying a point in the configuration space at which the net force on each atom vanishes. In other words, it is to find the coordinates where the first derivatives of the potential energy function equals zero. Such a conformation represents one of many different conformations that a molecule might assume at a temperature of 0°K. The potential energy function (or force field) is evaluated by a certain algorithm or minimizer (e.g., steepest descent or conjugate gradient) that moves the atoms in the molecule to a nearest local minimum (not necessarily the global minimum), whereas the selection of different minimization algorithms is important for various molecule systems, as discussed below.

Steepest Descent

Steepest descent method (32) is an optimization algorithm that approaches a local minimum of a function by taking steps proportional to the negative of the gradient (or the approximate gradient) of the function at the current point. Simply put, steepest descent uses the gradient to determine the direction and move down in one dimension parallel to the net force. Steepest descent will lead directly to the nearest local minimum by following a path that is determined by moving from the previous value to a new value (at some constant times) in the directions in which the energy is decreasing (Fig. 3.6). If the new movement decreases the energy, the new structure is accepted, and the process is repeated. If, on the other hand, the energy increases, the previous structure is restored. This algorithm converges fast in a steep place for correcting "bad" initial geometry, especially when systems are far from harmonic. It has poor convergence properties, however, and often jitters around the minimum area, because the gradient approaches zero near the minimum.

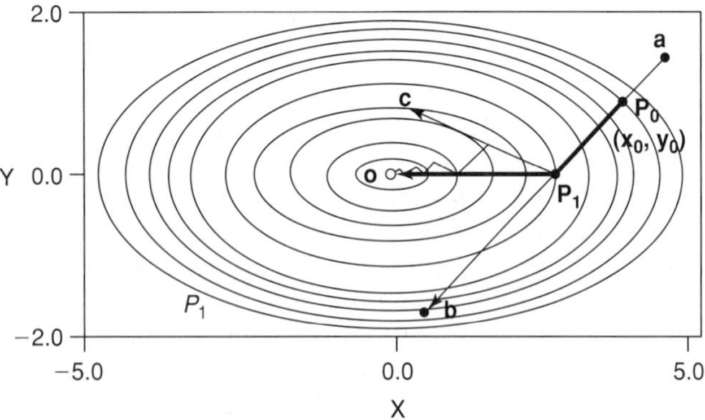

Fig. 3.6. Steepest descent algorithm (thin line): The derivative vector from the initial point P_0 (x_0,y_0) defines the line search direction. The derivative vector does not point directly toward the minimum (O). The negative gradient of the potential energy (the force) points into the direction ($P_0 \rightarrow b$, $P_1 \rightarrow c$) of the steepest descent of the energy hypersurface and is always oriented perpendicular to energy isosurfaces. Conjugate gradients algorithm (thick line): The search direction ($a \rightarrow P_1 \rightarrow$ O) is in one dimension for the minimum. The energy point P_1 takes the direction $P_1 \rightarrow$ O instead of the direction $P_1 \rightarrow c$. The direction $P_1 \rightarrow c$ of gradient conjugates to the direction $P_0 \rightarrow b$.

Conjugate Gradient

The conjugate gradient method (32,43) improves the step efficiency by minimizing only along directions that are mutually conjugate so that movement along one direction will not counteract progress made in earlier iterations. The conjugate gradient method takes the next search direction to be a linear combination of the current gradient and the previous ones (Fig. 3.6). Conjugate gradients require fewer energy evaluations and gradient calculations, and further convergence characterizations are better than with steepest descent. Conjugate gradient is the method of choice for large systems in which storing and manipulating a large second derivative matrix is impartial, such as the Newton-Raphson method.

Newton-Raphson Procedure

The Newton-Raphson procedure (32) is a powerful, convergent minimization procedure, but it requires the second derivative matrix to be available. The Newton-Raphson procedure is based on the assumption that the energy is quadratically dependent—in other words, that it behaves like a classical spring. Then, the new coordinates in each iteration can be found by the calculation of the matrix of the second derivative with respect to the coordinates and the first derivatives. The advantage of the Newton-Raphson procedure that the minimization could converge in one or two steps. The major drawback is that this method requires the calculation of the second derivatives. The minimization can then become unstable when a structure is far from the minimum (or the energy surface is anharmonic).

Criteria for Evaluating Convergence in Minimization Processes

Geometric optimization is an iterative procedure of computing the energy of a structure and then making incremental changes to reduce the energy. Minimization of a molecule involves two steps. First, an equation describing the energy of the system as a function of its coordinates must be defined and evaluated for a given conformation. Second, the conformation is adjusted to lower the value of the potential function. Minimization provides information complementary to that obtained from molecular dynamics. A minimum energy conformation can be found but may require thousands of iterations, depending on the nature of the algorithm, the form of the potential function, and the size of the molecule.

The efficiency of the minimization is judged by both the time to evaluate the target function and the number of structural adjustments (iterations) needed to converge on the minimum.

Zero Derivatives

Mathematically, a minimum is reached by the point at which the derivatives of the function are zero, as in Equation 3.9:

Eq. 3.9 $$\frac{\partial E}{\partial x} \longrightarrow 0, \frac{\partial E}{\partial y} \longrightarrow 0, \frac{\partial E}{\partial z} \longrightarrow 0$$

Several points may exist, however, where the net atomic forces are zero. The point of the lowest energy, or the global minimum, which usually is the conformation of interest, sometimes may not be found from a single starting point of energy minimization. Therefore, thorough conformation sampling (e.g., dynamics simulation) is critical to minimization studies. In theory, convergence occurs at a minimum point where all derivatives are zero and the second derivative matrix is positive-definite. In practice, however, it can be difficult to judge whether it is close enough to the true global minimum. To solve this problem, different algorithms and methods are chosen and combined to search for the global minimum.

Some minimization algorithms assume that the energy surface is approximately harmonic or, for nonharmonic surfaces, that the shape of the nonharmonic surface becomes harmonic in the limit as you converge on the minimum. The derivatives are proportional to the coordinates for the molecular energy surfaces where the force field is harmonic. The derivatives include the information regarding how far away you are from the minimum. The magnitude of the derivatives also is the most rigorous way to characterize the convergence to a minimization. In general, a minimization is converged when the derivatives are equal (or nearly equal) to zero.

Evaluation of the Atomic Derivatives

In molecular minimization, the results of minimization in terms of the atomic derivatives may be summarized either as an average, a root mean square, or the largest value of derivatives as the following. An average derivative is an average of the absolute value of the derivatives, because the distribution of derivatives is symmetric about zero. A root-mean-square derivative (RMS) weights larger derivatives more; therefore, it is less likely that a few large derivatives escape from the detection, which can occur with simple average derivatives. In most studies, the maximum derivative is used to evaluate the minimization convergence. There cannot be ambiguity about the quality of the minimum if all derivatives are less than a given value. For instance, minimizing until maximum derivative of 1.0 kcal/mol/Å normally is sufficient for relaxing overlapped atoms before a dynamics run. The acceptable maximum derivative, however, must be less than 0.001 kcal/mol if a normal mode of minimization analysis is performed.

Strategies for Selecting Minimization Algorithms

Numerous algorithms are available for geometric optimization, such as steepest descent, conjugate gradients, and Newton-Raphson, as discussed above. The proper selection of a minimization algorithm means selecting the most efficient one with good convergence. The choice of the algorithms depends on two factors, the size of the system and the current state of optimization. For example, when the derivatives are well above 100 kcal/mol/Å, it is likely that the structure is outside the quadratic region of the potential energy surface. So, the algorithms (conjugate gradients and Newton-Raphson) that assume the energy surface is quadratic can be unstable in this situation. Typically, two minimization algorithms are combined to achieve the good convergence effectively.

As a general rule for selecting minimization algorithms, when the derivative is larger than 10 kcal/mol/Å, the steepest descents algorithm should be used, and when derivative is less than 10 kcal/mol/Å, the conjugate gradients algorithm is used if the molecule is larger than 200 atoms and the Newton-Raphson algorithm if less than 200 atoms. The steepest descent algorithm often is the best minimizer to use for the first 10 to 100 steps, after which the conjugate gradients minimizer can be used to complete the minimization. The molecular structures built from default bond and angle geometry normally are heavily distorted structures. It is recommended to use the steepest descents with no Morse function and no cross-term options to minimize the structure near a minimum (e.g., maximum derivative <1 kcal/mol). Then, the conjugate gradients algorithm can be used with or without the Morse potential and cross-term as needed to do minimization. The Newton-Raphson minimizer is usually restricted to small molecules, because it requires analytically calculating the second derivatives. The advantage of this minimizer is its quadratic convergence close to the minimum. The Newton-Raphson method can give extremely good convergence to a much tighter criterion after running conjugate gradients to a near minimum.

As we described above, molecular mechanics is an approach of minimum-energy configuration calculations based on the certain force field and one or more minimization algorithms or minimizers. A common limitation of classical molecular mechanics minimization algorithms is that the molecules tend to locate at a local minimum close to the starting configuration and not necessarily at the global minimum, because the minimizers are specifically designed to ignore configurations if the energy increases. So, such minimazation algorithms do not push a system over barriers but, rather, down into the nearest valley. This problem can be solved using dynamics simulations in which kinetic energy gets over the local barrier, as described in the next section.

Molecular Dynamics Simulation

Exploring Molecular Dynamics

Molecular dynamics has been used to compute the dynamics of the molecular system, including time-averaged structural and energetic properties, structural fluctuations, and conformational transitions. The subsequent use of molecular mechanics energy minimizations revealed groups of conformations. In comparison, molecular mechanics, or empirical potential energy functions (Fig. 3.4), ignores the time evolution of the system and, instead, focuses on finding particular geometries and their associated energies or other static properties (31).

The dynamics of a system may be simplified as the movements of each of its atoms. If the velocities and the forces acting on atoms can be quantified, then their movement may be simulated. During the molecular dynamics process, the initial condition is specified by the analytical expression for the potential energy of a molecular system that includes coordinates, energies, and a set of velocities for each atom. Then, a force is applied on each atom, which is described by Newton's equation of motion (Eq. 3.10):

Eq. 3.10 $$F = ma$$

where F is the force on an atom, m is the atom's mass, and a is the acceleration. Because the negative of the first derivative of the potential energy (E) with respect to the coordinates (r) gives the force on each atom, Newton's equation (Eq. 3.10) can be used to describe the motion of a particular molecule:

Eq. 3.11 $$F = ma = -\frac{dE}{dr} = -m\frac{d^2r}{dt^2}$$

where t is the time and r represents the Cartesian coordinates of the atom. The forces are obtained from the energy expression by calculation of the analytical derivatives. The forces are applied for a small time step ($\sim 10^{-15}$ seconds), and the acceleration is calculated from Newton's Law (Eq. 3.11). Then, the velocity and position of each atom is updated to a new velocity and position using an integration algorithm, and the forces and accelerations are calculated once again at the new atomic positions. Next, this process is repeated to produce a trajectory. The positions of each atom in the system are recorded in the dynamics history file. The structures are retreated and then minimized with molecular mechanics and analyzed later. Above all, the solution of Eq. 3.11 using an empirical fit to the potential energy surface is known as molecular dynamics simulation.

It is then possible to approximate the movement of an atom a short time into the future, Δt, using a Taylor expansion:

Eq. 3.12 $$\vec{r}(t + \Delta t) = \vec{r}(t) + \vec{v}\Delta t + \vec{a}\,\frac{\Delta t^2}{2} + \ldots$$

This expression states that the position of an atom at some time in the future, $\vec{r}(t + \Delta t)$, may be found from its initial position ($\vec{r}$), velocity ($\vec{v}$) and acceleration ($\vec{a}$). The new position is now in terms of known quantities, because molecular dynamics calculations keep track of atomic positions and velocities at each step. Keeping this in mind, two important factors need to be considered in using dynamics simulation, simulation temperature and sampling time steps, in order to make sure that all conformers are sampled during the simulation.

Temperature and Time Steps in Dynamics Simulation

It is unique that molecular dynamics can simulate the molecular motion at high temperature. The simulation of molecular motion at high temperature increases the probability of overcoming energy barriers, giving the possibility of sampling all possible minimum conformations without being trapped in a local energy minimum. However, the temperature is expressed in terms of the atomic velocities, which are proportional to the kinetic energy of a system (31,42). The temperature setting is discussed in the given molecular dynamics simulation protocol below.

In addition, the molecular dynamics simulation requires using a value of time step Δt that is small enough to correctly simulate the fastest atomic motions. Choosing the proper simulation time step is very important to make sure all conformers are sampled during calculation. The C-H bonds vibrate with a period of about 10^{-14} seconds. To simulate these motions, the time step must be roughly one-tenth of that, or 10 to 15 seconds (1 femtosecond [fs]). Simulations become unstable with values much larger than this 1-fs time step. Simulations are also unstable when forces are applied for a longer time interval (Δt) than that for which they are really valid. For example, if the attractive force of a carbon acting on a hydrogen (in a C-H bond) is applied for too long a time interval or for a large time step, the hydrogen will have been repositioned too close to the carbon. During the next time step, a very strong repulsive force will lead to the hydrogen being repositioned well beyond its typical bond length. This oscillatory process will continue until the energy of the bond is no longer conserved and the molecular dynamics indicates an error condition. A typical molecular dynamics simulation protocol is given below.

Molecular Dynamics Simulation Protocol

As discussed above, in molecular dynamics, Newtonian equations of motion are solved numerically for all atoms as a function of time. A statistical average with time is obtained by applying initial velocities (i.e., kinetic energy), which allows the system to pass the energy barriers and sample all the local minima. An energy calculation, however, has to be carried out for each of a very large number of configurations. Only molecular mechanics can provide the necessary computational speed. So, molecular mechanics and molecular dynamics often are used together to achieve the target conformers with lowest energy configurations.

Several molecular dynamics simulation approaches are available, including regular simulation, constrained simulation, and simulated annealing techniques. In addition, the simulated annealing dynamics simulation also was popular in computational chemistry studies of proteins and drug molecules (34,44,45). A common experimental protocol has been widely used in molecular dynamics simulation as following (34,46,47):

1. *Build the target protein model.* The initial 3D protein structures can be constructed from an NMR or x-ray crystallographic structure or homology-predicted structure. For example, one can incorporate the NMR experimental data into the target structure by applying the distance constraints and/or dihedral constraints with a square-well potential and a force constant of 50 kcal/mol/Å. If it is to simulate the ligand–protein complex, the ligand should be placed into the putative binding site.
2. *Set up the simulation environment.* One can choose the simulation environment by selecting the proper dielectric constant or by adding counterions and immersing the protein into a periodic box of water, even in lipid bilayers.
3. *Perform energy minimization to relax the initial molecule.* It is important to remove any high-energy artifacts from the construction process to avoid the fault simulation.
4. *Heat up the system, and equilibrate at the selected temperature (e.g., 1,000K).* Typically, dynamics simulation will equilibrate at the temperature for 1 to 25 picoseconds (ps) to allow the total energy and core structures to be stabilized.
5. *Begin the molecular dynamics simulation at the desired temperature.* Typically, dynamics simulation is performed over a period of time 200 ps, with the sampling time step of 1 fs and the trajectories recorded every 1 ps. The dynamics sampling period is selected based on the target protein size and the available computer capacity (20–50 ps for large proteins and 200–300 ps for small molecules). With the time step of 1 fs, a total of 200,000 conformations or frames are sampled during the simulation. To reduce the volume of the output data to a more manageable level, conformer structures were recorded at 1-ps intervals, thus reducing the number of structures to 200 frames.
6. *Retrieve and energy-minimize the sampled conformers.* The 200 conformers recorded during the dynamics run were retrieved and energy-minimized with a two-step minimization, using the steepest descent method for the first 100 iterations and then the conjugate gradient method until the maximum derivative was less than 0.001 kcal/mol.

Furthermore, the molecular dynamics study also may be postprocessed in several ways. First, the study may attempt to locate the lowest-energy binding modes. In this case, the trajectories of the atoms may be sampled at 1-ps intervals and the resulting structures then subjected to energy minimization. The resulting structures could be ranked according to their energy and used to evaluate the expected binding mode. A second use would be to track the interatomic distances between residues of interest. A third use is to derive quantities, such as the free energy of binding, correlation functions, diffusion constants, or a potential of mean force. The full power of statistical thermodynamics may be applied to a simulation, because the time averaged quantities may be used to approximate the free energy.

An example of structure calculation of a G-protein-coupled receptor (GPCR) juxtamembrane domain is given here to illustrate the molecular dynamics simulation. The fourth cytoplasmic domain, the so-called C-terminal juxtamembrane segment, has been identified in numerous G protein–coupled receptors and exhibits unique functional characteristics. Xie and Chen (48) applied the molecular dynamics/molecular mechanics simulation with NMR-defined constraints to study the 3D structural conformations of a synthetic peptide

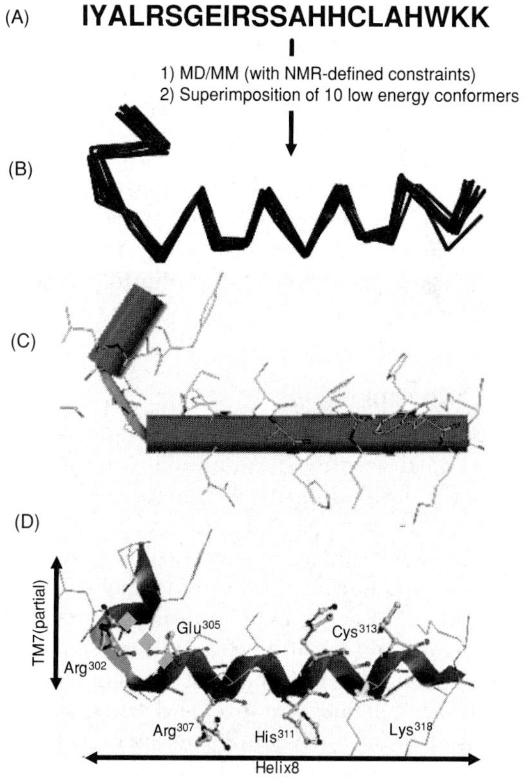

Fig. 3.7. NMR NOE-constrained MD/MM structure calculation of the polypeptides CB21298-K319 (A), the backbone superimposition of 10 low energy conformers (B), the cylinder representation with a turn at the fifth residue Arginine (C), and the ribbon display of the two helical segments (D), showing a curve side chain of Arg302 forming a salt bridge (green line) with Glu305. (See color plate.)

CB_2I298-K319 fragment of G protein–coupled CB_2 receptor (Fig. 3.7)

The initial structure was built by using SYBYL program and minimized to relieve any overly strained coordinates. Molecular dynamics simulation was carried out under the Kollman All Atom force field and Kollman charges for 200 ps with time steps of 1 fs at 1,000K. The NMR-determined Nuclear Overhauser Effect (NOE) distance constraints, with three boundaries of 1.8 to 2.8 Å (strong), 1.8 to 3.3 Å (medium), or 1.8 to 5.0 Å (weak), were applied during the dynamics simulation with a square-well potential and a force constant of 50 kcal/mol/Å. The distance restraints will be linearly released in 10 ps of dynamics. A total of 200,000 conformations or frames were sampled during the simulation with 1-fs time steps, and the sampled conformer structures were recorded at 1-ps intervals. The 200 frames recorded during the dynamics run were retrieved and minimized with a two-step minimization, using the steepest descent method for the first 100 iterations and then the conjugate gradient method until the maximum derivative was less than 0.001 kcal/mol. The superposition of the backbones of the 10 low-energy peptide conformers of the target peptide is illustrated in Fig. 3.7B. The calculated structures show two helical portions, the short helix segment and a long helix domain, which are assigned to the partial segment of transmembrane seven (TM7) and the cytoplasmic domain (Helix8), respectively, as displayed in cylinder representation in Fig. 3.7C with a turn at the fifth residue, arginine. In addition, the CB_2I298-K319 peptide fragment shows a curve side chain of Arg^{302} forming a salt bridge with Glu^{305}(Fig. 3.7D), which attributes to the specificity of the signal transduction activation by the C-terminal juxtamembrane region for the CB_2 receptor (48).

Monte Carlo simulation

Unlike the molecular dynamics techniques that evaluate forces to determine incremental atomic motions, Monte Carlo simulation simply imposes relatively large motions on the system and determines whether the altered structure is energetically feasible at the temperature simulated. Because Monte Carlo simulation samples conformation space by jumping abruptly from conformation to conformation rather than evolving smoothly through time, it cannot provide time-dependent quantities. It may, however, be much better than molecular dynamics in estimating average thermodynamics properties for which the sampling of many system configurations is important. Monte Carlo techniques (49,50) are stochastic methods in which a statistical ensemble of configurations are generated and the average structural features and thermodynamics properties are obtained by weighted averages. Monte Carlo makes use of Boltzmann probabilities, but not forces. The probability $P(x)$ of a configuration is calculated as the Eq. 13:

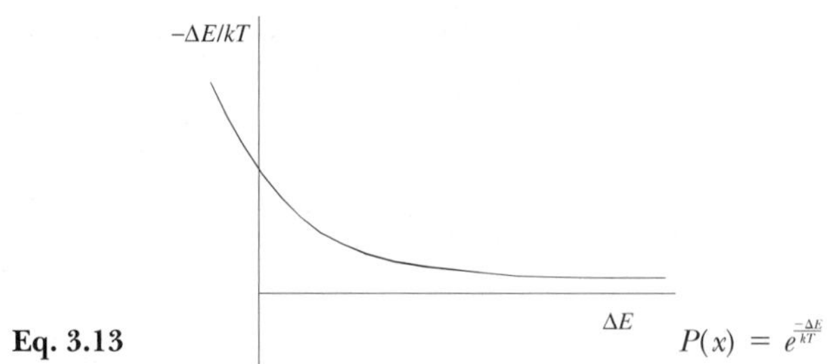

Eq. 3.13 $$P(x) = e^{\frac{-\Delta E}{kT}}$$

where the E is the energy of the configuration, k is the Boltzmann constant, and T is the temperature. The factor $e^{-E/kT}$ is the Boltzmann factor. The energy is calculated for each conformer or configuration generated, and a structural thermodynamics average is obtained according to the Boltzmann distribution. Unlike energy minimizations, Monte Carlo does not find an energy minimum but, rather, samples an ensemble of states, just as the actual molecular system does, with higher-energy states being sampled as temperature increases. As opposed to molecular dynamics techniques, in which the equations of motion are integrated numerically and the small time steps are necessary, in Monte Carlo simulation one can take larger time steps, which are then optimized independently. Monte Carlo calculations have been applied to a wide variety of biological problems, especially the study of solvent around peptides and proteins (51) and protein folding (52).

VIRTUAL DRUG SCREENING TECHNIQUES AND APPLICATIONS

Traditional molecular modeling methods discussed in the previous sections deal with a single or fewer number of molecules for structural properties at high resolution. Modern computational chemistry or cheminformatics tends to deal with massive amount of molecules or compounds for their biological behaviors at lower resolution. This is accomplished by using high-throughput virtual screening techniques, or 3D database search methods. The techniques are similar, however, in their attempt to improve their quality and generality by including as many of the principles of computational chemistry as possible. For example, scoring functions generally are based on simplified empirical force fields. Parameters for the scoring functions are increasingly derived from quantum mechanical calculations for improving the overall accuracy. Molecular dynamics or Monte Carlo sampling schemes are designed to explore as much of the relevant regions of conformation spaces as possible. In short, screening techniques attempt to incorporate as much of the molecular modeling methods discussed above as possible and still get the study completed within an acceptable amount of time.

Actually, the virtual screening and 3D database search techniques have been increasingly used in the pharmaceutical industry as lead generation, selection, and optimization are becoming a key bottleneck in drug discovery. The real-time experimental high-throughput drug screening (HTS) is the process to accelerate drug discovery by biologically screening large libraries of compounds

Table 3.2. Available Software Programs for Pharmacophore Identification and Ligand-Based Design

Software	Pharmacophore Identification Programs and Resources
GALAHALD	Genetic Algorithm with Linear Assignment for Hypermolecular Alignment of Datasets (GALAHAD), Tripos, Inc. http://www.tripos.com/data/SYBYL/GALAHAD_9-7-05.pdf
DISCO and DISCOtech	DIStance COmparison for multiple pharmacophores generations, Based on clique detection. The conformational search is separated. Tripos, Inc. www.tripos.com/data/SYBYL/DISCOTech_072505.pdf
GASP	Genetic Algorithm Similarity Program. A flexible genetic algorithm. The pharmacophoric features are defined by the SYBYL package. Tripos, Inc. www.tripos.com/data/SYBYL/GASP_072505.pdf
Catalyst	An integrated environment for database management and querying tasks for drug discovery. Accelrys, Inc. http://www.accelrys.com/products/catalyst/
HipHop	HipHop matches the chemical features of compounds without considering activity. The resulting hypotheses can be used to iteratively search chemical databases Accelrys, Inc. http://www.accelrys.com/products/catalyst/catalystproducts/cathypo.htm
HypoGen	HYpothesis GENerator uses ligand activity values and incorporates them into the scoring function. The conformational search is separated. Accelrys, Inc. www.accelrys.com/products/catalyst/catalystproducts/cathypo.html
PHASE	PHASE applys a novel, tree-based partitioning algorithm to exhaustively identify spatial arrangements of functional groups that are common and essential to the biologic activity of a set of high affinity ligands. Schrodinger Inc. http://www.schrodinger.com/
MOE/ pharmcophore modeling	Molecular Operating Environment (MOE). MOE's pharmacophore modeling module is to generate and use 3D geometric information to search for novel active compounds, particularly when no receptor geometry is available. Chemical Computing Group:http://www.chemcomp.com/software.htm
FlexS	Flexible Shape-Based Screening of Ligands http://www.biosolveit.de/FlexS/
MPHIL	Mapping Pharmacophores in Ligands. Relaxed MCS approach. A rigid alignment, based on clique detection and genetic algorithm. (141)
RAPID	Randomized Pharmacophore Identification. A rigid alignment based on mapping triangles of 3D atom coordinates. (142)
SCAMPI	Statistical classification of activities of molecules for pharmacophore identification. Handles large heterogeneous data sets. A random conformational search is combined. (144) Glaxo Wellcome, Inc. www.gsk.com/index.htm

(Adapted from Dror O, Shulman-peleg A, Nussinov R, Wolfson HJ: Predicting molecular interactions in silico: I. A guide to pharmacophore identification and its applications to drug design. *Current Medicinal Chemistry* 2004;11(1):71–90; with permission.)

(drug candidates) against targets (receptor or enzymes) using 96-, 384-, or 1,536-well microplate (250 μL at 1–10μM) at a rate of thousands of compounds per week. At screening rates of 500,000 compounds per week, however, a cost of $1 per well is still difficult for many companies or academic institutes to afford on a weekly basis (53). The costs of robotic equipment, compound purchasing, assay development, and radioactive material disposals also the main issues challenging the HTS method development and applications. Most importantly, the data show that only 1 in 100,000 HTS actives reaches the stage of becoming a drug candidate, which often also fails later because of the lack of good permeability, solubility, or ADME properties. In this regard, computational chemistry and a knowledge-based in silico design approach can play an important role in drug screening. It can be carried out as a "prescreen" or "virtual screen" before committing to the costly experimental testing of large numbers of compounds. The in silico methods will not only expedite the discovery of new leads but also generate a structurally diverse set of molecules or sublibraries of compounds that merit more detailed study.

Thus, the pressure to identify good leads and, therefore, drug candidates at an ever-increasing pace has led to the rapid advancement of molecular database or cheminformatics that manages information about small molecules, including the storage, display, and searching of chemical structures and their physical and biological properties. In general, four computer virtual screening techniques are available, which are related to each other in terms of the available structural information for the compounds and their targets: docking receptor–based design, ligand-based design, combinatorial computational chemistry, and de novo design techniques (2–10).

In Silico Drug Design Programs and Resources

Various virtual screening techniques have been developed as a result of the temptation to predict the geometries of

Table 3.3. Available Molecular Docking Software and Sources

Program	Source Information
Surflex-Dock	Tripos, Inc. http://www.tripos.com/resources/fileroot/surflex_final2.pdf Scientific and Software Partner with UCSF Cancer Center & Biopharmics (Prof. Ajay N. Jain)
FlexX	BioSolveIT GmbH, Sankt Augustine, Germany www.biosolveit.de/FlexX/ (previous:http://catan.gmd.de/flexx)
LigandFit	Accelrys, Inc., www.accelrys.com/products/cerius2/cerius2products/c2ligandfit.html
GOLD	Cambridge Crytallographic Data Center, Cambridge, UK www.ccdc.cam.ac.uk/products/life_sciences/gold/
DOCK	University of California, San Francisco (Irwin Kuntz) dock.compbio.ucsf.edu/
AUTODOCK	The Scripps Research Institute (David Goodsell) www.scripps.edu/pub/olson-web/doc/autodock
Glide	Schrödinger Inc. New York www.schrodinger.com/
Fred	OpenEye Scientific Software http://www.eyesopen.com/products/applications/fred.html
BiomedCAChe	CAChe Software http://www.cachesoftware.com/biomedcache\
MOE	Chemical Computing Group: http://www.chemcomp.com/software.htm
eHITS	SimBioSys http://www.simbiosys.ca/
ICM	Molsoft LLC, http://www.molsoft.com/
Molegro Virtual Docker	Molegro ApS, http://www.molegro.com/products.php
WHAT IF	Centre for Molecular and Biomolecular informatics, Radboud University, NIJMEGEN, Netherlands http://swift.cmbi.kun.nl/whatif

(Adapted from Seifert MHJ, Wolf K, Vitt D. Virtual high-throughput in silico screening. Biosilico 2003;1:143–149; with permission.)

biomolecular complex and to discover novel ligands as leads for drug design. Choices of various programs depend on the target goals and purposes of the performed computational chemistry, the capacity of computer facilities, and the availability of software programs.

The software programs used for ligand-based approach deal with the purpose of ligand pharmacophore identifications and 3D database search programs. The available pharmacophore identification programs are summarized in Table 3.2. New pharmacophore-generation programs, such as GALAHAD (Genetic Algorithm with Linear Assignment for Hypermolecular Alignment of Datasets) (54), are emerging with improved computational ability and capacity. GALAHAD assumes shared pharmacophore/shape, explores "all" of conformational space, and generates multiple partial-match constraints (or pharmacophore) for 3D database search. GALAHAD is an improvement over GASP in its multiobjective scoring capability and ability to deal with large numbers of molecules, and it is an improvement over DISCO in the simplicity of its interface and higher-quality molecular alignments. Other commonly used ligand-based virtual screening programs are UMOE (55), FlexS (56) and Catalyst (57,58), which are based on active ligand pharmacophore models, and ROCS (59), which is based on active ligand shape.

Most software programs, however, involve a large number of docking tools and score functions that have been developed for receptor-based virtual screening, as summarized in Table 3.3. The commonly used DOCK program (60) models receptor sphere centers to ligand atoms via either rigid or flexible docking to be scored by evaluation of empirical force field energy, using AMBER (61). Similarly, AUTODOCK (62) uses a simulated annealing or genetic algorithm and AMBER scoring method. FlexX (63), however, applies the fragment-based incremental buildup strategy and scores the docked ligands by an empirical algorithm based on the Bohm function (64). This strategy basically counts hydrogen bonds, salt bridges, aromatic-ring interactions, and hydrophobic interactions, and it effectively reduces the number of conformational possibilities (65,66). GOLD (67) applies a genetic algorithm for generating ligand-docked poses, and the results are scored by an empirical function based on interaction possibilities derived from atom–atom contact probabilities in the Cambridge Structural Database (CSD) (68). Other programs, including GLIDE(69), LigandFit (70), FFLD (71), Eudock (72), and ICM-DISCO (73), also are widely used for *in silico* drug screening.

In reviewing these drug available molecular docking programs used for in silico screening platforms (Table 3.3), their algorithms and advantages have been addressed in the literature (4). For example, DOCK (60) and Flexidock/UNITY (55) allow users to dock the ligand as flexible structures onto the target enzyme or receptor using the directed tweak algorithm (55). These methods are very time-consuming, however, because such "on-the-fly" conformational searches must be repeated for each pharmacophoric search query. The time will increase several-fold when van der Waals bump-check is included (74). For example, ChemDBS-3D/Chemical Design (75), Catalyst/MSI (57,76), and Merck Flexibase databases (77) use the method to generate a number of energetically reasonable representative conformations for each structure at the time of compound registration and stores these conformers in the database. This latter approach requires a sufficient coverage of the available conformational space such that at least one conformation of each active compound is sufficiently close to the active conformation to be considered a hit by a database query. FOUNDATION (78) and 3D search (79) have database queries consisting of pharmacophore models supplemented by steric constraints defined from protein crystallographic coordinates. Only a single conformation of a ligand is considered, however, and FOUNDATION only examines a single orientation of a ligand. The LUDI (80) software package has been applied to 3D database mining, but is restricted to single conformations of small, rigid molecules. Other programs, such as CLIX (81) and FLOG (82), essentially use the DOCK approach, although in FLOG, multiple conformations of each compound are explicitly stored in a database. So, many choices for docking programs are available either commercially or free for academics (Table 3.3).

In Silico Design and Virtual Screening Techniques

Several computational chemistry approaches are based on the availabilities of the target protein structures and known active ligands.

DOCK Receptor-Based Approach

When receptor and ligand structures are both known, the docking receptor-based approach is the most ideal situation (6,83–85). The ligand can be docked into the known receptor site and molecular mechanics used to simulate receptor–ligand interactions and dynamics. One can address highly specific receptor–ligand interactions using these techniques, but even here, there can be surprises in the form of alternative modes of binding and conformational changes in the receptor structure. It is frequently necessary (or of more interest) to study the binding of thousands of compounds at low resolution rather than fewer compounds at high resolution. This often is the case when searching for lead compounds. The GRID approach (86) maps the binding site by superimposing a grid and calculating the electrostatics, hydrogen-bonding sites, or lipophilicity at each grid point. Among the docking-related programs discussed above, classical DOCK program uses a similar approach (60) for scoring and also provides other tools for scoring compounds, attempting alternate orientations, and performing geometry optimization to include the flexibility of the ligand. A grid-based approach dramatically reduces the amount of computer time required. Each ligand's interaction is computed with the limited number of grid points and not all of the target's atoms. Several common programs, including AUTODOCK, Glide, LUDI, LigandFit, and FlexX/CSCores, also have been widely used in ligand docking and lead screening studies (6) (Table 3.3).

Ligand-Based Approach

When the receptor structure is unknown but the ligand structures are known, a ligand-based approach is used (7,87–90). This situation represents the most common case. An extension of the QSAR approach is taken to study the active ligands, also known as pharmacophore-based drug design. The pharmacophore refers to an ensemble of steric and electronic features (or 3D arrangement of the functional groups) that enables a molecule to exhibit a specific biological activity. The ligand-based approach is basically an indirect method of pharmacophore identifications. In general, pharmacophore-based virtual screening techniques depend on the application of descriptors of molecular structure and properties (2,91,92), including structure- or descriptor-based queries (or similarity search in two-dimensional (2D) and 3D substructures or pharmacophore models), fingerprint queries (or binary bit string-search based on Tanimoto coefficient, 2D/3D pharmacophore fingerprints), and clustering and partitioning (or intermolecular distances in chemical reference spaces and reference frame). The details descriptions of these techniques have been reviewed in literature (2,7,87) and summarized in Table 3.2.

Combinatorial-Based Approach

When receptor and ligand structures are both unknown, virtual combinatorial chemistry approaches are used. In this case, computational chemistry is used both to generate structures and in parallel to perform chemical similarity and diversity search analysis before and after combinatorial chemistry-based experimental HTS. For example, the combinatorial chemistry software package from Accelrys and Tripos companies provides the unique features to preanalyze and select diverse building blocks for the target libraries to help discover small molecule drug therapies. This promises a maximum range of drug-like compounds and increases the potential of finding active leads for the targets. The developments of combinatorial chemistry library have been described in the literature (93–95).

De Novo Design-Based Approach

When receptor structure is known and ligand structures are unknown, de novo design-techniques are used (10,96,97). In this situation, there is available information about the target receptor, or a similar receptor, but no existing leads that can interact with the active receptor sites. One can use recently developed de novo design- techniques to propose new ligands, which are complementary to the active site. These techniques use 3D searching of large databases to identify small molecule fragments that can interact with specific sites in the receptor, bridging fragments with the correct size and geometry, or framework structures that can support functional groups at favorable orientations. For example, programs such as GROW (98) or LEGEND (99)

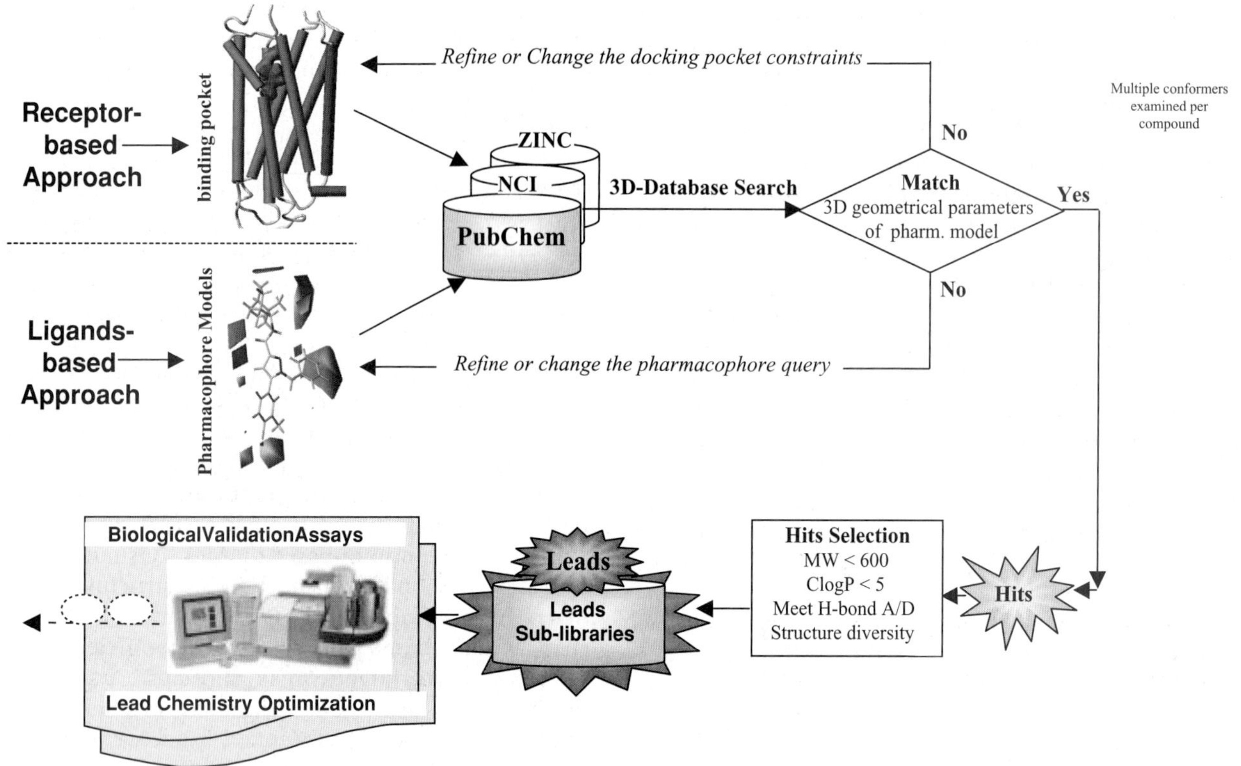

Fig. 3.8. A workflow of in silico virtual screening process: receptor-based and ligand-based approaches.

use "seed" structures through de novo design of a compound to fit the binding site and add functional groups to optimize the use of possible binding sites. These tools have been most effective when used to support rather than to automate drug design efforts (10).

Practical Aspects of Virtual Screening Applications

Given the recent advances in supercomputer clusters/CPU horsepower for new compute-intensive algorithms as well as the availability of public and proprietary databases, in silico drug design and virtual screening methods have been advanced to search large compound databases or hypothetical virtual libraries *in silico* by computer analysis and selection of a limited number of candidate molecules likely to be active against a biological target. The general methods of *in silico* design or virtual screening can be illustrated practically as in Fig. 3.8: protein structure-based compound screening or docking receptor-based design (100,101), and chemical-similarity searching based on small molecules or ligand-based design(102).

Basically, the virtual screening experimental protocol (Fig. 3.8) could be described as follows:

1. Build virtual compound database.
2. Generate the database search query, either ligand pharmacophore hypotheses or receptor-binding pockets.
3. Refine and modify the query through training databases.
4. Search the target compound databases for novel leads with new chemical scaffolds and better binding activities
5. Carry out the hit selection based on defined criteria.
6. Bio-validate the hit leads via HTS experiments and functional assays.
7. Conduct lead optimization virtually and experimentally to improve the novel lead bioactivity.

Build Virtual Compound Libraries

The first step of virtual screening is to build virtual compound collections that can be used for in silico virtual screening. Pharmaceutical companies treat the databases of compounds they have synthesized or purchased as a valued corporate asset. The National Institutes of Health (NIH) recently constructed a public compound library, PubChem, that consists of more than 11 million compounds (http://pubchem.ncbi.nlm.nih.gov/). In general, two major compound libraries are needed in virtual screening.

CONSTRUCT KNOWN COMPOUND TRAINING DATABASES. A training database is recommended to be constructed for the purposes of optimizing the query hypotheses to improve the hit accuracy in database search. Such a training database usually contains a thousand compounds typically, consisting of 980 random molecules and 20 known active ligands. For example, users can examine and refine the hypothetic pharmacophore (or query) against the test database in terms of hit precision rate, false-negative rate, and false-positive rate. The process is very important. It also helps to evaluate the qualities of pharmacophore queries and molecular alignments generated or the binding pocket defined in the target protein before searches in the large target database.

CONSTRUCT TARGET COMPOUND DATABASES. The 3D target virtual compound database can be constructed through single molecular entry or systematically importing from other public or commercial compound catalog sources (in either SFD, MOL2, or Smiles formats) (Table 3.4). For example, compound library catalogs can be converted from the 2D data format into a 3D searchable compound database by the CONCORD program (103) or Daylight Rubicon program (104) using artificial intelligence and geometry optimization. In addition, structurally diverse sublibrary or target-specific libraries also can be constructed from the large virtual libraries of millions of compounds. For example, the NIH PubChem database consists of approximately 11 million compounds. It will be reasonable to create one or several sublibraries from the PubChem database and then evaluate them by using software programs, such as Tripos' Diverse Solution (105), Selectors (106), or the TimTec's Diversity program (107). The diverse sublibraries are created to represent the parent libraries with the same diversities but much smaller datasets (usually ~10–20% compounds). The sublibraries are created mainly for the purpose of enhancing the computer screening. Although the virtual screening is much faster than the experimental HTS, especially with the high-horsepower computational facilities now available, it will still take a month to search through a 3D database with millions of compounds.

In addition, a quality-control procedure is required to ensure the 2D to 3D structure-converting accuracy and data integrity as well as further data portability. This includes randomly selecting the converted compounds

Table 3.4. Available Chemical and Drug Compound Databases

Database Name	No. of Compounds	Company/Web site
MDL®-ACD	435,000	MDL®- Available Chemicals Directory. MDL Information System, Inc. www.mdli.com/products/experiment/available_chem_dir/index.jsp
MDL®-SCD	3.5 million	MDL® Screening Compounds Directory (formerly ACD-SC). MDL Information System, Inc.www.mdli.com/products/experiment/screening_compounds/index.jsp
MDL®-PCD	1.5 million	MDL® Patent Chemistry Database. MDL Information System, Inc. www.mdli.com/products/knowledge/patent_db/index.jsp
MDL®-MDDR	132,726	MDL®-Drug Data Report. MDL Information System, Inc. www.mdli.com/products/knowledge/drug_data_report/index.jsp
MDL®-CMC	8,473	MDL® Comprehensive Medicinal Chemistry MDL Information System, Inc. www.mdl.com/products/knowledge/medicinal_chem/index.jsp
ZINC	2.67 million purchasable	Free database of commercially-available compounds. University of California @ San Francisco http://blaster.docking.org/zinc/, non-commercial database for virtual screening
NCID	213,628	National Cancer Institute Databases, NCI http://dtp.nci.nih.gov/docs/3d_database/Structural_information/structural_data. html distributed by MDL Information System, Inc. www.mdli.com/products/knowledge/cancer_db/index.jsp
CNPD	57,000	Chinese nature product database. Neotrident Technology Ltd. And Shanghai Institute of Materia Medica. www.neotrident.com/newpage/
ACX	500,000	Available Chemicals Xchange. CambridgeSoft Corporation. http://chemfinder.cambridgesoft.com/
CLP	260,000	ComGenex Library Portfolio (ComGenex,Ltd) www.comgenex.com
Menai Organics	4,000	Ryan Scientific, Inc. www.ryansci.com/
Pubchem	5,404,047	NCBI http://pubchem.ncbi.nlm.nih.gov/
BioSpecs	240,000	SPECS, Inc. http://www.specs.net
Chembank	110,000	Harvard university http://chembank.broad.harvard.edu/
CSD	400,000	Cambridge Crystallographic Data Center http://www.ccdc.cam.ac.uk/

(Adapted from Shen J, Xu X, Cheng F, et al. Virtual screening on natural products for discovering active compounds and target information. Curr Med Chem 2003;10:2327–2342; with permission.)

and examining them for the molecular structure (bond types/lengths, bond angles, atom types/charges, and carbon chirality), 3D molecular geometry (quick energy minimization, if needed), the compound catalog numbers versus their original numbers and the reference source, and the data export features to ensure portability of the data for sharing.

Build 3D Structure of the Target Protein

Knowledge of the 3D structure of a target protein is often a prerequisite for the receptor-based virtual screening and building a reliable 3D protein structure is a first important step for a successful receptor-based design. In general, protein structures are mainly derived from x-ray, NMR, or homology models. The experimental sources of 3D structures are available from Cambridge Structural Database (CSD) (~250,000 x-ray structures) and the Brookhaven Protein Data Bank (PDB; ~17,000 structures of proteins defined by x-ray, NMR, and computations). Several reviews of x-ray crystallography provide excellent overviews of ligand-free and ligand-bound protein crystallographic data for drug design (108). The x-ray crystallographic method, however, is limited by the available pure crystals of the target proteins, particularly for large membrane proteins. The GPCR membrane proteins do not generally crystallize in a form suitable for x-ray crystallography. In addition, the crystal protein conformation sometimes may be distorted by crystal packing force and may not be exactly relevant to its in vivo counterpart. Because of the difficulties in crystallizing membrane-bound protein for x-ray crystallography, the only GPCR that has been crystallized with high resolution x-ray is rhodopsin (109).

The NMR structures of target proteins generally are determined in a solution or membrane-like environment, which is similar to the physiological state of most systems. Often, however, the NMR-determined protein structures are studied at low pH, whereas the resulting structures sometimes can show significant pH-dependent variation and the protein backbone may display considerable motion and unfolding at different pH values (110).

Computer homology modeling provides an alternative way to predict 3D protein structure. The homology-generated models usually are refined further by incorporating experimental constraints measured by x-ray and NMR. Actually, if the sequence identity between the target protein and template is sufficiently high (>50%), the *in silico* design and virtual screening results using homology-predicted 3D models have been shown to be similar to those when x-ray structures are used (111). The homology-predicted 3D models have proven to be successful in docking receptor-based studies or receptor-based virtual screening. An example in Figure 3.9 is given here to illustrate that the computer homology and multiple sequence alignment techniques were used to build a 3D receptor structure (34,48). Xie et. al. constructed the 3D structural model of cannabinoid receptor CB2 by using multiple sequence alignment of 10 homologous GPCRs (34). Alignments were analyzed with mutation scores, pairwise hydrophobicity profiles, and Kyte-Doolittle plots. The 3D model of the transmembrane segment was generated by mapping the CB2 sequence onto the homologous residues of the x-ray crystallographic data of rhodopsin structure. The extra- and intracellular loop regions of the CB2 were generated by searching for homologous C_α backbone

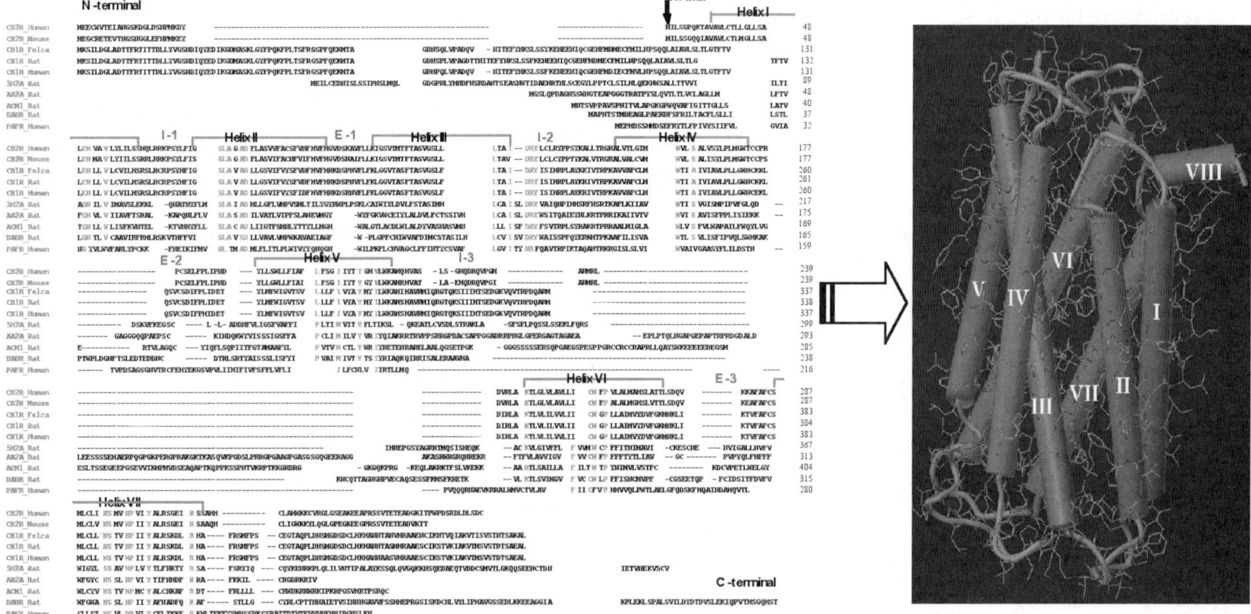

Fig. 3.9. Three-dimensional G protein–coupled CB2 receptor structure (right) constructed by homology and multiple sequence alignment method (left), including the seven transmembrane helices (cylinders, I-VII) and loop regions (ribbons) (See color plate.) (From Xie XQ, Chen JZ, Billings EM. 3D structural model of the G protein–coupled cannabinoid CB_2 receptor. Proteins: Structure, Function, and Genetics 2003;53:307–319; with permission.)

sequences of published structures in the Brookhaven Protein Databank (PDB). Residue side chains were positioned through a combination of rotamer library searches, simulated annealing and minimization.

Other successful homology models have been used in docking applications and have successfully resulted in the discovery of novel hits, include retinoic acid receptor (112), thyroid hormone receptor (113), CK2 kinase (114), SARS (severe acute respiratory syndrome) protease (115), CDK4 kinase (116), and SrC sH_2 (117) for the application of de novo design methods (117).

Predict the Binding Sites of the Target Proteins

After determination of the 3D target protein structure, identification of the target binding site is the next important step, which often depends on whether the ligand–receptor complex is known. Accordingly, binding sites generally are referred to as cavities or grooves (i.e., the depression in the protein surface). If the ligand–target complex structures are available through x-ray or NMR, identification of the binding site is straightforward. The experimental site-directed mutagenesis results will also be very informative to characterize the residues implicated in ligand binding or function.

Often, however, limited mutageneses data are available about the binding sites, and little is known about the protein or the protein complex, which requires using computational techniques to detect these surface features to predict the potential binding sites. Several geometry-based computational methods are available, including SiteID (118), LIGSITE (119), APROPOS (Automatic PROtein Pocket Search) (120), and PASS (Putative Active Site with Spheres) (121). Other programs, such as GRID (86), van der Waals–FFT (122), and XSITE (123), were used to search for complementarities between the ligand functional groups and site functionality and to identify the physicochemical properties of the different cavities to identify the site of interests.

In the 3D protein structure construction and binding site prediction above, drug binding pocket(s) should be mapped out for 3D database search using the docking program. An example is given here to illustrate the computer prediction of the protein binding pockets. Xie et al. (34) applied the MOLCAD solvent-accessible channel surfaces calculation (124) to predict the binding site of the cannabinoid CB2 receptor, as shown in Figure 3.10. The result was confirmed by Tripos SiteID program (118). The predicted binding site also is correlated well with known site mutagenesis data (except Phe87), as shown in Fig. 3.10. The data also showed an amphipathic binding contour (Fig. 3.10): The hydrophilic center (blue) is framed by polar residues, whereas the hydrophobic cleft (brown) is surrounded by aromatic residues. The computational chemistry approach offers an alternative avenue for understanding the receptor–ligand interactions in terms of hydrogen-bonding, hydrophobic centers, charged centers, and steric interactions that are defined in the pharmacophoric feature identification process and for assisting the in silico virtual screening.

Derive Active Pharmacophore Models

For a ligand-based design approach, generating reliable pharmacophore hypotheses is a prerequisite for the 3D pharmacophore database search. Several approaches are available for generating pharmacophore models, including programs to derive the active pharmacophore models or "virtual receptor" (e.g., 3D QSAR/CoMFA (125) and AAA [Active Analog Approach] (126)) and programs to generate hypothetical pharmacophore queries (e.g., DISCO (127) and GALLAHAD (54)) for database searches of the new chemical scaffolds that match the target pharmacophores. An example of the pharmacophore generations is given below.

The CoFMA (Comparative Molecular Field Analysis) is superior to classical QSAR in mapping out 3D QSAR models. The CoMFA program (128) provides tools to postulate a biological active conformation and to establish a set of alignment rules (129) to superimpose the molecules under consideration. It will generate a grid or lattice as a box of points around the molecules and calculate the electrostatic and steric fields that each molecule exerts on a probe atom positioned at each lattice point. Then, a statistical analysis of the data using partial least squares statistics is made to derive a linear correlation (3D QSAR) between the calculated values and the input biological data. Subsequently, it validates the predictability of the derived model by using cross-validation (r^2). Finally, active ligand CoMFA models are established that can be used to guide novel ligand design and to predict the biological activities. CoMFA analysis has been used to study the pharmacophoric requirements of cannabinoid antagonists (125) (Fig. 3.11), to study the effect of shape on binding of steroids to carrier proteins (130), to deduce active site geometries of angiotensin-converting enzyme (131), and to analyze a set of muscarinic agonists (132).

The DISCO (DIStance Comparison) program (133) often is used to generate multiple pharmacophore models by identifying common pharmacophoric features (e.g., H-bond donor atoms, H-bond acceptor atoms, charged centers, and centers of mass of hydrophobic rings) for a given set of active compounds, producing optimally aligned structures, and extracting the key features of the pharmacophores. Then, these pharmacophore hypotheses can be compared, refined, and used to guide lead generation and optimization and in performing 3D searches of databases for new leads. DISCO has been used in pharmacophore generation during studies of muscarinic M3 receptor antagonists (134), muscarinic agonists (135), and melatonin analogues (136).

Other pharmacophore identification approaches (7) include GALAHAD (54), GASP (137), HipHop (138), HypoGen (139), PHASE (140), MPHIL (141), RAPID (142), MOE (143), and SCAMPI (144), as well as AAA (126) and ensemble distance geometry (145).

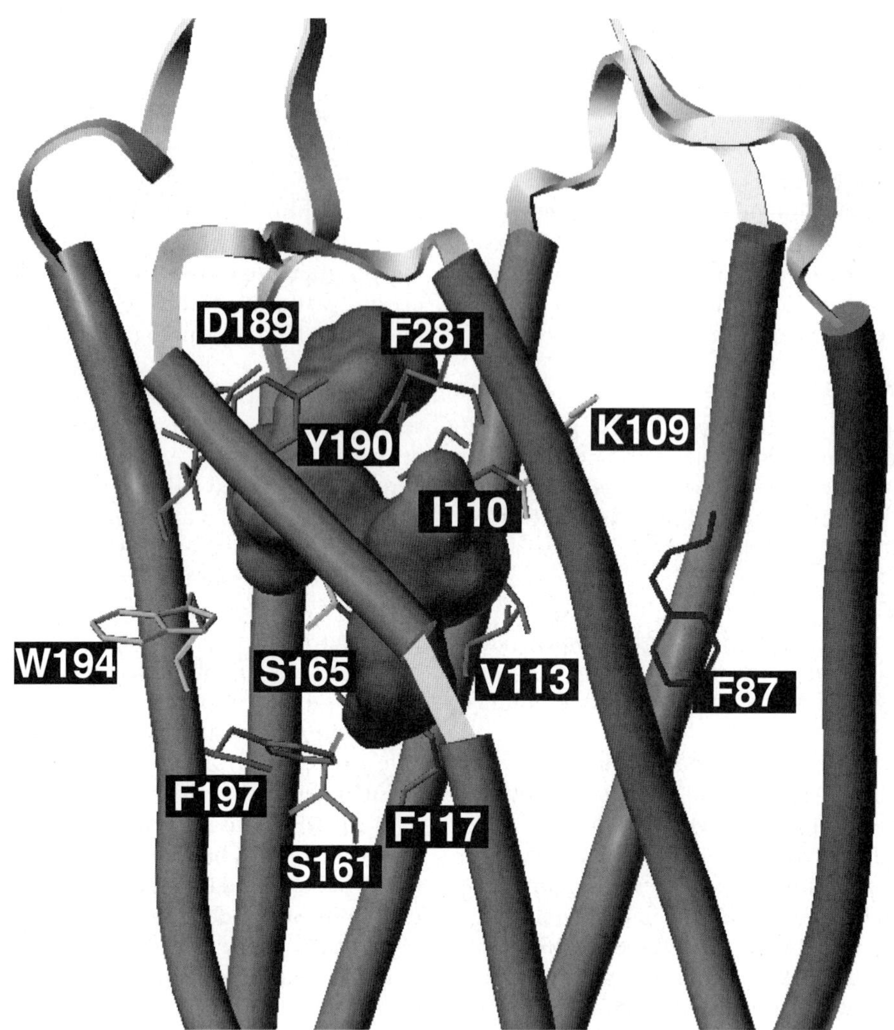

Fig. 3.10. MOLCAD-predicted CB_2-binding pocket surrounded by active amino acid residues, showing an amphipathic contour, hydrophilic center (blue), and hydrophobic cleft (brown). The site-directed mutagenesis–detected binding residues are color-coded in terms of their distance to the pocket (magenta > yellow > green > blue) as the interaction weakens. (See color plate.)

The generated various pharmacophore models will be used as hypothetic queries in the database search for lead discovery

To achieve a successful database search, one must ensure the quality of the derived pharmacophore models by considering the following issues while composing a 3D database query:

1. Which functional groups or set of topological constraints should be chosen?
2. What average distance should separate the pharmacophoric features, or by what average angle should the features be arranged?
3. Which type of geometric relationships should be imposed, and what are their tolerances (e.g., interatomic distances, angular relationships between two pendant substituents, and the angle of a lone pair to the plane of a phenyl ring)?

These factors often have influence on the false-positive or false-negative hits during the database search, as discussed later.

3D Database Search Protocol

The basic rationales of 3D database search methods are the same for either ligand-based or receptor-based approaches, as reviewed in literatures (2,6,53), whereas the search protocols may need to be changed as different approaches are used. In general, the docking receptor-based virtual screening techniques are based on the active defined receptor binding pockets as queries, whereas the ligand pharmacophore-based search is based on the active ligand pharmacophore models or shapes as database queries. Although 3D structures of target proteins are becoming increasingly available as search templates, small molecule virtual screening still dominates the field. This is particularly true for the receptors lacking 3D structures, except for

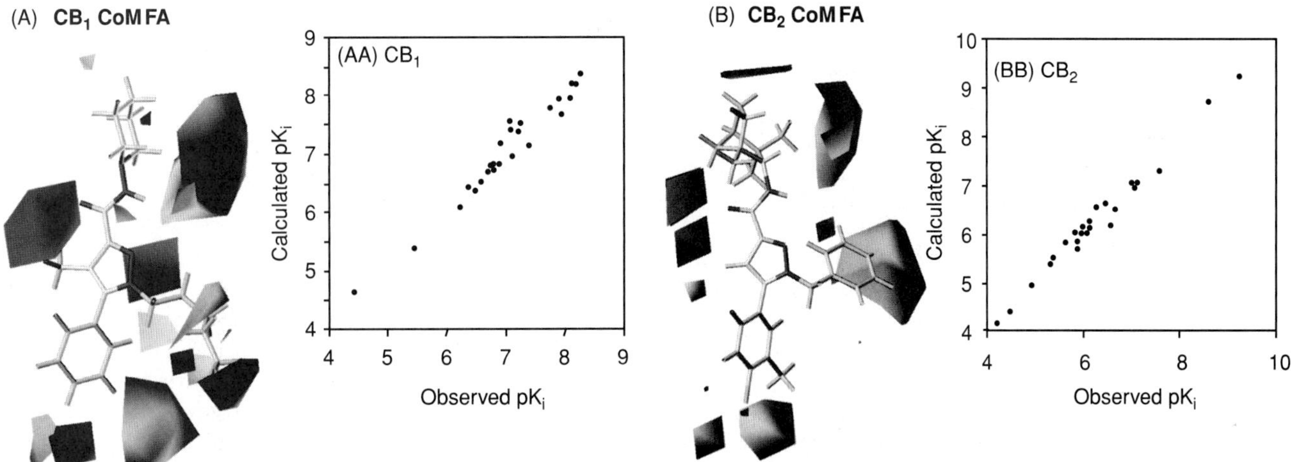

Fig. 3.11. CoMFA contour maps for arylpyrazole antagonists of cannabinoid receptor subtypes CB_1 (A) and CB_2 (B). Sterically favored areas (contribution level, 80%) are shown in green. Sterically unfavored areas (contribution level, 20%) are shown in yellow, and positive-potential favored areas (contribution level, 80%) are shown in blue. Positive-potential unfavored areas (contribution level, 20%) are shown in red. Plots of the corresponding CoMFA-calculated and experimental values of binding affinity (given as pK_i) of arylpyrazole compounds at CB_1 (AA) and CB_2 (BB) receptor, respectively are shown as well. (See color plate.) (Adapted with permission from Chen J, Han X, Lan R, et al. 3D-QSAR studies of arylpyrazole antagonists of cannabinoid receptor subtypes CB_1 and CB_2. A combined NMR and CoMFA approach. J Med Chem 2006;49:625–636; with permission.)

rhodopsin. In light of page limitations, we will illustrate the ligand pharmacophore database search and use the UNITY program as an example.

For a ligand-based search, a typical search query consists of the following types of information: a 2D pattern (representing important groups in the molecule; e.g., CC(C = O)N defines the backbone of an amino acid), 3D geometric features (e.g., name = hbond; atoms = 1,2,3; distance = 1.57; angle = 120.0; dihedral = 180.0), and 3D constraints (define the relationship between geometric features and excluded volumes). The common database search protocol is given here as an illustration:

1. A 2D similarity search is first carried out to find specific fragments in the database (e.g., CC(C=O)N for an amino acid). With the defined pharmacophore patterns, we will search the database using sub-/superstructure search, similarity search, Tanimoto coefficient (146), Tversky search (147), and so on. The search returned hit list will be grouped into a molecular spreadsheet for further studies. The 2D database searches usually are carried out as initial screening, followed by 3D searches.
2. A 3D geometric search is then performed to look for relationships between features in a molecule. The initial 2D pattern search takes into account only the composition of the molecule, such as atom types and bond types. The 3D portion is only concerned with the geometric relations between the features (e.g., distance, angle, exclusive van der Waals volume, overlapping van der Waals volume, and constraints). A 3D search makes use of the coordinates stored in the database for determining whether constraints are satisfied.
3. A flexible 3D search is subsequently conducted by altering the geometry of the molecule to determine any possibly satisfied geometric constraints without having to save every possible conformation in the database. The conformational flexibility can be explored by determining the geometries at search time without having to save every possible conformation, which is considered to be a unique feature for the UNITY database compared with other 3D databases (134,148).
4. The next step is database search hit evaluation and selection. Compounds that have at least one conformation satisfying the geometric requirements and possess functional groups residing within the respective tolerance spheres of the pharmacophoric features are considered to be "hits" (i.e., potential candidates for biological testing). A number of additional criteria are used in the selection of compounds for biological evaluation and experimental validations to achieve maximum efficiency in the discovery of lead compounds.

The hit selection strategy is initially established on the basis of Lipinski's rules (149). Hit selection criteria for a good lead compound have the following properties: simple chemical structure, easy synthesis, calculated logP (ClogP) of less than 5 (or measured logP <4.15), small molecule (molecular weight, <500 daltons), nonpeptidic, and chemical structure diversity. In addition, other drug-likeness parameters (e.g., ADME) also will be considered as hit selection. For example, the VolSurf program is used to predict ADME properties based on precalculated models, to compute unique ADME-relevant descriptors, and to create QSAR models of bioactivity (150), as discussed later.

5. No method is generally accepted to rank the hits of molecules obtained from pharmacophore-based database searches nor proper score functions are available, as for the docking receptor–based approach. Greenidge et al. (151) have reported use of the overall superimposition of functional groups of the molecules to the appropriate features of the pharmacophore to evaluate the hits (i.e., the better the superimposition, the higher the score of the fit). Van Drie (152) presented the DANTE approach, in which ranking candidate pharmacophores were used to evaluate the hit selection. For the FlexS/UNITY hits ranking approach (148), the evaluation of this potential is based on three values: strain energy of the hit, root mean square (RMS) of the hit features from their queries, and number of rotatable bonds in the hit (entropic term). The actual ranking could also be done by means of the simple scoring function:

$$\text{Score} = R_{\text{energy}} + \sqrt{R_{\text{bonds}} \times R_{\text{rms}}},$$

where R_{energy}, R_{bonds}, and R_{rms} are the ranks of the hits by energy, number of rotatable bonds, and RMS, respectively. Interested readers are encouraged to find these more detailed discussions in UNITY program (148) and the literature (7,87,152).

6. Often, one runs into the problem of too many hits (false positive) or too few hits (false negative) during a database search. One commonly used approach is to examine the following hypothesis by creating a training database (e.g., containing 980 random molecules plus 20 known active ligands) (90). The derived pharmacophore queries are examined and refined against the training database by carrying out the following investigations:

   a. *The influences of the numbers of pharmacophoric features and their tolerances on hit rates.* One should create a pharmacophore with different combinations of features and tolerances and examine those against the training database to find a reasonable balance between the number of pharmacophoric features and their tolerances to maximize the number of true positives and minimize the number of false positives. For example, if some ambiguity or uncertainty exists regarding whether an OH group is a hydrogen-bond donor or acceptor, two possible alternative hydrogen-bonding networks will be investigated in the defined pharmacophores.
   b. *The effects of pharmacophore tolerances versus weights on hit rates.* One could examine several variants of a pharmacophore model, such as one with the same feature tolerances but different feature weights (weight is a measure of its proposed importance to the pharmacophore as a whole) and another with the same feature weights but different feature tolerances to determine how altering tolerances and weights would affect hit rates, particularly how many known ligands structures are retrieved.
   c. *The effect of the receptor excluded volumes (REVs).* In addition, the ligand-generated REVs as additional search constraints can be combined with pharmacophoric features (numbers and tolerances) to reduce the number of false positives. In the actual experiments, one may consider several variants in the pharmacophoric search, such as the positions of the REVs and their scales according to the sizes of atoms delineating the putative binding cavity, the effects of the REV scale (volume radii to 25 and 50%) on the size of hit list or hit rates, and the effects of the REV radii on database search time (e.g., whether it significantly slows the search). Such studies will reveal unfavorable steric interactions between ligand and receptor, and uncover true positive hits at a given van der Waals scaling factor.

There are emerging examples of successful in silico design and virtual screening reports. The 3D pharmacophore database search methods have been successfully used to identify micromolar inhibitors of *Pneumocystis carinii* dihydrofolate reductase (82), to generate leads for muscarinic M3 receptor antagonists (134), and to search for novel protein kinase C agonists in the National Cancer Institute 3D database (153), HIV protease inhibitors (154), dopamine transporter inhibitors (90), thyroid hormone–receptor antagonists (151), and 5HT-2c agonists (155). The 3D pharmacophore database search to discover novel activities of existing compounds has emerged as a new tool for drug discovery in recent years, because in most cases, target receptor structures are unknown but the ligands are known.

The recent advances in virtual screening have revealed its particular efficiencies in discovering new and active lead compounds. For example, Doman et al. (156) reported a 1,700-fold higher hit rate of the virtual screening method over random HTS for the inhibitors of protein tyrosine phosphatase 1B (PTP1B), with a median inhibitory concentration (IC50) for enzymes of less than 100 μM. In their studies, the HTS bioassay showed that 400,000 compounds in the library generated a hit rate of 85 compounds (0.021%), whereas the *in silico* screening methods search of 235,000 compounds from the

Advanced Chemical Development (ACD) database (157) against the x-ray crystallographic structure of PTP1B gave a hit rate of 127 compounds (31.8%). Paiva et. al. (158) also demonstrated their studies between HTS and virtual screening on the Merck chemical collection against the tuberculosis target dihydrodipicolinate reductase, showing a hit rate of 0.2% for HTS and 6% for docking screening under the same threshold activity (IC50 <100 μM). Other successful virtual screening work includes 3D pharmacophoric searching in the discovery of VLA-4 integrin antagonists with submicromolar potency (159), 2D fingerprints QSAR (161), and flexible docking for discovery of novel carbonic anhydrase inhibitors (160). Clearly, computer modeling and 3D database virtual screening approaches have become an important drug discovery approach; many are carried out as "prescreening" before the beginning of costly experimental testing of large numbers of compounds.

CALCULATIONS OF ADME AND PHYSICOCHEMICAL PROPERTIES

As described previously, virtual screening and in silico design will accelerate the discovery of active lead compounds with new chemical scaffolds. The *in silico* prediction of physicochemical and ADME (absorption distribution metabolism elimination) properties, however, also are very critical for lead development. Actually, pharmacokinetics and toxicity have been identified as important causes of costly late-stage failures in drug development. The recently developed in silico approaches will increase model productivity in fine-tuned lead optimization to improve compound design and lead optimization.

The pharmacokinetic and metabolic behaviors in the body often are linked to the physical properties of a compound, as summarized by Lipinski et al. (149). Those authors analyzed a subset of 2,245 drugs from the World Drug Index by studies of QSAR structure permeability as a function of hydrophobicity, molecular size, and hydrogen-bonding capacity to better understand the common molecular features of orally available drugs. The results showed that a good oral drug absorption or permeation is more likely to occur when the molecular weight is less than 500 daltons, the ClogP (calculated octanol–water partition coefficient) is less than five, the number of hydrogen-bond donors is less than five (the sum of O-H and N-H groups), and the number of hydrogen-bond acceptors is less than 10 (the sum of N and O atoms).

Their computational results have been referred to as the "Rule of Five," and it had a major impact on drug discovery in the pharmaceutical industry. The Rule of Five was implemented early on in the drug discovery process for all the drug discovery stages, particularly medicinal chemistry design, to avoid a designed compound with potential absorption and permeability failure. In addition to oral drug absorption, blood-brain barrier (BBB) permeability is very important in medicinal chemistry design and virtual screening. A similar rule system (or "Rule of Two") was proposed by Norinder and Haeberlein (162) to evaluate the good permeability of a compound to cross the BBB: That is, the sum of nitrogen and oxygen (N + O) atoms must be less than or equal to five, and subtracting (N + O) from logP must yield a positive number. A lead compound satisfying these two rules is likely to have positive brain/blood concentration ratio. In summary, both the Rule of Five and the Rule of Two have provided a good starting point for computational and medicinal chemists in designing novel drug molecules. In the following sections, we will discuss the ADME prediction, logP, and solubility prediction methods.

ADME PREDICTION

In Silico ADME Prediction

Nearly 40% of drug candidates fail in clinical trials because of poor ADME. Today, it is widely accepted that ADME prediction plays a critical role in new drug development and that focusing on promising compounds will dramatically reduce the amount of wasted time and resources in the overall development process. Generally, two approaches exist for ADME prediction.

Structural Approach (Molecular Modeling)

The structural approach for ADME prediction is based on the 3D structure of the target protein as determined by x-ray, NMR, or homology modeling of related human protein. Quantum mechanical methods are used to assess the potential for interaction between the small molecules under consideration and the protein involved in the ADME processes. The structural approach can provide concrete and logic interpretation and enables us to understand the QSAR mechanism of drug–receptor interactions in systems. This method is limited, however, by the available 3D protein structures and long computation time. This approach has been used successfully for predicting cytochrome P450 drug metabolism (163) and p-glycoprotein substrates (164).

Data-Based Approach (Data Mining)

Multivariate statistical analyses are performed to search for the correlation between a given property and a set of molecular and structural descriptors of the molecules, including fragment descriptors, topological descriptors, and global physicochemical descriptors. Such a QSAR model was used to predict the property of unknown molecules. Although they are empirical methods, data-based approaches are useful for the prediction of complex physicochemical and biological phenomena. These approaches have been used successfully for predicting human intestinal absorption (165) and oral bioavailability (166). Because of the limited scope of this chapter, interested readers may turn to several reviews in the literature (167,168) regarding the subject of ADME prediction.

To illustrate the basic principle of the ADME prediction method, we give an example of computational protocol for prediction of percentage human intestinal absorption (%HIA) (165). First, the GRID program

(169) is used to create the 3D MIF (Molecular Interaction Fields) maps, which are a 3D matrix containing attractive and repulsive forces between a chemical probe and a target molecule. The VolSurf program (150,170) is then used to compress the information in the 3D maps into a few quantitative, numerical descriptors by multivariate analysis, including principal component analysis and partial least squares. Subsequently correlation between %HIA with the VolSurf descriptors will be established based on the "Training" database set. Furthermore, the HIA model will be used to calculate the %HIA for external compounds with unknown or imprecise human intestinal absorption values. Finally, once the model is created, the computational procedure will be fully automated and fast. Thus, the established protocol can be used a tool for fast virtual screening of lead compounds. Interested readers can find more detailed discussions on this subject in the literatures (165).

The ADME prediction method has been used to predict BBB permeation. As we know, the BBB separates the brain and central nervous system from the bloodstream. The BBB permeation remains a challenge in drug design. Crivori et al. (171) collected 40 agents containing a number of related, but chemically diverse, compounds, which are either high brain-penetrating (BBB+), have a moderate permeation BBB(±), or have little if any ability to cross the BBB (BBB-) (Fig. 3.12). The 3D structure of the compounds was built, and the GRID program was used to calculate the 3D molecular interaction fields. Molecular descriptors were calculated using the VolSurf program. Chemometric tools (principal component analysis and discriminant partial least squares) were used to correlate the data and to build a BBB permeation model. The calculated model is in good agreement with the known molecular factors influencing BBB permeation and predicts more than 90% of the BBB permeation data. The fully automatic and fast computational procedure provides a new tool for virtual screening. Recent review articles have provided detailed descriptions of the techniques and methodologies (170,172,173). Many computational programs are available for performing ADME prediction; popular commercial programs include VolSurf (150), ADME/Tox (174), ACD PhysChem (175), and ADMET (176).

In Silico Prediction of Partition Coefficient logP

The octanol-water partition coefficient, or logP, measures the partition of a compound to between 1-*n*-octanol and water, which in turn is a model for the propensity of a compound to cross membrane barriers via passive diffusion. Basically, logP is the log ratio of the concentrations of the chemicals in the two solvents, logP = log [O]/[W], where O is octanol and W is water. In addition, logP is a measure of the hydrophobicity and hydrophilicity of a chemical. Because the hydrophobic parameter is related to absorption, bioavailability, ligand–receptor

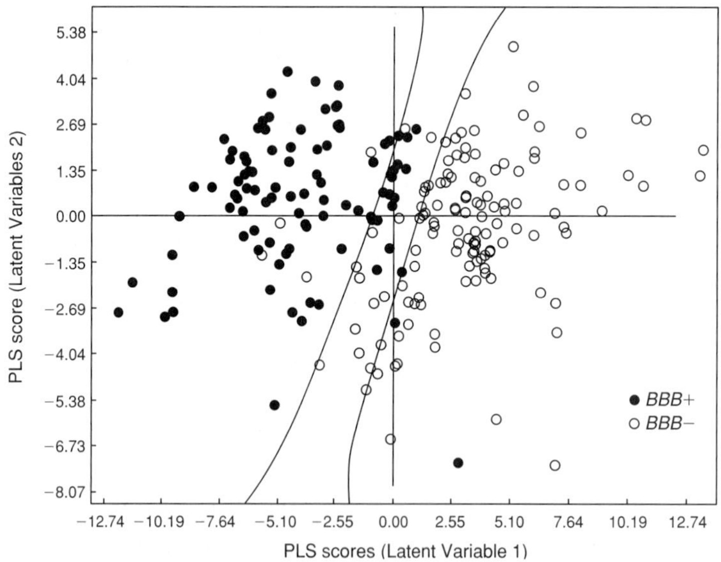

Fig. 3.12. Discriminant partial-least-squares score plot for the global model of blood-brain barrier (BBB) permeability prediction. The model offers a good discrimination and evaluation of a compound's ability to cross the BBB: good permeability, BBB+ (black circles); poor permeability, BBB− (open circles). The model assigned a correct BBB profile to more than 90% of the compounds. A confidence interval is built in the t1-t2 space, where BBB prediction can be borderline and doubtful. (From Crivori P, Cruciani G, Carrupt PA, et al. Predicting blood-brain barrier permeation from three-dimensional molecular structure. J Med Chem 2000;43:2204–2216; with permission.)

interactions, metabolism, and toxicity, logP has become a valuable parameter in many QSAR approaches that have been developed for pharmaceutical, environmental, biochemical, and toxicological sciences. In virtual screening and in silico drug design, logP values often are used to select the lead compounds. For example, Lipinski et. al. (149) has concluded that poor oral drug absorption of permeation are more likely to occur when the ClogP or logP is greater than five.

The value of logP can be measured experimentally or in silico predicted from structural data. Being more accurate than the prediction, measurement of this property is always recommended, but the experimental techniques are very time-consuming. So, it is important to be able to calculate reliable logP values of compounds that are not available for experimental determinations. A large number of different calculation methods have been derived for prediction of chemical logP values. The logP prediction methods can be distinguished into five major classes (177,178), including fragment-based, atomic contribution–based, molecular properties–based, solvatochromic parameters–based, and π-substituent–based methods.

Fragment-Based Method

The fragment-based methods of calculating logP was pioneered by Rekker (179) and further developed by Leo (177) into a widely used ClogP program. Briefly, the method is based on the assumption of the additive nature of hydrophobicity values from different molecular fragments, and the parameter values are calibrated by statistical analysis of a large experimental database. To estimate the logP value of a novel molecule, the chemical structure is first decomposed into smaller fragments that can be recognized by the ClogP program. The logP value of the molecule is simply the incremental sum of parameter values from the composite fragments and, in some cases, additional correction factors by employing the following general equation (180) shown in Figure 3.13,

$$\text{CLogP} = \Sigma fn + \Sigma Fm$$

where f denotes atomic or fragmental increments and F denotes correction factors. The simplified version of the logP calculation shown above was the basis of the hydrophilic–lipophilic values for organic fragments, as illustrated in Fig. 3.13. The main advantage of a fragment-based method is that it tends to be very accurate, because the correction factors play a crucial role in the success of the calculations. On the other hand, the approach suffers from two major problems. The first is that the molecular decomposition process often is very tricky. The second—and more serious—concerns missing parameter values when a given structure cannot be decomposed to structures for which fragment values are available.

The ClogP calculation methods have been widely used for predicting drug logP values in virtual screening studies. For example, ClogP was used to estimate the logP for

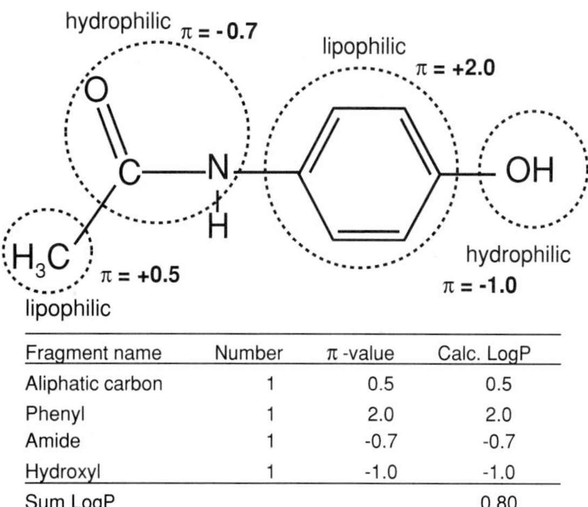

Fragment name	Number	π-value	Calc. LogP
Aliphatic carbon	1	0.5	0.5
Phenyl	1	2.0	2.0
Amide	1	-0.7	-0.7
Hydroxyl	1	-1.0	-1.0
Sum LogP			0.80

Fig. 3.13. LogP calculation gives LogP = 0.80 for acetaminophen (or Tylenol) based on the simplified fragment method (experimentally measured logP = 0.49).

the molecule of o-methylacetanilide (ClogP = 0.90) that is close to the experimental value (logP = 0.86) (181). The fragment-based logP prediction software programs include ClogP (177), ACD/logP (180), kLogP (182), and AB/logP (183).

Other Methods

The other LogP prediction methods include the π-substituent method, atomic contribution method, molecular properties method, and solvatochromic method. The atomic contribution method is similar to the fragment-based methods but uses atomic fragments instead of chemical group fragments (178). The contributions of each atom type and correction factor are derived by multivariate regression analysis of 1,853 organic compound with known experimental logP values. This method provides good estimation results, comparable to those of fragment-based approaches. The available software programs are MOLCAD (184), PrologP (185), SMIlogP (186), and XlogP (178). The π-substituent method (187,188) calculates logP by the replacement of a hydrogen atom on a parent compound of known logP with a π value of the given substituent based on the following equation (177): $\text{logP}_{(\text{Y-R-X})} = \text{logP}_{(\text{H-R-H})} + \pi_{(\text{Y})} + \pi_{(\text{X})}$. For example, the logP value of 3-cyanophenol is calculated to be 1.71, which is comparable with the experimental value of 1.70 (181). The molecular properties–based method (189) computes logP values as a function of different calculated molecular properties, including van der Waals molecular volume (V) and each functional group (N): $\text{logP} = a_1 V + a_2 N$. (Where a_1 and a_2 are coefficients determined by linear regression). The logP value is then determined by the oxygen- or nitrogen-containing functional groups in the molecule and correlates with hydrogen-bonding acceptor basicity. The software programs QlogP and BlogP have been used for studies of benzodiazepine γ-secretase inhibitors (190), Src tyrosine kinase inhibitor

(191), and the enzymatic hydrolysis of noncongener carboxylic esters (192). The solvatochromic approach (193) is, in essence, a molecular properties methodology but with more parameters, including a solute volume (V), solute polarity/polarizability (π^*), solute hydrogen-bond acceptor strength (β_H), solute hydrogen-bond donor strength (α_H), and the intercept (e): $\log P = aV + b\pi^* + c\beta_H + d\alpha_H + e$. The regression coefficients a, b, c, and d, reflect the relative contributions of each solute parameter to log P. The solvatochromic method has been used for predicting the oral absorption potential of peptides (194). Interested readers are encouraged to find more detailed discussions in literatures (195).

In Silico Prediction of Solubility LogS

Another important physicochemical parameter of a drug molecule is the aqueous solubility, often expressed as log units of molar solubility (mol/L), or logS. Aqueous solubility is a key property for all chemical compounds considered as drug lead molecules. Especially in drug discovery research, knowledge of a compound's aqueous solubility can lead to an understanding of its pharmacokinetics as well as an appropriate means of drug formulation. The solubility of organic compounds in water is related to the logP values discussed above and has become increasingly important for studies regarding the oral absorption of pharmaceuticals and the toxicity of chemical compounds.

Several computer programs have been developed for solubility prediction, as described in reviews (196–205). In this chapter, we only describe the commonly used prediction approaches based on logP values. Probably the best-known solubility model that includes crystal forces is the general solubility equation (GSE) (206): $\log(S_0) = -0.01(\text{MP} - 25°\text{C}) - \log P + 0.05$, where S_0 is the intrinsic aqueous solubility in the units of mol/L, logP is the octanol–water partition coefficient, and MP is the melting point (°C). The requirement of a measured melting point, however, has greatly limited use of the GSE in the pharmaceutical industry, because melting point measurements are no longer routine in modern medicinal chemistry. An extension from the GSE equation (e.g., ACD/solubility DB program) was made to use the pH-dependent solubility predictions of compounds with several functional groups (207): $\log S = a\log D + b\text{MW} + c\text{MV} + d\text{BP} + e\text{Hbond} + f\text{Polariz} + h\text{nd}_{20} + i\Sigma\text{Frg} + j$, where logS is solubility (mol/L), logD is the octanol–water partition coefficient for partially dissociated compounds, MW is the molecular weight, MV is McGowan molecular volume, BP is boiling point at 760 torr, Hbond is hydrogen-bond parameter, Polariz is polarizability, nd_{20} is refraction index, ΣFrg is the sum of fragmental increments, and j is the intercept. The regression coefficients a, b, c, and d reflect the relative contributions of each solute parameter to log P, and the interested readers can find the detailed description of various LogS value prediction methods in the recent literature (200,204,205).

In Silico Prediction of pK_a

Another important drug physicochemical phenomenon is the ionization of Brønsted acids and bases in aqueous solution that plays a central role in much of chemistry and biochemistry and that also affects drug in vitro stability and in vivo metabolism activity. The extent of ionization can be represented by the pK_a or ionization constant, which often is used in predicting drug–drug interaction because of the change of acid or base properties. For example, given a weak acid HA, its dissociation in water is subject to the chemical equilibrium:

$$HA \rightleftharpoons H^+ + A^-$$

The pK_a or ionization constant is defined as the negative logarithm of the equilibrium coefficient neutral and charged forms of HA concentration:

$$pK_a = -\log_{10} k_a = -\log_{10}\left[\frac{[H^+][A^-]}{[HA]}\right]$$

Often, pKa values are obtained through experimental measurement of associated and dissociated HA concentrations. Other situations exist, however, in which accurate measurements are difficult. Hence, theoretical prediction models were developed to calculate pK_a values in a variety of chemical systems by various computational techniques, including the classical method by Hammett (208) and Taft (209), the atom type-based pK_a prediction method (210), and the quantum chemistry–based pK_a prediction(211). The latter two methods, however, are more commonly used.

Prediction of pK_a by atom typing is a simple but surprisingly effective method. Typically, the two most influential factors governing pK_a are the atomic species undergoing protonation or deprotonation and the very local steric and electronic affects (210). Among many commercial programs, ACD/pK_a (212) allows rapid and automatic calculation of acid-base ionization constants (pK_a) for large sets of compounds at once. For example, the ACD/pK_a program was used to predict the pK_a of the drug atropine as 10.3 (experimental value of 9.9) (210). Another pK_a calculation is based on quantum chemistry, including density functional computations (211) on a series of aliphatic carboxylic acids, substituted benzoic acids, phenols, anilinium ions, and pyridinium ions (213). Comparison with accurate experimental values indicates that average unsigned errors of generally less than 0.2 pK_a units can be achieved in the calculation of relative pK_a values.

SUMMARY

Computational chemistry provides an array of valuable tools for in silico drug design and virtual screening, and it continues to expand its role in modern drug discovery. Computer molecular modeling, molecular graphic representations, and easy-to-access structural databases have become essential day-to-day components on the desktop of the medicinal chemist. In particular, virtual screening and in silico drug design techniques have become one of the important processes for medicinal chemists to conduct their rational design of novel scaffold compounds and can even predict their bioactivities before being synthesized. Furthermore, commercial software continues to expand on the core user interface, and new algorithms from both industry and academia are quickly incorporated into the high-end packages. Public domain packages are becoming more stable and offering functionality that rivals some of the commercial offerings. Computers continue to double in speed every year and a half as well as terabyte in data disk storage capacity as computational chemistry and cheminformatics become more sophisticated and intuitive.

In addition, emerging new techniques, such as computational enzymology as well as genomic and proteomic search engines, promise to extend the range of molecular modeling tools. The quality of the methods also is improving as greater computer power facilitates greater sampling, longer simulations, and improved statistics. Quantum mechanical calculations are improving the quality of empirical force field parameters and speeding the development of new parameters, such as those currently under development in carbohydrate chemistry for adjuvant studies and lipid bilayer simulations. All of these elements make molecular modeling an integral part of drug design, which is a synthetic, multidisciplinary research process rather than a linear process. As new insights regarding molecular interactions appear, new methods must be developed and incorporated. The extensibility of computational chemistry will ensure that it continues to play a vital role in visualizing and organizing our understanding of molecular interactions and designing novel drugs.

ACKNOWLEDGEMENTS

The author would like to thank Dr. Thomas Lemke for the invitation to write this chapter. Special thanks go to Dr. Eric Billings for his professional input on this chapter and Jian Wang and Dr. Jianzhong Chen for their help on this chapter.

References

1. Hendrickson JB. Molecular geometry. I. Machine computation of the common rings. J Am Chem Soc 1961;83:4537–4547.
2. Bajorath J. Integration of virtual and high-throughout screening. Nature Reviews Drug Discovery 2002,1:882–894.
3. Shen J, Xu X, Cheng F, et al. Virtual screening on natural products for discovering active compounds and target information. Curr Med Chem 2003;10:2327–2342.
4. Seifert MHJ, Wolf K, Vitt D. Virtual high-throughput in silico screening. Biosilico 2003;1:143–149.
5. Schneidman-Duhovny D, Nussinov R, et al. Predicting molecular interactions in silico: II. Protein–protein and protein–drug docking. Curr Med Chem 2004;11:91–107.
6. Kitchen DB, Decornez H, Furr JR, et al. Docking and scoring in virtual screening for drug discovery: methods and applications. Nature Reviews Drug Discovery 2004;3:935–949.
7. Dror O, Shulman-Peleg A, Nussinov R, et al. Predicting molecular interactions in silico: I. A guide to pharmacophore identification and its applications to drug design. Curr Med Chem 2004;11:71–90.
8. Shoichet BK. Virtual screening of chemical libraries. Nature (London) 2004;432:862–865.
9. Thiel KA. Structure-aided drug design's next generation. Nat Biotechnol 2004;22:513–519.
10. Schneider G, Fechner U. Computer-based de novo design of drug-like molecules. Nature Reviews Drug Discovery 2005;4:649–663.
11. Hehre WJ, Rasom L, Schleyer PR, et al. Ab-Initio Molecular Orbital Theory. New York: Wiley, 1986.
12. Frisch MJ, Trucks GW, Schlegel HB: Gaussian 03 (formerly Gaussian 98) online manual http://www.gaussian.com/g_ur/g03mantop.htm. Gaussian, Inc., Wallingford, CT 06492 USA. Accessed May 18, 2006.
13. Gordon MS, Schmidt MW: Advances in electronic structure theory: GAMESS a decade later. In: *Theory and Applications of Computational Chemistry: The First Forty Years* (*Editors,* Dykstra C, Frenking G, Kim K, et al.). Elsevier B.V., Amsterdam, Netherlands; 2005:1167–1189.
14. GAMESS: The General Atomic and Molecular Electronic Structure System. Available at: http://www.msg.ameslab.gov/GAMESS/GAMESS.html. GAMESS is maintained by the members of Mark Gordon's research group at Iowa State University. Accessed May 18, 2006.
15. Guest MF, Bush IJ, Van Dam HJJ, et al. The GAMESS-UK electronic structure packages: algorithms, developments, and applications. Mol Phys 2005;103: 719–747.
16. Salahub DR, Goursot A, Weber J, Koster AM, Vela A: Applied density functional theory and the deMon codes 1964–2004. In: *Theory and Applications of Computational Chemistry: The First Forty Years* (*Editors,* Dykstra C, Frenking G, Kim K, et al.). Elsevier B.V., Amsterdam, Netherlands; 2005:1079–1097.
17. Bickelhaupt FM, Baerends EJ. Kohn-Sham density functional theory: predicting and understanding chemistry. Reviews in Computational Chemistry 2000;15:1–86.
18. Sessler JL, Katayev E, Pantos GD, et al. Fine-tuning the anion-binding properties of 2,6-diamidopyridine dipyrromethane hybrid macrocycles. J Am Chem Soc 2005;127:11442–11446.
19. He X, Mei Y, Xiang Y, et al. Quantum computational analysis for drug resistance of HIV-1 reverse transcriptase to nevirapine through point mutations. Proteins: Structure, Function, and Bioinformatics 2005;61:423–432.
20. Patel MA, Deretey E, Csizmadia IG. Will ab initio and DFT drug design be practical in the 21st century? A case study involving a structural analysis of the β2-adrenergic G protein–coupled receptor. Theochem 1999;492:1–18.
21. Hoffmann M, Rychlewski J. Density functional theory (DFT) and drug design. Reviews of Modern Quantum Chemistry 2002;2:1767–1803.
22. Wrinn MC, Whitehead MA. PCILO: problems in predicting valid structure. Theochem 1986;30:197–205.
23. Pople JA, Segal GA. Approximate self-consistent molecular orbital theory. III. CNDO results for AB2 and AB3 systems. J Chem Phys 1966;44:3289–3296.
24. Sirichote O, Hansongnern K, Sudkeaw P. Vibrational frequencies and structure of estragole using semiempirical calculations. J Sci Soc Thai 1998;24:65–71.
25. Yadav JS, Barnickel G, Bradaczek H, et al. Quantum chemical studies on the conformational structure of bacterial peptidoglycan. II. PCILO calculations on the monosaccharides. J Theor Biol 1982;95:151–166.
26. Dewar MJS, Zoebisch EG, Healy EF, et al. Development and use of quantum mechanical molecular models. 76. AM1: a new general purpose quantum mechanical molecular model. J Am Chem Soc 1985;107:3902–3909.
27. Xie X-Q, Yang D-P, Melvin LS, et al. Conformational analysis of the prototype nonclassical cannabinoid CP-47,497 using 2D NMR and computer molecular modeling. J Med Chem 1994;37:1418–1426.
28. Saldanha JW, Howlin B, Du Toit L, et al. The dynamics of gallamine: a potent neuromuscular blocker. A determination by quantum mechanics and molecular dynamics. I. In vacuo studies. Journal of Computational Chemistry 1989;10:975–981.
29. Sipilae J, Taskinen J. CoMFA modeling of human catechol-O-methyltransferase enzyme kinetics. J Chem Inf Comput Sci 2004;44:97–104.
30. Burkert U, Allinger NL, eds. ACS Monograph 177: Molecular Mechanics. Washington, DC: American Chemical Society, 1986.
31. Hagler AT. Theoretical Stimulation of Conformation, Energetics, and Dynamics of Peptides, vol 7. New York: Academic Press, 1985.
32. Burt SK, Mackay D, Hagler AT. Chapter 3: Theoretical Aspects of Drug Design: Molecular Mechanics and Molecular Dynamics. In: Computer-Aided Drug Design. Methods and Applications. Edited by Perun TJ, Propst CL, New York and Basel: Marcel Dekker, Inc., 1989, pp 55–92.
33. Essmann U, Perera L, Berkowitz ML, et al. A smooth particle mesh Ewald method. J Chem Phys 1995;103:8577–8593.
34. Xie XQ, Chen JZ, Billings EM. 3D structural model of the G protein–coupled cannabinoid CB2 receptor. Proteins: Structure, Function, and Genetics 2003;53:307–319.
35. Dinur U, Hagler AT. New approaches to empirical force fields. Reviews in Computational Chemistry 1991;2:99–164.
36. Weiner SJ, Kollman PA, Nguyen DT, et al. An all-atom force field for simulations of proteins and nucleic acids. Journal of Computational Chemistry 1986;7:230–252.

37. Brooks BR, Bruccoleri RE, Olafson BD, et al. CHARMM: a program for macromolecular energy, minimization, and dynamics calculations. Journal of Computational Chemistry 1983;4:187–217.
38. Dauber-Osguthorpe P, Roberts VA, Osguthorpe DJ, et al. Structure and energetics of ligand binding to proteins: *Escherichia coli* dihydrofolate reductase–trimethoprim, a drug–receptor system. Proteins 1988;4:31–47.
39. Weiner SJ, Kollman PA, Case DA, et al. A new force field for molecular mechanical stimulation of nucleic acids and proteins. J Am Chem Soc 1984;106:765–784.
40. Wang J, Wolf RM, Caldwell JW, et al. Development and testing of a general Amber force field. Journal of Computational Chemistry 2004;25:1157–1174.
41. InsightII/Discover. Available at: http://www.accelrys.com; Accessed May 18, 2006.
42. Hagler AT, Lifson S, Dauber P. Consistent force-field studies of intermolecular forces in hydrogen-bonded crystals. 2. A benchmark for the objective comparison of alternative force fields. J Am Chem Soc 1979;101:5122–5130.
43. Fletcher R, Reeves CM. Function minimization by conjugate gradients. The Computer Journal 1964;7:149–154.
44. Goodsell DS, Olson AJ. Automated docking of substrates to proteins by simulated annealing. Proteins: Structure, Function, and Genetics 1990;8:195–202.
45. Kerr ID, Sankararamakrishnan R, Smart OS, et al. Parallel helix bundles and ion channels: molecular modeling via simulated annealing and restrained molecular dyanamics. Biophys J 1994;67:1501–1515.
46. Hagler AT, Osguthorpe DJ, Dauber-Osguthorpe P, et al. Dynamics and conformational energetics of a peptide hormone: vasopressin. Science 1985;227:1309–1315.
47. Xie X-Q, Melvin LS, Makriyannis A. The conformational properties of the highly selective cannabinoid receptor ligand CP-55,940. J Biol Chem 1996; 271:10640–10647.
48. Xie XQ, Chen JZ. NMR structural comparison of the cytoplasmic juxtamembrane domains of G protein–coupled CB1 and CB2 receptors in membrane-mimetic DPC mixelles. J Biol Chem 2005;280:3605–3612.
49. Metropolis N, Rosenbluth AW, Rosenbluth MN, et al. Equation-of-state calculations by fast computing machines. J Chem Phys 1953;21:1087–1092.
50. Hagler AT, Moult J, Osguthorpe DJ. Monte Carlo simulation of the solvent structure in crystals of a hydrated cyclic peptide. Biopolymers 1980;19: 395–418.
51. Hagler AT, Osguthorpe DJ, Robson B. Monte Carlo simulation of water behavior around the dipeptide N-acetylalanyl-N-methylamide. Science 1980;208:599–601.
52. Mirny L, Shakhnovich E. Protein folding theory: from lattice to all-atom models. Annu Rev Biophys Biomol Struct 2001;30:361–396.
53. Lengauer T, Lemmen C, Rarey M, et al. Novel technologies for virtual screening. Drug Discovery Today 2004;9:27–34.
54. GALAHAD: Genetic Algorithm with Linear Assignment for Hypermolecular Alignment of Datasets. SYBYL version 7.1. Tripos. http://www.tripos.com/data/SYBYL/GALAHAD_9-7-05.pdf. Accessed May 2, 2005.
55. MOE's Pharmacophore Modeling and Structure-Based Design modules are power means to perform ligand-based design and receptor-based design to screen ligand databases for novel lead discovery. Available at: http:/www.chemcomp.com/software.htm. *Molecular Operating Environment (MOE)*. Chemical Computing Group Inc. Montreal Quebec, Canada H3A 2R7. Accessed March 28, 2007.
56. FlexS: Rapid, Shape-Based Screening of Flexible Molecules. http://www.tripos.com/sciTech/inSilicoDisc/virtualScreening/flexs.html. Sybyl 7.01, Tripos, Inc., Accessed May 18, 2006.
57. Sprague PW, Hoffmann R. CATALYST pharmacophore models and their utility as queries for searching 3D databases. In: Computer Assisted Lead Finding and Optimization: Current Tools for Medicinal Chemistry. Edited by Van de Waterbeemd H. Testa, B., Folkers, G. Basel: VCHA, 1997, pp. 225–240.
58. Sprague PW. Automated chemical hypothesis generation and database searching with Catalyst. Perspect Drug Discovery Des 1995;3:1–20.
59. Evers A, Hessler G, Matter H, et al. Virtual screening of biogenic amine-binding G protein–coupled receptors: comparative evaluation of protein- and ligand-based virtual screening protocols. J Med Chem 2005;48: 5448–5465.
60. Kuntz ID, Blaney JM, Oatley SJ, et al. A geometric approach to macromolecule–ligand interactions. J Mol Biol 1982;161:269–288.
61. Cornell WD, Cieplak P, Bayly CI, et al. A second-generation force field for the simulation of proteins, nucleic acids, and organic molecules. J Am Chem Soc 1995;117:5179–5197.
62. Autodock. Autodock program: http://autodock.scripps.edu/. In: The Scripps Research Institute, MB-5, 10550 N. Torrey Pines Rd., La Jolla, CA 92037-1000 U.S.A.: Accessed May 18, 2006.
63. FlexX: Flexibly Dock Ligands into a Binding Site. http://www.biosolveit.de/FlexX/(FlexX was licensed through Tripos Inc.). BioSolveIT GmbH, An der Ziegelei 75, 53757 Sankt Augustin, Germany; Accessed May 18, 2006.
64. Kramer B, Metz G, Rarey M, et al. Ligand docking and screening with FLEXX. Med Chem Res 1999;9:463–478.
65. Rarey M, Kramer B, Lengauer T, et al. A fast, flexible docking method using an incremental construction algorithm. J Mol Biol 1996;261:470–489.
66. Rarey M, Kramer B, Lengauer T. Multiple automatic base selection: protein–ligand docking based on incremental construction without manual intervention. J Comput Aided Mol Des 1997;11:369–384.
67. GOLD: protein–ligand docking. Available at: http://www.ccdc.cam.ac.uk/products/life_sciences/gold/. Accessed May 18, 2006.
68. Jones G, Willett P, Glen RC, et al. Development and validation of a genetic algorithm for flexible docking. J Mol Biol 1997;267:727–748.
69. GLIDE—ligand–receptor docking program. Available at: http://www.schrodinger.com/ProductDescription.php?mID=6&sID=6&cID=0. Accessed May 18, 2006.
70. Accerlyr LigandFit program—the automatic docking of a flexible ligand into a protein active site is a critical step in the process of structure-based design. Available at: http://www.accelrys.com/products/cerius2/cerius2products/c2ligandfit.html. Accessed May 18, 2006.
71. Budin M. FFLD—fragment-based flexible ligand docking by evolutionary optimization (University of Zurich). Biol Chem 2001;382:1365–1372.
72. Pang YP. EUDOC: a computer program for identification of drug interaction sites in macromolecules and drug leads from chemical databases. J Comput Chem 2001;22:1750–1771.
73. Fernandez-Recio J. ICM-DISCO: docking by global energy optimization with fully flexible side chains. Proteins 2003;52:113–117.
74. Finn PW, Snarey M. Flexible three-dimensional database searching for the identification of novel lead compounds. In: Bioactive Compound Design. Ford, Martyn G. (ed), Oxford, UK: Bios Scientific Publishers, 1996; pp. 67–76.
75. Murrall NW, Davies EK. Conformational freedom in 3-D databases. I. Techniques. J Chem Inf Comput Sci 1990;30:312–316.
76. Catalyst. Catalyst is a database program package from Accelrys. 1998.
77. Kearsley SK, Underwood DJ, Sheridan RP, et al. Flexibases: a way to enhance the use of molecular docking methods. J Comput Aided Mol Des 1994;8:565–582.
78. Ho CMW, Marshall GR. FOUNDATION: a program to retrieve all possible structures containing a user-defined minimum number of matching query elements from three-dimensional databases. J Comput Aided Mol Des 1993;7:3–22.
79. Sheridan RP, Rusinko A III, Nilakantan R, et al. Searching for pharmacophores in large coordinate databases and its use in drug design. Proc Natl Acad Sci U S A 1989;86:8165–8169.
80. Bohm HJ. On the use of LUDI to search the Fine Chemicals Directory for ligands of proteins of known three-dimensional structure. J Comput Aided Mol Des 1994;8:623–632.
81. Lawrence MC, Davis PC. CLIX: a search algorithm for finding novel ligands capable of binding proteins of known three-dimensional structure. Proteins 1992;12:31–41.
82. Miller MD, Kearsley SK, Underwood DJ, et al. FLOG: a system to select "quasi-flexible" ligands complementary to a receptor of known three-dimensional structure. J Comput Aided Mol Des 1994;8:153–174.
83. Bissantz C, Folkers G, Rognan D. Protein-based virtual screening of chemical databases. I. Evaluation of different docking/scoring combination. J Med Chem 2000;43:4759–4767.
84. Claussen H, Buning C, Rarey M, et al. FlexE: efficient molecular docking considering protein structure variations. J Mol Biol 2001;308:377–395.
85. Humblet C, Dunbar JB Jr. 3D database searching and docking strategies. Annu Rep Med Chem 1993;28:275–284.
86. Goodford PJ. A computational procedure for determining energetically favorable binding sites on biologically important macromolecules. J Med Chem 1985;28:849–857.
87. Stahura FL, Bajorath J. New methodologies for ligand-based virtual screening. Curr Pharm Des 2005;11:1189–1202.
88. Van Drie JH. Strategies for the determination of pharmacophoric 3D database queries. J Comput Aided Mol Des 1997;11:39–52.
89. Mason JS, Cheney DL. Library design and virtual screening using multiple 4-point pharmacophore fingerprints. In: Pacific Symposium on Biocomputing 2000, Altman, Russ B. (ed) Honolulu: Publisher: World Scientific Publishing Co. Pte. Ltd., Singapore; 2000: 576–587.
90. Wang S, Sakamuri S, Enyedy IJ, et al. Discovery of a novel dopamine transporter inhibitor, 4-hydroxy-1-methyl-4-(4-methylphenyl)-3-piperidyl 4-methylphenyl ketone, as a potential cocaine antagonist through 3D-database pharmacophore searching. Molecular modeling, structure–activity relationships, and behavioral pharmacological studies. J Med Chem 2000;43:351–360.
91. Bajorath J. Selected concepts and investigations in compound classification, molecular descriptor analysis, and virtual screening. J Chem Inf Comput Sci 2001;41:233–245.
92. Livingstone DJ. The characterization of chemical structures using molecular properties: a survey. J Chem Inf Comput Sci 2000;40:195–209.
93. Spellmeyer DC, Grootenhuis PDJ. Recent developments i molecular diversity. Computational approaches to combinatorial chemistry. Annu Rep Med Chem 1999;34:287–296.
94. MacCuish J, Nicolaou C, MacCuish NE. Ties in proximity and clustering compounds. J Chem Inf Comput Sci 2001;41:134–146.
95. Oprea TI. Property distribution of drug-related chemical databases. J Comput Aided Mol Des 2000;14:251–264.
96. Moon JB, Howe WJ. 3D database searching and de novo construction methods in molecular design. Tetrahedron Computer Methodology 1990;3:697–711.
97. Joseph-McCarthy D. Computational approaches to structure-based ligand design. Pharmacol Ther 1999;84:179–191.

98. Moon JB, Howe WJ. Computer design of bioactive molecules: a method for receptor-based de novo ligand design. Proteins 1991;11:314–328.
99. Nishibata Y, Itai A. Automatic creation of drug candidate structures based on receptor structure. Starting point for artificial lead generation. Tetrahedron 1991;47:8985–8990.
100. Kuntz ID. Structure-based strategies for drug design and discovery. Science 1992;257:1078–1082.
101. Halperin I, Ma B, Wolfson H, et al. Principles of docking: an overview of search algorithms and a guide to scoring functions. Proteins: Structure, Function, and Genetics 2002;47:409–443.
102. Willett P, Barnard JM, Downs GM. Chemical similarity searching. J Chem Inf Comput Sci 1998;38:983–996.
103. Rusinko A III, Sheridan RP, Nilakantan R, et al. J Using CONCORD to construct a large database of three-dimensional coordinates from connection tables. Chem Inf Comput Sci 1989;29:251–255.
104. Daylight theory manual: Daylight 4.62. Chemical Information Systems; 1999.
105. Pearlman RS, Smith KM. Software for chemical diversity in the context of accelerated drug discovery. Drugs of the Future 1998;23:885–895.
106. Clark RD. OptiSim: an extended dissimilarity selection method for finding diverse representative subsets. J Chem Inf Comput Sci 1997;37:1181–1188.
107. Diversity and similarity analysis software program. Available at: http: //software.timtec.net/ched/ched_diversity.htm; Accessed May 18, 2006.
108. Davis AM, Teague SJ, Kleywegt GJ. Application and limitations of x-ray crystallographic data in structure-based ligand and drug design. Angewandte Chemie 2003;42:2718–2736.
109. Palczewski K, Kumasaka T, Hori T, et al. Crystal structure of rhodopsin: a G protein–coupled receptor. Science 2000;289:739–745.
110. Kasimova MR, Kristensen SM, Howe PWA, et al. NMR studies of the backbone flexibility and structure of human growth hormone: a comparison of high and low pH conformations. J Mol Biol 2002;318:679–695.
111. Oshiro C, Bradley EK, Eksterowicz J, et al. Performance of 3D-database molecular docking studies into homology models. J Med Chem 2004;47:764–767.
112. Schapira M, Raaka BM, Samuels HH, et al. In silico discovery of novel retinoic acid receptor agonist structures. Bio Med Central 2001;1:1.
113. Schapira M, Raaka BM, Das S, et al. Discovery of diverse thyroid hormone receptor antagonists by high-throughput docking. Proc Natl Acad Sci U S Am 2003;100:7354–7359.
114. Vangrevelinghe E, Zimmermann K, Schoepfer J, et al. Discovery of a potent and selective protein kinase CK2 inhibitor by high-throughput docking. J Med Chem 2003;46:2656–2662.
115. Xiong B, Gui C-S, Xu X-Y, et al. A 3D model of SARS_CoV 3CL proteinase and its inhibitors: design by virtual screening. Acta Pharmacol Sin 2003;24:497–504.
116. Honma T, Hayashi K, Aoyama T, et al. Structure-based generation of a new class of potent Cdk4 inhibitors: new de novo design strategy and library design. J Med Chem 2001;44:4615–4627.
117. Shakespeare W, Yang M, Bohacek R, et al. Structure-based design of an osteoclast-selective, nonpeptide Src homology 2 inhibitor with in vivo antiresorptive activity. Proc Natl Acad Sci U S A 2000;97:9373–9378.
118. Tripos SiteID: identify and visualize protein-binding sites Available at: http://www.tripos.com/data/SYBYL/SYBYLBH.pdf. Accessed March 28, 2007.
119. Hendlich M, Rippmann F, Barnickel G. LIGSITE: automatic and efficient detection of potential small molecule-binding in proteins. J Mol Graph Model 1997;15:359–363,389.
120. Peters KP, Fauck J, Froemmel C. The automatic search for ligand-binding sites in proteins of known three-dimensional structure using only geometric criteria. J Mol Biol 1996;256:201–213.
121. Brady GP Jr, Stouten PFW. Fast prediction and visualization of protein binding pockets with PASS. J Comput Aided Mol Des 2000;14:383–401.
122. Bliznyuk AA, Gready JE. Identification and energetic ranking of possible docking sites for pterin on dihydrofolate reductase. J Comput Aided Mol Des 1998;12:325–333.
123. Laskowski RA, Thornton JM, Humblet C, et al. X-SITE: use of empirically derived atomic packing preferences to identify favorable interaction regions in the binding sites of proteins. J Mol Biol 1996;259:175–201.
124. Tripos MOLCAD modules: sophisticated graphical rendering of molecular surfaces and properties. Available at: http://www.tripos.com/data/SYBYL/Molcad_072505.pdf. Accessed March 28, 2007.
125. Chen J, Han X, Lan R, et al. 3D-QSAR studies of arylpyrazole antagonists of cannabinoid receptor subtypes CB1 and CB2. A combined NMR and CoMFA approach. J Med Chem 2006;49:625–636.
126. Xie X-Q, Eissenstat M, Makriyannis A. Common cannabimimetic pharmacophoric requirements between aminoalkyl indoles and classical cannabinoids. Life Sci 1995;56:1963–1970.
127. Martin YC. Distance comparisons: a new strategy for examining three-dimensional structure–activity relationships. ACS Symp Ser 1995;606:318–329.
128. CoMFA (Comparative Molecular Field Analysis). Available at: http://www.tripos.com/admin/LitCtr/advcomfa.pdf. TRIPOS, Associates, Inc., St.Louis, MI 63144. Accessed March 28, 2007.
129. Sufrin JR, Dunn DA, Marshall GR. Steric mapping of the L-methionine binding site of ATP: L-methionine S-adenosyltransferase. Mol Pharmacol 1981;19:307–313.
130. Cramer RD III, Patterson DE, Bunce JD. Comparative molecular field analysis (CoMFA). 1. Effect of shape on binding of steroids to carrier proteins. J Am Chem Soc 1988;110:5959–5967.
131. DePriest SA, Mayer D, Naylor CB, et al. 3D-QSAR of angiotensin-converting enzyme and thermolysin inhibitors: a comparison of CoMFA models based on deduced and experimentally determined active site geometries. J Am Chem Soc 1993;115:5372–5384.
132. Greco G, Novellino E, Silipo C, et al. Comparative molecular field analysis on a set of muscarinic agonists. Quant Struct-Act Relat 1991;10:289–299.
133. DISCO (DIStance COmparison) was developed by Dr. Yvonne Martin and coworkers at Abbott Laboratories and distributed by Tripos Associates, St. Louis, MO. 2000.
134. Marriott DP, Dougall IG, Meghani P, et al. Lead generation using pharmacophore mapping and three-dimensional database searching: application to muscarinic M3 receptor antagonists. J Med Chem 1999;42:3210–3216.
135. Toy-Palmer A, Wu H, Liu X. Ligand docking in a muscarinic G protein–coupled receptor model. Med Chem Res 1999;9:565–578.
136. Spadoni G, Balsamini C, Diamantini G, et al. Conformationally restrained melatonin analogues: synthesis, binding affinity for the melatonin receptor, evaluation of the biological activity, and molecular modeling study. J Med Chem 1997;40:1990–2002.
137. Jones GW, P., Glen RC. Genetic algorithm superposition program. In: Pharmacophore Perception, Development, and Use in Drug Design. La Jolla, CA: International University Line, 2000:85–106.
138. Clement OO, Mehl AT. HipHop: pharmacophores based on multiple common-feature alignments. In: Pharmacophore Perception, Development, and Use in Drug Design. La Jolla, CA: International University Line, 2000:69–84.
139. Li H, Sutter J, Hoffmann R. HypGen: an automated system for generating 3D predictive pharmacophore models. In: Pharmacophore Perception, Development, and Use in Drug Design. La Jolla, CA: International University Line, 2000:171–189.
140. Dixon SL, Smondyrev AM, Rao SN: PHASE: a novel approach to pharmacophore modeling and 3D database searching. Chemical Biology & Drug Design 2006;67(5):370–372.
141. Holliday JD, Willett P. Using a genetic algorithm to identify common structural features in sets of ligands. J Mol Graph Model 1997;15:221–232.
142. Finn PW, Kavarki LE; Latombe JC, Motwani R, et al. Computational Geometry: Theory and Applications 1998,10:263–272.
143. MOE's Pharmacophore Modeling and Structure-Based Design modules are power means to perform ligand-based design and receptor-based design to screen ligand databases for novel lead discovery. Available at: http://www.chemcomp.com/software.htm. Molecular Operating Environment (MOE). Chemical Computing Group Inc. Montreal Quebec, Canada H3A 2R7. Accessed March 28, 2007.
144. Chen X, Rusinko A III, Tropsha A, et al. Automated pharmacophore identification for large chemical data sets. J Chem Inf Comput Sci 1999;39: 887–896.
145. Sheridan RP, Nilakantan R, Dixon JS, et al. The ensemble approach to distance geometry: application to the nicotinic pharmacophore. J Med Chem 1986;29:899–906.
146. Chuman H, Karasawa M, Sasaki M, et al. Exhaustive parallel conformational search of pyrethroids and structure similarity study. J Chem Software 1998;4:143–156.
147. Bradshaw J. Introduction to Tversky similarity measure. In: 11th Annual Daylight User Group Meeting. Available at http://www.daylight.com/meetings/mug97/Bradshaw/MUG97/tv_tversky.html. Accessed March 28, 2007.
148. Tripos UNITY module. Available at: http://www.tripos.com/data/SYBYL/Unity_072505.pdf. Accessed March 28, 2007.
149. Lipinski CA, Lombardo F, Dominy BW, et al. Experimental and computational approaches to estimate solubility and permeability in drug discovery and development settings. Drug Deliv Rev 1997;23:3–25.
150. VolSurf—calculate ADME properties and create predictive ADME models Available at: http://www.moldiscovery.com/soft_volsurf.php and http://www.tripos.com/data/SYBYL/volsurf_072505.pdf. Accessed March 28, 2007.
151. Greenidge PA, Carlsson B, Bladh L-G, et al. Pharmacophores incorporating numerous excluded volumes defined by x-ray crystallographic structure in three-dimensional database searching: application to the thyroid hormone receptors. J Med Chem 1998;41:2503–2512.
152. Van Drie JH. Pharmacophore discovery—lessons learned. Curr Pharm Des 2003;9:1649–1664.
153. Wang S, Zaharevitz DW, Sharma R, et al. The discovery of novel, structurally diverse protein kinase C agonists through computer 3D-database pharmacophore search: molecular modeling studies. J Med Chem 1994;37:4479–4489.
154. Carlson HA, Masukawa KM, Rubins K, et al. Developing a dynamic pharmacophore model for HIV-1 integrase. J Med Chem 2000;43:2100–2114.
155. Leysen D, Kelder J. Ligands for the 5-HT2C receptor as potential antidepressants and anxiolytics.Pharmacochem Libr 1998;29:49–61.
156. Doman TN, McGovern SL, Witherbee BJ, et al. Molecular docking and high-throughput screening for novel inhibitors of protein tyrosine phosphatase-1B. J Med Chem 2002;45:2213–2221.
157. Available Chemicals Directory:MDL® database is a chemical database providing access to pricing and supplier information for more than 400,000 research-grade and bulk chemicals. Available at: http://www.mdl.com. Accessed March 28, 2007.

158. Paiva AM, Vanderwall DE, Blanchard JS, et al. Inhibitors of hydrodipicolinate reductase, a key enzyme of the diaminopimelate pathway of *Mycobacterium tuberculosis*. Biochim Biophys Acta 2001;1545:67–77.
159. Singh J, van Vlijmen H, Liao Y, et al. Identification of potent and novel a4b1 antagonists using in silico screening. J Med Chem 2002;45:2988–2993.
160. Grueneberg S, Stubbs MT, Klebe G. Successful virtual screening for novel inhibitors of human carbonic anhydrase: strategy and experimental confirmation. J Med Chem 2002;45:3588–3602.
161. Stahura FL, Xue L, Godden JW, et al. Methods for compound selection focused on hits and application in drug discovery. J Mol Graph Model 2002;20:439–446.
162. Norinder U, Haeberlein M. Computational approaches to the prediction of the blood-brain barrier. Adv Drug Deliv Rev 2002;54:291–313.
163. Vermeulen NP. Prediction of drug metabolism: the case of cytochrome P450 2D6. Curr Top Med Chem 2003;3:1227–1239.
164. Cartmell J, Enoch S, Krstajic D, et al. Automated QSPR through competitive workflow. J Comput Aided Mol Des 2005;19:821–833.
165. Zhao YH, Le J, Abraham MH, et al. Evaluation of human intestinal absorption data and subsequent derivation of a quantitative structure–activity relationship (QSAR) with the Abraham descriptors. J Pharm Sci 2001;90:749–784.
166. Yoshida F, Topliss JG. QSAR model for drug human oral bioavailability. J Med Chem 2000;43:2575–2585.
167. Ekins S, Waller CL, Swaan PW, et al. Progress in predicting human ADME parameters in silico. J Pharmacol Toxicol Methods 2000;44:251–272.
168. Van de Waterbeemd H. Which in vitro screens guide the prediction of oral absorption and volume of distribution? Basic Clin Pharmacol Toxicol 2005;96:162–166.
169. Clementi S, Cruciano G, Fifi P, Riganelli D, et al. New set of principal properties for heteroaromatics obtained by GRID. Quant Struct-Act Relat 1995;15:108–120.
170. Ooms F, Weber P, Carrupt PA, et al. A simple model to predict blood-brain barrier permeation from 3D molecular fields. Biochim Biophys Acta 2002;1587:118–125.
171. Crivori P, Cruciani G, Carrupt PA, et al. Predicting blood-brain barrier permeation from three-dimensional molecular structures. J Med Chem 2000;43:2204–2216.
172. Narayanan R, Gunturi SB. In silico ADME modeling: prediction models for blood-brain barrier permeation using a systematic variable selection method. Bioorg Med Chem 2005;13:3017–3028.
173. Clark DE, Grootenhuis PD. Predicting passive transport in silico—history, hype, and hope. Curr Top Med Chem 2003;3:1193–1203.
174. Cerius2 ADME/Tox Package. Aviailable at: http://www.accelrys.com/products/datasheets/c2_adme_us_data.pdf:. Accessed March 28, 2007.
175. ACD/PhysChem batch program. Advanced Chemistry Development, Toronto, Ontario, Canada.
176. ADMET Modeler. Simulations Plus, Lancaster, CA.
177. Leo AJ. Calculating log Poct from structures. Chem Rev 1993;93:1281–1306.
178. Eros D, Kovesdi I, Orfi L, et al. Reliability of logP predictions based on calculated molecular descriptors: a critical review. Curr Med Chem 2002;9:1819–1829.
179. Rekker R. The Hydrophobic Fragmental Constant. Amsterdam: Elsevier Scientific Publishing; 1977.
180. Petrauskas AA, Kolovanov EA. Perspectives in drug discovery and design. ACD/Log P Method Description 2000,19:99–116.
181. Leo A, Jow PY, Silipo C, et al. Calculation of hydrophobic constant (logP) from pi and f constants. J Med Chem 1975;18:865–868.
182. Klopman G, Li J-Y, Wang S, et al. Computer automated logP calculations based on an extended group contribution approach. J Chem Inf Comput Sci 1994;34:735–744.
183. Japertas P, Didziapetris R, Petrauskas A. Fragmental methods in the design of new compounds. Applications of the advanced algorithm builder. Quant Struct-Act Relat 2002;21:23–37.
184. Broto P, Moreau G, Vandycke C. Molecular structures: perception, autocorrelation descriptor, and SAR studies. Systemic of atomic contributions for the calculation of the n-octanol/water partition coefficients. Eur J Med Chem 1984;19:71–78.
185. proLogP. Pallas PrologP. Sedona, AZ: CompuDrug International, Inc.
186. Convard T, Dubost J-P, Le Solleu H. SmilogP: a program for a fast evaluation of theoretical log P from the SMILES code of a molecule. Quant Struct-Act Relat 1994;13:34–37.
187. Fujita T. Substituent effects in the partition coefficient of disubstituted benzenes: bidirectional Hammett-type relationships. Progress in Physical Organic Chemistry 1983;14:75–113.
188. Fujita T, Iwasa J, Hansch C. A new substituent constant, π, derived from partition coefficients. J Am Chem Soc 1964;86:5175–5180.
189. Bodor N, Buchwald P. Molecular size–based approach to estimate partition properties for organic solutes. J Phys Chem B 1997;101:3404–3412.
190. Ravi KA, Ashok KB, Parthasarathy T, et al. QSAR studies–potent benzodiazepine γ-secretase inhibitors. Bioorg Med Chem 2005;13:1873–1878.
191. Kumar BA, Ramasree D, Parthasarathy T, et al. QSAR studies of amino propyl tetrahydro indole–based indolin-2-ones as potent inhibitor of Src tyrosine kinase. Journal of Teaching and Research in Chemistry 2004;11:20–24.
192. Buchwald P, Bodor N. Quantitative structure–metabolism relationships: steric and nonsteric effects in the enzymatic hydrolysis of noncongener carboxylic esters. J Med Chem 1999;42:5160–5168.
193. Kamlet MJ, Abboud J-LM, Abraham MH, et al. Linear solvation energy relationships. 23. A comprehensive collection of the solvatochromic parameters, p*, a, and b, and some methods for simplifying the generalized solvatochromic equation. J Org Chem 1983;48:2877–2887.
194. Paterson DA, Conradi RA, Hilgers AR, et al. A nonaqueous partitioning system for predicting the oral absorption potential of peptides. Quant Struct-Act Relat 1994;13:4–10.
195. Mannhold R. The impact of lipophilicity in drug research: a case report on β-blockers. Mini-Reviews in Medicinal Chemistry 2005;5:197–205.
196. McFarland JW, Du CM, Avdeef A. Factors influencing the water solubilities of crystalline drugs. Methods and Principles in Medicinal Chemistry 2003;55:1163–1183.
197. Polanski J. Prediction of physicochemical properties based on neural network modeling. Adv Drug Deliv Rev 2003;55:1149–1162.
198. Erös D, Kéri G, Kövesdi I, et al. Comparison of predictive ability of water solubility QSPR models generated by MLR, PLS, and ANN methods. Mini-Reviews in Medicinal Chemistry 2004;4:167–177.
199. Jorgensen WL, Duffy EM. Prediction of drug solubility from structure. Adv Drug Deliv Rev 2002;54:355–366.
200. Delaney JS. Predicting aqueous solubility from structure. Drug Discovery Today 2005;10:289–295.
201. Lombardo F, Gifford E, Shalaeva MY. In silico ADME prediction: data, models, facts, and myths. Mini-Reviews in Medicinal Chemistry 2003;3:861–875.
202. Lipinski CA. Aqueous solubility in discovery, chemistry, and assay changes. Methods and Principles in Medicinal Chemistry 2003;18:215–231.
203. Valko K. Measurements and predictions of physicochemical properties. High-Throughput ADMETox Estimation 2002;1–24:A1–A5.
204. Jónsdóttir SO, Jørgensen FS, Brunak S. Prediction methods and databases within chemoinformatics: emphasis on drugs and drug candidates. Bioinformatics 2005;21:2145–2160.
205. Johnson SR, Zheng W. Recent progress in the computational prediction of aqueous solubility and absorption. AAPS J 2006;8:E27–E40.
206. Sanghvi T, Jain N, Yang G, et al. Estimation of aqueous solubility by the general solubility equation (GSE): the easy way. QSAR and Combinatorial Science 2003;22:258–262.
207. ACD/solubilityDB. Advanced Chemistry Development, Toronto, Ontario, Canada.
208. Hammett LP. Physical Organic Chemistry. New York: McGraw-Hill, 1940.
209. Taft RWJ. Separation of polar, steric, and resonance effects in reactivity. In: Newman MS, ed. Steric effects in organic chemistry. New York: Wiley, 1956:556–675.
210. Sayle R. Physiological ionization and pK_a prediction. In: EuroMUG 2000. Available at: http://www.daylight.com/meetings/emug00/Sayle/pkapredict.html. Cambridge, England: 2000;19–20 September.
211. Adam KR. New density functional and atoms in molecules method of computing relative pK_a values in solution. J Phys Chem A 2002;106:11963–11972.
212. ACD/pKaBatch. Advanced Chemistry Development, Toronto, Ontario, Canada.
213. Barone V, Cossi MJ. Quantum calculation of molecular energies and energy gradients in solution by a conductor solvent model. J Phys Chem A 1998;102:1995–2001.

4. *Receptors and Drug Action*

TIMOTHY J. MAHER AND DAVID A. JOHNSON

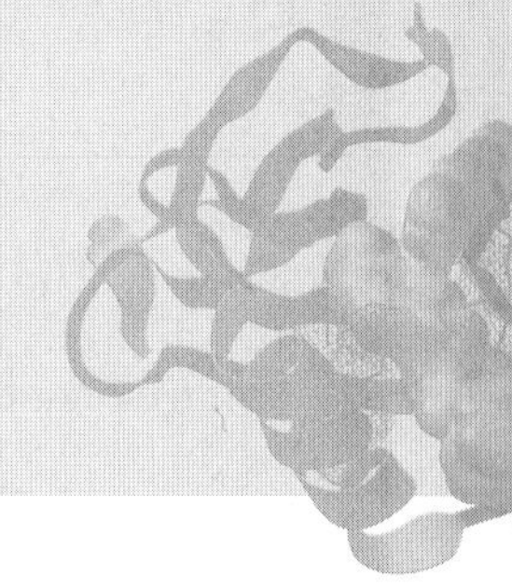

INTRODUCTION

The human body is an example of an exquisitely designed, extremely complex machine that functions day-in and day-out to allow for survival of the organism in response to a never-ending onslaught of external challenges. When one considers the enormous variety of environmental stressors to which the body is continually subjected, it is not surprising to anticipate the existence of a multitude of checks and balances associated with its physiological and biochemical systems. These systems, including endocrine, nervous, and enzymatic, typically function in concert to adapt to changing environmental conditions. Some systems are designed to respond quickly (i.e., within milliseconds) and for a short time; others are designed to act more slowly but usually have significantly longer durations (i.e., months to years). Together, these systems support the organism's survival. Often, however, malfunctioning of the control of such systems leads to disease and, potentially, the eventual demise of the individual.

The use of specific chemical compounds to treat disease dates back to early humans. Many primitive cultures used plants and other natural sources in an attempt to mitigate the influences of evil spirits and other factors rooted in superstition, which were believed to be the foundations of such illnesses. Over the centuries, a number of serendipitous observations involving the ability of largely botanical preparations to alter disease processes laid the foundation for the modern, more systematic approach to the discovery of medicinals for therapeutic use. The collaboration of chemical and biological scientists continue this quest for the "magic bullet" to treat those diseases that challenge the individual's well-being.

HISTORICAL PERSPECTIVES

For years, it had been known that some drugs were capable of producing their effects by acting at specific sites within the body. Claude Bernard was the first to demonstrate this in the mid-1800s, with his classical experiments involving curare (1). He showed that this neuromuscular blocking agent, which was used as an arrow poison by the South American natives, was capable of preventing skeletal muscle contraction following nerve stimulation, but was without effect when the muscle was stimulated directly. This work demonstrated for the first time a localized site of action for a drug and, most importantly, suggested that a gap, or synapse, existed between the nerve and the muscle. From these findings, he also postulated that some chemical substance normally communicated the information between the nerve and the target tissue—in this case, the muscle. These findings established the foundations for what is known today as "chemical neurotransmission," a process frequently disrupted by diseases and, likewise, the target of many therapeutic agents.

Investigations by J.N. Langley (2) in the early 1900s established the initial foundations for the interaction of drugs with specific cellular components, later to be identified and termed "receptors." Before this time, many leading experts believed that most drugs acted nonselectively on virtually all the cells in the body to produce their biological responses, with a response resulting from their general physical characteristics (e.g., lipid solubility) and not related to specific structural features of the compound. Langley noted that compounds like pilocarpine, which act to mimic the parasympathetic division of the autonomic nervous system, were very selective and also extremely potent. Additionally, a compound like atropine was capable of blocking, in a rather selective fashion, the effects of pilocarpine and parasympathetic nervous system stimulation. Importantly, he concluded that these two compounds interacted with the same component of the cell.

Paul Ehrlich (3), a noted microbiologist during the late 19th and early 20th centuries, is credited with coining the term "receptive substance," or "receptor." His observations that various organic compounds appeared to produce their antimicrobial effects with a high degree of selectivity led him to speculate that drugs produced their effects via binding to such a receptive substance. The interaction of the drug with the receptor was analogous to a "lock" and "key." Thus, certain organic compounds would fit properly into the receptor and activate it, leading to a high degree of specificity. Although such a situation might be considered to be ideal for drug therapy, few drugs actually interact only with their intended receptors. The frequency of side effects not associated with a simple extension of their desired pharmacological actions indicates that drug molecules also can combine with other receptors or nonreceptor entities on or within cells to produce a host of other—and often undesirable—effects.

Some drugs produce their desired effects without interaction with a specific receptor. For instance, osmotic diuretics produce their pharmacological effects simply by creating an osmotic gradient in the renal tubules and, thereby, foster the elimination of water in the urine. This is purely the result of a physical characteristic of the drug. Similarly, antacids produce their beneficial effects by chemically neutralizing the hydrochloric acid found in the gastrointestinal tract. No absorption of the drug is even required for its effects to be realized. Often, the failure of a drug to be absorbed and, thus, only act locally at the desired biological site constitutes a tremendous advantage regarding the safety of that compound. Unfortunately, from a practical standpoint, most pharmacological agents require absorption following administration to reach the intended target; thus, side effects typically are a serious consideration.

More sophisticated mechanisms also can be involved in the nonreceptor actions of therapeutic agents. For instance, the antineoplastic agent mechlorethamine, a nitrogen mustard, produces its beneficial (pharmacologic) and adverse (toxicologic) effects via interaction with many cellular components in both cancerous and normal cells. Via its conversion to a highly reactive electrophilic ethyleniminium ion intermediate, this agent reacts with nucleophilic cellular components, such as amino, hydroxyl, sulfhydryl, phosphate, carboxyl, and imidazole groups. In particular, by alkylating the N-7 position of guanine in DNA, this agent produces miscoding (cytosine normally base pairs with guanine in DNA; however, thymine now substitutes for cytosine) and the eventual death of the cell (4). When one realizes that all replicating cells contain an N-7 nitrogen in guanine in their DNA, it is easy to see why mechlorethamine produces nonselective destruction of cells throughout the body. Thus, no specific receptor is involved in the actions of this class of pharmacological agent.

AFFINITY—THE ROLE OF CHEMICAL BONDING

During the early 1900s, A.V. Hill used nicotine and curare in isolated muscle preparations and noted the effects of temperature in his experiments (1). He concluded that the ability of a drug to produce an effect must result from specific chemical interactions between the drug and specific sites. He also noted that the effects of many drugs were reversible, because washing the isolated tissue often restored the sensitivity of the tissue to nerve stimulation. These studies set the foundation for our understandings of the chemical interactions between drugs and receptors.

When a drug interacts with a receptor, a number of chemical attractive forces are believed to be responsible for the initial interaction. Compounds that are attracted to a receptor macromolecule are said to have affinity for that receptor and may be classified as agonists or antagonists. Additionally, compounds with affinity also are referred to as ligands. Agonists are those compounds that have affinity for the receptor and are capable of producing a biological response as a result of its interaction with the receptor (5). As will be noted later, the ability to produce a response is termed "efficacy," or "intrinsic activity." Drugs that are capable of interacting with the receptor but not of activating it to produce a response are classified as antagonists. This class of drug is said to have affinity, but it lacks intrinsic activity. The affinity of a compound for a receptor is dependent on its proper three-dimensional characteristics, such as its size, stereochemical orientation of its functional groups, and its physical and electrochemical properties (e.g., ionic and dipole interactions).

Assuming that a compound has been distributed to the general vicinity of a receptor, based on its physical characteristics, the binding of the drug to the receptor will then initially depend on the types of chemical bonds that can be established between the drug and its receptor. The overall strengths of these bonds will vary (Fig. 4.1) and will determine the degree of affinity between the drug and the receptor.

Covalent Bond

The strongest of bonds involved in drug–receptor interactions is the covalent bond, in which two atoms, one from the ligand and one from the receptor, share a pair of electrons. Because of the significant strength of the covalent bond (50–150 kcal/mol), covalent bonding often produces a situation in which the ligand is irreversibly bound by the receptor and, thus, leads to the receptor's eventual destruction via endocytosis and chemical destruction. Full recovery of cellular function therefore requires the synthesis of new receptors.

An example of an irreversible covalent bond formation between drug and receptor involves the long-lasting blockade of α-adrenoceptors by phenoxybenzamine (see Chapter 13). Once phenoxybenzamine is converted to a highly reactive carbonium ion intermediate, this haloalkylamine can covalently link, via alkylation with amino, sulfhydryl or carboxyl groups at the α-adrenoceptor. The receptor is thus rendered irreversibly nonfunctional and, eventually, destroyed. The synthesis of new receptor requires a number of days, thus accounting for the extremely prolonged duration of the block associated with this agent. As will be discussed below, this property of phenoxybenzamine to irreversibly bind the α-adrenoceptor was critical for the demonstration of spare receptors (6,7). Because other receptors and cellular components also contain molecular groups that are likewise capable of interacting with the activated phenoxybenzamine intermediate, it is not surprising to find that receptors that mediate the actions of other

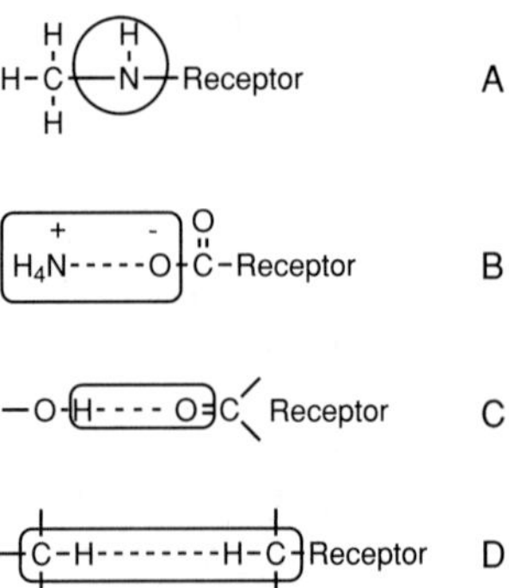

Fig. 4.1. Various drug–receptor bonds. (A) Covalent. (B) Ionic. (C) Hydrogen. (D) Hyrdophobic.

neurotransmitters (e.g., acetylcholine, serotonin, and histamine) also are subject to alkylation and blockade, demonstrating the lack of selectivity of phenoxybenzamine.

Another important example of a class of compounds that produces its effects via a covalent bond to its receptor are the organophosphate acetylcholinesterase inhibitors. Examples of such agents include the insecticides parathion and malathion and the nerve-gas agents sarin, soman, and tabun. These compounds are capable of alkylating the active site of this enzyme that normally is responsible for metabolizing acetylcholine, the neurotransmitter found at the neuromuscular junction and within many sites of the autonomic and central nervous systems. Reaction of the enzyme with its normal substrate acetylcholine leads to a readily hydrolyzable acetylated enzyme, which rapidly regenerates the active enzyme. Covalent bonding by the organophosphates, however, results in phosphorylation of a serine within the active site of the enzyme, which is extremely stable and essentially irreversible. Recovery of enzymatic function in the tissue requires the synthesis of new enzyme molecules.

Ionic Bond

When two ions of opposite charge are attracted to each other through electrostatic forces, an ionic bond is formed. The strength of this type of bond varies between 5 and 10 kcal/mol, and it decreases proportionally to the square of the distance between the two atoms. The ability of a drug to bind to a receptor via ionic interactions therefore increases significantly as the drug molecule diffuses closer to the receptor. Additionally, the strength associated with the ionic bond is strong enough to support an initial transient interaction between the receptor and the drug, but unlike the covalent bond, the ionic bond is not so strong as to prevent dissociation of the drug receptor complex.

The tendency of an atom to participate in ionic bonding is determined by its degree of electronegativity. Hydrogen, as a standard, has an electronegativity value of 2.1 (Linus Pauling Units). Fluorine and chlorine atoms as well as hydroxyl, sulfhydryl, and carboxyl groups form strong ionic bonds because of a stronger attraction for electrons compared with that of hydrogen. On the other hand, alkyl groups do not participate in ionic bonds because of a weaker tendency to attract electrons compared with that of hydrogen.

Hydrogen Bond

Hydrogen that is linked via a covalent bond to a strongly electronegative atom, such as oxygen, nitrogen, or sulfur, develops a relative positive charge and will be attracted to another atom possessing a relative negative charge via what is termed "hydrogen bonding." A water molecule that behaves as an electronic dipole (i.e., the hydrogens are relatively positive because of the attraction of electrons by the oxygen) can easily bond to other water molecule through hydrogen bonding. At 2 to 5 kcal/mol, a single hydrogen bond is relatively weak and would not be expected to support a drug–receptor interaction alone, but when multiple hydrogen bonds are formed between drugs and receptors, as typically is the case, a significant amount of stability is conferred on the drug–receptor interaction. Thus, hydrogen bonding most likely is an essential requirement for many drug–receptor interactions.

Hydrophobic Interactions

Hydrophobic interactions between nonpolar organic molecules also can contribute to the binding forces that attract a ligand to its receptor. Theorists have suggested that for these forces to operate, a momentary dipolar structure needs to exist to allow such association. This induced dipolar structure may result from a temporary imbalance of charge distribution within molecules. These forces are very weak (0.5–1 kcal/mol) and decrease proportionally to the seventh power of the interatomic distance. These bonds, also referred to as van der Waals forces or London forces, require that the two nonpolar molecules come in close proximity to one another.

AFFINITY—THE ROLE OF CONFORMATION

Most therapeutically useful drugs bind only transiently to their intended receptor. The combination of a variety of bonds, including ionic, hydrogen and van der Waals attractive forces, can contribute to the binding of a drug to the receptor. The critical portion of the structure of the drug that is believed to bind to the receptor is termed the "pharmacophore." Once the drug has bound, a biological response may result (e.g., especially if an agonist). Either following or during the process of binding to the receptor, a conformational change may occur in the receptor that initiates the activation of the biological response and changes the attractive environment between the drug and the receptor. This conformational change in the receptor also may allow the dissociation of the drug–receptor complex. This simple explanation of the interaction of a drug with a receptor producing a biological response is commonly referred to as the "occupancy theory," and it predicts that the response is directly related to the number of receptors bound by an agonist.

Another theory of drug–receptor interactions, termed the "rate theory," suggests that the number of drug–receptor interactions per unit time determines the intensity of the response. Thus, drugs that associate with and then rapidly dissociate from the receptor, thus allowing other drug molecules to subsequently interact with the receptor, would be expected to produce the most robust responses. The "induced-fit theory" suggests that as the drug approaches the receptor, a conformational change occurs in the receptor to allow effective binding (Fig. 4.2). According to this theory, the receptor does not normally exist in the proper conformation for drug binding. Following dissociation of the drug, the receptor can then

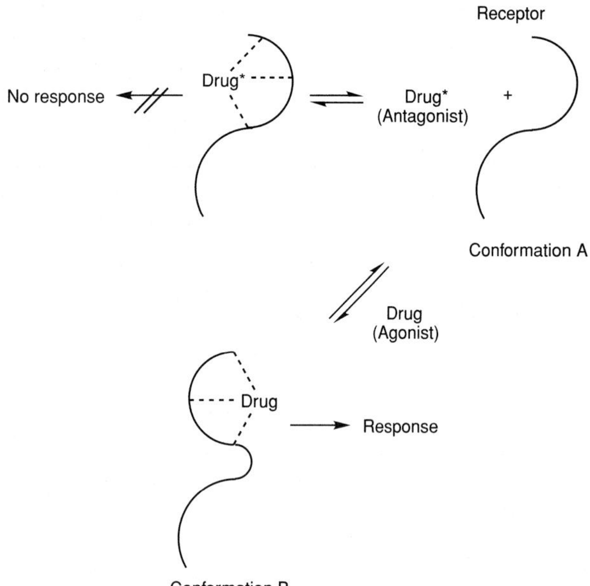

Fig. 4.2. Diagrammatic representation of drug-induced fit theory, in which an agonist (Drug) or antagonist (Drug*) interacts with two different conformations of the receptor.

revert to its original configuration. In this theory, an antagonist can induce a conformational change in the receptor; however, the change is not the proper change required for a biological response to be elicited. Combining the induced-fit and rate theories yields the "macromolecular pertubation theory," which suggests that two types of conformational changes exist and that the rate of their existence determines the observed biological response. Agonists produce the specific pertubation required for a biological response, whereas antagonists produce a nonspecific pertubation, which fails to yield a biological response. This theory can partially account for the activity of partial agonists. Finally, the "activation-aggregation theory" indicates that receptors are always in a dynamic equilibrium between active and inactive states. Agonists function by shifting the equilibrium toward the activated state, whereas antagonists prevent the activated state. This theory can account for the activity of inverse agonists, which produce neither a typical agonist response nor an antagonist response (i.e., blocking the receptor) but, rather, produce biological responses opposite to those of the agonist.

AFFINITY—THE ROLE OF STEREOCHEMISTRY

Very specific three-dimensional requirements must be satisfied for a compound to effectively act as an agonist. To elegantly demonstrate the specificity of a drug for its receptor, the unique three-dimensional characteristics of chiral compounds can be used as an example. As early as 1901, Pasteur (8) noted the significance of asymmetric compounds in biological systems. Since that time, much

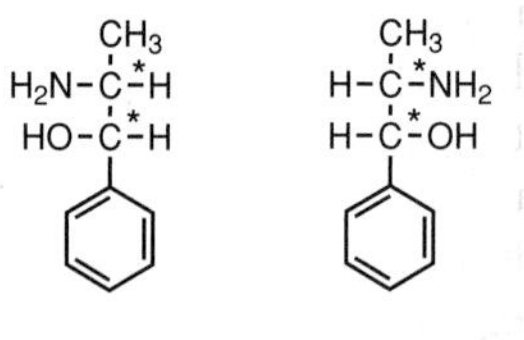

Fig. 4.3. Projection formulae of 2-amino-3-phenyl-1-propanol stereoisomers. (From Maher TJ, Johnson DA. Review of chirality and its importance in pharmacology. Drug Dev Res 1991;24:149–156; with permission.)

has been learned from chiral compounds regarding three-dimensional binding requirements of receptors. For instance, although the individual enantiomers (i.e., nonsuperimposable mirror images) of norephedrine (2-amino-3-phenyl-1-propanol) (Fig. 4.3) have identical molecular weights, melting points, lipid solubility, and empirical formulae, these compounds have significantly different α-adrenoceptor agonistic activities. The 1R,2S enantiomer (levo) is approximately 100-fold more potent than the 1S,2R enantiomer (dextro) both in vivo and in vitro (9,10). (Because there are two chiral centers, there also is another set of stereoisomers called diastereomers, 1S,2S and 1R,2R, that have an even different pharmacological profile.) Thus, the greater efficacy of the 1R,2S enantiomer most likely is dependent on its ability to bind and activate the receptor as a result of its preferential fit into the receptor.

Because labetalol, an adrenoceptor-blocking agent structurally related to epinephrine, has two asymmetric centers, four diastereomers exist (Fig. 4.4). The formulation available for use as a mixed α- and β-adrenoceptor blocker contains equal amounts of each diastereomer. The R,R isomer accounts for much of the β-adrenoceptor blocking activity, whereas the S,R isomer has the greatest effect on α-adrenoceptors. The S,S isomer has some α-adrenoceptor blocking activity but no activity at β-adrenoceptors. The R,S isomer is essentially devoid of activity at both α- and β-adrenoceptors.

Many synthetically prepared therapeutic agents are a mixture of two enantiomers (racemates), with one

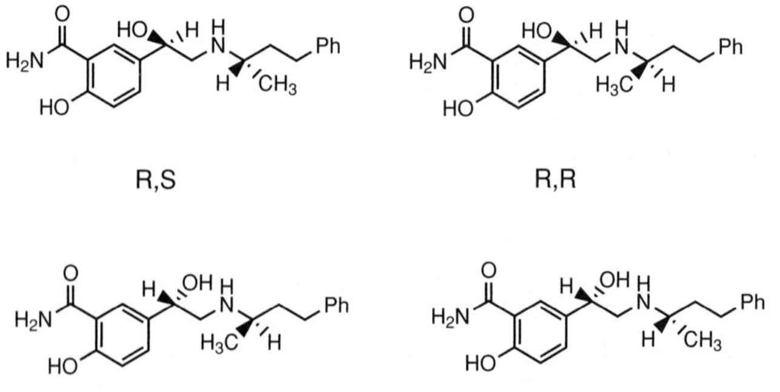

Fig. 4.4. Diastereomers of labetalol.

enantiomer, termed the "eutomer," being largely responsible for the desired pharmacological effect (11). The other enantiomer, termed the "distomer," may be inactive or even contribute more significantly to the toxicity of the therapeutic agent. Thus, in the future, knowledge of chirality should play a significant role in the advances gained in receptor theory as well as in therapeutics.

RECEPTOR BINDING AND DRUG DISCOVERY

The discovery of pharmacological agents by modern pharmaceutical companies and universities often involves the use of receptor–ligand binding techniques. Following the synthesis of a series of new chemically related compounds, which may constitute hundreds to thousands of compounds, the determination of the desired biological activity was once a rather daunting task. Before the advent of receptor–ligand binding techniques, the initial screening of these compounds involved individually injecting each agent into experimental animals or incubating each agent with isolated tissues (e.g., intestine, heart, and skeletal muscle), which are techniques that require a large investment of resources, including personnel, time, animals, and money. Today, receptor–ligand binding techniques are used to narrow large numbers of compounds down to those that display the greatest affinity for a receptor, thereby significantly decreasing the time and cost associated with identifying "lead" compounds. One danger associated with such an initial screening approach, however, is the failure to recognize potentially useful compounds that might require biotransformation before exerting a biological effect, such as a pro-drug. Additionally, it should be remembered that ligand binding based on the affinity of a drug for a receptor does not differentiate agonists from antagonists. Despite these potential pitfalls associated with receptor–ligand binding techniques, modern drug discovery relies heavily on these approaches.

DOSE–RESPONSE RELATIONSHIPS

A.J. Clark generally is given credit for being the first to apply the law of mass action principles to the concept of drug–receptor interactions, thus providing further evidence for the dose–effect phenomenon (12). This concept, as applied by Clark, states that the greater the number of agonist molecules at the site of the receptors, the greater the response (i.e., a direct relationship); however, these principles of the law of mass action in receptor–drug interactions have been questioned. The law of mass action applies to compounds dissolved in fluids that are allowed to diffuse freely. Now that much is known about the anchoring of most receptors to, or within, cell membranes where receptor–drug interactions are thought to occur, this environment would actually constitute a solid–liquid interface. Thus, the law of mass action as applied to compounds dissolved in fluids where they are allowed to diffuse freely might not be completely applicable.

Equation 4.1 illustrates the interaction of a drug ([D]) with a receptor ([R]), which results in a drug–receptor complex ([DR]) and a biological response. The interaction between most therapeutically useful drugs and its receptor generally is reversible:

Eq. 4.1 $$[D] + [R] \rightleftharpoons [DR] \rightarrow \text{Biological Response}$$

Following administration of a drug, one can monitor the biological responses produced. Plotting the dose or concentration of the drug versus the effect produced (% response) yields a rectangular hyperbolic function, as illustrated in Figure 4.5a. This type of function is mathematically difficult to accurately extrapolate quantitative information from because of the constantly changing slope of the curve. When the effect produced is plotted against the log of the drug concentration or the dose administered, however, a sigmoidal function results, as illustrated in Figure 4.5b. This function possesses a relatively linear portion of the curve about its central point, thereby making quantitative extrapolations more accurate.

Dose–response curves typically are plotted to determine both quantitative and qualitative parameters of potency and efficacy. Potency is inversely related to the dose required to produce a given response (typically half-maximum), and efficacy is the ability of a drug to produce a full response (100% maximum). In Figure 4.6, Drug X is equally efficacious to Drug Y, but Drug X is more potent than Drug Y. That is to say, both Drug X and Drug Y can produce a 100% response, but with Drug X reaching that response at a lower dose. Visual inspection of such dose–response curves allows easy qualitative interpretations (e.g., in a series of curves): Those positioned to the left are more potent than those positioned to the right. Additionally illustrated in Figure 4.6, Drug Z is more potent than Drug Y, and Drug Z is equipotent to Drug X. However, comparisons of efficacy are visually apparent, because the greater the maximum response (i.e., efficacy), the higher the maximum point on the dose–response curve. Thus, in Figure 4.6, Drug X and Drug Y are of equal efficacy, and Drug X and Drug Y are of greater efficacy than Drug Z.

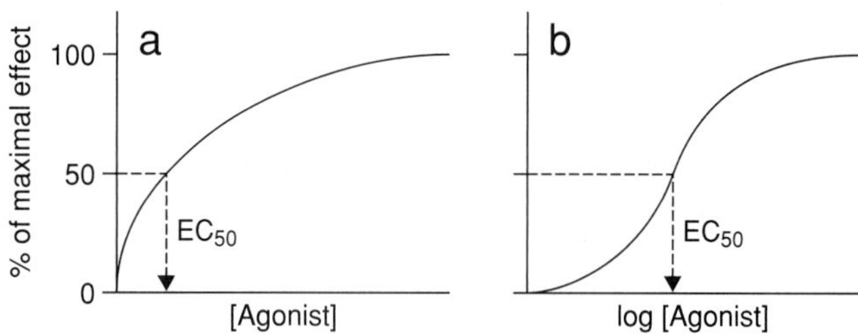

Fig. 4.5. Plot of (a) dose or concentration and (b) log of the dose or concentration of a drug versus the effect produced.

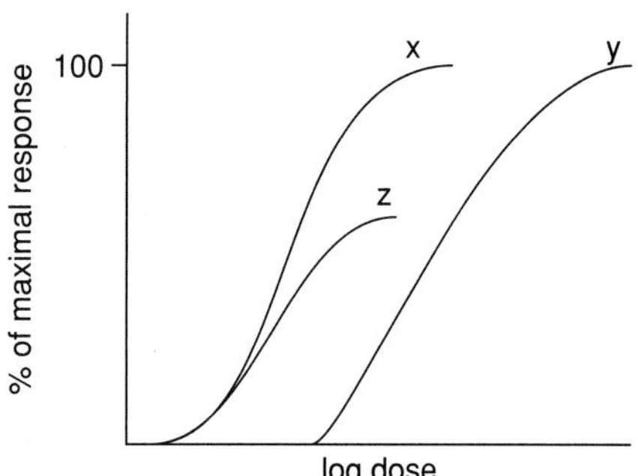

Fig. 4.6. Dose-response relationship.

PRESYNAPTIC AND POSTSYNAPTIC RECEPTOR LOCATIONS

When an action potential arrives at the nerve cell's axon, a depolarization-induced exocytosis of neurotransmitter from its storage sites in the presynaptic terminal occurs. Through this process, the action potential continues the flow of information to the target site, typically the postsynaptic cell. The neurotransmitter is believed to diffuse across the extracellular fluid filled space known as the synapse and to interact with postsynaptic receptors. The released neurotransmitter, however, also may be capable of interacting with presynaptic receptors located on the neurons that just released the neurotransmitter. The function of these receptors typically involve the regulation of nerve transmission and are termed "autoreceptors," because the neurotransmitters that activate them function to control their own release.

An exquisite example of both receptor locations and the action of autoreceptors in the control of neurotransmission is observed in norepinephrine-containing postganglionic neurons of the sympathetic nervous system (Fig. 4.7) (13). Norepinephrine, which is capable of stimulating both α- and β-adrenoceptors, initially is released and is present at low concentration in the synapse. Low concentrations of this agent are capable of preferentially stimulating β-adrenoceptors located presynaptically, which function to increase the release of more neurotransmitter and, thereby, to magnify the intended response. Additionally, the epinephrine released from the adrenal medulla during sympathetic stimulation also is thought to play an important role in facilitating neuronal norepinephrine release. This is an example of a positive-feedback system, which allows a rapid rise in the concentration of the neurotransmitter and, thus, the intended signal. Following this initial period of robust norepinephrine release, very high norepinephrine concentrations result in the synaptic cleft, which then is capable of stimulating other presynaptic autoreceptors, this time terminating the additional release of neurotransmitter. This negative-feedback system allows the signal to be terminated very quickly.

Together, the presynaptic facilitatory β-adrenoceptor–mediated mechanism and the presynaptic inhibitory α-adrenoceptor–mediated mechanism allow a rapid, robust,

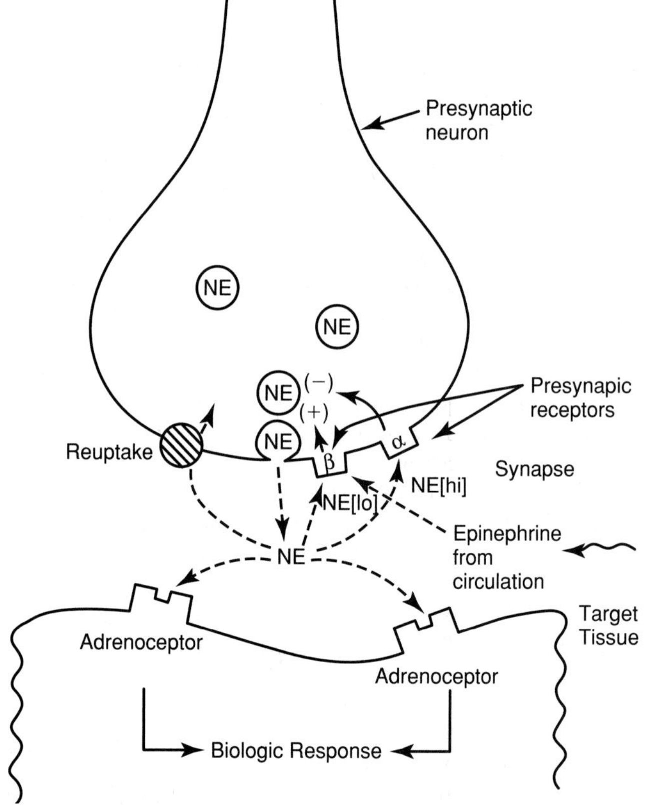

Fig. 4.7. Autoreceptor control of neurotransmission as observed in norepinephrine-containing postganglionic neurons of the sympathetic nervous system. NE, norepinephrine; NE[lo], low norepinephrine concentration; NE[hi], high norepinephrine concentration, α, α-adrenoceptor; β, β-adrenoceptor; (−), inhibit; (+), stimulate.

and well-controlled signal to be delivered. If one were to design a system that was to respond quickly to stressors, such as the sympathetic nervous system is believed to be designed to do, then a system that turns on rapidly and can be terminated quickly would be ideal and, presumably, an evolutionary advantage. Additionally, many other neurotransmitter autoreceptors have been identified, such as in the serotoninergic, dopaminergic, and histaminergic transmitter systems. Examples even exist whereby a neurotransmitter can interact with a presynaptic receptor to influence the release of a different neurotransmitter. For instance, norepinephrine released from neurons in the gastrointestinal tract can function to decrease acetylcholine release. This is termed a heteroreceptor.

DRUG RECEPTORS AND THE BIOLOGICAL RESPONSE

There are four major families of receptors that drugs, which mimic, modify, or antagonize endogenous neurotransmitters, hormones, or autocoids, are capable of interacting with in the body (Fig. 4.8). Some receptors allow a rapid response to a released neurotransmitter/

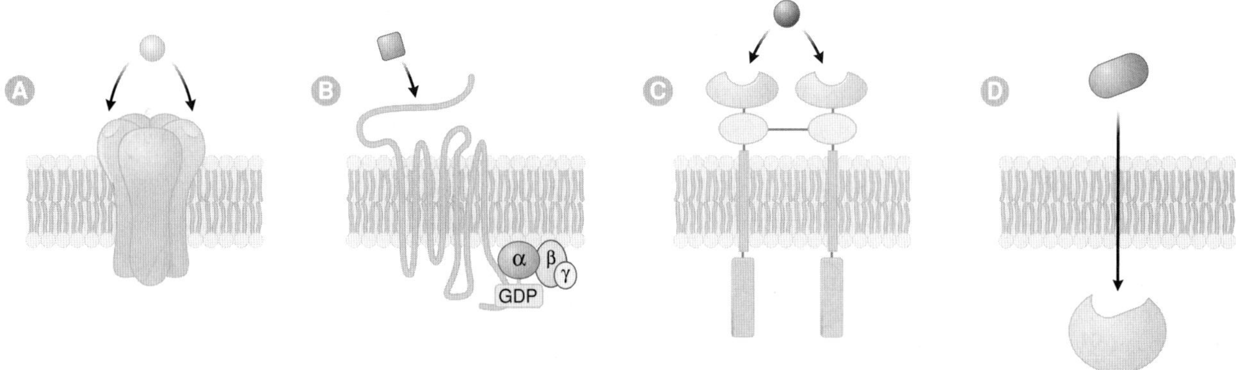

Fig. 4.8. Major classes of drug receptors. (A) Transmembrane ligand-gated ion channel receptor. (B) Transmembrane G protein–coupled receptor (GPCR). (C) Transmembrane catalytic receptor or enzyme-coupled receptors. (D) Intracellular cytoplasmic/nuclear receptor. (From Simon JB, Golan DE, Tashjian A, Armstrong E, et al., eds. Chapter 1, Drug-Receptor Interactions. In: Principles of Pharmacology: The Pathophysiologic Basis of Drug Therapy. Baltimore: Lippincott Williams & Wilkins, 2004, pp. 3–16, with permission.)

hormone or an administered drug. These responses generally are important for the immediate response to a significant homeostatic challenge to the individual. Both ion channel and G protein–coupled receptors tend to be rapid responders, with some catalytic receptors also characterized this way. These responses tend to be short-lived. On the other hand, many catalytic and just about all cytoplasmic/nuclear receptors tend to respond much more slowly, on the order of hours to days, and these responses are much longer in duration than the rapid-responding receptors.

Signal Transduction

Signal transduction is a communication process by which a cell converts an extracellular signal or stimulus by transmitting this signal across the cell membrane to the interior of the cell. Proteins on the cell's extracellular surface function as receptors for specific molecules, ligands, or agonists (first messengers). The binding of the ligand to the receptor initiates an interlinked series of processes, termed "signal transduction," that involve a sequence of biochemical reactions inside the cell, which are carried out by enzymes, proteins, and ions (especially calcium) that are linked through second messengers, such as cyclic AMP (cAMP) or inositol 1,4,5-trisphosphate (IP_3). This signal is relayed via a second messenger that results in specific cellular responses or changes in gene expression in the nucleus (Fig. 4.9). Such processes take place in as little as a millisecond or as long as a few seconds. Slower processes rarely are referred to as signal transduction.

The process of signal transduction serves several critical roles. First, it enables extracellular molecules to affect cellular function without entering the intracellular environment. This "long distance" communication is accomplished by the binding of a ligand (agonist) to the receptor protein and stabilizing the receptor structure in an active conformation. The active receptor conformation can then facilitate the flow of ions through a membrane

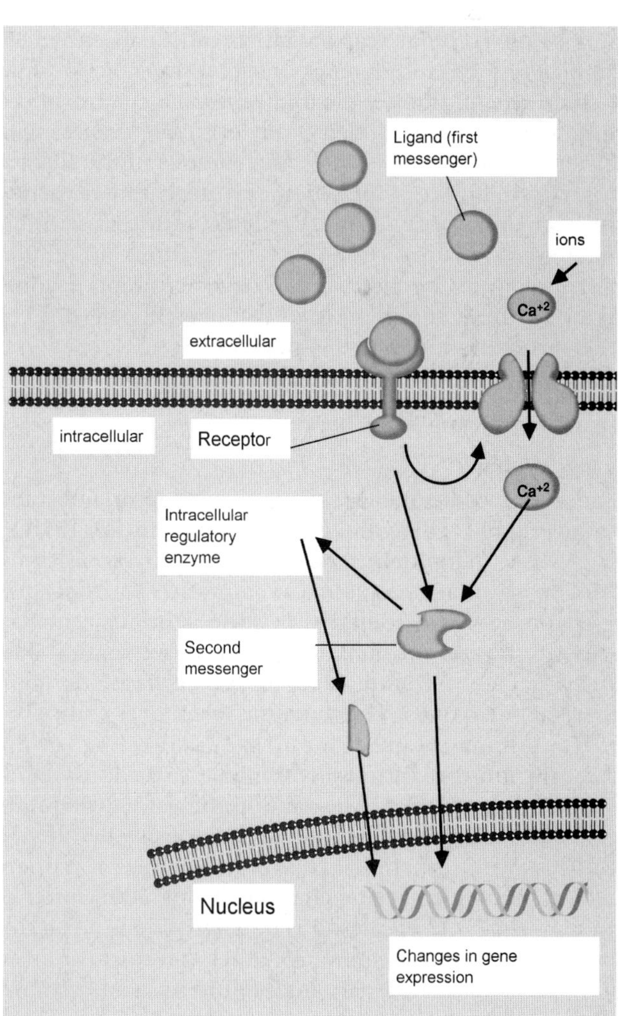

Fig. 4.9. Overview of signal transduction in cellular regulation and gene expression via second messengers.

channel by the removal of steric or electronic hindrances (opening of channel gates). For those receptors that produce signals via activation of intracellular metabolic pathways, the active state or conformation changes the intracellular molecular environment in such a way as to activate, directly or indirectly, intracellular regulatory enzymes. Second, several different signals may affect one another by facilitating or inhibiting the activation of regulatory enzymatic proteins via common or opposing metabolic pathways. Thus, signal transduction mechanisms can interact in such a way as to yield an integrated response to multiple stimuli. Third, via the activation of enzymes and the production of second messengers (e.g., cAMP, diacylglycerol [DAG], ad IP3), an initially weak signal can be amplified, and its duration prolonged, to produce a robust cellular response. This amplification can occur through several mechanisms. The kinetic time frame for enzyme activation and the presence of key metabolites may be much longer than the time of receptor activation itself. Thus, a brief activation of a small number of receptors may result in a magnified response by the cell. Amplification also can occur via a molecular "cascade," in which one initial signal can trigger a multitude of intracellular reactions that lead to an enhanced cellular response. Outcomes of signal transduction may include one or more of the following: 1) a change in cell membrane polarity in electrically excitable tissues, such as nerves and muscles, which then results in the facilitation or inhibition of an action potential, thus affecting the excitability of the tissue; 2) the activation of cytosolic metabolic cascades, resulting in alterations of cellular morphology or function; and 3) gene activation, leading to the synthesis of new proteins that may then modify cellular structures and physiology.

Transmembrane Ion Channels

Ligand-Gated Ion Channels

The most rapid cellular responses to receptor activation are mediated via ligand-gated ion channels (LGICs) (Fig. 4.8A). The main component of this signal transduction pathway is a plasma membrane–spanning protein composed of multiple peptide subunits, each of which contains four membrane-spanning domains. The nicotinic acetylcholine receptor is, perhaps, the best characterized LGIC. The nicotinic receptor is composed of five distinct subunits, two α and, depending on the receptor subtype, various combinations of additional α, β, γ, and δ subunits. The binding of an acetylcholine molecule to the binding site on each of two α subunits induces a conformational change in the receptor, opening a sodium-selective ion channel through the center of the protein (14). The result is depolarization of the surrounding plasma membrane. Other neurotransmitter-activated LGICs include γ-aminobutyric acid, glycine, glutamate, and some serotonin receptors (15). These receptors share a similar structural conformation and function to the nicotinic receptor, except for the specificity of the ligand-binding site and selectivity of the channel for particular ions. The primary reason for the rapidity (milliseconds) of the cellular response with LGICs is that the transduction of the signal requires the activation of a single molecule. Therefore, this transduction mechanism is especially suited for physiological processes necessitating an immediate response, such as the stimulation of nerves and muscles.

Voltage-Gated and Second Messenger–Gated Channels

Other ion channels are controlled by either voltage changes or second messenger molecules. An example of a voltage-gated channel includes the sodium channels responsible for impulse conduction in sensory nerve fibers that transmit information about pain and temperature. Following administration, the local anesthetic lidocaine enters the nerve cell via diffusion in its unprotonated form. Once inside the nerve cell, lidocaine is protonated, and in this charged form, it is capable of blocking the sodium channel from the intracellular side. Some second messenger molecules (e.g., cAMP and IP_3; discussed below) generated following the activation of G protein–coupled receptors can influence the degree of channel opening or closing. The most common channels influenced by these second messengers include those for calcium and potassium.

Transmembrane G Protein–Coupled Receptors

The G protein–coupled receptors (GPCRs) are a class of large membrane-bound proteins, which share a well-conserved structure and transduce their signal via the activation of an intracellular guanine nucleotide–binding protein (G protein). This family of proteins has seven hydrophobic (heptahelical) domains that span the plasma membrane; therefore, it sometimes is referred to as having a serpentine structure (Fig. 4.8B). The extracellular region of the protein is composed of the amino terminus and several loops, which comprise the ligand-binding site. Smaller ligands tend to bind deep within the extracellular loops, close to the plasma membrane, whereas larger molecules have binding sites that are more superficial. The carboxy end of the receptor is located in the area of the protein that protrudes into the cytoplasm. The intracellular side of the receptor also includes the binding site for the G protein, which usually binds to the third loop between the sixth and seventh transmembrane regions of the protein. Close to the carboxy terminus are serine and threonine residues, which are targets for ATP-dependent phosphorylation. Following prolonged activation, phosphorylation of these residues is hypothesized to occur via a negative-feedback regulatory metabolic pathway, which facilitates the binding of modulating molecules that subsequently impair the coupling of G proteins to the receptor. The result is receptor desensitization.

More than 100 different GPCRs bind to a variety of ligands encompassing biogenic amines, such as acetylcholine, norepinephrine, and serotonin; amino acid neurotransmitters, such as glutamate and glycine; and peptide hormones, such as angiotensin II and somatostatin. There are multiple GPCR types for a single ligand. The result is the possibility that a single ligand can activate a variety of transduction pathways and produce a multiplicity of cellular responses. Thus, a receptor is defined not just by which ligand binds to it but also by how the signal is transduced and the physiological response that results. As an example, at least nine different adrenergic receptor subtypes exist (16). Norepinephrine can bind to the β_1 receptor, which is coupled to a G protein (designated G_s). Following receptor stimulation of G_s, there is activation of the enzyme adenylyl cyclase, thus leading ultimately to an increase in heart rate and force of contraction. Norepinephrine binding to α_1-receptors, on the other hand, results in the binding to a different G-protein (G_q), which activates the production of the second messengers IP_3 and DAG, which then initiate a cascade of intracellular events leading to smooth muscle contraction. Therefore, a single ligand can induce a wide range of responses as a consequence of coupling to different G proteins. Which G protein is activated depends on factors such as the presence and availability of individual G proteins within a particular cell type, kinetic issues (e.g., the binding affinity of the G protein for the receptor protein), and finally, the affinity of the activated G-protein subunits for signal transduction enzymes.

G Proteins

G proteins are heterotrimeric in structure with the subunits (in decreasing size) designated as α, β, and γ. At least 13 types of G proteins have been identified, which are divided among four families, G_s, G_i, G_q, and G_{12}. Individual G proteins transduce the receptor activation signal via one of a number of second messenger systems discussed below. The best-understood second messenger systems associated with each G protein family are summarized in Table 4.1.

The characteristics of the α subunit are what determine the designation of the G protein. Receptor activation leads to a conformational change in the associated G protein, triggering the release of bound GDP from the α subunit, which is then replaced by a molecule of GTP. With the binding of GTP, the α-subunit GTP complex dissociates from the αβ subunits and binds to a particular target enzyme, resulting in its activation or inhibition. Within a short period of time, the α subunit catalyzes the dephosphorylation of the associated GTP molecule to GDP, resulting in the reassociation of the α subunit with the αβ subunits and, thus, the return of the G protein to the inactivated state (Fig. 4.10). Variations on this scheme include the activation of proteins such as G protein–gated ion channels by dissociated αβ subunits and the ability of receptor proteins to activate more than a single G protein. The simultaneous activation of more than one type of GPCR results in the initiation of multiple signals, which can then interact with one another (a phenomenon com-

Table 4.1. G-Protein Transducers and Second Messengers

G-Protein Transducer Family	Second Messenger System
G_s	Stimulates adenylyl cyclase activity and Ca^{2+} channels
G_i	Inhibits adenylyl cyclase activity and activates K^+ channels
G_q	Stimulate phospholipase C activity
G_{12}	Modulate sodium/hydrogen ion exchanger

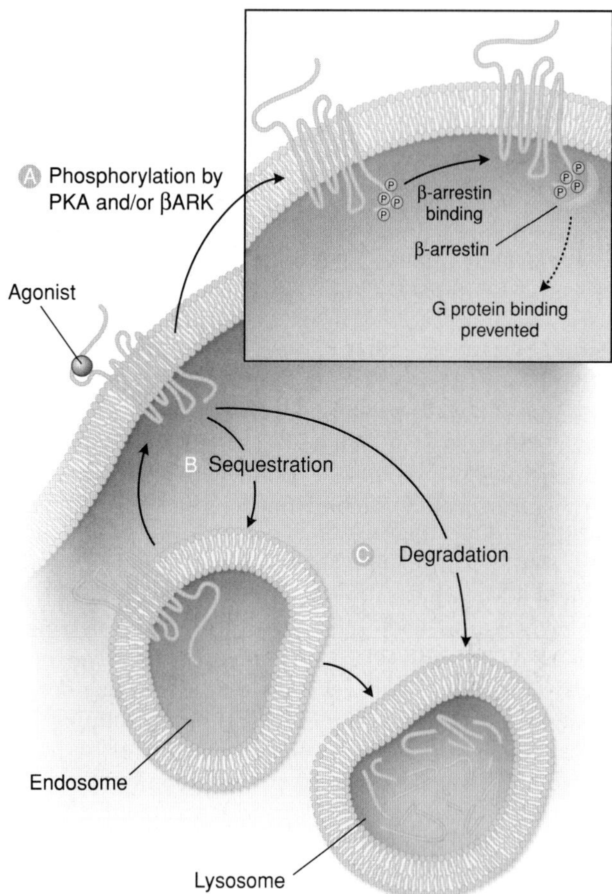

Fig. 4.10. β-Adrenoceptor regulation. Following repeated stimulation of the β-adrenoceptor by an agonist, phosphorylation of amino acids on the intracellular C-terminal domain by protein kinase A (PKA) and/or β-adrenergic receptor kinase (βARK) may (A) prevent subsequent G-protein binding, (B) enhance removal of the receptor from the membrane via sequestration into endosomes, or (C) enhance degradation via lysosomal internalization and cleavage. (From Simon JB, Golan DE, Tashjian A, Armstrong E, et al., eds. Chapter 1, Drug-Receptor Interactions. In: Principles of Pharmacology: The Pathophysiologic Basis of Drug Therapy. Baltimore: Lippincott Williams & Wilkins, 2004, pp. 3–16, with permission.)

*This enzyme is known by two names, *adenylate cyclase* (EC 4.6.1.1)- its official name from the International Union of Biochemistry and Molecular Biology Nomenclature Committee or its alternative name, adenylyl cyclase.

**This enzyme is known by two names, *guanylate cyclase* (EC 4.6.1.2)- its official name from the International Union of Biochemistry and Molecular Biology Nomenclature Committee or its alternative name, guanylyl cyclase.

monly referred to as cross-talk). This interaction can be of several types: If both receptors use a common signal transduction pathway, the activation can result in an additive response by the cell. Conversely, if simultaneous receptor activation triggers opposing signal transduction pathways, the outcome will be an attenuated cellular response. Other types of interactions may include the desensitization or activation of other receptor proteins or second messenger pathways. The final outcome of the activation of multiple signals is an integrated response by the cell.

Second Messenger Pathways

As discussed above, in response to receptor activation, G proteins activate plasma membrane-bound enzymes, which then trigger a metabolic cascade that results in a cellular response (17). The products of these enzymatic actions are termed "second messengers," because they mobilize other enzymatic and structural proteins, which then produce the cellular response. The enzymes that catalyze the synthesis of second messengers generally fall into two categories: those that convert the purine triphosphates ATP and GTP into their respective cyclic monophosphates, and enzymes that synthesize second messengers from plasma membrane phospholipids. The most thoroughly studied second messenger system is controlled by a family of 10 plasma membrane-bound isoenzymes of adenylyl cyclase, which catalyze the conversion of ATP to cAMP (Fig. 4.11). Adenylyl cyclase is activated by the G_s family of G proteins and inhibited by the G_i family. Following synthesis, cAMP activates cAMP-dependent protein kinases by triggering the dissociation of regulatory subunits from catalytic subunits. The catalytic subunits then activate other target proteins via phosphorylation, which then trigger the cellular response. The magnitude of the cellular response is proportional to the concentration of cAMP. Degradation of cAMP occurs via phosphodiesterases or by reducing cAMP concentration via active transport out of the cell. The result is termination of the signal.

A similar, although less ubiquitous, second messenger pathway is associated with guanylyl cyclase. Guanylyl cyclase is activated in response to catalytic receptors selective for ligands including atrial natriuretic factor and nitric oxide. When stimulated, guanylyl cyclase then catalyzes the synthesis of cyclic GMP (cGMP) from GTP. Cyclic GMP subsequently activates cGMP-dependent protein kinases, which then activate other proteins. The actions of cGMP are terminated by enzymatic degradation of the second messenger or the dephosphorylation of substrates. One effect of this second messenger pathway is the relaxation of smooth muscle via the dephosphorylation of myosin light chains.

The generation of second messengers from plasma membrane phospholipids is mediated primarily by G-protein activation of phospholipase C (PLC) (18). There are three families of PLC, designated PLC-β, PLC-γ, and PLC-δ. Phospholipase C-β can be activated by the α subunit of the G_q family of G proteins or the βγ subunits of other G proteins. Phospholipase C-γ is activated via tyrosine kinase receptors, but the mechanism for PLC-δ is not yet understood. On activation, PLC hydrolyzes phosphatidyl inositol-4,5-bisphosphate to DAG and IP_3 (Fig. 4.12). The water-soluble IP_3 diffuses into the cytoplasm, where it triggers the release of calcium from intracellular

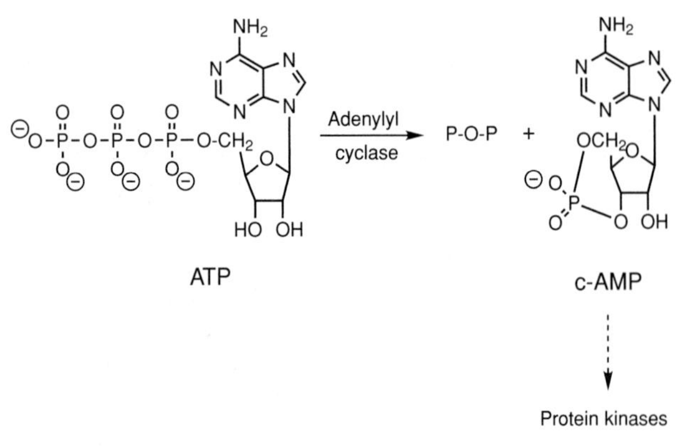

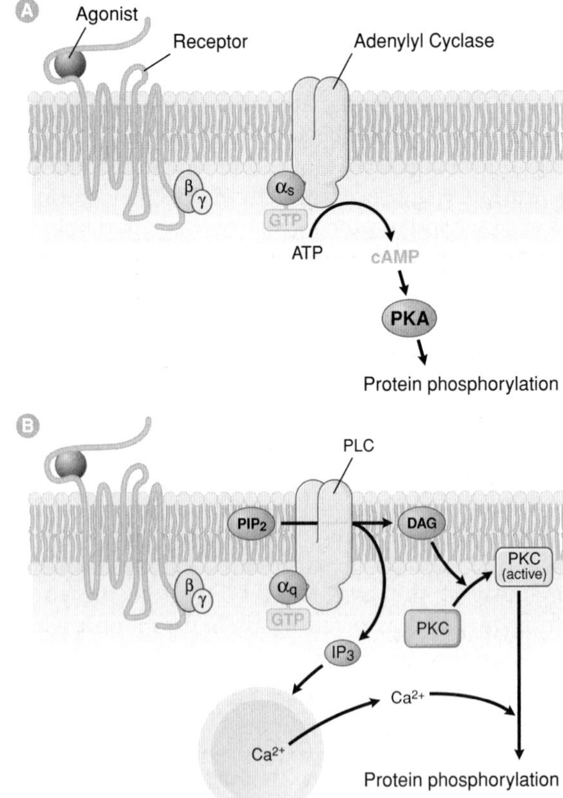

Fig. 4.12. Second messenger mechanisms for cyclic adenosine monophosphate (cAMP) and inositol trisphosphate. (From Simon JB, Golan DE, Tashjian A, Armstrong E, et al., eds. Chapter 1, Drug-Receptor Interactions. In: Principles of Pharmacology: The Pathophysiologic Basis of Drug Therapy. Baltimore: Lippincott Williams & Wilkins, 2004, pp. 3–16, with permission.)

ATP —Adenylyl cyclase→ P-O-P + c-AMP ⇢ Protein kinases

Fig. 4.11. Conversion of adenosine triphosphate (ATP) to cyclic adenosine monophosphate (c-AMP) catalyzed by adenylyl cyclase.

stores. Intracellular calcium then binds to the protein calmodulin and also to protein kinase C, both of which then stimulate, via protein phosphorylation, a broad range of enzymes and other proteins, including specific kinases. The other product of PLC, DAG, is lipid soluble and remains in the plasma membrane, where it facilitates the activation of protein kinase C by calcium. The signal is terminated via inactivation of IP_3 by dephosphorylation, whereas DAG is inactivated by phosphorylation to phosphatidic acid or deacetylation to fatty acids. The concentration of intracellular calcium is reduced by sequestration within cytoplasmic organelles or transport out of the cell. Activation of phospholipase D hydrolyzes phosphatidylcholine to phosphatidic acid, which can then be metabolized to DAG via phosphatidate phosphohydrolase. This pathway prolongs the duration of elevated levels of DAG. Phospholipase A_2 is activated by increased concentrations of intracellular calcium and metabolizes phosphatidylcholine to arachidonic acid. Arachidonic acid then functions as a substrate for the synthesis of autocoids, including prostaglandins, thromboxane A_2, and leukotrienes.

Transmembrane Catalytic Receptors

Catalytic receptors are a class of plasma membrane-bound receptors that are characterized by a monomer with a ligand-binding site in the extracellular domain, a single membrane-spanning domain, and an intracellular domain with enzymatic activity (Fig. 4.8C). This family of receptors is activated predominately by peptide hormones, such as insulin, epidermal growth factor, platelet-derived growth factor, and atrial natriuretic factor. The catalytic portion of the receptor functions as a protein kinase, targeting primarily tyrosine residues; however, the receptor for atrial natriuretic factor, rather than having kinase activity, activates guanylyl cyclase and metabolizes GTP to cGMP (19). Receptor activation occurs by ligand binding, which then triggers dimerization of receptor proteins via the cross-phosphorylation of tyrosine residues. The dimeric protein is the active form of the catalytic receptor. One consequence of activation via dimerization is that the intracellular signal can be maintained even after the ligand has dissociated from the binding site. The phosphorylation of intracellular proteins by this receptor type results in effects such as the opening of ion channels, changes in cytoplasmic function, or initiation of genomic expression. Other catalytic receptors, activated by transforming growth factor-β, use serine/threonine kinases in regulating cellular growth and differentiation.

Enzyme-Coupled Receptors

Enzyme-coupled receptors are similar in their function to catalytic receptors, except rather than inherent catalytic activity, enzyme-coupled receptors bind to separate enzymatic proteins (Fig. 4.8C). This class of receptor binds cytokines, including growth hormone, erythropoietin, and interferon. Like catalytic receptors, enzyme-coupled receptors are activated via dimerization following ligand binding. Kinase activity is accomplished by separate, noncovalently bound protein kinases of the Janus-kinase (JAK) family. Following dimerization, JAKs are activated and phosphorylate receptor tyrosine residues. The phosphorylated receptor then binds other molecules, termed "signal transducers and activators of transcription" (STATS), which are phosphorylated by the JAKs and, subsequently, dissociate into the cytoplasm. The STATS then translocate to the nucleus, where they initiate gene transcription.

Intracellular Cytoplasmic/Nuclear Receptors

Cytoplasmic/nuclear receptors differ from those described above in that they are not associated with the plasma membrane but, rather, are located within the cytoplasm or are bound to the surface of the nucleus (Fig. 4.8D). These receptors are composed of a single polypeptide with three functional domains. The amino terminal contains a binding site for a modulator protein, heat shock protein-90, which is associated with the receptor in the absence of agonist. In the middle of the receptor peptide is a binding site for DNA, and the carboxy terminus contains the ligand-binding site. Cytoplasmic/nuclear receptors are activated by lipid-soluble ligands, which passively diffuse through the plasma membrane (20). Agonists include nitric oxide, steroid hormones, and vitamin D. Ligand binding activates the receptor by inducing the dissociation of heat shock protein-90. The receptor then translocates to the nucleus and binds to a DNA response element, which then initiates translation of the target gene. The response to this type of signal transduction is relatively slow, requiring 30 minutes to several hours following protein binding. Moreover, the duration of the response can last long after the concentration of the ligand has fallen to zero. The duration of the response is related to turnover rate of the synthesized protein; however, it also may be affected by a ligand with extremely high binding affinity, possibly resulting in prolonged receptor activation.

RECEPTOR SUBTYPES

Careful examination of the effects of a series of sympathomimetics by Ahlquist (21) led him to postulate the existence of at least two types of adrenoceptors, which he termed α and β. Realizing that adrenoceptor agonists were capable of causing either relaxation or contraction of isolated smooth muscles, he noted that although a compound like norepinephrine had potent excitatory actions but weak inhibitory actions, another catecholamine, isoproterenol, had potent inhibitory actions but weak excitatory actions. When a series of related compounds were tested for potency in various tissues, it was demonstrated that for the α-adrenoceptor,

Table 4.2. Adrenoceptor Families

Receptor Type	Subtype	Transduction Mechanism	Tissue Function
α_1	1A	Activates $G_{q/11}$	Smooth muscle and myocardial contraction
α_1	1B	Activates $G_{q/11}$	Smooth muscle contraction
α_1	1D	Activates $G_{q/11}$	Smooth muscle contraction
α_2	2A	Activates $G_{i/o}$	Hypotension, sedation, analgesia, anesthesia
α_2	2B	Activates $G_{i/o}$	Vasoconstriction
α_2	2C	Activates $G_{i/o}$	Not established
β_1	—	Activates G_s	Increases heart rate and force of contraction
β_2	—	Activates G_s	Smooth muscle relaxation
β_3	—	Activates or inhibits adenylyl cyclase	Lipolysis, cardioinhibition

the order of potency was epinephrine ≥ norepinephrine >>> isoproterenol, and for the β-adrenoceptor, the order of potency was isoproterenol > epinephrine ≥ norepinephrine. Following the findings of Ahlquist, others used specific antagonists that had become available to further support this designation of receptor subtypes. Additionally, with the development of highly selective antagonists and procedures for cloning and determining the amino acid sequence of proteins, the classification of receptors into subtypes has expanded at a tremendous rate (22). For example, the α-adrenoceptor noted above can be subclassed as α_{1A}, α_{1B}, α_{1C}, α_{1D}, α_{2A}, α_{2B}, and α_{2C} based on cloning experiments (Table 4.2).

The therapeutic significance of such distinctions is not yet known, however, because of a lack of selective agonists or antagonists. Some therapeutic distinction can be made between α_1 and α_2 adrenoceptors in a general way, in that α_1 vasoconstriction antagonism by prazosin and central nervous system α_2-adrenoceptor stimulation by clonidine are useful in the treatment of hypertension. Similarly, β-adrenoceptor antagonists are available that antagonize β_1-adrenoceptors with some selectivity. Thus, the use of metoprolol, a selective β_1-antagonist, is effective and relatively safe in hypertensive patients with compromised airway function, whereas the use of a nonselective (β_1 and β_2) antagonist, such as propranolol, would be clearly contraindicated in such a patient.

A summary of the most important receptor subtypes from a therapeutic standpoint is presented in Table 4.3. The reader should realize that this is a simplification of what currently is known about the various receptor subtypes. For instance, within the general category of serotonin receptors, at least 13 subtypes can be identified from cloning experiments. The lack of selective agonists and antagonists to characterize the pharmacology of each of these subtypes, however, has hindered our understanding of their individual functions and importance from a therapeutic standpoint. Our ability to eventually develop drugs that selectively manipulate such receptor subtypes has enormous therapeutic implications.

SPARE RECEPTORS

Biological systems often have built-in safety factors to enhance the efficiency of receptor-stimulus coupling and, thereby, assure the desired neurotransmission. In many tissues containing α-adrenoceptors, only a small percentage of the available receptors need to be occupied to produce a maximum response. This depends on the particular tissue being studied and the agonist used. Therefore, 100% occupancy of the available receptors is not always required, because spare receptors (or a receptor reserve) are present. Studies using phenoxybenzamine, which alkylates the α-adrenoceptor and, therefore, irreversibly inactivates the receptor, indicate that only 5 to 10% of the available receptors need to be activated to elicit a maximum response to a full, or strong, agonist, such as norepinephrine or phenylephrine (6,7,23). To obtain a maximum response to a partial agonist like ephedrine, however, nearly 100% of the receptors need to be occupied. The explanation behind this difference may involve a less than ideal receptor–drug interaction for partial agonists. A partial agonist may function as an antagonist if it interferes with the ability of a full agonist to bind to its receptor and produce a response. In the absence of a full agonist, however, the partial agonist only displays agonistic activity.

DYNAMIC NATURE OF RECEPTORS

As is characteristic of most individual components of living systems, receptors are not static but, rather, are constantly in a state of dynamic adaptation. One could envision these protein molecules floating within the fluid mosaic of the biological membrane awaiting interaction with normal physiological signals. The function of such receptors, once stimulated, involves attempts to respond to perturbations of the normal physiology of the cell or organism. The role in maintaining homeostasis within the organism requires constant adaptation of receptor number and/or sensitivity in response to the changing environment in the vicinity of the receptor. One approach to controlling receptor activation is by regulating the concentration of neurotransmitter at the receptor binding

Table 4.3. Survey of Receptor Subtypes

Receptor Class	Subtype	Selective Agonist	Selective Antagonist	Effector	Cloned
Adrenoceptors	α_1	Phenylephrine	Prazosin	IP_3/DAG	Yes
	α_2	Clonidine	Yohimbine	↓cAMP	Yes
	β_1	Dobutamine	Atenolol	↑cAMP	Yes
	β_2	Terbutaline	Butoxamine	↑cAMP	Yes
Dopamine receptors	D_1	Fenoldopam	Dihydroxidine	↑cAMP	Yes
	D_2	Bromocriptine	(−) Sulpiride	↓cAMP	Yes
Excitatory amino acid receptors	NMDA	NMDA	D-AP5	↓Na^+/Ca^{2+}	Yes
	AMPA	AMPA	CNQX	↑Na^+	Yes
	Kainate	Kainate	?	↑Na^+/K^+	Yes
GABA receptors	$GABA_A$	Muscimol	Bicuculline	↑Cl^-	Yes
	$GABA_B$	Baclofen	Saclofen	↓cAMP	Yes
Histamine receptors	H_1	2-(m-Fluorophenyl) Histamine	Mepyramine	IP_3/DAG	Yes
	H_2	Dimapril	Ranitidine	↑cAMP	Yes
Muscarinic receptors	M_1	Oxotremorine	Pirenzepine	IP_3/DAG	Yes
	M_2	Oxotremorine	AF-DX116	↓cAMP	Yes
Nicotinic receptors	N_{muscle}	?	Decamethonium	↑Na^+/Ca^{2+}	Yes
	$N_{neuronal}$	?	Hexamethonium	↑Na^+/Ca^{2+}	Yes
Opioid receptors	Mu	Sufentanil	CTAP	↓cAMP	Yes
	Delta	[D-Ala^2]deltorphin	Naltrindole	↓cAMP	Yes
	Kappa	Dynorphin	Nor-binaltorphimine	↓cAMP	Yes
Serotonin receptors (5-HT)	5-HT_{1A}	8-OH-DPAT	Spiperone	↓cAMP	Yes
	5-HT_{2A}	α-Methyl-5-HT	Ketanserin	IP_3/DAG	Yes

?, no known selective compounds available; cloned, receptor subtype has been cloned and the amino acid structure is known. Chemical abbreviations used: AF-DX116, 11-([2-{(diethylamino)methyl}-1-piperidinyl]acetyl)-5-11-dihydro-6H-pyridol[2,3-b] [1,4]benzodiazepine-6-one; AMPA, D,L-α-amino-3-hydroxy-5-methyl-4-isoxalone propionic acid; cAMP, cyclic adenosine 3′,5′-monophosphate; CNQX, 6-cyano-7-nitroquinoxaline-2,3-dione; CTAP, D-Phe-Cys-Tyr-DTrp-Arg-Thr-Pen-Thr-NH2; DAG, diacyl glycerol; D-AP5, D-amino-5-phosphonopentanoate; GABA, γ-aminobutyric acid; 5-HT, 5-hydroxytryptamine, serotonin; IP_3, inositol 1,4,5-triphosphate; NMDA, N-methyl-D-aspartate; 8-OH-DPAT, 8-hydroxy-2-(di-n-propylamino)tetralin.

site. This is accomplished by the modulation of release via activation of presynaptic receptors, as described above. Altering the rate of synthesis, degradation, or efficiency of the enzymes that create or degrade neurotransmitter molecules also is used to regulate neurotransmitter concentrations at the receptor.

A second mechanism for modulating the cellular response to receptor activation is to alter receptor number and/or sensitivity. The process is best understood for GPCR but also has been characterized for ion channel receptors, such as the nicotinic receptor. The alteration in the availability or functional capacity of a given receptor constitutes an adaptive mechanism whereby the cell or organism is protected from agonist overload. For example, the chronic administration of a β-adrenoceptor agonist, such as isoproterenol, is known to produce a desensitization of the β-adrenoceptors in the heart (24). During the period of overstimulation, the receptor becomes desensitized to further activation via phosphorylation by G protein–coupled kinases, such as protein kinase A or β-adrenoceptor kinase, at serine and threonine residues on the C-terminal domain that interferes with G_S binding (Fig. 4.10). Desensitization also may occur at other receptors with analogous phosphorylation sites (heterologous desensitization). A more prolonged or powerful overstimulation typically results in a decrease in receptor number and is termed "downregulation." In these GPCRs, downregulation initiated by phosphorylation of amino acids near the intracellular C-terminal domain results in binding to β-arrestins that facilitate their internalization via a clathrin-dependent pathway. Following internalization, the receptor may either be recycled back into the plasma membrane via endosomes or degraded by lysosomes. Reduced receptor numbers also can be accomplished via changes in the transcription and/or translation of genes that code for the receptor. Changes in receptor number or efficiency of receptors that lead to diminished responses and, thus, the efficacy of a drug with repeated or long-term use is an example of pharmacodynamic tolerance. As a general principle, the body will always attempt to maintain homeostasis, whether perturbed by environmental challenges, disease processes, or even the administration of drugs. Actually, the body sees the administration of drugs as a pertubation of homeostasis and, usually, attempts to overcome the effects of the drug by invoking receptor adaptations. Often, however, with appropriate dosing schedules, drugs can be used with little observed receptor adaptation such that the desired pharmacological effect continues to be observed.

In a similar fashion to the example described above, chronic administration of the β-adrenoceptor antagonist propranolol leads to a state of receptor supersensitivity or upregulation. The cells within the tissue, such as the heart, sense an alteration in the normal rate of basal β-adrenoceptor stimulation and, thus, respond by either increasing the number or the affinity of the receptors for their natural agonists, norepinephrine and epinephrine. Additionally, an enhanced efficiency of the interaction between the receptor and its transducing systems also may account for a portion of the observed supersensitivity. The knowledge that such a receptor adaptation occurs has paramount practical therapeutic implications, because abrupt withdrawal of this class of agents may precipitate acute myocardial infarction. Thus, this practice should be scrupulously avoided.

Some pathophysiological states are characterized by perturbations in receptor dynamics. Prinzmetal's angina is thought to be characterized by an imbalance between vasodilatory β_2-adrenoceptor function and vasoconstrictor α_1-adrenoceptor function. In this disease state, the excessive alpha vasoconstriction of coronary arteries leads to myocardial ischemia and pain. The inadvertent use of a β-adrenoceptor antagonist, which is safely employed in typical angina pectoris to prevent β-adrenoceptor vasodilation, may leave unopposed alpha vasoconstrictor inputs and actually precipitate anginal pain. Thus, an understanding of the role that receptors play in physiology, pathophysiology, and pharmacology is essential for optimal therapeutic interventions.

FUTURE DIRECTIONS

Our understanding about the nature and role of receptors has increased tremendously since the early work of Langley and Ehrlich. Today, with the advances made in the field of molecular biology, it is possible to clone individual receptor subtypes (Table 4.3) and determine their function in cell culture. By modifying the amino acid structure at those sites believed to be involved in agonist binding, a better appreciation for the interaction of drugs currently available—and the rational design of those awaiting discovery—may be realized. Additionally, as we begin to be able to determine the structure of receptor subtypes through cloning techniques, we hopefully will better understand those disease processes that result from, or lead to, receptor adaptations or dysfunction.

References

1. Leake CD. A Historical Account of Pharmacology in the 20th Century. Springfield, IL: Charles C. Thomas, 1975.
2. Langley JN. On the reaction of cells and nerve endings to certain poisons. J Physiol 1905;33:374–413.
3. Ehrlich P. In: Himmelweit F, ed. Collected papers of Paul Ehrlich, vol III. London: Pergammon, 1957.
4. Price CC. Chemistry of alkylation. In: Sartorelli AC, Johns DG, eds. Antineoplastic and Immunosuppressive Agents, Part II—Handbuch der Experimentellen Pharmakologie, vol 38, Berlin: Springer-Verlag, 1975, pp. 1–5.
5. Nickerson M. Receptor occupancy and tissue response. Nature 1956;178: 697–698.
6. Minneman KP, Abel PW. Relationship between α_1-adrenoceptor density and functional response of rat vas deferens. Studies with phenoxybenzamine. Naunyn Schmiedebergs Arch Pharmacol 1984;327:238–246.
7. Besse JC, Furchgott RF. Dissociation constants and relative efficacies of agonists acting on α-adrenergic receptors in rabbit aorta. J Pharmacol Exp Ther 1976;197:66–78.
8. Pasteur L. On the asymmetry of naturally occurring organic compounds, the foundations of stereochemistry. In: Richardson GM, ed. Memoirs by Pasteur, Van't Hoff Le Bel, and Wislicenus. Stuttgart: Birkhauser, 1901, pp. 3–33.
9. Moya-Huff FA, Maher TJ. β-Adrenoceptor influences on the α_1- and α_2-mediated vasoconstriction induced by phenylpropanolamine and its two component isomers in the pithed rat. J Pharm Pharmacol 1988;40:876–878.
10. Johnson DA, Maher TJ. Vasoactive properties of phenylpropanolamine and its enantiomers in isolated rat caudal artery. Drug Dev Res 1991;23:159–169.
11. Maher TJ, Johnson DA. Review of chirality and its importance in pharmacology. Drug Dev Res 1991;24:149–156.
12. Parascandola J, Clark AJ. Quantitative pharmacology and the receptor theory. Trends Pharamcol Sci 1982;4:421–423.
13. Starke K. Presynaptic α-autoreceptors. Rev Physiol Biochem Pharmacol 1987;107:73–146.
14. Brisson A, Unwin PNT. Quaternary structure of the acetylcholine receptor. Nature 1985;315:474–477.
15. Kemp JA, Leeson PD. The glycine site of the NMDA receptor—five years on. Trends Pharmacol Sci 1993;14:20–25.
16. Kobilka BK. Adrenergic receptors as models for G protein–coupled receptors. Annu Rev Neurosci 1992;15:87–114.
17. Gilman AG. G proteins: transducers of receptor-generated signals. Annu Rev Biochem 1987;56:615–649.
18. Berridge MJ. Inositol triphosphate and diacylglycerol: two interacting second messengers. Ann Rev Biochem 1987; 56:159–193.
19. Chinkers M, Garbers DL, Chang MS, et al. A membrane form of guanylate cyclase is an atrial natriuretic peptide receptor. Nature 1989; 338:78–83.
20. Evans RM. The steroid and thyroid hormone receptor superfamily. Science 1988;240:889–895.
21. Ahlquist RP. A study of the adrenotropic receptors. Am J Physiol 1948;153: 586–600.
22. Minneman KP, Esbenshade TA. α_1-Adrenergic receptor subtypes. Annu Rev Pharmacol Toxicol 1994;34:117–133.
23. Furchgott RF. The use of β-haloalkylamines in the differentiation of receptors and in the determination of dissociation constants of receptor-agonist complexes. In: Harper NJ, Simmonds AB, eds. Advances in Drug Research, vol 3 New York, Academic Press, 1966, pp. 21–55.
24. Tattersfield AE. Tolerance to β-agonists. Bull Eur Physiopathol Respir 1985; 21:1S–5S.

Suggested Readings

Aranda A, Pascual A. Nuclear hormone receptors and gene expression. Physiol Rev 20018:1269–1304.
Ariens EJ. Affinity and intrinsic activity in the theory of competitive inhibition: problems and theory. Arch Int Pharmacodynam 1954;99:32–49.
Black JW, Leff P. Operational models of pharmacological agonists. Proc R Soc Lond Biol 1983;220:141–162.
Bylund DB. Subtypes of α_1- and α_2-adrenergic receptors. FASEB J 1992;6:832–839.
Kebabian JW, Neumeyer JL. The RBI Handbook of Receptor Classification. Natick, MA: Research Biochemicals International, 1998.
Kenakin T. Pharmacologic Analysis of Drug-Receptor Interaction, 2nd Ed. New York: Raven, 1993.
Liebmann C. G protein–coupled receptors and their signaling pathways: classical therapeutical targets susceptible to novel therapeutic concepts. Curr Pharm Design 2004:10:1937–1958.
Tallarida RJ, Jacobs LS. The Dose–Response Relation in Pharmacology. New York: Springer-Verlag, 1979.
Trends in Pharmacological Sciences. 2000 Receptor & Ion Channel Nomenclature Supplement. Oxford: Elsevier Science Ltd, 2000.

5. *Drug Discovery Through Enzyme Inhibition*

STEPHEN KERR

OVERVIEW OF ENZYMES AS CATALYTIC RECEPTORS

A Perspective

The concept of using small molecules that specifically target one or more enzymatic systems in the body is not new. Historically, compounds that were extracted from natural products have been used as medicinal agents (see Chapter 1). Subsequently, they have been shown to have their therapeutic effect by targeting certain systemic enzymes (1). A classic example is the bark of the willow tree, known since ancient days to have antipyretic and analgesic effects. Its active ingredient, salicin, a glycoside, is metabolized in vivo to salicylic acid, which is a known inhibitor of cyclooxygenase, a key enzyme in the formation of prostaglandins, which are mediators of pain and fever. Similarly, physostigmine, isolated from the West African Calabar bean, was used as a treatment for glaucoma in the mid-1800s.

Physostigmine's mechanism of action was only later determined to be inhibition of acetylcholinesterase (1).

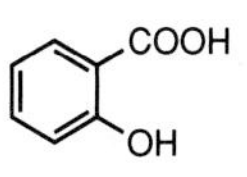

COOH OH
Salicylic acid

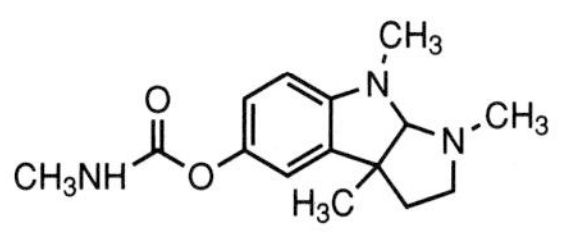

CH_3 O N N CH_3 CH_3NH O H_3C
Physostigmine

Inhibition of acetylcholinesterase in the eye leads to improved drainage and, thus, a decrease in the intraocular pressure giving relief to glaucoma patients. It was only in the 20th century, with the concept of the "magic bullet" having selective toxicity, introduced by Ehrlich as a rational approach to chemotherapy (1), that the concept of rational design and discovery of enzyme inhibitors followed. The discovery in 1935 of the antibacterial activity of the azo dye prontosil by Domagk (2), and the subsequent explanation in 1940 by Woods (3) of its metabolic reduction to sulfanilamide, an antimetabolite of *p*-aminobenzoic acid, finally paved the way for the rational design of enzyme inhibitors (Fig. 5.1). *p*-Aminobenzoic acid is an essential metabolite used in the bacterial synthesis of folic acid. Sulfanilamide, by its structural resemblance to *p*-aminobenzoic acid, competes for and selectively inhibits the bacterial enzyme dihydropteroate synthase (Fig. 5.2). In the absence of dihydropteroic acid, the bacteria are unable to synthesize tetrahydrofolic acid, an essential cofactor in one-carbon transfers that is involved in the de novo synthesis of purines and in the synthesis of thymidylate. This concept of designing drugs as antimetabolites, or structural analogues of essential metabolites, became the hallmark for the development of enzyme inhibitors. This was especially important in cancer therapy during the early days of rational drug design (4). As mechanisms of enzymes became better understood, the inhibitor design strategy grew more sophisticated, resulting in more potent and selective inhibitors being developed. The present-day focus on drug design through enzyme inhibition makes use of the antimetabolite theory as well as detailed kinetic and mechanistic information about the enzymatic pathways. These strategies use sophisticated assays, enzyme crystal structures and active site environments, site-directed mutagenesis experiments of catalytic residues of enzymes, and molecular docking experiments employing computers. It must be mentioned, however, that in the drug design process, designing a potent inhibitor of an enzyme is only the first step in the long and difficult process of drug development. Other factors, including pharmacokinetic profile of the inhibitor, toxicities and side effects, and animal and preclinical studies, must all be satisfactorily completed or addressed before the inhibitor can even enter clinical studies as a new drug candidate. Hence, even though an enormous amount of data exist regarding enzyme inhibitors, only a selected few turn out to be marketable drugs (Table 5.1). In succeeding paragraphs, an overview of enzymes as catalytic receptors and general concepts of enzyme inhibitors and their rational design into drugs will be discussed with selected examples.

Overview

Enzymes are biological catalysts. By interacting with substrates, they act as receptors and catalyze chemical reactions involved in the biosynthesis of many cellular products. Enzymes derive their name from Greek, in which the term means "in yeast" and was used mainly to distinguish the whole microorganism, such as yeast ("organized ferments"), from that of extracts of the whole microorganisms ("unorganized ferments"). The implication was that enzymes were unorganized ferments in yeast. Although the vast majority of enzymes are proteins, certain nucleic acids (RNAs) also possess enzymatic activity (i.e., ribozymes). Enzymes are the most efficient catalysts known in nature, because they have the ability to enhance reaction rates by enormous factors. Like all catalysts, enzymes have the ability to lower the activation energy of reactions, and the tremendous catalytic power they posses results from their inherent ability to provide stabilization to the reacting molecules at their activated complex states. A preliminary enquiry shows that enzymatic rates for reactions in aqueous solutions are limited

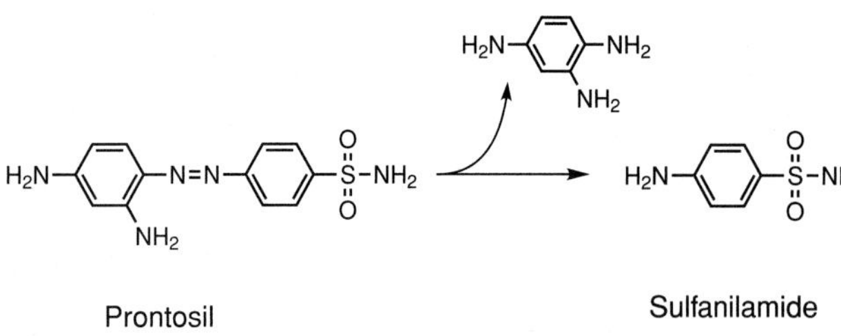

Prontosil

Sulfanilamide

Fig. 5.1. Metabolic reduction of prontosil to sulfanilamide.

by the diffusion rate constant so that the second-order rate constant of an enzyme (k_{cat}/K_m) is approximately $10^9\ M^{-1}s^{-1}$ (diffusion rate constant of water (5)). This implies that every collision of a reactant molecule (substrate) with the enzyme leads to product formation. Because for many enzymes K_m (the Michaelis or apparent substrate–enzyme dissociation constant) values are in the micro- or submicromolar range (10^{-4} M), one can compute the k_{cat} (the catalytic or first-order rate constant) value to be approximately 10^5/s. Estimates (6) for uncatalyzed reactions in water have ranged from 10^{-1} to 10^{-20}/s; thus, the rate enhancements for enzyme-catalyzed reactions over the noncatalyzed reaction (also referred to as the proficiency of an enzyme) can range from 10^6 to over 10^{25}—truly remarkable proficiencies. Moreover, enzymes display great specificity toward particular chemical bonds (bond specificity; e.g., peptidases for peptide bonds) or functional groups (group specificity; e.g., esterases for esters), or they display absolute specificity toward a single molecule (e.g., carbonic anhydrase, which catalyses the hydration of carbon dioxide). Furthermore, this specificity and catalytic proficiency is carried out, in most cases, at ambient temperatures and normal pressures in aqueous solutions. It is no wonder then that enzymes have intrigued scientists for many centuries.

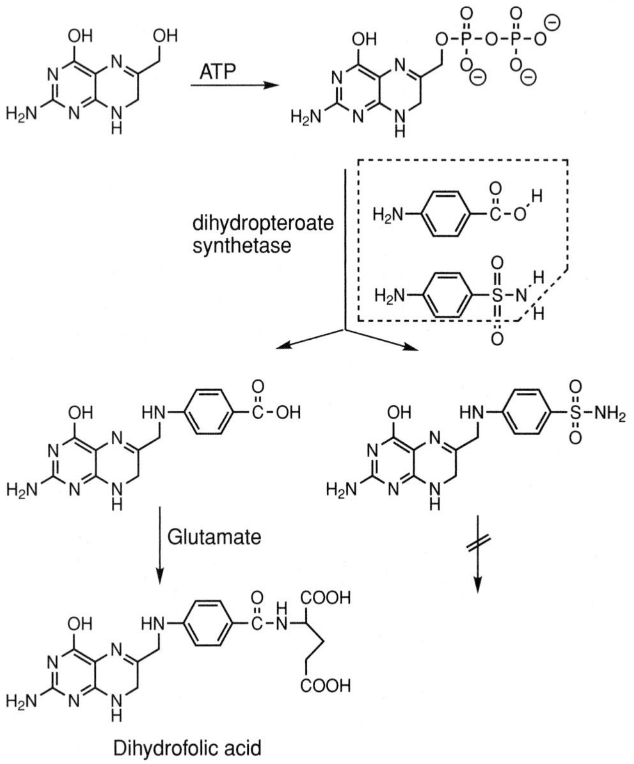

ATP

dihydropteroate synthetase

Glutamate

Dihydrofolic acid

Fig. 5.2. Metabolic pathway leading to dihydrofolic acid and its inhibition by sulfanilamide. This figure shows the structural resemblance to *p*-aminobenzoic acid.

Enzymes have been classified on the type of reaction catalyzed, and six major classes (families) of enzymes, numbered from 1 to 6, have been assigned by the Enzyme Commission (EC) of the International Union of Biochemistry and Molecular Biology (7). These classes are as follows: 1, oxidoreductases (e.g., dehydrogenases); 2, transferases (group transfer enzymes; e.g., kinases); 3, hydrolases (hydrolytic reactions; e.g., esterases); 4, lyases (formation or removal of double bonds; e.g., hydratase—addition of water across a double bond); 5, isomerases (e.g., mutarotation of glucose by mutases); and 6, ligases (joining of two substrates at the expense of energy, also referred to as synthetases). All presently discovered enzymes are identified by the prefix EC followed by an Arabic numeral based on the major class of reaction catalyzed, as indicated above. Furthermore, this is followed by a series of three more Arabic numerals, which indicate the subclass (functionality), sub-sub class (specific bond type), and serial number of the enzyme in that class, respectively. For example, the enzyme, acetylcholinesterase has been given the following assignment, EC 3.1.1.7. As can been seen in this example, the numeral 3 indicates that this enzyme belongs to the family of hydrolases, the first 1 indicates that the nature of the bond being hydrolyzed is an ester, the second 1 indicates that specific ester bond is a carboxylic acid ester, and the last number is the serial number of this enzyme in this sub-subclass.

Many enzymes make use of cofactors, which enable them to carry out the catalysis. These small molecules (including ions) are intimately bound to the enzyme and are essential to the functioning of the enzyme. As macromolecular receptors, enzymes have the inherent ability to bind ligands (substrates). In effecting the transformation of these substrates to products (catalyzing the chemical reaction), enzymes use all the necessary tools in the chemical bonding arsenal to hold these substrates extremely tightly as the transformation occurs. Because all chemical reactions require bond breakage and formation, the substrate must go through a transition state, or an "activated complex," which is a destabilizing event, because bonds are being polarized and there is partial charge development. It is the inherent ability of the enzyme to greatly stabilize such activated complexes that give them their role in nature and allows their phenomenal catalytic power.

Pauling (8) first proposed the stabilization theory of the activated complex by enzymes. He concluded that the active site of the enzyme is complementary to the

Table 5.1. A Partial Listing of Enzyme Inhibitor Drugs Presently Used as Drugs

Inhibitor (Drug)	Enzyme Inhibited	Use	Organism
Caspofungin	1,3-β-Glucan synthase	Antifungal	Fungal
Trilostane	3 (or 17)β-Hydroxysteroid dehydrogenase	Breast cancer	Human
Sildenafil	3',5'-Cyclic GMP phosphodiesterase	Erectile dysfunction	Human
Theophylline	3',5'-Cyclic nucleotide phosphodiesterase	Asthma	Human
Nitisinone	4-Hydroxyphenylpyruvate dioxygenase	Tyrosinemia	Human
Finasteride	Steroid 5α-reductase	Benign prostatic hyperplasia	Human
Pyridostigmine	Acetylcholinesterase	Myasthenia gravis	Human
Pentostatin	Adenosine deaminase	Cancer	Human
Cycloserine	Alanine racemase	Tuberculosis	Bacterial
Fomepizole	Alcohol dehydrogenase	Alcoholism	Human
Disulfiram	Aldehyde dehydrogenase	Alcoholism	Human
Acarbose	α-Amylase	Diabetes	Human
Miglitol	α-Glucosidase	Diabetes	Human
Ethambutol	Arabinosyltransferase	Tuberculosis	Bacterial
Zileuton	Arachidonate 5-lipoxygenase	Inflammation	Human
Carbidopa	Aromatic L-amino acid decarboxylase	Parkinson's disease	Human
Clavulinic acid	β-Lactamase	In combination with penicillins	Bacterial
Acetazolamide	Carbonate dehydratase (carbonic anhydrase)	Glaucoma	Human
Entacapone	Catechol O-methyltransferase	Parkinson's disease	Human
Miglustat	Ceramide glucosyltransferase	Gaucher's disease	Human
Methotrexate	Dihydrofolate reductase	Cancer	Human
Trimethoprim	Dihydrofolate reductase	Antibacterial	Bacterial
Sulfamethoxazole	Dihydropteroate synthase	Antibacterial	Bacterial
Topotecan	DNA topoisomerase	Cancer	Human
Ciprofloxacin	DNA gyrase	Antibacterial	Bacterial
Acyclovir	DNA-directed DNA polymerase	Antiviral (anti-HSV)	Viral
Rifampin	DNA-directed RNA polymerase	Antibacterial	Bacterial
Bacitracin	Dolichyl phosphatase	Antibacterial	Bacterial
Isoniazid	Fatty acid enoyl reductase	Tuberculosis	Bacterial
Oseltamivir	Viral neuraminidase	Anti-influenza	Viral
Fondaparinux	Factor Xa	Thrombosis	Human
Alendronate	Farnesyl-diphosphate farnesyltransferase	Osteoporosis	Human
Pyrazinamide	Mycobacterial fatty acid synthase	Tuberculosis	Bacterial
Valproic acid	Histone acetyltransferase	Seizures	Human
Nelfinavir	HIV protease	AIDS (Anti-HIV)	Viral
Esomeprazole	H^+/K^+-ATPase	Gastroesophageal reflux disease	Human
Atorvastatin	HMG-CoA reductase	Hyperlipidemia	Human
Mycophenolate	IMP dehydrogenase	Immune suppression	Human
Propylthiouracil	Iodide peroxidase	Hyperthyroid	Human
Cilastatin	Renal dehydropeptidase	In combination with imipenam	Human
Eflornithine	Ornithine decarboxylase	Trypanosomes	Parasitic
Allopurinol	Xanthine oxidase	Gout	Human
Captopril	Peptidyl-dipeptidase A (angiotensin-converting enzyme)	Hypertension	Human
Pemetrexed	Phosphoribosylglycinamide formyltransferase	Cancer	Human
Aprotinin	Plasma kallikrein	Thrombosis	Human
Aminocaproic acid	Plasmin	Thrombosis	Human
Etodolac	Prostaglandin-endoperoxide synthase (cyclooxygenase)	Inflammation	Human
Bortezomib	Proteasome endopeptidase complex	Myeloma	Human
Imatinib	Protein-tyrosine kinase	Cancer	Human
Gemcitabine	Ribonuleoside-diphosphate reductase	Cancer	Human
Ribavirin	IMP dehydrogenase	Anti-viral (Broad spectrum)	Viral
Azidothymidine	HIV reverse transcriptase	AIDS (Anti- HIV)	Viral
Lamuvidine	Reverse transcriptase	AIDS, Hepatitis B	Viral
Penicillin	Serine-type D-Ala—Ala carboxypeptidase	Antibiotic	Bacterial
Digitoxin	Na^+/K^+-ATPase	Congestive Heart Failure	Human
Terbinafine	Squalene monooxygenase	Antifungal	Fungal
Itraconazole	Sterol 14α-demethylase	Antifungal	Fungal
Lepirudin	Thombin	Thrombosis	Human
Floxuridine	Thymidylate synthase	Cancer	Human
Orlistat	Tricylglycerol lipase	Obesity	Human
Metyrosine	Tyrosine 3-monooxygenase	Pheochromocytoma	Human
Fosfomycin	UDP-N-acetylglucosamine 1-carboxyvinyltransferase	Antibacterial	Bacterial
Aminoglutethimide	Monooxygenase	Breast cancer	Human
Acetohydroxamic	Urease	Gastritis	Bacterial
Dicumarol	Vitamin K–epoxide reductase	Thrombosis	Human

(Adapted from Robertson J. Mechanistic basis of enzyme-targeted drugs. Biochemistry 2005;44:5561–5771; with permission.)

structure of the activated complex so that the binding of the enzyme to the activated complex is extremely tight. The ability to stabilize such complexes and correspondingly reduce the activation energy of the reaction and, thus, enhance the reaction rate is caused by many factors, both noncovalent as well as covalent (9). Noncovalent influences include entropic effects, such as proximity and orientation; restricted motion, where enzymes, by their evolvement, have the inherent ability to bring reacting molecules closer together and in the correct orientation for bonds to form; desolvation effects, to strip solvent (water) molecules from the reactants; transition state electrostatic stabilization, to stabilize the partial charges being developed in the activated complex; induced-fit effects, in which the flexibility of the enzyme can accommodate the substrate, intermediate, and/or product; strain and distortion effects, to increase the reactivity of compounds; and many other such ancillary effects. Moreover, covalent influences (effects) also play a vital role in the enzyme's catalytic role. "Covalent effects" imply a covalent bond being made by the enzyme (or its cofactor) to the substrate being transformed. These covalent effects would include general acid-base catalysis, in which amino acid residues partake in the overall reaction through proton donation (general acid) or proton abstraction (general base), as well as nucleophilic and electrophilic catalysis, in which there is bond formation with an amino acid side-chain residue (or cofactor) to the substrate.

It should be mentioned here that "covalent catalysis" has traditionally implied a group transfer reaction between one substrate and another being facilitated through an enzyme-residue intermediate (e.g., the enzyme sucrose phosphorylase transfers a glucose residue from sucrose to phosphate giving the products glucose-1-phosphate and fructose through an enzyme-glucosyl intermediate). Many amino acid side-chain residues (i.e., acidic and basic amino acids, e.g., Asp, Glu, His, Lys, Arg, Tyr, and Cys) as well as nucleophilic amino acid residues allow such covalent effects. Recent analysis of enzyme rate enhancements has postulated that noncovalent effects allow an increase of as many as 11 orders of magnitude over the noncatalyzed reaction, whereas for those enzymes with rate enhancements exceeding 11 orders of magnitude (over noncatalyzed reactions) it is covalent catalysis in the transition state that accounts for this exceptional increase in rate enhancement (10).

Noncovalent effects like proximity and orientation may be explained on the basis that enzymes have the inherent ability to affect the order of reactions by the "effective concentration" principle—for example, to change a second-order reaction to a first-order one by bringing the reacting molecules closer to each other so that there is a lower amount of entropic loss for the reacting substrates. In the example shown in Figure 5.3, which is taken from physical-organic chemical studies (11), one can consider the hydrolysis of a nitrophenyl ester by an amine in two scenarios: reaction (i), with two individual molecules reacting (i.e., amine and ester), versus reaction

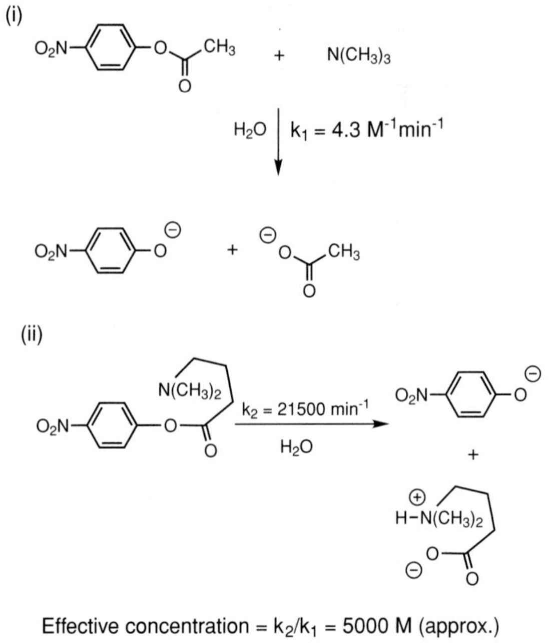

(i)

O_2N–C$_6$H$_4$–O–C(=O)–CH_3 + $N(CH_3)_3$ $\xrightarrow[H_2O]{k_1 = 4.3\ M^{-1}min^{-1}}$ O_2N–C$_6$H$_4$–$O^{\ominus}$ + $^{\ominus}O$–C(=O)–CH_3

(ii)

O_2N–C$_6$H$_4$–O–C(=O)–$CH_2CH_2CH_2N(CH_3)_2$ $\xrightarrow[H_2O]{k_2 = 21500\ min^{-1}}$ O_2N–C$_6$H$_4$–$O^{\ominus}$ + H–$\overset{\oplus}{N}(CH_3)_2$–$CH_2CH_2CH_2$–C(=O)–$O^{\ominus}$

Effective concentration = k_2/k_1 = 5000 M (approx.)

Fig. 5.3. Concept of proximity and effective concentration.

(ii), with a single molecule having an "in-built" amine on the ester molecule. If the reaction rate constants are compared (one needs to keep in mind that we are comparing a first-order rate constant for (ii), with a second-order rate constant for (i), which may not be a true comparison, because mechanisms are likely to be different), however, one finds that the first-order rate reaction (reaction (ii)) has a rate enhancement over the reaction (i) by a factor of ~5,000 M attributed to the fact that reaction (i) needs to give up more degrees of freedom (as compared to reaction (ii)) to react (i.e., form productive collision complexes, leading to product formation). This proximity effect indicates that by using such a system (bringing the reacting centers closer to each other), one can effectively increase the concentration of the reactants by this factor, resulting in a faster reaction. This enhancement factor of 5,000 M (i.e., effectively changing a second-order reaction to that of a first-order one) has been termed the "effective concentration," because this is an unrealistic increase in the concentration of the reactants, which gives rise to the higher rate constant (i.e., it is impossible to make a solution of 5,000 M of the reactants).

The next example, which is shown in Figure 5.4, illustrates that besides the proximity factor, one also can use "orientation" effects to bring about an increase in the reaction rate constant (12). For example, as shown in Fig. 5.4, one may use alkyl groups to sterically hinder rotation about single bonds, effectively freezing the molecule in a particular conformation to provide maximum orbital overlap for bonding. Thus, using a "dimethyl lock" system in molecule II, which restricts rotation, ensures that lactonization for molecule II is faster by a factor of 4×10^4 than molecule I. Both of these effects,

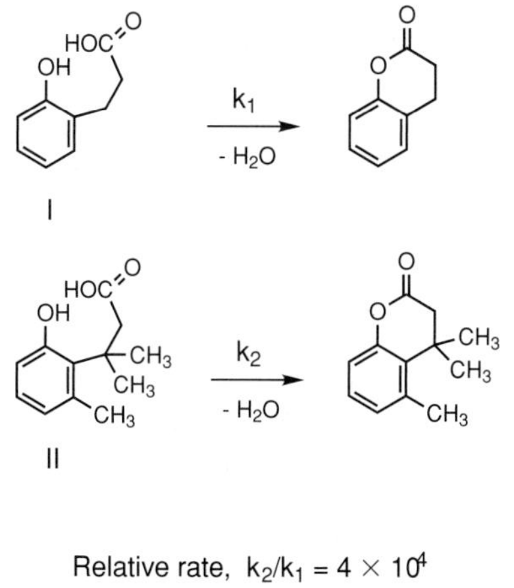

Fig. 5.4. Concept of orientation.

proximity and orientation, are thought to be part of an enzyme's arsenal of tools in allowing enzymes to lower the activation energy for reactions. Other noncovalent effects, such as desolvation of the reactant molecules, also can be effectively achieved by enzymes. Enzymes have the capacity, by lining their exterior and/or interior surfaces with appropriately situated hydrophobic amino acids, to effectively strip away water molecules from substrates as they enter into the active site of the enzyme through such channels. Thus, no further expense of energy is required to desolvate the substrate before the reaction.

As mentioned previously, enzymes also use covalent chemistry as a means to effect catalysis. Indeed, it has been recently postulated that covalent chemistry plays a far greater role in enzyme catalysis than previously thought (10). Nucleophilic catalysis by hydrolytic enzymes, such as the serine proteases or esterases, are classic examples of covalent effects in enzyme catalysis. In such systems, for example, as in the case of the serine protease chymotrypsin, which hydrolyzes peptide bonds containing aromatic amino acids (e.g., phenylalanine and tyrosine), the covalent effects occur at the level of general acid, general base, and nucleophilic covalent catalysis. Figure 5.5 illustrates an accepted mechanism for such enzymes. It should be noted that all serine proteases contain a "catalytic triad" of the amino acids, designated as Ser-195, His-57, and Asp-102 (numerals represent the amino acid position in the protein primary structure), which are present in the active sites of these proteases. The catalysis is effected by making the hydroxyl functionality of the serine residue more nucleophilic for attack at the carbonyl center of the peptide bond. One should recall that in general, hydroxyl groups have pK_a values in the range of greater than 14 and, as such, are not acidic and unable to ionize at physiological pH. Because of catalytic triad, however, the proton from the serine hydroxyl group is transferred to the aspartate residue through the histidine residue in a "charge relay system" such that the serine hydroxyl group is made into the highly nucleophilic alkoxide ion. This is achieved by the aspartate residue acting as a general base to pick up the proton from histidine, which also can abstract a proton from the serine-hydroxyl group (see I in Fig. 5.5). Thus, histidine behaves as a tautomeric catalyst in this enzyme (i.e., acts as both a general acid and a general base) and, in essence, relays the proton from serine to aspartate. The serine (as its alkoxide) is now a much more powerful nucleophile and can attack the peptidyl carbonyl group to generate a "tetrahedral oxy-anion intermediate" (see II in Fig. 5.5), which collapses to liberate a new amino terminus of the

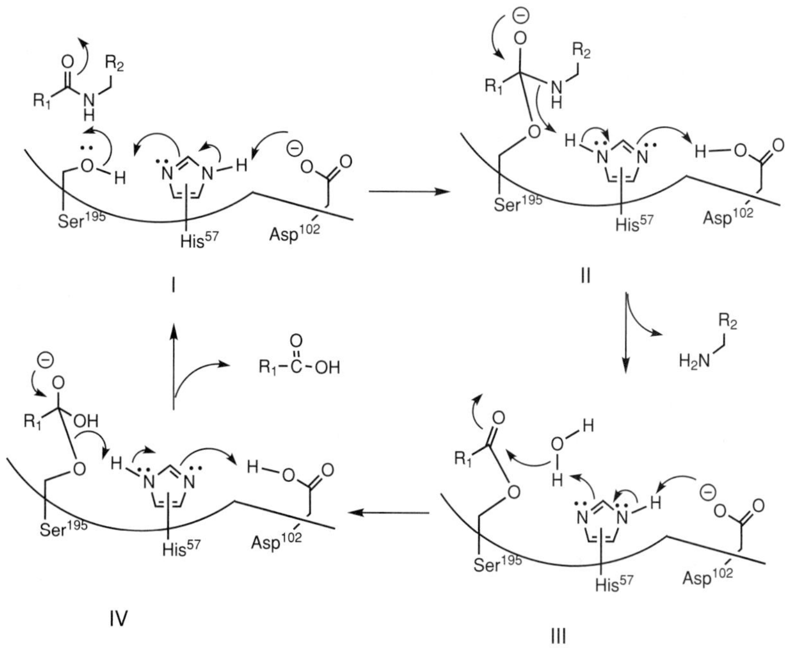

Fig. 5.5. Acid, base, and nucleophilic covalent catalysis by chymotrypsin.

peptide and the acylated serine enzyme (see III in Fig. 5.5). The next part of the reaction involves a water molecule (which also is made more nucleophilic by a similar mechanism; see III in Fig. 5.5) that goes on to hydrolyze, through a tetrahedral intermediate (see IV in Fig. 5.5), the serine-acyl bond to liberate the new carboxyl terminus of the peptide (R_1COOH) and the free enzyme, which can be recycled for another round of catalysis.

Knowledge of the mechanisms and interactions, both noncovalent and covalent, that allow enzymes to function as such efficient catalysts provides the medicinal chemist with insights to design molecules that achieve selective inhibition of the enzyme. Such knowledge also paves the way to the design and discovery of drugs.

GENERAL CONCEPTS OF ENZYME INHIBITION

The body is composed of thousands of different enzymes, many of them acting in concert to maintain homeostasis. Although disease states may arise from the malfunctioning of a particular enzyme, or the introduction of a foreign enzyme through infection by microorganisms, inhibiting a specific enzyme to alleviate a disease state is a challenging process. Most bodily functions occur through a cascade of enzymatic systems, and it becomes extremely difficult to design a drug molecule that can selectively inhibit an enzyme and result in a therapeutic benefit. To address the problem, however, the basic mechanism of enzyme action needs to be understand. Once knowledge of a particular enzymatic pathway is determined and the mechanism and kinetics are worked out, the challenge is then to design a suitable inhibitor that is selectively used by the enzyme causing its inhibition.

As outlined above, enzymes (E) represent the best-known chemical catalysts, because they are uniquely designed to carry out specific chemical reactions in a highly efficient manner (5). They initially act by binding a substrate (S) to form an enzyme–substrate complex [E·S], which undergoes specific chemistry (catalysis) to give the enzyme–product complex [E·P], followed by dissociation of product (P) and free enzyme (E). Equation 5.1 represents a simplified version of this scenario:

Eq. 5.1 $E + S \; K_d \text{ (or } K_m) \rightleftharpoons [E{\cdot}S] \; k_{cat} \rightleftharpoons [E{\cdot}P] \rightleftharpoons E + P$

where K_d is the enzyme–substrate dissociation constant and k_{cat} represents the rate constant for the catalytic step (chemical modification step or slowest step in the overall pathway). If the binding step of E + S to form [E·S] is relatively fast as compared to the catalytic step and one assumes steady-state conditions, then K_m, the Michaelis constant (the substrate concentration at half-maximum velocity [$V_{max}/2$]), may be equated to the K_d, as shown in Equation 5.2): where v = velocity of the reaction

Eq. 5.2 Michaelis-Menten equation: $v = \dfrac{V_{max}[S]}{K_m + [S]}$

Lineweaver-Burk equation: $\dfrac{1}{v} = \dfrac{K_m}{V_{max}} \cdot \dfrac{1}{[S]} + \dfrac{1}{V_{max}}$

The rate of the reaction can then be derived in terms of K_m and V_{max} (or $k_{cat} = V_{max}/[E]$). From the knowledge of the dissociation constant ($K_{m(d)}$) and the rate constant for catalysis (k_{cat}), it is then possible to compare inhibitors and the dissociation constant for the inhibitors, K_i, in relation to the natural substrates and the effect on the catalytic rates. These kinetic parameters, k_{cat} and $K_{m(d)}$ (or K_i) can then give an indication as to the affinity (K_i versus $K_{m(d)}$) and specificity (k_{cat}/K_i or $k_{cat}/K_{m(d)}$) of the inhibitor for a particular enzyme. Equation 5.3 represents the general scheme of reversible inhibition, and Figure 5.6 illustrates graphically and mathematically the relationship of the velocity of the enzyme reaction to the substrate [S] and inhibitor [I] concentration as well as the kinetic parameters K_m, k_i, and V_{max} (or $k_{cat} = V_{max}/[E]$):

Eq. 5.3(a) Competitive Inhibition

$$E + S \; K_m \rightleftharpoons [E{\cdot}S] \rightleftharpoons E + P$$
$$E + I \; K_i \rightleftharpoons [E{\cdot}I] \rightarrow P$$

Eq. 5.3(b) Noncompetitive Inhibition

$$E + S \overset{K_m}{\rightleftharpoons} [E{\cdot}S] \searrow + I$$
$$[E{\cdot}S{\cdot}I]$$
$$E + I \overset{K_i}{\rightleftharpoons} [E{\cdot}I] \nearrow + S$$

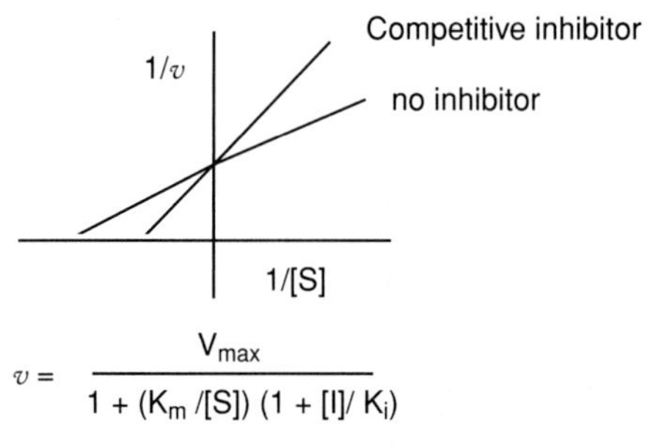

$$v = \frac{V_{max}}{1 + (K_m/[S])\,(1 + [I]/K_i)}$$

(K_m increases, V_{max} unchanged)

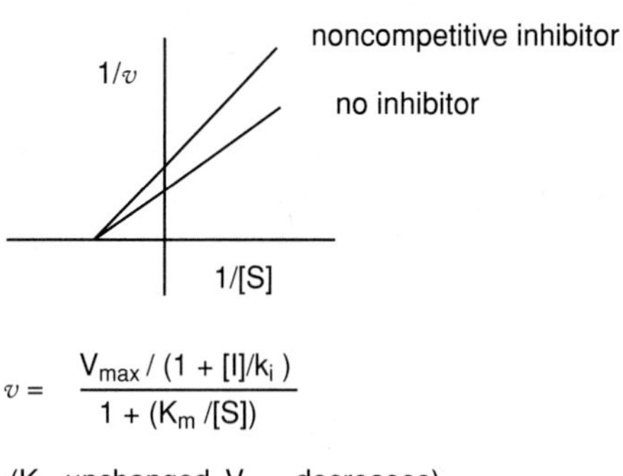

$$v = \frac{V_{max}/(1 + [I]/k_i)}{1 + (K_m/[S])}$$

(K_m unchanged, V_{max} decreases)

Fig. 5.6. Graphic representation of competitive and noncompetitive enzyme inhibition.

Inhibition of enzymes may be broadly classified under two categories—reversible and irreversible inhibitors—as shown in Equation 5.4:

Eq. 5.4 $E + I \; K_i \rightleftharpoons [E \cdot I]$ (reversible inhibition)
$E + I \; K_i \rightleftharpoons [E{-}I]$ (irreversible inhibition)

In the presence of inhibitor, the enzyme–substrate complex, [E·S], is replaced by the enzyme–inhibitor complex, [E·I], which may block or retard the formation of product. In the presence of a reversible inhibitor, the enzyme is tied up and the reaction retarded or stopped; however, the enzyme can be subsequently regenerated from the enzyme–inhibitor complex, [E·I], to react again with substrate and produce product (see Eq. 5.3). On the other hand, irreversible inhibition implies that the enzyme cannot be regenerated, and the only way for catalysis to proceed would be if new molecules of the enzyme are generated from gene transcription and translation. Irreversible inhibition is commonly associated with covalent bond formation between inhibitor and enzyme [E—I], which *cannot* be easily broken and often is defined as a time-dependent loss of enzyme activity. Reversible inhibition, on the other hand, does not necessarily imply noncovalent bond formation. In many instances, reversible inhibition can occur through covalent bond formation, but these bonds can be hydrolyzed to regenerate free enzyme and inhibitor. Thus, for a reversible enzyme inhibitor, there is no time-dependent loss of activity, and enzyme activity can always be recovered. There are instances when reversible inhibition tends to look kinetically like irreversible inhibition. This scenario results whenever there is a tight binding of a reversible inhibitor to the enzyme; consequently, the dissociation of the enzyme from this enzyme–inhibitor complex is extremely slow. Kinetically, it is extremely difficult to distinguish this type of inhibition from an irreversible inhibitor, because over time, the enzyme does tend to look like it loses its activity and, for all practical purposes, the enzyme behaves as if it were irreversibly tied up. To differentiate between tight-binding reversible and irreversible inhibitors, one can dialyze the enzyme–inhibitor complex. In case of the reversible inhibitor, on dialysis, the inhibitor will be removed from the enzyme, resulting in recovery of the enzyme activity; however, this is not so with the irreversible one.

Reversible Enzyme Inhibition

Reversible enzyme inhibition may be classified under two main headings, competitive and noncompetitive, with both following Michaelis-Menten kinetics. Competitive inhibition, by definition, requires that the inhibitor competes with the substrate for binding to the enzyme at the active site, and this binding is mutually exclusive. That is, if the inhibitor binds to the enzyme, the substrate will not be able to bind, and vice versa. Competitive inhibition also, however, suggests that the inhibition can be reversed in the presence of saturating amounts of substrate, because in this case, all enzyme active sites will be occupied by substrate-displacing inhibitor. In contrast, noncompetitive inhibition implies independent binding (i.e., both inhibitor and substrate may bind to the enzyme at different sites). Because binding of the inhibitor to the enzyme is at a site other than the active site, noncompetitive inhibition cannot be reversed by increasing the concentration of substrate. Graphing the kinetics of inhibition (Fig. 5.6), the Lineweaver-Burk plot of $1/V$ versus $1/[S]$ shows distinguishing characteristics between the two types of inhibition. In competitive inhibition, there is no change in the maximum velocity of the reaction (V_{max}; the intercept on the *y*-axis remains constant in the presence of inhibitor). However, the slope of the curve (K_m/V_{max}) is different with the inhibitor present, and K_m changes because of the presence of the competitive inhibitor (Fig. 5.6, competitive inhibition). In the case of noncompetitive inhibition, only the V_{max} of the reaction decreases, while the K_m remains unchanged (intercept on the *x*-axis unchanged with inhibitor, Fig. 5.6, noncompetitive inhibition).

Most of the rationally designed and clinically useful reversible inhibitors are competitive inhibitors. Table 5.1 gives a listing of several currently approved drugs that act as enzyme inhibitors. The majority of enzyme inhibitors generally bear some structural resemblance to the natural substrate of the enzyme. The design of such inhibitors would thus seem to be a logical and rational task which is uniquely suited to the medicinal chemist who can use the principles of bio-isosteric modification of natural enzyme substrates and metabolites, or modification of "lead" structures and structure activity relationships, to create selective and potent inhibitors. There are pitfalls in this endeavor, however, because even the most rationally designed drug must still overcome transport and other cellular barriers before exerting its effects. In the case of the noncompetitive inhibitors, the design is not as straightforward. These inhibitors can have widely differing structures, which in many instances bear no resemblance to the natural substrate. In general, inhibitors of the noncompetitive type have been obtained primarily through random screening of chemically novel molecules followed by further synthetic manipulation of the pharmacophore to optimize their inhibitory effects.

Examples of Reversible Inhibitors

The design of enzyme inhibitors has included random screening of synthetic chemical agents, natural products, and combinatorial libraries followed by molecular optimization or structure–activity relationships of so-called "lead" structures as well as bio-isosteric analogues of the enzyme substrates themselves. Drugs (e.g., finasteride) also have been developed for one indication but, based on observed side effects, have lead to other uses.

The rational approach in the design of enzyme inhibitors is greatly aided if the enzymatic reaction is characterized in

Uses of Finasteride

Finasteride (Proscar) an inhibitor of steroid 5α-reductase, an enzyme involved in the catalytic reduction of testosterone to dihydrotestosterone, was originally developed as an agent to treat prostate hyperplasia. In addition to this original use, finasteride also currently is indicated as an agent (Propecia) to stimulate hair growth for treatment of male pattern baldness. This benefit was recognized as a useful side effect during clinical trials of finasteride as an antiprostate agent.

terms of its kinetic mechanism. Such a characterization would include the knowledge of the kinetic parameters (rate constants and dissociation constants) of individual steps in the overall reaction pathway as well as the characterization of (any) intermediates involved in these individual steps. Examples of such "rational" inhibitors include both reversible and irreversible inhibitors of enzymes.

Antimetabolites

Antimetabolites are agents that interfere with the functioning of an essential metabolite and that most often are designed as structural analogues of the natural metabolite. As described earlier, the mechanism of action of sulfanilamide is that of a competitive inhibitor of *p*-aminobenzoic acid. In the case of the sulfanilamide, however, the mechanism was only determined after the bacterial inhibitory action was noted. This often is the case when a drug is discovered to have a certain therapeutic effect and, later, this effect is "rationalized" as being caused by an enzyme-inhibitory action (1). Other classic examples of a competitive inhibitor acting as an antimetabolite include a number of nucleoside analogues used as antiviral and anticancer agents. These agents again bear structural resemblance to natural nucleosides, which in their triphosphate form are substrates for nucleic acid polymerases involved in the synthesis of nucleic acids. Nucleic acid polymerases catalyze the condensation of the free 3′-hydroxy end of a nucleic acid with an incoming 5′-triphosphate derivative of a nucleoside (dNTP), resulting in a 3,′5′-phosphodiester linkage. Hence, nucleoside analogues, to compete with the natural substrate in the synthesis of nucleic acid, must be converted intracellularly to their mono-, di-, and finally, triphosphate derivative before exerting their inhibitory effects on nucleic acid synthesis. Certain drug design strategies incorporate a "masked" phosphate group on the nucleoside such that once absorbed, they enter into the systemic circulation as the monophosphate (13). The majority of these analogues are designed such that they lack the 3′-hydroxy group and are dideoxy derivatives of the natural substrate. These analogues thus ensure that once they are incorporated into nucleic acid, further extension of the nucleic acid is prevented because of the lack of a 3′-hydroxy group.

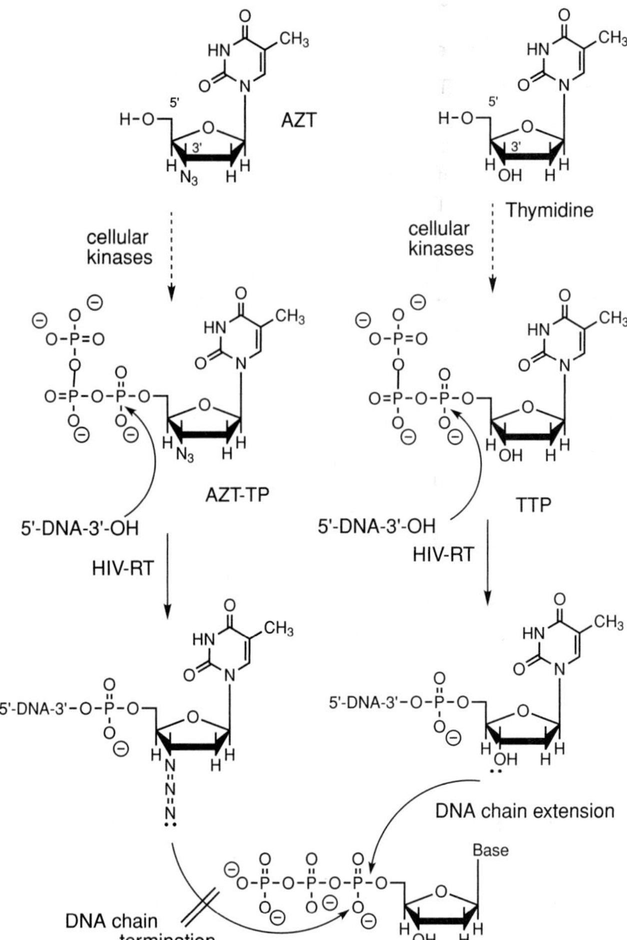

Fig. 5.7. Activation, incorporation, and chain-terminating action of azidothymidine (AZT), a thymidine analogue, as a reversible inhibitor of human immunodeficiency virus-reverse transcriptase (HIV-RT).

Inhibition of HIV-Reverse Transcriptase

Azidothymidine (AZT). The advent of AIDS stimulated a great interest in designing inhibitors against the essential viral polymerase—HIV-reverse transcriptase (HIV-RT). AZT is a potent inhibitor of HIV-RT (14), the retroviral polymerase that catalyzes the formation of proviral DNA from viral RNA. Structurally, AZT is similar to the natural nucleoside thymidine but has an azide group ($-N_3$) rather than a hydroxy group (—OH) at the 3′-position of the sugar deoxyribose (Fig. 5.7). AZT is activated intracellularly to its triphosphate and competes with thymidine triphosphate for uptake by HIV-RT into DNA (15). Once incorporated, further chain extension of the DNA is prevented, because there is no 3′-hydroxyl group to continue the DNA synthesis. In this fashion, AZT is an effective chain terminator of viral DNA synthesis.

Dideoxycytidine (ddC [Zalcitabine®]) and 3-thiacytidine (3-TC [Lamivudine®]). 2,′3′-Dideoxycytidine is another antiretroviral agent used against HIV-RT. In this case, ddC resembles the natural metabolite, deoxycytidine (dC),

Historical Development of AZT

Interestingly, AZT was originally synthesized as an anticancer agent to inhibit cellular DNA synthesis, but it was found to be too toxic. Subsequently, in the mid-1980s, during a random screening of nucleoside agents for potential inhibitory effects against HIV-RT, AZT was found to have selectivity for the HIV-RT (7). As such, its effects on host cell polymerases result in its dose-limiting bone marrow toxicity.

and as in the case of AZT, it is a 3′-deoxy analogue of dC, where the 3′-OH group of dC is replaced by a hydrogen atom. Similarly, 3-TC is another anti-HIV agent that resembles dC. In this example, however, rather than replacing the 3′-hydroxyl functionality as in ddC, the 3′-carbon position of the sugar has been substituted by a sulfur atom.

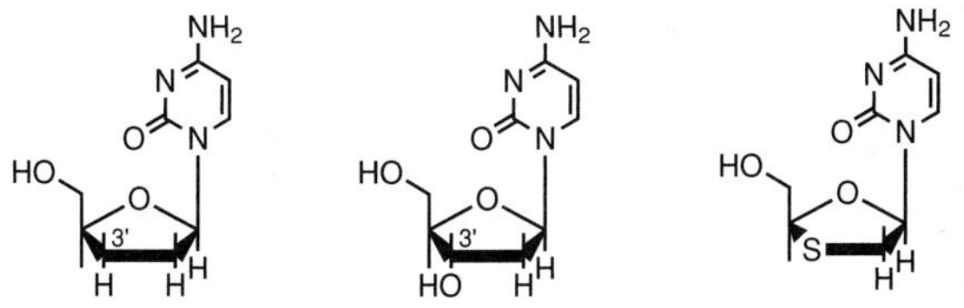

ddC dC 3-TC

Nevirapine. An example of a potent noncompetitive inhibitor of HIV-RT is the drug nevirapine, a benzodiazepine analogue (16), which is extremely tight-binding

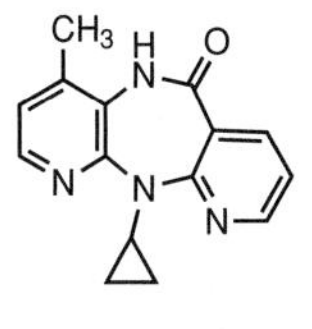

Nevirapine

to the enzyme, having a K_i in the nanomolar range. As can be seen in the structure of nevirapine, the drug bears no resemblance to any of the natural nucleotide substrates and was discovered through a random screening program. X-ray crystallographic studies of HIV-RT complexed with nevirapine have shown it binding in a hydrophobic pocket at a site adjacent to and slightly overlapping the nucleotide-binding site of HIV-RT (17). Kinetic studies with the enzyme have revealed an extremely slow binding rate for the drug; however, once bound, the polymerization rate for the reaction is effectively reduced (18).

A drawback for nevirapine, however, is that the virus can develop resistance very rapidly, through mutation of the amino acid residues in the binding pocket (19). Thus, its usefulness is limited to combination therapy with other antiretroviral agents rather than single-drug therapy.

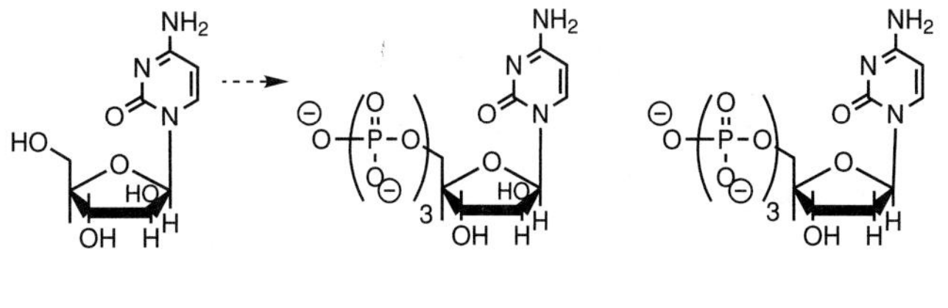

Ara-C Ara-CTP deoxyCTP

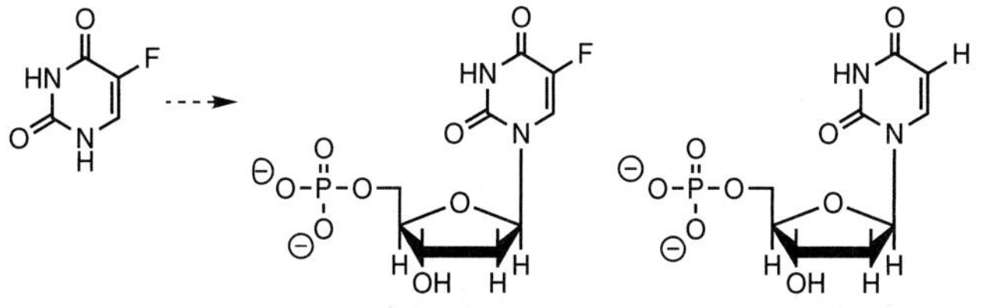

5-FU FUdR-monophosphate UdR-monophosphate

Fig. 5.8. Structures of pyrimidine antimetabolites used in cancer chemotherapy.

Reversible inhibitors used in cancer therapy. The design of several anticancer agents have been based on the antimetabolite theory. Because cancer results in overproliferation and uncontrolled cell growth, drugs designed against cancer have been based on inhibiting DNA synthesis in the cell. Thus, these drugs have been targeted against those enzymes, including nucleic acid polymerases, thymidylate synthase, and dihydrofolate reductase (DHFR), that play a role in DNA synthesis. Examples of drugs that have been designed against nucleic acid polymerases include cytosine arabinoside (Ara-C) and 5-fluorouracil (5-FU) (Fig. 5.8). Cytosine arabinoside is first converted to its triphosphate, and as such, it functions as an antimetabolite of deoxycytidine triphosphate (deoxy CTP) to inhibit DNA polymerase. As can be seen from its structure, Ara-C is the arabino isomer of cytidine. That is, the 2′-hydroxyl functionality in Ara-C is in the arabino configuration rather than the ribo configuration of cytidine. Because of this stereochemical change in the placement of the 2′-hydroxyl function, Ara-C tends to resemble deoxycytidine rather than cytidine. In this way, Ara-C inhibits DNA polymerases by competing with deoxycytidine. 5-FU is an analogue of the pyrimidine base uracil, where the hydrogen at the 5-position in uracil has been substituted by an isosteric fluorine (F) atom. This makes 5-FU look very similar to uracil. 5-FU, after conversion to 5-fluorodeoxyuridine monophosphate (FdUMP), is an inhibitor of thymidylate synthase, the enzyme involved in the de novo synthesis of thymidylate. In this case, FdUMP is an antimetabolite of deoxyuridine monophosphate.

Methotrexate is a potent inhibitor of DHFR, the enzyme responsible for the reduction of folic acid to dihydro- and tetrahydrofolic acid, precursors to one-carbon donation in purine and pyrimidine de novo synthesis. Methotrexate is

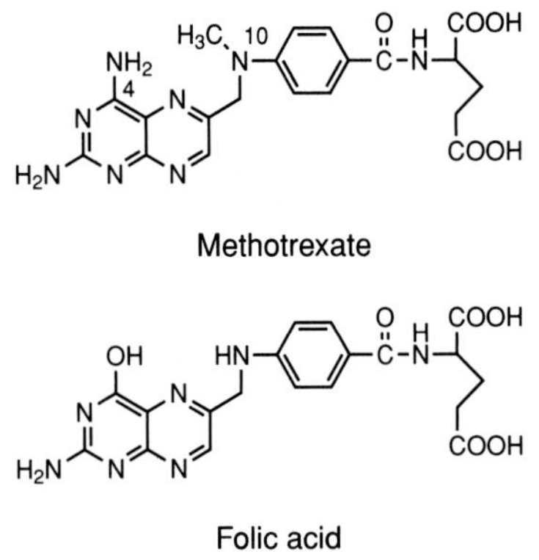

Methotrexate

Folic acid

Fig. 5.9. Methotrexate, the antimetabolite of folic acid.

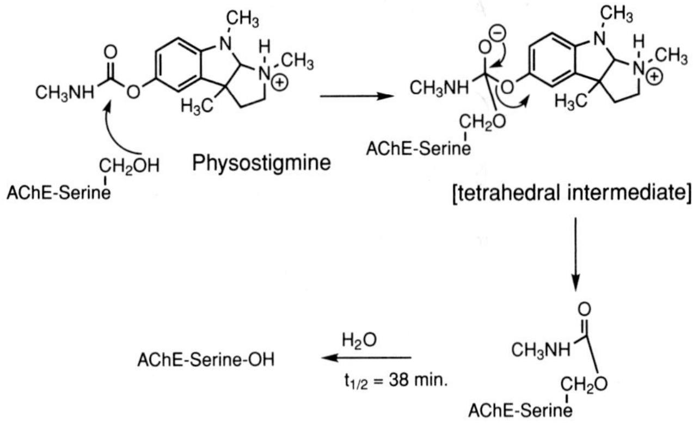

Physostigmine

[tetrahedral intermediate]

Fig. 5.11. Mechanism of inhibition of acetylcholine esterase by physostigmine.

an analogue of folic acid where the 4-hydroxyl group (—OH) on the pteridine ring of folic acid has been replaced by an amino (—NH_2) functionality and the nitrogen atom at the 10-position is methylated (Fig. 5.9). These substitutions led to methotrexate having an affinity for DHFR orders of magnitude greater than that for the natural metabolite, folic acid, and allows it to be an extremely potent inhibitor.

Inhibition of Acetylcholinesterase

Acetylcholinesterase (AChE) is the enzyme that catalyzes the catabolism of the neurotransmitter acetylcholine to acetate and choline (see Chapter 12). Thus, inhibition of AChE would lead to increased concentrations of acetylcholine and a prolonged action of the neurotransmitter. Inhibitors of AChE have found use in cases of myasthenia gravis, glaucoma, and Alzheimer's disease. To appreciate the design of these inhibitors, it is useful to first understand the mechanism of action of AChE. AChE has an anionic site that can bind the positively charged quaternary ammonium group of the choline functionality and an active esteratic site that contains a nucleophilic serine residue involved in the hydrolysis of the ester bond (Fig. 5.10). The mechanism involves the attack of the nucleophilic serine hydroxy group on the carbonyl group of acetylcholine to form a tetrahedral intermediate that breaks down, resulting in the release of choline and an intermediate, acetylated serine that subsequently hydrolyzes to release AChE.

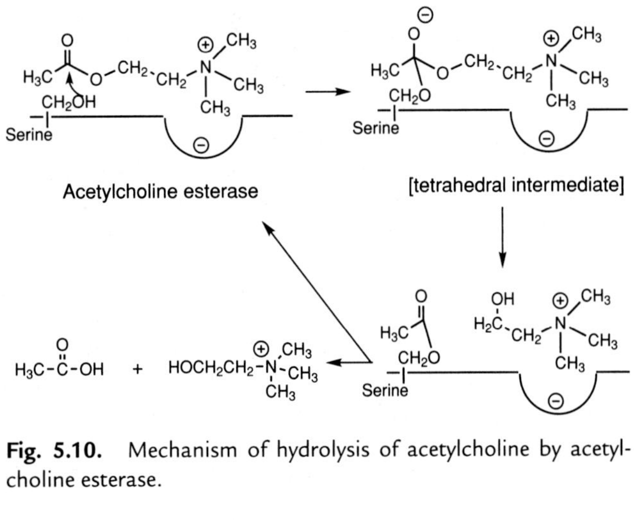

Acetylcholine esterase

[tetrahedral intermediate]

Fig. 5.10. Mechanism of hydrolysis of acetylcholine by acetylcholine esterase.

Physostigmine has been used in the treatment of glaucoma. It is an alkaloid with a carbamate moiety that resembles the ester linkage of acetylcholine. Being an alkaloid, it is protonated at physiological pH and, thus, can bind to the anionic site of AChE. Following the mechanism of AChE, the serine residue of the enzyme can attack the carbonyl group of physostigmine, and in the process, the serine is carbamylated (Fig. 5.11). This carbamyl serine intermediate is more stable, to enzymatic than is acetylated SER and subsequent hydrolysis by water occurs extremely slowly. The carbamylated enzyme is only slowly regenerated, with a half-life of 38 minutes—more than seven orders of magnitude slower than that for the natural substrate, acetylcholine. This is an example of a reversible inhibitor involved in covalent bond formation with the enzyme that ultimately gets hydrolyzed.

Inhibitors of Angiotensin-Converting Enzyme

Angiotensin-converting enzyme (ACE) is a carboxypeptidase having a zinc ion as a cofactor and is involved in the renin-angiotensin cascade of blood pressure control (20). The design of the antihypertensive drug captopril, a clinically important and potent reversible inhibitor of ACE, is an example of one of the early endeavors and successes of a rationally designed enzyme inhibitor (21) (see Chapter 28). The design of captopril was based on several factors. These included the knowledge that ACE was similar in its enzymatic mechanism to carboxypeptidase A, except that ACE cleaved off a dipeptide whereas carboxypeptidase A cleaved single amino acid residues from the carboxyl end of the protein; the discovery of L-benzylsuccinic acid as a potent inhibitor of carboxypeptidase A; and, studies of a potent pentapeptide inhibitor of ACE, $BPP_{5\alpha}$ (Glu-Lys-Trp-Ala-Pro), from the venom of the Brazilian viper (*Bothrops jararaca*), which showed that the N-terminal peptide fragments, including tetra-, tri-, and dipeptide fragments (Ala-Pro) of $BPP_{5\alpha}$, retained

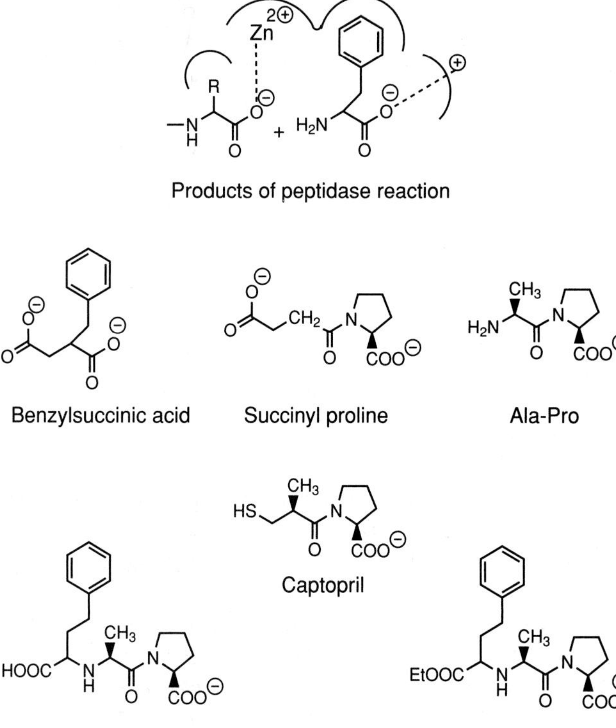

Fig. 5.12. Angiotensin-converting enzyme (ACE) inhibitors and efforts that led to their development.

some inhibitory activity. Benzylsuccinic acid has been described as a biproduct inhibitor of carboxypeptidase A, wherein its design was based on the combination of the products of the peptidase reaction (i.e., the two peptide fragments, one with a free carboxyl end that coordinates the zinc ion of the protease and the other with a free amino terminus) (Fig. 5.12) (22). In the case of benzylsuccinic acid, the amino ($-NH_2$) functionality is replaced by the isosteric methylene ($-CH_2-$) group. Using the above concepts, it was rationalized that succinyl amino acids could similarly behave as a biproduct inhibitors of ACE. Starting with a succinyl-proline moiety, the structural activity developmental effort finally resulted in captopril with the substitution of the stronger zinc coordinating mercapto functionality in place of the carboxylic residue (of succinic acid) and a stereospecific R methyl group on the succinyl function to represent the methyl group on the natural L-Ala residue in Ala-Pro (the dipeptide fragment that had previously shown inhibitory activity). Captopril soon became highly successful in the clinic as an antihypertensive agent and, in combination with diuretics, has proved to be the treatment of choice in controlling hypertension.

Following on the heels of captopril was another byproduct ACE inhibitor, enalaprilat. Enalaprilat incorporated a phenylethyl moiety with the S-configuration and made use of a hydrophobic binding pocket in ACE that was overlooked during the design of captopril (23). Recalling that the tripeptide fragment of $BPP_{5\alpha}$ (Trp-Ala-Pro) contained the aromatic tryptophan residue and showed weak inhibitory properties suggested the benefit of an aromatic binding site. Substituting the tryptophan residue with a phenyl group allowed the design of enalaprilat, which retained the carboxylic group as the coordinating ligand for zinc and resulted in a 20-fold increase in potency over captopril. However, enalaprilat, a diacid, was poorly absorbed from the gastrointestinal tract; thus, a pro-drug ethyl ester of enalaprilat, called enalapril, was developed. Enalapril had superior pharmacokinetics to enalaprilat and was rapidly metabolized to the active drug.

Transition-State Analogues

Transition-state analogues are compounds that resemble the substrate portion of the hypothetical transition state of an enzymatic reaction. All chemical reactions progressing from substrate to product must cross an energy barrier and proceed through a transition state or activated high-energy complex. This energy barrier is described as the activation energy. In the case of enzyme-catalyzed reactions, it is accepted that the enzyme reduces this energy barrier as compared to the nonenzyme catalyzed reaction. Factors contributing to this reduced energy barrier are several and include stabilization of the transition state and intermediate forms of the reaction during the course of transition from substrate to product as well as conformational effects of distortion of the substrate while traversing towards the product (5). In 1948, Pauling (8) initially suggested that compounds resembling the transition state of an enzyme-catalyzed reaction would be effective inhibitors of the enzyme, because the substrate transition state should have the greatest affinity for the enzyme. Later, Wolfenden (24) proposed that thermodynamically, it is possible to relate the hypothetical equilibrium dissociation constants between substrate and its transition state of an enzyme-catalyzed reaction with that of the nonenzyme-catalyzed one. Using such an analysis, he showed that the ratio of the hypothetical transition state dissociation constants of nonenzyme-catalyzed reaction to that of the enzyme-catalyzed one is equal to the ratio of the first-order rate constants of formation of transition state for enzyme-catalyzed reaction to noncatalyzed reaction. Because the ratio of the enzyme-catalyzed rate constant to that of the noncatalyzed one ranges from 10^7 to 10^{10}, it follows that the substrate transition state would bind the enzyme 10^7- to 10^{10}-fold more tightly than the substrate itself (25). Hence, transition-state analogues that resemble the substrate would be extremely tight-binding compounds. To design a transition-state inhibitor, knowledge of the enzyme chemistry and its mechanism is a basic requirement. It must be understood, however, that these substrate transition states are, by nature, unstable transient species existing for no longer than a few picoseconds. Nevertheless, experimental evidence

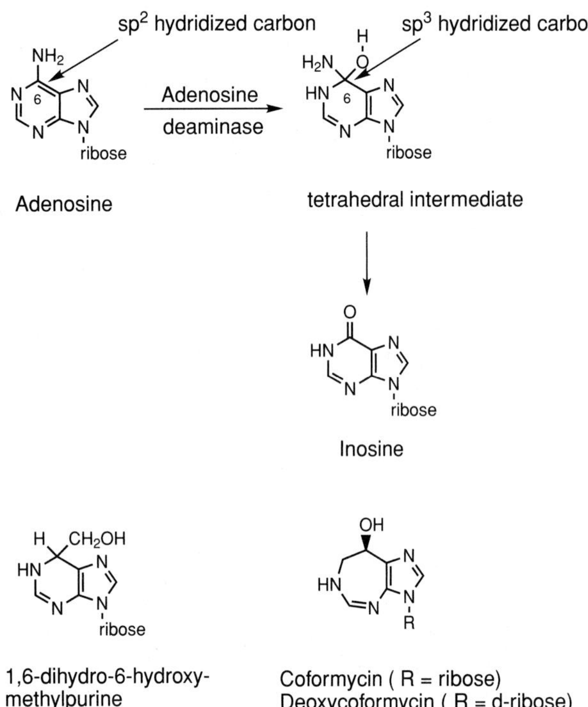

Fig. 5.13. Mechanism and transition-state inhibitors of adenosine deaminase.

has shown that even crudely designed transition-state inhibitors resembling the substrate are extremely potent inhibitors (25).

TRANSITION-STATE INHIBITOR OF ADENOSINE DEAMINASE. Adenosine deaminase is the enzyme that hydrolyzes adenosine (or deoxyadenosine) to inosine (or deoxyinosine) and is important for purine metabolism. High levels of adenosine are toxic to B cells of the immune system and can result in an immunocompromised state. Also, people who lack the gene for adenosine deaminase have the genetic condition of severe combined immunodeficiency and are extremely susceptible to opportunistic infections. Many cancer and antiviral agents also are degraded by this enzyme; hence, there is a role for the development of inhibitors of this enzyme (26). The mechanism proposed for adenosine deaminase is a nucleophilic attack of water at the 6-position of the purine base to form a tetrahedral intermediate (Fig. 5.13). The transition state presumably resembles this intermediate.

During the course of the deaminase reaction, the hybridization of the G-carbon changes from an sp^2-hybridized state to an sp^3 state. Subsequently, there is a loss of ammonia to give the product inosine. To develop a transition-state inhibitor for this enzyme, one would have to factor in this change in the hybridization of the substrate molecule; thus, molecules having an sp^3-hybridized carbon at this position and resembling the substrate would potentially be candidates for transition-state inhibitors. The compound 1,6-dihydro-6-hydroxymethylpurine has such geometry, and its potent inhibitory properties of adenosine deaminase ($K_i < 1$ μM, as compared to a K_m for adenosine of 31 μM) has been rationalized as being a transition-state inhibitor (27). Two compounds that nature has provided, coformycin and its deoxyribose analogue, deoxycoformycin (Fig. 5.13), are extremely potent inhibitors of adenosine deaminase (K_i = 0.002 nM). Both of these compounds contain a seven-member ring structure, which through its flexibility is presumed to resemble the hypothesized distorted sp^2–sp^3 transition state that forms during the addition of water to adenosine (28).

Irreversible Enzyme Inhibition

As previously described, irreversible enzyme inhibition is defined as "time-dependent inactivation of the enzyme," which implies that the enzyme has, in some way or form, been permanently modified, because it can no longer carry out its function. This modification is the result of a covalent bond being formed with the inhibitor and some amino acid residue in the protein. Furthermore, this bond is extremely stable and, for all practical purposes, is not hydrolyzed to give back the enzyme in its original state or structure. In most examples of irreversible inhibition, a new enzyme must be generated through gene transcription and translation for the enzyme to continue its normal catalytic action. Basically, there are two types of irreversible enzyme inhibitors, the affinity labels or active site–directed irreversible inhibitors and the mechanism-based irreversible enzyme inactivators.

Affinity Labels and Active Site–Directed Irreversible Inhibitors

The affinity labels are those chemical entities that are inherently reactive and can target any nucleophilic residue in the enzyme, especially those residing in and around the catalytic center of the protein. These agents generally resemble the substrate so that they may bind in the active site of the enzyme. In most examples, these agents also contain an electrophilic functional group, which includes groups such as halo-methyl ketones (X-CH_2C=O, where X = halide), sulfonyl fluorides (SO_2F), nitrogen mustards ($(ClCH_2CH_2)_2NH$), diazoketones ($COCHN_2$), and other such reactive groups, that can "label," or alkylate, a nucleophilic amino acid residue in the enzyme. They generally tend to be indiscriminate in their action and have little therapeutic value, because they are nonselective and, thus, inherently toxic. They have been used mainly as biochemical tools to probe active sites of enzyme to discern the types of amino acid residues both in and around the catalytic center of an enzyme. The classic example of an affinity label is TPCK (tosyl-phenylalanyl-chloromethyl-ketone), an irreversible inhibitor of the serine protease chymotrypsin (29). Because TPCK resembles the amino acid phenylalanine, it can bind to the active site of the chymotrypsin, the selectivity of which is for such hydrophobic amino acid residues (Phe and Tyr). During the course of normal peptide hydrolysis, the reactive chloromethyl-ketone

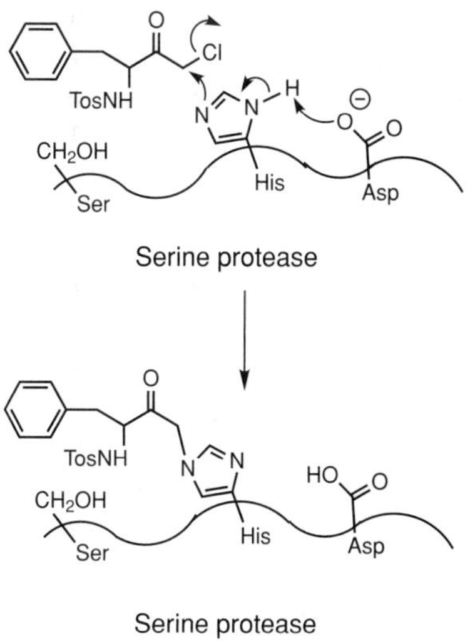

Serine protease

Serine protease

Fig. 5.14. Mechanism of affinity label of serine protease with TPCK (tosyl-phenylalanyl-chloromethyl-ketone).

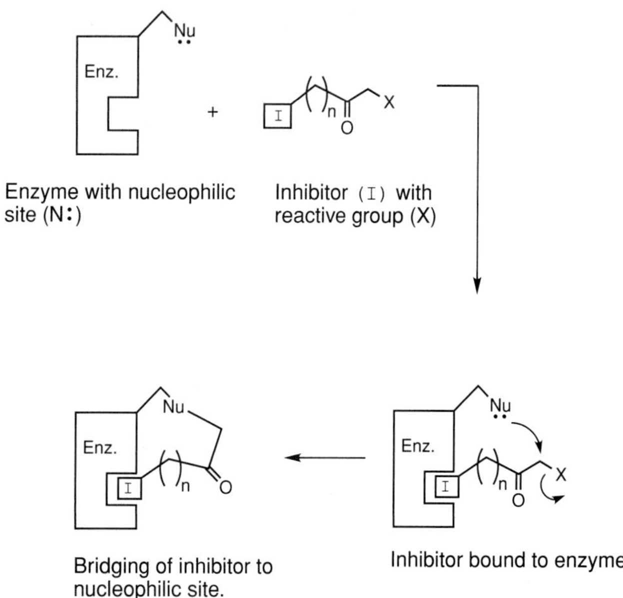

Fig. 5.15. Model showing Baker's (30 active site-directed irreversible inhibitors.

labels the nucleophilic histidine residue present as part of the catalytic triad (Ser-His-Asp) in the active site of the protease (Fig. 5.14). Another similarly designed affinity label is TLCK (tosyl-lysyl-chloromethyl-ketone), the specificity of which is for the protease trypsin. Trypsin cleaves peptide bonds adjacent to the basic amino acids, lysine and arginine. It was found that TLCK was a specific inhibitor of trypsin but had no activity for chymotrypsin. On the other hand, TPCK, although extremely specific for chymotrypsin, showed no activity for trypsin.

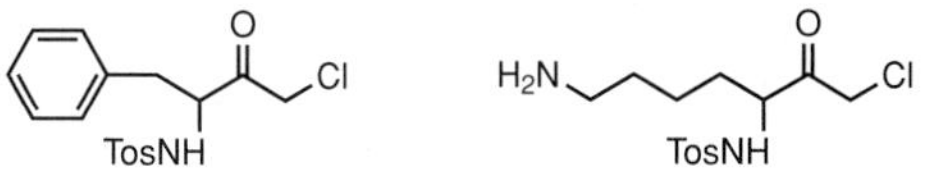

TPCK TLCK

Because of the inherent reactivity and nonselectivity of these affinity labels and their limited utility in drug therapy, the late B.R. Baker (30) extended this concept to design inhibitors that would have greater selectivity and specificity and, thus, be potential drug candidates. He designed several analogues, termed active site–directed irreversible inhibitors, targeted toward thymidylate synthase, a key enzyme involved in the de novo metabolism of thymidylate. These analogues contained a substrate-binding region linked to a reactive group, such as a halomethyl ketone, by a tether whose chain length could be manipulated. The substrate portion of the analogue ensures both affinity and rapid binding to the enzyme active site. Once bound, areas in and around the binding site and on the surface of the enzyme could be probed for nucleophilic amino acid residues. By manipulating the length of the tether, ideal inhibitors could then be designed such that any suitably located, sufficiently nucleophilic amino acid residue on the surface of the enzyme could potentially be alkylated by the halomethyl ketone (Fig. 5.15). Once alkylated, the tether "bridges" the active site with the labeled amino acid residue, thus "tying up" and preventing further catalysis by the enzyme.

Mechanism-Based Irreversible Enzyme Inactivators

Overview. The mechanism-based irreversible inhibitors also have been termed as suicide substrates," "k_{cat} inhibitors," "Trojan horse inhibitors," or "latent alkylating agents." These inhibitors are inherently unreactive but, on normal catalytic processing by the enzyme, are activated into highly reactive moieties (31–33). These reactive functionalities can then irreversibly alkylate a nucleophilic amino acid residue or cofactor in the enzyme and, in essence, cause the enzyme's death ("suicide"). Basically, these inhibitors have a latent reactive functionality that only becomes apparent after binding and acted on by the normal catalytic machinery of the enzyme. This type of inhibitor design differs from the preceding one in that these inhibitors have one more level of built-in selectivity. The kinetic scheme for such inhibition is shown in Equation 5.5, in which enzyme, E, binds with substrate (inhibitor), S, to give an [E–S] complex with dissociation constant of K_i:

Eq. 5.5 $$E + S \; K_i \rightleftharpoons [E{\cdot}S] \; k_{cat} \rightarrow [E{\cdot}S^*] \; k_{inact} \rightarrow [E\text{–}S]$$
$$\downarrow k_{diff}$$
$$E + S^* {}_{+} Nu: \rightarrow [Nu\text{–}S]$$

Next, the [E–S] complex is converted into a highly activated complex [E–S*] by the catalytic machinery (k_{cat}) of the enzyme, which can then go on to alkylate the enzyme, [E-S]. Note that it is possible for the reactive species [S*] to diffuse (dissociate) from the enzyme and react with some other target (nucleophilic species)—that is, the system is "leaky." If this happens, however, the inhibitor cannot be classified as a "true" suicide substrate, because specificity is lost.

Several requirements need to be met by these inhibitors for them to be classified as suicide substrates. These include the following: 1) Inactivation should be time dependent (reaction should be irreversible), 2) kinetics should be first order, 3) the enzyme should show saturation phenomenon, (4) the substrate should be able to protect the enzyme, and 5) stoichiometry of the reaction should be 1:1 (one active site to one inhibitor).

EXAMPLES OF SUICIDE SUBSTRATES. During the past three decades, besides the rational design of hundreds of molecules that have been synthesized and tested as suicide substrates, it also has come to light that nature itself has known about this mechanistic mode of enzyme inhibition and provided us with several extremely potent mechanism-based suicide inactivators. Below are a few selected examples to demonstrate the mode of action of these inhibitors.

Halo enol lactones. Halo enol lactones are an example of suicide inhibitors for serine proteases. These analogues were developed by Katzenellenbogen and coworkers at the University of Illinois (34). On normal catalytic processing by the serine hydroxyl functionality, they give rise to a reactive halo-methyl ketone, which subsequently alkylates a nearby nucleophilic residue on the enzyme (Fig. 5.16). Other suicide inactivators for the serine proteases have been designed by various researchers (32).

Clauvulinic acid. Clavulanic acid is a potent inhibitor of bacterial β-lactamase (35). This enzyme is a serine protease and can hydrolyze β-lactams, such as the penicillin antibiotics. It is the principal enzyme responsible for penicillin-resistant bacteria. Clavulanic acid itself is a β-lactam and, if given in combination with penicillin, is preferentially taken up by β-lactamase and hydrolyzed.

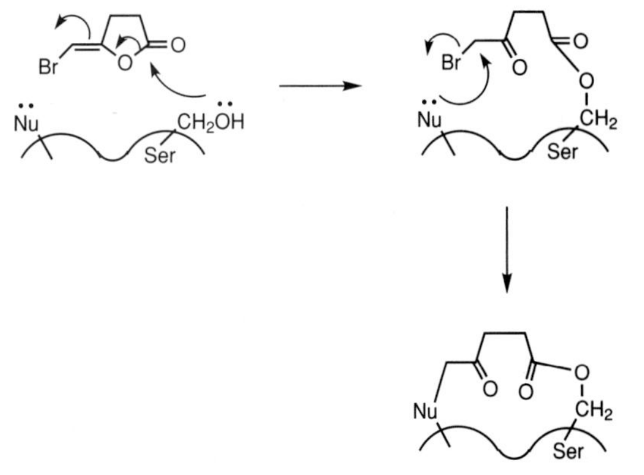

Fig. 5.16. Mechanism-based inhibition of serine proteases by Katzenellenbogen's halo enol lactone.

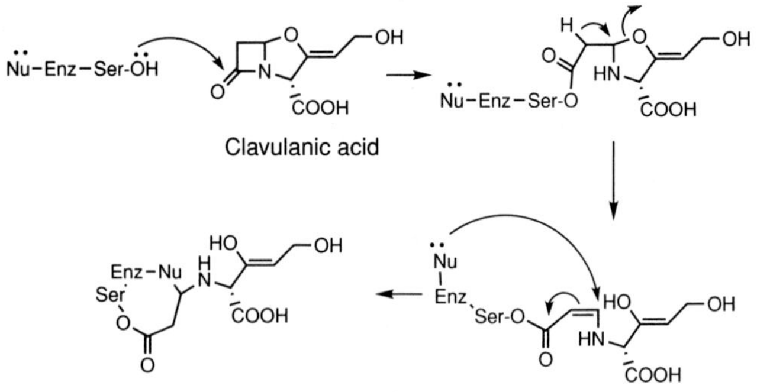

Fig. 5.17. Mechanism-based inhibition of β-lactamases by clavulinic acid.

During the process of hydrolysis, however, the molecule undergoes a cleavage, leading to the formation of a "Michael acceptor," which subsequently alkylates a nucleophilic residue on β-lactamase, causing irreversible inhibition (Fig. 5.17). Such combinations of a β-lactamase inhibitor and a penicillin have resulted in clinically useful agents [clavulanic acid plus amoxicillin (Augmentin)].

Gabaculin. Gabaculin, a naturally occurring neurotoxin, is a potent mechanism-based inhibitor of the enzyme γ-ainobutyric acid transaminase (GABA-T) with an interesting mechanism of action (36). GABA-T is a pyridoxal phosphate (PLP)–dependent enzyme involved in the catabolism (transamination) (Fig. 5.18) of the excitatory neurotransmitter, GABA, to succinate semialdehyde and pyridoxamine. As part of the normal catalytic mechanism of PLP-dependent enzymes, the amino group of gabaculin first forms a Schiff base with the aldehyde of PLP (Fig. 5.18). Next, this adduct undergoes an aromatization reaction, resulting in an extremely stable covalent bond with the cofactor, PLP. Hence, in this case, rather than an enzymatic nucleophilic residue being alkylated, the cofactor is "tied up," resulting in the inhibition.

Finasteride. Finasteride is a clinically useful agent in the treatment of prostate hyperplasia and male pattern baldness. It is a potent inhibitor of human steroid-5α-reductase, the enzyme responsible for the reduction of testosterone to dihydrotestosterone (Fig. 5.19). (see Chapter 45)The inhibitory action of finasteride has been attributed both to its similarity in structure to testosterone, which allows it to bind to the enzyme and be reduced to dihydrofinasteride in place of testosterone, as well as to its ability to act as a mechanism-based inhibitor, during which it can tie up the cofactor, NADPH, by forming a covalent NADP-dihydrofinasteride adduct (Fig. 5.19) (see Chapter 45). This adduct very slowly releases dihydrofinasteride with a half-life of one month (37).

CONCLUSION

This chapter has attempted to give the reader an overview of enzyme catalysis and the various ways in

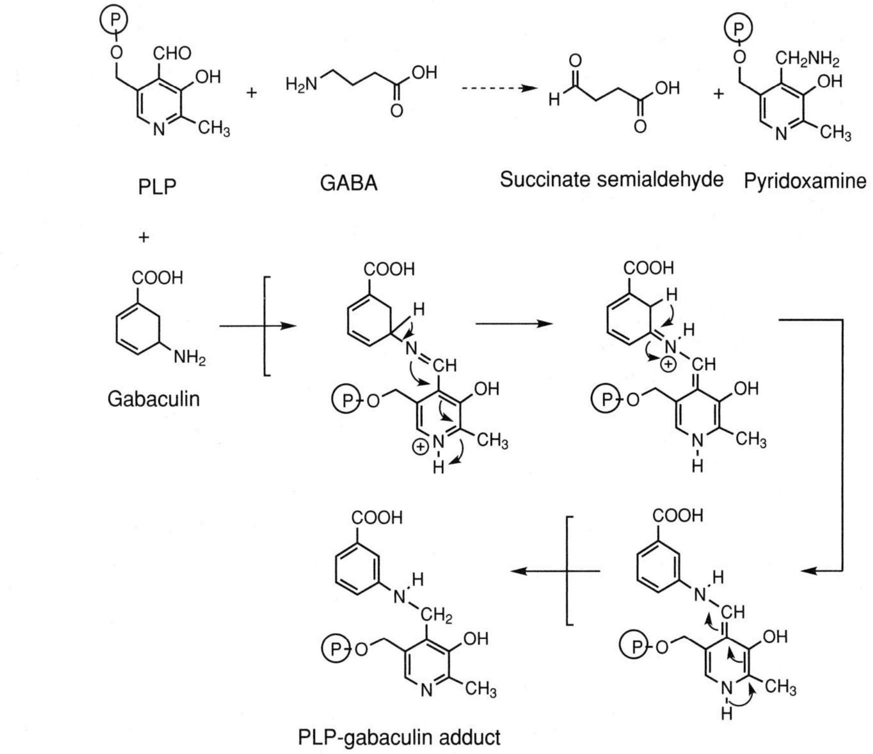

Fig. 5.18. Pyridoxal phosphate-dependent γ-ainobutyric acid transaminase (GABA-T) reaction and the mechanism of suicide inhibition by gabaculin.

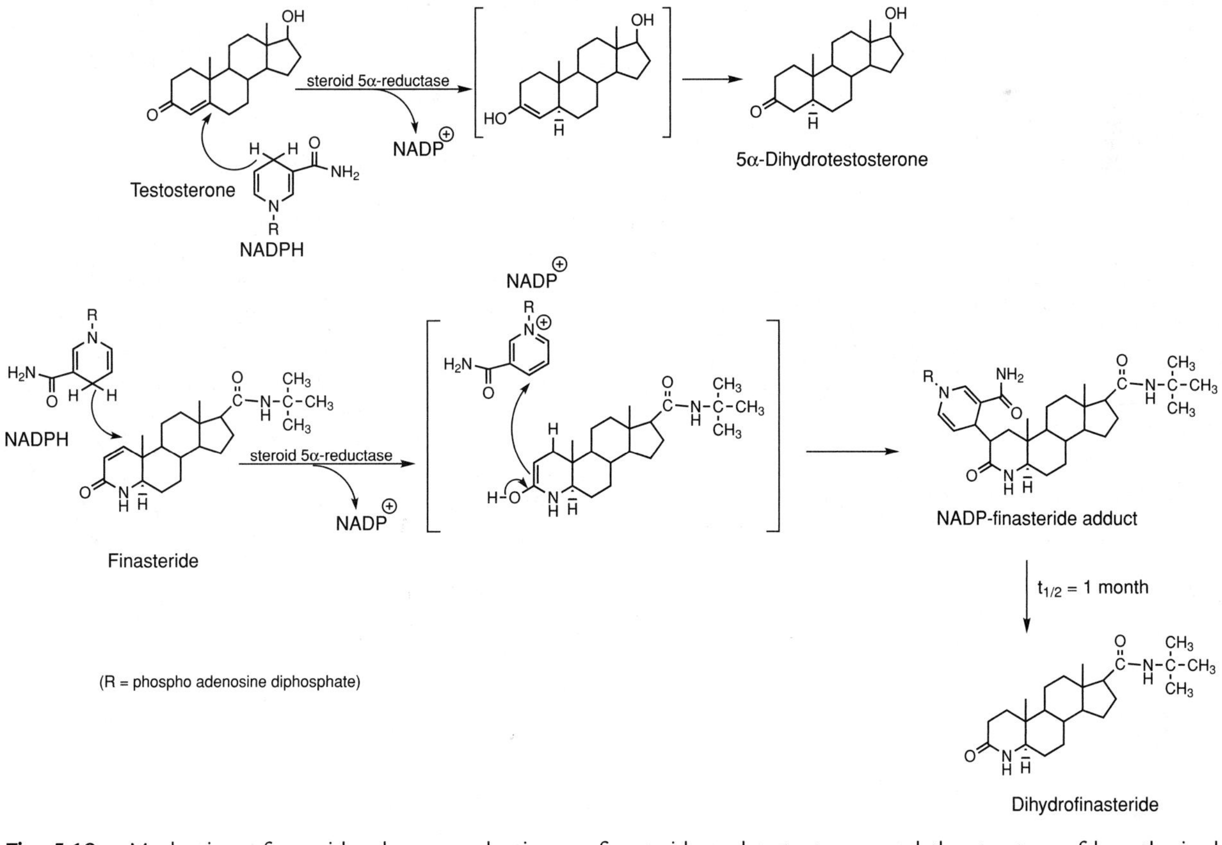

Fig. 5.19. Mechanism of steroid reductase reduction on finasteride and testosterone and the structure of hypothesized NADPH-dihydrofinasteride adduct (37).

which enzymes can act as catalytic receptors. Based on these properties and mechanisms of enzyme action, the essentials of drug design and discovery through enzyme inhibition with a few choice examples have been outlined. The reader is referred to suggested reading material for more detailed explanations and insights regarding the rationale and design strategies of enzyme inhibitors. In conclusion, drug design by enzyme inhibition is a continually developing enterprise. There will always be the need to discover more selective and more potent inhibitors in an effort to increase the therapeutic benefit to patients. This chapter has tried to give a brief insight into this fascinating area of medicinal chemistry and the various types of enzyme inhibitors that can be rationally designed.

References

1. Albert A. Selective Toxicity—The Physicochemical Basis of Therapy, 7th Ed. New York: Chapman & Hall, 1985.
2. Domagk G. Ein beitrag zur chemotherapie der bakteriellen infektionen. Dtsch Med Wochenschr 1935;61:250–253.
3. Woods DD. Relation of *p*-aminobenzoic acid to mechanism of action of sulfanilamide. Br J Exp Pathol 1940;21:74–90.
4. Albert A. Chapter 9. In: Selective toxicity—the physicochemical basis of therapy, 7th Ed. New York: Chapman & Hall, 1985.
5. Fersht A. Structure and Mechanism in Protein Science: A Guide to Enzyme Catalysis and Protein Folding, 3rd Ed.. New York: W.H. Freeman, 2000.
6. Lad C, Williams H, Wolfenden, R. The rate of hydrolysis of phosphomonoester dianions and the exceptional catalytic proficiencies of protein and inositol phosphatases. Proc Natl Acad Sci U S A 2003;100:5607–5610.
7. Available at: http://www.chem.qmul.ac.uk/iubmb/enzyme/. Accessed April 4, 2006.
8. Pauling L. The nature of forces between large molecules of biological interest. Nature 1948;161:707–709.
9. Garcia-Viloca M, Gao J, Karplus M, et al. How enzymes work: analysis by modern rate theory and computer simulations. Science 2004;303:186–195.
10. Zhang X, Houk KN. Why enzymes are proficient catalysts: beyond the Pauling paradigm. Acc Chem Res 2005;38:379–385.
11. Bruice TC, Benkovic SJ. A comparison of the bimolecular and intramolecular nucleophilic catalysis of the hydrolysis of substituted phenyl acylates by the dimethylamino group. J Am Chem Soc 1963;85:1–8.
12. Michael C, Gaston S. Formation and hydrolysis of lactones of phenolic acids. J Am Chem Soc 1980;102:4815–4821.
13. Sastry JK, Nehete PN, Khan S, et al. Membrane-permeable dideoxyuridine 5′-monophosphate analogue inhibits human immunodeficiency virus infection. Mol Pharmacol 1992;41:441–445.
14. Mitsuya H, Weinhold KJ, Furman PA, et al. 3′-Azido-3′-deoxythymidine (BW A509U): an antiviral agent that inhibits the infectivity and cytopathic effect of human T-lymphotropic virus type III/lymphadenopathy-associated virus in vitro. Proc Natl Acad Sci U S A 1985;82:7096–7100.
15. Furman PA, Fyfe JA, St. Clair MH, et al. Phosphorylation of 3′-azido-3′-deoxythymidine and selective interaction of the 5′-triphosphate with human immunodeficiency virus reverse transcriptase. Proc Natl Acad Sci U S A 1986;83:8333–8337.
16. Grob PM, Wu JC, Cohen KA, et al. Nonnucleoside inhibitors of HIV-1 reverse transcriptase: nevirapine as a prototype drug. AIDS Res Hum Retrovir 1992;8:145–152.
17. Kohlstaedt LA, Wang J, Friedman JM, et al. Crystal structure at 3.5 A resolution of HIV-1 reverse transcriptase complexed with an inhibitor. Science 1992;256:1783–1790.
18. Spence RA, Kati WM, Anderson KS, et al. Mechanism of inhibition of HIV-1 reverse transcriptase by nonnucleoside inhibitors. Science 1995;267:988–993.
19. Mellors JW, Dutschman GE, Im GJ, et al. In vitro selection and molecular characterization of human immunodeficiency virus-1 resistant to nonnucleoside inhibitors of reverse transcriptase. Mol Pharmacol 1992;41:446–451.
20. Harrold M. Calcium blockers; angiotensin-converting enzyme inhibitors; angiotensin antagonists. In: Lemke T, Williams DA eds. Foye's Principles of Medicinal Chemistry, 5th Ed. Philadelphia: Williams & Wilkins, 2001: 580–603.
21. Cushman DW, Cheung HS, Sabo EF, et al. Design of potent competitive inhibitors of angiotensin-converting enzyme. Carboxyalkanoyl and mercaptoalkanoyl amino acids. Biochemistry 1977;16:5484–5491.
22. Byers LD, Wolfenden R. Binding of the by-product analogue benzylsuccinic acid by carboxypeptidase A. Biochemistry 1973;12:2070–2078.
23. Patchett AA, Harris E, Tristram EW, et al. A new class of angiotensin-converting enzyme inhibitors. Nature 1980;288:280–283.
24. Wolfenden R. Transition-state analogues for enzyme catalysis. Nature 1969;223:704–705.
25. Wolfenden R. Transition-state analogues as potential affinity labeling agents. Methods Enzymol 1977;46:15–28.
26. Shannon WM, Schabel FM Jr. Antiviral agents as adjuncts in cancer chemotherapy. Pharmacol Ther 1980;11:263–390.
27. Evans BE, Wolfenden RJ. A potential transition-state analogue for adenosine deaminase. J Am Chem Soc 1970;92:4751–4752.
28. Nakamura H, Koyama G, Iitaka Y, et al. Structure of Coformycin, an unusual nucleoside of microbial origin. J Am Chem Soc 1974;96:4327–4328.
29. Walpole CSJ, Wrigglesworth R. Enzyme inhibitors in medicine. Nat Prod Rep 1989;63:311–346.
30. Baker BR. Design of Active Site Directed Irreversible Enzyme Inhibitors. New York: Wiley, 1967.
31. Walsh C. Recent developments in suicide substrates and other active site–directed inactivating agents of specific target enzymes. Horiz Biochem Biophys 1977;3:36–81.
32. Abeless RH. Suicide enzyme inactivators. Chem Eng News 1983;61(38):48–55.
33. Rando RR. Mechanism based irreversible enzyme inhibitors. Methods Enzymol 1977;46:28–41.
34. Kraft GA, Katzenellenbogen JA. Synthesis of halo enol lactones. Mechanism-based inactivators of serine proteases. J Am Chem Soc 1981;103:5459–5466.
35. Charnas RL, Knowles JR. Inactivation of RTEM β-lactamase from *Escherichia coli* by clavulanic acid and 9-deoxyclavulanic acid. Biochemistry 1981;20:3214–3219.
36. Rando RR. Mechanisms of naturally occurring irreversible enzyme inhibitors. Acc Chem Res 1975;8:281–288.
37. Bull HG, Garcia-Calvo M, Andersson S, et al. Mechanism-based inhibition of human steroid 5α-reductase by finasteride: enzyme-catalyzed formation of NADP-dihydrofinasteride, a potent bisubstrate analogue inhibitor. J Am Chem Soc 1996;118:2359–2365.

SUGGESTED READINGS

Abeless RH. Suicide enzyme inactivators. Chem Eng News 1983;61(38):48–55.
Albert A. Selective Toxicity—The physicochemical Basis of Therapy, 7th Ed. New York: Chapman & Hall, 1985.
Baker BR. Design of Active Site Directed Irreversible Enzyme Inhibitors. New York: Wiley, 1967.
Kalman TI, ed. Drug Action & Design—Mechanism-Based Enzyme Inhibitors. New York: Elsevier Science, 1979.
Seiler N, Jung MJ, Kock-Weser J, eds. Enzyme-Activated Irreversible Inhibitors. New York: Elsevier North Holland, 1978.
Silverman RB. The Organic Chemistry of Drug Design and Drug Action, 2nd Ed. New York: Elsevier–Academic Press, 2004.
Smith JS, ed. Smith and Williams' Introduction to the Principles of Drug Design and Action, 3rd Ed. Amsterdam: Harwood Academic Press, 1998.
Walpole CSJ, Wrigglesworth R. Enzyme inhibitors in medicine. Nat Prod Rep 1989;63:311–346.
Wolfenden R. Transition-state analogues as potential affinity labeling agents. Methods Enzymol 1977;46:15–28.

6. *Pharmaceutical Biotechnology—From Nucleic Acids to Personalized Medicine*

RONALD E. REID AND ROBERT D. SINDELAR

DRUGS COVERED IN THIS CHAPTER:

CYTOKINES
- Interferon α
- Concensus interferon
- Interferon β
- Interferon γ
- Interleukin-2/Aldesleukin
- IL-2 fusion protein
- Interleukin 11/Oprelvekin

DORNASE ALPHA

GONADOTROPINS
- Follitropin alpha
- Follitropin beta

HEMATOPOIETIC GROWTH FACTORS
- Erythropoietin (Epoetin alpha)
- Filgrastim
- Sargramostim

HUMAN GROWTH HORMONES

IMIGLUCDERASE

INSULIN AND ANALOGS

TISSUE PLASMINOGEN ACTIVATORS
- Alteplase
- Reteplase
- Tenecteplase

INTRODUCTION

Pharmaceutical biotechnology is advancing with unprecedented methodology and achievements. The early 1980s saw the products of modern pharmaceutical biotechnology come to the marketplace as the U.S. FDA approved recombinant DNA–produced insulin in 1982 and second-generation home pregnancy test kits containing monoclonal antibodies were developed. In an article entitled "Biotechnology: are you ready for it?", appearing as the cover story in the May 1990 issue of *Drug Topics,* Conlan (7) suggested that "pharmacists will skillfully ride the coming biotechnology drug wave into the 21st century, where they'll reign as the unchallenged drug therapy experts, designing, dispensing, counseling, and monitoring medicines in the brave new world of genetic engineering." Although a decade later this vision has yet to be fulfilled in its entirety, this is certainly an attractive scenario and represents an exciting opportunity for pharmacists (8). Pharmaceutical biotechnology generates basic scientific knowledge, useful therapeutic and diagnostic products, and promising methodologies for future research and clinical applications. There is little doubt that the techniques of biotechnology have led to the development and marketing of new and novel therapies residing on pharmacists' shelves today, improved methods of manufacturing pharmaceuticals, and significant contributions to our better understanding of disease etiology, pathophysiology, and biochemistry. Advances in biotechnology will have an increasing impact on pharmacy practice in the first decade of the 21st century and well into the future. Genomics, transcriptomics, proteomics, metabolomics, and enviromics—the core technologies of pharmaceutical biotechnology—are currently making major contributions to drug therapy in three areas (9):

1. Identification of new genes.
2. Identification of drug targets.
3. Development of "personalized medicine."

The human species is a product of millions of years of evolution. The living organism that has evolved is supported by complex chemical machinery that senses and responds to environmental signals, nourishes and protects the trillions of cells that are the basic unit of the living organism, determines and regulates cellular function, and finally, assures that cellular multiplication and organism reproduction will occur. Disruptions of this chemical machinery are the sources of disease and disability, and a detailed understanding of these mechanisms at the molecular level is critical to understanding disease pathology and developing an effective defense or aggressive therapy against disease and disability. Much information about the human condition to date arises from studies of simpler organisms like the bacteriophage and viruses, bacteria, yeasts, nematodes, fruit flies, and the more complex mouse. Through such studies, we seek understanding to be able to detect the damage potential of a particular internal or external environment, repair damage that has already occurred, or sustain the body in the presence of damage.

Current dogma places biochemical information and its transfer as the basis of the function of a living organism, regulating the nervous, immune, digestive, and reproductive systems. This information flow originates at the deoxyribonucleic acid (DNA) molecule and proceeds to ribonucleic acid (RNA), which is then translated into protein (10). Proteins are the main components of the functional organization of the cell and are critical to the relationship

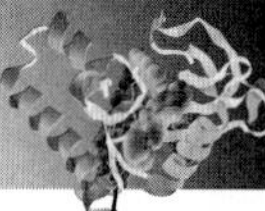

CLINICAL SIGNIFICANCE

The biotechnology industry has grown explosively over the past 30 years, with estimated 2005 revenues from human therapeutic and diagnostic products for the top 16 biotechnology companies reaching approximately $35.5 billion—more than twice the revenues for the entire industry five years ago (1). The nearly 375 publicly traded biotechnology and drug companies around the world have marketed more than 100 U.S. Food and Drug Administration (FDA)-approved biopharmaceuticals and vaccines (2). This is an impressive number, because only 39 products were approved by 1996.

Improved manufacturing of pharmaceuticals was the first major contribution of biotechnology to pharmaceutical care in the 1980s. Biotechnology-produced human insulin, growth hormone, and erythropoietin—all replacements of highly specific, endogenous molecules—were major advances in therapy. Since the late 1980s, however, pharmaceutical biotechnology also has helped to identify new compounds with new mechanisms of action. Significant contributions to our understanding about the mechanism of disease at the molecular level continue to be made by biotechnology researchers and will translate into newer, better pharmaceuticals. The impact of biotechnology on pharmaceutical care is expected to increase exponentially as advances in technology continue to yield novel medicinal agents, such as the colony-stimulating factors, tissue-type plasminogen activator, new vaccines, DNase, fusion protein drugs (e.g., leukin diftitox), and specific monoclonal antibodies, including trastuzumab. Products of biotechnology are playing a critical role in the discovery and design as well as in the production of treatments for life-threatening diseases, such as cancer, AIDS, and cardiovascular disease.

Pharmaceutical care using biotechnology-derived products requires (3,4):

1. An understanding of how the handling and stability of biopharmaceuticals differs from those of other drugs that pharmacists dispense.
2. A preparation of the product for patient use, including reconstitution or compounding, if required.
3. Patient education regarding their disease, benefits of the prescribed biopharmaceutical, potential side effects or drug interactions to be aware of, and the techniques to self-administer the biotechnology drug.
4. Patient counseling about the reimbursement issues involving an expensive product.
5. Monitoring of the patient for compliance.

The evolution of biotechnology medicine is gaining momentum. The techniques of pharmaceutical biotechnology will make it possible to prevent, cure, and treat more diseases than possible today; to anticipate and prevent disease symptoms; to eliminate the contamination risks of infectious pathogens found in human blood-derived biopharmaceuticals; to target drug therapy toward the underlying cause of diseases, not just the treatment of disease symptoms; to produce replacement human proteins on a large scale; and to develop more precise and effective medicines with fewer side effects (2). Key areas of future growth for biotechnology in the 21st century will include pharmacogenomics/pharmacogenetics; recombinant-based therapies, such as vaccines delivered by novel administrative routes; genetic modification of the patient; and cloning of human tissues and organs. The field has matured sufficiently with the first generic versions of original biotech drugs, called "Biogenerics" or "Follow-On Biologics," nearing regulatory approval (5,6). It will be interesting to view the impact of the breath of future biotechnological advances on the practice of pharmacy.

between the organism's DNA structure, or genotype, and the organism's functional organization, or phenotype. Therefore, intervention in the regulatory system to detect or repair disease or to sustain the organism in the event of disease may occur at any level between the genotype and the phenotype. Genetic intervention has many levels, from direct tinkering with the genes (the information source) to manipulating the many processes involved in the transcription and translation of the genetic information into proteins. Protein function may be altered through direct manipulation of proteins or through altering the many events occurring between protein production and the physical response noted by the organism. Regardless of the particular approach taken in any isolated instance, our understanding about the molecular mechanisms of the chemical-mediated information transfer will be the basis for rationalizing any therapeutic initiative. It is highly likely that any approach to disease therapy will use a mixture of techniques, only a few of which will involve the direct manipulation of genes in the form of gene replacement therapy. Further development of the knowledge of molecular processes involved in this information transfer and how it is related to disease may help us to make better use of the current therapeutic technologies and allow us to treat the individual patient rather than the disease symptoms (11).

The clinician of the future will have the tools to routinely screen for the genetic implications of new drugs, improving a patient's response to drug treatment and making therapeutics a true science. Although many of the first biotechnology-derived therapeutics were initially used in acutely ill, hospitalized patients, the products of today's pharmaceutical biotechnology increasingly have an impact on the chronic disease patient populations constituting much of ambulatory care practice.

THE CHEMICAL BASIS OF PHARMACEUTICAL BIOTECHNOLOGY

Pharmaceutical biotechnology is defined, at its most basic level, as the manipulation of nucleic acids in the production of therapeutic and diagnostic agents. Both DNA and RNA are the fundamental genetic material;

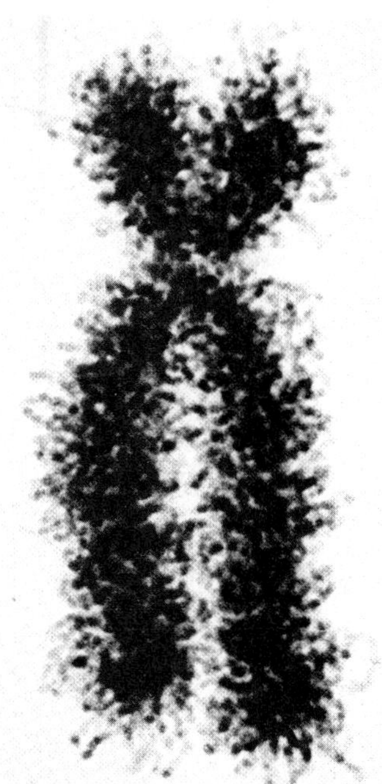

Fig. 6.1. Sister chromatids of a mitotic pair. The sister chromosomes are produced by the previous replication event and are still joined together at this stage of mitosis. Each of the chromosomes consists of a fiber with a diameter of approximately 30 nm. The DNA is 5- to 10-fold more condensed in chromosomes than it is at interphase. (Adapted from Lewin B. Genes IV, 4th Ed. Oxford: Oxford University Press and Cell Press, 1990; with permission.)

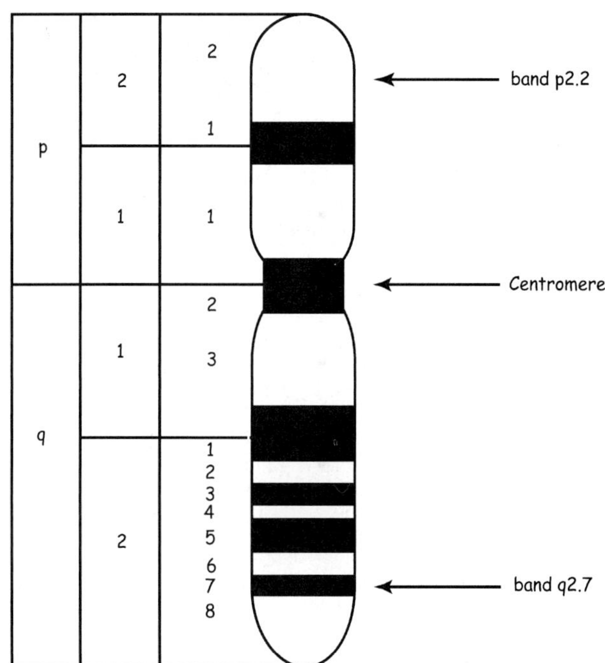

Fig. 6.2. The human X chromosome can be divided into distinct regions by its banding pattern. (Adapted from Lewin B. Genes IV, 4th Ed. Oxford: Oxford University Press and Cell Press, 1990; with permission.)

therefore, an understanding of the molecular composition of the genetic material and the structure and functional nature of the gene is basic knowledge on which to build the science of pharmaceutical biotechnology.

Nucleic Acids: DNA and RNA

The eukaryotic chromosome makes a brief appearance when the cell is actively dividing and can be seen as a pair of chromatids (daughter chromosomes produced during replication of DNA before mitosis) (Fig. 6.1). The individual chromosome can be divided along its length into many clear striations of dark bands and light interband regions (Fig. 6.2). The dark bands are dense clumps of protein and DNA; the interbands are regions with a lower density of protein and DNA. The reasons for this highly regular banding are not known. Each of these bands and interbands of the chromosome is composed of a well-defined mixture of protein and DNA called chromatin.

The main protein component of chromatin is histones, which are basic proteins associated with the DNA in the form of structures called nucleosomes (Fig. 6.3) (12). The DNA can be stored in very small, compact forms called condensed DNA, which is 10^4- to 10^6-fold less in volume than uncondensed DNA. The main force that must be overcome in the condensation process is charge repulsion because of the negatively charged phosphates in the polyanion. This repulsion may be overcome by DNA interaction with multivalent organic and inorganic cations. The histones, which are the major components of the nucleosome, are cationic organic proteins that interact with DNA in the compact nucleosome structure.

The nucleosome consists of a 200-base-pair (bp) DNA strand making two left-handed coils around an octamer of histone proteins consisting of two copies each of histones H2A, H2B, H3, and H4, and a single copy of the histone H1 (Fig. 6.3).

Separation of the protein spools from chromatin leaves a very long, string-like DNA molecule. The DNA is

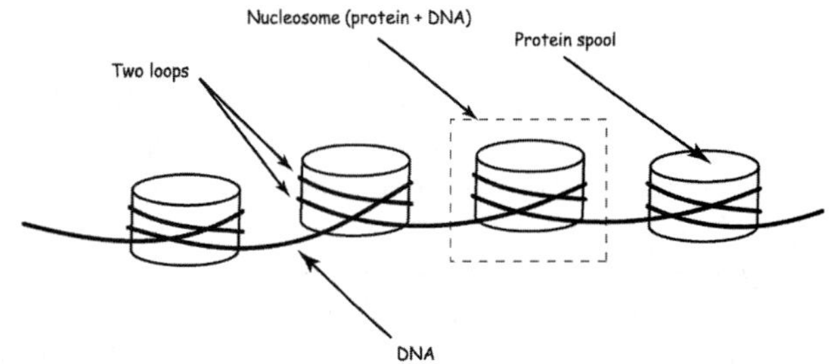

Fig. 6.3. A DNA thread making two left-handed coils around each of a series of protein spools. A single spool consists of an octamer of histone proteins, two each of H2A, H2B, H3, and H4. The ninth histone protein, H1, may be located in the linker region between spools immediately adjacent to the spool. The DNA and histones make up the nucleosome. (From Calladine CR, Drew HR. Understanding DNA: The Molecule and How It Works, 2nd Ed. New York: Academic Press, 1997; with permission.)

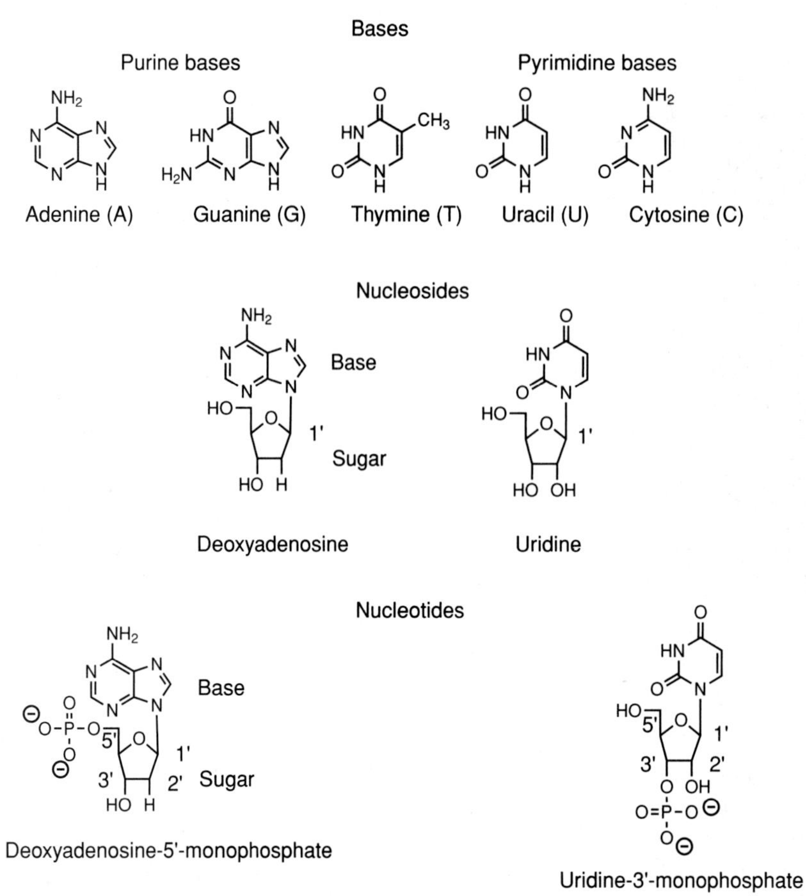

Fig. 6.4. Chemical structure of the purines and pyrimidine bases as well as representative nucleosides and nucleotides.

composed of purine bases (adenine [A] and guanine [G]), pyrimidine bases (cytosine [C] and thymine [T] or uracil [U], in the case of RNA), deoxyribose sugars (ribose sugars in the case of RNA), and phosphates (Fig. 6.4). The bases combine with the 1′ position of the ribose to form a nucleoside. The DNA structural unit, a nucleotide, is a 3′- or 5′-monophosphate ester of a nucleoside. Nucleotides are covalently linked through phosphate esters to form the DNA polymer chain. Each nucleotide is linked to one neighbor by a 5′,3′-phosphodiester bond and to the other neighbor by a 3′,5-phosphodiester bond (Fig. 6.5). All the 3′- and 5′-hydroxyl groups in the DNA molecule are involved in phosphodiester bonds except the first and last nucleotides in the chain. The first nucleotide in the chain has a 5′-phosphate nonbonded to a nucleotide, and the last nucleotide in the chain has a free 3′-hydroxyl group (Fig. 6.5). The DNA sugar-phosphate backbone chain has polarity, meaning it has a 5′ end and a 3′ end.

The structure of deoxyribonucleic acid was determined in 1953 by Watson and Crick to consist of two antiparallel strands of deoxyribonucleic acid coiled around a common axis in a "double helix" (Fig. 6.6). The purine and pyrimidine bases are on the inside of the helix, whereas the phosphate and deoxyribose units are on the outside. The planes of the bases are perpendicular to the axis of the helix. The planes of the sugars are at approximately 70° to those of the bases. The helix diameter is 20 Å; adjacent bases are separated by 3.4 Å along the

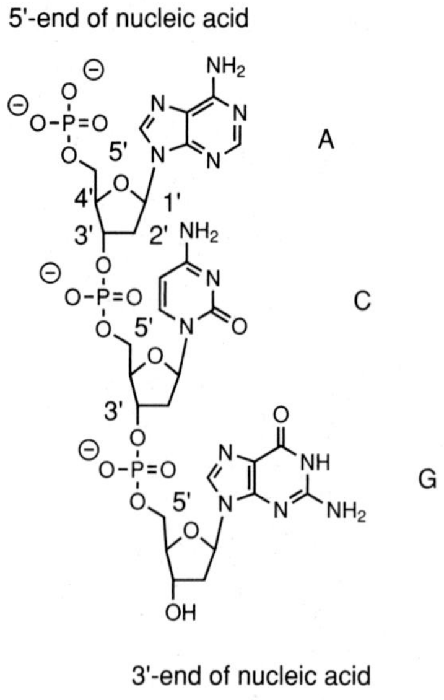

5'-end of nucleic acid

A

C

G

3'-end of nucleic acid

Fig. 6.5. Chemical structure of a DNA fragment ACG.

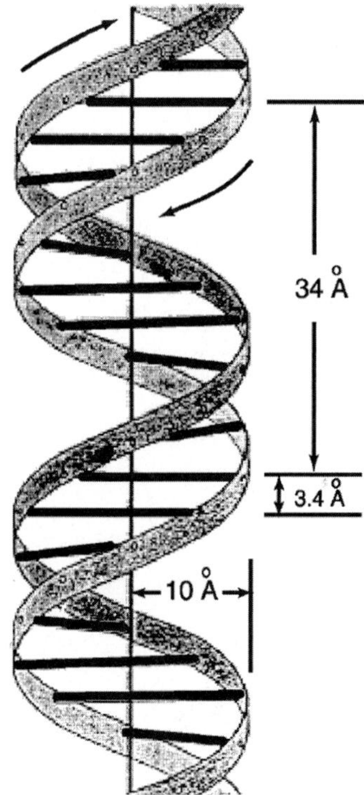

Fig. 6.6. Schematic representation of the Watson and Crick double helix model of DNA. The radius of the double helix is 10 Å, the vertical rise per base pair is 3.4 Å, and one complete turn of the double helix traverses 10 base pairs of 34 Å.

helical axis and related by a rotation of 36°. Hence, the helical structure repeats after 10 residues on each chain—that is, at intervals of 34 Å along the axis. The two chains are held together by hydrogen bonds between base pairs. Adenine is always paired with thymine, and guanine is always paired with cytosine, thus providing a specific interaction between the two DNA strands such that the nucleotide sequence of the strand can be exploited as a method of transmitting information (i.e., the amino acid sequence coded for by the nucleotide sequence in the nucleic acid).

The double helix stability is determined by a longitudinal interaction of neighboring bases, called base stacking, which results from complex interactions of π-electron orbitals of the planar bases, dipole, dipole-induced dipole, London dispersion forces, and hydrophobic interactions. The stability of base stacking is of the order purine-purine > purine-pyrimidine > pyrimidine-pyrimidine. The G/C pairs are more stable than A/T pairs, because they have three hydrogen bonds as opposed to two (Fig. 6.7). Therefore, stacked dimers high in G/C content are energetically preferred to those rich in A/T content (13).

Nucleic acids are water soluble because of the polyanionic character of the molecule. It is possible to obtain viscous aqueous solutions of DNA up to 1% (w/v). The long, thin DNA structure means that the molecule is very susceptible to cleavage by shearing or sonication in solution, which results in a reduction in solution viscosity.

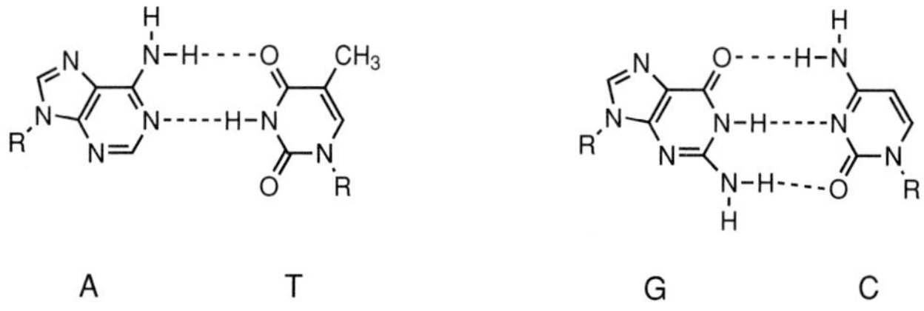

Fig. 6.7. Watson and Crick base pairing in double-stranded DNA. The purine A pairs with the pyrimidine T, and the purine G pairs with the pyrimide C.

The nucleic acids are precipitated from aqueous solution by the addition of alcohol.

Strong acid at high temperatures will result in complete hydrolysis of nucleic acids into their constituent bases, sugars, and phosphate. Milder acidic conditions (pH 3–4) at 37°C will result in hydrolysis of the most susceptible bonds, those being the glycosyl bonds linking the purine bases, A and G, to the sugar molecules, resulting in depurination of the nucleic acid. Depyrimidation is less frequently seen but also may occur.

Heterocyclic molecules containing nitrogen tautomerize to yield a mixture of molecular species in solution, because the hydrogens attached to nitrogen in the ring systems are able to migrate to other nitrogens or keto oxygens in the same molecule (Fig. 6.8).

Because correct base pairing is critical to information transfer in the replication, transcription, and translation of DNA structure, base tautomerization could be a disaster for living systems. Fortunately, the keto and amine structures are the predominant tautomeric structures, with less than 0.1% in the imino and enol tautomeric states. Increasing pH of the nucleic acid environment, however, will shift the keto/enol tautomeric equilibrium to the enol form due to ionization of the enolic hydroxyl group, with the net result being disruption of the hydrogen bonding in DNA and denaturation of the double-stranded molecule. The double helix structure of DNA also can be denatured through heat or relatively high concentrations of chemical agents, such as urea and formamide, that also disrupt the critical hydrogen bond system.

Helical regions of RNA are similarly denatured by alkali; however, hydrolysis of RNA is the predominant reaction occurring in alkali. The hydrolysis is assisted by the 2′-OH group on the ribose sugar (Fig. 6.9). The DNA is not as susceptible to the alkaline hydrolysis, because the 2′-OH group is missing.

The spectroscopic properties of DNA provide a wealth of information concerning concentration, structure, stability, and purity of a particular DNA preparation. Nucleic acids absorb ultraviolet (UV) light at λ_{max} = 260 nm because of the conjugated aromatic ring systems of the bases. The absorption intensity is greatest for single-stranded DNA (ssDNA) and RNA and least for double-stranded DNA (dsDNA) (Fig. 6.10). The hydrophobic environment of the stacked bases in dsDNA is responsible

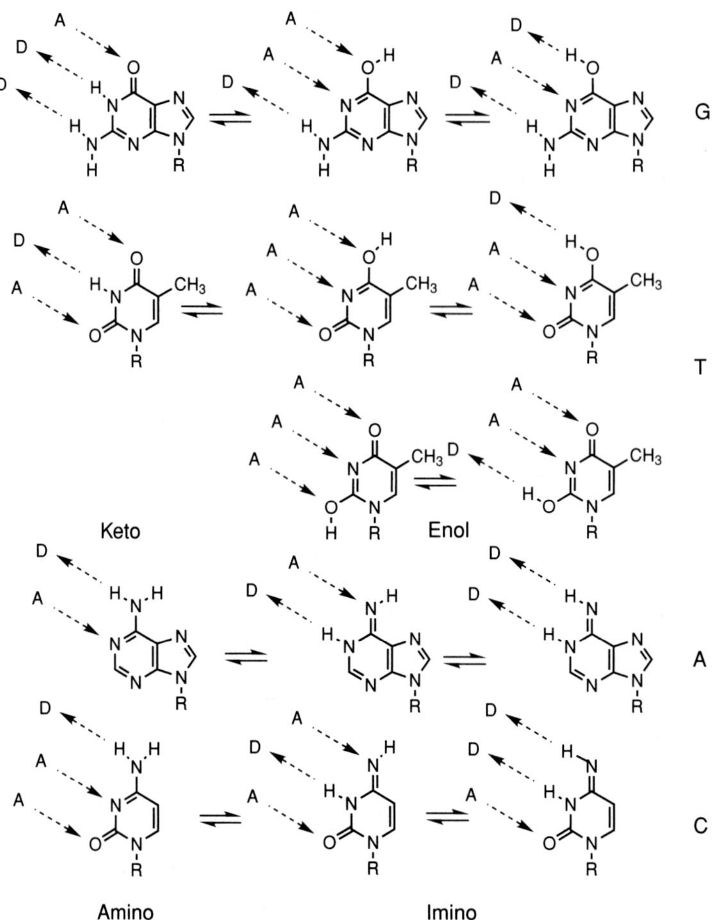

Fig. 6.8. Keto-enol and amino-imino tautomerism in nucleoside bases. Arrows denote A and D, which symbolize acceptor and donor sites for hydrogen bond formation. Note that in the enol forms, G becomes equivalent to A, and U becomes equivalent to C. In the imino forms, A is equivalent to U or G, and C is equivalent to U. The situation changes if the imino or enol groups rotate, giving rise to a diversity of hydrogen-bonding possibilities.

for the lower intensity of UV absorption of this molecule at 260 nm. The ssDNA is said to be hyperchromic relative to dsDNA; thus, dsDNA undergoes a hyperchromic shift during denaturation to ssDNA.

The extinction coefficient of a nucleic acid is not suitable for determination of the concentration of the nucleic acid, because it is dependent on the length of the molecule. The extinction coefficient is instead expressed in terms of concentration, where a 1 mg/ml solution of dsDNA has an A_{260nm} (absorbance at 260 nm) of 20. Similar concentrations of ssDNA or RNA have an A_{260nm} of approximately 25. This value is approximate for ssDNA and RNA, both because the absorbance of purines is greater than pyrimidines at 260 nm and because the ratio of purines to pyrimidines in ssDNA and RNA will vary (whereas the same ratio is one in dsDNA). Additionally, the A_{260nm} is dependent on base stacking, which also is variable in ssDNA and RNA but constant in dsDNA.

The spectroscopic properties of a DNA solution can be used to determine the approximate purity of the preparation as well. Because the shape and λ_{max} of the UV absorption spectra will vary depending on the environment of the bases, one can use the ratio of A_{260nm}/A_{280nm} to estimate the RNA and protein content of a dsDNA preparation. Pure dsDNA has a ratio of 1.8, and pure RNA has a ratio of 2.0. Because protein has a λ_{max} of around 280 nm, the A_{260nm}/A_{280nm} of a protein solution will always be less than one. Therefore, a sample of dsDNA with a A_{260nm}/A_{280nm} greater than 1.8 suggests RNA contamination, whereas a ratio less than 1.8 suggests protein contamination.

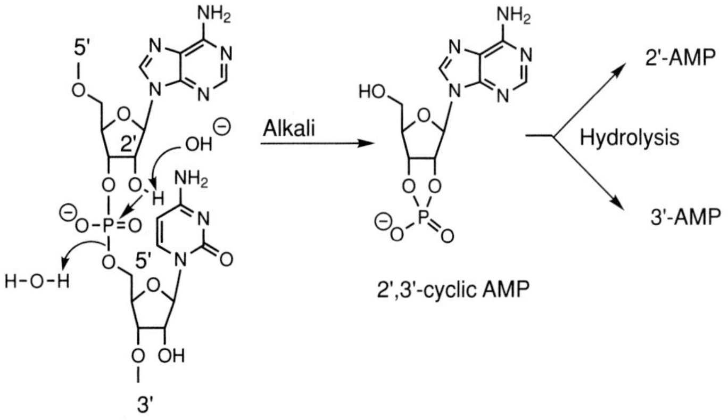

Fig. 6.9. Alkaline hydrolysis of RNA to produce the intermediate 2′, 3′-cyclic nucleotide monophosphate which undergoes further hydrolysis to 2′ and 3′ nucleotide monophosphates.

The stability of dsDNA can be determined through a temperature denaturation study. Native dsDNA will denature to ssDNA as the temperature of the solution is increased. This is a reversible process, and the ssDNA will anneal to dsDNA on slowly cooling the denatured solution. This behavior can be followed spectroscopically (Fig. 6.11) by noting the increase in A_{260nm} with temperature, indicating the hyperchromic shift as the dsDNA denatures to ssDNA. The midpoint of the sigmoid curve is termed the "melting temperature" of the dsDNA (T_m). Stability of different dsDNA molecules can be demonstrated by comparing the T_m values of the solutions (Fig. 6.11).

Replication

Replication of prokaryotic and eukaryotic DNA proceeds from the origin (single origins in prokaryotes and multiple origins in eukaryotes), which is a region high in A and T residues that make opening of the double helix easier because of fewer base-pairing hydrogen bonds

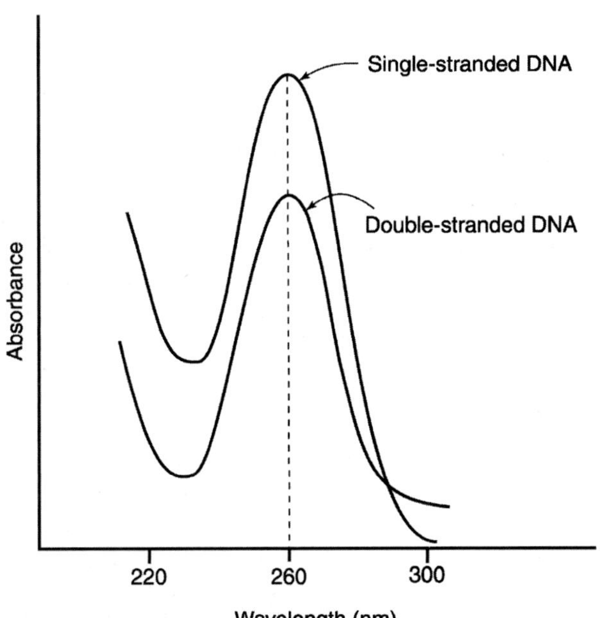

Fig. 6.10. Hyperchromic shift between double-stranded and single-stranded DNA. Single-stranded DNA has a higher ultraviolet absorbance at 260 nm than does double-stranded DNA.

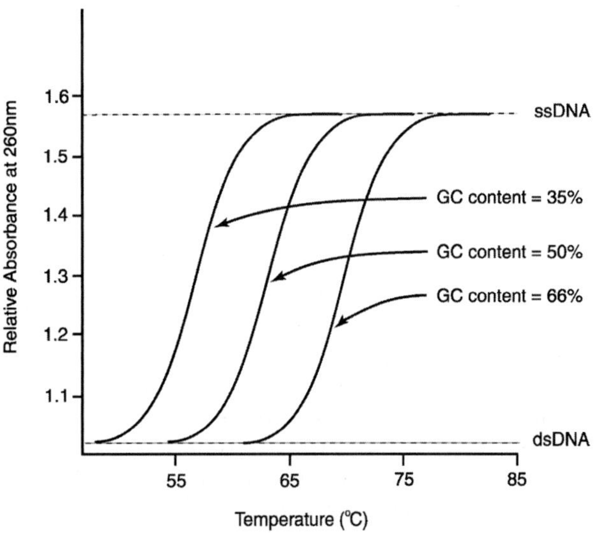

Fig. 6.11. Stability of double-stranded DNA (dsDNA) based on the GC content of the nucleic acid. The melting temperature is detected by a hyperchromic shift that occurs during the temperature-induced melting of dsDNA to single-stranded DNA and is shown to increase as the GC content of dsDNA increases.

between A/T compared to G/C. Because each strand of the DNA carries the same information, replication produces two daughter strands built from the parent strands acting as templates.

The process of replication takes place at the replication fork, where the parent strands are unwound and the daughter strands are synthesized in the $5' \rightarrow 3'$ direction (reading the parent template in the $3' \rightarrow 5'$ direction) (Fig. 6.12). Both daughter strands are synthesized at the same time. One is synthesized as a continuous strand called the leading strand. The other, called the lagging strand, must be made in the reverse direction to the leading strand starting at the replicating fork and proceeding $5' \rightarrow 3'$ back to the origin, resulting in the necessity of synthesizing blocks of nucleic acids (100–200 nucleotides in eukaryotes and 1,000–2,000 nucleotides in prokaryotes) known as Okazaki fragments. These fragments are subsequently joined into a continuous daughter strand by a DNA ligase. The DNA polymerase responsible for adding deoxynucleoside triphosphates to the growing strands requires short strands of nucleic acids as primers to start the synthetic process. These primer fragments are short RNA strands that are replaced with DNA by a proofreading exonuclease associated with the polymerase. The use of RNA primers assures the fidelity of DNA replication at the 5′ end of the newly synthesized strands, because the increased mobility of the "unanchored" base at the 5′ end of a DNA strand can never appear as a "correct" residue and, therefore, cannot be proofread. A short RNA strand, however, is recognized as low-fidelity material and replaced with DNA. The polymerases responsible for DNA replication are different in prokaryotes and eukaryotes. The DNA polymerase (pol) III synthesizes both the leading and lagging strands in prokaryotes but DNA pol I replaces the RNA primers in the lagging strand with DNA. Eukaryotic polymerases are more complex. The DNA pol α starts both the lagging and leading strands in eukaryotes but is replaced by DNA pol δ on the leading strand and DNA pol ϵ on the lagging strand.

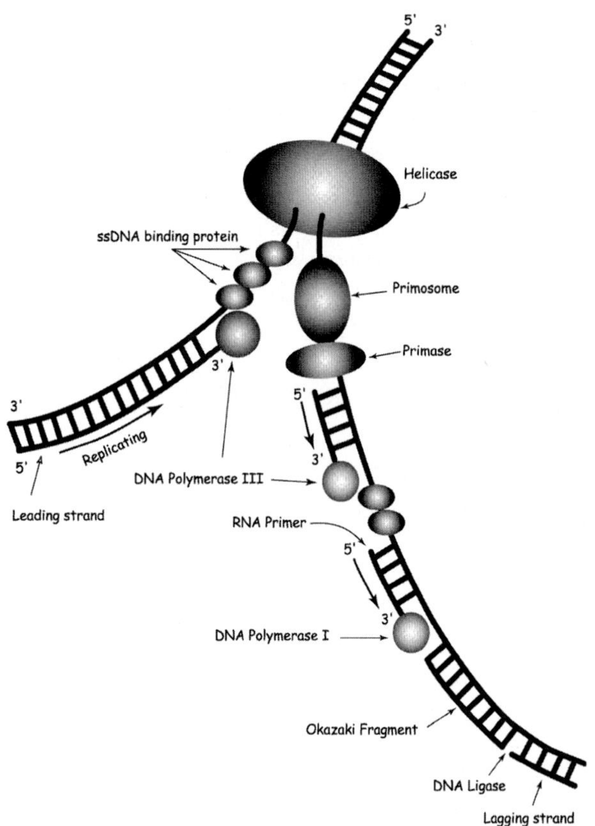

Fig. 6.12. Schematic representation of DNA replication. Helicase is responsible for unwinding the double-stranded DNA, and the single-stranded DNA is stabilized by single-stranded DNA-binding proteins. The leading strand is synthesized continuously by DNA polymerase III. A primase responsible for making the RNA primers that are used by DNA polymerase III to synthesize the initial fragments in the lagging strand, which are then elongated by DNA polymerase I to make the Okazaki fragments that are finally ligated by DNA ligase to complete the lagging strand. (Adapted from Watson JD, Gilman M, Witkowski J, et al. Recombinant DNA, 2nd Ed. New York: Scientific American Books, W.H. Freeman and Company, 1992; with permission.)

Transcription

It is impossible for DNA to act as a direct template in the ordering of amino acids in protein synthesis, because almost all DNA is located in the nucleus and protein synthesis occurs in the cytoplasm. The genetic information in DNA is transcribed to the intermediate RNA molecule that moves to the cytoplasm, where it directs the synthesis of the gene product on the ribosomes. The RNA differs chemically from the DNA in that the sugar molecule is ribose and thymine in DNA is replaced by uracil in RNA. Structurally, RNA is predominantly a single-stranded molecule with short, double helical regions providing some three-dimensional structure.

There are several types of RNA molecules in the cell, three of which play major roles in the message transcription and protein synthesis. Messenger RNA (mRNA) is transcribed from a particular DNA sequence and carries the specific message from DNA in the nucleus to the cytoplasm. The molecule is very unstable, with a relatively short half-life of only a few minutes. Transfer RNAs (tRNAs) are relatively small molecules of approximately 80 nucleotides in length. These molecules are covalently linked to specific amino acids, and they carry the anticodon triplet that recognizes a particular complementary trinucleotide sequence of mRNA specific for the amino acid that it carries. The tRNA is involved in protein synthesis and is metabolically unstable, being degraded once it has transferred its amino acid to the growing protein chain. Ribosomal RNA (rRNA) is a metabolically stable complex of ribonucleic acids and proteins. The rRNA provides the site of mRNA and tRNA interaction at which proteins are synthesized in the cytoplasm. Although several differences exist in the mechanism of transcription between prokaryotes and eukaryotes, the more complex eukaryotic system will be described here.

Transcription is carried out by RNA polymerases, of which there are three types in the eukaryote. RNA pol I catalyzes the synthesis of rRNAs, RNA pol II is responsible for the synthesis of mRNA, and RNA pol III synthesizes tRNA. All three polymerases are large enzymes containing 12 or more subunits.

Like prokaryotic RNA polymerase, each eukaryotic enzyme copies DNA from the 3′ end, thus catalyzing mRNA formation in the 5′ ⇒ 3′ direction and synthesizing RNA complementary to the antisense DNA template strand. The reaction requires the precursor nucleotides ATP, GTP, CTP, and UTP and does not require a primer for transcription initiation. Unlike the prokaryotic bacterial polymerases, the eukaryotic RNA polymerases require the presence of additional initiation proteins before they are able to bind to promoters and initiate transcription. The five stages of eukaryotic transcription include initiation, elongation and termination, capping, polyadenylation, and splicing.

Initiation. Eukaryotes have different RNA polymerase–binding promoter sequences than prokaryotes. The TATA consensus sequence of the eukaryotic promoter region is located 25 to 35 bp upstream from the transcription start site (Fig. 6.13). The low activity of basal promoters is greatly increased by the presence of other elements located upstream from the promoter called upstream regulatory elements. These elements are located 40 to 200 bp upstream of the promoter sequence and include the SP1 box, the CCAAT box, and the hormone response elements. Transcription from many eukaryotic promoters can be stimulated by control elements, called enhancers, located many thousands of base pairs away from the transcription start site and usually 100 to 200 bp in length.

The length of DNA between the enhancer and the promoter region loops out to allow the transcription factors bound to the enhancer to interact with the general transcription factors, other regulatory proteins, or the RNA polymerase itself to bring about initiation of polymerization. The RNA pol II requires a number of other proteins or protein complexes, called general transcription factors, to initiate transcription (Fig. 6.14). All these have the generic name of TFII (for transcription factor for RNA pol II). The first event in initiation is binding of TFIID to the TATA box. The key subunit of TFIID is TBP (TATA box-binding protein). After TFIID binding, TFIIA binds, followed by TFIIB and then RNA pol II already complexed with TFIIF, followed in turn by TFIIE, TFIIH, and TFIIJ. This final complex contains at least 40 polypeptides and is called the transcription initiation complex.

Elongation and termination. The RNA polymerase moves along the DNA template until a terminator sequence is reached. The RNA pol II does not terminate at specific sites but, rather, stops at varying distances downstream of the gene. Eukaryotic termination of transcription is not as well understood as that of prokaryotic transcription. The RNA molecule made from a protein-coding gene by RNA pol II in eukaryotes is called pre-mRNA. The pre-mRNA from a eukaryotic protein-coding gene is extensively processed en route to creating mRNA ready for translation.

Capping. At the end of polymerization, the 5′ end of the pre-mRNA molecule is modified by addition of a N-7-methyl guanine molecule (Fig. 6.15). The 5′ terminal phosphate is removed by a phosphatase, and the resulting diphosphate 5′ end reacts with the α-phosphate of GTP to form an unusual 5′,5′-triphosphate link (Cap 0). The 5′-cap also may be methylated by S-adenosylmethionine on the 2′-OH of the ribose sugar of the adjacent nucleotide (Cap 1) or on both ribose sugars in the 2 and 3 positions (Cap 2) (Fig. 6.15). This cap structure protects the 5′ end of the primary transcript against attack by ribonucleases

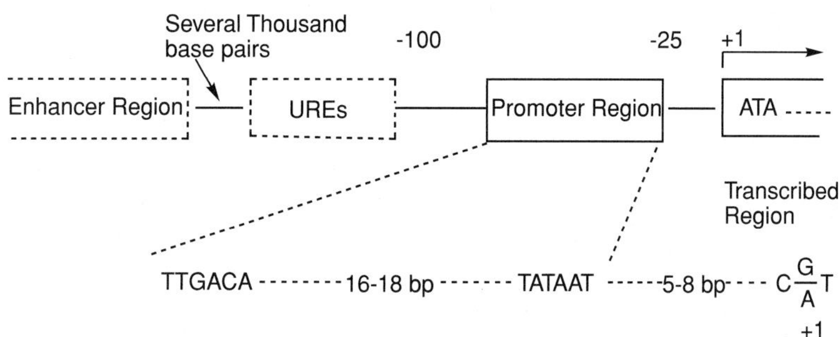

Fig. 6.13. Schematic representation of the eukaryotic transcription unit showing the relationship between the promoter, upstream regulatory elements, and enhancer region. Note that transcription usually starts with a purine base in the 1 position. (Adapted from Turner PC, McLennan AG, Bates AD, White MRH. Instant Notes in Molecular Biology. New York: BIOS Scientific Publishers Ltd, Springer-Verlag, 1997; with permission.)

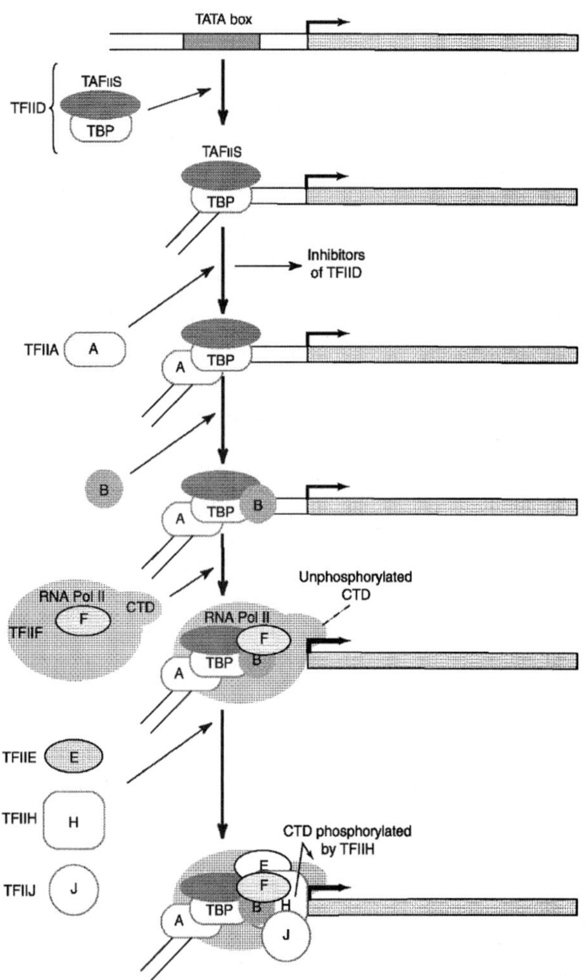

Fig. 6.14. Schematic representation of the assembly of the RNA polymerase II transcription initiation complex at a TATA box promoter. The transcription factors are labeled TFIIA, TFIIB, TFIIE, TFIIF, TFIIH, and TFIIJ. The TFIID is a complex of TATA-binding protein (TBP) and multiple accessory factors called TBP-associated factors of TFIIA. The TFIID binds to the TATA box, and this binding is enhanced by TFIIA, which appears to stop some inhibitory factors from binding to TFIID, thus preventing further assembly of the complex. The TFIIB binds to the complex and acts as a bridge for binding the RNA polymerase, which attaches itself to the complex along with TFIIF. When RNA polymerase II binding occurs, the transcription factors TFIIE, TFIIH and TFIIJ, which are required for transcription, bind in a defined sequence. The carboxyl-terminal domain (CTD) of RNA polymerase II is phosphorylated by TFIIH, thus allowing the polymerase to leave the promoter region. (Adapted from Turner PC, McLennan AG, Bates AD, White MRH. Instant Notes in Molecular Biology. New York: BIOS Scientific Publishers Ltd, Springer-Verlag, 1997; with permission.)

that have specificity for 3′,5′-phosphodiester bonds and so cannot hydrolyze the 5′,5′ bond in the cap structure. The cap structure also plays a role in the initiation step of protein synthesis in eukaryotes. Only RNA transcripts from eukaryotic protein-coding genes become capped;

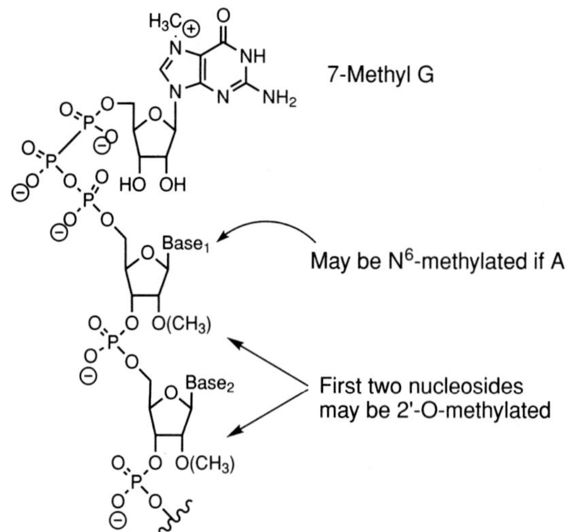

Fig. 6.15. Chemical structure of the 5′-cap of mRNA. Cap 0 consists of the 7-methylguanosine triphosphate attached to the 5′ end of the mRNA. Cap 1 consists of the 7-methylguanosine and 2′-O-methylation of the 5′ base. Cap 2 consists of the 7-methylguanosine and the 2′-O-methylation of the first two bases in the sequence.

prokaryotic mRNA and eukaryotic rRNA and tRNA are uncapped.

Polyadenylation. The 3′ end of the pre-mRNA is generated by cleavage by nucleases followed by the addition of a run, or tail, of 100 to 200 adenosine nucleotides, resulting in what is called the poly(A) tail. Cleavage and polyadenylation require specific sequences in the DNA and its pre-mRNA transcript that are part of the transcription termination signal (Fig. 6.16). A 5′-AAUAAA-3′ sequence followed by a 5′-PyA-3′ (Py = pyrmidine) within the next 11 to 20 nucleotides and a GU-rich sequence further downstream collectively make up the requirements for a polyadenylation site. The poly(A) tail is thought to help stabilize the molecule, because a poly(A)-binding protein interacts with the tail, reducing the pre-mRNA's sensitivity to 3′-nuclease activity. In addition, the poly(A) tail may have a role to play in the translation of mature RNA in the cytoplasm.

Splicing. The next step in pre-mRNA processing is the precise cutting out of the intron sequences and joining the ends of neighboring exons to produce a functional mRNA molecule, a process termed "RNA splicing." The exon–intron boundaries are marked by specific sequences. Introns are sequences that interrupt those sequences that will eventually become adjacent regions in mature RNA. Exons become the protein-coding regions of mRNA. The exon–intron boundary at the 5′ splice site always starts the intron with a GU sequence (Fig. 6.17a). The boundary at the 3′ splice site always ends the intron with an AG sequence. Each sequence at

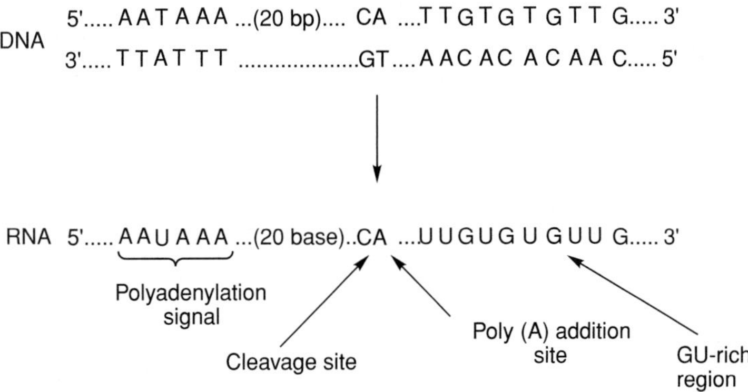

Fig. 6.16. Sequence of a typical polyadenylation site showing the polyadenylation signal, cleavage site, and GU-rich region. (Adapted from Turner PC, McLennan AG, Bates AD, White MRH. Instant Notes in Molecular Biology. New York: BIOS Scientific Publishers Ltd, Springer-Verlag, 1997; with permission.)

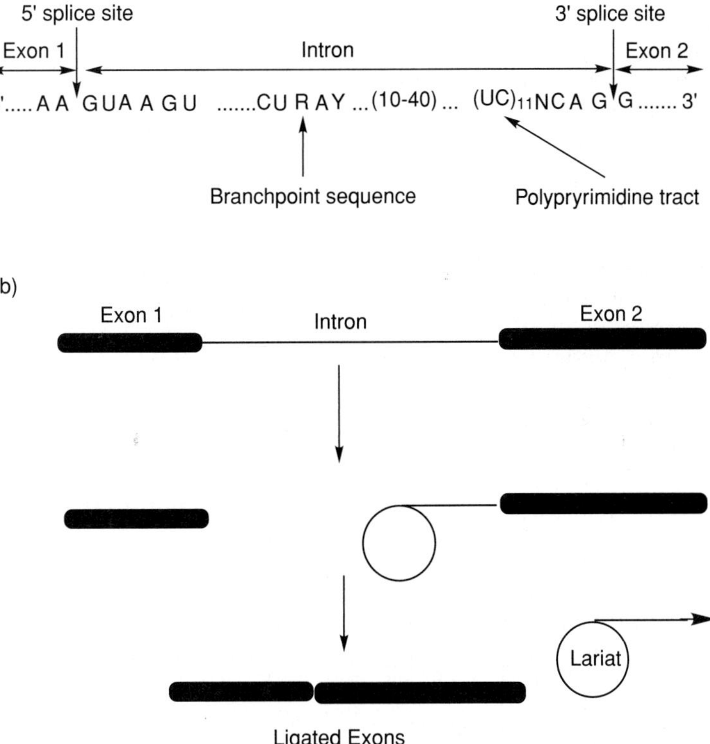

Fig. 6.17. (a) Splice-site concensus sequences showing the 5′ and 3′ splice sites. (b) Two steps in the splicing sequence showing formation of the lariat at the branchpoint sequence. R, purine; Y, pyrimidine. (Adapted from Turner PC, McLennan AG, Bates AD, White MRH. Instant Notes in Molecular Biology. New York: BIOS Scientific Publishers Ltd, Springer-Verlag, 1997; with permission.)

the 5′ and 3′ splice sites lie within a larger consensus sequence. The intron also has a stretch of 10 pyrimidines near the 3′ splice site and an internal branch site containing an important adenosine residue located approximately 20 to 50 nucleotides upstream of the 3′ splice site. Splicing takes place in a two-step reaction (Fig. 6.17b). First, the bond in front of the G at the 5′ splice site is attacked by the 2′ hydroxyl group of the A residue at the branch point sequence, creating a tailed, circular molecule called the lariat and a free exon. In the second step, cleavage of the 3′ splice site occurs after G of the AG sequence as the two exons are joined together.

Translation

Protein synthesis occurs when the triplet genetic code carried by mRNA is translated into a protein sequence on the ribosome. As mentioned earlier, tRNA carries a specific amino acid attached to its 3′ terminus based on the anticodon present in its structure. The anticodon complements the triplet codon sequence in mRNA. A triplet is the minimum number of nucleotides necessary to provide a unique sequence for each of the 20 amino acids. With a triplet code, there is a possibility of 64 different combinations, of which 61 actually code for amino acids (Table 6.1). The remaining three codons are nonsense or stop codons. Eighteen of the 20 common amino acids are coded for by more than one codon, meaning the code is degenerate or redundant. Two amino acids, Met (AUG) and Trp (UGG), each have one unique codon. From a fixed start point on the mRNA (start codon, AUG), which establishes the open reading frame, each group of three bases in the coding region of the mRNA represents a codon that is recognized by a complementary triplet on the end of a particular tRNA molecule. One triplet on an mRNA molecule is directly followed by the next one without any additional bases between them, indicating that the code is commaless and nonoverlapping. Because each triplet is independent of any other and there are no gaps between codons, any reading frame can be divided up in three ways. Once the start codon is found, the reading frame is fixed, and the protein sequence begins.

There are four stages in the protein synthesis in both prokaryotes and eukaryotes:

1. *Initiation*—assembly of the ribosome on an mRNA molecule.
2. *Elongation*—repeated cycles of amino acid addition.
3. *Termination*—recognition of the stop codon, release of the new protein chain, and breakdown of the synthetic complex.
4. *Posttranslational modification*—usually include protein cleavage by carboxy or amino peptidases, and chemical modification such as acetylation, sulfonylation, phosphorylation, hydroxylation, and/or addition of polysaccharides.

Table 6.1. The Genetic Code

First Position	Second Position				Third Position
	U	C	A	G	
U	**Phe** UUU	**Ser** UCU	**Tyr** UAU	**Cys** UGU	U
	Phe UUC	**Ser** UCC	**Tyr** UAC	**Cys** UGC	C
	Leu UUA	**Ser** UCA	**Stop** UAA	**Stop** UGA	A
	Leu UUG	**Ser** UCG	**Stop** UAG	**Trp** UGG	G
C	**Leu** CUU	**Pro** CCU	**His** CAU	**Arg** CGU	U
	Leu CUC	**Pro** CCC	**His** CAC	**Arg** CGC	C
	Leu CUA	**Pro** CCA	**Gln** CAA	**Arg** CGA	A
	Leu CUG	**Pro** CCG	**Gln** CAG	**Arg** CGG	G
A	**Ile** AUU	**Thr** ACU	**Asn** AAU	**Ser** AGU	U
	Ile AUC	**Thr** ACC	**Asn** AAC	**Ser** AGC	C
	Ile AUA	**Thr** ACA	**Lys** AAA	**Arg** AGA	A
	Met AUG	**Thr** ACG	**Lys** AAG	**Arg** AGG	G
G	**Val** GUU	**Ala** GCU	**Asp** GAU	**Gly** GGU	U
	Val GUC	**Ala** GCC	**Asp** GAC	**Gly** GGC	C
	Val GUA	**Ala** GCA	**Glu** GAA	**Gly** GGA	A
	Val GUG	**Ala** GCG	**Glu** GAG	**Gly** GGG	G

There are distinct differences in detail between the mechanism in prokaryotes and eukaryotes, most of which occur in the initiation stage.

GENES

Manipulation of genes is one of the major technologies in pharmaceutical biotechnology, so it is rather important to have an understanding of the techniques used in gene manipulation. A gene is not equated with the gene product. We have seen how several changes may occur to the gene product during the production process, and the final product seldom corresponds to a direct decoding of a linear nucleic acid chain. A gene is defined as the segment of DNA involved in producing a polypeptide chain; it includes regions preceding (the leader or 5′-untranslated region) and following (the trailer or 3′-untranslated region) the coding region as well as intervening sequences (introns) between individual coding segments (exons) (14). The details of cell function that are attainable using the current tools of molecular biology will find exceptions to the above definition.

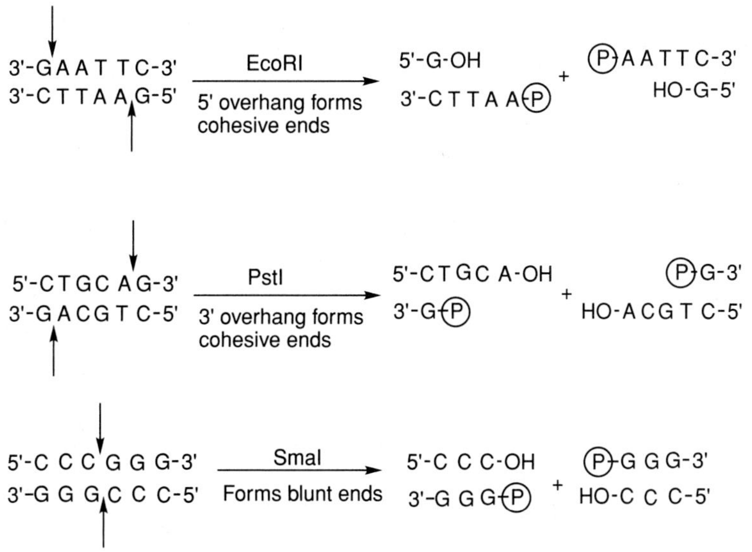

3'-G A A T T C-3'
3'-C T T A A G-5'
EcoRI
5' overhang forms cohesive ends
5'-G-OH
3'-C T T A A-P
+
P-A A T T C-3'
HO-G-5'
5'-C T G C A G-3'
3'-G A C G T C-5'
PstI
3' overhang forms cohesive ends
5'-C T G C A-OH
3'-G-P
+
P-G-3'
HO-A C G T C-5'
5'-C C C G G G-3'
3'-G G G C C C-5'
SmaI
Forms blunt ends
5'-C C C-OH
3'-G G G-P
+
P-G G G-3'
HO-C C C-5'

Fig. 6.18. Actions of restriction endonucleases *Eco*RI, *Pst*I, and *Sma*I at their recognition sequences. Note that *Eco*RI and *Pst*I enzymes produce "sticky ends," with overlapping sequences, whereas *Sma*I produces "blunt ends," or nonoverlapping sequences.

Cloning and the Preparation of DNA Libraries

Studies on the nature of DNA, genes and chromosomes ground to a near halt in the early 1960s, because DNA was just too large a molecule to work with and attempts to break it up into manageable pieces were thwarted by the inability to put the pieces back together in the correct order. The discovery in the early 1970s of bacterial enzymes capable of cleaving nucleic acids at specific, palindromic (symmetrical) base sequences was a major breakthrough in nucleic acid chemistry (Figs. 6.18 and 6.19). The second discovery in molecular biology that advanced genetic analysis was the use of bacterial plasmids as vehicles (vectors) to amplify gene fragments produced by restriction enzymes. Plasmids are small, circular, extrachromosomal nucleic acid molecules in bacteria that replicate independently within the bacterial cell. Restriction enzymes are used to produce relatively small DNA fragments that are inserted into bacterial plasmid vectors, forming recombinant DNA molecules (rDNA). The rDNA vectors are inserted into bacterial hosts, where the plasmid replicates with the bacteria, producing a large number of identical rDNA molecules known as clones, thus completing the process know as DNA cloning.

Phosphodiester
(site of cleavage by
restriction endonuclease)
3'-end
5'-end
Base
Restriction
endonuclease
Phosphomonoester
hydroxyl

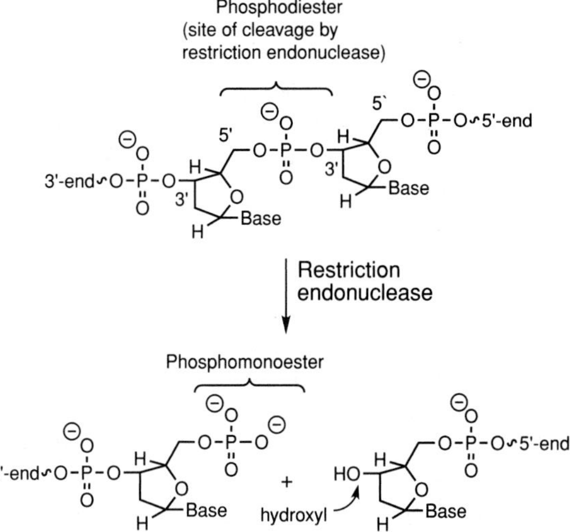

Fig. 6.19. Cleavage by restriction endonuclease.

Two sources of DNA are used to prepare fragments or libraries of DNA fragments. Genomic DNA isolated from the species of interest is digested with restriction enzymes, and the fragments are inserted into plasmids to produce a genomic DNA (gDNA) library. Alternatively, one can use mRNA fragments from restriction enzyme digests of mRNA from a cell or tissue and prepare DNA copies of the mRNA fragments using reverse transcription. The DNA fragment copies are complementary to the mRNA and are called complementary DNA (cDNA) fragments, thus producing a cDNA library. The two types of DNA libraries provide different genetic information. The gDNA library would have the gene regulatory sequences along with the introns in the gene coding sequence, whereas the cDNA would be missing these and other nontranscribed features of the gene sequence.

Finding a Gene in the Library

A well-prepared gene library has a high probability of containing a particular gene sequence. Library screening is the process through which one or more clones containing the gene of interest can be identified (15). If one wishes to screen for a particular gene, sufficient knowledge of that gene sequence must be available to allow synthesis of oligonucleotide fragments complementary to the gene or parts of it. These fragments can be radiolabeled or fluorescently labeled and used as nucleic acid probes to screen the library by hybridization. Assuming the library was made by ligating the gene fragments to bacterial vectors and inserting the vectors into *Escherichia coli,* the library is spread on several agar plates, and the bacteria are allowed to grow to form colonies such that each colony arises from a single bacteria carrying a single vector with a single gene fragment (Fig. 6.20).

After the colonies have grown to a size visible to the naked eye, nitrocellulose filters are carefully laid onto the surface of the agar plates to make an exact replica of the plate by blotting up a small amount of each colony on the plate (Fig. 6.20). The bacteria on the filter are lysed by soaking the filter in sodium dodecyl sulfate and a protease. The DNA is denatured using alkali (NaOH), and the ssDNA is bonded to the filter by baking. The filter is then incubated in a solution of radiolabeled or fluorescently labeled nucleic acid probe complementary to a portion of the gene of interest and allowed to hybridize to the ssDNA on the filter. The filters are carefully washed to remove the nonspecifically bound probe, and the specifically bound probes are located on the filter by exposing the filter to x-ray film (autoradiography) or laser excitation (fluorescence). The bacterial colony that specifically bound the probe likely contains a fragment of the gene in question. This colony will show up on the autoradiogram as a dark spot or a fluorescent band, and its position on the original agar plate can be located by comparing the nitrocellulose filter to the agar plate. Once located, the colony can be picked off the original plate and grown in culture to provide a large sample of the bacteria carrying the vector with the gene fragment.

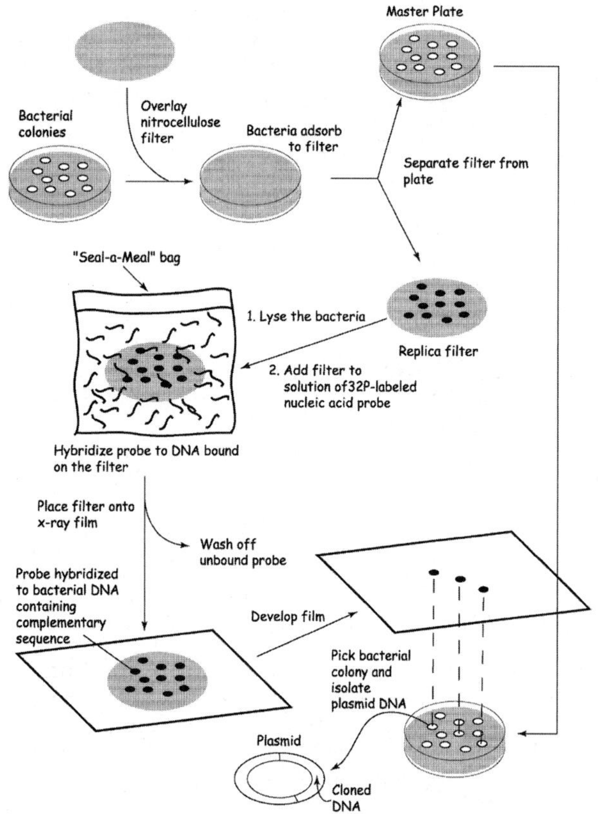

Fig. 6.20. Screening a library with a nucleic acid probe to find a clone of the pattern of bacterial colonies. (Adapted from Watson JD, Gilman M, Witkowski J, et al. Recombinant DNA, 2nd Ed. New York: Scientific American Books, W.H. Freeman and Company, 1992; with permission.)

Characterizing the Cloned Gene Fragment

Once the gene fragment has been cloned, the next step is characterization. Five techniques are critical to this characterization: size determination using agarose gel electrophoresis, restriction enzyme mapping to further reduce the size of the fragments, sequencing the fragments, synthesizing primers and probes used in the amplification and identification of the fragments, and amplification of the fragments through the polymerase chain reaction (PCR).

Agarose Gel Electrophoresis

The size of DNA fragments generally is determined by agarose gel electrophoresis. The dsDNA samples are placed in wells in the surface of the gel in separate lanes, and when an electric current is applied to an agarose gel in the presence of a buffer that will conduct electricity, the dsDNA fragments will travel through the gel toward the anode (positive electrode) at a rate dependent on the size of the linear molecule. Small fragments will travel faster than larger fragments, separating the mixture of DNA fragments according to size. The fragments generally are viewed by staining the gel with ethidium bromide, a chemical that intercalates into dsDNA. The molecular weight of fragments may be roughly determined by running a standard sample of DNA fragments with known molecular weights in a lane on the same gel as the unknown fragments.

Restriction Mapping and Southern Blotting

A DNA fragment isolated by the cloning technique described above may be characterized further by restriction enzyme mapping. This procedure consists of isolating the DNA fragment from the cloning vector and digesting it with one or more restriction enzymes, then separating the fragments on gel electrophoresis and staining them with ethidium bromide.

The number and size of the restriction fragments provide valuable information about the original DNA fragment. The individual restriction fragments may be extracted from the gels and the nucleotide sequence determined by Sanger's dideoxy method (see below) (16). When the nucleotide sequences of the restriction fragments are determined, overlapping fragments may be found and the fragments reassembled to determine the sequence of the original fragment. If examination of the sequence indicates the presence of a start and stop codon, an open reading frame exists in the sequence, and it is possible that the sequence codes for an expressed gene. Further studies are necessary, however, to determine if the sequence is expressed in the cell from which the original DNA fragment was isolated.

It also is possible to analyze DNA fragments by hybridization with particular radiolabeled or fluorescently labeled probes using a technique called Southern blotting (Fig. 6.21). The DNA solutions that have been digested with restriction enzymes are placed in wells at the top of the gel, and electrophoresis separates the fragments, which are then denatured with alkali and blotted onto nitrocellulose paper to make an exact replica of the gel. This is done by placing the agarose gel on a sponge in a tray of buffer. The nitrocellulose filter is placed over the gel and covered with a large stack of paper towels that act as a wick pulling the buffer through the gel and filter.

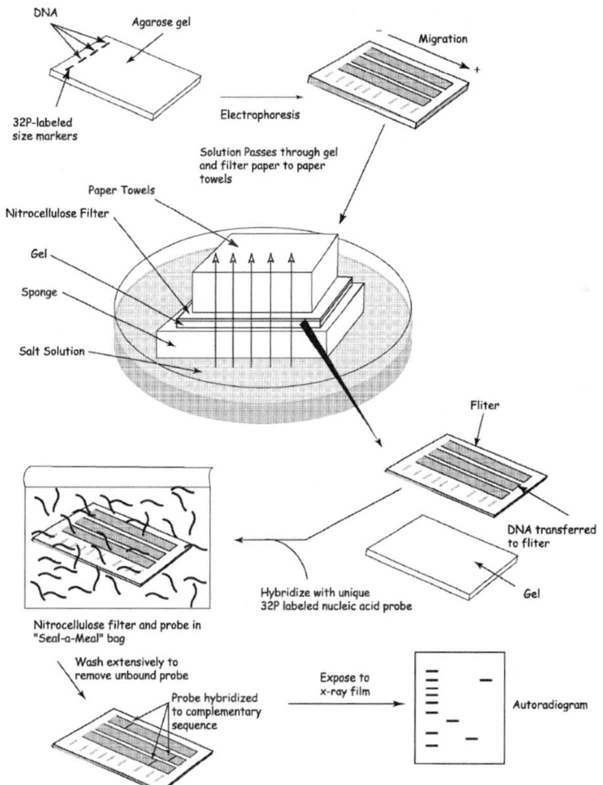

Fig. 6.21. Analyzing DNA by gel electrophoresis and Southern blotting. (Adapted from Watson JD, Gilman M, Witkowski J, et al. Recombinant DNA, 2nd Ed. New York: Scientific American Books, W.H. Freeman and Company, 1992; with permission.)

The DNA fragments are carried from the gel to the filter, where they stick. The filter is removed and hybridized with a radioactively labeled probe that specifically tags the sequence of interest through hybridization. The stringency with which the hybridization and washing is carried out is critical and is determined by temperature and salt concentration in the hybridization buffer, with high temperature and low salt being the most stringent conditions. If the conditions are not too stringent, then the probe may bind to too many nonhomologous sequences to be useful. Unbound probe is removed by washing, and the filter is placed on an x-ray film, where the bound probe appears as a band. A similar technique using RNA fragments is called Northern blotting.

Sequencing DNA Fragments

The two major methods of nucleic acid sequencing are the Maxam and Gilbert chemical method (17) and Sanger's dideoxy method (16). The dideoxy method of Sanger is largely the method of choice to sequence DNA fragments. It capitalizes on the use of DNA polymerase to catalyze the synthesis of a copy of the DNA fragment that one wishes to sequence. The method relies on the fact that when 2′,3′-dideoxynucleotide triphosphates (ddNTPs) are incorporated into growing nucleic acid chains, the growth ceases, because the dideoxynucleotide does not have a 3′-hydroxyl group on which to add the next nucleotide in the chain. The method consists of four reagent vials, each containing the ssDNA template fragment to be sequenced, DNA polymerase, a short radiolabeled oligonucleotide primer that hybridizes to the 3′ end of the template fragment, and the four nucleotide triphosphates (dATP, dGTP, dCTP, and dTTP). Each vial contains one of the four ddNTPs (either ddATP, ddGTP, ddCTP, or ddTTP), and the vial is labeled according to which ddNTP is present (Fig. 6.22). The ratio of the ddNTP to the normal dNTPs in the vial is carefully controlled such that the polymerase-catalyzed synthesis of the fragment will go to completion but a small, yet detectable, portion of the synthesis will be terminated each time a ddNTP is attached to the growing fragment. The reaction is initiated by the addition of the polymerase to the vials. When the synthesis is complete, a sample from each vial is applied to wells at the top of a polyacrylamide gel, and the gel is developed to separate the DNA fragments in each vial by size (Fig. 6.22). All fragments that arise in each of the vials as a result of termination of the synthesis at the incorporation of a ddNTP can be visualized on the gel by autoradiography, because the primer is radiolabeled (usually with a ^{32}P phosphate at the 5′- end) and all fragments will contain the primer sequence. The nucleotide sequence of the complementary strand of the fragment that acted as template in the DNA polymerase–catalyzed reaction can be read from the bottom of the gel starting with the sequence of the 5′ end primer and adding nucleotides based on the lane in which the next largest fragment occurs (Fig. 6.22). The smallest visible fragment will be

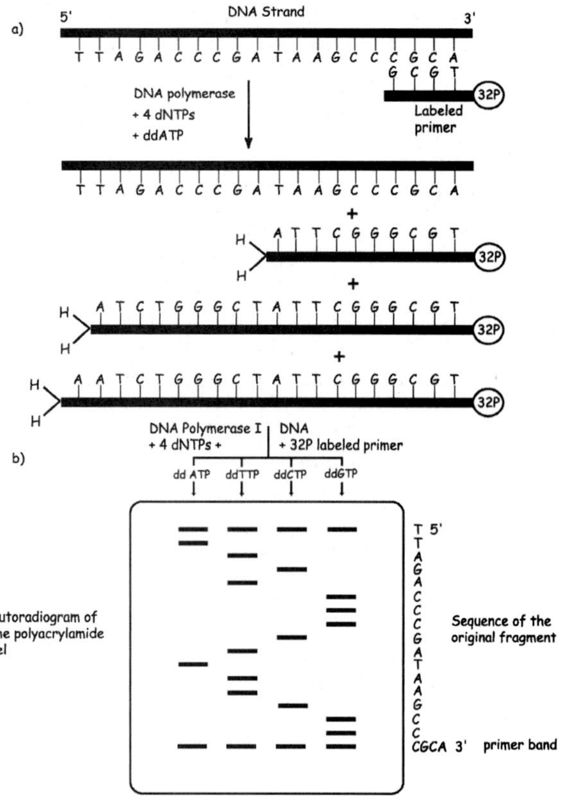

Fig. 6.22. The Sanger DNA-sequencing procedure. (a) The Sanger dideoxynucleotide sequencing reaction with ^{32}P-labeled primers. (b) Acrylamide gel separation of the labeled fragments. (Adapted from Watson JD, Gilman M, Witkowski J, et al. Recombinant DNA, 2nd Ed. New York: Scientific American Books, W.H. Freeman and Company, 1992; with permission.)

the primer, and the largest visible fragment will be the complete fragment, both of which will appear in all the vials. The intermediate fragment sizes will be different in each lane depending on the sequence of the template and which ddNTP was present.

This technique has been modified to use fluorescently labeled ddNTPs such that each NTP has a specific fluorescent label. The consequence of this change in protocol is that there is no need to use one reaction for each ddNTP. The sequencing reaction can be done in one vial, the separation of sequencing fragments run in one lane, and the terminal dNTP for each fragment identified by the color of the fluorescent label. After the gel is run, the lanes are scanned with an excitation laser, and the fluorescence detected is fed to a computer that records the data and provides a printout of the nucleic acid sequence.

Synthesizing Oligonucleotides

The need for short oligonucleotides of known sequence has grown tremendously with the need for radiolabeled and fluorescently labeled probes to isolate and characterize nucleic acids as well as the need for primers of the DNA polymerase–catalyzed synthesis of nucleic acids. It is now possible to synthesize an entire gene by enzymatically linking chemically synthesized oligonucleotide fragments making up the gene sequence. The phosphite triester (18) and the phosphotriester methods (19) are convenient solid-phase automated techniques for the synthesis of oligonucleotides. The solid-phase technique synthesizes the nucleic acid in the 3′ → 5′ direction by attaching the 3′-hydroxyl group of a 5′-O-dimethoxytrityl–protected deoxyribonucleoside to an insoluble solid support that may be polystyrene resin, silica gel, glass beads, polyamide, or cellulose paper. The subsequent 5′-protected nucleosides are coupled as 3′-phospho or phosphite triesters to the 5′-deprotected nucleic acid attached to the solid support. The 6-amino group of adenine and the 4-amino group of cytosine are protected as benzoyl amides, and the 2-amino group of guanine is protected by the isobutyryl amide.

The basic steps in the phosphite triester method are as follows (Fig. 6.23) (18):

1. Removal of the 5′-O-dimethoxytrityl group from the deoxyribonucleoside attached to the solid support is carried out by treatment of the reaction mixture with 3% dichloroacetic acid in dichloromethane.
2. The free 5′-OH group is coupled with excess 5′-O-dimethoxytrityl deoxyribounceloside-3′-phosphoramidite using tetrazole as an acid catalyst.

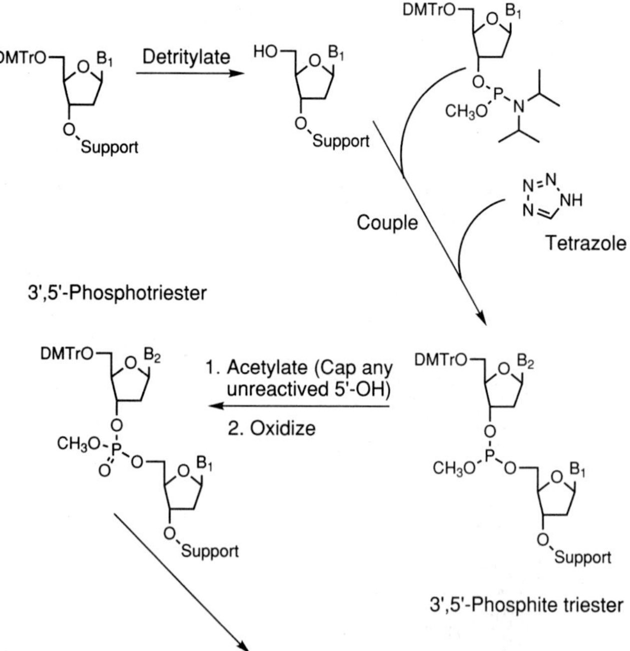

Fig. 6.23. Solid-phase phosphate triester method of oligodeoxyribonucleotide synthesis.

3. The new 3′,5′-phosphite triester linking the two nucleotides is converted to the more stable phosphotriester by iodine-catalyzed oxidation.
4. Any 5′-OH groups that failed to react are capped by acetylation with acetic anhydride.
5. The 5′-O-dimethoxytrityl protecting group is removed by treatment of the reaction mixture with 3% dichloroacetic acid in dichloromethane.
6. The sequence of deprotection, coupling, oxidation, and capping is repeated until the oligodeoxyribonucleotide of desired length is obtained.
7. The final product is deprotected, removed from the solid support, and purified.

Polymerase Chain Reaction

The problem of working with small quantities of nucleic acids isolated from cell and tissue sources was solved, to a certain extent, with the development of cloning techniques that would amplify a DNA fragment as part of a replicating vector in bacteria. The PCR was the second development that tremendously increased the ease with which a fragment of DNA could be amplified without the need for the complications of cloning (20). There was not even a need to isolate the fragment to be amplified. The only requirement was for DNA polymerase oligonucleotide primers at the boundaries of the fragment to be amplified.

The dsDNA fragment is targeted for amplification by designing oligonucleotide primers that anneal to the 3′ ends of the double-stranded fragment (Fig. 6.24). A DNA polymerase uses the oligonucleotides as primers to size the two strands from the 3′ ends, producing two new dsDNA strands carrying the DNA fragment bounded by the two primers. A series of cycles of denaturation, annealing primers, and DNA polymerization results in greatly amplified quantities of the fragment of interest (Fig. 6.24). The original technique used a DNA polymerase from *E. coli* that was heat sensitive and, hence, had to be replaced at every cycle of the reaction. The finding that thermophilic bacteria made DNA polymerases were resistant to the high temperatures used in the denaturation step of the polymerase cycle provided a source for the polymerase enzyme that would not have to be replaced each cycle, and the reaction could be automated without interruption. The most common temperature resistant enzyme used is *Taq* polymerase isolated from *Thermus aquaticus*. This enzyme survives a 1- to 2-minute exposure to 95°C temperature but lacks a 3′ → 5′ proofreading exonuclease activity, so it may introduce errors during DNA replication. Other enzymes with better features have been isolated and are being used in place of the *Taq* polymerase. The technique has many different applications in molecular biology and is really a cornerstone in the research on genetic structure/function relationships.

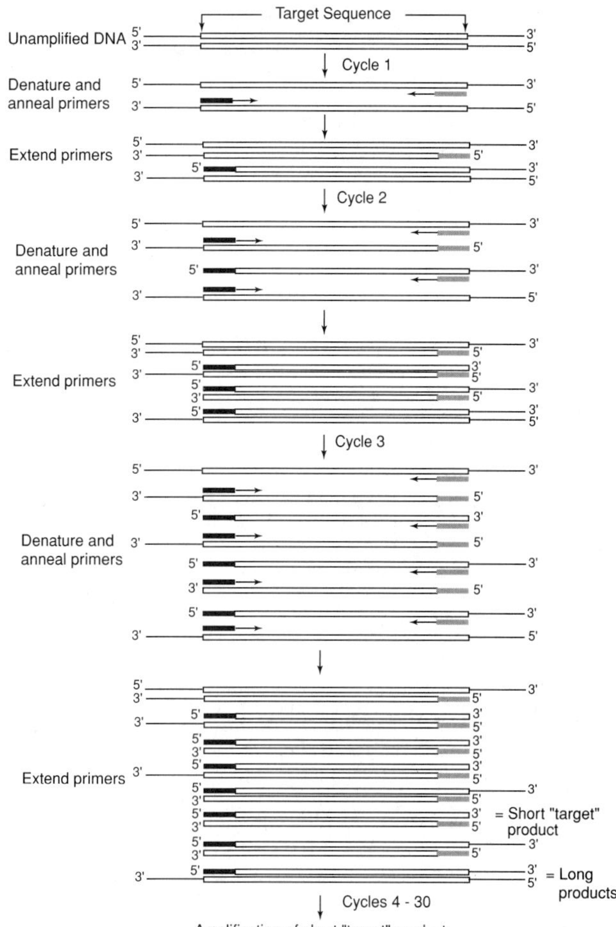

Fig. 6.24. The polymerase chain reaction.

Protein Synthesis through Recombinant DNA

Useful reviews detailing the process of rDNA are available (4–8,13–16). Applicable sections in any biochemistry or molecular biology textbook (21–24) provide more detailed reviews. Several reviews of rDNA technology have been written for practicing pharmacists (4,25–28). A general summary of the typical rDNA production of a protein follows and is schematically presented in Figure 6.25.

Once the gene coding for the desired protein has been identified and isolated (Fig. 6.25), the genetic material is introduced into cells using restriction endonucleases and a vector to enable DNA replication and to produce protein. The discovery of restriction endonuclease enzymes that recognize explicit sequences of bases in dsDNA and precisely hydrolyze the phosphodiester bonds of the nucleic acids at specific sites along the DNA strands offered a way of isolating predictable fragments of any DNA molecule. This family of "scissors-like" enzymes is used to provide the DNA fragment coding for the protein of interest by "cutting" or "clipping" the DNA (Figs. 6.18 and 6.19). The bacterial enzymes, numbering greater than 100 variations isolated

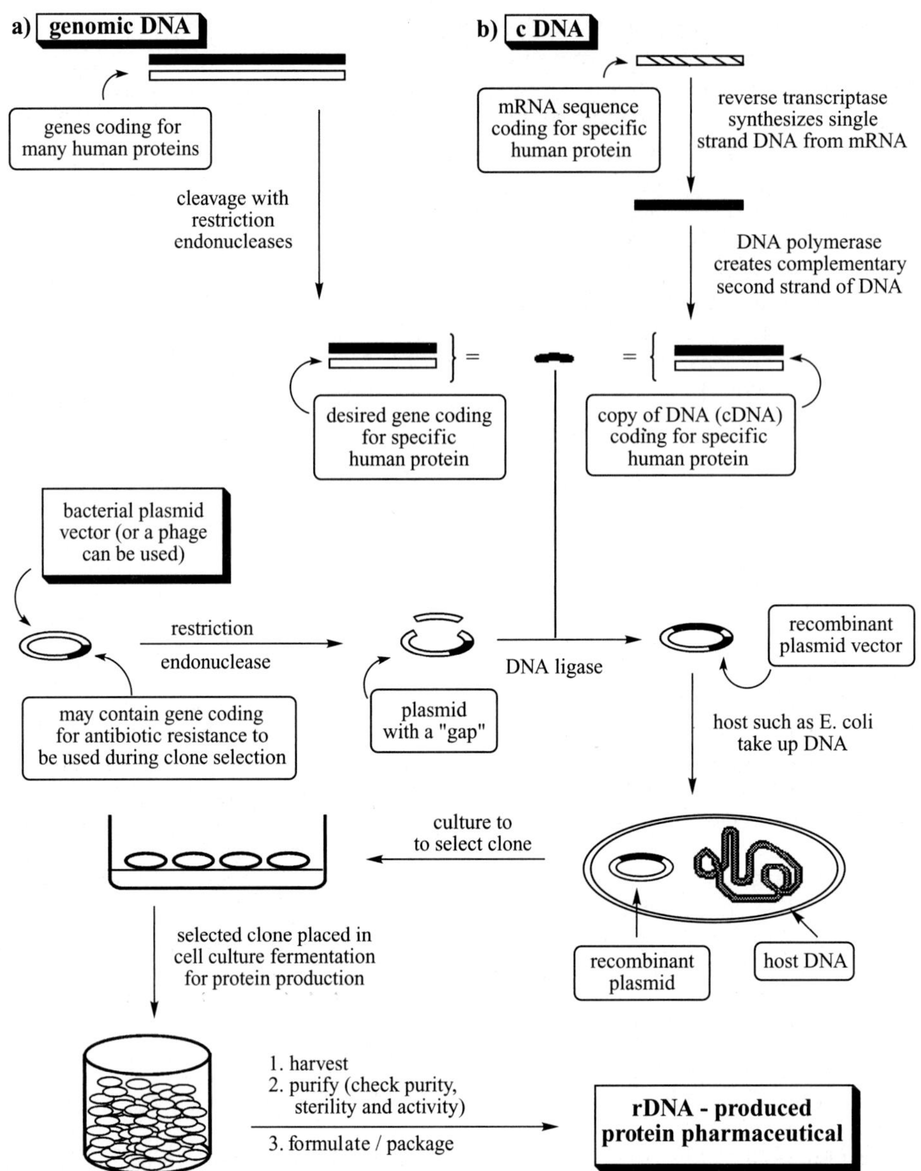

Fig. 6.25. Summary of typical rDNA production of a protein from either (a) genomic DNA or (b) cDNA.

(see Table 6.2 for representative examples), have led to the powerful techniques of DNA sequencing and rDNA technology. Most restriction endonucleases create two single-strand breaks, one in each strand generating a 5′-phosphomonoester and 3′-hydroxyl group from each cleavage. The breaks are not necessarily opposite one another, as can be seen in Table 6.2 (e.g., *Asu*II, *Bal*I, and *Eco*RV). For instance, Eco RI causes breaks that are not opposite one another, creating sticky (or cohesive or complementary) ends to the DNA strands. The DNA fragments can be isolated, purified, and identified.

A cloning vector is a carrier molecule, the vehicle that is used to insert foreign DNA into a host cell. Typically, vectors are genetic elements that can be replicated in a host cell separately from that cell's chromosomes. Bacterial plasmids, or circular DNA of only a few thousand base pairs outside of the nucleus that replicate freely within the cell, are ideal for carrying the gene into the host organism. In the first such rDNA experiments in early 1973, Cohen et al. (29) used the small *E. coli* plasmid pSC101 containing only a single Eco RI recognition site as the vector to insert foreign plasmid DNA into *E. coli.* Other vectors include the constructed plasmids pBR322 and pUC18 and bacteriophages. Bacteriophages are bacterial viruses modified to accept large pieces (7–20 kb) of exogenous DNA without altering their ability to infect and replicate inside the bacteria (30). Large genomic libraries have been created by fragmenting all

Table 6.2. Some Representative Examples of Restriction Endonucleases (15,39)

Restriction Endonucleases	Source	Recognition Sequence[a]	Cleavage Products	
AluI	*Arthrobacter luteus*	5′-TT/CGAA-3′ 3′-AAGC/TT-5′	-TT- -AAGC-	-CGAA- -TT-
AsuII	*Ananaena subcylindria*	5′-AG/CT-3′ 3′-TC/GA-5′	-AG- -TC-	-CT- -GA-
BalI	*Brevibacterium albidum*	5′-TGG/CCA-3′ 3′-ACC/GGT-5′	-TGG- -ACC-	-CCA- -GGT-
*Eco*RI	*Escherichia coli*	5′-G/AATTC-3′ 3′-CTTAA/G-5′	-G- -CTTAA-	-AATTC- -G-
*Eco*RV	*Escherichia coli*	5′-GAT/ATC-3′ 3′-CTA/TAG-5′	-GAT- -CTA-	-ATC- -TAG-
HhaI	*Haemophilus haemolyticus*	5′-GCG/C-3′ 3′-C/GCG-5′	-GCG- -C-	-C- -GCG-

[a]Illustrates the position where the DNA strands are cleaved.

of the embryonic or sperm cell DNA of an organism, inserting them into bacteriophage lambda, and screening with DNA probes to identify the gene sequences.

The DNA fragments coding for the desired protein can be cloned from genomic DNA or cDNA as described previously. The piece of DNA coding for the protein of interest is then inserted into the vector that carries the code to synthesize the protein in the host. The plasmid or bacteriophage DNA is opened with a restriction enzyme, and the exogenous gene is pasted into it by an enzyme called DNA ligase with the assistance of special sections of DNA called linkers. The DNA ligase seals the single-strand breaks in dsDNA. Also, promoter or enhancer DNA sequences are added to increase plasmid replication and increase protein synthesis by the gene. A promoter is a short DNA sequence that amplifies the expression of protein by the adjacent target gene. An enhancer is a viral DNA sequence that dramatically increases the level of transcription of adjacent DNA. A gene providing antibiotic resistance (as a selection tool) also may be placed in a plasmid that is inserted into a bacterial host. This gene confers a particular antibiotic resistance on the clone and may be used in the clone selection later in the rDNA process. This vector is now an rDNA molecule consisting of the gene, linker, promoter/enhancer, and vector DNA.

The vector containing the code for the target protein is then inserted into the host. Host cells are typically bacteria (e.g., *E. coli*), eukaryotic yeast (e.g., *Saccharomyces cerevisiae* [baker's yeast]), or mammalian cell lines. Examples of mammalian cell lines include CHO (Chinese hamster ovary), VERO (African green monkey kidney), and BHK (baby hamster kidney). The choice of host system is influenced primarily by the type of protein to be expressed and by the key differences among the various host cells (31). Bacterial and yeast cells are more easily cultured in large fermenters. Overall protein yields generally are much lower in mammalian cells, but in some cases, this may be the only system that produces some mammalian proteins. Another difference is that yeast and mammalian cells do not form toxins, whereas Gram-negative bacteria produce endotoxins. Finally, an important distinction is that posttranslational modification reactions, such as glycosylation, do not occur in bacteria.

The host cells containing the vector are grown in small-scale culture to select only for the correct clone that contains the desired gene and is able to express the best yields of the protein (32). The selected cloned cells (or cell bank cells) are used as inoculum first for a small-scale cell culture/fermentation, which is then followed by larger fermentations in bioreactors. The medium is carefully controlled to enhance cell reproduction and protein synthesis. The host cells divide, and the vectors within the hosts multiply. The host produces its natural proteins along with the desired protein, which may be secreted into the growth medium. The protein of interest can then be isolated from the fermentation, purified, and formulated to give a potential rDNA-produced pharmaceutical.

Protein Isolation and Purification

The isolation and purification of the final protein product from the complex mixture of cells, cellular debris, medium nutrients, and other host metabolites is a challenging task (31,32). The structure, purity, potency, and stability of the recombinant protein must be considered. Often, sophisticated filtrations, phase separations, precipitation, and complex multiple-column chromatographic procedures are required to obtain the desired protein. Although isolation of the recombinant protein, produced in culture in relatively large amounts, generally is easier than isolating the native protein, ensuring the stability and retention of the bioactive three-dimensional structure (correct protein folding) of any biopharmaceutical is a more arduous task. In addition, recombinant proteins from bacterial hosts require removal of endotoxins, whereas viral particles may need to be removed from mammalian cell culture products (33). A discussion of these techniques is beyond the scope of this chapter, however. Useful reviews on the extraction and purification (31,32,34) and the analysis and chromatography (35–39) of biotechnology products are available as a resource for further information.

THERAPEUTIC APPLICATION OF RECOMBINANT DNA

Overview

The techniques made available by advances in biotechnology that have provided new medicinal agents fall into several broad areas. First, rDNA technology, the ability to manipulate the genetic information inherent within the nucleus of living cells, provides the ability to take identified gene sequences from one organism and place them functionally into another to permit the production of protein medicines. Second, hybridoma techniques permit the production of monoclonal antibodies (MAbs), which are ultrasensitive hybrid immune system–derived proteins designed to recognize specific antigens. The MAbs are used as diagnostic agents for laboratory and home kits and for site-directed therapeutics. Additionally, the development of technologies to study DNA–DNA and DNA–RNA interactions has led to the formation of RNA and DNA probes (antisense technology) for a variety of research purposes with potential uses as diagnostics and therapeutics. Tools of modern pharmaceutical biotechnology also include PCR, genomics, proteomics, gene therapy, transgenics, glycobiology, and a host of other evolving techniques (Table 6.3).

Recombinant DNA Technology

The revolution in biology and genetics that has occurred over the past 30 years, affecting both the basic research and its practical aspects, has been fueled by rDNA technology. Sometimes also referred to as genetic engineering, gene cloning, or in vitro genetic manipulation, rDNA technology provides the ability to introduce genetic material from any source into cells (bacterial, fungal, plant, or animal) or even whole plants and animals (40). A general understanding of the technologies involved should readily help the pharmacist better gain insight regarding and comprehension of a biotechnology drug's use, stability, handling, side effects, and potential toxicity—in other words, how these agents differ from traditional drugs. Also, such an understanding should readily demonstrate the impact that rDNA technology is having on both current and future pharmacy practice.

Table 6.3. Major Techniques of Biotechnology

Recombinant DNA technology (rDNA)
Hybridoma technology (monoclonal antibodies)
Antisense technology
Polymerase chain reaction (PCR)
Genomics (including DNA microarrays)
Proteomics
Gene therapy
Transgenics
Glycobiology
Proteomics
Cloning
Molecular modeling
Peptidomimetics
Metabolomics
Pharmacogenomics
Toxicogenomics
Bioinformatics
RNA silencing

GENERAL PROPERTIES OF BIOTECHNOLOGY-PRODUCED MEDICINAL AGENTS

Although a majority of traditional medicinal agents are relatively small organic molecules, rDNA and hybridoma technologies have made it possible to produce large quantities of highly pure, therapeutically useful proteins. The rDNA-derived proteins and MAbs are not dissimilar to the other protein pharmaceuticals or biopharmaceuticals that pharmacists have dispensed in the past. As polymers of amino acids joined by peptide bonds, the properties of these proteins differ generally from those of small organic molecule pharmaceuticals. An overview of the general properties of biotechnology-produced medicinal agents actually is a review of the general physicochemical properties of proteins. Therefore, to study the stability, handling, storage, route of administration, and metabolism of biotechnology-produced pharmaceuticals, it is valuable to understand the chemical nature of proteins. Chapter 7 of this text and other publications (41–48) review the physical biochemistry of protein drugs; related chapters in any biochemistry textbook also review this topic.

Stability of Biotech Pharmaceuticals

Several detailed reviews on the stability of proteins and protein pharmaceuticals written for pharmaceutical scientists are available (43,45–50). A brief overview of these resources follows and provides additional information. The instability of proteins, including protein pharmaceuticals, can be separated into two distinct classes. Chemical instability results from bond formation or cleavage yielding a modification of the protein and a new chemical entity. Physical instability involves a change to the secondary or higher-order structure of the protein rather than a covalent bond-breaking modification.

Chemical Instability

A variety of reactions give rise to the chemical instability of proteins, including hydrolysis, oxidation, racemization, β-elimination, and disulfide exchange (Fig. 6.26). Each of these changes may cause a loss of biological activity.

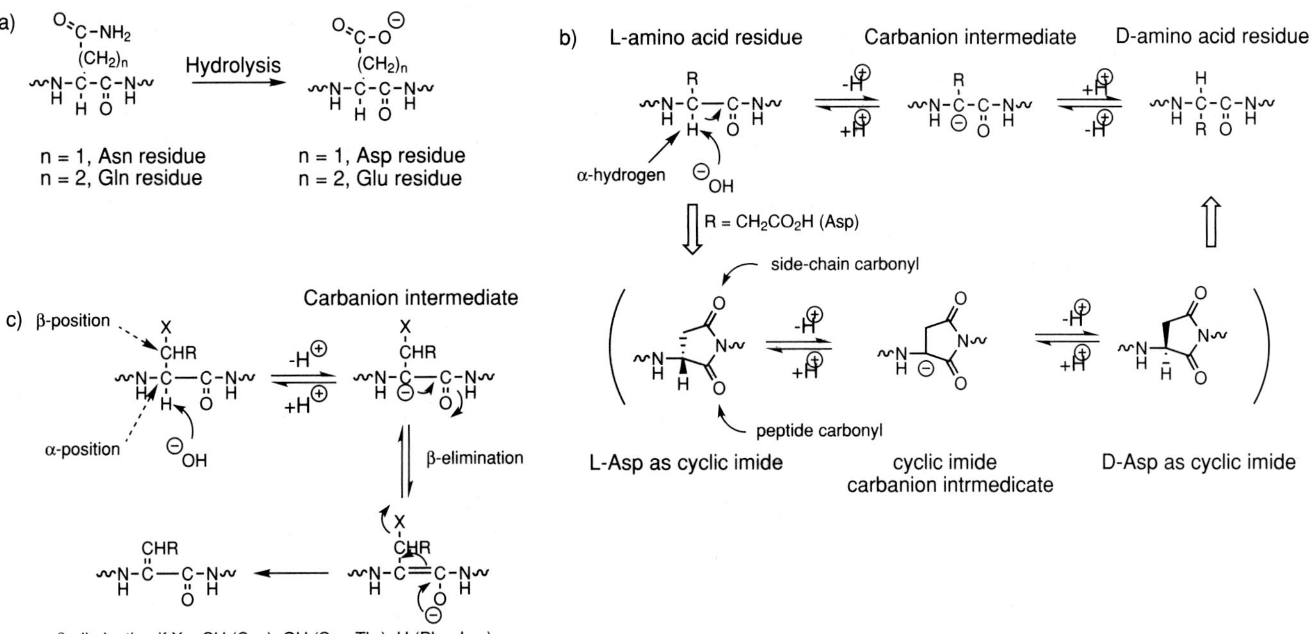

Fig. 6.26. Chemical instability of protein biopharmaceuticals. (a) Hydrolysis. (b) Base-catalyzed racemization. (c) β-Elimination.

Proteolytic hydrolysis of peptide bonds results in fragmentation of the protein chain. It is well established that in dilute acids, aspartic acid (Asp) residues in proteins are hydrolyzed at a rate at least 100-fold faster than that of other peptide bonds because of the mechanism of the reaction. An additional hydrolysis reaction is the deamidation of the neutral residue of asparagine (Asn) and glutamine (Gln) side-chain linkages, forming the ionizable carboxylic acid residues aspartic acid (Asp) and glutamic acid (Glu) (Fig. 6.26a). This conversion may be considered primary sequence isomerization.

Oxidative degradative reactions can occur to the side chains of sulfur-containing methionine (Met) and cysteine (Cys) residues and the aromatic amino acid residues histidine (His), tryptophan (Trp), and tyrosine (Tyr) in proteins during their isolation and storage. The weakly nucleophilic thioether group of Met (R-S-CH_3) can be oxidized at low pH by hydrogen peroxide as well as by oxygen in the air to the sulfoxide (R-SO-CH_3) and the sulfone (R-SO_2-CH_3). The thiol (sulfhydryl, R-SH) group of Cys can be successively oxidized to the corresponding sulfenic acid (R-SOH), disulfide (R-SS-R), sulfinic acid (R-SO_2H), and finally, sulfonic acid (R-SO_3H). A number of factors, including pH, influence the rate of this oxidation. Oxidation of His, Trp, and Tyr residues is believed to occur with a variety of oxidizing agents, resulting in the cleavage of the aromatic rings.

Base-catalyzed racemization reactions may occur in any of the amino acids except achiral glycine (Gly) to yield residues in proteins with mixtures of L- and D-configurations. The α-methine hydrogen is removed to form a carbanion intermediate (Fig. 6.26b). The degree of stabilization of this intermediate controls the rate of this reaction. Racemization generally alters the proteins' physicochemical properties and biological activity. Also, racemization generates nonmetabolizable D-configuration forms of the amino acids. Generally, most amino acid residues are relatively stable to racemization, with a notable exception. Aspartate residues in proteins racemize at 10^5-fold faster rate than when free, in contrast to the two- to fourfold increase for the other residues. The facilitated rate of racemization for Asp residues is believed to result from the formation of a stabilized cyclic imide.

Proteins containing cysteine (Cys), serine (Ser), threonine (Thr), phenylalanine (Phe), and lysine (Lys) are prone to β-elimination reactions under alkaline conditions (Fig. 6.26c). The reaction proceeds through the same carbanion intermediate as racemization. The reaction is influenced by a number of additional factors, including temperature and the presence of metal ions.

The interrelationships of disulfide bonds and free sulfhydryl groups in proteins are important factors influencing the chemical and biological properties of protein pharmaceuticals. Disulfide exchange can result in incorrect pairings and major changes in the higher-order structure (secondary and above) of proteins. The exchange may occur in neutral, acidic, and alkaline media.

Physical Instability

Generally not encountered in most small organic molecules, physical instability is a consequence of the polymeric nature of proteins. Proteins adopt secondary, tertiary, and quaternary structures, which influence their three-dimensional shape and, therefore, their biological activity. Any change to the higher-order structure of a protein may alter both. Physical instability includes denaturation, adsorption to surfaces, and noncovalent self-aggregation (soluble and precipitation). The most widely studied aspect of protein instability is denaturation. Noncovalent aggregation, however, is one of the primary mechanisms of protein degradation (43).

A protein, in principle, can be folded into a virtually infinite number of conformations. The combination of spatial arrangements and noncovalent intramolecular interactions of nearby amino acid residues providing the lowest-energy conformation is the most stable secondary structure. Longer-distance interactions cause the globular nature of proteins (tertiary structure), including their ability to fold so that hydrophilic amino acid side chains are directed toward the exterior surface of the protein exposed to an aqueous environment. In general, all molecules of any protein species adopt the same conformation, or native state. Denaturation occurs by disrupting the weaker noncovalent interactions that hold a protein together in its secondary and tertiary structures. Temperature, pH, and the addition of organic solvents and solutes may cause denaturation. The process can be reversible or irreversible. In general, denaturation affects the protein by decreasing aqueous solubility, altering three-dimensional molecular shape, increasing susceptibility to enzymatic hydrolysis, and causing the loss of the native protein's biological activity.

Handling and Storage of Biotechnology-Produced Products

The preparation and administration of drugs of recombinant or hybridoma origin are dissimilar to the other nonprotein pharmaceuticals that pharmacists have been dispensing in the past. Proteins generally have more limited shelf stability. The average shelf life for a biotechnology product is 12 to 18 months, compared with more than 36 months for a small molecule drug. Although each individual biotechnology drug may be different, several generalizations can be made.

Proper storage of the lyophilized and the reconstituted drug is essential. Most of these drugs are expensive, so special care must be taken not to inactivate the therapeutic protein during storage and handling. The human proteins have limited chemical and physical stability, which is shortened on reconstitution. Expiration dating ranges from 2 hours to 30 days. The self-association of either native state or misfolded protein subunits may readily occur under certain conditions. This can lead to aggregation and precipitation and results in a loss of biological activity. Self-association mechanisms depend on the conditions of formulation and may occur as a result of hydrophobic interactions.

Many of the biotechnology-produced drugs are stored refrigerated, but not frozen (2–8°C). In general, temperature extremes must be avoided. One example is the rDNA-produced, blood clot–dissolving drug alteplase. A recombinant version of a naturally occurring human tissue-type plasminogen activator, lyophilized alteplase is stable at room temperature for several years if protected from light (51). Freezing or exposure to excessive heat decreases the physical stability of the protein. Anything that causes denaturation or self-aggregation, even though labile peptide bonds are not broken, may inactivate the protein. Some pharmacy facilities may need to increase cold storage capacity to accommodate biotech storage needs. If the patient must travel any distance home after receiving the medication, the pharmacist should help package the biotechnology product according to the manufacturer's directions. This may mean supplying a reusable cooler for the patient's use. Because the protein drug should not be frozen, the cooler should contain an ice pack rather than dry ice.

Some rDNA-derived pharmaceuticals, particularly the cytokines (e.g., the interferons, interleukin-2, and colony-stimulating factors), require human serum albumin in their formulation to prevent adhesion of the protein drug to the glass surface of the vial, which results in loss of protein (51–53). The amount of human serum albumin added varies with the biotech product. The vials should not be shaken to prevent foaming of the albumin, which causes protein loss or inactivation of the biotechnology-derived proteins. Care must be exercised in reconstituting protein pharmaceuticals. The diluent used for reconstitution of biotechnology drugs varies with the product and is specified by the manufacturer. Diluents can include normal saline, bacteriostatic water, and 5% dextrose. Several reviews of biotechnology drugs written for pharmacists contain additional information on the subjects of handling and storage (4,26,52,54–57).

Biotechnology Drug Delivery

Protein-based pharmaceuticals, whether produced by biotechnology or isolated from traditional sources, present challenges to drug delivery because of the unique demands imposed by their physicochemical and biological properties. Although a detailed discussion of this topic is beyond the scope of this chapter, a brief overview follows. Useful reviews also are available for further information (46,58–62).

Delivery of large-molecular-weight, biotechnology-produced drugs into the body is difficult because of the poor absorption of these compounds, the acid lability of peptide bonds, and the rapid enzymatic degradation of these drugs in the body. In addition, protein pharmaceuticals are susceptible to physical instability, complex feedback control mechanisms, and peculiar dose–response relationships.

Given the limitations of today's technology, the strongly acidic environment of the stomach, the peptidases in the gastrointestinal tract, and the barrier to absorption presented by gastrointestinal mucosal cells preclude successful oral administration of most protein drugs. Therefore, administration of all the biotechnology-produced protein drugs currently is parenteral (by intravenous, subcutaneous, or intramuscular injections) to provide a better therapeutic profile. Manufacturers supply most of these drugs as sterile solutions without a preservative. In such cases, it is recommended that only one dose be prepared from each vial to prevent bacterial contamination. Novel solutions to overcome delivery problems associated with biotechnology protein products are being explored. Oral drug delivery approaches in development for various biotechnology-derived drugs include conjugated systems (e.g., with polyethylene glycol), liposomes, microspheres, erythrocytes as carriers, and viruses as drug carriers (45). Specialized delivery methods being examined include transdermal systems, pulmonary delivery, intranasal sprays, buccal administration, ocular delivery systems, rectal administration, iontophoresis, phonophoresis, metered pumps, protein pro-drugs, lymphatic uptake, coadministration of peptidase inhibitors, and penetration enhancers.

Some Pharmacokinetic Considerations of Biotechnology-Produced Proteins

The processes of adsorption into, distribution within, metabolism by, and excretion from the body (i.e., ADME) of biotechnology-produced pharmaceuticals are important factors affecting the time course of their pharmacologic effect. To deliver quality pharmaceutical care with biotech products, a pharmacist must be able to apply pharmacokinetic principles to establish and maintain a nontoxic, therapeutic effect. The pharmacokinetics of these protein drugs differ in some pharmacokinetic aspects from those of the small molecule organic agents with which we are most familiar. Although a lengthy discussion of this topic is beyond the scope of this chapter, a brief overview of metabolism follows. Useful reviews also are available for further information (63,64).

The plasma half-life of most administered proteins is relatively short, because they are susceptible to a wide variety of metabolic reactions. Rapid hydrolytic degradation of peptide bonds by both nonspecific enzymes and highly structurally selective aminopeptidases, carboxypeptidases, deamidases, and proteinases occurs at the site of administration, while crossing the vascular endothelia, at the site of action, in the liver, in the blood, in the kidney, and in fact, in most tissues and fluids of the body. Overall, the metabolic products of most proteins are not considered to be a safety issue. They generally are broken down into amino acids and reincorporated into new, endogenously biosynthesized proteins.

Metabolic oxidation reactions may occur to the side chains of sulfur-containing residues, similar to that observed for in vitro chemical instability. Methionine can be oxidized to the sulfoxide, whereas metabolic oxidation of cysteine residues forms a disulfide. Metabolic reductive cleavage of disulfide bridges in proteins may occur, yielding free sulfhydryl groups.

Adverse Effects

Overview

An important consideration in the pharmaceutical care of a patient being administered a biotechnology-produced medicinal agent is the potential for adverse reactions. Many of the protein agents are biotechnology-derived versions of endogenous human proteins normally present, on stimulus, in minute quantities near their specific site of action. Therefore, the same protein administered in much larger quantities may cause adverse effects not commonly observed at normal physiologic concentrations (63–65). Careful monitoring of patients administered biotechnology-produced drugs is critical for the health care team.

Immunogenicity

The immune system may respond to an antigen, such as a protein pharmaceutical, by triggering the production of antibodies. Biotechnology-derived proteins may possess a different set of antigenic determinants (i.e., regions of a protein recognized by an antibody) because of structural differences between the recombinant protein and the natural human protein (43,62,63). Factors that can contribute to this immunogenicity include lack of or incorrect glycosylation, amino acid modifications, and amino acid additions and deletions. A number of recombinant proteins produced with bacterial vectors contain an N-terminal methionine in addition to the natural human amino acid sequence. Bacterial vector-derived recombinant protein preparations also may contain small amounts of immunoreactive bacterial polypeptides as possible contaminants. Additionally, immunogenicity may result from proteins that are misfolded, denatured, or aggregated.

RECOMBINANT DNA-PRODUCED MEDICINAL AGENTS

Recombinant DNA technology provides a powerful tool for new pharmaceutical product development and production. Table 6.4 lists the rDNA-produced drugs and vaccines approved by the U.S. FDA through the year 2000. The biotech products include hormones, enzymes, cytokines, hematopoietic growth factors, other growth factors, blood clotting factors and anticoagulants, and vaccines.

Hormones

Insulin

Biotechnology has provided hormone replacement therapy with the introduction of human insulin (66–68), the first U.S. FDA–approved rDNA drug in 1982, for the treatment of insulin-dependent diabetes. The human insulin molecule has the structural characteristics of a large protein yet is only the size of a polypeptide, totaling 51 amino acid residues. Two disulfide bonds (cysteine [Cys] A7 to Cys B7 and Cys A20 to Cys B19) link two

Table 6.4. Drugs and Vaccines of Recombinant DNA Origin Approved by the U.S. Food and Drug Administration

Class	Generic Name	Indication
Hormone	Insulin (human)	Insulin-dependent diabetes mellitus
	Insulin (human) lispro	Insulin-dependent diabetes mellitus
	Insulin (human) aspart	Insulin-dependent diabetes mellitus
	Insulin (human) glargine	Insulin-dependent diabetes mellitus
	Glucagon	Treatment of hypoglycemia, diagnostic aid
	Somatrem	hGH deficiency in children
	Somatropin	hGH deficiency in children Growth failure in children because of chronic renal insufficiency Turner's syndrome hGH deficiency in adults Children with Prader-Willi syndrome
	Pegvisomant	Treatment of acromegaly
	Follitropin alpha	Infertility
	Follitropin beta	Infertility
	Thyrotropin alfa	Detection and treatment of thyroid cancer
	Teriparatide	Treatment of osteoporosis in postmenopausal women
Enzyme	Alteplase	Acute myocardial infarction Acute myocardial embolism Ischemic stroke
	Retavase	Acute myocardial infarction
	Tenecteplase	Acute myocardial infarction
	Dornase alpha	Cystic fibrosis
	Imiglucerase	Treatment of Gaucher disease
Cytokine	Interferon-α_{2a}	Hairy cell leukemia AIDS-related Kaposi's sarcoma Chronic myelogenous leukemia Hepatitis C
	Interferon-α_{2b}	Hairy cell leukemia Genital warts AIDS-related Kaposi's sarcoma Hepatitis B Hepatitis C Malignant melanoma Follicular lymphoma
	Peginterferon α_{2a}	Chronic hepatitis C
	Interferon alfacon-1	Treatment of chronic hepatitis C viral infection
	Interferon-β_{1a}	Relapsing multiple sclerosis
	Interferon-β_{1b}	Relapsing, remitting multiple sclerosis
	Interferon-γ_{1b}	Management of chronic granulomatous disease
	Aldesleukin	Renal cell carcinoma Metastatic melanoma
	Denileukin diftitox	Persistent or recurrent cutaneous T-cell lymphoma
	Oprrelvekin	Prevention of severe chemotherapy-induced thrombocytopenia
	Anakinra	Moderate to severe active rheumatoid arthritis
	Etanercept	Moderate to severe active rheumatoid arthritis
Hematopoietic growth factor	Epoetin alpha	Anemia related to AZT therapy in HIV-infected patients Anemia associated with chronic renal failure Anemia caused by chemotherapy in patients with nonmyeloid malignancies Prevention of anemia associated with surgical blood loss Anemia in children—chronic renal failure undergoing dialysis
	Darbepoetin alfa	Treatment of anemia
	Filgrastim	Decrease incidence of infection—patients with nonmyeloid malignancies receiving myelosuppressive drugs Autologous or allogeneic bone marrow transplantation Chronic severe neutropenia
	Sargramostim	Myeloid recovery in patients after autologous bone marrow transplantation Neutropenia—result of chemotherapy for acute myelogenous leukemia Allogeneic bone marrow transplantation Support for peripheral blood progenitor cell mobilization and transplantation
Other growth factors	Becaplermin	Lower extremity diabetic neuropathic ulcers
Blood clotting factor	Recombinant factor VIII	Hemophilia B
	Recombinant factor IX	Hemophilia A
Anticoagulant	Lepirudin	Heparin-inducer thrombocytopenia type II
Vaccine	Hepatitis B vaccine	Prevention of hepatitis B
	Lyme disease vaccine	Prevention of Lyme disease

polypeptide chains, with the A-chain consisting of 21 amino acids and the B-chain 30 residues. An additional disulfide loop is found in the A-chain between Cys A6 and Cys A11 (Fig. 7.17 and Fig. 32.1). Insulin formulation development focused on modifying the time-action profile (onset, peak plasma concentration, and duration of action) through the use of various levels of zinc and protamine. Also, the chemical stability of insulin was improved by moving from acidic to neutral formulations.

Before the availability of rDNA-produced human insulin, porcine and bovine insulin were the most commonly used pharmaceutical preparations. Both porcine and bovine insulin differ in primary structure from human insulin, with alanine (Ala) replacing threonine (Thr) at the C-terminal of the B-chain (B30). Bovine insulin also differs from human insulin by Ala replacing Thr at A8 and valine (Val) substituting for isoleucine (Ile) at A10 (Table 32.8). These subtle differences can result in immunologic responses to the nonhuman insulins, requiring a modification of the therapeutic regimen. The biotechnology solution has several advantages over insulin derived from animal sources:

1. It should have potentially fewer serious immune reactions.
2. It is pyrogen-free.
3. It is not contaminated with other peptide hormones, such as glucagon, somatostatin, and proinsulin, as found in isolated products.
4. It can be produced in larger amounts.

The first successful attempts to tailor a protein hormone for therapy by rDNA techniques has yielded interesting insulin analogues (66–68).

Human insulin rDNA origin is available commercially as Humulin, Novolin, and as several analogues. The Humulin and Novolin products are produced using genetically modified strains of two different microorganisms. Humulin is prepared using recombinant *E. coli* bacteria. The pharmaceutical preparation is reported to contain less than 4 ppm of immunoreactive bacterial polypeptides that act as possible contaminants. Baker's yeast (*S. cerevisiae*) serves as the recombinant organism for the production of Novolin. Before 1986, Humulin was produced by chemically joining together the separately rDNA-derived A-chain and B-chain. Today, the product is prepared by enzymatically cleaving the connecting peptide in recombinant proinsulin.

Studies in animals, healthy adults, and patients with type I diabetes mellitus have shown human insulin to have pharmacologic effects identical to those of purified porcine insulin. A comparable pharmacokinetic profile also has been shown. Human insulin, however, administered intramuscularly or intravenously, may have a slightly faster onset and slightly shorter duration of action when compared with purified porcine insulin in patients with diabetes. The usual precautions concerning toxic potentials observed with insulin of animal origin should be followed with rDNA human insulin. As would be expected, the recombinant product has been shown to be less immunogenic than animal insulins.

Insulin remains the only treatment option for type I diabetes and is still widely used to treat patients with type II diabetes who do not respond adequately to other pharmacotherapies. Recombinant DNA technology has lead recently to the development of insulin analogues that have greater utility in certain situations and may more closely resemble the normal diurnal pattern of insulin secretion (Table 32.10). The newly engineered analogues have specific amino acid sequence modifications that improve absorption properties and biological profiles (69). Insulin lispro (Humalog) has a more rapid onset and shorter duration of action than regular human insulin. Unlike regular insulin that must be injected 30 to 60 minutes before a meal, recombinant insulin lispro is effective when injected 15 minutes before a meal. The analogue differs from natural human insulin, because the B-chain amino acids B28 proline and B29 lysine are exchanged. Insulin aspart (Novolog), which is homologous with human insulin except for the single amino acid substitution of aspartic acid for proline at B28, is effective when injected 5 to 10 minutes before a meal. Insulin glargine (Lantus) is the newest rDNA-derived human insulin analogue. An ultra-long-acting agent, insulin glargine differs from human insulin in that the amino acid asparagine at residue A21 is replaced by glycine, and two arginines are added to the C-terminus of the B chain. When administered subcutaneously, insulin glargine has a duration of action up to 24 to 48 hours. This change in action profile resulted from structural modifications that enhanced the products basicity, thus causing the product to precipitate at neutral pH postinjection and, therefore, increasing its duration of action.

Glucagon (Glucagen)

Like insulin, glucagon is a hormone normally biosynthesized as a high-molecular-mass protein from which the mature peptide hormone is released by selective proteolytic cleavage. The single-chain, 29-amino-acid polypeptide has an overall catabolic effect that tends to oppose the actions of insulin. Interestingly, the amino acid sequence of human, bovine, and porcine glucagon are identical. Glucagon of rDNA origin is now available (67). Replacing the bovine product with the rDNA-derived drug would eliminate the risk of acquiring bovine spongiform encephalopathy from glucagon therapy.

Growth Hormones

The introduction of rDNA human growth hormone (hGH) (70), previously isolated from cadaver pituitaries, greatly improved the long-term treatment of children who have growth failure caused by a lack of adequate endogenous hGH. The major, circulating form of human pituitary hGH is a globular protein of 191 amino acids in

Table 6.5. Commercially Available rDNA hGH

Drug	Trade Name	Chemical Nature
Somatrem	Protropin	hGH + N terminal methionone
Somatoprotin	GenoTropin	hGH
	Humatrope	hGH
	Norditropin	hGH
	Nutropin	hGH
	Nutropin Depot	hGH-long acting
	Saizen	hGH
	Serostim	hGH
Pegvisomant	Somavert	hGH + polyethylene glycol

a single polypeptide chain with a molecular weight of 22,000 daltons. Pituitary hGH is a roughly spherical protein with a hydrophobic interior. It is nonglycosylated. Degradation pathways of hGH include typical proteolysis reactions; deamidation of Asn and Gln residues; oxidation of Met, Trp, His, and Tyr residues; disulfide exchange; and aggregation.

Somatrem, first introduced in 1985, contains the identical 191-amino-acid sequence found in the pituitary-derived hGH plus the addition of a methionine amino acid at the N-terminus of the peptide chain (resulting in a 192-amino-acid protein; also known as Met-rhGH) (Table 6.5). Somatropin products contain the 191-amino-acid sequence identical to that of hGH of pituitary origin. Marketed somatropin products are shown in Table 6.5. Actions of rDNA-derived hGHs include an increase in the linear growth of the patient, increased skeletal growth, increased protein synthesis, reduction in body fat stores, and increased organ growth (Table 6.4). Clearance and bioavailability do not appear to be clinically or statistically different from those for somatrem and somatropin. Although the direct clinical comparison of the efficacy of the two forms of hGH have yet to be performed, separate controlled studies of growth hormone–deficient patients were similar. Recombinant hGHs are safe and effective therapies with relatively few side effects. A long-acting dosage form of somatotropin is approval for use in children with Prader-Willi syndrome, a rare genetic disorder that causes short stature; an involuntary, continuous urge to eat that is lifelong and may be life threatening; low muscle tone; and cognitive disorders. The formulation was designed to reduce the frequency of injections to once or twice a month by encapsulating the agent in biodegradable microspheres.

Gonadotropins—Follitropin Alpha (Gonal-F) and Follitropin Beta (Fillistim)

The gonadotropins are a family of protein hormones that include follicle-stimulating hormone (FSH) and primarily target their actions to the gonads. Follicle-stimulating hormone is synthesized and released by the pituitary gland. The hormone enhances spermatogenesis in males and stimulates follicular growth in females, and it is a 34-kDa glycoprotein (approximately 14% carbohydrate) containing two polypeptide subunits, an α- and a β-chain. Follitropin alpha and follitropin beta are human FSH preparations produced by rDNA technology (71). Gonadotropin preparations are used for infertility treatments in men and women. The production of rhFSH in a CHO cell line has proved to be particularly challenging. Follitropin alpha was the first heterodimeric glycoprotein to be produced by rDNA technology. Before the product of rDNA origin was available for infertility treatment, FSH was isolated from urine at less than 5% purity.

Thyrotropin

Thyroid-stimulating hormone (thyrotropin) is a glycoprotein (molecular weight, 28,000–30,000 daltons) secreted by the anterior lobe of the pituitary gland that is necessary for the growth and function of the thyroid. A recombinant thyrotropin α useful for the detection and treatment of cancer was approved by the U.S. FDA in November 1998.

Enzymes

Tissue-Type Plasminogen Activator

The fibrinolytic system is activated in response to the presence of an intracellular thrombus or clot. The process of clot dissolution is initiated by the conversion of plasminogen to plasmin. Plasminogen activation is catalyzed by two endogenous highly specific serine proteases, urokinase-type plasminogen activator and tissue-type plasminogen activator (t-PA) (see Chapter 31).

The mature human t-PA is a glycoprotein consisting of a single chain of 527 amino acids. Its molecular weight is approximately 70,000 daltons. Human t-PA contains 35 cysteines assigned to 17 disulfide bonds (Fig. 31.22). A serine protease domain of approximately 260 residues is located at the carboxy-terminal end of this protein. A fibronectin "finger" domain, two kringle domains, and an epidermal growth factor domain also are present. The t-PA protease domain is approximately 35 to 40% homologous with typical serine protease, such as bovine trypsin and chymotrypsin.

Mammalian cells produce two t-PA variants of N-linked glycosylation, type 1 (at asparagines 117, 184, and 448) and type 2 (only as asparagines 117 and 448). The rate of fibrin-dependent plasminogen activation is two- to threefold faster for type 2 compared with type 1. The cDNA obtained from a human melanoma cell line was expressed in CHO cells to achieve glycosylation and a protein identical to the natural protein. Protein engineering studies have produced variant t-PA molecules with modified pharmacokinetics, affinity for fibrin, catalytic activity, and side effects.

Three rDNA thrombolytic agents are approved in the United States (31,72-74) (Table 6.6 and Fig. 31.22). The first is alteplase, an enzyme equivalent to human t-PA. It is supplied as vials of a white to off-white, lyophilized powder for injection. The powder should be stored at a

Table 6.6. Commercially Available rDNA Tissue-Type Plasminogen Activators

Generic Name	Trade Name	Chemical Nature
Alteplase	Activase	Human t-PA (527 amino acids)
Reteplase	Retavase	Modified human t-PA (355 amino acids)
Tenecteplase	TNKase, TNK-tPA	Modified human t-PA (527 amino acids)

room temperature of 15 to 30°C or refrigerated at 2 to 8°C. The expiration date is 2 years after manufacture. Reconstituted solutions (diluent supplied) contain no preservatives and should be stored at 2 to 30°C for no more than 8 hours.

Alteplase is indicated for the treatment of acute myocardial infarction (administered as a bolus), acute massive pulmonary embolism (administered by intravenous infusion), and ischemic stroke (Table 6.4). The mechanism of action of t-PA is unlike that of streptokinase and urokinase. It is the first fibrin-selective thrombolytic agent preferentially activating fibrinogen bound to fibrin. Thus, the thrombolytic effect is localized to a blood clot and avoids systemic activation of fibrinogen, preventing bleeding elsewhere in the body. Plasma t-PA concentrations are proportional to the rate of infusion. Alteplase is rapidly cleared from circulating plasma, with 50% cleared within 5 minutes after termination of infusion. The mechanisms for clearance of t-PA from the blood are poorly understood. Detectable levels of antibody against alteplase have been found in patients receiving the drug, although 12 days to 10 months later, antibody determinations have been negative.

The second, reteplase, a recombinant, is a nonglycosylated deletion mutation of human t-PA containing 355 of 527 amino acids of native t-PA. The drug is indicated for acute myocardial infarction and is given as a 10 U + 10 U double bolus.

The most recent addition to the marketed rDNA-derived t-PAs is tenecteplase. This recombinant protein contains three modifications from natural human t-PA. In the kringle 1 domain of natural t-PA, threonine(T)103 replaced by arginine(R); the kringle 1 domain asparagine (N) 117 is replaced by glutamine(Q); and in the protease domain, four amino acids (lysine [K], histadine [H], and two arginines [R]) are replaced by four alanines (A). The drug is indicated for acute myocardial infarction. Bleeding at the injection site is similar to that with alteplase, but there is a reduction in the noncerebral bleeding complications. It is administered as a single, 5-second bolus.

DNase—Dornase Alpha (Pulmozyme)

According to the Cystic Fibrosis Foundation, cystic fibrosis (CF) is the most common fatal genetic disorder, afflicting approximately 30,000 patients, most of whom die before the age of 30 years. They develop thick mucous secretions and suffer from severe, frequent lung infections. Studies during the 1950s and 1960s determined that CF-related secretions in the lungs contained large amounts of DNA. Mucus-thickening DNA release resulted from an inflammatory response and ensuing white blood cell death. The enzyme DNase I specifically cleaves extracellular DNA, such as that found in the mucous secretion of CF patients, and has no effect on the DNA of intact cells. The U.S. FDA has approved a recombinant human DNase (75).

The enzyme DNase I is a glycoprotein containing 260 amino acids with an approximate molecular weight of 37,000 daltons. The recombinant protein is expressed by genetically engineered CHO cells encoding for the native enzyme, although DNase I was not purified or sequenced from human sources at the time. A degenerate sequence, based on the sequence of bovine DNase (263 amino acids), was used to synthesize probes and screen a human pancreatic DNA library. The primary amino acid sequence of rhDNase is identical to native human DNase I.

The only U.S. FDA–approved DNase product, Dornase alpha (inhalation solution), has been developed as a therapeutic agent for the management of CF. The product is supplied in single-use ampules delivering 2.5 ml of a sterile, clear, colorless solution containing 1.0 mg/ml of dornase alpha with no preservative. Administration is by nebulizer aerosol delivery systems.

Dornase alpha is indicated for daily administration in conjunction with standard CF therapies to reduce the frequency of respiratory infections requiring parental antibiotics to improve pulmonary function. The breakdown of DNA in infected sputum results in improved airflow in the lung and reduced risk of bacterial infection. The medicinal agent has been shown in clinical trials to have a positive effect on pulmonary function, which returned to baseline on stopping therapy. Although effective for the management of the respiratory symptoms of CF, dornase alpha is not a replacement for antibiotics, bronchodilators, and daily physical therapy. Two short-term studies have reported no adverse reactions. The agent also is in early clinical trials for the treatment of chronic bronchitis, a disease afflicting 400,000 patients in the United States alone.

Imiglucerase (Cerezyme)

Type 1 Gaucher disease, the most common form, is an inherited disorder. Fewer than 1 in 40,000 people in the general population have Gaucher disease. Patients with the disease lack the normal form of the enzyme glucocerebrosidase. They cannot break down glucocerebroside, causing a buildup of the compound within the lysosomes. This leads to the poor functioning of macrophages and an accumulation of "Gaucher cells" in the spleen, liver, and bone marrow. Some individuals experience few symptoms; others develop life-threatening

Table 6.7. The Five families of Cytokine Receptors and Some Ligands

Receptor Families	Ligands
Class I cytokine receptors	IL-2, IL-7, IL-9, IL-11, IL-13, IL-15, CM-CSF, G-CSF
Class II cytokine receptors	INF-α, INF-β, INF-γ
Tumor necrosis factor receptors	TNF-α, TNF-β, CD30, CD40, FAS
Chemokine receptors	IL-8, RANTES, MIP-1, PF-4, MCAF
Immunoglobin superfamily receptors	IL-1, M-CSF

conditions. Imiglucerase is an analogue of glucocerebrosidase produced by rDNA technology. The drug consists of 497 amino acids with four glycosylation sites and differs from the human placental glucocerebrosidase by one amino acid (His 495 replaces Arg). Imiglucerase cares out the normal function of the missing enzyme.

Cytokines

Cytokine is a generic term for the soluble protein molecules released by participating and interacting cells in the innate and adaptive immune systems. Cytokines communicate in a dynamic cellular network during an immune/inflammatory response to an antigen (75–78). Lymphokine and monokine are the terms used for a cytokine derived from lymphocytes and macrophages, respectively. Chemokines are a group of at least 25 structurally homologous, low-molecular-weight cytokines that stimulate leukocyte movement and regulate the migration of leukocytes from the blood to tissues. Cytokines, usually released and targeted to produce a localized effect, regulate the growth, differentiation, and activation of the hematopoietic cells responsible for the maintenance of the immune response. A wide array of glycoproteins, including interferons, interleukins, hematopoietic growth factors, and tumor necrosis factors, are cytokines. Cytokines can only act on target cells that express receptors for that cytokine. There are five families of cytokine receptor proteins: Class I cytokine receptors, Class II cytokine receptors, TNF receptors, chemokine receptors, and immunoglobulin superfamily receptors (Table 6.7). Cytokine research has entered an exciting growth phase fueled by genomics, cancer research, and a growing understanding of apoptosis. More than 100 human cytokines are being studied. Among the many reviews discussing the cytokines, several written for pharmacists or pharmaceutical scientists are excellent sources for a readable overview of the area (31,79–85).

Interferons

The interferons (31,80) are a family of cytokines discovered in the late 1950s with broad-spectrum antiviral and potential anticancer activity, making them biological response modifiers. Biotherapy (the therapeutic use of any substance of biological origin) of cancer is different than standard chemotherapy. That is, biotherapeutic agents belong to a group of compounds that enhance normal immune interactions (therefore, they also are immunomodulators) with cells in a specific or nonspecific fashion. Chemotherapeutics interact directly with the cancer cells themselves. Three types of naturally occurring interferons have been found in small quantities: leukocyte interferon (IFN-α), produced by lymphocytes and macrophages; fibroblast interferon (IFN-β), produced by fibroblasts, epithelial cells, and macrophages; and immune interferon (IFN-γ), synthesized by CD4+, CD8+, and natural killer lymphocytes. Both IFN-α and IFN-β, also known as type I interferons, exhibit approximately 30% primary sequence homology but no structural similarity to IFN-γ, a type II interferon. All three are glycoproteins. Previously only available in low yields by chemical synthesis or isolation, several rDNA interferon pharmaceuticals now have been marketed in the United States, including three IFN-α products, two IFN-β agents, and an IFN-γ drug (Table 6.4).

Interferon-α. At least 24 different human genes producing 16 distinct mature IFN-α molecules with slight structural variations are known (31,80,86). Human IFN-α proteins generally are composed of either 165 or 166 amino acids. The two primary subtype, IFN-α_{2a} and IFN-α_{2b}, both contain 165 amino acids, differing only at position 23, with IFN-α_{2a} containing a lysine group and IFN-α_{2b} an arginine group at this position. They have molecular weights of approximately 19,000 daltons. Although cultures of genetically modified *E. coli* produce two recombinant U.S. FDA-approved IFN-α products, IFN-α_{2a} and IFN-α_{2b}, their method of purification differs. Purification of IFN-α_{2a} includes affinity chromatography using a murine MAb, whereas that of IFN-α_{2b} does not.

Interferon-α_{2a} is commercially available as a sterile solution or a sterile, white-to-beige, lyophilized powder to reconstitute for subcutaneous or intramuscular injection (Table 6.8). Interferon-α_{2b} is available as a sterile, white-to-cream, lyophilized powder to reconstitute for subcutaneous or intramuscular injection and in combination with the antiviral ribavirin. Storage of the lyophilized powders or the reconstituted solutions should be at 2 to 8°C. As lyophilized powders, IFN-α_{2a} and IFN-α_{2b} have expiration dates of 36 and 24 months, respectively, after manufacture. Reconstituted solutions, if stored properly, are stable for up to 30 days. During the manufacture of the rDNA IFN-α products, human albumin is added to minimize adsorption to glass and plastic by these cytokines. Solutions, therefore, should not be shaken.

Interferon-α possesses complex antiviral, antineoplastic, and immunomodulating activities. Approved indications are shown in Table 6.4. Although the precise mechanism of action of IFN-α is not known, it is believed to interact with cell surface receptors to produce the biological effects. The actions appear to result from a complex cascade of biological modulation and pharmacologic

Table 6.8. Commercially Available rDNA Cytokines

Generic Name	Trade Name	Chemical Nature
Interferon-α_{2a}	Roferon-A	Human interferon (165 amino acids)
Interferon-α_{2b}	Intron A	Human interferon (165 amino acids)
Interferon alfacon-1	Infergen, CIFN	Modified interferon (166 amino acids)
Interferon-β_{1ba}	Avonex	Human interferon (165 amino acids)
Interferon-β_{1b}	Betaseron	Modified interferon (165 amino acids)
Interferon-γ_{1b}	Actimmune	Human interferon (140 amino acids)
Aldesleukin	Proleukin	Modified human IL-2 (132 amino acids)
Denileuin diftitox	Ontak	Modified IL + modified diphtheria toxin
Oprelvekin	Neumega	Modified IL-11 (177 amino acids)
Etanercept	Enbrel	Modified TNF + human IgG1

effects that include the modulation of host immune responses; cellular antiproliferative effects; cell differentiation, transcription, and translation processes; and reduction of oncogene expression.

Interferon-α is filtered through the glomeruli in the kidney and undergoes rapid proteolytic degradation during tubular reabsorption. Toxicity generally is dose- and time-dependent, with fever, fatigue, myalgia, chills, and anorexia (all flu-like symptoms) generally occurring within 2 to 8 hours after administration of high doses.

CONCENSUS INTERFERON. Hepatitis C infection results in a chronic disease state in 50 to 70% of cases and is now the most important known cause of chronic liver disease (87). Following the acute phase, as many as 80% of patients may progress to the chronic phase of the infectious disease. An estimated 20% of patients with a chronic form of the disease progress to cirrhosis. The only agents shown to be effective in the treatment of hepatitis C are the interferons. A unique recombinant molecule, a concensus interferon, known as interferon alfacon-1, has been approved for the treatment of chronic hepatitis C infection. It contains 166 amino acids in a relationship in which each amino acid position in the molecule contains the most commonly occurring amino acid among all the natural IFN-α subtypes. Interferon alfacon-1 exhibits 5- to 10-fold higher biological activity when compared to either IFN-α_{2a} or IFN-α_{2b}.

INTERFERON-β. Normally produced by fibroblasts, human IFN-β (31,80,86) (Table 6.8) was first cloned and expressed in 1980; however, its instability made it unsuitable for clinical use. The more stable recombinant IFN-β_{1b}, a 165-amino-acid analogue of human IFN-β, differs from the native protein with a serine residue substituted for cysteine at position 17. The highly purified product of biotechnology has a molecular weight of 18,500 daltons. It is produced in a recombinant *E. coli*. Approved in December 1993 by the U.S. FDA, IFN-β_{1b} is indicated for the treatment of patients with exacerbating-remitting multiple sclerosis (MS). The National MS Society says that 250,000 to 300,000 Americans have this disease, with more than 60% of patients falling into the exacerbating-remitting category. A vial of recombinant IFN-β_{1b} contains 0.3 mg of protein with dextrose and human albumin as stabilizers. The sterile, white, lyophilized powder is reconstituted without preservative for single-use subcutaneous injection every other day. Before and after reconstitution, the preparation should be refrigerated at 2 to 8°C. The refrigerated solution should be administered within 3 hours of reconstitution.

Results from a large, double-blind, placebo-controlled study have found that 8 million IU subcutaneously (the low-dose treatment group) of IFN-β every other day brought the most promising results, with a one-third reduction in exacerbations and a decrease by half in the frequency of severe attacks. Cranial magnetic resonance imaging showed that treated patients did not develop new lesions in the central nervous system and had less active lesions than patients treated with placebo. The exact mechanism of action of IFN-β_{1b} is not known. Its immunomodulating effects, however, may benefit patients with MS by decreasing the levels of endogenous IFN-γ. Levels of IFN-γ are believed to rise before and during acute attacks in patients with MS.

As observed with other interferons, flu-like symptoms are common on administration. During clinical trials, a suicide and four attempted suicides were reported. Depression and suicide also have been reported with patients receiving IFN-α.

Whereas IFN-β_{1b} of rDNA origin was the first to the market, IFN-β_{1a} also is now available. Interferon-β_{1a} is produced in mammalian cells and has the same amino acid sequence and carbohydrate side chain as natural IFN-β. Recombinant IFN-β_{1a} is administered to patients once weekly by intramuscular injection (30 μg). This differs from the subcutaneous administration every other day of rDNA-produced IFN-β_{1b}. Similar to pharmacotherapy with IFN-β_{1b}, the most common side effects of IFN-β_1 therapy include flu-like symptoms.

INTERFERON-γ. Human IFN-γ (31,80,86,88) is a single-chain glycoprotein with a molecular weight of approximately 15,500 daltons. The cytokine mainly exists as a noncovalent dimer of differentially glycosylated chains in solution in vivo. Glycosylation does not appear to be necessary for biological activity. The 140-amino-acid IFN-γ_{1b} is produced by fermentation of a recombinant *E. coli.* Approved in 1990 by the U.S. FDA (Table 6.8), IFN-γ_{1b} is supplied as a sterile solution containing 100 μg of the drug for subcutaneous injection. Vials must be placed in a refrigerator at 2 to 8°C and neither frozen nor shaken.

Interferon-γ_{1b} possesses biological activity identical to the natural human IFN-γ derived from lymphoid cells. Although all the interferons share certain biological effects, IFN-γ differs distinctly from IFN-α and IFN-β by its potent capacity to activate phagocytes involved in host defense. These activating effects include the ability to enhance the production of toxic oxygen metabolites within phagocytes, resulting in a more efficient killing of various microorganisms. This activity is the basis for the use of IFN-γ_{1b} in the management of chronic granulomatous disease. Chronic granulomatous disease is a group of rare X-linked or autosomal genetic disorders of the phagocytic oxygen metabolite–generating system, leaving patients susceptible to severe infections. The drug extends the time that patients spend without being hospitalized for infectious episodes. Investigational applications of IFN-γ include the treatment of renal cell carcinoma, small-cell lung cancer, infectious disease, trauma, atopic dermatitis, asthma, allergies, rheumatoid arthritis, and venereal warts. Adverse reactions are similar to those reported for IFN-α.

Interleukins

Interleukins are cytokines involved in immune cell communication. Synthesized by monocytes, macrophages, and lymphocytes, interleukins serve as soluble messengers between leukocytes. Currently, at least 18 interleukins have been observed. One of the most studied cytokines is interleukin (IL)-2, originally called T-cell growth because of to its ability to stimulate growth of T lymphocytes.

INTERLEUKIN-2. Human IL-2 is a 133-amino-acid, 15,400-dalton protein that is O-glycosylated at a threonine in position 3. An intramolecular disulfide bond between cysteine 58 and cysteine 105 is essential for biological activity. A recombinant version of IL-2 is marketed as aldesleukin (Table 6.8) (31,80,86,89–92). Aldesleukin differs from the native protein by the absence of glycosylation, a lack of the N-terminal alanine residue at position 1 (132 amino acids), and the replacement of cysteine with serine at position 125 of the primary sequence. Sequence changes were accomplished by site-directed mutagenesis to the IL-2 gene before cloning and expression. Aldesleukin exists as noncovalent microaggregates with an average size of 27 recombinant IL-2 molecules. The recombinant drug does possess the biological activity of the native protein.

Aldesleukin is supplied as a lyophilized formulation of protein admixed with mannitol to provide bulk in the vial. Sodium dodecyl sulfate is present to ensure sufficient water solubility on reconstitution. The drug is administered as an intravenous infusion. Handling and storage considerations for aldesleukin are consistent with those of other cytokines. Recombinant IL-2 should be administered within 48 hours after reconstitution.

Aldesleukin is used in cancer biotherapy (i.e., the therapeutic use of any substance of biological origin) as a biological response modifier for the treatment of metastatic renal cell carcinoma and metastatic melanoma. Aldesleukin also recently has been studied in the management of HIV infection. Although the exact mechanism of action is not established, IL-2 is known to bind to an IL-2 receptor that has been well studied. In vitro, IL-2 induces killer cell activity, enhances lymphocyte mitogenesis and cytotoxicity, and induces IFN-γ production. The extent of its antitumor effect is directly proportional to the amount of IL-2 administered. Side effects are the major dose-limiting factor, because aldesleukin is an extremely toxic drug. The manufacturer's labeling should be consulted for full details. Careful patient selection and thorough patient monitoring are essential. The incidence of nonneutralizing anti-IL-2 antibodies in patients treated on an every-8-hour regimen is quite high (76% in one clinical study).

INTERLEUKIN-2 FUSION PROTEIN. Using ligation chemistry approaches during the preparation of recombinant proteins, researchers have created biologically active molecules that combine the activities of two individual proteins into "fusion molecules." These fusion technologies hold promise for developing custom molecules expressing a wide variety of dual activities. The U.S. FDA has approved the fusion protein denileukin diftitox for the treatment of patients with persistent or recurrent cutaneous T-cell lymphoma (CTCL) whose malignant cells express the CD25 component of the IL-2 receptor (93–95). Cutaneous T-cell lymphoma is a general term for a group of low-grade, non-Hodgkin's lymphomas affecting approximately 1,000 new patients/year. Malignant T cells manifest initially in the skin. Over time, there is systemic involvement. For many patients, CTCL is a persistent, disfiguring, and debilitating disease that requires multiple treatments. Malignant CTCL cells express one or more of the components of the IL-2 receptor. Thus, the IL-2 receptor may be a homing device to attract a "killer drug."

Denileukin diftitox is a rDNA-derived, cytotoxic IL-2 fusion protein that contains the first 389 amino acids of diphtheria toxin fused to amino acid residues 2 to 133 of human IL-2 (the IL-2 residues replace the amino acids of the receptor-binding domain of native diphtheria toxin). Thus, the biotech drug targets IL-2 receptors, and brings the diphtheria toxin directly to kill the CTCL target. Studies have shown that 30% of patients treated with this therapeutic fusion protein experience at least 50% reduction of tumor burden that is sustained for at least 6 weeks.

INTERLEUKIN-11. Interleukin-11 is a thrombopoietic growth factor that directly stimulates the proliferation of hematopoietic stem cells and megakaryocyte progenitor cells (96). This induces megakaryocyte maturation, resulting in increased platelet production. Interleukin-11 is a 178-amino-acid glycosylated cytokine produced by bone marrow stromal cells. Primary osteoblasts and mature osteoclasts express mRNAs for an IL-11 receptor (IL-11Rα). Thus, bone-forming cells and bone-resorbing cells are potential targets of IL-11. In 1997, the U.S. FDA approved an rDNA-derived version of IL-11 produced in *E. coli.* Oprelvekin (Table 6.8) contains only 177 amino acids, lacking the amino terminal proline of the native IL-11. Produced in *E. coli,* the cytokine analogue is nonglycosylated. Oprelvekin has potent thrombopoietic activity in animal models of compromised hematopoiesis. It is indicated for the prevention of thrombocytopenia following myelosuppressive chemotherapy. Pharmacists should monitor for possible fluid retention and electrolyte states when it is used with chronic diuretic therapy.

Tumor Necrosis Factor

Tumor necrosis factors (TNFs), a family of cytokines produced mainly by activated mononuclear phagocytes, have both beneficial and potentially harmful effects, mediating cytotoxic and inflammatory reactions (31). The TNFs are endogenous pyrogens capable of inducing chills, fever, and other flu-like symptoms. Tumor necrosis factor-α, also called cachectin (and commonly referred to as TNF), and TNF-β, also called lymphotoxin, both bind to the same receptor and induce similar biological activities. Biological effects of TNF-α include selective toxicity against a range of tumor cells, mediation of septic shock, activation of elements of the immune system in response to Gram-negative bacteria, and induction/regulation of inflammation. The TNF-α of rDNA origin has been studied extensively, but it has not been developed into a useful drug.

Etanercept is a rDNA-produced fusion protein that binds specifically to TNF and blocks its interaction with cell surface TNF receptors (97,98). It is indicated for the treatment of moderate to severe active rheumatoid arthritis in adults and for juvenile rheumatoid arthritis in patients who have had an inadequate response to one or more disease-modifying antirheumatic drugs. It is a genetically engineered protein that includes two components. The extracellular, ligand-binding portion (p75) of the human TNF receptor is linked as a fusion protein to the Fc portion of the human IgG1 antibody. Each etanercept molecule binds specifically to two TNF molecules found in the synovial fluid of patients with rheumatoid arthritis, blocking the interaction of TNF with the TNF receptor. The drug inhibits both TNF-α and TNF-β. The Fc portion of the fusion protein helps to clear the etanercept-TNF complex from the body.

Hematopoietic Growth Factors

Hematopoiesis is the complex series of events involved in the formation, proliferation, differentiation, and activation of red blood cells, white blood cells, and platelets. Hematopoietic growth factors are cytokines that regulate these events (31,99–102). Investigators have identified and cloned at least 20 factors, including IL-3 (or multi-CSF), IL-4, IL-5, IL-6, IL-7, erythropoietin (EPO), granulocyte-macrophage colony-stimulating factor (GM-CSF), granulocyte colony-stimulating factor (G-CSF), macrophage colony-stimulating factor (M-CSF), and stem cell factor. Figure 6.27 summarizes the elaborate hematopoietic cascade. All blood cells originate within the bone marrow from a single class of pluripotent stem cells. In response to various external and internal stimuli, regulated by hematopoietic growth factors, stem cells give rise to additional new stem cells (self-renewal) and differentiate into mature, specialized blood cells.

Erythropoietin–Epoetin Alpha (Epogen, Procrit)

Erythropoietin (31,99,103–107), a glycoprotein with a molecular weight of 30,000 to 34,000 dalton produced by the kidney, stimulates the division and differentiation of erythroid progenitors in the bone marrow, increasing the production of red blood cells. Epoetin alpha (sometimes called rHuEPO-α), a recombinant EPO prepared from cultures of genetically engineered mammalian CHO cells, consists of the identical 165 amino acid sequence of endogenous EPO. The molecular weight is approximately 30,400 daltons. The protein contains two disulfide bonds (linking cysteine 7 with 161 and 29 with 33) and four sites of glycosylation (one O-site and three N-sites); the disulfide bonds and glycosylation are necessary for the hormone's biological activity. Deglycosylated natural EPO or bacterial-derived EPO (without glycosylation) have greatly decreased in vivo activity, although in vitro activity is largely conserved. The sugars may play a role in thermal stability or the prevention of aggregation in vivo.

The marketed products are formulated as a sterile, colorless, preservative-free liquid for intravenous or subcutaneous administration. The vial should not be shaken, or the glycoprotein may become denatured, rendering it inactive. Epoetin alpha is indicated for the treatment of various anemias. Several of the conditions are listed in Table 6.4. Epoetin alpha represents a major scientific advance in the treatment of patients with chronic renal failure, serving as a replacement therapy for inadequate production of endogenous EPO by failing kidneys. Epoetin alpha may decrease the need for infusions in dialysis patients. By several mechanisms related to elevating the erythroid progenitor cell pool, epoetin alpha increases the production of red blood cells.

The manufacturer's full prescribing information should be consulted for dosing regimens, because the dose is titrated individually to maintain the patient's target hematocrit. The circulating half-life is 4 to 13 hours in patients with chronic renal failure. Peak serum levels are achieved within 5 to 24 hours following subcutaneous administration.

Colony-Stimulating Factors

The CSFs are glycoprotein cytokines that promote progenitor proliferation, differentiation, and some functional

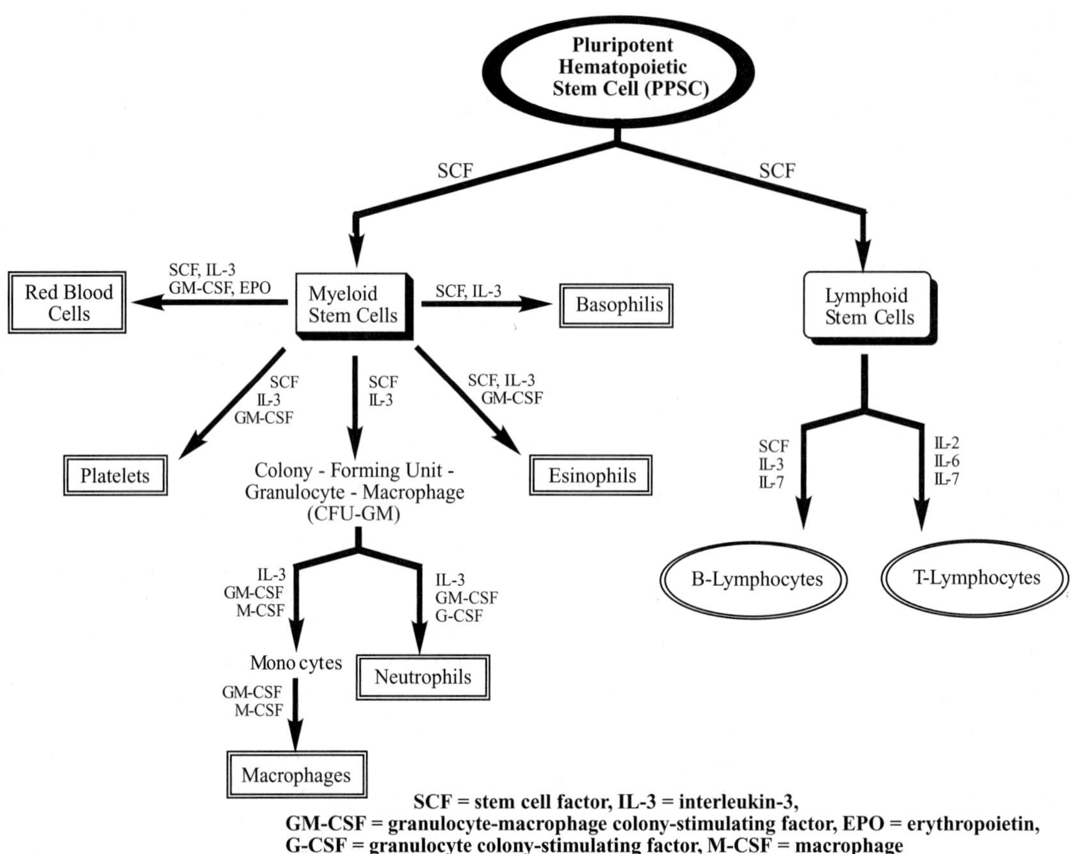

Fig. 6.27. Schematic overview of hematopoiesis.

activation. The name "colony-stimulating factor" results from the fact that these proteins often are assayed by their ability to stimulate the formation of cell colonies in bone marrow cultures. The names added to "CSF" reflect the types of cell colonies that arise in these assays.

GRANULOCYTE COLONY-STIMULATING FACTOR—FILGRATION (NEUPROGEN). Recombinant DNA–derived G-CSF (31,99,108–112), or filgrastim, was approved by the U.S. FDA in 1991 to decrease the incidence of infection in patients with nonmyeloid malignancies who are receiving myelosuppressive anticancer drugs. Additional indications are shown in Table 6.4. Filgrastim is a 175-amino-acid, single-chain protein with a molecular weight of 18,800 daltons. Filgrastim, produced by a recombinant bacteria, differs from the endogenous human protein by the addition of a methionine at the N-terminus (recombinant methionyl G-CSF is sometimes called r-metHuG-CSF) and the lack of glycosylation. Glycosylation, however, does not appear to be necessary for the biological activity.

Filgrastim injectable solution should be refrigerated at 2 to 8°C and is packaged with a patented indicator that turns red at temperatures below –4°C. The vials should never be shaken before the dose is withdrawn (contains human albumin). Administration is by intravenous infusion or by subcutaneous injection or infusion. The drug is rapidly absorbed, with perk serum concentrations in 4 to 5 hours. Elimination half-life is approximately 3.5 hours.

Filgrastim is lineage selective for the neutrophil lineage type of white blood cells, whereas GM-CSF is multilineage, stimulating progenitors of neutrophils, monocytes, basophils, and eosinophils. The drug reduces the period of neutropenia, the number of infections, and the number of days the patient is on antibiotics. Filgrastim generally is well tolerated, with medullary bone pain being the most frequently encountered side effect.

GRANULOCYTE-MACROPHAGE COLONY-STIMULATING FACTOR—SARGRAMOSTIM (LEUKINE). The GM-CSF (31,99,108–112) has been produced by rDNA technology in the yeast *S. cerevisiae*. Sargramostim is a glycoprotein of 127 amino acids, differing from the endogenous human GM-CSF by substituting leucine at position 23. Also, the glycosylation pattern may differ from that of the native protein.

Sargramostim is supplied in vials of lyophilized powder (with mannitol) for intravenous infusion. Reconstituted with 1 ml of Sterile Water for Injection, USP (without preservative), the drug should be administered within 6 hours. Vials are intended for single use only. The powder, reconstituted solution, and diluted solution require refrigeration at 2 to 8°C without being frozen or shaken.

Sargramostim's indications are shown in Table 6.4. Cellular division, maturation, and activation are induced through the binding of GM-CSF to specific receptors expressed on the surface of target cells. On 2-hour intravenous infusion, the alpha half-life is 12 to 17 minutes, followed by a slower decrease (beta half-life) of 2 hours. The manufacturer's label should be consulted for precautions. Additional indications for GM-CSF under study are as an adjuvant to chemotherapy and an adjuvant to AIDS therapy.

Other Growth Factors

Growth factors are cytokines responsible for regulating cell proliferation, differentiation, and function (31). They act as intercellular signals. Each cell type's response is specific for each particular growth factor and differs from growth factor to growth factor. Platelet-derived growth factor (PDGF) is an endogenous growth-promoting protein that is released from cells involved in the healing process and is evident at the cell proliferation stage of a healing open wound. A recombinant human PDGF B homodimer has been produced from genetically engineered *S. cerevisiae* cells (113). Becaplermin is the B-chain of the PDGF B protein. Thus, becaplermin also is referred to as rhPDGF-BB. The 25-kDa protein is formulated into a gel that mimics natural PDGF when applied to diabetic foot ulcers.

Clotting Factor VIII, Factor IX. and Anticoagulants

Antihemophiliac factor, or factor VIII, is required for the transformation of prothrombin (factor II) to thrombin by the intrinsic clotting pathway (31,74,114). Hemophilia A, a lifelong bleeding disorder, results from a deficiency of factor VIII. Conventional biotherapy for the treatment of hemophilia A includes protein concentrates from human plasma collected by transfusion services or commercial organizations. Therefore, the concentrates may contain other native human proteins and microorganisms, such as viruses (e.g., HIV and hepatitis), derived from infected blood. Four versions of recombinant factor VIII (antihemophiliac factor), highly purified, microorganism-free proteins are now available. All four therapeutic proteins are produced by the insertion of cDNA encoding for the entire factor VIII protein into mammalian cells. The mature, heavily glycosylated protein is composed of 2,332 amino acids (1–2 million daltons) and contains sulfate groups. Stability of the large protein is a concern. The products have proved to be safe and effective for reducing bleeding time in patients. There is the possibility, however, of induction of inhibitors in previously untreated patients.

Hemophilia B results when a patient is deficient in specific clotting factor IX (31). It affects males primarily and makes up approximately 15% of all hemophilia cases. A recombinant human factor IX is now available.

Surgeons have used medicinal leeches (*Hirudo medicinalis)* for years to prevent thrombosis in fine vessels of reattached digits. Hirudin is the potent, specific thrombin inhibitor isolated from the leech. Lepirudin is a rDNA-derived (recombinant yeast) polypeptide that differs from the natural polypeptide, having a terminal leucine instead of isoleucine and missing the sulfate group at Tyr 63 (115).

Vaccines

There are two types of immunization: active immunization, and passive immunization. Active immunization is the induction of an immune response either through exposure to an infectious agent or by deliberate immunization with a vaccine (vaccination) made from the microorganism or its products to develop protective immunity. Passive immunization involves the transfer of products produced by an immune animal or human (preformed antibody or sensitized lymphoid cells) to a previously nonimmune recipient host, usually by injection. Sufficient active immunity may take days, several weeks, or even months to induce (possibly including booster vaccinations), but it generally is long-lasting (even lifelong) through the clonal selection of genetically specific immunological memory B and T lymphocytes. Passive immunity, although often providing effective protection against some infection, is relatively brief, lasting only until the injected immunoglobulin or lymphoid cells have disappeared (a few weeks or months). Thus, vaccines enable the body to resist infection by diseases. In response to an injection of vaccine, the immune system makes antibodies, which recognize surface antigens found in the vaccine. If the subject is later exposed to a virulent form of the virus, the immune system is primed and ready to eliminate it. Many viral vaccines are produced from the antigens isolated from pooled human plasma of virus carriers. Vaccinations are among the most cost-effective and widely used public health interventions. Although generally safe, the minimal risk of vaccine-produced infections can be eliminated by administration of highly purified vaccine antigens of recombinant origin (31,115–117).

Two hepatitis B vaccines, Recombivax HB and Engerix-B, were marketed in 1986 and 1989 respectively. Both are derived from a hepatitis B surface antigen and are produced in yeast cells. The primary difference between the two appears to be in exact dosing regimens. The immunization regimen consists of three injections: initial, at 1 month, and at 6 months. The immune response and clinical reactions for both intramuscular and subcutaneous administration are comparable. Vials containing the vaccine in solution should be stored at 2 to 8°C; freezing destroys potency.

There also is a marketed Lyme disease vaccine containing recombinant OspA (31,115,116). The vaccine is a sterile suspension of a noninfectious recombinant vaccine containing an immunodominant outer surface protein of *Borrelia burgdorferi* known as lipoprotein OspA. The antigen is adsorbed onto aluminum hydroxide as an adjuvant. Vaccine efficacy against definite Lyme disease is 78% after three doses.

MONOCLONAL ANTIBODIES

Introduction to Antibodies

The human immune system is composed of two major branches or arms: the cell-mediated immune system, which includes macrophages, lymphocytes, and granulocytes, and the humoral immune system, which includes the antibody-secreting B cells or plasma cells (76–78). In contrast to the cell-mediated nature of the immune actions carried out by most lymphocytes, antibodies or immunoglobulins are soluble proteins that are produced in response to an antigenic stimulus. As part of the normal immune system, each B cell produces as many as 100 million antibody proteins (polyclonal antibodies) directed against bacteria, viruses, and other foreign invaders. Antibodies act by binding to a particular antigen, thereby "tagging" it for removal or destruction by other immune system components.

The production of antigen-"neutralizing" antibodies or immunoglobulins and the detection of a sufficient antibody titer are important concepts for an understanding of vaccinations and exposure to antigens. The humoral response to an antigen involves the creation of memory B cells and the transformation of B lymphocyte into plasma cells that serve as factories for the production of secreted antibodies. Approximately 4 days after initial contact with an antigen (immunization), IgM antibodies (one of five types of immunoglobulin structure) appear and then peak approximately 4 hours later. Approximately 7 days after exposure, IgG, the major class of circulating immunoglobulin, appears. The antibodies bind to the antigen and effect additional immune system-mediated events, "neutralizing" the antigen and leading to its elimination. The concentration of an immunoglobulin specific for a given antigen at a given time is referred to as the antibody titer and may be a measure of the effectiveness of the initial antigen exposure/vaccination to illicit immunologic memory

Antibody Structure

Antibodies are glycoproteins. The simplest structure of an immunoglobulin molecule consists of two identical long peptide chains (the heavy chains) and two identical short polypeptide chains (the light chains) interconnected by several disulfide bonds. The selectivity of any immunoglobulin for a particular antigen is determined by its structure and, specifically, by the variable or antigen-binding regions (Fig. 6.28). Enzymatic digestion of the antibody with papain yields the Fab fragment, which contains the antigen-binding sites, and the Fc fragment, which specifies the other biological activities of the molecule.

Hybridoma Technology

Monoclonal antibodies are ultrasensitive, hybrid immune system–derived proteins designed to recognize specific antigens. Nobel Laureates Kohler and Milstein first reported MAbs in 1975 (118). Monoclonal antibodies have been used in laboratory diagnostics, site-directed drugs, and home test kits (80,116,119–122). The B lymphocyte produces a wide range of structurally diverse antibody proteins with varying degrees of specificity in response to a single antigen stimulus. Because of their structural diversity, these antibodies would be called polyclonal antibodies. Monoclonal antibodies are homogeneous hybrid proteins produced by a selected, single clone of an engineered B lymphocyte. They are designed to recognize specific sites or epitopes on antigens.

Hybridoma technology (the technology used to produce MAbs) consists of combining or fusing two different cell lines: a myeloma cell (generally from a mouse) and a

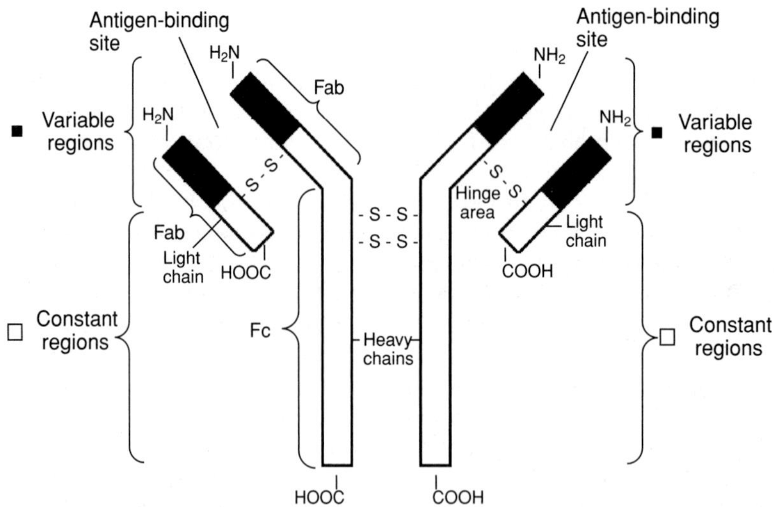

Fig. 6.28. Schematic model of an antibody molecule.

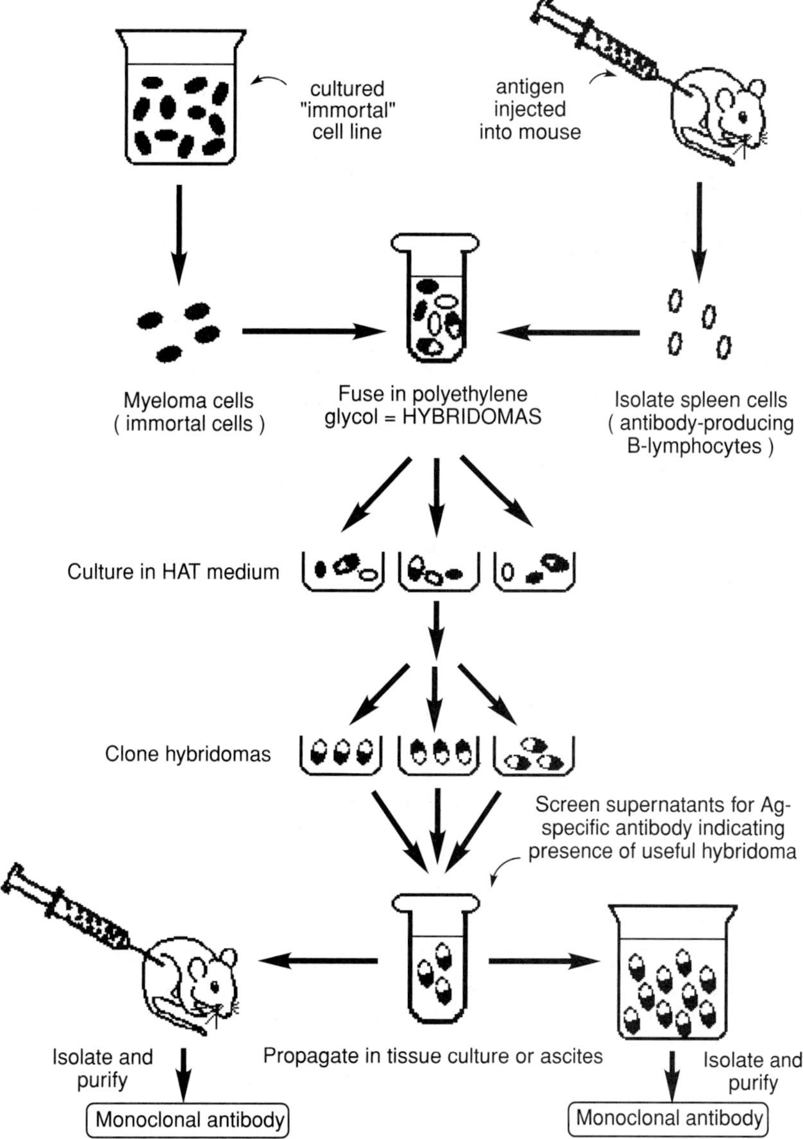

Fig. 6.29. Outline of hybridoma creation and monoclonal antibody (MAb) production.

plasma spleen cell (B lymphocyte) capable of producing an antibody that recognizes a specific antigen (Fig. 6.29). The resulting fused cell, or hybridoma, possesses some of the characteristics of both original cells: the myeloma cell's ability to survive and reproduce in culture (immortality), and the plasma spleen cell's ability to produce antibodies to a specific antigen.

Two myeloma variant cell lines with defects in nucleotide synthesis pathways are commonly used as fusion partners (80,119,120,123,124). One lacks the *HGPRT* gene coding for an essential enzyme in purine biosynthesis. The other lacks the *Tk* gene coding for a pyrimidine biosynthetic enzyme. Following fusion, the cells are cultured in a medium containing hypoxanthine, aminopterin, and thymidine (HAT medium). Correct hybridomas (one myeloma plus one spleen cell), although missing the gene from the myeloma partner, possess the gene from its spleen cell partner. Fused myeloma hybrids do not survive, because they lack the essential gene. Fused spleen cell hybrids do not grow in culture. Hybridomas, however, can be grown in large quantities, and clones producing antibodies with the appropriate specificity for the original antigen can be isolated from culture. Various techniques have been developed to select the single hybridoma clone producing the desired antibody (thus, MAb). Hybridomas are grown in in vitro cell culture or in vivo in mouse (murine) ascites to yield large amounts of MAbs (1–100 μg/mL in culture and 1 mg/mL in ascites).

Monoclonal antibodies are more attractive than polyclonal antibodies for diagnostic and therapeutic applications because of their increased specificity of antigen recognition. Thus, they can serve as target-directed "homing devices" to find and attach to the targeted antigen. Developments in hybridoma technology have led to highly specific diagnostic agents for home use in pregnancy testing and ovulation prediction kits; laboratory use in detection of colorectal cancer, ovarian cancer, and others; and design of site-directed therapeutic agents, such as trastuzumab to combat metastatic breast cancer and abciximab as an adjunct for the prevention of cardiac ischemic complications.

Monoclonal Antibody Immunogenicity

Nearly 25 years after the pioneering work of Kohler and Milstein, MAbs began to realize their therapeutic potential. Until recently, most MAbs were murine proteins based on their production. Initial clinical trials of murine MAbs showed that these mouse proteins were highly immunogenic in patients after just a single dose (125–127). Human patients formed antibodies to combat the foreign MAb that was administered. The human anti-mouse antibody response is known as HAMA. So, far from being the "magic bullets" that were proposed, immunogenic murine MAbs were useless in chronic therapy. Thus, a different approach was needed to eliminate the unwanted immune response (HAMA) in patients.

The variable regions of an immunoglobulin must be of a specific chemical structure with the ability to bind to the antigen they "recognize." The part within the variable region that forms the intermolecular interactions with the antigen is the complementarity-determining region (CDR). The variable domains of antibody light and heavy chains each contain three CDRs.

It was determined that immune responses against the mouse-produced MAbs were directed against both the variable and the constant regions of the antibody. Human and murine antibodies are very homologous in chemical structure. Thus, an MAb should be engineered to decrease the immunogenicity of an MAb by replacing the mouse constant regions of an IgG with human constant regions, making the antibody less mouse-like (119,128–132). In practice, what generally occurs is the variable heavy-chain and variable light-chain domains (CDRs) of human immunoglobulins are replaced with those of a murine antibody, which possesses the requisite antigen specificity. This "chimeric" MAb will retain its ability to recognize the antigen (a property of the murine MAb), retain the many effector functions of an immunoglobulin (both murine and human), but be much less immunogenic (a property of a human immunoglobulin). A chimeric MAb, containing approximately 70% human sequence, will have a longer half-life than its murine counterpart in a human patient. Therapeutic MAbs that are chimeric include abciximab, ritiximab, infliximab, and basiliximab.

The discovery of the conserved structure of antibodies, particular IgGs, across many species suggested the possibility of chimeric antibodies, and the realization that the homology extended to the antigen-binding site facilitated the engineering of humanized immunoglobulins. Advances in phage display technology and the production of transgenic animals has lead to the production of humanized or fully human MAbs (119,129–132). Functional human antibody fragments (e.g., Fab fragments) can be displayed on the surface of bacteriophages. A bacteriophage, also called a phage, is a virus that infects bacteria. The expression of these human antibody fragments on the phage surface has facilitated efficient screening of large numbers of phage clones (phage display) for antigen-binding specificity (133). Once a fragment with the requisite antigen specificity is selected, it can be isolated and engineered into a humanized MAb (replacing up to 95% of the murine protein sequence) or a fully human MAb (100% human sequence). Transgenic strains of mice have been genetically engineered to possess most or all of the essential human antibody genes. Thus, on immunization with a foreign antigen, the transgenic mice will develop humanized or fully human antibodies in response. Both of these techniques, although very complex and expensive, have yielded U.S. FDA–approved, humanized antibody pharmaceuticals, such as daclizumab, palivuzumab, and trastuzumab. The half-life of humanized antibodies is dramatically enhanced (from hours to weeks), and immunogenicity is drastically reduced.

Monoclonal Antibody Therapeutic Agents

Hybridoma technology and advanced antibody engineering has led to the design of an increasing number of site-directed therapeutic agents for the treatment and prevention of transplant rejection, therapy in rheumatoid arthritis, treatment of non-Hodgkin's lymphoma, and other indications. These products (Table 6.9) are examples of murine, chimeric, and humanized MAbs, and they represent significant advances in pharmacotherapy.

Monoclonal Antibody Diagnostic Agents

Several ultrasensitive diagnostic MAb-based products have enjoyed great success; these include a variety of imaging agents for the detection of blood clots and cancer cells. A monoclonal Fab fragment, technetium-99m-arcitumomab (CEA-Scan), can detect the presence and indicate the location of recurrent and metastatic colorectal cancer. Colorectal cancer and ovarian cancer can be detected with satumomab pendetide (OncoScint CR/OV). Capromab pentetate (ProstaScint) is used for detection, staging, and follow-up of patients with prostate adenocarcinoma. Small-cell lung cancer can be detected with nofetumomab (Verluma). The first imaging MAb for myocardial infarction is imiciromab pentetrate (MyoScint). Pharmaceutical Research Manufacturing of America (PhRMA) reports that 59 of the 369 biotechnology agents in testing are MAb-based products, and most are diagnostics.

Table 6.9. Some U.S. Food and Drug Administration–Approved MAb Therapeutic Agents

Generic Name	Trade Name	MAb Type	Indication
Trastuzumab	Herceptin	Humanized	Refractory breast cancer
Muromonab-CD3	Orthoclone-OKT3	Murine	Reversal of transplant rejection
Infliximab	Remicade	Chimeric	Crohn's disease
Abciximab	ReoPro	Chimeric	Adjunct to PTCA for prevention of acute cardiac complications
Ritiximab	Rituxan	Chimeric	Treatment of B-cell non-Hodgkin's lymphoma
Basiliximab	Simulect	Chimeric	Prevention of transplant rejection
Daclizumab	Zenapax	Humanized	Prevention of transplant rejection
Palivizumab	Synagis	Humanized	Respiratory syncytial virus prophylaxis
Gemtuzumab	Mylotarg	Fusion MAb	Treatment of CD33-positive cute myeloid leukemia
Alemtuzumab	Campath	Humanized	B-cell chronic lymphocytic leukemia
Adalimumab	Humira	Fully human	Rheumatoid arthritis
Omalizzumab	Xolair	Humanized	Asthma
Tositumomab	Bexxar	Murine	Non-Hodgkin's lymphoma
Efalizumab	Raptiva	Humanized	Psoriasis
Bevacizumab	Avastin	Humanized	Colorectal cancer
Cetuximab	Erbitux	Chimeric	Colorectal cancer
Natalizumab	Tysabri	Humanized	Multiple sclerosis

Monoclonal Antibody–Based, In-Home Diagnostic Kits

The strong trend toward self-care, coupled with a heightened awareness by the public of available technology and an emphasis on preventive medicine, has increased the use of in-home diagnostics (134–136). Sales of in-home diagnostics were predicted to exceed $3.7 billion by 2006. Monoclonal antibody specifically minimizes the possibilities of interference from other substances that might yield false-positive test results. The antigen being selectively detected by MAb-based pregnancy test kits is human chorionic gonadotropin, the hormone produced if fertilization occurs and that continues to increase in concentration during the pregnancy. Table 6.10 lists some examples of MAb-containing in-home pregnancy test kits. Luteinizing hormone in the urine is the antigen detected by MAb ovulation prediction in-home test kits. These test kits can help to determine when a woman is most fertile, because ovulation occurs 20 to 48 hours after the luteinizing hormone surge. Table 6.10 also provides some examples of MAb-based, in-home ovulation prediction kits.

Table 6.10. Some MAb-Based In-home Test Kits[a]

Manufacturer	Product Distributor	Positive End Point
Pregnancy		
Answer Plus	Carter Products	Plus in test window = +
Answer Quick & Simple	Carter Products	Plus in test window = +
Clear Blue Easy	Unipath	Blue line in large window = +
Clear Blue Easy One Min.	Unipath	Blue line in large window = +
Conceive	Quidel	Pink to purple test line = +
1 Step E.P.T.	Warner Lambert	Pink color in test and control = +
Fact Plus One Step	Advanced Care	Pink plus sign in window = +
Fact Plus	Advanced Care	Pink plus sign in window = +
First Response 1 Step	Carter Products	Two pink lines in window = +
Fortel Plus	Biomerica	Purple stick line darker than reference = +
One Step Fortel Early	Biomerica	Purple stick line darker than reference = +
Q Test	Quidel	Blue control line and pink plus sign = +
Ovulation		
Answer Quick & Simple	Carter Products	Purple stick line darker than reference = +
Conceive 1 Step	Quidel	Pink to purple test line darker than reference = +
First Response 1 Step	Carter Products	Purple test line darker than reference = +
ClearPlan Easy	Unipath	Blue test line in large window similar or darker than line in small window = +
Ovukit Self Test	Quidel	White to shades of blue compared to LH surge guide = +
OvuQuick	Quidel	Test spot appears darker than reference = +
Q Test	Quidel	Purple test line darker than reference = +

[a]Information from Pray W. Nonprescription Product Therapeutics, 2nd Ed. Philadelphia: Lippincott Williams & Wilkins, 2006:778–780; Quattrocchi E, Hove I. Ovulation & pregnancy home testing products. U.S. Pharmacist 1998;23:54–63; and Rosenthal WM, Briggs GC. Home testing and monitoring devices. In: Allen LV Jr., Berardi RR, DeSimone EM II, et al., eds. Handbook of Nonprescription Drugs. Washington, DC: American Pharmaceutical Association, 2000:917–942.

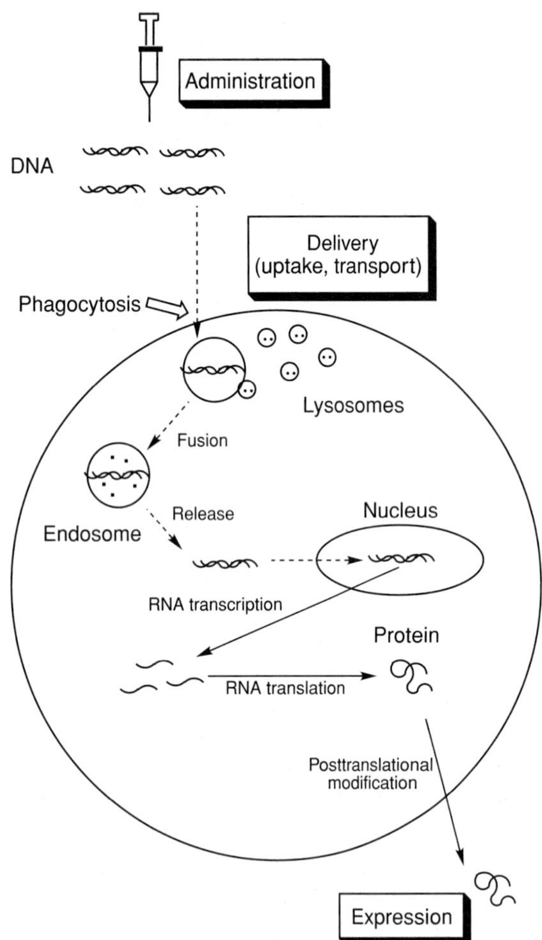

Fig. 6.30. Steps in gene therapy: administration, delivery, and expression. Dashed arrow represents uptake and transport.

GENE THERAPY

The premise of gene therapy is that genes can be used as pharmaceutical products to cause in vivo production of therapeutic proteins. There is considerable confidence that gene therapy, as a therapeutic paradigm, will provide a number of novel pharmaceutical products, diagnostics, and therapeutic approaches in the next decade (137).

A major problem in gene therapy is similar to the problem encountered in all forms of drug therapy, that being the assurance of drug efficacy through efficient delivery of the therapeutic agent to its biological target in a fully functional form (138). Gene delivery is unique in the sense that it is the product of gene function, the protein, and not the gene itself that is the therapeutic agent. Hence, we must not only deliver the gene to its proper target but also assure that when the gene reaches its target, it will arrive in a form that will produce the therapeutic agent in such a form that it, too, will be assured of reaching its specified target. What is most critical in gene delivery is the effective modulation of the production of the therapeutic protein. Constitutive expression of some proteins may occur without adversely affecting the therapeutic efficacy. Constitutive expression of most genes is not desirable, however, and can even be life-threatening. The proper, controlled delivery of the protein necessitates the previous delivery of the gene to the cell nucleus, and this special consideration for gene delivery compared to conventional drugs warrants the development of novel vehicles for the delivery of genes to the cell nucleus. Most gene therapy protocols involve the use of viruses as gene carriers or vectors; however, there also are nonviral methods of gene delivery appearing in the National Institutes of Health-approved gene therapy protocols. In both cases, the steps involved in the delivery of the therapeutic agent include the following (Fig. 6.30) (139):

1. **Administration** or introduction of the nucleic acid (DNA) into the body, which usually involves either in vivo or in vitro (ex vivo) techniques.
2. **Delivery** of the nucleic acid from the site of administration to the nucleus, which includes directing the bioavailability, uptake of the nucleic acid (DNA) into the cell, and translocation of the nucleic acid from the cytosol to the nucleus.
3. **Expression** of the nucleic acid product, including the normal steps in gene expression (transcription, translation, and posttranslational modification). Expression is vital to the therapeutic efficacy of the gene in the sense that controlled expression of genes is important for proper biological function. Current delivery technologies result in continuous gene expression.

The viral and nonviral vectors approach the problem of nucleic acid delivery from opposite directions. Viral vectors are reduced in complexity to make them less immunogenic yet maintain the efficient delivery properties, whereas nonviral vectors are altered to increase the complexity of their delivery systems to improve the specificity and efficiency of nucleic acid delivery. It is likely that the ideal vector will be a composite of viral and nonviral delivery vehicles. Some of the properties that might be features of the ideal delivery vector include:

1. No limit in the size of the gene that can be incorporated into the vector.
2. Absence of immunogenicity.
3. Ability to target specific tissue or cell populations.
4. Incorporation of elements that limit the expression of delivered genes to specific cell types.
5. Ability to modulate the levels of gene expression in response to exogenous and endogenous signals.
6. Stability and ease of productivity in large quantities at high concentrations.

Viral Vectors

Virus–based gene delivery arose from the attempt to exploit the highly evolved viral pathways for infection to achieve efficient delivery and expression of therapeutic genes in the body (137,140,141). Viral vectors

Table 6.11. Comparison of the Properties of Various Vector Systems[a]

Features	Retroviral	Adenoviral	AAV	Herpes
Maximum insert size	7.0–7.5 kb	~30 kb	3.5–4.0 kb	150 kb
Concentrations (viral particles/mL)	$>10^8$	$>10^8$	$>10^{12}$	$>10^8$
Route of gene delivery	Ex vivo	Ex/in vivo	Ex/in vivo	Ex/in vivo
Integration	Yes	No	Yes/no	No
Duration of expression in vivo	Short	Short	Long	Long
Stability	Good	Good	Good	Good
Ease of preparation (scale-up)	Pilot scale-up, up to 20–50 L	Easy to scale up	Difficult to purify, difficult to scale up	—
Immunological problems	Few	Extensive	Not known	—
Preexisting host immunity	Unlikely	Yes	Yes	—
Safety problems	Insertional mutagenesis	Inflammatory response, toxicity	Inflammatory response, toxicity	—

[a]Adapted from Verma IM, Somia N. Gene therapy—promises, problems, and prospects. Nature 1999;389:239–242; with permission.

are attenuated or defective viruses engineered to carry therapeutic genes. Several different viruses have been developed as vectors for gene therapy, including the murine C-type oncovirus and HIV (retroviruses), adenovirus, adeno-associated virus, and the herpes simplex virus (Table 6.11). Ultimately, the therapeutic gene vectors should target specific types of genetically damaged cells, insert into a specific position in the cell's genome, and produce large amounts of the corrective protein in a regulated fashion.

Retrovirus

The retroviruses (*Retroviridae*) have three subfamilies: the *Spumavirinae* (foamy viruses), the *Lentivirinae,* and the *Oncovirinae* (142). The oncoviruses based on the murine C-type oncovirus are the vector of choice for gene therapy protocols. The retrovirus enters the target cells, where its RNA genome is converted to proviral DNA and transported to the nucleus. In the nucleus, the proviral DNA becomes integrated into the host chromosomal DNA, thus ensuring long term persistence and stable transmission to all progeny of the transduced cell (Fig. 6.31).

The murine leukemia viruses have been the most widely used as vectors for gene therapy. Human retroviral gene therapy requires replication-defective vectors capable of delivering the therapeutic gene to the target cells without causing severe infection by further replication. The proviral genome has a complex sequence of essential components necessary for mRNA reverse transcription and integration of the viral RNA (142). These elements serve to carry out packaging to ensure encapsidation of vector RNA, portions of the genome directing reverse transcription, and regions necessary for the integration of the vector DNA into the host cell chromosome in the ordered and reproducible manner characteristic of retroviruses. The protein coding sequences *gag, pol,* and *env,* however, can be discarded and replaced with the therapeutic gene.

The modified vector carrying the cDNA of the therapeutic gene is incapable of forming viral particle, since the *gag, pol,* and *env* genes are missing. Therefore, a retroviral packaging cell line is required to provide the viral "helper" functions that have been deleted from the vector. The *gag, pol,* and *env* genes are stably expressed in the packaging cell from helper plasmids that lack the ψ packaging sequence; therefore, the transcripts from the helper plasmid are not packaged in viral particles (Fig. 6.32). The gag, pol, and env proteins are produced by the helper plasmid and form the viral core and envelope proteins. The vector transcript carrying the ψ packaging sequence and the therapeutic gene is recognized by the gag proteins and are incorporated into the core particle, which then buds off into a one-time-only infective particle delivering the therapeutic gene to the target cell. The *gag, pol,* and *env* genes are not packaged in a viral particle, because the sequence carrying these genes is lacking the packaging signal.

Adenovirus (AV)

Adenoviruses are DNA viruses that belong to the *Adenoviridae* family of viruses. They are the most widely used DNA viruses for gene transfer vectors. The primary target for AV infection is the respiratory epithelial cells. The AV are large viruses and, hence, can carry large DNA inserts (up to 35 kb) (Table 6.11). They can transduce nondividing cells and produce very high titers in culture. They also are human viruses and are able to transduce a large number of different human cell types at a very high efficiency. Unlike the retroviruses, the AV do not integrate into the host cell chromosome but remain in the nucleus as an extrachromosomal element or episome. Because of the extrachromosomal nature of the dsDNA insert, the therapeutic gene is eliminated over time.

The major problem with AV vectors is immunotoxicity. Because the recombinant AV vectors are attenuated (not defective) viruses, they express several viral proteins. The result is induction of cytopathic and immunogenic responses in vivo. Some of the attempts to improve the AV as a therapeutic gene vector include (137):

1. Reduction of immunogenicity by further mutation of the genome to reduce viral protein production.

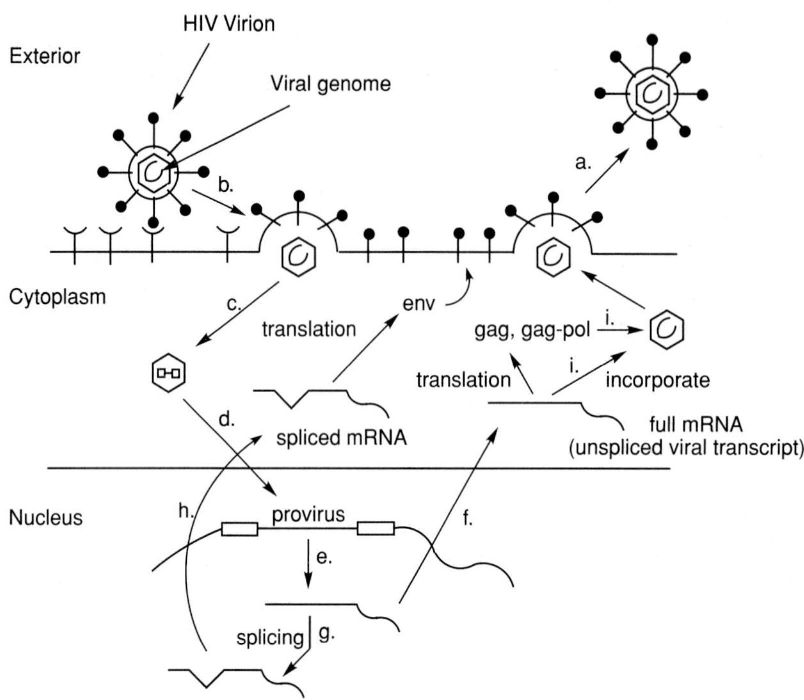

Fig. 6.31. Retroviral entry into target cells. The HIV virion is composed of a nucleoprotein core surrounded by an envelope. The core contains the viral genome, which consists of two identical positive, single-stranded RNA molecules and viral proteins. (a) The envelope is derived from the cell membrane when the virion buds from the cell. (b) Penetration into the cell is initiated by and dependent on specific interactions between the viral gp120 molecule, which is embedded in the viral envelope, and the cellular receptor, the CD4 molecule. (c) After partial uncoating of the virus, viral RNA is reverse transcribed to form a linear double-stranded DNA molecule. (d) This linear double-stranded DNA molecule is then translocated into the nucleus as part of a preintegration complex, where it integrates into the host genome. (e) The integrated viral DNA, called a provirus, is the template for transcription, a process that is under the strict regulation of the viral tat gene. (f and g) The initial viral transcript either is (f) transported to the cytoplasm without further processing to serve as genomic RNA or (g) remains in the nucleus, where it undergoes a series of splicing reactions regulated by the viral *rev* gene. (h) The viral *rev* gene generates mRNAs for viral protein synthesis. (i) The newly synthesized viral proteins (gag and gag-pol) associate with unspliced viral transcripts to form viral cores. (j) These viral cores bud through the cell membrane, acquiring the viral envelope.

2. Increasing the potency of the virus to reduce the immune challenge.
3. Coadministration of immunosuppressants with the vector therapy.

Adeno-associated Virus

The adeno-associated virus (AAV) is a nonpathogenic, ssDNA virus belonging to the *Parvoviridae* family of viruses. This virus has two genes: The *cap* gene encodes for three viral coat proteins, and the *rep* gene encodes for four proteins involved in viral replication and integration. This virus needs additional genes to replicate that are provided by the helper virus, which usually is the adenovirus or herpes virus. Interest in this virus as a vector arose from the discovery that the *rep* gene product directs the virus to integrate the viral DNA preferentially into human chromosome 19. The AAV vector is produced by replacing the *rep* and *cap* genes with the therapeutic gene. Without a helper virus, the AAV will integrate into the host genome and remain as a provirus. Because of the toxic nature of the *rep* gene products, it is difficult to develop a packaging cell line in which all of the protein can be stably produced, and this is a major problem with the AAV as a therapeutic gene vector. Also, because the rep proteins are missing in the therapeutic gene vector, the site-specific insertion in chromosome 19 is not observed. The AAV is a small vector that can only carry genes of approximately 4.8 kb. and the defective vector does not efficiently integrate into the genome of nondividing cells.

Herpes Simplex

Herpes simples virus (HSV) is a member of the alphaherpes virus family that are nuclear DNA viruses with large genomes capable of carrying therapeutic genes up to 150 kb. These viruses are able to establish lifelong latent infections in which the viral genome exists as a stable episome in the host cell (143,144). Genes delivered by the HSV vector can be maintained indefinitely as an episome in long-lived cells, such as those of the nervous system. Herpes simplex viruses made replication deficient by deleting the transcriptional regulator gene IE-3

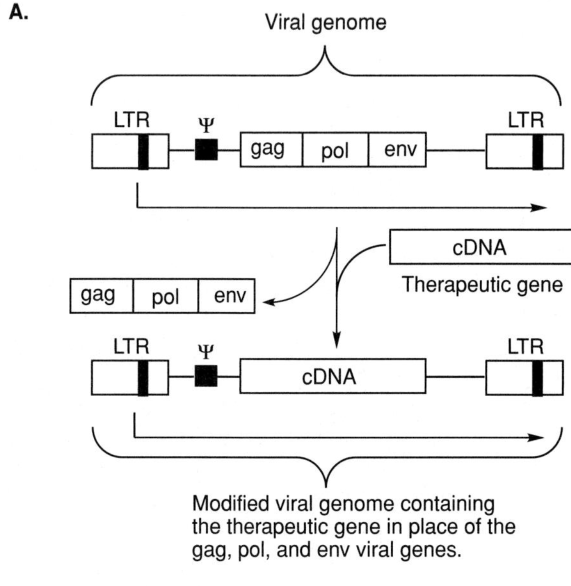

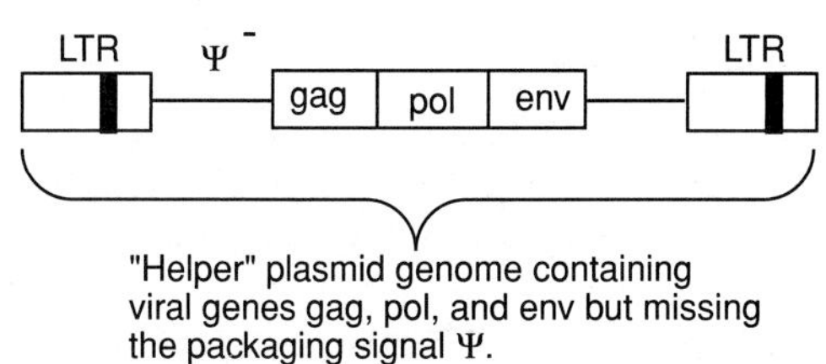

Fig. 6.32 (A) Schematic representation of the preparation of a single gene retroviral construct. The therapeutic gene replaces the retroviral *gag, pol,* and *env* genes. Expression of the therapeutic gene is driven off the viral long terminal repeat (LTR) containing the retroviral packaging signal sequence (ψ). (B) Schematic representation of a helper cell genome containing the retroviral *gag, pol,* and *env* genes but lacking the packaging signal sequence (ψ-).

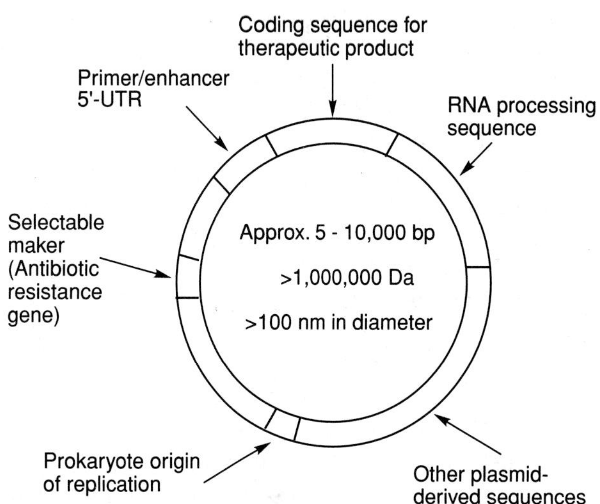

Fig. 6.33. Plasmid DNA constructed for gene delivery contains a therapeutic gene sequence, eukaryotic gene promoter regions, prokaryotic origins of replication, selectable markers, as well as RNA processing sequences and other plasmid-derived sequences. (Adapted from Ledley FD. Pharmaceutical approach to somatic gene therapy. Pharm Res 1996;13:1595–1614; with permission.)

are used as therapeutic gene vectors. Plasmids containing the HSV origin of replication and packaging signal are termed "amplicons." The amplicon also can be used as a vector in the presence of a helper virus, which usually is the IE-3–deficient HSV. In this case, the amplicon/helper virus requires a complementary cell line that provides the IE-3 gene products to assist in forming the replication-deficient viral vectors. Long-term expression is a major obstacle to routine use of this virus as a therapeutic vector.

Nonviral Vectors

Compared to the conventional small molecule drugs that are the mainstay of pharmaceutical care, the plasmids that are used to carry the therapeutic DNA (gene) in nonviral vectors are large, circular, hydrophilic macromolecules of bacterial origin with a hydrodynamic diameter between 100–200 nm and approximately 3,000 kDa in molecular weight (5–10 kbp) (Fig. 6.33) (137). Plasmids carry a net negative charge and are susceptible to nucleases, and their potential as a class of pharmaceuticals is limited by their colloidal and surface properties. The size and charge density of these particles are problematic when it comes to their delivery as therapeutic agents, and these properties depend on the number of base pairs and the DNA conformation. Supercoiled DNA has higher negative charge density than linear, or nicked-circular, DNA and, therefore, has a more negative zeta potential (electrophoretic mobility) than nicked-circular DNA that is slightly more negative than linear DNA (137). The zeta potential varies between −30 and −70 mV and effectively prevents the plasmid from crossing biological membranes. Plasmids contain the therapeutic gene of mammalian origin and other DNA sequences to control the gene expression in vivo. The plasmid also may contain genetic elements controlling mRNA stability and the timing of protein production, cell-specific promoters and enhancers to limit gene expression to specific sites in the body, as well as sequences to direct posttranslational processing and secretion of the gene product. Plasmids delivered by nonviral techniques do not integrate into the host genome at doses used but remain in the nucleus (extrachromosomal episomes). The plasmids will therefore persist in the target cells according to the biochemical half-life of the molecule, which can be anywhere from several months to a few hours. Therefore, as the transfected cells replicate, the DNA gradually is lost over time. The nonviral techniques thus provide a finite period of expression of the therapeutic gene. The advantage is that the techniques may be applied to both chronic and acute diseases, in which the dose and frequency of administration is controlled by the clinician and the level of expression may be quickly adjusted—or even terminated—in response to a patient's changing clinical needs. Plasmids also contain nucleic acid sequences that allow them to be grown in bacteria, including a prokaryotic origin of replication and selectable markers, thus allowing the plasmids to be amplified through cloning in bacteria.

Some of the specific barriers to the in vivo delivery of DNA can be identified (137):

1. Rapid degradation of DNA within tissues or blood by nucleases.
2. Limited dispersion of DNA from the site of interstitial administration.
3. The inability of DNA to cross intact basement membranes of the endothelium or epithelium effectively.
4. The rapid clearance of DNA from the vascular compartment by cells of the reticuloendothelial system.
5. The need for effective interaction with the surface of the target cell to induce internalization.
6. Destruction of DNA in the endosomal/lysosomal compartments by nuclease, acid, and/or reducing agents.
7. The need to penetrate to the nucleus of cells across the periplasmic membrane and nuclear membrane.

The elements of a nonviral gene delivery system include a gene coding for the therapeutic gene, a plasmid-based expression system, and a synthetic delivery system.

Direct Injection (30)

The microinjection of naked DNA in the form of circular plasmids often is used for introducing genes into embryos to engineer transgenic animals. Delivery is localized to the site of injection, and unless the injection is made directly into the cell, the problem of uptake of naked DNA into the cell limits the efficiency of the technique. There has been some success in using this technique to deliver genes to skeletal and cardiac muscle tissue; this success has been attributed to the possibility that the sarcoplasmic reticulum and transverse tubules found in muscle tissue are favorable structures for DNA uptake. The DNA uptake through the cavelolae in muscle via potocytosis involves invagination of the caveloae-rich membranes. There is potential for using direct injection of naked DNA in DNA vaccinations where delivery need not be widespread, because stimulation of the immune system is the goal of vaccination.

Electroporation

Electroporation is used in research for the transfection of a wide range of plant and animal cells, many of which are not amenable to transfection by other methods, such as calcium phosphate coprecipitation. Electroporation likely involves a physical interaction between the cell membrane and the applied electric field and, as such, may be relatively independent of cell type. The procedure involves charging a capacitor with a conventional power supply and then discharging the capacitor (2–10 kV/cm) through a cell suspension containing DNA over a very short time period (<5 microseconds [μs]). Mammalian cells have been transfected with a weaker pulse (0.53 kV/cm) and a longer duration (7,000 μs) (145). The DNA enters when the cells are exposed to a pulsed electric field, presumably disrupting the membrane lipids and creating pores in the cell membrane without damaging the membrane structure (146). The DNA concentration and voltage are critical parameters for electroporation. There is a sharply defined voltage for efficient transfection depending on the buffer and capacitance. The procedure should be applied over a range of voltages to determine the best voltage for the experimental conditions. The local potential difference across the cell is the driving force for membrane pore formation and is proportional to the product of the capacitor voltage and the cell diameter (147). Therefore, the voltage optimum for transfection will depend inversely on cell size (145).

Particle Bombardment

Particle bombardment involves the generation of a shockwave via an explosive device (148), compressed gas (149), or electrical discharge (150) to propel DNA-coated gold or tungsten particles into the target tissue. The gold particles usually are 1 to 3 μm in size; the tungsten particles are slightly larger (~4 μm). The particles are coated with DNA by precipitation through addition of calcium chloride and spermidine solutions to the plasmid DNA in the presence of a suspension of the gold or tungsten particles. The DNA-coated particles are deposited on macrocarrier disks, and a shockwave, generated as described above, accelerates the particles to a high velocity, enabling efficient penetration of target organs, tissues, or single cells in their path. Some acceleration devices can be finely tuned to adjust the velocity and resulting distribution of particles in various target tissues by varying the discharge voltage or gas pressure, bead density, and bead size. This technique is not likely to be widely used for gene delivery, because it is essentially a surgical procedure and the particles are only able to penetrate several millimeters into the target tissue. However, it may well have widespread use as a gene vaccine delivery vehicle (151).

Calcium Phosphate Precipitation

One of the early methods of facilitating the transport of DNA into cells was the coprecipitation of DNA with calcium phosphate or calcium chloride and application the precipitate to a monolayer of cells (152). The mechanism of uptake is not fully understood, but it is postulated that the particulate nature of the calcium phosphate/DNA complex adheres to the cell membrane and is taken up by endocytosis. The pH of the buffer during the formation of the precipitate, the gradual formation of the precipitate

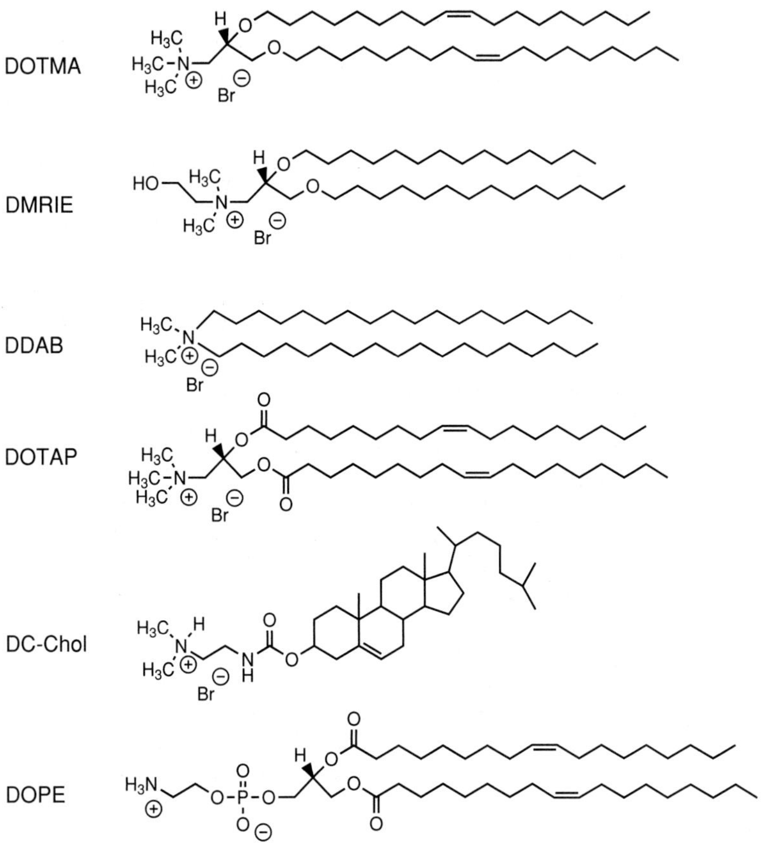

Fig. 6.34. Chemical structures of common cationic lipids: 1,2-dioleyl-oxyproply-3-trimethylammonium bromide (DOTMA), 1,2,-dimyristyl-oxypropyl-3,3-dimethyl-3(2-hydroxyethyl) ammonium bromide (DMRIE), N,N-dimethyl-N, N-dioctadecylammonium bromide (DDAB), 1,2-dioleoyloxy-proply-3-trimethylammonium bromide (DOTAP), 3β-[N-(N,N-dimethylaminoethyl)carbamoyl] cholesterol hydrobromide (DC-Chol), and 1,2-dioleoylpropyloxyphosphatidylethanolamine (DOPE).

(overnight incubation of the DNA in the calcium phosphate N,N-bis(2-hydroxyethyl)-2-aminoethane sulfonic acid–buffered saline, 2XBBS), and the concentration of the DNA are critical factors in determining the efficiency of the procedure in delivering DNA to the cell (153,154). A pH in the region of 7.0 and DNA concentrations of 40 μg/ml result in the most efficient uptake of DNA by the mammalian cells. Calcium is an efficient facilitator of DNA uptake for a number of reasons. It increases the concentration of DNA on the cell surface through precipitation and protects the DNA from digestion by serum and intracellular nucleases. Calcium phosphate itself also induces phagocytosis. Additionally, the calcium phosphate precipitate may neutralize the negative charge on the DNA molecule, thus facilitating penetration of the lipid membrane and reducing repulsion of the negatively charged DNA by the negatively charged cell membrane. Other cations, including polyornithine, polylysine, polybrene, and diethylaminoethylamine, also have been used as cationic facilitators for cellular uptake of DNA (155,156). The most efficient facilitated DNA uptake is observed in cells at the exponential stage of growth. This technique, however, depends on the phagocytosis of the DNA/calcium phosphate particle, resulting in endosome formation and the exposure of the DNA to the intracellular endosome/lysosome degradation process.

Cationic Lipids

Cationic lipids, or "cytofectins" as they sometimes are called, are positively charged amphiphilic molecules that interact with the negatively charged phosphate backbone of DNA molecules, neutralizing the charge and promoting the condensation of DNA into a more compact structure (157–159). The chemical composition of the cationic lipids consists of the following (Fig. 6.34):

1. A hydrophobic lipid anchor that aids in the formation of cationic liposomes that are critical components of the complex with DNA.
2. A linker group that is located between the cationic head group of the molecule and the lipid tail. The

linker determines the chemical stability and biodegradability of the cationic lipids. The most common link is the alkyl ether.

3. The cationic head group that is responsible for the complexation of the liposome with the negatively charged DNA. The cationic group is a singly or multiply charged primary, secondary, tertiary, or quaternary amine. The common counterions found with the cationic lipids are the bromide, chloride, or trifluoroacetate anion.

The cationic lipids are most frequently used in a 0.5 molar ratio with a neutral, zwitterionic phospholipid (usually dioleoylphophatidylethanolamine) called the colipid. The cationic lipid and colipid form unilamellar and multilamellar liposomes that are approximately 100 and 300–700 nm, respectively, in diameter. The role played by the cationic lipid in the cationic liposome is multifold and includes causing the condensation of DNA to form a particle with specific colloidal properties, controlling the distribution of DNA particles in the body, causing the particles to interact with the target cell, and finally, inducing cytosis to aid entry of the particle into the cell. The colipid may play an active role in the internalization of DNA into the cell through facilitating the fusion of the DNA/lipid complex with the cell membrane or endosome membrane, releasing the DNA into the cytoplasm (Fig. 6.35).

The cationic liposomes are absorbed onto the surface of the negatively charged cyclic polynucleotide (plasmid) to form aggregates that gradually surround the larger segments of the DNA. At a critical lipid concentration, the processes of lipid fusion and DNA collapse are initiated. Subsequent increase in the lipid concentration causes the collapsed DNA structures to become coated in the lipid bilayers. The final product is like a "condensed nanoparticle," with the lipid bilayers providing an internal structure that looks like the ridges of a fingerprint (160). Generally, the complexes formed with the larger multilamellar vesicles are more active than those formed with the smaller unilamellar vesicles.

The plasmid–lipid complexes tend to aggregate over time, and this aggregation is a function of a number of factors, which may include cationic lipid species, the DNA/cationic lipid ratio and concentrations, shearing force, temperature, solution viscosity, time, and salt and serum protein content. This instability necessitates that the plasmid–lipid complex be formed immediately before use and, therefore, limits the ability of the user to characterize and control the parameters of the formulations. The positive charge on the complex also results in an unfavorable interaction with negatively charged cellular proteins, leading to aggregation of the complex and premature release of the DNA. Additionally, cationic lipids interact with the complement system of the body and, therefore, are opsonized by the C3b/C4b components, resulting in rapid clearance by macrophages in the reticuloendothelial systems. The particle size and the

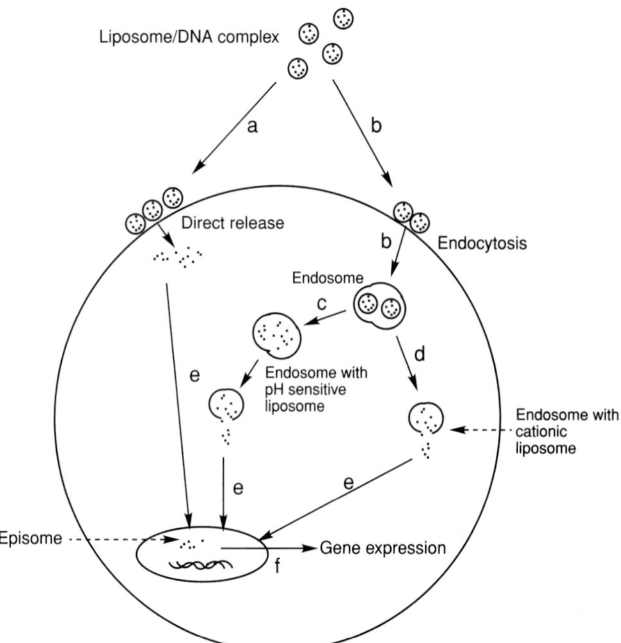

Fig. 6.35. Schematic representation of possible modes of interaction of liposomes with cells that lead to intracellular delivery. Liposomes can enter the cell by local destabilization of plasma membrane or fusion (a) or endocytosis (b). The releases of DNA by fusion is still not clear (c or d). The released DNA or cationic liposome-DNA complexes reach into the nucleus (e), and gene expression occurs (f). (Adapted from Singhal A, Huang L.Gene transfer in mammalian cells using liposomes as carriers. In: WolffJA, ed. Gene Therapeutics. Boston: Birkhauser, 1994:118; with permission.)

zeta potential of the plasmid–lipid complexes depends on various factors, including the cationic lipid species, the amount and type of colipid; the particle size and composition of the liposomes used in the preparation; the molecular weight, form, and type of plasmid; the stoichiometry of the cationic lipid and DNA; the concentration of lipid and DNA in the final preparation; and the mixing procedure.

Interaction of the plasmid–lipid complex with the target cell membrane occurs when the cationic lipid preparation has a high positive charge that results in an ionic interaction with the negatively charged cell membrane. The mechanism of transfer of the plasmid to the nucleus is poorly understood. Two hypotheses currently describe the mechanism, neither of which is mutually exclusive of the other (Fig. 6.35). One hypothesis suggests that the plasmid–lipid complex fuses with the target cell membrane and expels the plasmid into the cytosol, where it then makes its way to the nucleus, where it is taken up and remains as extrachromosomal material (episome). The second hypothesis suggests that the nanoparticle plasmid–lipid complex interacts with the target cell membrane and is absorbed through endocytosis. The colipid then aids in the fusion of the plasmid–lipid complex with the

Table 6.12. Actions of Cationic Lipids that Enhance Gene Delivery

- Protect the DNA against degradation by nucleases.
- Modify the size, charge, and surface characteristics of the DNA containing particulate to control its biodistribution within the body and access to the target cell.
- Improve the interaction of DNA with the surface of the target cell.
- Induce endocytosis.
- Improve release of DNA from the endosome.
- Improve the entry of DNA into the nucleus.

endosomal membrane and the disintegration of the endosome before interaction with the lysosome and destruction of the plasmid.

The presence of cationic lipids in the preparation may enhance gene delivery in several ways, including those indicated in Table 6.12.

Similar delivery systems have been designed using other cationic polymers, including lipopolyamines (161), amphipathic peptides (162), polylysine lipids (163), cholesterol (164), quaternary ammonium detergents (165), polyamidoamines called dendrimers, polyethylenimines or chitosan, diethylaminoethyl dextran (DEAE dextran), and polybrene.

Nonviral Targeted Gene Transfer

Receptor mediated uptake of nucleic acids is approached through the complexation of the DNA with protein ligands specific for cellular receptors. This technique is carried out by covalently linking the protein ligand to a positively charged polylysine polymer and then complexing the ligand/polymer unit to DNA by ionic interaction with the negatively charged phosphate groups. The interaction of polylysine with DNA causes the condensation of DNA into a compact torus-shaped (toroidal) protein/DNA structure that may be as small as 80 nm in diameter (166) and similar to that seen for the interaction of the cationic lipids with DNA. The protein retains its ability to interact with its receptor on the cell surface, and the resulting complex causes internalization of the DNA through endocytosis of the protein/receptor complex. The procedure for preparation of the covalent polylysine/ ligand complex is illustrated in Fig. 6.36. The amino groups on the lysine side chains of polymers of lysine containing 90, 270, or 450 lysine monomers ($pLys_{90}$, $pLys_{270}$, or $pLys_{450}$, respectively) are derivatized with 3-(2-pyridyldithio)propionate to give the pyridyldithiopropionate intermediate that is then reduced with dithiothreitol to give the 3-mercaptopropionate–modified polylysine containing approximately one mercaptopropionate group per 50 lysine residues in the polymer. A pyridyldithiopropionate derivative of the ligand also is prepared and conjugated with the mercaptopropionate polylysine polymer through disulfide bond formation. This procedure generally results in approximately one ligand linked to every 50 residues of the polylysine polymer.

The ligand/polylysine covalent complex is subsequently mixed with DNA plasmids containing the therapeutic gene to be targeted to the cells containing the ligand receptor to condense the DNA and form the ligand/polylysine/ DNA complex (Fig. 6.36). The targeted cells are exposed to the complex either in vitro through exposure of a cell culture to the complex or in vivo through intravenous injection of the complex into the animal. The following ligand/complexes have been used to deliver genes to specific cell targets:

- *Transferrin/polylysine/DNA*—hematopoietic cells, T-cells, pulmonary epithelial cells.
- *Asialoorosomucoid/polylysine/DNA*—liver cells.
- *Insulin/polylysine/DNA*—liver cells
- *Surfactant B/polylysine/DNA*—epithelial airway cells.
- *Antithromobomodulin/polylysine/DNA*—epithelial airway cells.

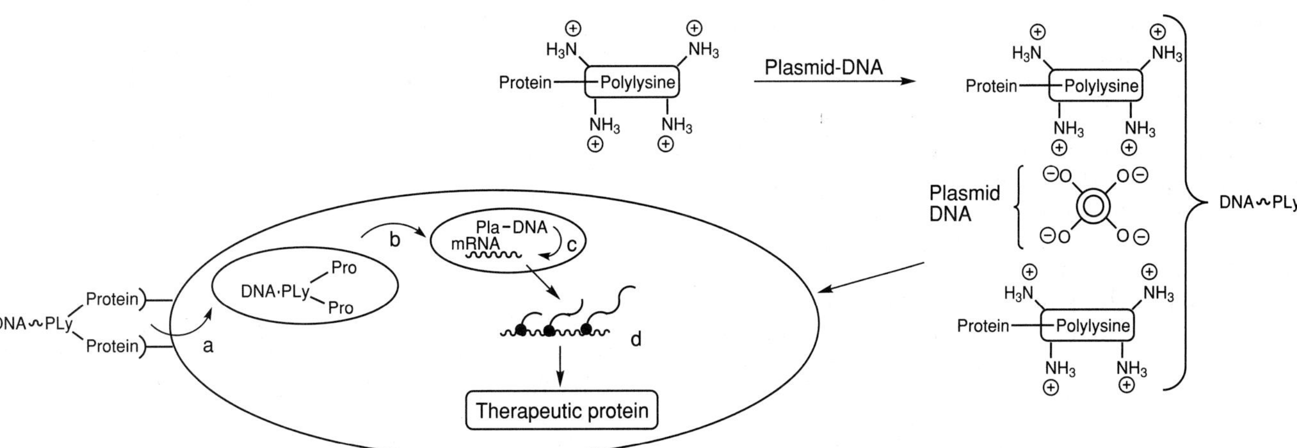

Fig. 6.36. Schematic representation of nonviral targeted gene transfer. The process involves complexation of a protein-polylysine component to plasmid-DNA (DNA~PLy) followed by protein-assisted cellular absorption (a) into hepatocytes, transfer into nucleus (b), transcription of the plasmid~DNA (Pla~DNA) into mRNA (c), and translation into therapeutic protein (d). Note that the protein is linked to the polylysine by a disulfide bond.

Several small molecules, including folate, galactose, lactose, and N-acetyl galactosamine, also have been used to prepare polylysine/DNA complexes for delivery of DNA by receptor-mediated endocytosis.

The major factors limiting the in vivo effectiveness of the protein/DNA complexes may be the poor bioavailability to many target cells and their colloidal instability in physiological media. The endocytotic uptake of the receptor complex also limits the effectiveness of the delivery system, because the DNA is quickly destroyed in the endosome/lysosome pathway.

Artificial Chromosomes—YACs and HACs

A more recent development in gene delivery that has potential for developing into a therapeutic gene delivery system is the artificial chromosome. Genetic manipulation of the yeast genome has resulted in the development of yeast artificial chromosomes (YACs). These linear structures use the same basic functional elements as the normal linear mammalian and yeast chromosomes.

The capacity for YACs to carry very large fragments of foreign DNA permits the cloning of genes with all their natural genomic elements in correct spatial orientation. The YACs have been used in the preparation of large DNA fragments for sequencing in the Human Genome Project (HGP). They also have been very useful in the analysis of gene function and the creation of chromosome transgenic mice.

The potential of artificial chromosomes for gene therapy is currently being investigated (167–169). The development of a properly segregating, autonomously replicating "minichromosome" has the potential to eliminate the disadvantages of viral vectors, such as genomic insertional position effects, gene size restrictions, and lack of proper regulation of gene function.

The human chromosome is far larger and more complex than the yeast chromosome. In spite of numerous complications, the human artificial chromosome (HAC, or MAC) is being developed and the potential applications to gene therapy investigated (170). Two approaches are currently being used to create the HAC (Fig. 6.37). Small human chromosomes (i.e., minichromosomes) are being developed through truncation of the normal chromosome mediated by insertion of human telomeres (the specialized structure of the ends of the chromosome) into the chromosomal arms, creating shortened chromosomes of 3.5 to 9.0 Mb (megabases) in size (170). Alternatively, many steps have been taken toward creating an artificial chromosome through assembly of the known functional elements of a human chromosome with genomic DNA containing a human gene (171).

Pharmacokinetics and Metabolism of DNA

Genes can be delivered using either ex vivo or in vivo strategy. The ex vivo strategy encounters intracellular barriers presented by the cell that include the cell, endosome, and nuclear membranes (Fig. 6.38).

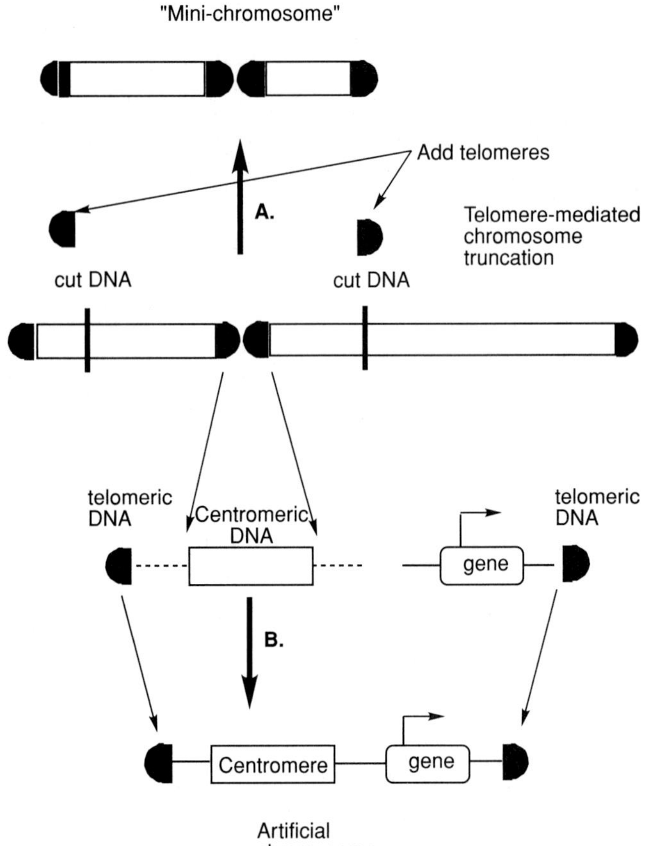

Fig. 6.37. Two approaches for manipulation of a human chromosome. (A) Minichromosomes can be generated in cultured cells by chromosome truncation mediated by the integration of telomeric sequences into chromosome arms. (B) Alternatively, artificial chromosomes might be constructed by combining the known functional elements of a human chromosome: telomeric DNA, centromeric DNA, and genomic DNA containing a human gene or selectable genetic marker.

Depending on the ex vivo vector used, the DNA can be delivered directly to the cell cytosol through fusion of the vector with the cell membrane, or the DNA may enter the cell through endocytosis, creating the endosomal membrane barrier. Endosomal DNA can be released from the endosome into the cytosol, or the endosome may fuse with the lysosome, resulting in degradation of the DNA by nucleases and the acidic environment of the lysosome. Cytosolic DNA is susceptible to a variety of nucleases found in cellular cytosol, and that which reaches the nuclear membrane is taken up by an active transport mechanism, possibly similar to that of protein uptake by the nuclear membrane (172). Once inside the nucleus, the transgene DNA is still susceptible to degradation by nucleases.

Delivery of DNA in vivo faces additional extracellular barriers posed by specific tissues and the immune system (Fig. 6.38). The blood-brain barrier, connective tissue, and epithelial cell linings are particular examples of cellular

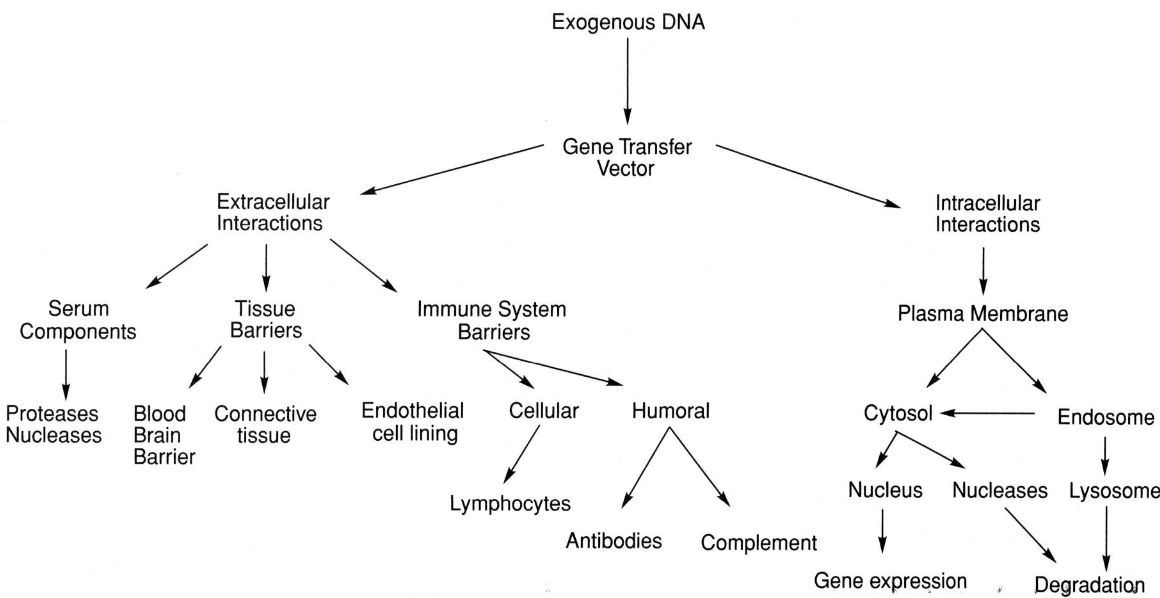

Fig. 6.38. Barriers to gene delivery.

structures that may impede delivery of DNA to the target cells. Humoral and cellular immune responses also pose serious barriers to successful delivery of DNA to target cells.

The DNA is rapidly eliminated from the compartment into which it is administered as a result of both degradation through endo- and exonucleases and distribution to other compartments. The DNA is eliminated from the blood compartment by interaction with Kuppfer cells through a specific scavenger/receptor interaction (173). An intravenously administered asialo-orosomucoid-polylysine-DNA complex is cleared from the blood with an apparent half-life of 2.5 min (174). The DNA taken up by the liver is eliminated with a half life of 1.0 to 1.3 hours, gene transcripts were evident for 1 to 12 hours, and the gene product persisted for 6 to 24 hours.

Different tissues have been shown to display different DNA pharmacokinetics. Genes and gene products have been observed as long as 19 months after direct injection without indication of plasmid integration or replication (175). Direct injection of the chloramphenicol acetyltransferase gene into the thyroid resulted in elimination of DNA from the gland with a half-life of 10 hours. The enzyme activity was maximal for 24 hours and eliminated through first-order kinetics with an apparent half-life of 40 hours (176). Similar results were recorded for synovial fluid intra-articular administration of plasmid DNA (177).

If the therapeutic gene is not incorporated into the host cell genome, adjusting the dose and administration schedule, as for any conventional drug therapy, can control the level of the therapeutic product. The formulation of the delivery vehicle and the design of the gene expression vector, however, affect the duration and level of therapeutic activity. Gene therapy also provides unique pharmacokinetic issues in that the apparent kinetic properties of the therapeutic agent are a combination of the intrinsic kinetic properties of the DNA vector, the RNA transcript, and the translated protein product (178). The intrinsic kinetic parameters are described by a six-compartment model of DNA pharmacokinetics (178). Flux between the compartments labeled Milieu, Endosome, Cell, RNA, Protein, and Product will reflect the biological process of uptake, endosomal transport into cells, transcription, translation, and secretion. Additionally, DNA will be subjected to degradation in each of the compartments. Although this model is a first approximation of the processes involved in using genes as medicines, a total description of DNA pharmacokinetics likely will include:

- Compartmental distribution and extracellular elimination of DNA after in vivo administration.
- Efficiency of DNA uptake into cells.
- Compartmentalization of DNA within the endosomal, cytoplasmic, and nuclear compartments of the cell.
- Rate of degradation of DNA within the cell.
- Rate of transcription of RNA from DNA.
- Stability of the mRNA.
- Rate of translation of the mRNA to create the new gene product.
- Rate of posttranslational modification of he gene product.
- Intracellular compartmentalization or secretion of the gene product.
- Pharmacokinetics of the gene product in the body.

PHARMACOGENETICS

With the completion of the HGP, there has been a visible shift from genomic research in gene structure to

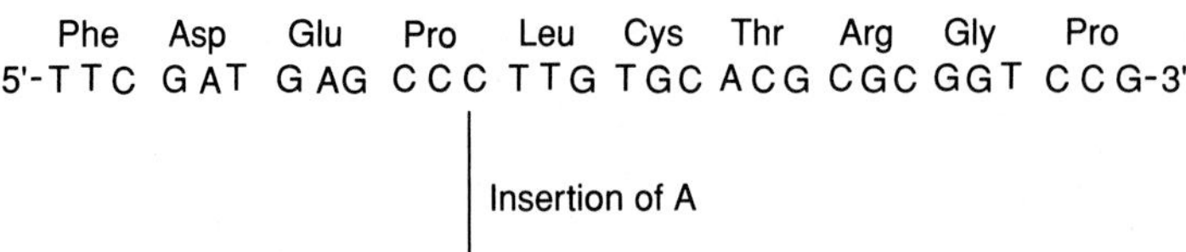

Phe Asp Glu **Thr** Leu Val His Ala Arg Ser
5'-TTC GAT GAG **ACC** CTT GTG CAC GCG CGG TCC-3'

Fig. 6.39. An example of a frameshift point mutation. Adenosine is inserted between guanosine, which is the last nucleotide in the glutamic acid triplet, and cytosine, which is the first nucleotide in the proline triplet. The reading frame is shifted to the left by one nucleotide, thereby changing the sequence of amino acids from glutamic acid onward.

research in gene function. The application of genetic information to disease diagnosis and drug therapy is a major development that will see tremendous changes over the next few years. The main benefit will be a reduction in the health care costs arising from drug toxicity and lack of efficacy in drug therapy.

Mutations are the result of heritable, permanent changes in the DNA base sequence. These usually come about by one of three mechanisms: substitution, addition, or deletion. The number of base pairs involved in a single gene mutation can vary from a single base pair change, called a point mutation, to a large number of gross changes in the gene structure involving insertion, deletion, or rearrangements of a very large number of base pairs.

Point mutations may result in a variety of changes to the gene product. If the base change occurs within the reading frame of the gene product and produces a single change in one amino acid in the amino acid sequence of the gene product, it is termed a "missense point mutation." Some of these point mutations result in no change in the amino acid sequence of the gene product and are termed "silent mutations." Generally speaking, a point mutation in a gene that does not result in functional change of the gene product is termed a "polymorphism." Mutations are defined as base changes causing a change in function of the gene product. This distinction is not rigidly adhered to, however, and many single base mutations causing changes in function of gene product frequently are called single-nucleotide polymorphisms (SNPs). In fact, SNPs have been defined as single base mutations that occur in 1% or more of the population (179). Many of these SNPs may be responsible for the production of a malfunctioning gene product that, in turn, is responsible for a serious disease. The well-used example here is the A → T mutation in the β-globin gene, in which the GAG glutamic acid codon is changed to the GTG valine codon, resulting in abnormal aggregation of the hemoglobin molecules and causing sickle cell anemia.

Point mutations occurring in the reading frame that convert an amino acid codon to a stop codon (TAA, TAG, or TGA) are termed "nonsense mutations" and result in the truncation of the gene product because of a premature stop in the translation process. These changes are very serious and may lead to loss of a large sequence of the carboxy terminus of the gene product especially if they occur in the 5′ region of the gene. One form of β-thalassemia results from a mutation of a CAG glutamine codon to the TAG stop codon early in the DNA sequence, resulting in premature termination of the translation process and total loss of the β subunit of the adult hemoglobin molecule.

A frameshift mutation occurs when, instead of changing a base pair, a base pair is inserted or deleted in the gene sequence. An insertion/deletion of more or less than three bases will result in a shift of the reading frame, and a different set of codons will be read 3′ (downstream) of the mutation (Fig. 6.39). These mutations have very serious effects and frequently result in the total loss of the gene product.

Point mutations occurring in the boundaries between the exons and introns may result in the inability of the pre-mRNA to splice properly and are termed "splice mutations." These mutations may result in the loss of many amino acids in the gene product sequence or may cause a frameshift, resulting in total loss of functional gene product. Mutations also may occur in introns with the resultant formation of splice sites that also cause the pre-mRNA to splice abnormally.

Point mutations in promoter regions, termed "promoter mutations," are responsible for reducing or eliminating the expression of a gene.

One of the gross changes in gene structure involves an unusual form of gene mutation termed the "trinucleotide repeat," in which a trinucleotide sequence undergoes a dramatic increase in the number of copies of the trinucleotide in a gene sequence. Fragile X syndrome and Huntington's disease are both the result of this unusual mutation.

In the early 1950s, at the time of Watson and Crick's seminal paper on the structure of DNA, it was discovered that some patients who were undergoing surgery and had been treated with the muscle relaxant succinyldicholine

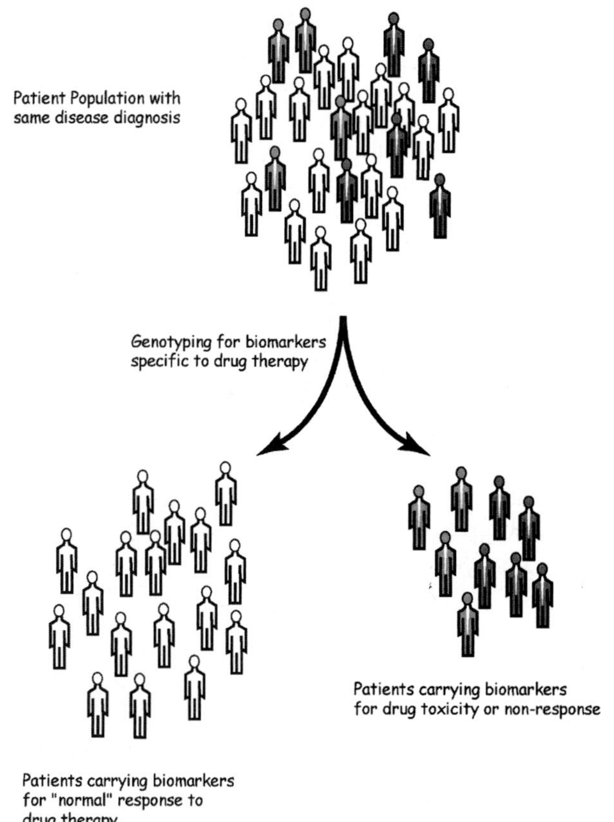

Fig. 6.40. Manipulating therapeutic outcomes: manipulating therapeutic outcomes through pharmacogenetic analysis of a population with the same disease diagnosis to eliminate those patients with genetic biomarkers indicating an adverse response to a particular drug therapy.

did not recover their respiratory function as quickly as expected. This problem eventually was traced to a lower-than-normal level of pseudocholinesterase activity in the patient's blood. The result was that the patient was not eliminating the muscle relaxant at the rate seen by "normal" patients; hence, the drug was acting longer than expected in a normal response. This problem was finally demonstrated to be a familial or hereditary problem. Similar "familial"-related abnormal responses to drug therapy were found in the use of primaquine therapy for the treatment of malaria and the use of isoniazid in the treatment of tuberculosis. In separate publications, Motulsky and Vogel coined the term "pharmacogenetics" to describe genetically determined variability in the effects of drugs on animal species, and the term then became defined as the study of interindividual variations in DNA sequences related to drug response.

In principle, one is able to manipulate the therapeutic outcome of a patient population by separating those patients who will not respond normally to a particular drug therapy from those who will, based on an analysis of established genetic biomarkers related to the drug's metabolic profile (Fig. 6.40). Patients who are homozygous for the genetic biomarkers indicating poor metabolism of the recommended therapeutic agent may, depending on the therapeutic window of the drug, exhibit a response resembling an overdose to the normal drug dose and require a reduced dose to achieve therapeutic levels (Patient A in Fig. 6.41), whereas those patients carrying the biomarkers indicating extensive metabolism may exhibit a lack of efficacy at normal doses and require an increased dose of the drug to achieve therapeutic activity (Patient D in Fig. 6.41). The patients who are homozygous or heterozygous for the normal (wild-type) genetic biomarker (Patients B and C, respectively, in Fig. 6.41) may require no alteration of the "normal" dose of the drug for adequate therapeutic outcome.

The application of genetic variation to drug therapy centered on the variations seen in a number of drug metabolism enzymes and much of the pharmacogenetic research have developed with the Phase I (oxidative) and

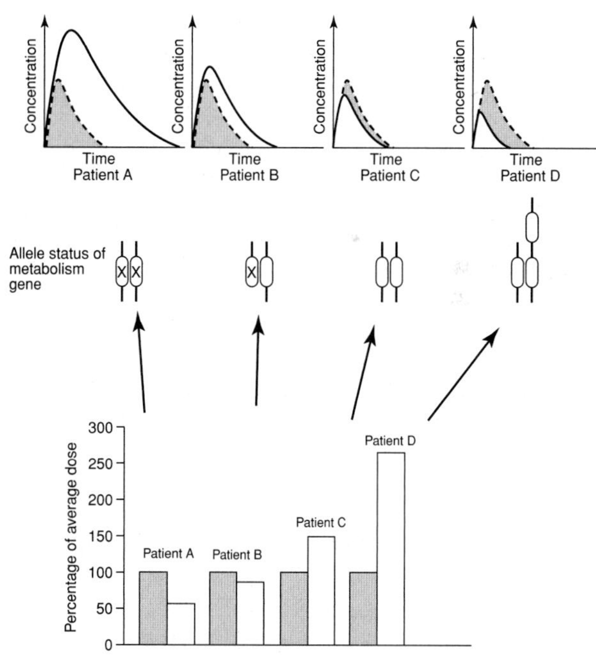

Fig. 6.41. Dose/Genotype Relationship: A schematic representation of the potential benefit of adjusting drug dose to patient genotype. The theoretical "normal" drug concentration/time curve is depicted by the dashed line in the concentration/time curves of Patients A-D at the top of the figure while the theoretical "genetic" drug concentration/time curve for each patient is expressed by the solid line. The allele status for each patient is shown below the theoretical plots. The oval containing the "X" indicates the presence of the detrimental allelic variation. The extra oval in Patient D indicates duplication of one of the normal alleles. The bar graph at the bottom of the figure indicates the normal doses (shaded) compared to the dose adjustments that should be made based on the patient's allele status (180).

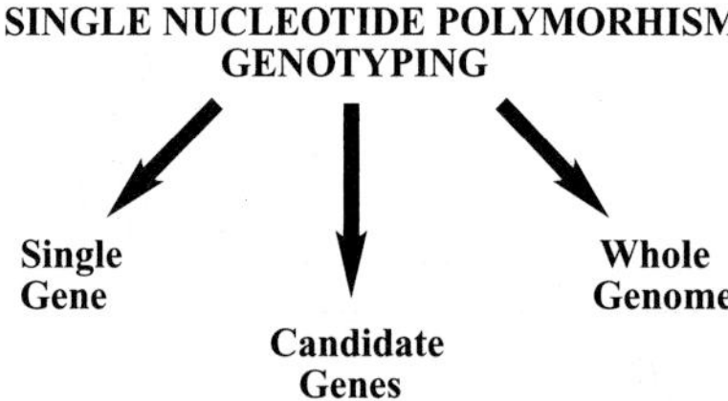

Fig. 6.42. Single-nucleotide polymorphism (SNP) genotyping: approaches to genotyping for drug therapy. The single gene approach has been used successfully in pharmacogenetic studies of a number of Phase I and Phase II metabolic enzymes. The candidate gene approach involves the selection of the genes for proteins that are demonstrated to be involved in a particular drug action, including metabolic enzymes, transport proteins, drug targets, and proteins involved in modular drug response pathways. The whole-genome approach uses SNPs evenly spaced throughout the genome.

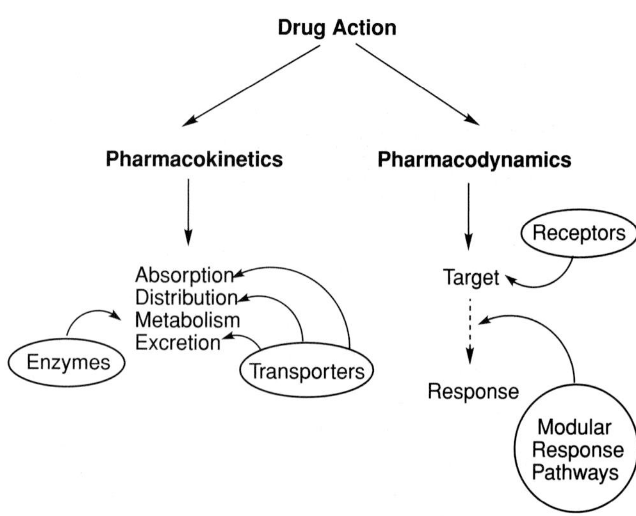

Fig. 6.43. Schematic representation of the multigenic therapeutic drug pathway.

Phase II (conjugative) metabolic enzymes. Currently, considerable data relate SNPs in the coding and regulatory regions of these genes to poor metabolism of particular drugs that have the potential to result in drug overdoses in those patients carrying the genetic variations and given the "normal" dose of drug (Fig. 6.42).

The action of a drug on the body is a more complex interaction involving the metabolism of drugs, the transport of drugs throughout the body, and the interaction of the drug with its target. These features are known as the pharmacokinetics (absorption, distribution, metabolism, and excretion) and pharmacodynamics (drug–target interaction) of drug therapy. These genes are known as the candidate genes for the application of genetic information to drug therapy (Fig. 6.42).

Transport proteins that move drugs through membrane barriers are critical in the absorption, distribution, and excretion of drugs and drug metabolites, while enzymes are critical in the metabolism of drugs in the body (Fig. 6.43). The pharmacodynamic pathway is represented most abundantly by the drug receptor pathway of drug response. This involves drug receptors as well as the numerous biochemical events that occur subsequent to drug–receptor interaction and before the measurement of the pharmacological response. The complexity of the pharmacodynamic pathway can be simplified if one takes the modular biology approach and considers the many biochemical pathways between the drug–receptor interaction and the drug response to be linked modules of biochemical systems.

Table 6.13. Specific Examples of the Application of Allelic Variation in Drug Therapy

Gene	Action	Drug	Therapy	Efficacy/Toxicity
CYP450 2D6	Drug metabolism	Codeine	Pain	Efficacy
CYP450 2C9	Drug metabolism	Warfarin	Coagulation	Toxicity (hemorrhage)
Thiopurine S-methyltransferase	Drug metabolism	Mercaptopurine	Acute lymphoblastic leukemia	Toxicity (myelotoxic)
HER2/neu	Drug target	Herceptin	Breast cancer	Efficacy
bcr/abl	Drug target	Gleevec	Chronic myelogenous leukemia	Efficacy
EFGR	Drug target	Erbitux	Colon cancer	Efficacy
Apolipoprotein E4	Marker	Tacrine	Alzheimer's disease	Efficacy
Cholesteryl ester transferase	Marker	Statins	Atherosclerosis	Efficacy
ATP-binding cassette B1	Drug transport	Saqinavir Indinavir Ritonavir Daunorubicin Etoposide	HIV Leukemia	Efficacy
UDP-glucuronosyl-transferase 1A1	Drug metabolism	Irinotecan	Cancer	Toxicity (myelotoxic)
N-acetyltransferase 2	Drug metabolism	Isoniazid	Tuberculosis	Toxicity (hepatotoxic)
Pseudocholinesterase	Drug metabolism	Suxamethonium	Muscle relaxation during surgery	Toxicity (prolonged apnea)

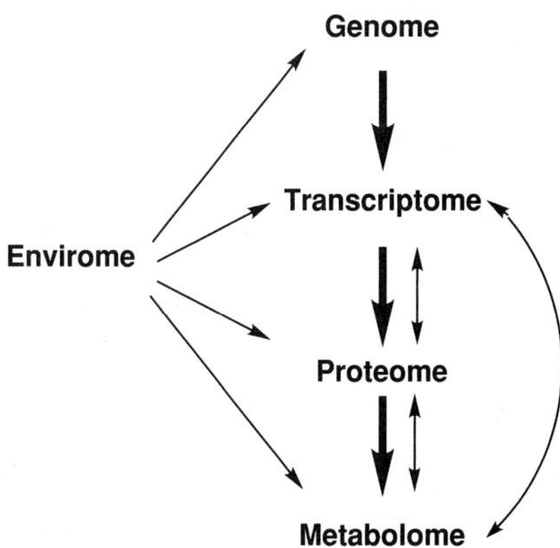

Fig. 6.44. A schematic representation of the biological organization of the '-omes'. This view represents the major flow of information from genome to transcriptome, to proteome and metabolome (⟶). Perturbation in this process can affect another (⟷). The environment has an affect on expression and concentrations of transcripts, proteins, and metabolites as well as the genome by selecting from adaptive changes in subpopulations of cells (┈➤). (Adapted from Griffin JL, Shockcor JP. Metabolic profiles of cancer cells. Nat Rev Cancer 2004;4: 551–561; with permission.)

Thus, the candidate genes for the therapeutic dry pathway includes the genes for drug metabolism, drug transport, and drug response (Table 6.13).

Finally, the whole-genome approach to SNP analysis on drug action suggested that a high density of coding and noncoding SNPs evenly spaced throughout the genome could be used to determine optimal drug therapy. In this case, the SNPs would be used as markers, as opposed to the functional SNPs of the individual gene approach. The use of linkage disequilibrium to map SNP loci that may be relevant to disease therapy indicated that linkage disequilibrium is highly variable in different parts of the genome, and those fragments appear to be inherited in blocks known as haplotype blocks. This has led to the international HapMap project, with the aim to map all the haplotype blocks in the human genome. The HapMap project has already demonstrated that haplotype blocks may contain several hundred SNPs, but also that only a few of these SNPs are needed to identify a particular block. These SNPs are known as haplotype tagged SNPs (htSNPs). Extension of the htSNP concept to candidate genes will reduce the number of htSNPs needed to characterize a drug therapy by limiting the htSNP variations to those SNPs in the candidate genes of the therapeutic drug pathway.

PHARMACOGENOMICS AND PERSONALIZED MEDICINE

To evaluate the effects of genetic variation on disease diagnosis and drug therapy, one must consider more than simply the genetics. The central dogma of gene function indicates that information flows from DNA to pre-mRNA to mRNA and finally protein. Therefore, it would be naïve to think that all the information in a cell is stored in the DNA. One also must consider the modifications to that message that may occur during the transcription of the DNA message to mRNA and the translation to protein. Additionally, consideration must be given to the subsequent modification that occur to proteins that also may alter their function in the cell. This complexity is summarized in Figures 6.44 and 6.45. The individual's phenotype is the result of gene expression, and this includes the genetic information (genome), the translated material (transcriptome), the transcribed proteins (proteome), and the effect that these translated proteins have on the metabolism within the cell (metabolome). It also is important to consider that the transcriptome, proteome, and metabolome are a direct result of genome expression; however, modifications to these components and to the genome occur as a result of environmental effects from the individual's envirome.

Personalized medicine is defined as the utilization of molecular biomarkers from an individual's genome, transcriptome, proteome, and metabolome under the influence of the individual's envirome in the assessment of predisposition to disease, screening and early diagnosis of disease, assessment of prognosis, pharmacogenomic prediction of therapeutic drug efficacy and risk of toxicity; and monitoring the illness until the final therapeutic outcome is determined (Fig. 6.45). A biomarker is a characteristic that is objectively measured and evaluated as an indicator of normal biological processes, pathogenic processes, or pharmacologic responses to a therapeutic intervention (182).

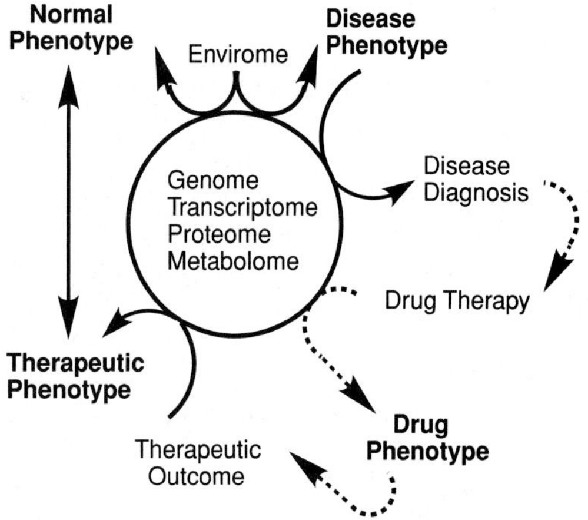

Fig. 6.45. Schematic representation of the concept of molecular profiling for personalized medicine. Dashed arrows indicate the critical components of pharmacogenomics; disease diagnosis, drug therapy, drug phenotype, and therapeutic outcome.

Table 6.14. Genotyping Technologies

Technique[a]	Mechanism of Allele Discrimination	Reaction Formate	Detection Mechanism	Reference
Reverse dot blot	Hybridization	Solid support	Colorimetric	183
Microarray	Hybridization	Solid support	Fluorescence	179,184,185
DASH	Hybridization	Solid support	Fluorescence	186,187
Molecular beacons	Hybridization	Homogeneous reaction	FRET	188
5′-Nuclease cleavage (TaqMan)	Hybridization	Homogeneous reaction	FRET or FP	189,190
Cleavase (Invader Assay)	Hybridization	Homogeneous reaction	FRET, FP, MS	191–194
Biosensor microchip	Hybridization	Solid support	Electrochemical and fluorescence	195–200
AS-PCR	Primer extension	Homogeneous reaction	Fluorescence or FRET	201–206
AS-PE	Primer extension	Solid support	Fluorescence	207
APEX	Primer extension	Solid support	Fluorescence	208–211
FP-TDI	Primer extension	Homogeneous reaction	FRET or FP	191,212,213
MALDI-TOF MS	Primer extension	Homogeneous reaction	MS	214–217
Pyrosequencing	Primer extension	Homogeneous reaction or solid support	Luminescence	218–222
BioBeads and TagArrays	Primer extension	Homogeneous reaction and solid support capture	Fluorescence	223–226
OLA	Ligation	Homogeneous and solid support	Colorimetric and Fluorescence	227–229
RCA	Ligation	Solid support	Fluorescence	229–232
Closed tube	Ligation	Homogeneous reaction	FRET	233
Microsphere/microarray ligation	Ligation	Homogeneous reaction	Fluorescence	224,234

[a]DASH, dynamic allele-specific hybridization; AS-PCR, allele-specific polymerase chain reaction; AS-PE, allele-specific primer extension; APEX, arrayed primer extension; FP-TDI, fluorescence polarization template directed dye terminator incorporation; MALDI-TOF-MS, matrix-assisted laser desorption/ionization time-of-flight mass spectrometry; OLA, oligonucleotide ligation assay; RCA, rolling circle amplification.

The application of genomic, transcriptomic, proteomic, and metabolomic technologies to the development of in vitro molecular biomarkers is molecular profiling. The molecular profiling of a patient's phenotype uses molecular biomarkers to provide a molecular basis to the normal or healthy patient phenotype in a particular envirome. Changes in molecular biomarkers in a disease state compared to the normal state provide a molecular characterization of the disease phenotype, which is used to provide a consistent, accurate diagnosis. The disease phenotype is used to choose the best therapy, which will alter the molecular biomarkers to a drug therapy phenotype (Fig. 6.45). The difference between the biomarkers used in the diagnosis and drug phenotype descriptions will be the result of drug therapy. A comparison of the therapeutic outcome with the patient's molecular biomarkers will provide a therapeutic phenotype for that particular therapeutic profile. The failure of many pharmacogenomic-based therapies are likely the result of inconsistencies in the disease diagnosis and/or assessment of therapeutic outcomes through a lack of sufficient molecular biomarkers or a lack of proper interpretation of the biomarkers. Further complicating factors include the fact that the interaction of the environment with the genome, transcriptome, proteome, and metabolome is poorly understood; genetic regulation of metabolic pathways may be polygenic or oligogenic, with many different genes interacting in the regulatory process; the regulatory genes may exhibit allelic heterogeneity with many different predisposing risk alleles; different individuals may exhibit locus heterogeneity with different or an overlapping set of genes being important in a particular pathway; genetic interactions may be additive, synergistic, or epistatic; and resulting individual pathologies may be qualitative rather than all-or-nothing traits with thresholds determining clinical manifestations.

Genomics

Genomics is the technology behind the study of the full complement of genetic information, both coding and noncoding, in a organism's genome. The main genomics technique is the use of known SNPs as biomarkers to inform clinicians about subtypes of disease that require differential treatments and provide pharmacists with information for selection of the best therapeutic methodology to effectively manage the disease as well as provide an indication of the patients at risk of experiencing adverse reactions or those who will not respond to a given drug dose.

The general genotyping procedure for detecting known SNPs consists of PCR amplification of the region of interest in the genome, discrimination of the alleles in that region, and detection of the discrimination products. Many genotyping technologies are available to choose from, and each has their advantages and disadvantages (Table 6.14). Discriminating between the alleles in the genomic region being examined generally fall into one of the five techniques illustrated in Figure 6.46:

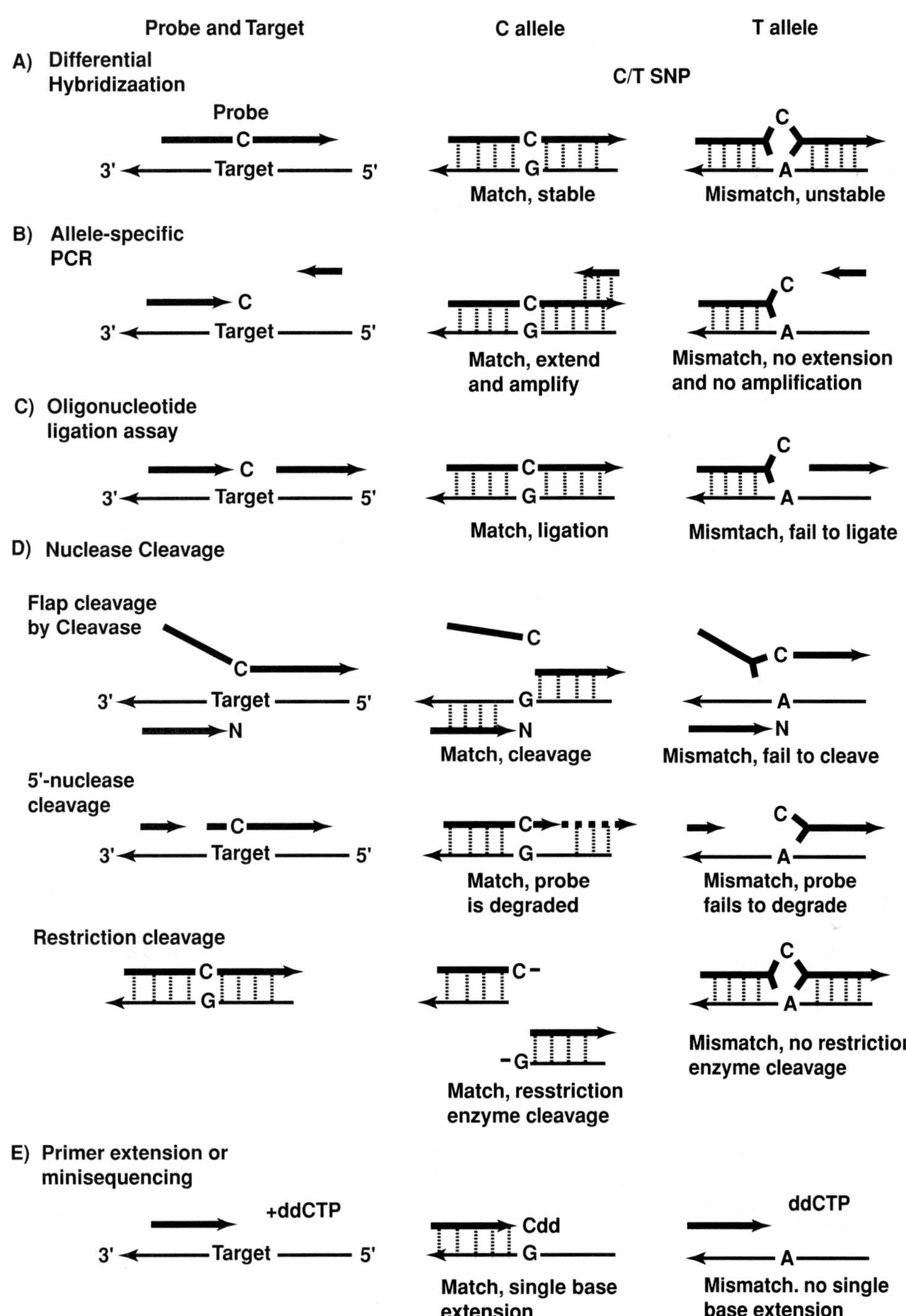

Fig. 6.46. Allele discrimination strategies for the detection of the C allele of a C/T transition. Figure summarizes the five main biochemical reaction principles that underlie the single-nucleotide polymorphism (SNP) genotyping technologies. Bold arrows indicate the probes; thinner arrows indicate the target. (From Syvanen AG. Accessing genetic variation: genotyping single-nucleotide polymorphisms. Nat Rev Genet 2001;2:930–942; Carlson CS, Newman TL, Nickerson DA. SNPing in the human genome. Curr Opin Chem Biol 2001; 5:78–85; with permission.)

1. Differential hybridization.
2. Allele-specific PCR.
3. Oligonucleotide ligation assay.
4. Nuclease cleavage (flap cleavage, 5′-nuclease cleavage, or restriction enzyme cleavage).
5. Minisequencing or primer extension.

Each of these detection techniques may be carried out in homogeneous reaction medium or on a solid support. Technology also is available that will carry out the detection reaction in homogeneous medium, then use a solid support to capture the product (see the discussion on minisequencing below).

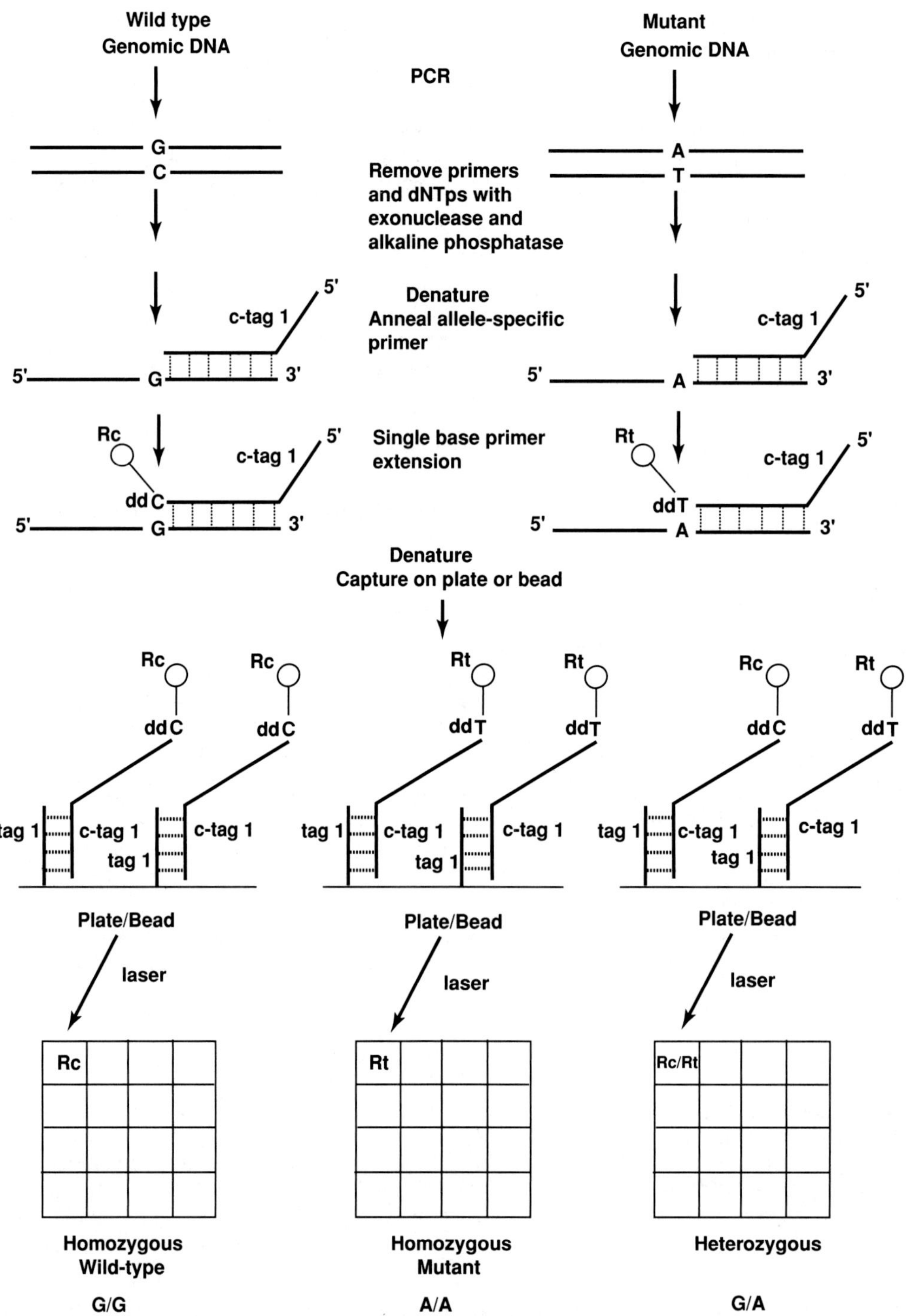

Fig. 6.47. Tag-Array and Bead technology. Tag 1 is specific for the G/A mutation at a particular position in the gene under investigation. Other tags can be designed for other single-nucleotide polymorphisms (SNPs) to permit multiplexing in the same well of the microtiter plate to produce and "array of arrays." R, reporter fluorescent label.

The technique of choice for high-throughput genotyping is the minisequencing/primer extension technique augmented with the 5′-tag technology to permit the purification of the extended products via specific tags (Fig. 6.47). The genomic region of interest is PCR amplified, and the amplified DNA is exposed to allele-specific primers with 5′-tags that are complementary to oligonucleotides immobilized at specific locations in the wells of microtiter plates or on specific colored beads. Single base extension using DNA polymerase and fluorescently labeled ddNTPs in solution is used to detect the SNP. The resulting fluorescently labeled and tagged DNA fragments are captured by complementary tags on microtiter plates or color-coded beads. Fluorescence resulting from laser excitation of the plates or beads is read by a detector and fed to a computer database for analysis and storage. Companies providing the single-base-extension tag–capture technology also provide a primer design service so that users can take advantage of multiplexing limited only by the capacity to design effective primers for the amplification and detection steps.

Transcriptomics

Transcriptomics is the technology behind the study of the full complement of mRNA transcripts in the cell's transcriptome and also is known as expression profiling. Methods of expression profiling are either "open" or "closed." Open systems do not require any advance knowledge of the sequence of the genome being examined; closed systems require some advance knowledge and usually involve the use of oligonucleotide or cDNA array hybridization technologies (the gene chip) and quantitative polymerase chain (Fig. 6.48).

The cDNA arrays are prepared by spotting gene-specific PCR products, including full-length cDNAs, collections of partially sequenced cDNAs, or randomly chosen cDNAs from any library of interest onto a glass, silicon, gel, or bead matrix or a nylon or nitrocellulose membrane. The matrix (most often glass) is coated with polylysine, amino silanes, or amino-reactive silanes to assist in the attachment of the cDNA probes. The PCR products of the clones are purified and spotted onto the matrix by robots through contact printing or noncontact piezo or ink-jet devices. After cross-linking the probe to the matrix by UV irradiation, the probe is made single stranded by heat or alkali treatment. The mRNA target is prepared from both a test and reference sample by reverse transcription to produce cDNA, which is then labeled with fluorescent probes (one for the test and another for the reference). The fluorescent targets are pooled and hybridized to the probe array under very stringent conditions. Laser excitation of the hybridized samples on the matrix and comparison of the fluorescence intensity of the reference sample with the fluorescence intensity of the test sample using computer algorithms yield an emission characteristic of the increase or decrease of mRNA expression under test conditions.

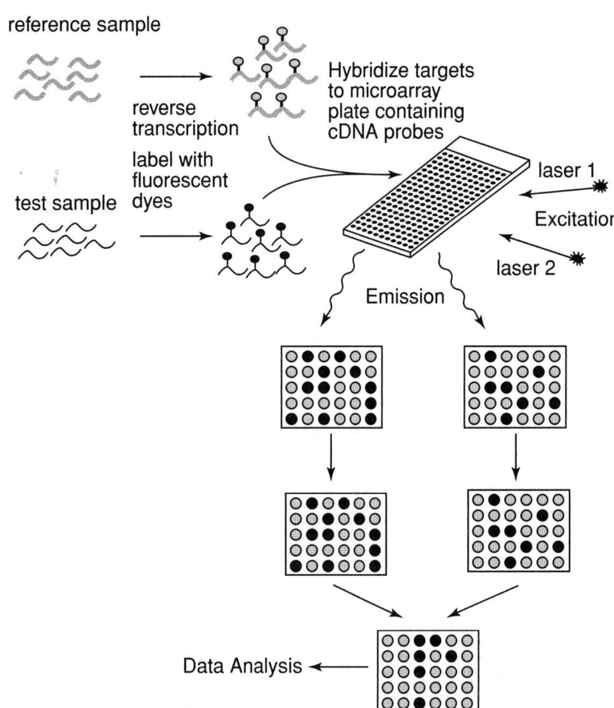

Fig. 6.48. (cDNA Chip): Schematic representation of a cDNA microarray chip. Probes of interest are obtained from DNA clones and printed on coated glass microscope slides. Analysis of mRNA expression is carried out by taking total mRNA from both a test and control sample; fluorescently labeling the samples with either Cye3- or Cye5-dUTP during a single round of reverse transcription; pooling the fluorescent targets and hybridizing to the immobilized probes on the array under very stringent conditions; laser excitation of the incorporated targets yields an emission with a characteristic spectra, which is measured using a scanning confocal laser microscope and analysed using a computer program (237).

Proteomics

Proteomics is the technology behind the study of the total protein complement of a genome, or the complete set of proteins expressed by a cell, tissue, or organism. The presence of an open reading frame in a DNA sequence indicates the presence of a gene, but it does not indicate gene transcription, RNA editing, translation, or posttranslational modification and the presence of isoforms. Analysis of the transcriptome does not indicate alteration of protein levels by proteolysis, recycling, and sequestration. Therefore, it is important to determine protein levels, protein expression, and protein–protein interactions directly.

Proteomics is divided into three main areas (238):

1. Microcharacterization for large-scale identification of proteins and posttranslational modifications (238).
2. Differential gel electrophoresis for comparison of protein levels (239).
3. Protein–protein interaction studies using protein chips (240), mass spectrometry isotope-coded affinity tag technology (241), and the yeast two-hybrid system (242).

Metabolomics

Metabolomics is the technology behind the measurement of metabolite concentrations, fluxes, and secretions in cells and tissues (metabolome). Metabolomics is at the cross-roads of genotype/phenotype interactions, where the interrelationship of metabolic pathways is considered to be the fundamental component of an organism's phenotype. Metabolomics is distinguished by the fact that metabolites are not directly linked to the genetic code but actually are products of a concerted action of many enzyme networks and other regulatory proteins (243). Metabolites also are more complex than nucleic acids, which are composed of four nucleotides, or proteins, which in turn are composed of 20 different amino acids. As a result, metabolites cannot be sequenced like genes and proteins so that their characterization requires that the structure of each metabolite be determined individually through description of elemental composition and stereochemical orientation of functional groups.

Metabolites are more than just products of enzyme-catalyzed reactions. They also are sensors and regulators of complex molecular interactions in the organism, and as a result, the composition of the metabolome can be altered by changes in the individual's environment. Therefore, a study of the metabolome is complicated not only by the uniqueness of the individual's genome but also by the uniqueness of the individual's environment. On the other side of the coin, however, one could consider the metabolome to be a very sensitive indicator of the individual's phenotype (244,245).

Metabolomics can be approached by using several different but related strategies:

1. Target analysis investigates the primary metabolic effect of a genetic variation, in which the analysis usually is limited to the substrate and/or product of the protein expressed by the altered gene.
2. Metabolic profiling limits the investigation to a number of predefined metabolites, usually in a specific metabolic pathway.
3. Metabolomics is a comprehensive analysis (both identification and quantification) of metabolites in a biological system, which investigates the effect of multiple genetic variations on many different biochemical pathways.
4. Metabolic fingerprinting is a strategy to screen a large number of metabolites for biological relevance in diagnostic or other analytical procedures in which it is important to rapidly distinguish between individuals in a population. Metabolic fingerprinting is the ultimate characterization of an individual's phenotype for disease diagnosis and drug therapy. Once the technological problems of high-throughput metabolic analysis is developed in this area, it will be a major competitor of SNP analysis in pharmacogenomics.

The analytical technologies used in metabolomic investigations are nuclear magnetic resonance and mass spectrometry alone or in combination with liquid or gas chromatographic separation of metabolites (243). Other techniques include thin-layer chromatography, Fourier-transform infrared spectrometry, metabolite arrays, and Raman spectroscopy.

Enviromics

Enviromics is the technology behind the measurement of environmental effects on disease diagnosis and drug therapy. This is a relatively new and undocumented area of pharmacogenomics, requiring considerable research to be carried out in the selection of environmental factors involved in personalized medicine and examining their effect on the genome, transcriptome, proteome, and metabolome in the production of molecular biomarkers.

The early concept of pharmacogenetics could be considered a very simple binary example of the gene–environment interaction, in which the environmental exposure is a drug and the genotype of the genes producing the metabolic enzymes involved in the metabolism of the particular drug are used to identify individuals at risk of adverse drug reactions or treatment failure. The population is then divided into the genotype that should avoid taking the drug and the genotype that should have the drug dose adjusted to avoid toxicity or treatment failure. It is, of course, naïve to assume that the drug is the only environmental factor playing a role in disease therapy. Indeed, under the holistic view of pharmacogenomics, a number of complicating factors lead to a successful drug therapy. Other examples of the binary gene–environment interaction are listed in Table 6.15.

SUMMARY

Genetic technology has evolved over the past 30 years to the stage where we have determined the entire sequence of the 3 billion base pairs in the human genome. The impact that such a scientific advance will have on our lives has yet to be determined, but the social, legal, ethical, and economic issues are certain to be extensive and complex. The HGP is developing scientific technology for the manipulation and analysis of the human genome. In turn, this analysis will provide valuable information concerning the relationship between genotype and potential for serious genetic disease. The HGP is already paying dividends in the analysis and therapy of monogeneic diseases, such as CF. The greatest killers of Western society, however, such as cancer, diabetes, cardiovascular disease, and many others, not only involve multiple genes but also are subject to environmental factors. As a result, many serious diseases will only be predicted with a certain potential. The possibility of preventative therapy that manipulates an individual's environment to reduce that potential will add another dimension to health care.

Table 6.15. Relative Risk Patterns in Gene-environment Interactions (246–248)

Gene Variant	Environmental Exposure	Relative Risk For: (XP)[a]	(PKU)[b]	(Emphysema)[c]
—	—	1.0	1.0	1.0
√	—	~1.0	1.0	Modest
—	√	Modest	1.0	Modest
√	√	Very high	Very high	High

Absent = —; Present = √;
[a]XP = Xeroderma pigmentosum, UV associated skin cancer in which incidence significantly increased with mutations and UV light exposure; XP mutations without UV exposure should reduce risk of skin cancer.
[b]PKU = Phenylketonuria, a condition associated with dietary phenylalanine and a deficiency of phenylalanine hydroxylase resulting from recessive mutations in the causative gene.
[c]Emphysema associated with a deficiency in the α-1 antitrypsin gene; highest risk seen in smokers at genetic risk; smokers and nonsmokers at genetic risk exhibit increased risk of emphysema.

We are likely to be inundated with information regarding the genetic composition of individuals and populations. Information management will be a daunting task after completion of the HGP. Already, the relatively new science of bioinformatics is developing methods for storing and retrieving the vast amounts of information that the HGP is generating. The social, legal, and ethical implications involved in the storage and release of information about the human individual must balance the individual's right to self-determination and the control of personal information against the interests of third parties and the public (11,249,250). One can see that the HGP is creating a revolution in the medical sciences, but the social, legal, and economic sciences also are being challenged to reevaluate their vision of the social structure. The future will see an altered form of health care using a genetic information infrastructure to contain costs and to predict outcomes, create advanced personalized therapies, and develop a predict-and-manage paradigm of health care (251).

References

1. Available at: http:/www.bioworld.com/servlet/com.accumedia.web.Dispatcher?next=TopDrugs51094. Accessed Sept. 2006.
2. Jacobs T. A rollercoaster ride. Nat Biotechnol 2006;24:284.
3. McKinnon B. Disease management—biotechnology and managed care pharmacy. Drug Benefit Trends, 1997(Dec):30–34.
4. Sindelar R. The pharmacy of the future—biotechnology and your practice. Drug Topics 1993;137:66–78.
5. Glassman RH, Sun AY. Biotechnology: identifying advances from the hype. Nat Rev 2004;3:177–183.
6. Young EA, ed. Beyond Borders—Global Technology Report 2005.
7. Conlan M. Biotechnology: are you ready for it? Drug Topics 1990; 134:34–41.
8. Scheindlin S. Update on biotechnology. Pharm Times 2003;65(5):42–48.
9. Drews II. Drug discovery today—and tomorrow. Drug Discov Today 2000;5:2–4.
10. Crick FH. On protein synthesis. Symposium of the Society for Experimental Biology 1957;**12**:138–163.
11. Kitcher P. The Lives To Come: The Genetic Relationship and Human Possibilities. New York: Simon and Schuster, 1997.
12. Calladine CR, Drew HR. Understanding DNA: The Molecule and How it Works, 2nd Ed. New York: Academic Press, 1997.
13. Saenger W. Principles of Nucleic Acid Structure. In: Cantor CR, ed. Springer Advanced Texts in Chemistry. New York: Springer-Verlag, 1994.
14. Lewin B. Genes IV, 4th Ed. Oxford: Oxford University Press and Cell Press, 1990.
15. Watson JD, Gilman M, Witkowski J, et al. Recombinant DNA, 2nd Ed. New York: Scientific American Books, W.H. Freeman and Company, 1992.
16. Sanger F, Nicklen S, Coulson AR. DNA sequencing with chain-terminating inhibitors. Proc Natl Acad Sci U S A 1977;74:5463–5467.
17. Maxam AM, Gilbert W. A new method of sequencing DNA. Proc Natl Acad Sci U S A 1977;74:560–564.
18. Atkinson A, Smith M. Solid-phase synthesis of oligodeoxyribonucleotides by the phosphite-triester method. In: Gait MJ, ed. Oligonucleotide Synthesis: A Practical Approach. Oxford: IRL Press Ltd, 1984:35–82.
19. Sproat BS, Gait MJ. Solid-phase synthesis of oligodeoxyribonucleotides by the phosphotriester method. In: Gait MJ, ed. Oligonucleotide Synthesis: A Practical Approach. Oxford: IRL Press Ltd, 1984:83–115.
20. Newton CR, Graham A. Introduction to biotechniques-PCR. Billington D, ed. PCR, 2nd Ed. New York: Springer-Verlag, 1997.
21. Alberts B, Bray D, Lewis J, et al., eds. Molecular Biology of the Cell, 3rd Ed. New York: Garland Publishing, 1994.
22. Freifelder D, MG, eds. Essentials of Molecular Biology, 2nd Ed. Boston: Jones & Bartlett Publishers; 1993.
23. Lodish H, Baltimore D, Berk A, eds. Molecular Cell Biology, 3rd Ed. New York: Scientific American Books, 1995.
24. Wolfe S. An introduction to Cell and Molecular Biology. Belmont, CA: Wadsworth Publishing Co., 1995.
25. Demuth J, ed. An Introduction to Pharmaceutical Biotechnology. Madison, Wisconsin: The Regents of the University of Wisconsin System, 1992.
26. Hall P. Pharmaceutical Biotechnology. New York: Global Medical Communications, 1992.
27. Hudson R., Black CD. Biotechnology—the new dimension in pharmacy practice. In: A Working Pharmacist's Guide. Toledo, OH: Council of Ohio Colleges of Pharmacy, 1999:1–14.
28. Tami JA. Recombinant DNA technology and therapeutics. Am Pharm 1991;NS31:63–69.
29. Construction of biologically functional bacterial plasmids in vitro. Proc Natl Acad Sci U S A 1973;70:3240–3244.
30. Davis HL, Whalen RG, Demeneix BA. Direct gene transfer into skeletal muscle in vivo: factors affecting efficiency of transfer and stability of expression. Hum Gene Ther 1993;4:151–159.
31. Walsh G. Biopharmaceutical: Biochemistry and Biotechnology. Chichester, UK: John Wiley & Sons Ltd., 1998:293–336.
32. Kadir F. Production of biotech compounds—cultivation and downstream processing. In: Crommelin DJA, Sindelar RD, eds. Pharmaceutical Biotechnology: An Introduction for Pharmacists and Pharmaceutical Scientists. Amsterdam: Harwood Academic Publishers, 1997:53–70.
33. Crommelin D. Formulation of biotech products, including biopharmaceutical considerations. In: Crommelin, DJA, Sindelar RD, eds. Pharmaceutical Biotechnology: An Introduction for Pharmacists and Pharmaceutical Scientists. Amsterdam: Harwood Academic Publishers, 1997: 71–99.
34. Seetharam R, Sharma SK, eds. Purification and Analysis of Recombinant Proteins. New York: Marcel Dekker, 1991.
35. Briggs J, Panfili PR. Quantitation of DNA and protein impurities in biopharmaceuticals. Anal Chem 1991;63:850–859.
36. Dwyer J, ed. Analytical chromatography of amino acids, peptides, and proteins. In: Franks F, ed. Protein Biotechnology. Totowa, NJ: Humana Press, 1993:49–90.
37. Hancock W, Willis B. The future of analytical chemistry in the characterization of biopharmaceuticals. Am Lab 1996:31–34.
38. Horvath C, Ettre LS, eds. Chromatography in Biotechnology. Washington, DC: American Chemical Society, 1993.
39. Prankerd R, Schulman SG. Analytical methods in biotechnology. In: Pezzuto JM, Johnson ME, Manasse HR, eds. Biotechnology and Pharmacy. New York: Chapman & Hall, 1993:71–96.
40. Gingold E. An introduction to recombinant DNA technology. In JM, Gingold EB, ed. Molecular Biology and Biotechnology, 3rd Ed. Cambridge, UK: Royal Society of Chemistry. 1993:13–32.

41. Franks FE. Solution properties of proteins. In: Protein Biotechnology. Totowa, NJ: Humana Press, 1993:133–189.
42. Arakawa T, Philo JS. Biophysical and biochemical analyses of recombinant proteins. In: Pharmaceutical Biotechnology: An Introduction for Pharmacists and Pharmaceutical Scientists, 2nd Ed. London: Taylor and Francis, 2002:25–52.
43. Oeswein J, Shire SJ. Physical biochemistry of protein drugs. In: Peptide and Protein Drug Delivery. New York: Marcel Dekker, 1991:167–202.
44. Samanen J. Physical biochemistry of peptide drugs: structure, properties, and stabilities of peptides compared with proteins. In: Peptide and Protein Drug Delivery. New York: Marcel Dekker, 1991:137–166.
45. Wang Y, Pearlman R, eds. Stability and Characterization of Protein and Peptide Drugs: Case Histories. New York: Plenum Press, 1993.
46. Burgess D. Drug Delivery Aspects of Biotechnology Products. In: Pezzuto JM, Johnson ME, Manasse HR, eds. Biotechnology and Pharmacy. New York: Chapman & Hall, 1993:116–151.
47. Lemke T. Review of Organic Functional Groups, 3rd Ed. Malvern, PA: Lea & Febiger, 1992.
48. Li S, Schoneich C, Borchardt RT. Chemical instability of proteins. Pharmaceut News 1995;12–16.
49. Frokjaer S, Otzen DE. Protein drug stability: a formulation challenge. Nature Reviews Drug Discovery 2005;4:298–306.
50. Powell M. Peptide stability in drug development: in vitro peptide degradation in plasma and serum. Annu Rep Med Chem 1993;28:285–294.
51. Genentech. Written Information on Storage, Reconstitution, compatibility, Stability, and Administration on File. South San Francisco: Genentech, Inc., 1995.
52. Banga A, Reddy IK. Biotechnology Drug: Pharmaceutical Issues. Pharm Times 1994;(March): 68–76.
53. Koeller J, Fields S. Biologic Response Modifiers. Contemp Pharm Issues 1991:4.
54. Evens R, Louie SG, Sindelar R, et al. Biotech Rx: Biotechnology in Pharmacy Practice: Science, Clinical Applications, and Pharmaceutical Care—Opportunities in Therapy Management. Washington, DC: American Pharmaceutical Association, 1997.
55. Fields S. Dispensing biotechnology products. Am Pharm 1993;NS33:28–29.
56. Kane B, Kuhn JG. Biotechnology: new roles and challenges for the pharmacist in ambulatory care. Drug Topics 1992:3–13.
57. Piascik P, Smith GH. Dispensing Biotechnology Products: Handling Professional Education and Product Information. In: Crommelin, D, Sindelar RD, eds. Pharmaceutical Biotechnology, An Introduction for Pharmacists and Pharmaceutical Scientists, 2nd Ed. London: Taylor and Francis, 2002:356–381.
58. Goldberg M, Gomezz-Orellana I. Challenges for the oral delivery of macromolecules. Nature Reviews Drug Discovery 2003;2:289–295.
59. Crommelin DJA, Storm G. Drug targeting. In Sammes G, Taylor JD, eds. Comprehensive Medicinal Chemistry. New York: Oxford Press, 1990; 661–701.
60. Bayley H. Protein therapy—delivery guaranteed. Nat Biotech 1999;17: 1066–1067.
61. Lee V. Peptide and Protein Drug Delivery. New York: Marcel Dekker, 1991.
62. Reddy I. Protein and peptide drug delivery. In: Zito SW, ed. Pharmaceutical Biotechnology: A Programmed Text. Lancaster, PA: Technomic Publishing, 1997:159–182.
63. Braeckman R. Pharmacokinetics and pharmacodynamics of peptide and proteins and drugs. In: Crommelin, DJA, Sindelar RD, eds. Pharmaceutical Biotechnology: An Introduction for Pharmacists and Pharmaceutical Scientists. Amsterdam: Harwood Academic Publishers, 1997:101–121.
64. Reddy I, Belmonte AA. Pharmacokinetics of Protein and Peptide Drugs. In: Zito SW, ed. Pharmaceutical Biotechnology: A Programmed Text. Lancaster, PA: Technomic Publishing, 1997:183–203.
65. Stewart, C., Fleming, RA., Biotechnology products: new opportunities and responsibilities for the pharmacist. Am J Hosp Pharm 1989:46(Suppl 2): S4–S8.
66. AHFS drug information. Am Soc Hospital Pharmacists 1999:2714–2728.
67. Facts and Comparisons. St. Louis: MO: 2000:287–290.
68. Beals J, Kovach PM. Insulin. In: Crommelin DJA, Sindelar RD, eds. Pharmaceutical Biotechnology: An introduction for Pharmacists and Pharmaceutical Scientists. Amsterdam: Harwood Academic Publishers, 1997:229–239.
69. Riley T, DeRuiter J. How effective are the new insulin analogs in regulating glucose metabolism? U.S. Pharmacist 2000;25(10):56–64.
70. Marian M. Growth hormones. In: Crommelin, DJA, Sindelar RD, eds. Pharmaceutical Biotechnology: An Introduction for Pharmacists and Pharmaceutical Scientists. Amsterdam: Harwood Academic Publishers, 1997:241–253.
71. Sam T, De Boer W. Follicle-stimulating hormone (FSH). In: Crommelin, DJA, Sindelar RD, eds. Pharmaceutical Biotechnology: An Introduction for Pharmacists and Pharmaceutical Scientists. Amsterdam: Harwood Academic Publishers, 1997:315–320.
72. Brixner D. Biotechnology products: an overview. In: Pezzuto JM, Johnson ME, Manasse HR, eds. Biotechnology and Pharmacy. New York: Chapman & Hall, 1993:392–395.
73. Higgins DL, Bennett WF. Tissue plasminogen activator: the biochemistry and pharmacology of variants produced by mutagenesis. Annu Rev Pharmacol Toxicol 1990;30:91–121.
74. Modi N. Recombinant tissue-type plasminogen activator and factor VIII. In: Crommelin DJA, Sindelar RD, eds. Pharmaceutical Biotechnology: An Introduction for Pharmacists and Pharmaceutical Scientists. Amsterdam: Harwood Academic Publishers, 1997:297–306.
75. Marian M, Sinicropi D. Recombinant human deoxyribonuclease. In: Crommelin DJA, Sindelar RD, eds. Pharmaceutical Biotechnology: An Introduction for Pharmacists and Pharmaceutical Scientists. Amsterdam: Harwood Academic Publishers, 2002:349–358.
76. Abbas AK, LA, Pober JS. Cellular and Molecular Immunology, 4th Ed. Philadelphia: WB Saunders, 2000:235–269.
77. Janeway CA, TP, Walport M, et al. Immunobiology: The Immune System in Health and Disease, 4th Ed. New York: Elsevier Science Ltd/Garland Publishing, 1999:288–292.
78. Roitt I, BJ, Male D. Immunology, 5th Ed. London: Mosby International, 1998:121–125.
79. Arai KI, et al. Cytokines: coordinators of immune and inflammatory responses. Annu Rev Biochem 1990;59:783–836.
80. Klegerman ME, PN. Lymphokines and monokines. In: Pezzuto JM, Johnson ME, Manasse HR, eds. Biotechnology and Pharmacy. New York: Chapman & Hall, 1993:53–70.
81. Louie SG, Jung B. Clinical effects of biologic response modifiers. Am J Hosp Pharm 1993;50(Suppl 3):S10–S18.
82. Pestka S, Krause CD, Walter MR. Interferons, interferon-like cytokines and their receptors. Immunol Rev 2004;202:8–32.
83. Rodriguez FH, Nelson S, Kolls JK. Cytokine therapeutics for infectious diseases. Curr Pharm Des 2000;665–680.
84. Urdal D. Cytokine receptors. Ann Rep Med Chem 1991;26:221–228.
85. Xing Z, WJ. Consideration of cytokines as therapeutic targets. Curr Pharm Design 2000;599–611.
86. Tami J. Interleukins and interferons. In: Crommelin, DJA, Sindelar RD eds. Pharmaceutical Biotechnology: An Introduction for Pharmacists and Pharmaceutical Scientists. Amsterdam: Harwood Academic Publishers, 1997:215–227.
87. Ebert S, De Muth JE. Hepatitis C: From Pathogenesis to Prognosis. Thousand Oaks, CA: Amgen, 1997.
88. Todd AV, et al. DzyNA-PCR: use of DNAzymes to detect and quantify nucleic acid sequences in a real-time fluorescent format. Clin Chem 2000;46: 625–630.
89. Romanelli F. Interleukin-2 for the management of HIV infection. J Am Pharm Assoc (Wash) 1999;39:867–868.
90. Rosenberg SA, Lotze M, Mule JJ. New approaches to the immunotherapy of cancer using interleukin-2. Ann Intern Med 1988;108:853–864.
91. Siegel JP, Puri RK. Interleukin-2 toxicity. J Clin Oncol 1991;9:694–704.
92. Solimando JD, Hanna WJ. Aldesleukin and levamisole. AMJ Hosp Pharm 1998;33:1172–1177.
93. Hussan D. New drugs of 1999 J Am Pharm Assoc 2000;40:181–221.
94. Mancano M. New drugs 1999. Pharm Times 2000;(March):67–91.
95. Piascik P. FDA approves fusion protein for treatment of lymphoma. J Am Pharm Assoc (Wash) 1999;39:571–572.
96. Vu K, Solimando DA Jr. Oprelvekin. AMJ Hosp Pharm 1998;33:387–389.
97. Cada DJ, Baker DE. AMJ Hosp Pharm 1999;34:462–481.
98. Newton RC, Decicco CP. Therapeutic potential and strategies for inhibiting tumor necrosis factor-alpha. J Med Chem 1999;42:2295–2314.
99. Flynn J, Rosman AW. Interleukins and interferons. In: Crommelin DJA, Sindelar RD, eds. Pharmaceutical Biotechnology: An Introduction for Pharmacists and Pharmaceutical Scientists. Amsterdam: Harwood Academic Publishers, 1997:185–214.
100. Huber SL, Yee G, Michau D. New Product Bulletin: Filgrastim. Washington, DC: American Pharmaceutical Association, 1993.
101. Kouides PA, DJ. The hematopoietic growth factors. In: Haskell CM, ed. Cancer Treatment. Philadelphia, WB Saunders, 1995:69–77.
102. Summerhayes M. Myeloid hematopoietic growth factors in clinical practice—a comparative review. Eur Hosp Pharm 1995(Parts 1 and II):1,30–36,67–74.
103. Faulds D, Sorkin EM. Epoetin (recombinant human erythropoietin). Drugs 1989;38:863–899.
104. Graber SE, Krantz SB. Erythropoietin: biology and clinical use. Hematol Oncol Clin North Am 1989;3:369–400.
105. Jensen JD, Madsen JK, Jensen LW, et al. Pharmacokinetics of epoetin in dialysis patients before and after Correction of the anemia. Drug Invest 1994; 8:278–287.
106. Johnson C. Epoetin alfa: a therapeutic achievement from pharmaceutical B biotechnology. U.S. Pharmacist 1989(Nov):1–11.
107. Mertelsmann R. Hematopoietins: biology, pathophysiology, and potentials therapeutic agents. Ann Oncol 1991;2:251–263.
108. Blackwell S, Crawford J. Colony-stimulating factors: clinical applications. Pharmacotherapy 1992;12(2 Pt 2):20S–31S.
109. Lieschke GJ, Burgess AW. Granulocyte colony-stimulating factor and granulocyte-macrophage colony-stimulating factor. N Engl J Med 1992;327:28–35.
110. Louie S, Rho J. Pharmacotherapeutics of biotechnology-produced drugs. In: Zito SW, ed. Pharmaceutical Biotechnology: A Programmed Text. Lancaster, PA: Technomic Publishing, 1997:224–231.
111. Petros WP. Pharmacokinetics and administration of colony-stimulating factors. Pharmacotherapy 1992;12(2 Pt 2):32S–38S.
112. Smith SP, Yee GC. Hematopoiesis. Pharmacotherapy 1992;12(2 Pt 2):11S–19S.
113. Becaplermin. Drugs Fut 1999;24:123–127.
114. Piascik P. Use of Regranex gel for diabetic foot ulcers. J Am Pharm Assoc (Wash) 1998;38:628–630.

115. Jiskoot W, Kersten GFA, Beuvery EC. Vaccines. In: Crommelin DJA, Sindelar RD, eds. Pharmaceutical Biotechnology: An Introduction for Pharmacists and Pharmaceutical Scientists. Amsterdam: Harwood Academic Publishers, 1997:255–278.
116. Glick BR, Pasternak J, eds, Molecular biotechnology. In: Principles and Applications of Recombinant DNA. Washington, DC: ASM Press, 1994: 207–233.
117. Hikal AH, Hikal EM. The ABCs of hepatitis. Drug Topics 1998;146:60–69.
118. Hoogenboom HR. Selecting and screening recombinant antibody libraries. Nat Biotechnol 2005;23:1105–1116.
119. Adair F. Immunogenicity: the last hurdle for clinically successful therapeutic antibodies. Pharm Tech 2000;24(10):50–56.
120. Adams VR, Karlix JL. Monoclonal antibodies. In: Concepts in Immunology and Immunotherapeutics. Bethesda, MD: American Society of Health-System Pharmacists, 1997:269–299.
121. Chamow SM, Ashkenazi A. Overview. In: Chamow SM, Ashkenazi A, eds. Antibody Fusion Proteins. New York: Wiley-Liss, 1999:1–12.
122. Shen W-C, Louie SG. Immunology for Pharmacy Students. Amsterdam: Harwood Academic Publishers, 1999:45–58.
123. Mayforth R. Designing Antibodies. San Diego, CA: Academic Press, 1993: 54–79.
124. Van Duijn G, Schram AW. Production and application of polyclonal and monoclonal antibodies. In: Franks F, ed. Protein Biotechnology. Totowa, NJ: Humana Press, 1993:365–393.
125. Chatenoud L, Baudrihaye MF, Chkoff N. Restriction of the human in vivo immune response against the mouse monoclonal antibody OKT3. J Immunol 1986;137:830–838.
126. Hakimi J, Mould D, Waldmann. TA. Development of Zenapax: a humanized anti-Tac antibody. In: Harris WJ, Adair JR, eds. Antibody Therapeutics. Boca Raton, FL: CRC Press, 1997:277–300.
127. Saleh MN, Khazaeli MB, Wheeler RH. Phase I trial of the murine monoclonal anti-GD2 antibody 14G2a in metastatic melanoma. Cancer Res 1992; 52:4342–4347.
128. Van Dijk MA, Vidarsson G. Monoclonal antibody-based pharmaceuticals. In: Crommelin D, Sindelar RD, eds. Pharmaceutical Biotechnology, An Introduction for Pharmacists and Pharmaceutical Scientists, 2nd Ed. London: Taylor and Francis, 2002:283–199.
129. Glover D. Fully human monoclonal antibodies come to fruition. Scrip Mag 1999:16–19.
130. Holliger P, Hoogenboom H. Antibodies come back from the brink. Nat Biotechnol 1998;16:1015–1016.
131. Kling J. Restoring magic to the bullets. Mod Drug Dis 1992;2:33–45.
132. Vaughan TJ, Osbourn JK, Tempest PR. Human antibodies by design. Nat Biotechnol 1998;16:535–539.
133. Huse W. Combinatorial antibody expression libraries in filamentous phage. In: Borrebaeck CAK, ed. Antibody Engineering—A Practical Guide. New York: W.H. Freeman and Company, 1992:103–120.
134. Pray W. Nonprescription Product Therapeutics, 2nd Ed. Philadelphia: Lippincott Williams & Wilkins, 2006:778–799.
135. Quattrocchi E, Hove I. Ovulation & pregnancy home testing products. U.S. Pharmacist 1998;23(9):54–63.
136. Rosenthal WM, Briggs GC. Home testing and monitoring devices. In: Allen LV Jr., Berardi RR, DeSimone EM II, et al., eds. Handbook of Nonprescription Drugs. Washington, DC: American Pharmaceutical Association, 2000:917–942.
137. Ledley FD. Pharmaceutical approach to somatic gene therapy. Pharm Res 1996;13:1595–1614.
138. Blau HM, Springer ML. Molecular medicine: gene therapy—a novel form of drug delivery. N Engl J Med 1995;333:1204–1207.
139. Ledley FD. Nonviral gene therapy: the promise of genes as pharmaceutical products. Hum Gene Ther 1995;6:1129–1144.
140. Verma IM, Somia N. Gene therapy—promises, problems, and prospects. Nature 1997;389:239–242.
141. Anderson WF. Human gene therapy. Nature 1998;392(Suppl):25–30.
142. Vile RG, Russel SJ. Retroviruses as vectors. BMJ 1995;51:12–30.
143. Efstathiou S, Minson AC. Herpes virus–based vectors. Br Med Bull 1995;51: 45–55.
144. Fink DJ, Glorioso JC. Engineering herpes simplex virus vectors for gene transfer to neurons. Nat Med 1997;3:357–359.
145. Chu G, Hayakawa H, Berg P. Electroporation for the efficient transfection of mammalian cells with DNA. Nucleic Acids Res 1987;15:1311–1326.
146. Kinosita K Jr., Tsong TY. Voltage-induced pore formation and hemolysis of human erythrocytes. Biochim Biophys Acta 1977;471:227–242.
147. Neumann E, Schaefer-Ridder M, Wang Y, et al. Gene transfer into mouse lyoma cells by electroporation in high electric fields. EMBO J, 1982;1: 841–845.
148. Klein TM, Wolf ED, Wu R, et al. High-velocity microprojectiles for delivering nucleic acids into living cells. Nature 1987;327:70–73.
149. Williams RS, Johnston SA, Riedy M, et al. Introduction of foreign genes into tissues of living mice by DNA-coated microprojectiles. Proc Natl Acad Sci U S A 1991;88:2726–2730.
150. Christou P, McCabeus DE, Martinelli BJ, et al. Soybean genetic engineering—commercial production of transgenic plants. Trends Biotechnol 1990; 8:145–151.
151. Tang D-C, DeVit M, Johnston SA. Genetic immunization is a simple method for eliciting an immune response. Nature 1993;356:152–154.
152. Graham FL, Van der Eb AJ. A new technique for the assay of infectivity of human adenovirus 5 DNA. Virology 1973;52:456-460.
153. Loyter A, Scangon GA, Ruddle FH. Mechanisms of DNA uptake by mammalian cells: fate of exogenously added DNA monitored by the use of fluorescent dyes. Proc Natl Acad Sci U S A 1982;79:422–426.
154. Chen C, Okayama H. High-efficiency transformation of mammalian cells by plasmid DNA. Mol Cell Biol 1987;7:2745–2752.
155. Kawai S, Nishizawa M. New procedure for DNA transfection with polycation and dimethyl sulfoxide. Mol Cell Biol 1984;4:1172–1174.
156. Farber FE, Melnick JL, Butel JS. Optimal conditions for uptake of exogenous DNA by Chinese hamster lung cells deficient in hypoxanthine-guanine phosphoribosyltransferase. Biochim Biophys Acta 1975;390:298–311.
157. Mahato RI, Rolland A, Thomlinson E. Cationic lipid-based gene delivery systems: pharmaceutical perspectives. Pharm Res 1997;14:853–859.
158. Felgner JH, Kumar R, Sridhar CN, et al. Enhanced gene delivery and mechanism studies with a novel series of cationic lipid formulations. J Biol Chem 1994;269:2550–2561.
159. Felgner PL, Gadek TR, Holm M, et al. Lipofection: a highly efficient, lipid-mediated DNA-transfection procedure. Proc Natl Acad Sci U S A 1987;84: 7413–7417.
160. Tomlinson E, Rolland AP. Controllable gene therapy. Pharmaceutics of non-vial gene delivery systems. Journal of Controlled Release 1996;39:357–372.
161. Behr J-P, Demeneix B, Loeffler J-P, et al. Efficient gene transfer into mammalian primary endocrine cells with lipopolyamine-coated DNA. Proc Natl Acad Sci U S A 1989;86:6982–6986.
162. Legendre J-Y, Szoka FCJ. Cyclic amphipathic peptide-DNA complexes mediate high-efficiency transfection of adherent mammalian cells. Proc Natl Acad Sci U S A 1993;90:893–897.
163. Zhou X, Huang L. DNA transfection mediated by cationic liposomes containing lipopolylysine: characterization and mechanism of action. Biochim Biophys Acta 1994;1189:195–203.
164. Li S, Gao X, Son K, et al. DC-Chol lipid system in gene transfer. Journal of Controlled Release 1996;39:373–381.
165. Pinnaduwage P, Schmit L, Huang L. Use of a quaternary ammonium detergent in liposome mediated DNA transfection of mouse L-cells. Biochim Biophys Acta 1989;985:33–37.
166. Wagner E, Cotton M, Foisner R, et al. Transferrin-polycation-DNA complexes: the effect of polycations on the structure of the complex DNA delivery to cells. Proc Natl Acad Sci U S A 1991;88:4255–4259.
167. Huxley C. Mammalian artificial chromosomes: a new tool for gene therapy. Gene Ther 1994;1:7–12.
168. Calos MP. The potential of extrachromosomal replicating vectors for gene therapy. Trends Genet 1996;12:463–466.
169. Vos J-MH. Mammalian artificial chromosomes as tools for gene therapy. Curr Opin Genet Dev 1998;8:351–359.
170. Willard HF. A systematic approach toward understanding human chromosome structure and function. Proc Natl Acad Sci U S A 1996;93: 6847–6850.
171. Willard HF. Human artificial chromosomes coming into focus. Nat Biotechnol 1998;16:415–416.
172. Melchior F, Gerace L. Mechanisms of nuclear protein import. Curr Opin Cell Biol 1995;7:310–318.
173. Kawabata K, Takakura Y, Hashida M. The fate of plasmid DNA after intravenous injection in mice: involvement of scavenger receptors in its hepatic uptake. Pharm Res 1995;12:825–830.
174. Stankovics J, Crane AM, Andrevos E, et al. Overexpression of human methylmalonyl CoA mutase in mice after in vivo gene transfer with asialoglycoprotein/polylysine/DNA complexes. Hum Gene Ther 1994;5:1095–1104.
175. Manthorpe M, Cornefort-Jensen F, Hartikka J, et al. Gene therapy by intramuscular injection of plasmid DNA: studies on firefly luciferase gene expression in mice. Hum Gene Ther 1993;4:419–431.
176. Sikes M, O'Malley BW Jr, Finegold MJ, et al. In vivo gene transfer into rabbit and thyroid follicular cells by direct DNA injection. Hum Gene Ther 1994;5:837–844.
177. Yovandich J, O'Malley BW Jr, Sikes M, et al. Gene transfer to synovial cells by intra-articular administration of plasmid DNA. Hum Gene Ther 1995;6: 603–610.
178. Ledley TS, Ledley FD. Multicompartment, numerical model of cellular events in the pharmacokinetics of gene therapies. Hum Gene Ther 1994;5:679–691.
179. Wang DG, Fan JB, Siao CJ, et al. Large-scale identification, mapping, and genotyping of single-nucleotide polymorphisms in the human genome. Science 1998;280:1077–1082.
180. Kirchheiner J, Brockmoller J. Clinical consequences of cytochrome P450 2C9 polymorphisms. Clin Pharmacol Ther 2005;77:1–16.
181. Griffin JL, Shockcor JP. Metabolic profiles of cancer cells. Nat Rev Cancer 2004;4:551–61.
182. Group BDW. Biomarkers and surrogate endpoints: preferred definitions and conceptual framework. Clin Pharmacol Ther 2001;69:89–95.
183. Saiki RK, Walsh PS, Levenson CH, et al. Genetic analysis of amplified DNA with immobilized sequence-specific oligonucleotide probes. Proc Natl Acad Sci U S A 1989;86:6230–6234.
184. Brockmoller J, Kirchheiner J, Meisel C, et al. Pharmacogenetic diagnostics of cytochrome P450 polymorphisms in clinical drug development and in drug treatment. Pharmacogenomics 2000;1:125–151.
185. Hacia JG, Brody LC, Collins FS. Applications of DNA chips for genomic analysis. Mol Psychiatry 1998;3:483–492.

186. Emahazion T, Feuk L, Jobs M, et al. SNP association studies in Alzheimer's disease highlight problems for complex disease analysis. Trends Genet 2001;17:407–413.
187. Howell WM, et al. Dynamic allele-specific hybridization. A new method for scoring single-nucleotide polymorphisms. Nat Biotechnol 1999;17:87–88.
188. Kostrikis S, Tyagi S, Mhlanga MM, et al. Spectral genotyping of human alleles. Science 1998;279:1228–1229.
189. Livak KJ. Allelic discrimination using fluorogenic probes and the 5′-nuclease assay. Genetic Analysis 1999;14:143–149.
190. Latif S, Bauer-Sardina I, Ranade K, et. al. Fluorescence polarization in homogeneous nucleic acid analysis. II: 5′-nuclease assay. Genome Res 2001;11:436–440.
191. Hsu TM, Chen X, Duan S, et al. A universal SNP genotyping assay with fluorescence polarization detection. BioTechniques 2001;31:560–570.
192. Kaiser MW, Lyamicheva N, Ma W, et al. A comparison of eubacterial and archaeal structure-specific 5′-exonucleases. J Biol Chem 1999;274:21387–21394.
193. Kwiatkowksi RW, Lyamichev VI, de Arruda M, et al. Clinical, genetic, and pharmacogenetic applications of the Invader assay. Mol Diagn, 1999;4:353–364.
194. Hall JG, Eis PS, Law SM, et al. Sensitive detection of DNA polymorphisms by the serial invasive signal amplification reaction. Proc Natl Acad Sci U S A 2000;97:8272–8277.
195. Edman CF, Raymond DE, Wu DJ, et al. Electric field directed nucleic acid hybridization by electric field control. Nucleic Acids Res 1997;25:4907–4914.
196. Cornell BA, Braach-Maksvytis VL, King LG, et al. A biosensor that uses ion channel switches. Nature 1997;387:580–583.
197. Wang J, Cai X, Rivas G, et al. Nucleic-acid immobilization, recognition, and detection at chronopotentiometric DNAchips. Biosens Bioelectron 1997;12: 587–599.
198. Heller MJ, Forster AH, Tu E. Active microelectronic chip devices which utilize controlled electrophoretic fields for multiplex DNA hybridization and other genomic applications. Electrophoresis 2000;21:157–164.
199. Radtkey R, Feng L, Muralhidar M, et al. Rapid, high-fidelity analysis of simple sequence repeats on an electronically active DNA microchip. Nucleic Acids Res 2000;28:E17; pp i–vi.
200. Westin L, Xu X, Miller C, et al. Anchored multiplex amplification on a microelectronic chip array. Nat Biotechnol 2000;18:199–204.
201. Mein CA, Barratt BJ, Dunn MG, et al. Evaluation of single-nucleotide polymorphism typing with invader on PCR amplicons and its automation. Genome Res 2000;10:330–343.
202. Myakishev MV, Khripin Y, Hu S, et al. High-throughput SNP genotyping by allele-specific PCR with universal energy-transfer-labeled primers. Genome Res 2001;11:163–169.
203. Germer S, Higuchi R. Single-tube genotyping without oligonucleotide probes. Genome Res 1999;9:72–78.
204. Beaudet L, Bedard J, Breton B, et al. Homogeneous assays for single-nucleotide polymorphism typing using AlphaScreen. Genome Res 2001;11: 600–608.
205. Nazarenko IA, Bhatnagar SK, Hohman RJ. A closed tube format for amplification and detection of DNA based on energy transfer. Nucleic Acids Res 1997;25:2516–2521.
206. Whitcombe D, Theaker J, Guy SP, et al. Detection of PCR products using self-probing amplicons and fluorescence. Nat Biotechnol 1999;17:804–807.
207. Pastinen T, Raitio M, Lindroos K, et al. A system for specific, high-throughput genotyping by allele-specific primer extension on microarrays. Genome Res 2000;10:1031–1042.
208. Tonisson N, et al. Unravelling genetic data by arrayed primer extension. Clin Chem Lab Med, 2000;38:165–170.
209. Shumaker JM, Metspalu A, Caskey CT. Mutation detection by solid-phase primer extension. Hum Mutat 1996;**7**:346–354.
210. Pastinen T, et al. Minisequencing: a specific tool for DNA analysis and diagnostics on oligonucleotide arrays. Genome Res 1997;**7**:606–614.
211. Dubiley S, Kirillov E, Mirzabekov A. Polymorphism analysis and gene detection by minisequencing on an array of gel-immobilized primers. Nucleic Acids Res 1999;27:E19; pp i–vi.
212. Chen X, Kwok P-Y. Template-directed dye-terminator incorporation (TDI) assay: a homogeneous DNA diagnostic method based on fluorescence energy transfer. Nucleic Acids Res 1997;25:347–353.
213. Chen J, Giovannucci EL, Hunter DJ. MTHFR polymorphism, methyl-replete diets, and the risk of colorectal carcinoma and adenoma among U.S. men and women: an example of gene-environment interactions in colorectal tumorigenesis. J Nutr 1999;129(Suppl 2):560S–564S.
214. Buetow KH, Edmonson M, MacDonald R, et al. High-throughput development and characterization of a genome wide collection of gene-based single-nucleotide polymorphism markers by chip-based matrix-assisted laser desorption/ionization time-of-flight mass spectrometry. Proc Natl Acad Sci U S A 1996;98:581–584.
215. Ross P, Hall L, Smirnov I, et al. High-level multiplex genotyping by MALDI-TOF mass spectrometry. Nat Biotechnol 1998;16:1347–1351.
216. Sauer S, Lechner D, Berlin K, et al. A novel procedure for efficient genotyping of single-nucleotide polymorphisms. Nucleic Acids Res 2000;28:E13; pp i–viii.
217. Braun A, Little DP, Koster H. Detecting *CFTR* gene mutations by using primer oligo base extension and mass spectrometry. Clin Chem 1997;43:1151–1158.
218. Nordstrom T, Nourizad K, Ronaghi M, et al. Method enabling pyrosequencing on double-stranded DNA. Anal Biochem 2000;282:186–193.
219. Ahmadian A, Gharizadeh B, Gustafsson AC. Single-nucleotide polymorphism analysis by pyrosequencing. Anal Biochem 2000;280:103–110.
220. Ronaghi M. Pyrosequencing sheds light on DNA sequencing. Genome Res 2001;11:3–11.
221. Alderborn A, Kristofferson A, Hammerling U. Determination of single-nucleotide polymorphisms by real-time pyrophosphate DNA sequencing. Genome Res 2000;10(8):p. 1249–1258.
222. Nyren P, Pettersson B, Uhlen M. Solid-phase DNA minisequencing by an enzymatic luminometric inorganic pyrophosphate detection assay. Anal Biochem 1993;208:171–175.
223. Fan JB, Chen X, Halushka MK, et al. Parallel genotyping of human SNPs using generic high-density oligonucleotide tag arrays. Genome Res 2000;10:853–860.
224. Chen J, Iannone MA, Li MS, et al. A microsphere-based assay for multiplexed single-nucleotide polymorphism analysis using single base chain extension. Genome Res 2000;**10**:549–557.
225. Cai H, White PS, Torney D, et al. Flow cytometry-based minisequencing: a new platform for high-throughput single-nucleotide polymorphism scoring. Genomics 2000;66:135–143.
226. Hirschhorn JN, Sklar P, Lindblad-Toh K, et al. SBE-TAGS: an array-based method for efficient single-nucleotide polymorphism genotyping. Proc Natl Acad Sci U S A 2000;97:12164–12169.
227. Nickerson DA, Kaiser R, Lappin S, et al. Automated DNA diagnostics using an ELISA-based oligonucleotide ligation assay. Proc Natl Acad Sci U S A 1990;87:8923–8927.
228. Grossman PD, Bloch W, Brinson E, et al. High-density multiplex detection of nucleic acid sequences: oligonucleotide ligation assay and sequence-coded separation. Nucleic Acids Res 1994;22:4527–4534.
229. Nilsson M, Malmgren H, Samiotaki M, et al. Padlock probes: circularizing oligonucleotides for localized DNA detection. Science 1994;265:2085–2088.
230. Baner J, Nilsson M, Mendel-Hartvig M, et al. Signal amplification of padlock probes by rolling circle replication. Nucleic Acids Res 1998;26:5073–5078.
231. Lizardi PM, Huang X, Zhu Z, et al. Mutation detection and single-molecule counting using isothermal rolling-cycle amplification. Nat Genet 1998;19: 225–232.
232. Zhang DY, Brandwein M, Hsuih TC, et al. Amplification of target-specific, ligation-dependent circular probe. Gene 1998;211:277–285.
233. Chen J, Stampfer MJ, Hough HL, et al. A prospective study of N-acetyltransferase genotype, red meat intake, and risk of colorectal cancer. Cancer Res 1998;58:3307–3311.
234. Gerry NP, Witowski NE, Day J, et al. Universal DNA microarray method for multiplex detection of low abundance point mutations. J Mol Biol 1999;292: 251–262.
235. Syvanen AC. Accessing genetic variation: genotyping single-nucleotide polymorphisms. Nat Rev Genet 2001;2:930–942.
236. Carlson CS, Newman TL, Nickerson DA. SNPing in the human genome. Curr Opin Chem Biol 2001;5:78–85.
237. Duggan DJ, Bittner M, Chen Y, et al. Expression profiling using cDNA microarrays. Nat Genet 1999;21(Suppl 1):10–14.
238. Pandey A, Mann M. Proteomics to study genes and genomes. Nature 2000;405:837–846.
239. Tonge R, Shaw J, Middleton B, et al. Validation and development of fluorescence two-dimensional differential gel electrophoresis proteomics technology. Proteomics 2001;1:377–396.
240. Zhu H, Snyder M. Protein arrays and microarrays. Curr Opin Chem Biol 2001;5:40–45.
241. Smolka MB, Zhou H, Purkayastha S, et al. Optimization of the isotope-coded affinity tag-labeling procedure for quantitative proteome analysis. Anal Biochem 2001;297:25–31.
242. Uetz P, Giot L, Cagney G, et al. A comprehensive analysis of protein–protein interactions in *Saccharomyces cerevisiae*. Nature 2000;403:623–627.
243. Saghatelian A, Cravatt BF. Global strategies to integrate the proteome and metabolome. Curr Opin Chem Biol 2005;9:62–68.
244. Bino RJ, Hall RD, Fiehn O, et al. Potential of metabolomics as a functional genomics tool. Trends Plant Sci 2004;9:418–425.
245. Fiehn O. Metabolomics—the link between genotypes and phenotypes. Plant Mol Biol 2002;48:155–171.
246. Chan AT, Tranah GJ, Giovannucci EL, et al. Genetic variants in the UGT1A6 enzyme, aspirin use, and the risk of colorectal adenoma. J Natl Cancer Inst 2005;97:457–460.
247. Khoury MJ, Adams MJ Jr, Flanders WD. An epidemiologic approach to ecogenetics. Am J Hum Genet 1988;42:89–95.
248. Botto LD, Khoury MJ. Commentary: facing the challenge of gene-environment interaction: the two-by-four table and beyond. Am J Epidemiol 2001;153: 1016–1020.
249. Wood-Harper J, Harris J. Ethics of human genome analysis: some virtues and vices. In: Marteau T, Richards M, eds. The Troubled Helix. Cambridge, UK: Cambridge University Press, 1996:274–294.
250. Harris J. Clones, Genes, and Immortality: Ethics and the Genetic Revolution. Oxford: Oxford University Press, 1998.
251. Bezold C, Halperin JA, Eng JL, eds. 2020 Visions: Health Care Information Standards and Technologies. Rockville, MD: The United States Pharmacopeial Convention, Inc., 1993.

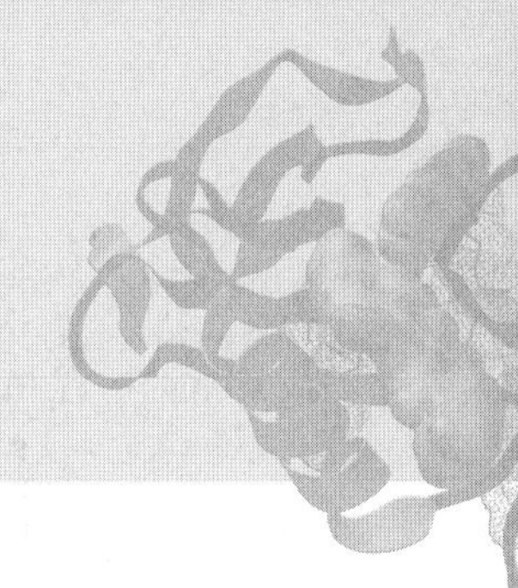

7. *Peptide and Protein Drugs*

MICHAEL MOKOTOFF

DRUGS COVERED IN THIS CHAPTER:

ADRENOCORTICOTROPIN HORMONES
- Cosyntropin

GONADOTROPIN-RELEASING HORMONES
- Abarelix
- Cetrorelix acetate
- Ganirelix acetate
- Goserelin acetate
- Histrelin acetate
- Leuprolide acetate
- Nafarelin acetate
- Triptorelin pamoate

GONADOTROPINS
- Follitropin alfa
- Follitropin beta
- Lutropin alfa
- Menotropins
- Urofollitropin

GROWTH HORMONES
- Pegvisomant
- Somatropin

PANCREATIC HORMONES
- Insulin
- Glucagon
- Amylin
- Pramlintide acetate

PARATHYROID HORMONES
- Teriparatide

PLACENTAL HORMONES
- Choriogonadotropin
- Human chorionic gonadotropin

PITUITARY HORMONES
- Desmopressin
- Oxytocin
- Vasopressin

SOMATOSTATINS
- Indium pentetreotide
- Octreotide acetate

THYROID HORMONES
- Calcitonin salmon

INTRODUCTION

Living cells produce a remarkable variety of macromolecules that serve as structural components, biocatalysts, hormones, receptors, or storehouse of genetic information. These macromolecules, proteins, nucleic acids, and polysaccharides are biopolymers constructed of monomer units or building blocks; for proteins the monomer units are α-amino acids. Proteins may contain substances other than α-amino acids, for example, glycoproteins also contain carbohydrates. The three-dimensional structure and the biological properties of proteins, however, are largely determined by the kinds of amino acids present, the order in which they are linked together in the polypeptide chain, and thus the spatial relationship of one α-amino acid to another.

Bacterial cells, plants, and animals contain a wide variety of peptides and proteins, consisting anywhere from 3 to 200 or more residues (each amino acid is considered to be a residue), many of which have profound biological activity. In humans, biological functions as varied as sexual reproduction, induction or augmentation of uterine contraction during labor, growth, calcium metabolism, formation of glucocorticoid and mineralocorticoid steroids, production of thyroid hormones, water balance, erythropoiesis, and glucose metabolism are known to be under the control of peptides and proteins. Proteins also are important as enzymes, as structural components of various tissues, and for receptor conformation. As a result, peptides and proteins are increasingly being used or investigated for their potential in drug therapy.

The production of many of these important peptides and proteins, via synthetic procedures as well as through biotechnology, very much involves the pharmaceutical industry. Of necessity, peptides of low to moderate molecular weight, chemically modified peptides, and those containing pseudopeptide bonds or fraudulent amino acids will continue to be made by synthetic procedures rather than through biotechnology. Therefore, this chapter discusses certain physicochemical properties of peptides and proteins, the limitations to their use as medicinal agents, the methodology used in their synthesis, and modifications aimed to improve their stability and biological action. With this backdrop, the chapter continues with a discussion of the importance of commercially available peptide and protein hormones that are used either diagnostically or in treating a variety of disease conditions. Many of these hormones are available as chemical analogues, and these also are discussed, particularly the chemical changes made and the implications of these changes to the resulting biological action.

History

Strange as it may seem to the reader, shortly before the end of the nineteenth century, it was not known that proteins consisted of peptide bonds between individual amino acids. The revelation that the linkages between amino acids were, indeed, amide bonds (peptide bonds) was not made until the early 1900s by two individuals, Hofmeister (1) and Fischer (2). The complexity of having multiple reactive functional groups in the amino acids, thus necessitating selective protection, led to great difficulty in the ability to synthesize peptides. The breakthrough came in 1932, when Bergmann and Zervas (3) developed a suitable blocking group for the α-amino function, the carbobenzoxy group (discussed later). Incentive for the further development of peptide synthesis came with the discovery in the 1940s of the peptide antibiotics as biologically important natural products. In the 1950s, two important discoveries involving peptide hormones, the structure elucidation and synthesis of oxytocin by du Vigneaud et al. (4) and the determination of the structure of insulin by Sanger (5), helped to solidify the importance of amino acids, peptides, and their synthesis. In the late 1960s and early 1970s, two independent groups, led by Drs. Guillemin and Schally, reported on the isolation, identification, and synthesis of several important hypothalamic hormones, such as thyrotropin-releasing hormone (6), luteinizing hormone releasing hormone (7), and growth hormone inhibiting factor (somatostatin) (8).

These discoveries led to further refinements in the synthesis of peptides, particularly such advances as the formation of the peptide bond via the coupling agent N,N′-dicyclohexylcarbodiimide (DCC) (9), the selective blocking of the α-amine functionality by the *tert*-butyloxycarbonyl (Boc) acid-sensitive group (10), and the 9-fluorenylmethyloxycarbonyl (Fmoc) base-sensitive group (11). Almost certainly, the ultimate achievement in peptide synthesis was the report by Merrifield (12) of his concept in which peptides could be more rapidly synthesized by "growing" the peptides on solid support. Merrifield's goals were to simplify and accelerate peptide synthesis in a way that would make the preparation of long peptides both practical and amenable to automation. These goals were realized in a few short years, and the solid-phase synthesis of a wide variety of peptides and proteins continues to appear in the literature.

The importance of these historical events can be measured, in part, by the fact that Nobel Prizes were awarded to those individuals most responsible for several of these advances. The following are quotes from the Nobel Prize Committee: Dr. du Vigneaud (Chemistry, 1955) "for his work on biochemically important sulfur compounds, especially for the first synthesis of a hormone"; Dr. Sanger (Chemistry, 1958) "for his work on the structure of proteins, especially that of insulin"; Drs. Guillemin and Schally (Medicine and Physiology, 1977, also with Dr. Yalow) for their work that "opened new vistas within biological and medical research far outside the border of their own spheres of interest"; Dr. Merrifield (Chemistry, 1984) for the development of a "simple and ingenious automated laboratory technique for rapidly synthesizing peptide chains in large quantities on a routine basis, called solid-phase peptide synthesis."

CHEMICAL AND PHYSICAL PROPERTIES OF PEPTIDES AND PROTEINS

Peptides and proteins are very similar in that they are made up of repeating units, or residues, of α-amino acids that are linked together by peptide bonds, also known as amide bonds. Peptides with fewer than 15 residues are known as oligopeptides (e.g., gonadotropin-releasing hormone [GnRH] contains 10 residues); those consisting of 15 to 50 residues (e.g., adrenocorticotropin hormone consists of 39 residues) are known as polypeptides. A polypeptide that contains more than 50 amino acid residues generally is referred to as a protein (e.g., parathyroid hormone contains 84 residues) (13).

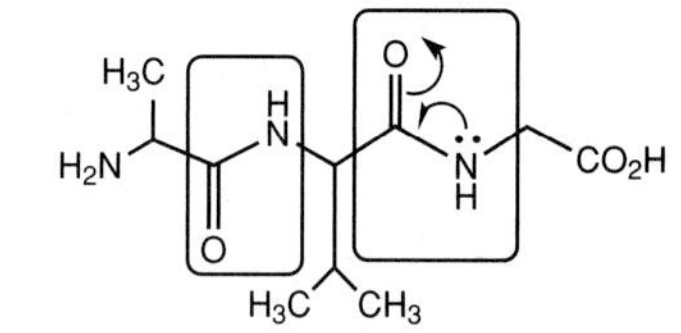

Fig. 7.1. A tripeptide, Ala-Val-Gly, indicating the planarity of the peptide bonds that are framed in the rectangles.

The Peptide Bond and Primary Structure of Peptides

A peptide consists of at least two amino acids linked by a peptide bond, an example of which is the tripeptide alanine-valine-glycine (Ala-Val-Gly) (Fig. 7.1). The properties of the peptide bonds that make up this tripeptide (framed in the rectangle of Fig. 7.1), like other amide bonds, are controlled by the conjugation that exists between the lone-pair electrons on the nitrogen and the adjacent carbonyl group. The major consequence of this conjugation is that peptide bonds are planar, as a result of the requirement that the nitrogen, carbon, and oxygen *p*-orbitals must lie in the same plane for the nitrogen lone-pair to conjugate with the carbonyl π-bond (14). It is this planarity and lack of free rotation about the C—N bond, which is so important for the three-dimensional shape of peptides and proteins, that accounts for the existence of two stable conformations, *cis* and *trans*. In natural peptides and proteins, however, the peptide bond largely exists in the *trans* form. The symbols for the natural, DNA-encoded amino acids found in human protein are shown in Table 7.1.

In the tripeptide shown in Figure 7.1, Ala-Val-Gly can be referred to as the primary structure of this peptide. That is, the primary structure of any peptide or protein is the number and sequence of the amino acids present (13). By convention, if the sequence is fully known, the peptide structures are written with the symbol for the α-amino, or N-terminal, residue at the left. This is followed, in order, with the symbols of all the other residues connected by hyphens and terminating on the right with the symbol for the carboxy or C-terminal residue. In the above example, Ala is the N-terminal residue and is understood, as written, to contain a free α-amino group, whereas Gly is the C-terminal residue and is understood, as written, to contain a free α-carboxylic acid. Several other conventions used in writing the primary structure of a peptide can be explained using the following model hexapeptide, Ac-Leu-Phe-Asp(OMe)-Lys(Ac)-Ser-Ile-NH_2. Ac-Leu is understood to mean that the α-amino group of the N-terminal amino acid is acetylated (Ac). When the symbol for an amino acid is followed in parentheses by an abbreviation, as is Asp(OMe) and Lys(Ac), this indicates

Table 7.1. Twenty, DNA Encoded, Amino Acids Found in Human Protein[a]

General structure: H_3N^+–C(H)(R)–C(=O)–O^-

Name[b]			R	pI[c]	Acidity/ Basicity[d]
Alanine	Ala	A	$-CH_3$	6.02	N
Glycine	Gly	G	$-H$	5.97	N
Isoleucine	Ile	I	$-CH(CH_3)-CH_2CH_3$	6.02	N
Leucine	Leu	L	$-CH_2-CH(CH_3)-CH_3$	5.98	N
Valine	Val	V	$-CH(CH_3)-CH_3$	5.97	N
Aspartic acid	Asp	D	$-CH_2\text{-}CO_2H$	2.98	A
Glutamic acid	Glu	E	$-CH_2\text{-}CH_2\text{-}CO_2H$	3.22	A
Arginine	Arg	R	$-(CH_2)_3-NH-C(=NH)-NH_2$	10.76	B
Lysine	Lys	K	$-(CH_2)_4\text{-}NH_2$	9.74	B
Histidine	His	H	$-CH_2$-(imidazolyl)	7.59	VWB
Cysteine	Cys	C	$-CH_2\text{-}SH$	5.02	VWA
Methionine	Met	M	$-CH_2\text{-}CH_2-SCH_3$	5.74	N
Serine	Ser	S	$-CH_2\text{-}OH$	5.68	N
Threonine	Thr	T	$-CH(OH)-CH_3$	5.60	N
Tyrosine	Tyr	Y	$-CH_2-C_6H_4-OH$	5.67	N
Asparagine	Asn	N	$-CH_2-C(=O)-NH_2$	5.41	N
Glutamine	Gln	Q	$-CH_2\text{-}CH_2-C(=O)-NH_2$	5.65	N
Phenylalanine	Phe	F	$-CH_2-C_6H_5$	5.48	N
Tryptophan	Trp	W	$-CH_2$-(indolyl, N–H)	5.89	N
Proline	Pro	P	(pyrrolidine ring, H_2N^+, $-CO_2^-$)	6.30	N

[a]Selenocysteine, Sec, U, is a rare 21st amino acid that is found in both prokaryotic and eukaryotic protein (e.g., glutathione peroxidase), but is not coded for directly in the genetic code. It differs from Cys by the presence of Se in place of S.

[b]Name of amino acid, 3-letter, 1-letter abbreviation.

[c]pI is the pH at which each amino acid is ionically balanced, carries no net charge, and exists entirely in its zwitterion form.

[d]Side-chains are acidic (A), very weakly acidic (VWA), basic (B), very weakly basic (VWB), or neutral (N).

Data from reference 14

that the side chain is protected by the group named in the parentheses. The Asp side-chain carboxylic acid is protected as its methyl ester (OMe), and the Lys side-chain amino group is acetylated. Finally, the representation Ile-NH_2 is understood to indicate that the C-terminal residue does not exist as a free carboxyl but, rather, as its C-terminal amide, —CO—NH_2. Many important biologically active peptides actually exist as C-terminal amides, examples of which include GnRH, oxytocin, and vasopressin.

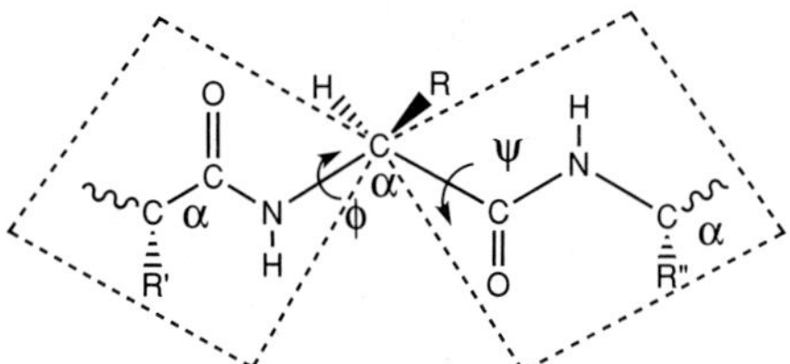

Fig. 7.2. Representation of a portion of a peptide backbone that indicates rotation about the N—C_α (angle ϕ, phi) and the C_α—C (angle φ, psi) bonds. Each C_α is a pivot point linking two adjacent peptide residues, as indicated by the dotted planes.

Stereochemical Features of Amino Acids, Peptides, and Proteins

Although some 300 different amino acids occur in nature, only 20 of these are DNA-encoded α-amino acids (selenocysteine, the twenty-first "natural" amino acid, is not actually coded for directly in the genetic code). The structures of the 20 natural amino acids can be found in Table 7.1. The amino acids in the table are not listed alphabetically; rather, they are tabulated according to properties determined by their side-chain (R) functionality. Interestingly, 19 of the DNA-encoded amino acids have the same stereochemistry and are chiral. The twentieth, Gly, is achiral, because its side-chain R-group is H. The 19 chiral amino acids are all configurationally related to L-glyceraldehyde and, therefore, are still known as L-amino acids, albeit this is an outdated nomenclature.

L-amino acid   L-Glyceraldehyde

A more informative system for indicating the stereochemistry of chiral carbon uses the Cahn-Ingold-Prelog system, in which the four groups on an asymmetric carbon are ranked according to a set of rules, the so-called *R/S* nomenclature (15). Using this nomenclature, one can show that 18 of the 19 chiral, DNA-encoded amino acids are of the *S*-configuration, and only Cys is *R*. This results from the sequencing rules, in which the side-chain CH_2SH (sulfur bonded to carbon) takes precedence over CO_2H (oxygen bonded to carbon). In addition, the side chains of Ile and Thr each have an additional chiral center, and the DNA-encoded forms exist as Ile (*S,S*) and Thr (*S,R*) (Table 7.1).

Conformational Features of Peptides and Proteins

The primary structure of a peptide or protein previously was defined simply as its sequence, but it should be recognized that this only describes its linear, or one-dimensional, structure. If one wants to know more about a polypeptide or protein's three-dimensional shape, it is necessary to have information about its secondary structure, or its well-defined conformation that is controlled by torsional angles (also called dihedral angles or rotations) and hydrogen bonds. The tertiary structure, or well-defined folding, of a polypeptide or protein affords its biologically active, three-dimensional structure. Finally, some proteins also can exist in a quaternary structure, which occurs when two or more protein monomers (subunits) combine into a multisubunit protein.

The conformation of a peptide is very much dependent on the spatial arrangement of the atoms that make up the bonds about each peptide residue of the backbone, which consists of repeating N—C_α—C units. These different conformations can vary by simple rotations without breaking a covalent bond or changing the chirality of atoms, in contrast to changing the configuration, which requires bond breaking. Consider Figure 7.2, which represents a section of a polypeptide chain containing two peptide units that can pivot about the central C_α, by rotation of the N—C_α and C_α—C bonds affording varying torsional angles ϕ (phi) and ψ (psi), respectively. As ϕ and ψ are rotated, varying conformations are formed, many of which are forbidden by steric interference caused by both backbone and side-chain atoms from adjacent residues (13,14,16). Those structures that have allowed ϕ and ψ values are further stabilized by hydrogen bonds formed between N—H····O=C of neighboring peptide bonds, giving rise to secondary structures.

The most common polypeptide and protein secondary structures found in nature are the α-helix and the β-pleated sheet. The α-helix involving L-amino acids, first proposed by Pauling et al. (17) in 1951, is a right-handed spiral structure that often is found in fibrous and globular proteins, wherein the torsion angles ϕ and ψ are ideal for most residues. The α-helix has very definite and regular properties and often is referred to as a 3.6_{13} helix (14). A 3.6_{13} helix contains 3.6 residues per turn and forms an hydrogen-bonded ring of 13 atoms between every carbonyl O^1 and peptide H^{13}. This means that each carbonyl oxygen of residue *n* is bonded to the hydrogen on α-amino nitrogen *n* + 4 (Fig. 7.3). Not shown in Figure 7.3 are the side chains that project out from the helix.

In a β-sheet conformation, unlike the α-helix coiled backbone, the polypeptide chain is nearly fully extended; two or more separate chains, or β-strands, can assemble side by side, wherein they are held together by hydrogen

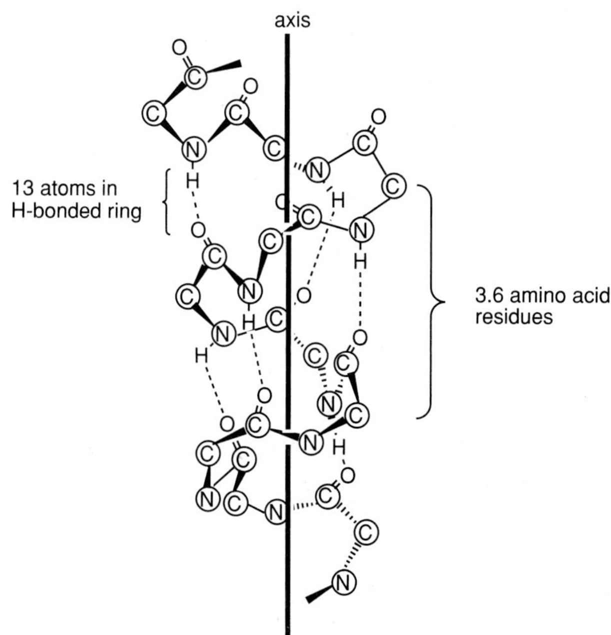

Fig. 7.3. Right-handed α-helix indicating H-bonds (dashed lines) that occur between each carbonyl oxygen and peptide N-H four residues removed; the ring formed by this H-bond contains 13 atoms. (From Horton HR, Moran LA, Ochs RS, et al. Principles of Biochemistry. Englewood Cliffs, NJ: Neil Patterson Publishers/ Prentice Hall, 1993; with permission.)

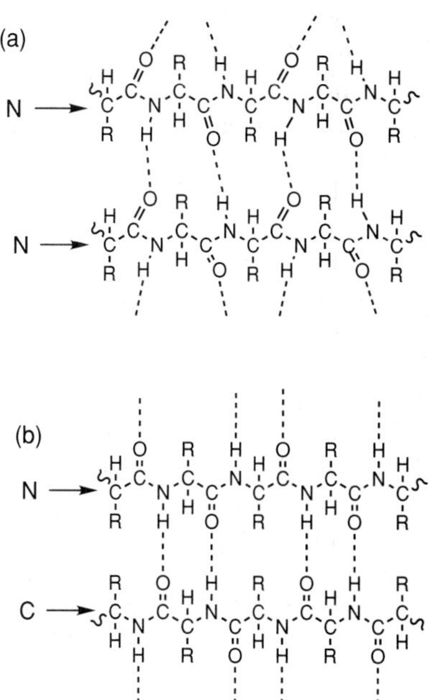

Fig. 7.4. Examples of (a) parallel and (b) antiparallel β-pleated sheets, shown with only two chains, that are held together by H-bonds (dashed lines). Note the difference in the H-bonds in the parallel (slanted and regularly spaced) and antiparallel (perpendicular with alternating wide and narrow spacing) sheets. (Adapted from Horton HR, Moran LA, Ochs RS, et al. Principles of Biochemistry. Englewood Cliffs, NJ: Neil Patterson Publishers/Prentice Hall, 1993; with permission.)

bonds. The hydrogen bonds are, again, between the carbonyl oxygen and the NH group of the backbone. The β-sheet can exist in two types, parallel and antiparallel, and in both cases, the torsional angles ϕ and ψ are sterically favorable. In the former case, the two stretches of polypeptide or protein are oriented in the same direction, whereas in the latter case, the chains are oriented in opposite directions (Fig. 7.4). The β-sheet is not completely planar, and when viewed along the backbone, it resembles that of a pleated sheet. Furthermore, the side chains protrude on alternating sides of the β-sheet.

Polypeptides and proteins can undergo other conformational changes, especially when they exist in relatively compact structures wherein the backbone can fold back on itself, or make a turn (i.e., a site where the polypeptide chain reverses its overall direction). It is these reverse turns (e.g., β-turn or hairpin bend) that afford proteins with globular properties (18). A further discussion of turns is beyond the scope of this chapter, but the interested reader can find many good discussions of this topic in other sources (16,19).

When a protein that exists as an α-helix, β-sheet, or combination of both folds into its biologically active globular shape, it becomes compacted and takes on a three-dimensional shape, or tertiary structure. In this case, amino acid residues, which might be far apart in the primary structure, may wind up quite close to each other, and this can be stabilized via noncovalent, usually hydrophobic interactions. That is, tertiary structures are formed and stabilized because of hydrophobic interactions between the side chains of amino acid residues. In some globular proteins, several subunits can combine with a well-defined stoichiometry and symmetry, giving rise to the quaternary structure of the protein. A good example of this is hemoglobin, the quaternary structure of which is a tetramer consisting of two α- and two β-chain subunits.

METABOLISM AND DRUG DELIVERY CONSEQUENCES

Peptides and proteins are metabolized quite extensively in the kidney, liver, and gastrointestinal (GI) tract via the enzymatic hydrolysis of the peptide bond. Metabolism also can occur in nasal mucosa, the lung, and blood. Because large proteins can assume complex tertiary structures, which thus better shields, or "hides," internal peptide bonds, they often are metabolized more slowly, or less completely, than smaller proteins or polypeptides (20).

The enzymes involved in peptide bond hydrolysis and, thus, the degradation of peptides and proteins are known as peptidases and can be found in the blood, in the vascular bed, in the interstitial fluid, on cell membranes, and within cells. These enzymes include carboxypeptidases (cleaves C-terminal residues), dipeptidyl carboxypeptidases (cleaves dipeptides from the C-terminus), aminopeptidases (cleaves N-terminal residues), and amidases (cleaves internal peptide bonds). The oral administration of protein or peptide drugs generally results in very extensive metabolism within the GI tract, the loss of biological activity, and little to no systemic absorption of the original drug. This results from the prevalence of peptidases within the GI tract, wherein the protein or peptide drugs undergo first-pass metabolism. Even if these drugs are administered parenterally, they still can undergo extensive metabolism because of their secretion across the intestinal mucosa and from hydrolyzing enzymes found in plasma and the vascular bed.

The fate of orally administered peptide drugs occur as follows. As the peptide drugs enter the stomach, wherein the gastric juice has a pH of approximately 2, they are acted on by pepsin, an enzyme secreted by the gastric mucosa. This enzyme is known as an endopeptidase, which means that it can hydrolyze "internal" peptide bonds at the carbonyl side of aromatic (Tyr, Phe, and Trp) and acidic (Asp and Glu) amino acid residues. Exiting the stomach, the contents continue on into the small intestine, where the pH rises to approximately 7 and the peptidases trypsin, chymotrypsin, and elastase continue the digestion. These enzymes are endopeptidases secreted by the pancreas. Trypsin generally cleaves at the carbonyl side of basic (Lys and Arg) residues, chymotrypsin at aromatic (Tyr, Phe, and Trp) residues, and elastase at small or sterically nonhindered (Ala, Gly, and Ser) residues. Finally, the oligopeptides that are remaining after endopeptidase hydrolysis are further acted on by two exopeptidases, carboxypeptidase and aminopeptidase. An exopeptidase is one that cleaves at the termini of peptides. The net result is a thorough breakdown of peptides and proteins into single amino acids and smaller dipeptides and tripeptides. For the most part, these enzymes are all specific for the natural amino acids of the L-configuration.

Chemical Methodology for Decreasing Proteolysis

The modification of peptides in a way that makes them more resistant to the onslaught of peptidases, thereby enhancing the biological activity and duration of action, is being pursued by peptide chemists. When metabolism studies indicate a predominant cleavage site, attempts can be made to replace that residue with another that retains the receptor-binding activity of the peptide while yielding enhanced resistance to peptidase activity. Often, this can be accomplished by replacing the offending L-residue with its enantiomer, the D-amino acid or another D-residue. Many peptidases are unable to cleave at peptide bonds consisting of a "fraudulent" D-amino acid, and peptides containing such changes can have enhanced biological activity because of an increase in their half-life. Such successes have been documented, as will be discussed later with the superagonists of GnRH. Also, the replacement of an L-amino acid with L-proline, or N-methylation of the amide nitrogen, offers the possibility of generating a peptide that is more resistant to enzymatic hydrolysis. The introduction of pseudo (ψ) peptide bonds (21) and the design of retro-inverso peptides (22) are two examples of strategies that can afford more peptidase-resistant peptides (discussed later).

Alternative Drug Delivery Methods for Peptides and Proteins

As evident from the previous discussion, a major barrier to the use of peptides as clinically useful drugs has to do with their poor delivery properties, because proteolytic enzymes present at most routes of administration are able to quickly metabolize most peptides. Peptides and proteins are, for the most part, hydrophilic in nature and, for this reason, do not readily penetrate lipophilic biomembranes. As well, they have short biological half-lives because of rapid metabolism and clearance, all of which deters from their efficient use in drug therapy. It is for these reasons that alternative drug delivery methods for peptides and proteins are an area of particular interest to the pharmaceutical industry.

An appreciation of the problems of drug absorption via different routes of administration was reported by Lee (23), wherein he compared the percentage of dose that is absorbed for two important peptides, insulin and an analogue of GnRH, leuprolide, when administered by the oral, nasal, buccal, rectal, vaginal, and subcutaneous (SC) routes. For example, dosing of insulin and leuprolide by the oral route afforded, in both cases, a mere 0.05% absorption; 30 and 2–3%, respectively, by the nasal route; and 80 and 65%, respectively, by the SC route. In addition to the above routes, alternative routes of administration for the delivery of peptide and protein drugs include transdermal, parenteral (including SC), targeted, and pulmonary routes (24). Space does not allow a detailed discussion of each of these routes, but several generalizations can be made.

Drug administration by the parenteral route, either intravenous (IV), intramuscular (IM), or SC injection, is certainly undesirable. Aside from the pain involved, it is a route that does not easily allow self-administration, especially when the drug has to be given IM or IV. In emergency situations, however, when rapid onset of action is warranted, the IV route is preferred. The peptide drug can act very fast, because it is placed directly into the bloodstream and no absorption is involved. On the other hand, when a more sustained action is desired, IM administration is preferred because of the ability to introduce larger volumes of fluid directly into skeletal muscle. The disadvantages of the IM route are pain after injection, possible degradation of the peptide at the injection site, slow absorption, and difficulty of self-injection. An SC injection of a peptide drug, which can be self-administered (e.g., insulin), affords a slower absorption rate when compared to the IM route and is useful for long-term therapy, but there is decreased drug potency because of degradation and poor absorption (25). There has been progress in improving parenteral dosage forms that allow better patient compliance, including biodegradable microspheres of poly(D,L-lactide-glycolide) for sustained-release IM injection of leuprolide acetate for up to 6 months and the administration of goserelin acetate dispersed in a copolymer matrix of D,L-lactic and glycolic acids. The latter is injected SC as a solid pellet for use up to 3 months (see later discussions on these GnRH analogues). More recently, pegylation, the attachment of a peptide or protein to various polyethylene glycol polymers, has gained in popularity as a way of improving the biological activity (26). For example, pegylated interferon-α_{2b} is commercially available as PEG-Intron and is used either alone or in combination with ribavirin for the treatment of patients with chronic hepatitis C.

The delivery of peptide and protein drugs by the nasal route has been studied extensively. Generally, the nasal route represents a significant improvement in bioavailability over the oral route, and it is noninvasive. Although the nasal route avoids first-pass hepatic metabolism, there is still a significant degree of enzymatic degradation that occurs in the nasal mucosa, especially by aminopeptidases (27). Also, the higher molecular weight of peptides and proteins, coupled with their more hydrophilic properties, generally affords compounds with poor absorptive properties. Therefore, to obtain successful nasal delivery of peptides and proteins, the coadministration of protease inhibitors and/or permeation enhancers generally is required. Still, only a very limited number of peptides, mostly of lower molecular weight, are commercially available for nasal use (e.g., calcitonin, desmopressin, and nafarelin).

The delivery of peptide and protein drugs via the pulmonary route (i.e., by inhalation therapy) is an area of considerable interest to the pharmaceutical industry (26). This method is noninvasive and allows the delivery of peptide and protein drugs to the lung epithelium, which is highly permeable and easily accessed via inhalation. That is not to say this methodology, which generally uses particles that are dry or liquid and delivers them with the use of dry-powder dispersers or liquid-aerosol generators, is not without problems (24). Issues such as protein stability, reproducible delivery devices, particle size, and bioavailability of the inhaled protein still need to be resolved before pulmonary delivery gains greater acceptance. Recently, however, studies regarding the systemic delivery of peptides and proteins via the lung, particularly with inhaled insulin (Exubera) for the treatment of diabetes, have sparked increased interest. Two other peptide hormones in development are Inhaled Leuprolide for prostate cancer and endometriosis and Inhaled Parathyroid Hormone for osteoporosis. A good treatise on inhalation therapy of peptide and protein drugs can be found in the book edited by Adjei and Gupta (27).

MAJOR METHODS OF PEPTIDE SYNTHESIS

Although there have been many advances in the chemistry of peptide synthesis, the problems that can occur during the large-scale synthesis of even a medium-size peptide (e.g., 20–35 residues) can be quite challenging and expensive, especially when using the classical solution-phase methodology. The alternative method of peptide synthesis, on solid phase, has certainly grown in popularity and eliminated some of these problems, but is not without its own limitations. A description of these two methodologies, the synthesis of peptides in solution or by solid phase, is described below.

Synthesis in Solution

The synthesis of peptides in solution, either by stepwise elongation or segment condensation, allows one to isolate the intermediates along the way and purify them to homogeneity. As a result of this, the eventual final products usually are less contaminated with by-products and are easier to isolate in a homogeneous form. This method also is more amenable to the preparation of bulk quantities of peptides compared with the solid-phase method. The trade-off, however, is that the solution method is laborious and time-consuming, especially as the size of the peptide grows, wherein the problem of maintaining the peptide in solution becomes formidable. Also, when using the segment method, there is always the danger that racemization will occur during the coupling of the segments. One of the more prolific laboratories that report outstanding achievements in the solution synthesis of complicated large peptides and proteins is that of Sakakibara (28) in Japan.

Selective Protection of the α-Amino Group

To be able to form a peptide bond between two amino acids (e.g., Ala-Val), the nucleophilicity of the amino function in Ala must be diminished. Thus, only the amino group of Val is nucleophilic, and only it can react with the activated carboxyl group (discussed later) of Ala. If this dipeptide is then to be elongated to a tripeptide (e.g., Gly-Ala-Val), the nucleophilicity of the Ala amine must be reinstated so that it now can react with an activated carboxyl group of Gly. The key then is to be able to easily protect and deprotect the amino functions of amino acids without inverting the chirality of the individual amino acids or disrupting any of the peptide bonds.

As mentioned previously, the first group that fit these criteria was the carbobenzoxy (Cbz) group discovered by Bergmann and Zervas (3) (Fig. 7.5). The advantages of the Cbz blocking group are that its amino acid derivatives are stable, crystalline, and therefore, commercially available for all the natural amino acids. When the Cbz group is bound to the α-amine, the resulting urethane functionality ($RO_2C{-}NH{-}$) imparts stability toward racemization (29). The Cbz group is stable to base, but it can be removed by treatment with hydrogen bromide in glacial acetic acid (HBr/AcOH) or liquid hydrogen fluoride (HF), both of

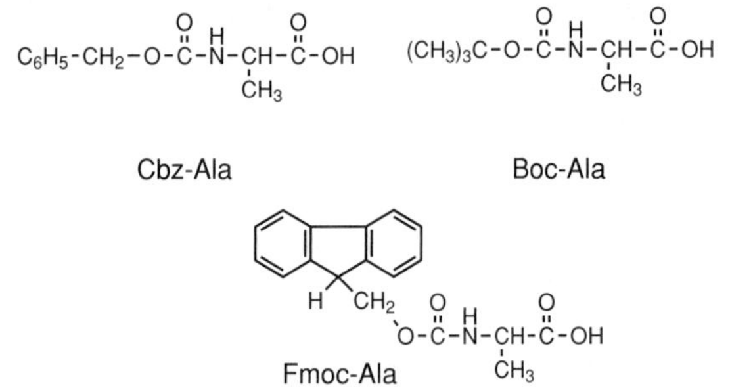

$C_6H_5-CH_2-O-C(=O)-NH-CH(CH_3)-C(=O)-OH$

Cbz-Ala

$(CH_3)_3C-O-C(=O)-NH-CH(CH_3)-C(=O)-OH$

Boc-Ala

Fmoc-Ala

Fig. 7.5. Three urethane-type amino protecting groups—Cbz. Boc, and Fmoc—shown attached to Ala.

which are examples of acidolytic, not hydrolytic, cleavage resulting from protonation of the urethane carbonyl oxygen. In addition, the Cbz group is readily cleaved by catalytic hydrogenation in the presence of palladium (Pd/H_2) except when also in the presence of the sulfur-containing amino acids, Cys and Met, wherein the sulfur poisons the Pd catalyst. Conversely, the Cbz group is not useful for α-amino protection in solid-phase peptide synthesis (SPPS), because the two acidolytic methods used in Cbz cleavage also would cleave the side-chain blocking groups of the trifunctional amino acids. Additionally, Pd/H_2 cleavage is not useful in SPPS, because Pd, being a solid, would contaminate the polymers used in SPPS. A further disadvantage of the Cbz group is that on acidolytic cleavage, benzyl (Bzl) cations can form and, potentially, alkylate the amino acids Trp and Met. Therefore, the addition of a scavenger agent (e.g., anisole) that can preferentially react with Bzl cations usually is added to the acid cleavage reagent.

The introduction of the Boc group (10) was a significant step forward as a protecting group for the α-amino function (Fig. 7.5). In addition to the advantages mentioned above for the Cbz group, including the urethane protection against racemization, the Boc group's ease of cleavage under milder acidic conditions, such as trifluoroacetic acid (TFA), broadens its use in peptide synthesis, especially in SPPS. Furthermore, its resistance to cleavage by Pd/H_2 but sensitivity to TFA allows differential blocking of trifunctional amino acids when using both Boc and Cbz groups. A disadvantage with the use of the Boc group is the possible formation of *tert*-butyl (Bu^t) cations which can alkylate the amino acids Trp and Met. Again, this can be minimized by the addition of a scavenger agent to the acidolytic cleavage reagent.

In the synthesis of peptides, the repeated use of acid in the cleavage of the α-amino protecting group can cause variable amounts of unwanted side products to occur. To circumvent the need for repeated acidolytic cleavages, Carpino and Han (11) introduced the now-popular Fmoc protecting group (Fig. 7.5). The main advantage of this urethane blocker is that it is stable to acid but readily cleaved by organic base, such as piperidine. Like Boc, it, too, is very useful in either solution or solid-phase synthesis. Because it is base labile, one can use various acid-labile blocking groups for the side chains of trifunctional amino acids. One disadvantage is that commercially available Fmoc amino acids are somewhat more expensive than the corresponding Boc or Cbz amino acids. Another disadvantage is that there can be some premature deblocking by the free amines that are the nucleophilic components of the coupling reaction.

Selective Protection of the α-Carboxyl Group

In the solution synthesis of peptides by the stepwise elongation method (the addition of one amino acid at a time) or segment condensation method (the synthesis of several segments, which are then joined to make the whole), the carboxyl function of the C-terminal residue must be blocked so that it does not partake in future coupling reactions. Clearly, the easiest to prepare and least expensive of the groups protecting the α-carboxyl function is the methyl or ethyl ester. These esters are only cleaved by alkaline hydrolysis, however, and that can lead to undesirable side reactions. Furthermore, these esters are not compatible with the conditions necessary to cleave the Fmoc group, in that piperidine can react with these simple esters.

The Bzl ester is another widely used blocker for the carboxyl function and is easily prepared with inexpensive reagents. It is readily cleaved with liquid HF or by Pd/H_2 yet is stable to TFA. The latter stability is the reason why the Bzl ester is especially useful when Boc amino acids are used. The TFA cleaves the Boc group but not the Bzl ester, whereas Pd/H_2 can cleave the Bzl group but not the Boc group.

The Bu^t ester is easily prepared with inexpensive reagents, is cleavable with TFA and other acidolytic reagents (HF), yet is stable to Pd/H_2. As a result, it is a very popular blocking group, because it is compatible with both Cbz and Fmoc amino acids. For example, the Cbz group can be cleaved via Pd/H_2, the Bu^t ester is stable. The converse, however, also is true: the Bu^t ester can be cleaved with TFA, and the Cbz group is stable. In the case of Fmoc amino acids, the Bu^t ester is stable under the basic conditions needed to cleave the Fmoc group.

Selective Protection of Trifunctional Amino Acids

A trifunctional amino acid, as seen in Table 7.1, has an additional functional group as part of its side chain. For ease of discussion, these can be divided into the following groups, as determined by their side-chain functionality: monoamino dicarboxylic acids (Asp and Glu), hydroxyl containing (Ser, Thr, and Tyr), sulfur containing (Cys and Met), basic (Arg, His, and Lys), and neutral (Asn, Glu, and Trp). In the discussion below, it is important to recognize that the goal is selective protection of the side-chain functionality so that it does not participate in any chemistry during the assembly of the peptide but, instead, undergoes cleavage at the end of the synthesis. That is, the side-chain protecting group should be stable to the conditions needed to cleave either the α-amino or α-carboxyl blocking groups during peptide chain elongation.

Irrespective of whether solution phase or SPPS is practiced, if Boc amino acids are used with monoamino dicarboxylic acids, then the side-chain carboxyl usually is protected as its Bzl ester. Because of the potential for intramolecular succinimide formation with Asp(Bzl) peptides, however, the replacement of Bzl with a cyclohexyl (cHex) ester reduces this undesirable side reaction (14). On the other hand, if Fmoc amino acids are used, then the side-chain carboxyl usually is protected as the Bu^t ester. Similarly, when using Boc-Ser and Boc-Thr, the hydroxyl function is protected as the Bzl ether. In the case of Tyr, however, the Bzl ether is not stable enough during repeated TFA treatments needed to cleave Boc groups. Therefore, in the case of Boc-Tyr, the preferred blocking group for the phenolic hydroxyl is the 2-bromo-carbobenzoxy (2Br-Z, $BrC_6H_4CH_2OCO$). When N^α-Fmoc is used, the hydroxyl groups of Ser, Thr, and Tyr usually are protected as the Bu^t ether.

The amino acid Cys contains a free sulfhydryl (SH) function that is very nucleophilic, easily oxidized, and must be protected. A discussion of the several different blocking groups used to protect the sulfur is beyond the scope of this chapter, but the interested reader should consult those references whose main thrust is peptide synthesis (29,30). The amino acid Met does not contain a free SH but, rather, a methylthio ether, $S\text{-}CH_3$, and as such, it most often is used unprotected. Some investigators prefer using Boc-Met protected as its sulfoxide, Boc-Met(O), to prevent alkylation of the sulfur and partial conversion to the sulfoxide during the synthesis. The sulfoxidation is most common during the acidic cleavage of other blocking groups. The use of the sulfoxide as a blocking group would, of course, necessitate a reduction step at the end of the synthesis to convert Met(O) back to Met, which can be accomplished by the low/high-HF cleavage procedure (31). When using Fmoc-Met, the side chain is left unprotected.

Of the three basic amino acids, Arg, Lys, and His, Arg is the most basic and is mainly used with the guanyl nitrogen (N^G) protected, even though at pH 9, the guanidino group (pK_a = 12.5) is virtually fully protonated. When N^α-Boc is used, the preferred protection for N^G is the tosyl (Tos) group, which is cleavable with HF at the end of the synthesis. On the other hand, when using N^α-Fmoc, the popular N^G-blocker 2,2,5,7,8-pentamethylchroman-6-sulfonyl (Pmc) group often is used, which like the Tos group is of the sulfonyl type (see structure below). The presence of the aromatic methyl groups and the chroman oxygen impart greater acidolytic lability, and the Pmc group is cleavable with TFA at the end of the synthesis. Similarly, N^G-protection as Fmoc-Arg(Pbf), where Pbf is 2,2,4,6,7-pentamethyldihydro benzofuran-5-sulfonyl (below), is now commonly used. The advantage of the Pbf group is greater TFA lability when compared to its structural analog Pmc (13).

Tos 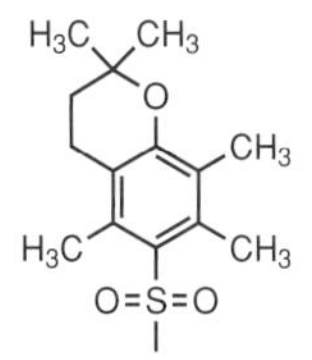 Pmc 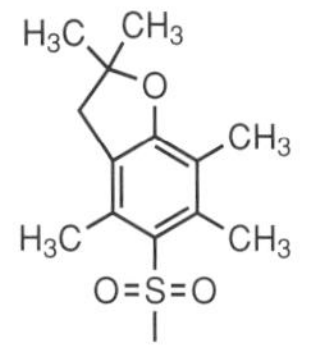 Pbf

The side chain of basic amino acid Lys usually is protected with the 2-chloro-carbobenzoxy (2Cl-Z, $ClC_6H_4CH_2OCO$) group when using N^α-Boc, because the presence of the 2-Cl increases the stability of the group to repeated treatments with TFA necessary for removing Boc groups. When N^α-Fmoc protection is used, the side-chain amine is protected with the Boc group. Finally, the least basic of the three, His, is always used with the imidazole ring protected; otherwise, it is susceptible to racemization during activation of the carboxyl for peptide coupling. There are two different ring nitrogens in the imidazole ring of His, N^π and N^τ. The N^π electrons, which do not participate in the aromaticity of the imidazole ring as the N^τ electrons do, are responsible for causing racemization (29).

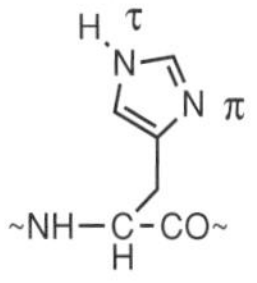

His residue

For this reason, Boc-His(N^π-Bom), wherein N^π is blocked with the benzyloxymethyl (Bom) group, is commercially available and widely used. When using Fmoc chemistry, however, peptide chemists often use Fmoc-His(N^τ-Trt), where Trt is the triphenylmethyl (trityl) group. Although the Trt group is attached at N^τ, it still suppresses racemization, both because it reduces the basicity of the imidazole ring and because its steric bulk hinders most racemization (13).

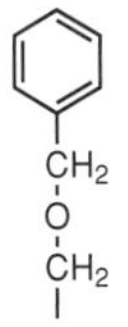

Bom 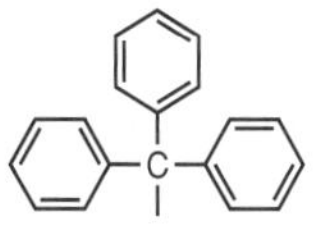 Trt

The aromatic, weakly nucleophilic Trp is susceptible to two side reactions, oxidation and alkylation of the indole ring by cations generated during acidolytic cleavage. Therefore, when using N^α-Boc chemistry, the formyl (For) group often is attached to the indole nitrogen (i.e., Boc-Trp(For)). The formyl group is removable at the end of the synthesis by cleavage treatment using the low/high-HF procedure (31). During peptide synthesis using N^α-Fmoc chemistry, Trp generally is used without side-chain

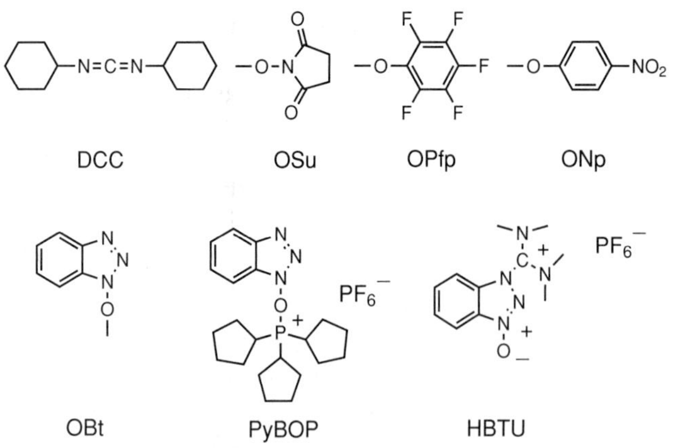

DCC OSu OPfp ONp

OBt PyBOP HBTU

Fig. 7.6. Structures of several of the reagents used in peptide bond formation.

protection. The use of Fmoc-Trp(Boc) is advantageous, because it prevents Trp-sulfonated by-products from occurring during final deprotection of peptides containing Arg(Pmc) and Arg(Pbf) residues (32).

Finally, the neutral amino acids Asn and Gln can be used in peptide synthesis without side-chain protection provided that the chemist is aware of the potential for carboxamide side-chain dehydration to a nitrile during peptide bond formation. This nitrile formation, which can occur in the presence of a variety of carboxyl activating reagents, is dramatically minimized by the addition of 1-hydroxybenzotriazole (HOBt) to the activating solution (Fig. 7.6) (33). During N^{α}-Fmoc chemistry with Asn and Gln, the use of the Trt group to block the amide nitrogen has gained in popularity. This is because it prevents nitrile formation, enhances solubility in dimethylformamide (an organic solvent commonly used in peptide synthesis), and can be removed by later treatment with TFA.

Major Methods of Peptide Bond Formation

To form a peptide bond, one must activate the α-carboxyl group of a suitably blocked amino acid so that it can react with the free α-amino group of another suitably blocked amino acid or growing peptide. The activation methodologies most often used can be divided into three main classes: 1) the carbodiimide coupling reagents, 2) the active esters, and 3) the phosphonium and uronium coupling reagents.

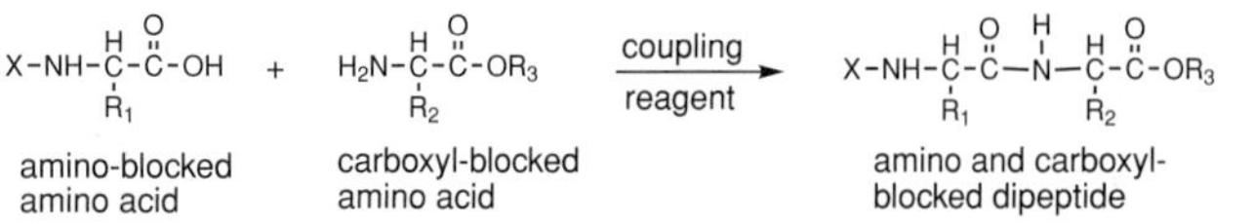

X-NH-CH(R$_1$)-C(=O)-OH + H$_2$N-CH(R$_2$)-C(=O)-OR$_3$ —coupling reagent→ X-NH-CH(R$_1$)-C(=O)-NH-CH(R$_2$)-C(=O)-OR$_3$

amino-blocked amino acid; carboxyl-blocked amino acid; amino and carboxyl-blocked dipeptide

The reagent DCC (Fig. 7.6), previously discussed as one of the important discoveries that helped to drive the field of peptide synthesis (9), probably is the most popular of the carbodiimide-type coupling reagents in use today. DCC is considered to be a dehydrating agent inasmuch as the results are a loss of a molecule of water from the amino and carboxyl groups involved in the coupling. Details of the mechanism can be found elsewhere (33). Advantages of the carbodiimides are their low cost, general insensitivity to moisture, and relatively fast coupling. Disadvantages are that extensive racemization can occur when coupling peptide segments, specifically the residue whose carboxyl is being activated, as well as nitrile formation from Asn and Gln residues, as mentioned above. The addition of HOBt to carbodiimide couplings, however, can very effectively minimize both of these disadvantages. Another annoying problem with DCC, more so with SPPS than with solution phase, is that its by-product, dicyclohexylurea (DCU), is highly insoluble in most solvents used in peptide coupling. Often, DCC is replaced with diisopropylcarbodiimide (DCI), because its by-product, diisopropylurea (DIU), is more soluble in the solvents used in SPPS and does not contaminate the solid phase.

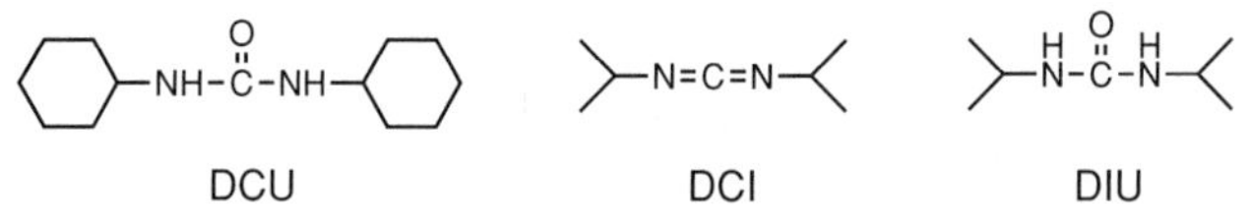

DCU DCI DIU

An active ester is a suitably protected amino acid whose carboxyl group has been esterified with a hydroxyl moiety that is easily eliminated on attack of the carbonyl group by the nucleophilic amino component. When the hydroxyl moiety is a phenol, it will contain either an electron withdrawing group (e.g., *para*-nitrophenol, ONp) or electronegative elements (e.g., pentafluorophenol, OPfp), which affords a better leaving group (Fig. 7.6). When using Boc-protected residues, two popular active esters employed are the ONp and N-hydroxysuccinimde (OSu) esters (Fig. 7.6). When using Fmoc-protected residues, the one active ester that is both commercially available and widely used is the OPfp ester (Fig. 7.6). These commercially available derivatives generally are crystalline and reasonably stable. On the other hand, the 1-hydroxybenzotriazole (OBt) active ester (Fig. 7.6) is very popular with both Boc and Fmoc chemistries. The OBt-esters, however, are not commercially available, because they usually are neither isolable nor stable and have to be prepared in situ from a protected amino acid, HOBt, and a carbodiimide. Still, this method finds wide use in both solution phase and SPPS.

More recently, the use of phosphonium (e.g., benzotriazole-1-yl-oxy-tris-pyrrolidino phosphonium hexafluorophosphate (PyBOP)) and uronium (e.g., 2-(1H-benzotriazole-1-yl)-1,1,3,3-tetramethyluronium hexafluorophosphate (HBTU)) coupling reagents have gained wide use in effecting peptide bond formation, particularly in SPPS (Fig. 7.6). The structures of PyBOP and HBTU both incorporate an equivalent of HOBt, and the final reactive Boc or Fmoc amino acid species is the corresponding OBt active ester (13).

Solid-Phase Peptide Synthesis

The Merrifield strategy of SPPS, as originally published in 1963 (12), consisted of attaching the N^{α}-Boc protected C-terminal amino acid of the peptide to be synthesized to a solid polymer support via an ester linkage (34). This ester linkage was designed to be stable to all chemical conditions involved in the elongation of the peptide but able to be cleaved from the polymer at the end of the synthesis without disturbing the integrity of the final peptide. An additional requirement was that the side-chain protecting groups should be stable during the synthesis but removable at the end, preferably at the same time that the final peptide was cleaved from the polymer. The original Merrifield solid support used to attach the growing peptide was a chloromethylated polystyrene polymer (resin). Today, several newer and more versatile polymers are popular and have, for the most part, replaced the original resin. A scheme that illustrates Merrifield's concept of SPPS is shown in Figure 7.7.

The following are some of the advantages gained when using the technique of SPPS. The attachment of the growing polypeptide to an insoluble polymer allows soluble reagents and by-products to be readily removed by simple filtering and washing of the insoluble polypeptide-bound polymer. This reduces the loss of valuable peptide that occurs, as the result of repeated isolation and purification of peptide intermediates, during solution-phase peptide synthesis. Another advantage is the ability to use excess soluble reagents to force reactions to completion and, thereby, achieve high yields, which then are readily removed by filtration of the growing insoluble peptide. The most valuable advantage is the ability to automate all the operations of the peptide synthesis, thus drastically reducing the time, labor, and cost involved in the synthesis. The disadvantages of SPPS are the inherent cost of using excess reagents and solvents to force the couplings to near completion and the actual purification of the final cleaved product, which can be difficult.

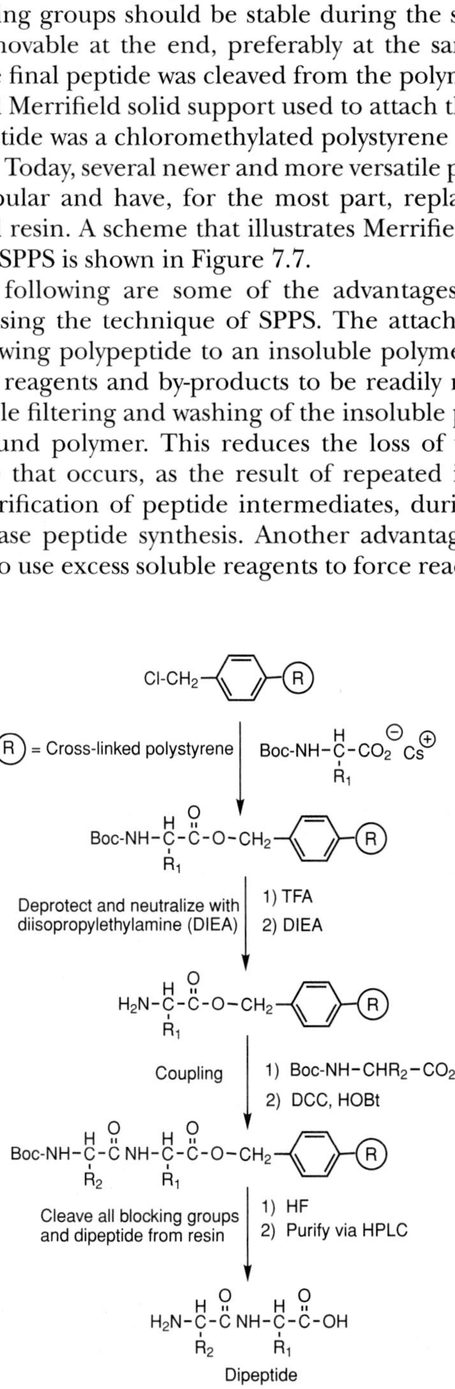

Cl-CH2-(C6H4)-(R)

(R) = Cross-linked polystyrene | Boc-NH-CH(R1)-CO2⁻ Cs⁺

Boc-NH-CH(R1)-C(=O)-O-CH2-(C6H4)-(R)

Deprotect and neutralize with diisopropylethylamine (DIEA) | 1) TFA 2) DIEA

H2N-CH(R1)-C(=O)-O-CH2-(C6H4)-(R)

Coupling | 1) Boc-NH-CHR2-CO2H 2) DCC, HOBt

Boc-NH-CH(R2)-C(=O) NH-CH(R1)-C(=O)-O-CH2-(C6H4)-(R)

Cleave all blocking groups and dipeptide from resin | 1) HF 2) Purify via HPLC

H2N-CH(R2)-C(=O) NH-CH(R1)-C(=O)-OH

Dipeptide

Fig. 7.7. A scheme based on Merrifield's methodology for Boc-based SPPS.

Boc Chemistry

The use of Boc-based SPPS for the synthesis of peptides with free C-terminal carboxylic acids generally requires that the peptide chains be linked to the resins as Bzl esters and that the side-chain protecting groups have a similar reactivity so that these bonds are stable to repeated TFA cleavage of the N^{α}-Boc group. The need for a more stable peptide Bzl ester linkage to the Merrifield solid support culminated in the development of the phenylacetamidomethyl (PAM) resin, and the need to synthesize peptide C-terminal amides gave rise to the 4-methylbenzhydrylamine (MBHA) resin (35) (Fig. 7.8). Merrifield, PAM, and MBHA resins linked to all the natural Boc-amino acids are now commercially available.

Fmoc Chemistry

The growth of N^{α}-Fmoc-based SPPS has been driven by the desire to avoid the repetitive acidolytic (TFA) treatment required in Boc-based SPPS as well as the final HF cleavage needed to remove the peptide from its resin and all remaining blocking groups. The repetitive TFA and final HF treatments often are the cause of unwanted by-products. The Fmoc-based SPPS allows the use of side-chain protection with Bu^t-derived esters, ethers, and urethanes that are stable to the recurring mild secondary base (piperidine) treatment necessary to cleave the N^{α}-Fmoc group. All the side-chain blockers can be cleaved, along with the peptide-to-resin linkage, via only one TFA treatment at the end of the synthesis. Problems that may be encountered during Fmoc-based SPPS are premature

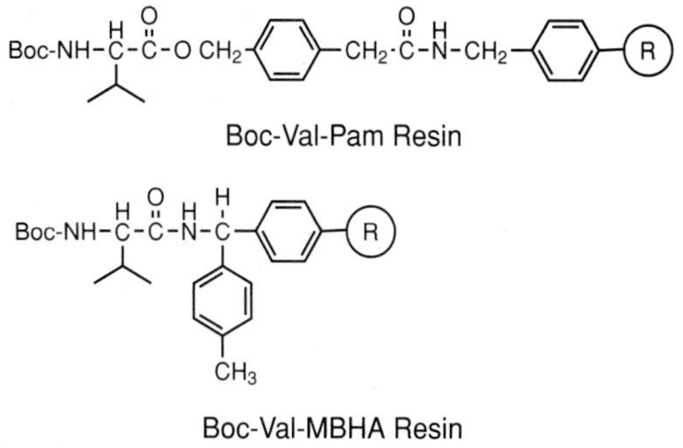

Boc-NH-CH(iPr)-C(=O)-O CH2-(C6H4)-CH2-C(=O)-NH-CH2-(C6H4)-(R)

Boc-Val-Pam Resin

Boc-NH-CH(iPr)-C(=O)-NH-CH(C6H4-CH3)-(C6H4)-(R)

Boc-Val-MBHA Resin

Fig. 7.8. Examples of Boc-Val attached to the phenylacetamidomethyl (PAM) resin and to the 4-methylbenzhydrylamine (MBHA) resin. The former is used to prepare peptides with a C-terminal carboxylic acid, whereas the latter is used for the preparation of peptide C-terminal amides.

cleavage of the Fmoc group and the potential for by-product formation during cleavage of the peptide from its resin when Met and Trp are present. These and other problems, as well as the resins most often used, are adequately addressed in the review by Wellings and Atherton (36).

Combinatorial Peptide Synthesis

Perhaps the reader can surmise from the above discourse on peptide synthesis that the preparation of a single peptide, its purification, and biological testing is an arduous and time-consuming task. Therefore, building on Merrifield's SPPS methodology, investigators in the 1980s began developing methods for synthesizing large numbers of peptides simultaneously and screening them for biological activity. These ideas, which have firmly taken root within the medicinal chemistry discipline and now expanded to small organic molecules, are collectively referred to as combinatorial chemistry, or the ability "to make a large number of chemical variants all at one time; to test them for bioactivity . . . and then to isolate and identify the most promising compounds for further development" (37). This gives rise to large numbers of biologically screenable compounds, usually referred to as a combinatorial library.

Two methods of combinatorial chemistry used in peptide and small molecule construction are known as parallel synthesis and split-and-mix synthesis. In the parallel synthesis approach, "all the products are assembled separately in their own reaction vessels," as in a single well of a microtiter plate (38). A typical plastic microtiter plate contains eight rows and 12 columns of small wells and, thus, 96 wells in which combinatorial parallel synthesis can take place. For example, if eight different amino acids (already attached to a polymeric support) were distributed into each of the eight rows, then their SPPS coupling with a different blocked amino acid in each of the 12 columns would afford a 96-member library of dipeptides (Fig. 7.9). Of course, after removing unreacted chemicals and "reloading" each well with a different blocked amino acid, a 96-member library of tripeptides could be prepared, and so forth. After cleaving these dipeptides, tripeptides, or larger peptides from the polymer, the entire plate of 96 different compounds could be screened for biological activity. If many microtiter plates were used, one could see how a large library of peptides could be constructed. Today, robotic machines are used to carry out these repetitive steps, and hundreds or even thousands of compounds can be made in a single day.

The split-and-mix technique first developed by Furka and colleagues has been reviewed elsewhere (39). In the parallel method previously described, each well contains only one peptide, whereas in the split-and-mix technique, a single vessel may contain a mixture of closely related peptides. This occurs because the technique requires the repetition of three operations: 1) dividing the polymer (on which the peptide is growing) into equal portions, 2) coupling each portion with a different amino acid, and 3)

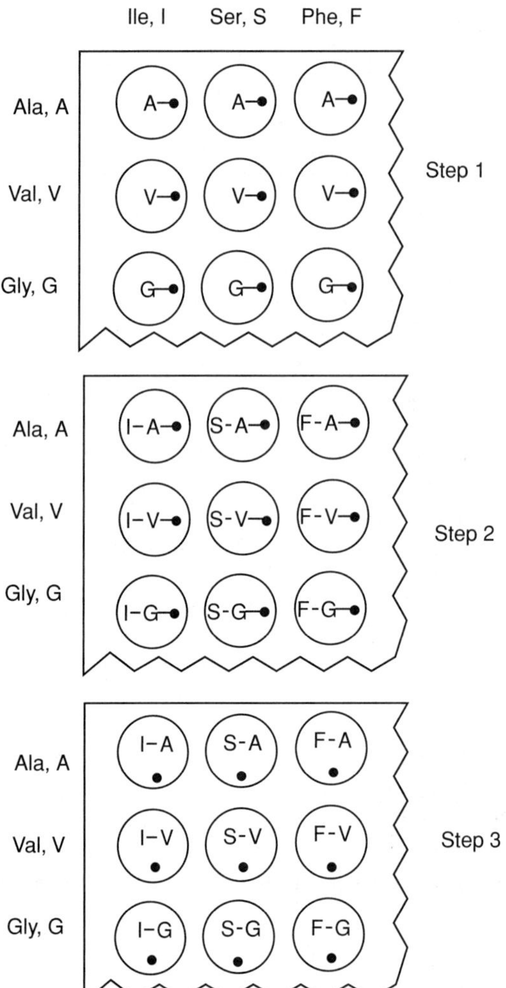

Fig. 7.9. Representation of a combinatorial parallel synthesis of a 96-member library of dipeptides in a typical plastic microtiter plate of eight rows and 12 columns; only the upper left three rows and three columns are shown. Step 1 shows three rows of wells containing three different amino acids that are already attached to a polymeric solid phase, as represented by the solid circles. In step 2, all eight rows are treated with the particular protected amino acids shown in each of the 12 columns, giving rise to 96 different polymer-bound dipeptides. In step 3, the dipeptides are cleaved from the solid support in preparation for testing them for biological activity.

homogenous mixing of these portions (Fig. 7.10). By using the method outlined in Figure 7.10, wherein one starts with only three amino acids bound to a polymer, the number of peptides obtained would triple after each coupling step, according to the formula 3^n. If all 20 of the natural amino acids were bound to a polymer, however, one could generate 3.2 million different peptides after only five couplings, according to the formula 20^n (40).

The biological activity of each vessel is then evaluated, and those with the most potent activity would be processed by a variety of techniques to determine which particular peptide(s) is responsible for the activity

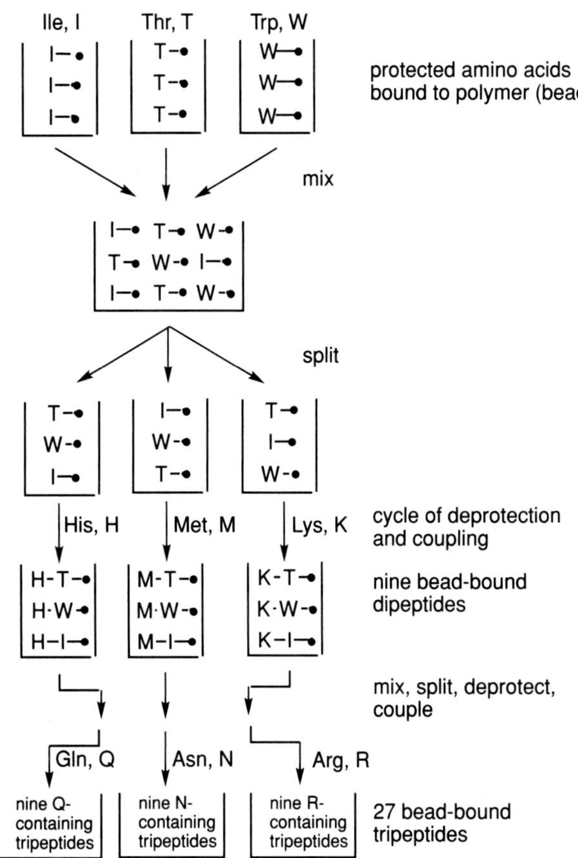

Fig. 7.10. Schematic representation of the split-and-mix technique.

(13,38). An important difference between the split-and-mix technique and parallel synthesis is that the former method affords small quantities of a large number of peptides, whereas the latter method yields larger quantities of a smaller number of peptides (37). A discussion of the many novel techniques and advances in combinatorial peptide synthesis is beyond the scope of this chapter; the interested reader may want to check recent current reviews on this topic (13,41).

TOPOLOGICAL MODIFICATIONS OF PEPTIDES

A common assumption is that the activity of a biologically active peptide depends on its three-dimensional structure. On the surface, where contact between ligand and receptor occurs, the relative spatial arrangements of the side-chain groups on the peptide pharmacophore are critical for receptor recognition and probably determine, in many cases, the affinity, selectivity, and activity of the peptide for a particular receptor protein. Therefore, side-chain modifications of a given peptide may provide important insights regarding the conformational and topological requirements for its activity (42).

Alternatively, other structure–activity studies of peptides have involved modifications of the peptide backbone. In this regard, there has been great interest in the replacement of some peptide bonds with pseudopeptide (ψ) bonds (21), because among other things, it may modify the backbone conformation as well as limit enzymatic degradation. Still another fascinating topological modification that has shown promise in limiting enzymatic degradation while retaining or enhancing biological activity is referred to as the retro-inverso modification (22). Both of these modifications, briefly mentioned above, will now be discussed in more detail.

Peptides Containing Pseudopeptide (ψ) Bonds

Replacement of the normal peptide bond (—CONH—) with an isosteric unit generally does not alter the overall dimensions of the modified peptide. The replacement unit is referred to as a pseudopeptide bond, and a peptide analogue containing the modified bond is referred to as a pseudopeptide. The symbol ψ was originally introduced (43) with specific reference to the sulfur-based CH_2S peptide bond replacement and was later used for various CH_2S-containing pseudopeptides. The pseudopeptide bond replacement term took on a broader meaning, however, and now is referred to by the symbols ψ[ ]. The ψ refers to the absence of the peptide bond, and the bracket, [ ], inserted between the named amino acid residue, specifies what the peptide bond replacement structure is. For example Alaψ[CH_2S]Gly refers to the pseudopeptide $NH_2CH(CH_3)CH_2SCH_2CO_2H$ (21). Several examples of the types of pseudopeptides that have been reported in the literature, as well as the nomenclature used to designate the replacements, are shown in Table 7.2. The ψ[CH_2NH] pseudopeptide replacement often has been used in attempts at modifying the peptide backbone (44). This unit has gained popularity because of its ready incorporation into peptides during conventional SPPS and the fact that it can afford receptor antagonists (45).

Table 7.2. Examples of Peptide Backbone Modifications

Unit-Replacing Peptide (—CONH—) Bond	Nomenclature Symbol
$-CH_2S-$	ψ[CH_2S]
$-CONCH_3-$	ψ[$CONCH_3$]
—COO—	ψ[COO]
—COS—	ψ[COS]
$-COCH_2-$	ψ[$COCH_2$]
—CSNH—	ψ[CSNH]
$-CH_2NH-$	ψ[CH_2NH]
—NHCO—	ψ[NHCO]
$-CH_2CH_2-$	ψ[CH_2CH_2]
—CHCH—	ψ[CHCH]
$-CH_2CONH-$	ψ[CH_2CONH]
—CONHO—	ψ[CONHO]
$-CHOHCH_2NH-$	ψ[$CHOHCH_2NH$]
$-COCH_2NH-$	ψ[$COCH_2NH$]
—CHOHNH—	ψ[CHOHNH]
$-CHOHCH_2O-$	ψ[$CHOHCH_2O$]
$-CHOHCH_2-$	ψ[$CHOHCH_2$]

Retro-Inverso Peptides

Another modified peptide approach used to transform biologically active peptides with short half-lives (and, thus, of little therapeutic use) into potentially novel and more enzymatically stable analogues is that of the retro-inverso modification. This modification involves reversing one or more amide groups within the peptide backbone. The reversal can be accomplished by using a correctly substituted gem-diaminoalkyl residue (gXaa, where Xaa refers to the 3-letter notation for any amino acid, e.g., Val, and g indicates gem-diaminoalkyl) as the N-terminal residue and a substituted malonic acid residue (mXaa, where m stands for malonic acid) as the C-terminal residue (22,46). The aim of this topological approach is to devise analogues wherein a particular reversed peptide bond (—NHCO—) still maintains its planarity and the spatial orientation of the side chains is retained as close as possible to that of the original peptide. This necessitates that the chirality of amino acids placed between the gem-diaminoalkyl and malonic acid residues must be reversed (rXaa, where r refers to a reversed direction of the peptide bond) (Fig. 7.11) (47). Retro-inverso analogues of several bioactive peptides, particularly partial retro-inverso analogues, generally have displayed enhanced enzymatic stability as well as increased bioavailability and potency (46).

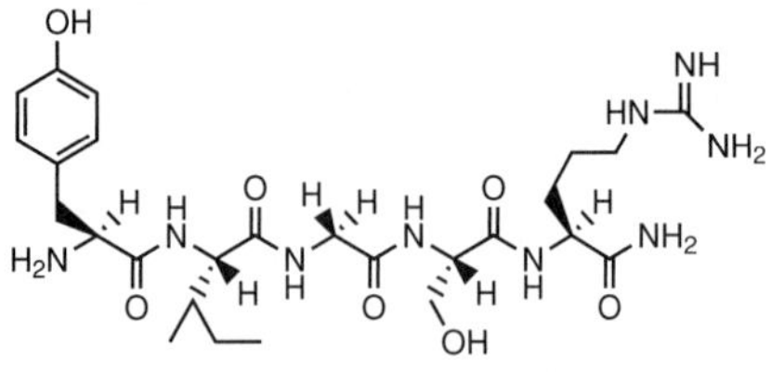

Tyr-Ile-Gly-Ser-Arg-NH_2

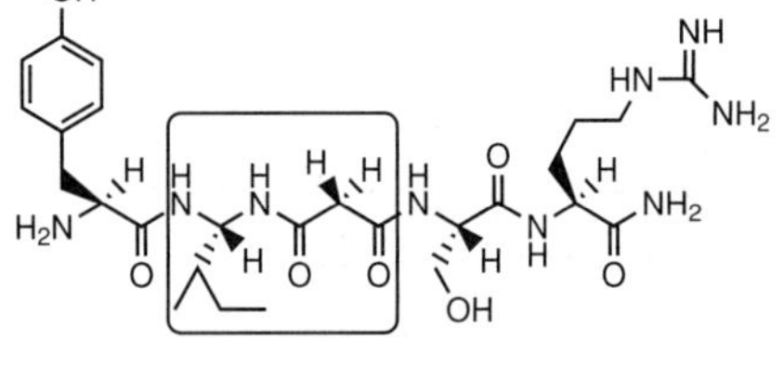

Tyr-gIle-mGly-Ser-Arg-NH_2

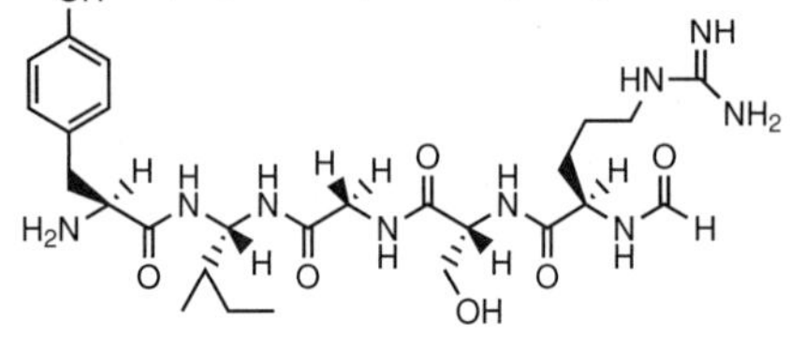

Tyr-gIle-rGly-D-rSer-D-rArg-CHO

Fig. 7.11. A spatial representation of the antimetastic peptide, Tyr-Ile-Gly-Ser-Arg-NH_2 (all L-configuration), and two types of partial retro-inverso analogues. The portion enclosed in the frame is the so-called "pairwise" modified segment (46). (Adapted from Zhao M, Kleinman HK, Mokotoff M. Synthesis and activity of partial retro-inverso analogs of the antimetastatic laminin-derived peptide, YIGSR-NH_2. J Peptide Res 1997;49:240–253; with permission.)

THERAPEUTIC PEPTIDE AND PROTEIN HORMONES AND ANALOGUES

The following sections introduce a variety of peptide and protein hormones, both natural and their analogues, that are commercially available for the treatment of various diseases or are used for diagnostic purposes. These hormones are obtained synthetically, from natural sources, or via genetic engineering. They are listed, for the most part, according to their endocrine organ of origin.

Hormones of Hypothalamic Origin

The hypothalamus, a relatively small organ that is located in the brain and is responsible for thermoregulation, among other functions, is the secretory source for a number of peptide hormones that are transported to the pituitary gland situated immediately below it. These hormones regulate the synthesis of other peptide hormones produced by the anterior pituitary (adenohypophysis) and are thus called releasing hormones, releasing factors, or inhibitory factors, as the case may be. The release of these hypothalamic hormones is regulated via cholinergic and dopaminergic stimuli from higher brain centers, and their synthesis and release are controlled by feedback mechanisms from their target organs.

Gonadotropin-Releasing Hormone

PHYSICOCHEMICAL PROPERTIES. Gonadotropin-releasing hormone (GnRH) is a decapeptide (Fig. 7.12) that causes the release of the gonadotropins, luteinizing hormone (LH) and follicle-stimulating hormone (FSH), from the anterior pituitary gland, but not in equal amounts (FSH release is partially inhibited by the gonadal protein inhibin). Therefore, GnRH is intimately involved in the control of both male and female reproduction. Medicinal chemists have capitalized on the relatively simple decapeptide structure of GnRH by preparing many analogues as potential fertility and antifertility agents, several of which are commercially available, especially those that are referred to as superagonists. It is known that GnRH can be degraded by enzymatic cleavage between Tyr^5-Gly^6 and Pro^9-Gly^{10} (48). Structure–activity relationship studies of GnRH analogues have shown that when Gly^6 is replaced with certain D-amino acids, as well as with changes in the peptide C-terminus, they generally are less susceptible to proteolytic enzymes, resulting in a longer-lasting action. For that reason, they are referred to as superagonists. Furthermore, when these D-amino acids at position 6 are hydrophobic, the half-life is enhanced (Fig. 7.12).

PHYSIOLOGICAL ACTION OF GNRH AGENTS. In physiological doses, GnRH agonists are able to induce ovulation and spermatogenesis by increasing LH and FSH levels and the resulting sex steroid levels, as does the normal hormone.

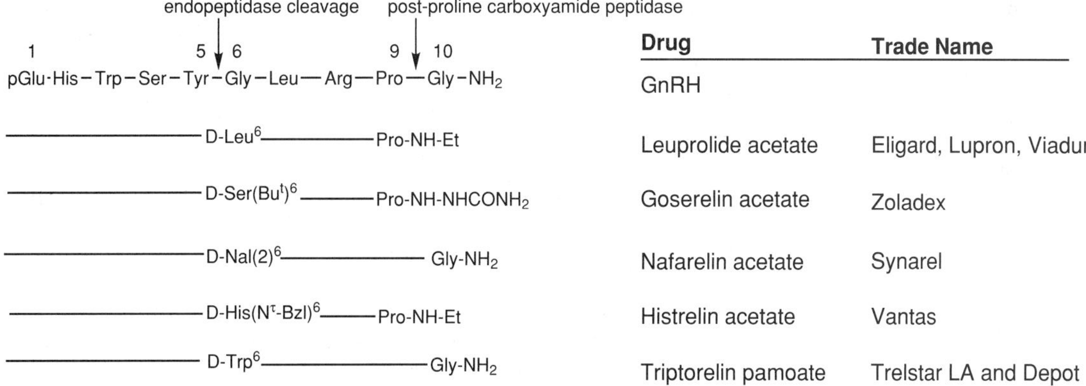

Fig. 7.12. GnRH-based drugs that are commercially available. Note that leuprolide, goserelin, nafarelin, histrelin, and triptorelin are all superagonists, contain a D-amino acid in place of Gly^6, and that three of the five are missing the C-terminal Gly (the line indicates an identical sequence of amino acids).

In larger pharmacological (therapeutic) doses, however, GnRH agonists, especially the superagonists, block implantation of the fertilized egg, cause luteolysis of the corpus luteum, and can act as postcoital contraceptive agents (although not approved for this latter use). This "paradoxical" antifertility effect seen with the superagonists has been attributed to the fact that GnRH must be administered in a low-dose, pulsatile manner for it to be therapeutically effective as a fertility agent. Natural GnRH release from the hypothalamus occurs in a pulsatile manner. When GnRH or, especially, a superagonist is administered in pharmacological doses each day, LH and FSH levels will initially rise but then begin to fall after a few days because of target tissue desensitization/downregulation of pituitary GnRH receptors. The continued use of these agents in a nonpulsatile manner will result in a drastic drop of the gonadal steroid levels to near castrate levels in both males and females, thereby giving rise to their use in such conditions as precocious puberty, endometriosis, and advanced metastatic breast and prostate carcinoma. Typically, however, the GnRH superagonists take approximately 2 weeks to finally desensitize the GnRH receptors, and during this time, there is a transient rise in LH and FSH levels, which often results in an initial "flare-up" of the original symptoms. The following discussion concerns the medicinal chemistry and medical use of the commercially available GnRH analogues (49).

SPECIFIC DRUGS

Leuprolide Acetate. Leuprolide acetate, a synthetic nonapeptide analogue of GnRH that possesses greater potency than the natural hormone, is a superagonist that is commercially available. Note that leuprolide acetate contains substitutions that hinder enzymatic degradation, D-Leu and NH-Et in place of Gly^6 and Gly^{10}-NH_2, respectively (Fig. 7.12). Leuprolide acetate is reportedly 15-fold the potency of natural GnRH. When given continuously and in therapeutic doses, leuprolide acetate inhibits LH and FSH secretion by desensitizing/downregulating the GnRH receptors, as discussed above. After an initial stimulation, chronic administration of leuprolide acetate results in suppression of ovarian and testicular steroidogenesis. In premenopausal females, estrogens are reduced to postmenopausal levels; in males, testosterone is reduced to castrate levels.

Leuprolide acetate is administered by daily injections or as depot injections every month, every 3 months, every 4 months, or every 6 months as a palliative treatment in advanced prostatic carcinoma (as an alternative to orchiectomy). An implant version (Viadur) also is available for long-term palliative therapy; after implantation of the device into the upper arm, leuprolide acetate is continuously released over a 12-month period. Because dihydrotestosterone, a metabolite of testosterone, is able to stimulate the growth of prostate cancer, the ability of leuprolide acetate to bring testosterone to near castrate levels is why this drug finds use as a palliative in the advanced disease. The addition of a nonpeptidyl antiandrogen, such as flutamide or bicalutamide, to the leuprolide acetate regimen inhibits adrenal and testicular synthesized androgens from binding to or being taken up by target prostate cancer tissue. This combination therapy helps to control the initial flare-up, by blocking all sources of androgen, and is referred to as maximal androgen blockade.

Leuprolide acetate, in monthly and every-3-months depot formulations, is useful in treating women diagnosed with endometriosis, but not for longer than six months because of the chance of developing osteoporosis. Endometriosis, a painful disorder of the female reproductive tract, occurs in women during their childbearing years. The disease involves the growth of endometrial tissue (normally shed monthly with menstruation) in areas outside the uterus, usually the pelvic region, where it swells and bleeds internally during the monthly menstrual cycle. The inability of the blood to leave the body leads to inflammation of the surrounding areas as well as formation of scar tissue. Several of the symptoms of endometriosis are painful urination and bowel movements, severe menstrual cramps, pain during sexual intercourse, and the potential for infertility. Because estrogens stimulate the growth of endometrial tissue, the ability of this drug to drastically reduce estrogen levels suggests why leuprolide acetate is useful in treating endometriosis.

Central precocious puberty that is idiopathic, or gonadotropin dependent, can cause the development of secondary sexual characteristics in girls before the age of 8 years and in boys before the age of 9 years. In addition to the psychological and physiological changes that occur because of entering puberty too early, there is the risk of the child failing to reach his or her full adult height. Therefore, leuprolide acetate's ability to suppress LH and sex steroid levels (testosterone and estradiol) to prepubertal levels is the reason that leuprolide acetate is approved for use in treating children with this disease. Use of this drug in a child with precocious puberty will slow or stop that child's secondary sexual development, slow linear growth and skeletal maturation, and in girls, will bring about the cessation of menstruation.

Uterine leiomyomas (fibroids), which are benign neoplasms derived from smooth muscle, can cause, among other problems, excessive vaginal bleeding that may progress to anemia. Leuprolide acetate, concomitant with iron therapy, is used in treating the anemia that arises from uterine leiomyoma. The decrease in the formation of the steroid sex hormones reduces fibroid and uterine volume, produces a relief in the clinical symptoms (pelvic pain), and stops the excessive vaginal bleeding, thus correcting the anemia.

Goserelin Acetate. Goserelin acetate, like leuprolide acetate, is a synthetic superagonist nonapeptide analogue of GnRH that possesses greater potency than the natural hormone. Note that it contains D-Ser(Bu^t) and NH-NHCONH$_2$ in place of Gly^6 and Gly^{10}-NH$_2$, respectively (Fig. 7.12). That is, the C-terminal modification simply has an NH substituting for the CH_2 of Gly, and like the C-terminal change in leuprolide acetate, this inhibits enzymatic degradation of the peptide by the postproline carboxyamide peptidase.

Goserelin acetate is available in the form of a small, solid pellet that is administered as an SC implant for the palliative treatment of advanced, metastatic breast cancer in pre- and perimenopausal women or, similarly, as a palliative in advanced prostatic cancer. The rationale for this drug's use is, as described above, its ability as a superagonist to bring the levels of estradiol or testosterone to near castrate levels, thus slowing the progression of breast or prostate carcinoma, respectively. Additionally, goserelin acetate is approved for use in treating endometriosis for up to 6 months.

Goserelin acetate also is used in combination with the antiandrogen flutamide for shrinking prostate carcinoma before radiation therapy. This maximal androgen blockade combination is used when the prostate carcinoma has been staged as locally confined to the prostate gland, with one or both lobes as well as the seminal vesicles involved. The treatment should start 8 weeks before radiation treatment begins and be continued throughout the radiation therapy.

Furthermore, women who are to undergo hysterectomy for menorrhagia can benefit from previous treatment with goserelin acetate, because it is able to induce endometrial thinning. This thinning of the endometrium improves the operating environment by causing less intrauterine bleeding, increased postoperative amenorrhea, and decreased dysmenorrhea following surgery, which is why goserelin acetate is approved for inducing endometrial thinning prior to a patient undergoing a hysterectomy for heavy menstrual bleeding.

Nafarelin Acetate. Nafarelin acetate, another synthetic superagonist decapeptide analogue of GnRH, contains D-Nal(2)^6 [Nal = 3-(2-naphthyl)-Ala] in place of Gly^6, but the C-terminus, Gly^{10}-NH$_2$, is identical with natural GnRH (Fig. 7.12). Nafarelin acetate is available as a 0.2% nasal spray for the relief of endometriosis. Estrogen, of course, is needed for the growth of endometrial tissue; thus, decreased estrogen leads to shrinkage of errant endometrial tissue. The observed side effects of nafarelin acetate are related to falling estrogen levels and include decreased libido, amenorrhea, hot flashes, and vaginal dryness. When used consistently, nafarelin acetate will inhibit ovulation and stop menstruation.

Nafarelin acetate also is used in children, male and female, for the treatment of central precocious puberty. By suppressing the release of LH, the estradiol or testosterone levels fall to prepubertal levels; early secondary sexual development is arrested, linear growth and skeletal maturation are slowed, and in girls, menstruation stops.

Histrelin Acetate. Histrelin acetate, a superagonist analogue of GnRH, contains D- His(N^τ-Bzl)^6 in place of Gly^6, and the C-terminus is identical with leuprolide acetate—namely, NH-Et in place of Gly^{10}-NH$_2$ (Fig. 7.12). This GnRH analogue is commercially available in the form of an implantable device (SC in the upper arm) that slowly releases the drug over a 12-month period, resulting in decreased testicular steroidogenesis, for the palliative treatment of advanced prostate cancer.

Triptorelin Pamoate. Triptorelin pamoate is another superagonist of GnRH, which like nafarelin acetate contains only a single amino acid substitution (D-Trp^6 for Gly^6) when compared to the natural hormone (Fig. 7.12). In the treatment of advanced prostate cancer, it is important to reduce serum testosterone levels to very low levels, which can be achieved surgically by orchiectomy. When this surgical method is unacceptable to the patient, an alternative approach is "chemical castration," which can be achieved by use of estrogen therapy, leupro-

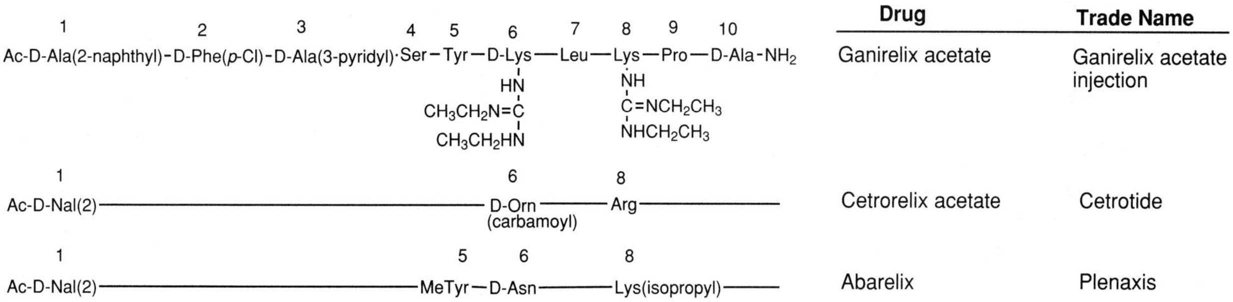

Fig. 7.13. GnRH-receptor antagonists.

lide, goserelin or histrelin acetates, and now, triptorelin pamoate. This product is available for IM depot injection (monthly or every 3 months), wherein serum testosterone concentration drops to a level generally seen in surgically castrated men.

Ganirelix Acetate. Ganirelix acetate is an analog of GnRH with substitutions at residues 1, 2, 3, 6, 8, and 10 (Fig. 7.13). It is not a superagonist but, rather, is a synthetic decapeptide with high antagonist activity and the first GnRH antagonist to be marketed. It is approved for the suppression of LH surges in women who are undergoing ovarian hyperstimulation fertility treatment; LH surges normally promote ovulation. The goal of this drug is to significantly reduce the number of medication days necessary to suppress the LH surge, thereby maintaining eggs in the ovaries. In vitro fertilization (IVF) treatment cycles were historically initiated by the administration of leuprolide acetate to suppress the premature release of LH. This inhibits ovulation so that the eggs remain available for retrieval by a fertility specialist. For this purpose, leuprolide acetate usually is injected for as many as 26 days. Clinical studies have shown that ganirelix acetate can shut down the LH surge in only 5 days of treatment, that the suppression of LH is more pronounced than that of FSH, and that the shorter treatment time minimizes unpleasant side effects, such as hot flashes and headaches.

Cetrorelix Acetate. Cetrorelix acetate is an analogue of GnRH with amino acid substitutions at residues 1, 2, 3, 6, and 10 and differing from ganirelix at amino acids 1, 6, and 8 (Fig. 7.13). Each of these substitutions are synthetic, non-DNA-directed amino acids and, like ganirelix acetate, impart GnRH antagonist activity to cetrorelix acetate. This drug also is marketed for use in women undergoing assisted reproductive therapy (ART) procedures, in which it is necessary to control their LH surge. This allows the follicles to develop to a size, as determined by ultrasound, that increases the success of timed insemination and oocyte retrieval for IVF. Like ganirelix acetate, cetrorelix acetate has an advantage over GnRH agonists, such as leuprolide acetate, because it reduces the fertility therapy cycle to days rather than weeks.

Abarelix. Abarelix is another GnRH receptor antagonist with substitutions or alterations of the natural hormone at seven residues; the amino acids at positions 4, 7, and 9 are identical with those in GnRH. Abarelix differs from ganirelix at amino acids 1, 5, 6, and 8 (Fig. 7.13). Unlike ganirelix and cetrorelix, however, abarelix is not used in women undergoing ART but, rather, as a palliative in men with advanced prostate cancer. Like the superagonists, abarelix affords a drop in testosterone to castrate levels. Abarelix does not, however, cause the initial rise in testosterone levels and resulting flare-up of symptoms often seen with the superagonists. Still, because of the risk of life-threatening allergic reactions associated with its use, this drug is specifically relegated to a select group of men with advanced symptomatic prostate cancer who are not candidates for other hormone therapies and who choose not to undergo orchiectomy. Abarelix is available only from health care providers who have participated in a special education program that allows them to identify allergic reactions associated with its use.

Somatostatin

PHYSIOLOGICAL ACTION. Somatostatin is a cyclic 14-peptide that was first isolated by Guillemin in 1973 and is probably the most thoroughly investigated and most important of the inhibitory factors produced by the hypothalamus (Fig. 7.14). The principal activity of somatostatin, which is of hypothalamic origin, is inhibition of the release of growth hormone (GH) from the anterior pituitary. Too much GH, as in pituitary tumors, causes acromegaly, a form of giantism. On the other hand, too little GH leads to dwarfism. Somatostatin also has been found in the pancreas and the GI tract, where it inhibits the secretion of both insulin and glucagon from the pancreas as well as the secretion of a variety of intestinal peptides (e.g., gastrin, secretin, pepsin, and renin). The short half-life of somatostatin, which is less than 3 minutes, has precluded its use as a therapeutic agent. Many derivatives of somatostatin have been prepared to increase its duration of action and/or to enhance its selectivity of action. The culmination of these structure–activity studies was the development of octreotide acetate.

SPECIFIC DRUGS

Octreotide Acetate. Octreotide acetate, a long-acting octapeptide analogue of somatostatin, has a half-life of approximately 100 minutes. A comparison of the primary structures of octreotide and somatostatin suggests little similarity, but from earlier work at the Salk Institute it was known that not all the residues in somatostatin were necessary to elicit its full biological activity. Other studies suggested that the essential fragment for its activity was the tetrapeptide Phe^7-Trp^8-Lys^9-Thr^{10} (Fig. 7.14). These earlier studies helped in the design of the potent drug now known as octreotide acetate (50). This drug suppresses the secretion of gastroenteropancreatic peptides, such as gastrin, vasoactive intestinal peptide (VIP), insulin, and glucagon, as well as pituitary GH. Furthermore, it is more potent than natural somatostatin in inhibiting the release of glucagon, insulin, and GH.

Octreotide acetate is used by SC injection in the palliative treatment of patients with metastatic carcinoid tumors, which are tumors of the endocrine system, GI tract, and lung (gastroenteropancreatic). Carcinoid tumors secrete increasing amounts of vasoactive substances, including histamine, serotonin, bradykinin, and prostaglandins. Octreotide acetate inhibits or suppresses the release of these vasoactive substances and, thus, is useful in treating the severe diarrhea, facial flushing, and wheezing episodes that accompany carcinoid tumors. In addition, it finds use in the palliative management of VIP-secreting tumors (VIPomas, usually pancreatic tumors). Patients with VIPomas suffer a profuse, watery diarrhea syndrome, and octreotide acetate is able to help by decreasing the release of damaging intestinal tumor cell secretions. Octreotide also helps to reduce hypokalemia by correcting electrolyte imbalances.

An excessive secretion of GH from the pituitary can cause the disorder known as acromegaly, which is characterized by a progressive enlargement of the head, face, hands, feet, and thorax. Inasmuch as octreotide acetate is able to decrease the secretion of GH from the pituitary, it is used in treating patients with acromegaly who are unresponsive to previous pituitary radiation therapy or surgery. It is used in the treatment of acromegaly, because it reduces the blood levels of both GH and insulin-like growth factor-I (IGF-I). The long-acting repository form of octreotide acetate also is used in treating acromegaly, carcinoid tumors, and VIPomas, but in monthly depot injections.

Octreotide for IV injection is used in the treatment of acute bleeding from esophageal varices. Variceal bleeding occurs in about half the patients with cirrhosis of the liver and is responsible for about one-third of deaths in these patients. Octreotide is a potent vasoconstrictor that reduces portal and collateral blood flow by constricting visceral vessels, which leads to reduced portal blood pressure and decreases the bleeding.

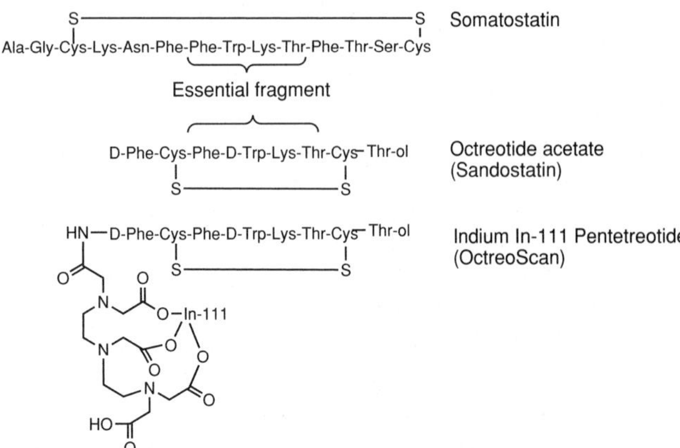

Fig. 7.14. Somatostatin and its analogue, octreotide.

Indium In-111 Pentetreotide (OctreoScan). Somatostatin receptors have a broad distribution in normal tissue as well as in a variety of human malignancies (e.g., small cell lung, brain, breast, pituitary, and endocrine pancreatic cancers). For this reason, octreotide, which binds to somatostatin receptors, was converted to a radionuclide-containing peptide by reacting the amino terminus with an active ester of diethylenetriaminepenta acetic acid (DTPA) to give DTPA-octreotide and then chelated to the radionuclide ^{111}In (Fig. 7.14). This radiopharmaceutical is used as a diagnostic agent for the early detection and localization of small tumors and their metastases in the body, especially tumors that originate from neuroendocrine cells.

Corticorelin Ovine Triflutate (Acthrel)

The primary function of corticotropin-releasing factor (CRF), a hypothalamic 41-peptide, is the regulation of the release of adrenocorticotropin hormone (ACTH) from the anterior pituitary gland, which then stimulates the release of hydrocortisone from the adrenal gland. The human peptide (hCRF) and the similar sequence found in sheep (oCRF) have been prepared by synthesis. The ovine form of the hormone, however, has replaced the human form because of its longer half-life and greater potency; hCRF is no longer commercially available.

Usually, ACTH deficiency in humans is associated with a pituitary disorder rather than with a deficiency of CRF, and oCRF can be used to distinguish between pituitary hypersecretion of ACTH (Cushing's disease) and ectopic ACTH secretion, both of which are conditions that cause a hypersecretion of hydrocortisone. In the case of ectopic ACTH secretion, the administration of oCRF will elicit little to no response in the production of ACTH and hydrocortisone. Therefore, synthetic oCRF trifluoroacetate salt is marketed as a diagnostic agent for patients with ACTH-dependent Cushing's syndrome.

Hormones Originating in the Anterior Lobe of the Pituitary Gland

The pituitary, lying just below the hypothalamus, is a small gland that can be divided into an anterior and a posterior lobe. This gland is responsible for the secretion of several important peptide hormones, two of which are released by the posterior lobe. The anterior pituitary peptide hormones control important functions such as growth, reproduction, metabolic and ion balance, as well as a number of others.

Growth Hormone (GH)

A protein containing 191 amino acids, GH is secreted by the anterior pituitary in response to the liberation of GH-releasing factor from the hypothalamus. This contrasts with somatostatin, which inhibits the release of GH. The primary function of GH in the body is to promote skeletal growth. When GH is absent during childhood, or if there is an inadequate supply, dwarfism results. Before 1985, children of short stature were sometimes treated with human GH (hGH) of pituitary origin, which was obtained from cadavers, but hGH of natural origin was discontinued by the U.S. FDA when several young adults, who had received hGH as children, died. Their deaths were attributed to contaminated hGH. The contaminant was an infective agent, known as a prion, that causes Creutzfeldt-Jakob disease, a rare and fatal neurodegenerative disease (51). Naturally occurring hGH has been replaced with material that is prepared by recombinant DNA (rDNA) methodology.

SPECIFIC DRUGS

Somatropin (Genotropin, Humatrope, Norditropin, Nutropin, Saizen, Serostim, Zorbtive). Somatropin, which is hGH that is prepared by rDNA procedures, contains exactly the same sequence of 191 amino acids as the natural hormone. Several of these products are indicated for the long-term treatment of children who fail to grow because of inadequate secretion of the body's normal endogenous GH and for growth problems associated with chronic renal failure. Even adults who are diagnosed with GH deficiency, which can arise as a result of pituitary or hypothalamic disease, surgery, radiation therapy, or other reasons, can benefit from hGH replacement therapy. Turner's syndrome, a genetic disease in which there is a complete or partial absence of one of the two X chromosomes in females, causes short stature as one of its many symptoms. Girls suffering from Turner's syndrome can benefit from the use of Humatrope, Norditropin, or Nutropin during their growth years.

The anabolic properties of hGH is the basis for the orphan drug uses of several of these recombinant products. It is used in AIDS-associated catabolism or weight loss, in cachexia resulting from AIDS, and as an anabolic agent in patients with severe burns. In addition, the anabolic property of rhGH is the reason for Zorbtive's use, along with specialized nutritional support, in the treatment of short-bowel syndrome.

Pegvisomant (Somavert). This product contains 191 amino acid residues (of recombinant origin), the same number as in GH, but there are substitutions at residues 18, 21, 120, 167, 168, 171, 172, 174, and 179. This product is then covalently linked to several polyethylene glycol molecules, and this pegylated protein is a GH-receptor antagonist. Thus, pegvisomant binds to the GH receptor and blocks endogenous GH from binding. The result is a blocking of the GH-stimulated overproduction of IGF-I that contributes to the disabling symptoms and long-term health problems associated with acromegaly.

Gonadotropins

CHEMISTRY. The gonadotropins, FSH and LH, are large glycoproteins released by the anterior pituitary on stimulation from GnRH produced by the hypothalamus. Both FSH and LH consist of two noncovalently associated α and β subunits. The α subunits both contain 92 amino acids and are identical in both hormones, whereas the β subunit in LH consists of 121 residues and 111 residues in FSH, with the β subunits being dissimilar (52). Thus, the β subunit gives each hormone its specific function.

PHYSIOLOGICAL PROPERTIES. Both LH and FSH are referred to as gonadotropins, because they act on the male and female gonads, which results in the production of the sex steroids testosterone and estradiol, respectively. In the female, FSH and LH act in concert in regulating ovarian function: egg maturation, ovulation, and transformation of the ruptured follicle into the corpus luteum. In males, spermatogenesis is dependent on these two hormones. Specifically, FSH in females facilitates the maturation of ovarian follicle cells and their secretion of estradiol, whereas in males, it stimulates the maturation of sperm in the testes. In females, LH promotes ovulation, formation of the corpus luteum, and progesterone secretion; in males, it enables the secretion of testosterone from the testes.

According to the Research Initiative Committee and the Public Communications Committee of the Endocrine Society, "[I]nfertility is the inability of a sexually active couple, who is not using any contraception, to achieve pregnancy in one year, the time in which 90% of couples succeed." In the case of male infertility, it generally is caused by the quality and/or quantity of the sperm produced. In the case of female infertility, however, it may be caused by several factors, such as the inability to produce an egg, to ovulate, for fertilization to occur, and for implantation of the fertilized ovum in the uterus. Several of the commercially available gonadotropins can help in enhancing both male and female fertility and are discussed below.

SPECIFIC DRUGS

Menotropins (Menopur, Repronex). Menotropins are a natural product that is obtained from the urine of postmenopausal women and then biologically standardized (international units [IU]) for FSH and LH activities in an approximate ratio of 1:1. Menotropins are used in males with primary (hypothalamic) or secondary (pituitary) hypogonadism to stimulate spermatogenesis, providing they have been treated previously with human chorionic gonadotropin (hCG; a peptide hormone of placental origin that has activity very similar to LH; discussed below) to effect masculinization (increased testosterone production). In females, menotropins and hCG are given sequentially for the purposes of inducing ovulation in women who are having difficulty ovulating as a result of either hypothalamic or pituitary hormonal dysfunction. The menotropins are given for 7 to 12 days, and after clinical evaluation (via ultrasound) indicates the presence of a mature follicle, a single dose of hCG is given to simulate the typical LH surge that normally triggers ovulation. Also, women use the combination of menotropins and hCG to promote the development of multiple follicles when they are participating in an IVF program requiring the recruitment of follicles.

Follitropins. Follitropins are hormonal products that consist entirely of FSH and are used to stimulate ovarian follicle growth in women who do not have primary ovarian failure. In the absence of an adequate endogenous LH surge, however, hCG must be given following the use of follitropins to stimulate ovulation.

Urofollitropins (Bravelle). Urofollitropin, a natural product like the menotropins, is obtained from the urine of postmenopausal women and then highly purified so as to contain only FSH, reportedly with only minute amounts of LH. Urofollitropin is used for its ability to stimulate follicle development, such as in women undergoing drug-induced pituitary suppression (GnRH antagonist or superagonist) for purposes of IVF (i.e., multiple follicle development or egg donation). When the number and size of the ovarian follicles are correct, as determined by ultrasound, hCG is administered so as to effect ovulation, and the oocytes are retrieved for IVF.

This drug also is indicated for women who have infertility caused by polycystic ovary syndrome, which generally is observed clinically as enlarged, cystic ovaries containing relatively small follicles. These patients often develop hirsutism, their androgen and LH levels appear elevated while their FSH levels are low, and the early exposure to these improper hormone levels may be causing the follicular atresia (53). The patient's monthly cycle is controlled by previous pituitary suppression via treatment with a GnRH superagonist or antagonist; urofollitropin, as an exogenous source of FSH, is administered and stimulates follicle maturation to preovulatory size, with little or no exposure of the follicles to additional LH. When the follicles have matured to preovulatory size, ovulation is assisted by the administration of hCG. The couple is then advised to engage in sexual intercourse daily, beginning on the day before hCG administration and until ovulation has occurred.

Lately, it has become desirable to have a nonnatural source of pure FSH. It is believed that exposure to increased amounts of LH early in follicular development, as would be the case with menotropins, is detrimental to fertility. Also, urofollitropin is derived from menopausal urine, and the supply of this natural product is limited. These problems are especially noteworthy in treating infertility in women with polycystic ovary syndrome and have given rise to recombinant forms of FSH.

Follitropin Alfa (Gonal-F, Gonal-F RFF, Gonal-F RFF Pen). Follitropin alfa is a human FSH preparation of rDNA origin. Because FSH is a glycoprotein, alterations in the carbohydrate side-chain attachments afford different isoforms, which leads to different pharmacokinetic and pharmacodynamic properties. Because it is of recombinant origin and not isolated from urine, it is free of any additional substances, such as urinary proteins and LH.

Like urofollitropin, it is marketed for enhancing the development of multiple follicles that can then be induced to ovulate, via hCG administration, so that the oocytes can be collected for IVF. It also is used in treating women who wish to become pregnant and are anovulatory because of polycystic ovary syndrome, in whom it can enhance follicle maturation before hCG administration for final ovulation. All commercial products can be administered by SC injection. The RFF notation signifies Revised Formulation Female, and the RFF Pen notation indicates a prefilled, ready-to-use device designed to make self administration easier.

Men with infertility also can benefit from therapy with follitropin alfa if their infertility is related to hypothalamic or pituitary hormonal dysfunction and not primary testicular failure, because it induces spermatogenesis. Just as with therapy using menotropins, pretreatment with hCG is performed for 3 months to achieve serum testosterone levels within the normal range, before hCG and follitropin alfa therapy.

Follitropin Beta (Follistim AQ). Follitropin beta is a human FSH preparation of rDNA origin, which differs chemically from natural FSH and follitropin alfa only by slight variances in the composition of the carbohydrate side chains. In fact, the primary and tertiary structures of both follitropins alfa and beta are indistinguishable from those of human FSH of natural origin. Furthermore, bioassays and physiochemical studies indicate that follitropins alfa and beta are indistinguishable from each other. Therefore, it is not surprising that follitropin beta is approved for the same medical uses as follitropin alpha.

Lutropin Alfa (Luveris). Lutropin alfa is the first pure human LH preparation and is of rDNA origin. According to physicochemical and biological assays, it is indistinguishable from human LH of natural origin. It is indicated for use in infertile women who are undergoing ART, specifically those with severe LH deficiency. It is meant to be coadministered with follitropin alfa so as to stimulate follicular growth in these women. When the follicles are of correct size, as determined by ultrasound examination, hCG would be administered to stimulate ovulation.

Adrenocorticotropin Hormone (H.P. Acthar Gel)

The anterior pituitary, under the influence of the hypothalamic hormone hCRF, releases ACTH, a single-chain peptide of 39 residues. ACTH is derived from a much larger precursor protein known as pro-opiomelanocortin, the latter of which is the precursor of the melanocyte-stimulating hormones, the lipotropins, and other biologically active peptides. The sequence of 24-amino-acid residues beginning from the amino terminus contains all the biological activity of the parent. The remaining 15 C-terminal residues confer species specificity as well as enhancing the stability of ACTH toward proteolytic cleavage. Consider the fact that residues 1 through 24 are identical in humans, pigs, sheep, and beef, whereas the species differ only slightly from each other in the final 15 residues. Furthermore, N-terminal residues 1 through 13 in ACTH are identical with the full structure of α-MSH. The main action of ACTH on the adrenal cortex involves the release of the glucocorticoid hormone hydrocortisone and the mineralocorticoid (electrolyte balance) hormone aldosterone.

Commercial ACTH is obtained from natural sources and is available in 16% gelatin (repository gel) to prolong its release after SC or IM injection. ACTH has both anti-inflammatory and immunosuppressant properties, which contributes to its use in the treatment of acute exacerbations of multiple sclerosis.

SYNTHETIC ACTH ANALOG

Cosyntropin (Cortrosyn). Cosyntropin is a synthetic polypeptide that consists of amino acid residues 1 through 24 of human ACTH, but that has the full biological activity of its parent. Because it is of synthetic origin, it is less allergenic than ACTH of natural origin. Cosyntropin is used as a diagnostic agent in the screening of patients suspected of having adrenocortical insufficiency. Normally, parenteral administration of cosyntropin acts rapidly on the adrenal cortex to effect release of plasma hydrocortisone; when performing the test, the hydrocortisone levels are compared to a control blood sample taken earlier.

Hormones Released from the Posterior Lobe of the Pituitary Gland

As previously discussed, the pituitary gland is responsible for the secretion of several peptide hormones, only two of which are released by the posterior lobe. Actually, these two hormones, oxytocin and vasopressin, are synthesized in neurons originating in the hypothalamus and are transported to the posterior pituitary for storage until release is required.

Oxytocin

Oxytocin is a cyclic 9-peptide that, like somatostatin, contains a ring that encompasses a disulfide bridge (Fig. 7.15). Oxytocin has uterotonic action, contracting the muscles of the uterus during gestation, and plays an important role in milk ejection (not milk secretion, which is regulated by the peptide hormone prolactin) from the mammary ducts into the nipples. Exogenous oxytocin most commonly is used for induction of labor, wherein it improves uterine contractions to achieve early vaginal delivery for fetal or maternal reasons (e.g., preeclampsia, Rh factor problems, pregnancy that has exceeded 42 weeks). It also finds use following delivery of the placenta, because it promotes contraction and vasoconstriction and helps to control postpartum bleeding.

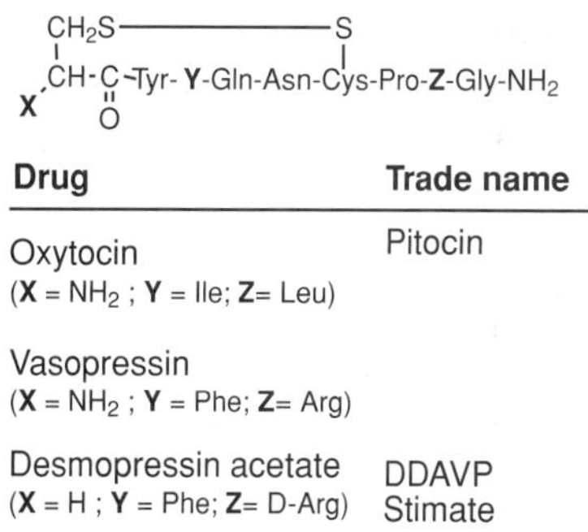

Fig. 7.15. Structural relationship between oxytocin, vasopressin, and its analogue.

Vasopressin

Human vasopressin, or Arg-vasopressin, is chemically very similar to oxytocin and therefore sometimes is referred to as [Phe^{3}, Arg^{8}]oxytocin (Fig. 7.15). The physiological role of vasopressin is the regulation of water reabsorption in the renal tubules (an antidiuretic action, thus often referred to as the antidiuretic hormone). In high doses, vasopressin promotes the contraction of arterioles and capillaries, resulting in an increase in blood pressure, thus the name vasopressin. An inadequate output of pituitary antidiuretic hormone can cause diabetes insipidus, which is characterized by the chronic excretion of large amounts of pale urine and results in dehydration and extreme thirst.

Desmopressin Acetate

Desmopressin, as its acetate salt, is a synthetic analogue of vasopressin in which the N-terminal Cys is devoid of its α-amino function (1-Deamino) and where Arg^{8} is present as its D-isomer (D-Arg^{8}), thus the commercial acronym DDAVP (Fig. 7.15). The presence of D-Arg and the absence of the N-terminal amine in the desmopressin structure have increased its half-life such that it is available for oral, parenteral, or nasal use. It is used by all three of these routes of administration to prevent or control polydipsia (excessive thirst), polyuria, and dehydration of patients with diabetes insipidus caused by a deficiency of vasopressin. It also has been approved for the treatment of nocturnal enuresis (bed-wetting), which is believed to be caused by an absence of the normal night time rise in vasopressin levels.

Desmopressin is known to cause an increase in both plasma factor VIII (antihemophilic factor) and plasminogen activator. It therefore is approved by the U.S. FDA for use, parenterally and nasally, in reducing spontaneous or trauma-induced bleeding episodes in patients with hemophilia A and type I Von Willebrand's disease, provided that their plasma factor VIII activity is greater than 5%. Stimate, the nasal spray used in treating patients with hemophilia A and type I Von Willebrand's disease, is 15-fold the concentration of DDAVP nasal spray; the latter is used in treating diabetes insipidus.

Hormone of Placental Origin

If, after ovulation occurs in females, the liberated ovum is fertilized and then implants in the endometrium, the resulting placenta that forms between mother and fetus begins to release a hormone, hCG, the function of which is to maintain and prolong the life of the ovarian corpus luteum. The corpus luteum is important for the continued production of progesterone. Progesterone is especially important because it prepares the uterus for pregnancy and helps in the maintenance of the placenta. Human chorionic gonadotropin begins to appear in the maternal bloodstream and urine shortly after conception and implantation of the fertilized ovum. As a result of this early release of hCG, its detection in the urine forms the basis for the home pregnancy kits that have become so popular in the early prediction of pregnancy.

Human Chorionic Gonadotropin (hCG, Pregnyl)

Placental hCG is a complex protein that consists of an α and β subunit. The α subunit consists of 92 amino acids that are identical in sequence with that found in both LH and FSH, whereas the β subunit contains 145 amino acids and is responsible for its biological specificity. The biological actions of hCG closely resemble those of LH, but the former has a longer half-life than the latter and has minimal FSH activity.

Like LH, hCG stimulates the production of testosterone by the testes; therefore, it is used in treating male hypogonadism and prepubertal cryptorchidism in young males (age, 4–9 years), in whom it stimulates testicular descent. In treating infertility caused by pituitary dysfunction, hCG, in combination with menotropins (as discussed previously) or clomiphene, can induce ovulation and pregnancy in anovulatory females. This hCG, which is of natural origin, is purified from the urine of pregnant women.

Choriogonadotropin Alfa (Ovidrel)

Choriogonadotropin alfa is obtained by rDNA technology and is biologically and chemically identical to hCG of natural origin. It is used, like hCG of natural origin, for inducing ovulation in women with anovulatory infertility. Following proper pretreatment with a GnRH antagonist or superagonist to desensitize the pituitary, women participating in ART are treated with a follicle-stimulating agent (e.g., menotropins) to effect the final maturation of the follicles within the ovaries. Ultrasonograms are used to determine proper follicle maturation before the administration of choriogonadotropin alfa to induce ovulation. A distinct advantage of this product is that it can be self-administered by the patient via SC injection.

Hormone of Parathyroid Origin

Overview

The parathyroid glands (four) exist as two pairs, one pair of which is embedded on the back surface of each lobe (two) of the thyroid gland. These very small glands are responsible for the secretion of parathyroid hormone (PTH), the action of which is the regulation of both calcium and phosphate metabolism within bone and kidney. In humans, the Ca^{2+} concentration is carefully regulated, and when it falls below a normal level, the parathyroid glands secrete PTH, an 84-residue, single-chain protein. Depending on whether PTH is administered intermittently or continuously, it can either stimulate bone formation or breakdown (resorption), respectively.

Teriparatide (Forteo)

Teriparatide, a polypeptide prepared by rDNA techniques, consists of the first 34 amino acid residues from the N-terminal end of PTH. It has been shown to contain all the structural requirements for the full biological activity of PTH. When teriparatide is administered daily by SC injection, it stimulates osteoblastic activity at the expense of osteoclastic activity, and this enhances bone formation. This is the basis for teriparatide's use in treating high-risk patients in danger of bone fracture resulting from osteoporosis, men with primary or hypogonadal osteoporosis, and women with postmenopausal osteoporosis.

Hormone Secreted by the Parafollicular C Cells of the Thyroid Gland

Overview

The majority of the thyroid gland contains follicular cells responsible for the production of the thyroid hormones. A second population of endocrine cells within the thyroid known as C (clear) cells, or parafollicular cells, produce the hormone calcitonin (CT), which has an opposing action to that of PTH in that it decreases the Ca^{2+} concentration in body fluids. It accomplishes this by inhibiting the activity of osteoclasts (i.e., decreasing Ca^{2+} release from bone by inhibiting bone resorption). The actual biosynthesis and release of CT is regulated by the concentration of Ca^{2+} in plasma (i.e., when it is high, CT secretion increases).

SALMON CALCITONIN (FORTICAL, MIACALCIN) Calcitonin is a single-chain polypeptide consisting of 32 amino acid residues (Fig. 7.16). Calcitonins as obtained from different species are identical at seven of the first nine residues, contain Gly at position 28, and all terminate with Pro-NH_2. The C-terminal proline amide (Pro-NH_2) is very important for the biological function of CT, as is the disulfide bridge between Cys residues at positions 1 and 7. In contrast, the residues from 10 through 27 can be varied and seem to influence CT's potency as well as its duration of action. Salmon CT differs from human CT at 16 amino acid residues

Only salmon CT is commercially available for medical use, because on a weight basis, it is approximately 45-fold more potent than human CT. Salmon CT, in parenteral form, is approved for treating Paget's disease of bone (generally seen in older persons; involves increased bone resorp-

S——————————S
Cys-Ser-Asn-Leu-Ser-Thr-Cys-Val-Leu-Gly-Lys-Leu-Ser-Gln-Glu-Leu-His-Lys-Leu-Gln—
1 5 10 15 20

Thr-Tyr-Pro-Arg-Thr-Asn-Thr-Gly-Ser-Gly-Thr-Pro-NH_2 Salmon CT
25 30

S——————————S
Cys-Gly-Asn-Leu-Ser-Thr-Cys-Met-Leu-Gly-Thr-Tyr-Thr-Gln-Asp-Phe-Asn-Lys-Phe-His—
1 5 10 15 20

Thr-Phe-Pro-Gln-Thr-Ala-Ile-Gly-Val-Gly-Ala-Pro-NH_2 Human CT
25 30

Fig. 7.16. Primary structures of salmon and human calcitonin (CT).

tion and softening of bones), postmenopausal osteoporosis, and hypercalcemia of malignancy (multiple myeloma or advanced breast carcinoma). Salmon CT also is available in a nasal spray formulation, which is used exclusively in the treatment of postmenopausal osteoporosis.

Hormones of Endocrine Pancreatic Origin

Overview

The exocrine pancreas consists mostly (~99%) of gland cells known as pancreatic acini, which are responsible for secreting several digestive enzymes. The endocrine pancreas, or the remaining 1% of the gland, consists of a group of cells known as pancreatic islets or islets of Langerhans. Each of these islets consists of four distinct cell types, designated as α, β, γ, and δ cells. The α cells secrete glucagon, the β cells insulin and amylin, the δ cells a peptide that is identical with somatostatin of hypothalamic origin, and the γ cells pancreatic polypeptide, of which little concerning its physiological action is known. Insulin, glucagon, and somatostatin are essential in regulating carbohydrate, lipid, and amino acid metabolism. Insulin is responsible for promoting the storage of glucose as glycogen and effecting hypoglycemia, whereas glucagon mobilizes glucose from its glycogen stores and causes hyperglycemia. The primary action of somatostatin of hypothalamic origin is to inhibit the release of GH from the pituitary, but pancreatic somatostatin suppresses the production of both insulin and glucagon. Amylin, which is cosecreted with insulin from the β cells, has physiological actions that include slowing of gastric emptying, suppression of postprandial glucagon secretion, reduction of food intake, and inhibition in the secretion of both stomach acid and pancreatic digestive enzymes.

Inasmuch as Chapter 32 is devoted primarily to a discussion of insulin and oral hypoglycemic agents, we will thus be brief in our coverage of the pancreatic polypeptides.

Insulin

Insulin has anabolic properties that include the stimulation of both skeletal muscle and liver cells to incorporate glucose and convert it to glycogen, to synthesize proteins from amino acids in the blood, and to act on fat cells to enhance their uptake of glucose and the synthesis of fat. In short, insulin encourages anabolism rather than catabolism, because it promotes the synthesis of glycogen, proteins, and lipids. A deficiency of insulin, which characterizes the disease diabetes mellitus (DM), causes extreme changes in the entire metabolic pattern of individuals with DM. Patients with DM often demonstrate elevated blood glucose levels, excess glucose in the urine, and failure to properly utilize carbohydrate and lipids. Untreated DM can be fatal. Even when treated, however, there can be numerous circulatory and renal complications, and some metabolic abnormalities may lead to blindness (diabetic retinopathy).

CHEMISTRY. Proinsulin, a single-chain protein of 86 amino acid residues, is synthesized in the β cells and enzymatically transformed therein to insulin. The conversion involves the cleavage of a connecting C-peptide, which contains between 30 and 35 residues, with the number and sequence varying among different species (human C-peptide consists of 35 residues). The resulting human insulin consists of two peptide chains, designated A (having 21 residues) and B (having 30 residues), which are interchain connected by two disulfide bonds. Furthermore, the A-chain also contains an intrachain disulfide bond between Cys^6 and Cys^{11} (Fig. 7.17).

The primary sequences of insulin from several species are known, and porcine insulin is the closest to that of humans. Their A-chains are identical, and they differ only in their B-chains, with Ala^{30} (porcine) in place of Thr^{30} (human). Human and bovine insulin differ in each chain, with Ala^8 and Val^{10} in the A-Chain (bovine) and

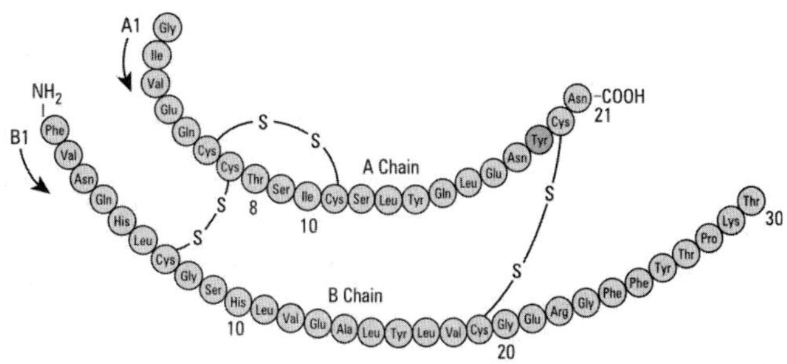

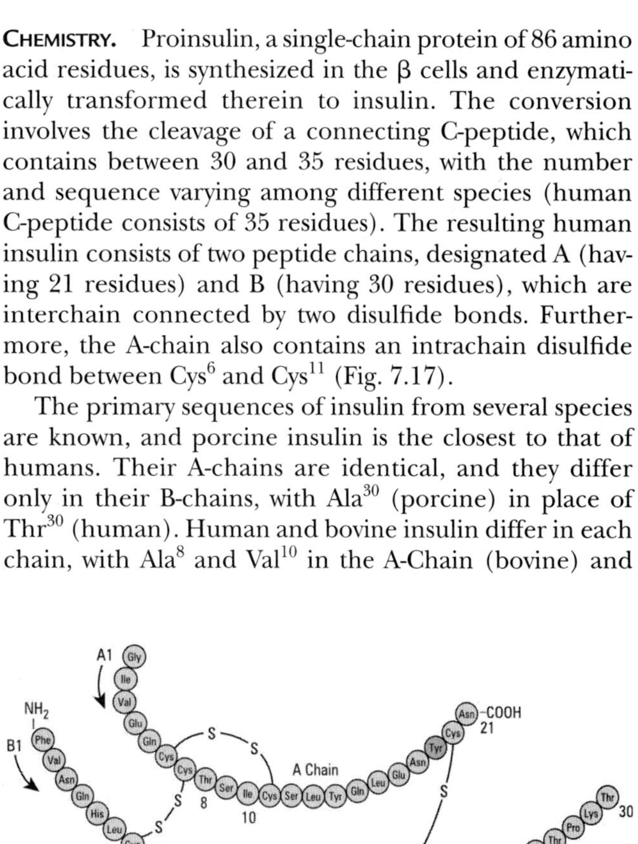

Fig. 7.17. Primary structure of human insulin chains A and B, including the interchain disulfide bonds A7-B7 and A20-B19 and intrachain disulfide bond A6-A11.

Ala^{30} in the B-chain (bovine). Nearly all human insulin is produced by rDNA technology, and insulin obtained from porcine sources is being phased out. Presently five genetically engineered human insulin products are marketed in which there have been small changes made in the amino acid composition, such as deletions, additions, reversal of order, or substitution, that determine if they are rapid-acting or long-acting. Further details of the chemistry and formulations of the commercially available insulin products are discussed in Chapter 32.

Specific drugs

Glucagon (GlucaGen).

```
1       5              10              15
His-Ser-Gln-Gly-Thr-Phe-Thr-Ser-Asp-Tyr-Ser-Lys-Tyr-Leu-Asp-Ser
        Thr-Asn-Met-Leu-Tyr-Gln-Val-Phe-Asp-Gln-Ala-Arg - Arg
                     25              20
```

Glucagon, a 29-amino-acid, straight-chain polypeptide of α-cell pancreatic origin, triggers liver glycogenolysis and gluconeogenesis, thereby elevating glucose levels. The principal action of glucagon is the liver-mediated release into the blood of abnormally high concentrations of glucose, which causes hyperglycemia. This means that glucagon has an effect on blood glucose levels that is opposite to what occurs with insulin.

Human glucagon of rDNA origin is marketed for the treatment of severe hypoglycemic reactions in patients with diabetes, as can occur when there is an overdose of insulin. In patients with type I diabetes, the increase in glucose, resulting from glucagon administration, may not be sufficient, and supplemental carbohydrates may need to be administered quickly, especially in children.

Amylin

Amylin is a 37-peptide that is structurally similar to CT. Amylin works together with insulin to regulate glucose concentrations after a meal. When in solution, amylin is viscous, unstable, and tends to aggregate; therefore it cannot be used parenterally and is not commercially available.

Pramlintide Acetate (Symlin). Pramlintide acetate is a synthetic analogue of amylin (a 37-peptide) with proline substitutions at residues 25, 28, and 29. These substitutions change its physical properties such that it is commercially available for SC injection. When pramlintide is used in combination with insulin, it slows gastric emptying, lowers blood glucose levels after meals, and affords a feeling of fullness that leads to decreased caloric intake and the potential for weight loss. Pramlintide has been approved for use in adults with type I or type II diabetes as an adjunct along with insulin. The dose is quite different for type I (15–60 μg SC before meals) and type II diabetes (60–120 μg). The drug should be refrigerated before opening and may be kept at room temperature for up to 28 days after opening.

OTHER BIOLOGICALLY SIGNIFICANT PEPTIDES AND PROTEINS

Space does not allow us to discuss other biologically significant peptides and proteins as well as peptides and proteins not directly used in medicine. Table 7.3, however, summarizes some of the more interesting peptides and proteins.

Table 7.3. Additional Significant Peptides and Proteins of Biological Interests

Name	Trade Name (If Applicable)	General Use or Action
Aldesleukin (Interleukin-2)	Proleukin	Protein of rDNA origin that is used in treating renal cell carcinoma and metastatic malignant melanoma.
Angiotensin II		8-peptide involved in blood pressure regulation.
Atrial natriuretic peptide		28-peptide, vasodilator, that increases glomerular filtration and diuresis.
Bradykinin		9-peptide, produced in response to tissue damage, inflammation, viral infections, etc. Produces pain, increased vascular permeability, and synthesis of prostaglandins.
Denileukin diftitox	Ontak	rDNA-derived fusion protein consisting of diphtheria toxin fragments A and B as well as interleukin-2. Used in treating cutaneous T-cell lymphoma.
Exenatide	Byetta	39-peptide known as an incretin mimetic; an agonist of glucagon-like peptide-1, used adjunctively in type II diabetes mellitus.
Insulin-like growth factor-I (human)		Protein of rDNA origin that has orphan drug status and is used in treating major burns requiring hospitalization.
Peginterferon Alfa-2a	Pegasys	Pegylated protein of rDNA origin containing 165 residues. Used either alone or in combination with antiviral agent ribavirin in chronic hepatitis C.
Secretin, synthetic human	Chirhostim	27-peptide used to evaluate exocrine pancreas function and in diagnosis of gastrinoma (Zollinger-Ellison syndrome).
Thymopentin	Timunox	Synthetic 5-peptide consisting of residues 32–36 of thymopoietin, an immunologically active polypeptide. It is an investigational drug used for its immunomodulating properties.
Thyrotropin Alfa	Thyrogen	Recombinant form of human thyroid-stimulating hormone (rhTSH). Used diagnostically for serum thyroglobulin testing.
Trastuzumab	Herceptin	Humanized monoclonal antibody that binds selectively to the epidermal growth factor receptor 2 (HER2) protein. Used in treating some breast carcinomas that overexpress HER2.
Vasoactive intestinal polypeptide		28-peptide that is structurally related to secretin and glucagon. It has a diverse biological actions. It has orphan drug status for the treatment of acute esophageal food impaction.

CASE STUDY

Victoria F. Roche and S. William Zito

PB is your favorite grandma, and you are her favorite grandchild. She is 78 years old this weekend, and you are visiting her at the nursing home, where they are celebrating her birthday with a small party. Grandma has had a history of vertebral fractures associated with osteoporosis but has only been treating herself with chewable calcium supplements and vitamin D. After the party, you have some quiet time, and your grandma confides in you that she has been experiencing severe back pain, which requires her to lie down frequently during the day. She recalls that the pain started one night during an outing to the symphony with your mom. You suspect that grandma has had a recurrence of a vertebral fracture, and you make an appointment for her to be evaluated by her physician. On physical examination, her physician notes tenderness directly over a couple of areas of her spine, and a series of plain-film radiographs show two classic wedge deformities correlating with the area of tenderness. Her physician recommends a short period of bed rest, but grandma should avoid prolonged inactivity. Chewable aspirin was recommended for the pain, because grandma has a great deal of trouble swallowing pills. The physician believes grandma to be at high risk for continued fractures, wants to prescribe a peptide hormone, and asks your opinion of the following peptides 1–4:

1. Identify the therapeutic problems in which the pharmacist's intervention may benefit the patient.
2. Identify and prioritize the patient-specific factors that must be considered to achieve the desired therapeutic outcomes.
3. Conduct a thorough and mechanistically oriented structure-activity analysis of all therapeutic alternatives provided in the case.
4. Evaluate the SAR findings against the patient-specific factors and desired therapeutic outcomes, and make a therapeutic decision.
5. Counsel your patient.

S——————————————S (disulfide bridge between Cys residues)

Ala-Gly-Cys-Lys-Asn-Phe-Phe-Trp-Lys-Thr-Phe-Thr-Ser-Cys

1

pGlu-His–Trp–Ser–Tyr–D-Nal(2)-Leu—Arg—Pro—Gly-NH_2

2

S——————————S (disulfide bridge between Cys residues)

Cys-Ser–Asn–Leu–Ser–Thr–Cys-Val—Leu–Gly–Lys–Leu–Ser–Gln–Glu–Leu–His—

Lys–Leu–Gln–Thr–Tyr–Pro–Arg–Thr–Asn–Thr–Gly–Ser-Gly–Thr—Pro-NH_2

3

Ser–Val–Ser·Glu–Ile–Glu–Leu–Met–His–Asp–Leu–Gly–Lys–His–Leu–Asp–Ser–Met–

Glu–Arg–Val–Glu–Tyr–Leu–Arg–Lys–Lys–Leu–Glu–Asp–Val–His–Asp–Phe

4

References

1. Hofmeister F. Ergeb Physiol Biol Chem Exp Pharmakol 1902;1:759–802.
2. Fischer E. Untersuchungen über aminosaüren, polypeptide, und proteine. Ber Dtsch Chem Ges 1906;39:530–610.
3. Bergmann M, Zervas L. A general process for the synthesis of peptides. Ber Dtsch Chem Ges 1932;65:1192–1201.
4. du Vigneaud V, Ressler C, Swan JM, et al. The synthesis of an octapeptide amide with the hormonal activity of oxytocin. J Am Chem Soc 1953;75:4879–4880.
5. Sanger F. A disulfide interchange reaction. Nature 1953;171:1025–1026.
6. Bøler J, Enzmann F, Folkers K, et al. The identity of chemical and hormonal properties of the thyrotropin releasing hormone and pyroglutamyl-histidyl-proline amide. Biochem Biophys Res Commun 1969;37:705–710.
7. Matsuo H, Baba Y, Nair RMG, et al. Structure of the porcine LH- and FSH-releasing hormone. I. The proposed amino acid sequence. Biochem Biophys Res Commun 1971;43:1334–1339.
8. Brazeau P, Vale W, Burgus R, et al. Hypothalamic polypeptide that inhibits the secretion of immunoreactive pituitary growth hormone. Science 1973;179:77–79.
9. Sheehan JC, Hess GP. A new method of forming peptide bonds. J Am Chem Soc 1955;77:1067–1068.
10. McKay FC, Albertson NF. New amine-masking groups for peptide synthesis. J Am Chem Soc 1957;79:4686–4690.
11. Carpino LA, Han GY. The 9-fluorenylmethoxycarbonyl amino-protecting group. J Org Chem 1972;37:3404–3409.
12. Merrifield RB. Solid-phase peptide synthesis. I: the synthesis of a tetrapeptide. J Am Chem Soc 1963;85:2149–2154.

13. Sewald N, Jakubke HD. Peptides: Chemistry and Biology. Weinheim, Germany: Wiley-VCH, 2002.
14. Bailey PD. An introduction to peptide chemistry. Chichester UK: John Wiley & Sons, 1990.
15. Cahn RS, Ingold C, Prelog V. Specification of molecular chirality. Angew Chem Int Ed Engl 1966;5:385–415.
16. Horton HR, Moran LA, Ochs RS, et al. Principles of Biochemistry. Englewood Cliffs: Neil Patterson Publishers/Prentice Hall, 1993.
17. Pauling L, Corey RB, Branson HR. The structure of proteins: two hydrogen-bonded helical configurations of the polypeptide chain. Proc Natl Acad Sci U S A 1951;37:205–211.
18. Chou K-C. Prediction of β-turns. J Peptide Res 1997;49:120–144.
19. Rose GD, Gierasch LM, Smith JA. Turns in peptides and proteins. In: Anfinsen CB, Edsall JT, Richards FM, eds. Advances in protein chemistry, vol 37. Orlando, FL: Academic Press, 1985;1–109.
20. Colburn WA. Peptide, peptoid, and protein pharmacokinetics/pharmacodynamics. In: Garzone PD, Colburn WA, Mokotoff M, eds. Peptides, Peptoids, and Proteins. Pharmacokinetics and Pharmacodynamics, vol 3. Cincinnati: Harvey Whitney, 1991.
21. Spatola AF. Peptide backbone modifications: a structure–activity analysis of peptides containing amide bond surrogates, conformational constraints, and replacement. In: Weinstein B, ed. Chemistry and Biochemistry of Amino Acids, Peptides, and Proteins. New York: Marcel Dekker, 1983.
22. Goodman M, Chorev M. On the concept of linear modified retro-peptide structures. Acc Chem Res 1979;12:1–7.
23. Lee VHL. Changing needs in drug delivery in the era of peptide and protein drugs. In: Lee VHL, ed. Peptide and Protein Drug Delivery. New York: Marcel Dekker, 1991.
24. Pettit DK, Gombotz WR. The development of site-specific drug delivery systems for protein and peptide biopharmaceuticals. Trends Biotechnol 1998;16:343–349.
25. Banerjee PS, Hosny EA., Robinson JR. Parenteral delivery of peptide and protein drugs. In: Lee VHL, ed. Peptide and Protein Drug Delivery. New York: Marcel Dekker, 1991.
26. Patton JS, Bossard MJ. Drug delivery strategies for proteins & peptides from discovery and development to life cycle management. Drug Development Technology 2004; 4(8).
27. Illum L, Fisher N. Intranasal delivery of peptides and proteins. In: Adjei AL, Gupta PK, eds. Inhalation Delivery of Therapeutic Peptides and Proteins. New York: Marcel Dekker, 1997;135–184.
28. Sakakibara S. Chemical synthesis of proteins in solution. Biopolymers 1999;51:279–296.
29. Bodanszky M. Principles of Peptide Synthesis, 2nd ed. Berlin: Springer-Verlag, 1993.
30. Annis I, Hargittal B, Barany G. Disulfide bond formation in peptides. In: Fields GB, ed. Solid-Phase Peptide Synthesis. Methods in Enzymology, vol 289. New York: Academic Press, 1997;10:198–221.
31. Tam JP, Heath WF, Merrifield RB. S_N2 deprotection of synthetic peptides with a low concentration of hydrogen fluoride in dimethyl sulfide: evidence and application in peptide synthesis. J Am Chem Soc 1983;105:6442–6455.
32. White P. Fmoc-Trp(Boc)-OH: a new derivative for the synthesis of peptides containing tryptophan. In: Smith JA, Rivier JE, eds. Peptides: Chemistry and Biology (Proceedings of the 12th American Peptide Symposium). Leiden: ESCOM, 1992;537–538.
33. Alberico F, Carpino LA. Coupling reagents and activation. In: Fields GB, ed. Solid-Phase Peptide Synthesis. Methods in Enzymology, vol 289. New York: Academic Press, 1997;7:104–126.
34. Merrifield B. Concept and early development of solid-phase peptide synthesis. In: Fields GB, ed. Solid-phase Peptide Synthesis. Methods in Enzymology, vol 289. New York: Academic Press, 1997;11–13.
35. Mokotoff M. Current state of the art in the preparation of synthetic peptides. In Garzone PD, Colburn WA, Mokotoff M, eds. Peptides, Peptoids, and Proteins. Pharmacokinetics and Pharmacodynamics, vol 3. Cincinnati: Harvey Whitney, 1991.
36. Wellings DA, Atherton E. Standard Fmoc protocols. In: Fields GB, ed. Solid-Phase Peptide Synthesis. Methods in Enzymology, vol 289. New York: Academic Press, 1997;4:44–67.
37. Borman S. Combinatorial chemists focus on small molecules, molecular recognition, and automation. Chem Eng News 1996; February 12:29–54.
38. Plunkett MJ, Ellman JA. Combinatorial chemistry and new drugs. Sci Am 1997;April:69–73.
39. Lam KS, Lebl M, Krchnák V. The "one-bead-one-compound" combinatorial library method. Chem Rev 1997;97:411–448.
40. Furka Á. Introduction to combinatorial chemistry. In: Advanced ChemTech Handbook of Combinatorial and Solid-Phase Organic Chemistry. Louisville: Advanced ChemTech, 1999.
41. Nicolaou KC, Hanko R, Hartwig W, eds. Handbook of Combinatorial Chemistry. Weinheim, Germany: Wiley-VCH, 2002.
42. Zhao M, Kleinman HK, Mokotoff M. Synthetic laminin-like peptides and pseudopeptides as potential antimetastatic agents. J Med Chem 1994;37:3383–3388.
43. Fok K-F, Yankeelov JA Jr. Peptide-gap inhibitors: I. Competitive inhibition of aminopeptidase M by a hydrolytically resistant dipeptide analogue of glycylleucine. Biochem Biophys Res Commun 1977;114:273–278.
44. Coy DH, Heinz-Erian P, Jiang NY, et al. Probing peptide backbone function in bombesin: a reduced peptide bond analogue with potent and specific receptor antagonist activity. J Biol Chem 1988; 263:5056–5060.
45. Mokotoff M, Ren K, Wong LK, et al. Synthesis and biological evaluation of novel potent antagonists of the bombesin/gastrin releasing peptide receptor. J Med Chem 1992;35:4696–4703.
46. Chorev M, Goodman M. A dozen years of retro-inverso peptidomimetics. Acc Chem Res 1993;26:266–273.
47. Zhao M, Kleinman HK, Mokotoff M. Synthesis and activity of partial retro-inverso analogs of the antimetastatic laminin-derived peptide, YIGSR-NH_2. J Peptide Res 1997;49:240–253.
48. Crowley WF Jr, Conn PM. Modes of Action of GnRH and GnRH Analogues. New York: Springer-Verlag, 1991.
49. Chengalvala MV, Pelletier JC, Kopf GS. GnRH agonists and antagonists in cancer therapy. Curr Med Chem 2003;3:399–410.
50. Bauer W, Briner U, Doepfner W, et al. SMS 201-995: a very potent and selective analogue of somatostatin with a prolonged action. Life Sci 1982; 31:1133–1140.
51. Hintz RL. Untoward events in patients treated with growth hormone in the USA. Horm Res 1992;38(Suppl):44–49.
52. Combarnous Y. Molecular basis of the specificity of binding of glycoprotein hormones to their receptors. Endocr Rev 1992;13:670–691.
53. Homburg R, Giudice LC, Chang RJ. Polycystic ovary syndrome. Hum Reprod 1996;11:465–466.

8. *Antisense Therapeutic Agents*

MARILYN SPEEDIE

INTRODUCTION

Principles

Antisense therapeutic agents are based on a simple and elegant concept, as illustrated in Figure 8.1. As genes are expressed to produce specific proteins, the two complementary strands of DNA begin uncoiling within the nucleus. The "sense" strand carries nucleic acid bases in an order that specifies which amino acids should be assembled to produce the protein. The complementary, or "antisense," strand is used as a template for assembling a complementary strand of messenger RNA (mRNA) in the process called transcription. The mRNA will have the same sequence as the sense strand of DNA but is made up of ribose sugars instead of deoxyribose sugars in the nucleotide backbone (ribonucleotides versus deoxyribonucleotides). In eukaryotes, the mRNA is further processed in the nucleus by capping and splicing and is transported into the cytoplasm, where ribosomes translate the mRNA into proteins. Antisense drugs are short stretches of deoxyribonucleotide analogues that bind to specific complementary areas of the mRNA (which have a "sense" sequence) by Watson-Crick base pairing. In doing so, they can induce a nuclease (RNase H) that cleaves the mRNA at the site of the binding or can physically block translation or other steps in mRNA processing and transport, thus stopping protein synthesis. Antisense drugs therefore work at an early stage in the production of a disease-causing protein and, theoretically, can be applied to a number of diseases for which the basic pathophysiology involves an overexpression or aberrant expression of a given protein molecule. Viral diseases, cancers, and inflammatory diseases are all examples of such diseases that potentially can be treated via antisense mechanisms.

Another use of antisense oligonucleotides is to modify mRNA splicing (1). Scientists were surprised when the human genome was sequenced and only approximately 30,000 human genes were found. To get the wide variety of proteins that humans produce, the pre-mRNAs produced from these genes are spliced in a variety of ways to produce several different mRNAs and, subsequently, several different proteins from each gene. It is estimated that up to 60% of human genes are alternatively spliced at the pre-mRNA stage. Aberrant splicing because of genetic mutations are estimated to cause approximately 50% of genetic disorders and lead to diseases such as β-thalassemia, cystic fibrosis, and a variety of cancers. Antisense oligonucleotides can be used to inhibit aberrant splicing, thus correcting the genetic defect. The oligonucleotides used for this purpose must not activate RNase H, which would destroy the pre-mRNA target before it could be correctly spliced, and must be able to effectively compete with splicing factors to gain access to the target pre-mRNAs.

Recently, a new approach to antisense therapeutics has emerged with the discovery that small interfering RNAs (siRNAs) can be used therapeutically. Naturally occurring siRNAs have been known as part of the defense by eukaryotic cells against invasion by double-stranded RNA viruses. In 1998, Fire et al. (2) discovered that double-stranded RNA could induce a potent silencing effect on homologous genes in the nematode *Caenorhabditis elegans.* Scientists have extensively applied this principle to genetic analysis in mammalian cell culture. More recently, the general principle has been applied to the design of externally administered siRNA therapeutic agents that can be used to target and silence specific target mRNA sequences involved in disease. As shown in Figure 8.2, double-stranded RNA molecules enter the cell and are cleaved by an enzyme called "Dicer" to generate 21 to 23 nucleotide fragments that contain two nucleotide 3′ overhangs and 5′-phosphate groups. Then, an ATP-dependent helicase recognizes these short duplexes and resolves siRNA into two single-stranded RNAs. One strand is incorporated into a high-molecular-weight protein complex termed "RNA-induced silencing complex" (RISC), where it serves to guide the RISC complex to the homologous target mRNA sequence, where cleavage occurs. Once one molecule of the mRNA is destroyed, the RISC complex moves on to other molecules of the same mRNA and is recycled to perform multiple rounds of catalysis. This property of RISC accounts for the potent nature of the silencing effect (3). The siRNA therapeutic agents are the most potent antisense agents available (4). In less than five years since the discovery of the silencing effect of double-stranded RNA molecules, the first potential agents are showing positive results in clinical trials for macular degeneration (5) and other diseases.

History

The beginning of antisense technology may be traced to a report of sequence-specific binding of a modified DNA to complementary mRNA in 1978 (6). The road from demonstration of the binding to an approved human therapeutic agent, however, has been one filled with alternating optimism and pessimism. Developmental steps included identifying the optimum chemistry for getting antisense molecules into cells and preventing nuclease destruction of the molecules while optimizing

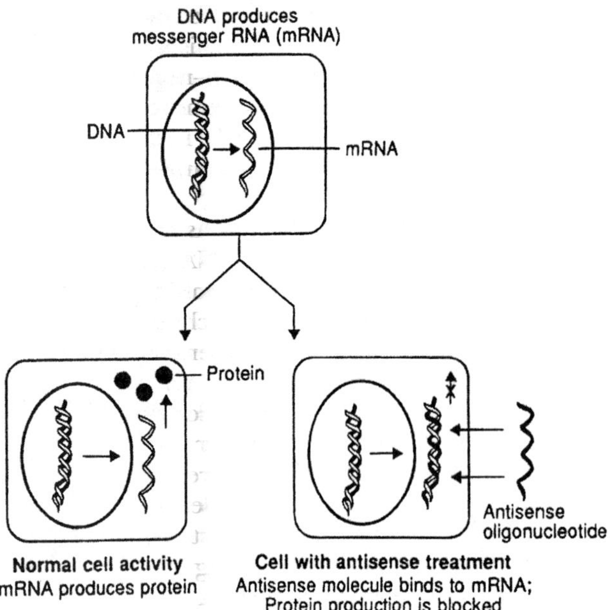

Fig. 8.1. Concept of antisense oligonucleotide inhibition of gene expression. The antisense oligonucleotide enters the cell and binds to specific complementary mRNA, causing it to be degraded or otherwise inhibiting synthesis of the corresponding protein.

binding to messenger. Design of antisense molecules to achieve selective binding to the target mRNA was essential if side effects were to be minimized. After several years of optimizing the parameters to improve efficacy in vitro (in tissue culture), scientists moved to testing antisense candidates in animal models. This did not prove to be an easy challenge, and it resulted in pessimism about the ultimate utility of the products. For a period, medical researchers were skeptical about the efficacy of the approach. Questions arose about the reproducibility of experiments and whether the pharmacological effects being observed in animal experiments were the result of sequence-specific antisense activity. Eventually, however, careful design of experiments to provide appropriate controls reversed the skepticism, and now scientists generally agree that antisense approaches can lead to useful medicinal agents (7,8).

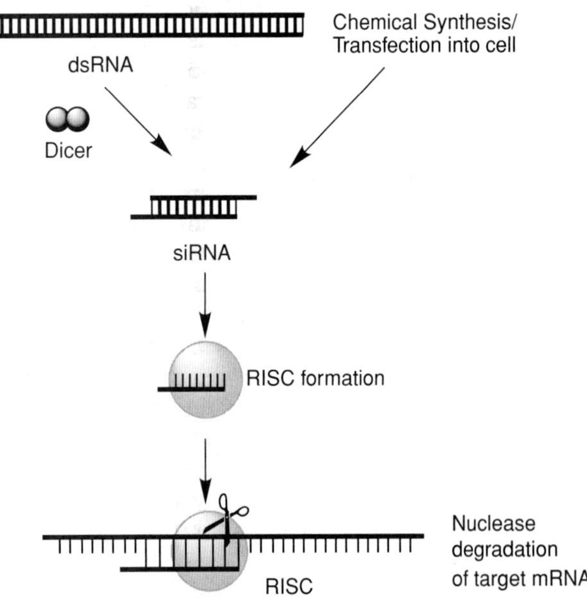

Fig. 8.2. Mechanism of action of siRNAs. The siRNAs are generated either from long, double-stranded RNA molecules processed by an enzyme called "Dicer" or by transfecting chemically synthesized double-stranded siRNA molecules into the cells. The siRNA is then incorporated into RNA-induced silencing complex (RISC), which guides a nuclease to the target mRNA, which is subsequently degraded, thus blocking protein synthesis.

Problems associated with the automated synthesis and cost of antisense molecules have been overcome. Initially, each compound could only be synthesized in small amounts, and the costs of each synthesis would have limited their clinical use. Improvements to the technology during scale-up, however, have resulted in prices between \$50 and \$100 per gram—well within a useful range for pharmaceutical agents (7).

Many people believe that we are only beginning to exploit the full potential of antisense drug development. The first-generation drugs were mostly of a single chemical design, and a wide variety of second-generation chemistries with improved properties have been designed and are being tested. The initial studies with siRNAs have infused excitement into the field as well. A wide variety of therapeutic agents are in Phase I or Phase II of clinical trial development, and a few are in Phase III testing. Yet, there remains only one marketed antisense drug, fomivirsen, and several seemingly promising agents have not held up when subjected to randomized clinical trials. The challenges of fulfilling the promise of this class of drugs are formidable. Only time will tell how useful this approach to drug design will be.

DESIGN OF FIRST-GENERATION ANTISENSE AGENTS

General Consideration

Conceptually, the design of an antisense strand is simple, but designing an antisense therapeutic agent that will function in human disease is quite complicated. Many conditions must be satisfied for an antisense drug to function. It must be administered in a manner that delivers it to the site of action in the body without the drug being degraded by nucleases, which are ubiquitous in human cells. It must get into the cell of the target tissue and colocalize with its target RNA at a sufficient concentration for a bimolecular reaction to occur. It must have a structure that favors association with the target RNA and be designed to bind to a RNA region that is vulnerable to binding. Identification of the molecule with optimum binding generally is performed in tissue culture experiments for which 30 or 40 oligonucleotides, each approximately 30 nucleotides in length, are synthesized. These oligonucleotides are complementary to different portions of the target mRNA and are used to determine where the binding can be best achieved, as indicated by inhibition of synthesis of the target protein. This "brute force" effort usually is quite successful, but it limits initial drug discovery, in general, to industrial laboratories that have the capability to efficiently synthesis large numbers of antisense molecules. Getting to the target cell, binding to the target mRNA and inhibiting protein synthesis are necessary—but still insufficient—to define successful antisense activity. For a target gene (and protein) to be suitable for an antisense approach, there must be sufficient turnover of the resultant protein that inhibiting its synthesis will have the desired effect within a reasonable period of time. This can be tested in tissue culture and in whole animals once the initial conditions are met.

Modifications in the base, sugar, and phosphate moieties as well as in the length of the polymer have been reported in attempts to create molecules with enhanced or more selective affinity for specific sites on the RNA, to enhance nuclease stability, to improve cellular uptake and distribution, and to optimize distribution and clearance. Much work remains in defining the medicinal chemistry of these molecules and correlating the chemistry with the biological effects. To date, the most detailed work has been done with phosphorothioate deoxyoligonucleotides, as described below, but even with this class of molecules, our current knowledge does not yet allow optimal structures to be predicted and developed without screening multiple drug candidates.

Site of Binding

It is known that at some sites, the binding of antisense oligonucleotides to mRNA creates a substrate for RNase H, leading to greater efficacy, because the mRNA actually is cleaved. The antisense deoxyoligonucleotide is released and can bind to yet another mRNA molecule, thus amplifying its effect (9). Screens incorporating RNase H–mediated cleavage offer the potential to improve identification of the optimal antisense drug molecules, although these cell-free systems still leave many critical parameters undefined in terms of achieving a drug that will be active in vivo (10). Phosphorothioate oligonucleotide complexes with mRNA can serve as substrates for RNase H, whereas many other oligonucleotides do not create RNase H–susceptible complexes. This appears to account, at least in part, for the efficacy of the phosphorothioates, and second-generation molecules attempt to maintain the ability to be a RNase H substrate while improving other properties.

Although many studies focus on antisense drugs creating substrates for RNase H, it is important to realize that a number of other mechanisms have been identified, including inhibition of translation, inhibition of splicing, and degradation of RNA via other mechanisms. Furthermore, studies, especially with antiviral antisense molecules, have shown antisense sequence–independent effects, such as decreasing the adsorption of the virus, in addition to the antisense sequence–dependent effects. Therefore, studies that attribute the effect of a given antisense molecule to an antisense mechanism must be carefully controlled to demonstrate dose–response effects, sequence-specific effects, and measurement of the loss of the target RNA or protein or both (11,12). Figure 8.3 illustrates some of the possible sites of antisense oligonucleotide action in the transcription, processing, and translation of a specific gene product. As shown in Figure 8.3, favorite targets have included RNA splice sites, 5′-capping, 3′-adenylation sites, and translation start and termination sites (13). In reality, the choice of the portion of a mRNA to be a target for antisense drug action is quite empirical. Little is known about the shape of the mRNA molecules within cells, and no common structure exists among the target sequences for a variety of successful antisense drugs. Therefore, there is no easy way to predict what portion of the mRNA molecule will be available for binding to the drug. Scientists make 30 to 40 oligonucleotides of appropriate length that complements different portions of the mRNA and use them to "march down the message" in tissue culture experiments to see where binding is best (7).

Structural Considerations

The generalized structures illustrating some of the first-generation antisense oligonucleotides that were tested are shown in Figure 8.4 (14). Each was designed and tested with the goal of optimizing and balancing the affinity of binding for mRNA, nuclease resistance, and uptake into the cells. As seen in Figure 8.4, the first-generation antisense oligonucleotide agents use methylphosphonate modifications, 2′-O-methylribonucleotides, and phosphorothioate linkages. The methylphosphonate backbone yields a molecule that is nonionic, has good nuclease resistance, and forms a stable duplex with mRNA. The duplex formed is not a substrate for RNase H, however, and uptake is via passive diffusion. Of the first-generation oligonucleotide antisense molecules, the class that has resulted in the broadest range of activities is the phosphorothioate class, in which one of the oxygen atoms in the phosphate group is replaced with a sulfur. The resulting compound is negatively charged, is chiral at each phosphorothioate, and is much more resistant to nuclease digestion than the parent phosphodiester compound. Compound length has been determined empirically. Molecules must have at least seven or eight complementary bases to bind to the target site and induce RNase H activity. Molecules less than 13 to 15 bases have lower specificity with complementary mRNA, and molecules longer than 20-mers result in more nonsequence specific interactions. Molecules in the range of approximately 15 to 20 bases (15- to 20-mers) are commonly synthesized, with 18 or 20 bases generally considered to be optimum (8).

Although the phosphorothioate molecules (unbound to mRNA) are relatively resistant to nucleases, some nuclease degradation occurs, primarily by exonucleases (which cleave the terminal bases) and, perhaps, with a

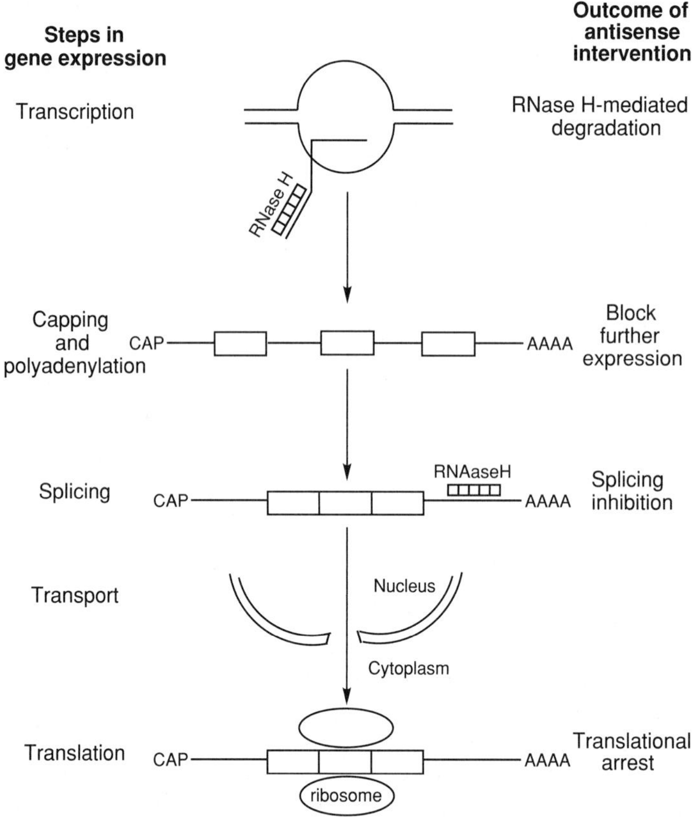

Fig. 8.3. Mechanism of action of antisense oligonucleotides. Each step in gene expression is a potential target for antisense oligonucleotide activity. Steps in gene expression are indicated on the left, and the outcome of antisense binding is shown on the right. (Adapted from Rawls RL. Optimistic about antisense: Promising clinical results and chemical strategies for further improvements delight antisense drug researchers. Chem Engin News 1997;75:35–38; with permission.)

modest contribution by endonucleases (which cleave within the chain) as well. Phosphorothioates are taken up by a wide range of cells in vitro, and it is thought that uptake is enhanced by the negative charge, which allows binding to specific uptake proteins, resulting in receptor-mediated endocytosis. Uptake is both time- and temperature-dependent and is influenced by the cell type as well as the specific sequence and length of the oligonucleotide. Cationic lipids have been used in vitro to enhance uptake of phosphorothioate oligonucleotides in cells that otherwise take up little of the compounds (15).

The negative charge also affects protein binding in vivo. The phosphorothiates exhibit a dissociation constant (kD) for albumin is approximately 150 micromolar, which is similar to that of aspirin or penicillin (16). Phosphorothioates are rapidly and extensively absorbed after parenteral administration and rapidly and extensively distributed to all peripheral tissues. No evidence indicates penetration of the blood-brain barrier. Clearance is primarily through metabolism by nucleases, with the degraded compounds being eliminated through the urine. Oral bioavailability is less than 5%, but the limiting factor may be degradation in the gut rather than absorption per se. Studies with a more stable 2′-methoxyphosphorothioate oligonucleotide showed a significant increase in oral bioavailability that appeared to be associated with improved stability of the analogs (14).

Potential Side Effects

Toxicological studies with phosphorothioate oligonucleotides have been performed with mice, monkeys, and to a lesser extent, humans. The dose-limiting effect in mice is a reversible immune stimulation observed as lymphoid hyperplasia, splenomegaly, and multiorgan monocellular infiltrate. These effects appear to be related to the terminal CpG dinucleotide that is cleaved by nucleases. In monkeys, the dose-limiting effect is sporadic drops in blood pressure associated with bradycardia and, at higher doses, abnormalities in blood clotting, perhaps resulting from interactions with thrombin. In humans, systemic intravenous administration of ISIS 2302 (a phosphorothioate that inhibits intercellular adhesion molecule 1 [ICAM-1]) caused no significant toxicities, including no

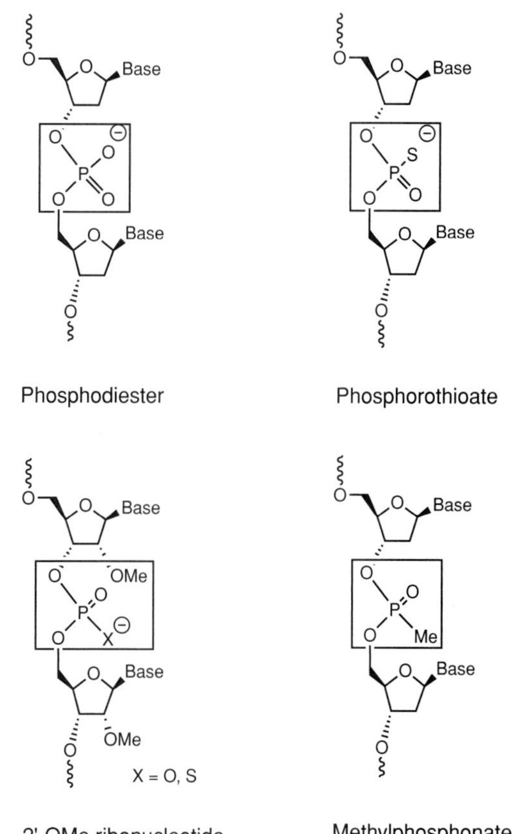

Fig. 8.4. First-generation generalized structures of natural DNA (phosphodiester) and three antisense oligonucleotide derivatives tested as antisense drugs. (Adapted from Agrawal S, Iyer RP. Perspectives in antisense therapeutics. Pharmacol Ther 1997;76:151–160; with permission.)

evidence of immune stimulation and no hypotension. A slight subclinical increase in activated partial thromboplastin time was observed at the highest dose (2 mg/kg) (17). Inflammation of the anterior chamber of the eye is the most common side effect of local (intravitreal injection) administration of fomivirsen (see below) for CMV retinitis.

The major disadvantages of commonly used phosphorothioates are their relatively low affinity for their target mRNA and toxic side effects, especially the immune stimulation and clotting abnormalities. Efforts to design newer compounds have yielded some with enhanced serum stability, higher target affinity, and lower toxicity (18). These molecules are discussed later in this chapter.

DRUG THERAPY

Fomivirsen (Vitravene)

The first antisense therapeutic agent to reach the market is fomivirsen (ISIS 2922) (19). Fomivirsen is a 21-mer phosphorothioate oligodeoxynucleotide (Fig. 8.5). It inhibits human cytomegalovirus (CMV), a ubiquitous herpesvirus that is the most common cause of viral retinitis in immunocompromised patients, especially those with HIV infection. Cytomegalovirus infection is characterized by the progressive destruction of retinal cells and, if untreated, leads to retinal detachment and blindness. Even with treatment, some degree of visual loss occurs in nearly all patients with a diagnosis of CMV retinitis. It can affect one or both eyes.

Mechanism of Action

Fomivirsen inhibits CMV by at least two mechanisms. The first is a sequence-specific antisense binding to inhibit expression of immediate-early genes, thus preventing viral replication. The second is sequence-independent and involves inhibition of adsorption of CMV to host cells, probably by direct binding to viral coat proteins (20,21). The reduction of immediate-early protein synthesis occurs in a dose-dependent manner. Although it does inhibit viral replication, fomivirsen does not eradicate the virus whose DNA, as for all herpesviruses, is integrated into the human genome. Therefore, treatment will have to continue for the life of the patient.

Pharmacokinetics

The series of clinical trials that led to approval by the U.S. Food and Drug Administration involved 430 eyes in 330 patients. Fomivirsen significantly delayed progression of CMV retinitis in patients with AIDS, including those who had failed treatment with ganciclovir or foscarnet, the first-line therapies. Fomivirsen is administered by intravitreal injection at doses of 165 μg once weekly for three weeks of induction and then once every two weeks. It also can be administered in a dose of 330 μg on days 1 and 15 and then once a month thereafter. Mean maximum retinal concentrations of fomivirsen occur at 2 days, and the elimination half-life after a single, 115-μg dose in monkey retina was 78 hours. There are no systemic side effects. Ocular side effects include increased intraocular pressure and mild to moderate intraocular inflammation that can be reversed with topical steroid treatment. It is important that side effects be minor, because treatment will be lifelong.

Therapeutics

The U.S. Food and Drug Administration approved fomivirsen as second-line treatment of CMV retinitis in patients with AIDS who are intolerant or unresponsive to previous treatment for the disease (22). Alternative treatments include intravenous or oral ganciclovir, ganciclovir implant, cidofovir, and foscarnet (23). All are virustatic and share a common mechanism, inhibition of DNA polymerase. The disadvantages of these agents include the need for an indwelling catheter for intravenous administration of ganciclovir or foscarnet and the high cost and repeated surgeries needed for the surgically implanted, controlled-release ganciclovir pellets. In cell culture assays, however, fomivirsen showed additive antiviral activity with ganciclovir or foscarnet, so further study may show some benefit to combination therapy in human patients who have not yet failed with these agents.

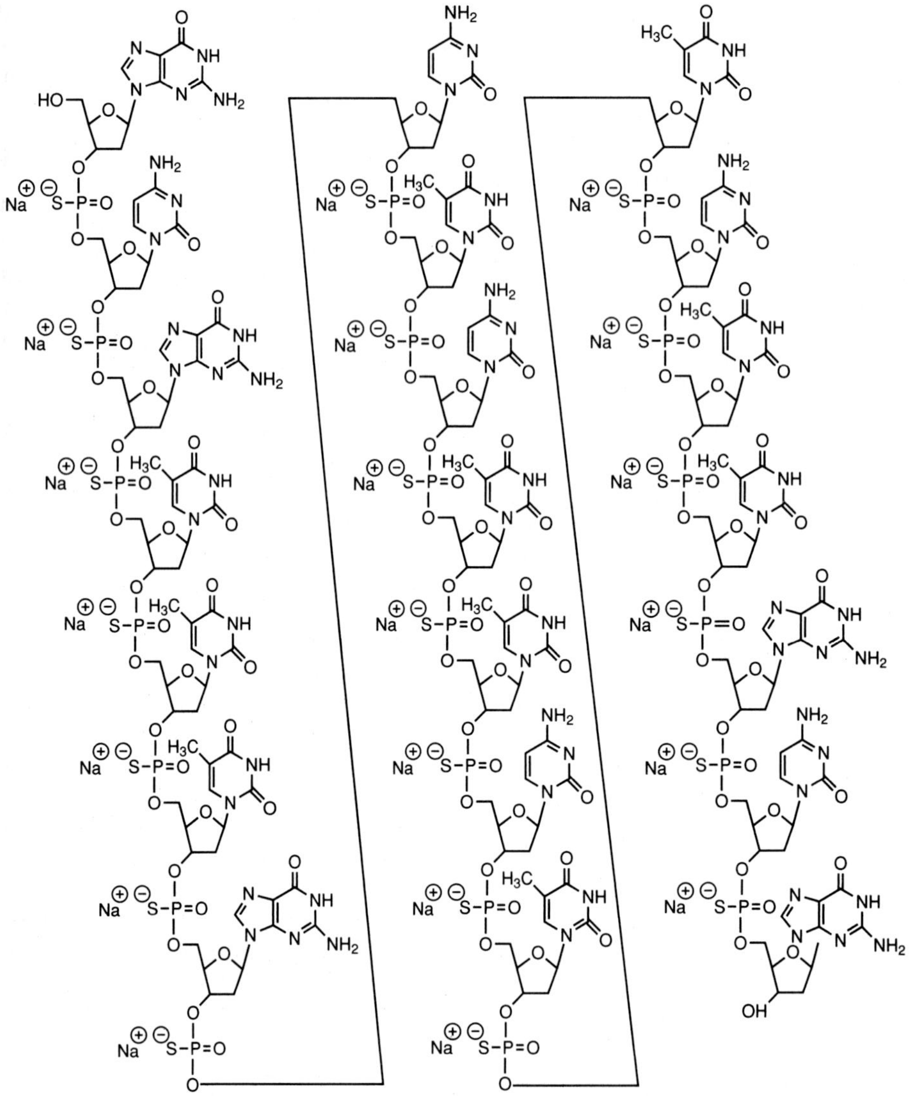

Fig. 8.5. Structure of fomivirsen, the first marketed antisense therapeutic agent. (Adapted from Field AK. Viral targets for antisense oligonucleotides: a mini review. Antiviral Res 1998;37: 67–81; with permission.)

The significance of fomivirsen goes beyond its efficacy for CMV retinitis. Fortunately, the better control of AIDS that is currently being achieved is decreasing the incidence of CMV retinitis. The impact of fomivirsen, however, on the quality of life of patients with the disease is dramatic. The further significance lies in the fact that it is the first antisense therapeutic agent. This achievement indicates that the concept can be developed into efficacious and safe drug products, including solving all the manufacturing, formulation, and analytical problems that this process entails.

Clinical Trials with Other Phosphorothioate Antisense Oligonucleotides

Alicaforsen (ISIS 2302)

Alicaforsen is a phosphorothioate oligodeoxynucleotide 20 bases in length with a sequence complementary to the 3′-untranslated region of the mRNA of human ICAM-1 (24). Hybridization of ISIS 2302 to mRNA inhibits expression of the ICAM-1 protein in response to inflammatory stimuli. Initial tests of activity were performed in mice using a analogous antisense oligonucleotide that is active against the analogous mouse ICAM molecule. Studies with this oligonucleotide showed that it had anti-inflammatory activity in models of organ transplant rejection, ulcerative colitis, and collagen-induced arthritis. Toxicities in the mouse model were similar to those observed with other antisense oligonucleotides and were independent of the suppression of ICAM-1 expression. Immune stimulation, kidney changes, liver abnormalities, and increased clotting times were observed, but all toxicities were reversible and occurred at doses well above those required for pharmacological activity. No genetic toxicity was observed (25). In a Phase II human trial, 47% of patients with Crohn's disease treated intravenously with ISIS 2302, but no patients treated with placebo, were in remission after 1 month of treatment. No clinically significant complications were observed (24). Illustrating the difficulty in actually getting a product to market, however, in two Phase III, randomized, double-blind, placebo-controlled trials, one with 150 patients and one with 180 patients, alicaforsen failed to show significant efficacy in inducing remission in patients with Crohn's disease and is not being further pursued by ISIS for this purpose (26). It is now being reinvestigated in a restructured, Phase III trial for use as an enema for treatment of ulcerative colitis.

Aprinocarsen (Affinitak, ISIS3521/LY900003)

Aprinocarsen is a phosphorothioate antisense agent targeted against protein kinase Cα, a protein that is implicated in malignant transformation and proliferation. It showed activity in Phase I and Phase II clinical trials against nonsmall-cell lung cancer when used in combination with cisplatin or the combination of cisplatin and gemcitabine (27). It proved to be disappointing, however, during initial Phase III trials. Eli Lilly was sponsoring Phase III trials to further explore its efficacy in combination with chemotherapeutic agents for lung cancer, but enrollment was terminated in March 2003, when a Phase III trial suggested that aprinocarsen did not have an added survival benefit when combined with paclitaxel and carboplatin therapy in patients with nonsmall-cell lung cancer (28).

Oblimersen sodium (Genasense, G-3139)

Genta is developing a phosphorothioate antisense drug called oblimersen sodium that is complementary to the first six codons of the open reading frame of the human bcl-2 mRNA sequence. Oblimersen turns off production of the apoptosis inhibitor Bcl2 in tumor cells. This appears to increase a tumor cell's sensitivity to a variety of other anticancer therapies and, ultimately, may lead to cell death. It is being investigated for use in treatment of myeloma and other cancers as well. In a recently reported Phase II trial (29), oblimersen was administered (3–7 mg/kg/d for 7 days) by continuous intravenous infusion. On day 4, patients started thalidomide (100–400 mg as tolerated) and dexamethasone (40 mg daily for 4 days) on 21-day cycles for three cycles. Oblimersen, dexamethasone, and thalidomide are well tolerated and result in encouraging clinical responses in patients with relapsed multiple myeloma. Phase III trials currently are underway with patients who have myeloma and chronic lymphocytic leukemia, as are earlier-stage trials with patients who have other cancers and other anticancer therapies (30).

These three drugs illustrate both the hope and the frustration that is experienced with this class of therapeutics. The antisense mechanism works in the cells, and protein synthesis can definitely be inhibited. Getting from cell culture observations to useful and effective therapies, however, is a long road, and several seemingly useful antisense agents have fallen by the wayside when tested in randomized, double-blind trials. Clearly, attention must be paid to getting the dosing schedule, formulation, and route of administration optimized.

FUTURE TARGETS AND DIRECTIONS

Design of Second- and Third-Generation Agents

Several alternative structures are being tested as second-generation antisense oligonucleotides. One of these involves a mixed backbone oligonucleotide (31). Studies have shown that the toxicity and immune stimulatory effects of phosphorothioates correlate with the nuclease cleavage of a terminal CG dinucleotide. The toxicity can be minimized by the use of 2′-O-methylribonucleosides in place of four deoxynucleotides at both the 3′ and 5′ end of the phosphorothioate oligonucleotide. These molecules have been termed "gapmers" (18). They retain the RNase H substrate properties of the original phosphorothioate molecule (oligonucleotides made up entirely of 2′-O-methylribonucleotides do not form RNase H susceptible duplexes) and have good duplex stability and better nuclease resistance. On intravenous administration, the hybrid oligonucleotides (or gapmers) exhibit rapid uptake and longer elimination half-lives, and analysis of tissues showed that mainly full-length oligonucleotides were present, consistent with the greater resistance to nuclease-mediated degradation compared to the nonhybrid phosphorothioate oligonucleotide. Excretion occurs primarily in the urine, and like phosphorothioates, the excretory products are mainly degraded products, with only trace amounts of the intact molecule. Studies in rats suggest that the mixed backbone oligonucleotides also may be orally bioavailable (25–30% of the administered dose), which would present a major advantage in the utility of antisense therapeutic agents, especially for chronic diseases.

Additional Developments

Mixed backbone hybrid oligonucleotides also have been made using methylphosphonate linkages at the ends. Methylphosphonates are nonionic, are resistant to nucleases, but do not lead to RNase H degradation. The reduced polyanionic nature of the mixed backbone oligonucleotide with methylphosphonate moieties have the potential to reduce the clotting abnormality associated with the use of phosphorothioate agents (14).

One goal for future development will be the design of orally available antisense products. Some attempts have included attaching a 2-methoxyethoxy group at the 2′ site of ribose on the bases at both ends of the oligonucleotide, creating 2′-methoxyphosphorothioate analogues and substituting aminopropoxy groups at the 2′ ribose site (7). Work will continue to develop orally available compounds, particularly for chronic diseases. The oral availability, however, must be balanced with penetration into target cells and tissues, binding to the mRNA, and RNase H induction.

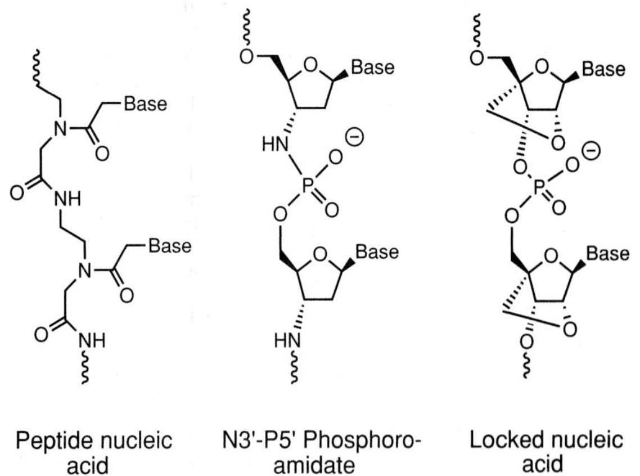

Fig. 8.6. Generalized structures of some second generation antisense oligonucleotides.

In some situations, RNase H induction is not desired, such as when inhibiting an aberrant splice site. The correctly spliced mRNA must be translated and not degraded if the desired effect is to be achieved. This approach has been used to treat the genetic blood disorder β-thalassemia, a disease in which a mutation in intron 2 of the β-globin gene causes aberrant splicing of the pre-mRNA and, as a consequence, β-globin deficiency. A phosphorothioate 2′-O-methyl oligonucleotide (that does not induce RNase H cleavage) was targeted to the aberrant splice site and restored correct splicing and β-globin production (1).

Another second-generation class of antisense molecules are the peptide nucleic acids, in which the deoxyribose backbone is replaced by polyamide linkages (Fig. 8.6). These molecules have favorable hybridization properties, are very stable in a biological environment, and seem to be nontoxic. They are electrostatically neutral, so solubility and cellular uptake are serious problems. They do not induce RNase H and, therefore, have been used to correct aberrant splicing (18).

Similarly, N3′-P5′ phosphoroamidates are another example of a modified phosphate backbone in which the 3′-hydroxy group of the 2′-deoxyribose ring is replaced by a 3′-amino group (Fig. 8.6). They have high affinity for the complementary RNA strand and are nuclease resistant. Additionally, they do not induce RNase H and, therefore, are most useful for correcting splicing (18).

One of the most promising second-generation modification is one called "locked nucleic acid" (LNA), in which the ribonucleotide contains a methylene bridge that connects the 2′-oxygen of the ribose with the 4′-carbon (Fig. 8.6). The LNAs have enhanced stability to nucleases and an extraordinarily high affinity for the target mRNA. They do not, however, activate RNase H. If degradation of the mRNA is desired, a chimeric DNA-LNA gapmer that contains a stretch of seven to eight DNA monomers in the center to induce RNase H activity should be used (18).

Finally, the newest molecules to induce excitement are the double-stranded siRNAs. The RNA interference is initiated by long, double-stranded RNA molecules that are processed into 21- to 23-nucleotide RNAs. These siRNAs are then incorporated into the RISC and serve to guide the nuclease that destroys the target RNA and stops protein synthesis. These molecules are extremely stable in the cell. In some experiments, they have been made even more stable by introducing two 2′-O-methyl RNA nucleotides at the 5′ end and four methylated monomers at the 3′ end. This modification resulted in a prolonged silencing effect in the cell culture. Because the basic effect of siRNA is the same as that of the other antisense technologies, researchers will be able to benefit from all the work that has gone on with antisense molecules, including the importance of proper controls to prove that the observed effect is, in fact, caused by specific reduction in target gene synthesis and the importance of looking for unspecific effects mediated by the immune system (18).

Future Targets and Products in Development

A number of molecules are in various phases of testing. In addition to the three phosphorothioates in Phase III trials, as already described, a number of second-generation products are undergoing testing in humans. Promising early results have been presented describing studies in patients with age-related macular degeneration who were treated with an injection into the eyes of a chemically modified siRNA that targets vascular endothelial growth factor receptor-1 (VEGFR-1). By targeting VEGFR-1, pathogenic angiogenesis is downregulated, and new vascularization is blocked (5).

Monarsen, an antisense oligonucleotide targeted to the acetylcholinesterase gene, is delivered orally to treat patients with myasthenia gravis and exhibits efficacy in early trials. Myasthenia gravis is a chronic and debilitating autoimmune disease in which the body's immune system attacks acetylcholine receptors at the neuromuscular junction, interfering with normal muscular function. Monarsen offers a novel mechanism of action for the control of an isoform of the acetylcholinesterase enzyme that is believed to play a key role in the onset and progression of myasthenia gravis (5).

Many other antisense and siRNA products are in various stages of early phase trials, including compounds targeted as antivirals, anti-inflammatory agents, and other approaches to cancer. In summary, the concept of antisense technology has been proven, one first-generation phosphorothioate oligonucleotide drug has reached the market, and second-generation drugs with improved properties are under development. It seems likely that the list of marketed antisense drugs will continue to grow.

References

1. Sazani P, Kole R. Therapeutic potential of antisense oligonucleotides as modulators of alternative splicing. J Clin Invest 2003,112:481–486.
2. Fire A, Xu S, Montgomery MK, et al. Potent and specific genetic interference by double-stranded DNA in *Caenorhabditis elegans*. Nature 1998;391:806–811.
3. Tomari Y, Zamore PD. Perspective: machines for RNAi. Genes Dev 2005;19: 517–529.
4. Finnegan EJ, Matske MA. The small RNA world. J Cell Sci 2003;116: 4689–4693.
5. Fredrickson RM. Nucleic acid medicines move toward the clinic. Mol Ther 2005;12:775–776.
6. Zamecnik PC, Stephenson ML. Inhibition of Rous sarcoma virus replication and cell transformation by a specific oligodeoxynucleotide. Proc Natl Acad Sci U S A 1978;75:280–284.
7. Rawls RL. Optimistic about antisense: Promising clinical results and chemical strategies for further improvements delight antisense drug researchers. Chem Engin News 1997;75:35–38.
8. Stein CA. How to design an antisense oligonucleotide experiment: a consensus approach. Antisense Nucleic Acid Drug Dev 1998;8:129–132.
9. Lavrovsky Y, Chen S, Roy AK. Therapeutic potential and mechanism of action of oligonucleotides and ribozymes. Biochem Mol Med 1997;62:11–22.
10. Branch AD. Antisense drug discovery: can cell-free screens speed the process? Antisense Nucleic Acid Drug Dev 1998;8:249–254.
11. Crooke ST. An overview of progress in antisense therapeutics. Antisense Nucleic Acid Drug Dev 1998;8:115–122.
12. Crooke ST. Molecular mechanisms of antisense drugs: RNase H. Antisense Nucleic Acid Drug Dev 1998;8:133–134.
13. Field AK. Viral targets for antisense oligonucleotides: a mini review. Antiviral Res 1998;37:67–81.
14. Agrawal S, Iyer RP. Perspectives in antisense therapeutics. Pharmacol Ther 1997;76:151–160.
15. Juliano RL, Alahari S, Yoo H, et al. Antisense pharmacodynamics: critical issue in the transport and delivery of antisense oligonucleotides. Pharm Res 1999;16:494–502.
16. Crooke ST, Graham MJ, Zuckerman JE, et al. Pharmacokinetic properties of several novel oligonucleotide analogs in mice. J Pharmacol Exp Ther 1996;277:923–937.
17. Glover JM, Leeds JM, Mant TGK, et al. Phase I safety and pharmacokinetic profile of an intercellular adhesion molecule-1 antisense oligodeoxynucleotide (ISIS 2302). J Pharmacol Exp Ther 1997;282:1173–1180.
18. Kurreck J. Antisense technologies: Improvement through novel chemical modifications. Eur J Biochem 2003;270(8):1628–1644.
19. Perry CM, Balfour JAB. Fomivirsen. Drugs 1999;57:375–380.
20. Azad RF, Driver VB, Tanaka K. Antiviral activity of a phosphorothioate oligonucleotide complementary to RNA of the human cytomegalovirus major immediate-early region. Antimicrob Agents Chemother 1993;37: 1945–1954.
21. Anderson KP, Fox MC, Brown-Driver V. Inhibition of human cytomegalovirus immediate-early gene expression by an oligonucleotide complementary to immediate early RNA. Antimicrob Agents Chemother 1996;40:2004–2011.
22. Crooke ST, Guest editorial: Vitravene®—another piece in the mosaic. Antisense Nucleic Acid Drug Dev 1998;8:vii–viii.
23. Piascik P. Fomivirsen sodium approved to treat CMV retinitis. J Am Pharm Assoc 1999;39:84–85.
24. Yacyshyn BR, Bowen-Yacyshyn MB, Jewell L, et al. A placebo-controlled trial of ICAM-1 antisense oligonucleotide in the treatment of Crohn's disease. Gastroenterology 1998;114:1133–1142.
25. Henry SP, Templin MV, Gillett N, et al. Correlation of toxicity and pharmacokinetic properties of a phosphorothioate oligonucleotide designed to inhibit ICAM-1. Toxicol Pathol 1999;27:95–100.
26. Available at: http://www.biospace.com/news_story.aspx?StoryID=18304620. Accessed April 2, 2006.
27. Villalona-Calero MA, Ritch P, Figueroa JA, et al. A phase I/II study of LY900003, an antisense inhibitor of protein kinase Cα, in combination with cisplatin and gemcitabine in patients with advanced nonsmall-cell lung cancer. Clin Cancer Res 2004:10(18 Pt 1):6086–6093.
28. Vansteenkiste J, Canon JL, Riska H, et al. Randomized phase II evaluation of aprinocarsen in combination with gemcitabine and cisplatin for patients with advanced/metastatic nonsmall-cell lung cancer. Invest New Drugs 2005:23: 263–269.
29. Meisenberg B, Takebe N, Heyman M, et al. Phase II study of G3139, a Bcl-2 antisense oligonucleotide, in combination with dexamethasone and thalidomide in relapsed multiple myeloma patients. J Clin Oncol 2005;23: 4089–4099.
30. Chanan-Khan A. Bcl-2 antisense therapy in hematological malignancies. Curr Opin Oncol 2004;16:581–585.
31. Agrawal S, Zhou Q. Mixed backbone oligonucleotides: Improvement in oligonucleotide-induced toxicity in vivo. Antisense Nucleic Acid Drug Dev 1998;8:135–139.

9. *Physicochemical and Biopharmaceutical Properties of Drug Substances and Pharmacokinetics*

SUNIL S. JAMBHEKAR

INTRODUCTION

Throughout its history, the pharmacy profession has been concerned primarily with the manner in which drugs produce their pharmacological effects and the dosage forms through which drugs are administered. Since the early twentieth century, efforts have been directed to determining, understanding, and providing rational explanations of drug effects on biological systems, but we have been limited by our ability to correlate the observed physiologic events with a reasonable hypothesis or concept. Pharmacists, at one time, were closely involved in formulating a prescription written by a physician for a patient. Today, most of the formulating is done by the pharmaceutical manufacturer.

Early descriptions of drug action were confined to their reference as tonic or toxic effects. This approach was followed by the concept of receptor theory, which for decades remained primarily an operational concept that was useful for discussing the new actions of drugs on a molecular level (1). Research in receptor theories, however, has provided evidence that the drug receptors do exist as distinct entities, and a limited success has been attained in the characterization of receptors (2,3).

An extension of the receptor theory of drug action is an increased emphasis on the importance of physicochemical properties of the drug and the relationship of such properties to the pharmacological responses. Because these properties play an important role in determining biological action of pharmaceuticals, it is appropriate to refer to these properties as biopharmaceutical properties of drug substances. Examples of such properties include solubility, partition coefficients, diffusivity, degree of ionization, and polymorphism, which in turn are determined by the chemical structure and stereochemistry of drug substances.

A consideration of these biopharmaceutical properties is fundamental to discussing several important aspects of the overall effects. For a given chemical entity (drug), there often will be a difference in physiological availability and, presumably, in clinical responses, primarily because drug molecules must cross various biological membranes and interact with intercellular and intracellular fluids before reaching the elusive region termed the "site of action." Under these conditions, the biopharmaceutical properties of the drug must contribute favorably to facilitate absorption and distribution processes to augment the drug concentration at various active sites. Furthermore, equally important is the fact that these biopharmaceutical properties of a drug must ensure a specific orientation on the receptor surface so that a sequence of events is initiated that leads to the observed pharmacological effects. Drug molecules that are deficient in the required biopharmaceutical properties may display generally marginal pharmacological action or be totally ineffective.

Biopharmaceutics may be defined as the study of the influence of formulation factors on the therapeutic activity of a drug product or dosage forms. It involves the study of the relationship between some of the physicochemical properties of a drug and the biological effects observed following the administration of a drug via various dosage forms or drug delivery systems. Almost any alteration in a drug delivery system is likely to alter the drug delivery rate and the amount of the drug delivered to the desired place in the body. This includes the chemical nature of the drug (e.g., ester, salts, and complexes), the particle size and surface area of the drug, the type of dosage forms (e.g., solution, suspension, capsule, and tablet), and the excipients and processes used in the manufacturing of the drug delivery systems.

Drugs, via drug delivery systems, most often are administered to human subjects by the oral route. Compared to other routes of drug administration, especially the intravenous route, the oral route is unusually complex with respect to the physicochemical conditions existing at the absorption site. Therefore, before we discuss how the biopharmaceutical properties of a drug in a dosage form may affect the availability and action of that drug, it is prudent to review the gastrointestinal physiology.

GASTROINTESTINAL PHYSIOLOGY

Figure 9.1 schematically represents the gastrointestinal tract and some of the problems encountered in a consideration of drug absorption from the site following administration of a drug via dosage forms (4). The stomach may be divided into two main parts: the body of the stomach, and the pylorus. Histologically, these parts correspond to the pepsin- and HCl-secreting area and the mucus-secreting area, respectively, of the gastric mucosa. In the human, the stomach contents usually are in the pH range of 1.0 to 3.5, with pH 1.0 to 2.5 being the most common range. Furthermore, there is a diurnal cycle of gastric acidity in humans. During the night, stomach contents usually are more acidic (pH ~1.3); during the day, because of food consumption, the pH is less acidic. The recovery of stomach acidity, however, occurs quite rapidly. The presence of protein, being amphoteric in nature, acts as an excellent buffer, and as digestion proceeds, the liberated amino acids increase the neutralizing capacity enormously.

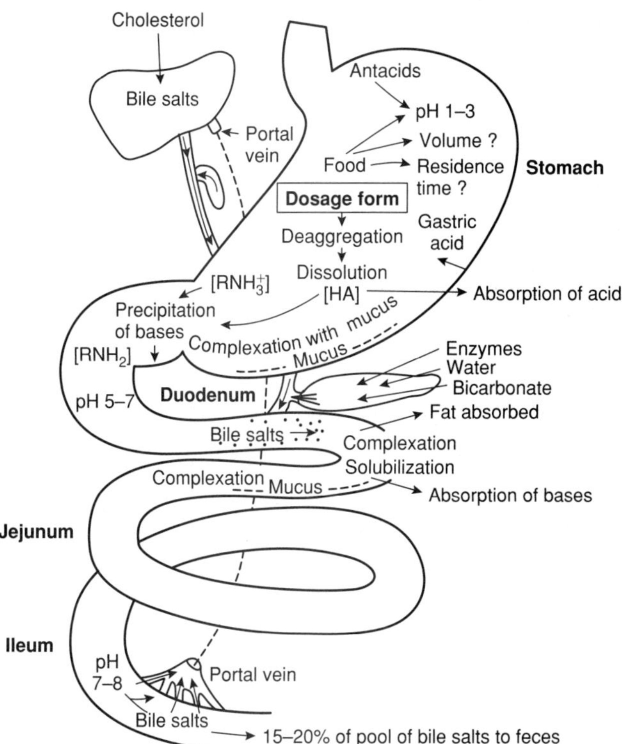

Fig. 9.1. Processes occurring along with drug absorption when drug molecules travel down the gastrointestinal tract and the factors that affect to drug absorption. (From Florence AT, Attwood D. Physiochemical Principles of Pharmacy, 2nd Ed. New York-Chapman and Hall, 1988, with permission).

The small intestine is divided anatomically into three sections: the duodenum, the jejunum, and the ileum. All three areas are involved in the digestion and absorption of food. The available absorbing area is increased by surface folds in the intestinal lining. The surface of these folds possesses villi and microvilli (Fig. 9.2). The duodenal contents in the human usually are in the pH range of 5 to 7. There is a gradual decrease in acidity along the length of the gastrointestinal tract, with the ultimate pH being 7 to 8 in the lower ileum. It has been estimated that approximately 8 L of fluid enter the upper intestine per day, with approximately 7 L of this arising from digestive juices and fluids and approximately 1 L arising from oral intake. Over the entire length of the large and small intestine and the stomach is the brush border, which consists of a uniform coating (thickness, 3 mm) of mucopolysaccharide. This coating layer serves to act as a mechanical barrier to bacteria or food particles.

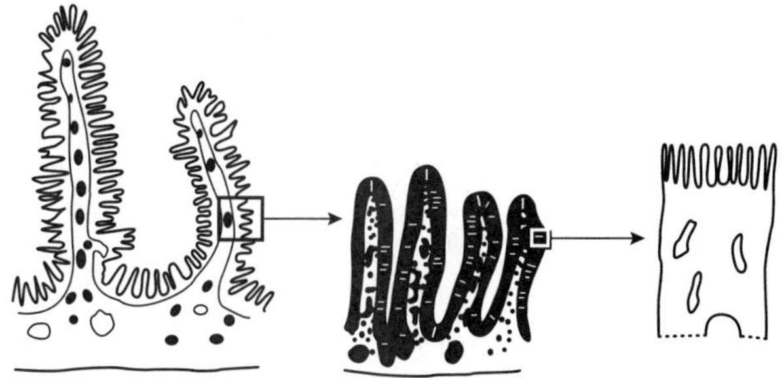

Fig. 9.2. The epithelium of the small intestine at different levels of magnification. From left to right: the intestinal villi and microvilli that constitute the brush border.

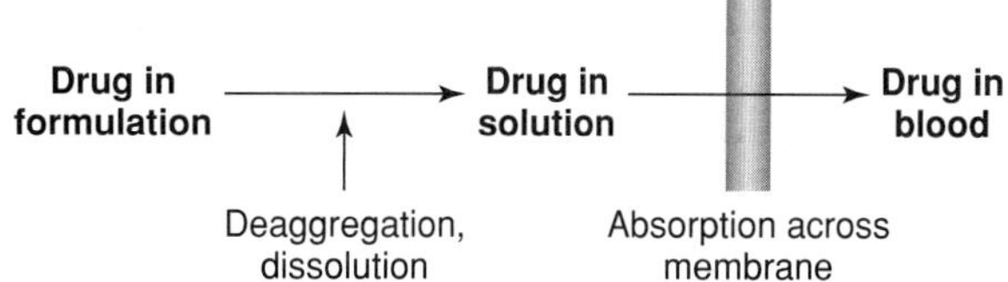

Fig. 9.3. Sequence of events in drug absorption from formulations of solid dosage forms.

When a dosage form containing a drug or drug molecules moves from the stomach through the pylorus into the duodenum, the dosage form encounters a rapidly changing environment with respect to pH. Furthermore, digestive juices secreted into the small bowel contain many enzymes not found in the gastric juices. Digestion and absorption of foodstuff occur simultaneously in the small intestine. Intestinal digestion is the terminal phase of preparing foodstuff for absorption and consists of two processes: completion of the hydrolysis of large molecules to smaller ones, which can be absorbed, and bringing the finished product of hydrolysis into an aqueous solution or emulsion.

Drug absorption, whether from the gastrointestinal tract or from other sites, requires the passage of the drug in a molecular form across the barrier membrane. Most drugs are presented to the body as solid or semi-solid dosage forms, and the drug particles must first be released from these dosage forms. These drug particles must dissolve, and if they possess the desirable biopharmaceutical properties, they will pass from a region of high concentration to a region of low concentration across the membrane into the blood or general circulation (Fig. 9.3). Knowledge of biological membrane structure and its general properties is pivotal in understanding absorption processes and the role of the biopharmaceutical properties of drug substances.

Biological Membrane

The prevalent view is that the gastrointestinal membrane consists of a bimolecular lipoid layer that is covered on each side by protein with the lipid molecule oriented perpendicular to the cell surface (Fig. 9.4). The lipid layer is interrupted by small, water-filled pores with a radius of approximately 4 A, and a molecule with a radius of 4 A or less may pass through these water-filled pores. Thus, membranes have a specialized transport system to assist the passage of water-soluble material and ions through the lipid interior, a process sometimes termed to as "convective absorption." The rate of permeation of such small molecules through the pore is affected not only by the relative sizes of the holes and the molecules but also by the interaction between permeating molecules

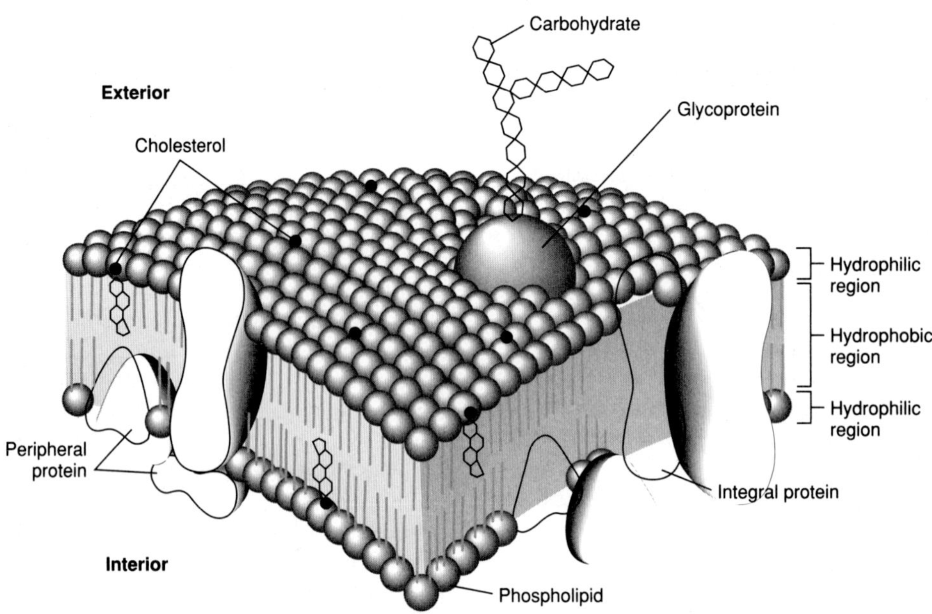

Fig. 9.4. Basic structure of an animal cell membrane. (From Smith C, Marks A, Lieberman M, eds. Basic Medical Biochemistry. Baltimore: Lippincott Williams & Wilkins, 2004:159–163, with permission.)

and the membrane. When permeation through the membrane occurs, the permeating substance is considered to have transferred from solution in the luminal aqueous phase to the lipid membrane phase, then to the aqueous phase on the other side of the membrane. Biological membranes differ from a polymeric membrane in that they are composed of small amphipathic molecules, phospholipids, and cholesterol. The protein layer associated with membranes is hydrophobic in nature. Therefore, biological membranes have a hydrophilic exterior and a hydrophobic interior. Cholesterol is a major component of most mammalian biological membranes, and its removal will render the membrane highly permeable. A cholesterol complexes with phospholipids, and its presence reduces the permeability of the membrane to water, cations, glycerides, and glucose. The shape of the cholesterol molecule allows it to fit closely with the hydrocarbon chains of unsaturated fatty acids in the bilayer. It is the general opinion that the cholesterol makes the membrane more rigid. The flexibility of the biological membrane to reform and adapt to a changed environment is its important feature. The details of membrane structure are still widely debated, and a more recent membrane model is shown in Figure 9.4.

In addition to biopharmaceutical factors, several physiological factors also may affect the rate and extent of gastrointestinal absorption. These factors are as follows: properties of epithelial cells, segmental activity of the bowel, degree of vascularity, effective absorbing surface area per unit length of gut, surface and interfacial tensions, electrolyte content and their concentration in luminal fluid, enzymatic activity in the luminal contents, and gastric emptying rate of the drug from stomach.

Mechanisms of Drug Absorption

Drug transfer often is viewed as the movement of a drug molecule across a series of membranes and spaces (Fig. 9.5), which, in aggregate, serve as a macroscopic membrane. The cells and interstitial spaces lying between the gastric lumen and the capillary blood or structure between sinusoidal space and the bile canaliculi are examples. Each of the cellular membranes and spaces may impede drug transport to varying degrees; therefore, any one of them can be a rate-limiting step to the overall process of drug transport. This complexity of structure makes quantitative prediction of drug transport difficult. A qualitative description of the processes of drug transport across functional membranes follows.

Passive Diffusion

The transfer of most drugs across a biological membrane occurs by passive diffusion, a natural tendency for molecules to move from a higher concentration to a lower concentration. This movement of drug molecules is caused by the kinetic energy of the molecules. The rate of diffusion depends on the magnitude of the concentration gradient (dC) across the membrane and can be represented by the following equation:

Eq. 9.1 $$-\frac{dC}{dt} = K \cdot dC = K(C_{abs} - C_b)$$

where $-dC/dt$ is the rate of diffusion across a membrane; K is a complex proportionality constant that includes the area of membrane, the thickness of the membrane, the partition coefficient of the drug molecule between the lipophilic membrane and the aqueous phase on each

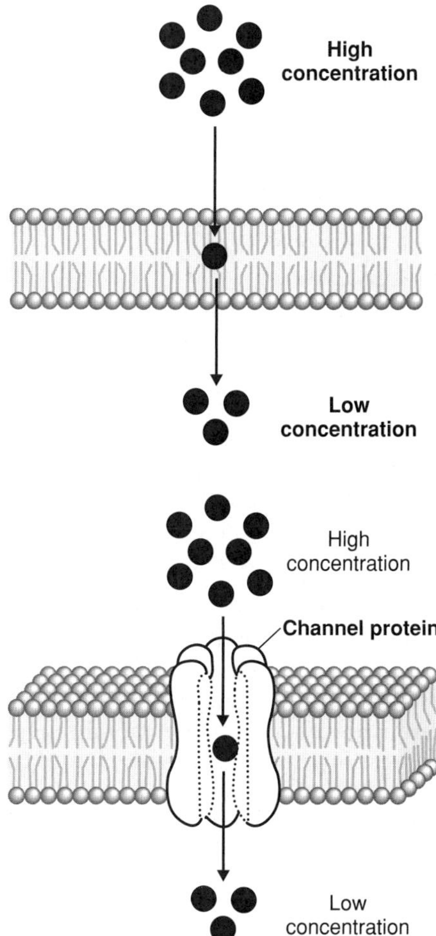

Fig. 9.5. (A) Simple diffusion. (B). Membrane channels. (From Smith C, Marks A, Lieberman M, eds. Basic Medical Biochemistry. Baltimore: Lippincott Williams & Wilkins, 2004:159–163, with permission.)

side of the membrane, and the diffusion coefficient of the drug; C_{abs} is the drug concentration at the absorption site; and C_b is the drug concentration in the blood.

The gastrointestinal absorption of a drug from an aqueous solution requires transfer from the lumen to the gut wall followed by penetration of the epithelial membrane by a drug molecule to the capillaries of the systemic circulation. On entering the blood, the drug distributes itself rapidly in the blood. Because of the volume differences at absorption and distribution sites, the drug concentration in blood (C_b) will be much lower than the concentration at the absorption site (C_{abs}). This concentration gradient is maintained throughout the absorption process—that is, ($C_{abs} - C_b$). As a result, the concentration gradient (dC in Eq. 9.1), is approximately equal to C_{abs}, so Equation 9.1 can be written as

Eq. 9.2
$$-\frac{dC}{dt} = K \cdot C_l$$

Because absorption by passive diffusion is a first-order process, the rate of absorption (dC/dt in Eq. 9.2) is

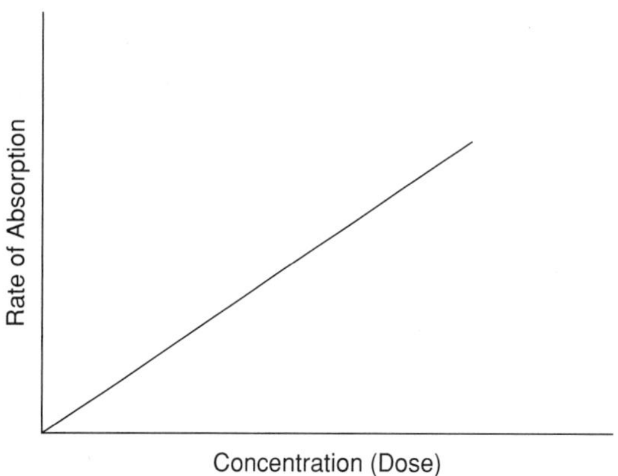

Fig. 9.6. Effect of drug concentration on the rate of absorption when passive diffusion is operative.

directly proportional to the concentration at the site of absorption (C_l). The greater the concentration of drug at the absorption site, the faster is the rate of absorption (Fig. 9.6). The percentage of dose absorbed at any time, however, remains unchanged.

A major source of variation is membrane permeability, which depends on the lipophilicity of the drug molecule. This often is characterized by its partition between oil and water. The lipid solubility of a drug, therefore, is a very important physicochemical property governing the rate of transfer through a variety of biological membrane barriers. Figure 9.7 illustrates the role of partition coefficients in the drug absorption process from the colon and that a good correlation exists between the percentage of

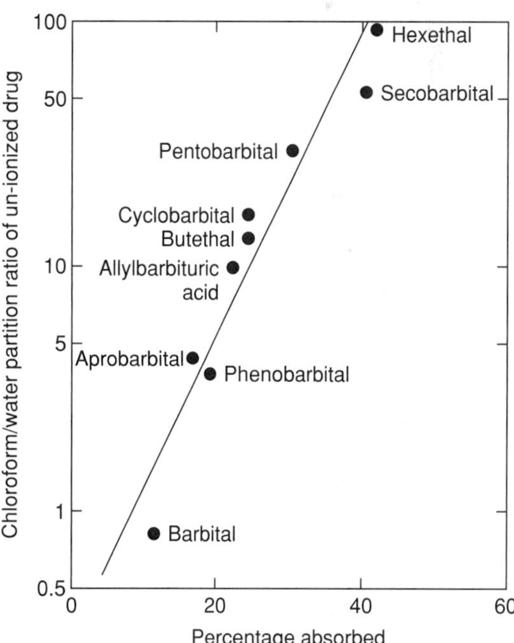

Fig. 9.7. Comparison between colonic absorption of barbiturates in the rat and lipid-to-water partition coefficient of the unionized form of the barbiturates. (From Schanker LS. Absorption of drugs from the colon. J Pharmacol Exp Ther 1959;126:283–294; with permission.)

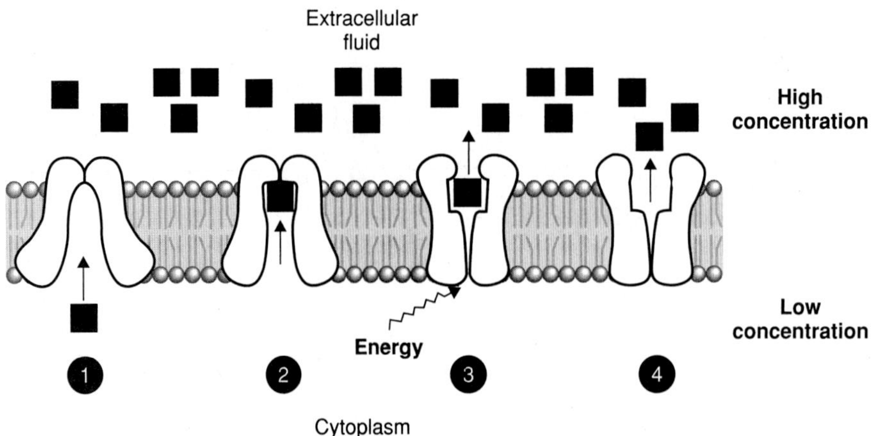

Fig. 9.8. Active transport. (From Smith C, Marks A, Lieberman M, eds. Basic Medical Biochemistry. Baltimore: Lippincott Williams & Wilkins, 2004:159–163, with permission.)

drug absorption and the partition coefficient of an unionized drug.

Carrier Mediated or Active Transport

Although most drugs are absorbed from the gastrointestinal tract by passive diffusion, some drugs of therapeutic interest and some chemicals of nutritional value, such as amino acids, di- and tripeptides, glucose, and folic acid, are absorbed by the action of transporter proteins (i.e., a carrier-mediated transport mechanism) (Fig. 9.8). In this type of transport, membranes have a specialized role. The usual requirement for active transport is structural similarities between the drug and the substrate normally transported across the membrane. Active transport differs from passive diffusion in the following ways: 1) The transport of the drug occurs against a concentration gradient, 2) the transport mechanism can become saturated at high drug concentration, and 3) a specificity for a certain molecular structure may promote competition in the presence of a similarly structured compound. This, in turn, may decrease the absorption of a drug. Active or facilitated absorption of a drug usually is explained by assuming that transporter proteins (i.e., carriers in membranes) are responsible for shuttling these solutes in mucosal or serosal direction. The number of apparent carriers in membranes, however, is limited. Therefore, the rate of transfer may be described by the following equation:

Eq. 9.3 $$\text{Absorption rate} = \frac{dC}{dt} = V_{max} \cdot C/K_m + C$$

where C is the solute concentration at the absorption site and V_{max} (the maximum theoretical transfer rate) and K_m (the concentration of drug at half the V_{max}) are constants. Low doses or concentrations, when $K_m \gg C$, reduce Equation 9.3 to

Eq. 9.4 $$\frac{dC}{dt} = \frac{V_{max}}{K_m \cdot C} = K \cdot C$$

Equation 9.4 indicates that the apparent first order kinetics is observed. Under these conditions, there are sufficient numbers of carriers available so that a constant proportion of solute molecules presented to the membrane are transported across the membranes. As the solute concentration increases, the number of free carriers is reduced, and the proportion of solute molecules transferred across the membrane is reduced until a maximum absolute number saturation is reached. When $C \gg K_m$,

Eq. 9.5 $$\text{Absorption rate} = \frac{dC}{dt} = V_{max}$$

Equation 9.5 indicates that a further increase in solute concentration will not result in any further increase in the rate of absorption (Fig. 9.9). The capacity-limited

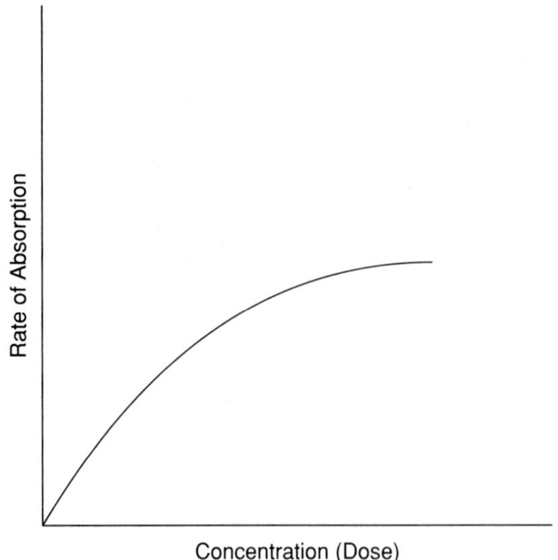

Fig. 9.9. Relationship between drug concentration and rate of absorption when an active transport process is operative.

characteristics of carrier-mediated processes suggest that the bioavailability of drugs absorbed in this manner should decrease nonlinearly with increasing doses. Therefore, the use of a large, single oral dose of these drugs is irrational, and if larger daily doses are necessary, one should use divided doses. Examples of substances that are actively transported include amino acids, methyldopa, 5-fluorouracil, penicillamine, and levodopa.

Convective Absorption

The absorption of small molecules (molecular radii less than ~4 A) through water-filled pores of biological membrane is referred to as convective absorption. The rate of absorption because of this mechanism is equated to the product of a sieving coefficient, the rate of fluid or water absorption, and the concentration of solute in the luminal content. The sieving coefficient is indirectly related to the relative sizes of the pores and the molecules.

Ion-Pair Absorption

In 1967, Higuchi suggested that highly ionized compounds, such as quaternary ammonium compounds, may possibly be absorbed by an ion pair mechanism (6). In vitro, a relatively large organic anion can combine with relatively large cation to form an ion pair of neutral properties, which will then cross a water–organic solvent interface and transfer to an organic phase.

PHYSICOCHEMICAL FACTORS AFFECTING DRUG ABSORPTION

The pH-Partition Hypothesis on Drug Absorption

Drug absorption is influenced by many physiological factors. Additionally, it also depends on many physicochemical properties of the drug itself. Shore, Brodie, Hogben, Schanker, Tocco, and others (5,7–12) concluded from their research that most drugs are absorbed from the gastrointestinal tract by a process of passive diffusion of the un-ionized moiety across a lipid membrane. Furthermore, the dissociation constant, lipid solubility, and pH of the fluid at the absorption site determines the extent of absorption from a solution. The interrelationship among these parameters is known as the pH-partition theory. This theory provides a basic framework for the understanding of drug absorption from the gastrointestinal tract and drug transport across the biological membrane. The principle points of this theory are as follows:

1. The gastrointestinal and other biological membranes act like lipid barriers.
2. The un-ionized form of the acidic or basic drug is preferentially absorbed.
3. Most drugs are absorbed by passive diffusion.
4. The rate of drug absorption and amount of drug absorbed are related to its oil–water partition coefficient (i.e., the more lipophilic the drug, the faster is its absorption).
5. Weak acidic and neutral drugs may be absorbed from the stomach, but basic drugs are not.

When a drug is administered intravenously, it is immediately available to body fluids for distribution to the site of action. All extravascular routes, however, can influence the overall therapeutic activity of the drug, primarily because of its dissolution rate, a step that is necessary for a drug to be available in a solution form. When a drug is administered orally in a dosage form such as a tablet, capsule, or suspension, the rate of absorption across the biological membrane frequently is controlled by the slowest step in the following sequence:

$$\text{Dosage form} \xrightarrow{\text{dissolution}} \text{Drug in solution} \xrightarrow{\text{absorption}} \text{Drug in general circulation}$$

In many instances, the slowest step, or the rate-limiting step, in the sequence is the dissolution of the drug. When dissolution is the controlling step, any factors that affect the rate of dissolution also must influence the rate of absorption. This, in turn, affects the extent and duration of action. Several factors can influence the dissolution rate of drug from solid dosage forms and, therefore, the therapeutic activity. These factors include solubility of a drug, particle size and surface area of drug particles, crystalline and salt form of a drug, and the rate of disintegration.

The absorption rate of drugs also can be affected by interaction or formation of complexes in the gastrointestinal tract. Generally, such complex formation reduces the concentration of free drug at the absorption site. Because the complexed drug is absorbed either slowly or not at all, the net effect is the reduction of concentration of drug at absorption site and slower rate of absorption.

Ionization and pH at Absorption Site

The fraction of the drug existing in its un-ionized form in a solution is a function of both the dissociation constant of a drug and the pH of the solution at the absorption site. The dissociation constant, for both weak acids and bases, often is expressed as the pK_a (the negative logarithm of a dissociation constant, K_a). The Henderson-Hasselbach equation for the ionization of a weak acid, HA, is derived from the following equation:

Eq. 9.6 $$HA + H_2O \rightleftharpoons A^- + H_3O^+$$

We may express the equilibrium constant as follows:

Eq. 9.7 $$K_a = \frac{[{}_aH_3O^+][{}_aA^-]}{[{}_aHA]}$$

where K_a is the equilibrium or dissociation constant and $_a$ is the activity coefficient. Assuming the activity coefficients approach unity in dilute solutions, the activity coefficient may be replaced by concentration terms, and Equation 9.7 becomes

Eq. 9.8 $$K_a = \frac{[H_3O^+][A^-]}{[HA]}$$

The negative logarithm of K_a is referred to as the pK_a. Thus,

Eq. 9.9 $$pK_a = -\log K_a$$

Taking the logarithm of the expression for the dissociation constant of a weak acid in Equation 9.8 yields

Eq. 9.10 $$-\log K_a = \frac{-\log [H_3O] - \log[A^-]}{[HA]}$$

where A^- is the ionized form of a weak acid and HA is the un-ionized form.

Eq. 9.11 $$pH - pK_a = \frac{\log [\text{Ionized}]}{[\text{Un-ionized}]}$$

Assuming that α is the fraction of ionized species and that 1−α is the fraction remaining as the un-ionized form, Equation 9.11 can be written as

Eq. 9.12 $$pH - pK_a = \log \frac{\alpha}{1 - \alpha}$$

or

Eq. 9.13 $$\frac{\alpha}{1 - \alpha} = \text{antilog} \longleftrightarrow (pH - pK_a)$$

From Equation 9.13, the fraction or percentage of the absorbable and nonabsorbable forms of a weak acid can be calculated if the pH condition at the site of administration is known. Analogously, the dissociation or basicity constant for a weak base is derived as follows:

Eq. 9.14 $$B + H_2O \longleftrightarrow BH^+ + OH^-$$

The dissociation constant, K_b, is derived as follows:

Eq. 9.15 $$K_b = \frac{[_aOH]\,[_aBH]}{[_aB]} = \frac{[OH^-][BH]}{[B]}$$

and

Eq. 9.16 $$pK_b = -\log K_b$$

The pK_a and pK_b values provide a convenient means of comparing the strength of weak acids and bases. The lower the pK_a, the stronger the acid, and the lower the pK_b, the stronger the base. The values for pK_a and pK_b of conjugate acid-base pairs are linked by the expression

Eq. 9.17 $$pK_a + pK_b = pK_w$$

where pK_w is the negative logarithm of dissociation constant of water. Taking the logarithm of Equation 9.15 and rearranging yields

Eq. 9.18 $$-\log K_b = \frac{-\log [OH^-] - \log [BH^+]}{[B]}$$

Although the dissociation constant of a weak base is described by the term K_b, it is conventionally expressed in terms of K_a, because of the relationship expressed in Equation 9.17.

Equation 9.18 can then be written as

Eq. 9.19 $$pH = pK_w - pK_b - \log \frac{[BH^+]}{[B]}$$

Because pK_w − pK_b − pK_a, Equation 9.19 takes the following form for a weak base (BH^+ is the ionized form, and B is the un-ionized form):

Eq. 9.20 $$pK_a - pH = \log \frac{[\text{Ionized}]}{[\text{Un-ionized}]}$$

Again, assuming that α is the fraction of ionized species and that 1 − α is the fraction of un-ionized species, Equation 9.20 becomes

Eq. 9.21 $$pK_a - pH = \log \frac{\alpha}{1 - \alpha}$$

or

Eq. 9.22 $$\frac{\alpha}{1 - \alpha} = \text{antilog } (pK_a - pH)$$

From Equation 9.22, one can calculate the fraction or percentage of absorbable and nonabsorbable form of a weak base if the pH condition at the site of drug absorption is known. Figure 9.10 shows the pK_a values of several drugs and the relative acid or base strength of these compounds.

The relationship between pH and pK_a and the extent of ionization is given by Equations 9.13 and 9.22 for weak acids and weak bases, respectively. Accordingly, most weak acidic drugs are predominantly in the un-ionized form at lower pH of the gastric fluid and, therefore, may be absorbed from the stomach as well as from the intestine. Some very weak acidic drugs, such as phenytoin and many barbiturates, the pK_a values of which are greater than 8.0, are essentially un-ionized at all pH values. Therefore, for these weak acidic drugs, transport is more rapid and independent of pH, provided that the un-ionized form is lipophilic or nonpolar. Furthermore, it is important to note that the fraction un-ionized changes dramatically only for weak acids with pK_a values between 3 and 7. Therefore, for the weak acids, a change in the rate of transport with pH is expected, as shown in Figure 9.11 (13). Although the transport of weak acids with pK_a values less than 3.0 should theoretically depend on pH, the fraction un-ionized is so low that transport across the gut membrane may be slow even under the most acidic conditions.

Most weak bases are poorly absorbed, if at all, in the stomach, because they are present largely in the ionized form at pH 1–2. Codeine, a weak base with a pK_a of

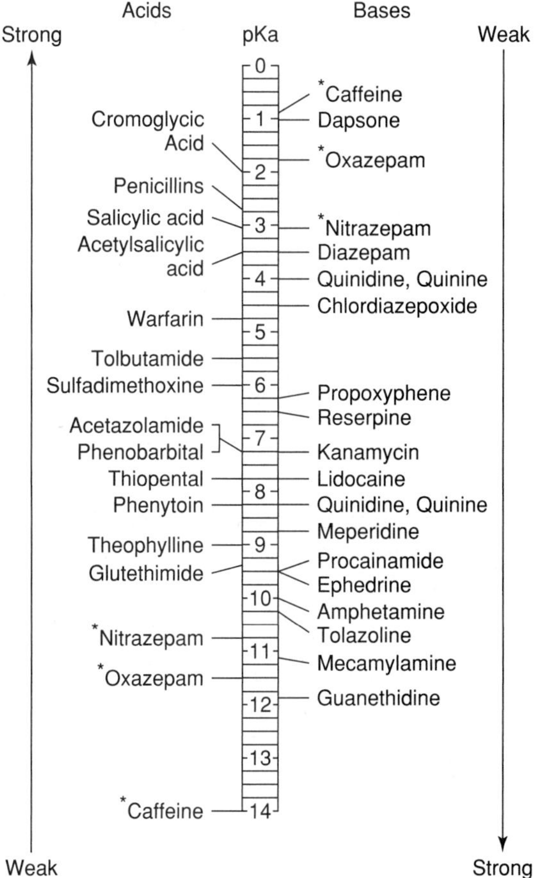

Fig. 9.10. The pK_a values of certain acidic and basic drugs. Drugs denoted with an asterisk are amphoteric (13). (From Rowland M, Tozer T. Clinical Pharmacokinetics: Concepts and Application, 2nd Ed. Philadelphia: Lea and Febiger, 1989, with permission.)

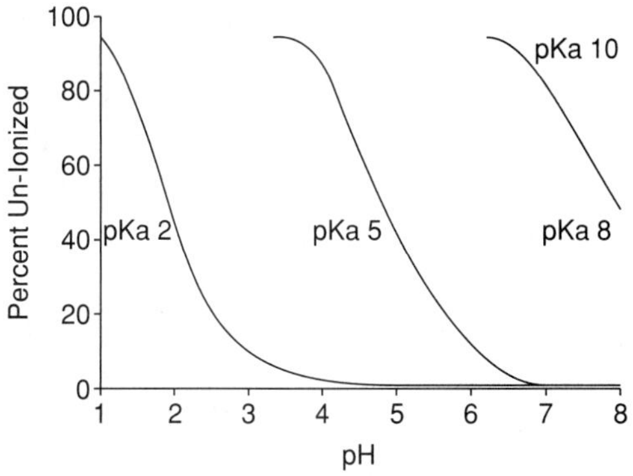

Fig. 9.11. For very weak acids, pK_a values greater than 8.0 are predominantly un-ionized at all pH values between 1.0 and 8.0. Profound changes in the un-ionized fraction occur with pH for an acid with a pK_a value that lies within the range of 2.0 to 8.0. Although the fraction un-ionized of even strong acids increases with hydrogen ion concentration, the absolute value remains low at most pH values shown. (From Rowland M, Tozer T. Clinical Pharmacokinetics: Concepts and Application, 2nd Ed. Philadelphia: Lea and Febiger, 1989, with permission.)

Table 9.1. Comparison of Gastric Absorption of Acids and Bases at pH 1 and 8 in the Rat

	pK_a	% Absorbed at pH 1	% Absorbed at pH 8
Acids			
5-Sulfosalicylic acid	<2.0	0	0
5-Nitrosalicylic acid	2.3	52	16
Salicylic acid	3.0	61	13
Thiopental	7.6	46	34
Bases			
Aniline	4.6	6	56
p-Toluidine	5.3	0	47
Quinine	8.4	0	18
Dextromethorphan	9.2	0	16

approximately eight, will have about 1 in every 1 million molecules in its un-ionized form at gastric pH 1.0. Weakly basic drugs with a pK_a of less than four, such as dapsone, diazepam, and chlordiazepoxide, are essentially un-ionized through the intestine. Strong bases, which are those with pK_a values between 5 and 11, show pH-dependent absorption. Stronger bases, such as guanethidine ($pK_a >$ 11) are ionized throughout the gastrointestinal tract and tend to be poorly absorbed.

The evidence of the importance of dissociation in drug absorption is found in the result of studies in which pH at the absorption site is changed (Tables 9.1 and 9.2). Table 9.2 clearly shows the decreased absorption of a weak acid at pH 8.0 compared to pH 1.0 (13). On the other hand, an increase to pH 8.0 promotes the absorption of a weak base with practically nothing absorbed at pH 1.0. The data in Table 9.2 also permits a comparison of intestinal absorption of acidic and basic drugs from buffered solutions ranging from pH 4.0 to 8.0 (14). These results are in agreement with the pH-partition hypothesis.

The pH-partition theory provides a basic framework for the understanding of drug absorption and, sometimes, is an oversimplification of a more complex process. For example, experimentally observed pH–absorption curves are less steep (Fig. 9.12) than that expected

Table 9.2. Comparison of Intestinal Absorption of Acids and Bases in the Rat at Several pH Values

		% Absorbed from Rat Intestine			
	pK_a	pH 4	pH 5	pH 7	pH 8
Acids					
5-Nitrosalicyclic acid	2.3	40	27	0	0
Salicylic acid	3.0	64	35	30	10
Acetylsalicylic acid	3.5	41	27	—	—
Benzoic acid	4.2	62	36	35	5
Bases					
Aniline	4.6	40	48	58	61
Amiopyrine	5.0	21	35	48	52
p-Toluidine	5.3	30	42	65	64
Quinine	8.4	9	11	41	54

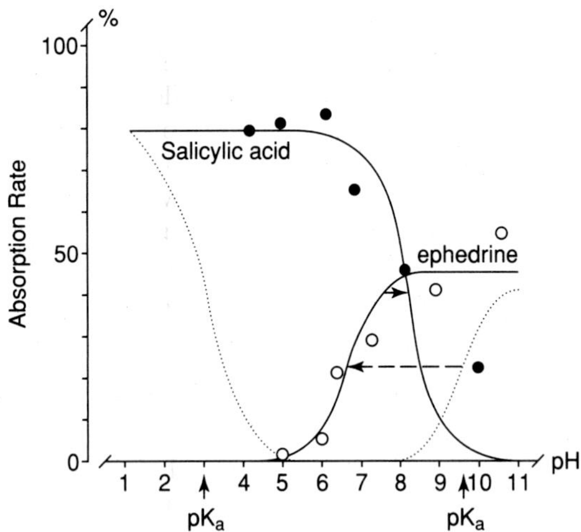

Fig. 9.12. Relationship between absorption rates of salicylic acid and ephedrine and bulk phase pH in the rat small intestine in vivo. Dashed lines represent curves predicted by the pH-partition theory in the absence of an unstirred layer. (From Winne D. The influence of unstirred layers on intestinal absorption in intestinal permeation. In: Kramer M, Lauterbach F, eds. Workshop Conference Hoechest, vol 4. Amsterdam: Excerpta Medica, 1977:58–64, with permission.)

theoretically and are shifted to higher pH values for bases and lower pH values for acids. This deviation, observed experimentally, has been attributed by several investigators to factors such as limited absorption of ionized species of drugs, the presence of an unstirred diffusion layer adjacent to the cell membrane, and a difference between lumenal pH and cell membrane surface pH.

Lipid Solubility

PARTITION COEFFICIENT. Some drugs may be poorly absorbed after oral administration even though they are available predominantly in the un-ionized form in the gastrointestinal tract. This is attributed to the low lipid solubility of the un-ionized molecule. A guide to lipid solubility or lipophilic nature of a drug is provided by a property called the partition coefficient (*P*). This parameter therefore influences the transport and absorption processes of drugs, and it is one of the most widely used properties in quantitative structure–activity relationships.

The movement of molecules from one phase to another is called partitioning. Drugs partition themselves between the aqueous phase and lipophilic membrane. Preservative emulsions partition between the water and oil phases; antibiotics partition from body fluids to microorganisms; and drug and other adjuvants can partition into the plastic and rubber stoppers of containers. It therefore is important that this process is understood.

If two immiscible phases are placed adjacent to each other, with one containing a solute soluble in both phases, the solute will distribute itself between two immiscible phases until equilibrium is attained; therefore, no further transfer of solute occurs. At equilibrium, the chemical potential of the solute (free energy of the solute in solvent) in one phase is equal to its chemical potential in the other phase. If we consider an aqueous (w) and an organic (o) phase, we write according to theory:

Eq. 9.23 $$\mu_w^\Theta + RT \ln a_w = \mu_o^\Theta + RT \ln a_o$$

where *a* represents the activity coefficient of a solute (effect of solute concentration on intersolute interactions). Rearranging Equation 9.23 yields

Eq. 9.24 $$\frac{\mu_w^\Phi - \mu_0^\Phi}{RT} = \ln \frac{a_w}{a_o}$$

The term on the left side of Equation 9.24 is a constant at a given temperature and pressure. Therefore,

Eq. 9.25 $$\frac{a_w}{a_o} = \text{constant or } \frac{a_o}{a_w} = \text{constant}$$

These constants are the partition (*P*) or distribution coefficients (*D*). Because most drugs are ionic, their partition coefficients are pH-dependent and usually reported at pH 7.4 and are therefore appropriately called distribution coefficients. If the solute under consideration forms an ideal solution in either phases or in solvent, the activity coefficient can be replaced by the concentration term, and Equation 9.25 becomes

Eq. 9.26 $$P = \frac{C_o}{C_w}$$

Equation 9.25 is used conventionally to calculate the partition coefficient of a drug. In Equation 9.25, C_o, the concentration of drug in the organic or oil phase, is divided by the concentration in the aqueous phase. The greater the value of *P*, the higher the lipid solubility of the solute. It has been demonstrated for several systems that the partition coefficient can be approximated by the solubility of the solute in the organic phase divided by the solubility in the aqueous phase. Therefore, the partition coefficient is a measure of the relative affinities of the solute for an aqueous or nonaqueous or oil phase. The effect of lipid solubility and, hence, the partition coefficient on the absorption of a series of barbituric acid derivatives is shown in Table 9.3. The term partition coefficient is more commonly expressed exponentially as log *P*.

Table 9.3. Comparison of Barbiturate Absorption in Rat Colon and Partition Coefficient (Chloroform/Water) of Undissociated Drug

Barbiturate	Partition Coefficient	% Absorbed
Barbital	0.7	12
Apobarbital	4.9	17
Phenobarbital	4.8	20
Allylbarbital	10.5	23
Butethal	11.7	24
Cyclobarbital	13.9	24
Pentobarbital	28.0	30
Secobarbital	50.7	40
Hexethal	>100	44

It must be clearly understood that even though drugs with greater lipophilicity and, therefore, partition coefficient are better absorbed, it is imperative that drugs exhibit some degree of aqueous solubility. This is essential, because the availability of the drug molecule in a solution form is a prerequisite for drug absorption and the biological fluids at the site of absorption are aqueous in nature. Therefore, from a practical viewpoint, drugs must exhibit a balance between hydrophilicity and lipophilicity. This factor is always taken into account while a chemical modification is being considered as a way of improving the efficacy of a therapeutic agent.

Examples of polar or hydrophilic molecules that are poorly absorbed following oral administration and, therefore, must be administered parenterally include gentamicin, ceftrixine, and streptokinase. Lipid-soluble drugs with favorable partition coefficients generally are well absorbed after oral administration. Very often, the selection of a compound with higher partition coefficient from a series of research compounds provides improved pharmacological activity. Occasionally, the structure of an existing drug is modified to develop a similar pharmacological activity with improved absorption. Chlortetracycline, which differs from tetracycline by the substitution of a chlorine at C-7, substitution of an n-hexyl (Hexethal) for a phenyl ring in phenobarbital, or replacement of the 2-carbonyl of pentobarbital with a 2-thio group (thiopental) are examples of enhanced lipophilicity (Fig. 9.13).

It is important to note that even a minor molecular modification of a drug also may promote the risk of altering the efficacy and safety profile of a drug. For this reason, medicinal chemists prefer the development of a lipid-soluble pro-drug of a drug with poor oral absorption characteristics.

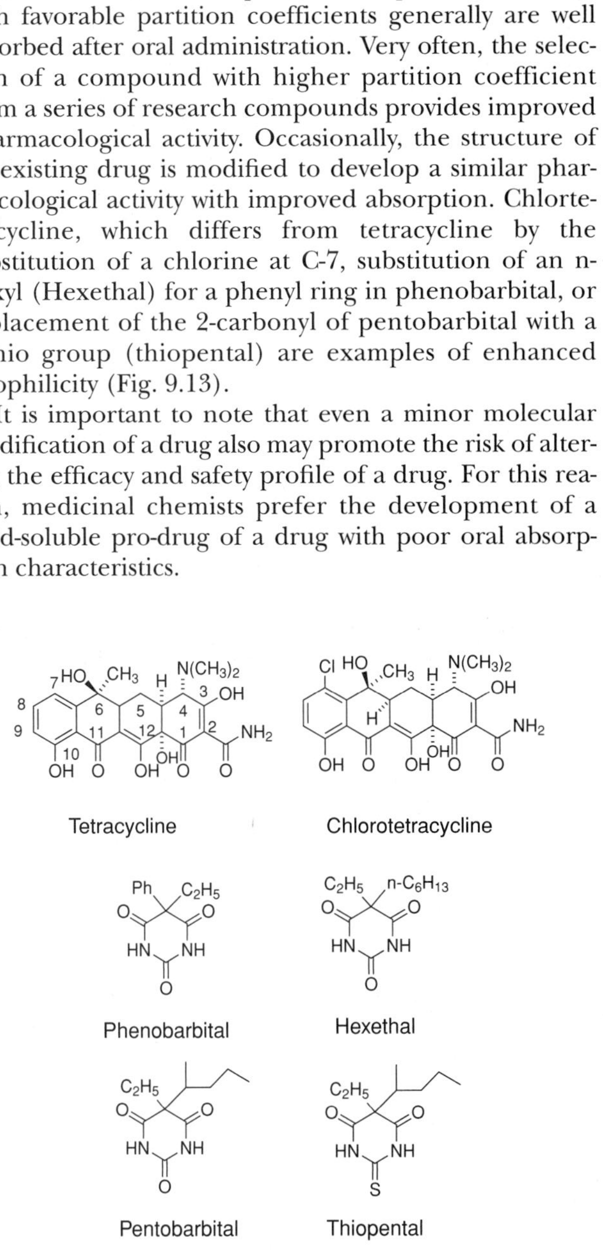

Tetracycline

Chlorotetracycline

Phenobarbital

Hexethal

Pentobarbital

Thiopental

Fig. 9.13. Drug pairs in which chemical modification enhances lipophilicity.

Estimation of Drug Absorption

When different chemical entities are being investigated for their potential as drug candidates, dosage form performance is one of the possible contributing factors to poor bioavailability. Historically, the concept of bioavailability is closely, if not solely, associated with dosage form performance. Because poor bioavailability in particular is increasingly an issue in the drug discovery and development process, application of the bioavailability principles and techniques has been extended to include animal studies in the selection of potential drug candidates for their full development.

As the drug travels down the gastrointestinal tract following its oral administration, part of the dose may not be available for absorption for a number of reasons. These include its chemical degradation, physical inactivation because of binding and complexation with substances in the intestinal tract, incomplete dissolution of the dosage form, microbial biotransformation, insufficient contact time in the gastrointestinal tract, poor solubility and poor permeability across the gastrointestinal mucosa, or metabolism within the gut wall. Of the absorbed dose, some of the drug may be metabolized in transit during its first passage through the gut wall and the liver. Unchanged drug that reaches the hepatic portal vein may be extracted by the liver via biotransformation or biliary excretion. Thus, the bioavailability (f) of an orally administered dose of a drug comprises the individual fractions that survive several barriers encountered by the drug during its first passage from gut lumen to the sampling site, and it is described (19), in general, by the following relationship.

Eq. 9.27 $$f = F_a F_g F_h$$

where F_a, F_g, and F_h are the fractions of intact drug absorbed (F_a) that escape irreversible elimination as the drug passes sequentially from the gastrointestinal tract across the gut wall (F_g) and traverses the liver (F_h) into systemic circulation. Thus, bioavailability of a drug can be equal to or less than the fraction absorbed, depending on the extent of metabolism and loss during the absorption process. Therefore, poor blood levels of a drug can be a consequence of poor absorption or of good absorption accompanied by extensive metabolism.

There appear to be several common misperceptions (20) regarding the nature of absorption. Among these is that intestinal absorption, permeability, fraction of drug absorbed, and in some cases, even bioavailability are equivalent properties and, consequently, can be used interchangeably. Another common misperception is that absorption, permeability, and so on are discrete fundamental properties of a drug molecule and can be predicted solely from its chemical structure. In reality, however, drug absorption is quite a complex process dependent on drug properties such as solubility and permeability, formulation factors, and physiological variables such as regional permeability differences, pH, luminal and mucosal enzymology, and intestinal motility, among others.

Publication of so-called "Rule of Five" (21) has generated widespread interest in regards to applying calculated physicochemical properties in the drug discovery process to separate out poor drug candidates before these go into clinical trials. According to the Rule of Five, poor intestinal absorption is associated with and attributed to the molecule possessing any two of the following properties: molecular weight greater than 750 daltons, number of hydrogen bond donors greater than five, number of hydrogen bond acceptors greater than 10, and calculated log P (partition coefficient) greater than five. These guidelines have been proven to be very useful for approximate predictions of intestinal drug absorption. The critical role of lipid solubility in drug absorption is a major guiding principle in the drug discovery and development process. Because the lipid-solubility of a drug molecule is the sum of the individual partition coefficients for each of its functional groups (see Chapter 2), the prediction of lipid solubility ($c \log P$) can be estimated.

A recent examination (22) of the relationship of molecular surface properties with biological performance of a molecule has been revealing. Most notably, it has been demonstrated that polar surface area (PSA) of a drug molecule has a strong correlation predicting drug transport from human intestine and across the drug membrane. The PSA is defined as the sum of the Van der Waals surface areas for the polar atoms, oxygens, nitrogens, and attached hydrogen atom (or the number of H-bond donors and H-bond acceptors). (See http://www.molinspiration.com for calculating the PSA). The PSA is a major determinant for oral absorption and brain penetration of drugs that are transported by the transcellular route (movement across cell membranes). This property should be considered in the early phase of drug screening. Another related parameter, dynamic PSA (PSAd), has surfaced (23) as a parameter of value in predicting membrane permeability and oral absorption in humans. Interpolation of the sigmoidal plot for 20 selected compounds suggests that when the PSAd is greater 140 Å^2, incomplete absorption (<10%) results, and when the PSAd value is less than 60 Å^2, drug absorption will be in excess of 90%.

A drug's absorption, as reflected in its bioavailability, is a fairly complex process, and although it is related to the drug structure, it is related in a complex manner. Failure to appreciate and understand these complexities, in an attempt to build models, may provide a prediction of marginal and low confidence. Both fraction absorbed and bioavailability are measures of the extent of absorption. Permeability, on the other hand, is related to the rate of absorption (20):

Eq. 9.28 $$J = P_e \cdot SA \cdot dC$$

where J is the absorptive flux and is equal to the permeability (P_e) of intestinal mucosa to the drug, the surface area available (SA), and the drug concentration gradient

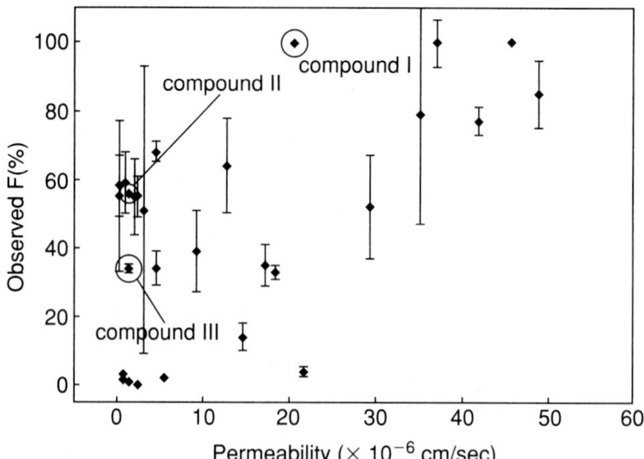

Fig. 9.14. Poor correlation between oral bioavailability and permeability as measured using Caco-2 cells for three compounds. (From Burton P, Goodwin J, Vidamas T, et al. Predicting drug absorption: how nature made it a difficult problem. J Pharm Exp Ther 2002;303:889–895 and from Hilgers AR, Smith DP, Biermacher JJ, et al. Predicting oral absorption of drugs: a case study with novel class of antimicrobial agents. Pharm Res 2003;20:1149–1155; with permission.)

(dC) across the mucosa. Factors that can influence permeability include structural characteristics of a drug, which include size, shape, solubility, charge, and surface area.

It has been argued (25), on a theoretical basis, that a fundamental relationship exists between the rate measured as a permeability coefficient and the extent of absorption. This has lead to the greater interest and increasing use of the in vitro permeability model to serve as an experimental surrogate for predicting oral absorption potential of drug candidates in drug discovery programs. Additionally, although in some instances (24,25) it has been possible to directly correlate absorption with permeability, more often poor correlation exists (20,26), as illustrated in Figure 9.14. At times, good absorption is observed for poorly permeable compounds. These poorly permeable but well-absorbed compounds exhibit high aqueous solubility, generally exceeding 2.5 mg/mL (20,22). This suggests that aqueous solubility may help to compensate for the poor in vitro permeability observed.

Estimating the extent of oral drug absorption and variation in drug absorption, therefore, can be of great value in the selection of a potential therapeutics agent and in identifying ways to optimize the oral drug delivery in patients. This may be facilitated by developing the predictive oral drug delivery models. In turn, these models permit the estimation of drug absorption without performing in vivo studies in humans and impart better understanding of the rate-limiting processes affecting drug absorption, which can assist in developing strategies for the development of oral drug delivery. There are three physical barriers to drug absorption: the dissolution resistance, the aqueous boundary layer resistance, and the membrane resistance (27,29).

Although physicochemical properties, such as solubility and permeability, and other properties, such as metabolic stability and toxicity, may be important individually, the interrelationship of these properties is what eventually determines the in vivo performance of a drug. In particular, the role of solubility is dependent on the potency, which will determine the dose. In other words, low solubility may be problematic for a high-dose drug; however, it may be more acceptable for a low-dose drug.

Measurement of Permeability

Although a variety of models (subcellular fraction, cell monolayer model, isolated intestinal tissue, and intestinal perfusion) are available to predict the permeability of a drug, the cell monolayer model and rat intestinal perfusion techniques are the most commonly used techniques.

Cell Monolayer

These models consist of cells grown on permeable inserts. Transport of compounds across the cell monolayer can be used to quantitate the permeability of a new chemical entity in a rapid manner. One of the most popular cell lines is Caco-2, derived from human colon adenocarcinoma cells. The monolayer exhibits ion conductance and possesses transepithelial electrical resistance indicative of fully formed tight junctions that restrict the paracellular transport of a chemical entity. Although Caco-2 cells are the most commonly used cells, Madin-Darby Canine Kidney (MDCK) cells are becoming more widespread in use, in part because of the shorter culture time (4–7 days versus 21–30 days for Caco-2 cells) needed for their use in permeability experiments.

Excellent correlation for permeability coefficient between MDCK and Caco-2 cells was observed for 55 compounds with known human intestinal absorption. Regardless of the type of cells used in determining permeability measurement, establishing the correlation between the permeability coefficient and the fraction of drug absorbed in vivo validates this approach.

Several clones of HT 29 cells have been used (30) to study different aspect of intestinal drug absorption. An enterocytic HT 29 clone, HT 29-18-C1, was proposed as a model to study intestinal permeability. The limitation of the cells is that these cells grow very slowly, and large number of cultured failed to develop acceptable barrier characteristics.

Biopharmaceutical Drug Classification

It is clear from the discussion thus far that the physicochemical properties, such as drug solubility and drug permeability, play a critical role in the drug absorption process. The following biopharmaceutical drug classification system (30,32) has been developed to optimize the development of an oral dosage form taking into consideration two rate-limiting factors, drug permeability and drug dissolution, the latter of which is related to drug solubility.

Class I Drugs (High Solubility and High Permeability)

Class I drugs provide both rapid dissolution and high membrane permeation. This class includes small molecule hydrophilic drugs that are not ionized in the gastrointestinal tract. Examples include acetaminophen, valproic acid, ketoprofen, dysopyramide, verapamil, propranolol, fluconazole, and metoprolol. Class I drugs are well absorbed and are affected by a limited set of interactions that alter drug absorption. Because gastric emptying frequently will control the rate of absorption for this class of drugs, interactions that delay gastric emptying will delay drug absorption. This can be important for class I analgesic drugs, for which a rapid rate of absorption and quick rise in the plasma level to within the therapeutic range is needed to alleviate pain quickly.

Class II Drugs (Low Solubility and High Permeability)

For immediate-release formulations of many poorly water-soluble drugs, the dissolution rate limits drug absorption. Along with this limitation, a greater impact on drug absorption will be observed with high oral doses. For example, the antifungal drug griseofulvin and the cardiac glycoside drug digoxin are both poorly water-soluble and possess similar dissolution profiles, which limit the rate of drug absorption. The extent of griseofulvin absorption, however, is incomplete for a typical dose of 500 mg, whereas a normal, 0.25-mg oral dose of digoxin usually provides a fairly complete absorption. Other examples are diazepam and nifedipine.

Any interactions that increase drug solubility and dissolution rate in the gastrointestinal tract will exert a positive effect on the gastrointestinal absorption of this class of drugs. The absorption of this class of drugs often is enhanced in proportion to the fat content of the coadministered meal. This is attributed to the increased gastrointestinal fluid volume from a coadministered meal, stimulated gastrointestinal secretions, and biliary solubilization effects that increase the dissolution rate. Furthermore, increased gastric residence time as a function of the caloric density permits greater time for drug dissolution.

Class III Drugs (High Solubility and Low Permeability)

For drugs possessing high water solubility, the intestinal membrane permeation rate often is the rate-limiting step in drug absorption from immediate-release dosage forms. Many drugs in this class (e.g., acyclovir and chloramphenicol) also show region-dependent absorption with better absorption in the upper small intestine. Therefore, any interactions that compromise upper intestinal absorption may result in a significant decrease in oral bioavailability. Consequently, these drugs show a sharp decrease in absorption with a coadministered meal that is independent of fat content. Meals tend to decrease the absorption of some drugs in this category as a result of simple physical barrier that compromises the availability of drug molecules to the upper intestinal membrane.

Class IV Drugs (Low Solubility and Low Permeability)

Poor aqueous solubility may not necessarily impart high lipophilicity and, therefore, high membrane permeation for a drug. Class IV drugs possess both low solubility and low permeability, both of which are undesirable for good drug absorption. Examples include furosemide and paclitaxel. Drugs in this class, however, still may be administered orally if the plasma concentrations obtained are sufficient to produce the desired therapeutic effect and the drugs do not possess a narrow therapeutic index.

Role of Transporters in Drug Absorption

The oral route of drug administration remains the most popular and convenient route of administration, despite its many shortcomings and challenges. Although the advantages associated with oral administration far outweigh the limitations, a major limitation for oral absorption relates to the interactions of drugs with intestinal membrane transporters and metabolizing enzymes (33). The rapidly growing awareness of transporters affecting the rate and extent of intestinal drug absorption has attracted attention in drug discovery and development. Intestinal membrane transporters affecting the rate of oral absorption are the influx peptide transporters (PepT1, PHTs, and HPT-1), bile salt transporter, phosphate transporter, nucleoside transporters, organic cation/anion transporters (OATP and OCTP), and fatty acid transporters. Transporters affecting drug efflux into the intestinal lumen include P-glycoprotein (P-gp), MRP2, BCRP, and MRP3. The primary intestinal enzyme affecting the absorption of drugs is CYP3A4, as well as the phase II enzymes, glutathione transferase, glucuronyltransferases, and sulfotransferases. Thus, inhibition of these membrane transporters and/or metabolizing enzymes and modulation of the expression of these membrane transporters and/or metabolizing enzymes are key factors affecting the rate and extent of drug absorption. Drug molecules recognized by OATP-B include bile acids, bilirubin and bilirubin glucuronides, estrogen and androgen sulfate conjugates, digoxin, pravastatin, fexofenadine, thyroid hormones, and other lipophilic organic anions. The PepT1 will transport peptide-like drugs, such as β-lactam antibiotics (penicillins and cephalosporins), angiotensin-converting enzyme inhibitors, rennin inhibitors, thrombin inhibitors, and di-/tripeptide pro-drugs of antivirals (valacyclovir).

Efflux Transporters

More recently (33,34,37), the role of efflux transporters in influencing the permeability as well as the overall bioavailability of drugs has emerged and gained considerable attention. Among these transporters is P-gp, which is expressed on the luminal surface of normal intestinal mucosa. Unlike absorptive transporters that increase the uptake of a substrate from intestinal lumen, P-gp impedes uptake by returning the portion of drug entering the mucosa back to the lumen in a concentration-dependent manner. Two types of P-gp have been observed in mammals: drug-transporting P-gp, and phospholipid-transporting P-gp.

The localization suggests that P-gp functionally can protect the body against toxic xenobiotics by excreting these compounds into bile, urine, and the intestinal lumen and by preventing their accumulation in brain and testes. Thus, P-gp may play a significant role in drug absorption and disposition in human and animals. An increasing number of drugs have been shown to be substrate for P-gp, including HIV protease inhibitors and verapamil, which also is an inhibitor of P-gp and, thus, can increase the intestinal permeability of other drugs

P-glycoprotein is a cell membrane–associated protein that transports a variety of substances. It has been studied extensively as a mediator of multidrug resistance in cancer, but only recently has the role of P-gp expressed in normal tissue as a determinant of drug pharmacokinetics and pharmacodynamics been investigated.

P-glycoprotein is 170-kDa protein product of the *MDRI* gene. It is a dimer consisting of 1280 amino acids, with 12 transmembrane segments and two adenosine 5′-triphosphate (ATP)–binding domains. P-glycoprotein requires binding of ATP to both ATP-binding domains for the transport function. A proposed mechanism by which P-gp secretes substrates is illustrated in Figure 9.15.

Unlike most other transport proteins that recognize a few structurally similar substrates, P-gp recognizes a broad range of pharmacologically and structurally diverse compounds. In general, P-gp substrates are large, lipophilic compounds that tend to be cationic at physiological pH. An evaluation of 100 structurally diverse compounds revealed that P-gp substrates have a relatively high number of electron-donating groups (i.e., O, N, S, F, Cl, or groups with a π-electron orbital of an unsaturated system).

In recent years, the role of drug transporters in the intestinal epithelium as major determinants of drug

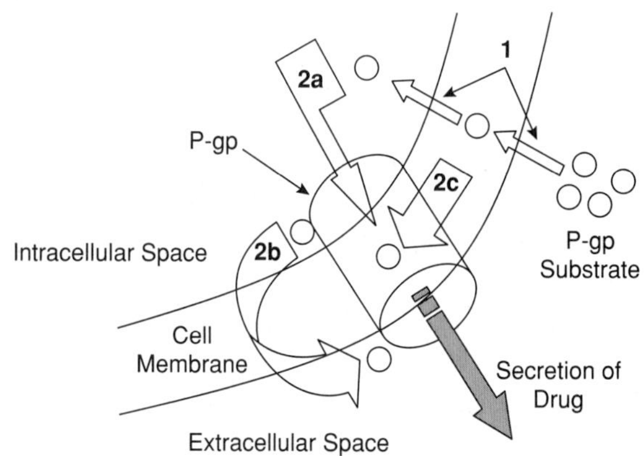

Fig. 9.15. Proposed mechanism by which P-glycoprotein (P-gp) secretes substrates. (1) Passive drug uptake across cell membrane. (2a) Formation of hydrophobic channel (pore) between the intracellular and extracellular space. (2b) Flippase activity, whereby the drug is flipped from the inner leaflet to the outer leaflet of the cell membrane. (2c) "Vacuum cleaner model," in which drug interacts with P-gp in the lipid bilayer and is subsequently secreted back into the extracellular space. (From Matheney C, Lamb M, Brouwer K, et al. Pharmacokinetics and pharmacodynamic implications of P-glycoprotein modulation. Reviews of Therapeutics 2001;21:778–796; with permission.)

absorption has been recognized, and P-gp and other transporters have been implicated in modulating the absorption and/or intestinal elimination of drugs. Reduction in the small intestinal transit time (SITT) of a drug can decrease the peak plasma concentration and area under the plasma concentration–time curve, the rate and extent of absorption, and therefore, the bioavailability of a drug. Another potential consequence of increased transit has been proposed for digoxin and, possibly, other drugs that are substrate for P-gp in the small intestine. Because intestinal permeability of such compounds may depend on the relative activity of P-gp in the intestine, factors affecting this activity also may affect absorption. One determinant is drug concentration, which will influence the degree of saturation of the transporters. Another consideration is the specific activity of the transporters with the intestine itself. Evidence suggests that P-gp is not homogenously distributed throughout the intestinal tract but, rather, increases in abundance from the proximal to the distal small intestine. Therefore, drugs that may be substrate for P-gp but that are partly permeable may be well absorbed in the duodenum and proximal jejunum, which have little P-gp. Drugs that inhibit P-gp can alter the absorption, disposition, and elimination of coadministered drugs and can enhance bioavailability or cause unwanted drug–drug interactions.

Pro-drugs

Pro-drugs are designed to improve the permeability and oral absorption of the parent drug. They are more lipid soluble than the parent drug and should be rapidly converted to the parent compound during absorption from the gut wall, liver, or site of action. Examples of pro-drugs include pivampicillin, the pivalate ester pro-drug of ampicillin that is more lipid soluble, and therefore, more efficiently absorbed than the parent compound (35); valacyclovir, a L-valyl ester pro-drug of acyclovir; lisdexamfetamine, a L-lysinylamide pro-drug of amphetamine that is slowly hydrolyzed to amphetamine, and methyldopa, a pro-drug of methyldopamine that is decarboxylated in the brain to methyldopamine. The recognition that di- and tripeptides are transported from the intestine by their PepT1 transporter has led to the development of pro-drugs designed as di- or tripeptide analogues (36). For example, the dipeptidyl analogue of methyldopa increased the intestinal absorption of methyldopa by more than 20-fold.

FACTORS AFFECTING THE ABSORPTION OF DRUGS FROM SOLID DOSAGE FORMS AND SUSPENSIONS

When a drug is administered orally via tablet, capsule, or suspension, the rate of absorption often is controlled by how fast the drug particles dissolve in the fluid at the site of administration. Hence, the dissolution

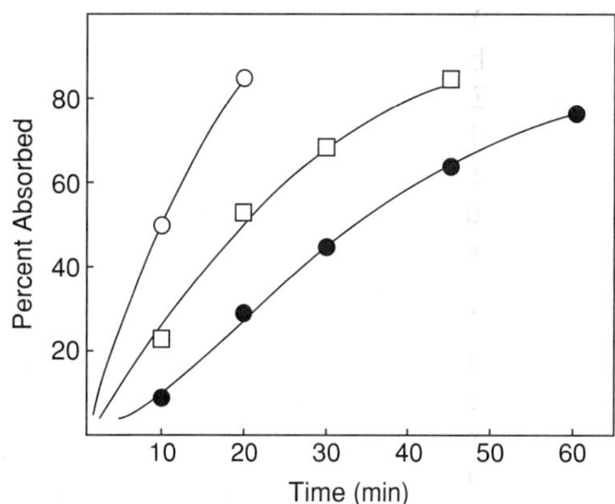

Fig. 9.16. Absorption of aspirin after oral administration of a 650-mg dose in solution (○), in buffered tablets (□), or in regular tablets (●). (From Kwan KC. Oral bioavailability and first-pass effects. Drug Metab Drug Dispos 1997;25:1329–1336, with permission.)

rate often is the rate-limiting (slowest) step in the following sequence:

$$\text{Solid drug} \xrightarrow[\text{Step I}]{\text{Dissolution}} \text{Drug in solution} \xrightarrow[\text{Step II}]{\text{Absorption}} \text{Drug in systemic circulation}$$

If the dissolution of the drug is slow or controlling the rate of absorption (Step I), then dissolution is the rate-determining step. Factors controlling dissolution, such as solubility, ionization, or surface area, will then control the overall dissolution process. Figure 9.16 describes the absorption of aspirin from solution and from two different types of tablets.

It is clear from Figure 9.16 that aspirin absorption is more rapid from solution than from tablet formulations. This rapid absorption of aspirin is an indication that the rate of absorption is dissolution rate limited. A general relationship describing the dissolution of a drug was first reported by Noyes and Whitney (38). The equation derived by those authors is as follows:

Eq. 9.29
$$\frac{dc}{dt} = KS(C_s - C_t)$$

where dc/dt is the dissolution rate, K is a constant, S is the surface area of the dissolution solid, C_s is the equilibrium solubility of drug in the solvent, and C is the concentration of drug in the solvent at time t.

The constant K in Equation 9.29 has been shown to be equal to D/h, where D is the coefficient of the dissolving material of the drug and h is the thickness of the diffusion layer surrounding the dissolving solid particles. This diffusion layer is a thin, stationary film of a solution adjacent to the surface of a solid particle (Fig. 9.17) and is saturated with drug (4); in other words, the drug concentration in the diffusion layer is equal to C_s, the equilibrium solubility. The term $(C_s - C_t)$ in Equation 9.29 represents the concentration gradient for the drug

Table 9.4. The Effect of Changing Parameters from the Dissolution Equation on the Rate of Solution

Equation Parameter	Comments	Effect on Rate of Solution
D (diffusion coefficient of drug)	May be decreased in presence of substances that increase viscosity of the medium	(−)
A (area exposed to solvent)	Increased by micronization and in "amorphous" drugs	(+)
δ (thickness of diffusion layer)	Decreased by increased agitation in gut or flask	(+)
C_s (solubility in diffusion layer)	That of weak electrolytes altered by change in pH by use of appropriate drug salt or buffer ingredient	(−) (+)
C (concentration in bulk)	Decreased by intake of fluid in stomach, by removal of drug by partition or absorption	(+)

between the diffusion layer and the bulk solution. If dissolution is the rate-limiting step in the absorption process, the term C_t in Equation 9.29 is negligible compared to C_s. Under this condition. Equation 9.29 is reduced to

Eq. 9.30
$$\frac{dc}{dt} = \frac{DSC_s}{h}$$

Equation 9.30 describes a diffusion-controlled dissolution process (4). It is visualized that when solid drug particles are introduced to the fluids at the absorption sites, the drug promptly saturates the diffusion layer (Fig. 9.17). This is followed by the diffusion of drug molecules from the diffusion layer into the bulk solution, which is instantly replaced in the diffusion layer by molecules from the solid crystal or particle. This is a continuous process. Although it oversimplifies the dynamics of the dissolution process, Equation 9.30 is a qualitatively useful equation and clearly indicates the effects of some important factors on the dissolution and, therefore, the absorption rate of drugs. When dissolution is the rate-limiting factor in the absorption, then bioavailability is affected. These factors are listed in Table 9.4.

The Noyes-Whitney equations (Eqs. 9.29 and 9.30) demonstrate that the equilibrium solubility (C_s) is one of the major factors determining the rate of dissolution. Changes in the characteristics of solvents, such as pH, affecting the solubility of the drug, affect its dissolution rate. Similarly, the use of a different salt or other physicochemical form of a drug, which exhibits a solubility different from the parent drug, usually affects the dissolution rate. Increasing the surface area of a drug exposed to the dissolution medium, by reducing the particle size, usually increases the dissolution rate. In the discussion to follow, some of the more important factors affecting dissolution and, therefore, absorption are presented in greater detail.

Dissolution

pH and Solubility of Weak Acids and Bases

Solubility is another factor determining the rate of dissolution. As solubility increases, so does the dissolution rate. One way of increasing solubility is to use salts. Salts of weak acids and weak bases generally have much higher aqueous solubility than the free acid or base; therefore, if the drug can be given as a salt, the solubility can be increased, and we should have improved dissolution (Fig. 9.18). This factor can lead to quite different peak plasma concentrations after oral administration.

The solubility of weak acids and bases is a function of the pH of the medium. Therefore, differences in the dissolution

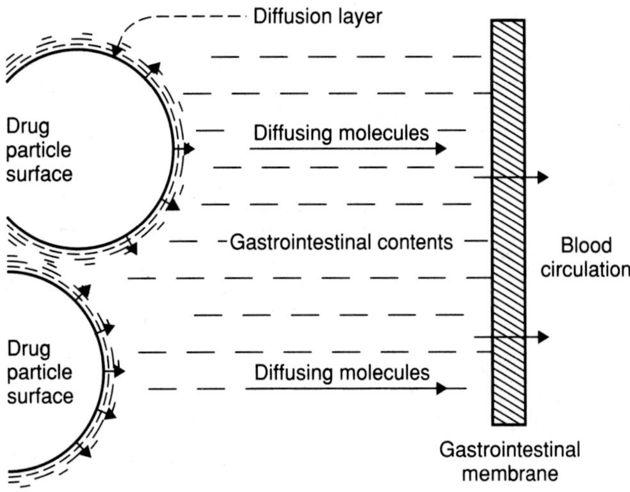

Fig. 9.17. Dissolution from a solid surface.

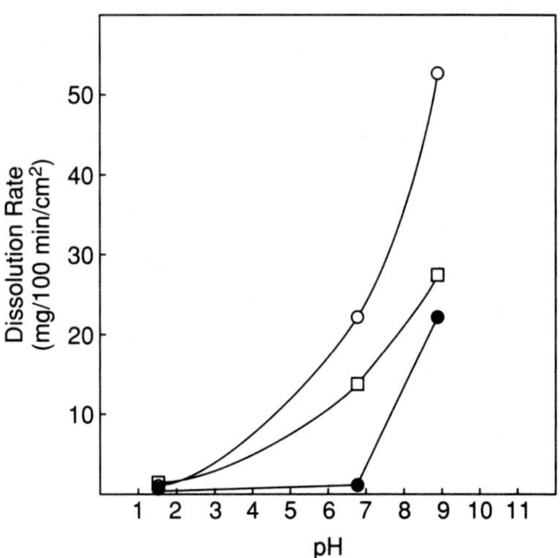

Fig. 9.18. The pH-dependent dissolution of salicylic acid (○), benzoic acid (□), and phenobarbital (●). (From Gibaldi M. Biopharmaceutics and Clinical Pharmacokinetics, 4th Ed. Philadelphia: Lea and Febiger, 1991, with permission.)

rate are expected to occur in different regions of the gastrointestinal tract. The solubility of weak acid is obtained by

Eq. 9.31 $$C_s = [HA] + [A^-]$$

where [HA] is the intrinsic solubility of the un-ionized acid (i.e., C_o) and $[A^-]$ is the concentration of its anion, which can be expressed in terms of its dissociation constant, K_a, and C_o; that is,

Eq. 9.32 $$C_s = C_o + \frac{K_a C_o}{[H^+]}$$

Analogously, the solubility of a weak base is obtained by

Eq. 9.33 $$C_s = C_o + \frac{C_o[H^+]}{K_a}$$

By substituting Equations 9.31 and 9.32 into Equation 9.30 for the term C_s, the following dissolution rate equations are obtained:

For weak acids:

Eq. 9.34 $$\frac{dc}{dt} = \frac{K'(C_o + K_a C_o)}{[H^+]}$$

or

Eq. 9.35 $$\frac{dc}{dt} = \frac{K' C_o(1 + K_a)}{[H^+]}$$

and for a weak base:

Eq. 9.36 $$\frac{dc}{dt} = \frac{K' C_o(1 + [H^+])}{K_a}$$

Equations 9.34 through 9.36 show that K' is equal to *DS/h*. Equations 9.35 and 9.36 clearly suggest that the dissolution rate of weak bases decreases with increasing pH. Hence, the dissolution rate of weak bases is optimum in gastric fluid, but for weak acids, it is at a minimum. Furthermore, the dissolution rate of weak acids increases as the solid drug particles move to the more alkaline regions of the gastrointestinal tract. Figure 9.18 illustrates the dissolution rates of weak acids as a function of pH (39). The absorption of a salt of weak acid or base can be explained by using the following figure:

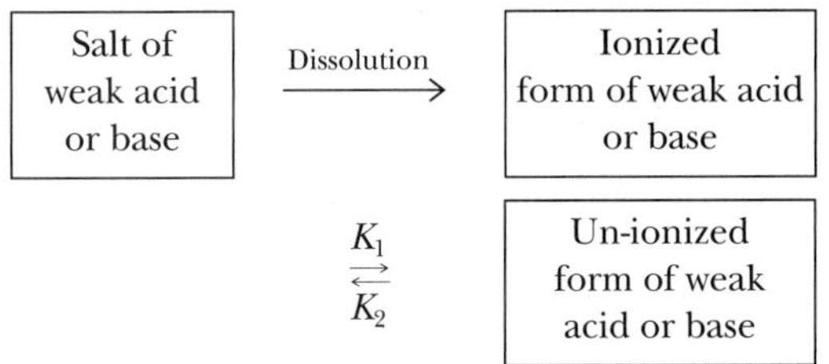

where K_1 and K_2 represent the rate constants associated with the formation of un-ionized and ionized species of a compound, respectively. The ratio of these two rate constants represents the dissociation constant of a compound. The absorption of the un-ionized species of a molecule disturbs the equilibrium of the process. To regain the equilibrium, some of the ionized species, therefore, is converted into un-ionized species, which are then absorbed through the membrane. This process, being a continuous one, permits the absorption of the un-ionized species to take place. Therefore, a drug molecule will eventually be absorbed.

The relatively poor dissolution of weak acids at the pH of gastric fluid further diminishes the importance of the stomach as a drug absorption site. Although gastric absorption of weak acids may occur from solution, it is unlikely that much of the drug dissolves and is absorbed during the short residence time as a solid dosage form in the stomach. A study by Ogata et al. (40) proposed that the critical value of solubility that separates acidic drugs from the absorption sites (stomach or intestine) is approximately 30 mg/mL in 0.1 N HCl when 1 g of drug is administered orally. Those authors found that if the solubility of a drug is less than 3 mg/mL, practically no absorption occurs in the stomach. Changes in the gastric pH also alter the solubility of certain drugs and may affect the dissolution and absorption rates. A patient with achlorhydria has a higher gastric pH and absorbs aspirin more rapidly than a normal subject. On the other hand, similar differences were not observed with respect to the absorption rates of acetaminophen, a much weaker acid, the solubility of which would be unaffected by changes in pH (41).

The relationships between dissolution rate and hydrogen ion concentration, described in Equations 9.35 and 9.36, are approximations and tend to overpredict the dissolution rate of both weak acids in the small intestine and weak bases in the stomach. In reality, the hydrogen ion concentration of the bulk is not equal to the hydrogen ion concentration of the diffusion layer.

Salts

The dissolution rate of a particular salt usually is different from that of a parent compound. Sodium or potassium salts of weak acids dissolve more rapidly than the free acid. The same is true with HCl or other salts of weak bases. Table 9.5

Table 9.5. Dissolution Rate of Weak Acids and Their Sodium Salts

		Dissolution Rate (mg/100 min/cm^2)		
Compound	pK_a	0.1 N HCl pH 1.5	0.1 M Phosphate pH 6.8	0.1 M Borate pH 9.0
Benzoic acid	4.2	2.1	14	28
Sodium salt		980	1770	1,600
Phenobarbital	7.4	0.24	1.2	22
Sodium salt		~200	820	1,430
Salicylic acid	3.0	1.7	27	53
Sodium salt		1,870	2,500	2,420
Sulfathiazole	7.3	<0.1	~0.5	8.5
Sodium salt		550	810	1,300

illustrates the dissolution rate differences between some weak acids and their sodium salts (39). The differences in the dissolution rates of salt and parent compound can be explained by taking into consideration the pH of the diffusion layer. At a given pH, regardless of salt or free acids/bases, a drug will have a fixed solubility. The classical dissolution equation predicts a slower dissolution of a salt of a drug, and the concept of a diffusion layer becomes useful.

For sodium or potassium salts of weak acids, the pH of the solution in a diffusion layer is greater than the pH of the diffusion layer for the corresponding weak acid. On the other hand, the pH of the solution in the diffusion layer for hydrochloride salts of weak bases is always smaller than the diffusion layer of the corresponding free base. Therefore, effective solubility and dissolution rate of soluble salts on drug absorption are available in the literature. The potassium salt of penicillin V yields a higher peak plasma concentration of antibiotic than the corresponding free acid (42). Sodium salts of barbiturates are reported by Anderson (43) to provide a rapid onset of sedation. Some salts have a lower solubility and dissolution rate than their parent compounds. Examples include aluminum salts of weak acids and pamoate salts of weak bases. In these particular examples, insoluble films of either weak acids or pamoic acid appear to form in the dissolving solids and further retard the dissolution rate.

Surface Area and Particle Size

The surface area per gram (or per dose) of a solid drug can be changed by altering the particle size. For example, a cube that is 1 cm on each side has a surface area of 6 cm^2. If this cube is broken into cubes with sides of 0.1 cm, the total surface area is 60 cm^2. If the particles are broken up by grinding, then irregular shapes with even larger surface areas are created. Generally, as the surface area increases, the drug will dissolve more rapidly. Therefore, many poorly soluble and slowly dissolving drugs currently are marketed in a micronized or microcrystalline form. The problems of low water solubility and particle size were not fully appreciated, but they have resulted in reducing the therapeutic dose of some drugs without sacrificing therapeutic efficacy. For example, since the original marketing of spironolactone, its dose has been reduced from 500 to 25 mg as a result of a reformulation that includes micronization. The bioavailability of digoxin increased from 40 to 80–97% by reducing the particle size from 100 to approximately 10 nm. A similar result has been obtained for griseofulvin.

Polymorphism

Many pharmaceutical solids can exist in two or more crystalline forms called polymorphs (44,45). Polymorphism is the ability of the same drug molecule to crystallize into more than one different crystal structure that has a different arrangement and/or conformation of molecules in the crystal lattice. However, once they are in the solution phase, polymorphs share a common form. The different arrangements of atoms within the crystal unit cell can have a profound effect on physical and chemical properties of the final crystallized compound and on the final drug product. Amorphous solids consist of disordered arrangements of molecules that do not possess a distinguishable crystal lattice. Solvates are crystalline solid adducts containing either stoichiometric or nonstoichiometric amounts of a solvent incorporated within the crystal structure (44,45). If the incorporated solvent is water, the solvates are commonly known as hydrates. Polymorphs and/or solvates of a pharmaceutical solid or pharmaceutical excipients (e.g., lactose) can have different physical and chemical properties, such as melting point, chemical reactivity, apparent solubility and dissolution rate. These properties of a drug substance can affect the intended shelf-life (stability), rate of dissolution, the bioavailability/bioequivalence of the drug product. A metastable (amorphous) pharmaceutical solid form can change crystalline structure or solvate/desolvate in response to changes in environmental conditions or shelf-life storage. When such differences in physical properties are sufficiently large, bioavailability is altered, and it often is difficult to formulate a bioequivalent drug product using a different polymorph. The Biopharmaceutics Classification criteria of high solubility and rapid dissolution should be considered in product development decisions when polymorphism exists. Drug substances with different physical form include warfarin sodium, famotidine, and ranitidine, and those with solvation or hydration state include terazosin hydrochloride, ampicillin, and cefadroxil.

Some drugs that exist as polymorphs may have different solubility properties and, thus, different dissolution characteristics. Chloramphenicol palmitate and ritonavir provide good examples of how polymorphism can influence drug dissolution and, thus, drug bioavailability. Chloramphenicol palmitate is a broad-spectrum antibiotic known to crystallize in at least three polymorphic forms and one amorphous (metastable) form, B. The most stable form, known as form A, is the polymorph that is marketed, whereas the metastable form B is approximately eight times more soluble than form A, thus providing an eightfold difference in bioavailability. This large difference in bioavailability creates the danger of fatal dosages when the unwanted polymorph is unwittingly administered because of alterations in process and/or storage conditions. The HIV protease inhibitor ritonavir (Norvir) was withdrawn from the market because an undesirable polymorph of ritonavir had been produced during its shelf-life. Ritonavir was found to exist in only one monoclinic form during development and early manufacturing. This form, called "form I", was not sufficiently bioavailable in the solid state by the oral route, requiring the initial product (Norvir) to be formulated as a capsule filled with a hydroalcoholic solution containing the dissolved drug. Two years after the product launch, several lots of Norvir capsules started failing dissolution specifications. Evaluation of the failed lots revealed that a second crystal form of ritonavir, "form II", had precipitated from the formulation during its shelf life. "Form II" was 50% less soluble compared to "form I", resulting in failure of batches in dissolution test affecting its bioavailability and eventual withdrawal of the product from the market. Substantial time and effort went in identifying and correcting the problem. To ensure a continuous supply of this life-saving drug, a liquid formulation had to be introduced in the market until the issue of the polymorphic form was resolved. Hence, an inadvertent production of the "wrong" polymorph at the crystallization stage, or any transformations of one form to another during dosage form during processing (e.g., drying, milling, granulation, compression, spray drying, or freeze-drying), storage, and scale-up, can result in pharmaceutical dosage forms that are either ineffective or toxic. This highlights that identification of different solid forms of a drug substance as well as determination of their physical and chemical properties, thermodynamic stabilities; and conditions kinetics of interconversion are essential for ensuring reproducible behavior of drug products.

Estimate of Dose Absorbed

Johnson and Swindell (46) proposed a simple predictive model that relates the aqueous solubility and absorption rate constant (K_a) to determine the maximum absorbable dose (MAD):

Eq. 9.37 $$\text{MAD} = K_a C_s V t$$

where K_a is the first-order absorption rate constant; $C_s V$ is a constant, and t is the time.

Hilgers et al. (27) argued that Equation 9.37, proposed by Johnson and Swindell (46), assumes that the drug absorption occurs under highly quixotic conditions, such as the intestine is exposed to a saturation solution of a compound of interest for a time equal to the normal SITT. For interrelating permeability and solubility of a drug to estimate the absorption potential (30) as MAD by employing the predictive model, Hilger et al. (27) proposed a modified equation:

Eq. 9.38 $$\text{MAD} = S \cdot K_a \cdot \text{SIV} \cdot \text{SITT}$$

where S is solubility and SIV is the small intestinal volume.

Briefly, the MAD calculates the total mass of drug that could theoretically be absorbed if a saturated solution of a compound with solubility S in the SIV were absorbed with a first-order absorption rate constant (K_a) for a time equivalent to SITT.

The absorption rate constant (K_a) was determined from Caco-2 permeability value with the assumption that the value of K_a and rat ileum permeability values are approximately equal and, consequently, that the estimated rat permeability (P_e) was converted to an absorption rate constant (K_a) from the following relationship:

Eq. 9.39 $$K_a = P_e(A/V)$$

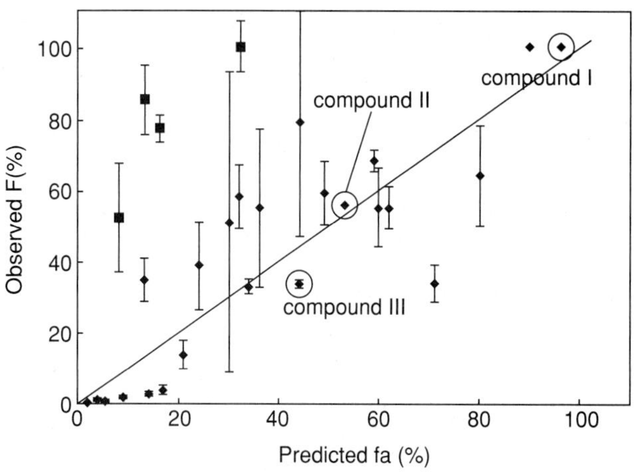

Fig. 9.19. A better correlation between observed bioavailability and predicted bioavailability when both aqueous solubility and permeability parameters of drugs are used to predict the fraction absorbed for three compounds. (From Burton P, Goodwin J, Vidamas T, et al. Predicting drug absorption: how nature made it a difficult problem. J Pharm Exp Ther 2002;303:889–895 and adapted from Hilgers AR, Smith DP, Biermacher JJ, et al. Predicting oral absorption of drugs: a case study with novel class of antimicrobial agents. Pharm Res 2003;20:1149–1155; with permission.)

where V is the volume of the intestinal lumen and A is the surface area. For the rats used in this study (27), A/V was equal to 10 cm^{-1}.

Employing Equations 9.37 and 9.38 for estimating the oral absorption of oxazolidinone antibiotics data obtained in rat and comparing the predicted MAD to the actually administered dose, Burton et al. (20) and Hilger et al. (27) reported the relationship illustrated in Figure 9.19.

It is clear from Figure 9.19 that better prediction of MAD is achieved when solubility, permeability, and dose are taken into consideration. In spite of this, drug permeability is an important determinant of drug absorption; therefore, it is informative to explore mechanisms contributing to permeability in the light of structure-based models for absorption prediction.

The relationship between the estimate of MAD and the fraction absorbed is hyperbolic (28); analogous to the relationship between drug permeability and fraction absorbed. Incorporating the solubility term in Equation 9.37 yields a more realistic value of estimate of MAD for poorly to moderately soluble compounds. The concept of MDA therefore serves to combine two major determinants of oral drug absorption (i.e., intestinal permeability and solubility). In turn, the value of MDA can provide a practical guideline in the early drug discovery program.

If the dose of a potential drug candidate is projected to be greater than the calculated estimated dose absorbed, this serves a cautionary notice that the following should be examined: the potential for solubilization in the gastrointestinal tract, and the formulation variables that could ultimately result in an increased solubility or drug dissolution during the gastrointestinal transit to increase the fraction absorbed.

To reach the systemic circulation, a drug must move from the intestinal lumen through an unstirred water layer and mucous coat adjacent to the epithelial cell structure. Movement across the epithelial layers takes place by two independent routes, transcellular flux (i.e., movement across the cells) and paracellular flux or movement between adjacent epithelial cells. The solute molecules then encounter a basement membrane, interstitial space, and mesenteric capillary wall to access the mesenteric circulation. Any and all of these microenvironments can be considered a resistance to solute molecule movement, each with an associated permeability coefficient. Therefore, the overall process consists of a number of resistances (i.e., reciprocal of permeability) in series. Furthermore, the influence of drug structure with permeability in these different domains may be different. For example, permeability in an unstirred water layer is inversely related to solute size, whereas paracellular permeability is a function of both size and charge. Furthermore, cations exhibit greater permeability than neutral species, which in turn manifest greater permeability than anions.

With respect to transcellular permeability, the relationship of solute structure with permeability depends on the mechanism. Historically, a passive diffusion pathway is assumed for most solutes. Nevertheless, a great number of solutes are identified as being associated with active absorption and secretary processes in intestinal epithelial cells. Additionally, although active transport involves specific interactions between a solute and transporter, passive diffusion is dependent on solute partitioning into the cellular plasma membrane and the diffusion coefficient within the membrane. Both processes, however, are influenced by the physicochemical and structural characteristics of the drug. Factors influencing plasma membrane partitioning are solute size, lipophilicity, hydrogen-bonding potential, and charge characteristics, whereas the diffusion coefficient is dependent on size or total molecular surface area. In general, a non-PSA favors partitioning.

For solutes that exhibit marginal (or a lack of) membrane affinity, permeability is low, resulting primarily from paracellular diffusion of the solute. As the propensity of the solute to partition into cell membrane increases, so does the permeability, as a result of the significant increase in surface area of the transcellular pathway relative to the paracellular route. This increase in permeability will approach a plateau, the so-called "aqueous boundary layer–limited situation," in which diffusion across the cell is very rapid relative to diffusion of the solute through the unstirred water/mucous layer.

In the case of ionizable solutes, permeability also is pH dependent. A neutral, uncharged species is capable of transcellular diffusion, whereas a charged species is restricted to the paracellular pathway. Thus, the observed permeability of such molecules is dependent on the relative concentrations of charged and neutral species.

Dressman et al. (47) developed an equation to determine the absorption potential (AP) of a drug by taking into consideration several of its physicochemical properties, including intrinsic solubility (S_o) of the un-ionized species of a drug, fraction of unionized form (F_{uni}) of a drug at a specific pH, volume of the luminal content (V_l), permeability of a drug in the gut wall (P_w), and the aqueous permeability (P_{aq}) of a drug. The equation is

Eq. 9.40 $$F_{abs} = \left(\frac{P_w}{P_{aq}}\right)(F_{uni})\left(\frac{S_o V_l}{X_o}\right)$$

where F_{abs} is the fraction absorbed and X_o is the administered dose. With the assumption that, in many cases, the permeability ratio (i.e., P_w/P_{aq}) of a drug is proportional to its membrane-water coefficient (P), which can be correlated to the 1-octanol–water partition coefficient (P), Equation 9.40 was simplified to

Eq. 9.41 $$AP = \log\left(P \cdot F_{uni} \cdot \frac{S_o V_l}{X_o}\right)$$

where AP is a dimensionless parameter

Employing Equation 9.41 and selecting drugs that represent a wide range of absorption characteristics, from poorly absorbed compounds to those that are virtually completely absorbed, the utility of the AP parameter as a predictor of the fraction absorbed was assessed (47). The physicochemical properties, such as the partition coefficient, solubility, fraction available in un-ionized form, dissociation constant, fraction of dose absorbed, and calculated dimensionless parameter AP for drugs selected in this study (47), are reported in Table 9.6. The observed

Table 9.6. Physicochemical Properties and Calculated Absorption Potential (AP) for Representative Drugs

Drug	P	S (mg/mL)	Dose (mg)	pK_a	F_{non} (pH 6.5)	AP	%ABS (range)
Acyclovir	0.018	1.3	200	9.5	1	−1.5	17 (12–23)
Chlorothiazide	0.54	0.4	250	6.7	0.6	−0.89	25 (10–40)
Griseofulvin	151	0.015	250	—	1	0.36	43 (35–51)
Hydrochlorothiazide	0.85	0.6	25	8.8	0.95	0.7	67 (50–90)
Phenytoin	295	0.014	100	9.2	0.99	1.0	90 (80–100)
Prednisolone	26	0.235	20	—	1	1.9	99
Digoxin	56	0.024	0.25	—	1	3.13	>90

P, partition coefficient; S, solubility; F_{non}, nonabsorbed fraction; %ABS, percentage of drug absorbed following an oral dose in human subjects.

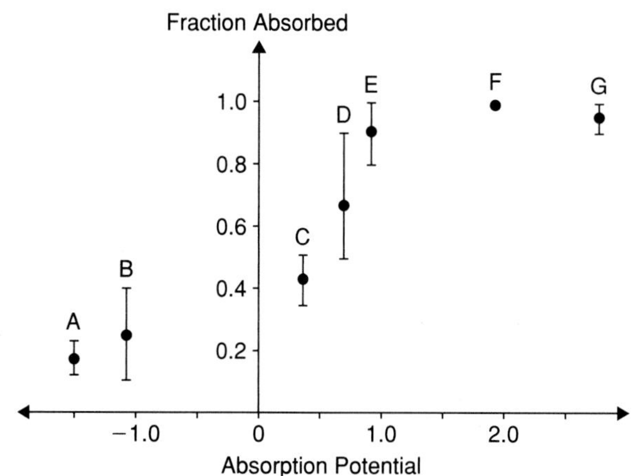

Fig. 9.20. The relationship between absorption potential (AP) and fraction absorbed for seven representative drugs (Table 9.6). A, acyclovir; B, chlorothiazide; C, micronized griseofulvin; D, hydrochlorothiazide; E, phenytoin; F, prednisolone; G, digoxin (Lanoxicap). (From Dressman JB, Amidon GL, Fleisher D. Absorption potential: estimating the fraction absorbed for orally administered compounds. J Pharm Sci 1985;74:588–589; with permission.)

correlation between the fractions absorbed and the AP is illustrated graphically in Figure 9.20.

From Table 9.6 and Figure 9.20, it is quite apparent that for the compounds selected in this study (47), the dimensionless parameter AP manifests a strong correlation to the fraction absorbed. Negative AP values correspond to poor drug absorption. For the range of AP values between zero and one, an increase in AP value correlates with an increase in fraction absorbed, whereas AP values greater than one indicate complete drug absorption.

Summary

At one time, it was common to assume that the biological response to a drug was simply a function of the intrinsic pharmacological activity of the drug molecule. Today, when assessing the potency of most drugs, consideration is given to plasma drug concentration–response rather than dose–response relationships. The concentration of a drug in the plasma is dependent on the rate and extent of absorption, which in turn is influenced by the physicochemical properties of drug substances. Drug absorption may markedly affect the onset and intensity of a biological response to a drug. Clinically significant differences in the absorption of closely related drugs, such as lincomycin and clindamycin, penicillin and pivampicillin, or secobarbital and sodium secobarbital, are invariably the result of significant differences in their physicochemical properties.

Dissolution is simply a process by which a solid substance goes into solution. The determination of dissolution rates of pharmaceutical substances from dosage forms does not predict their bioavailability or their in vivo performance; rather, it indicates the potential availability of drug substance for absorption. Therefore, it is essential for pharmacists and pharmaceutical scientists to know and understand the importance of dissolution and its potential influence on the rate and extent of absorption and availability for drugs.

Factors affecting the dissolution rate of a drug from a dosage form can be related to the physicochemical properties of a drug, formulation of a dosage form, and dissolution apparatus and test parameters. Additionally, a brief introduction of the role of intestinal transporters and metabolizing enzymes (CYP3A4) in drug absorption was provided. The role of intestinal permeability in drug absorption process, techniques of measuring intestinal permeability, and methods that permit the estimation of fraction of dose absorbed by taking into consideration the physicochemical properties of a drug also were discussed. Additionally, the biopharmaceutical drug classification based on the two physicochemical properties, solubility and permeability, of drugs and the implications of these properties on drug absorption were covered.

PHARMACOKINETICS

Introduction

The events following drug administration can be divided into two phases: a pharmacokinetic phase, in which the ability to adjust a dose, alter the dosage form, and alter the frequency and route of administration are related to drug concentration–time relationship in the body; and a pharmacodynamic phase, in which the drug concentration at the sites of action is related to the magnitude of effects produced. Once both of these phases have been defined for a drug, a dosage regimen for a drug can be established to achieve the optimum therapeutic goals in individual patients and to predict what may happen when a dosage regimen is changed.

The sites into which drugs are routinely administered are broadly classified as intravascular and extravascular. Intravascular administration refers to the placement of a drug directly into blood, either intravenously or intra-arterially. Because the drug is placed directly into blood, it is imperative that a drug administered intravascularly be given as a solution. The extravascular routes of administration include oral, intramuscular, sublingual, buccal, subcutaneous, dermal, rectal, and nasal routes. To enter the blood, a drug administered extravascularly must be absorbed from the site of administration. Additionally, if a drug is administered through solid dosage forms, such as tablets or capsules, then the drug must first dissolve at the site of administration. Therefore, the dissolution of a drug is essential before its absorption. On the other hand, no such absorption step is required when a drug is administered intravenously.

Pharmacokinetics is the scientific discipline that deals with the mathematical description of biological processes affecting drugs and affected by drugs. In addition to signifying the relationship of ADME (absorption, distribution, metabolism, and excretion) processes to the intensity and time course of pharmacological effects of drugs, pharmacokinetics describes the time course of a drug's ADME processes, which take place following the administration of a drug. It therefore is necessary to describe and analyze these processes and their effects in relation to their rates, rate constants, or time course. A qualitative description of these processes is quite insufficient and seldom leads to adequate and accurate characterizations of the effects of drugs on the body and effects of the body on the drugs. Pharmacokinetics is a quantitative study whose purposes are:

1. To develop mathematical expressions that permit one to describe the temporal changes of the drug concentration;
2. To determine constraints that describes ADME processes succinctly;
3. To make predictions and extrapolations based on the mathematical expressions; and
4. To help establish dosage regimen that, in turn, will result in improved drug utilization in patients.

At a fundamental level, pharmacokinetics is a useful tool of pharmacists and physicians for optimizing the dosage regimen of drugs for individuals who may differ in their intrinsic response and their ability to absorb and eliminate drugs. Adjustment of dosage regimen to account for individual differences and disease states is, in essence, an exercise in clinical pharmacokinetics and clinical pharmacy practice.

A basic tenet of pharmacokinetics is that the magnitude of both the desired response and toxicity are functions of drug concentration in the blood. Furthermore, it is not only the efficacy of a drug at the site of action that determines the intensity and duration of its pharmacological or therapeutic effects but also the amount of a drug and the rate at which the drug gets to the site of action. The vital processes of the body may delay the transport of drug molecules across membranes, convert drug molecules into metabolites, and remove them from the body as metabolites and/or the unchanged form. In turn, this may result in therapeutic failure as a result of drug concentrations being too low or unacceptable toxicity, as a consequence of too high a drug concentration. Between these concentration limits lies a region associated with therapeutic success. This region may be regarded as a therapeutic range, or "therapeutic window." Each drug may possess its own therapeutic window, and because the drug concentration rarely can be measured at the site of drug action, the drug concentration is measured at alternative and more accessible sites, such as plasma or serum and urine.

Figure 9.21 illustrates the concentration or therapeutic window for a drug. The terms "minimum toxic concentration" and "minimum effective concentration" describe the limits of the therapeutic range for a drug. If the administered dose of a drug produces the plasma concentration within this range, the drug will likely produce its therapeutic effect. The term "onset of action" is defined as the time at which the drug enters the therapeutic range (i.e., above the minimum effect concentration), and when the plasma concentration of a drug falls below the therapeutic range is defined as the termination of action. The time span between the termination and the onset of action is described as the duration of action.

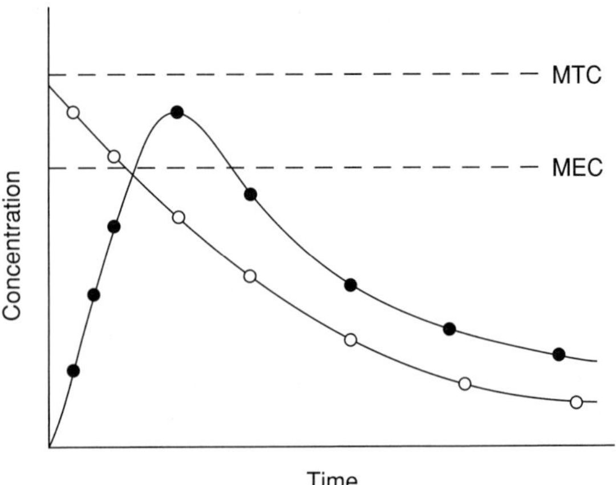

Fig. 9.21. Typical plasma concentration versus time profile following administration of a dose of a drug by intravascular (○) and extravascular routes (●).

It is clear from Figure 9.21 and the definitions above that an optimum dosage regimen might be defined as one that maintains the plasma concentration of a drug within the therapeutic range. Furthermore, it may be obvious from the above discussion that the success of a drug in providing the desired drug concentration depends on factors such as how rapidly the drug reaches the general circulation from the site of administration, particularly following the oral and other extravascular routes; whether the drug is reaching the general circulation in sufficient amounts to provide plasma concentration within the therapeutic range; and the pharmacokinetic properties of a drug.

The purpose of this section is to provide students with a brief overview and the functional understanding of basic pharmacokinetics and its application to how physicochemical properties of drug molecules affect pharmacokinetic properties. Emphasis is placed on how to carry out pharmacokinetic analysis of the data and on how to use the pharmacokinetic parameters for predictive purposes. The mathematical equations presented have been chosen because of their general utility for predicting the plasma concentrations following administration of a drug by intravascular and extravascular routes. Furthermore, this discussion attempts to review and illustrate how the chemical modification of a drug through molecular modifications may alter selected pharmacokinetic parameters of drugs and, therefore, possibly the pharmacological response in the drug discovery and development process.

Table 9.7 describes the dimensions of various pharmacokinetics parameters and provides examples of the corresponding typical dimensions reported in the literature, is provided at the end of the chapter.

Table 9.7. Dimensions of Measurement and Typical Dimensions for Important Pharmacokinetics Parameters

Pharmacokinetics Parameter	Dimension of Measurement	Examples of Typical Dimensions
Mass of drug (e.g., mass of drug in blood, mass of drug at the site of administration, mass of drug in urine, and mass of metabolite in urine)	Amount	mg, μg, etc.
Plasma and/or serum concentration	Amount per unit volume	$mg{\cdot}L^{-1}$, $\mu g{\cdot}mL^{-1}$, mg/L, μg/mL, etc.
Elimination half-life	Time	hr, min, etc.
All first-order rate constants (e.g., elimination, distribution, disposition, absorption, and intercompartmental transfer rate constants)	Reciprocal of time	hr^{-1}, min^{-1}, etc.
All the apparent volumes of drug distribution (e.g., V for one compartment model, and V_c and V_b for two-compartment model)	Volume or volume per unit weight of a subject	L, mL, etc. or $L{\cdot}kg^{-1}$, $mL{\cdot}kg^{-1}$ L/kg, mL/kg, etc.
Zero-order rate constant	Amount, concentration, or percentage per unit time	$mg{\cdot}hr^{-1}$, $\mu g{\cdot}mL{\cdot}hr^{-1}$, $\%{\cdot}hr^{-1}$, mg/hr, μg/hr, %/hr, etc.
All rates (zero as well as first order; e.g., absorption rate, elimination rate, and excretion rate)	Amount per time or concentration per time	$mg{\cdot}hr^{-1}$, $\mu g{\cdot}hr^{-1}$, $\mu g{\cdot}mL^{-1}{\cdot}hr^{-1}$, mg/hr, μg/hr, μg/mL/hr, etc.
All clearances (e.g., systemic, renal, metabolic, and creatinine clearance)	Volume per unit time or volume per unit time per unit weight	$mL{\cdot}hr^{-1}$, $L.hr^{-1}$, $mL{\cdot}hr^{-1}{\cdot}kg^{-1}$, $L{\cdot}hr^{-1}{\cdot}kg^{-1}$, mL/hr, L/hr, mL/hr/kg, etc.
Peak time	Time	hr, min, etc.
Dose administered (e.g., single intravenous or oral dose, loading dose, and maintenance dose)	Amount or amount per unit weight	mg, μg, $mg{\cdot}kg^{-1}$, mg/kg etc.
Peak concentration (e.g., for a single dose or multiple doses) etc.	Mass per unit volume	$mg{\cdot}L^{-1}$, $ng{\cdot}mL^{-1}$, mg/L, ng/mL
Area under the plasma concentration–time curve (AUC)	Mass per volume × time	$mg{\cdot}L^{-1}{\cdot}hr$, $ng{\cdot}mL^{-1}{\cdot}hr$, mg/L/hr ng/mL/hr, etc.
Dosing interval	Time	hr, min., etc.
Absolute or relative bioavailability	Dimensionless	
Blood flow rate	Volume per unit time	$L{\cdot}hr^{-1}$, $mL{\cdot}hr^{-1}$, L/hr, mL/hr, etc.
Extraction ratios	Dimensionless	
Infusion rate	Mass per unit time or mass per unit time per unit weight	$mg{\cdot}kg^{-1}$, $\mu g{\cdot}kg^{-1}$, $\mu g{\cdot}kg^{-1}{\cdot}hr^{-1}$, mg/kg, μg/kg, μg/kg//hr, etc.

Compartmental Concepts

The most commonly employed approach to pharmacokinetic characterization of a drug is to depict the body as a system of compartments, even though these compartments often do not have any apparent physiologic reality. These frequently used compartmental models are illustrated in Figure 9.22.

The one-compartment model considers the body as a single homogenous unit (central compartment). This simplest model is particularly useful for pharmacokinetic analysis of plasma concentration vs. time for drugs that are very rapidly distributed in the body. The two-compartments model consists of a central component, which includes the plasma and other highly perfused organs, connected to a peripheral or tissue compartment. Each compartment can be considered to include a group of tissues, fluids, or parts of organs. A somewhat more complex model, illustrated in Figure 9.23, is the three-compartment model, which consists of a central compartment connected to more than one peripheral compartment that differ in their relative accessibility to a drug. This model may be chosen if the available data warrant such a model.

The selection of a model depends greatly on the site and tissue being sampled, the frequency of sampling collection, and the ultimate goals of the study. The general operating rule in selecting a model for pharmacokinetic analysis of plasma concentration versus time data is to postulate the minimum number of compartments necessary to accurately describe the pharmacokinetics of a given drug. An approach to selecting the number of compartments should be parsimonious, unless experimental evidence dictates that such parsimony may lead to errors in estimating the pharmacokinetic parameters of drugs and, therefore, the use of equations for predicting blood levels of drugs.

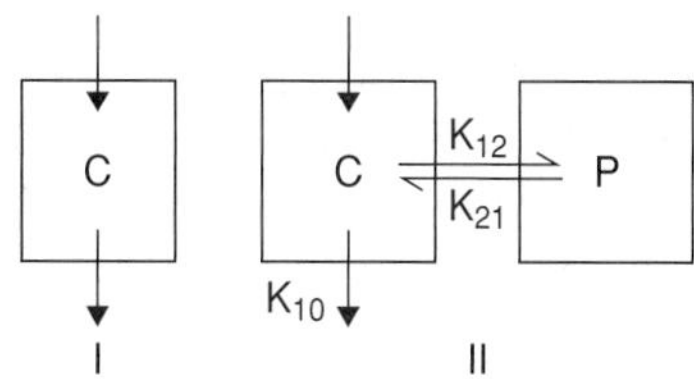

Fig. 9.22. Schematic representation of the one-compartment (I) and the two-compartment (II) models commonly used in pharmacokinetics. Arrows represent transfer of a drug because of the first-order process. C, central compartment (plasma, highly perfused organs); P, peripheral (tissue) compartment.

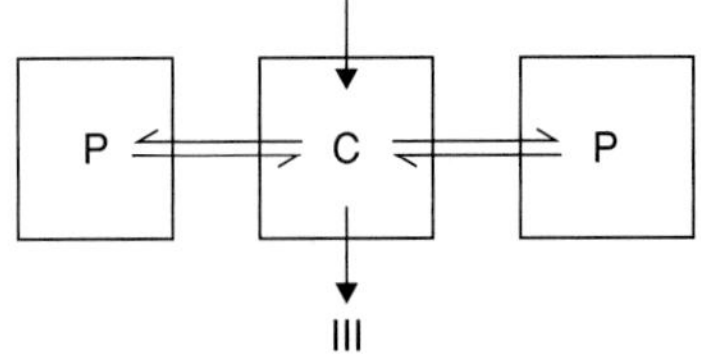

Fig. 9.23. Schematic representation of a three-compartment (III) model commonly used in pharmacokinetics. Arrows represent transfer of a drug because of the first-order process. C, central compartment; P, peripheral compartment.

Linear and Nonlinear Pharmacokinetics

Linear Pharmacokinetics

Many processes in pharmacokinetics can be described accurately by a first-order process. This means that the rate of drug biotransformation, the rate of transfer of a drug between compartments, and the rate of absorption and elimination of drugs from the body are directly proportional to the size of the dose administered. It also is true that passive diffusion is responsible for the transfer of a drug in the body and that a directly proportional relationship exists between the administered dose and the resulting drug concentration in the body. This dose proportionality often is used as an indicator of linear pharmacokinetics. It is important, however, to recognize that the pharmacokinetic parameters, such as the elimination half-life and the elimination rate constant, are independent of the size of the dose administered. Therefore, linear pharmacokinetics is regarded as dose-independent kinetics.

Nonlinear Pharmacokinetics

The rate of elimination of a few drugs (e.g., ethanol, salicylate, and phenytoin) by biotransformation and some other transfer processes involves protein carrier systems. These drugs are not removed from the body by a first-order process, which means that the elimination rate is not proportional to the concentration of drug or to the dose administered. In most of these cases, elimination follows zero-order kinetics—that is, the rate of change of drug concentration is independent of the drug concentration. A constant amount of a drug, rather than the constant percentage of the remaining amount of drug, is eliminated per unit time (i.e., mg/min or μg/ mL/min).

The most frequently reported reason for the use of nonlinear kinetics is that biotransformation and transfer processes require protein-carrier systems. These systems are specific with respect to substrates that have finite capacities. The kinetics of these processes often are described by the Michaelis-Menten equation (Eqs. 9.3–9.5).

This nonlinear, or dose-dependent, elimination kinetics also may be the result of effects other than the limited capacity of biotransformation or elimination processes. If a drug is partly reabsorbed from the renal tubules by a recycling process with limited capacity, then the elimination of large doses proceeds relatively more rapidly than the elimination of smaller doses. Similarly, lesser binding of drugs to plasma constituents or tissues at higher dosing may result in relatively more rapid drug elimination than is observed at lower drug concentrations.

Evidence suggests that some drug metabolites can inhibit their own formation. This process of product inhibition also can cause dose-dependent effects, with large doses being eliminated relatively more slowly than small doses. The rate of decline of a drug concentration in the postdistribution phase, at any given level of a drug in the body, will be independent of the dose in the case of simple Michaelis-Menten kinetics. In cases of product inhibition, this rate tends to decrease with increasing doses.

Intravascular Administration

Intravenous Bolus Administration and One-Compartment Model

Following the administration by intravenous injection, if a drug distributes very rapidly in the body, this confers on the body the characteristics of a one-compartment model, and if the drug elimination from the body can be described by a first-order process, then a plot of the logarithm of plasma drug concentration as a function of time yields a straight line, as shown in Figure 9.24.

The equation responsible for describing plasma drug concentration against time is as follows:

Eq. 9.42 $$C_p = (C_p)_0 e^{-Kt}$$

where C_p is the plasma drug concentration at time t, $(C_p)_0$ is the initial plasma drug concentration (i.e., $t = 0$)

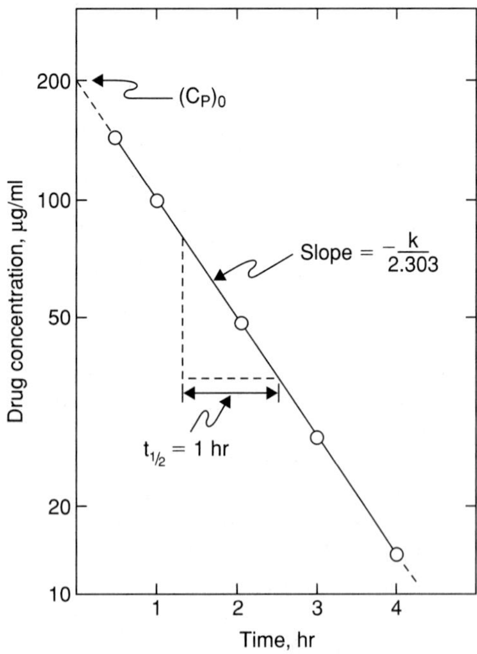

Fig. 9.24. Schematic representation of plasma concentration of drug in the body as a function of time following rapid intravenous injection.

immediately after the injection, K is the first-order elimination rate constant, and t represents time. Equation 9.42 also can be written as follows:

Eq. 9.43 $$\ln C_p = \ln(C_p)_0 - Kt$$

or

Eq. 9.44 $$\log C_p = \log(C_p)_0 - \frac{Kt}{2.303}$$

The initial plasma drug concentration, $(C_p)_0$, may be obtained by extrapolation of the line (Fig. 9.24) to $t = 0$ or the y-intercept of plasma drug concentration versus time plot. Figure 9.24 shows that a plot of the log of plasma drug concentration versus time will be linear under the stated condition.

Three primary factors determine the plasma concentration of the administered drug: 1) the route of administration, 2) the uptake of drug by body tissues, and 3) the elimination of the drug from the body. In the case of intravenous administration, because the drug is introduced directly into the blood, there is no delay as a result of the absence of the drug absorption process. The drug plasma level, however, depends on the size of the dose, and the maximum plasma drug concentration occurs immediately after completion of the dose administration.

The Elimination Rate Constant and Half-life

The half-life of a drug is a major factor in determining the dosing frequency, which is a function of the drug's clearance and apparent volume of distribution (V). The relationship of a drug's half-life to the prediction of human pharmacokinetics and dosing regimen is shown in Figure 9.25 (48–50). Drugs with short half-lives are more likely to require frequent administration, whereas those with long half-lives tend to require dosing once daily. The two pharmacokinetic parameters that determine the half-life of a drug are clearance and volume of distribution. Dosing regimen is also linked to other factors, such as the drug pharmacodynamics, and drug concentrations associated with side effects versus those minimally required for efficacy.

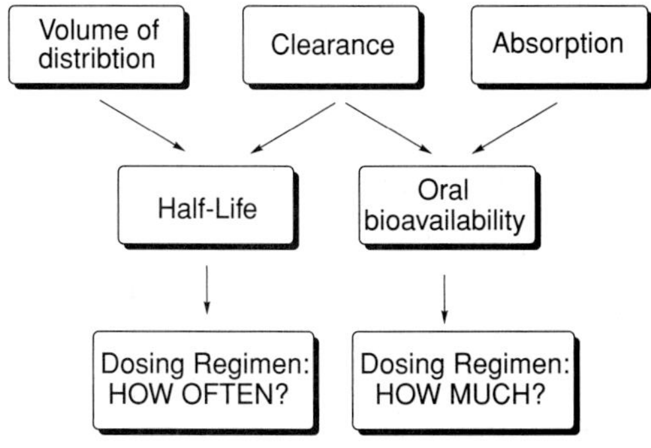

Fig. 9.25. The relationship of volume of distribution to the prediction of human kinetics.

The elimination rate constant (K) can be determined from the slope of the straight line as follows:

Eq. 9.45 $$(\text{slope})(2.303) = -K$$

It is, however, much easier to determine the elimination rate constant by making use of the following relationship:

Eq. 9.46 $$K = \frac{0.693}{t_{1/2}}$$

where $t_{1/2}$ is the time required for any drug concentration to decrease by half (i.e., 50%) and also is known as the biological or the elimination half-life. The elimination half-life is a pharmacokinetic property of a drug, and it is independent of the size of the administered dose when the administered drug exhibits the characteristics of a first-order process.

The elimination half-life ($t_{1/2}$) and the elimination rate constant (K) of a drug also play an important role in determining the plasma concentration of a drug at a given time. For instance, a drug with a short elimination half-life will be eliminated from the body much more quickly than a drug with a longer elimination half-life. These two parameters of a drug, therefore, become important in maintaining the desired drug blood levels in the body. In essence, these two parameters provide a quantifiable index of the presence of a drug in the body.

The process of drug elimination includes biotransformation and excretion, and it begins almost immediately, when circulation of blood distributes some of the drug to organs capable of metabolizing the drug or excreting it from the body. Among the organs of drug elimination, the liver is the principal site of biotransformation, and the kidney is primarily responsible for the excretion of unchanged drugs and their metabolites. Other organs, however, may also participate in the elimination of selected drugs.

The consequence of biotransformation of the drug to metabolite depends on the pharmacological activity of the individual metabolite(s). Metabolites may be active or completely inactive. Active metabolites may be more or less potent than the parent drug, and they may exhibit similar or dissimilar action. The kinetics of distribution and elimination of metabolites may differ from those of the parent drug, because each metabolite differs from the parent drug in its physicochemical properties as a result of functional group additions or changes.

The elimination rate constant (K) is the sum of the individual rate constants that characterize the elimination of a drug from the body and the form of metabolite or unchanged drug. Thus,

Eq. 9.47 $$K = K_u + K_m$$

where K_u and K_m represent the first-order rate constants associated with excretion and the form of metabolite or unchanged drug, respectively, removed from the blood.

The Apparent Volume of Distribution

Plasma or serum samples, collected immediately following the administration of equal doses (i.e., X_0) of two different drugs, may exhibit large differences in the drug concentration. This is because drug distribution in the body is largely a function of the physicochemical properties and, therefore, of the chemical structure of a therapeutic agent. The sole purpose of this parameter (V) is to relate the amount (mg) and the concentration (L^{-1}) of drug in the body at a given time. Therefore, it is important to recognize that knowledge of this parameter is essential for the determination of the dose of a drug required to attain the desired initial plasma concentration. The relationship of V to the prediction of human pharmacokinetics and dosing regiment is shown in Figure 9.25. Because it is not a true physical volume but, rather, a mathematical term that describes the behavior of a drug in the body with regard to its degree of partitioning between the plasma compartment and the remainder of the body, V is called "apparent." Drug partitioning into tissues represents a complex combination of physicochemical (lipophilicity, pK_a, plasma protein binding) and physiological parameters. Drugs that are equally bound to plasma proteins may yield different V values, because the drug with the greater tissue binding will yield the larger V. On the other hand, drugs with equal tissue binding may differ in V, with the compounds having the greater plasma protein binding yielding the smaller volume of distribution.

This relationship is shown in Equation 9.48:

Eq. 9.48 $$(X)_t = V(C_p)_t$$

where $(X)_t$ and $(C_p)_t$ are the dose of the drug and its plasma concentration, respectively, at a given time. The apparent volume of drug distribution (V) is determined by rearranging Equation 9.48 as follows:

Eq. 9.49 $$V = \frac{(X)_0}{(C_p)_t} = \frac{\text{Dose}}{(C_p)_0}$$

where X_0 is the administered dose of the drug and $(C_p)_0$ its initial plasma concentration.

V of a drug is usually a property of the drug rather than of a biological system, and it describes the extent to which a particular drug is distributed in the body tissues. The magnitude of V usually does not correspond to plasma, extracellular. or total body volume space but may vary from a few liters (7–10 L) to several hundred liters (≥200 L) in a 70-kg subject. The higher the value of V, the greater is the extent to which the drug is distributed in the body tissues, organs, or both. Furthermore, because body tissues, biological membranes, and organs are lipophilic in nature, the value of V is correlated with the lipophilicity of a drug, which in turn is influenced by the drug's chemical structure, pK_a, and protein binding. The more lipophilic the nature of the drug, the greater the value of V and the smaller the initial plasma concentration (assuming the administered doses of drugs are identical). Conversely, if the drug is hydrophilic, the drug will penetrate to a lesser extent into tissue; consequently, the plasma concentration will be higher and V smaller. It therefore is accurate to state that the value of V is influenced by the lipophilicity of the drug molecules.

In most situations, V is independent of the drug concentration, because doubling the amount of a drug in the body usually results in doubling of its plasma concentration (linear pharmacokinetics). This parameter, however, is constant for a drug. It remains independent of the dose administered and selected disease state. Other factors that may influence the blood composition, total body fluid, and the permeability characteristic of tissue may bring about changes in the value of V. Furthermore, because V reflects the extent to which a drug will penetrate into tissue, alteration in the permeability characteristics of tissue will alter V. Additionally, it is important to note that V of a drug may vary in infants, adults, and the geriatric population.

Many acidic drugs, including salicylates, sulfonamides, penicillins, and anticoagulants, are either highly bound to plasma proteins or are too water soluble to enter intracellular fluid and penetrate tissues in a significant amount. These drugs therefore have low volumes of distribution and low tissue to plasma concentration ratios. A given dose of these drugs will yield relatively higher plasma concentrations. It is tacitly assumed here that analytical problems in the determination of drug concentration are minimized or do not exist. Basic drugs, including tricyclic antidepressants and antihistamines, are extensively bound to extracellular tissues and are taken up by adipose tissues. The apparent volume of distribution for these drugs is large—often larger than the total body space. For example, the value of V for amphetamine is approximately 200 L (3 L/kg). The relatively small doses and large volume of distribution for amphetamine produces a low plasma concentration, which makes its quantitative detection in plasma a difficult task.

Theoretical limits for this parameter will be as low as 5 to 7 L (equivalent to the volume of the body fluid if the drug totally fails to penetrate the tissues or is extremely hydrophilic) to high as 200 L or greater. Because of differences in the magnitude of the apparent volume of distribution of a drug, a given dose of a drug with a relatively high V will provide low initial drug concentrations, and vice a versa (Eq. 9.48).

Clearance

One of the most important pharmacokinetic properties of a drug is clearance (Cl). In pharmacokinetic terms, clearance refers to the hypothetical volume of distribution from which the drug is entirely removed or cleared

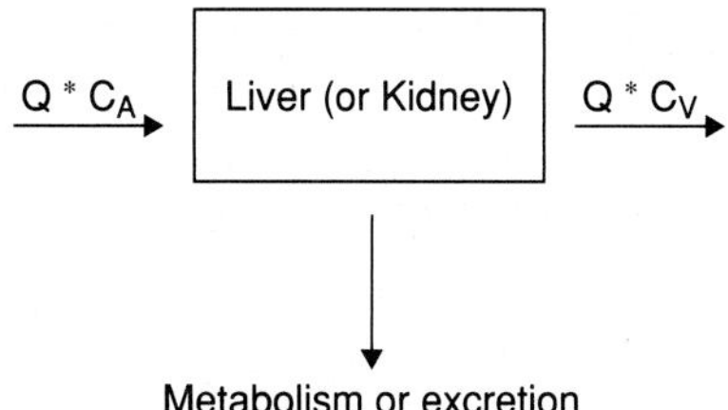

Fig. 9.26. Schematic representation of drug elimination by the liver (or kidney). $Q \cdot C_A$ is the rate at which the drug enters the liver (or kidney), and $Q \cdot C_V$ is the rate at which the drug leaves the liver (or kidney). The venous drug concentration (C_V) is less than the arterial drug concentration (C_A).

in unit time (mL/min or mL min^{-1}). In other words, it is an index of drug elimination from the body. Clearance is a function both of the intrinsic ability of certain organs, such as kidneys and liver, to excrete or metabolize a drug and of the blood flow rate to these organs. The concept of clearance can be illustrated by assuming the elimination in a single organ as depicted in Figure 9.26.

Under the conditions described in Figure 9.26, the venous concentration of drug (C_V) will always be less than the arterial concentration (C_A) because of the drug being eliminated or excreted during the passage of blood through the organ. The rate at which the drug enters the organ is the product of blood flow rate (Q) and the arterial concentration. The rate at which the drug leaves the organ, on the other hand, is equal to the product of blood flow rate and venous concentration:

Eq. 9.50 $$\text{The rate in} = QC_A$$

Eq. 9.51 $$\text{The rate out} = QC_V$$

The difference between the rate in and rate out is the rate of elimination of a drug by the organ:

Eq. 9.52 $$\text{Elimination rate} = Q(C_A - C_V)$$

The dimensionless ratio of elimination rate to the rate at which a drug enters the organ (QC_A) is defined as the extraction ratio (ER) and is obtained as follows:

Eq. 9.53 $$\text{ER} = \frac{Q(C_A - C_V)}{QC_A} = \frac{(C_A - C_V)}{C_A}$$

The extraction ratio (ER) of a drug ranges from zero to one depending on how well the organ eliminates or excretes the drug from the blood flowing through it. If an organ does not eliminate the drug, then $C_A = C_V$, and the extraction ratio is zero (low extraction ratio). If, on the other hand, the organ avidly removes the drug so that $C_V \cong 0$, then the extraction ratio is one (high extraction ratio). If liver is the organ responsible for metabolizing the drug, then the extraction ratio may be described by using the notation, E_H.

Using the extraction ratio number (i.e., ER of E_H), the drugs have been classified as having a low (ER < 0.3), intermediate (ER $= 0.3$–0.7) or high (ER > 0.7) extraction ratio drugs. Table 9.8 lists the representative drugs with their hepatic or extraction ratios. The influence of blood flow and intrinsic clearance of an organ on the clearance of a drug is determined by the extraction ratio of the drug.

The clearance of a drug (Cl) also may be viewed as a proportionality constant relating the elimination rate of a drug to its plasma concentrations at a given time and is expressed as

Eq. 9.54 $$(Cl) = \frac{\text{rate of elimination}}{\bar{C}_p}$$

where $\bar{C}_p$ is the average plasma concentration of a drug at a time that corresponds to the rate of elimination. It follows from an earlier equation (Eq. 9.54) that

Eq. 9.55 $$(Cl) = Q\text{ER}$$

where Q and ER have been previously defined and, because the drug elimination follows a first-order process, clearance is independent of the drug concentrations or the dose administered.

Table 9.8. Hepatic and Renal Extraction Ratios of Selected Drugs and Metabolites

Low (< 0.3)	Intermediate (0.3–0.7)	High (> 0.7)
Hepatic extraction[a]		
Carbamazepine	Aspirin	Alprenolol
Diazepam	Quinidine	Arabinosyl-cytosine
Digitoxin	Codeine	Desipramine
Indomethacin	Nortriptyline	Doxepin
Phenobarbital		Isoproterenol
Phenytoin		Lidocaine
Procainamide		Meperidine
Salicylic Acid		Morphine
Theophylline		Nitroglycerin
Tolbutamide		Pentazocine
Valproic Acid		Propoxyphene
Warfarin		Propranolol
Renal extraction[a]		
Atenolol	Cimetidine	(Many) Glucuronides
Cefazolin	Cephalothin	Hippurates
Chlorpropamide	Procainamide	(Some) Penicillins
Digoxin	(Some) Penicillins	(Many) Sulfates
Furosemide		
Gentamicin		
Lithium		
Phenobarbital		
Sulfisoxazole		
Tetracycline		

[a]At least 30% of the drug is eliminated by this route.

The total body clearance of a drug the from blood is equal to the ratio of the overall elimination rate to drug concentration (Eq. 9.54), where the overall elimination rate is comprised of the sum of the elimination processes occurring in all organs and the removal of a drug in all its forms. Therefore, the overall clearance, $(Cl)_s$, represents the renal clearance (i.e., unchanged form of a drug) and the metabolic clearance (i.e., removal of a drug as metabolic by kidney). It also is very useful to keep in mind that the clearance can be expressed as the product of the apparent volume of distribution (V) and the elimination rate constant (K) for drugs that exhibit characteristics of one compartment model. Thus,

Eq. 9.56 $$(Cl)_s = V_d K$$

Renal Clearance

Drug elimination occurs by renal excretion and an extrarenal pathway, usually hepatic metabolism. Renal clearance is defined as the proportionality constant between the urinary excretion rate and the plasma concentration:

Eq. 9.57 $$\left(\frac{dX_\mu}{dt}\right)_{\bar{t}} = (Cl)_r\overline{C_p}$$

where $(dX_\mu/dt)_{\bar{t}}$ is the average urinary excretion rate (mg/hr); $(Cl)_r$ is the renal clearance (mL/hr), and $\overline{C_p}$ is the plasma drug concentration. Equation 9.57, however, presents practical difficulty in measuring renal clearance, because the plasma drug concentration changes:

Eq. 9.58 $$(X_u)_t = (Cl)_r C_p dt$$

where $C_p dt$ corresponds to the area under the plasma concentration–time curve (AUC). The urine collection interval (dt) is composed of many such very small increments of time, and the amount of drug excreted in a collection interval is the sum of the drug amount excreted in each small time interval line. Then,

Eq. 9.59 $$(Cl)_r = \frac{\text{Total amount excreted (i.e., } (X_u)_\infty)}{(\text{AUC})_0^\infty \cdot}$$

where $(X_u)_\infty$ is the total amount excreted in the urine and $(\text{AUC})_0^\infty\cdot$ is the area under the plasma concentration–time curve from $t = 0$ to $t = \infty$.

To account for all the administered drugs in the urine when the drug is administered intravenously often is not possible. This may be caused by the excretion of some of the drug via an extrarenal route, excretion of a metabolite via an extrarenal route, further biotransformation of primary metabolite into chemical forms that are not identified by the analytical method used, or formation of unknown and unidentified primary metabolites. If the total amount of metabolites can be identified in the urine, then one can determine the metabolite clearance using the following equation:

Eq. 9.60 $$(Cl)_m = \frac{\text{Total amount excreted (i.e.,} (X_{mu})_\infty)}{(\text{AUC})_0^\infty}$$

where $(X_{mu})_\infty$ is the amount of matabolite in the urine at time infinity.

Hepatic Clearance

Although metabolism can take place in many organs, the liver frequently has the greater metabolic capacity and, therefore, has been the most thoroughly studied. The most direct quantitative measure of the liver's ability to eliminate a drug is hepatic clearance, $(Cl)_H$, which includes biliary excretion clearance and hepatic metabolic clearance:

Eq. 9.61 $$(Cl)_H = Q_H E_H$$

where Q_H is the sum of the hepatic portal and hepatic arterial blood flow rates, the values of which are 1,050 and 300 mL/min, respectively.

Under conditions of normal body functions, the pharmacokinetic behavior of most drugs can be established within reasonable limits, and optimal dosage regimens can be designed using the observed values of the pharmacokinetic parameters of the drug. When, however, the renal function is compromised as a result of acute or chronic renal diseases or the patient's age, drugs that are eliminated predominantly through the kidneys are likely to be retained in the body for a longer duration and accumulate to the extent of providing toxic drug levels with repeated dosing. If the drug is converted to a metabolite, the accumulation of active metabolite also may lead to toxic effect, and although most metabolites are inactive, their accumulation with repeated dosing may produce toxic reactions by displacement of the parent drug from plasma protein and by inhibiting further drug metabolism.

Renal failure can result from a variety of pathologic conditions. If renal impairment is rapid in onset and short in duration, then renal failure is described as acute. The primary cause of acute renal failure may be prerenal (i.e., acute congestive heart failure or shock), intrarenal (i.e., acute tubule necrosis) or postrenal (i.e., hypercalcemia). The condition generally is reversible; however, complete restoration of renal function may take 6 to 12 months.

Chronic renal failure almost always is caused by intrinsic renal diseases and is characterized by slow, progressive development. Unlike the acute condition, chronic renal impairment generally is irreversible. The degree or loss of kidney functional capacity in the chronic condition is best described in terms of the intact "nephron" hypothesis, in which the diseased kidney is comprised of nephrons that are essentially nonfunctional because of pathologic conditions together with normal nephrons. Progressive renal impairment is the result of an increasing fraction of nonfunctional nephrons.

The prolonged and progressive nature of chronic renal failure is of particular concern in older patients, who may require a variety of medications, both for their renal condition and for other unrelated conditions. The inability of these patients to excrete drugs and drug metabolites adequately and the influence of their uremic conditions on the functions of other physiological systems require careful adjustments of drug dosage to obtain accurate and adequate blood levels without increased toxicity.

Compounds (e.g., drugs) are cleared by kidneys because of passive filtration through the glomeruli or by active secretion in the kidney tubule. Once in the nephrons, compounds also may be reabsorbed into the circulation. The glomerular filtration rate can be measured using any compound that is filtered by glomeruli and not secreted and reabsorbed. Although exogenous compounds, such as urea and inulin, can be used for this purpose, the relative ease of using endogenous creatinine has made this the method of universal choice. In principle, the following equation determines the relationship between the creatine clearance, $(Cl)_{cr}$, the serum creatinine concentration, $(\bar{C}_s)_{cr}$, and creatinine excretion rate, $(dX_{\mu}/dt)_{\bar{t}}\cdot cr$:

Eq. 9.62
$$(Cl)_{cr} = \frac{(dX_{\mu}/dt)_{\bar{t}}\cdot cr}{(\bar{C}_s)_{cr}}$$

Serum creatinine concentration is constant unless there is a change in the rate of production of creatinine in the body or creatinine clearance. The creatinine clearance in normal kidneys is approximately 110 to 130 mL/min. This value declines with progressive renal impairment, and it drops to zero with severe renal impairment. Creatinine clearance values of 20 to 30 mL/min signify moderate renal impairment; values of less than 10 mL/min signify several renal impairment. Creatinine is poorly secreted and not subject to tubular reabsorption; therefore, its clearance is a useful measure of the glomerular filtration rate. Although creatinine clearance tells us about only one aspect of renal function (i.e., filtration), it is an excellent indicator for assessing the severity of renal impairment.

The extent to which decreased renal function influences drug elimination is a function of the percentage of circulating drug being cleared by the kidneys. From the literature, the influence of renal impairment on the elimination half-life of a drug clearly will be a direct function of the percentage of the drug cleared through the kidneys. If the elimination half-life of a drug that is cleared essentially unchanged via the kidneys is plotted against the endogenous creatinine clearance (Fig. 9.27), the result will be a hyperbola.

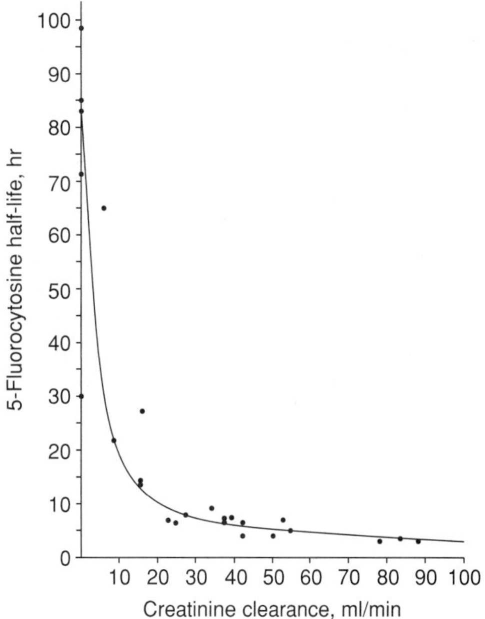

Fig. 9.27. Curvilinear relationship between the elimination half-life of 5-fluorocytosine and renal function (creatinine clearance). (from Gibaldi M. Biopharmaceutics and Clinical Pharmacokinetics, 4th Ed. Philadelphia: Lea and Febiger, 1991; with permission.)

Intravenous Bolus Administration (Two-Compartment Model)

Following the administration of a drug intravenously, it usually takes a finite amount of time before the distribution equilibrium is attained in the body. During this distribution phase, the drug concentration in the plasma will decline more rapidly than during the postdistribution phase, as shown in Figure 9.28. There are three possible types of two-compartment models. They differ in whether the elimination of the drug occurs from the central compartment, the peripheral compartment, or both. These three types of two-compartment models are, mathematically, indistinguishable on the basis of available concentration data. The type of two-compartment model illustrated in Figure 9.22 most often is used to describe the pharmacokinetics of drugs. In this model, it is assumed that drug elimination from a two-compartment model occurs exclusively from the central compartment, because the site of biotransformation and excretion (i.e., liver and kidney) are well perfused with blood and presumably, therefore, rapidly accessible to

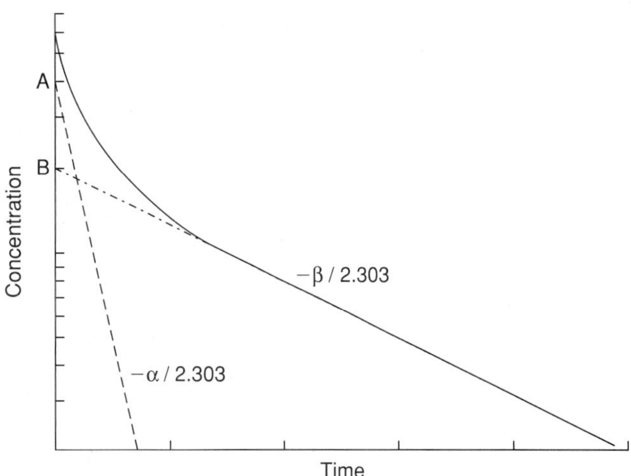

Fig. 9.28. Semilogarithmic plot of drug concentration in the plasma against time following administration of a rapid intravenous injection when the body may be represented as a two compartment open model. The dashed line is obtained by "feathering" the curve.

drug in the systemic circulation. Whether this distribution phase is apparent will depend on the early collection of blood samples. A distribution phase may last for only a few minutes or for several hours.

A semilogarithmic plot of plasma drug concentration as a function of time (Fig. 9.28) after rapid intravenous injection of a drug often can be resolved into two linear components. This can be done graphically by employing the residual, or "feathering," method, as shown in Figure 9.28, in which the slopes of rapid and slow disposition phases will permit the determination of α and β, respectively, in Eq. 9.63. The intercepts on the concentration axis are designated A and B. The entire plasma concentration–time curve may be described by the following equation:

Eq. 9.63 $$C_p = Ae^{-\alpha t} + Be^{-\beta t}$$

where α and β are the first-order distribution and disposition rate constants, respectively. A biexponential decline in the plasma drug concentration justifies, mathematically, the representation of the body as a two-compartment model.

The intercompartmental rate constants (K_{21} and K_{12}) (Eqs. 9.64 and 9.66) and the elimination rate constant (K_{10}) (Eq. 9.65) for a drug that exhibits the characteristics of a two-compartment model can be determined from the knowledge of α, β, A, and B (Fig. 9.28). This is achieved by employing the following equations:

Eq. 9.64 $$K_{21} = \frac{A\beta + B\alpha}{A + B}$$

where K_{21} is the rate constant associated with the transfer of a drug from compartment II to compartment I (i.e., from the peripheral to the central compartment):

Eq. 9.65 $$K_{10} = \frac{\alpha\beta}{K_{21}}$$

where K_{10} is the elimination rate constant of the drug.

Eq. 9.66 $$K_{12} = \alpha + \beta - (K_{21} + K_{10})$$

where K_{12} is the rate constant associated with the transfer of the drug from compartment I to compartment II (i.e., from the central compartment to the peripheral compartment). Determination of these rate constants permits an assessment of the relative contribution of distribution and the elimination processes to the drug concentration versus time profile. The knowledge of the transfer rate constant (K_{12}) also is required to calculate the amount of drug in the peripheral compartment (X_p) as a function of time after an intravenous administration:

Eq. 9.67 $$X_p = \frac{X_0 K_{12}}{(\beta - \alpha)}(e^{-\alpha t} - e^{-\beta t})$$

where X_0 is the administered dose.

Extravascular Route of Administration

When a drug is administered by extravascular routes, absorption is a requisite for a drug to reach the general circulation. Absorption is defined here as a process of a drug proceeding from the site of administration to the site of measurement within the body, generally blood, plasma, or serum. Figure 9.29 represents the passage of a drug through the gastrointestinal tract into the general circulation.

When a drug is administered orally, there are several possible sites for drug loss. One such site is the gastrointestinal lumen, where the decomposition of a drug may occur. If it is assumed that the drug survives destruction in

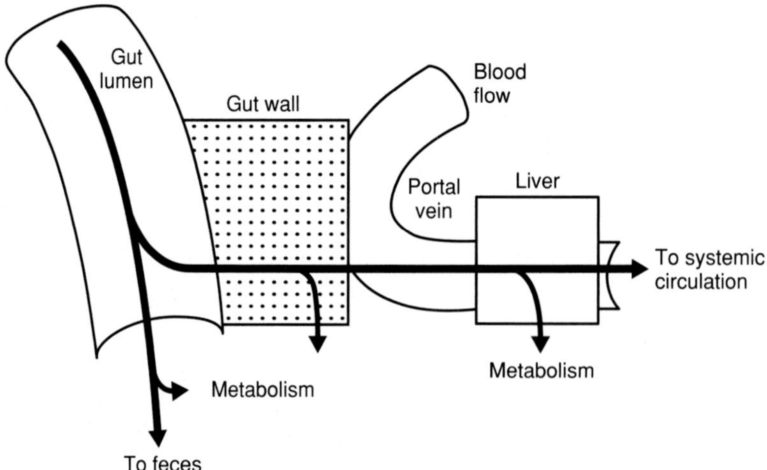

Fig. 9.29. After oral administration, a drug must pass sequentially through the gut lumen, gut wall, and then through the liver before reaching the general circulation. Metabolism may occur in the lumen before absorption, in the gut wall during the absorption, or in the liver after absorption and before reaching the systemic circulation. (From Rowland M, Tozer T. Clinical Pharmacokinetics: Concepts and Application, 2nd Ed. Philadelphia: Lea and Febiger, 1989; with permission.)

the gut lumen and is metabolized by enzymes as it passes through the membrane of the gastrointestinal tract, then even though the drug leaves the site of administration, it is considered not to be absorbed systemically. Indeed, loss at any site in the gastrointestinal tract before reaching the site of measurement may contribute to a decrease in the systemic absorption of the drug. The requirement for an orally administered drug to pass through the gastrointestinal tract makes the extent of absorption not always complete. The loss of a drug as it passes for the first time through gastrointestinal membrane and the lining, during absorption, is known as the first-pass effect. Figure 9.30 represents the time course of a drug and metabolite at each site in the body.

The rate or the change in the amount of drug in the body (dX/dt) following administration of a drug by an extravascular route is a function of both the absorption rate ($K_a X_a$) and the elimination rate (KX):

Eq. 9.68 $$\frac{dX}{dt} = K_a X_a - KX$$

where $K_a X_a$ is the first-order absorption rate, KX is the first-order elimination rate, and K_a and K are the first-order absorption and elimination rate constants, respectively.

When the absorption rate is greater than the elimination rate (i.e., $K_a X_a > KX$), the amount of drug in the body and the drug concentration in the plasma increase with time. Conversely, when the amount of drug remaining at the absorption site (X_a) is sufficiently small, the elimination rate exceeds the absorption rate (i.e., $KX > K_a X_a$); therefore, the amount of drug in the body and the drug concentration in the plasma decrease with time.

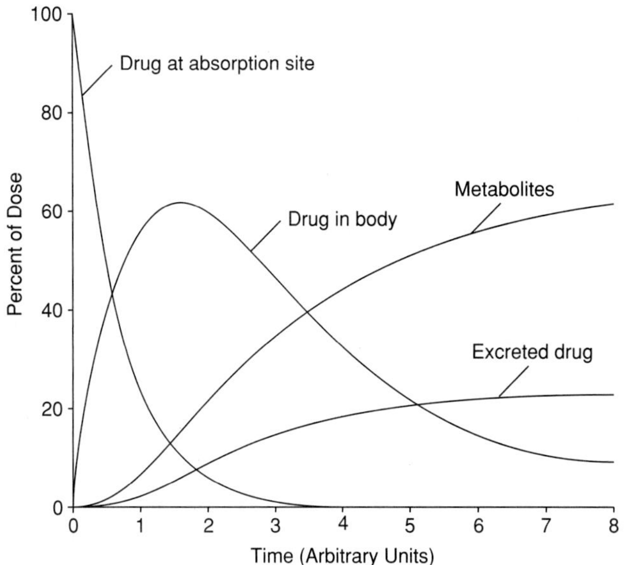

Fig. 9.30. Time course of a drug at each site following an extravascular administration.

The maximum, or peak, plasma concentration after drug administration occurs at the moment when the absorption rate equals the elimination rate (i.e., $K_a X_a = KX$). The faster the drug is absorbed, the higher the maximum plasma concentration and the shorter the time required following administration of a dose to observe the peak plasma concentration. Integration of Equation 9.68 from $t = 0$ to $t = t^*$ and converting the amount to the concentration results in the following equation:

Eq. 9.69 $$C_p = \frac{K_a F (X_a)_0}{V(K_a - K)}(e^{-Kt} - e^{-K_a t})$$

where $(X_a)_0$ is the administered dose and F is the fraction of the administered dose that is absorbed and available to reach the general circulation. Equation 9.69 often is used to determine plasma concentration after administration of a drug by an extravascular route when the administered drug manifests the characteristics of a one-compartment model.

The absorption rate constant (K_a) of a drug frequently is larger than the elimination rate constant (K). Under such a condition, at some time after drug administration, the value of the term e^{-Kt} in Equation 9.69 approaches zero, indicating that no more drug is available for absorption, and Equation 9.69 simplifies to

Eq. 9.70 $$C_p = \frac{K_a F (X_a)_0}{V(K_a - K)}(e^{-Kt})$$

Eq. 9.71 $$C_p = \text{Intercept}(e^{-Kt})$$

Eq. 9.72 $$\log C_p = \log \text{Intercept} - \frac{Kt}{2.303}$$

When the absorption is complete, the term $X_a K_a$ disappears from the Equation 9.68, and the equation is reduced to

Eq. 9.73 $$-\frac{dX}{dt} = KX$$

During the postabsorption phase, the decline in the plasma concentration with time follows first-order kinetics. A typical plot of plasma concentration versus time is shown in Figure 9.31, where the intercept of the extrapolated line (I^*) is a complex function of absorption and elimination rate constants (K_a and K, respectively) as well as the dose or amount absorbed, $F(X_a)_0$, and the apparent volume of distribution (V). It is, however, incorrect to assume that the intercept approximates the ratio of dose over the apparent volume of distribution unless the drug is rapidly and completely absorbed, which rarely occurs.

Importance of Absorption Rate

The influence of absorption on the drug concentration time profile is shown in Figure 9.32. Administration of an

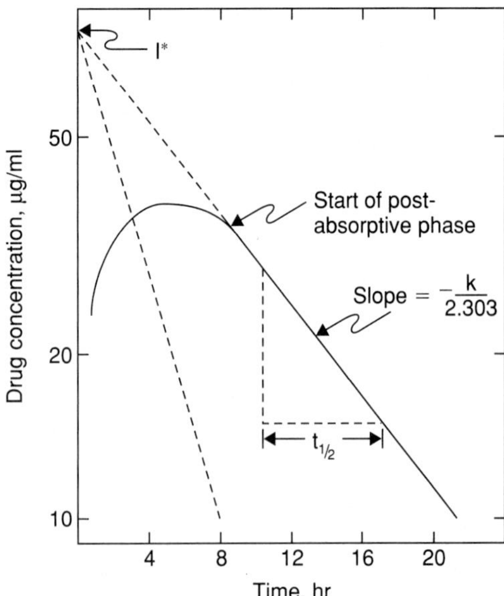

Fig. 9.31. Typical semilogarithmic plot of drug concentration versus time profile in plasma following the administration of a drug by an extravascular route. The dashed line represents the "feathered line" used to obtain the absorption rate constant (K_a).

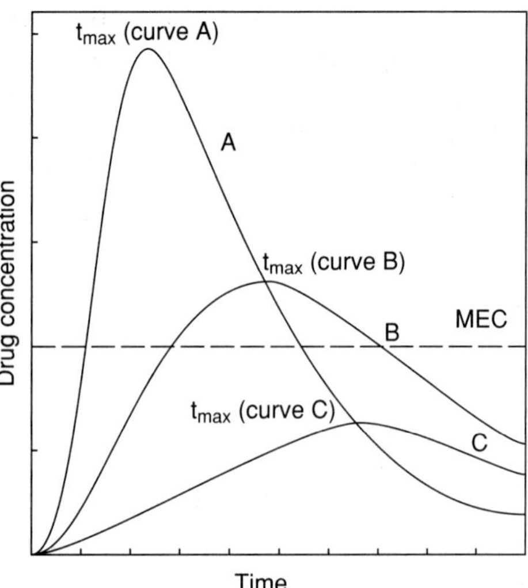

Fig. 9.32. A plasma concentration versus time profile illustrating the influence of absorption rate constant (K_a) on the rate of absorption as reflected in the peak time (t_{max}) and peak plasma concentration $(C_p)_{max}$.

equal dose of a drug in three different dosage forms or by three different extravascular routes or three different formations results in threefold the drug in the plasma. The faster the drug is absorbed (i.e., $K_a >>> K$), the greater the peak plasma concentration and the shorter the time required to achieve peak plasma drug concentration.

Many drugs do not exhibit demonstrable pharmacological effects or do not elicit a desired degree of pharmacological response unless a minimum concentration is reached at the site of an action and, therefore, a minimum therapeutic concentration in the plasma. Thus, the absorption rate of a drug may affect the clinical response if it fails to yield the minimum effective concentration. As evident in Figure 9.32, the more rapid the absorption of a drug, the faster its onset of response (i.e., curve A). When the drug is absorbed rather slowly (curve C), the minimum effective concentration is just barely attained. The intensity of maximum pharmacological effects is a function of the drug concentration. The data presented in Figure 9.32 suggest that the administered dose of a drug in curve A may produce a more intense response than observed in curves B and C.

The peak plasma drug concentration is always lower following administration of a drug by the extravascular route compared with its initial plasma concentration following administration of an identical dose by intravenous solution. In the former, at peak time, some drugs may still remain at the absorption site and some has been eliminated, whereas the entire dose is in the body immediately following the intravenous administration.

The delay between drug administration and a drug reaching the general circulation may be of particular importance when a rapid onset of effect is desired. This delay is termed "lag time," and it can be anywhere between a few minutes to many hours. Lag time generally is attributed to the slow and poor absorption of the drug, either because of slow disintegration and dissolution of the drug from the dosage form or because of slow removal of the coating material from coated tablets.

Determination of Peak Time

The determination of peak time (t_{max}) can be achieved by employing the following equation:

Eq. 9.74
$$t_{max} = \frac{\ln(K_a/K)}{(K_a - K)}$$

where K_a and K are the first-order absorption and elimination rate constants, respectively. Equation 9.74 shows that the peak time is a function only of the relative magnitude of the absorption and elimination rate constants. As the rate of absorption decreases (i.e., smaller K_a value), the peak time will be higher, as shown in Figure 9.32, progressing from curve C to curve A.

The rate of drug absorption varies when the extravascular route is changed, when the formulation of a drug is changed, or when the dosage form is changed. These changes will be reflected in different peak times for the same dose of a drug. The peak time will be unaffected, however, by a mere change in the size of the administered dose. In many disease states, the impairment in the renal function may affect the elimination rate constant, thereby producing a change in the peak time.

Determination of Peak Plasma Concentrations

The peak (maximum) plasma drug concentration, (C_p)max, in the body occurs at time t_{max}, which is described by substituting t_{max} for time t in Equation 9.69:

Eq. 9.75 $$(C_p)_{max} = \frac{K_a F(X_a)_0}{V(K_a - K)}(e^{-Kt_{max}} - e^{-K_a t_{max}})$$

Equation 9.75 is further simplified into

Eq. 9.76 $$(C_p)_{max} = \text{Intercept}(e^{-Kt_{max}} - e^{-K_a t_{max}})$$

where the intercept of the plasma drug concentration versus time is equal to $K_a F(X_a)_0/V(K_a - K)$, as described earlier in Equations 9.70 through 9.72.

A much simpler expression can be obtained as follows: At peak time,

Eq. 9.77 $$e^{-K_a t_{max}} = \frac{K}{K_a} e^{-Kt_{max}}$$

Substituting for $e^{-Kt_{max}}$ in Equation 9.75 yields

Eq. 9.78 $$(C_p)_{max} = \frac{K_a F(X_a)_0}{V(K_a - K)}\left(\frac{K_a - K}{K_a}\right)(e^{-Kt_{max}})$$

which, on the cancellation of terms, is readily simplified into

Eq. 9.79 $$(C_p)_{max} = \frac{F(X_a)_0}{V}(e^{-Kt_{max}})$$

where F is the fraction of the dose absorbed, $(X_a)_0$ is the administered dose, V is the apparent volume of distribution, and K and t_{max} are elimination rate constants and peak time, respectively. Equation 9.79 suggests that the peak plasma concentration of a drug is a function of a dose entering the general circulation, the apparent volume of distribution, and the first-order rate constants for absorption and elimination. Again, like the absorption rate constant, the fraction of the administered dose reaching the general circulation will depend on the route of administration, the formulation, and the dosage form. These factors therefore will contribute to the peak plasma concentration of a drug.

Bioavailability

The bioavailability of a drug is defined as the rate and extent to which the administered dose of a drug reaches the general circulation. Generally, rapid and complete absorption of a drug is desirable if it is used for pain, allergy response, insomnia, and other conditions for which a quick onset of action is desired. As indicated earlier (Fig. 9.32), the more rapid the absorption, the shorter the onset of action and the greater the intensity of a pharmacological response. Bioavailability determines the amount of administered dose that reaches the circulation, which also is related to rate of drug clearance (Fig. 9.25).

The efficacy of a single dose is a function of both the rate and the extent of absorption. Thus, for two dosage forms or two extravascular routes to be comparable with regard to the bioavailability following the administration of a drug, the absorption rate of a drug and the extent to which a drug reaches the general circulation from each dosage form or extravascular route must be comparable.

The useful estimate of relative absorption rates of a drug from different products, through different routes of administration or different conditions (i.e., with or without food or in the presence of other drugs, etc.) can be made by comparing the magnitude of time of occurrence of peak concentration, peak concentration, and area under the peak plasma concentration curve, $(AUC)_0^\infty$. The peak time and peak plasma concentration can be determined by employing Equations 9.74 and 9.76 or 9.79, respectively, and the extent of absorption can be determined as described below.

Estimating the Extent of Absorption

The extent of absorption can be estimated by determining the total area under the plasma drug concentration–time curve, $(AUC)_0^\infty$, or the total amount of an unchanged drug excreted in urine, $(X_u)_\infty$, after the administration of a drug. $(AUC)_0^\infty$ can be estimated by several methods, such as a planimeter, which is an instrument for measuring the area of a plan figure, and the cut-and-weight method, which weighs the paper of plasma concentration–time curve. The weight is converted to weight per unit area. The most common methods, however, are the application of trapezoidal rule and equation, when possible. In a single-dose study, we cannot determine the area under the plasma concentration time curve by the use of trapezoidal rule alone. In this case, a widely used practice is to determine the area under the plasma concentration–time curve from $t = 0$ to $t = t^*$ (the last sampling time) by means of trapezoidal rule and estimate the remaining area by employing the following equation:

Eq. 9.80 $$(AUC)_{t^*}^\infty = C_p^*/K$$

where $(AUC)_{t^*}^\infty$ is the area under the plasma concentration–time curve from the last sampling time to time ∞, C_p^* is the last observed plasma concentration, and K is the first-order elimination rate constant. This area under the curve, $(AUC)_{t^*}^\infty$, will be added to the area under the curve obtained from $t = 0$ to $t = t^*$ to calculate the total area under the plasma concentration–time curve:

Eq. 9.81 $$(AUC)_0^\infty = (AUC)_0^{t^\otimes} + (AUC)_t^{\infty\otimes}$$

When an intravenous administration of a drug exhibits the characteristics of a one-compartment model, the total area under the plasma concentration vs. time curve is estimated by the following equation:

Eq. 9.82 $$(AUC)_0^\infty = \frac{\text{dose}}{VK}$$

where VK is the systemic clearance of a drug.

Following the administration of a drug by an intravenous injection, if it is necessary to use a two-compartment model, the area under the plasma concentration–time curve from $t = 0$ to $t = t^*$ (the last sampling time) may be estimated by using trapezoidal rules, as mentioned earlier. Additionally, the area under plasma concentration–time curve from $t = t^*$ to $t = \infty$ may be computed using the following equation:

Eq. 9.83 $$(AUC)_{t}^{*\infty} = C_p^*/\beta$$

where C_p^* is the last observed plasma concentration and β is the first-order disposition rate constant.

When a drug is administered by an extravascular route, one may use the following equation to determine $(AUC)_0^\infty$:

Eq. 9.84 $$(AUC)_0^\infty = \frac{F(\text{dose})}{VK}$$

If it is desired to assess the relative extent of drug absorption from a product, the total area under the plasma concentration from the product to that obtained for a reference drug standard is compared. The reference standard may be an intravenous injection, an orally administered aqueous or water-miscible solution, or another product accepted as a standard.

When it is desired to assess the absolute bioavailability, the reference drug standard becomes an intravenous injection, and when it is desired to judge the bioequivalence, the reference standard is an innovator product. If the $(AUC)_0^\infty$ values are identical following the administration of equal doses of a drug through a test product and the reference intravenous solution, we conclude that the drug from the test product is completely absorbed and not subject to presystemic metabolism.

Frequently, however, the standard is an innovator product or another established product. If the $(AUC)_0^\infty$ values are identical following the administration of equal doses of the test and reference products, we conclude that the test product is completely bioavailable relative to the standard. It is essential to use the term "relative to the standard," because we do not know if the standard is completely absorbed or available. Additionally, when two products produce comparable peak plasma drug concentrations and t_{max} and the reference standard is an innovator product, then the products are judged to be bioequivalent.

By using the ratio of area under the plasma concentration–time curve for extravascular to intravenous routes, one can determine the absolute bioavailability of a drug from a test product as follows:

Eq. 9.85 $$F = \frac{(AUC)_0^\infty \text{ oral}}{(AUC)_0^\infty \text{ IV solution}}$$

where F is the absolute bioavailability of a drug or the fraction of the administered dose that reaches the general circulation following the administration of equal dose of a drug. If the administered doses of a drug are different then the AUC_0^∞, then estimates can be scaled approximately to permit comparison under identical conditions or equivalent doses—assuming, of course, that $(AUC)_0^\infty$ is directly proportioned to the administered dose. The relative bioavailability (F_{rel}) of a drug from a test product may be determined by using the following expression:

Eq. 9.86 $$F_{rel} = \frac{(AUC)_0^\infty \text{ test product}}{(AUC)_0^\infty \text{ reference standard}}$$

Equation 9.86 assumes that the doses administered from each product are identical, and if not, the $(AUC)_0^\infty$ values should be scaled for the dose differences.

The determination of bioavailability from the urinary excretion of an unchanged drug following administration by intravenous solution can be assessed using the following equations:

Eq. 9.87 $$(X_u)_\infty = \frac{(\text{dose})K_u}{K}$$

where $(X_u)_\infty$ is the amount of drug excreted in unchanged form in the urine after administration of a dose and K_u and K are the first-order excretion and the elimination rate constants, respectively. On the other hand, for drugs administered by an extravascular route, the amount of an unchanged drug excreted in urine, $(X_u)_\infty$, is obtained by

Eq. 9.88 $$(X_u)_\infty = \frac{F(\text{dose})K_u}{K}$$

where F is the fraction of the administered dose that reaches the general circulation. Therefore, the bioavailability of a drug following its extravascular administration can be expressed as

Eq. 9.89 $$F = \frac{(X_u)_\infty \text{ extravascular}}{(X_u)_\infty \text{ intravascular}}$$

To determine the assessment of relative bioavailability (F_{rel}), Equation 9.89 becomes

Eq. 9.90 $$F_{ref} = \frac{(X_u)_\infty \text{ test product}}{(X_u)_\infty \text{ standard product}}$$

and Equations 9.89 and 9.90 are applicable under the condition that the administered doses are identical. The utility of these equations depends on how much of the drug is eliminated by urinary excretion, the sensitivity of the analytical procedure, and the variability in urinary output of the drug. Many drugs are extensively metabolized, with little, if any, drug appearing in an unchanged form in the urine. In such cases, the bioavailability is estimated from the plasma concentration time data.

Presystemic or First-Pass Metabolism

Following oral administration, a drug must pass sequentially from the gastrointestinal lumen, through the gut wall, and through the liver before reaching the general circulation (Fig. 9.29). Because the gut wall and liver are the sites of drug metabolism, a fraction of the amount of drug absorbed may be eliminated or metabolized before reaching the general circulation. Therefore, an oral dose of a drug may be completely absorbed yet incompletely available to reach the general circulation because of presystemic or first-pass effect (metabolism) in the gut wall or liver. If such is the case, it will be reflected in the values of $(AUC)_0^\infty$ for the administered dose.

Criteria have been developed to identify and quantify the extent of presystemic metabolism and to indicate when it is occurring. The determination of presystemic metabolism requires only that the systemic availability of a drug is less than the fraction of the dose absorbed. The fraction absorbed may be determined from the urinary excretion of a drug and metabolite after oral administration of a drug relative to that after intravenous administration. Many drugs undergoing presystemic metabolism in humans have been identified on the basis of this type of information. Differentiation between the gut wall and the liver as the site of presystemic metabolism in humans is more difficult, though relatively easy in animals.

The liver is the most important site of presystemic elimination because of high levels of drug-metabolizing enzymes, its ability to rapidly metabolize different types of drugs, and its unique anatomical location. The following are selected examples of drugs that are subject to considerable hepatic first-pass metabolism: the β-blockers propranolol and metoprolol; the analgesics propoxyphene, meperidine, and pentazocine; the antidepressants imipramine and nortriptyline; and the antiarrhythmic lidocaine.

Hepatic presystemic metabolism is most easily understood when liver is the sole organ of drug elimination. Under these conditions, the clearance of the drug, as determined following intravenous administration of the drug, is equal to

Eq. 9.91
$$(Cl)_H = \frac{\text{dose}}{(AUC)_0^\infty}$$

Hepatic clearance, however, also is equal to

Eq. 9.92
$$(Cl)_H = Q_H \cdot E_H$$

where $(Cl)_H$ is the hepatic clearance, Q_H is the hepatic blood flow rate, and E_H is the dimensionless hepatic extraction ratio of the drug. Hepatic blood flow rate (Q_H) has a mean range from approximately 1.1 to 1.8 L/min, with an average of approximately 1.5 L/min. The hepatic extraction ratio (E_H) of a drug may range from zero to one, depending on the liver's ability to metabolize the drug. The maximum hepatic clearance of a drug, excluding hepatic metabolism, is equal to hepatic blood flow; this occurs when $E_H = 1.0$. The fraction of a drug eliminated from portal blood (Fig. 9.29) during the absorption phase is given by the hepatic extraction ratio (E_H); the remainder of the drug (i.e., $1 - E_H$) escapes into the systemic circulation and then is cleared from the circulation by the liver according to Equation 9.56.

If the fraction of the oral dose is absorbed and then subjected to hepatic presystemic metabolism, the AUC_0^∞ following oral administration of a drug is given by

Eq. 9.93
$$(AUC)_0^\infty = \frac{F(X_a)_0(1 - E_H)}{Q_H \cdot E_H}$$

Because $Q_H \cdot E_H$ is equal to hepatic clearance (Eq. 9.92), which under these conditions is given by the ratio of an intravenous dose to an area under the concentration–time curve, $(AUC)_0^\infty$ IV, Equation 9.93 can be rewritten as

Eq. 9.94
$$\frac{(AUC)_0^\infty \text{ oral}}{(AUC)_0^\infty \text{ IV}} = \frac{F(X_a)_0(1 - E_H)}{(X_a) \text{ IV}}$$

The ratio of $(AUC)_0^\infty$ after oral and intravenous administration of equal doses of drugs is the systemic availability (i.e., the fraction absorbed). If it is assumed that the drug is completely absorbed (i.e., $F = 1$), then Equation 9.94 reduces to

Eq. 9.95
$$F = (1 - E_H)$$

Equation 9.95 shows that the systemic availability of the drug depends on the hepatic extraction ratio of the drug, and those drugs with low hepatic extraction ratios, such as antipyrine, tolbutamide, and warfarin, undergo little presystemic metabolism.

An estimate of hepatic extraction ratio (E_H) may be made from determination of the clearance of a drug following intravenous administration and comparing this value to the mean value of liver blood flow according to Equation 9.92, when rearranged:

Eq. 9.96
$$E_H = \frac{(Cl)_H}{Q_H}$$

The intravenous clearance of propranolol is approximately 1.05 L/min. Assuming that the average liver blood flow is approximately 1.5 L/min, we can determine that the hepatic extraction for propranolol (E_H) is 0.7 and that the fraction absorbed (F) is 0.3. This means that even though propranolol is well absorbed, only 30% of the oral dose is available for systemic circulation.

This type of information, in conjunction with the value of the fraction absorbed (F), has been used to substantiate the predominantly hepatic presystemic elimination of several drugs, including propranolol, lidocaine, pentazocine, and so on. The plasma concentrations for pentazocine, following the oral administration of a 100-mg dose and an intravenous administration of a 30-mg dose, are shown in Figure 9.33. Figure 9.33 shows that

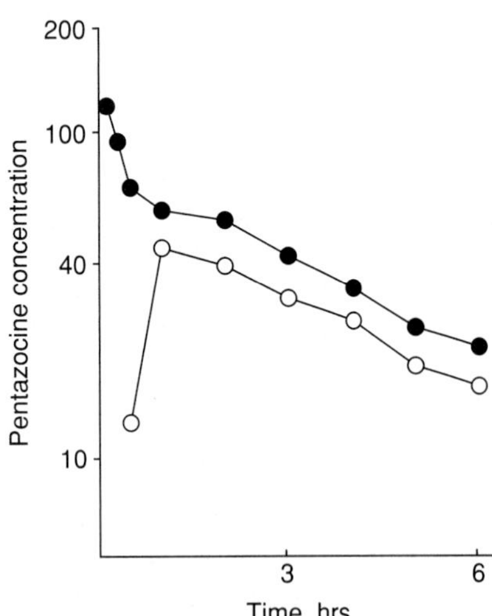

Fig. 9.33. Pentazocine concentration in plasma (ng/mL) after administration of 100 mg orally (○) or 30 mg intravenously (●). (From Ehrnebo M, Boreus L, Lonroth U. Bioavailability and first-pass metabolism of oral pentazocine in man. Clin Pharmacol Ther 1977;22:888–892; with permission.)

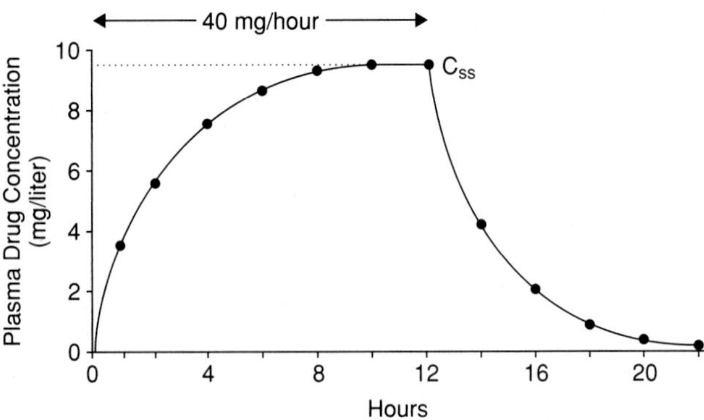

Fig. 9.34. Typical plasma concentration versus time profile following administration of a drug by intravenous infusion.

even though the intravenous dose is smaller, this route of administration provides higher plasma concentration than an oral dose. The systemic availability (F) of pentazocine after oral administration was reported to be 11 to 32%, with a mean of 18%. This low systemic availability is consistent with its high hepatic clearance.

Intravenous Infusion

If a drug is administered intravenously at a constant rate, its plasma concentration at any time will be provided by the following equation:

Eq. 9.97 $$C_p = \frac{Q}{VK}(1 - e^{-Kt})$$

where Q is the constant infusion rate (dose/unit time) and VK is the systemic clearance of the drug.

The plasma drug concentration will rise (Fig. 9.34) with time after the start of an infusion and will slowly approach a constant level, at which the rate of elimination of the drug from the body equals the rate of infusion.

After the commencement of an infusion, it takes approximately 4.32 elimination half-lives of the drug for the plasma concentration of the drug to be within 5% of the constant plateau level and seven elimination half-lives for the concentration to be within 1% of the plateau level. The plateau, or true steady-state, plasma concentration, $(C_p)_{ss}$, can be determined from Equation 9.97 by recognizing that the term (e^{-Kt}) approaches zero with increased time. Therefore,

Eq. 9.98 $$(C_p)_{ss} = \frac{Q}{VK}$$

Equation 9.98 permits one to calculate the infusion rate necessary to attain and then maintain the desired steady-state plasma concentration of a drug if the systemic clearance of the drug is available. Equation 9.98 also provides a convenient way to determine the apparent volume of distribution of a drug by means of intravenous infusion experiment if the infusion rate (Q), the elimination rate constant (K), and the steady-state plasma concentration $(C_p)_{SS}$ are known.

The decline of plasma concentration after the infusion is stopped can be calculated using the following equation:

Eq. 9.99 $$(C_p)_{t'} = (C_p)_T e^{-Kt'}$$

where $(C_p)t'$ is the plasma concentration at time t' following the cessation of infusion, and $(C_p)_T$ is the plasma concentration at the time the infusion is stopped.

Because the time required to reach the steady-state plasma drug concentration will be quite long for a drug with a long elimination half-life, the administration of an intravenous loading dose often is convenient to attain the desired drug concentration immediately and then maintain this concentration by the continuous infusion. The loading dose (D_L) required to attain the desired drug concentration is calculated as follows:

Eq. 9.100 $$D_L = (C_p)_{ss}V$$

Eq. 9.101 $$D_L = \frac{Q}{K}$$

Using Equation 9.98 or 9.101, one can determine the infusion rate (Q) needed to maintain the plasma concentration obtained by the administration of the loading dose (D_L).

Repetitive Drug Administration (Multiple Dosing)

If a fixed intravenous dose of a drug is administered repeatedly at a constant time interval (τ), the plasma

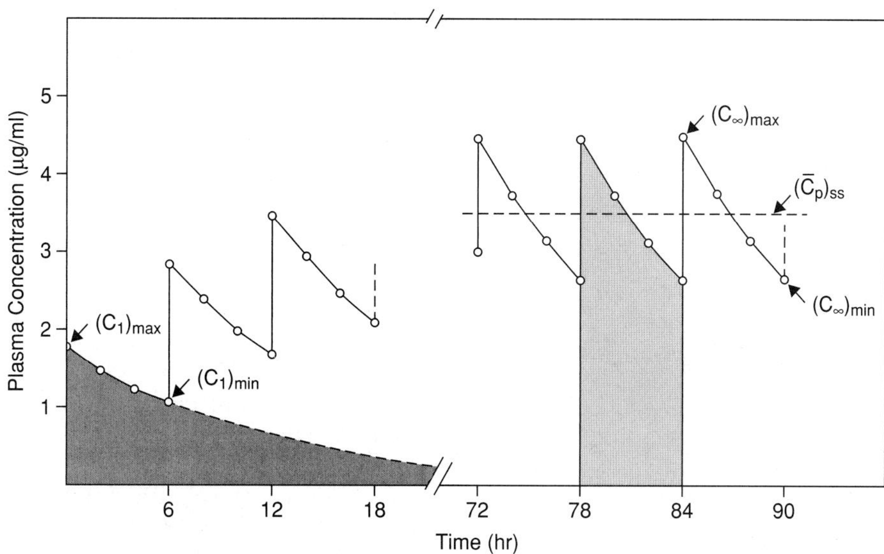

Fig. 9.35. A typical plasma concentration versus time profile for a drug administered intravenously as a fixed dose (X_0) at a fixed dosing interval (τ).

concentration of a drug at any time may be calculated using the following expression:

Eq. 9.102
$$(C_p)_t = \frac{X_0}{V}\left(\frac{1 - e^{-nK\tau}}{1 - e^{-K\tau}}\right)e^{-Kt}.$$

where n is the number of doses that have been administered, t is the time between $t = 0$ and $t = \tau$, τ is dosing interval, X_0 is the dose administered, V is the apparent volume of distribution of the drug, and K is the elimination rate constant. At the plateau, Equation 9.102 reduces to

Eq. 9.103
$$(C_p)_\infty = \frac{X_0}{V}\left(\frac{e^{-Kt}}{1 - e^{-K\tau}}\right)$$

where $(C_p)_\infty$ is the steady-state plasma concentration.

The maximum plasma concentration of a drug (Fig. 9.35) at the steady state, $(C_p)_\infty$ max, and its minimum plasma concentration at the steady state, $(C_p)_\infty$ min, can be determined by setting $t = 0$ and $t = \infty$, respectively. Equation 9.102 then becomes

Eq. 9.104
$$(C_p)_\infty \text{ max} = \frac{X_0}{V}\left(\frac{1}{1 - e^{-K\tau}}\right)$$

and

Eq. 9.105
$$(C_p)_\infty \text{ min} = \frac{X_0}{V}\left(\frac{1}{1 - e^{-K\tau}}\right)e^{-K\tau}$$

When drugs are administered as repetitive doses (multiple doses), it often is of practical use to determine the "average" plasma concentration at the plateau or steady state, $(\bar{C}_p)_{ss}$ average. This is obtained by

Eq. 9.106
$$(\bar{C}_p)_{ss} \text{ average} = \frac{X_0}{VK\tau}$$

where τ is the dosing interval, X_0 is the administered dose, and VK is its systemic clearance. Equation 9.106 clearly indicates that by knowing the apparent volume of distribution and the elimination rate constant, obtained from the administration of a single intravenous bolus dose, the average plasma concentration of a drug can be predicted for the intravenous bolus administration of a fixed dose (X_0) at a constant dosing interval (τ). Equation 9.106 clearly indicates that only the size of the dose (X_0) and the dosing interval (τ) may be adjusted to obtain the desired average steady-state plasma drug concentration.

It is important to recognize that the average steady-state plasma drug concentration, $(\bar{C}_p)_{ss}$ average, is neither the arithmatic nor geometric mean of $(C_p)_\infty$ max and $(C_p)_\infty$ min but, rather, the ratio of the area under the plasma concentration–time curve during the dosing interval (τ) at the plateau over the dosing interval (τ). We know from Equation 9.82 that the ratio of a dose over systemic clearance (VK) equals the area under the plasma concentration–time curve, $(\text{AUC})_0^\infty$. Therefore, substituting dose/clearance from Equation 9.82 into Equation 9.106 provides the following:

Eq. 9.107
$$(C_p)_{ss} \text{ average} = \frac{(\text{AUC})_0^\infty}{\tau}$$

where $(\text{AUC})_0^\infty$ represents the area under the plasma drug concentration–time curve following the administration of a single intravenous bolus dose.

When the drug is administered by oral route (Fig. 9.36), the mathematical expressions are more complex than analogous equations for intravenous administration:

Eq. 9.108
$$(C_p)_\infty = \frac{K_a F(X_a)_0}{V(K_a - K)}\left(\frac{e^{-Kt}}{1 - e^{-K\tau}} - \frac{e^{-K_a t}}{1 - e^{-K_a\tau}}\right)$$

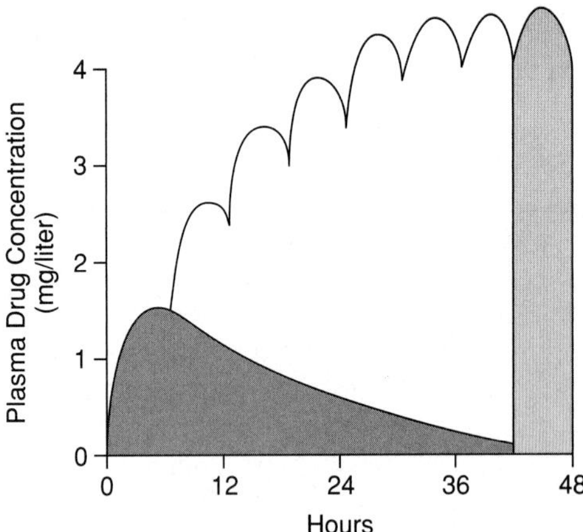

Fig. 9.36. A typical plasma concentration versus time profile for a drug administered orally as a fixed dose $(X_a)_0$ at a fixed dosing interval (τ).

where $(X_a)_0$ is the dose administered; F is the fraction absorbed; K_a and K are the first-order absorption and the elimination rate constants, respectively; V is the apparent volume of distribution; and t and τ are time and dosing intervals, respectively. Following the administration of each successive dose in the postabsorption period, Equation 9.100 reduces to

Eq. 9.109 $$(C_p)_\infty \min = \frac{K_a F (X_a)_0}{V(K_a - K)}\left(\frac{e^{-K\tau}}{1 - e^{-K\tau}}\right)$$

The average steady-state plasma concentration of a drug when administered by an extravascular route can be obtained using the following equation:

Eq. 9.110 $$(C_p)_{ss} \text{ average} = \frac{F(X_a)_0}{VK\tau}$$

or, by substituting Eq. 9.84 into Eq. 9.110,

Eq. 9.111 $$(C_p)_{ss} \text{ average} = \frac{(\text{AUC})_0^\infty}{\tau}$$

where F is the fraction absorbed or absolute bioavailability of a drug. Taking the ratio of Equations 9.110 over 9.106 following the attainment of the steady-state condition permits one to determine the bioavailability of a drug; of course, this assumes that the administered doses are identical.

Repeated administration of a fixed dose at a constant dosing interval (τ) produces a gradual increase of drug levels in the body until the steady-state condition is attained. This increase is the result of drug accumulation factor (R) because of the sequential dosing of the drug. Therefore, predicting the degree of accumulation of a drug under defined conditions becomes important. Multiplying each side of Equation 9.106 by the apparent volume of distribution and dividing by the administered dose, Equation 9.112 is obtained:

Eq. 9.112 $$\frac{X_{ss} \text{ average}}{X_0} = \frac{1}{K\tau} = \frac{1.44t_{1/2}}{\tau}$$

where

$$X_{ss} \text{ average}/X_0 = R = \text{drug accumulation factor}$$

where X_{ss} average is the "average" amount of drug in the body at the steady-state condition. The ratio of the average amount of a drug at its steady state and the administered dose is defined as drug accumulation (R). Equation 9.112 describes that the magnitude of drug accumulation is a function of the elimination half-life of a drug and the chosen dosing interval. For example, if a drug with an elimination half-life of 12 hours (i.e., $K = 0.0577$ hr^{-1}) is administered every 6 hours (τ), the ratio of X_{ss} average over dose is 2.9. This means that repeated administration of a fixed dose of a drug in the body is approximately 2.9-fold the amount administered in a single dose. It also is clear from Equation 9.112 that the drug accumulation ratio (R) is directly proportional to the elimination half-life of the drug ($t_{1/2}$) and inversely proportional to the dosing interval (τ); however, R is independent of the size of the administered dose.

Because considerable time may elapse before a steady-state condition is attained as a result of repeated drug administration, it often is desirable to administer a large dose initially (i.e., loading dose) to achieve the desired drug levels immediately. Equation 9.42, which describes the time course of drug concentration after a single intravenous bolus dose, may be written as

Eq. 9.113 $$(C_p)_1 \min = \frac{X_0}{V}(e^{-K\tau})$$

where $(C_p)_1$ min is the drug concentration immediately before administration of the second dose of the same size as the first one (i.e., the minimum concentration occurs at $t = \tau$ following administration of the first dose). The minimum steady-state plasma concentration, $(C_p)_\infty$ min, is given by Equation 9.105. Thus, the ratio of $(C_p)_\infty$ min to $(C_p)_1$ min (i.e., Eqs. 9.105 and 9.113) is another way to measure the drug accumulation (R). This ratio may be calculated by means of the following expression:

Eq. 9.114 $$R = \frac{(C_p)_\infty \min}{(C_p)_1 \min} = \frac{1}{1 - e^{-K\tau}}$$

This ratio of minimum drug concentrations, numerically, is not equal to the ratio of the "average" dose of a drug at steady state and the dose administered (Eq. 9.112).

If one wished to administer a loading dose (D_L) that produces the minimum concentration equal to $(C_p)_\infty$ min:

Eq. 9.115 $$(C_p)_1 \min = (C_p)_\infty \min = \frac{D_L}{V} e^{-K\tau}$$

Dividing the Equation 9.105 by Equation 9.115 will result in

Eq. 9.116 $$1 = \frac{D}{D_L(1 - e^{-K\tau})}$$

Equation 9.116, on rearrangement, yields an expression to determine the loading dose (D_L):

Eq. 9.117 $$\frac{D_L}{D} = \frac{1}{(1 - e^{-K\tau})}$$

In Equations 9.116 and 9.117, D_L is the loading dose and D is the maintenance dose. Equation 9.117 permits the calculation of loading dose for the chosen maintenance dose and dosing interval (τ) and is applicable for the administration of a drug not only by an intravenous bolus but also by the extravascular route. When a drug is administered by the extravascular route, however, it is essential that each maintenance dose be administered following the complete absorption of a drug from the previous dose. Conversely, Equation 9.117 also permits the determination of the maintenance dose required to maintain the minimum drug level produced by the administration of the initial dose for any chosen dosing interval.

Plasma Protein Binding in Pharmacokinetics

Drug binding to plasma proteins affects drug distribution and elimination as well as the pharmacological effect of a drug. The high molecular weight of plasma proteins restricts their passage across capillaries, and their low lipid solubility prevents them from crossing the cell membrane. Analogously, binding of drugs to plasma protein restricts their passage across cell membranes. Only that fraction of the drug concentration that is freely circulating or unbound can penetrate the cell membrane and be subject to glomerular filtration. Hepatic metabolism of most drugs is also limited by the availability of free fraction of drug in the blood. Because the interaction of drugs with plasma protein is a rapidly reversible process, one may view the plasma protein-binding phenomenon as being temporary storage of a drug, subject to instant recall.

Drug binding to plasma protein may be attributed to ionic, Van der Waals, and hydrogen bonding. The most important contribution to drug binding in the plasma is made by albumin, which comprises approximately 50% of the total plasma protein. In healthy subjects, albumin concentration in the plasma is approximately 4 g/100 mL. During pregnancy and other diseases, however, low levels of plasma protein may be observed. Albumin binds a wide variety of drug molecules; however, it plays a particularly important role in the binding of weak acidic and neutral drugs.

α_1-Acid glycoprotein is another important binding protein with an affinity for basic drugs. α_1-Acid glycoprotein is a low-molecular-weight protein. It is an acute-phase reactant, and its concentration in plasma rises in inflammation, malignant diseases, and stress. Conversely, its plasma concentration falls in hepatic diseases and nephrotic syndrome. The average concentration of α_1-acid glycoprotein is approximately 40 to 100 mg/100 mL. The presence of other plasma proteins plays a limited role in drug binding. The drug proteins interactions can be described by applying the law of mass action:

Eq. 9.118 $$D_F + \text{free sites} \underset{K_2}{\overset{K_1}{\rightleftharpoons}} D_B$$

where D_F and D_B represent the free and bound drug, respectively, and K_1 and K_2 are the rate constant of association and dissociation, respectively. Thus,

Eq. 9.119 $$K = \frac{K_1}{K_2} = \frac{[D_B]}{[D_F][\text{free sites}]}$$

Eq. 9.120 $$K = \frac{K_1}{K_2} = \frac{[D_B]}{[D_F][nP - D_B]}$$

where K is the equilibrium association constant, K_1 and K_2 are binding rate constants, n is the number of available binding sites per mole of protein, and $[D_F]$, $[D_B]$, and P are the molar concentration of free drug, bound drug, and protein, respectively.

The binding rate constants K_1 and K_2 appear to be large, because the equilibrium is established almost immediately. The value of the equilibrium constant (K) varies from zero, at which essentially no drug is bound, to greater than 10^6, at which almost all drug is bound to the protein. The fraction of drug in the plasma that is free or unbound (f_p) is then obtained as follows:

Eq. 9.121 $$f_p = \frac{[D_F]}{[D_F] + [D_B]}$$

Eq. 9.122 $$f_p = \frac{[D_F]}{[D_T]}$$

where $[D_T]$ is the total drug concentration in the plasma. In most cases, for a given amount of drug in the body, the greater the binding of drug to plasma protein and the larger is the total drug concentration of drug in the plasma. Changes in drug binding usually affect the blood level of total drug and play a role in pharmacokinetic variability.

The free fraction of drug in the plasma (f_p) depends on the magnitude of the equilibrium constant (K), the total drug concentration, $[D_T]$, and the protein concentration, $[P]$. In theory, there are limited numbers of binding sites on the protein. As the drug concentration in the plasma increases, the number of available free sites decreases; therefore, the fraction of available free drug increases. In reality, however, the fraction unbound drug in plasma for most drugs, when administered in therapeutic doses, is essentially constant over the entire drug concentration range. Concentration-dependent changes in the fraction of free drug in the plasma are most likely to occur with drugs exhibiting a high association constant ($K = 10^5$ to 10^6) administered in large doses.

The relationship between bioavailability and area under the plasma concentration–time curve is nonlinear and absorption rate dependent when the plasma protein binding of a drug is concentration dependent. Two drug products from which a drug is equally well absorbed will produce different values for the area under the plasma concentration–time curve if a difference exists in the absorption rate. Generally, such a comparison will overestimate the extent of drug absorption of the more slowly absorbed product.

The clearance of many drugs from blood is directly proportional to free fraction in the plasma (f_p). The steady-state concentrations of these drugs is inversely proportional to the free fraction in the plasma. On the other hand, clearance of some drugs is largely independent of plasma protein binding. The direction and magnitude of the effect of plasma protein binding on the elimination half-life of a drug depends on the size of the drug's apparent volume of distribution (V) and whether the drug exhibits restrictive clearance (i.e., has an intrinsic clearance less than the liver blood flow). The half-life of a restrictively cleared drug with relatively small apparent volume of distribution (i.e., $V < 0.25$ L/kg) may show a small decrease in elimination half-life when there is decrease in plasma protein binding (i.e., an increase in the free fraction in plasma. Conversely, the half-life of a nonrestrictively cleared drug with a small apparent volume of distribution may show a small increase in half life when the free fraction is increased. Drugs with a large value for the apparent volume of distribution (i.e., $V > 0.5$ L/kg) either will be essentially independent of the changes in plasma protein binding (restrictive clearance) or will show an increase in half-life that is directly proportional to the increase in free fraction (nonrestrictive clearance).

The classical methods of studying protein binding of drugs include equilibrium dialysis and ultrafiltration. The latter may provide quick measurements but is not necessarily as accurate as the equilibrium dialysis method. Detailed discussions on this may be found in textbooks listed in *Suggested Readings.*

Statistical Moment Analysis

Statistical moment analysis is a noncompartmental method, based on statistical moment theory, for calculation of the absorption, distribution, and elimination parameters of a drug. This approach to estimating pharmacokinetic parameters has gained considerable attention in recent years.

Table 9.9. Drug Concentration and Drug Concentration–Time Data During and After a 1-Hour, Constant-Rate Infusion

Time (hours)	Concentration (μg/mL)	Concentration-Time (μg/mL/hr)
0.5	3.2	1.6
1.0	5.9	5.9
2.0	4.2	8.4
3.0	3.0	9.0
4.0	2.1	8.4
5.0	1.5	7.5
6.0	1.1	6.6
8.0	0.5	4.0

The zero moment in the drug plasma concentration–time curve is the total area under the plasma concentration–time curve from $t = 0$ to $t = \infty$, $(\mathrm{AUC})_0^\infty$. Estimates of the area under this curve are useful in calculating bioavailability as well as drug clearance, which is the ratio of dose over area under the concentration–time curve for an intravenous dose.

The first moment of the plasma concentration–time profile is the total area under the concentration–time curve resulting from plot of the product of plasma concentration and time (i.e., $C_p t$) versus time, as illustrated in Table 9.9 and Figure 9.37 (39).

Column 2 of Table 9.9 shows the concentration vs. time data obtained following a 1-hour constant-rate infusion, and column 3 also includes concentration-time values for the product of concentration × time. These values are plotted against time in Figure 9.34. The area

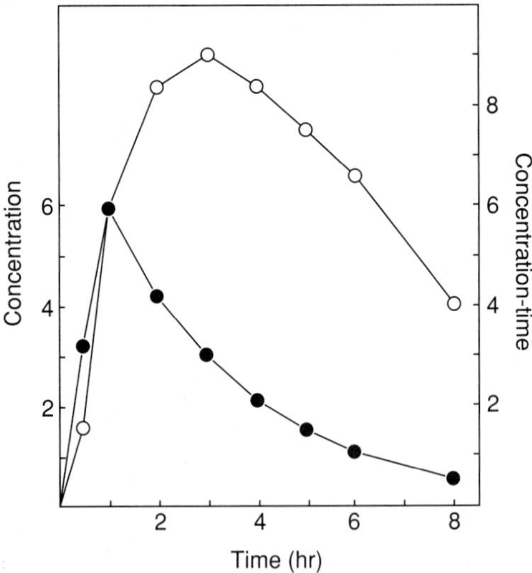

Fig. 9.37. Plots of drug concentration (μg/mL; ●) and drug concentration × time (μg/mL/hr; ○) versus time during and after 1 hour of a constant-rate infusion. The area under the concentration versus time plot to infinity is AUC; the area under the concentration × time versus time plot to infinity is AUMC. (From Gibaldi M. Biopharmaceutics and Clinical Pharmacokinetics, 4th Ed. Philadelphia: Lea and Febiger, 1991; with permission.)

under the curve for the concentration–time plot can be obtained by employing trapezoidal rule. The total area under the curve for the product of concentration × time is termed the "area under the first-moment curve" (AUMC).

The ratio of the AUMC over the area under the concentration–time curve for any drug, according to the theory, is the assessment of the mean residence time (MRT). The MRT provides a quantitative estimate of the persistence of a drug in the body, and like the half-life of a drug, MRT or persistence is a function of distribution and elimination of a drug. Comparison of MRTs following administration of a drug as an intravenous bolus or via any other extravascular route provides information regarding the mean absorption time (MAT).

One of the most useful properties of statistical moment analysis is that it permits estimation of the apparent volume of distribution that is independent of drug elimination (i.e. regardless of the model chosen to describe the concentration time data).

Mean Residence Time (MRT)

The MRT of a drug following administration of a single dose is provided by the following equation:

Eq. 9.123 $$\text{MRT} = \frac{\text{AUMC}}{\text{AUC}}$$

The MRT for a drug administered intravenously provides a useful estimate of the persistence time in the body. Therefore, in this sense, it is related to the half-life of a drug. When applied to a drug that distributes rapidly (i.e., one-compartment model), it has been shown that

Eq. 9.124 $$\text{MRT} = \frac{1}{K}$$

where K is the elimination rate constant.

Because the half-life of a drug is equal to $0.693/K$, half-life is a measurement of the time required to eliminate 50% of the administered dose. The MRT, on the other hand, indicates the time required to eliminate 63.2% of the administered dose.

When a drug is administered by an extravascular route, statistical moment analysis theory also can be employed for estimating the rate of absorption. This approach, however, requires the calculation of MRT for intravascular as well as extravascular routes, because the method is based on the differences in MRT for different modes of administration. In general,

Eq. 9.125 $$\text{MAT} = (\text{MRT})_{\text{EV}} - (\text{MRT})_{\text{IV}}$$

where $(\text{MRT})_{\text{EV}}$ is the MRT following administration of a drug by an extravascular route and $(\text{MRT})_{\text{IV}}$ is the MRT for the intravenous bolus dose. When the administered drug follows the first-order process,

Eq. 9.126 $$(\text{MRT})_{\text{EV}} = \frac{1}{K_a}$$

where K_a is the first-order absorption rate constant. Under these conditions,

Eq. 9.127 $$K_a = \frac{1}{\text{MAT}}$$

and the absorption half-life is obtained by 0.693/MAT.

The statistical moment theory offers an attractive alternative for the evaluation and estimation of the absorption data, and even in the absence of intravenous data, this method permits the ranking of several dosage forms, with respect to drug release and absorption, from the available MRT values.

SUMMARY

From this discussion, the efficacy of a drug is not determined by its pharmacodynamic characteristics alone, but efficacy also depends, to a large extent, on the pharmacokinetic parameters of the drug, because ADME processes control the rate and extent to which an administered dose of a drug reaches its site of action.

In light of a high degree of structural variability of drugs, multiplicity of kinetics and metabolite kinetics, the task of establishing a clear correlation between the structured chemistry of substituents and their pharmacokinetic properties appears somewhat daunting. The pharmacokinetic fate of a drug molecule, however, appears to be a consequence of its physicochemical properties and, therefore, may, to some extent, be predicted from its chemical structure.

Although the drug in the formulation has received considerable attention, many of the alterations in the formulation may be considered as chemical changes. Most of what has been reported applies primarily to the gastrointestinal absorption of drugs and may be viewed as attempts to:

1. Maximize the rate of absorption by increasing the rate of dissolution (i.e., micronization, salt of acid or bases, amorphous form and metastable polymorph, etc.).
2. Decrease the loss of a drug because of its degradation in the stomach (i.e., acid, insoluble esters or salt, and chemically stable derivatives of a drug).
3. Extend the duration of action by reducing the rate of a drug's release from a dosage form (e.g., timed release, depot-forming injectable, macrocrystals, and slowly dissolving salts).
4. Decrease the loss of a drug by reducing the complex formation.

These examples for enhancing gastrointestinal absorption represent the response to a particular problem with the parent compound and, therefore, may be viewed as "corrective" research. It is of considerable interest to see this aspect of research become "predictive and preventive," in which the pharmacokinetic parameters of drugs are required in the early phases of drug design to optimize the effectiveness of drugs.

An immediate problem facing those who would consider optimizing all factors of a drug is physically locating the receptor site and defining the ideal time course for the drug–receptor interaction, sustained effects, and so on. An ideal drug molecule should reach the site of action, arrive rapidly in sufficient quantity, remain at the site of action for sufficient time, be excluded from other sites, and be removed from the site, when appropriate. Such an ideal drug molecule rarely exists, however, and alternate approaches are chosen to optimize the effectiveness of a drug. Furthermore, if a correlation exists between a biological response and the blood levels of a drug in the biological fluid, then the pharmacokinetic parameters play an important role in influencing the biological response, because these parameters influence the magnitude of the blood level of a drug in the body. The task of examining the examples of drugs illustrating the connection between biological response and pharmacokinetics study is not an easy one, but the results do convey the important facts that:

1. Pharmacokinetic parameters influence the biological responses, which are critical in drug design, and
2. Pharmacokinetic parameters can be modified by subtle structural changes, which in turn may influence the desired blood level.

The ultimate goal is to design a drug molecule that exhibits the desired pharmacological effect as a result of the proper balance of ADME processes. Figure 9.37 illustrates how modification of a parent structure can influence the availability of a drug to the receptor site (53).

The following are some of the processes shown in Figure 9.38 that may be altered by changing a substituent group on the drug molecule:

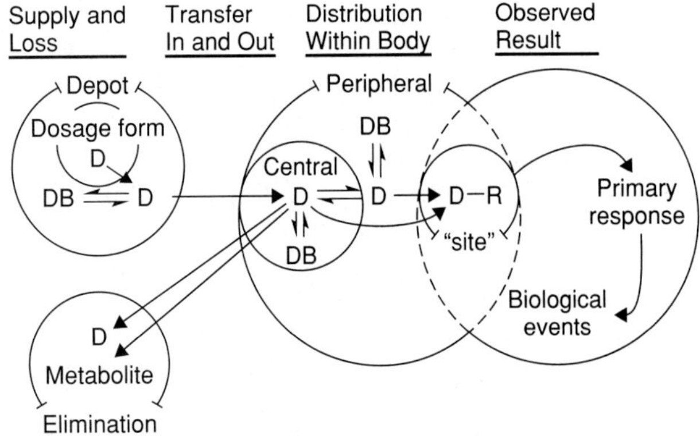

Fig. 9.38. How some of the processes can be altered by changing a substituent group on a drug molecule.

I. Supply and loss:
 A) Rate of transfer from the dosage form.
 B) Binding of a drug in the depot and
 C) Stability of a drug in the depot.
II. Distribution in the body:
 A) Binding of a drug in the central and peripheral compartments.
 B) Apparent volume of distribution and
 C) Transfer of a drug to the receptor sites.
III. Drug-receptor interaction.

Consider the following well-known example for the design of a urinary tract anti-effective. The site of infection is the urinary tract. The example selected is the prodrug, methenamine. In acidic pH, methenamine is converted to formaldehyde, which acts as an antibacterial agent (Fig. 9.39). Tablets of methenamine often are enteric coated to prevent conversion to formaldehyde in the stomach. Methenamine is cleared intact from the kidney into the urine, where it is hydrolyzed to formaldehyde if the pH is less than 6.5. The rate of hydrolysis is controlled by the urinary pH.

The influence of structural effects on pharmacokinetic parameters can be illustrated using the following examples: The steady-state levels of the antibiotic carbenicillin are twice those of ampicillin. These higher blood levels of carbenicillin following intravenous administration have been attributed to its efficacy in the treatment of relatively resistant infections, such as *Pseudomonas* sp. The reason for these differences in the higher steady-state plasma concentration is the larger apparent volume of distribution for ampicillin, because the elimination rate constants are similar. If all the factors were equal, one may argue that an increased value for the apparent volume of distribution is a clinical advantage, because bacteria germinate more frequently in the tissue than in the blood. The effectiveness of an antibiotic depends on its penetration into tissues, particularly inflamed tissue. Thus, if plasma protein binding is equal for both antibiotics, the antibiotic with a larger volume of distribution would appear to be reaching the site of action with better efficacy, but this is by no means unequivocal. Therefore, the spectrum of research activity in the area of antibiotics would imply that the following goals for molecular modifications are generally pursued:

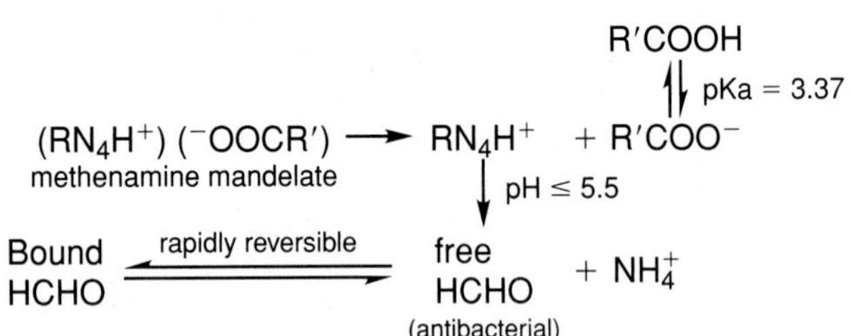

Fig. 9.39. Conversion of methenamine to formaldehyde in acidic pH.

1. Increased tissue distribution.
2. Longer half-life to maintain a higher blood level and decrease the frequency of dose administration.
3. Decreased binding capacity to foods and plasma protein.

ACKNOWLEDGMENT

The author would like to acknowledge Dr. Philip Breen, Associate Professor of Pharmaceutics, School of Pharmacy and the University of Arkansas for Medical Sciences, for helpful discussions and suggestions in preparing this chapter.

References

1. Ariens EJ. Intrinsic activity: partial agonists and partial antagonists. J Cardiovasc Pharmacol 1983;5:S8–S15.
2. Venter JC, Fraser CM. Mechanism of action and regulation. In: Kito S, Segawa T, Kuriyama K, eds. Neurotransmitter Receptors. New York: Plenum Press, 1984.
3. Lefkowitz RJ, Stadel JM, Caron MG. Adenylate cyclase–coupled β-adrenergic receptors: structure and mechanisms of activation and desensitization. Annu Rev Biochem 1983;52:159–186.
4. Florence AT, Attwood D. Physiochemical Principles of Pharmacy; 2nd Ed. New York: Chapman and Hall, 1988.
5. Schanker LS. Absorption of drugs from the rat colon. J Pharmacol Exp Ther 1959;126:283–294.
6. Wagner JG. Biopharmaceutics and Relevant Pharmacokinetics. Hamilton, IL: The Hamilton Press, 1971.
7. Shore PA, Brodie BB, Hogben CAM. The gastric secretion of drugs: a pH partition hypothesis. J Pharmacol Exp Ther 1957;119:361–369.
8. Hogben CAM, Tocco DJ, Brodie BB, et al. On the mechanism of intestinal absorption of drugs. J Pharmacol Exp Ther 1959;125:275–282.
9. Schanker LS. On the mechanism of absorption of drugs from the gastrointestinal tract. J Med Pharm Chem 1960;2:343–359.
10. Schanker LS. Mechanism of drug absorption and distribution. Annu Rev Pharmacol 1961;1:29–44.
11. Schanker LS. Passage of drugs across the gastrointestinal epithelium in drugs and membrane. In: Hogben CAM, ed. Proceedings of the First International Pharmacology Meeting, vol 4. New York: The Macmillan Company, 1963.
12. Schanker LS. Physiological transport of drug. In: Harper NJ, Simons AB, eds. Advances in Drug Research. London: Academic Press, 1966:71–106.
13. Rowland M, Tozer T. Clinical Pharmacokinetics: Concepts and Application, 2nd Ed. Philadelphia: Lea and Febiger, 1989.
14. Schanker LS. Absorption of drugs from the rat small intestine. J Pharmacol Exp Ther 1958;128:81–87.
15. Zimmerman JJ, Feldman S. Physical–chemical properties and biologic activity. In: Foye WO, ed. Principles of Medicinal Chemistry, 3rd Ed. Philadelphia: Lea and Febiger, 1988:7–38.
16. Winne D. The influence of unstirred layers on intestinal absorption in intestinal permeation. In: Kramer M, Lauterbach F, eds. Workshop Conference Hoechest, vol 4. Amsterdam: Excerpta Medica, 1977:58–64.
17. Levy G, Leonard JR, Procknal JA. Development of in vitro dissolution tests which correlate quantitatively with dissolution rate limited absorption. J Pharm Sci 1965;54:1319–1325.
18. Kwan KC. Oral bioavailability and first-pass effects. Drug Metab Drug Dispos 1997;25:1329–1336.
19. Burton P, Goodwin J, Vidamas T, et al. Predicting drug absorption: how nature made it a difficult problem. J Pharmacol Exp Ther 2002;303:889–895.
20. Lipinsky CA, Lombordo F, Dominy W, et al. Experimental and computational approaches to estimate solubility and permeability in drug discovery and development settings. Adv Drug Deliv Rev 1997;23:3–25.
21. Stewart B, Wang Y, Surendran N. Ex. In vivo approaches to predicting oral pharmacokinetics in humans. In: Ann Repts Med Chem. Trauma, 6 ed, Academic Press, 2000;35:299–307.
22. Ertl P, Rohde B, Selzer P. Fast calculation of molecular polar surface area as a sum of fragment-based contributions and its application to the prediction of drug transport properties. J Med Chem 2000;43:3714–3717.
23. Sinko PJ, Leesman GD, Amidon GL. Predicting fraction of dose absorbed in humans using a macroscopic mass-balance approach. Pharm Res 1991;8:979–988
24. Artusson P, Karlsson J. Correlation between oral drug absorption in humans and the apparent drug permeability coefficient in human intestinal epithelia (Caco-2) cells. Biochem Biophys Res Commun 1991;14:880–885.
25. Avdeef A. Absorption and Drug Development: Solubility, Permeability, and Charge State. New York: Wiley-Interscience, 2003.
26. Hilgers AR, Smith DP, Biermacher JJ, et al. Predicting oral absorption of drugs: a case study with novel class of antimicrobial agents. Pharm Res 2003;20:1149–1155.
27. Amidon GL, Sinko PJ, Fleisher D. Estimating human oral fraction dose absorbed: a correlation using rat intestinal permeability for passive and carrier-mediated compounds. Pharm Res 1988;5:651–654.
28. Dressman JB, Fleisher D. Mixing-tank model for predicting dissolution rate control oral absorption. J Pharm Sci 1986;75:109–116.
29. Johnson DA, Amidon GL. Determination of intrinsic transport parameters from perfused intestine experiments: a boundary layer approach to estimating the aqueous and unbiased membrane permeability. J Theor Biol 1988; 131:93–106.
30. Hidalgo I. Assessing the absorption of new pharmaceuticals. Curr Top Med Chem 2001;1:385–401.
31. Fleisher D, Cheng L, Zhou Y, et al. Drug, meal, and formulation interactions influencing drug absorption after oral administration: clinical implications. Clin Pharmacokinet 1999;36:233–254.
32. Amidon G, Lenncranas H, Shah V, et al. A theoretical basis for a biopharmaceutics drug classification: the correlation of in vitro drug product and in vivo bioavailability. Pharm Res 1995;12:413–420.
33. Kunta JR, Sinko PJ. Intestinal drug transporters: in vivo function and clinical importance. Curr Drug Metab 2004;5:109–124.
34. Matheney C, Lamb M, Brouwer K, et al. Pharmacokinetics and pharmacodynamic implications of P-glycoprotein modulation. Reviews of Therapeutics 2001;21:778–796.
35. Foltz EL. Clinical pharmacology of pivampicillin. Antimicrob Agents Chemother 1970;10:442–454.
36. Surendran N, Covits KMY, Han HK, et al. Evidence for overlapping substrate specificity between large neutral amino acid (LNAA) and dipeptide (hPEPT1) transporters for PD 158473, an NMDT antagonist. Pharm Res 1999;16:391–395.
37. Lin J, Chiba M, Baillie T. Is the role of the small intestine in first-pass metabolism overemphasized? Pharmacol Rev 1999;51:135–157.
38. Noyes NA, Whitney WR. The rate of solution of solid substances in their own solution. J Am Chem Soc 1897;19:930–942.
39. Gibaldi M. Biopharmaceutics and Clinical Pharmacokinetics, 4th Ed. Philadelphia: Lea and Febiger, 1991.
40. Ogata H, Shibazoki T, Inoue T, et al. Studies on dissolution tests of solid dosage forms. IV. Relation of absorption sites of sulfonamides administered orally in solid dosage forms to their solubilities and dissolution rates. Chem Pharm Bull 1979;27:1281–1286.
41. Pottage A, Nimmo J, Prescott LF. The absorption of aspirin and paracetamol in patients with achlorhydria. J Pharm Pharmacol 1974;26:144–145.
42. Juncher H, Raaschou F. Solubility of oral preparation of penicillin V. Antibiotic Med 1957;4:497–507.
43. Anderson KW. Oral absorption of quinalbarbitone and its sodium salt. Arch Int Pharmacodyn Ther 1964;147:171–177.
44. Grant DJW. Theory and origin of polymorphism. In: Brittain HG, ed. Polymorphism in Pharmaceutical Solids. New York: Marcel Dekker, 1999:1–34.
45. Brittain HG, Grant DJW. Effect of polymorphism and solid-state solvation on solubility and dissolution rate. In: Brittain HG, ed. Polymorphism in Pharmaceutical Solids. New York: Marcel Dekker, 1999:34–66.
46. Johnson KC, Swindell AC. Guidance in the setting of drug particle size specifications to minimize variability in drug absorption. Pharm Res 1996;13:1795–1798.
47. Dressman JB, Amidon GL, Fleisher D. Absorption potential: estimating the fraction absorbed for orally administered compounds. J Pharm Sci 1985;74:588–589.
48. Lombardo F, Obach RS, Dicapua FM, et al. A hybrid mixture discriminant analysis–random forest computational model for the prediction of volume of distribution of drugs in human. J Med Chem. 2006;49:2262–2267.
49. Lombardo F, Obach RS, Shalaeva MY, et al. Prediction of volume of distribution values in humans for neutral and basic drugs using physicochemical measurements and plasma protein binding data. J Med Chem 2002;45:2867–2876.
50. Lombardo F, Obach RS, Shalaeva MY, et al. Prediction of human volume of distribution values for neutral and basic drugs. 2. Extended data set and leave-class-out statistics. J Med Chem 2004;47:1242–1250.
51. Nelson E. Comparative dissolution rates of weak acids and their sodium salts. J Am Pharm Assoc (Sci Ed) 1958;47:297–299.
52. Ehrnebo M, Boreus L, Lonroth U. Bioavailability and first-pass metabolism of oral pentazocine in man. Clin Pharmacol Ther 1977;22:888–892.
53. Notari R. Pharmacokinetics and molecular modification: implications in drug design and evaluation. J Pharm Sci 1973;62:865–881.

Suggested Readings

Avdeef A. Absorption and Drug Development: Solubility, Permeability, and Charge State. New York: Wiley-Interscience, 2003.

Ganellin C, Roberts S. eds. Medicinal Chemistry: The Role of Organic Chemistry in Drug Research, 2nd Ed. New York: Academic Press, 1993.

Garrett E. Classical pharmacokinetics to frontiers. J Pharmacokinet Biopharm 1973;1:341–361.

Gibaldi M. Biopharmaceutics and Clinical Pharmacokinetics, 4th Ed. Philadelphia: Lea and Febiger, 1991.

Gibaldi M, Perrier D. Pharmacokinetics, 2nd Ed., vol 15: Drugs and the Pharmaceutical Sciences. New York: Marcel Dekker, 1982.

Horter D, Dressman JB. Influence of physiochemical properties on dissolution of drugs in the gastrointestinal tract. Adv Drug Deliv Rev 2001;46:75–87.

Hug C. Pharmacokinetics of drugs administered intravenously. Anesth Analg 1978;57:704–723.

Rowland M, Tozer T. Clinical Pharmacokinetics: Concepts and Application, 3rd Ed. Philadelphia: Lea and Febiger, 1994.

Taylor J, Kennewell P. Modern Medicinal Chemistry: Ellis Horwood Series in Pharmaceutical Technology. New York: Ellis Horwood, 1993.

Wagner J. A Modern view of pharmacokinetics. J Pharmacokinet Biopharm 1973;1:363–401.

Wagner J. Do you need a pharmacokinetic model, and, if so, which one? J Pharmacokinet Biopharm 1975;3:457–478.

Welling P. Pharmacokinetics: Processes and Mathematics. Monograph 185. Washington. DC: American Chemical Society, 1986.

Wermuth C, Koga N, Konig H, et al. Medicinal Chemistry for the 21st Century. Boston: Blackwell Scientific Publications, 1992.

10. *Drug Metabolism*

DAVID A. WILLIAMS

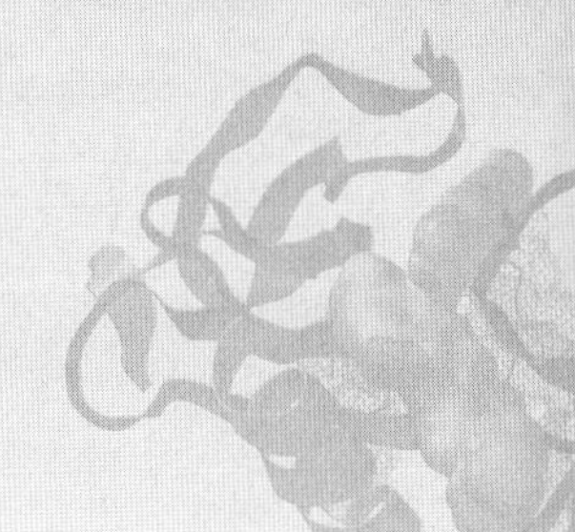

What is a poison?
All substances are poisons;
There is none that is not a poison.
The right dose differentiates a poison
from a drug.

—PARACELSUS (1493–1541)

INTRODUCTION

Humans are exposed throughout their lifetime to a large variety of drugs and nonessential exogenous (foreign) compounds (collectively termed "xenobiotics") that may pose health hazards. Drugs taken for therapeutic purposes as well as occupational or private exposure to the vapors of volatile chemicals or solvents pose possible health risks; smoking and drinking involve the absorption of large amounts of substances with potential adverse health effects. Furthermore, the ingestion of natural toxins in vegetables and fruits, pesticide residues in food, as well as carcinogenic pyrolysis products from fats and protein formed during the charbroiling of meat have to be considered. Most of these xenobiotics undergo enzymatic biotransformations by xenobiotic-metabolizing enzymes in the liver and extrahepatic tissues and are eliminated by excretion as hydrophilic metabolites. In some cases, especially during oxidative metabolism, numerous chemical procarcinogens form reactive metabolites capable of covalent binding to biopolymers, such as proteins or nucleic acids—critical components that can lead to mutagenicity, cytotoxicity, and carcinogenicity. Therefore, insight regarding the biotransformation and bioactivation of xenobiotics becomes an indisputable prerequisite for the assessment of drug safety and risk estimation of chemicals and drugs.

Detoxication and toxic effects of drugs and other xenobiotics have been studied extensively in various mammalian species. Frequently, differences in sensitivity to these toxic effects were observed and can now be attributed to genetic differences between species in the isoenzyme/isoforms of cytochrome P450 monooxygenases (CYP450). The level of expression of the CYP450 enzymes is regulated by genetics and a variety of endogenous factors, such as hormones, gender, age, and disease, as well as the presence of environmental factors, such as inducing agents. Drugs were developed and prescribed under the old paradigm that "one dose fits all," which largely ignores the fact that humans (both adults and children) are genetically and metabolically different, resulting in a variable response to drugs.

Drugs can no longer be regarded as chemically stable entities that elicit the desired pharmacological response and then are excreted from the body. Drugs undergo a variety of chemical changes in humans by enzymes of the liver, intestine, kidney, lung, and other tissues, with subsequent alterations in the nature of their pharmacological activity, duration of activity, and toxicity. Thus, the pharmacological and toxicological activity of a drug (or xenobiotic) is, in many ways, the consequence of its metabolism.

Drug therapy is becoming oriented more toward controlling metabolic, genetic, and environmental illnesses (e.g., cardiovascular disease, mental illness, cancer, and diabetes) rather than short-term therapy. In most of these cases, drug therapy lasts for months or even years, and the problem of drug toxicity from long-term therapy has become increasingly important.

The practice of prescribing several drugs simultaneously is common. Thus, an awareness of possible drug–drug interactions is essential to avoid catastrophic synergistic effects and chemical, enzymic, and pharmacokinetic interactions that may produce toxic side effects.

The study of xenobiotic metabolism has developed rapidly during the past few decades (1–9). These studies have been fundamental in the assessment of drug efficacy, safety, and the design of dosage regimens; in the development of food additives and the assessment of potential hazards of contaminants; in the evaluation of toxic chemicals; and in the development of pesticides and herbicides and their metabolic fate in insects, other animals, and plants. The metabolism of drugs and other xenobiotics is fundamental to many toxic processes, such as carcinogenesis, teratogenesis, and tissue necrosis. Often, the same enzymes involved in drug metabolism also carry out the regulation and metabolism of endogenous substances. Consequently, the inhibition and induction of these enzymes by drugs and xenobiotics may have a profound effect on the normal processes of intermediary metabolism, such as tissue growth and development, hematopoiesis, calcification, and lipid metabolism.

Familiarity with the mechanisms of drug metabolism often can predict the consequences of drug–drug interactions, drug–food interactions, and herbal drug–drug interactions to explain a patient's adverse responses to drug regimens. Incorporating pharmacogenomics into the selection of drug regimens will change the way in which drugs are chosen for patients. Selection based on the patient's individual genetic makeup could eliminate the unpredictable response of drug treatment because of genetic polymorphisms that effects metabolism, clearance, and tolerance. Pharmacogenomic testing to predict

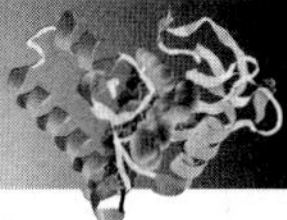

CLINICAL SIGNIFICANCE

The basic principles of drug metabolism may inform a wide variety of clinical decisions regarding pharmacotherapy. For example, a thorough understanding enables a careful assessment for drug-drug interactions in particular patient cases. Drugs, as chemical entities, can be substrates, inhibitors, or inducers of metabolic enzymes. The interplay of these roles potentially influences serum drug concentrations in ways that may directly affect the desired outcome, i.e., decreases in levels that may prevent therapeutic efficacy or increases that may enhance risks of toxicity. There are certainly many more theoretical pharmacokinetic interactions that invoke these mechanisms than are actually seen in clinical practice. Through careful observation and analysis of unexpected and possibly concentration-dependent events, one could more readily identify and document which interactions are of greater clinical significance by virtue of their actual occurrence in patients. The clinician would then be poised to recommend appropriate dosage adjustments or medication changes based on the actual outcomes of these interactions.

In addition, the biotransformation of drugs may produce reactive metabolites which, through basic chemical reactions, may interact with the components of cellular membranes and proteins in a manner that disrupts normal structure and function. A working knowledge of those functional groups within drug molecules that may be more susceptible to reactive metabolite formation could help explain toxic sequelae when they emerge during a medication trial. This could be useful information whenever alternative therapeutic agents within a given chemical class are being considered.

Ongoing discoveries from studies in the pharmacogenetics field are expanding the drug metabolism literature in directions that hint at the future prospect of truly individualized drug regimens. The need to keep abreast of these new developments is both compelling and exciting, and their application builds upon the principles presented in this chapter.

Mark D. Watanabe, PharmD, PhD, BCPP
Assistant Clinical Specialist
Department of Pharmacy Practice
Northeastern University
Boston, MA

a patient's phenotype (i.e., poor metabolizer) and, thus, their ability to metabolize drugs will become common in the future. Armed with such knowledge, improved selection of proper drug regimen and dose can be assured before therapy begins.

The increased knowledge of drug metabolism, fed by the need for greater safety evaluation of drugs and chemicals, has resulted in a proliferation of publications (e.g., *Drug Metabolism Reviews, Drug Metabolism and Disposition,* and *Xenobiotica*) and a series of monographs that present the current state of knowledge of foreign compound metabolism from biochemical and pharmacological viewpoints (3–9).

PATHWAYS OF METABOLISM

Drugs, plant toxins, food additives, environmental chemicals, insecticides, and other chemicals foreign to the body undergo enzymic transformations that usually result in the loss of pharmacological activity. The term "detoxication" describes the result of such metabolic changes. Although drug metabolism usually leads to detoxication, the processes of oxidation, reduction, glucuronidation, sulfation, and other enzyme-catalyzed reactions may lead to the formation of a metabolite having therapeutic or toxic effects. This process often is referred to as "bioactivation." One of the earliest examples of bioactivation was the reduction of Prontosil to the antibacterial agent sulfanilamide. Other examples of drug metabolism leading to therapeutically active drugs include the hydroxylation of acetanilid to acetaminophen as well as the N-demethylation of the antidepressant imipramine to desipramine and the anxiolytic diazepam to desmethyldiazepam. The insecticide parathion is desulfurized by both insects and mammals to paraoxon.

Most drugs and other xenobiotics are metabolized by enzymes normally associated with the metabolism of endogenous constituents (e.g., steroids and biogenic amines). The liver is the major site of drug metabolism, although other xenobiotic-metabolizing enzymes are found in nervous tissue, kidney, lung, plasma, and the gastrointestinal tract (digestive secretions, bacterial flora, and the intestinal wall).

Although hepatic metabolism continues to be the most important route of metabolism for xenobiotics and drugs, other biotransformation pathways play a significant role in the metabolism of these substances. Among the more active extrahepatic tissues capable of metabolizing drugs are the intestinal mucosa, kidney, and lung (see the discussion of extrahepatic metabolism). The ability of the liver and extrahepatic tissues to metabolize substances to either pharmacologically inactive or bioactive metabolites before reaching systemic blood levels is termed "first-pass metabolism" or the "presystemic first-pass effect." Other metabolism reactions occurring in the gastrointestinal tract are associated with the bacteria and other microflora of the tract. The bacterial flora can affect metabolism through the 1) production of toxic metabolites, 2) formation of carcinogens from inactive precursors, 3) detoxication, 4) exhibition of species differences in drug metabolism, 5) exhibition of individual differences in drug metabolism, 6) production of pharmacologically active metabolites from inactive precursors, and 7) production of metabolites not formed by animal tissues.

Phase 1 Reactions

The pathways of xenobiotic metabolism are divided into two major categories. Phase 1 reactions (biotransformations) include oxidation, hydroxylation, reduction, and hydrolysis. In these enzymatic reactions, a new functional group is introduced into the substrate molecule, an existing functional group is modified, or a functional group or acceptor site for Phase 2 transfer reactions is exposed, thus making the xenobiotic more polar and, therefore, more readily excreted.

Phase 2 Reactions

Phase 2 reactions (conjugation) are enzymatic syntheses whereby a functional group, such as alcohol, phenol, or amine, is masked by the addition of a new group, such as acetyl, sulfate, glucuronic acid, or certain amino acids, which further increases the polarity of the drug or xenobiotic. Most substances undergo both Phase 1 and Phase 2 reactions sequentially.

Those xenobiotics that are resistant to metabolizing enzymes or are already hydrophilic are excreted largely unchanged. This basic pattern of xenobiotic metabolism is common to all animal species, including humans, but species may differ in details of the reaction and enzyme control.

FACTORS AFFECTING METABOLISM

As indicated earlier, drug therapy is becoming oriented more toward controlling metabolic, genetic, and environmental illnesses rather than short-term therapy associated with infectious diseases. In most cases, drug therapy lasts for months or even years, and the problems of drug–drug interactions and chronic toxicity from long-term drug therapy have become more serious. Therefore, a greater knowledge of drug metabolism is essential. Several factors influencing xenobiotic metabolism include:

1. *Genetic factors.* Individual differences in drug effectiveness (drug sensitivity or drug resistance), drug interactions, and drug toxicity may depend on racial and ethnic characteristics with the population frequencies of the many polymorphic genes and the expression of the metabolizing enzymes. Pharmacogenetics focuses primarily on genetic polymorphisms (mutations) responsible for interindividual differences in drug metabolism and disposition (10). Genotype–phenotype correlation studies have validated that inherited mutations result in two or more distinct phenotypes causing very different responses following drug administration. The genes encoding for CYP2A6, CYP2C9, CYP2C19, and CYP2D6 are functionally polymorphic; therefore, at least 30% of CYP450-dependent metabolism is performed by polymorphic enzymes. For example, mutations in the *CYP2D6* gene result in poor, intermediate, or ultrarapid metabolizers of more than 30 cardiovascular and central nervous system drugs. Thus, each of these phenotypic subgroups experience different responses to drugs extensively metabolized by the CYP2D6 pathway ranging from severe toxicity to complete lack of efficacy. For example, ethnic specificity has been observed with the sensitivity of the Japanese and Chinese to ethanol as compared to Caucasians, CYP2C19 polymorphism (affects ~20% Asians and ~3% Caucasians) and the variable metabolism of omeprazole (proton pump inhibitor) and antiseizure drugs, and the polymorphic paraoxonase–catalyzed hydrolysis of the neurotoxic organophosphates and lipid peroxides (atherosclerosis) (see the discussion of genetic polymorphism).

   Incorporating pharmacogenomics, the study of heritable traits affecting patient response to drug treatment, into drug therapy will alter the way in which drug regimens are chosen for patients based on their individual genetic makeup (10), thus eliminating the unpredictable response of drug treatment because of genetic polymorphisms that effect metabolism, clearance, and tolerance. Understanding how individuals are genetically predisposed to differences in metabolism risk may result in new classes of drugs that are metabolized by nonpolymorphic CYP450 enzymes.
2. *Physiologic factors.* Age is a factor because the very young and the old have impaired metabolism. Hormones (including those induced by stress), sex differences, pregnancy, changes in the intestinal microflora, diseases (especially those involving the liver), and nutritional status also can influence drug and xenobiotic metabolism.

   Because the liver is the principal site for xenobiotic and drug metabolism, liver disease can modify the pharmacokinetics of drugs metabolized by the liver (11–13). Several factors identified as major determinants of the metabolism of a drug in the diseased liver are the nature and extent of liver damage, hepatic blood flow, the drug involved, the dosage regimen, and the degree of participation of the liver in the pharmacokinetics of the drug. Liver disease affects the elimination half-life of some drugs but not of others, although all undergo hepatic biotransformation (Table 10.1). Some results have shown that the capacity for drug metabolism is impaired in chronic liver disease, which could lead to drug overdosage. Consequently, because of the unpredictability of drug effects in the presence of liver disorders, drug therapy under these circumstances is complex, and more than the usual caution is needed (13).

Table 10.1. The Effect of Liver Disease in Humans on the Elimination Half-Life of Various Drugs[a]

Difference Reported	No Difference Reported
Acetaminophen	Chlorpromazine
Amylbarbital	Dicoumarol
Carbenicillin	Phenytoin
Chloramphenicol	Phenylbutazone
Clindamycin	Salicylic Acid
Diazepam	Tobutamide
Hexobarbital	
Isoniazid	
Lidocaine	
Meperidine	
Meprobamate	
Pentobarbital	
Phenobarbital	
Prednisone	
Rifamycin	
Tolbutamide	
Theophylline	

[a]Clearance is disputable but may be increased.

Substances influencing drug and xenobiotic metabolism (other than enzyme inducers) include lipids, proteins, vitamins, and metals. Dietary lipid and protein deficiencies diminish microsomal drug-metabolizing activity. Protein deficiency leads to a reduction in hepatic microsomal protein and lipid deficiency; oxidative metabolism is decreased because of an alteration in endoplasmic reticulum (ER) membrane permeability affecting electron transfer. In terms of toxicity, protein deficiency would increase the toxicity of drugs and xenobiotics by reducing their oxidative microsomal metabolism and clearance from the body.

3. *Pharmacodynamic factors.* Dose, frequency, and route of administration, plus tissue distribution and protein binding of the drug, affect its metabolism.
4. *Environmental factors.* Competition of ingested environmental substances with other drugs and xenobiotics for the metabolizing enzymes and poisoning of enzymes by toxic chemicals, such as carbon monoxide or pesticide synergists, alter metabolism. Induction of enzyme expression (the number of enzyme molecules is increased, but the activity is constant) by other drugs and xenobiotics is another consideration.

Such factors may change not only the kinetics of an enzyme reaction but also the whole pattern of metabolism, thereby altering the bioavailability, pharmacokinetics, pharmacological activity, or toxicity of a xenobiotic. Species differences in response to xenobiotics must be considered during the extrapolation of pharmacological and toxicological data from experiments in animals to humans. The primary factors in these differences probably are the rate and pattern of drug and xenobiotic metabolism in the various species.

DRUG BIOTRANSFORMATION PATHWAY (PHASE 1)

Human Hepatic Cytochrome P450 Enzyme System

Introduction

Oxidation probably is the most common reaction in xenobiotic metabolism. This reaction is catalyzed by a group of membrane-bound monooxygenases found in the smooth ER of the liver and other extrahepatic tissues, termed the "cytochrome P450 monooxygenase enzyme system" (14) (hereafter, the abbreviation CYP450 will be used for this enzyme system). Additionally, CYP450 has been called a mixed-function oxidase or microsomal hydroxylase. The tissue homogenate fraction containing the smooth ER is called the microsomal fraction. The CYP450 functions as a multicomponent electron-transport system responsible for the oxidative metabolism of a variety of endogenous substrates (e.g., steroids, fatty acids, prostaglandins, and bile acids) and exogenous substances (xenobiotics), including drugs, carcinogens, insecticides, plant toxins, environmental pollutants, and other foreign chemicals. Central to the functioning of this unique superfamily of heme proteins is a iron protoporphyrin. The iron protoporphyrin is coordinated to the sulfur of cysteine and has the ability to form a complex with carbon monoxide, the result of which is a complex that has its major absorption band at 450 nm (thus the title of these metabolizing CYP450 enzymes). The CYP450 has an absolute requirement for NADPH (reduced form of nicotinamide adenine dinucleotide phosphate) and molecular oxygen (dioxygen). The rate at which various compounds are metabolized by this system depends on the species, strain, nutritional status, tissue, age, and pretreatment of the animals. The variety of reactions catalyzed by CYP450 include (Table 10.2) the oxidation of alkanes and aromatic compounds; the epoxidation of alkenes, polycyclic hydrocarbons, and halogenated benzenes; the dealkylation of secondary and tertiary amines and ethers; the deamination of amines; the conversion of amines to N-oxides, hydroxylamine, and nitroso derivatives; and the dehalogenation of halogenated hydrocarbons. It also catalyzes the oxidative cleavage of organic thiophosphate esters, the sulfoxidation of some thioethers, the conversion of phosphothionates to the phosphate derivatives, and the reduction of azo and nitro compounds to primary aromatic amines.

The most important function of CYP450 is its ability to "activate" molecular oxygen (dioxygen), permitting the incorporation of one atom of oxygen into an organic substrate molecule concomitant with the reduction of the other atom of oxygen to water. The introduction of a hydroxyl group into the hydrophobic substrate molecule provides a site for subsequent conjugation with hydrophilic compounds (Phase 2), thereby increasing the aqueous solubility of the product for its transport and excretion from the organism. This enzyme system not only catalyzes xenobiotic transformations in ways that usually lead to detoxication but also, in some cases, in ways that lead to products

Table 10.2. Hydroxylation Mechanisms Catalyzed by Cytochrome P450

Aromatic hydroxylation

$$CH_3CO\text{-}\overset{H}{N}\text{-}C_6H_5 \xrightarrow{[OH]} CH_3CO\text{-}\overset{H}{N}\text{-}C_6H_4\text{-}OH$$

Aliphatic hydoxylation

$$R\text{-}CH_3 \xrightarrow{[OH]} R\text{-}CH_2\text{-}OH$$

Deamination

$$R\text{-}CH(NH_2)\text{-}CH_3 \xrightarrow{[OH]} (R\text{-}C(OH)(NH_2)\text{-}CH_3) \longrightarrow R\text{-}COCH_3 + NH_3$$

O-Dealkylation

$$R\text{-}O\text{-}CH_3 \xrightarrow{[OH]} (R\text{-}O\text{-}CH_2\text{-}OH) \longrightarrow R\text{-}OH + CH_2O$$

N-Dealkylation

$$R\text{-}N(CH_3)_2 \xrightarrow{[OH]} (R\text{-}N(CH_2OH)(CH_3)) \longrightarrow R\text{-}NHCH_3 + CH_2O$$

$$R\text{-}NH\text{-}CH_3 \xrightarrow{[OH]} (R\text{-}NH\text{-}CH_2OH) \longrightarrow R\text{-}NH_2 + CH_2O$$

N-Oxidation

$$(CH_3)_3\text{—}N \xrightarrow{[OH]} ((CH_3)_3\text{—}NOH) \longrightarrow (CH_3)_3\text{—}NO + H^{\oplus}$$

Sulfoxidation

$$R\text{-}S\text{-}R' \xrightarrow{[OH]} (R\text{-}\underset{OH}{S}\text{-}R') \longrightarrow R\text{-}\underset{O}{\overset{}{S}}\text{-}R' + H^{\oplus}$$

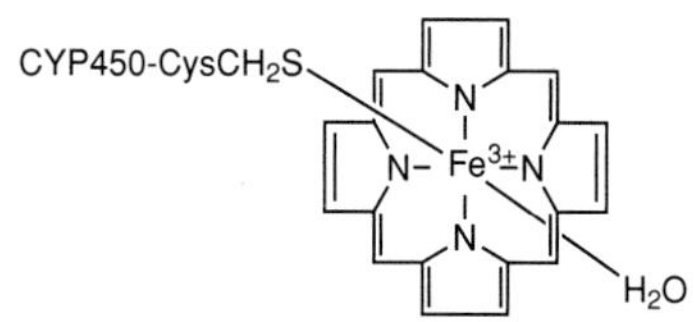

Fig. 10.1. Ferric heme thiolate catalytic center of CYP450. The porphyrin side chains are deleted for clarity.

having greater cytotoxic, mutagenic, or carcinogenic properties. A nonheme, microsomal flavoprotein monooxygenase is responsible for the oxidation of certain nitrogen- and sulfur-containing organic compounds.

Components of CYP450

The CYP450 consists of at least two protein components: a heme protein called cytochrome P450, and a flavoprotein called NADPH-CYP450 reductase, containing both flavin mononucleotide (FMN) and flavin dinucleotide (FAD). The CYP450 is the substrate- and oxygen-binding site of the enzyme system, whereas the reductase serves as an electron carrier, shuttling electrons from NADPH to CYP450. A third component essential for electron transport from NADPH to CYP450 is a phospholipid, phosphatidylcholine, that facilitates the transfer of electrons from NADPH-CYP450 reductase to CYP450 (14). Although the phospholipid does not function in the system as an electron carrier, it has great influence on the CYP450 monooxygenase system. The phospholipid makes up approximately one-third of the hepatic ER and contributes to a negatively charged environment at neutral pH.

Of the three components involved in microsomal oxidative xenobiotic metabolism, CYP450 is important because of its vital role in oxygen activation and substrate binding. The CYP450 is an integral membrane protein deeply imbedded in the membrane matrix. The environment surrounding the enzyme is negatively charged at neutral pH because of the phospholipids. The electron components of CYP450 are located on the cytoplasmic side of the ER and the hydrophobic active site toward the lumen of the ER (15). The active site of CYP450 consists of a hydrophobic substrate-binding domain in which is imbedded an iron protoporphyrin (heme) prosthetic group. This group is exactly like that of hemoglobin, peroxidase, and the b-type cytochromes. The iron in the iron protoporphyrin is coordinated with four nitrogens via a tetradentate to the porphyrin ring. X-ray studies reveal that in the ferric state, the two nonporphyrin ligands are water and cysteine (Fig. 10.1). The cysteine thiolate ligand (proximal) is present in all states of the enzyme and is absolutely essential for the formation of the reactive oxenoid intermediate. The sixth (distal) coordination position is occupied by an easily exchangeable ligand, most likely water, which is labile and easily exchanged for stronger ligands, such as cyanide, amines, imidazoles, and pyridines. The ferrous form loses the water ligand completely, leaving the sixth position open for binding ligands such as oxygen and carbon monoxide.

The vast array of xenobiotics presents a unique challenge to the human body to metabolize these lipophilic foreign compounds and makes it impractical to have one enzyme for each compound or each class of compounds. Therefore, whereas most cellular functions usually are very specific, xenobiotic oxidation requires CYP450s with diverse substrate specificities and regioselectivities (multiple sites of oxidation). Several types of CYP450 enzymes can be found in a single species of animal. For example, the rat has more than 40 different CYP450 genes, each coding for a different version of the enzyme (isoform) that can metabolize almost any lipophilic compound to which they are exposed.

Classification of the CYP450 Multigene Family

Nebert et al. (16,17) classified the CYP450 supergene family on the basis of their structural (evolutionary) relationships The CYP450 monooxygenases resulting from this supergene family have been subdivided into families with greater than 40% amino acid homology and subfamilies with greater than 55% homology (16,17). The CYP450s are named using the root symbol CYP (CYtochrome P450), followed by an Arabic numeral designating the family member (e.g., CYP1, CYP2, or CYP3), a letter denoting the subfamily (e.g., CYP1A, CYP2C, CYP2D, or CYP2E), and another Arabic numeral representing the individual gene. Names of genes are written in italics. The nomenclature system is based solely on sequence similarity

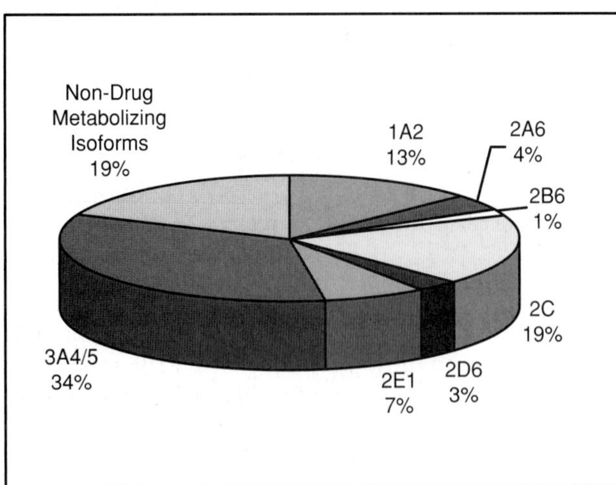

Fig. 10.2. Total human CYP450 isoforms expressed in the liver that metabolize drugs.

among the CYP450s and does not indicate the properties or function of individual P450s. Of the more than 17 CYP450 isoforms that have been identified to date, the major isoforms responsible for drug metabolism in the liver are presented in Figure 10.2 (18). It is quite evident that the CYP3A and CYP2C families are the isoforms most involved in the metabolism of clinically relevant drugs, and the CYP1A2 isoform is predominantly involved in the bioactivation of environmental substances.

The CYP450s probably evolved initially for the regulation of endogenous substances, such as for metabolization of cholesterol to maintain membrane integrity and for steroid biosynthesis and metabolism, rather than for metabolizing foreign compounds. The CYP450s are either involved in highly specific steroid hydroxylations located in the inner mitochondrial membrane or bound to the ER of the cell having broad substrate specificity. In evolutionary terms, CYP450s evolved from a common ancestor, and only more recently (during the last 100 million years) have CYP450 genes taken on the role of producing enzymes for metabolizing a vast array of lipophilic foreign compounds. The emergence of the xenobiotic CYP450 genes probably evolved from the steroidogenic CYP450s for enhancing animal survival by synthesizing new CYP450s for metabolizing plant toxins in the food chain. It is not surprising that animals and humans possess a large array of diverse CYP450 enzymes capable of handling a multitude of xenobiotics. Interindividual variation in the expression of xenobiotic CYP450 genes (genetic polymorphism) or their inducibility may be associated with differences, such as in individual susceptibility to cigarette smoke carcinogenesis. Certain CYP450 isoforms that clearly exhibit genetic polymorphism are known to metabolize and generally inactivate therapeutic agents. The extent of CYP450 polymorphisms in humans is being investigated to determine the risk or protection against cancer. Food mutagens typically are carcinogens in tissue, but they are activated by CYP1A2 in the liver and CYP3A. Specific forms of CYP450 in hepatic microsomes are regulated by hormones (e.g., CYP3A subfamily) and are induced or inhibited by drugs, food toxins, and other environmental xenobiotics (see the section on induction and inhibition of CYP450 isoforms). Identification of a specific CYP450 isoform as the major form responsible for metabolism of a drug in humans permits reconciliation of its toxicity or other pharmacological effects.

Substrate Specificity

No evidence exists that the active oxygenating species differ between CYP450s, suggesting that the substrate specificities, substrate affinity, regioselectivity, and rates of reaction probably are a consequence of topographic features of the active site of apoproteins (14,15,19,20). Because a primary function of these enzymes is the metabolism of hydrophobic substrates, it is likely that hydrophobic forces are important in the binding of many substrates to the apoproteins. Nonspecific binding is consistent with the multiple substrate orientations in the active site necessary for the broad regioselectivities observed. A specific binding requirement would decrease the diversity of substrates. Some CYP450 isoforms have constrained binding sites and, thus, metabolize small organic molecules (e.g., CYP2E1): CYP1A1/2 have planar binding sites and only metabolize aromatic planar compounds (i.e., polycyclic aromatic hydrocarbons [PAHs]); CYP2D6 exhibits high affinities with specific apoprotein interactions (hydrogen bonds, ion-pair formation) for specific substrates, such as lipophilic amines; and CYP3A4 has broader affinity for a variety of lipophilic substrates (molecular weight, 200–1,200 daltons). If the CYP450 isoforms are tightly membrane bound, substrate access to the active site would be limited to compounds that can diffuse through the membrane, whereas a different CYP450 isoform may be bound less tightly and will metabolize hydrophilic compounds.

In the past, the CYP450s often were referred to as having broad and overlapping specificities, but it became apparent that the broad substrate specificity can be attributed to multiple isoenzymic forms of CYP450. The phenotype of an individual with respect to the forms and amounts of the individual CYP450s expressed in the liver can determine the rate and pathway of the metabolic clearance of a compound (see the discussion of genetic polymorphism). Significant differences exist between humans and animal species with respect to the catalytic activities and regulation of the expression of the hepatic drug-metabolizing CYP450s. These differences often make it difficult to extrapolate to humans the results of CYP450-mediated metabolism studies performed experimentally in animal species. Caution is warranted in the extrapolation of rodent data to humans, because some isoforms are similar between species (e.g., CYP1A and CYP3A subfamilies) whereas others are different (e.g., CYP2A, CYP2B, CYP2C, and CYP2D).

The unique and diverse characteristics of the CYP450 ensure that predicting the metabolism of xenobiotics will be difficult. To date, no crystal structure for a mammalian membrane-bound CYP450 isoform has been described.

Other CYP450 Isoforms

The other CYP450 isoforms catalyzing the oxidation of steroids, bile acids, fat-soluble vitamins, and other endogenous substances include the following: CYP4, arachidonic acid or fatty acid metabolism; CYP5, thromboxane A_2 synthase converts arachidonic acid into thromboxane A_2, which causes platelet aggregation; CYP7A, 7α-hydroxylase catalyzes the rate-determining step in the biosynthesis of bile acids from cholesterol; CYP7B, brain-specific form of 7α-hydroxylase catalyzing the synthesis of the neurosteroids, 7α-hydroxy dehydroepiandrosterone, and 7α-hydroxy pregnenolone; CYP8A, prostacyclin synthase catalyzes the synthesis of prostaglandin I_2 and the regulation of hemostasis that opposes CYP5; CYP8B, 12α-hydroxylase in bile acid biosynthesis; CYP11A1, the first step in mitochondrial steroid biosynthesis that oxidatively cleaves the 17-side chain of cholesterol to pregnenolone, with defects in this enzyme lead to a lack of glucocorticoids, feminization, and hypertension; CYP11B1, a mitochondrial 11β- hydroxylase that hydroxylates 11-deoxycortisol to hydrocortisone or 11-deoxycorticosterone to corticosterone; CYP11B2, mitochondrial aldosterone synthase that hydroxylates corticosterone at the 18-position to aldosterone; CYP17, 17α-hydroxylase and 17,20-lyase (two enzymes in one) are required for production of testosterone and estrogen (lack of this enzyme affects sexual development at puberty); CYP19, aromatase, catalyzes the aromatization of ring A of testosterone to estrogen (lack of this enzyme causes an estrogen deficiency and failure of females to develop at puberty); CYP21, C21 steroid hydroxylase (lack of this enzyme prevents cortisol synthesis, diverting excess 17-hydroxy progesterone into overproduction of testosterone biosynthesis); CYP24, mitochondrial 25-hydroxyvitamin D_3 24-hydroxylase for the degradation/inactivation of vitamin D metabolites; CYP26A1, all-*trans*-retinoic acid hydroxylase, may be involved in terminating the retinoic acid signal and thus turning off a developmental switch.; CYP26B1, retinoic acid hydroxylase may hydroxylate the *cis*-retinoic acids not recognized by the CYP26A1; CYP26C, retinoic acid hydroxylase, function is not known; CYP27A1, 27-hydroxylase, oxidizes cholesterol 17-side chain as the first step in bile acid biosynthesis to the feedback inhibitors, cholic acid, and chenodeoxycholic acid, and 25-hydroxyvitamin D_3; CYP27B1, mitochondrial vitamin D_3 1-α-hydroxylase activates vitamin D_3; CYP27C1, unknown function; CYP39, 7-hydroxylase of 24-hydroxy cholesterol with unknown function; CYP46, cholesterol 24-hydroxylase with unknown function; CYP51, lanosterol 14α-demethylase, for converting lanosterol into cholesterol, inhibited by ketoconazole.

Cytochrome P450 Isoforms Metabolizing Drugs/Xenobiotics (18–20)

Figure 10.3 shows the participation (%) of hepatic CYP450 isoforms in the metabolism of drugs and xenobiotics (21). Outstanding is the fact that more than one-third of all the drugs are metabolized by one isoform, CYP3A4, increasing the potential for drug–drug interactions. When two drugs are metabolized by the same isoform, only one drug can serve as a substrate at one time, increasing the likelihood of a drug–drug interaction, especially if one drug has a lower therapeutic threshold.

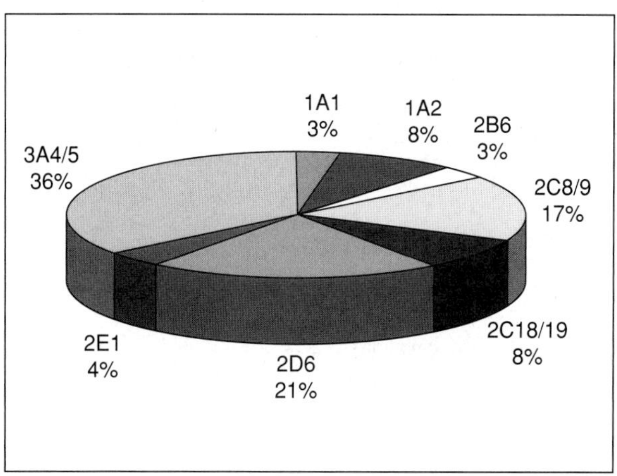

Fig. 10.3. Percentage of clinically important drugs metabolized by human CYP450 isoforms.

Family 1

The CYP1A subfamily plays an integral role in the metabolism of two important classes of environmental carcinogens, PAHs, and arylamines (Tables 10.3 and 10.4) (22). The PAHs commonly are present in the environment as a result of industrial combustion processes and in tobacco products. Several potent carcinogenic arylamines result from the pyrolysis of amino acids in cooked meats and can cause colon cancer in rats. Environmental and genetic factors can alter the expression of this subfamily of these enzymes.

CYP1A1. The CYP1A1 (also called aromatic hydrocarbon hydroxylase) is expressed primarily in extrahepatic tissues, small intestine, placenta, skin, and lung as well as in the liver in response to the presence of CYP1A1 inducers, such as PAHs (i.e., in cigarette smoke and the carcinogen 3-methylcholanthrene), α-naphthoflavone (a noncarcinogenic inducer related to dietary flavones), and indole-3-carbinol (found in Brussel sprouts and related vegetables). The CYP1A1 metabolizes a range of PAHs, including a large number of procarcinogens and promutagens. Diethylstilbestrol and 2- and 4-hydroxyestradiol (catecholestrogens) are oxidized by CYP1A1 to their quinone analogues, which normally are reduced to inactive metabolites (23). In the absence of a detoxifying reduction step, however, the quinones may accumulate and initiate carcinogenic processes or cell death by covalently damaging DNA or cellular proteins. Interindividual variation in the inducible expression of CYP1A1 might be related to a genetic difference in aromatic hormone (Ah) receptor expression, which could explain differences in individual susceptibility to cigarette smoke–induced lung cancer. Therefore, genetic factors appear to be important in the expression of the *CYP1A1* gene in humans and its involvement in human carcinogenesis. Women who smoke are at greater risk than men of developing lung cancer (adenocarcinoma) and chronic obstructive

Table 10.3. Some Substrates and Reaction Type for Human Subfamily CYP1A2[a]

Acetaminophen (imino quinone)
Amitriptyline (N-demethylation)
Caffeine (N^1- and N^3-demethylation)
Chlordiazapoxide
Cinacalcet
Clomipramine (N-demethylation)
Clopidogrel
Clozapine
Cyclobenzaprine
Desipramine (N-demethylation)
Diazepam
Duloxetine
Erlotinib
Estradiol (2- and 4-hydroxylation)
Flutamide
Fluoroquinolones (3′-hydroxylation of piperazine ring)
Fluvoxamine
Haloperidol
Imipramine (N-demethylation)
Levobupivacaine
Mexiletine
Mirtazepine
Naproxen
Nortriptyline
Olanzapine
Ondansetron
Propafenone
Propranolol
Ramelteon
Riluzole
Ropivacaine
Roprinirole
Tacrine
Theophylline
Tizanidine
Verapamil
R-warfarin
Zileuton
Zolmitriptan

[a]Drugs in bold italic have been reported to cause drug–drug interactions.

pulmonary diseases. The mechanism for the induction of the *CYP1A1* gene begins with binding of the inducing agents to a cytosolic receptor protein, the Ah receptor, which is translocated to the nucleus and binds to the DNA of the *CYP1A1* gene, thus enhancing its rate of transcription. The presence of the Ah receptor in hepatic and intestinal tissues may have implications beyond xenobiotic metabolism and may play a role in the induction of other genes for the control of cellular growth and differentiation. On the other hand, CYP1A1 may metabolize procarcinogens to hydroxylated inactive compounds that are not mutagenic. The question of how the bowel protects itself from ingested compounds known to be activated by CYP1A1 (i.e., PAH) remains unanswered (22).

CYP1A2. The CYP1A2 (also known as phenacetin O-deethylase, caffeine demethylase, or antipyrine N-demethylase) catalyzes the oxidation (and, in some cases, bioactivation) of arylamines, nitrosamines, and aromatic hydrocarbons and the bioactivation of promutagens and procarcinogens, caffeine, and other substances (Tables 10.3 and 10.4). It is expressed in the liver to the extent of 13% (range of up to 40%), intestine, and stomach and is induced by smoking, PAHs, and isosafrole (a noncarcinogenic dietary compound). CYP1A2 is primarily responsible for the activation of the carcinogen aflatoxin B1 under ordinary conditions of human exposure and the pneumotoxin ipomeanol. The latter activation occurs in the liver and not in the lungs by CYP2F1 and CYP4B1 as previously thought. Evidence for polymorphism of this isoform has been reported, and it is likely that low CYP1A2 activity will be associated with altered susceptibility to the bioactivation of procarcinogens, promutagens, and other xenobiotics known to be substrates for this enzyme. The expression of the *CYP1A2* gene in the stomach becomes an important issue for gastric carcinogenesis induced by smoking and the metabolic activation of the procarcinogens, arylamines, to mutagens (22).

Table 10.4. Some Procarcinogens and Other Toxins Activated by Human Cytochrome P450s

CYP1A1	CYP1A2	CYP2E1	CYP3A4
Benzo[a]pyrene and other polycyclic aromatic hydrocarbons	4-Aminobiphenyl	Benzene	Aflatoxin B1
	2-Naphthylamine	Styrene	Aflatoxin G1
	2-Aminofluorene	Acrylonitrile	Estradiol
	2-Acetylaminofluorene	Vinyl bromide	6-Aminochrysene
	2-Aminoanthracene	Trichloroethylene	Polycyclic hydrocarbon dihydrodiols
	Heteropolycyclic amines	Carbon tetrachloride	
	(2-aminoquinolines)	Chloroform	
	Aflatoxin B1	Methylene chloride	
	Ipomeanol	N-nitrosodimethylamine	
		1,2-Dichloropropane	
		Ethyl carbamate	

Table 10.5. Some Substrates for Human Subfamily CYP2B6

Bupropion	Sertraline
Cyclophosphamide	
Efavirenz	
Ifosfamide	
Methadone	

Clinical studies have suggested that the N-demethylation of imipramine is greater in smokers than in nonsmokers.

Family 2

CYP2A6. The CYP2A6 is the only member of this subfamily that is expressed primarily in the liver and also may be expressed in lung and nasal epithelium. It has a low level of hepatic expression and represents approximately 4% of the total hepatic CYP450 isoforms (Fig. 10.2). It catalyzes the 7-hydroxylation of coumarin (coumarin 7-hydroxylase), hydroxylation of aflatoxin B1, nicotine (C-oxidation to cotinine), naproxen, tacrine, clozapine, mexiletine, and cyclobenzaprine as well as the bioactivation of nitrosamines and procarcinogens. The CYP2A6 exhibits polymorphism with an incidence of 2% in the Caucasian population. This population is characterized as poor metabolizers. Smokers with a defective *CYP2A6* gene smoke fewer cigarettes, implicating a genetic factor in nicotine dependence.

CYP2B6. Limited data are available regarding the CYP2B6 isoform, and it represents less than 1% of the total hepatic CYP450 isoforms. Its level of expression is low, and phenobarbital appears to induce its formation. The role of CYP2B6 in human drug metabolism is questionable, although cyclophosphamide, ifosfamide, bupropion, sertraline and nicotine are metabolized by this isoform (Table 10.5).

CYP2C. The human CYP2C subfamily is the most complex family consisting of CYP2C8, CYP2C9, and CYP2C19, metabolizing approximately 25% of the clinically important drugs (Fig. 10.3), including S-warfarin, S-mephenytoin, and tolbutamide (Table 10.6). It represents

Table 10.6. Some Substrates and Reaction Type for Human Subfamily CYP2C[a]

CYP2C8	CYP2C9		CYP2C19
Amiodarone	Amitriptyline	Piroxicam	Amitriptyline
Amodiaquine	Carvedilol	***Ramelteon***	Carisoprodol
Benzphetamine	Celecoxib	Rosiglitazone	Cilostazol
Carbamzepine	Chlorpheniramine	Sertraline	Citalopram
Cerivastatin	Chloramphenicol	Sildenafil	Clomipramine
Docetaxel	Clomipramine	Sulfamethoxazole	Cyclophosphamide
Fluvastatin	Desogestrel	Sulfinpyrazone (aromatic hydroxylation)	Desipramine
Isotretinoin	Diclofenac (4′-hydroxylation)	Suprofen	***Diazepam*** (N-demethylation)
Paclitaxel	***Diazepam***	Tamoxifen	Escitalopram
Phenytoin	Dronabinol	Tienilic acid (thiophene ring hydroxylation)	Esomeprazole
Pioglitazone	Fluoxetine	Tolbutamide (*p*-methyl-hydroxylation)	Formoterol
Repaglinide	Flurbiprofen	Torsemide	Hexobarbital
Retinol	Fluvastatin	Δ^1-THC (7-hydroxylation)	Imipramine (N-demethylation)
Rosiglitazone	Formoterol	Testosterone (16α-hydroxylation)	Indomethacin
Tolbutamide	Glibenclamide	Valdecoxib	Lansoprazole
Torsemide	Glimepiride	Vardenafil	Loratidine (descarbethoxyation)
Verapamil	Glipizide	Valsartan	(*S*)-Mephenytoin (4′-hydroxylation)
Zopliclone	Glyburide	Voriconazole	(*R*)-Mephenytoin (N-demethylation)
	Hexobarbital (3′-hydroxylation)	*S*-Warfarin (7′-hydroxylation)	(*R*)-Mephobarbital
	Ibuprofen (*i*-butylmethyl-hydroxylation)	Zafirlukast	Moclobemide
	Imipramine	Zileuton	Nelfinavir
	Indomethacin		Nilutamide
	Irbesartan		Omeprazole (hydroxylation)
	Irinotecan		Pantoprazole
	Lomoxicam		Pentamidine
	Losartan		Phenobarbital
	Mefenamic acid		***Phenytoin*** (ring hydroxylation)
	Meloxicam		Progesterone
	(*R*)-Mephenytoin		Proguanil (cyclization)
	Montelukast		Propranolol (side chain hydroxylation)
	Nateglinide		Rabeprazole
	Omeprazole		Sertraline
	Phenytoin (4′-hydroxylation)		Teniposide
	Phenylbutazone (4-hydroxylation)		***Thioridazine***
			Tolbutamide
			Voriconazole
			(*R*)-Warfarin

[a]Drugs in bold italic have been reported to cause drug-drug interactions.

approximately 20% of the total CYP450 isoforms in the liver (Fig. 10.2). The CYP2C8 is expressed primarily in extrahepatic tissues (kidney, adrenal, brain, uterus, breast, ovary, and intestine) and metabolizes the tricyclic antidepressants, diazepam, and verapamil. Its level of expression is less than CYP2C9 and CYP2C19. Both CYP2C9 and CYP2C19 are found primarily in the liver and intestine. The expression of CYP2C19 in the liver is less than that for CYP2C9. Both CYP2C9 and CYP2C19 exhibit polymorphism (difference in the DNA sequence for the *CYP2C* gene) that changes the enzyme's ability to metabolize its substrates (i.e., poor metabolizer phenotype). Because of this genetic difference in expressing CYP2C isoforms, it is important to be aware of a person's race when prescribing drugs that are metabolized differently by different populations (see the section concerning genetic polymorphism). The CYP2C9 is involved in tolbutamide methyl hydroxylation and is a factor in the 4′-hydroxylation of phenytoin, 6/7–hydroxylation of S-warfarin, and R-mephenytoin. The CYP2C19 (S-mephenytoin hydroxylase) is the isoform associated with the 4′-hydroxylation of S-mephenytoin. The CYP2C subfamily apparently is not inducible in humans.

CYP2D6. The CYP2D6 polymorphism is, perhaps, the most studied CYP450 (see the section on genetic polymorphism). This enzyme is responsible for at least 30 different drug oxidations, representing approximately 21% of the clinically important drugs (Fig. 10.3). The CYP2D6 is only 3% expressed in the liver and minimally expressed in the intestine, and it does not appear to be inducible (Fig. 10.2). Because there may be no other way to clear drugs metabolized by CYP2D6 from the system, poor metabolizers of CYP2D6 substrates may be at severe risk for adverse drug reactions or drug overdose. The metabolism of debrisoquine by CYP2D6 is one of the most studied examples of metabolic polymorphism, with its molecular basis of defective metabolism being well understood (Table 10.7) (see the section on genetic polymorphism). This isoform metabolizes a wide variety of lipophilic amines and is probably the only CYP450 for which a charged or ion-pair interaction is important for substrate binding. It also appears to preferentially catalyze the hydroxylation of a single enantiomer (stereoselectivity) in the presence of enantiomeric mixtures. Quinidine is an inhibitor of CYP2D6, and concurrent administration with CYP2D6 substrates results in increased blood levels and toxicity for these substrates. If the pharmacological action of the CYP2D6 substrate depends on the formation of active metabolites, quinidine inhibition results in a lack of a therapeutic response. The interaction of two substrates for CYP2D6 can prompt a number of clinical responses. For example, depending on which substrate has the greater affinity for CYP2D6, the first-pass hepatic metabolism of the substrate (drug) with weaker affinity will be inhibited by a second substrate having greater affinity. The result of this will be a decrease and prolongation of elimination of the first substrate, leading to a higher plasma concentration and an increased potential for adverse toxicity.

CYP2E1. Few drugs are metabolized by CYP2E1, but it plays a major role in the metabolism of numerous halogenated hydrocarbons (including volatile general anesthetics) and a range of low-molecular-weight organic compounds, including dimethyformamide, acetonitrile, acetone, ethanol, and benzene, as well as in the activation of acetaminophen to its reactive metabolite, N-acetyl-p-benzoquinoneimine (Table 10.8) (24,25). The CYP2E1 is of most interest because of the toxicity and carcinogenicity of its metabolites. This isoform is expressed in the liver (7%), kidney, intestine, and lung, and it is inducible by ethanol, isoniazid, 4-methylpyrazole, and other chemicals (see Table 10.12). It also is known as microsomal ethanol-oxidizing system, benzene hydroxylase, or aniline hydroxylase. The CYP2E1 is induced in alcoholics, and there is a polymorphism associated with this isoform that is more common in Chinese people. This isoform also appears to be related to smoking-induced cancer (c.f., CYP1A2). Most of the same compounds that induce CYP2E1 also are substrates for the enzyme. The induction of this enzyme in humans can cause enhanced susceptibility to the toxicity and carcinogenesis of CYP2E1 substrates. Some evidence shows interindividual variation in the in vitro liver expression of this isoform. Diabetes and dietary alterations (i.e., fasting and obesity) result in the induction of CYP2E1. Ketogenic diets (increased serum ketone levels), including those deficient in carbohydrates or high in fat, are known to enhance the metabolism of halogenated hydrocarbons in rats (25). The mechanism of induction appears to be a combination of an increase in CYP2E1 transcription, mRNA translation efficiency, and stabilization of CYP2E1 against proteolytic degradation. The induction of CYP2E1 resulting from ketosis (i.e., starvation, a high-fat diet, uncontrolled diabetes, and obesity) or exposure to alcoholic beverages or other xenobiotics may be detrimental to individuals simultaneously exposed to halogenated hydrocarbons (increased hepatotoxicity from exposure to halothane, chloroform). Chronic alcohol intake is known to enhance the hepatotoxicity of halogenated hydrocarbons. Testosterone appears to regulate CYP2E1 levels in the kidney and pituitary growth hormone for regulating hepatic levels of CYP2E1. Kidney damage from halocarbons was greater for male rats but not for female rats. This finding may have implications for sexual differences in the nephrotoxicity of CYP2E1 substrates in humans.

Family 3

CYP3A4. The CYP3A subfamily includes the most abundantly expressed CYP450s in the human liver and intestine (extrahepatic metabolism). Although CYP3A4 is responsible for approximately two-thirds of CYP3A-mediated drug metabolism, the other minor isoforms (CYP3A5, CYP3A7, and CYP3A43) also contribute. The

Table 10.7. Some Substrates and Reaction Type for Human CYP2D6 Isoform[a]

Alprenolol (4-hydroxylation)
Amitriptyline (10-hydroxylation)
Amphetamine
Aripiprazole
Atomoxetine
Bifuralol (1′-hydroxylation)
Bisoprolol
Captopril
Carvedilol
Cevimeline
Chlorpheniramine (N-demethylation, ring hydroxylation, deamination)
Chlorpromazine
Chlorpropamide
Cinacalcet
Clemastine
Clomipramine (hydroxylation)
Clozapine (aromatic hydroxylation)
Codeine (O-demethylation)
Cyclobenzaprine
Darifenacine
Debrisoquine (4-hydroxylation)
Desipramine
Dexfenfluramine
Dextromethorphan (O-demethylation)
Diphenhydramine (N-demethylation, ring hydroxylation, cleavege ether bond)
Dolasetron (hydroxylation of indole ring)
Donepezil
Doxepin
Duloxetine
Encainide (N-demethylation, O-demethylation)
Fenfluramine
Fluphenazine
Fentanyl
Flecainide (O-dealkylation)
Fluoxetine(N-dealkylation)
Fluvoxamine
Formoterol
Galantamine
Guanoxan (6- and 7-hydroxylation)
Haloperidol
Hydrocodone
Hydroxyzine (ring hydroxylation)
Imipramine (2-hydroxylation)
Indoramin (6-hydroxylation)
Lidocaine (3-hydroxylation)
Maprotiline
Meperidine
Methadone
Methamphetamine
Methoxyamphetamine (4-hydroxylation, N-demethylation)
Metoclopramide
Metoprolol (O-demethylation)
Mexilletine (4-hydroxylation and methyl hydroxylation)
Minaprine
Mirtazepine
Morphine
Nebivolol
Nortriptyline (10-hydroxylation)
Olanzepine
Ondansetron (hydroxylation of indole ring)
Oxycodone
Paroxetine
Perhexiline (4′-hydroxylation)
Perphenazine (aromatic hydroxylation)
Phenacetin
Phenformin (4-hydroxylation)
Pindolol
Promethazine (ring hydroxylation, S-oxidation, N-demethylation)
Propafenone (4-hydroxylation)
Propoxyphene
Propranolol (4′-hydroxylation)
Quetiapine
Quinidine (hydroxylation)
Ranolazine
Risperidone
Ritonavir
Sertraline
S-Metoprolol
Sparteine (N-oxidation)
Tamoxifen
Thioridazine (aromatic hydroxylation)
Timolol (O-dealkylation)
Tolterodine (2-hydroxylation)
Tramadol
Trazodone
Tripelennamine
Tropisetron (hydroxylation of indole ring)
Venlafaxine

[a]Drugs in bold italic have been reported to cause drug–drug interactions.

CYP3A5 is the best studied of the minor CYP3A isoforms. Approximately 20% of human livers express CYP3A5. The expression of CYP3A5 shows interethnic differences, with the wild-type CYP3A5*1 allele being more common in Africans than in Caucasians and Asians. In individuals who express CYP3A5, 17 to 50% of the total hepatic CYP3A is this isoform. Additionally, CYP3A5 also is expressed in a range of extrahepatic tissues and is inducible via pregnane X receptor. Both CYP3A4 and CYP3A5 exhibit significant overlap in substrate specificity but can differ in catalytic activity and regioselectivity. Results from a comparison of CYP3A4 and CYP3A5 enzyme kinetics indicate that CYP3A5 has different enzymic characteristics from CYP3A4 in some CYP3A-catalyzed reactions. The enzyme kinetics for CYP3A5 suggest a faster substrate turnover than with CYP3A4.

Approximately one-third of the total CYP450 in the liver and two-thirds in the intestine is CYP3A4. This isoform is responsible for the metabolism of more than one-third of the clinically important drugs. The CYP3A4 is expressed in the intestine, lung, placenta, kidney, uterus, and brain and is glucocorticoid inducible. The CYP3A7 is predominantly expressed in fetal liver (~50% of total fetal CYP450 enzymes) but also is found in some adult livers and extrahepatically. The CYP3A7 has a specific role in hydroxylation of retinoic acid, 16α-hydroxylation of steroids, and hydroxylation of allylic and benzylic

Table 10.8. Some Substrates and Reaction Type for Human CYP2E1 Isoform[a]

Acetaminophen (*p*-benzoquinone imine)
Styrene (epoxidation)
Theophylline (C-8 oxidation)
Disulfiram
Halogenated Hydrocarbons
Dehalogenation of chloroform, methylene chloride
Volatile Anesthetics (fluorinated hydrocarbons)
Enflurane, Halothane, Methoxyflurane, Sevoflurane, Desflurane
Miscellaneous Organic Solvents
Ethanol (to acetaldehyde)
Glycerin
Dimethylformamide (N-demethylation)
Acetone
Diethylether
Benzene (hydroxylation)
Aniline (hydroxylation)
Acetonitrile (hydroxylation to cyanohydrin)
Pyridine (hydroxylation)

[a]Drugs in bold italics have been reported to cause drug–drug interactions.

carbons and, therefore, is of relevance both to normal development and to carcinogenesis. The most recently discovered CYP3A isoform is CYP3A3. In addition to a low level of expression in liver, it is expressed in prostate and testis. Its substrate specificity currently is unclear. Polymorphisms predicting absence of active enzyme have been identified.

The CYP3A4 subfamily metabolizes a wide range of clinically important drugs (Table 10.9) and is inhibited by a number of xenobiotics, including erythromycin (Table 10.10). It also appears to activate aflatoxin B1 and, possibly, benzo[a]pyrene metabolism. The interindividual differences reported for the metabolism of nifedipine, cyclosporine, triazolam, and midazolam probably are related to changes in induction and not to polymorphism. Binding of CYP3A is predominantly lipophilic (14). Drugs known to be substrates for CYP3A4 have a low and variable oral bioavailability that may be explained by prehepatic metabolism by a combination of intestinal CYP3A4 and P-glycoprotein in the enterocytes of the intestinal wall (see the section on oral bioavailability). Therefore, it is the expression and function of CYP3A4 that governs the rate and extent of metabolism of the substrates for the CYP3A subfamily. The induction of the CYP3A subfamily by phenobarbital in humans may ultimately be responsible for many of the well-documented interactions between barbiturates and other drugs (19,20).

Clearly, no one animal model or combination of animal models reflects the metabolic capabilities of humans. By having a complete understanding of the factors (e.g., inducers, inhibitors, and effect of disease state) that alter the expression and activity of the enzyme responsible for the metabolism of a particular compound, and by a determination of responsible isoforms and patient phenotyping, it may be possible to predict drug interactions and metabolic clearance.

An alphabetical listing of the clinically important drugs and their CYP450 isoforms catalyzing their oxidative metabolism is presented in Table 10.11.

Catalytic Cycle of Cytochrome P450: Steps of the Catalytic Cycle

The many variant CYP450 isoforms that have been isolated show a remarkable uniformity for the catalytic mechanism (21,26,27). The current view illustrating the cyclic mechanism for the reduction and oxygenation of CYP450 as it interacts stepwise with substrate molecules, electron donors, and oxygen is shown in Figure 10.4 and can be summarized as follows (26,27):

Step a. The ferric CYP450 binds reversibly with a molecule of the substrate (RH), resulting in a complex analogous to an enzyme–substrate complex. The binding of the substrate facilitates the first one-electron reduction step.

Step b. The substrate complex of ferric–CYP450 undergoes reduction to a ferrous–CYP450 substrate complex by an electron originating from NADPH and transferred by the flavoprotein, NADPH-CYP450 reductase, from the FNMH2/FADH complex.

Step c. The reduced CYP450 complex readily binds dioxygen as the ferrous iron sixth ligand to form oxy–CYP450 complex.

Step d. Oxy–CYP450 undergoes auto-oxidation to a superoxide anion.

Step e. The ferric superoxide anion undergoes further reduction by accepting a second electron from the flavoprotein (or possibly cytochrome b5) to form the equivalent of a two-electron-reduced complex,

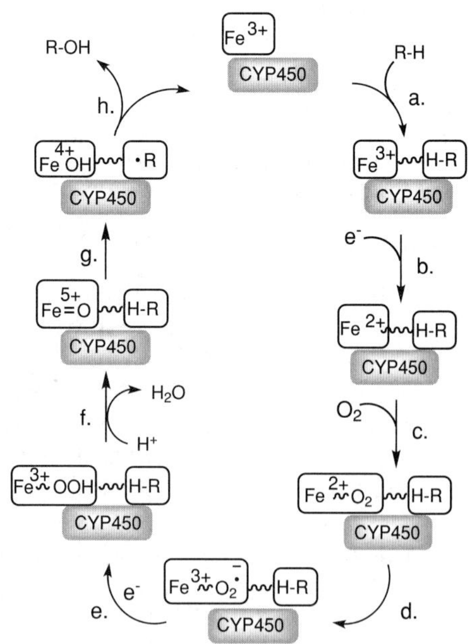

Fig. 10.4. Cyclic mechanism for CYP450. The substrate is RH, and the valence state of the heme iron in CYP450 is indicated.

Table 10.9. Substrates and Reaction Type for Human CYP3A4 Isoform[a]

Alfentanyl
Alfuzosin
Almotriptan
Alprazolam
Amitriptyline
Amiodarone (N-deethylation)
Amlodipine
Amprenavir
Aprepitant
Aripiprazole
Astemizole
Atazanavir
Atorvastatin
"Azole" antifungals
Bepridil
Bexarotene
Bromocriptine
Budesonide
Buprenorphine
Buspirone
Cafergot
Caffeine
Cannabinoids
Carbamzepine (epoxidation)
Cerivastatin
Cevimeline
Chlorpheniramine
Cilostazol
Cinacalcet
Citopram
Clarithromycin
Clindamycin
Clomipramine
Clonazepam
Clopidogrel
Clozapine
Cocaine
Codeine (N-demethylation)
Colchicine
Cyclophosphamide
Cyclosporine (N-demethylation and methyl oxidation)
Dapsone (N-oxide)
Darifenacin
Delavirdine
Desogestrel
Dextromethorphan (N-demethylation)
Diazepam (C-7 hydroxylation)
Dihydroergotamine
Diisopyramide
Diltiazem (N-deethylation)
Docetaxel
Dofetilide
Dolasetron (N-oxide)
Domperidone
Donepezil
Doxorubicin
Dronabinol
Duasteride
Efavirenz
Eplerenone
Ergotamine
Erlotinib
Erythromycin (N-demethylation)
Esomeprazole
Eszopiclone
Ethinylestradiol
Ethosuximide
Etonogestrel
Etoposide
Exemestane
Felodipine
Fentanyl
Finasteride
Fexofenadine
Flutamide
Fluticasone
Galantamine
Gleevec
Haloperidol
Hydrocodone
Imatinib
Imipramine (N-demethylation)
Isradipine (aromatization)
Indinavir
Irinotecan
Itraconazole
Keotconazole
Lansoprazole
Letrozole
Lercanidipine
Lidocaine (N-deethylation)
Loratidine
Lopinavir
Lovastatin (6-hydroxylation)
Methadone
Midazolam (methyl hydroxylation)
Mifepristone
Mirtazepine
Modafinil
Mometasone
Montelukast
Nateglinide
Nelfinavir
Nevirapine
Nicardipine (aromatization)
Nifedipine
Nisoldipine
Nitrendipine
Norethindrone
Odanestron
Omeprazole
Oral contraceptives/progestins
Oxybutynin
Paclitaxel
Pantoprazole
Pioglitazone
Propranolol
Quetiapine
Quinidine (not 3A5) (C-3 hydroxylation)
Quinine
Rabeprazole
Ramelteon
Ranolazine
Repaglinide
Rifampin, ***rifabutin***, and related compounds
Ritonavir
Salmeterol
Saquinavir
Sertraline
Sibuttramine
Sildenafil
Simvastatin
Sirolimus
Solifenacin
Sorafenib
Sunitinib
Steroids
  Testosterone (6β-hydroxylation)
  Progesterone (6β-hydroxylation)
  Estradiol (2- and 4-hydroxylation)
  17α-ethinyl estradiol (2- and 4-hydroxylation)
  Norethisterone (2-hydroxylation)
  Hydrocortisone (6-hydroxylation)
  Methylprednisolone
  Prednisone (6β-hydroxylation)
  Prednisolone (6β-hydroxylation)
  Dexamethasone
Tacrolimus
Tadalafil
Tamoxifen (N-demethylation)
Telithromycin
Temazepam
Δ^1-THC (6β-hydroxylation)
Theophylline (C-8 oxidation)
Tiagabine
Tinidazole
Tipranavir
Tolterodine (N-demethylation)
Toremifene
Tramadol
Trazodone
Triazolam
Trimetrexate
Valdecoxib
Valproic acid (hydroxylation and dehydrogenation)
Vardenafil
Verapamil (N-demethylation)
Vinblastine
Vincristine
Voriconazole
R-Warfarin
Zaleplon
Zileuton
Ziprasidone
Zolpidem
Zonisamide

[a]Drugs in bold italic have been reported to cause drug–drug interactions.

Table 10.10. Cytochrome P450 Inhibitors[a]

CYP1A2	CYP2B6	CYP2C8	CYP2C19	CYP2C9	CYP2D6	CYP2E1	CYP3A4/5/7
Amiodarone	Thiotepa	Anastrozole	Cimetidine	***Amiodarone***	***Amiodarone***	Diethyl dithiocarbamate	***Amiodarone***
Atazanavir	Ticlopidine	***Gemfibrozil***	Citalopram	Atazanavir	Bupropion	Disulfiram	***Amprenavir***
Cimetidine		Glitazones	Delavirdine	***Cimetidine***	Celecoxib		***Aprepitant***
Ciprofloxacin		Montelukast	Efavirenz	Clopidogrel	Chloroquine		***Atazanavir***
Citalopram		Nicardipine	Felbamate	Cotrimoxazole	Chlorpheniramine		***Cimetidine***
Clarithromycin		Sulfinpyrazone	Fluconazole	Delavirdine	Chlorpromazine		Ciprofloxacin
Diltiazem		Trimethoprim	***Fluoxetine***	Disulfiram	***Cimetidine***		***Clarithromycin***
Enoxacin			Fluvastatin	Efavirenz	***Cinacalcet***		***Cyclosporine***
Erythromycin			***Fluvoxamine***	Fenofibrate	Citalopram		Danazol
Ethinyl Estradiol			Indomethacin	***Fluconazole***	Clemastine		***Delavirdine***
Fluoroquinolones			Isoniazid	Fluorouracil	Clomipramine		Diethyl dithiocarbamate
Fluvoxamine			Ketoconazole	***Fluoxetine***	Cocaine		***Diltiazem***
Interferon			Lansoprazole	Fluvastatin	***Darifenacin***		***Efavirenz***
Isoniazid			Modafinil	***Fluvoxamine***	Desipramine		***Erythromycin***
Ketoconazole			Omeprazole	Gemfibrozil	Diphenhydramine		Ethinyl Estradiol
Methoxsalen			Oxcarbazepine	Imatinib	Doxepin		***Fluconazole***
Mibefradil			Probenicid	***Isoniazid***	Doxorubicin		Fluoxetine
			Ticlopidine	Itraconazole	***Duloxetine***		***Fluvoxamine***
			Topiramate	Ketoconazole	Escitalopram		Gestodene
				Leflunomide	***Fluoxetine***		Imatinib
				Lovastatin	Fluphenazine		***Indinavir***
				Methoxsalen	Halofantrine		***Isoniazid***
				Metronidazole	Haloperidol		***Itraconazole***
				Mexiletine	Hydroxychloroquine		***Ketoconazole***
				Modafinil	Hydroxyzine		Methylprednisolne
				Nalidixic acid	Imatinib		***Metronidazole***
				Norethindrone	Levomepromazine		Mibefradil
				Norfloxacin	Methadone		***Miconazole***
				Omeprazole	Metoclopramide		Mifepristone
				Oral Contraceptives	Mibefradil		***Nelfinavir***
				Paroxetine	Midodrine		Nicardipine
				Phenylbutazone	Moclobemide		***Nifedipine***
				Probenicid	Norfluoxetine		Norethindrone
				Sertraline	***Paroxetine***		***Norfloxacin***
				Sulfamethoxazole	Perphenazine		Norfluoxetine
				Sulfaphenazole	Propafenone		Oxiconazole
				Sulfonamides	Propoxyphene		Prednisone
				Tacrine	***Propranolol***		***Quinine***
				Teniposide	Quinacrine		***Ranolazine***
				Ticlopidine	***Quinidine***		***Ritonavir***
				Tipranavir	Ranitidine		***Roxithromycin***
				Troleandomycin	Ranolazine		***Saquinavir***
				Voriconazole	***Ritonavir***		***Sertraline***
				Zafirlukast	***Sertraline***		***Telithromycin***
				Zileuton	Terbinafine		***Troleandomycin***
					Thioridazine		***Verapamil***
					Ticlopidine		***Voriconazole***
					Tipranavir		***Zafirlukast***
					Tripelennamine		***Zileuton***

[a]CYP450 isoform inhibitors presented in bold italics have been associated with drug interactions of clinical relevance or with drug-drug interaction warnings that may require dosage adjustment. (Data from Stockley's Drug Interactions: A Source Book of Interactions, Their Mechanisms, Clinical Importance and Management. London and Chicago: Pharmaceutical Press, 2006.)

Table 10.11. Substrates for the CYP450 Isoforms Catalyzing Their Metabolism

Acetaminophen	1A2, 2E1, 3A4	Esomeprazole	2C19
Albendazole	3A4, 1A2	Estradiol	1A2
Alfentanil	3A4	Estrogens, oral	3A4
Alprazolam	3A4	Ethanol	2E1
Amiodarone	3A4, 2C8	Ethinyl estradiol	3A4
Amitriptyline	1A2, 2C9, 2D6, 3A4, 2C19	Ethosuximide	3A4
Amlodipine	3A4	Etoposide	3A4
Amphetamine	2D6	Felodipine	3A4
Anastrozole	3A4	Fenfluramine	2D6
Astemizole	3A4	Fentanyl	2D6, 3A4
Atomoxetine	2D6	Fexofenadine	3A4
Atorvastatin	3A4	Finasteride	3A4
Bepridil	3A4	Flecainide	2D6
Bisoprolol	2D6	Fluconazole	3A4
Bupropion	2B6	Flurbiprofen	2C9
Busulfan	3A4	Fluoxetine	2C9, 2D6
Caffeine	1A2	Fluvastatin	2C8, 2C9
Cannabinoids	3A4	Fluphenazine	2D6
Carbamazepine	2C8, 3A4	Flutamide	1A2, 3A4
Carisoprodol	2C19	Fluvoxamine	1A2, 2D6
Carvedilol	2C9, 2D6	Formoterol	2C9, 2C19, 2D6
Celecoxib	2C9	Galantamine	2D6
Cerivastatin	3A4	Glimepiride	2C9
Cevimeline	2D6	Glipizide	2C9
Chlordiazepoxide	1A2	Glyburide	2C9, 3A4
Chloroquine	3A4	Granisetron	3A4
Chlorpromazine	2D6, 3A4	Halofantrine	3A4
Chlorzoxazone	2E1	Haloperidol	1A2, 2D6
Cilostazol	2C19	Halothane	2E1
Cimetidine	3A4	Hexobarbital	2C19, 2C9
Cisapride	3A4	Hydrocodone	2D6, 3A4
Citalopram	2C19	Hydrocortisone	2D6, 3A4
Clarithromycin	3A4	Ibuprofen	2C9
Clindamycin	3A4	Ifosfamide	2B6, 3A4
Clomipramine	1A2, 2C9, 2C19, 2D6, 3A4	Imipramine	1A2, 2C19, 2C9, 2D6, 3A4
Clopidogrel	1A2	Indinavir	2D6, 3A4
Clonazepam	3A4	Indomethacin	2C9, 2C19
Clozapine	1A2, 2D6, 2A6	Irbesartan	2C9
Cocaine	3A4	Isoflurane	2E1
Codeine	2D6, 3A4	Isoniazid	2E1
Cyclobenzaprine	1A2, 2A6, 2D6, 3A4	Isotretinoin (retinoids)	1A2, 2C8, 3A4
Cyclophosphamide	2B6, 2C19, 3A4	Isradipine	3A4
Cyclosporine	3A4	Itraconazole	3A4
Dapsone	2C9, 3A4	Ketoconazole	3A4
Delavirdine	3A4	Labetalol	2D6
Desipramine	1A2, 2C19, 2D6	Lansoprazole	2C19, 3A4
Desogestrel	2C9	Lidocaine	2D6, 3A4
Dexamethasone	3A4	Losartan	2C9, 3A4
Dexfenfluramine	2D6	Lovastatin	3A4
Dextromethorphan	2D6, 3A4	Maprotiline	2D6
Diazepam	1A2, 2C19, 2C9, 3A4	Meclobemide	2C19
Diclofenac	2C8/9	Mefenamic acid	2C9
Diltiazem	3A4	Mefloquine	3A4
Disopyramide	3A4	Meloxicam	2C9
Divalproex sodium	2C19	Meperidine	2D6
Docetaxel	2C8, 3A4	Mephenytoin	2C19
Dolasetron	2D6, 3A4	Mephobarbital	2C9
Donepezil	2D6, 3A4	Methadone	1A2, 2D6
Doxepin	2D6	Methamphetamine	2D6
Doxorubicin	3A4	Metoprolol	2D6
Dronabinol	2C9	Mexiletine	1A6, 2D6, 2A6
Enalapril	3A4	Mibefradil	3A4
Encainide	2D6	Miconazole	3A4
Enflurane	2E1	Midazolam	3A4
Ergot alkaloids	3A4	Mirtazapine	1A2, 2D6, 3A4
Erythromycin	3A4	Montelukast	2C9

(Continued)

Table 10.11. *(Continued)*

Morphine	2D6	Ropivacaine	1A2, 2D6
Naproxen	1A2, 2C18, 2C9, 2A6	Rosiglitazone	2C8, 2C9
Nateglinide	2C9	Salmeterol	3A4
Navelbine	3A4	Saquinavir	3A4
Nefazodone	3A4	Selegiline	2D6
Nelfinavir	3A4	Sertindole	2D6
Nevirapine	3A4	Sertraline	2B6, 3A4, 2D6, 2C19, 2C9
Nicardipine	3A4	Sevoflurane	2E1
Nicotine	2A6, 2B6	Sildenafil	2C9, 3A4
Nifedipine	3A4/5	Simvastatin	3A4
Nilutamide	2C19	Sufentanil	3A4
Nimodipine	3A4	Sulfamethoxazole	2C9
Nisoldpine	3A4	Tacrine	1A2, 2A6
Nitrendipine	3A4	Tacrolimus	3A4
Nortriptyline	1A2, 2D6	Tamoxifen	1A2 , 2A6, 2B6, 2D6, 2E1, 3A4
Olanzapine	2D6	Temazepam	3A4
Omeprazole	2C19, 2C9, 3A4	Teniposide	3A4, 2C19
Ondansetron	1A2, 2D6, 2E1, 3A4	Terfenadine	3A4
Oral contraceptives	3A4	Testosterone	3A4
Oxycodone	2D6	Theophylline	1A2, 2E1, 3A4
Paclitaxel	2C8, 3A4	Thiabendazole	1A2
Pantoprazole	2C19	Thioridazine	2C19, 2D6
Paroxetine	2D6	Tiagabine	3A4
Perphenazine	2D6	Timolol	2D6
Phenacetin	1A2	Tolbutamide	2C8,2C9, 2C19
Phenformin	2D6	Tolteridine	2D6
Phenol	2E1	Torsemide	2C9
Phenytoin	2C19, 2C8, 2C9	Tramadol	2D6
Pimozide	3A4	Trazodone	2D6
Pindolol	2D6	Tretinoin	2C8, 3A4
Pioglitazone	2C8	Triazolam	3A4
Piroxicam	2C18, 2C9	Troleandomycin	3A4
Pravastatin	3A4	Tropisetron	2D6
Praziqantel	2B6, 3A4	Valsartan	2C9
Prednisone	3A4	Valproic acid	2C19
Progesterone	3A4, 2C19	Valdecoxib	2C9
Proguanil	2C18, 2C19	Vardenafil	3A4
Propafenone	1A2, 2D6, 3A4	Venlafaxine	2D6
Propoxyphene	2D6	Verapamil	1A2, 3A4,2C8
Propranolol	1A2, 2C18, 2C19, 2D6	Vinblastine	3A4
Quetiapine	2D6	Vinca alkaloids	3A4
Quinidine	3A4	Vincristine	3A4
Quinine	3A4	Voriconazole	2C9
Rabeprazole	2C19	Warfarin	2C18, 2C9
Rapaglinide	2C8	R-warfarin	1A2
Retinoic acid	2C8	S-warfarin	2C9, 2C18
Rifabutin	3A4	Yohimbine	2D6
Rifampin	3A4	Zafirlukast	2C9
Riluzole	1A2	Zaleplon	3A4
Risperidone	2D6	Zileuton	1A2, 2C9, 3A4
Ritonavir	2A6, 2C19, 2C9, 2D6, 2E1, 3A4	Zolpidem	3A4
Ropinirole	1A2	Zoplicone	2C8, 3A4

peroxy–CYP450. The cycle can be aborted (uncoupled) from subsequent substrate hydroxylation at this step by xenobiotics, which can cause the superoxide anion to disproportionate to hydrogen peroxide and dioxygen with regeneration of the starting point of the cycle, the ferric heme protein–substrate complex.

Step f. The ferric peroxy–CYP450 complex undergoes heterolytic cleavage of peroxide anion to water and to a highly electrophilic perferryl oxenoid intermediate ($Fe^{5+}{=}O$) or a perferryl oxygen–cysteine–porphyrin resonance-stabilized complex. This perferryl oxygen species represents the catalytically active oxygenation species.

Step g. Abstraction of a hydrogen from the substrate by the perferryl oxygen species gives rise to a carbon-centered radical–perferric hydroxide pair, radical addition to a π-bond, or electron abstraction from a heteroatom to form a heteroatom-centered radical–cation perferryl intermediate.

Step h. Subsequent radical recombination (oxygen rebound) or electron-transfer (deprotonation) yields the hydroxylated product and the regeneration of the ferric–CYP450 complex.

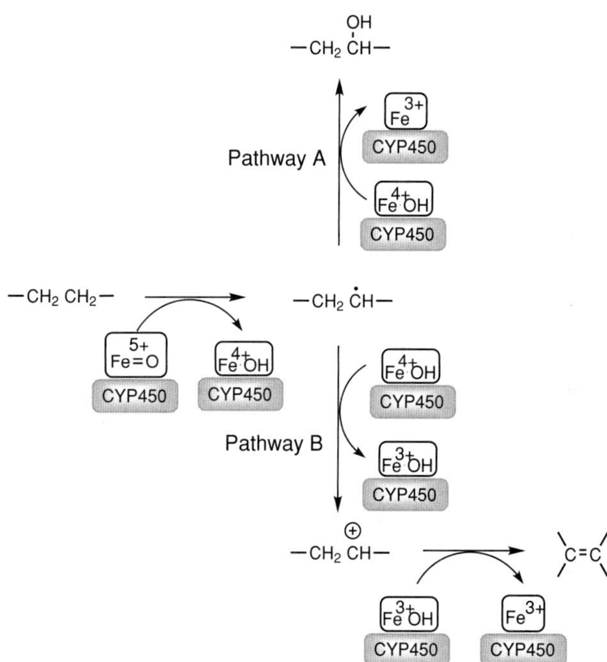

Fig. 10.5. Proposed mechanisms for the hydroxylation and dehydrogenation of alkanes.

Up to the final step, the oxidizable substrate has been an inactive spectator in the chemical events of oxygen activation. None of the preceding oxygenated intermediates has been sufficiently reactive to abstract hydrogen from the substrate. The perferryl–iron oxenoid complex (Step g), however, is a competent hydrogen abstractor, even for relatively inert terminal methyl groups on hydrocarbon chains. Evidence shows that the oxidant is selective in its choice of hydrogen atoms, balancing stability of the resulting carbon radical with stereochemical constraints. Because the inert aliphatic region of the substrate has been converted to a highly reactive radical, the process is described as substrate activation. Various studies have shown that the hydroxylation or alkene formation proceeds not by a direct one-step insertion of the oxygen atom but, rather, by a two-step, two-electron process involving radical or cationic substrate intermediates with subsequent radical recombination (oxygen rebound) to products (Fig. 10.5) (28).

Despite considerable experimental evidence, the proposed mechanism and intermediates of monooxygenation of unsaturated substrates (alkenes, alkynes, and aromatics) remains controversial (19,20,29–31). The

Oxygen Activation

Elemental oxygen (dioxygen) is a relatively unreactive form of oxygen that exists as an unpaired diradical in the triplet form. Alternatively, singlet oxygen is a form of dioxygen in which the diradical electrons are paired. In this form, oxygen is too reactive for biological systems. Free oxygen atoms (oxenes), formed by splitting dioxygen, are highly reactive but are not known to exist in biochemical processes. The solution to the problem of a reactive form of oxygen lies in the suggestion that the reduction of dioxygen occurs to one of the reactive oxygen species (ROS), such as superoxide radical anion, peroxide, hydroxyl radical, or oxygen atom.

Any of these ROS could oxidize an organic substrate with the net insertion of an oxygen atom. In each case, reductive reactions are required for activation of dioxygen to one of the ROS from electrons supplied by NADPH. The generation of a carbon-centered radical and a hydroxyl radical with triplet oxygen atom has been found to be relevant to a number of enzymatic and chemical reactions involving oxenoids (oxygen rebound mechanism) (28). The function of CYP450 monooxygenases usually is the hydroxylation of a substrate. A reactive radical-like iron oxenoid intermediate is generated that is reactive enough to split aliphatic C-H bonds, add to bonds α to heteroatoms, or remove single electrons from heteroatoms. The mechanisms of CYP450 are not fully understood, and the reactive oxygen intermediate has not been isolated or even spectroscopically observed.

$\cdot O{=}O \cdot$ ($\uparrow O{=}O \uparrow$) — Triplet oxygen; $\uparrow O{=}O \downarrow$ — Singlet oxygen (Dioxygen)

$\uparrow O \uparrow$ — Triplet; $\uparrow O \downarrow$ — Singlet (Oxenes)

$O_2 + e^- \rightarrow :O{=}O\cdot^{\ominus}$ Superoxide radical anion

$O_2 + 2e^- + 2H^+ \rightarrow H_2O_2$ Peroxide

$O_2 + 2e^- + 2H^+ \rightarrow 2\,HO\cdot + H_2O$ Hydroxyl radical

$O_2 + 2e^- + 2H^+ \rightarrow O + H_2O$ Oxygen atom

Reactive oxygen species (ROS)

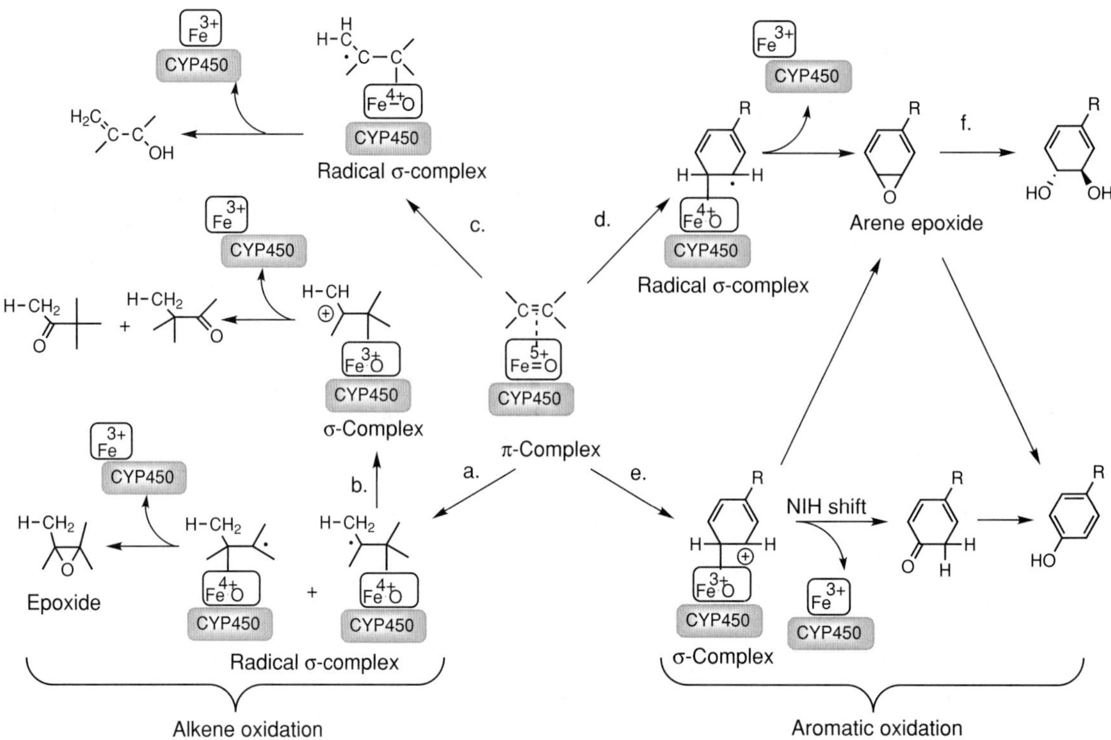

Fig. 10.6. Proposed mechanisms for the oxidation of alkene and aromatic compounds.

proposed mechanism for the oxidation of π-bonds in alkenes involves a stepwise sequence of one-electron transfer between the radical complex and the perferryl oxygen intermediate ([Fe^{5+}=O]) (alkene oxidation) (Fig. 10.6). Following the initial formation of an unsaturated CYP450 π-complex, the one-electron transfer yields a radical σ-complex which can either collapse to arene or alkene epoxide (steps a or d, Fig. 10.6), undergo a 1,2-group migration to a carbonyl product (steps a and b, Fig. 10.6), or give a vinyl hydroxylated product (step c, Fig. 10.6), or a σ-complex which can break down to a phenol (step e, Fig. 10.6). The presence of an oxygen radical in the porphyrin ring allows some substrate radicals to covalently bond through N-alkylation of a pyrrole nitrogen rather than recombining with $(Fe–OH)^{3+}$. This deviation from the normal course of reaction explains the suicide inhibition exhibited by some xenobiotics, such as the oral contraceptives, erythromycin, and paroxetine (32,33).

In the case of aromatic oxidations (Fig. 10.6), following the initial formation of an arene CYP450 π-complex, one-electron transfer yields either a π-complex or a radical σ-complex. The radical σ-complex can collapse to the arene epoxide (Fig. 10.6, step d), or the π-complex can proceed to a σ-complex followed by a NIH shift (1,2-group migration) to a phenolic product (Fig. 10.6, step e). Arene oxides are highly unstable entities and rearrange (NIH shift) nonenzymatically to phenols or hydrolyzed enzymatically with epoxide hydrolase to 1,2-dihydrodiols (trans configuration) (Fig. 10.6, step f), which subsequently are dehydrogenated to 1,2-diphenols. The oxidation of aromatic compounds can be highly specific to individual CYP450 isoforms, suggesting that substrate binding and orientation in the active site may dominate the mechanism of oxidative catalysis.

Heteroatom-containing substrates usually undergo hydroxylation adjacent (α) to the heteroatom, as compared to other positions. Reactions of this type include N-, O-, and S-dealkylation as well as dehydrohalogenations and oxidative deamination (dealkylation) reactions. Two mechanisms have been suggested (Fig. 10.7). One is the

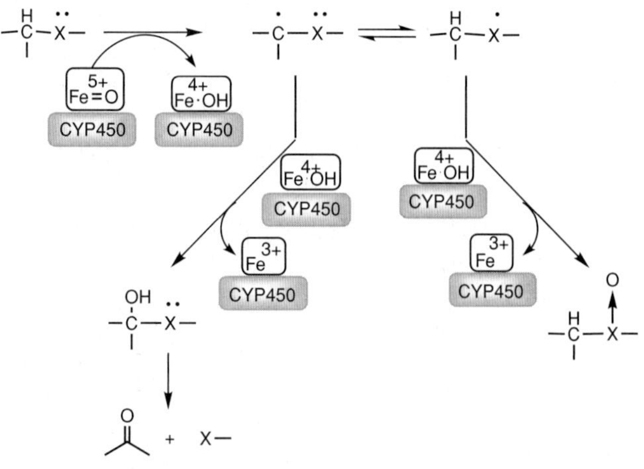

Fig. 10.7. Proposed mechanism for heteroatom-compound oxidation, dealkylation, and dehalogenation.

abstraction of a hydrogen atom from the carbon adjacent to the heteroatom, and the resultant carbon radical is stabilized by the heteroatom. Alternatively, abstraction of an electron from the heteroatom to form a heteroatom radical subsequently transfers a hydrogen atom from the more labile α-carbon to generate a carbon radical. Collapse of the carbon radical–perferric hydroxide radical pair hydroxylates the carbon adjacent to the heteroatom, generating an unstable geminal hydroxy heteroatom-substituted intermediate (e.g., carbinolamine, halohydrin, hemiacetal, hemiketal, or hemithioketal) that breaks down, releasing the heteroatom and forming a carbonyl compound (29–31).

Xenobiotics containing heteroatoms (N, S, P, and halogens) frequently are metabolized by heteroatom oxidation to its corresponding heteroatom oxide (tertiary amine to its N-oxide, sulfides to sulfoxides, or phosphines to phosphine oxides). Heteroatom oxidation also can be attributed to a microsomal flavin-containing monooxygenase. As is the case with heteroatom α-hydroxylation, one-electron oxidation of the heteroatom occurs as the first step to form the heteroatom cation perferric hydroxide radical intermediate, which collapses to generate the heteroatom oxide. This reaction is favored by the absence of α-hydrogens and stability of the heteroatom radical-cation (29–31).

All the known oxidative reactions catalyzed by CYP450 monooxygenase can be described in the context of a mechanistic scheme involving the ability of a high-valent iron oxenoid species to bring about the stepwise one-electron oxidation through the abstraction of hydrogen atoms, abstraction of electrons from heteroatoms, or addition to π-bonds. A series of radical recombination reactions completes the oxidation process.

Induction and Inhibition of Cytochrome P450 Isoforms

Induction

Many drugs, environmental chemicals, and other xenobiotics enhance the metabolism of themselves or of other coingested/inhaled compounds, thereby altering their pharmacological and toxicological effects (34–36). Prolonged administration of a drug or xenobiotic can lead to enhanced metabolism of a wide variety of other compounds. Enzyme induction is a dose-dependent phenomenon.

Drugs and xenobiotics exert this effect by inducing transcription of CYP450 mRNA and synthesis of xenobiotic-metabolizing enzymes in the smooth ER of the liver and other extrahepatic tissues (34,35). This phenomenon is termed "enzyme induction," which has been used to describe the process by which the rate of synthesis of an enzyme is increased relative to the rate of synthesis in the uninduced organism. In many older studies of mammalian systems, the term "induction" was inferred from the increase in enzyme activity, but the amount of enzyme protein had not been determined. Enzyme induction is important for interpreting the results of chronic toxicities, mutagenicities, or carcinogenesis and explaining certain unexpected drug interactions in patients.

Many drugs and xenobiotics stimulate the activity of the CYP450 isoforms, as shown in Table 10.12. These stimulators have nothing in common as far as their pharmacological activity or chemical structures are concerned, but they are all metabolized by one or more of the CYP450 isoforms. Most are lipid soluble at physiologic pH. Polycyclic aromatic hydrocarbons in cigarette

Table 10.12. Drugs that Induce the Expression of CYP450 Isoforms[a]

Drug	Isoforms	Drug	Isoforms
Amprenavir	3A4	4-Methylpyrazole	2E1
Aprepitant	2C9	Modafinil	3A4
Barbiturates	3A4, 2C9, 2C19, 2B6	Nevirapine	3A4
		Norethindrone	2C19
Carbamazepine	1A2, 3A4, 2C8, 2C9, 2D6	Omeprazole	1A1/2, 3A4
		Oxcarbazepine	3A4
Charbroiled meats	1A1/2,	***Phenobarbital***	3A4, 2C, 2B6, 2D6, 1A2
Cigarette smoke	1A1/2	***Phenytoin***	3A4, 1A2, 2B6, 2C8, 2C19, 2D6
Clotrimazole	1A1/2, 3A4	Primidone	3A4, 2C9, 1A2, 2B6, 2D6
Ethanol	2D6, 2E1	Psoralen	1A1/2
Efavirenz	3A4	***Ethosuximide***	3A4
Erythromycin	3A4	Polycyclic aromatic hydrocarbons	1A1/2
Glucocorticoids	3A4, 2A6,	Rifampin	2C8, 2C9,2C19, 2D6, 3A4
(Dexamethasone,		Rifampicin	2C8
prednisone)	2C19		Rifabutin 2C8, 3A4
		Rifapentine	3A4
Griseofulvin	3A4	Ritonavir	2D6, 3A4
Isoniazid	2E1	***St. Johns Wort***	1A2, 2C9, 3A4
Lansoprazole	1A1/2, 3A4	Troglitazone	3A4
Mephenytoin	2B6	Topiramate	3A4

[a]Drugs in bold italic have been reported to cause drug-drug interaction.

smoke, xanthines and flavones in foods, halogenated hydrocarbons in insecticides, polychlorinated biphenyls, and food additives are but a few of the environmental chemicals that alter the activity of CYP450 enzymes (37).

Enzyme induction can alter the pharmacokinetics and pharmacodynamics of a drug, with clinical implications for the therapeutic actions of a drug and increased potential for drug interactions. As a result of induction, a drug may be metabolized more rapidly to metabolites that are more potent, more toxic, or less active than the parent drug. Induction also can enhance the activation of procarcinogens or promutagens. Not all inducing agents enhance their own metabolism; for example, phenytoin induces CYP3A4 but is hydroxylated by CYP2C9, which is constitutive. Some of the more common enzyme inducers of CYP450 subfamilies, which also may be substrates for the same CYP450 isoform, include phenobarbital (CYP2B6, CYP2C, and CYP3A4), rifampicin (CYP3A4), and cigarette smoke (CYP1A1/2) (Table 10.12). The broad range of drugs metabolized by these CYP450 subfamilies (Table 10.11) and that also are affected by these enzyme inducers raises the issue of clinically significant drug interactions and their clinical implications. Examples of a clinical CYP450–drug interaction and an herbal drug–drug interaction include rifampin and oral contraceptives as well as St. John's wort and oral contraceptives. Both induce the expression of CYP3A4, thereby reducing the serum levels of the oral contraceptive because of increased oxidative metabolism of the oral contraceptives by CYP3A4 to less active metabolites, increasing the risk for pregnancy. Drugs poorly metabolized by CYP450 enzymes are less affected by enzyme induction. Inducers of CYP450 isoforms also stimulate the oxidative metabolism or synthesis of endogenous substances, such as the hydroxylation of androgens, estrogens, progestational steroids (synthetic oral contraceptives), glucocorticoids, vitamin D, and bilirubin, decreasing their biological activity. These enzyme inducers also might be implicated in deficiencies associated with these steroids. For example, the induction of C-2 hydroxylation of estradiol and synthetic estrogens by phenobarbital, dexamethasone, or cigarette smoking in women results in the increased formation of the principal and less active metabolite of these estrogenic substances, reducing their effectiveness (38). Thus, cigarette smoking in premenopausal women could result in an estrogen deficiency, increasing the risk of osteoporosis and early menopause. Postmenopausal women who smoke and take estrogen replacement therapy may lose the effectiveness of the estrogen.

In addition to enhancing metabolism of other drugs, many compounds, when chronically administered, stimulate their own metabolism, thereby decreasing their therapeutic activity and producing a state of apparent tolerance. This self-induction may explain some of the change in drug toxicity observed in prolonged treatment. The sedative action of phenobarbital, for example, becomes shorter with repeated doses and can be explained in part on the basis of increased metabolism.

The time course of induction varies with different inducing agents and different isoforms, except that CYP1A induction involves the Ah receptor. Increased transcription of CYP450 mRNA has been detected as early as 1 hour after the administration of phenobarbital, with maximum induction after 48 to 72 hours. After the administration of PAH, such as 3-methylcholanthrene and benzo[a]pyrene, maximum induction of the CYP1A subfamily is reached within 24 hours. Less potent inducers of hepatic drug metabolism may take as long as 6 to 10 days to reach maximum induction (34,35). Exposure to a variety of xenobiotics may preferentially increase the hepatic content of specific forms of CYP450 (34–36). Therefore, the process of enzyme induction involves the adaptive increase in the content of specific enzymes in response to the enzyme-inducing agent. Other inducible metabolizing enzymes include uridine diphosphate (UDP)–glucuronosyl transferase and glutathione transferase.

Specific Inducers

PHENOBARBITAL AND RIFAMPIN. Phenobarbital and rifampin probably are the enzyme inducers that have been studied most extensively. These drugs could alter the pharmacokinetics and pharmacodynamics of many concurrently administered drugs listed in Tables 10.6 (CYP2C) and 10.9 (CYP3A4), raising the issue of clinically significant drug interactions.

CIGARETTE SMOKE. Cigarette smoke has been shown to increase the hydrocarbon-inducible isoforms CYP1A1 and CYP1A2 in the lungs, liver, small intestine, and placenta of cigarette smokers. A decrease in the pharmacological action and stimulation of the metabolism of several drugs is the end result. Cigarette smoking has been reported to lower the blood levels of theophylline, imipramine, estradiol, pentazocine, and propoxyphene; to decrease the urinary excretion of nicotine; and to decrease drowsiness from chlorpromazine, diazepam, and chlordiazepoxide. The plasma levels, half-life, or total clearance for diazepam, however, are unchanged.

DIETARY SUBSTANCES. A diet containing Brussel sprouts, cabbage, and cauliflower was found to stimulate CYP450 activity in rat intestine (39). It was subsequently determined that indole derivatives (indole-3-carbinol) were responsible for the enzyme induction. Other examples of chemicals found naturally in foods that enhance metabolism in animals are flavones, safrole, eucalyptol, xanthines, β-ionone, and organic peroxides. Volatile oils in soft woods (e.g., cedar) have been shown to be enzyme inducers.

ALCOHOL. Sober alcoholics show an increase in CYP2E1 enzyme activity, leading to more rapid clearance of drugs and xenobiotics that are substrates for this isoform from the body. As discussed previously, hepatic CYP2E1 oxidizes ethanol, and chronic ethanol intake increases the activity of CYP2E1 through enzyme induction (24). When intoxicated, alcoholics are more susceptible to the action of various drugs because of inhibition of drug metabolism as a result of an excessive quantity of alcohol in the liver and an additive or synergistic effect in the central nervous system. The basis for this inhibition is unknown. Furthermore, moderate ethanol consumption reduces the clearance of some drugs, presumably because of competition between ethanol and the other drugs for hepatic biotransformation. The changes in drug metabolism in alcoholics also can be attributed to other factors, such as malnutrition, other drugs, and the trace chemicals that determine the flavor and odor of alcoholic beverages. Heavy drinkers metabolize phenobarbital, tolbutamide, and phenytoin more rapidly than nonalcoholics do, which may be clinically important because of problems in adjusting drug therapy in alcoholics.

Inhibition

Another method of altering the in vivo effects of xenobiotics metabolized by CYP450s is through the use of inhibitors (Table 10.10). The CYP450 inhibitors can be divided into three categories according to their mechanism of action: reversible inhibition, metabolite intermediate complexation of CYP450, or mechanism-based inactivation of CYP450 (36,40,41). The polysubstrate nature of CYP450 is responsible for the large number of documented interactions associated with the inhibition of drug oxidation and drug biotransformation.

Reversible inhibition. Reversible inhibition of CYP450 is the result of reversible interactions at the heme–iron active center of CYP450, the lipophilic sites on the apoprotein, or both. The interaction occurs before the oxidation steps of the catalytic cycle, and their effects dissipate quickly when the inhibitor is discontinued. The most effective reversible inhibitors are those that interact strongly with both the apoprotein and the heme–iron. It is widely accepted that inhibition has an important impact on the oxidative metabolism and pharmacokinetics of drugs with a metabolism that cosegregates with that of an inhibitor (Tables 10.3 and 10.6–10.9) (40,41). Drugs interacting reversibly with CYP450 include the fluoroquinolone antimicrobials, cimetidine, the azole antifungals, quinidine (specific for CYP2D isoforms), and diltiazem. Cimetidine is the only H-2 antagonist that inhibits CYP450 by interacting directly with the CYP450 heme–iron through one of its imidazole ring nitrogen atoms. Cimetidine is not a universal inhibitor of CYP450 oxidative metabolism, but it does bind differentially to several CYP450 isoforms (Table 10.10). Cimetidine inhibits the oxidation of theophylline (CYP1A), chlordiazepoxide (CYP2C), diazepam (CYP2C), propranolol (CYP2C and CYP2D), warfarin (CYP2C), and antipyrine (CYP1A) but not that of ibuprofen (CYP2C), tolbutamide (CYP2C), mexiletine (CYP2D), 6-hydroxylation of steroids (CYP3A), and carbamazepine (CYP3A) (36). The imidazole-based azole antifungals are potent inhibitors of CYP3A and of the CYP450-mediated biosynthesis of endogenous steroid hormones. The azole antifungals exert their fungiostatic effects through inhibition of fungal CYP450, inhibiting the oxidative biosynthesis of lanosterol to ergosterol, thereby affecting the integrity and permeability of the fungal membranes.

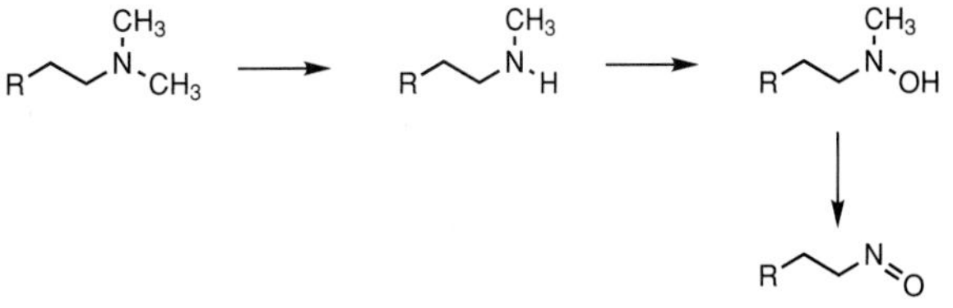

Fig. 10.8. Sequence of oxidation of dialkylamine to nitroso metabolite intermediate.

CYP450 complexation inhibition. Noninhibitory alkylamine drugs have the ability to undergo CYP450-mediated oxidation to nitrosoalkane metabolites (Fig. 10.9), which have a high affinity for forming a stable complex with the reduced (ferrous) heme intermediate for the CYP2B, CYP2C, and CYP3A subfamilies. This process is termed "metabolite intermediate complexation" (40,41). Thus, the CYP450 isoform is unavailable for further oxidation, and synthesis of the new enzyme is required to restore CYP450 activity. The process relies on at least one cycle of the CYP450 catalytic cycle to generate the required heme intermediate. The macrolide antibiotics, troleandomycin, erythromycin, and clarithromycin, as well as their analogues are selective inhibitors of CYP3A4 that are capable of inducing the expression of hepatic and extrahepatic CYP3A4 mRNA and induction of their own biotransformation into nitrosoalkane metabolites. The clinical significance of this inhibition with CYP3A4 is the long-lived impairment of the metabolism of a large number of coadministered substrates for this isoform and the potential for drug–drug interactions and time-dependent nonlinearities in their pharmacokinetics on long-term administration (Tables 10.9 and 10.10). For the macrolides to be so metabolized, they must possess an unhindered dimethylamino sugar, and the whole compound must be lipophilic. Other alkylamine-based drugs demonstrating this type of inhibition include orphenadrine (antiparkinson drug), the antiprogestin, mifepristone (CYP3A), and SKF525A (the original CYP450 inhibitor). Methylenedioxyphenyl compounds (i.e., the insecticide synergist piperonyl butoxide and the flavoring agent isosafrole) generate metabolite intermediates that form stable complexes with both the ferric and ferrous state of CYP450.

Mechanism-based inhibition. Certain drugs that are noninhibitory of CYP450 contain functional groups that, when oxidized by CYP450, generate metabolites that bind irreversibly to the enzyme. This process is termed "mechanism-based inhibition" ("suicide inhibition") and requires at least one catalytic CYP450 cycle either during or subsequent to the oxygen-transfer step, when the drug is activated to the inhibitory species. Alkenes and alkynes were the first functionalities found to inactivate CYP450 by generation of a radical intermediate that alkylates the heme structure (see the section on alkene and alkyne hydroxylation) (32,33,40,41). Iron is lost from the heme and abnormal N-alkylated porphyrins are produced. Drugs that are mechanism-based inhibitors of CYP450 include the 17α-acetylenic estrogen, 17α-ethinyl estradiol, the 17α-acetylenic progestin, norethindrone (norethisterone), and their radical intermediates that N-alkylate heme of CYP3A; chloramphenicol and its oxidative dechlorination to an acyl moiety that alkylates CYP450 apoprotein; cyclophosphamide (CYP3A) and its generation of acrolein and phosphoramide mustard; spironolactone and its 7-thio metabolite that alkylates heme; 8-methoxypsoralen (a furocoumarin) and its epoxide metabolite that alkylates the CYP450 apoprotein of CYP2A6; 21-halosteroids; halocarbons; and secobarbital. The selectivity of CYP450 isoform destruction by several of these inhibitors indicates the involvement of this isoform in its bioactivation of such drugs.

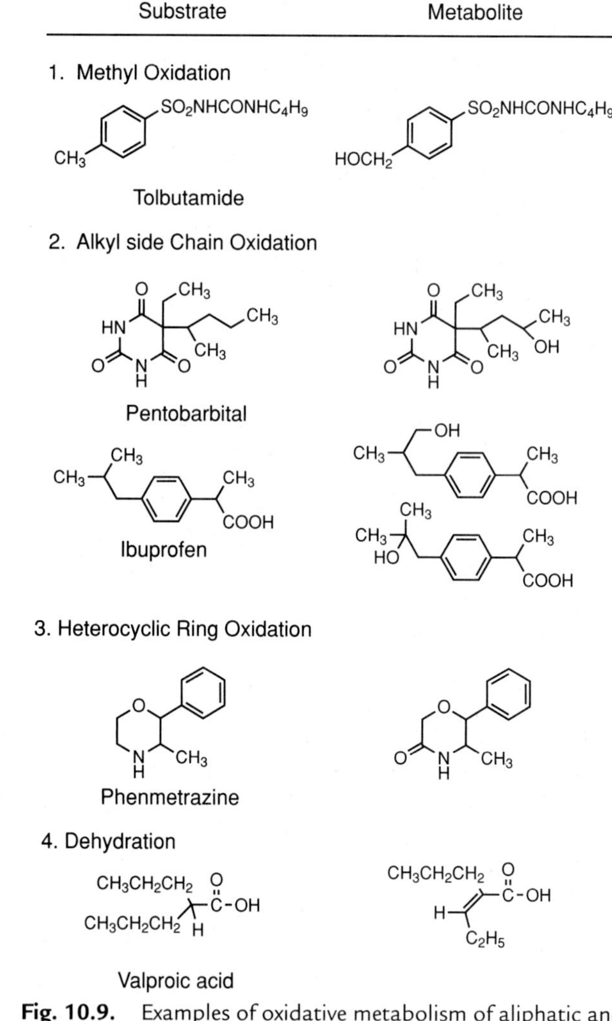

Fig. 10.9. Examples of oxidative metabolism of aliphatic and alicyclic hydrocarbons catalyzed by CYP450.

Oxidations Catalyzed by Cytochrome P450 Isoforms

ALIPHATIC AND ALICYCLIC HYDROXYLATIONS. The accepted mechanism for the hydroxylation of alkane C-H bonds is shown in Figure 10.5 and has been reviewed in detail elsewhere (29–31). The principal metabolic pathway for the methyl group is oxidation to the hydroxymethyl derivative followed by its nonmicrosomal oxidation to the carboxylic acid (e.g., tolbutamide) (Fig. 10.9). On the other hand, some methyl groups are oxidized only to the hydroxymethyl derivative, without further oxidation to the acid. Where there are several equivalent methyl groups, usually only one is oxidized. For aromatic methyl groups, the para methyl is the most vulnerable.

Alkyl side chains often are hydroxylated on the terminal or the penultimate carbon atom (e.g., pentobarbital) (Fig. 10.9). The isopropyl group is an interesting side chain that undergoes hydroxylation at the tertiary carbon and at either of the equivalent methyl groups (e.g., ibuprofen) (Fig. 10.9). Hydroxylation of alkyl side chains attached to an aromatic ring does not follow the general rules for alkyl side chains, because the aromatic ring influences the position of hydroxylation. Generally, oxidation occurs preferentially on the benzylic methylene group and, to a lesser extent, at other positions on the side chain.

The methylene groups of an alicycle are readily hydroxylated, generally at the least hindered position, or at an activated position—for example, α to a carbonyl (cyclohexanone), α to a double bond (cyclohexene), or α to a phenyl ring (tetralin). The products of hydroxylation often show stereoisomerism. Nonaromatic heterocycles generally undergo oxidation at the carbon adjacent to the heteroatom (e.g., phenmetrazine) (Fig. 10.9).

In addition to hydroxylation reactions, CYP450s can catalyze the dehydrogenation of an alkane to an alkene(olefin). The reaction is thought to involve the formation of a carbon radical, electron transfer to the perferryl complex of CYP450 giving a carbocation, and deprotonation to a dehydrogenated product alkene (Fig. 10.5) (29–31). An example of the ability of CYP450 to function as both a dehydrogenase and a monooxygenase has been demonstrated with the antiseizure valproic acid. Whereas the major metabolic products in humans are β-oxidation and acyl glucuronidation, several alkenes are formed, including (E)2-ene isomer (Fig. 10.9) (42). Presumably, the CYP3A subfamily catalyzes these reactions. The factors determining whether CYP450 catalyzes hydroxylation (oxygen rebound/recombination) or dehydrogenation (electron transfer) remain unknown, but hydroxylation generally is favored. In some instances, dehydrogenation may be the primary product (i.e., 6,7-dehydrogenation of testosterone).

ALKENE AND ALKYNE HYDROXYLATION. The oxidation of alkenes yields primarily epoxides and a series of products derived from 1,2-migration (see previous discussion) (Fig. 10.6). The stereochemical configuration of the alkene is retained during epoxidation. The epoxides can differ in reactivity. Those that are highly reactive either undergo pH-catalyzed hydrolysis to excretable vicinal dihydrodiols or react covalently (alkylate) with macromolecules, such as proteins or nucleic acids, leading to tissue necrosis or carcinogenicity. Moreover, the ubiquitous epoxide hydrolase can catalyze the rapid hydrolysis of epoxides to nontoxic vicinal dihydrodiols. Several drugs (carbamazepine, cyproheptadine, and protriptyline), however, were found to form stable epoxides at the 10,11-position during biotransformation (Fig. 10.10). The fact that these epoxides could be detected in the urine indicates that these oxides are not particularly reactive and should not readily react covalently with macromolecules.

The epoxidation of terminal alkenes is accompanied by the mechanism-based ("suicide") N-alkylation of the heme–porphyrin ring. If the π-complex attaches to the alkene at the internal carbon, the terminal carbon of the double bond can irreversibly N-alkylate the pyrrole nitrogen of the porphyrin ring (32,33). The heme adduct formation is mostly observed with monosubstituted, unconjugated alkenes (i.e., 17α-ethylenic steroids and 4-ene metabolite of valproic acid).

In addition to the formation of epoxides, heme adducts, and hydroxylated products, carbonyl products also are created. These latter products result from the migration of atoms to adjacent carbons (i.e., 1,2-group migration). For example, during the CYP450-catalyzed oxidation of trichloroethylene, a 1,2-shift of chloride occurred to yield chloral (Fig. 10.10).

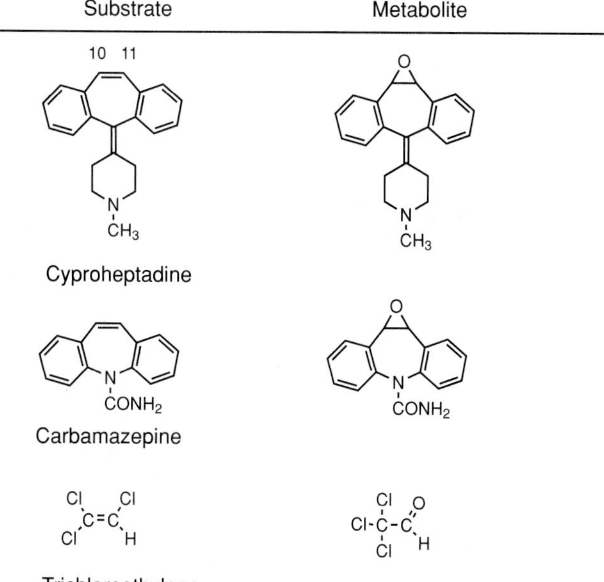

Fig. 10.10. Examples of oxidative metabolism of alkenes and alkynes catalyzed by CYP450.

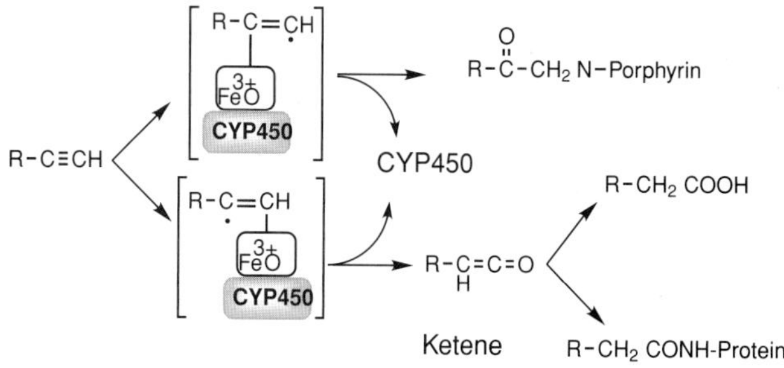

Fig. 10.11. Alkyne oxidation catalyzed by CYP450.

Like the alkenes, alkynes (acetylenes) are readily oxidized but usually faster. Depending on which of the two alkyne carbons are attacked, different products are obtained (32,33). If attachment of CYP450 occurs on the terminal alkyne carbon, a hydrogen atom migrates, forming a ketene intermediate that readily hydrolyzes with water to form an acid or that can alkylate nucleophilic protein side chains (i.e., lysinyl or cysteinyl) to form a protein adduct (Fig. 10.11). The effect of attaching the perferryl oxygen at the internal alkenyl carbon is N-alkylation of a pyrrole nitrogen in the porphyrin ring by the terminal acetylene carbon, with the formation of a keto heme adduct (Fig. 10.11). The latter mechanism has been proposed for the irreversible inactivation of CYP3A4 with 17α-alkenyl steroids (i.e., 17α-ethinyl estradiol).

AROMATIC HYDROXYLATION. The metabolic oxidation of aromatic carbon atoms by CYP450 depends on the isoform catalyzing the oxidation and the oxidation potential of the aromatic compound. The products usually are phenolic products, and the position of hydroxylation can be influenced by the type of substituents on the ring according to the theories of aromatic electrophilic substitution (Fig. 10.6). For example, electron-donating substituents enhance *p*- and *o*-hydroxylation, whereas electron-withdrawing substituents reduce or prevent *m*-hydroxylation. Moreover, steric factors also must be considered, because oxidation usually occurs at the least hindered position. For monosubstituted benzene compounds, parahydroxylation usually predominates, with some ortho product being formed (Fig. 10.12). When there is more than one phenyl ring, usually only one is hydroxylated (e.g., phenytoin).

Traditionally, the hydroxylation of aromatic compounds by CYP450 has been considered to be mediated by an arene oxide (epoxide) intermediate followed by the "NIH shift," as discussed previously (29–31) (Fig. 10.6). The formation of phenols and the isolation of urinary dihydrodiols, catechols, and glutathione conjugates (mercapturic acid derivatives) implicates arene oxides as intermediates in the metabolism of benzene and substituted benzenes in mammalian systems. The arene oxides

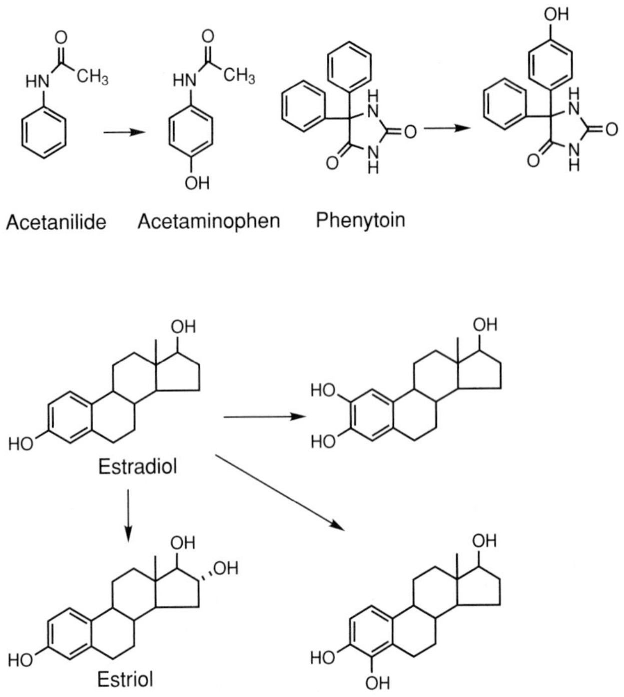

Fig. 10.12. Examples of oxidative metabolism of aryl compounds catalyzed by CYP450.

also are susceptible to conjugation with glutathione to form premercapturic acids (see the section on glutathione conjugation).

The CYP1A2 and CYP3A subfamilies are important contributors to 2- and 4-hydroxylation of estradiol, and CYP3A4 is an important contributor for the 2-hydroxylation of the synthetic estrogens (e.g., 17α-ethinyl estradiol) (38). The principal metabolite (as much as 50%) for estradiol is 2-hydroxyestradiol, with 4-hydroxy and 16α-hydroxyestradiol as the minor metabolites (Fig. 10.12). The 2-hydroxy metabolite of both estradiol and ethinyl estradiol have limited or no estrogenic activity, whereas the C-4 and C-16 α-hydroxy metabolites have a potency similar to estradiol. In humans, 16α-hydroxyestradiol is the major estrogen metabolite in pregnancy and in breast cancer. The metabolites 16α-hydroxyestrone and 4-hydroxyestrone may be carcinogenic in specific cells, because they are capable of damaging cellular proteins and DNA after their further activation to quinone intermediates.

Xenobiotic-metabolizing enzymes not only detoxify xenobiotics but also cause the formation of active intermediates (bioactivation), which in certain circumstances may elicit a diversity of toxicities, including mutagenesis, carcinogenesis, and hepatic necrosis (37). In addition to glutathione, some nucleophiles, such as other sulfhydryl compounds (most effective), alcohols, and phosphates, can react with arene oxides. Many of these nucleophiles are found in proteins and nucleic acids. The covalent binding of these bioactive epoxides to intracellular macromolecules provides a molecular basis for these toxic effects (see the discussion of toxicity from oxidative metabolism).

N-DEALKYLATION, OXIDATIVE DEAMINATION, AND N-OXIDATION

N-dealkylation. The dealkylation of secondary and tertiary amines to yield primary and secondary amines, respectively, is one of the most important and frequently encountered reactions in drug metabolism. The proposed mechanism for oxidative N-dealkylation involving α-hydrogen abstraction or an electron abstraction from the nitrogen by the perferryl oxygen has been discussed previously (29–31) (Fig. 10.7).

Typical N-substituents removed by oxidative dealkylation are methyl, ethyl, n-propyl, isopropyl, n-butyl, allyl, and benzyl. Usually, dealkylation initially occurs with the smaller alkyl group. Substituents that are more resistant to dealkylation include the tert-butyl (no α-hydrogen) and the cyclopropylmethyl. In general, tertiary amines are dealkylated to secondary amines faster than secondary amines are dealkylated to primary amines. This difference in rate has been correlated with lipid solubility. Appreciable amounts of secondary and primary amines therefore accumulate as metabolites that are more polar than the parent amine, thus slowing their rates of diffusion across membranes and reducing their accessibility to receptors. Frequently, these amine metabolites contribute to the pharmacological activity of the parent substance (e.g., imipramine) (Fig. 10.13) or produce unwanted side effects, such as hypertension, resulting from the N-dealkylation of N-isopropylmethoxamine to methoxamine. The design of an analogous drug without these unwanted drug metabolites can be achieved by proper choice of replacement substituents, such as substituting the N-isopropyl group in N-isopropylmethoxamine with a tert-butyl (N-tert-butylmethoxamine or butoxamine). N-dealkylation of substituted amides and aromatic amines occurs in a similar manner. N-substituted nonaromatic nitrogen heterocycles undergo oxidation on the α-carbon to a lactam (cotinine) as well as N-dealkylation (nicotine to nornicotine, cotinine, and norcotinine) (Fig. 10.13).

Oxidative deamination. The mechanism of oxidative deamination follows a pathway similar to that of N-dealkylation. Initially, oxidation to the imminium ion occurs, followed by decomposition to the carbonyl metabolite and ammonia. Oxidative deamination can occur with α-substituted amines, exemplified by amphetamine (Fig. 10.13). Disubstitution of the α-carbon inhibits deamination (e.g., phentermine). Some secondary and tertiary amines as well as amines substituted with bulky groups can undergo deamination directly, without N-dealkylation (e.g., fenfluramine). Apparently, this behavior is associated with increased lipid solubility.

N-oxidation. In general, N-oxygenation of amines form stable N-oxides with tertiary amines and amides, and hydroxylamines with primary and secondary amines,

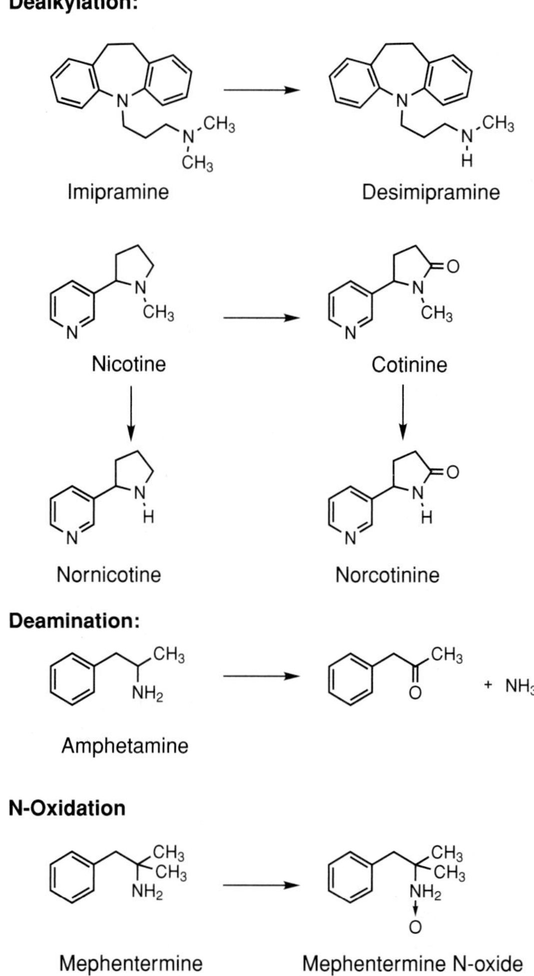

Fig. 10.13. Examples of N-dealkylation, oxidative deamination, and N-oxidation reactions catalyzed by CYP450.

when no α-protons are available (e.g., mephentermine and arylamines) (Fig. 10.13). Tertiary amines having one or more hydrogens on the adjacent carbon dealkylate via the N-oxide. Rearrangement of the N-oxide to a carbinolamine, which subsequently collapses, gives rise to the secondary amine. The amine metabolites can be N-conjugated, increasing their excretion.

O- AND S-DEALKYLATION. Oxidative O-dealkylation of ethers is a common metabolic reaction with a mechanism of dealkylation analogous to that of N-dealkylation; oxidation of the α-carbon, and subsequent decomposition of the unstable hemiacetal to an alcohol (or phenol) and a carbonyl product (29–31). Thioethers also are dealkylated by the same mechanism to hemithioacetals. The majority of ether groups in drug molecules are aromatic ethers (e.g., codeine, prazocin, and verapamil). For example, codeine is O-demethylated to morphine (Fig. 10.14). The rate of O-dealkylation is a function of chain length (i.e., increasing chain length or branching reduces the rate of dealkylation). Steric factors and ring substituents

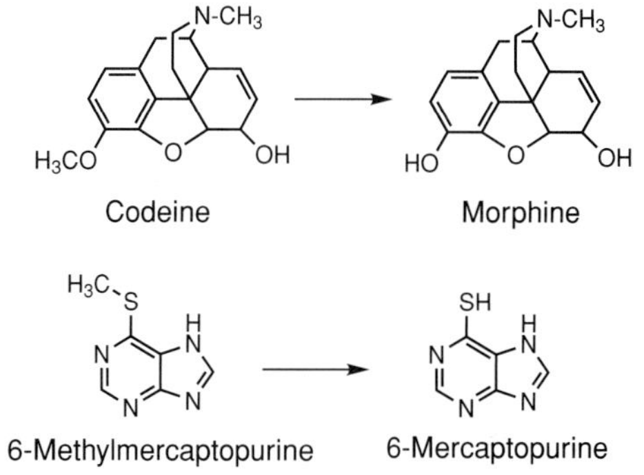

Codeine → Morphine

6-Methylmercaptopurine → 6-Mercaptopurine

Fig. 10.14. Examples of O- and S-dealkylations catalyzed by CYP450.

influence the rate of dealkylation but are complicated by electronic effects. Some drug molecules contain more than one ether group, in which case usually only one ether is dealkylated. The methylenedioxy group undergoes variable rates of dealkylation to the 1, 2-diphenolic metabolite. Metabolism of such a group also is being capable of forming a stable complex with and inhibiting CYP450.

Aliphatic and aromatic methyl thioethers undergo S-dealkylation to thiols and carbonyl compounds. For example, 6-methylthiopurine is demethylated to give the active anticancer drug 6-mercaptopurine (Fig. 10.14). Other thioethers are oxidized to sulfoxides (see N- and S-oxidations).

DEHALOGENATION. Many halogenated hydrocarbons, such as insecticides, pesticides, general anesthetics, plasticizers, flame retardants, and commercial solvents, undergo a variety of different dehalogenation biotransformations (24,25). Because of our potential exposure to these halogenated compounds as drugs and environmental pollutants in air, soil, water, or food, it is important to understand the interactions between metabolism and toxicity. Some halogenated hydrocarbons form glutathione or mercapturic acid conjugates, whereas others undergo dehydrohalogenation and reductive dehalogenation catalyzed by CYP2E1. In many cases, reactive intermediates, including radicals, anion, and cations, are produced that may react with a variety of tissue molecules.

Halogenated hydrocarbons differ in their chemical reactivity as a result of the electron-withdrawing properties of the halogens on adjacent carbon atoms, resulting in the α-carbon developing an electrophilic character. The halogen atoms also have the ability to stabilize α-carbon cations, free radicals, carbanions, and carbenes.

Oxidative dehydrohalogenation is a common metabolic pathway for many halogenated hydrocarbons (25,29–31). The CYP450-catalyzed oxidation generates the transient gem-halohydrin (analogous to alkane hydroxylation) that can eliminate the hydrohalic acid to form carbonyl derivatives (aldehydes, ketones, acyl halides, and carbonyl halides) (Fig. 10.7). This reaction

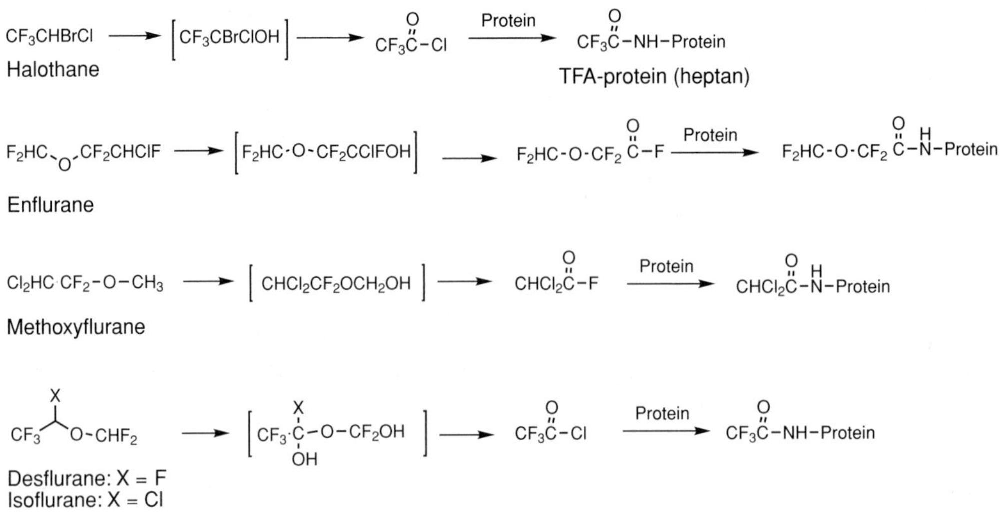

$CF_3CHBrCl$ → $[CF_3CBrClOH]$ → $CF_3C(=O){-}Cl$ —Protein→ $CF_3C(=O){-}NH{-}Protein$

Halothane; TFA-protein (heptan)

$F_2HC{-}O{-}CF_2CHClF$ → $[F_2HC{-}O{-}CF_2CClFOH]$ → $F_2HC{-}O{-}CF_2C(=O){-}F$ —Protein→ $F_2HC{-}O{-}CF_2C(=O){-}NH{-}Protein$

Enflurane

$Cl_2HC\,CF_2{-}O{-}CH_3$ → $[CHCl_2CF_2OCH_2OH]$ → $CHCl_2C(=O){-}F$ —Protein→ $CHCl_2C(=O){-}NH{-}Protein$

Methoxyflurane

$CF_3CHX{-}O{-}CHF_2$ → $[CF_3C(X)(OH){-}O{-}CF_2OH]$ → $CF_3C(=O){-}Cl$ —Protein→ $CF_3C(=O){-}NH{-}Protein$

Desflurane: X = F
Isoflurane: X = Cl

Fig. 10.15. CYP2E1-catalyzed metabolism of fluorinated volatile anesthetics to antigenic proteins.

requires the presence of at least one halogen and one α-hydrogen. gem-Trihalogenated hydrocarbons are more readily oxidized than are the gem-dihalogenated and monohalogenated compounds. The acyl and carbonyl halides formed are reactive metabolites that can react either with water to form carboxylic acids or nonenzymatically with tissue molecules (with a potential for eliciting increased toxicity). Chloramphenicol ($RNHCOCHCl_2$) is biotransformed into an acyl halide ($RNHCOCOCl$) that selectively acylates the apoprotein of CYP450 (40,41).

An excellent example of oxidative dehydrohalogenation leading to significant hepatotoxicity and nephrotoxicity is seen with the fluorinated inhalation anesthetics (Fig. 10.15). The toxicity of halothane and the fluranes is related to their metabolism to either an acid chloride (or fluoride) or a trifluoroacetate intermediate (see Fig. 18.7). The CYP2E1 has been identified as the isoform catalyzing the biotransformation of the fluranes (25,43,44). The hydroxylated intermediate decomposes spontaneously to reactive intermediates, an acid chloride (or fluoride) or trifluoroacetate, that can either react with water to form halide anions and a fluorinated carboxylic acid or bind covalently to tissue proteins to produce an acylated protein. The acylated protein becomes a "hapten," stimulating an immune response and a hypersensitivity reaction. Halothane has received the most attention because of its ability to cause "halothane-associated" hepatitis. This immunologic reaction occurs after repeated exposure in surgical patients to trifluoroacetylate protein. The patient is sensitized to future exposures of the volatile anesthetic. After subsequent exposure to a fluorinated anesthetic, the antigenic trifluoroacetylate protein stimulates an immune response, producing halothane-like hepatitis. Because of the common metabolic pathway involving CYP2E1 for enflurane, isoflurane, desflurane, and methoxyflurane, halothane-exposed patients who have halothane hepatitis can show cross-sensitization to one of the other fluranes, triggering an idiosyncratic hepatic necrosis. The formation of antigenic protein is related to the amount of CYP2E1-catalyzed metabolism for each agent: halothane (20–40%) > enflurane (2–8%) > isoflurane (0.2–1.0%) > desflurane (<0.1%). Enough fluoride ion is generated from oxidative dehalogenation during flurane anesthesia to produce subclinical nephrotoxicity. Interestingly, female rats metabolize halothane more slowly than males do and are less susceptible to hepatotoxicity than males are. For patients with preexisting liver dysfunction, isoflurane or desflurane may be a better choice of anesthetic.

In today's environment, most humans have been exposed to many CYP2E1-inducing agents (including recreational, industrial, agricultural chemicals, and alcohol), having an unknown effect on hepatic toxicity from volatile anesthetics. Enhanced activity for CYP2E1 has been observed in obesity, isoniazid therapy, ketogenic diets, and alcoholism.

AZO AND NITRO REDUCTION. In addition to the oxidative systems, liver microsomes also contain enzyme systems that catalyze the reduction of azo and nitro compounds to primary amines. A number of azo compounds, such as Prontosil and sulfasalazine (Fig. 10.16), are converted to aromatic primary amines by azoreductase, an NADPH-dependent enzyme system in the liver microsomes. Evidence exists for the participation of CYP450 in some reductions. Nitro compounds (e.g., chloramphenicol and nitrobenzene) are reduced to aromatic primary amines by a nitroreductase, presumably through nitrosamine and hydroxylamine intermediates. These reductases are not solely responsible for the reduction of azo and nitro compounds; reduction by the bacterial flora in the anaerobic environment of the intestine also may occur.

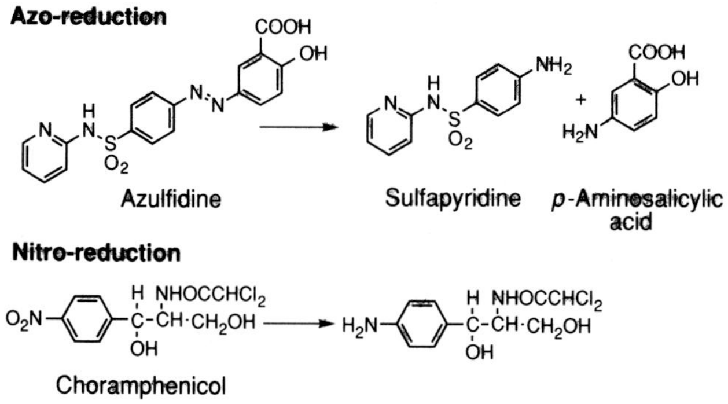

Azo-reduction

Azulfidine → Sulfapyridine + *p*-Aminosalicylic acid

Nitro-reduction

O_2N–C_6H_4–C(H)(OH)–CH(NHOCCHCl$_2$)–CH_2OH → H_2N–C_6H_4–C(H)(OH)–CH(NHOCCHCl$_2$)–CH_2OH

Choramphenicol

Fig. 10.16. CYP450-catalyzed reduction of azo and nitro compounds.

Nitrogen compounds:

Tert-acylic and cyclic amines to N-oxides

R_3N + Enz-FAD-OOH → $R_3N{\rightarrow}O$ + Enz-FAD-OH

Drugs: Amitriptyline, Atropine, Chlorpromazine, Diphenhydramine, Fluphenazine, Imipramine, Nicotine

Sec-acyclic and cyclic amines to hydroxylamines and nitrones

R_2NH + Enz-FAD-OOH → R_2N–OH + Enz-FAD-OH; R_2N–OH + Enz-FAD-OOH → R–N(⊕)(O⊖)=CH–R + Enz-FAD-OH

Drugs: Desmethylimipramine; Desmethyltrifluperazine

N-alkyl and N,N-dialkylaryl amines to hydroxylamines

R–NH–Ar + Enz-FAD-OOH → R–N(OH)–Ar + Enz-FAD-OH

1,1-Disubstituted hydrazines

R–N(R)–NH_2 + Enz-FAD-OOH → R–N(→O)(R)–NH_2 + Enz-FAD-OH

Sulfur compounds:

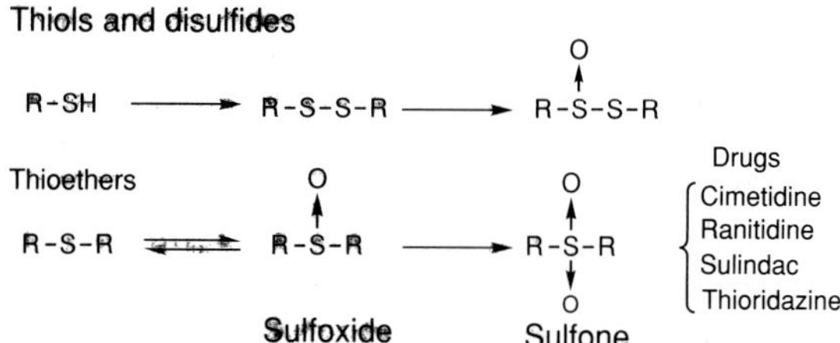

Fig. 10.17. Examples of flavin monooxygenase (FMO) oxidations.

N- and S-Oxidations Catalyzed by Flavin Monooxygenase

The major hepatic monooxygenase systems responsible for the oxidation of many drugs, carcinogens, pesticides, aromatic polycyclic hydrocarbons, and other xenobiotics containing nitrogen, sulfur, or phosphorus are CYP450 monooxygenase and microsomal flavin-containing monooxygenase (FMO) (45). The FMO exhibits broader substrate specificities than CYP450 monooxygenases and has a mechanism distinctly different from that of CYP450 monooxygenases. Because oxygen activation occurs before substrate addition, any compound binding to 4α-hydroperoxyflavin, the enzyme-bound monooxygenating FMO intermediate, is a potential substrate. Typically, FMO catalyzes oxygenation of the N- and S-heteroatoms ("soft nucleophiles") (Fig. 10.17) but not heteroatom dealkylation reactions. The products formed from FMO-catalyzed oxidation are consistent with a direct two-electron oxidation of the heteroatom. Thus, FMO constitutes an alternative biotransformation pathway for N- and S-containing lipophilic xenobiotics. Normally, FMO is not inducible by phenobarbital, nor is it affected by CYP450 inhibitors. With few exceptions, however, xenobiotic substrates for FMO also are substrates for the isoforms of CYP450, producing similar oxidation products. Which monooxygenase is responsible for the oxidation can be readily determined, because FMO is thermally labile in the absence of NADPH whereas CYP450 is stable.

Of the many nitrogen functional groups in xenobiotics, only secondary and tertiary acyclic, cyclic, and arylamines as well as hydroxylamines and hydrazines are oxidized by FMO and excreted in the urine (Fig. 10.17). The tertiary amines form stable amine oxides, and secondary amines are sequentially oxidized to hydroxylamines, nitrones, and a complex mixture of products. Secondary N-alkylarylamines can be N-oxygenated to reactive N-hydroxylated metabolites, which are responsible for the toxic, mutagenic, and carcinogenic activity of these aromatic amines. For example, the chemically unstable hydroxylamine intermediates of aromatic amines degrade into bladder carcinogens (see the discussion for this type of toxic mechanism under glucuronic acid conjugation), and the hydroxamic acid intermediates of N-arylacetamides are bioactivated into liver carcinogens. Hepatic FMO, however, will not catalyze the oxidation of primary alkyl- or arylamines, except for the carcinogenic N-hydroxylated derivatives of 2-aminofluorene, 2-aminoanthracene, and other amino PAHs.

S-oxidation occurs almost exclusively by FMO (Fig. 10.17). Sulfides are oxidized to sulfoxides and sulfones, thiols to disulfides, and thiocarbamates, mercaptopyrimidines, and mercaptoimidazoles (i.e., the antithyroid drug methimazole) via sulfenates (RSOH) to sulfinates (RSO_2H), all of which are eliminated in the urine.

The FMO does not catalyze epoxidation reactions or hydroxylation at unactivated carbon atoms of xenobiotics. Primary aromatic amines and amides, aromatic heterocyclic amines and imines, and the aliphatic primary amine phentermine are N-oxidized by CYP450 to hydroxylamines. The CYP450 oxidizes carbon disulfide to carbon dioxide and hydrogen sulfide and the antipsychotic phenothiazines to sulfoxides.

The major steps in the catalytic cycle for FMO are shown in Figure 10.18 (45,46). Like most of the other monooxygenases, FMO requires NADPH and oxygen as cosubstrates to catalyze the oxidation of the xenobiotic

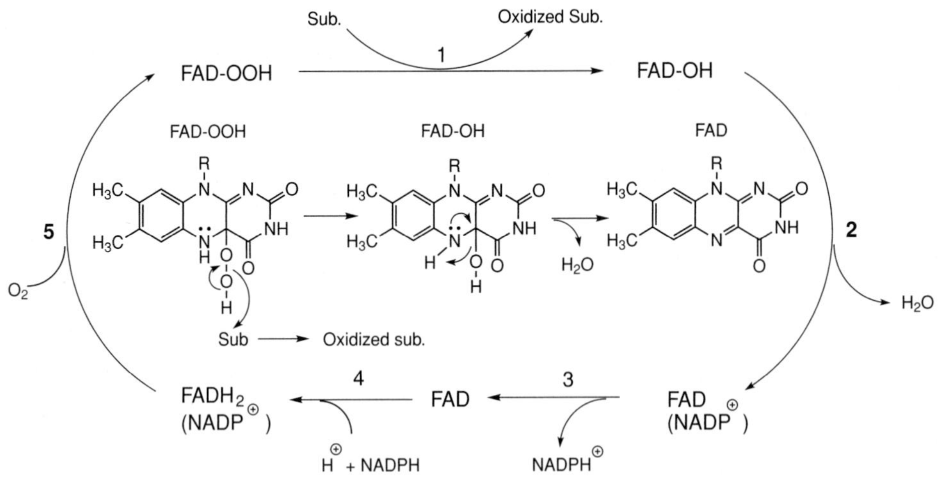

Fig. 10.18. Flavin monooxygenase (FMO) catalytic cycle. Oxygenated substrate is formed by nucleophilic attack of a substrate (Sub.) by the terminal oxygen of the enzyme-bound hydroperoxyflavin (FAD-OOH), followed by heterolytic cleavage of the peroxide (1). The release of H_2O (2) or of $NADP^+$ (3) is rate-limiting for reactions catalyzed by liver FMO. Reduction of flavin by NADPH (4) and addition of oxygen (5) complete the cycle by regeneration of the oxygenated FAD-OOH.

substrate. Unlike CYP450, however, the xenobiotic being oxidized does not need to be bound to the 4α-hydroperoxyflavin intermediate (FAD-OOH) for oxygen activation to occur. Apparently, FMO is present within the cell in its enzyme-bound activated hydroperoxide (Enz-FAD-OOH) state ready to oxidize any suitable lipophilic substrate that binds to it. The FMO uses a nonradical, nucleophilic displacement type of mechanism binding dioxygen with a reduced flavin. The reactive oxygen intermediate is a reactive derivative of hydrogen peroxide, flavin-4α-hydroperoxide (Fig. 10.18, insert), which is reactive enough to successfully attack a lone electron pair on a heteroatom, such as nitrogen or sulfur, but not reactive enough to attack a typical C-H bond. These studies suggest the xenobiotic substrate interacts with the 4α-hydroperoxyflavin form of FMO and is oxidized by oxygen transfer from Enz-FAD-OOH to form the oxidized product. Neither the substrate nor the oxidized substrate is essential for any other steps in the cycle. Steps 2 to 5 simply regenerate the oxygenating agent Enz-FAD-OOH from Enz-FAD-OH, NADPH, oxygen, and a proton. Any compound readily crossing cell membranes by passive diffusion and penetrating to the FMO-bound hydroperoxyflavin intermediate is a potential substrate, thus explaining the broad substrate specificity exhibited for FMO. The fact that the xenobiotic substrate is not required for activation of the FMO-hydroperoxyflavin state distinguishes FMO from CYP450 monooxygenases, in which substrate binding initiates the CYP450 catalytic cycle and activation of oxygen to the perferryl oxygenating agent. It is not unusual for FMO oxidation products to undergo reduction to the parent xenobiotic, which can enter into repeated redox reactions (termed "metabolic cycling").

Results of substrate specificity studies suggest that the number of ionic groups on endogenous substrate is an important factor enabling FMO to distinguish between xenobiotic and endogenous substrates, preventing the indiscriminate oxidation of physiologically important amine and sulfur compounds (47). Without exception, FMO readily catalyzes the oxidation of uncharged amines or sulfur compounds (in equilibrium with its respective monocation or monoanion; for sulfur compounds, the charge is on sulfur atom). The FMO will not catalyze the oxidation of dianions (e.g., thiamine pyrophosphate), dications (e.g., polyamines), dipolar ions (e.g., amino acids and peptides), or other polyionic compounds with one or more anionic groups (i.e., COO) distal to the heteroatom (e.g., coenzyme A).

Unlike the CYP450 system, only three isoforms of hepatic FMO have been characterized in the adult human liver (48,49): minor form I (or FMO 1A1), which is the major form in fetal tissue; major form II (FMO 1D1); and form III, of which little is currently known. The substrate specificities for these isoforms have not been reported. The availability of different forms of FMO may be of clinical importance in the pharmacological and toxicological properties of FMO-dependent drug oxidations.

Peroxidases and Other Monooxygenases

Peroxidases are hemoproteins and, perhaps, the most closely related enzymes to CYP450 monooxygenase (50,51). The normal course of peroxide (ROOH)-catalyzed oxidation involves the formation of the $[FeO]^{+3}$ intermediate, analogous to the perferryl complex in CYP450. It can perform heteroatom oxygenation and aromatization (oxidation) of 1,4-dihydropyridines (calcium channel blockers).

Other monooxygenases catalyzing oxidation reactions similar to CYP450 include dopamine β-monooxygenase, a mammalian copper-containing enzyme catalyzing carbon hydroxylation, epoxidation, S-oxygenation, and N-dealkylation reactions, and nonheme iron–containing enzymes from bacteria and plants.

Nonmicrosomal Oxidations

In addition to the microsomal monooxygenases, other oxidases and dehydrogenases that catalyze oxidation reactions are present in the mitochondrial and soluble fractions of tissue homogenates.

OXIDATION OF ALCOHOLS. Alcohol dehydrogenase is an NAD-specific enzyme located in the soluble fraction of tissue homogenates. It exhibits a broad specificity for alcohols. Most primary alcohols are readily oxidized to their corresponding aldehydes. Some secondary alcohols are oxidized to the ketones, whereas other secondary and tertiary alcohols are excreted either unchanged or as their conjugate metabolite. Some secondary alcohols also show mixed activity because of steric factors and a lack of substrate affinity for the enzyme.

$$C_2H_5{-}OH \longrightarrow H_3C{-}CHO$$

$$H_3C{-}CH(OH){-}CH_3 \longrightarrow H_3C{-}C(=O){-}CH_3$$

Oxidation by alcohol dehydrogenase is the principal pathway for ethanol metabolism, but the microsomal isoform CYP2E1 also plays a significant role in ethanol metabolism and tolerance. Apparently, two-thirds of ingested ethanol is oxidized by alcohol dehydrogenase and the remainder by CYP2E1; during intoxication, however, ethanol induces the expression of CYP2E1. The induction of CYP2E1 contributes to the activation of some xenobiotics, increasing the vulnerability of heavy drinkers to anesthetic drugs, over-the-counter analgesics, prescription drugs, and chemical carcinogens. In turn, the excessive amounts of acetaldehyde generated cause hepatotoxicity, lipid peroxidation of membranes, formation of protein adducts, and other cellular changes.

The toxicity of methanol and ethylene glycol in humans has long been recognized, but frequent reports of such toxicity are not surprising given the number of consumer products containing methanol and ethylene glycol (automotive antifreeze). Methanol (wood alcohol or methyl alcohol) is commonly used as a solvent in organic synthetic procedures, and is available to consumers in a variety of products, ranging from solid fuels (Sterno), paint removers, solvent for "ditto" copying machines, motor fuels, antifreeze, to alcoholic beverages (unintentional ingredient). Oral methanol toxicity in humans is characterized by its rapid absorption from the gut, followed by a latent period of many hours before metabolic acidosis (lowered blood pH and bicarbonate levels) and ocular toxicity are evident. The metabolic acidosis and blindness result from the excessive accumulation of formic acid and the inability of the hepatic tetrahydrofolate pathway to oxidize formate to carbon dioxide. The rate of elimination of methanol from the blood is relatively slow compared to that of ethanol, accounting for its long latency period. Its half-life ranges from 2 to 3 hours at low blood concentration to 27 hours at high blood concentration. Evidence supports the singular role of liver alcohol dehydrogenase in the metabolism of methanol to formaldehyde, although it is oxidized slowly by alcohol dehydrogenase (approximately one-sixth the rate of ethanol). The demonstration that methanol is a substrate for alcohol dehydrogenase provides a rational basis for the use of ethanol in the treatment of methanol toxicity. Ethanol depresses the rate of methanol oxidation by acting as a competitive substrate for alcohol dehydrogenase, reducing the formation of formaldehyde. On the other hand, formaldehyde is not usually detected in the blood because of its rapid metabolism by aldehyde dehydrogenase to formate. Although human exposure to methanol vapor is less prevalent, methanol is rapidly absorbed through the skin or by inhalation, and depending on the severity of exposure, this can result in methanol poisoning. Ethylene glycol is oxidized to hydroxyacealdehyde and glyoxal and, subsequently, to oxalate by aldehyde dehydrogenase. When eliminated into the urine, oxalate forms calcium oxalate crystals that can block the kidney tubules. 4-Methylpyrazole (Fomepizole) is an alcohol dehydrogenase inhibitor that is used as an antidote for the treatment of methanol or ethylene glycol poisoning. 1,4-Butanediol is a solvent that has became popular as a date-rape drug and drug-of-abuse because of its metabolism to γ-hydroxybutyrate (see Chapter 15), which binds to the γ-hydroxybutyrate receptor, which in turn produces central nervous system sedation with amnesia.

Alcohol dehydrogenase also functions as a reductase when it catalyzes the reduction of an aldehyde or ketone to an alcohol. In addition, other NADP- or NAD-dependent dehydrogenases in the cytosol are capable of reducing a variety of ketones. Ketones are stable to further oxidation and, consequently, yield reduction products as major metabolites. Examples of reduction include the sedative-hypnotic chloral hydrate to trichloroethanol, the opioid antagonist naltrexone to 6-β-hydroxynaltrexol, the opioid analgesic methadone to α-methadol, the antipsychotic haloperidol to hydroxyhaloperidol, and the antiemetic dolasetron to dihydrodolasetron. These alcohol metabolites are all pharmacologically active.

ALDEHYDE DEHYDROGENASE. A NAD-specific aldehyde dehydrogenase catalyzes the oxidation of endogenous aldehydes, such as those produced by the oxidation of primary alcohols or the deamination of biogenic amines, and of exogenous aldehydes to the corresponding carboxylic acids. By inhibiting this enzyme, disulfuram (Antabuse) and metronidazole produce an unpleasant set of reactions (flushing, abdominal cramping, and headache) when small amounts of alcohol are ingested. Antabuse is used therapeutically in controlling alcohol abuse. Aldehyde dehydrogenase deficiency exhibits significant polymorphic expression in Chinese patients.

$$H_3C\text{-}CHO \longrightarrow H_3C\text{-}COOH$$

MOLYBDENUM HYDROXYLASES. Molybdenum hydroxylases are additional non-CYP450 enzymes capable of catalyzing the oxidation of drugs. The molybdenum hydroxylases, which include aldehyde oxidase, xanthine oxidase, and xanthine dehydrogenase, are more commonly found in the cytosol of mammalian liver and carry out the oxidation and detoxification of a number of structurally different azaheterocycles (52). The efficient oxidation of endogenous purine nucleosides suggests that their metabolism and detoxification might be an important physiological role for the molybdenum hydroxylases. Among the azaheterocycles metabolized are derivatives of pyridine, quinoline, pyrimidine, purine, quinazoline, and pteridines. These hydroxylases generally oxidize the α-carbon to the nitrogen of the azaheterocycle to oxo metabolites (also known as lactams). The molybdenum hydroxylases contain a common electron-transfer system in each subunit: one molybdenum atom, two Fe/S clusters, and one flavin adenine dinucleotide molecule. The molybdenum hydroxylases catalyze their reactions differently than CYP450 and other hydroxylase enzymes, requiring water rather than molecular oxygen as the source of the oxygen atom incorporated into the metabolite, and with the concomitant reduction of molecular oxygen to superoxide (53,54). The active sites possess a catalytically labile Mo^{V}-OH (or, possibly, Mo^{VI}-OH_2) group that is transferred to the substrate during the course of the hydroxylation reaction.

Aldehyde oxidase In addition to metabolizing some aldehydes, aldehyde oxidase also oxidizes a variety of azaheterocycles but not thia- or oxaheterocycles. Of the various purine nucleosides metabolized by aldehyde oxidase, the 2-hydroxy- and 2-amino derivatives are more efficiently metabolized, and for the N^9-substituents, the typical order of preference is the acyclic nucleosides is as follows: 9-[(hydroxy-alkyloxy)methyl]-purines) > 2′-deoxyribofuranosyl > ribofuranosyl > arabinofuranosyl > H. The kinetic rate constants for purine analogues revealed that the pyrimidine portion of the purine ring system is more important for substrate affinity than the imidazole portion. Aldehyde oxidase is inhibited by potassium cyanide and menadione (synthetic vitamin K).

Aldehyde oxidase metabolizes an assortment of azaheterocycles including the short-acting sedative-hypnotic drug zaleplon (a pyrazolo[1,5α] pyrimidine derivative) to its 5-oxo metabolite; the anticancer drug thioguanine to 8-oxothioguanine; the α_2-adrenergic agonist brimonidine (a pyrimidine derivative) to its 2-oxo-, 3-oxo-, and 2,3-dioxo- metabolites; quinine and quinidine to their 2-quinolone metabolites; the pro-antiviral drug famiclovir (a purine derivative) to its active 6-oxo metabolite (penciclovir); O^6-benzylguanine to its 8-oxo metabolite (also formed primarily from CYP3A4); the metabolism of the anticancer drug DACA (an acridine-4-carboxamide derivative) to its 9-acridone metabolite; and the antiseizure drug zonisamide (a 1,2-benzisoxazole derivative) primarily by reductive cleavage of the 1,2-benzisoxazole ring to 2-sulfamoylacetylphenol. Although the azaheterocycles thiazole and oxazole are not metabolized by aldehyde oxidase, their carbocyclic analogues, benzothiazole, benzoxazole, and 1,2-benzisoxazole, are metabolized. On the other hand, the heterocycles, benzothiophene and benzofuran, which do not contain a nitrogen atom, are not metabolized by or inhibit aldehyde oxidase.

The hepatotoxic and neurotoxic 1-methyl-4-phenyl-1,2,3,6-tetrahydropyridine (MPTP) is metabolized by aldehyde oxidase to its nontoxic MP-2-pyridone metabolite (MPTP lactam). Although S-cotinine is formed primarily from S-nicotine in human smokers by CYP2A6, in vitro studies suggest that aldehyde oxidase contributes to S-nicotine metabolism by oxidizing the intermediate metabolite (S-nicotine Δ-1′,5′-imminium ion) to S-cotinine. These results suggest that hepatic aldehyde oxidase is a key detoxification enzyme for MPTP and S-nicotine.

Both aldehyde oxidase and xanthine oxidase contribute to the first-pass hepatic metabolism of orally administered methotrexate (a 2,4-diaminopteridine) to its 7-hydroxymethotrexate metabolite.

Xanthine oxidase and xanthine dehydrogenase. Xanthine oxidase and xanthine dehydrogenase represent different forms of the same gene product. Xanthine dehydrogenase and xanthine oxidase are interconvertable; thus, these two enzyme forms and their reactions often are referred to as xanthine oxidoreductase. Xanthine oxidase is the rate-limiting enzyme in purine catabolism of hypoxanthine to uric acid via xanthine. Both xanthine oxidase and xanthine dehydrogenase play important roles in the

6-Mercaptopurine → 6-Mercaptouric acid

metabolism of a number of purine anticancer drugs to their active and inactive metabolites. Although xanthine oxidase is strongly inhibited by the antigout drug allopurinol, aldehyde oxidase oxidizes it to oxypurinol. Only xanthine dehydrogenase requires NAD^+ as an electron acceptor for the oxidation of azaheterocycles. 6-Mercaptopurine is metabolized by xanthine oxidase to 6-mercapturic acid.

Oxidative Deamination of Amines

Monoamine oxidase (MAO) and diamine oxidase catalyze oxidative deamination of amines to the aldehydes in the presence of oxygen. The aldehyde products can be metabolized further to the corresponding alcohol or acid by aldehyde oxidase or dehydrogenase.

Monoamine oxidase. Monoamine oxidase is a mitochondrial membrane flavin-containing enzyme that catalyzes the oxidative deamination of monoamines according to the following equation:

$$R\text{-}CH_2\text{-}NH_2 + O_2 \longrightarrow [R\text{-}CH{=}NH] \longrightarrow R\text{-}CHO + NH_4^{\oplus}$$

Substrates for this enzyme include several monoamines, secondary and tertiary amines in which the amine substrates are methyl groups. The amine must be attached to an unsubstituted methylene group, and compounds having substitution at the α-carbon atom are poor substrates for MAO (e.g., aniline, amphetamine, and ephedrine) but are oxidized by the microsomal CYP450 enzymes rather than by MAO (Fig. 10.13). For secondary and tertiary amines, alkyl groups larger than a methyl and branched alkyl groups (i.e., isopropyl, t-butyl, or β-phenylisopropyl) inhibit MAO oxidation, but such substrates may function as reversible inhibitors of MAO. Nonselective irreversible inhibitors of MAO include hydrazides (phenelzine) and tranylcypromine and the MAO-B selective inhibitors pargyline and selegiline. Monoamine oxidase is important in regulating the metabolic degradation of catecholamines and serotonin in neural tissues, and hepatic MAO has a crucial defensive role in inactivating circulating monoamines or those that originated in the gastrointestinal tract and were absorbed into the systemic circulation (e.g., tyramine).

Two types of MAO are isolated: MAO-A, and MAO-B. They show dissimilar substrate preferences and different sensitivities to inhibitors. The type MAO-A is found mainly in peripheral adrenergic nerve terminals and shows substrate preference for 5-hydroxytryptamine, norepinephrine, and epinephrine. The type MAO-B is found principally in platelets and shows selectivity for nonphenolic, lipophilic β-phenethylamines. Common substrates to both MAO-A and MAO-B are dopamine, tyramine, and other monophenolic phenylethylamines.

A contaminant in the synthesis of reversed esters of meperidine, MPTP was discovered to be a highly selective neurotoxin for dopaminergic cells, producing parkinsonism (47). The neurotoxicity of MPTP is associated with cellular destruction in the substantia nigra along with severe reductions in the concentration of dopamine, norepinephrine, and serotonin. The remarkable neurotoxic action for MPTP involves a sequence of events beginning with the metabolic activation of MPTP to the toxic metabolite MPP^+ (1-methyl-4-phenylpyridinium ion) by MAO-B, specific uptake and accumulation of MPP^+ in the nigrostriatal dopaminergic neurons, and ending with the inhibition of oxidative phosphorylation (of NADH dehydrogenase in complex I). This inhibition results in mitochondrial injury depriving the sensitive nigrostriatal cells of oxidative phosphorylation with their eventual cell death (neurotoxic actions of MPP^+). The MAO-B inhibitors (e.g., deprenyl) blocked this biotransformation.

N-CH3 — MPTP

⊕ N-CH3 — MPP^+

Diamines, such as $H_2N\text{-}(CH_2)_n\text{-}NH_2$, in which n is less than six, are not attacked and show little affinity for MAO. If the intermolecular distance between the amine groups is increased, the rate of oxidation by MAO increases. Evidently, the second amine group interferes with attachment of the amine to the enzyme.

Diamine oxidase. Diamine oxidase attacks both diamines and histamine in much the same way that MAO attacks monoamines, forming aldehydes. This enzyme is inhibited by carbonyl-blocking reagents and produces hydrogen peroxide, supporting the role of pyridoxal phosphate and the flavin prosthetic groups in the catalytic action of the enzyme. Diamine oxidase is recovered in the supernatant after centrifugation and removal of particulate matter. It is present in kidneys, intestines, liver, lung, and nervous tissue. It limits the biological effects of histamine and the polymethylene amines putrescine and cadaverine. It also attacks monoamines, but at a higher substrate concentration.

$H_2N\text{-}(CH_2)_4\text{-}NH_2$ — Putrescine

$H_2N\text{-}(CH_2)_5\text{-}NH_2$ — Cadaverine

Plasma amine oxidases are in blood plasma of mammals and include spermine oxidase, which deaminates spermine and other polyamines.

Miscellaneous Reductions

Disulfides (e.g., disulfiram), sulfoxides (e.g., dimethylsulfoxide), N-oxides, double bonds such as those in progestational steroids, and dehydroxylation of aromatic and aliphatic hydroxyl derivatives are examples of reductions occurring in microsomal or nonmicrosomal (usually cytosol enzymes) fractions.

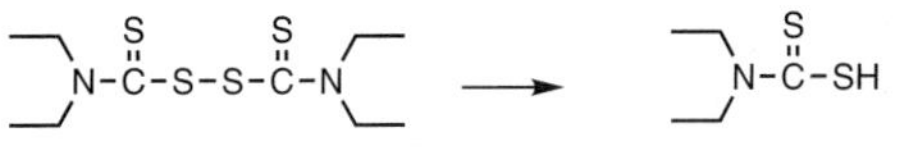

Disulfiram → Diethyldithiocarbamic acid

CH_3SOCH_3 → CH_3SCH_3

Dimethylsulfoxide → Dimethylsulfide

Various studies regarding the biotransformation of xenobiotic ketones have established that ketone reduction is an important metabolic pathway in mammalian tissue. Because carbonyl compounds are lipophilic and may be retained in tissues, their reduction to the hydrophilic alcohols and subsequent conjugation are critical to their elimination. Although ketone reductases may be closely related to the alcohol dehydrogenases, they have distinctly different properties and use NADPH as the cofactor. The metabolism of xenobiotic ketones to free alcohols or conjugated alcohols has been demonstrated for aromatic, aliphatic, alicyclic, and unsaturated ketones (e.g., naltrexone, naloxone, hydromorphone, and daunorubicin). The carbonyl reductases are distinguished by the stereospecificity of their alcohol metabolites.

β-Oxidation

Alkyl carboxylic acids, as their coenzyme A (CoA) thioesters, are metabolized by oxidation at the β–carbon to the carboxylic carbon (β-oxidation). This pathway involves the oxidative cleavage of two carbon units at a time (as acetate), beginning at the carboxyl terminus and continuing until no more acetate units can be removed. The reaction is terminated when a branch (e.g., valproic acid) or aromatic group is encountered. The metabolism of even and odd phenylalkyl acids can serve as an example:

$$C_6H_5-(CH_2)_{10}\text{-}COOH \longrightarrow C_6H_5-(CH_2)_8-\overset{\beta}{C}H_2\text{-}CH_2\text{-}\overset{O}{\overset{\|}{C}}\text{-}S\text{-}CoA \longrightarrow C_6H_5\text{-}COOH + 5\ H_3C\text{-}\overset{O}{\overset{\|}{C}}\text{-}S\text{-}CoA$$

$$C_6H_5-(CH_2)_{11}\text{-}COOH \longrightarrow C_6H_5-(CH_2)_{11}\text{-}CO\text{-}CoA \longrightarrow C_6H_5\text{-}CH_2\text{-}COOH + 5\ H_3C\text{-}\overset{O}{\overset{\|}{C}}\text{-}S\text{-}CoA$$

Hydrolysis

In general, esters and amides are hydrolyzed by enzymes in the blood, liver microsomes, kidneys, and other tissues. Esters and certain amides are hydrolyzed rapidly by a group of enzymes termed "carboxylesterases." The more lipophilic the amide, the more favorable it is as a substrate for this enzyme. In most cases, the hydrolysis of an ester or amide bond in a toxic substance results in bioinactivation to hydrophilic metabolites that are readily excreted. Some of these metabolites may yield conjugated metabolites (i.e., glucuronides).

Carboxylesterases include cholinesterase (pseudocholinesterase), arylcarboxyesterases, liver microsomal carboxylesterases, and other unclassified liver carboxylesterases. Cholinesterase hydrolyzes choline-like esters (succinylcholine) and procaine as well as acetylsalicylic acid. Genetic variant forms of cholinesterase have been identified in human serum (e.g., succinylcholine toxicity when administered as ganglionic blocker for muscle relaxation). Meperidine is hydrolyzed only by liver microsomal carboxylesterases (Fig. 10.19). Diphenoxylate is hydrolyzed to its active metabolite, diphenoxylic acid, within 1 hour (Fig. 10.19). Presumably, the peripheral pharmacological action of diphenoxylate is attributed to zwitterionic diphenoxylic acid, which is readily eliminated in the urine.

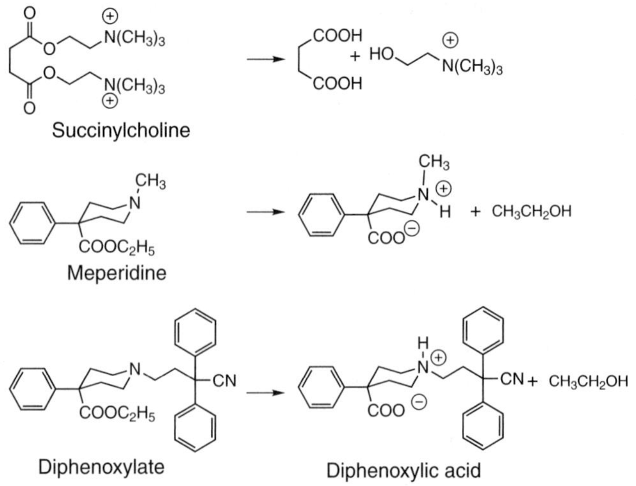

Succinylcholine → HOOC–CH₂CH₂–COOH + $HO\text{-}CH_2CH_2\text{-}N^{+}(CH_3)_3$

Meperidine → + CH_3CH_2OH

Diphenoxylate → Diphenoxylic acid + CH_3CH_2OH

Fig. 10.19. Examples of hydrolysis reactions.

A distinct type of esterase is the enzyme serum paraoxonase (PON1), which appears to act as an important guardian against the neurotoxicity of organophosphates and cellular damage from oxidized lipids in the LDL proteins (55). The PON1 (A-esterase) is similar to arylesterase in that it catalyzes the hydrolysis of phenyl acetate and other aryl esters. Without PON1, the organophosphate is free to react with, and irreversibly inhibit, acetylcholinesterse (see Chapter 12). Additionally, PON1 exhibits a substrate-dependent polymorphism. Individuals who are susceptible to the toxic effects of organophosphates such as paraoxon and chlorpyrifos (Dursban) are deficient in this isoenzyme.

Esters that are sterically hindered are hydrolyzed more slowly and may appear unchanged in the urine. For example, approximately 50% of a dose of atropine appears unchanged in the urine of humans. The remainder appears to consist of unhydrolyzed biotransformed products.

As a rule, amides are more stable to esterase hydrolysis than are esters, and it is not surprising to find amides excreted largely unchanged. This fact has been exploited in developing the antiarrhythmic drug procainamide. Procaine is not useful because of its rapid esterase hydrolysis, but 60% of a dose of procainamide was recovered unchanged from the urine of humans, with the remainder being mostly N-acetylprocainamide. On the other hand, the deacylated metabolite of indomethacin (a tertiary amide) is one of the major metabolites detected in human urine. Amide hydrolysis of phthalylsulfathiazole and succinylsulfathiazole by bacterial enzymes in the colon releases the antibacterial agent sulfathiazole.

Summary

In summary, Phase 1 metabolic transformations introduce new and polar functional groups into the molecule, which may produce one or more of the following changes:

1. Decreased pharmacological activity (deactivation)
2. Increased pharmacological activity (activation)
3. Increased toxicity (carcinogenesis, mutagenesis, cytotoxicity)
4. Altered pharmacological activity

Drugs exhibiting increased activity or activity different from the parent drug generally undergo further metabolism and conjugation, resulting in deactivation and excretion of the inactive conjugates.

DRUG CONJUGATION PATHWAYS (PHASE 2)

Conjugation reactions represent probably the most important xenobiotic biotransformation reaction (53,54). Xenobiotics usually are lipophilic, well absorbed in the blood, but slowly excreted in the urine. Only after conjugation (Phase 2) reactions have added an ionic hydrophilic moiety, such as glucuronic acid, sulfate, or glycine, to the xenobiotic is water solubility increased and lipid solubility decreased enough to make urinary elimination possible. The major proportion of the administered drug dose is excreted as conjugates into the urine and bile. Conjugation reactions may be preceded by Phase 1 reactions. For xenobiotics with a functional group available for conjugation, conjugation alone may be its fate.

Traditionally, the major conjugation reactions (glucuronidation and sulfation) were thought to terminate pharmacological activity by transforming the parent drug or Phase 1 metabolites into readily excreted ionic polar products. Moreover, these terminal metabolites would have no significant pharmacological activity (i.e., poor cellular diffusion and affinity for the active drug's receptor). This long-established view changed, however, with the discoveries that morphine 6-glucuronide has more analgesic activity than morphine in humans and that minoxidil sulfate is the active metabolite for the antihypertensive minoxidil. For most xenobiotics, conjugation is a detoxification mechanism. Some compounds, however, form reactive intermediates that have been implicated in carcinogenesis, allergic reaction, and tissue damage.

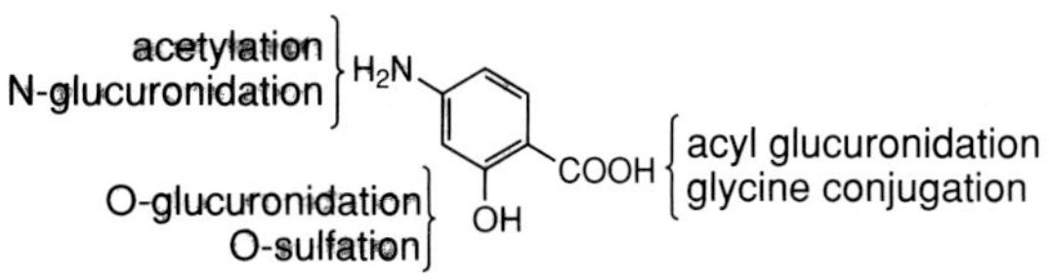

acetylation, N-glucuronidation — H_2N
O-glucuronidation, O-sulfation — OH
COOH — acyl glucuronidation, glycine conjugation

Fig. 10.20. Sequential conjugation pathways for *p*-aminosalicylic acid.

Sequential conjugation for the same substance gives rise to multiple conjugated products (see *p*-aminosalicylic acid in Fig. 10.20). The xenobiotic can be a substrate for more than one metabolizing enzyme. For example, different conjugation pathways could compete for the same functional group. The outcome is an array of metabolites excreted in the urine or feces. The factors determining the outcome of this interplay include availability of cosubstrates, enzyme kinetics (V_{max}), substrate affinity (K_m) for the metabolizing enzyme, and tissues. When a cosubstrate is low or depleted, the competing reactions can take over. The reactivity of the functional group determines all subsequent events. For example, major conjugation reactions are sulfation, ether glucuronidation, and methylation for the phenolic hydroxyl groups; acetylation, sulfation, and glucuronidation for amine groups; and amino acid conjugation and ester glucuronidation for carboxyl groups.

Conjugation enzymes may show stereospecificity toward enantiomers when a racemic drug is administered. The metabolite pattern of the same drug when administered orally may be different when administered intravenously because of presystemic intestinal conjugation. A current and in-depth review of the different Phase 2 conjugations is available in Mulder (56).

Glucuronic Acid Conjugation

Glucuronide formation probably is the major and most common route for xenobiotic Phase 2 metabolism to water-soluble metabolites, and it accounts for the major share of the conjugated metabolites found in the urine and bile (56). Its significance lies in the readily available supply of glucuronic acid in the liver and in the many functional groups forming glucuronide conjugates (e.g., phenols, alcohols, carboxylic acids, and amines).

Mechanism of Glucuronide Conjugation

The reaction involves the direct condensation of the xenobiotic (or its Phase 1 product) with the activated form of glucuronic acid, UDP–glucuronic acid (UDPGA). The overall scheme of reactions is shown in Figure 10.21. The reaction between UDPGA and the acceptor compound is catalyzed by UDP–glucuronosyl transferases (UGT), a multigene family of isozymes located along the ER of liver, epithelial cells of the intestine, and other extrahepatic tissues. Its unique location in the ER along with the CYP450 isoforms has important physiologic effects in the neutralization of reactive

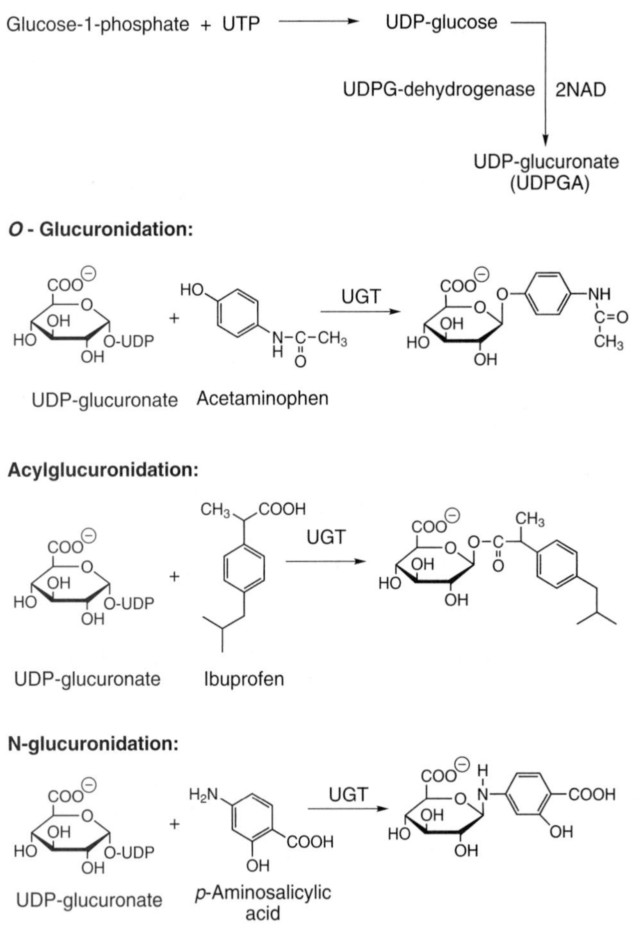

Glucose-1-phosphate + UTP → UDP-glucose

UDPG-dehydrogenase | 2NAD

UDP-glucuronate (UDPGA)

***O*- Glucuronidation:**

UDP-glucuronate + Acetaminophen → (UGT)

Acylglucuronidation:

UDP-glucuronate + Ibuprofen → (UGT)

N-glucuronidation:

UDP-glucuronate + *p*-Aminosalicylic acid → (UGT)

Fig. 10.21. Glucuronidation pathway catalyzed by UDP-glucuronosyl transferases (UGTs).

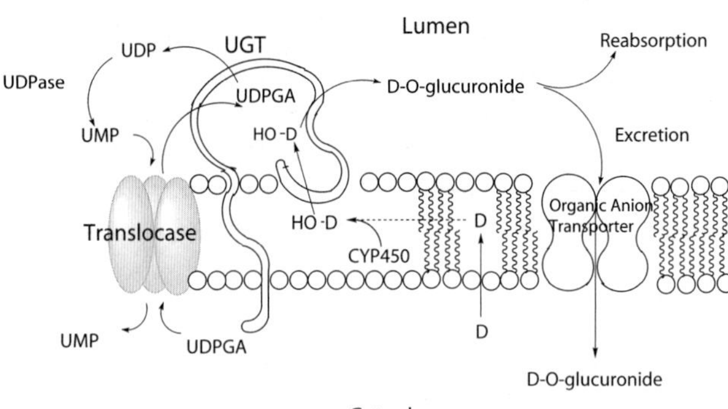

Fig. 10.22. Proposed topological model of UGT. A lipophilic drug (D) reaches the active site of CYP450 from the membrane or cytoplasm and is hydroxylated. The hydroxylated metabolite (D-OH) is transferred to UGT, where glucuronidation occurs, followed by release into the lumen and excretion from the cell via organic anion transporter. The UDPGA is synthesized in the cytoplasm and transported via translocase to UGT. (Adapted from Oesch F. Metabolic transformation of clinically used drugs to epoxides: new perspectives in drug-drug interactions. Biochem Pharmacol 1976;25 1935–1937; with permission.)

metabolites generated by the CYP450 isoforms and in controlling the levels of reactive metabolites present in these tissues.(Fig. 10.22). This cartoon depicts the spatial orientation and the interrelationship of the ER membrane–bound enzymes such as CYP450, UGTs, and membrane-bound transporters (57). The transporters carry the UDPGA and xenobiotics (D) from the cytosol into the ER lumen and transport the glucuronide metabolite from the ER lumen into the cytosol. The presence of the active site for UGT toward the ER lumen catalyzes the reaction between the substrate and UDPGA. The resultant glucuronide has the β-configuration about carbon 1 of glucuronic acid. With the attachment of the hydrophilic carbohydrate moiety containing an easily ionizable carboxyl group (pK_a = 3–4), a lipid-soluble substance is converted into a conjugate that is poorly reabsorbed by the renal tubules from the urine and is excreted more readily into the urine or, in some cases, into the bile. Endogenous substances conjugated with glucuronic acid include steroids, bilirubin, and thyroxine. Not all glucuronides are excreted by the kidneys. Some are excreted into the intestinal tract with bile (enterohepatic cycling), where β-glucuronidase in the intestinal flora hydrolyzes the C^1-O-glucuronide back to the aglycone (xenobiotic or their metabolites) for reabsorption into the portal circulation.

UGT Families

The UGTs have been classified into families according to similarities in amino acid sequences, analogous to the CYP450 family. The human UGT family is divided into two subfamilies, UGT1 and UGT2 (58). Considerable overlap in substrate specificities exists between the two families. The human UGT1A1 isoform is primarily responsible for the glucuronidation of bilirubin, estradiol, and other estrogenic steroids; UGT1A3 and UGT1A4 catalyze the glucuronidation of drugs with tertiary amines to form quaternary glucuronides and hydroxylated xenobiotics; UGT1A6 exhibits limited substrate specificity for planar phenolic substances; UGT1A9 has a wide range of substrate specificity and can glucuronidate nonplanar phenols, plant substances (e.g., anthraquinones and flavones), steroids, and other phenolic drugs; and UGT1A10 glucuronidates mycophenolic acid an inhibitor of inosine monophosphate dehydrogenase. Human family 2 isoform UGT2B4 is homologous to UGT2B7 and catalyzes the glucuronidation of the 6α-hydroxyl group of bile acids; UGT2B7 glucuronidates, the highest number of substrates, including the 3- and 6-glucuronidation of morphine and 6-glucuronidation of codeine; UGT2B11 glucuronidates a wide range of planar phenols, bulky alcohols, and polyhydroxylated estradiol metabolites; and UGT2B15 catalyzes the glucuronidation of the

17α-hydroxyl group of dihydrotestosterone and other steroidal compounds as well as phenolphthalein. The UGT1A isoforms are inducible with 3-methylcholanthrene and cigarette smoking, and the UGT2B family is inducible by barbiturates. Approximately 40% of the glucuronides are produced by UGT2B7, 20% by UGT1A4, and 15% by UGT1A1.

UGT Distribution

The human liver has been established as the most important tissue for all routes of metabolism, including glucuronidation. Studies have shown that the rate of glucuronidation is not uniform in the different sections of the liver: The UGT1A6 content was greatest in the middle but also found in the bile duct epithelium and in the endothelium of the hepatic artery and portal vein; UGT2B2 was uniformly distributed throughout the liver. The UGTs expressed in the intestine include UGT1A1 (bilirubin-glucuronidating isoform), UGT1A3, UGT1A4, UGT1A6, UGT1A8, UGT1A9, and UGT1A10. Substrate specificities of intestinal UGT isoforms are comparable to those in the liver. The UGT isoforms in the intestine can glucuronidate orally administered drugs, such as morphine, acetaminophen, α- and β-adrenergic agonists and other phenolic phenethanolamines, as well as other dietary xenobiotics, reducing their oral bioavailability (first-pass metabolism). Although UGT isoforms are found in kidney, brain, and lung, they are not uniformly distributed, with UGT1A6 being the isoform that is ubiquitous in extrahepatic tissue.

O-, N-, and S-Glucuronides

The xenobiotics forming glucuronides with alcohols and phenols are ether glucuronides. Aromatic and some aliphatic carboxylic acids form ester (acyl) glucuronides. Aromatic amines form N-glucuronides, and sulfhydryl compounds form S-glucuronides, both of which are more labile to acid compared with the O-glucuronides (Fig. 10.21). Some tertiary amines (e.g., tripelennamine) have been reported to form quaternary ammonium N-glucuronides. Substances containing a 1,3-dicarbonyl structure (e.g., phenylbutazone) can undergo formation of C-glucuronides by direct conjugation without previous metabolism. The acidity of the methylene carbon of the 1,3-dicarbonyl group determines the degree of C-glucuronide formation.

Acyl Glucuronides

Drug–acyl glucuronides are reactive conjugates at physiologic pH. The acyl group of the C^1-acyl glucuronide can migrate via transesterification from the original C-1 position of the glucuronic acid to the C-2, C-3, or C-4 positions (Fig. 10.21). The resulting positional isomers are not hydrolyzable by β-glucuronidase, giving the appearance of a new unknown conjugate. Under physiologic or weakly alkaline conditions, however, the C^1-acyl glucuronide can hydrolyze in the urine to the parent substance (aglycone) or undergo acyl migration to an acceptor macromolecule. The pH-catalyzed migration of the acyl group from the drug C^1-O-acyl glucuronide to a protein or other cellular constituent occurs with the formation of a covalent bond to the protein (59). The acylated protein becomes a "hapten" and could stimulate an immune response against the drug, resulting in the expression of an hypersensitivity reaction or other forms of immunotoxicity. A high incidence of anaphylactic reactions have been reported for several nonsteroidal anti-inflammatory drugs (NSAIDs; benoxaprofen, zomepirac, indoprofen, alclofenac, ticrynafen, and ibufenac) that have been removed from the market. All of these NSAIDs are metabolized by humans to acyl glucuronides. Similar reactions have been reported for other NSAIDs, including tolmetin, sulindac, ibuprofen, ketoprofen, and acetylsalicylic acid. The frequency of the immunotoxic response may be related to the stability of the acyl glucuronide, the chemical rate kinetics for the migration of the acyl group, and the concentration and stability/half-life of the antigenic protein. When the acyl glucuronide is the primary metabolite, in patients with decreased renal function (i.e., elderly individuals), or when probenecid is coadministered, renal cycling of the unconjugated (aglycone) parent drug or metabolite is likely to occur, resulting in the plasma accumulation of the aglycone. The reduced elimination of the acyl glucuronide increases its hydrolysis back to the aglycone or the migration of the C^1-O-acyl group to an acceptor macromolecule.

Bioactivation and Toxic Glucuronides

Generally, glucuronides are biologically and chemically less reactive than their parent molecules and are readily eliminated without interaction with intracellular substances. Some glucuronide conjugates, however, are more active than the parent drug (60). Morphine, for example, forms the 3-O- and 6-O-glucuronides in the intestine and in the liver. The 3-O-glucuronide is the primary glucuronide metabolite of morphine, with a blood concentration 20-fold that of morphine. Pharmacologically, it is an opiate antagonist. On the other hand, 6-O-glucuronide, with a blood concentration twice that of morphine, is a more potent μ-receptor agonist and, whether administered orally or parentally, is 650-fold more analgesic than morphine in humans. Thus, the analgesic effects of morphine are the result of a complex interaction of the drug and its two metabolites with the opiate receptor. Apparently, the 6-O-glucuronide can pass into the brain via an anion-transport system.

Glucuronidation also is capable of promoting cellular injury (e.g., hepatotoxicity and carcinogenesis) by facilitating the formation of reactive electrophilic (electron-deficient) intermediates and their transport into target tissues (37). The induction of bladder carcinogenesis by aromatic amines may result from the glucuronidation of N-hydroxylarylamine. These O-glucuronides become concentrated in the urine, where they are readily hydrolyzed by the acid pH of the urine back to the

N-hydroxylarylamines. Elimination of water under these conditions leads to the formation of electrophilic arylnitrenium species. This reactive species can bind covalently with endogenous cellular constituents (e.g., nucleic acids and proteins), initiating carcinogenesis.

Sulfation and glucuronidation occur side by side, often competing for the same substrate (most commonly phenols, i.e., acetaminophen). The balance between sulfation and glucuronidation is influenced by such factors as species, dose, availability of cosubstrates, and inhibition and induction of the respective transferases.

Sulfate Conjugation

Sulfate conjugation is an important reaction in the biotransformation of steroid hormones, catecholamine neurotransmitters, thyroxine, bile acids, phenolic drugs, and other xenobiotics (56). The major physiologic consequence of sulfate conjugation of a drug or xenobiotic is its increased aqueous solubility and excretion, because the pK_a of the sulfonate groups is approximately one to two. The sulfate conjugates are almost totally ionized in physiologic solutions and possess a smaller volume of distribution than unconjugated steroids and drugs. In certain instances, however, sulfate conjugation can result in bioactivation to reactive electrophiles or therapeutically active conjugates (e.g., minoxidil sulfate). The cytosolic sulfotransferases generally associated with the conjugation of phenolic steroids, neurotransmitters, and xenobiotics. The membrane-bound sulfotransferases are localized in the Golgi apparatus of most cells and are responsible for the sulfation of glycosaminoglycans, glycoproteins, and the tyrosinyl group of peptides and protein but generally are not associated with xenobiotic metabolism.

Mechanism of Sulfate Conjugation

A xenobiotic is sulfated by transfer of an active sulfate from 3′-phosphoadenosine-5′-phosphosulfate (PAPS) to the acceptor molecule, a cytosolic reaction catalyzed by a multigene sulfotransferases (Fig. 10.23); PAPS is formed enzymatically from adenosine triphosphate (ATP) and inorganic sulfate. Sulfate conjugation is a reaction principally of phenols and, to a lesser extent, of alcohols to form highly ionic and polar sulfates ($R\text{-}O\text{-}SO_2H$). The availability of PAPS and its precursor inorganic sulfate determines the reaction rate. The total pool of sulfate usually is limited and can be readily exhausted. With increasing doses of a drug, conjugation with sulfate becomes a less predominant pathway. At high doses with a competing substrate (i.e., acetaminophen), glucuronidation usually predominates over that of sulfation, which prevails at low doses. Other precursors for sulfate include L-methionine and L-cysteine. When PAPS, inorganic sulfate, or the sulfur amino acids are low or depleted, or when a substrate for sulfation is given in high doses, competing reactions with glucuronidation can take over. Additionally, O-methylation is a competing reaction for catecholamine.

Sulfotransferase Family

In humans, sulfotransferases are divided into two families, SULT1 and SULT2 (61). The isoforms SULT1A1, SULT1A2, and SULT1A3 catalyze the sulfation of many phenolic drugs, catecholamine, hormones, aromatic amines, and other xenobiotics (62). The SULT1A1/2 (formerly known as phenol sulfotransferase thermally stable) preferentially sulfates small planar phenols in the micromolar concentration range, estradiol and synthetic estrogens, phytoestrogens, acetaminophen, the N-oxide of minoxidil, and N-hydroxyaromatic and heterocylic amines; SULT1A3 (formerly known as phenol sulfotransferase thermally labile) selectively sulfates the catecholamines dopamine, norepinephrine, and epinephrine as well as the N-oxide of minoxidil, thyroid hormones, but not estrogenic steroids and other hydroxy steroids; SULT1B1 catalyzes the sulfation of the thyroid hormones; SULT1C1 is involved with the bioactivation of procarcinogens via sulfation; SULT1E1 (formerly known as estrogen sulfotransferase) preferentially sulfates estradiol in the nanomolar range; SULT2A1 (formerly known as dehydroepiandrosterone [DHEA] sulfotransferase) conjugates DHEA, estradiol (micromolar range), the synthetic estrogens, and other estrogen metabolites; and SULT2B1 (formerly known as hydroxysteroid sulfotransferase) sulfates DHEA and pregnenolone.

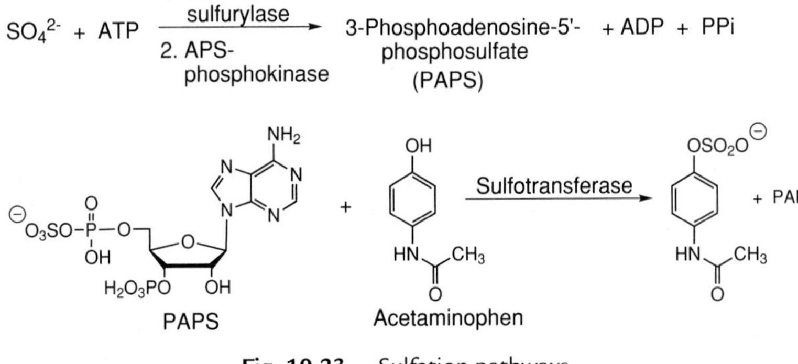

SO_4^{2-} + ATP —(1. ATP-sulfurylase; 2. APS-phosphokinase)→ 3-Phosphoadenosine-5′-phosphosulfate (PAPS) + ADP + PPi

PAPS + Acetaminophen —(Sulfotransferase)→ + PAP

Fig. 10.23. Sulfation pathways.

Sulfate conjugation appears to be an important reaction in the transport and metabolism of steroids. Sulfation decreases the biological activity of the steroid, because the steroid sulfates are not capable of binding to their receptors. It provides for the transport of an inactive form of the steroid to its target tissue, where the active steroid is regenerated by sulfatases at the target tissue.

Sulfotransferase Distribution

The SULT1A families are abundantly expressed in the liver, small intestine, brain, kidneys, and platelets (61). For example, phenol is sulfated by a sulfotransferase in the liver, kidneys, and intestines, whereas steroids are sulfated only in the liver. The broad diversity of compounds sulfated in human tissues results, in part, from the multi-isoforms of the cytosolic sulfotransferases and their overlapping substrate specificities. Sulfate conjugates are almost totally ionized and, therefore, are excreted mostly in the urine, but biliary elimination is common for steroids. On hydrolysis of biliary sulfate conjugates in the intestine by sulfatases, the parent drug (or xenobiotic) or its metabolites may be reabsorbed into the portal circulation for eventual elimination in the urine as a sulfate conjugate (enterohepatic cycling). The rate of sulfation appears to be age dependent, decreasing with age. An important site of sulfation, especially after oral administration, is the intestine. The result is a presystemic first-pass effect: decreasing drug bioavailability of several drugs for which the primary route of conjugation is sulfation. Drugs such as isoproterenol, albuterol, steroid hormones, α-methyldopa, acetaminophen, and fenoldopam are affected. Competition for intestinal sulfation between coadministered substrates may influence their bioavailability with either an enhancement of or a decrease in therapeutic effects. An example would be coadministration of acetaminophen and the oral contraceptive ethinyl estradiol.

Bioactivation and Toxicity

As with glucuronidation, sulfation is a detoxication reaction, although sulfate conjugates have been reported to be pharmacologically active (e.g., minoxidil sulfate, dehydroepiandrosterone sulfate, and morphine 6-sulfate) or to be converted into unstable sulfate conjugates that form reactive intermediates implicated in carcinogenesis and tissue damage. Sulfation of an alcohol generates a good leaving group and can be an activation process for alcohols to produce a reactive electrophilic species (37). Like the N-glucuronides, however, N-sulfates are capable of promoting cytotoxicity by facilitating the formation of reactive electrophilic intermediates. Sulfation of N-oxygenated aromatic amines is an activation process for some arylamines that can eliminate the sulfate to an electrophilic species capable of reacting with proteins or DNA (e.g., 2-acetylaminofluorene). The N-sulfation of arylamines to arylsulfamic acids ($R\text{-}NHSO_3H$) is a minor pathway.

Stereoselectivity

The SULT1A3 displays stereoselectivity in the sulfation of chiral phenolic phenethanolamines. This isoform may be responsible, in part, for the enantiomer-specific metabolism observed for the β-adrenergic agonists. For example, the (+)-enantiomers of terbutaline and isoproterenol and the (−)-enantiomer of albuterol are selectively sulfated.

Conjugation with Amino Acids

Conjugation with amino acids is an important metabolic route in the metabolism of xenobiotic carboxylic acids before elimination (56). Glycine, the most common amino acid, forms water-soluble ionic conjugates with aromatic, arylaliphatic, and heterocyclic carboxylic acids. These amino acid conjugates usually are less toxic than their precursor acids and are excreted readily into the urine and bile. These reactions involve the formation of an amide or peptide bond between the xenobiotic carboxylic acid and the amino group of an amino acid, usually glycine. The xenobiotic must first be activated to its CoA thioester before reacting with the amino group (Fig. 10.24). The formation of the xenobiotic acyl CoA thioester is of critical importance in intermediary metabolism of lipids as well as intermediate- and long-chain fatty acids.

The major metabolic biotransformations for xenobiotic carboxylic acids include conjugation with either glucuronic acid or glycine. The metabolic fate of these carboxylic acids depends on the size and type of substituents adjacent to the carboxyl group. Most unbranched aliphatic acids are completely oxidized and do not usually form conjugates, although branched aliphatic and arylaliphatic acids are resistant to β-oxidation and form glycine or glucuronide conjugates. Interestingly, substitution of the α-carbon

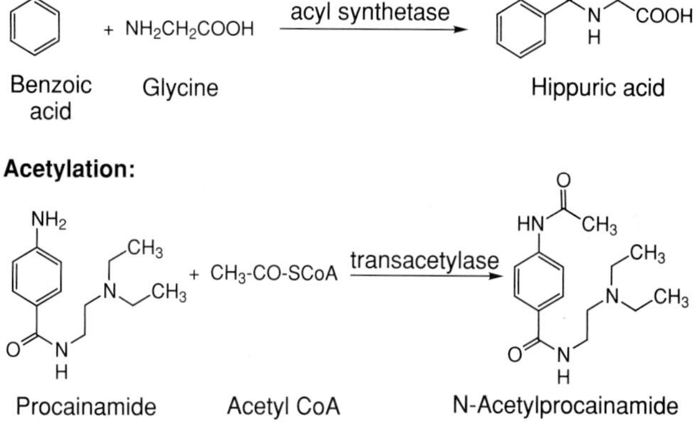

$$R\text{-}COOH + ATP + CoA \xrightarrow{\text{acyl synthetase}} R\text{-}CO\text{-}S\text{-}CoA + AMP$$

$$CH_3\text{-}CO\text{-}S\text{-}CoA + R'\text{-}NH_2 \xrightarrow{\text{transacetylase}} CH_3\text{-}CO\text{-}NH\text{-}R' + CoASH$$

Examples:

Glycine conjugation:

Benzoic acid (COOH) + NH_2CH_2COOH (Glycine) —acyl synthetase→ Hippuric acid

Acetylation:

Procainamide + $CH_3\text{-}CO\text{-}SCoA$ (Acetyl CoA) —transacetylase→ N-Acetylprocainamide

Fig. 10.24. Amino acid conjugation pathways of carboxylic acids with glycine and acetylation pathways.

favors glucuronidation rather than glycine conjugation. Benzoic and heterocyclic aromatic acids are principally conjugated with glycine. Glycine conjugation is preferred for xenobiotic carboxylic acids at low doses, and glucuronidation is preferred at high doses with broad substrate selectivity. In humans and some species of monkeys, glutamine forms a conjugate with phenylacetic acids and related arylacetic acids. Bile acids form conjugates with glycine and taurine by the action of enzymes in the microsomal fraction rather than in the mitochondria.

In contrast to the enhanced reactivity and toxicity of the various glucuronide, sulfate, acetyl, and glutathione conjugates, amino acid conjugates have not proven to be toxic. It has been proposed that amino acid conjugation is a detoxication pathway for reactive acyl CoA thioesters.

Conjugation with CoA

Several carboxylic acid–containing drugs (e.g., zomiperac and benzoxaprofen) have been implicated in rare but serious adverse reactions. These carboxylic acids were withdrawn in the late 1980s from the market because of unpredictable allergic reactions that may have been caused by carboxylic acid–protein adducts formed by reaction of their reactive acyl glucuronide or acyl CoA thioesters with endogenous proteins. The carboxylic acids can be bioactivated via two distinct pathways: UGT-catalyzed conjugation with glucuronic acid to acyl glucuronides, or acyl CoA synthetase–catalyzed formation of acyl CoA thioesters. The reactive CoA thioester intermediates of carboxylic acids are electrophilic and, therefore, can contribute to the acylation of target proteins. The acyl CoA thioester serves as an obligatory intermediate in the formation of glycine and carnitine ester. Therefore, their appearance in metabolism studies and urine is of significance, because they serve as biomarkers for the formation acyl CoA thioesters, which may provide the link between protein-reactive acyl CoA thioesters and the rare and unpredictable idiosyncratic drug reactions in humans.

A nontoxic reaction involving acyl CoA thioesters includes chiral inversions of the 2-arylpropionic acids ("profens"), a major group of NSAIDs that exist in two enantiomeric forms (59). The anti-inflammatory activity (inhibition of cyclooxygenase) for the NSAIDs resides with the S-(+)-enantiomer. The intriguing aspect for the metabolism of the NSAID is their unidirectional chiral inversion from the R-(−)- to the S-(+)-enantiomer (Fig. 10.25). The NSAID acyl CoA thioester is the critical intermediate for this chiral inversion of the 2-arylpropionic acids, and the formation of the thioester is stereospecific for the pharmacologically inactive R-enantiomer (61). Racemic ibuprofen and related anti-inflammatory 2-arylpropionic acids (e.g., benoxaprofen, carprofen, cicliprofen, clidanac, fenoprofen, indoprofen, ketoprofen, loxoprofen, and naproxen) undergo in vivo metabolic inversion to the more active S-enantiomer via the formation, epimerization, and hydrolysis of their respective acyl CoA thioesters (63). The unidirectional *R*- to *S*-inversion of ibuprofen is attributed to the stereoselective thioester formation of *R*-Ibuprofen

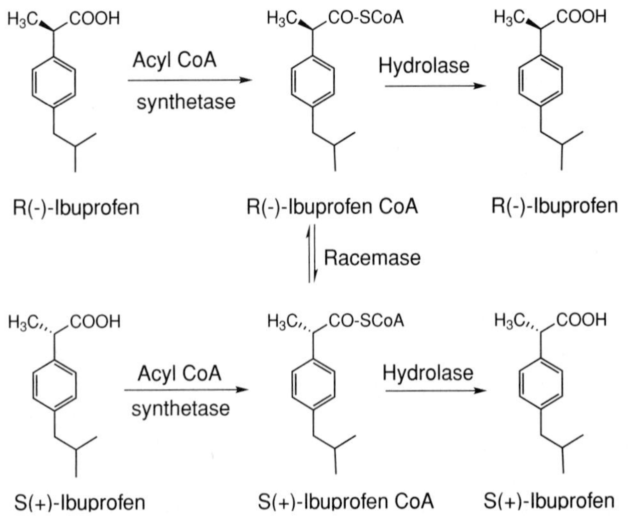

H$_3$C COOH — Acyl CoA synthetase → H$_3$C CO-SCoA — Hydrolase → H$_3$C COOH

R(-)-Ibuprofen R(-)-Ibuprofen CoA R(-)-Ibuprofen

Racemase

H$_3$C COOH — Acyl CoA synthetase → H$_3$C CO-SCoA — Hydrolase → H$_3$C COOH

S(+)-Ibuprofen S(+)-Ibuprofen CoA S(+)-Ibuprofen

Fig. 10.25. Coenzyme A (CoA) conjugation pathway: Stereospecific inversion of R(−)- to S(+)-ibuprofen.

CoA, not to the stereoselectivity of either the epimerization or hydrolysis steps (64). *S*-(+)-Ibuprofen does not form its CoA thioester in vivo. Because the formation of 2-arylpropionyl CoA thioester is analogous to the activation and metabolism of medium and long-chain fatty acids, it seems possible that conditions either elevating (e.g., diabetes or fasting) or depleting CoA may alter CoA thioester formation of the 2-arylpropionic acids and their in vivo metabolic inversion. Amino acid conjugation (i.e., CoA activation) is more sensitive to steric hindrance than is glucuronidation (e.g., arylacetic acids).

Acetylation

Acetylation is principally a reaction of amino groups involving the transfer of acetyl CoA to primary aliphatic and aromatic amines, amino acids, hydrazines, or sulfonamide groups (56). The liver is the primary site of acetylation, although extrahepatic sites have been identified. Sulfonamides, being difunctional, can form either N^1 or N^4 acetyl derivatives, and in some instances, the diacetylated derivative has been identified. Secondary amines are not acetylated. Acetylation may produce conjugates that retain the pharmacological activity of the parent drug (e.g., N-acetylprocainamide) (Fig. 10.24).

The existence of genetic polymorphism in the rate of acetylation has important consequences for drug therapy and tumorigenicity of xenobiotics. Acetylation polymorphism has been associated with differences in human drug toxicity between the two acetylator phenotypes, slow and fast acetylators. Slow acetylators are more prone to drug-induced toxicities and accumulate higher blood concentrations of the unacetylated drug (e.g., hydralazine and procainamide-induced lupus erythematous, isoniazid-induced peripheral nerve damage, and sulfasalazine-induced hematologic disorders) than fast acetylators do. Fast acetylators eliminate the drug more rapidly by

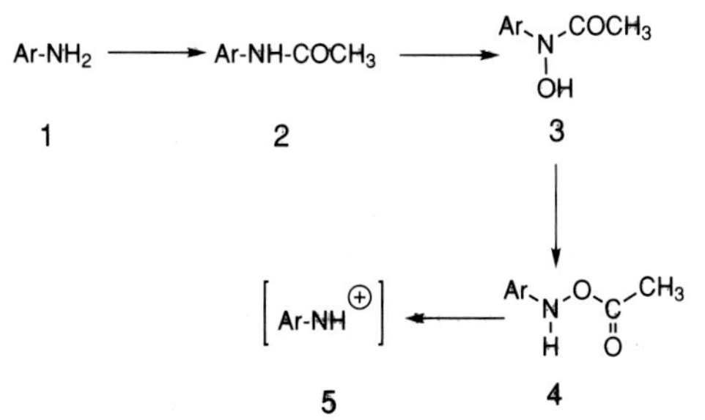

Fig. 10.26. Bioactivation of acetylated arylamines.

conversion to its relatively nontoxic N-acetyl metabolite. For some drug substances, however, fast acetylators may pose a greater risk of liver toxicity than slow acetylators, because fast acetylators produce toxic metabolites more rapidly (e.g., isoniazid forms the hepatotoxic monoacetylhydrazine metabolite). Thus, differences in acetylator phenotype can influence adverse drug reactions.

The possibility arises that genetic differences in acetylating capacity may confer differences in susceptibility to chemical carcinogenicity from arylamines. The tumorigenic activity of arylamines (1 in Fig. 10.26) may be the result of a complex series of sequential metabolic reactions commencing with N-acetylation (2 in Fig. 10.26), subsequent oxidation to arylhydroxamic acids (3 in Fig. 10.26), and metabolic transformation to acetoxyarylamines by N, O-acyltransferase (4 in Fig. 10.26). The acetoxyarylamine can eliminate the acetoxy group to form the reactive arylnitrenium ion (5 in Fig. 10.26), which is capable of covalently binding to nucleic acids and proteins, thus increasing the risk for development of bladder and liver tumors (65). The rapid acetylator phenotype is expected to form the acetoxyarylamine metabolite at a greater rate than the slow acetylator and, thereby, to present a greater risk for development of tumors compared with the slow acetylator.

Glutathione Conjugation and Mercapturic Acid Synthesis

Mercapturic acids are S-derivatives of N-acetylcysteine synthesized from glutathione (GSH) (53,54). It is generally accepted that most compounds metabolized to mercapturic acids first undergo conjugation with glutathione, catalyzed by the enzyme glutathione S-transferase (GST), a multigene isoenzyme family that is abundant in the soluble supernatant liver fractions. In humans, GSTs are divided into two isoforms, GSTM1 and GSTT1. The principal drug substrates for GSTM1 are the nitrosourea and mustard-type anticancer drugs. The GSTT1 isoform metabolizes small organic molecules, such as solvents, halocarbons, and electrophilic compounds (e.g., αβ-unsaturated carbonyl compounds). The reaction is depicted in Figure 10.27.

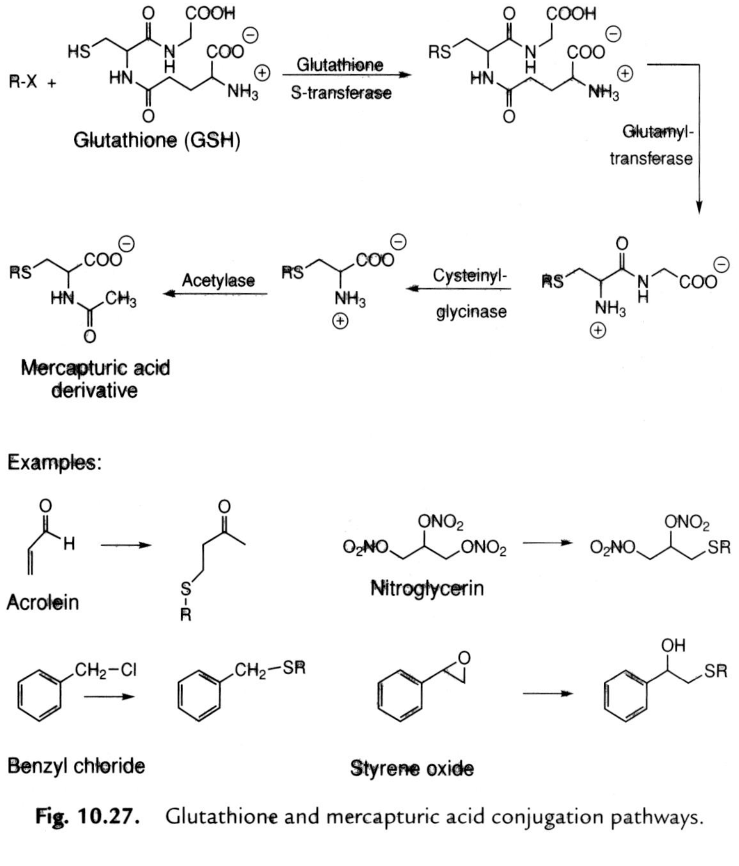

Fig. 10.27. Glutathione and mercapturic acid conjugation pathways.

The enzyme GST apparently increases the ionization of the thiol group of GSH, increasing its nucleophilicity toward electrophiles and conjugating with these potentially harmful electrophiles, thereby protecting other vital nucleophilic centers in the cell, such as nucleic acids and proteins. Glutathione also is capable of reacting nonenzymatically with nucleophilic sites on neighboring macromolecules. Once conjugated with GSH, the electrophiles usually are excreted in the bile and urine.

A range of functional groups yields thioether conjugates of GSH as well as products other than thioethers (Fig. 10.27). The nucleophilic attack by GSH occurs on electrophilic carbons with leaving groups (e.g., halogen [alkyl, alkenyl, aryl, or aralkyl halides], sulfate [alkylmethanesulfonates], and nitro [alkyl nitrates] groups), ring opening of small ring ethers (epoxides and β-lactones, e.g., β-propiolactone), and the Michael-type addition to the activated β-carbon of an α,β-unsaturated carbonyl compound (e.g., acrolein). Organic nitrate esters (e.g., the coronary vasodilator nitroglycerin) undergo a dismutation reaction that results in the oxidation of GSH to GSSG (through formation of the labile S-nitrate conjugation product) and reduction of the nitrate ester to an alcohol and inorganic nitrite. The lack of substrate specificity gives argument to the fact that glutathione transferase has undergone adaptive changes to accommodate the variety of xenobiotics to which it is exposed. Usually, the conjugation of an electrophilic compound with GSH is a reaction of detoxication, but some carcinogens have been activated through conjugation with GSH (29–31).

The enzymatic conjugation of GSH with epoxides provides a mechanism for protecting the liver from injury caused by certain bioactivated intermediates (see the subsequent Metabolic Bioactivation section). Not all epoxides are substrates for this enzyme, but the more chemically reactive epoxides appear to be better substrates. Important among the epoxides that are substrates for this enzyme are those produced from halobenzenes and PAHs through the action of CYP450 monooxygenase. Epoxide formation exemplifies bioactivation, because the epoxides are reactive and potentially toxic, whereas their GSH conjugates are inactive. Conjugation of GSH with the epoxides of aryl hydrocarbons eventually results in the formation of hydroxymercapturic acids (premercapturic acids), which undergo acid-catalyzed dehydration to the mercapturic acids. The halobenzenes usually are conjugated in the para position.

Monohalogenated, gem-dihalogenated, and vicinal dihalogenated alkanes undergo glutathione transferase–catalyzed conjugation reactions to produce S-substituted glutathione derivatives that are metabolically transformed into the more stable and less toxic mercapturic acids. This common route of metabolism occurs through nucleophilic displacement of a halide ion by the thiolate anion of glutathione (see the discussion on glutathione conjugation). The mutagenicity of the 1,2-dihaloethanes (e.g., the pesticide and fumigant ethylene dibromide) has been attributed to GSH displacing bromide with the formation of the S-(2-haloethyl) glutathione, which subsequently rearranges to a reactive episulfonium ion electrophile that, in turn, alkylates DNA. Many of the halogenated hydrocarbons exhibiting nephrotoxicity undergo the formation of similar S-substituted cysteine derivatives.

The mercapturic acid pathway appears to have evolved as a protective mechanism against xenobiotic-induced hepatotoxicity or carcinogenicity, serving to detoxify a large number of noxious substances that we inhale or ingest or that are produced daily in the human body. A correlation exists between the hepatotoxicity of acetaminophen and levels of GSH in the liver. The probable mechanism of toxicity that has emerged from animal studies is that acetaminophen is CYP1A2- and CYP2E1-oxidized to the N-acetyl-*p*-benzoquinonimine intermediate that conjugates with and depletes hepatic GSH levels (Fig. 10.28). This action allows the benzoquinonimine to bind covalently to tissue macromolecules. The mercapturic acid derivative of acetaminophen represents approximately 2% of the administered dose of acetaminophen. Thus, the possibility exists that those toxic metabolites that usually are detoxified by conjugating with GSH exhibit their hepatotoxicity (or, perhaps, carcinogenicity) because the liver has been depleted of GSH and is incapable of inactivating them. Pretreatment of animals with phenobarbital often hastens the depletion of GSH by increasing the formation of epoxides or other reactive intermediates.

Methylation

Methylation is a common biochemical reaction but appears to be of greater significance in the metabolism of

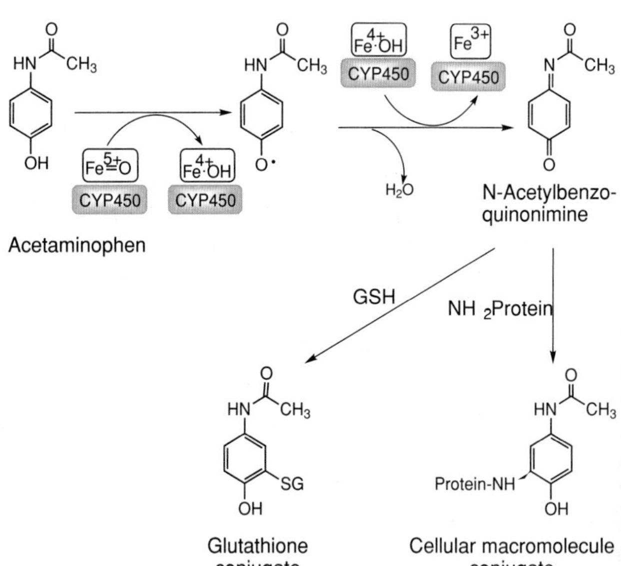

Fig. 10.28. Proposed mechanism for the CYP450-catalyzed oxidation of acetaminophen to its N-acetyl-*p*-benzoquinoneimine intermediate, which can further react with either glutathione (GSH) or cellular macromolecules (NH_2-protein).

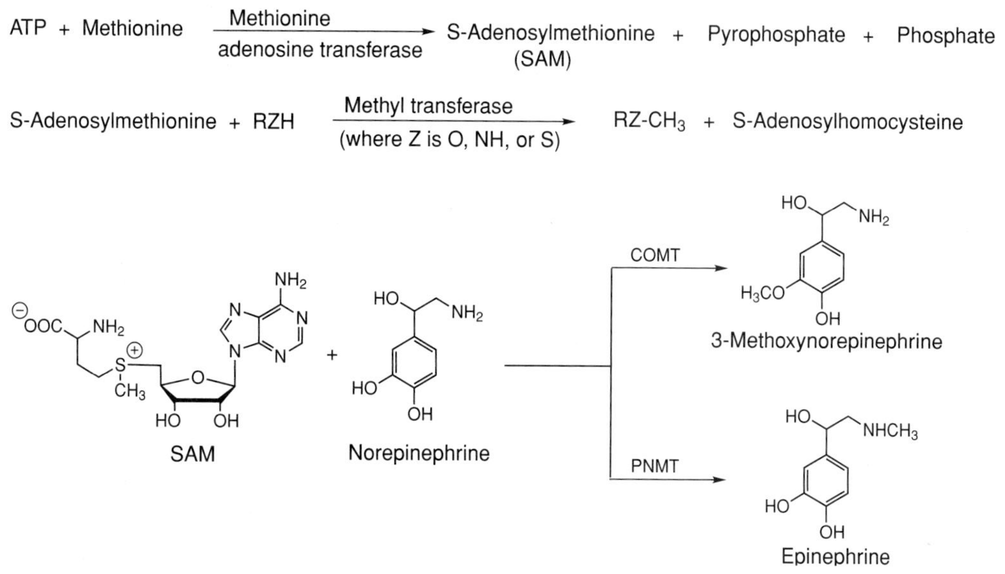

ATP + Methionine —Methionine adenosine transferase→ S-Adenosylmethionine (SAM) + Pyrophosphate + Phosphate

S-Adenosylmethionine + RZH —Methyl transferase (where Z is O, NH, or S)→ $RZ\text{-}CH_3$ + S-Adenosylhomocysteine

SAM + Norepinephrine → (COMT) 3-Methoxynorepinephrine; → (PNMT) Epinephrine

Fig. 10.29. Methylation pathways.

endogenous compounds than for drugs and other foreign compounds (56). Methylation differs from other conjugation processes in that the O-methyl metabolites formed may, in some cases, have as great or greater pharmacological activity and lipophilicity than the parent molecule (e.g., the conversion of norepinephrine to epinephrine). Methionine is involved in the methylation of endogenous and exogenous substrates, because it transfers its methyl group via the activated intermediate S-adenosylmethionine to the substrate under the influence of methyl transferases (Fig. 10.29). Methylation results principally in the formation of O-methylated, N-methylated, and S-methylated products.

O-Methylation

The process of O-methylation is catalyzed by the magnesium-dependent enzyme catechol-O-methyltransferase (COMT) transferring a methyl group to the meta- or, less frequently, the paraphenolic-OH (regioselectivity) of catecholamines (e.g., norepinephrine) as well as by their deaminated metabolites. It does not methylate monohydric or other dihydric phenols. The meta:para product ratio depends greatly on the type of substituent attached to the catechol ring. Substrates specific for COMT include the catecholamines norepinephrine, epinephrine, and dopamine; the catechol amino acids L-DOPA and α-methyl-DOPA; and 2- and 4-hydroxyestradiol metabolites of estradiol. The enzyme is thought to function in the biological inactivation of the adrenergic neurotransmitter norepinephrine as well as other endogenous and exogenous catechol-like substances. It is found in liver, kidneys, nervous tissue, and other tissues.

Hydroxyindole-O-methyltransferase, which is O-methylates N-acetylserotonin, serotonin, and other hydroxyindoles, is found in the pineal gland and is involved in the formation of melatonin. This enzyme differs from COMT in that it does not methylate catecholamines and has no requirement for magnesium iron.

N-Methylation

The N-methylation of various amines is among several conjugate pathways for metabolizing amines. Specific N-methyltransferases catalyze the transfer of active methyl groups from S-adenosylmethionine to the acceptor substance. Phenylethanolamine-N-methyltransferase methylates a number of endogenous and exogenous phenylethanolamines (e.g., normetanephrine, norepinephrine, and norephedrine) but does not methylate phenylethylamines. Histamine-N-methyl transferase specifically methylates histamine, producing the inactive metabolite N^1-methylhistamine. Amine-N-methyltransferase will N-methylate a variety of primary and secondary amines from a number of sources, including endogenous biogenic amines (serotonin, tryptamine, tyramine, and dopamine) and drugs (desmethylimipramine, amphetamine, and normorphine). Amine-N-methyl transferases seem to have a role in recycling N-demethylated drugs.

Thiol Methylation

Thiols generally are considered to be toxic, and the role of thiol S-methyl transferases is a nonoxidative detoxification pathway of these compounds (see the discussion of flavin-containing monooxygenases). The S-methylation of sulfhydryl compounds also involves a microsomal enzyme requiring S-adenosylmethionine. Although a wide range of exogenous sulfhydryl compounds are S-methylated by this microsomal enzyme, none of the endogenous sulfhydryl compounds (e.g., cysteine and GSH) can function as substrates. Clearly, S-methylation represents a detoxication step for thiols. Dialkyldithiocarbamates (e.g., disulfiram) and the antithyroid drugs (e.g., 6-propyl-2-thiouracil), mercaptans, and hydrogen sulfide (from thioglycosides as natural constituents of foods, mineral sulfides in water, fermented beverages, and bacterial digestion) are S-methylated. Other drugs undergoing S-methylation include captopril, thiopurine, penicillamine, and 6-mercaptopurine.

Conjugation of Cyanide

The toxicity of hydrogen cyanide is the result of its ionization to cyanide ion in biological tissues. It is a powerful metabolic inhibitor that arrests cellular respiration by inactivating cytochrome enzymes that are fundamental to the respiratory process as well as combining with hemoglobin to form cyanomethemoglobin, which is incapable of transporting oxygen to tissues. With the wide prevalence of cyanoglycosides in plant materials, the ability to detoxify cyanide is a vital function of the liver, erythrocytes, and other tissues. Rhodanase, a mitochondrial enzyme in liver and other tissues, catalyzes the formation of thiocyanate from cyanide rapidly in the presence of thiosulfate and colloidal sulfur, but cysteine and GSH are poor sulfur donors. The detoxification of cyanide depends on the availability of a physiologic pool of thiosulfate, the origin of which is not known. A possible source for thiosulfate is the transamination of cysteine to β-mercaptopyruvate and transfer of the mercapto group by a sulfur transferase to sulfite-producing thiosulfate. Depletion of this pool increases cyanide toxicity. In the presence of excess cyanide, however, minor pathways for cyanide metabolism may occur, including oxidation to cyanate (NCO^-), reaction with cobalamin (vitamin B_{12}) to form cyanocobalamin, and the formation of 2-iminothiazolidine-4-carboxylic acid from the nonenzymatic reaction between cysteine and cyanide (66).

$$S_2O_3^{2-} + CN^- \longrightarrow CNS^- + SO_3^{2-}$$

ELIMINATION PATHWAYS

Most xenobiotics are lipid-soluble and are altered chemically by the metabolizing enzymes, usually into less toxic and more water-soluble substances, before being excreted into the urine (or, in some cases, bile). The formation of conjugates with sulfate, amino acids, and glucuronic acid is particularly effective in increasing the polarity of drug molecules. The principal route of excretion of drugs and their metabolites is in the urine. If drugs and other compounds foreign to the body are not metabolized in this manner, substances with a high lipid–water partition coefficient could be reabsorbed readily from the urine through the renal tubular membranes and into the plasma. Therefore, such substances would continue to be recirculated, and their pharmacological or toxic effects would be prolonged. Very polar or highly ionized drug molecules often are excreted in the urine unchanged.

Urine

Tubular reabsorption is greatly reduced by conversion of a drug into a more polar substance with a lower partition coefficient. In general, the more resistance a drug is to the metabolizing enzymes, the greater the therapeutic action and the smaller the dose needed to achieve a particular therapeutic goal.

Urine is not the only route for excreting drugs and their metabolites from the animal body. Other routes include bile, saliva, lungs, sweat, and milk. The bile has been recognized as a major route of excretion for many endogenous and exogenous compounds.

Enterohepatic Cycling of Drugs

The liver is the principal organ for the metabolism and eventual elimination of xenobiotics from the human body in either the urine or the bile. When eliminated in the bile, steroid hormones, bile acids, drugs, and their respective conjugated metabolites are available for reabsorption from the duodenal–intestinal tract into the portal circulation, undergoing the process of enterohepatic cycling (EHC) (67). Nearly all drugs are excreted in the bile, but only a few are concentrated in the bile. For example, the bile salts are so efficiently concentrated in the bile and reabsorbed from the gastrointestinal tract that the entire body pool recycles several times per day. Therefore, EHC is responsible for the conservation of bile acids, steroid hormones, thyroid hormones, and other endogenous substances. In humans, compounds excreted into the bile usually have a molecular weight greater than 500 Da, whereas with rats, the critical molecular weight is 325 Da. Consequently, biliary excretion is more common in rats than in humans. Compounds with a molecular weight between 300 and 500 Da are excreted in both urine and bile. Some compounds would not be expected to be excreted in the bile because of a molecular weight of less than 300 Da and a relatively nonpolar structure. Compounds excreted into bile usually are strongly polar substances that may be charged (anionic; e.g., dyes) or uncharged (e.g., cardiac glycosides and steroid hormones). Biotransformation of this type of compound by means of Phase 1 and Phase 2 reactions would produce a conjugated metabolite, which usually is anionic, more polar, and has a molecular weight greater than that of the parent compound. They most often are present as their glucuronide conjugates, because glucuronidation adds 176 Da to the molecular weight of the parent compound. Unchanged drug in the bile is excreted with the feces, metabolized by the bacterial flora in the intestinal tract, or reabsorbed into the portal circulation.

Not unexpectedly, the bacterial intestinal flora is directly involved in EHC and the recycling of drugs through the portal circulation (see the discussion of extrahepatic metabolism). A conjugated drug and metabolites excreted via the bile may be hydrolyzed by enzymes of the bacterial flora, releasing the parent drug or its Phase I metabolite for reabsorption into the portal circulation (68). Among the numerous compounds metabolized in the enterohepatic circulation are the estrogenic and progestational steroids, digitoxin, indomethacin, diazepam, pentaerythritol tetranitrate, mercurials, arsenicals, and morphine. The oral ingestion of xenobiotics inhibiting the gut flora (i.e., nonabsorbable antibiotics) can effect the pharmacokinetics of the initial drug.

The impact of EHC on the pharmacokinetics and pharmacodynamics of a drug depends on the importance of biliary excretion of the drug relative to renal clearance and on the efficiency of gastrointestinal absorption. The EHC becomes dominant when biliary excretion is the major clearance mechanism for the drug. Because the majority of the bile is stored in the gallbladder and released on the ingestion of food, intermittent spikes in the plasma drug concentration is observed following reentry of the drug from the bile via EHC. From a pharmacodynamic point of view, the net effect of EHC is to increase the duration of a drug in the body and to prolong its pharmacological action.

Chronic treatment with the enzyme inducer phenobarbital enhances the biliary excretion of drug molecules and their metabolites by increasing liver size, bile flow, and more efficient transport into the bile. This behavior is not shared by all inducers of the CYP450 monooxygenases. The route of administration also may influence excretion pathways. Direct administration into the portal circulation might be expected to result in more biliary excretion than could be expected via the systemic route.

Table 10.13. Effect of Age on the Clearance of Some Drugs

No Change	Decrease
Acetaminophen*	Alprazolam
Aspirin	Amitriptylene
Diclofenac	Carbenoxolone
Digitoxin	Chlordiazepoxide
Diphenhydramine	Chlormethiazole
Ethanol	Clobazam
Flunitrazepam	Desmethyldiazepam
Heparin	Diazepam
Lormetazepam	Labetalol
Midazolam	Lidocaine
Nitrazepam	Lorazepam
Oxazepam	Morphine
Phenytoin*	Meperidine
Prazosin	Nifedipine and other dihydropyridines
Propylthiouracil	Norepinephrine
Temazepam	Nortriptyline
Thiopental*	Phenytoin
Tolbutamide*	Piroxicam
Warfarin	Propranolol
	Quinidine
	Quinine
	Theophylline
	Verapamil

*Drugs for which clearance is disputable but may be increased.

DRUG METABOLISM AND AGE

Approximately 30% of the population is older than 65 years of age and is responsible for more than 50% of the national drug expenditures. People older than 65 years represent a significant portion of the population; they are the most medicated and account for more than one-third of all prescription drugs dispensed. The average elderly patient in a health care facility could receive as many as 10 medications daily, which results in the potential for a greater incidence of adverse drug reactions. The widespread use of medications in the elderly will increase the potential for an increased incidence of drug-related interactions. Not unexpectedly, these interactions will be related to changes in drug metabolism and clearance from the body (Table 10.13). The interpretation of the age-related alteration in drug response must consider the contributions of absorption, distribution, metabolism, and excretion (69). Drug therapy in the elderly is expected to become one of the more significant problems for clinical medicine. It has been well documented that the metabolism of many drugs and their elimination is impaired in the elderly.

Metabolism in the Elderly

The decline in drug metabolism because of old age is associated with physiological changes that have pharmacokinetic implications affecting the steady-state plasma concentrations and renal clearance for the parent drug and its metabolites (70,71). Those changes relevant to the bioavailability of drugs in the elderly are decreases in hepatic blood flow, glomerular filtration rate, hepatic microsomal enzyme activity, plasma protein binding, and body mass. Because the rate of a drug's elimination from the blood through hepatic metabolism is determined by hepatic blood flow, protein binding, and intrinsic clearance, a reduction in hepatic blood flow can lead to an increase in drug bioavailability and decreased clearance, with the symptoms of drug overdose and toxicity as the outcome. Drugs for which elimination is dependent on hepatic blood flow have a high extraction ratio and undergo extensive first-pass metabolism when administered orally. Available evidence suggests that age is associated with a reduction in first-pass metabolism of some, but certainly not all, drugs. Those orally administered drugs exhibiting a reduction in first-pass metabolism in the elderly include the dihydropyridine calcium antagonists, chlormethiazole, diazepam, lorazepam, chlordiazepoxide, alprazolam, propranolol, verapamil, labetalol, theophylline, morphine, amitriptyline, and nortriptyline. The bioavailability of drugs with low extraction ratios depends on the percentage of drug–protein binding and not on first-pass hepatic metabolism. Inasmuch as drug binding to plasma proteins is an important factor in the rate of drug metabolism, it appears not to be a significant factor in the elderly.

Age-related changes in drug metabolism are a complicated interplay between the age-related physiological changes, genetics, environmental influences (diet and nutritional status, smoking, and enzyme induction), concomitant diseases states, and drug intake. In most studies, the elderly appear just as responsive to drug-metabolizing enzyme activity (Phase I and Phase II) as young individuals. All the common pathways of drug conjugation, including glucuronidation, sulfation, and glycine conjugation, are variably affected by aging. Given the number of factors that determine the rate of drug metabolism, it is not surprising that the effects of aging on drug elimination by metabolism has yielded variable results even for the same drug. Therefore, the bioavailability of a drug in the elderly and the potential for drug toxicity is largely dependant on its extraction ratio and mode of administration. The fact that drug elimination may be altered in old age suggests that initial doses of metabolized drugs should be reduced in older patients and then modified according to the clinical response (70,71). A decrease in hepatic drug metabolism coupled with age-related alterations in clearance, volume of distribution, and receptor sensitivity can lead to prolonged plasma half-life and increased drug toxicity (Table 10.13).

Drug Interactions

Although drug–drug interactions constitute only a small proportion of adverse drug reactions in the elderly, they are important, because they often are predictable and, therefore, avoidable or manageable. Their frequency is related to the age of the patient, the number of drugs prescribed, the number of physicians involved in the patient's care, and the presence of increasing frailty. The most important mechanisms for drug–drug interactions are the inhibition or induction of drug metabolism. Interactions involving a loss of action of one of the drugs are at least as frequent as those involving an increased effect. Although only approximately 10% of potential interactions result in clinically significant adverse events, death or serious clinical consequences are rare, but low-grade, clinical morbidity in the elderly may be much more common. Nonspecific complaints (e.g. confusion, lethargy, weakness, dizziness, incontinence, depression, and falling) should all prompt a closer look at the patient's drug list. A number of strategies can be adopted to decrease the risk of potential clinical problems. The number of drugs prescribed for each individual should be limited to as few as necessary. The use of drugs should be reviewed regularly, and unnecessary agents withdrawn if possible, with subsequent monitoring. Patients should be encouraged to engage in a "prescribing partnership" by alerting physicians, pharmacists, and other health care professionals to symptoms that occur when new drugs are introduced. Health care professionals should develop a strategy for monitoring their drug treatment looking for the drug–drug interactions that have been encountered.

Those CYP substrates reported to cause drug–drug interactions are shown in Tables 10.3 through 10.10 in bold italics.

Fetal Metabolism

The ability of the human fetus and placenta to metabolize xenobiotics is well established. A 1973 clinical study reported that women ingest an average of 10 drugs during pregnancy, not including anesthetics, intravenous fluids, vitamins, iron, nicotine, cosmetic products, artificial sweeteners, or exposure to environmental contaminants. The majority of these substances readily cross the placenta, thus exposing the fetus to a large number of xenobiotic agents. The knowledge regarding the effects of prenatal exposure to drugs, environmental pollutants (e.g., smoking), and other xenobiotics (e.g., ethanol) on the fetus has led to a decrease in the exposure to these substances during pregnancy. The human fetus is at special risk from these substances because of the presence of the CYP450 monooxygenase system, which is capable of metabolizing xenobiotics during the first part of gestation. Placentas of tobacco smokers have shown a significant increase in the rate of placental CYP450 monooxygenase activity (CYP1A subfamily). Concern for this type of enzyme activity is increasing, because this enzyme system is known to catalyze the formation of reactive metabolites capable of covalently binding to macromolecules producing permanent effects (e.g., teratogenic, hepatotoxic, or carcinogenic) in the fetus and newborn. A more disturbing fact is that the other conjugation enzymes (i.e., glucuronosyl transferases, epoxide hydrase, glutathione transferase, and sulfotransferase), which are important for the formation of Phase 2 conjugates of these reactive metabolites, are found in low to negligible levels, increasing the exposure of the fetus to these potentially toxic metabolites.

Fetal drug metabolism functions either as a protective mechanism against environmental xenobiotics to transform active molecules into inactive molecules or as a toxifying system when transforming innocuous substances into reactive molecules. The placenta is not a barrier protecting the fetus from xenobiotics; almost every drug present in the maternal circulation will cross the placenta and reach the fetus. For some drugs, however, the placental efflux transport protein, P-glycoprotein (P-gp; discussed later), functions as a maternofetal barrier, pumping drugs and P-gp substrates out of the fetal circulation back into the maternal circulation (72) and protecting the fetus from exposure to potentially harmful teratogenic xenobiotics/drugs and endogenous substances that have been absorbed through the placenta. The P-gp inhibitors should be carefully evaluated for their potential to increase fetal susceptibility to drug/chemical-induced teratogenesis. On the other hand, selective inhibition of P-gp could be used clinically to improve pharmacotherapy of the unborn child. Depending on the pharmacological activity of the parent substance or its metabolites, both fetal and adult maternal drug metabolism may be viewed as complimentary yet contradictory. Because metabolites generally are more water soluble than the parent substance, drug metabolites, when formed in the fetus, may be trapped and accumulate on the fetal side of the placenta. Such accumulation can result in drug-induced toxicities or developmental defects. The difference between fetal and adult metabolism, however, can be used advantageously and constitutes the rational for transplacental therapy (e.g., the administration of betamethasone several days before delivery can increase the production of surfactant in the fetal lung and prevent respiratory distress syndrome in the neonate).

The activity of CYP3A isoenzymes in the human fetal liver is similar to that seen in adult liver microsomes. The fetal activity for CYP3A7 isoenzyme is unusual as most other fetal isoenzymes of CYP450 exhibit 5 to 40% of the adult isoenzymes. Fetal and neonatal drug-metabolizing enzyme activities may differ from those in the adult.

Neonatal Metabolism

From the day of birth, the neonate is exposed to drugs and other foreign compounds persisting from pregnancy as well as those transferred via breast milk. Fortunately, many of the drug-metabolizing enzymes operative in the neonate developed during the fetal period. The routine use of therapeutic agents during labor and delivery, as well as during pregnancy, is widespread, and consideration must be given to the fact that potentially harmful metabolites can be generated by the fetus and newborn. Consequently, the use of drugs capable of forming reactive metabolic intermediates should be avoided during pregnancy, delivery, and the neonatal period. The activity of Phase 1 and Phase 2 drug-metabolizing enzymes is high at birth but decreases to normal levels with increasing age. Evidence suggests increased activity of drug-metabolizing enzymes in liver microsomes of neonates resulting from treatment of the mother during the pregnancy with enzyme inducers (e.g., phenobarbital).

GENETIC POLYMORPHISM

The reality of drug therapy is that many drugs do not work in all patients. By current estimates, the percentage of patients who will react favorably to a specific drug ranges from 20 to 80%. Drugs have been developed and dosage regimens prescribed under the old paradigm that "one dose fits all," which largely ignores the fact that humans are genetically different, resulting in interindividual differences in drug metabolism and disposition (10). It is widely accepted that genetic factors have an important impact on the oxidative metabolism and pharmacokinetics of drugs. Genotype–phenotype correlation studies (pharmacogenetics) have shown that inherited mutations in CYP450 genes (alleles) result in distinct phenotypic subgroups. For example, mutations in the *CYP2D6* gene result in poor (PM), intermediate (or extensive [EM]), and ultrarapid (UM) metabolizers of CYP2D6 substrates (73) (Table 10.7). Each of these phenotypic subgroups experience different responses to drugs extensively metabolized by the CYP2D6 pathway, ranging from severe toxicity to complete lack of efficacy. Genetic studies confirm that "one dose does not fit all," leaving the question of why we would continue to develop and prescribe drugs under the old paradigm. As early as 1997, the U.S. Food and Drug Administration (FDA) recognized that identifying genetic polymorphisms might allow the safe dosing, marketing, and approval of drugs that would otherwise not be approved and advised pharmaceutical companies to incorporate the knowledge of genetic polymorphisms into drug development (see sidebar below). Importantly, pharmacogenomic testing (the study of heritable traits affecting patient response to drug treatment) can significantly increase the likelihood of developing drug regimens that benefit most patients without severe adverse events.

> **U.S. FDA Advisory on Genetic Polymorphism**
>
> "When a genetic polymorphism affects an important metabolic route of elimination, large dosing adjustments may be necessary to achieve the safe and effective use of the drug... indeed in some cases understanding how to adjust the dose to avoid toxicity may allow the marketing of a drug that would have an unacceptable level of toxicity were its toxicity unpredictable and unpreventable."
>
> —U.S. FDA, *Guidance of Industry, Drug Metabolism/Drug Interaction Studies in the Drug Development Process: Studies in Vitro,* April 1997.

Polymorphisms are expressed for a number of metabolizing enzymes, but the polymorphic CYP450 isoforms that are most important for drug metabolism include CYP2A6, CYP2C9, CYP2C19, and CYP2D6. These polymorphic isoforms give rise to phenotypic subgroups in the population differing in their ability to perform clinically significant biotransformation reactions with obvious clinical ramifications (74). Metabolic polymorphism may have several consequences; for example, when enzymes that metabolize drugs used either therapeutically or socially are deficient, adverse or toxic drug reactions may occur in these individuals. The discovery of genetic polymorphism resulted from the observation of increased frequency of adverse effects or no drug effects after normal doses of drugs to some patients (e.g., hyper–central nervous system response from the administration of the antihistamine doxylamine or no analgesic response with codeine). A polymorphism is a difference in DNA sequence found at 1% or greater in a population and expressed as an amino acid substitution in the protein sequence of an enzyme resulting in changes in its rate of activity (V_{max}) or affinity (K_m). Thus, mutant DNA sequences can lead to interindividual differences in drug metabolism. Furthermore, the polymorphisms do not occur with equivalent frequency in all racial or ethnic groups. Because of these differences, it is important to be aware of a person's race and ethnicity

Table 10.14. Impact of Human CYP450 Polymorphisms on Drug Treatment in Poor Metabolizers

Polymorphic Enzyme	Decreased Clearance	Adverse Effects (overdosage)	Reduced Activation of Prodrug
CYP2C9	*S*-Warfarin	Bleeding	Losartan
	Phenytoin	Ataxia	
	Losartan		
	Tolbutamide	Hypoglycemia	
	NSAIDs	GI bleeding?	
CYP2C19	Omeprazole		Proguanil
	Diazepam	Sedation	
CYP2D6	TC antidepressants	Cardiotoxicity	Tramadol
	SSRIs	Serotonin syndrome	Codeine
	Anti-arrythmic drugs	Arrythmias	Ethylmorphine
	Perhexiline	Neuropathy	
	Haloperidol	Parkinsonism?	
	Perphenazine		
	Zuclopenthixol		
	S-Mianserin		
	Tolterodine		
CYP2A6	Nicotine		

when giving drugs that are metabolized differently by different populations (73,75). Because no other way exists to adequately clear these drugs from the body, PMs may be at greater risk for adverse drug reactions or toxic overdoses. The signs and symptoms of these overdoses are primarily extensions of the drug's common adverse effects or pharmacological effects (Table 10.14) (75). The level of adverse reactions or overdosage depends very much on the overall contribution of the mutant isoform to the drug's metabolism. Perhaps the most interesting explanation for the various mutant isoforms is that they evolved as protective mechanisms against alkaloids and other common substances in the food chain for the different ethnicities. Although much effort has gone into finding polymorphisms of CY*P3A4* and *CYP1A2* genes, none has yet to be discovered.

Occasionally, one derives benefit from an unusual CYP phenotype. For example, cure rates for peptic ulcer treated with omeprazole are substantially greater in individuals with defective CYP2C19 because of the sustained high plasma levels achieved.

CYP2C9 and CYP2C19

The CYP2C9 and CYP2C19 are the main isoforms for the metabolism of the antiseizure drug phenytoin and for the anticoagulant S-warfarin. Although CYP2C19 metabolizes fewer drugs than CYP2D6 does, the drugs CYP2C19 does metabolize are clinically important (Table 10.6). Deficit of CYP2C19 is found in the PM phenotype, which is only seen in 8 to 13% of Caucasians, 20 to 30% of the Asian population (11–23% of Japanese and 5–37% of Chinese), up to 20% of the black African-American population, 14 to 15% of Saudi Arabians and Ethiopians, and up to 70% of Pacific Islanders (73,75). The more common mutant allele in these individuals is *CYP2C19*2,* which expresses an inactive enzyme. The large interindividual variability observed in the therapeutic response to the antiseizure drug mephenytoin is attributed to CYP2C19 polymorphism, which catalyzes the *p*-hydroxylation of its S-stereoisomer (74). The R-enantiomer is N-demethylated by CYP2C8 with no difference in its metabolism between PMs and EMs.

The CYP2C9 is the primary isoform for the metabolism of the antiseizure drug phenytoin, the anticoagulant S-warfarin, and the hypoglycemic drug tolbutamide. Other clinically important drugs are listed in Table 10.6. At least six different mutant *CYP2C9* alleles have been identified; of these, the two alleles primarily responsible for CYP2C9 deficiency are *CYP2C9*2* and *CYP2C9*3* and code for enzymes with reduced affinity for substrates (73,75). A deficiency of this isoform, however, is seen in 8 to 13% of Caucasians, 2 to 3% of African Americans, and 1% of the Asians. Individuals with the PM phenotype who possess this deficient isoform variant are ineffective in clearing S-warfarin (so much so that they may be fully anticoagulated on just 0.5 mg of warfarin per day) and in the clearance of phenytoin, which has a potentially very toxic narrow therapeutic range. On the other hand, the pro-drug losartan will be poorly activated and ineffective.

CYP2D6

The CYP2D6 is of particular importance, because it metabolizes a wide range of commonly prescribed drugs, including antidepressants, antipsychotics, β-adrenergic blockers, and antiarrhythmics (Table 10.7). The CYP2D6 deficiency is a clinically important genetic variation of drug metabolism characterized by three phenotypes: UM, EM and PM. The PM phenotype is inherited as an autosomal recessive trait, with 5 of 30 of the known *CYP2D6* gene mutations leading to either zero expression or the expression of a nonfunctional enzyme (73). Approximately 12 to 20% of Caucasians express the *CYP2D6*4* allele, and 5% express the other *CYP2D6* alleles. Up to 34% of African Americans express the *CYP2D6*17* allele, and 5% express the other *CYP2D6* alleles. Up to 50% of Chinese express the *CYP2D6*10* allele, and 5% express the other *CYP2D6* alleles (these individuals are referred to as PM) (73,75). Conversely, the 20 to 30% of Saudi Arabians and Ethiopians who express the *CYP2D6*2XN* allele are known as UMs of CYP2D6 substrates, because they express excess enzyme as a result of having multicopies of the gene (73). Inasmuch as CYP2D6 is not inducible, individuals of Ethiopian and Saudi Arabian descent have genetically developed a different strategy to cope with the (presumed) high load of alkaloids and other substances in their diet; thus, the high expression of CYP2D6 using multiple copies of the gene. Those individuals who are deficient in CYP2D6 will be predisposed to adverse effects or drug toxicity from antidepressants or neuroleptics caused by inadequate metabolism or long half-lives, but the metabolism of pro-drugs in these patients will be ineffective because of lack of activation (e.g., codeine, which must be metabolized by O-demethylation to morphine). Those with the UM phenotype will require a dose that is much higher than normal to attain therapeutic drug plasma concentrations (e.g., one patient required a daily dose of ~300 mg of nortryptyline to achieve therapeutic plasma levels) or a lower dose for pro-drugs that require metabolic activation. Individuals with the PM phenotype also are characterized by loss of CYP2D6 stereoselectivity in hydroxylation reactions. It can be anticipated that large differences in steady-state concentration for CYP2D6 substrates will occur between individuals with the different phenotypes when they receive the same dose. Depending on the drug and reaction type, a 10- to 30-fold difference in blood concentrations may be observed in the PM-phenotype debrisoquine polymorphism (76).

CYP2A6

The CYP2A6 is of particular importance, because it activates a number of procarcinogens to carcinogens and is the major isoform metabolizing nicotine to cotinine. Approximately 15% of Asians express the *CYP2A6*4del* allele, and 2% of Caucasians express the other *CYP2AD6*2* allele. Both these alleles express zero or a nonfunctional enzyme; these individuals are referred to as having the PM phenotype (73,75). A benefit from being a PM of CYP2A6 substrates might be the protection from some carcinogens and smoking because of the high plasma levels of nicotine achieved with fewer cigarettes.

Acetylation

Acetylation, a nonmicrosomal form of metabolism, also exhibits polymorphisms and was first demonstrated in the acetylation of isoniazid (see the section on acetylation). Several forms of acetyl transferase occur in humans. Some clinically used drugs undergoing polymorphic acetylation include isoniazid, procainamide, hydralazine, phenelzine, dapsone, caffeine, some benzodiazepines, and possibly, the carcinogenic secondary N-alkylarylamines (2-aminofluorene, benzidine, and 4-aminobiphenyl). Intestinal acetyl transferase appears not to be polymorphic (i.e., 5-aminosalicylic acid). The proportion of the fast acetylation phenotype is approximately 30 to 45% in Caucausians, 89 to 90% in the Oriental population, and 100% in Canadian Eskimos. Drug-induced systemic lupus erythematosus from chronic procainamide therapy is more likely to appear with slow acetylators.

Other Polymorphic Metabolizing Enzymes

The polymorphism for CYP2E1 is expressed more in Chinese than in Caucasians. Those with the CYP2E1 PM phenotype exhibit tolerance to alcohol and less toxicity from halohydrocarbon solvents.

The only FMO pathway exhibiting polymorphism is the genetic disease trimethylaminuria, in which individuals excrete diet-derived free trimethylamine in the urine. Usually, trimethylamine undergoes extensive FMO N-oxidation.

In human populations, serum PON1 exhibits a substrate-dependent polymorphism to the neurotoxic effects of organophosphates in those susceptible individuals that are deficient in PON1 (i.e., PM phenotype) (55). The PON1 catalyzes the hydrolysis of paraoxon, chlorpyrifos (Dursban), and other organophosphates.

Polymorphism has been associated with serum cholinesterases (particularly succinyl cholinesterase, causing skeletal muscle paralysis), alcohol dehydrogenases, aldehyde dehydrogenases, epoxide hydrolase, and xanthine oxidase (74). Approximately 50% of the Oriental population lack aldehyde dehydrogenase, resulting in high levels of acetaldehyde following ethanol ingestion and causing nausea and flushing. People with genetic variants of cholinesterase respond abnormally to succinylcholine, procaine, and other related choline esters. The clinical consequence of reduced enzymic activity of cholinesterase is that succinylcholine and procaine are not hydrolyzed in the blood, resulting in prolongation of their respective pharmacological activities.

A suggestion has been made that those with EM phenotypes may be more prone than those with PM phenotypes to develop cancers, because they are better able to activate procarcinogens. Such interindividual variations may have a major influence in determining the risk of cancer. The activity of a particular CYP450 isoform may be a rationale for predicting the individual risk from exposure to carcinogenic compounds.

Our increasing knowledge of genetic polymorphism has contributed a great deal to our understanding about interindividual variation in the metabolism of drugs, including how to change dose regimens accordingly to minimize drug toxicity and improve therapeutic efficacy. In humans, drugs not subject to polymorphic metabolism also exhibit substantial interindividual variation in their disposition, which is attributed to a great extent to environmental factors (e.g., inducing agents, smoking, and alcohol ingestion).

ORAL BIOAVAILABILITY

Oral bioavailability (see Chapter 9) is the fraction of the total dose of a drug that reaches the systemic circulation. The low oral bioavailability for a drug may be the result of disintegration and dissolution properties of the drug formulation, solubility of the drug molecule in the gastrointestinal environment, membrane permeability, presystemic intestinal metabolism, hepatic first-pass metabolism, or susceptibility to membrane transporters, such as P-gp efflux. Other routes of administration (e.g., subcutaneous, intravenous, inhalation, and nasal) for susceptible drugs have been investigated in an attempt to overcome the pronounced presystemic metabolism. The extent of first-pass metabolism depends on the drug delivery system, because a formulation may increase or decrease the rate of dissolution, the residence time of a drug in the gastrointestinal tract, and the dose. The more prolonged the residence time, the greater the efficiency of first-pass metabolism. The drug form and delivery system should yield optimal bioavailability and pharmacokinetic profiles, resulting in a reproducible clinical response.

Studies are being performed to determine the effect of presystemic and hepatic first-pass metabolism on the toxicity and carcinogenicity of xenobiotics. For a nontherapeutic toxic substance, the existence of a first-pass effect is desirable, because the liver can bioinactivate it, preventing its distribution to other parts of the body. On the other hand, first-pass metabolism may increase its toxicity by biotransforming the toxicant to a more toxic metabolite, which can reenter the blood and exert its toxic effect.

Presystemic First Pass Metabolism

Although hepatic metabolism continues to be the most important route of metabolism for xenobiotics, the ability of the liver and intestine to metabolize substances to either pharmacologically inactive or bioactive metabolites before reaching systemic blood levels is called prehepatic or presystemic first pass metabolism, which results in the low systemic availability for susceptible drugs. Sulfation and glucuronidation are major pathways of presystemic intestinal first-pass metabolism in humans for acetaminophen, phenylephrine, terbutaline, albuterol, fenoterol, and isoproterenol.

The discovery that CYP3A4 is found in the mucosal enterocytes of the intestinal villi signifies its role as key determinant in the oral bioavailability of its numerous drug substrates (Table 10.9) (77). Drugs known to be substrates for CYP3A usually have a low and variable oral bioavailability that may be explained by presystemic first-pass metabolism by the small intestine CYP450 isoforms. The concentration of functional intestinal CYP3A is influenced by genetic disposition, induction, and inhibition, which to a great extent determines drug blood levels and therapeutic response. Xenobiotics when ingested orally can modify the activity of intestinal CYP3A enzymes by induction, inhibition, and stimulation. By modulation of the isoform pattern in the intestine, a xenobiotic could alter its own metabolism and that of others in a time- and dose-dependent manner. Its concentration in the intestine is comparable to that of the liver. The oral administration of dexamethasone induces the formation of CYP3A and erythromycin inhibits it. The glucocorticoid inducibility of CYP3A4 also may be a factor in differences of metabolism between males and females. Studies have suggested that intestinal CYP3A4 C-2 hydroxylation of estradiol contributed to the oxidative metabolism of endogenous estrogens circulating with the enterohepatic recycling pool (38). Norethisterone has a low oral bioavailability of 42% because of oxidative first-pass metabolism (CYP3A), but levonorgestrel is completely available in women with no conjugated metabolites.

Several clinically relevant drug interactions between orally coadministered drugs and CYP3A4 can be explained by a modification of drug metabolism at the CYP450 level. If a drug has high presystemic elimination (low bioavailability) and is metabolized primarily by CYP3A4, then coadministration with a CYP3A4 inhibitor can be expected to alter the drug's pharmacokinetics by reducing its metabolism, thus increasing its plasma concentration. Drugs and some foods (e.g., grapefruit juice) that are known inhibitors, inducers, or substrates for intestinal CYP3A4 can potentially interact with the metabolism of a coadministered drug, affecting its area under the curve and rate of clearance (Tables 10.10 and 10.12) (78). Inducers can reduce absorption and oral bioavailability, whereas these same factors are increased by inhibitors. For example, erythromycin can enhance the oral absorption of another drug by inhibiting its metabolism in the small intestine by CYP3A4. By virtue of being competitive substrates for CYP3A4, prednisone, prednisolone, and methylprednisolone (but not dexamethasone) are competitive inhibitors of synthetic glucocorticoid metabolism. This is because a major metabolic pathway for synthetic glucocorticoids involves CYP3A4. In addition to coadministered drugs, metabolic interactions with exogenous CYP3A4 substrates secreted in the bile are possible. The poor oral bioavailability for cyclosporine is attributed to a combination of intestinal metabolism by CYP3A4 and efflux by P-gp (79).

Because the intestinal mucosa is enriched with glucuronosyltransferases, sulfotransferases, and glutathione transferases, presystemic first-pass metabolism for orally administered drugs susceptible to these conjugation reactions results in their low oral bioavailability (65). Presystemic metabolism often exceeds liver metabolism for some drugs. For example, more than 80% of intravenously administered albuterol is excreted unchanged in urine, with the balance as glucuronide conjugates, whereas when albuterol is administered orally, less than 5% is systemically absorbed because of intestinal sulfation and glucuronidation. Presystemic metabolism is a major pathway in humans for most β-adrenergic agonists, such as glucuronides or sulfates for terbutaline, fenoterol, albuterol, and isoproterenol, morphine (3–O-glucuronide), acetaminophen (O-sulfate), and estradiol (3–O-sulfate). The bioavailability of orally administered estradiol or ethinyl estradiol in females is approximately 50%. Mestranol (3-methoxyethinyl estradiol) has greater bioavailability, however, because it is not significantly conjugated. Levodopa has a low oral bioavailability because of its metabolism by intestinal L-aromatic amino acid decarboxylase. The activity of this enzyme depends on the percentage bound of its cofactor pyridoxine (vitamin B_6). Tyramine, which occurs in fermented foods such as cheeses and red wines, ripe bananas, and yeast extracts, is metabolized by both MAO-A and MAO-B in the gut wall.

The extensive presystemic first-pass sulfation of phenolic drugs, for example, can lead to increased bioavailability of other drugs by competing for the available sulfate pool, resulting in the possibility of drug toxicity (56). Concurrent oral administration of acetaminophen with ethinyl estradiol resulted in a 48% increase in ethinyl estradiol blood levels. Ascorbic acid, which is sulfated, also increases the bioavailability of concurrently administered ethinyl estradiol. Sulfation and glucuronidation occur side by side, often competing for the same substrate, and the balance between sulfation and glucuronidation is influenced by several factors, such as species, doses, availability of cosubstrates, inhibition, and induction of the respective transferases.

First-Pass Metabolism

Several orally administered drugs are known to undergo liver first-pass metabolism during their transport to the systemic circulation from the gastrointestinal tract (e.g., metoprolol). Thus, the liver can remove substances from the blood after their absorption from the gastrointestinal tract, thereby preventing distribution to other parts of the body. This effect can seriously impair the bioavailability of an orally administered drug, reducing the amount of the drug that reaches the systemic circulation and, ultimately, its receptor to produce its pharmacological effect. Drugs subject to first-pass metabolism are included in Table 10.15.

Table 10.15. Examples of Drugs Exhibiting First-Pass Metabolism

Acetaminophen	Isoproterenol	Oxprenolol
Albuterol	Lidocaine	Pentazocine
Alprenolol	Meperidine	Propoxyphene
Aspirin	Methyltestosterone	Propranolol
Cyclosporin	Metoprolol	Salicylamide
Desmethylimipramine	Dihydropyridines (Nifedipine)	Terbutaline
Fluorouracil		Verapamil
Hydrocortisone	Nortriptyline	
Imipramine	Organic nitrates	

P-Glycoprotein

Description of P-Glycoprotein

P-glycoprotein is a transmembrane ATP-dependent active transport protein that is strategically expressed in the luminal endothelial cells of organs associated with lipophilic xenobiotic absorption and distribution. For example, in the intestinal mucosa, P-gp functions to move xenobiotics into the intestine to block their absorption into the portal circulation; in the endothelial cells of the brain, as a blood-brain barrier to move substances out of the brain into systemic circulation; and in the endothelial cells of the renal proximal tubules of the kidney and in the canicular membranes of hepatocytes, to increase xenobiotic elimination into the urine and bile, respectively (81). Additionally, P-gp is expressed in the endothelial cells of the adrenal cortex and medulla, of the testis and ovaries, of the peripheral nerves (functions as a blood-nerve barrier), and of the pancreas; in the epithelial cells of the placenta, where it serves as the maternofetal barrier for the fetus; and in the stem cells of the bone marrow. The particular localization of P-gp suggests that this transmembrane transporter protein probably evolved as a protective mechanism against the absorption of xenobiotics to increase their transport out of these organs and tissues. It appears that the substrates, inhibitors, or inducers are nonselective for various P-gps. P-glycoprotein should exhibit saturation/nonlinear kinetics; at or near saturation concentrations, an increase in drug absorption can result in a two- to threefold increase in plasma drug concentration. Activity of P-gp is controlled by a variety of endogenous and environmental stimuli that evoke stress responses, including cytotoxic agents, heat shock, irradiation, genotoxic stress, inflammation, inflammatory mediators, cytokines, and growth factors.

Another factor that must be considered in the oral bioavailability of many CYP3A4 substrates is intestinal P-gp (80). Originally discovered as a transmembrane transporter protein associated with the resistance (elimination) of anticancer drugs, P-gp also can play a role in how a drug is absorbed, distributed, metabolized, and eliminated from the body (79,80). Considering its role as a transporter protein (efflux pump), it is logical that it should exhibit saturable (nonlinear) kinetics. P-glycoprotein exhibits a broad specificity for a large number of substrates, inhibitors, and inducers (Table 10.16). The common link between P-gp substrates is that most of the same compounds also are substrates for CYP3A4. The close physical location of P-gp and CYP3A4 in the endothelial cells of the intestinal mucosa allows these proteins to work in concert with each other to decrease drug plasma concentrations of CYP3A4 substrates, suggesting a complementary protective mechanism for these two proteins, forming a barrier to the absorption intestinal of CYP3A4 substrates. Hepatic and renal P-gp also appear to function in a complementary manner, promoting the elimination of substrates into the bile and urine, respectively. For example, if a drug is a substrate for intestinal P-gp, its oral absorption will be

Table 10.16. Some Substrates, Inhibitors, and Inducers for P-Glycoprotein

Substrate		**Inhibitors**		**Foods**
Acetolol	Lidocaine*	Amiodarone*	Lovastatin*	Daidzein
Amiodarone*	Loperamide*	Amitriptyline*	Maprotiline	Genistein
Atorvastatin*	Methotrexate	Astemizole*	Mefloquine*	Grapefruit juice*
Celiprolol	Mibefradil	Atorastatin*	Mibefradil*	Orange juice
Cimetidine*	Nadolol	Carvedilol	Midazolam*	Isoflavones
Ciprofloxacin	Nelfinavir*	Chlorpromazine*	Mifepristone*	
Colchicine	Nicardipine*	Clarithromycin*	Nelfinavir*	**Inducers**
Cyclosporin*	Ondansetron*	Cyclosporin*	Nicardipine*	Dexamethasone*
Daunorubicin*	Paclitaxel*	Desipramine	Nifedipine*	Prazosin
Debrisoquine	Pravastatin*	Dexverapamil*	Nitrendipine*	Progesterone*
Dexamethasone*	Quinidine*	Diltiazem*	Ofloxacin	Quercetin
DHEA	Quinolones	Dipyridamole	Prochlorperzine	Rifampin
Digoxin*	Ranitidine	Disulfiram	Progesterone*	St. John's Wort*
Diltiazem*	Rifampin*	Doxepin	Propanolol	
Docetaxel*	Ritonavir*	Erythromycin*	Propafenone*	
Domperidone*	Saquinaivr*	Flupenthixol	Quinidine*	
Doxorubicin*	Tacrolilmus*	Felodipine*	Quinine*	
Enoxacin	Taxol*	Fluphenazine	Reserpine	
Erthromycin*	Teniposide*	Glibenclamide	Rifampin*	
Estradiol*	Terfenadine*	Haloperidol*	Ritonavir*	
Etoposide*	Timolol	Hydrocortisone*	Saquinavir*	
Fexofenadine*	Verapamil*	Imipramine*	Tacrolimus*	
Hydrocortisone*	Vinblastine*	Itraconazole*	Testosterone*	
Idarubicin	Vincristine *	Ivermectin	Tamoxifen*	
Indinavir*	Vindesine*	Ketoconazole*	Trimipramine	
Ivermectin		Lidocaine*	Verapamil*	

*CYP3A4 substrate, inhibitor or inducer.

incomplete, and this same drug will be actively transported by the renal tubules into the urine, enhancing its elimination. On the other hand, inhibiting P-gp would be expected to improve the oral bioavailability of P-gp substrates, but if the inhibitor also is a substrate for CYP3A4, increased metabolism (presystemic) would occur. Drugs with low oral bioavailability or high first-pass metabolism may be particularly susceptible to alterations in the transport kinetics of P-gp. Because P-gp exhibits saturation (nonlinear) kinetics, drugs with low dosages can have their oral bioavailability enhanced by increasing its oral dosage, thus saturating the P-gp pump. As with CYP3A4, there is significant interindividual variation (4- to 10-fold) in the intestinal expression of P-gp, which could explain the variance observed in the pharmacokinetics for CYP3A4 substrates. The interactive nature of CYP3A4 and P-gp will be of importance in controlling and improving the oral bioavailability of CYP3A4 substrates and drug regimens. The presence of inhibitors of P-gp in grapefruit juice (e.g., 6,7-dihydroxybergamottin and other furanocoumarins) has confirmed that the inhibition of efflux transport of drugs and of drug metabolism by CYP3A4 could be an important cause of drug–grapefruit juice interaction (82).

In summary, oral bioavailability for xenobiotics is dependent on a combination of factors, including physical properties of the drugs and formulation and biological factors such as metabolizing enzymes, membrane permeability, and the membrane efflux pump, P-gp.

EXTRAHEPATIC METABOLISM

Because the liver is the primary tissue for xenobiotic metabolism, it is not surprising that our understanding of mammalian CYP450 monooxygenase is based chiefly on hepatic studies. Although the tissue content of CYP450s is highest in the liver, CYP450 enzymes are ubiquitous, and their role in extrahepatic tissues remains unclear. The CYP450 pattern in these tissues differs considerably from that in the human liver (83). In addition to liver tissue, CYP450 enzymes are found in lung, nasal epithelium, intestinal tract, kidney and adrenal tissues, and brain. It is possible that the expression of the polymorphic genes and induction of the isoforms in the extrahepatic tissues may affect the activity of the CYP450 isoforms in the metabolism of drugs, endogenous steroids, and xenobiotics. Therefore, characterization of CYP450, UGT, SULT, and other polymorphic drug-metabolizing enzymes in extrahepatic tissues is important to our overall understanding about the biological importance of these isoform families to improved drug therapy, design of new drugs and dosages forms, toxicity, and carcinogenicity.

The mucosal surfaces of the gastrointestinal tract, the nasal passages, and the lungs are major portals of entry for xenobiotics into the body and, as such, are continuously exposed to a variety of orally ingested or inhaled airborne xenobiotics, including drugs, plant toxins, environmental pollutants, and other chemical substances. As a consequence of this exposure, these tissues represent a major target for necrosis, tumorigenesis, and other chemically induced toxicities. Many of these toxins and chemical carcinogens are relatively inert substances that must be bioactivated to exert their cytotoxicity and tumorigenicity. The epithelial cells of these tissues are capable of metabolizing a wide variety of exogenous and endogenous substances, and these cells provide the principal and initial source of biotransformation for these xenobiotics during the absorptive phase. The consequences of such presystemic biotransformation is either a decrease in the amount of xenobiotics available for systemic absorption by facilitating the elimination of polar metabolites or toxification by activation to carcinogens, which may be one determinant of tissue susceptibility for the development of intestinal cancer. The risk of colon cancer may depend on dietary constituents that contain either procarcinogens or compounds modulating the response to carcinogens.

Intestinal Metabolism

Mounting evidence shows that many of the clinically relevant aspects of CYP450 may, in fact, occur at the level of the intestinal mucosa and could account for differences among patients in dosing requirements. The intestinal mucosa is enriched especially with CYP3A4 isoform, glucuronosyl transferases, sulfotransferases, and GSTs, making it particularly important for orally administered drugs susceptible to oxidation (77), glucuronidation or sulfation conjugation pathways (56), or glutathione conjugation pathways. The highest concentrations of CYP450s occur in the duodenum, with gradual tapering into the ileum. In the human intestine, CYP2E, CYP3A, CYP2C8, CYP2C9, CYP2C19, and CYP2D6 have been identified. Therefore, intestinal CYP450 isoforms provide potential presystemic first-pass metabolism of ingested xenobiotics affecting their oral bioavailability (e.g., hydroxylation of naloxone) or bioactivation of carcinogens or mutagens. It is not surprising that dietary factors can affect the intestinal CYP450 isoforms. For example, a two-day dietary exposure to cooked Brussel sprouts significantly decreased the 2α-hydroxylation of testosterone yet induced CYP1A2 activity for PAH. An 8-oz. glass of grapefruit juice inhibited the sulfoxidation metabolism of omeprazole (CYP3A4) but not its hydroxylation (CYP2C19), thus increasing its systemic blood concentration. These types of interactions between a drug and a dietary inhibitor could result in a clinically significant drug interaction.

In the intestine, UGT isoforms can glucuronidate orally administered drugs, such as morphine, acetaminophen, α- and β-adrenergic agonists and other phenolic phenethanolamines, and other dietary xenobiotics. This is a result of reduction in their oral bioavailability (increasing first-pass metabolism), thus altering their pharmacokinetics and pharmacodynamics. The UGTs expressed in the intestine include UGT1A1 (bilirubin-glucuronidating isoform), UGT1A3, UGT1A4, UGT1A6, UGT1A8, UGT1A9, and UGT1A10. Substrate specificities of intestinal UGT isoforms are comparable to those in the liver. Glucuronidase hydrolysis of biliary glucuronide conjugates in the intestine can contribute to EHC of the parent drug.

Likewise, the sulfotransferases in the small intestine can sulfate orally administered drugs and xenobiotics for which the primary route of conjugation is sulfation (e.g., isoproterenol, albuterol, steroid hormones, α-methyldopa, acetaminophen, and fenoldopam), decreasing their oral bioavailability and, thus, altering their pharmacokinetics and pharmacodynamics. Competition for intestinal sulfation between coadministered substrates may influence their bioavailability with either an enhancement or a decrease of therapeutic effects. Sulfatase hydrolysis of biliary sulfate conjugates in the intestine can contribute to EHC of the parent drug.

The occurrence of intestinal CYP450 enzymes and bacterial enzymes in the microflora allows the metabolism of relatively stable environmental pollutants and food-derived xenobiotics (i.e., plants contain a variety of protoxins, promutagens, and procarcinogens) into mutagens and carcinogens (68). For example, cruciferous vegetables (Brussel sprouts, cabbage, broccoli, cauliflower, and spinach) are all rich in indole compounds (e.g., indole 3-carbinol), which with regular and chronic ingestion are capable of inducing some intestinal CYP450s (CYP1A subfamily) and inhibiting others (CYP3A subfamily). It is likely that these vegetables also would alter the metabolism of food-derived mutagens (e.g., heterocyclic amines produced during charbroiling of meat are CYP450 N-hydroxylated and become carcinogenic in a manner similar to arylamines) and carcinogens.

The extent of a drug's metabolism in the small bowel and its role in clinically relevant drug interaction remain to be evaluated and must be taken into account during oral pharmacokinetics analysis of future drug interaction studies. Clinically significant interaction will not always occur when a drug is combined with other isoform subfamily substrates. Oral coadministration of a drug with drugs that interact with its metabolism need not be avoided. The blood concentration of the drug must be monitored closely, however, and the dose should be adapted to avoid adverse drug reactions.

Intestinal Microflora

When drugs are orally ingested or there is considerable biliary excretion of a drug or its metabolites into the gastrointestinal tract, such as with a parentally administered drug (EHC or recirculation), the intestinal bacterial microflora can have a role in the metabolism of these drugs. The microflora plays an important role in the enterohepatic recirculation of xenobiotics via their conjugated metabolites (e.g., digoxin, the oral contraceptives norethisterone and ethinyl estradiol, and chloramphenicol) and endogenous substances (steroid hormones, bile acids, folic acid, and cholesterol), which reenter the gut via the bile (68). Compounds eliminated in the bile are conjugated with glucuronic acid, glycine, sulfate, and glutathione, and once secreted into the small intestine, the bacterial β-glucuronidase, sulfatase, nitroreductases, and various glycosidases catalyze the hydrolysis of the conjugates. The activity of orally administered conjugated estrogens (e.g., Premarin) involves the hydrolysis of the sulfate conjugates by sulfatases, releasing estrogens to be reabsorbed from the intestine into the portal circulation. The clinical use of oral antibiotics (e.g., erythromycin, penicillin, clindamycin, and aminoglycosides) has a profound effect on the gut microflora and the enzymes responsible for the hydrolysis of drug conjugates undergoing EHC. Bacterial reduction includes nitro reduction of nitroimidazole, azo reduction of azides (sulfasalazine to 5-aminosalicylic acid and sulfapyridine), and reduction of the sulfoxide to its sulfide. The sulfoxide of sulindac is reduced by both gut microflora and hepatic CYP450s. Other ways in which bacterial flora can affect metabolism include the following: 1) production of toxic metabolites, 2) formation of carcinogens from inactive precursors, 3) detoxication, 4) exhibition of species differences in drug metabolism, 5) exhibition of individual differences in drug metabolism, 6) production of pharmacologically active metabolites from inactive precursors, and 7) production of metabolites not formed by animal tissues. In contrast to the predominantly hepatic oxidative and conjugative metabolism of the liver, gut microflora is largely degradative, hydrolytic, and reductive, with a potential for both metabolic activation and detoxication of xenobiotics.

Lung Metabolism

Some of the hepatic xenobiotic biotransformation pathways also are operative in the lung (84,85). Because of the differences in organ sizes, the total content of the pulmonary xenobiotic-metabolizing enzyme systems generally is lower than in the liver, creating the impression of a minor role for the lung in xenobiotic elimination. The CYP2E1 is the CYP450 isoform that is expressed in the lung to the greatest extent. The other CYP450s, FMO, epoxide hydrolase, and the Phase 2 conjugation pathways, however, are comparable to those in the liver. Thus, the lungs may play a significant role in the metabolic elimination or activation of small-molecular-weight inhaled xenobiotics. When drugs are injected intravenously, intramuscularly, or subcutaneously, or after skin absorption, the drug initially enters the pulmonary circulation, after which the lung becomes the organ of first-pass metabolism for the drug. The blood levels and therapeutic response of the drug are influenced by genetic disposition, induction, and inhibition of the pulmonary metabolizing enzymes. By modulation of the CYP450 isoform pattern in the lung, a xenobiotic could alter its own metabolism and that of others in a time- and dose-dependent manner. Because of its position in the circulation, the lung provides a second-pass metabolism for xenobiotics and their metabolites exiting from the liver, but it also is susceptible to the cytotoxicity or carcinogenicity of hepatic activated metabolites. Antihistamines, β-blockers, opioids, and tricyclic antidepressants are among the basic amines known to accumulate in the lungs as a result of their binding to surfactant phospholipids in lung tissue. The significance of this relationship to potential pneumotoxicity remains to be seen.

Nasal Metabolism

The nasal mucosa is recognized as a first line of defense for the lung against airborne xenobiotics, because it is constantly exposed to the external environment (86). Drug metabolism in the nasal mucosa is an important consideration not only in drug delivery but also for toxicological implications because of xenobiotic metabolism of inhaled environmental pollutants or other volatile chemicals. The CYP450 enzymes in the nasal epithelial cells can convert some of the airborne chemicals to reactive metabolites, increasing the risk of carcinogenesis in the nasopharynx and lung (e.g., nitrosamines in cigarette smoke). The most striking feature of the nasal epithelium is that CYP450 catalytic activity is higher than in any other extrahepatic tissue, as well as the liver. Nasal decongestants, essences, anesthetics, alcohols, nicotine, and cocaine have been shown to be metabolized in vitro by CYP450 enzymes from the nasal epithelium. Because the CYP450s in the nasal mucosa are active, first-pass metabolism should be considered when delivering susceptible drugs to the nasal tissues. Flavin monooxygenases, carboxylesterases, aldehyde dehydrogenase, and other conjugation (Phase 2) enzymes also are active in the nasal epithelium.

Metabolism in Other Tissues

The isoforms of CYP450s and their regulation in the brain are of interest in defining the possible involvement of CYP450s in central nervous system toxicity and carcinogenicity. The CYP450s in the kidney and adrenal tissues include isoforms primarily involved in the hydroxylation of steroids, arachidonic acid, and 25-hydroxycholcalciferol.

STEREOCHEMICAL ASPECTS OF DRUG METABOLISM

In addition to the physicochemical factors that affect xenobiotic metabolism, stereochemical factors play an important role in the biotransformation of drugs. This involvement is not unexpected, because the xenobiotic-metabolizing enzymes also are the same enzymes that metabolize certain endogenous substrates, which for the most part are chiral molecules. Most of these enzymes show stereoselectivity but not stereospecificity; in other words, one stereoisomer enters into biotransformation pathways preferentially but not exclusively. Metabolic stereochemical reactions can be categorized as follows: substrate stereoselectivity, in which two enantiomers of a chiral substrate are metabolized at different rates; product stereoselectivity, in which a new chiral center is created in a symmetric molecule and one enantiomer is metabolized preferentially; and substrate-product stereoelectivity, in which a new chiral center of a chiral molecule is metabolized preferentially to one of two possible diastereomers (87). An example of substrate stereoselectivity is the preferred decarboxylation of S-α-methyldopa to S-α-methyldopamine, with almost no reaction for R-α-methyldopa. The reduction of ketones to stereoisomeric alcohols and the hydroxylation of enantiotropic protons or phenyl rings by monooxygenases are examples of product stereoselectivity. For example, phenytoin undergoes aromatic *p*-hydroxylation of only one of its two phenyl rings to create a chiral center at C-5 of the hydantoin ring, methadone is reduced preferentially to its α-diastereometric alcohol, and naltrexone is reduced to its 6-β-alcohol. An example of substrate-product stereoselectivity is the reduction of the enantiomers of warfarin and the β-hydroxylation of S-α-methyldopamine to (1*R*,2*S*)-α-methylnorepinephrine, whereas *R*-α-methyldopamine is hydroxylated only to a negligible extent. In vivo studies of this type often can be confused by the further biotransformation of one stereoisomer, giving the false impression that only one stereoisomer was formed preferentially. Moreover, some compounds show stereoselective absorption, distribution, and excretion, which proves the importance of also performing in vitro studies. Although studies regarding the stereoselective biotransformation of drug molecules are not yet extensive, those that have been done indicate that stereochemical factors play an important role in drug metabolism and, in some cases, could account for the differences in pharmacological activity and duration of action between enantiomers (see the discussion of chiral inversion of the NSAIDs).

METABOLIC BIOACTIVATION: ROLE IN HEPATOTOXICITY, IDIOSYNCRATIC REACTIONS, AND CHEMICAL CARCINOGENESIS

Drug-Induced Hepatotoxicity

Drug-induced hepatotoxicity is the leading cause of hepatic injury, accounting for approximately half of all cases of acute liver failure in the U.S. (88,89). Recent studies have shown that drug-induced hepatotoxicity represents a larger percentage of adverse drug reactions than reported previously and that the incidence and severity of drug-induced liver injury is underestimated among the general population.

Acetaminophen overdose is the leading cause for calls to Poison Control Centers (>100,000 calls/year) and accounts for more than 56,000 emergency room visits, 2,600 hospitalizations, and an estimated 458 deaths from acute liver failure each year. Among the listed drugs in Table 10.17, acetaminophen is the most frequent hepatotoxic agent and can cause extensive hepatic necrosis with as little as 10 to 12 g (30–40 tablets). Chronic alcohol intake enhances acetaminophen hepatotoxicity more than five times as compared to acute alcohol intake, yet acetaminophen is heavily marketed for its safety as compared to nonsteroidal analgesics. U.S. drug manufacturers continue to market and promote Extra-strength acetaminophen products (500–750 mg/tablet) and a variety of Extra-strength acetaminophen-drug combination products. Self-poisoning with acetaminophen (paracetamol) also is a common cause of hepatotoxicity in the Western World. To reduce the number of acetaminophen poisonings in the UK, OTC sales of acetaminophen are limited to 16 tablets per packet.

Drug-induced hepatic damage is also the most frequent reason that new therapeutic agents are not approved by the U.S. FDA (e.g., ximelagatran in 2004) and the most common adverse drug reaction leading to withdrawal of a drug from the market (Table 10.17). Hepatotoxicity almost always involves metabolism with Phase I CYP450 enzymes rather than Phase II enzymes. More than 600 drugs, chemicals, and herbal remedies can cause hepatotoxicity, of which more than 30 drugs have either been withdrawn from the U.S. market

Table 10.17. Some Drugs Causing Hepatic Injury[a]

Acarbose	Meloxicam
Acetaminophen	Methotrexate
Allopurinol	Methsuximide
Amiodarone	Methyldopa
Amprenavir	Nabumetone
Anagrelide	Naproxen
Atomoxetine	*Nefazodone (2005)*
Atorvastatin	**Nevirapine**
Azathioprine	Niacin (SR)
Bicalutamide	Nitrofurantoin
Bosentan	Olanzapine
Bromfenac (1998)	Oxaprozin
Carbamazepine	Peg-interferon-α_{2a}
Celecoxib	*Pemoline (2005)*
Dapsone	Pentamidine
Deferasirox	Pioglitazone
Diclofenac	Piroxicam
Disulfiram	Pravastatin
Duloxetine	**Pyrazinamide**
Efavirenz	Ribavirin
Ethotoin	Rifabutin
Ethosuximide	**Rifampin**
Felbamate	Riluzole
Fenofibrate	Ritonavir
Fluconazole	Rosiglitazone
Flutamide	Rosuvastatin
Fluvastatin	**Saquinavir**
Gemfibrozil	Simvastatin
Gemtuzumab	Sulindac
Griseofulvin	**Tacrine**
Halothane	Tamoxifen
Imatinib	*Tasosartan (1998)*
Indinavir	**Terbinafine**
Infliximab	Testosterone
Interferon-β_{1a}	Thioguanine
Interferon-β_{1b}	Tizanidine
Isoflurane	**Tolcapone**
Isoniazid	*Troglitizone (2000)*
Isotretinoin	**Trovafloxacin**
Itraconazole	**Valproic acid**
Ketoconazole	Voriconazole
Ketorolac	*Ximelagatran (2004)*
Lamivudine	**Zileuton**
Leflunomide	**Zifirlukast**
Lovastatin	

[a]Drugs in italics have exhibited severe drug-induced hepatotoxicity were withdrawn either voluntarily or by a regulatory agency (year given). Drugs in bold have exhibited moderate–severe drug-induced hepatotoxicity requiring a black box warning restricting their use. The other drugs have exhibited mild to moderate drug-induced hepatotoxicity that may need frequent liver transaminase testing for those at risk (see Table 10.18).

because of hepatotoxicity or have carried a black box warning for hepatotoxicity since 1990. Table 10.17 includes some of the more common drugs that have exhibited drug-induced hepatotoxicity ranging from severe, requiring the drug's regulatory withdrawal from the market (italics in Table 10.17); moderate to severe, requiring black box warning restrictions (bold in Table 10.17); or mild to moderate, requiring frequent liver function monitoring.

Some Drugs Exhibiting Drug-induced Hepatotoxicity Never Approved for Use in United States

Drugs with reactive metabolites that were used in other countries but never approved in the United States include: alpidem, amineptine, amodiaquine, cinchophen, dihydralazine, dilevalol, ebrotidine, glafenine, ibufenac, isoxicam, niperotidine, perhexiline, pirprofen, and tilbroquinol.

However, Watkins (90) recently reported in the Journal of the American Medical Association that 1/3 of 106 patients taking a maximum daily acetaminophen dose of 4 grams for 8 days, either alone or in combination with Hydrocodone, exhibited a 3-fold increase in liver enzymes associated with acetaminophen-induced liver injury. This 3-fold increase in transminase levels is a signal for potential liver safety concerns in those individuals who are at risk of acetaminophen-induced liver toxicity. Drug-induced injury is most common and includes hepatic necrosis and steatosis, which can affect significant portions of the liver (88). Drugs reported to cause hepatocellular necrosis include acetaminophen, methyldopa, valproic acid, trazodone, nefazodone, venlafaxine, and lovastatin. Drug-induced liver damage occurs after a prolonged period of drug administration.

The most commonly used indicators of hepatotoxicity (i.e., liver injury) are increased levels of the liver transaminases, aspartate aminotransferase (AST) and alanine aminotransferase (ALT) (88,89). Drug-induced hepatotoxicity can develop rapidly, often before abnormal laboratory tests are noticed, which are characterized by rapid elevations in ALT and AST of 8 to 500 times the upper normal limit, with variable elevations in bilirubin. Drugs causing acute liver injury (hepatocellular necrosis) exhibit elevations in hepatic transaminases ranging from 50 to 100 times higher than the normal level. On the other hand, the elevations of ALT and AST in alcoholic liver disease are two- to three times higher than normal. Some hepatotoxins, however, do not elevate transaminases, whereas nonhepatic toxins can elevate ALT.

Most drug-induced hepatotoxicity is of an idiosyncratic nature, occurring in a small percentage of patients (1 in 5,000) who ingest the drug (88,89). These reactions tend to be of two distinct types: 1) hypersensitivity reactions that are immune mediated, occurring within the first 4 to 6 weeks, and are associated with fever, rash, eosinophilia, and a hepatitis-like picture (e.g., phenytoin, sulindac and allopurinol); and 2) metabolic idiosyncratic reactions that tend to occur at almost any time during the first year of treatment (e.g., troglitazone and isoniazid). The incidence of overt idiosyncratic liver diseases varies with the drug, ranging from approximately 1 in 100 with isoniazid to 1 in 1,000 with phenytoin, to 1 in 10,000 or more with sulindac and troglitazone, and 1 in 100,000 with diclofenac. To detect a single case of drug-induced hepatotoxicity with 95% confidence requires the number of patients studied to be threefold the incidence of the reaction. For one adverse drug reaction in 10,000 patients, at least 30,000 patients need to be evaluated. Thus, many drugs are approved before liver toxicity is observed. It is the responsibility of postmarketing surveillance and monitoring of liver transaminases to identify potential cases of liver-adverse drug reactions.

Risk factors (Table 10.18) for drug-induced liver injury, such as age, gender, genetic predisposition, multiple drugs or dietary supplements, and degree of alcohol consumption, appear to increase the susceptibility to drug-induced hepatotoxicity (88,89). Patients with mild to moderate chronic liver disease do not appear to be at increased risk for idiosyncratic hepatic injury from drugs. However, the drugs in Table 10.17 should be used with caution in these patients, because such patients may have altered metabolism of these drugs and, therefore, may be at increased risk for liver injury. The coadministration of drugs in Table 10.17 with enzyme inducers, such as phenobarbital, phenytoin, ethanol, and/or cigarette smoke, can induce hepatic enzymes, resulting in the enhancement of hepatotoxicity.

Most hepatic adverse effects associated with drugs occur in adults rather than children. Drug-induced liver injury occurs at a higher rate in patients older than 50 years, and drug-associated jaundice also occurs more frequently in the geriatric population (88,89). This age-risk may be the result of increased frequency of drug exposure, multidrug therapy, and age-related changes in drug metabolism.

For reasons that are unclear, drug-induced liver injury affects females more than males: Females accounted for approximately 79% of all reactions to acetaminophen and 73% of all idiosyncratic drug-induced reactions (88). Females exhibit increased risk of hepatic injury from drugs such as atorvastatin, nitrofurantoin, methyldopa, and diclofenac.

Genetic factors as a result of enzyme polymorphism in affected individuals may decrease the ability to metabolize or eliminate drugs, thus increasing their duration of action and the drug exposure and/or decreasing the ability to modulate the immune response to drugs or metabolites. Chronic ingestion of alcohol may also predispose many patients to increased hepatotoxicity from drugs by lowering the store of glutathione (a detoxifying mechanism), which prevents trapping of the toxic metabolites as mercapturate conjugates that are excreted in the urine.

Table 10.18. Risk factors for drug-induced liver injury

Race	Some drugs exhibit different toxicities based on race because of individual CYP450 polymorphism. For example, blacks and Hispanics may be more susceptible to isoniazid (INH) toxicity.
Age	Elderly persons are at increased risk of hepatic injury because of decreased clearance, drug-to-drug interactions, reduced hepatic blood flow, variation in drug binding, and lower hepatic volume. In addition, poor diet, infections, and multiple hospitalizations are important reasons for drug-induced hepatotoxicity. Hepatic drug reactions are rare in children (e.g., acetaminophen, halogenated general anesthetics).
Gender	Although the reasons are unknown, hepatic drug reactions are more common in females. Females are more susceptible to acetaminophen, halothane, nitrofurantoin, diclofenac, and sulindac.
Alcohol	Alcoholics are susceptible to drug toxicity, because alcohol induces liver injury and cirrhotic changes that alter drug metabolism. Alcohol causes depletion of glutathione (hepatoprotective) stores, making the person more susceptible to toxicity by drugs (e.g., acetaminophen, statins).
Liver disease	Patients with chronic liver disease are not uniformly at increased risk of hepatic injury. Although the total CYP450 level is reduced, some patients may be affected more than others. The modification of doses in persons with liver disease should be based on knowledge of the specific CYP450 isoform involved in the metabolism. Patients with HIV infection who are coinfected with hepatitis B or C virus are at increased risk for hepatotoxic effects. Similarly, patients with cirrhosis are at increased risk to hepatotoxic drugs (e.g., methotrexate, methyldopa, valproic acid).
Genetic factors	Genetic (polymorphic) differences in the formation of CYP450 isoforms (2C family and 2D6) can result in abnormal reactions to drugs, including idiosyncratic reactions (see Table 10.18).
Other comorbidities	Patients with AIDS, renal disease, diabetes mellitus, persons who are malnourished, and persons who are fasting may be susceptible to drug reactions because of low glutathione stores.
Pharmacokinetics	Long-acting drugs may cause more injury than shorter-acting drugs, as well as sustained-release drug product formulation.
Drug adulterants	Contaminants are often found in noncertified herbal supplements (e.g., hepatitis C).

Other factors include the effect of drug formulation (sustained vs. rapid release; increased exposure) on pharmacokinetics, e.g., elimination half-life of the drug or adulterants (e.g., enzyme inducers) in dietary supplements.

Drug-induced hepatotoxicity can be categorized as intrinsic (predictable) or idiosyncratic (unpredictable) drug reactions (89). Most drugs involved in hepatotoxicity belong to the idiosyncratic group. Intrinsic heptotoxins produce liver injury in a dose-related manner when the toxic amount of drug is ingested without bioactivation, such as these toxins found in the *Amanita* mushroom. Fortunately, few drugs are intrinsic heptotoxins. Idiosyncratic hepatotoxicity is the result of the toxic effects of a drug's metabolites.

The common trigger for both mild and severe forms of hepatotoxicity is bioactivation of relatively inert functional groups to reactive electrophilic intermediates, which is considered to be an obligatory event in the etiology of many drug-induced idiosyncratic hepatotoxicity (91–92). A great deal of evidence now shows that reactive metabolites are formed from drugs known to cause idiosyncratic hepatotoxicity, but how these toxic species initiate and propagate tissue damage remains poorly understood. However, the relationship between bioactivation and the occurrence of hepatic injury is not simple. For example, many drugs at therapeutic doses undergo bioactivation in the liver but are not hepatotoxic. The tight coupling of bioactivation with bioinactivation pathways may be one reason for the lack of hepatotoxicity with these drugs. Examples of bioinactivation (detoxification) pathways include glutathione conjugation of quinones by glutathione S-transferases (GSTs) and hydration of arene oxides to dihydrodiols by epoxide hydrolases. When reactive metabolites are poor substrates for such detoxifying enzymes, they can escape bioinactivation and, thereby, damage proteins and nucleic acids, prompting hepatotoxicity.

Most drugs, however, are not directly chemically reactive but, through the normal process of drug metabolism, may form electrophilic, chemically reactive metabolites (90–92). Formation of chemically reactive metabolites is mainly catalyzed by CYP450 enzymes (Phase I), but products of Phase II metabolism (e.g., acylglucuronides, acyl CoA thioesters, or N-sulfonates) also can lead to toxicity. However, if Phase I drug bioactivation is closely coupled with Phase II bioinactivation (e.g. glutathione conjugation to mercapturates), then the net chemical process is one of detoxification if the final product is rapidly cleared. Toxicity may accrue when accumulation of a chemically reactive metabolite that, if not detoxified, can lead to covalent modification of biological macromolecules. The identity of the target macromolecule and the functional consequence of its modification will dictate the resulting toxicological response. The CYP450 enzymes are present in many organs, mainly the liver but also the kidney and lung, and thus can bioactivate chemicals to cause organ-specific toxicity. Evidence for the formation of reactive metabolites was found for five of the six drugs that have been withdrawn from the marketplace since 1995 and for 8 of the 15 drugs that have black box warnings. Evidence for reactive metabolite formation has been found for acetaminophen, bromfenac, diclofenac, clozapine, and troglitazone (91–93). Acetaminophen is the most studied hepatotoxin. The current hypotheses of how reactive metabolites leads to liver injury suggests that hepatic (target) proteins can be modified by reactive metabolites. Much more important may be the identification of the target proteins modified by these toxic metabolites and how this reactions alters the function of

Hard/Soft Acids/Bases

The nonenzymatic reaction of an electrophilic metabolite with a nucleophilic molecule usually occurs via a substitution or addition mechanism involving the donation of an electron pair by the nucleophile to an acceptor molecule, an electrophile, with subsequent formation of a covalent bond and an adduct product (Coles B. Effects of modifying structure on electrophilic reactions with biological nucleophiles. Drug Metab Rev. 1984–1985; 15:1307–34). The most accepted concept classifies electrophiles and nucleophiles according to Pearson's "hard-soft acid-bases" (HSAB) model. Thus, hard electrophiles have a formal positive charge at the electrophilic center, and the valence electrons are not easily delocalized or polarized (e.g., acylonium ions, carbocations, nitrenium ions, Figs. 10.30 and 10.33), whereas soft electrophiles have a partial positive charge density and valence electrons that are delocalized (polarized), such as activated double bonds of α,β-unsaturated carbonyl compounds as shown in Fig. 10.32. Hard nucleophiles have high electronegativity (oxygen and nitrogen groups) and low polarization of valence electrons, whereas soft nucleophiles have low electronegativity and are more polarizable. The softest biological nucleophilic sites are cysteine thiol groups on proteins and glutathione (GSH). The primary and secondary amino groups of lysine and histidine or the hydroxyl groups of serine or threonine on proteins are hard nucleophiles, whereas the hardest nucleophiles are the oxygen atoms of purines and pyrimidines on DNA and RNA.

Based on the HSAB theory, the reaction rates and selectivities of electrophiles and nucleophiles are dependent upon comparable states of "hardness." Specifically a soft electrophile such as quinoneimine will react predominantly with a soft nucleophile such as the thiol group of cysteine. A hard electrophile such as the acylonium ion formed from acyl glucuronide will react with hard nucleophiles such as the hydroxyl group of serine. This preferential non-enzymatic reactivity is due primarily to the high-energy transition state that acts as a barrier to the reaction of a hard electrophile with a soft nucleophile such as, the delocalized double bonds of p-benzoquinoneimines, p-benzoquinonemethides, and other α,β-unsaturated carbonyl intermediates which react by Michael- Type addition of the nucleophile to the polarized (partial positive charge) located on the β-carbon.

Adduct formation is dependent not only upon the physiochemical nature of the electrophilc but also upon the microenvironment of the nucleophilic center, which can vary significantly even among centers of the same elemental type (e.g., sulfur or amino groups). Thus, nucleophilic reactivity among free sulfhydryl groups on proteins can be diverse and, consequently, soft electrophilic metabolites will form adducts with the more reactive thiol groups on a given protein or free thiols on glutathione. This diversity in nucleophilic reactivity is a function of both steric and electronic factors mediated primarily by the tertiary structure of a protein. For example, adjacent acidic and basic amino acids on a protein significantly influence the reactivity of the target nucleophilic group. Depending upon the physiochemical nature of the electrophile, the resulting electrophilic metabolite can produce toxicity by reacting with either a soft thiol nucleophilic sites on proteins and free thiols such as GSH or harder nucleophilic centers on DNA and RNA to produce adducts.

For example, metabolic epoxidation of an aromatic ring produces an epoxide, a relatively hard electrophilic metabolite that will form a ring-opened hydroxyl adduct primarily with hard nucleophilic centers on guanine and adenine on DNA, and not with soft thiol nucleophiles. On the other hand, a soft electrophile such as the N-acetyl p-benzoquinone imine metabolite of acetaminophen will form adducts with thiol groups on proteins and free thiols on GSH, but not with hard nucleophilic groups on lysine or serine on proteins or with those on guanine and adenine on DNA. Glutathione offers little protection against carcinogens, most of which are hard nucleophiles. These examples show that the bioactivated metabolite can exhibit distinct electrophilic characteristics and different nucleophilic target molecules. Thus, soft electrophiles are associated with organ-specific toxicities, e.g., heptatotoxicity, renal toxicity, and hard electrophiles with carcinogenicity.

the target proteins. Additionally, it is important to note that the toxicity of reactive metabolites also may be mediated by noncovalent binding mechanisms, which may have profound effects on normal liver physiology. Technological developments in the wake of the genomic revolution now provide unprecedented power to characterize and quantify covalent modification of individual target proteins and their functional consequences (93). Such information should dramatically improve our understanding of drug-induced hepatotoxic reactions. Moreover, covalent binding per se does not necessarily lead to drug hepatotoxicity. The regioisomer of acetaminophen, 3-hydroxyacetanilide, becomes covalently bound to hepatic proteins in rodents without inducing hepatotoxicity (94).

It therefore is necessary to identify targets for these reactive metabolites (i.e., covalently modified macromolecules) that are critical to the toxicological process. Hard electrophiles generally react with hard nucleophiles, such as the basic groups in DNA and lysine ω-amino residues in proteins. Soft electrophiles react with soft nucleophiles, which include cysteine residues in proteins and in glutathione. Unfortunately, no simple rules predict the target macromolecules for a particular chemically reactive metabolite or the biological consequences of a particular modification. Furthermore, noncovalent interactions also play a role, because covalent binding of hepatotoxins is not indiscriminate with respect to proteins. Even within a single protein, there can be selective modification of an amino acid side chain found repeatedly in the primary structure. Thus, the microenvironment (e.g., pK_a and hydrophobicity) of the amino acid in the tertiary structure appears to be the crucial determinant of selective binding and, therefore, the impact of covalent binding on protein function. In turn, the extent of binding and the biochemical role of the protein will determine the toxicological insult of drug bioactivation. The resulting pathological consequences will be a balance between the rates of protein damage and the rates of protein replacement and cellular repair.

Drug-Induced Idiosyncratic Reactions

Idiosyncratic drug reactions (IDR; type B adverse drug reactions) occur in from 1 in 1,000 to 1 in 50,000 patients, are not predictable from the known pharmacology or toxicology of the drug, are not produced experimentally in vitro and in vivo, and are dose independent. The occurrence of IDRs during late clinical trials or after a drug has been released can lead to severe restriction of its use and even its withdrawal. The IDRs usually do not result from the drug itself, because most people can tolerate the drug, but, rather, from a unique set of patient characteristics, including gender, age, genetic predisposition, and a lack of drug-metabolizing enzymes, that may increase the risk of these adverse drug reactions. Most IDRs are caused by hypersensitivity reactions and can result in hepatocellular injury. The hepatic injury occurs within 1 week to 12 months after initiation of drug therapy and often is accompanied by systemic characteristics of allergic drug reactions, such as rash and fever. Signs of hepatic injury reappear with subsequent administration of the same drug with only one or two doses. Hypersensitivity reactions can be severe and associated with fatal reactions as a multiorgan clinical syndrome usually characterized by the following: 1) fever; 2) rash; 3) gastrointestinal symptoms (e.g., nausea, vomiting, diarrhea, or abdominal pain); 4) generalized malaise, fatigue, or achiness; and 5) respiratory symptoms (e.g., dyspnea, cough, or pharyngitis). Examples of drugs causing IDRs through a hypersensitivity mechanism include penicillin, methyldopa, chlorpromazine, erythromycin, azathioprine toxicity in thiopurine methyltransferase–deficient individuals, sulfonamide and acetaminophen hepatotoxicity in alcoholics and in UGT1A6 deficient cats, ivermectin neurotoxicity in Collie dogs deficient in P-gp, perhexilene hepatotoxicity in CYP2D6-deficient individuals, phenytoin toxicity in CYP2C9-deficient individuals, and valproic acid hepatotoxicity.

The clinical features of some cases of drug-induced idiosyncratic hepatotoxicity strongly suggest an involvement of the immune system (95). These clinical characteristics include the following: 1) concurrence of rash, fever, and eosinophilia; 2) delay of the initial reaction (1–8 weeks) or requirement of repeated exposure to the culprit drug; 3) rapid recurrence of toxicity on reexposure to the drug; and 4) presence of antibodies specific for native or drug-modified hepatic proteins. Our current understanding of drug-induced adaptive immune responses is largely based on the hapten hypothesis.

Idiosyncratic drug reactions that are connected with hepatotoxicity involve the formation of reactive metabolites (91,92). Such reactions are not predictable, but current bioanalytical technology have enabled the in vivo identification of the formation of reactive metabolites, as evidenced by the detection of biomarkers (i.e., mercapturate or cysteine adducts) in urine, drug-specific antibodies, or antibodies to CYP isoforms (93). As a result, some drugs known to cause hepatic injury continue to be used, because the drug's benefit outweighs its risk and no alternative efficacious drug exists. For example, isoniazid, a drug commonly used to treat tuberculosis, is implicated in approximately 15 to 20% of the individuals who show increased serum transaminases after receiving the drug as a single agent for tuberculosis prophylaxis. Of these individuals, an estimated 1 in 1,000 patients may develop severe hepatic necrosis. Additionally, NSAIDs, including cyclooxygenase-2 inhibitors, commonly are associated with idiosyncratic liver injury. Most of the idiosyncratic toxins listed in Table 10.19 that have been studied to date produce reactive metabolites.

Current hypotheses regarding IDRs suggest that metabolic activation of a drug to a reactive metabolite is a

Table 10.19. Some Examples of Idiosyncratic Toxins

Abacavir	Hypersensitivity
Acetaminophen	Hepatotoxicity
Amiodarone	Hepatotoxicity
Aromatic anticonvulsants	Hypersensitivity
Cefaclor	Hepatotoxicity
Clozapine	Agranulocytosis
Diclofenac	Hepatotoxicity
Felbamate	Aplastic anemia
Fibrates	Hepatotoxicity
Halothane	Hepatotoxicity
Indomethacin	Hepatotoxicity
Isoniazid	Hepatotoxicity
Levamisole	Hepatotoxicity
Nefazodone	Hepatotoxicity
Nevirapine	agranulocytosis
Oral contraceptives	Hepatotoxicity
Paroxetine	Hepatotoxicity
Phenytoin	Hepatotoxicity
Statins	Hepatotoxicity
Sulfonamides	Stevens-Johnson syndrome
Tamoxifen	Hepatotoxicity
Tacrine	Hepatotoxicity
Tienilic acid	Hypersensitivity
Ticlopidine	Agranulocytosis
Troglitazone	Hepatotoxicity
Valproic acid	Hepatotoxicity
Vesnarinone	Agranulocytosis
Penicillinamine[a]	Hypersensitivity

[a]Does not produce reactive metabolites.

necessary yet insufficient step in the generation of an idiosyncratic reaction (91,92). Evidence for this hypothesis comes from drugs that are associated with hepatotoxicity (Table 10.19) and the detection of a drug-metabolite specific antibodies in affected patients.

For the other drugs that have been associated with idiosyncratic hepatotoxicity but that do not have black box warnings, either evidence for hepatotoxicity was not available or suitable studies had not been carried out. High doses increase the risk for an IDR (e.g., cloazapine at 300 mg/day vs. olanzapine 20 mg/day). Strong evidence also exists that T cells play an important role in immune-mediated IDR and can trigger cell death. In patients exhibiting IDR, pretreatment with immunosuppressants prevented the IDR (rash). The incidence of IDRs also appears to be lower in patients with low T-cell counts.

The hapten hypothesis proposes that the reactive metabolites of the drugs act as haptens and covalently bind to endogenous proteins to form immunogenic drug–protein adducts triggering either antibody or cytotoxic T-cell responses (92,96). The hapten hypothesis is supported by the detection of antibodies that recognize drug-modified hepatic proteins in the sera of drug-induced liver injury (DILI) patients. For example, antibodies that recognize trifluoroacetate-altered hepatic proteins have been detected in the sera of patients with halothane-induced hepatitis. Such drug-specific antibodies or autoantibodies that recognize native liver proteins also have been found in patients with liver injury caused by other drugs, such as diclofenac. In patients who developed IDRs of the liver and other organs, drug-specific T cells have been detected, and in some cases, T-cell clones were generated. Most drugs are small molecules and are unlikely to form haptens. Electrophilic acylators (hard electrophiles) can react with the lysine ω-amino residues (hard nucleophiles) of the target protein or guanosine residues of DNA. How much chemical modification is required to trigger an IDR remains unknown. Halothane is the most studied molecule for supporting this hypothesis regarding IDRs (91). Therefore, it is not surprising that irreversible chemical modification of a protein, which has a profound effect on function, is a mechanism of idiosyncratic hepatotoxicity. However, it is important to note that a number of drugs (e.g., penicillins, aspirin, and omeprazole) rely on covalent binding to proteins for their efficacy; thus, prevention of their covalent binding through chemical modification of the compound also may, inadvertently, lead to loss of efficacy.

Drug-induced stress and/or damage of hepatocytes may trigger activation and inflammatory responses of the immune system within the liver (95,96). Evidence to support this idea has been obtained mainly from studies of liver injury induced by overdoses of acetaminophen, which is one of the few drugs that provide an experimental animal model of drug-induced liver injury. Evidence is growing that the initial benzoquinoneimine-induced hepatocyte damage may lead to activation of immune cells within the liver, thereby stimulating hepatic infiltration by inflammatory cells. Activated T cells of the immune system produce a range of inflammatory mediators, including cytokines, chemokines, and reactive oxygen and nitrogen species, that contribute to the progression of liver injury. On the other hand, the immune cells also represent a major source of hepatoprotective factors.

Reactive Metabolites Resulting from Bioactivation

Electrophiles

The concept that small organic molecules can undergo bioactivation to electrophiles and free radicals and elicit toxicity by chemical modification of cellular macromolecules has its basis in chemical carcinogenicity and the pioneering work of the Millers (97) and Gillette et al. (98–100). A number of different types of reactive metabolites exist; however, they may be broadly classified as either electrophiles (Fig. 10.30) or free radicals (Fig. 10.31) (93,101). These reactive metabolites are short-lived, with half-lives of generally less than 1 minute, and usually are not detectable in plasma or urine except as phase 2 conjugates or other biomarkers. Electrophiles are reactive because they possess electron-deficient centers (polarization-activated double bonds or positive-charge acylators) (Figs. 10.30 and 10.32) and can form covalent bonds with electron-rich biological nucleophiles. They are either soft electrophiles that react directly with soft nucleophiles (:Nuc), such as the thiol groups in either glutathione or cysteine residues within proteins, or hard electrophiles that react with hard nucleophiles, such as basic groups in DNA and lysine ω-amino residues in proteins, or are mediated by bioinactivation enzymes, such as glutathione transferase or epoxide hydrase. Softness or hardness are associated with the polarizability of the electrophilic/nucleophilic species (see Hard/Soft Acids/Bases). Activated double bonds are soft electrophilic intermediates as shown in Fig. 10.32.

Examples of activated double bond electrophiles include α, β-unsaturated carbonyl compounds, quinones, quinoneimines, quinonemethides and diiminoquinones as shown in Fig. 10.32B. These electrophilic intermediates are highly polarized and can react with nucleophiles in a 1,4-Michael-type addition at the more electrophilic or β-carbon of the activated double bond intermediate to the addition product (Fig. 10.32A). Specific examples of activated double bond electrophiles that have been proposed for the anticancer drug leflunamide, the food antioxidant butylated hydroxytoluene, acetaminophen, the antiandrogen flutamide, the anticonvulsant felbamate and the cytotoxic cyclophosphamide as shown in Fig. 10.32C. The bioinactivation pathways for these electrophilic intermediate can involve either direct addition, with or without transferases, depending upon the degree of polarization and reactivity of the electrophilic intermediate (hard vs soft electrophiles).

Other commonly found electrophilic intermediate for drug molecules in Fig. 10.30 include the formation of ketenes from the bioactivation of acetylenic groups (e.g.,

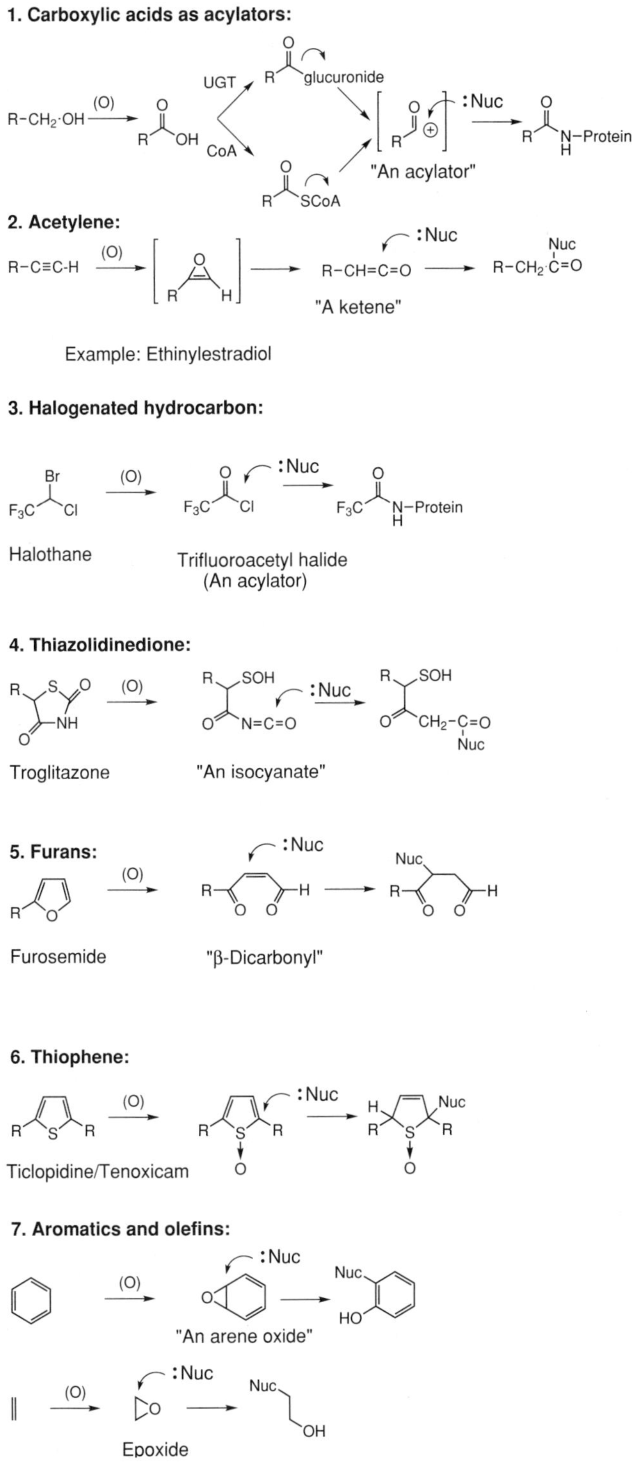

1. Carboxylic acids as acylators:

2. Acetylene:

Example: Ethinylestradiol

3. Halogenated hydrocarbon:

Halothane — Trifluoroacetyl halide (An acylator)

4. Thiazolidinedione:

Troglitazone — "An isocyanate"

5. Furans:

Furosemide — "β-Dicarbonyl"

6. Thiophene:

Ticlopidine/Tenoxicam

7. Aromatics and olefins:

"An arene oxide"

Epoxide

Fig. 10.30. Some examples of electrophilic intermediates resulting from bioactivation. NUC = nucleophiles.

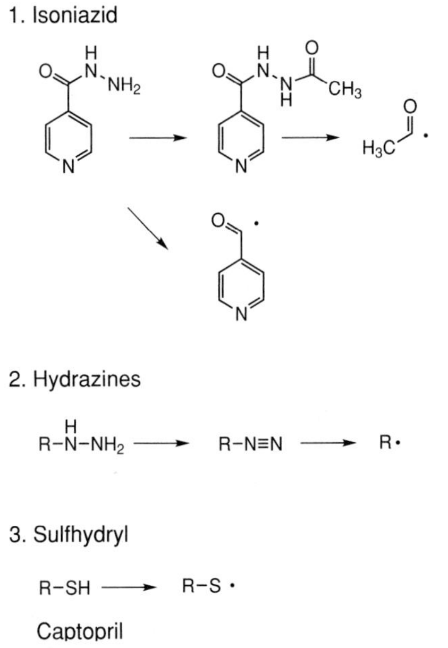

1. Isoniazid

2. Hydrazines

3. Sulfhydryl

Captopril

Fig. 10.31. Drug bioactivation to free radicals.

ethinylestradiol) (Fig. 10.30-2), isocyanates from thiazoldinediones (e.g., the "glitazones") (Fig. 10.30-4) (93), acylonium ions from halogenated hydrocarbons (e.g., halothane) (Fig. 10.30-3) (93) and carboxylic acids, β-dicarbonyl from furans (e.g., furosemide) (Fig. 10.30-5) (93), activated thiophene-S-oxide from thiophenes, such as ticlopidine, tenoxicam which cause an IDR, agranulocytosis (Fig. 10.30-6) (93), and epoxides and arene oxides from olefins and aromatic compounds (Fig10.30-7) (93). Drug possessing structural features prone to metabolic epoxidations are abundant. Therefore the incidence of epoxide metabolites in mediating adverse biologic effects has aroused concern about clinically used drugs known to be metabolized to epoxides. Metabolically produced epoxides have been reported for allobarbital, secpbarbital, protriptyline, carbamazepine, cyproheptadine, and are implicated with 8-methoxypsoralen and other furanocoumarins (6,7-dihydroxybergamottin in grapefruit juice), phenytoin, phensuximide, phenobarbital, mephobarbital, lorazepam, and imipramine (81). The alarming biologic effects of some epoxides, however, do not imply that all epoxides have similar effects. Epoxides vary greatly in molecular geometry, stability, electrophilic reactivity, and relative activity as substrates for epoxide-transforming enzymes (e.g., epoxide hydrolase, glutathione S-transferase, and other).

Some carboxylic acid–containing drugs have been implicated in rare IDRs, which was the basis for the market withdrawal of the NSAIDs, zomiperac, and benzoxaprofen. These drugs (e.g., NSAIDs, fibrates, "statins," and valproic acid) can be bioactivated to acyl glucuronides or acyl CoA thioesters (Fig. 10.30A). These products are electrophilic acylators that can acylate target proteins if they escape inactivation by S-glutathione–thioester formation. A crucial factor is the concentration of acyl glucuronides in hepatocytes because of their transport by conjugate export pumps, where acylglucuronides may selectively acylate canalicular membrane proteins. Acyl CoA esters may be either rapidly hydrolyzed or further metabolized in hepatocytes. Evidence is accumulating that acyl glucuronides can alter cellular function by haptenation of

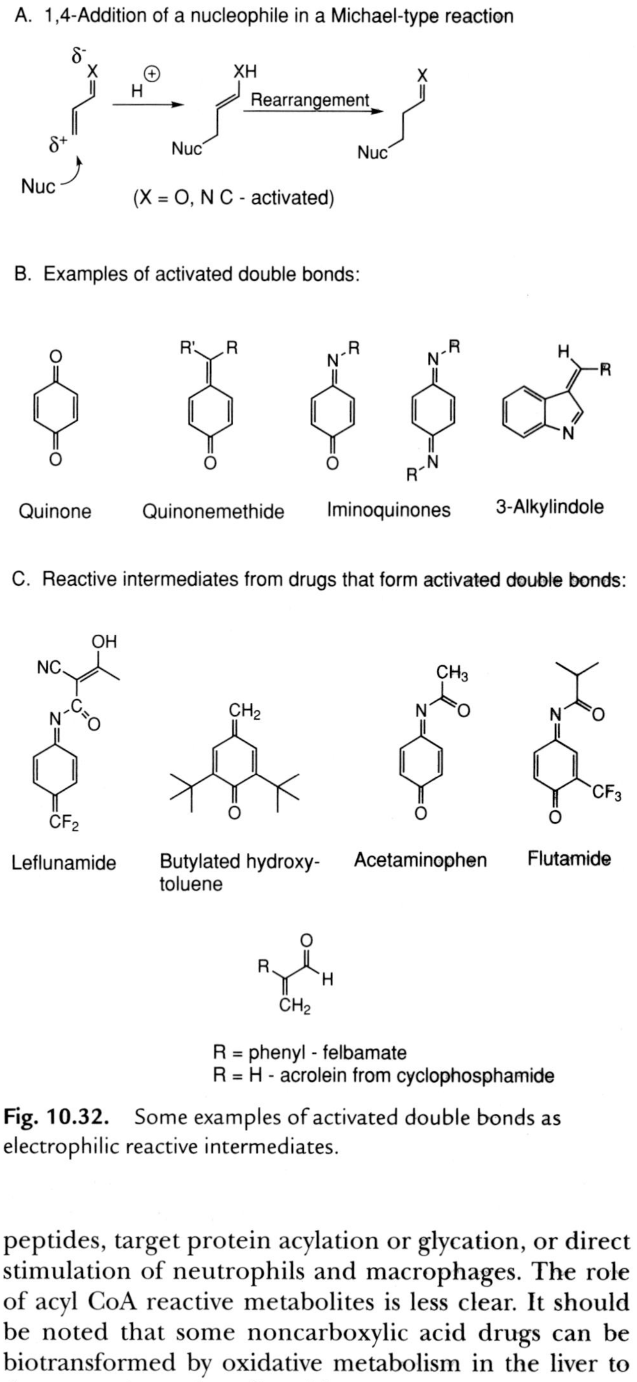

A. 1,4-Addition of a nucleophile in a Michael-type reaction

(X = O, N C - activated)

B. Examples of activated double bonds:

Quinone Quinonemethide Iminoquinones 3-Alkylindole

C. Reactive intermediates from drugs that form activated double bonds:

Leflunamide Butylated hydroxy-toluene Acetaminophen Flutamide

R = phenyl - felbamate
R = H - acrolein from cyclophosphamide

Fig. 10.32. Some examples of activated double bonds as electrophilic reactive intermediates.

peptides, target protein acylation or glycation, or direct stimulation of neutrophils and macrophages. The role of acyl CoA reactive metabolites is less clear. It should be noted that some noncarboxylic acid drugs can be biotransformed by oxidative metabolism in the liver to the respective carboxylic acids.

Free Radicals

Cytochrome P450 activates molecular dioxygen to generate reactive oxygen species (ROS), such as singlet oxygen ($^1O_2$) or superoxide (see Oxygen Activation p. 269). Reactive metabolites that possess unpaired electrons are free radicals (molecular species which contain an odd unpaired electron) which can react with molecular oxygen (ground state triplet) to generate intracellular oxidative stress damage (93,98–100). Free radicals usually abstract a hydrogen atom from other molecules rather than becoming covalently bound. Free radical reactions can be self-propagating by abstracting a hydrogen atom from the double bond of a lipid that initiates a chain reaction leading to lipid peroxidation, oxidative stress or other types of modification of biological molecules.

Some examples of free-radicals generated by the bioactivation of drug molecules are shown in Fig. 10.31. Isoniazid is acetylated to its major metabolite acetylisoniazid, which is hydrolyzed to acetylhydrazine and isonicotinic acid (Fig. 10.31-1). Acetylhydrazine is further metabolized by the CYP2E1 to an N-hydroxy intermediate that hydrates into an acetyl radical, which can then initiate the process that leads to hepatic necrosis. Other carbon-centered radicals are formed from hydrazines such as the antihypertensive hydralazine, and thio-radicals from the ACE inhibitor captopril (Fig. 10.31-2 and -3).

Bioinactivation Mechanisms

Several enzyme systems exist as cellular defense (detoxification) pathways against the chemically reactive metabolites generated by CYP metabolism (91,92,102,103). These include GST, epoxide hydrolase, and quinone reductase, as well as catalase, glutathione peroxidase, and superoxide dismutase, which detoxify the peroxide and superoxide by-products of metabolism. The efficiency of the bioinactivation process is dependent on the inherent chemical reactivity of the electrophilic intermediate, its affinity and selectivity of the reactive metabolite for the bioinactivation enzymes, the tissue expression of these enzymes, and the rapid upregulation of these enzymes and cofactors mediated by the cellular sensors of chemical stress. The reactive metabolites that can evade these defense systems may damage target proteins and nucleic acids by either oxidation or covalent modification.

The most abundant agents of cellular defense are thiols. Glutathione is a soft electrophile and, therefore, will only react noncatalytically with soft electrophiles, such as activated double bonds (Fig. 10.32). Glutathione conjugation to mercapturates is one of the most important defenses against hepatocellular injury. Glutathione protects cellular enzymes and membranes from toxic metabolites, and its inadequate stores can compromise efficient detoxification of the reactive metabolites. The subsequent inability to detoxify the reactive metabolites can result in hepatocellular injury. The rate-limiting factor for glutathione synthesis is the intracellular concentration of cysteine. N-acetylcysteine is often used as an alternative to glutathione to trap the iminoquinone intermediate in the treatment of acute acetaminophen toxicity. Glutathione plays a protective role in the hepatic tissue injury produced by acetaminophen but not by furosemide.

The relationship between bioactivation, bioinactivation, and DNA adduct formation has been well established for a number of hepatocarcinogens. Glutathione conjugation of hard electrophiles becomes more efficient when catalyzed by GSTs, an important example being the detoxication of the hepatocarcingen aflatoxin. Aflatoxin, a hepatocarcinogen and a hepatotoxin found in mold grow-

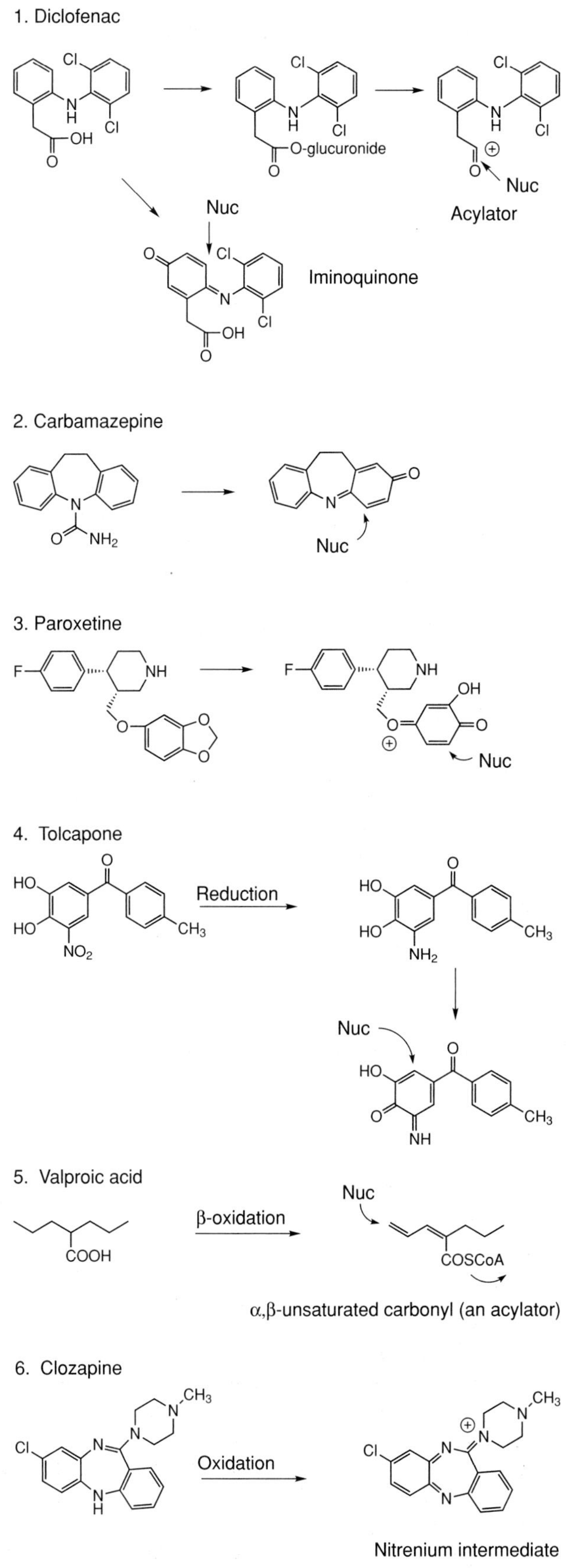

Fig. 10.33. Some examples of drug bioactivation to their hepatotoxic intermediates.

ing on peanuts, is converted into aflatoxin B1 epoxide in rodents, which is more readily detoxified by GST enzymes than by epoxide hydrolase. The balance between these transferase reactions explains the greater DNA damage in humans compared with rodents, because human forms of GST are less able to catalyze the conjugation of aflatoxin epoxide compared with the rodent forms. Transgenic knockout mice have been used to establish the role of bioactivation by CYP450 and bioinactivation by GSTs for a number of carcinogenic polyaromatic hydrocarbons.

Substances that detoxify free radicals include the antioxidants vitamin C, vitamin E, and carotene, which scavenge free radicals, including reactive metabolites and reactive oxygen species generated as a consequence of chemical stress.

Specific Examples

Some examples of bioactivation to hepatotoxic or IDR electrophilic intermediates are shown in Fig. 10.33. Bioactivation may occur by both oxidation and conjugation reactions, such as those with diclofenac, which undergoes the formation of an acyl glucuronide and/or acyl CoA (acylator intermediates) or to produce iminoquinones via formation of a phenol intermediator (Fig. 10.33-1) (92). The anticonvulsant carbamazepine is 2-hydroxylated and the elimination of the amide group yields the reactive quinoneimine intermediate (Fig. 10.33-2), and the antidepressant paroxetine and other xenobiotics with the common methylenedioxyphenyl nucleus undergo methylene oxidation to a *p*-quinoid intermediate (Fig. 10.33-3). The COMT inhibitor used in the treatment of Parkinsonism, tolcapone, the nitro group is first reduced to an amine, then oxidized to a *o*-quinoneimine (Fig. 10.33-4). The mitochondrial/hepatotoxocity of the anticonvulsant valproic acid results from the formation of an activated α,β-unsaturated CoA thioester via mitochrondrial β-oxidation, most commonly associated with the oxidation of fatty acids (Fig. 10.33-5). The agranulocytosis resulting from the ingestion of the antipsychotic clozapine is bioactivated by its oxidation by hypochlorous acid in neutrophils to a nitrenium intermediate (Fig. 10.33-6) (93). The effect of structure modification for troglitazone that reduced its hepatotoxicity is shown in Fig. 10.34. The *p*-dihydroxy elements of the chroman ring nucleus (outlined in bold bonds in Fig. 10.34) of troglitazone is bioactivated to an activated double bond (*p*-quinone) and has been replaced with a pyridine ring that is not bioactivated, although the thiazolidone ring can be bioactivated to an isocyanate (Fig. 10.30) (92).

The oxidation of acetaminophen to the chemically reactive N-acetyl-*p*-benzoquinoneimine (Fig. 10.32), is catalyzed by the isoforms CYP1A2 and CYP2E1, which can either react covalently with glutathione to form an inactive product or with cellular macromolecules, initiating the processes leading to hepatic necrosis (Fig. 10.28) (93). The usual route for acetaminophen metabolism is either glucuronidation. If insufficient UDP-glucuronic acid is present, then bioactivation will dominate.

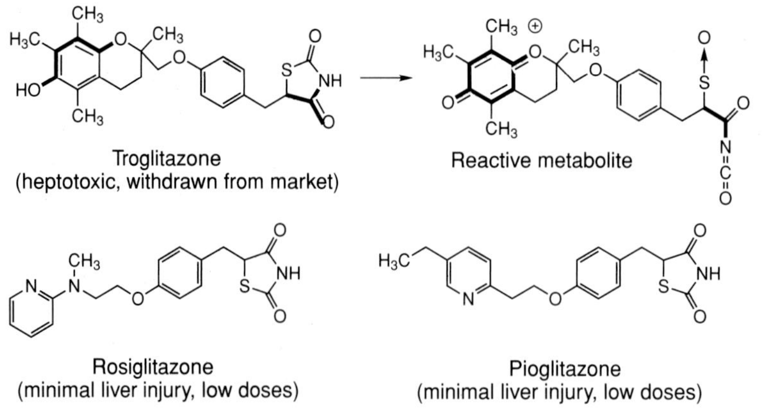

Troglitazone
(heptotoxic, withdrawn from market)

Reactive metabolite

Rosiglitazone
(minimal liver injury, low doses)

Pioglitazone
(minimal liver injury, low doses)

Fig. 10.34. The effect of structure modification on the drug-induced hepatotoxicity of troglitazone.

Furosemide, a frequently used diuretic drug, is reportedly a human hepatocarcinogen. The hepatic toxicity apparently results from metabolic activation of the furan ring to a β-dicarbonyl intermediate (Fig. 10.30-5) (93). Ticlopidine and tenoxicam, reported to cause agranulocytosis, do so via metabolic activation of the thiophene ring to an S-oxide (Fig. 10.30-6) (93). The agranulocytosis resulting from the ingestion of clozapine is via its bioactivation to a nitrenium ion intermediate (Fig. 10.33-6) (96–101).

Drug-Induced Chemical Carcinogenesis

The mechanism whereby xenobiotics are transformed into chemical carcinogens is generally accepted as bioactivation to reactive metabolites, which are responsible for initiating carcinogenicity (98–100). Many carcinogens elicit their cytotoxicity through a covalent linkage to DNA. This process can lead to mutations and, potentially, to cancer. Most chemical carcinogens of concern are chemically inert but require activation by the xenobiotic-metabolizing enzymes before they can undergo reaction with DNA or proteins (cytotoxicity). There are many ways to bioactivate procarcinogens, promutagens, plant toxins, drugs, and other xenobiotics (37) (Fig. 10.35). Oxidative bioactivation reactions are by far the most studied and common. Conjugation reactions (Phase 2), however, are also capable of activating these xenobiotics to produce electrophiles, in which the conjugating derivative acts as a leaving group. These reactive metabolites are mostly electrophiles, such as epoxides, quinones, or free radicals formed by the CYP450 enzymes or FMO. The reactive metabolites tend to be oxygenated in sterically hindered positions, making them poor substrates for subsequent bioinactivation transferases, such as epoxide hydrolase and GST. Therefore, their principal fate is formation of covalent linkage to intracellular macromolecules, including enzyme proteins and DNA. Experimental studies indicate that the CYP1A subfamily can oxygenate aromatic hydrocarbons (e.g., PAHs) in sterically hindered positions to arene oxides. Activation by N-hydroxylation of polycyclic aromatic amines (e.g., aryl N-acetamides) appears to depend on either FMO or CYP450 isoforms. The formation of chemically reactive metabolites is important, because they frequently cause a number of different toxicities, including tumorigenesis, mutagenesis, tissue necrosis, and hypersensitivity reactions.

Our understanding of these reactions was advanced by the studies of the Millers (97) and Gillette et al. (98–100). They proposed that the proportion of the dose that binds covalently to critical macromolecules could depend on the quantity of the reactive metabolite is formed.

A scheme illustrating the complexities of drug-induced chemical carcinogenesis is shown in Fig. 10.35. Reactions that proceed via the open arrows eventually lead to neoplasia. Some carcinogens may form the "ultimate carcinogen" directly through CYP450 isoform bioactivation; others, like the PAHs (e.g., benzo[a]pyrene), appear to involve a multistep reaction sequence forming an epoxide, reduction to a diol by axpoxide hydrase and perhaps, the formation of a second epoxide group on another part of the molecule.

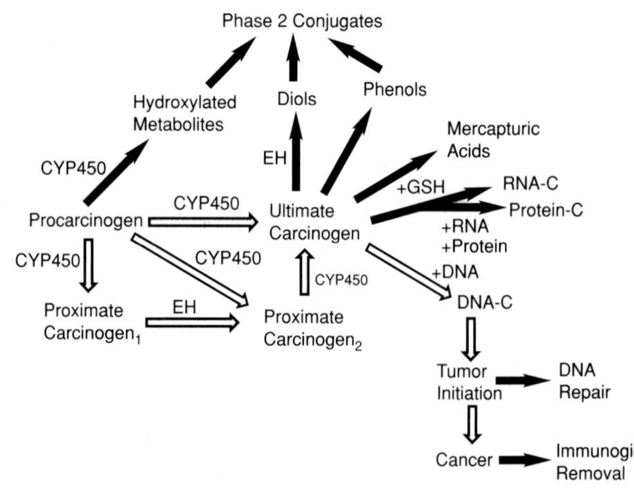

Fig. 10.35. The bioactivation of procarcinogens and a proposed mechanism of chemical carcinogenesis.

Other procarcinogens form the N-hydroxy intermediate that requires transferase-catalyzed conjugation (e.g., O-glucuronide and O-sulfate) to form the "ultimate carcinogen." The quantity of "ultimate carcinogen" formed should relate directly to the proportion of the dose that binds or alkylates DNA.

The solid-arrow reaction sequences in Figure 10.35 are intended to show detoxification mechanisms, which involve several steps. First, the original chemical may form less active products (phenols, diols, mercapturic acids, and other conjugates). Second, the "ultimate carcinogen" may rearrange so as to be prevented from its reaction with DNA (or whatever the critical macromolecule is). Third, the covalently bound DNA may be repaired. Fourth, immunologic removal of the tumor cells may occur. Several mechanisms within this scheme could regulate the quantity of covalently bound carcinogen: 1) The activity of the rate-limiting enzyme, such as epoxide hydrolase, CYP450 isoform, or one of the transferases, could be involved; 2) the availability of cosubstrates, such as glutathione, UDP-glucuronic acid, or PAPS, may be rate-limiting; 3) relative CYP450 activities for detoxification and activation must be considered; 4) availability of alternate reaction sites for the ultimate carcinogen (e.g., RNA and protein may be involved); 5) and possible specific transport mechanisms that deliver either the procarcinogen or its ultimate carcinogen to selected molecular or subcellular sites.

It is now well established that numerous organic compounds that are essentially nontoxic as long as their structure is preserved can be converted into cytotoxic, teratogenic, mutagenic, or carcinogenic compounds by normal biotransformation pathways in both animals and humans (37). The reactive electrophilic intermediate (hard acids) involves its reaction with cellular constituents (hard bases) forming either detoxified products or binding covalently with essential macromolecules, initiating processes that eventually lead to the toxic effect. A better understanding of the mechanisms underlying these reactions may lead to more rational approaches to the development of nontoxic therapeutic drugs. For the present, it seems that new advances in drug therapy cannot occur without some risk of causing structural tissue lesions. Special attention to risk factors is required for drugs that will be used for long periods in the same patient.

Some toxic chemicals exert their toxic action by lethal injury or biological auto-oxidation (radical lipid peroxidation). Lethal injury involves the disruption of cellular energy metabolism by inhibition of oxidative phosphorylation or adenosine triphosphatase, resulting in disruption of subcellular organelles, cell death, and tissue necrosis. Because the early stages of lethal injury are reversible, complete recovery may occur. Auto-oxidation is the process whereby cellular components are irreversibly oxidized and damaged by free radicals or free radical–generating systems. This results in the oxidation and depletion of glutathione, various thiol enzymes, or lipid peroxidation, which in turn leads to the disruption of cellular membranes and to cell death, tissue necrosis, and death of the organism. When cell death does not occur, nonlethal changes, such as mutations and malignant transformations, are likely.

DRUG–DRUG INTERACTIONS

Drug–drug interactions represent a common clinical problem, which has been compounded by the introduction of many new drugs and the expanded the use of herbal medicines. Between 1999 and 2005, approximately 100 drug–drug interactions were reported, of which approximately 50% involved CYP450 inhibition. Drug–drug interactions occur when the efficacy or toxicity of a medication is changed by coadministration of another substance, drug, food (i.e., grapefruit), or herbal product (103,104). Pharmacokinetic interactions often occur as a result of a change in drug metabolism. For example, CYP3A4 oxidizes more than 60% of the clinically used drugs with a broad spectrum of structural features, and its location in the small intestine and liver permits an effect on both presystemic and systemic drug disposition. Some interactions with CYP3A4 substrates/inhibitors also may involve inhibition of P-gp. Other clinically important drug interactions resulting from coadministration of CYP3A4 substrates or inhibitors include rhabdomyolysis with the coadministration of some 3-hydroxy-3-methylglutaryl–CoA reductase inhibitors ("statins"), symptomatic hypotension with some dihydropyridine calcium antagonists, excessive sedation from benzodiazepine or nonbenzodiazepine hypnosedatives, ataxia with carbamazepine, and ergotism with ergot alkaloids.

The clinical importance of any drug–drug interaction depends on factors that are drug-, patient-, and administration-related. Drugs with low oral bioavailability or high first-pass metabolism are particularly susceptible to drug–drug interactions as a result of coadministration of inhibitors that alter absorption, distribution, and elimination. Generally, a doubling or more in the plasma drug concentration has the potential for enhanced adverse or beneficial drug response. Less pronounced pharmacokinetic interactions may still be clinically important for drugs with a steep concentration–response relationship or narrow therapeutic index. In most cases, the extent of drug interaction varies markedly among individuals; this is likely to be dependent on interindividual differences in CYP450 content (polymorphism), preexisting medical conditions, and possibly, age. Interactions may occur under single-dose conditions or only at steady state. The pharmacodynamic consequences may or may not closely follow pharmacokinetic changes. Drug–drug interactions may be most apparent when patients are stabilized on the affected drug and the CYP450 substrates or inhibitors are then added to the regimen (103). One reason for the increased incidence of drug–drug interactions is the practice of simultaneously prescribing several potent drugs as well as concurrently ingesting nonprescription products and herbal products.

Although drug–drug interactions constitute only a small proportion of adverse drug reactions, they have become an important issue in health care. Many of the drug–drug interactions can be explained by alterations in the metabolic enzymes in the liver and other extrahepatic tissues, and many of the major pharmacokinetic interactions between drugs are caused by hepatic CYP450 isoenzymes being affected by coadministration of other drugs. Some drugs act as potent enzyme inducers, whereas others are inhibitors. Drug–drug interactions involving enzyme inhibition, however, are much more common. Understanding these mechanisms of enzyme inhibition or induction is extremely important to give appropriate multidrug therapies. In the future, individuals at greatest risk for drug–drug interactions and adverse events need to be identified. Cytochrome P450s play a dominant role in the metabolism and elimination of drugs from the body, and their substrates are shown in Tables 10.3 and 10.6 through 10.9. Drugs in bold italics have been associated with drug interactions (103). Inhibitors of CYP450 are shown in Table 10.10. Pharmacokinetic interactions may arise when the biotransformation and elimination of a drug are impaired by coadministered drugs. Thus, drugs may compete for biotransformation by a common CYP450. Adverse drug reactions, including toxicity, can occur if elimination is dependent on a CYP450 that exhibits defective gene variants. Thus, the genetic makeup of the individual (see the section on genetic polymorphism) has a major influence on the duration of drug action as well as on drug efficacy and safety. CYP450 pharmacogenetics affects the tendency for certain drug–drug interactions to occur. Thus, the future safe use of drug combinations in patients may require genotyping and phenotyping of individuals before the commencement of therapy. Identification of subjects who metabolize drugs in a different fashion from the general population should minimize the impact of pharmacogenetic variation on drug pharmacokinetics.

Many drug–drug interactions are a result of inhibition or induction of CYP450 enzymes. Metabolism-based enzyme inhibition usually involves competition between two drugs for the enzyme-active site. Metabolic drug–drug interactions occur when drug A (or its metabolite) alters the pharmacokinetics of a coadministered drug B by inhibiting, activating, or inducing the activity of the enzymes that metabolize drug B. Inhibitory drug–drug interactions could result in serious adverse effects, including fatalities in patients receiving multiple medications. This process is usually competitive, begins with the first dose of the inhibitor, and the extent of inhibition correlates with their relative affinities for the enzymes and the metabolic half-lives of the drugs involved. On the other hand, mechanism-based (irreversible) inhibition results from a metabolite that binds irreversibly with a covalent bond to the enzyme, rendering the enzyme inactive. Enzyme-specific CYP450 inhibitors, including metabolism- and mechanism-based inhibitors, or are metabolized by specific CYP450 isoforms and are usually excluded from further consideration for new drug development. Not only is CYP3A4 the most abundant isoform in human liver, it also metabolizes more than 60% of the drugs in clinical use, which renders CYP3A4 highly susceptible to both metabolism- (reversible) and mechanism-based inhibition. The CYP3A subfamily is involved in many clinically significant drug–drug interactions, including those involving nonsedating antihistamines and cisapride, that may result in cardiac dysrhythmias. For example, inhibitors of CYP1A2 can increase the risk of toxicity from clozapine or theophylline. Inhibitors of CYP2C9 can increase the risk of toxicity from phenytoin, tolbutamide, and oral anticoagulants (e.g., warfarin). Inhibitors of CYP3A4 can increase the risk of toxicity from many drugs, including carbamazepine, cisapride, cyclosporine, ergot alkaloids, lovastatin, pimozide, protease inhibitors, rifabutin, simvastatin, tacrolimus, and vinca alkaloids. Inhibitors of CYP2D6 can increase risk of toxicity of many antidepressants, opiate analgesics, and psychotherapeutic agents. An excellent example of a metabolism-based inhibition drug–drug interaction that resulted in a life-threatening ventricular arrhythmia associated with QT prolongation (torsades de pointes) occurred when CYP3A4 substrates or inhibitors were coadministered with terfenadine, astemizole, cisapride, or pimozide. This potentially lethal drug interaction led to the withdrawal of terfenadine and cisapride from clinical use and to the introduction of fexofenadine, the metabolite of terfenadine, which does not have this interaction. Examples of enzyme inducers include barbiturates, carbamazepine, glutethimide, griseofulvin, phenytoin, primidone, rifabutin, and rifampin. Some drugs, such as ritonavir, may act as either an enzyme inhibitor or an enzyme inducer, depending on the situation. Drugs metabolized by CYP3A4 or CYP2C9 are particularly susceptible to enzyme induction.

Mechanism-based inhibition is characterized by NADPH-, time-, and concentration-dependent enzyme inactivation, occurring when some drugs are converted by CYP450s to reactive metabolites (103). Mechanism-based inactivation of CYP3A4 by drugs can be the result of chemical modification of the heme, the apoprotein, or both, as a result of covalent binding of the modified heme to the protein. The clinical pharmacokinetic effect of a CYP3A4 inactivator is a function of its enzyme kinetics (i.e., K_m and V_{max}) and the synthesis rate of new or replacement enzyme. Predicting drug–drug interactions involving CYP3A4 inactivation is possible when pharmacokinetic principles are followed. Such prediction may become difficult, however, because the clinical outcomes of CYP3A4 inactivation depend on many factors associated with the enzyme, the drugs, and the patients.

Some of the clinically important drugs that have been identified to be mechanism-based CYP3A4 inhibitors include antibiotics (e.g., erythromycin), anticancer drugs (e.g., irinotecan), antidepressants (e.g., fluoxetine and paroxetine), anti-HIV agents (e.g., ritonavir and delavirdine), antihypertensives (e.g., dihydralazine and verapamil), steroids and their receptor modulators (e.g., ethinyl estradiol, gestodene, and raloxifene), dihydrotestosterone reductase inhibitors (e.g., finasteride), and some herbal constituents (e.g., bergamottin and glabridin). Compared to the more common metabolism-based (reversible) inhibition, mechanism-based inhibitors of CYP3A4 usually are the cause for unfavorable drug–drug interactions, because the inactivated CYP3A4 must be replaced by newly synthesized CYP3A4 protein. Most CYP3A4 inactivators also are P-gp substrates/ inhibitors, confounding the in vitro–to–in vivo extrapolation. Clinicians should have good knowledge about these CYP3A4 inactivators and avoid their combination use.

The clinical significance of CYP3A inhibition for drug safety and efficacy warrants closer understanding of the mechanisms for each inhibitor. Furthermore, such inactivation may be exploited for therapeutic gain in certain circumstances.

By understanding the unique functions and characteristics of these enzymes, health care practitioners may better anticipate and manage drug interactions. They also may predict or explain an individual's response to a particular therapeutic regimen.

Beneficial Drug–Drug Interactions

A beneficial drug interaction, for example, is the coadministration of a CYP3A4 inhibitor with cyclosporine, which allows reduction of the dosage and cost of the immunosuppressant. Certain HIV protease inhibitors, such as saquinavir, have a low oral bioavailability because of intestinal CYP3A4 metabolism. The oral bioavailability of saquinavir can be profoundly increased by the addition of a low dose of a CYP3A4 inhibitor, such as ritonavir. This concept of altering drug pharmacokinetics by adding a low, subtherapeutic dose of a CYP3A4 inhibitor (ritonavir) to increase the oral bioavailability of another protease inhibitor, lopinavir (CYP3A4 substrate), led to the marketing of Kaletra, a new drug combination of lopinavir and ritinavir.

Grapefruit Juice–Drug Interactions

Historical Significance of Grapefruit Juice

The discovery that grapefruit juice can markedly increase the oral bioavailability of CYP3A4 drugs was based on an unexpected observation from an interaction study between the dihydropyridine calcium channel antagonist felodipine and ethanol in which grapefruit juice was used to mask the taste of the ethanol. Subsequent investigations confirmed that grapefruit juice significantly increased the oral bioavailability of felodipine by reducing presystemic felodipine metabolism through selective inhibition of CYP3A4 expression in the intestinal wall (106).

Grapefruit juice is a beverage often consumed at breakfast for its health benefits and to mask the taste of drugs or foods. Unlike other citrus fruit juices, however, grapefruit juice can significantly increase the oral bioavailability of drugs that are metabolized primarily by intestinal CYP3A4, causing an elevation in their serum concentrations (Table 10.20). Those drugs with high oral bioavailabilities (>60%), however, are all likely safe to take with grapefruit juice, because their high oral bioavailability leaves little room for elevation by grapefruit juice. The importance of the interaction appears to be influenced by individual patient susceptibility, type and amount of grapefruit juice, and administration-related factors.

Grapefruit juice can alter oral drug pharmacokinetics by different mechanisms. Irreversible inactivation of intestinal CYP3A4, which can persist up to 24 hours, is produced by grapefruit juice given as a single, normal, 200- to 300-mL drink or by whole fresh fruit segments (Table 10.20). As a result, presystemic metabolism is reduced, and oral drug bioavailability increased. Enhanced oral drug bioavailability can occur up to 24 h after juice consumption. Inhibition of P-gp is a possible mechanism that increases oral drug bioavailability by reducing intestinal and/or hepatic efflux transport. Inhibition of organic anion–transporting polypeptides by grapefruit juice and apple juice has been observed; intestinal uptake transport appeared to be decreased as oral drug bioavailability was reduced. Numerous medications used in the prevention or treatment of coronary artery disease and its complications have been observed or predicted to interact with grapefruit juice. Such interactions may increase the risk of rhabdomyolysis when dyslipidemia is treated with the HMG-CoA reductase inhibitors ("statins"). Such interactions also might cause excessive vasodilatation when hypertension is managed with the dihydropyridines felodipine, nicardipine, nifedipine, nisoldipine, or nitrendipine. An alternative agent could be amlodipine. The therapeutic effect of the angiotensin II type I receptor antagonist losartan may be reduced by grapefruit juice. Grapefruit juice interacting with the antidiabetic agent repaglinide may cause hypoglycemia, and interaction with the appetite suppressant sibutramine may cause elevated blood pressure and heart rate. In angina pectoris, administration of grapefruit juice could result in atrioventricular conduction disorders with verapamil or attenuated antiplatelet activity with clopidrogel. Grapefruit juice may enhance the drug toxicity for antiarrhythmic agents, such as amiodarone, quinidine, disopyramide, or propafenone, and for the congestive heart failure drug carvediol. Some drugs for the treatment of peripheral or central vascular disease also have the potential to interact with grapefruit juice. Interaction with sildenafil, tadalafil, or vardenafil for erectile dysfunction may cause serious systemic vasodilatation, especially when combined with a nitrate. In stroke, interaction with nimodipine may cause systemic hypotension.

Table 10.20. Some CYP3A4 Substrates and Interactions with Grapefruit Juice (78)

Drug	Interaction[a]	Drug	Interaction[a]
Calcium channel blocker		HMG-CoA reductase inhibitors	
Amlodipine	Y	Atorvastatin	Y
Felodipine	Y	Cerivastatin	Y?
Nifedipine	Y	Fluvastatin	N?
Nimodipine	Y	Lovastatin	Y
Nisoldipine	Y	Pravastatin	N?
Nitrendipine	Y	Simvasta	Y
Pranidipine	Y	CNS Drugs	
Antiarrhythmics		Buspirone	Y
Diltiazem	N	Carbamazepine	Y
Verapamil	N	Diazepam	Y
Quinidine	N	Midazolam	Y
Antihistamines		Triazolam	Y
Ebastine	Y?	Immunosuppressants	
Loratidine	Y?	Cyclosporine	Y
HIV protease inhibitors		Tacrolimus	Y?
Indinavir	N?	Other	
Nelfinavir	N?	Methadone	Y
Ritonavir	N?	Sildenafil	Y
Saquinavir	Y		
Macrolides			
Clarithromycin	N		

[a]Y (yes) and N (no) indicate published evidence of the presence or absence of an interaction with grapefruit juice. Y? and N? indicate expected findings based on available data. Those drugs with Y or Y? should not be consumed with grapefruit juice in an unsupervised manner.

If a drug has low inherent oral bioavailability from presystemic metabolism by CYP3A4 or efflux transport by P-gp and the potential to produce serious overdose toxicity, avoidance of grapefruit juice entirely during pharmacotherapy appears mandatory. Although altered drug response is variable among individuals, the outcome is difficult to predict, and avoiding the combination will guarantee that toxicity is prevented. The elderly are at particular risk, because they often are prescribed medications and frequently consume grapefruit juice.

The mechanism by which grapefruit juice produces its effect is through inhibition of the enzymatic activity and a decrease in the intestinal expression of CYP3A4. The P-gp efflux pump also transports many CYP3A4 substrates; thus, the presence of inhibitors of P-gp in grapefruit juice (e.g., 6′,7′-dihydroxybergamottin and other furanocoumarins) could be a related factor for drug–grapefruit juice interactions (82). Numerous studies have shown that grapefruit juice acts on intestinal CYP3A4, not at the hepatic level.

Does the quantity of juice matter? The majority of the presystemic CYP3A4 inhibition is obtained following ingestion of one glass of grapefruit juice; however, 24 hours after ingestion of a glass of grapefruit juice, 30% of its effect is still present (78). The reduction in intestinal CYP3A4 concentration is rapid: a 47% decrease occurred in a healthy volunteer within 4 hours after consuming grapefruit juice. Daily ingestion of grapefruit juice results in a loss of CYP3A4 from the small intestinal epithelium. Consumption of very large quantities of grapefruit juice (six to eight glasses/day) may lead to inhibition of hepatic CYP3A4.

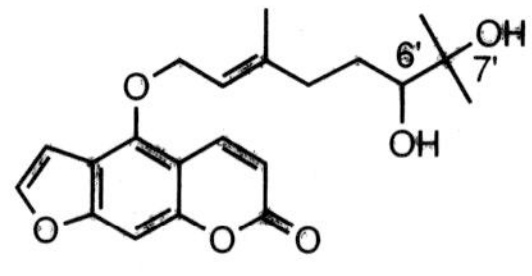

6′,7′-Dihydroxybergamottin

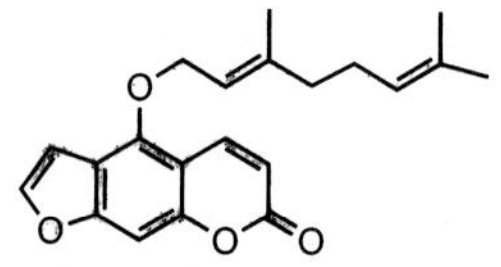

Bergamottin

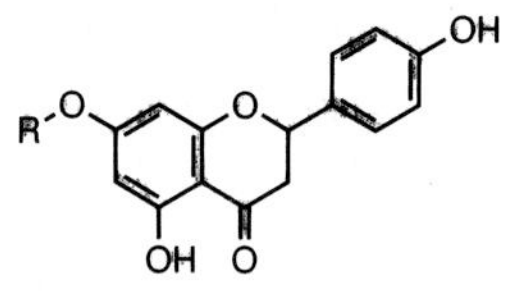

Naringin R: rhamnose-glucoside-
Naringinin R: H-

The active constituents found in grapefruit juice responsible for its effects on CYP3A4 include flavonoids (e.g., naringenin and naringin) and furanocoumarins (e.g., bergamottin and 6′,7′-dihydroxybergamottin) (82). Of particular interest are the effects of naringin and 6′,7′-dihydroxybergamottin on the activity of intestinal CYP3A4. The majority of studies to date have used either freshly squeezed grapefruit juice, reconstituted frozen juice, commercial grapefruit juice, grapefruit segments, or grapefruit extract; all are capable of causing drug–drug interactions with CYP3A4 substrates (blended grapefruit juices have not yet been investigated). The active constituents in grapefruit juice are present not just in the juice but also in the pulp, peel, and core of the fruit and are responsible for its flavor. Bergamottin and 6′,7′-dihydroxybergamottin are potent mechanism-based inhibitors of CYP3A4, and naringenin isomers are competitive inhibitors of CYP3A4 (82). Higher concentrations of 6′,7′-dihydroxybergamottin and naringin are present in grapefruit segments. Thus, any therapeutic concern for a drug interaction with grapefruit juice should now be extended to include whole fruit and other products derived from the grapefruit peel. The difference in the in vitro CYP3A4 inhibition between grapefruit juice and orange juice is that orange juice contained no measurable amounts of 6′,7′-dihydroxybergamottin.

If a patient has been taking medication with grapefruit juice for some time without ill effects, is it safe to continue to do so? Much of this unpredictability results from the inconsistency of the juice concentrations and the sporadic manner in which grapefruit juice is consumed, suggesting that this approach may not be entirely safe (106). Given the unpredictability of the effect of grapefruit juice on the oral bioavailability of the drugs in Table 10.20, patients should be advised to avoid this combination, thus preventing the onset of potential adverse effects. Each patient's situation should be considered, and advice should be based on consumption history and the specific medications involved. The benefits of increased and controlled drug bioavailability by grapefruit juice may, in the future, be achieved through either standardizing the constituents or coadministration of the isolated active ingredients. This would then lead to a safe, effective, and cost-saving means to enhance the absorption of many therapeutic agents.

P-glycoprotein–Drug Interactions

From the earlier discussion regarding P-gp, it is obvious that P-gp–mediated transport plays an important role in pharmacokinetic-mediated drug–drug interactions (79). Thus, inhibition of P-gp–mediated transport could dramatically increase the systemic bioavailability of an otherwise poorly absorbed drug. Similar consequences could be expected with a reduction in renal or biliary clearances (e.g., digoxin). Numerous investigations with drugs such as digoxin, etoposide, cyclosporine, vinblastine, taxol, loperamide, domperidone, and ondansteron demonstrate that P-gp has an important role in determining the pharmacokinetics of substrate drugs (79). For example, if drug A is a substrate for both P-gp and *only* for CYP3A4, and if a second drug B is added that is an inhibitor for both P-gp and CYP3A4 (Table 10.16), then the plasma drug concentration for unmetabolized drug A will be elevated, with increased potential for drug–drug interactions as adverse effects or for causing a drug overdose. If drug A is a substrate for multiple CYP450 isoforms, however, then drug A will be metabolized by these other isoforms, with minimal effect on plasma drug concentrations. On the other hand, if the second drug B is only an inhibitor for P-gp, then drug A will be subject to CYP3A4 metabolism, thus decreasing the plasma concentration for drug A to subtherapeutic levels. The effect of P-gp inhibition is to increase the oral bioavailability so that the later actions of CYP3A4 inhibition will be increased. One of the best examples is the interaction between digoxin and quinidine. Quinidine blocks P-gp in the intestinal muscosa and in the proximal renal tubule; thus, digoxin elimination into the intestine and urine is inhibited, increasing the plasma digoxin concentration to toxic levels. Another example is loperamide, which is an opiate antidiarrheal normally kept out of the brain by the P-gp pump; however, inhibition of P-gp allows accumulation of loperamide in the brain, leading to respiratory depression. Increasingly, the relevant clinical data for drug interactions can be found on the World Wide Web.

The components of grapefruit juice reportedly inhibit P-gp, and this may be one of the mechanisms for the increase in bioavailability of drugs that are substrates for P-gp (Table 10.16). Although fexofenadine is a P-gp substrate, rather than a decrease in its plasma levels when it is coadministered with grapefruit juice, the blood levels are increased as a result of fexofenadine being a substrate of the anion transporter (OATP) in the intestine. Studies have shown that apple and other fruit juices are more potent inhibitors of OATP than of P-gp.

Food–Drug Interactions

Drug pharmacokinetics can be altered by the fat content of food through changes in drug solubility as well as the nutritional status of a patient (107). The fact that grapefruit juice can increase the bioavailability of certain drugs by their reducing presystemic intestinal metabolism has led to renewed interest in the area of "food–drug interactions," with particular interest regarding the effects of grapefruit constituents. Specific naturally occurring chemicals in food have been associated with drug interactions. For example, severe hypertensive reactions have occurred when patients treated with antidepressant MAO inhibitors have ingested cheeses and other foods rich in the biogenic amine tyramine (see Chapter 21).

Drug–Dietary Supplement Interactions

The increasing use of dietary supplements presents a special challenge in health care; thus, there is an increasing need to predict and avoid these potential adverse drug–dietary supplement interactions. The present interest and widespread use of herbal remedies has created the possibility of interaction between them and over-the-counter or prescription drugs if they are used simultaneously. As herbal medicines become more popular, herbal hepatotoxicity is being increasingly recognized. Females appear to be predisposed to hepatotoxicity, and coadministered agents that induce CYP450 enzymes (e.g., St. Johns wort) also may increase individual susceptibility to some dietary supplements. Currently, nearly one in five adults taking prescription medicines also are taking at least one dietary supplement. The mechanisms for drug–dietary supplement interactions are similar to those for drug–drug interactions affecting the pharmacokinetics of the respective drug. Little is known regarding the pharmacokinetic properties of many of the substances in dietary supplements. Therefore, the potential for drug–dietary supplement interactions has greatly increased. Licorice, when taken with steroids, can reduce their metabolism and elimination.

St. John's Wort

A commonly reported drug–dietary supplement interaction is between St. John's Wort and HIV protease inhibitors, leading to drug resistance and treatment failure. St. John's wort is a popular dietary supplement often used for depression. Of the two substances found in St. John's wort, hypericin and hyperforin, hyperforin appears to be the main constituent, with in vitro selective serotonin reuptake inhibitor (SSRI) activity (see Chapter 21). Hyperforin also appears to be the more potent inducer of CYP3A enzymes based on in vitro and in vivo studies.

The U.S. FDA has issued a statement that "concomitant use of St. John's wort with protease inhibitors or nonnucleoside reverse transcriptase inhibitors is not recommended." St. John's wort appeared to have minimal effects on the CYP3A4 enzymes after acute administration; however, chronic administration (≥2 weeks) of St. John's wort selectively induced CYP3A4, with a greater effect in the small intestine than in the liver. Administration of St. John's wort for 8 weeks decreased the plasma levels of norethindrone, a low-dose oral contraceptive, and reduced the half-life of ethinyl estradiol, consistent with increased CYP3A activity, increase breakthrough bleeding, and reduce contraceptive efficacy. Based on the these in vivo and in vitro studies, the efficacy of drugs that are substrates for the CYP3A family or P-gp may be reduced on coadministration of St. John's wort. St. John's wort should be listed along with other known CYP3A inducers (e.g., rifampin and rifabutin) as possibly decreasing plasma levels of CYP3A substrates. The drug products Kaletra (lopinavir and ritonavir), Mifeprex (mifepristone, RU-486), Nuvaring (etonogestrel/ethinyl estradiol), Gleevec (imatinib), Neoral (cyclosporine), Rapamune (sirolimus), and Prograf (tacrolimus) include information about drug interactions with St. John's wort in their labeling. Thus, patients ingesting St. John's wort products should be advised that St. John's wort can have potentially dangerous interactions with some prescription drugs and to consult a physician before taking St. John's wort if currently taking anticoagulants, oral contraceptives, antidepressants, antiseizure medications, drugs to treat HIV or prevent transplant rejections, or any other prescription drug.

St. John's Wort also decreases the absorption of digoxin and fexofenadine, apparently by inducing P-gp in the intestinal and renal endothelium, increasing their elimination in the intestine and urine, respectively, and their plasma concentrations.

Echinacea

In vitro or in vivo chronic administration studies of Echinacea, an herbal product used for the treatment of colds and viral infections, inhibited hepatic CYP1A2 and intestinal CYP3A activities and induced hepatic CYP3A. Based on these preliminary findings, the effect of Echinacea on various CYP3A substrates may vary depending on the relative contribution to a given drug's overall clearance by intestinal CYP3A versus hepatic CYP3A in the individual substrate's clearance pathway.

Ginkgo Biloba

In vitro studies with Ginkgo biloba, often used for memory improvement, exhibited induction of CYP2C19. The extent of induction appears to be CYP2C19 genotype dependent.

Kava

Reports of hepatotoxicity have been associated with the use of kava, a popular drug in Europe and North America. Hepatotoxicity was not observed when kava was prepared as a water infusion but was with solvent-extracted products available in stores and on the World Wide Web. The three kava lactones (methysticin, desmethoxyyangonin, and yangonin; active principles) are potent inhibitors of CYP1A2, CYP2C9, CYCYP2C19, CYP2E1, and CYP3A4, with methysticin being the most potent enzyme inhibitor as well as the most cytotoxic. The potent inhibition of CYP450 enzymes suggests a high potential for interactions with drugs and other herbs that are metabolized by the same CYP450 enzymes. Long-term use or use in individuals with liver disorders should be avoided, and liver function transaminases need to be checked frequently.

Other Dietary Supplements Exhibiting Drug-Induced Heptatotoxicity

DHEA and androstenedione are testosterone precursors that have been associated with hepatic toxicity and should be avoided in those with hepatic disease or coingestion with other potentially hepatotoxic products or enzyme inducers that might increase the risk of liver damage. Liver enzymes should be monitored once or twice a year. Boldo can cause hepatotoxicity and exacerbate existing liver disease. Because chaparral, comfrey, germander, skullcap, valerian root can cause acute and chronic liver injury, these products should be considered unsafe. Pennyroyal oil can cause acute hepatotoxicity liver injury, which has been attributed to the bioactivation of the terpine, R (+) pulegone resulting in depletion of hepatic glutathione. In some cases, unknown adulterants found in these herbal products may be responsible for the hepatotoxicity. Black cohosh, commonly used by women for menopausal symptoms, including hot flashes and sleep disorders, formed quinone metabolites in vitro, but no mercapturate conjugates were detected in urine samples from women who consumed multiple oral doses of up to 256 mg of a standardized black cohosh extract. At moderate doses of black cohosh, the risk of liver injury is minimal.

Silybum marianum (milk thistle) is used in the treatment of chronic or acute liver disease as well as in protecting the liver against toxicity (109). Silybum is cited as one of the oldest known herbal medicines. The active constituents of milk thistle are flavonolignans, which are known collectively as silymarin. The most remarkable use of silymarin is in the treatment of *Amanita* mushroom poisoning. *Amanita* mushrooms possess two extremely powerful hepatotoxins, amanitin and phalloidin (the median lethal dose of amanitin is 0.1 mg/kg body weight). Severe liver damage (and death) is avoided if silymarin is administered within 24 hours following ingestion of *Amanita*. It also is a hepatoprotective on chronic exposure to ethanol and acetaminophen toxicity.

Miscellaneous Drug Interactions

The ability of drugs and other foreign substances to stimulate (induction) metabolism of other drugs has already been discussed. Phenobarbital, for example, stimulates metabolism of a variety of drugs (e.g., phenytoin and coumarin anticoagulants). Stimulation of bishydroxycoumarin metabolism can create a problem in patients undergoing anticoagulant therapy. If phenobarbital administration is stopped, the rate of metabolism of the anticoagulant decreases, resulting in greater plasma concentrations of bishydroxycoumarin and enhanced anticoagulant activity, increasing the possibility of hemorrhage. Serious side effects have resulted from this type of interaction. These observations indicate that combined therapy of a potent drug (e.g., bishydroxycoumarin) and a inducer of drug metabolism (e.g., phenobarbital) can create a hazardous situation if the enzyme inducer is withdrawn and therapy with the potent drug is continued without an appropriate decrease in dose.

Some drugs are competitive inhibitors of nonmicrosomal metabolic pathways. Serious reactions have been reported in patients treated with an MAO inhibitor, such as trancypromine or iproniazid, because they usually are sensitive to a subsequent dose of a sympathomimetic amine (e.g., amphetamine) or a tricyclic antidepressant (e.g., amitriptyline), which is metabolized by MAO.

Allopurinol, a xanthine oxidase inhibitor used for the treatment of gout, inhibits metabolism of 6-mercaptopurine and other drugs metabolized by this enzyme. A serious drug interaction results from the concurrent use of allopurinol for gout and 6-mercaptopurine to block the immune response from a tissue transplant or as antimetabolite in neoplastic diseases. In some cases, however, allopurinol is used in conjunction with 6-mercaptopurine to control the increase in uric acid elimination from 6-mercaptopurine metabolism. The patient should be supervised closely, because when given in large doses, allopurinol, an inhibitor of purine metabolism, may have serious effects on bone marrow.

GENDER DIFFERENCES IN DRUG METABOLISM

The role of gender as a contributor to variability in xenobiotic metabolism and IDRs, which are more common in women than in men, is not clear, but increasing numbers of reports show differences in metabolism between men and women, raising the intriguing possibility that endogenous sex hormones, hydrocortisone, or their synthetic equivalents may influence the activity of inducible CYP3A. For example, N-demethylation of erythromycin was significantly higher in females than males. Nevertheless, the N-demethylation was persistent throughout adulthood. In contrast, males exhibited unchanged N-demethylation values.

Gender-dependent differences of metabolic rates have been detected for some drugs. Side-chain oxidation of propranolol was 50% faster in males than in females, but no differences between genders were noted in aromatic ring hydroxylation. N-demethylation of meperidine was depressed during pregnancy and for women taking oral contraceptives. Other examples of drugs cleared by oxidative drug metabolism more rapidly in men than in women included chlordiazepoxide and lidocaine. Diazepam, prednisolone, caffeine, and acetaminophen are metabolized slightly faster by women than by men. No gender differences have been observed in the clearance of phenytoin, nitrazepam, and trazodone, which interestingly are not substrates for the CYP3A subfamily. Gender differences in the rate of glucuronidation have been noted.

More investigation is warranted, and future pharmacokinetic studies examining the alteration in drug metabolism in one gender need to be reexamined with respect to the other gender. Even in postmenopausal women, CYP3A function may be altered and influenced by the lack of estrogen or the presence of androgens.

MAJOR PATHWAYS OF METABOLISM

Table 10.10 contains an extensive list of commonly used drugs and the CYP450 isoforms that catalyze their metabolism. In addition, Phase 1 and Phase 2 metabolic pathways for some common drugs are listed in Table 10.21.

Table 10.21. Metabolic Pathways of Common Drugs

Drug	Pathway	Drug	Pathway
Amphetamines 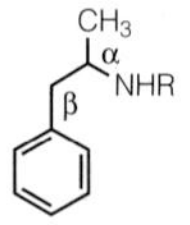	Deamination (followed by oxidation and reduction of the ketone formed) N-oxidation N-dealkylation Hydroxylation of the aromatic ring Hydroxylation of the β-carbon atom Conjugation with glucuronic acid of the acid and alcohol products from the ketone formed by deamination	Barbiturates 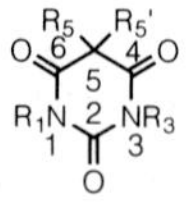	Oxidation and complete removal of substituents at carbon 5 N-dealkylation at N^1 and N^3 Desulfuration at carbon 2 (thiobarbiturates) Scission of the barbiturate ring at the 1:6 bond to give substituted malonylureas
Phenothiazines 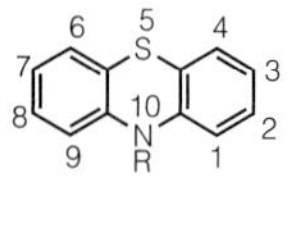	N-dealkylation in the N^{10} side chain N-oxidation in the N^{10} side chain Oxidation of the heterocyclic S atom to sulfoxide or sulfone Hydroxylation of one or both aromatic rings Conjugation of phenolic metabolites with glucuronic acid or sulfate Scission of the N^{10} side chain	Sulfonamides 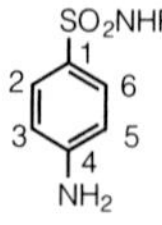	Acetylation at the N^4 amino group Conjugation with glucuronic acid or sulfate at the N^4 amino group Acetylation or conjugation with glucuronic acid at the N^1 amino group
Phenytoin 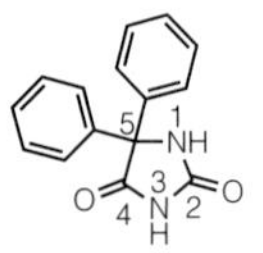	Hydroxylation of one aromatic ring Conjugation of phenolic products with glucuronic acid or sulfate Hydrolytic scission of the hydantoin ring at the bond between carbons 3 and 4 to give 5,5-diphenylhydantoic acid	Meperidine 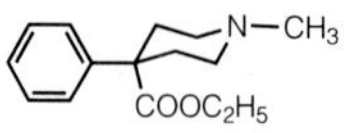	Hydroxylation and conjugation in the heterocyclic ring, R Hydrolysis of ester to acid N-dealkylation Hydroxylation of aromatic ring N-oxidation Both N-dealkylation and hydrolysis Conjugation of phenolic products
Pentazocine 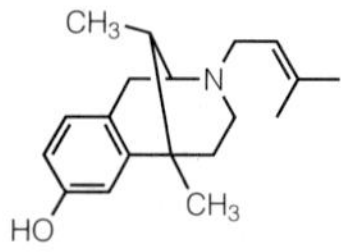	Hydroxylation of terminal methyl groups of the alkenyl side chain to give cis and trans (major) alcohols Oxidation of hydroxymethyl product of the alkenyl side chain to carboxylic acids Reduction of alkenyl side chain and oxidation of terminal methyl group	Cocaine 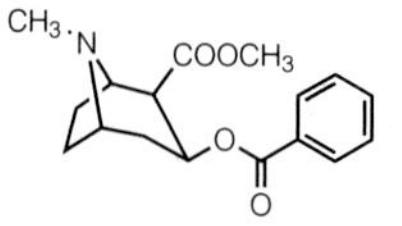	Hydrolysis of methyl ester Hydrolysis of benzoate ester N-dealkylation Both hydrolysis and N-dealkylation
Phenmetrazine 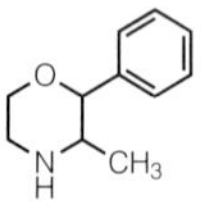	Oxidation to lactam Aromatic hydroxylation N-oxidation Conjugation of phenolic products	Ephedrine 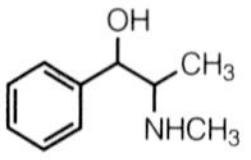	N-dealkylation Oxidative deamination Oxidation of deaminated product to benzoic acid Reduction of deaminated product to 1,2-diol
Propranolol 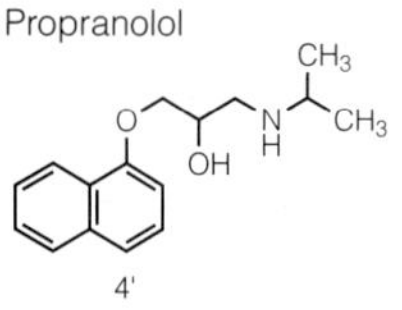	Aromatic hydroxylation at C-4' N-dealkylation Oxidative deamination Oxidation of deaminated product to naphthoxylactic acid Conjugation with glucuronic acid O-dealkylation	Indomethacin 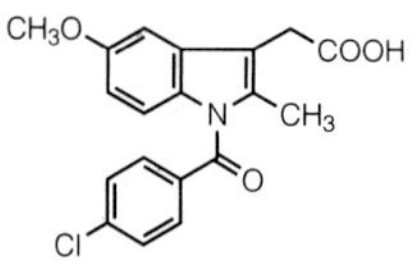	O-demethylation N-deacylation of *p*-chlorobenzoyl group Both O-dealkylation and N-deacylation Conjugation of phenolic products with glucuronic acid Other conjugation products
Diphenoxylate 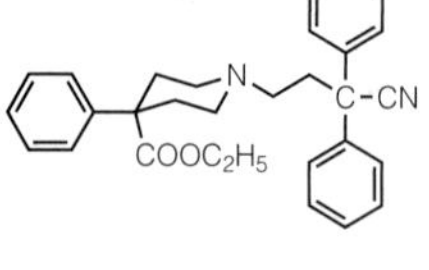	Hydrolysis of ester to acid Hydroxylation of one aromatic ring attached to the N-alkyl side chain	Diazepam 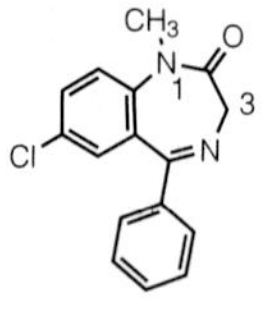	N-dealkylation at N1 Hydroxylation at carbon 3 Conjugation with glucuronic acid Both N-dealkylation of N1 and hydroxylation at carbon 3
Prostaglandins 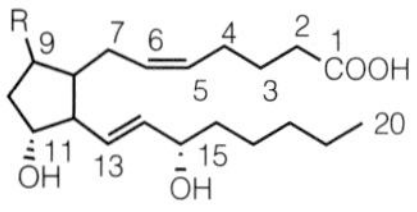	Reduction of double bonds at carbons 5 and 6, and 13 and 14 Oxidation of 15-hydroxyl to ketone β-Oxidation of carbons 3, 5 and 7 ω-Oxidation of carbon 20 to acid	Cyproheptadine 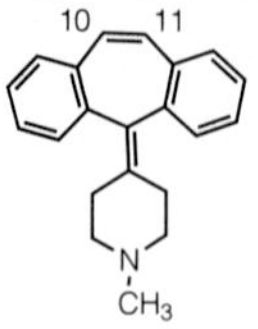	N-dealkylation 10,11-Epoxide formation Both N-dealkylation and 10,11-epoxidation
Hydralazine 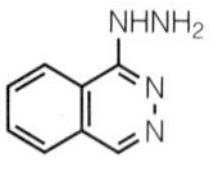	N-acetylation with cyclization to a methyl-s-triazolophthalazine N-formylation with cyclization to an s-triazolo-phthalazine Aromatic hydroxylation of benzene ring Oxidative loss of hydrazinyl group to 1-hydroxy Hydroxylation of methyl of methyl-s-triazolophthalazine Conjugation with glucuronic acid	Methadone 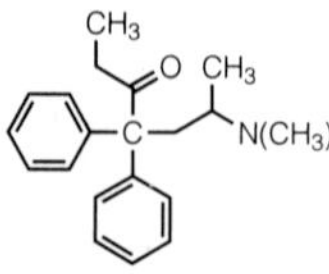	Reduction of ketone to hydroxyl Aromatic hydroxylation of one aromatic ring N-dealkylation of alcohol product N-dealkylation with cyclization to pyrrolidine

(Continued)

Table 10.21. *(Continued)*

Drug	Pathway	Drug	Pathway
Lidocaine 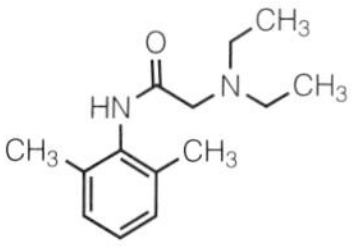	N-dealkylation Oxidative cyclization to a 4-imidazolidone N-oxidation of amide N Aromatic hydroxylation ortho to methyl Hydrolysis of amide	Imipramine 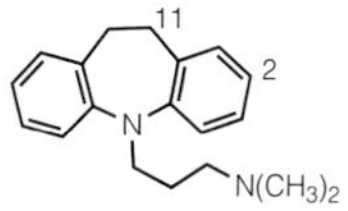	N-dealkylation Hydroxylation at C-11 Aromatic hydroxylation (C-2) N-oxidation Both N-dealkylation and hydroxylation
Cimetidine 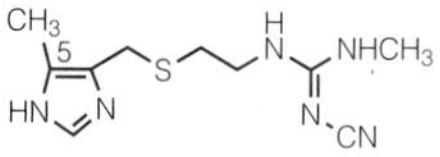	S-oxidation Hydroxylation of 5-methyl	Valproic acid 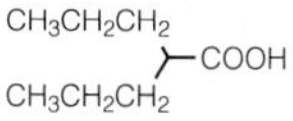	CoA thioester Dehydrogenation to (E) 2-ene Dehydrogenation to (E) 2,4-diene Dehydrogenation to 4-ene 3-Hydroxylation
Piroxicam 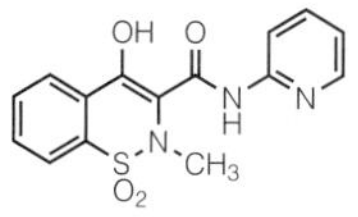	Pyridine 3'-hydroxylation Hydrolysis of amide Decarboxylation	Caffeine 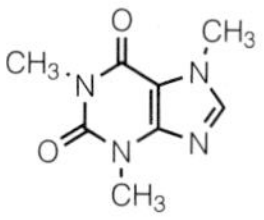	N^3-demethylation N^1-demethylation N^7-demethylation to theophylline C-8 oxidation to uric acids Imidazole ring opened
Theophylline 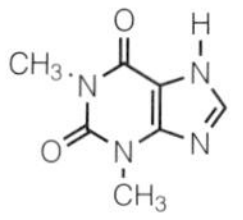	N^3-demethylation N^1-demethylation C-8 oxidation to uric acids Imidazole ring opened 1-Me xanthine to 1-Me uric acid - xanthine oxidase	Nicotine 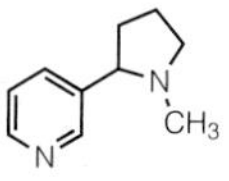	Pyrrolidine 5'-hydroxylation to cotinine Pyrrolidine N-oxidation (FMO) N-demethylation (nornicotine and norcotinine) Pyridine N-methylation 3'-Hydroxylation of cotinine
Ibuprofen 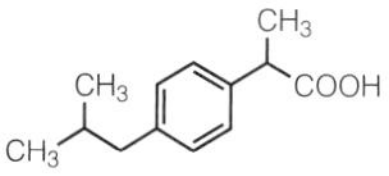	CoA thioester and epimerization of R- to S+ enantiomer Methyl hydroxylation to CH_2OH CH_2OH to COOH Acylglucuronide	Tamoxifen 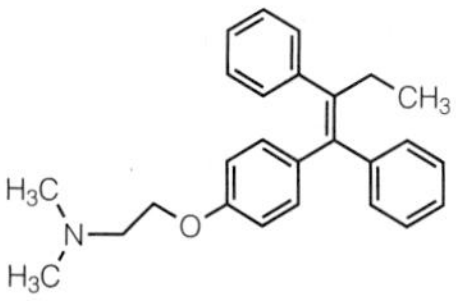	N-demethylation 4'-Hydroxylation N-oxidation (FMO) 4'-O-sulfate 4'-O-glucuronide
Lovastatin 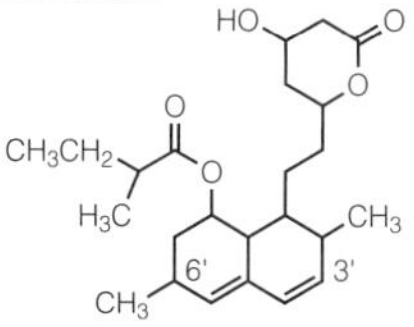	6'-Hydroxylation 3'-Side chain hydroxylation 3'-Hydroxylation β-oxidation of lactone O-glucuronides	Ciprofloxacin 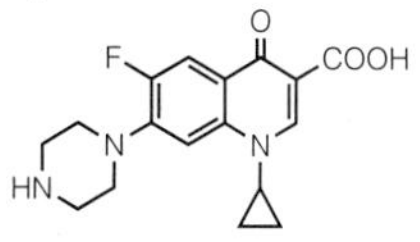	Piperazine 3'-hydroxylation N-sulfation
Labetalol 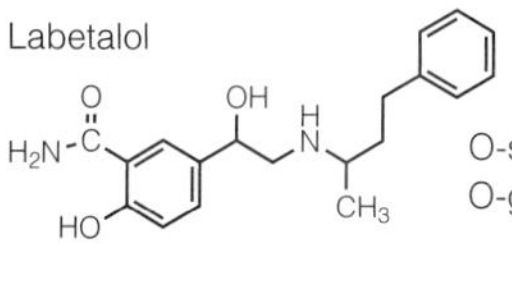	O-sulfate (major) O-glucuronide	Acetaminophen 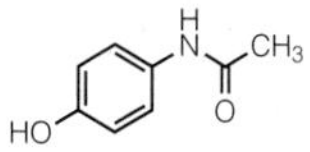	O-glucuronide O-sulfate Oxidation to N-acetyl-*p*-benzoquinoneimine Conjugation of N-acetyl-*p*-benzoquinoneimine with glutathione
Tripelennamine 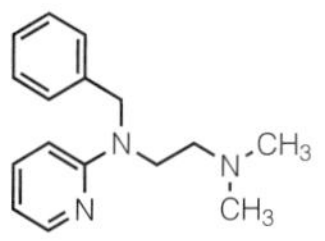	*p*-Hydroxylation Benzylic C-hydroxylation N-depyridinylation N-debenzylation	Felodipine 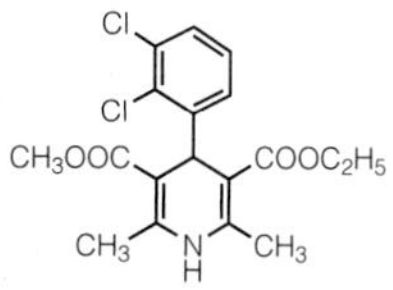	Aromatization Ester hydrolysis Methyl hydroxylation

CASE STUDY

Victoria F. Roche and S. William Zito

WH-L is a 62-year-old, Beijing-born scientist attending an international scientific meeting in your hometown. While delivering his groundbreaking paper on the neuroprotective action of some unique bicyclic molecules he has synthesized, WH-L experienced a very rapid and irregular heart rate, followed by a tight, gripping pain in his chest. Recognizing that he was having a myocardial infarction (MI), WH-L immediately took an aspirin tablet while his colleagues called an ambulance to take him to a nearby hospital. Fortunately, his quick action has averted a fatality, although the medical staff cannot get his heartbeat to stabilize. His situation is considered dire, and the decision is made to put him on an antiarrhythmic agent until he is well enough to return home to consult with his personal physician. It also is decided that β-adrenergic blocking therapy is in order. WH-L has evidence of coronary artery disease and elevated blood pressure. He is taking rosuvastatin calcium (Crestor 20 mg q.d.) to keep his serum cholesterol levels in check and flurbiprofen potassium (Ansaid, 50 mg q.i.d.) for mild-moderate arthritis pain.

As the pharmacist-in-charge on the drug therapy decision team, you consult with WH-L and learn that he recently had an oral abscess that resulted in a tooth extraction and used codeine sulfate to treat his significant, but short-term, postsurgical pain. A few years ago, he experienced a deep vein thrombosis that was treated for 12 weeks with standard doses of warfarin sodium (Coumadin). A decision is made to initiate warfarin therapy again post-MI. WH-L does not consume alcohol but loves grapefruit juice, which he always has for breakfast and often once or twice again during the course of the day. He has asked for it routinely while in the hospital. Given this medical history, and keeping the drug metabolism pathways firmly in mind, select one antiarrhythmic agent and one β-blocker that would best suit the needs of this patient. Assume that all drug choices would be therapeutically effective for the disease they are intended to treat.

1. Identify the therapeutic problem(s) for which the pharmacist's intervention may benefit the patient.
2. Identify and prioritize the patient-specific factors that must be considered to achieve the desired therapeutic outcomes.
3. Conduct a thorough metabolic analysis of all therapeutic alternatives provided in the case.
4. Evaluate the metabolic findings against the patient-specific factors and desired therapeutic outcomes and make a therapeutic decision.
5. Counsel your patient.

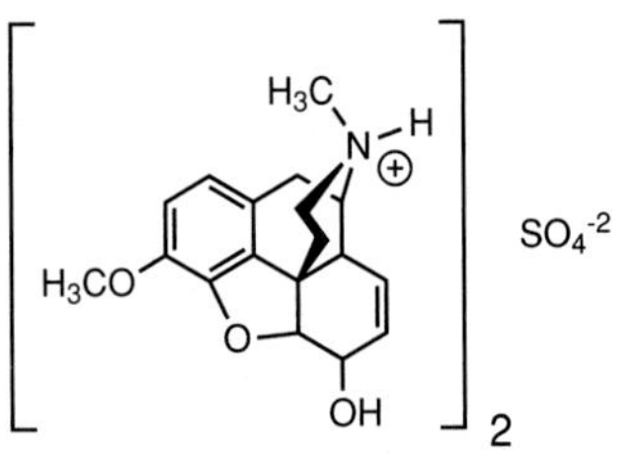

Codeine sulfate

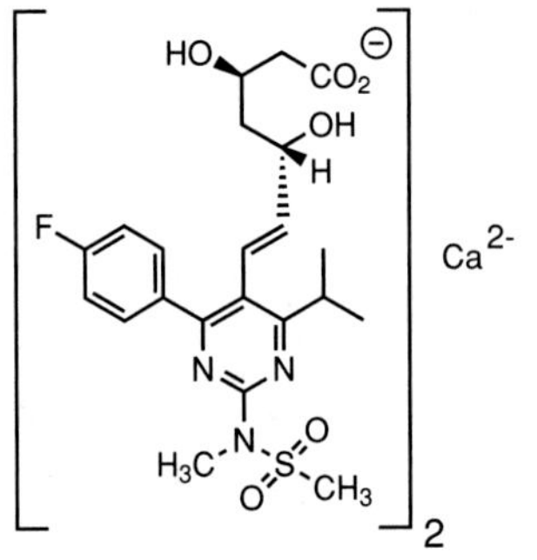

Rosuvastatin calcium

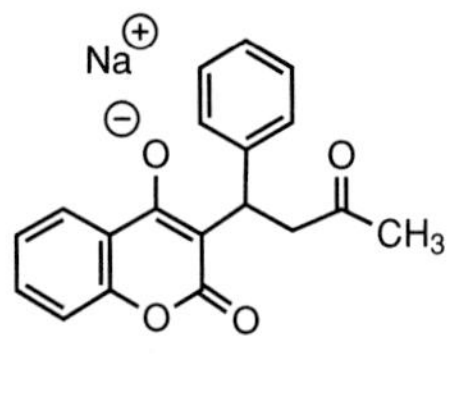

Warfarin

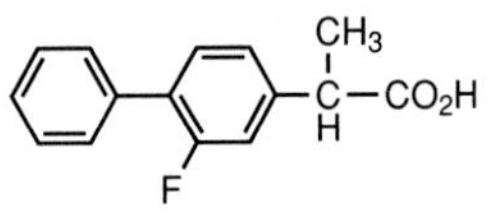

Flurbiprofen

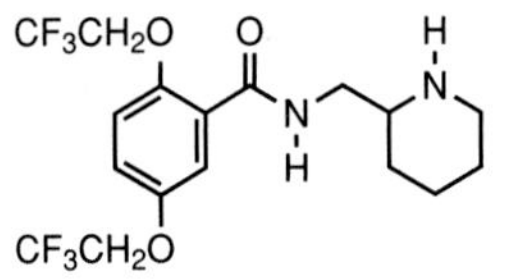

Flecainide

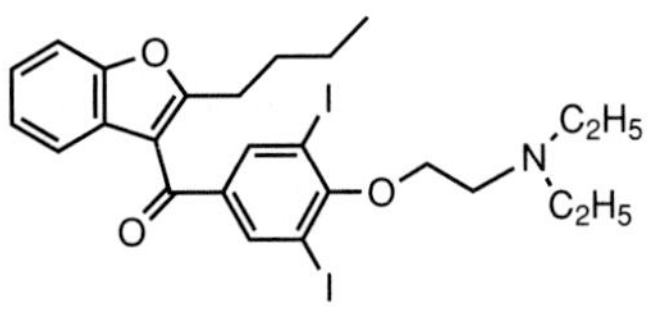

Amiodarone

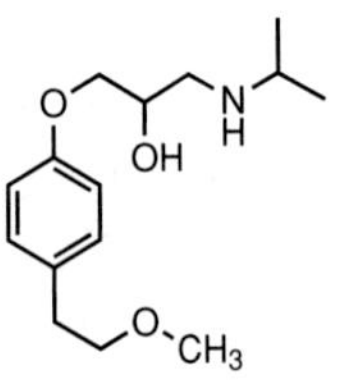

Metoprolol

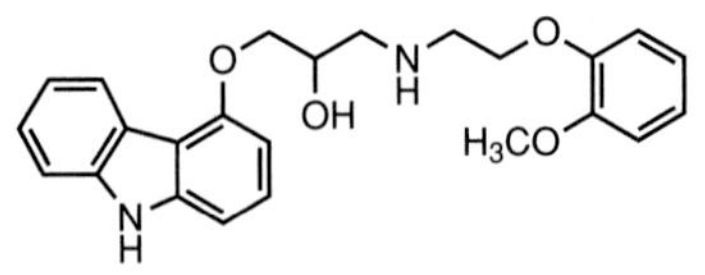

Carvedilol

References

1. Williams RT. Detoxication Mechanisms, 2nd Ed. New York: John Wiley and Sons, 1959.
2. Anders M, ed. Bioactivation of Foreign Compounds. New York: Academic Press, 1985.
3. Caldwell J, Jakoby W, eds. Biological Basis of Detoxication. New York: Academic Press, 1983.
4. Jakoby W, ed. Enzymatic Basis of Detoxication, vols I and II. New York: Academic Press, 1980.
5. Jakoby W, Bend JR, Caldwell J, eds. Metabolic Basis of Detoxication—Metabolism of Functional Groups. New York: Academic Press, 1982.
6. Mulder GJ, ed. Conjugation Reactions in Drug Metabolism: An Integrated Approach. London: Taylor and Francis, 1990.
7. Ortiz de Montellano PR, ed. Cytochrome P450: Structure Mechanism and Biochemistry, 2nd Ed. New York: Plenum Press, 1995.
8. Testa B, Jenner P, eds. Drug Metabolism: Chemical and Biochemical Aspects. New York: Marcel Dekker, 1976.
9. Testa B, Jenner P, eds. Concepts in Drug Metabolism. New York: Marcel Dekker, 1981.
10. Murphy MP. Pharmacogenomics: a new paradigm for drug development. Drug Discovery World 2000;1:23–32.
11. Wilkinson GR, Schenker S. Drug disposition and liver disease. Drug Metab Rev 1975;4:139–175.

12. McLean AJ, Morgan DJ. Clinical pharmacokinetics in patients with liver disease. Clin Pharmacokinet 1991;21:42–69.
13. Rodighiero V. Effects of liver disease on pharmacokinetics. An update. Clin Pharmacokinet 1999;37:399–443.
14. Groves JT. Models and mechanisms of cytochrome P450. In: Ortiz de Montellano PR, ed. Cytochrome P450: Structure Mechanism and Biochemistry, 3rd Ed. New York: Plenum Press, 2005, pp1–44..
15. Nielson KA, Moller BL. Cytochrome P450 in plants. In: Ortiz de Montellano PR, ed. Cytochrome P450: Structure Mechanism and Biochemistry, 3rd Ed. New York: Plenum Press, 2005, p553.
16. Nebert DW, Nelson DR, Coon MJ, et al. The P450 superfamily: update on new sequences, gene mapping, and recommended nomenclature. DNA Cell Biol 1991;10:1–14.
17. Gonzalez FJ, Gelboin HV. Human cytochromes P450: evolution and cDNA-directed expression. Environ Health Perspect 1992;98:810–885.
18. Rendic S, DiCarlo FJ. Human cytochrome P450 enzymes: a status report summarizing their reactions substrates inducers and inhibitors. Drug Metab 1997;29:413–580.
19. Guengerich FP. Enzymatic oxidation of xenobiotic chemicals. Crit Rev Biochem Mol Biol 1990;25:97–153.
20. Wighton SA, Stevens JC. The human hepatic cytochromes P450 involved in drug metabolism. Crit Rev Toxicol 1992;22:1–21.
21. Makris TM, Denisov I, SchlichTing I, et al. Activation of molecular oxygen by cytochrome P450. In: Ortiz de Montellano PR, ed. Cytochrome P450: structure mechanism and biochemistry, 3rd Ed. New York: Plenum Press, 2005, pp149–182.
22. Traber PG, McDonnell WM, Wang R. Expression and regulation of cytochrome P450I genes (CYP1A1 and CYP1A2) in the rat alimentary tract. Biochim Biophys Acta 1992;1171:167–175.
23. Roy D, Bernhardt A, Strobel H, et al. Catalysis of the oxidation of steroid and stilbene estrogens to estrogen quinone metabolites by the β-naphthoflavone-inducible cytochrome P450 1A family. Arch Biochem Biophys 1992;296: 450–456.
24. Koop DR. Oxidative and reductive metabolism of cytochrome P4502E1. FASEB J 1992;6:724–730.
25. Raucy JL, Kraner JC, Lasker JM. Bioactivation of halogenated hydrocarbons by cytochrome P4502E1. Crit Rev Toxicol 1993;23:1–20.
26. White RE, Coon MJ. Oxygen activation by cytochrome P450. Ann Rev Biochem 1980;49:315–356.
27. White RE. The involvement of free radicals in the mechanisms of monooxygenases Pharmacol Ther 1991;49:21–42.
28. Groves JT. Key elements of the chemistry of cytochrome P450. The oxygen rebound mechanism. J Chem Educ 1985;62:928–931.
29. Guengerich FP, MacDonald TL. Chemical mechanisms of catalysis by cytochromes P450: a unified view. Acc Chem Res 1984;17:9–16.
30. Guengerich FP, MacDonald TL. Mechanisms of cytochrome P450 catalysis. FASEB J 1990;4:2453–2459.
31. Ortiz de Montellano PR. Cytochrome P-450 catalysis: radical intermediates and dehydrogenation reactions. Trends Pharmacol Sci 1989;10:354–359.
32. Correia MA, Ortiz de Montellano PR. Inhibition of cytochrome P450 enzymes. In: Ortiz de Montellano PR, ed . Cytochrome P450: Structure Mechanism and Biochemistry, 3rd Ed. New York: Plenum Press, 2005, pp247–322.
33. Ortiz de Montellano PR. Alkenes and alkynes. In: Anders M, ed. Bioactivation of Foreign Compounds. New York: Academic Press, 1985:121–155.
34. Williams SN, Dunkan E, Bradfield CA. Induction of cytochrome P450 enzymes. In: Ortiz de Montellano PR, ed. Cytochrome P450: Structure Mechanism and Biochemistry, 3rd Ed. New York: Plenum Press, 2005, pp323–346.
35. Okey AB. Enzyme induction in the cytochrome P450 system. Pharmacol Ther 1990;45:241–298.
36. Barry M, Feely J. Enzyme induction and inhibition. Pharmacol Ther 1992; 48:71–94.
37. Guengerich FP. Metabolic activation of carcinogens. Pharmacol Ther 1992; 54:17–61.
38. Martucci CP, Fishman J. P450 enzymes of estrogen metabolism. Pharmacol Ther 1993;57:237–257.
39. Conney AH, Pantuck EJ, Kuntzman R, et al. Nutrition and chemical biotransformations in man. Clin Pharmacol Ther 1977;22:707–711.
40. Murray M, Reidy GF. Selectivity in the inhibition of mammalian cytochromes P-450 by chemical agents. Pharmacol Rev 1990;42:85–101.
41. Murray M. P450 enzymes. Clin Pharmacokinet 1992;23:132–146.
42. Ballie TA. Metabolism of valproate to hepatotoxic intermediates. Pharm Weekbl [Sci] 1992;14:122–125.
43. Thummel KE, Kharasch ED, Podoll, et al. Human liver microsomal enflurane defluorination catalyzed by cytochrome P-450 2E1. Drug Metab Dispos 1993;21:350–356.
44. Elliot RH, Strunun L. Hepatotoxicity of volatile anesthetics. Br J Anaesth 1993;70:339–348.
45. Zeigler DM. Flavin-containing monooxygenases. Drug Metab Rev 1988; 19:1–32.
46. Zeigler DM. Flavin-containing monooxygenases: enzymes adapted for multisubstrate specificity. Trends Pharmacol Sci 1990;11:321–324.
47. Singer TP, Ramsay RR. Mechanism of neurotoxicity of MPTP. FEBS Lett 1990;274:1–8.
48. Krueger SK, Williams DE. Mammalian flavin-containing monooxygenases: structure/function, genetic polymorphisms and role in drug metabolism. Pharmacol Thera 2005;106:357–387.
49. Cashman JR, Wang Z, Yang L, et al. Stereo- and regioselective N- and S-oxidation of tertiary amines and sulfides in the presence of adult liver microsomes. Drug Metab Dispos 1993;21:492–501.
50. Hollenberg PF. Mechanism of cytochrome P450 and peroxide-catalyzed xenobiotic metabolism. FASEB J 1992;6:686–694.
51. Ortiz de Montellano PR, De Voss J. Substrates oxidation by cytochrome P450 engymes. In: Ortiz de Montellano PR, ed. Cytochrome P450: structure mechanism and biochemistry, 3rd Ed. New York: Plenum Press, 2005, pp183–246.
52. Hille R. Molybdenum enzymes. Essays Biochem 1999;34:125–137.
53. Kitamura S, Sugihara K, Ohta S. Drug-metabolizing ability of molybdenum hydroxylases. Drug Metab Pharmacokinetics 2006;21:83–98.
54. Lang D, Kalgutkar AS. Non-P450 mediated oxidative metabolism of xenobiotics. In: Lee JS, Obach RS, Fisher MB, Drug Metabolizing Enzymes: Cytochrome P450 and Other Enzymes in Drug Discovery and Development. New York: FontisMedia-Marcel Dekker, 2003, pp483–539.
55. Costa LG, Li WF, Richter RJ, et al. The role of paraoxonase (PON1) in the detoxication of organophosphates and its human polymorphism. Chemico-Biological Reactions 1999;119–120:429–439.
56. Mulder GJ, ed. Conjugation Reactions in Drug Metabolism: An Integrated approach. New York: Taylor and Francis, 1990.
57. Jansen PLM, Mulder PJ, Burchell B, et al. New developments in glucuronidation research: report of a workshop on "Glucuronidation its role in health and disease." Hepatology 1992;15:532–544.
58. Burchell B, Mcgurk K, Brierly CH, et al. UDP-glucuronosyltransferases. In: Guengerich FP, ed. Comprehensive Toxicology, vol 3. New York: Pergamon–Elsevier Science, 1997, pp449–473.
59. Spahn-Langguth H, Benet LZ. Acylglucuronides revisited: is the glucuronidation process a toxification as well as a detoxication mechanism. Drug Metab Rev 1992;24:5–48.
60. Mulder GJ. Pharmacological effects of drug conjugates: is morphine 6-glucuronide an exception. Trends Pharmacol Sci 1992;13:302–304.
61. Falani CN. Enzymology of human cytosolic sulfotransferases. FASEB J. 1997; 11:206–216.
62. Raftigianis RB, Wood TC, Weinshilboum RM. Human phenolsulfotransferases SULT1A2 and SULT1A1. Biochem Pharmacol 1999;58:605–616.
63. Caldwell J, Hutt AJ, Fournel-Gigleux S. The metabolic chiral inversion and dispositional enantioselectivity of the 2-arylpropionic acids and their biological activity. Biochem Pharmacol 1988;37:105–115.
64. Tracy TS, Wirthwein DP, Hall SD. Metabolic inversion of R-ibuprofen. Drug Metab Dispos 1993;21:114–119.
65. Nelson SD. Arylamines and arylamide: oxidation mechanisms. In: Anders M, ed. Bioactivation of foreign compounds. New York: Academic Press, 1985:349–375.
66. Ahmed AE. Nitriles. In: Anders M, ed. Bioactivation of foreign compounds. New York: Academic Press, 1985:485–489.
67. Dobrinska MR. Enterohepatic circulation of drugs. J Clin Pharmacol 1989; 29:577–580.
68. Ilett KF, Tee LBG, Reeves PT, et al. Metabolism of drugs and other xenobiotics in the gut lumen and wall. Pharmacol Ther 1990;46:67–93.
69. Schmucker DL. Aging and drug disposition: an update. Pharmacol Rev 1985;37:133–145.
70. Durnas C, Loi CM, Cusack BJ. Hepatic drug metabolism and aging. Clin Pharmacokinet 1990;19:359–389.
71. Woodhouse K, Wynne HA. Age-related changes in hepatic function: implications for drug therapy. Drugs Aging 1992;2:243–246.
72. Smit JW, Huisman MT, van Tellingen O, et al. Absence or pharmacological blocking of placental P-glycoprotein profoundly increases fetal drug exposure. J Clin Invest 1999;104:1441–1447.
73. Ingelmann-Sundberg M, Oscarson M, McLellan RA. Polymorphic human cytochrome P450 enzymes: an opportunity for individualized drug treatment. Trends Pharmacol Sci 1999;20:342–349.
74. Daly AK, Cholerton S, Gregory W, et al. Metabolic polymorphisms. Pharmacol Ther 1993;57:129–160.
75. Gaedigk A. Interethic differences of drug-metabolizing enzymes. Int J Clin Pharmacol Ther 2000;38:61–68.
76. Myer UA, Skoda RC, Zanger UM. The genetic polymorphism of debrisoquine/sparteine metabolism—molecular mechanisms et al. Pharmacol Ther 1990; 46:297–308.
77. Kaminsky LS, Fasco MJ. Small intestinal cytochromes P450. Crit Rev Toxicol 1991;21:407–422.
78. Kane GC, Lipsky JJ. Drug–grapefruit juice interactions. Mayo Clin Proc 2000;75:933–942.
79. Yu Dk. The contribution of P-glycoprotein to the pharmacokinetics of drug–drug interactions. J Clin Pharmacol 1999;39:1203–1211.
80. Silverman JA. Multidrug resistance transporters. Pharm Biotechnol 1999;12: 353–386.
81. Oesch F. Metabolic transformation of clinically used drugs to epoxides: new perspectives in drug–drug interactions. Biochem Pharmacol 1976;25:1935–1937.
82. Ohnishi A, Matsuo H, Yamada S, et al. Effect of furanocoumarin derivatives in grapefruit juice on the uptake of vinblastine by Caco-2 cells and on the activity of cytochrome P450 3A4. Br J Pharmacol 2000;130:1369–1377.

83. Watkins PB. Role of cytochrome P450 in drug metabolism and hepatotoxicity. Semin Liver Dis 1990;10:235–250.
84. Roth RA, Vinegar A. Action by the lungs on circulating xenobiotic agents, with a case study of physiologically based pharmacokinetic modeling of benzo[a]pyrene disposition. Pharmacol Ther 1990;48:143–155.
85. Reed CJ. Drug metabolism in the nasal cavity. Drug Metab Rev 1993;25:173–205.
86. Sarkar MA. Drug metabolism in the nasal mucosa. Pharmacol Res 1992;9: 1–8.
87. Testa B, Jenner P, eds. Drug metabolism: chemical and biological aspects. New York: Marcel Dekker, 1976.
88. Lee WM. Drug-induced hepatotoxicity. N Engl J Med 2003;349:474–485.
89. Navarro VJ, Senior JR. Drug-related hepatotoxicity. N Engl J Med. 2006:354: 731–739.
90. Watkins, PB, Kaplowitz, N, Slattery JT, et al. Aminotransferase elevations in healthy adults receiving 4 grams of acetaminophen daily. JAMA 2006;296:87–93.
91. Park BK, Kitteringham NR, Maggs JL, et al. The role of metabolic activation in drug-induced hepatotoxicity. Annu Rev Pharmacol Toxicol 2005;45: 177–202.
92. Williams DP, Kitteringham NR, Naisbitt DJ, et al. Are chemically reactive metabolites responsible for adverse reactions to drugs? Curr Drug Metab 2002;3:351–366.
93. Kalgutkar AS, Gardner I, Obach RS, et al. A comprehensive listing of bioactivation pathways of organic functional groups. Curr Drug Metab 2005;6: 161–225.
94. Myers TG, Dietz EC, Anderson N, et al. A comparative study of mouse liver proteins arylated by reactive metabolites of acetaminophen and its nonhepatotoxic regioisomer, 3'-hydroxyacetanilide. Chem Res Toxicol 1995;8:403–413.
95. Holt MP, Ju C. Mechanisms of drug-induced liver injury. AAPS J 2006;3; 8:E48–E54.
96. Ju C, Uetrecht JP. Mechanism of idiosyncratic drug reactions: reactive metabolite formation, protein binding, and the regulation of the immune system. Curr Drug Metab 2002;3:367–377.
97. Miller EC, Miller JA. Mechanisms of chemical carcinogenesis. Cancer 1981; 47:1055–1064.
98. Gillette JR. The problem of chemically reactive metabolites. Drug Metabolism Reviews 1982;13:941–961.
99. Reed DJ. Cellular defense mechanisms against reactive metabolites. In: Anders M, ed. Bioactivation of Foreign Compounds. New York: Academic Press, 1985:71–108.
100. Nelson SD, et al. Role of metabolic activation in chemical-induced tissue injury. In: Jerina DM, ed. Drug Metabolism Concepts. ACS Symposium Series 44. Washington, DC: American Chemical Society, 1977:155–185.
101. Uetrecht J. Bioactivation. In: Lee JS, Obach RS, Fisher M, eds. Drug-Metabolizing Enzymes: Cytochrome P450 and Other Enzymes in Drug Discovery and Development. Weimar, TX: Culinary and Hospitality Industry Publications Services, 2003, pp87–145.
102. Boelsterli UA. Xenobiotic acyl glucuronides and acyl CoA thioesters as protein-reactive metabolites with the potential to cause idiosyncratic drug reactions. Curr Drug Metab 2002;3:439–450.
103. Zhou S, Yung Chan S, Cher Goh B, et al. Mechanism-based inhibition of cytochrome P450 3A4 by therapeutic drugs. Clin Pharmacokinet 2005;44: 279–304.
104. Dressor GK, Spence JD, Bailey DG. Pharmacokinetic–pharmacodynamic consequences and clinical relevance of cytochrome P450 3A4 inhibition. Clin Pharmacokinet 2000;38:41–57.
105. Michalets EL. Update: clinically significant cytochrome P450 interactions. Pharmacotherapy 1998;18:84–112.
106. Bailey DG, Dresser GK, Kreeft JH, et al. Grapefruit–felodipine interaction: effect of unprocessed fruit and probable active ingredients. Clin Pharmacol Ther 2000;68:468–477.
107. Evans AM. Influence of dietary components on the gastrointestinal metabolism and transport of drugs. Ther Drug Monit 2000;22:131–136.
108. Johnson BM, Van Breemen RB. In vitro formation of quinoid metabolites of the dietary supplement cimicifuga racemosa (black cohosh). Chem Res Toxicol 2003;16:838–846.
109. Saller R, Meier R, Brignoli R. The use of silymarin in the treatment of liver diseases. Drugs 2001;61:2035–2063.

Suggested Readings

Anders M, ed. Bioactivation of Foreign Compounds. New York: Academic Press, 1985.
Caldwell J, Jakoby W, eds. Biological Basis of Detoxication. New York: Academic Press, 1983.
Jakoby W, ed. Enzymatic Basis of Detoxication, vols I and II. New York: Academic Press, 1980.
Jakoby W, Bend JR, Caldwell J, eds. Metabolic Basis of Detoxication—Metabolism of Functional Groups. New York: Academic Press, 1982.
Lee JS, Obach RS, Fisher M, eds., Drug-Metabolizing Enzymes :Cytochrome P450 and Other Enzymes in Drug Discovery and Development. Weimer, TX: Culinary and Hospitality Industry Publications Services, 2003.
Mulder GJ, ed. Conjugation Reactions in Drug Metabolism: An Integrated Approach. London: Taylor and Francis, 1990.
Ortiz de Montellano PR, ed. Cytochrome P450: Structure Mechanism and Biochemistry, 2nd Ed. New York: Plenum Press, 1995.
Testa B, Jenner P, eds. Concepts in Drug Metabolism. New York: Marcel Dekker, 1981.
Testa B, Jenner P, eds. Drug Metabolism: Chemical and Biochemical Aspects. New York: Marcel Dekker, 1976.
Williams RT, ed. Detoxication Mechanisms, 2nd Ed. New York: John Wiley and Sons, 1959.
Wolf TF, ed. Handbook of Drug Metabolism. New York: Marcel Dekker, 1999.

11. *U.S. Drug Regulation: An Overview*

Douglas J. Pisano

INTRODUCTION

Regulations and laws are central, social constructs that provide guidance for all societies around the globe. Governments create laws in a number of ways and with various intents for a myriad of purposes. In the United States, laws are created by the Congress, a body of officials elected by the citizenry and charged with the governance of the country by representing the common, public good. The Congress proposes and passes laws that are relatively general in nature and intended to address some particular issue in a fashion that can be consistently applied by all who are affected by them. Once passed, laws are remanded to the appropriate government or administrative agency, which then decides how these laws are to be applied. These applications of law are termed "regulations." Regulations serve as the practical foundation from which citizens adhere to the law as it was originally intended.

In the United States, all food, drugs, cosmetics and medical devices, for both humans and animals, are regulated under the authority of the U.S. Food and Drug Administration (FDA). The U.S. FDA and all its regulations were created by the federal government in response to the pressing need to address the safety of the public with respect to its foods and medicinals. The purpose of this chapter is to describe and explain the nature and extent of these regulations as they apply to drugs in the United States. A historical perspective is offered as a foundation for regulatory context. In addition, the chapter will discuss the U.S. FDA's regulatory oversight and that of other agencies, the drug approval and development process, the mechanisms used to regulate manufacturing and marketing, as well as various violation and enforcement schema.

BRIEF HISTORY OF DRUG LAWS AND REGULATIONS

Before 1902, the U.S. government took a hands-off approach to the regulation of drugs. Many of the drugs available were so-called "patent medicines," which were so named because each had a more or less descriptive or patent name that was protected by a trademark, the contents of which were incompletely disclosed. No laws, regulations, or standards existed to regulate drugs, their purity, and their strength to any noticeable extend, even though the U.S. Pharmacopeia (USP) became a reality in 1820 as the first official compendia of the United States. The USP set standards for drug strength and purity that could be used by physicians and pharmacists who needed centralized guidelines to extract, compound, and otherwise use drug components that existed at the time (1).

Biologics Control Act

In 1848, however, the first U.S. drug law, the Drug Importation Act, was enacted when American troops serving in Mexico became seriously ill from the quinine that was administered to treat malaria. The quinine was subsequently discovered to be adulterated. This law required laboratory inspection, detention, and even destruction of drugs that did not meet acceptable standards. Later, in 1902, the Virus, Serum, and Toxins Act (Biologics Control Act) was passed in response to tetanus-infected diphtheria antitoxin serum that was manufactured by a small laboratory in St. Louis, Missouri. Ten schoolchildren died as a result of the infected serum. No national standards were as yet in place for establishing purity or potency of medicinal products.

Wiley Act

The Biologics Control Act authorized the U.S. Public Health Service to license and regulate the interstate sale of serum, vaccines, and related biological products used to prevent or treat disease. This Act also spurred Dr. Harvey W. Wiley, Chief Chemist for the Bureau of Chemistry, a branch of the U.S. Department of Agriculture and the forerunner for today's U.S. FDA, to investigate the country's foods and drugs. He established the Hygienic Table, a group of young men who volunteered to serve as human guinea pigs, which would allow Dr. Wiley to feed them a controlled diet laced with a variety of preservatives and artificial colors. More popularly known as the "Poison Squad," they helped Dr. Wiley gather enough data to prove that many of America's foods and drugs were either "adulterated" and that the products' strength or purity were suspect or "misbranded" with inadequate or inaccurate labeling. Dr. Wiley's efforts, along with publication of Upton Sinclair's *The Jungle* (a book revealing the putrid conditions in America's meat industry), were rewarded when Congress passed America's first food and drug law in 1906, the Pure Food and Drug Act (USPFDA; also known as the Wiley Act). The Wiley Act prohibited interstate commerce of misbranded foods or drugs based on their labeling. This act did not affect unsafe drugs, however, in that its legal authority would only come to bear when a product's ingredients were falsely labeled. Even intentionally false therapeutic claims were not prohibited.

Sherley Amendment

Changes in the labeling of drugs began to occur in 1911 with the enactment of the Sherley Amendment, which was intended to prohibit the labeling of medications with false therapeutic claims that were meant to defraud the purchaser. The Sherley Amendment, however, required the government to find proof of intentional labeling fraud. Later, in 1937, a sentinel event occurred that changed the entire regulatory picture. Sulfa (e.g., sulfanilamide) became the miracle drug of the time and was used to treat many life-threatening infections. It tasted bad and was hard to swallow, which led entrepreneurs to seek a palatable solution. S.E. Massingill Co. of Bristol, Tennessee, developed what they thought was a palatable, raspberry-flavored liquid product. They used diethylene glycol to solubilize the sulfa, however, and six gallons of this dangerous mixture ("Elixir of Sulfanilamide") killed approximately 107 people, mostly children.

Federal Food, Drug, and Cosmetic Act

The result of these unnecessary deaths from ingestion of diethylene glycol was the passage of one of the most comprehensive statutes in the history of U.S. health law, the Federal Food, Drug, and Cosmetic Act of 1938 (FDCA). The enactment of this act repealed the Sherley Amendment and required that all new drugs be tested by their manufacturers for human safety and that results then be submitted to the government for marketing approval via a New Drug Application. The FDCA also mandated that drugs be labeled with adequate directions if they were shown to have had harmful effects. In addition, the FDCA authorized the U.S. FDA to conduct unannounced inspections of drug manufacturing facilities. Though amended many times since 1938, the FDCA is still the broad foundation of the statutory authority for the U.S. FDA as it exists today.

A new crisis loomed, however. Throughout the late 1950s, European and Canadian physicians began to encounter a number of infants born with a curious birth defect called phocomeglia, which resulted in limbs that resembled "flippers" similar to those found on seals. These birth defects were traced back to mothers who had been prescribed the drug thalidomide in an effort to relieve morning sickness while pregnant. The manufacturer of this drug applied for U.S. marketing approval as a sleep aid. Because of the efforts of Dr. Frances O. Kelsey, however, who was the U.S. FDA's chief medical officer at the time, the case was made that the drug was not safe for human consumption and, therefore, not effective for release in the U.S. marketplace.

Kefauver-Harris Act

Dr. Kelsey's efforts and decisive work by the Congress resulted in yet another necessary amendment to the FDCA in 1962, the Kefauver-Harris Act. This Act essentially closed many of the loopholes regarding drug safety in U.S. law. These "Drug Efficacy Amendments" now required manufacturers to prove the safety and efficacy of their drug products registered with the U.S. FDA, to be inspected at least every 2 years, to have their prescription drug advertising approved by the U.S. FDA (this authority being transferred from the Federal Trade Commission), to provide and obtain documented "informed consent" from research subjects before human clinical trials, and to have increased controls over drug manufacturing and testing to determine drug effectiveness.

To address these new provisions of the Act, the U.S. FDA contracted the National Academy of Sciences, along with the National Research Council, to examine some 3,400 drug products approved between 1938 and 1962 based on safety alone. Called the Drug Efficacy Study Implementation Review of 1966 (DESI), it charged these organizations with making a determination as to whether post-1938 drug products were "Effective," "Probably Effective," "Possibly Effective," or "Ineffective" for the indications claimed in their labeling. Those products not deemed "Effective" were either removed from the marketplace, reformulated, or sold with a clear warning to prescribers that the product was deemed not to be effective.

Over-The-Counter Product Review

Later, in 1972, the U.S. FDA began to examine over-the-counter (OTC) drug products. Phase II of the Drug Efficacy Amendments required the U.S. FDA to determine the efficacy of OTC drug products. This project was much larger in scope than the analysis of prescription drugs. During the 1970s, American consumers could choose from more than 300,000 OTC drug products. The U.S. FDA soon realized that it did not have the resources to evaluate each and every OTC drug product and, hence, created advisory panels of scientists, medical professionals, and consumers who were charged with evaluating the active ingredients used in OTC products within 80 defined therapeutic categories. After examining both the scientific and medical literature of the day, the advisory panels made decisions regarding active ingredients and their labeling. The result was a "monograph" that described, in detail, acceptable active ingredients and labeling for products within a therapeutic class. Products that complied with monograph guidelines were deemed "Category I: Safe and Effective, Not Misbranded." Products not in compliance with monograph guidelines, however, were deemed "Category II: Not Safe and Effective" or "Misbranded." Category II products were removed from the marketplace or reformulated. Products for which data was insufficient for classification were deemed "Category III" and allowed to continue on the market until substantive data could be established or until they were reformulated and in compliance with the monograph. The OTC Drug Review took approximately 20 years to complete.

Federal Controlled Substances Act

Though numerous other federal laws and regulations were passed throughout the 1970s, many were based on regulating the professional practice of medical professionals or for the direct protection of consumers. For example, the Federal Controlled Substances Act, part of the Comprehensive Drug Abuse and Prevention Act of 1970, placed drugs with a relatively high potential for abuse into five federal schedules along with a "closed record keeping system" designed to track federally controlled substances via a definite paper trail as they were ordered, prescribed, dispensed, and used throughout the health care system.

Orphan Drug Act

The 1980s also saw significant regulatory change. Biotechnology had begun on a grand scale, and the pharmaceutical industry was on its cutting edge. Many of the medicinal compounds being discovered were shown to be very expensive and to have limited use in the general U.S. population. These compounds could prove lifesaving, however, to demographically small patient populations (less than 200,000) who suffered from diseases and conditions considered to be rare. In an effort to encourage these biotech pharmaceutical companies to continue developing these and other products, Congress passed the Orphan Drug Act in 1983. The Act continues to allow manufacturers to gain incentives for research, development, and marketing of drug products used to treat rare diseases or conditions that otherwise would be unprofitable via a system of breaks and deductions in a manufacturer's corporate taxes. Though the success of the Orphan Drug Act provided great medical benefit for a few, a scandal was looming in other parts of the pharmaceutical industry.

Price Competition and Patent Restoration Act (Waxman-Hatch Act)

The generic pharmaceutical industry experienced steady growth as many of the exclusive patents enjoyed by major pharmaceutical companies for brand-named products were beginning to expire. Generic versions of these now freely copied products were appearing much more frequently in the marketplace. These generic copies, however, were required to undergo the same rigorous testing that brand name, pioneer, or innovator products did. This led to a very public scandal in which a few unscrupulous generic pharmaceutical companies took shortcuts in reporting data, submitted fraudulent samples, and offered bribes to U.S. FDA officials to gain easy and rapid market approval of their products. As a result, Congress passed the Price Competition and Patent Restoration Act of 1984. This Act, also called the Waxman-Hatch Act after its sponsors, was designed to level the playing field in the prescription drug industry with regard to pioneer/innovator/brand name prescription drug products and their generic copies. The Act was composed of two distinct parts, or "Titles." Title I was for the benefit of the generic pharmaceutical industry and extended the scope of the Abbreviated New Drug Application to cover generic versions of drug products approved after 1962. It required that generic versions of pioneer or innovator drugs have the same relevant properties regarding bioequivalence (rate and extent of absorption of the active drug in the human body) and pharmaceutical equivalence (same dosage form as the pioneer drug to which it is compared). Though somewhat simplified, the Waxman-Hatch Act permitted easier market access to generic copies of pioneer drugs provided they were not significantly different from the pioneer drug in its absorption, action, and dosage form. In addition, Title II was designed to aid and encourage research-based or innovator pharmaceutical companies in continuing their search for new and useful medicinal compounds by extending the patent life of pioneer drug products while in the U.S. FDA "review period."

Prescription Drug User Fee Act

The patent extension benefit has become somewhat moot, however, because of an overall reduction in U.S. FDA review time as a result of prescription drug user fees. In 1992, Congress passed the Prescription Drug User Fee Act (PDUFA). The Act was intended to help the U.S. FDA generate additional funds to upgrade and modernize its operations and to accelerate drug approval. It authorized the U.S. FDA to charge pharmaceutical manufacturers a "user fee" to accelerate drug review. As a result of the PDUFA legislation, the U.S. FDA has been able to reduce approval time of new pharmaceutical products from more than 30 months to approximately 13 to 15 months. The Act had a "sunset" provision, however, that limited the authority of the U.S. FDA to charge user fees until the year 1997.

U.S. FDA Modernization Act

After reviewing the successes of the PDUFA legislation, Congress extended the user fee provisions during passage of the U.S. FDA Modernization Act (FDAMA) of 1997. The FDAMA reauthorized the fees until the year 2002 in an effort to further reduce prescription drug approval time. The Act, however, not only extended user fee provisions. It also gave the U.S. FDA the authority to conduct "fast-track" product reviews to further speed lifesaving drug therapies to market, permitted an additional 6-month patent exclusivity for pediatric prescription drug products, and required the National Institutes of Health to build a publicly accessible database of clinical studies involving investigational drugs or life-threatening diseases.

Summary

American drug law has come quite far since the early 1900s. Today, the U.S. FDA continues to work with Congress and the pharmaceutical industry to regulate and evaluate new and existing drug, biologic, and device products. The overriding regulatory challenge that the U.S. FDA will face will be to keep current, through regulation and policy, with future technological advances by the science and the industry.

REGULATORY OVERSIGHT OF PHARMACEUTICALS

The primary responsibility for the regulation and oversight of pharmaceuticals and the pharmaceutical industry lies with U.S. FDA, created in 1931 and one of several branches within the U.S. Department of Health and Human Services. The U.S. FDA's counterparts within that department include agencies such as the Centers for Disease Control and Prevention, the National Institutes of Health, and the Health Care Financing Administration.

U.S. Food and Drug Administration

The U.S. FDA is organized into a number of Offices and Centers headed by a Commissioner who is appointed by the President with consent of the Senate. It is a scientifically based law enforcement agency whose mission is to safeguard the public health and to ensure honesty and fairness between health regulated industries (i.e., pharmaceutical, device, biologic, and the consumer) (2). It licenses and inspects manufacturing facilities, tests products, evaluates claims and prescription drug advertising, monitors research, and creates regulations, guidelines, standards and policies. It does all this through its Office of Operations, which contains component Offices and Centers such as the Center for Drug Evaluation and Research (CDER), Center for Biologics Evaluation and Research, Center for Devices and Radiological Health (CDRH), Center for Food Safety and Applied Nutrition, Center for Veterinary Medicine, Office of Orphan Products Development, Office of Biotechnology, Office of Regulatory Affairs, and National Center for Toxicological Research. Each of these entities has a defined role, but sometimes their authorities overlap. For example, if a pharmaceutical company submits a drug that is contained and delivered to a patient during therapy by a device not comparable to any other, the CDER and CDRH may need to coordinate that product's approval. Most prescription drugs are evaluated by CDER, but any other Center or Office may become involved with its review. One of the most significant resources to industry and consumers is the U.S. FDA's website (http://www.fda.gov) and its FDA approved drug products website (http://www.accessdata.fda.gov/scripts/cder/drugsatfda/index.cfm). Easily accessible and navigable, each Center and Office has its own HTML page within the site.

Other Governmental Agencies

The U.S. FDA is not the only agency within the U.S. government with a stake in pharmaceutical issues. The Federal Trade Commission has authority over general business practices in general, such as deceptive and anticompetitive practices (i.e., false advertising). In addition, the Federal Trade Commission regulates the advertising of OTC drugs, medical devices, and cosmetics. To a lesser degree, the Consumer Product Safety Commission regulates hazardous substances and the containers of poisons and other harmful agents, the U.S. Environmental Protection Agency regulates pesticides used in agriculture, the U.S. FDA regulates food products; the Occupational Safety and Health Administration regulates the working environment of employees who may use U.S. FDA–regulated commodities (i.e., syringes, chemotherapy, and chemical reagents); the Health Care Financing Administration regulates the federal Medicaid and Medicare programs, and the Drug Enforcement Administration enforces the Federal Controlled Substances Act and is charged with controlling and monitoring the flow of licit and illicit controlled substances. Additionally, various state and local drug control agencies establish their own regulations and procedures for manufacturing, research, and development of pharmaceuticals.

NEW DRUG APPROVAL AND DEVELOPMENT

Before any discussion of how pharmaceuticals make their way through the U.S. FDA for market approval, one needs to have an understanding of what constitutes a "drug." A drug is a substance that exerts an action on the structure or function of the body by chemical action or metabolism and is intended for use in the diagnosis, cure, mitigation, treatment, or prevention of disease (3). The concept of "new drug" stems from the Kefauver-Harris Amendments to the FDCA. A new drug is defined as one that is not generally recognized as safe and effective for the indications proposed. This definition has much greater reach, however, than simply a "new" chemical entity. The term "new drug" also refers to a drug product already in existence but never approved by U.S. FDA for marketing in the United States, a new therapeutic indication, a new dosage form, a new route of administration, a new dosing schedule, or any other significant clinical differences than those previously approved (4). Therefore, any chemical substance intended for use in humans or animals for medicinal purposes, or any existing chemical substance that has some significant change associated with it, is considered not safe or effective and to be a new drug until proper testing is performed and U.S. FDA approval is granted.

Approval by the U.S. FDA can be a fairly lengthy and expensive process. For a pharmaceutical manufacturer to place a product on the market for human use, a multiphase procedure must be followed. Remember that the mission of U.S. FDA is to protect the public, and they take that charge very seriously. Hence, all drug products must at least follow the stepwise process.

Preclinical Investigation

The testing of new drugs in humans cannot begin until solid evidence exists that the drug product can be used with reasonable safety in humans. This phase is termed "preclinical investigation." The basic goal of preclinical investigation is to assess the potential therapeutic effects of the substance on living organisms and to gather sufficient data to determine reasonable safety of the substance in humans through laboratory experimentation and animal investigation (5). The U.S. FDA requires no previous approval for investigators or pharmaceutical industry sponsors to begin a preclinical investigation on a potential drug substance. Investigators and sponsors are, however, required to follow Good Laboratory Practices (GLP) regulations (6). The GLPs govern laboratory facilities, personnel, equipment, and operations. Compliance with GLPs requires procedures and documentation of training, study schedules, processes, and status reports, which are submitted to facility management and are included in the final study report to the U.S. FDA. Preclinical investigation usually takes from 1 to 3 years to complete. If at that time enough data are gathered to reach the goal showing a potential therapeutic effect and reasonable safety, the product sponsor must formally notify the U.S. FDA of their wishes to test the potential new drug on humans.

Investigational New Drug Application

Overview

Unlike the preclinical investigation stage, the Investigational New Drug Application (INDA) phase has much more direct U.S. FDA activity throughout. Because a preclinical investigation is designed to gather significant evidence of reasonable safety and efficacy of the compound in live organisms, the INDA phase is the clinical phase in which all activity is used to gather significant evidence of reasonable safety and efficacy data about the potential drug compound in humans. Clinical trials in humans are carefully scrutinized and regulated by the U.S. FDA to protect the health and safety of human test subjects and to ensure the integrity and usefulness of the clinical study data (7). Numerous meetings between both the agency and sponsor will occur during this time. As a result, the clinical investigation phase may take as many as 12 years to complete. Only one in five compounds tested may actually demonstrate clinical effectiveness and safety and reach the U.S. marketplace.

The sponsor will submit the INDA to the U.S. FDA. The INDA must contain information regarding the compound itself and information about the study. All INDAs must have the same basic components: a detailed cover sheet, a table of contents, an introductory statement and basic investigative plan, an investigators' brochure, comprehensive investigation protocols, the compound's actual or proposed chemistry, manufacturing and controls, any pharmacology and toxicology information, any previous human experience with the compound, and any other pertinent information that the U.S. FDA deems necessary. After submission, the sponsor company must wait 30 days to commence clinical trials. If the U.S. FDA does not object within that period, the trials may begin.

Institutional Review Board

Before the actual commencement of the clinical investigations, however, a few ground rules must be established. For example, a clinical study protocol must be developed, proposed by the sponsor, and reviewed by an Institutional Review Board (IRB). An IRB is required by regulation (8) and is a committee of medical and ethical experts designated by an institution, such as a University Medical Center, in which the clinical trial will take place. The charge of the IRB is to oversee the research to ensure that the rights of human test subjects are protected and that rigorous medical and scientific standards are maintained (9). The IRBs must approve the proposed clinical study and monitor the research as it progresses. It must develop written procedures of its own regarding its study review process and its reporting of any changes to the ongoing study as they occur. In addition, an IRB must review and approve documents for informed consent before commencement of the proposed clinical study. Regulations require that potential patients in a clinical study are informed adequately about the risks, benefits, and treatment alternatives before participating in experimental research (10). The membership of an IRB must be sufficiently diverse to review the study in terms of the specific research issue, community and legal standards, and professional conduct and practice norms. All its activities must be well documented and open to U.S. FDA inspection at any time.

Once the IRB is satisfied that the proposed trial is ethical and proper, the clinical trial phase will begin. The clinical trial phase has three steps or phases. Each phase has a purpose, requires numerous patients, and can take more than 1 year to complete.

Phase I. A Phase I study is relatively small (<100 subjects) and brief (≤1 year). The purpose is to determine toxicology, metabolism, pharmacological actions, and if possible, any early evidence of effectiveness. The results of the Phase I study are used to develop the next step.

Phase II. Phase II studies are the first controlled clinical trials using several hundred subjects afflicted with the disease or condition being studied. The purpose of Phase II is to determine the compound's possible effectiveness against the targeted disease or condition and its safety in humans. Phase II may be divided into two subparts: Phase IIa, a pilot study that is used to determine initial efficacy, and Phase IIb, which uses controlled studies on several hundred patients. At the end of the Phase II studies, the sponsor and the U.S. FDA usually will confer to discuss the data and plans for Phase III.

Phase III. Phase III studies are considered to be "pivotal" trials that are designed to collect all the necessary data to meet the safety and efficacy standards the U.S. FDA requires to approve the compound for the U.S. marketplace. Phase III studies usually are very large, consisting of several thousand patients in numerous clinical study centers and a large number of investigators who conduct

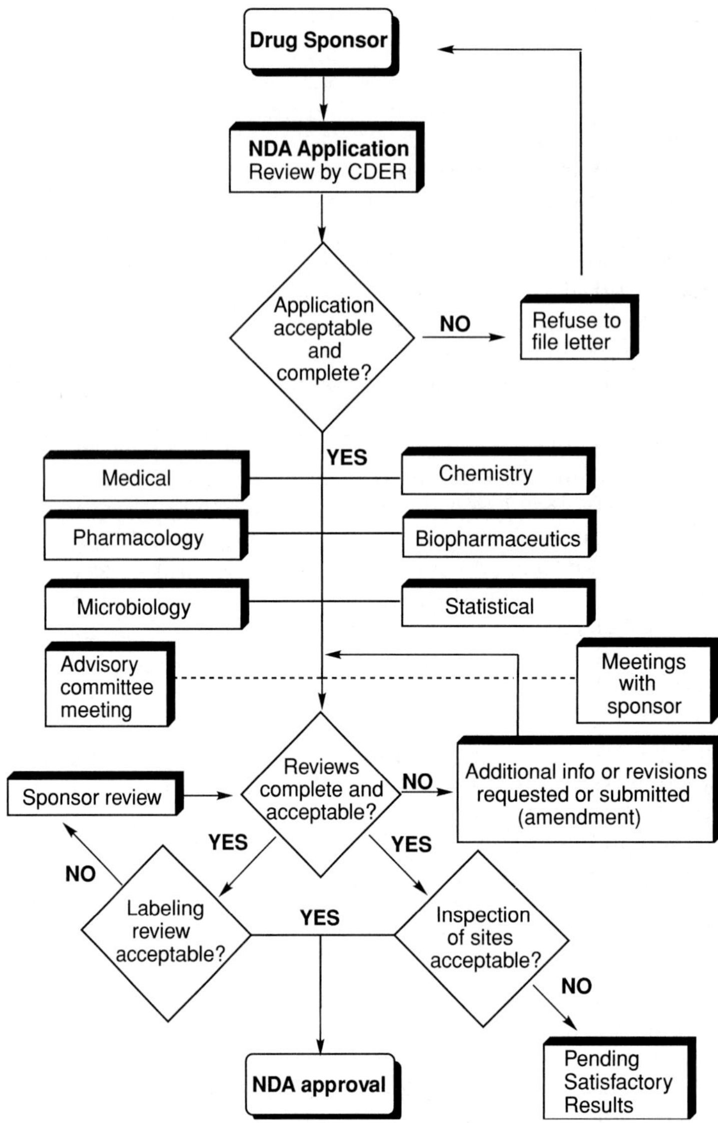

Fig. 11.1. New Drug Application (NDA) review process. (Adapted from http://www.fda.gov/cder/handbook/nda.htm. Accessed March 2007.)

long-term trials over several months or years. Additionally, Phase III studies establish the final formulation, marketing claims, product stability, packaging, and storage conditions. On completion of Phase III, all clinical studies are complete, all safety and efficacy data have been analyzed, and the sponsor is ready to submit the compound to the U.S. FDA for market approval. This process begins with submission of a New Drug Application.

New Drug Application

Overview

A New Drug Application (NDA) is a regulatory mechanism that is designed to give the U.S. FDA sufficient information to make a meaningful evaluation of a new drug (11) (see Fig. 11.1 for an overview of the NDA review process). All NDAs must contain the following information: preclinical laboratory and animal data; human pharmacokinetic and bioavailability data; clinical data; methods of manufacturing, processing, and packaging; a description of the drug product and substance; a list of relevant patents for the drug; its manufacture or claims; and any proposed labeling. In addition, an NDA must provide a summary of the application's contents and a presentation of the risks and benefits of the new drug (12). Traditionally, NDAs have consisted of hundreds of volumes of information, in triplicate and all cross-referenced. Since 1999, the U.S. FDA has issued final guidance documents that allow sponsors to submit NDAs electronically in a standardized format. These electronic submissions facilitate ease of review and possible approval (13).

The NDA must be submitted complete, in the proper form, and with all critical data. If "accepted," the U.S. FDA will then determine the applications completeness. If "complete," the agency considers the application "filed" and will begin the review process within 60 days (14). The purpose of an NDA from the U.S. FDA's perspective is to ensure that the new drug meets the criteria to be "safe and effective." Safety and effectiveness are determined through the Phase III pivotal studies based on "substantial evidence" gained from a well-controlled clinical study. Because there are no absolutely safe drugs, the U.S. FDA looks to the new drug's efficacy as a measure of its safety. It weighs the risks versus benefits of approving the drug for use in the U.S. market.

Additionally, the NDA must be very clear about the manufacture and marketing of the proposed drug product. The application must define and describe the manufacturing processes, validate Current Good Manufacturing Practices, and provide evidence of quality, purity, strength, identity, and bioavailability (a preinspection of the manufacturing facility will be conducted by the U.S. FDA). Finally, the U.S. FDA will review all product packaging and labeling for content and clarity. Statements on a product's package label, package insert, media advertising, or professional literature must be reviewed. Of note, "labeling" refers to all of the above and not just the label on the product container.

The U.S. FDA is required to review an application within 180 days of filing. At the end of that time, the agency is required to respond with an "action letter." There are three kinds of action letters. An "Approval Letter" signifies that all substantive requirements for approval are met and that the sponsor company can begin marketing the drug as of the date on the letter. An "Approvable Letter" signifies that the application substantially complies with the requirements but has some minor deficiencies that must be addressed before an approval letter is sent. Generally, these deficiencies are minor in nature, and the product sponsor must respond within 10 days of receipt. At this point, the sponsor may amend the application and address the agency's concerns, request a hearing with the agency, or withdraw the application entirely. A "Non-Approvable Letter" signifies that the U.S. FDA has major concerns with the application and will not approve the proposed drug product for marketing as submitted. The remedies that a sponsor can take for this type of action letter are similar to those for the "Approvable Letter."

Effects of PDUFA and FDAMA

The NDA review has been significantly affected by both the PDUFA and FDAMA legislation. The PDUFA allows the U.S. FDA to collect fees from sponsor companies who submit applications for review. The fees are used to update facilities and to hire and train reviewers. The fees only apply to NDA drug submissions, biological drug submissions, and any supplement thereto. The fees do not apply to generic drugs or medical devices. The results of the PDUFA legislation were significant: Approval rates have increased from approximately 50 to nearly 80%, and review times have decreased to under 15 months for most applications (15).

Later, in 1997, the FDAMA reauthorized the PDUFA until the year 2002. It waives the user fee to small companies who have fewer than 500 employees, are submitting their first application, allows payment of the fee in stages, and permits a certain percentage of refund if the application is refused. Additionally, it exempts applications for drugs used in rare conditions (i.e., orphan drugs), supplemental applications for pediatric indications, and applications for biologicals used as precursors for other biologics manufacture. The FDMA also permits a "fast-track" approval of compounds that demonstrate significant benefit to critically ill patients, such as those who suffer from AIDS (16).

Biologics

Biologics are defined as substances derived from or made with the aid of living organisms and include vaccines, antitoxins, serums, blood, blood products, therapeutic protein drugs derived from natural sources (i.e., antithrombin III), biotechnology (i.e., recombinantly derived proteins), and gene or somatic cell therapies (17). As with the more traditionally derived drug products, biologics follow virtually the same regulatory and clinical testing schema with regard to safety and efficacy. A Biologics License Application is used rather than an NDA, although the official U.S. FDA Form is designated "356h" and is one and the same. The sponsor merely indicated in a check box if the application is for a drug or a biologic. Compounds characterized as biologics are reviewed by the Center for Biologics Evaluation and Research (18).

Orphan Drugs

Orphan drugs are approved using many of the same processes as any other application; however, there are several significant differences. An orphan drug, as defined under the Orphan Drug Act of 1993, is a drug used to treat a "rare disease" that normally would not be of interest to commercial manufactures during the ordinary course of business. A "rare disease" is defined in the law as any disease that affects fewer than 200,000 persons in the United States or one for which a manufacturer has no reasonable expectation of recovering the cost of its development and availability in the United States. The Act creates a series of financial incentives for these manufacturers. For example, the Act permits grant assistance for clinical research, tax credits for research and development, and a 7-year market exclusivity to the first applicant who obtains market approval for a drug designated as an orphan. This means that if a sponsor gains approval for an orphan drug, the U.S. FDA will not approve any application by any other sponsor for the same drug for the same disease or condition for 7 years from the date of the first applicant's approval provided that certain conditions are met, such as an assurance of sufficient availability of drug to those in need or a revocation of the drug's orphan status (19,20).

Abbreviated New Drug Applications

Abbreviated New Drug Applications (ANDAs) are used when a patent has expired for a drug product that has been on the U.S. market and another pharmaceutical company wishes to market a generic copy. In the United States, a drug patent is good for 20 years. After that time, a manufacturer is able to submit an abbreviated application for the pioneer product provided the manufacturer certifies that the product patent in question has already expired, is invalid, or will not be infringed.

The generic copy must meet certain other criteria as well. The drug's active ingredient must already have been approved for the conditions of use proposed in the ANDA, and nothing must have changed to call into question the basis for approval of the original drug's NDA (21). Sponsors of ANDAs are required to prove that their version meets with standards of bioequivalency and pharmaceutical equivalence. This is accomplished using an abbreviated clinical study that serves to validate, within reasonable parameters, that the generic copy acts in a therapeutic way similar to the action of the original product. This abbreviated study may use several hundred patients or less and may be completed in 1 to 3 years. Once bioequivalency and pharmaceutical equivalency are established, the sponsor company may then submit the ANDA to the U.S. FDA for approval (see Fig. 11.2 for an overview of the ANDA generic drug review process).

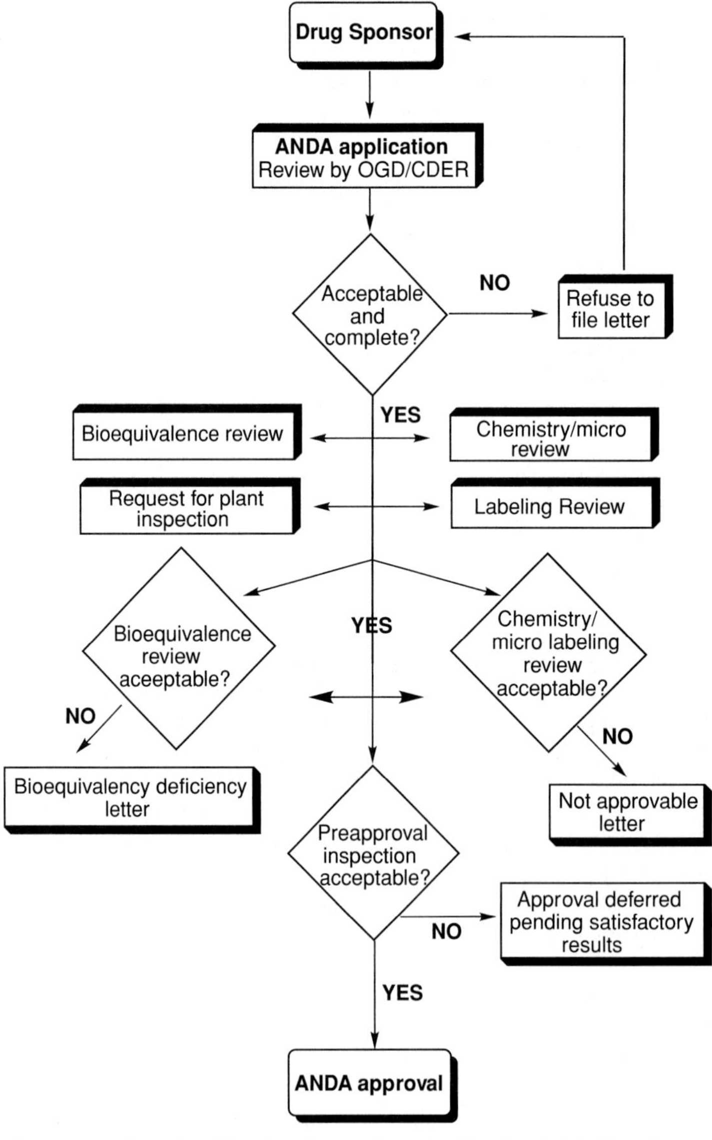

Fig. 11.2. Generic Abbreviated New Drug Application (ANDA) review process. (Adapted from http://www.fda.gov/cder/handbook/generic.htm. Accessed March 2007.)

The U.S. FDA publishes a list of all approved drugs called "Approved Drug Products with Therapeutic Equivalence Evaluations," which is also called the "Orange Book" because of its orange-colored cover. It lists marketed drug products that are considered by the U.S. FDA to be safe and effective, and it provides monthly information about therapeutic equivalence evaluations for approved multisource prescription drug products (22). The Orange Book rates drugs based on their therapeutic equivalence. For a product to be considered therapeutically equivalent, it must be both pharmaceutically equivalent (i.e., same dose, dosage form, strength, etc.) and bioequivalent (i.e., rate and extent of its absorption not significantly different from the rate and extent of absorption of the drug with which it is to be interchanged) (Fig. 11.2)

Realizing that there may be some degree of variability in patients, the U.S. FDA allows pharmaceuticals to be considered bioequivalent using either of two methods. The first method studies the rate and extent of absorption of a test drug that may or may not be a generic variation and a reference or brand-name drug under similar experimental conditions and in similar dosing schedules where the test results do not show significant differences. The second approach uses the same method. The results, however, determine that there is a difference in the test drug's rate and extent of absorption, except the difference is considered to be medically insignificant for the proper clinical outcome of that drug. In other words,

> bioequivalence of different formulations of the same drug substance involves equivalence with respect to the rate and extent of drug absorption. Two formulations whose rate and extent of absorption differ by 20% or less are generally considered bioequivalent. The use of the 20% rule is based on a medical decision that, for most drugs, a 20% difference in the concentration of the active ingredient in blood will not be clinically significant. (23)

The U.S. FDA's Orange Book uses a two-letter coding system that is helpful in determining which drug products are considered to be therapeutically equivalent. The first letter, either an A or a B, indicates a drug product's therapeutic equivalence rating. The second letter describes the dose forms and can be any one of a number of different letters.

The "A" codes are described in the "Orange Book" as follows:

> Drug products that FDA considers to be therapeutically equivalent to other pharmaceutically equivalent products, i.e., drug products for which:
>
> 1. There are no known or suspected bioequivalence problems. These are designated **AA, AN, AO, AP,** or **AT,** depending on the dose form; or
> 2. Actual or potential bioequivalence problems have been resolved with adequate in vivo and/or in vitro evidence supporting bioequivalence. These are designated **AB.** (24)

The B codes are a much less desirable rating when compared to the A codes. Products that are rated with a B code may still be commercially marketed; however, they may not be considered therapeutically equivalent. The Orange Book describes B codes as follows:

> Drug products that FDA at this time does not consider to be therapeutically equivalent to other pharmaceutically equivalent products, i.e., drug products for which actual or potential bioequivalence problems have not been resolved by adequate evidence of bioequivalence. Often the problem is with specific dosage forms rather than with the active ingredients. These are designated BC, BD, BE, BN, BP, BR, BS, BT, or BX. (25)

The U.S. FDA has adopted an additional subcategory of B codes. The designation, B* is assigned to former A-rated drugs "if [the] FDA receives new information that raises a significant question regarding therapeutic equivalence" (26). Not all drugs are listed in the Orange Book. Drugs obtainable only from a single manufacturing source, DESI drugs, or drugs manufactured before 1938 are not included. Those that do appear in the Orange Book are listed by generic name.

Phase IV, Postmarketing Surveillance, and Supplemental NDAs

Pharmaceutical companies that successfully gain marketing approval for their products are NOT exempt from further regulatory requirements. Many products are approved for market on the basis of a continued submission of clinical research data to the U.S. FDA. This data may be required to further validate efficacy or safety, to detect new uses or abuses for the product, or to determine the effectiveness of labeled indications under conditions of widespread usage (27). Additionally, the U.S. FDA may require a Phase IV study for drugs approved under the "fast-track" provisions of the FDAMA.

Any changes to the approved product's indications, active ingredients, manufacture, or labeling require the manufacturer to submit a Supplemental NDA (SNDA) for agency approval. Additionally, "adverse drug reports" are required to be reported to the agency. All reports must be reviewed by the manufacturer promptly, and if found to be serious, life-threatening, or unexpected (i.e., not listed in the product's labeling), the manufacturer is required to submit an "alert report" within 15 working days of receiving the information. All adverse reactions thought not to be serious or unexpected must be reported quarterly for 3 years after the application is approved and annually thereafter (28).

OVER-THE-COUNTER REGULATIONS (1951 DURHAM-HUMPHREY AMENDMENTS)

The 1951 Durham-Humphrey Amendments of the FDCA specified three criteria to justify prescription-only status. If the compound is shown to be habit forming, requires a prescriber's supervision, or has a NDA prescription-only limitation, it will require a prescription. The principles used to establish OTC status (no prescription required) are a wide margin of safety, method of use, benefit-to-risk

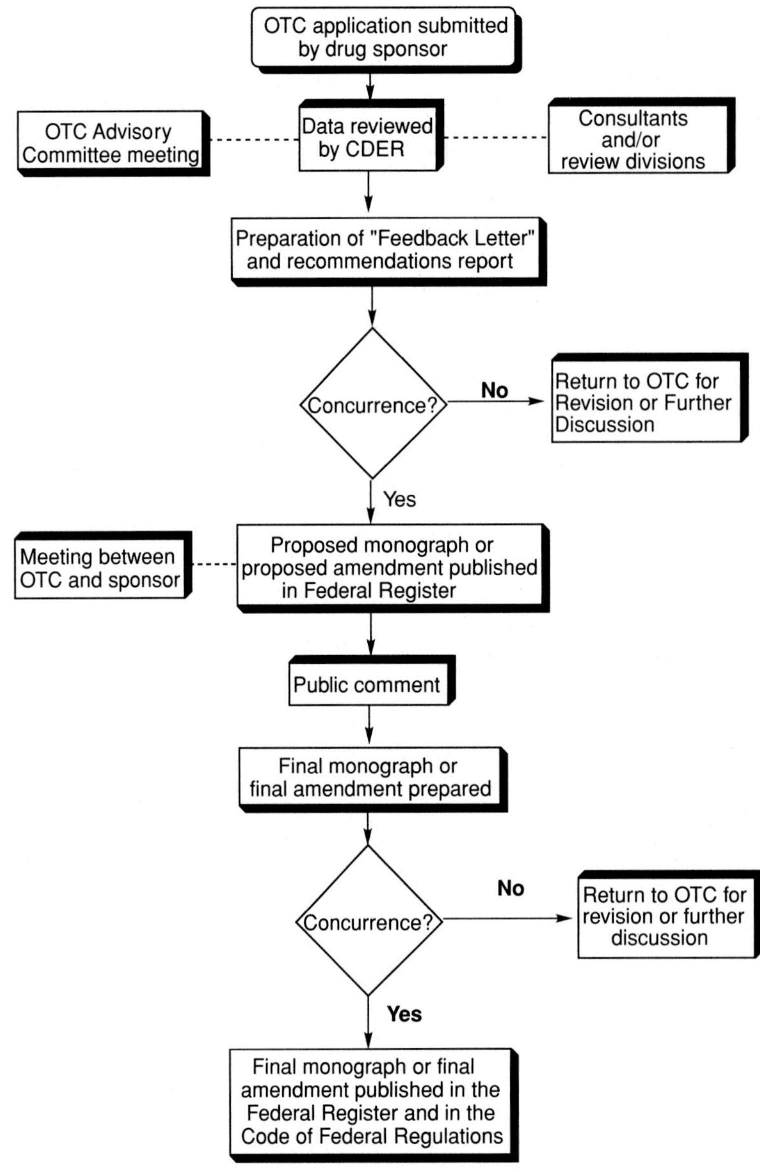

Fig. 11.3. Over-the-counter (OTC) drug monograph review process. (Adapted from http://www.fda.gov/cder/handbook/otc.htm. Accessed March 2007.)

ratio, and adequacy of labeling for self-medication. For example, injectable drugs may not be used OTC with certain exceptions (e.g., insulin). Entry into the OTC market is less restrictive than that into the prescription market and does not require premarket clearance. They pose many fewer safety hazards than prescription drugs, because they are designed to alleviate symptoms rather than disease. Easier access to OTC drugs far outweighs the risks of side effects that can be adequately addressed through proper labeling.

As previously discussed, OTC products underwent an efficacy review in 1972. Though reviewing the therapeutic efficacy of the more than 30,000 OTC drug products in existence at the time would have been virtually impossible, the U.S. FDA created OTC Advisory Panels to review data based on some 26 therapeutic categories. The OTC drugs would only be examined by active ingredient within a therapeutic category. Inactive ingredients would only be examined provided they were shown to be safe and suitable for the product and not to interfere with effectiveness and quality.

This review of active ingredients would result in the promulgation of a regulation or a "monograph," which is a "recipe" or set of guidelines applicable to all OTC products within a therapeutic category (see Fig. 11.3 for an overview of the OTC application review process). The OTC monographs are general and require that OTC products be shown to have "general recognition of the safety and effectiveness of the active ingredient." The OTC products do not fall under prescription status if their active ingredients (or combinations) are deemed by the U.S. FDA to be "Generally Recognized as Safe and Effective" (GRASE). The monograph system is a public system with a public comment component included after each phase of the process. Any products for which a final monograph has not been established may remain on the market until one is determined.

The OTC monograph system has four phases. In Phase I, an expert panel is selected to review data for each active ingredient in each therapeutic category for safety, efficacy, and labeling. Their recommendations are made in the *Federal Register.* A public comment period of 30 to 60 days is permitted, and supporting or contesting data are accepted for review. Then, the panel reevaluates the data and publishes a "proposed monograph" in the *Federal Register* that publicly announces the conditions for which the panel believed OTC products in a particular therapeutic class are GRASE and not misbranded. A "Tentative Final Monograph," the U.S. FDA's position on safety and efficacy of a particular ingredient within a therapeutic category and acceptable labeling for indications, warnings, and directions for use, is then developed and published. Active ingredients are deemed as follows: Category I, GRASE for claimed therapeutic indications and not misbranded; Category II, Not-GRASE and or misbranded; and Category III, insufficient data for determination.

After public comment, the final monograph is established and published with the U.S. FDA's final criteria for which all drug products in a therapeutic class become GRASE and not misbranded. Following the effective date of the final monograph, all covered drug products that fail to conform to its requirements are considered to be misbranded and an unapproved new drug (29).

Because the monograph panels are no longer convened, however, many current products are switched from prescription to OTC status. A company that wishes to make this switch and offer an OTC product to the U.S. marketplace can submit an amendment to a monograph to the U.S. FDA, which will act as the sole reviewer. The company also may file an SNDA provided that they have 3 years of marketing experience as a prescription product, can demonstrate a relatively high use during that period, and can validate that the product has a mild profile of adverse reactions. The last method involves a "Citizens Petition," which rarely is used (30).

REGULATING MARKETING

The U.S. FDA has jurisdiction over prescription drug advertising and promotion. The basis for these regulations lies within the 1962 Kefauver-Harris Amendments. Essentially, any promotional information in any form must be truthful, balanced, and fully disclosed. The U.S. FDA views this information as either "advertising" or "labeling." Advertising includes all traditional outlets in which a company places an ad. Labeling includes everything else, including brochures, booklets, lectures, slide kits, letters to physicians, company-sponsored magazine articles, and so on. All information must be truthful and not misleading. All material facts must be disclosed in a manner that is balanced and accurate. If any of these requirements are violated, the product is considered to be "misbranded" regarding the indications for which it was approved under its NDA. Additionally, the U.S. FDA also is sensitive to the promotion of a product for "off-label use," which occurs when a product is in some way presented in a manner that does not agree with or is not addressed in its approved labeling. Also, provisions of the Prescription Drug Marketing Act of 1987 apply. The Act prohibits company representatives from directly distributing or reselling prescription drug samples. Companies are required to establish a closed system of record keeping that will be able to track a sample from their control to that of a prescriber to prevent diversion. Prescribers are required to receive these samples and to record and store them appropriately (31).

VIOLATIONS AND ENFORCEMENT

The U.S. FDA has the power to enforce the regulations for any product as defined under the FDCA. It has the jurisdiction to inspect a manufacturer's premises and their records. After a facilities inspection, an agency inspector will issue a U.S. FDA Form 483s, which describes observable violations. Response to the finding as described on this form must be made promptly. A "Warning Letter" may be used when the agency determines that one or more of a company's practices, products, or procedures are in violation of the FDCA. The U.S. FDA district office has 15 days to issue a warning letter after an inspection. The company has 15 days in which to respond to this warning letter. If the company response is satisfactory to the U.S. FDA, no other action is warranted. If the response is not, the U.S. FDA may request a "recall" of the violated products. However, the U.S. FDA has no authority to force a company to recall a product but may force removal of a product through the initiation of a seizure.

Recalls

Recalls can fall into one of three classes. A Class I recall exists when a reasonable possibility exists that the use of a product will cause either serious adverse effects on health or death. A Class II recall exists when the use of a product may cause temporary or medically reversible adverse effects on health or when the probability of serious adverse effects on health is remote. A Class III recall exists when the use of a product is not likely to cause adverse health consequences. Recalls also are categorized as consumer level, where the product is requested to be recalled from the consumers' homes or control; retail level, where the products are to be removed from retail shelves or control; and wholesale level, where the product is to be removed from wholesale distribution. Companies that conduct a recall of their products are required to conduct "Effectiveness Checks" to determine the effectiveness of recalling the product from the marketplace.

An Injunction

If a company refuses to recall the product, the U.S. FDA will seek an injunction against the company (32). An injunction is recommended by the U.S. FDA to the U.S. Department of Justice, which takes the request to federal court and issues the order that forbids a company from carrying out a particular illegal act, such as marketing a product that the U.S. FDA considers a violation of the FDCA. Companies can either comply with the order and sign a "consent agreement," which will specify changes required by the U.S. FDA for the company to continue operations, or litigate.

Seizure of Products

The U.S. FDA also may initiate a seizure of violative products (33). A seizure is ordered by the federal court in the district that the products are located. The seizure order specifies products, their batch numbers, and any records determined by the U.S. FDA as violative. The U.S. Marshals carry out this action. The U.S. FDA institutes a seizure to prevent a company from selling, distributing, moving, or otherwise tampering with the product.

Additionally, the U.S. FDA may debar individuals or firms from assisting or submitting an ANDA or from directly providing services to any firm with an existing or pending drug product application. Debarment may last for up to 10 years (34).

One of the more powerful deterrents that the U.S. FDA uses is adverse publicity. The U.S. FDA has no authority to require a company to advertise adverse publicity, but it does publish administrative actions against a company in any number of federal publications, such as the *Federal Register, FDA Enforcement Report, FDA Medical Bulletin,* and *FDA Consumer* (35).

SUMMARY

The laws and regulations that govern the U.S. pharmaceutical industry are both vast and complicated. Interpretation of the FDCA is in a constant state of flux. The U.S. FDA is charged with this interpretation based on the rapid technological changes that are occurring each day within the industry. Many may suggest that more rapid drug approval places the citizenry in greater danger of adverse events. Others may reply that technology offers newer and more effective therapies for deadly diseases.

Historically, Congress has passed laws governing our medication based on a reaction to a crises. The USPFDA, the FDCA, and the Price Competition and Patent Restoration Act are just a few. One hopes that this method of regulation will not continue as the norm. We can be proud of proactive legislation, such as the Kefauver-Harris Act, the Orphan Drug Act, the PDUFA, and FDAMA. These Acts have paved the way for meaningful change within the drug investigation process as we continue in our battle against disease. The U.S. system of investigating new drugs is one that continues to have merit by allowing enough time to investigate benefit versus risk. The American public can look forward to great advances from the industry and should be comfortable that the U.S. FDA is watching.

References

1. Valentino J. Practical Uses for the USP: A Legal Perspective. In: Strauss's Federal Drug Laws and Examination Review, 5th Ed. Lancaster, PA: Technomic Publishing Co., 1999:38.
2. Strauss S. Food and Drug Administration: An Overview. In: Strauss's Federal Drug Laws and Examination Review, 5th Ed. Lancaster, PA: Technomic Publishing Co., 1999:323.
3. FDCA, Sec.21(g)(1).
4. Strauss S., ibid., p. 176, 186.
5. Pinna K, Pines W. The Drugs/Biologics Approval Process. In: A Practical Guide to Food and Drug Law and Regulation. Washington, DC: Food, Drug Law Institute, 1998:96.
6. 21 CFR 58.
7. Pinna K, et al., ibid., p. 98.
8. 21 CFR 56.
9. Pinna K, et al., ibid., p. 98.
10. 21 CFR 50.
11. 21 CFR 314.
12. Pinna K, et al., ibid., p. 102–103.
13. *Federal Register,* V.64(18), January 28, 1999.
14. Pinna K, et al., ibid., p. 103.
15. Strauss S, ibid., p. 280.
16. Food and Drug Administration Modernization Act of 1997, PL 105, 1997.
17. 42 U.S. Code 262.
18. Form FDA 356h.
19. The Orphan Drug Act of 1982, PL 97-414.
20. The Orphan Drug Amendments of 1985, PL 99-91.
21. Pinna K, et al., ibid., p. 119.
22. Preface. In: USP/DI, vol III, 16th Ed. Rockville, MD: U.S. Pharmacopeia, 2000:v.
23. Preface. In: USP/DI, vol III, 16th Ed. Rockville, MD: U.S. Pharmacopeia, 2000:I/7.
24. Preface. In: USP/DI, vol III, 16th Ed. Rockville, MD: U.S. Pharmacopeia, 2000:I/9.
25. Preface. In: USP/DI, vol III, 16th Ed. Rockville, MD: U.S. Pharmacopeia, 2000:I/10.
26. Preface. In: USP/DI, volume III, 16th Ed. Rockville, MD: U.S. Pharmacopeia, 2000:I/12.
27. Pinna K, et al., ibid., p. 111.
28. Pinna K, et al., ibid., p. 111.
29. Strauss S, ibid., p. 285.
30. Strauss S, ibid., p. 285.
31. 21 U.S. Code 301, et seq.
32. 21 U.S. Code 302, et seq.
33. 21 U.S. Code 304, et seq.
34. Fundamentals of Regulatory Affairs, Regulatory Affairs Professions Society, 1999, p. 199.
35. Fundamentals of Regulatory Affairs, p. 200.

PART II

DRUG RECEPTORS AFFECTING NEUROTRANSMISSION AND ENZYMES AS CATALYTIC RECEPTORS

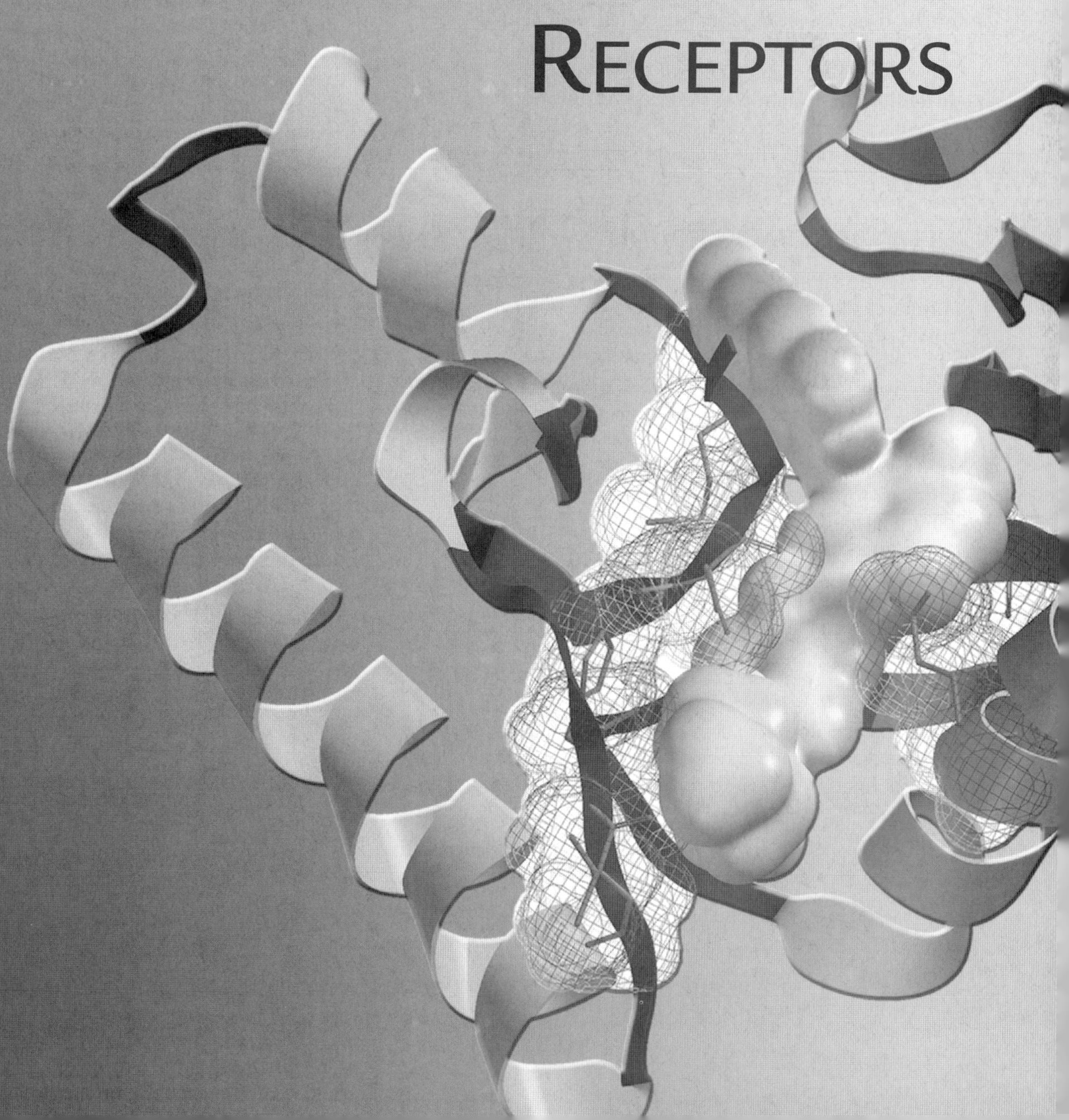

Overview of Drug Receptors: A Perspective

DAVID J. TRIGGLE

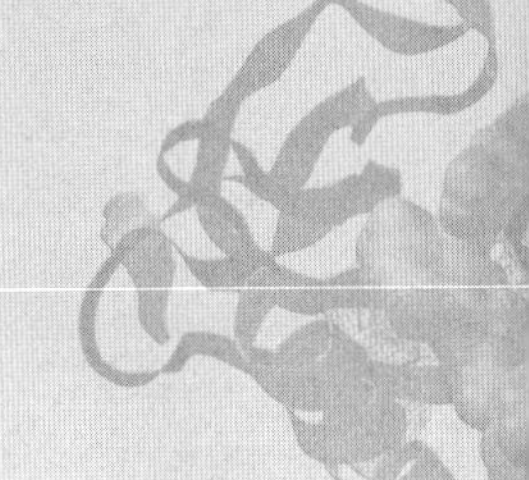

Pharmacodynamics is the study of drug action principally in terms of the structure of the drug, its site of action, and the biological consequences of the drug–receptor interaction. Pharmacodynamics defines the selectivity, sites of action, concentration– and time–response relationships of a drug. These relationships are determined in turn by several pharmacokinetic processes, including absorption, metabolism, distribution, and excretion: these processes are profoundly important in determining drug action, including the therapeutic and contraindications profile of a given agent, and they can significantly modify the consequences of drug action at the specific site of action—the pharmacological receptor. In this chapter, a broad overview of the pharmacological receptor is presented in terms of classification, recognition and transduction events, structures, and the relationship between structure and function as well as the alterations of receptor structure in discrete disease states. Separate chapters will provide more detailed application of these general concepts to specific receptors and classes of drugs.

HISTORICAL BACKGROUND

During the late nineteenth century, several separate but ultimately complementary lines of evidence led the postulate regarding the existence of receptors serving as specific sites of interaction with which drugs interacted selectively to initiate or block a particular biological event—physiological or pathological. From his work on immunology and the chemotherapy of protozoan infections, Paul Ehrlich speculated that the cell possessed specific protoplasmic side chains of defined and unique chemical and steric architecture and that these interacted specifically with complementary groups of a chemotherapeutic agent or antibody:

> "For the sake of brevity in what follows we shall in general always designate as **receptor** that binding group of the protoplasmic molecule to which a foreign, newly introduced group binds" (1).

The concept of "lock-and-key" action, which is critical to the issue of specificity in the drug-receptor interaction, had been defined previously by Emil Fischer, who observed:

> " . . . I will say that enzyme and glucoside must fit together like lock and key in order to be able to exercise a chemical action on each other" (2).

Prior to these speculations, John Newton Langley wrote:

> "We may, I think, without much rashness assume that there is some substance or substances in the nerve endings or gland cells with which both atropine and pilocarpine are capable of forming compounds. On this assumption, then, the atropine or pilocarpine compounds are formed according to some law of which their relative mass and chemical affinity for the substance are factors" (3).

The existence of structure–function relationships in biologically active materials had been noted as early as 1869 by the Edinburgh physicians Crum-Brown and Fraser (4), who were studying a variety of alkaloids, including strychnine, brucinem and nicotin. Langley also recognized the receptor as a transducer that "receives the stimulus and, by transmitting it causes contraction" (response) (5), thus serving to convert one form of information—the drug–receptor interaction—into another—the physiologic response. Later, and contemporaneously with the writings of Ehrlich, Langley used the term "receptive substance" for these compounds and speculated that separate receptors existed for atropine, pilocarpine, curare, and other "autonomic agents" with which his physiologic research had been concerned.

Thus, by the beginning of the twentieth century, the foundation had been laid for a definition of receptors that embodied the concepts of specificity, including stereoselectivity, dose–response relationships, and transduction. These components of the definition are those that we use today, although they have been substantially refined and quantitated, notably with respect to definition of the location, structure, and chemistry of the drug-binding site and the coupling of this site to response. Indeed, by the end of the twentieth century, the structures of many receptors had been delineated and three-dimensional models established, either by modeling or by direct determination, that serve both to define drug action and to facilitate new drug discovery.

RECEPTOR CLASSIFICATION

In principle, receptors may be classified in a variety of ways: 1) by the physiological ligand that interacts with the receptor, 2) by the response that activation of the receptor induces, 3) by the biochemical changes that may link receptor activation to response, and 4) by the structure of the receptor protein. Each of these schemes, however, has its own limitations. It is of little help to refer to the receptor that elevates blood pressure or increases heart rate, because these are properties common to many receptor activation processes. Similarly, many receptors share a common biochemical cascade—for example, activation of adenylyl cyclase—yet may produce similar or different physiologic responses. Furthermore, agonists at many receptors are pleiotropic, producing multiple biochemical consequences that may have different effects according to cell type. Additionally, because the coupling between receptor and effector depends on intrinsic properties of the ligand, the biochemical effect induced at the same receptor in the same cell can be agonist specific. Physiological ligands may interact with multiple receptors that are clearly unrelated: For example, acetylcholine interacts with both the nicotinic and muscarinic classes of acetylcholine that are, by all other criteria, quite distinct receptor families, belonging to the transmitter-gated ion channel and guanine nucleotide binding protein–coupled (G protein–coupled receptors) classes, respectively. Furthermore, acetylcholine is the physiological substrate for acetylcholinesterase, the synaptic clearing enzyme for this transmitter. Similar divisions occur with γ-aminobutyric acid (GABA) where $GABA_A$ and $GABA_B$ receptors belong to the transmitter-gated channel and G protein–coupled classes, respectively. Of particular interest, all receptors $5\text{-}HT_{1-7}$ for serotonin belong to the G protein–coupled class, save for the $5\text{-}HT_3$ category, which is a ligand-gated ion channel. Finally, the same receptor may interact with ligands that are totally unrelated both structurally and functionally. A prominent example is the chemokine family of receptors that recognize both the physiologic chemokine class of ligands, including interleukin-8, monocyte chemoattractant protein, and other cytokines, and that also is a coreceptor of the pathological HIV.

The use of nonphysiological ligands, notably selective agonists and antagonists, has permitted the subclassification of receptor families and allowed the characterization of receptor subtypes. Thus, atropine and curare are classically known drugs and receptor antagonists that permitted the early subdivision of acetylcholine receptors into the "muscarinic" and "nicotinic" families. Today, these families have been established, by structural information, to be quite distinct, although they do share a common physiological ligand—acetylcholine. Finally, it must be recognized that receptors exist that recognize signals other than chemical and that these receptors belong to the same classes as those for physiological ligands. Thus, rhodopsin, the visual light–recognizing pigment, is a member of the G protein–coupled class of receptors (Table II.1), and the visual cascade bears many similarities to the events initiated by, for example, catecholamine interaction at β-adrenoceptors. Similarly, ion channels that are opened or closed by changes in membrane potential—that is, voltage-gated channels—are similar in their fundamental construction to ligand/transmitter-gated ion channels. Finally, receptors for odorant molecules, of which there may be many thousands, also belong to the G protein–coupled receptor class.

Receptor structure (i.e., the linear amino acid sequence of the receptor protein inferred from the gene) provides a definitive identification and basis for classification of receptors. The degree of similarity between these sequences permits the establishment of receptor families and, through the techniques of molecular biology, has made possible the identification of receptors—so-called "orphan receptors"—for which physiological ligands may still remain unidentified. Even linear and, ultimately, three-dimensional structure, however, is not without its limitations. Posttranslational modifications that are cell- or tissue-specific may contribute to the properties of the expressed receptor, including its coupling to effector systems. Additionally, receptors that are oligomeric assemblies of individual subunits may be heteromeric assemblies; thus, the properties of the total receptor complex may depend on the subunit composition. Because of the importance of receptor classification to the science and practice of pharmacology, the International Union of Pharmacology has established a set of committees designed to report on receptor classification schemes and protocols (6). The total functional classification is dependent on consideration of structural, recognition, and transduction components (Fig. II.1). From these considerations, four principal classes of pharmacological receptors may be recognized (Table II.1).

Table II.1. Classification of Pharmacological Receptors[a]

Class	Receptor Type	Characteristics
1	1-Transmembrane protein	Enzyme associated
2	Transcriptional regulators	Nonmembrane, cytosolic protein with DNA-binding domains
3	Ion channels	Integral membrane; subunit composition; each subunit or domain has two or more membrane inserts as a pore region, and four or more form the central pore of the channel
4	7-Transmembrane proteins	G protein–coupled receptors

[a]For further explanations, see text.

1-Transmembrane Proteins

This first major class of pharmacological receptors contains those that are intrinsically enzyme-associated, including those with guanylate cyclase activity or tyrosine kinase activity or that associate directly with a diffusible tyrosine kinase. These receptors include those for a number of growth factors, neurotrophins and cytokines (Table II.2). In these receptors, there is only a single membrane-spanning domain, and the receptor and the enzyme are components of the same peptide chain. In a variation on this structural theme, the receptor and enzyme complexes are on separate but closely associated chains. Activation of these receptors occurs through a process of dimerization (Fig. II.2). Several growth factors, including platelet-derived growth factor, can induce cross-linking of their corresponding receptors because

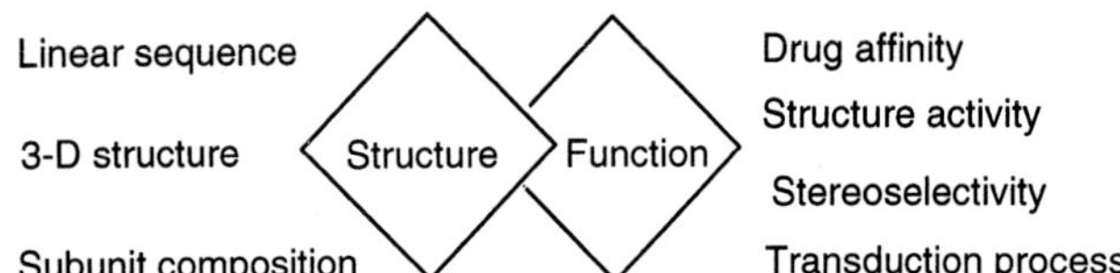

Fig. II.1. Defining structure–function factors that affect ligand-binding sites and the transduction process.

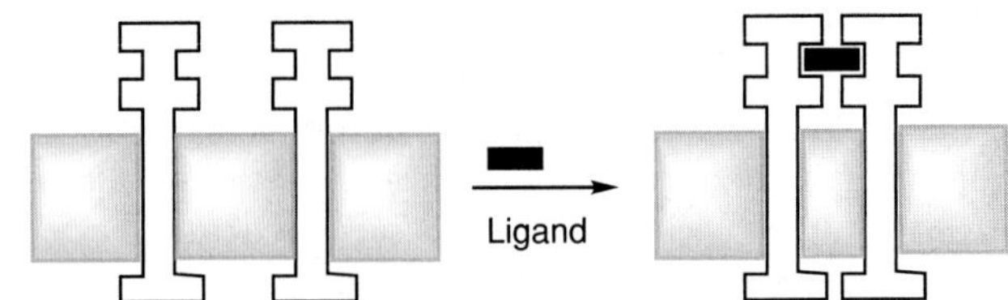

Fig. II.2. The dimerization process subsequent to ligand binding to a tyrosine kinase.

they contain two binding sites. Other growth factors recruit accessory molecules to induce receptor oligomerization. This dimerization process is an integral component of the activation of many cell surface receptors associated with kinase activities. In contrast, the activity of tyrosine phosphatases also is controlled by dimerization, but dimerization decreases the enzyme activity.

Transcriptional Regulators

The intracellular hormone receptors constitute the second major class and include the receptors for steroid hormones, including estrogens and androgens, the glucocorticoids (e.g., corticosterone), vitamin D, thyroxine, and retinoic acid (Fig. II.3). There are in excess of 150 members of this receptor family that serve as transcription factors. This receptor superfamily shares a number of common characteristics, including the possession of multiple functional domains—ligand-binding, DNA-binding, and transcriptional activation (Fig. II.4). Type I receptors for steroid hormones are localized in the cytoplasm and nucleus and form large macromolecular complexes with heat shock and other proteins: Ligand binding induces dissociation of the complex to form monomeric receptors, which then homodimerize and bind to hormone response elements in the nuclear DNA. Type II receptors for vitamin D, thyroid hormone, and retinoic acid are exclusively localized in the nucleus and form heterodimers capable of binding to DNA in the absence of ligand (Fig. II.5). These nuclear receptors may be associated with corepressor proteins that inhibit basal transcription of the target genes. Several processes, including the tissue-specific expression of receptors and the sequence and organization of the DNA target sequences, presumably ensure selectivity of target gene activation.

Ion Channels

The ion channel category of pharmacological receptors includes voltage-gated channels and transmitter-gated channels (Table II.3); the latter include receptors for acetylcholine (nicotine), glycine and GABA, glutamate, serotonin, ATP, cyclic nucleotides, and inositol *tris*-phosphate. These channels differ in the nature of their physiological ligands—membrane potential and neurotransmitter or neuropeptide, respectively—but they share a common oligomeric subunit construction, ion permeation pathways, and multiple drug-binding sites. Additionally, ion channels exhibit "state-dependent binding" of ligands, whereby the access and/or affinity of the ligand depends on the state of the channel—resting, open, phosphorylated, and so on. State-dependent binding is extremely important in modulating the selectivity of action of drugs active at ion channels.

A large number of drugs and toxins interact at ion channels to produce their therapeutic and toxicologic effects. Among the therapeutic agents are the calcium channel drugs (cardiovascular agents), local anesthetics interacting at sodium channels (antiarrhythmic agents), potassium channel antagonists (type II diabetes), drugs at nicotinic receptors (skeletal muscle relaxants), and GABA receptors (benzodiazepine antianxiety agents). Nature has capitalized on the central role of ion channels in cellular excitability

Table II.2. Receptors for Growth Factors and Related Ligands

Receptor Type	Ligand
Tyrosine kinase	Platelet-derived growth factor (PDGF)
	Epidermal growth factor (EGF)
	Insulin-like growth factor (IGF)
	Fibroblast growth factor (FGF)
	Neurotrophins
Cytokines	Growth hormone
	Erythropoietin
	Interleukin-2, -3, and -6
	Interferon
Tumor necrosis	Tumor necrosis factor
	Low-affinity growth factor receptor
Serine/threonine kinase	Transforming growth factor β (TGFβ)
	Activin

Vitamin D_3 Thyroxine Estradiol Corticosterone Retinoic acid

Fig. II.3. Hormonal ligands that act as "nuclear receptors" of the transcriptional regulator receptors.

A/B Variable transactivation	C Zn fingers DNA binding	D Hinge	E Ligand binding	F Variable

Fig. II.4. Structure of the nuclear hormone receptor made up of discrete regions or domains, such as the C-terminal region for ligand binding and receptor dimerization (A/B), the central DNA binding region that contacts critical nucleotide sequences termed hormone-response elements (C–E), and a variable region at the N-terminal domain (F).

and function by directing toxins at many ion channels. Toxin species include the sodium channel blockers tetrodotoxin from the Japanese puffer fish and scorpion toxin from the scorpion, potassium channel toxins from snakes, and of particular interest, a multiplicity of toxins directed at a variety of voltage- and ligand-gated channels from mollusks of the *Conus* genus (see Chapter 28).

7-Transmembrane Proteins (G Protein–Coupled Receptors)

The G protein–coupled receptors represent the largest single class of pharmacological receptors. Almost 200 human receptors are known, and there are an additional number for which no physiological function has yet been defined—the so-called "orphan receptors." Additionally, odorant receptors, of which there are several hundred, also belong to this class. The G protein–coupled receptors are of major therapeutic significance, because they are an established target of many therapeutic agents (Tables II.4 and II.5): It has been estimated that approximately 60% of existing therapeutically active drugs act on this class of receptor. Furthermore, an increasing number of structural and expression defects in these receptors are linked to defined disease states (see *Receptors as Regulated Species*). The G protein–coupled receptors also have the ability to dimerize, either homologously or heterologously, thus providing further complexity to their physiological properties and functions (7). An example of such complexity is revealed by the interaction of the opioid agent 6′-guanidinonaltrindole that interacts selectively in the spinal cord with the hetero-oligomer δ-κ-opioid receptor, but not with the homo-oligomers to produce an analgesic response (8).

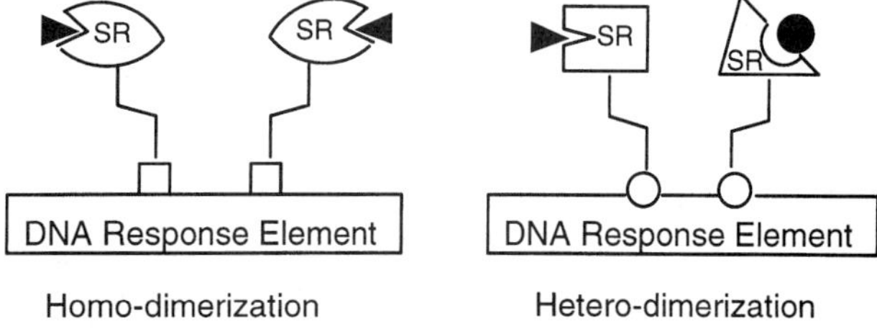

Fig. II.5. Representation of nuclear hormone receptor dimers and their interaction with DNA. SR, steroid receptor.

6'-Guanidinonaltrindole

The ability of receptors to form homo- or heterodimers provides but one example of receptor complexity. It is now quite apparent that the dogma "one gene = one protein = one receptor" is quite wrong. Alternative splicing, oligomerization, multiple ligand sensitivity, and constitutive activity all yield biological and pharmacological selectivity beyond that envisaged by any simple dogma. These overall considerations permit the broad classification of receptors into several major classes. It is instructive to note that the detailed subclassification of receptors, which is critical to understanding the pharmacological selectivity and therapeutic efficacy of drugs, depends on the simultaneous application of a number of considerations. This is seen with the receptors for the transmitter acetylcholine and for which two major structural classes exist—muscarinic and nicotinic receptors, which represent two major classes of receptors—the G protein–coupled receptors and the transmitter-gated channels.

Table II.3. Classification of Ion Channels

Family	Ions	Functional Characteristics
Voltage-gated	Na^+, K^+, Ca^{2+}	Opened and closed by changes in membrane potential. Members of one structural superfamily. Target of many toxins and therapeutic agents.
Transmitter-gated	Na^+, K^+, Ca^{2+}, Cl^-	Opened by interaction with transmitter. Members of several structural classes.
ACh (nicotinic)	Cation (Na^+, Ca^{2+}) channel	
Glycine	Anion (Cl^-) channel	
$GABA_A$	Anion (Cl^-) channel	
Glutamate	Cation (Na^+, Ca^{2+}) channel	
Serotonin	Cation channel	
ATP (purinergic)	Cation (K^+) channel	
Cyclic-nucleotide	Cation channel	
IP_3	cation (Ca^{2+}) channel	

Table II.4. G protein–coupled Receptors As Therapeutic Targets

Receptor	Drug	Indication
Acetylcholine (muscarinic)	Bethanchol	Gastrointestinal
	Ipratropium	Pulmonary
Norepinephrine		
β_1	Atenolol	Cardiovascular
β_1/β_2	Propranolol	Cardiovascular
β_2	Albuterol	Pulmonary
α_1	Terazosin	Cardiovascular
α_2	Clonidine	Cardiovascular
Angiotensin (AT_1)	Losartan	Cardiovascular
Dopamine (D_2)	Haloperidol	Central nervous system
Serotonin (5-HT_{ID})	Sumatriptan	Central nervous system
Histamine (H_2)	Cimetidine	Gastrointestinal
Opiod (μ)	Morphine	Central nervous system

Table II.5. Drugs (Including Those Under Development) for Peptide G-Protein–Coupled Receptors

Receptors	Clinical Status	Drugs	Indication
Opiod	In use	Morphine	Pain
Angiotensin II	In use	Losartan Valsartan	Hypertension
Endothelin [ETA, ETB]	In development	—	Heart failure
Tachykinin (NK1)	In development	—	Depression Asthma
Vasopressin (V_2)	In development	—	Heart failure
Cholecystokinin	In development	—	Anxiety Appetite
Neuropeptide (Y, Y1, Y5)	In development		Appetite
Neuropeptide (Y, Y_2)	In development	—	Depression
Chemokine (CCR5, $CXCR_4$)	In development	—	HIV

Muscarinic receptors are of five major classes—M_1 to M_5—coded by separate genes, with differential expression, function, coupling, and drug sensitivity (Table II.6). They are all members of the G protein–coupled receptor family that is characterized by a single protein with seven transmembrane-spanning regions (see *Receptor Structure*). Synthetic drugs differentially recognize them, although the greatest differential selectivity is demonstrated by antagonists rather than by agonists. Atropine is a nonselective antagonist. Pirenzepine has selectivity for M_1 receptors, methoctramine and AF-DX 384 for M_2 receptors, and darifenacin for M_3 receptors. None of these antagonists (Fig. II.6), however, exhibits absolute selectivity against a receptor subtype. In contrast, the nicotinic receptor is a transmitter-gated channel made up of a pentameric structure with α, β, γ and δ subunits.

The classic curare-sensitive nicotinic acetylcholine receptor of skeletal muscle is made up of two α, one β, one γ, and one δ subunit, with the acetylcholine-binding sites being carried on the α subunit. Nicotinic receptors found in the central and peripheral nervous system have a considerable diversity of subunit combination, with α_{1-9} and β_{2-4} expressed in combination (heteromeric) or, in a few cases, alone (homomeric). The major permutations found in the nervous system include $\alpha_4\beta_2$ that is widespread in the central nervous system and α_7, which also is widespread in the central nervous system and found in ganglia and several other combinations (Table II.7).

Consideration of the classification of voltage-gated ion channels provides a further useful comparison. These channels respond to an electrical signal rather than an endogenous chemical signal, but they also can be classified according to the specific toxins and synthetic chemicals with which they interact. A significant number of therapeutically useful drugs interact with both transmitter-gated and voltage-gated ion channels (Table II.8). Ion channels that permeate, with varying

Table II.6. Classification of Muscarinic Acetylcholine Receptors[a]

	Receptor Subtype				
	M_1	M_2	M_3	M_4	M_5
G-protein coupling	√ Simulation	√ Inhibition	√ Stimulation	√ Inhibition	√ Stimulation
Second messenger	PLC/IP_3/DAG	cAMP	PLC/IP_3/DAG	cAMP	PLC/IP_3/DAG
Locations	CNS DNS Glands	CNS Heart Smooth muscle	CNS Glands Smooth muscle	CNS	CNS
Function	K^+ (M) current inhibition	Decrease heart rate and force	Glandular secretion	—	—
Antagonist	Atropine	Atropine	Atropine	Atropine	Atropine
	Pirenzepine	—	—	—	—
	—	Methoctramine	—	Methoctramine	—
	—	—	Darifenacin	—	—
	—	AF-DX 384	—	AF-DX-384	—

[a]PLC, phospholipase C; IP_3, 1,4,5-inositol triphosphate; DAG, diacylglycerol; cAMP, 3,5-cyclic adenosine monophosphate; CNS, central nervous system.

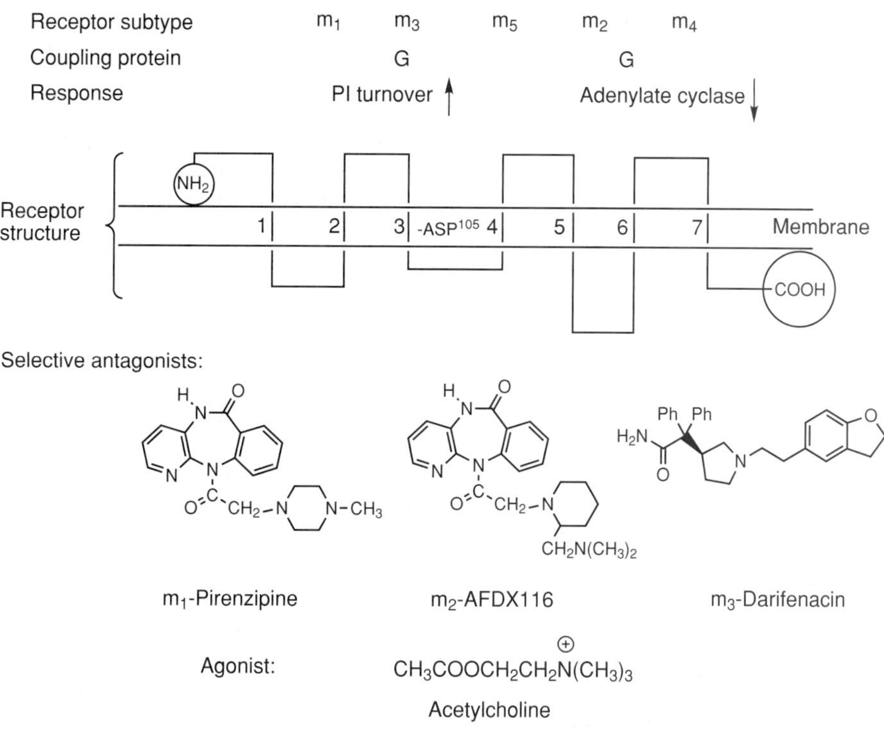

Fig. II.6. Schematic representation of the G protein–coupled muscarinic receptor family (m_1–m_5) and the selective antagonists that interact with the receptor.

degrees of selectivity, Na^+, K^+, Ca^{2+} and Cl^- may be subclassified according to a number of criteria:

a. Structure and subunit composition
b. Voltage-gated or transmitter-gated
c. Ionic selectivity
d. Electrophysiological properties—conductance, kinetics of opening and closing, voltage-dependence and voltage-range of opening and closing
e. Sensitivity to drugs and toxins.

This classification scheme is shown in Table II.9 for voltage-gated Ca^{2+} channels. The L-type channel is the site of action of a major group of cardiovascular drugs, the calcium channel blockers, that are antihypertensive, antianginal, and selectively antiarrhythmic and that interact at discrete receptors on the channel (Fig. II.7). Generally, all ion channels are oligomeric assemblies that possess multiple drug-binding sites for both physiological and pharmacological ligands.

Hijacked Receptors

An increasing number of examples are known in which a receptor for a physiological ligand and with a defined physiological event has been adopted, or "hijacked," by a totally unrelated ligand for a pathological purpose (9,10). Such hijacking represents an important mechanism by which viruses achieve cellular entry (Table II.10). Of particular interest is HIV, which gains entry through simultaneous occupancy of two receptors on T cells—the CD4 and a chemokine receptor. It is of clinical and therapeutic significance that individuals with specific mutations in the CCR5 receptor exhibit enhanced resistance to this virus. Of related interest is the fact that the coronavirus, which is responsible for severe acute respiratory syndrome,

Table II.7. Classification of Nicotinic Acetylcholine Receptors[a] (14)

	Receptor Subtype				
Subunit composition	$\alpha_1\beta_1\delta_1$	$\alpha_4\beta_2$	α_7	$\alpha_3\beta_2\beta_4$ (?)	$\alpha_3\alpha_5\beta_4$
Localization	Skeletal muscle	CNS	CNS	CNS	PNS
Function	Muscle contraction	Cognition NT release	Cognition neuroprotection	NT release	Synaptic transmission
Selective drugs	α-Bungarotoxin	Nicotine Epibatidine Cytosine	α-Bungarotoxin	Dihydro-β-erythroidine	hexamethonium -n-bungarotoxin

[a]CNS, central nervous system, NT, neurotransmitter.

Table II.8. Therapeutic Agents that Interact with Ion Channels

Drug	Channel	Therapeutic Use
Ligand-gated ion channels		
Diazepam	$GABA_A$	Antianxiety
Phencyclidine	Glutamic acid	Tranquilizer
Minoxidil	K^+_{ATP}	Hair growth[a]
Glibenclamide	K^+_{ATP}	Diabetes
Pinacidil	K^+_{ATP}	Hypertension
Voltage-gated ion channels		
Nifedipine	Ca^{2+}	Hypertension
Diltiazem	Ca^{2+}	Angina
Lidocaine	Na^+	Antianxiety Local anesthetic
Phenytoin	Na^+	Anticonvulsant
DDT	Na^+	Insecticide
Sotalol	K^+	Antiarrhythmic
Quinidine	K^+	Antiarrhythmic

[a]Not established to be related to any activity at the K^+_{ATP} channel.

employs a homologue of angiotensin-converting enzyme (ACE), known as ACE-2, that converts angiotensin II to $angiotensin_{1-7}$ by removing the terminal phenylalanine, as its receptor for cellular entry. Recombinant ACE-2 administration affords protection against severe acute respiratory syndrome (11), and presumably, selective ACE-2 blockers will block corona virus entry when available. The ability to recognize known and pharmacologically well-characterized receptors as viral entry points offers obvious potential for the design of small molecule antiviral agents.

Drugs Without Receptors?

Although general anesthetics have been in use for some 150 years, only comparatively recently have their sites and mechanisms of actions been defined. The wide range of structures—chloroform and ether, alkanes, fluorocarbons, alcohols, and so on—as well as a general association of anesthetic potency with the hydrophobic nature of the anesthetic molecule focused attention on a general membrane "stabilization" mode of action. It was assumed, therefore, that general anesthetics might be drugs that did not act at specific pharmacological receptors. More recently, however, it has been concluded that the complex pharmacology exhibited by these agents likely results from their actions at multiple pharmacological receptors, most prominently at synaptic and extrasynaptic receptors for a variety of neurotransmitters. Consistent with this, appropriately structured general anesthetics do demonstrate chirality of interaction. Thus, general anesthetics are polyreceptor ligands (12).

RECEPTOR STRUCTURE

The majority of the pharmacological receptors under discussion are integral membrane proteins and have not, until very recently, been amenable to high-resolution structural studies. Considerable progress, however, has been made in three areas: 1) the structure of rhodopsin as a model for G protein–coupled receptors, 2) the structure of the nicotinic acetylcholine receptor as an example of a ligand-gated ion channel, and 3) bacterial and other K^+ channels that serve to define the conductivity and ionic selectivity mechanisms of ion channels. In addition to such structural studies are an increasing number of biochemical and mutational studies that serve to delineate particular protein regions and residues associated with ligand interaction. Regardless of the receptor type under consideration, structural studies have followed closely parallel pathways—biochemical studies that gave evidence of size and subunit composition, genomic and sequencing studies that described the primary structure of the proteins, modeling studies that provided descriptions of potential membrane organization, and the final three-dimensional experimental structural analyses.

Bacteriorhodopsin and G Protein–Coupled Receptors

The G protein–coupled receptor superfamily is an extremely large family of integral membrane proteins that receive chemical information from odorants, neuro-

Table II.9. Classification of Voltage-Gated Ca^{2+} Channels

	Channel Class			
Property	T	L	N	P
Conductance	Low	High	High	High
Voltage-activating threshold	Low	High	High	High
Ion selectivity	$Ba^{2+} = Ca^{2+}$	$Ba^{2+} > Ca^{2+}$	$Ba^{2+} > Ca^{2+}$	$Ba^{2+} > Ca^{2+}$
Function	Pacemaking; cardiac and neuronal cells	Smooth muscle and cardiac contractibility	← Neurotransmitter release →	
Pharmacology	Mibefradil[a]	Verapamil Diltiazem Nifedipine and 1, 4-dihydropyridines	Conotoxins[b]	Agatoxins[c]

[a]Cardiovascular drug now withdrawn.

[b]Polypeptide disulfide-bridged toxins from mollusks of the *Conus* genus.

[c]Polypeptide toxins from spiders, including *Agelenopsis aperta*.

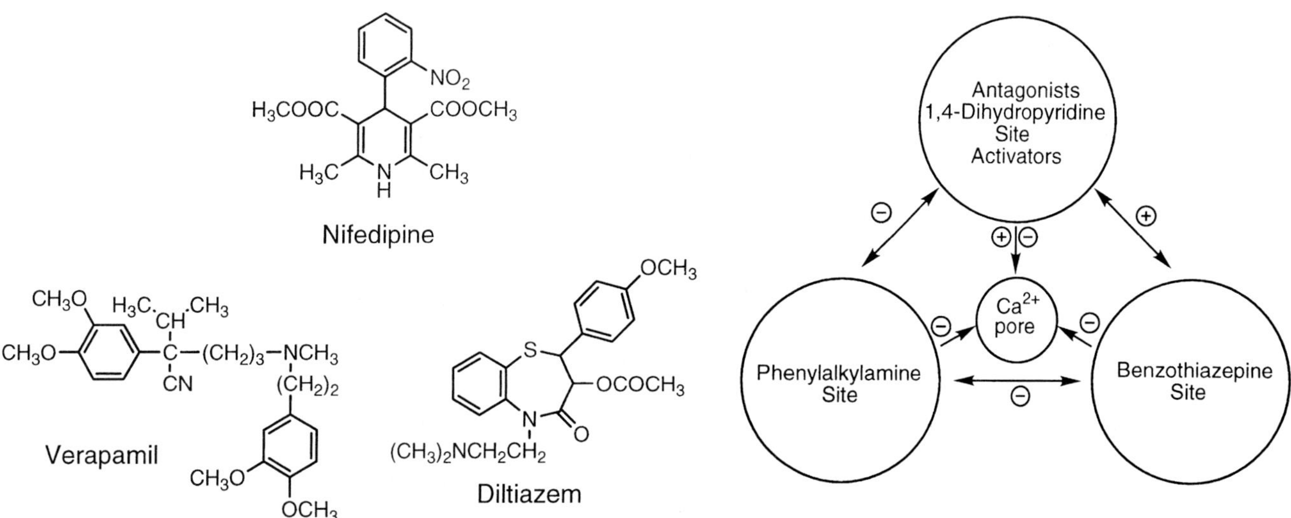

Fig. II.7. Interaction of calcium channel antagonists with the binding sites of the L-type voltage-gated calcium channel. Three distinct receptors interact with specific drug classes represented by the prototypical diltiazem, verapamil, and nifedipine. The 1,4-dihydropyridine receptor also is the binding site for the 1,4-dihydropyridine activators and second-generation dihydropyridines.

transmitters, and polypeptide hormones and translate that information through the family of heterotrimeric G proteins into biological response. This protein superfamily has a common 7-transmembrane helical (7-TM) structure that apparently evolved early in evolution, because it is widely distributed from bacteria onward. Three principal subfamilies exist—rhodopsin/β-adrenergic, secretin/vasointestinal peptide, and metabotropic glutamate—of which the rhodopsin/β-adrenergic is both the largest and the most extensively studied.

The basic model of the 7-TM receptor (>700 sequences have been reported) is based on the established structures of bacteriorhodopsin and vertebrate rhodopsin. The structure of the template protein bacteriorhodopsin is shown in Figure II.8, and from this, a number of models of G protein–coupled receptors have been constructed. The addition of mutagenesis studies to these model-building exercises has permitted the construction of several models of ligand interaction with their specific receptors. Such models do not, however, permit the full realization of the necessary dynamics of the receptor activation process. The availability of structures for G protein–coupled receptors is a major advance for our understanding of receptor function (13).

Table II.10. Receptors for Viruses

Receptor	Virus
ICAM	Human rhinovirus
nAChR	Rabies
Integrin VLA-2	Echovirus 1
Complement	Epstein-Barr
CD4/CCR5	HIV-1
EphrinB2	Nipah
Serotonin (5-HT_{2a})	Human polyoma

The biogenic amine neurotransmitter receptors have been analyzed in some detail to generate models defining the critical interacting residues. Thus, for example, the β-adrenoceptor critical interacting residues are defined as aspartate-113 on helix III, serine-204 and -207 on helix V, and phenylalanine-290 on helix VI (Fig. II.9). These and related studies have defined an homologous ligand "binding pocket" for cationic neurotransmitters and other small ligands that is shared by the catecholamines, histamine,

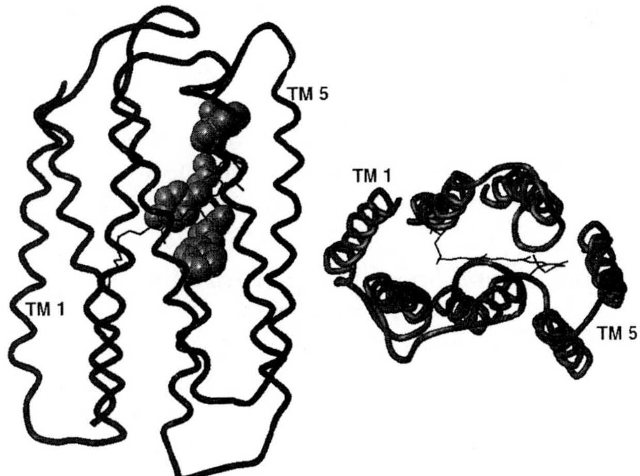

Fig. II.8. Representations of the structure of bacteriorhodopsin, a template protein for G protein–coupled receptors. The left representation depicts retinal covalently bound to transmembrane segment 7 (TM 7), and the right representation depicts the helical arrangement of the protein. (Reproduced with permission from Bikker JA, Trump-Kallmeyer S, Humblet C. G-Protein coupled receptors: models, mutagenesis, and drug design. J Med Chem 1998; 41: 2911–2927. Copyright 1998 American Chemical Society.)

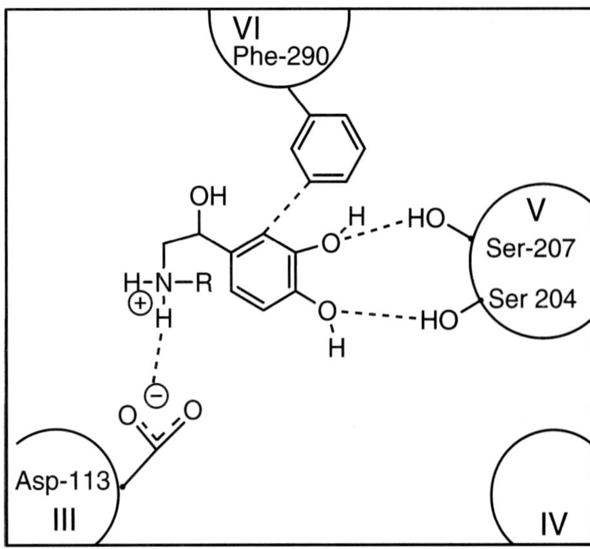

Fig. II.9. Schematic representation of the "amine binding pocket" of the β-adrenergic G protein-coupled receptors (GPCR) with interactions at residues of three of the seven transmembrane helices. (Reproduced with permission from Bikker JA, Trump-Kallmeyer S, Humblet C. G- Protein coupled receptors: models, mutagenesis, and drug design. J Med Chem 1998; 41: 2911–2927. Copyright 1998 American Chemical Society.)

serotonin, acetylcholine, as well as by other ligands. Similarly, these modeling and mutagenesis studies can produce models that accommodate the known stereoselectivity of interaction of the chiral species.

The interaction of peptides and small proteins with G protein–coupled receptors presents, given the disparity in size, a scaling problem relative to the small neurotransmitter ligands. Small peptides, with as few as six residues, appear to define the minimally active fragment. The loop regions of the receptor may play a larger role in defining ligand interactions, although the binding site still shows similarity to the binding site for biogenic amines.

Nicotinic Acetylcholine Recepter (nAChR) and Ligand-Gated Channel Receptors

This ligand-gated channel receptor was the first to have its amino acid sequence determined, and it has been the subject of particularly intensive biochemical, electrophysiological, and pharmacological analysis (14). Early work revealed the nicotinic acetylcholine receptor as a heteromeric association of five subunits—α_2, β, γ, and δ. The α subunit bears the acetylcholine-binding site. The sequence analysis revealed the three types of subunits to be significantly homologous to each other and to have likely originated from an ancestral subunit by gene duplication and independent mutation. Differential combination of these subunits provides for differential distribution of nAChR subtypes with distinctive biophysical and pharmacological properties (Fig. II.10).

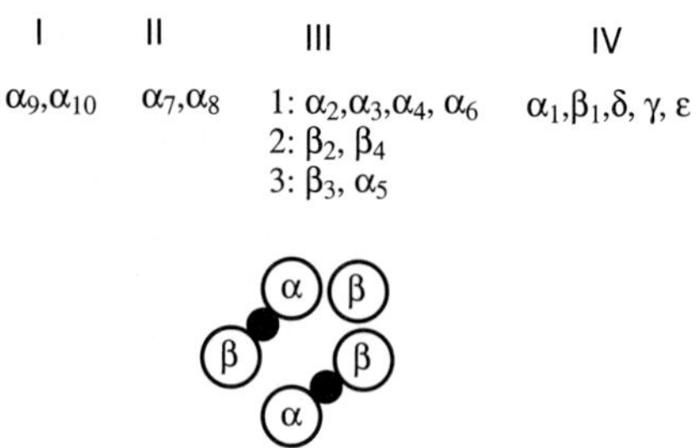

Fig. II.10. Organization of the subunits of the nAChR depicting the four principal subclasses (I–IV) and the pentameric organization of subunits. The acetylcholine-binding site is located on the interface between the α and β subunits.

Ion channels are molecular machines, and a great interest exists regarding how they perform the conformational changes associated with opening, closing, and the translocation of ions. In the case of the nAChR, high-resolution electron micrographs of tubular arrays of receptors isolated from the electric organs of *Torpedo* sp. have revealed major differences between the open and closed states. Although little change occurs in the wide outer mouth of the channel, a substantial change occurs in the orientation of the M_2 helices that form the permeation pathway. At rest, these helices are in a bent shape, thus providing a narrow "stricture" in the path. In the open state, the lower halves of the helices move to replace the hydrophobic leucine residues from the axis of the pore and replace them with smaller polar residues, which results in an "opening" of the channel. Because clear homologies exist between the nAChR and other ligand-gated channels, including GABA, glycine, and 5-HT_3, this activation mechanism may be quite general.

Voltage-Gated Ion Channel Permeation and Selectivity

A long series of electrophysiological studies, starting with the classic work of Hodgkin and Huxley, served to establish conceptually the key features of ion channel function and organization. These are summarized in Figure II.11. There must be a pore through which ions

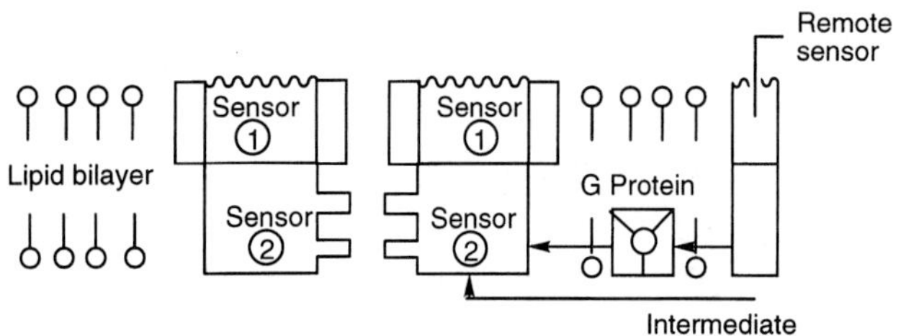

Fig. II.11. Schematic representation of an ion channel depicting the presence of gates that open and close in response to stimuli, sensors or receptors that respond to physical or chemical stimuli, and "remote" receptors linked to the channel via indirect pathways using cytosolic or membranal "second" messengers.

permeate, and this pore must have an ionic selectivity filter, because channels can distinguish ions with remarkable fidelity: K^+ channels select for K^+ over Na^+ by a factor of approximately 10^3 to 10^4. Channels open and close in response to specific signals, typically changes in membrane or chemical potential; hence, there are specific sensors that both recognize these signals and signal channel gates. Additional work has shown that these sensors may be integral to or remote from the channel structure proper and, if the latter, are linked to the channel machinery by diffusible or membrane-associated signals.

Recent studies have established the three-dimensional structure of a number of K^+ channels, and this has contributed significantly to our understanding of channel function not only for K^+ channels but also by extrapolation to other voltage-gated channels and to channel permeation in general (15,16). A principal feature is that of oligomeric association with identical or nonidentical subunits. A schematic representation of the voltage-gated Ca^{2+} channel is sketched in Figure II.12. The principal α_1 subunit carries the major molecular machinery of the channel, including the permeation and gating machinery, together with the binding sites for drugs of the Ca^{2+} channel antagonist class. The expression and properties of this subunit, however, are significantly affected by the presence of the β, γ, and α_2- δ subunits.

GENOME STUDIES

Finding New Receptors

Until very recently, the identification of receptors as targets for drug action, whether of physiologic or other origin, had followed the process depicted in Figure II.13, in which the initial characterization of a functional activity and identification of the responsible ligand (e.g., a neurotransmitter or hormone) led to the ultimate definition of the physiologic role of the receptor, its protein characterization, and finally, its gene identification. This process then permits the characterized and expressed receptor to be used as a screen for the identification of novel structures. The genome project has now permitted the genomics-based process (Fig. II.13), whereby receptors can be identified and shown to have homology to existing receptors even though there may be no currently known physiological ligand with which these newly identified receptors interact. The cloned and expressed receptor, however, can now be used to identify the putative physiological ligand and to identify novel structures—a process that is the reverse of that historically employed (17).

The G protein–coupled receptor class is of particular importance as a source of such "orphan receptors," because this class has a proven history of providing major therapeutic targets (Table II.5). At least 140 such receptors have been characterized from the human genome.

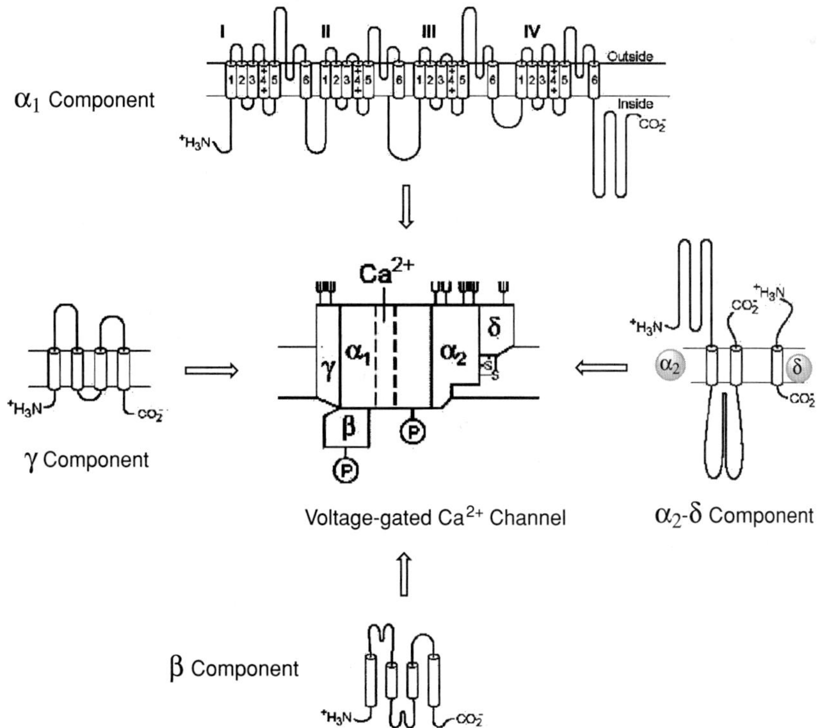

Fig. II.12. Representation of the structure of the voltage-gated Ca^{2+} channel composed of several subunits (α_1, α_2-δ, β, and γ) organized as depicted in the central area.

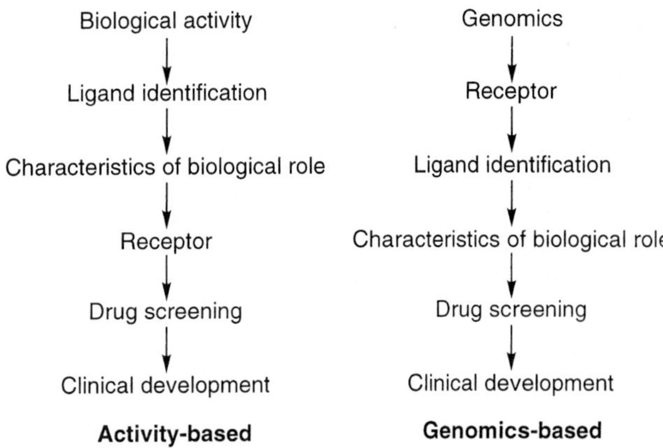

Fig. II.13. Comparison of "activity-based" and "genomics-based" drug discovery process. In activity-based, biologic, physiologic, or pathologic activity is chosen, which forms the "discovery target." Genomics-based discovery arises from a gene sequence discovery of a new putative receptor, which is used to search for a physiological ligand from which derived the physiologic function.

Furthermore, an increasing number of diseases have been specifically associated with mutations in this class of receptors. The identification of a new human opiate receptor called ORL1 (opioid receptor-like) that does not interact with known opiate ligands is an excellent example of this approach. This receptor has a specific endogenous agonist called nociceptin, a 17-amino-acid peptide with some similarity to the physiologic peptide dynorphin A (Fig. II.14). Consistent with the widespread distribution of the ORL1 receptor in the brain, nociceptin appears to have correspondingly widespread actions, including nociception and stress reduction. Similarly, the orexins—orexin-A and orexin-B—are hypothalamic peptides involved in the complex process of regulation of feeding behavior and were discovered by screening brain extracts against the expressed orphan receptors, OX_1 and OX_2.

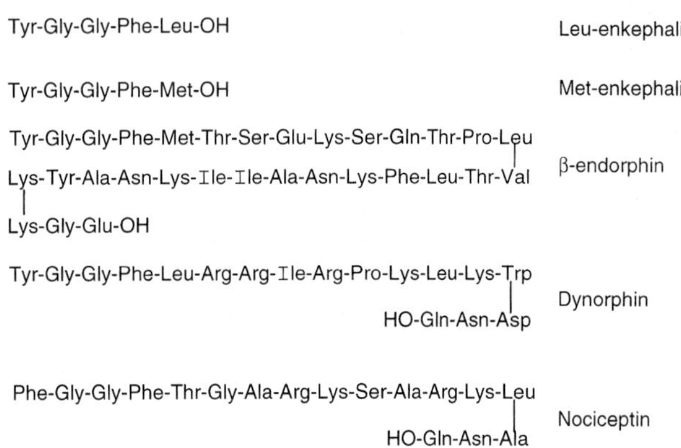

Fig. II.14. The physiological ligands for the opiate-receptor—leu-enkephalin, met-enkephalin, β-endorphin, and dynorphin. Nociceptin is the physiological agonist for the human opioid receptor known as ORL1 (opioid receptor-like-1).

In a similar fashion, the steroid hormone receptor family also has generated a large number of orphan receptors—more than 70 in all. For the great majority of these, no physiological ligand or function has yet been described. The retinoic acid receptor was first identified as an orphan species. These orphan receptors are widely expressed throughout animal species. Their widespread distribution indicates a fundamental importance to the processes of cellular activity. Thus, the RXR (retinoid-X-receptor) family of receptors does not bind the endogenous ligand, all-*trans*-retinoic acid, for the retinoic acid receptor, although these receptors share structural homology. Rather, the RXRs bind 9-*cis*-retinoic acid, and from this discovery has come the development of new selective RXR ligands, including bexarotene.

Finding Receptor Differences: From Pharmacology To Polygamy

Genome studies have been extremely important in establishing receptor structures, the classification of receptors, and the definition of orphan receptors for which ligands and physiological function have yet to be found. Genome studies also have been critical in establishing that very small differences in sequence or expression levels may accompany profound intra- and interspecies differences in function and behavior. Three examples will be illustrative.

Good evidence exists for the role of 5-HT_6 receptors in cognitive function. These receptors are distributed quite differently, however, in mouse, rat, and human, and the mouse receptor has a quite different pharmacological profile based on two amino acid differences only in transmembrane regions 5 and 6 in this G protein–coupled receptor (18). Thus, a mouse knockout of this receptor may not be a good model with which to validate a receptor as a human drug target. Similarly, the 5-HT_{1B} receptor in rat and human shows major pharmacological distinction that is conferred by residue 355; when the threonine of the human receptor is replaced by the asparagine of the rodent receptor, the pharmacology becomes essentially indistinguishable (19) (Table II.11). A single arginine residue determines the species specificity of the human growth hormone receptor: Arg^{43} in the human

Table II.11. Ligand-Binding Properties of Human and Rodent 5-HT_{1B} Receptors (Wild-Type) and the Mutant Human Receptor (19)

	Receptor K_inM		
Ligand	Human	Rat	Mutant
5-HT	10	16	8
DHE	6	4	2
Metergoline	25	129	200
Sumatriptan	38	465	560
Methsergide	130	1823	970
8-HO-DPAT	1,600	>10,000	25,000
RU 24909	44	2	10

growth hormone receptor interacts with asp^{171} of the hormone. In nonprimates, these residues are leucine and histidine, respectively, and it is the noncomparability of arg^{43} in the human receptor and his^{171} in the nonprimate hormone that determines the lack of interaction and, hence, the species specificity. There are important implications to these observations both for drug discovery, in which the use of human receptors becomes increasingly important (*"The proper study of mankind is man."* [Alexander Pope,1688–1744]), and in the determination of individual human variability to drugs, in which single nucleotide polymorphisms may control drug sensitivity. Thus, some 10% of the human population express an $A^{118} \rightarrow G$ nucleotide substitution at position 118 of the μ-opiod receptor gene, and the expressed variant receptor binds β-endorphin with some three times higher affinity.

Finally, differences in receptor expression may have very important social consequences, at least in the area of vole fidelity and promiscuity. Prairie voles exhibit monogamous behavior, whereas the closely related meadow voles are solitary and polygamous. This profound and important behavioral difference apparently results from the differential expression of the vasopressin 1a receptor in the ventral forebrain (20).

RECEPTOR QUANTITATION

The receptor represents the locus of drug action, and analysis of the kinetics of drug–receptor interaction is important from the perspective of defining the ability of a drug to interact with the receptor (affinity) and to activate the information encoded within the receptor (efficacy). The quantitation of drug–receptor interaction is based on the occupancy–response relationship that states the more receptors occupied by a drug, the larger the response to the drug. The concentration of the drug at the receptor site in vivo, however, is determined by the amount of drug administered and by the various pharmacokinetic processes, including metabolism, tissue binding, and excretion, as shown in Figure II.15. In this model, drugs are thought to interact with receptors via two mechanisms: drugs that stimulate the receptor and produce a biological response (agonists), and drugs that bind to the receptor and do not produce an effect but, rather, prevent agonists from binding (antagonists). Thus, agonists are drugs with affinity and efficacy, whereas antagonists are drugs with affinity and zero efficacy. The principal issue is the definition of the parameters and mechanisms that define "efficacy."

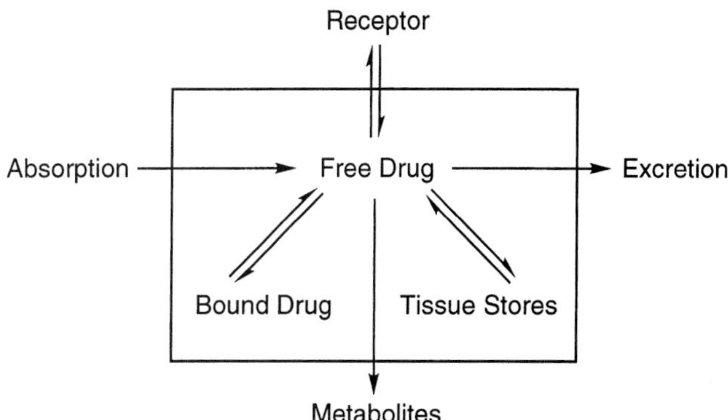

Fig. II.15. Concentration of drug at the receptor is greatly influenced by a number of pharmacokinetic processes, including absorption, metabolism, distribution, storage, and excretion.

The analysis of antagonists thus appears to be straightforward—they are simply agents that bind, do not activate, and prevent agonists from exerting their efficacy. Antagonists may be subdivided into competitive and noncompetitive antagonists. Competitive antagonists can have their blocking effect overcome by addition of more agonist, but this will not hold true for noncompetitive antagonists. Almost all the antagonists in clinical use are competitive antagonists. Noncompetitive antagonists can be further subdivided into irreversible and allosteric antagonists, with the latter being agents that interact at a site distinct from the agonist-binding site but coupled to it through an "allosteric" linkage. The latter are a particularly important class of drugs as well, because many drugs that are active at ion channels exert their effects on permeation and gating through allosteric mechanisms.

The simple distinction between agonists and antagonists is complicated, however, by the existence of "partial" agonists. These are compounds that elicit a cellular response that is less than that observed with other agonists. Partial agonists possess affinity and efficacy, but the efficacy is less than that of a "full" agonist. The implications of this observation are that the total number of receptors becomes important for the overall generation of a biological response but also that some drug–receptor couplings are very efficient, whereby maximum response can be generated from occupancy of a small fraction of receptors. Thus, the fraction of receptors not occupied for response generation is termed the "receptor reserve," or "spare receptors." An agonist may, according to the density of receptors within a cell and the efficiency of receptor–effector coupling, be an agonist, partial agonist, or antagonist, according to the tissue and its physiologic or pathologic state.

An extension of the simple division of receptor-active drugs into agonists/partial agonists and antagonists is provided by the recognition that receptors are considered as two-state devices (or, more accurately, as multistate devices) that are conformationally mobile between activated and inactivated states (Fig. II.16). The function of ligands active at such receptors is then to influence the equilibrium between active and inactive receptor states. Accordingly, agonists shift the equilibrium to the activated state, and antagonists do not exhibit selective affinity for either state and, thus, do not shift equilibria. This model recognizes the existence of a third class of receptor-active drugs, those that preferentially stabilize the inactive conformation; these are termed "inverse agonists" (21,22). These agents exert their efficacy in constitutively active G

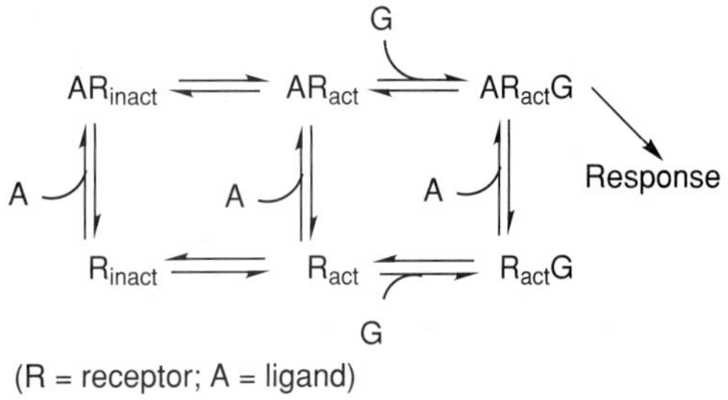

$$
\begin{array}{ccccc}
AR_{inact} & \rightleftharpoons & AR_{act} & \overset{G}{\rightleftharpoons} & AR_{act}G \rightarrow \text{Response} \\
A \updownarrow & & A \updownarrow & & A \updownarrow \\
R_{inact} & \rightleftharpoons & R_{act} & \underset{G}{\rightleftharpoons} & R_{act}G
\end{array}
$$

(R = receptor; A = ligand)

Fig. II.16. A schematic representation of a two-state model of a G protein-coupled receptor (GPCR). The receptor can exist in an inactive state (R_{inact}) and in active liganded and unliganded states (AR_{act} and R_{act}, respectively). Equilibrium between these forms can be shifted by the presence of agonist, antagonist, and inverse agonist.

protein–coupled receptor systems, in which the receptor system is functionally active in the absence of a ligand. Receptors that are overexpressed or mutated can show such constitutive behavior. Accordingly, ligands can exert efficacy at receptors that range from +1 through 0 to –1, constituting the range of full agonist, partial agonist, neutral antagonist, and partial and full inverse antagonist. In fact, many drugs simply referred to as antagonists likely have inverse agonist properties.

RECEPTORS AS RECOGNITION ENTITIES

The specificity of drug interaction, including stereoselectivity, at pharmacological receptors has long been recognized as a distinguishing characteristic of both drug and receptor. The basic assumption in the analysis of structure–activity relationships is the existence of a definable mutual complementarity between the structure of a drug and its corresponding binding site. The specifics of such interactions are a central theme of the discipline of medicinal chemistry and are a major focus of this volume: Structure–activity relationships are discussed individually for specific drug classes. The absence of such specificity, including stereoselectivity of recognition, frequently is employed as an argument against a biological response being mediated through a receptor process. The definition of the action of general anesthetics has, for example, been intimately involved with questions of chemical specificity of the anesthetic interaction. Until the mid-1980s, the attempted correlation of chemical structure and biological activity was the only available approach to the definition of receptor site structure. This has changed dramatically, however, with the ability to determine protein sequences and the three-dimensional structures of proteins in both the native state and liganded with substrates and antagonists.

Quantitative Structure–Activity Relationships

Quantitative structure–activity relationships (QSARs) for drug–receptor interactions are a subset of structure–property correlations in which a variety of chemical and

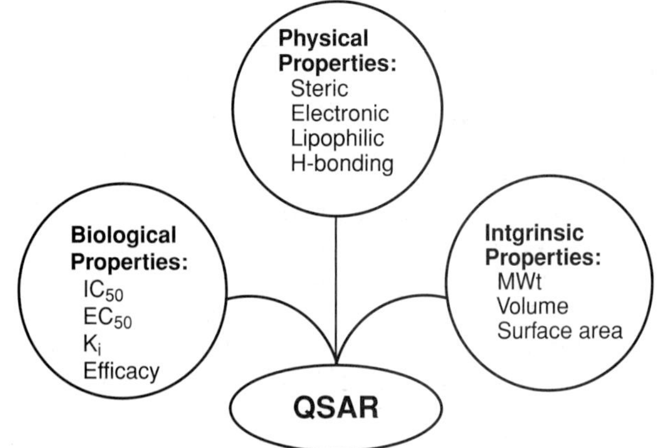

Fig. II.17. The definition of quantitative structure-activity relationships (QSARs) is defined by physical properties, intrinsic properties, and biological properties.

physical molecular properties is employed to define the association between structure and property. Such QSARs have become widespread in medicinal chemistry since the advent of cheap, high-speed computing technologies during the past 20 years. They rely on the ability to examine multiple relationships between physical properties and biological activities (Fig. II.17).

Classic QSARs, such as Hansch-type analyses, provide an equation defining biological activity as a linear free energy relationship, such as in the description of cyclooxygenase inhibition by substituted phenylpropionic acids. Six variables as shown in Figure II.18 are used to describe the biological activity, and an optimal compound occurs when R_1 = Cl, R_2 = Me, and R_3 = H. This approach is clearly useful in probing, albeit indirectly, the nature of the interaction forces between drug and receptor as well as for predicting active compounds ahead of simple cumulative synthesis.

The QSAR approach can be extended with the recognition that the ligand occupies three-dimensional space. The ability to determine or predict a pharmacophore map by the use of molecular modeling techniques and the synthesis of rigid analogues then generates a hypothesis of bioactive conformation, from which comparative molecular field analysis can be used to calculate the intermolecular interaction fields that surround each molecule. Subsequently, the relationship between the biological activity and the calculated fields is determined.

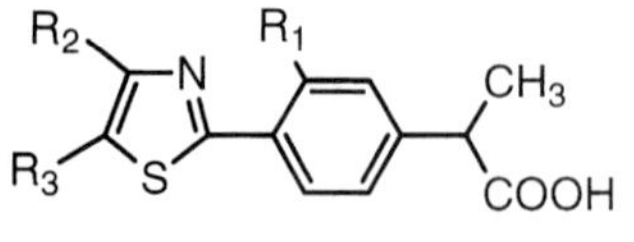

R_2, R_1, N, CH_3, R_3, S, COOH

$$
\begin{aligned}
pI_{50} &= 1.03\,\pi(R_1) - 4.48\,\sigma_R(R_2) - 0.86\,\Delta L(R_2) \\
&\quad + 0.44\,\pi(R_3) - 0.40\,\Delta L(R_3) - 1.48\,I_{180} + 6.11
\end{aligned}
$$

Fig. II.18. Quantitative structure-activity relationship (QSAR) for inhibition of cyclooxygenase by substituted propionic acid derivatives.

Structural Approaches

The increasing availability of protein and DNA structures determined by x-ray crystallographic and solution nuclear magnetic resonance (nmr) approaches has greatly accelerated both the interpretation of structure–activity relationships and the structure– assisted design of drugs (23). The availability of these structures has not only permitted the analysis of key structural features that contribute to the activity of an enzyme or receptor but also identified binding areas for drug molecules that can be explored by in silico techniques to permit the more efficient synthesis of potentially active molecules. The majority of receptors are membrane proteins that until recently have been very resistant to three-dimensional structure determination. This situation is rapidly changing, however, and the recent elucidation of the structure of a number of ion channels should greatly expedite our understanding of drug action at this important group of pharmacological receptors.

Ion channels have become particularly important and exploited targets for drug action in recent years. Many agents, from animal toxins to natural and synthetic insecticides, cardiovascular drugs (Ca^{2+} channel antagonists and K^+ channel activators), antiarrhythmic agents, and local anesthetics, are active at one or more classes of ion channels. The properties of ion channels in terms of their ion selectivity, translocation properties, conductance, opening and closing kinetics, and voltage-dependence of activation and inactivation have been well established from electrophysiological studies and have led to the construction of models of channel structure and function. Until recently, integral membrane proteins ion channels have defied direct structural characterization. The recent elucidation of the structure of several K^+ channels, however, has confirmed the essentials of the previous structural models and revealed this channel to have a flat outer mouth lined with negatively charged residues, a pore that progressively narrows, and a "selectivity filter," consisting of a small sequence of amino acids that coordinate the translocating ion through their carbonyl residues. Interestingly, the inward portion of the pore is lined by hydrophobic residues, and the selectivity filter holds two K^+ ions. The selectivity filter provides the discriminating capacity of this channel for Na^+ over K^+ or Ca^{2+}, and the multiple occupancy provides rapid transit, approximately diffusion-controlled, through mutual electrostatic repulsion. Although the K^+ channel is the smallest of the cation channels, it is highly probable that the larger and more complex Na^+ and Ca^{2+} channels will mimic closely this fundamental structure, thus permitting advances in structure-based drug discovery for these membrane effectors. Although the direct structures of these larger channels remain undetermined, advances have been made in the elucidation of the localization and function of drug-binding sites. Local anesthetics serve as antiarrhythmics by interacting in a state-dependent manner with the voltage-gated Na^+ channel: The drug prefers to bind to the open or inactivated states of the ion channel. The binding site for etidocaine has been localized close to the pore-forming region and involves specific interactions with the aromatic residues phenylalanine and tyrosine (Fig. II.19). Presumably, conformational changes during channel opening (activation) position these residues such that they make tighter interactions than in the resting state (24).

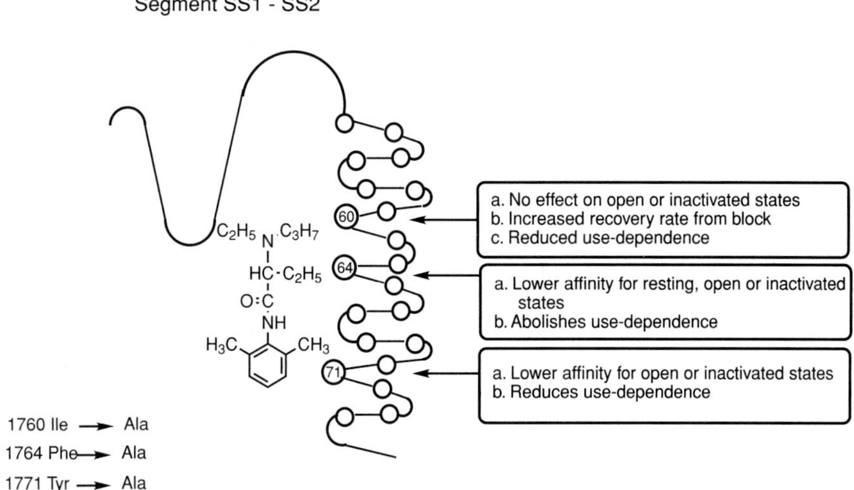

Fig. II.19. The binding of a local anesthetic, etidocaine, to the voltage-gated Na^+ channel. Deduced from site-directed mutagenesis studies, critical interactions of etidocaine depend on residues 60, 64, and 71, and their replacement by alanine results in loss of specific site-dependent properties of etidocaine block. (Reproduced with permission from Ragsdale S, McPhee JC, Scheuer T, et al. Molecular determinants of state-dependent block of Na^+ channels by local anesthetics. Science 1994; 265:1724–1728. Copyright 1994 AAAS.)

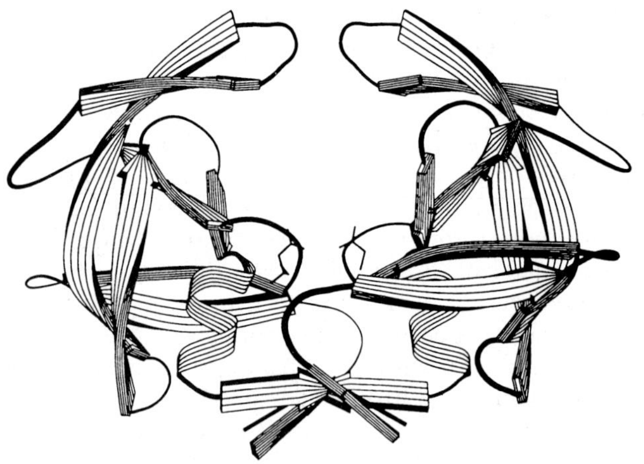

Fig. II.20. Structure of HIV protease-1 depicted as a ribbon backbone structure. The twofold axis of symmetry is vertical, and the active site aspartate residues are depicted in the middle of the cleft. (Reproduced with permission from Greer J, Erickson JW, Baldwin JJ, et al. Application of the three-dimensional structures of protein target molecules—structure-based drug design. J Med Chem 1994; 37: 1035–1054. Copyright 1994 American Chemical Society.)

The introduction of the "protease inhibitors" effective against HIV infection represents one of the recent triumphs of structure-based drug design. A critical component of the HIV genome codes for an aspartate protease. Inactivation of this enzyme resulted in the crippling of viral reproduction; hence, this protease was recognized early on as a likely target for drug action. The structure reveals a dimer composed of two identical aspartate protease-like domains, and it is thus essentially a symmetric structure (Fig. II.20).

This symmetry guided development of the first inhibitors of the enzyme (Fig. II.21), leading ultimately to the nonsymmetric clinically available agents. A particularly interesting feature of the structural studies of the enzyme–inhibitor complex is the presence of a water molecule that serves, through hydrogen-bonding interactions, to mediate contacts between enzyme and inhibitor. Potent protease inhibitors have been designed that include in the ligand, groups that serve as a replacement for this water molecule, DMP-450 (Fig. II.21), an interesting and possibly unique example of structure–activity relationship around a water molecule.

Stereochemistry of Drug–Receptor Interactions

Chirality is a fundamental property of biological systems, reflecting the underlying asymmetry of matter. Drug–receptor interactions have long been recognized as stereoselective, and it is increasingly recognized that both pharmacokinetic and pharmacodynamic processes contribute to the clinically observed stereoselectivity. In fact, stereoselective drug–receptor interactions are so widely observed that they frequently are considered to be a defining component of the overall process of drug stereoselectivity (25).

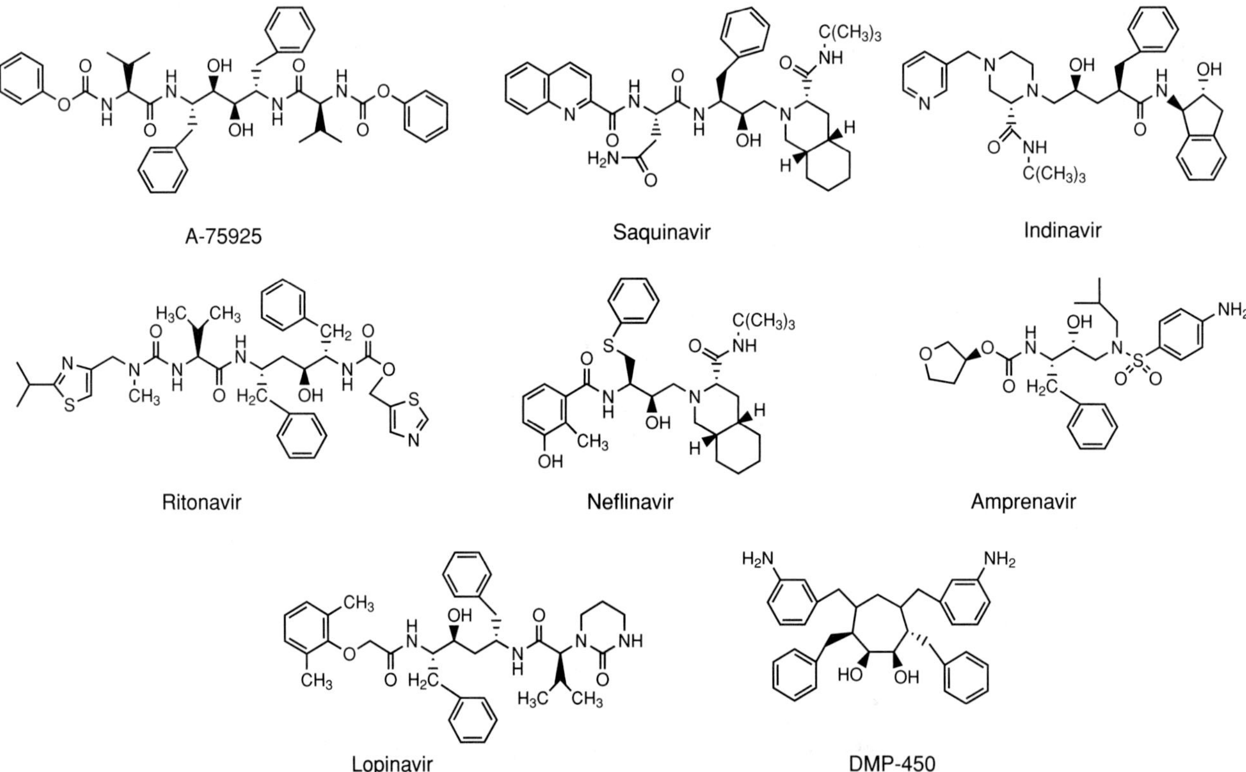

Fig. II.21. Inhibitors of HIV-1 protease. A-75925: Early symmetric inhibitor. Nonsymmetric clinically available molecules: Saquinavir, Indinavir, Ritonavir, Neflinavir, Amprenavir, and Lopinavir. DMP-450: Molecule that replaces bound water in protease active site.

In principle, stereoisomers may differ in several ways in their pharmacological activities:

1. Both [all] enantiomers are equally active, and there is no observed stereoselectivity of action. This situation is rare, but in some cases, such as general anesthetics, the stereoselectivity may be very modest.
2. The enantiomers differ quantitatively in their pharmacological activities: In the extreme situation, one enantiomer is totally devoid of pharmacological activity.
3. The enantiomers differ qualitatively in their pharmacological activities and exhibit discrete activities at the same or different receptors.

In recognition of these differences, drug regulatory agencies are issuing guidelines for drug evaluation and development that explicitly recognize racemic drugs as being composed of distinct chemical entities. Examples of all these differences are known and are common (Fig. II.22). Thus, β-blockers exhibit stereoselectivity at β-adrenoceptors, whereby S-propranolol is some 40-fold more potent than its R-enantiomer. In local anesthetic and antiarrhythmic properties, however, the enantiomers are essentially equipotent. The enantiomers of the Ca^{2+} channel antagonist verapamil, marketed as a racemate, exhibit stereoselectivity of interaction at its receptors in both vascular and cardiac tissue, but the stereoselectivity ratios are different in each tissue. Thus, S-verapamil has both vasodilating and cardiodepressant properties, whereas R-verapamil is dominantly a vasodilating drug. The 1,4-dihydropyridine Bay K 8644 has Ca^{2+} channel activator and antagonist properties associated with the S- and the R-isomers respectively.

Until recently, the issue of stereoselectivity of drug action was largely scientific. Increasingly, however, it has become a regulatory matter. In particular, the use of single enantiomers may reduce undesired side effects that may be present in one enantiomer—the "inactive" enantiomer. The elimination or reduction of pharmacokinetic complexities that may arise from the differential metabolism, transport, protein binding, or elimination of the enantiomers may constitute a further—and significant—advantage. Additionally, advances in synthetic chemistry, translatable to the process scale, have greatly simplified the production of enantiomerically pure chemicals. Although there is no current regulatory prohibition on the development of racemic agents, it is increasingly likely that single enantiomer drugs will be the overwhelming future therapeutic choice.

Common Characteristics of Drug Structures

Until recently, the process of new drug discovery typically involved random screening of new compounds, either synthetic or of natural origin, followed by the manual synthesis of modified structures, typically "one molecule at a time" and with directed evaluation of pharmacological activity. Associated with this process has been a significant component of "chemical intuition," although this has been increasingly expanded with the advent of receptor structure availability and molecular modeling. With the advent of combinatorial chemistry and high-throughput screening, opportunities exist for the quick synthesis and evaluation of tens of millions of molecules on a rapid timescale. In practice, such methodologies need to be focused to ensure that the "most profitable" chemical

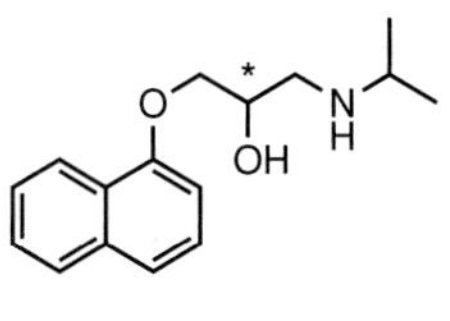

Propranolol
(S - β-antagonist)
(R - Inactive)

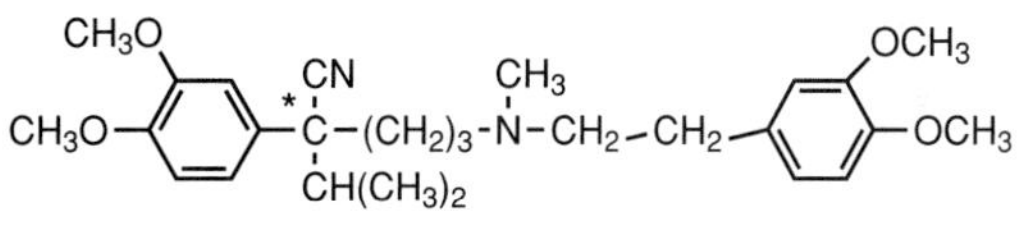

Verapamil
(S-vasodilating and cardiodepressant)
(R -vasodilating)

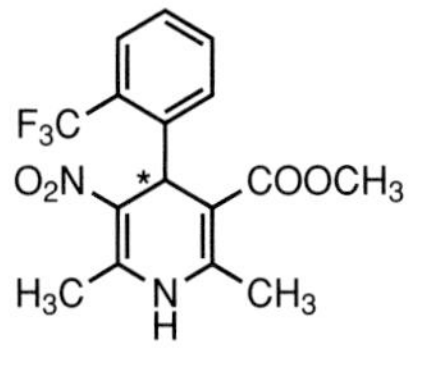

Bay K 8644
(S - agonist)
(R - antagonist)

Fig. II.22. Stereoselectivity of drug action at a variety of discrete receptor classes.

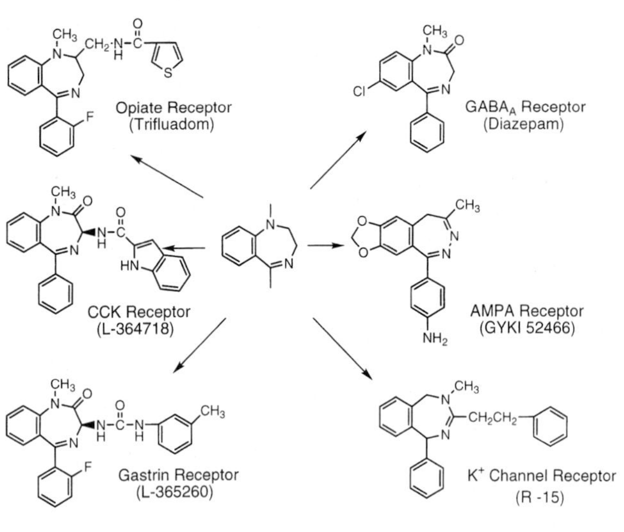

Fig. II.23. Benzodiazepine nucleus as a basic pharmacophore, or "privileged," structure capable of being directed, with appropriate molecular modification, against a number of discrete and nonrelated receptors.

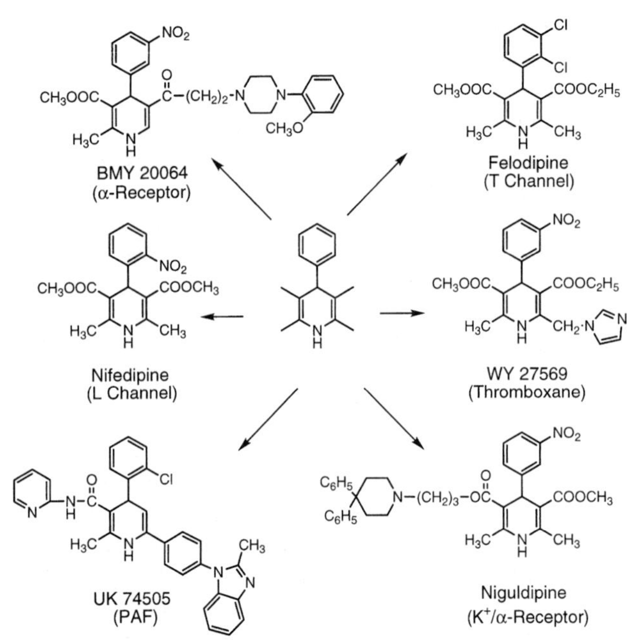

Fig. II.24. 1,4-Dihydropyridine nucleus as a "privileged" structure.

space is the most extensively exploited. The ability to delineate structural features that characterize "drug-like" molecules and distinguish these from "nondrug" molecules therefore is an important factor in the contemporary paradigm of drug discovery.

Several methodologies have been advanced that classify molecules in terms of sets of molecular descriptors, including molecular weight, functional groups, partition coefficients, hydrogen-bonding groups, charge, atom type, and so on. These methodologies have been reasonably successful in "predicting" drug-like molecules in large chemical databases, such as the Available Chemicals Directory, the World Drug Index, and the Comprehensive Medicinal Chemistry Database. Before the development of these methodologies, it had been realized that certain structures were, indeed, "pharmacophoric" and that when appropriately "decorated" with molecular features, they functioned as drugs active at a number of discrete receptors. One such early recognized pharmacophore is the benzodiazepine nucleus, which is active at receptors as diverse as GABA, opiate, and cholecystokinin (Fig. II.23). A more recently recognized pharmacophore is the 1,4-dihydropyridine nucleus, which also is active at a wide variety of receptors and ion channel types (Fig. II.24).

It is in fact likely that a number of basic pharmacophoric structures, or "scaffolds," exist (Fig. II.25) and onto which are grafted the functional groups that define specific individual drugs and drug families. It has been suggested that these scaffolds or templates are to be considered as structures that resist "hydrophobic collapse"—that is, they resist, through their conformational nonflexibility, the ability to self-associate to inactive species. This property is seen in the diphenylmethyl group, a popular molecular substructure of many active drugs of diverse classes.

From Proteins and Peptides to Small Molecule Drugs

One of the most challenging issues in both drug–receptor recognition and drug development is the translation of the receptor recognition properties of proteins and peptides to small molecules—"peptide mimetics" or "peptidomimetics"—without loss of the potency and specificity of action of the large parent molecule. Among the best-known examples of this process are morphine and its various synthetic congeners that mimic the actions of the various opiate peptides (Fig. II.26). It is important to note, however, that in this instance, the small molecule mimetics were known long before the opiate peptides were discovered and that the structural resemblance between the peptides and their nonpeptide mimics is not immediately clear.

Peptide mimetics have been discovered by a variety of processes, including routine screening and structure-based approaches designed to minimize the protein or

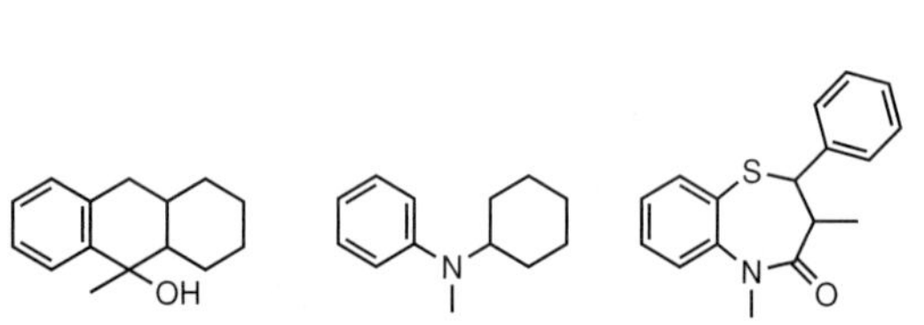

Fig. II.25. A number of basic pharmacophoric structures, or "scaffolds," onto which may be grafted the functional groups that direct the ligand against a specific receptor type or subtype.

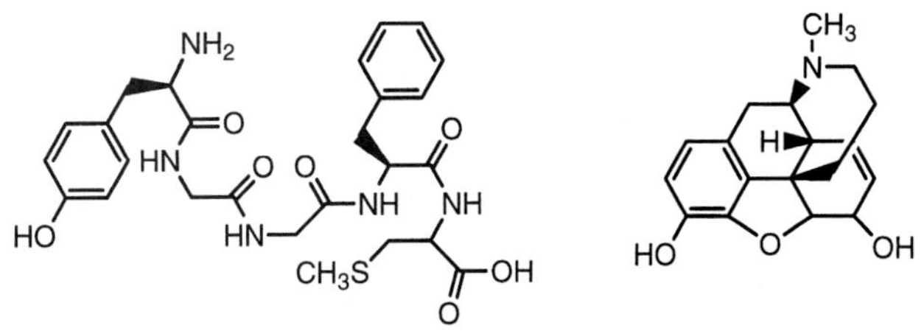

Met-Enkephalin Morphine

Fig. II.26. Structures of the physiologic peptide, met-enkephalin, and the nonpeptide morphine, both of which are potently active at opiate receptors.

polypeptide size or to reproduce in nonpeptide molecules the essential conformation and functional characteristics of the binding epitopes (protein surface-binding sites) of the polypeptide or protein. From the former process has been derived the benzodiazepine-based cholecystokinin (CCK) and gastrin antagonists depicted in Figure II.23. Similarly, a small molecule mimetic agonist, SB 247,464, was discovered for the granulocyte colony-stimulating factor receptor activation, which stimulates the growth of white blood cells (26,27). This receptor, a member of the growth factor receptor family, is activated by oligomerization, and the symmetric nature of this synthetic agonist suggests that it may be acting by mimicking the cross-linking capacity of the physiological ligand.

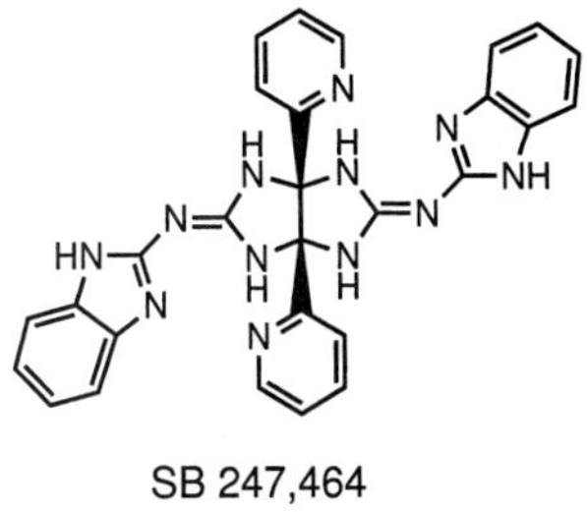

SB 247,464

RECEPTORS AS TRANSDUCTION MACHINES

As recognized by John Newton Langley as early as 1906, a critical function of the receptor is to translate the information of the ligand–receptor interaction into a biological response. With this translation comes very substantial amplification of the input information, whereby a single ligand–receptor interaction is amplified in gain by several orders of magnitude. This is achieved by a variety of biochemical processes involving direct or indirect roles for second messengers—ions, cyclic nucleotides, lipid metabolites, and the activation of protein kinases. The G protein–coupled receptors and ion channels, representing the largest categories of membrane receptors, are increasingly well understood from a molecular standpoint and represent systems that frequently cross-communicate.

In the large family of G protein–coupled receptors, heterotrimeric G proteins serve to translate the agonist–receptor interaction into a biological response. The G proteins are a large "superfamily" of regulatory GTP hydrolase proteins and one that includes the receptor linked α subunits, Ras, and elongation factors. The interaction of an activated 7-TM receptor with the heterotrimeric G protein stimulates the G protein to release bound GDP and to associate with GTP, leading to dissociation of the β and γ subunits and liberation of the activated GTP-associated G protein α subunit. This activated subunit and the dissociated β and γ subunits then interact with a number of effector systems, including adenylyl cyclase, phospholipases, phosphodiesterases, and ion channels. Dissociation of the subunits from these effector systems and hydrolysis of the bound GTP by an intrinsic or extrinsic GTPase activity terminates the transduction process (Fig. II.27). This process can be further modulated by desensitization events (see following section).

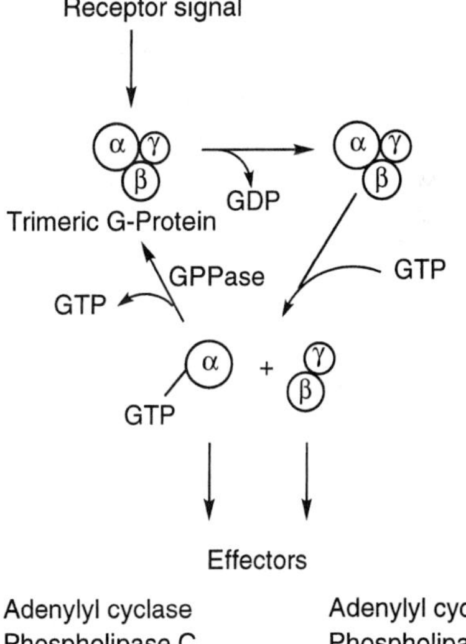

Adenylyl cyclase	Adenylyl cyclase
Phospholipase C	Phospholipase C
	Phospholipase A_2
c-GMP phosphodiesterase	
	Receptor kinases
K^+ channel	K^+ channel
Ca^{2+} channel	

Fig. II.27. Transduction pathways for G protein–coupled receptors. The formation of the activated receptor (constitutively or through ligand interaction) interacts with the trimeric G protein in its GDP-ligated state. An exchange for GDP by GTP permits the formation of the GTP-bound α subunit and the β and γ subunits that are activators or inhibitors of a variety of biological effectors. GTP hydrolysis and reassociation of the subunits terminates the process.

RECEPTORS AS REGULATED SPECIES

Although the principal physiologic function of a receptor is to be activated by a physiological ligand to generate the corresponding biological response, receptors also are controlled on a longer time frame through processes of desensitization and downregulation. These processes may be viewed as elements of a homeostatic control system, whereby the potentially deleterious effects of persistent receptor activation are reduced. In contrast, persistent occupancy of a receptor by an antagonist results in upregulation of receptor number and function, and this also may be viewed as a component of the same homeostatic control process designed to maintain balance between receptor number and receptor output or gain. Mutational defects in the structure of receptors or associated components are increasingly well characterized. These defects may cause persistent receptor activation in the absence of a ligand ("constitutively active receptors"), may render the receptor unable to respond to a ligand ("constitutively silent receptors"), or may simply shift the dose–response curve for the activated receptor in the directions of greater or lesser sensitivity to the ligand.

Desensitization and downregulation appear to be common components to all receptor processes from bacterial chemotaxis, olfaction, and neurotransmission to T-cell activation and may well be considered as a further characteristic property of receptors, together with specific ligand recognition and transduction mechanisms. Desensitization may be specific (homologous) or nonspecific (heterologous), whereby the receptor is desensitized only to its receptor-specific ligand or to a series of unrelated ligands respectively (Fig. II.28). The processes of desensitization and downregulation have, however, been particularly well described for G protein–coupled receptors, in which a series of biochemical events and cellular internalization processes operate to sequentially regulate receptor activity on the acute timescale of seconds or minutes. Longer-term control processes operate at the protein, translation, and transcriptional levels to regulate the rates of degradation and synthesis of receptors.

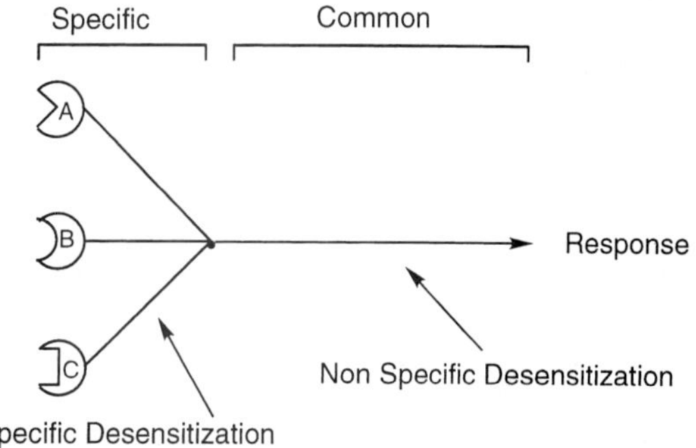

Fig. II.28. Process of specific and nonspecific desensitization. Depicted are three discrete receptors—A, B, and C—linked to a common or shared transduction system and biological response. The process of specific desensitization is assumed to be directed at the specific and discrete receptor components, whereas the process of nonspecific desensitization is assumed to be directed through the common components of the receptor response pathway.

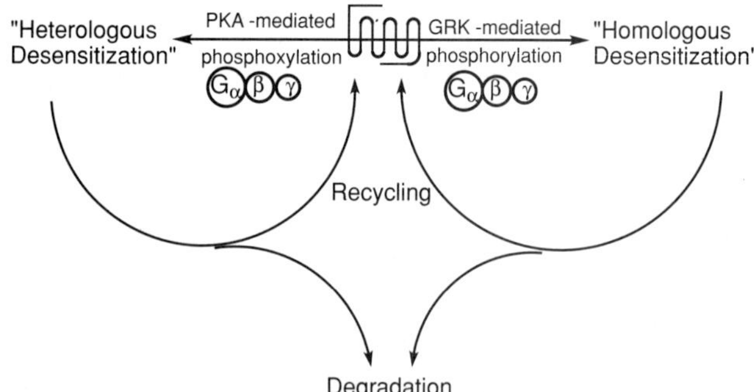

Fig. II.29. Biochemical events during desensitization and downregulation of G protein–coupled receptors. In nonspecific desensitization, receptor phosphorylation uncouples the receptor from the G protein; in contrast, during specific desensitization, the agonist-occupied receptor is phosphorylated by a G protein–receptor kinase (GRK_{1-6}). Subsequent to phosphorylation receptors may be recycled to a patent form in the plasma membrane or may be subjected to degradation through the lysosomal machinery to generate receptor downregulation.

Figure II.29 demonstrates a typical cycle of desensitization for a G protein–coupled receptor, in which receptor phosphorylation mediated by a kinase activated by a second-messenger product of receptor activation, cAMP or Ca^{2+}, renders the receptor uncoupled from the G protein. This process generates nonspecific or heterologous regulation. In contrast, phosphorylation of the agonist-occupied receptor by a G protein–coupled receptor kinase (GRK_{1-6}), followed by association of the receptor with a member of the arrestin protein family, yields agonist-specific or homologous desensitization. Subsequently, these receptors may be internalized and recycled to be reinserted into the plasma membrane, or they may be subject to lysosomal degradation processes. In the latter event, receptor restoration will be dependent on de novo protein synthesis and export.

An increasing number of receptor diseases are known, many of which fall into the G protein–receptor and ion channel families (28,29). Mutations in the receptor protein or in associated signaling components may produce either loss-of-function or gain-of-function disorders. In loss-of-function mutations, the receptor protein may not be delivered to the cell membrane, or it may have impaired agonist binding or receptor coupling with G proteins. In contrast, gain-of-function mutations produce receptors that may be constitutively active, even in the absence of the physiological ligand. A

Table II.12. G Protein–Coupled Receptor Inherited Disorders

Receptor	Disease	Mutation Type
Cone opsins	Color blindness	Loss
V_2 vasopressin	Nephrogenic diabetes insipidus	Loss
ACTH	Familial ACTH resistance	Loss
LH	Male precocious puberty	Gain
TSH	Pseudohermaphroditism	Loss
Ca^{2+}	Familial hypoparathyroidism	Gain
Thromboxane A_2	Congenital bleeding	Loss
Endothelin B	Hirschsprung's disease	Gain

number of these receptor and ion channel inherited disorders are listed in Tables II.12 and II.13. In addition, defects in the associated coupling components of these receptors may similarly alter the capacity of the receptor to achieve its signaling mission. Thus, a loss of function of the G protein α_s subunit is associated with type 1a pseudohypoparathyroidism, and a gain of function in this subunit is associated with acromegaly, hyperfunctional thyroid nodules, and other disorders. Similarly, over- or underexpression of the GRKs can produce systems that show attenuated responses to agonists or that are not capable of showing homologous desensitization, respectively.

Similar diseases are known to be associated with mutational defects in both ligand- and voltage-gated ion channels. Long QT syndrome, associated with ventricular arrhythmias and sudden death, is actually a group of diseases associated with defects in both K^+ and Na^+ channels, cystic fibrosis with defects in a Cl^- channel, hypokalemic periodic paralysis with defects in the L-type voltage-gated Ca^{2+} channel, and hyperinsulinemic hypoglycemia of infancy with defects in an ATP-sensitive K^+ channel. The form of long QT syndrome associated with defects in the HERG K^+ channel has assumed particular significance, because this channel is blocked by a number of common drugs, including some antibiotics, antihistamines, and antifungal agents, that increase the chances of cardiac arrhythmias and sudden death.

Table II.13. Ion Channel Inherited Disorders

Channel	Disease
Voltage-gated Na^+	Hypokalemic periodic paralysis
	Long QT syndrome
Voltage-gated K^+	Episodic ataxia
	Periodic paralysis
Inward rectifier K^+	Familial hyperinsulinemia
ATP-K^+	Hypoglycemia of infancy
Voltage-gated Ca^{2+}	Muscular dysgenesis (murine)
	Familial hemiplegic migraine
CFTR Cl^- channel	Cystic fibrosis

REDEEMED RECEPTORS

The major focus for the ultimate treatment of inherited disorders has been gene therapy to replace the mutant gene. A significant number of inherited mutations in receptors and ion channels, however, are associated with loss of function because of trafficking errors—that is, the receptor or channel proteins fail to be incorporated in the plasma membrane because of protein misfolding. Some of these misfolded proteins may be rescued, or "redeemed," through the intervention of an appropriate ligand that binds to the misfolded protein, corrects its conformation, and permits export to the appropriate locus in the cell. Such an approach has actually been demonstrated for a number of systems, including the gonadotropin-releasing hormone receptor, in which a putative gonadotropin-releasing hormone antagonist is capable of entering the cell and binding to the mutant protein (30).

References

1. Ehrlich P. Chemotherapeutics: scientific principles, methods and results. Lancet 1913;ii:Aug:445–451.
2. Fischer E. Einfluss der konfiguration auf die wirkung der enzyme. Ber Dtsch Chem Ges 1894;27:2985–2993.
3. Langley JN. On the physiology of salivary secretion. J Physiol 1878;1:339–367.
4. Crum-Brown A, Fraser TR. On the connection between chemical constitution and physiological action. Part 1. On the physiological actions of the salts of the ammonium bases, derived from strychnia, brucia, thebia, codeia, morphia, and nicotia. Trans R Soc Edinburgh 1868;25:151–203.
5. Langley JN. Royal Society Croonian Lecture. On nerve endings and on special excitable substances in cells. Proc R Soc London Ser B 1906;78:170–184.
6. International Union of Pharmacology. Available at: http://www.iuphar-db.org/iuphar-rd/. Accessed March 30, 2007.
7. Milligan G. G protein–coupled receptor dimerization: function and ligand pharmacology. Mol Pharmacol 2004;66:1–7.
8. Waldhoer M, Fong J, Jones RM, et al. A heterodimer-selective agonist shows in vivo relevance of G protein–coupled receptor dimers. Proc Natl Acad Sci U S A 2005;102:9050–9055.
9. Triggle DJ. Hijacked receptors. Pharm Acta Helv 2000;74:287–290.
10. Smith AE, Helenius A. How viruses enter animal cells. Science 2004;304: 237–257.
11. Imai Y, Rao S, Huan Y, et al. Angiotensin-converting enzyme protects from severe acute lung failure. Nature 2005;436:112–116.
12. Hemmings HC, Akabas MH, Goldstein PA, et al. Emerging molecular mechanisms of general anesthetic action. Trends Pharmacol Sci 2005;26: 503–510.
13. Bikker JA, Trump-Kallmeyer S, Humblet C. G protein–coupled receptors: models, mutagenesis, and drug design. J Med Chem 1998;41:2911–2927.
14. Jensen AA, Frolind B, Liljefors T, et al. Neuronal nicotinic acetylcholine receptors: structural revelations, target identification, and therapeutic inspirations. J Med Chem 2005;48:4705–4745.
15. Jiang Y, Chait BT, Lee A, et al. X-ray structure of a voltage-dependent K^+ channel. Nature 2003;423:33–41.
16. Triggle DJ, Gopalakrishnan M, Rampe D, et al., eds. Voltage-Gated Ion Channels as Drug Targets. Weinheim, Germany: Wiley-VCH, 2006.
17. Howard AD, McAllister G, Feishner SD, et al. Orphan G protein–coupled receptors and natural ligand discovery. Trends Pharmacol Sci 2001;22: 132–140.
18. Hirst WD, Abrajamsen B, Blaney FE, et al. Differences in the central nervous system distribution and pharmacology of the mouse 5-hydroxytryptamine-6 receptor compared with rat and human receptors investigated by radioligand binding, site-directed mutagenesis, and molecular modeling. Mol Pharmacol 2003;64:1295–1308.
19. Oksenberg D, Marrsters SA, O'Doud F, et al. A single amino-acid difference confers major pharmacologic variation between human and rodent 5-HT_{1B} receptors. Nature 1992;360:161–163.
20. Lim MM, Wang Z, Olazabai DE, et al. Enhanced partner preference in a promiscuous species by manipulating the expression of a single gene. Nature 2004:429:754–757.
21. Milligan G. Constitutive activity and inverse agonists of G protein–coupled receptors: a current perspective. Mol Pharmacol 2003;64:1271–1276.
22. Kenakin T. Efficacy as a vector: the relative prevalence and paucity of inverse agonism. Mol Pharmacol 2004;65:2–11.

23. Greer J, Erickson JW, Baldwin JJ, et al. Application of the three-dimensional structures of protein target molecules—structure-based drug design. J Med Chem 1994;37:1035–1054.
24. Ragsdale S, McPhee JC, Scheuer T, et al. Molecular determinants of state-dependent block of Na^+ channels by local anesthetics. Science 1994;265: 1724–1728.
25. Lough WJ, Wainer IW, eds. Chirality: Natural and Applied Science. Boca Raton, FL: CRC Press, 2002.
26. Tian S-S, Lamb P, King AG, et al. A small nonpeptidyl mimic of granulocyte colony-stimulating factor. Science 1998;281:257–259.
27. Toogood PL. Inhibition of protein-protein association by small molecules: approaches and progress. J Med Chem 2002;45:1543–1558.
28. Spiegel AM, Weinstein LS. Inherited diseases involving proteins and G protein–coupled receptors. Annu Rev Med 2004;55:27–39.
29. Ashcroft FM. Ion Channels and Diseases. San Diego: Academic Press, 2000.
30. Brothers SP, Cornea A, Janovick JA, et al. Human loss-of-function gonadotropin-releasing hormone receptor mutants retain wild-type receptors in the endoplasmic reticulum: molecular basis of the dominant-negative effect. Mol Endocrinol 2004;18:1787–1797.

12. *Drugs Affecting Cholinergic Neurotransmission*

E. KIM FIFER

DRUGS COVERED IN THIS CHAPTER:

ACETYLCHOLINE MIMETICS—MUSCARINIC AGONIST
- Methacholine chloride
- Carbachol chloride
- Bethanechol chloride
- Pilocarpine
- Cevimeline

ACETYLCHOLINESTERASE INHIBITORS (ANTICHOLINESTERASES)
- Physostigmine
- Neostigmine
- Pyridostigmine
- Carbaryl
- Edrophonium
- Echothiophate iodide

ACETYLCHOLINESTERASE INHIBITORS FOR THE TREATMENT OF ALZHEIMER'S DISEASE
- Tacrine
- Donepezil
- Rivastigmine
- Galantamine

INSECTICIDAL ACETYLCHOLINESTERASE INHIBITORS
- Parathion
- Malathion

ACETYLCHOLINE ANTAGONISTS—MUSCARINIC ANTAGONISTS
- Atropine
- Scopolamine
- Propantheline
- Oxybutynin
- Solifenacin
- Darifenacin

NICOTINIC ANTAGONISTS—NEUROMUSCULAR BLOCKING AGENTS
- Decamethonium bromide
- Succinylcholine chloride
- *d*-Tubocurarine
- Metocurine
- Pancuronium bromide
- Vecuronium bromide
- Pipecuronium bromide
- Rocuronium bromide
- Atracurium besylate
- Mivacurium chloride
- Doxacurium chloride

INTRODUCTION

It is likely that no other mammalian system or chemical neurotransmitter has been studied as exhaustively as the parasympathetic nervous system and acetylcholine. Acetylcholine functions as the neurotransmitter for many different neurons (Fig. 12.1) (1). In the autonomic nervous system, it is released by pre- and postganglionic fibers of the parasympathetic division, preganglionic fibers of the sympathetic division, and a few postganglionic fibers of the sympathetic division (e.g., sweat and salivary glands). It also is released by neurons of the somatic (voluntary) nervous system and by some neurons in the central nervous system (CNS). Neurons that release acetylcholine are referred to as cholinergic, as are the receptors on which these neurons synapse. These receptors are further classified as either muscarinic or nicotinic, depending on their ability to bind the naturally occurring alkaloid muscarine or nicotine, respectively. Parasympathetic nerve impulses stimulate contraction of smooth muscle in the gastrointestinal tract and urinary tract, contraction of the ciliary muscle of the eye, relaxation of smooth muscle of the blood vessels, and decreased heart contractility and rate.

H_3C–C(=O)–O–CH_2CH_2–$N^{\oplus}(CH_3)_3$ $Cl^{\ominus}$

(-) - Muscarine chloride

S(-) - Nicotine

Chemical compounds that cause stimulation of the parasympathetic nervous system are called cholinomimetic or, more specifically, parasympathomimetic agents. Cholinomimetic agents might be agonists that act directly on cholinergic receptors or function as inhibitors of acetylcholinesterase (AChE), the enzyme responsible for hydrolysis of acetylcholine. Those compounds that possess affinity for cholinergic receptors but exhibit no intrinsic activity are called cholinergic antagonists, cholinolytic, or parasympatholytic agents. This chapter is devoted to the discussion of cholinergic agonists and antagonists and to the biochemistry of cholinergic neurotransmission.

Studies of the parasympathetic nervous system and cholinergic agents led to the concept of neurochemical transmission and were instrumental in the development of early drug receptor hypotheses and our understanding of the stereochemical influence on drug action. An excellent summary of this history is presented by Holmstedt (2).

In 1914, Dale defined two subdivisions of the parasympathetic nervous system when he observed that ethers and esters (including acetylcholine) of choline produced effects similar to those of muscarine (muscarinic effects) or nicotine (nicotinic effects) (2). The initial experiments were performed using an ergot extract contaminated with acetylcholine, although Dale was unaware of this contamination. Ewins, a chemist who collaborated with Dale, isolated acetylcholine from the ergot extract and subsequently synthesized acetylcholine, thus allowing Dale to show that the unexpected muscarinic effects observed with the ergot preparation were the result of acetylcholine. He proposed the term "parasympathomimetic" to describe

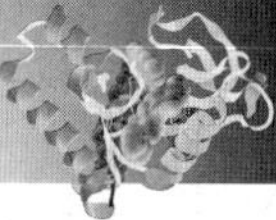

CLINICAL SIGNIFICANCE

Agents affecting cholinergic neurotransmission are some of the most widely studied agents to date. It also is one of the most intriguing classes of study in that the clinical utility of these compounds runs the gamut from the life-saving potential of atropine given to patients undergoing cardiac life support to the life-threatening capacity of chemical warfare agents, such as sarin. Advancements in our understanding of muscarinic and nicotinic receptor activity and compounds that modulate these effects have led to decreased morbidity and mortality and increased quality of life for millions of individuals throughout the world. Additionally, those agents employed as insecticides or pesticides have had tremendous economic impact as well. Agents affecting cholinergic neurotransmission are used to treat a variety of clinical conditions, including impaired or excessive gastric motility/secretion, glaucoma, bradycardia, Alzheimer's disease, Parkinson's disease, and myasthenia gravis. Nicotinic antagonists are used to facilitate surgical procedures by reducing the amount of anesthetic or sedative agent required, thus reducing risk to the patient.

A thorough understanding of the structure–activity relationships of these compounds has led to an ability to enhance their desired pharmacodynamic effects while minimizing unwanted or harmful adverse effects. The impact of the application of this knowledge is multifaceted for the clinician. Examples include the synthesis of newer chemical compounds used to treat Alzheimer's disease that provide greater affinity for acetylcholinesterase in the brain than in the periphery, decrease the frequency of dosing required, and alleviate the risk of hepatotoxicity that was associated with the first Alzheimer's agent, tacrine. These advances have increased the utility of these agents and given hope to countless individuals and families affected by this devastating disease. Modifications to the neuromuscular blocking agents have resulted in differences in onset and length of activity, reduction in adverse effects (e.g., hypotension), and alternate routes of elimination, which increase their utility for patients with certain comorbid conditions (e.g., cardiac disease or renal dysfunction). Finally, it also is important for the clinician to recognize the capacity of certain chemical configurations to be allergenic or more prone to producing adverse effects so that the best agent for a particular patient can be selected.

Kathryn Neill, Pharm.D.
Assistant Professor
Critical Care Specialist
Department of Pharmacy Practice
College of Pharmacy
University of Arkansas for Medical Sciences

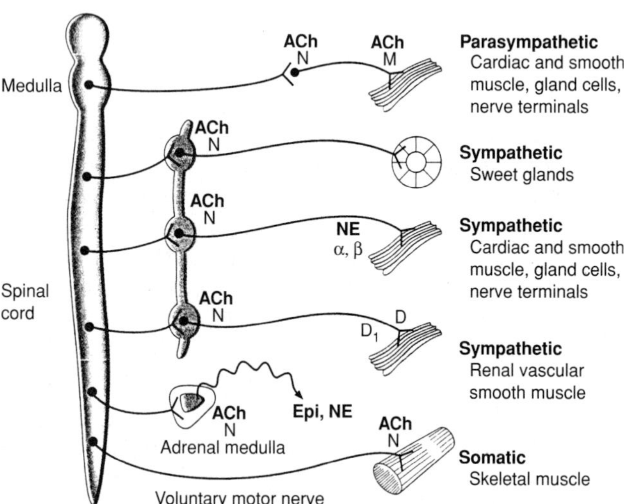

Fig. 12.1. Schematic representation of autonomic and somatic motor nerves. The sites of action of acetylcholine (ACh), norepinephrine (NE), epinephrine (Epi), and dopamine (D) are indicated. Cholinergic receptors are designated as nicotinic (N) or muscarinic (M). (From Katzung BG. Introduction to autonomic pharmacology. In: Katzung BG, ed. Basic and Clinical Pharmacology, 9th Ed. New York: McGraw-Hill, 2004, pp. 75–93; with permission.)

the ability of acetylcholine to produce the same effects as electrical stimulation of parasympathetic nerves, and he suggested that acetylcholine was a chemical neurotransmitter in the parasympathetic nervous system. Dale also observed that the action of acetylcholine was short-lived, and he proposed that tissues contained an esterase that hydrolyzed acetylcholine. In 1921, Loewi (3) demonstrated that a chemical compound mediated impulses between nerves; he referred to the chemical substance in his preparation as *vagusstoff.* In 1926, Loewi and Navratil (4) provided experimental evidence suggesting that vagusstoff was acetylcholine.

These classic studies are the foundation of our current understanding about the role of acetylcholine in cholinergic nerve transmission and our recognition of muscarinic and nicotinic cholinergic receptors. They provided the stimulus for subsequent studies of acetylcholine biochemistry, synthesis of new organic compounds (e.g., cholinergic and anticholinergic drugs), and purification of cholinergic receptors.

The concept that muscarinic and nicotinic receptors may explain the different physiologic responses produced by acetylcholine was derived from this early research of Dale and Loewi. Although it currently is recognized that there are multiple subclasses of both muscarinic and nicotinic receptors, the general classification of these two types of cholinergic receptors continues to effectively explain the different physiologic responses produced by acetylcholine.

Because of the important role of acetylcholine as a chemical neurotransmitter in the autonomic nervous system, an imbalance in parasympathetic tone can lead to serious consequences. Conceptually, deficiencies in acetylcholine could be treated by administering the neurotransmitter itself, but acetylcholine is a poor therapeutic agent. Its actions are nonselective, producing effects at all cholinergic receptor sites, which could result in serious consequences for the patient. Because acetylcholine is a quaternary ammonium salt, it is poorly absorbed across biological membranes, resulting in poor bioavailability regardless of the route of administration. Furthermore, its ester functional group is rapidly hydrolyzed in the acidic conditions of the gastrointestinal tract and by esterases in plasma.

Muscarinic cholinergic agents are used postsurgically to reestablish smooth muscle tone of the gastrointestinal and urinary tracts to relieve abdominal distention and urinary retention. They also are used to treat some forms of glaucoma by enhancing the outflow of aqueous humor, thereby reducing intraocular pressure. Cholinomimetic compounds with CNS activity are being evaluated for the treatment of cognitive disorders (e.g., Alzheimer's disease). Those that exhibit nicotinic effects are commonly used to treat myasthenia gravis.

Cholinergic muscarinic antagonists (anticholinergic drugs) are sometimes referred to as antispasmodics because of their ability to reduce smooth muscle spasms resulting from overstimulation of the gastrointestinal smooth muscles. Newer drugs in this class have found use in the treatment of overactive bladder.

Many synthetic cholinergic agonists have been designed using structure–activity relationships (SARs) based on the structure of acetylcholine. To design cholinergic agents that are selective for specific cholinergic receptors, it is necessary to have a thorough understanding of acetylcholine neurochemistry as well as the chemical nature and role of cholinergic receptors.

CHOLINERGIC RECEPTORS

History

Much effort has gone into understanding how cholinergic receptors carry out the two primary functions of all receptors—molecular recognition and signal transduction. A thorough understanding of these phenomena is essential to achieving rational, efficient, and selective drug therapy.

Knowledge regarding the structure and function of cholinergic receptors has increased substantially since the concept of distinct muscarinic and nicotinic receptors was first postulated. Early efforts to describe these receptors were hindered in that receptors were only a concept. Indeed, their existence was not established until 1973, when Pert and Snyder (5) provided demonstrable evidence for the existence of opiate receptors.

Early attempts to characterize cholinergic receptors were based on SAR and stereochemical studies of cholinergic agonists and antagonists. This led to synthesis of agonists and antagonists with exceptionally high affinity and selectivity for cholinergic receptors as well as to synthesis of radiolabeled cholinergic ligands with high specific radioactivity. These advances were paralleled by advances in biochemistry, molecular pharmacology, and molecular biology that made possible the purification and sequencing of small quantities of protein, the measurement of ligand binding to cell membranes and subcellular components, and the cloning and sequencing of genes. This led to isolation, purification, and amino acid sequencing of one of the nicotinic cholinergic receptors—the first acetylcholine receptor and the first neurotransmitter receptor to be fully characterized (6,7). Subsequently, muscarinic receptors were isolated, purified, and sequenced using these techniques.

Current pharmacological and molecular biological research indicates that multiple muscarinic and nicotinic acetylcholine receptor subtypes exist (8,9). The traditional classification of muscarinic and nicotinic receptors, however, adequately describes the actions of most cholinergic medicinal agents and is used throughout this chapter. Furthermore, most of the current therapeutic agents acting at muscarinic receptors exhibit little selectivity for the receptor subtypes, with the exception of a few recently introduced anticholinergic agents for treatment of overactive bladder.

Muscarinic Receptors

The SAR regarding the affinity and efficacy of cholinergic agonists provided the basis for early models of muscarinic receptor structure. An early model of the muscarinic receptor, depicted in Fig. 12.2, illustrates the importance of muscarinic agonists having an ester functional group and a quaternary ammonium group separated by two carbons. This model depicts ionic bonding between the positively charged quaternary nitrogen of acetylcholine and a negative charge at the anionic site of the receptor. The negative charge was suggested to result from a carboxylate ion from the free carboxyl group of a dicarboxylic amino acid (e.g., aspartate or glutamate) at the binding site of the receptor protein. This model also involved a hydrogen bond between the ester oxygen of acetylcholine and a hydroxyl group contributed by the esteratic site of the receptor.

Although this early muscarinic receptor model accounted for two important SAR requirements for muscarinic agonists, it failed to explain the following: 1) At least two of the alkyl groups bonded to the quaternary nitrogen must be methyl groups, 2) the known stereo-

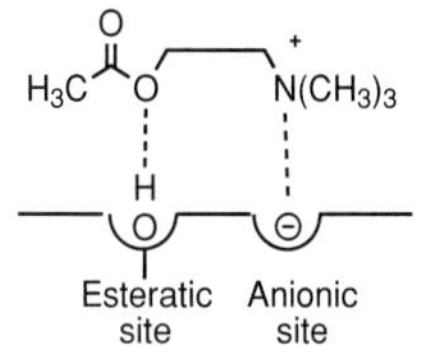

H_3C O O $\overset{+}{N}(CH_3)_3$ H O ⊖ Esteratic site Anionic site

Fig. 12.2. Original representation of the muscarinic receptor.

chemical requirements for agonist binding to the receptor, and 3) the fact that all potent cholinergic agonists have only five atoms between the quaternary nitrogen and the terminal hydrogen atom. This last point is known as Ing's "Rule of Five" (10).

Subsequent models of the cholinergic muscarinic receptor depicted the receptor as a binding site on a protein molecule and explained more completely the structural and stereochemical requirements for cholinergic agonist activity. Some scientists proposed that the muscarinic receptor and AChE were the same entity, but this proposal was dispelled by experiments demonstrating that interaction of cholinergic ligands with the muscarinic receptor did not lead to hydrolysis of the ligand. None of these models, however, completely explained the diverse pharmacological effects produced by all muscarinic agonists and antagonists.

Subsequent developments suggested that the effects of muscarinic receptor stimulation are mediated by second messengers that are biosynthesized by at least two important events: 1) inhibition of adenylyl cyclase*, and 2) activation of phospholipase C. Both involve a guanosine triphosphate (GTP)–dependent mechanism. Two other important developments were the synthesis of radiolabeled muscarinic ligands and the utilization of molecular biology techniques in the study of muscarinic receptors.

Heterogeneity in the muscarinic receptor population was first suggested in the late 1970s during pharmacological studies using the muscarinic antagonist pirenzepine. At the time, pirenzepine was the only muscarinic antagonist to block gastric acid secretion at concentrations that did not block the effects of muscarinic agonists. This observation initiated research that ultimately led to discovery of muscarinic receptor subtypes, designated as M_1, M_2, and M_3 based on their pharmacological responses to various ligands. Rapid advances in molecular biology led to the cloning of cDNAs that encoded for five muscarinic receptors, designated as m1 through m5; m1, m2, and m3 correspond to the respective M_1 through M_3 receptors identified by their pharmacological specificity. The International Union of Pharmacology Committee on Receptor Nomenclature and Drug Classification has recommended that the uppercase nomenclature M_1 through M_5 be used to designate both pharmacological as well as molecular subtypes (8).

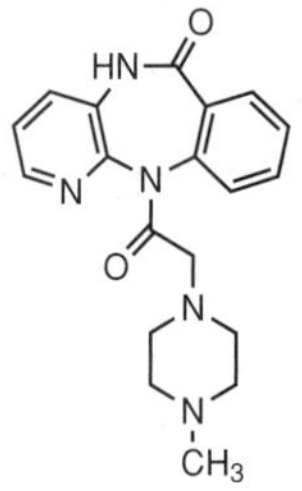

Pirenzepine

*This enzyme is known by two names, *adenylate cyclase (EC 4.6.1.1)*, its official name from the International Union of Biochemistry and Molecular Biology Nomenclature Committee, or its alternative name, adenylyl cyclase.

All the muscarinic receptor subtypes (M_1–M_5) are found in the CNS, and other tissues may contain more than one subtype. These receptors are summarized in Table 12.1 (11). As more muscarinic receptor subtypes have been discovered, it has become apparent that there is a lack of known antagonists exhibiting "very high subtype selectivity" and that there "are no muscarinic agonists with high selectivity" (8). Thus, proof for involvement of any one receptor subtype in a given system currently requires use of more than one antagonist. Additionally, if the selectivity of a novel muscarinic antagonist or putative agonist is to be assessed, it should be through the use of recombinant muscarinic receptors expressed in cell lines rather than with native receptors.

Cloning and sequencing of genes encoding muscarinic receptors have led to major advances in understanding of their chemical nature and function (8,12–14). These experiments demonstrated that muscarinic receptors belong to a group of receptors that are coupled to guanine nucleotide–binding proteins and are referred to as G protein–coupled receptors (GPCR) (8,15,16). The guanine nucleotide regulatory protein to which the receptors are coupled has three subunits (α, β, and γ), which link the receptor to effectors that produce second messenger molecules within the cell. Binding of muscarinic agonists to GPCRs leads to a variety of effector responses (see below). The ultimate observable response is a function of the tissue where the receptor is located.

The amino acid sequences (primary structures) of muscarinic receptor proteins expressed by cloned genes for the GPCRs have been deduced from the base sequence of the respective genes. These GPCRs are components of the cell membrane and consist of seven hydrophobic transmembrane helical domains as well as hydrophilic extracellular and intracellular domains (17). The N-terminus of the GPCR protein is extracellular, and the C-terminus is intracellular. This proposed arrangement for the human type 1 muscarinic receptor, including its deduced amino acid sequence, is illustrated in Fig. 12.3 (12). Computer-assisted molecular modeling also has made it possible to obtain three-dimensional models of the muscarinic receptor (17); a proposed top-view model of the M_1 muscarinic receptor is shown in Fig. 12.4 (18). It is interesting to observe that this model suggests that the quaternary nitrogen of acetylcholine participates in an ionic bond with the free carboxylate group of an aspartate residue (D105)—one of the receptor functional groups that was hypothesized to be involved in receptor binding of acetylcholine almost 60 years ago using only SAR data and the powers of deduction.

The current model for muscarinic receptors is much more descriptive than earlier models, and it better describes ligand binding (molecular recognition) and its effect (signal transduction) (Fig. 12.5) (14). In this model, acetylcholine binds to the muscarinic receptor located in the cell membrane, and this ligand–receptor interaction is translated, presumably by a conformational perturbation, through the receptor protein to

Table 12.1. Muscarinic Acetylcholine Receptor Subtypes[a]

Receptor	G Protein	Tissue Location	Cellular Response	Function
M_1	$G_{q/11}$	CNS, gastric and salivary glands, autonomic ganglia, enteric nerves	PLC activation (↑IP_3 & ↑DAG → ↑Ca^{2+} & PKC); depolarization and excitation (↑sEPSP); PLA_2 and PLD_2 activation; ↑AA	↑ Cognitive function ↑ Seizure activity ↑ Secretions ↑ Autonomic ganglia depolarization ↓ DA release and locomotion
M_3	$G_{q/11}$	CNS (< other mAChRs), smooth muscle, glands, heart	Same as M_1	↑ Smooth muscle contraction (e.g., bladder) ↑ Salivary gland secretion ↑ Food intake, body fat deposits Inhibits dopamine release Synthesis of nitric oxide
M_5	$G_{q/11}$	Low levels in CNS & periphery; predominate mAChRs in dopaminergic neurons of substantia nigra & ventral tegmentum area	Same as M_1	Mediates dilation of cerebral arteries Facilitates dopamine release Augments drug seeking behavior and reward
M_2	G_i/G_o	Autonomic nerve terminals; CNS; heart; smooth muscle	Inhibition of adenylyl cyclase (↓cAMP) & voltage gated Ca^{2+} channels; activation of inwardly rectifying K^+ channels	↓ Heart rate ↑ Smooth muscle contraction Neural inhibition in periphery via autoreceptors and heteroreceptor ↓ Ganglionic transmission Neural inhibition in CNS ↑ Tremors hypothermia & analgesia
M_4	G_i/G_o	CNS	Same as M_2	Inhibition of autoreceptor- and heteroreceptor-mediated transmitter release in CNS Analgesia Cataleptic activity; Facilitates dopamine release

[a]CNS, central nervous system; PLC, phospholipase C; IP_3, inositol-1, 4, 5-triphosphate; DAG, diacylglycerol; PLD_2, phospholipase D; AA, arachidonic acid; PKC, protein kinase C; sEPSP, slow excitatory postsynaptic potential; mAChRs, muscarinic acetylcholine receptor subtypes; PLA, phospholipase A; cAMP, cyclic adenosine monophosphate; VTA, ventral tegmentum area.

Adapted from Westfall TC, Westfall DP. Neurotransmission: the autonomic and somatic motor nervous systems. In: Brunton LL, Lazo JS, Parker KL, eds. Goodman and Gilman's The Pharmacological Basis of Therapeutics, 11th Ed. New York: McGraw-Hill, 2006, pp. 137–181; with permission.

the receptor-coupled guanine nucleotide regulatory protein (G protein). A relationship between the guanine nucleotide regulatory protein and the effector is illustrated in Fig. 12.6. In this scheme, the G protein is in the inactive state, with guanosine diphosphate (GDP) bound to its α subunit. On interaction of an agonist with the muscarinic receptor, the α subunit releases GDP and binds GTP. The α subunit–GTP complex then dissociates from the βγ subunits. Both the α subunit–GTP complex and the βγ subunits interact with membrane-bound effectors (phospholipase C or adenylate cyclase) or ion channels (K^+ and Ca^{2+}), either independently or in a parallel manner. The α subunit possesses GTPase activity and quickly hydrolyzes the GTP to GDP to terminate signal transmission, at which time the α, β, and γ subunits reassociate and migrate back to the receptor protein. Characteristics of the α subunit determine the classification of the particular G protein:

Gsincreases adenylyl cyclase activity and increases Ca21 currents

G_i decreases adenylyl cyclase activity and increases K^+ currents

G_o decreases Ca^{2+} currents

G_q increases phospholipase C activity

The βγ subunits are involved with receptor-operated K^+ currents and with activity of adenylyl cyclase and phospholipase C.

Signal transduction at the stimulatory "odd-numbered" muscarinic receptors (i.e., M_1, M_3, and M_5) is via coupling with a $G_{q/11}$ protein that is involved with mobilization of intracellular calcium. Agonist binding to these receptors results in activation of phospholipase C, with subsequent production of the second messengers, diacylglycerol and inositol-1,4,5-triphosphate (IP_3). Stimulation of IP_3 ion channel receptors leads to the release of intracellular calcium from the endoplasmic reticulum. The diacylglycerol produced, along with calcium, activates protein kinase C, which phosphorylates proteins to afford various physiological responses. The M_1, M_3, and M_5 receptors also stimulate phospholipase A_2 and phospholipase D. Activation of phospholipase A_2 results in release of arachidonic acid, with subsequent synthesis of eicosanoids (C_{20} fatty acids).

The "even-numbered" muscarinic receptor subtypes (i.e., M_2 and M_4) are coupled to G_i/G_o proteins, the activation of which results in inhibition of adenylyl cyclase.

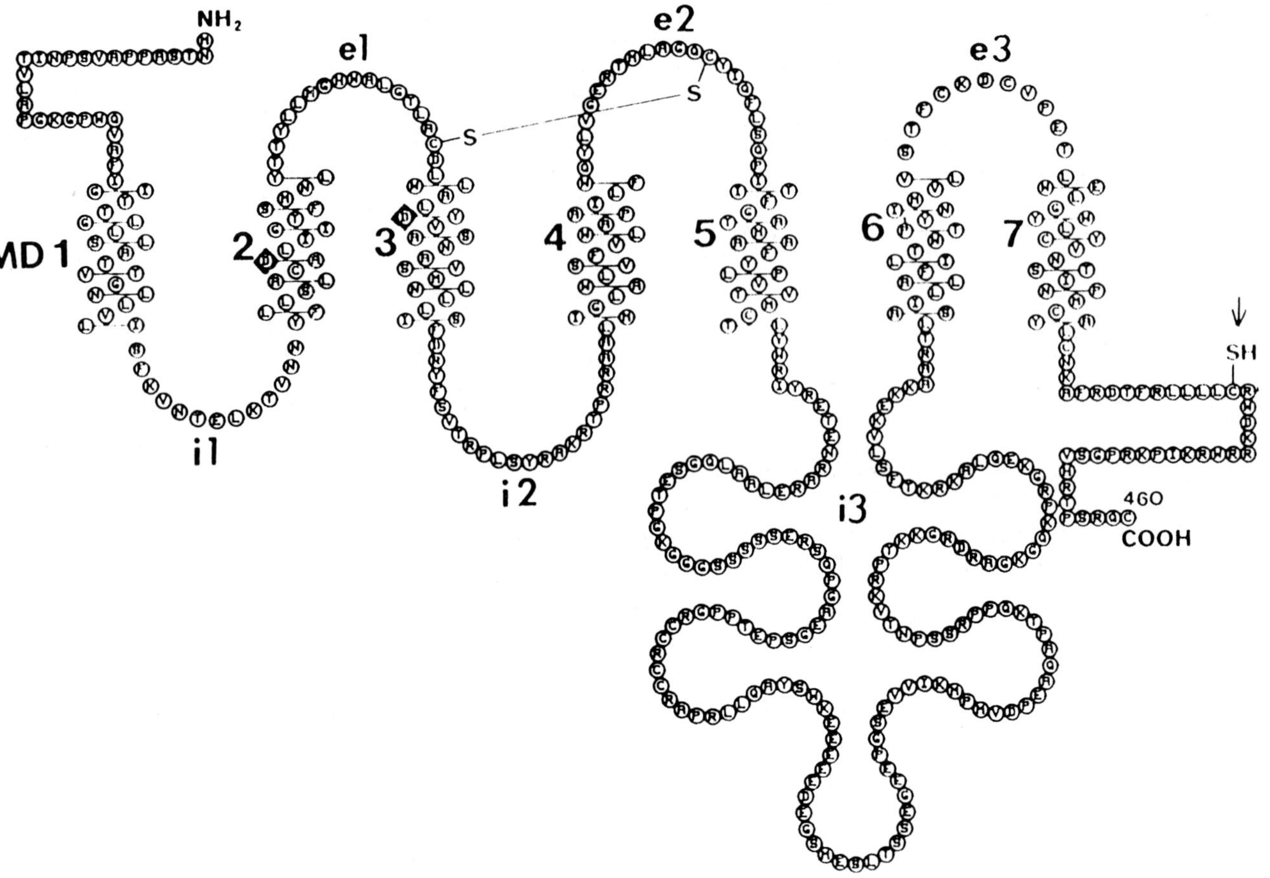

Fig. 12.3. Deduced amino acid sequence of human muscarinic acetylcholine receptor M_1 and putative arrangement of the seven transmembrane domains, three intracellular domains (i_1–i_3), and three extracellular domains (e_1–e_3). (From Lameh J, Cone RI, Maeda S, et al. Structure and function of G protein coupled receptors. Pharm Res 1990;7:1213–1221; with permission.)

This results in a decrease in cyclic adenosine monophosphate, inhibition of voltage-gated calcium channels, and activation of inwardly rectifying potassium channels (19). The result is hyperpolarization and inhibition of these excitable membranes.

The M_1 receptors sometimes are termed "neural" because of their abundance in the cerebral cortex, hippocampus, and striatum. The M_1 receptors have been implicated in Alzheimer's disease and are thought to be involved with such functions as memory and learning. Early studies suggested that the agonist McN-A-343 was selective for the M_1 receptor, but more recent evidence indicates otherwise. It may show moderate selectivity for

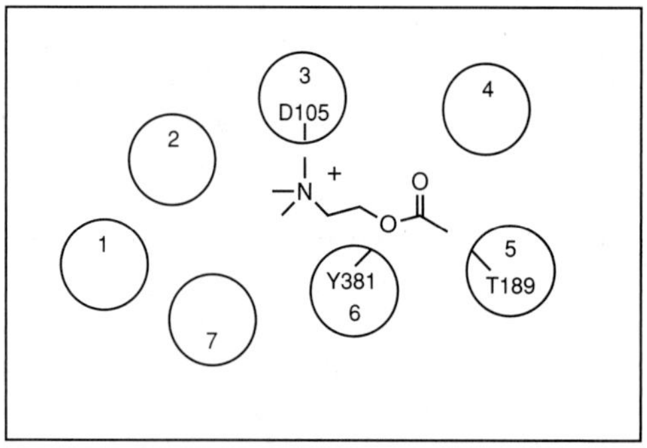

Fig. 12.4. Model of acetylcholine interaction with muscarinic M_1 receptor. Circles represent seven transmembrane domains; D105, T189, and Y381 are aspartate, threonine, and tyrosine residues, respectively.

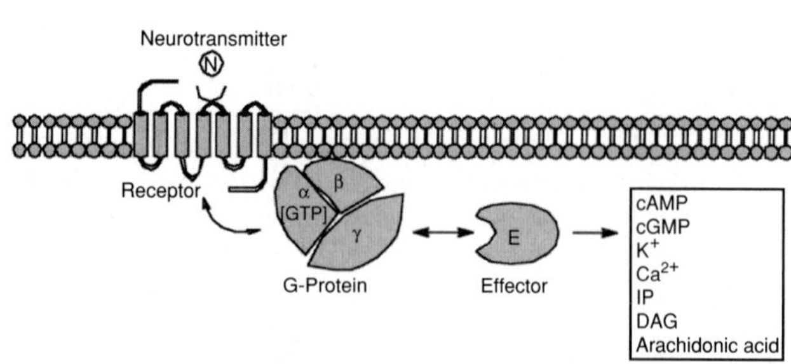

Fig. 12.5. Model of signal transduction by a G protein-coupled receptor. This illustrates a proposed relationship between receptor, G protein, effector, and various second messengers.

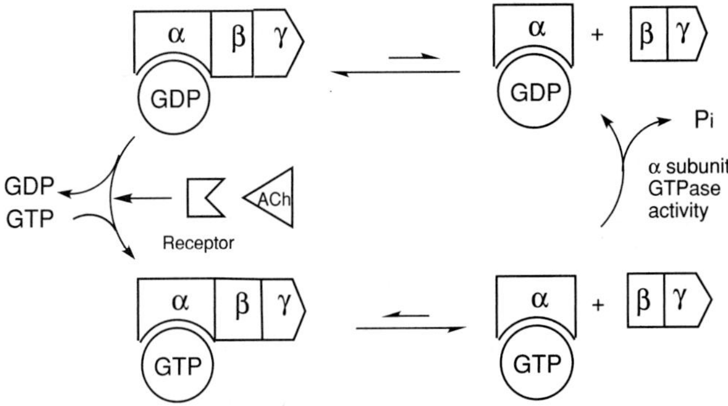

Fig. 12.6. Diagram of a GTPase cycle and subunit association/dissociation proposed to control signal transduction between muscarinic G protein-coupled receptors and the effector. The ACh-receptor interaction facilitates GTP binding and activates the α subunit. The α subunit-GTP complex then dissociates from the βγ subunit, and each is free to activate effector proteins. The duration of separation is determined by the rate of α subunit-mediated GTP hydrolysis.

M_4 receptors. Additionally, M_1 receptors are found at autonomic ganglia, enteric nerves, and salivary and gastric glands. Agonists at M_1 receptors show the greatest promise for treatment of the cholinergic deficit associated with Alzheimer's disease.

Cl–C$_6$H$_4$–NH–C(=O)–O–CH_2–C≡C–CH_2–$N^{\oplus}(CH_3)_3$ $Cl^{\ominus}$

McN-A-343

The M_2 receptors are found in abundance in the heart, where their activation exerts both negative chronotropic and inotropic actions. In smooth muscle, they stimulate contraction. Activation of M_2 autoreceptors located on nerve terminals affords neural inhibition by decreasing acetylcholine release.

The M_3 receptors are found in abundance in smooth muscle and glands, where their stimulation leads to contraction and secretion, respectively. Knowledge of this effect on smooth muscle of the bladder has led to the development and subsequent approval of several M_3 receptor antagonists for the treatment of overactive bladder (see below). Although widely distributed in the CNS, their concentration there is lower than those of other muscarinic receptors. They function to decrease neurotransmitter release.

The M_4 receptors are found in the striatum and basal forebrain, where they decrease transmitter release in both the CNS and periphery. Their activation in smooth muscle and secretary glands leads to inhibition of potassium and calcium channels.

The M_5 receptors are the least characterized of the muscarinic receptors. There is evidence for their existence in the CNS and the periphery, and they may regulate dopamine release in the CNS.

Nicotinic Receptors

Nicotinic acetylcholine receptors are found at the skeletal neuromuscular junction, adrenal medulla, and autonomic ganglia. They have been the focus of intensive research interest, even though the majority of clinically effective cholinergic medicinal agents are either muscarinic agonists or antagonists (20). This interest in nicotinic receptors is the result of both the availability of the receptor protein from the electric organs of the electric eel *(Electrophorus electricus)* and the marine ray *(Torpedo californica)* and the important role they play in myasthenia gravis, an autoimmune disease.

The concept of multiple nicotinic receptors is based on the different structural requirements for agonists and antagonists acting at the autonomic ganglia and the skeletal neuromuscular junction. This multiplicity of nicotinic receptors also is supported by molecular biology research (20).

Both neuronal and muscular nicotinic receptors are classified as ligand-gated ion channel receptors, and they are structurally and functionally related to other ligand-gated ion channel receptors, such as γ-aminobutyric acid receptors, 5-hydroxytryptamine receptors, and glycine receptors (21). The receptor creates a transmembrane ion channel (the gate), and acetylcholine (the ligand) serves as a gatekeeper by binding with the receptor to modulate passage of ions, principally K^+ and Na^+, through the channel.

A nicotinic receptor was the first neurotransmitter receptor to be isolated and purified in the active form using the same molecular biological techniques described above for isolation and purification of muscarinic receptors. The primary sequence of nicotinic receptors has been deduced from cloning and sequencing of genes that encode their receptor proteins (22,23). Nicotinic receptors are pentameric transmembrane proteins made up of α, β, δ, and/or γ subunits (24).

The nicotinic receptor of muscle tissue is a transmembrane glycoprotein consisting of four types of subunits—α, β, γ(or ϵ), and δ. Only the α_1 subtype of the α subunit is present in muscle. In a mature muscle end plate, the γ subunit is replaced by an ϵ subunit. This change in gene expression encoding the γ and ϵ subunits affects ligand selectivity along with receptor turnover and/or tissue location.

One class of neuronal nicotinic receptors exists as a heteromeric pentamer composed of α (α_2–α_6) and β (β_2–β_4) subunits (25–27)—for example, $\alpha_4\beta_3$ with a stoichiometry of two α_4 and three β_3 subunits. Another class of functional homomeric nicotinic receptors is composed of α_7 through α_{10} subunits. The diversity of the subunits and the pentameric structure suggest that a large number of nicotinic receptor subtypes may exist.

The five subunits of each receptor protein in muscle tissue are arranged around a central pore that serves as

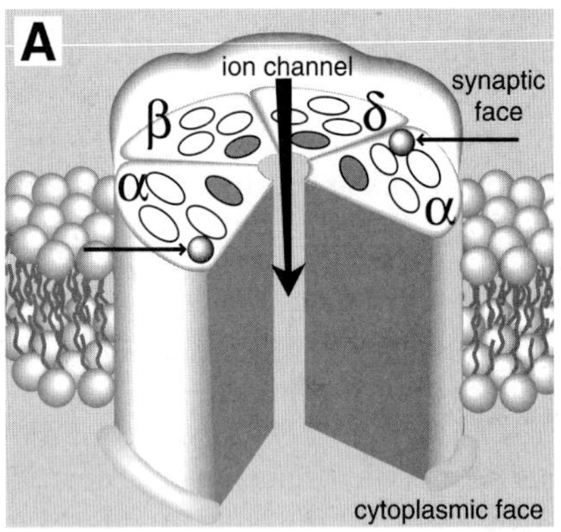

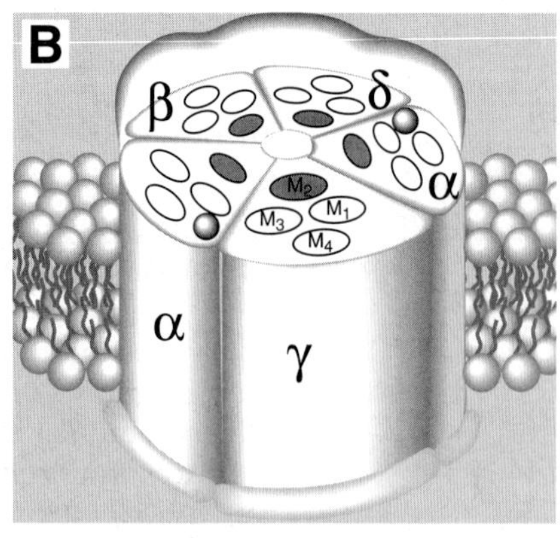

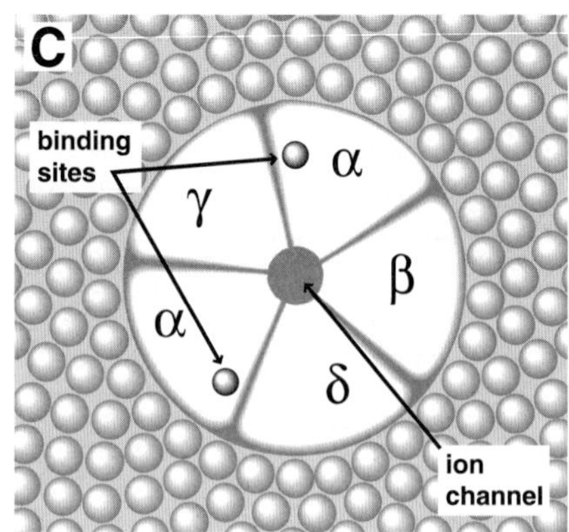

Fig. 12.7. Nicotinic cholinergic receptor. (A) Longitudinal view (γ subunit removed) showing the internal ion channel. Acetylcholine binding sites on the α subunits are indicated by the arrows. These are located at the αγ and αδ interfaces. (B) Each of the five transmembrane subunits (α, α, β, δ, and γ) are composed of four hydrophobic membrane spanning segments (M_1–M_4). (C) Top view of the nicotinic receptor showing the subunits surrounding the ion channel.

the ion channel. Based on molecular modeling of the deduced primary structure of the individual subunits, it has been proposed that each subunit (α, β, γ, δ, or ϵ) possesses a hydrophilic extracellular N-terminus, a hydrophilic intracellular C-terminus, and four α helical hydrophobic transmembrane domains (M_1–M_4) (Fig. 12.7) (26,28). A pentameric arrangement of these five amphipathic subunits makes up the walls of the ion channel. Two acetylcholine binding sites exist on the extracellular domain of each receptor molecule. In Figure 12.7, one binding site is located on each α subunit at the αγ and αδ interfaces (28). The binding sites show a positive cooperativity, even though the two binding sites are not adjacent to each other in the pentameric receptor. Some central and peripheral nicotinic receptor subtypes are summarized in Table 12.2 (11).

Our knowledge and understanding of the muscarinic and nicotinic receptors have advanced tremendously from the time when these receptors were only ethereal concepts. This understanding provides the basis for the rational design of new selective therapeutic agents to treat diseases associated with cholinergic neurons.

Table 12.2 Nicotinic Acetylcholine Receptor Subtypes

Receptor	Location	Membrane Response	Molecular Mechanism	Agonists	Antagonists
Skeletal muscle (N_M) $(\alpha_1)_2\beta_1\epsilon\delta$ $(\alpha_1)_2\beta_1\gamma\delta$	Skeletal neuromuscular junction (postjunctional)	Excitatory; end plate depolarization; contraction (skeletal muscle)	Increased Na^+ & K^+ permeability	ACh; nicotine; succinylcholine	Atracurium; vecuronium; *d*-tubocurarine; pancuronium; α-conotoxin; α-bungarotoxin
Peripheral neuronal (N_N) $(\alpha_3)_2(\beta_4)_3$	Autonomic ganglia; adrenal medulla	Excitatory; depolarization firing of postganglionic neuron; depolarization & secretion of catecholamines	Increased Na^+ & K^+ permeability	ACh; nicotine; epibatidine; dimethylphenylpiperazinium	Trimethaphan; mecamylamine; dihydro-β erythrodine; erysodine lophotoxin
Central neuronal (CNS) $(\alpha_4)_2(\beta_4)_3$ (α-bungarotoxin insensitive)	CNS; pre- & postjunctional	Pre- & postsynaptic excitation; prejunctinal control of transmitter release	Increased Na^+ & K^+ permeability	Cytisine; epibatidine; Anatoxin A	
$(\alpha_7)_5$ (α-bungarotoxin sensitive)	CNS; pre- and postsynaptic	Same as central neuronal	Increased CA^{2+} permeability	Anatoxin A	Methyllycaconities; α-conotoxin; α-bungarotoxin

Adapted from Westfall TC, Westfall DP. Neurotransmission: the autonomic and somatic motor nervous systems. In: Brunton LL, Lazo JS, Parker KL, eds. Goodman and Gilman's The Pharmacological Basis of Therapeutics, 11th Ed. New York: McGraw-Hill, 2006, pp. 137–181; with permission.

DRUGS AFFECTING CHOLINERGIC NEUROTRANSMISSION

Acetylcholine Neurochemistry

The neurochemistry of acetylcholine includes its biosynthesis, storage, release, and metabolism. These are illustrated in Figure 12.8.

Biosynthesis

Acetylcholine is biosynthesized in cholinergic neurons by the enzyme-catalyzed transfer of the acetyl group from acetyl coenzyme A (acetyl-S-CoA) to choline, a quaternary ammonium alcohol (29). The enzyme catalyzing this reaction, choline acetyltransferase, is also biosynthesized in the cholinergic neuron. Some choline is biosynthesized from the amino acid serine (Fig. 12.9), but most of the choline used to form acetylcholine is recycled following AChE-catalyzed hydrolysis of acetylcholine in the synaptic space. Extracellular choline is actively transported into the presynaptic nerve terminal by both high-affinity and low-affinity uptake sites. The high-affinity sites are responsible for the uptake of most of the choline recycled from the synapse. Uptake is considered to be the rate-determining step in biosynthesis of acetylcholine. This uptake is inhibited by hemicholinium.

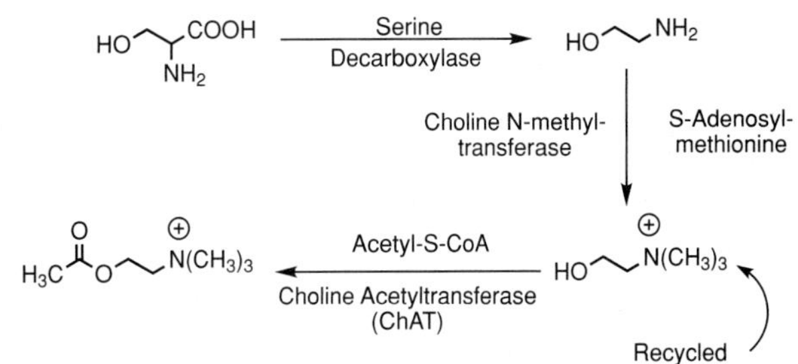

Fig. 12.9. Biosynthesis of acetylcholine.

Hemicholinium chloride

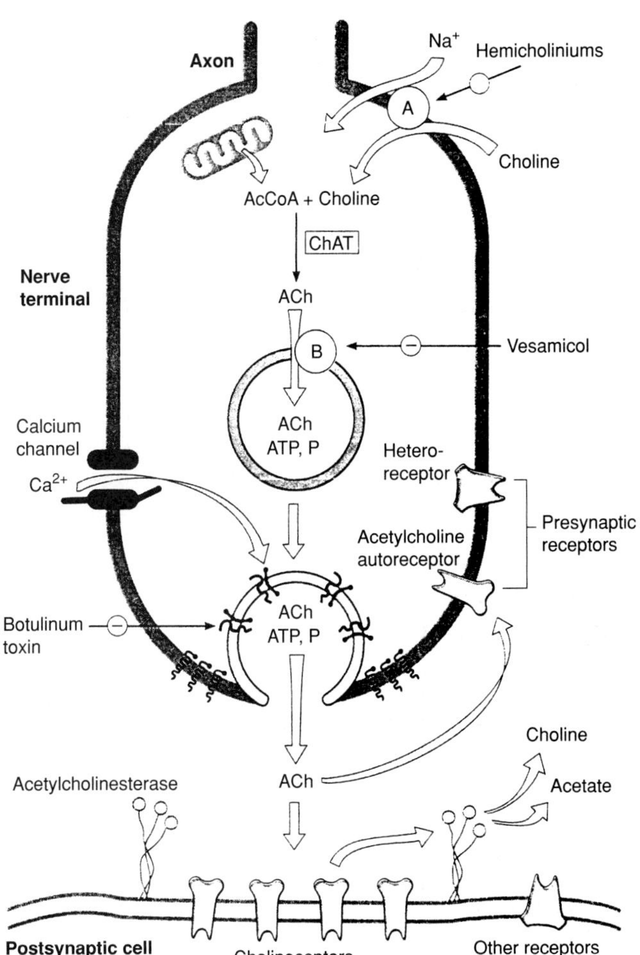

Fig. 12.8. General cholinergic nerve junction showing location of receptor sites and biosynthesis, storage, release, and hydrolysis of acetylcholine. (Katzung BG. Introduction to autonomic pharmacology. In: Katzung BG, ed. Basic and Clinical Pharmacology, 9th Ed. New York: McGraw-Hill, 2004, pp. 75–93; with permission.)

Efforts to Modulate Acetylcholine Biosynthesis

Efforts to develop therapeutic agents based on regulation of acetylcholine biosynthesis have not been successful. Dexpanthenol, the dextrorotatory enantiomer of the alcohol derived from pantothenic acid (a vitamin), was once used as a cholinomimetic agent to help reestablish normal smooth muscle tone in the gastrointestinal tract following surgery. Pantothenic acid is essential for the biosynthesis of coenzyme A (CoA). The apparent rationale for the therapeutic use of dexpanthenol was that it would be biotransformed to pantothenic acid, which would be incorporated into CoA. This would lead to increased intracellular levels of acetyl CoA, which would facilitate increased biosynthesis of acetylcholine. The limited therapeutic success of dexpanthenol, difficulty with administration, and effectiveness of synthetic cholinergic agonists led to its discontinuation. The quaternary pyridinium salt, *trans*-N-methyl-4-(1-naphthylvinyl)pyridinium iodide, is an effective inhibitor of choline acetyltransferase in vitro, but it has proven to be a poor inhibitor in whole animal experiments.

Although efforts have been made to design cholinergic agents based on the mechanism of biosynthesis of acetylcholine, such agents would be expected to have nonselective effects, because it currently is thought that acetylcholine is biosynthesized by the same mechanism in all cholinergic neurons.

Storage

Most newly biosynthesized acetylcholine is actively transported into cytosolic storage vesicles located in presynaptic nerve endings, where it is maintained with ATP (10:1 ratio) along with calcium and magnesium ions until it is released. Some acetylcholine remains in the cytosol and eventually is hydrolyzed. Only the stored form of acetylcholine serves as the functional neurotransmitter.

Release

Release of acetylcholine from the storage vesicles is initiated by an action potential that has traveled down the axon to the presynaptic nerve membrane. This action potential leads to opening of voltage-dependent calcium channels, affording an influx of Ca^{2+} and exocytotic release of acetylcholine into the synapse. The increase in intracellular Ca^{2+} may induce fusion of acetylcholine storage vesicles with the presynaptic membrane before release of the neurotransmitter. Each synaptic vesicle contains a quantum of acetylcholine; one quantum represents between 12,000 and 60,000 molecules of acetylcholine. A single action potential causes the release of several hundred quanta of acetylcholine into the synapse.

Metabolism

Acetylcholine in the synapse can bind with cholinergic receptors on the postsynaptic or presynaptic membranes to produce a response. Free acetylcholine that is not bound to a receptor is hydrolyzed by AChE. This hydrolysis is the physiologic mechanism for terminating the action of acetylcholine. Enough AChE is present in the synapse to hydrolyze approximately 3×10^8 molecules of acetylcholine in 1 millisecond; thus, adequate enzyme activity exists to hydrolyze all the acetylcholine ($\sim 3 \times 10^6$ molecules) released by one action potential. A number of useful therapeutic cholinomimetic agents have been developed based on the ability of the compounds to inhibit AChE; these agents are addressed later in this chapter.

Stereochemistry

One shortcoming of early models for cholinergic receptors was that they did not account for the observed stereoselectivity of the receptors for agonist and antagonist ligands. Even though acetylcholine is achiral, many synthetic and naturally occurring agonists and antagonists possess chirality; usually, one enantiomer is many times more active than the other. It was apparent to early receptor investigators that the stereochemistry of cholinergic ligands was important for receptor binding. In this regard, the stereochemical–activity relationships of cholinergic ligands have been studied extensively to provide a rational basis for design of cholinergic drugs as well as to describe the properties and functions of cholinergic receptors.

The stereochemistry of acetylcholine resides in the different arrangements in space of its atoms by virtue of rotation about σ bonds (i.e., conformational isomerism). Because of relatively unrestricted rotation about these single covalent bonds, acetylcholine can exist in an infinite number of conformations. Most studies of the conformational isomerism of acetylcholine have focused on torsion angles between the ester oxygen atom and the quaternary nitrogen resulting from rotation about the Cα-Cβ bond. Four of these conformations are illustrated by Newman projections in Fig. 12.10.

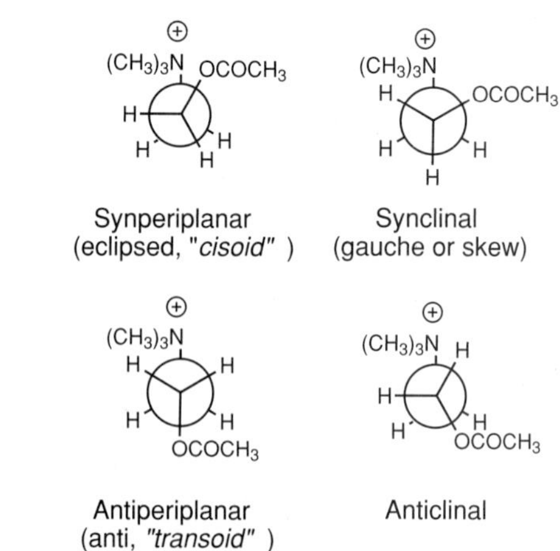

Fig. 12.10. Conformational isomers of acetylcholine.

Nuclear magnetic resonance (NMR) studies in aqueous solution revealed that the preferred conformation between the ester oxygen and the quaternary nitrogen of acetylcholine was synclinal (gauche or skew). Using x-ray data, the synclinal conformation was observed for acetylcholine in the solid crystalline state as well. The same conclusion was also obtained for the preferred conformation of acetylcholine using molecular orbital calculations. These experimental and theoretical determinations of the acetylcholine conformation differ from the antiperiplanar conformation that might be expected when using molecular models to visualize minimum steric interactions. The synclinal conformation would be stabilized by intramolecular electrostatic interactions between the quaternary nitrogen and the carbonyl oxygen.

It must be emphasized that the experimentally determined synclinal conformation of acetylcholine is only that measured in aqueous solution (NMR) or the crystalline state (x-ray). This may not be the conformation preferred by the receptors. Indeed, the conformation of receptor-bound acetylcholine could be much different and might not be a thermodynamically preferred conformation.

In recognition of this possibility, conformationally restricted acetylcholine analogues have been synthesized and pharmacologically evaluated in an effort to determine the conformation of acetylcholine when it binds to cholinergic receptors. The most significant study in this regard is that of Armstrong et al. (30). They synthesized and evaluated the muscarinic and nicotinic activity of *cis-* and *trans-*isomers of a conformationally rigid model of acetylcholine, *cis-* and *trans*-2-acetoxycyclopropyl-1-trimethylammonium iodide. Because this model is based on the cyclopropane ring, the ester and quaternary ammonium functional groups cannot change their relative positions by bond rotation. The *cis-* and *trans*-isomers are rigidly constrained to the conformations shown. The *cis*-isomer is similar to the synperiplanar conformation of acetylcholine, and the *trans*-isomer approximates the anticlinal conformation. The (+)-*trans*-enantiomer was observed to be equally as or more potent, depending on the pharmacological test used, than acetylcholine at muscarinic receptors; it was much more potent than the (−)-*trans*-enantiomer. The racemic *cis*-compound had almost no activity in the same muscarinic receptor test system, and all compounds were very weak nicotinic agonists.

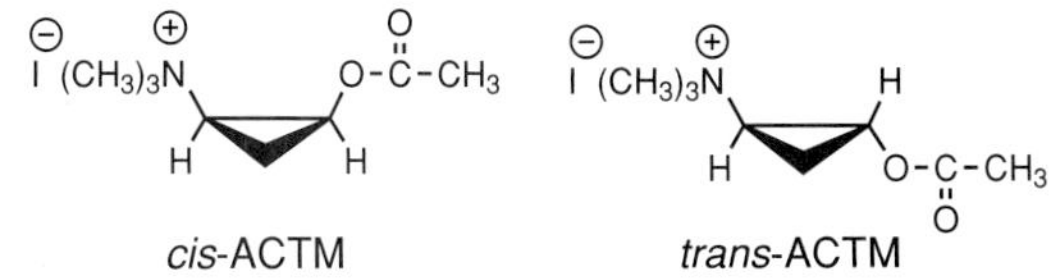

$\overset{\ominus}{I}\ (CH_3)_3\overset{\oplus}{N}$ ... $O-\overset{O}{\overset{\|}{C}}-CH_3$ (H, H)

cis-ACTM

$\overset{\ominus}{I}\ (CH_3)_3\overset{\oplus}{N}$ ... H ... $O-\underset{O}{\underset{\|}{C}}-CH_3$ (H)

trans-ACTM

The important conclusion drawn from this study (30) was that acetylcholine would most probably interact with muscarinic receptors in its less favored anticlinal conformation. The most active isomer, the (+)-*trans*-enantiomer, of these cyclopropane analogues was found to have a torsion angle of 137° (anticlinal) between the ester oxygen and the quaternary nitrogen. This is significantly different from the 60° torsion angle in the synclinal conformation found by NMR and x-ray determinations to be the preferred conformation.

Stereochemistry of cholinergic ligands and stereoselectivity of receptors has played an important role in design of cholinergic ligands as therapeutic agents. This role becomes apparent in subsequent sections.

Acetylcholine Mimetics—Muscarinic Agonists

Interaction of cholinergic agonists with muscarinic receptors leads to well-defined pharmacological responses depending on the tissue or organ in which the receptor is located. These responses include contractions of smooth muscle, vasodilation, increased secretion from exocrine glands, miosis, and decreased heart rate and force of contraction.

Acetylcholine

Acetylcholine is the prototypical muscarinic (and nicotinic) agonist, because it is the physiologic chemical neurotransmitter. It is a poor therapeutic agent, however, both because of its lack of nicotinic or muscarinic receptor specificity and because of the chemical and physicochemical properties associated with its ester and quaternary ammonium salt functional groups. It is quite stable in the solid crystalline form but undergoes rapid hydrolysis in aqueous solution. This hydrolysis is accelerated in the presence of catalytic amounts of either acid or base. For this reason, acetylcholine cannot be administered orally because of rapid hydrolysis in the gastrointestinal tract. Even when administered parenterally, its pharmacological action is fleeting as a result of hydrolysis by butyrylcholinesterase (pseudocholinesterase) in serum. The quaternary ammonium functional group of acetylcholine imparts excellent water solubility, but quaternary ammonium salts are poorly absorbed across lipid membranes because of their high hydrophilic and ionic character. Thus, even if acetylcholine were stable enough to be administered orally, it would be poorly absorbed. When used during ocular surgery to produce complete miosis within seconds, acetylcholine must be directly instilled into the anterior chamber. It cannot be administered topically, because it is not lipophilic enough to penetrate the cornea. It requires aqueous reconstitution immediately before instillation because of its chemical hydrolytic lability.

Structure–Activity Relationship

The necessity to design compounds that would serve as therapeutic alternatives to acetylcholine and as probes to study the role of acetylcholine in neurotransmission led to an exhaustive study of the structural features required for the action of acetylcholine. Structure–activity relationships that developed from these studies have provided the basis for the design of all muscarinic agonists currently used as therapeutic agents.

To review the SAR, it is logical to divide the structure of acetylcholine into the three components shown below to examine the effects of chemical modification of each group:

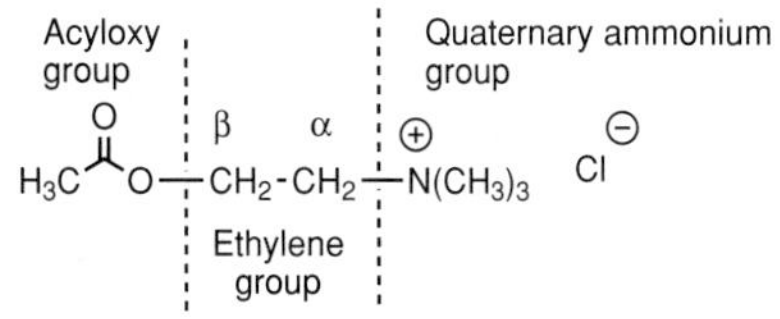

Acyloxy group | Ethylene group | Quaternary ammonium group

$H_3C-\overset{O}{\overset{\|}{C}}-O-\overset{\beta}{C}H_2-\overset{\alpha}{C}H_2-\overset{\oplus}{N}(CH_3)_3\quad \overset{\ominus}{Cl}$

Modification of the Quaternary Ammonium Group. Analogues of acetylcholine in which the nitrogen atom was replaced by arsenic, phosphorus, or sulfur have been synthesized (10,31). Although they exhibited some of the activity of acetylcholine, these compounds are less active and are not used clinically. It was concluded that only compounds possessing a positive charge on the atom in the position of the nitrogen had appreciable muscarinic activity.

Compounds in which all three methyl groups on the nitrogen are replaced by larger alkyl groups are inactive as agonists. When the methyl groups are replaced by three ethyl groups, the resulting compound is a cholinergic antagonist. Replacement of only one methyl group by an ethyl or propyl group affords a compound that is active, but much less so than acetylcholine (32). Furthermore, successive replacement of one, two, or three of the methyl groups with hydrogen atoms to afford a tertiary, secondary, or primary amine, respectively, leads to successively diminishing muscarinic activity (33,34).

Modification of the Ethylene Bridge. Synthesis of acetic acid esters of quaternary ammonium alcohols of greater length than choline led to a series of compounds with activity that was rapidly reduced as the chain length increased. This observation led Ing (10) to postulate his Rule of Five. This rule suggests that there should be no more than five atoms between the nitrogen and the terminal hydrogen atom for maximal muscarinic potency. Present concepts suggest that the muscarinic receptor cannot successfully accommodate molecules larger than acetylcholine and still produce its physiologic effect. Although larger molecules may bind to the receptor, they lack efficacy and demonstrate antagonist properties.

Replacement of the hydrogen atoms of the ethylene bridge by alkyl groups larger than methyl affords compounds that are much less active than acetylcholine. Introduction of a methyl group on the carbon β to the quaternary nitrogen affords acetyl-β-methylcholine (methacholine), which has muscarinic potency almost equivalent to that of acetylcholine and much greater muscarinic than nicotinic selectivity.

A methyl group on the carbon α to the quaternary nitrogen affords acetyl-α-methylcholine. Although activity relative to acetylcholine is reduced at both muscarinic and nicotinic receptors, it exhibits greater nicotinic than muscarinic potency. This compound is not currently used as a therapeutic agent.

Addition of methyl groups to either one or both of the ethylene carbons results in chiral molecules. Muscarinic receptors (see below) display stereoselectivity for the enantiomers of methacholine. The S-(+)-enantiomer is equipotent with acetylcholine, and the R-(−)-enantiomer is approximately 20-fold less potent. Acetylcholinesterase hydrolyzes the S-(+)-isomer much slower (approximately half the rate) than acetylcholine. The R-(−)-isomer is not hydrolyzed by AChE and even acts as a weak competitive inhibitor of the enzyme. This stability toward AChE hydrolysis as well as the AChE inhibitory effect of the R-(−)-enantiomer may explain why racemic methacholine produces a longer duration of action than acetylcholine. The nicotinic receptor and AChE exhibit little stereoselectivity for the optical isomers of acetyl-α-methylcholine.

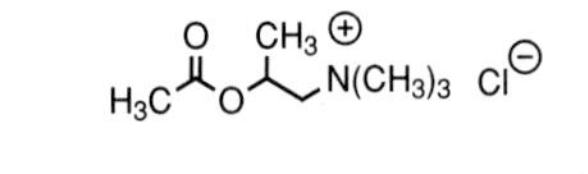

$H_3C-C(=O)-O-CH(CH_3)-CH_2-N^{\oplus}(CH_3)_3\ Cl^{\ominus}$

Acetyl-β-methylcholine chloride (Methacholine)

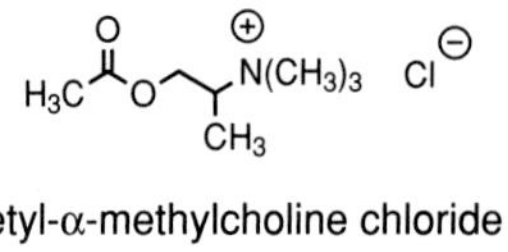

$H_3C-C(=O)-O-CH_2-CH(CH_3)-N^{\oplus}(CH_3)_3\ Cl^{\ominus}$

Acetyl-α-methylcholine chloride

Modification of the Acyloxy Group. As would be predicted by the Rule of Five (10), when the acetyl group is replaced by higher homologues (i.e., the propionyl or butyryl groups), the resulting esters are less potent than acetylcholine. Choline esters of aromatic or higher-molecular-weight acids possess cholinergic antagonist activity.

Because the fleeting pharmacological action and chemical instability of acetylcholine result from its rapid hydrolysis, a logical approach to the development of better muscarinic therapeutic agents was to replace the acetyloxy functional group with a functional group more resistant to hydrolysis. This led to synthesis of the carbamic acid ester of choline (carbachol), a potent cholinergic agonist possessing both muscarinic and nicotinic activity. Esters derived from carbamic acid are referred to as carbamates, and because their carbonyl carbon is less electrophilic, they are more stable than carboxylate esters to hydrolysis. Carbachol is less readily hydrolyzed by gastric acid, AChE, or butyrylcholinesterase than acetylcholine is, and it can be administered orally.

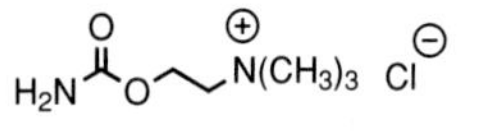

$H_2N-C(=O)-O-CH_2-CH_2-N^{\oplus}(CH_3)_3\ Cl^{\ominus}$

Carbachol

$H_2N-C(=O)-O-CH(CH_3)-CH_2-N^{\oplus}(CH_3)_3\ Cl^{\ominus}$

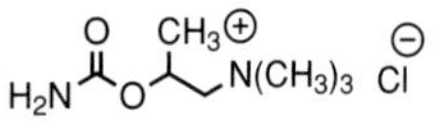

Bethanechol

This same chemical logic was extended to methacholine and led to synthesis of its carbamate ester, bethanechol, an orally effective potent muscarinic agonist with almost no nicotinic activity at therapeutic doses. Muscarinic receptors exhibit stereoselectivity for the two optical isomers of bethanechol, and similar to methacholine, the S-(+)-enantiomer exhibits greater binding affinity at muscarinic receptors than the R-(−)-enantiomer in isolated receptor preparations.

The profound muscarinic activity of the alkaloid muscarine provided substantial rationale for synthesizing ethers of choline. Muscarine, which is obtained from the red variety of mushroom (*Amanita muscaria*) and other mushrooms is one of the oldest known cholinergic agonists and is the compound for which muscarinic receptors were named. It was used in many pharmacological experiments during the latter 19th century and the early part of the 20th century, and its use preceded the discovery and chemical characterization of acetylcholine (2). The chemical structure of muscarine (see above), however, was not completely characterized until 1957. Muscarine possesses three chiral centers (C2, C3, and C5). Thus, eight optical isomers (four enantiomeric pairs) are possible. Of these, only the naturally occurring alkaloid, (2S,3R,5S)-(+)-muscarine (also called L-(+)-muscarine), is correctly referred to as muscarine. The C5 carbon of (+)-muscarine has the same absolute configuration as the analogous chiral β carbon in S-(+)-methacholine.

Other choline ethers as well as alkylaminoketones have been synthesized and evaluated for muscarinic activity. Choline ethyl ether exhibits significant muscarinic activity and is chemically stable, but it has not been used clinically. The most potent ketone derivatives possess the carbonyl on the carbon δ to the quaternary nitrogen; this is the same relative position as the carbonyl in acetylcholine. This suggests that these carbonyl groups bind by either a hydrogen bond or other dipole–dipole interaction with an appropriate group on the muscarinic receptor. Furthermore, the activity of these ethers and ketones demonstrates that neither the ester functional group nor a carbonyl is required for muscarinic agonist activity.

H_3C–O–$N(CH_3)_3^{\oplus}$ $Cl^{\ominus}$

Choline ethyl ether

H_3C–CO–$(CH_2)_n$ - $N(CH_3)_3^{\oplus}$ $X^{\ominus}$

Alkylaminoketones

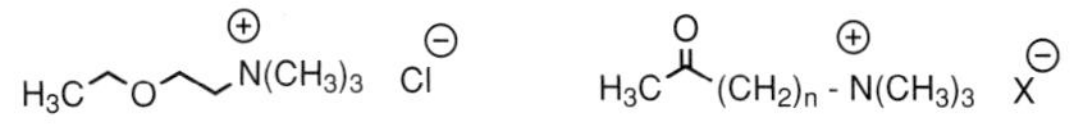

The classic SAR for muscarinic agonist activity can be summarized as follows:

1. The molecule must possess a nitrogen atom capable of bearing a positive charge, preferably a quaternary ammonium salt.
2. For maximum potency, the size of the alkyl groups substituted on the nitrogen should not exceed the size of a methyl group.
3. The molecule should have an oxygen atom, preferably an ester-like oxygen, capable of participating in a hydrogen bond.
4. There should be a two-carbon unit between the oxygen atom and the nitrogen atom.

It is important to note that this SAR was based on in vitro and in vivo pharmacological evaluations performed over a 60-year period. Scientists conducting this research did not have the luxury of modern, highly refined biological testing systems (i.e., protein-binding assays, cell membrane–binding assays, and single-cell models) that are considered to be state-of-the-art today for pharmacological evaluation of new medicinal agents. This is why some classic muscarinic agonists and many of the more modern agents do not adhere to this SAR. Indeed, SAR rules are not static; they should change as new experimental data refine the structural and stereochemical requirements for muscarinic agonist activity.

Specific Muscarinic Agonists

METHACHOLINE CHLORIDE (PROVOCHOLINE). Methacholine, acetyl β-methylcholine, (see previous structure and SAR discussion) is marketed as the racemic mixture. It is a selective muscarinic agonist with very little activity at nicotinic receptors. Although methacholine chloride is marketed as the racemic mixture, the S-(+)-enantiomer is 240-fold more potent than the R-(−)-isomer at muscarinic receptors. In addition, AChE hydrolyzes S-(+)−methacholine at approximately 54% the rate of acetylcholine, whereas the R-(−)− enantiomer is a weak inhibitor. Methacholine chloride is used via inhalation for the diagnosis of asthma. The resulting bronchospasm may be relieved with bronchodilators. Methacholine chloride is available as a powder that is reconstituted for inhalation.

CARBACHOL CHLORIDE (ISOPTO CARBACHOL). Carbachol (see structure above), the carbamate analogue of acetylcholine, shows no selectivity for muscarinic or nicotinic receptors. Because it is a carbamate ester, carbachol is more resistant toward acid-, base-, or enzyme (AChE)-catalyzed hydrolysis than acetylcholine. It also is reported to exhibit weak anticholinesterase activity. Both of these actions work to prolong the duration of action of carbachol. Because of erratic absorption and its actions at nicotinic receptors, use of carbachol has been limited to the treatment of glaucoma and for the induction of miosis in ocular surgery. Carbachol is available as an intraocular solution and an ophthalmic solution.

BETHANECHOL CHLORIDE (URECHOLINE). Bethanechol (see structure above), the carbamate analogue of methacholine, is selective for muscarinic receptors and exhibits almost no activity at nicotinic receptors. It is used to treat postsurgical and postpartum urinary retention and abdominal distention. Bethanechol is administered orally, because there is danger of a cholinergic crisis if it is given by intravenous or intramuscular injection.

PILOCARPINE HYDROCHLORIDE (ISOPTO CARPINE). Pilocarpine, the salt of an alkaloid obtained from *Pilocarpus jaborandi*, is an example of a muscarinic agonist that does not adhere to the traditional SAR. In 1876, Langley reported that extracts containing the alkaloid stimulated the end organs of parasympathetic neurons. The structure of pilocarpine was reported in 1901.

Pilocarpine is marketed as tablets (Salogen), an ophthalmic solution, and gel. It penetrates the eye well and is the miotic of choice for open-angle glaucoma and to terminate acute angle closure attacks. It also is used for the treatment of xerostomia (dryness of the mouth) caused by radiation therapy of the head and neck, Sjogren's syndrome, or as a side effect of some psychotropic drugs.

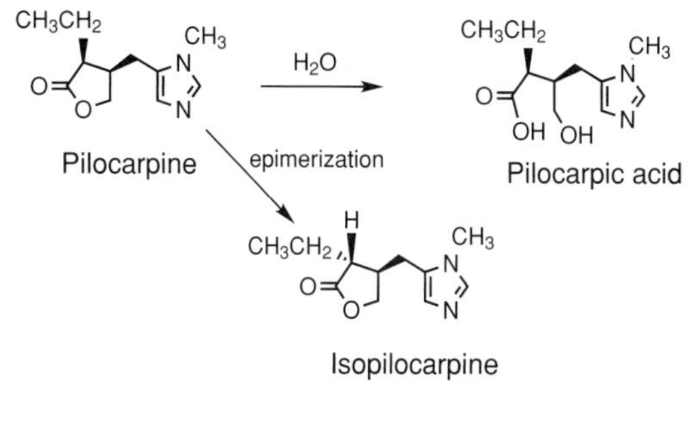

CH_3CH_2 CH_3 N N O O — H_2O → CH_3CH_2 CH_3 N N O OH OH

Pilocarpine — epimerization → Pilocarpic acid

H CH_3CH_2 CH_3 N N O O

Isopilocarpine

Because pilocarpine is a lactone, its solutions are subject to hydrolysis to afford the pharmacologically inactive pilocarpic acid and to base-catalyzed epimerization at C3 in the lactone to give isopilocarpine, an inactive stereoisomer of pilocarpine. Epimerization is not believed to be a serious problem if the drug is properly stored. Its solutions can be stored at room temperature, but the gel should be refrigerated and labeled with a 2-week expiration date when dispensed.

Cevimeline hydrochloride (Evoxac). Cevimeline is a nonclassical muscarinic agonist. It is a quinuclidine derivative that exhibits partial direct M_1 receptor agonist activity in the CNS and affinity for M_3 receptors in epithelial tissue of lacrimal and salivary glands. Its elimination half-life is 3 to 5 hours. It is metabolized by CYP2D6, CYP3A3, and CYP3A4 to inactive metabolites, the *cis*- and *trans*-sulfoxide, N-oxide, and glucuronide. Cevimeline hydrochloride is available as an oral capsule for the treatment of xerostomia (dry mouth) associated with Sjogren's syndrome. Before its approval, pilocarpine was the only drug for this condition.

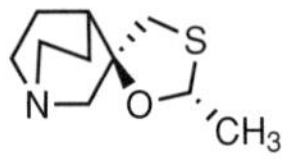

Cevimeline

Future Muscarinic Agonists

Current research interest in the design and synthesis of new muscarinic agonists is focused on discovering agents that might be effective in the treatment of Alzheimer's disease and other cognitive disorders. Investigators are searching actively for muscarinic agonists that exhibit selectivity for muscarinic receptors in the brain. Among these compounds are analogues of arecoline, oxotremorine, and McN-A-343 as well as many other novel chemical structures possessing muscarinic agonist activity.

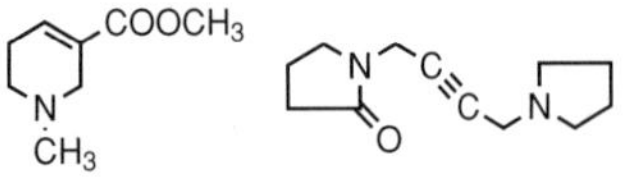

Arecoline Oxotremorine

Arecoline is of historical interest, because its structure, like those of many other early medicinal agents, was determined and confirmed by a 19th-century German pharmacist, E. Jahns (2). Xanomeline may be viewed as a nonclassical bio-isostere of the ester moiety of arecoline. It is a muscarinic M_1/M_4 agonist that is showing promise in clinical trials for the treatment of Alzheimer's disease (35). Although it is not tolerated at orally effective doses, transdermal delivery systems are showing promise.

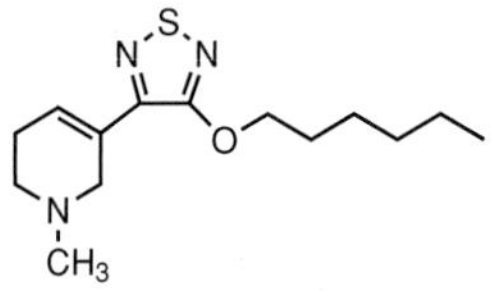

Xanomeline

Acetylcholinesterase Inhibitors

Another means of producing a cholinergic response is to interfere with the mechanism by which the action of acetylcholine is terminated. Thus, inhibition of its rapid hydrolysis by AChE increases the concentration of acetylcholine in the synapse and results in production of both muscarinic and nicotinic effects.

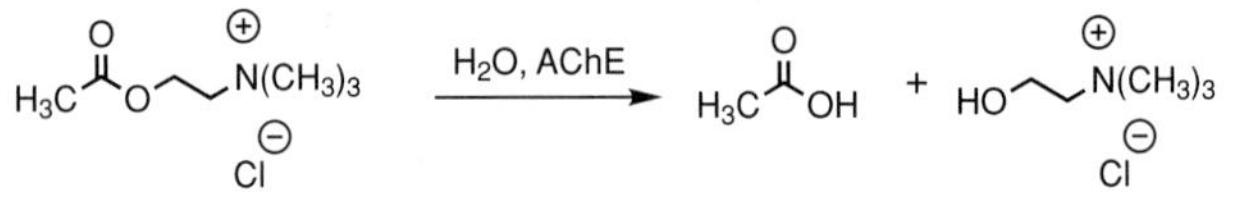

$$H_3C-C(=O)-O-CH_2CH_2-\overset{\oplus}{N}(CH_3)_3\ Cl^{\ominus} \xrightarrow{H_2O,\ AChE} H_3C-C(=O)-OH + HO-CH_2CH_2-\overset{\oplus}{N}(CH_3)_3\ Cl^{\ominus}$$

Therapeutic Application

Acetylcholinesterase inhibitors (AChEIs), sometimes referred to as anticholinesterases, are classified as indirect cholinomimetics, because their principle mechanism of action does not involve binding to cholinergic receptors. These agents are used therapeutically to improve muscle strength in myasthenia gravis. They also are used in open-angle glaucoma to decrease intraocular pressure by stimulating contraction of the ciliary muscle and sphincter of the iris. This facilitates outflow of aqueous humor via the canal of Schlemm. Recently, AChEIs have found use in the treatment of symptoms of Alzheimer's disease and similar cognitive disorders (36,37), which are conditions characterized by a cholinergic deficiency in the cortex and basal forebrain. They are used extensively as insecticides and are in military arsenals for use as chemical warfare agents.

Mechanism of Acetylcholinesterase Hydrolysis

Extensive studies of AChE have resulted in the purification and amino acid sequencing of the enzyme from several sources as well as the description of its quaternary structure from x-ray crystallographic and molecular modeling studies (38). To understand the mode of action of AChEIs, it is necessary to examine the mechanism by which AChE catalyzes hydrolysis of acetylcholine. This enzymatically controlled hydrolysis parallels the two chemical mechanisms for hydrolysis of esters. The first mechanism is acid-catalyzed hydrolysis, in which the initial step involves protonation of the carbonyl oxygen. The transition state is formed by the attack of a molecule of water at the electrophilic carbonyl carbon atom. Collapse of the transition state affords the carboxylic acid and the alcohol (Fig. 12.11). The second mechanism, base-catalyzed hydrolysis, involves the nucleophilic attack

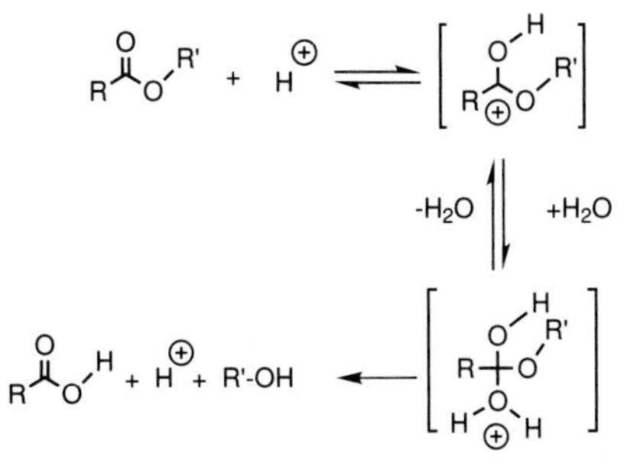

Fig. 12.11. Mechanism of acid-catalyzed hydrolysis of an ester.

of hydroxide anion on the electrophilic carbonyl carbon (Fig. 12.12).

Both mechanisms for ester hydrolysis are proposed to be involved in the mechanism for AChE-catalyzed hydrolysis of acetylcholine. Fig. 12.13 is a schematic illustration of the binding of acetylcholine to the catalytic (active) site of AChE, which consists of an ester-binding site and an "anionic-binding site." This figure reflects binding of the quaternary nitrogen of acetylcholine to an area that has been described as an "anionic site" on the enzyme. Originally, this "anionic site" was proposed to be contributed by the free carboxylate group of a glutamate residue. Current evidence using selective mutagenesis, however, suggests that rather than ionic bonding between the quaternary nitrogen and an anionic site, there is a cation–pi interaction between the quaternary nitrogen and the aromatic rings of tryptophan and phenylalanine of the enzyme (39). In Fig. 12.13, there is a concerted protonation of the carbonyl oxygen by an imidazole proton from a histidine residue and nucleophilic attack on the partial positive carbon of the carbonyl group by the hydroxyl group of a serine residue. The remainder of the hydrolysis mechanism is described in Fig. 12.14: Transition state B is unstable and collapses to form choline and acetylated AChE (C); this form of the enzyme is referred to as the acetylated enzyme. As long as the enzyme is acetylated, it cannot bind another molecule of acetylcholine; the enzyme is in an inactive state. The acetylated enzyme undergoes rapid hydrolysis to regenerate the original, active form of AChE and a molecule of acetic acid.

The latter step in the mechanism—the regeneration of the active enzyme—is important in the development

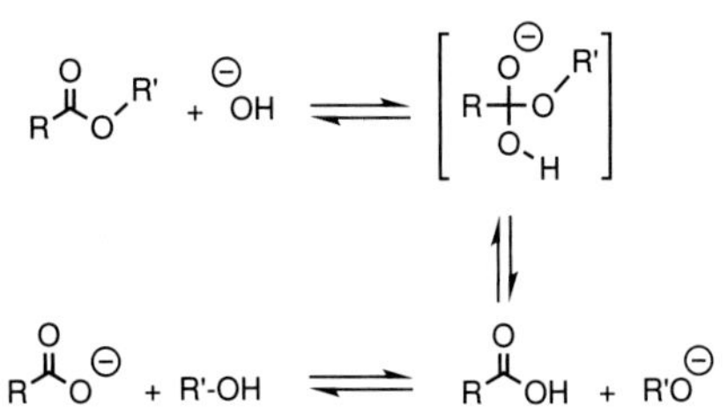

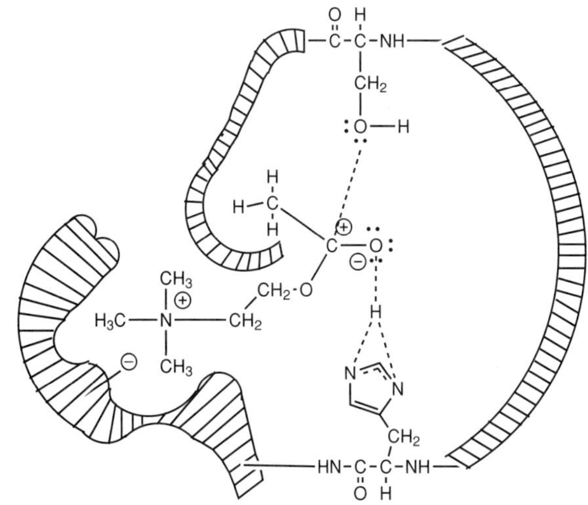

Fig. 12.13. Binding of acetylcholine to catalytic site of acetylcholinesterase; role of serine and histidine residues is illustrated.

of AChEIs. If the enzyme becomes acylated by a functional group (i.e., carbamyl or phosphate) that is more stable to hydrolysis than a carboxylate ester, the enzyme remains inactive for a longer period of time. Application of this chemical principle regarding rates of hydrolysis led to discovery and design of two classes of AChEIs, the reversible inhibitors and the irreversible inhibitors.

Reversible Inhibitors of Acetylcholinesterase

MECHANISM OF ACTION. Reversible AChEIs are those compounds that are substrates for and react with AChE to form an acylated enzyme, which is more stable than the acetylated enzyme but still capable of undergoing hydrolytic regeneration, or that bind to AChE with greater affinity than acetylcholine but do not react with the enzyme as a substrate. Inhibitors of both types have found clinical application. Those that acylate AChE include the aryl carbamates, such as esters of carbamic acid and phenols (e.g., physostigmine). Alkyl carbamates (esters of carbamic acid and alcohols), such as carbachol and bethanechol, both of which are structurally related to acetylcholine, also are substrates for and competitively inhibit AChE, because they are hydrolyzed very slowly by AChE. For reasons previously discussed, carbachol and

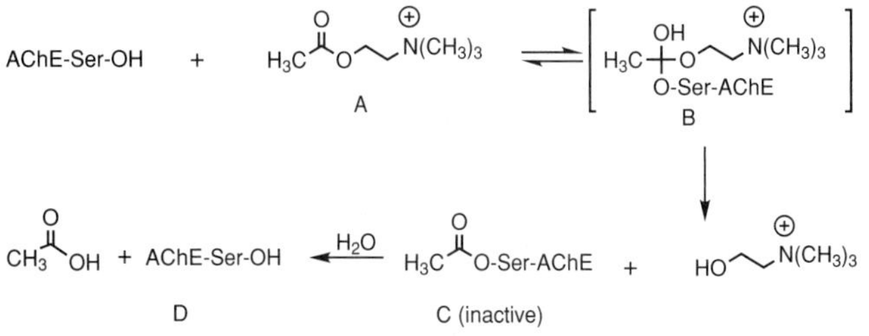

Fig. 12.12. Mechanism of base-catalyzed hydrolysis of an ester.

Fig. 12.14. Mechanistic steps in the hydrolysis of ACh.

bethanechol are more resistant than acetylcholine to AChE-catalyzed hydrolysis.

When aryl carbamate AChEIs, such as physostigmine and its analogues, bind to the catalytic site of AChE, hydrolysis of the carbamate occurs. This transesterifies the serine residue with carbamic acid, forming what is termed a "carbamylated enzyme." The rate of carbamylation follows the order of carbamic acid esters > methylcarbamic acid esters > dimethylcarbamic acid esters (40).

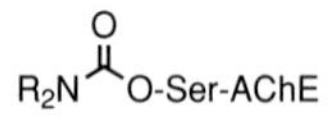

R_2N–C(=O)–O-Ser-AChE

Carbamylated AChE

Regeneration of active AChE by hydrolysis of the carbamylated enzyme is much slower than hydrolysis of the acetylated enzyme. The rate for hydrolytic regeneration of the carbamylated AChE is measured in minutes (e.g., the half-life for methyl carbamylated enzyme is ~15 minutes); the rate of hydrolytic regeneration of acetylated AChE is measured in milliseconds (e.g., the half-life for acetylated enzyme is ~0.2 milliseconds). Despite the longer time required to regenerate the carbamylated enzyme, the active form of AChE eventually is regenerated. Therefore, these inhibitors are considered to be reversible.

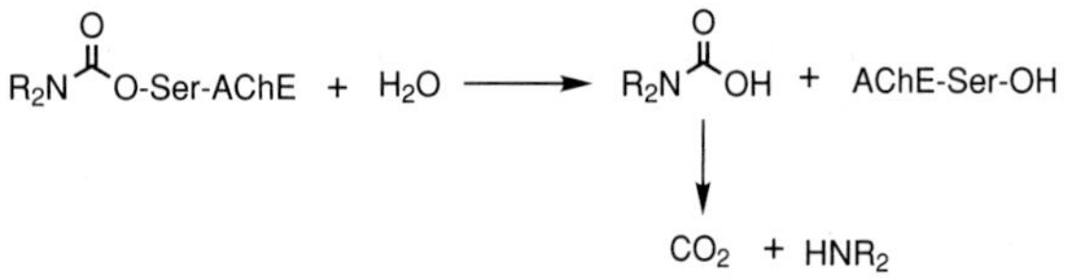

R_2N–C(=O)–O-Ser-AChE + H_2O ⟶ R_2N–C(=O)–OH + AChE-Ser-OH

↓

CO_2 + HNR_2

Aryl carbamates are superior to alkyl carbamates as AChEIs, because they have better affinity for AChE and, therefore, carbamylate AChE more efficiently. Physostigmine and other aryl carbamates exhibit inhibition constants (K_i) on the order of 10^{-9} to 10^{-8} M and are three to four orders of magnitude more effective than alkyl carbamates, such as carbachol ($K_i \sim 10^{-5}$ M). This is to be expected, because phenoxide anions are more stable than and, hence, are better leaving groups than alkoxide anions. Phenoxide anions are stabilized through resonance with the aromatic ring. Thus, the therapeutically effective carbamate inhibitors of AChE are derived from phenols.

Specific Agents

Reversible Acetylcholinesterase Inhibitors

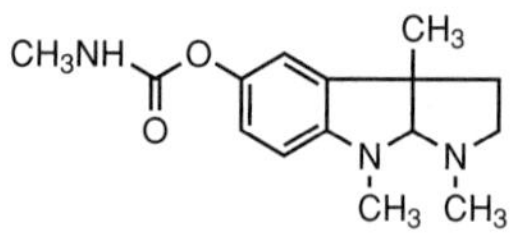

Physostigmine

Physostigmine. The classic AChEI, physostigmine, is an alkaloid obtained from seeds of the Calabar bean (*Physostigma venenosum*) (37). Its parasympathomimetic effects were recognized long before its structure was elucidated in 1923. In 1929, Stedman found that the mechanism of the parasympathomimetic effects of physostigmine was inhibition of AChE; it inhibits AChE by acting as a substrate and carbamylating the enzyme. Acetylcholinesterase is carbamylated at a slow rate, but physostigmine has exceptionally high affinity ($K_i \sim 10^{-9}$ M) for the catalytic site of the enzyme. By comparison, the K_s for acetylcholine is on the order of 10^{-4} M. Thus, physostigmine is classified as a reversible AChEI that carbamylates the enzyme at a slow rate; the carbamylated AChE also is regenerated quite slowly. Because physostigmine is a tertiary amine with a pK_a of 8.2 (^+BH) rather than a quaternary ammonium salt, it is more lipophilic than many other AChEIs and can diffuse across the blood-brain barrier. The tertiary amine also imparts pH dependence to its ability to inhibit AChE, because its affinity for AChE is greater when the amine is protonated. Physostigmine is metabolized in vivo by esterases to the phenol and has an elimination half-life of 1 to 2 hours. Its aqueous solutions are subject to hydrolytic decomposition to form eseroline, which undergoes light-catalyzed oxidation to form rubreserine, a red-colored compound (Fig. 12.15). Both degradation products are inactive as AChEIs.

Physostigmine has been used for many years in ophthalmology for the treatment of glaucoma. More recently, the salicylate salt has been used in hospital emergency rooms to treat overdoses of compounds possessing significant anticholinergic CNS effects (for example, antidepressants), such as atropine and tricyclic antidepressants. Physostigmine's ability to cross the

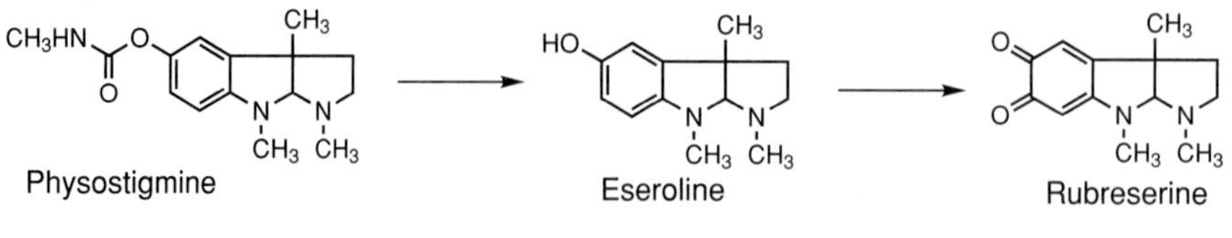

Physostigmine ⟶ Eseroline ⟶ Rubreserine

Fig. 12.15. In vitro degradation of physostigmine.

blood-brain barrier has led to renewed interest in this molecule, and it also is one of a number of centrally active AChEIs being investigated as indirect cholinomimetics for use in the treatment of Alzheimer's disease and other cognitive disorders.

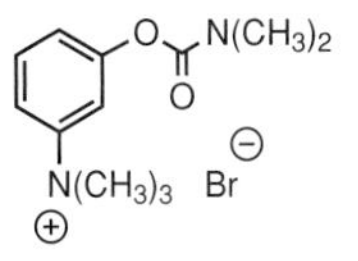

Neostigmine bromide

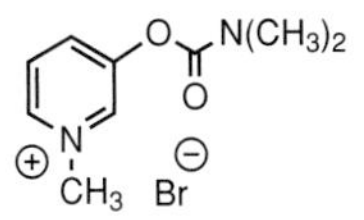

Pyridostigmine bromide

Neostigmine (Prostigmin). The discovery that physostigmine and other aryl carbamates inhibit AChE reversibly led to research to find other AChEIs possessing this activity. Most of this research involved incorporation of the required structural features of both physostigmine and acetylcholine into the new molecules. This led to synthesis of neostigmine, a compound resembling physostigmine but having a much simpler structure. Neostigmine retains the substituted carbamate group, the benzene ring, and the nitrogen atom of the first heterocyclic ring of physostigmine. The distance between the ester and the quaternary ammonium group is approximately the same as that found in acetylcholine and physostigmine. Because of its quaternary ammonium group, it lacks central activity. Neostigmine is metabolized to 3-hydroxyphenyltrimethylammonium, 3-hydroxyphenyldimethylamine, and its glucuronide conjugate, and it has an elimination half-life of 15 to 90 minutes. Neostigmine is indicated for prophylaxis of postoperative abdominal distension and urinary retention, myasthenia gravis, reversal of neuromuscular blockade.

Pyridostigmine (Mestinon). Pyridostigmine, a closely related structure to neostigmine that incorporates the charged nitrogen into a pyridine ring, acts by the same mechanism as physostigmine, but it lacks CNS activity. It is orally effective and, compared to neostigmine, has a longer duration of action and a lower incidence of side effects. Thus, it is a better choice for oral therapy of myasthenia gravis. It is approved for U.S. military use as an adjunct for prophylaxis of soman nerve gas exposure. It is also administered parenterally to reverse the effects of nondepolarizing neuromuscular blocking agents. Its elimination half-life is 1 to 2 hours.

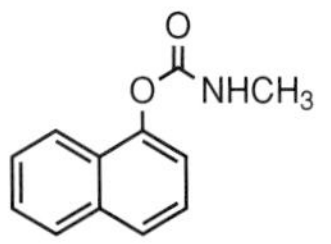

Carbaryl

Carbaryl. Carbaryl is a reversible, carbamate-derived AChEI that has tremendous economic impact as an insecticide for use on houseplants and vegetables as well as for control of fleas and ticks on pets. Its structural relationship to physostigmine and neostigmine is readily apparent. A number of other carbamate AChEIs also are commercially available for this use.

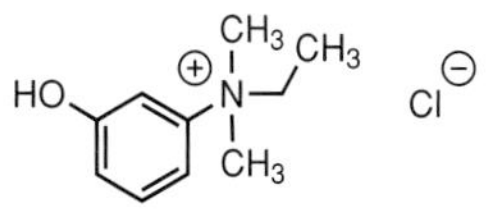

Edrophonium chloride

Edrophonium chloride (Enlon, Reversol). Edrophonium is a quaternary ammonium-substituted phenol. Because it is a phenol derivative rather than a carbamate ester of a phenol, it does not carbamylate AChE. It does, however, inhibit AChE in a reversible manner, and it also exhibits a direct cholinomimetic effect at skeletal muscle. Edrophonium is used intravenously for the diagnosis of myasthenia gravis, where it acts rapidly to increase muscle strength. It also is administered intramuscularly to rapidly reverse the effects of nondepolarizing neuromuscular blocking agents like *d*-tubocurarine and gallamine. It is not effective, however, at reversing the effects of the depolarizing blockers such as succinylcholine and decamethonium. Its elimination half-life 1.3 to 2.4 hours.

Reversible Acetylcholinesterase Inhibitors for Treatment of Alzheimer's Disease. Of all the age-related disorders in which dementia is a component, Alzheimer's disease (AD) is probably the best known. Much effort has been expended to discover the cause of AD. Autopsy examination of the brains of patients who had AD has revealed microscopic structural changes characteristic of the disease. In addition, neurotransmitter dysfunction involving reduction in acetylcholine, serotonin, norepinephrine, dopamine, and glutamate levels have been reported. For a review of AD and the search for therapies, see Rzeszotarski (41). It is known that in AD patients, there is widespread atrophy in the primary motor and sensory cortices and cerebellum. There is a disruption in cholinergic innervation in these areas of the brain, along with decreases in choline acetyltransferase, high-affinity nicotinic acetylcholine receptor binding, and choline transporter sites (42–45). Impairment of short-term memory is the first observable symptom of the disease, and progressive memory impairment, severe mood changes, and depression coupled with loss of judgment and reasoning ability follow. The U.S. Food and Drug Administration has approved four AChEIs for the treatment of AD: tacrine, donepezil, rivastigmine, and galantamine. Although these four AChEIs are not without problems, they do provide some benefit in early to mild AD. Their clinical effectiveness in advanced AD is yet to be shown.

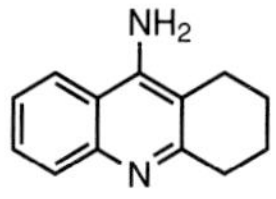

Tacrine

Tacrine hydrochloride (Cognex). Tacrine, an aminoacridine synthesized in the 1930s, is a nonclassic cholinesterase inhibitor that binds to both AChE or butyrylcholinesterase (46). It was approved in 1993 for the treatment of AD. Approximately 20% of tacrine-treated patients may show improvement, but its use has been limited because of hepatotoxicity. Use of tacrine has greatly decreased because of the recent development of safer AChEIs. Tacrine is extensively metabolized by CYP450 to at least three metabolites. The major metabolite, 1-hydroxy-tacrine, is active. Its elimination half-life is between 1.5 and 4 hours, with metabolites being are excreted via the urine.

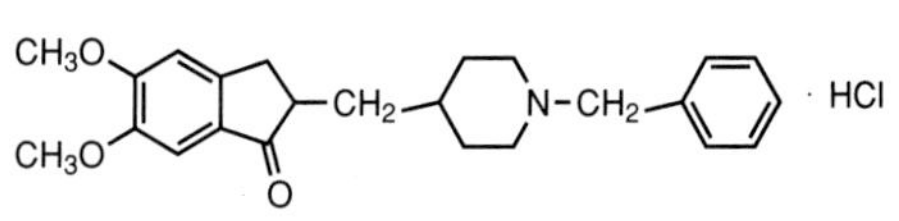

Donepezil hydrochloride

Donepezil (Aricept). Donepezil is another "nonclassic," centrally acting, reversible, noncompetitive AChEI that was approved in 1997 for treatment of mild-to-moderate AD and dementia. Its selectivity for AChE is 570- to 1,250-fold that for butyrylcholinesterase, and it also exhibits greater affinity for brain AChE than for AChE in the periphery (47). When compared to tacrine, donepezil exhibits greater CNS AChE selectivity, longer elimination half-life (70–104 hours in subjects older than 55 years) and little or no potential for hepatotoxicity. Donepezil is metabolized by CYP2D6 and CYP3A4 via demethylation, debenzylation, hydroxylation, oxidation to the *cis*-N-oxide, and glucuronidation. The 6-O-desmethyl metabolite accounts for 11% of a dose, and it exhibits AChE inhibitory activity comparable to that of the parent compound.

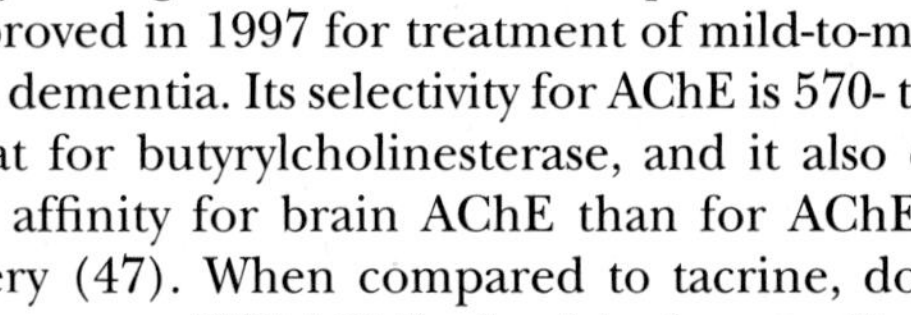

Rivastigmine tartrate

Rivastigmine (Exelon). Rivastigmine is a centrally selective, arylcarbamate AChEI that was approved in 2000 for oral administration in the treatment of AD. It has an elimination half-life of 1.4 to 1.7 hours but is able to inhibit AChE for up to 10 hours. Because of the slow dissociation of the carbamylated enzyme, it has been referred to as a pseudo-irreversible AChEI (47). Like donepezil, rivastigmine exhibits a low level of hepatotoxicity. It is rapidly and extensively hydrolyzed in the CNS by cholinesterase with minimal involvement of CYP450. The phenolic metabolite is excreted primarily via the kidneys.

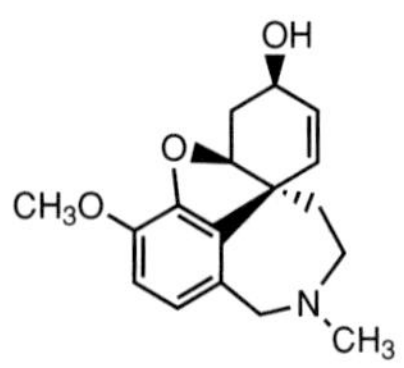

Galantamine

Galantamine hydrobromide (Razadyne). Galantamine, which was introduced in 2001, is an alkaloid found in plants of the family Amaryllidaceae, which includes the daffodil (*Narcissus pseudonarcissus*) and snowflake (*Leucojum aestivum*). It is a reversible inhibitor of AChE, but it does not appear to inhibit butyrylcholinesterase. Because it is a tertiary amine and can cross the blood-brain barrier, it is indicated for treatment of mild-to-moderate AD and dementia. It has been used outside the U.S. for more than 30 years as an anticurare agent in anesthesia. Galantamine differs from other cholinesterase inhibitors, because it allosterically binds to nicotinic receptors, giving it a dual cholinergic action. It is metabolized (75%) by CYP2D6 and CYP3A4 to afford the normethyl, O-desmethyl, and O-desmethylnormethyl metabolites, along with some other minor metabolites. Unlike tacrine, galantamine is not associated with hepatotoxicity. Its elimination half-life is 5.7 hours.

Irreversible Inhibitors of Acetylcholinesterase

Mechanism of Action. The chemical logic involved in the development of effective AChEIs was to synthesize compounds that would be substrates for AChE and result in an acylated enzyme more stable to hydrolysis than a carboxylate ester. Phosphate esters are very stable to hydrolysis, being even more stable than many amides. Application of this chemical property to the design of AChEI compounds led to derivatives of phosphoric, pyrophosphoric, and phosphonic acids that are effective inhibitors of AChE. These act as inhibitors by the same mechanism as the carbamate inhibitors, except that they leave the enzyme esterified as phosphate esters. The rate of hydrolytic regeneration of the phosphorylated enzyme is much slower than that of the carbamylated enzyme, and its rate is measured in hours (e.g., the half-lives for diethyl phosphates are ~8 hours). Because the duration of action of these compounds is much longer than that of carbamate esters, they are referred to as irreversible inhibitors of AChE.

An important difference between irreversible phosphoester-derived AChEIs and reversible AChEIs is that the phosphorylated AChE can undergo a process known as aging (Fig. 12.16). The aging process plays an

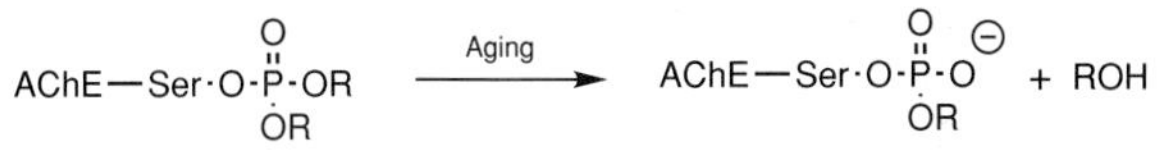

AChE—Ser·O-P(=O)(OR)-OR —Aging→ AChE—Ser·O-P(=O)(OR)-O⊖ + ROH

Fig. 12.16. Aging of phosphorylated AChE.

important role in the toxicity of these irreversible AChEIs. Aging is the result of cleavage of one or more of the phosphoester bonds while the AChE is phosphorylated. This reaction affords an anionic phosphate that possesses a phosphorus atom that is much less electrophilic and, therefore, much less likely to undergo hydrolytic regeneration than the original phosphoester. Thus, the aged phosphorylated enzyme does not undergo nucleophilic attack and regeneration by antidotes (see next section) for phosphate ester AChEIs. This aging process occurs over a period of time, which depends on the rate of the P-O bond cleavage reaction; during this time, the antidotes to phosphate ester poisoning may be effective.

Only those phosphorus-derived AChEIs that have at least one phosphoester group undergo the aging process. Knowledge of the chemical mechanisms associated with irreversible inhibition of AChE and the aging process led to the development of deadly phosphorus-derived chemical warfare agents, one of which is sarin (GB is the two letter NATO designation for this nerve agent). When this compound phosphorylates AChE, only one aging reaction takes place, and then the enzyme becomes refractory to regeneration by the currently available antidotal agents.

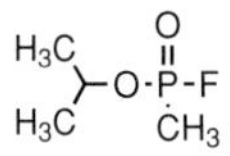

$(H_3C)_2CH$-O-P(=O)(F)-CH_3

Sarin

SPECIFIC AGENTS

$(CH_3CH_2O)_2$-P(=O)-S-CH_2CH_2-$N^{\oplus}(CH_3)_3$ $I^{\ominus}$

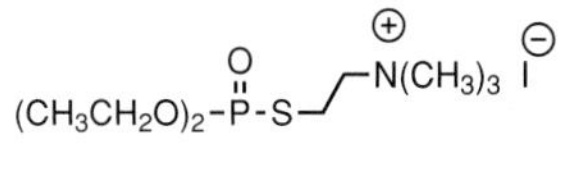

Echothiophate iodide

Echothiophate iodide (Phospholine Iodide). Echothiophate iodide has found therapeutic application for the treatment of glaucoma and strabismus. Echothiophate is applied topically as a solution and is the only irreversible AChEI for the treatment of glaucoma. The decrease in intraocular pressure observed can last up to 4 weeks. Phosphoester AChEIs exhibit cataractogenic properties; thus, their use should be reserved for patients who are refractory to other forms of treatment (i.e., short-acting miotics, β-blockers, epinephrine, and possibly, carbonic

Malathion: CH_3O-P(=S)(OCH_3)-S-CH($COOCH_2CH_3$)-$CH_2COOCH_2CH_3$

Parathion: CH_3CH_2O-P(=S)(OCH_2CH_3)-O-C_6H_4-NO_2

Paraoxon: CH_3CH_2O-P(=O)(OCH_2CH_3)-O-C_6H_4-NO_2

Schradan: $[(CH_3)_2N]_2$-P(=O)-O-P(=O)-$[N(CH_3)_2]_2$

Dichlofenthion: CH_3CH_2O-P(=S)(OCH_2CH_3)-O-$C_6H_3Cl_2$

Chlorpyrifos: CH_3CH_2O-P(=S)(OCH_2CH_3)-O-(3,5,6-trichloropyridin-2-yl)

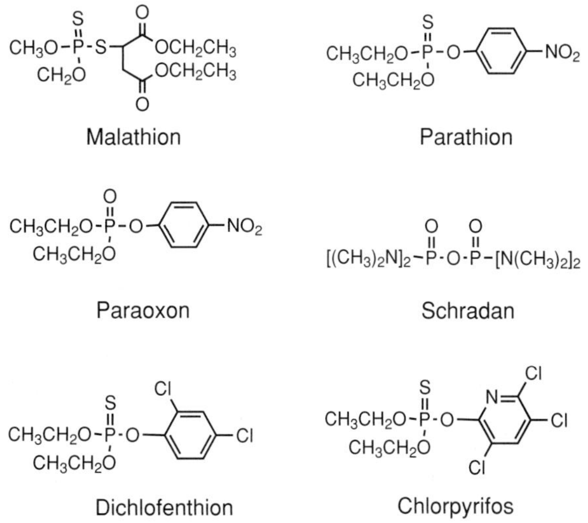

Fig. 12.17. Irreversible acetylcholinesterase inhibitors used as insecticides.

anhydrase inhibitors). Because of its toxicity, echothiophate is not used for its systemic action. Selectivity of echothiophate for the AChE catalytic site was enhanced by incorporation in the molecule of a quaternary ammonium salt functional group two carbons removed from the phosphoryl group.

Insecticidal AChEIs. A number of lipophilic derivatives of phosphoester AChEIs have been designed as insecticides; the structures of some of these are shown in Fig. 12.17. This group of irreversible AChEI insecticides is beneficial to agricultural production throughout the world. In addition to being extremely lipophilic, another physicochemical property common to these compounds is a high vapor pressure. This combination of physicochemical properties makes it imperative that these compounds be used with extreme caution in the presence of humans and other mammals to prevent inhalation of the vapors and their absorption through the skin. Both routes of exposure cause a number of poisoning accidents every year, some of which are fatal.

Some of these irreversible AChEI insecticides have a sulfur atom bonded to the phosphorus atom with a coordinate-covalent bond. These compounds exhibit little AChEI activity, but they are rapidly bioactivated via desulfurization by microsomal oxidation in insects to afford the corresponding oxo derivatives (phosphate esters), which are quite potent. A good example of this bioactivation phenomenon is illustrated by the commercially available insecticide parathion and its bioactivation to a toxic metabolite paraoxon.

Malathion (Ovide). Malathion (Fig. 12.17) is a dithiophosphate ester that has found use both as an aerial insecticide and clinically as a mitocide for topical treatment of lice infestations of the hair and scalp. It will kill both hatched lice and their eggs (nits) within 3 seconds after application. Compared to other organophosphate AChEIs, malathion exhibits lower transdermal absorption. On intact skin, less than 10% of a topical dose is systemically absorbed. Similar to parathion, malathion is bioactivated in insects to its toxic phosphate ester metabolite. It is much less toxic in humans, mammals, and birds than in insects. Selective toxicity with malathion is achieved because plasma esterases hydrolyze the carboxylate esters to less toxic carboxylic acid metabolites that are rapidly eliminated in urine as carboxylate anions in humans but not in insects. Acute toxicity with malathion is rare and usually occurs only after oral ingestion. The lethal dose in mammals is approximately 1 g/kg.

Antidotes for Irreversible AChEIs

Background. The marked toxicity of the phosphate ester irreversible AChEIs, their widespread use as insecticides, and their proliferation as chemical warfare agents posed serious problems that stimulated research to develop antidotes for these agents. This required rational use of reaction kinetics, organic reaction mechanisms, and synthetic organic chemistry. Water is a nucleophile capable of rapidly hydrolyzing acetylated AChE and regenerating the active enzyme. Phosphorylated AChE (irreversibly inhibited), however, was known to involve a phosphate ester of serine. It is well established from reaction kinetic studies that the rate of hydrolysis is much slower for organic phosphate esters than for carboxylate esters and that a significantly stronger nucleophile than water would be required for efficient hydrolysis of phosphate esters. The problem required the design of reagents capable of efficiently catalyzing phosphate ester cleavage to regenerate active AChE while being safe enough for use as therapeutic agents. The resolution of this problem is an elegant example of the application of chemical principles to the solution of a therapeutic problem (48–50).

Hydroxylamine (NH_2OH) is a strong nucleophilic compound that efficiently cleaves phosphate esters. It significantly increases the rate of hydrolysis of phosphorylated AChE, but only at toxic concentrations (51). This prompted the development of a number of structurally related compounds in the hope of eliminating toxicity. The toxicity inherent in hydroxylamine would most probably be present in any structurally related compound, but this toxicity might be minimized if sufficiently small doses could be used. It would be logical to design a compound that would have a high degree of selectivity and strong binding affinity for AChE and also carry a hydroxylamine-like nucleophile into close proximity to the phosphorylated serine residue. This was achieved by synthesis of hydroxylamine derivatives of organic compounds possessing a functional group bearing a positive charge.

Reaction of hydroxylamine with aldehydes or ketones affords oximes, which possess the desired nucleophilic oxygen atom. A pyridine ring was considered an attractive carrier for the oxime function, because such groups are common in a number of biochemical systems (e.g., NAD and NADP), indicating a possible low order of toxicity. Furthermore, three readily available positional isomers of pyridine aldehyde can be converted easily to oximes. Finally, the nitrogen atom of the pyridine ring can be converted to a quaternary ammonium salt by treatment with methyl iodide. This cationic charge would be expected to increase affinity of the compound for the anionic-binding site of the phosphorylated AChE.

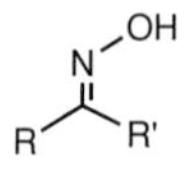

OH
N
R R'

Oxime

The three isomeric pyridine aldoxime methiodides were synthesized and biologically evaluated. Of these, the most effective is the isomer derived from 2-pyridinylaldehyde. This compound, known as pralidoxime chloride (2-PAM, or 2-pyridine aldoxime methyl chloride) currently is the only available agent proven to be clinically effective as an antidote for poisoning by phosphate ester AChEIs. The proposed mechanism for regeneration of AChE by 2-PAM is illustrated in Fig. 12.18. The initial step involves binding of the quaternary ammonium nitrogen of 2-PAM to the anionic-binding site of phosphorylated AChE. This places the nucleophilic oxygen of 2-PAM in close proximity to the electrophilic phosphorus atom. Nucleophilic attack of the oxime oxygen results in breaking of the ester bond between the serine oxygen atom and the phosphorus atom. The final products of the reaction are the regenerated active form of AChE and phosphorylated 2-PAM.

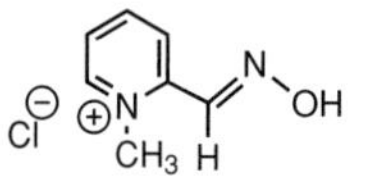

Cl^- N OH
CH_3 H

Pralidoxime chloride (2-PAM)

Pralidoxime is administered subcutaneously, intramuscularly, or intravenously, and it must be given within a short

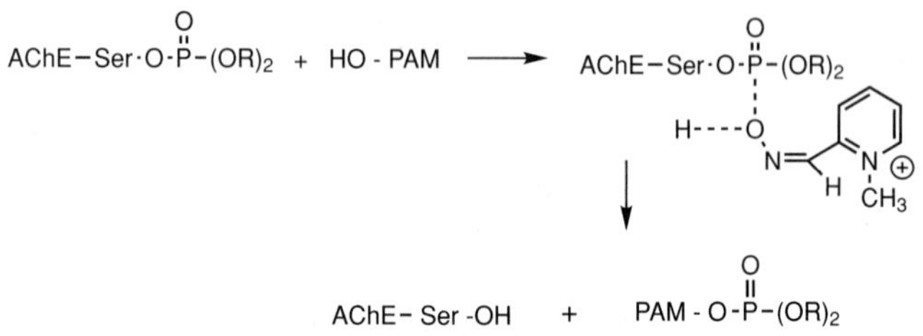

AChE−Ser·O·P(=O)−$(OR)_2$ + HO - PAM ⟶ AChE−Ser·O·P(=O)−$(OR)_2$ ··· H----O N= H N⊕ CH_3

AChE− Ser -OH + PAM - O-P(=O)−$(OR)_2$

Fig. 12.18. Reactivation of AChE with 2-PAM.

period of time after enzyme phosphorylation, generally a few hours after exposure, for it to be effective because of the aging process of the phosphorylated enzyme. Little reactivation is likely if given 36 hours after exposure. If the phosphorylated AChE has aged, 2-PAM will not regenerate the enzyme. For this reason, as well as because new phosphate ester AChEIs capable of aging rapidly are being developed as insecticides and chemical warfare agents, there is a continuing effort to discover new and better substitutes for 2-PAM. This research is focused on finding substitutes for 2-PAM that are better nucleophiles and, therefore, more effective generators of active AChE as well as compounds that cross the blood-brain barrier to regenerate phosphorylated AChE in the brain.

Acetylcholine Antagonists—Muscarinic Antagonists

Muscarinic antagonists are compounds that have high binding affinity for muscarinic receptors but have no intrinsic activity. When the antagonist binds to the receptor, it is proposed that the receptor protein undergoes a conformational perturbation that is different from that produced by an agonist. Therefore, antagonist binding to the receptor produces no response. Muscarinic antagonists commonly are referred to as anticholinergics, antimuscarinics, cholinergic blockers, antispasmodics, or parasympatholytics. The term "anticholinergic" refers, in a pure sense, to medicinal agents that are antagonists at both muscarinic and nicotinic receptors. Common usage of the term, however, has become synonymous with muscarinic antagonist, and it is used as such in this section.

Therapeutic Application

Muscarinic antagonists frequently are employed as both prescription drugs and over-the-counter medications. Because they act as competitive (reversible) antagonists of acetylcholine, these compounds have pharmacological effects that are opposite those of muscarinic agonists. Responses of muscarinic antagonists include decreased contractions of smooth muscle of the gastrointestinal and urinary tracts, dilation of the pupils, and reduced gastric, mucociliary, and salivary secretions. It follows that these compounds have therapeutic value in treating smooth muscle spasms associated with increased tone of the gastrointestinal tract or with overactive bladder, in ophthalmologic examinations, and in treatment of gastric ulcers. Compounds possessing muscarinic antagonist activity are common components of cold and flu remedies that act to reduce nasal and upper respiratory tract secretions.

In addition to reducing gastric motility, anticholinergic agents decrease gastric acid secretion and were once widely used to manage peptic ulcers. Histamine H_2 antagonists and, more recently, the proton pump inhibitors have largely replaced them for this use. When used systemically, they tend to produce undesirable side effects, such as blurred vision, photophobia, dry mouth, and difficulty in urination. These side effects tend to reduce patient compliance.

Anticholinergic agents exhibit a mydriatic action and, thus, must be used with caution because of their effect on intraocular pressure. Drainage of the canal of Schlemm is restricted by the iris when the pupil is dilated, and this can cause an increase in intraocular pressure. Hence, muscarinic antagonists are contraindicated in patients with glaucoma.

The aforementioned side effect of causing difficulty in urination has been used to advantage with the recent approval of several anticholinergic agents—darifenacin trospium, solifenacin, tolterodine, and oxybutynin—for the treatment of overactive bladder.

Centrally acting belladonna alkaloids, such as scopolamine, have been used in transdermal delivery systems for the prevention of motion sickness. They are most effective when used prophylactically; they have less effect when used after nausea and vomiting have begun. Several of the synthetic muscarinic antagonists have been used to treat parkinsonism and to block the extrapyramidal effects of antipsychotic agents. The anticholinergic alkaloid atropine is used for treatment of central and peripheral symptoms associated with poisoning by organophosphorus anticholinesterase agents.

Specific Agents—Solanaceous Alkaloids

The earliest known anticholinergic agents were alkaloids found in the family Solanaceae, a large family of plants that includes potatoes. *Atropa belladonna* (deadly nightshade), *Hyoscyamus niger* (black henbane), and *Datura stramonium* (jimsonweed, thorn apple) are plants that have significant historical importance to our understanding of the parasympathetic nervous system. Pharmacological effects of extracts from these plants have been recognized since the Middle Ages, although these effects were not associated with the autonomic nervous system until the latter part of the 19th century. (−)-Hyoscyamine, isolated as atropine, and scopolamine are the two alkaloids that have found the widespread clinical applications.

CH_3 N CH_2OH O O

Atropine

CH_3 N O CH_2OH O O

Scopolamine

Atropine. Atropine is the tropic acid ester of tropine and is marketed as the sulfate salt. The naturally occurring alkaloid, (−)-hyoscyamine, undergoes base-catalyzed racemization during isolation from plants of the Solanaceae to give (±)-hyoscyamine or atropine. It was the first compound shown to block the effects of electrical stimulation and muscarine on the parasympathetic nervous system. Atropine sulfate has a number of clinical uses; two of the most common are treatment of bradycardia and as a preoperative agent to reduce secretions before surgery. Its use for management of parkinsonism has been supplanted by newer agents with fewer peripheral side effects. It has been used in ophthalmology as a cycloplegic agent to paralyze the iris and ciliary muscle in the treatment of iritis and uveitis and as a cycloplegic/ mydriatic agent. Atropine is contraindicated in glaucoma because of its ability to increase intraocular pressure during mydriasis. Its prolonged duration of mydriasis makes other drugs more attractive for this purpose. In poisoning by organophosphate nerve agents and insecticides, atropine is used to decrease the muscarinic cholinergic actions (e.g., lacrimation, salivation, sweating, bradycardia, and breathing problems) associated with this poisoning. It only treats the symptoms and does not reverse the underlying AChE inhibition. Atropine undergoes nonenzymatic ester hydrolysis in vivo and has an elimination half-life of 4 hours in adults and 6.5 hours in children.

SCOPOLAMINE. Scopolamine, another Solanaceous alkaloid, is chemically and pharmacologically similar to atropine. Scopolamine is the generic name given to (−)-hyoscine, the naturally occurring alkaloid. The racemic compound, isolated during extraction of the alkaloid from plants, is atroscine. Scopolamine is marketed as the hydrobromide salt, because it is less deliquescent than some of its other salts. Scopolamine is a CNS depressant at usual therapeutic doses, whereas atropine and other antimuscarinic agents are CNS stimulants. It has been used for the treatment of uveitis, iritis, and parkinsonism, but its most widespread use is for the treatment of motion sickness. For this indication, scopolamine is used in a transdermal patch applied behind the ear. It is almost completely metabolized in the liver and is excreted via the kidneys. Its elimination half-life is approximately 8 hours.

Structure–activity relationship. Atropine, the prototype anticholinergic agent, provided the structural model that guided the design of synthetic muscarinic antagonists for almost 70 years. The circled portion of the atropine molecule depicts the segment resembling acetylcholine.

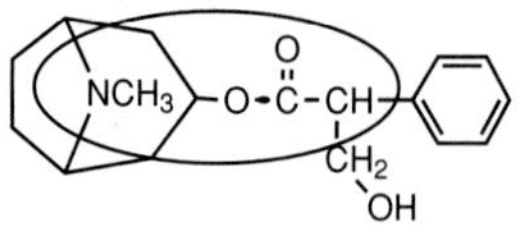

NCH3 –O–C(=O)–CH–(phenyl)
CH2
OH

Although the amine functional group is separated from the ester oxygen by more than two carbons, the conformation assumed by the tropine ring orients these two atoms such that the intervening distance is similar to that in acetylcholine. One important structural difference between atropine and acetylcholine, both of which are esters of amino alcohols, is the size of the acyl portion of the molecules. Based on the assumption that size was a major factor in blocking action, many substituted acetic acid esters of amino alcohols were prepared and evaluated for biological activity.

It became apparent that the most potent compounds were those that possessed two lipophilic ring substituents on the carbon α to the carbonyl of the ester moiety. This is the first of the classic SARs for muscarinic antagonist activity, and this SAR became defined more precisely as research on these antagonists continued. The SAR for muscarinic antagonists can be summarized as follows:

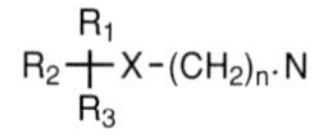

$$R_2-\overset{R_1}{\underset{R_3}{C}}-X-(CH_2)_n-N$$

1. Substituents R_1 and R_2 should be carbocyclic or heterocyclic rings for maximal antagonist potency. The rings may be identical, but the more potent compounds have different rings. Generally, one ring is aromatic and the other saturated or possessing only one olefinic bond. Substituents R_1 and R_2, however, may be combined into a fused aromatic tricyclic ring system, such as that found in propantheline (Table 12.1). The size of these substituents is limited. For example, substitution of naphthalene rings for R_1 and R_2 affords compounds that are inactive, apparently because of steric hindrance of the binding of these compounds to the muscarinic receptor.
2. The R_3 substituent may be a hydrogen atom, a hydroxyl group, a hydroxymethyl group, or a carboxamide, or it may be a component of one of the R_1 and R_2 ring systems. When this substituent is either a hydroxyl group or a hydroxymethyl group, the antagonist usually is more potent than the same compound without this group. The hydroxyl group presumably increases binding strength by participating in a hydrogen bond interaction at the receptor.
3. The X substituent in the most potent anticholinergic agents is an ester, but an ester functional group is not an absolute necessity for muscarinic antagonist activity. This substituent may be an ether oxygen, or it may be absent completely.
4. The N substituent is a quaternary ammonium salt in the most potent anticholinergic agents. This is not a requirement, however, because tertiary amines also possess antagonist activity, presumably by binding to the receptor in the cationic (conjugate acid) form. The alkyl substituents usually are methyl, ethyl, propyl, or isopropyl.
5. The distance between the ring-substituted carbon and the amine nitrogen apparently is not critical; the length of the alkyl chain connecting these may

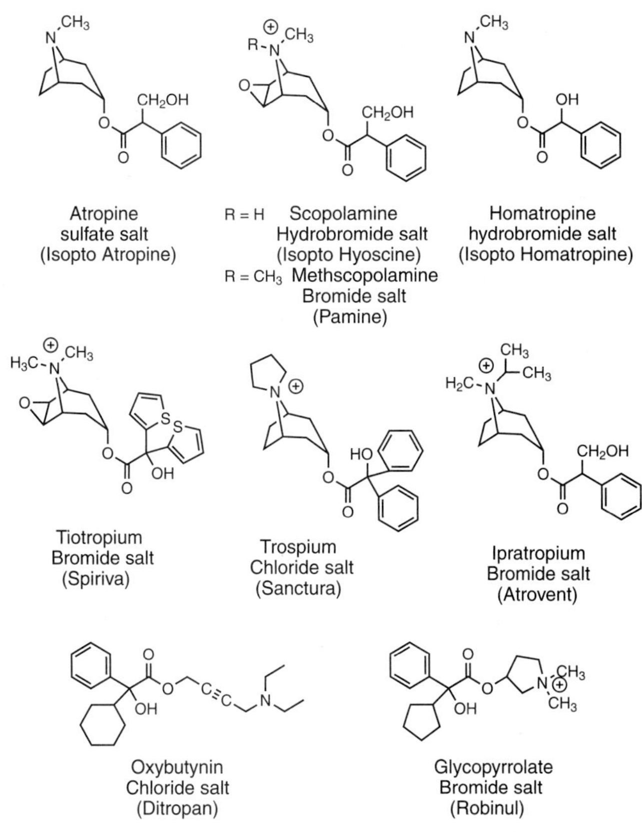

Fig. 12.19. Anticholinergic aminoalcohol esters.

be from two to four carbons. The most potent anticholinergic agents have two methylene units in this chain.

Muscarinic antagonists must compete with agonists for a common receptor. Their ability to do this effectively is because the large groups R_1 and R_2 enhance binding to the receptor. Because antagonists are larger than agonists, this suggests that groups R_1 and R_2 bind outside the binding site of acetylcholine. It has been suggested that the area surrounding the binding site of acetylcholine is hydrophobic in nature (52). This accounts for the fact that in potent cholinergic antagonists, groups R_1 and R_2 must be hydrophobic (usually phenyl, cyclohexyl, or cyclopentyl). This concept also is supported by the current models for muscarinic receptors.

Figures 12.19 and 12.20 and Table 12.3 include structures and pharmacological properties of some of the anticholinergic agents that have found clinical application. These compounds reflect the SAR features that have been described. All these compounds are effective when administered orally or parenterally. Anticholinergic agents possessing a quaternary ammonium functional group generally are not well absorbed from the gastrointestinal tract because of their ionic character. These drugs are useful primarily in the treatment of ulcers or other conditions for which a reduction in gastric secretions and reduced motility of the gastrointestinal tract

Anticholinergic aminoalcohols:

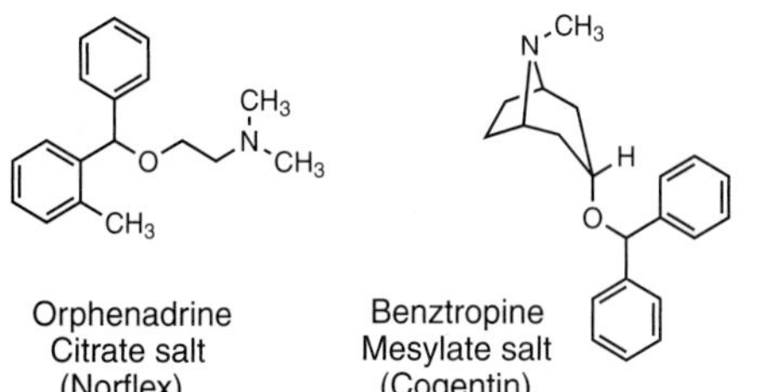

Anticholinergic aminoethers:

Orphenadrine
Citrate salt
(Norflex)

Benztropine
Mesylate salt
(Cogentin)

Miscellaneous anticholinergic agnets:

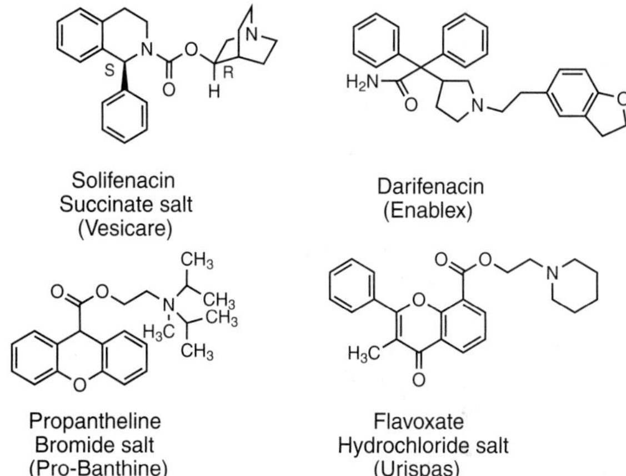

Fig. 12.20. Aminoalcohol, aminoether, and miscellaneous anticholinergic agents.

are desired. Those antagonists having a tertiary nitrogen are much better absorbed and distributed following all routes of administration and are especially useful when systemic distribution is desired. The tertiary amino-derived anticholinergic agents readily cross the blood-brain barrier. These have proven to be particularly beneficial in the treatment of Parkinson's disease and other diseases requiring a central anticholinergic effect.

All these drugs display pronounced selectivity for muscarinic receptors; however, some of those possessing the quaternary ammonium functional group exhibit nicotinic antagonist activity at high doses. With the exception of the M_3 antagonists, solifenacin and darifenacin, these agents display no marked selectivity for muscarinic receptor subtypes.

Recent Muscarinic Antagonists. More recently discovered muscarinic antagonists display a higher affinity for

Table 12.3. Anticholinergic Agents

Name	Calculated[a] Log P Log D (pH 7)	Half-life	Metabolism	Indications	Comments
Atropine	1.53 −1.21	3.5 ± 1.5 hours	Hydrolysis; N-dealkylation; N-oxide	Bradycardia; parkinsonism; cycloplegic/mydriatic	Nonselective muscarinic antagonist; stimulates the CNS
Scopolamine	0.76 0.29	8 hours	Almost completely metabolized (liver)	Uveitis; iritis; parkinsonism; motion sickness	Nonselective muscarinic antagonist; CNS depressant
Homatropine (Isopto Homatropine)	1.57 −1.17	—	—	Cycloplegic/mydriatic	Nonselective muscarinic antagonist; less potent an shorter duration than atropine
Ipratropium bromide (Atrovent)	—	2 hours	Hydrolysis	Bronchodilator (oral inhalation); seasonal rhinitis (nasal spray)	Nonselective muscarinic antagonist; slow onset after inhalation
Tiotropium bromide (Spiriva)	—	5–6 days	CYP2D6 and CYP3A4 Hydrolysis; N-dealkylation; glucuronide conjugation	Chronic obstructive pulmonary disease (oral inhalation)	Equal affinity for M_1, M_2 and M_3 receptors
Trospium Chloride (Sanctura)	—	20 hours	Hydrolysis; conjugation	Urinary and gastrointestinal antispasmodic	High affinity for M_1 and M_3 receptors, lesser affinity for M_2.
Oxybutynin (Oral: Ditropan and Ditropan XL) Oxybutynin (transdermal: Oxytrol)	5.19 3.93	2–5 hours	CYP3A4 Hydrolysis; N-dealkylation	Overactive bladder	Nonselective muscarinic antagonist
Solifenacin (Vesicare)	3.70 1.70	55 hours	4 R-Hydroxy (active); N-glucuronide; N-oxide; 4R-hydroxy-N-oxide	Overactive bladder	Selective M_3 antagonist
Tolterodine (Detrol)	5.77 2.79	2–4 hours (extensive metabolizers) 9.6 (poor metabolizers)	Primary pathway: CYP2D6 (primary); 7% of Caucasians & 2% of African Americans lack CYP2D6; CYP3A4 is the primary pathway in the latter. Metabolites: 5-hydroxymethyl (active), 5-carboxylic acid, N-dealkylated-5-carboxylic acid	Overactive bladder	Nonselective muscarinic antagonist
Darifenacin	4.50 2.25	—	CYP2D6 (primary; see tolterodine above); hydroxylation of the dihydrobenzofuran; ring opening (dihydrobenzofurna); N-dealkylation	Overactive bladder	Selective M_3 antagonist

[a]Values calculated using ACD Lab Solarius, Chemical Abstracts Service, 2006, Columbus, OH (values for quaternary compounds are not listed).

the receptors compared with the older agents, as exemplified by quinuclidinylbenzilate (QNB), which has structural features common to the classic anticholinergic agents. Radiolabeled QNB was instrumental in the development of muscarinic receptor labeling techniques as well as the discovery of subtypes of muscarinic receptors. This latter research also depended on the M_1-selective antagonist pirenzepine, a compound having a novel structure for muscarinic antagonist activity. A number of compounds structurally related to pirenzepine have demonstrated a similar M_1 selectivity; among these is telenzepine (53). Because of their selectivity for muscarinic M_1 receptors, pirenzepine and telenzepine have been evaluated in clinical trials for the treatment of duodenal ulcers. It is of interest to note that AFDX-116, structurally similar to pirenzepine, is a muscarinic antagonist exhibiting selectivity for cardiac M_2 receptors.

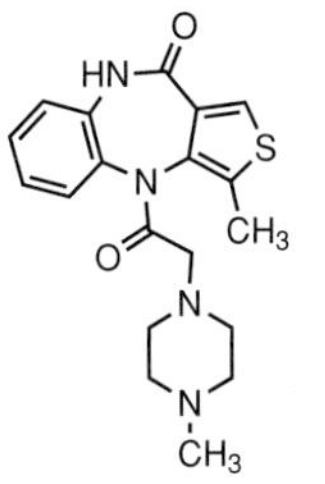

Telenzepine 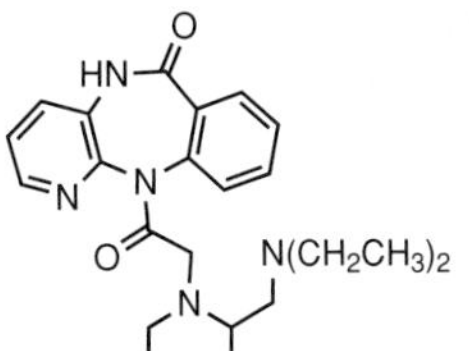 AFDX - 116 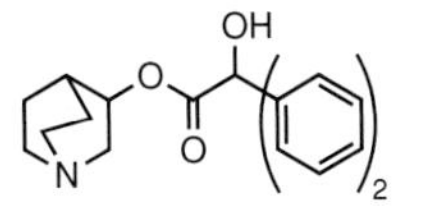 3-Quinuclidinylbenzilate (QNB)

NICOTINIC ANTAGONISTS—NEUROMUSCULAR BLOCKING AGENTS

Nicotinic antagonists are chemical compounds that bind to cholinergic nicotinic receptors but have no efficacy. All therapeutically useful nicotinic antagonists are competitive antagonists; in other words, the effects are reversible with acetylcholine. There are two subclasses of nicotinic antagonists—skeletal neuromuscular blocking agents and ganglionic blocking agents—classified according to the two populations of nicotinic receptors. This section emphasizes nicotinic antagonists used clinically as neuromuscular blocking agents. These medicinal agents should not be confused with those skeletal muscle relaxant compounds that produce their effects through the CNS.

History

In terms of the historical perspective, tubocurarine, the first known neuromuscular blocking drug, was as important to the understanding of nicotinic antagonists as atropine was to that of muscarinic antagonists. The neuromuscular blocking effects of extracts of curare were first reported as early as 1510, when explorers of the Amazon River region of South America found natives using these plant extracts as arrow poisons. Early research with these crude plant extracts indicated that the active components caused muscle paralysis by effects on either the nerve or the muscle (remember that the concept of neurochemical transmission was not introduced until the late 19th century). In 1856, however, Bernard (54) described the results of his experiments, which demonstrated unequivocally that curare extracts prevented skeletal muscle contractions by an effect at the neuromuscular junction, rather than the nerve innervating the muscle or the muscle itself.

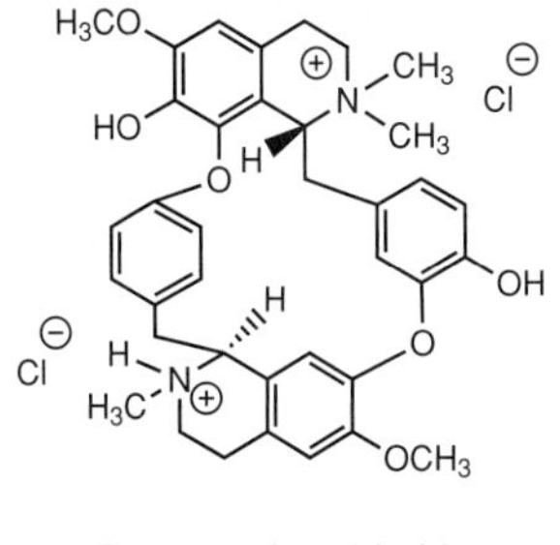

d-Tubocurarine chloride

Much of the early literature concerning the effects of curare is confusing and difficult to interpret. This is not at all surprising considering that this research was performed using crude extracts, many of which came from different plants. It was not until the late 1800s that scientists recognized that curare extracts contained quaternary ammonium salts. This knowledge prompted the use of other quaternary ammonium compounds to explore the neuromuscular junction. In the meantime, curare extracts continued to be used to block the effects of nicotine and acetylcholine at skeletal neuromuscular junctions and to explore the nicotinic receptors.

In 1935, King (55) isolated a pure alkaloid, which he named *d*-tubocurarine, from a tube curare of unknown botanical origin. The word "tube" refers to the container in which the South American natives transported their plant extract. It was almost 10 years later that the botanical source for *d*-tubocurarine was clearly identified as *Chondodendron tomentosum*. The structure that King assigned to tubocurarine possessed two nitrogen atoms, both of which were quaternary ammonium salts (e.g., a *bis*-quaternary ammonium compound). It was not until 1970 that the correct structure was reported by Everett et al. (56). The correct structure, shown here, has only one quaternary ammonium nitrogen; the other nitrogen is a tertiary amine salt. Nevertheless, the incorrect structure of tubocurarine served as the model for the synthesis of all the neuromuscular blocking agents in use today. These compounds have been of immense therapeutic value for surgical and orthopedic procedures and have been essential to research that led to the isolation and purification of nicotinic receptors.

The potential therapeutic benefits of the neuromuscular blocking effects of tubocurarine as well as the difficulty in obtaining pure samples of the alkaloid encouraged medicinal chemists to design structurally related compounds possessing nicotinic antagonist activity. Using the incorrectly assigned *bis*-quaternary ammonium structure of tubocurarine (as reported by King) as a guide, a large number of compounds were synthesized and evaluated. It became apparent that a *bis*-quaternary ammonium compound having two quaternary ammonium salts separated by 10 to 12 carbon atoms (similar to the distance between the nitrogen atoms in tubocurarine) was a requirement for neuromuscular blocking activity. The rationale for this structural requirement was that in contrast to muscarinic receptors, nicotinic receptors possessed two anionic-binding sites, both of which had to be occupied for a neuromuscular blocking effect. It is important to observe that the current transmembrane model for the nicotinic receptor protein has two anionic sites in the extracellular domain.

Some of the new *bis*-quaternary ammonium agents produced depolarization of the postjunctional membrane at the neuromuscular junction before causing blockade; other compounds, such as tubocurarine, did not produce this depolarization. Thus, the structural features of the remainder of the molecule determined whether the nicotinic antagonist was a depolarizing or a nondepolarizing neuromuscular blocker.

Therapeutic Application

Neuromuscular blocking agents are used primarily as an adjunct to general anesthesia. They produce skeletal muscle relaxation that facilitates operative procedures such as abdominal surgery. Furthermore, they reduce the depth requirement for general anesthetics; this decreases the overall risk of a surgical procedure and shortens the postanesthetic recovery time. Muscles producing rapid movements are the first to be affected by neuromuscular blocking agents. These include muscles of the face, eyes, and neck. Muscles of the limbs, chest, and abdomen are affected next, with the diaphragm (respiration) being affected last. Recovery generally is in the reverse order.

Neuromuscular blocking agents also have been used in the correction of dislocations and the realignment of fractures. Short-acting neuromuscular blocking agents, such as succinylcholine, are routinely used to assist in tracheal intubation. When choosing a neuromuscular blocking agent, four questions must be considered:

1. Will the compound produce the desired neuromuscular blockade?
2. What is its duration of action?
3. What are its adverse effects?
4. What is its relative cost?

Side Effects

Adverse reactions to most, but not all, of the neuromuscular blocking agents may include hypotension, bronchospasm, and cardiac disturbances. The depolarizing agents also cause an initial muscle fasciculation before relaxation. Many of these agents cause release of histamine and subsequent cutaneous (flushing, erythema, urticaria, and pruritus), pulmonary (bronchospasm and wheezing), and cardiovascular (hypotension) effects.

Specific Depolarizing Neuromuscular Blocking Agents

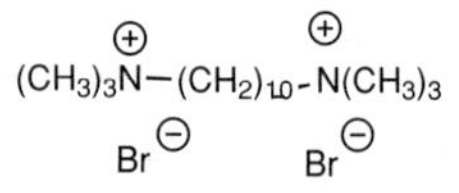

$$(CH_3)_3\overset{\oplus}{N}-(CH_2)_{10}-\overset{\oplus}{N}(CH_3)_3 \quad Br^{\ominus} \quad Br^{\ominus}$$

Decamethonium bromide

DECAMETHONIUM BROMIDE. Decamethonium was one of the first neuromuscular blocking agents to be synthesized. An SAR study on a series of *bis*-quaternary ammonium compounds with varying numbers of methylene groups separating the nitrogen atoms demonstrated that maximal neuromuscular blockade occurred with 10 to 12 unsubstituted methylene groups. Activity diminished as the number of carbons was either decreased or increased. The compound with six methylene groups, hexamethonium, is a nicotinic antagonist at autonomic ganglia (ganglionic blocking agent). All the compounds in this series that possessed neuromuscular blocking activity also caused depolarization of the postjunctional membrane.

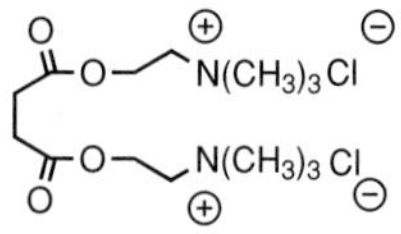

Succinylcholine chloride

SUCCINYLCHOLINE CHLORIDE (ANECTINE). Succinylcholine is a depolarizing neuromuscular blocking agent that represents a dimer of acetylcholine bonded through their α carbons. The molecule can exist in an extended conformation (antiperiplanar), as shown in the Newman projection. This would account for the appropriate separation of the quaternary nitrogens. Succinylcholine is rapidly hydrolyzed and rendered inactive both in aqueous solution and by plasma esterases; this chemical instability must be considered when preparing solutions for parenteral administration. This same chemical property, however, gives the compound a brief duration of action. As a result, succinylcholine is frequently used for the rapid induction of neuromuscular blockade and when blockade of short duration is desired (Table 12.4). As such, it is used primarily to produce muscle relaxation during endotracheal intubation or endoscopic procedures. The depolarizing property is undesirable in neuromuscular blockers, so most research efforts have been directed toward the design of nondepolarizing agents.

Specific Nondepolarizing Neuromuscular Blocking Agents

Compounds in this class have one or two quaternary ammonium groups. Those with only one quaternary ammonium group, however, exist as *bis*-cations in vivo because of the second positive charge being on a protonated tertiary amine. The various structures of these compounds serve primarily as a "scaffold" to position two

Table 12.4. Properties of Clinically Useful Neuromuscular Blocking Agents

Agent	Time of Onset (min)	Duration of Action (min)	Half-life (min)	Mode of Elimination
Succinylcholine	1–1.5	6–8	<1	Hydrolysis by plasma cholinesterases
d-Tubocurarine	4–6	80–120	173	Renal elimination, liver clearance
Vecuronium	2–4	30–40	65–80	Liver metabolism and clearance, renal elimination
Pancuronium	4–6	120–180	89–140	Renal elimination, liver metabolism and clearance
Pipecuronium	2–4	80–100	137–161	Renal elimination, liver metabolism and clearance
Rocuronium	1–2	30–40	84–131	Liver metabolism and clearance
Atracurium	2–4	30–40	16–20	Hofmann degradation, hydrolysis by plasma cholinesterases
Mivacurium	2–4	12–18	1.8–2.0	Hydrolysis by plasma cholinesterases
Doxacurium	4–6	90–120	72–96	Renal elimination, liver metabolism and clearance

Adapted from Taylor P. Agents acting at the neuromuscular junction and autonomic ganglia. In: Brunton LL, Lazo JS, Parker KL, eds., Goodman and Gilman's The Pharmacological Basis of Therapeutics, 11th Ed. New York: McGraw-Hill, 2006, pp. 217–236; with permission.

positive charges in the correct three-dimensional orientation for interaction with the transmembrane nicotinic receptors.

d-Tubocurarine chloride (R = H, X = Cl)
Metocurine iodide (R = CH_3, X = I)

d-TUBOCURARINE AND METOCURINE (METUBINE IODIDE). The prototype of this class is *d*-tubocurarine. It is administered intravenously and has a relatively long duration of action. Only approximately 1% of a dose is demethylated in the liver, and it is excreted primarily as unchanged drug in the urine and bile. *d*-Tubocurarine preparations contain bisulfites and, thus, may potentiate allergic reactions in patients with bisulfate allergy. It is the most potent inducer of histamine release of all the nondepolarizing neuromuscular blockers.

Reaction of *d*-tubocurarine with methyl iodide affords metocurine iodide (see above), in which the two phenolic hydroxyl groups of *d*-tubocurarine are changed to the methyl ethers and the tertiary amine becomes quaternary. This agent is approximately fourfold more potent than *d*-tubocurarine in neuromuscular blocking activity. Like *d*-tubocurarine, it has a long duration of action and is eliminated (predominantly unchanged) via the kidney.

STEROID-BASED NEUROMUSCULAR BLOCKING AGENTS. An ideal neuromuscular blocking agent would be a nondepolarizing compound that is metabolically inactivated and rapidly eliminated. Efforts to design such a neuromuscular blocker have resulted in the development of several synthetic neuromuscular agents. Those that have found clinical use are either aminosteroids derived from (+)-malouetine (an aminosteroid found in the rain forest of central Africa) (Fig. 12.21) or tetrahydroisoquinoline derivatives (Fig. 12.22).

Pancuronium bromide (Pavulon). Pancuronium, a long-acting agent, is more active than tubocurarine. It may cause increases in heart rate and blood pressure and should not be used in patients with coronary artery disease. Pancuronium undergoes hydrolysis in the liver to the active 3-hydroxy metabolite and the inactive 17-hydroxy and 3,17-dihydroxy metabolites; it is excreted primarily in the urine, with small amounts in the bile.

Vecuronium bromide (Norcuron). Removal of the methyl group from the quaternary piperidinium group at position 3 of pancuronium affords vecuronium, an intermediate-acting agent. Vecuronium has the advantage of not inducing histamine release at normal doses and of not exhibiting significant cardiovascular effects. One-third of an administered dose of vecuronium is hydrolyzed to the 3-hydroxy, 17-hydroxy, and 3,17-dihydroxy metabolites, all of which are active. Accumulation of the 3,17-dihydroxy metabolite is responsible for prolonged neuromuscular blockade in patients receiving long-term therapy with vecuronium.

Pipecuronium bromide (Arduan). Pipecuronium bromide, a long-acting neuromuscular blocking agent, exhibits minimal cardiovascular effects. Like pancuronium and vecuronium, pipecuronium undergoes some hydrolysis but is excreted primarily unchanged in the urine with very small amounts in the bile. Pipecuronium may be used in patients with coronary artery disease, but neuromuscular blockade is prolonged in patients with renal failure.

Rocuronium bromide (Zemuron). Rocuronium bromide is an intermediate-acting agent with a duration of action similar to vecuronium and atracurium but with a more rapid onset. It does not appear to cause significant histamine release.

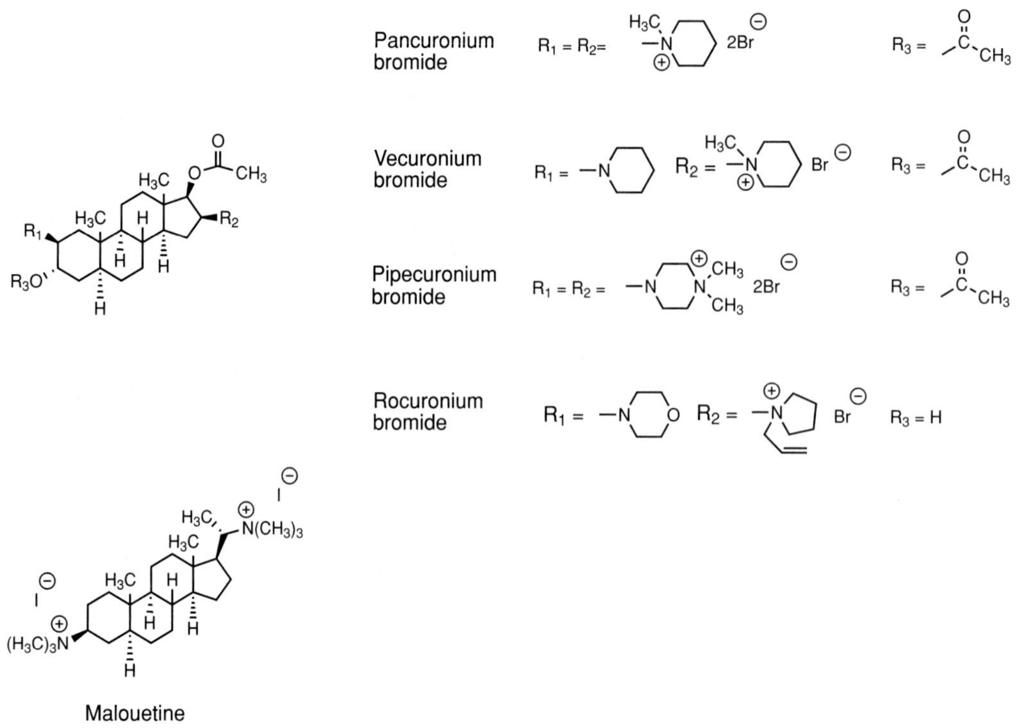

Fig. 12.21. Amino steroid-based neuromuscular blocking agents.

TETRAHYDROISOQUINOLINE-BASED NEUROMUSCULAR BLOCKING AGENTS

Atracurium besylate (Tracrium). Atracurium besylate is a nondepolarizing neuromuscular blocker in which the quaternary ammonium groups are located in two substituted tetrahydroisoquinoline rings separated by an aliphatic diester. It has a duration of action slightly longer than that of succinylcholine. Atracurium is not metabolized in the liver; rather, it undergoes hydrolysis of the ester functional groups that connect the two quaternary nitrogens. It also undergoes Hofmann elimination, a nonenzymatic, base-catalyzed decomposition, to yield laudanosine, which is inactive (Fig. 12.23) (57,58). Thus, termination of the effects of atracurium are independent of renal elimination. Because of this unusual metabolic profile, it is useful in patients with hepatic or renal disease.

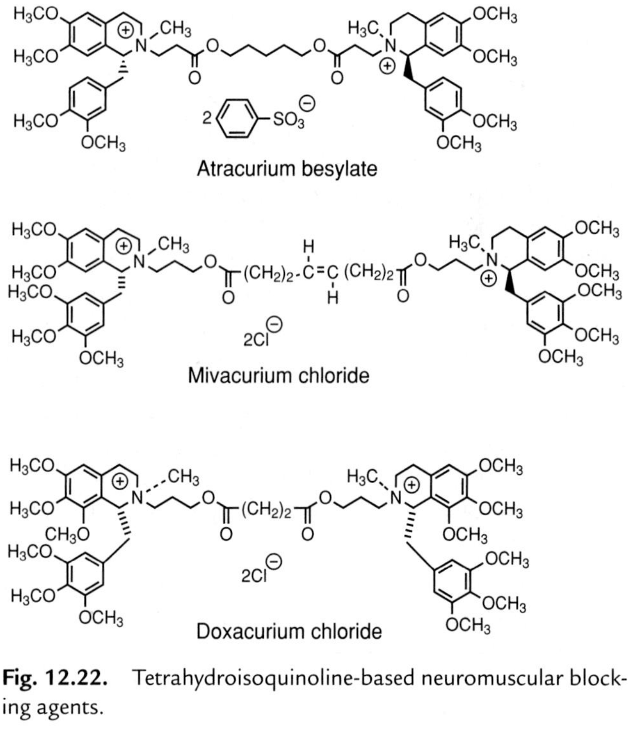

Fig. 12.22. Tetrahydroisoquinoline-based neuromuscular blocking agents.

Mivacurium chloride (Mivacron). Mivacurium chloride is a mixture of three stereoisomers, with the *trans-trans* (92–96%) and the *cis-trans* diesters being equipotent. The *cis-cis* diester produces only minimal (<5%) neuromuscular blockade. It is hydrophilic, has a small volume of distribution, and is distributed primarily to extracellular fluids. Mivacurium is short acting (Table 12.4), with mean elimination half-lives for the *trans-trans* and *cis-trans* stereoisomers of 2.0 and 1.8 minutes, respectively, in adults receiving opioid/ nitrous oxide/oxygen anesthesia. It is rapidly hydrolyzed and does not undergo Hofmann elimination like atracurium.

Doxacurium chloride (Nuromax). Doxacurium is a mixture of three *trans, trans*-stereoisomers, a *dl* pair [(1R,1′R,2S,2′S) and (1S,1′S,2R,2′R)] and a meso form (1R,1′S,2S,2′R). Doxacurium is hydrophilic, has a small volume of distribution, and is distributed primarily to extracellular fluids. It is not metabolized by plasma cholinesterase or hepatic enzymes and does not undergo Hofmann elimination.

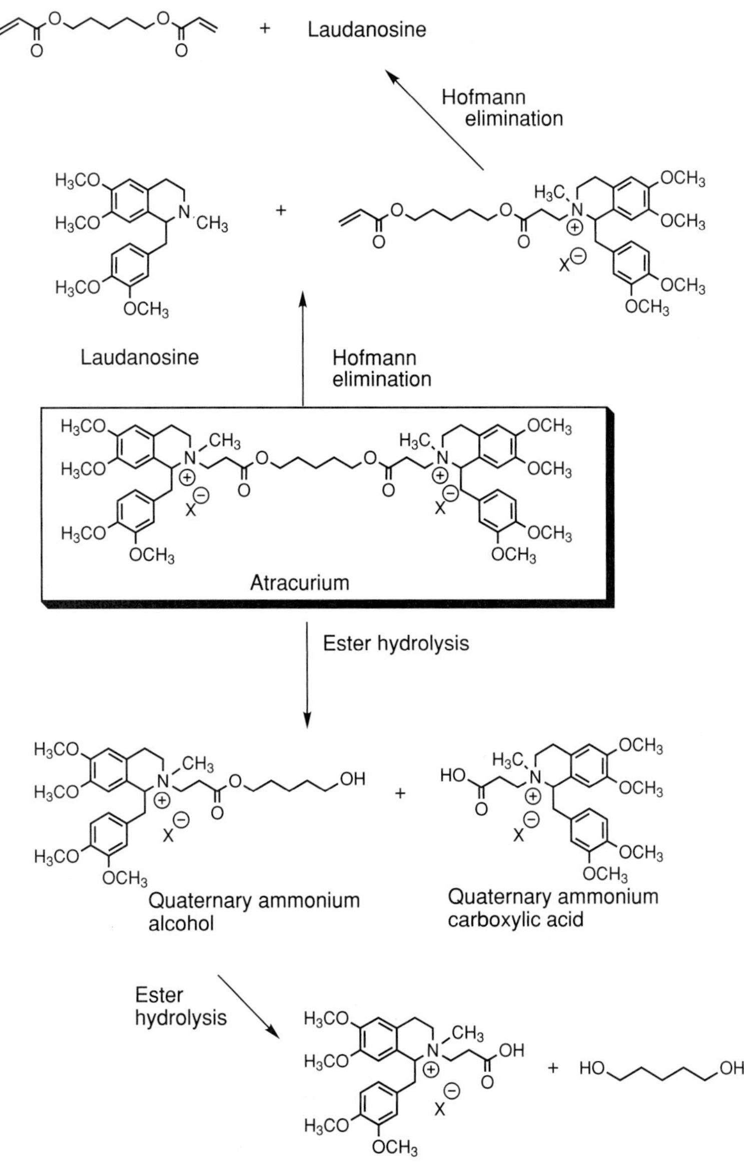

Fig. 12.23. Inactivation of atracurium by Hofmann elimination and hydrolysis.

CASE STUDY

Victoria F. Roche and S. William Zito

PJ was brought to the emergency department where you work by his fellow housemates. PJ is a 29-year-old graduate student at the local university who has been studying for his Ph.D. in anthropology for the past 7 years. His housemates say he is a devotee of "natural highs" and is known to consume 6 to 12 beers per day and for his stash of natural substances, including marijuana. In the emergency department, he is extremely agitated, confused, and combative. His friends say he became that way soon after he ingested a handful of brown, kidney-shaped seeds. On examination, PJ's vital signs showed a temperature of 102°F, with tachycardia, hypertension, and unresponsive, dilated pupils. Urine was collected for routine drug screening and serum for liver function tests. Test results determined that he had elevated aspartate aminotransferase and lactate dehydrogenase, a prolongation of his prothrombin time, and atropine and scopolamine (structures 1 and 2, respectively) in the urine. A diagnosis of anticholinergic overdose was made, and PJ was administered gastric lavage with 2.5 L of normal saline followed by activated charcoal. The physician wants to administer a cholinergic agonist to counter the effects of the anticholinergic overdose. Evaluate structures 3 to 5 for possible use in this case.

1. Identify the therapeutic problem(s) where the pharmacist's intervention may benefit the patient.
2. Identify and prioritize the patient-specific factors that must be considered to achieve the desired therapeutic outcomes.
3. Conduct a thorough and mechanistically oriented SAR analysis of all therapeutic alternatives provided in the case.
4. Evaluate the SAR findings against the patient-specific factors and desired therapeutic outcomes, and make a therapeutic decision.
5. Counsel your patient.

CH_3 N CH₂OH O O 1

H-N CH_3 O CH₂OH O O 2

CH_3HN O O CH_3 N N CH_3 CH_3 3

O $(CH_3CH_2O)_2$-P-S $N(CH_3)_3$ 4

O $N(CH_3)_2$ O $N(CH_3)_3$ 5

References

1. Katzung BG. Introduction to autonomic pharmacology. In: Katzung BG, ed. Basic and Clinical Pharmacology, 9th Ed. New York: McGraw-Hill, 2004, pp. 75–93.
2. Holmstedt G. Pages from the history of research on cholinergic mechanisms. In: Waser PG, ed. Cholinergic Mechanisms. New York: Raven Press, 1975:1–21.
3. Loewi O. Humoral transfer of heart action. Arch Ges Physiol 1921;189: 237–242.
4. Loewi O, Navratil E. Mechanism of the action of physostigmine and of ergotamine on vagus action. Arch Ges Physiol 1926;214:689–696.
5. Pert CB, Snyder SH. Opiate receptor: demonstration in nervous tissue. Science 1973;179:1011–1114.
6. Changeaux JP, Devillers-Thiery A, Chemouilli P. Acetylcholine receptor: an allosteric protein. Science 1984;225:1335–1345.
7. Mishina M, Kurodaki T, Tobimatsu T, et al. Expression of functional acetylcholine receptor from cloned cDNAs. Nature 1984;307:604–608.
8. Caulfield JP, Birdsall NJM. International Union of Pharmacology. XVII. Classification of muscarinic acetylcholine receptors. Pharmacol Rev 1998;50:279–290.
9. Lukas RJ, Bencherif M. Heterogeneity and regulation of nicotinic acetylcholine receptors. Int Rev Neurobiol 1992;34:25–131.
10. Ing HR. The structure–action relationships of the choline group. Science 1949;109:264–266.
11. Westfall TC, Westfall DP. Neurotransmission: the autonomic and somatic motor nervous systems. In: Brunton LL, Lazo JS, Parker KL, eds. Goodman and Gilman's The Pharmacological Basis of Therapeutics, 11th Ed. New York: McGraw-Hill, 2006, pp 137–181.
12. Lameh J, Cone RI, Maeda S, et al. Structure and function of G protein coupled receptors. Pharm Res 1990;7:1213–1221.
13. Drubbisch V, Drubbisch V, Lameh J, Philip M, et al., Mapping the ligand binding pocket of the human muscarinic cholinergic receptor Hm1: contribution of tyrosine-82. Pharm Res 1992;9:1644–1647.
14. Dixon RAF, Strader CD, Sigal IS. Structure and function of G protein–coupled receptors. Annu Rep Med Chem 1988;23:221–233.
15. Linder ME, Gilman AG. G Proteins. Sci. Am 1992;267:56–65.
16. Ehlert FJ, Ostrom RS, Sawyer GW. Subtypes of the muscarinic receptor in smooth muscle. Life Sci 1997;61:1729–1740.
17. Nordvall G, Hacksell U. Binding-site modeling of the muscarinic m_1 receptor: a combination of homology-based and indirect approaches. J Med Chem 1993;36:967–976.
18. Humblet C, Mirzadegan T. Three-dimensional models of G protein–coupled receptors. Annu Rep Med Chem 1992;27:291–300.
19. van Koppen CJ, Kaiser B. Regulation of muscarinic acetylcholine signaling. Pharmacol Ther 2003;98:197–220.
20. Lindstrom J, Anand R, Peng X, et al. Neuronal nicotinic receptor subtypes. Ann N Y Acad Sci 1995;757:100–116.
21. Le Novere N, Changeux JP. Molecular evolution of the nicotinic acetylcholine receptor: an example of multigene family in excitable cell. J Mol Evol 1995;40:155–172.
22. Changeux JP. The nicotinic acetylcholine receptor: an allosteric protein prototype if ligand-gated ion channels. Trends Pharmacol Sci 1990;11:485–492.
23. Luyten WHML, Heinemann SG. Molecular cloning of the nicotinic acetylcholine receptor: new opportunities in drug design. Annu Rep Med Chem 1987;22:281–291.
24. Arias HR. Localization of agonist and competitive antagonist binding sites on nicotinic acetylcholine receptors. Neurochem Int 2000;36:595–645.
25. Picciotto MR, Caldarone BJ, Brunzell DH, et al. Neuronal nicotinic acetylcholine receptor subunit knockout mice: physiological and behavioral phenotypes and possible clinical implications. Pharmacol Ther 2001;92: 89–108.
26. Taylor P. Agents acting at the neuromuscular junction and autonomic ganglia. In: Brunton LL, Lazo JS, Parker KL, eds., Goodman and Gilman's The Pharmacological Basis of Therapeutics, 11th Ed. New York: McGraw-Hill, 2006, pp. 217–236.
27. Holladay MW, Dart MJ, Lynch JK. Neuronal nicotinic receptors as targets for drug discovery. J Med Chem 1997;40:4170–4194.
28. Changeux JP. Chemical signaling in the brain. Sci Am 1993;269(5):58–62.
29. Tucek S. Choline acetyltransferase and synthesis of acetylcholine. In: Wittaker VP, ed. The Cholinergic Synapse: Handbook of Experimental Pharmacology. Berlin: Springer-Verlag, 1988, pp. 125–165.
30. Armstrong PD, Cannon JG, Long JP. Conformationally rigid analogues of acetylcholine. Nature 1968;220:65–66.
31. Ing HR, Kordik P, Williams DPHT. The structure–action relationships of the choline group. Br J Pharmacol 1952;7:103–116.
32. Welch AD, Roepke MH. A comparative study of choline and certain of its analogues. I. The pharmacological activity of acetylphosphocholine and acetylarsenocholine relative to acetylcholine. J Pharmacol Exp Ther 1935;55: 118–126.
33. Hotlon P, Ing HR. The specificity of the trimethylammonium group in acetylcholine. Br J Pharmacol 1949;4:190–196.
34. Stehle RL, Melville KI, Oldham FK. Choline as a factor in the elaboration of adrenaline. J Pharmacol Exp Ther 1936;56:473–481.
35. Bocick NC, Offen WW, Levey AI, et al. Effects of xanomeline, a selective muscarinic receptor agonist, on cognitive function and behavioral symptoms in Alzheimer's disease. Arch Neurol 1997;54:465–473.
36. John V, Lieberburg I, Thorsett ED. Alzheimer's disease: current therapeutic approaches. Annu Rep Med Chem 1993;28:197–206.
37. Karczmar AG. Anticholinesterase agents: In: Raduoco-Thomas C, ed. International Encyclopedia of Pharmacology and Therapeutics, Section 13, vol 1. New York: Pergamon Press, 1970, pp. 1–44.
38. Sussman JL, Harel M, Frolow F, et al. Atomic structure of acetylcholinesterase from *Torpedo californica*: a prototypic acetylcholine-binding protein. Science 1991;253:872–879.
39. Ordentlich A, Barak D, Kronman C, et al. Dissection of the human acetylcholinesterase active center determinants of substrate specificity. Identification of residues constituting the anionic site, the hydrophobic site, and the acyl pocket. J Biol Chem 1993;268:17083–17095.
40. Wilson IB, Harrison MA, Ginsberg S. Carbamyl derivatives of acetylcholinesterase. J Biol Chem 1961;236:1498–1500.
41. Rzeszotarski WJ. Alzheimer's disease: search for therapeutics. In: Abraham DJ, ed., Burger's Medicinal Chemistry & Drug Discovery, vol 6, 6th Ed. Hoboken, NJ: John Wiley & Sons, 2003, pp. 743–777.
42. Schroder H, Giacobini E, Strubble RG, et al. Nicotinic cholinoceptive neurons of the frontal cortex are reduced in Alzheimer's disease. Neurobiol Aging 1991; 12:259–262.
43. Nordberg A, Winblad B. Reduced number of $[H^3]$nicotine and $[H^3]$ acetylcholine binding sites in the frontal cortex of Alzheimer brains. Neurosci Lett 1986;72:115–119.
44. Sugaya K, Giacobini E, Chiappinelli VA. Nicotinic acetylcholine receptor subtypes in human frontal cortex: changes in Alzheimer's disease. J Neurosci Res 1990;27,349–359.
45. Whitehouse PJ, Martino AM, Antuono PG, et al. Nicotinic acetylcholine binding sites in Alzheimer's disease. Brain Res 1986;371:146–151.

46. Shutske GM, Pierrat FA, Kapples KJ, et al. 9-Amino-1,2,3,4-tetrahydroacridin-1-ols: synthesis and evaluation as potential Alzheimer's disease therapeutics. J Med Chem 1989;32:1805–1813.
47. Galatsis P. Market to market—1997. Annu Rep Med Chem 1998;33:327–353.
48. Wilson IB, Ginsburg S. A powerful reactivator of alkylphosphate-inhibited acetylcholinesterase. Biochim Biophys Acta 1955;18:168–170.
49. Wilson IB. Molecular complementarity and antidotes for alkyl phosphate poisoning. Fed Proc 1959;18:752–758.
50. Wilson IB. Acetylcholinesterase. XI. Reversibility of tetraethylpyrophosphate inhibition. J Biol Chem 1951;190:111–117.
51. Hestrin S. Acetylation reactions mediated by purified acetylcholine esterase. J Biol Chem 1949;180:879–881.
52. Ariens EJ. Receptor theory and structure–activity relationships. Adv Drug Res 1966;3:235–285.
53. Mihm G, Wetzel B. Peripheral actions of selective muscarinic agonists and antagonists. Annu Rep Med Chem 1988;23:81–90.
54. McIntyre AR. History of curare. In: Cheymol J, ed. International Encyclopedia of Pharmacology and Therapeutics, Section 14, vol 1. Oxford: Pergamon Press, 1972:187–203.
55. King H. Curarie alkaloids. I. Tubocurarine. J Chem Soc 1935:1381–1389.
56. Everett AJ, Lowe AJ, Wilkinson S. Revision of the structures of (+)-tubocurarine chloride and (+)-chondrocurine. J Chem Soc 1970;16:1020–1021.
57. Stenlake JB, Waigh RD, Urwin J, et al. Atracurium: conception and inception. Br J Anaesth 1983;55:3S–10S.
58. Basta SJ, Ali HH, Savarese JJ, et al. Clinical pharmacology of atracurium besylate (BW33A): a new nondepolarizing muscle relaxant. Anesth Analg 1983; 61:723–729.

Suggested Readings

Belleau B. In: Harper NJ, Simmons AR, eds. Conformational perturbation in relation to the regulation of enzyme and receptor behaviour. Advances in Drug Research, vol 2. New York: Academic Press, 1965:143, pp. 89–126.

Cannon JG. Cholinergics. In: Abraham, DJ, ed. Burger's Medicinal Chemistry & Drug Discovery, vol 6, 6th Ed. New York: John Wiley & Sons, 2003, pp. 39–108.

Rama Sastry BV. Anticholinergic drugs. In: Abraham, DJ, ed. Burger's Medicinal Chemistry & Drug Discovery, vol 6, 6th Ed. New York: John Wiley & Sons, 2003, pp. 109–165.

13. *Adrenergic Receptors and Drugs Affecting Adrenergic Neurotransmission*

ROBERT K. GRIFFITH

DRUGS COVERED IN THIS CHAPTER:

NONSELECTIVE ADRENERGIC AGONISTS
- Norepinephrine
- Epinephrine

SELECTIVE α_1-ADRENERGIC AGONISTS
- Metaraminol
- Methoxamine
- Phenylephrine
- Oxymetazoline
- Tetrahydrozoline

SELECTIVE α_2-ADRENERGIC AGONISTS
- Clonidine
- Tizanidine
- Apraclonidine
- Brimonidine
- Guanfacine
- Guanabenz
- Methyldopa

β_1-ADRENERGIC AGONISTS
- Dopamine
- Dobutamine

β_2-ADRENERGIC AGONISTS
- Isoproterenol
- Albuterol
- Pirbuterol
- Terbutaline
- Bitolterol
- Ritodrine
- Salmeterol
- Formoterol

MIXED-ACTING SYMPATHOMIMETICS
- Phenylpropanolamines
  - (−)-Ephedrine
  - (+)-Pseudoephedrine
  - (+)-Phenylpropanolamine
- Phenylisopropylamines
  - Amphetamine
  - Methamphetamine

NONSELECTIVE α-ADRENERGIC ANTAGONISTS
- Phenoxybenzamine
- Tolazoline
- Phentolamine

SELECTIVE α_1-ADRENERGIC ANTAGONISTS (SEE CHAPTER 45)
- Alfuzosin
- Prazosin
- Doxazosin
- Terazosin
- Tamsulosin

SELECTIVE α_2-ADRENERGIC ANTAGONISTS
- Yohimbine

β-ADRENERGIC ANTAGONISTS (ALSO CHAPTER 29)

MIXED α/β-ADRENERGIC ANTAGONISTS (ALSO CHAPTER 29)

ERGOT ALKALOIDS
- Ergotamine
- Dihydroergotamine
- Ergonovine
- Methylergonovine
- Methysergide

INTRODUCTION

Adrenergic drugs are a broad class of agents employed in the treatment of disorders of widely varying severity. Adrenergic drugs include popular prescription drugs, such as albuterol for asthma and atenolol for hypertension (Table 13.1), as well as many common over-the-counter cold remedies, such as the nasal decongestant pseudoephedrine.

Adrenergic drugs act on effector cells through adrenoceptors that normally are activated by the neurotransmitter norepinephrine (noradrenaline), or they may act on the neurons that release the neurotransmitter. The term "adrenergic" stems from the discovery early in the twentieth century that administration of the hormone adrenaline (epinephrine) had specific effects on selected organs and tissues similar to the effects produced by stimulation of the sympathetic (adrenergic) nervous system. For a number of years, adrenaline was thought to be the neurotransmitter in the sympathetic nervous system, but it also was recognized that the effects of administered epinephrine were not quite identical to those of sympathetic stimulation. Finally, in the 1940s, norepinephrine was identified as the true neurotransmitter at the terminus of the sympathetic nervous system (1,2). Adrenoceptors are widely located in various organs and tissues as well as on neurons of both the peripheral nervous system (PNS) and central nervous system (CNS).

Norepinephrines, R = H
Epinephrine, R = CH_3

Norepinephrine and epinephrine are members of a class of pharmacologically active substances known as catecholamines, because they contain within their structures both an amine and ortho-dihydroxybenzene, which is known by the common chemical name of catechol. Many adrenergic drugs also are catecholamines, and their structure-activity-relationships (SARs) will be discussed.

Neurons at the terminus of an adrenergic neuron fiber release norepinephrine to influence the target tissue through binding to receptors on cells of the tissue or organ. The cells bearing the receptors are called effector cells, because they produce the effect seen by adrenergic stimulation.

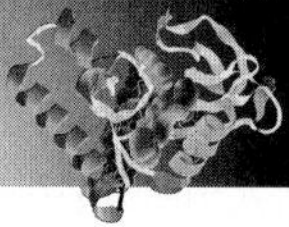

CLINICAL SIGNIFICANCE

Through the years, an increased understanding of adrenergic receptors and compounds that modulate their activity has led to decreased morbidity and mortality as well as increased quality of life for millions of patients worldwide with multiple drugs in this category on the Top 200 list of prescriptions dispensed. Agents affecting adrenergic neurotransmission are used to treat a variety of clinical conditions, including hypertension, hypotension, angina, heart failure, arrhythmias, and asthma. In fact, our understanding of structure-activity relationships led to an ability to alter the pharmacodynamic effects of various agents even before the specific receptor types were identified.

A thorough understanding of the structure-activity relationships of these compounds and application of the principles of medicinal chemistry to alter their pharmacodynamic effects has enhanced the desired properties and diminished the incidence and/or severity of associated unwanted adverse effects. Furthermore, therapeutic utility and patient compliance has been improved with the advent of orally active agents with longer elimination times and decreased frequency of dosing. For clinicians, a thorough understanding of the resultant pharmacodynamic properties of these agents is necessary to substantiate therapeutic decision making for an individual patient. For example, a patient with hypotension resulting in shock is treated with an adrenergic agonist that will increase blood pressure. If the patient's hypotension results from distributive shock, an agent with α_1-stimulant properties is necessary. If the hypotension results from cardiogenic shock, however, a β_1-agonist drug would be most effective, and in actuality, an α_1-stimulant agent may cause the patient to further decompensate by increasing cardiac workload without lending support to the failing heart. Manipulation of three sites on the basic phenylethanolamine structure alter these receptor specificities, which allows a clinician to tailor drug selection for an individual patient based on the specific desired pharmacological effects of each compound. A second example would be selection of a β_1-selective receptor blocking agent like metoprolol as opposed to a nonspecific β-antagonist like propranolol to treat a patient with asthma who has experienced a myocardial infarction. This allows the patient to benefit from the potential mortality reduction associated with the β-blocking agent while minimizing the risk of decreasing β_2-agonist utility for bronchospasm. These are only a couple of simple illustrations of altering the structure-activity relationship of adrenergic compounds to increase their utility for specific disease processes and outlining the importance of understanding the pharmacodynamic impact of these alterations.

Kathryn Neill, Pharm.D.
Assistant Professor
Critical Care Specialist
Department of Pharmacy Practice
College of Pharmacy
University of Arkansas for Medical Sciences

Table 13.1. Adrenergic Prescription Drugs in the Top 200 for 2005

Drug	Application
Albuterol (Ventolin)	Bronchodilator
Atenolol (Tenormin)	Antihypertensive
Metoprolol (Lopressor)	Antihypertensive
Clonidine (Catapress)	Antihypertensive
Doxazosin (Cardura)	Antihypertensive, benign prostatic hyperplasia
Bisoprolol (Zebeta)	Antihypertensive
Propranolol (Inderal)	Antihypertensive
Terazosin (Hytrin)	Antihypertensive, benign prostatic hyperplasia
Labetolol (Normodyne)	Antihypertensive
Nadolol (Corgard)	Antihypertensive
Timolol (Timoptic)	Glaucoma therapy
Sotalol (Betapace)	Antiarrhythmic

In general, stimulation of the sympathetic nervous system causes what is known as "fight-or-flight" responses. These effects include an increased rate and force of heart contraction, a rise in blood pressure, a shift of blood flow to skeletal muscles, dilation of bronchioles and pupils, and an increase in blood glucose levels through gluconeogenesis and glycogenolysis. These responses are what one might predict in a mammal that is enraged and preparing to fight or in one that is frightened and preparing to flee. Drugs can influence adrenergic responses through a variety of mechanisms, and an understanding of these mechanisms requires knowledge regarding the details of norepinephrine biosynthesis, storage, release, and fate following release.

BIOSYNTHESIS, STORAGE, AND RELEASE OF NOREPINEPHRINE

Biosynthesis of norepinephrine takes place within adrenergic neurons near the terminus of the axon and junction with the effector cell. The biosynthetic pathway (Fig. 13.1) begins with the active transport of the amino acid L-tyrosine into the adrenergic neuron cell (1). In the first step within the cytoplasm, the enzyme tyrosine hydroxylase (tyrosine-3-monooxygenase) oxidizes the 3′ position of tyrosine to form the catechol amino acid L-dopa. This is the rate-limiting step in norepinephrine biosynthesis, and the activity of tyrosine hydroxylase is carefully controlled (3). The enzyme is under feedback inhibition control by product catecholamines and is controlled through a complex pattern of phosphorylation/

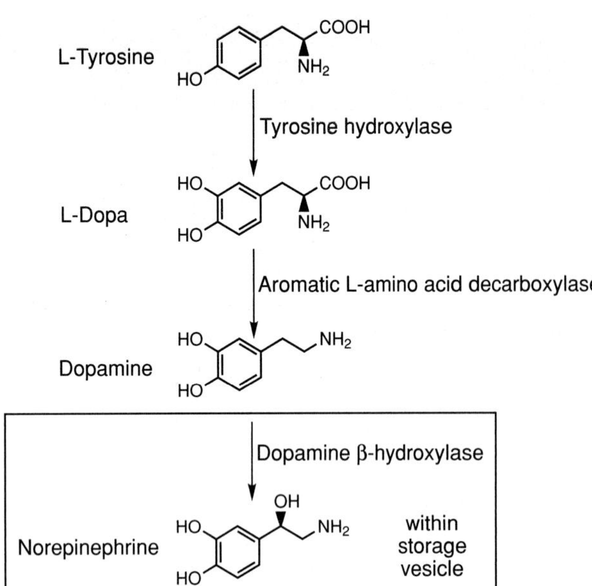

Fig. 13.1. Biosynthesis of norepinephrine.

dephosphorylation, in which phosphorylation by protein kinases activates the enzyme and dephosphorylation by phosphatases decreases activity.

In the second step, L-dopa is decarboxylated to dopamine by aromatic L-amino acid decarboxylase, another cytoplasmic enzyme. Aromatic L-amino acid decarboxylase was discovered in the 1930s and originally named dopa decarboxylase. Researchers subsequently discovered that dopa decarboxylase is not specific for dopa and decarboxylates other aromatic amino acids having the L (or S) absolute configuration, such as 5-hydroxytryptophan, tryptophan, and tyrosine. Nevertheless, the enzyme often still is referred to by the older name.

The dopamine formed in the cytoplasm by decarboxylation of L-dopa is then taken up by active transport into storage vesicles or granules located near the terminus of the adrenergic neuron. Within these vesicles, the enzyme dopamine β-hydroxylase stereospecifically introduces a hydroxyl group in the R absolute configuration on the carbon atom β to the amino group to generate the neurotransmitter norepinephrine. Norepinephrine is stored in the vesicles in a 4:1 complex with ATP in such quantities that each vesicle in a peripheral adrenergic neuron contains between 6,000 and 15,000 molecules of norepinephrine (4). The norepinephrine remains in the vesicles until released into the synapse during signal transduction. When a wave of depolarization reaches the terminus of an adrenergic neuron, it triggers the transient opening of voltage-dependent calcium channels, causing an influx of calcium ions. This influx of calcium ions triggers fusion of the storage vesicles with the neuronal cell membrane, spilling the norepinephrine and other contents of the vesicles into the synapse through exocytosis (Fig. 13.2). The pathway for epinephrine biosynthesis in the adrenal medulla is the same as for norepinephrine with the additional step of conversion of norepinephrine to epinephrine by the enzyme phenylethanolamine-N-methyltransferase.

REUPTAKE AND METABOLISM OF NOREPINEPHRINE FOLLOWING RELEASE

Following its release, norepinephrine diffuses through the intercellular space to bind reversibly to adrenoceptors (α or β) on the effector cell, inducing a conformational change in the receptor. This conformational change triggers a biochemical cascade that results in a physiologic response by the effector cell. In addition to the receptors on effector cells are adrenoreceptors that respond to norepinephrine (α_2-receptors) on the presynaptic neuron,

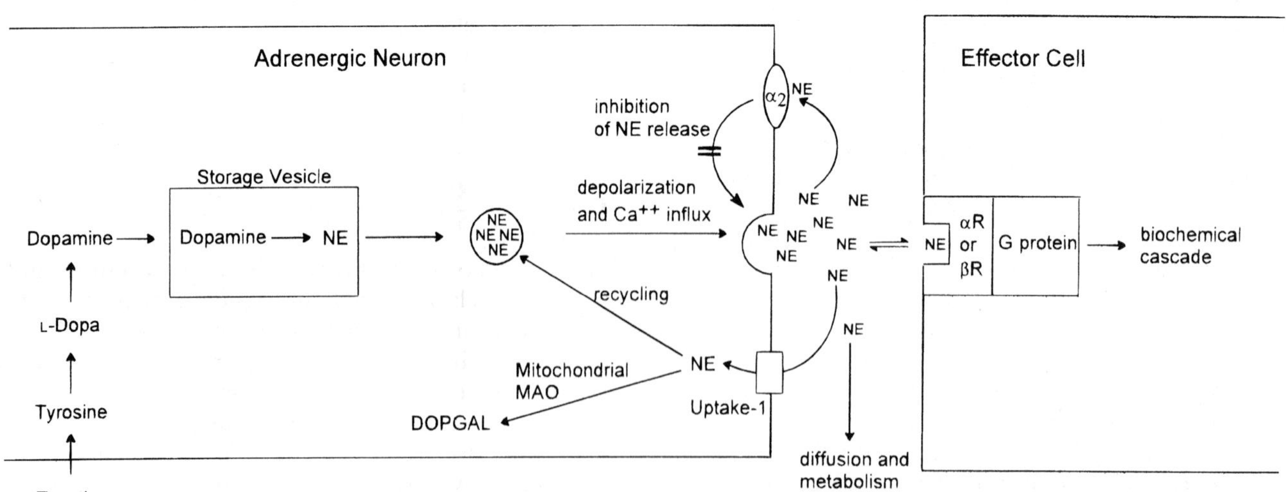

Fig. 13.2. Neurotransmission events in an adrenergic neuron and effector cell. NE, norepinephrine; αR, α adrenoceptor; βR, β adrenoceptor; MAO, monoamine oxidase; DOPGAL, 3,4-dihydroxyphenylglycolaldehyde.

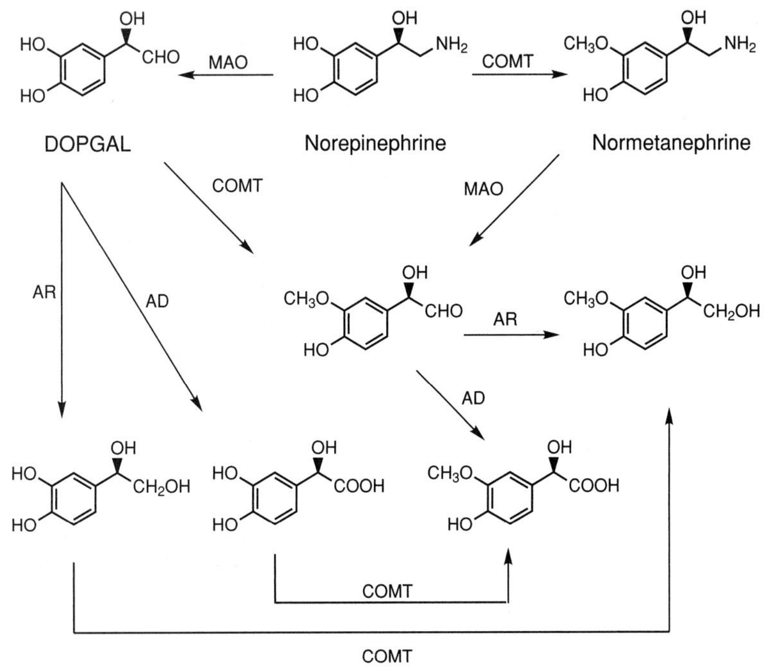

Fig. 13.3. Metabolism of norepinephrine. MAO, monoamine oxidase; COMT, catechol-O-methyltransferase; AR, aldehyde reductase; AD, aldehyde dehydrogenase.

which, when stimulated by norepinephrine, act to inhibit the release of additional norepinephrine into the synapse. Once it has been released and is stimulating its various receptors, there must be mechanisms for removing the norepinephrine from the synapse and terminating the adrenergic impulse. By far the most important of these mechanisms for removing the norepinephrine is transmitter recycling through active transport uptake into the presynaptic neuron. This process, called uptake-1, is efficient, and in some tissues, up to 95% of released norepinephrine likely is removed from the synapse by this mechanism (5). Part of the norepinephrine taken into the presynaptic neuron by uptake-1 is metabolized to 3,4-dihydroxyphenylglycolaldehyde (DOPGAL) by mitochondrial monoamine oxidase (MAO) (Fig. 13.3), and part of it is sequestered in the storage vesicles to be used again as neurotransmitter. A less efficient uptake process, called uptake-2, operates in a variety of other cell types but only in the presence of high concentrations of norepinephrine. That portion of released norepinephrine that escapes uptake-1 diffuses out of the synapse and is metabolized in extraneuronal sites by catechol-O-methyltransferase (COMT), which methylates the meta hydroxyl group. Norepinephrine also is metabolized to DOPGAL by MAO at extraneuronal sites, principally the liver and blood platelets. Both DOPGAL and normetanephrine are subject to further metabolism, as outlined in Figure 13.3 (6). These pathways also are important to drugs that are structural analogues of norepinephrine. In particular, drugs that are catechols (a 1,2-diphenolic moiety) are subject to metabolism by COMT, and drugs with unsubstituted aliphatic amino groups often are substrates for MAO.

In summary (Fig. 13.3), following biosynthesis and storage in a vesicle, norepinephrine release into the synapse is triggered by depolarization-induced calcium influx. The norepinephrine in the synapse interacts with postsynaptic G protein–linked α- or β-receptors on the effector cell, triggering effector cell response, or with presynaptic α_2-receptors on the neuron, which inhibit release of more norepinephrine. Most of the synaptic neurotransmitter is taken back into the presynaptic neuron by uptake-1 active transport. Some of the norepinephrine is metabolized by MAO, and the remainder is stored in a vesicle to be used again. That portion of norepinephrine not captured by uptake-1 diffuses out of the synapse and is metabolized by COMT and MAO.

CHARACTERIZATION OF ADRENERGIC RECEPTOR SUBTYPES

The discovery of subclasses of adrenergic receptors and the ability of relatively small molecule drugs to stimulate differentially or block these receptors represented a major advance in several areas of pharmacotherapeutics. Adrenergic receptors were subclassified by Ahlquist (7) in 1948 into α- and β-adrenoreceptor classes according to their responses to different adrenergic receptor agonists, principally norepinephrine, epinephrine, and isoproterenol. These catecholamines are able to stimulate α-adrenoceptors in the following descending order of potency: epinephrine > norepinephrine > isoproterenol.

In contrast, β-adrenoceptors are stimulated in the following descending order of potency: isoproterenol > epinephrine > norepinephrine.

Isoproterenol

In the years since Ahlquist's original classification, additional small molecule agonists and antagonists have been used to allow further subclassification of α- and β-receptors into α_1 and α_2 subtypes of α-receptors and the β_1, β_2, and β_3 subtypes of β-adrenoceptors. The powerful tools of molecular biology have been used to clone, sequence, and identify even more subtypes of alpha receptors for a total of six. Currently, three types of α_1-adrenoceptor, called α_{1A}, α_{1B}, and α_{1D}, are known. (There is no α_{1C}, because identification of a supposed α_{1C} was found to be incorrect.) Currently, three subtypes of α_2, known as α_{2A}, α_{2B}, and α_{2C}, also are known (8). The data derived from molecular biology provides a wealth of information on the structures and biochemical properties of both α- and β-receptors. Intensive research continues in this area, and the coming years may provide evidence of additional subtypes of both α- and β-receptors. At this time, however, only the α_1-, α_2-, β_1-, and β_2-receptor subtypes are sufficiently well differentiated by their small molecule binding characteristics to be clinically significant in pharmacotherapeutics, although therapeutic agents acting selectively on β_3-adrenoceptors to induce fat catabolism may become available in the near future (9).

The adrenoceptors, both α and β, are members of a receptor superfamily of membrane-spanning proteins, including muscarinic, serotonin, and dopamine receptors, which are coupled to intracellular GTP-binding proteins (G proteins), which determine the cellular response to receptor activation (10). All these receptors exhibit a common motif of a single polypeptide chain that is looped back and forth through the cell membrane seven times with an extracellular N-terminus and intracellular C-terminus. The human β_2-adrenoceptor was one of the first to be cloned and thoroughly studied (Fig. 13.4) (11). The seven transmembrane domains, TMD1 through

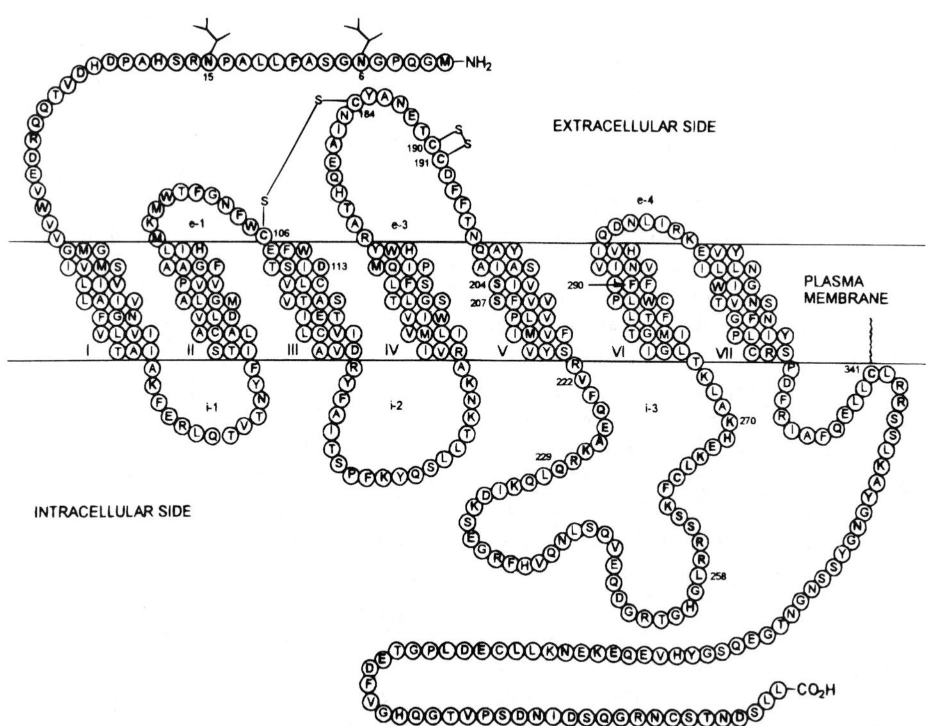

Fig. 13.4. Human β_2-adrenergic receptor: amino acid sequence of the human β_2-receptor showing the seven transmembrane domains (I–VII), the connecting intracellular and extracellular loops, extracellular glycosylation sites at asparagines 6 and 15, and intrachain disulfide bonds between cysteines 106–184 and 190–191. Also indicated are the amino acids identified as participating in neurotransmitter binding—aspartate 113 in transmembrane domain III, which binds the positively charged amine of the neurotransmitter, and serines 204 and 207 of transmembrane domain V, which form hydrogen-bonds with the catechol hydroxyls. Phenylalanine 290 may participate in agonist binding as well. Amino acids 222–229 and 258–270 of the third intracellular loop are critical for G protein-coupling, and palmitoylated cysteine 341 is critical for proper adenylyl cyclase activation. (From Ostrowski J, Kjelsberg MA, Caron MG, et al. Mutagenesis of the β_2-adrenergic receptor: how structure elucidates function. Annu Rev Pharmacol Toxicol 1992;32:167–183; with permission.)

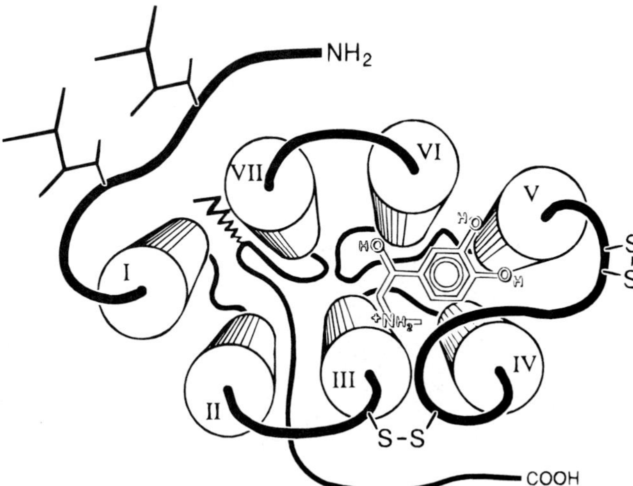

Fig. 13.5. Proposed arrangement for the transmembrane helices of the β_2-adrenergic receptor depicting the binding site for epinephrine as viewed from the extracellular side. (From Ostrowski J, Kjelsberg MA, Caron MG, et al. Mutagenesis of the β_2-adrenergic receptor: how structure elucidates function. Annu Rev Pharmacol Toxicol 1992;32:167–183; with permission.)

TMD7, are composed primarily of lipophilic amino acids arranged in α-helices connected by regions of hydrophilic amino acids. The hydrophilic regions form loops on the intracellular and extracellular faces of the membrane. In all the adrenoceptors, the agonist/antagonist recognition site is located within the membrane-bound portion of the receptor. This binding site is within a pocket formed by the membrane-spanning regions of the peptide, as illustrated in Figure 13.5 for epinephrine bound to the human β_2-receptor. All the adrenoceptors are coupled to their effector systems through a G protein, which is linked through reversible binding interactions with the third intracellular loop of the receptor protein.

Salient features of the extensively studied β_2-adrenoreceptor are indicated in Figure 13.4. Binding studies with selectively mutated β_2-receptors have provided strong evidence for binding interactions between agonist functional groups and specific residues in the transmembrane domains of adrenoceptors. Such studies indicate that Asp113 in transmembrane domain 3 (TMD3) of the β_2-receptor is the acidic residue that forms a bond, presumably ionic or a salt bridge, with the positively charged amino group of catecholamine agonists. An aspartic acid residue also is found in a comparable position in all the other adrenoceptors as well as other known G protein–coupled receptors that bind substrates having positively charged nitrogens in their structures. Elegant studies with mutated receptors and analogues of isoproterenol demonstrated that Ser204 and Ser207 of TMD5 are the residues that form hydrogen bonds with the catechol hydroxyls of β_2-agonists (12). Furthermore, the evidence indicates that Ser204 interacts with the meta hydroxyl group of the ligand, whereas Ser207 interacts specifically with the para hydroxyl group. Serine residues are found in corresponding positions in TMD5 of the other known adrenoceptors. Evidence indicates that the phenylalanine residue of TMD6 also is involved in ligand-receptor bonding with the catechol ring. Studies such as these and others that indicated the presence of specific disulfide bridges between cysteine residues of the β_2-receptor led to the binding scheme shown in Figure 13.5.

Structural differences exist among the various adrenoceptors with regard to their primary structure, including the actual peptide sequence and length. Each of the adrenoceptors is encoded on a distinct gene, and this information was crucial to the proof that each adrenoreceptor is, indeed, distinct although related. The amino acids that make up the seven transmembrane regions are highly conserved among the various adrenoreceptors, but the hydrophilic portions are quite variable. The largest differences occur in the third intracellular loop connecting TMD5 and TMD6, which is the site of linkage between the receptor and its associated G protein. Compare the diagram of the β_2-receptor in Figure 13.4 with that of the α_2-receptor in Figure 13.6 (13).

Effector Mechanisms of Adrenergic Receptors

ATP —(Adenylyl cyclase)→ cAMP —(Phosphodiesterase)→ AMP

Each adrenoceptor is coupled through a G protein to an effector mechanism. Effector mechanisms are proteins that are able to translate the conformational change caused by activation of the receptor into a biochemical event within the cell. All the β-adrenoceptors are coupled via specific G proteins (G_s) to the activation of adenylyl cyclase* (14). Thus, when the receptor is stimulated by an agonist, adenylyl cyclase is activated to catalyze the formation of cyclic AMP (cAMP) from ATP. Called a second

*This enzyme is known by two names, *adenylate cyclase (EC 4.6.1.1)*, its official name from the International Union of Biochemistry and Molecular Biology Nomenclature Committee, or its alternative name, adenylyl cyclase.

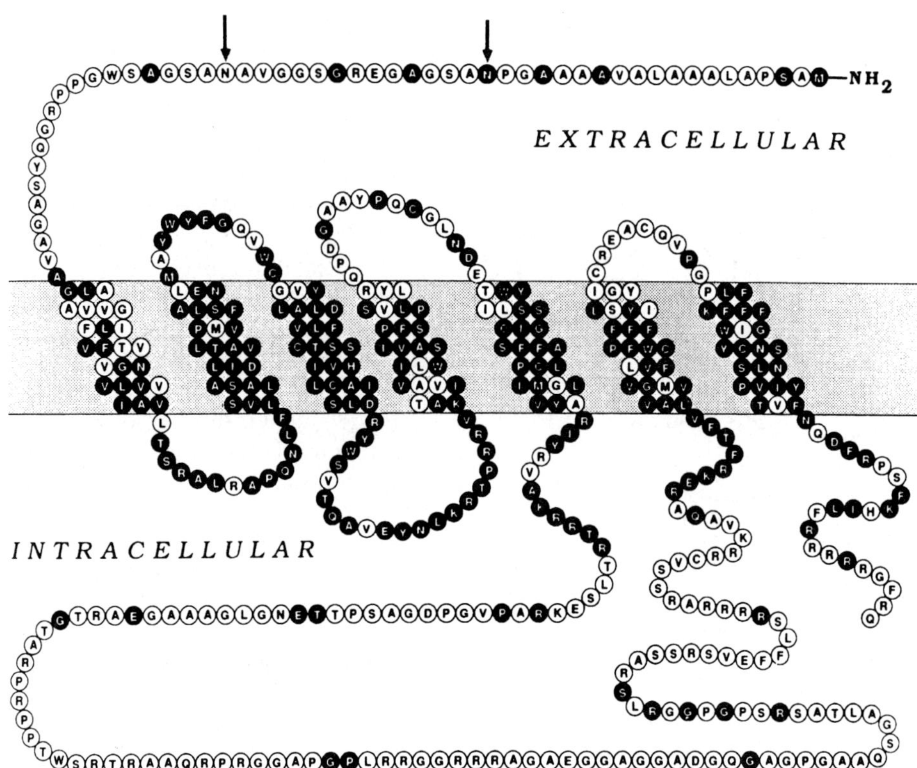

Fig. 13.6. Human kidney α_2-adrenergic receptor: amino acid sequence of the human kidney α_2-receptor showing the seven transmembrane domains and the connecting intracellular and extracellular loops. Note particularly the large third intracellular loop, which is the G protein–binding site. The arrows point to the sites of glycosylation. Amino acids in black circles are those identical to the amino acids in the human platelet α_2-receptor. (From Regan JW, Kobilka TS, Yang-Feng TL, et al. Cloning and expression of a human kidney cDNA for an α_2-adrenergic receptor subtype. Proc Natl Acad Sci U S A 1988;85:6301–6305; with permission.)

messenger for the β-adrenoceptors, cAMP is known to function as a second messenger for a number of other receptor types. cAMP is considered to be a messenger, because it can diffuse through the cell for at least short distances to modulate biochemical events remote from the synaptic cleft. Modulation of biochemical events by cAMP includes a phosphorylation cascade of other proteins. Additionally, cAMP is rapidly deactivated by hydrolysis of the phosphodiester bond by the enzyme phosphodiesterase. The α_2-receptor may use more than one effector system depending on the location of the receptor. To date, however, the best-understood effector system of the α_2-receptor appears to be similar to that of the β-receptors, except that linkage via a G protein (G_i) leads to inhibition of adenylyl cyclase instead of activation.

The α_1-adrenoreceptor is linked through yet another G protein to a complex series of events involving hydrolysis of polyphosphatidylinositol (15). The first event set in motion by activation of the α_1-receptor is activation of the enzyme phospholipase C. Phospholipase C catalyzes the hydrolysis of phosphatidylinositol-4,5-biphosphate. This hydrolysis yields two products, each of which has biological activity as second messengers of the α_1-receptor (see Chapter 4). These two products are 1,2-diacylglycerol (DAG) and inositol-1,4,5-triphosphate (IP_3). The latter, IP_3, causes the release of calcium ions from intracellular storage sites in the endoplasmic reticulum, resulting in an increase in free intracellular calcium levels. Increased free intracellular calcium is correlated with smooth muscle contraction. The other product, DAG, is thought to activate cytosolic protein kinase C, which may induce slowly developing contractions of vascular smooth muscle. The end result of a complex series of protein interactions triggered by agonist binding to the α_1-receptor includes increased intracellular free calcium, which leads to smooth muscle contraction. When the smooth muscle innervated by α_1-receptors is in vascular walls, stimulation leads to vascular constriction.

Receptor Localization

The generalization made in the past about synaptic locations of adrenoreceptor subtypes was that all α_1-, β_1-, β_2-, and β_3-receptors are postsynaptic receptors that are linked to stimulation of biochemical processes in the postsynaptic cell. Presynaptic β-receptors, however, are known to occur, although their function is unclear. Traditionally, the α_2-receptor has been viewed as a presynaptic receptor that resides on the outer membrane of the nerve terminus or presynaptic cell and reacts with released neurotransmitter. The α_2-receptor serves as a sensor and modulator of the quantity of neurotransmitter present in the synapse at any given moment. Thus, during periods of rapid nerve firing and neurotransmitter release, the α_2-receptor is stimulated and causes an inhibition of further release of neurotransmitter. This is a well-characterized mechanism for modulation of neurotransmission. Not all α_2-receptors are presynaptic, but the physiologic significance of postsynaptic α_2-receptors is less well understood (16).

Table 13.2. Selected Tissue Responses to Stimulation of Adrenoceptor Subtypes

Organ or Tissue	Major Receptor Type	Response
Arterioles,		
vascular bed	α_1, α_2	Constriction
to skeletal muscle	β_2	Dilation
Eye (radial muscle)	α_1	Contraction (papillary dilation)
Heart	β_1	Increased rate and force
Lungs	β_2	Relaxation (bronchodilation)
Liver	α_1, β_2	Increased gluconeogenesis and glycogenolysis
Fat cells	α_1, β_3	Lipolysis
Uterus (pregnant)	α_1	Contraction
	β_2	Relaxation
Intestine	α_1, β_2	Decreased motility

THERAPEUTIC RELEVANCE OF ADRENERGIC RECEPTOR SUBTYPES

The clinical utility of receptor-selective drugs becomes obvious when one considers the adrenoreceptor subtypes and effector responses of only a few organs and tissues innervated by the sympathetic nervous system. The major adrenoceptor subtypes are listed in Table 13.2. For example, the predominant response to adrenergic stimulation of smooth muscle of the peripheral vasculature is constriction causing a rise in blood pressure. Because this response is mediated through α_1-receptors, an α_1-antagonist would be expected to cause relaxation of the blood vessels and a drop in blood pressure with clear implications for treating hypertension. In addition, the presence of α_1-adrenoceptors in the prostate gland leads to the use of α_1-antagonists in treating benign prostatic hyperplasia. The principal therapeutic uses of adrenergic agonists and antagonists are shown in Table 13.3. A smaller number of β_2-receptors on vascular smooth muscle mediate arterial dilation, particularly to skeletal muscle, and a few antihypertensives act through stimulation of these β_2-receptors. (Adrenergic antihypertensives are discussed more thoroughly in Chapter 29.) Adrenergic stimulation of the lungs causes smooth muscle relaxation and bronchodilation mediated through β_2-receptors. Drugs acting as β_2-agonists are useful for alleviating respiratory distress in persons with asthma or other obstructive pulmonary diseases (see Chapter 44). Activation of β_2-receptors in the uterus also causes muscle relaxation, and so some β_2-agonists are used to inhibit uterine contractions in premature labor. Adrenergic stimulation of the heart causes an increase in rate and force of contraction, which is mediated primarily by β_1-receptors. Drugs with β_1-blocking activity slow the heart rate and decrease the force of contraction. These drugs have utility in treating hypertension, angina, and certain cardiac arrhythmias (see Chapters 26 and 29).

From the preceding discussions of the biosynthesis, storage, release, and fate of norepinephrine, one can readily conceive of a number of possible sites of drug action for adrenergic drugs. As mentioned, there are drugs that act

Table 13.3. Principal Therapeutic Uses of Adrenergic Agonists and Antagonists

Adrenoceptor	Drug Action	Therapeutic Uses
α_1	Agonists	Shock, hypotension (to raise blood pressure)
		Nasal decongestants
	Antagonists	Antihypertensives
		Benign prostatic hyperplasia (BPH)
α_2	Agonists	Antihypertensives
		Glaucoma
		Analgesia
		Sedatives
β_1	Antagonists	Antihypertensives
		Antiarrythmics
β_2	Agonists	Bronchodilators (asthma and COPD)
		Glaucoma
β_3	Agonists	Weight loss (investigational drugs)

directly on the receptors as agonists and antagonists, drugs that affect storage and release from vesicles, drugs that affect neurotransmitter biosynthesis, and drugs that affect uptake and catabolism of norepinephrine and epinephrine. These categories are discussed in turn. Most adrenergic drugs fit into well-defined classes with readily defined SARs, but a few adrenergic drugs do not permit such straightforward structural definition of their activity. We begin with a discussion of phenylethanolamine (or phenethanolamine) agonists, which do have reasonably clear SARs. Although many of these drugs directly stimulate adrenoceptors, others exhibit what is termed "indirect activity." Indirect agonists do not directly bind to and activate adrenergic receptors; rather, they are taken up into the presynaptic neuron, where they cause the release of norepinephrine, which can diffuse into the receptor causing the observed response. Mixed-acting drugs have both a direct and an indirect component to their action, and the relative amount of direct versus indirect activity for a given drug varies considerably with its chemical structure, the tissue preparation examined, and the experimental animal species.

STRUCTURE-ACTIVITY RELATIONSHIPS OF ADRENERGIC AGONISTS

Phenylethanolamine Agonists

The structures of many clinically useful phenylethanolamine-type adrenergic agonists are summarized in Table 13.4. Agents of this type have been extensively studied over the years since discovery of the naturally occurring prototypes, epinephrine and norepinephrine, and the structural requirements and tolerances for substitutions at each of the indicated positions have been established (2). In general, a primary or secondary aliphatic amine separated by two carbons from a substituted benzene ring is minimally required for high agonist activity in this class. Because of the basic amino groups (pK_a range, ~8.5–10), all these agents are highly positively charged at physiologic pH. By definition, agents in this class have a hydroxyl group on C1 of the side chain, β to the amine, as in epinephrine and norepinephrine. This hydroxyl-substituted carbon must be in the R absolute configuration for maximal direct activity as in the natural neurotransmitter, although most drugs currently are sold as mixtures of both (R) and (S) stereoisomers at this position (racemates). Given these features in common, the nature of the other substituents determines receptor selectivity and duration of action. In the following discussions, keep in mind that saying a drug is selective for a given receptor does not mean it has no activity at other receptors and that the clinically observed degree of selectivity is frequently dose-dependent.

R^1, Substitution on the Amino Nitrogen

We have already seen that as R^1 is increased in size from hydrogen in norepinephrine to methyl in epinephrine to isopropyl in isoproterenol, that activity at α-receptors decreases, and that activity at β-receptors increases. These

Table 13.4. Phenylethanolamine Adrenergic Agonists

Drug	R_1	R_2	R_3	Receptor Activity
Norepinephrine	H	H	3′,4′-diOH	α + β
Epinephrine	CH_3	H	3′,4′-diOH	β ≥ α
α-Methylnorepinephrine	H	CH_3	3′,4′-diOH	α + β
Ethylnorepinephrine	H	CH_2CH_3	3′,4′-diOH	β > α
Isoproterenol	$CH(CH_3)_2$	H	3′,4′-diOH	General β
Isoetharine	$CH(CH_3)_2$	CH_2CH_3	3′,4′-diOH	Selective β_2
Colterol	$C(CH_3)_3$	H	3′,4′-diOH	Selective β_2
Metaproterenol	$CH(CH_3)_2$	H	3′,5′-diOH	Selective β_2
Terbutaline	$C(CH_3)_3$	H	3′,5′-diOH	Selective β_2
Albuterol	$C(CH_3)_3$	H	3′-CH_2OH, 4′-OH	Selective β_2
Phenylephrine	CH_3	H	3′-OH	α
Metaraminol	H	CH_3	3′-OH	α
Methoxamine	H	CH_3	2′,5′-diOCH_3	α
Ephedrine, pseudoephedrine	CH_3	CH_3	H	α + β
Phenylpropanolamine	H	CH_3	H	α + β
Salmeterol	-$(CH_2)_6$-O-$(CH_2)_4$-C_6H_5	H	3′-CH_2OH, 4′-OH	$\beta_2 > \beta_1$
Formoterol	-$CH(CH_3)CH_2$-C_6H_4-4-OCH_3	H	3′-NH-COH, 4′-OH	$\beta_2 > \beta_1$

compounds were used to define α- and β-activity long before receptor proteins could be isolated and characterized. The activity at both α- and β-receptors is maximal when R^1 is methyl as in epinephrine, but α-agonist activity is dramatically decreased when R^1 is larger than methyl and is negligible when R^1 is isopropyl, as in isoproterenol, leaving only β-activity. In fact, the β-activity of isoproterenol actually is enhanced over norepinephrine and epinephrine. Presumably, the β-receptor has a large lipophilic binding pocket adjacent to the amine-binding aspartic acid residue, which is absent in the α-receptor. As R^1 becomes larger than *t*-butyl into aryl-α-methylalkyl groups, affinity for α_1-receptors, but not intrinsic activity, returns, which means large lipophilic groups can afford compounds with α_1-blocking activity (e.g., labetalol, a mixed α/β-antagonist). In addition, the N-substituent also can provide selectivity for different β-receptors, with a *t*-butyl group affording selectivity for β_2-receptors. For example, with all other features of the molecules being constant, colterol is a selective β_2-agonist, whereas isoproterenol is a nonselective β-agonist. When considering use as a bronchodilator, a nonselective β-agonist, such as isoproterenol, has undesirable cardiac stimulatory properties because of its β_1-activity, which is greatly diminished in a selective β_2-agonist, such as albuterol. Also, an arylalkyl group (where the alkyl chain ranges from 2–11 carbon/oxygen atoms) can provide β-selectivity with increased lipophilicity and cell penetration for longer duration of action.

R^2, Substitution α to the Basic Nitrogen, Carbon-2

Small alkyl groups, methyl or ethyl, may be present on the carbon adjacent to the amino nitrogen, carbon-2 in Table 13.4. Such substitution slows metabolism by MAO but has little overall effect on duration of action in catecholamines, because they remain substrates for COMT. Resistance to MAO activity is more important in noncatechol, indirect-acting phenylethylamines. An ethyl group in this position diminishes α-activity far more than β-activity, affording compounds with β-selectivity, such as ethylnorepinephrine. Substitution on this carbon also introduces another asymmetric center into these molecules producing pairs of diastereomers, which can have significantly different biological and chemical properties. For example, maximal direct activity in the stereoisomers of α-methylnorepinephrine resides with the erythro stereoisomer with the 1R,2S absolute configuration (17). The configuration of C2 has a great influence on receptor binding, because the 1R,2R diastereomer of α-methylnorepinephrine has primarily indirect activity, even though the absolute configuration of the hydroxyl-bearing C1 is the same as in norepinephrine. In addition, with respect to α-activity, this additional methyl group makes the direct-acting 1R,2S stereoisomer of α-methylnorepinephrine more selective for α_2-adrenoceptors than for α_1-adrenoceptors. This has important consequences in the antihypertensive activity of α-methyldopa, which is discussed later and in Chapter 29. The same stereochemical relationships hold for metaraminol and other phenylethanolamines, in which stereochemical properties have been investigated.

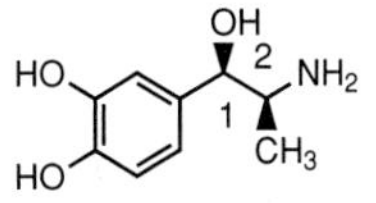

HO, HO, OH, 2, NH2, 1, CH3

α–Methylnorepinephrine
direct acting stereoisomer

R^3, Substitution on the Aromatic Ring

The natural 3′,4′-dihydroxy–substituted benzene ring in norepinephrine provides excellent receptor activity for both α- and β-sites. Such catechol-containing compounds have poor oral activity, however, because they are rapidly metabolized by COMT. Alternative substitutions have been found that retain good activity but are more resistant to COMT metabolism. In particular, 3′,5′-dihydroxy compounds are not good substrates for COMT and, in addition, provide selectivity for β_2-receptors. Thus, because of its ring substitution pattern, metaproterenol is an orally active bronchodilator with little of the β_1 cardiac stimulatory properties possessed by isoproterenol.

Other substitutions are possible that enhance oral activity and provide selective β_2-activity, such as the 3′-hydroxymethyl and 4′-hydroxy substitution pattern of albuterol, the 3′-amino or 3′-formylamino, which also are resistant to COMT. At least one of the groups must be capable of forming hydrogen bonds, and if there is only one, it should be at the 4′ position to retain β-activity. For example, ritodrine has only a 4′-OH for R3 yet retains good β-activity, with the large substituent on the nitrogen making it β_2 selective. Ritodrine has been administered to pregnant women to prevent premature labor, consistent with β_2-adrenoceptor stimulation relaxing the uterus.

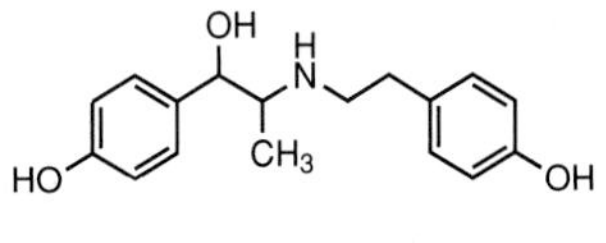

OH, H, N, CH3, HO, OH

Ritodrine

If R3 is only a 3′-OH or 3′-sulfonamide, however, activity is reduced at α sites but almost eliminated at β sites, thus affording selective α-agonists, such as phenylephrine and metaraminol. Further indication that α sites have a wider range of substituent tolerance for agonist activity is shown by the 2′,5′-dimethoxy substitution of methoxamine, which is a selective α-agonist that also has β-blocking activity at high concentrations. In keeping with the presence of α-adrenoceptors in the peripheral vasculature, all three of these agents cause vasoconstriction.

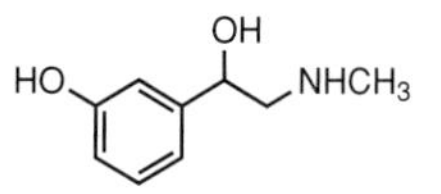

Phenylephrine 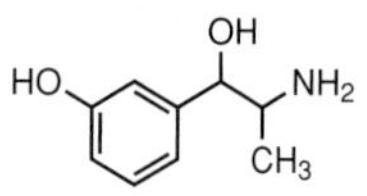 Metaraminol 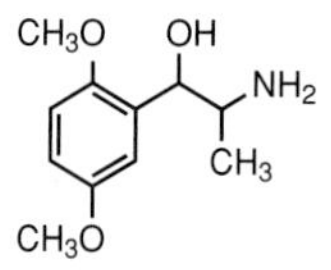 Methoxamine

When the phenyl ring has no phenolic substituents (i.e., R3 = H), these phenylethanolamines may have both direct and indirect activity. Direct activity (i.e., agonist) is the stimulation of an adrenoceptor by the drug itself; indirect activity is the result of displacement of norepinephrine from its storage granules or reuptake inhibition, resulting in nonselective stimulation of the adrenoceptors by the displaced norepinephrine. Because norepinephrine stimulates both α- and β-adrenoceptors, indirect activity cannot be selective. Stereochemistry of the various substituents also may play a role in determining the extent of direct/indirect activity.

For example, ephedrine and pseudoephedrine have the same substitution pattern, but substitution of both carbons 1 and 2 means four stereoisomers are possible. Racemic (±)-ephedrine is a mixture of the erythro enantiomers 1R,2S and 1S,2R, whereas the threo pair of enantiomers, 1R,2R and 1S,2S, are known as racemic pseudoephedrine (ψ-ephedrine). As discussed for α-methylnorepinephrine, (−)-ephedrine is the naturally occurring stereoisomer and has the 1R,2S absolute configuration with a mixed direct activity on both α- and β-receptors and some indirect activity. Its 1S,2R-(+)-enantiomer exhibits primarily indirect activity. 1S,2S-(+)-Pseudoephedrine has virtually no direct receptor activity and is mostly indirect acting.

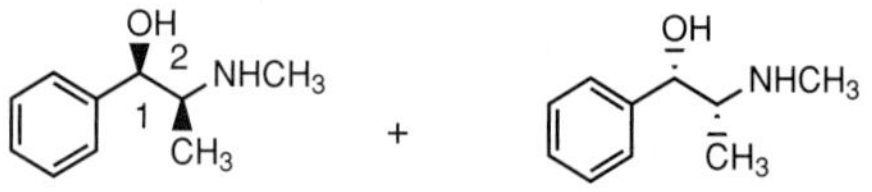

(1R:2S) Ephedrine (1S:2R)

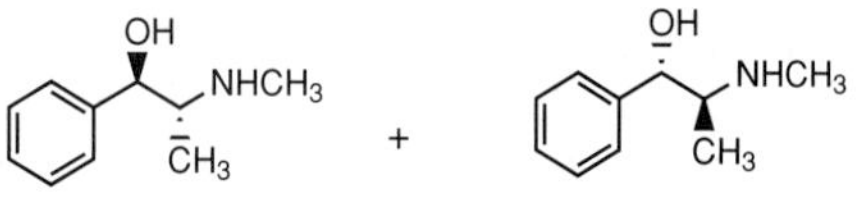

(1R:2R) (1S:2S)
Pseudoephedrine

Norepinephrine and Epinephrine

Norepinephrine has limited clinical application because of the nonselective nature of its action, which causes both vasoconstriction and cardiac stimulation. In addition, it must be given intravenously, because it has no oral activity (poor oral bioavailability) as a result of its rapid metabolism by intestinal and liver COMT and MAO, 3′-O-glucuronidation/sulfation in the intestine, and low lipophilicity. Rapid metabolism by MAO and COMT limits its duration of action to only 1 or 2 minutes, even when given by infusion. The drug is used to counteract various hypotensive crises, because its α-activity raises blood pressure and as an adjunct treatment in cardiac arrest, where its β-activity stimulates the heart.

Epinephrine is far more widely used clinically than norepinephrine, although it also lacks oral activity for the same reasons as norepinephrine. Epinephrine, similar to norepinephrine, is used to treat hypotensive crises and, because of its greater β-activity, to stimulate the heart in cardiac arrest. The β_2-activity of epinephrine leads to its administration intravenously and in inhalers to relieve bronchoconstriction in asthma and to application in inhibiting uterine contractions. Because it has significant α-activity, epinephrine has been used in nasal decongestants. Constriction of dilated blood vessels in mucous membranes shrinks the membranes and reduces nasal congestion, although significant aftercongestion may limit its utility.

Selective α-Adrenergic Agonists

α_1-Agonist Phenylethanolamines: Metaraminol, Methoxamine, and Phenylephrine

Metaraminol, methoxamine, and phenylephrine are selective for α_1-receptors and have minimal cardiac stimulatory properties. Because they are not substrates for COMT, their duration of action is significantly longer than that of norepinephrine. Their α_1-agonist activity makes them strong vasoconstrictors, however, and their primary systemic use is limited to treating hypotension during surgery or severe hypotension accompanying shock. Methoxamine is bioactivated by O-demethylation to an active m-phenolic metabolite. The β-blocking activity of methoxamine, which is seen at high concentrations, affords some use in treating tachycardia. Phenylephrine, which also is a selective α_1-agonist, is used similarly to metaraminol and methoxamine for hypotension. It also has widespread use as a nonprescription nasal decongestant in both oral and topical preparations. Its oral bioavailability is less than 10% because of its hydrophilic properties and intestinal 3′-O-glucuronidation/sulfation. Phenylephrine preparations applied topically to the eye constrict the dilated blood vessels of bloodshot eyes and, in higher concentrations, are used to dilate the pupil during eye surgery.

2-Arylimidazoline α_1-Agonists

In addition to phenylethanolamine derivatives, α-adrenoceptors accommodate a diverse assortment of structures. The imidazoline derivatives in Figure 13.7 also are selective α_1-agonists and, therefore, are called vasoconstrictors/vasopressors. They all contain a one-carbon bridge between C2 of the imidazoline ring (pK_a range, 10–11) and a phenyl substituent; therefore, the general skeleton of a phenylethylamine is contained within the structures. Lipophilic substitution on the phenyl ring *ortho* to the methylene bridge appears to be required for agonist activity at α_1- and α_2-receptors (15). Presumably, the bulky lipophilic groups attached to the phenyl ring at the meta or para positions provide selectivity for the α_1-receptor by

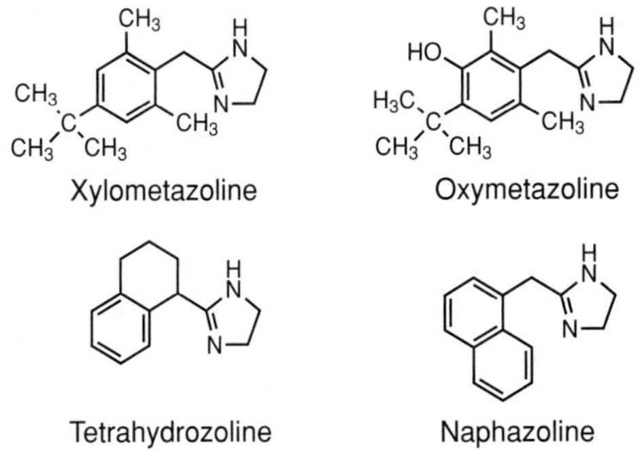

Fig. 13.7. Imidazoline α_1-adrenergic agonists.

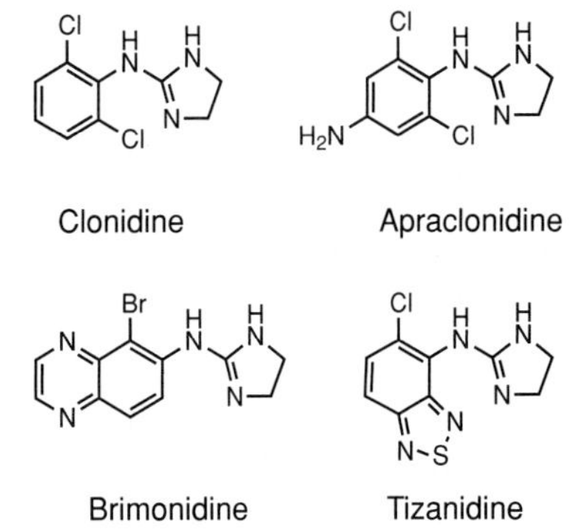

Fig. 13.8. Imidazoline α_2-adrenergic agonists.

diminishing affinity for α_2-receptors. These highly ionic compounds are widely used only in topical preparations as nasal decongestants and eye drops (Table 13.5). Systemically, they are potent vasoconstrictors.

α_2-Adrenergic Agonists: 2-Aminoimidazolines and Other α_2-Agonists

Three subtypes of α_2-adrenoceptors, α_{2A}, α_{2B}, and α_{2C}, are recognized. Each plays a role in the different clinical applications of α_2-agonists, which include use as antihypertensives (see Chapter 29), antiglaucoma drugs, and analgesics. The first of these drugs, clonidine, was introduced as an antihypertensive, an effect attributed to central α_{2A}-adrenoceptors in cardiovascular control areas of the brain (18).

CLONIDINE (CATAPRES). Closely related structurally to the imidazoline nasal decongestants is clonidine and other developed analogues (Fig. 13.8). Clonidine was originally synthesized as a vasoconstricting nasal decongestant but, in early clinical trials, was found to have dramatic hypotensive effects—in contrast to all expectations for a vasoconstrictor (19). Subsequent pharmacological investigations showed that clonidine not only has some α_1-agonist (vasoconstrictive) properties in the periphery but also that it is a powerful α_2-adrenergic agonist and exhibits specific binding to nonadrenergic imidazoline binding sites in the CNS (mainly in the medulla oblongata) causing inhibition of sympathetic output (sympathoinhibition) (see Chapter 29). Because of its peripheral activity on extraneuronal vascular postsynaptic α_{2B}-receptors (18), initial doses of clonidine may produce a transient vasoconstriction and an increase in blood pressure that is soon overcome by vasodilation as clonidine penetrates the blood-brain barrier and interacts with CNS α_{2A}-receptors.

Similar to the imidazoline α_1-agonists, clonidine has lipophilic *ortho*-dichloro substituents on the phenyl ring, but the most readily apparent difference between clonidine and the α_1-agonists in Figure 13.7 is the replacement of the CH_2 bridge on C1 of the imidazoline by an amine NH. This makes the imidazoline ring part of a guanidino group, and the uncharged form of clonidine exists as a pair of tautomers as shown.

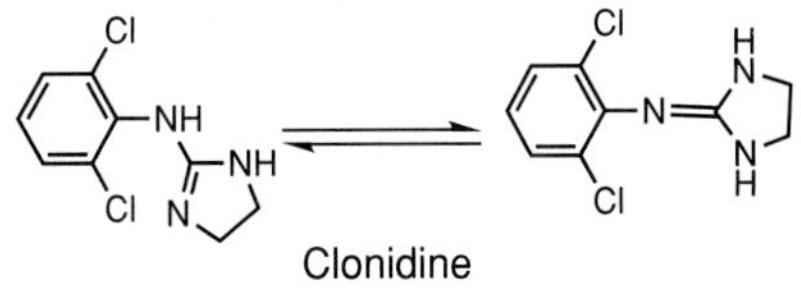

Clonidine has a pK_a of 8.3 and is approximately 80% ionized at physiologic pH. Its experimental log P is 1.6 (log D at pH 7.4 is 0.8). The positive charge is shared through resonance by all three nitrogens of the guanidino group. Steric crowding by the bulky *ortho*-chlorine groups does not permit a coplanar conformation of the two rings, as illustrated in Figure 13.9.

The o,o′-dichloro-substituents in clonidine can be replaced by a methyl group without losing any potency or selectivity. A methyl group is approximately similar in size (volume) as a chlorine atom; thus, it will exhibit similar steric interactions to force the phenyl ring to assume proper conformation for binding to the α_2-receptors similar to Figure 13.9. Thus, replacement of the o-dichlorines by bulky groups in clonidine will retain its agonist potency. The aromatic methyl group, however, will be readily

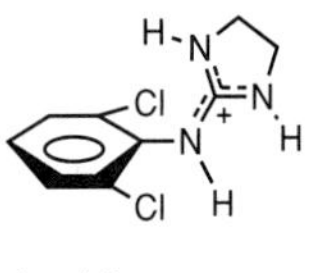

Fig. 13.9. Protonated clonidine.

Table 13.5 Imidazoline α_1-Agonists in Over-the-Counter Vasoconstrictors

Drug	Nasal Decongestant	Eye drops
Xylometazoline	Otrivin, Inspire	—
Oxymetazoline	Afrin, Duration, Neo-Synephrine, Vicks Sinex	Visine L.R. Ocu Clear
Tetrahydrozoline	—	Murine, Visine, Soothe
Naphazoline	4-Way Fast Acting, Privine	Naphcon, Clear Eyes

metabolized by the cytochrome P450 enzyme to the corresponding hydroxymethyl and then to the carboxylic acid group, both of which are inactive at the α_2-receptors. Thus, the methyl analogue will have a shorter duration of action.

In addition to its use as an antihypertensive, clonidine has been proven useful in a wide variety of conditions. Clonidine has sedative properties and has been used to treat attention-deficit hyperactivity disorder, nicotine and opiate withdrawal, and glaucoma among other uses. Epidural anesthesia has been found to be enhanced by α_2-agonists (20), and clonidine is available in an injectable form for epidural administration.

TIZANIDINE Tizanidine (Fig. 13.8) is a centrally active muscle relaxant analogue of clonidine that is approved for use in reducing spasticity associated with cerebral or spinal cord injury. Its mechanism of action for reducing spasticity suggests presynaptic inhibition of motor neurons at the α_2-adrenergic receptor sites, reducing the release of excitatory amino acids and inhibiting facilitatory ceruleospinal pathways, thus resulting in a reduction in spasticity. Tizanidine only has a small fraction of the antihypertensive action of clonidine, presumably because of action at a selective subgroup of α_{2C}-adrenoceptors, which appear to be responsible for the analgesic and antispasmodic activity of imidazoline α_2-agonists(20).

APRACLONIDINE (IOPIDINE) AND BRIMONIDINE (ALPHAGAN). The other imidazoline α_2-agonists in Figure 13.8 that are clinically used for treatment of glaucoma are apraclonidine ($pK_a = 9.22$, $\log P = 1.53$) and brimonidine ($pK_a = 7.4$, $\log P = 0.78$). Stimulation of α_2-receptors in the eye reduces production of aqueous humor and enhances outflow of aqueous humor, thus reducing intraocular pressure, and also has a neuroprotective effect apparently through α_{2A}-receptors located in the retina (21,22). Animal and human studies suggest that apraclonidine's primary mechanism of action may be related to a reduction of aqueous formation, whereas brimonidine lowers intraocular pressure by reducing aqueous humor production and increasing uveoscleral outflow. Brimonidine is approximately 1,000-fold more selective for α_2-receptors than are clonidine or apraclonidine and is a first-line agent for treating glaucoma. It exhibited minimal effect on blood pressure and heart rate. Although both are applied topically to the eye, measurable quantities of these drugs are detectable in plasma, so caution must be employed when cardiovascular agents also are being coadministered to the patient. Plasma brimonidine levels peaked within 1 to 4 hours and declined with a systemic half-life of approximately 3 hours. Brimonidine has been reported to enter the brain and can potentially cause fatigue and/or drowsiness in some patients. Brimonidine is primarily metabolized by aldehyde oxidase.

GUANFACINE (TENEX) AND GUANABENZ (WYTENSIN). Following the discovery of clonidine, extensive research into the SAR of central α_2-agonists showed that the imidazoline ring was not necessary for activity in this class but that the phenyl ring required at least one ortho chlorine or methyl group. Two clinically useful antihypertensive agents resulting from this effort are guanfacine and guanabenz (see Chapter 29). These are ring-opened analogues of clonidine, and their mechanism of action is the same as that of clonidine.

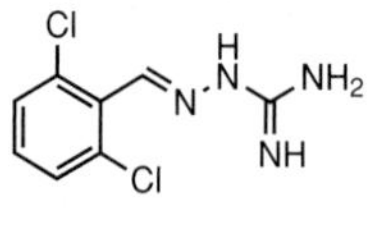

Guanabenz

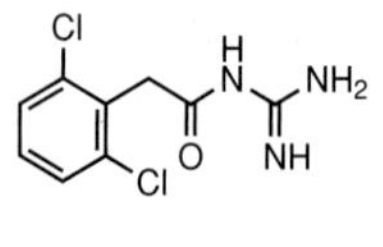

Guanfacine

METHYLDOPA (ALDOMET). Although structurally unrelated to the aminoimidazolines or the guanidines, the pro-drug L-α-methyldopa (methyldopa) is an α_2-agonist acting in the CNS via its active metabolite, α-methylnorepinephrine (Fig. 13.10). Methyldopa is transported across the blood-brain barrier, where it is decarboxylated by aromatic L-amino acid decarboxylase in the brain to α-methyldopamine, which is then stereospecifically hydroxylated to 1R,2S-α-methylnorepinephrine. This stereoisomer is a selective α_2-agonist and acts as an antihypertensive agent much like clonidine to inhibit sympathetic neural output from the CNS, thus lowering blood pressure. α-Methylnorepinephrine and α-methyldopamine do not cross the blood-brain barrier because of their hydrophilicity. Originally synthesized as a norepinephrine biosynthesis inhibitor, methyldopa was thought to act through a combination of inhibition of norepinephrine biosynthesis through dopa decarboxylase inhibition and metabolic decarboxylation to generate α-methylnorepinephrine. The latter was thought to replace norepinephrine in the nerve terminal and, when released, to have less intrinsic activity than the natural neurotransmitter. This latter mechanism is an example of the concept of a false neurotransmitter. (The antihypertensive properties for methyldopa are further described in Chapter 29.)

β-Adrenergic Agonists

β_2-Agonist Phenylethanolamines

Most of the β_2-selective adrenergic agonists listed in Table 13.4 are used primarily as bronchodilators in

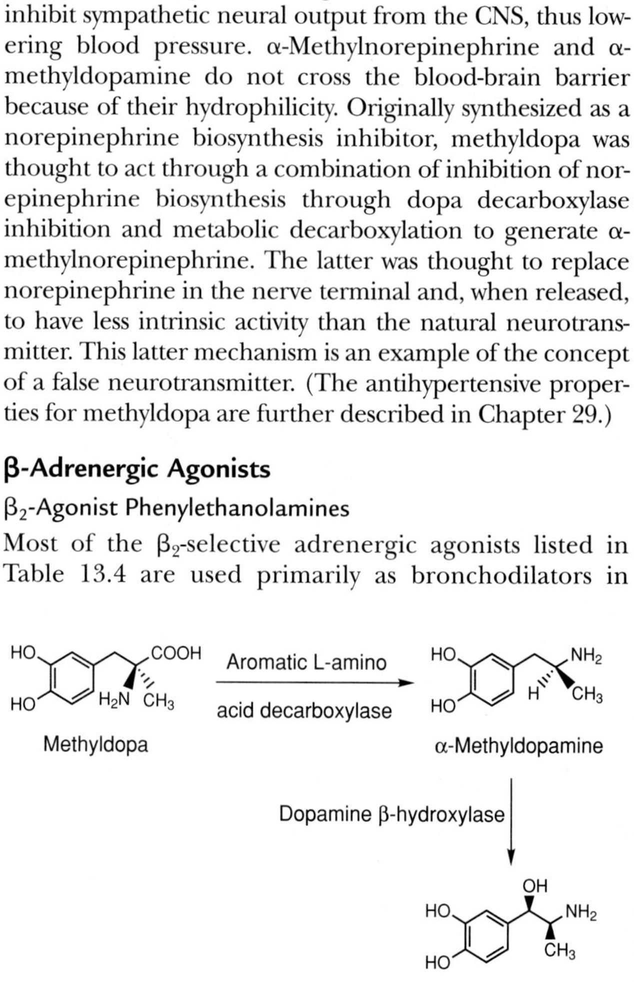

Methyldopa → (Aromatic L-amino acid decarboxylase) → α-Methyldopamine → (Dopamine β-hydroxylase) → α-Methylnorepinephrine

Fig. 13.10. Methyldopa bioactivation.

Table 13.6. Pharmacologic Effects and Pharmacokinetic Properties of Sympathomimetic Bronchodilators

Sympathomimetic	Adrenergic Receptor Activity	β_2-potency	Route of Administratio Onset (min)	Duration (hr)
Salmetero[2]	β1<<β2	0.5 Inh	within 20	12
(Serevent)				
Albuterol[2]	β1<<β2	2 PO Inh[3]	within 30	4–8
(Ventolid, Airet, Proventil)			within 5	3–6
Levalbuterol	β1<<<β2	3–4 Inh[3]	within 5	3–6
R-albuterol (Xopenex)				
Bitolterol[2]	β1<β2	5 Inh	2–4	5–8
(Tomalate)				
Isoetharine[2]	β1<β2	6 Inh[3]	within 5	2–3
Metaproterenol[2]	β1<β2	15 PO	≈30	4
(Alupent)		Inh[3]	5–30	1–6
Pirbuterol[2]	β1<β2	5 Inh	within 5	5
(Maxair)				
Terbutaline[2]	β1<β2	4 PO	30	4–8
(Bricanyl, Brethine, Brethaire)		SC	5–15	1.5–4
Isoproterenol	β1= β2	1 Inh	5–30	3–6
(Isuprel, Medihaler-Iso)		IV	immediate	<1
		Inh[3]	2–5	1–3
Ephedrine	α β1 β2	PO	15–60	3–5
		SC	>20	≤1
		IM	10–20	≤1
		IV	immediate	—
Epinephrine	α β1 β2	SC	5–10	4–6

[1]Relative molar potency: 1= potent.
[2]These agents all have minor β activity.
[3]May be administered via aerosol or bulb nebulizer or IPPB administration. Table modified from Drug Facts and Comparisons 2000.

asthma and other constrictive pulmonary conditions. Their pharmacological and pharmacokinetic properties are described in Table 13.6. Isoproterenol is a nonselective β-agonist ($\beta_2/\beta_1 = 1$), and the cardiac stimulation caused by its β_1-activity and its lack of oral activity have led to its diminished use in favor of more selective β_2-agonists.

SHORT-ACTING β_2-ADRENERGIC AGONISTS

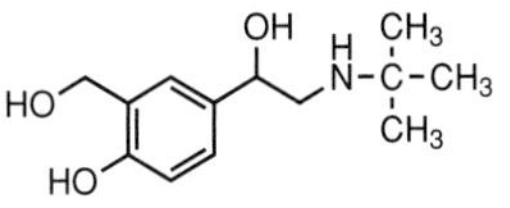

Albuterol 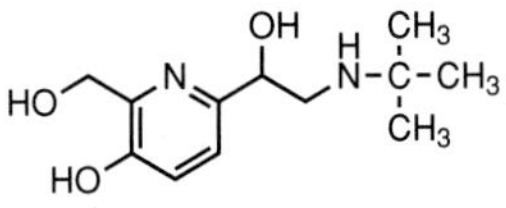   Pirbuterol

Albuterol, pirbuterol, terbutaline. The noncatechol selective β_2-agonists, such as racemic albuterol ($\beta_2/\beta_1 = 60$), metaproterenol, and terbutaline, are available in oral dosage forms as well as in inhalers. All have similar activities and durations of action. Pirbuterol is an interesting analogue of albuterol in which the benzene ring has been replaced by a pyridine ring, altering its pharmacokinetic properties. Similar to albuterol, pirbuterol is a selective β_2-agonist currently available only for administration by inhalation.

Studies with the R/S enantiomers of albuterol have shown that the (S)-enantiomer may be proinflammatory, exacerbating airway reactivity to a variety of spasmogens and, thereby, enhancing bronchial muscle contraction, thus opposing the bronchodilation effects of the (R)-enantiomer levoalbuterol. Moreover, racemic albuterol exhibits enantioselective presystemic metabolism. Levalbuterol undergoes more rapid metabolism (sulfation) than the (S)-(+)-isomer, resulting in a lower oral bioavailability and rapid elimination. Because of its slower metabolism, (S)-albuterol thus has a higher and prolonged tissue concentrations than levalbuterol, increasing airway reactivity. These adverse effects of (S)-albuterol are completely avoided by using the (R)-enantiomer, levalbuterol (Xopenex®). Thus, the removal of (S)-albuterol from racemic albuterol increases the clinical potency of levalbuterol, such that bronchodilator efficacy is achieved at one-fourth the dose of racemic albuterol along with a marked reduction in side effects.

Bitolterol. Bitolterol is a pro-drug form of colterol in which the catechol hydroxyl groups have been converted to 4-methylbenzoic (p-toloyl) acid esters, providing increased lipid solubility and prolonged duration of action. Bitolterol is administered by inhalation, and the ester groups are hydrolyzed by esterases to liberate the active drug, colterol. Colterol is then subject to metabolism by COMT, but the duration of action of a single dose of the pro-drug bitolterol, up to 8 hours, is twice that of a single dose of colterol, permitting less frequent administration and greater convenience to the patient.

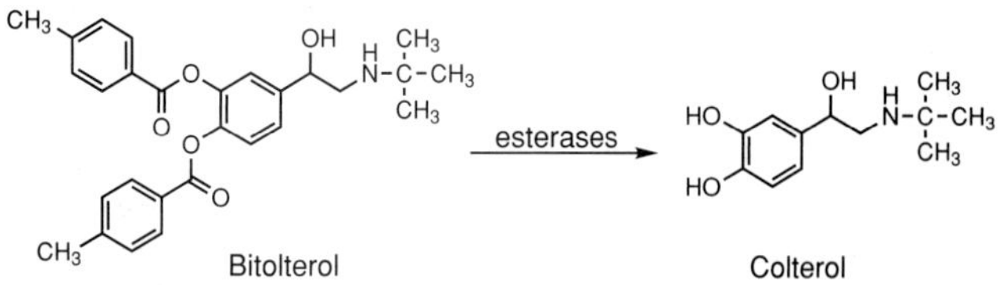

Bitolterol → esterases → Colterol

Ritodrine. The previously mentioned ritodrine is a selective β_2-agonist that is used exclusively for relaxing uterine muscle and inhibiting the contractions of premature labor. Terbutaline, in addition to its use as a bronchodilator, also has been used for halting the contractions of premature labor.

LONG-ACTING β_2-ADRENERGIC AGONISTS. The mechanisms behind the long duration of the bronchodilating effect of the β_2-adrenoceptor agonists formoterol and salmeterol are only partially understood. The long duration of action for formoterol and salmeterol is attributed to their higher lipophilicity and greater receptor affinity compared to those of the short-acting agonists at the β_2-adrenoceptor. Lipophilicity determines the amount of drug entering into the cell membrane of the β_2-adrenoceptor and how much β_2-adrenoceptor agonist must remain at the receptor for maximal sustained activity.

Salmeterol (Serevent). A β_2-agonist with a slow onset and extended duration of action is salmeterol. Salmeterol has the same phenyl ring substitution R^3 as albuterol but also an unusually long and lipophilic group R^1 on the nitrogen. The octanol–water partition coefficient, log P, for salmeterol is 3.88, compared with 0.66 for albuterol. Salmeterol is approximately 50-fold more selective than albuterol for the β_2-receptor. Substantial evidence indicates that its long duration of action results from a specific binding interaction ("anchoring") of the phenyl group at the end of the extended lipophilic side chain with a specific region of the β_2-receptor, affording salmeterol a unique binding mechanism (Fig. 13.11) .

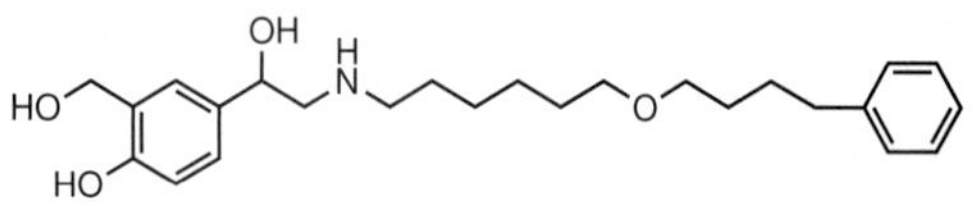

Salmeterol

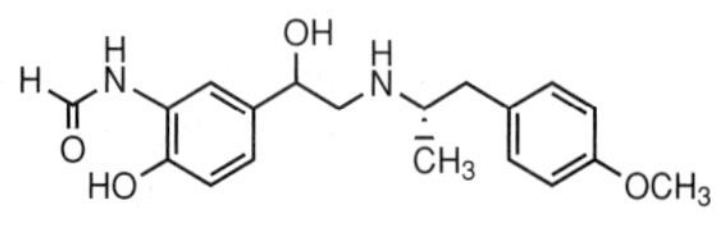

Formoterol

Salmeterol usually is prescribed for severe persistent asthma following previous treatment with a short-acting β-agonist, such as albuterol. The noticeable differences between salmeterol and albuterol are the onset of action and their duration of action (Table 13.6). When used regularly every day as prescribed, inhaled albuterol decreases the number and severity of asthma attacks. It is not used, however, for relieving an asthma attack that has already started.

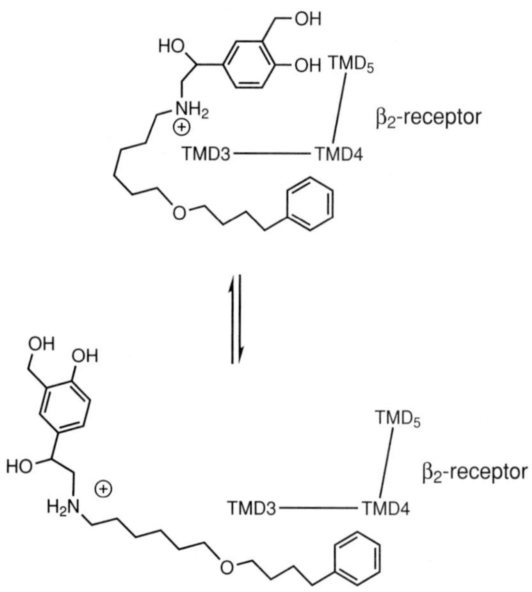

Fig. 13.11. Mechanism of action for salmeterol.

Formoterol (Foradil). Formoterol has 3′-formylamino and 4′-hydroxy ring R^3 substitution pattern but also an alkoxyphenylethyl lipophilic group R^1 on the nitrogen, similar to ritodrine. Although it is less lipophilic (log P = 1.6) than salmeterol, it has a 12-hour duration of action similar to that for salmeterol. It is administered as an inhaled dry powder, because it is unstable to heat and moisture. It is a mixture of (R,R)-(−)- and (S,S)-(+)-stereoisomers, with the (R,R)-isomer having approximately 1,000-fold more affinity for the β_2-receptor than the (S,S)-isomer. Because of its high potency and low dose, however, there is no clinical advantage for using (R,R)-formoterol as bronchodilator compared to the racemate. Unlike salmeterol, formoterol has a faster onset of action as a result of its lower lipophilicity. It is also more potent; a 12-μg dose of formoterol has been demonstrated to be equivalent to a 50-μg dose of salmeterol.

β_1-Adrenergic Agonists

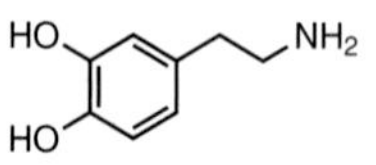

Dopamine 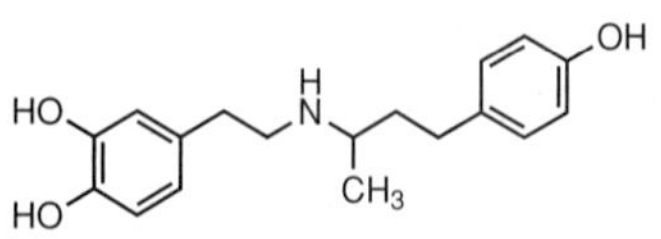 Dobutamine

DOPAMINE. Although not strictly an adrenergic drug, dopamine is a catecholamine with properties related to the cardiovascular activities of the other agents in this chapter. Dopamine acts on specific dopamine receptors to dilate renal vessels, increasing renal blood flow.

Dopamine also stimulates cardiac β_1-receptors through both direct and indirect mechanisms. It is used to correct hemodynamic imbalances induced by conditions such as shock, myocardial infarction, trauma, or congestive heart failure. As a catechol and primary amine, dopamine is rapidly metabolized by COMT and MAO and, similar to dobutamine, has a short duration of action with no oral activity. It is administered as an intravenous infusion.

DOBUTAMINE (DOBUTREX). Not all the adrenergic agonists with direct activity have an aliphatic β-hydroxyl group such as the agents discussed so far. One of these is the catechol dobutamine. Dobutamine is a dopamine analogue with a bulky arylalkyl group on the nitrogen and one chiral (asymmetric) center. Racemic (±)-dobutamine has direct activity on both α_1- and β_1-receptors, but because of some unusual properties of its two enantiomers, the overall pharmacological response looks similar to that of a selective β_1-agonist. The (S)-(−)-enantiomer of dobutamine exhibits β_1-agonist activity and also is a powerful α_1-agonist and vasopressor. The (R)-(+)-isomer is an α_1-antagonist; thus, when the racemate is used clinically, the α-effects of the enantiomers cancel each other, leaving primarily the β_1-effects. The stereochemistry of the methyl substituent does not affect the ability of the drug to bind to the α_1-receptor but does affect the ability of the molecule to activate the receptor. That is, the stereochemistry of the methyl group affects intrinsic activity but not affinity. Because both stereoisomers are β_1-agonists with the (−)-isomer approximately one-tenth the potency of the (+)-isomer, the net effect is β_1 stimulation. Dobutamine is used as a cardiac stimulant after surgery or congestive heart failure. As a catechol, dobutamine is readily metabolized by COMT and has a short duration of action with no oral activity.

Mixed-Acting Sympathomimetics

Phenylpropanolamines

(−)-EPHEDRINE. As discussed earlier, ephedrine is a natural product isolated from several species of ephedra plants, which have been used for centuries in folk medicines in a variety of cultures worldwide (23). Its occurrence in ephedra is approximately 80 to 90%. Other substances also found include (+)-pseudoephedrine (10–15%) and N-methylephedrine (2–5%). Pure ephedrine was first isolated and crystallized in 1887 from a Chinese herbal medicine called Ma Huang. Its sympathomimetic activity was not recognized until 1917, and the pure drug was used clinically even before epinephrine and norepinephrine were isolated and characterized. Ephedrine does not have any phenolic substituents on the phenyl ring, giving it a mixed-acting response and good oral activity, because it is not a substrate for COMT. Lacking hydrogen-bonding phenolic substituents, ephedrine is less polar than the other compounds discussed thus far and crosses the blood-brain barrier far better than the catechols do. Because of its ability to penetrate the CNS, ephedrine has been used as a stimulant and exhibits side effects related to its action in the brain. Ephedrine is widely used for many of the same indications as epinephrine, including use as a bronchodilator, vasopressor, cardiac stimulant, and nasal decongestant.

(+)-PSEUDOEPHEDRINE. Pseudoephedrine, as previously discussed, is the threo diastereomer of ephedrine, with virtually no direct activity and fewer CNS side effects than ephedrine. (+)-Pseudoephedrine is widely used as a nasal decongestant.

(+)-PHENYLPROPANOLAMINE. Phenylpropanolamine (Table 13.4) is the N-desmethyl analogue of ephedrine that has many of the same properties. Lacking the N-methyl group, however, phenylpropanolamine has none of the β_2-agonist activity of ephedrine, is slightly less lipophilic, and therefore, does not enter the CNS as well as ephedrine. Phenylpropanolamine, similar to ephedrine, is a mixture of erythro enantiomers with mixed direct and mostly indirect activity. The drug had been the active ingredient of a number of nasal decongestants and used as a nonprescription appetite suppressant (anorexiant) until its U.S. Food and Drug Administration (FDA)–mandated recall in 2000 because of cerebral hemorrhages in women.

Phenylisopropylamines

AMPHETAMINE AND METHAMPHETAMINE. Other methyl-substituted phenylethylamines (phenylisopropylamines), such as (S)-(+)-amphetamine and (S)-(+)-methamphetamine, which lack both ring substituents and a side-chain hydroxyl, are sufficiently lipophilic to cross the blood-brain barrier readily and cause dramatic CNS stimulation, which gives them serious abuse potential. The clinical utility of (S)-(+)-amphetamine and its derivatives is entirely based on CNS stimulant and central appetite suppressant effects. The only amphetamine product available that is used for the treatment of attention-deficit disorder combines the sulfate, saccharate, and aspartate salts of dextroamphetamine and amphetamine (total amphetamine base, 3.1 mg; Adderal®). (These agents as well as the methoxylated amphetamines are discussed in Chapter 23.)

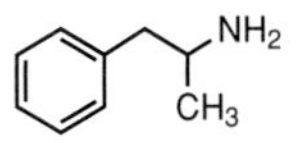

NH_2 CH_3

Amphetamine

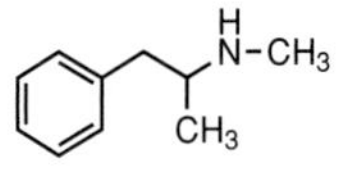

H N-CH_3 CH_3

Methamphetamine

STRUCTURE–ACTIVITY RELATIONSHIPS OF ADRENERGIC ANTAGONISTS

Nonselective α-Antagonists

Phenoxybenzamine

Because α-agonists cause vasoconstriction and raise blood pressure, one would expect α-antagonists to be therapeutically used as antihypertensive agents. An old

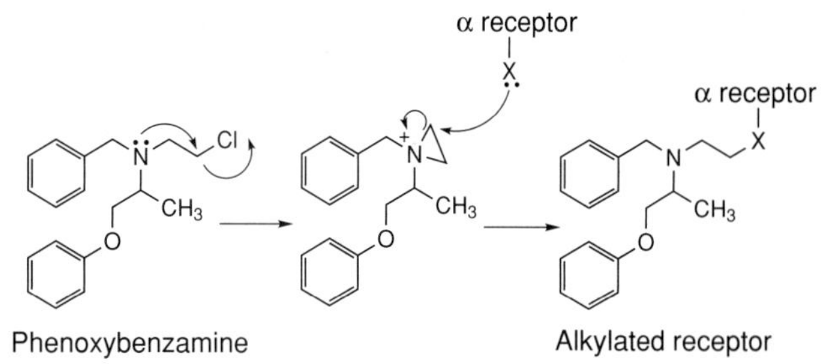

Fig. 13.12. Phenoxybenzamine alkylation of α-adrenoceptors. X is a nucleophile, such as S, N, or O.

but powerful drug in this class is phenoxybenzamine (dibenzyline), a β-haloalkylamine that alkylates α-receptors. β-haloalkylamines are present in nitrogen mustard anticancer agents and are highly reactive alkylating agents. The acid salt of phenoxybenzamine is stable, but at physiologic pH, equilibrium exists between the protonated drug and free base. The unshared electrons of the unprotonated amino group are nucleophilic and displace the β-chlorine atom in an intramolecular reaction to form a highly reactive aziridinium ion (Fig. 13.12). If this occurs in the vicinity of an α-receptor, a nucleophile group X on the receptor can open the aziridinium ion in a nucleophilic reaction to form a covalent bond between the receptor and the drug. The substituents attached to the haloalkylamine provide selectivity for binding to α-adrenoceptors so that the nucleophile generally is part of the target receptor. The nucleophile X is presumably part of an amino acid side chain, such as a cysteine thiol, serine hydroxyl, or lysine amino group, but the specific site of covalent attachment to the α-receptor has not been determined. Because the reaction in which phenoxybenzamine forms covalent bonds with the receptors is irreversible, new receptors must be synthesized before the effects can be overcome. Therefore, the α-blockade is long-lasting.

Unfortunately, other biomolecules besides the target α-receptor also are alkylated. Because of its receptor nonselectivity and toxicity, the use of phenoxybenzamine largely is limited to alleviating the sympathetic effects of pheochromocytoma. This tumor of chromaffin cells of the adrenal medulla produces large amounts of epinephrine and norepinephrine, which are released into the bloodstream, producing hypertension and generalized sympathetic stimulation.

Tolazoline and Phentolamine

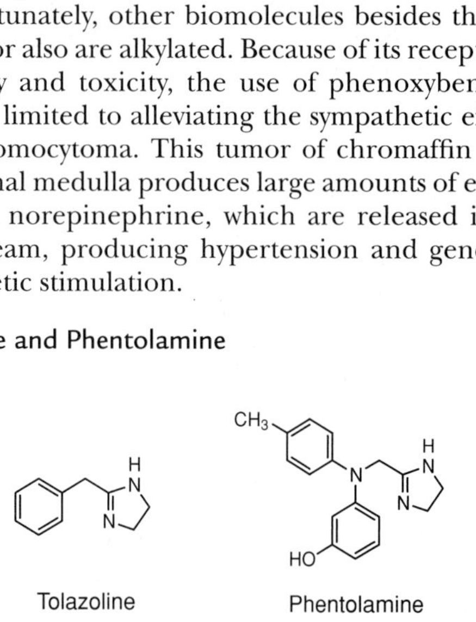

Tolazoline and phentolamine are two imidazoline α-antagonists that also have antihypertensive activity, although they have been replaced in general clinical use by far better agents. Tolazoline has clear structural similarities to the imidazoline α_1-agonists, such as naphazoline and xylometazoline (Fig. 13.7), but does not have the lipophilic substituents required for agonist activity. The resemblance of phentolamine is not as readily apparent, but extensive molecular modeling studies have provided a topologic scheme for α_1-antagonist SAR (19). This pattern, however, cannot be readily visualized without computer graphics and is beyond the scope of this chapter.

Both phentolamine and tolazoline are potent but rather nonspecific α-antagonists. Both drugs stimulate gastrointestinal smooth muscle, an action blocked by atropine, which would indicate cholinergic activity, and they both stimulate gastric secretion, possibly through release of histamine. Because of these and other side effects, the clinical applications of tolazoline and phentolamine also are limited to treating the symptoms of pheochromocytoma.

Selective α_1-Antagonists

Prazosin, Doxazosin, Terazosin, Tamsulosin, and Alfuzosin

Prazosin, the first known selective α_1-blocker, was discovered in the late 1960s (24) and is now one of a small group of selective α_1-antagonists that includes three other quinoxaline antihypertensives terazosin, doxazosin, and alfuzosin and the nonquinazoline benzensulfonamide tamsulosin (Fig. 13.13). Prazosin, doxazosin, and terazosin contain a 4-amino-6,7-dimethoxyquinazoline ring system attached to a piperazine ring except for alfuzosin, which has a rotatable propylenediamine group (an open piperazine ring). The other structural differences are the heterocyclic acyl groups attached to the second nitrogen of the piperazine or the propyl chain. The differences in these groups afford dramatic differences in some of the pharmacokinetic properties of these agents (Table 13.7). For example, reduction of the furan ring for prazosin to the tetrahydrofuran ring of terazosin increases its duration of action by altering its rate of metabolism. Some of the important clinical parameters of the quinazolines are shown in Table 13.6. Perhaps most significant are the long half-lives and durations of action for terazosin, doxazosin, and tamsulsin, which permit once-a-day dosing and generally lead to increased patient compliance.

Prazosin is an antihypertensive agent, as are terazosin and doxazosin. The latter two were subsequently discovered to block α_1-receptors in the prostate gland and alleviate the symptoms of benign prostatic hyperplasia (BPH) (see Chapter 45). The more recently developed tamsulosin and alfuzosin are more selective for the subtype of α_1-adrenoceptor found in the prostate gland, α_{1A}, over those found in vascular tissue. Thus, tamsulosin and alfuzosin are first-line drugs for the treatment of BPH and have no utility in treating hypertension. They have fewer cardiovascular side effects than terazosin and doxazosin

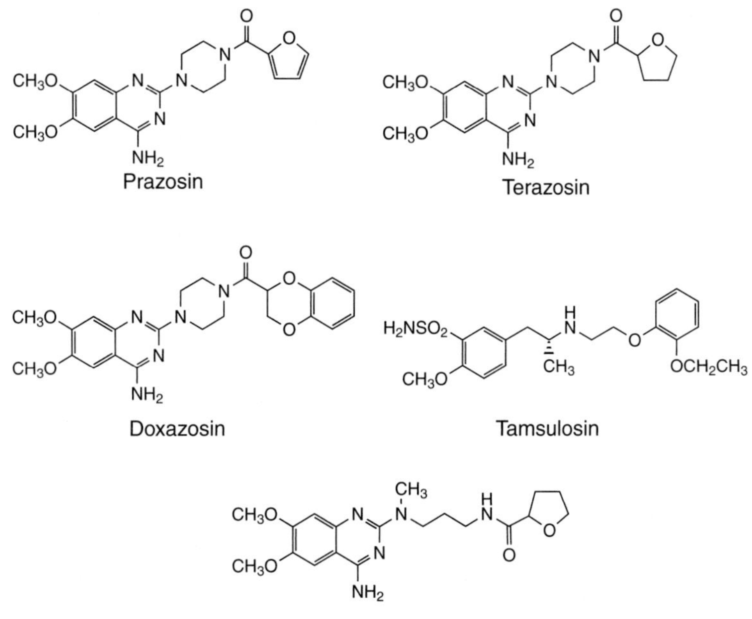

Fig. 13.13. Selective α_1-adrenergic antagonists.

in treating BPH. (Details on the use and pharmacokinetics of α_1-antagonists in treating hypertension and BPH are provided in Chapters 29 and 45, respectively.)

Selective α_2-Adrenergic Antagonists

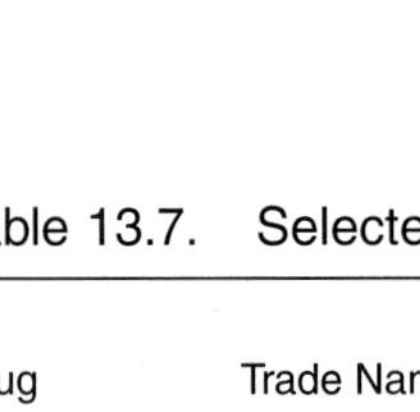

Yohimbine

Yohimbine, an indole alkaloid isolated from *Pausinystlia yohimbe* bark and *Rauwolfia* roots is an α_2-antagonist with greater selectivity for α_2- than for α_1-adrenoceptors, but it also is a serotonin antagonist. It has actions both in the CNS and in the periphery, inducing hypertension and increases in heart rate. Yohimbine has no indications sanctioned by the U.S. FDA, but it has been used to treat male impotence and postural hypotension. Yohimbine also has been used in research to induce anxiety. As was the case with ephedrine and the herbal Ma Huang, the purified chemical yohimbine is regulated by the U.S. FDA. Herbal remedies and dietary supplements containing yohimbe bark are not regulated,

Table 13.7. Selected Clinical Parameters of α_1-Adrenergic Antagonists

Drug	Trade Name	cLogP/LogD[a] (pH 7)	Half-life (hours)	Duration of Action (hours)	Bioavailability (%)
Prazosin	Minipres	− 1.1/ − 1.3	2–3	4–6	45–65
Terazosin	Hytrin	− 1.0/ − 1.0	12	>18	90
Doxazosin	Cardura	0.7/0.5	22	18–36	65
Tamsulosin	Flomax	2.2/0.5	14–15	>24	<50 with food 50–90 fasting
Aflusosin	Uroxatral	− 1.0/ − 2.7	3–5	>48	65

[a]Chemical Abstracts, American Chemical Society, calculated using Advanced Chemistry Development (ACD/Labs) Software V8.14 for Solaris (1994–2006 ACD/Labs).

however, even though the active ingredient is the same chemical entity.

Dichloroisoproterenol

Pronethalol

Propranolol

β-ADRENERGIC ANTAGONISTS

In the 1950s, dichloroisoproterenol (DCI), a derivative of isoproterenol in which the catechol hydroxyls had been replaced by chlorines, was discovered to be a β-antagonist that blocked the effects of sympathomimetic amines on bronchodilation, uterine relaxation, and heart stimulation (25). Although DCI had no clinical utility, replacement of the 3,4-dichloro substituents with a carbon bridge to form a naphthylethanolamine derivative did afford a clinical candidate, pronethalol, which was introduced in 1962 only to be withdrawn in 1963 because of tumor induction in animal tests.

Structure–Activity Relationships

Shortly thereafter, a major innovation in drug development for the β-adrenergic antagonists was introduced when it was discovered that an oxymethylene bridge, OCH_2, could be inserted into the arylethanolamine structure of pronethalol to afford propranolol, an aryloxypropanolamine and the first clinically successful β-blocker. Note that along with the introduction of the oxymethylene bridge, the side chain has been moved from C2 of the naphthyl group to the C1 position. In general, the aryloxypropanolamines are more potent β-blockers than the corresponding arylethanolamines, and most of the β-blockers currently being used clinically are aryloxypropanolamines. β-Blockers have found wide use in treating hypertension (Chapter 29) and certain types of glaucoma. Several β-blockers are in the Top 200 prescription drugs in the United States (Table 13.1).

Initially, it might appear that lengthening the side chain would prevent appropriate binding of the required functional groups to the same receptor site. Molecular models, however, show that the side chains of aryloxypropanolamines can adopt a conformation that places the hydroxyl and amine groups into approximately the same position in space (Fig. 13.14). Although the simple two-dimensional drawing in Figure 13.14 exaggerates the true degree of overlap, elaborate molecular modeling studies confirm that the aryloxypropanolamine side chain can

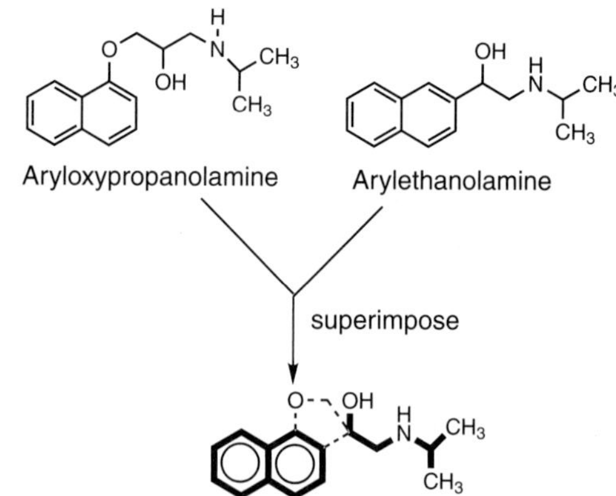

Fig. 13.14. Overlap of aryloxypropanolamines and arylethanolamines. The structures of prototype β-antagonists propranolol and pronethalol may be superimposed so the critical functional groups occupy the same approximate regions in space, as indicated by the bold lines in the superimposed drawings. The dotted lines are those parts that do not overlap but are not necessary to receptor binding.

adopt a low-energy conformation that permits close overlap with the arylethanolamine side chain (26).

Propranolol

Propranolol was initially introduced for the treatment of angina pectoris and later underwent trials as an antiarrhythmic. During clinical trials as an antianginal, propranolol was discovered to have antihypertensive properties, and it has been widely employed for that purpose for decades (27). Propranolol rapidly became widely used for a variety of cardiac arrhythmias as well. In addition, because of its high lipophilicity and ability to penetrate the CNS, propranolol has found use in treating disorders of the CNS, such as anxiety.

At approximately this same time, a new series of 4-substituted phenyloxypropanololamines emerged that selectively inhibited sympathetic cardiac stimulation. These observations led to the recognition that not all β-receptors were the same, which in turn led to the introduction of β_1 and β_2 nomenclature to differentiate cardiac β_1-receptors from others. Development of β-blockers proceeded rapidly, and today, a large number of additional drugs, both nonselective β-antagonists and selective β_1-antagonists, are available on the world market. (Clinical use of β-blockers as antihypertensives are covered in Chapter 29.) Of those antagonists that are selective for the cardiac β_1-receptor, most also have some β_2-antagonist properties at the higher levels of therapeutic dosing (dose dependent). With the exception of sotalol, all the drugs shown in Figures 13.15 and 13.16 are aryloxypropanolamines. Metipranolol (Fig. 13.15) is an exception to the general rule that 4-substituted aryloxypropanolamines are selective β_1-blockers.

Other than β_1-selectivity of 4-substituted aryloxypropanolamines, little obvious structural pattern relates

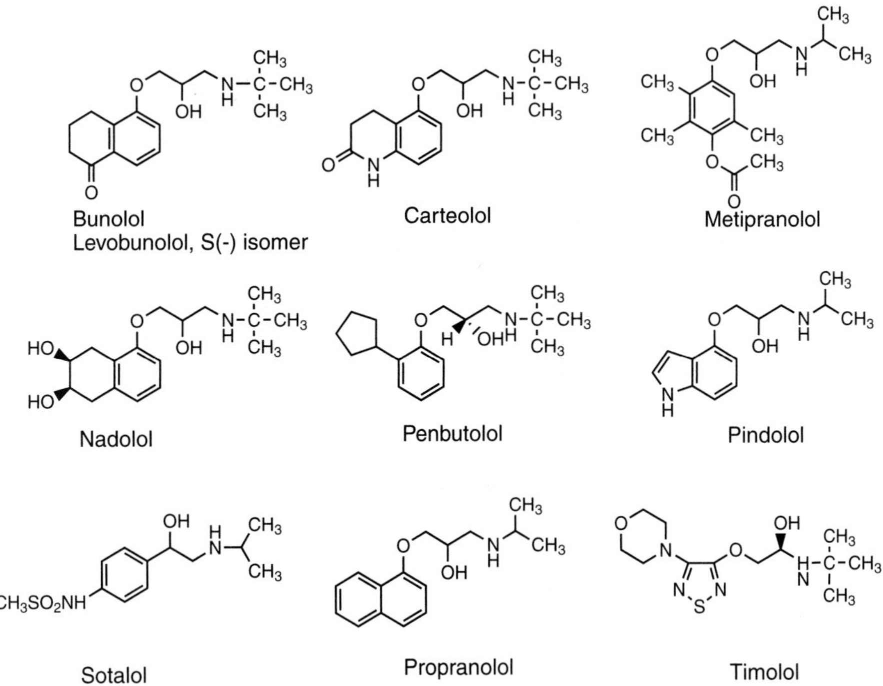

Fig. 13.15. Nonselective β-adrenergic antagonists.

β-blockers to specific clinical applications, with the exception of esmolol. Esmolol is the methyl ester of a carboxylic acid, which makes it is susceptible to hydrolysis by serum esterases. The acid metabolite generated by hydrolysis is essentially inactive and readily excreted as its zwitterion. For this reason, esmolol has a half-life of only approximately 8 minutes and is used to control supraventricular tachycardia during surgery when a short-acting β_1-adrenergic antagonist is desirable.

Another physicochemical parameter with some clinical correlation is the relative lipophilicity of different agents. Propranolol is by far the most lipophilic of the available β-blockers, and it enters the CNS far better than the less lipophilic agents, such as atenolol or nadolol. Lipophilicity as measured by octanol–water partitioning also correlates with the primary site of clearance, as seen in Table 13.8. The more lipophilic drugs are primarily cleared by the liver, whereas the more hydrophilic agents are cleared by the kidney. This could influence the choice of agents in cases of renal failure or liver disease. Several of the β-blockers must be dose adjusted in patients with impaired renal function, as indicated in Table 13.7.

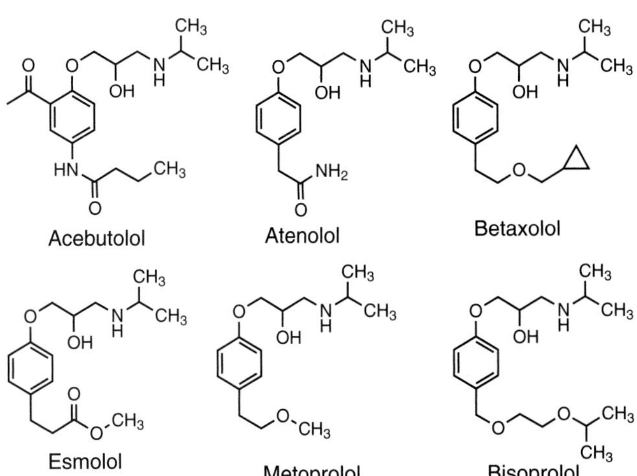

Fig. 13.16. Selective β_1-adrenergic antagonists.

β-Blockers also have found extensive use in treating glaucoma, although the mechanism of action in treating glaucoma is more difficult to explain. The β-blockers lower intraocular pressure by decreasing the amount of aqueous humor fluid produced in the eye by the ciliary body, and β_2-receptors have been found in that tissue. Observations have shown, however, that the ciliary body has no adrenergic innervation, that the effect is not stereoselective, and that a correlation of activity exists with decreased ciliary blood flow and decreased dopamine levels, indicating that the mechanism of action of β-blockers in treating glaucoma is unusual (28).

Mixed α/β-Adrenergic Antagonists

Labetalol and carvedilol are antihypertensives with α_1-, β_1-, and β_2-blocking activity (Fig. 13.17) (see Chapter 29). In terms of SAR, recall from the earlier discussion of phenylethanolamine agonists that the type of N-substituents, such as N-isopropyl and N-t-butyl, eliminated α-receptor activity; however, arylalkyl groups with α-methyl substituent returned α_1-affinity but not intrinsic activity (c.f., dobutamine). Thus, these two drugs have

Table 13.8. Pharmacologic/Pharmacokinetic Properties of β-Adrenergic Blocking Agents

Drug	Adrenergic Receptor Blocking Activity	Membrane Stabilizing Activity	Intrinsic Sympath omimetic Activity	cLog Pa /Log D (pH 7)	Extent of Absorption (%)	Absolute Oral Bioavailability (%)	Half-life (hours)	Protein binding (%)	Metabolism/Excretion
Acebutolol (Sectral)	β_1[1]	+	+	2.67/0.52	90	20–60	3–4	26	Hepatic; renal excretion, 30–40%; nonrenal excretion, 50–60% (bile)
Atenolol (Tenormin)	β_1[1]	0	0	0.1/−2.0	50	50–60	6–9	16–16	~50% excreted unchanged in feces
Betaxolol (Kerlone, Betoptic)	β_1[1]	+	0	2.7/0.6	~100	89	14–22	~50	Hepatic; >80% recovered in urine, 15% unchanged
Bisoprolol (Zebeta)	β_1[1]	0	0	2.2/0.1	≥90	80	9–12	~30	~50% excreted unchanged in urine, remainder as inactive metabolites; <2% excreted in feces.
Esmolol (Brevibloc)	β_1[1]	0	0	1.9/−0.22	na[5]	na[5]	0.15	55	Rapid metabolism by esterases in cytosol of red blood cells
Metoprolol (Lopressor) Metoprolol, LA	β_1[1]	0[2]	0	1.8/−0.34	95	40–50 77	3–7	12	Hepatic; renal excretion, <5% unchanged
Carteolol (Cartrol, Ocupress)	β_1 β_2	0	++	1.7/−0.4	80	85	6	23–30	50–70% excreted unchanged in urine
Nadolol (Corgard)	β_1 β_2	0	0	1.3/0.84	30	30–50	20–24	30	Urine, unchanged
Penbutolol (Levatol)	β_1 β_2	0	+	4.2/2.1	~100	~100	5	80–98	Hepatic (conjugation, oxidation); renal excretion of metabolites (17% as conjugate)
Pindolol (Visken)	β_1 β_2	+	+++	1.97/−0.2	95	~100	3–4[3]	40	Urinary excretion of metabolites (60–65%) and unchanged drug (35–40%)
Propranolol (Inderal) Propranolol, LA	β_1 β_2	++	0	3.1/1	90	30 9–18	3–5 8–11	90	Hepatic; <1% excreted unchanged in urine
Sotalol (Betapace)	β_1 β_2	0	0	0.3/−1.8	nd[6]	90–100	12	0	Not metabolized; excreted unchanged in urine
Timolol (Blocadren, Timoptic)	β_1 β_2	0	0	−4.3/−2	90	75	4	10	Hepatic; urinary excretion of metabolites and unchanged drug
Labetalol[4] (Normodyne)	β_1 β_2 α_1	0	0	2.9/0.99	100	30–40	5.5–8	50	55–60% excreted in urine as conjugates or unchanged drug
Carvedilol (Coreg)	β_1 β_2 α_1	0	0	4.2/3.2	>90	25–35	7–10	98	

[a]Chemical Abstracts, American Chemical Society, calculated using Advanced Chemistry Development (ACD/Labs) Software V8.14 for Solaris (1994–2006 ACD/Labs).
[1]Inhibits β_2-receptors (bronchial and vascular) at higher doses.
[2]Detectable only at doses much greater than required for β-blockade.
[3]In elderly hypertensive patients with normal renal function, half-life is variable (7–15 hours).
[4]Not labetalol monograph.
[5]Not applicable (available IV only).
[6] No data.
0 = none; + = low; ++ = moderate; +++ = high.

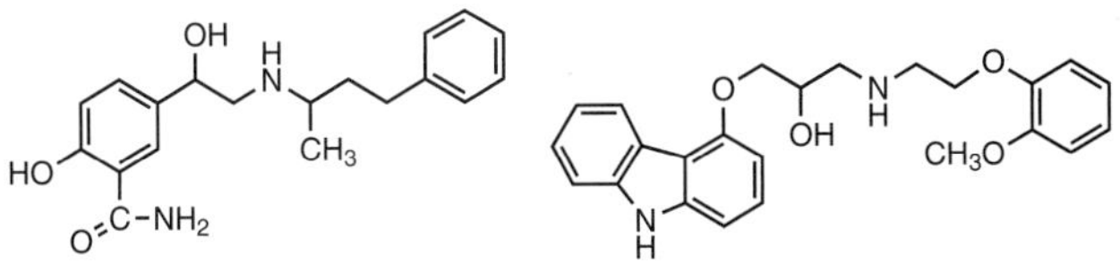

Labetalol Carvedilol

Fig. 13.17. Mixed α/β-adrenergic antagonists.

structural features that permit binding to the α_1-receptor and nonselectively to both β-receptors. The β-blocking activity of labetalol is approximately 1.5-fold that of its α-blocking activity. Carvedilol has an estimated β-blocking activity 10- to 100-fold its α-blocking activity.

Stereochemistry of the β-Adrenergic Antagonists

A factor that sometimes causes confusion when comparing the structures of arylethanolamines with aryloxypropanolamines is the stereochemical nomenclature of the side-chain carbon bearing the hydroxyl group. For maximum effectiveness in receptor binding, the hydroxy group must occupy the same region in space as it does for the phenylethanolamine agonists in the R absolute configuration. Because of the insertion of an oxygen atom in the side chain of the aryloxypropanolamines, the Cahn-Ingold-Prelog priority of the substituents around the asymmetric carbon changes, and the isomer with the required special arrangement now has the S absolute configuration. This is an effect of the nomenclature rules; the groups still have the same spatial arrangements (Fig. 13.18).

DRUGS AFFECTING NOREPINEPHRINE/ EPINEPHRINE BIOSYNTHESIS

Hypothetically, inhibitors of any of the three enzymes involved in the conversion of L-tyrosine to norepinephrine could be used as drugs to moderate adrenergic transmission. Inhibitors of the rate-limiting enzyme tyrosine hydroxylase would be the most logical choice. One inhibitor of tyrosine hydroxylase, metyrosine or α-methyl-L-tyrosine, is in limited clinical use to help control hypertensive episodes and other symptoms of catecholamine overproduction in patients with the rare adrenal tumor pheochromocytoma (29). Metyrosine, a competitive inhibitor of tyrosine hydroxylase, inhibits the production of catecholamines by the tumor. Although metyrosine is useful in treating hypertension caused by excess catecholamine biosynthesis in pheochromocytoma tumors, it is not useful for treating essential hypertension. The drug metyrosine is the (S)-stereoisomer of α-methyltyrosine. The enantiomer, (R)-α-methyltyrosine, does not bind to the active site of tyrosine hydroxylase and, thus, has no useful pharmacological activity.

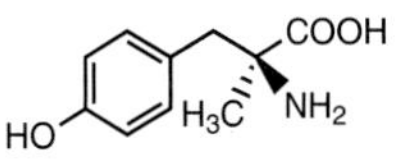

R absolute configuration S absolute configuration

Fig. 13.18. Stereochemical nomenclature for arylethanolamines versus aryloxypropanolamines. The relative positions in space of the four functional groups are the same in the two structures; however, one is designated (R) and the other (S). This is because the introduction of an oxygen atom into the side chain of the aryloxypropanolamine changes the priority of two of the groups used in the nomenclature assignment.

Metyrosine

Powerful inhibitors of the next enzyme in the pathway, aromatic L-amino acid decarboxylase (e.g., carbidopa), have proven clinically useful, but not as modulators of peripheral adrenergic transmission. Rather, these agents are used to inhibit the metabolism of exogenous L-dopa administered in the treatment of Parkinson's disease (see Chapter 25).

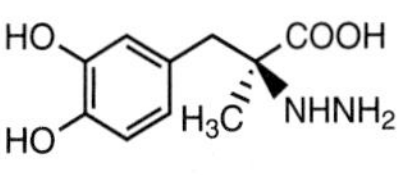

Carbidopa

The next enzyme in the biosynthetic pathway to norepinephrine and epinephrine, dopamine β-hydroxylase, has been the subject of extensive research into its chemical mechanism and the subject of many enzyme inhibition studies. The inhibitors known to date, however, are primarily of basic biochemical research interest and have no therapeutic relevance. The same is true of phenylethanolamine-N-methyltransferase, the last enzyme in the biosynthesis of epinephrine in the adrenal medulla.

DRUGS AFFECTING NOREPINEPHRINE RELEASE, REUPTAKE, AND METABOLISM

Two drugs that act by inhibiting the release of norepinephrine from the nerve terminal and depleting stored norepinephrine are guanethidine and guanadrel, which have been used as antihypertensives but have largely been replaced by more effective agents and discontinued in the United States.

Drugs that selectively block the reuptake of norepinephrine can exert an acute and powerful sympathomimetic effect by prolonging the amount of time that released norepinephrine remains in the synaptic cleft. Cocaine is a powerful inhibitor of catecholamine reuptake (see Chapter 23). The tricyclic secondary amines, such as the antidepressants desipramine, nortriptyline,

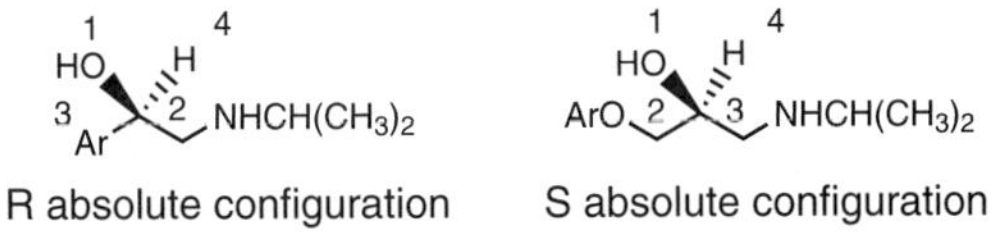

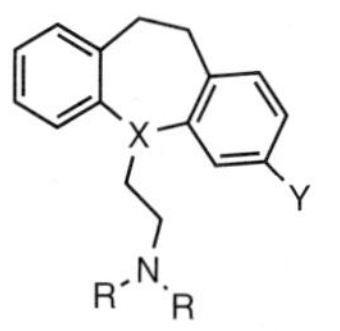

Tricyclic antidepressants

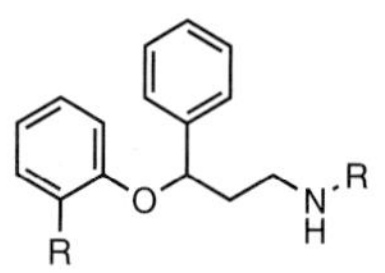

Phenoxyphenylpropylamine antidepressent

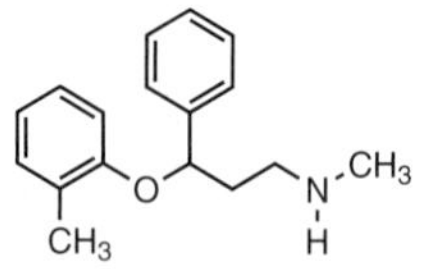

Atomoxetine

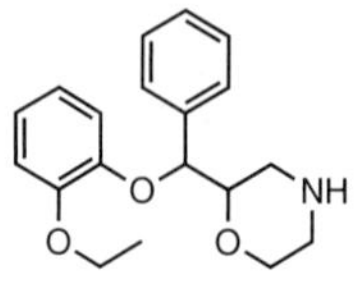

Reboxetine

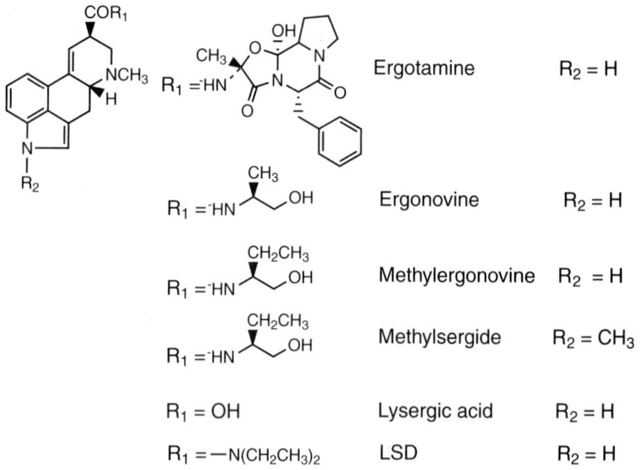

R_1		R_2
(peptide moiety)	Ergotamine	R_2 = H
R_1 = HN–CH(CH_3)CH_2OH	Ergonovine	R_2 = H
R_1 = HN–CH(CH_2CH_3)CH_2OH	Methylergonovine	R_2 = H
R_1 = HN–CH(CH_2CH_3)CH_2OH	Methylsergide	R_2 = CH_3
R_1 = OH	Lysergic acid	R_2 = H
R_1 = —N(CH_2CH_3)$_2$	LSD	R_2 = H

Fig. 13.19. Ergot alkaloids.

or the phenoxypropylamines reboxetine and atomoxetine, block the reuptake of norepinephrine into the presynaptic terminals, whereas the tricyclic tertiary amine antidepressants amitriptyline, doxepin, and imipramine block both norepinephrine and serotonin reuptake in their respective presynpatic terminals (see Chapter 21). The tertiary tricyclic antidepressants are promiscuous antagonists at muscarinic, α-adrenergic, and H_1-histaminic receptors. (Clinical application of these and other antidepressant drugs is discussed in more detail in Chapter 21.)

Inhibitors of the enzymes that degrade norepinephrine, MAO and COMT, have application as antidepressants and anti-Parkinson's agents, respectively. These drugs are covered in Chapters 21 and 25.

ERGOT ALKALOIDS

The ergot alkaloids have been recognized for more than 2,000 years, but their effects are varied and complex. Because of their structural similarities with the neurotransmitters, the ergot alkaloids exhibit affinity for α-adrenergic, dopaminergic, and serotonergic receptor systems. They also block the release of vasoactive neuropeptides, such as substance P. In general, their pharmacological effects result from their action as partial agonists and antagonists on these biogenic amine receptors. Their spectrum of effects varies with their structural features. Thus, the ergot alkaloids have been largely displaced by other more selective and effective drugs, except for methysergide, which remains the gold standard for the treatment of migraine headaches. They are discussed in this chapter because of their effects on the adrenergic nervous system.

The ergot alkaloids are a large group of indole alkaloids isolated from the ergot fungus, *Claviceps purpurea,* which is a plant parasite principally infecting rye. Eating grain contaminated with ergot caused a severely debilitating and painful disease during the Middle Ages called St. Anthony's Fire (ergotism), but in small doses, ergot was known to midwives for centuries for its ability to stimulate uterine contraction. Gangrene with burning pain in the extremities was one of two common presentations of ergot poisoning, which also could produce convulsions, hallucinations, severe psychosis, and death. St. Anthony was the patron saint of those who were stricken, and the Order of St. Anthony provided care for these patients. Outbreaks of "dancing mania," which occurred between the thirteenth and sixteenth centuries, sometimes have been attributed to ergotism, and one appealing—if unprovable—theory proposes that the women accused of witchcraft in the Salem trials of 1692 were suffering from ergot-induced psychosis and convulsions. The pharmacology of the various ergot alkaloids is complex, involving actions on the adrenergic nervous system as well as a number of others. The structures of several ergot alkaloids are shown in Figure 13.19.

Ergotamine and dihydroergotamine are structurally related to biogenic amines and, because of this structural relationship, exert a broad range of pharmacological effects mediated by the adrenergic, the dopaminergic, and particularly, the serotonergic receptor systems. These are the serotonin (5-HT) 1A, 1B, 1D, and 1F receptor agonists, and they also block the release of two important vasoactive neuropeptides currently thought to be involved in migraine, substance P and calcitonin gene-related peptide. They exhibit mixed agonist/antagonist effects at the adrenergic and dopaminergic receptors. Ergotamine is a potent vasoconstrictor but also can produce vasodilatory effects depending on the degree of resistance of the vasculature. When preexisting resistance is low, vasoconstriction occurs, resulting in increased arterial blood pressure. When there is increased resistance of the vascular bed, vasodilation may occur, whereas ergotamine binding to serotonin receptors result in vasoconstrictor effects. In migraine headache, ergotamine most likely relieves cranial vascular pressure by selective vasoconstriction of arterial cranial vessel beds, thus reducing carotid blood flow, as well as by depression of central serotonergic neurons, thus mediating pain transmission. The uterine stimulant properties (oxytocic) of ergotamine result from its strong induction of contractions in the pregnant uterus, which appears to be partially an α-adrenergic effect, because it is blocked by phentolamine. Ergotamine is more potent than dihydroergotamine as a uterine stimulant. It also is used to contract the postpartum uterus to prevent excessive bleeding. The bioavailability of ergotamine following oral, sublingual, inhalation, and rectal administration is less than 5%., but oral bioavailability is improved when ergotamine is coadministered with caffeine Its elimination half-life is 1.5 to 2.5 hours. These medications may cause nausea and vomiting via direct stimulation of the chemoreceptor trigger zone.

Dihydroergotamine mesylate (Migranal) is a 5-HT_{1D} receptor agonist used to treat migraine headache with or without aura. Its clinical efficacy in treatment of migraine is thought to be related to the activation of 5-HT_{1D} receptors in the intracranial blood vessel bed, resulting in vasoconstriction. Dihydroergotamine also inhibits the release of pro-inflammatory neuropeptides, such as substance P release caused by the activation of the 5-HT_{1D} receptors found on sensory nerve endings. The oral bioavailability is less than 1%, whereas with an intranasal spray, the bioavailability is 32%. It also is administered intramuscularly, subcutaneously and intravenously.

Ergonovine (Ergotrate) and methylergonovine (Methergen) produce arterial vasoconstriction by stimulating the α-adrenergic and serotonin receptors and inhibiting the release of endothelial-derived relaxation factor. As vasoconstrictors, they are less potent than ergotamine. Ergonovine causes vasoconstriction of coronary arteries. In the CNS, it exhibits weak dopaminergic antagonist actions in certain blood vessels and partial agonist actions at serotonin receptors in umbilical and placental blood vessels, but it does not possess significant α-adrenergic blocking activity. Its duration of action as uterine stimulant is approximately 3 hours. Ergonovine is a strong inducer of uterine contractions and, because of its better oral absorption, has largely replaced ergotamine for this purpose. Methylergonovine is rapidly and completely absorbed following oral or intramuscular administration, with an oral bioavailability of 60%, even though it undergoes extensive first-pass metabolism to ergonovine.

Methysergide (Sansert), which is structurally identical to methylergonovine except for the addition of a methyl group to the indole nitrogen, has far less of the uterine stimulatory properties of the other agents and, instead, is used exclusively for treatment of migraine headache as a serotonin antagonist at 5-HT_1/5-HT_2 receptors. Methysergide is a potent peripheral inhibitor of 5-HT receptors in the blood vessel, which inhibits vessel-wall permeability. Methysergide also inhibits the release of histamine from mast cells and stabilizes platelets against the release of 5-HT, which may be responsible for the onset of the migraine attack. In contrast to its peripheral effects, methysergide appears to be a central 5-HT_1 agonist, resulting in alleviation of the central hyperalgesia effect that occurs in patients with migraine. Its oral bioavailability of less than 13% suggests extensive first-pass N-demethylation to its primary metabolite, methylergonovine, which has a longer elimination half-life than methysergide. The fact that the metabolite has a higher concentration and a longer half-life than the parent drug may be relevant to the treatment of migraine if methylergonovine contributes to the antimigraine effect of methysergide.

All these ergot alkaloids are amide derivatives of lysergic acid, but only the diethylamide LSD produces the profound hallucinatory effects for which it is so well-known.

CASE STUDY

Victoria F. Roche and S. William Zito

CB is a 57-year-old female independent real estate agent with mild persistent asthma who recently moved to your community after the traumatic breakup of her 25-year marriage and the death of her beloved mother. She and her mother grew very close during the last years of her stormy marriage, and while she felt the need for this new start, she is feeling quite lost and alone. She is currently taking the antidepressant duloxetine hydrochloride (Cymbalta, 20 mg b.i.d.) to assist in managing her emotional stress and has initiated psychotherapy with a qualified counselor. She is in the process of finding a realty company with which to affiliate to ease her way into the market, but thus far, she has not had a firm offer of employment. She has a modest inheritance from her mother that will tide her over for a time, but she is definitely anxious about her situation and wonders whether she did the right thing in leaving her old hometown. She claims to have lost 20 pounds over the past several months because of the stress and still is not able to eat very well.

CB's asthma is currently being treated with a low-dose of the inhaled corticosteroid beclomethasone dipropionate (QVAR, 40 μg b.i.d.). She is in your pharmacy now with prescriptions for both chronic medications written by her new provider. After taking her medical history and reviewing her psychosocial situation, you recognize that she has many risk factors for "near-fatal asthma" and believe she should have ready access to rescue therapy in case she experiences an acute episode of severe bronchoconstriction. Consider the structures of the adrenergic agents drawn below, and prepare to make a therapeutic recommendation to CB's new physician.

1. Identify the therapeutic problems in which the pharmacist's intervention may benefit the patient.
2. Identify and prioritize the patient-specific factors that must be considered to achieve the desired therapeutic outcomes.
3. Conduct a thorough and mechanistically oriented structure–activity analysis of all therapeutic alternatives provided in the case.
4. Evaluate the SAR findings against the patient specific factors and desired therapeutic outcomes, and make a therapeutic decision.
5. Counsel your patient.

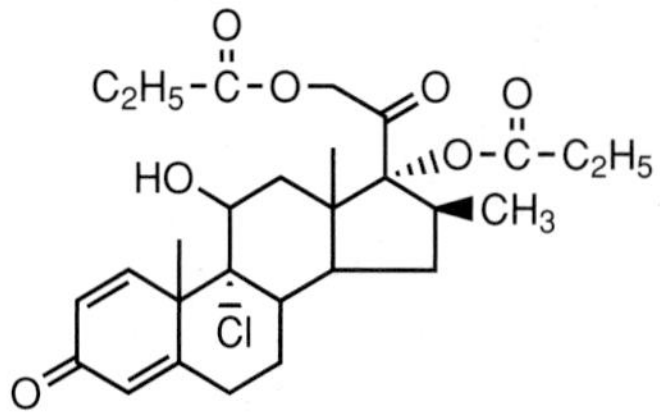

Beclomethasone dipropionate

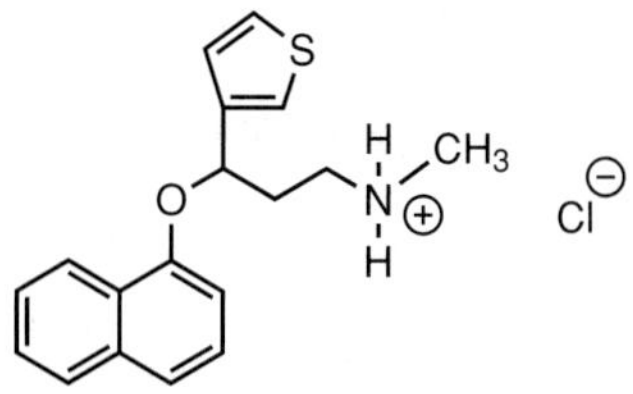

Duloxetine hydrochloride

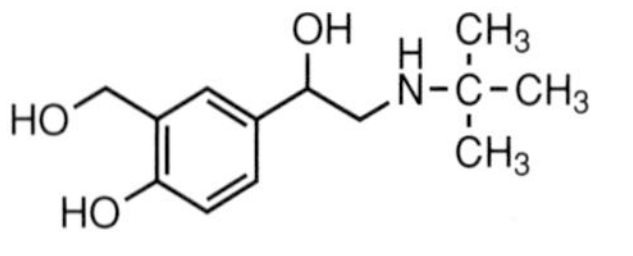

1

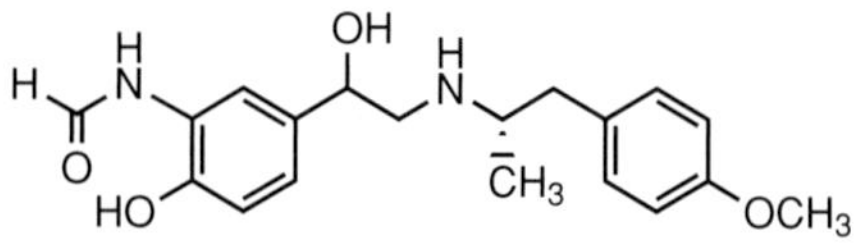

2

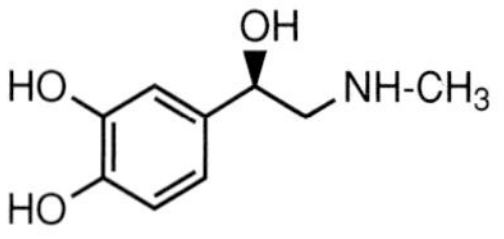

3

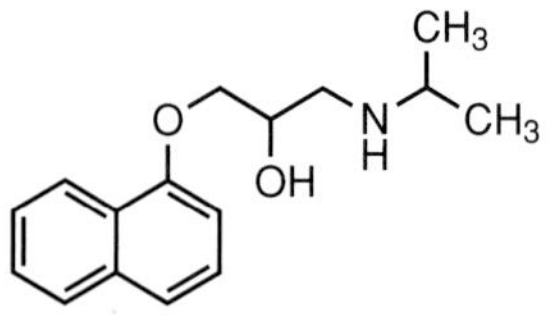

4

References

1. Von Euler US. Synthesis, uptake, and storage of catecholamines in adrenergic nerves: the effect of drugs. In: Blaschko H, Marshall E, ed. Catecholamines. New York: Springer, 1972:186–230.
2. Griffith RK. Adrenergics and adrenergic-blocking drugs. In: Abraham DJ, ed. Burger's Medicinal Chemistry and Drug Discovery. Hoboken, NJ: John Wiley and Sons, 2003:1–37.
3. Kaufman S, Nelson TJ. Studies on the regulation of tyrosine hydroxylase activity by phosphorylation and dephosphorylation. In: Dahlstrom A, Belmaker RH, Sandler M, eds. Progress in Catecholamine Research. Part A: Basic Aspects and Peripheral Mechanisms. New York: Alan R Liss, 1988:57–60.
4. Philippu A, Matthaei H. Transport and storage of catecholamines in vesicles. In: Trendelenburg U, Weiner N, eds. Catecholamines I. New York: Springer, 1988:1–42.
5. Trendelenburg U. Factors influencing the concentration of catecholamines at the receptors. In: Blaschko H, Marshall E, eds. Catecholamines. New York: Springer, 1972:726–761.
6. Kopin IJ. Metabolic degradation of catecholamines. In: Blaschko H, Marshall E, eds. Catecholamines. New York: Springer, 1972:270–282.
7. Ahlquist RP. A study of the adrenotropic receptors. Am J Physiol 1948; 153:586–600.
8. Harrison JK, Pearson WR, Lynch KR. Molecular characterization of α_1- and α_2-adrenoceptors. Trends Pharmacol Sci 1991;12(2):62–67.
9. De Souza CJ, Burkey BF. β_3-Adrenoceptor agonists as antidiabetic and antiobesity drugs in humans. Curr Pharm Des 2001;7:1433–1449.
10. Trumpp-Kallmeyer S, Hoflack J, Bruinvels A, et al. Modeling of G protein–coupled receptors: application to dopamine, adrenaline, serotonin, acetylcholine, and mammalian opsin receptors. J Med Chem 1992;35:3448–3462.
11. Ostrowski J, Kjelsberg MA, Caron MG, et al. Mutagenesis of the β_2-adrenergic receptor: how structure elucidates function. Annu Rev Pharmacol Toxicol 1992;32:167–183.
12. Strader CD, Candelore MR, Hill WS, et al. Identification of two serine residues involved in agonist activation and the β-adrenergic receptor. J Biol Chem 1989;264:13572–13578.
13. Regan JW, Kobilka TS, Yang-Feng TL, et al. Cloning and expression of a human kidney cDNA for an α_2-adrenergic receptor subtype. Proc Natl Acad Sci U S A 1988;85:6301–6305.
14. Kobilka B. Adrenergic receptors as models for G protein–coupled receptors. Annu Rev Neurosci 1992;15:87–114.
15. Nichols AJ, Ruffolo RR Jr. Structure–activity relationships for α-adrenoceptor agonists and antagonists. In: Ruffolo RR Jr., ed. α-Adrenoceptors: Molecular Biology, Biochemistry, and Pharmacology. New York: Karger, 91:75–114.
16. Timmermans PB, van Zwieten PA. α_2-Adrenoceptors: classification, localization, mechanisms, and targets for drugs. J Med Chem 1982;25:1389–1401.
17. Patil PN, Jacobowitz D. Steric aspects of adrenergic drugs. IX. Pharmacologic and histochemical studies on isomers of cobefrin (α-methylnorepinephrine). J Pharmacol Exp Ther 1968;161:279–295.
18. Kanagy NL. α_2-Adrenergic receptor signaling in hypertension. Clin Sci (Lond) 2005;109:431–437.
19. Kobinger W. Central α-adrenergic systems as targets for hypotensive drugs. Rev Physiol Biochem Pharmacol 1978;81:39–100.
20. Fairbanks CA, Stone LS, Kitto KF, et al. α_{2C}-Adrenergic receptors mediate spinal analgesia and adrenergic-opioid synergy. J Pharmacol Exp Ther 2002;300:282–290.
21. Wheeler LA, Woldemussie E. α_2-Adrenergic receptor agonists are neuroprotective in experimental models of glaucoma. Eur J Ophthalmol 2001;11 (Suppl 2):S30–S35.
22. Wheeler L, WoldeMussie E, Lai R. Role of α_2-agonists in neuroprotection. Surv Ophthalmol 2003;48(Suppl 1):S47–S51.
23. Chen KK, Schmidt CF. Ephedrine and related substances. Medicine 1930;9:1–117.
24. Scriabine A, Constantine JW, Hess HJ, et al. Pharmacological studies with some new antihypertensive aminoquinazolines. Experientia 1968;24(11):1150–1151.
25. Moran NC. New adrenergic blocking drugs: their pharmacological, biochemical, and clinical actions. Ann N Y Acad Sci 1967;139:545–548.
26. Jen T, Frazee JS, Schwartz MS, et al. Adrenergic agents. 8.1. Synthesis and β-adrenergic agonist activity of some 3-tert-butylamino-2-(substituted phenyl)-1-propanols. J Med Chem 1977;20:1263–1268.
27. Evans DB, Fox R, Hauck FP. β-Adrenergic receptor blockers as therapeutic agents. Ann Rep Med Chem 1979;14:81–90.
28. Lesar TS. Comparison of ophthalmic β-blocking agents. Clin Pharm 1987; 6:451–463.
29. Brogden RN, Heel RC, Speight TM, et al. α-Methyl-p-tyrosine: a review of its pharmacology and clinical use. Drugs 1981;21(2):81–89.

Suggested Reading

Westfall TC, Westfall DP. Adrenergic agonists and antagonists. In: Brunton LL, Lazo JS, Parker KL, eds. Goodman and Gilman's The Pharmacological Basis of Therapeutics, 11th Ed. New York: McGraw-Hill, 2006:237–295.

14. *Serotonin Receptors and Drugs Affecting Serotonergic Neurotransmission*

RICHARD A. GLENNON AND MALGORZATA DUKAT

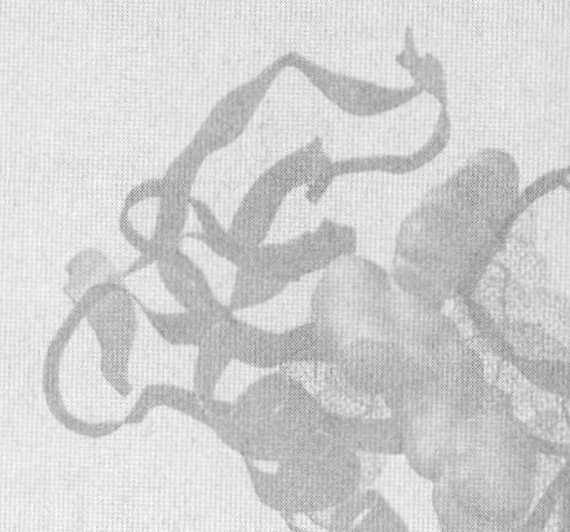

DRUGS COVERED IN THIS CHAPTER:

DRUGS FOR THE TREATMENT OF MIGRAINE ($5\text{-}HT_1$ agonists)
- Almotriptan
- Frovatriptan
- Eletriptan
- Naratriptan
- Rizatriptan
- Sumatriptan
- Zolmitriptan

ANTIEMETIC DRUGS ($5\text{-}HT_3$ antagonists)
- Alosetron
- Dolasetron
- Granisetron
- Ondansetron
- Palonosetron
- Tropisetron

DRUG FOR THE TREATMENT OF IRRITABLE BOWEL SYNDROME ($5\text{-}HT_4$ agonists)
- Tegaserod

DRUGS FOR THE TREATMENT OF NEUROPSYCHIATRIC DISORDERS
- Buspirone
- Clozapine
- Fluoxetine
- Olanzapine
- Risperidone
- Trazodone
- Tranyclypromine

SEROTONIN

Serotonin is the "baby boomer" of neurotransmitters: It was identified in the late 1940s, its adolescence was troubled and turbulent, it made the drug scene in the 1960s, and it nearly died of an overdose in the early 1970s. At one point, the remark was made that "serotonin doesn't do anything" (1). On reaching its middle years, serotonin has matured and become an important topic of study, a household name, and more complicated than ever. Serotonin has been associated with, among other things, anxiety, depression, schizophrenia, drug abuse, sleep, dreaming, hallucinogenic activity, headache, cardiovascular disorders, and appetite control, and it is now dabbling in acupuncture and transcendental meditation. This has prompted the comment that "it almost appears that serotonin is involved in everything" (1). A review of the patent literature provides an indication of some of the claims being made for novel serotonergic agents (Table 14.1). Tens of thousands of papers have been published on serotonin. Much is known—but an incredible amount remains to be learned.

Serotonin (5-HT)

Historical Perspectives

(+) Lysergic acid diethylamide (LSD)

Serotonin was independently identified in the late 1940s by two groups of investigators: In the United States, it was called serotonin, whereas in Italy, it was called enteramine. Its total synthesis in the early 1950s confirmed that both substances were 5-hydroxytryptamine (5-HT). Serotonin (5-HT) was detected in numerous plant and animal species and, in the mid-1950s, was identified in the central nervous system (CNS) of animals. A neurotransmitter role was subsequently proposed for this substance. Later, 5-HT was implicated in a variety of central and peripheral physiologic actions. It seemed to be involved in vasoconstriction and vasodilation, regulation of body temperature, sleep, and hormonal regulation, and evidence suggested that it might be involved in depression. The structural similarity between 5-HT and the then recently discovered hallucinogenic agent (+)-lysergic acid diethylamide (LSD) intrigued investigators. This observation led to speculation that 5-HT might be involved in the mechanism of action of psychoactive substances and that it might play a seminal role in various mental disorders. The hallucinogenic agent LSD was shown to behave as a potent 5-HT agonist in some peripheral assays and as a potent antagonist in others. The late 1960s and early 1970s, however, witnessed a decline in 5-HT research as the result of three factors: 1) sophisticated techniques were still lacking for the investigation of the central actions of 5-HT: 2) apart from ergolines (LSD-related agents), only a few potent 5-HT agonists or antagonists had been developed: and 3) it was becoming increasingly difficult to understand how a single putative neurotransmitter substance could be involved in so many different central and peripheral actions. The development of histochemical fluorescence techniques and radioligand binding methodology led to the mapping of serotonergic pathways, to identifying binding sites in the brain, and to measuring the affinity (i.e., K_i values) of serotonergic agents for their respective serotonergic receptors. Much of the earlier work on serotonin and on most of the more established serotonergic agents has been reviewed (2); the interested reader is urged to consult this review for references to the primary literature.

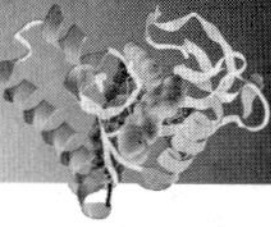

CLINICAL SIGNIFICANCE

Discovery of the different types of serotonin receptors during the past few years has created the potential to target these receptors. Altering the chemical structures may improve tolerability, reduce the risk for side effects, improve efficacy, enhance compliance, or simply provide an alternative drug should another in the class fail to provide relief for a given patient.

The clinical effects of serotonin receptors are multifaceted. At this time, only a few of the identified receptors have drugs that are currently marketed for use in humans. Buspirone stimulates the 5-HT_{1A} receptor to cause antianxiety effects. The 5-HT_{1D} agonists, or the "triptans," vary by side chains on essentially the same core structure to create compounds with different affinities for the 5-HT_{1D} receptors and, likely, for other serotonin receptors as well. The varying affinities of each triptan for receptors change the profiles of their effectiveness and adverse or complimentary effects. As a rule, the triptans work to treat migraine headaches by causing vasoconstriction. Unfortunately, they also may cause coronary vasoconstriction, making them contraindicated in patients with underlying coronary artery disease. Antagonists of the 5-HT_3 receptor, ondansetron and granisetron, work to lessen emesis in chemotherapy-induced and radiation-associated emesis as well as postoperative nausea and vomiting. A variety of drugs work to inhibit selective serotonin reuptake without acting on any specific serotonin receptor. Drugs such as fluoxetine, paroxetine, sertraline, fluvoxamine, and others have been effective in the treatment of depression, obsessive-compulsive disorder, and panic disorder with varying degrees of side effects like weight gain, weight loss, and drowsiness.

Jill T. Johnson, Pharm.D., BCPS
Associate Professor
Department of Pharmacy Practice
College of Pharmacy
University of Arkansas for Medical Sciences

Table 14.1. Some Indications and Treatment Claims for Novel Serotonergic Agents in Recent Patent Literature

Aggression disorders	Esophagitis	Obsessive-compulsive
Alcoholism	Gastric motility	Pain
Alzheimer's disease	Head injury	Panic disorders
Amnesia	Headache	Parkinson's disease
Anorexia	Hypertension	Psychosis
Bulimia	Impotence	Raynaud's disease
Cardiac failure	Irritable bowel syndrome	Schizophrenia
Cardiovascular disorders	Ischemia	Sedation
Cerebrovascular disorders	Migraine	Sexual dysfunction
Cognition	Movement disorders	Sleep disorders
Depression	Nausea	Substance abuse
Drug abuse	Neurodegenerative disease	Substance dependence
Emesis	Obesity	Thromobembolism

RADIOLIGANDS

Radioligand binding techniques measure the affinity of agonists and antagonists for their respective receptors (i.e., K_i values). Radioligands are receptor agonists or antagonists to which a radioactive atom (label) is covalently attached.

Serotonin Biosynthesis, Catabolism, and Function as Targets for Drug Manipulation

Serotonin, or 5-HT, is biosynthesized (3) from its dietary precursor L-tryptophan (Fig. 14.1). Serotonergic neurons contain tryptophan hydroxylase (L-tryptophan-5-monooxygenase) that converts tryptophan to 5-hydroxytryptophan (5-HTP) in what is the rate-limiting step in 5-HT biosynthesis and aromatic L-amino acid decarboxylase (previously called 5-HTP decarboxylase) that decarboxylates 5-HTP to 5-HT. This latter enzyme also is responsible for the conversion of L-DOPA to dopamine (see Chapter 12). The major route of metabolism for 5-HT is oxidative deamination by monoamine oxidase (MAO-A) to the unstable 5-hydroxyindole-3-acetaldehyde, which is either reduced to 5-hydroxytryptophol (~15%) or oxidized to 5-hydroxyindole-3-acetic acid (~85%). In the pineal gland, 5-HT is acetylated by 5-HT N-acetyltransferase to N-acetylserotonin, which undergoes O-methylation by 5-hydroxyindole-O-methyltransferase to melatonin.

Each of the steps in 5-HT biosynthesis, metabolism, and function is a theoretical target for drug manipulation (Fig. 14.2). Tryptophan depletion, by reducing or eliminating dietary tryptophan, can result in decreased 5-HT biosynthesis. Conversely, tryptophan "loading," by increasing dietary tryptophan, can result in the overproduction of 5-HT. This latter effect also can occur in nonserotonergic neurons, such as dopaminergic neurons, because of the nonselective nature of aromatic amino acid decarboxylase. Inhibitors of tryptophan hydroxylase, such as *para*-chlorophenylalanine, are used as pharmacological tools; they are not used therapeutically.

Therapeutically exploited serotonergic targets include the postsynaptic receptors, reuptake mechanisms, and metabolism. The monoamine oxidase (MAO) inhibitors effectively interfere with the oxidative deamination of 5-HT to increase synaptic concentrations of 5-HT. The

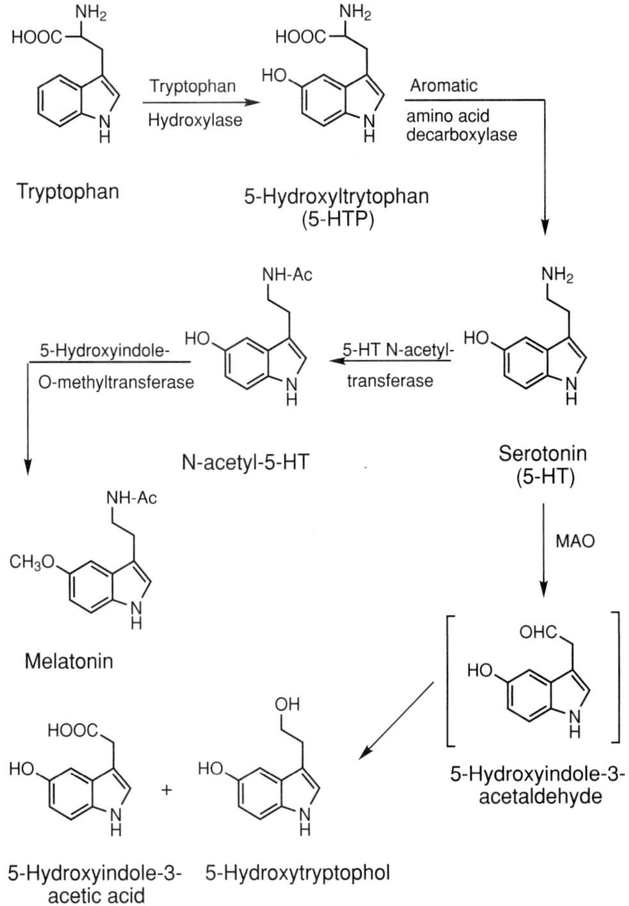

Fig. 14.1. Biosynthesis and catabolism of serotonin. In the pineal, serotonin is converted to melatonin. Ac = acetyl.

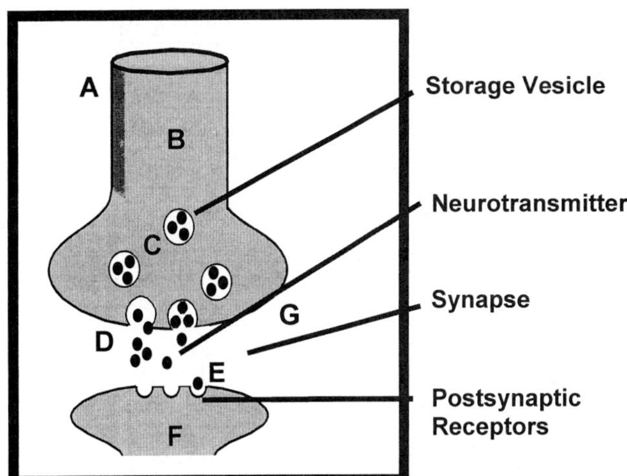

Fig. 14.2. Steps involved in serotonergic neurotransmission. The serotonin precursor tryptophan is taken up into the neuron (A) and converted to 5-HT (B). Synthesized 5-HT is stored in synaptic vesicles (C). Under the appropriate conditions, the synaptic vesicles migrate to and fuse with the cell membrane, releasing their store of 5-HT (D). Released neurotransmitter interacts with postsynaptic receptors (E) and, in the case of G protein–coupled receptors, activates second messenger systems (F). The action of 5-HT is terminated (G) either by diffusion of 5-HT away from the synapse, with subsequent metabolism, or by the 5-HT being taken back up by a 5-HT transporter into the presynaptic neuron (i.e., reuptake), where it can be stored or metabolized.

MAO inhibitor tranylcypromine, for example, has been used since the 1960s as an antidepressant. A problem associated with many MAO inhibitors is that they are notoriously nonselective and can interfere with the metabolism of other neurotransmitters, amines found in certain foods, and exogenously administered amine-containing therapeutic agents.

Tranylcypromine

SEROTONIN RECEPTORS

Seven families or populations of serotonergic receptors have been identified, 5-HT_1 through 5-HT_7, and several are divided into distinct subpopulations (Table 14.2). The discovery of the individual populations and subpopulations of 5-HT receptors follows the approximate order of their numbering, and as a consequence, more is known about 5-HT_1 and 5-HT_2 receptors than about 5-HT_6 and 5-HT_7 receptors. Other factors contributing to our current lack of knowledge about certain receptor populations (i.e., 5-HT_{1E} or 5-HT_5 receptors) is the absence of agonists/antagonists with selectivity for these receptors.

History

Tritiated LSD ([^{3}H]LSD) was the first radioligand used to identify a brain 5-HT binding site, suggesting it to be a "hallucinogen receptor." Tritiated 5-HT ([^{3}H]5-HT)–labeled serotonergic sites displayed high affinity for LSD. Thus, not only did 5-HT and LSD share structural similarity, there was now evidence that these agents might be acting via a common receptor type. According to the interconvertible receptor conformation hypothesis that was popular at the time, 5-HT (known to be an agonist) interacted with the agonist conformation of the receptor, whereas [^{3}H]LSD (LSD being known to be a partial agonist) labeled both the agonist and antagonist conformations. A search was initiated for 5-HT antagonists that could be used as radioligands for studying serotonergic receptors. Following the serendipitous discovery that a tritiated version of the dopamine antagonist spiperone not only labeled dopaminergic receptors but also labeled nondopaminergic receptors in other brain regions, it was shown that 5-HT displayed modest affinity for these sites

Table 14.2. Classification and Nomenclature for the Various Populations of 5-HT Receptors

Populations and Subpopulations	Second Messenger System[a]	Currently Accepted Name[b]	Comments
5-HT_1			
5-HT_{1A}	AC(−)	5-HT_{1A}	Cloned and pharmacological 5-HT_{1A} receptors
5-HT_{1B}	AC(−)	5-HT_{1B}	Rodent homologue of 5-HT_{1B} receptors
$5\text{-HT}_{1B\beta}$			A mouse homologue of $h5\text{-HT}_{1B}$ receptors
5-HT_{1D}			Sites identified in binding studies using human and calf brain homogenates
$5\text{-HT}_{1D\alpha}$	AC(−)	$h5\text{-HT}_{1D}$	A cloned human 5-HT_{1D} subpopulation
$5\text{-HT}_{1D\beta}$	AC(−)	$h5\text{-HT}_{1B}$	A second cloned human 5-HT_{1D} subpopulation; human counterpart of rat 5-HT_{1B}
5-HT_{1E}	AC(−)	5-HT_{1E}	Sites identified in binding studies using brain homogenates and cloned receptors
$5\text{-HT}_{1E\alpha}$			An alternate name that has been used for cloned human 5-HT_{1e} receptors
$5\text{-HT}_{1E\beta}$	AC(−)	5-ht_{1F}	A cloned mouse homologue of 5-HT_{1F} receptors
5-HT_{1F}			A cloned human 5-HT_1 receptor population
5-HT_2			
5-HT_2	PI	5-HT_{2A}	Original "5-HT_2" (sometimes called $5\text{-HT}_{2\alpha}$) receptors
5-HT_{2F}	PI	5-HT_{2B}	5-HT_2-like receptors originally found in rat fundus
5-HT_{1C}	PI	5-HT_{2C}	Originally described as 5-HT_{1C} ($5\text{-HT}_{2\beta}$) receptors
5-HT_3			
5-HT_3	Ion channel	5-HT_3	An ion channel receptor
5-HT_4	AC(+)	5-HT_4	5-HT_4 population originally described in functional studies
5-HT_{4S}			Short form of cloned 5-HT_4 receptors
5-HT_{4L}			Long form of cloned 5-HT_4 receptors
$5\text{-HT}_{4(b)\text{–}4(d)}$			Recently identified human 5-HT_4 receptor isoforms
5-HT_5			
5-HT_{5A}	?	5-HT_{5A}	Cloned mouse, rat and human 5-HT_5 receptors
5-HT_{5B}	?	5-HT_{5A}	Cloned mouse and rat 5-HT_{5A}-like receptor
5-HT_6			
5-HT_6	AC(+)	5-HT_6	Cloned rat and human 5-HT receptor
5-HT_7			
5-HT_7	AC(+)	5-HT_7	Cloned rat, mouse, guinea pig and human 5-HT receptors

[a]AC = adenylate cyclase; (−) = negatively coupled; (+) = positively coupled; PI = phospholipase coupled.
[b]Currently accepted names are taken from Hoyer et al. (8).

and that they might represent 5-HT receptors. Spiperone also was shown to antagonize some of the pharmacological effects of 5-HT. These data, coupled with the additional observation that 5-HT agonists, tended to display higher affinity for [^{3}H]5-HT–labeled sites, whereas 5-HT antagonists displayed higher affinity for [^{3}H]spiperone-labeled sites, led to the conclusion that [^{3}H]5-HT and [^{3}H]spiperone labeled two distinct populations of sites, termed 5-HT_1 and 5-HT_2 receptors, respectively (5). Soon thereafter, 5-HT_1 receptors were found to consist of 5-HT_{1A} and 5-HT_{1B} subpopulations. During the 1950s, Gaddum and Picarelli had demonstrated the existence of two populations of serotonergic receptors in isolated guinea pig ileum and called these receptors 5-HT-D (because the phenoxybenzamine dibenzyline blocked 5-HT at this receptor) and 5-HT-M (because morphine and cocaine blocked the actions of 5-HT at the second population). Later, 5-HT-D receptors were found to be identical with 5-HT_2 receptors, and 5-HT-M receptors were eventually renamed 5-HT_3 receptors. By the early 1980s, 5-HT_{1A}, 5-HT_{1B}, 5-HT_2, and 5-HT_3 receptors had been identified, and interest in 5-HT research exploded. Molecular biology intervened in the late 1980s and early 1990s, which allowed new populations of serotonergic receptors to be cloned and expressed. This led to attempts to develop selective agonists and antagonists for each subpopulation (2,6).

Table 14.2 lists the receptor classification and nomenclatures that have been employed for serotonergic receptors. Other 5-HT orphan receptors that have not yet been cloned include the 5-HT_{1P} receptors, which are found only in the gastrointestinal tract. Care should be used when reading the older primary literature, because 5-HT receptor nomenclature has changed so dramatically and often can be confusing and very frustrating to comprehend.

All of the seven serotonergic receptor populations have been cloned and, together with the cloning of other neurotransmitter receptors, has led to generalizations regarding amino acid sequence homology (7). Any two receptors with amino acid sequences that are approximately 70 to 80% identical in their transmembrane-spanning segments are called the intermediate-homology

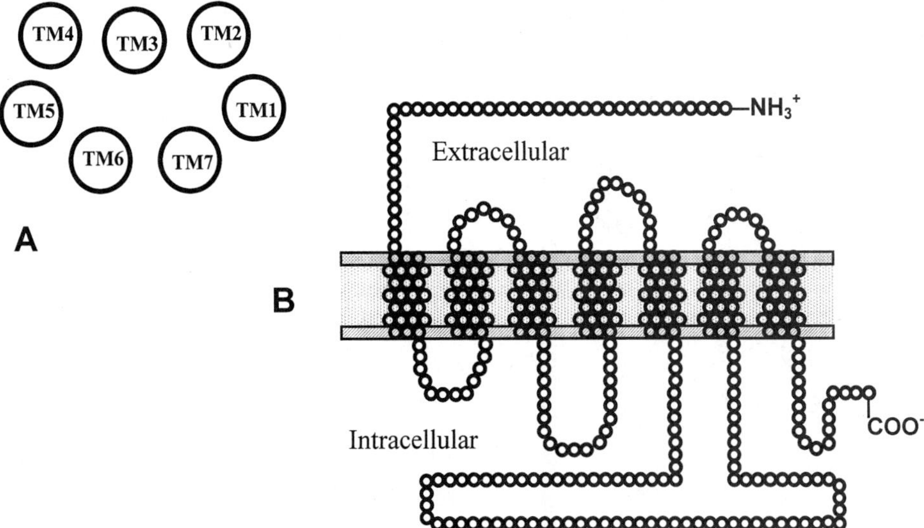

Fig. 14.3. Top (A) and side (B) views of a schematic representation of a typical G protein–coupled receptor. In B, the transmembrane-spanning helical portions are numbered, from left to right, as TM1 to TM7. The seven helices are connected by extracellular and intracellular loops. The large intracellular loop between TM5 and TM6 is believed to be associated with coupling to a second messenger system. The helices are arranged in such a manner that TM1 is adjacent to TM7, as shown in A. Molecular graphics studies suggest that agonists might bind in a manner that utilizes an aspartate residue in TM3 (common to all G protein–coupled 5-HT receptors) and residues in the TM4, TM5, and TM6 regions, whereas antagonists likely utilize the aspartate moiety but residues in the TM6, TM7, and TM1 regions.

group. This group of receptors may be members of the same subfamily and have highly similar to nearly indistinguishable pharmacological profiles or second messenger systems. A low-homology group (~35–55% transmembrane homology) consists of distantly related receptor subtypes from the same neurotransmitter family, and a high-homology group (~95–99% transmembrane homology) consists of species homologues from the same gene in different species (7). Species homologues of the same gene reveal high sequence conservation in regions outside the transmembrane domains, whereas intraspecies receptor subtypes usually are quite different (7). Current 5-HT receptor classification and nomenclature require that several criteria be met before a receptor population can be adequately characterized. Receptor populations must be identified on the basis of drug binding characteristics (operational or recognitory criteria), receptor–effector coupling (transductional criteria), and gene and receptor structure sequences for the nucleotide and amino acid components, respectively (structural criteria) (6–8).

5-HT$_1$ Family

The 5-HT$_1$ receptors were one of the first two populations of 5-HT receptors to be identified (5), and 5-HT$_{1A}$, 5-HT$_{1B}$, 5-HT$_{1C}$ (later renamed 5-HT$_{2C}$), 5-HT$_{1D}$, 5-HT$_{1E}$, and 5-HT$_{1F}$ receptor subfamilies have been subsequently defined and cloned. With the exception of 5-HT$_{1E}$ receptors, all 5-HT$_1$ receptors exhibit high affinity for 5-carboxamidotryptamine (5-CT).

NH2 O H2N N H

5-CT

5-HT$_{1A}$ Receptors and Agents

The 5-HT$_{1A}$ receptors are G protein–coupled receptors that consist of seven transmembrane-spanning helices connected by intracellular and extracellular loops (see Fig. 14.3 for a schematic representation of a generalized G-protein receptor structure). The receptors are negatively coupled to an adenylate cyclase* second messenger system, and the 5-HT$_{1A}$ receptors located in the raphe nuclei correspond to somatodendritic autoreceptors (Fig. 14.4). The 5-HT$_{1A}$ receptors differ significantly in structure from most other 5-HT receptors and exhibit a substantial similarity to adrenergic receptors, which probably explains why a number of adrenergic agents bind at 5-HT$_{1A}$ receptors with high affinity. Cloned 5-HT$_{1A}$ receptors and 5-HT$_{1A}$ ligands have been extensively reviewed (8–18).

*This enzyme is known by two names, *adenylate cyclase (EC 4.6.1.1)*- its official name from the International Union of Biochemistry and Molecular Biology Nomenclature Committee or its alternative name, adenylyl cyclase.

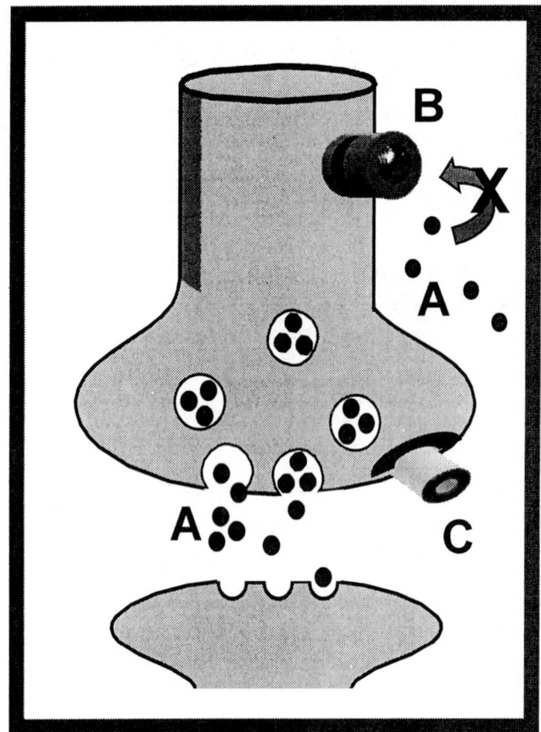

Fig. 14.4. Typical nerve ending showing the cell body (i.e., somatodendritic) autoreceptors (B) and the terminal autoreceptors (C). Neurotransmitter molecules also are shown (A). Neurotransmitters can interact with cell body autoreceptors (B) to regulate synthesis and with terminal autoreceptors (C) to regulate release. Shown above is a drug molecule blocking the cell body autoreceptor and preventing an interaction with the neurotransmitter.

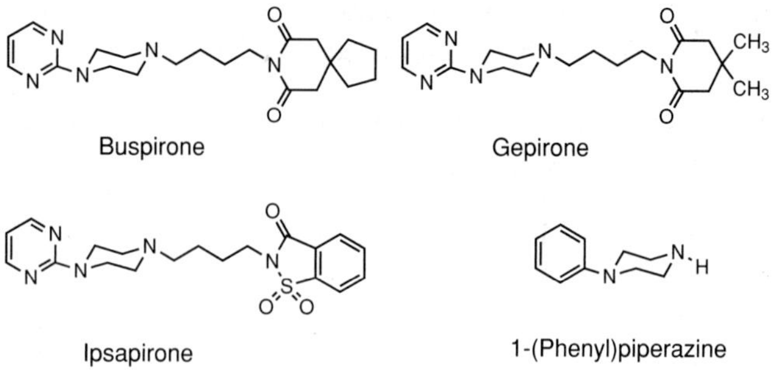

Buspirone Gepirone

Ipsapirone 1-(Phenyl)piperazine

Fig. 14.5. 5-HT_{1A} agonists (arylpiperazines).

STRUCTURE–ACTIVITY RELATIONSHIP OF 5-HT_{1A} AGONISTS

Overview. Numerous tryptamines bind with high affinity at 5-HT_{1A} receptors, but most are notoriously nonselective. One of the most selective 5-HT_{1A} receptor agonists is the aminotetralin derivative 8-hydroxy-2-(di-n-propylamino)tetralin (8-OH DPAT), and its early discovery was significant in advancing an understanding of 5-HT_{1A} receptors. Furthermore, because the structure of 8-OH DPAT is similar to that of 5-HT (8-OH DPAT/serotonin), its activity indicated that an intact indole nucleus was not required for 5-HT_{1A} actions. Although numerous 8-OH DPAT derivatives have been reported, none is used therapeutically because of low oral bioavailability. This has led to efforts to develop novel aminotetralins with greater oral availability.

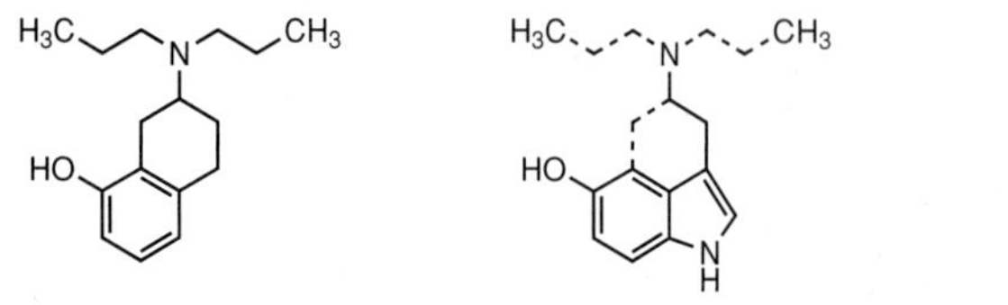

8-OH DPAT 8-OH DPAT superimposed on Serotonin

Long-chain arylpiperazines. Simple arylpiperazines (i.e., those bearing no N_4-substituent or only a small N_4-substituent), such as 1-(phenyl)piperazine (Fig. 14.5), bind with modest to reasonably high affinity at a multitude of receptor types and are nonselective agents. Long-chain arylpiperazines (LCAPs), which are those piperazines possessing an elaborated N_4 substituent, probably represent the largest class of 5-HT_{1A} ligands (13). Buspirone (Fig. 14.5), the first arylpiperazine approved for clinical use as an anxiolytic agent, and the structurally related gepirone and ipsapirone bind at 5-HT_{1A} receptors and behave as agonists or partial agonists. Structure–activity relationships (SARs) and structure–affinity relationships have been formulated, and this has led to LCAPs with enhanced affinity and selectivity for 5-HT_{1A} receptors (12–14). With the LCAPs, there seems to be substantial structural latitude for 5-HT_{1A} binding (14).

The aryl portion of these agents (Fig. 14-6) typically is a phenyl, substituted phenyl, or a heteroaryl group, such as 2-pyrimidinyl. The intact piperazine ring seems to be optimal for binding to 5-HT_{1A} receptors. A spacer or linker separates the N_4-nitrogen atom of the piperazine and the terminus. There has been controversy as to whether the spacer actively participates in binding to the receptor or whether it acts simply as a connector; in any event, a chain of two to five atoms is common. The terminus typically is an amide or imide, but it has been shown that neither is required for binding. Alternatively, it may be a phenyl or some other aryl or heteroaryl substituent (14). With respect to spacer length, when the spacer is -$(CH_2)_n$–, two to four methylene groups appear optimal. Chain length (n) can influence affinity and selectivity. When the terminus contains a heteroarylamide, $n = 4$ seems to be optimal, whereas when the terminus is an alkylamide, optimal affinity is associated with $n = 2$. A region of bulk tolerance is associated with the terminus, or at least a portion thereof, and very bulky groups have been introduced into this part of the molecule (12–14). Some LCAPs are nonselective and may

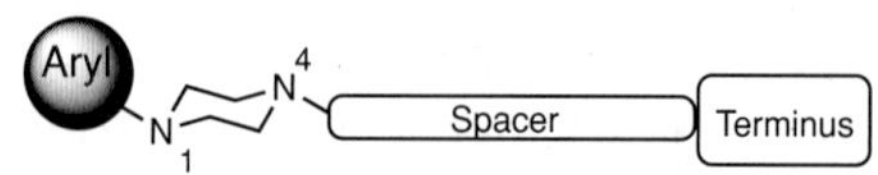

Fig. 14.6. General structure of long-chain arylpiperazines.

variously bind at other populations of 5-HT receptors, dopamine receptors, or adrenergic receptors.

STRUCTURE–ACTIVITY RELATIONSHIP OF 5-HT_{1A} ANTAGONISTS. Many 5-HT_{1A} antagonists possess a 2-methoxyphenyl group with structural similarity to buspirone. BMY 7378 and NAN-190 were among the first agents shown to be very-low-efficacy partial agonists at 5-HT_{1A} receptors and were used as antagonists (Fig. 14.7). Certain aminotetralins (e.g., S(−)UH-301) and arylpiperazines (e.g., WAY 100135 and WAY 100635) represent new classes of 5-HT_{1A} antagonists that are termed "silent antagonists," because they are without any 5-HT_{1A} agonist action. The alkylpiperidine spiperone is a 5-HT_{1A} antagonist, but it displays even greater affinity for D_2-dopamine receptors and 5-HT_{2A} receptors.

Molecular graphics studies suggest (15,16) that 5-HT and 5-HT_{1A} agonists typically interact with amino acid residues associated with helices 4, 5 and 6 (Site 1), whereas 5-HT_{1A} antagonists likely interact with amino acid residues in helices 1, 2, 7 and perhaps, 6 (Site 2). The basic primary amine for both types of agents are thought to bind at a common aspartate residue found in TM helix (TM) 3 (Fig. 14.3). The 5-hydroxy group of 5-HT forms a hydrogen bond with threonine residue in TM5 (15,16).

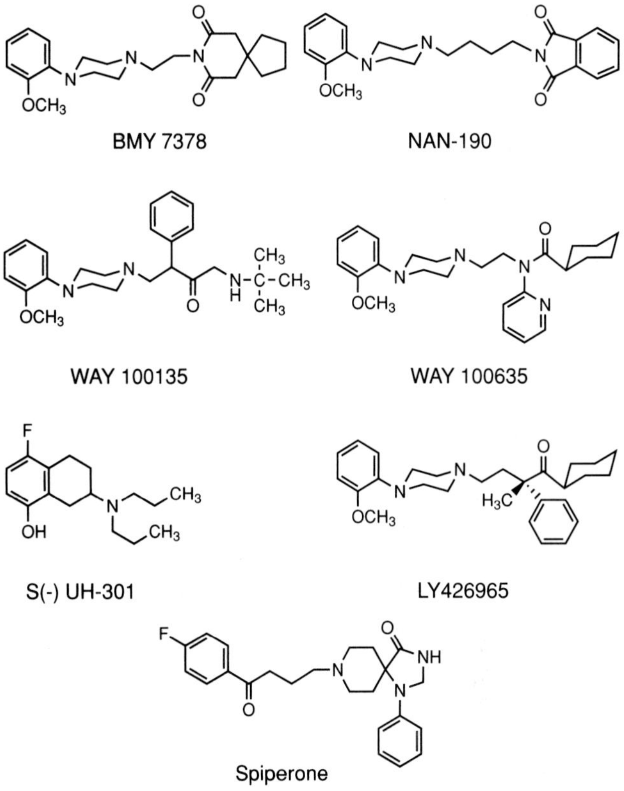

BMY 7378

NAN-190

WAY 100135

WAY 100635

S(-) UH-301

LY426965

Spiperone

Fig. 14.7. 5-HT_{1A} antagonists.

5-HT_{1A} RECEPTOR AGONISTS: CLINICAL SIGNIFICANCE. In preclinical studies, 5-HT_{1A} agonists have demonstrated antianxiety, antidepressant, antiaggressive, and perhaps, anticraving, anticataleptic, antiemetic, and neuroprotective properties (17). Evidence also exists that indicates 5-HT_{1A} receptors might be involved in sleep, impulsivity, alcoholism, sexual behavior, appetite control, thermoregulation, and cardiovascular function (17,19–21). The main focus of drug development for 5-HT_{1A} receptors is their therapeutic potential for the treatment of anxiety and depression (19). Buspirone (Buspar) was the first LCAP to become clinically available as an anxiolytic agent, and a number of structurally related agents hold promise as novel anxiolytics (11,12,22). Additionally, 5-HT_{1A} agents might be useful in the treatment of depression, and there may be a relationship between 5-HT metabolism, depression, and violent behavior. The antianxiety actions of 5-HT_{1A} (partial) agonists may involve primarily presynaptic somatodendritic 5-HT_{1A} receptors, whereas the antidepressant actions of 5-HT_{1A} agents may primarily involve postsynaptic 5-HT_{1A} receptors (17). Gepirone produced marked improvement in depressed patients, and buspirone was effective in the treatment of mixed anxious-depressive patients. The 5-HT_1 and, possibly, 5-HT_{1A} receptors have been implicated in obsessive-compulsive disorders.

5-HT_{1A} RECEPTOR ANTAGONISTS: CLINICAL SIGNIFICANCE. A new direction in 5-HT_{1A} research targets the development of 5-HT_{1A} antagonists (23). Agents such as the dopaminergic antagonist spiperone and the β-adrenergic antagonist propranolol were among the first to see application as 5-HT_{1A} antagonists. These agents are obviously nonselective, however, and bind at other populations of neurotransmitter receptors with higher affinities than they display at 5-HT_{1A} receptors. The next generation of 5-HT_{1A} antagonists, the LCAPs BMY 7378 and NAN-190, possessed postsynaptic antagonist character but also some presynaptic agonist action (14,23) (Fig. 14.7). A third generation of agents—the "silent" 5-HT_{1A} antagonists—has been developed and includes WAY 100635, WAY 100135 (a structural relative of BMY 7378 and NAN-190), and S(−)UH-301 (a derivative of the 5-HT_{1A} agonist 8-OH DPAT); these are both presynaptic and postsynaptic 5-HT_{1A} antagonists (23,24). The silent 5-HT_{1A} antagonists, such as WAY 100135 and S(−)UH-301, are not intrinsically inactive and can indirectly produce non-5-HT_{1A} serotonin-mediated actions (25,26). These antagonists presumably block presynaptic 5-HT_{1A} autoreceptors, increasing the synaptic concentration of 5-HT, which results in the activation of other serotonergic receptor populations. Human evaluation of silent and selective 5-HT_{1A} antagonists should prove interesting and could open new vistas in 5-HT_{1A} research and therapeutics. For example, pretreatment of patients with 5-HT_{1A} antagonists could accelerate the effects of selective 5-HT reuptake inhibitors (SSRIs) and enhance their clinical efficacy as antidepressants (27). The 5-HT_{1A} antagonist WAY 100635 enhances the anorectic effect of citalopram in animals (28) and, thus, may be of benefit in weight reduction. Combination therapy using an SSRI plus a 5-HT_{1A} antagonist, including the β-blocker pindolol, which binds at 5-HT_{1A} receptors, has been reported (29). A new

LCAP, LY426965, is more metabolically stable than WAY 100635 and is orally available. In combination with fluoxetine, LY426965 has been shown to increase extracellular levels of 5-HT beyond that achievable by fluoxetine alone, and it is being examined for the treatment of depression and as a smoking cessation agent (30). The therapeutic potential of 5-HT_{1A} antagonists is quite intriguing.

5-HT_{1B} Receptors and Agents

Overview. Early studies identified 5-HT_{1B} receptors in rodent brain using radioligand binding techniques but failed to find them in human brain. The 5-HT_{1B} receptors are located both presynaptically, where they regulate the release of 5-HT (Fig. 14.4), and postsynaptically (31). Like 5-HT_{1A} receptors, they are negatively coupled to adenylate cyclase. (See 5-HT_{1D} Receptors for further related discussion.)

5-HT_{1B} receptors: clinical significance. Rodent 5-HT_{1B} receptors have been implicated as playing roles in thermoregulation, respiration, appetite control, sexual behavior, aggression, locomotor activity, sleep regulation, sensorimotor inhibition, and anxiety (32).

5-HT_{1D} Receptors

The 5-HT_{1D} receptors were first identified by radioligand binding techniques, and they are widely distributed throughout the CNS (33). They are G protein–linked and are coupled to inhibition of adenylate cyclase. Two human subpopulations of 5-HT_{1D} receptors, 5-$HT_{1D\alpha}$ and 5-$HT_{1D\beta}$ receptors, display approximately 77% sequence homology, and their pharmacological properties are nearly indistinguishable. Because of the high degree of species homology with rat and mouse 5-HT_{1B} receptors, human 5-$HT_{1D\beta}$ receptors have been renamed h5-HT_{1B} receptors. Human 5-$HT_{1D\alpha}$ receptors have been renamed h5-HT_{1D}. Most agents that bind at 5-HT_{1B} receptors typically bind at 5-HT_{1D} receptors. Curious exceptions have been observed with certain aryloxyalkylamines, however, such as the β-blockers, propranolol, and pindolol, which exhibit very low affinity (K_i > 5,000 nM) for h5-HT_{1D} receptors (34,35). The major functional difference between rat 5-HT_{1B} receptors and human h5-HT_{1B} receptors has been attributed to both the presence of a threonine residue at position 355 (i.e., Thr 355) in TM7 of the latter and the presence of an asparagine residue at the corresponding position in 5-HT_{1B} receptors; site-directed mutagenesis studies have demonstrated that conversion of Thr 355 to an asparagine (i.e., a T355N mutant) accounts for the binding differences of certain ligands (e.g., aryloxyalkylamines such as propranolol). Combined ligand SAR, site-directed mutagenesis, and molecular modeling studies have led to the conclusion that although most typical serotonergic agonists bind in the central cavity formed by TM3, TM4, TM5, and TM6 (Site 1) (Fig. 14.3), propranolol most likely occupies the region defined by TM1, TM2, TM3, and TM7 (Site 2). The higher affinity of propranolol for the T355N mutant 5-HT_{1B} receptors relative to the wild-type receptors was specifically attributed to the formation of two hydrogen bonds between the receptor asparagine and the ether and hydroxyl oxygen atoms of propranolol (35).

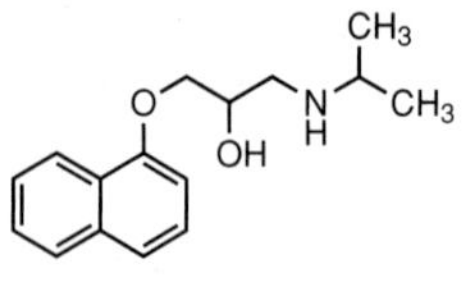

Propranolol 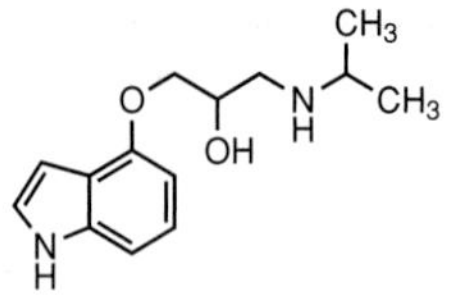 Pindolol

5-HT_{1D} agonists and antagonists. There are few 5-HT_{1D}-selective agonists, but one agent commonly referred to as a prototypical 5-HT_{1D} agonist is sumatriptan (Imitrex). Sumatriptan, however, exhibits only 2- to 20-fold greater selectivity for the 5-HT_{1D} receptors than for certain other populations of 5-HT_1 receptors, binds at h5-HT_{1D} and h5-HT_{1B} receptors with nearly identical affinity, and also binds at 5-HT_{1F} receptors (36). Structure–activity relationships for 5-HT_{1D} agonists have been reported for many indolealkylamines or tryptamine derivatives, which bind with high affinity but with little selectivity. New agents displaying high affinity and reasonable selectivity for h5-HT_{1D}/h5-HT_{1B} receptors over other populations of 5-HT receptors (37) include, for example, zolmitriptan (Zomig), naratriptan (Amerge), rizatriptan (Maxalt), and alniditan. Of these, all are tryptamine derivatives or sumatriptan-related structures except for the benzopyran alniditan. Many of these are commercially available or currently undergoing clinical trials. Other investigational agonists are shown in Figure 14.8.

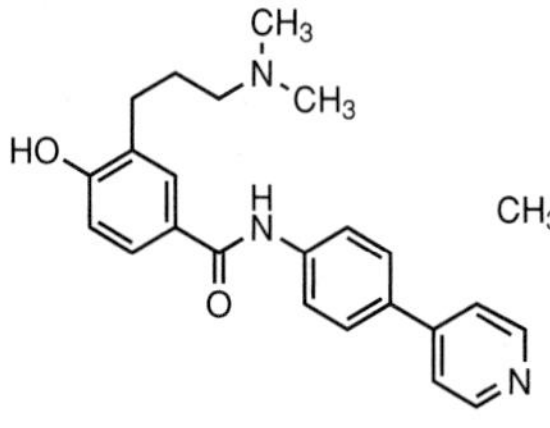

GR 55562 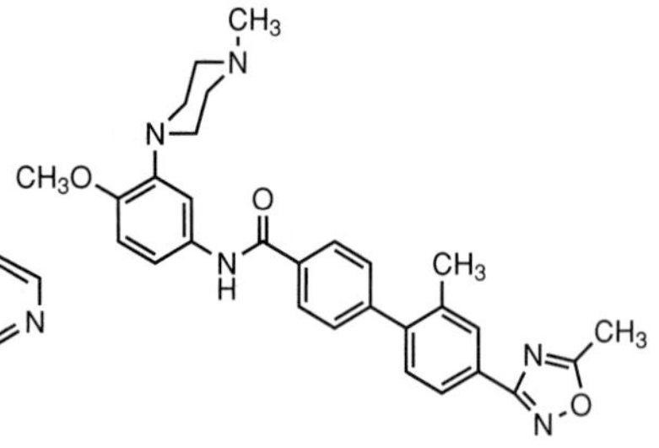 GR 127935

Several 5-HT_{1D} receptor antagonists have been developed, including GR127935 (high affinity for h5-HT_{1D}/h5-HT_{1B} receptors but possibly a low-efficacy partial agonist) and GR55562. Both of these agents antagonize many of the effects of sumatriptan.

5-HT_{1D} receptors: clinical significance. The clinical significance of 5-HT_{1D} receptors remains largely unknown. These receptors are speculated to be involved in anxiety, depression, and other neuropsychiatric disorders, but this remains to be substantiated. Recent studies show, however, that 5-HT_{1D} receptors are the dominant species in human cerebral blood vessels. Sumatriptan and several closely related agents are clinically effective in the treatment of migraine, and logical extrapolation implies a role for 5-HT_{1D} receptors in this disorder. Agents with 5-HT_{1D} agonist activity that have found application in the treatment of migraine are, as a group, termed "triptans," because the first agent introduced was sumatriptan. As efficacious as the triptans may be, however, it is unknown if their activity involves action only in the periphery or in the CNS as well (38). Sumatriptan is a h5-HT_{1B} and h5-HT_{1D} agonist. It also is an agonist at 5-HT_{1F} receptors. Most triptans share a similar binding profile. The vasoconstrictor properties of sumatriptan probably are mediated by its action on arterial smooth muscle. The triptans also are believed to inhibit the activation of peripheral nociceptors (38), and this might be related to the localization of 5-HT_{1D} receptors on peptide nociceptors.

Relatively little sumatriptan normally penetrates the blood-brain barrier. Although it has been speculated that transient changes in blood-brain barrier permeability might occur during migraine attacks, agents with greater lipophilicity (and, hence, enhanced ability to penetrate the blood-brain barrier) have been introduced, including zolmitriptan and rizatriptan (Table 14.3), Their greater lipophilicity, however, does not seem to correlate with significantly improved clinical efficacy over sumatriptan (38). Other triptans (Fig. 14.8) currently being examined include eletriptan, almotriptan, donatriptan, and frovatriptan (37).

In general, the newer triptans (e.g. zolmitriptan, rizatriptan, and naratriptan) have a higher oral bioavailability and longer plasma half-life than sumatriptan (39,40) (Table 14.3). Additionally, most triptans bind at 5-HT_{1F} receptors, and 5-HT_{1F} receptor agonists have demonstrated efficacy in the treatment of migraine (41). At this time, it is not known whether 5-HT_{1D} (i.e., h5-HT_{1B} and h5-HT_{1D}), 5-HT_{1F}, or a combination of 5-$HT_{1D/1F}$ actions are most important for the treatment of migraine. The 5-HT receptor binding characteristics of various triptans have been compared (37).

The safety of the triptans has been established, with more than 8 million patients treating greater than 340 million attacks with sumatriptan alone. All triptans narrow coronary arteries by 10 to 20% at clinical doses and should not be administered to patients with coronary or cerebrovascular disease. Triptans having the potential for significant drug–drug interactions include sumatriptan, naratriptan, rizatriptan, almotriptan, and MAO inhibitors; rizatriptan and propanolol; zolmitriptan and cimetidine; and zolmitriptan, naratriptan, and eletriptan and CYP3A4-metabolized drugs and P-glycoprotein pump inhibitors.

The rational employment of triptans should be governed by the use of these medications for patients with disability associated with migraine. Patients with greater than 10 days of at least 50% disability during 3 months have benefited from treatment with triptans as their first-line treatment for acute attacks. When the decision has been made to treat with a triptan, the patient should be instructed to treat early in the attack, when the pain is at a mild phase. This approach increases the likelihood of achieving a pain-free response, with fewer adverse events and lower likelihood of the headache recurring.

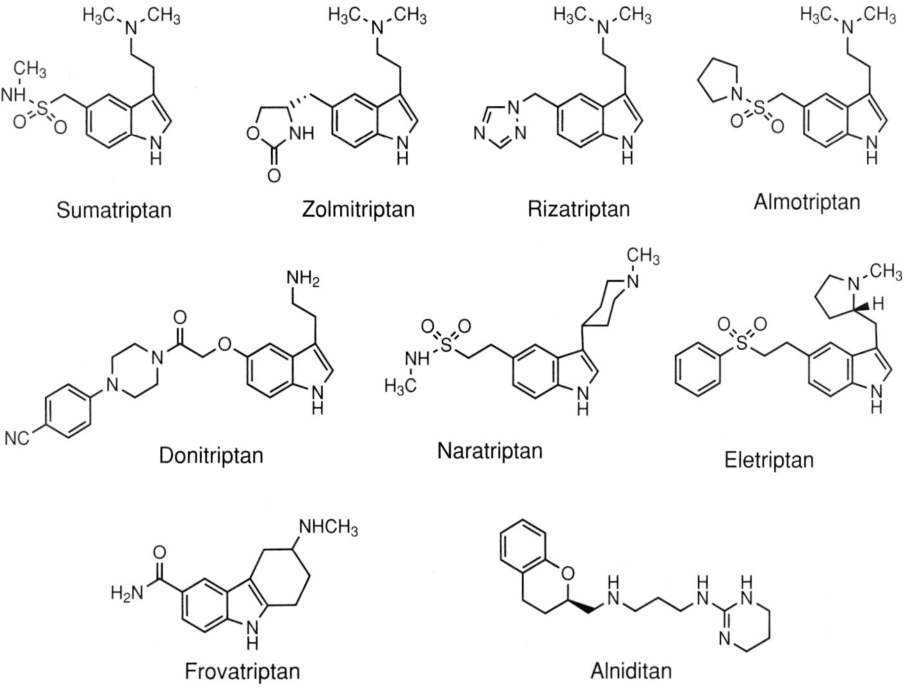

Fig. 14.8. 5-HT_{1D} receptor agonists.

Table 14.3. Pharmacokinetics of the 5-HT_1 Agonists (the Triptans)

Parameters	Sumatriptan	Zolmitriptan	Naratriptan	Rizatriptan	Almotriptan	Frovatriptan	Eletriptan
Trade name	Imitrex	Zomig	Amerge	Maxalt	Axert	Frova	Relpax
Log P (calc)[a]	0.7 ± 0.6	1.6 ± 0.4	1.4 ± 0.6	0.9 ± 0.6	1.9 ± 0.6	0.9 ± 0.4	3.1 ± 0.6
Log D (pH 7) (calc)[a]	−1.7	−0.8	−1.2	−1.4	−0.5	−2.1	0.18
Bioavailability (%)							
Oral	14–15[b]	40–50[b]	70[c] Female: 75 Male: 60	40–50[b]	70–80	20–30[b] Female: ~30 Male: ~20	50[cd]
Nasal	17	102	—	—	—	—	—
SQ (subcutaneous)	97		—	—	—	—	—
Protein binding (%)	14–20	25	28–30	14	35	15	85
Volume of distribution (L/kg)	50	PO: 7 Nasal: 4	170	110–140	180–200	3–4	2.0–2.5
Elimination half-life (h)	PO: 2.5 SC: 2.5	PO: 2–3 Nasal: 3–4	5–6	2.3	PO: 3–4 SC: 3–4	25	4–5 Elderly: 6
Major metabolites (%)	Indoleacetic acid Glucuronides Hepatic: 60%	N-demethyl (act): 4 Indoleacetate: 31	Hepatic: 50%	Indolacetate N-demethyl (act) 6-OH	Indolacetate GABA N-demethyl Hepatic: 60%	N-demethyl (act) N-Ac demethyl	N-demethyl (act)
Metabolizing enzymes	MAO-A	CYP3A4	CYP3A4 MAO-A	MAO-A CYP3A4	CYP3A4/ CYP2D6:12% MAO-A: 27%	CYP1A2	CYP3A4
Excretion (%)	PO: Urine metab: ~60 Feces metab: ~40 Unchanged: 3–22	Urine metab: 60 Feces metab: 30 Unchanged: <10	Urine metab: 30 Feces metab: ~15	Urine metab: 80 Feces metab: 12 Unchanged: 14	Urine metab: 75 Feces metab: 10 Unchanged: 40–50	Urine metab: 10–30 Feces metab: 60	Urine metab: ~ 90% Unchanged: <10
Time to peak concentration (min)	SQ: 12 (5–20) Nasal: 60–90 PO: 60–120	PO: 120–240 Nasal: 180–240	PO: 60–180	PO: 60–90	PO: 60–240 SC: <30	120–240	60–90
Onset (min)	SQ: <10 Nasal: <15 PO: <30	PO: 60	PO: 60–180	PO: 30–120	PO: 60–120 SC: 60–120	PO: 120	PO: <60
Dosage range (mg)	SQ: 6 Nasal: 5–20 PO: 25–100 Max PO: 200/24 h Duration PO: 2–4 h	PO: 1.25–5.00 Max PO: 10/24 h	PO: 1.0–2.5 Max PO: 5/24 h Duration PO: <24 h	PO: 5–10 Max PO: 25/24 h Duration PO: 14–16 h	6.25–12.5 Max PO: 25/24 h	PO: 2.5–5.0 Max PO: 7.5/24 h Duration PO: <24 h	PO: 20–40 Max PO: 80/24 h Duration PO: 18 h

[a]Chemical Abstracts, American Chemical Society, calculated using Advanced Chemistry Development (ACD/Labs) Software V8.14 for Solaris (1994-2006 ACD/Labs).
[b]First-pass metabolism.
[c]Delayed by food.
[d]Slower onset during migraine attack.

5-HT_{1E} Receptors and Agents

The masking of brain 5-HT_{1A} and 5-HT_{1B} receptors in radioligand binding studies using [^{3}H]5-HT as radioligand resulted in biphasic competition curves, providing evidence for additional 5-HT_1-like receptor populations. One of these was the 5-HT_{1D} receptors, and the other was termed 5-HT_{1E}. The low affinity of 5-CT and ergotamine for 5-HT_{1E} receptors allowed their differentiation from 5-HT_{1D} receptors. Simple O-methylation of 5-HT reduces the affinity of 5-HT for this receptor by approximately 100- to 300-fold (42,43). The receptors have been cloned, and typically, ergolines, such as ergonovine and methylergonovine, bind to 5-HT_{1E} receptors with K_i values in the 100 nM range. Studies indicate that these receptors are negatively coupled to adenylate cyclase. No 5-HT_{1E}-selective agonists or antagonists have been reported.

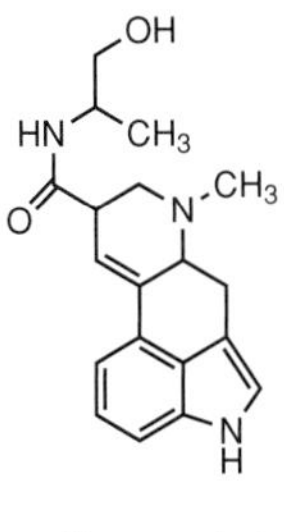

Ergonovine

5-HT_{1F} Receptors

Overview. The newest 5-HT_1 receptor subpopulation to be cloned is the human 5-HT_{1F} receptor (44), which exhibits intermediate (~50–70%) amino acid sequence homology with other 5-HT_1 receptor subpopulations. The receptors are coupled to inhibition of adenylate cyclase. Detection of these receptors in the uterus and mesentery suggest a possible role in vascular contraction. Although their distribution in the brain appears to be limited, distributional similarities with h5-HT_{1B} receptors are observed. A 4-(3-indolyl)piperidine, LY-334370, and an aminocarbazole, LY-344864, have been identified as the first 5-HT_{1F}-selective agonists (45). The nonselective 5-HT_1 antagonist methiothepin also has been shown to act as a 5-HT_{1F} antagonist.

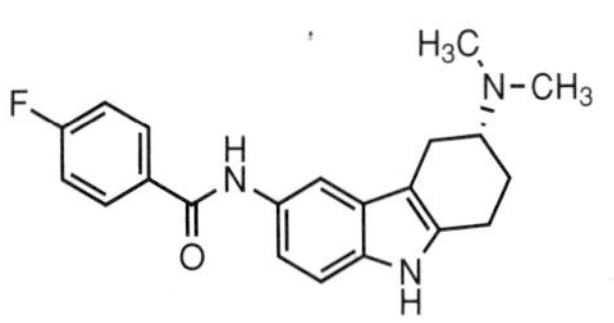

LY-344864 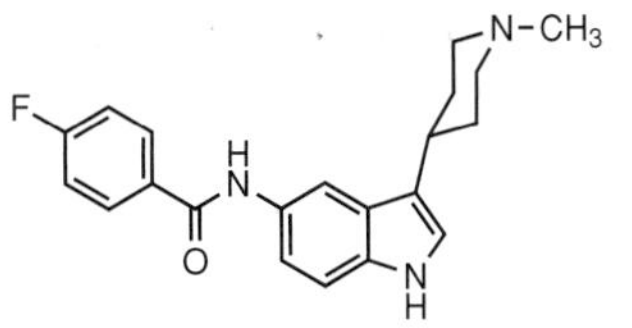 LY-334370

5-HT_{1F} Receptors: Clinical Significance. The clinical significance of 5-HT_{1F} receptors is unknown at this time. The binding of sumatriptan to this receptor population suggests a relationship between 5-HT_{1F} receptor binding and antimigraine activity. Other antimigraine agents, including naratriptan, rizatriptan, and zolmitriptan, also bind at 5-HT_{1F} receptors (37). Recent studies show that 5-HT_{1D} receptors are the dominant species in human cerebral blood vessels and that 5-HT_{1F} receptors also are expressed in both neural and vascular tissue; however, 5-HT_{1F} agents might play a role in migraine as well (41).

5-HT_2 Family

Serotonin receptors were first divided into 5-HT_1 and 5-HT_2 receptor families in 1979 (5), and the latter was subsequently divided into the subfamilies 5-HT_{2A}, 5-HT_{2B}, and 5-HT_{2C} (formerly 5-HT_{1C}) receptors. The term "5-HT_2" now refers to a receptor family, not to an individual population of receptors. Ketanserin (Fig. 14.9) was identified early as a 5-HT_2 antagonist with no affinity for 5-HT_1 receptors, and [^{3}H]ketanserin was introduced as a radioligand to label 5-HT_2 receptors. 1-(2,5-Dimethoxy-4X-phenyl)-2-aminopropane, where X = -Br and -I (DOB and DOI, respectively) were introduced as 5-HT_2 agonists. A significant amount of pharmacology was published, and structure–activity studies led to the development of many novel agents (46). Many of the original agents thought to be 5-HT_2-selective, including standard antagonists such as ketanserin and the agonists DOB and DOI, were later shown to bind nonselectively both to 5-HT_{2A} and 5-HT_{2C} receptors. Consequently, pharmacological actions originally thought to be 5-HT_2-mediated might actually involve 5-HT_{2A} receptors, 5-HT_{2C} receptors, or a combination of 5-HT_{2A} and 5-HT_{2C} receptors. The structures of the three 5-HT_2 receptor subpopulations were found to be consistent with those of transmembrane-spanning G protein–coupled receptors, and the receptors all utilize a phospholipase C second messenger system. Approximately 70 to 80% sequence homology is found among the three receptor subtypes. Only very recently have novel agents with subpopulation selectivity been reported.

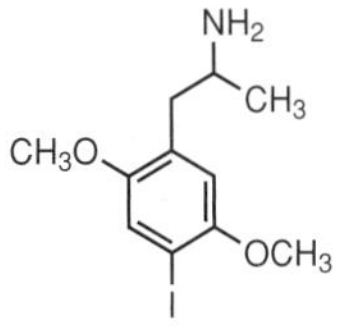

DOI 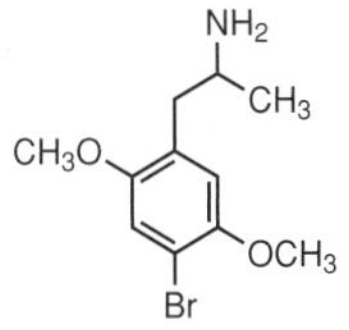 DOB

5-HT_{2A} Receptors

The 5-HT_{2A} receptors, formerly called the 5-HT_2 receptors, have been extensively reviewed (10,46–50). The 5-HT_{2A} receptors have been cloned from various species, including human, and exhibit a high degree (>90%) of species homology. Significant (78%) amino acid sequence homology is found between the transmembrane portions of 5-HT_{2A} receptors and cloned 5-HT_{2C} receptors, which may explain the observed similarities in the binding of various ligands at the two receptor populations. Evidence was provided that 5-HT_{2A} receptors exist in a high-affinity state and a low-affinity state (sometimes referred to as the 5-HT_{2H} and 5-HT_{2L} state, respectively). Under normal conditions, the low-affinity state predominates. The tritiated antagonist [^{3}H]ketanserin has comparable affinity for both states, whereas agonists display higher affinity for the high-affinity state (e.g., when a tritiated agonist is employed as radioligand).

5-HT_{2A} AGONISTS. The SARs for 5-HT_{2A} binding have been reviewed (8,13,46,50). Most indolealkylamines are nonselective 5-HT_{2A} ligands, and they typically bind with higher affinity at the tritiated agonist–labeled high-affinity state. Recent investigations suggest that all indolealkylamines may not bind in the same manner at 5-HT_{2A} receptors (51). Phenylalkylamines, such as DOB and DOI, act as 5-HT_{2A} agonists or high-efficacy partial agonists (see Chapter 23) and are significantly more selective than the indolealkylamines because of their low affinity for non-5-HT_{2A} sites, but they do not differentiate between 5-HT_2 subpopulations.

5-HT_{2A} ANTAGONISTS. One of the largest and more selective classes of 5-HT_{2A} antagonists are the N-alkylpiperidines. The best-known examples are ketanserin and ritanserin. Although numerous ketanserin-related derivatives have been reported, their SARs still have not been well defined. Nevertheless, far less than the entire structure of ketanserin is required for high affinity. Spiperone (Fig. 14.7) has been employed as a 5-HT_{2A} antagonist with 1,000-fold selectivity for 5-HT_{2A} versus 5-HT_{2C} receptors, but it also is a dopamine antagonist, a 5-HT_{1A} antagonist, and a 5-HT_7 antagonist. Other structurally-related agents, such as the piperazine derivative irindalone, also act as 5-HT_{2A} antagonists. Many 5-HT_{2A} antagonists, although fairly selective for 5-$HT_{2A/2C}$ receptors versus most other populations of 5-HT receptors, bind with modest to high affinity at dopaminergic, histaminergic, or adrenergic neurotransmitter receptors. The tricyclic antipsychotics, atypical antipsychotics (risperidone, clozapine, and olanzapine) (Fig. 14.9), and tricyclic antidepressants also bind at 5-HT_{2A} receptors. Current research is focused on 5-HT_2 subtype-selective antagonists, and the most popular 5-HT_{2A}-selective antagonist is MDL 100,907 (also called M100907).

5-HT_{2A} RECEPTORS: CLINICAL IMPLICATIONS

Overview. The potential therapeutic roles of 5-HT_{2A} ligands and the possible involvement of 5-HT_{2A} receptors in modulating normal physiologic functions and various pathologic and psychopathologic conditions have been extensively reviewed (10,20,21). The 5-HT_{2A} receptors appear to play a role in thermoregulation and sleep, and they might be involved in appetite control, learning , and along with various other serotonergic receptor populations, cardiovascular function and muscle contraction. Many of the clinical implications of 5-HT_{2A} receptors actually may involve 5-HT_{2C} receptors or a combination of 5-HT_{2A} and 5-HT_{2C} receptors, both because of the high homology between the two populations and because the investigations were conducted before the discovery of subpopulations of 5-HT_2 receptors. With the recent development of subpopulation-selective agents, this is currently an important area of research.

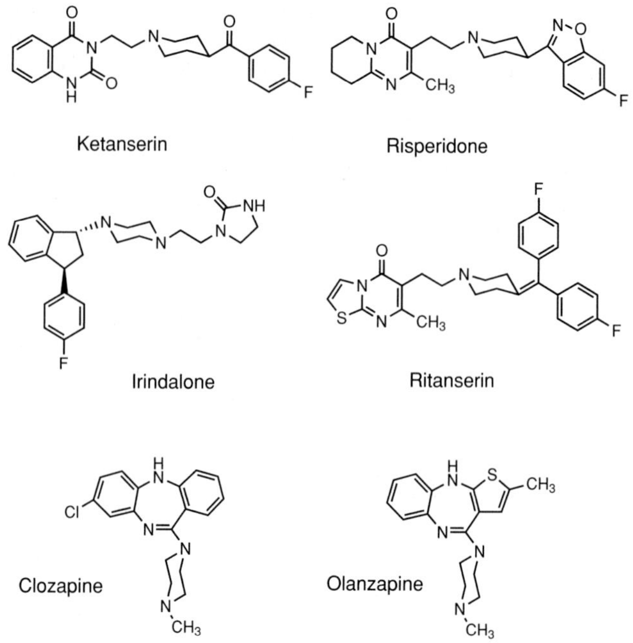

Ketanserin

Risperidone

Irindalone

Ritanserin

Clozapine

Olanzapine

Fig. 14.9. 5-HT_{2A} antagonists.

Antipsychotic agents and antidepressants. Various typical and atypical antipsychotic agents (see Chapter 22) and antidepressants (see Chapter 21) bind with relatively high affinity at 5-HT_{2A} receptors as antagonists (52,53). Although no direct correlation exists between their receptor affinities and clinically effective doses, strong evidence suggests that these disorders involve, at least to some extent, 5-HT_{2A} receptors. For example, chronic administration of 5-HT_{2A} antagonists results in a paradoxical downregulation of 5-HT_{2A} receptors. Such a downregulation would be of benefit in the treatment of depression. Several 5-HT_{2A} antagonists, such as risperidone, seem to possess antipsychotic activity. Many 5-HT_{2A} antagonists also bind at dopamine receptors. Although this may obfuscate the role of 5-HT_{2A} antagonism versus dopamine antagonism as being the more important for antipsychotic activity, it has been suggested that certain types of schizophrenia might actually be more responsive to the combined effect. That is, D_2-dopaminergic antagonists seem to be more effective for treating the positive symptoms of schizophrenia, whereas the 5-HT_{2A} antagonists might be more effective in treating the negative symptoms. Certain atypical antipsychotic agents (e.g., clozapine, olanzepine quetiapine, risperidone, and ziprasidone) bind both to dopamine and to 5-HT_{2A} receptors, suggesting an atypicality theory of psychosis (52,54). This theory suggests that the 5-HT_{2A} component of binding may be related to the decrease in extrapyramidal side effects associated with these types of agents. Those drugs that display a D_2/5-HT_{2A} ratio of greater than one seem to produce fewer extrapyramidal effects than those with ratios of less than one. The atypical antipsychotic agent clozapine, for example, has a D_2/5-HT_{2A} ratio of 10 to 20. From preclinical studies, there are indications that 5-HT_{2A} antagonists possess anxiolytic properties; for example, ritanserin (Fig. 14.9) has been demonstrated to produce both antipsychotic and antianxiety effects in humans. The role of 5-HT receptors in anxiety has been reviewed elsewhere (22).

The 5-HT_{2A} receptors may be involved in the actions of the classical hallucinogens (55) (see Chapter 23). Although indolealkylamine (e.g., 5-methoxy-N,N-dimethyltryptamine [5-OMe DMT]) and ergot-related (e.g., LSD) classical hallucinogens are fairly nonselective ligands that bind to multiple populations of serotonergic receptors, the phenylalkylamine hallucinogens (e.g., DOB, and DOI) are much more 5-HT_2-selective agonists. Furthermore, a significant correlation exists between the human hallucinogenic potencies of classical hallucinogens and their 5-HT_{2A} receptor affinities (55). Interestingly, phenylalkylamine hallucinogens also bind at 5-HT_{2B} and 5-HT_{2C} receptors, and here, too, a significant correlation is found between human potency and receptor affinity for 17 different agents (56). Recent studies suggest that 5-HT_{2A} receptors may play a more prominent role than 5-HT_{2B} or 5-HT_{2C} receptors for the behavioral actions of hallucinogens (56), and differences may exist in the manner in which hallucinogens activate the different receptor populations (57,58).

5-HT_{2B} Receptors

The rat fundus preparation is a peripheral tissue assay that has been used as a functional assay for serotonergic action for approximately 50 years. Long-standing questions concerning the pharmacological similarity of serotonergic fundus receptors (now called 5-HT_{2B} receptors) to the 5-HT_2 family of receptors were answered once they were cloned (59). The 5-HT_{2B} receptors exhibit approximately 70% homology to 5-HT_{2A} and 5-HT_{2C} receptors, and like 5-HT_{2A} receptors, they appear to couple functionally to phosphoinositol hydrolysis. Nevertheless, rat and human 5-HT_{2B} receptors display more than 90% transmembrane sequence homology. Therefore, most agents that bind at rat 5-HT_{2B} receptors also bind with similar affinity at human 5-HT_{2B} receptors. There are, however, some exceptions (60). The standard 5-HT_{2A} antagonist ketanserin and the 5-HT_{2A} agonists DOI and DOB display higher affinity for 5-HT_{2A} and 5-HT_{2C} receptors than for 5-HT_{2B} receptors (56). Nevertheless, a number of DOI-related hallucinogens have been shown to bind at 5-HT_{2B} receptors with modest affinity (56). Evidence suggests that human 5-HT_{2B} receptors, like human 5-HT_{2A} receptors, also exist in high-affinity and low-affinity states (60). The 5-HT_{2B} receptors are found on cardiovascular tissue. Activation of such receptors by agents with a 5-HT_{2B} agonist character might result in cardiac valvulopathy; valvular heart disease associated with the anorectic agent fenfluramine might involve its metabolism to norfenfluramine—a high affinity 5-HT_{2B} agonist (61). The designer drug MDMA (Ecstasy) and its N-desmethyl analogue MDA also show a 5-HT_{2B} agonist character (62).

5-HT_{2C} Receptors

The 5-HT_{2C} receptors, formerly called 5-HT_{1C} receptors, originally were identified in various regions of the brain using autoradiographic and radioligand binding techniques. Cloned human 5-HT_{2C} receptors display a high amino acid sequence homology with 5-HT_{2A} receptors, and like 5-HT_{2A} receptors, they are coupled to phosphoinositol hydrolysis. As previously mentioned, some pharmacological functions once attributed to 5-HT_{2A} receptors actually might involve a 5-HT_{2C} mechanism. For example, the hyperthermic activity of a series of phenylisopropylamines is significantly correlated not only with 5-HT_{2A} but also with their 5-HT_{2C} receptor affinity. Numerous atypical antipsychotic agents bind at 5-HT_{2C} receptors as well as at 5-HT_{2A} receptors; however, no significant correlation exists between their atypical properties and binding affinity. The 5-HT_{2C} receptors may play a greater role than 5-HT_{2A} receptors in migraine. Other preclinical studies also suggest that 5-HT_{2C} receptors might be involved in anxiolytic activity (63) or be targeted for the treatment of obesity (64). The 5-HT_{2C} agonist 1-(3-chlorophenyl)piperazine (*m*CPP) produces an appetite suppressant effect in rodents.

Newer 5-HT_2 Subpopulation-Selective Agents

Although numerous SARs for overall 5-HT_2 binding and pharmacology have been published, very few agents at present can discriminate between subpopulations of 5-HT_2 receptors. In fact, relatively few agents have even been examined in all three 5-HT_2 subpopulations. Spiperone, MDL 100,907, and AMI-193 are among the most 5-HT_{2A}-selective antagonists available (65) (Fig. 14.10). Spiperone and AMI-193 bind at 5-HT_{2A} receptors with 1,000- to 3,000-fold selectivity relative to 5-HT_{2C} receptors but display higher affinity for 5-HT_{1A} and D_2 dopamine receptors. A newer member of this series, KML-010, is a spiperone-related derivative that lacks affinity for 5-HT_{2C} and 5-HT_{1A} receptors and binds at D_2-dopamine receptors with low affinity (65). MDL 11,939 displays more than 300-fold selectivity for 5-HT_{2A} versus 5-HT_{2C} receptors, and its affinity and selectivity are primarily associated with its R-(−)-enantiomer, MDL 100,907 (66). The latter agent is one of the best-investigated 5-HT_{2A}-selective antagonists, and it has been examined as a novel antipsychotic agent in humans. A series of 1-substituted β-carbolines (e.g., LY-23728, LY-287375, and LY-266097) has been reported to be the first 5-HT_{2B}-selective antagonists. SB-221284 shows 100-fold selectivity for 5-HT_{2C} versus 5-$HT_{2A/2B}$ receptors and is probably the most 5-HT_{2C}-selective antagonist to date.

Much less work has been done with 5-HT_2 subpopulation-selective agonists. Mounting evidence suggests that many of the behavioral properties of DOB-like

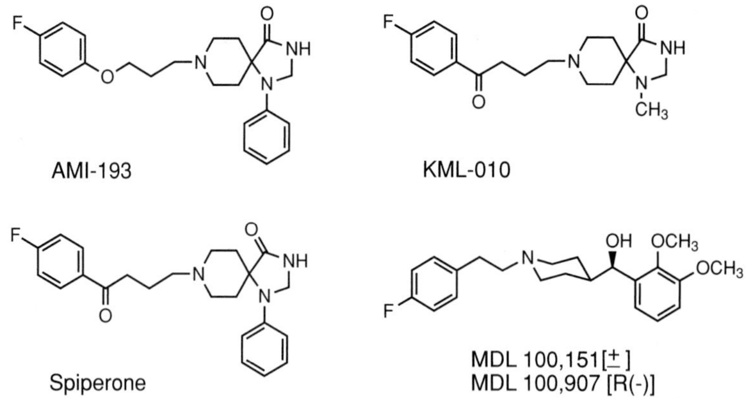

AMI-193

KML-010

Spiperone

MDL 100,151[±]
MDL 100,907 [R(-)]

Fig. 14.10. Typical examples of newer 5-HT_2 subpopulation selective agents.

phenylisopropylamines are mediated by 5-HT_{2A} receptors. A series of isotryptamine derivatives, including Ro 60-0175 (ORG-35030), has been shown to display up to 1,000-fold selectivity for 5-HT_{2C} versus 5-HT_{2A} receptors and to possess 5-HT agonist activity; structurally related tricyclic analogues, such as Ro 60-0332 (ORG-35035), also have been examined and display more than 100-fold selectivity (67). 10-Methoxy-9-methylpyrazino[1,2-a]indole, Ro 60-0175, and Ro 60-0332 all were active in animal models predictive of therapeutic utility for obsessive-compulsive disorders, panic disorders, and depression (67).

It is still not known with confidence specifically what pharmacological effects are related to what 5-HT_2 subpopulation. Nevertheless, results with the newer agents indicate that 5-HT_{2A} receptors might be involved in psychosis, depression, and hallucinogenic activity and that 5-HT_{2C} receptors may play a role in obsessive-compulsive disorders, panic, anxiety, depression, and eating disorders. In the periphery, 5-HT_{2B} receptors seem to be involved in muscle contraction; however, their function in the CNS is still a matter of speculation. On the basis of some preliminary studies and considering their central distribution in brain, 5-HT_{2B} receptors might be involved in anxiety, cognition, food intake, neuroendocrine regulation, locomotor coordination, and balance (68). Several novel approaches may assist in further elucidating the roles of these subpopulations and in the development of site-selective agents. For example, site-directed mutagenesis and synthesis of chimeric receptors, coupled with the use of molecular graphics modeling studies, are beginning to identify what portions of the receptors are important for ligand binding (49).

5-HT_3 Receptors

Unlike most 5-HT receptor populations, early 5-HT_3 pharmacology relied almost exclusively on functional assays. It took a number of years before radioligands were available to identify 5-HT_3 receptors in brain. The 5-HT_3 receptors are unique among the families of serotonergic receptors in that they are nonselective Na^+/K^+ ion channel receptors (Fig. 14.11). They are found in the periphery and in the CNS, and they bear greater structural and functional similarity to nicotinic acetylcholinergic receptors than to other members of the 5-HT receptor family (69,70). Evidence indicates that 5-HT_3 receptors modulate release of other neurotransmitters, including dopamine, acetylcholine, GABA, and serotonin (71).

Structure–Activity Relationships of 5-HT_3 Agonists

Only a few 5-HT_3 agonists have been identified, and the topic has been comprehensively reviewed (72). Many

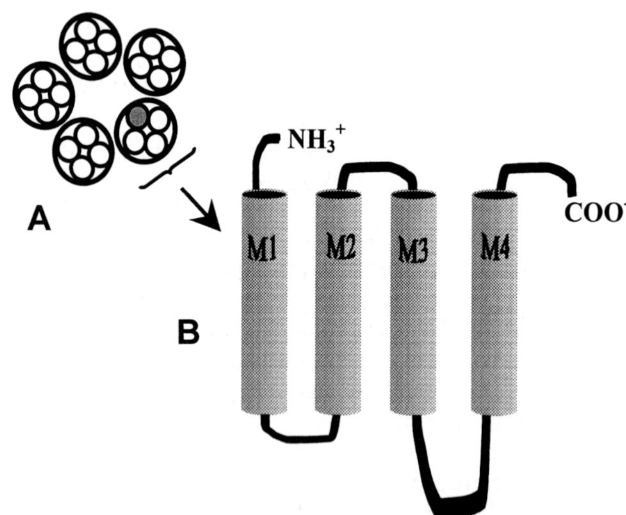

Fig. 14.11. Top (A) and side (B) views of a schematic representation of an ion channel receptor. Ion channel receptors are pentameric units arranged to form a pore or ion channel. Each subunit consists of four transmembrane-spanning amino acid chains (M_1–M_4) constructed such that the M_2 chain faces the channel. The transmembrane portions are connected by extracellular and intracellular loops. In the serotonin family, only 5-HT_3 receptors have been identified as ion channel receptors.

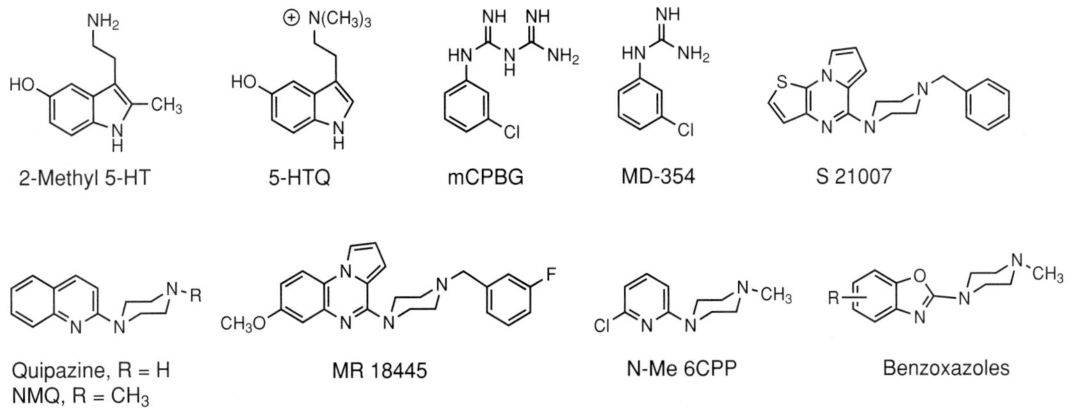

2-Methyl 5-HT
5-HTQ
mCPBG
MD-354
S 21007
Quipazine, R = H
NMQ, R = CH_3
MR 18445
N-Me 6CPP
Benzoxazoles

Fig. 14.12. 5-HT_3 agonists or partial agonists.

indolealkylamine or tryptamine derivatives bind at 5-HT_3 receptors in a nonselective manner. Simple O-methylation of 5-HT, however, significantly decreases its affinity for 5-HT_3 receptors. Ergolines either do not bind or bind only with very low affinity. 5-HT is a nonselective 5-HT_3 agonist that binds only with modest affinity ($K_i \sim$ 500–1,000 nM). Its 2-methyl analogue, 2-methyl 5-HT (K_i = 1,200 nM) (Fig. 14.12) is somewhat more selective but binds with slightly lower affinity than 5-HT. Although 2-methyl 5-HT may be only a partial agonist, it has found widespread application in 5-HT_3 research because of its greater selectivity over 5-HT. Recently, however, 2-methyl 5-HT was shown to bind at 5-HT_6 receptors. The N,N,N-trimethyl quaternary amine analogue of 5-HT, 5-HTQ, binds with approximately 10-fold greater affinity than 5-HT and is much more selective than 5-HT; however, because of its quaternary nature, it might not readily penetrate the blood-brain barrier when administered systemically. Using cloned mouse 5-HT_3 receptors, 5-HT and 5-HTQ act as full agonists, suggesting that the quaternary nature of 5-HTQ has little effect on efficacy, whereas 2-methyl 5-HT and tryptamine act as partial agonists. Another example of a low-affinity ($K_i \sim$ 1,000 nM) 5-HT_3 agonist is phenylbiguanide. *meta*-Chlorophenylbiguanide (*m*CPBG), which binds in the low nanomolar range ($K_i \sim$ 20–50 nM) and retains agonist character, has largely replaced phenylbiguanide. Because of its polar nature, *m*CPBG does not readily penetrate the blood-brain barrier. *meta*-Chlorophenylguanidine (MD-354; *m*CPG) shows that the entire biguanide moiety is not required for serotonergic activity. Adding multiple chloro groups to *m*CPBG or *m*CPG increases their lipophilicity and affinity (72).

Simple arylpiperazines were among the first serotonergic agents investigated at 5-HT_3 receptors. Many are nonselective 5-HT_3 ligands (see previous discussion of 5-HT_{1A} receptors). Depending on the particular substitution pattern, they can behave as 5-HT_3 agonists, partial agonists, or antagonists (72). This nonselectivity probably accounts for the initial lack of interest in arylpiperazines as 5-HT_3 ligands, but today, there is renewed interest in these types of agents. Quipazine was the first arylpiperazine shown to bind at 5-HT_3 receptors, even though it also is a 5-HT_{2A} agonist. It binds with much higher affinity than 5-HT at 5-HT_3 receptors ($K_i \sim$ 1 nM), and was subsequently shown to act as an agonist in certain assays and as an antagonist in others. Interestingly, its structure was quite different from that of other 5-HT_3 antagonists known at that time. Early structure–affinity studies showed that its (pyridine-ring) centroid to N_4-piperazine nitrogen distance (~5.5 Å) was similar to that of 5-HT. Other findings indicated that 1) the N_4-piperazine nitrogen atom, but not the N_1-piperazine nitrogen atom, was important for binding; 2) the quinoline ring nitrogen atom was a major contributor to binding; 3) the benzene ring portion of the quinoline nucleus was not required for binding, but its presence was optimal for high affinity; and 4) N_4-methylation (N-methylquipazine) enhances 5-HT_3 receptor selectivity (Fig. 14.12) (72). With the availability of newer arylpiperazines, it has been possible to conduct more comprehensive structure–activity studies. A summary of quipazine SAR is shown in Figure 14.13; results of other SAR studies and several pharmacophoric models have been described (72). Appropriate structural modification of arylpiperazines can result in rather selective 5-HT_3 agonists (Fig. 14.12). For example, ring-fused quipazine-related analogues, such as the pyrrolo[1,2-a]quinoxalines, represent novel 5-HT_3 agonists. Some are full agonists, whereas other (e.g., MR 18445) are partial agonists (72–75).

Structure–Activity Relationship of 5-HT_3 Antagonists

Bemestron (MDL-72222) was the first selective 5-HT_3 antagonist (Fig. 14.14). Its development stems from the structural modification of cocaine, an agent that had been previously shown to be a weak 5-HT-M antagonist. Since then, many hundreds of 5-HT_3 antagonists have been identified (75,76). Many of these agents belong to the structural

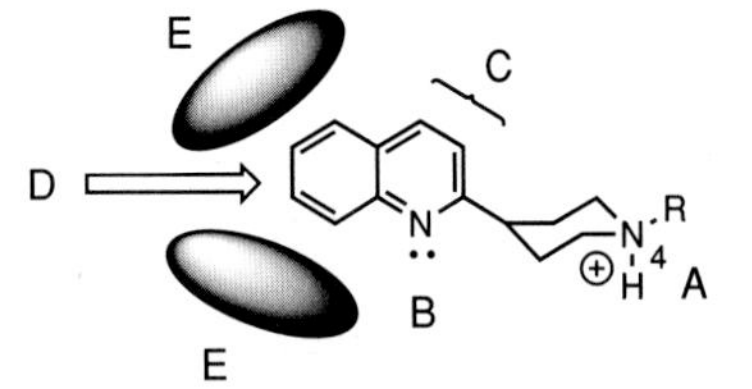

Fig. 14.13. Structure-activity composite for quipazine binding at 5-HT_3 receptors (4,97,100,105). (A) The N_4-piperazine nitrogen atom, but not the N_1-piperazine nitrogen atom, is important for binding; an R_5-CH_3 is tolerated and results in somewhat greater 5-HT_3 selectivity. (B) The quinoline nitrogen atom is required for high affinity, and its replacement by an sp2-hybridized carbon atom results in a more than 100-fold decrease in affinity. (C) Substituents in this region are tolerated and can influence intrinsic activity (105). (D) An aromatic moiety (e.g., benzene ring or isosteric structure), although not required for binding, results in optimal affinity. (E) Regions of limited bulk tolerance.

class of compounds broadly referred to as keto compounds and contain an amide, reverse amide, ester, reverse ester, carbamoyl, or ketone function. Typical of these 5-HT_3 antagonists is retention of the bulky tropane or tropane-like amine group. Some of the more widely used or newer agents include dolasetron (Anzemet), granisetron (Kytril), itasetron, renzapride, ricasetron, tropisetron, WAY-100289, zacopride, and zatosetron. It should be noted that some of these keto compounds also bind at 5-HT_{1P} and 5-HT_4 receptors.

A related group of antagonists that possess an imidazole or related heterocyclic terminal amine include ondansetron (Zofran), alosetron (Lotronex), fabesetron, and ramosetron (Fig. 14.15). Many others have been described (75,76). The SARs of 5-HT_3 antagonists have been reviewed in detail elsewhere (75–77).

Molecular modeling studies have identified a pharmacophore (Fig. 14.16) that is common to many 5-HT_3 antagonists (75,78). The 5-HT_3 antagonists remain a very important area of research, and refinements of 5-HT_3 pharmacophores (76) are very likely to lead to the development of novel therapeutic agents.

5-HT_3 Receptors: Clinical Implications

Preclinical studies suggest that 5-HT_3 antagonists may enhance memory and be of benefit in the treatment of anxiety, depression, pain, and dementia (71,79,80). There have been claims that 5-HT_3 antagonists may represent a novel class of atypical antipsychotics. Additional clinical trials, however, are required to substantiate these claims (80). Finally, evidence suggests that 5-HT_3 antagonists may suppress the behavioral consequences of withdrawing chronic treatment with drugs of abuse, including alcohol, nicotine, cocaine, and amphetamine (75,80). It has been mentioned that one of the most attractive features of 5-HT_3 antagonists is their general lack of the undesirable side effects characteristic of many psychotherapeutic agents. Very little is known about the possible therapeutic application of 5-HT_3 agonists (72).

One of the most noteworthy clinical success stories in 5-HT research relates to the antiemetic properties of 5-HT_3 receptor antagonists. Ondansetron was introduced as an antiemetic in the 1990s, and 5-HT_3 receptor antagonists are now the "gold standard" for treatment of chemotherapy- and radiation-induced nausea and vomiting (81). Twenty or so years ago, nausea and vomiting were inevitable side effects that forced many patients to delay or avoid chemotherapy (82). With the current antiemetic therapy, nausea and vomiting can be prevented

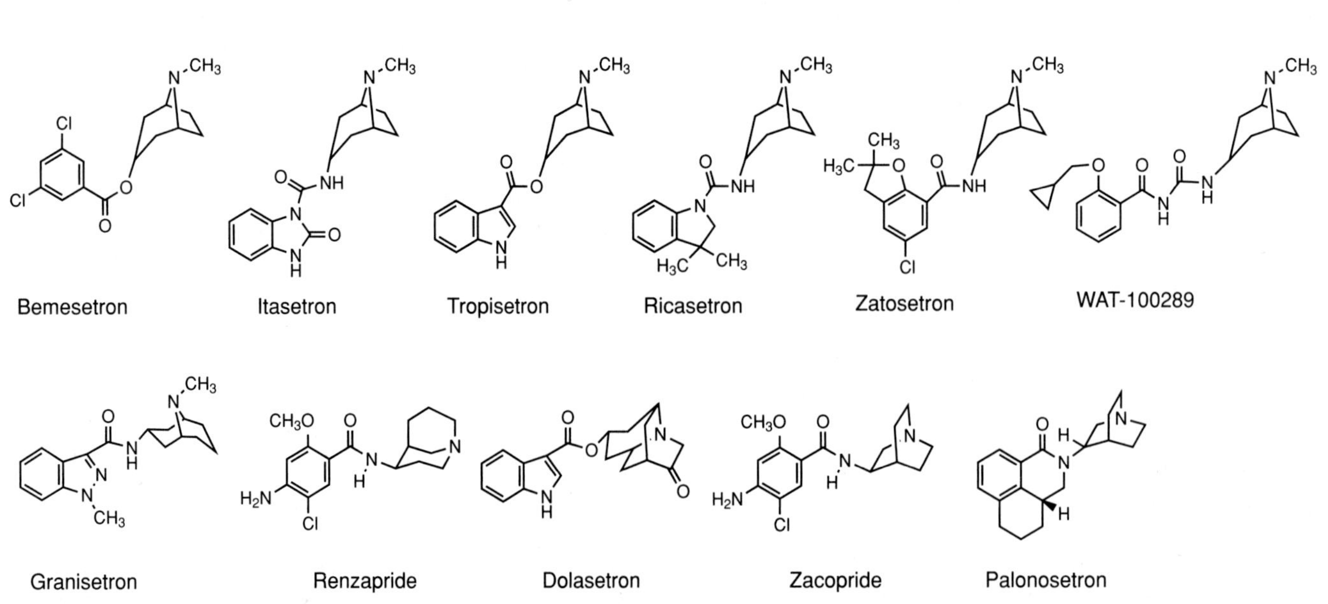

Fig. 14.14. 5-HT_3 antagonists.

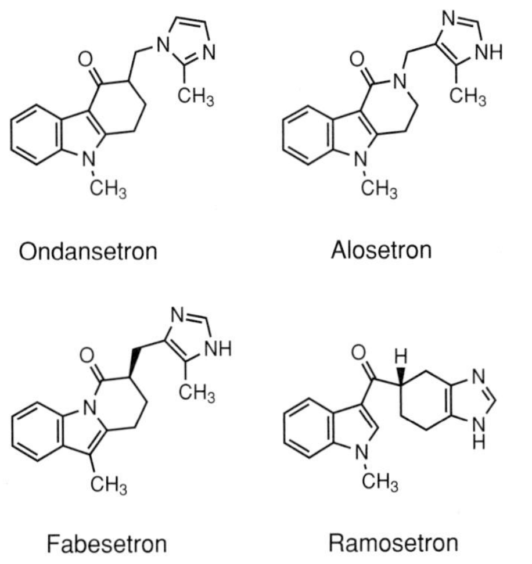

Ondansetron Alosetron

Fabesetron Ramosetron

Fig. 14.15. Imidazole-containing 5-HT_3 antagonists.

in nearly 80% of patients (82). The most commonly employed 5-HT_3 receptor antagonists are ondansetron, granisetron, dolasetron, and in Europe, tropisetron; a new 5-HT_3 antagonist in clinical use in the United States is palonosetron (83). The various 5-HT_3 antagonists are commonly perceived as being of comparable efficacy and safety (84); however, they vary widely in their pharmacological and pharmacokinetic properties (81–84) (Table 14.4). For example, their duration of action and elimination half-lives differ considerably. Ondansetron displays the shortest half-life (~4 hours), whereas the half-life of palonosetron has been reported to be up to 128 hours (84). Another difference in their pharmacology is that ondansetron is a competitive 5-HT_3 antagonist, whereas granisetron and tropisetron (and, perhaps, palonosetron) produce an insurmountable antagonism (83,84). Selection of a particular 5-HT_3 antiemetic follows specific guidelines that are related, at least in part, to such factors as the emeticity of the chemotherapeutic regimen, side effect tolerability, patient history, and financial considerations. Patients who are refractory to the effect of a particular antiemetic may benefit by switching antiemetic agents—improvement might be related to different routes of metabolism (81) (Table 14.4).

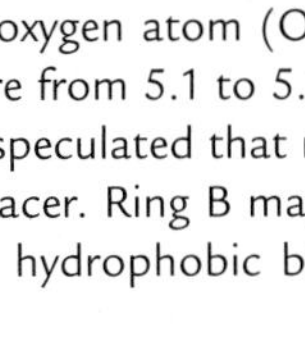

Fig. 14.16. A general pharmacophore model for 5-HT_3 antagonists. An aromatic centroid (A) to oxygen (O) distance of 3.3 to 3.5 Å is thought to be optimal. Distances calculated from the terminal amine (N) to the oxygen atom (O) and from the terminal amine N to centroid A are from 5.1 to 5.2 and from 6.7 to 7.2 Å, respectively. It has been speculated that ring A is not required for binding and acts as a spacer. Ring B may be more important for binding, and associated hydrophobic binding regions has been proposed (74,147).

5-HT_4 Receptors and Agents

A novel population of serotonergic receptors, originally identified in primary cell cultures of mouse embryo colliculi neurons and later termed 5-HT_4 receptors, have broad tissue distribution and are positively coupled to adenylate cyclase (85). In the brain, 5-HT_4 receptors appear to be localized on neurons and may mediate the slow excitatory responses to 5-HT. Peripherally, these receptors facilitate acetylcholine release in guinea pig ileum and may play a role in peristalsis. The uniqueness of this receptor type and its potential therapeutic utility spurred initial interest in drug development. Human 5-HT_4 receptors have been cloned and display low transmembrane sequence homology (<50%) with other 5-HT receptors. In fact, two 5-HT_4 isoforms have been isolated, a long form (5-HT_{4L}) and a short form (5-HT_{4S}). These isoforms are splice variants and differ only in their C-terminus ends, with identical transmembrane regions (86). In general, the potency of agonists to stimulate cyclic adenosine monophosphate (cAMP) was greater for the 5-HT_{4S} receptor than for the 5-HT_{4L} receptor. It has been suggested that 5-HT_4 receptors might exist in high- and low-affinity states, as previously described for 5-HT_2 receptors (87). A mouse 5-HT_{4L} receptor has been cloned, and a human pseudogene has been identified that codes for a 5-HT_4-like receptor. Indeed, several new human 5-HT_4 receptor isoforms have been recently cloned and expressed (88). The new 5-HT_4 receptors have been termed 5-$HT_{4(b)}$, 5-$HT_{4(c)}$, and 5-$HT_{4(d)}$; the stimulatory pattern of cAMP formation in response to the 5-HT_4 agonist renzapride was found to be different for the various isoforms, suggesting that the splice variants might differ in the manner by which they trigger signal transduction following receptor activation (88). In the rat gastrointestinal tract, both 5-HT_{4L} and 5-HT_{4S} receptors are expressed, whereas only 5-HT_{4S} receptors are found in the heart, with localization almost exclusively in the atrium. The 5-HT_{4a} receptors have been cloned from human atrium and appear to correspond to the rodent 5-HT_{4S} isoform. It has been proposed that the cardiac effects of 5-HT are mediated by this short splice variant, whereas 5-HT_{4L} determines the neuronal effects of 5-HT (88).

Although 5-HT_3 receptors are ion channel receptors and 5-HT_4 receptors represent G protein–coupled receptors (Table 14.2), a number of 5-HT_3 ligands are active at 5-HT_4 receptors. Even more interesting is that a number of 5-HT_3 antagonists, or what were considered at one time to be 5-HT_3-selective antagonists (e.g., renzapride and zacopride), actually exhibited 5-HT_4 agonist activity. Even today, there is considerable structural similarity among the various 5-HT_3 and 5-HT_4 ligands. In addition to their lack of selectivity for 5-HT_4 versus other 5-HT

Table 14.4. Pharmacokinetics of the 5-HT_3 Antagonists (Setrons)

Parameters	Ondansetron	Dolasetron	Granisetron	Alosetron	Palonosetron	Tropisetron
Trade name	Zofran	Anzemet	Kytril	Lotronex	Aloxi	Navoban
CLog P (calc)[a]	2.1 ± 0.5	2.8 ± 0.5	1.5 ± 0.5	0.88 ± 0.8	2.6 ± 0.5	3.6 ± 0.3
Log D (pH 7) (calc.)[a]	1.5	2.8	−1.5	0.4	0.01	0.8
Bioavailability (%)	56–70[d]	Hydrodolasetron: 60–80	60[d]	50–60[bc]	IV	60 (60–100)
Protein binding (%)	70–76	Hydrodolasetron: 70–80	65	82	62	71
Volume of distribution (L/kg)	IV: 160 PO: 2.2–2.5	Hydrodolasetron: 5.8–10 Women: 7 Men: 6	3.9	70 (65–95)	6.8–12.5	IV: 500
Elimination half-life (h)	3–6 Elderly: 11	<10 min Hydrodolastron: 4–9	IV: 4–5 PO: ~6	1.5–2.0	30–40	EM: 6–8 PM: 30
Major metabolites (%)	Hydroxylation Glucuronidation Hepatic	Hydrodolastron Hydroxylation N-demethyl	N-demethyl Hepatic	6-Hydroxylation N-demethyl	N-oxide 6S-hydroxy Hepatic: 50%	Hydrolyation Glucuronides
Metabolizing enzyme(%)	CYP3A4 CYP2D6	Carbonyl reductase CYP2D6 CYP3A4(N-oxide)	CYP3A4	CYP2C9: 30 CYP3A4: 20 CYP1A2: 10	CYP2D6 CYP3A4 CYP1A2	CYP2D6
Time to peak plasma concentration (h)	PO: 1–2 IM: <0.5 Suppository: 3–4	Hydrodolasetron: IV: <0.5 Hydrodolasetron oral: <1	2–3	0.5–2	IV: 30 sec	EM: 3 PM: 4
Excretion (%)	Urine metab: 40–60 Feces metab: 25 Unchanged: <10	Urine metab: 45 Feces: 30 Unchanged hydrodolasetron: 60	Urine metab: 48 Feces metab: 38 Unchanged: <10	Urine metab: 70 Feces metab: 25 Unchanged: <10	Urine metab: 80 Unchanged: 40	Urine metab: ~70 Feces metab: ~15 Unchanged: <10
Duration (h)	—	—	8–24	1–10	>24	—

[a]Chemical Abstracts, American Chemical Society, calculated using Advanced Chemistry Development (ACD/Labs) Software V8.14 for Solaris (1994–2006 ACD/Labs).
[b]First-pass metabolism.
[c]Food delays absorption and peak plasma concentrations.
[d]Food increase extent of absorption.

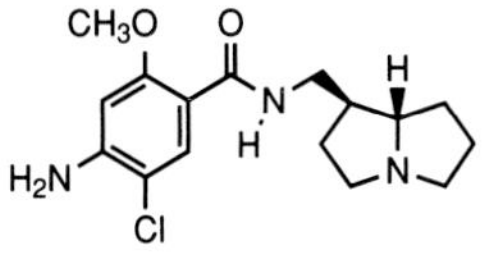

SC 53116 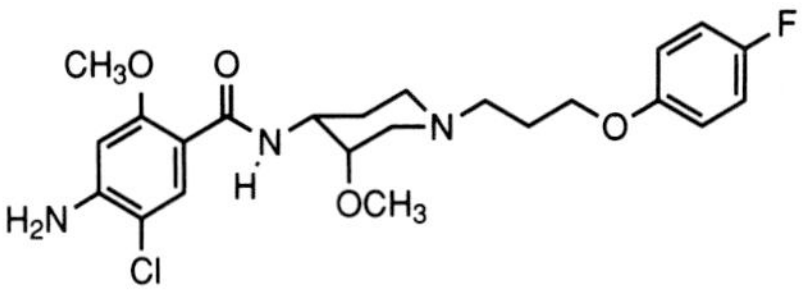 Cisapride 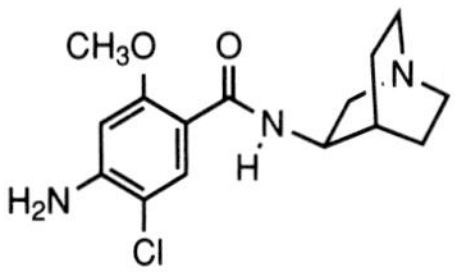 Zacopride 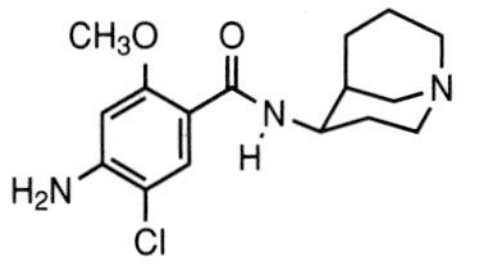 Renzapride

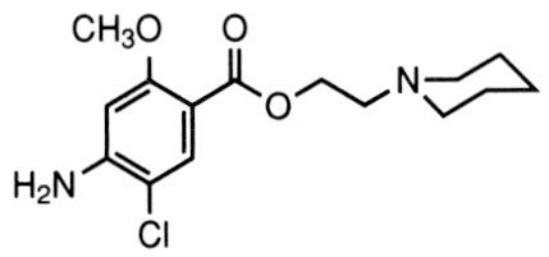

ML-10302 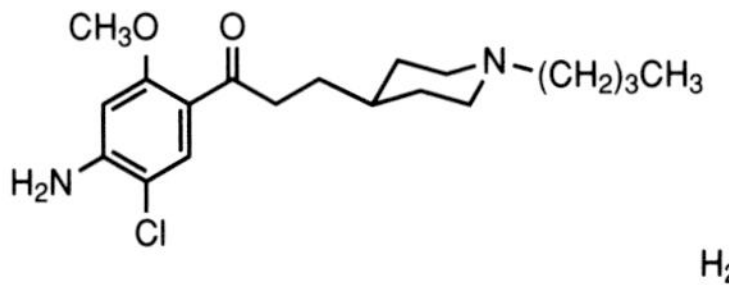 RS 67333 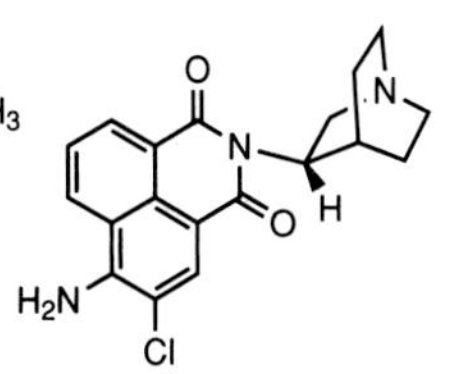 (S)-RS 56532 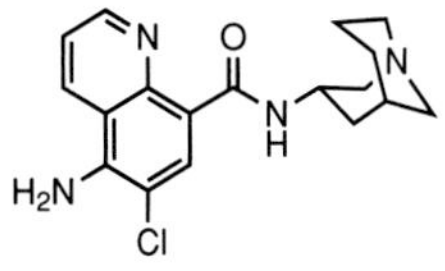 SDZ 216,908 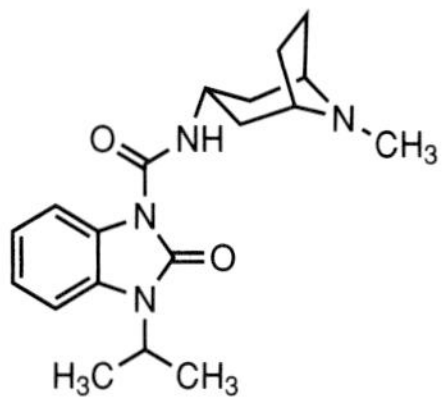 BIMU 8

Fig. 14.17. 5-HT_4 agonists.

receptors, many early 5-HT_4 ligands suffered from several other disadvantages, such as their affinity for other receptor types, inability or difficulty in penetrating the blood-brain barrier, and hydrolytic instability (89).

Structure–Activity Relationships of 5-HT_4 Agonists

In general terms, 5-HT_4 agonists can be divided into several different categories (Fig. 14.17) (90): tryptamines (e.g., 5-HT and 5-CT, with 2-methyl 5-HT and 5-methoxy-N, N-dimethyltryptamine being nearly inactive), benzamides (particularly those bearing a 2-methoxy-4-amino-5-chloro substitution pattern, e.g., SC 53116, renzapride, zacopride, and cisapride), benzimidazolones (e.g., BIMU 8), quinolines (e.g., SDZ 216,908), naphthalimides (e.g., *S*-RS 56532), benzoates (ML-10302), and ketones (e.g., RS 67333).

Structure–Activity Relationships of 5-HT_4 Antagonists

The 5-HT_3 antagonist tropisetron was the first agent to see application as a 5-HT_4 antagonist, and its low affinity for 5-HT_4 receptors prompted a search for higher-affinity agents. Various agents now have been identified (76,90–92), and 5-HT_4 antagonists are derived from structural classes similar to those from which the 5-HT_4 agonists are derived. These include indole esters and amides (e.g., GR 113,808), benzoates (e.g., SB 204070), benzimidazolones (e.g., DAU 6285), imidazoles (e.g., SC 53606), and ketones (e.g., RS 100235) (Fig. 14.18). These are just a few representative examples of the many agents that have been examined as 5-HT_4 antagonists. Structure–activity details for several different receptor preparations have been reviewed (76,90–92). It is worth noting that apart from 5-HT_3 receptors, 5-HT_4 receptors

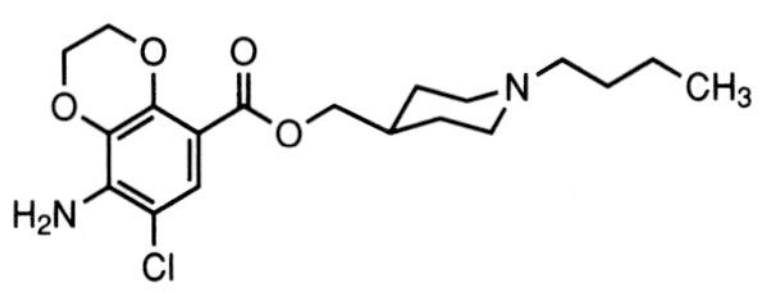

SB 204070 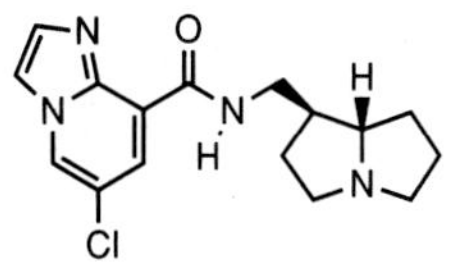 SC 53606

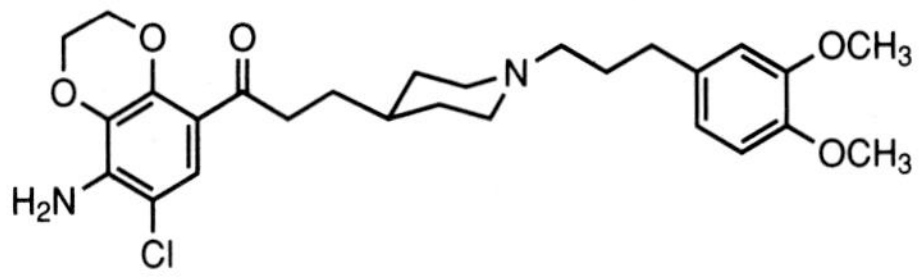

RS 100235 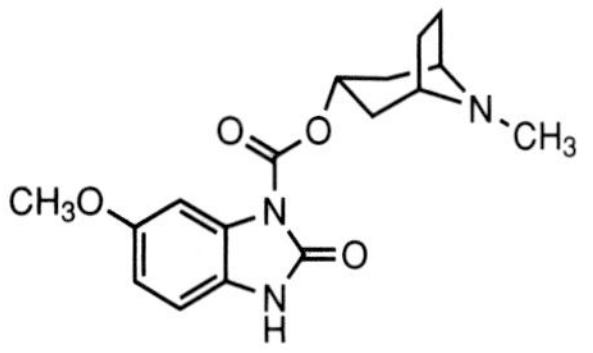 DAU 6285

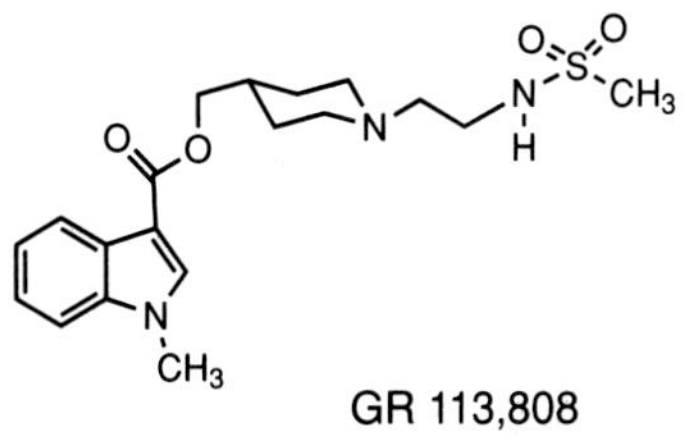

GR 113,808

Fig. 14.18. 5-HT_4 antagonists.

are the only other population of serotonergic sites that seem to accommodate quaternary amines.

5-HT_4 Receptors: Clinical Implications

Only relatively recently have selective 5-HT_4 agents been developed, and studies regarding the clinical potential of 5-HT_4 agents are still in their infancy. Peripheral actions currently being examined include irritable bowel syndrome (IBS), gastrointestinal tract motility, bladder contraction, gastroesophageal reflux, corticosteroid secretion, and atrial contractility (90). Cisapride was available as a prokinetic agent. With respect to their central effects, it has been suggested that 5-HT_4 agonists may restore deficits in cognitive function and that 5-HT_4 antagonists may be useful as anxiolytics or in the treatment of dopamine-related disorders. It is further speculated that 5-HT_4 receptors may be involved in memory and learning, and it has been noted that 5-HT_4 receptors are markedly decreased in patients with Alzheimer's disease (93,94). A high density of 5-HT_4 receptors in the nucleus accumbens has led some to speculate that these receptors may be involved in the reward system and that they might influence drug self-administration behavior. Other central roles also are beginning to emerge; for example, repeated administration of antidepressants decreases the responsiveness of central 5-HT_4 receptors to activation (95). It would appear that therapeutic roles exist for both 5-HT_4 antagonists and 5-HT_4 agonists. It has been cautioned, however, that the use of highly potent and selective 5-HT_4 agonists might result in cardiovascular side effects (94). If different 5-HT_4 receptor isoforms can be shown to mediate the various effects for which 5-HT_4 receptors have been implicated, the potential exists for the development of selective agents. Another problem associated with 5-HT_4 agents is their lack of oral bioavailability; progress is now being made in this area (96).

Irritable bowel syndrome is one of the most common gastrointestinal disorders in the United States accounting for more than 3.5 million doctor visits per year (97). Irritable bowel syndrome is characterized by abdominal discomfort or pain associated with altered bowel function (i.e., constipation [IBS-C]), diarrhea (IBS-D), or alternating constipation and diarrhea (IBS-A). Until recently, treatment has been limited by the poor efficacy or side effects of available agents. Agents commonly employed to treat IBS include laxatives, antispasmodics and smooth muscle relaxants (e.g., dicyclomine and hyoscyamine), and tricyclic antidepressants, but only 40% of patients are satisfied with these medications (97). Because more than 95% of all serotonin in the body is found in the gut, it would seem logical that serotonergic agents should be of benefit in the treatment of IBS.

In general, peristaltic and secretory reflexes are initiated by 5-HT acting at 5-HT_{1P} receptors (98). The 5-HT_3 receptors are associated with excitation of the gastrointestinal tract resulting in increased motility, secretion, and excitation (97) as well as signaling to the CNS (98); 5-HT_3 antagonists reduce colonic transit and improve fluid absorption (97). The 5-HT_3 antagonists tend to be constipating (98). The 5-HT_4 receptors mediate both excitatory and inhibitory effects on gut function (97).

Alosetron (Fig. 14.15), a 5-HT_3 antagonist, and tegaserod (Zelnorm®), a 5-HT_4 agonist, are two of the most recent entries for the treatment of IBS. Recent clinical trials have found that both agents are more effective than placebo for the treatment of IBS-C and IBS-D (97). Tegaserod acts by accelerating small bowel and colonic transit in patients with IBS. It is rapidly absorbed following oral administration, with a bioavailability of approximately 10%, except that food reduces the bioavailability by 40 to 65%. Peak plasma concentrations are reached in approximately 1 hour. Tegaserod is approximately 98% bound to plasma proteins, primarily to α_1-acid glycoprotein. Its volume of distribution is approximately 368 L/kg. Tegaserod undergoes presystemic acid-catalyzed hydrolysis in the stomach, followed by hepatic oxidation to its principal inactive metabolite (5-methoxyindole-3-carboxylic acid), its acyl glucuronide, and three isomeric N-glucuronides. The terminal half-life is approximately 11 hours following intravenous administration. Approximately two-thirds of the orally administered dose of tegaserod is excreted unchanged in feces, with the remainder excreted in urine, primarily as glucuronide. Tegaserod exhibits dose-proportional kinetics when given twice daily at therapeutic doses for 5 days, with no relevant accumulation. No dosage adjustment is required in elderly patients or those with mild to moderate hepatic or renal impairment. No clinically relevant drug–drug interactions have been identified with tegaserod.

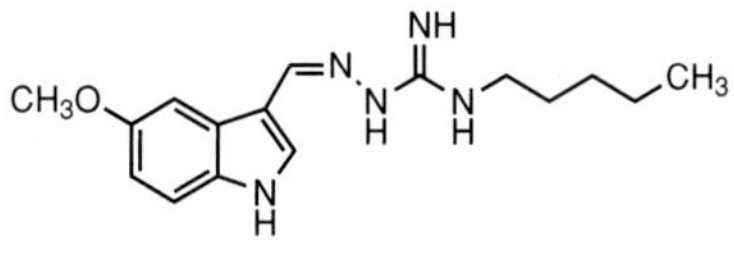

CH_3O NH N N H N H N H CH_3

Tegaserod

NOTE: Investigational drug as of August 2007 (limited access).

5-HT_5 Receptors and Agents

Overview

Two 5-HT_5 receptors, expressed primarily in the mouse CNS, have been identified as 5-HT_{5A} and 5-HT_{5B} receptors (99). The two 5-HT_5 receptors exhibit 77% amino acid sequence homology but less than 50% homology with other cloned serotonergic receptors. To some extent, the 5-HT_5 receptors appear to resemble 5-HT_1 receptors (e.g., high affinity for 5-HT and 5-CT); however, their low homology with other 5-HT_1 receptors suggest that they represent a distinct family of receptors. Only 5-HT_{5A} receptors have been identified in humans (99). Recent studies provide evidence that human 5-HT_{5A} receptors are G protein–coupled receptors that are coupled in a complex manner to multiple signaling cascades; apparently, they are coupled to adenylate cyclase and also can transiently open K^+ channels after formation of inositol 1,4,5-triphosphate (100).

Radiolabeled LSD binds to both HT_{5A} and 5-HT_{5B} receptors, with 5-CT having 10-fold greater affinity for human 5-HT_{5A} receptors than 5-HT, which binds with modest affinity (K_i = 100–250 nM). The SAR for the binding of various ligands at 5-HT_{5A} receptors has been reviewed elsewhere (101). Ergotamine and methiothepin bind with high affinity at human 5-HT_{5A} receptors, whereas agents such as spiperone, sumatriptan, yohimbine, ketanserin, propranolol, zacopride, and clozapine bind with much lower affinity (K_i > 1,000 nM) . To date, no 5-HT_{5A}-selective agonists or antagonists have been reported.

5-HT_5 Receptors: Clinical Implications

Pharmacological functions of 5-HT_5 receptors are currently unknown. It has been speculated, on the basis of their localization, that they may be involved in motor control, feeding, anxiety, depression, learning, memory consolidation, adaptive behavior, and brain development (99). The 5-HT_{5A} receptors also may be involved in a neuronally driven mechanism for regulating astrocyte physiology with relevance to gliosis; disruption of 5-HT neuronal–glial interactions may be involved in the development of certain CNS pathologies, including Alzheimer's disease, Down's syndrome, and some drug-induced developmental deficits. Recent evidence indicates that genes that encode for the human 5-HT_{5A} receptor might be involved in schizophrenia (102) and that spinal 5-HT_{5A} receptors could play a role in nociception and control of pelvic floor musculature (103).

5-HT_6 Receptors and Agents

Overview

A novel G protein–coupled serotonergic receptor that appears to be localized exclusively in the CNS was cloned from rat brain (104) and named 5-HT_6. This receptor exhibits only 40% transmembrane homology with 5-HT_{1A}, 5-HT_{1B}, 5-HT_{1D}, 5-HT_{1E}, 5-HT_{2A}, and 5-HT_{2C} receptors. Both LSD and 5-HT display modest affinity for 5-HT_6 receptors (K_i ~ 50–150 nM). Of interest is that a number of typical and atypical antipsychotic agents and tricyclic antidepressants bind with K_i values in the nM range. For example, Lisuride acted as a partial agonist, and amoxapine, clozapine, and methiothepin acted as antagonists (104).

More recently, the human 5-HT_6 receptor has been cloned, and its gene structure, distribution, and pharmacology are similar to those of the rat receptor (105). Like the rat receptor, the human receptor is positively coupled to adenylate cyclase. 5-HT binds at human 5-HT_6 receptors with moderate affinity (K_i = 65 nM), and one of the highest-affinity, albeit nonselective, agents is methiothepin (K_i = 0.4 nM). Agents that bind at human 5-HT_6 receptors with K_i < 50 nM include 5-methoxytryptamine, bromocriptine, octoclothepin, and the antipsychotic agents clozapine, olanzapine, chlorpromazine, loxapine, and fluphenazine (106). Agents with K_i >500 nM include 5-CT, sumatriptan, quipazine, ketanserin, 8-OH DPAT, haloperidol, risperidone, and mesulergine (106). A number of other antipsychotic agents, both typical and atypical, as well as antidepressants bind with low nanomolar affinity (101,105,106).

5-HT_6 Agonists and Antagonists

Just a few years ago, there were no 5-HT_6-selective agents; however, tremendous progress has been made recently. 2-Ethyl-5-methoxy-N,N-dimethyltryptamine (EMDT) represented the first reasonably selective 5-HT_6 agonist (107), and Ro 04-6790 and Ro 63-0563 represented the first 5-HT_6-selective antagonists (108) (Fig. 14.19). These were soon followed by the antagonists SB-271046 (109), MS-245 (107,110) and PMDT (2-phenyl-5=mutroxy-N,N-

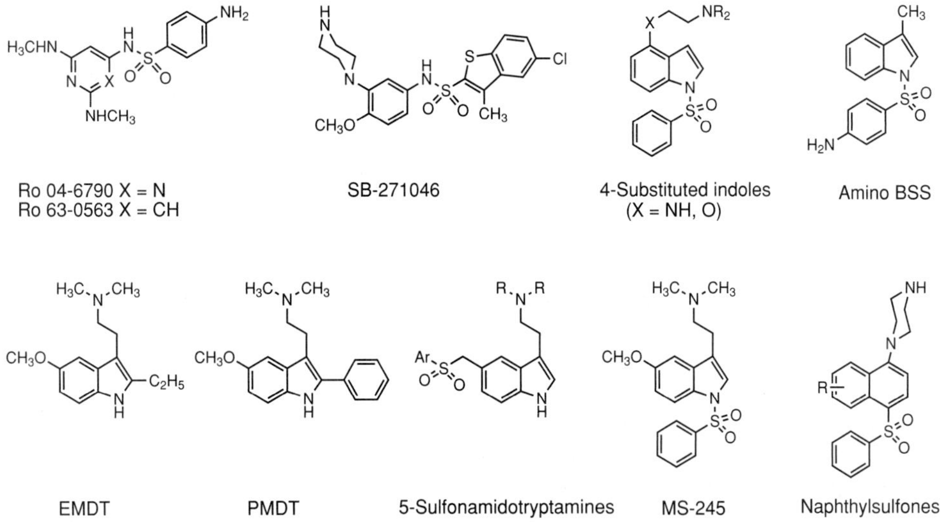

Ro 04-6790 X = N
Ro 63-0563 X = CH

SB-271046

4-Substituted indoles (X = NH, O)

Amino BSS

EMDT

PMDT

5-Sulfonamidotryptamines

MS-245

Naphthylsulfones

Fig. 14.19. 5-HT_6 agonists and antagonists.

dimethyl tryptamine, also known as BGC20-761) (107). Since then, work has continued on related structure-types, leading to agents with greater metabolic stability and bioavailability (101). It might be noted that most of the early 5-HT_6 antagonists contained an arylsulfonamide moiety. Interestingly, the importance of this functionality was an independent discovery from several different laboratories, and this structural feature is now commonplace among many 5-HT_6 agents. In some cases, the sulfonamido moiety can be replaced by a sulfone (e.g., naphthylsulfones) (Fig. 14.19). Numerous structural modifications have now been reported, and among some of the interesting findings are that the basic side chain of MS-245–type compounds can be moved to the indole 4-position (Fig. 14.19) (111,112) or removed altogether (e.g., amino-BSS) (101) with retention of antagonist action. 5-Sulfonamidotryptamines also bind with high affinity at 5-HT_6 receptors and, depending on the nature of their pendent substituents, act as 5-HT_6 agonists, partial agonists, or antagonists (113,114).

5-HT_6 Receptors: Clinical Implications

The exact clinical significance of 5-HT_6 receptors is unknown at this time. The high affinity of various antipsychotics, particularly atypical antipsychotics, and antidepressants suggests a possible connection between 5-HT_6 receptors and certain psychiatric disorders (115). The different binding profiles of atypical antipsychotics may be responsible for their atypical nature (e.g., D_2:5-HT_{2A} ratio); for example, certain agents, such as clozapine, may be classified as atypical on the basis of their binding with higher affinity at 5-HT_{2A} than at D_2 receptors. However, antipsychotics that produce the fewest extrapyramidal side effects in humans (e.g., clozapine, olanzapine, and fluperlapine) also possess high affinity for 5-HT_6 receptors (106). The atypical antipsychotic agent risperidone, which produces some extrapyramidal symptoms, binds with 1,000-fold higher affinity at 5-HT_{2A} than at 5-HT_6 receptors; thus, the affinity of agents for 5-HT_6 receptors may contribute to the difference between typical and certain atypical antipsychotics (106). Furthermore, preclinical studies indicate that combinations of a 5-HT_6 antagonist and a 5-HT_{2A} antagonist were effective in models of psychosis and cognition (116). PMDT differs from most other 5-HT_6 antagonists in that it combines both types of antagonist action in the same molecule (101). The 5-HT_6 knockout mice produce a behavioral syndrome that seems to involve an increase in cholinergic function. Blocking the receptors in rats with 5-HT_6 antagonists produces a similar effect. This has led to speculation that one of the roles of 5-HT_6 receptors may be to control cholinergic neurotransmission and that 5-HT_6-selective antagonists could be useful in the treatment of anxiety and memory deficits. Other studies have shown that although 5-HT_6 antagonists might not influence basal levels of dopamine by themselves, they apparently increase amphetamine-induced increases in brain dopamine and can potentiate certain dopamine-mediated behavioral effects (117,118). The exact mechanisms underlying this process are not understood, but 5-HT_6 receptors play a role in neuronal plasticity (119) and can influence the actions of dopaminergic agents. Evidence also suggests that 5-HT_6 receptors might be involved in motor function, mood-dependent behavior, anxiety disorders, appetite control, anticonvulsant activity, and early growth processes involving 5-HT (105,107,111). With the newly identified 5-HT_6 agonists and antagonists, interest in the therapeutic potential of such agents is on the upswing.

5-HT_7 Receptors and Agents

Overview

Like 5-HT_5 receptors, 5-HT_7 receptors were once considered to be orphan receptors. Rat, mouse, guinea pig, and human 5-HT_7 receptors have now been cloned and are expressed mainly in the CNS (101,120). Hydropathic analysis suggests a seven transmembrane-spanning G protein–coupled receptor. The 5-HT_7 receptors are positively coupled to adenylate cyclase, and several splice variants have been identified. Alternative splicing in rat and human receptors results in four 5-HT_7 receptor isoforms that vary with respect to the length of their C-terminus chains (101,121). In rat, the isoforms are named 5-HT_{7a}, 5-HT_{7b}, and 5-HT_{7c}. Two of the isoforms are homologous in rat and human (5-HT_{7a} and 5-HT_{7b}). The third human isoform is named 5-HT_{7d}. These different isoforms could have important functional consequences, such as different distribution or G protein–coupling efficiency, or different susceptibility to desensitization (121,122). Apparently, however, the three human isoforms are pharmacologically indistinguishable and show similar affinity for various ligands. Evidence suggests that 5-HT_7 receptors are constitutively active and that the degree of constitutive activity might vary among the isoforms. Nonselective agents with K_i values at 5-HT_7 receptors of 10 nM or less include 5-HT, 5-methoxytryptamine, LSD, methiothepin, and mesulergine; those with K_i values in the range of 10 to 100 nM include 8-OH DPAT (long considered a 5-HT_{1A}-selective agonist!), spiperone, ritanserin, metergoline, mianserin, and chlorpromazine; those with K_i values in the range of 100 to 1,000 nM include NAN-190, sumatriptan, and haloperidol; and those with K_i values of greater than 1,000 nM include 2-methyl 5-HT, tropisetron, pindolol, and ketanserin. Reportedly, 5-HT, 5-CT, and 8-OH DPAT act as agonists, whereas methiothepin, mianserin, mesulergine, ritanserin, spiperone (a 5-HT_{1A}, 2-HT_{2A}, and D_2 antagonist), NAN-190 (a 5-HT_{1A} antagonist), and clozapine act as antagonists. Numerous antidepressants and antipsychotic agents bind at 5-HT_7 receptors with nanomolar or subnanomolar affinity ($K_i \leq 10$ nM) include fluphenazine, acetophenazine, chlorprothixene, zotepine, clorotepine, clozapine, fluperlapine, pimozide, tiospirone, and risperidone (101,122).

5-HT_7 Antagonists

Only during the last few years have reasonably selective 5-HT_7 agents been identified. The first reported 5-HT_7

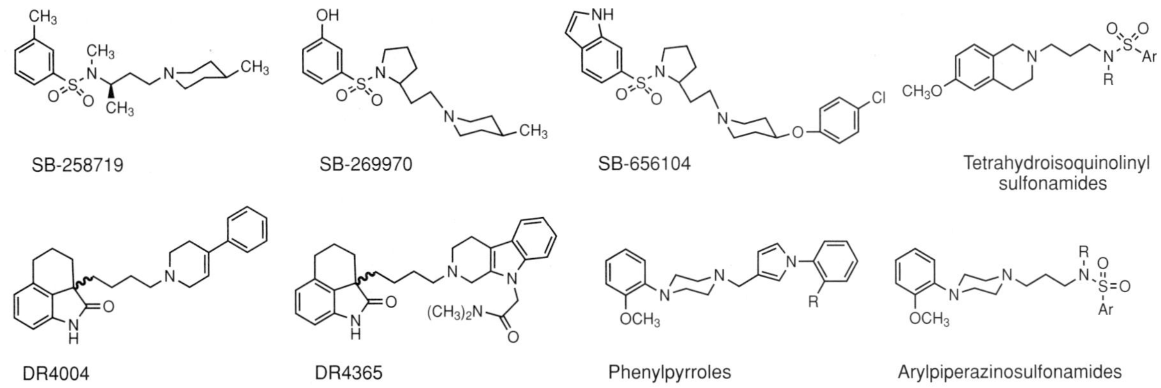

Fig. 14.20. 5-HT_7 antagonists.

antagonist was SB-258719 (K_i ~ 30 nM) (123), and attempts to optimize binding affinity and selectivity led to SB-269970 (*S*-isomer, K_i = 1.3 nM) (Fig. 14.20). Both compounds displayed some inverse agonist action. The high in vivo blood clearance of SB-269970 resulted in further structural modification, leading to compounds such as SB-656104 (*S*-isomer, K_i = 2 nM) (101). Another early series of 5-HT_7 antagonists was the DR-compounds: DR4004 was the first of these to show activity as a competitive antagonist; structural modification resulted in others, including DR4365 (K_i = 4 nM) (124). Other antagonists (Fig. 14.20) include phenylpyrrole-containing LCAPs (Fig. 14.20), which because of their structural similarity to other 5-HT_{1A} ligands might have been expected to—and do—bind at 5-HT_{1A} receptors (125), as well as arylpiperazinosulfonamides and tetrahydroisoquinolinylsulfonamides (126). Actually, the latter two types of compounds have been demonstrated to act as inverse agonists (126).

5-HT_7 Agonists

N-Arylaminoimidazolines (Fig. 14.21) were identified as the first 5-HT_7 agonists (127); however, they have not been pursued because of their profound effects on blood pressure and heart rate, which is probably a consequence of their affinity for α-adrenoceptors. Several new 5-HT_7 agonists have been recently reported, including the piperazinylhexanones (128) and 2-aminotetralins (129) (Fig. 14.21); the later can function either as agonists (e.g., R = *n*Pr) or antagonists (e.g. R = Me) depending on the nature of the R group. Pharmacophore models have been proposed for 5-HT_7 agonists (130), antagonists (131), and inverse agonists (126).

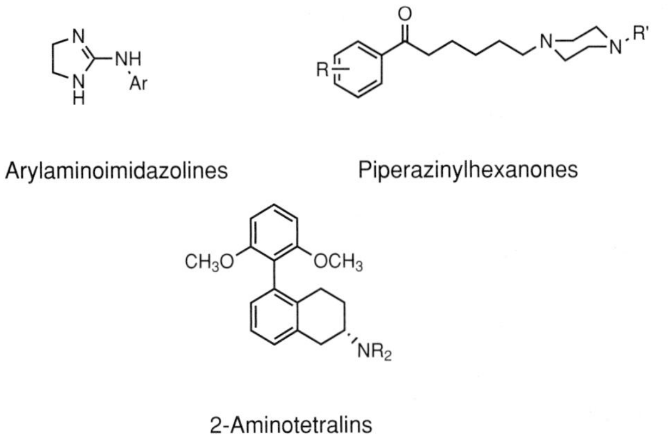

Fig. 14.21. 5-HT_7 agonists.

5-HT_7 Receptors: Clinical Implications

Because of the previous unavailability of 5-HT_7-selective agents, the pharmacology of the 5-HT_7 system is still relatively unexplored. Nevertheless, studies with nonselective agents, 5-HT_7 receptor knockout animals, and some of the first few selective agents that were identified have provided some tantalizing clues (101,122,132–134). The 5-HT_7 receptors might be involved in mood and learning as well as in neuroendocrine and vegetative behaviors. The 5-HT_2 ligand ritanserin, certain tricyclic antidepressants (e.g., amitriptyline), classical antipsychotic agents (e.g., chlorpromazine), and nonclassical antipsychotic agents (e.g., clozapine) bind with K_i values of less than 100 nM (115). On this basis, it has been speculated that 5-HT_7 receptors may play a role in certain neuropsychiatric disorders. Consistent with these suggestions, 5-HT_7 receptors are sensitive to antidepressant treatment (135). The 5-HT_7 receptors have been implicated in serotonergic-regulation of circadian rhythm, leading to suggestions that 5-HT_7-selective agents might be effective in the treatment of jet lag or sleep disorders of a circadian nature (136). Additionally, 5-HT_7 receptors might be involved in sleep disorders, anxiety, memory and cognition, epilepsy, pain, migraine, and thermoregulation. In the periphery, 5-HT produces both contraction and relaxation of coronary artery from various species (137). It has been proposed that relaxation of coronary artery may be mediated by 5-HT_7 receptors. Agents active at 5-HT_7 receptors might thus be effective in the treatment of coronary heart disease. Now that newer, more selective agents are finally available, many of these hypotheses can be further tested.

THE SEROTONIN TRANSPORTER

The actions of a neurotransmitter are terminated by diffusion away from the synapse, by enzymatic degradation, and by reuptake into the presynaptic terminal. Following reuptake, once the neurotransmitter is inside the neuron, it can be re-stored in storage vesicles or metabolized. The reuptake process involves a high-affinity transporter protein that is localized in the presynaptic terminal membrane. The transporter appears to regulate the duration and magnitude of postsynaptic response to the neurotransmitter. A different transporter is associated with different neurotransmitters. The 5-HT transporter (or SERT) has been cloned and expressed (138), and its putative structure is roughly similar to the general receptor structure shown in Figure 14.3 except that 1) it consists of 12 membrane-spanning helices, 2) both the amino terminus and the carboxy terminus are located on the intracellular side, and 3) it has an exaggerated extracellular loop between TM3 and TM4 (Fig. 14.22). The 5-HT transporter possesses approximately 50% homology with the norepinephrine transporter (NET) and the dopamine transporter. For 5-HT transport, a ternary complex of protonated 5-HT, Na^+, and Cl^- binds to the transporter protein to form a quaternary complex; the transporter undergoes a conformational change to release 5-HT into the cytoplasm of the neuron (138).

The 5-HT transporter has been implicated as playing a role in affective disorders (53). Agents that block the transporter and, thereby, increase synaptic levels of 5-HT are useful for the treatment of depression, obsessive-compulsive behavior, and panic disorders (53). Tricyclic antidepressants block the 5-HT transporter and the NET to varying degrees. Some display a preference for one transporter over the other, but most are nonselective (139). The SSRIs display greater selectivity for the 5-HT transporter over the NET. The first SSRI to be used clinically was fluoxetine; several other agents have since become available. The SARs of SSRIs have been reviewed elsewhere (140); see Chapter 21 for further discussion and examples. Certain drugs of abuse (e.g., cocaine) also block the 5-HT transporter, although cocaine's primary mechanism of action likely involves the dopamine transporter.

Fluoxetine

Trazodone

Various tricyclic antidepressants and SSRIs, including fluoxetine, also bind at 5-HT_{2A} and 5-HT_{2C} receptors (141,142). The role, if any, that is derived from a direct interaction of these agents with 5-HT_2 receptors versus their interaction at the 5-HT transporter remains to be elucidated. In general, 5-HT_2 antagonists downregulate

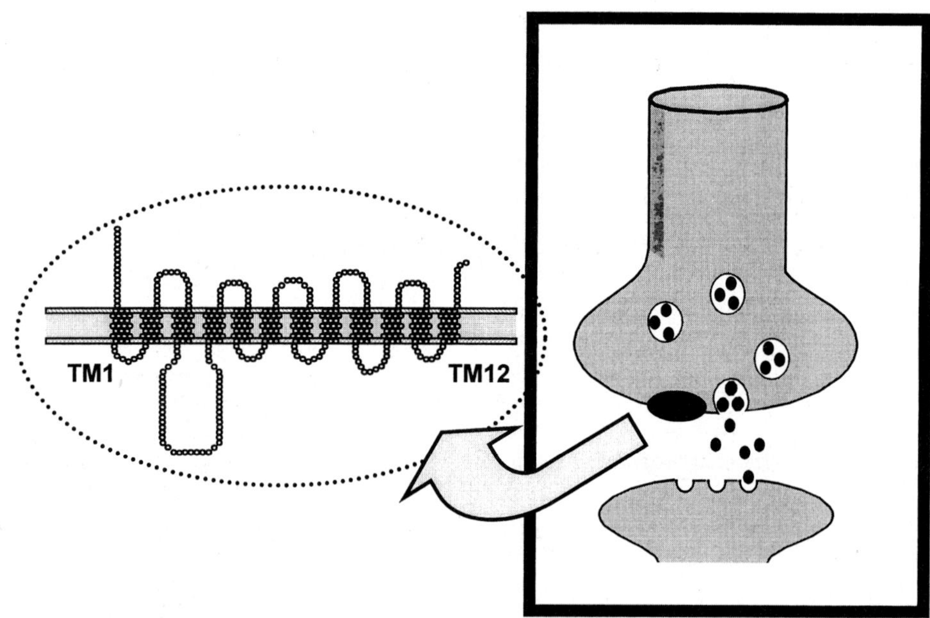

Fig. 14.22. Schematic of a neuron showing the general location and basic structure (inset) of a serotonin transporter (SERT). Note that the transporter possesses 12 transmembrane-spanning helices (TM1–TM12). Both the amine terminus (attached to TM1) and the carboxy terminus (attached to TM12) are on the intracellular side.

5-HT_2 receptors. The antidepressant trazodone, for example, is a weak reuptake blocker but binds at 5-HT_2 receptors and is a 5-HT_2 antagonist (142). The 5-HT_{2C} agonist *m*CPP induces panic attacks in patients with panic disorder and increases obsessive compulsions in patients with obsessive-compulsive disorder (143), implicating a role for this specific 5-HT_{2C} subpopulation. The 5-HT_{2C} receptor antagonists might be useful targets for the development of novel agents to treat these disorders (53). This issue is complicated, however, by findings that trazodone is metabolized to *m*CPP and that, in some instances, trazodone possesses 5-HT_{2C} agonist properties (144). In any event, long-term treatment with tricyclic antidepressants (and MAO inhibitors) leads to a down-regulation in the number of 5-HT_2 receptors, the time course for which approximates the clinical response in depressed patients (139). Some SSRIs produce adaptive changes involving decreased responsiveness of 5-HT_2 receptors, whereas electroconvulsive therapy increases the number of 5-HT_2 receptors (139). Several 5-HT receptor populations have been implicated in the actions of antidepressants (e.g., 5-HT_1, 5-HT_2, 5-HT_6, and 5-HT_7), but the 5-HT transporter remains an attractive target for the development of novel psychotherapeutic agents (53).

SUMMARY

Serotonin is a major neurotransmitter in the brain and also is involved in a number of peripheral actions. Seven families or populations of 5-HT receptors have been identified (5-HT_1–5-HT_7), and several are divided into distinct subpopulations (Table 14.2). Excluding splice variants, 14 different populations and subpopulations of 5-HT receptors have been cloned. Over the past 20 years, selective agonists and antagonists have been developed and identified for some of the subpopulations, but subpopulations remain for which selective agents have yet to be synthesized. The availability of such agents is important, because it aids functional investigations of the different 5-HT receptors. In addition to acting directly on 5-HT receptors, therapeutic agents with other mechanisms are available for influencing serotonergic transmission, including SSRIs and MAO inhibitors. Studies with 5-HT receptors have led to the introduction of agents useful for treating anxiety (e.g., buspirone), migraine (e.g., sumatriptan), IBS (e.g. tegaserod), and chemotherapy-induced emesis (e.g., ondansetron); numerous other agents are currently in clinical trials for the treatment of depression, schizophrenia, and obsessive-compulsive and other disorders (21). Investigations also have led to a greater understanding of cardiovascular pharmacology, obesity, neurodegenerative disorders, aggression, sexual behavior, and drug abuse, just to mention a few examples. Serotonin may even play an indirect role in techniques as diverse as acupuncture (145) and transcendental meditation (146). To reiterate a phrase from the introduction, "[I]t almost appears that serotonin is involved in everything" (1).

References

1. Rapport MR. The discovery of serotonin. Perspect Biol Med 1997;40: 260–273.
2. Glennon RA, Dukat M. Serotonin receptors and drugs affecting serotonergic neurotransmission. In: Williams DA, Lemke TL, eds. Foye's Principles of Medicinal Chemistry, 5th Ed. Philadelphia: Lippincott Williams & Wilkins, 2002:315–337.
3. Frazer A, Hensler JG. Serotonin. In: Siegel GJ, Agranoff BW, Albers RW, et al, eds. Basic Neurochemistry. New York: Raven Press, 1993:283–308.
4. Kroeze WK, Kristiansen K, Roth BL. Molecular biology of serotonin receptors: structure and function at the molecular level. Curr Top Med Chem 2002;2:507–528.
5. Peroutka SJ, Snyder SH. Multiple serotonin receptors: differential binding of [^{3}H]5-hydroxytryptamine, [^{3}H]lysergic acid diethylamide and [^{3}H]spiroperidol. Mol Pharmacol 1979;16:687–699.
6. Hoyer D, Hannon JP, Martin GR. Molecular, pharmacological, and functional diversity of 5-HT receptors. Pharmacol Biochem Behav 2002;71:533–534.
7. Hartig PR, Branchek TA, Weinshank RL. A subfamily of 5-HT_{1D} receptor genes. Trends Pharmacol Sci 1992; 3:152–159.
8. Hoyer D, Clarke DE, Fozard JR, et al. International Union of Pharmacology Nomenclature and Classification of receptors for 5-hydroxytryptamine (serotonin). Pharmacol Rev 1994;46:157–203.
9. Saudou F, Hen R. 5-HT receptor subtypes: Molecular and functional diversity. Med Chem Res 1994;4:16–84.
10. Zifa E, Fillion G. 5-Hydroxytryptamine receptors. Pharmacol Rev 1992;44: 401–458.
11. van Wijngaarden I, Soudijn W, Tulp MTM. 5-HT_{1A} receptor ligands. In: Olivier B, van Wijngaarden I, Soudin W, eds. Serotonin Receptors and Their Ligands. Amsterdam: Elsevier, 1997:17–43.
12. Glennon RA, Dukat M. 5-HT_1 receptor ligands: Update 1997. Invest Drugs Res Alerts 1997;2:351–372.
13. Glennon RA, Dukat M. 5-HT receptor ligands—Update 1992. Current Drugs: Serotonin 1993;1:1–45.
14. Glennon RA. Concepts for the design of 5-HT_{1A} serotonin agonists and antagonists. Drug Dev Res 1992;6:251–274.
15. Kuipers W, van Wijngaarden I, Ijzerman AP. A model of the serotonin 5-HT_{1A} receptor: agonist and antagonist binding sites. Drug Design Discov 1994;11:231–249.
16. Kuipers W. Structural characteristics of 5-HT_{1A} receptors and their ligands. In: Olivier B, van Wijngaarden I, Soudin W, eds. Serotonin receptors and their ligands. Amsterdam: Elsevier, 1997:45–64.
17. De Vry J. 5-HT_{1A} receptor agonists: recent developments and controversial issues. Psychopharmacology 1995;121:1–26.
18. Caliendo G, Santagada V, Perissutti E, et al. Derivatives as 5-HT_{1A} receptor ligands—past and present. Curr Med Chem 2005;12:1721–1753.
19. File SE. Recent developments in anxiety, stress, and depression. Pharmacol Biochem Behav 1996;54:3–12.
20. Saxena P. Serotonin receptors: subtypes, functional responses, and therapeutic relevance. Pharmacol Ther 1995;66:339–368.
21. Jones BJ, Blackburn TP. The medical benefit of 5-HT research. Pharmacol Biochem Behav 2002;71:555–568.
22. Perregaard J, Sanchez C, Arnt J. Recent developments in anxiolytics. Curr Opin Ther Pat 1993;3:101–126.
23. Fletcher A, Cliffe I, Dourish CT. Silent 5-HT_{1A} receptor antagonists: utility as research tools and therapeutic agents. Trends Pharmacol Sci 1993;14: 441–448.
24. Assie M-B, Koek W. Effects of 5-HT_{1A} receptor antagonists on hippocampal 5-hydroxytryptamine levels: (S)-WAY100135, but not WAY100635, has partial agonist properties. Eur J Pharmacol 1996;304:15–21.
25. Darmani NA, Reeves SL. The mechanism by which the selective 5-HT_{1A} receptor antagonist S-(−)-UH-301 produces head-twitches in mice. Pharmacol Biochem Behav 1996;55:1–10.
26. Mundey MK, Fletcher A, Marsden CA. Effects of 8-OH DPAT and 5-HT_{1A} antagonists WAY 100135 and WAY 100635 on guinea pig behavior and dorsal raphe 5-HT neurone firing. Br J Pharmacol 1996;117:750–756.
27. Arborelius L, Nomikos GG, Hertel P, et al. The 5-HT_{1A} receptor antagonist (S)-UH-301 augments the increase in extracellular concentrations of 5-HT in the frontal cortex produced by both acute and chronic treatment with citalopram. Naunyn-Schmiedeberg's Arch Pharmacol 1996;353:630–640.
28. Grignaschi G, Invernizzi RW, Fanelli E, et al. Citalopram-induced hypophagia is enhanced by blockade of 5-HT_{1A} receptors: role of 5-HT_{2C} receptors. Br J Pharmacol 1998;124:1781–1787.
29. Segrave R, Nathan PJ. Pindolol augmentation of selective serotonin reuptake inhibitors: accounting for the variability of results of placebo-controlled double-blind studies in patients with major depression. Human Psychopharmacol 2005;20:163–174.
30. Rasmussen K, Calligaro DO, Czachura JF, et al. The novel 5-hydroxytryptamine$_{1A}$ antagonist LY426965: effects on nicotine withdrawal and interactions with fluoxetine. J Pharmacol Exp Ther 2000;294:688–700.
31. Schoeffter P, Hoyer D. Interaction of arylpiperazines with 5-HT_{1A}, 5-HT_{1B}, 5-HT_{1C}, and 5-HT_{1D} receptors. Do discriminatory 5-HT_{1B} receptor ligands exist? Naunyn-Schmiedeberg's Arch Pharmacol 1989;339:675–683.

32. Glennon RA, Westkaemper RB. 5-HT_{1D} receptors: a serotonin receptor population for the 1990s. Drug News Perspect 1993;6:390–405.
33. Middlemiss DN, Beer MS, Matassa VG. 5-HT1D receptors. In: Olivier B, van Wijngaarden I, Soudin W, eds. Serotonin Receptors and Their Ligands. Amsterdam: Elsevier, 1997:101–138.
34. Adham N, Tamm JA, Salon JA, et al. A single point mutation increases the affinity of serotonin $5\text{-HT}_{1D\alpha}$, $5\text{-HT}_{1D\beta}$, 5-HT_{1E}, and 5-HT_{1F} receptors for β-adrenergic antagonists. Neuropharmacology 1994;33:387–391.
35. Glennon RA, Dukat M, Westkaemper RB, et al. The binding of propranolol at $5\text{-hydroxytryptamine}_{1D\beta}$ T355N mutant receptors may involve formation of two hydrogen bonds to asparagine. Mol Pharmacol 1996;49:198–206.
36. Hamel E. 5-HT_{1D} receptors: pharmacology and therapeutic potential. Serotonin 1996;1:19–29.
37. Saxena PR, Tfelt-Hansen P. Success and failure of triptans. J Headache Pain 2001;2:3–11.
38. Ahn AH, Basbaum AI. Where do triptans act in the treatment of migraine? Pain 2005;115:1–4.
39. Villalon CM, Centurion D, Valdivia IF, et al. Migraine: pathophysiology, pharmacology treatment, and future trends. Curr Vasc Pharmacol 2003;1:71–84.
40. Mathew NT, Loder EW. Evaluating the triptans. Am J Med 2005;118(Suppl 1): 28S–35S.
41. Ramadan NM, Skljarevski V, Phebus LA, et al. 5-HT_{1F} receptor agonists in acute migraine treatment: a hypothesis. Cephalgia 2003;23:778–785.
42. Gudermann T, Levy FO, Birnbaumer M, et al. Human S31 serotonin receptor clone encodes a $5\text{-hydroxytryptamine}_{1E}$-like serotonin receptor. Mol Pharmacol 1993;43:412–418.
43. Zgombick JM, Schechter LE, Macchi M, et al. Human gene S31 encodes the pharmacologically defined serotonin $5\text{-hydroxytryptamine}_{1E}$ receptor. Mol Pharmacol 1992;42:180–185.
44. McAllister G, Castro JL. 5-HT_{1E} and 5-HT_{1F} receptors. In: Olivier B, van Wijngaarden I, Soudin W, eds. Serotonin Receptors and Their Ligands. Amsterdam: Elsevier, 1997:141–157.
45. Phebus LA, Johnson KW, Zgombick JM, et al. Characterization of LY344864 as a pharmacological tool to study 5-HT_{1F} receptors: Binding affinities, brain penetration, and activity in the neurogenic dural inflammation model of migraine. Life Sci 1997;61:2117–2126.
46. Sanders-Bush E, Fentress H, Hazelwood L. Serotonin 5-HT_2 receptors: molecular and genomic diversity. Mol Interventions 2003;3:319–330.
47. Leysen JE, 5-HT_2 receptors. Curr Drug Targets CNS Neurol Disord 2004;3:11–26.
48. Gavarini S, Becamel C, Chanrion B, et al. Molecular and functional characterization of proteins interacting with the C-terminal domains of 5-HT_2 receptors: emergence of 5-HT_2 "receptorsomes." Biol Cell 2004;96:373–381.
49. Roth B, Willins DL, Kristiansen K, et al. 5-hydroxytryptamine2-family receptors ($5\text{-hydroxytryptamine}_{2A}$, $5\text{-hydroxytryptamine}_{2B}$, $5\text{-hydroxytryptamine}_{2C}$): where structure meets function. Pharmacol Ther 1998;79:231–257.
50. van Wijngaarden I, Soudijn W. 5-HT_{2A}, 5-HT_{2B}, and 5-HT_{2C} receptor ligands. In: Olivier B, van Wijngaarden I, Soudin W, eds. Serotonin Receptors and Their Ligands. Amsterdam: Elsevier, 1997:161–197.
51. Johnson MP, Wainscott DB, Lucaites VL, et al. Mutations of transmembrane IV and V serines indicate that all tryptamines do not bind to rat 5-HT_{2A} receptors in the same manner. Mol Brain Res 1997;49:1–6.
52. Meltzer HY, Li Z, Kaneda Y, et al. Serotonin receptors: their key role in drugs to treat schizophrenia. Prog Neuropsychopharmacol Biol Psychiat 2003;27: 1159–1172.
53. Iversen L, Glennon RA. Antidepressants, In: Abraham DJ, ed. Burger's Medicinal Chemistry and Drug Discovery, Vol 6, Nervous System Agents. Wiley: New York, 2003:483–524.
54. Reynolds GP. Receptor mechanisms in the treatment of schizophrenia. J Psychopharmacol 2004;18:340–345.
55. Glennon RA. Do hallucinogens act as 5-HT_2 agonists or antagonists? Neuropsychopharmacology 1990;56:509–517.
56. Nelson DL, Lucaites VL, Wainscott DB, et al. Comparison of hallucinogenic phenylisopropylamine binding affinities at cloned human 5-HT_{2A}, 5-HT_{2B}, and 5-HT_{2C} receptors. Naunyn-Schmiedeberg's Arch Pharmacol 1999;359:1–6.
57. Smith RL, Canton H, Barrett RJ, et al. Agonist properties of N,N-dimethyltryptamine at serotonin 5-HT_{2A} and 5-HT_{2C} receptors. Pharmacol Biochem Behav 1998;61:323–330.
58. Newton RA, Phipps SL, Flanigan TP, et al. Characterisation of human $5\text{-hydroxytryptamine}_{2A}$ and $5\text{-hydroxytryptamine}_{2C}$ receptors expressed in the human neuroblastoma cell line SH-SY5Y: comparative stimulation by hallucinogenic drugs. J Neurochem 1996;67:2521–2531.
59. Nelson DL. The serotonin2 (5-HT_2) subfamily of receptors: pharmacological challenges. Med Chem Res 1993;3:306–316.
60. Wainscott DB, Sasso DA, Kursar JD, et al. [^{3}H]Rauwolscine: an antagonist radioligand for the cloned human $5\text{-hydroxytryptamine}_{2B}$ (5-HT_{2B}) receptor. Naunyn-Schmeideberg's Arch Pharmacol 1998;375:17–24.
61. Rothman RB, Baumann MH, Savage JE, et al. Evidence for possible involvement of 5-HT_{2B} receptors in the cardiac valvulopathy associated with fenfluramine and other serotonergic medications. Circulation 2000;102:2836–2841.
62. Setola V, Hufeisen SJ, Grande-Allen KJ, et al. 3,4-Methylenedioxymethamphetamine (MDMA, "Ecstasy") induces fenfluramine-like proliferative actions on human cardiac valvular interstitial cells in vitro. Mol Pharmacol 2003; 63:1223–1229.
63. Kennett GA, Bailey F, Piper DC, et al. Effect of SB 200646A, a $5\text{-HT}_{2C}/5\text{-HT}_{2B}$ antagonist in two conflict models of anxiety. Psychopharmacology 1995;118:178–182.
64. Bickerdike MJ, Vickers SP, Dourish CT. 5-HT_{2C} receptor modulation and the treatment of obesity. Diabetes Obes Metab 1999;1:207–214.
65. Metwally KA, Dukat M, Egan CT, et al. Spiperone: Influence of spiro ring substituents on 5-HT_{2A} serotonin receptor binding. J Med Chem 1998; 41:5084–5093.
66. Kehne JH, Baron BM, Carr AA, et al. Preclinical characterization of the potential of the putative atypical antipsychotic MDL 100,907 as a potent 5-HT_{2A} antagonist with a favorable CNS safety profile. J Pharmacol Exp Ther 1996;277:968–981.
67. Martin JR, Bos M, Jenck F, et al. 5-HT_{2C} receptor agonists: pharmacological characteristics and therapeutic potential. J Pharmacol Exp Ther 1998;286: 913–924.
68. Duxon MS, Flanigan TP, Reavley AC, et al. Evidence for expression of the 5-hydroxytryptamine-2B receptor system in the rat central nervous system. Neuroscience 1997;76:323–329.
69. Lummis SC. The transmembrane domain of the 5-HT_3 receptors: its role in selectivity and gating. Biochem Soc Trans 2004;32(Part 3):535–539.
70. Morreale A, Iriepa I, Galvez E. The 5-HT_3 and nACh ionotropic receptors: a perspective from the computational chemistry point of view. Curr Med Chem 2002;9:99–125.
71. Farber L, Haus U, Spath M, et al. Physiology and pathophysiology of the 5-HT_3 receptor. Scand J Rheumatol Suppl 2004;119:2–8.
72. Dukat M. 5-HT_3 serotonin receptor agonists: a pharmacophoric journey. Curr Med Chem 2004;4:77–94.
73. Campiani G, Cappelli A, Nacci V, et al. Novel and highly potent 5-HT_3 receptor agonists based on a pyrroloquinozaline structure. J Med Chem 1997;40: 3670–3678.
74. Katounina T, Besret L, Dhilly M, et al. Synthesis and biological investigations of [^{18}F]MR 18445, a 5-HT_3 receptor partial agonist. Bioorg Med Chem 1998;6:789–795.
75. Gozlan H. 5-HT_3 receptors. In: Olivier B, van Wijngaarden I, Soudin W, eds. Serotonin receptors and their ligands. Amsterdam: Elsevier, 1997: 221–258.
76. Gaster LM, King FD. Serotonin 5-HT_3 and 5-HT_4 receptor antagonists. Med Res Rev 1997;17:163–214.
77. Heidempergher F, Pillan A, Pinciroli V, et al. Phenylimidazolidin-2-one derivatives as selective 5-HT_3 receptor antagonists and refinement of the pharmacophore model for 5-HT_3 receptor binding. J Med Chem 1997; 40:3369–3380.
78. Evans SM, Huang B-S, Feng D, et al. Probing the 5-HT_3 receptor site using novel indole-3-glyoxylic acid derivatives. Med Chem Res 1993;3:386–406.
79. Gyermek L. 5-HT_3 receptors: pharmacologic and therapeutic aspects. J Clin Pharmacol 1995;35:845–855.
80. Greenshaw AJ. Behavioral pharmacology of 5-HT_3 receptor antagonists: a critical update on therapeutic potential. Trends Pharmacol Sci 1993;14: 265–270.
81. De Wit R, Aapro M, Blower PR. Is there a pharmacological basis for differences in 5-HT_3-receptor antagonist efficacy in refractory patients? Cancer Chemother Pharmacol 2005;56:231–238.
82. Jordin K, Kasper C, Schmoll H.-J. Chemotherapy-induced nausea and vomiting: current and new standards in antiemetic prophylaxis and treatment. Eur J Cancer 2005;41:199–205.
83. Aapro M, Blower P. 5-Hydroxytryptamine type-3 antagonists for chemotherapy-induced and radiotherapy-induced nausea and vomiting. Cancer 2005;104:1–13.
84. Aapro M. Optimizing antiemetic therapy: what are the problems and how can they be overcome? Curr Med Res Opin 2005;21:885–897.
85. Bockaert J, Claeysen S, Compau V, et al. 5-HT_4 receptors. Curr Drug Targets CNS Neurol Disord 2004;3:39–51.
86. Gerald C, Adham N, Kao H-T, et al. The 5-HT_4 receptor: molecular cloning and pharmacological classification of two splice variants. EMBO J 1995;14:2806–2815.
87. Adham N, Gerald C, Schechter L, et al. [^{3}H]5-hydroxytryptamine labels the agonist high-affinity state of the cloned rat 5-HT_4 receptor. Eur J Pharmacol 1996;304:231–235.
88. Blondel O, Gastineau M, Dahmoune Y, et al. Cloning, expression, and pharmacology of four human $5\text{-hydroxytryptamine}_4$ receptor isoforms produced by alternative splicing in the carboxyl terminus. J Neurochem 1998;70: 2252–2261.
89. Eglen RM, Bonhaus DW, Clark RD, et al. (R) and (S) RS 56532: mixed 5-HT_3 and 5-HT_4 receptor ligands with opposing enantiomeric selectivity. Neuropharmacology 1994;33:515–526.
90. Dumuis A, Ansanay H, Waeber C, et al. 5-HT_4 receptors. In: Olivier B, van Wijngaarden I, Soudin W, eds. Serotonin Receptors and Their Ligands. Amsterdam: Elsevier, 1997:261–308.
91. Langlois M, Fischmeister R. 5-HT_4 receptor ligands: applications and new prospects. J Med Chem 2003;30:319–344.
92. Lopez-Rodriguez ML, Benhamu B, Morcillo MJ, et al. 5-HT_4 receptor antagonists: structure–affinity relationships and ligand receptor interactions. Curr Top Med Chem 2002;2:625–641.

93. Maillet M, Robert SJ, Lezoualch F. New insights into serotonin 5-HT_4 receptors: a novel therapeutic target for Alzheimer's disease? Curr Alzheimer Res 2004;1:79–85.
94. Eglen RM, Wong EHF, Dumuis A, et al. Central 5-HT_4 receptors. Trends Pharmacol Sci 1995;16:391–398.
95. Bijak M, Tokarski K, Maj J. Repeated treatment with antidepressant drugs induces subsensitivity to the excitatory effect of 5-HT_4 receptor activation in the rat hippocampus. Naunyn-Schmeideberg's Arch Pharmacol 1997;355: 14–19.
96. Schaus JM, Thompson DC, Bloomquist WE, et al. Synthesis and structure–activity relationships of potent and orally active 5-HT_4 receptor antagonists: indazole and benzimidazolone derivatives. J Med Chem 1998;41:1943–1955.
97. Johanson JF. Options for patients with irritable bowel syndrome: contrasting traditional; and novel serotonergic therapies. Neurogastroenterol Motil 2004;16:701–711.
98. Gershon MD. Review article: serotonin receptors and transporters—roles in normal and abnormal gastrointestinal motility. Aliment Pharmacol Ther 2004;20(Suppl 7):3–14.
99. Nelson DL. 5-HT_5 receptors. Curr Drug Targets CNS Neurol Disord 2004; 3:53–58.
100. Noda M, Higashida H, Aoki S, et al. Multiple signal transduction pathways mediated by 5-HT receptors. Mol Neurobiol 2004;29:31–39.
101. Glennon RA. Higher-end serotonin receptors: 5-HT_5, 5-HT_6, and 5-HT_7. J Med Chem 2003;46:2795–2812.
102. Dubertret C, Hanoun N, Ades J, et al. Family-based association studies between 5-HT_{5A} receptor gene and schizophrenia. J Psychiat Res 2004;38: 371–376.
103. Doly S, Fischer J, Brisorgueh M-J, et al. 5-HT_{5A} receptor localization in the rat spinal cord suggests a role in nociception and control of pelvic floor musculature. J Comp Neurol 2004;476:316–329.
104. Monsma FJ, Shey Y, Ward RP, et al. Cloning and expression of a novel serotonin receptor with high affinity for tricyclic psychotropic drugs. Mol Pharmacol 1993;43:320–327.
105. Woolley ML, Marsden CA, Fone KC. 5-HT6 receptors. Curr Drug Targets CNS Neurol Disord 2004;3:59–79.
106. Kohen R, Metcalf MA, Khan N, et al. Cloning, characterization, and chromosomal localization of a human 5-HT6 serotonin receptor. J Neurochem 1996;66:47–56.
107. Glennon RA, Lee M, Rangisetty JB, et al. 2-Substituted tryptamines: agents with selectivity for 5-HT_6 serotonin receptors. J Med Chem 2000;43: 1011–1018.
108. Sleight AJ, Boess FG, Bos M, et al. Characterization of Ro 04-6790 and Ro 63-0563; Potent and selective antagonists at human and rat 5-HT_6 receptors. Br J Pharmacol 1998;124:556–562.
109. Bromidge SM, Brown AM, Clarke SE, et al. 5-Chloro-N-(4-methoxy-3-piperazin-1-yl-phenyl)-3-methyl-2-benzothiophenesulfonamide (SB-271046): A potent, selective, and orally bioavailable 5-HT_6 receptor antagonist. J Med Chem 1999;42:202–205.
110. Tsai Y, Dukat M, Slassi A, et al. N1-(Benzenesulfonyl)tryptamines as novel 5-HT_6 antagonists. Bioorg Med Chem Lett 2000;10:2295–2299.
111. Russell MGN, Baker RJ, Barden L, et al. N-Arylsulfonylindole derivatives as serotonin 5-HT_6 receptor ligands. J Med Chem 2001;44:3881–3895.
112. Zhou P, Yan Y, Bernotas R, et al. 4-(2-Aminoethoxy)-N-(phenylsulfonyl) indoles as novel 5-HT_6 receptor ligands. Bioorg Med Chem Lett 2005; 15:1393–1396.
113. Holenz J, Merce R, Diaz JL, et al. Medicinal chemistry driven approaches toward novel and selective 5-HT_6 receptor ligands. J Med Chem 2005;48:1781–1795.
114. Cole DC, Lennox WJ, Lombardi S, et al. Discovery of 5-arylsulfonamido-3-(pyrrolidin-2-ylmethyl)-1H-indole derivatives as potent, selective 5-HT_6 receptor agonists and antagonists. J Med Chem 2005;48:353–356.
115. Roth BL, Craigo SC, Choudhary MS, et al. Binding of typical and atypical antipsychotic agents to 5-hydroxytryptamine-6 and 5-hydroxytryptamine-7 receptors. J Pharmacol Exp Ther 1994;268:1403–1410.
116. Hedley L, Kamphuis S, Secchi R, et al. The combined effects of the 5-HT_{2A} antagonist MDL 100,907 and the selective 5-HT_6 receptor antagonist Ro 4368554 in rat models of psychosis and cognition. Behav Pharmacol 2005;16(Suppl 1):S23.
117. Frantz KJ, Hannson KJ, Stouffer DG, et al. 5-HT_6 receptor antagonism potentiates the behavioral and neurochemical effects of amphetamine but not cocaine. Neuropharmacology 2002;42:170–180.
118. Dawson LA, Nguyen HQ, Li P. Potentiation of amphetamine-induced changes in dopamine and 5-HT by a 5-HT_6 receptor antagonist. Brain Res Bull 2003;59:513–521.
119. Svenningsson P, Tzavara ET, Liu F, et al. DARPP-32 mediates serotonergic neurotransmission in the forebrain. Proc Nat Acad Sci U S A 2002;99: 3188–3193.
120. Eglen RM, Jasper JR, Chang DJ, et al. The 5-HT_7 receptor: orphan found. Trends Pharmacol Sci 1997;18:104–107.
121. Heidmann DE, Metcalf MA, Kohen R, et al. Four 5-hydroxytryptamine$_7$ (5-HT_7) receptor isoforms in human and rat produced by alternative splicing. Species differences due to altered intron–exon organization. J Neurochem 1997;68:1372–1381.
122. Vanhoenacker P, Haegeman G, Leysen JE. 5-HT_7 receptors: current knowledge and future prospects. Trends Pharmacol Sci 2000;21:70–77.
123. Forbes IT, Dabbs S, Duckworth DM, et al. *R*-3,N-Dimethyl-N-[1-methyl-3-(4-methylpiperidin-1-yl)propyl]benzenesulfonamide: The first selective 5-HT_7 receptor antagonist. J Med Chem 1998;41:655–657.
124. Kikuchi C, Ando T, Watanabe T, et al. 2α-[4-(Tetrahydropyrodoindol-2-yl)butyl]tetrahydrobenzindole derivatives: new, selective, antagonists of the 5-hydroxytryptamine$_7$ receptor. J Med Chem 2002;45:2197–2206.
125. Paillet-Loilier M, Fabis F, Lepailleur A, et al. Phenylpyrroles, a new chemolibrary virtual screening class of 5-HT_7 receptor ligands. Bioorg Med Chem Lett 2005;15:3753–3757.
126. Vermeulen ES, van Smeden M, Schmidt AW, et al. Novel 5-HT7 receptor inverse agonists. Synthesis and molecular modeling of arylpiperazine- and 1,2,3,4-tetrahydroisoquinolin-based arylsulfonamides. J Med Chem 2004;47:5451–5466.
127. Parikh V, Welch WM, Schmidt AW. Discovery of a series of (4,5-dihydroimidazol-2-yl)biphenylamine 5-HT_7 agonists. Bioorg Med Chem Lett 2003;13: 269–271.
128. Perrone R, Berardi F, Colabufo NA, et al.. Synthesis and structure–affinity relationships of 1-[ω-(4-aryl-1-piperazinyl)alkyl]-1-aryl ketones as 5-HT_7 receptor ligands. J Med Chem 2003;46:646–649.
129. Holmberg P, Sohn D, Leideborg R, et al. Novel 2-aminotetralin and 3-aminochroman derivatives as selective serotonin 5-HT_7 receptor agonists and antagonists. J Med Chem 2004;47:3927–3930.
130. Vermeulen ES, Schmidt AW, Sprouse JS, et al. Characterization of the 5-HT_7 receptor. Determination of the pharmacophore for 5-HT_7 receptor agonism and CoMFA-based modeling of the agonist binding site. J Med Chem 2003;46:5365–5374.
131. Lopez-Rodriguez ML, Porras E, Morcillo MJ, et al. Optimization of the pharmacophore model for 5-HT_7R antagonism. Design and synthesis of new naphtholoactam and naphthosultam derivatives. J Med Chem 2003;46: 5638–5650.
132. Pouzet B. SB-258741: a 5-HT_7 receptor antagonist of potential clinical interest. CNS Drug Rev 2002;8:90–100.
133. Thomas DR, Hagan JJ. 5-HT_7 receptors. Curr Drug Targets CNS Neurol Diord 2004;3:81–90.
134. Hedlund PB, Sutcliffe JG. Functional, molecular and pharmacological advances in 5-HT_7 receptor research. Trends Pharmacol Sci 2004;25:481–486.
135. Sleight AJ, Carolo C, Petit N, et al. Identification of 5-hydroxytryptamine$_7$ receptor binding sites in rat hypothalamus: sensitivity to chronic antidepressant treatment. Mol Pharmacol 1995;47:99–103.
136. Lovenberg TW, Baron BM, de Lecea L, et al. A novel adenylyl cyclase–activating serotonin receptor (5-HT_7) implicated in the regulation of mammalian circadian rhythms. Neuron 1993;11:449–458.
137. Cushing DJ, Zgombick JM, Nelson DL, et al. LY215840, a high-affinity 5-HT_7 receptor ligand blocks serotonin-induced relaxation in canine coronary artery. J Pharmacol Exp Ther 1996;277:1560–1566.
138. Barker EL, Blakely RD. Norepinephrine and serotonin transporters. In: Bloom FE, Kupfer DJ, eds. Psychopharmacology: The Fourth Generation of Progress. New York: Raven Press, 1995:321–333.
139. Maes M, Meltzer HY. The serotonin hypothesis of major depression. In: Bloom FE, Kupfer DJ, eds. Psychopharmacology: The Fourth Generation of Progress. New York: Raven Press, 1995:933–944.
140. Soudjin W, van Wijngaarden I. 5-HT transporter. In: Olivier B, van Wijngaarden I, Soudin W, eds. Serotonin receptors and their ligands. Amsterdam: Elsevier, 1997:327–361.
141. Stanford SC. Prozac: panacea or puzzle? Trends Pharmacol Sci 1996;17: 150–154.
142. Jenck F, Moreau JL, Mutel V, et al. Brain 5-HT_{1C} receptors and antidepressants. Prog Neuropsychopharmacol Biol Psychiat 1994;18:563–574.
143. Broekkamp CLE, Leysen D, Peeters BWMM, et al. Prospects for improved antidepressants. J Med Chem 1995;38:4615–4633.
144. Marcoli M, Maura G, Tortarolo M, et al. Trazodone is a potent agonist at 5-HT_{2C} receptors mediating inhibition of the N-methyl-D-aspartate/nitric oxide/cyclic GMP pathway in rat cerebellum. J Pharmacol Exp Ther 1998; 285:983–986.
145. Murray J. Evidence for acupuncture's analgesic effectiveness and proposals for the physiological mechanisms involved. J Psychol 1995;129:443–461.
146. Walton KG, Pugh ND, Gelderloos P, et al. Stress reduction and preventing hypertension: preliminary support for a psychoneuroendocrine mechanism. J Altern Complement Med 1995;1:263–283.
147. Heidempergher F, Pillan A, Pinciroli V, et al. Phenylimidazolidin-2-one derivatives as selective 5-HT_3 receptor antagonists and refinement of the pharmacophore model for 5-HT_3 receptor binding. J Med Chem 1997;40: 3369–3380.

15. *Amino Acid Neurotransmitters in the Central Nervous System*

TIMOTHY J. MAHER

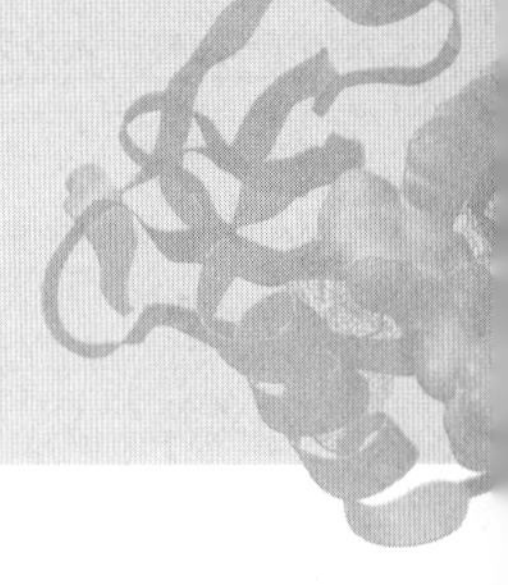

HISTORICAL BACKGROUND

In the late 1800s and early 1900s, scientists studying the physiology of the body began to postulate that drugs produced their responses by interacting with a special group of structures termed "receptive substances." This suggestion was based on the observation that seemingly very minor changes in the chemical structures of a series of compounds greatly altered the biological responses observed following administration of these compounds to animals or people. Later, it was recognized that many of these drugs typically were acting as mimics or antagonists of endogenous compounds and that their responses were caused by interactions with what we today term "receptors." Thus was born the era of chemical neurotransmission, which challenged the long-accepted dogma that communication between cells was the result of electrical transmission.

Acetylcholine released from the parasympathetic nerves innervating the heart and termed "vagustuff" was one of the first neurotransmitters to be recognized. Drugs that acted similarly to the then-unknown acetylcholine, including muscarine and nicotine, led to the eventual characterization of muscarinic cholinergic and nicotinic cholinergic receptors, respectively. Epinephrine found in adrenal gland extracts and termed "adrenaline" also was described in those early days of discovery in the field of neurotransmitter pharmacology. Each of these compounds could produce very powerful responses when released from nerves or tissues or when applied exogenously to isolated tissues or intact animals. Today, we know that these compounds serving as neurotransmitters, neuromodulators, and/or hormones are normal mediators of information transfer throughout the body.

The earliest characterizations of chemical compounds as neurotransmitters involved studies of physiological systems in the periphery and used both chemical and physiological techniques. Later, investigators started to apply some of the same techniques used in characterizing these peripheral neurotransmitters and their receptors to the central nervous system (CNS), which is comprised of the brain and spinal cord. These investigations often were much more difficult because of the complex structures and functions in the CNS. The seemingly less well defined and more ambiguous areas (e.g., limbic system, temporal lobe, and prefrontal cortex) in the CNS as well as the smaller and more diverse synaptic connections (e.g., axo-axonal and somato-dendritic) presented significant challenges to early investigators. In the periphery, stimulation of a nerve innervating a target tissue often led to an easily observable end point (e.g., changes in heart rate or blood pressure, hormone release), but stimulation of nerves in the brain or spinal cord often failed to produce easily observable and quantifiable endpoints (e.g., sensations of warmth, fear, memory, and hallucinations), making such studies very challenging, especially when performed in experimental animals.

Early studies by Falk and Hillarp used formaldehyde to visualize neurons containing the monoamines dopamine, norepinephrine, and epinephrine (fluoresces green) as well as serotonin (fluoresces yellow) in brain slices. With improvements in the chemical techniques for measuring these classical monoamines and acetylcholine and, eventually, the enzymes involved with their synthesis and degradation, investigators began to map the neurons in the CNS that used these neurotransmitters and began to appreciate the neurochemical basis of drug action in the brain and spinal cord. In the late 1950s and early 1960s, however, investigators began to observe the neuronal effects of simple amino acids in these brain tissues. The suggestion that simple amino acids could be sophisticated neurotransmitters was met with considerable resistance and skepticism. These compounds usually are reserved for protein synthesis and serve many metabolic functions, and they did not appear to have the same unique functional characteristics of the classical monoamine neurotransmitters and acetylcholine. As studies continued to support the neurotransmitter role of amino acids such as γ-aminobutyric acid (GABA), glutamic acid (glutamate [Glu]) and glycine, however, overwhelming evidence has led to their nearly universal acceptance as the major neurotransmitters in the CNS. Quantitatively, the amino acids are the most prevalent neurotransmitters in the CNS. For example, it has been estimated that more than 40% of all neurons in the CNS use GABA as a neurotransmitter substance and that less than 10% use one of the other monoamines, such as norepinephrine and serotonin, or acetylcholine.

Although neuronal functioning is very complex, a simplistic view of the two major effects of neurotransmitters involve changes in membrane potential toward states of depolarization and hyperpolarization (Fig. 15.1). Such changes in membrane potential usually result from alterations in membrane conductance to ions such as Na^+, K^+, Ca^{2+}, and Cl^-, which typically flow down their electrochemical gradients when a selective ion channel is opened. Ion channels need only open for 0.1 to 100 milliseconds to effect this change. Thus, when a neuron is to be depolarized, Na^+ or Ca^{2+} typically enters the cell, making the membrane potential more positive and more likely to reach the threshold potential and exhibit an action potential (Fig. 15.1A). On the other hand, when a neuron is hyperpolarized, typically either K^+ moves out of the cell into the extracellular space or Cl^- moves

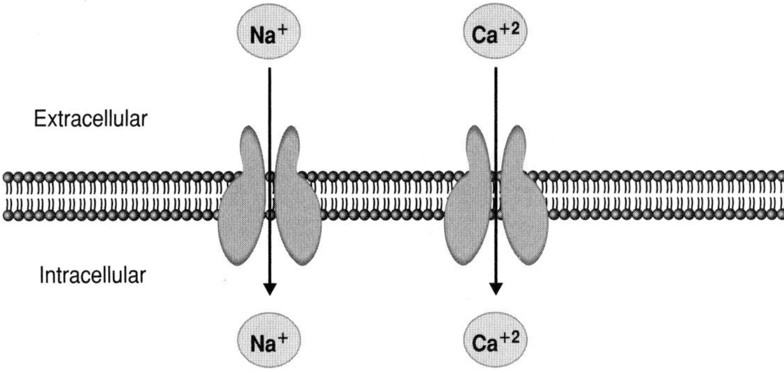

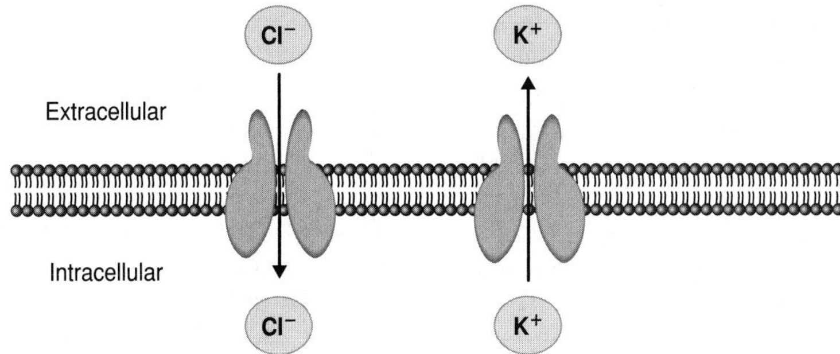

Fig. 15.1. Electrophysiology of excitatory and inhibitory neurotransmitters. The tendency of an ion to move across the membrane depends on the difference in its electrochemical gradient on either side of the membrane. The electrochemical gradient depends on the difference in the concentration of the ion between the two sides of the membrane, the charge of the ion, and the transmembrane potential (the difference in voltage between the two sides of the membrane).

into the cell (Fig. 15.1B). Both of these ion fluxes result in a hyperpolarization of the membrane, which decreases the likelihood that a neuronal cell will fire. Thus, these two opposing alterations in neuronal membrane potentials commonly are referred to as excitatory (depolarization) and inhibitory (hyperpolarization). When amino acid neurotransmitters produce their effects on neuronal function, they commonly are categorized as either excitatory amino acids (EAAs) or inhibitory amino acids (IAAs) (Fig. 15.2). The major established EAA neurotransmitter in the CNS is Glu. Other endogenous EAAs include aspartate (Asp), cysteine, and homocysteine. The major endogenous IAAs in the CNS include GABA and glycine, but much evidence also supports a role for taurine and β-alanine.

Excitatory amino acids:

L-Glutamate L-Aspartate L-Cysteine L-Homocysteine

Inhibitory amino acids:

GABA Glycine β-Alanine Taurine

Fig. 15.2. Endogenous excitatory and inhibitory amino acids.

NEUROTRANSMITTER CRITERIA

For a compound to be classified as a neurotransmitter substance, a number of criteria must be satisfied. Firstly, the neurotransmitter must be present. Usually, the concentrations of the neurotransmitter in various parts of the CNS will vary such that a unique and unequal distribution results. For some amino acids, this unequal distribution is difficult to demonstrate, because most of these compounds also are used to support protein synthesis and for intermediary metabolism, unlike the monoamine neurotransmitters, for which an unequal distribution is relatively easy to demonstrate. Although compounds such as glucose and sodium are present in the CNS, their regional distribution is rather uniform, and few would consider either of these to be a classical neurotransmitter substance. Besides determining the concentration of the neurotransmitter itself, evidence that also can be used to support this criterion include the distribution of specific receptors, reuptake systems, and enzymes involved with synthesis and/or degradation of the particular amino acid neurotransmitter. Today, with the aid of molecular biological techniques (e.g., mRNA, cloning techniques, and in situ hybridization), the location and quantification of proteins that serve as receptors, transporters, or metabolizing enzyme is more readily achieved. Second, the compound must be released when the nerve cell is stimulated. To date, the vast majority of amino acid neurotransmitter release, like that of the monoamines and acetylcholine, has been found to be Ca^{2+}-dependent and originating from presynaptic storage vesicles. Release can be determined using brain slices prelabeled with radioactive neurotransmitter or with in vivo microdialysis, in which the extracellular fluid surrounding neurons is continuously sampled. Additionally, there should be a mechanism in place that terminates the action of the neurotransmitter compound (e.g., reuptake, removal into astroglia or other cells, metabolism, or some other form of inactivation). Finally, for a compound to be considered a neurotransmitter, the exogenous administration or application of the suspected neurotransmitter compound must mimic the effects (e.g., depolarization, hyperpolarization, activation of protein kinase C, or inhibition of adenylyl cyclase) that are observed when the neurotransmitter is released endogenously following nerve cell stimulation.

EXCITATORY AMINO ACID NEUROTRANSMITTERS

Glutamate

The major EAA neurotransmitter in the CNS is L-Glu. (Note that all amino acids with the exception of glycine mentioned in this chapter are considered to be in the "L" configuration; thus, the "L" will be omitted, unless specifically indicated as "D"). Early studies in invertebrates demonstrated the potent actions of the acidic amino acid Glu, as well as another acidic amino acid, Asp. Acceptance of Glu as a neurotransmitter in the CNS was delayed for many years as neuroscientists attempted to distinguish its role as a component of protein and peptides (e.g., glutathione), an important intermediate in numerous metabolic processes, and as a precursor to the inhibitory neurotransmitter GABA. Whereas Glu is found in all cells within the CNS, an unequal distribution of this amino acid as well as of Asp has been demonstrated.

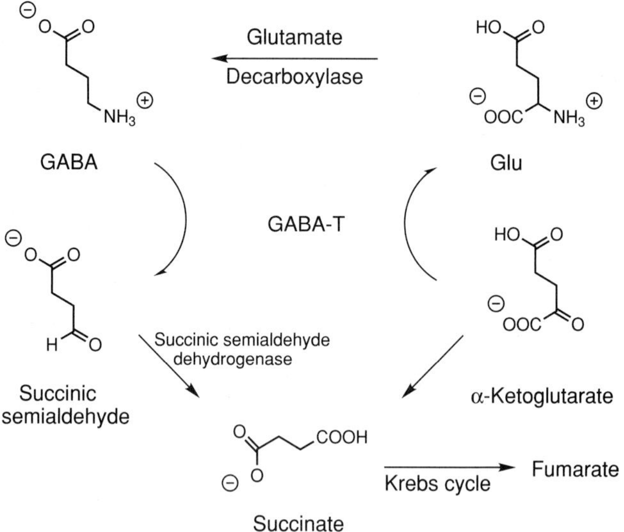

Fig. 15.3. GABA biosynthesis.

Glutamate Synthesis, Storage, and Release

Glutamate is synthesized in the CNS via the transamination of α-ketoglutarate (Fig. 15.3), which is produced from glucose in the Krebs cycle. Additionally, Glu can be synthesized from glutamine via glutaminase. Once produced, Glu can be stored in vesicles. With the vast number of compounds that can feed into the Krebs cycle and the various sources of glucose, it is not surprising that the control of Glu synthesis in the CNS is still poorly understood.

The oral ingestion of Glu in protein, as the individual amino acid in the form of a dietary supplement or in the form of the flavor enhancer monosodium glutamate (MSG), fails to significantly increase CNS levels of this amino acid neurotransmitter. Following its ingestion, blood Glu levels do increase transiently, but largely because of the ability of the blood-brain barrier to regulate the entry of Glu into the CNS, no significant changes in brain Glu are observed. This ability to regulate synaptic Glu levels in brain despite fluctuations in peripheral levels is very important, because uncontrolled variations in CNS Glu would lead to serious consequences, ranging between seizures and coma for increases and decreases of Glu, respectively. Within the blood-brain barrier, there exists transport proteins that are responsible for controlling the influx of amino acids into the CNS. Of the three major types—acidic, basic, and neutral amino acid transporters—it is the acidic amino acid transporter that carries Glu. These transporters act via facilitated diffusion and cannot operate against a concentration gradient (active transport). In actuality, the acidic amino acid transporter normally functions to move Glu out of the

CNS. There have been studies in which Glu, often in the form of MSG, has been injected subcutaneously to neonatal mice or nonhuman primates and hypothalamic lesions noted. The lesions are mostly restricted to the circumventricular organs (those near the fourth ventricle), where the blood-brain barrier is significantly diminished. Additionally, when MSG is directly injected into the brains of laboratory animals, cellular necrosis is observed. When MSG is given in very high doses orally, however, the homeostatic processes in liver and other tissues help to regulate plasma Glu concentrations, and large changes are not observed. Additionally, the blood-brain barrier functions to keep CNS Glu at appropriate levels. The studies in which Glu is injected do not reflect the chemical changes that occur following oral ingestion and should not be interpreted as an indicator of toxicity of MSG (1).

Similar concerns have been voiced regarding the safety of the acidic amino acid Asp in the artificial sweetener aspartame (L-aspartyl-L-phenylalanine methylester). As with MSG, however, the homeostatic mechanisms regulating

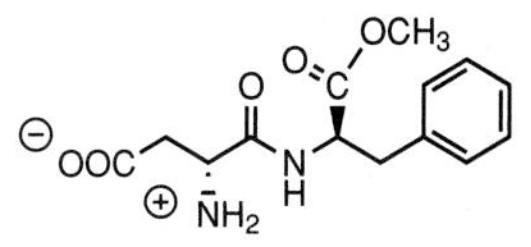

Aspartame

plasma Asp levels following Asp consumption do not allow for large increases in plasma Asp that could alter CNS function. In fact, the concern regarding the safety of aspartame results from the other amino acid phenylalanine, which much more readily crosses the blood-brain barrier and can alter CNS function. This is especially important for people who unknowingly are heterozygous for phenylketonuria (2).

The transporter, VGLUT1, transports Glu into storage vesicles in preparation for the Ca^{2+}-mediated release of this neurotransmitter that uses adenosine triphosphate (ATP) to concentrate Glu against its concentration gradient (ATP-dependent transporter). Unrelated to any of the other families of neurotransmitter vesicle transporters, VGLUT1 originally was thought to be an inorganic phosphate membrane transporter. Today, it is known that VGLUT1 uses a vacuolar ATPase to cleave ATP to provide the energy required to generate and maintain an electrochemical proton gradient that allows the concentration of Glu to remain extremely high in synaptic vesicles compared to that in the cytoplasm—and especially compared to that in the synapse. Although probably not the basis of their main pharmacological actions, known inhibitors of VGLUT1 include the ergot bromocriptine (a dopamine agonist used in the treatment of Parkinson's disease and hyperprolactinemia) and some of the azo-dyes, including Evans Blue (3). Recently, a family of endogenous inhibitory proteins has been identified that not only blocks Glu vesicular transport but also GABA vesicular transport. The significance of the role that these proteins, known as IPF_α, IPF_β, and IPF_γ, play in regulating glutamatergic neurotransmission is still poorly understood (4). As more is learned about such proteins and other yet unknown regulatory mechanism, a better appreciation regarding the pathology of various disease states may be realized and therapeutic interventions designed based on this knowledge.

Like most other recognized neurotransmitter substances, vesicular release of Glu occurs in a Ca^{2+}-dependent manner following depolarization of the presynaptic terminal. In cell culture or isolated tissue studies, agents that bind Ca^{2+}, such as ethylenediamine tetra-acetic acid (EDTA) or Ca^{2+}-free perfusion solutions, the vesicular release of Glu can be diminished or prevented. Thus, this is one of the techniques that can be employed to distinguish, in part, between the neurotransmitter and metabolic roles of Glu in a particular biological system.

Glutamate Reuptake and Metabolism

Transporter proteins that regulate the synaptic concentrations of Glu are essential in keeping the basal levels of this EAA neurotransmitter low and in helping to terminate the responses to neuronally released Glu. These high-affinity, sodium-dependent transporters are so efficient at sequestering Glu from the synaptic cleft that the concentration of Glu inside the presynaptic terminal usually is several thousand-fold greater than that found in the synapse (5).

These EAA transporters (EAATs) have been identified and characterized into five major subtypes: EAAT1, EAAT2, EAAT3, EAAT4 and EAAT5 (Table 15.1 and Fig. 15.4). Their distribution tends to be primarily cellular, and relative anatomical distribution of the subtypes in brain for each subtype is such that EAAT1 and EAAT2 are mostly found in astroglial cells in the cerebellum and forebrain, respectively. The astroglial reuptake of neuronally released Glu is believed to be very important in terminating the Glu-mediated synaptic signal. The EAAT3 and EAAT4 subtypes are highly concentrated in the cortical and cerebellar Purkinje neurons, respectively, whereas the EAAT5 is most abundant in the retina. The reuptake of Glu or Asp via any of the EAAT subtypes is coupled to the cotransport of H^+ and $3Na^+$ into astroglia or neurons, with the extrusion of K^+, as shown in Figure 15.4.

Table 15.1. Excitatory Amino Acid Transporters

Subtype	Predominant Brain Distribution
EAAT1	Cerebellar glia
EAAT2	Forebrain glia
EAAT3	Cortical neurons
EAAT4	Cerebellar Purkinje neurons
EAAT5	Retina

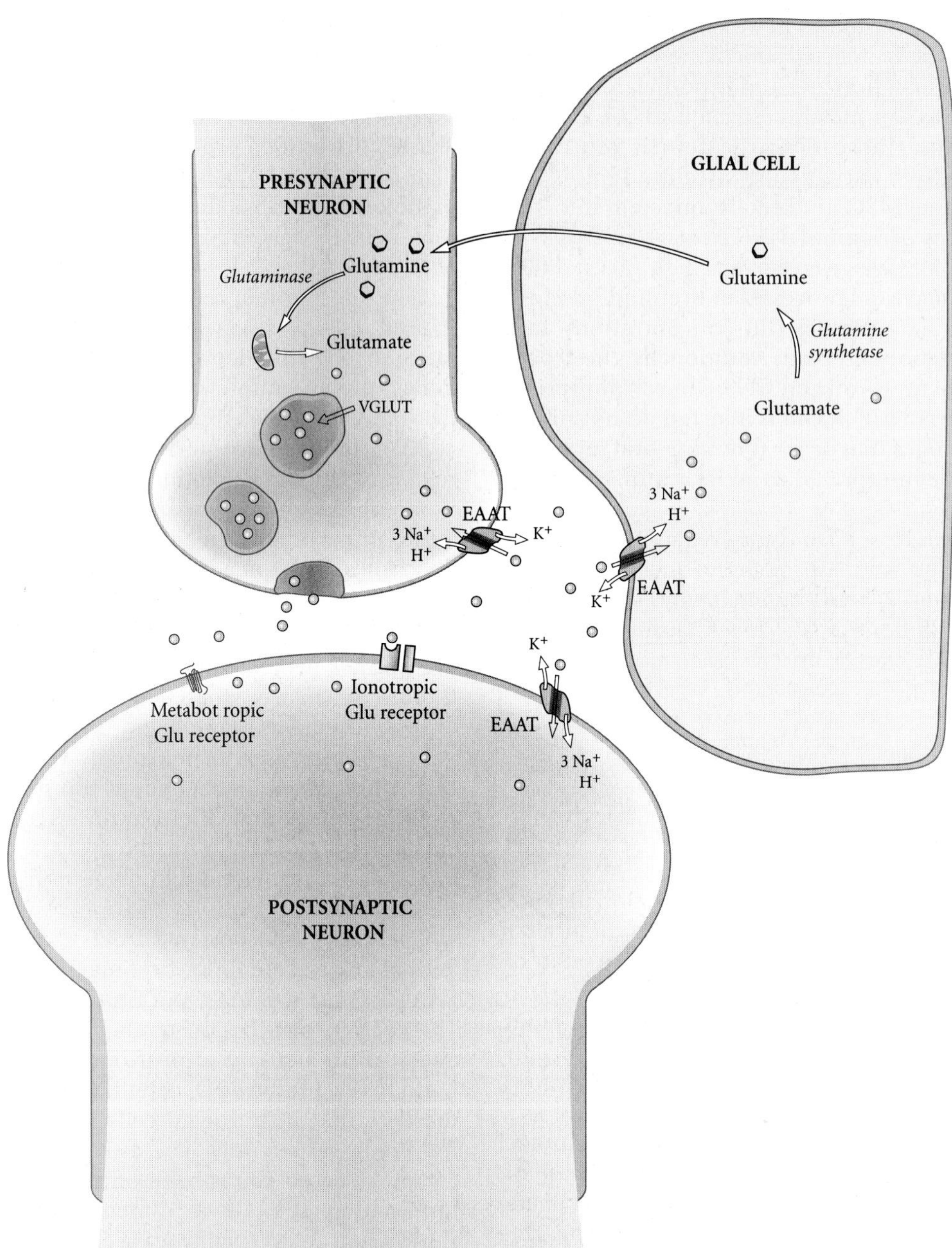

Fig. 15.4. The glutamate neuron showing the formation of glutamate (o) from glutamine (◊), ionotropic and metabotropic receptors, storage vesicles, and reuptake transporters.

The EAATs are capable of transporting D-Asp, L-Asp, and L-Glu but do not transport D-Glu. The known inhibitors of Glu reuptake transport are classified as either competitive (these usually act as substrates and are transported) or noncompetitive (these are nontransported), but no therapeutically useful agents have yet been discovered. The actions of Glu are terminated via its reuptake into the presynaptic neuron, from where it originally was released, into the surrounding glia and into the postsynaptic neuron, as demonstrated, that houses the various target EAA receptors (6). Following its release, Glu that is taken up via EAATs into neurons or astroglial cells may be recycled, in part, directly into vesicles for subsequent release or, more likely, is converted to glutamine via glutamine synthetase and is available for eventual recycling to Glu via the activity of the enzyme glutaminase, as shown in Figure 15.4.

EAA Receptors

The receptors for Glu and the other EAAs are categorized into major two groups: ionotropic, and metabotropic (Fig. 15.4). The three ionotropic receptor types are classified based on their selective affinity for the EAA ligands: N-methyl-D-aspartate (NMDA), α-amino-3-hydroxy-5-methyl-4-isoxazole propionic acid (AMPA), and kainite

Table 15.2. Ionotropic Glutamate Receptor Subtypes

Subtype	Subunits	Agonists	Actions
AMPA	GluR1 GluR2 GluR3 GluR4	Glutamate or AMPA	Increases Na^+ and Ca^{2+} influx, increases K^+ efflux
Kainate	GluR5 GluR6 GluR7 KA1 KA2	Glutamate or kainate	Increases Na^+ influx, increases K^+ efflux
NMDA	NR1 NR2A NR2B NR2C NR2D	Glutamate or NMDA and glycine	Increases Ca^{2+} influx, increases K^+ efflux

(Table 15.2). AMPA is a homologue of the neurotoxin ibotenic acid found in *Amanita* mushrooms. Kainate is a neurotoxin isolated from red algae.

NMDA L-AMPA Kainate

These ligand-gated ion channel receptors are composed of homo- or heterotetramers of individual subunits that confer cation-selectivity. Each subunit has an extracellular N-terminus with three transmembrane domains, an intramembrane reentrant "p-loop" between the first and third transmembrane domains, and an intracellular C-terminus (Fig. 15.5) (7). The metabotropic Glu receptors belong to the larger family of G protein–coupled receptors (GPCRs). When activated, these metabotropic receptors can alter the activity of effector proteins, such as adenylyl cyclase and

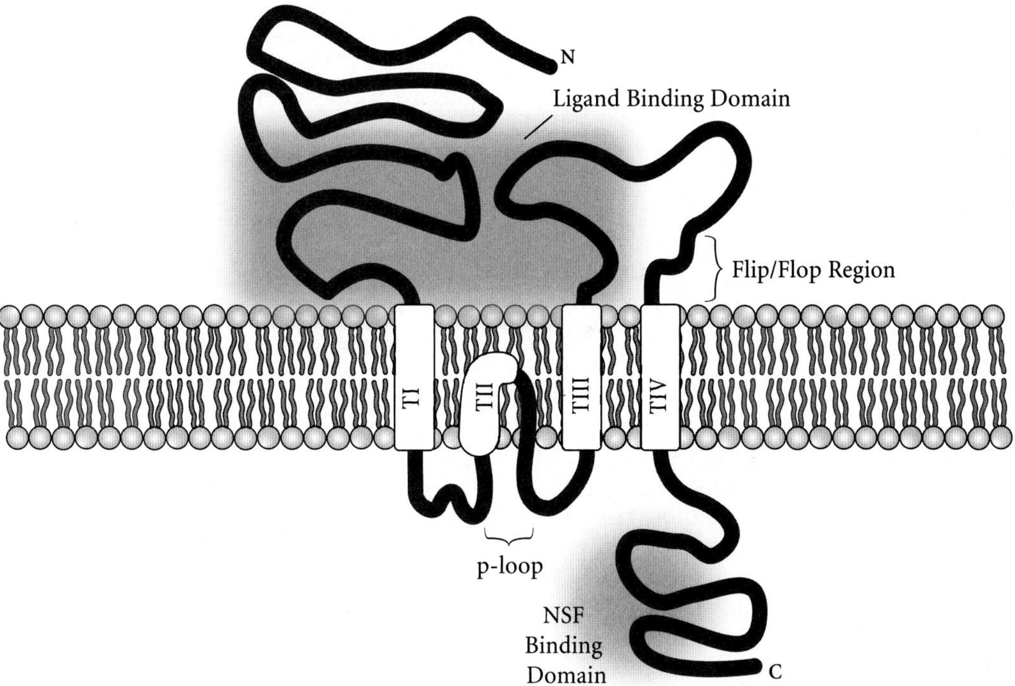

Fig. 15.5. The ionotropic glutamate receptor showing the p-loop, ligand binding domain, N-ethylmaleimide-sensitive fusion protein (NSF) binding domain (shaded area), flip/flop region, and the N- and C-terminal regions.

phospholipase C (PLC). To date, at least eight distinct EAA metabotropic receptor subtypes appear to exist. The EAA receptors, in balance with the receptors for the IAAs, likely are crucial for the regulation of neuronal plasticity involving dynamic changes of neurons in response to environmental stimuli. Neuronal plasticity accounts for the ability of an organism to learn and adapt, which includes both long-term potentiation and long-term depression.

Ionotropic Receptors

NMDA RECEPTOR. The NMDA receptor is a heterotetramer comprised of a number of subunit forms—GLU_{N1}, GLU_{N2A}, GLU_{N2B}, GLU_{N2C}, GLU_{N2D}, GLU_{N3A}, and GLU_{N3B}—that can confer unique pharmacology to individual receptors (Table 15.2). Additionally, splice variants can lead to a number of isoforms of the above subunits with the potential of changing the binding characteristics and functions on the receptor. Activation of the NMDA receptor requires the binding of two agonists: Glu to the GLU_{N2} subunit, and glycine to a binding site on the GLU_{N1} subunit (8). Glycine appears to act as an important coagonist positive modulator at a unique recognition site on the GLU_{N1} subunit, and unlike the actions of glycine as an IAA neurotransmitter, this recognition site is not sensitive to blockade by strychnine (see the following section on glycine). Thus, this glycine binding site often is referred to as the strychnine-insensitive receptor or site. Agonists at the Glu binding site on the GLU_{N2} subunit include NMDA, Glu, Asp, and homoquinolinic acid. The best-characterized antagonist at this site is D-2-aminophosphonopentanoate. D-Serine is a well-known agonist

Homoquinolinate D-AP5 D-Serine

at the GLU_{N1} glycine site. D-Serine, which normally is found only in glia and astrocytes, is synthesized from L-serine via serine racemase and is thought to be one of the important modulators of NMDA receptor activity.

The NMDA receptor also has many sites for channel modulation by pharmacological agents. Endogenous inhibitory channel modulators include Mg^{2+}, Zn^{2+}, and protons. Neurosteroids can either inhibit or potentiate NMDA receptor channel function depending on how the subunits comprising the tetrameric structure are assembled. For instance, the neurosteroid pregnenolone sulfate inhibits NMDA receptors that are assembled as GLU_{N1}/GLU_{N2C} but potentiates those assembled as GLU_{N1}/GLU_{N2A} and GLU_{N1}/GLU_{N2B} (9). Polyamines, such as spermine and spermidine, are known to be positive channel modulators.

Spermine Spermidine Pregnenolone sulfate

A number of important NMDA channel antagonists (Fig. 15.6) also exist, and these include amantadine (an antiviral agent that also releases dopamine and is used in Parkinson's disease), ketamine (a dissociative anesthetic agent that acts via the NMDA receptor), phencyclidine (a psychoactive drug of abuse also known as PCP), and memantine (recently approved for the treatment of Alzheimer's disease). Whereas the antitussive agent dextromethorphan, via its metabolite dextrorphan, is known to block within the NMDA channel, its cough-suppressant activity likely is not the result of action at this site. The psychotomimetic effects observed with the abuse of this compound, however, are likely mediated by the NMDA receptor. An endogenous antagonist of the NMDA receptor is Mg^{2+}, which normally prevents the flow of Ca^{2+} through the channel. When both Glu or another suitable agonist binds, along with glycine, the inhibition normally maintained by Mg^{2+} is relieved, Ca^{2+} can flow, and the cell can depolarize. Some studies in experimental animals have demonstrated the NMDA receptor–mediated neuroprotective effects of Mg^{2+} in models of stroke and other CNS insults.

One of the first NMDA receptor antagonists to be identified was dizocilpine, commonly known as MK-801 (Fig. 15.6). Initially, much excitement was generated with the discovery of MK-801, because the ability to block the excessive intracellular cation flow (Ca^{2+}, Na^{+}) that follows neuronal hypoxic insults, as are seen following cerebral vascular accidents (stroke) or head trauma, might lead to effective treatments for such pathological conditions. Whereas MK-801 was very effective in decreasing infarct size in various rodent models of stroke, poor efficacy was

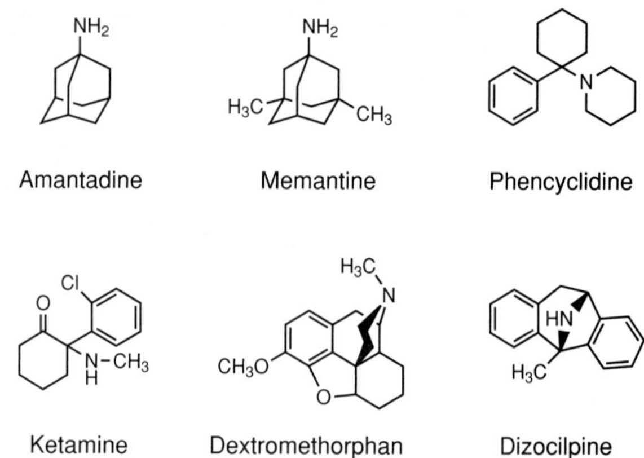

Fig. 15.6. NMDA channel antagonists.

noted in humans. Additionally, the generation of severe psychotic behaviors was deemed to be unacceptable.

The strychnine-insensitive binding site on the NMDA receptor also has been a target for researchers, because an agent that would antagonize this binding site might be useful in preventing the neuronal damage that occurs following hypoxic insults that lead to excessive Glu release or in controlling electrical neuronal dysfunction associated with epilepsy. One agent, R-(+)-3-amino-1-hydroxypyrrolidin-2-one ((R)-HA-966), is a glycine receptor antagonist that, unfortunately, has not been used

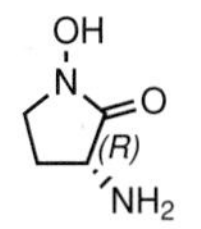

(R)-HA-966

therapeutically because of its hepatotoxic properties unrelated to the NMDA receptor. Whereas the dicarbamate anticonvulsant felbamate (see Chapter 20) produces part of its activity by inducing conformational (allosteric) changes in the receptor (allosterism) that alters the binding of glycine at the NMDA glycine binding site. Felbamate also has interactions at the AMPA and kainate receptors that contribute to its anticonvulsant activity (10,11).

AMPA Receptors

Another ionotropic EAA receptor is preferentially activated by AMPA. While at one time, this receptor was referred to as the quisqualate receptor, but the AMPA receptor mediates fast synaptic activity via the influx of Na^+ and, in some neurons, K^+ efflux (Table 15.2). The AMPA receptor, which is found in high abundance in the cerebral cortex and hippocampus, is comprised of four subunits: GluR1, GluR2, GluR3, and GluR4. One of these subunits, GluR2, when present prevents the formation of an ionophore that can efficiently conduct Ca^{2+}. When the AMPA receptor does not contain a GluR2 subunit, however, Ca^{2+} can be conducted through the ion channel. On the extracellular loop between transmembrane segments III and IV exists a region termed the "flip-flop" that is sensitive to splice variants of the gene coding for each subunit. Such splice variants can lead to significant differences in the desensitization kinetics of the receptor (12). Additionally, intracellular sites on the C-terminus, where modulatory proteins such as N-ethylmaleimide-sensitive fusion protein and protein interacting with C kinase can bind, allow another important site where regulation of receptor trafficking can be influenced.

Recently, the discovery that some of the 2,3-benzodiazepines (e.g., GYK1 53655) can selectively bind the AMPA receptor has aided in studies to understand its location and functions, especially where mixed populations of EAA receptors are present (13). Agents known to potentiate AMPA receptor activity include piracetam (a

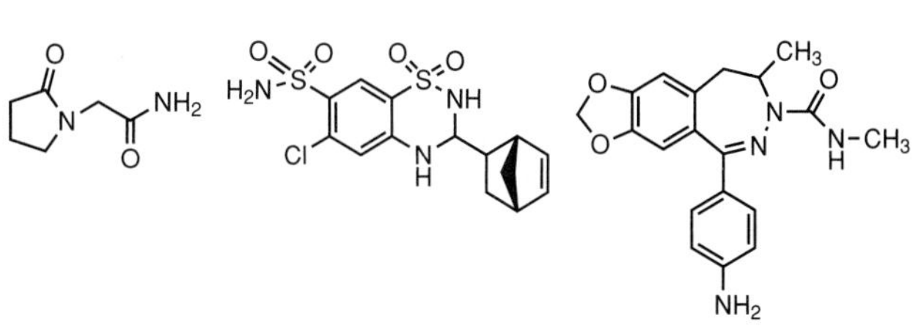

Piracetam Cyclothiazide GYKI 53655

Fig. 15.7. AMPA agonists.

drug for improving mental performance), a cyclic derivative of GABA, and the benzothiazide diuretic, cyclothiazide (Fig. 15.7). Additionally, some evidence suggests that certain barbiturates and volatile anesthetics have binding sites on the AMPA receptor. Agents that act to cause conformational changes that positively modulate the AMPA receptor have been termed "ampakines" and have been suggested to improve memory, to enhance the activity of certain antipsychotic agents, to improve attention-deficit hyperactivity disorder, to improve Parkinson's disease symptoms, and to provide neuroprotection following CNS ischemic insults (14).

Kainate Receptors

The ionotropic kainate receptor is a heterotetramer comprised of subunits GluR5, GluR6, GluR7, KA1, and KA2 (Table 15.2). The subunits GluR5, GluR6, and GluR7 can form functional homo- and heteromeric receptors; the KA1 and KA2 subunits require the presence of the GluR5, GluR6, and GluR7 subunits to properly assemble into functional receptors. Similarities exist between the binding characteristics of AMPA receptors and kainite receptors such that few pharmacological agents are available that effectively differentiate between the two (15). Kainate receptors tend to be more sensitive to the phycotoxin domoic acid, an EAA found in red algae (*Pseudonitzschia* sp.), than are AMPA receptors. Domoic acid causes Amnesic shellfish poisoning that may cause in humans nausea, vomiting, abdominal cramps, short-term memory loss, seizures, arrhythmias, and death in severe cases of ingestion. Domoic acid bioaccumulates in shellfish that feed on the red algae phytoplankton.

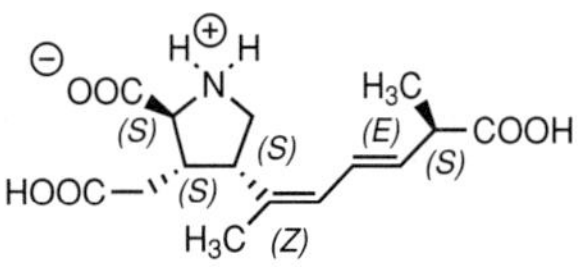

Domoic acid

Kainate receptors are located postsynaptically and mediate neuronal excitation, as do NMDA and AMPA receptors, but kainate receptors also have been found to be located presynaptically. Such presynaptic receptors appear to regulate the release of GABA in the hippocampus and Glu in other brain regions. Additionally, some kainate receptors have been shown to be linked to a pertussis toxin–sensitive G protein, which via interaction with PLC may in turn act to influence nearby voltage-dependent Ca^{2+} channels (16). This dual signaling capability of kainate receptors appears to be unique for an EAA ionotropic receptor and may facilitate the role of this receptor subtype in influencing both short- and long-term synaptic plasticity (adaptive changes to the synapse affecting the efficacy of neurotransmission) in the CNS.

Metabotropic Glutamate Receptors

Another class of EAA receptors are the G protein–coupled metabotropic receptors (m), which are categorized into one of three groups based on their pharmacology, sequence similarity, and intracellular effector signaling systems. Group I, which includes mGlu1 and mGlu5, are positively coupled to PLC via $G_{q/11}$, whereas Group II, which includes mGlu2 and mGlu3, and Group III, which includes mGlu4, mGlu6, mGlu7, and mGlu8, are negatively coupled via $G_{i/o}$ to adenylyl cyclase (17). The term "metabotropic" is used to indicate that activation of these receptors results in alterations in metabolic processes within the cell. All of the metabotropic receptors are activated by Glu and ibotenate, but none is activated by NMDA, AMPA, or kainate.

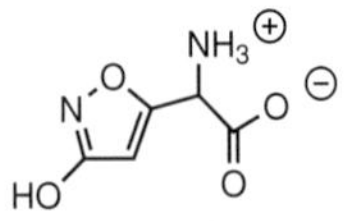

Ibotenate

Few useful selective agonists or antagonists are available for these receptors subtypes, but some researchers have used knockout mice to explore the role of a particular metabotropic receptor. For instance, mice lacking the mGlu5 receptor fail to display the reinforcing and locomotor stimulant effects of cocaine, suggesting that an agent that is selective at antagonizing the mGlu5 receptor might find utility in treating patients dependent on cocaine (18). Additionally, because the mGlu5 receptor is located in areas of the brain thought to be involved with anxiety, compounds that negatively modulate this receptor subtype have been shown to be anxiolytic in animal studies. The Group II mGlu receptors also are highly concentrated in areas involved with anxiety such that agents that are selective positive modulators for this receptor subtype are found to act as anxiolytics. Finally, positive modulators of the mGlu4 receptor subtype have been suggested as an approach for treating Parkinson's disease (19). As more information is revealed about the distribution, function, binding characteristics, and trafficking of the metabotropic receptor subtypes in the CNS, advances in the therapy of disease states such as Parkinson's, schizophrenia, chronic pain, epilepsy, depression, and drug dependence may be realized (20).

A steady accumulation of evidence supports a role for Glu and its mGlu1 and mGlu5 receptors in depression and antidepressant activity. Furthermore, evidence also implicates Glu release, which can result in activation of NMDA and mGlu1 and mGlu5 receptors, an underlying cause for depression and anxiety. Studies with NMDA receptor antagonists of mGlu1 and mGlu5 receptors as well as positive modulators of AMPA receptors have antidepressant-like activity in a variety of preclinical models. The concept of NMDA antagonists as antidepressants has generated considerable interest in the NMDA receptor as a target for new antidepressant therapies (see Chapter 21). Several studies have shown that chronic antidepressant treatment can modulate NMDA receptor expression and function. Preclinical studies with NMDA receptor antagonists have demonstrated their potential antidepressant properties.

INHIBITORY AMINO ACID NEUROTRANSMITTERS

γ-Aminobutyric Acid

The major IAA neurotransmitter in the mammalian CNS is GABA (Fig. 15.2). Initially found to be involved with neuromuscular transmission in the lobster, GABA has since been well characterized as a neurotransmitter in the brain and spinal cord of mammals. In the periphery, in tissues such as the liver, spleen, sympathetic ganglia, and splenic nerve, GABA and its receptors also are found. The levels are very low, however, and their function in these non-CNS tissues is poorly understood. While levels of GABA in the CNS are very high (millimoles per gram tissue) compared to those of the classical monoamine neurotransmitters (nanomoles per gram tissue), the distribution of GABA in the CNS is unique, with an unequal distribution, thus supporting a neurotransmitter role. Unlike many of the other putative amino acid neurotransmitters that also are components of CNS proteins, GABA is not known to be incorporated into proteins, thus making it easier to support a role for GABA as a neurotransmitter.

The synthesis of GABA uses Glu and the enzyme glutamic acid decarboxylase (GAD), the levels of which closely parallel those of GABA (Fig. 15.3). Although Glu itself functions as an important neurotransmitter, the control of GABA synthesis appears to be dependent on the activity of GAD and its cofactor, pyridoxal phosphate. Glutamic acid can be synthesized from α-oxoglutaric acid, α-ketoglutarate, and glutamine (Fig. 15.3). Glucose and pyruvate also can be converted to Glu via metabolism involving the Krebs cycle. Two isoforms of GAD derived from different genes have been characterized: GAD-65, and GAD-67. The lower-molecular-weight GAD-65 has a much higher affinity for its pyridoxal cofactor than does the larger GAD-67. Additionally, there appears to be different cellular and subcellular distribution patterns between the two GAD isoforms, but the significance of their unique roles in GABAergic neurotransmission is not fully understood (21).

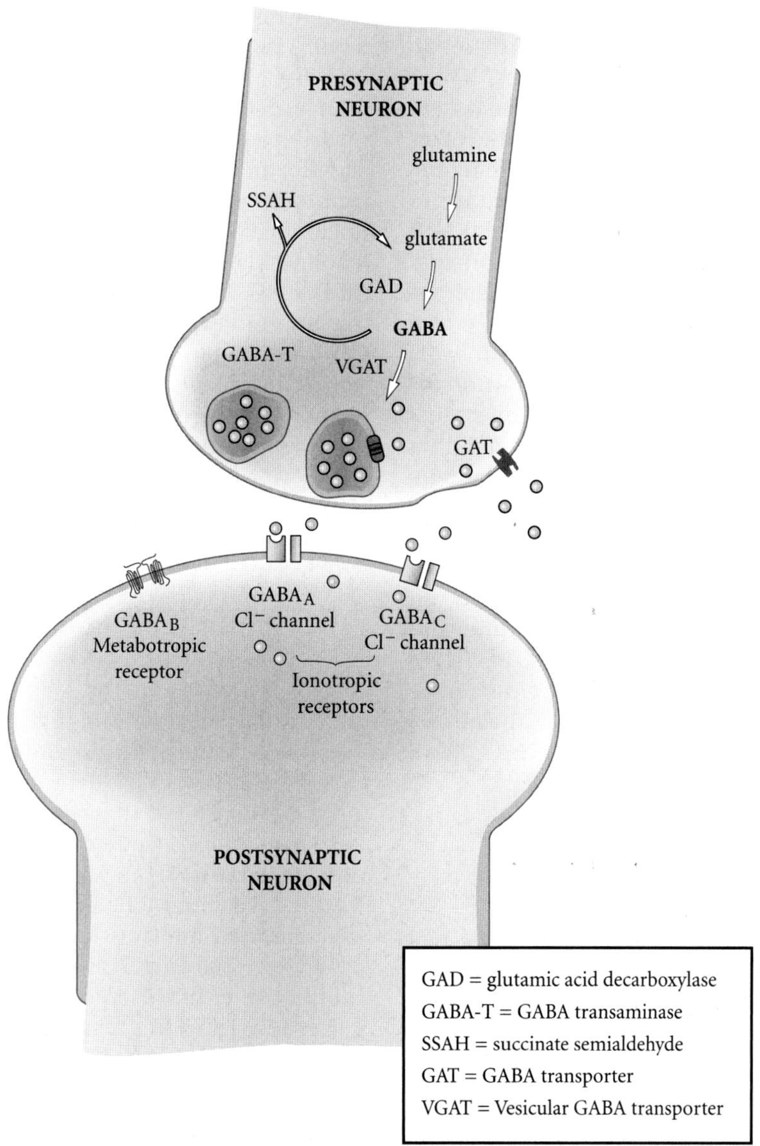

Fig. 15.8. The GABA neuron, showing the formation of GABA, ionotropic and metabotropic receptors, and reuptake transporters.

In a similar manner to most other classical neurotransmitters, GABA, once synthesized, is stored in vesicles located in the presynaptic nerve terminals, as shown in Figure 15.8. A specific vesicular transporter protein (VGAT) has been identified that transports largely GABA into the storage vesicles (22). The VGAT lacks complete selectivity, because the other major IAA neurotransmitter glycine also appears to be a substrate for VGAT, which has been shown to be present in glycinergic terminals. Unlike the well-defined vesicular transporters for the monoamine neurotransmitters, which are characterized by 12 transmembrane-spanning segments, VGAT only contains 10 such transmembrane-spanning segments. Similar to the monoamine vesicular transporters, however, VGAT appears to be driven by a H^+ electrochemical gradient generated by an ATP-dependent H^+ pump in the vesicle plasma membrane. Whereas vigabatrin potently inhibits and nipecotic acid weakly inhibits VGAT, the role of VGAT inhibition in the overall pharmacological actions of these agents is not

Vigabatrin Nipecotate

known, because both agents probably act largely via other mechanisms involving GABA.

Nerve stimulation leading to depolarization of GABAergic presynaptic terminals cause the Ca^{2+}-mediated exocytosis of vesicles containing GABA. Once released, GABA diffuses across the synapse to the postsynaptic side, where interaction with GABA receptors takes place, leading to hyperpolarization of the postsynaptic neuron, as shown in Figure 15.8 (these receptor subtypes are described in detail below). Some regulation of GABA release occurs via presynaptic $GABA_B$ autoreceptors that decrease subsequent neurotransmitter release. The termination of the GABA-mediated signal takes place as a result of reuptake transporter systems that transport GABA back into the presynaptic neuron or into surrounding glial cells and astrocytes. This dual neuronal–glial reuptake process is distinct from that observed with the classical monoamines, for which neuronal reuptake predominates. Four transporters with 12 transmembrane-spanning segments have been identified and cloned: GAT-1, GAT-2, GAT-3, and BGT-1 (23). All four are capable of transporting GABA, but they also can transport other IAAs, particularly glycine, β-alanine, and taurine (Fig. 15.2). One of the transporters, BGT-1, is capable of transporting the dimethylated glycine derivative betaine and also is known as the betaine transporter. A number of inhibitors of these transporters are known,

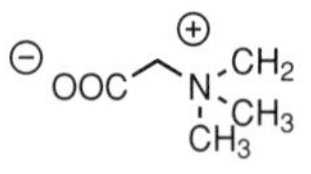

Betaine

but only one currently is available for therapeutic use. Tiagabine, by selectively inhibiting GAT-1, which may be the major GABA neuronal reuptake transporter, is an approved agent for the treatment of partial seizures (see Chapter 20). Clinical trials are underway for its use in the treatment of anxiety, neuropathic pain, and insomnia (24). Two GABA analogues that have been shown to interact with GAT-1 include gabapentin and pregabalin. The concentrations required to inhibit GAT, however, are very high, and a GABAergic mechanism of action

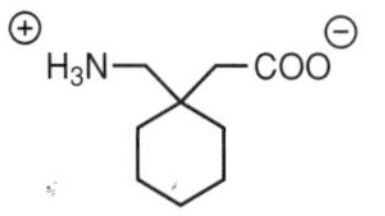

Gabapentin 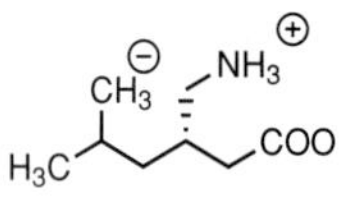 Pregabalin

most likely does not explain their anticonvulsant activity (25). Despite their close structural similarity to GABA, inhibition of a voltage-gated calcium channel containing the $\alpha_2\delta_1$ subunit is believed to be responsible for their pharmacological actions.

Metabolism of GABA occurs via a series of enzymatic steps starting with GABA transaminase (GABA-T), as shown in Figure 15.3. This reversible mitochondrial enzyme uses pyridoxal phosphate as a cofactor and is widely distributed throughout the CNS. Transamination results in the formation of succinic semialdehyde (SSA), which can be further metabolized to succinate via SSA dehydrogenase (SSADH) or, alternatively, reduced to γ-hydroxybutyrate (GHB). Other metabolites of unknown significance include carnitine, homoanserine, homopantothenic acid, and a number of γ-butyryl derivatives, including γ-butyryllysine, γ-butyrylhistidine, and γ-butyrylcholine. Vigabatrin (γ-vinyl-GABA), an irreversible inhibitor of GABA-T, increases the levels of GABA by inhibiting its metabolism and is used for the treatment of seizure disorders in some countries. Other inhibitors of GABA-T include gabaculline and acetylenic GABA. These agents display anticonvulsant activity in experimental animal models of epilepsy.

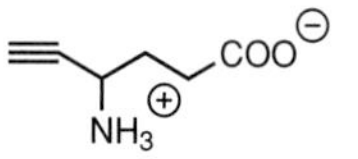

Acetylenic GABA 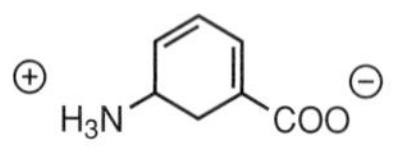 Gabaculine

$GABA_A$ Receptors

The initial observations that application of GABA was capable of hyperpolarizing neurons, as well as the lack of activity of structurally related amino acids and other compounds, suggested that a receptor likely mediated this response. At least three different families of GABA receptors have been identified to date: $GABA_A$, $GABA_B$, and $GABA_C$ (Fig. 15.9). The $GABA_A$ receptor was the first to be identified and was found to be a neurotransmitter-gated ion channel (ionotropic) that, when activated, allows the entry of chloride ion into the cell, thereby hyperpolarizing the neuron and making cell firing less likely to occur. The $GABA_A$ receptor (Fig. 15.9) is a member of the Cys-loop (cysteine–cysteine loop located on the N-terminal region) family of receptors that also include the strychnine-sensitive glycine, nicotinic acetylcholine, and serotonin $5\text{-}HT_3$ receptors. The pentameric $GABA_A$ receptor is composed of various combinations of subunits (α, β, γ, δ, ϵ, π, ρ, and θ). Various subunit isoforms have been identified with 6α, 3β, 3γ, and 3ρ subunits (some have suggested that the ρ subunits are found only in the $GABA_C$ receptor). Each subunit is a four transmembrane-spanning protein that, when arranged in a circle, forms the ion channel with a diameter of approximately 8 nm that remains closed until GABA binds to its ligand recognition site. One of the most common $GABA_A$ receptor conformations in the mammalian CNS consists of a pair of α_1 subunits, a pair of β subunits, and a single γ_2 subunit, as shown in Figure 15.10. Other commonly identified receptors contain α_1, α_2, α_3, and α_5 as well as forms of the β subunit and, typically, the γ_2 subunit, and always in a 2:2:1 stoichiometry (26). The binding of two molecules of GABA, as shown in Figure 15.10, probably to the individual β subunits near the α–β interface, is believed to be required for normal receptor activation. In fact, among $GABA_A$ receptors, 17 different

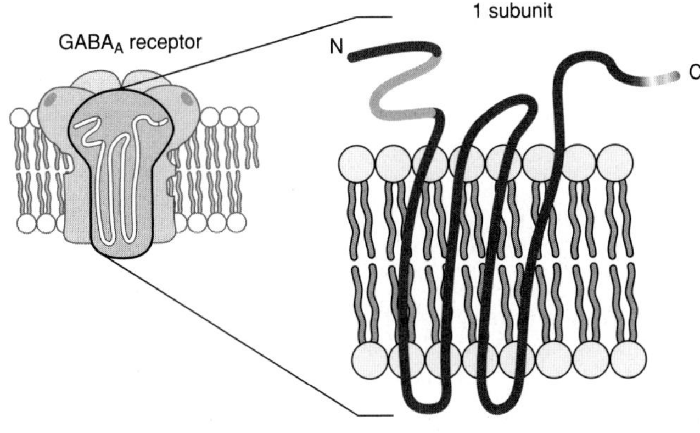

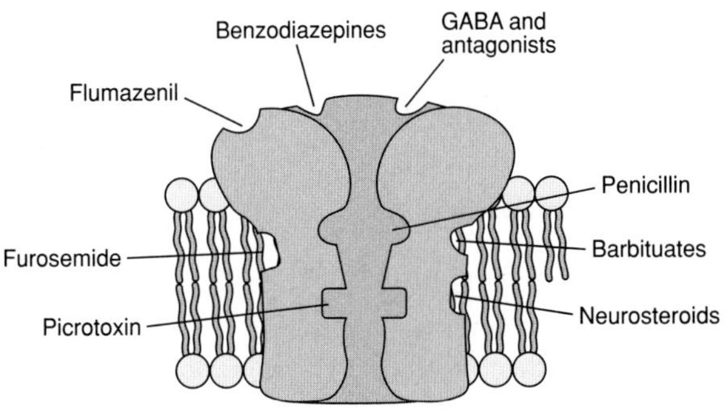

Fig. 15.9. GABA$_A$ receptor. (A) The structure of the GABA$_A$ receptor, showing the N- and C-terminal regions of the four membrane-spanning regions for each of the five subunits. (B) The major binding sites on the GABA$_A$ receptor. (From Chou J, Strichartz GR, Lo EH. Pharmacology of excitatory and inhibitory neurotransmitters, Chapter 10. In: Golan DE, Tashjian A, Tashjian A, et al. Principles of Pharmacology: The Pathophysiologic Basis of Drug Therapy. Baltimore: Lippincott, Williams & Wilkins, Baltimore, 2004: pp139-160; with permission.)

combinations of subunits have been identified. Having a family of receptors that all share the same basic structure but that differ in specific subunit composition allows greater levels of functional diversity. Each of the receptor varieties vary in binding affinity, channel activity, and the degree to which GABA binding is affected by different endogenous modulators. As a result, inhibitory neurotransmission can be more finely controlled. Such receptor heterogeneity also allows more control at the genomic level, in turn allowing postsynpatic cells to respond to changing environmental needs or variable activity at the synapse (plasticity).

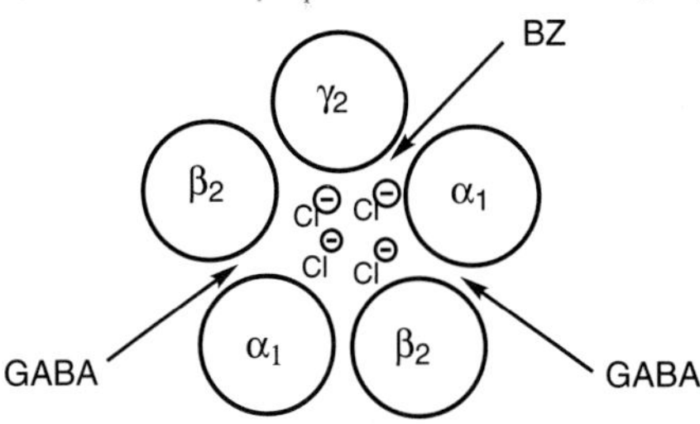

Fig. 15.10. Extracellular view of the GABA$_A$ receptor showing the location of benzodiazepine (BZ) and low-affinity GABA binding sites.

A major class of compounds that modulate GABA$_A$ receptor function is that of the benzodiazepines (e.g., diazepam). The binding site for benzodiazepines likely is the α subunit in proximity to the β subunit, as shown in Figure 15.10. The form of the γ subunit appears to help to determine the affinity of the individual benzodiazepine to the receptor. The benzodiazepines appear to bind better to receptors containing γ_2 than to the γ_1

Diazepam

Ro-19-4603

subunit, as shown in Table 15.3. Similarly, very low-affinity binding is observed if a receptor contains the α_6 subunit. In fact, the α_6 subunit seems to confer binding preference to inverse agonists (agents that stabilize the inactive/resting receptor), such as Ro194603. The benzodiazepines do not bind to the GABA (ligand-recognition) site on the receptor and can only produce effects if presynaptic GABA has been released and is present at the receptors. Benzodiazepines are allosteric modulators, or ligands that bind at a secondary binding site on a receptor that is distinct from the primary ligand binding site, resulting in conformational changes in the structure of the receptor that either activates or, sometimes, inhibits the receptor. Thus, the benzodiazepines allosterically modulate the GABA$_A$ receptor, increasing the frequency of the chloride channel opening when GABA is bound, thus potentiating the response of exogenously released GABA. The benzodiazepines are very safe when used alone in the absence of CNS depressants, because they are not active on GABA receptors alone. This is in contrast to the barbiturates that can directly activate the GABA$_A$ receptor when present at higher concentration and, thus, have a much lower therapeutic index. Flumazenil, a benzodiazepine receptor antagonist, is used for the treatment of severe overdoses of benzodiazepines. Flumazenil competitively antagonizes the binding and allosteric effects of benzodiazepine agonists as well as benzodiazepine inverse agonists, such as the β-carbolines.

Flumazenil

β-Carboline

Gaboxadol

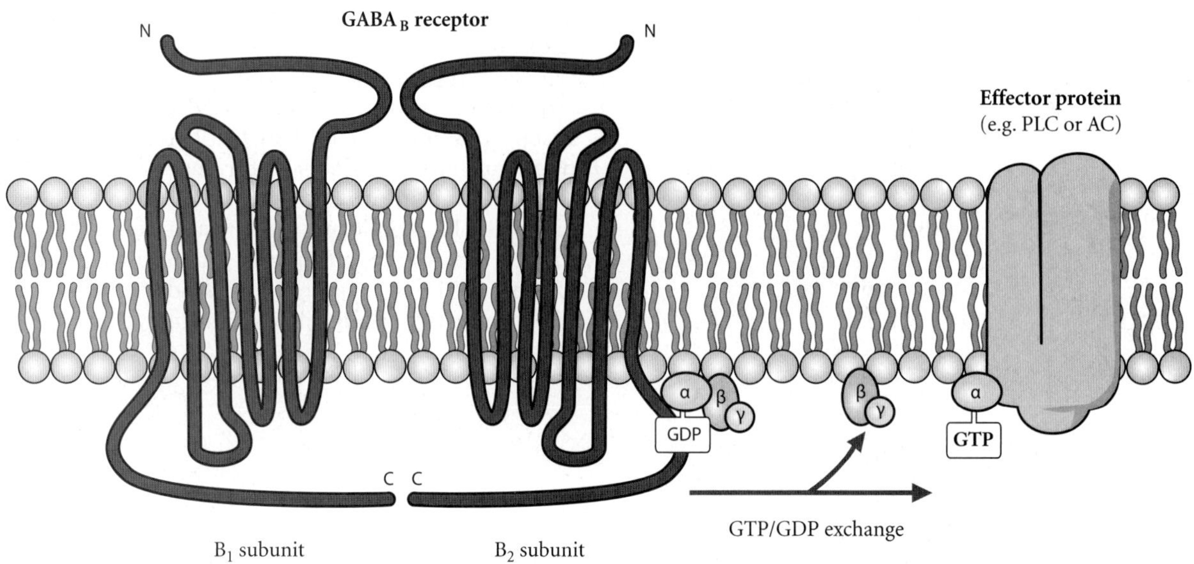

Fig. 15.11. The $GABA_B$ receptor, showing its B_1 and B_2 subunits and its mechanism of signal transduction.

Using molecular biological techniques, point mutations of the α subunits have revealed that the sedative effects of the benzodiazepines likely result from an interaction with the α_1 subunit, whereas the anxiolytic effects result from an interaction at the α_2 subunit (27,28), as shown in Figure 15.10 and Table 15.3. Nonbenzodiazepine receptor agonists, such as the sedative-hypnotics indiplon, zaleplon, zolpicone, and zolpidem (see Chapter 19), are α_1 subunit–preferring ligands, as shown in Table 15.3 (29).

An agent that acts on the $GABA_A$ receptor that does not interact with the benzodiazepine binding site is gaboxadol (previously called THIP). This sedative-hypnotic binds with high affinity to the extrasynaptic $\alpha_4\beta_x\delta$ $GABA_A$ receptor and does not alter sleep onset or REM sleep as do the benzodiazepines. On the other hand, gaboxadol increases slow-wave sleep (30).

The barbiturates bind to a different portion of the $GABA_A$ receptor and, similar to the benzodiazepines, enhance the activity of GABA. The binding of a barbiturate leads to an increase in the duration of ion channel opening. Higher concentrations of the barbiturates can directly open the chloride channel; thus, overdoses of barbiturates can lead to life-threatening, CNS-mediated respiratory and cardiovascular depression.

A number of compounds are known to directly activate the $GABA_A$ receptor. Of these compounds, muscimol, the decarboxylated metabolite of ibotenate, and

Table 15.3. A Comparison of the Binding Affinities (nM) of Benzodiazepine and Nonbenzodiazepine Ligands for $GABA_A$ Receptor Subtypes (45)

	$GABA_A$ Receptor Subtypes					
Compound	$\alpha_1\beta\gamma_2$	$\alpha_2\beta\gamma_2$	$\alpha_3\beta\gamma_2$	$\alpha_4\beta\gamma_2$	$\alpha_5\beta\gamma_2$	$\alpha_6\beta\gamma_2$
Benzodiazepines						
Diazepam	16	17	17	>10,000	15	>10,000
Clonazepam	1.3	1.7	2.0	—	—	>10,000
Triazolam	1.8	1.2	3.0	—	1.2	—
Flumazenil	1.0	1.1	1.5	107	2.4	90
Nonbenzodiazepines						
Zaleplon	130	1,820	1,530	>10,000	490	>10,000
Zolpidem	17	290	357	—	>15,000	—
Zoplicone	19	33	—	—	—	—

isoguvacine are the most well known. Unlike GABA, which does not cross the blood-brain barrier, these agents do cross the blood-brain barrier and display GABA-mimetic activity following peripheral administration. Additionally, a number of compounds can bind to the $GABA_A$ receptor and antagonize the actions of GABA. Bicuculline, by binding to the GABA recognition site and preventing GABA from binding, produces convulsions in experimental animals. Picrotoxin, via its active metabolite picrotoxinin, binds in the chloride channel to prevent ion flow when the receptor is activated by GABA. Picrotoxin does not alter GABA binding but, instead, prevents ions from flowing and is a potent convulsant.

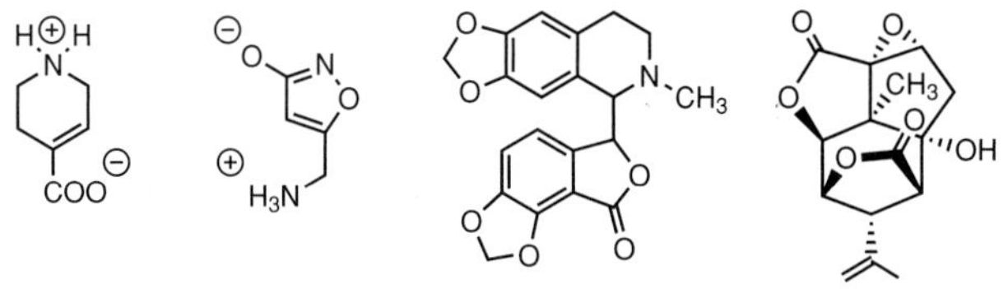

Isoguvacine Muscimol Bicuculline Picrotoxinin

With the many possible subunit assembly sequences of $GABA_A$ receptors, advances in medicinal chemistry may someday lead to the design of compounds that target specific pentameric subunit assemblies to preferentially produce specific effects (31). For instance, located on the base of the dendritic spines of hippocampal pyramidal cells are $GABA_A$ receptors with an α_5 subunit composition. These receptors are thought to counteract the excitatory input because of glutamatergic NMDA receptor activation involved in learning and memory. Activation of $GABA_A$ receptors in this area disrupt learning and memory, whereas NMDA receptor activation improves learning and memory. Administration of an inverse agonist of the $GABA_A$ receptor with selectivity for the α_5 subunit improves memory performance in experimental animals (32). Additionally, α_3-selective agonists may be useful in treating schizophrenia, because this subtype of $GABA_A$ receptor appears to play a role in decreasing the release of dopamine from overactive neurons in the mesolimbic system (33).

General anesthetics (see Chapter 18) also appear to have interactions with the $GABA_A$ receptor in producing their various anesthetic effects, including immobilization, respiratory depression, and hypnosis via binding to hydrophobic pockets within the receptor. Using point-mutated knock-in mice, general anesthetic agents, such as enflurane, etomidate, and propofol, have been found to interact with the β_3 subunit of the $GABA_A$ receptor to produce immobilization and hypnosis (33). The heart rate and body temperature depressant effects of etomidate and propofol, however, do not appear to be mediated by the sub-β_3 subunit. Studies are underway to improve our understanding of the molecular mechanisms of this chemically varied group of agents used as general anesthetics.

Neurosteroids also are capable of modulating the activity of GABA at the $GABA_A$ receptor by binding to a site distinct from that used by GABA, benzodiazepines, and barbiturates. These steroids, including the progesterone metabolites pregnanolone, allopregnanolone, and allotetrahydrodeoxycorticosterone, enhance GABA- mediated inhibitory activity. The presence of the δ subunit in the pentameric $GABA_A$ receptor greatly increases the affinity of steroid binding and efficacy. High concentrations of these steroids also can result in direct activation of the receptor.

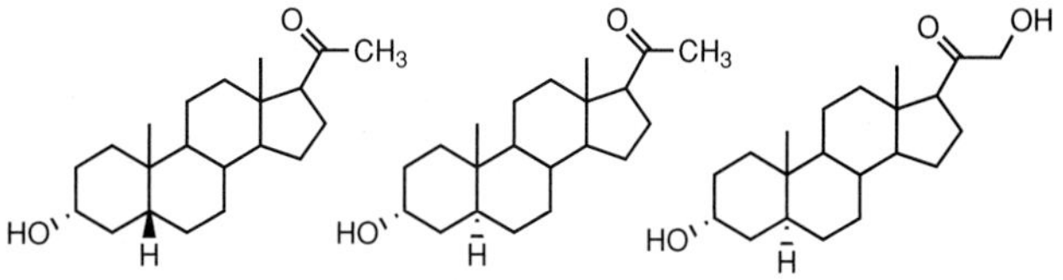

Pregnanolone Allopregnanolone Allotetrahydrodeoxy-corticosterone

Thus, it may be possible in the future to selectively target the various modulatory sites on the $GABA_A$ receptor to produce preferential pharmacological effects—for example, benzodiazepines that are anxiolytic without sedative effects, antischizophrenic agents that lack sedation and extrapyramidal side effects, and general anesthetics that do not alter respiratory and/or heart rates.

$GABA_B$ Receptors

As studies continued, the application of GABA to cells occasionally was found to produce effects that were not blocked by the standard GABA receptor antagonist bicuculline. Additionally, standard GABA agonists, such as muscimol and isoguvacine, were ineffective as agonists in such systems. This led to the suggestion that a different subtype of GABA receptor mediated these observed effects. In 1998, the structure of the $GABA_B$ receptor was elucidated and found to be a GPCR heterodimer comprised of $GABA_{B1}$ and $GABA_{B2}$ subunits (Fig. 15.11). Each subunit had a 7-membrane spanning segment, which allowed their intracellular C-termini to connect in a 1:1 stoichiometric fashion (34). The $GABA_{B1}$ subunit also was found to exist in two isoforms, $GABA_{B1a}$ and $GABA_{B1b}$. Some have suggested that the $GABA_{B1a}$ subunit is preferentially located presynaptically, whereas the $GABA_{B1b}$ subunit is located postsynaptically. Within this metabotropic receptor, the $GABA_{B1}$ subunits contain the GABA binding domain extracellularly, whereas the $GABA_{B2}$ subunit couples to the G-protein mechanism intracellularly. Both subunits are required for normal receptor function, as shown in Figure 15.11. Knockout mice lacking either of these subunits typically display epileptiform seizures, hyperalgesia, hyperlocomotion, and impaired memory function (35). Besides the normal endogenous agonist GABA, a structural analogue, (−)-baclofen, acts stereoselectively as an agonist at the $GABA_B$

Baclofen

CGP 36742

receptor. (±)-Baclofen, which enters the brain via a selective transporter, has been approved for therapeutic use since 1972 for the treatment of spasticity as a muscle relaxant (36). Besides relaxing skeletal muscles, baclofen is capable of exacerbating absence seizures, decreasing cognitive function, increasing food intake, and decreasing drug-seeking behaviors. Drug development of selective $GABA_B$ receptor antagonists may someday lead to therapeutically useful agents for the treatment of absence seizures, depression, anxiety, and cognitive impairments. One such compound currently undergoing clinical trials is the orally bioavailable $GABA_B$ receptor antagonist CGP-36742, which is in clinical trials for the treatment of mild cognitive impairment and Alzheimer's disease. The inhibition of $GABA_B$ receptors is believed to cause disinhibition of somatostatin (a peptide neurotransmitter in the CNS) release, which then allows activation of NMDA receptors in the hippocampus that normally are required for memory and cognitive functions (37).

γ-Hydroxybutyrate

Another endogenous compound that binds to and weakly activates the $GABA_B$ receptor is GHB (38). This compound, which can be formed as a result of the metabolism of GABA, has a unique distribution in the CNS, but it does not parallel closely that of GABA, as shown in Figure 15.12. Levels of GHB are increased significantly in patients and knockout mice lacking the enzyme SSADH, which is responsible for the conversion of SSA to succinic acid, with eventual entry into the citric acid cycle. A deficiency of this enzyme in patients is caused by a rare, autosomal recessive inheritance and is termed "GHB aciduria" (39).

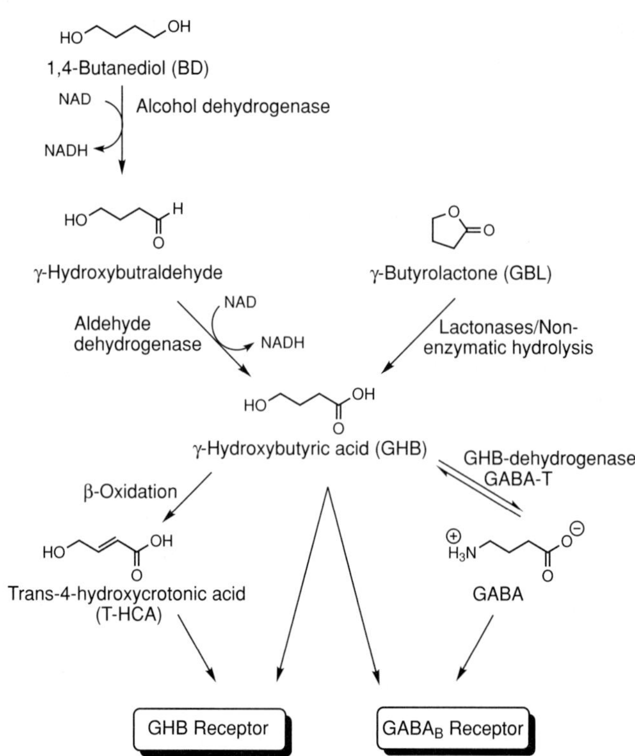

Fig. 15.12. The Biotransformation of 1,4-butanediol (BD) and γ-butyrolactone (GBL) and the receptor sites for their metabolites, γ-hydroxybutyrate (GHB), GABA, and trans-4-hydroxycrotonic acid (T-HCA).

Endogenous GHB likely interacts with a recently discovered GHB receptor, but the function of GHB in the CNS is not completely understood. A specific GHB receptor was reportedly cloned in 2003 and found to have no sequence homology with the $GABA_B$ receptor—or with any other known GPCR (40). This putative receptor is a member of the GPCR family and is distributed in most brain regions known to bind GHB. The association is not perfect, however, because high levels of mRNA for the GHB receptor are found in the cerebellum even though little GHB normally binds here.

In the United States, GHB is approved for the treatment of cataplexy associated with the sleeping disorder narcolepsy (41). Narcolepsy usually is characterized by a lack of the CNS 11-amino-acid polypeptide orexin (also known as hypocretin) or, possibly, its receptors. Patients with narcolepsy experience excessive bouts of sudden-onset daytime sleepiness and have been treated in the past with stimulants, such as methylphenidate and amphetamine, or with modafinil (see Chapter 23) or antidepressants. The use of GHB in narcolepsy takes a different approach in that dosing is at bedtime and, being a CNS depressant, it acts to enhance sleep quality. Patients then awake the following morning and experience a rebound insomnia, which counteracts any propensity for daytime sleepiness. Exogenously administered GHB appears to produce its clinical and toxic effects via interaction with $GABA_B$ receptors, because most studies have been able to block its effects with $GABA_B$ receptor antagonists but not with the GHB receptor antagonist NCS-382 (although NCS-382 is not an ideal antagonist as it can function as a partial agonist).

NCS-382

Additionally, GHB has been used for illicit purposes. Because GHB produces CNS sedation with amnesia, some have used this compound for drug-facilitated sexual assault (e.g., "date rape"). As regulations on the availability of GHB became tighter, the use of GHB precursors, such as γ-butyrolactone and 1,4-butanediol, became popular (42). Figure 15.12 shows the biotransformation of γ-butyrolactone and 1,4-butanediol to GHB and GABA, explaining their relationship to GHB and $GABA_B$ receptors. They are popular as drugs-of-abuse because they are readily available as solvents. Furthermore, GHB can be further metabolized by β-oxidation to trans-4-hydroxycrotonic acid, which also can bind to the GHB receptor. Body builders use these compounds as well in an attempt to enhance the release of growth hormone. Usually, however, chronic abuse leads to tolerance, with a need to increase dosing and a propensity to produce physical dependence (43). A serious and difficult-to-treat withdrawal syndrome from GHB abuse has been documented.

$GABA_C$ Receptor

Another receptor that binds GABA but is not antagonized by bicuculline ($GABA_A$) or phaclofen ($GABA_B$) and is not

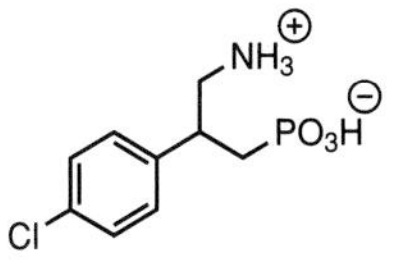

Phaclofen

influenced by either the benzodiazepines or barbiturates is known as the $GABA_C$ receptor. The endogenous neurotransmitter GABA is an order of magnitude more potent on the $GABA_C$ receptor as compared with the $GABA_A$ receptor, and the responses to activation of the $GABA_C$ receptor are much slower and sustained as compared with the rapid and brief responses following $GABA_A$ receptor activation. The $GABA_C$ receptor is most abundant in the retina, with significant levels in the spinal cord and pituitary gland. This ligand-gated ion chloride channel is a pentamer of subunits that form the ion channel. Some have suggested that the ρ subunit is unique to the $GABA_C$ receptor (44). On the extracellular domain are binding sites for zinc, which is a potent modulator of receptor activity. The most well-described antagonist is TPMPA. Interestingly, isoguvacine, an agonist at the $GABA_A$ receptors, acts as an antagonist at the $GABA_C$ receptor. Much information regarding the location, function, and pharmacology of the $GABA_C$ receptor is needed to begin to take advantage of this receptor for therapeutic purposes.

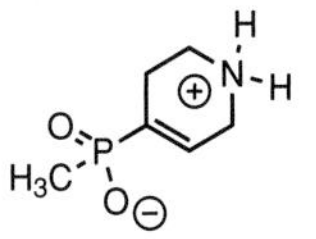

TPMPA

GLYCINE

The simplest of all amino acids, glycine, which classically causes hyperpolarization of neurons in the CNS, satisfies all the required criteria for neurotransmitter candidacy (45). Glycine in the CNS is unevenly distributed, with the highest concentrations found in the ventral gray areas of the spinal cord and in the medulla oblongata in the brainstem (46). The retina also is a structure with high concentrations of glycine (47). The synthesis of glycine in glycinergic neurons appears to be from L-serine and to be regulated by the enzyme serine hydroxymethyltransferase (SHMT), the concentrations of which in the CNS parallel those of glycine. Another substrate of SHMT, however, is L-threonine, which also can serve as a precursor of glycine. Administration of large doses of L-serine to animals fails to alter CNS glycine levels, but administration of L-threonine, which passes the blood-brain barrier much better than L-serine does, increase CNS glycine

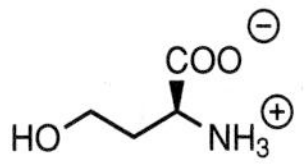

L-Threonine 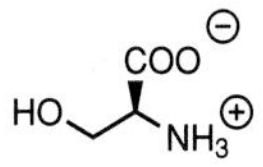 L-Serine

levels (48). L-Threonine has been used to treat a rare form of spasticity, familial spastic paraparesis in humans (49). The synthesis of glycine also could occur via a transamination reaction involving Glu in which glycine and α-ketoglutarate are produced. The understanding of the synthesis of glycine in the CNS for its neurotransmitter functions has been a difficult hurdle to overcome, likely because of the varied roles of glycine in the synthesis of protein, porphyrin, bile salts, and nucleic acids in addition to intermediary metabolic processes involving one-carbon fragments.

Glycine is stored in vesicles, and its uptake is mediated via VGAT, which also is capable of transporting GABA. Release of glycine occurs from presynaptic terminals in a Ca^{2+}-dependent fashion and, similarly, is taken back up into these terminals and, possibly, nearby glial cells (50,51). Reuptake is via Na^+/Cl^--dependent neurotransmitter transporters known as GLYT-1 and GLYT-2. These 12 transmembrane-spanning transporters are located in areas where glycine is believed to act as a neurotransmitter. Few pharmacological tools are available to examine the role of either form of the membrane transporters.

The glycine receptor mediating the inhibitory actions of glycine is similar to the $GABA_A$ receptor and other members of the Cys-loop family in being a pentameric, circular ion channel that allows the conduction of chloride (52). Unlike the GABA receptor, however, the inhibitory glycine receptor can be a homopentamer of α subunits or a heteropentamer comprised of two α subunits and three β subunits. Four isoforms of the α subunits have been identified, whereas only one β subunit is known. The neurotransmitter glycine, in addition to taurine, D-alanine, L-alanine, β-alanine, hypotaurine, serine, and β-aminobutyric acid can bind to any of three sites on the receptor to lead to activation. Positive modulators of the inhibitory glycine receptor include zinc, neurosteroids, propofol, ethanol, and volatile anesthetics, such as isoflurane (53,54).

The best-described antagonist of the inhibitory glycine receptor is the convulsant strychnine. Strychnine binds to a

Anandamide Strychnine

different site than that which recognizes glycine. Sometimes, the inhibitory glycine receptor is referred to as the "strychnine-sensitive" glycine receptor to distinguish it from the glycine modulatory site on the glutamatergic NMDA receptor. The $GABA_A$ receptor antagonist picrotoxin also can inhibit the glycine receptor. More recently, the endocannabinoids, such as anandamide and 2-arachidonylglycerol, also have been shown to antagonize the activity of glycine at this receptor. Agents that act as agonists at the IAA glycine receptor may find utility as anticonvulsants, muscle relaxants, sedatives, and general anesthetics.

As more information regarding the control of the synthesis of the neurotransmitter pool of glycine becomes available and the development of compounds with selectivity for the IAA glycine receptor are discovered, useful therapeutic agents that take advantage of modulating the glycinergic neurotransmitter system may be realized.

FUTURE DIRECTIONS

The amino acids play an essential role in the normal control of neurotransmission in the CNS, but during pathological conditions, these same amino acids may mediate a number of the adverse effects that are observed. Many desired agents are available that take advantage of one or more aspects of amino acidergic neurotransmission to produce their pharmacological effects. As agents are developed that are more specific for a particular isoform configuration of an amino acid receptor, the more effectively the treatment of various diseases likely will become. Additionally, associations between disease states and receptor isoform configurations, transporter density, and activity of enzymes involved in the synthesis and degradation of amino acid neurotransmitters may help to improve our understanding of the pathology of these diseases and lead to improved therapies.

References

1. Raiten DJ, Talbot JM, Fisher KD, eds. Analysis of adverse reactions to monosodium glutamate (MSG). Report prepared for Center for Food Safety and Applied Nutrition, Food and Drug Administration. Bethesda, MD: Life Sciences Research Office, Federation of American Societies for Experimental Biology, 1995.
2. Maher TJ. Effects of phenylalanine or aspartame on catecholamine synthesis and catecholamine-mediated behaviors. In: Belmaker R, Sandler M, Dahlstrom A, eds. Progress in Catecholamine Research. Part C: Clinical Aspects. New York: Liss, 1988:55–60.
3. Carlson MD, Kish PE, Ueda T. Glutamate uptake into synaptic vesicles: competitive inhibition by bromocriptine. J Neurochem 1989;53:1889–1894.
4. Ozkan ED, Lee FS, Ueda T. A protein factor that inhibits ATP-dependent glutamate and GABA accumulation into synaptic vesicles: purification and initial characterization. Proc Natl Acad Sci U S A 1997;94:4137–4142.
5. Zerangue N, Kavanaugh MP. Flux coupling in a neuronal glutamate transporter. Nature 1996;383:634–637.
6. Dunlop J. Glutamate-based therapeutic approaches: targeting the glutamate transport system. Curr Opin Pharmacol 2006;6:103–107.
7. Dingdledine R, Borges K, Bowie D, et al. The glutamate receptor ion channels. Pharmacol Rev 1999;51:7–61.
8. Erreger K, Chen PE, Wyllie DJ, et al. Glutamate receptor gating. Crit Rev Neurobiol 2004;16:187–224.
9. Malejev A, Gibbs TT, Farb DH. Inhibition of the NMDA response by pregnenolone sulfate revels subtype selective modulation of NMDA receptors by sulfated steroids. Br J Pharmacol 2002;135:901–909.
10. Subramaniam S, Rho JM, Penix L, et al. Felbamate block of the N-methyl-D-aspartate receptor. J Pharmacol Exp Ther 1995;273:878–886.
11. De Sarro G, Ongini E, Bertorelli R, et al. Excitatory amino acid neurotransmission through both NMDA and non-NMDA receptors is involved in the anticonvulsant activity of felbamate in DBA/2 mice. Eur J Pharmacol 1994;262:11–19.
12. Brorson JR, Li D, Suzuki T. Selective expression of heteromeric AMPA receptors driven by flip-flop differences. J Neurosci 2004;24:3461–3470.
13. Paternain AV, Morales M, Lerma J. Selective antagonism of AMPA receptors unmasks lainate receptor–mediated responses in hippocampal neurons. Neuron 1995;14:185–189.
14. Lynch G. Glutamate-based therapeutic approaches: ampakines. Curr Opin Pharmacol 2006;6:82–88.
15. Lerma J, Paternain AV, Rodriguez-Moreno A, et al. Molecular physiology of kainate receptors. Physiol Rev 2001;81:971–998.
16. Lerna J. Kainate receptor physiology. Curr Opin Pharmacol 2006;6:89–97.
17. Foster AC, Kemp JA. Glutamate- and GABA-based CNS therapeutics. Curr Opin Pharmacol 2006;6:7–17.
18. Chiamulera C, Epping-Jordan MP, Zocchi A. Reinforcing and locomotor stimulant effects of cocaine are absent in mGluR5 null mutant mice. Nature Neurosci 2001;4:873–874.
19. Valenti O, Marino MJ, Wittmann M, et al. Group II metabotropic glutamate receptor–mediated modulation of the striatopallidal synapse. J Neurosci 2003;23:7218–7226.
20. Marino MJ, Conn PJ. Glutamate-based therapeutic approaches: allosteric modulators of metabotropic glutamate receptors. Curr Opin Pharmacol 2006;6:98–102.
21. Sheikh SN, Martin SB, Martin DL. Regional distribution and relative amounts of glutamate decarboxylase isoforms in rat and mouse brain. Neurochem Int 1999;35:73–80.
22. McIntire SL, Reimer RJ, Schuske K, et al. Identification and characterization of the vesicular GABA transporter. Nature 1997;389:870–876.
23. Soudijin W, Van Wijingaarden I. The GABA transporter and its inhibitors. Curr Med Chem 2000;7:1063–1079.
24. Foster AC, Kemp JA. Glutamate- and GABA-based CNS therapeutics. Curr Opin Pharmacol 2006;6:7–17.
25. Sills GJ. The mechanisms of action of gabapentin and pregabalin. Curr Opin Pharmacol 2006;6:108–113.
26. Rudolph U, Mohler H. GABA-based therapeutic approaches: $GABA_A$ receptor subtype functions. Curr Opin Pharmacol 2006;6:18–23.
27. Rudolph U, Crestani F, Benke D, et al. Benzodiazepine actions mediated by specific γ-aminobutyric acid(A) receptor subtypes. Nature 1999;401: 796–800.
28. Low K, Crestani F, Keist R, et al. Molecular and neuronal substrates for the selective attenuation of anxiety. Science 2000;290:131–134.
29. Foster AC, Pelleymounter MA, Cullen MJ, et al. In vivo pharmacological characterization of indipion, a novel pyrazolopyrimidine sedative-hypnotic. J Pharmacol Exp Ther 2004;311:547–559.
30. Lancel M, Langebartels A. γ-aminobutyric acid(A) agonist 4,5,6,7-tetrahydroisoxazolo[4,5-c]pyridine-3-ol persistently increases sleep maintenance and intensity during chronic administration to rats. J Pharmacol Exp Ther 2000;293:1084–1090.
31. Whiting PJ. GABA-A receptors: a viable target for novel anxiolytics? Curr Opin Pharmacol 2006;6:24–29.
32. Sternfeld F, Carling RW, Jelly RA, et al. Selective, orally active γ-aminobutyric acid(A) α_5 receptor inverse agonists as cognition enhancers. J Med Chem 2004;47:2176–2179.
33. Yee BK, Keist R, von Boehmer L, et al. A schizophrenia-related sensorimotor deficit links α_3-containing $GABA_A$ receptors to a dopamine hyperfunction. Proc Natl Acad Sci U S A 2005;102:17154–17159.
34. Jurd R, Arras M, Lambert S, et al. General anesthetic actions in vivo strongly attenuated by point mutation in the GABA(A) receptor β_3 subunit. FASEB J 2003;17:250–252.
35. White JH, Wise A, Main M et al. Heterodimerization is required for the formation of a functional $GABA_B$ receptor. Nature 1998;396:679–682.
36. Bowery NG. $GABA_B$ receptor: a site of therapeutic benefit. Curr Opin Pharmacol 2006;6:37–43.

37. Van Bree JB, Heijligers-Feijen CD, de Boer AG, et al. Stereoselective transport of baclofen across the blood-brain barrier in rats as determined by the unit impulse response methodology. Pharm Res 1991;8:259–262.
38. Malcangio M, Bowery NG. Possible therapeutic application of GABAB receptor agonists and antagonists. Clin Neuropharmacol 1995;18:285–305.
39. Crunelli V, Emri Z, Leresche N. Unravelling the brain targets of γ-hydroxybutyric acid. Curr Opin Pharmacol 2006;6:44–52.
40. Gibson KM. γ-Hydroxybutyric aciduria: a biochemist's education from a heritable disorder of GABA metabolism. J Inherit Metab Dis 2005;28: 247–265.
41. Andrianmampandry C, Taleb O, Viry S, et al. Cloning and characterization of a rat brain receptor that binds the endogenous neuromodulator γ-hydroxybutyrate (GHB). FASEB J 2003;17:1691–1693.
42. Lemon MD, Strain JD, Farver DK. Sodium oxybate for cataplexy. Ann Pharmacother 2006;40:433–440.
43. Quang LS, Desai MC, Shannon MW, et al. Pretreatment of CD-1 mice with 4-methylpyrazole blocks toxicity from the γ-hydroxybutyrate precursor, 1,4-butanediol. Life Sci 2002;71:771–778.
44. Carai MAM, Quang LS, Atzeri S, et al. Withdrawal syndrome from γ-hydroxybutyric acid (GHB) and 1,4-butanediol (1,4-BD) in Sardinian alcohol-preferring rats. Brain Res Brain Res Protoc 2005;15:75–78.
45. Seighart W, Sperk G. Subunit composition, distribution, and function of GABA(A) receptor subtypes. Curr Topics Med Chem 2002;2:795–816.
46. Werman R, Davidoff RA, Aprison MH. Inhibitory action of glycine on spinal neurons in the cat. J Neurochem 1968;31:81–95.
47. Boehme DH, Fordice MW, Marks N, et al. Distribution of glycine in human spinal cord and selected regions of the brain. Brain Res 1973;50:353–359.
48. Berger SJ, McDaniel ML, Carter JC, et al. Distribution of four potential transmitter amino acids in the monkey retina. J Neurochem 1977;28:149–163.
49. Maher TJ, Wurtman RJ. L-Threonine administration increases glycine concentrations in the rat central nervous system. Life Sci 1980;26:1283–1286.
50. Nader TM, Gowdeu JH, Maher TS, et al. L-Threonine administration increases CSF glycine levels and suppresses spasticity. Neurology 1987(Suppl 1);375:125.
51. Shank RP, Aprison MH. Method for multiple analysis of concentration and specific radioactivity of individual amino acids in nervous tissue extracts. Anal Biochem 1970;35:136–145.
52. Neal MJ, Pickles H. Uptake of ^{14}C-glycine by spinal cord. Nature (Lond) 1969;222:679–680.
53. Breitinger HG, Becker CM. The inhibitory glycine receptor—simple views of a complicated channel. Chem Bio Chem 2003;3:1042–1052.
54. Lobo IA, Harris RA. Sites of alcohol and volatile anesthetic action on glycine receptors. Int Rev Neurobiol 2005;65:53–87.

16. *Inhibitors of Nerve Conduction: Local Anesthetics*

MATTHIAS C. LU

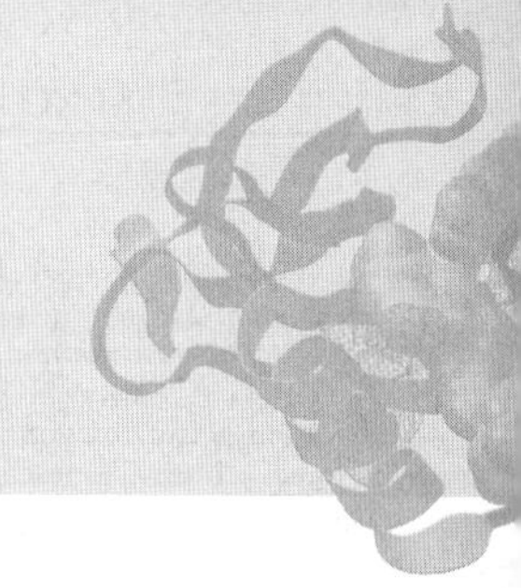

DRUGS COVERED IN THIS CHAPTER:

- Articaine
- Benzocaine
- Bupivacaine
- Chloroprocaine
- Mepivacaine
- Levobupivacaine
- Lidocaine
- Ropivacaine

INTRODUCTION

A local anesthetic agent is a drug that, when given either topically or parenterally to a localized area, produces a state of local anesthesia by reversibly blocking the nerve conductances that transmit the feeling of pain from this locus to the brain. The term "anesthesia" is defined as a loss of sensation with or without loss of consciousness. According to this definition, wide ranges of drugs with diverse chemical structures are anesthetics. The list includes not only the classic anesthetic agents, such as the general and local anesthetics, but also many central nervous system (CNS) depressants, such as analgesics, barbiturates, benzodiazepines, anticonvulsants, and muscle relaxants.

What Is the Difference between a Local Anesthetic and Other Anesthetic Drugs?

Both general and local anesthetic drugs produce anesthesia by blocking nerve conductance in both sensory and motor neurons. This blockade of nerve conduction leads to a loss of pain sensation as well as to impairment of motor functions. Generally, however, the anesthesia produced by local anesthetics is without loss of consciousness or impairment of vital central functions. It is accepted that a local anesthetic blocks nerve conductance by binding to selective sites on the sodium channels in the excitable membranes, thereby reducing sodium passage through the pores and, thus, interfering with the action potentials. Therefore, a local anesthetic decreases the excitability of nerve membranes without affecting the resting potential. By contrast, a general anesthetic agent alters physical properties of nerve membranes through rather nonspecific interactions with the lipid bilayer or the receptor/ionic channel proteins. These, in turn, reduce membrane excitability through a number of possible mechanisms, including changes in membrane fluidity, permeability, and receptor/channel functions. Furthermore, local anesthetics, in contrast to analgesic compounds, do not interact with the pain receptors or inhibit the release or the biosynthesis of pain mediators.

The Discovery of Local Anesthetics

Similar to many modern drugs, the initial leads for the design of clinically useful local anesthetics were derived from natural sources. As early as 1532, the anesthetic properties of coca leaves (*Erythroxylon coca* Lam) became known to Europeans from the natives of Peru, who chewed the leaves for a general feeling of well-being and to prevent hunger. Saliva from chewing the leaves often was used by the natives to relieve painful wounds. The active principle of the coca leaf, however, was not discovered until 1860 by Niemann, who obtained a crystalline alkaloid from the leaves, to which he gave the name cocaine, and who noted the anesthetic effect on the tongue. Although Moréno y Maiz in 1868 first asked the question of whether cocaine could be used as a local anesthetic, it was Von Anrep in 1880 who, after many animal experiments, recommended that cocaine be used clinically as a local anesthetic. The first report of successful surgical use of cocaine appeared in 1884 by Koller, an Austrian ophthalmologist. This discovery led to an explosive development of new anesthetic techniques and local anesthetic agents (1).

Although the structure of cocaine was not known until 1924, many attempts were made to prepare new analogues of cocaine without its addicting liability and other therapeutic shortcomings, such as allergic reactions, tissue irritations, and poor stability in aqueous solution. Also, cocaine is easily decomposed when the solution is sterilized (Fig. 16.1).

Initially, analogues of ecgonine and benzoic acid, the hydrolysis products of cocaine, were prepared. When the chemical structure of ecgonine became known, the preparation of active compounds accelerated. It was soon realized that a variety of benzoyl esters of amino alcohols, including benzoyltropine, exhibited strong local anesthetic properties without any addicting liability. Thus, removal of the 2-carbomethoxy group of cocaine also abolished the addicting liability. This discovery eventually led to the synthesis of procaine (N,N-diethylaminoethyl ester of *p*-aminobenzoic acid [PABA]) in 1905, which became the prototype for local anesthetics for nearly half a century, largely because it did not have the severe local and systemic toxicities of cocaine.

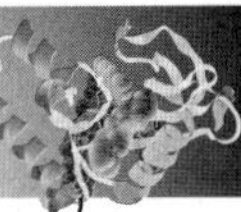

CLINICAL SIGNIFICANCE

Local anesthetics are widely used clinically in surgery, dentistry, ophthalmology, and in other clinical procedures in which temporary relief of pain is warranted. Some local anesthetics also can be used to treat or prevent cardiac arrhythmias because of their action on cardiac sodium channels.

Before using a local anesthetic, clinicians must take into account the physical properties of the drug, such as its lipid solubility and protein binding as well as the degree of vascularization, the rate of blood flow at the site of application, and the total dosage administered, because these factors govern local anesthetic activity and its associated toxicities. For example, increasing the lipid solubility of an anesthetic may produce an increased penetration into a nerve membrane, but it also can enhance the ability of the drug to pass through a blood vessel wall. This then leads to reduction in anesthetic potency because of the more rapid removal of the agent from the site, which thereby increases its systemic toxicity. Another complicating factor affecting local anesthetic action is distribution of the drug into adipose tissue, because this reduces local anesthetic activity. Additionally, if the protein binding affinity of the local anesthetic is too great, the ability of the drug to reach its target site can be impeded.

Extraneuronal blood vessels near the site of drug application affect the amount of drug that reaches the nerve trunk to establish anesthesia; thus, a larger dosage is required to elicit local anesthesia, which also contributes to toxicity. After the establishment of anesthesia, a contributing factor to loss of the drug from the nerve may be caused by the intraneuronal blood vessels. Finally, a reduction in local blood flow also slows systemic uptake of the drug from the injection site and, thus, minimizes any potential toxicity, but it increases the amount of drug available to the nerve and, thus, the duration of anesthesia

Therefore, a sound understanding of how local anesthetics work as well as their relative potencies, duration of action, metabolism, and excretion, along with their relative central nervous system and cardiovascular toxicities, significantly affects clinical practice in which local anesthetics are administered.

Matthias C. Lu
University of Illinois at Chicago
Professor, Assistant Head for Curricular Affairs
Department of Medicinal Chemistry and Pharmacognosy

Benzoylatropine

Procaine

Although the intrinsic potency of procaine was low and its duration of action relatively short compared with that of cocaine, it was found that these deficiencies could be remedied when procaine was combined with a vasoconstrictor, such as epinephrine. Apparently, a vasoconstrictor agent reduces the local blood supply and, thereby, prolongs the residence time of the local anesthetic.

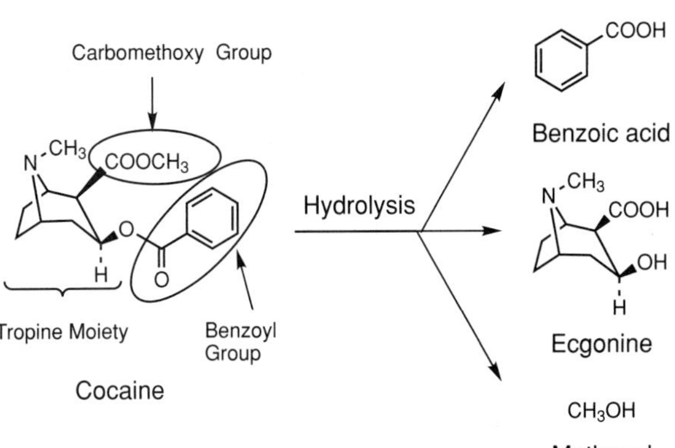

Fig. 16.1. Structures of cocaine and its hydrolysis products.

Following the introduction of procaine, hundreds of structurally related analogues were prepared and their local anesthetic properties examined. Most of these compounds were prepared for the purposes of enhancing the intrinsic potency and the duration of action of procaine. Among these compounds, tetracaine remains the most potent, long-acting ester-type local anesthetic agents used in spinal anesthesia.

Benzocaine, an effective topical anesthetic agent, was synthesized by Ritsert in 1890 and was found to have good anesthetizing properties and low toxicity. Benzocaine, however, has limited water solubility except at low pH values because of the lack of a basic aliphatic amino group, thereby disallowing the preparation of pharmaceutically acceptable parenteral solutions.

Tetracaine

Benzocaine

The next major turning point in the development of clinically useful local anesthetic agents was the serendipitous discovery of the local anesthetic activity of another natural alkaloidal product, isogramine, in 1935 by von Euler and Erdtman. This observation led to the synthesis of lidocaine (Xylocaine) by Löfgren in 1946; lidocaine was the first nonirritating, amide-type local anesthetic agent with good local anesthetic properties yet less prone to allergenic reactions than procaine analogues. A further practical advantage of lidocaine was its stability in aqueous solution because of the more stable amide functionality. Structurally, lidocaine can be viewed as an open-chain analogue of isogramine and, thus, is a bio-isoteric analogue of isogramine.

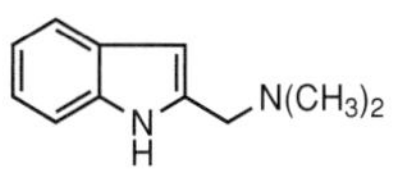

Isogramine

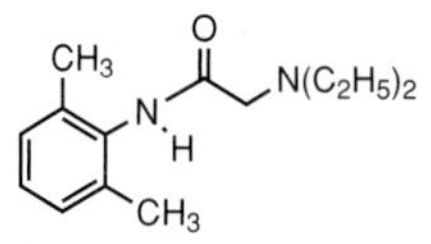

Lidocaine

In the years since 1948, extensive progress has been achieved primarily in the fields of neurophysiology and neuropharmacology rather than that of synthetic medicinal chemistry. Most of this research has significantly increased our understanding of how nerve conduction occurs and how compounds interact with the neuronal membranes to produce local anesthesia. It should be noted, however, that although a number of current clinically useful local anesthetic agents have been introduced into the market, an ideal local anesthetic drug has, unfortunately, not been realized.

Characteristics for an Ideal Local Anesthetic

An ideal local anesthetic should produce reversible blockade of sensory nerve fibers with a minimal effect on the motor fibers. It also should possess a rapid onset and have a sufficient duration of action for the completion of major surgical procedures without any systemic toxicity.

This goal, however, can be attained only through further structure–activity relationship studies, particularly with regard to their selective actions on the voltage-gated sodium channels. Additional leads for the design of ideal local anesthetics also could come from a more systematic metabolic and toxicity study of currently available agents. To understand the chemical aspects of local anesthetics and, thus, to provide a proper background for practical uses of these compounds, it is necessary to have a working knowledge of basic neuroanatomy and electrophysiology of the nervous system.

NEUROANATOMY AND ELECTROPHYSIOLOGY OF THE NERVOUS SYSTEM

Neuroanatomy

As can be seen in Figure 16.2, the sensory fibers (afferent neurons) course together in bundles with the motor fibers (efferent neurons) from the periphery to the spinal cord (2). The cell bodies of the sensory fibers are found at the point at which the nerve enters the vertebra, and they are seen as enlargements on the nerve bundles. The cell bodies of the motor fibers are found within the spinal cord. The bundles of sensory and motor fibers outside the spinal cord are wrapped in a connective tissue sheath, the epineurium. Groups of fibers are found within this "nerve" in small bundles, each of which is surrounded by connective tissue known as perineurium and, in even smaller tubes of connective tissue, called endoneurium.

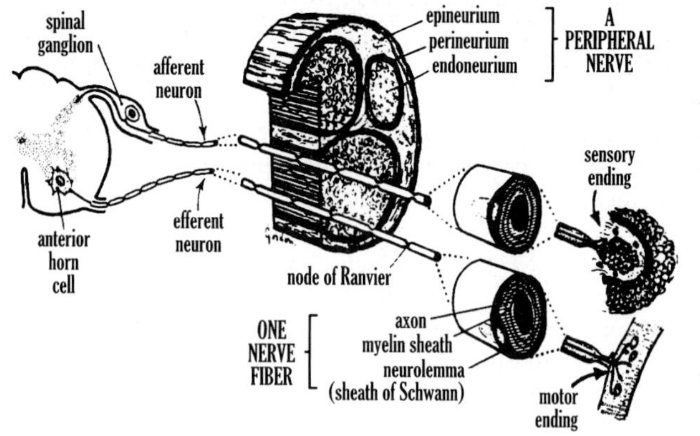

Fig. 16.2. Diagram showing the various parts of a peripheral nerve. (Adapted from Ham AW. Histology, 6th Ed. Philadelphia: JB Lippincott, 1969: p. 524; with permission.)

Figures 16.2 and 16.3 also show that each nerve axon has its own membranous covering, often called the nerve membrane, tightly surrounded by a myelin sheath called a Schwann cell covering. The myelin is not continuous along the fiber. The interruptions are the nodes of Ranvier, which are of great importance for nerve functioning.

Electrophysiology of Nerve Membrane

Resting Potential

Most nerves have resting membrane potentials of approximately −70 to −90 mV as a result of a slight imbalance of electrolytes across the nerve membranes (i.e., between the cytoplasm and the extracellular fluid) (3). The origin of this membrane potential has been of great interest to neurophysiologists. The main electrolytes in nerve axons and cell bodies are sodium, potassium, calcium, magnesium, and chloride.

At resting potential, the nerve membrane was believed to be impermeable to sodium because of the low sodium ion concentration in the excitable cell. Potassium ions may flow in and out of the cell with ease, indicating that the membrane is highly permeable to potassium ions. A high potassium ion concentration is retained intracellularly by the attractive forces provided by the negative charges on the protein molecules. Thus,

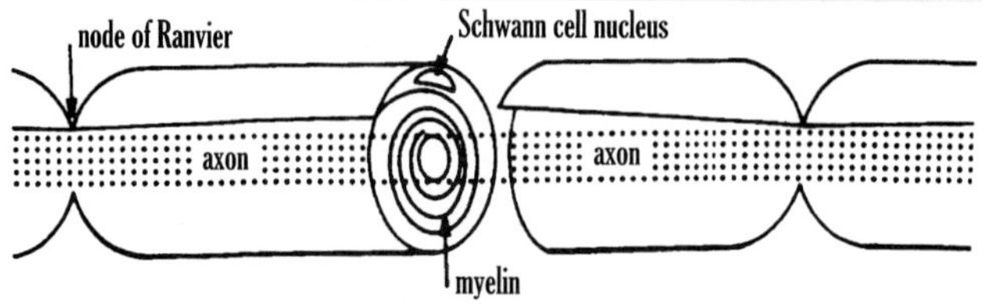

Fig. 16.3. Single myelinated nerve fiber.

the predominant intracellular cation is potassium (~110 to 170 mmol/L), and the predominant extracellular ions are sodium (~140 mmol/L) and chloride (~110 mmol/L).

It would appear that changes in the intracellular or extracellular concentration of potassium ions markedly alter the resting membrane potential. For this reason, neurophysiologists treated an excitable cell as if it were an electrochemical, or Nernst, cell. The resting potential for one permeant species could therefore be explained by the familiar Nernst equation:

$$E = -RT/zF \ln [K^+]_i/[K^+]_o$$

in which E = membrane potential, inside minus outside; R = gas constant; T = temperature; z = valence of ion; F = Faraday's constant; $[K^+]_i$ = activity of potassium intracellularly, and $[K^+]_o$ = activity of potassium extracellularly.

Action Potential

Action potentials are transient membrane depolarizations that result from the influx of sodium ions through a brief opening of the voltage-gated sodium channels on excitation of the cell (3). The transmembrane potential during an action potential goes from −70 to approximately +40 mV (a total net change of 110 mV) and promptly returns to the resting potential; the event lasts approximately 1 millisecond (Fig. 16.4).

The transmembrane potential at the peak of the action potential can be predicted from the Nernst equation by substituting appropriate sodium ion concentrations for those of potassium ions. Thus, it appears that the excitable membrane can be transformed from a potassium electrode to a sodium electrode during the active process (4).

As the cell approaches its peak action potential, the permeability to sodium again decreases (sodium inactivation or repolarization). If no other event occurred, this cell would slowly return to its resting potential, but the cell again becomes highly permeable to potassium ions, allowing potassium ions to flow out and quickly restore the membrane potential. After an action potential, the cell would therefore be left with a small increase in sodium ions and a decrease in potassium ions. To explain how the nerve is restored to its original electrolyte composition at the resting potential, it was necessary to postulate a mechanism by which sodium ions could be extruded and potassium ions could probably be accumulated. It has been suggested that by using the energy derived from splitting adenosine triphosphate, an adenosine triphosphatase system could serve this function and act as a sodium pump (5). Other investigators believe that during excitation, the membrane goes from one stable state to another, functioning more like an ion exchanger (6). Koketsu (7) suggests that during excitation, the membrane goes from a calcium-associated to a calcium-dissociated state, triggered by the depolarizing pulse, and that during recovery, the membrane returns to the resting state by the reassociation as a result of outward movement of potassium ions.

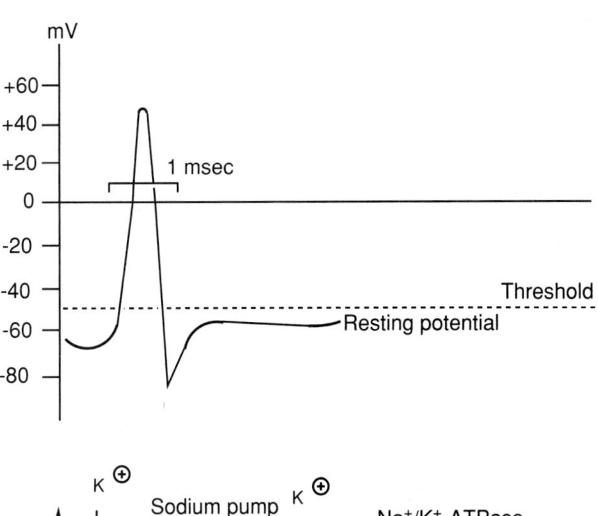

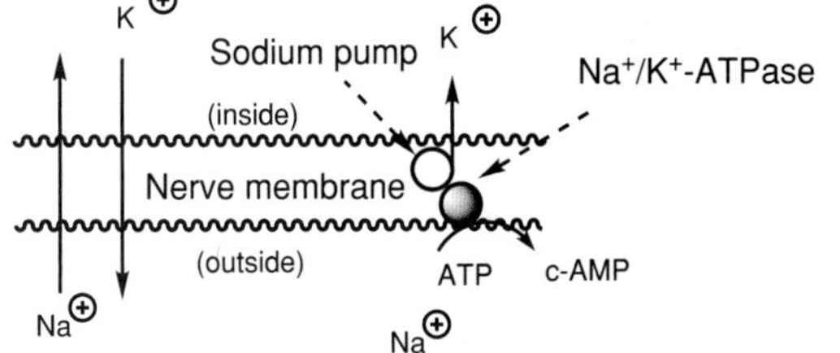

Fig. 16.4. Relationship between membrane action potential and ionic flux across the nerve membrane.

Threshold

An electrical stimulus of less than a certain voltage can result in only local electronegativity and cannot elicit a propagated action potential. The voltage necessary to change localized electronegativity into a propagated action potential is called the threshold voltage, which is closely related to the stimulus duration—the longer the stimulus, the lower the threshold voltage.

Refractoriness

Immediately after an impulse has been propagated, the axon is absolutely refractory, or completely inexcitable, and no stimulus, no matter how strong or long, can excite it. Shortly thereafter, the axon becomes relatively refractory; it responds with a propagated impulse only to stimulation that is greater than the normal threshold. The length of the refractory period is affected by the frequency of stimulation and by many drugs (Fig. 16.5).

Conductance Velocity

The conductance velocity is the velocity at which an impulse is conducted along the nerve and is proportional to the diameter of the fiber.

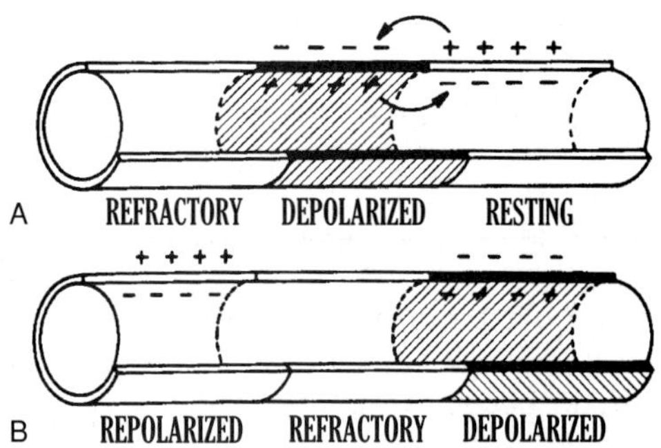

Fig. 16.5. Impulse propagation. (A) The wave of depolarization passes down the nerve, followed by a wave of refractoriness. (B) The wave of refractoriness is followed by a wave of repolarization. (Adapted from De Jong RH, Freund FG. Physiology of peripheral nerve and local anesthesia. Int Anesthesiol Clin 1970;8:35–53; with permission.)

Nodal Conduction

Because longitudinal resistance is inversely proportional to cross-sectional area, impulses are conducted faster in large-diameter fibers. The squid axon is unmyelinated and exceptionally large (~800 μμ); therefore, impulses are conducted rapidly along it. Contraction of the mantle of a squid, however, is an uncomplicated procedure that does not require a complex sensorimotor system. Perhaps, during evolution, vertebrates developed a complicated input–output system of many fibers collected in bundles, as shown in Figure 16.2.

Conduction in these fibers would be slow if they were not insulated with a myelin coat, interrupted at intervals by the nodes of Ranvier, where current enters and exits. Ionic fluxes occur at these nodes. The impulse jumps along the fiber from node to node faster than in unmyelinated fiber (8).

Sodium Channel

The voltage-gated sodium channels are discrete, membrane-bound glycoproteins that mediate sodium permeability and, thus, are responsible for the generation of action potentials in skeletal muscle, nerve, and cardiac tissues (9–16). Our understanding of the structural domains and binding sites on voltage-gated sodium channels have evolved considerably since the first cloning and expression studies of the channel protein by Noda (9). The channel gating kinetics have been extensively studied with the use of selective blockers of sodium channels, such as tetrodotoxin (TTX) and saxitoxin (STX), and by site-directed mutagenesis (15). Both TTX and STX bind stoichiometrically to the outer opening of the channels and are detected with patch-clamp electrophysiological techniques on the cut-open squid giant axon (16). Neher and Sakmann, two German scientists, were awarded the 1991 Nobel Prize in physiology and medicine for their work on ion channels with these neurotoxins (16).

(Lactone form) (Hemiacetal form)

Tetrodotoxin (TTX)

Saxitoxin (STX) Batrachotoxin

Recent mapping of receptor binding sites within the channel protein for lipid soluble neurotoxins, such as batrachotoxin (BTX), and for local anesthetics using site-directed mutagenesis has provided further insight regarding these channels (15). For example, mammalian voltage-gated sodium channel contain one large α subunit and one or two smaller β subunits (15). The primary structure of the α subunit is composed of four homologous domains (D1–D4), each with six transmembrane segments (S1–S6) and a hydrophobic loop thought to dip into the membrane to line the aqueous pore in a pseudotetrameric arrangement (Fig. 16.6) (13–15).

Furthermore, the voltage sensor for activation gating and the structure for fast inactivation gating have been delineated to involve the positively charged S4 segments of each domain (also known as the ion selectivity filter, because it contains positively charged amino acid residues). The selective filter is needed to discriminate sodium ions from other ions (i.e., sodium ions pass

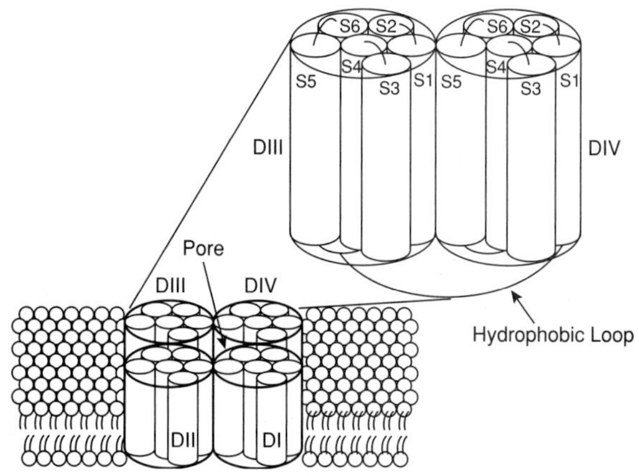

Fig. 16.6. A schematic representation of the α subunit of the sodium channel and the pore-forming unit. (From Anger T, Madge DJ, Mulla M, et al.. Medicinal chemistry of neuronal voltage-gated sodium channel blockers. J Med Chem 2001;44:115–137; with permission.)

What Are the Sources of These Neurotoxins?

Tetradotoxin is a potent neurotoxin isolated from the ovaries and liver of many species of Tetradodontidae, especially the Japanese fugu (or puffer fish). Saxitoxin is a mussel or clam poison produced by certain marine dinoflagellates, *Gonyaulax catenella* or *G. tamarensis,* the consumption of which cause the mussels or clams to become poisonous. These poisonous shellfish were connected to a toxic "red tide" environmental condition on the coastal region of California in early 1970. Batrachotoxin is a cardiotoxic and neurotoxic steroid isolated originally from the poison dart frog, *Phyllobates terribilis*. It is a lipid soluble neurotoxin that is at least 10-fold more toxic than tetradotoxin.

through this pore approximately 12-fold faster than the potassium ions). Sodium channels open and close as they switch between several conformational states: the resting/closed form (nonconducting state), the open channel (conducting), and the inactivated form (nonconducting state).

It generally is agreed that at resting potential, the sodium channels are in a rest/closed state and are impermeable to the passage of sodium ions. On activation, the channels undergo conformational changes to an open state, allowing rapid influx of sodium ions across the axonal membrane.

Thus, when threshold potential is exceeded, most of the sodium channels are in an open, or conducting, state. At the peak of the action potential, the open channels spontaneously convert to an inactivated state (i.e., nonconducting and nonactivatable), leading to a decrease in sodium permeability. When a sodium channel is in the inactivated state, it cannot be opened without first transforming to the normal resting/closed form.

THERAPEUTIC CONSIDERATIONS FOR USING LOCAL ANESTHETIC DRUGS

Since the discovery of cocaine in 1880 as a surgical local anesthetic, several thousand new compounds have been tested and found to produce anesthesia by blocking nerve conductance. Among these agents, only approximately 20 are clinically available in the United States as local anesthetic preparations (Table 16.1). Table 16.2 contains chemical structures of the different types of agents in current or recent use.

Pharmaceutical Preparations

Local anesthetic agents generally are prepared in various dosage forms: aqueous solutions for parenteral injection, and creams and ointments for topical applications. Thus, chemical stability and aqueous solubility become primary factors in the preparations of suitable pharmaceutical dosage forms.

Table 16.1. Clinically Available Local Anesthetics

Generic Name	Trade Name	Recommended Application
Articaine[a]	Septocaine, Septanest	Parenteral (dental)
Benoxinate[b]	Oxybuprocaine	Mainly in ophthalmology
Benzocaine[ab]	Americaine, Anbesol, Benzodent, Orajel, Oratect, Rid-A-Pain, Hurricaine	Topical
Bupivacaine[ab]	Marcaine, Sensorcaine	Parenteral
Butamben[ab]	Butesin	Topical
Chloroprocaine[ab]	Nesacaine	Parenteral
Dibucaine[ab]	Nupercainal, Cinchocaine	Topical
Dyclonine[ab]	Sucrets	Topical (mucosal only)
Etidocaine[a]	Duranest	Parenteral
Levobupivacine[a]	Chirocaine	Parenteral
Lidocaine[ab]	Xylocaine, L-Caine, DermaFlex, Dilocaine, Lidoject, Lignocaine, Octocaine,	Parenteral, topical
Mepivacaine[ab]	Carbocaine, Polocaine, Isocaine	Parenteral, topical
Pramoxine[ab]	Prax, Tronothane	Topical
Prilocaine[ab]	Citanest	Parenteral, topical
Procaine[ab]	Novocain	Parenteral
Proparacaine[ab]	Alcaine, Ophthaine, Ak-Taine	Mainly in ophthalmology
Propoxycaine[b]	Blockaine, Ravocaine	Parenteral
Ropivacaine[ab]	Naropin	Parenteral
Tetracaine[ab]	Pontocaine, Amethocaine, Prax	Parenteral, topical
Benzyl alcohol[b]		Topical, mainly in combination with pramoxine
Eugenol[b]		Topical, especially in dentistry
Menthol[ab]	Chloraseptic lozenges, Dermoplast, Pramegel, Pontacaine ointment	Topical, mainly in combination with benzocaine or pramoxine or tetracaine
Phenol[ab]	Anbesol	Topical, mainly in combination with benzocaine
Ethyl chloride[b]		Extracutaneous, temperature decreasing

[a]USP DI (2004), Vol I: Drug Information for the Health Care Professional, United States Pharmacopeial Convention, Inc. Rockville, MD.
[b]United States Pharmacopoeia 29 — National Formulary 24 (2006), United States Pharmacopeial Convention, Inc. Rockville, MD.

Table 16.2. Structures of Local Anesthetics

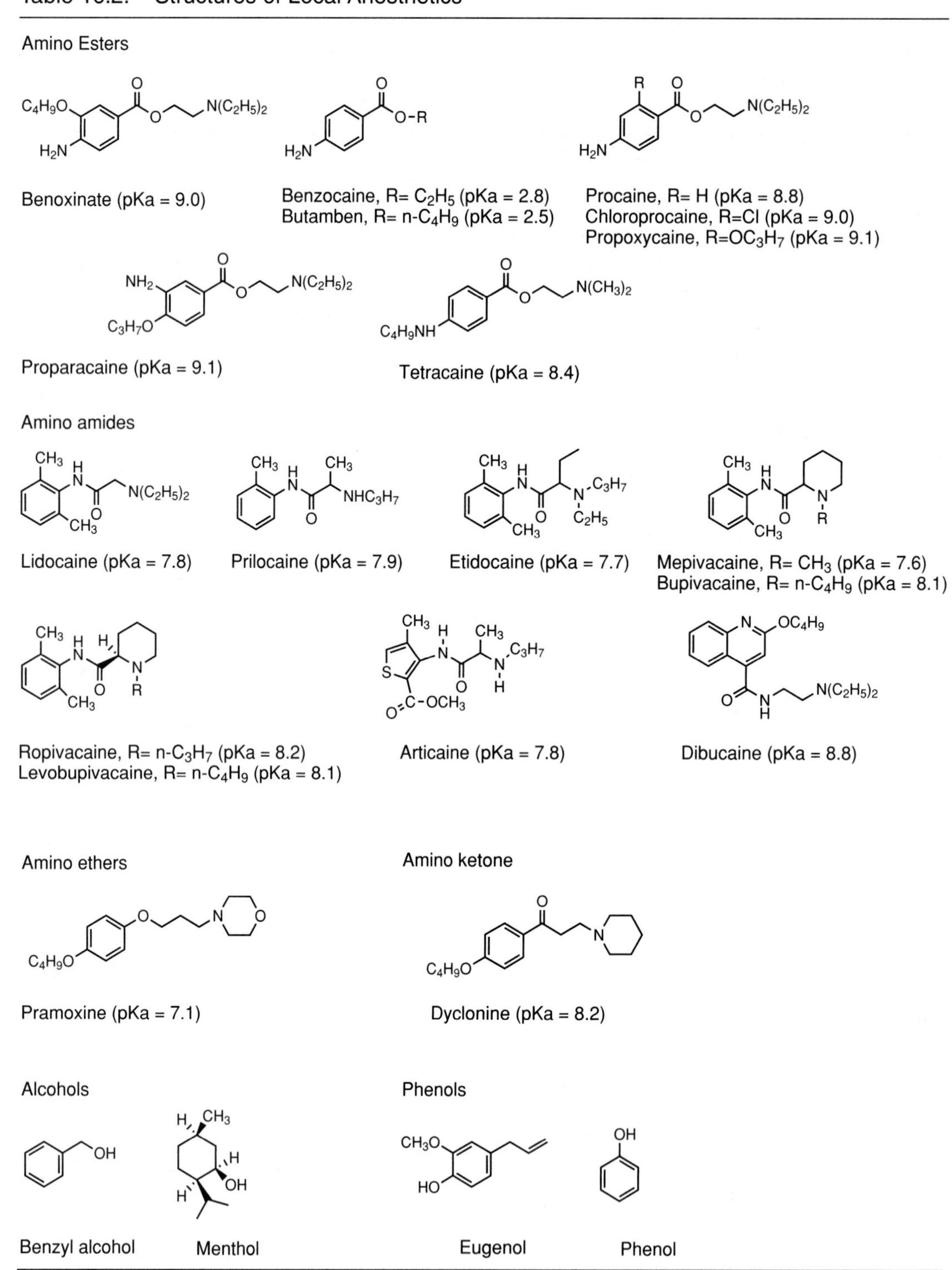

As a rule, compounds containing an amide linkage have greater chemical stability than the ester types do. In this regard, an aqueous solution of an amino ester-type local anesthetic is more likely to decompose under normal conditions and cannot withstand heat sterilization because of base-catalyzed hydrolysis of the ester.

Local anesthetic activity usually increases with increasing lipid solubility. Unfortunately, this increase in lipid solubility is often inversely related to water solubility. For this reason, a suitable parenteral dosage form may not be available for these agents because of poor water solubility under acceptable conditions. For example, benzocaine, which lacks a sufficiently basic aliphatic amino group needed for salt formation, is practically insoluble in water at a neutral pH. Protonation of the aromatic amino group in benzocaine results in a salt with a pK_a of 2.78,

Study Question 1

Question: What is the biochemical and pharmacological basis for the observation that coadministration of epinephrine with procaine leads to an increase in the duration of action as well as a decrease in systemic toxicity of procaine?

which is too acidic and, therefore, unsuitable for the preparation of a parenteral dosage form for injection. For this reason, benzocaine and its closely related analogue, butamben, are used mostly in creams or ointments to provide topical anesthesia of accessible mucous membranes or skin for burns, cuts, or inflamed mucous surfaces.

Many attempts have been made to substitute oils, fats, or fluid polymers for the aqueous vehicle commonly used in injectable local anesthetics. Unfortunately, the pharmacological results of these experiments have been quite disappointing, often as a result of the undesirable toxicity of the nonaqueous vehicle.

The only commonly accepted organic additives to local anesthetics are vasoconstrictors, such as epinephrine. These compounds often increase the frequency of successful anesthesia and, to a limited degree, increase the duration of activity by reducing the rate of drug loss from the injection site. These agents are believed to function by constricting arterioles that supply blood to the area of the injection.

The effect of these vasoconstrictors is less pronounced if the agents are added to a local anesthetic solution that is to be injected in an area that has profuse venous drainage but is remote from an arterial supply.

Administration of a local anesthetic in a carbonic acid–carbon dioxide aqueous solution rather than the usual solution of a hydrochloride salt appreciably improves the time of onset and duration of action. This change in solution form is apparently not associated with local or systemic toxicity.

Current theories suggest that carbon dioxide potentiates the action of local anesthetics by initial indirect depression of the axon, followed by diffusion trapping of the active form of the local anesthetic within the nerve. Use of the carbonate salt appears to be one pharmaceutical modification of the classic local anesthetic agents that may result in significant clinical advantages.

A eutectic mixture of a local anesthetic cream (EMLA cream) containing 2.5% lidocaine and 2.5% prilocaine (or etidocaine) also is available for topical application of local anesthetic through the keratinized layer of the intact skin to provide dermal or epidermal analgesia. This mode of administration allows the use of higher concentrations with minimal local irritation and lower systemic toxicity. The use of EMLA creams, especially those containing prilocaine, on mucous membranes is not recommended, however, because of the faster absorption of the drugs and, therefore, the increasing risk of systemic toxicity, such as methemoglobinemia (17).

Study Question 2

Question: Why is the alkalinization of local anesthetics to improve onset time theoretically sound but clinically impractical?

Toxicity and Side Effects

The side effects and toxicity of local anesthetics seem to be related to their actions on other excitable membrane proteins, such as in the sodium and potassium channels in the heart, the nicotinic acetylcholine receptors in the neuromuscular junctions, and the nerve cells in the CNS. In general, neuromuscular junctions and the CNS are more susceptible than the cardiovascular system to the toxic effects of local anesthetics.

The actions on skeletal muscles are transient and reversible, whereas the CNS side effects can be deleterious. The primary effect of the toxicity seems to be convulsions, followed by severe CNS depression, particularly of the respiratory and cardiovascular centers. This may be related to an initial depression of inhibitory neurons, such as GABAergic systems, causing convulsions, followed by depression of other neurons, leading to general depression of the CNS.

Amino amide-type local anesthetics (i.e., lidocaine derivatives) are, in general, more likely to produce CNS side effects than the amino ester-type compounds (procaine analogues). It should be noted, however, that the toxic effects observed depend heavily on the route and site of administration as well as on the lipid solubility and metabolic stability of a given local anesthetic molecule. For example, most amide-type local anesthetics, such as lidocaine, are first degraded via N-dealkylations by the hepatic enzymes (see Fig. 16.10). Unlike lidocaine, however, the initial metabolic degradation of prilocaine in humans is hydrolysis of the amide linkage to give o-toluidine and N-propylalanine. Formation of o-toluidine and its metabolites are said to cause methemoglobinemia in some patients (17). For this reason, prilocaine is more likely than other local anesthetics to cause methemoglobinemia.

In contrast, allergic reactions to local anesthetics, although rare, are known to occur exclusively with *p*-aminobenzoic ester-type local anesthetics (18). Whether the formation of PABA on ester hydrolysis is solely responsible for this hypersensitivity remains to be investigated. However, the preservative compounds, such as methyparaben, used in the preparation of amide-type local anesthetics are metabolized to PABA-like substance, *p*-hydroxybenzoic acid. Thus, patients who are allergic to amino ester-type local anesthetics should be treated with a preservative-free amino amide-type local anesthetic.

Amide-type local anesthetics (e.g., procainamide and lidocaine) also possess antiarrhythmic activity when given parenterally and at a subanesthetic dosage. Although this action can be attributed to their actions on sodium channels in cardiac tissues, current evidence suggests a distinctly different mechanism of action with respect to the modulation of channel receptors and the location of binding sites for these compounds (19,20).

CHEMICAL AND PHARMACODYNAMIC ASPECTS OF LOCAL ANESTHETICS

Mechanism of Action

Local anesthetics decrease the excitability of nerve cells without affecting the resting potential. Because the action potential, or the ability of nerve cells to be excited, seems to be associated with the movement of sodium ions across the nerve membranes, anything that interferes with the movement of these ions interferes with cell excitability. For this reason, many hypotheses have been suggested to explain how local anesthetics regulate the changes in sodium permeability that underlie the nerve impulse. These hypotheses include direct action on ionic channels that interferes with ionic fluxes and interaction with phospholipids and calcium that reduces membrane flexibility and responsiveness to changes in electrical fields.

The nonspecific membrane actions of local anesthetics can be easily ruled out, because most clinically useful agents, in contrast to general anesthetics, possess a defined set of structure–activity relationships. As mentioned earlier, local anesthetic agents block nerve conductance and produce anesthesia as a result of their selective actions on membrane-bound sodium channels. It should be pointed out that at much higher drug concentrations, local anesthetics also bind and block potassium channels.

Interaction with Phospholipids and Calcium

Calcium exists in the membrane in a bound state. Many investigators believe that the release of the bound calcium is the first step in membrane depolarization and that this release leads to the changes in ionic permeability described previously. It has been suggested that local anesthetics displace the bound calcium from these sites and form more stable bonds, thereby inhibiting ionic fluxes. The following evidence has been offered in support of this theory: Both calcium and local anesthetics bind to phospholipids in vitro, reducing their flexibility and responsiveness to changes in electrical fields (21–23). Also, membrane excitability and instability increase in calcium-deficient solutions. Local anesthetics counteract this abnormal increase in excitability, and more local anesthetic is necessary to block excitation in calcium-poor solutions (24). Direct proof of this hypothesis, however, is lacking because of the difficulty in measuring calcium movements in vivo. It also is possible that the aforementioned cause-and-effect relationship between intracellular free calcium and membrane excitability is the result of a sodium-calcium exchange reaction; that is , the influx of sodium ions displaces the membrane-bound calcium, which leads to an increase of intracellular free calcium and, thereby, increases cellular excitability.

Local anesthetics interact differently, however, with neuronal phospholipids with or without the presence of cholesterol. Thus, the interactions of local anesthetics with the cellular membranes actually may contribute to their observed differences in toxicity (25).

Action on Voltage-Sensitive Sodium Channels

As mentioned, the voltage-sensitive sodium channels are membrane-bound glycoproteins that mediate sodium permeability. On excitation, these channels undergo conformational changes from a closed to an open state, thus allowing a rapid influx of sodium. The movement of sodium ions is blocked by the neurotoxins TTX and STX and by local anesthetics (26). Most electrophysiologists and neuropharmacologists now agree that the mechanism of action of local anesthetics results primarily from their binding to one or more sites within the sodium channels, thus blocking the sodium conductance (27). The exact location of these binding sites, however, and whether all local anesthetics interact with a common site remain matters of dispute.

Action on Sodium Conductance

Local anesthetics block sodium conductance by two possible modes of action: tonic inhibition, and phasic inhibition (28,29). Tonic inhibition results from the binding of local anesthetics to nonactivated closed channels and, thus, is independent of channel activation. Phasic inhibition may be accomplished when local anesthetics bind to activated, open states (conducting) or to inactivated states (nonconducting) of the channels. Thus, it is not surprising that a greater phasic inhibition usually is obtained with repetitive depolarization.

Two reasons have been suggested to explain this observation. First, channel inactivation during depolarization increases the number of binding sites that normally are inaccessible to local anesthetics at resting potential. Second, both the open and the inactivated channels possess binding sites with a higher affinity; therefore, local anesthetics bind more tightly and result in stronger nerve block.

Furthermore, it generally is agreed that most of the clinically useful local anesthetics exert their actions by binding to the inactivated forms of the channels and, thus, prevent their transition to the original rest state (29). Because most of these drugs exhibit both tonic and phasic inhibitions, however, whether tonic and phasic block results from drug interaction at the same or different sites remains unclear.

Local Anesthetics Binding to Sodium Channels

Most of the clinically useful local anesthetics are tertiary amines with a pK_a of 7.0 to 9.0. Thus, under physiological conditions, both protonated forms (onium ions) and the un-ionized, molecular forms are available for binding to the channel proteins. In fact, the ratio between the onium ions $[BH^+]$ and the un-ionized molecules [B] can be easily calculated based on the pH of the medium and the pK_a of the drug molecule by the Henderson-Hasselbach equation:

$$pH = pK_a - \log [BH^+]/[B]$$

The effect of pH changes on the potency of local anesthetics has been extensively investigated (30). Based on these studies, it was concluded that local anesthetics block the action potential by first penetrating the nerve membrane in their un-ionized forms and then binding to a site within the channels in their onium forms. Perhaps the most direct support for this hypothesis comes from the experimental results of Narahashi et al. (31,32), who studied the effects of internal and external perfusion of local anesthetics (both tertiary amines and quaternary ammonium compounds), at different pH values, on the sodium conductance of the squid axon. The observation that both tertiary amines and quaternary ammonium compounds produce greater nerve blockage when applied internally indicates an axoplasmic site for these compounds.

Furthermore, only the tertiary amines exhibit a reduction in their local anesthetic activities when the internal pH is raised from 7.0 to 8.0. Because the increase of internal pH to 8.0 favors the existence of the un-ionized forms, this result again suggests that the onium ions are required for binding to the channel receptors. Narahashi and Frazier (33) further estimated that approximately 90% of the blocking actions of lidocaine may be attributed to onium forms of the drug molecule, whereas only approximately 10% may result from un-ionized molecule and, perhaps, at a hydrophobic binding site other than the primary binding site. Benzocaine, because of its lack of a basic amine group (pK_a = 2.78), and other neutral anesthetics, such as benzyl alcohol, have been suggested to bind to this hydrophobic binding site.

In 1984, Hille (34) proposed a unified theory involving a single receptor in the sodium channels for both onium ions (protonated tertiary amines and quaternary ammonium compounds) and un-ionized forms of local anesthetics. As depicted in Figure 16.7, a number of pathways are available, depending on the size, pK_a, and lipid solubility of the drug molecules as well as the voltage and frequency-dependent modulation of the channel states, for a drug to reach its receptor binding sites. Protonated anesthetic molecules $[BH^+]$ and quaternary ammonium compounds reach their target sites via the hydrophilic pathway externally (pathway b in Fig. 16.7), which is available only during channel activation.

The lipid-soluble anesthetic molecules, on the other hand, diffuse across the neuronal membrane in their un-ionized forms. They can interact with the same receptors from either the hydrophilic pathway (pathway b′ in

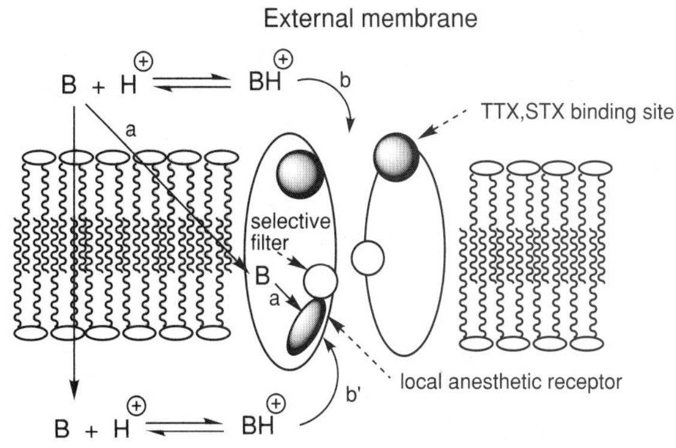

Fig. 16.7. Model of a sodium channel, as suggested by Hille (34), depicting a hydrophilic pathway (denoted by b and b′) and a hydrophobic pathway (denoted by a) by which local anesthetics may reach their receptor sites.

Fig. 16.7) on reprotonation to their onium ions [BH+] or via the hydrophobic pathway (pathway a in Fig. 16.7) in their un-ionized forms [B]. Benzocaine and other nonbasic local anesthetic molecules use this hydrophobic pathway and, thus, bind to the same receptor, although at the hydrophobic site of the receptor, to produce their actions. Again, this hypothesis is purely speculative, and its acceptance remains open for further debate. Recent site-directed mutagenesis studies (35–38) suggest that local anesthetics bind to the hydrophobic amino acid residues near the center and the intracellular end of the S6 segment in the domain D4, whereas the BTX receptor is within segment S6 in domain D1, of the α subunit of the sodium channels (Fig. 16.7) (15).

Structure–Activity Relationships

A quick perusal of Table 16.2 reveals that many diverse chemical structures possess local anesthetic properties: amino esters (procaine analogues), amino amides (lidocaine analogues), amino ethers (pramoxine), amino ketones (dyclonine), alcohols (benzyl alcohol and menthol), and phenols (eugenol and phenol). It would seem that there is no obvious structure–activity relationship among these agents. Most of the clinically useful local anesthetics, however, are tertiary amines with pK_a values of 7.0 to 9.0. These compounds exhibit their local anesthetic properties by virtue of the binding of the onium ions to a selective site within the sodium channels (Fig. 16.7). For this reason, any structural modifications that alter the lipid solubility, pK_a, and metabolic inactivation have a pronounced effect on the ability of a drug molecule to reach or bind to the hypothetical receptor sites, thus modifying its local anesthetic properties.

Lipophilic Portion

The lipophilic portion of the molecule is essential for local anesthetic activity. For most of the clinically useful local

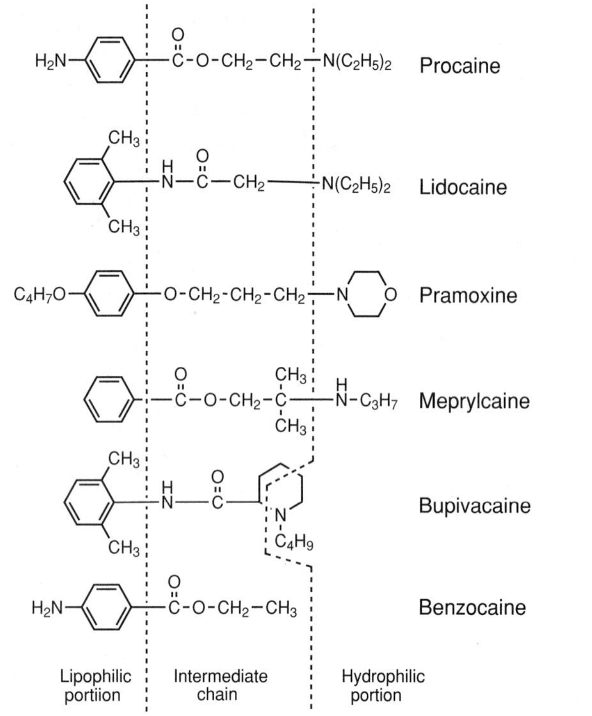

Fig. 16.8. Structure-activity relationship comparison of local anesthetics.

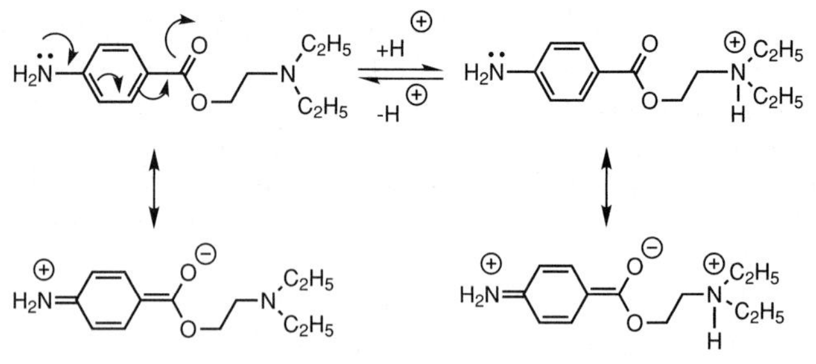

Fig. 16.9. Possible zwitterionic forms for procaine.

anesthetics, this portion of the molecule consists of either an aromatic group directly attached to a carbonyl function (the amino ester series) or a 2,6-dimethylphenyl group attached to a carbonyl function through an —NH— group (the amino amide series) (Fig. 16.8).

Both of these groups are highly lipophilic and appear to play an important role in the binding of local anesthetics to the channel receptor proteins. Structural modification of this portion of the molecule has a profound effect on its physical and chemical properties, which in turn alters its local anesthetic properties.

In the amino ester series, an electron-donating substituent in the ortho or para (or both) positions increases local anesthetic potency. Such groups as an amino (procaine, chloroprocaine, and propoxycaine), an alkylamino (tetracaine), or an alkoxy (proparacaine and propoxycaine) group can contribute electron density to the aromatic ring by both resonance and inductive effects, thereby enhancing local anesthetic potency over nonsubstituted analogue (meprylcaine).

As illustrated in Figure 16.9, resonance is expected to give rise to a zwitterionic form; (i.e., the electrons from the amino group can be resonance delocalized onto the carbonyl oxygen). Although neither drawn structure of procaine in Figure 16.9 may accurately represent the structure of procaine when it binds to the local anesthetic receptors, it is reasonable to assume that the greater the resemblance to the zwitterionic form, the greater the affinity for the receptor (i.e., binding from both the hydrophilic pathway b′ and hydrophobic pathway a in Fig. 16.7). This is particularly true for the binding of benzocaine to its receptors, because it lacks a basic amine group. Therefore, it can only bind from the hydrophobic pathway a. Thus, addition of any aromatic substitution that can enhance the formation of the resonance form through electron donation or inductive effects will produce more potent local anesthetic agents. Electron-withdrawing groups, such as nitro (—NO_2), reduce the local anesthetic activity.

Insertion of a methylene group between the aromatic moiety and the carbonyl function in the procaine molecule, which prohibits the formation of the zwitterionic form, has led to a procaine analogue with greatly reduced

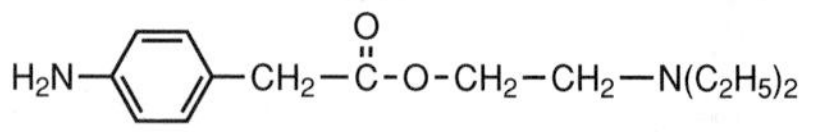

anesthetic potency. This observation lends further support for the involvement of the resonance form when an ester-type local anesthetic binds to the receptor. When an amino or an alkoxy group is attached to the meta position of the aromatic ring, however, no resonance delocalization of their electrons is possible. The addition of this function only increases (alkoxy group) or decreases (amino group) the lipophilicity of the molecule (e.g., benoxinate and proparacaine).

Furthermore, tetracaine is approximately 50-fold more potent than procaine. Experimentally, this increase in potency cannot be correlated solely with the increase of lipid solubility of the n-butyl group. Perhaps part of this potentiation of local anesthetic activity can be attributed to the electron-releasing property of the n-butyl group via the inductive effect, which indirectly enhances the electron density of the *p*-amino group, which in turn increases the formation of the zwitterionic form available for binding to the receptor proteins via both the hydrophobic and the hydrophilic pathways of the receptor.

Another important aspect of aromatic substitution has been observed from structure–activity relationship studies. In the amino amides (lidocaine analogues), the o,o′-dimethyl groups are required to provide suitable protection from amide hydrolysis to ensure a desirable duration of action. Similar conclusions can be made to rationalize the increase in the duration of action of propoxycaine by the o-propoxy group. The shorter duration of action, however, observed with chloroprocaine when compared with that of procaine can only be explained by the inductive effect of the o-chloro group, which pulls the electron density away from the carbonyl function, thus making it more susceptible for nucleophilic attack by the plasma cholinesterases.

Intermediate Chain

The intermediate chain almost always contains a short alkylene chain of one to three carbons in length linked to the aromatic ring via several possible organic functional groups. The nature of this intermediate chain determines the chemical stability of the drug. It also influences the duration of action and relative toxicity. In general, amino amides are more resistant to metabolic inactivation than the amino esters and, thus, are longer-acting local anesthetics. The placement of small alkyl groups (i.e., branching), especially around the ester function (e.g., meprylcaine) or the amide function (e.g., bupivacaine, etidocaine, prilocaine, and ropivacaine), also hinders esterase- or amidase-catalyzed hydrolysis, prolonging the duration of action (Fig. 16.8 and Table 16.2). It should be mentioned, however, that prolonging the duration of action of a compound usually also increases its systemic toxicities unless it is more selective toward local anesthetic receptor, as in the case of levobupivacaine (39,40).

In the lidocaine series, lengthening of the alkylene chain from one to two or three increases the pK_a of the terminal tertiary amino group from 7.7 to 9.0 or 9.5, respectively. Thus, lengthening of the intermediate chain effectively reduces local anesthetic potency as a result of a reduction of onium ions under physiological conditions. As mentioned earlier, the onium ions are required for effective binding of the amino amide-type local anesthetics to the channel receptors.

Hydrophilic Portion

Most clinically useful local anesthetics have a tertiary alkylamine, which readily forms water-soluble salts with mineral acids, and this portion commonly is considered to be the hydrophilic portion of the molecule (Fig. 16.9). The necessity of this portion of the molecule for amino ester-type local anesthetics remains a matter of debate. The strongest opposition for requiring a basic amino group for local anesthetic action comes from the observation that benzocaine, which lacks the basic aliphatic amine function, has potent local anesthetic activity. For this reason, it often is suggested that the tertiary amine function in procaine analogues is needed only for the formation of water-soluble salts suitable for pharmaceutical preparations. With the understanding of the voltage-activated sodium channel and the possible mechanism of action of local anesthetics discussed previously, however, it is quite conceivable that the onium ions produced by protonation of the tertiary amine group also are required for binding to the receptors (Fig. 16.7).

From Table 16.2, the hydrophilic group in most of the clinically useful drugs can be in the form of a secondary or tertiary alkyl amine or part of a nitrogen heterocycle (e.g., pyrrolidine, piperidine, and morpholine). As mentioned earlier, most of the clinically useful local anesthetics have pK_a values of 7.5 to 9.0. As we learned in organic chemistry, the effects of an alkyl substituent on the pK_a depend on the size, length, and hydrophobicity of the group; it is difficult to see a clear structure–activity relationship among these structures. Generally, however, it is accepted that local anesthetics with higher lipid solubility and lower pK_a values appear to exhibit more rapid onset and lower toxicity.

Stereochemistry

Are there any stereochemical requirements of local anesthetic compounds when they bind to the sodium channel receptors? A number of clinically used local anesthetics do contain a chiral center (i.e., bupivacaine, etidocaine, mepivacaine, and prilocaine) (Table 16.2), but in contrast to cholinergic drugs, the effect of optical isomerism on isolated nerve preparations revealed a lack of stereospecificity. In a few cases (e.g., prilocaine, bupivacaine, and etidocaine), however, small differences in the total pharmacological profile of optical isomers have been noted when administered in vivo (41–43). Whether these differences result from differences in uptake, distribution, and metabolism or from direct binding to the receptor has not been determined. When structural rigidity has been imposed on the molecule, however, as in the case of some aminoalkyl spirotetralin succinimides (44), differences in local anesthetic potency of the enantiomers have been observed (range, 1:2 to 1:10). Although these differences in enantiomers clearly are not as pronounced as those in other pharmacological agents, such as adrenergic blocking agents or anticholinergic drugs, steric requirements are necessary for effective interaction between a local anesthetic agent and its proposed channel receptors.

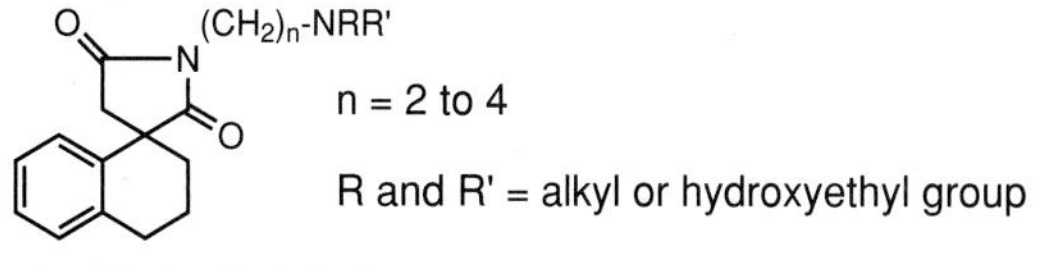

$(CH_2)_n$-NRR'

n = 2 to 4

R and R' = alkyl or hydroxyethyl group

N-Aminoalkyl spirotetralin succinimides

Stereochemistry of the local anesthetics, however, plays an important role in their observed toxicity and pharmacokinetic properties. For example, ropivacaine and levobupivacaine, the only optically active local anesthetics currently being marketed, have considerably lower cardiac toxicities than their close structural analogue, bupivacaine (45). Furthermore, the degree of separation between motor and sensory blockade is more apparent with ropivacaine and levobupivacaine relative to bupivacaine at a lower end of the dosage scale (46). Thus, the observed cardiac toxicity of bupivacaine has been attributed to the *R*-(+)-bupivacaine enantiomer (41–43). The exact mechanisms for this enantiomeric

Study Question 3

Question: Patients who are dibucaine-resistant homozygotes or heterozygotes are more likely to experience toxic reactions to amino ester-type local anesthetics. Explain.

difference remain unknown. Longobardo and colleagues observed a stereoselective blockade on the cardiac hKv1.5 channels by the *R*-(+)-enantiomers of bupivacaine, ropivacaine, and mepivacaine (47,48). It should be noted that the *S*-(−)-bupivacaine, which was recently approved by the U.S. Food and Drug Administration (FDA) and is marketed under the name of Chirocaine, has even less CNS toxicity than ropivacaine.

Metabolism of Local Anesthetics

An understanding of the metabolism of local anesthetics is important in clinical practice, because the overall toxicity of a drug depends not only on its uptake and tissue distribution but also on how it is deactivated in vivo. The amino ester-type local anesthetics are rapidly hydrolyzed by plasma cholinesterase (also known as pseudocholinesterase), which is widely distributed in body tissues. These compounds can therefore be metabolized in the blood, kidneys, and liver and, to a lesser extent, at the site of administration. For example, both procaine and benzocaine are easily hydrolyzed by cholinesterase into PABA and the corresponding N,N′-diethylaminoethyl alcohol.

It is not surprising that potential drug interactions exist between the amino ester-type local anesthetics and other clinically important drugs, such as cholinesterase inhibitors or atropine-like anticholinergic drugs. These compounds either inhibit or compete with local anesthetics for cholinesterases, therefore prolonging local anesthetic activity or toxicity. Another potential drug interaction with clinical significance may be envisioned between benzocaine and sulfonamides; that is, the hydrolysis of benzocaine to PABA may antagonize the antibacterial activity of sulfonamides.

Study Question 4

Question: The metabolism of ropivacaine in human is mediated by CYP1A2 and, to a minor extent, by CYP3A4 (50). The major metabolite is 3-hydroxyropivacaine, and the minor metabolite is (S)-2′,6′-pipecoloxylidide (a N-dealkylated product). Explain, based on your knowledge of drug metabolism, why severe drug-drug interactions between ropivacaine and fluvoxamine, a serotonin reuptake inhibitor, were observed whereas ketoconazole, a known hepatic enzyme inhibitor, causes only a minor decrease in ropivacaine renal clearance.

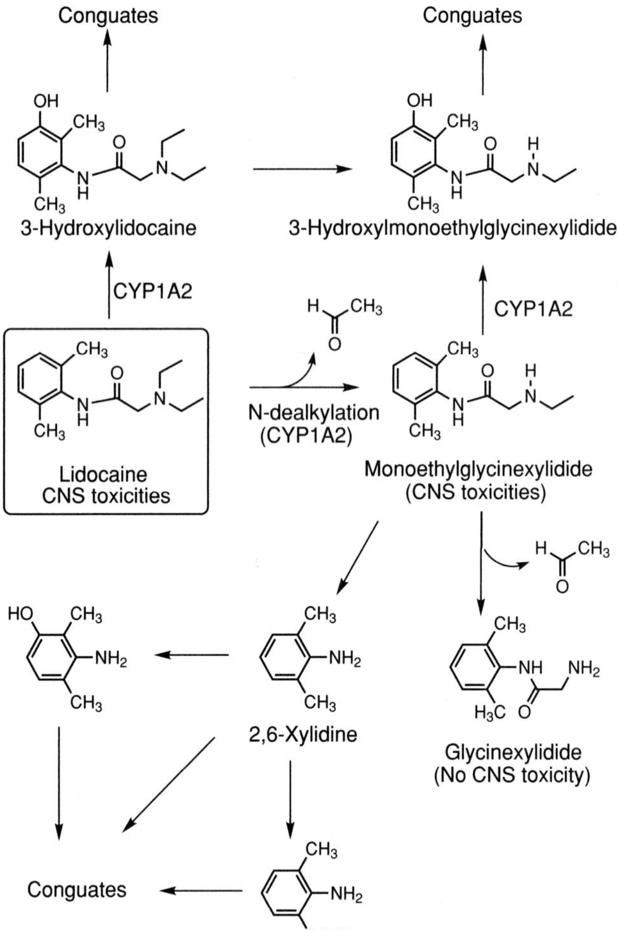

Fig. 16.10. Metabolic scheme for lidocaine.

The amino amide-type local anesthetics, however, are metabolized primarily in the liver, involving CYP1A2 isozymes (49). A general metabolic scheme for lidocaine is shown in Figure 16.10.

Marked species variations occur in the quantitative urinary excretion of these metabolites. For example, rats produce large quantities of the 3-hydroxy derivatives of both lidocaine and monoethylglycinexylidide, which subsequently are conjugated and recycled in the bile. Significant quantities of these two metabolites, however, are not produced by guinea pigs, dogs, or humans. It therefore is unlikely that biliary excretion is a major pathway for excretion in these species. Species variability is important primarily when the acute and chronic toxicity of nonester-type local anesthetic agents is being evaluated.

Although the exact mechanism for the CNS toxicity of lidocaine remains unclear, the metabolic studies of lidocaine provide some insight for future studies. Of all the metabolites of lidocaine, only monoethylglycinexylidide (and not glycinexylidide) contributes to some of the CNS side effects of lidocaine. This observation suggests that the toxicities of lidocaine are, perhaps, related to the removal of the N-ethyl groups of lidocaine after crossing

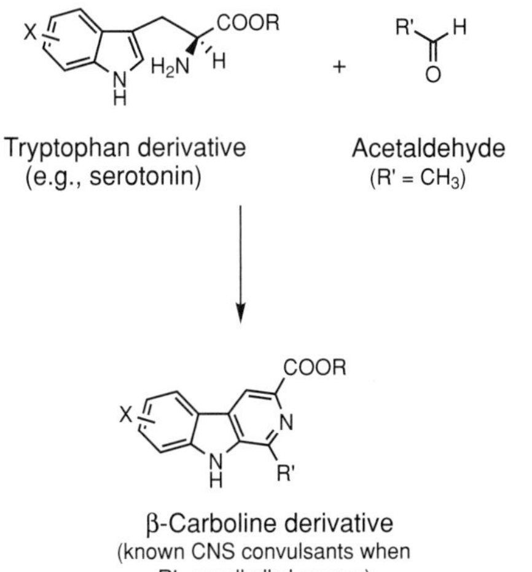

Fig. 16.11. Reaction of a tryptophan derivative with acetaldehyde under physiological conditions.

the blood-brain barrier. Support for this hypothesis can be obtained from the fact that reaction of a tryptophan derivative with formaldehyde under physiological conditions will give a β-carboline derivative, which is a CNS convulsant (Fig. 16.11). Recent advances in the $GABA_A$ receptor–benzodiazepine receptor–chloride ion channels and their role in the mechanism of action of benzodiazepine anticonvulsants lends further support to this hypothesis (i.e., β-carbolines are inverse agonists of benzodiazepines).

To minimize these unwanted side effects of lidocaine, tocainide and tolycaine have been prepared and found to possess good local anesthetic activity without any appreciable CNS side effects. Tocainide, which lacks the vulnerable N-ethyl group but has a α-methyl group to prevent degradation of the primary amine group from amine oxidase, has desirable local anesthetic properties. Tolycaine has an o-carbomethoxy substituted for one of the o-methyl group of lidocaine. The carbomethoxy group is fairly stable in tissues but is rapidly hydrolyzed in the blood to the polar carboxylic function and, thus, is unable to cross the blood-brain barrier.

For this reason, tolycaine lacks any CNS side effects, even though it still contains the N-ethyl groups. It should be noted, however, that both tocainide and tolycaine are primarily used clinically as antiarrhythmic agents.

Tocainide

Tolycaine

Furthermore, nonester-type drugs, especially lidocaine derivatives, also are known to be more prone to enzyme induction or inhibition of other medications (e.g., cimetidine and barbiturates).

Common Agents Used for Local Anesthesia

Local anesthetics are widely used in many primary care settings. Techniques for their administration in these settings include topical application, local infiltration, field block, and peripheral nerve block. Their use can be maximized by an understanding of their potencies, durations of action, routes of administration, and their pharmacokinetic and side effect profiles. The generic, trade name, and recommended application are given in Table 16.1, and the chemical structures of these agents can be found in Table 16.2.

Articaine

Articaine [4-methyl-3-(2-propylaminopropionamido) thiophene-2-carboxylic acid methyl ester hydrochloride] has been widely used in dentistry since its approval by the U.S. FDA in the year 2000 because of its quick onset and short duration of action. The structure of articaine differs from those of all other amino amide-type local anesthetics in that it contains a thiophene ring instead of a benzene ring and a carbomethoxy group. This renders the molecule more lipophilic and, thus, easier to cross any lipoidal membranes.

Its local anesthetic potency is approximately 1.5-fold that of lidocaine, even though it has similar pK_a (7.8) and plasma protein binding (76%) properties. Articaine also is metabolized primarily by plasma cholinesterases because of the presence of an ester group and, therefore, has a much shorter duration of action than lidocaine (i.e., only approximately one-fourth that of lidocaine). Articaine undergoes rapid hydrolysis of the carbomethoxy group to give articainic acid, which is eliminated either unchanged (75%) or as its glucuronides (25%). Compared with to other short-acting, amino amide-type local anesthetics, such as mepivacaine, lidocaine, or prilocaine, articaine is said to be a much safer drug for regional anesthesia and is the drug of choice for dental procedures.

Benzocaine

Benzocaine (ethyl *p*-aminobenzoate) is used topically by itself or in combination with menthol or phenol in nonprescription dosage forms such as gels, creams, ointments, lotions, aerosols, and lozenges to relieve pain or irritation caused by such conditions as sunburn, insect bites, toothache, teething, cold sores or canker sores in or around the mouth, and fever blisters. Benzocaine is a lipophilic local anesthetic agent with a short duration of action.

Like most amino ester-type local anesthetics, it is easily hydrolyzed by plasma cholinesterase. Because of its low

Study Question 5

Articaine, a dental anesthetic, is said to lack the CNS and cardiovascular toxicity associated with lidocaine and other amide-type local anesthetics. Explain.

Study Question 6

Question: Explain, with your knowledge of acid-base chemistry, why benzocaine can only be used for topical applications.

pK_a, however, it is un-ionized under most physiological conditions and, therefore, can only bind to the lipid side of the local anesthetic receptor (Fig. 16.7). It also can easily cross membranes into systemic circulation to cause systemic toxicities. Furthermore, being a PABA derivative, it has similar allergenic properties to procaine and is contraindicated with sulfonamide antibacterial agents.

Chloroprocaine

Chloroprocaine (N,N′-diethylaminoethyl 4-amino-2-chlorobenzoate) is a very short-acting, amino ester-type local anesthetic used to provide regional anesthesia by infiltration as well as by peripheral and central nerve block, including lumbar and caudal epidural blocks. The presence of a chlorine atom ortho to the carbonyl of the ester function increases its rate of hydrolysis by plasma cholinesterase at least threefold compared to procaine and benzocaine. Thus, chloroprocaine may be used in maternal and neonatal patients with minimal placental passage of chloroprocaine. The lower plasma cholinesterase activity in the maternal epidural space must still have sufficient activity for degrading chloroprocaine and, thus, not allowing it to cross the placenta barrier.

Like PABA, the hydrolysis product of chloroprocaine, 4-amino-2-chlorobenzoic acid, also inhibits the action of sulfonamides. Therefore, its use with sulfonamides should be avoided.

Lidocaine

Lidocaine [2-(diethylamino)-N-(2, 6-dimethylphenyl) acetamide monohydrochloride] is the most commonly used amino amide-type local anesthetic. Lidocaine is very lipid soluble and, thus, has a more rapid onset and a longer duration of action than most amino ester-type local anesthetics, such as procaine and tetracaine. It can be administered parenterally (with or without epinephrine) or topically either by itself or in combination with prilocaine or etidocaine as a eutectic mixture that is very popular with pediatric patients. The use of lidocaine–epinephrine mixtures should be avoided, however, in areas with limited vascular supply to prevent tissue necrosis. Lidocaine also frequently is used as a class IB antiarrhythmic agent for the treatment of ventricular arrhythmias, both because it binds and inhibits sodium channels in the cardiac muscle and because of its longer duration of action than amino ester-type local anesthetics.

Central nervous system changes are the most frequently observed systemic toxicities of lidocaine. The initial manifestations are restlessness, vertigo, tinnitus, slurred speech, and eventually, seizures. Subsequent manifestations include CNS depression with a cessation of convulsions and the onset of unconsciousness and respiratory depression or cardiac arrest. This biphasic effect occurs because local anesthetics initially block the inhibitory GABAergic pathways, resulting in stimulation, and eventually block both inhibitory and excitatory pathways (i.e., block the sodium channels associated with the NMDA receptors, resulting in overall CNS inhibition) (51).

Lidocaine is extensively metabolized in the liver by N-dealkylation and aromatic hydroxylations catalyzed by CYP1A2 isozymes (Fig. 16.10). Lidocaine also possesses a weak inhibitory activity toward the CYP1A2 isozymes and, therefore, may interfere with metabolism of other medications (52).

Mepivacaine

Mepivacaine hydrochloride [N-(2, 6-dimethylphenyl)-1-methyl 2-piperidinecarboxamide monohydrochloride] is an amino amide-type local anesthetic agent widely used to provide regional analgesia and anesthesia by local infiltration, peripheral nerve block, and epidural and caudal blocks. The pharmacological and toxicological profile of mepivacaine is quite similar to that of lidocaine, except that mepivacaine has a slightly longer duration of action and lacks the vasodilator activity of lidocaine. For this reason, it serves as an alternate choice for lidocaine when addition of epinephrine is not recommended in patients with hypertensive vascular disease.

Mepivacaine undergoes extensive hepatic metabolism catalyzed by CYP1A2, with only a small percentage of the administered dosage (<10%) being excreted unchanged in the urine. The major metabolic biotransformations of mepivacaine are N-dealkylation (to give the N-demethylated compound 2′,6′-pipecoloxylidide) and aromatic hydroxylations. These metabolites are excreted as their corresponding glucuronides.

Bupivacaine and Levobupivacaine

Bupivacaine hydrochloride [N-(2,6-dimethylphenyl)-1-n-butyl 2-piperidinecarboxamide monohydrochloride] contains a racemic mixture of the S-(−)- and R-(+)-enantiomers. Bupivacaine has higher lipid solubility and a much decreased rate of hepatic degradation compared with lidocaine. For this reason, bupivacaine has greater tendency than lidocaine to produce cardiotoxicity. Because of its greater affinity for voltage-gated sodium channels, the R-(+)-enantiomer confers greater cardiotoxicity to racemic bupivacaine.

It was not surprising to see the approval of levobupivacaine, the S-(-)-enantiomer of (±)-bupivacaine, as the second optically active, amino amide-type local anesthetic for parenteral applications. Like ropivacaine, levobupivacaine has a lower cardiotoxicity than bupivacaine, but it also has a lower CNS toxicity than both ropivacaine and lidocaine.

Answer for Study Question 1

Answer: With the exception of cocaine (itself a vasoconstrictor), all local anesthetics are associated with arteriolar dilatation. Thus, to decrease the rate of removal of local anesthetics from the site of administration and to maintain an effective drug concentration at the site of action, a vasoconstrictor, such as epinephrine, frequently is used to reduce regional blood supply. Epinephrine is a potent adrenergic agonist at the α- and β-adrenergic receptors; however, its vasoconstricting action results primarily from its action on the α1-adrenergic receptors. A reduction of regional blood flow into and out of the site of action greatly reduces the systemic toxicity of procaine. Furthermore, as procaine and other ester-type local anesthetics are inactivated predominantly by plasma esterase, a reduction of local blood flow also lowers the plasma esterase concentrations and, thereby, prolongs the duration of action of the local anesthetic.

Answer for Study Question 2

Answer: Many in vitro studies have demonstrated that addition of sodium bicarbonate to solutions of local anesthetics decreases the ratio of ionized to un-ionized molecules, thereby allowing more rapid penetration of the local anesthetic through the lipid membrane (Fig. 16.7) and, thus, shortening the onset time. Addition of too much bicarbonate, however, will cause precipitation of the drug molecules, and this may result in the injection of particulate un-ionized drug along with the solution. For this reason, routine alkalization of local anesthetics is not desirable.

Answer for Study Question 3

Answer: Patients with genetic anomalies of plasma cholinesterase in so-called dibucaine-resistant homozygotes (lacks one such gene) or heterozygotes (lacks both genes) are unable to efficiently hydrolyze local anesthetics. Thus, an increased drug level in the blood circulation would lead to increased cardiac and CNS toxicity. For this reason, an individual with atypical plasma cholinesterase should wear a Medic-Alert bracelet so that complications can be avoided.

Answer for Study Question 4

Answer: 3-Hydroxyropivacaine is produced via the microsomal aromatic hydroxylation catalyzed by CYP1A2 isozymes. This enzymatic reaction introduces a hydroxy group ortho to one of the methyl group of ropivacaine. Because CYP1A2 is the most important isozyme for the degradation of ropivacaine, a potent inhibitor of this isozyme, such as fluvoxamine, will greatly reduce the renal plasma clearance of ropivacaine. On the other hand, (S)-2′,6′-pipecoloxylidide is formed by removal of N-propyl group of ropivacaine by CYP3A4 isozyme. Because this is only a minor metabolite, an inhibitor of CYP3A4, such as ketoconazole, will have no relevance in the total clearance of ropivacaine.

Answer for Study Question 5

Answer: Articaine lacks the CNS and cardiovascular toxicity of lidocaine, because it has a carbomethoxy group instead of a methyl group at the ortho position. It will protect amide hydrolysis at the site of local anesthetic action because of a lower tissue esterase concentration. When articaine is absorbed into the blood circulation, however, this carbomethoxy group is rapidly hydrolyzed to provide a carboxylic acid function. The presence of this carboxylic acid function with a basic amine group in the molecule will greatly decrease the concentration of neural un-ionized molecules needed to cross the lipoidal membranes in heart and the blood-brain barrier. Furthermore, any unprotonated drug molecules in the blood circulation will probably exist as an internal salt similar to that of amino acid, thus greatly reducing their ability to cross lipid membranes.

Answer to Study Question 6

Answer: Benzocaine, which lacks an aliphatic amino group needed for salt formation, is practically insoluble in water. Protonation of the aromatic amino group in benzocaine results in a salt with a pK_a of 2.78, which is too acidic and, therefore, unsuitable for preparation of a parenteral dosage form for injection. Based on the acid-base chemistry principle, an aromatic amino group is a weak base, because its nonbounded elections are delocalized into the aromatic ring. Thus, an aromatic amine salt, such as benzocaine, will not hold onto its proton as tightly as an aliphatic amine salt and, therefore, will readily release the proton when dissolved in water.

Possible pathways for metabolism of bupivacaine include aromatic hydroxylation, N-dealkylation, and to a minor extent, the amide hydrolysis. Only the N-dealkylated product, however, has been identified in urine after epidural or spinal anesthesia.

Ropivacaine

Ropivacaine hydrochloride [*S*-(−)-N-(2, 6-dimethylphenyl)-1-n-propyl 2-piperidine-carboxamide monohydrochloride] is the first optically active, amino amide-type local anesthetic marketed in recent years. It combines the anesthetic potency and long duration of action of (±)-bupivacaine with a side-effect profile intermediate between those of bupivacaine and lidocaine. Although ropivacaine has a pK_a nearly identical to that of bupivacaine, it is two- to threefold less lipid soluble and has a smaller volume of distribution, a greater clearance, and a shorter elimination half-life than bupivacaine in humans.

The metabolism of ropivacaine in human is mediated by hepatic CYP1A2 isozymes and, to a minor extent, by CYP3A4 (50). The major metabolite is 3-hydroxyropivacaine, and the minor metabolite is (S)-2′,6′-pipecoloxylidide (a N-dealkylated product).

CASE STUDY

Victoria F. Roche and S. William Zito

BJ is a 58-year-old woman who is undergoing the novel method of transesophageal echocardiography in preparation for use in determining the correct placement of a central vein catheter for long-term parenteral nutrition. To assist in the insertion of the tube, BJ's esophagus was sprayed with 20% benzocaine solution, and oxygen was delivered via nasal route (1.5 L/min). During the procedure, BJ's arterial oxygen saturation, as determined by pulse oximetry, dropped from 99 to 88%, and her lips appeared cyanotic. The procedure was stopped and 100% oxygen administered by face mask with no effect. At this point, co-oximetry was used to measure arterial blood gas and hemoglobin with the following results: pH 7.47; partial pressure oxygen, 292 mm Hg; partial pressure of carbon dioxide, 32 mm Hg; bicarbonate, 24 mEq/L; and arterial oxygen saturation, 67%. The diagnosis of methemoglobinemia was confirmed by determination of a methemoglobin level of 31%. BJ was treated with IV methylene blue (1 mg/kg body wt) and recovered promptly. Her physician wants to perform the procedure again with another local anesthetic. Evaluate structures 2 through 4 for possible use in this case.

H_2N OCH_2CH_3 O

Benzocaine (1)

CH_3 H N CH_3 NHC_3H_7 O

2

O N C_4H_9O

3

CH_3 H N H O N C_3H_7 CH_3

4

1. Identify the therapeutic problem(s) in which the pharmacist's intervention may benefit the patient.
2. Identify and prioritize the patient-specific factors that must be considered to achieve the desired therapeutic outcomes.
3. Conduct a thorough and mechanistically oriented structure–activity analysis of all therapeutic alternatives provided in the case.
4. Evaluate the structure–activity relationship findings against the patient-specific factors and desired therapeutic outcomes, and make a therapeutic decision.
5. Counsel your patient.

References

1. Liljestrand G. The historical development of local anesthesia in local anesthetics. In: Lechat P, ed. International Encyclopedia of Pharmacology and Therapeutics. Oxford: Pergamon Press, 1971:1–38.
2. Arey LB, Developmental Anatomy, 7th Ed. Philadelphia: WB Saunders, 1965.
3. De Jong RH, Freund FG. Physiology of peripheral nerve and local anesthesia. Int Anesthesiol Clin 1979;8:35–53.
4. Hodgkin AL, Huxley AF. The dual effect of membrane potential on sodium conductance in the giant axon of *Loligo*. J Physiol (Lond) 1952;116:497–506.
5. Skou JC. Further investigations on a Mg^{2+}- and Na^+-activated adenosine triphosphatase, possibly related to the active, linked transport of Na^+ and K^+ across the nerve membrane. Biochim Biophys Acta 1960;42:6–23.
6. Tasaki I, Singer I, Takenaka T. Effects of internal and external ionic environment on excitability of squid giant axon. A macromolecular approach. J Gen Physiol 1965;48:1095–1123.
7. Koketsu K. Calcium and the excitable cell membrane. Neurosci Res 1969;2: 2–39.
8. Tasaki I. Nerve Transmission. Springfield, IL: Charles C Thomas, 1953.
9. Noda M, Shimizy S, Tanabe T, et al. Primary structure of *Electrophorus electricus* sodium channel deduced from complimentary DNA sequence. Nature 1984;312:121-127.
10. Catterall WA. Structure and function of voltage-sensitive ion channels. Science 1988;242:50–61.
11. Catterall WA. Cellular and molecular biology of voltage-gated sodium channels. Physiol Rev 1992;72(Suppl):15–48.
12. Balser JR. The molecular interaction between local anesthetic/antiarrhythmic agents and voltage-gated sodium channels. Trends Cardiovasc Med 1998;8:83–88.
13. Clare JJ, Tate SN, Nobbs M, et al. Voltage-gated sodium channels as therapeutic targets. Drug Discovery Today 2000;5:506–520.
14. Anger T, Madge DJ, Mulla M, et al.. Medicinal chemistry of neuronal voltage-gated sodium channel blockers. J Med Chem 2001;44:115–137.
15. Yang S-Y, Wang GK. Voltage-gated sodium channels as primary targets of diverse lipid-soluble neurotoxins. Cellular Signaling 2003;15:151–159.
16. Hamill OP, Marty A, Neher E, et al. Improved patch-clamp techniques for high-resolution current recording from cells and cell-free membrane patches. Pflügers Arch 1981;391:85–100.
17. Arthur GR. Pharmacokinetics of local anesthetics. In: Strichartz GR, ed. Local Anesthetics. Handbook of Experimental Pharmacology. Berlin: Springer, 1987;81:165–186.
18. Eggleston ST, Lush LW. Understanding allergic reactions to local anesthetics. Ann Pharmacother 1996;30: 851–857.
19. Bean BP, Cohen CJ, Tsien RW. Lidocaine block of cardiac sodium channels. J Gen Physiol 1983;81:613–642.
20. Makielski JC, Sheets MF, Hanck DA, et al. Sodium current in voltage clamped internally perfused canine Purkinje cells. Biophys J 1987;52:1–11.
21. Welin-Berger K, Neelissen JAM. Engblom J. Physicochemical interaction of local anesthetics with lipid model systems—correlation with in vitro permeation and in vivo efficacy. J Control Release 2002;81:33–43.
22. Feistein MB. Reaction of local anesthetics with phospholipids. A possible chemical basis for anesthesia. J. Gen Physiol 1964;48:357–374.
23. Blaustein MP, Goldman DE. Competitive action of calcium and procaine on lobster axon. J Gen Physiol 1966;49:1043–1063.
24. Ritchie JM, Greengard P. On the mode of action of local anesthetics Annu Rev Pharmacol 1966;6:405–430.
25. Pardo L, Blanck TJJ, Recio-Pinto E. The neuronal lipid membrane permeability was markedly increased by bupivacaine and mildly affected by lidocaine and ropivacaine. Eur J Pharmacol 2002;455:81–90.
26. Tamkun MM, Talvenheimo JA, Catterall WA. The sodium channel from rat brain: reconstitution of neurotoxin-activated ion flux and scorpion toxin binding from purified components. J Biol Chem 1984;259:1676–1688.
27. Butterworth JF IV, Strichartz GR. Molecular mechanisms of local anesthetics: a review. Anesthesiology 1990;72:711–734.
28. Strichartz GR. The inhibition of sodium currents in myelinated nerve by quaternary derivatives of lidocaine. J Gen Physiol 1973;62:37–57.
29. Courtney KR. Mechanism of frequency-dependent inhibition of sodium currents in frog myelinated nerve by the lidocaine derivative GEA 968. J Pharmacol Exp Ther 1975;195:225–236.
30. Narahashi T, Frazier DT. Site of action and active form of local anesthetics. Neurosci Res (NY), 1971;4:65–99.
31. Narahashi T, Yamada M, Frazier DT. Cationic forms of local anesthetics block action potentials from inside the nerve membrane. Nature 1969;223:748–749.
32. Narahashi T, Frazier DT, Yamada M. The site of action and active form of local anesthetics. I. Theory and pH experiments with tertiary compounds. J Pharmacol Exp Ther 1970;171:32–44.
33. Narahashi T, Frazier DT. Site of action and active form of procaine in squid giant axons. J Pharmacol Exp Ther 1975;194:506–513.
34. Hille B. Mechanisms of Blocks. In: Hille B. ed. Ionic channels of excitable membranes, Chapter 12. Sunderland MA, Sinauer Associates, 1984:272–302.
35. Ragsdale DR, McPhee JC, Scheuer T, et al. Molecular determinants of state-dependent block of Na^+ channels by local anesthetics. Science 1994;265: 1724–1728.
36. Wang GK, Quan C, Wang SY. Local anesthetic block of batrachotoxin-resistant muscle Na^+ channels. Mol Pharmacol 1998;54:389–396.
37. French RJ, Zamponi GW, Sierralta IE. Molecular and kinetic determinants of local anesthetic action on sodium channels. Toxicol Lett 1998;100–101: 247–254.
38. Scheuer T. A revised view of local anesthetic action: what channel state is really stabilized? J Gen. Physiol 1999;113:3–6.

39. Mather LE, Chang DH. Cardiotoxicity with modern local anesthetics. Is there a safer choice? Drugs 2001;61 333–342.
40. Rood JP, Coulthard P, Snowdon AT, et al. Safety and efficacy of levobupivacaine for postoperative pain relief after the surgical removal of impacted third molars: a comparison with lignocaine and adrenaline. Br J Oral Maxillofac Surg 2002;40:491–496.
41. Rutten AJ, Mather LE, McLean CF. Cardiovascular effects and regional clearances of IV bupivacaine in sheep: enantiomeric analysis. Br J Anaesth 1991;67:247–256.
42. Denson DD, Behbehani MM, Gregg RV. Enantiomer-specific effects of an intravenously administered arrhythmogenic dose of bupivacaine on neurons of the nucleus tractus solitarius and the cardiovascular system in the anesthetized rat. Reg Anesth 1992;17:311–316.
43. Rutten AJ, Mather LE, McLean CF, et al. Tissue distribution of bupivacaine enantiomers in sheep. Chirality 1993;5:485–491.
44. Aåkerman SBA, Camougis G, Sandburg RV. Stereoisomerism and differential activity in excitation block by local anesthetics. Eur J Pharmacol 1969;8:337–347.
45. McClure JH. Ropivacaine. Br J Anesth 1996;76:300–307.
46. Markham A, Faulds D. Ropivacaine. A review of its pharmacology and therapeutic use in regional anesthesia. Drugs 1996;52:429–449.
47. Longobardo M, Delpon E, Caballero R, et al. Structural determinants of potency and stereoselective block of hKv1.5 channels induced by local anesthetics. Mol Pharmacol 1998;54:162–169.
48. Franqueza L, Longobardo M, Vicente J, et al. Molecular determinants of stereoselective bupivacaine block of hKv1.5 channels. Circ Res, 1997;81: 1053–1064.
49. Imaoka S, Enomotl K, Oda Y, et al. Lidocaine metabolism by human cytochrome P-450s purified from hepatic microsomes: comparison of those with rat hepatic cytochrome P-450s. J Pharmacol Exp Ther 1990;255: 1385–1391.
50. Arlander E, Ekstrom G, Alm C, et al. Metabolism of ropivacaine in humans is mediated by CYP1A2 and to a minor extent by CYP3A4: an interaction study with fluvoxamine and ketoconazole as in vivo inhibitors. Clin Pharmacol Ther 1998;64:484–491.
51. Castaneda-Castellanos DR, Nikonorov I, Kallen RG, et al. Lidocaine stabilizes the open state of CNS voltage-dependent sodium channels. Mol Brain Res 2002;99:102–113.
52. Wei X, Dai R, Zhai S, et al. Inhibition of human liver cytochrome P-450 1A2 by the class 1B antiarrhythmics mexiletine, lidocaine, and tocainide. J. Pharmacol Exp Ther 1999;289:853–858.

Suggested Readings

Akeson M, Deamer DW. Anesthetics and membranes: a critical review. In: Aloia RC, Curtain CC, Gordon LM, eds. Drug and Anesthetic Effects on Membrane Structure and Function. New York: Wiley-Liss, 1991:71–89.

Arthur GR. Pharmacokinetics of local anesthetics. In: Strichartz GR, ed. Local Anesthetics. Handbook of Experimental Pharmacology. Berlin: Springer, 1987;81:165–186.

Courtney KR, Strichartz GR. Structural elements which determine local anesthetic activity. In: Strichartz GR, ed. Local Anesthetics. Handbook of Experimental Pharmacology. Berlin: Springer, 1987; 81:53–94.

Covino BG. Local anesthetics. In: Feldman SA, Scurr CF, Paton W, eds. Drugs in Anesthesia: Mechanisms of Action. London: Edward Arnold, 1987:261–291.

Covino BG. Toxicity and systemic effects of local anesthetic agents. In: Strichartz GR. ed. Local Anesthetics. Handbook of Experimental Pharmacology. Berlin: Springer, 1987:81:187–212.

Strichartz R, Ritchie JM. The action of local anesthetics on ion channels of excitable tissues. In: Strichartz GR. ed. Local Anesthetics. Handbook of Experimental Pharmacology. Berlin: Springer, 1987;81:21–52.

Vandam LD. Some aspects of the history of local anesthesia. In: Strichartz GR. ed. Local Anesthetics. Handbook of Experimental Pharmacology. Berlin: Springer, 1987;81:1–19.

17. *Phosphodiesterase Inhibitors*

KEVIN DALBY

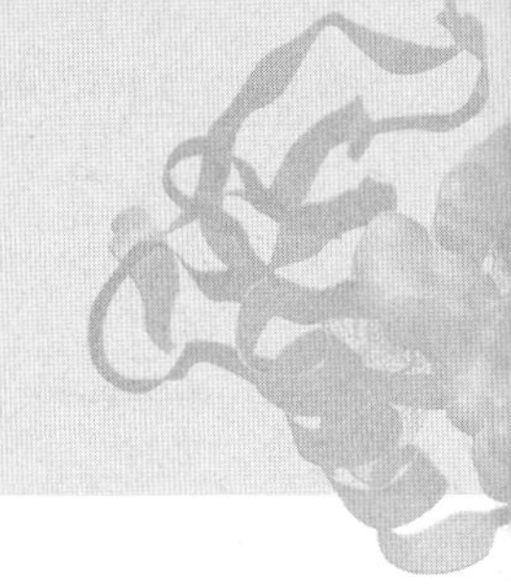

DRUGS COVERED IN THIS CHAPTER:

PHOSPHODIESTERASE INHIBITOR 5
- Sildenafil
- Tadalafil
- Vardenafil

PHOSPHODIESTERASE INHIBITOR 4
- Cilomilast
- Roflumilast

PHOSPHODIESTERASE ENZYME SYSTEM

Cyclic Nucleotide Signaling

The cyclic nucleotides cyclic adenosine 3′,5′-monophosphate (cAMP) and cyclic guanosine 3′,5′-monophosphate (cGMP) play critical roles in mediating cellular signals in response to hormones, neurotransmitters, chemokines, and cytokines (Fig. 17.1) (1–3). These signals usually begin through binding of a hormone neurotransmitter to a G protein–coupled receptor with subsequent triggering of adenylyl and guanylyl cyclases* that synthesize cAMP or cGMP, respectively. In turn, these newly synthesized nucleotides bind and activate effectors, such as protein kinase A and protein kinase G. These protein kinases phosphorylate a variety of substrates, including ion channels and transcription factors. The resulting signaling can lead to changes in gene expression and cell metabolism and, ultimately, to the regulation of a wide variety of cellular functions, such as immune responses, cardiac and smooth muscle contraction, visual response, glycogenolysis, apoptosis, and growth control (4).

Phosphodiesterases (PDEs) hydrolyze the cyclic nucleotides to their inactive linear forms (5′-AMP and 5′-GMP) (Fig. 17.1) and may be considered as negative regulators of cyclic nucleotide signaling. Their activity is regulated by multiple signals, however, suggesting a higher level of complexity in function that reflects their roles in compartmentalizing cyclic nucleotide signaling and integrating these signaling events with other pathways (4–10).

Therapeutic Use of Phosphodiesterase Inhibitors

Nomenclature

Human PDEs comprise a family of 21 genes, the products of which fall into 11 families with as many as 60 isoforms (4–10). In the most widely accepted nomenclature, the PDE family is indicated by an Arabic numeral, followed by a capital letter indicating the gene within a family and a second Arabic numeral indicating the splicing variant derived from a single gene (e.g., PDE4D2: family 4, gene D, splicing variant 2) (11).

Despite the complexity of cyclic nucleotide signaling pathways, PDE inhibitors have emerged as an attractive drug class with the potential to treat a number of human conditions. For example, PDE inhibitors may potentially serve as anti-inflammatory agents, vasodilators, smooth muscle relaxants, antidepressants, antithrombotics, cardiotonic agents, and agents for improving cognitive functions (12). These enzymes are widely distributed throughout the body, exhibiting isoform-specific tissue concentrations. Thus, therapeutic strategies have focused on targeting specific PDE isoforms in efforts to limit their drug effects on cellular cAMP or cGMP levels within localized tissues.

PDE5 Inhibitors

The most successful area of intervention to date has been in treating erectile dysfunction, in which PDE5 selective competitive inhibitors, such as sildenafil, vardenafil, and the more discriminatory tadalafil (Fig. 17.2), have proven to be highly efficacious (13,14). These drugs work by enhancing and prolonging smooth muscle relaxation and vasodilation as a result of sexual stimulation. Normally, sexual stimulation causes the release of nitric oxide by endothelial cells as well as cavernous nerves, activating the enzyme guanylate cyclase (EC 4.6.1.2), thus stimulating the production of cGMP (13,14). This leads to a decrease in cellular levels of calcium, the relaxation of smooth muscle cells in the cavernosal bodies, and ultimately, erection (15). Erectile dysfunction results from a disruption in this sequence of events and can be the result of a number of different factors, such as hormonal imbalance and neurologic or vascular impairment (14). Because the degradation of cGMP in the penile corpora is catalyzed primarily by PDE5, the inhibition of PDE5 leads to the maintenance of an increased level of cGMP in the corpus cavernosum and an improved ability to obtain or maintain an erection (13).

*These enzymes are known by two names, *adenylate cyclase (EC 4.6.1.1)* and *guanylate cyclase (EC 4.6.1.2),* their official names from the International Union of Biochemistry and Molecular Biology Nomenclature Committee, or their alternative names, adenylyl cyclase and guanylyl cyclase.

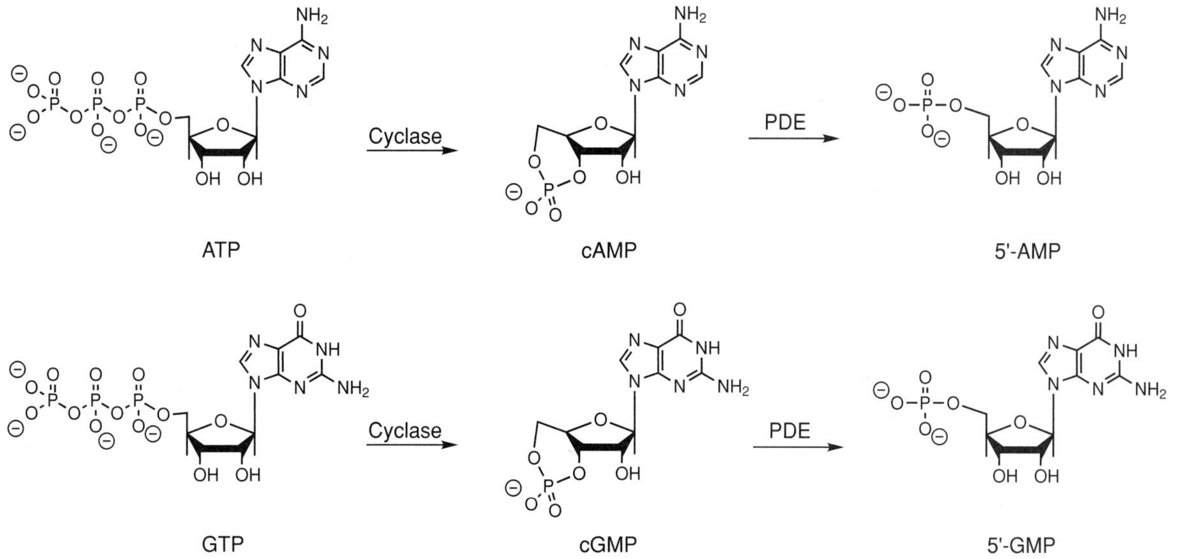

Fig. 17.1. Enzymatic interconversion of cyclic and linear nucleotides.

PDE4 Inhibitors

The PDE4 isozymes have been known since the early 1980s to regulate cAMP signaling pathways that are affected by antidepressants (16). In addition, intracellular elevations of cAMP are associated with broad anti-inflammatory effects, in which the PDE4A, PDE4B, and PDE4D isoforms are thought to be the major cAMP-hydrolyzing PDEs in most inflammatory cells (17,18). Currently, the clinical utility of PDE4 selective inhibitors for the treatment of a number of inflammatory-related conditions is still in development (19,20). It is thought that nausea and emesis, the most common side effects of PDE4 inhibitors, results from the inhibition of PDE4D in the brain (21). Therefore, much research effort currently is directed toward the design of subtype selective inhibitors which might show better profiles.

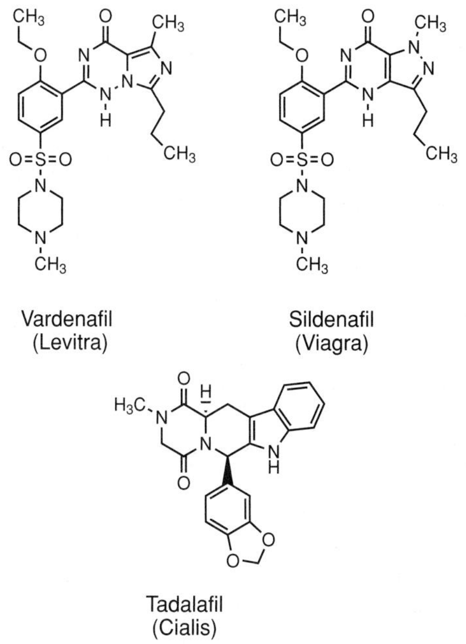

Fig. 17.2. Competitive inhibitors of PDE5.

PDE3 Inhibitors

The inhibition of platelet activation is a critical component in the treatment and prevention of cardiovascular diseases and cerebral ischemia/thrombotic disorders. Nitric oxide and prostacyclins inhibit platelet activation by elevating intracellular levels of both cGMP and cAMP, respectively. In platelets, the most abundant PDE is PDE3A, which lowers the intracellular concentration of cAMP. Inhibitors of PDE3A serve as potential antiplatelet agents by elevating cAMP levels. One PDE3-type selective inhibitor cilostazol, which has both antiplatelet, antithrombotic, and vasodilatory effects, is used for the treatment of intermittent claudication and for the prevention of short- and medium-term vessel closure (22).

Specificity of Cyclic Nucleotide Phosphodiesterases

The PDEs catalyze the hydrolysis of the 3′-phosphate diester bond of the cyclic nucleotides to give the acyclic 5′-phosphate monoesters (Fig. 17.1). They can be distinguished according to their primary structure, tissue distribution, intracellular localization, regulation, and specificity: Families 4, 7, and 8 hydrolyze cAMP; families 5, 6, and 9 hydrolyze cGMP; and families 1, 2, 3, 10, and 11 hydrolyze both cyclic nucleotides (Table 17.1).

All human PDEs are modular (Fig. 17.3) composed of a conserved C-terminal catalytic domain and various signal transduction domains that are thought to be sensors of intracellular signals, the reception of which leads to changes in conformation of the PDE and, thus, its activity (8). The catalytic domain contains a core of 16 α-helices

Table 17.1. Specificity and Potency of PDE Inhibitors

PDE	Specificity	Inhibitor	IC_{50}[a] (nM)	PDE	Specificity	Inhibitor	IC_{50}[a] (nM)
PDE1B	Duel	Rolipram	>200,000	PDE6	cGMP	Sildenafil	50[b]
		Cilomilast	87,000			Vardenafil	11[c]
		Roflumilast	>200,000			Tadalafil	2,000[b]
		Sildenafil	1,500	PDE7B	cAMP	Rolipram	>200,000
		Vardenafil	300			Cilomilast	44,000
		Tadalafil	50,000			Roflumilast	>200,000
PDE2A	Duel	Rolipram	>200,000			Sildenafil	78,000
		Cilomilast	160,000			Vardenafil	1,900
		Roflumilast	>200,000			Tadalafil	74,000
		Sildenafil	35,000	PDE8A	cAMP	Rolipram	>200,000
		Vardenafil	3,100			Cilomilast	7,000
		Tadalafil	130,000			Roflumilast	>200,000
PDE3B	cAMP > cGMP	Rolipram	>200,000			Sildenafil	>200,000
		Cilomilast	87,000			Vardenafil	57,000
		Roflumilast	>200,000			Tadalafil	>200,000
		Sildenafil	15,000	PDE9A	cGMP	Rolipram	>200,000
		Vardenafil	580			Cilomilast	>200,000
		Tadalafil	280,000			Roflumilast	>200,000
PDE4B	cAMP	Rolipram	570			Sildenafil	5,600
		Cilomilast	25			Vardenafil	680
		Roflumilast	0.84			Tadalafil	150,000
		Sildenafil	20,000	PDE10A	cAMP<cGMP	Rolipram	140,000
		Vardenafil	3,800			Cilomilast	73,000
		Tadalafil	9,200			Roflumilast	>200,000
PDE4D	cAMP	Rolipram	1,100			Sildenafil	6,800
		Cilomilast	11			Vardenafil	880
		Roflumilast	0.68			Tadalafil	19,000
		Sildenafil	14,000	PDE11A	Duel	Rolipram	>200,000
		Vardenafil	3,900			Cilomilast	21,000
		Tadalafil	19,000			Roflumilast	25,000
PDE5A	cGMP	Rolipram	>200,000			Sildenafil	6,100
		Cilomilast	53,000			Vardenafil	240
		Roflumilast	17,000			Tadalafil	10
		Sildenafil	2.2				
		Vardenafil	1.0				
		Tadalafil	1.2				

[a]Data are from Sutherland and Rall (28) unless stated otherwise. The numbers shown in the table are the 50% inhibition concentration (IC50). The cAMP and cGMP concentrations used were far below the K_m of all the PDEs assayed except for PDE9A, in which case it was close to the K_m. The IC50s obtained are good approximations of the inhibition constant K_i. Selectivities of an inhibitor may be determined by taking ratios of the numbers given in the table.
[b]K_i values are from Card et al. (30).
[c]Value from Hatzelmann and Schudt (34).

in a compact arrangement (Fig. 17.4) of three subdomains comprised of αH1-7, αH8-11, and αH12-16, respectively (23). The active site at the intersection of these three domains forms a deep hydrophobic pocket with a narrow opening and a wide inner space (Fig. 17.5). Eleven of 16 invariant amino acids are present in the active site and facilitate recognition and catalysis through four key interactions: 1) the binding of two divalent metal ions, 2) the coordination to the phosphate diester moiety, 3) the hydrophobic clamping of the nucleotide ring by highly conserved hydrophobic residues that sandwich the substrate in the active site, and 4) a hydrogen-bonding network that helps to determine nucleotide specificity (Fig. 17.6A and B).

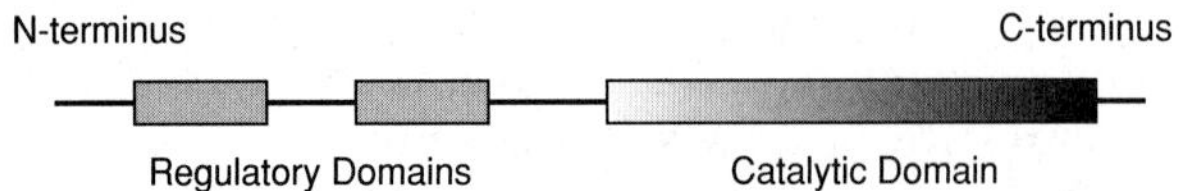

Fig. 17.3. Schematic representation of the domain organization of PDEs. The conserved catalytic domain is found toward the C-terminal half of the PDE (8). The number and function of the regulatory domains differ between the different PDE subfamilies. These domains include calcium-sensing domains as well as signaling domains that mediate interactions with other signaling proteins.

Several structures of PDEs complexed to various ligands are available and have been reviewed (24). The structure of 5′-AMP bound to PDE4D2 (25) (Fig. 17.7) reveals direct coordination of the phosphate to two divalent metal ions as well as His-160, Asp-201, and Asp-318. This enzyme product complex is suggestive of a potential catalytic mechanism in which the cyclic phosphate diester undergoes nucleophilic attack from a metal-bound hydroxide ion (Fig. 17.8), which then displaces the 3′-hydroxyl leaving group. According to this mechanism, His-160 is

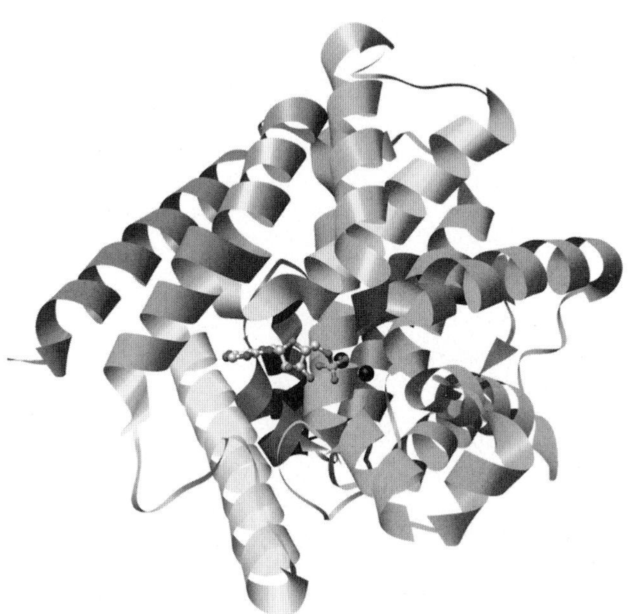

Fig. 17.4. Ribbon diagram of monomeric PDE4D2 (PDB 1PTW). 5′-AMP is shown as balls-and-sticks, whereas two divalent metal icons are shown as solid spheres (24). (See color plate.)

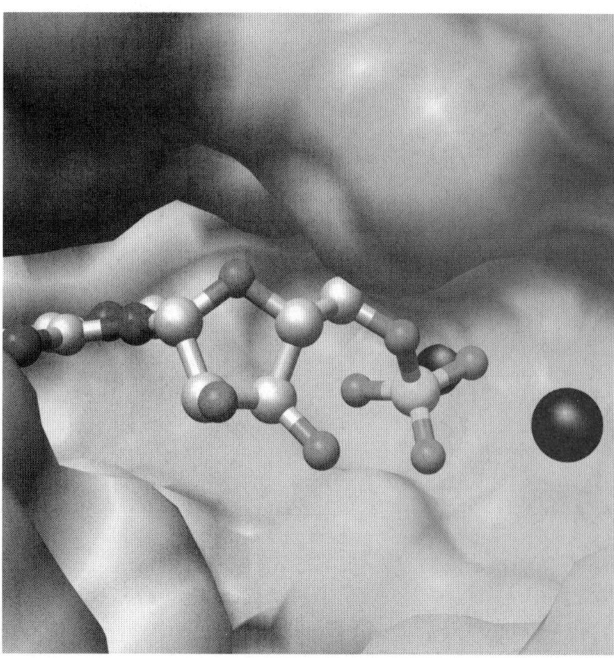

Fig. 17.5. Surface representation showing 5′-AMP in the nucleotide binding pocket of PDE4D2 (PDB 1PTW). 5′-AMP is shown as balls-and-sticks, while two divalent zinc icons are shown as solid spheres (24). (See color plate.)

predicted to serve as a general acid to protonate and, thus, stabilize developing negative charge on the 3′-hydroxyl leaving group. This mechanism is consistent with the observed structure as well as studies on other enzymes that catalyze similar processes using a binuclear strategy.

Recognition of the nucleotide base is mediated by π-π interactions with a conserved phenylalanine (Phe-372 in PDE4D2) that shapes the roof of the hydrophobic pocket and van der Waals interactions that line both the roof and the base. Additional hydrophobic interactions to the ribose ring, which has a C3′-endo puckering configuration, contributes to substrate recognition.

An important question, given the high degree of conservation between the PDE active sites, is what determines their substrate specificity (26). Current theory points toward the role of a key glutamine conserved in all PDEs (Gln-369 in PDE4D2), which can adopt either an adenine- or a guanine-specific binding conformation (27). The specificity of the PDEs is thus derived from

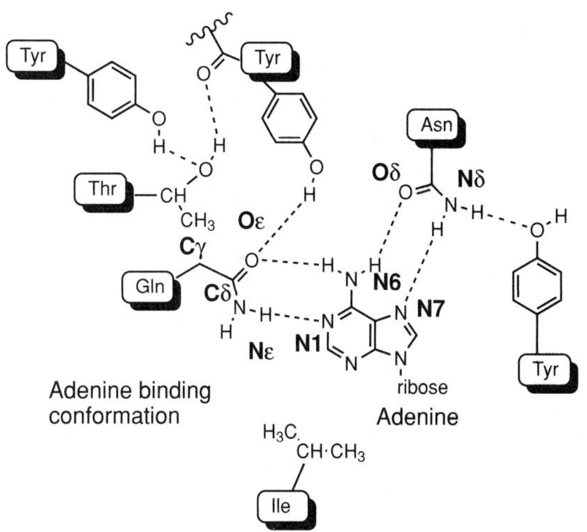

A. PDE4 active siter which specifies adenine recognition

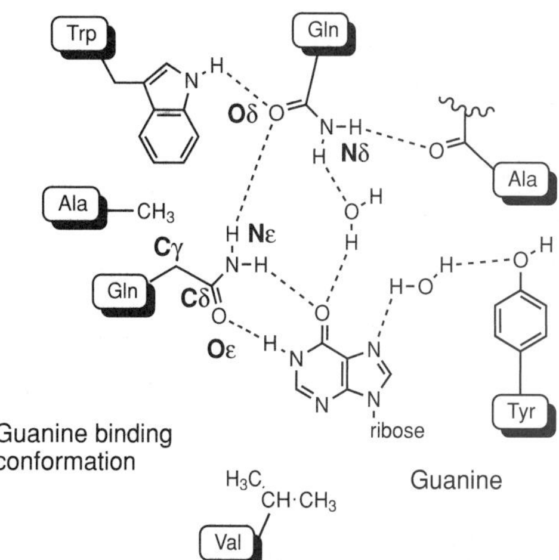

B. PDE5 active siter which specifies guanine recognition

Fig. 17.6. Schematic representation of the hydrogen-bonding network in the active site of PDEs.

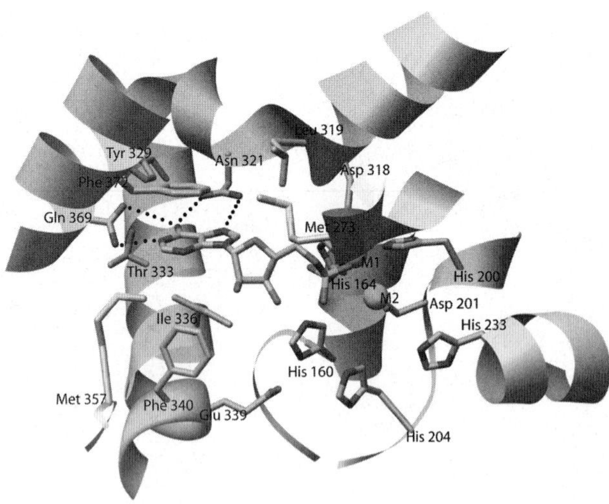

Fig. 17.7. Ribbon diagram of the active site of PDE4D2. The AMP phosphate group binds two divalent zinc icons and forms hydrogen bonds with His-160, Asp-201, and Asp-318. The adenine group of AMP adopts an anticonformation and orients toward the hydrophobic pocket made up of residues Tyr-159 (not shown), Leu-319, Asn-321, Thr-333, Ile-336, Gln-369, and Phe-372. It forms three hydrogen bonds with Gln-369 and Asn-321 and buttresses against Phe-372. The ribose of AMP has a C3′-endo puckering configuration and makes van der Waals contacts with residues His-160, Met-273, Asp-318, Leu-319, Ile-336, Phe-340, and Phe-372 (24). (See color plate.)

hydrogen-bond networks within the active site, which strongly favor either the cAMP-specific (26) or the cGMP-specific (27) conformation (Fig. 17.6A and B). These two conformations differ essentially by rotation about the Cγ-Cδ bond of the glutamine, which switches the positions of the Nε and Oε atoms to accommodate the hydrogen-bonding requirements of either adenine or guanidine (Fig. 17.6). It has been suggested that the ability of PDEs 1, 2, 3, 10, and 11 to hydrolyze both cAMP and cGMP reflects the ability of the glutamine to adopt either conformation.

Specificity of Phosphodiesterase Inhibitors

The first PDE inhibitor described was theophylline, the activity of which toward PDE was first reported some 50 years ago (28). Like all PDE inhibitors, theophylline and other xanthines, such as 3-isobutyl-1-methylxanthine (IBMX), have a planar structure that mimics the planarity of the cAMP and cGMP bases. They are nonselective, however, and adopt multiple binding modes in the active sites of the PDEs (24).

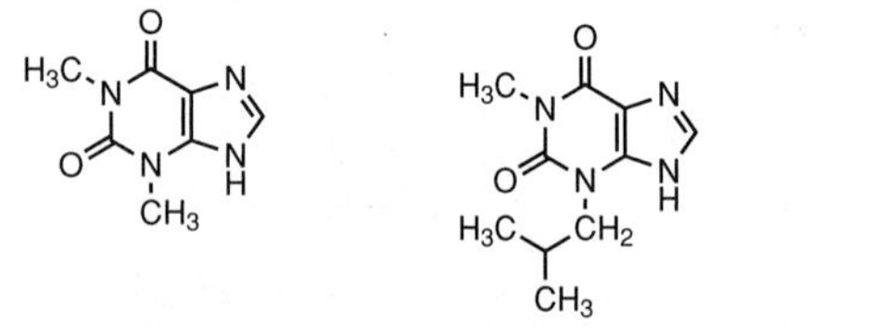

Theophyline 3-Isobutyl-1-methylxanthine (IBMX)

Recent years have seen the development of a number of selective PDE inhibitors that compete with cyclic nucleotides for binding. Notably, the solved structures of a number of PDE inhibitor complexes have been instrumental in allowing researchers to delineate some of the reasons for the selectivity of various inhibitors (29,30). These structures have clearly shown that the uniformly important planar property of PDE inhibitors supports binding in the hydrophobic cleft of the active site that normally is reserved for the nucleotide base. They also allude to further specificity, resulting from an array of hydrogen-bonding interactions and the extension of inhibitors into unique regions of space. Notably, the conformation of the conserved active site glutamine, that specifies nucleotide binding, also is a key determinant of inhibitor selectivity.

PDE5 Selective Inhibitors

Sildenafil (7) and its analogue, vardenafil (Fig. 17.2), are substituted azaguanine analogues, the pyrazolopyrimidinone group of which mimics the binding mode of guanine in cGMP, whereas the 3′-n-propyl substituent binds in a similar region to the ribose ring (Fig. 17.9). The

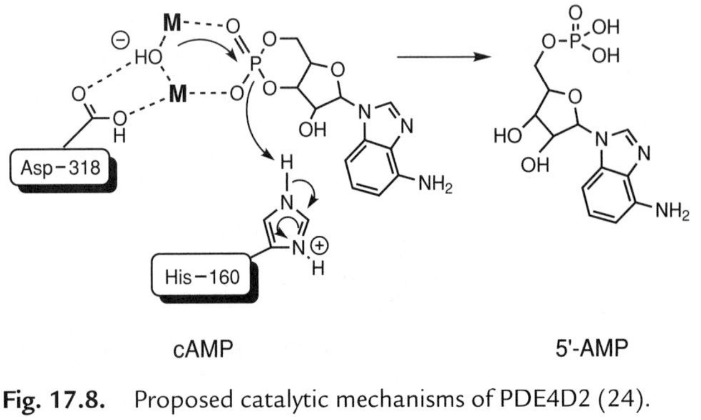

Asp−318 His−160

cAMP 5′-AMP

Fig. 17.8. Proposed catalytic mechanisms of PDE4D2 (24).

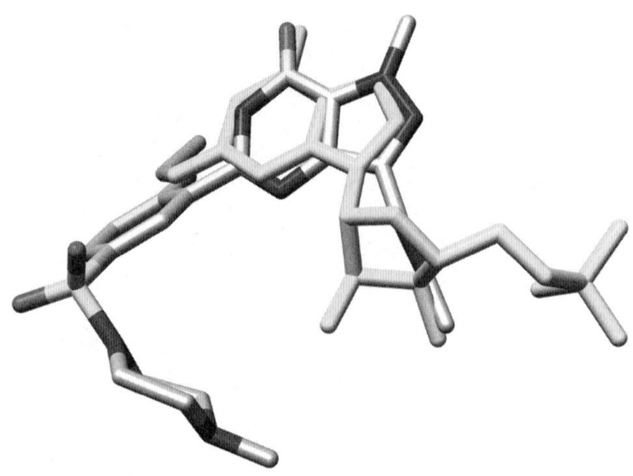

Fig. 17.9. Overlay of sildenafil with 5′-GMP in the active site of PDE5 (35). (See color plate.)

PDE5/PDE selectivity of sildenafil and vardenafil appears to revolve in part around the conserved glutamine residue (Gln-817), which interacts with the pyrimidine ring of cGMP in the guanine selective conformation. Further specificity may result from the alkylpiperazine ring, which has no overlap with the nucleotide and is exposed at the protein surface through the opening to the active site. Its interactions with surrounding hydrophobic residues are not found in the equivalent regions of PDE4, for example, suggesting that they may contribute to the specificity (24). Whereas sildenafil and vardenafil show good PDE5/PDE selectivity against the cAMP selective PDEs (PDEs 4, 7, and 8), they do inhibit other cGMP selective PDEs (1,6,9–11), and their low PDE5/PDE6 selectivity (22- and 11-fold respectively) (Table 17.1) is a particular issue that is thought to be a factor in certain side effects related to transient aberrations in vision. This lack of selectivity can be explained by the high homology between the active sites of PDE5 and PDE6. The basis for the high PDE5/PDE2 and PDE5/PDE3 selectivities of sildenafil and vardenafil are unclear.

The newer drug tadalafil (Fig. 17.2) is structurally unrelated to sildenafil, and it displays an approximately 1,000-fold PDE5/PDE6 selectivity ratio (Table 17.1). Interestingly, whereas the binding mode of tadalafil clearly is different from that of sildenafil, the reasons for its high PDE5/PDE6 selectivity are currently unclear (24).

PDE4 Selective Inhibitors

The PDE4 is inhibited by rolipram (Fig. 17.10), with a PDE4/PDE (all forms) selectivity of more than 100-fold (Table 17.1) (31). Like all PDE inhibitors, rolipram adopts a binding mode that resembles the cyclic nucleotide substrate (Fig. 17.11). In the adenosine binding conformation, Gln-369 of PDE4 bisects the two ether oxygens of rolipram, providing a specific binding interaction (32). In addition, the cyclopentyl ring of rolipram interacts with Mrt-357 and Phe-340 of PDE4D. Interestingly, the lactam ring does not make any specific interactions with the binding site. On the basis of Gln-369 binding, the cGMP selective enzymes (PDEs 5, 6, and 9) may be excluded. The high PDE4/PDE selectivities for PDEs 1, 2, 3, 10, and 11, however, in which the conserved glutamine side chain is free to rotate, are difficult to explain on this basis. In this regard, it has been suggested that the selectivity may be the result of a prohibitive cost in freezing the rotation of the glutamine in these PDEs. Similar arguments have been made to explain the high PDE4/PDE7 and PDE4/PDE8 selectivities of rolipram (24).

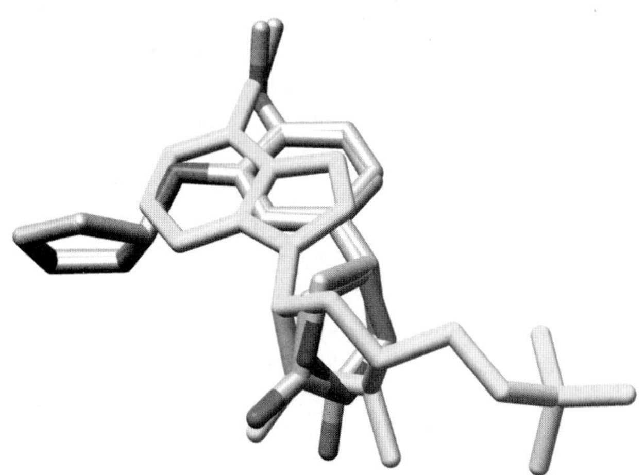

Fig. 17.11. Overlay of (R,S)-rolipram with 5′-AMP in the active site of PDE4D (31). (See color plate.)

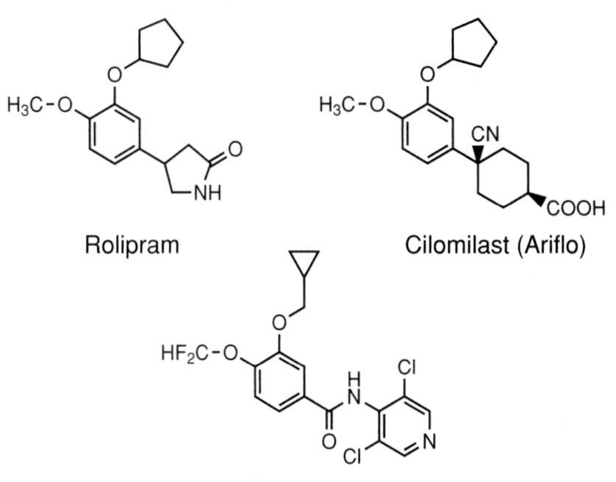

Fig. 17.10. Competitive inhibitors of PDE4.

Cilomilast (33) and roflumilast (34) are newer PDE4 selective inhibitors that are related to rolipram, but they display enhanced potency toward PDE4 (Fig. 17.10) (Table 17.1). They bind similarly, with the substituted aromatic ring occupying the hydrophobic clamp and the substituents making differential contacts with hydrophobic residues that line the pocket. Interestingly, these inhibitors also interact with the active-site metal ions via a water molecule, a potential source of additional potency (30).

PDE3 Selective Inhibitors

Presently, no structures of cilostazol or dipyridamole are bound to a PDE. Therefore, the precise mechanism of inhibition and the basis for their selectivity are unknown.

Summary

Two common features of inhibitor binding to PDEs define the scaffold for all known PDE inhibitors (29,30). A planar ring structure is held tightly in the active site by interactions with hydrophobic residues that line the nucleotide-binding pocket, facilitating hydrogen-bond interactions with an invariant glutamine, which is essential for nucleotide recognition and selectivity. In addition to these features, further hydrophobic interactions near the invariant purine selective glutamine also are important for inhibitor binding, and potency also is improved through interactions with residues near the metal ions and through indirect, water-mediated interactions with the metals. Furthermore, the selectivity of inhibitors is enhanced by exploiting the differences in shape and hydrophobicity of the binding pockets near the invariant glutamine.

DRUGS INHIBITING PHOSPHODIESTERASES

Clinical Experience

PDE5 Selective Inhibitors

As indicated earlier, the selective PDE5 inhibitors developed for the treatment of male erectile dysfunction resulting from organic or mixed organic-psychogenic origin have been the most successful PDE inhibitors. The three marketed drugs are sildenafil, vardenafil, and tadalafil (Fig. 17.2). In addition to the treatment of erectile dysfunction, sildenafil has been indicated for the treatment of pulmonary hypertension and female sexual dysfunction. These latter uses are unlabeled uses.

SILDENAFIL. Sildenafil is rapidly absorbed and peaks in concentration (127–560 ng/mL) after 0.5 to 2.0 hours, displaying a half-life of 3 to 4 hours for the full therapeutic dose (25–100 mg). It is 96% bound to plasma proteins and is metabolized by the liver CYP3A4 (13). The metabolite N-desmethylsildenafil possesses approximately 50% of the activity of the parent molecule.

VARDENAFIL. Vardenafil also is rapidly absorbed and peaks in concentration (9.05 μg/mL after a 10-mg dose) after 0.9 hours, displaying a half-life of 4 to 5 hours. The absorption rate of both sildenafil and vardenafil are reduced when taken with a high-fat diet (13). The drug also is metabolized by hepatic CYP3A4, and a potential for drug–drug interaction with inhibitors or enhancers of CYP3A4 exists. Biochemical studies demonstrate a significant increase in selectivity of vardenafil over sildenafil for PDE5 versus PDE6. Whether this translates into a significant improvement in side effects must await studies in a greater population of patients.

TADALAFIL. Tadalafil is different in structure from both sildenafil and vardenafil. It is rapidly absorbed and peaks in concentration (378 μg/L after a 20-mg dose) after 2 hours, displaying a long half-life of 17.5 hours. It also is metabolized by the liver (CYP3A4). Notably, its pharmacokinetics is not clinically influenced by alcohol or food intake or by factors such as diabetes or impaired hepatic or renal function (13).

Adverse effects related to oral therapy for erectile function are primarily concerned with adverse cardiovascular effects, because PDE5 inhibitors promote vasodilation and, therefore, have an inherent potential to cause hypotension. This is a particular concern for elderly patients with a preexisting condition (13).

Additional discussion on the pharmacodynamics of the PDE5 inhibitors can be found in Chapter 45.

PDE4 Selective Inhibitors

Considerable interest in PDE4 inhibitors is based on the recognition that of the four gene-produced PDE4s, three (PDE4A, PDE4B, and PDE4D) are abundant in inflammatory and immune cells, which include T and B cells, monocytes, macrophages, neutrophils, and eosinophils. The fourth PDE4 (PDE4C) is localized in testis, skeletal muscle, and brain. Inhibition of PDE4 has been shown to suppress production of cytokines, cell proliferation and chemotaxis, and release of inflammatory mediators. Thus, the interest in PDE4 inhibitors for treatment of asthma, chronic obstructive pulmonary disease (COPD), and the intestinal conditions of Crohn's disease and inflammatory bowel disease (20). Two PDE4 inhibitors are proceeding through clinical studies. Cilomilast is an investigational drug being studied in the United States for use in COPD (asthma studies have been discontinued), and roflumilast is moving forward in Europe for the treatment of asthma and COPD (Fig. 17.10) (see Chapter 44).

ROFLUMILAST. Roflumilast is the more potent of the two drugs, and along with its active metabolite, roflumilast-N-oxide, it is nonselective in its inhibitory action on PDE4B and PDE4D. The PDE4B appears to be the most closely

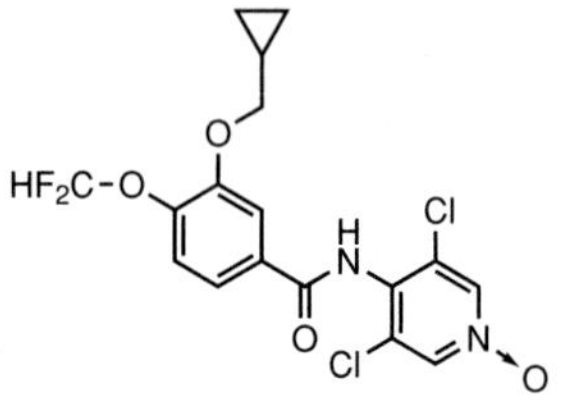

HF_2C-O, O, H, N, Cl, O, Cl, N, O

Roflumilast-N-oxide

linked to anti-inflammatory effects, whereas the PDE4D receptor subtype is thought to be linked to nausea, possibly through a central effect (21). Roflumilast exhibits 80% oral bioavailability and has an elimination half-life of 10 hours, whereas the N-oxide has an elimination half-life of 20 hours and has shown no drug interactions. Clinical trials in patients with asthma or COPD are quite promising.

CILOMILAST. Cilomilast is rapidly absorbed following oral administration (96% bioavailability), has an elimination half-life of 7 hours, and is extensively metabolized, but not by cytochrom P450 enzymes. The drug shows considerably more selectivity than roflumilast toward PDE4D, and this might account for the common side effects of nausea and emesis (20). Studies regarding the benefits of cilomilast versus placebo in the treatment of asthma have not been very encouraging, but significant improvement was seen in clinical trials of cilomilast in the treatment of COPD. The side effects of diarrhea and nausea have been considerably higher with cilomilast versus placebo, but these effects generally are tolerable and self limiting.

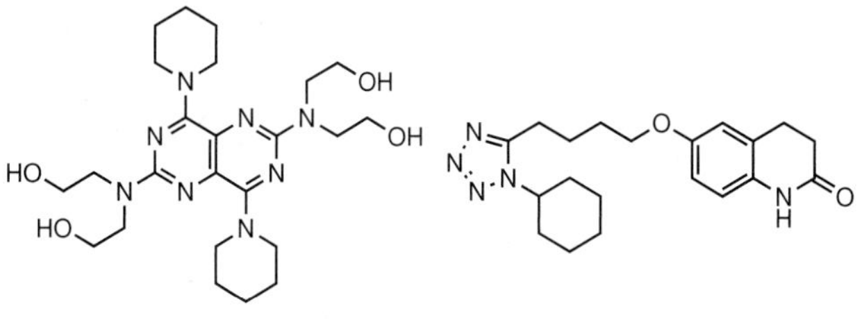

Dipyridamole Cilostazol

Fig. 17.12. Antiplatelet competitive inhibitors of PDE3.

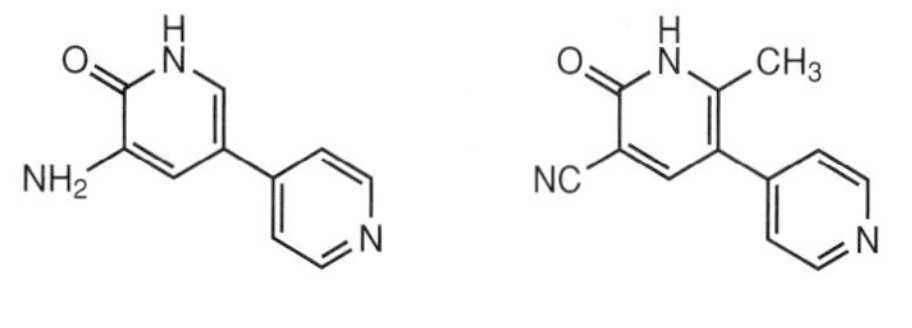

Inamrinone Milrinone (Primacor)

Fig. 17.13. PDE3 inhibitors with cardiac and pulmonary effects.

PDE3 Selective Inhibitors

ANTIPLATELET DRUGS. A site for regulating blood coagulation and subsequent thrombus formation is at the level of the platelets. Antiplatelet drugs work by inhibiting platelet activation via a number of different mechanisms. The major role of antiplatelet drugs is in the prevention of ischemic complications in patients with coronary diseases. They also are effective in combination with moderate-intensity anticoagulants for patients with atrial fibrillation (see Chapter 31). Rapid platelet aggregation and thrombus formation at the site of vascular injury is the main mechanism of hemostasis (i.e., stoppage of bleeding, a normal process of wound healing). When platelets are activated on the ruptured atherosclerotic plaques or in regions of restricted blood flow, however, it can lead to thromboembolic complications that contribute to common diseases, such as myocardial infarction or ischemic stroke.

Mechanism of action of antiplatelet drugs. Most of the currently available antiplatelet drugs exert their actions by affecting only the secondary platelet aggregation pathways, and in the case of dipyridamole and cilostazol (Fig. 17.12), interruption of platelet function through increasing cellular concentration of cAMP by inhibiting PDE serves as the mechanism of action. The PDE3 is an enzyme responsible for degradation of cAMP to AMP in platelets and blood vessels. Selective cAMP PDE3 inhibitors, such as dipyridamole and cilostazol, inhibit the degradation of cAMP, thereby increasing cellular concentration of cAMP, leading to inhibition of platelet aggregation and vasodilation.

Dipyridamole and cilostazol. Dipyridamole is a pyrimidopyrimidine derivative with vasodilatory and antiplatelet properties, whereas cilostazol is a quinolinone derivative, which is a potent, orally active antiplatelet with a higher degree of selectivity than dipyridamole for PDE3. The latter drug appears to possess greater therapeutic potential. It is rapidly absorbed following oral administration and is extensively metabolized. Several of the metabolites also possess antiplatelet activity. (For a more in-depth discussion of these drugs, see Chapter 31.)

CARDIAC DRUGS

Inamrinone and milrinone. Inamrinone and milrinone (Fig. 17.13) have been available for some time and have been used for the treatment of cardiac heart failure. Their action is based on a positive inotopic response and a concentration-dependent vasodilatory effect (Chapter 26). These drugs are selective PDE3 inhibitors, resulting in increased levels of cAMP. To what extent this inhibition contributes to the clinical effects of the drugs is not totally clear. Recent studies have shown that milrinone exhibits pulmonary vasodilation, which might prove to be beneficial in the treatment of pulmonary hypertension, although the same studies suggested that the use of zaprinast, a PDE5 inhibitor, has greater potential for such use (35).

References

1. Conti M, Jin SL. The molecular biology of cyclic nucleotide phosphodiesterases. Prog Nucleic Acid Res Mol Biol 1999;63:1–38.
2. Soderling SH, Beavo JA. Regulation of cAMP and cGMP signaling: new phosphodiesterases and new functions. Curr Opin Cell Biol 2000;12:174–179.
3. Mehats C, Andersen CB, Filopanti M, et al. Cyclic nucleotide phosphodiesterases and their role in endocrine cell signaling. Trends Endocrinol Metab 2002;13:29–35.
4. Francis SH, Turko IV, Corbin JD. Cyclic nucleotide phosphodiesterases: relating structure and function. Prog Nucleic Acid Res Mol Biol 2001;65:1–52.
5. Muller T, Engels P, Fozard JR. Subtypes of the type 4 cAMP phosphodiesterases: structure, regulation, and selective inhibition. Trends Pharmacol Sci 1996;17:294–298.
6. Manganiello VC, Degerman E. Cyclic nucleotide phosphodiesterases (PDEs): diverse regulators of cyclic nucleotide signals and inviting molecular targets for novel therapeutic agents. Thromb Haemost 1999;82:407–411.
7. Corbin JD, Francis SH. Cyclic GMP phosphodiesterase-5: target of sildenafil. J Biol Chem 1999;274:13729–13732.
8. Conti M. Phosphodiesterases and cyclic nucleotide signaling in endocrine cells. Mol Endocrinol 2000;14:1317–1327.
9. Houslay M, Adams DR. PDE4 cAMP phosphodiesterases: modular enzymes that orchestrate signaling cross-talk, desensitization, and compartmentalization. Biochem J 2003;370:1–18.
10. Conti M, Richter W, Mehats C, et al. Cyclic AMP-specific PDE4 phosphodiesterases as critical components of cyclic AMP signaling. J Biol Chem 2003; 278:5493–5496.
11. Beavo JA, Conti M, Heaslip RJ. Multiple cyclic nucleotide phosphodiesterases. Mol Pharmacol 1994;46:399–405.
12. Corbin JD, Francis SH. Pharmacology of phosphodiesterase-5 inhibitors. Int J Clin Pract 2002;56:453–459.
13. Rosen RC, Kostis JB. Overview of phosphodiesterase 5 inhibition in erectile dysfunction. Am J Cardiol 2003;92:9M–18M.
14. Fazio L, Brock G. Erectile dysfunction: management update. Canadian Med Assoc J 2004;170:1429–1437.
15. Lue TF, Tanagho EA. Physiology of erection and pharmacological management of impotence. J Urol 1987;137:829–836.
16. Wachtel H. Potential antidepressant activity of rolipram and other selective cyclic adenosine 3′,5′-monophosphate phosphodiesterase inhibitors. Neuropharmacology 1983;22:267–272.
17. Torphy TJ. Phosphodiesterase isozymes: molecular targets for novel antiasthma agents. Am J Respir Crit Care Med 1998;157:351–370.
18. Houslay MD, Sullivan M, Bolger GB. The multienzyme PDE4 cyclic adenosine monophosphate-specific phosphodiesterase family: intracellular targeting,

regulation, and selective inhibition by compounds exerting anti-inflammatory and antidepressant actions. Adv Pharmacol 1998;44:225–342.
19. Spina D. Phosphodiesterase-4 inhibitors in the treatment of inflammatory lung disease. Drugs 2003;63:2575–2594.
20. Banner KH, Trevethick MA. PDE4 inhibition: a novel approach for the treatment of inflammatory bowel disease. Trends Pharmacol Sci 2004;25:430–436.
21. Robichaud A, Savoie C, Stamatiou PB, et al. Assessing the emetic potential of PDE4 inhibitors in rats. Br J Pharmacol 2002;135:113–118.
22. Dawson DL. Comparative effects of cilostazol and other therapies for intermittent claudication. Am J Cardiol 2001;87:19D–27D.
23. Xu RX, Hassell AM, Vanderwall D, et al. Atomic structure of PDE4: insights into phosphodiesterase mechanism and specificity. Science 2000;288:1822–1825.
24. Manallack DT, Hughes RA, Thompson PE. The next generation of phosphodiesterase inhibitors: structural clues to ligand and substrate selectivity of phosphodiesterases. J Med Chem 2005;48:3449–3462.
25. Huai Q, Colicelli J, Ke H. The crystal structure of AMP-bound PDE4 suggests a mechanism for phosphodiesterase catalysis. Biochemistry 2003;42: 13220–13226.
26. Conti M. A view into the catalytic pocket of cyclic nucleotide phosphodiesterases. Nat Struct Mol Biol 2004;11:809–810.
27. Zhang KY, Card GL, Suzuki Y, et al. A glutamine switch mechanism for nucleotide selectivity by phosphodiesterases. Mol Cell 2004;15:279–286.
28. Sutherland EW, Rall TW. Fractionation and characterization of a cyclic adenine ribonucleotide formed by tissue particles. J Biol Chem 1958;232: 1077–1091.
29. Card GL, Blasdel L, England BP, et al. A family of phosphodiesterase inhibitors discovered by cocrystallography and scaffold-based drug design. Nat Biotechnol 2005;23:201–207.
30. Card GL, England, BP, Suzuki Y, et al. Structural basis for the activity of drugs that inhibit phosphodiesterases. Structure (Camb) 2004;12:2233–2247.
31. Maurice DH, Palmer D, Tilley DG, et al. Cyclic nucleotide phosphodiesterase activity, expression, and targeting in cells of the cardiovascular system. Mol Pharmacol 2003;64:533–546.
32. Huai Q, Wang H, Sun Y, et al. Three-dimensional structures of PDE4D in complex with rolipram and implication on inhibitor selectivity. Structure (Camb) 2003;11:865–873.
33. Barnette MS, Christensen SB, Essayan DM, et al. SB 207499 (Ariflo), a potent and selective second-generation phosphodiesterase 4 inhibitor: in vitro anti-inflammatory actions. J Pharmacol Exp Ther 1998;284:420–426.
34. Hatzelmann A, Schudt C. Anti-inflammatory and immunomodulatory potential of the novel PDE4 inhibitor roflumilast in vitro. J Pharmacol Exp Ther 2001;297:267–279.
35. Matot I, Gozal Y. Pulmonary responses to selective phosphodiesterase-5 and phosphodiesterase-3 inhibitors. Chest 2004;125:644–651.

PART III

PHARMACODYNAMIC AGENTS

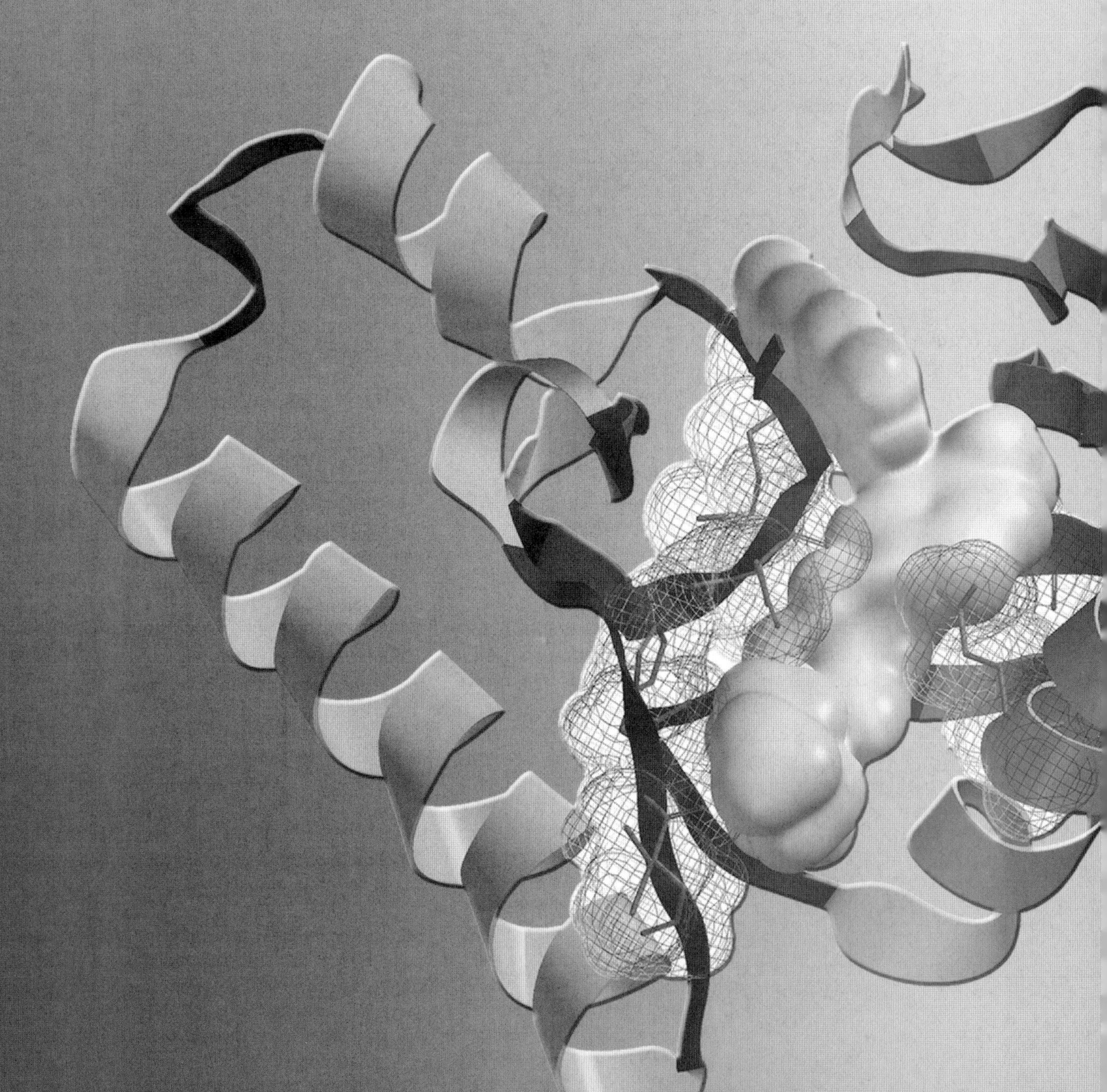

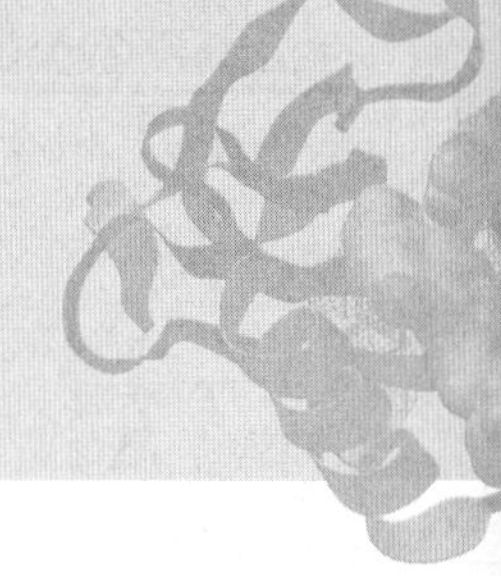

18. *General Anesthetics*

TIMOTHY J. MAHER

DRUGS COVERED IN THIS CHAPTER:

INHALED GENERAL ANESTHETICS
- Ether
- Halothane
- Desflurane
- Enflurane
- Isoflurane
- Methoxyflurane
- Sevoflurane
- Nitrous oxide

INTRAVENOUS GENERAL ANESTHETICS
- Etomidate
- Ketamine
- Propofol
- Thiopental

INTRODUCTION

Before the mid-1800s, pain-producing surgical and dental procedures typically were undertaken without the aid of acceptable anesthetic agents. Chemical methods available at the time included intoxication with ethanol, hashish, or opium, whereas physical methods included packing a limb in ice, creating ischemic conditions with tourniquets, inducing unconsciousness by a blow to the head, or the most common technique, employing strong-armed assistants to hold down the helpless patient during the entire surgical procedure. Additionally, at this time, many practicing physicians had been taught that pain was a requirement for effective healing; therefore, the observation of a patient in terrible pain was viewed as part of the normal healing process. These factors, along with the lack of knowledge regarding sterile techniques or the availability of suitable infection-fighting agents, made surgical procedures a method of last resort.

There have been many accounts of the first demonstration by the Hartford dentist Horace Wells of the use of nitrous oxide as a surgical anesthetic in 1844. Wells first observed the anesthetic actions of nitrous oxide at a public demonstration of "laughing gas." One of the volunteers, a pharmacy clerk named Samuel Cooley, injured his leg while under the influence of this gas and appeared to experience no pain. The next day, Wells inhaled the gas himself and, with the aid of a colleague, had one of his own teeth extracted without any sensation of pain. Wells then began routinely using nitrous oxide for dental procedures in his own practice. In 1845, he attempted to demonstrate the anesthetic effects of nitrous oxide at the Massachusetts General Hospital in Boston. This demonstration was considered to be a failure, however, because the patient cried out during the procedure. Following this unfortunate incident, use of nitrous oxide was minimal until it resurfaced in dental practice during the mid-1860s, when it was combined with oxygen and made available in steel cylinders. This gas is still commonly used today, especially in combination with other anesthetic and analgesic agents.

The anesthetic that gained greatest popularity shortly after the failed demonstration of Wells was diethyl ether. William Morton, a Boston dentist, was familiar at the time with the use of nitrous oxide by Wells. He also had heard of the interesting effects of diethyl ether and began to experiment on animals and himself with this volatile liquid. In 1846, he was allowed an opportunity to demonstrate the anesthetic actions of diethyl ether at, again, Massachusetts General Hospital. In the famed "Ether Dome," which still stands today, Morton administered the diethyl ether with a specially designed delivery device to the nervous patient, and the surgical procedure was performed without apparent pain. Following this demonstration, word of its success spread quickly, and soon, dental and medical practices throughout the United States and Europe were employing diethyl ether as an anesthetic agent. Today, diethyl ether is no longer used in procedures because of its toxicity and dangerous physical properties (e.g., it is flammable and explosive).

Another anesthetic agent that enjoyed some early popularity was cyclopropane. Like diethyl ether, however, it also is explosive and is no longer used. As described below, the inhalational anesthetic agents used today generally are hydrocarbons and ethers with halogen (Cl, Br, or F) substitutions. Nitrous oxide is the exception. Table 18.1 lists the characteristics of the "ideal" general anesthetic agent. Currently, the agent that fulfills all these characteristics is not known.

STAGES OF ANESTHESIA

The ideal anesthetic state is characterized by a loss of all sensations and includes analgesia and muscle relaxation. Neuronal depression in specific areas of the central nervous system is believed to be largely responsible for such an anesthetic state. The areas involved include many cortical regions that are represented by excitatory pyramidal

Table 18.1. Characteristics of the Ideal Anesthetic

Rapid and pleasant induction of surgical anesthesia
Rapid and pleasant withdrawal from anesthesia
Adequate relaxation of skeletal muscles
Potent enough to permit adequate oxygen supply in mixture
Wide margin of safety
Nontoxic
Absence of adverse effects
Nonflammable/nonexplosive
Chemically compatible with anesthetic devices
Nonreactive
Inexpensive

cells and inhibitory/excitatory stellate cells. Excitation of the pyramidal cells helps to maintain consciousness, whereas the degree of inhibition or excitation of stellate cells determines the overall activity level of the pyramidal cells with which they synapse. As the concentration of anesthetic increases in the central nervous system, the degree of overall neuronal depression also increases, resulting in progressively deeper stages of anesthesia. Based on observations using diethylether, Guedel in 1920 originally described this progression into four distinct stages, and Gillespie subsequently further subdivided these stages (Fig. 18.1), as described below.

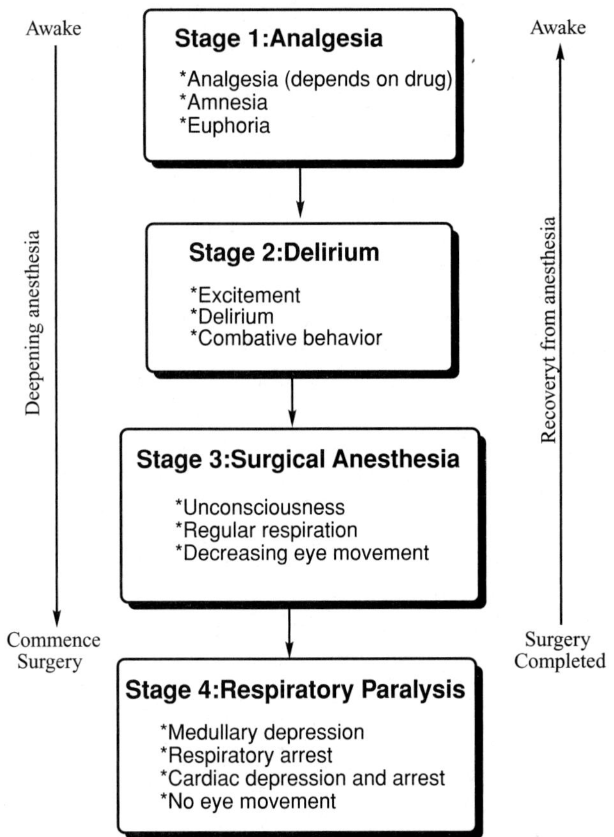

Fig. 18.1. Stages of anesthesia.

Stage 1: Analgesia

Characterized by a mild depression of higher cortical neurons, this stage is suitable for minor surgical procedures that do not require significant neuromuscular relaxation. Depression of thalamic centers probably accounts for the observed analgesia, because many of the neuronal systems that mediate pain sensation traverse through this anatomic area. Some general anesthetic agents do not possess significant analgesic activity, but they all produce a loss of consciousness that, in turn, may produce some degree of insensitivity to painful stimuli.

Stage 2: Delirium

As depression of inhibitory neurons in the central nervous system progresses, especially in the reticular formation, a resultant excitation of cortical motor neurons leads to significant involuntary muscle activity. This paradoxical response is caused by inhibition of inhibitory neurons that normally function to closely regulate such neuronal activity. Typically, urination, delirium, and uncontrolled muscular movements occur that may be accompanied by increased heart rate, blood pressure, and respiration. Ideally, an anesthetic agent should produce little or no excitatory phase. Together, stages 1 and 2 comprise the induction period, which ideally should be of short duration.

Stage 3: Surgical Anesthesia

This stage is divided into four planes characterized by increasing central nervous system depression: first, loss of spinal reflexes; second, decreased muscle reflexes; third, paralysis of intercostal muscles; and fourth, loss of most muscle tone. Stage 3 also is characterized by regular breathing, a loss of many reflexes, and roving eyeball movements.

Stage 4: Respiratory Paralysis

Characterized by respiratory and vasomotor paralysis, this stage represents an overdose or toxic level that should be avoided. Normally, this stage is never reached, because the anesthesiologist is careful to monitor abdominal respiration to prevent apnea, blood pressure to prevent hypotension, and heart rate to prevent asystole.

MODERN ANESTHETIC AGENTS

Although these stages have been described for diethylether, an anesthetic agent not used today, some of today's clinically useful anesthetic agents fail to follow this described pattern of anesthetic progression. Some attempts have been made to correlate changes in the electroencephalograph (EEG) with the depth of anesthesia. Most of these studies, however, have failed to yield a reliable predictor for anesthesiologists to utilize. Additionally, concomitant drugs used as preanesthetic agents may alter the EEG while not altering the depth of anesthesia. Rather than describing specific stages or using EEG patterns, a number of useful signs that more accurately reflect the depth of anesthesia for most of the anesthetic agents currently are employed. When during the initial period of anesthetic administration a patient has irregular respiratory depth and rate, is still swallowing, blinks the eyes when the eyelashes are touched, the desired surgical stage of anesthesia likely has not been reached. When a loss of the eyelash reflex occurs along with rhythmic breathing, however, a level of adequate surgical anesthesia generally has begun. If a patient at this stage exhibits elevations in blood pressure, increased respiration rate, or increased jaw tension when a surgical incision is attempted, the subject is considered to be "light" and typically requires additional anesthesia to facilitate further surgical manipulations. These responses decrease further—until they are abolished—as the depth of anesthesia progresses. By monitoring reflexes, blood pressure, and respiration rate and depth, today's anesthesiologist is capable of effectively maintaining an appropriate depth of surgical anesthesia without producing unwanted medullary depression.

PHARMACOKINETIC PRINCIPLES OF VOLATILE ANESTHETICS

The production and maintenance of the anesthetic state is believed by most to be dependent on the concentration, or partial pressure, of the anesthetic agent in yet unknown areas of the brain. Obviously, the concentration of the anesthetic agent in the gas mixture administered, as well as the rate and depth of respiration of the patient, will influence the rate of anesthesia induction. The rate at which delivery of anesthetic agents to these sites occurs is dependent on their physicochemical properties, particularly their solubility in lipid and blood.

Administration of Volatile Anesthetics

The administration of gaseous or volatile liquid anesthetics involves a number of sophisticated devices that have been refined over the years to aid the anesthesiologist in carefully controlling the amount of anesthetic delivered to the patient. Early systems used a gauze pad in a mask placed over the nose and mouth of the patient. The anesthesiologist would then put drops of the volatile anesthetic on the gauze pad, and as the patient breathed, the anesthetic was delivered to the lungs. This procedure was somewhat effective, but it allowed little or no control over the amount of anesthetic and oxygen delivered to the patient. Additionally, the anesthetic not inhaled was allowed to penetrate the surrounding area and posed a significant risk to the surgical personnel. Today, flowmeters, vaporizers, and absorber devices are routinely available, allowing precise determination and control of the amount of volatile anesthetic, oxygen, and carbon dioxide administered while preventing significant exposure to workers. Typically, oxygen is bubbled through a volatile anesthetic liquid, and the resultant gas mixture is delivered to the patient for continual inhalation. Many of these devices are described in greater detail elsewhere (1).

The inhaled anesthetic concentration is controlled by the anesthesiologist, who can increase or decrease this concentration depending on the observed depth of anesthesia. Eventually, with continued administration, the concentration of anesthetic in the bronchiolar alveoli reaches equilibrium with that in the inspired gas mixture (Fig. 18.2). Transfer from the alveolar space to the blood proceeds quickly, and depending on the concentrations of anesthetic used and its physiochemical characteristics, equilibrium with the arterial blood is achieved. Before appreciable amounts of anesthetic dissolved in the blood will enter tissues, however, the blood must be saturated with the anesthetic. Therefore, anesthetics that are highly soluble in the blood will require a longer time to achieve saturation of the blood compartment. In such cases, the time for induction will be prolonged. On the other hand, an anesthetic that is poorly soluble in blood will quickly saturate the blood compartment and then rapidly enter the tissues to produce a short induction period. Similarly, agents with high blood/gas partition coefficients (i.e., high blood solubility) will require a longer time for recovery from anesthesia. The solubility of an agent in the blood usually is expressed as the blood/gas partition coefficient, which is the ratio of the concentration of anesthetic in blood to that in the gas phase at equilibrium (Table 18.2). These values correspond well with the oil/gas partition coefficient, which is easier to determine experimentally. The blood/gas partition coefficient can be very high (e.g., 12) for soluble agents, such as methoxyflurane, and extremely low (e.g., 0.47) for poorly soluble agents, such as nitrous oxide.

The solubility of the anesthetic in tissue is expressed as the tissue/blood partition coefficient. Because the concentration of the anesthetic in the brain is probably of most interest, however, the brain/blood partition coefficient is more useful. Additionally, because the solubility of the anesthetic in lean tissues is essentially equal to that in blood, the tissue/blood or brain/blood partition coefficient typically is close to one. In fatty tissues, however, the partition coefficient can be much larger. The rate of blood flow to a particular organ also will influence the rate at which anesthetics reach their sites of action. The brain, liver, and kidneys have relatively high blood flows, whereas skeletal muscle at rest and fat tissues have relatively poor blood flows.

Reversal of the anesthetic state and recovery requires a reduction in the concentration of the anesthetic in the brain. This is achieved by stopping the delivery of the

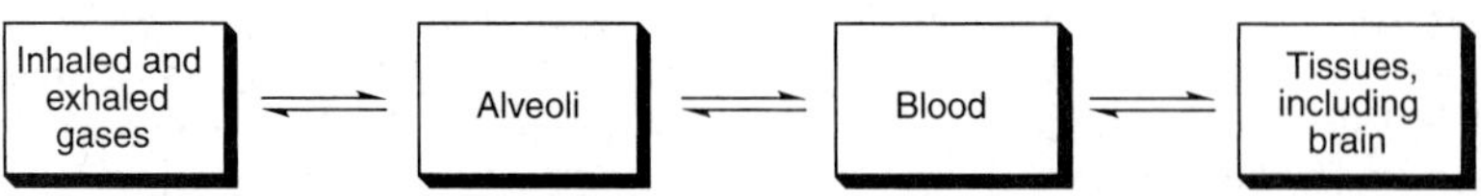

Fig. 18.2. Dynamic equilibria existing during the state of anesthesia.

Table 18.2. Partition Coefficients, MACs, and Metabolism of Some General Anesthetics

	Partition Coefficients at 37°C		MAC (vol %)[a]			
Anesthetics	Oil/Gas	Blood/Gas	Without N_2O	With N_2O (%)	MAC-Awake (Vol %)	% Metabolism
Methoxyflurane	970	12	0.16	0.07 (56)	—	50
Halothane	224	2.3	0.77	0.29 (66)	0.4	20
Enflurane	98.5	1.1	91.7	0.60 (70)	0.4	2.4
Isoflurane	90.8	1.4	1.15	0.50 (70)	0.4	0.17
Sevoflurane (2)	53.4	0.60	1.71	0.66 (64)	0.6	4–6
Desflurane (3)	16.7	0.42	6.0	2.83 (60)	2.4	0.02
Nitrous oxide	1.4	0.47	104	—	60	None

[a]MAC = minimum alveolar concentration, expressed as volume %, that is required to produce immobility in 50% of middle-aged humans.

anesthetic through the lungs. As the patient continues to breathe, the anesthetic is continually removed, which favors diffusion from the brain to the blood, to the alveoli, and finally, to the expired air. The rate at which this occurs generally parallels that of induction, because the solubility of an agent in the brain and in the blood determines how quickly these compartments will return to a preanesthetic state. The main route of elimination is via the expired air, which can be mostly captured by gas-scavenging devices with absorbers, but some metabolism of these agents does take place (discussed below).

Minimum Alveolar Concentration

The minimum alveolar concentration (MAC) is defined as the concentration at 1 atmosphere of anesthetic in the alveoli that is required to produce immobility in 50% of adult patients subjected to a surgical incision. A further increase to 1.3 MAC frequently will cause immobility in 99% of patients. At equilibrium, the concentration (or partial pressure) of an anesthetic in the alveoli is equal to that in the brain, and it is this concentration in the brain that probably most closely reflects the concentration at the site responsible for the anesthetic actions. Thus, the MAC often is used as a measure of the potency of individual anesthetic agents. The MAC of many of the volatile and gaseous anesthetics in use today is shown in Table 18.2.

When used in combinations, the MACs for inhaled anesthetics are additive. For instance, the anesthetic depth achieved with 0.5 MAC of enflurane plus 0.5 MAC of nitrous oxide is equivalent to that produced by 1.0 MAC of either agent alone. The combination of two anesthetics is a very common practice, because this technique allows a reduction in the patient exposure to any one of the individual agents, thereby decreasing the likelihood of adverse reactions.

Many factors can influence the MAC via a number of different mechanisms (Table 18.3). Factors that have been shown to increase the MAC for many volatile anesthetics include elevated catecholamines in the central nervous system following pharmacological treatments, hypernatremia, and hyperthermia. Factors known to decrease MAC include alcohol ingestion, clonidine, lithium, lidocaine, centrally administered opioids, and drugs that decrease central catecholamine levels. Additionally, hyponatremia, hypotension, hypothermia, hypoxia, increasing age, and pregnancy also have been shown to decrease MAC. Plasma potassium, hypertension, gender, and the duration of anesthesia typically have minimal effect on the MAC (2).

Another term, the "MAC-Awake," is used to describe the concentration of anesthetic at which appropriate responses to verbal commands are lost in 50% of the patients tested. At this concentration, amnesia and a loss of awareness are evident, and the patient is said to be in a state of hypnosis. The MAC-Awake occurs at concentrations significantly lower (e.g., 50–75% lower) than those required for surgical anesthesia.

THEORIES ABOUT THE MECHANISMS OF ANESTHESIA

Meyer-Overton Theory

In the early 1900s Hans Meyer and Charles Overton suggested that the potency of a substance as an anesthetic was directly related to its lipid solubility, or oil/gas partition coefficient (4,5). This has commonly been referred

Table 18.3. Factors That May Alter MAC

Increase MAC	Increased catecholamine levels in CNS Hypernatremia Hyperthermia	
Decrease MAC	Decreased catecholamine levels in CNS Alcohol ingestion Clonidine Lidocaine Lithium Opioids	 Hyponatremia Hypotension Hypothermia Hypoxia Increased age Pregnancy
No effect on MAC	Plasma potassium Gender Hypertension Duration of anesthesia	

to as the "unitary theory of anesthesia." They used olive oil, octanol, and other "membrane-like" lipids to determine the lipid solubility of the agents available at the time. Compounds with high lipid solubility required lower concentrations (i.e., lower MAC) to produce anesthesia. Later, it was postulated that the interaction of the anesthetic molecules with a hydrophobic portion of the membrane caused a distortion of the membrane near the channels that conducted sodium ions, those that mediated the fast action potentials and neuronal cell firing. The presence of this critical volume of anesthetic dissolved within the membrane caused the membrane to "bloat" and "squeeze" in on the channel to interfere with sodium conductance and normal neuronal depolarization. In support of this theory, it was found that at high pressures (40–100 atmospheres), the anesthetic actions of many of these agents could be partially reversed, presumably by compressing membranes back to their original conformation. Arguing against this theory, however, is the finding that not all highly lipid-soluble substances are capable of producing anesthesia. Additionally, more recent work involving protein–drug interactions has seriously challenged this theory. Today, more than 150 years after the first demonstration of the use of a volatile anesthetic agent, most theories about the mechanisms of anesthesia suggest that multiple selective lipid–protein membrane interactions, involving numerous receptor types, are responsible for the anesthesia produced and that no reason exists to believe that all anesthetic agents need to produce their effects via identical actions. Thus, a single molecular target for anesthetic actions is no longer required (6).

Stereochemical Aspects

The volatile anesthetics isoflurane, desflurane, enflurane, and halothane each contain an asymmetric carbon and, thus, can exist as (+)- or (−)-enantiomers. Although all of the commercially available preparations are racemates, some researchers have been able to determine the anesthetic properties of individual enantiomers. The (+)-enantiomer of isoflurane is at least 50% more potent as an anesthetic in the rat than the (−)-enantiomer is (7). In that study, the MAC values were 1.06 and 1.62% for the (+) and (−)-enantiomers, respectively. In another study, however, the potency of the individual isoflurane enantiomers to depress myocardial activity was not found to be different, suggesting possible involvement of mechanisms dissimilar from that responsible for producing anesthesia (8). These findings argue against the original and simple lipid-solubility theory of anesthesia, and they support a more complex mechanism, probably likely involvement of proteins in the form of receptor–anesthetic interactions (9).

Ion Channel and Protein Receptor Hypotheses

More recently, investigators have determined the effects of anesthetics on a number of protein receptors within the central nervous system. Features that support the likelihood of an interaction with a protein include 1) the steep dose–response curves observed, 2) the stereochemical requirements of various anesthetics, 3) the finding that increasing the molecular weight and corresponding lipid solubility of an anesthetic may actually decrease or abolish anesthetic activity, and 4) the finding that specific ion channels and neurotransmitter receptor systems are required for most of the observed effects of the anesthetics. What appears to be emerging as a central theme for the mechanism of action of general anesthetics involves the interaction of the anesthetics with receptors that allosterically modulate the activity of ion channels (e.g., chloride and potassium) or with the ion channel directly (e.g., sodium). Many other mechanisms also are emerging to help explain the mechanisms of action of the general anesthetics.

Chloride Channel

The ion channel that has received the most investigative attention is that for chloride (Fig. 18.3). Both the γ-aminobutyric $acid_A$ ($GABA_A$) and the $glycine_A$ (strychnine-sensitive) receptors are ligand-gated ion channels and linked to chloride channels that normally mediate inhibitory responses within the central nervous system. Halothane, isoflurane, and other volatile anesthetics are capable of inhibiting the synaptic destruction of GABA, thereby increasing the GABAergic neurotransmission, which typically is inhibitory in nature (10). Additionally, studies have demonstrated the ability of these anesthetics to enhance the binding of GABA or other allosteric modulators within the GABA receptor complex (11). In one such study, (+)-isoflurane was significantly more potent than the (−)-enantiomer at enhancing GABAergic function (12). The volatile anesthetics, and many of the intravenous anesthetic agents, bind to discrete cavities within the $GABA_A$ receptor complex to enhance GABA neurotransmission (13,14), Studies using mutant chimeric $GABA_A$ receptors have identified a specific binding site for general anesthetics located between transmembrane segments 2 and 3 (15). At therapeutic concentrations, just about all of the inhalational general anesthetics are capable of enhancing GABAergic function, whereas at considerably higher concentrations, many also may act directly as GABA mimetics (16). Recent studies have demonstrated an effect of these agents not only on the synaptic $GABA_A$ receptor function that mediates phasic neuronal responses but also on those extrasynaptic $GABA_A$ receptors that mediate tonic neuronal activity (17). Other specific anesthetic agents may alter $GABA_A$ receptor function via different mechanisms. For instance, propofol, an intravenous anesthetic, appears to slow the desensitization of the $GABA_A$ receptor during bouts of rapid, repetitive activation at inhibitory synapses (18). Most of these agents also potentiate the actions of glycine, the other important inhibitory amino acid neurotransmitter (16). The combination of GABAergic and glycinergic potentiation by the general anesthetics probably accounts for the

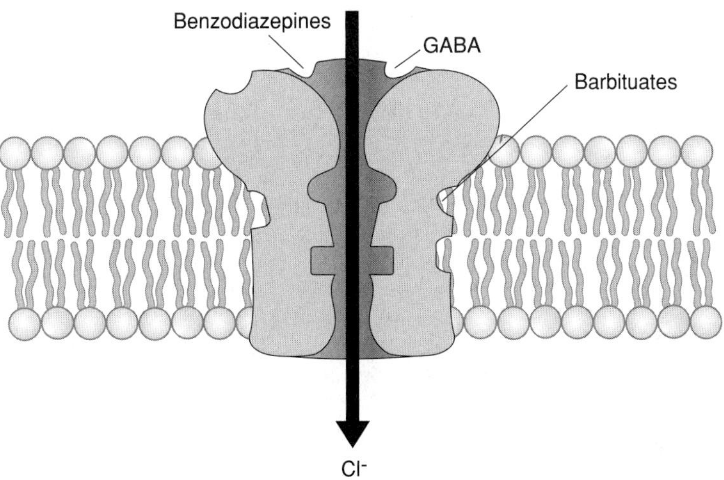

Fig. 18 3. The $GABA_A$ receptor controls the chloride ion channel. GABA binds to its receptor, opening the chloride ion channel and resulting in hyperpolarization of the neuron. Benzodiazepines and barbiturates may produce anesthesia by allosterically enhancing GABA opening of chloride channels, which are located at inhibitory synapses on pyramidal cells. ECF = extracellular fluid; ICF = intracellular fluid.

vast majority of the observed activity of the inhalational agents as well as that of the barbiturates.

Sodium Channels

One channel that has received much attention regarding the mediation of drug-induced anesthetic actions is the ligand-gated sodium channel within the N-methyl-D-aspartate (NMDA) receptor complex. When activated by the excitatory amino acid neurotransmitter, glutamate, an increase in the conductance to sodium occurs that promotes neuronal depolarization (Fig. 18.4) (19). Compounds known to stimulate NMDA receptors typically are capable of increasing alertness and of acting as convulsants, whereas pharmacological agents that act as antagonists at this site usually are sedatives, anticonvulsants, and dissociative anesthetics (e.g., ketamine). Halothane has been demonstrated to specifically antagonize the glutamate-stimulated depolarization of neurons (20), whereas isoflurane has been shown to decrease glutamate release and enhance its removal from the synaptic cleft (21). Glutamate acting at NMDA and other non-NMDA receptors within the central nervous system probably is one of the most important excitatory inputs that supports consciousness. It is not surprising that the general anesthetics would act via altering neurotransmission in this system (22). Others have reported an interaction of general anesthetics with the neuronal nicotinic acetylcholine receptor–linked sodium ion channel (23). Voltage-gated sodium channels in small, nonmyelinated hippocampal axons also appear to be inhibited by general anesthetics, such as isoflurane (24).

Potassium Channels

Potassium channels also have been suggested as a site for general anesthetic agents. Increasing K^+ conductance normally functions to maintain the polarized state of neurons and to assist in the repolarization of neurons following their stimulation-induced depolarization (Fig. 18.5). Thus, enhancing the activity of certain K^+ channels would be expected to result in a decreased likelihood of neuronal excitation. A novel, anesthetic-sensitive K^+ current ($I_{K(an)}$) has been identified that is stereoselectively activated by isoflurane (25). Mice with a targeted deletion of the TREK-1 two-pore-domain K^+ channel show significantly reduced sensitivity to general anesthetics compared to wild-type controls (26). Additionally, certain α_2-adrenoceptor agonists (e.g., dexmedetomidine) when injected produce an anesthetic state that is mediated by a G protein–coupled receptor that allosterically modulates K^+ channels. These responses can be antagonized by pertussis toxin and 4-aminopyridine, agents that inactivate G proteins and block K^+ channels, respectively, lending further support to the role of this ion channel (27). Similarly, G protein–mediated mechanisms appear to be involved with the action of morphine via the μ-receptor (Fig. 18.5).

Dexmedetomidine

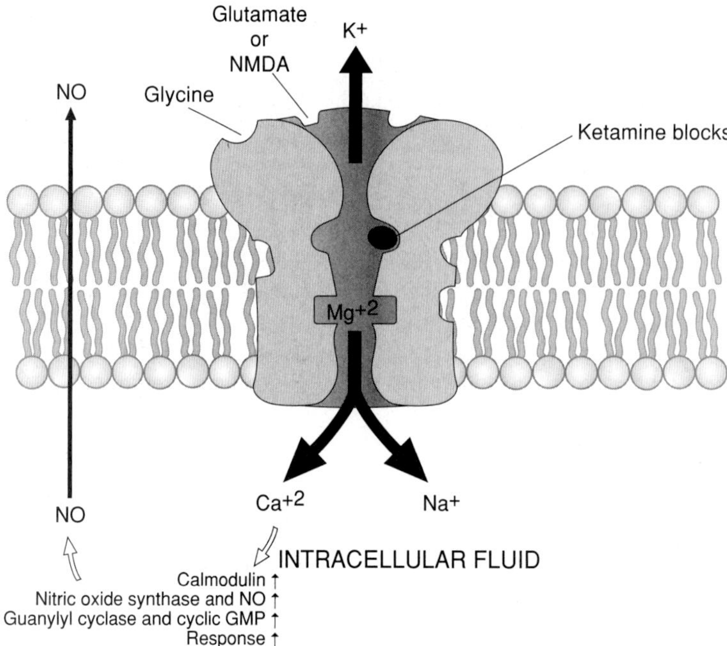

Fig. 18.4. Glutamate or NMDA receptors in the central nervous system. Binding of agonists (glutamate or NMDA) opens the channel, allowing potassium ions to flow outward to extracellular fluid (ECF) and sodium and calcium ions to flow into the nerve cells. Increased intracellular (ICF) calcium ion concentration triggers a cascade that produces a response and liberates the neuronal messenger nitric oxide (NO). Ketamine may produce anesthesia by blocking these NMDA-controlled channels, which are located at excitatory synapses on pyramidal cells (3). Glycine acts as a positive allosteric modulator at the NMDA receptor.

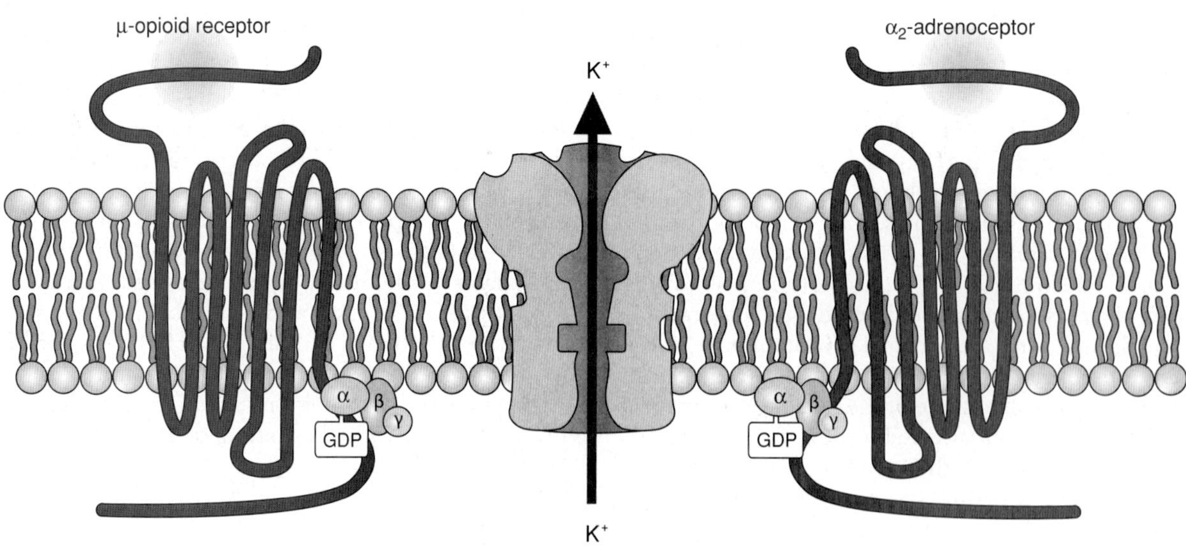

Fig. 18.5. Morphine and α_2-agonists activate their respective G proteins, which hyperpolarize neurons by lowering intracellular fluid (ICF) potassium ion concentration.

HALOGENATED HYDROCARBONS AND ETHERS

Historical Aspects

Ether

The useful volatile anesthetics, with the exception of nitrous oxide, are halogenated hydrocarbons and ethers. Diethyl ether (Fig. 18.6), one of the first agents to be introduced as an anesthetic, has high potency with significant analgesic and neuromuscular relaxing effects. This agent is flammable, and when mixed with air, oxygen, or nitrous oxide, it is explosive. Induction with diethyl ether is very slow; significant time can be spent progressing through the delirium stage. Irritation of the respiratory tract by diethyl ether may lead to excessive bronchial secretions complicating adequate ventilation. In addition to the unpleasant induction and adverse effects, recovery is similarly prolonged and may be accompanied by vomiting. These pharmacological and physical characteristics of diethyl ether limit the utility of this anesthetic in humans.

Short-Chain Hydrocarbons

Many of the short-chain alkanes, alkenes, and alkynes are capable of producing an anesthetic state when administered to patients. Potency generally increases as chain length increases. Because of their flammability and increased propensity to cause cardiovascular toxicity, however, these nonsubstituted hydrocarbons are not useful as anesthetic agents.

Chloroform

Another of the earlier anesthetic agents to be employed was chloroform. This halogenated hydrocarbon was first officially used in the United States in 1847; however, its toxicity seriously limited its utility. The addition of halogens to the hydrocarbon backbone increases potency and decreases flammability. Similar effects also are observed with such substitutions on ethers. As an anesthetic agent, chloroform is very potent and possesses significant analgesic and neuromuscular relaxing activity. Chloroform, a known carcinogen, has the disadvantage of being both hepatotoxic and nephrotoxic, in addition to producing adverse cardiovascular effects, such as arrhythmias and severe hypotension. As a result of these toxicities, chloroform has an unacceptable therapeutic index that prohibits its use in anesthesia. Knowledge regarding the influence of the halogen substitutions on the potency and flammability of hydrocarbons and ethers, however, has significantly contributed to our understanding of the structure–activity relationship of volatile anesthetics and the eventual design of substantially improved agents.

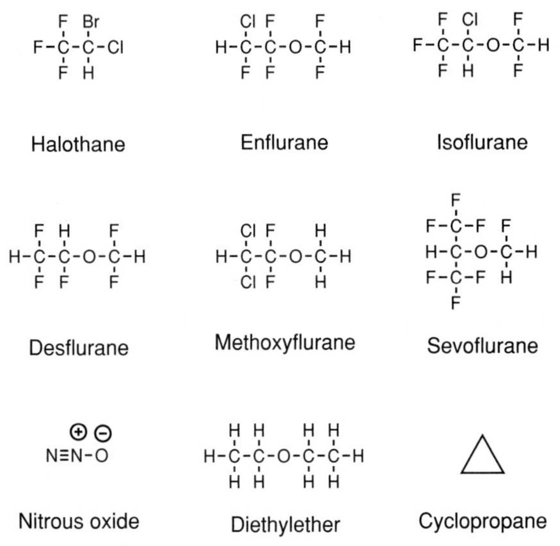

```
  F Br            Cl F    F          F  Cl   F
F-C-C-Cl        H-C-C-O-C-H        F-C-C-O-C-H
  F H             F F    F           F H    F

Halothane       Enflurane          Isoflurane

                                       F
  F H    F        Cl F    H          F-C-F F
H-C-C-O-C-H     H-C-C-O-C-H          H-C-O-C-H
  F F    F        Cl F    H          F-C-F H
                                       F

Desflurane      Methoxyflurane     Sevoflurane

 ⊕ ⊖              H H    H H
N≡N-O           H-C-C-O-C-C-H          △
                  H H    H H

Nitrous oxide   Diethylether       Cyclopropane
```

Fig. 18.6. General anesthetics.

Table 18.4. Relative Flammability of "Nonflammable" Anesthetics

	Halothane (%)	Enflurane (%)	Isoflurane (%)
Minimum flammable conc (MFC) of agent in 30% O_2 with remaining atmosphere N_2O	4.75	5.75	7.0
Minimum effective alveolar conc. (MAC) of agent given in above atmosphere	0.28	0.65	0.46
MAC in humans in the absence of N_2O	0.75	1.68	1.15
MFC/MAC in N_2O	17	8.9	15.2

Flammability

The occurrence of fires in operating rooms is of great concern to all participants in the surgical procedure. Although the introduction of "nonflammable" agents, such as halothane, enflurane, and isoflurane, has substantially decreased this hazard, such fires still occur. Three essential ingredients are required for any combustion: 1) an ignition source (e.g., a laser), 2) a combustible material (e.g., gauze, drapes, or rubber tubes), and 3) an oxidizing agent (e.g., O_2 or N_2O). Many substances are flammable in pure oxygen, N_2O, or mixtures but not air. Certain substances are flammable in N_2O at concentrations that are too low to permit ignition in pure oxygen (28). The concentrations required for combustion, as indicated in Table 18.4, are higher than those generally encountered, except possibly during induction.

CLINICALLY USEFUL INHALATION AGENTS

Fluorinated Hydrocarbons

The structure and physical properties of the volatile anesthetics are given in Table 18.5. Toxic degradation products are formed by reaction of the anesthetic agent with the

Table 18.5. Physicochemical Properties of Clinically Useful Volatile Anesthetics

Generic Name (Trade and Structure Name)	Boiling Point (°C)	Chemically Stable[a]
Desflurane (Suprane) $F_2HC\text{–}O\text{–}CHF\text{–}CF_3$	23.5	Yes
Enflurane (Ethrane) $F_2HC\text{–}O\text{–}CF_2\text{–}CHFCl$	56.5	Yes
Halothane (Fluothane) $F_3C\text{–}CHBrCl$	50.2	No
Isoflurane (Forane) $F_2HC\text{–}O\text{–}CHCl\text{-}CF_3$	48.5	Yes
Methoxyflurane (Penthrane) $H_3C\text{–}O\text{–}CF_2\text{–}CHCl_2$	104.7	No
Nitrous oxide N_20	–*8.0	Yes
Sevoflurane (Ultane) $(CF_3)_2CH\text{–}O\text{–}CH_2F$	58.5	No

[a]Indicates stability to soda lime, ultraviolet light, and common metals.

bases used as carbon dioxide absorbents during anesthesia. This reaction results in the conversion of halothane to 2-bromo-2-chloro-1,1-difluoroethylene, sevoflurane to 2-(fluoromethoxy)-1,1,3,3,3-pentafluoro-1-propene (Compound A), and desflurane, isoflurane, and enflurane to carbon monoxide. Compound A forms a glutathione S-conjugate, which undergoes hydrolysis to cysteine S-conjugates and bioactivation of the cysteine S-conjugates by renal cysteine conjugate β-lyase to give nephrotoxic metabolites.

Halothane

Halothane (Fig. 18.6) was introduced into medical practice in the United States in 1956 as a nonflammable, nonexplosive, halogenated volatile anesthetic that usually is mixed with air or oxygen. The presence of the carbon–halogen bonds contributes to its nonflammability. This clear liquid with a sweet odor was developed based on predictions that its halogenated structure would provide chemical stability, an intermediate blood solubility, and significant anesthetic potency. Halothane is the only useful volatile anesthetic possessing a bromine atom, which has been suggested to contribute to its potency. Similarly, the addition of fluorine atoms, of which halothane has three, is thought to contribute to the increased potency, volatility, and increased chemical stability of the hydrocarbon skeleton (Table 18.5).

Halothane produces rapid onset and recovery from anesthesia with high potency when used alone or in combination with nitrous oxide. Most metals, with the exception of chromium, nickel, and titanium, are easily tarnished by halothane. Although halothane is relatively stable, it is subject to spontaneous oxidative decomposition to hydrochloric acid, hydrobromic acid, and phosgene. For this reason, it is available in dark, amber glass containers with thymol added as a preservative to minimize decomposition. Halothane may permeate into the rubber components of the anesthetic delivery devices, which might account for some slowing of the induction onset and recovery. Approximately 20% of an administered dose is metabolized, which accounts, in part, for the increased hepatotoxicity observed with this agent (Fig. 18.7).

Enflurane

Enflurane (Fig. 18.6) was introduced into medical practice in the United States in 1973 and is a clear, colorless, nonflammable general liquid with a mild, sweet odor. Although relatively stable chemically, enflurane does not attack aluminum, copper, iron, or brass and is soluble in rubber (partition coefficient = 74), which can prolong induction/recovery times, as seen with halothane (Table 18.5). Enflurane has an intermediate solubility in blood and significant potency. Most of its pharmacological properties are similar to those of halothane, although there may be slightly less nausea, vomiting, arrhythmias, and postoperative shivering than observed with halothane. High concentrations of enflurane, however, are more likely to produce convulsions and circulatory depression. Enflurane also relaxes the uterus and, thus, should not be used as an anesthetic during labor. Metabolism via CYP2E1 accounts for 2% of an inhaled dose and includes transformation to the fluoride ion and fluoromethoxydifluoroacetic acid (Fig. 18-7) (30). During recovery, enflurane leaves the fatty tissues rapidly and, therefore, is not available for a prolonged period of time for significant metabolism to proceed.

Isoflurane

Isoflurane (Fig. 18.6) was introduced in the United States in 1981 and is a potent anesthetic agent with many similarities to its isomer enflurane (potent, nonflammable, and intermediate blood solubility). It does produce significantly fewer cardiovascular effects than enflurane, however, and it can be used safely with epinephrine without as great a concern for arrhythmia production. Isoflurane has a more pungent odor than halothane and, thus, can cause irritation to the throat and respiratory tract, triggering coughing and laryngospasm. To overcome this problem, it often is supplemented with intravenous agents. Less than 0.2% of an administered dose is metabolized, mostly to fluoride and trifluoroacetic acid (Fig. 18.7). As discussed below, some minimal potential for hepatotoxicity is associated with a trifluoroacetyl halide metabolite.

A comparative assessment of the volatile anesthetic properties of enflurane, halothane and isoflurane are shown in Table 18.6.

Desflurane

Desflurane (Fig. 18.6) was introduced in the United States in 1992 and is a pungent, volatile agent that is nonflammable and noncorrosive to metals. With a poor blood solubility similar to that of nitrous oxide, desflurane rapidly induces anesthesia. Because the boiling point of desflurane is close to room temperature, a specially designed, heated vaporizer is used to deliver the anesthetic with appropriate concentrations of oxygen either alone or in combination with nitrous oxide. Recovery from the anes-

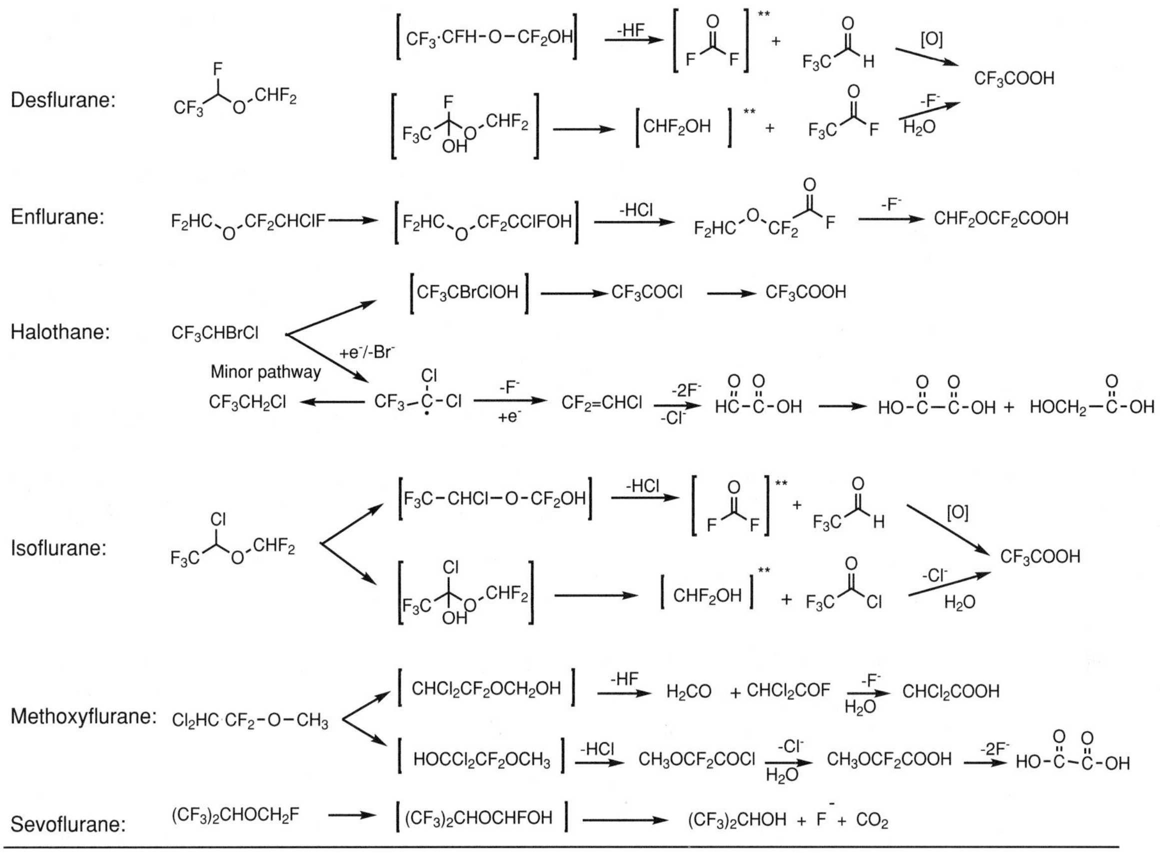

Desflurane: $CF_3CHFOCHF_2$ → $[CF_3\text{-}CFH\text{-}O\text{-}CF_2OH]$ $\xrightarrow{-HF}$ $[CF_2O]^{**}$ + CF_3CHO $\xrightarrow{[O]}$ CF_3COOH; → $[CF_3CF(OH)OCHF_2]$ → $[CHF_2OH]^{**}$ + CF_3COF $\xrightarrow[H_2O]{-F^-}$ CF_3COOH

Enflurane: $F_2HC\text{-}O\text{-}CF_2CHClF$ → $[F_2HC\text{-}O\text{-}CF_2CClFOH]$ $\xrightarrow{-HCl}$ $F_2HC\text{-}O\text{-}CF_2COF$ $\xrightarrow{-F^-}$ CHF_2OCF_2COOH

Halothane: $CF_3CHBrCl$ → $[CF_3CBrClOH]$ → CF_3COCl → CF_3COOH; $\xrightarrow{+e^-/-Br^-}$ $CF_3\text{-}\dot{C}Cl\text{-}Cl$ $\xrightarrow[+e^-]{-F^-}$ $CF_2{=}CHCl$ $\xrightarrow[-Cl^-]{-2F^-}$ $HC(O)\text{-}C(O)\text{-}OH$ → $HO\text{-}C(O)\text{-}C(O)\text{-}OH$ + $HOCH_2\text{-}C(O)\text{-}OH$; Minor pathway: → CF_3CH_2Cl

Isoflurane: $F_3CCHClOCHF_2$ → $[F_3C\text{-}CHCl\text{-}O\text{-}CF_2OH]$ $\xrightarrow{-HCl}$ $[CF_2O]^{**}$ + CF_3CHO $\xrightarrow{[O]}$ CF_3COOH; → $[F_3CCCl(OH)OCHF_2]$ → $[CHF_2OH]^{**}$ + CF_3COCl $\xrightarrow[H_2O]{-Cl^-}$ CF_3COOH

Methoxyflurane: $Cl_2HC\,CF_2\text{-}O\text{-}CH_3$ → $[CHCl_2CF_2OCH_2OH]$ $\xrightarrow{-HF}$ H_2CO + $CHCl_2COF$ $\xrightarrow[H_2O]{-F^-}$ $CHCl_2COOH$; → $[HOCCl_2CF_2OCH_3]$ $\xrightarrow{-HCl}$ CH_3OCF_2COCl $\xrightarrow[H_2O]{-Cl^-}$ CH_3OCF_2COOH $\xrightarrow{-2F^-}$ $HO\text{-}C(O)\text{-}C(O)\text{-}OH$

Sevoflurane: $(CF_3)_2CHOCH_2F$ → $[(CF_3)_2CHOCHFOH]$ → $(CF_3)_2CHOH + F^- + CO_2$

*Data from references 28 and 29.

**Decomposition of unstable intermediates: $CF_2O \longrightarrow 2F^- + CO_2$; $CHF_2OH \longrightarrow 2F^- + HCOOH$;

Fig. 18.7. Proposed metabolites of fluorinated anesthetics.

thetic state also is rapid, being approximately twice as rapid as that with isoflurane. Because of the rapid induction and recovery associated with desflurane, this anesthetic has gained popularity in outpatient surgical procedures. Desflurane is rather pungent, so patients often are induced with an intravenous anesthetic agent and then maintained with desflurane. Desflurane is not metabolized to any great extent and, therefore, has not been associated with hepatotoxicity or nephrotoxicity (31). Metabolites, mostly trifluoroacetate, account for less than 0.02% of the administered dose (Fig. 18.7). Whereas desflurane can react with soda lime or Baralyme to form carbon monoxide, no reports of adverse outcomes in patients have appeared.

Table 18.6. Comparative Assessment of Enflurane (E), Halothane (H), and Isoflurane (I)

Property	Superior	Intermediate	Inferior
Stability	I = E	—	H
Blood solubility	I	E	H
Pungency	H	I	E
Respiratory depression	H	I	E
Circulatory depression	I	H	E
Induction of arrhythmias	I	E	H
Muscle relaxation	I = E	—	H
Increased intracranial pressure/cerebral blood flow	I	E	H
Seizure activity	H = E	—	E
Metabolism	I	E	H
Toxicity	I	E	H

Adapted from Wade JG, Stevens WC. Isoflurane; an anesthetic for the eighties? Anesth Analg 1981;60:666–682; with permission.

Sevoflurane

Sevoflurane (Fig. 18.6) is a nonflammable, nonirritating, pleasant-odored volatile anesthetic available for use in the United States. Similar to desflurane in many of its pharmacological actions, sevoflurane has low blood solubility, higher potency, and the advantage of not being irritating to the respiratory tract. Induction and recovery are rapid. Sevoflurane undergoes significantly more metabolism (CYP2E1) than desflurane, however, and as much as 3% of an administered dose can be recovered as hexafluoroisopropanol (Fig. 18.7). Some fluoride ion also can be produced, but the incidence of nephrotoxicity or hepatotoxicity appears low, especially when used infrequently for short periods of time. There have been concerns regarding the reactivity of sevoflurane with soda lime or Baralyme, in which a potentially toxic olefin by-product termed "Compound A" (2-(fluoromethoxy)-1,1,3,3,3-pentafluoro-1-propene) can be formed. With appropriate precautions, however, sevoflurane can be used safely in both children and adults.

Methoxyflurane

Methoxyflurane (Fig. 18.6) is seldom used because of its propensity to cause renal toxicity. It is the most potent of the agents discussed here, and it has the highest solubility in blood. Induction and recovery would be expected to be slow. Chemically, it is rather unstable, and as much as 50% of an administered dose can be metabolized. Toxic metabolites significantly limit its utility as a general anesthetic (Fig. 18.7).

Toxicity of Fluorinated General Anesthetics

Although few signs of toxicity usually are observed during the short-term, infrequent administration of general anesthetics, a few well-defined toxic effects have been noted. For instance, halothane and methoxyflurane are known to produce hepatotoxicity and nephrotoxicity, respectively. Both of these toxic reactions are believed to result from highly reactive metabolites of the parent compound. Overall, however, the therapeutic ratio for most of the general anesthetics approaches 4:1 (32).

Hepatotoxicity. Hepatitis caused by halothane occurs in 1 in 20,000 patients exposed to this anesthetic. It is thought to result from the binding of a reactive free radical metabolite to liver tissue (Fig. 18.7). The resultant abnormal molecular product in the liver is viewed by the immune system as a foreign substance (e.g., an antigen), which then sensitizes cells to produce antibodies. Some have suggested that the trifluoroacetyl halide metabolite is responsible for the initiation of halothane hepatitis. Interestingly, both enflurane and isoflurane can be metabolized to the acylated halides and produce a similar immune-mediated syndrome, although to a much lesser extent. Additionally, there appears to be cross-reactivity among these three agents, because the antigen formed is similar enough in structure to elicit the immune system response. Some investigations have suggested that a genetic susceptibility factor may be responsible, in part, for this serious form of hepatitis.

Halothane also can produce another form of hepatotoxicity. This is a self-limiting hepatic dysfunction characterized by elevated liver transaminase enzymes, which probably results from impaired oxygenation of the hepatocytes during exposure to this anesthetic. Isoflurane and enflurane also have been reported to produce a similar elevation of liver enzymes, although to a lesser extent than halothane.

Malignant Hyperthermia. This rare (1 per 15,000 anesthetic uses) but potentially fatal complication associated with the use of certain anesthetics (e.g., halothane) is characterized by a rapid rise in core body temperature associated with hypermetabolic reactions in the skeletal muscle of genetically susceptible subjects. Such individuals appear to have an autosomal dominant mediated defect in the Ca^{2+}-release channel commonly referred to as the ryanodine receptor. The large amounts of heat generated, massive increase in oxygen consumption, and production of carbon dioxide may quickly lead to death or permanent neurological damage unless appropriate supportive treatment, including rapid cooling, 100% oxygen, and control of acidosis, is promptly initiated. The administration of the skeletal muscle relaxant dantrolene, which blocks release of Ca^{2+} from the sarcoplasmic reticulum, reduces muscle rigidity and heat production, which significantly improves the prognosis of the patient. Besides the fluorinated volatile anesthetics, some depolarizing neuromuscular blocking agents (e.g., succinylcholine) and some neuroleptics (e.g., haloperidol) also are reportedly associated with similar malignant hyperthermic syndromes, although the underlying mechanism mediating these may differ somewhat from those associated with the general anesthetics.

Nephrotoxicity. Fluorinated anesthetics that undergo metabolism to inorganic fluoride have the potential to produce damage to the renal tubular cells. Of the fluorinated anesthetics, methoxyflurane is the only agent commonly associated with nephrotoxicity. Methoxyflurane is subject to metabolism (Fig. 18.7), yielding plasma fluoride ion levels in excess of the threshold value for renal damage of 40 μM. Others, such as sevoflurane, have only very rarely been associated with nephrotoxicity—and then usually in patients with severe renal compromise. Plasma levels of fluoride only reach 15 to 20 μM following 2.5 MAC-hour exposure to enflurane (33). The rates of metabolic defluorination of the useful anesthetic agents are as follows: methoxyflurane > enflurane = sevoflurane > isoflurane > desflurane = halothane.

Low-Level Chronic Exposure. Typically, patients are exposed to greater-than-MAC concentrations of the volatile anesthetics for limited periods of time, such as a number of hours during a surgical procedure and not for extended periods of time (e.g., days or weeks). Because surgical and dental personnel, however, may be exposed to low levels of the general anesthetics for prolonged periods over many years or even decades, the ability of such agents to produce chronic toxicity is of paramount concern. Although the occupational exposure to these agents has been minimized with improved waste gas–scavenging devices, some epidemiological studies have demonstrated increased levels of spontaneous abortions, congenital birth defects in offspring, and increased rates of certain cancers in chronically exposed medical personnel (34).

Nitrous Oxide

Commonly called "laughing gas," nitrous oxide (dinitrogen monoxide, or N_2O) is a gas at room temperature and is the least potent of the inhalation anesthetics used today (Table 18.5). With an MAC value in excess of 105%, this colorless, tasteless, and odorless to slightly sweet-smelling gas is not normally capable of producing surgical anesthesia when administered alone. The MAC for nitrous oxide has been demonstrated to be between 105 and 140% and, thus, cannot achieve surgical anesthesia under conditions at standard barometric pressure. To demonstrate that the MAC was greater than 100%, Bert in 1879 used a mixture of 85% nitrous oxide with oxygen at 1.2 atmospheres in a pressurized chamber. Only at this elevated pressure could an MAC adequate for surgical anesthesia be achieved. Decreasing the oxygen content of a nitrous oxide mixture to values less than 20% to allow an increase in the concentration of nitrous oxide to greater than 80% can be dangerous, because hypoxia would be expected to result. Thus, when administered alone, nitrous oxide finds utility as an anesthetic agent during certain procedures (e.g., dental) in which full surgical anesthesia is not required. Most commonly, however, nitrous oxide is used in combination with other general anesthetics, because it is capable of decreasing the concentration of the added anesthetic required to produce an adequate depth of anesthesia for surgical procedures.

While no firm underlying mechanisms have been demonstrated, some authors have suggested that irreversible oxidation of the cobalt atom in vitamin B_{12} by nitrous oxide can lead to inactivation of enzymes dependent on this vitamin, with resultant metabolic aberrations. Such examples have included methionine synthetase and thymidylate synthetase, which are essential in the synthetic pathways leading to the production of myelin and thymidine, respectively. Should these enzymes be impaired during the sensitive periods of in utero development, the potential for malformations may unfortunately be realized. To date, no studies have been able to demonstrate conclusively that low-level exposure to nitrous oxide is associated with a meaningful disruption of crucial metabolic functions to produce the above-described toxicity; however, measures including improved waste gas–scavenging systems should be taken to minimize exposure of personnel.

CLINICALLY USEFUL INTRAVENOUS AGENTS

Propofol

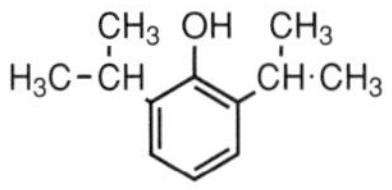

CH_3 OH CH_3
H_3C-CH $CH \cdot CH_3$

Propofol

The most commonly used parenteral anesthetic used in the United States is propofol. Used intravenously, propofol is not chemically related to the barbiturates or other intravenous anesthetics. Propofol appears to act via enhancing GABAergic neurotransmission within the central nervous system. This occurs most likely at the GABA receptor complex, but at a site distinct from where the benzodiazepines bind. Because of its poor water solubility, propofol is formulated as a 1 or 2% emulsion with soybean oil, egg lecithin, and glycerol. Sodium metabisulfite or ethylenediaminetetra-acetic acid also is included in the parenteral dosage form. Because of the likelihood of bacterial contamination of open containers, propofol should be either administered or discarded shortly after sterility seals are broken. Following intravenous administration of a dose of 2.0 to 2.5 mg/kg, a state of hypnosis is achieved within 1 minute, which lasts for approximately 5 minutes. A longer anesthetic state can be achieved by additional propofol dosing or, as typically is the case, maintenance with a volatile anesthetic agent. Blood pressure and heart rate usually are decreased following propofol administration. Metabolism of propofol proceeds rapidly via hepatic conversion to its glucuronide and sulfate conjugates, with less than 0.3% excreted unchanged. Because this agent produces a rapid induction and recovery and is infrequently associated with episodes of vomiting, propofol has found utility as an anesthetic agent in outpatient surgical environments.

Ketamine

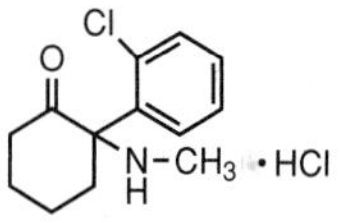

Cl O
N-CH_3 •HCl
H

Ketamine

Ketamine hydrochloride is an injectable, very potent, rapidly acting anesthetic agent. As with propofol above, its duration of anesthetic activity also is relatively short (10–25 minutes). Ketamine does not relax skeletal muscles and, therefore, can only be used alone in procedures of short duration that do not require muscle relaxation. Recovery from anesthesia may be accompanied by "emergence delirium," which is characterized by visual, auditory, and confusional illusions. Disturbing dreams and hallucinations can occur up to 24 hours after the administration of ketamine. Its elimination half-life is 2 to 3 hours, and its volume of distribution is 2 to 3 L/kg. Ketamine has an oral bioavailability of less than 16%. Termination of the acute action of ketamine is largely a result of its redistribution from the brain into other tissue; however, the formation of the glucuronide conjugate and metabolism in the liver to a number of metabolites does occur. One of these metabolites of interest, norketamine, is formed via the action of CYP2B6. This N-demethylated derivative retains significant activity at the NMDA receptor and may account for some of the longer-lasting effects of this anesthetic agent. Eventual conversion of norketamine to hydroxylated metabolites and subsequent conjugation leads to metabolites that can be renally eliminated. Less than 4% of a dose is excreted unchanged in the urine.

Ketamine is capable of producing a "dissociative" anesthesia, which is characterized by EEG changes indicating a dissociation between the thalamocortical and limbic systems (35). These neuronal systems, which normally are associated with one another, help to maintain the neuronal connections required for consciousness. When disassociated, the subject will appear to be cataleptic, with the eyes open in a slow, nystagmic gaze (1). A potent analgesic and amnesic effect is produced, as is an increase in muscle tone in some areas. Although patients may appear to be awake, they are incapable of communicating and do not remember the event or the people around them. Blood pressure and heart rate usually are increased following ketamine administration.

Ketamine appears to act similarly to phencyclidine (PCP; also known as Angel Dust), which acts as an antagonist within the cationic channel of the NMDA receptor complex (36). By preventing the flow of cations through this channel, ketamine prevents neuronal activation, which normally is required for the conscious state. The analgesic activity of ketamine, however, is more likely the result of an interaction with an opioid receptor or the less-well-understood σ-receptor. Other studies have suggested a possible involvement of serotonin receptors and muscarinic receptors (37). Ketamine, like PCP, has a significant potential for abuse.

Etomidate

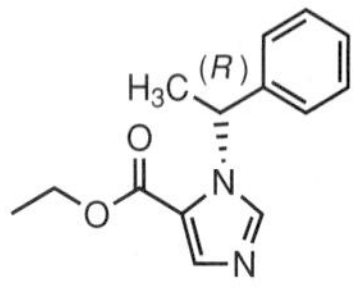

R-Etomidate

Etomidate is the ester of a carboxylated imidazole, with a log P of 3 and a weak base pK_a of 4.5, that is available as the D-isomer solubilized in 35% propylene glycol for intravenous injection in addition to being available for rectal administration. It is a potent, short-acting hypnotic agent (<3 min) without analgesic activity and with a rapid onset of action. This agent is useful for the induction of anesthesia in hemodynamically unstable patients prone to hypotension because of hypovolemia, coronary artery disease, or cardiomyopathies. Recovery is similarly rapid following discontinuance of the drug. Etomidate is hydrolyzed by hepatic esterases to the corresponding inactive carboxylic acid, with subsequent renal and biliary excretion terminating its action. Its apparent elimination half-life is approximately 5 to 6 hours, with a volume of distribution of 5 to 7 L/kg. Changes in hepatic blood flow or hepatic metabolism will have only moderate effects on etomidate disposition. Concerns regarding the ability of etomidate to precipitate myoclonic jerks and inhibit adrenal steroid synthesis have been reported.

Ultrashort-Acting Barbiturates

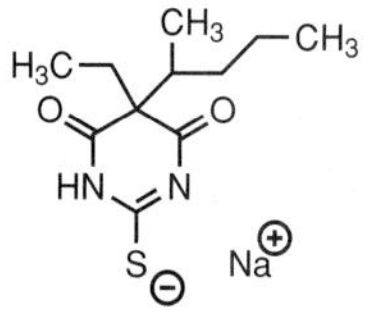

Thiopental

The ultrashort-acting barbiturates (e.g., thiopental) are used intravenously to produce a rapid unconsciousness for surgical and basal anesthesia. These agents may be used initially to induce anesthesia, which then can be maintained during the surgical procedure with a general anesthetic agent. The induction typically is very rapid and pleasant. (These ultrashort-acting barbiturates are discussed in Chapter 19.)

CASE STUDY

Victoria F. Roche and S. William Zito

JA is a brought to the emergency department where you work. He is a 58-year-old street person. His clothes are disheveled, he needs a bath and a shave, and he smells of alcohol. JA is in extreme pain and grumpily complains that he was pushed down hard by a couple of young "punks" who were after his shopping cart, which contained all of his worldly possesions. The pain is radiating from his right hip, and radiographs reveal that he has an intertrochanteric hip fracture just below the femoral neck of his right leg. This type of fracture is treated by repairing the fracture with a metal plate and screws. Tests reveal that JA has slightly low blood pressure (105/70 mm Hg), and his liver enzymes and creatinine clearance are indicative of decreased liver and kidney function, most likely

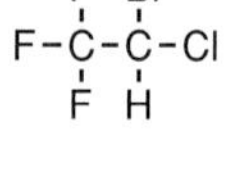

1

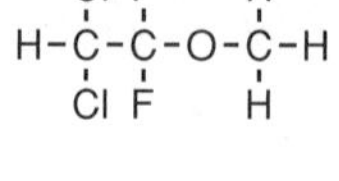

2

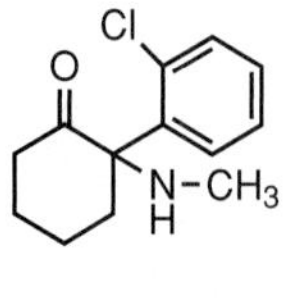

3

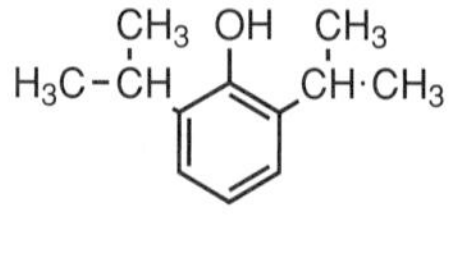

4

because of alcohol and the hard life on the streets. Evaluate structures 1 to 4 for use as the general anesthetic for JA's surgery.

1. Identify the therapeutic problem(s) in which the pharmacist's intervention may benefit the patient.
2. Identify and prioritize the patient-specific factors that must be considered to achieve the desired therapeutic outcomes.
3. Conduct a thorough and mechanistically oriented structure–activity analysis of all therapeutic alternatives provided in the case.
4. Evaluate the structure–activity relationship findings against the patient-specific factors and desired therapeutic outcomes, and make a therapeutic decision.
5. Counsel your patient.

References

1. Stoelting RK. Pharmacology and Physiology of Anesthetic Practice, 3rd Ed. Philadelphia: Lippincott Williams & Wilkins, 1999.
2. Stevens WC, Kingston HGG. Inhalation anesthesia. In: Barash PG, Cullen BF, Stoelting RK, eds. Clinical Anesthesia, 2nd Ed. Philadelphia: JB Lippincott, 1992, pp. 439–465.
3. Harrison NL, Flood P. Molecular mechanisms of general anesthetic action. Sci Med 1998;(May:June):50:18–27.
4. Meyer HH. The theory of narcosis. JAMA 1906;26:1499–1502.
5. Overton E. Studien ueber die narkose, zugleich ein beitrag zur allgemeinem pharmakologie. Jena: Gustav Fischer, 1901.
6. Hemming HC, Akabas MH, Goldstein PA, et al. Emerging molecular mechanisms of general anesthetic action. Trends Pharmacol Sci 2005:26:503–510.
7. Lysco GS, Robinson JL, Casto R, et al. The stereospecific effects of isoflurane isomers in vivo. Eur J Pharmacol 1994;263:25–29.
8. Graf BM, Boban M, Stowe DF, et al. Lack of stereospecific effects of isoflurane and desflurane isomers in isolated guinea pig hearts. Anesthesiology 1994;81:129–136.
9. Sidebotham DA, Schug SA. Stereochemistry in anesthesia. Clin Exp Pharmacol Physiol 1997;24:126–130.
10. Cheng S-C, Brunner EA. Effects of anesthetic agents on synaptosomal GABA disposal. Anesthesiology 1981;55:34–40.
11. Olsen RW. The molecular mechanism of action of general anesthetics: structural aspects of interactions with $GABA_A$ receptors. Toxicol Lett 1998;100–101:193–201.
12. Moody EJ, Harris BD, Skolnick P. Stereospecific actions of the inhalation anesthetic isoflurane at the $GABA_A$ receptor complex. Brain Res 1993;615:101–106.
13. Tomlin SL. Stereoselective effects of etomidate optical isomers on γ-aminobutyric acid type A receptors and animals. Anesthesiology 1998:88:708–717.
14. Krasowski MD, Harrison NL. General anesthetic actions at ligand-gated ion channels. Cell Mol Life Sci 1999:55:1278–1303.
15. Koltchine VV. Agonist gating and isoflurane potentiation in the human $GABA_A$ receptor determined by the volume of a TM2 residue. Mol. Pharmacol 1999:56:1087–1093.
16. Belelli D, Pistis M, Peters JA, et al. General anesthetic action at transmitter-gated inhibitory amino acid receptors. Trends Pharmacol Sci 1999;20: 496–502.
17. Bai D. Distinct functional and pharmacological properties of tonic and quantal inhibitory postsynaptic currents mediated by γ-aminobutyric acid A receptors in hippocampal neurons. Mol Pharmacol 2001:59:814–824.
18. Bai D. The general anesthetic propofol slows deactivation and desensitization of $GABA_A$ receptors. J Neurosci 1999:19:10635–10646.
19. Flohr H, Glade U, Motzko D. The role of the NMDA synapse in general anesthesia. Toxicol Lett 1998;100–101:23–29.
20. Perouansky M, Kirson ED, Yaari Y. Mechanism of action of volatile anesthetics: effects of halothane on glutamate receptors in vitro. Toxicol Lett 1998; 100–101:65–69.
21. Larsen M, Langmoen IA. The effect of volatile anesthetics on synaptic release and uptake of glutamate. Toxicol Lett 1998; 100–101:59–64.
22. Hudspith MJ. Glutamate: a role in normal brain function, anesthesia, analgesia and CNS injury. Br J Anaesth 1997;78:731–747.
23. Narahashi T, Aistrup GL, Lindstrom JM, et al. Ion modulation as the basis for general anesthetics. Toxicol Lett 1998;100–101:185–191.
24. Shiraishi M, Harris RA. Effects of alcohol and anesthetics on recombinant voltage-gated NA^+ channels. J Pharmacol Exp Ther 2004:309:987–994.
25. Franks NP, Lieb WR. Stereospecific effects of inhalational general anesthetic optical isomers on nerve ion channels. Science 1991;25:427–430.
26. Heurteaux C. TREK-1, a K+ channel involved in neuroprotection and general anesthesia. EMBO J 2004:23:2684–2695.
27. Doze VA, Chen BX, Ticklenberg JA, et al. Pertussis toxin and 4-aminopyridine differentially affect the hypnotic-anesthetic action of dexmedetomidine and pentobarbital. Anesthesiology 1990;73:304–307.
28. Perry LB, Gould AB, Leonord PE. Case history number 82: "nonflammable" fires in the operating room. Anesth Analg 1975;54:152–154.
29. Eger EI II. Anesthetic Uptake and Action. Baltimore: Williams & Wilkins, 1974.
30. Christ DD, Kenna JG, Kammerer W, et al. Enflurane metabolism produces covalently bound liver adducts recognized by antibodies from patients with halothane hepatitis. Anesthesiology 1988;69:833–888.
31. Koblin DD. Characteristics and implications of desflurane metabolism and toxicity. Anesth Analg 1992;75:S10–S16.
32. Dodds C. General anesthesia: practical recommendations and recent advances. Drugs 1999;58:453–467.
33. Mazze RI, Calverely RK, Smith NT. Inorganic fluoride nephrotoxicity: prolonged enflurane and halothane anesthesia in volunteers. Anesthesiology 1977;46:265–271.
34. Lane GA Nahrwold ML, Tait AR. Anesthetics as teratogens: nitrous oxide is fetotoxic, xenon is not. Science 1980;210:899–901.
35. Reich DL, Silvay G. Ketamine: an update on the first twenty-five years of clinical experience. Can J Anaesth 1989;36:186–197.
36. Yamamura T, Harada K, Okamura A, et al. Is the site of action of ketamine anesthesia the N-methyl-D-aspartate receptor? Anesthesiology 1990;72:704–710.
37. Toro-Matos A, Redon-Platas AM, Avila-Valdez E, et al. Physostigmine antagonizes ketamine. Anesth Analg 1980;59:764–767.

Suggested Readings

Cooper JR, Bloom FE, Roth RH. The Biochemical Basis of Neuropharmacology, 7th Ed. New York: Oxford University Press, 1996.

Ezekiel MR. Handbook of Anesthesiology. 2004–2005 Edition. Laguna Hills, CA: CCS Publishing, 2004.

Hardman JG, Limbird LE, Molinoff PB, et al. The Pharmacological Basis of Therapeutics, 9th Ed. New York: McGraw Hill, 1996.

Mashour GA, Forman GA, Campagna SA, et al. Mechanisms of general anesthesia: from molecules to mind. Best Pract Res Clin Anesthesiol 2005;19:349–364.

Stoelting RK. Pharmacology and Physiology of Anesthetic Practice, 3rd Ed. Philadelphia: Lippincott Williams &Wilkins, 1999.

Tung A. New anesthesia techniques. Thoracic Surg Clin 2005;15:27–38.

19. *Sedative-Hypnotics*

WILLIAM SOINE

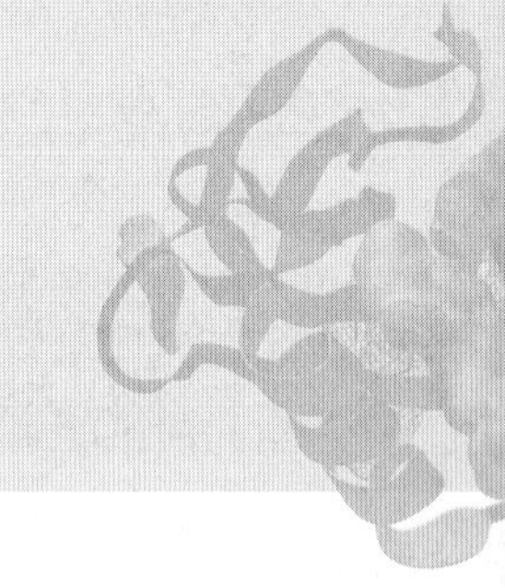

DRUGS COVERED IN THIS CHAPTER:

BENZODIAZEPINE SEDATIVE-HYPNOTICS
- Estazolam
- Flurazepam
- Quazepam
- Temazepam
- Triazolam

NONBENZODIAZEPINE SEDATIVE-HYPNOTICS
- Zolpidem
- Zaleplon
- Eszopiclone

BARBITURATE
- Amobarbital
- Aprobarbital
- Butabarbital
- Pentobarbital
- Phenobarbital
- Secobarbital

MELATONIN RECEPTOR AGONIST
- Ramelteon

CHLORAL HYDRATE

ANTIHISTAMINES
- Diphenhydramine
- Doxylamine

INTRODUCTION

Hypnotics often are referred to as sleeping pills, sedative medications, soporifics, and sedative-hypnotics and are used to treat insomnia. This class of drugs causes drowsiness and facilitates the initiation and maintenance of sleep. The observed pharmacological effects of most drugs in this class usually are dose related. Small doses cause sedation, larger doses cause hypnosis (sleep), and still larger doses may bring about surgical anesthesia. Drugs used as hypnotics often are sedative and anxiolytic (depending on the dose), but not all anxiolytic drugs cause sedation. See Chapter 22 for more information concerning sedative/anxiolytic use of the benzodiazepines. This chapter will emphasize the concepts important in sleep and wakefulness, then present current drugs used to initiate and maintain sleep.

Clinical situations commonly are encountered that require the use of hypnotics. Insomnia can be classified as primary (pathogenesis unknown) or secondary (from other causes). Secondary insomnia is more common and can be the result of situational stress, lifestyle habits, drugs, and psychiatric or medical disorders (1). There are effective nonpharmacological treatments for insomnia; however, a need remains to use hypnotics on both a short-term and a long-term basis to facilitate sleep (2). The drugs currently used as hypnotics are effective, but there is ample need for newer and safer hypnotics. The introduction of supposedly a newer yet safer and more effective hypnotic drug has always been greeted with optimism, such as the piperidinedione thalidomide (3). Thalidomide was proposed to be a substitute for the barbiturates in the 1950s. Similar to most other drugs used as hypnotics or sedatives, however, only after its introduction and extensive clinical use did its limitations become better understood. The ideal hypnotic should 1) cause a transient decrease in the level of consciousness for the purpose of sleep without lingering effects (sleep induction and sleep maintenance), 2) have no potential for decreasing or arresting respirations (even at relatively high doses), and 3) produce no abuse, addiction, tolerance or dependence (4). A search for newer and better hypnotics continues.

PHYSIOLOGY OF SLEEP

Sleep Cycle

At the start of the 20th century, sleep was considered to be a passive process. During the late 1920s and 1930s, it was possible to monitor human electrical brain activity using the electroencephalogram (EEG). Using the EEG, it was established that there occurred a passive nature of sleep that alternated with wakeful activity (5). This was followed by the discovery by Moruzzi and Magoun of the ascending reticular activating system and its relationship to the EEG (6). This discovery provided the basis for the modern theories of sleep and was validated by finding that sleeping animals could be awakened through stimulation of electrodes implanted in the midbrain reticular formation. Sleep is studied using related techniques that permit electronic monitoring of the head and neck muscles (electromyogram) and eye movements (electrooculogram). From these and related studies, three states have been defined: 1) wakefulness, 2) slow-wave sleep (nonrapid eye movement [NREM] sleep), and 3) paradoxic sleep (PS; rapid eye movement [REM] sleep). Wakefulness is characterized by low-voltage fast activity of the EEG, high muscle activity, and numerous REMs, indicating intensive interaction with the environment.

The two states of sleep, NREM and REM, have been characterized primarily using EEG. The NREM sleep has been subdivided by Dement and Kleitman into four stages, which are precisely defined (although somewhat arbitrarily) using the EEG (5). Stages 1 through 4 follow a sleep continuum, with the ability to arouse an individual

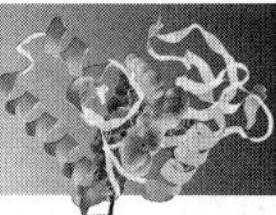

CLINICAL SIGNIFICANCE

The pharmacotherapy of insomnia has improved dramatically, and the recent development of novel agents has continued to grow thanks to the drug discovery process.

Older medications, such as the barbiturates, are used as sedative-hypnotics, but toxicity limits their widespread use. For example, they can cause significant central nervous system (CNS) depression, physical dependence, and tolerance. Additionally, they are potent inducers of liver enzymes, which can lead to clinically significant drug interactions when these medications are administered with other drugs extensively metabolized by the liver.

The benzodiazepines are much safer for the treatment of insomnia and are commonly used for this purpose. Within the benzodiazepine class, drug discovery has resulted in medications with improved pharmacokinetic profiles for the treatment of insomnia. For example, the newer triazolobenzodiazepines posses a much shorter elimination half-life, and this feature can be used clinically to improve sleep while at the same time inducing less daytime sedation.

The nonbenzodiazepine agents also are effective and, thus far, appear to be even safer than the benzodiazepines. The three medications belonging to this class are known as the "Z" drugs and are zolpidem, zopiclone (i.e., eszopiclone), and zaleplon. With these drugs, the basic sciences have provided clinicians with medications that are both safe and effective.

The most recent addition to the armamentarium is the melatonin receptor agonist ramelteon. Molecular modifications to melatonin resulted in this potent and selective melatonin receptor agonist. This medication is very unique in that it does not appear to posses any abuse liability and is not a controlled substance like most other sedative-hypnotics. Also, it does not appear to interfere with cognitive function or memory.

The drug discovery process and an understanding of structure–activity relationships has taken us from very toxic medications that were dangerous at high doses and caused physical dependence (i.e., barbiturates) to medications that are safe and apparently free from any abuse liability (i.e., ramelteon). These newer medications, brought to us by basic science techniques, will improve the quality of life for many who suffer from insomnia.

Christian Teter, Pharm.D.
Assistant Professor
Northeastern University
Department of Pharmacy Practice
Bouvé College of Health Sciences

being lowest in stage 1 and highest in stage 4 sleep. When sleep overtakes wakefulness, the transition is gradual; indeed, not one single measure is reliable all of the time.

The simplest pattern of sleep is that associated with a normal young adult. The normal adult enters sleep through NREM sleep. After approximately 90 minutes of NREM sleep, the first REM sleep occurs, with a mean duration of approximately 20 minutes. Thereafter, NREM and REM sleep alternate cyclically through the night, with the average length of the NREM-REM sleep cycle being approximately 90 to 120 minutes. REM sleep tends to be greatest during the last third of the night. Therefore, a normal young adult displays a sleep pattern of 75 to 80% NREM and 20 to 25% REM sleep. The length of nocturnal sleep is dependent on a number of factors, of which voluntary control is the most significant. Other important factors are genetic determinants and processes associated with circadian rhythms. As sleep is extended, the amount of REM sleep is increased.

A number of factors modify sleep stage distribution: age, previous sleep history, drug ingestion, circadian rhythms, temperature, and pathology. Only the first four factors will be discussed in this chapter.

Age

Age related differences are seen in infants. The cyclic alteration of NREM-REM sleep at birth has a period of 50 to 60 minutes versus 90 minutes in adults. Infants gradually develop normal nocturnal slow-wave sleep after 2 to 6 months of life. Slow-wave sleep becomes maximal in young children and decreases markedly with age. Slow-wave sleep may no longer be present by 60 years of age, but this is more common in men than in women. The interindividual variability in the elderly is greatly increased, and the generalizations made for young adults concerning "normal" sleep are no longer applicable.

Previous Sleep History and Drug Ingestion

Previous sleep history and the effects of drug ingestion on sleep history are important when comparing hypnotics. An individual experiencing sleep loss on one or more nights will show a sleep pattern of increased slow-wave sleep during the first recovery night, with REM sleep showing a rebound on the second or subsequent nights. When an individual becomes deprived of REM sleep by being awakened every time the electro-oculogram and EEG indicated that dreaming has begun, the individual becomes selectively deprived of REM sleep, and a pressure for REM sleep builds. A preferential rebound of REM sleep will occur. The cyclic patterns of sleep states and sleep stages can be affected by many common drugs, including the hypnotics. The ability of drugs to differentially affect one sleep stage over another can, on withdrawal, produce rebound effects leading to exacerbation of the sleep disorder, comparable to deprivation of REM sleep.

Circadian Rhythms

The importance of the circadian phase at which sleep occurs and its effect on the distribution of sleep stages has become of interest because of the current popularity of melatonin. It has been shown that with individuals sleeping in situations free of all time cues, circadian phase can influence the timing of sleep onset and length of sleep. If sleep onset is delayed until the peak REM phase of circadian rhythm (early morning), REM sleep can predominate and even may occur at the onset of sleep. This abnormal sleep-onset pattern or phase shift can occur because of a work-shift change or a change resulting from jet travel across a number of time zones.

As a brief summary, the normal adult human enters sleep through NREM sleep. After approximately 80 minutes or longer, the individual starts REM sleep after which NREM-REM sleep alternates through the remainder of the sleep period. Any situation that causes an alteration of this normal sleep cycle leads to compensation of REM or NREM sleep in subsequent nights.

Sleep Factors

The involvement of many autonomic, physiologic, and biochemical changes are associated with wakefulness, NREM sleep, and REM sleep. The relationship of cause and effect in relation to these systems is still somewhat controversial and a rapidly changing area of research. Several brain regions that regulate sleep have now been identified; however, the specific contribution on any one region to sleep is still controversial (7). The roles of the major systems are important to be familiar with in relation to sleep. This not only helps one to understand the mechanism by which hypnotics work but also provides some understanding of why unrelated drugs, such as neuroleptics, antihistamines, antidepressants, and antimanic drugs, occasionally are used as hypnotics to facilitate sleep.

Neurotransmitter/Neuromodulator

Every neurotransmitter has, at one time or another, been implicated in sleep or wakefulness. The assumption is that if a neurotransmitter is involved in wakefulness, it may be involved in initiation or maintenance of REM sleep. In contrast, an antagonist of the neurotransmitter would be anticipated to initiate or maintain NREM sleep. Studies of this type rarely are unambiguous because of the integration of the neural pathways. Some of the evidence for the involvement of these neurotransmitters in sleep or wakefulness is presented; however, the reader should consult Kales (7) for details.

Catecholamines. It would be anticipated that catecholamines (originating from the locus ceruleus) would be involved in wakefulness and REM sleep (8). Initial experiments with reserpine suggested that a decrease in catecholamines involved in neurotransmission caused a decrease in REM sleep. Contradictory and inconsistent findings with other compounds that modulate catecholamine synthesis, however, gave ambiguous results concerning the relationship between monoamine levels and stages of sleep. The only consistent finding is that an intact catecholamine transmission system is needed for the REM component of sleep.

The catecholaminergic effects on sleep and wakefulness can be broken down in the following manner:

a. Drugs interfering with catecholaminergic transmission via the depletion or inhibition of the synthesis of the catecholamines.
b. α_1- and α_2-agonists and antagonists and β-adrenergic agonists and antagonists.
c. Dopamine 1 and 2 agonists and antagonists.

Studies support the hypothesis that norepinephrine neurons aid in regulating wakefulness and REM sleep. For example, an α_1-agonist (e.g., methoxamine) decreased REM sleep, whereas an α_1-antagonist increased REM sleep. Clonidine, primarily an α_2-agonist is associated with a sleep induction but inhibits deep NREM (stages 3 and 4) sleep. Involvement of the β-adrenergic receptors for regulation of sleep is ambiguous. Propranolol in humans often is associated with the side effect of insomnia that can be reversed by β-agonists and has been interpreted as suggesting these receptors are involved in regulation of REM sleep. It has been proposed that dopamine has a facilitative and active role in the sleep-wakefulness cycle. Waking appears to be a state maintained by D2 activation, whereas decreased D2 activity appears to promote sleep. The D1 receptor may be important in the regulation of REM sleep, but it is not important in initiation or timing of REM sleep.

Serotonin. Initially, serotonin was thought to be a sleep-promoting neurotransmitter or an "antiwaking" agent (9). The recognition of the numerous 5-HT receptor subtypes, often with unique anatomical distribution, has required that a more complex role for serotonin be developed. Current studies indicate that conditions for sleep are now met when the serotoninergic system becomes inactive. The serotonin agonists for the 5-HT_1 (via the 5-HT_{1A} and 5-HT_{1B} types at the hypothalamic level), 5-HT_2, and 5-HT_3 receptors cause wakefulness and inhibit sleep. Blockade of the 5-HT_2 receptors (e.g., the 5-HT_2 antagonist ritanserin) results in increased NREM sleep and inhibition of REM sleep. It has been proposed that the 5-HT_{1A} and 5- HT_2 may be involved in sleep by regulation of sleep-promoting substances in the hypothalamus. With the development of newer and more selective ligands for use in studying the numerous serotonin receptor subtypes (see also Chapter 14), a better understanding of the role of serotonin in sleep will evolve.

Histamine. It is proposed that histamine may have an involvement in wakefulness and REM sleep (10). Histamine-related functions in the CNS are regulated at post-synaptic sites by both the H_1 and H_2 receptors, whereas the H_3 receptors appear to be a presynaptic autoreceptor regulating the synthesis and release of histamine. These three receptors differ in molecular structure, distribution in the CNS, and physiologic responses. The H_1 receptor agonists and the H_3 receptor antagonists increase wakefulness, whereas the H_1 receptor antagonists (e.g., diphenhydramine) and H_3 receptor agonists have the opposite effect. The H_2 receptor agonists and antagonists have not been shown to have any effect on wakefulness or sleep parameters. The H_1 receptor agonists do not modify sleep induction or maintenance, although it does increase stage 4 NREM sleep and sleep latency. In controlled sleep laboratory studies, the H_1 receptor antagonists (e.g., diphenhydramine), when given before bedtime to normal subjects, have little effect on wakefulness. In equal doses given during the day, however, they increase drowsiness, with an increased tendency to sleep and impair performance.

Acetylcholine. The cholinergic system was the first neurotransmitter system shown to have a role in wakefulness and initiation of REM sleep (11). Because of the poor penetration of the cholinergic drugs into the CNS, the role of this system in sleep has relied on animal studies using microinjection into the brain, primarily in the area of the dorsal pontine tegmentum. Acetylcholine, cholinergic agonists (e.g., arecoline or bethanechol), and cholinesterase inhibitors are effective in the initiation of REM sleep from NREM sleep after microinjection. Conversely, administration of anticholinergic drugs (e.g., atropine or scopolamine) hinders the transition to REM sleep. Increase in the rate of discharge of these cholinergic cells (that activate the thalamus, cerebral cortex, and hippocampus) during REM sleep parallel the same pattern seen with arousal and alertness.

Adenosine. Adenosine acts as neurotransmitter in the mammalian nervous system (12). Because of the highly polar nature of adenosine, it also has to be injected into the brain (intracerebroventricular and preoptic). The stimulation of the adenosine A1 receptors with adenosine causes a hypnotic effect. It has been proposed that the hypnotic effect occurs via suppressing calcium efflux into presynaptic nerve terminals and decreasing the amount of neurotransmitters released into the synapse in brain regions critical for sleep. This apparent induction and maintenance of sleep is associated with increases in both NREM and REM sleep. Consistent with the above proposal is that blocking of the central adenosine receptors with methylxanthines (e.g., caffeine or theophylline) is associated with wakefulness and a reduction in total sleep time. Studies also suggest that some of the actions of the benzodiazepines may be related to their ability to inhibit adenosine uptake, leading to downregulation of central adenosine receptors.

γ-Aminobutyric acid. γ-Aminobutyric acid (GABA) probably represents the most important inhibitory transmitter of the mammalian CNS (also see Chapter 15) (13). Both types of GABAergic inhibition (pre- and postsynaptic) use the same $GABA_A$ receptor subtype, which acts by regulation of the chloride channel of the neuronal membrane. A second GABA receptor type, $GABA_B$, that is a G protein–coupled receptor is not considered to be important in understanding the mechanism of hypnotics. Activation of a $GABA_A$ receptor by an agonist increases the inhibitory synaptic response of central neurons to GABA through hyperpolarization. Because many, if not all, central neurons receive some GABAergic input, this leads to a mechanism by which CNS activity can be depressed. For example, if the GABAergic interneurons are activated by an agonist that inhibits the monoaminergic structures of the brainstem, hypnotic activity will be observed. The specific neuronal structures in different brain regions affected by $GABA_A$ agonist continues to be better defined.

Neurohumoral Modulators

Sleep and circadian rhythmicity, both of which are controlled by the CNS, can exhibit significant effects on hormonal release. Many of the hypophyseal hormones follow a circadian rhythm; however, both growth hormone (GH) and prolactin (PRL) appear to be the most closely linked with sleep. This suggests that these hormones may affect sleep and contribute to the maintenance and quality of sleep.

Growth hormone and prolactin. In normal adult subjects, the plasma level of GH remains very stable at a low level; however, a secretory pulse of GH occurs in association with the first phase of NREM sleep (14). Most of the GH pulse secretions occur during NREM sleep, and a good correlation has been observed between the amount of GH secreted and the duration of NREM sleep. Studies in healthy elderly men (age, 67–84 years) have observed that a decreased secretion of GH in the elderly parallels the decrease in NREM sleep and may be related to the decrease in sleep observed in the elderly.

Regardless of the time of day, sleep onset has a stimulatory effect on PRL release (14). Maximal effect is observed, however, when sleep and circadian effects are superimposed. Because of pulse-like secretions of PRL, there seems to be a relationship between the low PRL levels and initiation of REM sleep or nocturnal awakenings, especially in the elderly.

Melatonin

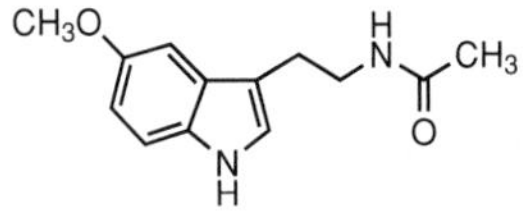

CH_3O — N–H — CH_3 — O — N–H

Melatonin, at times referred to as the "hormone of darkness," normally is secreted during the night (15–17). It is synthesized in the pineal gland, and its secretion is controlled by the suprachiasmatic nucleus, following an endogenous circadian rhythm. Studies indicate that melatonin may have effects on circadian rhythm and sleep processes. The presence of a pharmacologically specific receptor for melatonin in which the molecular structure is known are referred to as MT_1, MT_2, and MT_3 receptors. The MT_1 and MT_2 receptors are high-affinity G protein–coupled receptors, whereas MT_3 is a form of quinone reductase. The MT_1 receptor appears to be primarily involved in initiating sleep, whereas the MT_2 receptor appears to mediate melatonins effect in the eye, circadian rhythm, and vascular effects (18). The importance of MT_3, although widely distributed in different tissues, is currently unknown. The normal physiological concentration of melatonin observed at night is approximately 100 to 200 pg/mL, and oral doses of 0.1 to 0.3 mg of melatonin are adequate to obtain these concentrations even though melatonin frequently is given at doses of 1 to 10 mg to obtain "supraphysiological" levels. These higher doses may be the reason for some of the side effects not currently associated with the melatonin receptors. Melatonin is most effective in young individuals and appears to be less effective in elderly individuals (possibly because of a decreased number of receptors). Melatonin causes a phase shift of approximately 1 hour per day. This means that the use of melatonin in the morning can delay the onset of evening sleepiness, whereas melatonin taken in the evening has been associated with faster onset of sleep and increased total sleep time. Melatonin is sold as a food supplement in the United States, but it has become popular for use as a hypnotic and for alleviating jet lag (a flight across five or more time zones) and helping to resynchronize individuals who have difficulty adapting to night-shift work.

CNS PEPTIDES. Several CNS peptides have been associated with regulation of sleep and wakefulness. Currently, the hypocretins (orexins) are of greatest interest (19,20). They consist of two neuropeptides, Hcrt-1 and Hcrt-2, that are synthesized by neurons in the posterolateral hypothalamus. Initially, these peptides were shown to be involved in the regulation of arousal, motor tone, locomotion, regulation of appetite, and neuroendocrine and autonomic functions. Recent research has indicated that these peptides also are involved in the regulation of sleep and wakefulness, especially in relation to narcolepsy. It has been observed that approximately 80% of patients with narcolepsy had low or undetectable levels of Hcrt-1, suggesting that a deficiency or abnormality in hypocretin neurotransmission may play a pivotal role in this disease. The Hcrt-1 is a 33-amino-acid, carboxy-amidated peptide with an N-terminal pyroglutamyl residue and two intrachain disulfide bonds, whereas the Hcrt-2 is a C-terminally amidated, linear peptide of 28 amino acids. The hypocretins bind at two G protein–coupled receptors with high affinity and have excitatory effects on the neurons. It has been proposed that hypocretin receptor antagonists may be useful in the treatment of insomnia, although no drug is currently in clinical studies based on this concept.

TESTING AND DEVELOPMENT OF NEW HYPNOTICS

As presented in the earlier section, a number of potential receptors can be identified that are associated with causing sleep and have the potential to be developed into a hypnotic. Initially, animal tests have been used for identifying new hypnotic drugs. In vitro receptor binding studies can then be used for screening of drugs that bind with improved specificity. The animal assays basically measure varying levels of CNS depression instead of sleep. The assumption is that CNS depression will relate to clinical hypnosis, although exceptions commonly occur. Common assays in mice or rats include an increase in sleeping time, a loss of righting reflex, rotorod impairment, decreased activity in an activity cage, or potentiation of other CNS depressants. The observed pharmacological effects of many drugs in this class usually are dose related such that small doses cause sedation, larger doses cause hypnosis, and still larger doses may bring about surgical anesthesia.

Larger animals, including rats, cats, and monkeys, are studied in a sleep laboratory. In these studies, electrophysiologic and electroencephalographic measurements are obtained and often are helpful in gaining information about the site of action of CNS depressants as well as about induced sleep patterns. Drug discrimination studies also have been useful in differentiating sites of action of CNS depressants.

Guidelines for the clinical evaluation of hypnotic drugs have been developed by the U.S. Food and Drug Administration for specific evaluation of this class of drugs. Human sleep laboratory studies have become increasingly valuable in determining a range of efficacy and defining an optimal dose. Because sleep laboratory studies are under closely controlled conditions, they are capable of continuous electrophysiologic measurement throughout the night. This is then followed by objective measurement of pre- and postsleep results to assess effectiveness and withdrawal effects of new hypnotics. The sleep laboratory studies coupled with clinical studies based on patients' subjective estimates of efficacy provide a thorough and clinically relevant approach for developing a new hypnotic (21).

CLASSIFICATION OF HYPNOTICS

Introduction to Classes of Hypnotics

The hypnotic drugs are not characterized by common structural features. Instead, a wide variety of chemical compounds have been used in clinical therapy. An arbitrary classification is as follows:

- $GABA_A$ receptor agonists
  - Benzodiazepines
  - Imidazopyridines and cyclopyrrolones
  - Pyrazolopyrimidines
  - Barbiturates

Chloral
Melatonin receptor agonists
Antihistamines
Antidepressants
Herbal preparations

Benzodiazepines

Benzodiazepines are used as daytime anxiolytics, sleep inducers, anesthetics, anticonvulsants (also known as antiseizure agents), and muscle relaxants; they will be discussed in depth in Chapters 20 and 22. Examination of the basic pharmacodynamic properties of the benzodiazepines (defined as receptor-specific binding activity) show that the clinically useful benzodiazepines exhibit comparable sedative activity at therapeutically comparable doses (Fig. 19.1) (13). The use of a specific benzodiazepine as a hypnotic is based primarily on pharmacokinetic properties and marketing considerations. Hypnotics are unusual in that they normally are given as a single dose. The following variables will determine how well a benzodiazepine will work as a hypnotic: 1) Is acute tolerance developed to the benzodiazepine that will diminish CNS effects before the drug is eliminated from the CNS, 2) is redistribution of the benzodiazepine from the CNS to other tissues very rapid, and 3) is there a rapid drug elimination by biotransformation and the metabolite active? The benzodiazepines that are specifically promoted as sleep inducers are listed in Table 19.1 (22); however, it is important to keep in mind that depending on the dose, any benzodiazepine may be used for its hypnotic effect.

Mechanism of Action

The initial studies suggesting a possible involvement of the benzodiazepines with GABA provided a basis for understanding the pharmacological effects of this class of

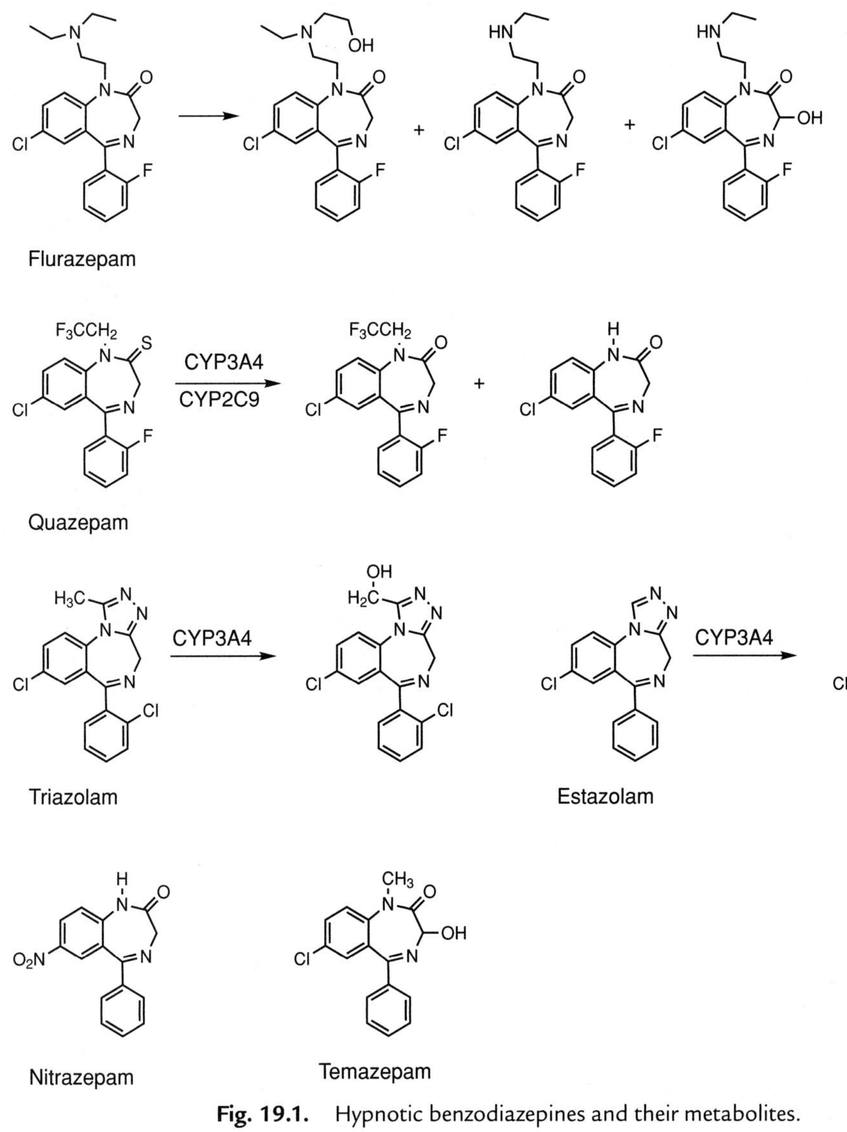

Flurazepam

Quazepam

CYP3A4
CYP2C9

Triazolam

CYP3A4

Estazolam

CYP3A4

Nitrazepam

Temazepam

Fig. 19.1. Hypnotic benzodiazepines and their metabolites.

Table 19.1. Some Properties and Pharmacokinetics of the Benzodiazepine Sedative-Hypnotics

Parameters	Estazolam	Flurazepam	Quazepam	Temazepam	Triazolam
Trade name	Prosom	Dalmane	Doral	Ristoril	Halcion
Log P (calc)[a]	3.3 ± 0.9	4.0 ± 0.7	4.1 ± 0.8	2.2 ± 0.6	2.7 ± 0.1
Log D (pH 7)[a]	3.3	1.4	4.1	2.2	2.7
Oral bioavailability (%)	Rapid	Rapid	Rapid	>80	86 (75–95)
Protein binding (%)	93	97	95	>96	89
Volume of distribution (L/kg)			5.0–8.6	0.8–1.4	0.8–1.3
Elimination half-life (hours)	10–24	2.4	39 (25–41)	8–15	4 (1.5–5.5) ~7 (obese)
Major metabolites (half-life hours)	4-OH (inactive)	N-desethyl (47–100) N-1-OH-ethyl (2–4)	2-oxo (39) N-desalkyl (47–100)	O-glucuronide	Hydroxymethyl (50% active)
T_{max} (hours)	0.5–6.0	0.5–1.0	<2	1–2	<2
Excretion (%)	Urine as O-glucuronide <5 unchanged	Urine as O-glucuronides	Urine as O-glucuronides feces 23	80 urine as O-glucuronide feces 12 <2 unchanged	80 urine as O-glucuronides <2 unchanged
Cytochrome isoforms	3A4	3A4	3A4 2C9	—	3A4
Hypnotic dose (mg)	5–10	5–10	1–3	15–30	0.125–0.5
IC50 (nmol/L)	9	15	30	16	4

[a]Chemical Abstracts, American Chemical Society, calculated using Advanced Chemistry Development (ACD/Labs) Software V8.14 Ser Solaris (1994–2006 ACD/Labs).

drugs. The identification of specific, high-affinity binding sites for the benzodiazepines on the $GABA_A$ receptors was an important advance (23,24). The majority of $GABA_A$ receptors are made up of a mixture to subunit types (α_{1-6}, β_{1-3}, γ_{1-3}, θ, ε, δ, and π) with the majority of receptors composed of α, β, and γ subunits in the ratio of 1:2:1 (13). The major combinations of subunits are $\alpha_1\beta_2\gamma_2$ (~60%) and $\alpha_2\beta_3\gamma_2$ (~15–20%) of the $GABA_A$ receptors. Studies suggest that drugs interacting with the α_1 subunit receptor are involved in the modulation of sedative, amnesic, and seizure protection, whereas drugs binding with the α_2 subunits receptors provide anxiolytic and myorelaxant properties. The current generation of benzodiazepines bind with comparable affinity at both $GABA_A$ receptor subtypes. It has been proposed that compounds specific for the α_2 subunit would be "nonsedative," whereas compounds specific for α_1 would primarily be sedative-hypnotic (13). All of the benzodiazepines affect the normal sleep stages. They increase total sleep and EEG fast activity, and they decrease nocturnal wakefulness, body movements, number of awakenings, sleep latency (the time required to fall asleep), and stages 3 and 4 sleep (NREM). On withdrawal of the drug, a gradual return to baseline values of NREM sleep returns. They also cause a mild suppression of REM sleep, especially during the first third of the night, with rapid return to baseline on withdrawal.

Pharmacodynamic/Pharmacokinetic Balance

The onset of sedative or hypnotic activity of intravenously administered benzodiazepines is rapid, with a range of 15 to 30 seconds (a single circulation time) to a few minutes, depending on the patient's sensitivity, pharmacological response, and size of the dose. The speed of onset of action by orally administered benzodiazepines can be very dependent on the drug dosage form. For example, when first introduced in the United States, temazepam was formulated as a hard gelatin capsule. This formulation had a very slow rate of absorption following oral administration, with peak plasma levels reaching on average of 1.8 to 4.7 hours after dosing and exhibiting little effect on sleep induction, with most of its effect on sleep maintenance. Total wake time was slightly decreased with short-term drug administration and was similar to baseline with intermediate and long-term use. Temazepam has since been reformulated as a tablet or in a soft gelatin form. These formulations are now more effective in improving sleep by decreasing the time to sleep induction and improved sleep maintenance (25). Among the oral benzodiazepines, formulations specifically indicated for the treatment of insomnia, flurazepam is absorbed most rapidly, triazolam has an intermediate rate of absorption, and temazepam is absorbed slowly and may be given 1 to 2 hours before bedtime.

Hypnotics can be used for short-term (1 week), intermediate-term (2 weeks), and long-term (≥4 weeks) periods. The vast majority of the benzodiazepines are effective for inducing and maintaining sleep when used initially or for a short term Differences are observed when they are used for longer terms. and the proper balance between pharmacodynamics and pharmacokinetic effects become very important.

The pharmacokinetic profile for each of the benzodiazepines is shown in Table 19.1. The benzodiazepines that are slowly eliminated or are metabolized to slowly eliminated active metabolites can be used as hypnotics. For example, flurazepam is primarily metabolized by

N-dealkylation and 1-hydroxylation (26), and quazepam is metabolized by oxidative loss of sulfur to oxygen and N-dealkylation (Fig. 19.1) (27). Both drugs form active metabolites that are slowly eliminated and are associated with the slow development of tolerance to the hypnotic effects. These compounds exhibit good efficacy as hypnotics with long-term use and are associated with little loss of initial effectiveness. Minimal rebound insomnia or rebound anxiety is observed when the drug is withdrawn because of the presence of the active metabolite. As a result of their slow elimination, however, the presence of active drug or active metabolite in blood and brain tissue is responsible for the residual effects of hypnotics in the daytime. These effects may consist of "hangover" effects and oversedation, which may be so severe, especially in elderly patients, as to cause tremors, ataxia, and confusion. A good example of this is flurazepam, which undergoes N-dealkylation to N-desethylflurazepam (26). This metabolite has its own antianxiety and sedative activities and a long plasma half-life of 47 to 100 hours. Nitrazepam, a hypnotic drug used in Europe, has a moderately long elimination half-life of approximately 30 hours and may cause hangover effects as well as accumulation on repeated use. The presence of active drug or active metabolite in blood and brain tissue is responsible for the residual effects of hypnotics in the daytime.

On development of the newer triazolobenzodiazepines, such as triazolam and estazolam, with high receptor binding affinity and more rapid elimination, it was anticipated that the problem of daytime sedation would be eliminated. The duration of action for triazolam, which has an ultrashort half-life of less than 4 hours because of biotransformation to inactive metabolites (primarily hydroxylation of the triazole methyl group) and elimination as O-glucuronides (Fig. 19.1) (28). The average oral bioavailability for triazolam was 86%; however, its mean absolute oral bioavailability is 44%. This difference is suggestive of first-pass metabolism in the gut wall by CYP3A4. Moreover, because triazolam is metabolized primarily by hepatic and intestinal CYP3A4, coadministration with grapefruit juice increased its peak plasma concentration by 30%, which was associated with increased drowsiness. Temazepam is rapidly metabolized because of direct conjugation of the 3-hydroxyl with glucuronic acid (29). Triazolam and estazolam have gained popularity as sleep inducers, especially in elderly individuals. Sleep laboratory studies, however, show that these compounds rapidly lose much of their initial effectiveness, often after only 1 week of continuous nightly administration. Estazolam is metabolized primarily by CYP3A4 to its 4-hydroxy metabolite, which is excreted in urine as its O-glucuronide (Fig. 19.1). The effectiveness of other benzodiazepines have been shown to decrease when used long term. In addition, these compounds are associated with hyperexcitability that is exhibited as daytime anxiety, tenseness, or panic and early morning insomnia (25).

Although there exist some disadvantages to using the benzodiazepines as hypnotics, they have other advantages, primarily their relative safety. Fatalities resulting from benzodiazepine overdosage alone are rare. When taken together with other drugs, intoxication probably depends largely on the type and quantity of the benzodiazepine (30). Caution must be taken when coadministering oral benzodiazepines with CYP3A4 inhibitors, particularly in patients with other causes for increases in bioavailability, such as advanced age and liver cirrhosis. In addition, benzodiazepines do not cause significant hepatic enzyme induction in humans; therefore, their tendency to interact with other drugs is less than that seen with other hypnotics. The benzodiazepines are still extensively used and are well tolerated as hypnotics. Because of the modest side effects discussed, however, the use of the benzodiazepines as hypnotics has decreased, and the use of the newer nonbenzodiazepine drugs has been increasing (1).

Nonbenzodiazepine $GABA_A$ Agonists

Historically, benzodiazepines have been the mainstay for treatment of sleeping disorders, yet they have many shortcomings. A new group of sedative-hypnotic agents similar to the benzodiazepines—zaleplon, zolpidem, and zopiclone—have been developed with affinity for the GABA receptor complex (31). This produces a more efficacious clinical profile with fewer side effects than the benzodiazepines. Zolpidem, zopiclone, and zaleplon (the "Z" drugs) are structurally distinct, nonbenzodiazepine structures (see Figs. 19.3–19.4) (32) and are being used as short-acting sedative-hypnotics in the United States and Europe. They act at the $GABA_A$ high-affinity receptors comparable to the benzodiazepines but with different subunit specificity (Table 19.2) (31). Because of variation in binding to the GABA receptor subunits, these three compounds show subtle differences in their effect on sleep stages and as antiepileptics, anxiolytics, and amnestics.

Some generalities associated with these "Z" compounds is that they are very lipophilic, facilitating their rapid absorption and the absence of active metabolites in the plasma and brain tissue. They can be administered orally without regard to meals, but administration with a high-fat meal before sleep should be avoided because of a potential decreased rate of drug absorption and, therefore, decreased (delayed onset) efficacy in initiating sleep. These drugs are dependent on the liver for metabolism to more water-soluble ionic metabolites for their rapid renal clearance, minimizing any accumulation or residual drug effect. Their duration of action and plasma levels can be related to their individual pharmacokinetic profile, which subsequently determines the time course of drug effect and their dosages in elderly patients, in patients with hepatic insufficiency, or in patients with renal compromise. Each of these compounds has a unique pharmacokinetic profile, with different bioavailabilities, volume of distributions, and elimination half-lives (Table 19.2).

Table 19.2. Some Properties and Pharmacokinetics of the Nonbenzodiazepine Sedative-Hypnotics

Parameters	Zolpidem	Zaleplon	Eszopiclone	Ramelteon
Trade name	Ambien	Sonata	Lunesta	Rozerem
cLog P[a]	3.1 ± 0.6	0.9 ± 1.2	0.7 ± 0.8	2.6 ± 0.3
Log D (pH 7)[a]	2.9	0.9	0.5	2.6
Oral bioavailability (%)	72	31	75–80	<2
Protein binding (%)	90	60	52–60	82
Volume of distribution (L/kg)	0.54–0.68	1.3	1.3–1.6	
Elimination half-life (hours)	1.7–2.6 ~10 hepatic insufficiency	~1	3.5–6.5	~2
Major metabolites	Oxidation to carboxylic acids	N-deethylation 5-oxo	N-desmethyl N-oxide	Oxid alcohol
T_{max} (hours)	1.5	~1	~1	~1
Excretion (%)	56 urine 37 feces <1 unchanged	Urine <1 unchanged	75 urine 10 unchanged	84 urine 4 feces
Cytochrome isoforms	3A4 2C9, 1A2 minor	3A4	2E1 (40%) 3A4 (60%)	1A2 2C,3A4
Hypnotic dose (mg)	5–10	5–10	1–3	
IC50 (nmol/L)	13 $\alpha_1\beta_2\gamma_2$ 131 $\alpha_2\beta_1\gamma_2$	66 $\alpha_1\beta_2\gamma_2$ 830 $\alpha_2\beta_1\gamma_2$	19 $\alpha_1\beta_2\gamma_2$ 33 $\alpha_2\beta_1\gamma_2$ (racemic zopiclone)	

[a]Chemical Abstracts, American Chemical Society, calculated using Advanced Chemistry Development (ACD/Labs) Software V8.14 Ser Solaris (1994–2006 ACD/Labs).

Zaleplon has a rapid elimination, so fewer residual side effects occur after taking a single dose at bedtime. By comparison, zolpidem and zopiclone have a more delayed rate of elimination, which may result with a prolonged drug effect. This can produce residual sedation and side effects but may be useful for sustained treatment of insomnia, with less waking during the night. There also are differences in potency based on plasma concentrations, suggesting that differences exist in binding to the GABA receptor complex. Although zaleplon has a much lower bioavailability (~30%), the treatment dose is similar to those of zolpidem and zopiclone (bioavailability, ~70%) because of the increased potency of zaleplon. The pharmacokinetics and pharmacodynamics of zaleplon, zolpidem, and zopiclone are significantly different from those of benzodiazepines (Table 19.2). Zaleplon may be best indicated for the delayed onset of sleep, zolpidem and zopiclone may be better indicated for maintaining a complete night's sleep. Only the patient's symptoms and response to treatment will dictate the best course of treatment.

Although these compounds show differences from the benzodiazepines in some pharmacological tests, with a reduced ability to cause physical dependence and minimal abuse potential, these drugs are listed as Schedule IV controlled substances.

Specific Drugs

IMIDAZOPYRIDINE

Zolpidem tartrate. Zolpidem exhibits a high selectivity for the α_1 subunit. Its good bioavailability of 72% and rapid onset of action of approximately 1.4 hours following oral absorption can be attributed to its weak base ($pK_a = 6.2$) and high lipophilicity (mlog P = 3.85). Its pharmacokinetic profile is characterized by rapid absorption from the gastrointestinal tract and a short elimination half-life because of rapid oxidative metabolism to inactive carboxylic acid metabolites (Fig. 19.2). Zolpidem undergoes CYP3A4 (major), CYP2D9, and CYP1A2 hydroxylation of the aryl methyl groups, followed by further oxidation by aldehyde

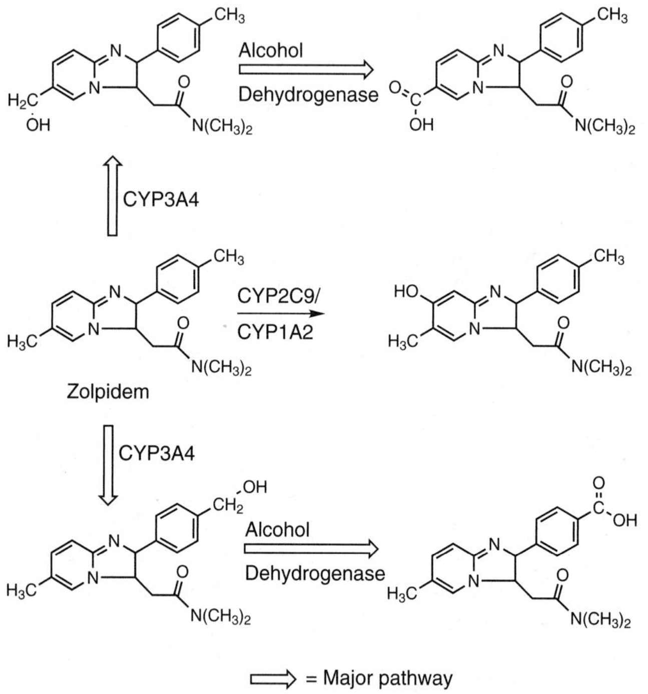

Zolpidem
CYP3A4
Alcohol Dehydrogenase
CYP2C9/ CYP1A2
⟹ = Major pathway

Fig. 19.2. Zolpidem and its metabolism pathways.

dehydrogenase to the ionic carboxylic acids, which are readily eliminated in the urine (33). Zolpidem demonstrates linear (dose-proportional) kinetics in the dose range of 5 to 20 mg. Although protein binding was 90%, no drug accumulation was observed following nightly dosing with 20-mg zolpidem tartrate tablets for 2 weeks. Food can prolong the time to peak concentration from 1.4 to 2.2 hours without affecting the half-life. These results suggest that for faster sleep onset, zolpidem should not be administered with or immediately after a meal. In the elderly, the dose should be 5 mg, because the elimination half-life is increased by 50% (from ~2 to ~3 hours). No accumulation was observed in elderly subjects following nightly oral dosing of 10 mg for 1 week. In patients with hepatic insufficiency, the plasma concentration doubled with an increase in the elimination half-life from approximately 2 to approximately 10 hours (range, 4–25 hours). Therefore, dosing should be modified in patients with hepatic insufficiency. No dosage adjustment should be necessary in patients with compromised renal function. Zolpidem is not hemodialyzable, but it does cross the placenta and into breast milk. Because of its longer elimination half-life (when compared to zaleplon), it may be preferred when sleep maintenance is a primary concern.

PYRAZOLOPYRIMIDINE

Zaleplon. Zaleplon displays a unique binding profile with $GABA_A$ that is distinct from the benzodiazepines but similar to that of zolpidem (31). Because of it greater potency for $GABA_A$, the starting dose for zaleplon is comparable to that of zolpidem. It is rapidly absorbed, with a log P of 1.23, although only 30% of the dose is bioavailable because of rapid first-pass metabolism via liver cytosolic aldehyde oxidase/xanthine oxidase (molybdenum hydroxylases) to its major ring oxidation product, 5-oxo-zaleplon metabolite (Fig. 19.3) (34). The minor metabolism pathways include N-dealkylation from microsomal oxidation via CYP3A4 to N-desethyl-zaleplon and N-desethyl-5-oxo-zaleplon. It is rapidly metabolized by the liver, with an elimination half-life of approximately 1 hour. The oxidative metabolites are inactive, conjugated with glucuronic acid, and eliminated in the urine. Inhibitors of CYP3A4 and aldehyde oxidase can increase the plasma concentration of zaleplon significantly, although this usually does not require dosage modification. Zaleplon does not accumulate with once-daily administration and displays linear pharmacokinetics in the therapeutic range. The elimination half-life of zaleplon is increased in patients with hepatic insufficiency, requiring an adjustment in dosage. High-fat meals increase the time to peak concentration and decrease the plasma concentration without affecting the half-life. These results suggest that for faster sleep onset, zaleplon should not be administered either with or immediately after a meal, which increases the time to reach peak plasma concentrations. In short-term studies (2–5 weeks), zaleplon has been shown to improve sleep quality with minimal adverse effects and no significant rebound insomnia on stopping the drug. Because of its short elimination half-life, zaleplon is quite good at getting people to sleep but is not as good at keeping people asleep. Unlike with zolpidem and eszopiclone, it has been proposed that if the patient awakens in the middle of the night (with ≥4 hours of sleep time remaining), another dose of zaleplon can be taken (35).

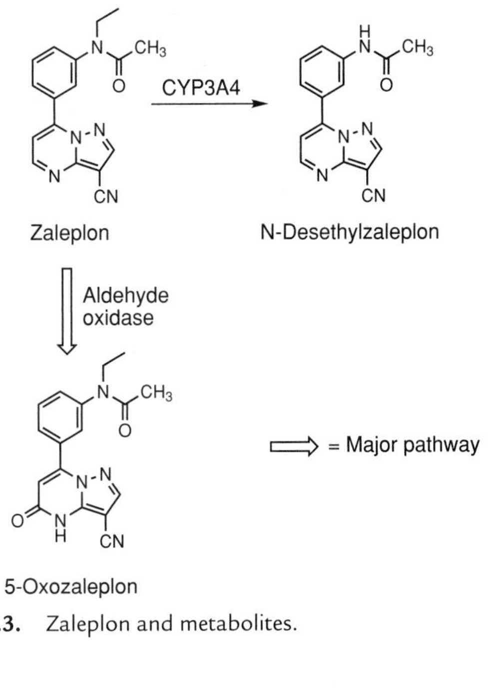

Zaleplon —CYP3A4→ N-Desethylzaleplon

Zaleplon ⇓ Aldehyde oxidase → 5-Oxozaleplon

⟹ = Major pathway

Fig. 19.3. Zaleplon and metabolites.

CYCLOPYRROLONE

Eszopiclone. Zoplicone was originally marketed as a racemic mixture; however, because the sedative activity is primarily associated with the S-isomer, only the S-isomer is currently marketed in the United States (as esozopliclone) (36). It is soluble in dilute mineral acids. Unlike zolpidem and zaleplon, eszoplicone is not as specific for the α_1 subunit of $GABA_A$, but it binds broadly, like the benzodiazepines (Table 19.2). Its pharmacological and pharmacodynamic activities, however, are more closely related to those of the nonbenzodiazepines (32,37). It is rapidly absorbed, with an oral bioavailability of approximately 80%, reaching peak concentrations in 1 h and having a relatively long elimination half-life of approximately 6 hours (Table 19.2). Eszopliclone is primarily metabolized to (S)-zoplicone N-oxide and (S)-N-desmethylzoplicone by the CYP3A4 (Fig. 19.4). (S)-N-desmethylzopiclone binds to GABA receptors with substantially lower potency than eszopiclone, and (S)-zopiclone-N-oxide shows no significant binding to this receptor. It does not accumulate with once-daily administration, and it exhibits linear (dose-proportional) pharmacokinetics over the range of 1 to 6 mg. Eszopiclone is weakly bound to plasma protein (52–60%), suggesting that eszopiclone distribution should not be affected by drug–drug interactions caused by protein binding. Up to 75% of an oral dose of racemic zopiclone is excreted in the urine, primarily as metabolites. A similar excretion

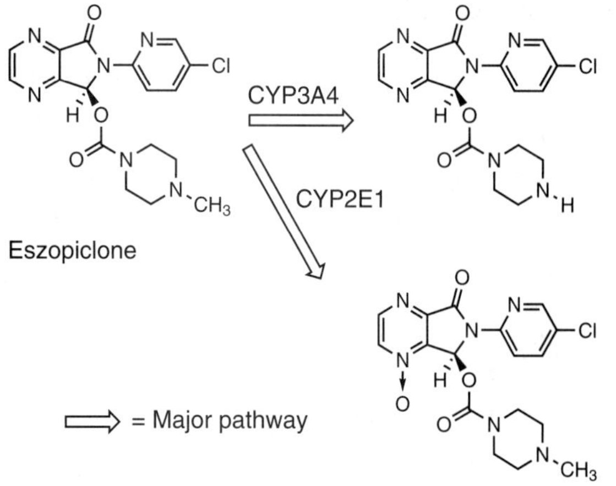

Fig. 19.4. Eszopliclone and its metabolites.

profile would be expected for eszopiclone. Less than 10% of the orally administered eszopiclone dose is excreted in the urine as unchanged drug. After a high-fat meal, peak plasma concentrations can be delayed by approximately 1 hour without affecting its half-life. The effects of eszoplicone on sleep onset may be reduced if it is taken either with or immediately after a high-fat/heavy meal. In elderly subjects, the elimination half-life was prolonged to approximately 5 to 9 hours. Therefore, in elderly patients, the starting dose should be decreased to 1 mg, and the dose should not exceed 2 mg. No dose adjustment is necessary in patients with renal impairment, because less than 10% of the orally administered eszopiclone dose is excreted in the urine as parent drug. Although no pharmacokinetic or pharmacodynamic or drug interactions have been reported for eszopiclone, potent inhibitors of CYP3A4 could increase plasma levels of eszopiclone. Eszopiclone does not alter the clearance of drugs metabolized by common CYP450 enzymes. Potential pharmacodynamic interactions (additive pharmacological effects) with CNS depressants such as alcohol, anticonvulsants, antihistamines, antidepressants, or other psychotropic drugs could occur. Dosage adjustment may be necessary when eszopiclone is administered with CNS depressants; concomitant use with alcohol should be avoided.

The primary advantage of eszoplicone is that it has been shown to be effective in chronic insomnia (long-term treatment) in measures of sleep latency, total sleep time, and wake time after sleep onset without development of tolerance (38). Eszoplicone would appear to be most effectively used for patients who tend to awaken during the night rather than patients for whom the primary problem is initiating sleep (35).

Barbiturates

The barbiturates have a different pharmacological and binding profile from that of the benzodiazepines. They exert a depressant effect on the cerebrospinal axis and depress neuronal activity as well as skeletal muscle, smooth muscle, and cardiac muscle activity. Depending on the compound, dose, and route of administration, the barbiturates can produce different degrees of CNS depression and have found use as sedatives, hypnotics, anticonvulsants, or anesthetics.

Currently, the barbiturates get minimal use as sedatives and hypnotics (especially compared to the benzodiazepines) because of higher toxicity. This is associated with their ability to cause greater CNS depression and their ability to induce many of the liver drug-metabolizing enzymes. In addition, the barbiturates cause tolerance and, often, dependence. Even with all these disadvantages, the barbiturates continue to find occasional clinical applications as sedatives and hypnotics. Their primary use, however, is as general anesthetics (see Chapter 18) and as antiseizure drugs (see Chapter 20). Primarily because of historical convention, the general chemistry, structure–activity relationships, and metabolism of the barbiturates will be covered in this section.

Barbiturates exert their action on the central synaptic transmission process associated with $GABA_A$ (13). A paradoxical effect of barbiturates occurs in which small doses bring about hyperexcitation and agitation instead of sedation. This is because the barbiturate concentration is not sufficient to depress the reticular activating system but is able to impede the inhibitory synapses that normally are present within the cortex. The barbiturates act on the reticular activating system and on the limbic, hypothalamic, and thalamic synaptic systems (39).

Mechanism of Action

The effects of the barbiturates is marked by a decrease in functional activities in the brain. At therapeutic doses, the barbiturates enhance the GABAergic inhibitory response in a mechanism similar to that of the benzodiazepines (i.e., by influencing conductance at the chloride channel). At higher concentrations, the barbiturates can potentiate the $GABA_A$-mediated chloride ion conductance and enhance both GABA and benzodiazepine binding. Therefore, the barbiturates and benzodiazepines display cross-tolerance, and this can be seen with the barbiturates exhibiting weak anxiolytics and muscle relaxant properties. The barbiturate binding site is different from the benzodiazepines and is believed to occur at the picrotoxin binding site on the chloride channel. These drugs affect the transport of sugars and are noted for their ability to induce liver microsomal enzymes that lead to an increased rate of biotransformation of many commonly used drugs, including the barbiturates. The biochemical effects of these drugs have been summarized elsewhere (40).

Pharmacological Effects

The effects of barbiturates on the sleep pattern are comparable to those of benzodiazepines. In short-term studies, the barbiturates are equally effective as the benzodiazepines. Again, the importance of the pharmacokinetic properties of the barbiturates determines their usefulness

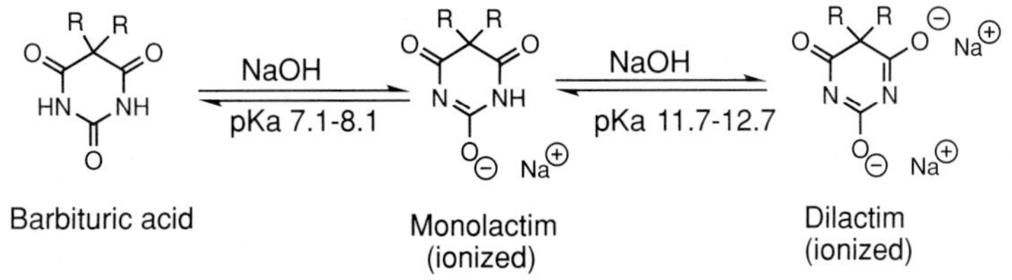

Fig. 19.5. pH-dependent tautomerization of barbiturates.

as hypnotics. The barbiturates that are slowly eliminated are capable of producing hangover and persistent psychomotor impairment. For example, amobarbital was once extensively used as a hypnotic but is no longer commercially available for oral dosing as a hypnotic (although it remains available in Tuinal, a combination of amobarbital and secobarbital) because of excessive daytime sedation. Even amobarbital, however, still finds clinical application as a parenteral formulation when used in the "intracarotid amobarbital procedure" to determine lateralization of language and memory before surgery (41).

The barbiturates also cause a physical dependence different from the opioid narcotics. In an individual addicted to barbiturates, the barbiturates should not be withdrawn abruptly but, rather, tapered slowly. Sudden withdrawal of the barbiturates can precipitate extreme agitation and grand mal seizures. This can lead to a spasm of the respiratory musculature, producing impaired respiration, cyanosis, and possibly, death (42). As a rule, drug dependence is followed by tolerance, in which increasing doses are required to obtain the same pharmacological effect. Because barbiturates cause tolerance and, often, dependence, their use as a hypnotic rarely is justified.

Structure–Activity Relationships

Hundreds of barbiturates have been synthesized on a trial-and-error basis. Although many structural features required for hypnotic activity have been recorded, no clear correlation between structure and activity has emerged. In 1951, Sandberg (43) made his fundamental postulation that to possess good hypnotic activity, a barbituric acid must be a weak acid and must have a lipid/water partition coefficient between certain limits. Therefore, only the 5,5,-disubstituted barbituric acids, the 5,5,-disubstituted thiobarbituric acids, and the 1,5,5-trisubstituted barbituric acids possess acceptable hypnotic, anticonvulsant, or anesthetic activity. All other substitution patterns, such as 5-monosubstituted barbituric acids, 1,3-disubstituted barbituric acids, or 1,3,5,5-tetrasubstituted barbituric acids, are inactive or produce convulsions.

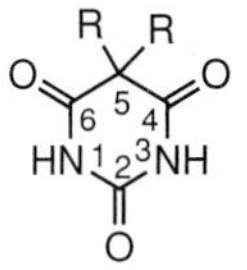

pK$_A$ AND STRUCTURE OF THE BARBITURATES. The 5,5-disubstituted barbituric acid contains three lactam groups that can undergo pH dependent lactim–lactam tautomerization, as shown in Figure 19.5.

Ultraviolet spectroscopic studies with 5,5-disubstituted barbituric acids (44) indicated that in aqueous solutions, the dominant forms are either the dioxo tautomeric form (i.e., monolactam in alkaline medium) or the trioxo tautomeric form (barbituric acid structure in acid medium). The acidity of barbiturates in aqueous solution depends on the number of substituents attached to barbituric acid. The 5,5-disubstituted barbituric acids, 5,5-disubstituted thiobarbituric acids, and 1,5,5-trisubstituted barbituric acids are relatively weak acids, and salts of these barbiturates are easily formed by treatment with bases. The pK_a of 5,5-disubstituted barbituric acids ranges from 7.1 to 8.1 (44). The 5,5-disubstituted barbituric acids can undergo a second ionization, having pK_a values in the range of 11.7 to 12.7. The alkali metal salts of the barbiturates coupled with their highly lipophilic character will cause chemical incompatibility reactions (precipitation) when these compounds are mixed with acid salts of weakly basic amines.

5,5-DISUBSTITUTION. As the number of carbon atoms at the fifth carbon position increases, the lipophilic character of the substituted barbituric acids also increases (44). Branching, unsaturation, replacement of alicyclic or aromatic substituents for alkyl substituents, and introduction of halogen into the alkyl substituents all increase the lipid solubility of the barbituric acid derivatives. A limit is reached, however, because as the lipophilic character increases, the hydrophilic character decreases. Although lipophilic character determines the ability of compounds to cross the blood-brain barrier, hydrophilic character also is important, because it determines solubility in biological fluids and ensures that the compound reaches the blood-brain barrier. Introduction of polar groups into the alkyl substituent decreases lipid solubility below desirable levels. Modifications at this position by variation of the alkyl substituents were of primary importance in the development of barbiturates with short (3–4 hours) to intermediate (6–8 hours) duration of action. These barbiturates were once extensively used as sedatives and hypnotics.

SUBSTITUTION ON NITROGEN. Substitution of one imide hydrogen by alkyl groups increases lipid solubility (44). The result is a quicker onset and a shorter duration of activity. As the size of the N-alkyl substituent increases (methyl → ethyl → propyl), the lipid solubility increases

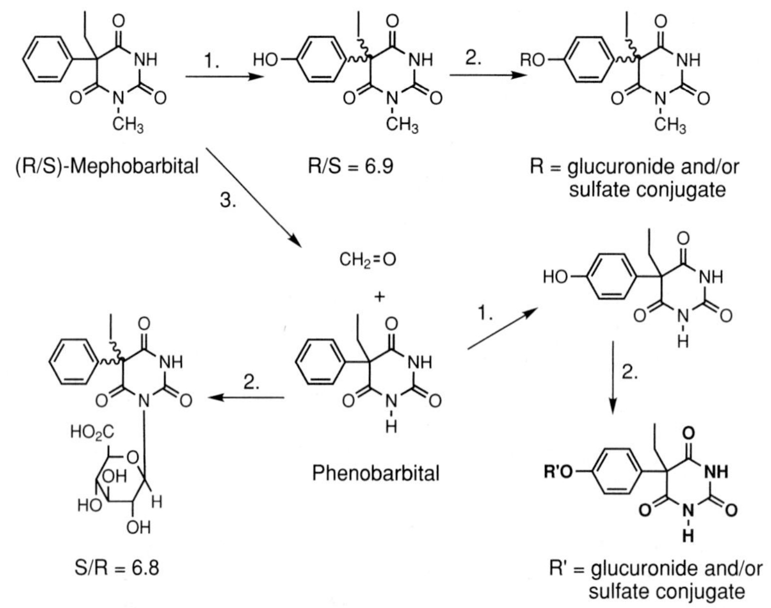

Fig. 19.6. Metabolism of mephobarbital and phenobarbital.

and the hydrophilic character decreases beyond limits. Furthermore, attachment of large alkyl groups (starting with the ethyl group) to the nitrogen imparts convulsant properties to barbiturates. Attachment of alkyl substituents to both N^1 and N^3 renders the drugs nonacidic, making them inactive. Modifications at this position are of primary importance in the barbiturates used as anticonvulsants and anesthetics.

Modification of oxygen. Replacement of C^2 oxygen by sulfur increases lipid solubility (44). Because maximal thiobarbiturate brain levels are quickly reached, onset of activity is rapid. As a result, these drugs (i.e., thiopental) are used as intravenous anesthetics.

Metabolism

Barbiturates lose their activities through metabolic transformations and redistribution. The metabolism of the barbiturates takes place primarily in the liver, in the endoplasmic reticulum (45). After metabolism, the lipophilic character of barbiturates decreases, and this is associated with a loss in depressant activity. Although not used as a hypnotic, the metabolic pathway for mephobarbital (Fig. 19.6) is representative of the metabolic pathway for the barbiturates. The major pathways by which the activity of the barbiturates are terminated include the following:

1. Oxidation of substituents at carbon 5 occurs by CYP2C19. The initial products are alcohols or phenols that form glucuronide and sulfate conjugates. The alcohols can undergo further oxidation to ketones or carboxylic acids, but these pathways generally are of minor importance in the biodisposition of the barbiturates. A pronounced product enantioselectivity often is observed for the chiral barbiturates. The barbiturates containing a propene at the 5-position (e.g., secobarbital) have been shown to inactivate CYP450 by alkylation of the porphyrin ring of CYP450 (46).
2. Conjugation of the heterocyclic nitrogen with glucosides. This unusual conjugation pathway can be as important as oxidative metabolism in the biotransformation of 5,5-disubstituted barbiturates (phenobarbital, amobarbital, pentobarbital). In humans, a pronounced product enantioselectivity is observed for excretion of these metabolites (47).
3. Oxidative N-dealkylation at the nitrogen. The CYP450 oxidation does not proceed rapidly. Introduction of an alkyl group on a barbiturate nitrogen introduces a site of asymmetry at the 5-position. The S-isomers of the these barbiturates primarily undergo N-dealkylation, and the R-isomer primarily undergoes oxidation at the 5 position. The dealkylated products, however, may be excreted more slowly and, therefore, accumulate in the course of therapy with N-alkylated barbiturates. For example, a definite blood level of phenobarbital has been established in the course of mephobarbital therapy (48).
4. Oxidative desulfurization of 2-thiobarbiturates takes place readily to yield the more hydrophilic barbiturates. This occurs primarily following redistribution of the thiobarbiturate anesthetics.

Clinical Applications

The currently available barbiturates are listed in Table 19.3. It must be concluded that a prescription for long-term use of the barbiturates as hypnotics rarely is indicated.

Table 19.3 Barbiturates Used Clinically as Hypnotics

Barbiturate	R_5	R_5	Hypnotic Dose (mg)	Onset (min)	Duration (hours)
Amobarbital	C_2H_5	$(CH_3)_2CHCH_2CH_2$	100–200	45–60	6–8
Aprobarbital	$CH_2{=}CHCH_2$	$(CH_3)_2CH$	40–160	45–60	6–8
Butabarbital	C_2H_5	$CH_3CH_2CH(CH_3)$	50–100	45–60	6–8
Pentobarbital	C_2H_5	$CH_3(CH_2)_2CH(CH_3)$	100	10–15	3–4
Phenobarbital	C_2H_5	C_6H_5	100–320	30–60	10–16
Secobarbital	$CH_2{=}CHCH_2$	$CH_3(CH_2)_2CH(CH_3)$	100	10–15	3–4

Chloral Derivative

During the 1950s and 1960s, chloral hydrate was widely promoted as a hypnotic (doses of 500 mg), because it did not significantly suppress REM sleep (44). Today, it still finds use as a sedative in nonoperating room procedures for pediatric patients (49). Chloral hydrate does demonstrate initial and short-term effectiveness for sleep induction and maintenance. Sleep occurs within 1 hour and lasts from 4 to 8 hours. After 2 weeks of drug administration, however, a marked decrease in effectiveness is observed. Chloral hydrate has no analgesic or tranquilizing effect, and it is devoid of adverse respiratory effects at therapeutic doses.

Chloral is a unique aldehyde because of the electron-withdrawing effect of the CCl_3 group. When chloral (an oily liquid) is treated with water or alcohol, a crystalline solid, chloral hydrate or chloral alcoholate, is formed. Chloral hydrate is stable, but as indicated in Figure 19.7, when it is dissolved in water, it is in equilibrium with the chloral form (equilibrium strongly favoring the chloral hydrate structure). The CCl_3 group is sufficiently electron-withdrawing that chloral hydrate is a weak acid (pK_a = 10.04) (44). A 10% solution of chloral hydrate in water has pH 3.5–4.4. This acidity makes it quite irritating to mucous membranes, such as in the stomach. Therefore, it is not surprising that gastrointestinal upset commonly occurs with chloral if it is undiluted or taken on an empty stomach. This led to the development of adducts or complexes, or pro-drugs, that were widely used but are now no longer available. Only chloral hydrate as a capsule, syrup, or suppository is currently available.

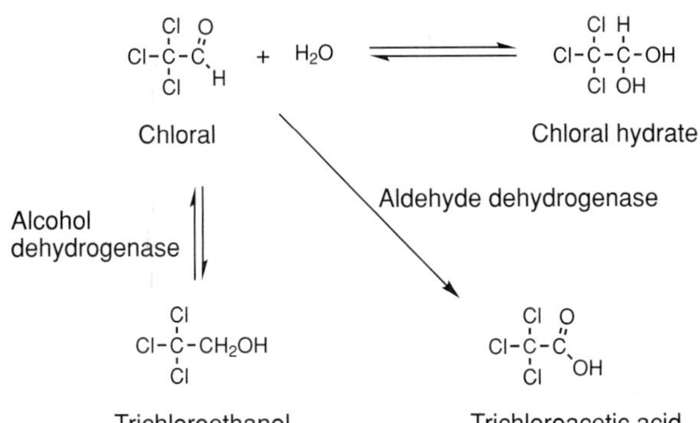

Fig. 19.7. Reactions and metabolism of chloral.

Chloral hydrate is readily absorbed from the gastrointestinal tract following oral or rectal doses of 500 mg to 2 g and is quickly reduced to trichloroethanol, its active metabolite, by alcohol dehydrogenase in the liver and erythrocytes. The plasma half-life of trichloroethanol is approximately 8 to 11 hours. Oral administration of 500 mg to 1 g of chloral hydrate usually produces sleep within 30 minutes to 1 hour; this sleep lasts for 4 to 8 hours. The metabolic transformation to trichloroethanol is so fast that it is difficult to detect appreciable chloral hydrate blood levels. It is believed that the initial hypnotic effect of chloral hydrate is exerted by the drug, but the more prolonged effect is caused by trichloroethanol. In vitro, it has been shown that trichloroethanol can exert barbiturate-like effects on the $GABA_A$ receptor channels. Trichloroethanol is metabolized by alcohol dehydrogenase oxidation to chloral and then to the inactive metabolite, trichloroacetic acid, via aldehyde dehydrogenase (Fig. 19.7), which also is extensively metabolized to acyl glucuronides via conjugation with glucuronic acid and then excreted into the urine (50). Chloral hydrate is not excreted in the urine unchanged; the quantities of metabolites excreted in the urine appear to be variable not only between different individuals but even in the same individual on different days. Trichloroethanol can cross the placenta as well as into the cerebrospinal fluid, but only clinically insignificant amounts are found in breast milk.

Other, older hypnotic drugs are believed to act at the $GABA_A$ receptor and are clinically similar to the barbiturates (e.g., glutethimide, ethychlorvynol, and methaprylon). These drugs are still available and have been reviewed in previous editions of this text. Rarely, however, is the use of these drugs indicated because of their limited effectiveness, tendency of patients to develop tolerance to their effect, depression of cognitive effects, physical dependence, ability to induce microsomal metabolism, and lethal toxicity.

Melatonin Receptor Agonist

As a neurohormone, melatonin is a poor drug because of its poor absorption, low oral bioavailability (<10%), rapid first-pass metabolism by CYP1A2 to 6-hydroxymelatonin (its primary metabolite), and ubiquitous effects. In their

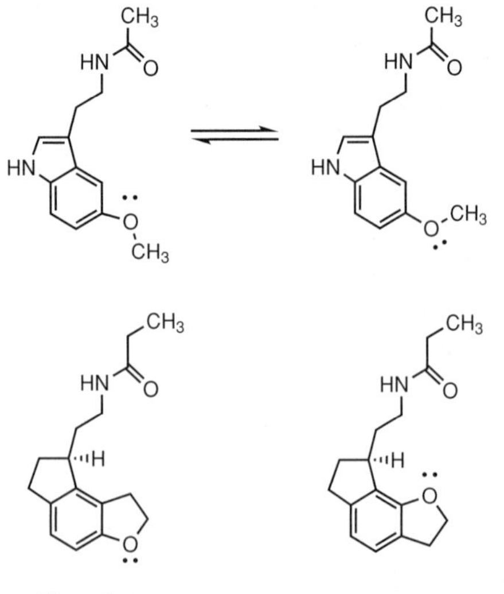

Fig. 19.8. Constrained analogues of melatonin.

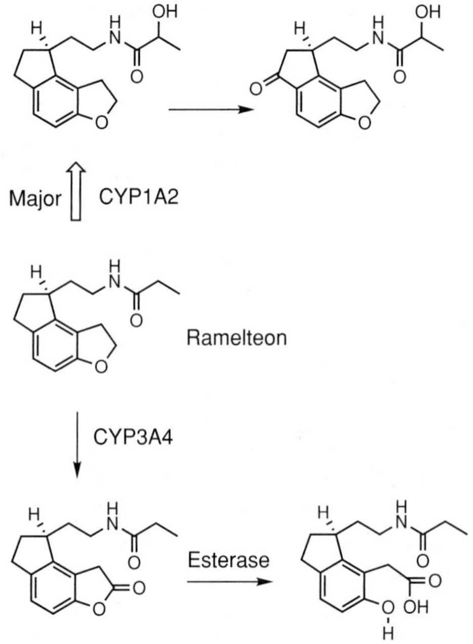

Fig. 19.9. Ramelteon and metabolites.

search for melatonin agonists as sedatives, the melatonin molecule was reengineered by substituting the nitrogen of the indole ring with a carbon to give an indane ring bio-isostere of melatonin and by constraining the conformational flexibility of the 5-methoxyl group into a furan ring to form either an angular indeno[5,4-b]furan or a linear indeno[5,6-b]furan heterocyclic ring systems (Fig. 19.8) (51,52). Subsequent M_1 receptor testing revealed that the binding constant (K_i) for the indeno[5,4-b]furan derivative was 0.017 nM, whereas that for the indeno[5,6-b]furan derivative was 255 nM—an approximately 15,000-fold weaker affinity for the M_1 receptor. Furthermore, the S-enantiomer showed approximately 500-fold greater affinity than the R-isomer for this receptor. Molecular modeling of the indeno[5,4-b]furan derivative with the M_1 receptor showed that by fixing the orientation of the 5-methoxyl group of melatonin into an angular furan ring plays a major factor for reinforcing the binding of the nonbonding pair oxygen electrons to a histidine residue in the ligand binding pocket of the receptor. Thus, the methyl orientation of the 5-methoxyl group of melatonin (conformer B) is critical for the optimal orientation of the oxygen lone pairs for optimal ligand binding to the receptor. This approach culminated in the discovery and approval of ramelteon (Fig. 19.8) as a very potent and very selective ligand for the MT_1 receptor, with superior in vivo activity and safety profile for use in the treatment of insomnia.

Because it does not contain a basic nitrogen (nor is the amide hydrolyzed once absorbed), ramelteon binds primarily with the melatonin M_1 receptor and does not bind with other receptors associated with sleep (e.g., $GABA_A$, dopamine, or opiate receptors). Its greater selectivity for the human MT_1 receptor (K_i = 0.014 nM) versus the MT_2 receptor (K_i = 0.112 nM) is consistent with its ability to primarily shorten sleep onset rather than to readjust the circadian rhythm (51–53). Ramelton is rapidly absorbed and undergoes extensive first-pass metabolism with an oral bioavailability of less than 2% and an elimination half-life of approximately 2 hours (Table 19.3). Metabolism is primarily hydroxylation of the propionamide side chain to an active metabolite (Fig. 19.9). Metabolism primarily occurs with CYP1A2, with minor contributions from CYP2C and CYP3A4. The overall mean systemic exposure of the hydroxylated metabolite is 20- to 100-fold greater than ramelton but 17- to 25-fold less potent than ramelton in binding assays (54). Additional oxidative metabolism by the CYP enzymes occurs on the indane ring and the dihydrofuran ring to form a lactone ring and esterase hydrolysis of the lactone to a carboxylic acid. These metabolites are inactive.

Ramelton has been shown to be effective in initiating sleep (shortening sleep latency) but not in maintaining sleep (promoting night time sleep maintenance; short half-life) (51,52). The recommended dose is 8 mg taken 30 minutes before bedtime. In contrast to the $GABA_A$ agonist drugs, ramelton does not depress cognitive function, memory, or ability to concentrate at normal doses. Ramelton does not appear to have any abuse liability, and it is not listed as a Schedule II to V controlled substance.

Antihistamines and Anticholinergics

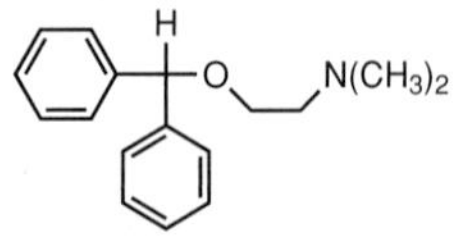

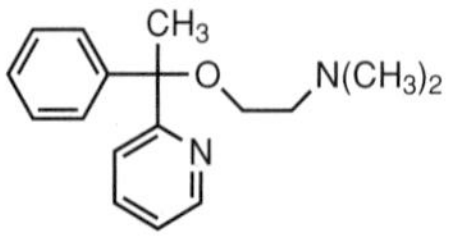

Some of the antihistamine (H_1)-receptor antagonists that can cross the blood-brain barrier are used for their hypnotic activity. The primary antihistamines used for their sedative effect are diphenhydramine and doxylamine, which belong to the ethanolamine class of antihistamines (see Chapter 37). Both drugs are sold without prescription. Sleep laboratory-controlled studies indicate that the antihistamines (H_1-receptor antagonists) have little effect on normal subjects when given before bedtime. The same doses given during the day, however, lead to drowsiness, increased tendency to sleep, and impaired performance (10).

Antidepressants

Antidepressants with sedation as a side effect often are used to treat insomnia. The antidepressants most frequently associated with sedation as a side effect are the tricyclics (amitryptyline, imipramine, nortriptyline, trimipramine, doxepin, amoxapine, and protriptyline), nontricyclics (maprotiline and mirtazepine), trazodone, and nefazodone (55), which are discussed in greater detail in Chapter 21. Of these drugs, trazodone, doxepin, and mirtazepine have been shown to be effective in the treatment of insomnia in patients with depression (1). The effectiveness of these drugs to treat insomnia in nondepressed patients, however, has not been proven. The mechanism by which this occurs is unknown, but most of these drugs have some activity as H_2 antagonists that may contribute to the effect (56).

Herbal Preparations

A number of herbal preparations are used as sedatives for the treatment of sleep disorders, including valerian, German camomile, kava, lavender, hops, lemon balm, and passiflora (57). Kava is no longer recommended because of potential hepatotoxicity (58). Of the other preparations, valerian has been most extensively studied for its effectiveness in treating insomnia, but the evidence verifying its sedative effect is still inconclusive (59). The fraction associated with the sedating effects of valerian is the aqueous extract, which contains no valepotriates or volatile oils. Clinical studies suggest that 450 mg of extract is an adequate dose to induce sleep (dose range, 60–900 mg), and effects may not be seen until valerian has been used for a few weeks. When taken at night, valerian does not appear to affect cognitive or motor performance the following day (i.e., comparable to placebo), and no addiction to valerian has been reported. At high doses, disturbance of cardiac function and CNS depression may occur. No data are available regarding the long-term use of valerian. One of the problems in studying valerian is similar to that observed for most herbal preparations. It is unknown exactly what active component(s) is responsible for its proposed sedative effect, and the variability between species and types of extract makes the study of valerian very difficult.

CASE STUDY

Victoria F. Roche and S. William Zito

PQ is a 45-year-old mother of four healthy young children. Her husband died suddenly 6 months ago from a heart attack. PQ's husband was a patent lawyer and left her and the children in an adequate financial state. During the last 4 weeks, however, PQ has had trouble falling asleep, finding herself worrying about the future and staring at the ceiling as she imagines her children being injured in all sorts of weird accidents. PQ needs to drive her children to school each day, and she has taken a part-time job so that she is free each afternoon to pick her children up from school. She misses her husband terribly, and the bedroom has become a lonely place—one that she is becoming fearful to enter. Once asleep, PQ sleeps through the night and wakes rested. PQ is otherwise healthy and has no history of any physical ailments or medication use. She is diagnosed with situational insomnia stemming from the loss of her husband and the change in her responsibilities. Evaluate the following benzodiazepines, and recommend an appropriate one for the treatment of PQ's insomnia.

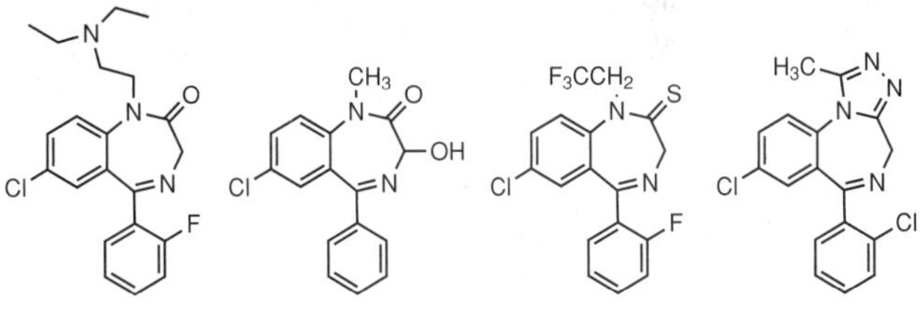

Flurazepam Temazepam Quazepam Triazolam

1. Identify the therapeutic problem(s) in which the pharmacist's intervention may benefit the patient.
2. Identify and prioritize the patient-specific factors that must be considered to achieve the desired therapeutic outcomes.
3. Conduct a thorough and mechanistically oriented structure-activity analysis of all therapeutic alternatives provided in the case.
4. Evaluate the structure-activity relationship findings against the patient specific factors and desired therapeutic outcomes, and make a therapeutic decision.
5. Counsel your patient.

References

1. Silber MH. Chronic insomnia. N Engl J Med 2005;353:803–810.
2. Sateia MJ, Nowell PD. Insomnia. Lancet 2004;364:1959–1973.
3. Mellin GW, Katzenstein M. The saga of thalidomide. N Eng J Med 1962;267: 1184–1192.
4. Miller NS, Gold MS. Sedative-hypnotics: pharmacology and use. J Fam Pract 1989;29:665–670.
5. Carskadon MA, Dement WC. Normal human sleep: an overview. In: Kryger MH, Roth T, Dement WC, eds. Principles and Practices of Sleep Medicine, 2nd Ed. Philadelphia: WB Saunders, 1994:16–25.
6. Moruzzi G, Magoun H. Brainstem reticular formation and activation of the EEG. Electroencephalogr Clin Neurophys 1949;1:455–473.
7. Kales A, ed. The Pharmacology of Sleep, v. 116. Berlin: Springer-Verlag, 1995.
8. Wauquier A. Pharmacology of the catecholaminergic system. In: Kales A, ed. The Pharmacology of Sleep. Berlin: Springer-Verlag, 1995;116:65–90.
9. Adrien J. The serotoninergic system and sleep-wakefulness regulation. In: Kales A, ed. The Pharmacology of Sleep. Berlin: Springer-Verlag, 1995;116:91–116.
10. Monti JM. Pharmacology of the histaminergic system. In: Kales A, ed. The Pharmacology of Sleep. Berlin: Springer-Verlag, 1995;116:117–142.
11. Tononi G, Pompeiano O. Pharmacology of the cholinergic system. In: Kales A, ed. The Pharmacology of Sleep. Berlin: Springer-Verlag, 1995;116:143–210.
12. Radulovacki M. Pharmacology of the adenosine system. In: Kales A, ed. The Pharmacology of Sleep. Berlin: Springer-Verlag, 1995;116:307–322.
13. Bateson AN. The benzodiazepine site of the $GABA_A$ receptor: an old target with new potential? Sleep Med 2004;5(Suppl 1):S9–S15.
14. Van Cauter E. Hormones and sleep. In: Kales A, ed. The pharmacology of sleep. Berlin: Springer-Verlag, 1995;116:279–306.
15. Zhdanova IV. Melatonin as a hypnotic: pro. Sleep Med Rev 2005;9:51–65.
16. Van den Heuval CJ, Ferguson SA, Macchi MM, et al. Melatonin as a hypnotic: con. Sleep Med Rev 2005;9:71–80.
17. Turek FW, Gillette MU. Melatonin, sleep, and circadian rhythms: rationale for development of specific melatonin agonists. Sleep Med 2004;5:523–532.
18. Dubocovich ML, Masana MI, Benloucif S. Molecular Pharmacology and function of melatonin receptor subtypes. In: Olcese J, ed. Melatonin After Four Decades. New York: Kluwer Academic, 2000:181–190.
19. Taheri S, Zeitzer JM, Mignot E. The role of hypocretins (orexins) in sleep regulation and narcolepsy. Annu Rev Neurosci 2002;25:282–313.
20. Baumann CR, Bassetti CL. Hypocretins (orexins) and sleep-wake disorders. Lancet Neurol 2005;4:673–682.
21. Bixler EO, Vgontzas AN, Kales A. Methodological issues in pharmacological studies of sleep. In: Kales A, ed. The Pharmacology of Sleep. Berlin: Springer-Verlag, 1995;116:323–344.
22. Threlkeld DS, ed. Drug Facts and Comparisons. St. Louis: Wolters Kluwer Health, 2006, pp. 969–971.
23. Squires RF, Braestrup C. Benzodiazepine receptors in rat brain. Nature 1977; 266:732–734.
24. Mohler H, Okada T. Benzodiazepine receptor: demonstration in the central nervous system. Science 1977;198:849–851.
25. Kales A, Vgontzas AN, Bixler EO. Hypnotic drugs. In: Kagan F, Hatwood T, Rickels K, et al., eds., Hypnotics. New York: Spectrum Publications, 1975:345–385.
26. Clatworthy AJ, Jones LV, Whitehouse MJ. The gas chromatography–mass spectrometry of the major metabolites of flurazepam. Biomed Mass Spectrom 1977;4:248–254.
27. Zampaglione N, Hilbert JM, Ning J, et. al. Disposition and metabolic fate of ^{14}C-quazepam in man. Drug Metab Dispos 1985;13:25–29.
28. Eberts FS Jr, Philopoulos Y, Reineke LM, et al. Triazolam disposition. Clin Pharmacol Ther 1981;29:81–93.
29. Schwarz HJ. Pharmacokinetics and metabolism of temazepam in man and several animal species. Br J Clin Pharmacol 1979;8:23S–29S.
30. Greenblatt DJ, Allen MD, Noel BJ, et al. Acute overdosage with benzodiazepine derivatives. Clin Pharmacol Ther 1977;21:497–514.
31. Damgen A, Luddens H. Zaleplon displays a selectivity to recombinant $GABA_A$ receptors different from zolpidem, zopiclone, and benzodiazepines. Neurosci Res Commun 1999;25:139–148.
32. Drover DR. Comparative pharmacokinetics and pharmacodynamics of short-acting hypnosedatives zaleplon, zolpidem, and zopiclone. Clin Pharmacokinet 2004;43:227–238.
33. Pichard L, Gillet G, Bonfils C, et al. Oxidative metabolism of zolpidem by human liver cytochrome P450s. Drug Metab Disp 1995; 23:1253–1262.
34. Kawashima K, Hosoi K, Naruke T, et. al. Aldehyde oxidase-dependent marked species difference in hepatic metabolism of the sedative-hypnotic, zaleplon, between monkeys and rats. Drug Metab Dispos 1999;27:422–428.
35. George CFP. Pyrazolopyrimidines. Lancet 2001;358:1623–1626.
36. Carlson JN, Haskew R, Maisonneuve IM, et al. Sedative and anxiolytic effects of zopiclone's enantiomers and metabolite. Eur J Pharmacol 2001;414:181–189.
37. Dundar Y, Dodd S, Strobyi J, et al. Comparative efficacy of newer hypnotic drugs for the short-term management of insomnia: a systematic review and meta-analysis. Hum Psychopharmacol Clin Exp 2004;19:305–322.
38. Krystal AD, Walsh JK, Laska E, et al. Sustained efficacy of eszoplicone over 6 months of nightly treatment: results of a randomized, double-blind, placebo-controlled study of adults with chronic insomnia. Sleep 2003;23:1087–1096.
39. Richter JA, Holtman JR. Barbiturates: their in vivo effects and potential biochemical mechanisms. Prog Neurobiol 1982;18:275–319.
40. Knoll R. Selective actions of barbiturates on synaptic transmission. In: Lipton MA, DiMascio A, Killam AF, eds. Psychopharmacology: A Generation of Progress. New York: Raven Press, 1978:1337–1348.
41. Acharya JN, Dinner DS. Use of the intracarotid amobarbital procedure in the evaluation of memory. J Clin Neurophysiol 1997;14:311–325.
42. Wang RIH. Dependence liability of sedatives and hypnotics. In: Kagan F, Hatwood T, Rickels K, et al., eds., Hypnotics. New York: Spectrum Publications, 1975:297–310.
43. Sandberg F. Anesthetic properties of some new N-substituted and N,N′-disubstituted derivatives of 5,5-diallylbarbituric acid. Acta Physiol Scand 1951;24: 7–26.
44. Vida JA. Central nervous system depressants: sedative-hypnotics. In: Foye WO, Lemke TL, Williams DA, eds., Principles of Medicinal Chemistry, 4th Ed. Baltimore: Williams & Wilkinson, 1995:154–180.
45. Freudenthal RI, Carroll FI. Metabolism of certain commonly used barbiturates. Drug Metab Rev 1973;2:265–278.
46. He K, He YA, Szklarz GD, et al. Secobarbital-mediated inactivation of cytochrome P450 2B1 and its active site mutants. Partitioning between heme and protein alkylation and epoxidation. J Biol Chem 1996;271:25864–25872.
47. Soine WH, Soine PJ, England TM, et al. Identification of the diastereomers of pentobarbital N-glucosides excreted in human urine. Pharm Res 1994;11: 1536–1540.
48. Lim WH, Hooper WD. Stereoselective metabolism and pharmacokinetics of racemic methylphenobarbital in humans. Drug Metab Dispos 1989;17: 212–217.
49. Warner TM. Clinical applications for pediatric sedation. CRNA 1997;8: 144–151.
50. Breimer DD. Clinical pharmacokinetics of hypnotics. Clin Pharmacokinet 1977;2:93–109.
51. Osamu Uchikawa O, Fukatsu K, Tokunoh R, et al., Synthesis of a novel series of tricyclic indan derivatives as melatonin receptor agonists. J Med Chem 2002;45:4222–4239.
52. Cajochen C. TAK-375 Takeda. Curr Opin Invest Drugs 2005;6:114–121.
53 Nguyen NN, Yu SS, Song JC. Ramelton: a novel melatonin receptor agonist for the treatment of insomnia. Formulary 2005;40:146–155.
54. Rozerem. Package insert.
55. Pagel JF. Medications and their effect on sleep. Prim Care Clin Office Pract 2005;32:491–509.
56. Ringdahl EN, Pereira SL, Delzell JE. Treatment of primary insomnia. J Am Board Fam Pract 2004;17:212–219.
57. Gyllenhaal C, Merritt SL, Peterson SD, et al. Efficacy and safety of herbal stimulants and sedatives in sleep disorders. Sleep Med Rev 2000;4:229–251.
58. Zhardova IV. Advances in the management of insomnia. Expert Opin Pharmacother 2004;5:1573–1579.
59. Stevenson C, Ernst E. Valerian for insomnia: a systematic review of randomized clinical trials. Sleep Med 2000;1:91–99.

20. *Antiseizure Drugs*

BARBARA LEDUC

DRUGS COVERED IN THIS CHAPTER:

PRIMARY DRUGS FOR TREATMENT OF SEIZURES
- Carbamzepine
- Clonazepam
- Diazepam
- Ethosuximide
- Phenytoin

ALTERNATIVE DRUGS FOR TREATMENT OF SEIZURES
- Phenobarbital
- Primidone

ADJUNCT DRUGS FOR TREATMENT OF SEIZURES
- Felbamate
- Gabapentin
- Lamotrigine
- Levetiracetam
- Oxcarbazepine
- Tiagabine
- Topiramate
- Valproic acid
- Zonisamide

INTRODUCTION

As early as 2000 BC, it was recognized that some people suffered from convulsive seizures. The term "epilepsy," based on the Greek word *epilambanein* (meaning "to seize"), was first used by Hippocrates. In the world's first scientific monograph on epilepsy, entitled *On the Sacred Disease* (~400 BC), Hippocrates disputed the myth that the cause of epilepsy is supernatural and the cure magic. He described epilepsy as a disease of the brain, which should be treated by diet. At the same time, Hippocrates provided the first classification of epilepsy, which is still used. He distinguished true (idiopathic) epilepsy (i.e., a disorder for which the cause is unknown) from symptomatic (organic) epilepsy (i.e., a disorder resulting from a physiologic abnormality, e.g., brain injury, tumor, infection, intoxication or metabolic disturbances).

Two opinions were put forward as to the causes of epilepsy. One was that epilepsy is a single disease entity, and all forms of it have a common cause. On the other hand, it was proposed that different types of epilepsy result from different chemical, anatomic, or functional disorders. At the Symposium on Evaluation of Drug Therapy in Neurologic and Sensory Disease, the general opinion was that "epilepsy is a symptom complex characterized by recurrent paroxysmal aberrations of brain functions, usually brief and self-limited" (1).

All forms of epilepsy originate in the brain and appear to be the result of changes in neuronal activity. In turn, these changes, such as an excessive neuronal discharge, may be brought about by a disturbance of physicochemical function and electrical activity of the brain. The cause of this abnormality, however, is not clearly understood.

The most important property of the nerve cell is its excitability. It responds to excitation by generating an action potential, which may lead to repeated discharges. All normal neurons may become epileptic if subjected to excessive excitation. DeRobertis et al. (2) list two possible mechanisms for convulsive disorders: a loss of the normal inhibitory control mechanism, and a chemical supersensitivity that increases excitability of neuronal elements.

The origin of the seizures was established as early as the 19th century by Jackson (3). According to him, an intense discharge of gray matter in various regions of the brain initiates the seizures. As a result, it is only a normal reaction of the brain to initiate convulsive seizures. The discharge of excessive electrical (nervous) energy has, indeed, been substantiated by brain-wave studies made possible by electroencephalography (EEG).

Attempts to classify epileptic seizures have been only partially successful, primarily because of limited knowledge regarding the pathological processes of the brain. At the turn of the century, a classification of seizures had been published (4), and even more attempts appeared during the 1950s and 1960s. (5–9). In 1981, the Commission on Classification and Terminology of the International League Against Epilepsy put forward a new proposal (10). The classification outlined in Table 20.1 is a short version of this proposal, which is based on clinical seizure type, ictal (seizure-induced) EEG expression, and interictal (occurring between attacks or paroxysms) EEG expression.

SEIZURE CLASSIFICATION

Seizures result from the sudden, excessive firing of neurons. They are classified broadly as either partial seizures, in which the abnormal firing initially occurs in a small number of neurons but may spread to adjacent areas, or generalized seizures, in which virtually the entire brain is affected simultaneously (11). Seizures can be characterized by clinical symptoms and by EEG patterns. In addition, computed tomography and magnetic resonance imaging of the head are used in virtually all patients with suspected epilepsy to aid in identifying the seizure type.

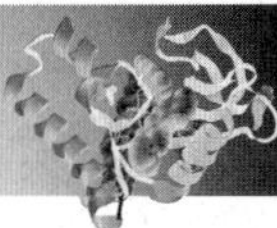

CLINICAL SIGNIFICANCE

Seizure disorders can be devastating to a patient's quality of life. Restrictions placed on patients with epilepsy include revocation of driver's licenses, potential physical limitations, work absenteeism, and various emotional and mental issues related to the disease and to the side effects from many of the medications these patients require. Because of the nature of the pathophysiology of seizures (i.e., abnormal neuron firing involving ion channels and an imbalance between excitatory and inhibitory synaptic function), medicinal chemistry plays a vital role in the understanding of this disease and, particularly, in its treatment. Molecular agents used to treat seizures exert varying effects on neuronal function through their structure–activity relationships and chemical interactions with ion channels (carbamazepine, phenytoin, ethosuximide, and zonisamide) and their similarities to naturally occurring neurotransmitters, such as γ-aminobutyric acid (GABA; benzodiazepines, barbiturates, topiramate, gabapentin, and tiagabine).

Approximately 60% of patients with epilepsy can be controlled with monotherapy, but a significant number of patients will require drug combinations. An understanding of basic chemical principles of antiseizure drugs is critical in making appropriate clinical recommendations regarding drug dosing and other issues, such as combination and concomitant therapies. The pharmacokinetics of antiseizure medications are very complex and require a strong foundational knowledge base routed in medicinal chemistry. Monitoring of side effects (and, specifically, the multitude of drug interactions associated with these agents) is extremely important to ensure patient safety and efficacy in the clinical setting, with the ultimate goals to keep patients seizure-free and to maintain their quality of life.

Michael Gonyeau, Pharm.D.
Associate Clinical Specialist
Northeastern University
Department of Pharmacy Practice
Bouvé College of Health Sciences

Partial (Local, Focal) Seizures

Partial seizures are divided into three categories: simple partial, complex partial, and partial progressing to generalized seizures. The key distinction between simple and complex partial seizures is the level of consciousness of the person undergoing the seizure. In partial seizures, the initial neuronal discharge originates from a specific, limited cortical area, which is termed a "focus." Development of the focus is thought to be caused by scarring after head trauma, infection, or oxygen deprivation. The abnormal EEG seizure patterns are restricted to one region of the brain, at least at the onset. These types of seizures are possible at all ages but are most frequent in the elderly. Partial seizures respond fairly well to antiseizure drugs (most commonly referred to as AEDs) (Fig. 20.1) (12).

Table 20.1. Classification of Epileptic Seizures

- I. Partial (local, focal) seizures
  - A. Simple (consciousness not impaired)
  - B. Complex partial seizures (psychomotor seizures)
    1. Beginning as simple partial seizures, progressing to complex seizures
    2. With impairment of consciousness at onset
  - C. Partial seizures evolving to secondarily generalized tonic-clonic convulsions
- II. Generalized seizures (convulsive or nonconvulsive)
  - A. Absence seizures
    - Typical (petit mal)
    - Atypical
  - B. Myoclonic
  - C. Clonic
  - D. Tonic
  - E. Tonic-clonic (grand mal)
  - F. Atonic
- III. Unclassified epileptic seizures (includes some neonatal seizures)

Medications to combat partial seizures are effective against secondary or generalized tonic-clonic seizures as well. These seizures respond well to carbamazepine, hydantoins, and barbiturates, although this latter group unfortunately displays substantial sedative effects. The newer AEDs (gabapentin, lamotrigine, levetiracetam, oxcarbazepine, tiagabine, topiramate, and zonisamide) are useful for either monotherapy or as adjunctive drugs. On the other hand, oxazolidinediones and succinimides are ineffective in the treatment of partial seizures. Valproate is appropriate when tonic-clonic seizures are combined with either myoclonic or absence seizures.

Simple Partial Seizures

The specific symptoms displayed during a simple partial seizure will depend on the area of the brain that is affected, and they will occur on the opposite side of the body from the lesion. Combinations of symptoms are frequent, making accurate diagnosis a challenge. The temporal lobes are the most common origination site for partial seizures. Seizure foci located within the temporal lobe result in psychic symptoms, such as fear, panic, or hallucinations; autonomic signs, such as flushing and sweating; or unpleasant smells or tastes. Frontal lobe foci usually present with motor symptoms. Focal motor attacks most commonly start in one hand, one foot, or one side of the face. Often, however, the onset of focal seizures is not specific. Should the focal motor seizures spread to contiguous cortical areas, there may be an

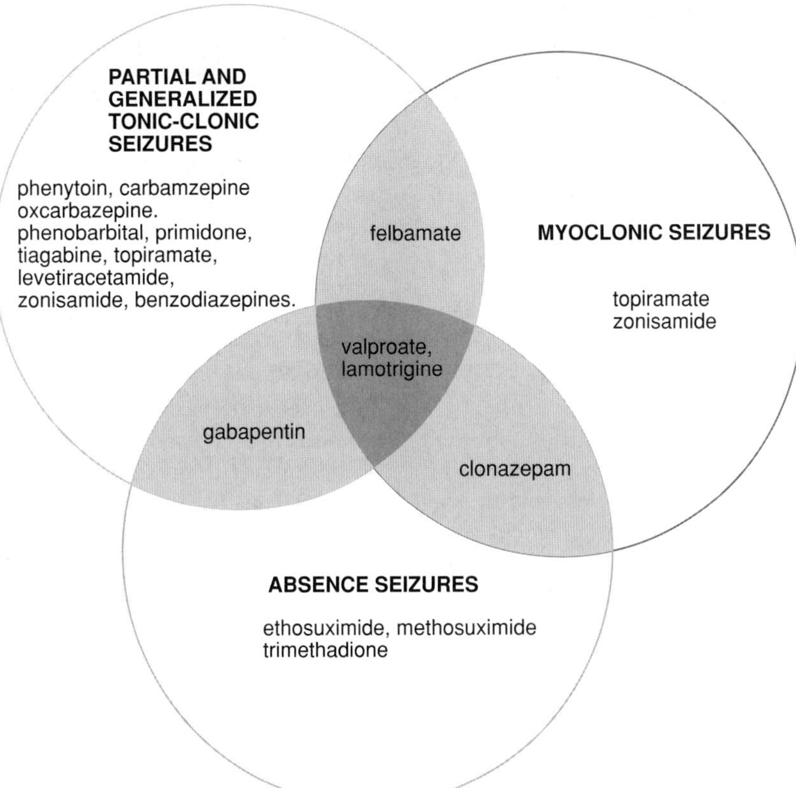

Fig. 20.1. The antiseizure drugs used in treatment of the various seizures.

orderly sequence of repeated events (movement of hands, face, and legs) known as an epileptic march. This type of seizure is termed a "jacksonian seizure." If the unilateral movements characteristic of focal motor or jacksonian seizures steadily spread to the other half of the body, a generalized seizure may follow. In contrast, seizures beginning in the parietal lobes are termed "sensory seizures" and present with altered sensations, tingling, numbness, or pain. Foci in the occipital lobes produce nystagmus, blinking, or visual disturbances, such as flashing lights or the appearance of strange colors.

In simple partial seizures, the patient's consciousness is not impaired. Thus, the person remains able to respond to simple commands, perform simple deliberate movements, and recall events that occurred during the seizure.

Complex Partial Seizures

When consciousness is impaired, the seizure is classified as a complex partial seizure. Impaired consciousness will be manifested by the person's staring, inability to respond to simple commands, by inaccurate recall or amnesia of events occurring during the seizure. Clouding of consciousness may be apparent initially or may appear subsequent to the start of a simple partial seizure. With the exception of the mental status, the other symptoms of complex partial seizures are similar to those outlined above. Many complex seizures have bilateral hemispheric involvement and frequently are accompanied by automatisms (i.e., repetitive involuntary movements, including chewing, swallowing, or wringing the hands).

Partial Seizures Evolving to Secondarily Generalized Seizures

The abnormal electrical activity responsible for any type of partial seizure can generalize throughout the brain, thus evolving into a secondary generalized tonic-clonic seizure. The diagnosis of partial seizures is therefore difficult to establish. The generalization may occur rapidly, or it may occur slowly enough that the symptoms of the partial seizure are experienced by the patient as an "aura" before the generalized tonic-clonic phase. Auras are comprised of symptoms such as seeing blinking lights or hearing unusual sounds, and they serve as an important warning for the patient. The symptoms of tonic-clonic seizures are described below.

Generalized Seizures (Convulsive or Nonconvulsive)

These disorders are generalized from the outset, and they show simultaneous involvement of both cerebral hemispheres and loss of consciousness. It is not possible to single out one anatomic or functional system in one hemisphere of the brain that is responsible for the clinical symptoms. The initial neuronal discharge spreads quickly into the entire (or at least the greater part of) the gray matter. The EEG pattern consists of bilateral, essentially synchronous and symmetric discharges from the start and indicates the widespread nature of neuronal discharge. The cause rarely is known, but it usually is attributed to diffuse lesions, to toxic and metabolic disturbances, or to constitutional genetic factors. People of all ages are affected by generalized convulsions. There are several classes of generalized seizures, and useful drugs are selected according to the seizure type that transpires (Fig. 20.1).

Absence (Petit Mal) Seizures

Both typical and atypical absence seizures bring about brief loss of consciousness. Typical absence seizures have a rapid onset and cessation, which may cause them to be misinterpreted as daydreaming; however, the person cannot be alerted or awakened during the seizures. Absence seizures often begin with a change in facial expression, which is followed by a period of motionless, blank staring. After the brief interruption in consciousness (typically ~10 seconds), the activity that was in progress before the seizure is resumed. The individuals have neither memory of events during the seizure nor postictal confusion. Typical absence seizures (petit mal) are more common in children than in adults. They are particularly disabling, because they tend to occur very many times daily. Most children will respond to drug treatment, but a small percentage will go on to develop generalized tonic-clonic seizures as adults. Complex typical absence seizures may include additional phenomena, such as clonic or myoclonic motions, automatisms, or more elaborate behaviors. Between 25 and 40% of affected children have a family history of absence seizures.

Atypical absence seizures have a slower onset and cessation, and they last longer (up to several minutes) than typical absence seizures. They may include clonic motions, automatisms, or autonomic symptoms. Differential diagnosis between these types is made on the basis of the EEG. Typical absence seizures display a 3-Hz spike-and-wave EEG pattern, but the pattern of atypical absence seizures is slower, usually in the range of 1.5 to 2.5 Hz.

Both forms of absence seizure often occur as part of one of the recognized epilepsy syndromes. Typical absence seizures respond fairly well to AEDs; ethosuximide and valproate are first-choice drugs. Clonazepam is effective but sedating, and tolerance to the antiabsence effects may develop. Lamotrigine may be useful. Treatment of atypical absence seizures with AEDs is less successful.

Lennox-Gastaut syndrome is a mixed seizure disorder combining the atypical absence seizures with tonic, tonic-clonic, or myoclonic motor patterns. The syndrome begins in childhood and usually includes mental retardation. Although adequate control of the seizures rarely is achieved, valproate, phenytoin, felbamate, lamotrigine, topiramate, and clonazepam have been useful.

Myoclonic Seizures

Myoclonic seizures consist of sudden, very brief, jerking contractions that may involve the entire body or be confined to limited areas, such as the face and neck. The contractions may affect individual muscles or groups, with simultaneous contraction of both extensor and flexor muscles. These seizures occur in all age groups, with symptoms ranging from rapid tremors to falling down. No loss of consciousness is detectable because of the brief duration of the seizure. Myoclonic seizures often occur in combination with other seizure types. Valproate and clonazepam are used most often to treat myoclonic seizures; lamotrigine and topiramate also have shown some efficacy.

Tonic Seizures

Tonic seizures occur mostly in children and are characterized by increased tone in extensor muscles, resulting in falling to the ground. Although brief, the duration of contractions is somewhat longer than in myoclonic seizures. Vocalization may occur as a result of contraction of thoracic muscles, forcing air past the larynx. Brief periods of apnea and postictal tiredness may be associated.

Atonic Seizures

In atonic seizures, a very sudden decrease in muscle tone occurs, leading to a head drop, drooping of a limb, or loss of all muscle tone, resulting in falling. The risk of injury is high in these sudden "drop attacks." Atonic seizures are more common in children.

Attaining good control of tonic or atonic seizures is difficult. Valproate, felbamate, lamotrigine, benzodiazepines, and topiramate have proven to be effective in some individuals.

Clonic Seizures

Clonic seizures nearly always occur in babies or young children. A loss or impairment of consciousness occurs simultaneously with a decrease in muscle tone or with a generalized tonic contraction, and it is followed by period of asymmetric jerking motions.

Tonic-Clonic (Grand Mal) Seizures

Generalized tonic-clonic seizures represent a maximal epileptic response of the brain. These seizures are characterized by the absence of an aura and by tonic stiffening of all muscle groups, causing the patient to fall. The initial contraction may be flexor and is rapidly followed by prolonged extension. Subsequently, there is a period of bilateral symmetric jerking of the extremities. The seizure may be associated with loss of bladder control and biting of the tongue or inside of the mouth. There is a pronounced postictal state following the seizure, and the person may pass directly into sleep before waking several hours later.

Status Epilepticus

Status epilepticus is a condition in which there is a single prolonged seizure lasting more than 5 minutes or in which there is insufficient time between multiple seizures to permit recovery. Several types exist, depending on the type of seizure involved (i.e., tonic-clonic, simple partial, complex partial, or absence). Tonic-clonic status epilepticus is both the most common and the most life-threatening. Pharmacological treatment of most forms of status epilepticus may include intravenous (IV) administration of diazepam or lorazepam, fosphenytoin, and lastly, phenobarbital. Although lorazepam is not approved by the U.S. Food and Drug Administration (FDA) for this purpose, it sometimes is preferred because of its longer half-life.

Absence status epilepticus is a condition of impaired consciousness, perhaps including mild motor symptoms, that lasts from 30 minutes to 12 hours. It can be distinguished from ongoing seizures because of organic or toxic causes by the spike-and-wave EEG pattern that is characteristic of absence seizures. The usual pharmacological treatment of absence status employs diazepam or lorazepam, followed by ethosuximide.

MECHANISMS OF ACTION FOR THE ANTISEIZURE DRUGS

Seizures result from bursts of abnormal synchronous discharging by a network of neurons. Although the mechanisms of seizure generation are still poorly understood, the causes of abnormal firing appear to involve neuronal ion channels and an imbalance between excitatory and inhibitory synaptic function. Various AEDs exhibit different mechanisms of action on neuronal function, causing them to show selective efficacy against different seizure types (Fig. 20.2).

Ion Channels

Sodium and chloride ions are present at greater concentration outside the cell, whereas potassium, organic cations, and charged proteins are more numerous within the cell. Because the membrane is permeable only to small ions and not large ions or proteins, the neuronal membranes maintain a charge separation, resulting in a "resting potential" in the range −50 to −80 mV versus the outside of the cell.

An increase in interior negativity, termed "hyperpolarization," decreases the resting potential (e.g., to −90 mV), thus making it more difficult for a neuron to reach threshold and subsequently fire. A reduction in interior negativity, termed "depolarization," can result in generation of an action potential if the depolarization is sufficient to reach threshold (approximately −40 mV). Neuronal firing is initiated by an influx of sodium ions.

After each depolarization, voltage-dependent sodium channels adopt an inactive state and remain refractory to reopening for a period of time. While those channels are unable to open, rapid repetitive firing is diminished, and spread of electrical seizure activity to adjacent brain regions is suppressed (14). Stabilization and prolongation of this inactive state appears to be the primary mechanism of action of phenytoin, carbamazepine, and lamotrigine and may be instrumental in the antiseizure actions of phenobarbital, oxcarbazepine, valproate, topiramate, and zonisamide (Fig. 20.2).

Alterations in the structure or function of an ion channel caused by mutations in a gene encoding one of the channel's subunits are termed "channelopathies." Initially, these abnormalities were associated with cardiac and muscular disorders, but today, it is recognized that channelopathies are responsible for several forms of epilepsy (15,16). Presently, most of the discovered channel mutations appear to be associated with the development of idiopathic generalized epilepsy; most partial seizures are believed to be acquired. Minor alterations in gene structure or expression, however, may predispose a given individual to partial seizures. It is estimated that 40% of adult and childhood epilepsy may result from genetic factors.

Mutations in sodium and potassium channels are most common, because they give rise to hyperexcitability and burst firing. Mutations in the sodium channel subunit gene *SCN2A1* have been associated with benign familial neonatal epilepsy; in *SCN1A* with severe myoclonic epilepsy of infancy, and in *SCN1A* and *SCN1B* with generalized epilepsy with febrile seizures. Mutation of the *SCN1B* gene has been shown to reduce the channel's response to phenytoin (17). The potassium channel genes *KCNQ2* and *KCNQ3* are implicated in some cases of benign familial neonatal epilepsy. Chloride channels have been implicated as well. Mutations of the *CLCN2* gene have been found to be altered in several cases of classical idiopathic generalized epilepsy subtypes: Childhood and juvenile absence epilepsy, juvenile myoclonic epilepsy, and epilepsy with grand mal on awakening. Mutations of $GABA_A$ receptor subunits also have been detected. The gene encoding the α_1 subunit, *GABRG1*, has been linked to juvenile myoclonic epilepsy; mutated *GABRG2*, encoding an abnormal γ subunit, has been associated with generalized epilepsy with febrile seizures and childhood absence epilepsy. Lastly, mutations of calcium channel subunits have been identified in juvenile absence epilepsy (mutation in *CACNB4*; the B4 subunit of the L-type calcium channel) and idiopathic generalized epilepsy (*CACN1A1*) (15,16).

Synaptic Inhibition and Excitation

For a neuron, whether an action potential is generated depends on the balance between excitatory and inhibitory stimulation. The predominant inhibitory neurotransmitter in the brain is GABA. It is synthesized from an amino acid, glutamic acid, by glutamic acid decarboxylase and is inactivated by GABA-transaminase. GABA binds to two receptor types, $GABA_A$ and $GABA_B$. $GABA_A$ receptors occur on chloride ion channels, and the binding of GABA causes chloride influx and neuronal hyperpolarization. $GABA_B$ receptors are linked via G proteins and second messengers to potassium and calcium channel activity, also mediating inhibition in the central nervous

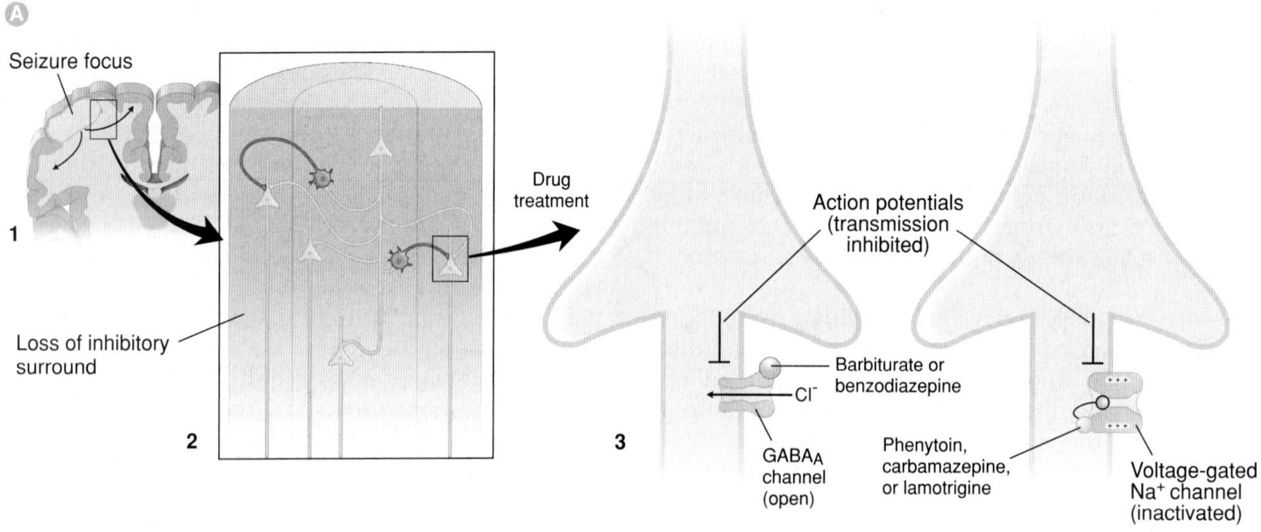

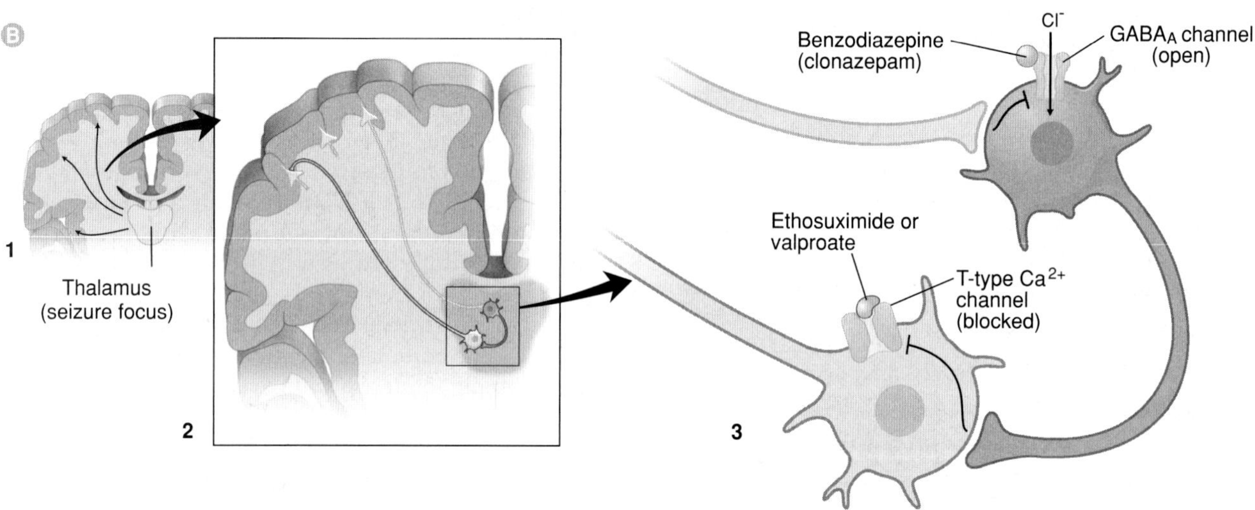

Fig. 20.2. Mechanisms of antiseizure drugs. (A) Drugs for partial seizures: 1) Seizure activity spreads because of loss of surround inhibition; 2) drugs act in the surrounding region to 3) enhance γ-aminobutyric acid (GABA) inhibition or prolong Na^+ channel inactivation. (B) Drugs for absence seizures: 1) The seizure activity results from cyclic activity between the thalamus and the cortex; 2) drugs prevent synchronization by either 3) deactivating the inhibitory reticular neurons and decreasing hyperpolarization of the thalamic relay neurons or blocking T-type Ca^{2+} channels to prevent burst firing by the thalamic relay neurons. (From Griffin EA Jr, Lowenstein DH. Pharmacology of abnormal electrical neurotransmission in the central nervous system. In: Golan DE, Tashjian A, Armstrong E, et al., eds. Principles of Pharmacology: The Pathophysiologic Basis of Drug Therapy. Baltimore: Lippincott Williams & Wilkins, 2004, pp. 193–203; with permission.)

system (CNS) (18). $GABA_B$ receptors also may play a role in oscillatory rhythms in some forms of epilepsy (19) (Fig. 20.3).

A number of AEDs augment GABA-mediated inhibition or affect GABA concentration. Benzodiazepines, barbiturates, and perhaps, topiramate enhance the action of GABA on the $GABA_A$ chloride channel. Tiagabine decreases the reuptake of GABA and, perhaps, gabapentin decrease its metabolism.

The ionotropic neurotransmitter glutamate provides excitatory neurotransmission via two types of receptors, the N-methyl-D-aspartate (NMDA) and L-α-amino-3-hydroxy-5-methyl-4-isoxazole propionate (AMPA) and kainate (KA) receptors (see Chapter 15). NMDA, AMPA, and KA are specific agonists for these receptor that are used in experiments to distinguish the glutamate ionotropic receptors.

AMPA Kainate

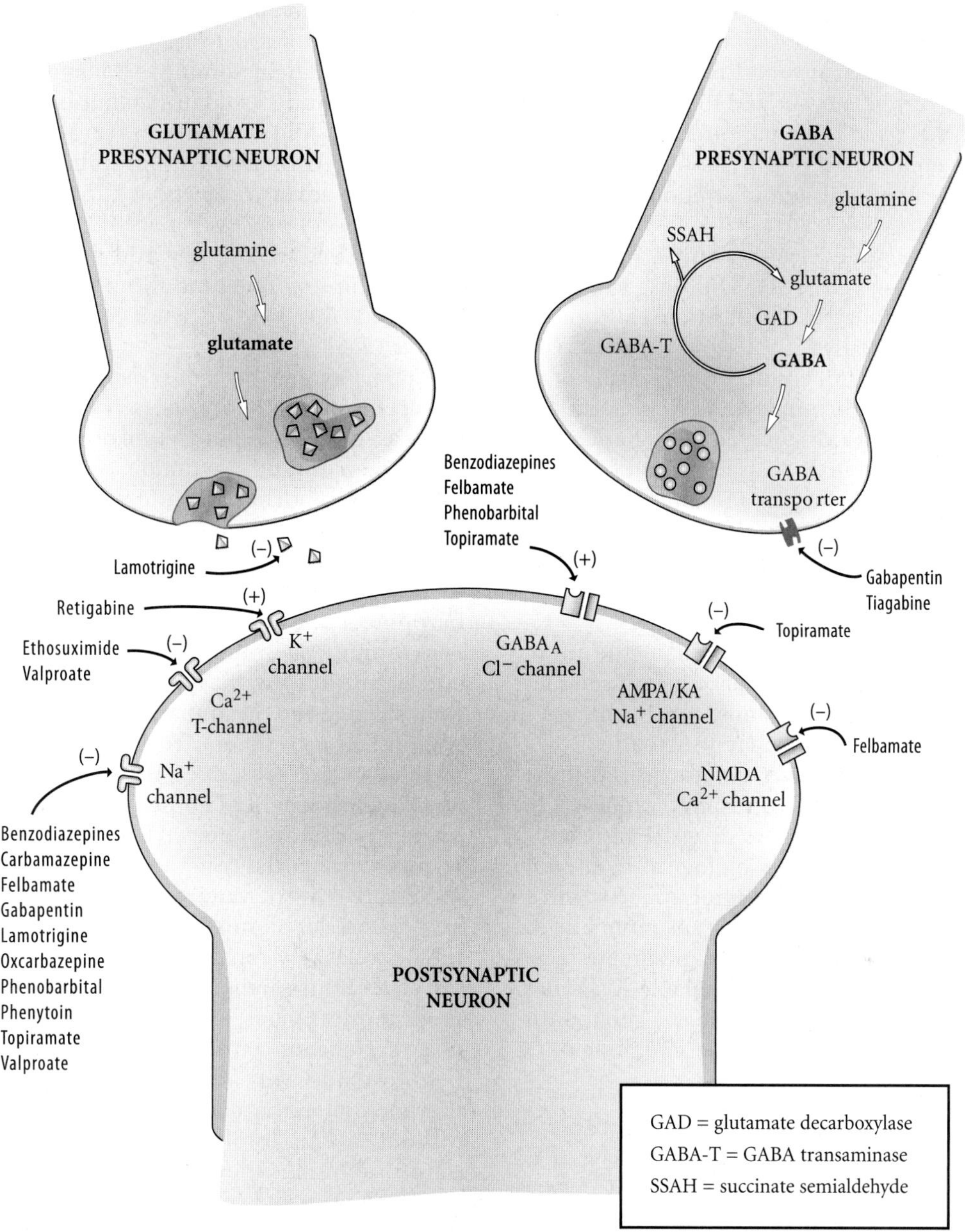

Fig. 20.3. A summary of the sites of action for the antiepileptic drugs (Adapted from Taylor CP. Mechanisms of new antiepileptic drugs. In: Delgado-Escueta AV, Wilson WA, Olsen RW, et al., eds. Jasper's Basic Mechanisms of the epilepsies, 3rd Ed. (Advances in Neurology, vol 79.) Philadelphia: Lippincott Williams & Wilkins, 1999:1012–1027; with permission.)

Activation of these ligand-gated channels enables sodium and calcium influx and potassium efflux, facilitating depolarization. Blockade of the NMDA receptor by felbamate or of the AMPA/KA receptor by phenobarbital and topiramate inhibits depolarization (Fig. 20.3).

Aberrant Calcium Signaling

Low-threshold T-type calcium currents act as pacemakers for normal brain activity, particularly the thalamic oscillatory currents thought to be involved in the generation of absence seizures (19,20). Drugs such as ethosuximide, the oxazolidinediones, and zonisamide, which inhibit T-type currents, are effective against absence seizures but ineffective against partial or other seizure types.

ANTISEIZURE DRUGS

Introduction

The primary use of AEDs is in the prevention and control of epileptic seizures. Theoretically, the ideal AED should, among other things, completely suppress seizures in doses that do not cause sedation or other undesired CNS toxicity. It should be well tolerated and highly effective against various types of seizures and be devoid of undesirable side effects on vital organs and functions. Its onset of action should be rapid after parenteral injection for control of status epilepticus, and it should have a long duration of effect after oral administration for prevention of recurrent seizures.

The first effective remedy, potassium bromide, was introduced by Locock in 1857 (21). This drug was largely replaced by phenobarbital in 1912, when Hauptmann tried this sedative in epilepsy (22). Its great value was recognized at once, and it is still commonly prescribed.

The usefulness of both bromide and phenobarbital in convulsive disorders was discovered by chance, but phenytoin was developed in 1937 as the result of a study of potential AEDs in animals by Putnam and Merritt (23,24). Bromide is highly effective in humans and is relatively nonsedating. Treatment of convulsive disorders using bromide, phenobarbital, and phenytoin constitutes an important advance in clinical therapy.

Many of the standard AEDs that contain the ureide structure, as shown in Figure 20.4, have been used clinically for more than 30 years without much change in their ureide structures. Small changes in the X substituent of the ureide structure can cause significant changes in the type of seizures controlled, which will be discussed for each of the respective drugs. As a result of rapid developments in molecular biological techniques for the study of the neurophysiology of epilepsy and in the interactions of AEDs with neurotransmitters at ion channels or brain receptors (AMPA/KA glutamate receptors), a new generation of clinically available AEDs have emerged. These AEDs include felbamate, gabapentin, lamotrigine, levetiracetam, oxcarbazepine, tiagabine, topiramate, and zonisamide. Their mechanisms of action are targeted toward ion channels and brain receptors either by enhancing brain GABA activity (e.g., tiagabine) or by inhibiting excitatory amino acids (L-Glu; e.g., lamotrigine and felbamate) (Fig. 20.2). These new-generation AEDs also exhibit limited drug interactions with fewer adverse effects. A rational approach to the drug discovery process is necessary to develop new leads to novel effective therapy and to use structure–activity relationships to fine-tune the pharmacology of existing AEDs with the same or better efficacy and fewer adverse effects (25).

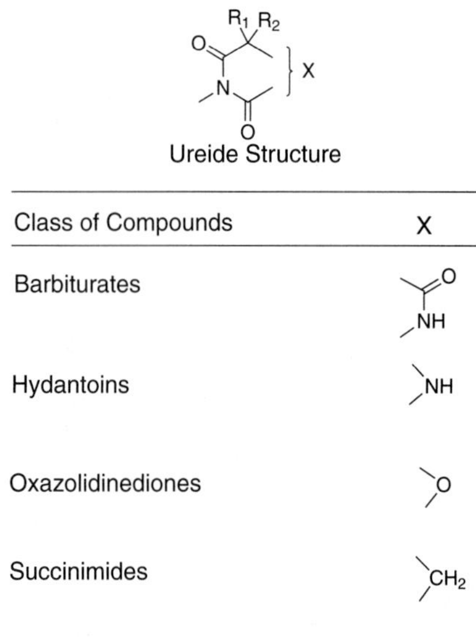

Fig. 20.4. Structure of anticonvulsant drugs containing the ureide structure.

Approximately 60% of patients with epilepsy become seizure-free with monotherapy using frontline drugs, such as carbamazepine, benzodiazepine (clonazepam and diazepam), ethosuximide, or phenytoin. Alternative monotherapy drugs include phenobarbital and primidone. Another 20% have their epilepsy controlled with more than one AED called adjunct drugs (e.g., felbamate, gabapentin, lamotrigine, levetiracetam, oxcarbazepine, tiagabine, topiramate, valproic acid, and zonisamide). Despite recent advances in neurobiology and significant insight regarding the molecular dysfunction of epilepsy, the remaining 20% do not completely respond to the current frontline therapeutic drugs and most often are prescribed more than two AEDs without any obvious benefit (11). Recently, much effort has been made to discover new AEDs effective in refractory seizures and partial complex seizures.

Seizure control requires continuous antiseizure action and is not achievable unless plasma concentrations remain relatively consistent at therapeutic levels throughout all 24 hours of the day. Therefore, a knowledge of the therapeutic ranges of plasma concentrations, time to peak serum concentrations, and elimination half-lives help to guide AED administration to achieve consistent therapeutic serum concentrations that control seizures without causing intolerable toxicity (26). Enzymatic biotransformation is the principal determinant of the pharmacokinetic properties for most AEDs, although some drugs are excreted by the kidneys predominantly as unchanged drug. Most AEDs exhibit linear enzyme kinetics, in which changes in daily dose lead to proportional changes in serum concentration if clearance remains constant. The traditional concept of administering a drug at intervals equal to one elimination half-life, however, does not apply to some drugs, in which the half-life of biological activity may exceed its elimination half-life. The standard AEDs have the greatest potential to be involved in pharmacokinetic drug interactions when they are coadministered with other AEDs or other drugs (27). These interactions usually involve changes in the rate of biotransformation or in the protein binding of one or both coadministered drugs (26). Drug-induced changes in the pharmacokinetics for many of the AEDs are particularly pronounced in children, requiring a higher oral dose per kilogram body weight than in adults to obtain an effective plasma concentration (28).

Table 20.2. Mechanism(s) of Action and Pharmacokinetics for Antiseizure Drugs

Drug	Mechanism of Action[a]	Elimination Half-life in Children (hours)	Elimination Half-life in Adults (hours)	Time to Steady -state Plasma Concentration (hours)	Protein Binding (%)	Log P (pH 7.4)
Carbamazepine (Tegretol)	A	14–27 (children), 8–28 (neonates)	14–27	2–8	66–89	2.2
Clonazepam (Klonopin)	A,B	20–40	20–40	—	95–98	2.3
Diazepam (Diastat)	A,B	17	36	—	40	2.6
Ethosuximide (Zarontin)	C	20–60	20–60	7–10	0	0.38
Gabapentin (Neurontin)	E	—	5–7	—	0	−1.3[d]
Lamotrigine (Lamictal)	A,D	—	See text	—	55	−0.2[d]
Oxcarbazepine (Trileptal)	A	—	7–11[b]	2–3	40	1.25[d]
Phenobarbital	A,B	37–73	40–136	12–21	40–60	1.53
Phenytoin (Dilantin)	A	5–14 (children), 10–60 (neonates)	12–36	7–28	69–96	2.39 p-OH metabolite1.72
Primidone (Mysoline)	A,B	5–11	6–18	4–7	0	0.91
Tiagabine (Gabitril)	A	—	4–7	2	96	3.2[d]
Topiramate (Topamax)	A,B,D	10–15, 6–8[c]	20–30 12–15[c]	—	15	2.9[d]
Valproic acid (Depakene, Depakote, Depacon)	A,B	8–15	6–15	1–4 3–5 (sustained release)	80–95	0.13
Zonisamide (Zonegran)	A,C	—	27–46	10–12	40	−0.10[d]

[a]See the *Mechanism of Action* sections of this chapter for discussion. A, sodium currents; B, γ-aminobutyric $acid_A$ receptor currents; C, T-calcium currents; D, glutamate receptor antagonist; E, unknown.
[b]Monohydroxy metabolite.
[c]In the presence of enzyme-inducing drugs, such as carbamazepine, phenobarbital, or primidone.
[d]clogP calculated using Advanced Chemistry Development (ACD Labs) Software V8.14, accessed Chemical Abstracts, American Chemical Society, June 16, 2006.

This chapter surveys the structure–activity relationship, mechanism of action, metabolism, and pharmacokinetic parameters for the new generation of AEDs (felbamate, gabapentin, lamotrigine, oxcarbazepine, levetiracetam, tiagabine, topiramate, zonisamide, and vigabatrin) and the standard AEDs (phenytoin, carbamazepine, phenobarbital, primidone, valproate, ethosuximide, and the benzodiazepines) as well as for several of the older AEDs that are less commonly used today. The application of AEDs in the treatment of various kinds of epilepsies is shown in Figure 20.1; this illustration is based on AEDs used in clinical therapy. Table 20.2 lists the AED, its mechanism of action, and some of the pharmacokinetic properties.

Drugs Effective Against Partial and Generalized Tonic-Clonic Seizures

Hydantoins

The hydantoins have a 5-membered ring structure containing two nitrogens in an ureide configuration (Fig. 20.4) and were tested as antiepileptics by Merritt and Putnam (23,24). These drugs suppressed electrically induced convulsions in animals but were ineffective against convulsions induced by pentylenetetrazole, picrotoxin, or bicuculline. The structures for the clinically available hydantoins are listed in Figure 20.5.

Phenytoin (Diphenylhydantoin). Phenytoin is the prototype and most commonly prescribed member of the hydantoin family of drugs. Bioequivalency is a problem with the hydantoins because of their very poor water solubility (~32 mg/L) and a low therapeutic ratio. Phenytoin exhibits nonlinear pharmacokinetics that exaggerate the effects of changes in the fraction of dose absorbed. Its apparent pK_a is in the range of 8.06 to 8.33 and, thus, can form a water-soluble sodium salt (~15 mg/mL at solution pH >11).

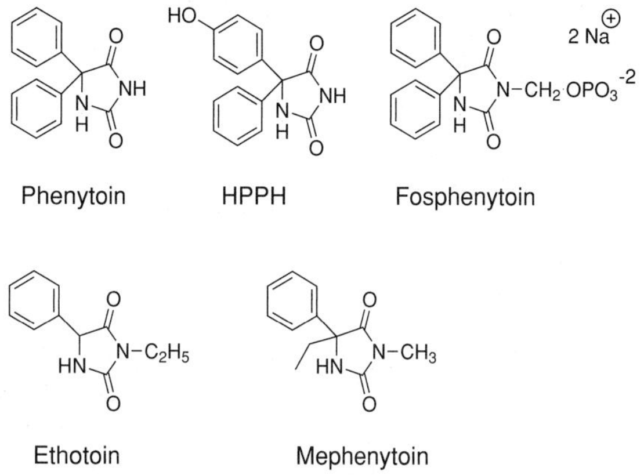

Phenytoin HPPH Fosphenytoin

Ethotoin Mephenytoin

Fig. 20.5. Hydantoins.

Aqueous solutions of phenytoin sodium (pH 11–12) gradually absorb carbon dioxide, neutralizing the alkalinity of the solution and causing partial hydrolysis and crystallization of free phenytoin resulting in turbid solutions. When phenytoin sodium is administered intramuscularly (IM), its absorption may be erratic as a result of crystallization of insoluble phenytoin at the injection site because of the decrease in pH from 11.5. Phenytoin sodium injection is physically and chemically incompatible in D5W, normal saline, or with parenteral solutions of many drugs, especially salts of basic drugs. The nature of the incompatibility depends on several factors, including the type of salt, concentrations of the drugs, diluents used, resulting pH of the final admixture (must be pH >11), and temperature. Phenytoin sodium capsules also will absorb carbon dioxide overtime, resulting in the formation of free phenytoin with a different dissolution profile.

Mechanism of action. Phenytoin is indicated for initial monotherapy or adjunct treatment of complex partial or tonic-clonic seizures, convulsive status epilepticus, and prophylaxis. It often is selected for initial monotherapy because of its high efficacy and relatively low incidence of side effects (29). Phenytoin is not used in the treatment of absence seizures, because it may increase their frequency of occurrence (30,31). Phenytoin binds to and stabilizes the inactivated state of sodium channels, thus producing a use-dependent blockade of repetitive firing and inhibition of the spread of seizure activity to adjacent cortical areas.

Pharmacokinetics. Phenytoin sodium from immediate-release capsules is rapidly absorbed and generally attains peak serum concentration in 1.5 to 3.0 hours; extended-release phenytoin sodium is absorbed more slowly, attaining peak serum concentration in 4 to 12 hours. The oral bioavailability for sodium phenytoin (70–100%) may vary enough among formulations from different manufacturers to result in a subtherapeutic serum concentration and, therefore, are ineffective in controlling seizures or a toxic blood concentration. Capsules of sodium phenytoin will absorb carbon dioxide, causing dissociation or neutralization to free phenytoin, thus altering its oral bioavailability (gastrointestinal dissolution), pharmacokinetics, and plasma concentrations that could cause breakthrough seizures. Therapeutic plasma concentrations for phenytoin usually are 7.5 to 20.0 μg/mL, although in some patients, seizure control is not achieved at these plasma concentrations. Phenytoin is highly protein bound (Table 20.2).

Phenytoin is metabolized predominately by CYP2C9 to its primary metabolite, 5-(4′-hydroxyphenyl)-5-phenylhydantoin (HPPH) (Fig. 20-5) (32). Approximately 60 to 75% of an oral dose is excreted as HPPH glucuronide or sulfate metabolites. Approximately 1% is excreted unchanged in urine, and some undergoes enterohepatic circulation. Other minor metabolites also appear in urine. Up to 10% of the oral phenytoin may be excreted unchanged by the kidneys at toxic doses. Phenytoin is notorious for displaying nonlinear pharmacokinetics, because the route of metabolism is a saturable process. Therefore, small increases in dosage may produce substantial increases in plasma phenytoin concentrations; the steady-state plasma concentration (C_p) may double or triple as a result of a 10% or more increase in dosage, possibly resulting in toxicity. Phenytoin also induces CYP3A4 and uridine diphosphate–glucuronyltransferases (UGTs; increased glucuronidation). Therefore, plasma concentrations for drugs metabolized by these isoforms will be affected (see Chapter 10). Thus, the addition of phenytoin to an AED regimen can reduce their plasma levels by inducing their CYP3A4 metabolism for carbamazepine, felbamate, lamotrigine, oxcarbazepine, tiagabine, valproate, and zonisamide. Other drugs for which metabolism is induced by phenytoin include methadone, theophylline, warfarin, and oral contraceptives. On the other hand, plasma phenytoin levels are increased by carbamazepine, felbamate, cimetidine, warfarin, chloramphenicol, isoniazid, and disulfiram. Plasma phenytoin levels are decreased by rifampin, antacids, and valproate (free phenytoin levels remain the same).

The pharmacokinetics of phenytoin is significantly affected by age. Its rate of elimination is strongly dose-dependent (nonlinear) at all ages. The elimination half-life for phenytoin in children increases with age because of an age-dependent decrease in its rate of metabolism (28). The combination of these factors makes it difficult to predict the phenytoin plasma concentrations following the dose (dose/kg) adjustments in neonates and children, particularly when phenytoin is coadministered with other liver enzyme-inducing AED, such as phenobarbital and carbamazepine.

Adverse effects. Drug interactions, especially with other AEDs and CYP3A4 substrates, are extensive. Although toxic effects may begin in the upper normal plasma range (>20 μg/mL), serious toxicity is rare. Central nervous system effects are most frequent and include nystagmus, ataxia, dysarthria, and sedation. Gingival hyperplasia, usually reversible, is common. Aromatic anticonvulsants, such as phenytoin, have been associated with a number of toxic effects, including a drug-induced hypersensitivity syndrome that manifests with a triad of reactions, such as rash, agranulocytosis, thrombocytopenia, lymphadenopathy, Stevens-Johnson syndrome, and hepatitis that have occurred in affected individuals. Although anticonvulsant-induced hypersensitivity reactions are relatively rare events, occurring with an incidence of between 1:1,000 and 1:10,000 exposures, these idiosyncratic reactions can be potentially life-threatening. The hypersensitivity syndrome is consistent with an immune etiology, with symptoms typically appearing within 2 to 8 weeks after the initiation of therapy and generally abate on discontinuation of phenytoin. Dermal metabolism of phenytoin by CYP2C18 to reactive metabolites may be related to the occurrence of hypersensitivity rashes (33). Although the mechanism by which the aromatic anticonvulsants induce hypersensitivity reactions has not been well characterized, recent studies have suggested that the immune response elicited by phenytoin may be caused, at least in part, by its metabolism into chemically reactive metabolites and may be the critical step in the formation of protein adducts and subsequent immune responses. Identification of the reactive metabolite(s) for phenytoin has been difficult, because the rate at which human liver microsomes convert phenytoin to metabolites capable of binding to proteins is quite low. It also is important to note that phenytoin typically is administered in doses ranging from hundreds of milligrams to grams per day, suggesting that a substantial amounts of reactive metabolites could be formed on a daily basis. Therefore, it is conceivable that individuals with a low capacity to detoxify reactive metabolites via glucuronidation or other secondary pathways may represent individuals at risk for idiosyncratic toxicity.

The incidence of phenytoin toxicity may be increased in the elderly, or in those patients with hepatic or renal impairment, because of alterations in its pharmacokinetics. Plasma level determinations may be indicated in these cases. Although a role for P-glycoprotein transporter alleles in the development of phenytoin toxicity remains controversial, phenytoin is a robust substrate for the non-ABC efflux transporter RLIP76. Because RLIP76 has been found to be overexpressed in excised human epileptic foci, its action may account for treatment failures; conversely, inhibition of transport may cause toxicity (34). There is a 2 to 3% increase in the risk of fetal epilepsy syndrome if the mother is taking phenytoin. Phenytoin is contraindicated in cardiac patients with bradyarrhythmias. Induction of CYP2C19 by ginkgo biloba may increase phenytoin clearance and precipitate serious seizures (35).

Fosphenytoin (Cerebyx). Fosphenytoin sodium (Fig. 20.5) is a soluble pro-drug disodium phosphate ester of phenytoin (142 mg/mL) that was developed as a replacement for parenteral phenytoin sodium to circumvent the pH and solubility problems associated with parenteral phenytoin sodium formulations (36,37). Unlike phenytoin, fosphenytoin is freely soluble in aqueous solutions and is rapidly absorbed by the IM route. It is rapidly metabolized (conversion half-life, 8–15 minutes) to phenytoin by in vivo phosphatases. Therapeutic free (unbound) and total plasma phenytoin concentrations are consistently attained following IM or IV administration of fosphenytoin (26). It is administered IV following benzodiazepines for control of status epilepticus or whenever there is a need to rapidly achieve therapeutic plasma concentrations. Severe bradycardiac adverse events to fosphenytoin, including some fatalities, have been reported (38). A dose reduction in patients who are elderly or have renal or hepatic impairment has been suggested.

Ethotoin (Peganone). Ethotoin differs from phenytoin in that one phenyl substituent at position 5 has been replaced by hydrogen, and the N-H at position 3 is replaced by an ethyl group (Fig. 20.5). It may be indicated for treatment of tonic-clonic and complex partial (psychomotor) seizures. Because it is considered to be less toxic but also less effective and more sedating than phenytoin, ethotoin usually is reserved for use as an add-on drug (39). Ethotoin does not share phenytoin's profile of antiarrhythmic action. The metabolism of ethotoin, like phenytoin, is saturable and nonlinear. Its administration is contraindicated in patients with hepatic abnormalities and hematologic disorders.

Mephenytoin. Mephenytoin is N-methylated at position 3 with an ethyl group replacing one of the phenyl substituents at position 5 (Fig. 20.5). It is indicated for focal and jacksonian seizures in patients refractory to less toxic AEDs. Mephenytoin produces more sedation than phenytoin and should be used only when safer drugs have failed, because it is associated with an increased incidence of serious toxicities, such as severe rash, agranulocytosis, and hepatitis (40). Its N-desmethyl metabolite, 5-phenyl-5-ethylhydantoin, contributes to both efficacy and toxicity for mephenytoin. The drug is no longer commercially available inside but is still available outside the United States

Iminostilbenes

Carbamazepine. Carbamazepine (CBZ; Tegretol) (Fig. 20.6) was approved by the U.S. FDA in 1968, and it is presently indicated as initial or adjunct therapy for complex partial, tonic-clonic, and mixed-type seizures. It is one of the two safest and most effective older AEDs for these seizure types (phenytoin is the other) and is chosen for monotherapy because of its high effectiveness and relatively low incidence of side effects (40). Its tricyclic structure resembles that of the psychoactive drugs imipramine, chlorpromazine, and maprotiline and also

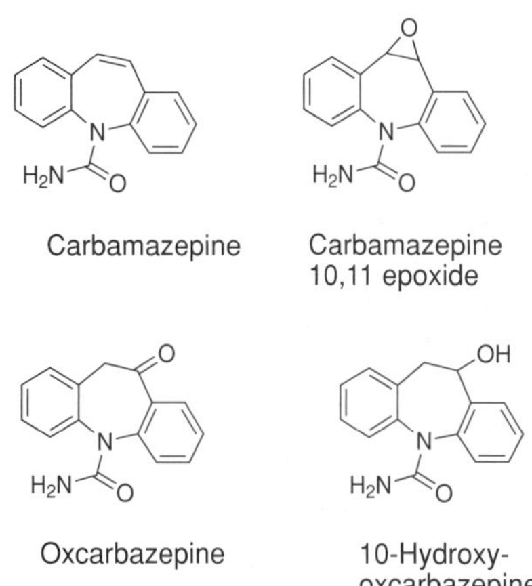

Fig. 20.6. Iminostilbenes.

shares some structural features with the AEDs phenytoin, clonazepam, and phenobarbital. In addition, CBZ has been found to be effective for treatment of bipolar disorder and trigeminal neuralgia.

Mechanism of action. In animals, the profile of antiseizure properties for CBZ is similar to that of phenytoin. CBZ is effective in the maximal electroshock (MES) test (electrically induced seizure test) but is ineffective against pentylenetetrazole-induced seizures. It is not effective for absence or myoclonic seizures and, indeed, may exacerbate their onset (30,41). Like phenytoin, CBZ acts on voltage-dependent sodium channels to prevent the spread of seizures. CBZ depresses synaptic transmission in the reticular activating system, thalamus, and limbic structures. In a double-blind, crossover study in patients whose seizures were not controlled completely by combinations of AED, CBZ was equal in efficacy to phenobarbital and phenytoin in controlling seizure frequency, and side effects were minimal.

Pharmacokinetics. Following the administration of an oral dose, CBZ is slowly absorbed, with the attainment of peak concentration from immediate-release tablets in 4 to 5 hours and from extended-release tablets in 3 to 12 hours. The normal half-life averages between 12 and 17 hours; however, because of autoinduction, the half-life may range from 8 to 29 hours. The half-life for CBZ-10,11-epoxide is 5 to 8 hours. Therapeutic plasma concentrations range from 4 to 12 μg/mL (in adults) and may require a month to achieve a stable therapeutic concentration for the desired antiseizure effect because of induction of hepatic metabolizing enzymes.

CBZ is principally metabolized by CYP3A4 its 10,11-epoxide, with CYP2C8 and CYP1A2 having minor roles. CBZ epoxide is hydrolyzed to inactive 10,11-dihydroxy CBZ by epoxide hydrolase. CBZ epoxide is active and appears to be more toxic than CBZ (42,43). However, CBZ not only induces CYP3A4 activity but also its own metabolism (an autoinducer) as well as UGT and the increased formation of glucuronide metabolites. Like phenytoin, CBZ has been associated with a number of toxic effects, including a drug-induced hypersensitivity syndrome. Although phenytoin-induced hypersensitivity reactions are relatively rare events, they can be potentially life-threatening. Although the mechanism by which CBZ induces hypersensitivity reactions has not been well characterized, recent studies have suggested that the immune reaction may be caused, at least in part, by its metabolism into chemically reactive metabolites, which may be the critical step in the formation of protein adducts and subsequent immune responses. Identification of the reactive metabolite(s) has been difficult, because the rate at which human liver microsomes convert CBZ to metabolites capable of binding to proteins is quite low. Furthermore, it also is important to note that CBZ typically is administered in doses ranging from hundreds of milligrams to grams per day, suggesting that a substantial amounts of reactive metabolites may be formed on a daily basis. Therefore, it is conceivable that individuals with a low capacity to detoxify reactive metabolites via glucuronidation or other pathways may present individuals at risk for idiosyncratic toxicity. Although an arene oxide was originally proposed as the reactive species and an iminoquinone metabolite derived from the CBZ metabolite (CBZ-IQ) or 2-hydroxyiminostilbene (2-OHIS) are potential candidates for the reactive metabolite, because quinone- and iminoquinone-type metabolites have been implicated in drug-induced hepatotoxicity (see Chapter 10). CYP3A4-catalyzed secondary metabolism of 2-hydroxycarbamazepine to 2-OHIS or to CBZ-IQ, followed by nonenzymatic reduction to 2-hydroxyiminostilbene, may well underlie subsequent development of drug-induced hypersensitivity to CBZ (Fig. 20.7) (44). Based on the formation of glutathione and N-acetylcysteine conjugates, it has been suggested that 2-OHIS is the target for the formation of protein adducts, which could lead to localized idiosyncratic toxicities. Like phenytoin, CBZ is highly protein bound (Table 20.2) and is extensively transformed. Approximately 72% of an oral dose is excreted in the urine as metabolites and 3% as unchanged drug. The 28% found in the feces may be the result of incomplete absorption and enterohepatic cycling. As previously mentioned, interindividual variability in apparent plasma half-life and total body clearance is related to the phenomenon of autoinduction.

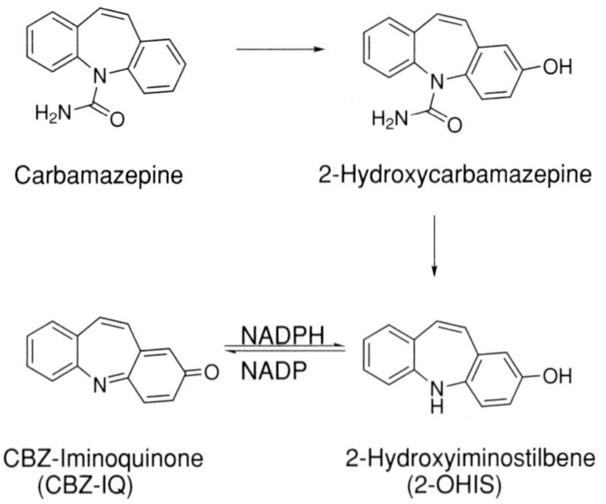

Carbamazepine → 2-Hydroxycarbamazepine → 2-Hydroxyiminostilbene (2-OHIS) ⇌ (NADPH / NADP) CBZ-Iminoquinone (CBZ-IQ)

Fig. 20.7. Bioactivation pathway for carbamazepine.

Adverse effects. Gastric upset from CBZ may be diminished by taking the drug after meals. Common toxicities include blurred vision, dizziness, drowsiness, and ataxia. Tremor, depression, hyponatremia, and cardiac disturbances are seen at high serum concentrations. Idiosyncratic rashes are common; rarer severe idiosyncratic effects include aplastic anemia, agranulocytosis, thrombocytopenia, and jaundice. Therefore, patients receiving CBZ should have periodic blood count determinations and liver function tests. Both CBZ and oxcarbazepine can reduce plasma 25-hydroxy vitamin D levels (45). CBZ increases levels of phenytoin and decreases levels of felbamate, lamotrigine, oral contraceptives, theophylline, valproate, and zonisamide. CBZ levels are increased by propoxyphene, erythromycin, chloramphenicol, isoniazid, verapamil, and cimetidine. CBZ levels are decreased by phenobarbital, phenytoin, felbamate, and primidone. Lamotrigine and valproic acid may elevate CBZ epoxide levels. Administration of the extended-release form has been associated with fewer side effects and with improved seizure control (46).

Macrolide antibiotics inhibit CBZ metabolism, thus increasing CBZ plasma levels and decreasing clearance with the potential for toxicity effects. Drug-induced changes in CBZ pharmacokinetics are particularly pronounced in children (28).

CBZ should be used with caution in patients with a history of congestive heart failure or cardiac arrhythmias (because it may aggravate them) and with a history of hematologic reactions to other drugs or hypersensitivity to tricyclic antidepressants. Blood levels should be monitored in patients with renal or hepatic impairment.

OXCARBAZEPINE. Oxcarbazepine (Trileptal®) is the 10-keto analogue of carbamazepine (Fig. 20.6). It is indicated as monotherapy or adjunctive therapy for partial seizures in adults with epilepsy, as monotherapy for the treatment of partial seizures in children 4 years of age or older, and as adjunct therapy in children 2 to 4 years of age.

Mechanism of action. Although oxcarbazepine is less potent that CBZ, its mechanism of action is similar (47). The majority of the pharmacological activity for oxcarbazepine is attributed to its primary metabolite, 10-monohydroxycarbazepine (MHD) (Fig. 20.6), the plasma levels of which may be ninefold higher than those for CBZ. Both oxcarbazepine and MHD produce a blockade of voltage-dependent sodium channels, thus decreasing repetitive firing and spread of electrical activity. An additional action on calcium and potassium channels may contribute to the therapeutic effect. Like carbamazepine, oxcarbazepine may worsen juvenile myoclonic or absence seizures (41).

Pharmacokinetics. Oxcarbazepine is completely absorbed, and food has no effect on its absorption. Unlike CBZ, it does not cause autoinduction of its own metabolism. The metabolism of oxcarbazepine is different from that of CBZ. Oxcarbazepine is reduced by cytosolic enzymes to MHD before its O-glucuronidation. More than 95% of its oral dose is excreted as conjugated metabolites, with approximately 4% of the drug converted to inactive 10,11-dihydroxy CBZ. Unlike CBZ, no epoxide nor aromatic hydroxylation metabolites are formed. The half-life is 2 hours for oxcarbazepine and 9 hours for the active 10-monohydroxy metabolite. In patients with impaired renal function, the half-life for MHD is prolonged to 19 hours, with a doubling in its area under the plasma concentration curve. Peak plasma concentration following an oral dose occurs at approximately 4.5 hours.

Oxcarbazepine induces CYP3A4/5 and UTP, and it also inhibits CYP2C19, producing significant effects on the plasma concentration of other drugs. Therefore, oxcarbazepine decreases felodipine bioavailability and lowers plasma levels for lamotrigine, CBZ, CBZ epoxide, calcium channel blockers, and oral contraceptives (48). Oxcarbazepine increases plasma levels of phenobarbital and phenytoin. Unlike carbamazepine, oxcarbazepine has no effect on plasma levels of risperidone or olanzepine (49,50). The plasma levels for oxcarbazepine or MHD are decreased by CBZ, phenobarbital, phenytoin, valproate, and verapamil. Serum MHD may decrease during pregnancy but increase following delivery (51). Oxcarbazepine clearance is decreased in renal impairment and the elderly. In children, a higher dose/kg for oxcarbazepine than in adults is required to obtain an effective plasma concentration.

Adverse effects. Patients with hypersensitivity reactions to carbamazepine can be expected to show cross-sensitivity (e.g., rash) or related problems to oxcarbazepine. The improved toxicity profile for oxcarbazepine when compared to CBZ may result from absence of the epoxide or CBZ-iminoquinone metabolites (47). The most common side effects are headache, dizziness, nystagmus, blurred vision, somnolence, nausea, ataxia, and fatigue. The incidence of adverse effects has been related to elevated serum MHD concentrations (52). Adverse effects on cognitive status, hyponatremia, and serious dermatological reactions have been reported, as has hyponatremia (53).

Barbiturates

The barbiturates are substituted pyrimidine derivatives with an ureide configuration (Fig. 20.4). They are lipophilic weak acids (pK_a 7–8) that are well distributed into brain (see Appendix A for the respective pK_a values). Although many barbiturates display sedative-hypnotic activity (see Chapter 19), only a few have antiseizure properties. Paradoxically, many barbiturates cause convulsions at larger doses. The barbiturates clinically useful as AEDs are phenobarbital, mephobarbital, and primidone (Fig. 20.8). In laboratory animals, phenobarbital is effective by several tests in nontoxic doses. It is active against electrically induced seizures (MES), and it elevates the threshold for pentylenetetrazole stimulation. The mechanism of antiseizure action for the barbiturates

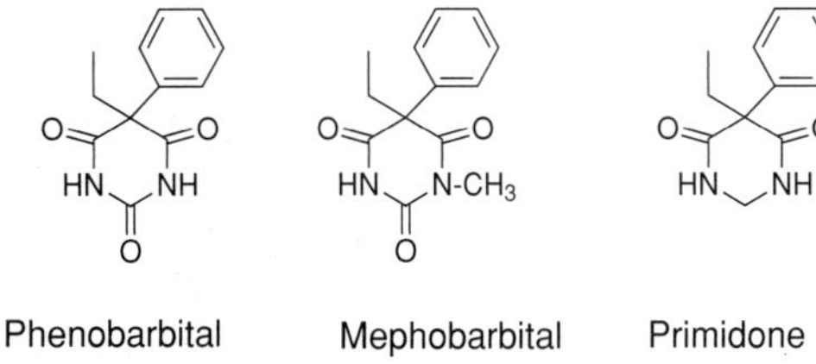

Phenobarbital Mephobarbital Primidone

Fig. 20.8. Barbiturates.

is unknown but is thought to involve blockade of sodium channels and enhancement of GABA-mediated inhibitory transmission.

PHENOBARBITAL. Phenobarbital is commonly used for convulsive disorders and is the drug of choice for seizures in infants up to 2 months of age. Phenobarbital is indicated for the treatment of partial and generalized tonic-clonic seizures in all age groups, although it is less effective than phenytoin or CBZ in adults (40). Although occasionally used as monotherapy, it usually is combined with another AED. Phenobarbital may be administered parenterally, as its sodium salt, for emergency control of acute convulsive disorders associated with eclampsia (although magnesium sulfate is the standard treatment), meningitis, tetanus, and toxic reactions to strychnine or local anesthetics. Because of its slow onset of action, it is administered after benzodiazepines for the treatment of status epilepticus.

Pharmacokinetics. Phenobarbital is a weak acid (pK_a 7.4, log P = 1.53 at pH 7.4) that is approximately 50% ionized at physiologic pH and is well distributed into the CNS. Its oral absorption is slow but nearly complete, with an oral bioavailability of 80–100%, and it shows linear kinetics. Phenobarbital is 40 to 60% protein bound and exhibits a long plasma half-life of 2 to 6 days, which yields an extremely stable plasma concentration. Approximately 25 to 50% of a phenobarbital dose is excreted unchanged in the urine. The remainder is metabolized primarily by hydroxylation to its inactive metabolite, 5-p-hydroxyphenyl-5-ethyl-barbituric acid, which is then conjugated as its glucuronide or sulfate and is excreted in the urine. Some of the conjugated metabolites may appear in the feces from enterohepatic cycling. Alkalinizing the urine or increasing the urine flow substantially increases the rate of excretion of unchanged phenobarbital and its metabolites. Phenobarbital is a potent liver enzyme–inducing drug of CYP3A4 and increases the ability of the liver to metabolize many drugs, when taken concurrently, that normally are metabolized by CYP3A4. It also induces UGTs and increased formation of glucuronidation. No conclusive evidence, however, shows that phenobarbital induces its own metabolism (autoinducer), as does CBZ.

Because of its inducing effect on hepatic enzymes, phenobarbital has many drug interactions, decreasing plasma levels of CBZ, valproate, lamotrigine, tiagabine, zonisamide, warfarin, theophylline, cimetidine, and those of other CYP3A4 substrates. Serum concentrations of phenobarbital are increased by valproate.

Adverse effects. Serious toxicity is rare; however, drowsiness is the most common side effect reported for phenobarbital. Of the barbiturates, only phenobarbital, mephobarbital, and primidone are antiseizure at subhypnotic doses. The sedative effect of phenobarbital limits its use in older children and adults, although tolerance to the sedative effects often develops. When compared to phenytoin or CBZ, phenobarbital shows more sedation, irritability, paradoxical hyperactivity, and impaired intellectual function. This may prove to be particularly troublesome in children, especially those of school age, and in the elderly. Quite rare are idiosyncratic hypersensitivity reactions to phenobarbital that include rash, agranulocytosis, aplastic anemia, and hepatitis. Although the mechanism by which the phenobarbital and other aromatic anticonvulsants induce hypersensitivity reactions has not been well characterized, recent studies have suggested that the immune response elicited may be caused, at least in part, by the metabolism of phenobarbital into chemically reactive metabolites, which may be the critical step in the formation of protein adducts and subsequent immune responses (see discussion for CBZ). Long-term use of phenobarbital may precipitate folate, vitamin K, or vitamin D deficiencies.

Phenobarbital should be used with caution in patients with hepatic impairment; therefore, a dose reduction may be needed. It should be avoided in patients with renal impairment. Barbiturates are known to cause fetal abnormalities and a neonatal coagulation defect responsive to vitamin K.

MEPHOBARBITAL (MEBARAL). Mephobarbital is a barbiturate-derivative AED with a pK_a of 7.7 (log P = 1.84 at pH 7.4). Approximately 50% of an oral dose of mephobarbital is absorbed from the gastrointestinal tract. The plasma concentrations required for its therapeutic effects are unknown. The principal route of mephobarbital metabolism is N-demethylation by the liver to form phenobarbital, which may be excreted in the urine unchanged and as its p-hydroxy metabolite and glucuronide or sulfate conjugates (see Fig. 19.6). Conversion to the 4-hydroxy metabolite is stereoselective, being catalyzed by either CYP2C19 (R-enantiomer) or CYP2B6 (S-enantiomer); individuals who are CYP2C19 poor metabolizers show decreased clearance (54). Approximately 75% of a single oral dose of mephobarbital is converted to phenobarbital. It has not been determined whether mephobarbital contributes to the antiseizure effect or whether it results from its active metabolite, phenobarbital. Similarly, it is unclear whether mephobarbital, like phenobarbital, is a potent inducer of the enzymes involved in the metabolism of other drugs, but because the drug is chemically and pharmacologically similar to phenobarbital and is metabolized to phenobarbital, this possibility is likely.

Mephobarbital is less commonly used in the treatment of generalized and partial seizures. Like phenobarbital, it is classified as a long-acting barbiturate. No evidence exists that it is more effective than phenobarbital in equivalent doses; however, it may be less sedating in children.

PRIMIDONE (MYSOLINE). Primidone is the 2-deoxy derivative of phenobarbital (Fig. 20.8) and is approved by the U.S. FDA for initial or adjunctive treatment of simple partial, complex partial, and tonic-clonic seizures. It is less effective against these types of seizures than is phenytoin or CBZ, and it shares the antiseizure and sedative actions of phenobarbital. Although not approved for the purpose, it often is used to treat benign familial tremor (essential tremor).

Pharmacokinetics. Approximately 60 to 80% of an oral dose of primidone is absorbed and slowly metabolized by the liver to phenobarbital and phenylethylmalonamide (PEMA) (55,56). All three molecules have antiseizure effects, but PEMA appears to be weaker and to be the more toxic metabolite. During chronic therapy, approximately 15 to 25% of an oral dose of primidone is excreted in the urine unchanged, 15 to 25% metabolized to phenobarbital, and 50 to 70% excreted as PEMA (half-life, 24–48 hours). The phenobarbital metabolite may be excreted in the urine unchanged, as its p-hydroxy metabolite, and as glucuronide or sulfate conjugates. Following an oral dose, the peak plasma levels for primidone are reached in approximately 4 hours, with a reported half-life of 10 to 12 hours. Plasma concentrations in the range of 8 to 12 μg/mL control seizures and minimize adverse effects. Primidone shows antiseizure activity before the phenobarbital levels reach therapeutic range. Only after chronic dosing of primidone are the levels of phenobarbital significant, suggesting autoinduction. Serum levels of chronically administered primidone exceed those of its metabolite, phenobarbital, thus demonstrating that it has antiseizure activity independent of phenobarbital. When primidone is coadministered with enzyme-inducing AEDs, the levels of its phenobarbital metabolite may be two- to threefold higher than those in the noninduced state. Protein binding of primidone and PEMA is negligible, and the phenobarbital metabolite is approximately 50% protein bound.

Primidone use is associated with decreases in CBZ, lamotrigine, valproate, tiagabine, and zonisamide serum levels. Primidone levels are increased by nicotinamide and isoniazid. Hydantoins increase the plasma concentrations of primidone, phenobarbital, and PEMA. CBZ increases levels of phenobarbital derived from primidone. Primidone levels are decreased by succinimides, CBZ, and acetazolamide.

Adverse effects. As with phenobarbital, serious toxicity for primidone is rare, although it may cause disabling sedation, irritability, and decreased mental functioning in a number of persons. Ataxia, dysphoria, idiosyncratic rash, leukopenia, agranulocytosis, lymphadenopathy, hepatitis, and a systemic lupus erythematosus–like syndrome have been reported adverse effects for primidone. Deficiencies of folic acid and of vitamins D and K are possible with long-term therapy of primidone, as is a folate-responsive megaloblastic anemia. Measurement of the complete blood cell count should be performed at 6-month intervals (40).

Benzodiazepines

This class of drugs has been widely used as sedative-hypnotics and antianxiety drugs (see Chapters 19 and 22). In

Diazepam Clonazepam Lorazepam

Clorazepate dipotassium Midazolam

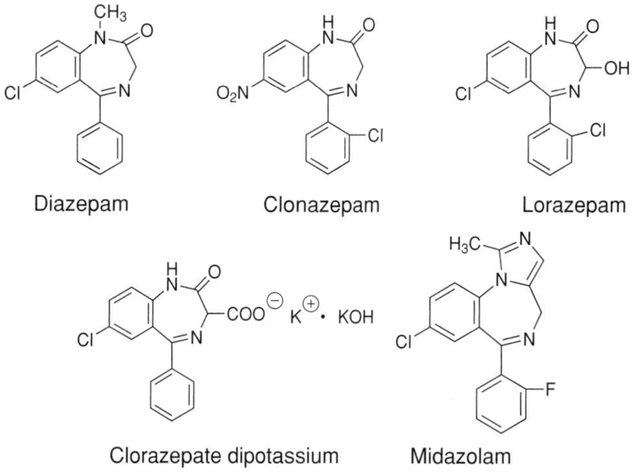

Fig. 20.9. Benzodiazepines.

laboratory animals, benzodiazepines display outstanding antiseizure properties against seizures induced by maximal electroshock and pentylenetetrazole. The benzodiazepines diazepam, lorazepam, clonazepam, clorazepate dipotassium, and midazolam are effective for seizure control (Table 20.2 and Fig. 20.9). All benzodiazepines enter cerebral tissue rapidly. Although the duration of action is short for diazepam (2 hours) and midazolam (3–4 hours), longer for clonazepam (24 hours), and much longer for lorazepam (up to 72 hours), no correlation exists with the plasma concentration–time profiles for these drugs (57,58). Diazepam and lorazepam can be administered either IV or IM for control of status epilepticus; however, absorption is slower from the IM site. Midazolam is particularly useful for treating status epilepticus, because its imidazole ring is open at low pH, allowing it to be dissolved in aqueous solution for IM injection, but is closed at physiologic pH, increasing lipophilicity with rapid IM absorption, brain penetration, and fast onset of action. When administered IM, midazolam has a faster onset of action than diazepam and lorazepam because of its rapid absorption from the injection site, with an efficacy at least equal to that of IV diazepam (57,58). Seizure arrest usually is attained within 5 to 10 minutes. In addition, the use of midazolam by the buccal route for initial treatment of acute seizure activity has been shown to be more effective and without increased respiratory depression as compared to the use of rectal diazepam (59). Midazolam has been used intranasally as well (60,61). Lorazepam, although not approved by the U.S. FDA for this purpose, is preferred by some clinicians for the treatment of status epilepticus because of its longer duration of action.

Mechanism of Action. The benzodiazepines are thought to produce their antiseizure effects primarily by enhancing the effect of the inhibitory neurotransmitter GABA on the $GABA_A$ chloride channel (Figs. 20.1 and 20.2).

Additional evidence suggests that the benzodiazepines may diminish voltage-dependent sodium, potassium, and calcium currents in a manner independent of the $GABA_A$/ benzodiazepine receptor complex.

DIAZEPAM (VALIUM). Diazepam is given orally for adjunctive control of convulsive disorders, as a rectal gel (Diastat) for refractory patients with epilepsy on a stable regimen of AEDs who require intermittent use of diazepam to control bouts of increased seizure activity, and parenterally as part of the regimen for the treatment of status epilepticus or other severe, recurrent seizures. Rectal diazepam gel is an effective and well-tolerated therapy for acute repetitive seizures (59).

Pharmacokinetics. Orally administered diazepam is less effective as an AED, because tolerance to the antiseizure effects of diazepam develops within a short period. Diazepam gel is rapidly absorbed rectally, having greater than 90% bioavailability. In addition to cluster seizures, it has been proven to be useful to control prolonged febrile seizures in children.

Intravenously administered diazepam is the route of choice for rapid control of status epilepticus (62). Because of its high lipid solubility, IV diazepam enters the CNS rapidly. However, the initial high brain concentration is reduced quickly because of its redistribution; thus, status epilepticus may return. To prevent the return of status epilepticus, the initial dose of diazepam is followed sequentially by parenteral phenytoin (fosphenytoin) and phenobarbital as needed for control of tonic-clonic status epilepticus. For absence status epilepticus, diazepam usually is followed by ethosuximide.

The half-life for diazepam is 46 hours and is metabolized by CYP2C19 and CYP3A4 to desmethyldiazepam, an active metabolite with a half-life of 71 hours. Diazepam is 95% protein bound. Cimetidine, by inhibiting CYP3A4, decreases the metabolism and clearance of diazepam. Drugs that affect the activity of CYP2C19 or CYP3A4 may alter diazepam kinetics, and vice versa.

Adverse effects. The most frequent side effect for diazepam is somnolence; dizziness, ataxia, headache, nervousness, euphoria, and rash occur less frequently. Excessive use of rectal diazepam may produce rebound seizures (63). Intravenous administration may produce infrequent respiratory depression and hypotension. Other sedative drugs, such as barbiturates, valproate, narcotics, phenothiazines, monoamine oxidase inhibitors, and antidepressants, can potentiate the effects of diazepam.

Because diazepam clearance is decreased in the elderly and in patients with hepatic insufficiency, a dosage reduction may be warranted. Intravenous diazepam should be used cautiously in patients who are elderly, very ill, or have limited pulmonary reserve, because respiratory depression has occurred. Rarely, IV diazepam is given to patients for absence status (typical and atypical), because it will precipitate tonic status epileptic.

CLONAZEPAM. Clonazepam (Klonopin) was approved in 1975 for monotherapy or adjunctive treatment of akinetic (atonic), myoclonic, and absence variant seizures (64). Clonazepam also was found to be effective in controlling absence seizures, but because of the high incidence of side effects, it is rated second to ethosuximide. It may be useful, however, in absence seizures when succinimide therapy has failed. It is considered to be a third-line drug after 1) ethosuximide or valproate and 2) lamotrigine or valproate for the treatment of absence seizures. It is ineffective for treatment of generalized clonic-tonic seizures.

Clonazepam is well absorbed, 95 to 98% protein bound, and extensively metabolized by CYP3A4. Clonazepam displays a wide spectrum of antiseizure activities and is one of the most potent AEDs. Side effects are common, however, and the development of tolerance is more frequent than with ethosuximide or valproate. Sedation is prominent, especially early in treatment. Drowsiness, ataxia, and behavioral changes may be disabling, but slowly increasing its dose over a 2-week period is recommended to minimize adverse effects. Diplopia, headaches, nystagmus, and other neurologic effects have been reported with the use of clonazepam.

Serum levels of clonazepam are decreased by the enzyme-inducing properties of phenobarbital, phenytoin, and CBZ. Concurrent administration of amphetamines, methylphenidate, ethanol, antianxiety drugs, or antipsychotics may cause CNS depression or altered respiration. The combined administration of clonazepam and valproate may cause absence status, and in patients displaying a mixed seizure pattern, clonazepam may precipitate grand mal seizures.

CLORAZEPATE DIPOTASSIUM. Clorazepate dipotassium (Tranxene) was approved for use as an AED by the U.S. FDA in 1981. It is less commonly used as adjunct therapy for the management of partial seizures in adults and children older than 9 years. Clorazepate is decarboxylated by the acidity of the stomach to desmethyldiazepam, which also is the major active metabolite of diazepam. Therefore, clorazepate exhibits the profile and properties of diazepam.

LORAZEPAM (ATIVAN). Lorazepam is a benzodiazepine (Fig. 20.6), with pK_a values of 1.3 and 11.5. Its parenteral solutions are formulated with polyethylene glycol and dilution with diluents may cause its crystallization from solution. Lorazepam also is used IV or IM for the management of status epilepticus. Although IV diazepam has been used more extensively, some clinicians prefer IV lorazepam because of its more prolonged duration of effect. It has been recommended for initial treatment of generalized convulsive status epilepticus in the elderly (65). A long-acting AED, such as IV phenytoin or fosphenytoin, can be added to IV benzodiazepine therapy for the management of recurring seizures associated with status epilepticus.

Intramuscular lorazepam is slowly absorbed, with peak plasma concentrations reached in approximately 60 to 90 minutes. The half-life for unconjugated lorazepam is approximately 16 hours when given IV or IM, and it is eliminated in the urine as its major metabolite, lorazepam 3-O-glucuronide. Lorazepam glucuronide has no demonstrable CNS activity in animals but has a half-life of approximately 18 hours. Lorazepam is 85% bound to plasma proteins. Drugs that inhibit or induce the oxidative metabolism of benzodiazepines (CYP3A4) are less likely to affect lorazepam, because it undergoes only glucuronide conjugation.

OTHER BENZODIAZEPINES. In addition to their anxiolytic and sedative-hypnotic properties, several other benzodiazepines also display antiseizure activity. They include clobazam and nitrazepam, which are used outside the United States.; they have not demonstrated any clinical advantage over clonazepam.

Bis-Carbamates

FELBAMATE (FELBATOL)

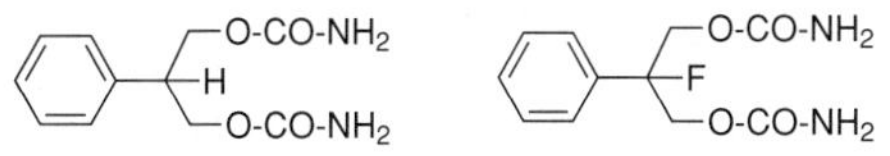

Felbamate is a dicarbamate that is structurally similar to the antianxiety drug meprobamate. It was approved by the U.S. FDA for antiseizure use in 1993. Following the occurrence of rare cases of aplastic anemia and of severe hepatotoxicity associated with the use of felbamate during early 1994, however, a black box warning was added to the drug's package insert (53). Despite this, felbamate continues to be used in many patients, although not as a first-line treatment. These toxicity effects may be attributed to the formation of toxic metabolites (66). Although felbamate use is now uncommon, it is used for severe refractory seizures, either partial, myoclonic, or atonic, or in Lennox-Gastaut syndrome.

Mechanism of action. Although its mechanism of action is unknown, felbamate antagonizes the NMDA receptor by binding to the glycine recognition site, preventing the usual glycine-induced increase in calcium channel opening frequency and lowering calcium currents (Fig. 20.2) (67).

Metabolism and pharmacokinetics. Although the metabolism of felbamate has not been fully characterized, felbamate is esterase hydrolyzed to its monocarbamate metabolite, 2-phenyl-1,3-propanediol monocarbamate, which subsequently is oxidized via aldehyde dehydrogenase to its major human metabolite 3-carbamoyl-2-phenylpropionic acid (Fig. 20.10). Other metabolites include the p-hydroxy and mercapturic acid metabolites of felbamate, which have been identified in human urine. Felbamate is a substrate for CYP2C19, with minor activity for CYP3A4 and CYP2E1. Thompson et al. (68) has provided evidence for the formation of the reactive metabolite, 3-carbamoyl-2-phenylpropionaldehyde (CBMA), from the alcohol oxidation of 2-phenyl-1,3-propanediol monocarbamate. CBMA then undergoes spontaneous elimination to another reactive intermediate, 2-phenylpropenal (more commonly known as atropaldehyde), which is proposed to play a role

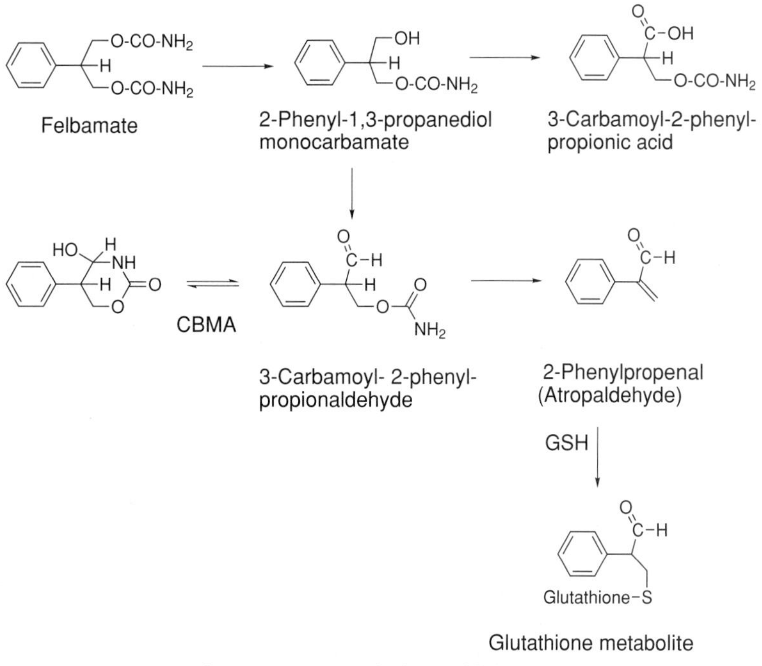

Fig. 20.10. Metabolism of felbamate.

in the development of toxicity during felbamate therapy. CBMA or a further product has been shown to provoke an immune response in mice (69). Evidence for in vivo atropaldehyde formation was confirmed with the identification of its mercapturic acid conjugates in human urine after felbamate administration. This is consistent with the hypothesis that atropaldehyde reacts rapidly with thiol nucleophiles, such as glutathione, to form mercapturates (see Chapter 10). More recently, a fluorine analogue of felbamate was synthesized in which the benzylic C_2 hydrogen of the propane chain was replaced with fluorine, preventing the formation of atropaldehyde and confirming that the acidic benzylic hydrogen plays a pivotal role in its formation (70). This analogue is presently undergoing drug development. Felbamate administration exhibited linear kinetics, with a half-life of 20 to 23 hours in the absence of enzyme-inducing AEDs. Approximately 50% of an oral dose of felbamate is excreted unchanged.

Adverse effects. Felbamate has exhibited the rare occurrence of aplastic anemia and of severe hepatotoxicity, which may be associated with the in vivo formation of reactive metabolites. Felbamate increases phenytoin and valproate serum levels but decreases the level of CBZ. The increase in valproate plasma concentrations by felbamate is through the inhibition of β-oxidation. No clinically relevant pharmacokinetic interactions have been noted between felbamate and lamotrigine, clonazepam, vigabatrin, or the active monohydroxy metabolite of oxcarbazepine. The enzyme inducers phenytoin, phenobarbital, and CBZ decrease felbamate plasma levels by increasing its clearance.

GABAPENTIN (NEURONTIN)

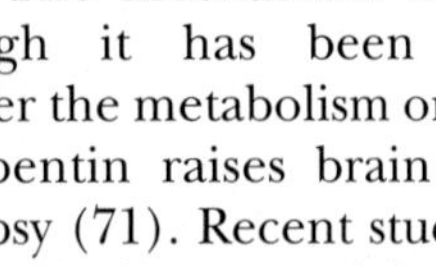

$H_3N^{\oplus}$—C(cyclohexane)—CH_2—C(=O)—$O^{\ominus}$

Mechanism of action. Gabapentin is a water-soluble amino acid originally designed to be a GABA-mimetic analogue capable of penetrating the CNS. Surprisingly, it has no direct GABA-mimetic activity, nor is it active on sodium channels. The mechanism of action remains unknown, although it has been suggested that gabapentin may alter the metabolism or release of GABA (Fig. 20.2). Gabapentin raises brain GABA levels in patients with epilepsy (71). Recent studies have demonstrated gabapentin binding to calcium channels in a manner that can be allosterically modulated (72).

Gabapentin is indicated as an adjunct for use against partial seizures with or without secondary generalization, in patients older than 12 years, and as adjunct for the treatment of partial seizures in children 3 to 12 years of age. It also is approved for the treatment of postherpetic neuralgia.

Pharmacokinetics. The pharmacokinetic properties for gabapentin generally are favorable, with a bioavailability of 60% when given in low doses and somewhat less when given at higher doses because of saturable intestinal uptake by the L-amino-acid transporter (73). The L-amino-acid transporter is very susceptible to substrate saturation (low K_m value). Its absorption and distribution into the CNS appears to be dependent on this amino acid transporter. Following the administration of an oral dose, gabapentin reaches peak plasma concentration in 2 to 3 hours. Additionally, it exhibits linear pharmacokinetics. Moreover, it is not extensively metabolized, nor is it an inducer of hepatic metabolizing enzymes. The elimination of unmetabolized gabapentin occurs by the renal route. Although its therapeutic range is not well characterized, gabapentin has a broad therapeutic index. This implies that a wide range of doses can be used, based on individual patient needs, without significant limitation because of dose-dependent side effects. Protein binding is negligible. Its elimination half-life of 5 to 7 hours is not affected by the dose or by other drugs, and its short half-life necessitates multiple daily administration.

Adverse effects. Adverse effects of gabapentin are uncommon and not serious. The CNS effects include mild to moderate sedation, fatigue, ataxia, headache, dizziness, and diplopia. Gabapentin may exacerbate myoclonus, but the effect is mild and does not require discontinuance of the drug (53,74). It has been associated with the development of neuropsychiatric adverse events in children.

Drug interactions are infrequent with gabapentin. It does not induce hepatic metabolizing enzymes, nor do other AEDs affect its metabolism and elimination. Antacids may decrease absorption. Gabapentin dosage may need to be decreased in patients with renal disease or in the elderly.

LAMOTRIGINE (LAMICTAL)

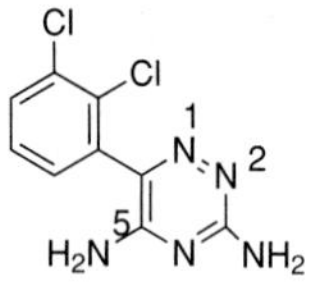

Cl, Cl, 1, N, N, 2, 5, H_2N, N, NH_2

Lamotrigine is a 5-phenyl-1,2,4-triazine derivative indicated as monotherapy or as an adjunct for partial seizures in adults, as adjunct in patients with Lennox-Gastaut syndrome, and as adjunct for partial seizures in children 2 years of age and older. Lamotrigine may have additional benefit in combating myoclonic and typical absence seizures. It is approved for use in the maintenance treatment of bipolar disorder.

Mechanism of action. The most probable explanation for lamotrigine's efficacy is its ability to produce a blockade of sodium channel repetitive firing. In addition, lamotrigine appears to reduce glutaminergic excitatory transmission, although the mechanism for this action remains unclear (75,76).

Pharmacokinetics. Following oral administration, lamotrigine is absorbed rapidly and completely, exhibiting linear pharmacokinetics and modest protein binding (55%). Lamotrigine is metabolized predominantly by N-glucuronidation and subsequent urinary elimination of its major metabolite, the quaternary 2-N-glucuronide (80–90%), the minor 5-amino-N-glucuronide (8–10%), and unchanged drug (8–10%) (77). Lamotrigine's usual elimination half-life of 24–35 hours is reduced to 13–15 hours in patients taking enzyme-inducing AEDs. The presence of valproate increases the lamotrigine half-life substantially by inhibiting N-glucuronidation, necessitating a reduction in dose to avoid toxicity. Hepatic disease patients may demonstrate a reduced capacity to for lamotrigine glucuronidation, thus reducing its rate of clearance.

Adverse effects. The usefulness of lamotrigine is limited by the increased incidence of serious rashes, particularly in children or patients taking valproate (53). This increase, however, may be attenuated by very slow dose escalation, because most rashes appear within the first 8 weeks of treatment. The drug should be discontinued if a rash appears at any time. Additionally, lamotrigine may be associated with development of myoclonus after 2 to 3 years of drug treatment (78). Additional common side effects associated with lamotrigine therapy include dizziness, diplopia, headache, ataxia, blurred vision, somnolence, and nausea.

S-(–)-LEVETIRACETAM (KEPPRA)

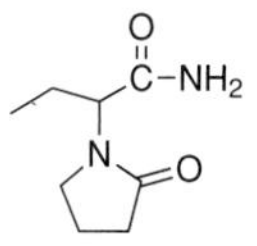

S-(–)-levetiracetam is a pyrrolidone derivative unrelated to the structures of other AEDs. It is indicated as an adjunct in the treatment of partial onset seizures in adults, and it has shown some benefit in clinical trials for generalized tonic-clonic seizures (GTC) and myoclonic seizures in adults and children (79,80).

Mechanism of action. The mechanism of action for S-(–)-levetiracetam is unknown. It does not appear to interact with any of the recognized excitatory or inhibitory neural mechanism. A CNS-specific binding site for S-(–)-levetiracetam has been identified as the synaptic vesicle protein (SV2A). Knockout animals without SV2A proteins accumulated presynaptic Ca^{2+} during consecutive action potentials that destabilized synaptic circuits and induced epilepsy. Thus, it appears that SV2A plays a major role in the antiepileptic properties of S-(–)-levetiracetam, which acts by modulating the function of SV2A and the regulation of Ca^{2+}-mediated synaptic transmission. These data support previous indications that S-(–)-levetiracetam possesses a mechanism of action distinct from that of other antiepileptic drugs. Three SV2 isoforms (SV2A, SV2B, and SV2C) have been identified, each of which has a unique distribution in brain, suggesting synapse-specific functions (81) as well as antagonism of neuronal synchronization (74,82).

Pharmacokinetics. S-(–)-levetiracetam displays rapid and complete absorption, although food slows the rate but not the extent of absorption. It exhibits linear pharmacokinetics and is minimally protein bound (83). Approximately 60% of an oral dose is excreted into the urine unchanged and 24 to 30% as its carboxylic acid metabolite, with an elimination half-life in adults of approximately 7 hours. Although S-(–)-levetiracetam is not metabolized by hepatic CYP450, UGT, or epoxide hydrolase, it is esterase hydrolyzed to its carboxylic acid metabolite (loss of amido group), which is not affected by the hepatic metabolizing enzymes.

Adverse effects. The risk of clinically relevant drug interactions is minimal with S-(–)-levetiracetam, because it does not alter the pharmacokinetics of coadministered drugs by inhibition or induction of hepatic enzymes (84). Toxic effects include mild to moderate somnolence, asthenia, ataxia, and dizziness; these effects seldom require discontinuance. An increase in the incidence of behavioral abnormalities in children and in adults having a previous history of neuropsychiatric problems has been noted (85). Its use in the elderly or in patients with renal impairment will require an individualization of dose, and an additional dose is needed after renal dialysis. Levetiracetam was associated with developmental toxicity in the offspring of pregnant animals.

RETIGABINE

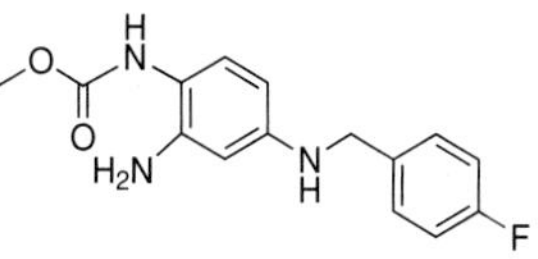

Retigabine is an investigational antiepileptic drug with a novel mechanism of action that involves opening of neuronal voltage-activated K^+ channels that serves to stabilize the membrane potential and to control neuronal excitability. Thus, retigabine also may prove to be useful in the treatment of other diseases associated with neuronal hyperexcitability.

TIAGABINE (GABITRIL®)

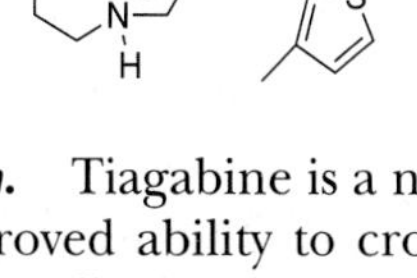

Mechanism of action. Tiagabine is a nipecotic acid derivative with an improved ability to cross the blood-brain barrier. It was rationally designed to be a GABA uptake inhibitor based on the fact that nipecotic acid (piperidine-3-carboxylic acid) inhibits GABA uptake by glial cells. Tiagabine binds to the GABA transporter GAT1, blocking the uptake of GABA into both neurons and glia, thus enhancing GABA-mediated inhibition (Fig. 20.2) (52,86). Tiagabine is presently approved for adjunct use in patients with epilepsy who are older than 12 years and have partial seizures not controlled by first-line drugs.

Pharmacokinetics. Tiagabine is well absorbed, with an oral bioavailability of 90 to 95%. It displays linear pharmacokinetics, with a plasma half-life of 5 to 8 hours, necessitating a multiple daily dosing regimen (87). It also is highly protein bound (96%). The major pathway of metabolism for tiagabine is oxidation by CYP3A4, followed by glucuronidation. Its pharmacokinetics are altered by the coadministration of enzyme-inducing AEDs, even though tiagabine does not appear to induce or inhibit hepatic microsomal metabolizing enzymes.

Adverse effects. Side effects are more common with tiagabine than with other adjunct drugs and most often involve the CNS. They include somnolence, headache, dizziness, tremor, abnormal thinking, depression, and psychosis. Furthermore, recent reports have implicated tiagabine in the development of nonconvulsive status epilepticus (88,89). There is an increased risk of seizure in patients being treated for off-label psychiatric indications. Tiagabine may interfere with visual color perception (90).

Tiagabine does not affect the hepatic metabolism of other AEDs, but its half-life is decreased by enzyme-inducing AEDs, such as CBZ, phenytoin, and barbiturates. Other CYP3A4-inducing drugs may act similarly. Valproate decreases the protein binding of tiagabine. increasing its plasma concentration in these patients.

Hepatic disease causes decreased clearance of tiagabine, and a dose reduction may be required. Renal disease does not affect elimination.

Topiramate (Topamax)

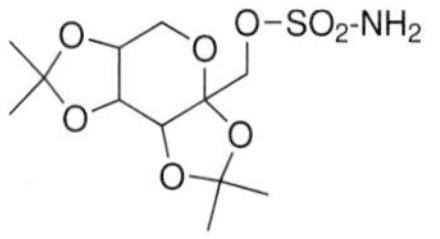

O–SO_2–NH_2

Topiramate is a sulfamate-substituted monosaccharide derived from fructose with a broad spectrum of AED activity. It is approved for monotherapy or as an adjunct drug for partial or primary generalized tonic-clonic seizures in patients older than 10 years, as adjunct therapy in children aged from 2 to 10 years with partial-onset seizures, and in persons older than 2 years with Lennox-Gastaut syndrome (40,53). Topiramate also is approved for the prophylaxis of migraine headaches.

Mechanism of action. The mechanism of action for topiramate is unknown, but several actions are thought to contribute to its AED activity (91). It blocks repetitive firing by acting on sodium channels, may enhance $GABA_A$-mediated chloride flux, and appears to be an antagonist at the AMPA and KA receptors, thus blocking the effect of glutamate (Fig. 20.2) (92,93). In addition, recent evidence suggests inhibition of L-type calcium currents (94).

Pharmacokinetics. Topiramate is rapidly absorbed, with at least an 80 to 95% oral bioavailability that is unaffected by food. Following an oral dose of topiramate, peak plasma concentration is reached in 1 to 4 hours, exhibiting linear pharmacokinetics (95). Protein binding is minimal (<20%), and the usual elimination half-life is 20 to 30 hours, allowing a twice-daily dosing regimen. In the absence of enzyme-inducing drugs, approximately 70 to 80% of the drug is excreted unchanged in the urine, with the remainder as metabolites resulting from oxidation and hydrolysis. Enzyme-inducing AEDs alter the pharmacokinetics of topiramate by reducing its plasma levels and increasing its rate of elimination.

In children from 4 to 17 years of age, topiramate exhibits linear pharmacokinetics, with a 50% increase in clearance rate compared to adults (95). Topiramate may require up to a 50% dose reduction in patients with renal insufficiency, and a replacement dose may be needed after renal dialysis. Topiramate has demonstrated teratogenicity in animal studies.

Adverse effects. Common CNS side effects associated with topiramate therapy include drowsiness, dizziness, impaired concentration and memory, speech and language difficulties, and confusion. These effects develop during the first weeks of therapy and may decline over time. Acute closed-angle glaucoma caused by topiramate requires immediate evaluation (96). Only rare hepatic or bone marrow effects have been noted thus far; however, an increased incidence of renal stones is troublesome and probably related to the drug's activity as a carbonic anhydrase inhibitor, reducing citrate excretion and increasing urinary pH. Use of additional carbonic anhydrase inhibitors, a ketogenic diet, or a family history of nephrolithiasis may be considered as contraindications for using topiramate.

Topiramate is not devoid of potential interaction properties: It induces CYP3A4 and inhibits CYP2C19, thus significantly increasing plasma phenytoin levels. Topiramate also may decrease the effectiveness of oral contraceptives.

Valproic acid and its derivatives

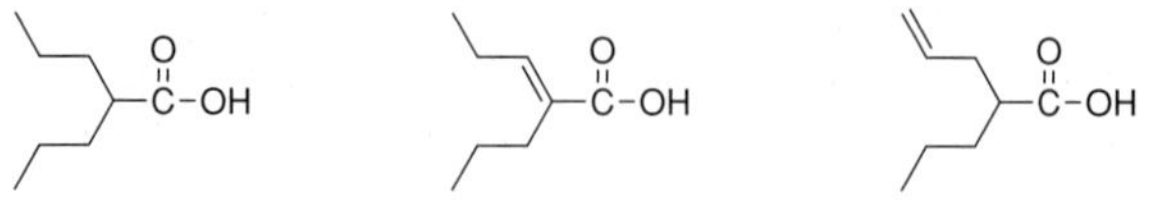

Valproic acid (dipropylacetic acid)

(E)-2-ene-valproic acid

4-ene-valproic acid

Valproate is available as valproic acid (Depakene), divalproex sodium (Depakote), and valproate sodium (Depacon) for IV use. Its AED properties were discovered serendipitously when it was used as a solvent for potential new AEDs undergoing testing. It is effective against both MES test- and pentylenetetrazole-induced seizures in animals and possesses a satisfactory margin of safety. Because the pK_a of valproic acid is 4.7, the drug is completely ionized at physiologic pH; thus, the valproate ion is almost certainly the pharmacologically active species.

Mechanism of action. Although its mechanism of action is not clearly established, valproate appears to increase the inhibitory effect of GABA, possibly by activation of glutamic acid decarboxylase or inhibition of GABA-transaminase (Fig. 20.2). The high drug concentrations required, however, cast doubt on the clinical relevance of this effect. Furthermore, valproate recently has been shown to decrease the uptake of GABA into cultured astrocytes; this action may contribute to the AED efficacy (97). Valproate is known to produce a blockade of high-frequency repetitive firing by slowing the rate of Na^+ recovery from inactivation, a mechanism consistent with the actions of phenytoin and CBZ. Valproate blocks the low-threshold T-type Ca^{2+} channel. Consequently, the overall therapeutic utility of valproate is likely caused by multiple effects.

Valproate is indicated for initial or adjunct treatment of absence seizures or as an adjunct when absence seizures occur in combination with either tonic-clonic seizures, myoclonic seizures, or both. For patients with unambiguous idiopathic generalized epilepsy, valproate often is the drug of choice, because it controls absence, myoclonic, and generalized tonic-clonic seizures well (98). It also is approved by U.S. FDA for use in complex partial seizures, occurring with or without other seizure types in adults or children 10 years of age or older. In new patients with typical absence seizures, ethosuximide is preferred to valproate because of the latter drug's risk of producing hepatotoxicity. In a comparative trial, sodium valproate and ethosuximide were equally effective when either drug was given alone or in combination with other AEDs in children with typical absence seizures. In atypical absence seizures (Lennox-Gastaut syndrome), sodium valproate is more effective, whereas in myoclonic seizures, it is less effective than clonazepam. Valproate is approved by the U.S. FDA for use in bipolar disorder and against migraine headaches.

PHARMACOKINETICS. Valproate undergoes rapid and complete absorption, which is only slightly slowed by food. It is 90% protein bound, and its clearance is dose-dependent because of an increase in the free fraction of the drug at higher doses. It is metabolized almost entirely by the liver, with 30 to 50% of an orally administered dose being eliminated in the urine as its acyl glucuronide conjugate, 40% from mitochondrial β-oxidation, approximately 15 to 20% by ω-oxidation, and less than 3% is excreted unchanged in urine. Its major active metabolite is (E)-2-ene valproate (*trans* 2-ene valproate). Its 4-ene metabolite has been proposed to be a reactive metabolite responsible for the hepatotoxicity of valproate (see Chapter 10). Other metabolites found in the urine include 3-oxo- and 4-hydroxyvalproate. The elimination half-life for valproate ranged from 9 to 16 hours following oral dosing regimens of 250 to 1,000 mg. Patients who are not taking enzyme-inducing AEDs (carbamazepine, phenytoin, and phenobarbital) will clear valproate more rapidly; therefore, monitoring of AED plasma concentrations should be intensified whenever concurrent AEDs are introduced or withdrawn.

Adverse effects. The most commonly observed side effects for valproate are gastrointestinal (anorexia, nausea, and indigestion). These effects can be minimized by selecting divalproex sodium, which is enterically coated, and by initiating therapy at a low dose. More importantly, however, valproate is associated with the development of fatal hepatotoxicity, especially in children or when coadministered with other AEDs. Frequent monitoring of liver function tests is mandatory for determining the onset of toxicity, particularly during the first 6 months of treatment. Tremors, hematologic dyscrasias, pancreatitis, stupor, depression, behavioral anomalies, and coma also have been observed with valproate therapy.

Valproate, a substrate for hepatic CYP2C19 and CYP2C9, has an extensive pattern of drug interactions. It increases the plasma concentrations of lamotrigine, CBZ, and phenobarbital and the free fraction of phenytoin by either displacing these drugs from plasma proteins or inhibiting their metabolism. Phenytoin, phenobarbital, and CBZ cause decreased plasma concentrations of valproate, whereas felbamate increases valproate levels.

Because of its propensity for causing liver damage, valproate therapy should be avoided in persons with liver disease. It should be used with caution before surgery, because it can produce thrombocytopenia and inhibition of platelet aggregation. In pregnancy, it has been associated with an increased risk of fetal epilepsy syndrome and spina bifida.

ZONISAMIDE (ZONEGRAN)

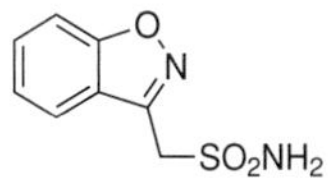

O N SO_2NH_2

Mechanism of action. Zonisamide is a sulfonamide derivative that is indicated as an adjunct for partial seizures in patients older than 16 years whose seizures are not controlled by first-line drugs. In Japan, it is used for myoclonic seizures as well. Apparently, it has more than one mechanism of action—all as yet unidentified. It is known to produce blockade of both sodium and T-type calcium channels (Fig. 20.2) (99,100). Because it also affects dopaminergic transmission, bipolar or schizoaffective disorder patients may improve.

Pharmacokinetics. The absorption for orally administered zonisamide is slow but nearly complete. Its pharmacokinetics are nonlinear, with a half life of 50 to 70 hours when administered alone or 27 to 46 hours when administered concurrently with enzyme-inducing AEDs. Protein binding is moderate (<50%). An oral dose of zonisamide is completely absorbed, with peak plasma concentration occurring in 2 to 6 hours. Although the presence of food will delay the attainment of its peak plasma concentration, oral bioavailability does not appear to be altered. More than one-third of each oral dose is excreted in the urine in an unchanged form. The routes of metabolism for zonisamide include acetylation to form its N-acetyl metabolite, reduction by CYP3A4/CYP2D6, and the formation of an open-ring metabolite, 2-sulfamoylacetyl phenol. These metabolites subsequently are eliminated unconjugated or glucuronidated in the urine, with an elimination half-life of 63 hours. Its coadministration with enzyme-inducing AEDs, such as phenytoin, CBZ, or phenobarbital, and with valproate will alter its pharmacokinetics by reducing its half-life and serum concentration. The half-life for zonisamide is decreased to 27 hours in the presence of phenytoin, to 38 hours in the presence of either CBZ or phenobarbital, and to 46 hours with valproate. Other drugs that inhibit or induce CYP3A4 could affect the metabolism of zonisamide.

Zonisamide should be used with caution in patients with hepatic or renal disease. It also has shown to be teratogenic in animal studies.

Adverse effects. Zonisamide is contraindicated in patients with a history of allergy to sulfonamides. The most frequent side effects include somnolence, anorexia, dizziness, agitation, confusion, headache, cognitive impairment, and memory loss. In addition, an incidence of drug-induced psychosis has been noted (101). Reports from both the United States and Europe have indicated that development of renal stones may occur with use of this drug. A family history of nephrolithiasis may be a contraindication, and urinary monitoring for hypercalciuria may be warranted in bedridden patients or those receiving multiple AEDs (102). Although the incidence of severe rashes attributable to zonisamide is low, sulfonamides are associated with Stevens-Johnson syndrome. Thus, it is recommended to discontinue the drug immediately should a rash occur.

Drugs Effective Against Absence Seizures

Drugs that are effective against absence seizures include the 5-membered ureides, the oxazolidinediones and the succinimides (Fig. 20.11), and clonazepam and lamotrigine, which have been previously discussed. An examination of the structure–activity relationship for the 5-membered heterocyclic ureides (Fig. 20.4) reveals that a small substructural difference between ring N (hydantoins), ring O (oxazolidinediones), and ring CH_2 (methylene and succinimides) results in switching from AEDs effective against partial and generalized tonic-clonic seizures to those effective against absence seizures.

Trimethadione Dimethadione

Phensuximide Methsuximide Ethosuximide

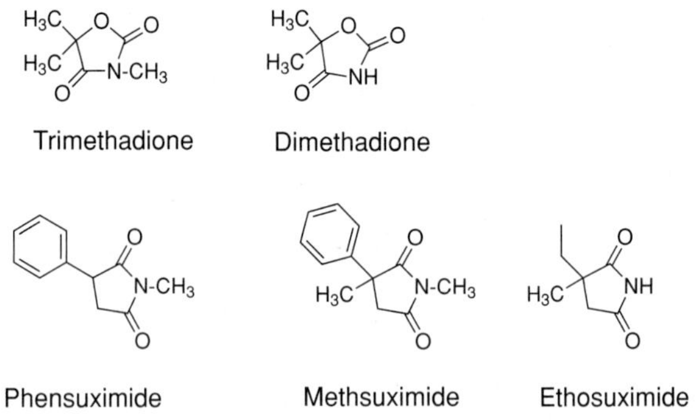

Fig. 20.11. Drugs effective against absence seizures.

Oxazolidinediones

These compounds are some of the oldest AEDs in use, having been introduced into antiseizure therapy between 1946 and 1948. At that time, no effective drugs were available to control absence seizures (petit mal disorders). Therefore, the acceptance of trimethadione in 1946 and of paramethadione in 1948 for the control of absence seizures was rapid. At present, trimethadione (Tridione) (Fig. 20.11) is indicated only for control of absence seizures refractory to treatment with other AEDs. It is ineffective against other seizure types. Trimethadione is a pro-drug and is metabolized by N-demethylation to dimethadione, which is effective in the pentylenetetrazole test, which acts by decreasing T-type calcium currents. Trimethadione is rapidly absorbed, is not protein bound, and has a half-life of 16 to 24 hours. The half-life of dimethadione, however, is substantially longer (i.e., 6–13 days), and dimethadione accumulates to concentrations greater than the parent drug. Because of its potentially fatal side effects. including aplastic anemia, nephrosis, idiosyncratic rashes, and exfoliative dermatitis, trimethadione rarely is used today. It causes malformations or fetal death in up to 87% of pregnancies. Paramethadione is no longer clinically available in the United States.

Succinimides

Because oxazolidinediones are toxic, an extensive search was undertaken to replace them with less toxic drugs. Substituting the ring O in the oxazolidinediones with a methylene group gave the antiseizure succinimides. The clinically used succinimides include ethosuximide, methsuximide, and phensuximide, which were introduced between 1951 and 1958 (Fig. 20.11) and widely accepted for the treatment of absence seizures.

Mechanism of Action. Succinimides suppress the paroxysmal 3-Hz spike-and-wave activity associated with the lapses of consciousness associated with absence (petite mal) seizures, thus reducing the frequency of seizures and raising the threshold to seizures. The proposed mechanism of action involves a decrease in T-type calcium channel activity (Fig. 20.2).

Succinimides are indicated for the monotherapy of absence seizures or with concomitant therapy when additional forms of seizures occur in combination with absence seizures. These drugs are readily absorbed from the gastrointestinal tract and display very low protein binding. The drug interactions for the succinimides are less extensive than with the oxazolidinediones. They may increase plasma phenytoin levels, decrease plasma primidone levels, and either increase or decrease valproate levels, although the changes may not be clinically significant.

Renal/hepatic disease does not appear to enhance their toxicity. Extreme caution is advised, however, because succinimides can cause morphological changes to kidneys and liver. Periodic monitoring of the blood count, hepatic function, and urinalysis are recommended with the use of succinimides.

Ethosuximide (Zarontin). Although ethosuximide is the drug of choice for treatment of simple absence seizures, it is not effective against partial complex or tonic-clonic seizures and may increase the frequency of grand mal attacks. Thus, it must be administered in combination with other AEDs when treating persons with mixed seizure types. Ethosuximide is a substrate for both CYP3A4 and CYP2E1. The major metabolite for ethosuximide is 3-(1-hydroxyethyl) succinimide, which is inactive and excreted unconjugated into the urine. Several additional metabolites have been characterized recently (103). Approximately 20% of an oral dose is excreted unchanged.

Although ethosuximide is thought to be the least toxic of the succinimides, it can cause gastrointestinal disturbances and dose-related CNS effects, such as drowsiness, dizziness, ataxia, sleep disturbances and depression. Idiosyncratic hypersensitivity reactions include severe rashes, leukopenia, agranulocytosis (some fatal), systemic lupus erythematosus, and parkinsonian-like symptoms. In addition to being less toxic than trimethadione, ethosuximide offers a wider range of protection against different kinds of absence seizures.

Methsuximide. Although methsuximide is less commonly used, it may be indicated for the control of absence seizures refractory to other drugs. Although it does not precipitate tonic-clonic convulsions, it often is combined with phenytoin or phenobarbital when absence seizures coexist with tonic-clonic symptoms. Much of the efficacy of methsuximide is attributed to its desmethyl metabolite. The half-life of methsuximide is between 2.6 and 4.0 hours, but the half-life for N-desmethylsuximide is 25 hours, causing it to accumulate substantially. Concentrations of greater than 40 g/mL may be associated with toxicity. Methsuximide is considered to be more toxic than ethosuximide.

Phensuximide. Phensuximide occasionally is used for the treatment of absence seizures refractory to other drugs, although it is considered to be less effective than ethosuximide. It is excreted in both urine and bile, and it may cause harmless pink to red discoloration of the urine. It should be used with caution in patients with acute intermittent porphyria.

Drugs Effective Against Myoclonic Seizures

Clonazepam and valproate commonly are used to control myoclonic seizures. Studies suggest that lamotrigine and topiramate may be effective as well, although neither is approved by the U.S. FDA for this indication.

Drugs for Status Epilepticus

Diazepam, administered IV or IM, is a drug of choice for rapid control of status epilepticus. Lorazepam, although not approved by the U.S. FDA for the purpose, is preferred by some clinicians for its longer duration of action (40), and midazolam is preferred for its more rapid onset of action (67). Because of its high lipid solubility, IV diazepam enters the CNS rapidly. The initially high brain concentration is quickly reduced, however, because of its redistribution, increasing the chance of recurring status epilepticus (62). Concomitant IV injection of diazepam and phenobarbital or fosphenytoin has been suggested to overcome this difficulty (104).

ANTIEPILEPTIC DRUGS IN PHASE III CLINICAL TRIALS

Antiepileptic drugs in Phase III clinical trials are shown in Figure 20.12. Talampanel is a 2,4-benzodiazepine that is a AMPA/KA receptor antagonist. RWJ-333369 is a monocarbamate antagonist at KA receptors. Rufinamide is a 1,2,3-triazole carboxamide that blocks sodium channels. Soretilide has a mechanism of action similar to that of CBZ, and brivaracetam and seletracetam are derivatives of S-(−)-levetiracetam for treatment of myoclonic seizures.

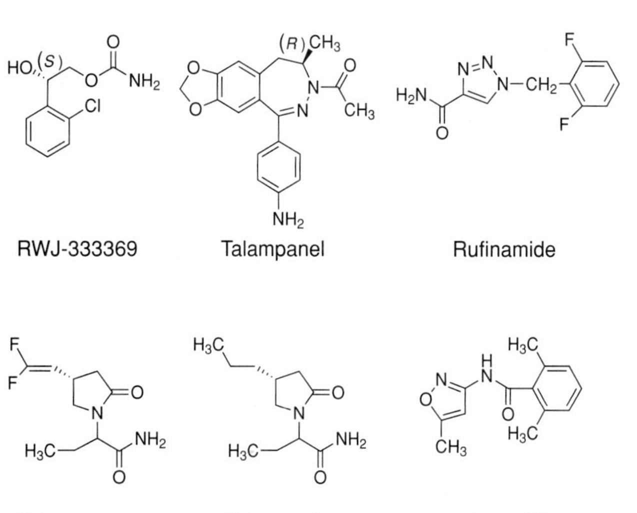

RWJ-333369 Talampanel Rufinamide

Seletracetam Brivaracetam Soretolide

Fig. 20.12. Antiepileptic drugs in Phase III clinical trials.

CASE STUDY

Victoria F. Roche and S. William Zito

FP is a 63-year-old physician practicing in a rural, sparsely populated county in northeast Arkansas. Although he works two days a week out of a clinic in one of his county's larger communities, he is on the road the other three days, often driving long distances to see patients who live in the more remote areas. Despite his health issues and advancing years, FP will not retire, because the patients he treats have very few alternatives for care.

FP has a history of cardiovascular disease, having survived a myocardial infarction that occurred in his mid-50s and, more recently, a stroke. Currently, he is on extended-release diltiazem (Cardiazem, 420 mg q.i.d.) and betaxolol HCl (Kerlone, 10 mg q.i.d.) for chronic stable angina coupled with hypertension. He also takes one baby aspirin each day. FP is troubled by rheumatoid arthritis, for which he takes diclofenac (Voltaren, 50 mg t.i.d.), and he has a documented allergy to sulfonamides.

FP is now facing a diagnosis of complex partial seizure disorder. The etiology of his newly acquired epilepsy is unknown, but he believes that it is related to the stroke he recently experienced. An animal lover, he is trying to acquire a "seizure dog" (a dog that can sense the onset of seizures and warn patients in time to seek care or safety) to take with him on his rural rounds. Regarding antiseizure therapy, FP has his opinions (of course) but is seeking you out to select an anticonvulsant for oral maintenance therapy. Consider the choices below, and advise this practitioner colleague.

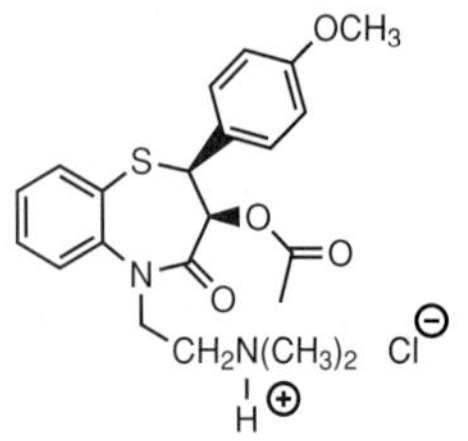

Diltiazem HCl

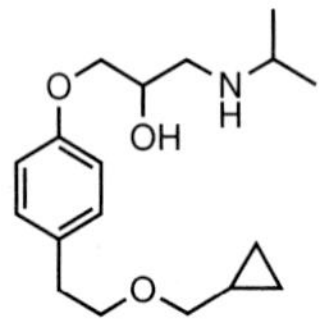

Betaxolol

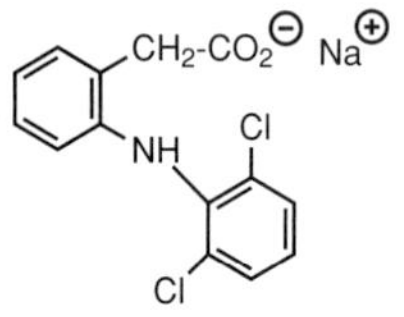

Diclofenac sodium

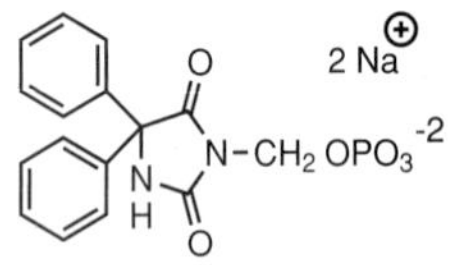

1

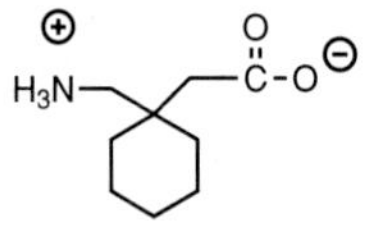

2

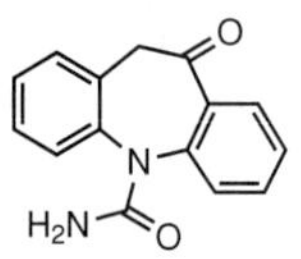

3

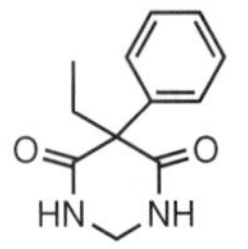

4

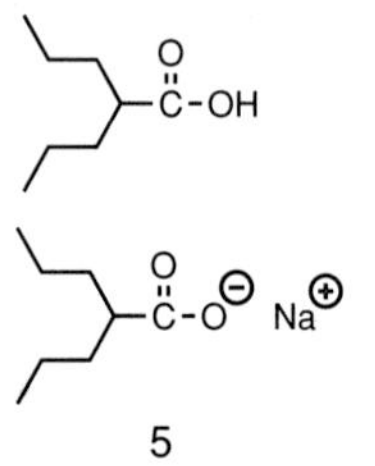

5

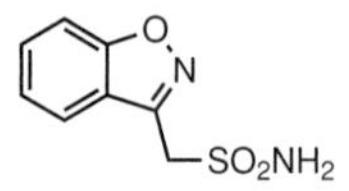

6

1. Identify the therapeutic problem(s) in which the pharmacist's intervention may benefit the patient.
2. Identify and prioritize the patient-specific factors that must be considered to achieve the desired therapeutic outcomes.
3. Conduct a thorough and mechanistically oriented structure–activity analysis of all structures provided in the case.
4. Evaluate the structure–activity relationship findings against the patient-specific factors and desired therapeutic outcomes, and make a therapeutic decision.
5. Counsel your patient.

References

1. Forster FM, ed.. Report of the Panel on Epilepsy. Madison, WI: University of Wisconsin Press, 1961:91.
2. DeRobertis E, DeLores-Arnaiz GR, Alberici M. Ultrastructural neurochemistry. In: Jasper HH, Pope A, Ward AA. eds. Basic Mechanisms of the Epilepsies. Boston: Little, Brown and Co., 1969:137–158.
3. Jackson JH. On the anatomical and physiological localization of movements in the brain. In: Taylor J, ed. Selected Writings of John Hughlings Jackson, vol 1. London: Hodder and Stoughton, 1958:52.
4. Gowers WR. Epilepsy and Other Chronic Convulsive Diseases: Their Causes, Symptoms, and Treatment, 2nd Ed. London: J. and A. Church, 1901.
5. Gastaut H. A Proposed International Classification of Epileptic Seizures. Epilepsia (Amst) 1964;5:297–303.
6. Lennox WG. Epilepsy and Related Disorders. Boston: Little, Brown and Co., 1960.
7. Penfield W, Jasper HH. Epilepsy and the Functional Anatomy of the Human Brain. Boston, Little, Brown and Co., 1954:20.
8. Gastaut H. Classification of the epilepsies. Proposal for an international classification. Epilepsia 1969;10(Suppl):14–21.
9. Masland RL. Comments on the classification of epilepsy. Epilepsia 1969;10(Suppl):22–28.
10. Proposal for Revised Clinical and Electroencephalographic Classification of Epileptic Seizures. Epilepsia 1981;22:489–501.

11. Browne TR, Holmes GL. Types of seizures. In: Handbook of Epilepsy, 2nd Ed. New York: Lippincott Williams & Wilkins, 1999:19–41.
12. Golan, DE, Tashjian AH, Armstrong EJ, et al., eds. Principles of Pharmacology: The Pathophysiologic Basis of drug Therapy. Philadelphia: Lippincott Williams &Wilkins, 2005.
13. Taylor CP. Mechanisms of new antiepileptic drugs. In: Delgado-Escueta AV, Wilson WA, Olsen RW, et al., eds. Jasper's Basic Mechanisms of the epilepsies, 3rd Ed. (Advances in Neurology, vol 79.) Philadelphia: Lippincott Williams &Wilkins, 1999:1012–1027.
14. MacDonald RI, Meldrum B. Principles of antiepileptic drug action. In: Levy RH, Meldrum BS, eds. Antiepileptic Drugs, 4th Ed. New York: Raven Press, 1995:61–78.
15. Armijo JA, Shushtarian M, Valdizan EM, et al. Ion channels and epilepsy. Curr Pharm Des 2005;11:1975–2003.
16. Lerche H, Weber YG, Jurkat-Rott K, et al. Ion channel defects in idiopathic epilepsies. Curr Pharm Des 2005;11:2737–2752.
17. Lucas PT, Meadows LS, Nicholls J, et al. An epilepsy mutation in the β_1 subunit of the voltage-gated sodium channel results in reduced channel sensitivity to phenytoin. Epilepsy Res 2005;64:77–84.
18. Jones KA, Tamm JA, Craig DA, et al. Signal transduction by $GABA_B$ receptor heterodimers. Neuropsychopharmacology 2000;23(Suppl 4):S41–S49.
19. Bal T, Debay D, Destexhe A. Cortical feedback controls the frequency and synchrony of oscillations in the visual thalamus. J Neurosci 2000;20: 7478–7488.
20. Browne TR, Holmes GL. Epilepsy: definitions and background. In: Handbook of Epilepsy, 2nd Ed. New York: Lippincott Williams & Wilkins, 1999:1–18.
21. Swinyard EA,Woodhead JH, White HS, et al. General principles, experimental selection, quantification, and evaluation of anticonvulsants. In: Levy R, Mattson, RH, Meldrum B, et al., eds. Antiepileptic Drugs, 3rd Ed. New York: Raven Press, 1989:85–102.
22. Vida JA. In: Foye WO, ed. Central Nervous System Depressants: Sedative-Hypnotics. Principles of Medicinal Chemistry, 2nd Ed. Philadelphia: Lea & Febiger, 1981. pp 173–188.
23. Swinyard EA, Brown WC, Goodman LS. Comparative assays of antiepileptic drugs in mice and rats. J Pharmacol Exp Ther 1952;106:319–330.
24. Woodbury LA, Davenport VD. Design and use of a new electroshock seizure apparatus, and analysis of factors altering seizure threshold and pattern. Arch Int Pharmacodyn 1952;92:97–106.
25. Emilien G, Maloteaux JM. Pharmacological management of epilepsy. Mechanism of action, pharmacokinetic drug interactions, and new drug discovery possibilities. Int J Clin Pharmacol Ther 1998;36:181–194.
26. Browne, TR. Pharmacokinetics of antiepileptic drugs. Neurology 1998;51(Suppl 4):S2–S7.
27. Benedetti MS. Enzyme induction and inhibition by new antiseizure drugs: a review of human studies. Fundam Clin Pharmacol 2000;14:301–319.
28. Battino D, Estienne M, Avanzini G. Clinical pharmacokinetics of antiseizure drugs in pediatric patients. Part II. Phenytoin, carbamazepine, sulthiame, lamotrigine, vigabatrin, oxcarbazepine, and felbamate. Clin Pharmacokinet 1995;29:341–369.
29. Mattson RH and the Department of Veterans Affairs Epilepsy Cooperative Study No. 118 Group. A comparison of carbamazepine, phenobarbital, phenytoin, and primidone in partial and secondarily generalized tonic-clonic seizures. N Engl J Med 1985;313:145–151.
30. Osorio I, Reed RC, Peltzer JN. Refractory idiopathic absence status epilepticus: a probable paradoxical effect of phenytoin and carbamazepine. Epilepsia 2000;41:887–894.
31. Thomas P, Valton L, Genton P. Absence and myoclonic status epilepticus precipitated by antiepileptic drugs in idiopathic generalized epilepsy. Brain 2006;129:1281–1292.
32. Cuttle L, Munns AJ, Hogg NA, et al. Phenytoin metabolism by human cytochrome P450: involvement of P450 3A and 2C forms in secondary metabolism and drug-protein adduct formation. Drug Metab Dispos 2000;28:945–950.
33. Kinobe RT, Parkinson OT, Mitchell DJ, et al. P450 2C18 catalyzes the metabolic bioactivation of phenytoin. Chem Res Toxicol 2005;18:1868–1875.
34. Awasthi S, Hallene KL, Fazio V, et al. RLIP76, a non-ABC transporter, and drug resistance in epilepsy. BMC Neurosci 2005;6:61–76.
35. Kupiec T, Raj V. Fatal seizures due to potential herb–drug interactions with Ginkgo biloba. J Anal Toxicol 2005;29:755–758.
36. DeToledo JC, Ramsay RE. Fosphenytoin and phenytoin in patients with status epilepticus: improved tolerability versus increased costs. Drug Saf 2000;22:459–466.
37. Browne TR, Kugler AE, Eldon MA. Pharmacology and pharmacokinetics of fosphenytoin. Neurology 1996;46(Suppl 1):S3–S7.
38. Adams BD, Buckley NH, Kim JY, et al. Fosphenytoin may cause hemodynamically unstable bradydysrhythmias. J Emerg Med 2006;30:75–79.
39. Biton V, Gates JR, Ritter FJ, et al. Adjunctive therapy for intractable epilepsy with ethotoin. Epilepsia 1990;31:433–437.
40. Browne TR, Holmes GL. Antiepileptic drugs. In: Handbook of Epilepsy, 2nd Ed. New York: Lippincott Williams & Wilkins, 1999:163–196.
41. Gelisse P, Genton P, Kuate C, et al. Worsening of seizures by oxcarbazepine in juvenile idiopathic generalized epilepsies. Epilepsia 2004;45: 1282–1286.
41. Potter JM, Donnelly A. Carbamazepine-10, 11-epoxide in therapeutic drug monitoring. Ther Drug Monit 1998;20:652–657.
42. Bu H, Kang P, Deese AJ, et al. Human in vitro glutathionyl and protein adducts of carbamazepine-10,11-epoxide, a stable and pharmacologically active metabolite of carbamazepine. Drug Metab Dispos 2005;33: 1920–1924.
44. Pearce RE, Uetrecht JP, Leeder JS. Pathways of carbamazepine bioactivation in vitro: II. The role of human cytochrome P450 enzymes in the formation of 2-hydroxyiminostlibene. Drug Metab Dispos 2005;33: 1819–1826.
45. Mintzer S, Boppana P, Toguri J, et al. Vitamin D levels and bone turnover in epilepsy patients taking carbamazepine and oxcarbazepine. Epilepsia 2006;47:510–515.
46. Ficker DM, Privitera M, Krauss G, et al. Improved tolerability and efficacy in epilepsy patients with extended-release carbamazepine. Neurology 2005;65: 593–595.
47. Benes J, Parada A, Figueiredo AA, et al. Anticonvulsant and sodium channel–blocking properties of novel 10,11-dihydro-5H-dibenz[b,f]azepine-5-carboxamide derivatives. J Med Chem 2000;42:2582–2587.
48. Perucca E. Clinically relevant drug interactions with antiepileptic drugs. Br J Clin Pharm 2005;61:246–255.
49. Muscatello MR, Pacetti M, Cacciola M, et al. Plasma concentrations of risperidone and olanzepine during coadministration with oxcarbazepine. Epilepsia 2005;46:771–774.
50. Besag FMC, Berry D. Interactions between antiepileptic and antipsychotic drugs. Drug Saf 2006;29:95–118.
51. Mazzucchelli I, Onat FY, Ozkara C, et al. Changes in the disposition of oxcarbazepine and its metabolites during pregnancy and the puerperium. Epilepsia 2006;47:504–509.
52. Striano S, Striano P, DiNocera P, et al. Relationship between serum mono-hydroxy-carbazepine concentrations and adverse effects in patients with epilepsy on high-dose oxcarbazepine therapy. Epilepsy Res 2006; 69:170–176.
53. Wong IC, Lhatoo SD. Adverse reactions to new anticonvulsant drugs. Drug Saf 2000;23:35–56.
54. Kobayashi K, Morita J, Chiba K, et al. Pharmacogenetic roles of CYP2C19 and CYP2B6 in the metabolism of R- and S-mephobarbital in humans. Pharmacogenetics 2004;14:549–556.
55. Goodman LS, Swinyard EA, Brown WC, et al. Anticonvulsant properties of 5-phenyl-5-ethyl-hexandropyrimidine-4,6-dione (Mysoline), a new antiepileptic. J Pharmacol Exp Ther 1953;108:428–434.
56. Butler TC, Waddell WJ. Metabolic conversion of pyrimidone (Mysoline) to phenobarbital. Proc Soc Exp Biol Med 1956;93:544–546.
57. Fountain NB, Adams RE . Midazolam treatment of acute and refractory status epilepticus. Clin Neuropharmacol 1999;22:261–267.
58. Towne AR, DeLorenzo RJ. Use of intramuscular midazolam for status epilepticus. J Emerg Med 1999;17:323–328.
59. McIntyre J, Robertson S, Norris E, et al. Safety and efficacy of buccal midazolam versus rectal diazepam for emergency treatment of seizures in children: a randomized controlled trial. Lancet 2005;366:205–210.
60. Harbord MG, Kyrkou NE, Kyrkou MR, et al., Use of intranasal midazolam to treat acute seizures in pediatric community settings. J Paediatr Child Health 2004;40:556–558.
61. Pang T, Hirsch LJ. Treatment of convulsive and nonconvulsive status epilepticus. Current Treatment Options in Neurology 2005;7:247–259.
62. Gastaut H, Alaquet R, Poire R, et al. Epilepsia (Amst) 1965;13:167–182.
63. Brodtkorb E, Aamo T, Henricksen O, et al. Rectal diazepam: pitfalls of excessive use in refractory epilepsy. Epilepsy Res 1999;35:123–133.
64. Schmidt D, Bourgeois B. A risk–benefit assessment of therapies for Lennox-Gastaut syndrome. Drug Saf 2000;22:467–477.
65. Treiman DM, Walker MC. Treatment of seizure emergencies: convulsive and nonconvulsive status epilepticus. Epilepsy Res 2006;68(Suppl 1): S77–S82.
66. Thompson CD, Barthen MT, Hopper DW, et al. Quantification in patient urine samples of felbamate and three metabolites: acid carbamate and two mercapturic acids. Epilepsia 1999;40:769–776.
67. Mazarati AM, Baldwin RA, Sofia RD, et al. Felbamate in experimental model of status epilepticus. Epilepsia 2000;41:123–127.
68. Thompson CD, Gulden PH, Macdonald TL. Identification of modified atropaldehyde mercapturic acids in rat and human urine after felbamate administration. Chem Res Toxicol 1997;10:457–462.
69. Popovic M, Nierkens S, Pieters R, et al. Investigating the role of 2-phenylpropenal in felbamate-induced idiosyncratic drug reactions. Chem Res Toxicol 2004;17:1568–1576.
70. Parker RJ, Hartman NR, Roecklein BA, et al. Stability and comparative metabolism of selected felbamate metabolites and postulated fluorofelbamate metabolites by postmitochondrial suspensions. Chem Res Toxicol 2005;18:1842–1848.
71. Petroff OA, Hyder F, Rothman DL, et al. Effects of gabapentin on brain GABA, homocarnosine, and pyrrolidinone in epilepsy patients. Epilepsia 2000;41:675–680.
72. Taylor MT, Bonhaus DW. Allosteric modulation of [^{3}H]gabapentin binding by ruthenium red. Neuropharmacology 2000;39:1267–1273.

73. Luer MS, Hamani C, Dujovny M, et al. Saturable transport of gabapentin at the blood-brain barrier. Neurol Res 1999;21:559–562.
74. Asconape J, Diedrich A, DellaBadia J. Myoclonus associated with the use of gabapentin. Epilepsia 2000;41:479–481.
75. Calabresi P, Centonze D, Marfia GA, et al. An in vitro electrophysiological study on the effects of phenytoin, lamotrigine, and gabapentin on striatal neurons. Br J Pharmacol 1999;126:689–696.
76. Lingamanemi R, Hemmings HC Jr. Effects of anticonvulsants on veratridine- and KCl-evoked glutamate release from rat cortical synaptosomes. Neurosci Lett 1999;276:127–130.
77. Magdalou J, Herber R, Bidault R, et al. In vitro N-glucuronidation of a novel antiepileptic drug, lamotrigine, by human liver microsomes. J Pharmacol Exp Ther 1992;260:1166–1173.
78. Jansky J, Rasonyi G, Halasz P, et al. Disabling erratic myoclonus during lamotrigine therapy with high serum level—report of two cases. Clin Neuropharmacol 2000;23:86–89.
79. Grunewald R. Levetiracetam in the treatment of idiopathic generalized epilepsies. Epilepsia 2005;46(Suppl 9):154–160.
80. Vigevano F. Levetiracetam in pediatrics. J Child Neurol 2005;20:87–93.
81. Noyer M, Gillard M, Matagne A, et al. The novel antiepileptic drug levetiracetam (ucb LO59) appears to act via a specific binding site in CNS membranes. Eur J Pharmacol 1995;286:137–146.
82. Margineanu GD. Inhibition of neuronal hypersynchrony in vitro differentiates levetiracetam from classical antiepileptic drugs. Pharmacol Res 2000;42:281–285.
83. Patsalos PN. Pharmacokinetic profile of levetiracetam: toward ideal characteristics. Pharmacol Ther 2000;85:77–85.
84. Gidal BE, Baltes E, Otoul C, et al. Effect of levetiracetam on the pharmacokinetics of adjunctive antiepileptic drugs: a pooled analysis of data from randomized clinical trials. Epilepsy Res 2005;64:1–11.
85. Briggs DE, French JA. Levetiracetam safety profiles and tolerability in epilepsy. Expert Opin Drug Saf 2004;3:415–424.
86. Soudijn W, van Wijngaarden I. The GABA transporter and its inhibitors. Curr Med Chem 2000;7:1063–1079.
87. Gustavson LE, Mengel HB. Pharmacokinetics of tiagabine, a γ-aminobutyric acid–uptake inhibitor, in healthy subjects after single and multiple doses. Epilepsia 1995;36:605–611.
88. Knake S, Hamer HM, Schomburg U, et al. Tiagabine-induced absence status in idiopathic generalized epilepsy. Seizure 1999;8:314–317.
89. Koepp MJ, Edwards M, Collins J, et al. Status epilepticus and tiagabine therapy revisited. Epilepsia 2005;46:1625–1632.
90. Sorri I, Kalviainen R, Mantyjarvi M. Color vision and contrast sensitivity in epilepsy patients treated with initial tiagabine monotherapy. Epilepsy Res 2005;67:101–107.
91. Shank RP, Gardocki JF, Streeter AJ, et al. An overview of the preclinical aspects of topiramate: pharmacology, pharmacokinetics, and mechanism of action. Epilepsia 2000;41(Suppl 1):S3–S9.
92. Skradski S, White HS. Topiramate blocks kainate-evoked cobalt influx into cultured neurons. Epilepsia 2000;41(Suppl 1):S45–S47.
93. DeLorenzo RJ, Sombati S, Coulter DA. Effects of topiramate on sustained repetitive firing and spontaneous recurrent seizure discharges in cultured hippocampal neurons. Epilepsia 2000;41(Suppl 1):S40–S44.
94. Zhang X, Velumian AA, Jones OT, et al. Modulation of high-voltage–activated calcium channels in dentate granule cells by topiramate. Epilepsia 2000;41(Suppl 1):S52–S60.
95. Garnett WR. Clinical pharmacology of topiramate: a review. Epilepsia 2000;41(Suppl 1):S61–S65.
96. Craig JE, Ong TL, Lousi DL, et al. Mechanism of topiramate-induced acute-onset myopia and angle closure glaucoma. Am J Ophthalmol 2004;137:193–195.
97. Fraser CM, Sills GJ, Butler E, et al. Effects of valproate, vigabatrin, and tiagabine on GABA uptake into human astrocytes cultured from fetal and adult brain tissue. Epileptic Disord 1999;1:153–157.
98. Benbadis SR. Practical management issues for idiopathic generalized epilepsies. Epilepsia 2005;46(Suppl 9):125–132.
99. Leppik IE. Zonisamide: chemistry, mechanism of action, and pharmacokinetics. Seizure 2004;13(Suppl 1):S5–S9.
100. Oommen KJ, Mathews S. Zonisamide: a new antiepileptic drug. Clin Neuropharmacol 1999;22:192–200.
101. Miyamoto T, Kohsaka M, Koyama T. Psychotic episodes during zonisamide treatment. Seizure 2000;9:65–70.
102. Kubota M, Nishi-Nagase M, Sakakihara Y, et al. Zonisamide-induced urinary lithiasis in patients with intractable epilepsy. Brain Dev 2000;22:230–233.
103. Millership JS, Mifsud J, Galea D, et al. Chiral aspects of the human metabolism of Ethosuximide. Biopharm Drug Dispos 2005;26:225–232.
104. Gallagher BB. Anticonvulsants. In: Vida JA, ed. Neuropharmacology and Treatment of Epilepsy. New York: Academic Press, 1977:11–55.

21. *Antidepressants*

DAVID A. WILLIAMS

DRUGS COVERED IN THIS CHAPTER:

SELECTIVE NOREPINEPHRINE REUPTAKE INHIBITORS (SNRIs)
- Desipramine
- Nortriptyline
- Amoxepine
- Protriptyline
- Maprotiline
- Reboxetine
- Nisoxetine
- R-(2)-Atomoxetine

SELECTIVE 5-HT REUPTAKE INHIBITORS (SSRIs)
- Fluoxetine
- Paroxetine
- Citalopram
- Escitalopram
- Sertraline
- Fluvoxamine

NONSELECTIVE REUPTAKE INHIBITORS (NSRIs)
- Amitriptyline
- Imipramine
- Doxepin
- Clomipramine
- Trimipramine
- Dothiepin
- Lofepramine
- Venlafaxine
- Milnacipran
- Duloxetine

DOPAMINE AND NOREPINEPHRINE REUPTAKE INHIBITORS (DNRIs)
- Bupropion

SEROTONIN ANTAGONIST/REUPTAKE INHIBITORS (SARIs)
- Trazodone

NORADRENERGIC SPECIFIC SEROTONERGIC ANTIDEPRESSANTS (NaSSAs)
- Mirtazapine

MONOAMINE OXIDASE INHIBITORS (MAOIs)
- Phenelzine
- Tranylcypromine
- Moclobemide

MOOD STABILIZERS
- Lithium carbonate

Canst thou not minister to a mind diseas'd
Pluck from the memory a rooted sorrow,
Raze out the written troubles of the brain
And with some sweet oblivious antidote
Cleanse the stuff'd bosom of that perilous stuff
Which weighs upon the heart?

—WILLIAM SHAKESPEARE

INTRODUCTION

Depression is an ancient and prevalent mental condition that has been referenced throughout history in song, poetry, and literature. In a depressed state, one feels hopeless and experiences an overwhelming sense of despair. Depression immobilizes a person, afflicting men and women, rich and poor, and young and old alike. Depression makes one feel exhausted, worthless, helpless, and hopeless. It is an illness that involves the body, mood, and thoughts and affects the way one eats and sleeps, the way one feels about oneself, and the way one thinks about things. It often interferes with normal functioning, causing pain and suffering not only to themselves but also to those around them. Serious depression can destroy family life as well as the life of the person who is ill. A depressive disorder is not the same as a passing blue mood. Without treatment, symptoms can last for weeks, months, or years. Appropriate treatment, however, can help most people who suffer from depression. Negative thinking fades as treatment begins to take effect. Unfortunately, many people do not recognize that depression is a treatable illness. Much of this suffering is unnecessary, because *depression is one of the most treatable mental illnesses.*

> "Depression is the flaw in love. The meaninglessness of every enterprise and every emotion, the meaninglessness of life itself, becomes self-evident. The only feeling left in this loveless state is insignificance."
>
> "My depression had grown on me as that vine had conquered the oak; it had been a sucking thing that had wrapped itself around me, ugly and more alive than I. It had a life of its own that bit by bit asphyxiated all of my life out of me. My moods belonged to the depression as surely as the leaves on that oak tree's high branches belonged to the vine."
>
> "Drug therapy hacks through the vine. You can feel it happening, how the medication seems to be poisoning the parasite so that bit by bit it withers away. You feel the weight going, feel the way that the branches can recover much of their natural bent. But even with the vine gone, you may still have a few leaves and shallow roots, and the rebuilding of your self cannot be achieved with any drugs that now exist. Rebuilding of the self in and after depression requires love, insight, and most of all, time."
>
> *—Andrew Solomon, The Noonday Demon: An Atlas of Depression*

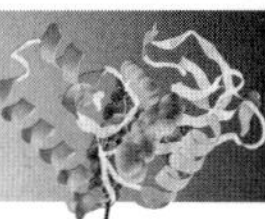

CLINICAL SIGNIFICANCE

The antidepressant class of drugs are well-known and widely used today not only for the treatment of mood disorders, such as depression and bipolar disorders, but also for the treatment of neuropathic pain, smoking cessation, and obsessive-compulsive disorders, among others. The application of medicinal chemistry in the development of newer antidepressants, such as selective serotonin uptake inhibitors (SSRIs), in the past 20 years has significantly affected the treatment of depression. The SSRIs have become first-line therapy in the treatment of major depressive disorder, and they also are used as adjunct treatment in other mood disorders. This new generation of antidepressants has more favorable side effect and pharmacokinetic profiles than the older generations of antidepressants, such as tricyclic antidepressants (TCAs) and monoamine oxidase inhibitors (MAOIs). This has resulted in improved patient compliance and therapeutic outcomes for patients with major depressive disorder.

Modifications of the structure-activity relationships of the antidepressant drugs have produced medications with multiple indications. For example, both duloxetine and buproprion are indicated for major depressive disorder, but duloxetine also is used for diabetic neuropathic pain and buproprion for smoking cessation. With a growing number of antidepressants on the market, it is more important than ever for the clinician to be knowledgeable about the drug's structure-activity relationships, adverse effects, drug interactions, and pharmacokinetic properties to properly select the optimal drug regimen for the patient.

Nancy Ordonez, Pharm.D.
Clinical Assistant Professor
University of Houston
College of Pharmacy

Depression affects approximately 10 to 12% percent of the Western population (United States, ~10%; Europe, 9–12%; Australia, ~18%), with females outnumbering males 2:1: One in four women and 1 in 10 men can expect to develop depression during their lifetime. Thus, depression ranks among the Top 5 diseases in these countries. In the United States alone, approximately 19 million adults will be afflicted yearly with depression, and at least 50% of those with major depression will suffer one or more repeated episodes of depression during their adult lifetime (1–3). Depression affects at least 1 in 50 children under the age of 12 years and 1 in 20 teenagers, mostly girls. The increase in the rate of depression among adolescent girls is related more to physical changes that occur during puberty, suggestive of hormonal changes. Premenstrual syndrome (PMS) and postpartum depression are additional conditions involving depression that specifically affect women and are suggestive of hormonal involvement in the pathogenesis of depression. About half of all cases of depression go unrecognized and untreated, and approximately 10 to 15% of those with depression will take their own lives yearly.

Depression in the elderly (17–35%) often is dismissed as a normal part of aging and may go undiagnosed and untreated, causing needless suffering for the family and for the individual who could otherwise live a fruitful life. Often, the symptoms described usually are physical, and the older person often is reluctant to discuss feelings of hopelessness, sadness, loss of interest in normally pleasurable activities, or extremely prolonged grief after a loss. Some symptoms may be the result of adverse (side) effects of medication that the elderly person is taking for other physical problems, or they may be caused by a concurrent illness. Improved recognition and treatment of depression will make life more enjoyable and fulfilling for the depressed elderly person, the family, and the caretakers.

The economic cost for depressive illnesses in the United States is estimated to be $53 billion per year, (2005), but the cost in human suffering cannot be estimated. In 2005, antidepressants drugs (primarily selective serotonin reuptake inhibitors [SSRIs]) ranked in the Top 50 drugs dispensed, first in total prescriptions written and third in total dollar prescription sales, at approximately $12.5 billion (~5% of total prescription drug sales) (4).

TYPES OF DEPRESSIVE DISORDERS

Why are some people more susceptible to depression than others? Hippocrates, the father of medicine, theorized that we are born into one of four primary temperament styles and that each style has its own unique outlook on life: Choleric (aggressive), Sanguine (emotional), Phlegmatic (passive), and Melancholy (analytical). Of these four styles, the introverted Melancholy is the most perfection driven and depression prone. The analytical Melancholy influence gives one tremendous attention to detail, but it also can create stress, anxiety, and depression. In fact, the term "melancholy" has become synonymous with depression. People with the Melancholy temperament style are by their very nature sensitive, judgmental, and critical. This temperament style becomes depressed primarily from the fact that they fail to reach their own incredibly high standards. This depression often leads to suicide, violence against others, or both.

Major Depression (MDD)

Major depression (also called unipolar depression) is the most serious type of depression; is manifested by a combination of symptoms that interfere with the ability to work, study, sleep, eat, and enjoy once-pleasurable activities; and may reoccur several times during a lifetime (5). Many people with major depression cannot continue to function normally. Major depression seems to run in families, suggesting that depressive illnesses can be inherited. Early signs (prodromal symptoms) of major depression include changes in brain function in those individuals having low self-esteem, who consistently view themselves and the world with pessimism or who are readily overwhelmed by stress. The treatments for major depression are medication, psychotherapy, and in extreme cases, electroconvulsive therapy.

Dysthymia

This is a mild, chronic depression that lasts for 2 years (1 year for children and adolescents) or longer and is characterized by chronic symptoms that do not disable but that keep one from functioning well or from feeling good about themselves (5). Many of those with dysthymia also experience major depressive episodes at some point in their lives. Most people may not realize that they are depressed and continue to function at work or school, but often with the feeling that they are "just going through the motions." Antidepressants or psychotherapy can help.

Bipolar Disorder (Manic-Depressive Illness)

Bipolar disorders can be divided into bipolar I (manic-depressive episodes), bipolar II (hypomanic-depressive episodes or cyclothymia [low grade bipolar II]) (5). Clinical studies over the years have provided evidence that monoamine signaling and hypothalamic-pituitary-adrenal axis disruption are integral to the pathophysiology of bipolar disorder (6). Bipolar disorders also appear to run in families and affect men and women equally. Not nearly as prevalent as the other forms of depressive disorders, bipolar disorders are characterized by cyclical periods of depression (lows) with periods of abnormal behavior (highs) known as hypomanic or mania. Sometimes, the mood switches are dramatic and rapid, but most often, they are gradual. When in the depressed cycle, an individual can exhibit the symptoms of a depressive disorder. When in the hypomanic manic cycle, the individual may be overactive, overtalkative, and have a great deal of energy. The hypomanic/manic cycle often affects thinking, judgment, and social behavior in ways that cause serious problems and embarrassment. For example, the individual in the hypomanic/manic cycle may feel elated, full of grand schemes that might range from unwise business decisions to romantic sprees. Lithium, carbamazepine, topiramide, and valproic acid are effective mood-stabilizing treatments for bipolar disorders. Also, the atypical antipsychotic, olanzepine (see Chapter 22) is used as a mood stabilizer for acute bipolar mania or in conjunction with antidepressants (e.g., Symbyax, a combination of olanzepine and fluoxetine).

Other Types of Depressive Disorders

Other, less common types of depression include seasonal affective disorder, a popular name that describes a type of depression that happens during particular seasons of the year (seasonal pattern) but that it is not a Diagnostic and Statistical Manual of Mental Disorder (DSM IV) (5) diagnosis. This disorder involves symptoms of depression that occur during the fall and winter seasons, when the days are shorter and there is less exposure to natural sunlight. When the spring and summer seasons begin and there is greater exposure to longer hours of daylight, the symptoms of depression disappear. Adjustment disorder with depressed mood is a type of depression that results when a person has something bad happen that depresses them (e.g., loss of one's job can cause this type of depression). It generally fades as time passes and the person gets over whatever it was that happened (5). Additional factors involved in its onset include stresses at home, work, or school, and symptoms may persist for as long as six months.

BIOLOGICAL BASIS OF DEPRESSION

Current theories regarding the causes of depression support the role of the neurotransmitters serotonin (also known as 5-HT) and norepinephrine (NE) in depression and their interrelationships with each other and with dopamine (Fig. 21.1). Although the precise nature of the depression is not fully understood at the level of the chemistry in the brain, several theories explain the role of NE and 5-HT in the causes of depression (7).

Monoamine Hypothesis

The monoamine hypothesis proposes that depression results from a deficiency in 5-HT and/or NE (8,9) and that antidepressant therapy aims to correct these deficiencies. The role of dopamine in depression remains unclear. Schildkraut et al. (8) postulated that depression arises as a consequence of a deficiency of NE and that the effects caused by catecholamine depletion can be reversed by the tricyclic antidepressants (TCAs). Depression in animals following reserpine administration can be reversed by TCAs, suggesting that the stimulating effects for desipramine (a secondary amine TCA) and monoamine oxidase inhibitors (MAOIs) were NE based.

During the late 1960s, Kielholz, a Swiss psychiatrist, argued that different antidepressants did quite different things and that it was important to select the right antidepressant for the right patient. He differentiated the TCAs based on whether they possessed the ability to sedate (e.g., trimipramine), to stimulate (e.g.,

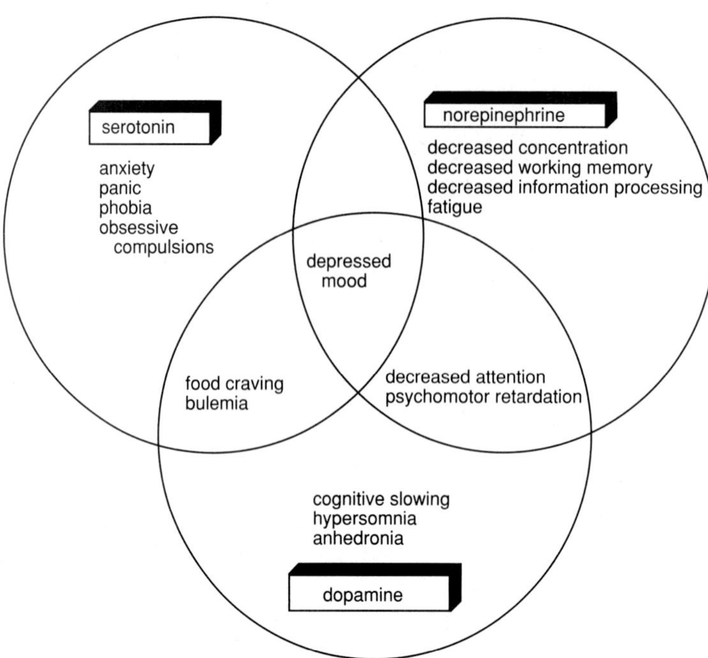

Fig. 21.1. Neurotransmitter deficiency syndromes and their interactions.

desipramine or nortriptyline), or to improve mood (e.g., clomipramine). By the end of the decade, the broad consensus was that secondary amine TCAs (like desipramine or nortriptyline) inhibited the reuptake of NE into noradrenergic neurons and that blocking 5-HT reuptake by tertiary amine TCAs (such as clomipramine), gave an explanation for the mood elevation of some antidepressants.

The catecholamine hypothesis was then modified to include 5-HT in the etiology of depression (9,10). It should be noted, however, that not all inhibitors of monoamine reuptake are antidepressants, because cocaine, a potent inhibitor of NE and dopamine reuptake, is not an antidepressant but, rather, an addictive stimulant. Subsequent studies with inhibitors of monoamine biosynthesis appear to confirm Kielholz's opinion and Schildkraut's modified theory that clinical depression is the result of a deficiency in both 5-HT and NE and that the antidepressive mechanism of action most likely affects levels of both.

Inhibition of 5-HT biosynthesis reverses the therapeutic effects of treatment with antidepressants that have predominantly 5-HT reuptake inhibitory activity (e.g., fluoxetine) but less so with those that have predominantly NE reuptake inhibitory activity (e.g., desipramine) (11,12). Also, inhibition of 5-HT biosynthesis produced a relapse in depressed patients who had their depression successfully treated with imipramine or tranylcypromine, whereas inhibitors of dopamine or NE synthesis had no effect on these depressed patients (13,14). A depletion of catecholamines reverses the therapeutic effects of desipramine more than that of fluoxetine or sertraline. These studies appear to confirm that the antidepressive action of antidepressants is, indeed, a function of their monoamine activity.

Kielholz further reasoned that because NE reuptake inhibitors (activating antidepressants) were likely to trigger suicide, the greatest hazard of an antidepressant, such as the 5-HT reuptake inhibitors would be less likely to lead to suicide. These observations led to the proposition that it would be worth developing drugs that selectively inhibited the reuptake of 5-HT, producing agents more useful for the treatment of depression.

Changes in NE and 5-HT levels do not affect mood in everyone. Some evidence also suggests that for a subset of patients, dopamine plays a role in depression. Dopaminergic substances have been used as antidepressants when other measures have failed. The dopamine hypothesis of schizophrenia and the emphasis on other neurotransmitters, most notably NE and 5-HT, in the pathogenesis of depression have focused attention away from dopamine and its role in affective disorders. Recent clinical evidence suggests the involvement of dopamine in several subtypes of depression, psychomotor retardation and diminished motivation, and in seasonal mood disorder (11). The biochemical evidence in patients with depression indicates diminished dopamine turnover. In addition, a considerable amount of pharmacological evidence exists regarding the efficacy of antidepressants with dopaminergic effects in the treatment of depression. However, the role of dopamine in depression must be understood, in the context of existing theories involving other neurotransmitters that may act independently and interact with dopamine and other neurochemicals to contribute to depression (12).

Receptor Sensitivity Hypothesis

The receptor sensitivity hypothesis proposes that it is not simply the level of NE or 5-HT in the synapse that matters but, rather, the sensitivity of the postsynaptic receptors to these neurotransmitters. Those with depression, it is speculated, possess postsynaptic receptors that have grown hypersensitive to NE and 5-HT because of their depletion in the synaptic cleft. Thus, a low level of NE and 5-HT at their respective receptors can lead to changes in the receptors themselves, even if there are no clinical signs of depression. Increased receptor sensitivity (hypersensitivity) and an increase in receptor numbers on the neuronal cell membrane are events that may correlate with the start of depression. This theory is an important step toward understanding the long delay between administration of antidepressant drugs and their clinical response. According to this hypothesis, relief from the symptoms of depression following chronic administration of antidepressants comes from a normalization of receptor sensitivity (reducing receptor hypersensitivity) by increasing the concentration of NE and 5-HT in the synaptic cleft. Therefore, the use of reuptake inhibitors and the MAOIs as antidepressants increases the concentration of NE and/or 5-HT in the synaptic cleft and, over time, causes the postsynaptic neuron to compensate by decreasing receptor sensitivity (desensitization) and the number of receptor sites (decrease in the expression of NE and 5-HT receptors: downregulation). About one-third of depressed patients, however, fail to respond to antidepressant therapy. For some unknown reason, the increased concentration of NE and/or 5-HT fail to desensitize the postsynaptic receptors.

Permissive Hypothesis

The permissive hypothesis (10) emphasizes the importance of the balance between 5-HT and NE in regulating mood, not the absolute levels of these neurotransmitters or their receptors. If 5-HT levels are too low, the balanced control of the NE system is lost, permitting abnormal levels of NE to cause mania, as seen in bipolar disorders. If the NE levels fall, the balanced control of the 5-HT system is lost, allowing abnormal levels of 5-HT to cause the person to exhibit the symptoms of depression.

Hormonal Hypothesis

The hormonal hypothesis suggests that changes in the hypothalamus-pituitary-adrenal axis (HPA) can influence the levels of 5-HT and NE released by nerve cells in the brain and, subsequently, their function (15). In the event of stress, the hypothalamus produces a hormone locally in the brain called corticotrophin-releasing factor, which in turn stimulates the pituitary gland to secrete adrenocorticotropic hormone into the blood, where it stimulates the adrenal glands to release hydrocortisone (cortisol), which prepares the body for dealing with stress. Stress also directly stimulates the adrenal gland to secrete epinephrine and NE. Hydrocortisone can cause depression, especially when released in higher-than-usual amounts. The release of hydrocortisone may push the individual over the edge into depression or contribute to the component of anxiety, which so often accompanies depressive illnesses. Approximately 50% of those with major depression have elevated hydrocortisone levels.

Living organisms operate in a state of imbalance, and the neural (autonomic) and endocrine systems have evolved to modify the rates of biochemical pathways to maintain homeostasis. One of the hallmarks of these regulatory systems is the short-lived nature of the nerve signals produced. The half-life of neurotransmitters is measured in seconds, whereas those of the circulating hormones may be minutes or hours. A rationale for the short-lived nature of the neurotransmitters is to permit these signaling pathways to quickly reset themselves to meet the next challenge. Readjustments (i.e., plasticity) in these systems include uncoupling of receptor responses from signaling events, degradation of receptors, and up- and downregulation of signaling molecules that affect the primary signaling pathway. These hypotheses are not mutually exclusive and in each it is assumed that the more extreme the event, the more severe the clinical outcome.

GENERAL APPROACHES TO TREATMENT OF DEPRESSION

Before 1950, there were no antidepressants—at least not as we know them today. The two treatments for depressive illness were either amphetamine stimulants, which often were ineffective and had the general affect of increasing energy and activity (16), or electroconvulsive therapy, which was effective but had the disadvantage of terrifying and often endangering the patient. Not until the late 1950s were the first generation of antidepressants discovered (the TCAs and MAOIs), not by design but by chance. While searching for "chlorpromazine-like" compounds to treat schizophrenia, imipramine was recognized by Kuhn (16) for its antidepressant properties, thus becoming the forerunner for the tricyclic class of monoamine reuptake inhibitor antidepressants (i.e., the TCAs). The second compound to be discovered was the antitubercular drug isoniazid (17), which proved to have powerful mood-enhancing properties, becoming the forerunner of the MAOIs. With the introduction of imipramine and isoniazid, the theory and treatment of depression changed. These early studies still summarize much of our current knowledge regarding the therapeutic effects of antidepressant treatments.

Between 1960 and 1980, TCAs were the major pharmacological treatment for depression (18). The TCAs, however, have many other actions in addition to blocking monoamine reuptake, including anticholinergic, antihistaminergic, and cardiotoxic side effects that are related to their affinity for muscarinic, histamine, and α_1-adrenergic receptors as well as their action on cardiac and central nervous system (CNS) Na^+ channels in membranes. The improved safety, tolerability, and reuptake selectivity of the newer antidepressants (i.e., SSRIs, selective NE reuptake inhibitors [SNRIs], and nonselective NE and 5-HT reuptake inhibitors [NSRIs]) have resulted in displacement of the TCAs as the first choice for prophylactic treatment of major depression. The TCAs occupy a narrower—but still important—role in the psychopharmacological therapy.

The early MAOIs irreversibly inhibited the oxidative deamination of the neurotransmitter monoamines, the proposed mechanism of their antidepressant activity. The biggest liability for these MAOIs was their potential to cause life-threatening hypertensive reactions, resulting from the nonselective irreversible inhibition of MAO-A and MAO-B, which decreases the intestinal and hepatic degradation of dietary sources of tyramine. This inhibition of MAO allows excessive amounts of dietary tyramine, a weak sympathomimetic vasoconstrictor, to be absorbed from the food, resulting in increased blood pressure (refer to the section of MAOIs in this chapter for more details). Inhibition of monoamine oxidases also can alter the pharmacokinetics of monoamine over-the-counter and prescription drugs, allowing them to accumulate in the blood and, thus, increasing their potential for causing adverse drug effects and drug–drug interactions. Minimizing drug and food interactions of these early MAOIs inspired the development of a new generation of MAOIs that are both reversible and selective for MAO-A. The demise of the early MAOIs allowed the TCAs to become the gold standard for the treatment of depressive disorders.

The discovery that certain antihistaminic agents without the condensed aromatic ring systems are selective inhibitors of 5-HT reuptake with little affinity for the other neuroreceptors and almost devoid of cardiotoxicity questioned the need for the 10,11-ethylene bridge for the TCAs. Thus, the search for inhibitors that selectively blocked 5-HT reuptake without the 7-membered central ring of the TCAs resulted in the synthesis of the diarylpropylamine analogues of the TCAs (Fig. 21.2). Thus, during the late 1960s and early 1970s, antihistamine molecules were structurally manipulated in the search for compounds that selectively inhibited 5-HT reuptake with greater potency. The initial breakthrough came with the synthesis of *Z*-zimeldine (the *cis*-isomer) (a.k.a., zimelidine, Zemid, patented in 1971), the first SSRI that selectively inhibited the presynaptic reuptake of 5-HT without the adverse events associated with the multireceptor activities of the TCAs (19,20). Zimeldine was synthesized from the manipulation of the antihistamine pheniramine into a diary allylamine, the *cis*-isomer (rigid analogue) of the propylamine group (Fig. 21.2).

Other structural changes that enhanced its potency and selectivity for blocking 5-HT reuptake was moving the regional position of the 2-pyridyl ring of pheniramine to the 3-pyridyl position and substitution of a halogen into the 4-position of the phenyl ring (2-substitutions selectively block NE reuptake). The secondary amine and primary metabolite, norzimeldine, was 15 times more potent than zimeldine for blocking 5-HT reuptake. On the other hand, (*E*)-zimeldine (the *trans*-isomer) is a nonselective inhibitor of 5-HT and NE reuptake, whereas its corresponding secondary amine is a potent and selective inhibitor of NE reuptake. It is not unusual for geometric isomers to differ markedly from each other with regard to their receptor

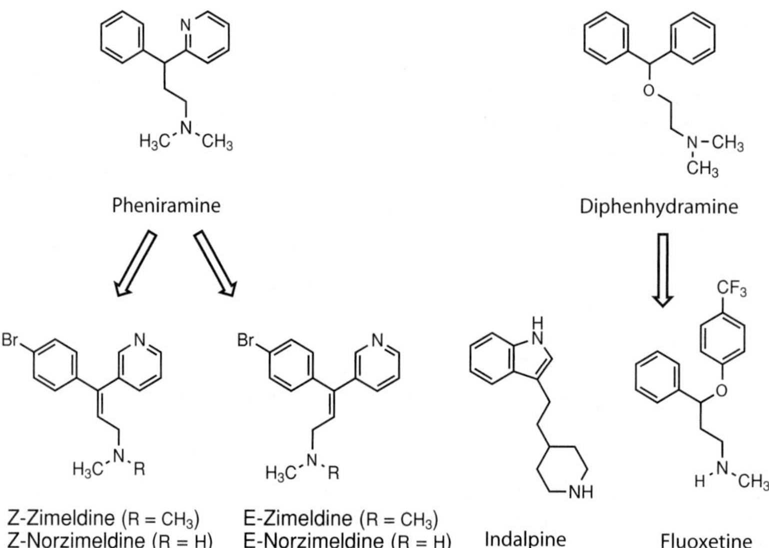

Fig. 21.2. Structural relationship between antihistamines and antidepressants that block the reuptake of 5-HT.

or transporter selectivity, affinity, and pharmacodynamic properties. Thus, zimeldine became the first SSRI to be marketed as an antidepressant, but unfortunately, several cases of Guillain-Barre syndrome (an autoimmune disorder attacking the peripheral nervous system) were associated with the use of this drug and led to its withdrawal from the market in 1983. During postmarketing clinical studies, zimeldine showed an increase in the number of suicide attempts than had been expected—this adverse event was to become a major issue with the SSRIs 20 years later.

The success of zimeldine as an SSRI, however, led to the discovery and marketing of several nontricyclic SSRIs from multiple pharmaceutical companies worldwide. Another manipulation of the antihistamines produced indalpine (patented 1977 by Rhône Poulenc) (Fig. 21.2). It produced responses in patients who had not responded to the TCAs or MAOIs but then ran into trouble, because clinical trials suggested that it might cause agranulocytopenia (a lowering of the white blood cell count). For the most part, this is not a serious problem, but in rare cases, if undetected, it can be fatal. It was removed from the European market in 1985 and was never marketed in the United States.

Other SSRIs developed during this period that have become household words include paroxetine (patented 1975 by Ferrosan to SmithKlineBeecham to GlaxoKline), citalopram (patented 1979 Lindberg, licensed to Forest Labs), fluoxetine (patented 1982 Lilly), and sertraline (patented 1985 Pfizer).

Scientists at Lilly Research Laboratories synthesized more than 50 phenoxypropylamines derived from the antihistamine diphenhydramine (Benadryl) before discovering fluoxetine (21,22) (Fig. 21.2). The first of these compounds was nisoxetine, a potent SNRI (see Fig. 21.8) that was clinically developed but never marketed. Other derivatives that have since been marketed by Lilly include atomoxetine (a SNRI) and duloxetine (a NSRI).

Fluoxetine (Prozac) was heralded as the prototype for the next generation of SSRI antidepressants possessing fewer adverse effects and with a greater margin of safety when overdoses are consumed compared with the TCAs and also lacking the food-interaction toxicity of MAOIs. Fluoxetine was marketed in 1987, and within a few years, it boasted worldwide sales of nearly $1.2 billion a year. During the past 20 years, nontricyclic selective and nonselective NE and 5-HT reuptake inhibitors as well as reversible selective MAOIs have been approved for use in depression. These newer additions allow exploration of the roles of NE versus 5-HT using treatments that are devoid of confounding receptor activities. Conscious targeting of more than one neurotransmitter activity (e.g., of serotonergic and noradrenergic mechanisms or of NE and dopamine), while retaining specificity, is the target for the development of the next generation of antidepressants.

The majority of antidepressants in current use selectively inhibit the reuptake of 5-HT and/or NE. Based on the previously neglected role proposed for dopamine in depression, it has been hypothesized that a "broad-spectrum" antidepressant will produce a more rapid onset and/or higher efficacy than agents inhibiting the reuptake of 5-HT and/or NE (23). Broad-spectrum antidepressants are compounds that inhibit the reuptake of NE, 5-HT, and dopamine, the three biogenic amines most closely linked to depression. The pharmacological profile of one such compound, DOV 21947, an azabicyclo[3.1.0]hexane, has recently been described and is in Phase III clinical trials (23,24). It is a potent inhibitor of NE, 5-HT, and dopamine reuptake by their corresponding membrane transporter proteins. The plasma concentrations of DOV 21947, following both single and multiple doses, appear to be sufficient to inhibit NE, 5-HT, and dopamine reuptake.

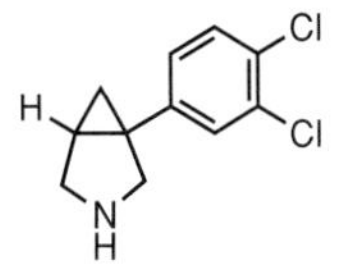

DOV 21947

The antiobesity agent, racemic (*R*, *S*)-sibutramine is a 5-HT and NE reuptake inhibitor and has an antidepressant profile similar to that of a "triple-acting" antidepressant in animals (25). It has two active metabolites, desmethylsibutramine and didesmethylsibutramine (the terms "desmethyl" and "demethyl" are used interchangeably). The IC50 for the R-enantiomers of these metabolites were more potent as in vitro inhibitors of dopamine and NE reuptake than 5-HT (25). Both *R*-enantiomers had significantly greater anorectic effects than those of their respective *S*-enantiomers as well as that of (*R*,*S*) sibutramine. The results suggest that these enantioselective metabolites of sibutramine could be safe and effective treatments for binge-eating disorder in obese patients.

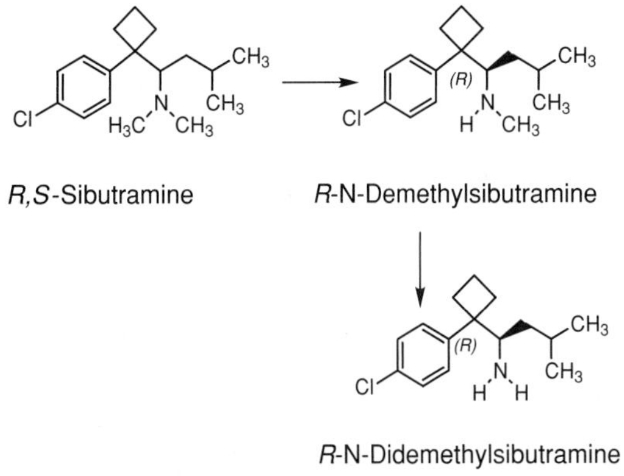

R,*S*-Sibutramine

R-N-Demethylsibutramine

R-N-Didemethylsibutramine

Table 21.1. Antidepressant Classes with Examples of Generic and Trade Names

Drug Classes	Abbreviation	Drug Examples	Trade Names
Selective norepinephrine reuptake inhibitors	SNRIs	Amoxapine	Asendin
		Desipramine	Norpramin
		Maprotiline	
		Nortriptyline	Aventyl, Pamelor
		Roboxetine	Vestra
		Atomoxetine	Strattera
Selective serotonin reuptake inhibitors	SSRIs	Citalopram	Celexa
		Escitalopram	Lexapro
		Fluoxetine	Prozac
		Fluvoxamine	
		Paroxetine	Paxil
		Sertraline	Zoloft
Norepinephrine and serotonin reuptake inhibitors	NSRIs	Amitriptyline	Elavil
		Clomipramine	Anafranol
		Doxepine	Sinequan
		Imipramine	Tofranil
		Milnacipran	Ixel
		Trimipramine	Surmontil
		Venlafaxine	Effexor
		Duloxetine	Cymbalta
Dopamine and norepinephrine reuptake inhibitors	DNRIs	Bupropion	Wellbutrin, Zyban
Serotonin receptor modulators	SRMs		
Serotonin-2 antagonists/serotonin reuptake inhibitors	SARIs	Trazodone	Desyrel
α_2-Noradrenergic antagonists/serotonin antagonists	NaSSAs	Mirtazepine	Remeron
Monoamine oxidase inhibitors	MAOIs	Meclobemide	
		Phenelzine	
		Nardil	
		Tranylcypramine	Parnate
Mood stabilizers		Lithium	Eskalith, Lithobid
		Valproic acid	Depakote, Depakene, Depacon
		Carbamazepine	Tegretol

Traditionally, antidepressants have been classified according to their structure (i.e., secondary or tertiary amine TCAs) or their principal mechanism of action (i.e., MAOIs and SSRIs). With the appearance of increasing numbers of second- and third-generation antidepressants, however, a better way of classifying and describing the antidepressants was necessary. For the purposes of this chapter, the antidepressants are organized into eight classes (Table 21.1) and discussed according to their distinct and different mechanisms of action (Fig. 21.3). Considerable overlap exists in their mechanism of actions and uses, but these different classes of antidepressants work by distinct mechanisms, have different side-effect profiles, and may be favored for different types of depressive illnesses.

A key step that determines the intensity and duration of monoamine signaling at synapses is the reuptake of the released neurotransmitter into nerve terminals through high-affinity plasma membrane transporters (26). Reuptake is the process of rapidly removing the monoamine neurotransmitters from the synaptic cleft and allowing most of the released neurotransmitter to be recycled for further use. The advantage of reuptake is that it is faster than passive diffusion through the membrane. Any monoamine neurotransmitter remaining in the synaptic cleft is then absorbed and metabolized into inactive metabolites. The monoamine reuptake transporter protein binds the released neurotransmitter in the extracellular fluid and transports the monoamine across the presynaptic plasma membrane back into the intracellular fluid of the presynaptic neuron (Fig. 21.4). Monoamine transporters (Fig. 21.5 and sidebar for more detail) are embedded in the plasma membrane of the nerve terminals (perisynaptically) of dopaminergic, noradrenergic, and serotonergic neurons rather than intrasynaptically (along the portion of the nerve terminal forming the synapse). They are members of a larger sodium-dependent transporter family and represent a major mechanism terminating the action of released monoamine neurotransmitters in the synaptic cleft. These transporters are important targets for many antidepressive drugs and substances of abuse (i.e., cocaine). Transporter proteins are specific to their respective neurotransmitter: SERT for 5-HT (serotonin reuptake transporter), NET (NE reuptake transporter) for NE, and DAT for dopamine. None of the reuptake antidepres-

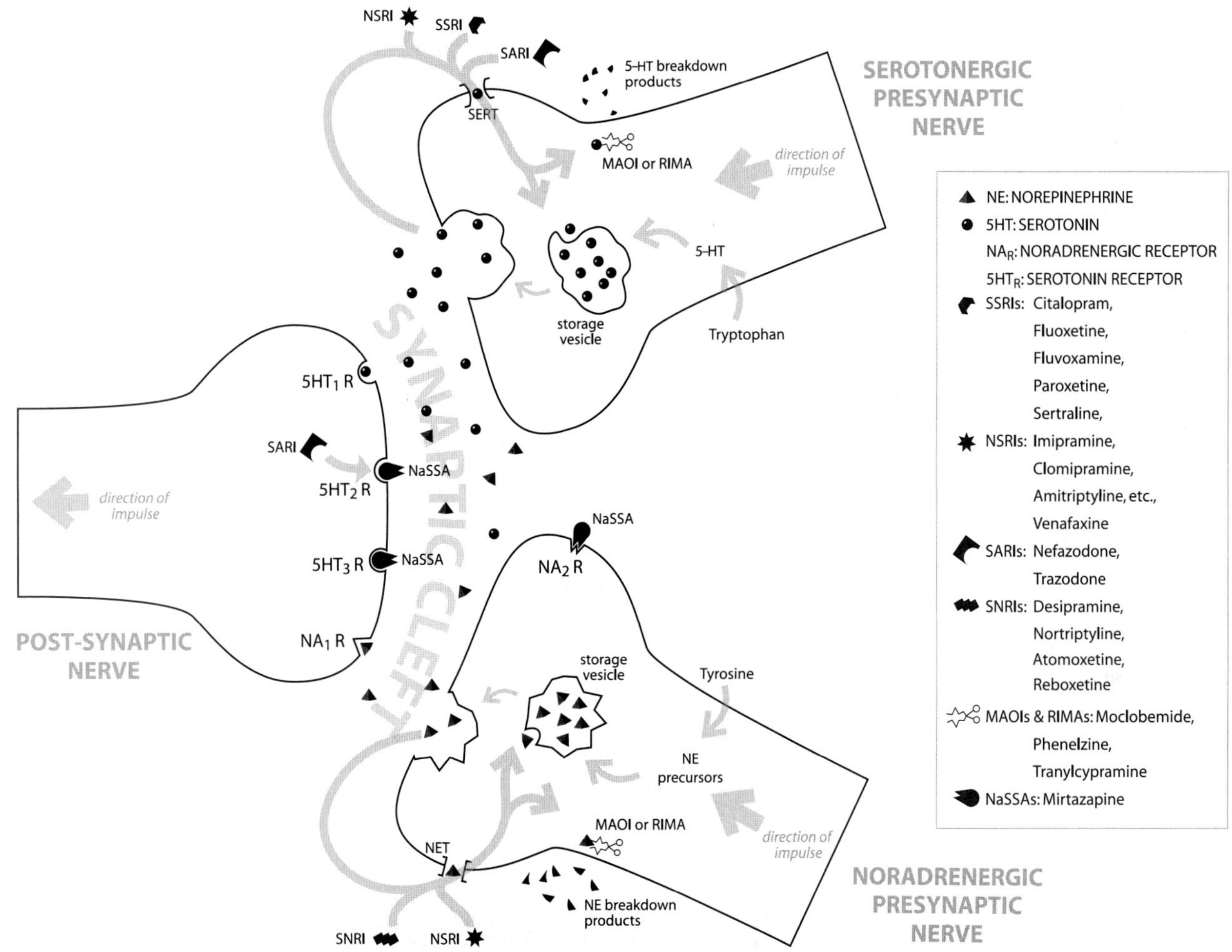

Fig. 21.3. Sites of action of the antidepressants.

sants exhibit significant affinity for dopamine transporters, which may be related to their ineffectiveness in types of depression that is resistant to the SNRIs, SSRIs, and NSRIs. The TCAs and nontricyclic NSRIs nonselectively block the reuptake transporters for both NE and 5-HT, the SSRIs selectively block SERT, and SNRIs selectively block NET. The antidepressant reuptake inhibitors also may contribute to relief of depression by decreasing the expression of their respective transporter proteins.

Figure 21.6 graphically illustrates the selectivity of the reuptake inhibitors for their respective transporters. The selectivity ratios for inhibiting SERT (ratio, >1) is obtained by dividing the affinity of the inhibitor (K_i) for inhibiting SERT with its affinity (K_i) for inhibiting NET, whereas the selectivity ratio for inhibiting NET (ratio <1) is obtained by dividing its affinity (K_i) for inhibiting NET with the affinity (K_i) for inhibiting SERT. For example, a value of approximately one for amitriptyline means that amitriptyline will inhibit both NET and SERT at the same concentration (i.e., no selectivity with regard to their mechanism of antidepressant activity). The value of -30 for desipramine means that desipramine is 30 times more potent at inhibiting the NET than the SERT, although the SSRIs with selectivity ratio values of greater than 100 are more than 100 times more potent at inhibiting the SERT than the NET. Furthermore, because the selectivity ratio for most SSRIs is more than 100, a plasma concentration of any SSRI that will produce inhibition of the SERT will produce no physiologically meaningful inhibition of NET (27–29). The converse will be true regarding selectivity for the NET. Clinically, such selectivity ratios of greater than 100 translate into being able to produce all the physiological effects mediated by inhibiting one transporter without causing any effects that will be produced by inhibiting the other uptake transporter. When the selectivity ratio is less than 30, such as with fluoxetine, the difference is small enough that inhibition of both reuptake transporters may occur under therapeutic doses and, thus, can contribute to the broad antidepressant activity of the drug.

Transporter Proteins

The monoamine transporter protein (molecular weights, 60-80 kDa) is a string of amino acids that weaves in and out of the presynaptic membrane 12 times (Fig. 21.4)—that is, 12 transmembrane domains (TMs) with a large extracellular loop between TM3 and TM4. Both the N- and C-termini of the transporters are located within the cytoplasm. There are six potential sites of phosphorylation by protein kinase A and protein kinase C, which regulate the transporters. The large extracellular loop and the cytoplasmic parts of the N- and C-termini do not appear to be the target sites for the transporter inhibitors (i.e., antidepressants). Rather, the areas important for selective monoamine affinity appear to be localized within TM1 to TM3 and TM8 to TM12 that project into the synapse, and these areas of the transporters have a common binding site for the monoamine and many of its inhibitors (Fig. 21.4). To transport protonated 5-HT^+, SERT cotransports a sodium ion and a chloride ion while countertransporting a potassium ion (Fig. 21.5). The SERT then flips inside the cell, releasing the 5-HT^+ and the ions into the cytoplasm of the neuron. On releasing the 5-HT^+ and the ions, SERT flips back out, with the unoccupied binding site exposed to the synaptic cleft, ready to receive and transport another 5-HT^+ molecule. To transport protonated NE^+, NET also cotransports sodium and chloride ions with intracellular potassium stimulation and no potassium efflux. The initial complex of the monoamine, Na^+, and Cl^- with the transporter protein creates a conformational change in the transporter protein. The driving force (electrical potential) for the energetically unfavorable transport of the monoamine is the Na^+ concentration gradient. The Na^+, K^+ transporter (Na^+, K^+-ATPase) maintains the extracellular Na^+ concentration as well as the intracellular K^+ concentration. The Na^+, K^+-ATPase transport three Na^+ ions for each two K^+ ions pumped into the cell. Unlike channels that stay open or closed, transporters undergo conformational changes (changes in their three-dimensional shape) and move one monoamine molecule in each cycle.

Most scientists agree that MAOIs, SSRIs, SNRIs, and NSRIs improve depression by boosting the levels of NE and/or 5-HT in the brain, but what is not established is how increased concentrations of NE and 5-HT translate into reducing depression. One problem with the original monoamine model was that whereas plasma concentrations of the antidepressant and binding to the monoamine transporter occur almost immediately, chronic administration of antidepressants is needed before clinical efficacy is attained (18). The therapeutic effect of an antidepressant is almost always observed after a period of 3 to 6 weeks of treatment. This suggests that certain adaptive changes are occurring with chronic administration of these drugs that may be important for their antidepressant action (see Receptor Sensitivity Hypothesis). This concept has been the motivating force for much of the refinement of the monoamine theory. Over the years, mechanisms such as downregulation of β-adrenergic receptors, desensitization of presynaptic α_2-adrenoceptors, increased postsynaptic 5-HT receptor sensitivity, downregulation of 5-HT_2 receptors, and desensitization of presynaptic 5-HT_{1A} receptor have been cited either as the final common pathway or as one of many possible final common pathways.

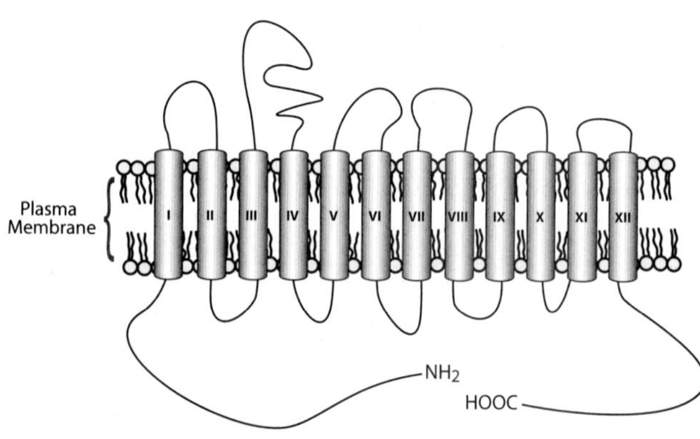

Fig. 21.4. Monoamine reuptake transporter.

It should be remembered that the neurotransmitter and downregulation hypotheses are incomplete explanations for how antidepressants work. Antidepressants most likely set off an intricate chain of reactions that occur

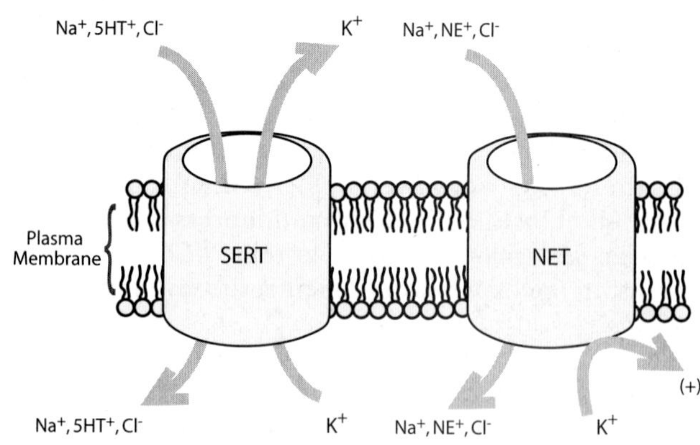

Fig. 21.5. Model of the NET and SERT and the ion-coupled NE and 5-HT reuptake. Reuptake of 5-HT is dependent on the cotransport of Na^+ and Cl^- and countertransport of K^+. Reuptake of NE is dependent on the cotransport of Na^+ and Cl^- with intracellular K^+ stimulation but without K^+ efflux.

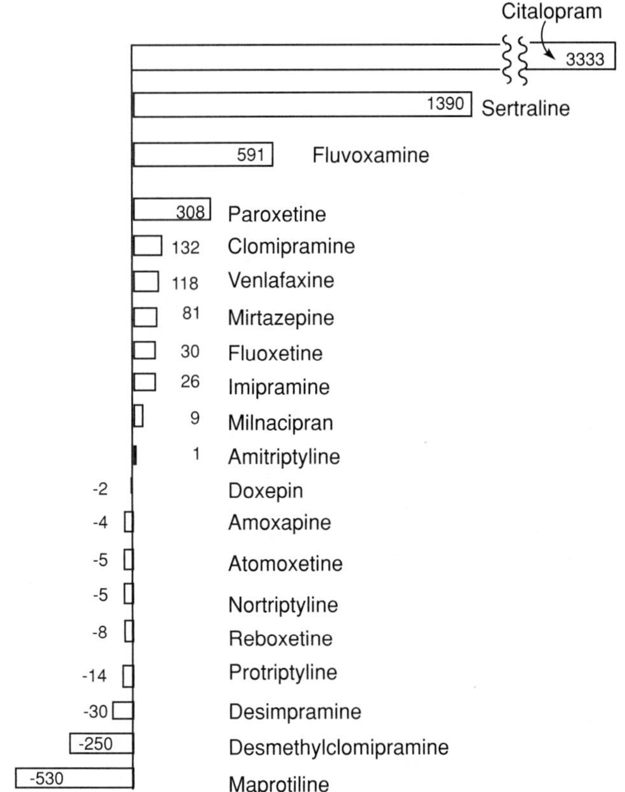

Fig. 21.6. In vitro selectivity ratios for reuptake inhibitors.

between the time the patient first takes them and the following few weeks, when they finally produce their effect. What the neurotransmitter and downregulation hypotheses do provide are useful—if simplistic—models for comprehending at least some of the basic biochemical processes triggered by antidepressants.

ANTIDEPRESSANTS IN PSYCHOTHERAPY

The introduction of the second-generation classes of antidepressants in the 1980s and 1990s (SSRIs, SNRIs, NSRIs, and serotonin receptor modulators [serotonin antagonist/reuptake inhibitors (SARIs) and noradrenergic specific serotonergic antidepressants (NaSSA)]) (Table 21.1) has been regarded as the major pharmacological advance in the treatment of depression since the appearance of the TCAs and MAOIs. The SSRIs, SNRIs, and NSRIs have proven to be effective for a broad range of depressive illnesses, dysthymia, several anxiety disorders, and bulimia. The SSRIs are the most widely prescribed antidepressant drugs and rank in the Top 50 drugs in terms of total United States sales for 2004. In addition to being the usual first-line treatments for major depression, the SSRIs also are first-line treatments for panic disorder, obsessive-compulsive disorder, social phobia, posttraumatic stress disorder, and bulimia. They also may be the best medications for treatment of dysthymia and generalized anxiety disorder.

Differences in general tolerability of the different classes of antidepressants and in their side-effect profiles are well known and generally accepted. Compared with the TCAs, the SSRIs cause significantly more nausea, diarrhea, agitation, sexual dysfunction, anorexia, insomnia, nervousness, and anxiety, whereas the TCAs cause more cardiotoxicity, dry mouth, constipation, dizziness, sweating, and blurred vision (18). Consistent evidence also indicates that SSRIs, as a group, are better tolerated than TCAs. Despite pharmacological differences in their mechanisms of actions, the general view has been that all antidepressants are of equal efficacy. Only within the last 10 years has this general assumption come under serious challenge from comparisons of antidepressants with dual mechanisms of action versus those with a single mechanism of action (11).

Often, a variety of antidepressants will be prescribed and the dosage adjusted before the most effective antidepressant or combination of antidepressants is found. Although some improvements may be seen during the first few weeks, the antidepressants must be taken regularly for 3 to 4 weeks (and, in some cases, for as many as 8 weeks) before the full therapeutic effect occurs. Patient compliance can become an issue, because they often are tempted to stop medication too soon as a result of feeling better and, thus, thinking they no longer need the medication. Additionally, they may have problems with the adverse effects, or they may think the medication is not helping at all. It is important for the patient to keep taking the antidepressant until it has a chance to work, although side effects often appear before antidepressant activity does. Once the individual is feeling better, it is important to continue the medication for at least 4 to 9 months (or longer) to prevent a recurrence of the depression. Antidepressants alter the brain chemistry; therefore, they must be stopped gradually to give the brain time to adjust. For some individuals with bipolar disorder or chronic major depression, antidepressant therapy may need to be maintained indefinitely (30). All patients who are prescribed antidepressants should be informed that although the drugs are not associated with tolerance and craving, discontinuation/withdrawal symptoms may occur on stopping, missing doses, or occasionally, on reducing the dose of the drug. These symptoms usually are mild and self-limiting, but occasionally, they can be severe, particularly if the drug is stopped abruptly. Symptoms of antidepressant withdrawal include nausea, vomiting, anorexia, headache, restlessness, agitation, "chills," insomnia, and sometimes, hypomania, panic-anxiety, and extreme motor restlessness, especially if an antidepressant (particularly an MAOI) is stopped suddenly after regular administration for 8 weeks or more.

Clinical trials have concluded that 2 or 3 of every 100 children and teenagers treated with antidepressants might be at higher risk of suicidal behavior. Data regarding suicidal behavior varies among the antidepressants, which leads to the conclusion that no antidepressant is free from risk at this time. Most of the suicides have occurred with the SSRIs, especially paroxetine (Paxil) and fluoxetine (Prozac); only fluoxetine has been proven to be effective and is approved for treating pediatric depression. Approximately 7% of antidepressant prescriptions are written for children. Thus, the U.S. Food and Drug Administration (FDA) in 2007 approved that "black box labeling" be included on antidepressant product packaging, alerting physicians to avoid prescribing antidepressants to children because of possible risks of suicidal behavior and to watch for signs of worsening depression or suicidal thoughts in children who are taking any antidepressant.

Guidelines for Managing Depression

The following guidelines apply to all antidepressants, including SSRIs, SNRIs, and NE/serotonin reuptake inhibitors (NSRIs):

- For most SSRIs used for treating depression, recommended daily dosages should not be exceeded, because no evidence indicates any additional benefit from higher amounts.
- Patients who are taking antidepressants should be monitored carefully and frequently during the early stages of treatment, especially if symptoms worsen or if new symptoms appear.
- Adverse drug reactions should be considered if a patient does not do well after treatment begins; if restlessness or agitation occur, increasing antidepressant doses can be detrimental.
- Although the relationship between suicidality and increasing or decreasing antidepressant doses is not clear, patients should be monitored during such periods for changes in symptoms. Data supporting a link with suicidality have come from studies of patients younger than 18 years of age; however, because people mature at different rates, young adults who are being treated with these agents should be monitored especially carefully.
- Pharmacists should expect to hear questions from patients regarding the safety and continued use of their antidepressant medication. Pharmacists can help patients and other health care professionals to evaluate the situation to determine the most appropriate action for the patient.
- Patients should talk to their pharmacist or physician about any concerns they may have before making any changes to the way they take their medication.
- Patients should not abruptly stop taking or lower the dosage of their antidepressant medication and should continue with their current medication plan until a decision is made with their health care provider because of the possibility of withdrawal symptoms, especially if the patient has been on extended therapy for 6 weeks or more. If a patient is taken off antidepressant medication, he or she should be advised of a tapered approach and should watch for increased dizziness, restlessness, agitation, anxiety, nervousness, headache, nausea and vomiting, mood changes, and fatigue. If a patient feels that these symptoms are severe or there is a reemergence of depression, the patient should immediately contact the health care provider. Patients should be carefully monitored for reemergence of depression or severe symptoms. If antidepressant therapy is discontinued, the dosage should be tapered gradually, over at least a 2-week time frame, to minimize withdrawal reactions.

EFFECT OF PHYSICOCHEMICAL PROPERTIES AND STEREOCHEMISTRY ON ANTIDEPRESSANT EFFICACY

Small substituent changes in molecular structure can affect the pharmacokinetic and pharmacodynamic (clinical) properties of antidepressant drug molecules, resulting in profound differences between their transporter selectivity and their antidepressant effect—for example, a difference of a 2-chloro group between the structurally related antidepressants imipramine and clomipramine or the *o*- versus *p*-substituents between duloxetine (NSRI) and atomoxetine (SNRI) (Fig. 21.7). Furthermore, a seemingly simple isosteric replacement of a sulfur atom in the central ring of chlorpromazine with an ethylene group to give a 7-membered azepine ring (clomipramine), or the replacement of the methylpiperidylidene at the 5-position for the antihistamine/5-HT antagonist cyproheptadine with a dimethylaminopropylidene for the antidepressant reuptake inhibitor amitriptyline, has profound effects on the physicochemical properties, pharmacokinetics, mechanisms of action, and therapeutic activities (Fig. 21.7). On the other hand, the physicochemical differences can translate into differences in in vitro and in vivo pharmacological and clinical properties, as exemplified between mianserin and mirtazapine (Fig. 21.7) (31). The isosteric replacement of a benzene ring (mianserin) with a pyridine (mirtazapine) resulted in significant changes in their dipole moments, lipophilicity (log P), pK_a values, and electronegativity, resulting in different mechanisms of action and regioselectivity in formation of hydroxylated metabolites.

Many antidepressants are stereoisomers and contain either a chiral center or a center of unsaturation by which chiral metabolites could result (32,33). Often, such drugs are marketed as a mixture of the resultant enantiomers (racemates) or of geometric isomers. These enantiomers or geometric isomers may differ markedly from each other with regard to their pharmacodynamic and/or pharmacokinetic properties. Increased knowledge about the molecular structure of specific drug targets and an awareness of several possible advantages to using single enantiomers rather than racemic mixtures of drugs have led to an increased emphasis on understanding the role of chirality in drug development of antidepressant drugs. Several notable examples of antidepressants (the SSRIs) currently are available in which the individual enantiomers or geometric isomers differ considerably with regard to factors such as binding to SERTs and NETs, interactions with receptors and metabolizing enzymes, and clearance rates from the body.

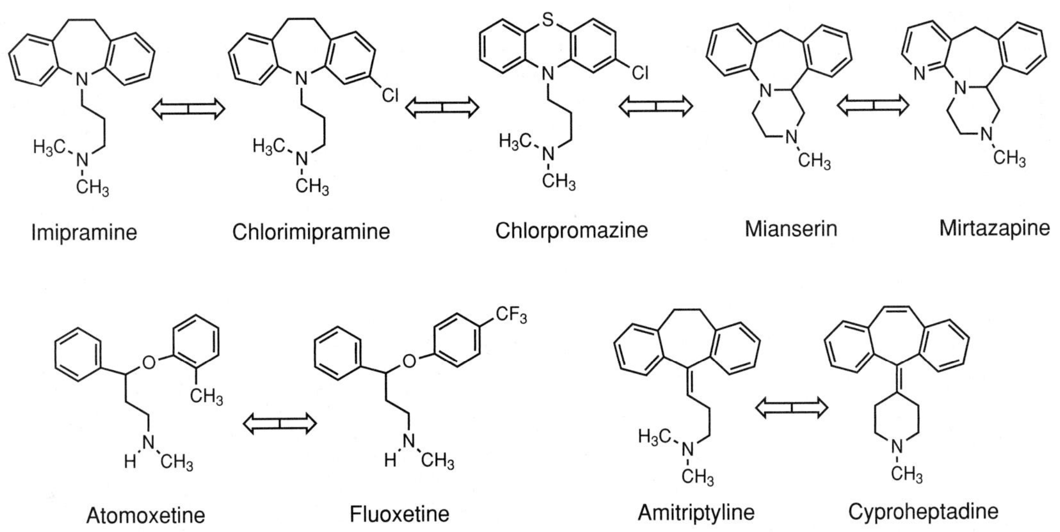

Imipramine Chlorimipramine Chlorpromazine Mianserin Mirtazapine

Atomoxetine Fluoxetine Amitriptyline Cyproheptadine

Fig. 21.7. Structural relationship between selected molecular structures.

Examples of the effects of chiral centers or geometric centers on such properties include racemic mixtures (e.g., fluoxetine, citalopram, bupropion, and trimipramine), single enantiomers (e.g., (+)-sertraline, (−)-paroxetine, (−)-escitalopram, and (−)-atomoxetine), or geometric isomers (e.g., *Z*-zimeldine, *Z*-dioxepin, *E*-dothiepin, and *E*-fluvoxamine). Recent developments in analytical and preparative resolution of racemic and geometric drug mixtures as well as increased interest in developing new drugs that interact with specific targets, which have been described in detail at the molecular level, have resulted in increased emphasis on stereochemistry in antidepressant drug development.

DRUG METABOLISM AND DRUG–DRUG INTERACTIONS

Antidepressant treatment carries increased risks of adverse drug events because of age-related physiologic changes, polypharmacotherapy, and individual variability in drug metabolism (e.g., genetic factors, concurrent disease, diet, and eating habits). Pharmacokinetic drug–drug interactions occur when one medication (the precipitant drug) significantly affects the plasma concentration, half-life, or both of another medication (the object drug) by altering its absorption, distribution, metabolism, or elimination. For object drugs with narrow therapeutic indices, even small elevations in plasma drug concentration can cause potentially serious adverse reactions. Pharmacodynamic drug–drug interactions occur when the precipitant drug affects the ability of the object drug to bind with its therapeutic target (e.g., transporter protein) or receptor. Some compounds compete directly for binding to a receptor; others indirectly affect the ability of an object drug to interact with its site of action. Many medications can bind to multiple receptor types (e.g., first-generation TCAs), causing diverse adverse reactions. Thus, before adding a new drug to an existing antidepressant regimen, it is wise to determine whether any medications can be eliminated. Reduction of total drug burden, adjustment of dose levels, and careful selection of an appropriate agent are important steps toward avoiding adverse drug interactions. In addition, the documented and potential drug interactions of the various classes of antidepressants—and of the specific drugs within each class—should be considered. Each patient should be treated individually and monitored carefully during the initiation and maintenance of antidepressant therapy.

The infamous drug–drug interactions between mibefradil (Propulsid) and terfenadine (Seldane) and other drugs metabolized by cytochrome P450 (CYP) 3A4 resulted in these drugs being withdrawn from the market, which placed a spotlight on hepatic drug metabolism as a significant participant in drug–drug interactions. Nearly all the antidepressants are metabolized by at least one CYP isoform, and these drugs and their metabolites may be substrates or inhibitors for the CYPs (Table 21.2).

When an antidepressant is metabolized by more than one CYP isoform in parallel, it is unlikely to be affected by drug interactions or genetic polymorphisms and to cause clinically significant drug interactions via CYP isoform inhibition (34). However, if the drug is metabolized primarily by CYP3A4 or the polymorphic CYP2C18 or CYP2D6 isoforms, the potential for drug–drug interactions increases. Therefore, knowledge regarding the metabolic pathways of antidepressants as well as knowledge about substrates and inhibitors of the CYP isoforms can assist in the selection of a proper drug and its dose, thus minimizing the risks of drug–drug interactions (37).

Table 21.2. Cytochrome P450 (CYP) Metabolism[a]

Antidepressant	Major CYP	Minor CYP	Metabolism Pathway	CYP Inhibitor
Amitriptyline	2D6	3A4, 2C19, 2C9, 1A2, and 2B6	2D6, 3A4, 2C19, and 1A2 N-demethylation 2D6 and 2B6 E-10-hydroxylation	2D6, 2C19, 1A2, and 2C9[b]
Clomipramine	2D6	3A4, 2C19, 1A2, and 2C9	2D6, 3A4, 2C19, 2C9, and 1A2 N-demethylation 2D6 2- and 8-hydroxylation	2D6
Desipramine	2D6	1A2 and 2C19	1A2 and 2C19 N-demethylation 2D6 and 2C19 2-hydroxylation	2D6 and 2C19[b]
E-Doxepine	2D6 and 2C9	3A4, 1A2, and 2C19	2D6 and 2C9 hydroxylation 3A4 and 1A2 N-demethylation	
Z-Doxepine	2C19	2C9, 3A4, and 1A2	2C19 and 2C9 N-demethylation 3A4 and 1A2 N-demethylation	
Imipramine	2D6	3A4, 2C19, 1A2, 2B6, and 2C9	1A2 and 2C19 N-demethylation 2D6, 1A2, 3A4, and 2C19 2- and 10-hydroxylation	1A2, 2D6, and 2C19
Maprotiline	2D6	1A2	2D6 and 1A2 N-demethylation	
Nortriptyline	2D6	3A4, 2C19, and 1A2	2D6, 3A4, 2C19, and 1A2 N-demethylation 2D6 E-10-hydroxylation	2D6 and 2C19[b]
Trimipramine	2D6	2C9 and 2C19	2-hydroxyl, 10-hydroxyl, and N-demethylation	2D6
(±)-Citalopram	2D6	1A2 and 2C19	2D6, 2C19, and 3A4 N-demethylation 2D6 N-oxidation	1A2[b] and 2D6[b]
Escitalopram	2D6	1A2 and 2C19	2D6, 2C19, and 3A4 N-demethylation 2D6 N-oxidation	
(±)-Fluoxetine	2D6	3A4, 2C9, 2C19, and 1A2	2D6 and 2C19 N-dealkylation 1A2 and 2C9 O-dealkylation	2D6 (S-fluoxetine) 1A2,[b] 2C19,[b] 3A4,[b] 2C9,[b] and 2D6[b]
Sertraline	2B6 and 3A4	2D6, 2C9, and 2C19	3A4 and 2C19 Deamination 2B6, 2C19, 2D6, and 3A4 N-demethylation	2C19,[b] 3A4,[b] and 2D6[b]
Fluvoxamine	1A2	3A4, 2C19, and 2D6	2D6 and 1A2 O-dealkylation	2C19, 1A2,[b] and 3A4[b]
Paroxetine	2D6	3A4, 1A2, and 2C9	2D6 cleavage methylene dioxy	2D6,[c] 2C19,[b] and 3A4[b]
Venlafaxine	2D6	3A4, 2C19, and 2C9	2D6, 2C19, and 2C9 O-demethylation 2C19, 2C9, and 3A4 N-demethylation	2D6[b]
Reboxetine	3A4		O-dethylation, aromatic ring hydroxylation	2D6 and 3A4
Atomoxetine	2D6	3A4, 2C19, and 1A2	2D6, 1A2, 2B6, and 2C19 4-hydroxylation 2C19, 3A4, and 2B6 N-demethylation	
Duloxetine	2D6		4- and 6-hydroxylation	2D6
Mirtazepine	2D6	3A4 and 1A2	2D6 and 1A2 8-hydroxylation 3A4 N-demethylation 3A4 and 1A2 N-oxidation	3A4[b] and 2D6[b]
Bupropion	2B6	2E1, 3A4, and 2D6	Hydroxylation t-butyl group	2D6[b]
Trazodone	3A4	2D6	N-dealkylation to chlorophenylpiperazine Aromatic ring hydroxylation	
Trancypromine		3A4, 2A6, 2D6, 2C19, and 2C9	Aromatic ring hydroxylation	2A6[c]
Meclobemide	2C19	2D6 and 1A2	Aromatic ring hydroxylation Morpholine ring oxidation	2D6[b]

[a]Rendic S. Human P450 metabolism database. Available at: http://www.gentest.com/human_p450_database. Accessed July 11, 2003.
[b]Weak CYP inhibitor.
[c]Mechanism-based inhibition.

P-Glycoprotein Transporters

P-glycoprotein (P-gp) is a member of the ATP-binding cassette superfamily of membrane transport proteins responsible for the efflux of many drugs. It represents a major component of the blood-brain barrier and the intestinal barrier, and contributes to renal and biliary elimination of drugs. At the blood-brain barrier, P-gp is localized in the apical membrane of brain capillary endothelial cells and transports substrates into the blood. Therefore, P-gp limits the penetration into and retention of numerous compounds, including the antidepressants, within the brain and, thus, modulate their effectiveness and CNS toxicity.

Inhibition of P-gp could significantly increase drug concentrations in the CNS. Additionally, P-gp is highly expressed in the apical membrane of epithelial cells in the small and large intestine, where it transports drugs out of the cells into the intestinal lumen, thus limiting the bioavailability of compounds such as paclitaxel and HIV protease inhibitors.

The role of P-gp for affecting the pharmacokinetic parameters of antidepressants and contributing to numerous pharmacokinetic drug–drug interactions with coadministered drugs has not been thoroughly elucidated. Antidepressants, particularly TCAs, have a significant potential for inducing adverse drug reactions and, therefore, are subject to numerous drug–drug interactions. The role of P-gp in causing clinically relevant drug interactions is becoming more and more obvious (35). Concentrations of paroxetine and venlafaxine increased two to three times in the brains of mice without P-gp (i.e., knockout mice) after single-dose administration and after treatment for 11 days (34), suggesting that these antidepressants are P-gp substrates and that their pharmacokinetics might be influenced by coadministered P-gp inhibitors. In contrast, fluoxetine exhibited no P-gp substrate characteristics (34), indicating that not all antidepressants share these properties. For citalopram, the results are contradictory.

The potency of sertraline and its N-demethylated metabolite, desmethylsertraline, and paroxetine for inhibiting P-gp was comparable with that of quinidine (35). Fluoxetine, norfluoxetine, fluvoxamine, reboxetine, and O-demethylparoxetine showed intermediate inhibition, and citalopram, desmethylcitalopram, venlafaxine, and N-desmethylvenlafaxine showed only weak inhibition. No inhibition was found for O-desmethylvenlafaxine.

Inhibition of P-gp by drugs may play an important role in drug safety by increasing plasma and brain concentrations of coadministered drugs and, thus, causing adverse drug reactions. No evidence for a potent drug–drug interaction was found with fluoxetine, although sertraline and paroxetine exhibited the greatest potential for affecting the pharmacokinetics of coadministered drugs at the level of P-gp (35,36). At usual therapeutic doses of paroxetine and sertraline, however, the IC50 for the inhibition of P-gp is approximately 250 times higher than the plasma concentration for paroxetine and approximately 500 times higher than that for sertraline (36), suggesting that even if the accumulation of sertraline within the cell (e.g., in the biliary or renal system) is taken into account, the P-gp inhibition observed in vitro might not be clinically relevant. This is substantiated by the fact that neither sertraline, fluvoxamine, nor citalopram had a clinically relevant influence on the pharmacokinetic parameters of digoxin, a P-gp prototype substrate. On the other hand, in addition to being an inhibitor of CYP2D6, paroxetine is a substrate for this same isoform, the activity of which is regulated by a genetic polymorphism. In individuals who lack this active enzyme (i.e., poor metabolizers), plasma paroxetine concentrations are up to 25 times higher than those in individuals who are extensive metabolizers. Therefore, one cannot exclude that in patients who are poor metabolizers, administration of high doses of paroxetine may translate into clinically relevant changes in the pharmacokinetics of concomitantly administered P-gp substrates.

It remains to be studied whether the inhibition of P-gp by the newer antidepressants might lead to drug–drug interactions in patients. Such interactions might, for instance, be relevant when drugs with low oral bioavailability because of substantial transport back into the gut lumen are to be coadministered, as has been shown for loperamide when given in combination with quinidine (38).

SPECIFIC DRUGS

Selective Norepinephrine Reuptake Inhibitors (SNRIs)

Despite the current popularity of the SSRIs for the treatment of depression, the noradrenergic neurons should not be overlooked, because they also influence the depressed mood (39). The noradrenergic system appears to be associated with increased drive, whereas the serotonergic system relates more to changes in mood (Fig. 21.1). Thus, the different symptoms of depression may benefit from drugs acting mainly on one or other of the neurotransmitter systems (18). The SNRIs (Fig. 21.8) seem to be at least as effective as the SSRIs in the treatment of depressive illness (39) by acting specifically at noradrenergic sites. Thus, the SSRIs and SNRIs influence depression by parallel, independent pathways. The SNRIs have a role in the treatment of depression, either alone or as adjunct therapy. The SNRI antidepressants are well tolerated but possess different adverse-event profiles.

The selectivity ratios (Fig. 21.6) show that the SNRIs, as a group, are potent selective inhibitors of the NET and that the secondary amine TCAs are substantially more potent with regard to their inhibition of NE reuptake in comparison to the SSRIs. Their in vitro affinity for inhibiting the NET essentially mirrors more or less their clinical efficacy as SNRIs (11): desipramine > protriptyline > amitriptyline = nortriptyline > reboxetine > maprotiline > amoxapine > imipramine > paroxetine. The level of affinity of the SNRIs for NET is not predictive for antidepressant activity.

Tricyclic Secondary Amine Antidepressants

STRUCTURE–ACTIVITY RELATIONSHIP OF THE TCAs. The tricyclic ring structure can be found in a variety of different drugs and, for the most part, represents a method for medicinal chemists to restrict the conformational mobility of two phenyl rings attached to a common carbon or hetero atom. The tricyclic ring structure is formed by joining the two phenyl rings into 6-6-6 or 6-7-6 ring systems, in which the central ring is either a 6–membered or

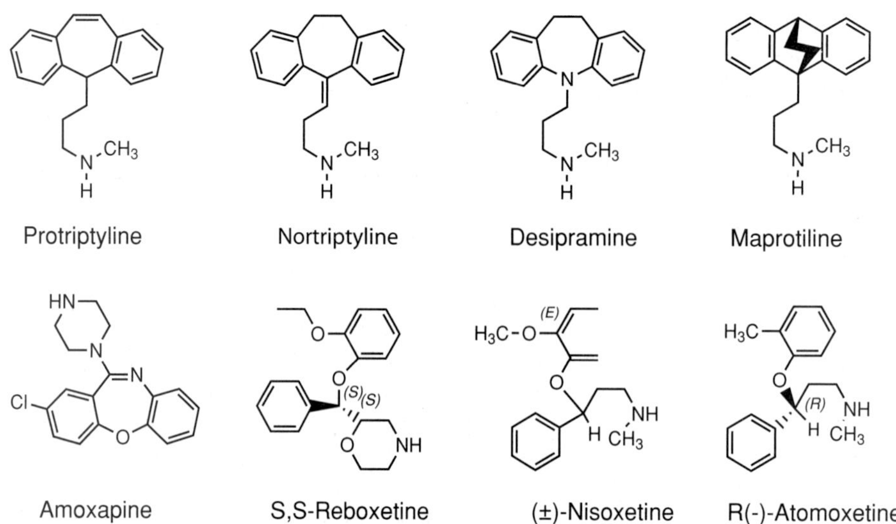

Fig. 21.8. Selective norepinephrine reuptake inhibitors (SNRI).

7-membered carbocyclic or heterocyclic ring, respectively. Small molecular changes, such as ring flexibility, substituents, or heteroatoms in the tricyclic ring structure, can bring about significant changes in physicochemical, electronegativity (dipole moments), and pharmacodynamic properties (e.g., anticholinergics [antimuscarinic], cholinesterase inhibitors, antihistamine, antipsychotics, and antidepressants). This suggests that the tricyclic structure is not associated with affinity for any particular receptor but, rather, contributes to a range of multiple CNS pharmacodynamic (adverse) effects because of increased lipophilicity. The most common tricyclic ring found in drugs is the near-planar phenothiazine ring common to most of the antipsychotic drugs (Fig. 21.9). The TCAs are classified as such because they contain a 6-7-6 ring arrangement in which the central 7-membered ring is either carbocyclic or heterocyclic, saturated or unsaturated, which is fused to two phenyl rings (Fig. 21.8; also see Fig. 21.15 for NSRIs). The side chain may be attached to any one of the atoms in the central 7-membered ring, but it must be three carbon atoms, either saturated (propyl) or unsaturated (propylidine), and have a terminal amine group (secondary or tertiary). The TCAs differ structurally from the antipsychotic phenothiazines in that the two phenyl (aromatic) rings are connected by a 2-carbon link to form a central 7-membered ring instead of a sulfur bridge.

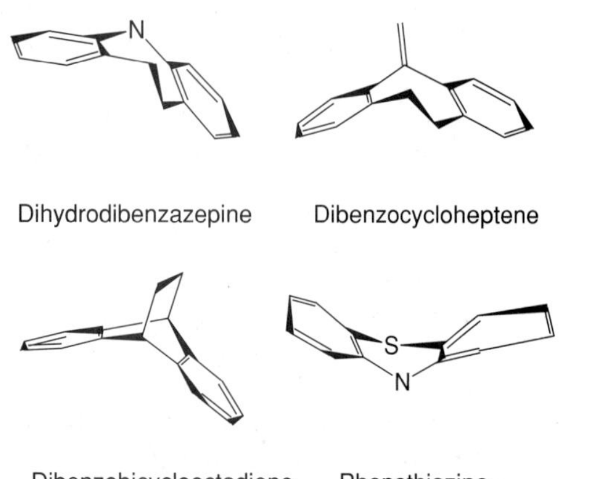

Fig. 21.9. Three-dimensional models of the tricyclic and tetracyclic ring systems.

The TCAs are subdivided into a dihydrodibenzazepine ring (a.k.a., iminodibenzyl, from which the name imipramine is derived), a dibenzocycloheptene ring (e.g., amitriptyline), a dibenzoxepin ring (e.g., doxepin), a dibenzocycloheptriene ring (e.g., protriptyline), or a tetracyclic (bicyclic ring, e.g., maprotiline) derivatives. The tricyclic ring system has little significance regarding selectivity for inhibiting the NET or SERT, but it appears to be important for dopamine transporter inhibition.

The secondary and tertiary amine TCAs differ markedly with regard to their selectivity ratios (Fig. 21.6) and their pharmacodynamic and/or pharmacokinetic properties (Table 21.3; see Table 21.8). Substituting a halogen (i.e., chlorine; clomipramine) or cyano group into the 3-position of the dihydrodibenzazepine ring enhances preferential affinity for SERT. 3-Cyanoimipramine was investigated as a potent, SSRI but was never marketed as an antidepressant agent. It is used as a research probe for studying 5-HT transporters. Branching the propyl side chain with a 2-methyl group (as in trimipramine) significantly reduces the affinity (~100 times) of imipramine for both the SERT and NET. The *Z* (*cis*) geometry for the propylidine group in chiral TCAs appears to be important for transporter selectivity and affinity (e.g., doxepin).

Studies correlating the binding of the TCAs with the SSRIs found that the TCAs and SSRIs bind to different

Table 21.3. Pharmacokinetics of the Selective Norepinephrine Reuptake Inhibitors

Parameters	Desipramine	Nortriptyline	Amoxapine	Protriptyline	Maprotiline	Roboxetine	Atomoxetine
Oral bioavailability (%)	60–70	32–79	ND	77–93	66–75	95	>70%
Protein binding (%)	91	92	92	92	88	>97	>97
Volume of distribution (L/kg)	17–42	14–22	ND	22	15–28	12–28	93–328 (250)
Elimination half-life (hours)	30 (12–30)	30 (18–44)	8 (8–30)	67–89	43 (27–58)	12	4 (3–6) (EM) 17–21 (PM)
Major active metabolites	None	10-E-hydroxy-	8-OH (30 hours) 7-OH (6.5 hours)	None	(60–90 hours)	None	4-hydroxy
Peak plasma concentration (hours)	4–6	7–9	90 min	24–30	8–24	12	1–2
Excretion (%)	Urine Feces	Urine 40 Feces minor	Urine 60 (6 d) Feces 7–18	Urine 50 (16 d) Feces minor	Urine 65 (21 d) Feces 30	Urine ~90% Feces minor	Urine Feces
Plasma half-life (hours)	14–62	18–93	8	54–198	21–52	2–4	4.3
Time to steady-state concentration	ND	ND	ND		7 days	ND	ND

ND, not determined.

sites on the transporter and that the TCAs may act as a modulator of monoamine reuptake by producing conformational changes in the transporter, affecting affinity of the monoamine neurotransmitter (40).

Although similar in a two-dimensional plane to the antipsychotic (neuroleptic) phenothiazines, the ethylene bridge linking the two phenyl rings of the TCAs causes the two phenyl rings to be twisted out of the plane, leading to a less rigid and more conformationally mobile molecular structures than the phenothiazines (Fig. 21.9). The conformational mobility for the TCAs, including ring inversion of the tricyclic ring system, flexing of the CH_2-X bridge (X= CH_2, O, N, or S) in the central 7-membered ring, and flexibility of the alkyl side chain, can result in substantial changes in the overall shape of the molecules, affecting transporter affinity and selectivity, diverse neuroreceptor affinity, and their physicochemical properties. The rate of ring flexibility seems to be correlated with their differences in clinical potency. A dibenzazepine ring system exhibits a greater degree of conformational ring flexing, whereas the dibenzocycloheptene ring system and inserting heteroatoms into the benzylic position reduces the rate of ring flexing in TCAs and their potency (41). Thus, the differences in the pharmacological activity between these TCAs allows selective binding to their respective transporter proteins. The angle between the two aromatic rings ranges from 106 to 110° for the TCAs, and the large lipophilic ring enhances the affinity of TCA to block the CNS muscarinic, H_1-, and α_1-adrenergic receptors and to block sodium channels, contributing to its multiple pharmacodynamic effects.

PHARMACOKINETICS COMMON TO SECONDARY AMINE TCAS. The secondary amine TCAs are rapidly and well absorbed following oral administration. Although the pharmacokinetics are approximately similar within the tertiary and secondary amine groups, the pharmacokinetics are different between the two groups (Table 21.3; also see Table 21.9 for NSRIs). The secondary amine TCAs have relatively high bioavailability. Their primary routes of hepatic metabolism are N-demethylation to inactive primary amine metabolites and aromatic ring hydroxylation (Table 21.2). Despite the fact that serum plasma levels are reached with 1 to 2 days, their onset of antidepressant action typically is at least 2 to 3 weeks or longer. Their volume of distribution is very high, suggesting distribution into the CNS and protein binding. Elimination is primarily as metabolites and their conjugates via renal elimination. Renal and liver function can affect the elimination and metabolism of the parent secondary amine TCA and its metabolites, leading to increased potential for adverse effects, especially in those patients (i.e., the elderly) with renal disease.

MECHANISMS OF ACTION COMMON TO SECONDARY AMINE TCAS. The exact mechanism of action for the secondary TCAs is unclear, but the secondary amine TCAs exhibit substantially more affinity than the SSRIs and the tertiary TCAs for inhibiting the NE transporter. None of the secondary TCAs has significant affinity for the dopamine transporter. Blocking the reuptake of NE increases its concentration in the synaptic cleft and its ability to interact with synaptic NE receptors. When drugs are selective for a transporter, differences in potency become clinically irrelevant, because the plasma concentration can be dose-adjusted to achieve inhibition of the desired transporter without affecting the other transporters. During chronic therapy with the TCAs, adaptive changes at the noradrenergic receptor occur (i.e., downregulation) as a result of neurotransmitter hypersensitivity from low concentrations of NE at the postsynaptic receptor. These changes involve the α_1-adrenergic receptor.

THERAPEUTIC USES COMMON TO ALL TCAS. The efficacy of the secondary and tertiary amine TCAs in the clinical treatment of depressive illness is recommended for various conditions, including major depressive episodes, dysthymia, panic disorder, social phobia, bulimia, narcolepsy, attention-deficit disorder with or without hyperactivity, migraine headache and various other chronic pain syndromes, enuresis in children, and obsessive-compulsive disorder (clomipramine). The TCAs possibly are useful as well for a broader range of depressive conditions described as dysthymia or depressive neurosis and even for prolonged or pathological mourning, agoraphobia without panic attacks, and some of the symptoms (e.g., nightmares) in posttraumatic stress disorder.

ADVERSE EFFECTS COMMON TO ALL TCAS. The family of TCAs has many undesirable side effects and behaves like "five drugs wrapped into one." They not only block the reuptake of NE and 5-HT but also block muscarinic receptors (anticholinergic), α_1-adrenergic receptors, H_1-receptors (antihistamine), and sodium channels. The common side effects and appropriate responses are given in Table 21.4.

DRUG–DRUG INTERACTIONS COMMON TO THE SECONDARY AMINE TCAS. The secondary amine TCAs were once first-line therapy for depression because of their efficacy in a broad range of depressive disorders. Today, however, these agents generally are reserved for second-line treatment because of their narrow therapeutic-to-toxicity ratios and troublesome adverse-effect profiles. Even the better-tolerated nortriptyline is fatal in overdose and may have significant adverse effects at therapeutic dose levels. Most TCAs are metabolized by multiple CYP enzymes and, thus, are likely to be object drugs for many common medications. Because these TCAs have narrow therapeutic indices, any interference with their metabolism can lead to serious adverse reactions resulting from increased plasma concentrations (e.g., arrhythmias, seizures, and confusion). Such reactions are both more common and more likely to be life-threatening in elderly patients because of age-related pharmacokinetic alterations. Therefore, although specific secondary amine TCAs are useful for some conditions (e.g., major depression), coadministration with other drugs should be done cautiously.

Table 21.4. Common Side Effects with Secondary Amine Tricyclic Antidepressants and Recommendations

Side Effects	Treatment Recommendations
Dry mouth	Drink sips of water; chew sugarless gum; clean teeth daily
Constipation	Diet rich in bran cereals, prunes, fruit, and vegetables
Bladder complaints (weak urine stream, emptying difficulty, painful urination)	Consult physician
Sexual problems	Consult physician
Blurred vision	Should pass with time
Dizziness	Rise slowly from the bed or chair
Daytime drowsiness	Do not drive; take medication at bedtime; commonly will pass with time

Concurrent administration of these TCAs and MAOIs is contraindicated, and at least two weeks should elapse between discontinuance of TCA therapy and initiation of MAOI therapy, and vice versa, to allow washout. Coadministration of SNRIs, TCAs, and MAOIs is potentially hazardous and may result in severe adverse effects associated with hypertension.

Because protein binding of secondary amine TCAs is high, displacement interactions with other highly protein-bound drugs with narrow therapeutic indices, although not yet fully evaluated, may be important. Concurrent use of the secondary amine TCAs with anticholinergic or sympathomimetic drugs requires close supervision and careful adjustment of the dosage because of potential additive anticholinergic effects (i.e., spastic colon) and increased blood pressure and heart rate. An additional disadvantage of these TCAs is their toxicity from overdosage, especially in those being treated for depression who may have suicidal thoughts.

In addition, the secondary amine TCAs are inhibitors of sodium channels and, thus, can slow ventricular conduction at therapeutic doses. If the patient overdoses or drug interactions result in increased plasma concentration of the TCA, severe conduction block contributing to cardiotoxicity may result in ventricular arrhythmias. Also, changes in CNS conduction can result in seizures. Patients who are sensitive to one TCA may be sensitive to other TCAs.

The effect of smoking on the activity of CYP1A2 does not appear to have an affect on the plasma concentrations of the secondary TCAs. This is because CYP1A is not involved with the N-dealkylation to their primary amine metabolites.

For common patient information and recommendations, see Table 21.5.

UNIQUE PROPERTIES FOR THE SPECIFIC SECONDARY AMINE TCAS

Desipramine. Desipramine is a dihydrodibenzazepine secondary amine TCA that also is the active metabolite of imipramine (Fig. 21.8). Desipramine appears to have a bioavailability comparable to the other secondary TCAs (Table 21.3). Desipramine is distributed into milk in concentrations similar to those present at steady state in maternal plasma. This drug is metabolized primarily by CYP2D6 to its 2-hydroxy metabolite and by CYP1A2 and CYP2C19 to its N-demethylated (primary amine) metabolite (Table 21.2).

Desipramine exhibits a greater potency and selectivity for the NET than the other secondary TCAs do (Fig. 21.6). Its antidepressant effect results from increases in the level of NE in CNS synapses, and long-term administration

Table 21.5. Patient Information and Recommendations for Secondary Amines Tricyclic Antidepressants (TCAs)

Patient Information	Recommendations
Potential drug–drug and drug–health interactions	Share medical conditions, other medicines (including over-the-counter and herbal medicines), allergies to TCAs, fertility status, or breast-feeding with pharmacist
Seizures, breathing difficulties, fever and sweating, loss of bladder control, muscle stiffness, unusual weakness or tiredness	Discontinue therapy, and consult physician (TCAs may increase risk of seizures)
Course of therapy	Complete full course of therapy
Discontinuance of therapy	Consult physician; abrupt discontinuance not recommended, because it may cause nausea, headache, and malaise
Alcohol use	Avoid alcohol
Central nervous system depressants	May exacerbate TCAs
Drowsiness, dizziness, blurred vision	Avoid driving or performing tasks requiring alertness and coordination
Sun/sunlamp exposure	Avoid prolonged exposure because of photosensitivity

causes a downregulation of α_1-adrenoceptors and desensitization of presynaptic α_2-receptors, equilibrating the noradrenergic system and, thus, correcting the dysregulated output of depressed patients. The SSRIs do not produce this effect. Desipramine also downregulates the NET, but not the 5-SERT. Substantial loss of NE transporter–binding sites takes 15 days to occur and is accompanied by a marked reduction of NET function in vivo. Desipramine has weak effects on 5-HT reuptake.

Nortriptyline. Nortriptyline is a secondary amine dibenzocycloheptene TCA (Fig. 21.8) as well as the major metabolite of amitriptyline. Similar to desipramine, nortriptyline appears in mother's milk and is metabolized by CYP2D6 to the primary amine and by ring hydroxylation to its E-10-hydroxy metabolite (Table 21.2). Approximately one-third of a dose of nortriptyline is excreted in urine as metabolites within 24 hours, and small amounts are excreted in feces via biliary elimination.

Amoxepine. Amoxapine is a dibenzoxazepine TCA (Fig. 21.8) with antidepressant and antipsychotic effects that has shown therapeutic effectiveness in patients with delusional depression. Additionally, it is the N-desmethyl metabolite of the antipsychotic loxapine. Amoxapine differs structurally from the other secondary TCAs in that it has both a nitrogen and an oxygen atom in its 7-membered central ring and a piperazinyl ring rather than a propylamino side chain attached to the central ring.

Amoxapine is a less potent inhibitor of neuronal NE reuptake compared with the other secondary TCAs, with a mechanism of action similar to that of desipramine. Amoxapine shares the toxic potentials of the TCAs, and the usual precautions of TCA administration should be observed. Amoxapine resembles the atypical antipsychotic drugs in its intermediate affinity as an antagonist of dopamine-2 and of 5-HT_2 receptors.

Amoxapine is rapidly and almost completely absorbed from the gastrointestinal (GI) tract. Its pharmacokinetics are shown in Table 21.3. Amoxapine and its 8-hydroxyamoxapine metabolite have been detected in human milk at concentrations below steady-state therapeutic concentrations. Amoxapine has the shortest elimination time (~8 hours) of the secondary TCAs. It is metabolized in the liver principally to 8-hydroxyamoxapine and to 7-hydroxyamoxapine. Both of these metabolites are pharmacologically active and have half-lives of 30 and 6.5 hours, respectively. The hydroxylation of amoxapine is inhibited by ketoconazole, suggesting the involvement of CYP3A4.

Protriptyline. Protriptyline is a dibenzocycloheptriene TCA that differs from the other tricyclics by having an unsaturated ethylene bridge joining the two aromatic rings and a secondary aminopropyl side chain (Fig. 21.8). Protriptyline is completely absorbed from the GI tract and slowly eliminated. Its pharmacokinetics are shown in Table 21.3. Metabolism data are limited for protriptyline, but it is most likely to be metabolized via the same pathways as the other TCAs are (Table 21.2). Very little drug is excreted in the feces via the bile.

Protriptyline exhibits high selectivity for the NE transporter, but with less potency than desipramine. Its mechanism of action is similar to that of desipramine. Minimal effect on 5-HT reuptake has been observed.

Maprotiline. Maprotiline is a secondary amine dibenzobicyclooctadiene (a tetracyclic antidepressant) that differs structurally from the TCAs by having an ethylene bridge in its central ring, resulting in a rigid bicyclo-molecular skeleton (Fig. 21.8).

Maprotiline exhibits the highest affinity and selectivity for the NE transporter (Fig. 21.6). Its antidepressant mechanism of action is similar to that of desipramine, with an onset of action of up to 2 to 3 weeks.

Maprotiline is slowly but completely absorbed from the GI tract, and like the other TCAs, it is metabolized by the polymorphic CYP2D6 and CYP2C19 isoforms in the liver, primarily to pharmacologically active N-desmethylmaprotiline and to maprotiline-N-oxide. Its pharmacokinetics are shown in Table 21.3. Maprotiline is distributed into breast milk at concentrations similar to those found at steady state in maternal blood. The elimination half-life of maprotiline averages 43 hours (60–90 hours for its N-desmethyl metabolite).

Maprotiline shares the toxic potentials of the TCAs, and the usual precautions of TCA administration should be observed. Although most of the TCAs have been reported to induce seizures, it is generally recognized that maprotiline may be associated with a higher incidence of dose-dependent seizures compared with the other secondary TCAs. Maprotiline has been reported to produce sedation in depressed patients and to reduce aggressive behavior in animals. Maprotiline also shares the anticholinergic and cardiovascular effects of the secondary TCAs and may cause electrocardiographic changes, tachycardia, and postural hypotension.

Nontricyclic Secondary Amine Antidepressants

REBOXETINE. Reboxetine is a nontricyclic SNRI in which the propylamine side chain of the TCAs is constrained into a morpholine ring (Fig. 21.8). It is a potent and selective ligand for the NET, with a mechanism of action is similar to that of desipramine. Reboxetine is used for the treatment of major depressive disorders. It is a chiral compound that is marketed as a racemic mixture of *R,R*- and *S,S*-reboxetine. The antidepressant activity for reboxetine appears to reside with the *S,S*-(+)-enantiomer, which has approximately twofold the inhibition potency of the *R,R*-enantiomer (42). It is well tolerated, with different adverse-event profiles, and it appears to be at least as effective as the SSRIs in the treatment of depressive illness. Currently, it is available only in Europe and is under U.S. FDA review. It preferentially inhibits the reuptake of NE (5-HT:NE ratio, 8). Reboxetine is not metabolized by the polymorphic isoforms, CYP2D6 or CYP2C19, and may offer a valuable alternative to the secondary amine TCAs in the treatment of major depression. Reboxetine is likely to become a promising alternative for patients who have failed treatment with or do not tolerate serotonergic antidepressants. Reboxetine has been shown to be effective and well tolerated in the treatment of panic disorder.

Reboxetine's oral bioavailability is greater than 90% for both *R,R*-(−)-reboxetine and *S,S*-(+)-reboxetine, indicating that stereoisomerism has no significant effect on absorption and first-pass metabolism. The pharmacokinetics of reboxetine are linear following multiple oral doses of 12 mg/day (Table 21.3). Food affects the rate but not the extent of absorption. In human liver microsomes, each reboxetine enantiomer was metabolized to one primary metabolite, O-desethylreboxetine, and three minor metabolites, two arising via oxidation of the ethoxy aromatic ring and a third yet-unidentified metabolite (43). The metabolism of both reboxetine enantiomers in humans is mediated principally via CYP3A4 and are a competitive inhibitors of CYP2D6 and CYP3A4. Less than 10% of the unmetabolized drug is cleared renally, with the other 90% being excreted hepatically.

After a single, 4-mg dose, the plasma concentration in the elderly (mean age, 81 years) was twice that of younger subjects, although in both groups, the plasma concentration was similar after 2 hours. The area under the curve (AUC) was nearly four times greater in the elderly than in the younger subjects, and the elimination half-life was twice as long (24 ± 6 vs. 12 ± 3 hours). Renal clearance also was reduced. The increased plasma concentrations of reboxetine observed in elderly subjects supports a reduction of the starting dose to 4 mg/day (in two divided doses) for elderly patients (44). Because of reduced metabolic clearance, reboxetine plasma concentrations also are increased in those patients with hepatic or renal dysfunction. In these populations, reboxetine should be used with caution, and a dosage reduction is indicated. No ethnic differences have been observed with *R,R*-(−)- or *S,S*-(+)-reboxetine.

Drug interactions. Reboxetine seems to be an antidepressant that has negligible interference with the pharmacokinetics of other drugs; thus, fewer drug–drug interactions are expected. It also may be possible to use reboxetine in combination with MAOIs, because it has no inhibitory effect on this enzyme, which would avoid tyramine-induced hypertensive reactions.

Adverse effects. Reboxetine is relatively well tolerated, with insomnia, sweating, constipation, and dry mouth being commonly reported adverse events. Hypotension and urinary hesitancy occur at lower rates than with the TCAs. When compared with the SSRIs, reboxetine is associated with lower rates of nausea, somnolence, and diarrhea.

STRUCTURE–ACTIVITY RELATIONSHIPS FOR THE PHENOXYPHENYLPROPYLAMINES

(±)-Nisoxetine. Nisoxetine (Fig. 21.8) was the initial phenoxyphenylpropylamine synthesized in the Lilly research laboratories during the early 1970s from the rearrangement of an oxygen atom in diphenyhydramine, a diphenylmethoxyethylamine, to a phenoxyphenylpropylamine (Figs. 21.2). Nisoxetine was discovered to be a potent and very selective SNRI, with little affinity for other receptors. It underwent clinical studies as an alternative to Lilly's best-selling antidepressant, nortriptyline, but without the adverse effects associated with the tricyclic secondary amines. It was never marketed, however, because of a greater interest in developing its 4-trifluoromethyl analogue, fluoxetine, an SSRI.

The type and position of the ring substitution plays a critical role in the mechanism of action for these phenoxyphenylpropyamines (see Table 21.6 for structure–activity relationships of the phenoxypropylamines). The unsubstituted molecule is a weak SSRI. However, 2-substitutions into the phenoxy ring (except for the 2-trifluoromethyl) yields compounds with high potency and selectivity for blocking NE reuptake (an SNRI), whereas the 4-substitution results in compounds having potent SSRI activity, with the 4-trifluormethyl group (fluoxetine) being the most potent and selective for SERT (28,29). The substantial changes in transporter selectivity for NET and SERT and the differences in affinity is more likely attributed to the bulky 2-(ortho)-substituted groups, which restricts the flexibility of the aromatic rings, thereby enhancing alignment of the hydrogen-bond acceptor group (the

Table 21.6. Structure Activity Relationships for Phenoxyphenyl-propylamines

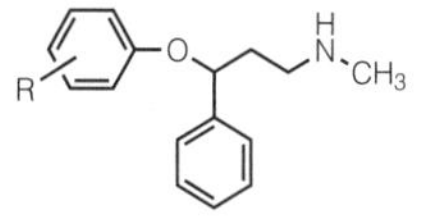

R (drug)	Inhibition of Re-Uptake (Ki nM) (20)	
	5-HT	NE
H	102	200
2-OCH_3 (nisoxetine)	1371	2.4
2-SCH_3 (thionisoxetine)	130	0.2
2-CH_3 (atomoxetine)	390	3.4
2-F	898	5.3
2-I	25	0.4
2-CF_3	1489	4467
3-CF_3	16	1328
4-CF_3 (fluoxetine)	17	2703
4-CF_3 (norfluoxetine, NH_2)	17	2176
4-CH_3	95	570
4-OCH_3	71	1207
4-Cl	142	568
4-F	638	1276

methoxy) with a donor group on the binding site on the NET for NE that is not available for the 5-HT binding site. The *R*-isomer of nisoxetine has 20 times greater affinity than its *S*-isomer for NET. The NET K_i for nisoxetine is 0.8 nM and is 40 times more selective for NET than for SERT. Its tertiary amine is approximately 100 times less effective at inhibiting NET. Increasing the size of the dimethylamino with ethyl or larger alkyl eliminates all activity. The 2- and 4-analogues exhibited weak effects on neuronal uptake of dopamine and lack affinity for other neuroreceptors at therapeutic concentrations. Substituting the 2-methoxy with the isosteric 2-methylthio (thionisoxetine) produced a more potent SNRI (K_i = 0.2 nM for the *R*-enantiomer) and 600 times more selective for NET than for SERT. Thionisoxetine is approximately 10 times more potent than nisoxsetine at inhibiting NET, and unlike nisoxetine, it reduces food consumption in rodents and has been studied for the treatment of obesity and eating disorders. Substitution of the phenoxy group with a naphthyloxy group and the phenyl ring with the isosteric thienyl (thiophene) group results in a drug with dual inhibition of NE and 5-HT reuptake (i.e., duloxetine) (see Fig. 21.18 and the discussion of nonselective inhibitors of NE and 5-HT for a description of duloxetine).

R-(−)-ATOMOXETINE. *R*-(−)-atomoxetine, a 2-methylphenoxyphenylpropylamine, was marketed in 2003 as a "nonstimulant" treatment for attention-deficit hyperactivity disorder (ADHD) in both adults and children and for treatment of adult depression. The 2-methyl substitution (c.f., nisoxetine) (Fig. 21.8) confers selectivity for inhibiting NE reuptake (Table 21.6) (21,22,45). The *R*-enantiomer is 10 times more potent than the *S*-enantiomer as a NET reuptake inhibitor. Atomoxetine has a low propensity for anticholinergic and adverse cardiovascular effects.

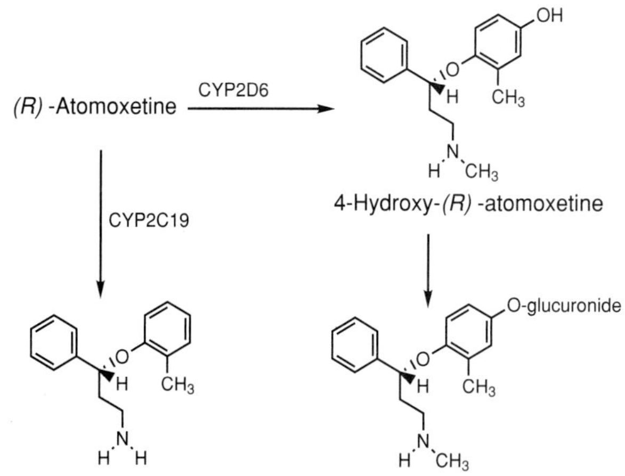

(R)-Atomoxetine —CYP2D6→ 4-Hydroxy-(R)-atomoxetine → O-glucuronide; (R)-Atomoxetine —CYP2C19→ N-desmethyl

Fig. 21.10. Metabolism of *R*-atomoxetine.

Pharmacokinetics. Atomoxetine is well absorbed from the GI tract and cleared primarily by metabolism, with the majority of the dose being excreted into the urine. Atomoxetine is metabolized primarily by CYP2D6 to its major active metabolite, 4-hydroxyatomoxetine, which is eliminated as its glucuronide (Fig. 21.10). Peak plasma concentrations of atomoxetine occur 1 to 2 hours after oral administration. Significant differences are seen in the elimination half-life between normal metabolizers, extensive metabolizers, and poor metabolizers (Table 21.3). Atomoxetine exhibited an elimination half-life of 3 to 6 hours for normal and extensive metabolizers and 17 to 21 hours for poor metabolizers (46). CYP2C19 is the other enzyme primarily responsible for the formation of its minor metabolite N-desmethylatomoxetine (46).

Adverse effects. At therapeutic doses, no serious drug-related adverse effects have been encountered. Adverse effects have included modest increases in diastolic blood pressure and heart rate, anorexia, weight loss, somnolence, dizziness, GI effects (nausea), dry mouth, and skin rash.

Therapeutic uses. Atomoxetine is used as a safe and well-tolerated "nonstimulant" treatment of ADHD in both adults and children and of depression. Among children and adolescents aged 8 to 18 years, atomoxetine was superior to placebo in reducing symptoms of ADHD and in improving social and family functioning symptoms. Oral atomoxetine is promoted as an alternative to conventional ADHD therapy with methylphenidate, dextroamphetamine, and pemoline. It also can be a replacement for bupropion or for TCAs. Onset of action is approximately 7 days.

Selective 5-HT Reuptake Inhibitors (SSRIs)

Serotonin Hypothesis of Depression

5-HT is a major player in depressive illness, and serotonergic pathways are closely related to mood disorders, especially depression (Fig. 21.1) (11,47). Thus, drugs affecting the 5-HT levels in the neural synapse and serotonergic pathways may lead to effective therapy of depression.

5-HT is synthesized from tryptophan, packaged into vesicles, and released into the synaptic cleft following an action potential (see Chapter 14). Once in the synaptic cleft, 5-HT interacts with both the pre- and postsynaptic serotonergic receptors. Evidence implicating multiple abnormalities in serotonergic pathways as a cause of depression include:

1. Low urinary concentrations of 5-HT's major metabolite, 5-hydroxyindoleacetic acid.
2. A low density of brain and platelet 5-HT transporters in depressed individuals.
3. A high density of brain and platelet 5-HT binding sites.
4. A low synaptic concentration of tryptophan, which is used in 5-HT synthesis.

Of these, the low level of SERTs in depressed patients has received the most attention in the development and synthesis of the SSRIs. The precise antidepressant mechanism of action for the SSRIs eludes neuroscientists, but the SSRIs have been shown to alleviate depression and are the most commonly used drugs in the therapy for depression. Claims of decreased adverse effects (adverse drug reactions) and less toxicity in overdose than both the MAOIs and the TCAs, together with increased safety, have led to their extensive use, and several are ranked in the Top 50 prescription drugs dispensed in the United States during the year 2005.

The SSRIs are proven treatments for depression, obsessive-compulsive disorder, and panic disorder and are helpful in a variety of other conditions as well. The most substantial benefit to the SSRIs compared with the TCAs is their reduced adverse-effect profile and the fact that they are better tolerated. Although the SSRIs have become the most commonly prescribed drugs for depression, there are clinical situations in which TCAs may be more appropriate (e.g., melancholic depression). Meaningful differences between the individual SSRIs are largely related to their pharmacokinetics, metabolism to active metabolites, inhibition of CYP isoforms, effect of drug–drug interactions, and the half-life of the individual SSRI.

The SSRIs are expensive, and it has been common to have noncompliant patients (especially elderly) relapse because they cannot afford their medications. Persuading the patient to take his or her medication as prescribed is extremely important for potentially suicidal patients with depression. Because of this, it is exceedingly important that patients receive the lowest effective (and, thereby, the most cost-effective) dose of any drug they are prescribed. Also, the SSRIs have a history of increased risk of suicide for reasons that are not clearly understood.

The Discovery of SSRIs

Although the TCAs, as a group, are effective antidepressants, their adverse-event profile and high potential for toxicity have limited their use. The early antidepressants indicated that 5-HT might play a significant role in depression. Therefore, medicinal chemists set out in search of the ideal SSRI with the goal for developing drugs with:

- High affinity and selectivity for the 5-HT uptake transporter.
- Ability to slow or inhibit the transporter when bound to it.
- Low affinity for the multiple neuroreceptors known to be responsible for many of the adverse effects of the TCAs (e.g., acetylcholine, histamine, and adrenergic receptors).
- No inhibition of the fast sodium channels. which cause the cardiotoxicity problems associated with TCAs.

Initial success occurred with the synthesis of zimeldine, in which the central ring of amitriptyline was opened to form a diphenylpropylidine analogue. *Z*-zimeldine displayed selective inhibition of 5-HT reuptake, with minimal inhibition of NE reuptake. Most importantly, zimeldine was without the adverse-event profile exhibited by the TCAs. Thus, zimeldine became the template for the second-generation SSRIs shown in Figures 21.11 to 21.13.

Mechanisms of Action Common to the SSRIs

The SSRIs preferentially act to inhibit SERT (the reuptake transporter for 5-HT) with minimal or no affinity for NE and dopamine transporters (11). These drugs have a high and selective affinity for SERT (Fig. 21.6) and, therefore, block 5-HT from binding to SERT and being absorbed into presynaptic cells. The excess 5-HT in the synaptic cleft means overactivation of the postsynaptic receptors. Over an extended period of time, this causes downregulation of pre- and postsynaptic receptors, a reduction in the amount of 5-HT produced in the CNS, and a reduction in the number of SERTs expressed. Long-term administration of SSRIs causes downregulation of the SERT, but not the NET. Substantial loss of 5-HT transporter binding sites takes 15 days to occur and is accompanied by a marked reduction of SERT function in vivo. These compensatory responses at receptors and transporters are thought to produce the antidepressant effects of SSRIs. This onset delay may, in part, explain the delayed onset of action of SSRIs in the treatment of depression (48). Similar to the binding of 5-HT, SSRIs likely bind to SERT at the same site as 5-HT does, although it has not been determined conclusively. Although not as selective as the SSRIs, drugs of abuse, such as cocaine, fenfluramine, and 3,4-methylenedioxymethamphetamine ("Ecstasy"), are inhibitors of SERT.

The affinity data for the SSRIs show that the SSRIs, as a group, are very potent and selective inhibitors for SERT compared with their affinity for NE and dopamine reuptake transporters (Fig. 21.6) and are more potent inhibitors of 5-HT reuptake than are the tertiary amine TCAs, with the exception of clomipramine. None of the SSRIs has substantial effect on the NET or dopamine transporter. Of the SSRIs, sertraline exhibits the most potent inhibition of dopamine reuptake transporter, although it is still 100 times less potent in terms of inhibiting the dopamine versus the SERT. Therefore, the plasma concentration of sertraline would have to be increased by as much as 100 times to inhibit the dopamine reuptake transporter. When drugs are this selective for the reuptake transporters, differences in potency become clinically irrelevant, because the plasma concentration can be dose-adjusted to achieve inhibition of the desired transporter without affecting the other transporters. Clomipramine displays less affinity for SERT than citalopram, fluvoxamine, paroxetine, or sertraline does and is more potent than fluoxetine. In terms of the ability to inhibit the NET, the SSRIs are two to three times less potent than the SNRI TCA, desipramine.

Their in vitro potency for selectively inhibiting the 5-HT transporter more or less mirrors their clinical efficacy as SSRIs (11): paroxetine> sertraline> clomipramine> fluoxetine> citralopram> fluvoxamine> imipramine> amitriptyline> roboxetine> venlafaxine = milnacipran> desipramine. Clinically, however, all the SSRIs are equally effective over time, suggesting that these variations in potency do not affect efficacy or adverse effects. The SSRIs have less affinity for α_1, α_2, H_1, and muscarinic receptors, which may explain the adverse-effect profile differences between TCAs and SSRIs.

The results in Table 21.7 show the therapeutic doses that produce approximately 70 to 80% inhibition of the SERT (48). The inhibition of SERT is relevant to the antidepressant efficacy of the SSRIs and suggests that approximately 70 to 80% inhibition of this transporter usually is necessary to produce an antidepressant effect. Higher doses of these drugs do not produce a greater antidepressant response on average (i.e., a flat dose–response curve for antidepressant efficacy) but do increase the incidence and severity of adverse effects mediated by excessive 5-HT reuptake inhibition. Obviously, the results shown in Table 21.7 pertain to the average patient. A patient who has a rapid clearance of the SSRI may need a higher-than-average dose to achieve an effective concentration, whereas a patient who has a slow clearance may do better in terms of the ratio of efficacy to adverse effects on a minimum dose.

The β-adrenergic blocker pindolol blocks the presynapatic 5-HT_{1A} receptors, thereby increasing 5-HT neuronal transmission. The 5-HT_{1A} receptors do not require prolonged exposure (several weeks) to excessive amounts of 5-HT to promote downregulation. This results in augmentation and acceleration of the antidepressant effect of the SSRIs when combined with a 5-HT_{1A} inhibitor. Bordet et al. (49) demonstrated the accelerated antidepressant response of pindolol with paroxetine.

Pharmacokinetics Common to the SSRIs

The SSRIs share a number of pharmacokinetic characteristics (48,50) (Table 21.8). They are well absorbed orally, although the presence of food in the stomach may alter the absorption of some SSRIs. Food, however, does not affect the AUC and does not appear to affect clinical efficacy. The SSRIs are highly lipophilic and are highly plasma protein bound.

Current SSRIs tend to be characterized by high volumes of distribution, which results in relatively long plasma concentration (typically 4–8 hours). The SSRIs display a range of elimination half-life values for the parent drugs, from half-life values of approximately 20 hours for paroxetine and fluvoxamine to 2 days for fluoxetine. Only sertraline and citalopram exhibit linear pharmacokinetics, whereas fluvoxamine, fluoxetine, and paroxetine exhibit nonlinear pharmacokinetics (i.e., changes in plasma concentration are not proportional to dose) as a result of their longer plasma half-lives within the usual therapeutic ranges (Table 21.8). Sertraline stands out as having the best effects on depression among all antidepressants. Fluoxetine and fluvoxamine are least likely to penetrate into breast milk. Thus, the SSRI antidepressants best suited for pharmacokinetic optimization of therapy are the following: sertraline, fluvoxamine, and citalopram. All the SSRIs are extensively metabolized by CYP isoforms to pharmacologically active N-demethylated metabolites, which are then excreted in urine and feces. Except for sertraline, the drugs fluoxetine, paroxe-

Table 21.7. Relationship Between Dose, Plasma Level, Potency, and Serotonin Uptake

SSRI	Dose (mg/day)	Plasma Level	In Vitro Potency (IC50)	Inhibition of SERT
Citalopram	40	85 ng/mL (260 nM)	1.8	60%
Fluoxetine	20	200 ng/mL (300 nM)[a]	3.8	70%
Fluvoxamine	150	100 ng/mL (300 nM)	3.8	70%
Paroxetine	20	40 ng/mL (130 nM)	0.29	80%
Sertraline	50	25 ng/mL (65 nM)	0.19	80%

[a]Plasma level for fluoxetine represents the total of fluoxetine plus norfluoxetine given comparable effects on SERT; parent SSRI alone shown for all others. Also, plasma levels are a total of both enantiomers for citalopram and fluoxetine. Values for the parent drug and for the respective major metabolite are in parentheses.

Table 21.8. Pharmacokinetics of the Selective Serotonin Reuptake Inhibitors

Parameters	(±)-Fluoxetine	(−)-Sertraline	(−)-Paroxetine	E-Fluvoxamine	(±)-Citalopram [(+)-Escitalopram]
Oral bioavailability (%)	70	20–36	50	>50	80 (51–93)
Protein binding (%)	95	96–98	95	77	~56 (70–80)
Volume of distribution (L/kg)	12–18	17 (9–25)	25 (12–28)	15–31	12–16
Elimination half-life (hours)	50	24 (19–37)	22	15–20	36 (27–32) Elderly ~48
Cytochrome P450 major isoform	2D6	3A4	2D6	2D6	2C19, 2D6, and 3A4
Major active metabolites	O-desmethyl-fluoxetine (240 hours) Norfluoxetine (96–364 hours)	N-desmethyl (62–104 hours)	None	None	Desmethylcitalopram (30 hours)
Peak plasma concentration (hours)	6–8	4–8	2–8	3–8	4 (1–6)
Excretion (%)	Urine 25–50	Urine 51–60	Renal ~50%	Urine ~ 40% (24 hrs)	Feces 80–90%
	Feces minor	Feces 24–32	Feces minor	Feces minor	Urine<5%
Plasma half-life (hours)	1–4 days (norfluoxetine 7–15 days)	22–35	24	7–63	36 (23–75)
Time to steady-state concentration (days)	~4 weeks	7–10 d Elderly 2–3 weeks	7–14 d	10 d	7 d

tine, and fluvoxamine are metabolized by polymorphic CYP isoforms, a matter of concern for poor and extensive metabolizers who may need dose adjustments. Citalopram is metabolized almost equally by CYP2C19, CYP2D6, and CYP3A4 (Table 21.7). Peak plasma levels usually are reached in approximately 6 to 8 hours and steady-state plasma levels in approximately 7 to 10 days except for fluoxetine (~4 weeks). The half-lives are variable depending on the specific SSRI and the presence and plasma concentration of an active metabolite, but the half-lives tend to be prolonged. No evidence indicates that serum drug monitoring of SSRIs is a useful strategy to predict response. The SSRIs in general exhibit a flat, dose-independent antidepressant response curve (i.e., the antidepressant activity does not improve with increasing dose, only side effects increase) (50).

Some of the key differences among the SSRIs are the result of differences in their pharmacokinetic properties and metabolism to active metabolites (Table 21.8). Fluoxetine is unique because of its long half-life and the long half-life of its active metabolite norfluoxetine (48,50). Although sertraline also has an active metabolite, it is 10 times less potent than sertraline and probably is not clinically relevant (51). Fluvoxamine and paroxetine have no active metabolites. Because of the differences in half-lives and activities of metabolites, a much longer washout period is necessary when switching from fluoxetine (a long-acting SSRI) to another SSRI or MAOI. These differences can cause considerable therapeutic delays in the treatment of refractory patients.

Adverse Effects Common to the SSRIs

The SSRIs are reported to have fewer side effects than the TCAs, which have strong anticholinergic and cardiotoxic properties (50). Among the SSRIs, there are few differences in adverse effects. The adverse effects observed for the SSRIs include nausea, diarrhea, anxiety, agitation, insomnia, and sexual dysfunction. Fewer patients have discontinued SSRIs than TCAs (amitriptyline and imipramine, and not nortriptyline, desipramine, doxepin, and clomipramine).

Sexual dysfunction is reported in both men and women, such as of decreased libido, anorgasmia, ejaculatory incompetence, ejaculatory retardation, or inability to obtain or maintain an erection. The basic pharmacological similarities among the SSRIs suggest that the effects on sexual function should be similar for each drug and that no one SSRI was more likely to cause the reported sexual adverse effects than another. Moreover, evidence suggests that SSRI-induced sexual dysfunction may be dose-related and may be treated by simply lowering its dose. In patients who cannot have their SSRI dosage reduced, another option is simply to wait and reassess sexual function after several months. If the above measures are ineffective in managing SSRI-induced sexual dysfunction, the next step is to consider an alternative antidepressant without serotonergic activity (e.g., bupropion). Orgasm difficulties and impotence occurred more frequently with paroxetine as compared with sertraline and fluoxetine. The addition of amantadine, cyproheptadine, yohimbine, or sildenafil has been reported to be effective in some patients with SSRI-induced sexual dysfunction.

Drug Interactions Common to the SSRIs

The most serious drug–drug interaction for the SSRIs is their potential to produce the "serotonin syndrome" (i.e., hyperserotonergic effect), which typically develops within hours or days following the addition of another serotonergic agent to a drug regimen that already includes serotonergic-enhancing drugs. Symptoms of the 5-HT syndrome include agitation, diaphoresis, diarrhea, fever, hyperreflexia, incoordination, confusion, myoclonus, shivering, or tremor.

The 5-HT syndrome interaction between MAOIs and SSRIs is the most important drug interaction for the SSRIs, necessitating a washout ranging from 2 to 5 weeks depending on the plasma half-life of the SSRI. These differences in washout times for the SSRIs when switching to an MAOI are key differences between SSRIs and should be remembered if an MAOI is planned as a possible subsequent treatment in the event of SSRI failure. The differences among SSRIs are not important, when a patient is switched from an MAOI to an SSRI. However, in this case, a 10- to 14-day washout for the MAOI is necessary, regardless of which SSRI is used, to allow regeneration of monoamine oxidase. The drug interaction between TCAs and SSRIs is of particular importance because of the potential for the development of toxic TCA concentrations, 5-HT syndrome, and subsequent adverse effects (48,50).

Coadministration of the antihistamine cyproheptadine or other 5-HT antagonists with SSRIs might be expected to result in a pharmacodynamic interaction (i.e., reduced effectiveness for the SSRI). Cyproheptadine acts to block postsynaptic 5-HT. Lack of antidepressant efficacy has been reported when cyproheptadine was given concurrently with fluoxetine and paroxetine.

Clinically, the potency of the SSRIs to inhibit CYP2D6 decreases from paroxetine to fluoxetine to norfluoxetine and then to fluvoxamine, with sertraline and citalopram being metabolized by CYP3A4 and CYP2C19, respectively, explaining the extent of differences in pharmacokinetic interactions between the SSRIs and other CYP2D6 substrates. Fluvoxamine is associated with drug interactions from its inhibition of CYP1A2, CYP2C9, CYP2C19, and CYP3A4 (see Table 10.10 for inhibition drug interactions). Because all the SSRIs are extensively metabolized in the liver, it is possible that other drugs that inhibit or induce hepatic CYP microsomal enzyme systems may alter SSRI plasma concentrations (AUCs) (Table 21.7). The SSRIs may inhibit or interfere with the metabolism of other frequently prescribed drugs that are CYP hepatically metabolized, increasing the potential for drug–drug interactions (Table 21.2; see also Tables 10.5 and 10.6). Although similar drug interactions are possible with other SSRIs, there is considerable variability among the drugs in the extent to which they inhibit CYP2D6. Fluoxetine and paroxetine appear to be more potent in this regard than sertraline. The extent to which this potential interaction may become clinically important depends on the extent of inhibition of CYP2D6 by the SSRI and the therapeutic index of the concurrently administered drug. The drugs for which this potential interaction is of greatest concern are those that are metabolized principally by CYP2D6 and have a narrow therapeutic index. Caution should be exercised whenever concurrent therapy with fluoxetine and other drugs metabolized by CYP2D6 is considered. The clinical significance of these possible interactions with the CYP isoforms is questionable, however, because there is no known correlation between plasma concentration and therapeutic response for any of the SSRIs (50). If an interaction is suspected, the patient's SSRI dosage can be easily adjusted.

The SSRIs are highly protein bound and may affect the pharmacodynamic effect of other protein-bound drugs with narrow therapeutic indices (e.g., warfarin). The changes appear to be clinically significant, however, only for fluoxetine, fluvoxamine, and paroxetine (50). Close monitoring of prothrombin time and international normalized ratio is necessary if these drugs are used together.

The SSRIs have a high toxic to therapeutic ratio and, therefore, are safer than the TCAs or MAOIs in acute overdose. The SSRI overdoses can result in drowsiness, tremor, nausea, and vomiting, including seizures, electrocardiographic changes, and coma. Fatalities are uncommon with pure SSRI overdoses.

Therapeutic Uses Common to the SSRIs

The primary uses for the SSRIs include MMD and bipolar depression (fluoxetine, paroxetine, sertraline, and citalopram), "atypical" depression (i.e., depressed patients with unusual symptoms, e.g., hypersomnia, weight gain, and interpersonal rejection sensitivity; fluoxetine, paroxetine, sertraline, and citalopram), anxiety disorders, panic disorder (sertraline and paroxetine), dysthymia, premenstrual syndrome, postpartum depression, dysphoria, bulimia nervosa (fluoxetine), obesity, borderline personality disorder, obsessive-compulsive disorder (fluvoxamine, fluoxetine, paroxetine, and sertraline), alcoholism, rheumatic pain, and migraine headache. Among the SSRIs, there are more similarities than differences; however, the differences between the SSRIs could be clinically significant.

The SSRIs, such as paroxetine and fluoxetine, need stronger pediatric use warnings because of the possible risks of suicidal thoughts and behavior in some children and teenagers. Such risks may be unrelated to any specific SSRI. Recent clinical trials have concluded that 2 or 3 of every 100 young people treated with antidepressants might be at higher risk of suicidal behavior. Only fluoxetine has been proven to be effective and is approved for the treatment of pediatric depression

Phenoxyphenylalkylamines

(±)-Fluoxetine

Structure–activity relationship. Fluoxetine is a 3-phenoxy-3-phenylpropylamine that exhibits selectivity and high affinity for human SERT and low affinity for NET (Fig. 21.11). It is marketed as a racemic mixture of *R*- and *S*-fluoxetine. Its selectivity for SERT inhibition depends on the position of the substituent in the phenoxy ring (Table

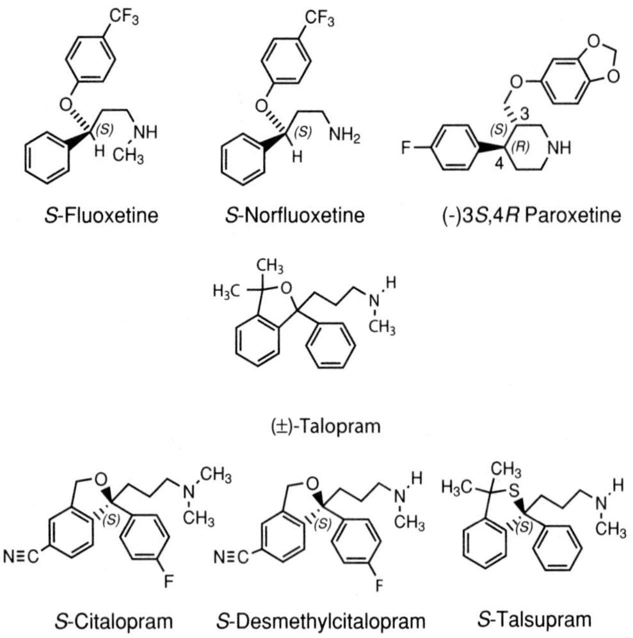

S-Fluoxetine S-Norfluoxetine (-)3S,4R Paroxetine

(±)-Talopram

S-Citalopram S-Desmethylcitalopram S-Talsupram

Fig. 21.11. Phenoxyphenylalkylamine SSRIs.

21.6). Mono-substitution in the 4-(para) position of the phenoxy group (with an electron-withdrawing group, e.g., trifluoromethyl group, as in fluoxetine) results in selective inhibition of 5-HT reuptake. Disubstitution (2,4- or 3,4-substitution) results in loss of SERT selectivity. Constraining fluoxetine into semirigid analogues, such as MDL28618A or a phenylpiperidine (i.e., femoxetine), maintains selectivity for SERT, but both have approximately 10% of the affinity of fluoxetine for SERT (52) (Fig. 21.12). The *trans*-(1S,2S)-MDL 28618A stereoisomer is approximately 10 times more potent than the *cis*-(−)enantiomer (52,53). The *trans*-(3*R*,4*S*)-(+)-enantiomer of femoxetine has approximately 10% the affinity of fluoxetine for SERT (54). N-demethylation of femoxetine to its secondary amine enhances affinity for SERT by 10 times (comparable to fluoxetine). Femoxetine is not only an analogue of fluoxetine and paroxetine but also the (3*R*,4*S*)-diastereomer of a paroxetine analogue.

Mechanism of action. Fluoxetine is a potent and selective inhibitor of 5-HT reuptake, but not of NE or dopamine uptake in the CNS. Its mechanism of action is common to the SSRIs. Fluoxetine does not interact directly with postsynaptic 5-HT receptors and has weak affinity for the other neuroreceptors. Both enantiomers of fluoxetine display similar affinities for human SERT. The NE:5-HT selectivity ratio, however, indicates that the *S*-enantiomer is approximately 100 times more selective for SERT inhibition than the *R*-enantiomer. The *R*-(+)-stereoisomer is approximately eight times more potent an inhibitor of SERT together with a longer duration of action than the *S*-(−)-isomer. However, the *S*-(−)-norfluoxetine metabolite is seven times more potent as an inhibitor of the 5-HT transporter than the *R*-(+)-metabolite, with a selectivity ratio approximately equivalent to that of *S*-fluoxetine (55,56).

PHARMACOKINETICS. The pharmacokinetics of fluoxetine fit the general characteristics of the SSRIs (Table 21.8). Of particular importance is its long half-life contributing to its nonlinear pharmacokinetics. In vitro studies show that fluoxetine and norfluoxetine are potent inhibitors of CYP2D6 and CYP3A4 and less potent inhibitors of CYP2C9, CYP2C19 and CYP1A2. Fluoxetine is metabolized primarily by CYP2D6 N-demethylation to its active metabolite norfluoxetine and, to a lesser extent, O-dealkylation to form the inactive metabolite *p*-trifluoromethylphenol. Following oral administration, fluoxetine and its metabolites are excreted principally in urine, with approximately 73% as unidentified metabolites, 10% as norfluoxetine, 10% as norfluoxetine glucuronide, 5% as fluoxetine N-glucuronide, and 2% as unmetabolized drug.

Both *R*- and *S*-Norfluoxetine were less potent than the corresponding enantiomers of fluoxetine as inhibitors of NE uptake. Inhibition of 5-HT uptake in cerebral cortex persisted for more than 24 hours after administration of *S*-norfluoxetine similarly to fluoxetine. Thus, *S*-norfluoxetine is the active N-demethylated metabolite responsible for the persistently potent and selective inhibition of 5-HT uptake in vivo (55).

The pharmacokinetics of fluoxetine in healthy geriatric individuals do not differ substantially from those in younger adults. Because of its relatively long half-life and nonlinear pharmacokinetics, the possibility of altered pharmacokinetics in geriatric individuals could exist, particularly those with systemic disease and/or in those receiving multiple medications concurrently. The elimination half-lives of fluoxetine and norfluoxetine do not appear to be altered substantially in patients with renal or hepatic impairment.

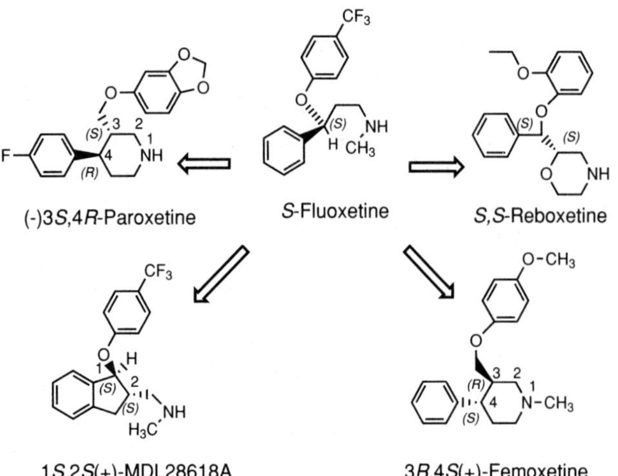

Fig. 21.12. Derivatives of fluoxetine.

Drug interactions. Fluoxetine and its norfluoxetine metabolite, like many other drugs metabolized by CYP2D6, inhibit the activity of CYP2D6 and, potentially, may increase plasma concentrations of concurrently administered drugs that also are metabolized by this enzyme. Fluoxetine may make normal CYP2D6 metabolizers resemble poor metabolizers. Fluoxetine can inhibit its own CYP2D6 metabolism, resulting in higher-than-expected plasma concentrations during upward dose adjustments. Therefore, switching from fluoxetine to another SSRI or other serotonergic antidepressant requires a washout period of at least 5 weeks or a lower-than-recommended initial dose with monitoring for adverse events.

Fluoxetine is highly protein bound and may affect the free plasma concentration and, thus, the pharmacological effect of other highly protein-bound drugs (e.g., warfarin sodium).

Paroxetine

Structure–activity relationship. Paroxetine is a constrained analogue of fluoxetine in which the linear phenylpropylamine group has been folded into a piperidine ring (Fig. 21.11). Paroxetine contains two chiral centers, with the possibility of four stereoisomers. One of these stereoisomers, the (3*S*,4*R*)-(−)-enantiomer is marketed as paroxetine. Paroxetine is a potent and selective inhibitor of SERT and displays high affinity for human SERT and little affinity for NE and dopamine transporters (Fig. 21.6). Converting the secondary amine of the piperidine ring into a tertiary amine with a methyl group reduces affinity for SERT by 100 times. Substituting the 4-fluoro with either a hydrogen or methyl reduces affinity for human SERT by approximately 10 times; replacing the 3,4-methylenedioxy group with a 4-methoxy group in the phenoxy ring also reduces affinity by a factor of 10. Stereochemical factors affect affinity of the paroxetine molecule for SERT. Therefore, substitution into the 2-(ortho) position of either aromatic ring decreases affinity for rat SERT by as much as 10- to 100 times, with the greatest loss occurring in the phenoxy ring. In vitro binding studies suggest that paroxetine is a more selective and potent inhibitor of 5-HT reuptake than fluoxetine. The drug essentially has no effect on NE or dopamine reuptake, nor does it show affinity for other neuroreceptors. Its onset of action is 1 to 4 weeks.

Pharmacokinetics. Paroxetine appears to be slowly but well absorbed from the GI tract following oral administration with an oral bioavailability of approximately 50%, suggesting first-pass metabolism (Table 21.8), reaching peak plasma concentrations in 2 to 8 hours. Food does not substantially affect the absorption of paroxetine. Paroxetine is distributed into breast milk. Approximately 80% of an oral dose of paroxetine is oxidized by CYP2D6 to a catechol intermediate, which is then either O-methylated or O-glucuronidated. These conjugates are then eliminated in the urine.

Paroxetine exhibits a preincubation-dependent increase in inhibitory potency of CYP2D6 consistent with a mechanism-based inhibition of CYP2D6 (56). The inactivation of CYP2D6 occurs via the formation of an o-quinonoid reactive metabolite.

Paroxetine —CYP2D6→

o-Quinoid metabolite of paroxetine

The methylenedioxy has been associated with mechanism-based inactivation of other CYP isoforms (57,58). In contrast, fluoxetine, a potent inhibitor of CYP2D6 activity, did not exhibit a mechanism-based inhibition of CYP2D6. As a result of mechanism-based inhibition, saturation of CYP2D6 at clinical doses appears to account for its nonlinear pharmacokinetics observed with increasing dose and duration of paroxetine treatment, which results in increased plasma concentrations of paroxetine at low doses. The elderly may be more susceptible to changes in doses and, therefore, should be started off at lower doses. Following oral administration, paroxetine and its metabolites are excreted in both urine and feces.

Oral administration of a single dose resulted in unmetabolized paroxetine accounting for 2% and metabolites accounting for 62% of the excretion products. The effect of age on the elimination of paroxetine suggests that hepatic clearance of paroxetine can be reduced, leading to an increase in elimination half-life (e.g., to ~36 hours) and increased plasma concentrations. The metabolites of paroxetine have been shown to possess no more than 2% of the potency of the parent compound as inhibitors of 5-HT reuptake; therefore, they are essentially inactive.

Because paroxetine is a potent mechanism-based inhibitor of CYP2D6, this type of inhibition yields nonlinear and long-term effects on drug pharmacokinetics, because the inactivated or complexed CYP2D6 must be replaced by newly synthesized CYP2D6 protein. Thus, coadministration of paroxetine with CYP2D6-metabolized medications should be closely monitored or, in certain cases, avoided, as should upward dose adjustment of paroxetine itself.

(±)-Citalopram. In trying to create a new antidepressant to inhibit NE reuptake, Lundbeck chemists accidentally synthesized two new compounds (talopram and tasulopram) having the phenylspiro-isobenzofuran nucleus (Fig. 21.11). These compounds were potent SNRIs, but considering that a number of suicide attempts were reported during clinical studies with these compounds, Lundbeck discontinued the studies. Undeterred, the chemists subsequently converted talopram into citalopram by a single 6-cyano substitution. (±)-Citalopram also can be viewed as a constrained analogue of paroxetine (Fig. 21.11). Therapeutic activity for (±)-citalopram resides in the *S*-(+)-isomer. Isosteric substitution of the isobenzofuran ring in citalopram with an isobenzothiophene yields talsupram which changes selectivity from an inhibitor of SERT to a potent inhibitor of NET (Fig. 21.11). Citalopram was marketed in the United States in 1996 as the most selective SSRI and, therefore, as the least likely to cause the adverse effects observed with most of the other antidepressants (Fig. 21.6).

Mechanism of action. Citalopram, primarily through its *S*-enantiomer, blocks 5-HT reuptake, leading to potentiation of serotonergic activity in the CNS. Citalopram exhibits the greatest in vitro selectivity for 5-HT reuptake inhibition compared with the other SSRIs (Fig. 21.6). The drug essentially has no effect on NE or dopamine reuptake, nor does it show affinity for other neuroreceptors.

Pharmacokinetics. The pharmacokinetics of citalopram are shown in Table 21.8. Unlike several of the other SSRIs, citalopram does not undergo first-pass metabolism; it has an oral bioavailability of approximately 80%. The drug is metabolized via hepatic N-demethylation to its major metabolite, N-desmethylcitalopram, almost equally by CYP2C19, CYP2D6, and CYP3A4 (Table 21.7). The major metabolite exhibits approximately 50% of the potency of citalopram as an inhibitor of 5-HT reuptake. Because the metabolite concentration in the plasma is lower than that of citalopram, it should not add significantly to citalopram's antidepressant effects. Citalopram exhibits dose-proportional linear pharmacokinetics in a dosage range of 10 to 60 mg/day; plasma levels increase proportionately with each increasing dose. Approximately 10 to 12% of an oral dose was recovered in the urine as unmetabolized drug. The clearance of orally administered citalopram was reduced by 37 and 17% in patients with hepatic and renal function impairment, respectively.

Citalopram and its desmethyl metabolite are weak inhibitors of the CYP isoforms, suggesting a low potential for drug interactions. Although no relevant in vivo interactions between citalopram and CYP2D6-metabolized medications have been reported, caution is advised when coadministering citalopram with potential object drugs, especially those having narrow therapeutic indices, in elderly patients. Because citalopram is metabolized in parallel by CYP2C19, CYP2D6, and CYP3A4, it would have little inhibitory effect on the metabolism of other drugs metabolized by these isoenzymes. Citalopram is less highly protein bound than the other SSRIs, reducing the potential for drug interactions with protein-bound drugs having narrow therapeutic indices.

ESCITALOPRAM. Escitalopram is the *S*-enantiomer of citalopram that binds with high affinity and selectivity to the human SERT equivalent to (±)-citalopram. It has been reported that nearly all the activity resides in the *S*-enantiomer and that *R*-citalopram actually counteracts the action of the *S*-enantiomer (59,60). Studies show that escitalopram exhibits twice the activity of citalopram and is at least 27 times more potent than the R-enantiomer. The *R*-enantiomer inhibits the *S*-enantiomer at the transporter (59,60). Escitalopram's mechanism of action is common to the SSRIs.

The pharmacokinetics for escitalopram does not exhibit stereoisomer selectivity and, therefore, is similar to that for citalopram (Table 21.7). Likewise, it exhibits linear pharmacokinetics so that plasma levels increase proportionately and predictably with increased doses, and its half-life of 27 to 32 hours is consistent with once-daily dosing. It also has been found that *R*-citalopram is cleared more slowly than the *S*-enantiomer. Therefore, when the drug is used as a racemic mixture (citalopram), the inactive isomer predominates at steady state. This is an added incentive for use of the enantiomerically pure escitalopram. Escitalopram has negligible effects on CYP isoforms, suggesting a low potential for drug–drug interactions. Escitalopram is indicated for patients with major depressive disorder, generalized anxiety disorder, panic disorder, and social anxiety disorder.

Escitalopram is metabolized to *S*-desmethylcitalopram by CYP2C19 (37%), CYP2D6 (28%), and CYP3A4 (35%) and to *S*-didesmethylcitalopram (only by CYP2D6) in human liver microsomes and in expressed cytochromes. Escitalopram and its desmethyl metabolite were negligible inhibitors of CYP1A2, CYP2C9, CYP2C19, CYP2E1, and CYP3A and were weakly inhibited by CYP2D6. *R*-citalopram and its metabolites had properties very similar to those of the corresponding *S*-enantiomers. Because escitalopram is biotransformed by three CYP isoforms in parallel, escitalopram is unlikely to be affected by drug interactions or genetic polymorphisms and is unlikely to cause clinically important drug interactions via CYP inhibition.

Phenylalkylamine

SERTRALINE. Although sertraline appears to differ structurally from the other SSRIs, it is a phenylaminotetralin, in which the diphenylpropylamine nucleus is constrained into a rigid bicyclic ring system (Fig. 21.13). In the early work with the discovery of SSRIs at Pfizer, tametraline was initially synthesized in 1978. Animal studies showed it to be a stimulant and to block NE and DA uptake, a use that Pfizer was not interested in pursuing. Subsequently, one or two chlorine atoms were introduced into tametraline to produce new molecules that were potent inhibitors of 5-HT reuptake in the brain. One of the dichloro compounds was to become known as sertraline.

Sertraline contains two chiral centers, and only the *S,S*-(+)-diastereomer is marketed. The *R,R*-, *R,S*-, and *S,R*-diastereomers are significantly weaker as inhibitors of 5-HT reuptake. Sertraline was marketed in the United States in 1992, emphasizing its pharmacokinetic differences from the other SSRIs.

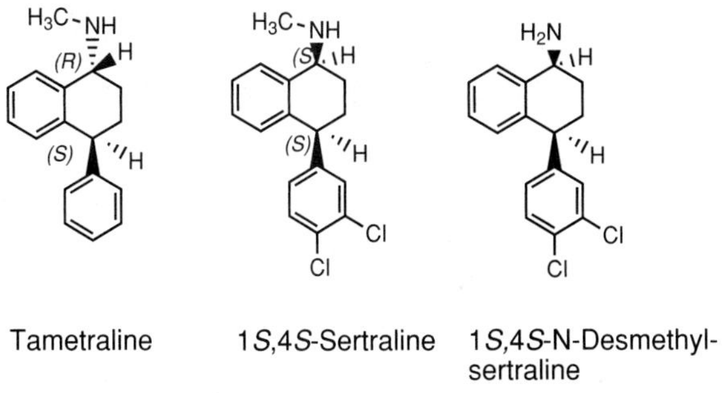

Tametraline 1*S*,4*S*-Sertraline 1*S*,4*S*-N-Desmethyl-sertraline

Fig. 21.13. Phenylalkylamine SSRIs.

Mechanism of Action. Sertraline is a potent and selective inhibitor of the neuronal reuptake 5-HT transporter. In vitro binding studies suggest that sertraline has a substantially higher selectivity for inhibiting 5-HT reuptake than other SSRIs or TCAs, including clomipramine (Fig. 21.6). It has only weak effects on neuronal uptake of NE and dopamine. Its mechanism of action is common to the SSRIs. Sertraline is very selective, lacking affinity for other neuroreceptors at therapeutic concentrations.

Pharmacokinetics. Sertraline appears to be slowly but well absorbed from the GI tract following oral administration. The oral bioavailability of sertraline in humans ranges from 20 to 36% (Table 21.8), suggesting extensive first-pass metabolism to its N-desmethylated metabolite. Food enhances its oral absorption decreasing the time to achieve peak plasma concentrations from approximately 8 to 6 hours. Following multiple dosing, steady-state plasma sertraline concentrations are proportional and linearly related to dose (half-life: single dose, 24 hours; multiple dose, 24 hours). N-desmethylsertraline, sertraline's principal metabolite, exhibits dose-dependent pharmacokinetics. Sertraline and N-desmethylsertraline are distributed into breast milk. Although in elderly patients the elimination half-life is increased to approximately 36 hours, this effect does not appear to be clinically important and does not warrant dosing alterations. Sertraline is primarily metabolized by CYP3A4 N-demethylation in the intestine and liver to its principal metabolite N-desmethylsertraline and several other metabolites. N-desmethylsertraline is approximately 5- to 10 times less potent as an inhibitor of 5-HT reuptake than sertraline. Sertraline and N-desmethylsertraline undergo further metabolism via oxidative deamination and ring hydroxylation and glucuronide conjugation. N-desmethylsertraline has an elimination half-life approximately 2.5 times that of sertraline. Following oral administration, sertraline and its conjugated metabolites are excreted in both urine and feces, and unmetabolized sertraline accounts for less than 5% of oral dose. Plasma clearance of sertraline was approximately 40% lower in geriatric patients. The elimination half-life of sertraline in patients with hepatic disease was prolonged to a mean of 52 hours, compared with 22 hours in individuals without hepatic disease.

Drug Interactions. Sertraline is not a potent inhibitor of CYP3A4, and because CYP2D6 metabolism is a minor pathway for sertraline, drug–drug interactions with these isoforms is unlikely to be of clinical importance. Sertraline is metabolized by more than one CYP isoform in parallel; therefore, drug interactions or genetic polymorphisms are unlikely to cause clinically significant drug interaction via CYP isoform inhibition. Caution is advised, however, when coadministering sertraline with potential object drugs, especially those with narrow therapeutic indices in elderly patients. For example, sertraline has been shown to reduce the clearance of desipramine and imipramine as a result of CYP2D6 inhibition.

Because sertraline is highly protein bound, patients receiving it concurrently with any highly protein-bound drug should be observed for potential adverse effects associated with combined therapy.

Additional SSRIs

FLUVOXAMINE. Fluvoxamine is a nontricyclic SERT inhibitor that is structurally unique among the SSRIs by being the (*E*)-isomer of a 2-aminoethyl oxime ether of an aralkylketone (Fig. 21.14). The C=N double bond is isosteric with the propylidene group in amitriptyline and, thus, imparts geometric *E* or *Z* stereoisomerism to fluvoxamine. The oxime ether is found in a previously marketed analogue of amitriptyline called noxiptilin (1966 by Bayer AG [Germany]). Thus, fluvoxamine may be considered to be an open-chain analogue of the tricyclic noxipitilin. The 4-trifluoromethyl group or other electronegative group is essential for SERT affinity and selectivity. The C=N double bond also enhances the susceptibility of fluvoxamine to photoisomerization by ultraviolet (UV)-B light (290–320 nm). When fluvoxamine solutions were exposed to UV-B light, photoisomerization to the pharmacologically inactive *Z*-isomer occurred. Thus, fluvoxamine solutions should be protected from sunlight to prevent loss of antidepressant efficacy. No studies have been reported regarding its solid-state stability to UV-B light.

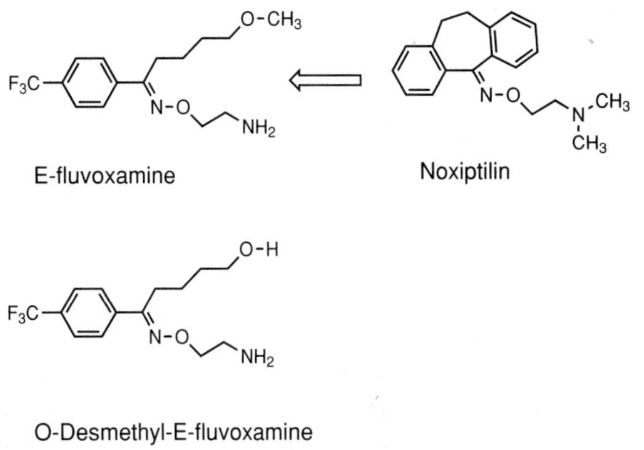

E-fluvoxamine Noxiptilin

O-Desmethyl-E-fluvoxamine

Fig. 21.14. Miscellaneous SSRIs.

Mechanism of action. Fluvoxamine is a highly selective inhibitor of 5-HT reuptake at the presynaptic membrane. Potency data from in vitro affinity studies suggest that fluvoxamine is less potent than the other SSRIs (e.g., paroxetine, sertraline, and citalopram). Its mechanism of action is similar to that of the other SSRIs. Fluvoxamine appears to have little or no effect on the reuptake of NE or dopamine. In vitro studies have demonstrated that fluvoxamine possesses virtually no affinity for other neuroreceptors. Its onset of action is similar to the other SSRIs (2–4 weeks).

Pharmacokinetics. Fluvoxamine is well absorbed, with a bioavailability of approximately 50%, probably because of first-pass metabolism (Table 21.8). At steady-state doses, fluvoxamine demonstrates nonlinear pharmacokinetics over a dosage range of 100 to 300 mg/day, which results in higher plasma concentrations at higher doses than would be predicted by lower-dose kinetics (single dose, 15 hours; multiple dosing, 22 hours). Food does not significantly affect oral bioavailability. The mean apparent volume of distribution for fluvoxamine reflects its lipophilic nature, extensive tissue distribution, and protein binding. Fluvoxamine is distributed into breast milk. Fluvoxamine is preferentially metabolized by CYP2D6 in the liver by O-demethylation to its alcohol metabolite, which subsequently is oxidized to a carboxylic acid. Oxidative deamination and nine other metabolites have been identified, none of which shows significant pharmacological activity.

Adverse effects. The adverse effects for fluvoxamine include symptoms of drowsiness, nausea or vomiting, abdominal pain, tremors, sinus bradycardia, and mild anticholinergic symptoms. Toxic doses could produce seizures and severe bradycardia.

Drug interactions. In vitro studies have shown fluvoxamine to be a potent inhibitor of CYP1A2, to inhibit CYP3A4 and CYP2C19, and to weakly inhibit CYP2D6. The bioavailability of fluvoxamine is significantly decreased in smokers compared with nonsmokers, possibly because of induction of CYP1A metabolism of fluvoxamine. Therefore, interactions with drugs that inhibit CYP1A2 also should be considered (e.g., theophylline and caffeine).

Therapeutic uses. Fluvoxamine is approved for use in obsessive-compulsive disorders.

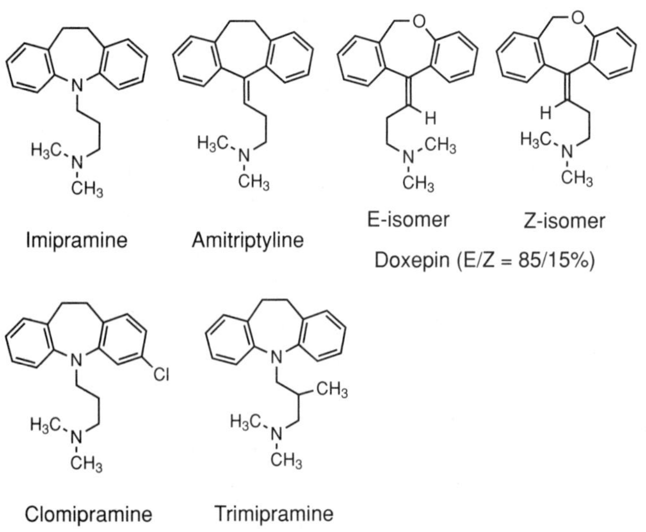

Norepinephrine and Serotonin Reuptake Inhibitors (NSRI)

The NSRI antidepressant drugs in this class block both the NET and SERT (i.e., they combine the mechanisms of action for both the SSRIs and SNRIs), exhibiting dual affinity for NET and SERT (low NE:5-HT potency ratio). These dual inhibitors, as a group, do not show a significant separation in selectivity for the NET and SERT reuptake transporter. Historically, the tertiary amine TCAs displayed dual inhibition of 5-HT and NE presynaptic reuptake, but they also bind to other types of neuroreceptors, which is responsible for their narrow therapeutic window and adverse effects. Clinical studies suggest that dual-acting inhibitors of 5-HT and NE reuptake may be more beneficial than selective inhibitors in managing depression. This has given impetus to the search for nontricyclic NSRIs and has lead to a second group of NSRIs, such as venlafaxine and duloxetine.

Imipramine, Amitriptyline, Doxepin (E/Z = 85/15%) (E-isomer, Z-isomer), Clomipramine, Trimipramine

Fig. 21.15. Tricyclic nonselective reuptake inhibitors.

Tricyclic Tertiary Amine Antidepressants

The TCAs in this class belong to the tertiary amine TCAs (Fig. 21.15). The relatively low bioavailability for the tertiary amine TCAs suggests first-pass metabolism (N-demethylation) to their secondary amine active metabolites (nor or desmethyl metabolites) and aromatic ring hydroxylation (Table 21.2). Despite the fact that steady-state serum plasma levels are reached within 1 to 2 days, their onset of antidepressant action typically is at least 2 to 3 weeks or longer. Their volume of distribution is very high, suggesting distribution into the CNS and protein binding. Excretion is primarily as metabolites via renal elimination. Renal and liver function can affect the elimination and metabolism of the parent TCA and its metabolites, leading to increased potential for adverse effects, especially in those patients (i.e., elderly) with renal disease.

Meaningful differences between the tertiary TCAs is largely related to their pharmacokinetics, metabolism to active metabolites, inhibition of CYP isoforms, potential for drug-drug interactions, and half-life of the tertiary TCA.

MECHANISMS OF ACTION COMMON TO THE TERTIARY AMINE TCAs. The exact mechanism of action for the tertiary TCAs is unclear, but it is known that the parent tertiary amine TCA exhibits dual inhibition of the NET and

SERT. The result is an increase in both NE and 5-HT concentrations in the synaptic cleft. The in vivo antidepressant activity for these TCAs is more complex, however, because of the formation of secondary amine TCA metabolites, which in many cases annuls the 5-HT affinity of the parent TCA, leading to NE transport selectivity. The plasma concentrations for the secondary amine metabolites usually are higher than that of their parent tertiary amine TCA because of rapid N-demethylation metabolism. Note that none of the tertiary amine TCAs have any significant affinity for the DA transporter. During chronic therapy with the tertiary amine TCAs, downregulation of the noradrenergic and serotonergic receptors occurs, which is a result of neurotransmitter hypersensitivity caused by the continued high concentrations of NE and 5-HT at the postsynaptic receptor. The tertiary TCAs are less potent inhibitors than the SSRIs for SERT.

THERAPEUTIC USES COMMON TO TRICYCLIC TERTIARY ANTIDEPRESSANTS. For the most part, the therapeutic uses for the tertiary amine TCAs are very similar as a group, but these TCAs may be used in different cases of depression because of their variability in their dual mechanism of action as SNRIs and SSRIs. Their efficacy in treating depression suggests that mixed inhibition of NET and SERT influence depression by parallel and independent pathways. The tertiary TCAs may offer an option in the treatment of major depression for patients who have failed treatment with or who do not tolerate SNRIs or SSRIs.

ADVERSE EFFECTS COMMON TO TERTIARY TCAS. Because of their potent and multiple pharmacodynamic effects at histamine H_1, muscarinic, and α_1-adrenergic receptors, the tertiary TCAs exhibit greater anticholinergic, antihistaminic, and α_1-antiadrenergic adverse effects than the secondary TCAs do. Increased cardiotoxicity or frequency of seizures is higher for the tertiary TCAs than for the secondary TCAs, because they are potent inhibitors of sodium channels, leading to changes in nerve conduction. Cardiotoxicity can occur at plasma concentrations approximately 5- to 10 times higher than therapeutic blood levels. These concentrations can occur in individuals who take an overdose of the TCA or who are slow metabolizers and develop higher plasma concentrations on what usually are therapeutic doses.

DRUG–DRUG INTERACTIONS COMMON TO TERTIARY TCAS. For the most part, drug–drug interactions for the tertiary amine TCAs are very similar to those for the secondary amine TCAs. These reactions, however, may be more pronounced.

The concurrent use of tertiary amine TCAs with SSRIs and other serotonergic drugs may result in 5-HT syndrome (see the discussion of drug interactions of SSRIs). Coadministration of a tertiary amine TCA with an MAOI is potentially hazardous and may result in severe adverse effects associated with 5-HT syndrome.

Because protein binding of the tertiary amine TCAs are high, displacement interactions with other highly protein-bound drugs and drugs with narrow therapeutic indices, although not fully evaluated, may be important. Concurrent use of tertiary amine TCAs with anticholinergic drugs requires close supervision and careful adjustment of the dosage because of potential additive anticholinergic effects (i.e., spastic colon). An additional disadvantage of TCAs is their toxicity from overdosage, especially in those who are being treated for depression having suicidal thoughts.

The plasma concentrations of tertiary amine TCAs usually are lower, and plasma concentrations of their secondary amine metabolites higher, as a result of CYP1A induction.

PATIENT INFORMATION COMMON TO THE TERTIARY AMINE TCAS. Common patient information and recommendations are similar to those given to patients who are prescribed secondary TCAs (Table 21.5).

UNIQUE PROPERTIES OF SPECIFIC TERTIARY AMINE TCAS

Amitriptyline. Amitriptyline is a tertiary amine dibenzocycloheptadiene TCA with a propylidene side chain extending from the central carbocyclic ring (Fig. 21.15). The diarylpropylideneamine moiety for amitriptyline makes it sensitive to photo-oxidation; therefore, its hydrochloride solutions should be protected from light to avoid ketone formation and precipitation.

Pharmacokinetics. Amitriptyline is rapidly absorbed from the GI tract and from parenteral sites. Its pharmacokinetics are shown in Table 21.9. Amitriptyline and its active metabolite, nortriptyline, are distributed into breast milk. Amitriptyline is primarily (65%) metabolized by N-demethylation by CYP2D6 to nortriptyline and hydroxylation to its *E*-10-hydroxy metabolite. Nortriptyline is pharmacologically active as a secondary amine TCA. Amitriptyline shows approximately equal affinity for 5-HT and NE transporters.

Imipramine. Imipramine is a 10,11-dihydrodibenzazepine tertiary amine TCA (Fig. 21.15) that is marketed as hydrochloride and pamoate salts, both of which are administered orally. Although the hydrochloride salt may be administered in divided daily doses, imipramine's long duration of action suggests that the entire oral daily dose may be administered at one time. On the other hand, imipramine pamoate usually is administered as a single daily oral dose. Imipramine preferentially inhibits 5-HT reuptake over NE; however, the formation of its N-desmethyl metabolite removes whatever 5-HT activity imipramine had, with the net result of enhanced noradrenergic activity from inhibition of NE reuptake at the presynaptic neuronal membrane. Imipramine shares the pharmacological and adverse-effect profile of the other tertiary TCAs.

Table 21.9. Pharmacokinetics of the Tricyclic Nonselective Reuptake Inhibitors (NSRIs)

Parameters	Amitripytline	Clomipramine	Doxepin	Imipramine	Trimipramine
Oral bioavailability (%)	31–61	~50	13–45	29–77	44
Protein binding (%)	95	96–98	ND	89–95	95
Volume of distribution (L/kg)	12–18	17 (9–25)	12–28	23 (15–31)	~31
Elimination half-life (hours)	10–26	32 (19–37)	11–16	11–25	9–11
Cytochrome P450 major isoform	2D6	2D6	2D6 and 2C19	2D6 and 2C19	2D6 and 2C19
Major active metabolites	Nortriptyline	Desclomipramine (54–77 hours)	Nordoxepin (~30 hours)	Desipramine	Desmethyltrim-ipramine (30 hours)
Peak plasma concentration (hours)	2–12	2–6 (4.7)	<2	1–2	<2
Excretion (%)	Urine 25–50	Urine 51–60 (14 days)	Renal ~50	Urine ~40 (24 hours)	Feces 80–90
	Feces minor	Feces 24–32	Feces minor	Feces minor	Urine<5
Plasma half-life (hours)	21 (10–46)	34 (22–84)	8–24	18 (9–24)	9
Time to steady-state concentration	—	1–2 weeks	ND	ND	ND

ND = not determind.

The pharmacokinetics for imipramine are shown in Table 21.9. Imipramine is completely absorbed from the GI tract. Imipramine is primarily metabolized by CYP2D6 to its 2- and 10-hydroxylated metabolites and N-demethylated via CYP2C19 and CYP1A2 to desipramine, its N-monodemethylated metabolite, an SNRI.

Therapeutic uses. Besides being used in the clinical treatment of depression, imipramine also has been used for the treatment of functional enuresis in children who are at least 6 years of age (25 mg daily administered 1 hour before bedtime, not to exceed 2.5 mg/kg daily).

Doxepin. Doxepin is a tertiary amine dibenzoxepine derivative with an oxygen replacing one of the ethylene carbons in the bridge. The oxygen introduces asymmetry into the tricyclic ring system, resulting in the formation of two geometric isomers: *E* (*trans*) and *Z* (*cis*) (Fig. 21.15). No commercial attempt was made to separate the isomers; thus, doxepin is administered as a 85:15 mixture of *E*- and *Z*-stereoisomers, with the *Z*-isomer being the more active stereoisomer for inhibiting the reuptake of 5-HT (61). The E-isomer, on the other hand, inhibits the reuptake of NE. Unless otherwise specified, the reported in vitro and in vivo studies with dioxepin were done with the 85:15 geometric mixture.

Mechanism of action. Because doxepin is administered as an 85:15 mixture of geometric isomers, its mechanism of action and antidepressant properties reflects this ratio. Therefore, dioxepin's selectivity for inhibiting presynaptic NE reuptake is most likely caused by the 85% presence of the *E*-isomer in the geometric mixture. Its antidepressant activity is similar to amitriptyline. Data suggest NE reuptake inhibitory potency comparable to imipramine and clomipramine; the fact that doxepin is an 85:15 mixture of *E*- and *Z*-geometric isomers clouds its true efficacy for SERT or NET. The formation of N-desmethyldoxepin results in inhibition of NE reuptake with enhanced noradrenergic activity. As a result of these mixed effects on the 5-HT and NE transporters, doxepin shares the pharmacological and adverse-effect profile of the other TCAs.

The pharmacokinetics for oral doxepin are described in Table 21.9. After oral dosing, no significant difference was found between the bioavailability of the *E*- and *Z*-isomers. The plasma concentrations of the doxepin isomers remained roughly those of the administered drug, whereas the ratio for the metabolites, *E*-N-desmethyldoxepin and *Z*-N-desmethyldoxepin, were approximately 1:1 (61,62). This similarity in ratios of metabolites is attributed to *E*-doxepine being primarily metabolized in parallel by CYP2D6 and CYP2C19, whereas *Z*-doxepine is primarily metabolized only by CYP2C19 and not at all by CYP2D6 (Table 21.2) (61). Its *Z*-N-demethylated metabolite is pharmacologically more active than its *E*-metabolite as an inhibitor of 5-HT and NE reuptake (61). Both isomers of doxepin showed large volumes of distribution and relatively short half-lives in plasma, suggestive of extensive distribution and/or tissue binding. Renal clearances did not differ for the isomers.

Clomipramine. Clomipramine is considered to be the most powerful antidepressant ever made. This dihydrodibenzazepine TCA, with actions on both the NE and 5-HT transporters, was the last of the major TCAs to come to market. Initially, the U.S. FDA regarded it as another "me-too" drug, and accordingly, they did not license it. Subsequently, however, it was licensed for the treatment of obsessive-compulsive disorders. Clomipramine differs from imipramine only by the addition of a 3-chloro group (Fig. 21.15).

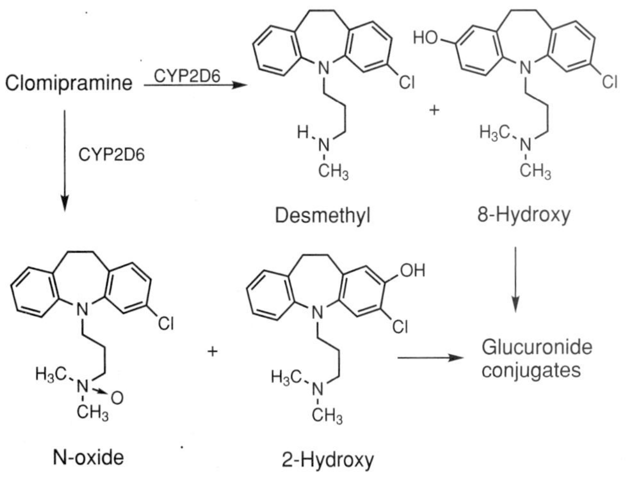

Mechanism of Action. Clomipramine is different from the other TCAs, exhibiting preferential selectivity for inhibiting the reuptake of 5-HT at the presynaptic neuronal membrane. Its antidepressant mechanism of action as an inhibitor of the 5-HT transporter is reduced in vivo, however, because of the formation of its active metabolite, N-desmethylclomipramine, which inhibits the reuptake of NE. As a result of its common structure with the other TCAs, clomipramine shares the pharmacological and adverse-effect profile of the other TCAs.

The efficacy of clomipramine relative to the other TCAs in the treatment of obsessive-compulsive disorder may be related to its potency in blocking 5-HT reuptake at the presynaptic neuronal membrane, suggesting a dysregulation of 5-HT for the pathogenesis of obsessive-compulsive disorder. Clomipramine appears to decrease the turnover of 5-HT in the CNS, probably because of a decrease in the release and/or synthesis of 5-HT.

Although in vitro studies suggest that clomipramine is approximately four times more potent than fluoxetine as a 5-HT reuptake inhibitor, in vivo studies suggest the opposite. This difference has been attributed to the relatively long elimination half-lives for fluoxetine and its principal serotonergic metabolite norfluoxetine. In addition, metabolism of clomipramine to its N-desmethyl secondary amine metabolite decreases the potency and selectivity of 5-HT-reuptake inhibition of clomipramine, but not fluoxetine.

Pharmacokinetics. Clomipramine appears to be well absorbed from the GI tract following oral administration, with an oral bioavailability of approximately 50%, suggesting some first-pass metabolism (Table 21.9). Food does not appear to substantially affect its bioavailability. Clomipramine and its active metabolite, N-desmethylclomipramine, exhibit nonlinear pharmacokinetics at 25 to 150 mg daily. At dosages exceeding 150 mg daily, their elimination half-lives may be considerably prolonged, allowing plasma concentrations of both to accumulate, which may increase the incidence of plasma concentration-dependent adverse effects, particularly seizures. Because of the relatively long elimination half-lives of clomipramine and N-desmethylclomipramine, their steady-state plasma concentrations generally are achieved within approximately 1 to 2 weeks. Plasma concentrations of N-desmethylclomipramine generally are greater than those for chlomipramine at steady-state conditions. Clomipramine crosses the placenta and is distributed into breast milk.

Clomipramine is primarily metabolized by CYP2D6 N-dealkylation to its pharmacologically active metabolite, the 2- and 8-hydroxylated metabolites and their glucuronides, and clomipramine N-oxide (Fig. 21.16). N-dealkylation also involves CYP3A4, CYP2C19, CYP2C9, and CYP1A2. Like all the other secondary amine TCAs, N-desmethylclomipramine is significantly more potent as an inhibitor of NE reuptake than clomipramine is. Although N-desmethylclomipramine is pharmacologically active, its efficacy in obsessive-compulsive disorder is not known. 8-Hydroxyclomipramine and 8-hydroxydesmethylclomipramine also are pharmacologically active, but their clinical importance remains unknown. The hydroxylation and N-demethylation of clomipramine highlight CYP2D6 polymorphism in healthy adults who were phenotyped as either extensive metabolizers or poor metabolizers of clomipramine. Interindividual variation in plasma concentrations may be caused by genetic differences in the metabolism of the drug. In addition, CYP1A2 ring hydroxylates clomipramine. Less than 1% of an oral dose of clomipramine was excreted unmetabolized into the urine, with 8-hydroxyclomipramine glucuronide as the principal metabolite found in the urine. The effects of renal clearance suggest that clomipramine and desmethylclomipramine should be decreased in patients with renal impairment.

Fig. 21.16. Metabolism of clomipramine.

Pharmacogenetic differences in the metabolism of clomipramine after a single oral dose are apparent as increased plasma clomipramine concentrations in Indian and Pakistani patients compared with Caucasians. In Japanese patients, substantial interindividual variation in demethylation and hydroxylation of clomipramine was observed, although the prevalence of poor demethylators and poor hydroxylators of clomipramine has been estimated to be less than 1%.

If inhibition of SERT is critical to the desired clinical effect for clomipramine, then a patient may fail to respond, because he or she develops higher levels of N-desmethylclomipramine as opposed to the parent drug. On the other hand, if a patient who had responded well and was stabilized to a dose of clomipramine, the drug might lose efficacy if exposed to an environmental agent that is capable of inducing CYP1A or CYP3A4.

Adverse effects. Male patients taking clomipramine should be informed of sexual dysfunction as a side effect associated with antidepressants having significant serotonergic activity. Sexual dysfunction in men appears as ejaculatory incompetence, ejaculatory retardation, decreased libido, or inability to obtain or maintain an erection. Sexual dysfunction is dose-related and may be treated by simply lowering the drug dose.

Trimipramine. Trimipramine also is a dihydrodibenzazepine TCA that differs structurally from imipramine in that the 5-propyl side chain is branched by a methyl group creating a chiral center (Fig. 21.15). Trimipramine is marketed as a racemic mixture. No data are available regarding the activity of the enantiomers. Apparently, branching the propyl side chain reduces affinity by 100 times for both 5-HT and NE transporters, but the selectivity ratio favors the 5-HT transporter. Although trimipramine has the weakest binding affinity for the monoamine transporters, it shares the pharmacological and toxicity actions of the other TCAs and is used primarily in the treatment of depression.

The pharmacokinetics for trimipramine are shown in Table 21.9. Trimipramine is rapidly absorbed. Trimipramine demonstrates stereoselectivity in its metabolism to its three major metabolites. (−)-Trimipramine is primarily metabolized via CY2D6 hydroxylation to 2-hydroxytrimipramine, whereas (+)-trimipramine is preferentially metabolized by CYP2C19 N-demethylation to desmethyltrimipramine. Desmethyltrimipramine is further hydroxylated to 2-hydroxydesmethyltrimipramine. (−)-Trimipramine is metabolized by CYP3A4/5 to an unknown metabolite (63,64). Most of the oral dose is excreted in urine in 72 hours, primarily as N-demethylated or hydroxylated and conjugated metabolites. The pharmacokinetics of trimipramine in geriatric individuals (≥65 years of age) do not differ substantially from those in younger adults.

Trimipramine is one of the antidepressants with the most pronounced differences in pharmacokinetics caused by the CYP2D6 genetic polymorphism (63,64). Its bioavailability and systemic clearance depended significantly on the CYP2D6 isoform with a linear dose relationship. Its mean bioavailability was 44% in individuals without CYP2D6 (poor metabolizers) but 16 and 12% in those individuals with two and three active genes of CYP2D6 (fast and ultrafast metabolizers), respectively. Consequently, the mean total clearances of the oral dose were 27, 151, and 253 L/hour in poor, extensive, and ultrarapid metabolizers, respectively. The 44% bioavailability combined with low systemic clearance of trimipramine in poor metabolizers of CYP2D6 substrates results in a very high exposure to trimipramine with the risk of adverse drug reactions. On the other hand, the presystemic elimination may result in subtherapeutic drug concentrations in carriers of CYP2D6 gene duplications with a high risk of poor therapeutic response (63,64).

OTHER TRICYCLIC NSRIs. Figure 21.17 shows two tricyclic serotonin/NE reuptake inhibitors. One is an analogue of imipramine, and the second is an isostere of doxepin.

Dothiepin. Dothiepin (Dosulepin) is the thio isostere of doxepin and is marketed in Europe as its single E-geometric isomer (Fig. 21.17), in contrast to the active Z-geometric isomer for doxepin. Its antidepressant activity is mediated by inhibition of both the NET and SERT, with preferential affinity for SERT (65). It exhibits greater overall in vitro affinity for NET and SERT than its oxygen isostere doxepin, consistent with its greater potency. Its overall therapeutic efficacy is similar to that of amitriptyline.

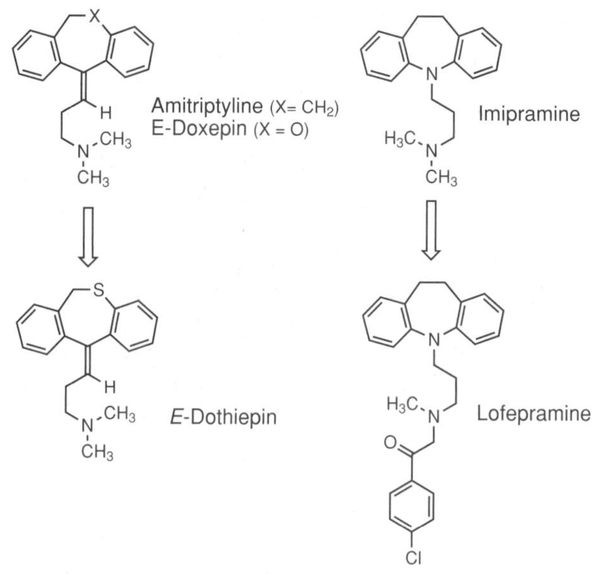

Fig. 21.17. Future tricyclic NSRIs.

Although dothiepin is readily absorbed from the GI tract, it is extensively first-pass metabolized by *S*-oxidation in the liver to its primary active metabolite, dothiepin S-oxide, and by N-demethylation to its minor metabolite, desmethyldothiepin (northiaden) (65). Dothiepin is excreted in the urine, mainly in the form of its metabolites; small amounts of the drug also are excreted in the feces and distributed into breast milk.

The incidence of anticholinergic side effects is less among patients treated with dothiepin than with amitriptyline and without cardiotoxicity at therapeutic doses. The sedative/anxiolytic activity of dothiepin is similar to that of amitriptyline. Dothiepin is an effective treatment for patients with depressive symptoms of varying severity and coexisting anxiety (65).

Lofepramine. Lofepramine differs from imipramine by the attachment of a p-chlorophenacyl moiety to the N-aminopropyl side chain (Fig. 21.17). This change confers enhanced lipophilicity and the potential of more rapid distribution into the CNS with greater in vitro affinity and selectivity for NET. Its mechanism of antidepressant action is attributed to its rapid metabolism to the secondary amine metabolite, desipramine, which selectively inhibits the neuronal uptake of NE (66).

Lofepramine has an oral bioavailability of less than 10% as a result of the extensive first-pass metabolism. Most of a dose of lofepramine is excreted via the urine as metabolites, with a mean elimination half-life of approximately 2 hours. The adverse effects of lofepramine are similar to the secondary TCAs. Lofepramine displays reversible hepatotoxicity (jaundice and hepatitis), usually within 8 weeks of initiation of therapy.

Oral lofepramine is effective in the treatment of various types of depression and is similar in efficacy to imipramine and amitriptyline while inducing fewer adverse effects. This suggests its potential use in patients who are unable to tolerate other antidepressants.

Nontricyclic Serotonin and Norepinephrine Reuptake Inhibitors

Clinical studies suggest that compounds which increase the synaptic availability of both NE and 5-HT have greater efficacy than single-acting drugs in the treatment of major depression. Thus began the efforts to design a drug that combined the properties of SSRIs and SNRIs that only blocked SERTs and NETs and without the unwanted adverse effects of TCAs (67). Currently, the nontricyclic dual inhibitors of 5-HT and NE uptake are venlafaxine, milnacipran, and duloxetine (Fig. 21.18). A structurally related nontricyclic SNRI is atomoxetine. Based on preclinical studies, venlafaxine, milnacipran, and duloxetine inhibit the reuptake of 5-HT and NE both in vitro and in vivo in the following order of decreasing potency: duloxetine> milnacipran> venlafaxine. All the dual reuptake inhibitors exhibit low affinity at neuronal receptors of the other neurotransmitters, suggesting a low side-effect potential. Venlafaxine, milnacipran, and duloxetine have repeatedly shown to be as efficacious as TCA drugs in treating major depressive disorders. These nontricyclic antidepressants reported to produce a faster and greater antidepressant response than an SSRI alone, suggesting that these two mechanisms of action can be synergistic in terms of mediating antidepressant efficacy. Meaningful differences between the nontricyclic NSRIs are largely related to their pharmacokinetics, metabolism to active metabolites, inhibition of CYP isoforms, effect of drug–drug interactions, and the half-life of the nontricyclic NSRI.

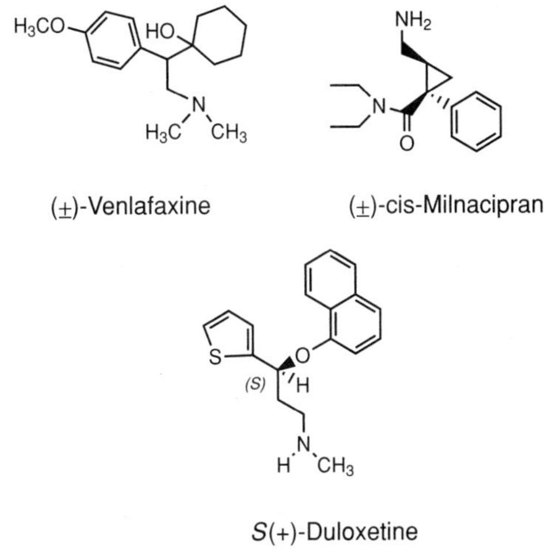

H_3CO HO N H_3C CH_3

(±)-Venlafaxine

NH_2 N O

(±)-cis-Milnacipran

S O (S) H N H CH_3

S(+)-Duloxetine

Fig. 21.18. Nontricyclic NSRIs.

VENLAFAXINE. Venlafaxine is a methoxyphenylethylamine antidepressant that resembles an open TCA with one of the aromatic rings replaced by a cyclohexanol ring and a dimethylaminoethyl group rather than a dimethylaminopropyl chain (Fig. 21.18).

Venlafaxine and its active metabolite, O-desmethylvenlafaxine (ODV), have dual mechanisms of action, with preferential affinity for 5-HT reuptake and weak inhibition of NE and dopamine reuptake. Venlafaxine is approximately 30 times more potent as an inhibitor of SERT than of NET (68). Because of the 30 times difference in transporter affinities, increasing the dose of venlafaxine from 75 to 375 mg/day can sequentially inhibit SERT and NERT. Thus, venlafaxine displays an ascending dose-dependent antidepressant response in contrast to the flat dose–antidepressant response curve observed with the SSRIs. This sequential action for venlafaxine also is consistent with its dose-dependent adverse-effect profile. Its mechanism of action is similar to imipramine.

Venlafaxine is rapidly and well absorbed, but with a bioavailability of 45%, which has been attributed to first-pass metabolism (Table 21.10). Food delays its absorption but does not impair the extent of absorption. Venlafaxine is distributed into breast milk. Venlafaxine is primarily metabolized in the liver by CYP2D6 to its primary metabolite, ODV, which is approximately equivalent in pharmacological activity and potency to

Table 21.10. Pharmacokinetics of the Nontricyclic Nonselective Reuptake Inhibitors (NSRIs)

Parameters	Venlafaxine	Milnacipran	Duloxetine
Oral bioavailability (%)	45	90	>70%
Protein binding (%)	25–30	15–30	>90
Volume of distribution (L/kg)	8 (5–19) ODV 5.7	17 (9–25)	1,940
Elimination half-life (hours)	4 (2–7) ODV 11	~8	11–16
Cytochrome P450 major isoform	2D6	None	2D6 and 1A2
Major active metabolites	ODV	None	4-Hydroxy
Peak plasma concentration (hours)	2 ODV 3–4	32–48	6–10
Excretion (%)	Urine 87 (48 hours) Feces 2 (35 days)	Urine 90 Feces minor	Urine >70 Feces 15
Plasma half-life (hours)	2	—	6
Time to steady-state concentration (hours)	3	32–48	3–7

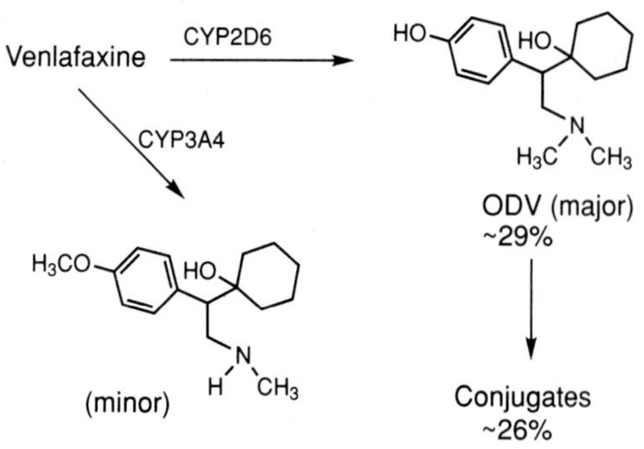

Fig. 21.19. Metabolism of venlafaxine.

venlafaxine. In vitro studies indicate that CYP3A4 also is involved in the metabolism of venlafaxine to its minor and less active metabolite, N-desmethylvenlafaxine (Fig. 21.19). Protein binding for venlafaxine and ODV is low and is not a problem for drug interactions. In patients with hepatic impairment, elimination half-lives were increased by approximately 30% for venlafaxine and approximately 60% for ODV (Table 21.10). In patients with renal function impairment, elimination half-lives were increased by approximately 40 to 50% for venlafaxine and for ODV. At steady-state doses, venlafaxine and ODV exhibit dose-proportional linear pharmacokinetics over the dose range of 75 to 450 mg/day. Steady-state concentrations of venlafaxine and ODV are attained within 3 days with regular oral dosing. Venlafaxine and its metabolites are excreted primarily in the urine (87%).

The potential for cardiotoxicity with venlafaxine during normal use and for various toxicities in overdose situations are key concerns. Venlafaxine displays minimal in vitro affinity for the other neural neurotransmitter receptors and, thus, a low probability for adverse effects. To minimize GI upset (e.g., nausea), venlafaxine can be taken with food without affecting its GI absorption. Venlafaxine should be administered as a single daily dose with food at approximately the same time each day. The extended-release capsules should be swallowed whole with fluid and should not be divided, crushed, chewed, or placed in water.

Whenever venlafaxine is being discontinued after more than 1 week of therapy, it generally is recommended that the patient be closely monitored and the dosage of the drug be tapered gradually to reduce the risk of withdrawal symptoms.

Although venlafaxine is a weak inhibitor of CYP2D6, variability has been observed in the pharmacokinetic parameters of venlafaxine in patients with hepatic or renal function impairment. As a precaution, elderly patients taking venlafaxine concurrently with a drug that has a narrow therapeutic index and also is metabolized by CYP2D6 should be carefully monitored. Concurrent use of CYP3A4 inhibitors with venlafaxine has been shown to interfere with its metabolism and clearance. Similar to the other antidepressants that block 5-HT reuptake, venlafaxine may interact pharmacodynamically to cause toxic levels of 5-HT to accumulate, leading to the 5-HT syndrome.

MILNACIPRAN. (±)-Milnacipran is the *cis*-aminomethyl derivative of phenylcyclopropanecarboxamide (Fig. 21.18) that acts by inhibiting both NE and 5-HT reuptake. It is structurally different from the other NSRIs and currently is only available in Europe as a racemic mixture, with both enantiomers exhibiting antidepressant activity. Substituting the aminomethyl group of milnacipran with an aminopropyl gives a milnacipran homologue that exhibits antidepressant activity as a potent N-methyl-D-aspartate (NMDA) receptor antagonist. A glutamate hypothesis is being investigated as an alternative mechanism of depression (see the subsection on NMDA antagonists).

Milnacipran selectively inhibits the reuptake of 5-HT (selectivity ratio, 9) at the presynaptic membrane site, thus increasing the concentration of 5-HT in the synaptic cleft (69). Although milnacipran is not a TCA, its mechanism of action is similar to that of imipramine, and its binding and reuptake inhibition profile more closely resembles that of the TCAs. Milnacipran has weak affinity for adrenergic, muscarinic, and H_1 receptors and, therefore, is expected to be devoid of the prominent side effects observed for the TCAs. In clinical studies, milnacipran showed antidepressant efficacy similar to that of TCAs and SSRIs.

In humans, milnacipran distinguishes itself from many other antidepressants by its simple pharmacokinetics. It is rapidly absorbed, with a high oral bioavailability, and it exhibits linear pharmacokinetics over a dose range of 25 to 200 mg/day (Table 21.10) (70). It circulates in the blood and distributes in the body principally as unmetabolized drug. Steady-state plasma levels are reached within 32 to 48 hours after twice-daily oral administration, and its metabolism does not involve the CYP enzyme system. Approximately 50% of the dose is excreted in urine as unmetabolized drug, and another 14% is excreted as its N-glucuronide conjugate. The remaining eliminated drug is composed of conjugated Phase I inactive metabolites. Because the unmetabolized drug is the only compound responsible for the activity of milnacipran, no dosage adjustment is needed in patients presenting liver impairment.

Milnacipran has proven to be a very safe drug, with an adverse-event profile clearly superior to that of TCAs and, to a certain extent, that of SSRIs. Only approximately 10% of patients experience side effects, and only dysuria occurred more frequently (2%) with milnacipran than with TCAs or SSRIs. Milnacipran therefore appears to be an antidepressant with a very favorable benefit:risk ratio, although with a slower onset of action than the TCAs.

DULOXETINE. Duloxetine (Fig. 21.18) has been approved for the treatment of depression and diabetic peripheral neuropathic pain. It is another analogue in the line of fluoxetine-based products from Lilly, in which the phenyl and phenoxy groups of fluoxetine have been respectively replaced with the benzene isostere, thiophene, and a naphthyloxy group (previously described under fluoxetine). Duloxetine exhibits dual inhibition with high affinity for the SERTs and NETs, with a five times preferential inhibition of the SERT (68). Duloxetine appears to be a more potent in vitro blocker of SERTs and NETs than venlafaxine. In humans, duloxetine has a low affinity for the other neuroreceptors, suggesting low incidence of unwanted adverse effects.

Duloxetine appears to be fairly well absorbed after oral doses, with peak plasma levels in 6 to 10 hours and linear pharmacokinetics (Table 21.10) (71). The drug is extensively metabolized in the liver to active metabolites, with 72% of an oral dose primarily excreted in the urine as conjugated metabolites and up to 15% appearing in the feces. Its elimination half-life, time to steady-state blood levels, and mean volume of distribution are shown in Table 21.10.

N-demethylation to an active metabolite (CYP2D6) and hydroxylation of the naphthyl ring (CYP1A2) at either the 4-, 5-, or 6-positions are the main metabolic pathways for duloxetine. Its metabolites are primarily excreted into the urine as glucuronide, sulfate, and O-methylated conjugation products (Fig. 21.20). The major metabolites found in plasma also were found in the urine (71). Preclinical data for 4-hydroxyduloxetine suggests it has a similar pharmacological profile to duloxetine, with selective inhibition of SERT but less activity at the NET.

Adverse effects have included insomnia, somnolence, headache, nausea, diarrhea, and dry mouth. Mild withdrawal symptoms on abrupt discontinuation have been described in studies with healthy subjects.

Duloxetine is a moderately potent CYP2D6 inhibitor (intermediate between paroxetine and sertraline). Thus, duloxetine should be used with caution when CYP2D6 substrates and inhibitors are coadministered.

Viloxazine, originally developed for the treatment of depression and nocturnal enuresis, was withdrawn from consideration for business reasons. It deserves some discussion because of its early relationship with the development of the nonselective reuptake inhibitors.

Research scientists at ICI in England (now Zeneca) recognized that some β-blockers exhibited CNS 5-HT antagonist activity at high doses. To improve the CNS distribution for the β-blockers, the medicinal chemists at ICI constrained the ethanolamine side chain of the β-blockers into a morpholine ring, resulting in the synthesis of viloxazine.

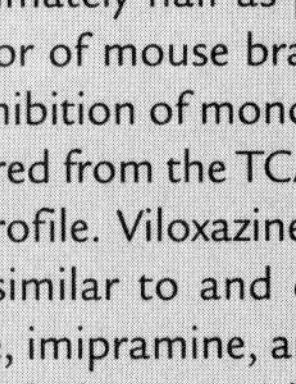

Viloxazine

Viloxazine selectively inhibits the presynaptic reuptake of NE reuptake (approximately half as potent as imipramine) and is a weak inhibitor of mouse brain 5-HT reuptake. No appreciable in vivo inhibition of monoamine oxidase activity was observed. It differed from the TCAs in not exhibiting the TCA adverse-effect profile. Viloxazine produces antidepressant activities both similar to and different from the tricyclics desimipramine, imipramine, and amitriptyline. These actions appear to be of relevance with respect to the antidepressant action of this drug.

Presently, viloxazine is classified as an orphan drug, under the trade name of Catatrol, for the treatment of narcolepsy and cataplexy.

Dopamine and Norepinephrine Reuptake Inhibitors

Bupropion. Bupropion (amfebutamone) is a phenylisopropylaminoketone that is structurally related to the phenylisopropylamine CNS stimulant, methamphetamine, and the phenylisopropylaminoketone, cathinone (a constituent in khat), and the anorexiant, diethylpropion (Fig. 21.21). Although structurally similar to the CNS stimulants, bupropion exhibits distinctive different pharmacologic and therapeutic effects. The absence of the tricyclic ring system in bupropion results in a better adverse-effect profile than with the TCAs. The tertiary butyl group in bupropion prevents its N-dealkylation to metabolites that could possess sympathomimetic and/or anorexigenic properties.

Wellbutrin and Zyban (an aid in smoking cessation treatment) are trade name products for bupropion. Therefore, the potential exists for an overdose toxicity in a patient receiving multiple brand name and generic prescriptions containing bupropion for the treatment of depression, smoking cessation, and other off-label uses.

Mechanism of action. Although the mechanism of antidepressant action for bupropion is unclear, in vitro binding studies show bupropion to be a selective inhibitor of dopamine reuptake at the dopamine presynaptic neuronal membrane and minimal inhibition of NE and 5-HT reuptake (Table 21.2). Bupropion does not exhibit clinically significant anticholinergic, antihistaminic, α_1-adrenergic blocking activity, or MAO inhibition.

The mechanism of its antidepressant action is more complex because of bupropion's metabolism to its three principal metabolites (Fig. 21.21), which likely contribute to the mechanism of action for bupropion because their plasma concentrations are as high or higher than those of bupropion, with a longer duration of action (see the discussion of pharmacokinetics below).

Bupropion reduces the discomfort and craving associated with smoking cessation, which suggests that the principal mode of action by bupropion as an aid in smoking cessation is on the withdrawal symptoms following smoking cessation. Its precise mechanism of action, however, remains unclear. The efficacy of bupropion in smoking cessation does not appear to depend on the presence of underlying depression. Bupropion increases extracellular

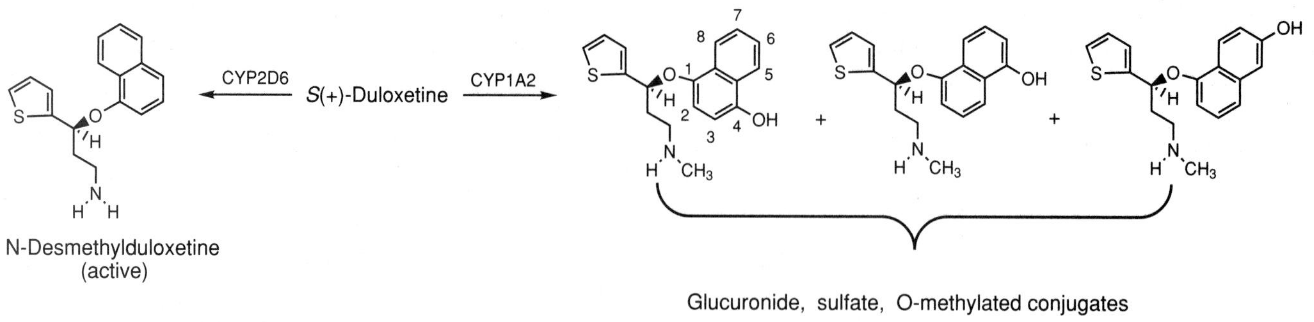

Fig. 21.20. Metabolism of duloxetine.

dopamine concentrations in the CNS, most likely as a result of its inhibition of dopamine and noradrenaline reuptake transporters (Table 21.2). It also has been shown to be an antagonist at the nicotinic receptor at clinically relevant concentrations of bupropion (72). As nicotine concentrations in the CNS drop with smoking cessation, the firing rates of noradrenergic neurons increase, which may be the basis for the withdrawal symptoms. Thus, during withdrawal, bupropion and its active metabolite, hydroxybupropion, reduce the firing rates of these noradrenergic neurons in a dose-dependent manner, attenuating the symptoms of smoking cessation. Furthermore, its ability to antagonize nicotinic receptors also may prevent relapse by attenuating the reinforcing properties of nicotine but probably cannot acutely reduce smoking. Bupropion is extensively metabolized in humans with its major hydroxylated metabolites reaching plasma levels higher than those of bupropion itself. These hydroxylated metabolites share many of the pharmacological properties of bupropion, so they may play a greater role in attenuating the withdrawal and relapse by which bupropion exerts its activity in smoking cessation (73).

Pharmacokinetics. Bupropion is absorbed from the GI tract, with a low oral bioavailability as a result of first-pass metabolism. The pharmacokinetic properties of bupropion are shown in Table 21.11. Food does not appear to substantially affect its peak plasma concentration or AUC. Following oral administration, peak plasma concentrations usually are achieved within 2 hours for bupropion and 3 hours for sustained-released bupropion products, followed by a biphasic decline for bupropion. Plasma concentrations are dose-proportional (linear pharmacokinetics) following single doses of 100 to 250 mg/day. The fraction of a dose excreted unmetabolized was less than 1%.

Bupropion hydroxylation of the tert-butyl group to hydroxypropion is mediated almost exclusively by CYP2B6 and, to a lesser extent, by CYP2E1 (74). Other metabolites include reduction of the aminoketone to amino-alcohol isomers, threo-hydrobupropion and erythro-hydrobupropion (Fig. 21.21). Further oxidation of the bupropion side chain results in the formation of m-chlorobenzoic acid, which is eliminated in the urine as its glycine conjugate. Hydroxybupropion is approximately 50% as potent as bupropion, whereas threo-hydrobupropion and erythro-hydrobupropion have 20% of the potency of bupropion. Peak plasma concentrations for hydroxybupropion are approximately 10 times the peak level of the parent drug at steady state, with an elimination half-life of approximately 20 hours. The times to

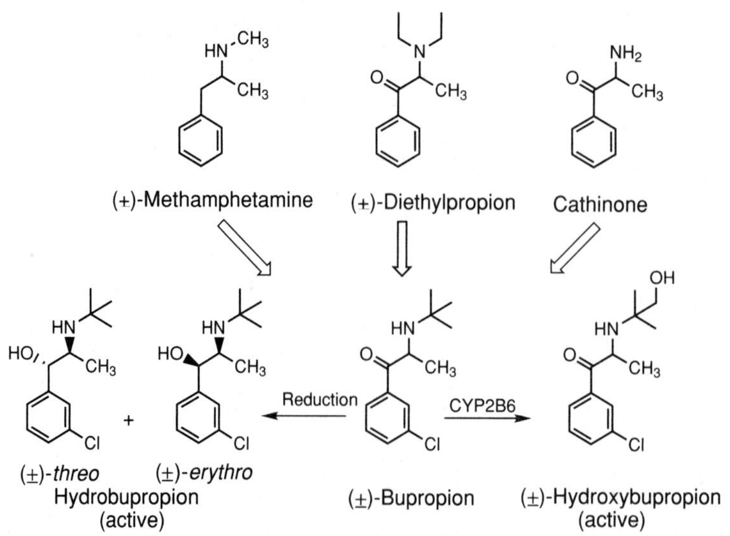

Fig. 21.21. Bupropion, related derivatives, and metabolites.

Table 21.11. Pharmacokinetics of the Dopamine and Norepinephrine Reuptake Inhibitors (DNRIs) and Serotonin Receptor Modulators (SRMs)

Parameters	Bupropion	Trazodone	Mirtazapine
Oral bioavailability (%)	5–20	65 (60–70)	~50
Protein binding (%)	80	90–95	85
Volume of distribution (L/kg)	19–21	0.84 (0.5–1.2)	107
Elimination half-life (hours)	21 (14–24) ~20 (S,S)-hydroxy	7 (4–9)	16–40
Cytochrome P450 major isoform	2B6	3A4	3A4 and 2D6
Major active metabolites	(S,S)-Hydroxyl	m-chlorophenyl piperazine	None
Peak plasma concentration (hours)	2–3 8 (S,S)-hydroxy	1–2	2
Excretion (%)	Urine 87 Feces 10	Urine 70–75 Feces 25–30	Urine 75 Feces 15
Plasma half-life (hours)	3–4 20 (S,S)-hydroxy	6 (4–8)	2
Time to steady-state concentration (days)	5 8 (S,S)-hydroxy	3–7	5

peak concentrations for the erythro-hydrobupropion and threo-hydrobupropion metabolites are similar to that of the hydroxybupropion metabolite. The plasma levels of the erythro-hydrobupropion correlate with several side effects, such as insomnia and dry mouth. Their elimination half-lives, however, are longer (~33 and 37 hours, respectively), and steady-state AUCs are 1.5- and 7.0 times that of bupropion, respectively. The hepatic clearance in patients with liver disease was increased from 19 to 29 hours. The median observed t_{max} was 19 hours for hydroxybupropion and 31 hours for threo/erythro-hydrobupropion. The mean half-lives for hydroxybupropion and threo/erythro-hydrobupropion were increased by five- and two times, respectively, in patients with severe hepatic cirrhosis compared with healthy volunteers Bupropion and its metabolites are distributed into breast milk.

In geriatric patients, the apparent half-life of hydroxybupropion averaged approximately 34 hours. Reduction in renal or hepatic function may affect elimination of the major metabolites, because these compounds are moderately polar and are likely to be metabolized further or conjugated in the liver before urinary excretion.

The pharmacokinetic parameters for bupropion and hydroxybupropion did not differ between smokers and nonsmokers, but adolescent females exhibited increased AUCs and volume of distribution (normalized to body weight) and longer elimination half-life than do males for bupropion and its major metabolite, hydroxybupropion. No differences in clearance between males and females, however, were observed.

Drug Interactions

Inhibition studies with the SSRIs and bupropion suggest that bupropion is a potent CYP2D6 inhibitor (74). Bupropion hydroxylation was strongly inhibited by, in the following order, paroxetine> fluvoxamine> sertraline> desmethylsertraline> norfluoxetine> nefazodone> fluoxetine and only weakly inhibited by venlafaxine, ODV, citalopram, and desmethylcitalopram. The inhibition of bupropion hydroxylation in vitro by SSRIs suggests the potential for clinical drug interactions. Therefore, coadministration of drugs that inhibit CYP2D6 warrants careful monitoring. Because of its selective inhibition of DA reuptake, pharmacodynamic interactions with dopamine agonists (e.g., levodopa) and antagonists should be anticipated. Coadministration of bupropion with drugs that lower the seizure threshold should be avoided because of the risk of serious seizures.

Drugs that affect metabolism by CYP2B6 (e.g., orphenadrine and cyclophosphamide) also have the potential to interact with bupropion.

Therapeutic Uses

Besides being used to treat depression, bupropion is a nonnicotine aid in the cessation of smoking. The efficacy of bupropion in smoking cessation is comparable to that of nicotine replacement therapy and should be considered as a second-line treatment in smoking cessation. (72,73). It possesses a broad spectrum of infrequent

Miscellaneous Norepinephrine and Dopamine Reuptake Inhibitors

Nomifensine is a substituted phenylpiperidine (an aminophenyltetrahydroisoquinoline) structurally related to sertraline that was marketed as a stimulatory antidepressant in the mid-1970s but later withdrawn because of a high incidence of hemolytic anemia. Nomifensine inhibits the NE and dopamine reuptake transporters. It displays high affinity for NET (human pK_i = 7.8), moderate affinity for dopamine transporter (pK_i = 6.6), and a low affinity for SERT (5-HT:NE ratio, 65).

Nomifensine Mazindol

Mazindol (Sanorex®) is a phenyl-substituted imidazobenzoisoindole that inhibits both NE and dopamine reuptake transporters. It exhibits high affinity for the NET (rat pK_i = 9.3), good affinity for dopamine transporter (rat pK_i = 7.8), and a 5-HT:NE ratio of 224. Dopamine reuptake inhibitors suppress appetite; thus, mazindol is approved to be marketed as an appetite suppressant.

adverse effects, however, with potential drug metabolism interactions with TCAs, β-adrenergic blocking drugs, and class Ic antiarrhythmics.

Serotonin Receptor Modulators

SEROTONIN ANTAGONIST/REUPTAKE INHIBITORS

General mechanism of action. Serotonin receptor modulators are a class of antidepressants, the function of which is to modulate the concentration of 5-HT in the brain. A neuromodulator functions as a "volume control in the brain and nervous system," regulating the other neurotransmitters through its receptors in the brain in response to external stimuli. As previously described, the serotonergic system modulates a large number of physiological events, such as temperature regulation, sleep, learning and memory, behavior, sexual function, hormonal secretions, and immune activity, and is implicated in stress, anxiety, aggressiveness, and depression disorders. Of the various types of 5-HT receptors (see Chapter 14) mediating serotonergic activity, the 5-HT_{1B} receptors play an important role in modulating the serotonergic system. The 5-HT_{1B} receptors are autoreceptors localized on serotonergic neuron terminals, where they inhibit the release of 5-HT and its biosynthesis; they also are heteroreceptors located on nonserotonergic terminals, where they inhibit the release of other neurotransmitters, such as acetylcholine, γ-aminobutyric acid (GABA), and NE. Excessive amounts of 5-HT in the brain may cause relaxation, sedation, and a decrease in sexual drive; inadequate amounts of 5-HT can lead to psychiatric disorders. Therefore, the 5-HT receptor modulator antidepressants exert their antidepressant effects by mechanisms that enhance noradrenergic or serotonergic transmission by acting as mixed 5-HT_2 antagonists/5-HT reuptake inhibitors (SARI; trazodone), and α_2 adrenergic antagonists/5-HT_2 and 5-HT_3 antagonists (NaSSA; mirtazapine). Chronic antidepressant treatment with SARIs and NaSSAs modulate 5-HT receptor expression and, in turn, 5-HT functioı

Trazodone. Trazodone is a phenylpiperazine–triazolopyridine antidepressant that is structurally unrelated to most of the other antidepressant classes (Fig. 21.22).

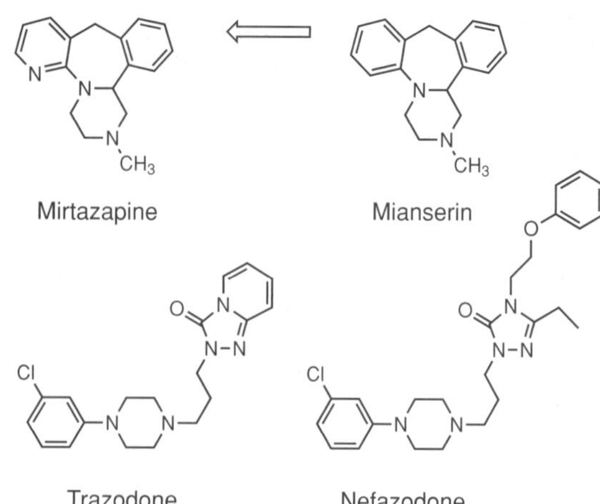

Fig. 21.22. Serotonin receptor modulators.

Mechanism of action. Trazodone acts as an antagonist at 5-HT_{2A} receptors and is a weak inhibitor of 5-HT reuptake at the presynaptic neuronal membrane, potentiating the synaptic effects of 5-HT. Its mechanism of action is complicated by the presence of its metabolite, m-chlorophenylpiperazine (Fig. 21.23), which is a 5-HT_{2C} agonist. At therapeutic dosages, trazodone does not appear to influence the reuptake of dopamine or NE within the CNS. It has little anticholinergic activity and is relatively devoid of toxic cardiovascular effects. The increase in serotonergic activity with long-term administration of trazodone decreases the number of postsynaptic serotonergic (i.e., 5-HT_2) and β-adrenergic binding sites in the brains of animals, decreasing the sensitivity of adenylate (or adenylyl) cyclase to stimulation by β-adrenergic agonists. It has been suggested that postsynaptic serotonergic receptor modification is mainly responsible for the antidepressant action observed during long-term administration of trazodone. Trazodone does not inhibit MAO and, unlike amphetamine-like drugs, does not stimulate the CNS.

Trazodone is rapidly and almost completely absorbed from the GI tract following oral administration, with an oral bioavailability of approximately 65% (Table 21.11). Peak plasma concentrations of trazodone occur approximately 1 hour after oral administration when taken on an empty stomach or 2 hours when taken with food. At steady state, its plasma concentrations exhibit wide interpatient variation.

Trazodone is extensively metabolized in the liver by N-dealkylation to its primary active metabolite, m-chlorophenylpiperazine (m-CPP), which subsequently undergoes aromatic hydroxylation to p-hydroxy-m-CPP (Fig. 21.23) (75). In vitro studies indicate that CYP3A4 is the major isoform involved in the production of m-CPP from trazodone (and CYP2D6 to a lesser extent). The p-hydroxy-m-CPP and oxotriazolopyridine-propionic acid (the major metabolite excreted in urine) are conjugated with glucuronic acid. Less than 1% of a dose is excreted unmetabolized.

Trazodone therapy has been associated with several cases of idiosyncratic hepatotoxicity (see Chapter 10). Although the mechanism of hepatotoxicity remains unknown, the generation of an iminoquinone, an epoxide reactive metabolite or both may play a role in the initiation of trazodone-mediated hepatotoxicity (Fig. 21.23) (75). Studies have shown that the bioactivation of trazodone involves, first, aromatic hydroxylation of the 3-chlorophenyl ring, followed by its oxidation to a reactive iminoquinone intermediate, which then reacts with glutathione or, oxidation of the triazolopyridinone ring to an electrophilic epoxide and ring opening by either a Nucleophile (:Nu) or to generate the corresponding hydrated trazodone–Nucleophile conjugate or the stable

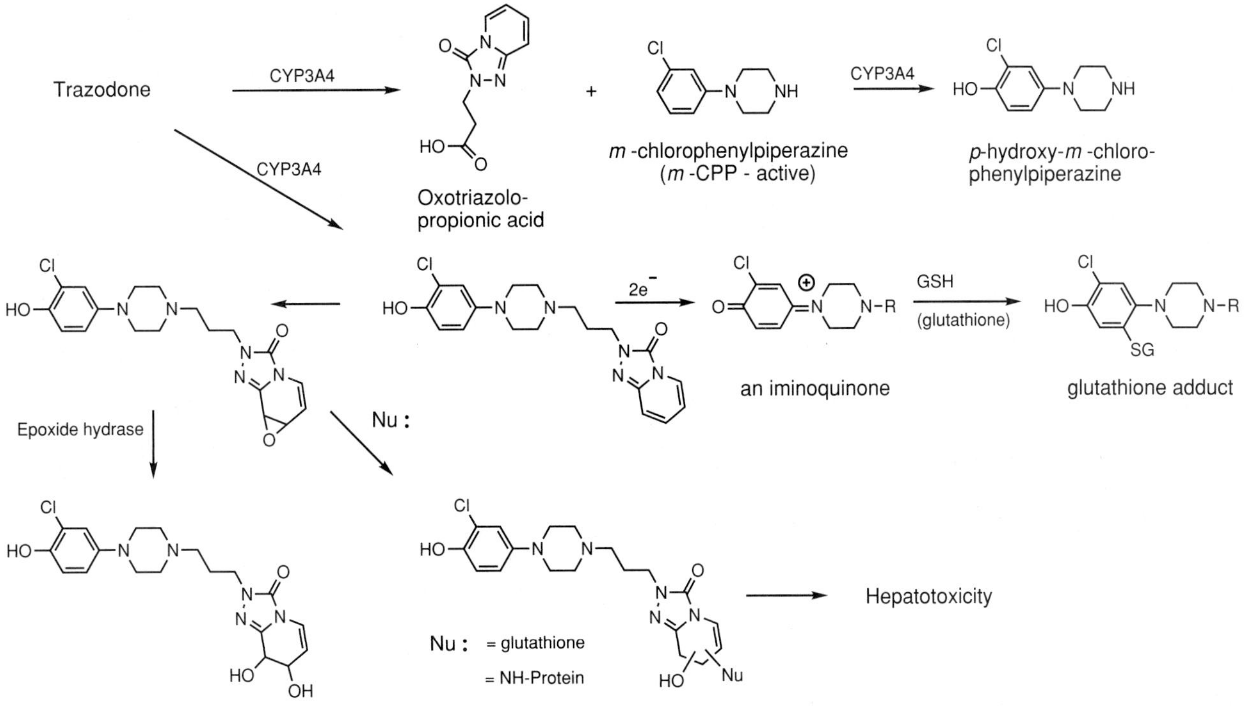

Fig. 21.23. Metabolism of trazodone.

diol metabolite, respectively. The pathway involving trazodone bioactivation to the iminoquinone also has been observed with many para-hydroxyanilines (e.g., acetaminophen) (see Chapter 10). including the structurally related antidepressant nefazodone. The reactive intermediates consume the available glutathione, allowing the reactive intermediate to react with hepatic tissue leading to liver damage.

Unlike the TCAs, trazodone does not block the fast sodium channels and, thus, does not have significant arrhythmic activity. Compared with the SSRIs, it has a lesser tendency to cause drug-induced male sexual dysfunction as a side effect. Although trazodone displays α_1-adrenergic blocking activity, hypotension is relatively uncommon. Signs of overdose toxicity include nausea, vomiting, and decreased level of consciousness. Trazodone produces a significant amount of sedation in normal and mentally depressed patients (principally from its central α_1-adrenergic blocking activity and antihistaminic action).

Drug interactions. Trazodone possesses serotonergic activity; therefore, the possibility of developing 5-HT syndrome should be considered in patients who are receiving trazodone and other SSRIs or serotonergic drugs concurrently. When trazodone is used concurrently with drugs metabolized by CYP3A4, caution should be used to avoid excessive sedation. Trazodone can cause hypotension, including orthostatic hypotension and syncope; concomitant administration of antihypertensive therapy may require a reduction in dosage of the antihypertensive agent.

The possibility of drug–drug interactions with trazodone and other substrates, inducers, and/or inhibitors of CYP3A4 exists (75).

Therapeutic uses. Trazodone is used primarily in the treatment of insomnia, mental depression, or depression/anxiety disorders. The drug also has shown some efficacy in the treatment of benzodiazepine or alcohol dependence, diabetic neuropathy, and panic disorders.

Noradrenergic Specific Serotonergic Antidepressants

MIRTAZAPINE. Mirtazapine is a piperazinodibenzoazepine antidepressant that is an isostere of the antidepressant mianserin (Fig. 21.22). A seemingly simple isosteric replacement of an aromatic methine group (CH) in mianserin with a nitrogen to give a pyridine ring (mirtazapine) has profound effects on the physicochemical properties, pharmacokinetics, mechanisms of action, and antidepressant activities (Table 21.12) (31). Profound differences between receptor affinity and transporter affinity, pharmacokinetics, regioselectivity in the formation of metabolites, and toxicity are observed for mianserin and mirtazapine and their antidepressant mechanisms of action. The pyridine ring increases the polarity of the molecule and decreases the measured partition coefficient and the basicity. Mianserin is a potent inhibitor of NET, whereas mirtazapine has negligible effects on the inhibition of NET (pK_i = 7.1 vs. 5.8 respectively).

Mianserin is currently marketed in Europe as an antidepressant. Mianserin has not been approved for use in the United States because of its serious adverse effects of

Nefazodone is a phenylpiperazine antidepressant structurally related to trazodone, but it differs pharmacologically from trazodone, the SSRIs, the MAOIs, and the TCAs (Fig. 21.22). When compared with trazodone, nefazodone displays approximately twice the affinity potency for SERT. Nefazodone therapy, however, was associated with life-threatening cases of idiosyncratic hepatotoxicity, and as a result, nefazodone was withdrawn from both the North American and European markets in 2003. The mechanism of hepatotoxicity remains unknown, but nefazodone, being structurally similar to trazodone (Fig. 21.23), is metabolized to p-hydroxynefazodone, m-CPP, and phenoxyethyltriazoledione. In turn, p-hydroxynefazodone is thought to be oxidized to an iminoquinone and/or an epoxide reactive metabolite, which may play a role in the initiation of nefazodone-mediated hepatotoxicity (76).

agranulocytosis and leukopenia. Mirtazapine has not exhibited this adverse effect

Mechanism of action. Animal studies indicate that the efficacy of mirtazapine as an antidepressant results from enhancing central noradrenergic possibly through blocking central presynaptic α_2-adrenergic receptors. Blocking these receptors inhibits the negative feedback loop, which increases the release of NE into the synapse. Mirtazapine also is a potent antagonist at 5-HT_2 and 5-HT_3 receptors, and it shows no significant affinity for 5-HT_{1A} or 5-HT_{1B} receptors. Additionally, it displays some anticholinergic properties, and it produces sedative effects (because of potent histamine H_1 receptor antagonism) and orthostatic hypotension (because of moderate antagonism at peripheral α_1-adrenergic receptors). Its antidepressant effect is comparable to the TCAs and may be better than some SSRIs, especially in patients with depression of the melancholic type, but at higher doses, it may cause drowsiness and weight gain. The drug generally is well tolerated, producing no more adverse events (including anticholinergic events) than the SSRIs and fewer adverse events than the TCAs.

The pharmacokinetics for mirtazepine are shown in Table 21.11. Mirtazapine absorption is rapid and complete, with a bioavailability of approximately 50% as a result of first-pass metabolism. The rate and extent of mirtazapine absorption are minimally affected by food. Dose and plasma levels are linearly related over a dose range of 15 to 80 mg. The elimination half-life of the (−)-enantiomer is approximately twice that of the (+)-enantiomer. In females of all ages, the elimination half-life is significantly longer than in males (mean half-life, 37 versus 26 hours).

Following oral administration, mirtazapine undergoes first-pass metabolism by N-demethylation and ring hydroxylation to its 8-hydroxy metabolite, followed by O-glucuronide conjugation (77). In vitro studies indicate that CYP2D6 and CYP1A2 are involved in the formation of the 8-hydroxy metabolite and that CYP3A4 is responsible for the formation of the N-desmethyl and N-oxide metabolites (Fig. 21.24). The 8-hydroxy and N-desmethyl metabolites possess weak pharmacological activity, but their plasma levels are very low and, thus, are unlikely to contribute to the antidepressant action of mirtazapine. Clearance for mirtazapine may decrease in patients with hepatic or renal impairment, increasing its plasma concentrations. Therefore, it should be used with caution in these patients. In vitro studies have shown mirtazapine to be a weak inhibitor of CYP1A2, CYP2D6, and CYP3A4.

Monoamine Oxidase Inhibitors

The discovery of MAOIs resulted from a search for derivatives of isoniazid (isonicotinic acid hydrazide) (Fig. 21.25) with antitubercular activity. During clinical trials with this hydrazine derivative, a rather consistent beneficial effect of mood elevation was noted in depressed patients with tuberculosis. Although no longer used clinically, iproniazid (Fig. 21.25), the first derivative to be synthesized, was found to be hepatotoxic at dosage levels required for antitubercular and antidepressant activity. The antidepressant activity of iproniazid, however, prompted a search for other MAOIs, which resulted in

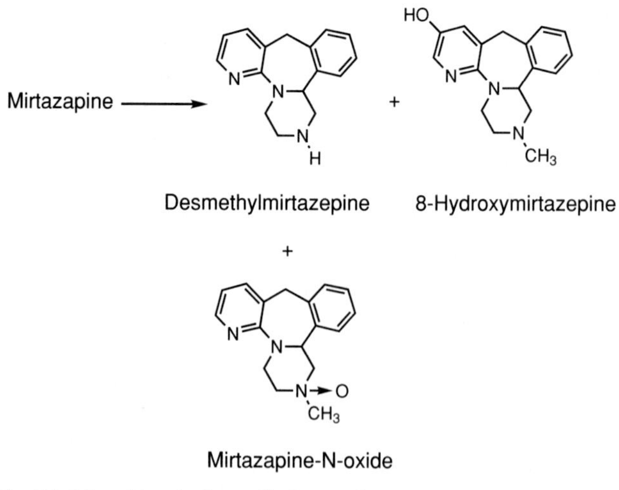

Table 21.12. Physicochemical and Properties of Mirtazapine and Mianserin

Properties	Mirtazapine	Mianserin
pK_a	7.1	7.4
Lipophilicity[a]	3.3	4.0
Polarity	2.63 debye	0.82 debye
NERT affinity (pK_i)	5.8	7.1
5-HT release	Yes	No

[a]Partition coefficient (log P) experimental determination.

Mirtazapine → Desmethylmirtazepine + 8-Hydroxymirtazepine + Mirtazapine-N-oxide

Fig. 21.24. Metabolism of mirtazepine.

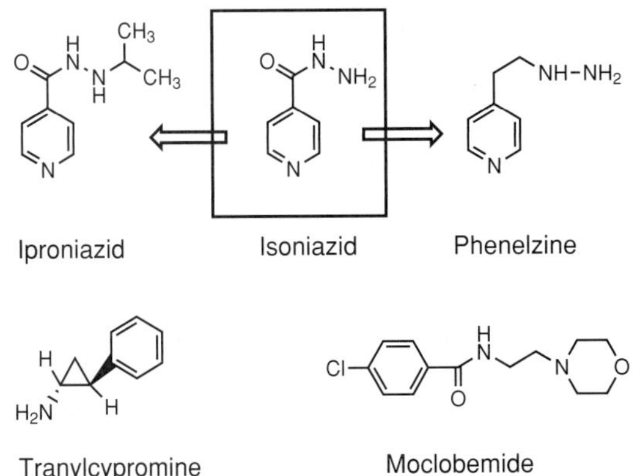

Fig. 21.25. MAOI antidepressants.

the synthesis of hydrazine and nonhydrazine MAOIs that were relatively less toxic than iproniazid.

The MAOIs can be classified as hydrazines (e.g., phenelzine) and nonhydrazines (e.g., tranylcypromine), which can block the oxidative deamination of naturally occurring monoamines. MAOIs can also be classified according to their ability to selectively or nonselectively inhibit MAO. The currently available MAOI antidepressants (phenelzine and tranylcypromine) (Fig. 21.25) are considered to be irreversible nonselective inhibitors of MAO. The mechanism of antidepressant action of the MAOIs suggests that an increase in free 5-HT and NE and/or alterations in other amine concentrations within the CNS is mainly responsible for their antidepressant effect.

Mechanisms of Action Common to MAOIs

An enzyme found mainly in nerve tissue and in the liver and lungs, MAO catalyzes the oxidative deamination of various amines, including epinephrine, NE, dopamine, and 5-HT. At least two isoforms of MAO exist, MAO-A and MAO-B, with differences in substrate preference, inhibitor specificity, and tissue distribution. The MAO-A substrates include 5-HT, and the MAO-B substrates include phenylethylamine. Tyramine, epinephrine, NE, and dopamine are substrates for both MAO-A and MAO-B. The cloning of MAO-A and MAO-B has demonstrated unequivocally that these enzymes consist of different amino acid sequences and also has provided insight regarding their structure, regulation, and function (51). Both MAO-A and -B knockout mice exhibit distinct differences in neurotransmitter metabolism and behavior (51). The MAO-A knockout mice have elevated brain levels of 5-HT, NE, and dopamine, and they manifest aggressive behavior similar to human males with a deletion of MAO-A. In contrast, MAO-B knockout mice do not exhibit aggression, and only levels of phenylethylamine are increased. Both MAO-A and -B knockout mice show increased reactivity to stress. These knockout mice are valuable models for investigating the role of monoamines in psychoses and in neurodegenerative and stress-related disorders.

The pharmacological effects of MAOIs are cumulative. A latent period of a few days to several months may occur before the onset of the antidepressant action, and effects may persist for up to 3 weeks following discontinuance of therapy.

Adverse Effects Common to MAOIs

Common side effects for the nonselective MAOIs include difficulty getting to sleep and broken sleep, daytime insomnia, agitation, dizziness on standing that results in fainting (orthostatic hypotension), dry mouth, tremor (slight shake of muscles of arms and hands), syncope, palpitations, tachycardia, dizziness, headache, confusion, weakness, overstimulation including increased anxiety, constipation, GI disturbances, edema, dry mouth, weight gain, and sexual disturbances.

Drug Interactions Common to MAOIs

The most significant drug interaction limiting the efficacy of the nonselective MAOIs is with certain foods that have the potential to cause hypertensive crisis because of the release and potentiation of catecholamines. The severity and consequences of such interactions vary among individuals from only minor increases in blood pressure to substantial and rapid increases in blood pressure within 20 minutes. These patients may experience symptoms associated with brain hemorrhage or cardiac failure.

Hypertensive crises with MAOIs have occurred in some patients following ingestion of foods containing large amounts of tyramine or tryptophan. In general, patients taking MAOIs should avoid protein foods that have undergone protein breakdown by aging, fermentation, pickling, smoking, or bacterial contamination. Some of the common foods to avoid are shown in Table 21.13. Patients should be warned against eating foods

Table 21.13. Foods To be Avoided Due to Potential Monoamine Oxidase Inhibitor–Food Interactions

Cheeses	Cheddar	**Meats**	Chicken livers
	Camembert		Genoa salami
	Stilton		Hard salami
	Processed cheese		Pepperoni
	Sour cream		Lebanon bologna
Spirits	Chianti	**Fruit**	Figs (overripe/canned)
	Champagne		Raisins
	Alcohol free/reduced wines		Overripe bananas
Fish	Pickled herring	**Dairy product**	Yogurt
	Anchovies	**Vegetable products**	Yeast extract
	Caviar		Pods-broad beans
Miscellaneous	Shrimp paste		Bean curd
	Chocolate		Soy sauce
	Meat tenderizers (papaya)		Avocado

Table 21.14. Common Information for Patients taking Monoamine Oxidase Inhibitors (MAOIs)

Patient Information	Recommendation
Discontinuance of therapy or dose adjustment	Consult physician
Adding medication (prescription/ over- the-counter)	Consult physician
Tyramine containing foods and over- the-counter products	Avoid
Drowsiness, blurred vision	Avoid driving or performing tasks requiring alertness or coordination
Dizziness, weakness, fainting	Arise from sitting position slowly
Alcohol use	Avoid alcohol
Onset of action	Effects may be delayed for a few weeks
Severe headache, palpitation, tachycardia, sense of constriction in throat or chest, sweating, stiff neck, nausea, or vomiting	Consult physician
New physician or dentist	Inform practitioner of MAOI use

with a high tyramine content, because hypertensive crisis may result. Excessive amounts of caffeine also reportedly may precipitate hypertensive crisis.

The MAOIs interfere with the hepatic metabolism of many prescription and nonprescription (over-the-counter) drugs and may potentiate the actions of their pharmacological effects (i.e., cold decongestants, sympathomimetic amines, general anesthetics, barbiturates, and morphine).

Therapeutic Uses Common to MAOIs

The MAOIs are indicated in patients with atypical (exogenous) depression and in some patients who are unresponsive to other antidepressive therapy. They rarely are a drug of first choice. Unlabeled uses have included bulimia (having characteristics of atypical depression), treatment of cocaine addiction (phenelzine), night terrors, posttraumatic stress disorder; some migraines resistant to other therapies, seasonal affective disorder (30 mg/day), and treatment of some panic disorders.

A list of information that should be transmitted to the patient concerning use of MAOIs is shown in Table 21.14.

Nonselective MAOI antidepressants

Phenelzine. Phenelzine is a hydrazine MAOI (Fig. 21.25). Its mechanism of action is the prolonged, nonselective, irreversible inhibition of MAO. Phenelzine has been used with some success in the management of bulimia nervosa. The MAOIs, however, are potentially dangerous in patients with binge eating and purging behaviors, and the American Psychiatric Association states that MAOIs should be used with caution in the management of bulimia nervosa.

Table 21.15. Pharmacokinetics of the Monoamine Oxidase Inhibitors (MAOIs)

Parameters	Phenelzine (Nardil)	Tranylcypromine (Parnate)	Meclobemide
Oral bioavailability (%)	NA	~50	50–90
Protein binding (%)	NA	NA	50
Volume of distribution (L/kg)	NA	1.1–5.7	1.2
Elimination half-life (hours)	NA	2.5 (1.5–3.2)	1.5
Peak plasma concentration (hours)	2–3	1.5 (0.7–3.5)	0.82
Excretion route	Urine	Urine Feces	Renal Feces

NA, not available.

Limited information is available regarding MAOI pharmacokinetics of phenelzine (Table 21.15). Phenelzine appears to be well absorbed following oral administration; however, maximal inhibition of MAO occurs within 5 to 10 days. Acetylation of phenelzine to its inactive acetylated metabolite appears to be a minor metabolic pathway (78). Phenelzine is a substrate as well as an inhibitor of MAO, and major identified metabolites of phenelzine include phenylacetic acid and p-hydroxyphenylacetic acid. Phenelzine also elevates brain GABA levels, probably via its β-phenylethylamine metabolite. The clinical effects of phenelzine may continue for up to 2 weeks after discontinuation of therapy. Phenelzine is excreted in the urine mostly as its N-acetyl metabolite. Interindividual variability in plasma concentrations have been observed among patients who are either slow or fast acetylators. Slow acetylators of hydrazine MAOIs may yield exaggerated adverse effects after standard dosing. If adverse neurological reactions occur during phenelzine therapy, phenelzine-induced pyridoxine deficiency should be considered. Pyridoxine supplementation can correct the deficiency while allowing continuance of phenelzine therapy.

Tranylcypromine. Tranylcypromine is a nonhydrazine, irreversible MAO inhibitor antidepressant agent that was designed as the cyclopropyl analogue of amphetamine (Fig. 21.25). Instead of exhibiting amphetamine-like stimulation, its mechanism of action is nonselective, irreversible inhibition of MAO. Its onset of antidepressant action is more rapid than for phenelzine. Tranylcypromine is well absorbed following oral administration (Table 21.15). Metabolism occurs via aromatic ring hydroxylation and N-acetylation (78). It is a competitive inhibitor of CYP2C19 and CYP2D6 and a noncompetitive inhibitor of CYP 2C9. Most metabolism studies suggest that tranylcypromine is not metabolized to amphetamine contrary to debate. Maximal MAO inhibition, however, occurs within 5 to 10 days. The GI absorption of the tranylcypromine shows interindividual variation and may be biphasic in some individuals, achieving an initial peak within approximately 1 hour and a secondary peak within 2 to 3 hours. It has been suggested that this apparent biphasic absorption in some individuals may represent different absorption rates. Following discontinuance of tranylcypromine, the drug is excreted within 24 hours. On withdrawal of tranylcypromine, MAO activity is recovered in 3 to 5 days (possibly in up to 10 days). Concentrations of urinary tryptamine, an indicator of MAO-A inhibition return to normal, however, within 72 to 120 hours.

Reversible MAO-A Inhibitor Antidepressants

The major goal for developing new reversible MAO-A inhibitors (RIMAs) is to avoid the severe, life-threatening hypertensive reactions that can occur with irreversible inhibitors. Irreversible inhibition of intestinal and hepatic MAO-A can lead to inhibition of tyramine degradation, thus allowing excessive amounts of naturally occurring tyramine to be absorbed from the food. Because these reversible compounds form unstable complexes with the MAO-A subtype, they can be easily displaced from MAO-A by tyramine. Thus, it becomes possible for ingested tyramine to be metabolized, diminishing the need for the dietary restrictions that plague the use of older irreversible nonselective MAOIs. This new class of selective and reversible inhibitors of MAO-A includes moclobemide (Fig. 21.25).

MOCLOBEMIDE. Moclobemide is a benzamide derivative containing a morpholine ring with a pK_a of 6.2 and a partition coefficient of 40 in a octanol/pH 7.4 buffer solution. Moclobemide is not currently available commercially in the United States, but is available in the United Kingdom and Australia.

Mechanism of action. Moclobemide is an RIMA that preferentially inhibits MAO-A (~80%) and, to a lesser extent, MAO-B (20–30% inhibition), thereby increasing the concentration of 5-HT, NE, and other catecholamines in the synaptic cleft and in storage sites. During chronic therapy with the MAOIs, adaptive changes at the noradrenergic and serotonergic receptors occur ("downregulation") as a result of neurotransmitter hypersensitivity because of prolonged concentrations of NE and 5-HT at the postsynaptic receptor (see the discussion of the receptor sensitivity hypothesis for details). This mechanism is likely the basis for its antidepressant activity. Inhibition of MAO-A by moclobemide is short-acting (maximum, 24 hours) and reversible. This is in contrast to phenelzine, which is nonselective, long-acting, and irreversible in its binding to MAO-A and MAO-B.

The pharmacokinetics (Table 21.15) for moclobemide are linear only up to 200 mg; at higher doses, nonlinear pharmacokinetics are observed (79). Although well absorbed from the GI tract, the presence of food reduces the rate but not the extent of absorption of moclobemide. Small quantities of moclobemide are distributed into human breast milk. Moclobemide undergoes a complex metabolism, initially involving morpholine carbon and nitrogen oxidation, deamination, and aromatic hydroxylation. The N-oxide and ring-opened metabolites retain some in vitro MAO-A inhibition. Moclobemide is a weak inhibitor of CYP2D6 in vitro. It is extensively metabolized in the liver by oxidation and is eliminated primarily into the urine as conjugates. Less than 1% of an administered dose of moclobemide is eliminated unmetabolized.

Because moclobemide is partially metabolized by the polymorphic isozymes CYP2C19 and CYP2D6, plasma concentrations of moclobenmide may be affected in patients who are poor metabolizers. In patients who are slow metabolizers, the AUC for moclobemide was 1.5 times greater than the AUC in patients who are extensive metabolizers and receiving the same dose. This increase is within the normal range of variation (up to twofold) typically seen in patients.

Drug interactions for the RIMAs include interaction with SSRI antidepressants, which can cause the 5-HT syndrome (see the discussion of SSRIs). The effect of stimulant drugs, such as methylphenidate and dextroamphetamine (used to treat ADHD), may be increased. Some over-the-counter cold and hay fever decongestants (i.e., sympathomimetic amines) can have increased stimulant effects. Selegiline, a selective MAO-B used for Parkinson's disease, should not be used concurrently with the RIMAs. Unlike the irreversible MAOIs, no significant interactions with foods occur, because the selective inhibition of MAO-A does not stop the metabolism of tyramine. The RIMAs must not be taken concurrently with a nonreversible MAOI.

Mood Stabilizers

Manic-depression, or bipolar affective disorder, is a prevalent mental disorder with a global impact. Mood stabilizers have acute and long-term effects and, at a minimum, are prophylactic for manic or depressive disorders. Lithium is the classic mood stabilizer and exhibits significant effects on mania and depression but may be augmented or substituted by some antiepileptic drugs. The biochemical basis for mood stabilizer therapies or the molecular origins of bipolar disorder is unknown. Lithium ion directly inhibits two signal transduction pathways. It suppresses inositol trisphosphate signaling through depletion of intracellular inositol and inhibits glycogen synthase kinase-3 (GSK-3), a multifunctional protein kinase. A number of GSK-3 substrates are involved in neuronal function and organization and, therefore, present plausible targets for manic-depression. Despite these intriguing observations, it remains unclear how changes in inositol trisphosphate signaling underlie the origins of bipolar disorder (80,81).

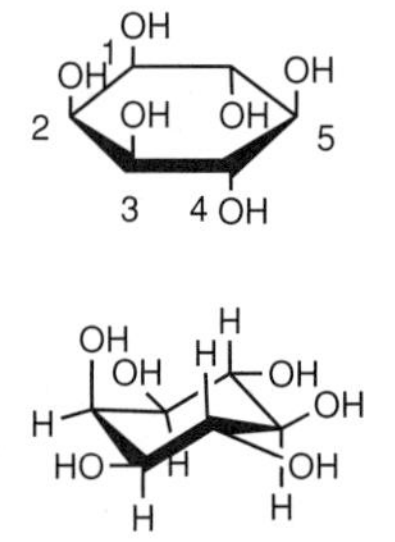

myo - inositol

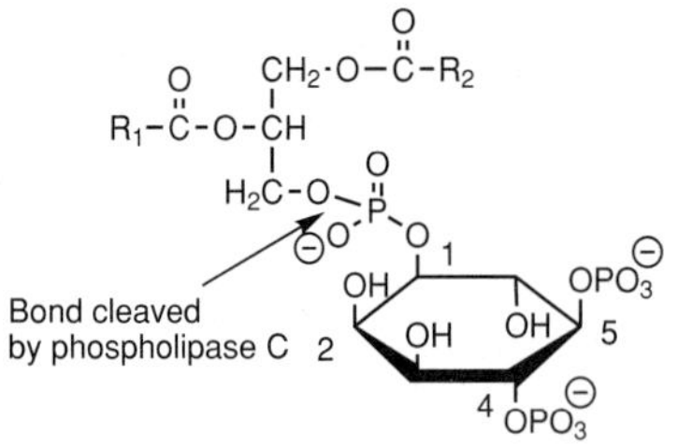

Bond cleaved by phospholipase C

Phosphatidylinositol-4,5-triphosphate

Inositol (myo-inositol), a naturally occurring isomer of glucose, is a key intermediate of the phosphatidylinositol signaling pathway, a second messenger system used by noradrenergic, serotonergic, and cholinergic receptors. The suggestion that lithium might treat mania via its reduction of inositol levels led to experiments showing that oral doses of inositol reverse the behavioral effects of lithium in animals and the side effects of lithium in humans. Cerebrospinal fluid levels of inositol are low in depressed individuals (82). The effectiveness of inositol in treating manic-depression was shown in a double-blind trial that large doses of inositol (12 g) increased inositol concentrations in human cerebrospinal fluid by 70% and led to improvement in depressed patients compared to placebo (82). Valproic acid and carbamazepine are antiepileptic drugs with mood-stabilizing properties that also inhibit inositol trisphosphate signaling through the inositol-depletion mechanism.

Inositol significantly reduced the number of panic attacks per week in patients as compared to fluvoxamine and without the nausea and tiredness that are common with fluvoxamine. Inositol has few known side effects, thus making it attractive for administration to patients with manic-depression who are ambivalent about taking other antidepressant drugs (82).

Lithium

Lithium (from the Greek word *lithos*, meaning "stone") is a monovalent cation that competes with sodium, potassium, calcium, and magnesium ions at intracellular binding sites; at sugar phosphatases; at protein surfaces; at carrier binding sites; and at transport sites. Lithium readily passes through sodium channels, and high concentrations can block potassium channels. In the 1870s, claims for the healthful effects of lithium fueled the markets for products such as Lithia Beer and Lithia Springs Mineral Water (in 1887, analysis of Lithia Springs Mineral Water proved the water to be rich not only in lithium but also in potassium, calcium, magnesium, fluoride, and other essential trace minerals). In 1890, the Lithia Springs Sanitorium (Georgia) was established using natural lithium water to treat alcoholism, opium addiction, and compulsive behavior, even though manic depression had not been identified as a form of mental illness until the early 1900s.

Lithium's mood-stabilizing properties were revitalized in the 1940s when an Australian physician, John Cade, hypothesized that a toxin in the blood was responsible for bipolar illness. Believing that uric acid would protect individuals from this toxin, he began studying the effects of a mixture of uric acid and lithium in rats. Lithium carbonate was used to dissolve the uric acid. He observed a calming effect of this combination on the rats and subsequently determined that the lithium, rather than the uric acid, was responsible for this calming effect. He then speculated that lithium might be useful in humans as a mood attenuator, subsequently administered lithium to a sample of patients with bipolar disorder, and discovered that lithium not only decreased the symptoms of mania but also prevented the recurrence of both depression and mania when taken regularly by these patients. After a decade of clinical trials, the U.S. FDA approved lithium for treatment of mania in 1970.

Lithium carbonate (Eskalith) is the most commonly used salt of lithium to treat manic depression. Lithium carbonate dosage forms are labeled in mg and mEq/dosage unit, and lithium citrate (Lithobid) is labeled as mg equivalent to lithium carbonate and mEq/dosage unit. Lithium is effectively used to control and prevent manic episodes in 70 to 80% of those with bipolar disorder as well as to treat other forms of depression. Those who respond to lithium for depression often are those who have not responded to TCAs after several weeks of treatment. When giving lithium in addition to their antidepressants, some of these people have shown significant improvement.

MECHANISM OF ACTION. Lithium therapy for disorders is believed to be effective because of its ability to reduce signal transduction through the phosphatidylinositol signaling pathway (Fig. 21.26) (83,84). In this pathway, the second messengers diacylglycerol and inositol 1,4,5-trisphosphate are produced from the enzymatic hydrolysis of phosphatidylinositol-4,5-bisphosphate (a membrane phospholipid) by the receptor-mediated activation of the membrane-bound, phosphatidylinositol-specific phospholipase C. The second messenger activity for inositol 1,4,5-trisphosphate is terminated by its hydrolysis in three steps by inositol monophosphatases to inactive inositol, thus completing the signaling pathway. To recharge the signaling pathway, inositol must be recycled back to phosphatidylinositol bisphosphate by inositol phospholipid–synthesizing enzymes in the CNS, because inositol is unable to cross the blood-brain barrier into the CNS in sufficient concentrations to maintain the signaling pathway. By uncompetitive inhibition of inositol phosphatases in the signaling pathway, the therapeutic plasma concentrations of lithium ion deplete the pool of inositol available for the resynthesis of phosphatidylinositol-4,5- bisphosphate, ultimately decreasing its cellular levels and, thereby,

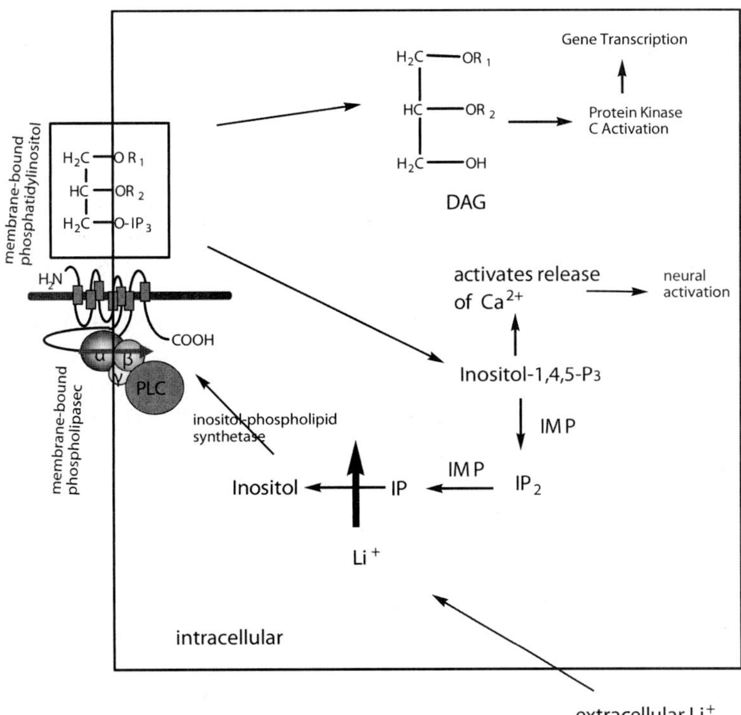

Fig. 21.26. Intracellular phosphatidylinositol signaling pathway and site of action for lithium. Phospholipase (PLC) is a membrane-bound enzyme. IP, inositol monophosphate; DAG, diacylglyceride; IMP, inositol monophosphatase.

reducing the enzymatic formation of the second messengers. Thus, lithium ion restores the balance among aberrant signaling pathways in critical regions of the brain.

The effects of lithium ion on disorders are surprisingly specific because of the inability of inositol to cross the blood-brain barrier and replenish depleted inositol levels. Lithium ion exerts its greatest influence on this signaling pathway when the lithium ion concentration is at saturation conditions.

The clinical efficacy of lithium in the prophylaxis of recurrent affective episodes in bipolar disorder is characterized by a lag in onset and remains for weeks to months after discontinuation. Thus, the long-term therapeutic effect of lithium likely requires reprogramming of gene expression. Protein kinase C and GSK-3 signal transduction pathways are perturbed by chronic lithium at therapeutically relevant concentrations and have been implicated in modulating synaptic function in nerve terminals (84).

Pharmacokinetics. The absorption of lithium is rapid and complete within 6 to 8 hours. The absorption rate of slow-release capsules is slower and the total amount of lithium absorbed lower than with other dosage forms. Lithium is not protein bound. The elimination half-life for elderly patients (39 hours) is longer than that for adult patients (24 hours), which in turn is longer than that for adolescent patients (18 hours). The time to peak serum concentration for lithium carbonate is dependent on the dosage form (tablets, 1–3 hours; extended tab, 4 hours; slow release, 3 hours). Steady-state serum concentrations are reached in 4 days, with the desirable dose targeted to give a maintenance lithium ion plasma concentration range of 0.6 to 1.2 mEq/L, with a level of 0.5 mEq/L for elderly patients. The risk of bipolar recurrence was approximately threefold greater for patients with lithium dosages that gave plasma concentrations of 0.4 to 0.6 mEq/L. Adverse reactions are frequent at therapeutic doses, and adherence is a big problem. Toxic reactions are rare at serum lithium ion levels of less than 1.5 mEq/L. Mild to moderate toxic reactions may occur at levels from 1.5 to 2.5 mEq/L, and severe reactions may be seen at levels from 2.0 to 2.5 mEq/L, depending on individual response. The onset of therapeutic action for clinical improvement is 1 to 3 weeks. Renal elimination of lithium ion is 95%, with 80% actively reabsorbed in the proximal tubule. The rate of lithium ion urinary excretion decreases with age. Fecal elimination is less than 1%.

Drug interactions. Lithium pharmacokinetics may be influenced by a number of factors, including age. Elderly patients require lower doses of lithium to achieve serum concentrations similar to those observed in younger adults as a result of reduced volume of distribution and reduced renal clearance. Lithium ion clearance decreases as the glomerular filtration rate decreases with increasing age. Reduced lithium ion clearance is expected in patients with hypertension, congestive heart failure, or renal dysfunction. Larger lithium ion maintenance doses are required in obese compared with nonobese patients. The most clinically significant pharmacokinetic drug interactions associated with lithium involve drugs that are commonly used in the elderly and that can increase serum Li^+ concentrations. People who are taking lithium should consult their physician before taking the following drugs: acetazolamide, antihypertensives, angiotensin-converting enzyme inhibitors, nonsteroidal anti-inflammatory drugs, calcium channel blockers, carbamazepine, thiazide diuretics, hydroxyzine, muscle relaxants, neuroleptics, table salt, baking powder, tetracycline, TCAs, MAOIs, and caffeine. The tolerability of lithium is lower in elderly patients. Lithium toxicity can occur in the elderly at concentrations considered to be "therapeutic" in the general adult populations. Serum concentrations of lithium ion need to be markedly reduced in the elderly population—and particularly so in the very old and frail.

Adverse effects. Common side effects of lithium include nausea, loss of appetite, and mild diarrhea, which usually taper off within first few weeks. Dizziness and hand tremors also have been reported. Increased production of urine and excessive thirst are two common side effects that usually are not serious problems, but patients with kidney disease should not be given lithium. Taking the day's dosage of lithium at bedtime also seems to help with the problem of increased urination. Other side effects of lithium include weight gain, hypothyroidism, increased white blood cell count, skin rashes, and birth defects.

While on lithium, a patient's blood level must be closely monitored. If the blood level of lithium ion is too low, the patient's symptoms will not be relieved. If the blood level of lithium ion is too high, there is a danger of a toxic reaction.

Therapeutic uses. For many years, lithium has been the treatment of choice for bipolar disorder, because it can be effective in smoothing out the mood swings common to this condition. Its use must be carefully monitored, however, because the range between an effective and a toxic dose is small.

N-Methyl-D-Aspartate Antagonists

In spite of intensive research, the problem of treating antidepressant-resistant patients has not yet been solved. The past decade has seen a steady accumulation of evidence supporting a role for the excitatory amino acid neurotransmitter, glutamate, and its mGluR1 and mGluR5 receptors in depression and antidepressant activity (85,86). Glutamate plays an essential role as a neurotransmitter in many physiological functions, and an increase in glutamate release can result in activation of NMDA receptors, an underlying cause for depression and anxiety. The NMDA receptor is a ligand-gated ion channel that mediates excitatory synaptic transmission in the CNS. This channel opening and receptor activation are triggered by synaptically released glutamate and require the binding of glycine, which is a coagonist. Studies with NMDA receptor antagonists of mGluR1 and mGluR5 receptors, as well as positive modulators of α-amino-3-hydroxy-5-methyl-4-isoxazolepropionic acid (AMPA) receptors, have antidepressant-like activity in a variety of preclinical models. Furthermore, evidence implicates disturbances in glutamate metabolism, NMDA, and mGluR1/5 receptors in depression and suicidality.

Moreover, antidepressant-like activity can be produced not only by drugs modulating the glutamatergic synapse but also by agents that affect subcellular signaling systems linked to excitatory amino acid neurotransmitter receptors (e.g., nitric oxide synthase). These studies suggest that an intimate relationship exists between regulation of monoaminergic and excitatory amino acid neurotransmission and antidepressant effects.

The concept of NMDA antagonists as antidepressants has generated considerable interest in the NMDA receptor as a target for new antidepressant therapies (85–87). Recent data indicate that *cis*-1-phenyl-2-[1-aminopropyl]-N,N-diethylcarboxamide, a NMDA receptor antagonist and homologue of milnacipran, produces sustained relief from depressive symptoms. Several studies have shown that chronic antidepressant treatment can modulate NMDA receptor expression and function. Preclinical studies with this and other NMDA receptor antagonists have demonstrated their potential antidepressant properties.

The combination of traditional antidepressant drugs (e.g., imipramine) and uncompetitive NMDA receptor antagonists (e.g., memantine) may produce enhanced antidepressive effects as a result of synergism. This observation may be of particular importance for the treatment of antidepressant-resistant patients. Most interesting was the observation that fluoxetine, which was inactive in the forced swimming test in rats when given alone, showed a positive effect when combined with memantine (2.5 and 5 mg/kg).

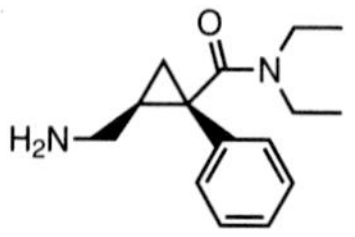

cis-Milnacipram 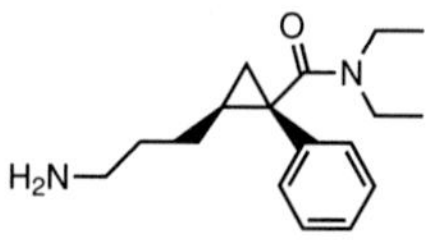   *cis*-1-Phenyl-2-[1-aminopropyl]-N,N-diethylcyclopropanecarboxamide   Memantine

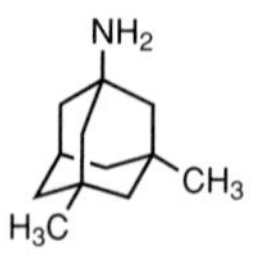

Neuropeptides

The pharmacological treatment of depressive illness has been dominated by drugs that directly target monoamine neurotransmitter systems. Monoamine transport inhibitors are first-line treatments for depression. Current antidepressants exhibit a delayed onset of therapeutic action, and a significant number of patients are nonresponsive to this treatment regimen (54). Moreover, many patients discontinue treatment because of adverse side effects, including nausea, sexual dysfunction, anorexia, mouth dryness, and cardiotoxicity. A complementary strategy is to identify other treatments that target other neurotransmitter and neuromodulators in the brain. Neuropeptides have been shown to be attractive targets for depression (88,89). Neuropeptides are short-chain amino acid neurotransmitters and neuromodulators often localized in brain regions that mediate emotional behaviors and the response to stress (88,89). The neuropeptides that have been identified in stress include the tachykinins (substance P and neurokinin A), corticotropin-releasing factor, vasopressin, galanin, brain-derived neurotrophic factor (BDNF) and melanocyte-inhibiting factor. Thus, drugs that are antagonists at these neuropeptide receptors might exhibit a lower incidence of adverse effects, because such antagonists would not be expected to bind to the NE and 5-HT neurotransmitter receptors. The expression of BDNF in individuals with MDD is decreased suggesting that BDNF plays a role in the pathophysiology of depression as a regulator of neuronal signaling pathways. Antidepressant drugs increase the BDNF brain levels, and therefore, enhance the mechanism of action of the antidepressant drugs. Drugs that boost the levels of BDNF may lead to the development of novel therapeutic agents for the treatment of MDD and bipolar disorders.

Corticotropin-Releasing Factor

Increasing evidence suggests that the neuroendocrine changes seen in patients suffering from affective disorders may be causally related to the course of depression. The most robustly confirmed neuroendocrine finding among patients with affective disorders is hyperactivity of the hypothalamic-pituitary-adrenocortical (HPA) system, resulting from hyperactive hypothalamic corticotropin-releasing factor (CRF) neurons. Abnormal HPA activity has been implicated in conditions related to stress, including HPA overactivation in depression, eating and substance abuse disorders, irritable bowel syndrome, inflammation, and cardiovascular dysfunction. Preclinical and clinical evidence suggests that both genetic and environmental factors contribute to the development of these HPA system abnormalities. Corticotropin-releasing factor is a 41-amino-acid neuropeptide that initiates and regulates the HPA-axis response to stress, and it has been intensively studied in the pathophysiology and treatment of depression (90). In humans, the CRF system consists of CRF and two G protein–coupled CRF receptors (CRF_1 and CRF_2). The CRF_1 receptors play an important role in mediating the HPA response to stress. Additionally, CRF is capable of reproducing the hormonal changes that are characteristically seen in depressed patients. Postmortem and endocrine studies suggest that both hypothalamic and extrahypothalamic concentrations of CRF are elevated in proportion to antidepressant treatment. High CRF concentrations tend to reestablish the HPA imbalance. The careful manipulation of CRF concentrations with high-affinity CRF_1 antagonists, such as R121919, may hold therapeutic promise for sufferers of depression.

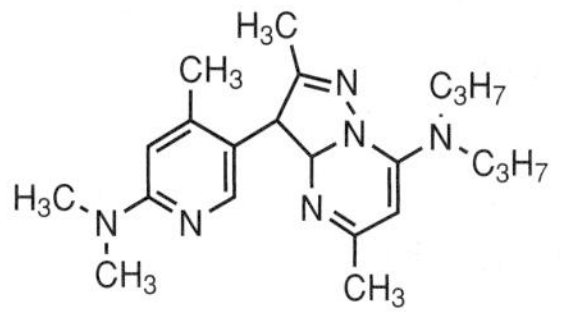

R121919

Substance P

Substance P is an 11-amino-acid neuropeptide belonging to the tachykinin family, mediating its biological actions through activation of G protein–coupled tachykinin (neurokinin-1 [NK_1]) receptors. Its proposed physiological roles include inflammation, pain, GI and respiratory function, stress responses, and emesis. Substance P is uniquely associated with the monoamine neurotransmitters, 5-HT and NE. The 5-HT neurons coexpress substance P, and the firing of NE neurons is modulated by substance P. Preclinical studies have supported a role of the substance P–NK_1 receptor system in stress-related disorders, which has guided the antidepressant development of centrally active NK_1 receptor antagonists, such as aprepitant (91). The NK_1 antagonists are generally well tolerated and exhibit less nausea and sexual dysfunction than some currently used antidepressants.

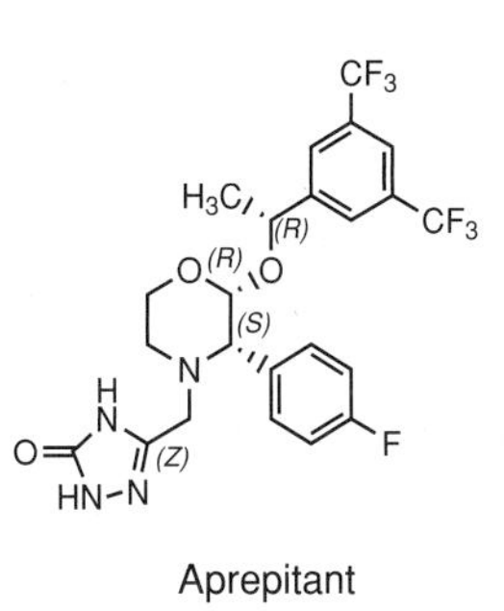

Aprepitant

Vasopressin

The nonapeptide vasopressin is well known for its role on fluid metabolism (see Chapter 7), but it also is a key regulator of the HPA axis. Stress stimulates the release of vasopressin in the pituitary gland, where it strongly potentiates the effects of CRF on adrenocorticotropic hormone release. These findings suggest that HPA axis dysregulation in depression might be associated with the development of centrally acting vasopressin receptor antagonists for the treatment of depression.

Galanin

Since its discovery in 1983, the neuropeptide galanin has been found to be involved in a wide range of functions, including pain sensation, sexual activity, feeding, and learning and memory (92). Galanin is widely distributed in the central and peripheral nervous systems and in the endocrine system, and it acts as a inhibitory neuromodulator of NE and 5-HT in the brain. The 29- to 30-amino-acid sequence of galanin is conserved (almost 90% among species), indicating the importance of the molecule among species. Galanin is colocalized with acetylcholine, 5-HT, and NE in neurons or in brain regions implicated in cognitive and affective behavior, suggesting a possible role in the regulation of 5-HT and NA neurotransmission in depressive states and during the course of antidepressant therapy. Three galanin receptor subtypes have been cloned and studied, but little is known about their specific contributions to behavioral processes. In the CNS, galanin inhibits acetylcholine release, suggesting a possible role for galanin in cholinergic dysfunction; inhibits neurotransmitter release and neuronal firing rate; and inhibits signal transduction by inhibition of phosphatidyl inositol hydrolysis, leading to symptoms of depression. Thus, blocking the inhibitory effects of galanin on monoamine neurotransmitters with galanin receptor antagonists would be predicted to mimic or augment the action of the other monoamine classes of antidepressants.

Melanocyte-Inhibiting Factor

Nemifitide is a peptide analogue of melanocyte-stimulating hormone release–inhibiting factor currently in clinical development for the potential treatment of moderate to severely depressed patients (93). It is rapidly absorbed, with a peak plasma concentration of 10 min and an elimination half-life of 15 to 30 minutes in most subjects. The pharmacokinetic results indicate that the dose is proportional in the dose range investigated. No evidence indicated systemic accumulation of drug following five daily doses. No serious adverse events or clinically significant systemic adverse events occurred at any of the doses investigated in the more than 100 subjects dosed in these studies. Drug-related adverse events were limited to local and transient skin reactions (pain and/or erythema) at the injection site, especially at the high doses administered. Melanocyte-stimulating hormone release–inhibiting factor-1 (MIF-1) has been shown to have antidepressant activity when administered subcutaneously (10 mg for 5 consecutive days) in a double-blind study to 20 depressed patients who all met the DSM-IIIR criteria for major depression. After the 5-day treatment with MIF-1, these patients all exhibited substantial improvement in their symptoms of depression (94). Moreover, the potential clinical efficacy of combining MIF-1 (0.01 mg/kg IP) with small doses of the TCAs amitriptyline (5 mg/kg IP) or desipramine (1.25 mg/kg IP) may be of benefit in the therapy of depressed patients.

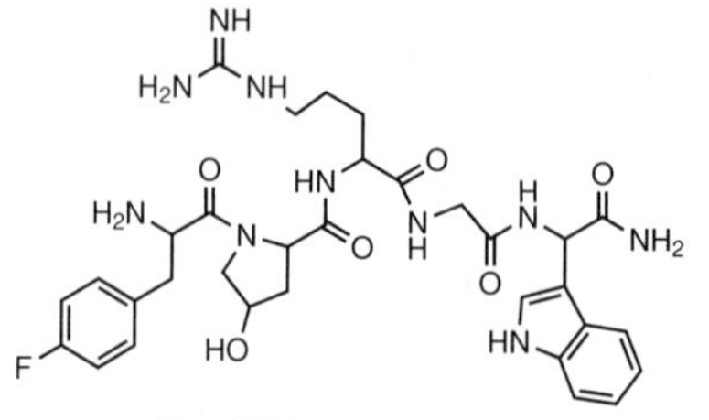

Nemifitide

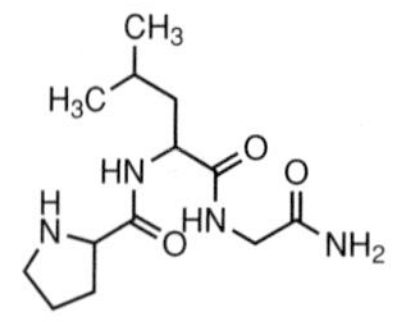

MIF-1

Herbal Therapy

In the past few years, much interest has been generated regarding the use of herbs in the treatment of both depression and anxiety (95). Recent studies, however, have revealed potentially fatal interactions between herbal remedies and traditional drugs.

St. John's wort (*Hypericum perforatum*), an herb used extensively in the treatment of mild to moderate depression in Europe, has aroused interest in the United States. A bushy, low-growing plant covered with yellow flowers in summer, St. John's wort has been used for centuries in many folk and herbal remedies. In Germany, hypericum is used in the treatment of depression more than any other antidepressant. The scientific studies that have been conducted regarding its use have been short-term, however, and have used several different doses. St. John's Wort works like the SSRIs, in that it not only increases the availability of 5-HT in synaptic clefts by blocking its reuptake but also increases the availability of NE, which increases energy and alertness, and dopamine, which increases the feeling of well-being.

Ingestion of St John's wort increases the expression (i.e., upregulation) of intestinal P-glycoprotein and of CYP3A4 in the liver and intestine, which impairs the absorption and stimulates the metabolism of other CYP3A4 substrates (e.g., the protease inhibitors indinavir and nevirapine, oral contraceptives, and TCAs [e.g., amitriptyline]), resulting in their subtherapeutic plasma levels. Hyperforin, the principal component in St. John's wort (2–4% in the fresh herb) contributes to the induction of CYP3A4. Furthermore, it not only inhibits the neuronal reuptake of 5-HT, NE, and dopamine, like many other antidepressants, but also inhibits GABA and L-glutamate uptake. This broad-spectrum effect is obtained by an elevation of the intracellular sodium ion concentration, probably resulting from activation of sodium conductive pathways not yet finally identified but most likely to be ionic channels. This makes hyperforin the first member of a new class of compounds with a preclinical antidepressant profile because of a completely novel mechanism of action (95,96). Hypericin, the other component in St. John's wort, also may exhibit inhibitor action on key neuroreceptors and may be responsible for the phototoxicity/photosensitivity of St. John's wort.

The National Institutes of Health conducted a double-blind, 3-year study in patients with major depression of moderate severity using St. John's wort and sertraline. This study did not support the use of St. John's wort in the treatment of major depression, but a possible role for St. John's wort in the treatment of milder forms of depression was suggested. Health care providers should alert their patients about potential drug interactions with St. John's Wort. Some other frequently used herbal supplements that have not been evaluated in large-scale clinical trials are ephedra, gingko biloba, echinacea, and ginseng. Any herbal supplement should be taken only after consultation with the physician or other health care provider.

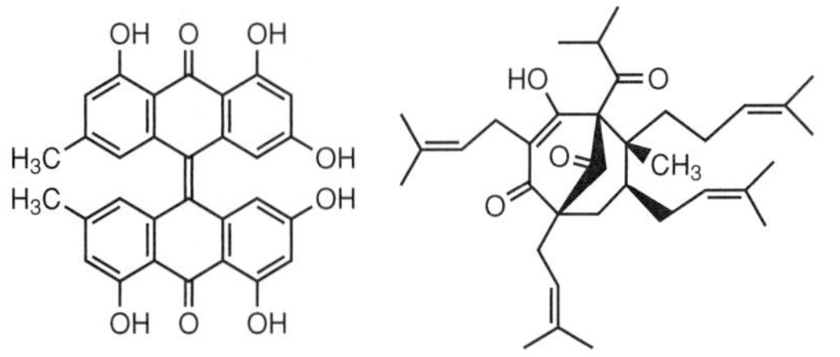

Hypericin Hyperforin

ELECTROCONVULSIVE THERAPY

Electroconvulsive therapy (ECT) has been in use since the late 1930s to treat a variety of severe mental illnesses, most notably major depression. Use of ECT is beneficial particularly for individuals whose depression is severe or life threatening or who cannot take antidepressant medication. Often, ECT is effective in cases where antidepressant drugs do not provide sufficient relief of symptoms.

Electroconvulsive therapy remains the "gold standard" for the treatment of major depression and a variety of other psychiatric and neurologic disorders (97). Because of the effectiveness and resurgence of ECT, more patients are considered to be good candidates for this treatment option. Overall, these patients are medication refractory and elderly and, thus, are more sensitive to polypharmacy. Additionally, these patients tend to have more coexisting medical problems.

In recent years, ECT has been much improved. A muscle relaxant is given before treatment, which is done under brief anesthesia. Electrodes are placed at precise locations on the head to deliver electrical impulses. The stimulation causes a brief (~30 seconds) seizure within the brain. The person receiving ECT does not consciously experience the electrical stimulus. For full therapeutic benefit, at least several sessions of ECT, typically given at the rate of three per week, are required. Electroconvulsive therapy appears to increase the sensitivity of postsynaptic 5-HT receptors and upregulation of 5-HT_{1A} postsynaptic receptors.

Side effects may result from the anesthesia, the ECT treatment, or both. Common side effects include temporary short-term memory loss, nausea, muscle aches, and headache. Some people may have longer-lasting problems with memory after ECT. Sometimes, a person's blood pressure or heart rhythm changes. If these changes occur, they are carefully watched during the ECT treatments and are immediately treated.

CASE STUDY

Victoria F. Roche And S. William Zito

NL is an 84-year-old female who had to move to a retirement community after losing her husband to a prolonged battle with cancer. She desperately misses her home and the life they shared there, and the move was made all the more devastating because of the need to find good homes for their beloved cats. NL has experienced symptoms of depression regularly during her adult life but never sought medical assistance until her husband fell ill. She has been taking escitalopram (Lexapro, 10 mg q.d.) for 3 years, although it has not totally controlled the despair and anxiety that she experiences, especially at night. After being off cigarettes for 20 years, she has started smoking again, which is adding to her distress. She is embarrassed by her need for antidepressant medication and finds it hard to talk with her physician about her feelings. Recently, she has become restless and agitated, both at bedtime and during the day, and is considering self-medicating with St. John's wort, which has been highly recommended by a member of the bridge club she has joined. She is in your pharmacy now, carrying a bottle of Kaopectate and trying to select a St. John's wort product.

NL has osteoporosis that is being managed with sodium alendronate (Fosamax), and fortunately, the recent falls she experienced after losing her balance on standing did not result in any broken bones. In addition to thyroid hormone replacement therapy, her other current medications include metoprolol for high blood pressure and clonazepam for restless leg syndrome. Turn your attention to the antidepressant choices shown below, and prepare to make a recommendation to NL and her physician.

1 Identify the therapeutic problem(s) in which the pharmacist's intervention may benefit the patient.
2. Identify and prioritize the patient-specific factors that must be considered to achieve the desired therapeutic outcomes.
3. Conduct a thorough and mechanistically oriented structure-activity analysis of all therapeutic alternatives provided in the case.
4. Evaluate the structure-activity relationship findings against the patient specific factors and desired therapeutic outcomes and make a therapeutic decision.
5. Counsel your patient.

Escitalopram Clonazepam Adendronate sodium Metoprolol

1 2 3 4

References

1. Depression. National Institutes of Health Publication 00-3561. 2000.
2. Real men; real depression. National Institutes of Health Publication 03-4972. 2003.
3. Depression—management of depression in primary and secondary care. Clinical Guideline 23. National Institute for Clinical Excellence (UK), December 2004.
4. Commonly requested therapeutic class and product information (update February 2006). Available at: 7 IMS Health.com. Accessed July 11, 2006.
5. Diagnostic and Statistical Manual of Mental Disorders, 4th Ed., Text Revision (DSM-IV-TR). Washington, DC: American Psychiatric Association, 2002.
6. Manji HK, Lenox RH. Signaling: cellular insights into the pathophysiology of bipolar disorder. Biol Psychiatry 2000 48:518–530.
7. Duman RS, Heninger GR, Nestler EJ. A molecular and cellular theory of depression. Arch Gen Psychiatry 1997;54:597–606.
8. Schildkraut JJ, Klerman GL, Hammond R, et al. Excretion of 3-methoxy-mandelic acid (VMA) in depressed patients treated with antidepressant drugs. J Psychiatr Res 1965;2:257–266.
9. van Praag HK, Korf J. Endogenous depression with and without disturbance of 5-hydroxytryptamine metabolism: a biochemical classification? Psychopharmacology 1971;19:148–152.
10. Coppen A, Prange AJ Jr, Whybrow PC, et al. Abnormalities of indoleamines in affective disorders. Arch Gen Psychiat 1972;26:474–478.
11. Lenox RH, Frazer A. Mechanism of action of antidepressants and mood stabilizers. In: Davis KL, Charney D, Coyle JT, et al., eds. Neuropsychopharmacology: The Fifth Generation of Progress. Baltimore: Lippincott Williams & Wilkins, 2002;1139–1164.
12. Brown AS, Gershon S. Dopamine and depression. J Neural Transm 1993;91:75–109.
13. Shopsin B, Gershon S, Goldstein M, et al. Use of synthesis inhibitors in defining a role for biogenic amines during imipramine treatment in depressed patients. Psychopharmacol Commun 1975;1:239–249.
14. Shopsin B, Friedman, E, Gershon S. Parachlorphenylalanine reversal of tranylcypromine effects in depressed patients. Arch Gen Psychiatry 1976;33:811–819.
15. Mitchell AJ. The role of corticotropin-releasing factor in depressive illness: a critical review Neurosci Biobehav Rev 1998;22:635–651.
16. Kuhn R. Uber Die Behandlung Depressives Zustande Mit Einem Iminobenzylderivat (G 22,355). Schweiz Med Wschr 1957;87:1135–1140.
17. Loomer HP, Saunders JC, Kline NS. A clinical and pharmacodynamic evaluation of iproniazid as a psychic energizer. Psychiatr Res Rep Am Psychiatr Assoc 1957;8:129–141.
18. Baldessarini RJ. Drug therapy of depression and anxiety disorders. In: Brunton LL, Lazo JS, Parker KL eds. Goodman & Gilman's The Pharmacological Basis of Therapeutics, 11th Ed. New York: McGraw-Hill, 2006; 429–460.
19. Hogberg T, Ulff B, Renyi AL, et al. Synthesis of pyridylallylamines related to zimelidine and their inhibition of neuronal monoamine uptake. J Med Chem 1981;24:1499–1507.
20. Ogren SO, Ross SB, Hall H, et al. The pharmacology of zimelidine: a 5-HT selective reuptake inhibitor. Acta Psychiatr Scand Suppl 1981;290: 127–151.
21. Wong DT, Bymaster FP, Horng JS, et al. A new selective inhibitor for uptake of serotonin into synaptosomes of rat brain: 3-(p-trifluoromethylphenoxy). N-methyl-3-phenylpropylamine. J Pharmacol Exp Ther 1975;193:804–811.
22. Wong DT, Bymaster FP, Engleman EA. Prozac (Fluoxetine, Lilly 110140), the first selective serotonin uptake inhibitor and an antidepressant drug: twenty years since its first publication. Life Sci 1995;57:411–441.
23. Skolnick P, Popik P, Janowsky A, et al. "Broad spectrum" antidepressants: is more better for the treatment of depression? Life Sci 2003;73:3175–3179.
24. Skolnick P, Popik P, Janowsky A, et al. Antidepressant-like actions of DOV 21,947: a "triple" reuptake inhibitor. Eur J Pharmacol 2003;461:99–104.
25. Glick SD, Haskew RE, Maisonneuve IM, et al. Enantioselective behavioral effects of sibutramine metabolites. Eur J Pharmacol 2000;397:93–102.
26. Torres GE, Gainetdinov RR, Caron MG. Plasma membrane monoamine transporters: structure, regulation, and function. Nat Rev Neurosci 2003;4: 13–25.
27. Owens MJ, Morgan WN, Plott SJ, et al. Neurotransmitter receptor and transporter binding profile of antidepressants and their metabolites. J Pharmacol Exp Ther 1997;283:1305–1322.
28. Hyttel J. Pharmacological characterization of selective serotonin reuptake inhibitors (SSRIs). Int Clin Psychopharmacol 1994;9(Suppl 1):19–26.
29. Sanchez C, Hyttel J. Comparison of the effects of antidepressants and their metabolites on reuptake of biogenic amines and on receptor binding. Cell Mol Neurobiol 1999;19:467–489.

30. Brunello N, Mendlewicz J, Kasper S, et al. The role of noradrenaline and selective noradrenaline reuptake inhibition in depression. Eur Neuropsychopharmacol 2002;12:461–475.
31. Kelder J, Funke C, De Boer T, et al. A comparison of the physicochemical and biological properties of mirtazapine and mianserin. J Pharm Pharmacol 1997;49:403–411.
32. Baker GB, Prior TI. Stereochemistry and drug efficacy and development: relevance of chirality to antidepressant and antipsychotic drugs. Ann Med 2002;34:537–543.
33. Lane RM, Baker GB. Chirality and drugs used in psychiatry: nice to know or need to know? Cell Mol Neurobiol 1999;19:355–372.
34. Venkatakrishnan K, Von Moltke LL, Greenblatt DJ. Human drug metabolism and the cytochromes P450: application and relevance of in vitro models. J Clin Pharmacol 2001;41:1149–1179.
35. Weiss J, Dormann SM, Martin-Facklam M, et al. Inhibition of P-glycoprotein by newer antidepressants. J Pharmacol Exp Ther 2003;305:197–204.
36. Ekins S, Kim RB, Leake BF, et al. Three-dimensional quantitative structure–activity relationships of inhibitors of P-glycoprotein. Mol Pharmacol 2002;61:964–973.
37. Preskorn SH. Clinically relevant pharmacology of selective serotonin reuptake inhibitors. An overview with emphasis on pharmacokinetics and effects on oxidative drug metabolism. Clin Pharmacokinet 1997;32(Suppl 1):1–21.
38. Sadeque AJ, Wandel C, He H, et al. Increased drug delivery to the brain by P-glycoprotein inhibition. Clin Pharmacol Ther 2000;68:231–237.
39. Eriksson E. Antidepressant drugs: does it matter if they inhibit the reuptake of noradrenaline or serotonin? Acta Psychiatr Scand Suppl 2000;402:12–17.
40. Norregaard L, Gether U. The monoamine neurotransmitter transporters: structure, conformational changes, and molecular gating. Curr Opin Drug Discov Dev 2001;4:591–601.
41. Casarotto MG, Craik DJ. Ring flexibility within tricyclic antidepressant drugs. J Pharm Sci 2001;90:713–721.
42. Fleishaker JC. Clinical pharmacokinetics of reboxetine, a selective norepinephrine reuptake inhibitor for the treatment of patients with depression. Clin Pharmacokinet 2000;39:413–427.
43. Wienkers LC, Allievi C, Hauer MJ, et al. Cytochrome P-450–mediated metabolism of the individual enantiomers of the antidepressant agent reboxetine in human liver microsomes. Drug Metab Dispos 1999;27:1334–1340.
44. Bergmann JF, Laneury JP, Duchene P, et al. Pharmacokinetics of reboxetine in healthy, elderly volunteers. Eur J Drug Metab Pharmacokinet 2000;25: 195–198.
45. Zerbe RL, Rowe H, Enas GG, et al. Clinical pharmacology of tomoxetine, a potential antidepressant. J Pharmacol Exp Ther 1985;232:139–143.
46. Sauer JM, Ponsler GD, Mattiuz EL, et al. Disposition and metabolic fate of atomoxetine hydrochloride: the role of CYP2D6 in human disposition and metabolism. Drug Metab Dispos 2003;31:98–107.
47. Cowen PJ. Serotonin hypothesis. In: Feighner JP, Boyer WR, eds. Selective Serotonin Reuptake Inhibitors, 2nd Ed. 1996;63–86.
48. Preskorn SH. Clinical pharmacology of SSRIs. Available at: http://www.preskorn.com. Accessed August 3, 2004.
49. Bordet R, Thomas P, Dupuis B. Effect of pindolol on onset of action of paroxetine in the treatment of major depression: intermediate analysis of a double-blind, placebo-controlled trial. Reseau de Recherche et d'Experimentation Psychopharmacologique. Am J Psychiatr 1998;155:1346–1351.
50. Brosen K, Rasmussen BB. Selective Serotonin Reuptake Inhibitors: Pharmacokinetics and Drug Interactions. In: Feighner JP, Boyer WR, eds. Selective Serotonin Reuptake Inhibitors, 2nd Ed. 1996;87–108.
51. Shih JC, Chen K, Ridd MJ. MAO: from genes to behavior. Annu Rev Neurosci 1999;22:197–217.
52. Olivier B, Soudjin W, van Wijngaarden I. Serotonin, dopamine, and norepinephrine transporters in the CNS and their inhibitors. In: Jucker E, ed. Progress in Drug Research, vol 54. Basel, Switzerland: Birkhäuser-Verlag, 2000;59–120.
53. Wong DT, Threlkeld PG, Robertson DW. Affinities of fluoxetine, its enantiomers, and other inhibitors of serotonin uptake for subtypes of serotonin receptors. Neuropsychopharmacology 1991;5:43–47.
54. Frazer A, Benmansour S. Delayed pharmacological effects of antidepressants. Mol Psychiatry 2002;7(Suppl 1):S23–S28.
55. Wong DT, Bymaster FP, Reid LR, et al. Norfluoxetine enantiomers as inhibitors of serotonin uptake in rat brain. Neuropsychopharmacology 1993;8:337–344.
56. Bertelsen KM, Venkatakrishnan K, Von Moltke LL, et al. Apparent mechanism-based inhibition of human CYP2D6 in vitro by paroxetine: comparison with fluoxetine and quinidine. Drug Metab Dispos 2003;31:289–293.
57. Nakajima M, Suzuki M, Yamaji R, et al. Isoform selective inhibition and inactivation of human cytochrome P450s by methylenedioxyphenyl compounds. Xenobiotica 1999;29:1191–1202.
58. Bolton JL, Acay NM, Vukomanovic V. Evidence that 4-allyl-o-quinones spontaneously rearrange to their more electrophilic quinone methides: potential bioactivation mechanism for the hepatocarcinogen safrole. Chem Res Toxicol 1994;7:443–450.
59. Sanchez C, Bogeso KP, Ebert B, et al. Escitalopram versus citalopram: the surprising role of the R-enantiomer. Psychopharmacology 2004;174:163–176.
60. Owens MJ, Knight DL, Nemeroff CB. Second-generation SSRIs: human monoamine transporter binding profile of escitalopram and R-fluoxetine. Biol Psychiatry. 2001;50:345–350.
61. Haritos VS, Ghabrial H, Ahokas JT, et al. Role of cytochrome P450 2D6 (CYP2D6) in the stereospecific metabolism of E- and Z-doxepin. Pharmacogenetics 2000;10:591–603.
62. Yan JH, Hubbard JW, McKay G, et al. Absolute bioavailability and stereoselective pharmacokinetics of doxepin. Xenobiotica 2002;32:615–623.
63. Eap CB, Bender S, Gastpar M, et al. Steady-state plasma levels of the enantiomers of trimipramine and of its metabolites in CYP2D6-, CYP2C19-, and CYP3A4/5-phenotyped patients. Ther Drug Monit 2000;22:209–214.
64. Kirchheiner J, Muller G, Meineke I, et al. Effects of polymorphisms in CYP2D6, CYP2C9, and CYP2C19 on trimipramine pharmacokinetics. J Clin Psychopharmacol 2003;23:459–466.
65. Lancaster SG, Gonzalez JP. Dothiepin: a review of its pharmacodynamic and pharmacokinetic properties, and therapeutic efficacy in depressive illness. Drugs 1989;38:123–147.
66. Lancaster SG, Gonzalez JP. Lofepramine: a review of its pharmacodynamic and pharmacokinetic properties, and therapeutic efficacy in depressive illness. Drugs 1989;37:123–140.
67. Wong DT, Bymaster FP. Dual serotonin and noradrenaline uptake inhibitor class of antidepressants potential for greater efficacy or just hype? Prog Drug Res 2002;58:169-222.
68. Bymaster FP, Dreshfield-Ahmad LJ, Threlkeld PG, et al. Comparative affinity of duloxetine and venlafaxine for serotonin and norepinephrine transporters in vitro and in vivo, human serotonin receptor subtypes, and other neuronal receptors. Neuropsychopharmacology 2001;25:871–880.
69. Vaishnavi SN, Nemeroff CB, Plott SJ, et al. Milnacipran: a comparative analysis of human monoamine uptake and transporter binding affinity. Biol Psychiatry 2004;55:320–322.
70. Puozzo C, Panconi E, Deprez D. Pharmacology and pharmacokinetics of milnacipran. Int Clin Psychopharmacol 2002;17(Suppl 1):S25–S35.
71. Lantz RJ, Gillespie TA, Rash TJ, et al.. Metabolism, excretion, and pharmacokinetics of duloxetine in healthy human subjects. Drug Metab Dispos 2003;31:1142–1150.
72. Haustein KO. Bupropion: pharmacological and clinical profile in smoking cessation. Int J Clin Pharmacol Ther 2003;41:56–66.
73. Warner C, Shoaib M. How does bupropion work as a smoking cessation aid? Addict Biol 2005;10:219–231.
74. Hesse LM, Venkatakrishnan K, Court MH, et al. CYP2B6 mediates the in vitro hydroxylation of bupropion: potential drug interactions with other antidepressants. Drug Metab Dispos 2000;28:1176–1183.
75. Rotzinger S, Fang J, Baker GB. Trazodone is metabolized to m-chlorophenylpiperazine by CYP3A4 from human sources. Drug Metab Dispos 1998;26:572–575.
76. Rotzinger S, Baker GB. Human CYP3A4 and the metabolism of nefazodone and hydroxynefazodone by human liver microsomes and heterologously expressed enzymes. Eur Neuropsychopharmacol 2002;12:91–100.
77. Stormer E, von Moltke LL, Shader RI, et al. Metabolism of the antidepressant mirtazapine in vitro: contribution of cytochromes P-450 1A2, 2D6, and 3A4. Drug Metab Dispos 2000;28:1168–1175.
78. Baker GB, Urichuk LJ, McKenna KF, et al. Metabolism of monoamine oxidase inhibitors. Cell Mol Neurobiol 1999;19:411–426.
79. Bonnet U. Moclobemide: evolution, pharmacodynamic, and pharmacokinetic properties. CNS Drug Rev 2002;8:283–308.
80. Harwood AJ. Neurodevelopment and mood stabilizers. Curr Mol Med 2003;3:472–482.
81. Harwood AJ, Agam G. Search for a common mechanism of mood stabilizers. Biochem Pharmacol 2003;66:179–189.
82. Benjamin J, Agam G, Levine J, et al. Inositol treatment in psychiatry. Psychopharmacol Bull 1995;31:167–175.
83. Berridge MJ. The Albert Lasker Medical Awards. Inositol trisphosphate, calcium, lithium, and cell signaling. JAMA 1989;262:1834–1841.
84. Lenox RH, Wang L. Molecular basis of lithium action: integration of lithium-responsive signaling and gene expression networks. Mol Psychiatry 2003;8:135–144.
85. Paul IA, Skolnick P. Glutamate and depression: clinical and preclinical studies. Ann N Y Acad Sci 2003;1003:250–272.
86. Skolnick P. Modulation of glutamate receptors: strategies for the development of novel antidepressants. Amino Acids 2002;23:153–159.
87. Ono S, Ogawa K, Yamashita K, et al. Conformational analysis of the NMDA receptor antagonist (1S,2R)-1-phenyl-2-[S-1-aminopropyl]-N,N-diethylcyclopropanecarboxamide (PPDC) designed by a novel conformational restriction method based on the structural feature of cyclopropane ring. Chem Pharm Bull (Tokyo). 2002;50:966–968.
88. Holmes A, Heilig M, Rupniak NM, et al. Neuropeptide systems as novel therapeutic targets for depression and anxiety disorders. Trends Pharmacol Sci 2003;24:580–588.
89. Hokfelt T, Bartfai T, Bloom F. Neuropeptides: opportunities for drug discovery. Lancet Neurol 2003;2:463–472.
90. De Souza EB, Grigoriadis DE. Corticotropin-releasing factor: physiology, pharmacology, and role in central nervous system disorders. In: Davis KL,

Charney D, Coyle JT, et al., eds. Neuropsychopharmacology: The Fifth Generation of Progress. Baltimore: Lippincott Williams & Wilkins, 2002;91–109.
91. Kramer MS, Cutler N, Feighner J, et al. Distinct mechanism for antidepressant activity by blockade of central substance P receptors. Science 1998;281: 1640–1645.
92. Vrontakis ME. Galanin: a biologically active peptide. Curr Drug Targets CNS Neurol Disord 2002;1:531–541.
93. Feighner JP, Nicolau G, Abajian H, et al. Clinical pharmacokinetic studies with INN 00835 (nemifitide), a novel pentapeptide antidepressant. Biopharm Drug Dispos 2002;23:33–39.
94. Ehrensing RH, Kastin AJ, Wurzlow GF, et al. Improvement in major depression after low subcutaneous doses of MIF-1. J Affect Disord 1994;31:227–233.
95. Ioannides C. Pharmacokinetic interactions between herbal remedies and medicinal drugs. Xenobiotica 2002;32:451–478.
96. Muller WE, Singer A, Wonnemann M. Hyperforin—antidepressant activity by a novel mechanism of action. Pharmacopsychiatry 2001;34(Suppl 1): S98–S102.
97. Christopher EJ. Electroconvulsive therapy in the medically ill. Curr Psychiatry Rep 2003;5:225–230.

22. *Psychotherapeutic Drugs: Antipsychotic and Anxiolytic Agents*

RAYMOND G. BOOTH

DRUGS COVERED IN THIS CHAPTER:

PHENOTHIAZINE CLASS

THIOXANTHINES CLASS

BENZAMIDE CLASS

BENZAZEPINES
- Clozapine
- Loxapine
- Olanzapine
- Quetiapine

BENZISOXAZOLE AND BENZISOTHIAZOLES
- Risperidone
- Ziprasidone

MISCELLANEOUS ANTIPSYCHOTIC AGENTS
- Aripiprazole
- Molindone
- Sertindole

BENZODIAZEPINES
- Chlordiazepoxide
- Diazepam
- Flurazepam
- Oxazepam

MISCELLANEOUS ANXIOLYTIC AGENTS
- Eszopiclone
- Zalpidem
- Zolpidem

OVERVIEW OF MENTAL ILLNESSES

Mental illnesses that can be treated with psychotropic drugs are broadly categorized as psychoses, neuroses, and mood (depression, bipolar) disorders. Different classes of psychotropic agents differ in their ability to modify symptoms of these mental illnesses; thus, an appropriate diagnosis is critical to selecting an efficacious psychotropic drug. This chapter is focused on the medicinal chemistry of drugs that are used to treat psychosis and anxiety disorders. The definitive diagnostic criteria for psychiatric disorders in the United States are well described in the *Diagnostic and Statistical Manual of Mental Disorders of the American Psychiatric Association* (DSM-IV-TR) (1). The psychoses (e.g., schizophrenia) are among the most severe mental illnesses and commonly include symptoms of delusions and sensory hallucinations. In anxiety disorders (neuroses), the ability to comprehend reality is retained, but mood changes (anxiety, panic, dysphoria) and thought (obsessions, irrational fears) and behavioral (rituals, compulsions, avoidance) dysfunction can be disabling. Mood and panic disorders usually include dysfunction of the autonomic nervous system (e.g., altered patterns of sleep and appetite) in addition to psychic abnormalities. Depression can lead to self-harm and suicide. In general, antipsychotic agents, which can have severe neurological side effects, should be used to treat only the most severe mental illnesses (i.e., psychoses such as schizophrenia).

SCHIZOPHRENIA

Definition

An historical definition of schizophrenia may begin approximately 100 years ago, with the German psychiatrist Emil Kraepelin's description of a type of dementia that was characterized as a severe, chronic mental disorder without known external causation wherein functional deterioration progresses with the symptoms of hallucinations, delusions, thought disorder, incoherence, blunted affect, negativism, stereotyped behavior, and lack of insight (2). The deterioration progresses to catatonia and hebephrenia (illogical, incoherent, and senseless thought processes and actions, delusions, and hallucinations). Meanwhile, the Swiss psychiatrist Eugen Bleuler coined the term "schizophrenia" to take into account the perceived "schism" or splitting in mental functioning (3).

A modern definition of schizophrenia comes from DMS-IV (1). The diagnostic criteria for schizophrenia require two or more of the following characteristic symptoms to be present for a significant proportion of time during a 1-month period: delusions, hallucinations, disorganized speech, or grossly disorganized or catatonic behavior. There is, however, flexibility in the diagnostic criteria that leaves room for professional psychiatric judgment. For example, it is enough if hallucinations consist of a voice maintaining a running commentary on the patient's behavior or there are two or more voices that converse with each other. Also, for a significant proportion of time, one or more areas of social functioning, such as work, interpersonal relationships, or self-care, are markedly below the level achieved before the onset of symptoms. Continuous symptoms must persist for 6 months. Finally, before a diagnosis of schizophrenia is made, affective disorders as well as, drug/alcohol abuse or other medical conditions must be ruled out.

Etiology of Schizophrenia

A neurobiological basis for schizophrenia and related psychotic syndromes remains elusive. Compelling evidence linking genetic factors to the etiology of schizophrenia is not apparent despite enormous progress in

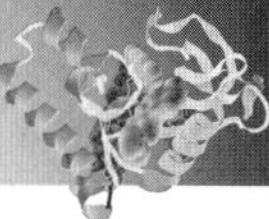

CLINICAL SIGNIFICANCE

There is probably no greater contribution to morbidity in life than those disorders that affect the mind. The burden of depression, psychosis, anxiety, and other related disorders take a significant toll on individuals and society as a whole. The ability to effectively address these maladies in clinical practice relies on an understanding of neuropharmacology and the chemical characteristics of psychotropic agents used to treat patients. Although certain agents may be effective, they also may convey significant adverse effects. Case in point, 25 years ago we had effective agents to treat psychosis. Their effectiveness came at a high price, however, because in many patients, these agents produced severe extrapyramidal symptoms. As the understanding of neuropharmacology and structure–activity relationship evolved, the introduction of atypical antipsychotics to the treatment armamentarium came about. The ability of these agents to influence serotonergic and dopaminergic activity is thought by many to convey additional effectiveness while limiting extrapyramidal symptoms. Consequently, these agents have revolutionized the treatment of psychosis and related disorders. As a class, the atypical antipsychotics are fairly heterogeneous, and clinicians may choose certain agents based on their activities at various receptors. As you read this chapter, pay particular attention to the receptor affinity of all the psychotropic agents and how it is thought to translate into effectiveness and/or toxicity. This will help you in your practice to make rational treatment decisions based on inherent characteristics of these agents, their performance in clinical trials, and your clinical understanding of the patient.

David Hayes, Pharm.D.
Clinical Assistant Professor
Department of Clinical Sciences & Administration
University of Houston College of Pharmacy

the field of molecular genetics and numerous investigations of hereditary factors associated with psychotic illnesses. Current epidemiological evidence suggests that individual variation in susceptibility to schizophrenia involves alleles of moderate to small effect in multiple genes. Investigations of environmental causative factors have focused on prenatal and perinatal risk factors for brain damage. For example, studies have examined the incidence of schizophrenics who were born under conditions of obstetrical complications, influenza epidemics, food shortages, and Rh factor incompatibility. Neuroanatomical hypotheses include increased ventricular volume; however, neuropathological changes associated with schizophrenic brains are not obvious as in, for example, Parkinson's disease. In contrast, neurochemical abnormalities are well documented. Alterations of brain dopaminergic neurotransmission in psychoses have been studied for more than 30 years, and this field of psychobiological research generally revolves around the "dopamine hypothesis" of schizophrenia.

The connection between dopaminergic neurotransmission and schizophrenia is an example of a "pharmacocentric" approach to characterizing the etiology and neuropathology of mental illnesses (4–6). The dopamine hypothesis of schizophrenia arose from observations that the first relatively safe and effective antipsychotic drugs, the phenothiazines, such as chlorpromazine, used in the early 1950s affected brain dopamine metabolism (7). Simply put, the dopamine hypothesis of schizophrenia suggests that schizophrenia results from increased dopaminergic neurotransmission and that approaches which decrease dopaminergic neurotransmission will alleviate psychotic symptoms (8). Most antipsychotic agents have activity to limit dopaminergic neurotransmission, providing some indirect evidence to support the dopamine hypothesis of schizophrenia. In a seminal study by Seeman et al. (9), the average daily dose of antipsychotic was found to correlate well with affinity for dopamine D_2-type receptors. Moreover, extrapyramidal side effects of antipsychotic drugs certainly correlates with their dopamine D_2 antagonism effect. It should be noted, however, that functional interaction of antipsychotic drugs with the D_2 receptor is complex, involving antagonism, inverse agonism, and partial agonism. For example, recent studies show that essentially all clinically used antipsychotic drugs are D_2 inverse agonists (10), suggesting that biochemical as well as clinical effects may not be explained by simple blockade of agonist (dopamine) access to the D_2 receptor.

The dopamine hypothesis of schizophrenia and pharmacotherapy involving antagonism of dopamine receptors (especially the D_2-type) has dominated research directions, but it should be noted that the entire argument is somewhat circular. Consideration of potential new drugs as antipsychotic agents usually is limited to compounds that have demonstrated behavioral or biochemical evidence of antidopaminergic actions. Of course, this somewhat conservative and exclusive approach is practical considering the lack of proven alternative neuropharmacological explanations of antipsychotic drug activity. Nevertheless, in light of the nearly 50 years of research focusing on brain dopaminergic systems, uncontested evidence linking the etiology of psychotic illnesses to the neurobiology of dopaminergic systems has remained elusive. Alternative explanations, especially those involving adrenergic and serotonergic receptor systems, probably will gain popularity as more atypical antipsychotic drugs (e.g., clozapine) are introduced and also found to have actions at these receptor systems, perpetuating and expanding the pharmacocentric approach to antipsychotic drug design and development.

Role of Dopamine Receptors in Schizophrenia

Modern molecular biological methods involving recombinant DNA techniques have led to cloning and characterization of five different dopamine receptors: D_1 (446 amino acids), $D_{2\ short}$ (414 amino acids) and $D_{2\ long}$ (443 amino acids), D_3 (400 amino acids), D_4 (387 amino acids), and D_5 (477 amino acids) [for a review, see Hartman and Civelli (11)]. The amino acid sequence, as deduced from their established nucleotide sequence, shows that dopamine receptors are a member of the G protein–coupled receptor (GPCR) superfamily that is structurally characterized by a 7-transmembrane-spanning region. Currently, no medicinal chemical probes with high selectivity to distinguish between the five subtypes are available; thus, dopamine receptors often are classified as two major types, according to the functional effect on adenylyl cyclase (12): The D_1-types that stimulate adenylyl cyclase are D_1 and D_5; the D_2-types that inhibit adenylyl cyclase are $D_{2\ short}$, $D_{2\ long}$, D_3, and D_4.

Several chemical probes are available that can distinguish between the general D_1-type and D_2-type receptor families (Fig. 22.1). The R-(+)-isomer of the benzazepine derivative, SKF 38393, is used for research as a selective D_1-type partial agonist. Meanwhile, the structurally related benzazepine derivative, R-(+)-SCH 23390, is used as a selective D_1-type receptor antagonist. Although not very selective for D_1-type over D_2-type receptors, the rigid benzophenanthridine derivative (−)-dihydrexidine is a useful research tool, because it is a D_1-type full efficacy agonist (produces stimulation of adenylyl cyclase equivalent to dopamine itself) (13,14). Selective D_2-type full agonists, such as the pyrazole derivative (−)-quinpirole, and D_2-type antagonists, such as (−)-sulpiride, also are available to researchers. Currently, the dopamine D_3 receptor subtype is of particular neuropharmacological interest because of its preferential distribution in certain limbic regions of mammalian brain, notably in the nucleus accumbens of the basal forebrain. It is proposed that highly D_3-selective drugs might be developed as antipsychotic agents with preferential limbic antidopaminergic actions while sparing the extrapyramidal basal ganglia, presumably decreasing the neurological movement disorder side effects associated with antipsychotic drug therapy (vide infra). The tetrahydronaphthalene, (+)-7-hydroxy-N,N-di-n-propyl-2-aminotetralin (7-OH-DPAT), and some of its congeners are particularly promising D_3-selective lead agents. The benzazepine clozapine, which is proposed to have a superior antipsychotic clinical profile with a low incidence of extrapyramidal side effects, shows relatively greater affinity for the D_4 dopamine receptor subtype in addition to its relatively high affinity for serotonin 5-HT_2, adrenergic α_1 and α_2, muscarinic M_1, and histamine H_1 receptors (15).

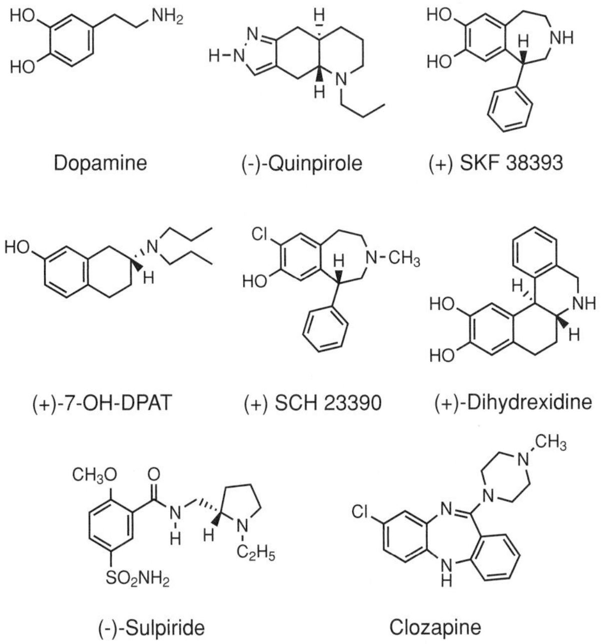

Dopamine (-)-Quinpirole (+) SKF 38393

(+)-7-OH-DPAT (+) SCH 23390 (+)-Dihydrexidine

(-)-Sulpiride Clozapine

Fig. 22.1. Structures of compounds useful for characterizing dopamine receptors.

Dopamine Receptors and Functional Selectivity

It is now realized that the same GPCR can couple to different Gα proteins to result in "multifunctional" signaling (16). Molecular mechanisms to account for GPCR multifunctional signaling involve the concept of "GPCR permissiveness," which assumes a high degree of flexibility in the interactions between a ligand, receptor, and G protein (17). These interactions occur mainly between the G proteins and the second and third intracellular loops and carboxy-terminal tail of the receptor. Some factors that influence this interaction include receptor:G protein ratios and amounts, alternative GPCR splicing, and conformational changes in the G protein and/or receptor. A critical assumption of GPCR multifunctional signaling theory is that a heterogeneity of active receptor conformations exists and that agonist ligands differ in their ability to induce, stabilize, or select among receptor conformations, as described in the "stimulus trafficking" hypothesis (18). Of particular relevance to the medicinal chemist, it follows that on binding, agonist ligand chemical structural parameters are among the most important determinants of GPCR conformation that influences type of Gα protein and signaling pathway activated. Thus, ligand stereochemistry or other more subtle structural parameters may influence GPCR conformation to affect the type of G protein and intracellular signaling pathway activated, resulting in ligand-specific functional outcomes (19,20). Ligands that show such "functional selectivity" (21–23) can be exploited for drug design purposes. A

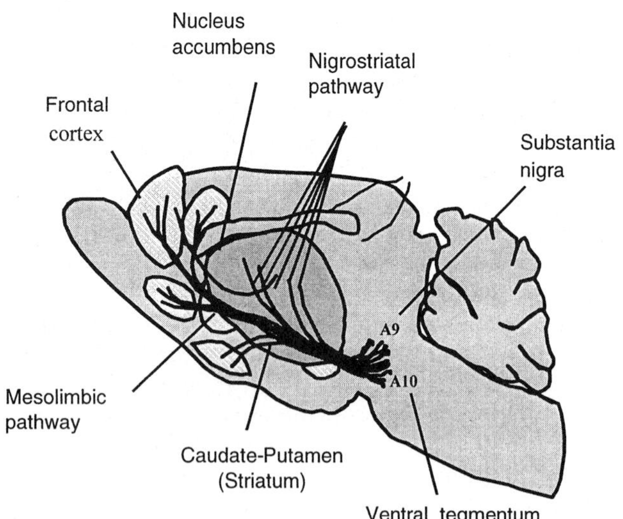

Fig. 22.2. Some dopamine pathways in mammalian brain.

clinically relevant example is the antipsychotic drug aripiprazole, which interacts with the dopamine D_2 receptor to produce antagonist, inverse agonist, or agonist functional effects, depending on the D_2 receptor cellular milieu (e.g., G-protein complement and concentration) and particular location (e.g., presynaptic vs. postsynaptic and extrapyramidal vs. limbic brain regions).

The dopamine D_1-type and D_2-type receptor families are differentially distributed in mammalian forebrain dopaminergic pathways. The extrapyramidal nigrostriatal pathway, which plays a key role in locomotor coordination, consists of neurons with cell bodies in the A9 pars compacta of the substantia nigra in the midbrain. These neurons project to the basal ganglia structures caudate nucleus and putamen (collectively referred to as striatum) in the forebrain (Fig. 22.2). Degeneration of neurons in the nigrostriatal pathway is the hallmark pathological feature of Parkinson's disease, clinically manifested as bradykinesia, muscular rigidity, resting tremor, and impairment of postural balance. Blockade of dopamine receptors on cholinergic neurons in striatum is associated with the sometimes severe extrapyramidal, parkinsonian-like side effects (muscular rigidity, bradykinesia, akathisia) that frequently occur with antipsychotic drug treatment.

The mesolimbic and mesocortical pathway, involved in integration of emotions, behaviors, and higher thought processes, consists of neurons with cell bodies in the A10 ventral tegmentum. These neurons project to limbic forebrain structures, including the nucleus accumbens and amygdala, and to higher levels of cerebral function, such as the frontal cortex (Fig. 22.2). According to the dopamine hypothesis, increased dopaminergic neurotransmission in limbic pathways contributes to the "positive" symptoms (e.g., hallucinations and excited delusional behavior that can be reduced with typical antipsychotic drugs) but not necessarily to the "negative" symptoms (e.g., catatonia) observed in the clinical manifestation of schizophrenia.

Typical antipsychotic drugs act in both extrapyramidal and limbic brain regions at D_2-type dopamine receptors that can be located postsynaptically (on cell bodies, dendrites, and nerve terminals of other neurons) as well as presynaptically on dopamine neurons. Dopamine receptors located presynaptically on dopamine cell bodies and nerve terminals are called autoreceptors and act to negatively modulate neuronal firing and dopamine synthesis and release (Fig. 22.3) (24). Low concentrations of certain

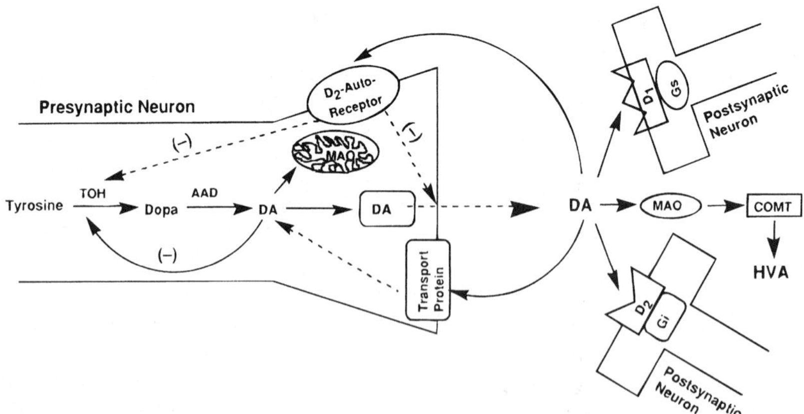

Fig. 22.3. Tyrosine is hydroxylated in a rate-limiting step by tyrosine hydroxylase (TOH) to form dihydroxylphenylalanine (DOPA), which is decarboxylated by L-aromatic amino acid decarboxylase (AAD) to form dopamine (DA). Newly synthesized DA is stored in vesicles, from which release occurs into the synaptic cleft by depolarization of the presynaptc neuron in the presence of Ca^{2+}. The DA released into the synaptic cleft may go on to stimulate postsynaptic D_1- and D_2-type autoreceptors that negatively modulate DA synthesis (via inhibition of TOH) and release. The action of synaptic DA is inactivated largely via reaccumulation into the presynaptic neuron by high-affinity DA neurotransport proteins located on the nerve terminal membrane. Free cytoplasmic DA negatively modulates DA synthesis via end-product (feedback) inhibition of TOH by competition with biopterin cofactor. Cytoplasmic pools of DA may undergo metabolic deamination by monoamine oxidase (MAO), an enzyme bound to the outer membrane of mitochondria, to form dihydroxyphenylacetaldehyde, which oxides to didydroxyphenylacetate (DOPAC). The DA or DOPAC may undergo methylation by catechol-O-methyltransferase (COMT), ultimately forming homovanillic acid (HVA), a metabolite excreted in urine.

dopamine agonists can stereospecifically activate dopamine D_2-type autoreceptors to decrease dopamine synthesis (25,26) and release (27), thus reducing dopaminergic neurotransmission. Therefore, consistent with the dopamine hypothesis of schizophrenia, selective dopamine autoreceptor agonists could, theoretically, be pharmacotherapeutic agents in schizophrenia and related mental illnesses. In fact, activation of dopamine autoreceptors may form an integral part of the therapeutic action of the most recently developed antipsychotic drugs, such as the D_2 receptor partial agonist aripiprazole (28).

In addition to postsynaptic dopamine receptors and presynaptic dopamine D_2-type autoreceptors, heteroreceptors, such as adenosine (A_2) (29), histamine (H_1) (30,31), and serotonin ($5\text{-}HT_{1A}$) (32), located on or near presynaptic dopaminergic nerve terminals in the striatum (extrapyramidal) or nucleus accumbens (limbic) regions of brain can modulate dopamine synthesis (and release) by altering the activity of tyrosine hydroxylase, the rate-limiting step in catecholamine biosynthesis. Similarly, activation of adrenergic (α_2) autoreceptors in the limbic structure hippocampus negatively modulates the release of the neurotransmitter norepinephrine (33). It is proposed that atypical antipsychotic drugs, such as clozapine, may interact with these other neurotransmitter receptor systems (i.e., histamine, serotonin, and adrenergic) instead of (or in addition to) dopamine receptor systems. Preceding the introduction of the first clinically successful phenothiazine-type neuroleptic, chlorpromazine, the first phenothiazine to be used to treat psychiatric patients in the 1940s (unsuccessfully) was promethazine, an "antihistamine" H_1 antagonist.

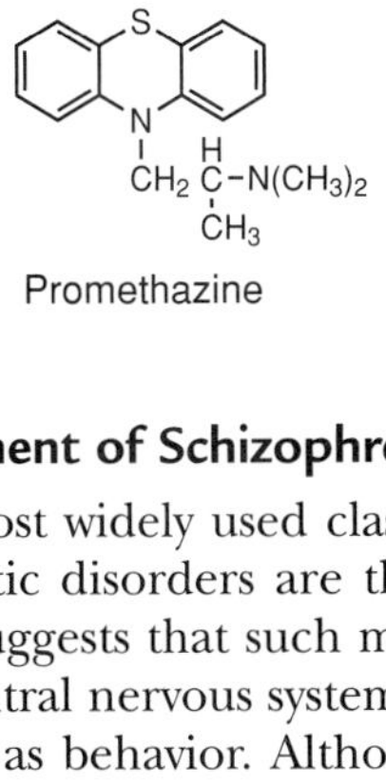

Promethazine

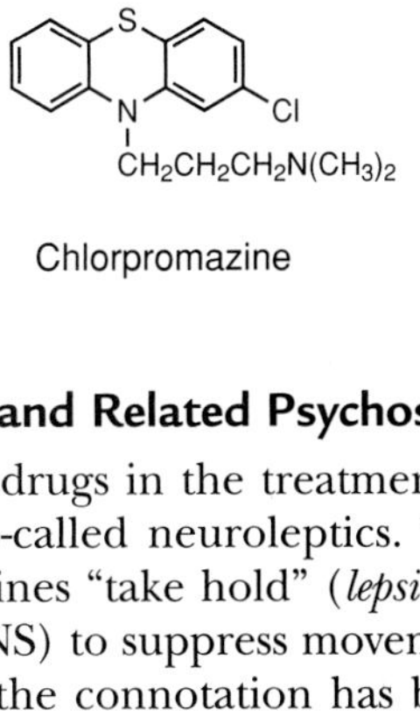

Chlorpromazine

Treatment of Schizophrenia and Related Psychoses

The most widely used class of drugs in the treatment of psychotic disorders are the so-called neuroleptics. This term suggests that such medicines "take hold" (*lepsis*) of the central nervous system (CNS) to suppress movement as well as behavior. Although the connotation has been stretched to include biochemical and clinical antagonism of dopamine D_2 receptors, debilitating extrapyramidal movement side effects are implicit in the clinical definition of neuroleptic antipsychotic drugs. Indeed, the term "neuroleptic" is so synonymous with neurologic side effects that newer antipsychotic drugs, without substantial risk of extrapyramidal effects, are referred to as atypical neuroleptic drugs. Also implied in the term "atypical" is a mechanism of antipsychotic action other than (or in addition to) postsynaptic D_2 receptor blockade.

In general, neuroleptic therapy benefits patients with schizophrenia or other psychiatric illnesses marked by agitation, aggressive and impulsive behavior, and impaired reasoning. Positive symptoms respond to treatment with typical neuroleptics, whereas negative symptoms are not appreciably affected. In general, neuroleptics provide calming, mood-stabilizing, and antihallucinatory effects, and their beneficial impact on psychiatric medicine is unquestioned in spite of their sometimes severe extrapyramidal side effects. Chemical classes of neuroleptics include the phenothiazines, thioxanthenes, and butyrophenones. The dibenzodiazepines and benzisoxazoles are examples of atypical neuroleptics that have less potential for extrapyramidal side effects and have activity at brain serotonin $5\text{-}HT_2$, adrenergic α_1/α_2, and/or histamine H_1 receptors, in addition to dopamine receptors.

Mechanism of Action of Antipsychotic Drugs

Given that the pathogenesis of schizophrenia and related psychiatric disorders is unknown, it is perhaps naïve to suggest how drugs act at the molecular level to relieve the symptoms of these disorders. Nevertheless, it generally is agreed that the antipsychotic mechanism of action of neuroleptics involves modulation of dopamine neurotransmission in the mesolimbic–mesocortical pathways. This may be achieved via direct interaction with D_2-type receptors and include the functional spectrum of antagonism, inverse agonism, and/or partial agonism. Antipsychotic drug clinical efficacy, however, is not solely accounted for by D_2-type receptor interactions; other CNS receptor systems (acetylcholine, histamine, norepinephrine, and serotonin) appear to be involved, especially for the atypical drugs described below.

Side Effects of Neuroleptics

Many of the side effects associated with antipsychotic agents can be attributed to their antagonist activity at a variety of CNS receptors, which include histamine H_1, adrenergic α_1/α_2, cholinergic M_1 receptors, serotonin $5\text{-}HT_2$, and dopamine D_2 receptors in the brain. For example, antipsychotic drug side effects such as sedation, hypotension, sexual dysfunction, and other autonomic effects reflect blockade of adrenergic and histamine receptors. Meanwhile, the anticholinergic actions of neuroleptics in cardiac, ophthalmic, gastrointestinal, bladder, and genital tissue result from antagonism of muscarinic acetylcholine receptors. Such anticholinergic actions also are characteristic of atypical antipsychotics such as clozapine, and it has been proposed that anticholinergic activity may be beneficial in controlling negative symptoms in schizophrenics. The parkinsonian-like movement side effects of neuroleptics clearly result from antagonism of dopamine D_2 receptors in the nigrostriatal pathway, and the severity of these extrapyramidal side effects increases with the ratio of their antidopaminergic to anticholinergic potency. Extrapyramidal side effects occur in 30 to 50% of patients receiving standard doses of typical neuroleptics and tend to occur during the first to eighth week of therapy. Extrapyramidal side effects include acute dystonias (e.g., facial grimacing, torticollis, and oculogyric crisis), akathisia (motor restlessness), and parkinsonian-type symptoms, such as bradykinesia, cogwheel rigidity, tremor, masked face, and shuffling gait. The higher the D_2 potency of the neuroleptic, the worse the side effects, some of which can be reversed using anticholinergic drugs. Tardive dyskinesia occurs in 15 to 25% of patients after prolonged treatment with typical neuroleptics and is characterized by stereotyped, involuntary, repetitive, choreiform movements of the face, eyelids, mouth (grimaces), tongue, extremities, and trunk. There also are metabolic and endocrine side effects of neuroleptics, such as weight gain, hyperprolactinemia, and gynecomastia. Relatively common dermatologic reactions (e.g., urticaria and photosensitivity) also are observed especially with the phenothiazines. Interestingly, anticholinergic and dopaminergic agents worsen tardive dyskinesia, whereas antidopaminergic agents tend to suppress the symptoms. The pathophysiology of tardive dyskinesia is not known, and the disorder essentially is irreversible.

Meanwhile, antagonism of dopamine D_2-type receptors in the chemoreceptor trigger zone in the brainstem is responsible for beneficial antiemetic effects produced by neuroleptics. Several phenothiazines (e.g., promethazine and prochlorperazine) are marketed to exploit this pharmacological effect.

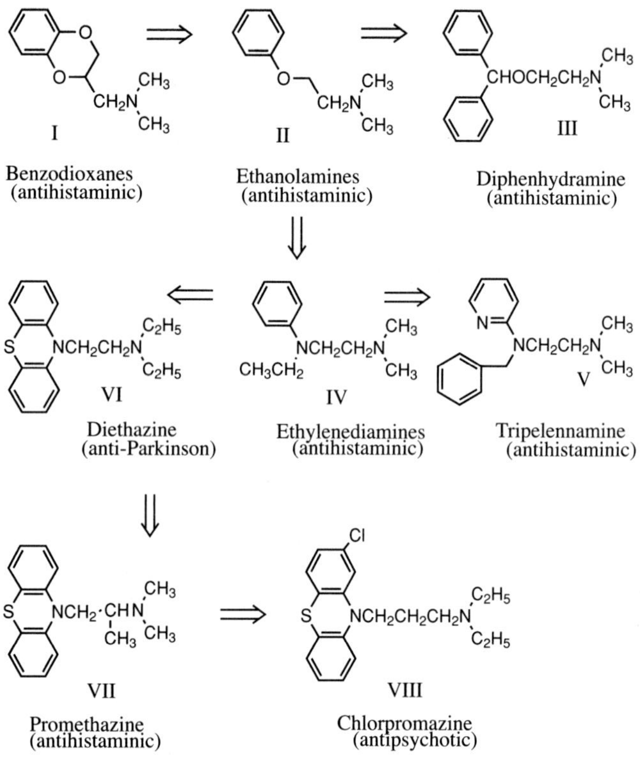

Development of Phenothiazine and Related Neuroleptics

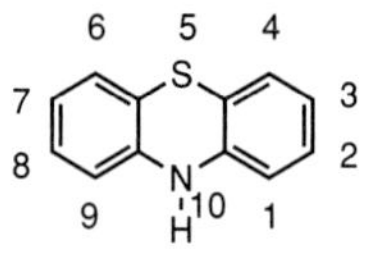

6 5 4 S 7 3 8 2 N 9 H 10 1

Phenothiazine

Although the phenothiazine nucleus was synthesized in 1883, and although it was used as an anthelmintic for many years, it has no antipsychotic activity. The basic structural type from which the phenothiazine antipsychotic drugs trace their origins is the antihistamines of the benzodioxane type I (Fig. 22.4). In 1937, Bovet (34) hypothesized that specific substances antagonizing histamine ought to exist, tried various compounds known to act on the autonomic nervous system, and was the first to recognize antihistaminic activity. With the benzodioxanes as a starting point, many molecular modifications were carried out in various laboratories in a search for other types of antihistamines. The benzodioxanes led to ethers of ethanolamine of type II, which after further modifications led to the benzhydryl ethers (type III), which are characterized by the clinically useful antihistamine diphenhydramine, or to ethylenediamine (type IV), which led to antihistamine drugs, such as tripelennamine (type V). Further modification of the ethylenediamine type of antihistamine resulted in the incorporation of one of the nitrogen atoms into a phenothiazine ring system, which produced phenothiazine

O O CH_2N CH_3 CH_3 I Benzodioxanes (antihistaminic)
O CH_2N CH_3 CH_3 II Ethanolamines (antihistaminic)
$CHOCH_2CH_2N$ CH_3 CH_3 III Diphenhydramine (antihistaminic)
S NCH_2CH_2N C_2H_5 C_2H_5 VI Diethazine (anti-Parkinson)
NCH_2CH_2N CH_3CH_2 CH_3 CH_3 IV Ethylenediamines (antihistaminic)
N NCH_2CH_2N CH_3 CH_3 V Tripelennamine (antihistaminic)
S $NCH_2 \cdot CHN$ CH_3 CH_3 CH_3 VII Promethazine (antihistaminic)
Cl S $NCH_2CH_2CH_2N$ C_2H_5 C_2H_5 VIII Chlorpromazine (antipsychotic)

Fig. 22.4. Development of phenothiazine-type antipsychotic drugs.

(type VI), a compound that was found to have antihistaminic properties and, similar to many other antihistaminic drugs, a strong sedative effect. Diethazine (type VI) is more useful in the treatment of Parkinson's disease (because of its potent antimuscarinic action) than in allergies, whereas promethazine (type VII) is clinically used as an antihistaminic. After the ability of promethazine to prolong barbiturate-induced sleep in rodents was discovered, the drug was introduced into clinical anesthesia as a potentiating agent.

To enhance the sedative effects of such phenothiazines, Charpentier and Courvoisier synthesized and evaluated many modifications of promethazine. This research effort eventually led to the synthesis of chlorpromazine (type VIII) in 1950 at the Rhône-Poulenc Laboratories (35). Soon thereafter, the French surgeon Laborit and his coworkers described the ability of this compound to potentiate anesthetics and produce artificial hibernation (36). They noted that chlorpromazine, by itself, did not cause a loss of consciousness but did produce only a tendency to sleep and a marked disinterest in the surroundings. The first attempts to treat mental illness with chlorpromazine alone were made in Paris in 1951 and early 1952 by Paraire and Sigwald. In 1952, Delay and Deniker began their important work with chlorpromazine (37). They were convinced that chlorpromazine achieved more than symptomatic relief of agitation or anxiety and that this drug had an ameliorative effect on psychosis. Thus, what initially involved minor molecular modifications of an antihistamine that pro-

Table 22.1. Phenothiazine and the Thioxanthene Derivatives Used as Neuroleptics*

Phenothiazines Generic name	Trade name	R_{10}	R_2	Adult Antipsychotic Oral Dose Range (mg/day)	Side Effects** Sedative Effects	Extra-pyramidal Effects	Hypotensive Effects	Other Effects
Chloropromazine hydrochloride	Thorazine	$(CH_2)_3N(CH_3)_2{\cdot}HCl$	Cl	300-800	+++	++	Oral ++ IM +++	Antiemetic dose 10-25 mg every 4-6 hrs
Triflupromazine hydrochloride	Vesprin	$(CH_2)_3N(CH_3)_2{\cdot}HCl$	CF_3	100-150	++	+++	++	Antiemetic dose 5-15 mg every 4-6 hrs
Thioridazine hydrochloride	Mellaril	$(CH_2)_2$-(N-methylpiperidin-2-yl)·HCl	SCH_3	200-600	+++	+	++	
Mesoridazine mesylate	Serentil	$(CH_2)_2$-(N-methylpiperidin-2-yl)·$C_6H_5SO_3H$	$S(=O)CH_3$	75-300	+++	+	++	
Perphenazine	Trilafon	$(CH_2)_3$-N(piperazine)N-CH_2CH_2OH	Cl	8-32	++	+++	+	
Prochlorperazine edisylate maleate	Compazine	$(CH_2)_3$-N(piperazine)N-CH_3	Cl	75-100	++	+++	+	Antiemetic dose 5-10 mg every 4-6 hrs
Fluphenazine hydrochoride	Permitil, Prolixin	$(CH_2)_3$-N(piperazine)N-CH_2CH_2OH·2HCl	CF_3	1-20	+	+++	+	
Trifluperazine hydrochoride	Stelazine	$(CH_2)_3$-N(piperazine)N-CH_3·2HCl	CF_3	6-20	+	+++	+	
Acetophenazine maleate	Tindal	$(CH_2)_3$-N(piperazine)N-CH_2CH_2OH	$COCH_3$	60-120	++	++	+	
Thiethylperazine maleate	Torecan	$(CH_2)_3$-N(piperazine)N-CH_3	SCH_2CH_3		+	+	+	Antiemetic dose 10-30 mg daily
Thioxanthene								
Thiothixene hydrochoride	Navane	thioxanthene, 2-$SO_2N(CH_3)_2$, =CH-$(CH_2)_2$-N(piperazine)N-CH_3·HCl		6-30	++	++	++	

*The phenothiazine derivatives that are effective in the treatment of nausea and vomiting are included in this listing. ** +++, high; ++, medium; +, low.

duced sedative side effects resulted in the development of a major class of drugs that initiated a new era in the drug therapy for the mentally ill. More than anything else in the history of psychiatry, the phenothiazines and related drugs have positively influenced the lives of schizophrenic patients, enabling them to assume a greatly improved role in society.

More than 24 phenothiazine and the related thioxanthene derivatives are used in medicine, most of them for psychiatric conditions. The structures, generic and trade names, dose, and side effects of phenothiazines and thioxanthenes currently used as neuroleptics are listed in Table 22.1.

STRUCTURE–ACTIVITY RELATIONSHIPS OF PHENOTHIAZINE AND THIOXANTHENE NEUROLEPTICS. It is presumed that phenothiazine and thioxanthene neuroleptics mediate their pharmacological effects mainly through interactions at D_2-type dopamine receptors. Examination of the x-ray structures of dopamine (in the preferred *trans* α-rotamer conformation) and chlorpromazine shows that these two structures can be partly superimposed (Fig. 22.5) (38). In the preferred conformation of chlorpromazine, its side chain tilts away from the midline toward the chlorine-substituted ring.

The electronegative chlorine atom on ring "a" is responsible for imparting asymmetry to this molecule, and the attraction of the amine side chain (protonated at physiologic pH) toward the ring containing the chlorine atom indicates an important structural feature of such molecules. Phenothiazine and related compounds lacking a chlorine atom in this position are, in most cases, inactive as neuroleptic drugs. In addition to the ring "a" substituent, another major requirement for therapeutic efficacy of phenothiazines is that the side-chain amine contain three carbons separating the two nitrogen atoms (Fig. 22.5). Phenothiazines with two carbon atoms separating the two nitrogen atoms lack antipsychotic efficacy. Compounds such as promethazine (Fig. 22.4, VII) are primarily antihistaminic and are less likely to assume the preferred conformation.

When thioxanthene derivatives that contain an olefinic double bond between the tricyclic ring and the side chain

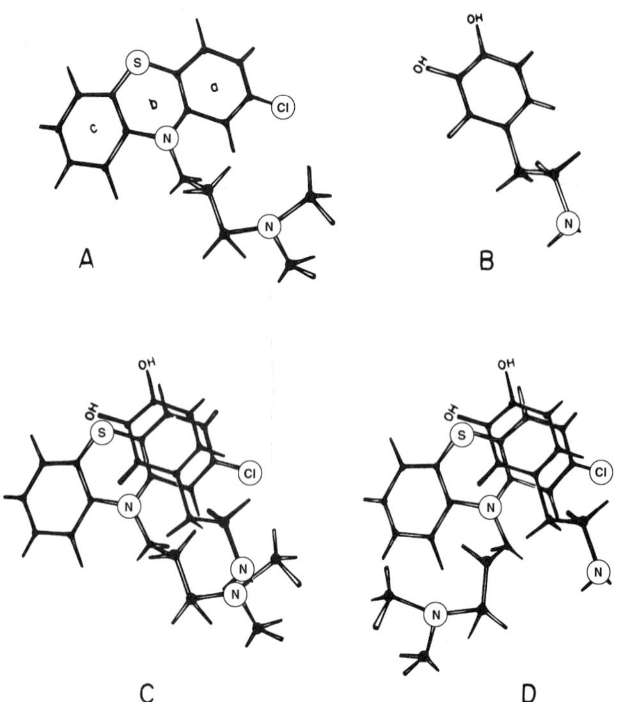

Fig. 22.5. Conformations of chlorpromazine (A), dopamine (B), and their superposition (C) as determined by x-ray crystallographic analysis. The a, b, and c in (A) designate rings. Also shown (D) is another conformation in which the alkyl side chain of chlorpromazine is in the trans conformation (ring a and amino side chain), which is not superimposable on to dopamine. (Adapted from Horn AS, Snyder SH. Chlorpromazine and dopamine: Conformational similarities that correlate with the antischizophrenic activity of phenothiazine drugs. Proc Natl Acad Sci U S A 1971;68:2325–2328; with permission.)

are examined, it can be seen that such structures can exist in either the *cis* or *trans* isomeric configuration. The *cis* isomer of the neuroleptic thiothixene is several-fold more active than both the *trans* isomer and the compound obtained from saturation of the double bond. Structure D in Figure 22.5 shows that the active structure of dopamine does not superimpose with a *trans*-like conformer of chlorpromazine that would be predicted to be inactive.

Cis isomer — *Trans* isomer

Thiothixene

Long-acting neuroleptics.

The duration of action of many of the neuroleptics with a free hydroxyl (OH) moiety can be considerably prolonged by the preparation of long-chain fatty acid esters (Table 22.2). Thus, fluphenazine decanoate and fluphenazine enanthate were the first of these esters to appear in clinical use and are longer acting, with fewer side effects, than the unesterified precursor. The ability to treat patients with a single intramuscular injection every 1 to 2 weeks with the enanthate or every 2 to 3 weeks with the decanoate ester means that problems associated with patient compliance to the drug regimens and with drug

Table 22.2. Long-acting Neuroleptics for IM Depot Injection

Phenothiazines Generic name	R	R_2	Dosage Range (mg)	Typical Duration of Action (weeks)
Fluphenazine enanthate	$(CH_2)_3$–N(piperazine)N–CH_2CH_2O–C(=O)–$(CH_2)_5CH_3$	CF_3	25-100	1-2
Fluphenazine decanoate	$(CH_2)_3$–N(piperazine)N–CH_2CH_2O–C(=O)–$(CH_2)_8CH_3$	CF_3	25-200	2-3
Perphenazine enanthate	$(CH_2)_3$–N(piperazine)N–CH_2CH_2O–C(=O)–$(CH_2)_5CH_3$	Cl	25-100	1-2
Thioxanthene				
Flupenthixol decanoate	Thioxanthene, $SO_2N(CH_3)_2$; =CH–$(CH_2)_2$–N(piperazine)N–$(CH_2)_2$–O–C(=O)–$(CH_2)_8CH_3$		100-200	1-2

Adapted from Simpson and Lee (41) and Baldessarini (4).

malabsorption can be reduced. Table 22.2 lists long-acting forms of phenothiazine and thioxanthene, which are derivatives available in the United States and other countries.

METABOLISM OF PHENOTHIAZINES AND THIOXANTHENES. Increasing evidence suggests that the metabolism of neuroleptic drugs is of major significance in the effects of these drugs. Although considerable information about the metabolism of the extensively studied chlorpromazine is available, information about many of the other drugs administered for prolonged periods is scant. Generally, however, the liver microsomal cytochrome P450–catalyzed metabolic pathways for neuroleptics are similar to those for many other drugs. Some metabolic pathways for chlorpromazine are shown in Figure 22.6. It should be kept in mind that during metabolism, several processes can and do occur for the same molecule. For example, chlorpromazine can be demethylated, sulfoxidized, hydroxylated, and glucuronidated to yield 7-O-glu-nor-CPZ-SO. The combination of such processes leads to more than 100 identified metabolites. Evidence indicates that the 7-hydroxylated derivatives and, possibly, other hydroxylated derivatives as well as the mono- and didesmethylated products (nor_1-CPZ, nor_2-CPZ) are active in vivo and at dopamine D_2 receptors, whereas the sulfoxide (CPZ-SO) is inactive. Although the thioxanthenes are closely related to the phenothiazines in their pharmacological effects, there seems to be at least one major difference in metabolism: Most of the thioxanthenes do not form ring-hydroxylated derivatives. Metabolic pathways for phenothiazines and thioxanthenes are significantly altered, both quantitatively and qualitatively, by a number of factors, including species, age, gender, interaction with other drugs, and route of administration.

Development of Butyrophenone Neuroleptics

In the late 1950s, Janssen and coworkers synthesized the propiophenone and butyrophenone analogues of meperidine in an effort to increase its analgesic potency (39). The propiophenone analogue had 200-fold the

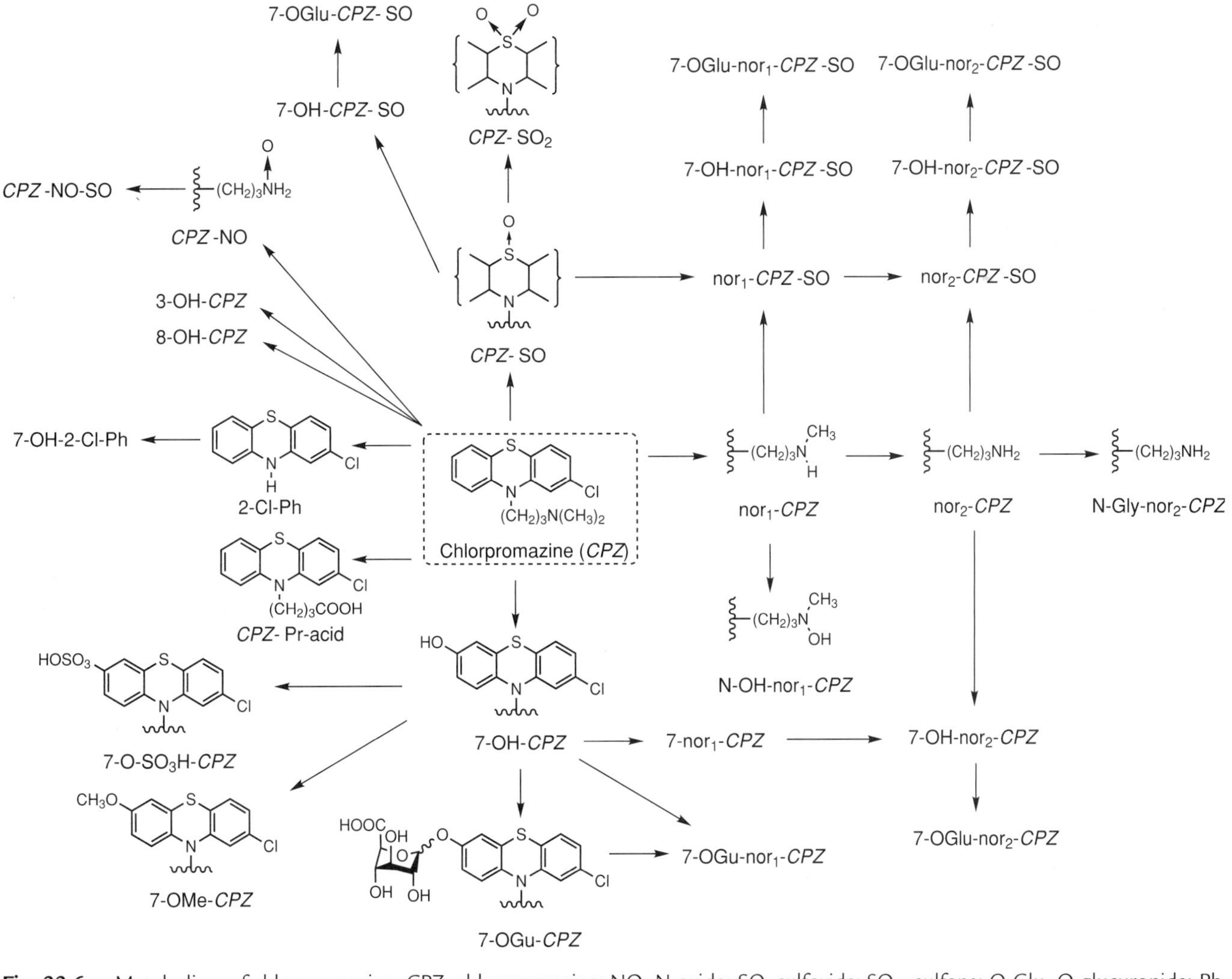

Fig. 22.6. Metabolism of chlorpromazine. CPZ, chlorpromazine; NO, N-oxide; SO, sulfoxide; SO_2, sulfone; O-Glu, O-glucuronide; Ph, phenothiazine; Pr-acid, propionic acid; $O\text{-}SO_3H$, sulfate.

analgesic potency of meperidine, but the butyrophenone analogue also displayed activity resembling that of chlorpromazine. Janssen and coworkers found that it was possible to eliminate the morphine type of analgesic activity and, simultaneously, to accentuate the chlorpromazine type of neuroleptic activity in the butyrophenone series, provided that certain structural changes are made.

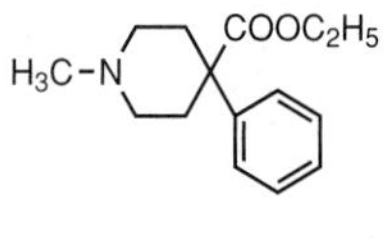

Meperidine

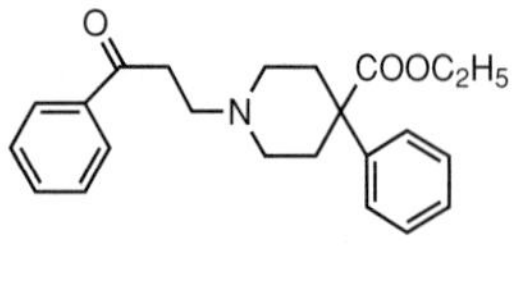

Propiophenone analog

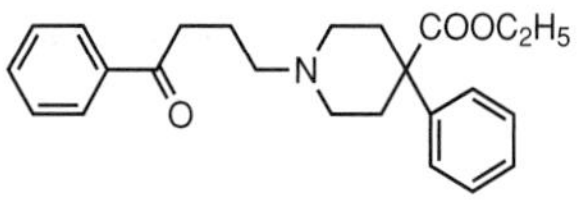

Butyrophenone analog

Structure–Activity Relationships. Haloperidol binds with equally high affinity to dopamine D_2, and serotonin 5-HT_2 receptors in mammalian brain tissue, and both of these receptor systems may be involved in mediating the antipsychotic activity of the butyrophenones. In most respects, the pharmacological effects of haloperidol and other butyrophenones differ in degree, but not in kind, from those of the piperazine phenothiazines. Haloperidol produces a high incidence of extrapyramidal reactions, but its sedative effect in moderate doses is less than that observed with chlorpromazine. Haloperidol has less prominent autonomic effects than the other antipsychotic drugs do, and only mild hypotension occurs with the use of haloperidol, even in high doses.

All butyrophenone derivatives displaying high neuroleptic potency have the following general structure:

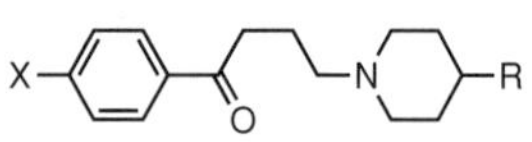

X = F or OCH_3

The attachment of a tertiary amino group to the fourth carbon of the butyrophenone skeleton is essential for neuroleptic activity; lengthening, shortening, or branching of the three-carbon propyl chain decreases neuroleptic potency. Replacement of the keto moiety (e.g., with the thioketone group as in the butyrothienones, with olefinic or phenoxy groups, or reduction of the carbonyl group) decreases neuroleptic potency. In addition, most potent butyrophenone compounds have a fluorine substituent in the para position of the benzene ring. Variations are possible in the tertiary amino group without loss of neuroleptic potency; for example, the basic nitrogen usually is incorporated into a 6-membered ring (piperidine, tetrahydropyridine, or piperazine) that is substituted in the para position.

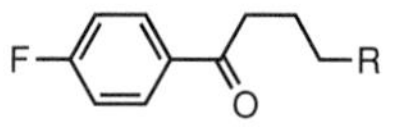

Generic names	Trade names	R
Haloperidol	Haldol	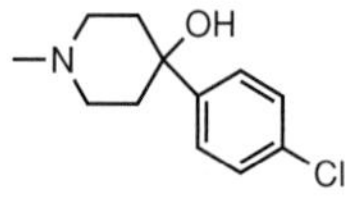
Haloperidol decanoate		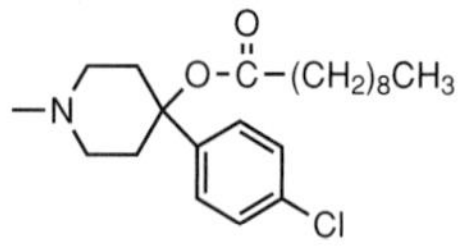
Spiperone		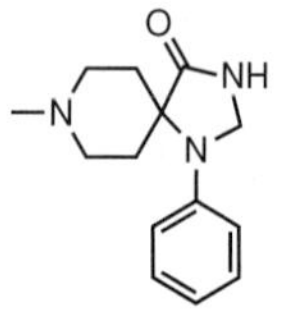
Trifluperidol		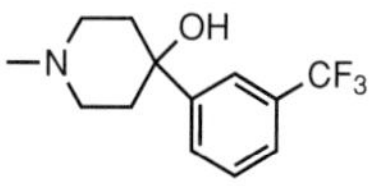
Droperidol	Inapsine	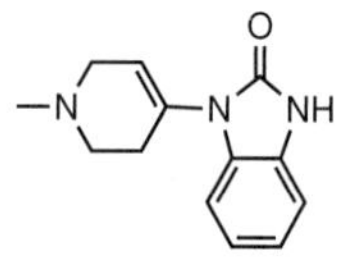

Fig. 22.7. Haloperidol and it analogues.

Haloperidol was introduced for the treatment of psychoses in Europe in 1958 and in the United States in 1967 (Fig. 22.7). It is an effective alternative to more familiar antipsychotic phenothiazine drugs and also is used for the manic phase of bipolar (manic-depressive) disorder. Haloperidol decanoate has been introduced as depot maintenance therapy. When injected every 4 to 6 weeks, the drug appears to be as effective as daily orally administered haloperidol. Other currently available (mostly in Europe) butyrophenones include the very potent spiperone (spiroperidol) as well as trifluperidol and droperidol. Droperidol, a short-acting, sedating butyrophenone, is used in anesthesia for its sedating and antiemetic effects and, sometimes, in psychiatric emergencies as a sedative-neuroleptic. Droperidol often is administered in combination with the potent narcotic analgesic fentanyl for preanesthetic sedation and anesthesia.

Modification of the haloperidol butyrophenone side chain by replacement of the keto function with a di-4-flurophenylmethane moiety results in diphenylbutyl piperidine neuroleptics, such as pimozide, penfluridol, and fluspirilene. The diphenylbutyl piperidines neuroleptics have a longer duration of action than the butyrophenone analogues. All are effective in the control of

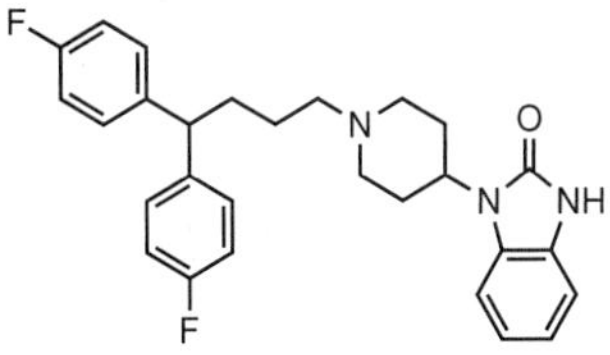

Pimozide

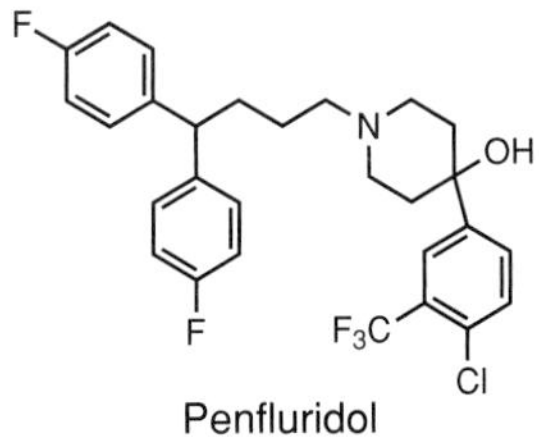

Penfluridol

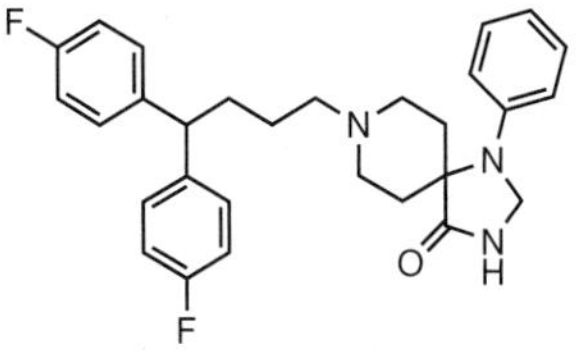

Fluspirilene

schizophrenia, and pimozide in particular has been shown to be useful in treating acute exacerbation of schizophrenia and in reducing the rate of relapse in chronic schizophrenic patients (40). Pimozide also is used for treatment of Tourette's syndrome, a movement disorder that is characterized by facial tics, grimaces, strange and uncontrollable sounds, and sometimes, involuntary shouting of obscenities. This disorder may be misdiagnosed by clinicians as schizophrenia. Typically, the onset of Tourette's syndrome occurs at age 10, and standard treatment for Tourette's syndrome in the past has been the neuroleptics, such as haloperidol. Chronic treatment of Tourette's syndrome with haloperidol as well as with pimozide carries the risk of producing potentially irreversible tardive dyskinesia. Penfluridol and fluspiriline, although not currently available in the United States, are other examples of long-acting neuroleptics in this structure class.

METABOLISM. Haloperidol is readily absorbed from the gastrointestinal tract. Peak plasma levels occur 2 to 6 hours after ingestion. The drug is concentrated in the liver and CNS. Approximately 15% of a given dose is excreted in the bile, and approximately 40% is eliminated through the kidney. Figure 22.8 shows the typical oxidative metabolic pathway of butyrophenones as exemplified by haloperidol (41).

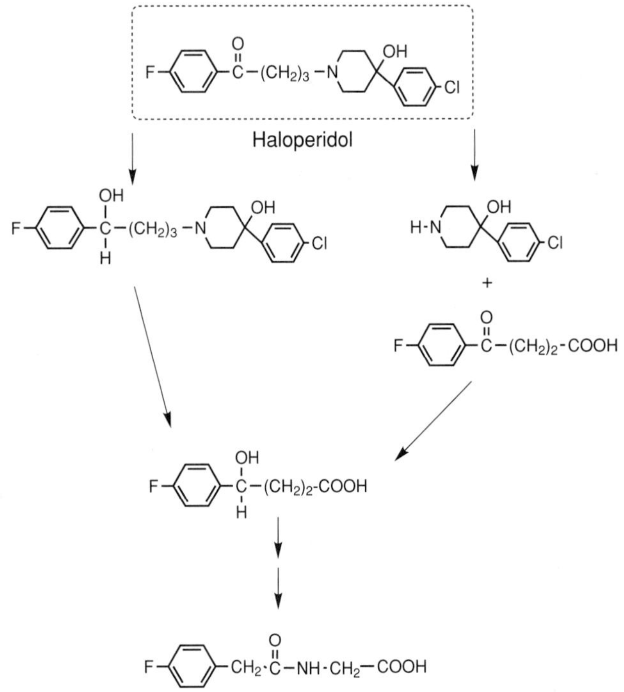

Haloperidol

Fig. 22.8. Metabolism of haloperidol.

Additional Classes of Antipsychotic Agents

BENZAMIDE DERIVATIVES. Certain benzamide derivatives have both local anesthetic and antiemetic properties (47). The benzamide metoclopramide has limited local anesthetic activity but is an efficacious antiemetic drug that modifies gastric motility. Similar to the phenothiazine antiemetics (e.g., promethazine), metoclopramide was found to antagonize dopamine D_2-type receptors in the chemoreceptor trigger zone of the brainstem and, subsequently, was shown to be neuroleptic (48). Metoclopramide has relatively low affinity and selectivity for several receptors in addition to D_2/D_3 antagonism. It blocks muscarinic M_3 and serotonin 5-HT_{1A} GPCRs as well as the 5-HT_3 ligand-operated ion channel. Moreover, numerous studies have documented its anticholinesterase activity. The weak affinity and lack of selectivity of metoclopramide likely is explained by the large number of permissible conformers arising from the flexible 2-(diethylamino)ethyl moiety.

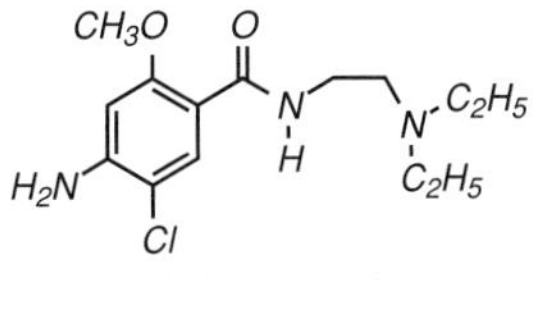

Metoclopramide (Reglan)

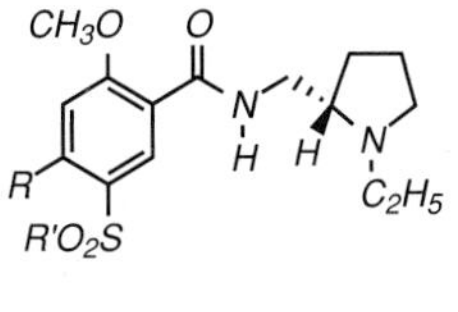

S-(-)-Sulpiride, R = H, R' = NH_2
Amisulpride, R = NH_2, R' = Et

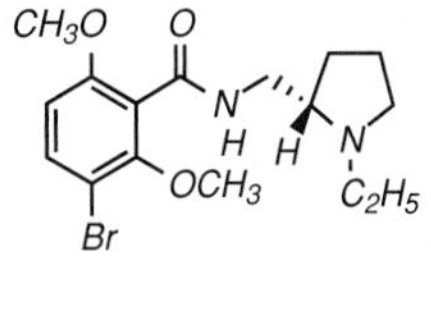

S-(-)-Remoxipride (Roxiam)

Toxicology

As described in the text (see the discussion regarding side effects of neuroleptics), extrapyramidal side effects occur in 30 to 50% of patients receiving standard doses of typical neuroleptics. Extrapyramidal side effects include acute dystonias, akathisia, and parkinsonian-type symptoms, such as bradykinesia, cogwheel rigidity, tremor, masked face, and shuffling gait. Tardive dyskinesia is a severe extrapyramidal side effect that occurs in 15 to 25% of patients after prolonged treatment with typical neuroleptics. Tardive dyskinesia is characterized by stereotyped, involuntary, repetitive, choreiform movements of the face, eyelids, mouth, tongue, extremities, and trunk. The pathophysiology of tardive dyskinesia is not known, and the disorder essentially is irreversible.

Haloperidol-induced dyskinesias may involve neurotoxicological mechanisms similar to the dopaminergic toxicant MPTP.

HP → HPTP → → HPP+

R = $-(CH_2)_3-C(=O)-C_6H_4-F$

MPTP —MAO-B→ MPDP+ → MPP+

Haloperidol (Fig. 22.7) is a potent neuroleptic associated with a high incidence of tardive dyskinesia. Microsomal-catalyzed dehydration of haloperidol yields the corresponding 1,2,3,6-tetrahydropyridine derivative, HPTP, which is a close analogue of the parkinsonian-inducing neurotoxin 1-methyl-4-phenyl-1,2,3,6-tetrahydropyridine (MPTP). Long-term (58-week) administration of HPTP to nonhuman primates alters both presynaptic and postsynaptic dopaminergic neuronal function, which may contribute to the neurotoxicologic effects of haloperidol (42). In baboons treated chronically with HPTP, animals developed orofacial dyskinesia, and histopathological studies revealed volume loss in the basal forebrain and hypothalamus, along with other neuronal cell loss that may be relevant to the pathophysiology of tardive dyskinesia (43). In humans and baboons, HPTP is oxidized in vivo to the corresponding pyridinium species, HPP^+, similar to the oxidation of MPTP to its ultimate neurotoxic species MPP^+. HPP^+ is neurotoxic to dopaminergic and, especially, serotonergic neurons in vivo in rats (44), and HPP^+ has been identified in the urine of humans treated with haloperidol (45). Furthermore, in a recent study involving psychiatric patients who were treated chronically with haloperidol, the severity of tardive dyskinesia and parkinsonism was associated with an increased serum concentration ratio of HPP^+ to haloperidol (46), providing compelling clinical evidence for the neurotoxicity of HPP^+. Investigations continue to determine if neuroleptic-induced pathology of the extrapyramidal motor system, such as that associated with tardive dyskinesia, may be related to production of MPP^+/HPP^+-type species in humans.

See Chapter 25 for a related discussion of Parkinson's disease caused by MPTP.

Several analogues of metaclopramide in which the side chain is incorporated into a pyrrolidine ring include S-(−)-sulpiride and S-(−)-remoxipride. Both drugs display neuroleptic properties. Sulpiride produces a relatively low incidence of extrapyramidal side effects, putatively because of a preferential effect on limbic versus extrapyramidal (striatum) tissue. The hydrophilic properties of sulpiride may account for its poor oral absorption, limited penetration into the CNS, and resulting low potency. The racemic para-amino congener of sulpride, amisulpride, is used as an antipsychotic agent outside the United States. Remoxipride was a promising neuroleptic that is comparable to haloperidol in potency and efficacy and has less incidence of extrapyramidal and autonomic side effects. Life-threatening aplastic anemia, however, was reported with remoxipride use, which prompted its withdrawal from the market.

Benzazepine derivatives. Clozapine, olanzapine, loxapine, and quetiapine are benzazepine-type derivatives with antipsychotic activity and atypically low risk of extrapyramidal side effects (Fig. 22.9).

Mechanism of action. Currently, it generally is agreed that the mechanism of benzazepine-type and other recently introduced atypical antipsychotic drugs (e.g., risperidone, ziprasidone, and aripiprazole) involves occupancy of both D_2 and 5-HT_{2A} receptors. Meanwhile, activity at other dopamine and serotonin receptor subtypes as well as at adrenergic, histamine, and muscarinic receptors may contribute to psychotherapeutic effects, such as modulation of negative symptoms, and certainly may cause autonomic (cardiovascular, sedative, sexual) and other peripheral antimuscarinic side effects (gas-

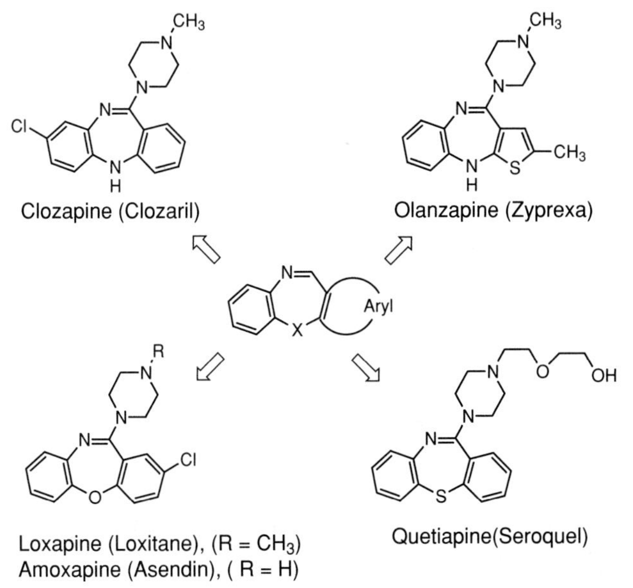

Clozapine (Clozaril)

Olanzapine (Zyprexa)

Loxapine (Loxitane), (R = CH_3)
Amoxapine (Asendin), (R = H)

Quetiapine(Seroquel)

Fig. 22.9. Benzazepine derivatives.

trointestinal, urinary, ophthalmic). Short-term weight gain for both typical and atypical antipsychotic drugs likely correlates to high H_1 receptor affinity (49). The high 5-HT_{2A} receptor affinity of atypical antipsychotic agents (e.g., clozapine and olanzapine) led to the proposal that 5-HT_{2A} antagonism accounts for the lower propensity of these drugs to cause extrapyramidal side effects, but reduced affinity for D_2 receptors also likely plays a role. Nevertheless, antagonism of presynaptic 5-HT_{2A} receptors that inhibit dopamine release from striatal dopaminergic nerve terminals could increase dopaminergic neurotransmission in the striatum to modulate postsynaptic D_2 blockade and reduce extrapyramidal symptoms.

Specific drugs

Clozapine. The dibenzazepine clozapine is representative of the new generation of antipsychotic drugs that have greatly reduced or minimal extrapyramidal side effects and do not produce tardive dyskinesia with long-term use. Clozapine also appears to effectively alleviate the negative symptoms of schizophrenia and has proven to be beneficial in treating patients who do not respond adequately to classical neuroleptic agents, such as the phenothiazines or butyrophenones. A serious drawback to the use of clozapine, however, is the potentially fatal agranulocytosis that is reported to occur in 1 to 2% of unmonitored patients (50), necessitating weekly white blood cell counts for at least the first 6 months of pharmacotherapy. Clozapine is orally active and metabolized mainly by CYP3A4 to inactive desmethyl, hydroxyl, and N-oxide derivatives, with a half-life of approximately 12 hours. Clozapine has relatively low affinity for brain dopamine D_1 and D_2 receptors (moderate affinity for D_4) in comparison to its affinity at adrenergic α_1 and α_2, histamine H_1, muscarinic M_1 and serotonin 5-HT_{2A} receptors (15,51).

Olanzapine. The thienobenzodiazepine olanzapine is an effective atypical antipsychotic agent that is close in structure to clozapine but has a somewhat different neuropharmacological profile, in that it is a more potent antagonist at dopamine D_2 and, especially, serotonin 5-HT_{2A} receptors (15). Olanzapine is well absorbed after oral administration and is metabolized mainly by CYP1A2 to inactive metabolites, with a variable half-life of approximately 20 to 50 hours.

Loxampine. The dibenzo-oxazepine loxapine is another antipsychotic in this structural class that has a more typical neuroleptic biochemical profile with mainly antidopaminergic activity at D_2-type receptors. Loxapine undergoes Phase I aromatic hydroxylation to yield several phenolic metabolites that have higher affinity for D_2 receptors than the parent. Loxapine also undergoes N-demethylation to form amoxapine, which is used clinically as an antidepressant. Amoxapine binds to D_2 receptors and inhibits the norepinephrine neurotransporter to block neuronal norepinephrine reuptake, a correlate of antidepressant activity.

Quetiapine. Quetiapine is a dibenzothiazepine with a brain receptor–binding profile similar to that of clozapine. Quetiapine binds most effectively to histaminergic H_1, adrenergic α_1 and α_2, and serotonergic 5-HT_{2A} receptors in the brain and has even lower affinity than clozapine for dopaminergic D_2 receptors. Unlike clozapine, however, quetiapine also has very low affinity for muscarinic receptors. Quetiapine is 100% bioavailable, but first-pass metabolism yields at least 20 metabolites via CYP3A4, with a half-life of approximately 6 hours. Quetiapine is about as effective as haloperidol in treating the positive symptoms of schizophrenia, but it also manages negative symptoms and induces a lower incidence of extrapyramidal side effects.

BENZISOXAZOLE AND BENZISOTHIAZOLE DERIVATIVES. Neuroanatomical and neurophysiologic interactions between dopaminergic and serotonergic systems, together with evidence that several benzazepine-type antipsychotic agents (e.g., clozapine and olanzapine) have high affinity for 5-HT_{2A} receptors, led to the proposal that combination D_2/5-HT_{2A} antagonists may produce atypical antipsychotic effects (52,53). Combining the chemical features present in the potent benzamide D_2 antagonists (e.g., remoxipride) with those of the benzothiazolyl piperazine 5-HT_{2A} antagonists (e.g., tiospirone) led to the development of the 3-(4-piperidinyl)-1,2-benzisoxazole nucleus present in the 5-HT_{2A}/D_2 antagonist risperidone and ziprasidone, which also have relatively high affinity at histamine H_1 and adrenergic α_1/α_2 receptors (Fig. 22.10).

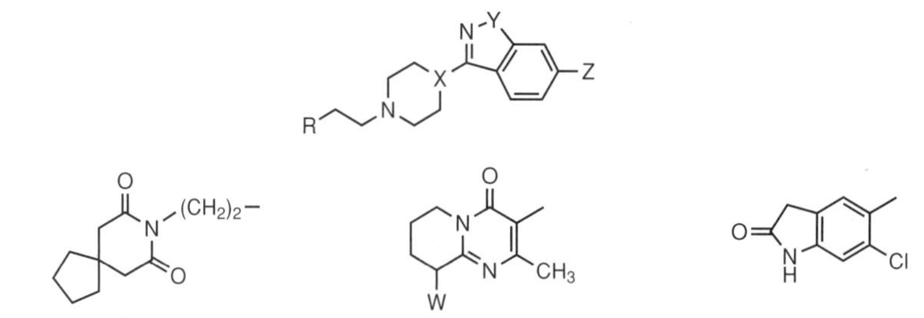

Tiospirone
(Y = S, X = N, Z = H)

Risperidone (Risperdal)
(Y = O, X = CH, Z = F, W = H)
Risperidone (active metabolite)
(Y = O, X = CH, Z = F, W = OH)

Ziprasidone (Geodon)
(Y = S, X = N, Z = H)

Fig. 22.10. Benzisoxazole and benzisothiazole antipsychotic agents.

Specific drugs

Risperidone. Risperidone has antiserotonergic effects similar to the benzazepine-type antipsychotic drugs. It is proposed that the 5-HT_{2A} antagonist activity of risperidone uninhibits dopaminergic neurotransmission in the striatum and cortex, reducing the severity of D_2 antagonist-induced extrapyramidal side effects and alleviating negative symptoms of schizophrenia while maintaining a blockade of limbic system D_2 receptors (54). Risperidone is well absorbed orally and undergoes hepatic CYP2D6-catalyzed 9-hydroxylation (active metabolite) and N-dealkylation (Fig. 21.10). The half-life of risperidone (as well as of hydroxyrisperidone) is approximately 22 hours.

Ziprasidone. Ziprasidone is chemically similar to risperidone but with a substitution of piperzinyl and benzisothiazole for piperidinyl and benzisoxazole and with minor aromatic modification. Like risperidone, ziprasidone is a high-affinity antagonist at 5-$HT_{2A/C}$ and D_2 receptors as well as at adrenergic α_1/α_2 and histamine H_1 receptors. Moreover, ziprasidone can activate 5-HT_{1A} receptors (55) that regulate dopaminergic neurotransmission in brain regions involved in critical cognitive functions. Thus, in addition to D_2 partial agonism (see below), 5-HT_{1A} agonism is now thought to be an important pharmacological property for atypical antipsychotic drug efficacy (56). Ziprasidone (half-life, 6 hours) has an oral bioavailability of approximately 60%, which can be enhanced in the presence of fatty foods. It is extensively metabolized (<5% excreted unchanged) by aldehyde oxidase, which results in reductive cleavage of the S–N bond, and then by S-methylation. Ziprasidone also can undergo CYP3A4-catalyzed N-dealkylation and S-oxidation (Fig. 22.11) (57).

Miscellaneous derivatives

Aripiprazole (Abilify)

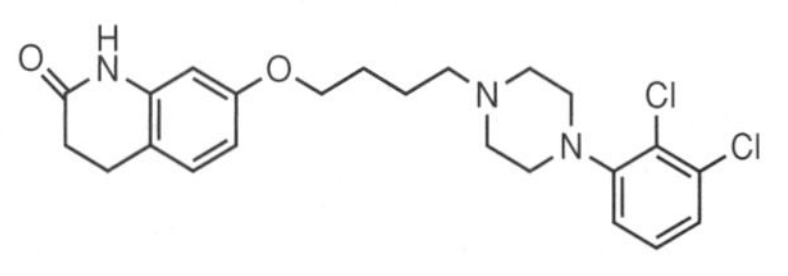

Aripiprazole is an arylpiperazine quinolinone derivative that has complex functional activity at several aminergic receptors currently thought to be important in the pathophysiology and pharmacotherapy of schizophrenia, including dopamine D_2 and serotonin 5-HT_{1A} and 5-$HT_{2A/C}$ receptors. The affinity of aripiprazole for D_2 receptors is relatively high; however, it has a low propensity to cause untoward extrapyramidal symptoms and hyperprolactinemia (58). This may be explained by the ability of aripiprazole to show partial agonist activity at some D_2 receptors, depending on the cell type expression—that is, it is a functionally selective drug (59). Aripiprazole also is a high-affinity partial agonist at 5-HT_{2A} receptors and a low-affinity agonist at 5-HT_{2C} receptors, and it has moderate affinity for α_1-adrenergic and histamine H_1 receptors. As with other atypical antipsychotic drugs, such as the benzazepines, molecular mechanisms related to efficacy are presumed to include a balanced

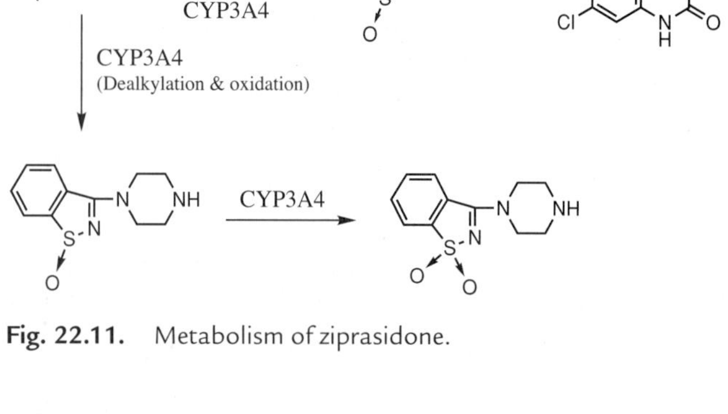

Dehydroziprasidone
Aldehyde oxidase
Ziprasidone
CYP3A4
CYP3A4
(Dealkylation & oxidation)
CYP3A4

Fig. 22.11. Metabolism of ziprasidone.

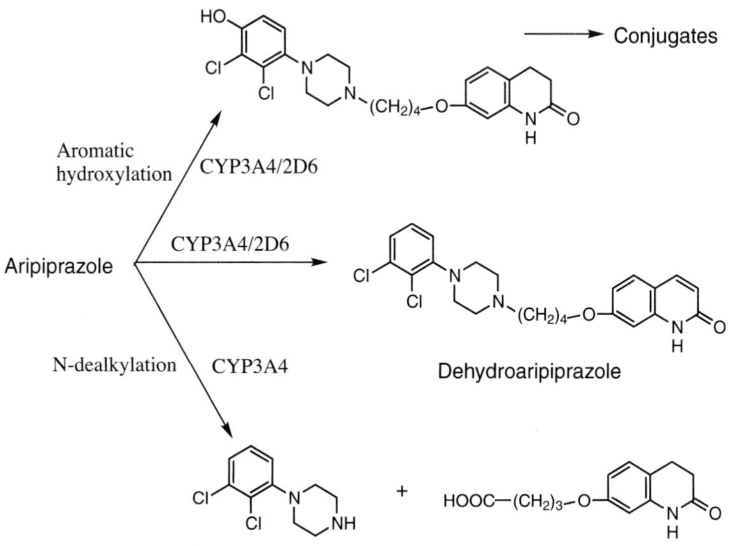

Fig. 22.12. Metabolism of aripiprazole.

occupancy of 5-HT_{2A} receptors and D_2 receptors. Interestingly, the incidence of clinically significant weight gain is relatively low for aripiprazole as well as for risperidone (58), likely because of the relatively moderate histamine H_1 receptor affinity of these agents. In addition, the agonist properties of aripiprazole at 5-HT_{2C} receptors may reduce its potential for weight gain, because 5-HT_{2C} activity is associated with satiety (60). Aripiprazole (half-life, 75 hours) is orally bioavailable (90%) and undergoes hepatic CYP3A4- and CYP2D6-catalyzed N-dealkylation and hydroxylation as well as dehydrogenation to dehydroaripiprazole (half-life, 90 hours), which is an active metabolite (Fig. 22.12) (61).

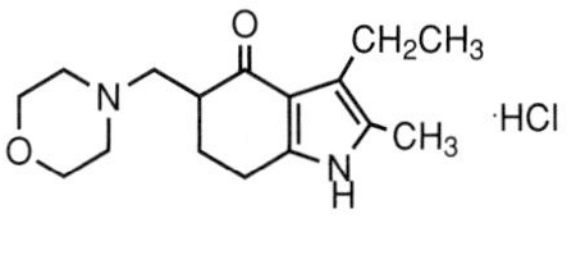

Molindone (Moban)

Molindone. Molindone hydrochloride, a tetrahydroindolone derivative, is a neuroleptic agent that is structurally unrelated to any of the other marketed neuroleptics. Molindone is less potent than haloperidol at blocking D_2 receptors; however, it nonetheless can produce extrapyramidal side effects. Metabolism studies in humans show molindone to be rapidly absorbed and metabolized when given orally. There are 36 recognized metabolites, with less than 2 to 3% unmetabolized molindone being excreted in urine and feces. Clinical studies show that the antipsychotic effects of molindone last more than 24 hours, suggesting that one or more metabolites may contribute to its activity in vivo (62).

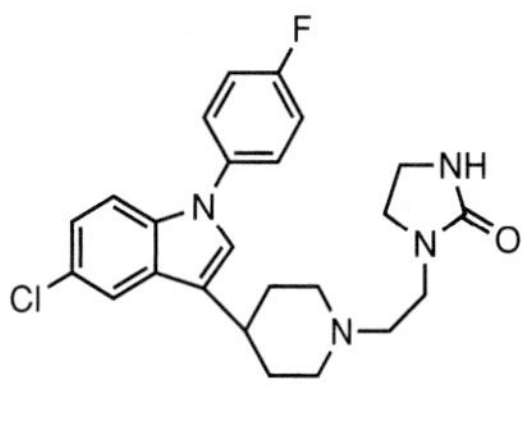

Sertindole (Serdolect)

Sertindole. Sertindole is an indole-containing compound that behaves as a high-affinity serotonin 5-HT_2 receptor antagonist, with weak affinity for adrenergic α_1 receptors and almost no affinity for dopaminergic D_2 receptors. It is about as effective as haloperidol in the treatment of acute and chronic schizophrenia, but with much lower incidence of extrapyramidal side effects. Sertindole is relatively nonsedating, and its effects are long lasting (several days) (63).

ANXIETY AND ANXIETY DISORDERS

Definitions

Anxiety can be defined as a sense of apprehensive expectation. In reasonable amounts and at appropriate times, anxiety is helpful (e.g., anxiety before an examination may cause a student to initiate an appropriate study plan). Too much anxiety, however, can be deleterious. Anxiety can be considered pathological when it is either completely inappropriate to the situation or is in excess of what the situation normally should call for. An example of the former is nocturnal panic attacks—episodes of extreme anxiety that arise out of one of the most physiologically quiet times of the day, stage III/IV sleep (64). An example of the latter is specific phobias—for example, an irrational fear to venture outside of one's home.

According to the DMS-IV (1), abnormal anxiety is that level of anxiety that interferes with normal social or occupational functioning. This definition is helpful to distinguish between normal and pathologic levels of anxiety. To meet general DSM-IV criteria, anxiety symptoms must not be caused by an exogenous factor (e.g., caffeine) or a medical condition (e.g., hyperthyroidism). Examples of anxiety disorders include specific phobias, generalized anxiety disorder (chronic abnormally high level of worry), social phobia (e.g., fear of public speaking), obsessive-compulsive disorder, panic disorder with or without agoraphobia (avoidance of situations believed by the patient to precipitate panic attacks), and posttraumatic stress disorder.

Etiology of Anxiety Disorders

Studies of patients with anxiety disorders have not revealed a general gross neuroanatomical lesion. In vivo functional imaging studies, however, show altered blood flow or utilization of glucose in certain brain areas in patients with anxiety conditions, including obsessive-compulsive disorder (65,66), panic disorder (67,68), specific phobia (69), generalized anxiety disorder (70), and posttraumatic stress disorder (71), mostly implicating the prefrontal cortex and hippocampus (and other limbic areas) as being involved in the anatomy of pathologic anxiety. It is important to note that there is significant comorbidity for anxiety and major depressive disorders, and it is not clear if one illness has primacy or is part of the other (72). Likewise, although there may be genetic predisposition to general distress that can lead to anxiety and/or depression, no clear genetic evidence suggests specific symptoms of either disorder.

A variety of neurotransmitters, neuromodulators (e.g., adenosine), and neuropeptides (e.g., cholecystokinin, corticotropin-releasing factor, and neuropeptide Y) are suggested to be involved in the pathophysiology of anxiety. Currently, abundant evidence exists to document the involvement of the neurotransmitters γ-aminobutyric acid (GABA), norepinephrine, and serotonin in anxiety, and research increasingly is revealing that these neurotransmitter systems have complex anatomical and functional interrelationships. For example, stimulation of the locus ceruleus, which contains the highest concentration of norepinephrine cell bodies in the CNS, generates a state of agitation and fear behaviors in laboratory animals (73). Meanwhile, data suggest that benzodiazepines influence norepinephrine release by stimulating inhibitory GABA receptors located on noradrenergic neurons (74).

GABA Receptors

The major inhibitory neurotransmitter in the mammalian CNS, GABA is widespread, with approximately one-third of all synapses in the CNS utilizing this neurochemical for intercellular communication (75). The two major classes of GABA receptors are inotropic $GABA_A$ and metabotropic $GABA_B$ receptors. There also exist $GABA_C$ inotropic receptors that activate chloride channels, similar to $GABA_A$. The $GABA_C$ receptors may play a role in cognitive and memory functions (76); however, there currently are no drugs that target these receptors.

$GABA_A$ Receptor

The $GABA_A$ receptor is a member of the gene superfamily of ligand-gated ion channels that is known as the "cys-loop" family because of the presence of a cysteine loop in their N-terminal domain (77–79). These receptors exist as heteropentameric subunits arranged around a central ion channel (Fig. 22.13). The five polypeptide subunits are composed of an extracellular region, four membrane-spanning α-helical cylinders, and a large intracellular cytoplasmic loop. The $GABA_A$ ion channel conducts chloride and is defined by the second of the

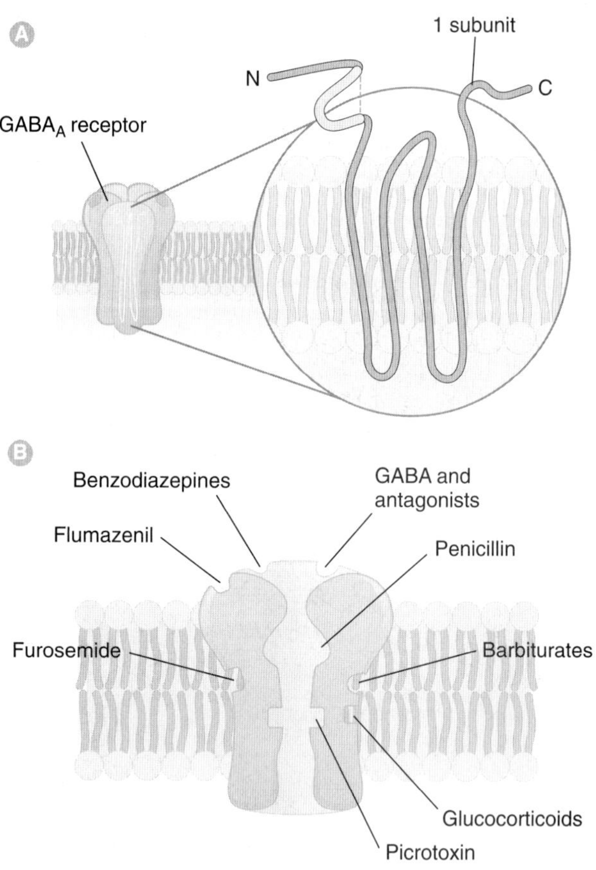

Fig. 22.13. Schematic representation of the γ-aminobutyric $acid_A$ ($GABA_A$) receptor. The $GABA_A$ receptors have a pentameric structure composed predominantly of α, β, and γ subunits arranged, in various proportions, around a central ion channel that conducts chloride. Each subunit has four membrane-spanning regions and a cysteine loop in the extracellular N-terminal domain (dashed line). The type and proportion of α and γ subunit composition affects affinity, pharmacological activity, and efficacy of ligands. (Chou J. Strichartz GR, Lo EA. Pharmacology of Excitatory and Inhibitory Neurotransmission. In: Golan DE, ed. Principles of Pharmacology. Philadelphia: Lippincott Williams & Wilkins, 2005:142; with permission.)

four membrane-spanning α-helical cylinders. The first $GABA_A$ polypeptide subunit was sequenced in 1987 (80), and so far, 19 different subunits have been isolated. These polypeptides are denoted as α_{1-6}, β_{1-3}, γ_{1-3}, δ, ε, π, θ, and ρ_{1-3}. The subunits can combine in varied proportions (81) and alternatively spliced variants are common. Thus, many possible receptor subtypes may exist. The major (60%) $GABA_A$ receptor isoform in the adult mammalian (rat) brain consists of α_1, β_2, and γ_2 subunits ($GABA_{A1a}$) (82).

The $GABA_A$ extracellular N-terminal region contains a number of distinct binding sites for neuroactive drugs (e.g., barbiturates, benzodiazepines, β-carolines, and neurosteroids). The benzodiazepines, among the most commonly prescribed anxiolytic agents, bind to the benzodiazepine receptor (BZR), which is defined mostly by the α and γ subunits. The α and γ subunit composition can dramatically affect affinity and efficacy of BZR ligands (83,84). Early research on the BZR gave rise to the pharmacological concept of inverse agonism in addition to the better known concepts of agonism and antagonism. Inverse agonist compounds bind to the BZR on the $GABA_A$ receptor complex and negatively modulate GABA binding and neurophysiological activity (i.e., agonists decrease chloride conductance), producing physiological effects opposite that of GABA (e.g., anxiogenesis and proconvulsant action). The BZR agonist ligands potentiate GABA binding and activity to increase chloride conductance, enhancing physiological effects of GABA (e.g., sedation and anticonvulsant activity). The BZR antagonists occupy the receptor but have no intrinsic activity to modulate GABA binding and function. A clinical example of a BZR antagonist is the compound flumazenil, which is used to reverse benzodiazepine-induced sedation in overdose. There also have been developed agents that are partial agonists and inverse partial agonists at the BZR/$GABA_A$ receptor complex. The existence of a $GABA_A$ receptor complex that recognizes benzodiazepines has implications for our understanding of both normal and pathologic anxiety states and suggests the existence of endogenous $GABA_A$ receptor ligands. Thus, anxiety could conceivably be either a lack of an endogenous $GABA_A$ receptor agonist or a relative excess of a $GABA_A$ receptor antagonist or inverse agonist.

$GABA_B$ Receptors

The $GABA_B$ receptors are GPCRs that exist as two major subtypes, $GABA_{B(1)}$ and $GABA_{B(2)}$. The $GABA_{B(1)}$ subtype can be expressed as $GABA_{B(1a)}$ and $GABA_{B(1b)}$ isoforms that differ in their extracellular NH_2-terminal domains but are derived from the same gene (85). Interestingly, it was discovered early on that compared to native $GABA_B$ receptors, recombinant $GABA_{B(1a)}$ and $GABA_{B(1b)}$ receptors expressed in heterologous cells display 100- to 150-fold lower affinity for agonist ligands. Likewise, recombinant $GABA_{B(1a)}$ and $GABA_{B(1b)}$ receptors were shown to couple inefficiently to their effector systems (predominantly via $G\alpha_i$ and $G\alpha_o$). These surprising pharmacological findings were explained by the discovery that recombinant $GABA_{B(1a)}$ and $GABA_{B(1b)}$ receptors expressed in heterologous cells are retained in the endoplasmic reticulum (84). In fact, it turned out that $GABA_{B(1)}$ receptors do not traffic to the cell membrane surface in the absence of $GABA_{B(2)}$ receptors. This remarkable discovery that the $GABA_{B(2)}$ receptor coexpresses on the cell surface with the $GABA_{B(1a)}$ or $GABA_{B(1b)}$ receptor to form a functional heterodimeric GPCR was reported simultaneously by three industry research groups in 1998 (85–88). The $GABA_B$ receptors were the first GPCR shown to function not as a single protein but, rather, as two distinct subunits, neither of which is functional by itself (Fig. 22.14). Homo- and/or heterodimerization (and oligomerization) now is documented for many GPCRs and may account for the diverse signaling functionality for this protein family.

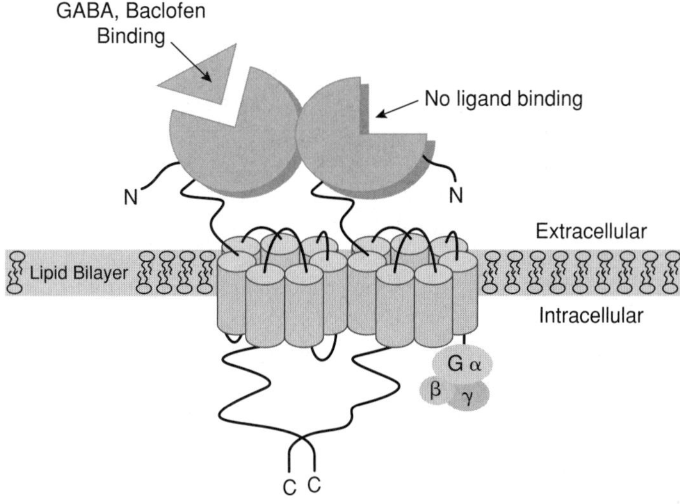

Fig. 22.14. Schematic representation of the γ-aminobutyric $acid_B$ ($GABA_B$) receptor.

The structure of functional heterodimeric $GABA_{B(1)}/GABA_{B(2)}$ GPCRs (Fig. 22.14) is assumed to be very different and considerably more complex in comparison to other aminergic GPCRs that are able to function as monomers. Functional $GABA_B$ receptors are proposed to contain a binding pocket that consists of two globular lobes separated by a hinge region. According to the Venus flytrap model, the two lobes close on ligand binding; however, it is thought that ligands bind in only one of the lobes (89–91). The individual $GABA_{B(1)}$ and $GABA_{B(2)}$ subunits can affect a number of other membrane and cytoplasmic proteins to result in complex signaling and a diverse array of pharmacological and physiological effects. For example, $GABA_B$ receptors modulate activity of calcium channels, potassium channels, adenylyl cyclase, and phospholipase C via $G\alpha_i$, $G\alpha_o$, and $G_{\beta\gamma}$ proteins. Meanwhile, preclinical data suggests that drugs which affect $GABA_B$ receptor function may produce, for example, anxiolytic, anticonvulsant, and antidepressant effects as well as muscle relaxant and analgesic effects (90,91).

Cl
H_2N
O
OH

R(-)-Baclofen

The only drug currently in clinical use that selectively interacts with the $GABA_B$ receptor is baclofen (β-p-chlorophenyl-GABA). Baclofen was first synthesized in 1962 and was shown to have potent muscle relaxant and analgesic activity. In 1972, the racemate was marketed to treat spasticity disorders (92). In 1980, the R-(−)-enantiomer of baclofen was shown to stereoselectively interact (as an agonist) with what is now known as the $GABA_B$ receptor (93). The role of $GABA_B$ receptors in anxiety, however, is not clear, and baclofen (racemate) is approved only for use as a spasmolytic agent (see Chapter 25).

Drugs Used in the Treatment of Anxiety

Benzodiazepines

The benzodiazepines are the prototypic antianxiety agents. They target the $GABA_A$ receptor, and although other molecular targets (e.g., serotonin neuroreceptors) now are exploited for anxiolytic pharmacotherapy, none of the alternative approaches has been shown to match either the efficacy or the rapid onset of the benzodiazepines (84). Chlordiazepoxide was the first benzodiazepine to be marketed for clinical use in 1960. Its effectiveness and wide margin of safety were major advances over compounds, such as barbiturates, used previously. A variety of new benzodiazepines followed, each with some minor differences from the competition. The major factors considered when selecting an agent include rate and extent of absorption, presence or absence of active metabolites, and degree of lipophilicity. These factors help to determine how a benzodiazepine is marketed and used; for example, an agent that is rapidly absorbed, highly lipid soluble, and without active metabolites would be useful as a hypnotic but less useful for treatment of a chronic anxiety state. On the other hand, a compound with slower absorption, active metabolites, and low lipophilicity would be a more effective antianxiety agent but less helpful as a soporific.

Despite their efficacy in a variety of pathologic anxiety syndromes, the benzodiazepines are not perfect anxiolytics. Such a hypothetical agent would selectively ameliorate anxiety without inducing other behavioral effects. Future efforts to enhance the efficacy of benzodiazepine anxiolytics may depend on a greater understanding of the heterogeneity of the $GABA_A$ receptor—for example, which specific clinical actions (anxiolytic, muscle relaxation, sleep facilitation) reside with which specific subunit composition.

Development of Benzodiazepine Anxiolytics. In the 1950s, the medicinal chemist Sternbach noted that "basic groups frequently impart biological activity," and in accordance with this observation, he synthesized a series of compounds by treating various chloromethylquinazoline N-oxides with amines to produce what he hoped would be products with "tranquilizer" activity at the New Jersey laboratories of Hoffman LaRoche (94,95). Sternbach's studies included the reaction of 6-chloro-2-chloromethyl-4-phenylquinazoline-3-oxide with methylamine, which yielded the unexpected rearrangement product 7-chloro-2-(N-methylamino)-5-phenyl-3H-1, 4,-benzodiazepin-4-oxide (Fig. 22.15). This product was given the code name RO 50690 and screened for pharmacological activity in 1957. Subsequently, Randall et al. (96, 97) reported that RO 50690 was hypnotic and sedative and had antistrychnine properties similar to the propanediol meprobamate, a sedative that has tranquilizer (anxiolytic) properties only at intoxicating doses. Renamed chlordiazepoxide, RO 50690 was marketed in 1960 as Librium, a safe and effective anxiolytic agent.

Chlordiazepoxide turned out to have rather remarkable pharmacological properties and tremendous potential as a pharmacotherapeutic product, but it possessed a number of unacceptable physical chemical properties. In an effort to enhance its "pharmaceutical elegance," structural modifications of chlordiazepoxide were undertaken that eventually led to the synthesis of diazepam in 1959. In contrast to the maxim that basic groups impart biological activity, diazepam contains no basic nitrogen moiety. Diazepam, however, was found to be 3- to 10-fold more potent than chlordiazepoxide and was marketed in 1963 as the still enormously popular anxiolytic drug Valium. Subsequently, thousands of benzodiazepine derivatives were synthesized, and more than two dozen benzodiazepines are in clinical use in the United States (Fig. 22.16).

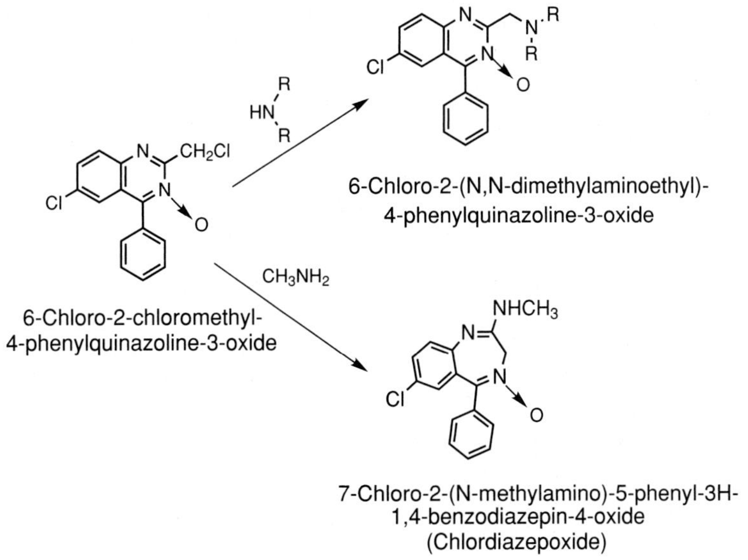

6-Chloro-2-chloromethyl-4-phenylquinazoline-3-oxide

CH_3NH_2

6-Chloro-2-(N,N-dimethylaminoethyl)-4-phenylquinazoline-3-oxide

7-Chloro-2-(N-methylamino)-5-phenyl-3H-1,4-benzodiazepin-4-oxide (Chlordiazepoxide)

Fig. 22.15. Synthesis of chlordiazepoxide.

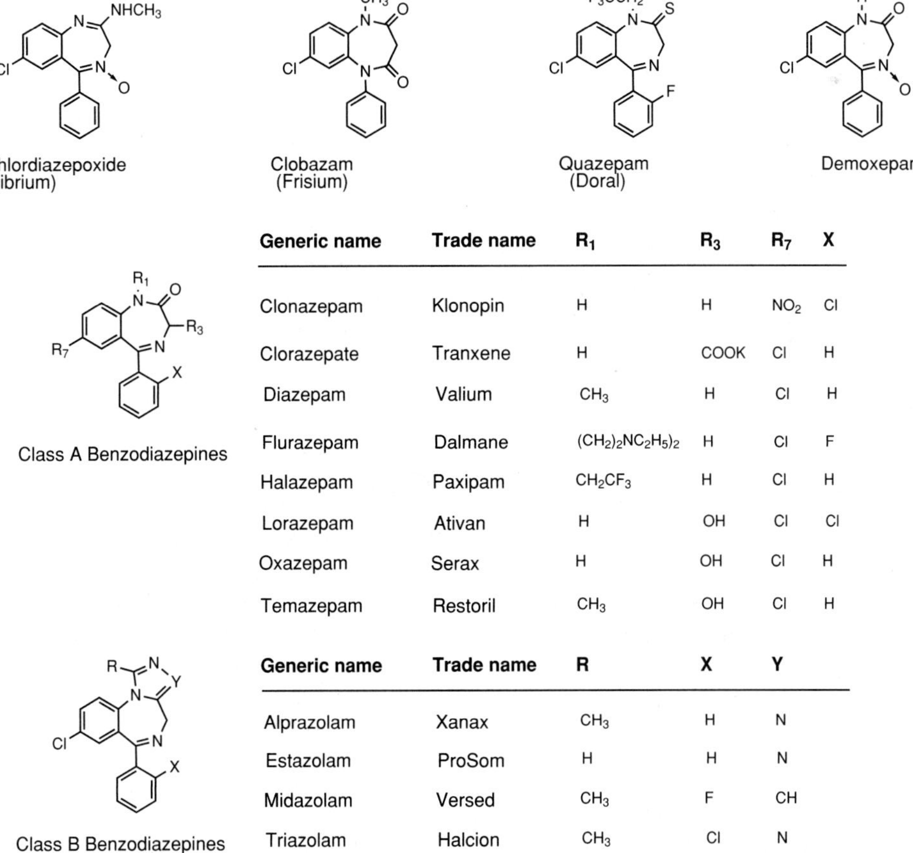

Generic name	Trade name	R_1	R_3	R_7	X
Clonazepam	Klonopin	H	H	NO_2	Cl
Clorazepate	Tranxene	H	COOK	Cl	H
Diazepam	Valium	CH_3	H	Cl	H
Flurazepam	Dalmane	$(CH_2)_2NC_2H_5)_2$	H	Cl	F
Halazepam	Paxipam	CH_2CF_3	H	Cl	H
Lorazepam	Ativan	H	OH	Cl	Cl
Oxazepam	Serax	H	OH	Cl	H
Temazepam	Restoril	CH_3	OH	Cl	H

Generic name	Trade name	R	X	Y
Alprazolam	Xanax	CH_3	H	N
Estazolam	ProSom	H	H	N
Midazolam	Versed	CH_3	F	CH
Triazolam	Halcion	CH_3	Cl	N

Fig. 22.16. Structures of some commercially available benzodiazepines.

Endogenous BZR Ligands

An endogenous ligand with affinity for the CNS benzodiazepine receptor (BZR) of the $GABA_A$ receptor complex has not been conclusively identified. Several compounds of endogenous origin, however, that inhibit the binding of radiolabeled benzodiazepines to the BZR have been reported. In 1980, Braestrup et al. (98) reported the presence in normal human urine of β-carboline-3-carboxylic acid ethyl ester (βCCE), which has very high affinity for the BZR complex. It was subsequently shown, however, that βCCE formed as an artifact from Braestrup's extraction procedure, during which the urine extract was heated with ethanol at pH 1, a condition favoring formation of the ethyl ester from β-carboline-3-carboxylic acid, a tryptophan metabolite.

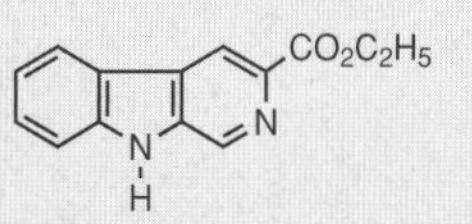

βCCE

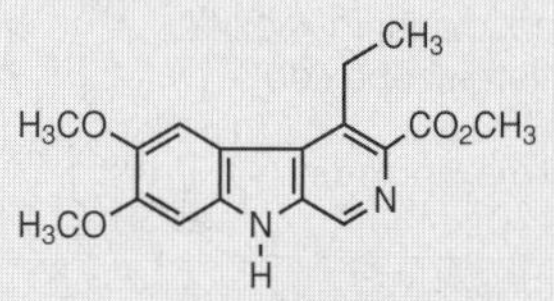

DMCM

Although βCCE actually was shown not to be of endogenous origin, its discovery as a high-affinity BZR ligand stimulated research that led to the synthesis of a series of β-carboline derivatives with a variety of intrinsic activities, presumably mediated through the BZR that is associated with the $GABA_A$ receptor complex. For example, although βCCE is considered to be a partial inverse agonist at this site, 6,7-dimethoxy-4-ethyl-β-carboline-3-carboxylic acid methyl ester (DMCM) appears to be a full inverse agonist (99). In fact, βCCE blocks the convulsions produced by the very potent convulsant DMCM (100). These effects are even more complex and interesting in light of the approximately 10-fold higher affinity that βCCE shows for the BZR labeled by [^{3}H]diazepam when compared to DMCM (101). The β-carbolines currently are important research tools to probe the agonist, competitive antagonist, inverse agonist, and partial agonist/inverse agonist pharmacophores of the BZR/GABA receptor complex

A major advance in the BZR field was made in 1981 with the first report that the imidazobenzodiazepinone derivative, flumazenil, binds with high affinity to the BZR and blocks the pharmacological effects of the classical benzodiazepines in vitro and in vivo (102). Unlike agonists, binding of [^{3}H]flumazenil

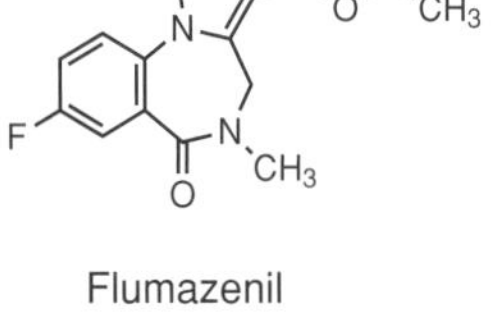

Flumazenil

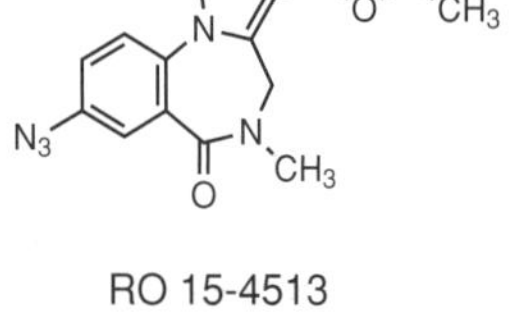

RO 15-4513

to the BZR is not affected by modulators such as GABA and several ions that induce changes in receptors (103). The insensitivity of flumazenil to changes in BZR conformation suggests that the ligand does not induce a conformational change in the receptor to trigger a biological response and is a pure antagonist (104). Such benzodiazepine antagonists are being used to characterize the pharmacological nature of the BZR, and several of these agents, including flumazenil, are used to treat benzodiazepine overdose. Other imidazobenzodiazepinone derivatives are not true BZR antagonists but, rather, have inverse agonist activity. For example, RO 15-4513, is reported to be a partial inverse agonist that produces anxiogenic-like effects in rats (105), a pharmacological activity quite different from a true BZR competitive antagonist, such as flumazenil.

Mechanism of Action of Anxiolytic Benzodiazepines. The BZR ligands, regardless of intrinsic activity, do not directly alter transmembrane chloride conduction to produce their observed characteristic physiologic anxiolytic or anxiogenic effects. The BZR is an allosteric modulator of GABA binding to the $GABA_A$ receptor complex that, in turn, modulates the transmembrane conductance of chloride. In the presence of BZR agonists or partial agonists, affinity and functional potency of GABA at $GABA_A$ receptors is enhanced maximally or submaximally, respectively, and conductance of chloride is increased. Inverse agonists and partial inverse agonists reduce the effect of GABA and $GABA_A$ receptor–mediated conductance of chloride is accordingly decreased. The $GABA_A$ receptor–chloride channels thus become either more or less sensitive to GABA in the presence of BZR agonists or inverse agonists, respectively. BZR competitive antagonists block access of agonists to the BZR but have no intrinsic activity to affect GABA-modulated conductance of chloride.

A representation of the relationship between ligand interaction with the BZR and intrinsic activity to modulate $GABA_A$ receptor function is shown in Figure 22.17. The interaction of agonists, competitive antagonists, and inverse agonists with the BZR, as shown in the figure, is a simplistic rendering of the proposed three-state model of the BZR and $GABA_A$ receptor interrelationship (106,107). This model is based on the hypothesis that the BZR and $GABA_A$ receptor exist in three spontaneously oscillating conformational states, functionally described as "active" or agonist, "neutral" or "resting," and "inactive" or inverse agonist. The BZR agonists and partial agonists bind to and stabilize the "active" state, inducing a conformational change in the $GABA_A$ receptor complex that results in chloride channel opening, which may lead to an anticonvulsant or anxiolytic effect. The BZR inverse agonists and partial inverse agonists bind to and stabilize the "inactive" state, resulting in the chloride channel remaining closed, that may lead to a convulsant or anxiogenic effect. The BZR competitive antagonists

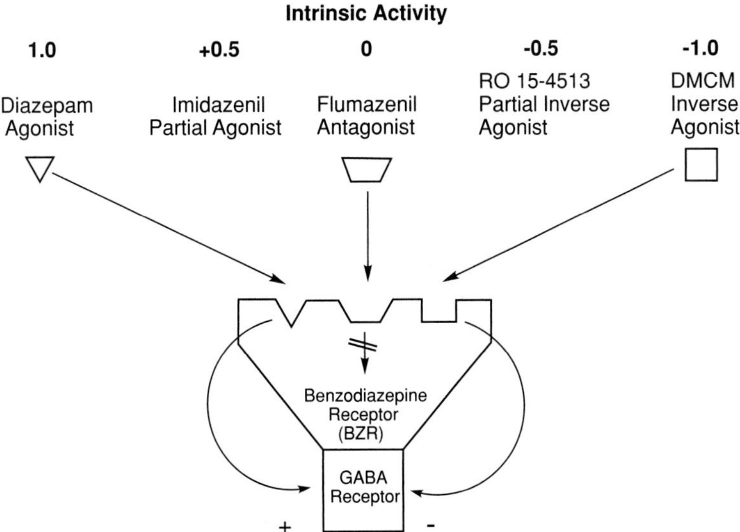

Fig. 22.17. Ligand interaction with the γ-aminobutyric $acid_A$ ($GABA_A$)/ benzodiazepine receptor complex.

presumably bind equally well to both states (hence, they bind to a "neutral" state) and affect no change in $GABA_A$ receptor function or chloride conductance, but access of agonists to the BZR is blocked.

The classical BZR is located on the $GABA_A$ receptor complex mainly at the interface of the α and γ subunits that can be rendered benzodiazepine-insensitive by a point mutation in the α subunit, replacing a critical histidine residue for arginine (108). Different α and γ subunit compositions give rise to subtypes of the BZR receptor that are pharmacologically distinct with regard to ligand affinity and intrinsic activity (109–111), providing a mechanistic basis for development of ligands that are anxioselective (i.e., anxiolysis in the absence of sedation, muscle relaxation, amnesia, and ataxia). Thus, current drug discovery approaches target specific α and γ molecular subunits of the $GABA_A$ receptor complex in the quest for benzodiazepine and nonbenzodiazepine (see below) drugs that demonstrate anxioselectivity. As a group, currently used benzodiazepines are not α subtype-selective. Interestingly, in recent studies using nonhuman primates, it has been suggested that $GABA_A$ α_2, α_3, and α_5 subunits mediate anxiolytic and muscle relaxant effects of benzodiazepines, whereas α_1 receptors mediate the sedative effects (112). Several putative anxioselective compounds have reached the clinic; however, they have not exhibited the degree of anxioselectivity predicted from preclinical testing and, usually, have lower efficacy than standard benzodiazepines (84). Of possible clinical importance, "uncoupling" of the BZR/$GABA_A$ receptor complex has been observed in response to chronic benzodiazepine exposure both in vitro (113) and in vivo (114). In the absence of exogenous influences, however, coupling efficiency appears to be determined by the composition and stoichiometry of the α subunits (109), whereas benzodiazepine affinity, intrinsic activity, and efficacy is determined by the nature of both the α and γ subunits (84,110,111).

STRUCTURE–ACTIVITY RELATIONSHIPS. The structure–activity relationship for classical 5-phenyl-1,4-benzodiazepine-2-one anxiolytic agents has been described by Sternbach and other investigators (94,104,106,115). Thousands of benzodiazepine derivatives with a variety of substituents have been synthesized that interact with the BZR; however, classical quantitative structure–activity relationship and molecular modeling techniques have been used to reduce this myriad of structures to the minimal common molecular features necessary for binding (116–118). The pharmacological activity continuum (agonist, antagonist, inverse agonist) displayed by BZR ligands would seem to suggest that such diverse functional activity be mediated by ligand interaction with different sites on the $GABA_A$ receptor-chloride channel complex. This continuum of activity, however, is displayed by ligands within the same chemical class, and small modifications in the chemical structure of a ligand can shift the intrinsic activity from agonist to antagonist to inverse agonist. Moreover, each functional class of BZR ligands can competitively inhibit the binding of the other two classes as well as functionally antagonize each other. These observations suggest that the binding sites of functionally diverse BZR receptor ligands, at least, overlap. Nevertheless, most BZR pharmacophore models that describe ligand functional activity are based initially on the BZR pharmacophore for ligand binding activity at a single binding domain, and this approach is used here to summarize the structure–activity relationship for benzodiazepine derivatives at the BZR receptor.

Ring A. In general, the minimum requirements for binding of 5-phenyl-1,4-benzodiazepin-2-one derivatives to the BZR includes an aromatic or heteroaromatic ring (ring A), which is believed to participate in π-π stacking with aromatic amino acid residues of the receptor. Substituents on ring A have varied effects on binding of benzodiazepines to the BZR, but such effects are not predictable on the basis of electronic or (within reasonable limits) steric properties. It is generally true, however, that an electronegative group (e.g., halogen or nitro) substituted at the 7-position markedly increases functional anxiolytic activity, albeit effects on binding affinity in vitro are not as dramatic. On the other hand, substituents at positions 6, 8, or 9 generally decrease anxiolytic activity. Other 1,4-diazepine derivatives in which ring A is replaced by a heterocycle generally show weak binding affinity in vitro and even less pharmacological activity in vivo when compared to phenyl-substituted analogues.

Ring B. A proton-accepting group is believed to be a structural requirement of both benzodiazepine and nonbenzodiazepine ligand binding to the $GABA_A$ receptor, putatively for interactions with a histidine residue that serves as a proton source in the $GABA_A$ α_1 subunit (119). For the benzodiazepines, optimal affinity occurs when the proton-accepting group in the 2-position of ring B (i.e., the carbonyl moiety) is in a coplanar spatial orientation with the aromatic ring A. Substitution of sulfur for oxygen at the 2-position (as in quazepam) may affect selectivity for binding to GABA BZR subpopulations, but anxiolytic activity is maintained. Substitution of the methylene 3-position or the imine nitrogen is sterically unfavorable for antagonist activity but has no effect on agonist (i.e., anxiolytic) activity (e.g., clobazam). Derivatives substituted with a 3-hydroxy moiety have comparable potency to nonhydroxylated analogues and are excreted faster. Esterification of a 3-hydroxy moiety also is possible without loss of potency. Neither the 1-position amide nitrogen nor its substituent is required for in vitro binding to the BZR, and many clinically used analogues are not N-alkylated (Fig. 22.16). Although even relatively long N-alkyl side chains do not dramatically decrease BZR affinity, sterically bulky substituents like tert-butyl drastically reduce receptor affinity and in vivo activity. Neither the 4,5-double bond, nor the 4-position nitrogen (the 4,5-[methyleneimino] group) in ring B is required for in vivo anxiolytic activity, albeit in vitro BZR affinity is decreased if the C=N bond is reduced to C−N. It is proposed that in vivo activity of such derivatives results from oxidation back to C=N (69). It follows that the 4-oxide moiety of chlordiazepoxide can be removed without loss of anxiolytic activity.

Ring C. The 5-phenyl ring C is not required for binding to the BZR in vitro. This accessory aromatic ring may contribute favorable hydrophobic or steric interactions to receptor binding, however, and its relationship to ring A planarity may be important. Substitution at the 4′-(para)-position of an appended 5-phenyl ring is unfavorable for agonist activity, but 2′-(ortho)-substituents are not detrimental to agonist activity, suggesting that limitations at the para position are steric, rather than electronic, in nature.

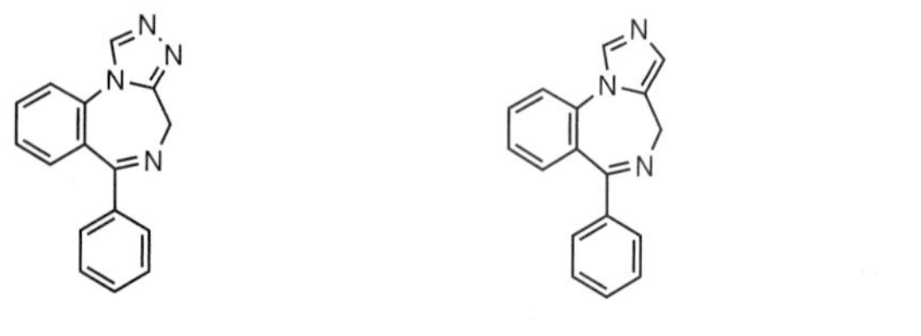

s-Triazolo[4,3a][1,4]benzodiazepine Imidazo[1,5a][1,4]benzodiazepine

Annelating the 1,2-bond of ring B with an additional "electron-rich" (i.e., proton acceptor) ring, such as *s*-triazole or imidazole, also results in pharmacologically active benzodiazepine derivatives with high affinity for the BZR (Fig. 22.17). For example, the *s*-triazolo-benzodiazepines triazolam, alprazolam, and estazolam and the imidazobenzodiazepine midazolam are popularly prescribed, clinically effective anxiolytic agents (Fig. 22.16).

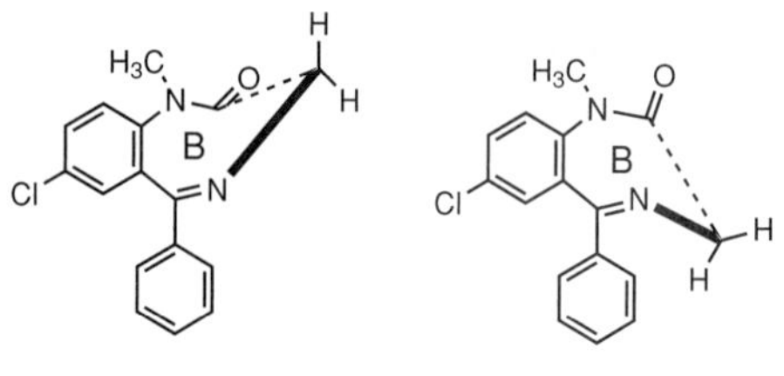

a b

STEREOCHEMISTRY. Most clinically useful benzodiazepines do not have a chiral center; however, the 7-membered ring B may adopt one of two possible boat conformations, *a* and *b*, that are "enantiomeric" (mirror images) to each other. Nuclear magnetic resonance studies indicate that the two conformations can easily interconvert at room temperature, making it impossible to predict which conformation is active at the BZR, a priori. Evidence for stereospecificity for binding to the BZR was provided by introducing a 3-substituent into the benzodiazepine nucleus to provide a chiral center and enantiomeric pairs of derivatives (104). In vitro BZR binding affinity and in vivo anxiolytic activity of several 3-methylated enantiomers was found to reside in the *S*-isomer. Moreover, the *S*-enantiomer of 3-methyldiazepam was shown to stabilize conformation *a* for ring B, whereas the *R*-enantiomer stabilizes conformation *b*. Also, the 3-*S* configuration and *a* conformation for ring B is present in both the crystalline state (120) and in solution (121) for 3-methyldiazepam. In spite of the enantioselectivity demonstrated for benzodiazepines, the commonly used 3-hydroxylated derivatives (e.g., lorazepam and oxazepam) are commercially available only as racemic mixtures.

Physiochemical and pharmacokinetics. The physiochemical and pharmacokinetic properties of the various benzodiazepines vary widely, and these properties have clinical implications. For example, depending on the nature of substituents, particularly with regard to electronegative substituents, the lipophilicity of the benzodiazepines may vary by more than three orders of magnitude, affecting absorption, distribution, and metabolism of individual agents. In general, most benzodiazepines have relatively high lipid:water partition coefficients (log P values) and are completely absorbed after oral administration and rapidly distributed to the brain and other highly perfused organs. A notable exception is clorazepate, which is rapidly decarboxylated at the 3-position to N-desmethyldiazepam and, subsequently, quickly absorbed. Also, most benzodiazepines and their metabolites bind to plasma proteins. The degree of protein binding is dependent on lipophilicity of the compound and varies from approximately 70% for more polar benzodiazepines, such as alprazolam, to 99% for very lipophilic derivatives, such as diazepam.

Hepatic microsomal oxidation, including N-dealkylation and aliphatic hydroxylation, accounts for the major metabolic disposition of most benzodiazepines. Subsequent conjugation of microsomal metabolites by glucuronyl transferases yields polar glucuronides that are excreted in urine. In general, the rate and product of benzodiazepine metabolism varies, depending on route of administration and the individual drug.

Chlordiazepoxide. Chlordiazepoxide is well absorbed after oral administration, and peak blood concentration usually is reached in approximately 4 hours. Intramuscular absorption of chlordiazepoxide, however, is slower and erratic. The half-life of chlordiazepoxide is variable but usually quite long (6–30 hours). The initial N-demethylation product, N-desmethylchloridiazepoxide, undergoes deamination to form the demoxepam (Fig. 22.18), which is extensively metabolized, and less than 1% of a dose of chlordiazepoxide is excreted as demoxepam. Demoxepam can undergo four different metabolic fates. Removal of the N-oxide moiety yields the active metabolite, N-desmethyldiazepam (desoxydemoxepam). This product is a metabolite of both chlordiazepoxide and diazepam and can be hydroxylated to yield oxazepam, another active metabolite that is rapidly glucuronidated

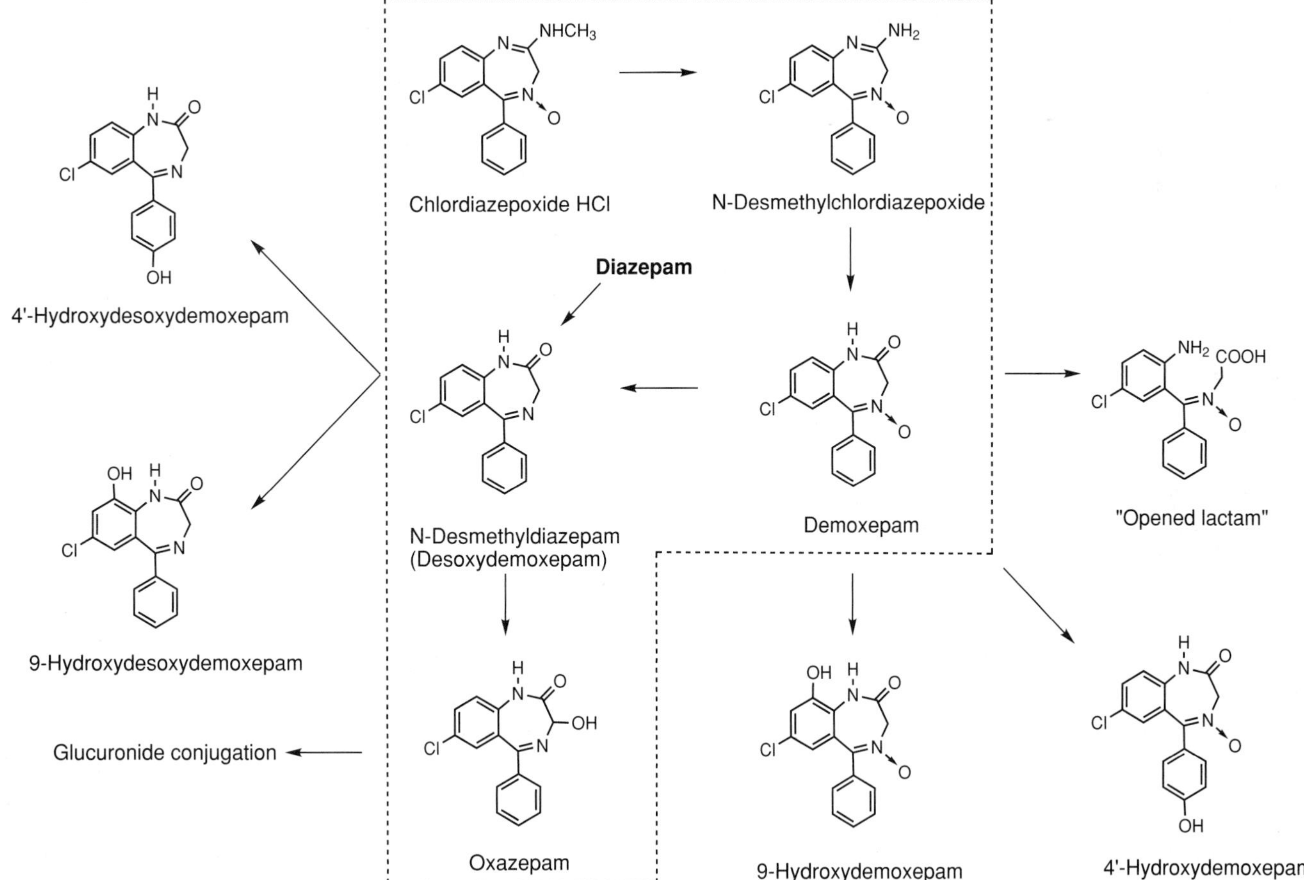

Fig. 22.18. Metabolism of chlordiazepoxide and related benzodiazepines.

and excreted in the urine. Another possibility for metabolism of demoxepam is hydrolysis to the "opened lactam," which is inactive. The two other metabolites of demoxepam are the products of ring A hydroxylation (9-hydroxydemoxepam) or ring C hydroxylation (4′-hydroxydemoxepam), both of which are inactive. The majority of a dose of chlordiazepoxide is excreted as glucuronide conjugates of oxazepam and other phenolic (9- or 4′-hydroxylated) metabolites. As with diazepam (vide infra), repeated administration of chlordiazepoxide can result in accumulation of parent drug and its active metabolites, which may have important clinical implications, including excessive sedation (4,5).

Diazepam. Diazepam is rapidly and completely absorbed after oral administration. Maximum peak blood concentration occurs in 2 hours, and elimination is slow, with a half-life of approximately 20 to 50 hours. As with chlordiazepoxide, the major metabolic product of diazepam is N-desmethyldiazepam, which is pharmacologically active and undergoes even slower metabolism than its parent compound. Repeated administration of diazepam or chlordiazepoxide leads to accumulation of N-desmethyldiazepam, which can be detected in the blood for more than 1 week after discontinuation of the drug. Hydroxylation of N-desmethyldiazepam at the 3-position gives the active metabolite oxazepam (Fig. 22.18).

Oxazepam. Oxazepam is an active metabolite of both chlordiazepoxide and diazepam and is marketed separately, as a short-acting anxiolytic agent. Oxazepam is rapidly inactivated to glucuronidated metabolites that are excreted in the urine (Fig. 22.18). The half-life of oxazepam is approximately 4 to 8 hours, and cumulative effects with chronic therapy are much less than with long-acting benzodiazepines, such as chlordiazepoxide and diazepam. Lorazepam is the 2′-chloro derivative of oxazepam and has a similarly short half-life (2–6 hours) and pharmacological activity.

Flurazepam. Flurazepam is administered orally as the dihydrochloride salt. It is rapidly ^{1}N-dealkylated to give the 2′-fluoro derivative of N-desmethyldiazepam, and it subsequently follows the same metabolic pathways as chlordiazepoxide and diazepam (Fig. 22.18). The half-life of flurazepam is fairly long (~7 hours); consequently, it has the same potential as chlordiazepoxide and diazepam to produce cumulative clinical effects and side effects (e.g., excessive sedation) and residual pharmacological activity, even after discontinuation. Chlorazepate is yet another benzodiazepine that is rapidly metabolized (3-decarboxylation) to N-desmethyldiazepam and so shares similar clinical and pharmacokinetic properties to chlordiazepoxide and diazepam.

Detailed pharmacokinetic analysis. Detailed pharmacokinetic analysis for most benzodiazepines is complex. Two-compartment models may be adequate to describe the disposition of most derivatives, but three-compartment models are necessary for highly lipophilic agents, such as diazepam. The distribution of such lipophilic drugs is further complicated by enterohepatic circulation. Thus, the usually stated elimination half-life of benzodiazepines may not adequately account for the pharmacodynamics of the distributive phase of the drug, which can be clinically important. For example, the distributive (α) half-life of diazepam is approximately 1 hour, whereas the elimination (β) half-life is approximately 1.5 days, acutely, and even longer after chronic dosing that results in accumulation of drug (4,5). Furthermore, plasma concentration and clinical effectiveness of benzodiazepines is difficult to correlate, and only a two-fold increase in clinically effective levels produces sedative side effects. Consequently, in spite of the long half-life of many benzodiazepines, they are not safe or effective when given in one daily dose and usually are divided into two to four doses per day for treatment of daytime anxiety (4,5). Both therapeutic and toxic effects may persist several days after discontinuation of chronically administered, long-acting benzodiazepines, such as chlordiazepoxide and diazepam. Thus, short-acting benzodiazepines, such as oxazepam, that are rapidly metabolized to inactive products should be considered in elderly or hepatocompromised patients.

Nonbenzodiazepine Agonists at the Benzodiazepine Receptor

Relatively few structural classes of nonbenzodiazepine compounds have clinically relevant affinity for the BZR and show pharmacological activity in vivo. Examples of these classes include the β-carbolines, triazolopyridazines, cyclopyrrolones, pyrazolopyrimidines, and imidazopyridines. Representative drugs of these classes in current clinical use are the pyrazolopyrimidine zaleplon, the cyclopyrrolone eszopiclone, and the imidazopyridazine zolpidem. These nonbenzodiazepine BZR ligands show greater selectivity for $GABA_A$ receptors containing the α_1 subunit; however, it should be noted that the α_2, α_3, α_5, and γ subunits may be important in mediating anxiolytic effects of BRZ agonists (84).

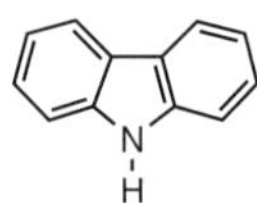

β-Carboline

β-Carboline. Several β-carbolines have approximately 10-fold higher affinity for the BZR when compared to diazepam. The ethyl ester of β-carboline-3-carboxylic acid (βCCE), identified in human urine extracts as an artifact of the extraction procedure, has very high affinity for the BZR. Although βCCE and other β-carbolines are not endogenous BZR ligands (vide supra) and are not currently approved for clinical use, they are used to characterize different $GABA_A$/BZR subtypes (based on α and γ subunit composition) and function (e.g., the partial agonist abecarnil) toward the discovery of anxioselective drugs. In this regard, the β-carboline ring system is planar in comparison to the boat conformation of the 1,4-benzodiazepines (see the discussion of stereochemistry); thus, β-carbolines have been useful to extend structure–activity relationship information for the agonist, antagonist, and inverse agonist pharmacophores of the various $GABA_A$/ BZR subtypes.

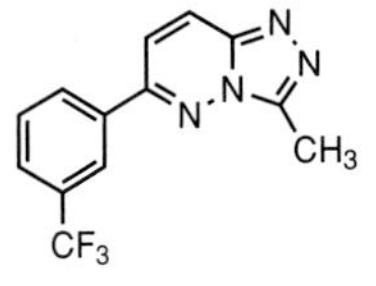

CL 218,872

CL 218,872. The triazolopyridazine CL 218,872 is another research tool used to probe BZR heterogeneity, because it is known to have selective high affinity at BZR subtypes containing the a1 subunit, hypothesized to mediate anxioselective actions (84,122). CL 218,872 has lower efficacy than benzodiazepines in potentiating GABA-gated chloride currents, but it produces anxiolytic effects in animal models at substantially lower doses than those required to produce untoward side effects (e.g., sedation, ataxia, and muscle relaxation) (78,122).

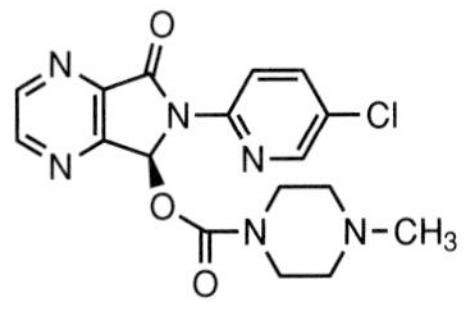

Eszopiclone
(Lunesta)

Eszopiclone. The cyclopyrrole zopiclone is described as a "superagonist" at BZRs with the subunit composition $\alpha_1\beta_2\gamma_2$ and $\alpha_1\beta_2\gamma_3$ (Table 15.3), because it potentiates the GABA-gated current more than the benzodiazepine (flunitrazepam) reference agonist (123). Racemic zopiclone has been available in Europe since 1992 and the higher affinity *S*-enantiomer (eszopiclone) was marketed in the United States in 2005, primarily to treat insomnia, because of its rapid onset and moderate duration (half-life, ~6 hours) of hypnotic-sedative effect (124). Less than 10% of orally administered eszopiclone is excreted unchanged, because it undergoes extensive CYP3A4- and CYP2E1-catalyzed oxidation and demethylation to metabolites excreted primarily in urine.

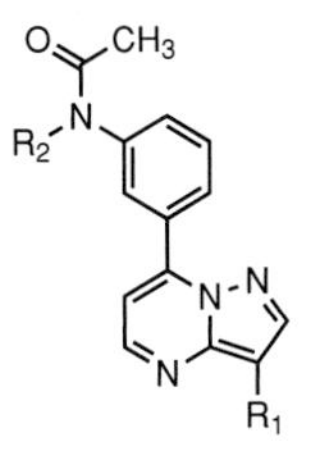

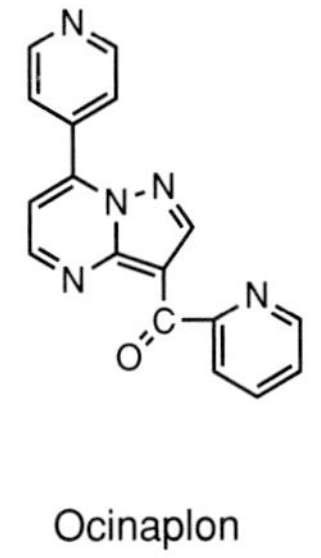

Zaleplon (Sonata) R_1 = CN, R_2 = CH_2CH_3

Indiplon R_1 = 2-thienylcarbonyl, R_2 = CH_3

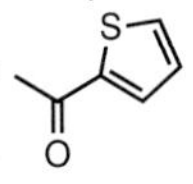

Ocinaplon

Pyrazolopyrimidines. The pyrazolopyrimidines zaleplon, indiplon, and ocinaplon have selective high affinity for α_1-containing BZRs but also produce effects at other BZR/$GABA_A$ subtypes. Animal studies show that both zaleplon and indiplon are effective sedative-hypnotics (125). In patients with insomnia, zaleplon is effective to decrease sleep latency and does not appear to induce withdrawal symptoms or rebound insomnia on discontinuation. Indiplon is similar and currently under review by the U.S. FDA. Zaleplon is absorbed rapidly and reaches peak plasma concentrations in approximately 1 hour, with a half-life approximately 1 hour as well. Less than 1% of a dose of zaleplon is excreted unchanged, because most is oxidized by aldehyde dehydrogenase and CYP3A4 to inactive metabolites, which are converted to glucuronides and eliminated in urine.

Ocinaplon, on the other hand, is being studied for its putative anxioselective activity rather than for its sedative effects. In rats, ocinaplon produces muscle relaxation, ataxia, and sedation only at doses 25-fold higher than the effective anxiolytic dose (122). Likewise, in patients with generalized anxiety disorder, ocinaplon produces anxiolytic effects at doses that do not cause greater incidence of sedation or dizziness than placebo. As a group, the pyrazolopyrimidines may be useful compounds to study discrepancies observed using molecular ($GABA_A$ subunit-selective) approaches versus transgenic animals and other in vivo models in the quest for anxioselective drugs. For example, for some compounds, partial agonism at a particular α subunit may be sufficient to produce a full anxiolytic activity in vivo, whereas other compounds must be full agonists for clinically relevant anxiolysis. Currently, it appears that high relative potency and high relative efficacy at multiple receptor subtypes can account for anxioselective properties of certain compounds, including for ocinaplon (122), which currently is under U.S. FDA review.

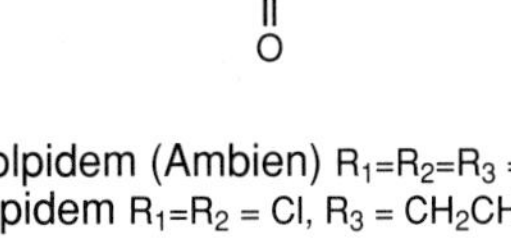

Zolpidem (Ambien) R_1=R_2=R_3 = CH_3
Alpidem R_1=R_2 = Cl, R_3 = $CH_2CH_2CH_3$

Imidazopyridines. The imidazopyridines, zolpidem and alpidem, represent another example of α_1 subunit-selective BZR/$GABA_A$ ligands that have clinical profiles different from those of typical benzodiazepines. For example, although the agonist effects of zolpidem on $GABA_A$ receptors qualitatively resemble those of benzodiazepines, clinically it shows a weaker anticonvulsant effect and a stronger sedative effect, which may mask anxiolytic effects. Zolpidem was marketed as a sedative-hypnotic in the United States in 1993, and it appears to be effective in shortening sleep latency and prolonging total sleep time, without affecting sleep stages, in patients with insomnia (126). Zolpidem is readily absorbed from the gastrointestinal tract and is extensively metabolized by the liver to inactive oxidized products, with a half-life of approximately 2 hours. Alpidem is similar to zolpidem in that it apparently induces no significant changes in sleep parameters (127) and has no effect on memory or muscle tone (128). Alpidem was found to be of at least equal efficacy to lorazepam in the treatment of patients with generalized anxiety disorder (129); however, it recently was withdrawn because of hepatotoxicity (130).

$GABA_A$ Partial Allosteric Modulators

Partial agonists of the $GABA_A$ receptor complex offer some theoretical and practical advantages over full agonists. For example, compared to the benzodiazepine-type full agonists, partial agonists seem to have lesser side effects, such as sedation, ataxia, and potentiation of alcohol. Also, there may be less abuse potential associated with partial agonists. Three partial agonists of $GABA_A$ receptors currently are being investigated: imidazenil, bretazenil, and abecarnil (Fig. 22.19). Abecarnil is reported by some investigators to have preferential affinity for BZR/$GABA_A$ α_1 subunits, whereas imidazenil and bretazenil are not subtype selective. In any event, abecarnil as well as bretazenil exhibit anxioselectivity in animal models, but data from clinical trials do not support the anxioselective profile predicted from preclinical results (84).

Imidazenil is an imidazobenzodiazepine carboxamide that has higher BZR affinity than diazepam but is only about half as efficacious at modulating GABA effects on chloride currents. Consistent with the general pharmacological principle that partial agonists may show antagonist functional effects in competition with a more efficacious agonist, imidazenil blocks the sedative and ataxic effects of diazepam (131). Interestingly, however, imidazenil does not block the anticonvulsant effects of diazepam; accordingly, it has been proposed as an alternative to flumazenil in the alleviation of benzodiazepine-induced withdrawal symptoms (131). Bretazenil has qualitatively similar binding and clinical characteristics as imidazenil (132). Its anxiolytic activity comes with significant sedation, however, and this led to discontinuation of its development. Abecarnil is a β-carboline with anxiolytic properties. Typical of other partial allosteric modulators, abecarnil demonstrates antianxiety and anticonvulsant activities, with little or no development of tolerance to these effects (133). Like bretazenil, however, doses of abecarnil required to produce anxiolysis also produce sedation, and it is unlikely that this drug lead will be developed (84).

Miscellaneous Anxiolytic Agents

Serotonin Receptor–Active Agents. In the development of anxiolytic agents that do not act via the $GABA_A$ receptor complex, serotonin receptors have been the focus of intensive research in recent years, because preclinical and clinical evidence supports the involvement of serotonin in anxiety (134,135). For example, serotonin 5-HT_{1A} receptors are found in relatively high density in the septohippocampal region of the brain, which is involved in the modulation of anxiety (136). In the structures of the limbic system, 5-HT_{1A} receptors are predominantly postsynaptic, whereas presynaptic 5-HT_{1A} are found in the dorsal and median raphe nuclei. Presynaptic 5-HT_{1A} receptors function as autoreceptors to inhibit serotonergic neurotransmission, and postsynaptic receptor activation also results in decreased neuronal activity.

The pyrimidinylbutylpiperazines (azapirones), buspirone, ipsaperone, and gepirone (Fig. 22.20) partial agonists at brain 5-HT_{1A} receptors and have anxiolytic activity in humans (135,137). Their anxiolytic effects appear only after several days of treatment, and although it is well

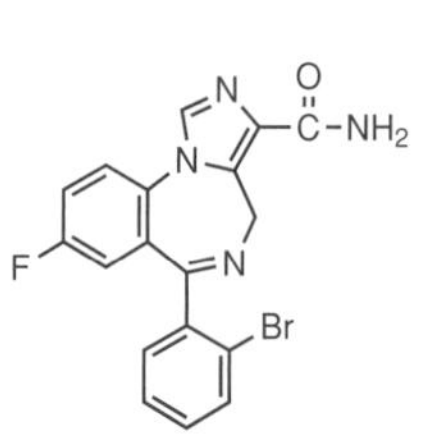

Imidazenil 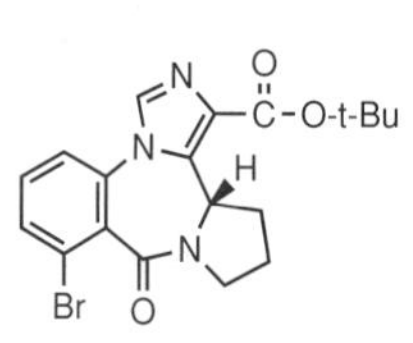 Bretazenil 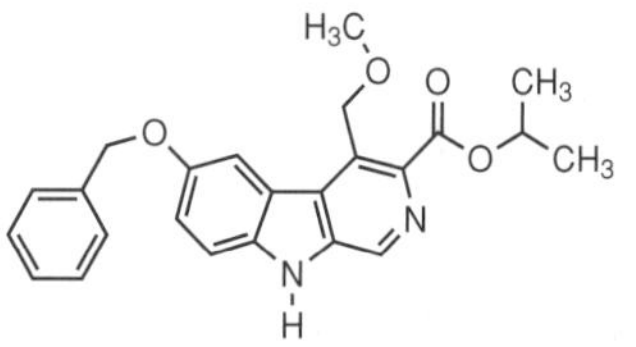 Abecarnil

Fig. 22.19. Structures of γ-aminobutyric $acid_A$ ($GABA_A$) receptor partial agonists.

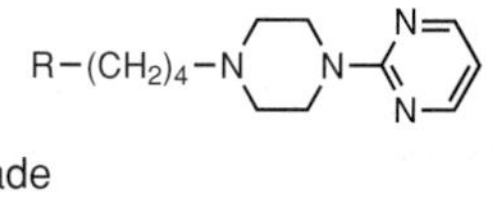

R–$(CH_2)_4$–N(piperazine)N–pyrimidinyl

Generic name	Trade name	R
Buspirone	Buspar	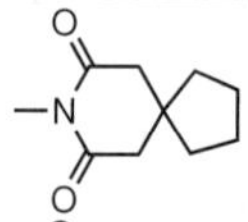
Gepirone		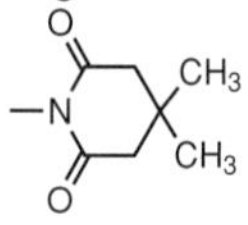
Ipsapirone		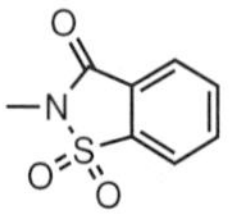

Fig. 22.20. Structures of 5-HT_{1A} partial agonists.

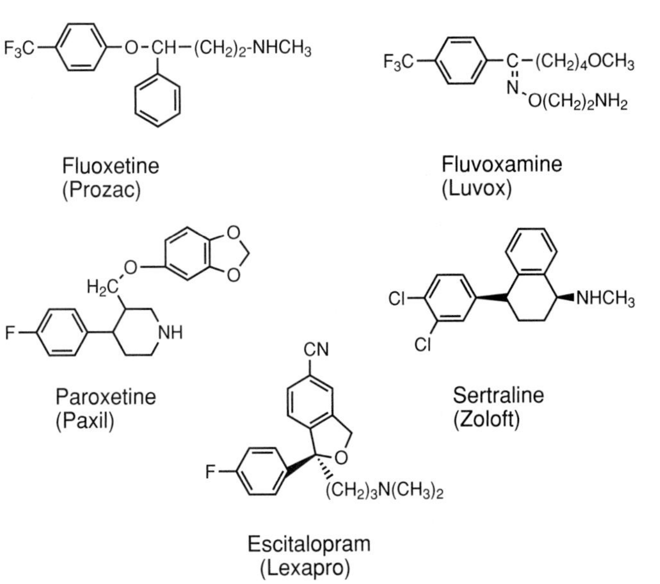

Fluoxetine (Prozac)

Fluvoxamine (Luvox)

Paroxetine (Paxil)

Sertraline (Zoloft)

Escitalopram (Lexapro)

Fig. 22.21. Structures of the selective serotonin reuptake inhibitors (SSRIs) fluoxetine, fluvoxamine, paroxetine, sertraline, and escitalopram.

established that agonistic activity is required, the optimal level of intrinsic activity is still a matter of debate. Thus, it is unclear whether their mechanism of action is to acutely increase serotonergic activity or chronically decrease serotonergic activity (138). Buspirone is the only one of these agents currently marketed in the United States. It also has antidopaminergic activity that complicates interpretation of its interaction with 5-HT_{1A} receptors regarding anxiolytic effects. In any event, busiprone is shown to be effective in the treatment of generalized anxiety disorders that are mild to moderate in severity, but it is not useful for severe anxiety (e.g., with panic attacks).

Serotonin reuptake inhibitors. Several selective serotonin reuptake inhibitors (SSRIs), including escitalopram, fluoxetine, fluvoxamine, paroxetine, and sertraline (Fig. 22.21), are effective as first-line treatment of some anxiety disorders, with the purported advantage that they lack the addictive properties of benzodiazepines (135). Specifically, the SSRIs have been shown to be effective in obsessive-compulsive disorder (139), panic disorder (140), and social phobia (141). The mechanism of action of these agents in anxiety may differ with their role in the treatment of depression; however, current understanding centers on functional imaging studies that show SSRI treatment can dampen brain excitability (135).

ACKNOWLEDGMENT

The author wishes to express his gratitude to Drs. John L. Neumeyer and Ross J. Baldessarini for the training and guidance involved in preparing this chapter.

CASE STUDY

Victoria F. Roche and S. William Zito

RP is a 45-year-old Caucasian male whose increasingly impulsive, agitated, and antisocial behaviors have culminated in a diagnosis of schizophrenia. This is a particularly difficult situation given that for the past several years, he has been exhibiting symptoms of premature Parkinson's disease, with gait and balance being his most adversely affected abilities. RP's Parkinson's disease is currently being treated with levodopa/carbidopa (Sinemet 25/100 t.i.d.), although he is still experiencing periods of rigidity and unsteadiness in his movements. He is of the poor 2D6 metabolizer phenotype but the compounds in Sinemet (the only drug he is taking) are known to be metabolized by CYP2D6.

RP is single and, since the onset of the Parkinson's disease, has lived with his brother's family, which includes his wife and 6-year-old twin boys. He has a high school education and contributes to the household income through his job as a host at a nearby pancake restaurant. In the small Midwestern community in which he lives, he has received emotional support from his friends and neighbors (including those who frequent the restaurant), but there is concern about the impact of this new diagnosis on his ability to retain his job, particularly because he has recently had his first auditory hallucination. In addition, RP's sister-in-law is becoming concerned about the impact of his behavior on her two young sons. Consider the structures of the antipsychotic agents drawn below, and prepare to make a recommendation to RP's psychiatrist.

1. Identify the therapeutic problem(s) in which the pharmacist's intervention may benefit the patient.
2. Identify and prioritize the patient-specific factors that must be considered to achieve the desired therapeutic outcomes.
3. Conduct a thorough and mechanistically oriented structure-activity analysis of all therapeutic alternatives provided in the case.
4. Evaluate the structure–activity relationship findings against the patient-specific factors and desired therapeutic outcomes, and make a therapeutic decision.
5. Counsel your patient.

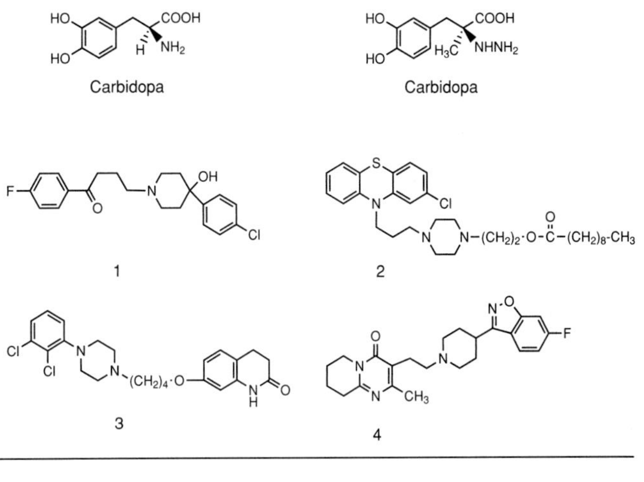

Carbidopa

Carbidopa

1

2

3

4

References

1. American Psychiatric Association. Diagnostic and Statistical Manual of Mental Disorders, 4th Ed. Washington, DC: APA Press, 1994. Revised text, 2000.
2. Kraepelin E. Dementia Praecox and Paraphrenia (Barclay RM, Roberston GM, trans.). Edinburgh: Livingstone, 1919.
3. Bleuler E. Dimentia Praecox oder Gruppe der Schizophrenien. In: Aschaffenberg G, ed. Handbuch der Psychiatric (Spezieller Teil, 4. Abteilung). Leipzig: Denticke, 1911.
4. Baldessarini RJ, Tarazi FI. Chemotherapy in Psychiatry: Principles and Practice, 3rd Ed. Cambridge, MA: Harvard University Press, 1996.
5. Baldessarini RJ, Tarazi FI. Drugs and the treatment of psychiatric disorders: psychosis and mania. In: Hardman JG, Limbird LE, Gilman AG, eds. The Pharmacological Basis of Therapeutics, 9th Ed. New York: McGraw-Hill, 2001:485–520.
6. Baldessarini RJ, Tarazi FI. Brain dopamine receptors: a primer on their current status, basic and clinical. Harv Rev Psychiatry 1996;3:301–325.
7. Carlsson A, Lindquist M. Effect of chlorpromazine and haloperidol on formation of 3-methoxytyramine and normetanephrine in mouse brain. Acta Pharmacol Toxicol 1963;20:140–144.
8. Seeman P. Dopamine receptors and the dopamine hypothesis of schizophrenia. Synapse 1987;1:133–152.
9. Seeman P, Lee T, Chau-Wong M, et al. Antipsychotic drug doses and neuroleptic/dopamine receptors. Nature 1976;261:717–719.
10. Akam E, Strange PG. Inverse agonist properties of atypical antipsychotic drugs. Biochem Pharmacol 2004;6:2039–2045.
11. Hartman DS, Civelli O. Dopamine receptor diversity: molecular and pharmacological perspectives. Prog Drug Res 1997;48:173–194.
12. Kebabian J, Calne D. Multiple receptors for dopamine. Nature 1979;277:93–96.
13. Lovenberg TW, Brewster WK, Motolla DM, et al. Dihydrexidine, a novel selective high potency full dopamine D_1 receptor agonist. Eur J Pharmacol 1989;166:111–113.
14. Knoerzer TA, Nichols DE, Brewster WK, et al. Dopaminergic Benzo[*a*]phenanthridines: Resolution and pharmacological evaluation of the enantiomers of dihyrexidine, the full efficacy D_1 dopamine receptor agonist. J Med Chem 1994;37:2453–2460.
15. Richelson E. Preclinical pharmacology of neuroleptics: focus on new generation compounds. J Clin Psychiatry 1996;57(Suppl 11):4–11.
16. Milligan G. Mechanisms of multifunctional signaling by G protein–linked receptors. Trends Pharmacol Sci 1993;14:239–244.
17. Raymond JR. Multiple mechanisms of receptor–G protein signaling specificity. Am J Physiol 1995;269:F141–F158.
18. Kenakin T. Inverse, protean, and ligand-selective agonism: matters of receptor conformation. FASEB J 2001;15:598–611.
19. Gay EA, Urban JD, Nichols DE, et al. Functional selectivity of D_2 receptor ligands in a Chinese hamster ovary hD_{2L} cell line: evidence for induction of ligand-specific receptor states. Mol Pharmacol 2004;66:97–105.
20. Moniri NH, Covington-Strachan D, Booth RG. Ligand-directed functional heterogeneity of histamine H_1 receptors: novel dual-function ligands selectively activate and block H_1-mediated phospholipase C and adenylyl cyclase signaling. J Pharmacol Exp Ther 2004;311:274–281.
21. Lawler CP, Prioleau C, Lewis MM, et al. Interactions of the novel antipsychotic aripiprazole (OPC-14597) with dopamine and serotonin receptor subtypes. Neuropsychopharmacology 1999;20:612–627.
22. Kilts JD, Connery HS, Arrington EG, et al. Functional selectivity of dopamine receptor agonists. II. Actions of dihydrexidine in D2L receptor-transfected MN9D cells and pituitary lactotrophs. J Pharmacol Exp Ther 2002;301:1179–1189.
23. Mottola DM, Kilts JD, Lewis MM, et al. Functional selectivity of dopamine receptor agonists. I. Selective activation of postsynaptic dopamine D_2 receptors linked to adenylate cyclase. J Pharmacol Exp Ther 2002;301: 1166–1178.
24. Wolf, ME, Roth RH. Autoreceptor regulation of dopamine synthesis. Ann N Y Acad Sci 1990;604:323–342.
25. Tissari AH, Atzori L, Galdieri MT. Inhibition of dopamine synthesis in striatal synaptosomes by lisuride: Stereospecific reversal by (−)-sulpiride. Naunyn-Schmiedeberg Arch Pharmacol 1983;322:89–91.
26. Booth RG, Baldessarini R J, Kula NS, et al. Presynaptic inhibition of dopamine synthesis in rat striatal tissue by enantiomeric mono- and dihydroxyaporphines. Mol Pharmacol 1990;38:92–101.
27. Arbilla S, Langer SZ. Stereoselectivity of presynaptic autoreceptors modulating dopamine release. Eur J Pharmacol 1981;76:345–351.
28. Bolonna AA, Kerwin RW. Partial agonism and schizophrenia. Br J Psychiatry 2005;186:7–10.
29. Booth RG, Baldessarini RJ. Adenosine A_2 stimulation of tyrosine hydroxylase activity in rat striatal minces is reversed by dopamine D_2 autoreceptor activation. Eur J Pharmacol 1990;185:217–221.
30. Booth RG, Owens CE, Brown RL, et al. Putative σ3 sites in mammalian brain have histamine H_1 receptor properties: Evidence from ligand binding and distribution studies with the novel H_1 radioligand [^{3}H]-(−)-*trans*-1-phenyl-3-aminotetralin (PAT). Brain Res 1999;837:95–105.
31. Choksi NY, Nix William B, Wyrick SD, et al. A novel phenylaminotetralin recognizes histamine H1 receptors and stimulates dopamine synthesis in vivo in rat brain. Brain Res 2000;852:151–160.
32. Johnson EA, Tsai CE, Shahan YH, et al. Serotonin 5-HT_{1A} receptors mediate inhibition of tyrosine hydroxylase in rat striatum. J Pharmacol Exp Ther 1993;266:133–141.
33. El Tamer A, Prokopenko I, Wulfert E, et al. Mivazerol, a novel α_2-agonist and potential anti-ischemic drug, inhibits KC1-stimulated neurotransmitter release in rat nervous tissue preparations. J Neurochemistry 1996;67:636–644.
34. Bovet D, Staup AM. Action protectrice des éthers phénoliques au cours da l'intoxication histaminique. C R Soc Biol (Paris) 1937;124:547–549.
35. Charpentier P, Gailliot P, Jacob R, et al. Rescherches sur les di methylaminopropyl-N-phenothiazines substituees. C R Acad Sci (Paris) 1952;235:59–60.
36. Laborit H, Huguenard P, Alluaume R. A new vegetative stabilizer. Presse Med 1952;60:206–208.
37. Delay J, Deniker P, Harl J. Utilization therapeutique psychiatrique d'une phenothiazine d'action centrale elective. Ann Med Psychol (Paris) 1952;110:112–117.
38. Horn AS, Snyder SH. Chlorpromazine and dopamine: Conformational similarities that correlate with the antischizophrenic activity of phenothiazine drugs. Proc Natl Acad Sci U S A 1971;68:2325–2328.
39. Janssen PA. The butyrophenone story. In: Ayd FI, Blackwell B, eds. Discoveries in Biological Psychiatry. Philadelphia: Lippincott, 1970;165–179.
40. Simpson GM, Lee JH. A ten-year review of antipsychotics. In Lipton MA, ed. Psychopharmacology: A Generation of Progress. New York: Raven Press, 1978:1131–1137.
41. Janssen PAJ, Van Bever FM. Applications. In: Usdin E, Forrest IS, eds. Psychotherapeutic Drugs. Part II. New York: Marcel Decker, 1977:839–921.
42. Subramanyam B, Pond S, Eyles D, et al. N. Identification of a potentially neurotoxic pyridinium metabolite in the urine of schizophrenic patients treated with haloperidol. Biochem Biophys Res Commun 1990;181: 573–578.
43. Halliday GM, Pond SM, Cartwright H, et al. Clinical and neuropathological abnormalities in baboons treated with HPTP, the tetrahydropyridine analogue of haloperidol. Exp Neurol 1999;158:155–163.
44. Igarashi K, Matsubara K, Kasuya F, et al. Effect of a pyridinium metabolite derived from haloperidol on the activities of striatal tyrosine hydroxylase in freely moving rats. Neurosci Lett 1996;214:183–186.
45. Rollema H, Skolnick M, D'Engelbronner J, et al. MPP-like neurotoxicity of a pyridinium metabolite derived from haloperidol: in vivo microdialysis and in vitro mitochondrial studies. J Pharmacol Exp Ther 1994;268:380–387.
46. Ulrich S, Sandmann U, Genz A. Serum concentrations of haloperidol pyridinium metabolites and the relationship with tardive dyskinesia and parkinsonism: a cross-section study in psychiatric patients. Pharmacopsychiatry 2005;38:171–177.
47. Augrist BM. The neurobiologically active benzamides and related compounds: some historical aspects. In: Rotrosen J, Stanley M, eds. The Benzamides: Pharmacology, Neurobiology, and Clinical Effects. New York: Raven Press, 1982:1–6.
48. Jenner P, Marsden CD. Neuroleptic agents; acute and chronic receptor actions. In: Horwell DC, ed. Drugs in Central Nervous System Disorders. New York: Marcel Dekker, 1985:149–262.
49. Kroeze WK, Hufeisen SJ, Popadak BA, et al. H_1-histamine receptor affinity predicts short-term weight gain for typical and atypical antipsychotic drugs. Neuropsychopharmacology 2003;28:519–526.
50. Alvir JMJ, Jeffrey PH, Lieberman JA, et al. Clozapine-induced agranulocytosis. Incidence and risk factors in the United States. N Engl J Med 1993;329:162–167.
51. Kinon BJ, Lieberman JA. Mechanisms of action of atypical antipsychotic drugs: a critical analysis. Psychopharmacology 1996;124:2–34.
52. Meltzer HY, Matsubara S, Lee JC. The ratios of $serotonin_2$ and $dopamine_2$ affinities differentiate atypical and typical antipsychotic drugs. Psychopharmacol Bull 1989;25:390–392.
53. Busatto GF, Kerwin RW. Perspectives on the role of serotonergic mechanisms in the pharmacology of schizophrenia. J Psychopharmacol 1997;11:3–12.
54. Kapur S, Remington G. Serotonin–dopamine interaction and its relevance to schizophrenia. Am J Psychiatry 1996;153:466–476.
55. Newman-Tancredi A, Gavaudan S, Conte C, et al. Agonist and antagonist actions of antipsychotic agents at 5-HT_{1A} receptors: a [^{35}S]GTPγS binding study. Eur J Pharmacol 1998;55:245–256.
56. Meltzer HY, Li Z, Kaneda Y, et al. Serotonin receptors: their key role in drugs to treat schizophrenia. Prog Neuro-Psychopharmacol Biol Psychiatry 2003;27:1159–1172.
57. Beedham C, Miceli JJ, Obach RS. Ziprasidone metabolism, aldehyde oxidase, and clinical implications. J Clin Psychopharmacol 2003;23:229–232.
58. Potkin SG, Saha AR, Kujawa MJ, et al. Aripiprazole, an antipsychotic with a novel mechanism of action, and risperidone vs placebo in patients with schizophrenia and schizoaffective disorder. Arch Gen Psychiatry 2003;60:681–690.
59. Shapiro DA, Renock S, Arrington E, et al. Aripiprazole, a novel atypical antipsychotic drug with a unique and robust pharmacology. Neuropsychopharmacology 2003;28:1400–1411.
60. Vickers SP, Clifton PG, Dourish CT, et al. Reduced satiating effect of D-fenfluramine in serotonin 5-HT_{2C} receptor mutant mice. Psychopharmacology (Berl) 1999;143:309–314.

61. Winans E. Aripiprazole. Am J Health Syst Pharm 2003;60:2437–2445.
62. Owen RR Jr, Cole JO. Molindone hydrochloride: a review of laboratory and clinical findings. J Clin Psychopharmacol 1989;9:268–276.
63. Galatsis P. Market to market. In Bristol JA, ed. Annual Reports in Medicinal Chemistry, vol. 32. San Diego: Academic Press, 1997:305–326.
64. Mellman TA, Uhde TW. Electroencephalographic sleep in panic disorder. Arch Gen Psychiatry 1989;46:178–184.
65. Rapoport JL. The neurobiology of obsessive-compulsive disorder. JAMA 1988;260:2888–2890.
66. Baxter L. Positron-emission tomography studies of cerebral glucose metabolism in obsessive-compulsive disorder. J Clin Psychiatry 1994; 55:54–59.
67. Nordahl TE, Semple WE, Gross M, et al. Cerebral glucose metabolic differences in patients with panic disorder. Neuropsychopharmacology 1990;3: 261–272.
68. Nickell PV, Uhde TW. Dose–response effects of intravenous caffeine in normal volunteers. Anxiety 1995;4:161–168.
69. Rauch S, Savage C, Alpert N, et al. A positron-emission tomographic study of simple phobic symptom provocation. Arch Gen Psychiatry 1995;52: 20–28.
70. Wu JC, Buchsbaum MS, Hershey TG, et al. PET in generalized anxiety disorder. Biol Psychiatry 1991;29:1181–1199.
71. Semple WE, Goyer P, McCormick R. Preliminary report: brain blood flow using PET in patients with posttraumatic stress disorder and substance abuse histories. Biol Psychiatry 1993;34:115–118.
72. Gershenfeld HK, Philibert RA, Boehm GW. Looking forward in geriatric anxiety and depression: implications of basic science for the future. Am J Geriatr Psychiatry 2005;13:1027–1040.
73. Redmond DEJ, Huang YH. New evidence for a locus ceruleus–norepinephrine connection with anxiety. Life Sci 1979;25:2149–2162.
74. Harary N, Kellogg C. The relationship of benzodiazepine binding sites to the norepinephrine projection of the adult rat. Brain Res 1989;492: 293–299.
75. Haefely W. Actions and interactions of benzodiazepine agonists and antagonists at GABAergic synapses. In Bower NG, ed. Actions and Interactions of GABA and Benzodiazepines. New York: Raven Press, 1984:263–285.
76. Gibbs ME, Johnston GA Opposing roles for $GABA_A$ and $GABA_C$ receptors in short-term memory formation in young chicks. Neuroscience 2005;131: 567–576.
77. Olsen RW, Tobin AJ. Molecular biology of $GABA_A$ receptors. FASEB J 1990;4:1469–1480.
78. Wafford KA, Whiting PJ, Kemp JA. Differences in affinity and efficacy of benzodiazepine receptor ligands at recombinant γ-aminobutyric $acid_A$ receptor subtypes. Mol Pharmacol 1993;43:240–244.
79. Wafford KA. $GABA_A$ receptor subtypes: any clues to the mechanism of benzodiazepine dependence? Curr Opin Pharmacol 2005;5:47–52.
80. Schofield PR, Darlison MG, Fujita N, et al. Sequence and functional expression of the $GABA_A$ receptor shows a ligand gated ion channel family. Nature 1987;328:221–227.
81. DeLorey TM, Olsen RW. γ-Aminobutyric $acid_A$ receptor structure and function. J Biol Chem 1992;267:16747–16750.
82. Wisden W, Laurie DJ, Monyer H, et al. The distribution of 13 $GABA_A$ receptor subunit mRNAs in the rat brain: I. Telencephalon, diencephalon, mesencephalon. J Neurosci 1992;12:1040–1062.
83. Sanger DJ, Benavides J, Perrault G, et al. Recent developments in the behavioral pharmacology of benzodiazepine (ω) receptors: evidence for the functional significance of receptor subtypes. Neurosci Biobehav Rev 1994;18: 355–372.
84. Basile AS, Lippa AS, Skolnick P. Anxioselective anxiolytics: can less be more? Eur J Pharmacol 2004;500:441–451.
85. Kaupmann K, Malitschek B, Schuler V, et al. GABA-B receptor subtypes assemble into functional heteromeric complexes. Nature 1998;396:683–687.
86. Couve A, Filippov AK, Connolly CN, et al. Intracellular retention of recombinant GABA-B receptors. J Biol Chem 1998;273:26361–26367.
87. Jones KA, Borowsky B, Tamm JA, et al. GABA-B receptors function as a heteromeric assembly of the subunits GABA-BR1 and GABA-BR2. Nature 1998;396:674–679.
88. White JH, Wise A, Main MJ, et al. Heterodimerization is required for the formation of a functional GABA-B receptor. Nature 1998;396:679–682.
89. Quiocho FA, Ledvina PS. Atomic structure and specificity of bacterial periplasmic receptors for active transport and chemotaxis: variation of common themes. Mol Microbiol 1996;20:17–25.
90. Bettler B, Kaupmann K, Mosbacher J, et al. Molecular structure and physiological functions of $GABA_B$ receptors. Physiol Rev 2004;84:835–867.
91. Cryan JF, Kaupmann K. Don't worry 'B' happy!: a role for $GABA_B$ receptors in anxiety and depression. Trends Pharmacol Sci 2005;26:36–43.
92. Froestl W, Bettler B, Bittiger H, et al. Ligands for expression cloning and isolation of $GABA_B$ receptors. Farmaco 2003;58:173–183.
93. Bowery NG, Hill DR, Hudson AL, et al. (−)-Baclofen decreases neurotransmitter release in the mammalian CNS by an action at a novel GABA receptor. Nature 1980;238:92–94.
94. Sternbach LH. Chemistry of 1,4-benzodiazepines and some aspects of the structure-activity relationship. In: Garattini S, Mussini E, Randall LD, eds. The Benzodiazepines. New York: Raven Press, 1973:1–25.
95. Sternbach LH. The benzodiazepine story. J Med Chem 1979;22:1–7.
96. Randall LO, Schallek W, Heise GA, et al. The psychosedative properties of methaminodiazepoxide. J Pharmacol Exp Ther 1960;129:163–171.
97. Randall LO, Scheckel CL, Banziger RF. Pharmacology of the metabolites of chlordiazepoxide and diazepam. Current Therapeutic Research, Clinical & Experimental 1965;7:590–606.
98. Braestrup C, Nielsen M, Olsen CE. Urinary and brain β-carboline-3-carboxylates as potent inhibitors of brain benzodiazepine receptors. Proc Natl Acad Sci U S A 1980; 121:2288–2292.
99. Cole BJ, Hillman M, Seidelmann D, et al. Effects of benzodiazepine receptors partial inverse agonists in the elevated plus mase test of anxiety in the rat. Psychopharmacology 1995;121:118–126.
100. Braestrup C, Schmiechen R, Neef G, et al. Interaction of convulsive ligands with benzodiazepine receptors. Science 1982;216:1241–1243.
101. Haefely W, Kyburz E., Gerecke M, et al. Recent advances in the molecular pharmacology of benzodiazepine receptors and the structure-activity relationships of these agonists and antagonists. Advances in Drug Research, vol 14. London: Academic Press, 1985:166-322.
102. Hunkeler W, Möhler H, Pieri L, et al. Selective antagonists of benzodiazepines. Nature 1981;290:514–516.
103. Möhler H, Richards JG. Agonist and antagonist benzodiazepine receptor interaction in vitro. Nature 1981;294:763–765.
104. Haefely W, Kyburz E, Gerecke M, et al. Recent advances in the molecular pharmacology of benzodiazepine receptors and the structure-activity relationships of these agonists and antagonists. Advances in Drug Research, vol 14. London: Academic Press, 1985:166–322.
105. Cole BJ, Hillman M, Seidelmann D, et al. Effects of benzodiazepine receptor partial inverse agonists in the elevated plus maze test of anxiety in the rat. Psychopharmacology 1995; 121:118–126.
106. Fryer RI. Ligand interaction at the benzodiazepine receptor. In Hansch C, ed. Comprehensive Medicinal Chemistry, vol. 3. New York: Pergamon Press, 1990:539–566.
107. Haefely W. The GABA-benzodiazepine interaction fifteen years later. Neurochemical Res 1990;15:169–174.
108. Wieland HA, Lüddens H, Seeburg PH. A single histidine in $GABA_A$ receptors is essential for benzodiazepine agonist binding, J Biol Chem 1992;267:1426–1429.
109. Huh KH, Delorey TM, Endo S, et al. Pharmacological subtypes of the γ-aminobutyric $acid_A$ receptors defined by a gamma-aminobutyric acid analogue 4,5,6,7-tetrahydroisoxazolo[5,4-c] pyridin-3-ol and allosteric coupling: characterization using subunit-specific antibodies. Mol Pharmacol 1995;48: 666–675.
110. Pritchett DB, Sontheimer H, Shivers BD, et al. Importance of a novel $GABA_A$ receptor subunit for benzodiazepine pharmacology. Nature 1989;338: 582–585.
111. Pritchett DB, Seeburg PH. γ-Aminobutyric $acid_A$ receptor α_5 subunit creates novel type II benzodiazepine receptor pharmacology. J Neurochem 1990;54:1802–1804.
112. Rowlett JK, Platt DM, Lelas S, et al. Different $GABA_A$ receptor subtypes mediate the anxiolytic, abuse-related, and motor effects of benzodiazepine-like drugs in primates. Proc Natl Acad Sci U S A 2005;102: 915–920.
113. Wong G, Lyon T, Skolnick P. Chronic exposure to benzodiazepine receptor ligands uncouples the γ-aminobutyric acid type A receptor in WSS-1 cells. Mol Pharmacol 1994;46:1056–1062.
114. Tietz EI, Chiu TH, Rosenberg HC. Regional GABA/benzodiazepine receptor/chloride channel coupling after acute and chronic benzodiazepine treatment. Eur J Pharmacol 1989;167:57–65.
115. Crippen GM. Distance geometry analysis of the benzodiazepine binding site. Mol Pharmacol 1982;22:11–19.
116. Zhang W, Koehler KF, Zhang P, et al. Development of a comprehensive pharmacophore model for the benzodiazepine receptor. Drug Des Discov 1995;12:193–248.
117. Diaz-Arauzo H, Koehler KF, Hagen TJ, et al. Synthetic and computer assisted analysis of the pharmacophore for agonists at benzodiazepine receptors. Life Sci 1991;49:207–216.
118. Villar HO, Davies MF, Loew GH, et al. Molecular models for recognition and activation at the benzodiazepine receptor: a review. Life Sci 1991;48: 593–602.
119. Falco JL, Lloveras M, Buira I, et al. Design, synthesis and biological activity of acyl substituted 3-amino-5-methyl-1,4,5,7-tetrahydropyrazolo[3,4-b]pyridin-6- ones as potential hypnotic drugs. Eur J Med Chem 2005;40: 1179–1187.
120. Blount JF, Fryer RI, Gilman NW, et al. Quinazolines and 1,4-benzodiazepines. 92. Conformational recognition of the receptor by 1,4-benzodiazepines. Mol Pharmacol 1983;24:425–428.
121. Sunjic V, Lisin A, Sega A, et al. Conformation of 7-chloro-5-phenyl-d5-3(s)-methyldihydro-1,4-benzodiazepine-2-one in solution. Heterocyc Chem 1979;16:757–761.
122. Lippa A, Czobor P, Stark J, et al. Selective anxiolysis produced by ocinaplon, a $GABA_A$ receptor modulator. Proc Natl Acad Sci U S A 2005;102:7380–7385.
123. Davies M, Newell JG, Derry JM, et al. Characterization of the interaction of zopiclone with γ-aminobutyric acid type A receptors. Mol Pharmacol 2000;58:756–762.

124. Rosenberg R, Caron J, Roth T, et al. An assessment of the efficacy and safety of eszopiclone in the treatment of transient insomnia in healthy adults. Sleep Med 2005;6:15–22.
125. Foster AC, Pelleymounter MA, Cullen MJ, et al. In vivo pharmacological characterization of indiplon, a novel pyrazolopyrimidine sedative-hypnotic. J Pharmacol Exp Ther 2004;311:547–559.
126. Herrmann WM, Kubicki ST, Boden S, et al. Pilot controlled double-blind study of the hypnotic effects of zolpidem in patients with chronic "learned" insomnia: psychometric and polysomnographic evaluation. J Int Med Res 1993;21:306–322.
127. Saletu B, Schultes M, Grunberger J. Sleep laboratory study of a new antianxiety drug, alpidem: short-term trial. Curr Ther Res 1986;40: 769–779.
128. Bartholini G. Nonbenzodiazepine anxiolytics and hypnotics: concluding remarks. Pharmacol Biochem Behav 1988;29:833–834.
129. Diamond BI, Nguyen H, et al. A comparative study of alpidem, a nonbenzodiazepine, and lorazepam in patients with nonpsychotic anxiety. Psychopharmacol Bull 1991;27:67–71.
130. Berson A, Descatoire V, Sutton A, et al. Toxicity of alpidem, a peripheral benzodiazepine receptor ligand, but not zolpidem, in rat hepatocytes: role of mitochondrial permeability transition and metabolic activation. J Pharmacol Exp Ther 2001;299:793–800.
131. Auta J, Costa E, Davis JM, et al. Imidazenil: an antagonist of the sedative but not the anticonvulsant action of diazepam. Neuropharmacology 2005;49: 425–429.
132. Puia G, Ducic I, Vicini S, et al. Molecular mechanisms of the partial allosteric modulatory effects of bretazenil at γ-aminobutyric acid type A receptor. Proc Natl Acad Sci U S A 1992;89:3620–3624.
133. Ozawa M, Sugimachi K, Nakada-Kometani Y, et al. Chronic pharmacological activities of the novel anxiolytic β-carboline abecarnil in rats. J Pharmacol Exp Ther 1994;269:457–462.
134. Lucki I. Serotonin receptor specificity in anxiety disorders. J Clin Psychiatry 1996;57(Suppl 6):5–10.
135. Gross C, Hen R. The developmental origins of anxiety. Nat Rev Neurosci 2004;5:545–552.
136. Gray JAG. The Neuropsychology of Anxiety: An Enquiry Into the Functions of the Septo-Hippocampal System. New York: Oxford University Press, 1982.
137. Traber J, Glaser T. 5-HT_{1A} receptor–related anxiolytics. Trends Pharmacol Sci 1987;8:432–437.
138. Peroutka SJ. 5-Hydroxytryptamine receptors. J Neurochem 1993;60:408–416.
139. Pigott TA, Pato BT, Bernstein SE, et al. Controlled comparisons of clomipramine and fluoxetine in the treatment of obsessive-compulsive disorder. Arch Gen Psychiatry 1990;47:926–932.
140. Schneirer FR, Liebowitz MR, Davies SO, et al. Fluoxetine in panic disorder. J Clin Psychopharmacol 1990;10:119–121.
141. Black B, Uhde TW, Tancer ME. Fluoxetine for the treatment of social phobia. J Clin Psychopharmacol 1992;12:293–295.
142. Orr G, Munitz H, Hermesh H, Low-dose clozapine for the treatment of Parkinson's disease in a patient with schizophrenia. Clin Neuropharmacol 2001;24:117–119.

23. *Hallucinogens, Stimulants, and Related Drugs of Abuse*

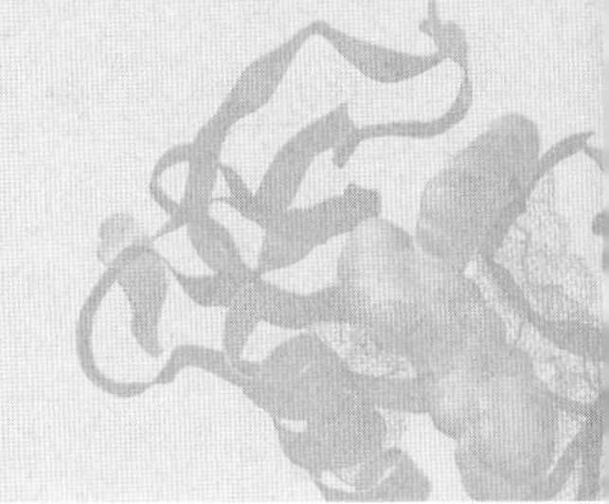

RICHARD A. GLENNON

PSYCHOTOMIMETIC/HALLUCINOGENIC AGENTS

Introduction

Why study psychotomimetic agents? In the past, it was argued that investigations of such agents might shed light on mental illness and its treatment. Although studies with psychotomimetic agents have certainly contributed to our understanding of these disorders, it is now recognized that there are many kinds of mental illnesses and that the actions—and putative mechanisms of action—of psychotomimetic agents are only tangentially related to their etiology or treatment. It also has been argued that investigations of psychotomimetic agents might contribute to a greater general understanding of basic neurochemical mechanisms and neurotransmitter function. This research approach has been more rewarding. Studies with psychotomimetic agents have contributed significantly to what is currently known about G protein–coupled receptors (e.g., cannabinoid receptors and serotonin receptors) and ion channel receptors (e.g., phencyclidine [PCP] receptors and excitatory amino acid receptors). Subsequent work with these receptors has identified new receptor subtypes that are being targeted for the development of novel therapeutic agents. Indeed, the past 10 years have witnessed an explosion of interest in the investigation of psychoactive substances because of their relevance to neurochemical mechanisms. Perhaps the most important reason to study psychotomimetic agents, however, is because these agents represent a large group of abused substances, and pharmacists generally serve as one of the first lines of defense for the dissemination of drug abuse prevention and treatment information. In addition, the past one or two decades have seen the popularization of controlled substance analogues (i.e., designer drugs), and the future will likely witness the introduction of yet more designer drugs. So, a second reason to study these agents is to prepare for the future: An understanding of the presently available agents and their structure–activity relationships (SARs) will be instructive, because many designer drugs result from the clandestine application of these same structure–activity principles at the street level. Lastly, some agents currently in clinical use possess an abuse liability that should be recognized. An understanding of how these drugs of abuse work can lead to new treatment modalities.

Definitions and Classification

"Psychotomimetic" and "hallucinogenic" are commonly used terms, and they frequently are used interchangeably. Little agreement, however, exists regarding what constitutes such agents or exactly what they do. Because the actions of these agents are largely subjective, the best information should come from those who are experiencing the agents, yet by experiencing their effect, one may not be in a position to accurately describe the effects they produce (1). In contrast, an outside observer can never fully and accurately describe the effects of the agents. This has led to problems of definition. Perhaps the best and most widely accepted definition of a psychotomimetic substance is that provided by Hollister (2): Psychotomimetic/hallucinogenic agents are those that on administration of a single effective dose consistently produce changes in thought, mood, and perception with little memory impairment; produce little stupor, narcosis, or excessive stimulation; produce minimal autonomic side effects; and are nonaddicting. Although certain opioid analgesics occasionally produce psychotomimetic effects, they are effectively eliminated from this category of agents, because they do not meet the necessary criteria (e.g., they can be addicting). Likewise, chronic administration of high doses of stimulants, such as amphetamine and cocaine, sometimes produce hallucinogenic episodes (i.e., amphetamine psychosis and cocaine psychosis). These agents are not considered to be hallucinogens, however, because multiple doses typically are required to produce this effect. The Hollister criteria have served a very useful function in narrowing the list of agents that belong to this category of drugs. Nevertheless, Hollister was still able to identify several classes of psychotomimetic agents: lysergic acid derivatives (e.g., lysergic acid diethylamide [LSD]), phenylethylamines (e.g., mescaline), indolealkylamines (e.g., N,N-dimethyltryptamine), other indolic derivatives (e.g., ibogaine and the harmala derivatives), piperidyl benzilate esters (e.g., JB-329), phenylcyclohexyl compounds (e.g., PCP), and miscellaneous agents (e.g., kawain, dimethylacetamide, and cannabinoids) (2).

Over time, it has been demonstrated that psychotomimetic agents represent a behaviorally heterogeneous class of psychoactive agents. For example, human subjects can differentiate between the actions produced by certain compounds in this category, and cross-tolerance develops among some of these agents but not between others. Likewise, it is possible to differentiate between certain of these agents using various animal procedures. Subcategorization was necessary. Today, it is recognized that some hallucinogens act primarily via a serotonergic mechanism, that the cannabinoids probably produce their behavioral effects via cannabinoid receptors, and that PCP likely produces its effects via PCP receptors. This is not to imply that a full understanding of how these agents work now exists, but it does support the concept that the agents do not belong to a homogeneous mechanistic class.

Human Versus Animal Studies: Applicability of Animal Models

Human subjects should be best suited to provide the most reliable assessment of the actions and potency of psychotomimetic agents, and considerable human data are available for some agents. Much less information, however, is available for most. Often, what information is available comes from studies that were not well controlled, that included limited subject populations, or that investigated only a few drug doses. Some of what is known even comes from anecdotal reports. Very few clinical studies with psychotomimetic agents were sanctioned following the early 1960s. Although some limited human evaluation has been allowed since in the early 1990s, for a period of approximately 30 years information concerning psychotomimetic substances relied—and continues to rely—heavily on the use of animal studies. This raises several questions: Do animal models exist that can accurately reflect human hallucinogenic activity? Indeed, do animals hallucinate? Many attempts have been made to develop animal models of psychotomimetic or hallucinogenic activity, but to date, no single animal model accounts for the actions of these agents as a class (3).

DRUG DISCRIMINATION PARADIGM. One animal technique that has seen widespread application for the investigation of psychoactive agents is the drug discrimination paradigm (4). It must be emphasized at the outset that this method does not represent a model of psychotomimetic activity. Indeed, the technique has general applicability and has been employed to study a wide variety of centrally acting agents, including stimulants, barbiturates, anxiolytics, opiates, and many other drug classes. The technique may be viewed as a "drug detection" procedure. Specifically, animals (typically rats, pigeons, or monkeys) are trained to recognize or discriminate the stimulus effects of a training drug from vehicle; humans also have been used as subjects in some drug discrimination studies. Many centrally acting agents produce an interoceptive cue or stimulus that that subjects recognize. When animals are used, they are taught to make a particular response (e.g., to respond on one lever of a two-lever operant apparatus or Skinner box) when administered a training drug and to make a different response (e.g., to respond on the second of the two levers) when administered saline vehicle. After a period of time, the animals learn the stimulus cue and associate it with one of the two levers; that is, the animals make more than 80% of their responses on the training-drug lever (i.e., >80% drug-appropriate responding) when administered the training dose of the training drug and less than 20% of their responses on the same lever when administered vehicle. Doses of training drug less than those of the training dose result in a decrease in percentage drug-appropriate responding. The effect is dose related, and a dose–response curve can be constructed. A median effective dose (ED50) also can be calculated as a measure of potency.

Once trained, these animals can be used in what are referred to as tests of substitution or stimulus transfer or, more commonly, as tests of stimulus generalization. In such tests, other agents (i.e., challenge drugs) are administered to the animals to determine if they produce stimulus effects similar to those of the training drug. Stimulus generalization is said to have occurred when animals make more than 80% of their responses on the training drug–appropriate lever following administration of some dose of challenge drug. Stimulus generalization or substitution implies that the challenge drug and the training drug are producing similar stimulus effects in the animals. It should be noted that no claim has ever been made that the agents—the training drug and a challenge drug—are producing identical effects; rather, there is an implication that the agents are capable of producing a common stimulus effect or a behavioral cue common to the two agents (e.g., a drug that produces effects A and B may be recognized by animals trained to a drug that produces effects B and C; although this may not be a common occurrence, it should be recognized that it is possible). Thus, not only is it possible to determine if two agents are producing similar stimulus effects, it also is possible to compare their relative potencies by calculating an ED50 for the challenge drug.

Other studies that can be conducted are tests of stimulus antagonism. That is, a specific training drug can be administered together with another agent; if the combination results in less than 20% training drug–appropriate responding, stimulus antagonism is said to have occurred. Although this technique can be employed in the development of novel antagonists for a series of agents for which an antagonist is unknown, it is more common to use a receptor-selective antagonist to investigate mechanisms of action. Drug discrimination, then, is a very powerful tool for investigating the actions and mechanisms of action of many different kinds of centrally acting agents. Specific examples of stimulus generalization and stimulus antagonists will be described later.

The drug discrimination procedure has seen broad application in the investigation of centrally acting agents, and a wide variety of different training drugs has been employed. When a psychotomimetic agent is used as the training drug, it should be possible to identify other agents that produce similar stimulus effects (5). In this manner, it has been demonstrated that the psychotomimetics represent a behaviorally heterogeneous group of agents, much in the same way that humans have been able to differentiate the effects of these agents. Animals trained to discriminate LSD, for example, do not recognize PCP, and animals trained to discriminate PCP do not recognize LSD. Neither LSD-nor PCP-trained animals recognize tetrahydrocannabinol (THC). However, LSD-trained animals recognize mescaline, 1-(2,5-dimethoxy-4-methylphenyl)-2-aminopropane (DOM), and certain other hallucinogens. Using this technique, then, it has been possible to identify what are termed the "classical hallucinogens" (6). The classical hallucinogens are LSD-like agents that share common stimulus properties and that may act via a common mechanism of action. The remaining psychotomimetic agents will be referred to here as nonclassical agents; these groups of agents act by different mechanisms and produce distinct effects common to members within each group.

Psychoactive Drugs of Abuse: Nonclassical Hallucinogens

The term "nonclassical hallucinogen" is used here to differentiate these psychoactive agents from the classical hallucinogens that will be discussed later in this chapter. Several categories of agents are described, but there is no implication that these classes produce similar effects or act via similar mechanisms.

Cannabinoids

The marijuana or cannabis plant represents one of the oldest and most widely used psychoactive substances in the world. Botanically, there are three major species of the plant—*Cannabis sativa, Cannabis indica,* and *Cannabis ruderalis*—and cannabis has been cultivated since approximately 6,000 BC. Reference is made to three preparations, listed here in order of increasing potency: bhang, ganja, and hashish. Bhang typically refers to the leaves and stems of the plant, ganja is prepared from the flowering tops of the plant, and hashish is the pure resin. Although marijuana is active orally, inhalation by smoking is a more frequently used route of administration. One of the major active constituents of the plant is Δ^9-THC (often referred to simply as THC). THC is rapidly and efficiently absorbed by inhalation; it is absorbed into body tissue and slowly released back into circulation. Deuterium-labeled THC has been detected in human plasma up to nearly 2 weeks postadministration. A major metabolite of THC is 11-hydroxy-Δ^9-THC. Evidence suggests that tolerance develops to THC and that THC does not generally lead to physical dependence. Marijuana can produce impairment of performance, memory, and learning; controversy exists over whether it produces an amotivational syndrome. There are many claims for the medicinal use of marijuana and THC.

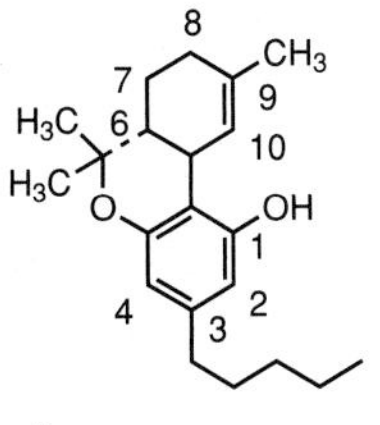

Δ^9-Tetrahydrocannabinol (Δ^9-THC)

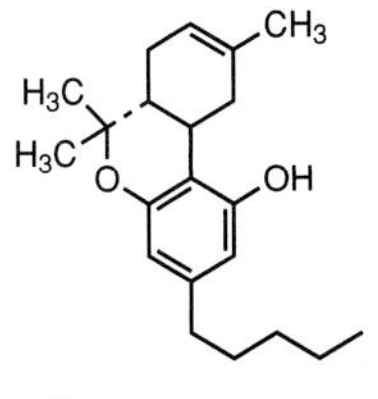

Δ^8-Tetrahydrocannabinol

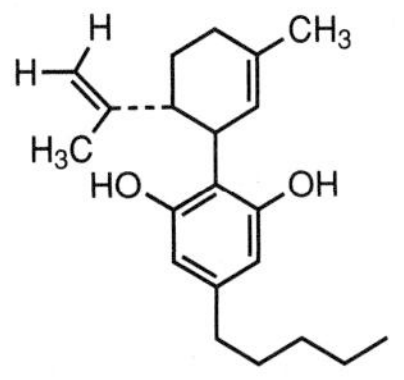

Cannabidiol

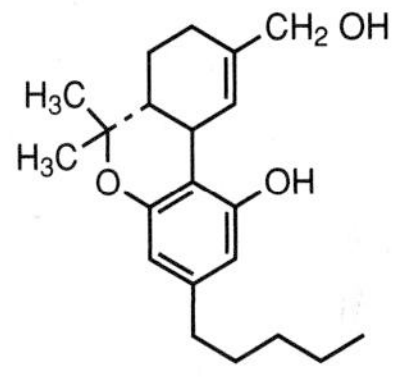

11-Hydroxy-Δ^9-Tetrahydrocannabinol (11-OH-Δ^9-THC)

Over the years, many cannabinoids and related structures, such as CP-55,940, were synthesized and evaluated. Noncannabinoids, such as WIN-55,212-2, also were shown to possess THC-like actions. Few compounds displayed cannabinoid antagonist properties, and an extensive search was conducted to find possible candidates that would be useful for better defining the actions of THC. A number of compounds were explored, and the pyrazole analogue SR141716A (rimonabant) has been found to be one of the most effective. SR141716A attenuates the effects of WIN-55,212-2 and THC (7) as well as the stimulus effects of THC. Thus, in addition to cannabinoids and cannabinoid-related structures such as CP-55,940, there are other structural classes of cannabinoid ligands, including indolic derivatives such as WIN-55,212–2, pyrazoles such as SR141716A, and fatty acid derivatives such as anandamide (discussed below).

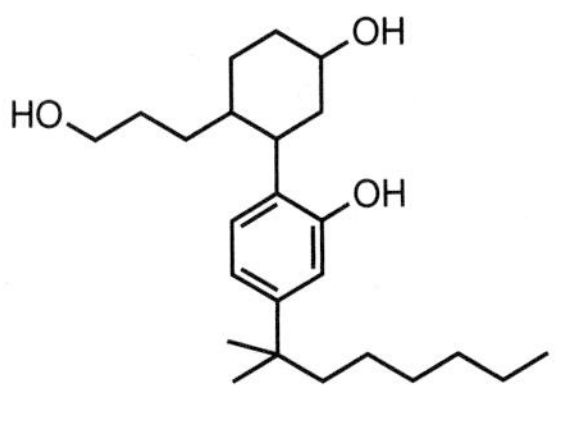

CP-55,940

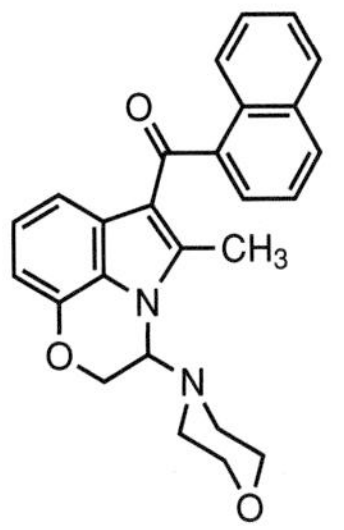

WIN-55,212-2

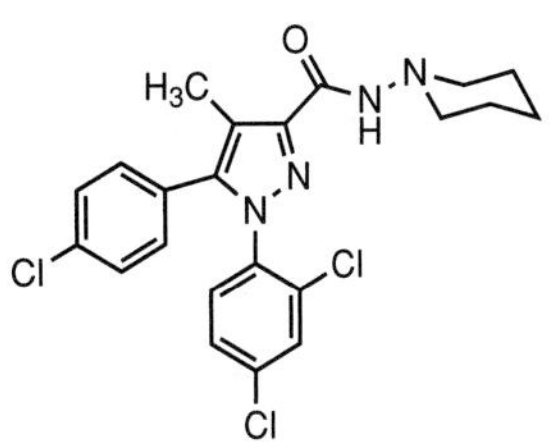

SR141716A

MECHANISM OF ACTION. For many years, it was thought that cannabinoids were acting in a nonspecific manner, but in the early 1990s, two populations of cannabinoid receptors were identified: CB-1, and CB-2 (8,9). Human forms of these receptors have been cloned. Both types are G protein–coupled, seven-helix transmembrane-spanning receptors. These receptors are differentially expressed: CB-1 receptors, which may mediate the psychoactive effects of THC-related agents, are found primarily in the brain, whereas CB-2 receptors, which possibly are involved in immunomodulatory actions, are found almost exclusively in the periphery. The identification of such receptors suggested the possible existence of endogenous ligands, and claims for several have been published. The best investigated of these is the eicosanoid derivative arachidonylethanolamide or anandamide, which initially was isolated from porcine brain. Anandamide (K_i = 52 nM) binds at CB-1 receptors with an affinity similar to that of THC (46 nM) (10). Related structures also have been detected in brain, including docosatetraenylethanolamide (K_i = 34.4 nM) and homo-γ-linolenyllathanolamide (K_i = 53.4 nM) (10). A related compound, palmitoylethanolamide, may show selectivity for CB-2 receptors. Anandamide seems to be a THC-like agent. Although the actions of anandamide may not be identical to those of THC, particularly regarding in vivo studies, differences may be related to the metabolic instability of anandamide. For example, in drug discrimination studies, a THC stimulus failed to consistently or reliably generalize to anandamide; however, the more metabolically stable methanandamide, a chain-methylated analogue of anandamide, produced THC-like effects. Furthermore, methanandamide has been used as a training drug, and the methanandamide stimulus generalizes to THC (11).

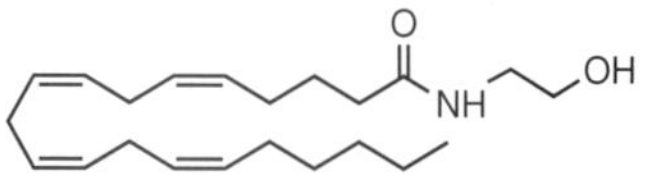

O NH OH

Anandamide

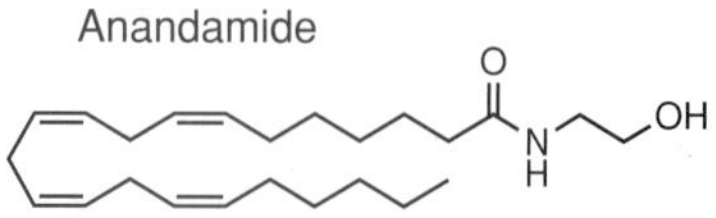

O N H OH

Docosatetraenoylethanolamide

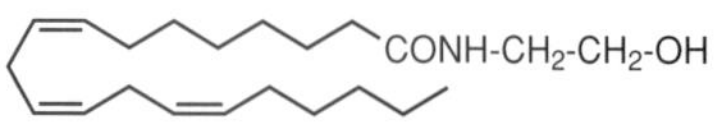

$CONH\text{-}CH_2\text{-}CH_2\text{-}OH$

Homo-γ-linolenylethanolamide

STRUCTURE–ACTIVITY RELATIONSHIPS. Structure–activity relationships both for THC-like actions and for CB receptor binding have been formulated (7). Structure–activity studies can be discussed on the basis of several different types of behavioral assays in rodents, and it has been shown for 60 cannabinoids that behavioral potencies are highly correlated with receptor binding affinities (12). THC-like discriminative effects probably offer a more specific method of detecting and measuring cannabimimetic effects and are particularly useful for formulating SARs (4). Using this approach, it has been demonstrated that SARs for THC-like stimulus effects are not necessarily identical to those for the analgesic, antiemetic, or anticonvulsant actions of cannabinoids. An early study showed that animals trained to discriminate intraperitoneal dosing of THC recognized hashish smoke and that animals trained to discriminate hashish smoke recognized THC, supporting the concept that THC likely accounts for the stimulus actions of hashish. A number of cannabinoids now have been evaluated. Cannabidiol, for example, does not produce THC-like stimulus effects. Relative to Δ^9-THC (ED50 = 0.43 mg/kg IP), some 11-hydroxy metabolites are quite potent, such as 11-OH Δ^9-THC (ED50 = 0.10 mg/kg) and 11-OH Δ^8-THC (ED50 = 0.38 mg/kg). One of the more potent cannabinoids is Δ^8-THC-DMH (ED50 = 0.05 mg/kg), in which the 4-pentyl moiety of THC has been replaced with a 1,1-dimethylheptyl (i.e., DMH) group; its 11-hydroxyl analogue, 11-OH Δ^8-THC-DMH (ED50 = 0.002 mg/kg), is even more potent (4). One of the most extensively studied cannabinoid ligands is WIN-55,212-2 (13). Molecular modeling and site-directed mutagenesis studies suggest that cannabinoids, CP-55,940, and anandamide bind in a similar fashion but in a manner that differs from the binding of WIN-55,212-2. Two distinct pharmacophores have been proposed (13,14). Attempts also are being made to identify CB-1 versus CB-2 pharmacophoric features (14).

The discovery of CB receptors, and novel chemical tools with which to investigate these receptors (7,15), has generated renewed interest in the cannabinoids; in fact, during the past 18 months as of this writing, more than 600 scientific papers have been published regarding cannabinoid research. In particular, the discovery of cannabinoid antagonists, endogenous cannabinoids, subpopulations of CB receptors, and agents showing selectivity for the two subpopulations finally promise that the mechanism of action of THC will be unraveled and that novel therapeutic agents lacking THC's psychoactive effects will be developed. For example, cannabinoid receptor agents might be of value in the treatment of glaucoma, spasticity associated with multiple sclerosis, Tourette's syndrome, neuropathic pain, Parkinson's disease, epilepsy, drug abuse, immune disorders, and several types of neuropsychiatric disorders (16). Because THC has been shown to result in decreased appetite, cannabinoids also have been examined for the control of appetite. Currently, SR141716A (rimonabant) is in late-phase clinical trials for the treatment of obesity (17).

PCP-Related Agents

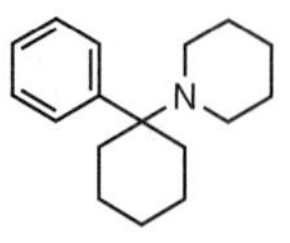

N Cl CH_3 NH O

Phencyclidine (PCP) Ketamine

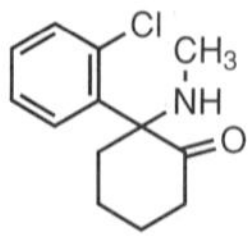

Phencyclidine, or 1-(1-phenylcyclohexyl)piperidine (PCP), was introduced as a dissociative anesthetic during the late 1950s. Shortly after its introduction, clinical studies were terminated because of the occurrence of schizophrenic-like psychotomimetic effects, particularly during emergence from anesthesia. This might have been the end of the story except that 1) additional attempts were made to exploit the anesthetic effects of PCP, leading to the development of novel agents, such as ketamine; 2) it was theorized that PCP-like states might provide a good model for investigating schizophrenia, leading to studies of PCP's mechanism of action; and 3) PCP (e.g., "Angel Dust"), administered by inhalation, injection, or smoking (as with PCP-laced parsley, tobacco, or marijuana), and ketamine (e.g., "Special K") emerged as drugs of abuse, leading to investigations of their abuse liability. Shortly thereafter, it was discovered that PCP behaves as an N-methyl-D-aspartate (NMDA) antagonist. Because NMDA receptors had been implicated in seizures and trauma, PCP and related arylcycloalkylamines were explored as potential antiepileptics and neuroprotective agents.

ACTIONS. In humans, PCP can produce disorientation, confusion, incoordination, delirium, impaired memory, and euphoria (18). Additionally, PCP has a history of producing aggression and violent behavior. Because PCP often is consumed together with other substances, however, it sometimes has been difficult to establish exactly which effects are produced by PCP and which may be related to possible drug interactions. PCP has seen extensive investigation in animals, and it appears to produce effects similar to those of amphetamine-like stimulants and central depressants. PCP is self-administered by animals, and tolerance develops to the behavioral effects of PCP on repeated exposure to the drug (18). PCP has both direct and indirect effects on dopaminergic systems; this may account, at least in part, for some of the amphetamine-like effects of PCP and may contribute to the production of its schizophrenic-like actions. The PCP model of schizophrenia was particularly attractive, because PCP seemed to produce both the positive and negative symptoms associated with this disorder. PCP also has been widely investigated as a training drug in animals during drug discrimination studies.

MECHANISM OF ACTION. N-Allylnormetazocine (NANM; SKF-10047) produces some effects reminiscent of those produced by PCP. At one time, NANM was considered a prototypic σ opiate receptor ligand. It is now recognized that the σ receptors likely are not a class of opioid receptors and that the low-affinity NANM is only one of very few opiates that bind at these receptors. Subsequent structure–activity studies showed that NANM simply possesses certain minimal pharmacophoric features that are required for σ receptor binding (19). Nevertheless, the behavioral similarities between NANM and PCP led to early investigations regarding the binding of PCP at σ receptors. and because of its affinity (albeit low) for

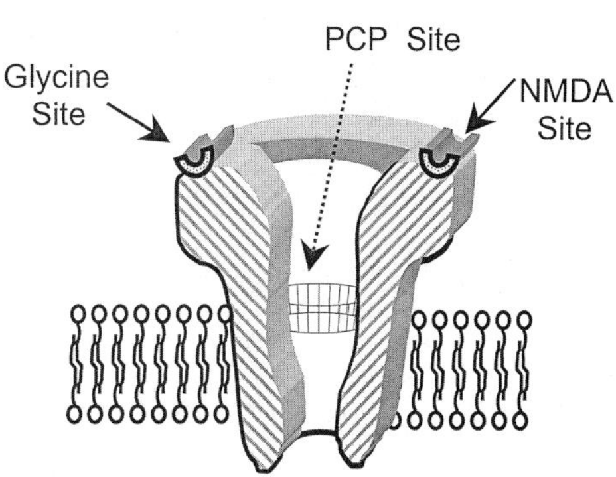

Fig. 23.1. NMDA ion channel receptor showing binding sites for glycine, NMDA, and PCP.

these receptors, the σ receptors were renamed NANM-PCP receptors, or σ/PCP receptors. This confusion continued for several years, until it was demonstrated that agents with much higher affinity and selectivity than PCP for σ receptors failed to produce PCP-like actions in animals (18). Later, it was shown that PCP antagonizes the effects of the excitatory amino acid NMDA. [^{3}H]PCP has been used to label putative PCP binding sites, and PCP binding and NMDA binding has displayed similar regional distribution in brain. It is established that PCP is a noncompetitive NMDA receptor antagonist.

The NMDA receptor (Fig. 23.1) is a ligand-gated ion channel receptor that regulates the flow of cations (Na^+, Ca^{2+}) into certain neurons. The receptor complex possesses multiple binding sites, similar to the benzodiazepine/γ-aminobutyric acid (GABA) receptor complex, that allows the binding of glutamate, glycine, polyamines, and other ligands that can modulate the actions of NMDA. Like the NMDA antagonist dizocilpine (MK-801), PCP binds at a site (i.e., the PCP site) that is believed to be located within the ion channel. Drug discrimination studies have shown that PCP-trained animals recognize NMDA antagonists that bind at PCP receptors; for example, MK-801 is nearly 10-fold more potent than PCP. Furthermore, animals trained to discriminate MK-801 recognize PCP and other PCP-related agents. Consistent with early findings that PCP produces a psychotic state in humans, PCP has been shown to produce a pattern of metabolic, neurochemical, and behavioral changes in animals that reproduce almost exactly those seen in patients with schizophrenia. Consequently, this provides new insight regarding the mechanisms underlying such disorders, and it offers an animal model for the evaluation of novel antipsychotic agents (20).

STRUCTURE–ACTIVITY RELATIONSHIPS. Structure–activity relationships for PCP-like actions have not been particularly well defined, and what little is known stems primarily from drug discrimination studies. The PCP stimulus does not generalize to opioids, sympathomimetic stimulants, anticholinergic agents, or classical hallucinogens and only partially generalizes to depressants, such as barbiturates; in general, the stimulus properties of PCP are not shared by members of other drug classes (21). The PCP stimulus generalizes to ketamine and other structurally related derivatives of PCP, such as TCP, an analogue of PCP in which the phenyl ring has been replaced by the isosteric 2-thienyl group.

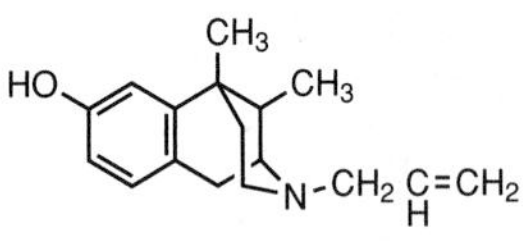

N-Allylnormetazocine (NANM) 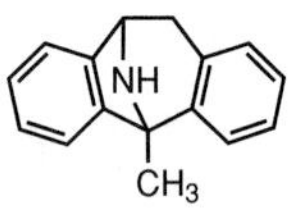 Dizocilpine (MK-801) 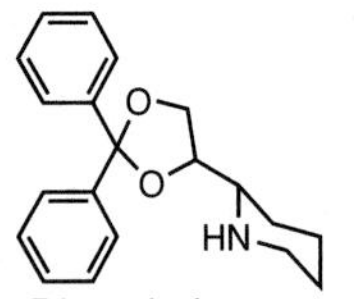 Dioxadrol

PCP does not possess a chiral center. Several 1,3-dioxolanes possessing an asymmetric center produce PCP-like effects and have proven to be useful for investigating PCP-like actions. Dioxadrol, or 2-(2,2-diphenyl-1,3-dioxolan-4-yl) piperidine, and etoxadrol (i.e., dioxadrol in which one of the phenyl groups has been replaced by an ethyl group) are examples of such dioxolanes. The (+)-isomer of dioxadrol, dexoxodrol, but not the (−)-isomer levoxadrol, binds at PCP receptors and is recognized by PCP-trained animals (21).

Psychoactive Drugs of Abuse: Classical Hallucinogens

Classical hallucinogens are agents that meet the Hollister definition (2) and, in addition, bind at 5-HT_2 serotonin receptors and are recognized by DOM-trained animals in tests of stimulus generalization (5). The classical hallucinogens all possess the general structure Ar-C-C-N, where Ar is a substituted phenyl, 3-indolyl, or substituted 3-indolyl moiety; C-C is an ethyl or branched ethyl chain; and N is a primary, secondary, or tertiary amine. This will be further discussed. (See Chapter 14 for additional information on serotonin receptors.)

Classification

There are two major structural categories of classical or arylalkylamine hallucinogens: the indolealkylamines, and the phenylalkylamines. The indolealkylamines are further divided into the simple N-substituted tryptamines, the α-alkyltryptamines, the ergolines (or lysergamides), and tentatively, the β-carbolines. The phenylalkylamines consist of the phenylethylamines and the phenylisopropylamines. In humans, examples from the different categories seem to produce similar effects. It should be noted, however, that relatively few agents have been examined in comprehensive and carefully controlled clinical situations. Furthermore, no claim is made that these agents produce identical effects in humans. Each category—and, indeed, even certain examples from within a given category—may produce effects that make them somewhat different from the others. As if to underscore the behavioral similarity among these agents, however, examples from each of the above categories produce common DOM-like stimulus effects in animals (Table 23.1).

Table 23.1. Results of Stimulus Generalization Studies with Examples from the Various Categories of Classical Hallucinogens Using Animals Trained to Discriminate DOM from Vehicle

Category	Example[a]	ED50 Value for DOM-Stimulus Generalization (mg/kg)[b]
N-Alkyltryptamines	DMT	5.8
α-Alkyltryptamines	α-MeT	3.1
Lysergamides	(+)LSD	0.05
β-Carbolines	Harmaline	6.2
Phenylethylamines	Mescaline	14.6
Phenylisopropylamines	DOB	0.2

[a]See text for explanation of abbreviations.
[b]Data from Glennon et al. (4) and from Glennon (5).

INDOLEALKYLAMINES

N-Alkyltryptamines. One of the best-investigated hallucinogens is N,N-dimethyltryptamine (DMT) (Table 23.2), which is considered to be the prototype of this subclass of agents. Although readily synthesized in the laboratory, DMT also is a naturally occurring substance. Its actions are characterized by a rapid onset (typically <5 minutes) and short duration of action (~30 minutes). Like some other members of this family, DMT is not active via oral administration; it generally is administered by inhalation or by smoking. Although less common, DMT also can be injected. Some indolealkylamines are sensitive to the acidic conditions of the stomach. The corresponding secondary amine, N-monomethyltryptamine, and primary amine, tryptamine, are inactive as psychoactive substances, both because they are not sufficiently lipophilic to readily penetrate the blood-brain barrier and because what little does get into the brain is rapidly metabolized by monoamine oxidase (MAO). Other tertiary amine derivatives, such as the N-ethyl-N-methyltryptamine, N,N-diethyltryptamine (DET), N,N-di-n-propyltryptamine (DPT), and some secondary amines, also are hallucinogenic in humans. If the N-alkyl or N,N-dialkyl substituents are bulky and lipophilic enough, these tryptamines can be orally active (Table 23.2).

The effect of substitution in the pyrrole portion of DMT has not been extensively investigated in humans. In contrast, substitution in the benzenoid ring can enhance or diminish potency depending on the specific nature and location of the substituents. Table 23.2 shows some of the more frequently encountered derivatives of DMT, their common names, and their approximate human potency. Serotonin is not hallucinogenic and does not readily penetrate the blood-brain barrier when administered systemically. N,N-Dimethylserotonin (bufotenine [5-OH DMT]) has been reported to be a weak hallucinogen, but the results of human studies are controversial. It, too, likely does not readily penetrate the blood-brain bar-

Table 23.2. Psychoactive Indolealkylamine and Related Agents

Agent	Common Name	R_1/R_2	R	X	Approximate Hallucinogenic Dose (mg)*	DOM Stimulus Generalization Potency (mg/kg)**
Tryptamine		H/H	H	H	Likely inactive	Inactive
N-Methyltryptamine	NMT	CH_3/H	H	H	Likely inactive	Inactive
(±)α-Methyltryptamine	α-Me	H/H	CH_3	H	5–20 (smoked) 15–30 (po)	3.13
N,N-Dimethyltryptamine	DMT	CH_3/CH_3	H	H	60–100 (smoked) 4–30(iv)	5.80
N,N-Diethyltryptamine	DET	C_2H_5/C_2H_5	H	H	50–100 (po)	2.45
N-Ethyl-N-methyltryptamine	Met	C_2H_5/CH_3	H	H	Unknown	---
N,N-Di-n-propyltryptamine	DPT	n-C_3H_7/n-C_3H_7	H	H	100–250 (po)	2.20
N,N-Di-isopropyltryptamine	DIPT	i-C_3H_7/i-C_3H_7	H	H	25–100 (po)	2.60
(±)α-Ethyltryptamine	α-EtT	H/H	C_2H_5	H	100–150 (po)	6.62
4-Hydroxy DMT	Psilocin	CH_3/CH_3	H	4-OH	10–20 (po)	---
4-Methoxy DMT	4-OMe DMT	CH_3/CH_3	H	4-OCH_3	Unknown	3.53
5-Hydroxytryptamine	5-HT	H/H	H	5-OH	Inactive	Inactive
5-OH DMT	Bufotenine	CH_3/CH_3	H	5-OH	Likely inactive	Inactive
5-Methoxy DMT	5-OMe DMT	CH_3/CH_3	H	5-OCH_3	6–20 (smoked) 2–3 (iv)	1.22
(±)5-Methoxy-α–MeT	5-OMe α-MeT	H/H	CH_3	5-OCH_3	2.5–4.5 (po)	0.50
6-Methoxy DMT	6-OMe DMT	CH_3/CH_3	H	6-OCH_3	Likely inactive	Inactive
7-Methoxy DMT	7-OMe DMT	CH_3/CH_3	H	7-OCH_3	Likely inactive	Inactive

*Data primarily from reference 22. Key: po = oral, iv = intravenous.
** Drugs were administered via the ip route reference 5.

rier and produces considerable peripheral effects (e.g., facial flushing and cardiovascular actions) that prevent evaluation of an extended dose range. O-Methylation of bufotenine results in 5-OMe DMT, one of the more potent N-alkyltryptamines. A naturally occurring substance, 5-OMe DMT is a constituent of a number of plants used in various concoctions prepared by South American Indians for ceremonial and visionary purposes. Bufotenine and 5-OMe DMT also are found in the skin of certain frogs and may have given rise to the phenomenon of "toad licking." Psilocin is 4-hydroxy DMT. Like bufotenine, with a polar hydroxyl group, psilocin might not have been expected to enter the brain, yet it is hallucinogenic. Although this phenomenon has never been adequately explained, it has been speculated that the 4-hydroxyl group forms a hydrogen bond with the terminal amine and that this reduces polarity just enough that psilocin penetrates the blood-brain barrier. Psilocin and its phosphate ester, psilocybin, are widely found in certain species of mushrooms and have given rise to the terms "shrooms" and "shrooming." There are no reports that 6-methoxy DMT or 7-methoxy DMT are hallucinogenic. It is quite difficult to make strict potency comparisons within this series because the different routes of administration that have been used (Table 23.2).

In tests of stimulus generalization, the DOM stimulus has been shown to generalize to DMT, DET, DPT, 4-OMe DMT, 5-OMe DMT, and a number of other DMT analogues, but not to 5-OH DMT, 6-OMe DMT, or 7-OMe DMT.

The metabolism of these agents has not been well investigated. The indolealkylamine 5-HT is a substrate for oxidative deamination by MAO. What evidence exists suggests that other indolealkylamines also are substrates for this enzyme system.

α-Alkyltryptamines. Tryptamine is not psychoactive. Introduction of an α-methyl group seemingly enhances lipophilicity and sufficiently protects against metabolism such that α-methyltryptamine (α-MeT) (Table 23.2) is approximately twice as potent as DMT. As a general rule of thumb, α-methyltryptamines, when such agents have been investigated, typically are twice as potent as their corresponding DMT counterpart. Otherwise, their SAR is essentially the same as that of the DMT analogues. For example, 5-methoxy-α-methyltryptamine (5-OMe α-MeT) is approximately twice as potent as 5-OMe DMT. Introduction of the α-methyl group results in the creation of an asymmetric center and the S-(+)-isomers of α-methyltryptamines are more potent than their R-(−)-enantiomers. Homologation of the α-methyl group to an α-ethyl group affords α-ethyltryptamines. α-Ethyltryptamine (α-EtT) has been reported to be hallucinogenic, with effects somewhat distinguishable by human subjects from those of LSD and mescaline (23). Interestingly, α-EtT was clinically available during the early 1960s as an antidepressant because of its actions as an MAO inhibitor; however, it was removed from the market about a year after its introduction. It may be the MAO inhibitory effect that allowed the actions of α-EtT to be distinguished from those of LSD and mescaline (see also the section below on designer drugs). During the mid-1990s, α-ET made an appearance on the clandestine market as a designer drug (i.e., "ET"). (±)-α-Methyltryptamine, (±)-5-methoxy-α-methyltryptamine and both of its optical isomers, and (±)-α-ethyltryptamine are recognized by DOM-trained animals in tests of stimulus generalization.

Ergolines or lysergamides. (+)-LSD is perhaps the best known—and, certainly, one of the most potent—of the classical hallucinogens. Although LSD itself is not naturally occurring, many related ergolines are found in nature. In terms of potency, LSD is at least 3,000-fold more potent than mescaline, with doses of 100 μg showing activity. Certain structurally modified analogues of LSD retain hallucinogenic activity; although many derivatives are possible, relatively few have been investigated in humans. Structural changes often can reduce the activity of a pharmacologically active substance. Here is an instance in which a structural change resulting in even a 1,000-fold decrease in potency can afford a very active agent. Some work has been reported on the SARs of LSD (24,25).

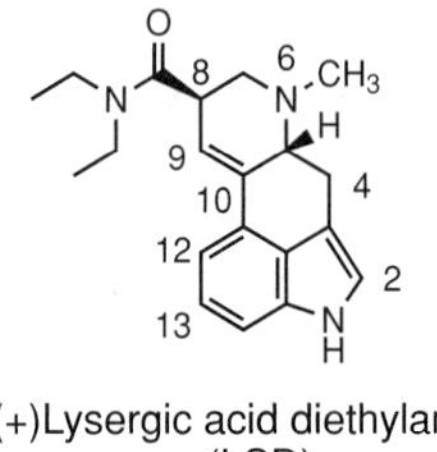

(+)Lysergic acid diethylamide (LSD)

In humans, LSD has been thoroughly investigated (24); no other hallucinogen has been as extensively studied as this agent. Its actions in humans can be divided into three major categories: perceptual (altered shapes and colors, heightened sense of hearing), psychic (alterations in mood, depersonalization, visual hallucinations, altered sense of time), and somatic (nausea, blurred vision, dizziness). In terms of principal effects, there seems to be little difference between LSD, psilocybin, and mescaline.

Although LSD has been sold on the clandestine market in tablet form, it is not uncommon to find this material available on "blotter paper" because of its high potency. A sheet of porous paper is impregnated with a solution of LSD, and the sheet can later be cut to afford the appropriate dose.

β-Carbolines. The β-carbolines represent a very interesting class of agents generally referred to as the harmala alkaloids. Several are naturally occurring. In South America, β-carbolines are found in certain vines and lianas (e.g., *Banisteriopsis caapi*), and in the Old World, β-carbolines are constituents of Syrian Rue (*Pegnum harmala*). South American Indians prepare a variety of concoctions and snuffs, the most notable of which is Ayahuasca, that are used for their hallucinogenic and visionary healing properties. In fact, the first written account of the use of these substances was made by a member of the Columbus expedition in 1493. There is little question that the concoctions are psychoactive; however, these plant preparations usually consist of admixtures in which certain tryptamines, such as DMT or 5-OMe DMT, sometimes have been identified. Some β-carbolines possess activity as MAO inhibitors; thus, the MAO inhibitory effect of the β-carbolines might be simply potentiating the effect of any tryptaminergic hallucinogens possibly present in an admixture by interfering with their metabolism. Studies with individual β-carbolines, especially under carefully controlled clinical settings, have been very limited. The three most commonly occurring β-carbolines are harmine, harmaline, and tetrahydroharmine, and evidence suggests that harmine and harmaline are hallucinogenic in humans (with potencies not greater than that of DMT) (27). Harmaline has seen some limited experimental application as an adjunct to psychotherapy (28). Like other classical hallucinogens, certain β-carbolines bind at $5\text{-}HT_{2A}$ receptors, and in animal studies, DOM stimulus generalization occurs to harmaline (28). Using harmaline-trained animals, harmaline stimulus generalization occurs to DOM. To date, however, very few β-carbolines have been investigated, so they are only tentatively categorized as classical hallucinogens.

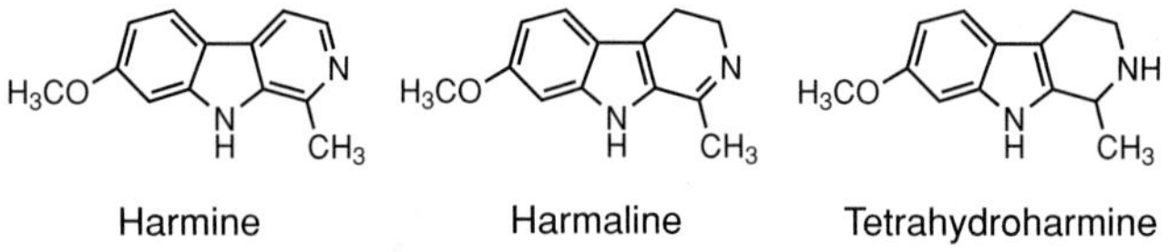

Harmine Harmaline Tetrahydroharmine

Although the scientific community has been aware of the psychoactive effects of the β-carbolines or β-carboline–containing natural substances for more than 100 years, only in the past decade or so have they become popular "on the street." The use of β-carboline–containing plants has moved out of the jungle and given rise to a variety of religious movements in some South American cities. Recent books and movies also are helping to popularize the use of these preparations, and they are now being encountered in North America.

PHENYLALKYLAMINES. Phenylalkylamines, the phenylethylamines and the phenylisopropylamines, represent the largest group of classical hallucinogens (29,30). The phenylethylamines are the α-desmethyl counterparts of the phenylisopropylamines; as with the indolealkylamines, the presence of the α-methyl group increases the agent's lipophilicity and reduces its susceptibility to metabolism by MAO. As a consequence, the phenylethylamines typically produce effects that are qualitatively similar to those of their corresponding phenylisopropylamines but typically less potent. Phenylethylamine counterparts of weak phenylisopropylamines might be inactive. Literally hundreds of analogues have been examined in human and in animal studies (29).

Phenylethylamines. Phenylethylamines are usually less-potent analogues of the phenylisopropylamines. Some hallucinogenic phenylisopropylamines are claimed to possess some stimulant character that may be minimized or altogether absent in the corresponding phenylethylamines. The phenylisopropylamines also possess a chiral center that is absent in the phenylethylamines. Otherwise, the SARs of the two groups of agents are relatively similar; consequently, the phenylethylamines will not be discussed in detail here. The most common—and, indeed, one of the oldest known—phenylethylamine hallucinogens is mescaline. A constituent of peyote (and other) cactus, mescaline is a relatively weak hallucinogenic agent (total human dose ~ 350 mg). Like many of the hallucinogens, mescaline is listed as a Schedule I substance; however, the use of peyote in certain native American Indian religious practices is sanctioned.

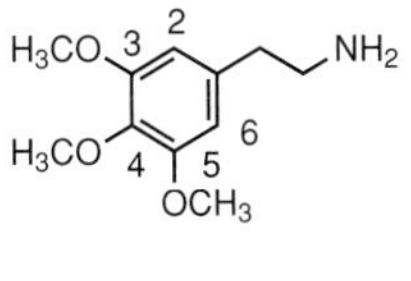

Mescaline

Phenylisopropylamines. Structural modification of mescaline and related substances by introduction of an α-methyl group and by deletion or rearrangement of the position of its methoxy groups results in a series of agents known as the phenylisopropylamines. As might have been expected, introduction of an α-methyl group, to afford 3,4,5-TMA or α-methylmescaline, doubles the potency of mescaline. Although different nomenclatures exist for the dimethoxy- and trimethoxyphenylisopropylamines, the one used herein is a commonly used nomenclature: The position of methoxy groups is given by indicating its position, and the number of methoxy groups is indicated by a prefix. For example, α-methylmescaline is 3,4,5-TMA, indicating that it is a trimethoxy analogue and that the methoxy groups are situated at the 3-, 4-, and 5-positions. Dimethoxy analogues are referred to as DMAs.

There are three possible monomethoxyphenylisopropylamines: the ortho-methoxy analogue OMA, the meta-methoxy analogue MMA, and the para-methoxy analogue PMA (Table 23.3). Although PMA is specifically listed as a Schedule I substance, none of these three analogues is hallucinogenic. PMA possesses weak central stimulant actions and is an abused substance; several deaths have been attributed to PMA overdose within the past few years.

There are six isomeric DMA analogues. These have not been thoroughly investigated in humans, and few produce DOM-like stimulus effects in animals (Table 23.3). None is more potent than DOM. The most potent agent, and one that has been evaluated in humans, is 1-(2,5-dimethoxyphenyl)-2-aminopropane, or 2,5-DMA. There also are six different TMA analogues (Table 23.3). Here, most show some activity, but the 2,4,5-timethoxy analogue 2,4,5-TMA (sometimes referred to simply as TMA) is the most potent of the series. Most of the trimethoxy analogues are recognized by DOM-trained animals, but none is more potent than DOM itself (5). The presence of the 2,5-methoxy substitution pattern in 2,5-DMA and 2,4,5-TMA might be noted.

The DMAs and TMAs are methoxy-substituted derivatives of the parent phenylisopropylamine known as amphetamine (Fig. 23.2). Amphetamine undergoes several different routes of metabolism; one of these is para-hydroxylation (a route that seems more important in rodents than in humans). Initially, it was thought that the greater potency of 2,4,5-TMA over that of 2,5-DMA might be related to the 4-position of the former being blocked to metabolism by para-hydroxylation. Keeping the 2,5-dimethoxy substitution intact, different 4-position substituents were examined. This led to a series of agents, such as DOM and DOB (Table 23.3). These 4-substituted 2,5-dimethoxy analogues represent some of the most potent members of the series.

1-(2,5-Dimethoxy-4-methylphenyl)-2-aminopropane (DOM) represents the prototype member of this family of agents. Increasing the length of this 4-methyl group to an ethyl or n-propyl group (i.e., DOET and DOPR, respectively) results in enhanced potency on a molar basis. Further extension of the alkyl chain results in a decrease in potency or loss of action. Substitution at the 4-position by electron-withdrawing groups, particularly those with hydrophobic character, also results in active agents, such as DOB (Table 23.3), which is quite a potent agent and has been misrepresented on the clandestine market as LSD both in tablet and "blotter" form.

When optical isomers have been examined, activity resides primarily with the R-(−)-isomer; the S-(+)-isomers typically are less active, inactive, or have received little study. For example, although not well investigated, it appears that R-(−)-DOM and R-(−)-DOB show activity at total human doses of less than 4 and less than 1 mg, respectively. N-monomethylation reduces potency or abolishes activity; for example, the N-monomethyl analogues of DOM and DOB are approximately 10% as potent as their primary amine counterparts. The SARs for the DOM-like actions of phenylisopropylamines are summarized in Table 23.3 and Figure 23.2.

Table 23.3 also provides a comparison of the approximate human doses of various phenylisopropylamines when administered via the oral route. These agents represent a mere sampling of the agents that have been

Table 23.3. Psychoactive Phenylisopropylamines and Related Agents

Agent	R_2	R_3	R_4	R_5	R_6	Human Hallucinogenic Dose (mg)*	DOM-stimulus Gen. Potency (umol/kg)†
Amphetamine	H	H	H	H	H	NH	NSG
OMA	OCH_3	H	H	H	H	NH	NSG
MMA	H	OCH_3	H	H	H	NH	NSG
PMA	H	H	OCH_3	H	H	NH	NSG
2,3-DMA	OCH_3	OCH_3	H	H	H	(?)	NSG
2,4-DMA	OCH_3	H	OCH_3	H	H	>60(?)	21.0
2,5-DMA	OCH_3	H	H	OCH_3	H	120 (80–160)	23.8
2,5-DMA, R(-)	OCH_3	H	H	OCH_3	H	(?)	14.0
2,6-DMA	OCH_3	H	H	H	OCH_3	(?)	NSG
3,4-DMA	H	OCH_3	OCH_3	H	H	>500 (?)	NSG
3,5-DMA	H	OCH_3	H	OCH_3	H	(?)	NSG
2,3,4-TMA	OCH_3	OCH_3	OCH_3	H	H	>100 (?)	29.8
2,3,5-TMA	OCH_3	OCH_3	H	OCH_3	H	>80 (?)	63.0
2,3,6-TMA	OCH_3	OCH_3	H	H	OCH_3	>30 (?)	---
2,4,5-TMA	OCH_3	H	OCH_3	OCH_3	H	30 (20–40)	13.7
2,4,6-TMA	OCH_3	H	OCH_3	H	OCH_3	38 (25–50)	13.9
3,4,5-TMA	H	OCH_3	OCH_3	OCH_3	H	175 (100–250)	24.2
MEM	OCH_3	H	OC_2H_5	OCH_3	H	35 (20–50)	22.9
DOM	OCH_3	H	CH_3	OCH_3	H	7 (3–10)	1.8
DOM, R(-)	OCH_3	H	CH_3	OCH_3	H	(?)	0.9
DOM, S(+)	OCH_3	H	CH_3	OCH_3	H	(?)	6.9
DOET	OCH_3	H	C_2H_5	OCH_3	H	4 (2.5–5)	0.9
DOPR	OCH_3	H	nC_3H_7	OCH_3	H	4 (3–4.5)	0.6
DOIP	OCH_3	H	iC_3H_7	OCH_3	H	(?)	2.9
DOBU	OCH_3	H	nC_4H_9	OCH_3	H	(?)	3.2
DOAM	OCH_3	H	nC_5H_{11}	OCH_3	H	(?)	NSG
DOT	OCH_3	H	SCH_3	OCH_3	H	8 (5–10)	---
DON	OCH_3	H	NO_2	OCH_3	H	4 (3–4.5)	2.7
DOF	OCH_3	H	F	OCH_3	H	(?)	5.8
DOC	OCH_3	H	Cl	OCH_3	H	2.5 (1.5–3)	1.2
DOB	OCH_3	H	Br	OCH_3	H	2 (1–3)	0.6
DOB, R(-)	OCH_3	H	Br	OCH_3	H	1.0–1.5 (?)	0.3
DOI	OCH_3	H	I	OCH_3	H	2.5 (1.5–3)	1.2
DOOC	OCH_3	H	COOH	OCH_3	H	(?)	NSG
DOOH	OCH_3	H	OH	OCH_3	H	(?)	NSG

*Data are primarily from reference 29. Where a dose range was reported in the literature, the arithmetic mean is also provided here for comparison (original range is fiven in parenthesis). The values should not be taken as a measure of precision. Doses are approximate and no implication is made that the different agents produce an identical effect. Key: NH = not hallucinogen, (?) = material has not been well studied or that its actions or potency are unknown.
†Drug discrimination data represent ED50 values and are from 5,30. NSG = so stimulus generalization.

Position	Amphetamine-like action	DOM-like actions
A: Terminal amine	N-Methyl > NH_2 > NHR > NR_2	NH_2 > NHR > NR_2
B: Chiral center	S(+) > (±) > R(-)	R(-) > (±) > S(+)
C: α-Methyl group	Homologation decreases potency Replacement by H decreases potency	Homologation decreases potency Replacement by H decreases potency
D: β-Position	β-OH: reduces potency β =O: retains activity and potency	β-OH: not well investigated β =O: not well investigated
E: Aromatic substitution	Unsubstituted aromatic ring prefered	2,5-Dimethyl-substitution preferred 4-Substitution further modulates activity

Fig. 23.2. Comparative SAR for the amphetamine-like stimulant actions and the DOM-like action of the phenylisopropylamines (30).

examined; it can be imagined, using only those functional groups shown in the table, how many different analogues are possible on the basis of structural rearrangement. There is no reason to suspect that each of these agents produces identical effects. In fact, the actions of some of these agents have been reported to be quite unique, ranging from hallucinations and closed-eye imagery to intellectual and sensory enhancement to erotic arousal (29).

Classical Hallucinogens: Mechanism of Action

Given that the arylalkylamines may not be producing identical effects, a common mechanism of action may not be expected. LSD was one of the first hallucinogens to be investigated mechanistically; another agent to see extensive investigation is mescaline. Interestingly, from a potency perspective, these two agents seem to represent opposite extremes. LSD has been proposed to produce its effects via numerous mechanisms, including those involving serotonergic, dopaminergic, histaminergic, adrenergic, and other receptors. LSD binds with high affinity at many different receptor populations and acts as an agonist at some, an antagonist at others, and a partial agonist at yet others. For many years, it was supposed that mescaline might be acting via a dopaminergic or adrenergic mechanism because of its structural similarity to dopamine and norepinephrine. As early as the late 1950s, it was speculated, because of its structural similarity to 5-HT, that LSD might be working through a serotonergic mechanism. Significant experimental evidence supported this claim. Controversy exists, however, regarding whether LSD was a serotonergic agonist or antagonist. Furthermore, later studies revealed the existence of at least 14 populations of 5-HT receptors (see Chapter 14). With the subsequent availability of 5-HT_2 selective antagonists, it was demonstrated that several of these antagonists (e.g., ketanserin and pirenperone) were particularly effective in blocking the stimulus effects of DOM, and of DOM stimulus generalization to other hallucinogens, such as LSD, in tests of stimulus antagonism. It was later shown that the classical hallucinogens bind at 5-HT_2 serotonin receptors and that their receptor affinities were significantly correlated with both their DOM stimulus generalization potencies and their human hallucinogenic potencies (30). The classical hallucinogens are now thought to produce their effect by acting as agonists at 5-HT_2 receptors in the brain (i.e., the 5-HT_2 hypothesis of hallucinogen action). Radiolabeled analogues of DOB and DOI (e.g., [^{3}H]DOB and [^{125}I]DOI, respectively) are now available for the investigation of 5-HT_2 pharmacology.

More recently, it has been demonstrated that 5-HT_2 receptors actually represent a family of 5-HT receptors that consist of 5-HT_{2A}, 5-HT_{2B}, and 5-HT_{2C} receptor subpopulations. Fewer than three dozen arylalkylamines have been compared, but it appears that they show little selectivity for one subpopulation versus another. Various pharmacological studies with selective antagonists or employing antagonist correlation analysis, however, suggest that it may be the 5-HT_{2A} subtype that plays a predominant role in the behavioral actions of these agents (30,31). Although the 5-HT_{2A} receptors might be responsible for those actions that the classical hallucinogens have in common, other neurochemical mechanisms may account for their differences. For example, LSD is a very promiscuous agent that binds with high affinity at many receptor populations for which most other classical hallucinogens show little to no affinity. Many of the indolealkylamines bind with high affinity at multiple populations of 5-HT receptors, and some display comparable or higher affinity at these receptors (e.g., 5-HT_{1A}, h5-HT_{1D}, and 5-HT_6) than they do at 5-HT_{2A} receptors. The phenylalkylamines are quite selective for 5-HT_2 receptors but, as mentioned above, display little selectivity for the three 5-HT_2 subpopulations. Some β-carbolines, although they bind at 5-HT_2 receptors, also possess activity as MAO inhibitors. Thus, these differences might account for their somewhat different actions. The one feature that all the classical hallucinogens have in common (i.e., the common component hypothesis) is that they bind at 5-HT_{2A} receptors (5).

CENTRAL STIMULANTS

Introduction, Classification, and Definitions

Stimulants can be divided into several categories. The term "stimulant," or "behavioral stimulant," typically refers to agents with a central stimulatory effect for which the actions are manifested mostly in motor activity, whereas the term "analeptics" refers to agents that have a stimulant effect primarily on autonomic centers, such as those involved in the regulation of respiration and circulation. Nicotine and related nicotinic agents also possess stimulant properties but are best discussed with other cholinergic agents. Analeptics include agents such as pentylenetetrazol, nikethamide, and strychnine. The boundary between analeptics and behavioral stimulants is not sharply defined. Caffeine, for example, has been classified as an analeptic, but high doses produce a stimulant effects. Caffeine is probably the best known of a series of xanthines; in fact, caffeine, which is found in coffee, tea, chocolate, and other naturally occurring substances, is probably the most widely used psychoactive substance in the world. Although most analeptics do not represent significant abuse problems, evidence does exist for caffeine abuse (32). However, because caffeine, particularly in the form of its naturally occurring products, is not subject to legal constraints, it will not be discussed here.

The term "stimulant" typically conjures up substances such as the phenylisopropylamine amphetamine and the tropane analogue cocaine. The following discussion will focus primarily on such substances.

Phenylisopropylamine Stimulants: Amphetamine-Related Agents

The simplest unsubstituted phenylisopropylamine is 1-phenyl-2-aminopropane, or amphetamine. Amphetamine possesses central stimulant, anorectic, and sympathomimetic actions, and it is the prototype member of this class (33). It is common to refer to amphetaminergic structures and amphetaminergic activity, but amphetamine may be more of an exception than a rule. Most substituted derivatives of amphetamine (i.e., phenylisopropylamine) lack central stimulant activity; in fact, pharmacologically, there are a greater number of "non-amphetamine-like" derivatives of amphetamine than there are "amphetamine-like" derivatives of amphetamine. Relatively few derivatives of amphetamine retain the activity of amphetamine; still fewer retain the potency of amphetamine. The present section will focus almost exclusively on the central stimulant actions of amphetamine, and it should be recognized that these SARs are not necessarily identical to those for anorectic or sympathomimetic actions.

Structure–Activity Relationships for Amphetamine-like Stimulant Action

In general, the SARs for amphetamine-like actions of the phenylisopropylamines are quite distinct from those for the DOM-like actions of the phenylisopropylamines, even though both share a common structural skeleton. The SARs for the two actions are summarized in Figure 23.2. The stimulus effects of amphetamine analogues have been reviewed elsewhere (34).

ARYL-SUBSTITUTED DERIVATIVES. In general, incorporation of substituents into the aromatic ring of amphetamine reduces or abolishes amphetamine-like stimulant activity. The sympathomimetic agent 4-hydroxyamphetamine lacks central stimulant action and is unlikely to penetrate the blood-brain barrier because of the presence of the polar aromatic hydroxyl group. Masking of the hydroxyl group in the form of its methyl ether affords the Schedule I substance PMA (para-methoxyamphetamine, also known as 4-methoxyamphetamine). PMA is a weak central stimulant with approximately 10% of the potency of amphetamine. 4-Methylamphetamine (1-(para-tolyl)-2-aminopropane [pTAP]) also has been found on the clandestine market and is, at best, a weak central stimulant. Incorporation of electron-withdrawing substituents results in agents that generally lack central stimulant properties. For example, PCA, or para-chloroamphetamine, is a 5-HT–releasing agent that saw evaluation as a potential antidepressant. Another related analogue is the 5-HT–releasing agent fenfluramine, which was used for some time as an appetite suppressant. Both of these latter agents are still widely employed as pharmacological tools in basic neuroscience research.

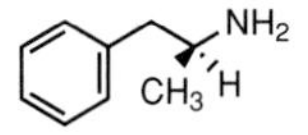

NH_2, CH_3, H — S(+)Amphetamine

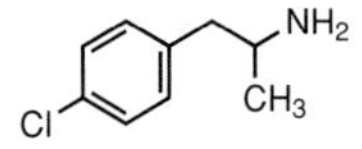

NH_2, CH_3, Cl — *p*-Chloroamphetamine (PCA)

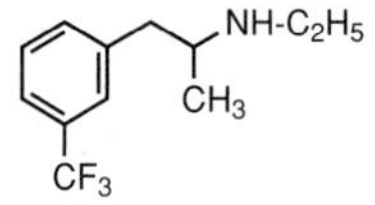

NH-C_2H_5, CH_3, CF_3 — Fenfluramine

AMINE SUBSTITUTION. In general, the primary amines are more potent than the secondary amines, and the secondary amines are more potent than the tertiary amines, as central stimulants. With regard to secondary amines, as the length of the amine substituent increases, activity decreases; the N-monoethyl and N-mono-n-propyl amines retain stimulant character but are somewhat less potent than amphetamine itself. Larger substituents typically result in agents with little to no stimulant character. The one exception is the N-monomethyl derivative methamphetamine. Methamphetamine (e.g., "crystal," "ice," or "meth") is at least as potent as amphetamine as a central stimulant; in most studies, it may be two- to threefold more potent than amphetamine. Methamphetamine is the most widely abused synthetic substance in the world. N-Hydroxylation of amphetamine has little effect on stimulant action. N,N-Dimethylamphetamine has been seized from clandestine laboratories, but it has never been certain whether this agent was being prepared for its possible stimulant actions or as a by-product of methamphetamine synthesis.

α-Substituents. Amphetamine possesses an α-methyl group. As already mentioned at the beginning of this chapter, α-demethylation (to afford phenylethylamine or 2-phenyl-1-aminoethane in the case of amphetamine) results in agents with decreased lipophilicity and increased susceptibility to metabolism. Phenylethylamine lacks central stimulant activity. Homologation of the α-methyl group to, for example, an α-ethyl or α-n-propyl group results in a decrease or loss of central stimulant activity. The presence of the α-methyl group in amphetamine creates a chiral center; hence, amphetamine exists as a pair of optical isomers. With respect to central stimulant actions, the S-(+)-isomer (i.e., dextroamphetamine) is several-fold more potent than its R-(−)-enantiomer (i.e., levamphetamine); this is not necessarily the case with other actions produced by amphetamine, particularly those produced in the periphery, such as its cardiovascular actions.

β-Substituents. The β-position has not been particularly well investigated. Perhaps the best-studied derivatives are ephedrine and norephedrine—and even these agents have not been especially well investigated. Ephedrine and norephedrine are phenylpropanolamines that may be viewed as the β-hydroxy analogues of methamphetamine and amphetamine, respectively. Actually, β-hydroxylation of amphetamine or methamphetamine results in the creation of a new chiral center; hence, a total of four optical isomers result from hydroxylation in each case. These eight structures are shown in Figure 23.3. Relatively little comparative information is available regarding the central stimulant actions of these phenylpropanolamine isomers.

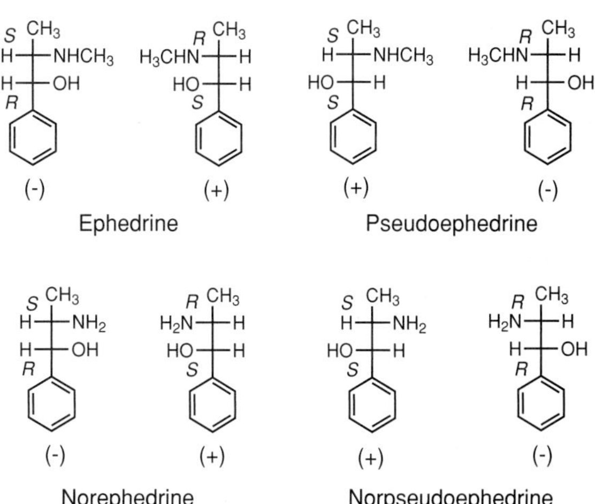

Fig. 23.3. Structures of β-oxidized analogues of methamphetamine (ephedrine and pseudoephedrine) and amphetamine (norephedrine and norpseudoephedrine). Note that norpseudoephedrine also is known as cathine.

During the 1970s, there was a problem with what were termed "look-alike drugs." Look-alikes available on the clandestine market were made to resemble amphetamine and methamphetamine, both in action and physical appearance, to circumvent the control of amphetamine. The major constituents of these agents were various combinations of ephedrine, norephedrine, and caffeine. Although the look-alikes are no longer a major problem, the 1990s witnessed the introduction of "herbal dietary supplements." These supplements were—and still are—legally available in some health food and herbal shops; several dozen such preparations have appeared on the market. The major ingredients of many of these preparations are various combinations of ephedrine and caffeine (or of ephedrine-containing natural products [e.g., ma huang or ephedra] or caffeine-containing natural products [e.g., guarana or kola nut]). Interestingly, although ephedrine and caffeine possess stimulant character of their own, evidence suggests that these agents may potentiate one another's actions (35). The exact mechanism by which they do so, however, is unknown.

Although β-hydroxylation of amphetamine results in decreased central stimulant actions, this may be the result of the decreased ability of norephedrine to penetrate the blood-brain barrier, or it may be a clue that the presence of a β-oxygen substituent is inherently detrimental to activity. Support for the former possibility is derived from the shrub *Catha edulis*. Commonly known as khat or kat, *C. edulis* is a plant indigenous to certain regions of the Middle East and eastern portion of Africa. The fresh shrub is sold openly in local markets and is used for its central stimulant character, much in the same way as the West uses coffee. Khat is used to prepare an infusion, or the fresh leaves are simply chewed. For more than 50 years, it was thought that the active constituent was the phenylpropanolamine cathine or (+)-norpseudoephedrine (Fig. 23.3). In the late 1970s, however, a more potent compound was isolated from fresh leaves and shown to be what is now called cathinone. Cathinone, which is simply β-ketoamphetamine or an oxidized analogue of norephedrine, is at least as potent as amphetamine as a central stimulant. Certain anorectic agents, such as diethylpropion, also possess a benzylic keto group. The anorectic agent phenmetrazine or 3-methyl-2-phenylmorpholine and aminorex possess a benzylic oxygen atom in the form of an ether. All three of these agents possess stimulant character. A related stimulant is pemoline (available as a magnesium salt). Hence, it is specifically the hydroxyl analogues that seem to possess weak stimulant actions, and this is likely a result of their reduced lipophilicity and not because they simply possess an oxygen atom at the β or benzylic position.

Cathinone Diethylpropion Phenmetrazine

Aminorex Pemoline

Metabolism of Amphetamine

In humans, (+)-amphetamine has a half-life of approximately 7 hours. Some of the metabolic products of amphetamine metabolism are shown in Figure 23.4. Although a significant portion of amphetamine is excreted unchanged, it also undergoes both Phase I (functionalization to more polar derivatives) and Phase II (conjugation) metabolism (36). The Phase I metabolism of amphetamine analogues is catalyzed by two enzyme systems: cytochrome P450, and flavin monooxygenase. The latter system oxidizes secondary and tertiary amine analogues of amphetamine. Amphetamine undergoes hydroxylation on the α-carbon, the β-carbon, the terminal amine, and on the aromatic ring. These metabolites are subsequently oxidized, where possible, or conjugated.

Amphetamine is oxidized to phenylacetone via a presumed carbinolamine intermediate. The phenylacetone is further oxidized directly to benzoic acid or, first, to a hydroxy keto analogue that is subsequently converted to benzoic acid. Amphetamine also can undergo aromatic hydroxylation to parahydroxyamphetamine.

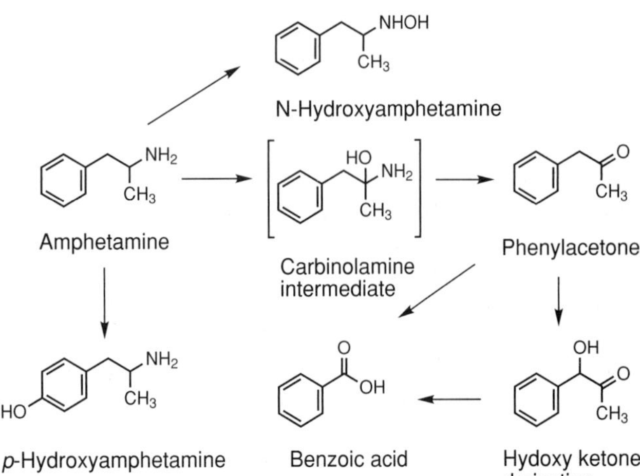

Fig. 23.4. Some products of amphetamine metabolism.

Initial work with rats indicated that para-hydroxylation is a major route of metabolism; however, subsequent studies showed that benzoic acid is the major metabolite in humans. Subsequent oxidation at the benzylic position by dopamine β-hydroxylase affords parahydroxynorephedrine. Alternatively, direct oxidation of amphetamine by dopamine β-hydroxylase can afford norephedrine. Amphetamine and related derivatives also undergo N-hydroxyalation, and the N-hydroxy derivatives can be further oxidized to nitroso, nitro, and oximino compounds. Some evidence suggests that the oximino derivative is hydrolyzed to phenylacetone. Additional metabolites are possible as well. In Phase II reactions, ring-hydroxylated metabolites are conjugated to their corresponding glucuronides. Sulfation of the enol form of phenylacetone has been reported. Approximately 23% of methamphetamine is excreted unchanged, 18% as parahydroxymethamphetamine, and 14% as the demethylated product (36).

Mechanism of Action of Amphetamine

Amphetamine is an indirect-acting dopaminergic and noradrenergic agonist; that is, amphetamine causes an increase in the synaptic concentrations of these neurotransmitters. The central stimulant actions of amphetamine primarily involve the dopamine system; amphetamine enhances the release of dopamine and, to a lesser extent, prevents the reuptake of dopamine into presynaptic terminals (Fig. 23.5). The stimulant actions of amphetamine can be attenuated by the administration of dopamine antagonists, such as the antipsychotic phenothiazine chlorpromazine and the butyrophenone haloperidol. Chronic administration of high doses of amphetamine may result in "amphetamine psychosis," which exhibits symptoms similar to those of acute paranoid psychosis. This is consistent with a role for dopamine in the central actions of amphetamine and,

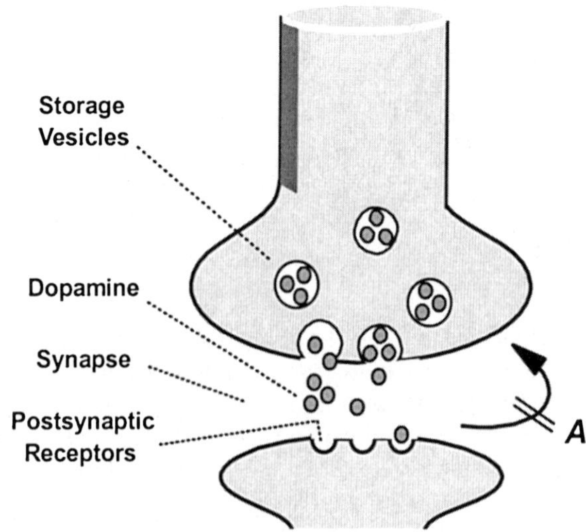

Fig. 23.5. Schematic of a dopaminergic nerve terminal. Amphetamine increases synaptic concentration of dopamine primarily by causing its release from presynaptic terminals, whereas cocaine increases synaptic concentration by preventing its reuptake (*A*).

further, with the dopamine antagonist mechanisms proposed for certain antipsychotic agents. Similar psychotic episodes have been associated with khat ("khat psychosis" or "cathinone psychosis") and cocaine ("cocaine psychosis").

Clinical Applications

Although phenylisopropylamines generally are known for their abuse liability, several have gained clinical acceptance. Indeed, certain of these agents display reduced stimulant character and/or are infrequently abused. Ephedrine (and, later, phenylpropanolamine) and amphetamine were two of the first agents used to treat obesity. Caffeine also has been used to treat obesity, and when given in combination with ephedrine, the combination has a supra-additive effect (37,38). Alternatives to the synthetic products include herbal preparations that contain ephedrine (e.g., ma huang) or caffeine (e.g., guarana). Recent studies indicate that ephedrine–caffeine combinations are associated with an increased risk of psychiatric, autonomic, cardiovascular, and other side effects (38). The central stimulant actions of the phenylispropylamines led to their structural modification and the subsequent introduction of anorectic agents, such as diethylpropion, phenmetrazine, and phentermine. Despite a lack of widespread abuse, many of these agents retain central stimulant properties. (±)-Fenfluramine was developed in the 1960s and marketed as Pondimin®. Although structurally related to amphetamine, fenfluramine is devoid of stimulant character. Unlike amphetamine-related agents that act primarily via noradrenergic and dopaminergic mechanisms, fenfluramine is primarily a serotonin-releasing agent. The more potent isomer in reducing food intake, (+)-fenfluramine (i.e., dexfenfluramine), was introduced clinically during the 1980s. Fenfluramine also was available in combination with phentermine (i.e., phen-fen). Unfortunately, some patients treated with this combination displayed symptoms of valvular heart disease, resulting in the voluntary withdrawal from the market in 1997 of fenfluramine-containing anorectic agents. (±)-Fenfluramine is metabolized to its primary amine norfenfluramine, and evidence suggests that valvulopathy might be the result of the agonist action of norfenfluramine on cardiac 5-HT_{2B} receptors (39,40). Today, it is not unusual for new drug candidates to be examined for 5-HT_{2B} agonist action during the early stages of their development.

Other serotonergic agents have been evaluated for their antiobesity actions including selective serotonin reuptake inhibitors (SSRIs; e.g., fluoxetine) (37) (see Chapter 21). Sibutramine, an agent with an amphetamine-like structural skeleton that was initially developed as an antidepressant, is an inhibitor of serotonin and norepinephrine reuptake. Animal studies indicate that sibutramine reduces food intake by decreasing meal duration rather than feeding frequency, suggesting an effect on satiation mechanisms (37). Sibutramine stimulates thermogenesis and effectively reduces amounts of visceral fat (41). Side effects of sibutramine include increased heart rate and blood pressure that have been attributed to its adrenergic action. These and other approaches and strategies to the treatment of obesity have been recently reviewed elsewhere (37,41).

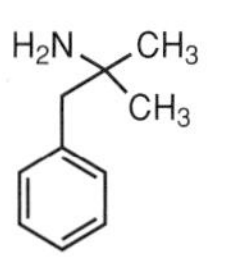

Phentermine 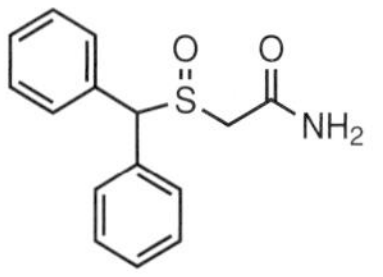 — Modafinil (Provigil) 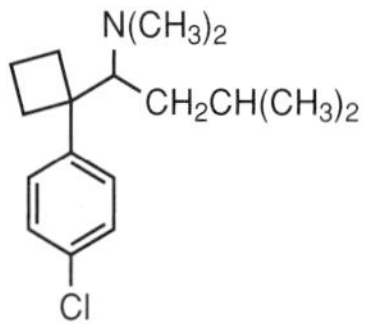 — Sibutramine (Merida)

Causes of excessive daytime sleepiness are numerous and include intrinsic sleep disorders, such as obstructive sleep apnea/hypopnea syndrome and narcolepsy; circadian rhythm sleep disorders, such as jet lag; and sleep disorders associated with neuropsychiatric conditions, such as anxiety and depression (42). In many instances, excessive daytime sleepiness is treated by addressing the underlying cause; however, the specific etiology of narcolepsy is unknown. Narcolepsy also can be characterized by brief periods of muscle paralysis (cataplexy). Hence, a need exists for agents that can effectively treat narcolepsy and cataplexy. Because of the increased behavioral activation (i.e., arousal, alertness, and motor activity) caused by psychostimulants, their use has been the mainstay for the treatment of narcolepsy. Agents such as methylphenidate and amphetamine frequently are used, and methamphetamine and caffeine are used less commonly. Pemoline (Cyclert) also has seen some application but has been reported to produce liver toxicity (42-44). Adderall, a combination of amphetamine salts (equal amounts of (+)-amphetamine saccharate, (+)-amphetamine sulfate, amphetamine aspartate, and amphetamine sulfate), was introduced in 1996; although used primarily for the treatment of attention-deficit hyperactivity disorder (ADHD), it also is used in the treatment of narcolepsy. Newer agents include sodium oxybate ($HO\text{-}CH_2CH_2CH_2COO^-\ Na^+$; presumed to act through a gabaminergic mechanism) and modafanil. Modafinil (Provigil) is a new agent that seems to promote wakefulness without producing the arousing effects associated with many other stimulants; it also has been approved for the treatment of obstructive sleep apnea/hypopnea syndrome (45). The exact mechanism of action of modafinil is unknown but has been shown by various investigators to involve dopamine, norepinephrine, histamine, serotonin, and/or GABA receptors; modafinil also binds at hypocretin (orexin receptors) (46,47). Modafinil showed reduced stimulant character relative to methylphenidate, and its potential for abuse in patients with narcolepsy has been demonstrated to be low (42). Hepatic metabolism responsible for the clearance of modafinil include amide hydrolysis to modafinil acid, its primary inactive metabolite. S-oxidation and aromatic ring hydroxylation occurred via CYP2C9. Less than 10% is excreted as unchanged drug.

Motor suppression seen in patients with cataplexy is similar to the motor suppression seen in healthy individuals during REM sleep. Consequently, agents previously found to decrease REM sleep have been evaluated for the treatment of cataplexy (44,46). Agents that suppress REM sleep include those that increase noradrenergic, serotonergic, and dopaminergic signaling. Tricyclic antidepressants, certain SSRIs, selective norepinephrine–serotonin reuptake inhibitors (e.g., venlafaxine) and MAO inhibitors have found application in the treatment of cataplexy, as has sodium oxybate (46,47). Psychostimulants also might be of some anticataplexic benefit, but modafinil generally produces little improvement (46).

Cocaine-Related Agents

There are eight possible stereoisomeric forms of methyl 3-(benzoyloxy)-8-methyl-azabicyclo[3.2.1]octan-2-carboxylate, of which one, R-cocaine, is simply referred to as "cocaine." Chemically, cocaine is known as 2R-carbomethoxy-3S-benzyloxy-1R-tropane. Cocaine is naturally occurring in a variety of plants belonging to the *Erythroxylon coca* species, which is indigenous to some countries in South America. In addition to its stimulant actions, cocaine possesses vasoconstrictor actions and is a local anesthetic; it has served as a template for the development of other therapeutically useful agents, including local anesthetics and 5-HT_3 serotonin antagonists.

Cocaine has a very interesting history. The coca plant was used by South American Indians for religious and mystical purposes and as a stimulant both to increase endurance and to alleviate hunger. It was introduced into Europe during the 1800s, and at the end of the 19th century, cocaine use was popular and socially acceptable. Various cocaine-containing preparations were available, and it also was used to "fortify" wines (e.g., Vin Coca). For a period of approximately 20 years, until just after the turn of the century, it was a constituent of the soft drink Coca-Cola. Additionally, cocaine was used for therapeutic reasons but was later supplanted by amphetamine.

Cocaine is active via nearly every possible route of administration; however, insufflation of "snow" or "coke" represents one of the most popular routes. Administered in this manner, peak effects and plasma levels are achieved within 30 minutes (48). Smoking the freebase form of cocaine ("crack") results in an even more rapid effect. The freebase form rather than the hydrochloride salt is used for smoking, because the temperatures required for vaporization of the salt result in considerable decomposition (48). Intravenously administered cocaine can achieve peak blood levels within a few minutes. Cocaine is metabolized to benzoylecgonine, the methyl ester of ecgonine, and to a lesser extent, to ecgonine, norcocaine, and hydroxylated derivatives.

Mechanism of Action of Cocaine

Cocaine has been shown to block the reuptake of norepinephrine, serotonin, and dopamine; however, the reinforcing and stimulant nature of cocaine seems to be related primarily to blockade of dopamine reuptake, leading to the "dopamine hypothesis" of cocaine's actions (49). [^{3}H]Cocaine was used in an attempt to identify the "cocaine receptor," and this was later shown to be similar to the dopamine transporter. Currently, it is thought that cocaine produces it reinforcing effects by interfering with dopamine reuptake (Fig. 23.5) by blocking the dopamine transporter (50). Although the human dopamine transporter has been cloned, it is unknown if the dopamine and cocaine binding domains are identical or how much they overlap (49).

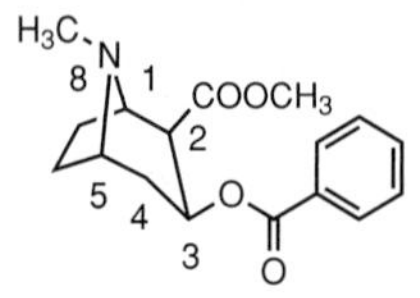

H_3C N 8 1 $COOCH_3$ 2 5 4 3 O O

Cocaine

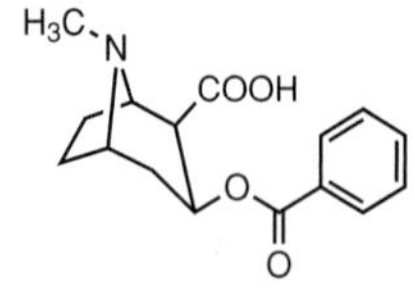

H_3C N COOH O O

Benzoylecgonine

H_3C N COOH O H

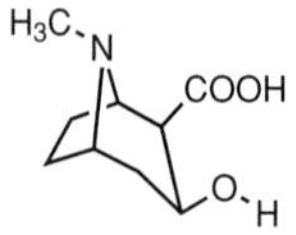

Ecgonine

COCAINE-LIKE STRUCTURE–ACTIVITY RELATIONSHIPS AND COCAINE-LIKE AGENTS. Because cocaine binds at the dopamine transporter, this provides a convenient method for the investigation and formulation of SARs; these have been recently reviewed elsewhere (48,49). Important features for the binding of cocaine analogues include configuration, substituent at C_2, stereochemistry at C_2, substituent at N_8, and substituents at C_3. With respect to cocaine analogues, inversion of configuration can decrease activity. The C_2-position is quite important: Epimerization from β to α reduces activity by 30- to 200-fold, and hydrolysis of the ester to the acid (i.e., benzoylecgonine) reduces activity by more than 1,500-fold. Although an ester function seems to be important, the methyl group can be replaced by other substituents (e.g., phenyl or benzyl) with relatively little effect. A basic nitrogen atom appears to be optimal. Replacement of the N_8-methyl group by other substituents, such as small alkyl or benzyl, has only a small negative influence on activity, whereas quaternization or acylation (of norcocaine) reduces activity by 33- and 111-fold, respectively (49).

Other dopamine transport blockers are known, and their SARs have been investigated (50). One of the oldest and most widely investigated is WIN 35,428, and [^{3}H]WIN 35,428 is available as a radioligand. Others include benztropine, GBR 12909, mazindol, and methylphenidate (50,51). These latter compounds produce varying degrees of cocaine-like actions and, thus, are being examined as structural leads for the development of therapies for the treatment of cocaine abuse (50). Because there are currently more than 1.7 million cocaine users in the United States, various novel pharmacotherapies are being pursued, including gabaminergic agents, dopaminergic agents, adrenoceptor antagonists, vasodilators, and cocaine vaccines (52).

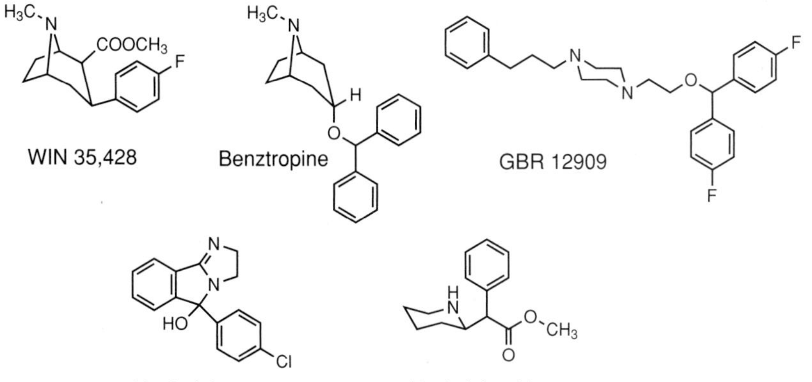

WIN 35,428 Benztropine GBR 12909

Mazindol Methylphenidate

DESIGNER DRUGS

Introduction

Designer drugs, or controlled substance analogues, are the end result of the application of SARs at the clandestine level. That is, knowledge of the established SARs of a particular class of abused substances can be applied at the clandestine level for the development of novel agents of abuse. What is particularly frightening about this concept is that the novel agents are not necessarily—or even commonly—examined for action or toxicity before they are put on the illicit market. The term "designer drug" was first introduced in reference to novel opiate-related analogues that appeared on the clandestine market approximately three decades ago; today, the term is applied more generically to any class of abusable substance. Furthermore, the term is now commonly applied to nearly any substance, novel or not, that is new to the street scene. Designer drugs have appeared that are structurally related to the hallucinogens and stimulants discussed above; the present discussion will focus on some of these agents.

Specific Examples

Because some designer drugs result from the clandestine application of SARs, it should be possible to legitimately forecast the actions and, perhaps, even the approximate potencies of novel street drugs on the basis of the same SAR data. In fact, this sometimes is the case. For example, "Nexus" made an appearance on the east coast of the United States in the early 1990s. Nexus is α-desmethyl DOB, or 2-(4-bromo-2,5-dimethoxyphenyl)-1-aminoethane. Knowing that DOB is a potent phenylisopropylamine hallucinogen and that α-demethylation typically reduces the potency of phenylisopropylamines, it might be suspected that Nexus would be a DOB-like agent with reduced potency. This has been supported by the results of drug discrimination studies in animals. Furthermore, this material, also known as 2C-B, has been shown to be active in humans at 12 to 24 mg relative to approximately 2 mg for DOB (29). In the last year or two, a number of related agents have been found on the clandestine market and, like 2C-B, are phenylethylamine analogues of their phenylisopropylamine counterparts; for example, 2C-C, 2C-I, 2C-N, 2C-E, and 2C-P are the phenylethylamine analogues of DOC, DOI, DON, DOET, and DOPR, respectively (Table 23.3) (Fig. 23.6). Another agent attracting recent attention is 2C-T-7 (e.g., "Blue Mystic" or "Tripstasy") (53), which has been recently controlled as a Schedule I substance. Recently controlled indolealkylamine analogues include α-MeT (AMT), α-EtT ("ET"), and 5-methoxy-N,N-diisopropyltryptamine ("Foxy Methoxy") (Fig. 23.6); these agents had been previously shown to produce DOM-like stimulus effects in animals (54).

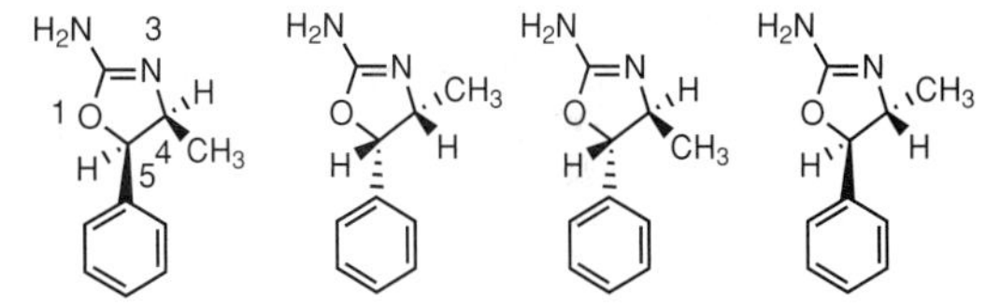

cis(4S,5R) cis(4R,5S) trans(4S,5S) trans(4R,5R)

4-Methylaminorex

Stimulant designer drugs also have appeared. For example, CAT, or methcathinone, has been found on the illicit American market. Interestingly, it seems that methcathinone was a popular drug of abuse in the former Soviet Union (where it was known under a variety of names including ephedrone), but reports of this agent were never published in either the scientific or lay literature of that time. Methcathinone is the N-monomethyl analogue of cathinone. Indeed, structurally, methcathinone is to cathinone what methamphetamine is to amphetamine. Methcathinone, which may be viewed as an oxidation product of ephedrine (hence the name ephedrone) is a potent central stimulant that is at least as potent as methamphetamine. Another example of a stimulant designer drug is 4-methylaminorex (U4Euh), which has been misrepresented on the illicit market as cocaine or methamphetamine. 4-Methylaminorex, an alkylated version of the anorectic/stimulant aminorex,

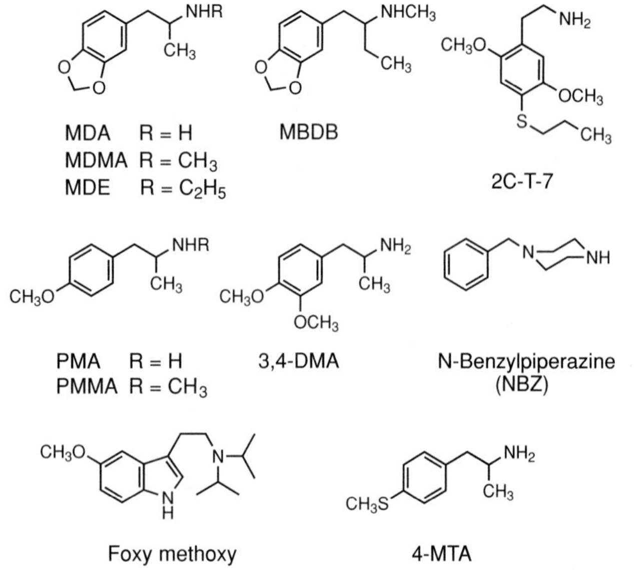

Fig. 23.6. Designer drugs.

contains two chiral centers and, hence, exists as four optical isomers. Typically, it is a mixture of the two *cis* isomers that has been confiscated by law enforcement officials, and *cis* 4-methylaminorex is now classified as a Schedule I substance. Interestingly, all four isomers behave as amphetamine-like agents, with the *trans*-(4S,5S) isomer being the most active, having a potency slightly greater than that of (+)-amphetamine itself. Yet other examples include the piperazines. Several piperazine analogues have been reported to produce amphetamine-like effects in humans, and one in particular, N-benzylpiperazine (known either alone or in combination with other piperazines as "Rapture"), has been recently classified as a Schedule I substance (Fig. 23.6).

Not all designer drugs result in actions that are entirely predictable. One of the most popular of such agents is MDMA, or N-methyl-1-(3,4-methylenedioxyphenyl)-2-aminopropane (e.g., "Ecstasy," "XTC," or "Adam") (Fig. 23.6). MDMA is the N-monomethyl analogue of MDA, or 1-(3,4-methylenedioxyphenyl)-2-aminopropane. MDA was popular during the 1960s, when it was known on the street as the "Love Drug." It was reported to produce effects in humans akin to a combination of cocaine and LSD. It has since been shown that MDA produces both amphetamine-like and DOM-like stimulus effects in animals and, furthermore, that animals trained to discriminate MDA recognize central stimulants, such as amphetamine and cocaine, as well as classical hallucinogens, such as LSD, mescaline, and DOM. Interestingly, the stimulant actions of MDA appear to be associated with the S-(+)-isomer, whereas the DOM-like actions are associated with the R-(−)-isomer. Knowing that N-monomethylation of phenylisopropylamine stimulants enhances their potency, whereas the corresponding change is detrimental to DOM-like actions, it would have been predicted that MDMA would probably behave as an amphetamine-like stimulant. Consistent with this prediction, amphetamine-trained (but not DOM-trained) animals recognized MDMA in tests of stimulus generalization. Furthermore, animals trained to discriminate MDMA recognized amphetamine but not DOM. However, MDMA was claimed to produce empathogenic effects in humans (i.e., increased empathy and sociability and enhanced feelings of well being) and was used for several years as an adjunct to psychotherapy before emergency scheduling under the Controlled Substances Act as a Schedule I substance. It was argued that MDMA produced a unique, nonamphetamine-like effect (55). Although both optical isomers are active, the S-(+)-isomer is the more active of the two. A closely related agent is its N-ethyl homologue MDE ("Eve"). The general consensus today is that MDMA is probably an empathogen with amphetamine-like stimulant side effects. Homologation of the α-methyl group of phenylisopropylamine stimulants and hallucinogens typically diminishes their potency or abolishes their activity; however, the α-ethyl analogue of MDMA (MBDB, or N-methyl-1-(3,4-methylenedioxyphenyl)-2-aminobutane) retains MDMA-like actions (56) (Fig. 23.6). Another agent, sold as a substitute for MDMA, is 4-MTA (e.g., "Flatliners" or "Golden Eagles") (Fig. 23.6); this agent produces MDMA-like stimulus effects in animals but did not produce either DOM-like or cocaine-like effects (53).

A closely related agent is PMMA, or N-methyl-1-(4-methoxyphenyl)-2-aminopropane. PMMA is a hybrid structure of two phenylisopropylamine stimulants: PMA, and methamphetamine (Fig. 23.6) Surprisingly, PMMA lacks significant central stimulant actions, and unlike PMA and methamphetamine, PMMA is not recognized by (+)-amphetamine–trained animals. Because PMMA is structurally related to metabolites of MDMA, it was examined in MDMA-trained animals and found to be several-fold more potent than MDMA. Animals have been trained to discriminate PMMA from vehicle, and PMMA stimulus generalization occurred to (±)-MDMA and S-(+)-MDMA, but not to DOM, (+)-amphetamine, R-(−)-MDMA, or R-(−)-PMMA. Another psychoactive agent that has not been well investigated is 3,4-DMA (Table 23.3). 3,4-DMA may be viewed as an O-methyl ring-opened analogue of MDA (Fig. 23.6). Although 3,4-DMA was not recognized by either DOM- or (+)-amphetamine–trained animals, it was recognized by MDA- and PMMA-trained animals. These results, coupled with the above discussion of MDMA, suggest that phenylisopropylamines may not be best described as merely central stimulants or hallucinogens; a third action needs to be accounted for. Although MDMA is widely abused, a contributing factor may be related to its amphetaminergic actions. It is not yet known if agents that fall into this third pharmacological category possess abuse potential; consequently, they have been referred to simply as "other" agents. It has been proposed that the behavioral actions of the phenylisopropylamines can be described by the Venn diagram shown as Figure 23.7. As depicted in that figure, the three types of actions are classical hallucinogen (*H*), stimulant (*S*), and PMMA-like (*P*) (57). Because MDMA

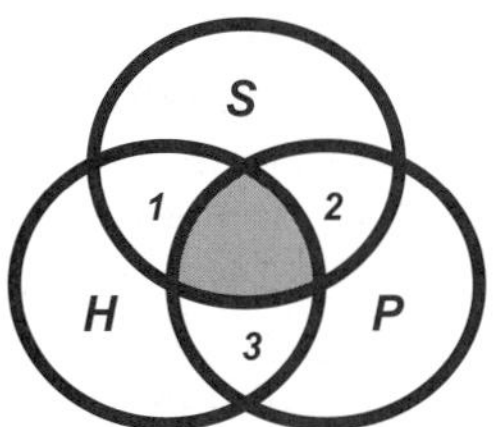

Fig. 23.7. The behavioral effects of arylalkylamines may be described as falling into one or more of three different stimulus categories: classical hallucinogen (*H*), central stimulant (*S*) or PMMA-like (*P*). See text for further discussion.

possesses both PMMA-like and (+)-amphetamine–like activity, it is perhaps best represented by Intersect 2. As mentioned above, R-(−)-MDA is hallucinogenic, and S-(+)-MDA is a stimulant. Both isomers possess PMMA-like activity. Thus, R-(−)-MDA is best represented by Intersect 3, whereas S-(+)-MDA is best represented by Intersect 2. The common intersect (shaded area) describes the actions of (±)-MDA. Using this classification system, it should be possible to classify the various phenylisopropylamines as falling into one or more categories. Furthermore, there is no reason to suspect that this classification system will be limited to the phenylisopropylamines; that is, there is evidence that the indolealkylamines might be classified in a similar manner. For example, S-(+)-α-EtT produces both DOM- and PMMA-like effects, but not (+)-amphetamine–like effects, whereas R-(−)-α-EtT produces (+)-amphetamine– and PMMA-like effects, but not DOM-like effects (58). The classification scheme suggests that there will be three different SARs and three different mechanisms of action. Certain agents, because they fall into more than one category, may represent mechanistic and structure–activity composites. The same may be said of arylalkylamine designer drugs; indeed, it may be the particular "mix" of actions that makes certain designer drugs so attractive as drugs of abuse.

Perhaps the most worrisome things about designer drugs are that almost none has been investigated under controlled clinical settings, that relatively little is known about their toxicity or long-term effects, and that medical professionals generally are unfamiliar with them (or with the treatment of their overdose) in emergency room settings. The situation is further exacerbated by the broad availability of Web sites describing such agents to potential users (59).

NEURONAL PLASTICITY AND DRUGS OF ABUSE

Release of neurotransmitter from presynaptic terminals results in the activation of postsynaptic neurotransmitter receptors that can be coupled to complex effector mechanisms. Through modulation of postsynaptic pathways, the state of the neuron can be altered such that neurons become more or less responsive to the neurotransmitter (60). This process is referred to as functional plasticity. One of the most exciting recent findings with implications for the treatment of drug abuse (as well as other neuropsychiatric disorders) involves the regulation of DARPP-32, an integrator of intracellular signaling. Interaction of dopamine at D_1-like receptors (D_1/D_5) activates adenylate cyclase, which increases cyclic adenosine monophosphate (cAMP) levels; this, in turn, can regulate phosphorylation of DARPP-32 (dopamine- and cAMP-regulated phosphoprotein of 32 kDa) by protein kinase A

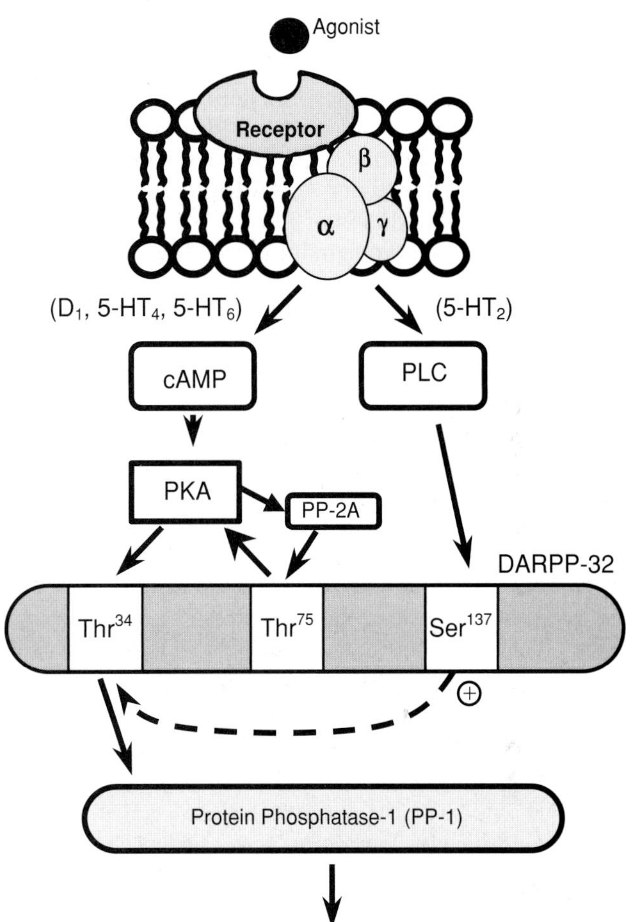

Fig. 23.8. A simplistic schematic showing the proposed involvement of DARPP-32 in neurotransmission. Agonists (e.g., DA and 5-HT) can interact with certain postsynaptic G protein–coupled receptors to activate second messenger systems. Agonist action at D_1 receptors increases cAMP levels and causes PKA to phosphorylate DARPP-32 at Thr^{34}; activation of D_1 receptors also decreases the phosphorylation state of DARPP-32 at Thr^{75} by what appears to involve PKA-dependent activation of a protein phosphatase (PP-2A). Likewise, the action of 5-HT at $5\text{-}HT_4$ and $5\text{-}HT_6$ receptors increases phosphorylation of Thr^{34} and decreases phosphorylation of Thr^{75}. Interaction of 5-HT at $5\text{-}HT_2$ receptors activates phospholipase C (PLC) and promotes phosphorylation of DARPP-32 at Ser^{137}. Phosphorylation at Thr^{34} inhibits protein phosphatase-1 (PP-1). Inhibition of PP-1 enhances signaling. Phosphorylation of Thr^{75} has an inhibitory effect on Thr^{34} phosphorylation (conversely, decreased Thr^{75} phosphorylation disinhibits PKA to increase Thr^{34} phosphorylation), whereas phosphorylation of Ser^{137} prevents dephosphorylation of Thr^{34}. Other receptors can impinge on this mechanism (60–65).

(PKA). Interaction of dopamine at D_2-like receptors ($D_2/D_3/D_4$, which are negatively coupled to cAMP) has an effect that is essentially opposite that of activation of D_1 receptors. Phosphorylation of a specific amino acid residue (threonine[34] [Thr[34]]), induced by D_1 agonists, converts DARPP-32 to an inhibitor of protein phosphatase-1 (PP-1); thus, when phosphorylated at Thr[34], DARPP-32 behaves as an amplifier of PKA-mediated signaling through its ability to inhibit PP-1. The actions of DARPP-32 also can be modulated by phosphorylation (or dephosphorylation) of Thr[75] (Fig. 23.8). Activation of D_1 receptors decreases the phosphorylation state of DARPP-32 at Thr[75] by a process that involves PKA-dependent activation of protein phosphatase-2A (PP-2A); this disinhibits phosphorylation of Thr[34] by PKA (i.e., results in enhanced phosphorylation of Thr[34]). The result is potentiation of dopaminergic signaling. Together, PKA and PP-1 regulate the phosphorylation state of downstream neuronal effector proteins. Additionally, DARPP-32 can be phosphorylated at serine[137] (Ser[137]), and this phosphorylation decreases the rate of dephosphorylation of Thr[34].

Serotonin causes an increase in phosphorylation of Thr[34] (via activation of 5-HT_4 and 5-HT_6 receptors, which are positively coupled to cAMP) and Ser[137] (via activation of 5-HT_2 receptors–receptors coupled to phospholipase C), and a decrease in the phosphorylation of Thr[75] (via activation of 5-HT_4 and 5-HT_6 receptors). Hence, serotonin inhibits PP-1 through what might be considered a synergistic mechanism (61). Other receptors that might modulate DARPP-32 include glutamate, GABA, adenosine, nitrous oxide, and opioid receptors. Hence, it has been speculated that various drugs of abuse, including amphetamine, methamphetamine, cocaine, caffeine, opioids (e.g., morphine), nicotine, and ethanol involve a DARPP-32 mechanism; furthermore, agents such as antidepressants, antipsychotics, and antiparkinsonian drugs have been shown to influence phosphorylation of DARPP-32. Classical hallucinogens, as described above, are thought to act by activation of 5-HT_{2A} receptors. It has been shown that LSD increases phosphorylation of Ser[137] (62). In theory, DARPP-32 should be modulated by various designer drugs that act via a dopaminergic or serotonergic mechanism. Only selected aspects of intracellular integration have been mentioned here, and others already have been implicated. The state of the art has been recently described (61–65). Nevertheless, the actions of many drugs of abuse might involve such postsynaptic events and certainly require further attention.

ACKNOWLEDGEMENT

Work from the author's laboratory was supported by PHS grant DA 01642.

CASE STUDY

Victoria F. Roche and S. William Zito

EW, a 25-year-old wildhair who has always been "just this side" of the law, is on a solo motorcycle trip through the desert Southwest with an ultimate destination of Mendocino, California. He is traveling light, but he did take care to pack enough grass to last the trip—or so he thought. Somewhere around Gallup, New Mexico, he met up with some other "born to be wild" folks heading south to Mexico, and they pooled their stashes and partied together until everything was gone. As he crossed into Arizona and entered the Navajo Nation a few hours later (still half-stoned), he was wondering how in the heck he was going to make it to California without the aid of illicit pharmaceuticals. When he rode by a Native-American church building, he exercised some very poor judgment in turning around, breaking in, and stealing a small quantity of botanical intended to be used in a sacred manner to facilitate spiritual communion with the Creator.

Afraid of being caught with his stolen property, EW decided to consume what he had taken and, a few hours later, began to have visual hallucinations that distorted his image of the road ahead. The mesas appeared to be on fire and, feeling dizzy and abruptly "seeing" the ocean right in front of him, he turned sharply, ran off the road at 75 mph, and was thrown from his bike into a wash. The tribal police now have him in custody, and he was taken to the health care facility in Chinle for treatment of his injuries. As the IHS pharmacist in charge, you and your rotation student are now about to see him as you make your morning rounds. You ask your student to take the lead on the consultation, beginning by identifying the hallucinogenic substance from the structural choices provided below.

1. Identify the therapeutic problem(s) where the pharmacist's intervention may benefit the patient.
2. Identify and prioritize the patient-specific factors that must be considered to achieve the desired therapeutic outcomes.
3. Conduct a thorough and mechanistically oriented SAR analysis of all structures provided in the case.
4. Counsel your patient

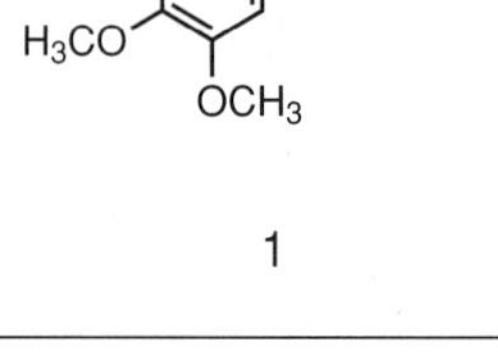

1 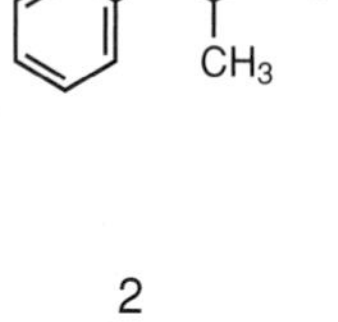 2 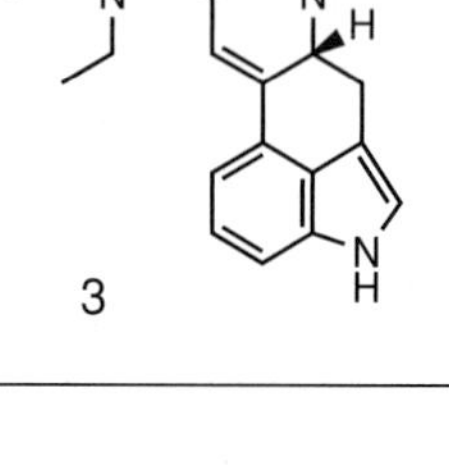 3 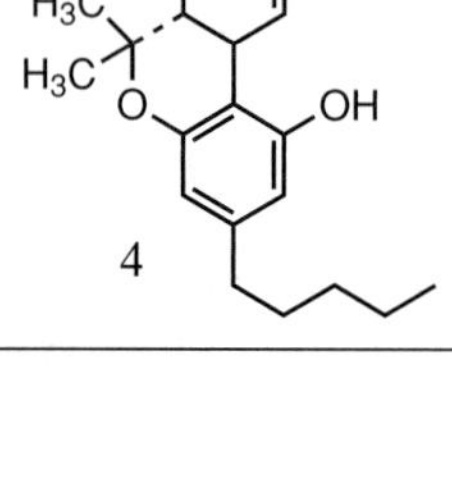 4

References

1. Brimblecombe RW, Pinder RM. Hallucinogenic Agents. Bristol, UK: Wright-Scientechnica, 1975.
2. Hollister LE. Chemical Psychoses. Springfield, IL: Charles C. Thomas, 1968.
3. Glennon RA. Animal models for assessing hallucinogenic agents. In: Boulton AA, Baker GB, Wu PH, eds. Animal Models of Drug Addiction. Totowa, NJ: Humana Press, 1992:345–381.
4. Glennon RA, Jarbe TUC, Frankenheim J, eds. Drug Discrimination: Applications to Drug Abuse Research. Rockville, MD: National Institute on Drug Abuse, 1991.
5. Glennon RA. Discriminative stimulus properties of hallucinogens and related designer drugs. In: Glennon RA, Jarbe TUC, Frankenheim J, eds. Drug Discrimination: Applications to Drug Abuse Research. Rockville, MD: National Institute on Drug Abuse, 1991:25–44.
6. Lin JC, Glennon RA, eds. Hallucinogens: An Update. Rockville, MD: National Institute on Drug Abuse, 1994.
7. Padgett LW. Recent developments in cannabinoid ligands. Life Sci 2005;77:1767–1798.
8. Matsuda L, Lolait SJ, Brownstein MJ, et al. Structure of a cannabinoid receptor and functional expression of the cloned cDNA. Nature 1990;246:561–564.
9. Munro S, Thomas KL, Abu-Shaar M. Molecular characterization of a peripheral receptor for cannabinoids. Nature 1993;365:61–64.
10. Hanus L, Gopher A, Almog S, et al. Two new unsaturated fatty acid ethanolamides in brain that bind to the cannabinoid receptor. J Med Chem 1993;36:3032–3034.
11. Jarbe TUC, Lamb RL, Makriyannis A, et al. (R)-methanandamide as a discriminative stimulus in rats: tests with anandamide and Δ^9-THC. Behav Pharmacol 1998;9:S47.
12. Martin BR. Marijuana. In: Bloom FE, Kupfer DJ, eds. Psychopharmacology: The Fourth Generation of Progress. New York: Raven Press, 1995:1757–1765.
13. Reggio PH, Wang T, Brown AE, et al. Importance of the C-1 substituent in classical cannabinoids to CB_2 receptor selectivity: synthesis and characterization of a series of O,2-propano-Δ^8-tetrahydrocannabinol analogues. J Med Chem 1997;40:3312–3318.
14. Lagu SG, Varona A, Chambers JD, et al. Construction of a steric map of the binding pocket for cannabinoids at the cannabinoid receptor. Drug Des Discov 1995;12:179–192.
15. Huffman JW. CB_2 receptor ligands. Mini Rev Med Chem 2005;5:641–649.
16. Corey S. Recent development in the therapeutic potential of cannabinoids. P R Health Sci J 2005;24:19–26.
17. Fernandez JR, Allison DB. Rimonabant Sanofi-Synthelabo. Curr Opin Invest Drugs 2004;5:430–435.
18. Balster RL, Willetts J. Phencyclidine: a drug of abuse and a tool for neuroscience research. In: Schuster CR, Kuhar MJ, eds. Pharmacological Aspects of Drug Dependence. Handbook of Experimental Pharmacology Series, vol 118. Berlin: Springer, 1996:233–262.
19. Glennon RA. Pharmacophore identification for sigma-1 (σ_1) receptor binding-application of the "deconstruction-reconstruction-elaboration" approach. Mini Rev Med Chem. 2005;5:927–940.
20. Morris BJ, Cochran SM, Pratt JA. PCP: from pharmacology to modeling schizophrenia. Curr Opin Pharmacol 2005;5:101–106.
21. Balster RL. Discriminative stimulus properties of phencyclidine and other NMDA antagonists. In: Glennon RA, Jarbe TUC, Frankenheim J, eds. Drug Discrimination: Applications to Drug Abuse Research. Rockville, MD: National Institute on Drug Abuse, 1991:163–180.
22. Shulgin AT, Shulgin A. Tihkal. Berkeley, CA: Transform Press, 1997.
23. Murphree HB, Dippy RH, Jenney EH, et al. Effects in normal man of α-methyltryptamine and α-ethyltryptamine. Clin Pharmacol Ther 1961;2:722–726.
24. Siva Sankar DV. ed. LSD: a total study. Westbury, NY: PJD Publications, 1975.
25. Pfaff RC, Huang X, Marona-Lewicka D, et al. Lysergamides revisited. In: Lin JC, Glennon RA, eds. Hallucinogens: an update. Rockville, MD: National Institute on Drug Abuse, 1994:52–73.
26. Naranjo C. Psychotropic properties of harmala alkaloids. In: Efron DK, Holmstedt B, Kline NS, eds. Ethnopharmacologic search for psychoactive drugs. Washington, DC: U.S. Government Printing Office, 1967:385–391.
27. Naranjo C. The Healing Journey. New York: Pantheon Books, 1973.
28. Grella B, Dukat M, Young R, et al. Investigation of hallucinogenic and related β-carbolines. Drug Alcohol Depend 1998;50:99–107.
29. Shulgin AT, Shulgin A. Pihkal. Berkeley, CA: Transform Press, 1991.
30. Glennon RA. Classical hallucinogens. In: Schuster CR, Kuhar MJ, eds. Pharmacological Aspects of Drug Dependence. Handbook of Experimental Pharmacology Series, vol 118. Berlin: Springer, 1996:343–371.
31. Nelson DL, Lucaites VL, Wainscot DB, et al. Comparisons of hallucinogenic phenylisopropylamine binding affinities at cloned human $5\text{-}HT_{2A}$, $5\text{-}HT_{2B}$, and $5\text{-}HT_{2C}$ receptors. Naunyn-Schmeideberg's Arch Pharmacol 1998;359:1–6.
32. Griffiths RR, Mumford GK. Caffeine reinforcement, discrimination, tolerance, and physical dependence in laboratory animals and humans. In: Schuster CR, Kuhar MJ, eds. Pharmacological Aspects of Drug Dependence. Handbook of Experimental Pharmacology Series, vol 118. Berlin: Springer, 1996:315–341.
33. Cho AK, Segal DS, eds. Amphetamine and its analogues. San Diego: Academic Press, 1994:43–77.
34. Young R, Glennon RA. Discriminative stimulus properties of amphetamine and structurally related phenalkylamines. Med Res Rev 1986;6:99–130.
35. Young R, Gabryszuk M, Glennon RA. (−)-Ephedrine and caffeine mutually potentiate one another's amphetamine-like stimulus effects. Pharmacol Biochem Behav 1998;61:169–173.
36. Cho AK, Kumagai Y. Metabolism of amphetamine and other arylisopropylamines. In: Cho AK, Segal DS, eds. Amphetamine and its analogues. San Diego: Academic Press, 1994:43–77.
37. Finer N. Pharmacotherapy of obesity. Best Pract Res Clin Endocrinol Metab 2002;16:717–742.
38. Linne Y, Rossner S. Pharmacotherapy of obesity. Clin Dermatol 2004;22: 319–324.
39. Rothman RB, Baumann MH, Savage JE, et al. Evidence for possible involvement of $5\text{-}HT_{2B}$ receptors in the cardiac valvulopathy associated with fenfluramine and other serotonergic medications. Circulation, 2000;102:2836–2841.
40. Setola V, Dukat M, Glennon RA, et al. Molecular determinants for the interaction of the valvulopathic anorexigen norfenfluramine with the $5\text{-}HT_{2B}$ receptor. Mol Pharmacol 2005;68:20–33.
41. van Gaal L, Mertens I, Ballaux D, et al. Modern, new pharmacotherapy for obesity. Best Pract Res Clin Endocrinol Metab 2004;18:1049–1072.
42. Banerjee D, Vitiello MV, Grunstein RR. Pharmacotherapy for excessive daytime sleepiness. Sleep Med Rev 2004;8:339–354.
43. Boutrel B, Koob GF. What keeps us awake: the neuropharmacology of stimulants and wakefulness-promoting medications. Sleep 2004;27:1181–1194.
44. Black J, Guilleminault C. Medications for the treatment of narcolepsy. Expert Opin Emerg Drugs 2001;6:239–247.
45. Schwartz JR. Modafinil: new indications for wake promotion. Expert Opin Pharmacother 2005;6:115–129.
46. Houghton WC, Scammell TE, Thorpy M. Pharmacotherapy for cataplexy. Sleep Med Rev 2004;8:355–366.
47. Mignot E. An update on the pharmacotherapy of excessive daytime sleepiness and cataplexy. Sleep Med Rev 2004;8:333–338.
48. Fischman MW, Johanson CE. Cocaine. In: Schuster CR, Kuhar MJ, eds. Pharmacological Aspects of Drug Dependence. Handbook of Experimental Pharmacology Series, vol 118. Berlin: Springer, 1996:159–195.
49. Carroll FI, Lewin AH, Boja JW, et al. Cocaine receptor: biochemical characterization and structure–activity relationships of cocaine analogues at the dopamine transporter. J Med Chem 35:969–981.
50. Newman AH. Novel dopamine transporter ligands: the state of the art. Med Chem Res 1998;8:1–11.
51. Deutsch HM, Shi Q, Gruszecka-Kowalik E, et al. Synthesis and pharmacology of potential cocaine antagonists. 2. Structure–activity relationship studies of aromatic ring-substituted methylphenidate analogues. J Med Chem 1996;39: 1201–1209.
52. Sofuoglu M, Kosten TR. Novel approaches to the treatment of cocaine abuse. CNS Drugs 2005;19:13–25.
53. Khorana N, Pullagurla M, Dukat M, et al. Stimulus effects of three sulfur-containing psychoactive agents. Pharmacol Biochem Behav 2004;78: 821–826.
54. Glennon RA, Young R, Jacyno JM, et al. DOM-stimulus generalization to LSD and other hallucinogenic indolealkylamines. Eur J Pharmacol 1983;86: 453–459.
55. Nichols DE, Oberlender R. Structure–activity relationships of MDMA-like substances. In: Ashgar K, De Souza E, eds. Pharmacology and toxicology of amphetamine and related designer drugs. Washington, DC: U.S. Government Printing Office, 1989:1–29.
56. Oberlender R, Nichols DE. (+)-N-methyl-1-(1,3-benzodioxol-5-yl)-2-butanamine as a discriminative stimulus in studies of 3,4-methylenedioxyamphetamine-like behavioral activity. J Pharmacol Exp Ther 1990;255:1098–1106.
57. Glennon RA, Young R, Dukat M, et al. Initial characterization of PMMA as a discriminative stimulus. Pharmacol Biochem Behav 1997;57:151–158.
58. Glennon RA. Arylalkylamine drugs of abuse: an overview of drug discrimination studies. Pharmacol Biochem Behav 1999;64:251–256.
59. Wax PM. Just a click away: recreational drug web sites on the internet. Pediatrics 2002;109:96–100.
60. Benavides DR, Bibb JA. Role of Cdk5 in drug abuse and plasticity. Ann N Y Acad Sci 2004;1025:335–344.
61. Svenningsson P, Tzavara ET, Liu F, et al. DARPP-32 mediates serotonergic neurotransmission in the forebrain. Proc Natl Acad Sci U S A 2002;99: 3188–3193.
62. Svenningsson P, Tzavara ET, Carruthers R, et al. Diverse psychotomimetics act through a common signaling pathway. Science 2003;302:1412–1415.
63. Svenningsson P, Nishi A, Fisone G, et al. DARPP-32: an integrator of neurotransmission. Ann Rev Pharmacol Toxicol 2004;44:269–296.
64. Nairn AC, Svenningsson P, Nishi A, et al. The role of DARPP-32 in the actions of drugs of abuse. Neuropharmacology 2004;47(Suppl 1):14–23.
65. Gould TD, Manji HK. DARPP-32: a molecular switch at the nexus of reward pathway plasticity. Proc Natl Acad Sci U S A 2005;102:253–254.

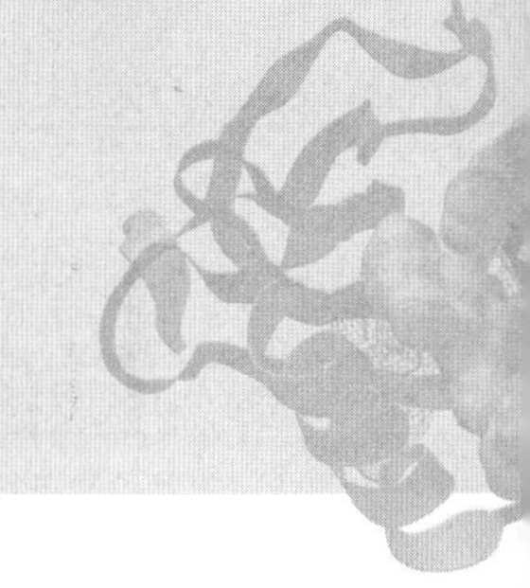

24. *Opioid Analgesics*

DAVID S. FRIES

DRUGS COVERED IN THIS CHAPTER:

μ AGONISTS
- Morphine
- Codeine
- Dihydromorphone
- Dihydrocodeinone
- Oxymorphione
- Oxycodone
- Levorphanol
- Meperidine
- Methadone
- Fentanyl
- Alfentanyl
- Sufentanil
- Remifentanil

OTHER ANALGESICS
- Tramadol
- Propoxyphene

MIXED AGONIST/ANTAGONIST ANALGESICS
- Buprenorphine
- Butorphanol
- Nalbuphine
- Pentazocine
- Dezocine

μ ANTAGONISTS
- Naloxone
- Naltrexone

ANTIDIARRHEAL AGENTS
- Diphenoxylate
- Loperamide

COUGH SUPPRESSANTS
- Dextromorphan

INTRODUCTION

Agents that decrease pain are referred to as analgesics, or analgetics. Although analgetic is grammatically correct, common use has made analgesic preferable to analgetic for the description of the pain-killing drugs. Pain relieving agents also are called antinociceptives.

A number of classes of drugs are used to relieve pain. The nonsteroidal anti-inflammatory agents have primarily a peripheral site of action, are useful for mild to moderate pain, and often have an anti-inflammatory effect associated with their pain-killing action. Local anesthetics inhibit pain transmission by inhibition of voltage-regulated sodium channels. These agents often are highly toxic when used in concentrations sufficient to relieve chronic or acute pain in ambulatory patients. Dissociative anesthetics (ketamine), and other compounds that act as inhibitors of N-methyl-D-aspartate (NMDA)–activated glutamate receptors in the brain, are effective antinociceptive agents when used alone or in combination with opioids. Compounds, such as the antiseizure drug pregabulin, which inhibits voltage regulated Ca^{2+} ion channels, are useful in treating neuropathic pain. Most central nervous system (CNS) depressants (e.g., ethanol, barbiturates, and antipsychotics) will cause a decrease in pain perception. Inhibitors of serotonin and norepinephrine reuptake (i.e., antidepressant drugs) are useful either alone and in combination with opioids in treating certain cases of chronic pain. Current research into the antinociceptive effects of centrally acting α-adrenergic-, cannabinoid-, and nicotinic-receptor agonists may yield clinically useful analgesics working by nonopioid mechanisms. Research in one or more of the above areas may lead to new drugs, but at present, severe acute or chronic pain generally is treated most effectively with opioid agents.

Historically, opioid analgesics have been called narcotic analgesics. Narcotic analgesic literally means that the agents cause sleep or loss of consciousness (narcosis) in conjunction with their analgesic effect. The term "narcotic" has become associated with the addictive properties of opioids and other CNS depressants. Because the great therapeutic value of the opioids is their ability to induce analgesia without causing narcosis, and because not all opioids are addicting, the term "narcotic analgesic" is misleading and will not be used further in this chapter.

History

The juice (*opium* in Greek) or latex from the unripe seed pods of the poppy *Papaver somniferum* is among the oldest recorded medications used by humans. The writings of Theophrastus around 200 BC describe the use of opium in medicine; however, evidence suggests that opium was used in the Sumerian culture as early as 3500 BC. The initial use of opium was as a tonic, or it was smoked. The pharmacist Surtürner first isolated an alkaloid from opium in 1803. He named the alkaloid morphine, after Morpheus, the Greek god of dreams. Codeine, thebaine, and papaverine are other medically important alkaloids that were later isolated from the latex of opium poppies.

Morphine was among the first compounds to undergo structure modification. Ethylmorphine (the 3-ethyl ether of morphine) was introduced as a medicine in 1898. Diacetylmorphine (heroin), which may be considered to be the first synthetic pro-drug, was synthesized in 1874 and marketed as a nonaddicting analgesic, antidiarrheal, and antitussive agent in 1898.

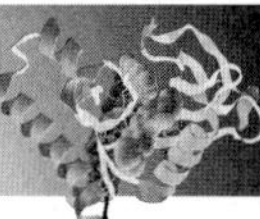

CLINICAL SIGNIFICANCE

Opioid agonists and partial agonist/antagonists generally act on δ, μ, and κ receptors. All of these receptors have subtypes that provide varying degrees of analgesia, euphoria or dysphoria, central nervous system depression, and perhaps, the potential for tolerance. By modifying their structures, properties can be changed to develop agents that require more or less hepatic metabolism and, thus, affect the duration of action and the bioavailability. Other changes in the chemical structures can yield agents with much higher affinity for analgesic receptors, which corresponds to more potency on a milligram-to-milligram basis. Other alterations of the chemical structures can lead to improved profiles regarding respiratory depression, emesis, tolerance, and allergenicity. By altering the affinities for some receptors more than others, the addictive properties also may be manipulated.

Through an understanding of the relationship of chemical structures to biological activity, the clinician can improve the selection of drug to the specific patient.

Jill T. Johnson, Pharm.D., BCPS
Associate Professor
Department of Pharmacy Practice
College of Pharmacy
University of Arkansas for Medical Sciences

Opiate/Opioid

The use of the terms "opiate" and "opioid" requires clarification. Until the 1980s, the term "opiate" was used extensively to describe any natural or synthetic agent that was derived from morphine. One could say an opiate was any compound that was structurally related to morphine. In the mid-1970s, the discovery of peptides in the brain with pharmacological actions similar to morphine prompted a change in nomenclature. The peptides were not easily related to morphine structurally, yet their actions were like those produced by morphine. At this time, the term "opioid," meaning opium- or morphine-like in terms of pharmacological action, was introduced. The broad group of opium alkaloids, synthetic derivatives related to the opium alkaloids, and the many naturally occurring and synthetic peptides with morphine-like pharmacological effects are called opioids. In addition to having pharmacological effects similar to morphine, a compound must be antagonized by an opioid antagonist, such as naloxone, to be classed as an opioid. The neuronal-located proteins to which opioid agents bind and initiate biological responses are called opioid receptors.

ENDOGENOUS OPIOID PEPTIDES AND THEIR PHYSIOLOGICAL FUNCTIONS

Scientists had postulated for some time, based on structure–activity relationships (SARs), that opioids bind to specific receptor sites to cause their actions. It also was reasoned that morphine and the synthetic opioid derivatives are not the natural ligands for the opioid receptors and that some analgesic substance must exist within the brain. Techniques to prove these two points were not developed until the mid-1970s. Hughes et al. (1) used the electrically stimulated contractions of guinea pig ileum and the mouse vas deferens, which are very sensitive to inhibition by opioids, as bioassays to follow the purification of compounds with morphine-like activity from mammalian brain tissue. These researchers were able to isolate and determine the structures of two pentapeptides, Tyr-Gly-Gly-Phe-Met (Met-enkephalin) and Tyr-Gly-Gly-Phe-Leu (Leu-enkephalin), that caused the opioid activity. The compounds were named enkephalins after the Greek word *Kaphale,* which translates as "from the head."

At about the same time as Hughes and coworkers were making their discoveries, three other laboratories, using a different assay technique, were able to identify endogenous opioids and opioid receptors in the brain (2–4). These scientists used radiolabeled opioid compounds (radioligands), with high specific activity, to bind to opioid receptors in brain homogenates (5). They demonstrated saturable binding (i.e., the tissue contains a finite number of binding sites that can all be occupied) of the radioligands and that the bound radioligands could be displaced stereoselectively by nonradiolabeled opioids. Discovery of the enkephalins was soon followed by the identification of other endogenous opioid peptides, including β-endorphin (6), the dynorphins (7), and the endomorphins (8).

The opioid peptides isolated from mammalian tissue are known collectively as endorphins, a word that is derived from a combination of endogenous and morphine. The opioid alkaloids and all of the synthetic opioid derivatives are exogenous opioids. Interestingly, the isolation of morphine and codeine in small amounts has been reported from mammalian brain (9). The functional significance of endogenous morphine remains unknown.

Opioid Peptides

The endogenous opioid peptides are synthesized as part of the structures of large precursor proteins (10). There is a different precursor protein for each of the major types of opioid peptides (Fig. 24.1). Proopiomelanocortin is the precursor for β-endorphin. Proenkephalin A is the precursor for Met- and Leu-enkephalin. Proenkephalin B (prodynorphin) is the precursor for dynorphin and

Met-enkephalin	= Tyr-Gly-Gly-Phe-Met
Leu-Enkephalin	= Tyr-Gly-Gly-Phe-Leu
β-Endorphin	= Tyr-Gly-Gly-Phe-Met-Thr-Ser-Glu-Lys-Ser^{10}-Gln-Thr-Pro-Leu-Val-Thr-Leu-Phe-Lys- Asn^{20}-Ala-Ile-Ile-Lys-Asn-Ala-Tyr-Lys-Lys-Gly-GluOH^{31}
Dynorphin(dyn$^{1-17}$)	= Tyr-Gly-Gly-Phe-Leu-Arg-Arg-Ile-Arg-Pro-Lys-Leu-Lys-Trp-Asp-Asn-Gln
Dynorphin(dyn$^{1-8}$)	= Tyr-Gly-Gly-Phe-Leu-Arg-Arg-Ile
Dynorphin(dyn$^{1-13}$)	= Tyr-Gly-Gly-Phe-Leu-Arg-Arg-Ile-Arg-Pro-Lys-Leu-Lys
α-Neoenodorphin	= Tyr-Gly-Gly-Phe-Leu-Arg-Lys-Tyr-Pro-Lys
β-Neoendorphin	= Tyr-Gly-Gly-Phe-Leu-Arg-Lys-Tyr-Pro
Nociceptin	= Phe-Gly-Gly-Phe-Thr-Gly-Ala-Arg-Lys-Ser-Ala-Arg-Lys-Leu-Ala-Asn-Gln

Fig. 24.1. Precursor proteins to the endogenous opioid peptides.

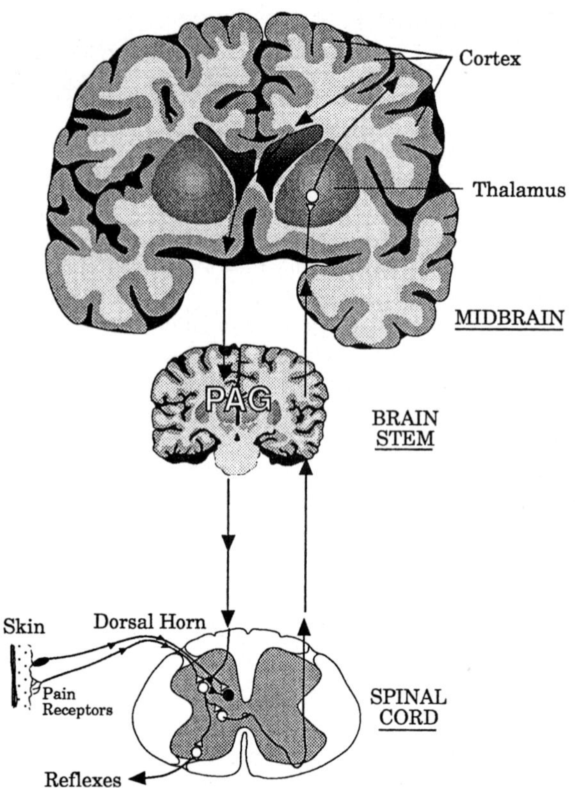

Fig. 24.2. Location of endogenous opioid nerve tracts in the central nervous system. Endorphins and opioid receptors in the dorsal horn of the spinal cord, thalamus, and periaqueductal gray (PAG) areas are associated with the transmission of pain signals.

α-neoendorphin. The pronociceptin protein has been identified and contains only one copy of the active peptide, whereas the precursor protein for the endomorphins remains to be identified. All of the pro-opioid proteins are synthesized in the cell nucleus and transported to the terminals of the nerve cells from which they are released. The active peptides are hydrolyzed from the large proteins by processing proteases that recognize double basic amino acid sequences positioned just before and after the opioid peptide sequences.

Peptides with opioid activity have been isolated from sources other than mammalian brain. The heptapeptide β-casomorphin (Tyr-Pro-Phe-Pro-Gly-Pro-Ile), found in cow's milk, is a μ opioid agonist (11). Dermorphin (Tyr-D-Ala-Phe-Gly-Tyr-Pro-Ser-NH2), a μ-selective peptide isolated from the skin of South American frogs, is approximately 100-fold more potent than morphine in in vitro tests (12).

The endogenous opioids exert their analgesic action at spinal and supraspinal sites (Fig. 24.2). They also produce analgesia by a peripheral mechanism of action associated with the inflammatory process. In the CNS, the opioids exert an inhibitory neurotransmitter or neuromodulator action on afferent pain-signaling neurons in the dorsal horn of the spinal cord and on interconnecting neuronal pathways for pain signals within the brain. In the brain, the arcuate nucleus, periaqueductal gray, and the thalamic areas are especially rich in opioid receptors and are sites at which opioids exert an analgesic action. In the spinal cord, concentrations of endogenous opioids are high in laminae 1, laminae 2, and trigeminal nucleus areas. All of the endogenous opioid peptides and the three major classes of opioid receptors appear to be at least partially involved in the modulation of pain. The actions of opioids at the synaptic level are described in Figure 24.3.

Analgesia that results from acupuncture or is self-induced by a placebo or biofeedback mechanisms is caused by release of endogenous endorphins. Analgesia produced by these procedures can be prevented by the previous dosage of a patient with an opioid antagonist. Electrical stimulation from electrodes properly placed in the brain causes endorphin release and analgesia. This procedure is used for the "self-stimulated" release of endorphins in patients with chronic pain who do not respond to any other medical treatment. As with exogenously administered opioid drugs, tolerance develops to all procedures that work by release of endogenous opioids.

OPIOID RECEPTORS

There are the three major types of opioid receptors: μ, κ (13), and δ (14). All three of the receptor types have been well characterized and cloned (15). A nomenclature adopted by the International Union of Pharmacology (IU PHAR) in 1996 classifies the three opioid receptors by the order in which they were cloned (16). By this classification, δ opioid receptors are OP_1 receptors, κ opioid receptors are OP_2 receptors, and μ opioid receptors are OP_3 receptors. The IUPHAR approved a new nomenclature in 2000, naming the receptors as MOP-μ, DOP-δ, and KOP-κ. In current literature, however, the opioid receptors often are referred to as DOR (δ), KOR (κ), and MOR (μ). There is evidence for subtypes of each of these receptors; however, the failure of researchers to find genomal evidence for

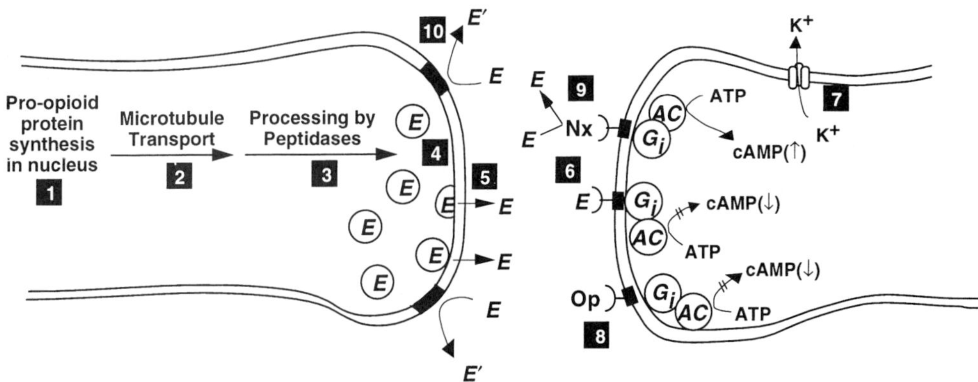

Fig. 24.3. Schematic representation of a δ enkephalinergic nerve terminal. (1) Pro-opioid proteins (proenkephalin A) are synthesized in the cell nucleus. (2) Pro-opioid proteins undergo microtubular transport to the nerve terminal. (3) Active endogenous opioids (E) are cleaved from the pro-opioid proteins by the action of "processing" proteases. (4) The active peptides (E) are taken up and stored in presynaptic vesicles. (5) The peptides are released when the presynaptic neuron fires. (6) The endogenous opioid peptides bind to postsynaptic receptors and activate second messenger systems. (7) For all opioid receptors, the second messenger effect is primarily mediated by a G-inhibitory ($G_{i/o}$) protein complex, which promotes the inactivation of adenylate cyclase (AC), a decrease in intracellular cyclic-adenosine-3′,5′-monophosphate (cAMP), and finally, an efflux of potassium ions (K^+) from the cell. The net effect is the hyperpolarization of the postsynaptic neuron and inhibition of cell firing. (8). Exogenous opioids (Op), such as morphine, combine with opioid receptors and mimic the actions of E. (9) Opioid antagonists, such as naloxone (Nx), combine with opioid receptors and competitively inhibit the actions of E or Op. (10) The action of E is terminated by a membrane-bound endopeptidase [EC3.4.24.11] (enkephalinase), which hydrolyze the Gly3-Phe4 peptide bond of enkephalin. Other endopeptidases may be employed in the metabolism of different endogenous opioid peptides.

additional receptors indicates that the receptor subtypes are posttranslational modifications (splice variants) of known receptor types (17). Receptor subtypes also may be known receptor types that are coupled to different signal transduction systems. Table 24.1 lists the opioid receptor types and subtypes, their known physiological functions, and selective agonists and antagonists for each of the receptors. All three of the opioid receptor types are located in human brain or spinal cord tissues, and each has a role in the mediation of pain. At this time, only μ and κ agonists are in clinical use as opioid analgesic drugs.

Orphan Opioid Receptor

A fourth receptor has been identified and cloned (OP_4) based on homology with cDNA sequence of the known (μ, δ, and κ) opioid receptors (18). Despite the homology in cDNA sequence with known opioid receptors, this new receptor did not bind the classical opioid peptide or nonpeptide agonists or antagonists with high affinity. Thus, the receptor was called the orphan opioid receptor (NOP). In subsequent studies, two research groups found a heptadecapeptide (Phe-Gly-Gly-Thr-Gly-Ala-Arg-Lys-Ser-Ala-Lys-Ala-Asn-Gln) to be the endogenous peptide for the orphan opioid receptor. One of the research groups (19) named the heptadecapeptide nociceptin, because they determined that it caused hyperalgesia (nociception) after intracerebral ventricular injection into mice. The other research group (20) named the heptapeptide orphanin FQ, after its affinity for the orphan opioid receptor and the first and last amino acids in the peptides sequence (i.e., F = Phe and Q = Gln) Nociceptin/orphanin FQ resembles dynorphin-A in structure, with the most notable difference being the replacement of Tyr at the N-terminus with Phe. Conflicting results have now been published regarding the ability of nociceptin/orphanin FQ to produce hyperalgesia versus analgesia in rodent pain assay models. One study has established this compound to be a potent initiator of pain signals in the periphery, where it acts by releasing substance P from nerve terminals (21). Injection of a nociceptin/orphanin antagonist into the brains of laboratory animals results in an analgesic effect, raising hope for the use of these agents in the management of pain (22).

Identification and Activation of Opioid Receptors

Identification of multiple opioid receptors has depended on the discovery of selective agonists and antagonists, the identification of sensitive assay techniques (23), and ultimately, the cloning of the receptor proteins (15). The techniques that have been especially useful are the radioligand binding assays on brain tissues and the electrically stimulated peripheral muscle preparations. Rodent brain tissue contains all three opioid receptor types, and special evaluation procedures (computer-assisted line fitting) or selective blocking (with reversible or irreversible binding

Table 24.1. Opioid Receptor Types and Subtypes

Receptor Type (Natural Ligand)	Selective Agonists	Agonist Properties	Selective Antagonists
μ, mu, MOP, OP_3 (endomorphin 1) (endomorphin 2) (β-endorphin)	Morphine Sufentanil DAMGO (Tyr-D-Ala-MePhe-NH-$(CH_2)_2OH$ PLO17 (Tyr-Pro-MePhe-D-Pro-NH_2 BIT (affinity label)	Analgesia (morphine-like) Euphoria Increased gastrointestinal transit time Immune suppression Respiratory depression (volume)	Naloxone Naltrexone CTOP Cyprodime β-FNA (affinity label)
μ_1 (high affinity)	Meptazinol Etonitazene	Emetic effects Tolerance Physical dependence	Naloxonazine
μ_2 (low affinity)	TRIMU-5 (Tyr-D-Ala-Gly-NH-$(CH_2)_2$-CH-$(CH_3)_2$		
κ, kappa, KOP, OP_2 (dynorphins) (β-endorphin)	Ethylketocyclazocine (EKC) Bremazocine Mr2034 dyn (1–17) Trifluadom	Analgesia Sedation Miosis Diuresis Dysphoria	TENA nor-BNI
κ_1 (high affinity)	U-50,488 Spiradoline (U-62,066) U-69,593 PD 117302		UPHIT
κ_2	dyn 1–17		
κ_3	NalBzOH		
δ, delta, DOP, OP_1 (enkephalins) (β-endorphin)	DADLE (D-Ala[2]-D-Leu[5]-enkephalin) DSLET (Tyr-D-Ser-Gly-Phe-Leu-Thr) DPDPE (D-Pen[2]-D-Pen[5]-Convulsions (?) Enkephalin)	Analgesia Immune stimulation Respiratory depression (rate)	ICI 174864 FIT (affinity label) SUPERFIT (affinity label)
δ_2	DADLE		Naltrindole (NTI) BNTX
δ_2	D-Ala[2]-deltorphin II		Naltriben (NTB) Naltrindol isothiocyanate (NTII)

agents) of some of the receptor types must be used to sort out the receptor selectivity of test compounds. The myenteric plexus–containing longitudinal strips of guinea pig ileum contain μ and κ opioid receptors. The contraction of these muscle strips is initiated by electrical stimulation and is inhibited by opioids. The vas deferens from mouse contains μ, δ, and κ receptors and reacts similarly to the guinea pig ileum to electrical stimulation and to opioids. Homogenous populations of opioid receptors are found in rat (μ), hamster (δ), and rabbit (κ) vas deferentia.

The signal transduction mechanism for μ, δ, and κ receptors is through $G_{i/o}$ proteins. Activation of opioid receptors is linked through the G protein to an inhibition of adenylate cyclase* activity. The resultant decrease in cAMP production, efflux of potassium ions and closure of voltage-gated Ca^{2+} channels causes hyperpolarization of the nerve cell (24,25), and a strong inhibition of nerve firing.

*This enzyme is known by two names, *adenylate cyclase (EC 4.6.1.1)* – its official name from the International Union of Biochemistry and Molecular Biology Nomenclature Committee or its alternative name, adenylyl cyclase.

μ Opioid Receptors

Endomorphin-1 (Tyr-Pro-Trp-Phe-NH_2) and endomorphin-2 (Try-Pro-Phe-Phe-NH_2) are endogenous opioid peptides with a high degree of selectivity for μ (MOP) receptors (8). A number of therapeutically useful compounds have been found that are selective for μ opioid receptors (Fig. 24.4). All of the opioid alkaloids and most of their synthetic derivatives are μ-selective agonists. Morphine, normorphine, and dihydromorphinone have 10- to 20-fold μ receptor selectivity and were particularly important in early studies to differentiate the opioid receptors. Sufentanil and the peptides DAMGO (26) and dermorphin (27), all with 100-fold selectivity for μ over other opioid receptors, frequently are used in the laboratory studies to demonstrate μ receptor-selectivity in cross-tolerance, receptor binding, and isolated smooth muscle assays. Studies with μ receptor knockout mice have confirmed that all the major pharmacological actions observed on injection of morphine (e.g., analgesia, respiratory depression, tolerance, withdrawal symptoms, decreased gastric motility, and emesis) occur by interactions with μ receptors (28).

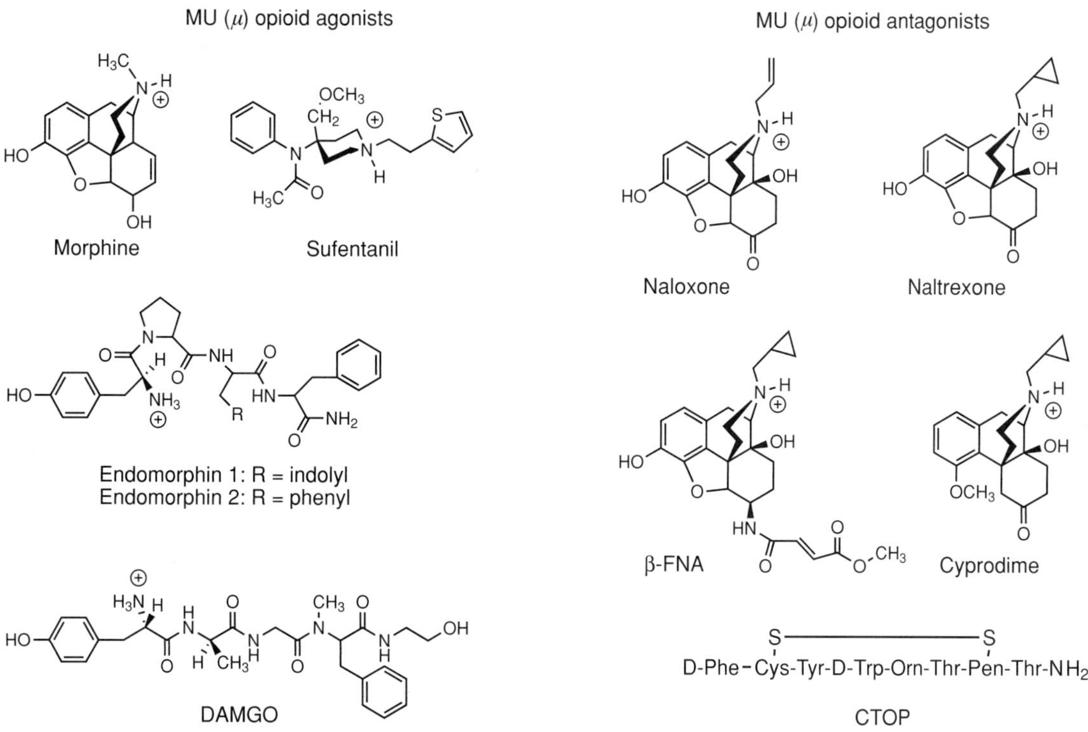

Fig. 24.4. Structures of compounds selective for μ (OP_3) opioid receptors.

Naloxone and naltrexone are antagonists that have weak (5 to 10 times) selectivity for μ receptors. Cyprodime is a selective nonpeptide μ antagonist (~30-fold selective for μ over κ and 100-fold selective for μ over δ) available for laboratory use (29). CTOP, a cyclic peptide analogue of somatostatin, is a selective μ antagonist (30). There is evidence that μ_1 receptors are high-affinity binding sites that mediate pain neurotransmission, whereas μ_2 receptors control respiratory depression. Naloxoneazine is a selective inhibitor of μ_1 opioid receptors (31).

κ Opioid Receptors

Ethylketazocine and bremazocine are 6,7-benzomorphan derivatives with κ opioid receptor selectivity (Fig. 24.5). These two compounds were used in early studies to investigate κ (KOP) receptors. They are not highly selective, however, and their use in research has diminished. A number of arylacetamides derivatives, having a high selectivity for κ over μ or δ receptors, have been discovered. The first of these compounds, (±)-U50488, has a 50-fold selectivity for κ over μ receptors and has been extremely important in the characterization of κ opioid activity (32). Other important agents in this class are (±) PD-117302 (33) and (-) CI-977 (34). Each of these agents has 1,000-fold selectivity for κ over μ or δ receptors. Evidence suggests that the arylacetamides bind to a subtype of κ receptors. In general, κ agonists produce analgesia in animals, including humans. Other prominent effects are diuresis, sedation, and dysphoria. Compared to μ agonists, κ agonists lack respiratory depressant, constipating, and strong addictive (euphoria and physical dependence) properties. It was hoped that κ agonists would become useful strong analgesics that lacked addictive properties; however, clinical trials with several highly selective and potent κ agonists were aborted because of the occurrence of unacceptable sedative and dysphoric side effects. κ-Selective opioids with only a peripheral action have been shown to be effective in relieving inflammation and the pain associated with it (35). The scientific evidence suggesting κ_1, κ_2, and κ_3 subtypes of κ receptors; however, the physiological effects initiated by the κ receptor subtypes are not well defined (36).

The peptides related to dynorphin are the natural agonists for κ receptors. Their selectivity for κ over μ receptors is not very high. Synthetic peptide analogues have been reported that are more potent and more selective than dynorphin for κ receptors (37,38).

The major antagonist with good selectivity for κ receptors is nor-binaltorphimine (39). This compound has approximately 100-fold selectivity for κ over δ receptors and an even greater selectivity for κ over μ receptors when tested during competitive binding studies in monkey brain homogenate. No medical use for a κ antagonist has been found.

δ Opioid Receptors

Enkephalins, the natural ligands at δ (DOP) receptors, are only slightly selective for δ over μ receptors. Changes

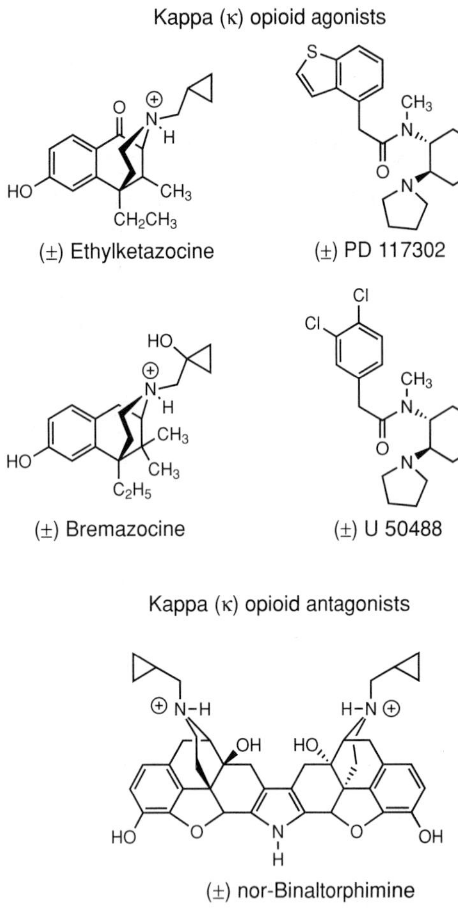

Kappa (κ) opioid agonists

(±) Ethylketazocine (±) PD 117302

(±) Bremazocine (±) U 50488

Kappa (κ) opioid antagonists

(±) nor-Binaltorphimine

Fig. 24.5. Structures of compounds selective for κ (OP_2) opioid receptors. (−)-Stereoisomers are the most active compounds.

in the amino acid composition of the enkephalins can give compounds with high potency and selectivity for δ receptors. The peptides most often used as selective δ receptor ligands (Fig. 24.6) are [D-Ala^2, D-Leu^5] enkephalin (DADLE) (40), [D-Ser^2, Leu^5] enkephalin-Thr (DSLET) (41), and the cyclic peptide [D-Pen^2, D-Pen^5] enkephalin (DPDPE) (42). These and other δ receptor selective peptides have been useful for in vitro studies, but their metabolic instability and poor distribution properties (i.e., penetration of the blood-brain barrier is limited by their hydrophilicity) has limited their usefulness for in vivo studies. Nonpeptide agonists that are selective for δ receptors have been reported. Derivatives of morphindoles were the first nonpeptide molecules to show δ selectivity in in vitro assays (43). SNC-80 is a newer and more selective δ opioid receptor agonist (44). This compound produces analgesia after oral dose in several rodent models and side effects appear minimal. Clinical trials with SCN-80 and other nonpeptide δ receptor agonists were attempted and aborted, primarily because of the convulsant action of δ receptor agonists. Radioligand binding studies in rodent brain tissue and in electrically stimulated vas deferentia have provided evidence of δ_1 and δ_2 receptors (45). The functional significance of this differentiation has not been determined.

Naltrindol and naltriben are highly selective nonpeptide antagonist for δ receptors (46,47). Naltrindol penetrates the CNS and displays antagonist activity that is selective for δ receptors in in vitro and in vivo systems. Peptidyl antagonists TIPP and TIPP-ψ are selective for δ receptors (48,49); however, their usefulness for in vivo studies and as clinical agents is limited by their poor pharmacokinetic properties. The δ opioid receptor antagonists have shown clinical potential as immunosuppressants and in treatment of cocaine abuse.

Receptor Affinity Labeling Agents

A number of opioid receptor selective affinity labeling agents (i.e., compounds that form an irreversible covalent bond with the receptor protein) have been developed (Fig. 24.7). These compounds have been important

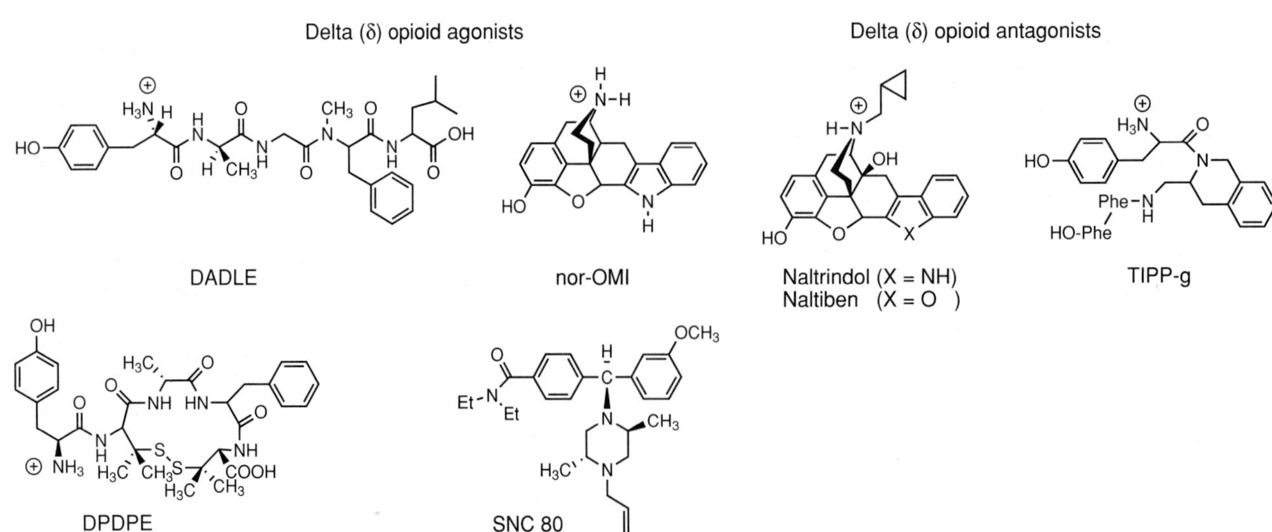

Fig. 24.6. Structures of compounds selective for δ (OP_1) opioid receptors.

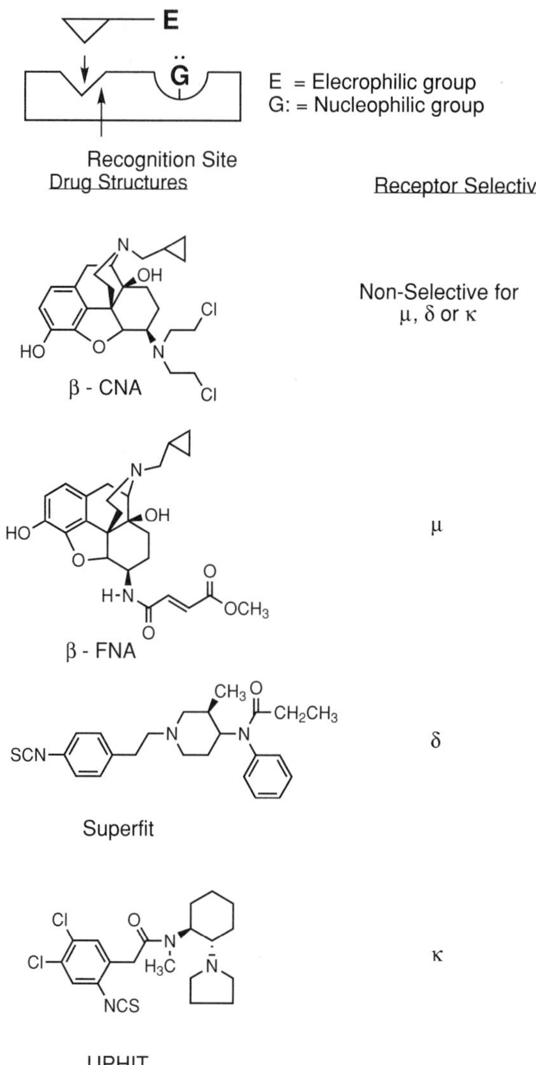

Fig. 24.7. A representation of the concept of affinity labeling of receptors and affinity labeling agents for opioid receptors.

in the characterization and isolation of the opioid receptor types. Each of the affinity-labeling agents contains a pharmacophore that allows initial reversible binding to the receptor. Once reversibly bound to the receptor, an affinity labeling agent must have an electrophilic group positioned so that it can react with a nucleophilic group on the receptor protein. The receptor selectivity of these agents is dependent on 1) the receptor type selectivity of the pharmacophore, 2) the location of the electrophile within the pharmacophore structure so that when bound to the receptor it is positioned near a nucleophile, and 3) the relative reactivities of the electrophilic and nucleophilic groups.

Examples of important affinity labeling agents are β-CNA, which because of its highly reactive 2-chloroethylamine electrophilic group irreversibility binds to all three opioid receptor types (50). The structurally related compound β-FNA has a less reactive fumaramide electrophilic group and reacts irreversibly with only μ receptors (51). Derivatives of the fentanyl series, FIT and SUPERFIT, bind μ and δ receptors, but only the δ receptor is bound irreversibly (52,53). Apparently, when these agents are bound to μ receptors, the electrophilic isothiocyanate group is not oriented in proper juxtaposition to a receptor nucleophile for covalent bond formation to occur. Incorporation of the electrophilic isothiocyanate into the structure of the highly κ receptor–selective arylacetamides has provided affinity labeling agents (UPHIT and DIPPA) for κ receptors (54,55).

NEUROBIOLOGY OF DRUG ABUSE AND ADDICTION

The factors that drive some individuals to abuse drugs, with resultant tolerance and psychological and physical dependence, remains unknown. It has been proposed that a deficiency exists in the opioid-mediated self-reward system of individuals who have a predisposition to abuse addictive drugs (56). In the United States, the use of highly addictive drugs, such as heroin and cocaine, is treated as a crime rather than as a medical problem. New insights regarding the neurobiology of drug addiction is now providing an understanding of why individuals abuse drugs and how drug abuse and addiction can be avoided and treated.

Self-Reward Response

It is now evident that most forms of drug addiction are driven by the stimulation of the brain's self-reward system (57), which originates in the ventral tegmental nucleus (VTN) and extends to the nucleus accumbens (NAC) area of the midbrain (Fig. 24.8). Self-reward is initiated by the release of dopamine (DA) from the mesocorticolimbic DA neurons originating in the VTN and stimulating D_1 and D_2 receptors in the NAC. Cocaine acts by inhibiting the reuptake of DA at nerve terminals, thus increasing the intensity and duration of the reward response. Amphetamine, methamphetamine, and similar indirect acting adrenergic stimulants cause inhibition of DA reuptake, DA release, and inhibition of monoamine oxidase–mediated metabolism of DA at this site. The μ opioid agonists work upstream in the reward neuronal system by exerting an inhibitory action on GABAergic neurons, thus removing the inhibitory GABAergic tonus on DA neurons and initiating the self-reward response. The κ opioid agonists work at a site more downstream in the system and cause the opposite effect of the μ agonists. The κ neurons synapse directly onto the DA nerve terminal in the NAC and exert an inhibitory effect (negative tonus) on DA release. Thus, a μ agonist will cause a self-reward and euphoric stimulus, and a κ agonist will cause an aversive and dysphoric stimulus. Alcohol (ethanol) also causes a stimulation of the self-reward system, partially by acting on the μ opioid neurons to facilitate the release of endogenous opioids

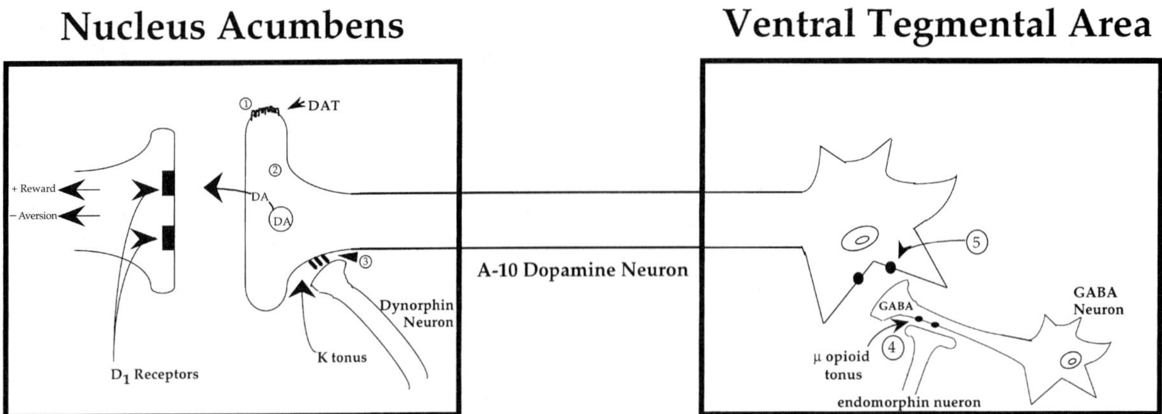

Fig. 24.8. The neurochemical basis of drug abuse and addiction. The diagram is a representation of the brain's self-reward system. According to this theory, any agent that promotes stimulation of type-1 dopamine (D_1) receptors in the nucleus accumbens (NCA) potentiates self-reward and has the potential to be abused. Major drugs of abuse exert their actions at various sites within the self-reward system to increase dopamine (DA) in the NCA and stimulate D_1 receptors. Site 1: Cocaine blocks DA reuptake by the DA transporter (DAT) and greatly enhances DA action at D_1. Site 2: Amphetamine, methamphetamine, and related drugs cause DA release with the resultant stimulation of D_1. Site 3: Opioid κ agonists exert an inhibitory effect on DA neuronal firing, resulting in a decrease in DA release and aversion in animals. Site 4: Opioid μ agonists, such as morphine and heroin, exert an inhibitory action on γ-aminobutyric acid (GABA) interneurons in the VAT, thus removing the GABAergic inhibition on DA neuronal firing. Site 5: GABA agonists, such as gabapentin, enhance DA neuronal firing and DA release, and these agents may be useful in treating or preventing drug abuse and addiction.

(58). Nicotine, acting through nicotinic cholinergic receptors, also has been shown to stimulate the DA self-reward system (59).

Thus, the common driving pathway in drug addiction is the euphoria experienced when a drug is taken and the self-reward system is activated by DA release. The self-reward response tends to be self-limiting, because feedback (adaptive) mechanisms in the nerve cells attenuate the reward delivered after prolonged or repeated activation of the system. Agents that slowly distribute to the brain have minor abuse potential, because the adaptive mechanisms in the self-reward neuronal system are able to respond quickly enough to attenuate the euphoric response. Highly abused substances tend to have high potency, full efficacy, and a fast onset of action so that the reward signal is initiated and fully activated before the adaptive process can take effect. Factors that contribute to fast onset of action are high lipophilicity of the drug and a dosing method that allows rapid distribution to the brain. Most abused drugs are highly lipophilic so that they rapidly cross the blood-brain barrier. The dosage routes preferred by drug addicts (smoking and intravenous injection) meet the criteria for fast distribution to the brain. Of course, agents that are rapidly distributed to and absorbed by the brain also are rapidly redistributed from the brain to other body tissues. Because of the redistribution phenomenon, the intense euphoric rush experienced by the addict is short-lived and must be frequently reinduced. Repeated exposure of the reward system to the drugs activates the adaptive mechanisms, which results in desensitization (tolerance) of the system to the abused substance. The addict must take a larger dose of the drug to get the euphoric high that she or he seeks, which results in increased tolerance and propagation of the addiction cycle.

Opioid Tolerance and Withdrawal

Tolerance to and withdrawal from the opioids is explained by the cellular adaptation that occurs on repeated activation of μ opioid receptors (60). When an agonist binds to the μ receptor, $G_{i/o}$ second messenger proteins are activated, and inhibition of adenylate cyclase occurs. Continual activation of the receptors results in an upregulation of adenylate cyclase to compensate for the decrease in cellular concentrations of cAMP. In addition, cellular mechanisms are activated that result in a decrease in the synthesis of $G_{i/o}$ protein subunits and an internalization of the μ receptor protein. Together, these adaptations cause a decrease in the magnitude of the opioid response to a given dose of agonist and explain the development of tolerance in the system and the need for ever-higher doses to get the same degree of euphoric response.

When the nerve cells are pushed into a highly tolerant state, they have a great capacity to make cAMP because of the upregulation in adenylate cyclase; however, the capacity is held in check by inhibitory effect of the opioids on adenylate cyclase. On cessation of dosing the opioid (~4–6 hours with heroin), the inhibitory effect on the upregulated adenylate cyclase system is removed, and the cells overproduce cAMP. The increase in cellular cAMP induces a number of abnormal and unpleasant effects that are recognized collectively as opioid withdrawal symptoms. The acute phase of withdrawal lasts for days (i.e., the time required for cAMP levels and receptor mechanisms to return to a normal state). The long-term effect of drug addiction is a learned drug-craving behavior, which can last for a lifetime and is thought to be responsible for the high incidence of stress-induced relapses into drug abuse.

Interestingly, not all μ opioid agonists have the same capacity to initiate receptor internalization and downregulation, which are typical occurrences in the development of tolerance. Morphine has a high capacity to induce tolerance, whereas methadone has a much lower tolerance capacity. Clinical studies are in progress to see if coadministration of morphine and methadone will result in lower tolerance development (61).

Rehabilitation of Opioid Addiction

Therapeutic programs that employ drugs in the rehabilitation of drug addicts have been in use for some time. The best-known treatment is the use of methadone maintenance in the rehabilitation of the opioid addict. In a well-run program, daily treatment with oral methadone maintains the addicted (tolerant) state while allowing minimal euphoric/aversive mood swings, attenuates drug craving, decreases the spread of HIV (by decreasing needle sharing), and minimizes the social destructive behavior (e.g., prostitution and theft) of the addicted patient (62). Other agents, such as the μ agonist L-α-acetylmethadol (levomethadyl) and the partial μ agonist buprenorphine, can be substituted for methadone and offer the advantage of dosing every third day (63,64). The biggest problem with addiction treatment programs is their failure to alleviate the drug-craving behavior of the recovering addict, and she or he resumes the habit of drug abuse. Evidence suggests that treatment of a detoxified opioid addict (i.e., an individual who has been weaned from opioid dependence through a methadone or other treatment program) with a long-acting opioid antagonist, such as naltrexone, can not only pharmacologically block readdiction but also curb the addict's drug-craving urge (65). Interestingly, naltrexone treatment has been shown to inhibit alcohol craving in recovering alcoholics (66). Naltrexone and buprenorphine have shown promise in treatment of cocaine abuse (67,68).

A number of possible neurobiological mechanisms have been identified by which drug intervention might prevent drug abuse or aid in the recovery of the addict (Fig. 24.8). The use of μ opioid agonists, partial agonists, and antagonists has been described in the preceding paragraph. Additional opioid-related mechanisms may be effective in the prevention of drug abuse and addiction. When a δ opioid agonist is given in combination with a μ opioid agonist, analgesia is enhanced, and there is minimal induction of tolerance and physical dependence (69). It also has been shown that administration of a μ agonist along with a δ antagonist to rodents resulted in analgesia without inducing tolerance and physical dependence (70). α-Adrenergic agonists are known to interact with many of the same neuronal systems as the opioids. The centrally acting μ-agonist clonidine works through the same $G_{i/o}$ second messenger system as the opioids, and it is used clinically to inhibit withdrawal symptoms in patients addicted to opioids. Testing of the long-acting indirect GABAergic agent vigabatrin (a suicide inhibitor of GABA aminotransferase) has been proposed for the treatment of drug addiction (71). One additional area of promise is the proposal that a high-affinity, slow-onset inhibitor of the DA transporter will be effective for the treatment of cocaine abuse (72).

STRUCTURE–ACTIVITY RELATIONSHIPS OF μ RECEPTOR AGONISTS

Morphine

Morphine is the prototype opioid (Table 24.2). It is selective for μ opioid receptors. The structure of morphine is composed of five fused rings, and the molecule has five chiral centers with absolute stereochemistry 5(*R*), 6(*S*), 9(*R*), 13(*S*) and 14(*R*). The naturally occurring isomer of morphine is levo-[(−)] rotatory. (+)-Morphine has been synthesized, and it is devoid of analgesic and other opioid activities (73).

It is important to remember that a minor change in the structure of morphine (or any other opioid) will likely cause a different change in the affinity and intrinsic activity of the new compound at each of the opioid receptor types. Thus, the opioid receptor selectivity profile of the new compound may be different than the structure from which it was made or modeled (i.e., a selective μ agonist may shift to become a selective κ agonist, etc.). In addition, the new compound will have different physicochemical properties than its parent. The different physicochemical properties (e.g., solubility, partition

Table 24.2 Structure, Numbering and Selected SAR for (-)-Morphine)

(-)-Morphine

Substituent Change	Analgesic Activity
3-H for -OH	10× Decrease
6-OH to 6-keto	Decrease activity or increase w/7,8-dihydro
6-OH to 6-H	Increase activity
7,8-dihydro	Increase activity
14 β-OH	Increase activity
3-OCH_3 for OH	Decrease activity
CH_3CO-ester at 3	Decrease activity
CH_3CO-ester at 6	Increase activity
NCH_2CH_2Ph for NCH_3	Increase activity (10×)
$NCH_2CH{=}CH_2$ for NCH_3	Becomes a μ antagonist

coefficient, and pK_a) will result in different pharmacokinetic characteristics for the new drug and can affect its in vivo activity profile. For example, a new drug (Drug A) that is more lipophilic than its parent may distribute better to the brain and appear to be more active, whereas in actuality, it may have lower affinity or intrinsic activity for the receptor. The greater concentration of Drug A reaching the brain is able to overcome its decreased agonist effect at the receptor. The SARs discussed in the following paragraphs describe the relative therapeutic potencies of the compounds and are a combination of pharmacokinetic and receptor binding properties of the drugs.

The A ring and the basic nitrogen, which exists predominantly in the protonated (ionized) form at physiological pH, are the two most common structural features found in compounds displaying opioid analgesic activity. The aromatic A ring and the cationic nitrogen may be connected either by an ethyl linkage (9,10-positions of the B ring) or a propyl linkage (either edge of the piperidine ring that forms the D ring). The A ring and the basic nitrogen are necessary components in every potent μ agonist known. These two structural features alone are not sufficient for μ opioid activity, however, and additional pharmacophoric groups are required. In compounds having rigid structures (i.e., fused A, B, and D rings), the 3-hydroxy group and a tertiary nitrogen either greatly enhance or are essential for activity. A summary of other important SAR features for morphine is given in Table 24.2.

Nitrogen Atom

The substituent on the nitrogen of morphine and morphine-like structures is critical to the degree and type of activity displayed by an agent. A tertiary amine usually is necessary for good opioid activity. The size of the N-substituent can dictate the compound's potency and its agonist versus antagonist properties. Generally, N-methyl substitution results in a compound with good agonist properties. Increasing the size of the N-substituent to three to five carbons (especially where unsaturation or small carbocyclic rings are included) results in compounds that are antagonists at some or all opioid receptor types. Larger substituents on nitrogen return agonist properties to the opioid. An N-phenylethyl–substituted opioid usually is on the order of 10-fold more potent as a μ agonist than the corresponding N-methyl analogue.

Ideal Opioid

Thousands of derivatives of morphine and other μ agonists have been prepared and tested (74,75). The objective of most of the synthetic efforts has been to find an analgesic with improved pharmacological properties over known μ agonists. Specifically, one would like to have an orally active drug that retains the strong analgesic properties of morphine yet lacks its ability to cause tolerance, physical dependence, respiratory depression, emesis, and constipation. The success of this search has been limited. Many compounds that are more potent than morphine have been discovered. Also, compounds with pharmacodynamic properties different from those of morphine have been discovered, and some of these compounds are preferred to morphine for selected medical uses. The ideal analgesic drug, however, is yet to be discovered. Research to find new centrally acting analgesics has turned away from classic μ agonists and now is focused on agents that act through other types or subtypes of opioid receptors or through nonopioid neurotransmitter systems.

3-Phenolic Hydroxy Group

The SARs of compounds structurally related to morphine are outlined in Table 24.2. A number of the structural variations on morphine have yielded compounds that are available as drugs in the United States. The most important of these agents, in terms of prescription volume, is the alkaloid codeine. Codeine, the 3-methoxy derivative of morphine, is a relatively weak μ agonist, but it undergoes slow metabolic O-demethylation to morphine, which accounts for much of its action. Codeine also is a potent antitussive agent and is used extensively for this purpose.

Heroin

The 3,6-diacetyl derivative of morphine is commonly known as heroin. It was synthesized from morphine in 1874 and was introduced to the market in 1898 by the Friedrich Bayer Co. in Germany. The 1906 Squibb's *Materia Medica* listed 10-mg tablets of heroin at $1.20 per 1,000. At the time of its introduction, heroin was described as "preferable to morphine because it does not disturb digestion or produce habit readily." Heroin itself has relatively low affinity for μ opioid receptors; however, its high lipophilicity compared to morphine results in enhanced penetration of the blood-brain barrier. Once in the body (including the brain), serum and tissue esterases hydrolyze the 3-acetyl group to produce 6-acetylmorphine. This latter compound has μ agonist activity in excess of morphine. The combination of rapid penetration by heroin into the brain after intravenous dose and rapid conversion to a potent μ agonist provides a "euphoric rush" that makes this compound a popular drug of abuse. Repeated use of heroin results in the development of tolerance, physical dependence, and acquisition of a drug habit that often is destructive to the user and society. In addition, the use of unclean or shared hypodermic needles for self-administering heroin often results in the transmission of the HIV, hepatitis, and other infectious diseases.

C Ring

Changes in the C-ring chemistry of morphine or codeine can lead to compounds with increased activity. Hydromorphone is the 7,8-dihydro-6-keto derivative of morphine,

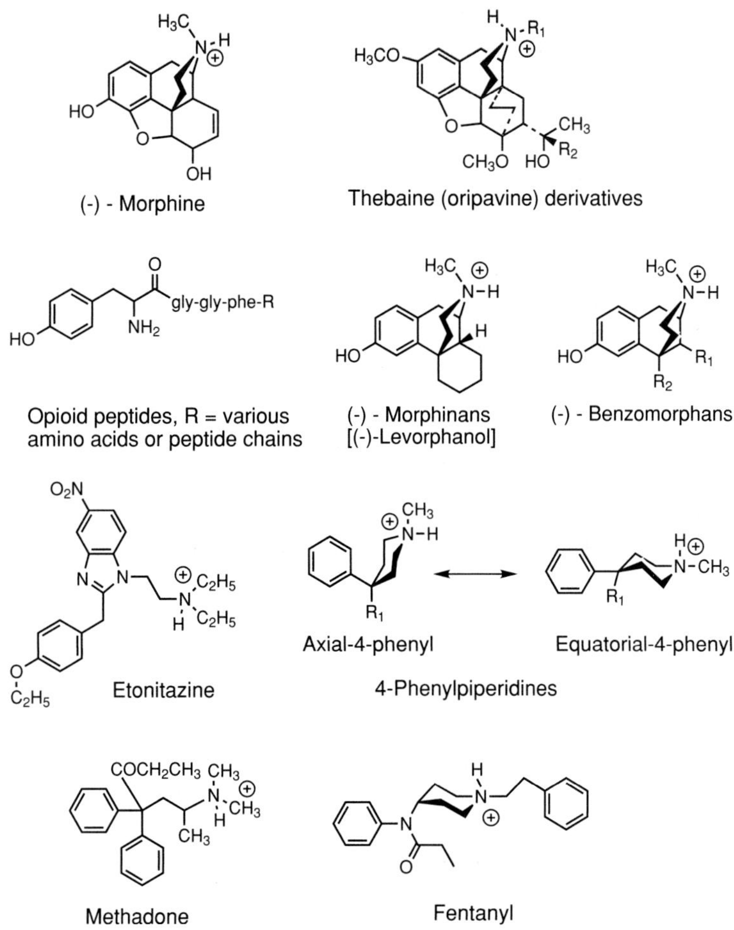

Fig. 24.9. Diverse structural families that yield potent opioid agonists.

and it is 8 to 10 times more potent than morphine on a weight basis. Hydrocodone, the 3-methoxy derivative of hydromorphone, is considerably more active than codeine.

14α-Hydroxy-6-Keto Derivatives

The opium alkaloid thebaine can be synthetically converted to 14α-hydroxy-6-keto derivatives of morphine. The 14α-hydroxy group generally enhances μ agonist properties and decreases antitussive activity, but activity varies with the overall substitution on the structure. Oxycodone, the 3-methoxy-N-methyl derivative, is about as potent as morphine when given parenterally, but its oral to parenteral dose ratio is better than that for morphine. Oxymorphone is the 3-hydroxy-N-methyl derivative, and it is 10 times as potent as morphine on a weight basis. Substitution of an N-cyclobutylmethyl for N-methyl and reduction of the 6-keto group to 6α-OH of oxymorphone gives nalbuphine, which acts through κ receptors and has approximately half the analgesic potency of morphine. Nalbuphine is an antagonist at μ receptors. Interestingly, N-allyl- (naloxone) and N-cyclopropylmethyl- (naltrexone) noroxymorphone are "pure" opioid antagonists. Naloxone and naltrexone are slightly μ receptor selective and are antagonists at all opioid receptor types.

Figure 24.9 contains some of the diverse chemical structures that produce μ agonist activity. The structures shown in the figure illustrate that the morphine structure may be built up or broken down to yield compounds that produce potent agonist activity. Reaction of thebaine with dienophiles (i.e., Diels-Alder reactions) results in 6, 14-endo-ethenotetrahydrothebaine derivatives, which are commonly called oripavines (76). Some of the oripavine derivatives are extremely potent μ agonists. Etorphine and buprenorphine are the best known of these derivatives. Etorphine is approximately 1,000 times more potent than morphine as a μ agonist. Etorphine has a low therapeutic index in humans, and its respiratory depressant action is difficult to reverse with naloxone or naltrexone. Thus, the compound is not useful in medical practice. Etorphine (M-99) is available for use in veterinary medicine for the immobilization of large animals. The oripavine structure–based antagonist diprenorphine is used to reverse the tranquilizing effect of etorphine. Buprenorphine, a marketed oripavine derivative, is a partial agonist at μ receptors, with a potency of 20 to 30 times that of morphine. The compound's uses and properties are described in the section on clinically available agents.

3,4-Epoxide Bridge and the Morphinans

Removal of 3,4-epoxide bridge in the morphine structure results in compounds that are referred to as morphinans. One cannot remove the epoxide ring from the morphine structure by simple synthetic means. Rather, the morphinans are prepared by total synthesis using a procedure described by Grewe (77). The synthetic procedure yields compounds as racemic mixtures and only the levo-(−)-isomers possess opioid activity. The dextro isomers have useful antitussive activity. The two morphinan derivatives that are marketed in the United States are levorphanol and butorphanol. Levorphanol is approximately eight times more potent than morphine as an analgesic in humans. Levorphanol's increased activity results from an increase in affinity for μ opioid receptors and its greater lipophilicity, which allows higher peak concentrations to reach the brain. Butorphanol is a μ antagonist and a κ agonist. The mechanism of action of the mixed agonist/antagonists is described in more detail later in this chapter.

Benzomorphans

Synthetic compounds that lack both the epoxide ring and the C ring of morphine retain opioid activity. Compounds having only the A, B, and D rings are named chemically as derivatives of 6,7-benzomorphan (Fig. 24.9) or, using a different nomenclature system, of 2,6-methano-3-benzazocine. They are commonly referred to simply as benzomorphans. The only agent from this structural class that is marketed in the United States is pentazocine, which has an agonist action on κ opioid receptors—an effect that produces analgesia. Pentazocine is a weak antagonist at μ receptors. The dysphoric side effects that are produced by higher doses of pentazocine result from actions at κ opioid receptors and also at σ (PCP) receptors. The benzomorphan-derivative phenazocine (N-phenylethyl) is approximately 10 times as potent as morphine as a μ agonist and is marketed in Europe.

Aminotetralins represent A- and B-ring analogues of morphine. A number of active compounds in this class have been described, but only dezocine, a mixed agonist/antagonist, has been marketed.

4-Phenylpiperidines

Analgesic compounds in the 4-phenylpiperidine class may be viewed as A- and D-ring analogues of morphine (Fig. 24.9). The opioid activity of these agents was discovered serendipitously. The first of these agents, meperidine, was synthesized in 1937 by Eislab (78), who was attempting to prepare antispasmodic agents. The compound produced an S-shaped tail (Straub tail) in cats, an effect that had been recognized as a response caused by morphine and its derivatives. Meperidine proved to be a typical μ agonist, with approximately one-fourth the potency of morphine on a weight basis. It is particularly useful in certain medical procedures because of its short duration of action because of esterases hydrolysis to a zwitterionic metabolite. Reversed esters of meperidine have greater potency, and several of these derivatives have been marketed. The 3-methyl reversed ester derivatives of meperidine, α- and β-prodine, were available in the United States but have been removed from the market because of their low prescription volume and their potential to undergo elimination reactions to compounds that resemble the neurotoxic agent MPTP (see Chapter 25). Trimeperidine or γ-promedol, the 1,2,5-trimethyl reversed ester of meperidine, is used in Russia as an analgesic.

Anilidopiperidines

Structural modification of the 4-phenylpiperidines has led to discovery of the 4-anilidopiperidine, or the fentanyl, group of analgesics (Fig. 24.9). Fentanyl and its derivatives are μ agonists, and they produce typical morphine-like analgesia and side effects. Structural variations of fentanyl that have yielded active compounds are substitution of an isosteric ring for the phenyl group, addition of a small oxygen containing group at the 4-position of the piperidine ring, and introduction of a methyl group onto the 3-position of the piperidine ring. Newer drugs that illustrate some of these structural changes are alfentanil and sufentanil. Both of these drugs have higher safety margins than other μ agonists. For unknown reasons, the compounds produce analgesia at much lower doses than is necessary to cause respiratory depression.

Diphenylheptanone

In the period just before or during the Second World War, German scientists synthesized another series of open-chain compounds as potential antispasmodics. In a manner analogous to that of meperidine, animal testing showed some of the compounds to possess analgesic activity. Methadone was the major drug to come from this series of compounds (Fig. 24.9). Methadone is especially useful for its oral activity and its long duration of action. These properties make methadone useful in maintenance therapy for opioid addicts and for pain suppression in the terminally ill (i.e., hospice programs). Methadone is marketed in the United States as a racemic mixture, but the (−)-isomer possesses almost all of the analgesic activity. Many variations on the methadone structure have been made, but little success in finding more useful drugs in class has been achieved. Reduction of the keto and acetylation of the resulting hydroxyl group gives the acetylmethadols (see below). Variations of the methadone structure have led to the discovery of the useful antidiarrheal opioids diphenoxylate and loperamide.

Propoxyphene is an open-chain compound that was discovered by structural variation of methadone. Propoxyphene is a weak μ opioid agonist having only one-fifteenth the activity of morphine. The (+)-isomer produces all of the opioid activity.

μ Antagonists

The SAR for μ antagonists is relatively simple if one focuses just on marketed compounds. All of the marketed, rigid-structured opioid analogues that have the 3-phenolic group and an N-allyl, N-cyclopropylmethyl (N-CPM), or N-cyclobutylmethyl (N-CBM) substituent replacing the N-methyl are μ antagonists (Fig. 24.5). Compounds behaving as μ antagonists may retain agonist activity at other opioid receptor types. The only exception to this rule is buprenorphine, which has an N-CPM substituent and is a potent partial agonist (or partial antagonist) at μ receptors. Only two compounds are pure antagonists (i.e., act as antagonists at all opioid receptors). These compounds are the N-allyl (naloxone) and N-CPM (naltrexone) derivatives of noroxymorphone. The 14α-hydroxyl group is believed to be important for the pure antagonistic properties of these compounds. It is not understood how the simple change of an N-methyl to an N-allyl group can change an opioid from a potent agonist into a potent antagonist. The answer may lie in the ability of opioid receptor protein to effectively couple with signal transduction proteins (G proteins) when bound by an agonist but not to couple with the G proteins when bound by an antagonist. This explanation infers that an opioid having an N-substituent of three to four carbons in size induces a conformational change in the receptor or blocks essential receptor areas that prevent the interaction of the receptor and the signal transduction proteins.

Those interested in an in-depth understanding of the SAR for μ receptor antagonists should be aware that properly substituted N-methyl-4-phenylpiperidines, N-methyl-6,7-benzomorphans, and even nonphenolic opioid derivatives that have good antagonist activity are known.

STRUCTURE–ACTIVITY RELATIONSHIPS OF κ RECEPTOR AGONISTS

The SAR for marketed κ agonists is somewhat related to that of μ antagonists (Fig. 24.5). All of the marketed κ agonists have structures related to the rigid opioids and N-allyl, N-CPM or N-CBM substitutions. The compounds are all μ receptor antagonists and κ receptor agonists. The κ agonist activity is enhanced if there is an oxygen group placed at the 8-position (e.g., ethylketazocine) or into the N-substituent (e.g., bremazocine). The oxygen group in a N-furanylmethyl substituent also enhances κ activity.

Potent and selective κ agonists that lack antagonistic properties at any of the opioid receptors are found in a number of *trans*-1-arylacetamido-2-aminocyclohexane derivatives. There are not enough compounds reported in this class to develop strong trends in SARs. The relative mode of receptor binding for the morphine-related verses the arylacetamide κ agonists is not known. Evidence exists for the selective binding of the arylacetamides to κ_1 and of the benzomorphan compounds (e.g., bremazocine) to κ_2 and κ_3 opioid receptor subtypes.

STRUCTURE–ACTIVITY RELATIONSHIPS OF δ RECEPTOR AGONISTS

Structure–activity relationships for δ receptor agonists are the least developed among the opioid compounds. Peptides with high selectivity for δ receptors are known. The SARs for some of these peptides are discussed in the following paragraphs. Nonpeptide δ selective agonists (Fig. 24.6) have been discovered, and SARs are being developed (79). Several selective δ agonists entered clinical trials but were withdrawn because of the potential convulsive (80) action of the agents.

STRUCTURE–ACTIVITY RELATIONSHIPS OF OPIOID PEPTIDES

Thousands of derivatives related to the endogenous opioid peptides have been prepared since the discovery of the enkephalins in 1975 (81) (Fig. 24.1). A thorough discussion of the SAR of these peptides would be a major task; however, some major trends have emerged and easily can be discussed. Some selected general SAR points for peptide opioids are:

1. All of the endogenous opioid peptides, except for the endomorphans, have Leu- or Met-enkephalin as their first five amino acid residues.
2. The tyrosine at the first amino acid residue position of all the endogenous opioid peptides is essential for activity. Removal of the phenolic hydroxyl group or the basic nitrogen (amino terminus group) will abolish activity. The Tyr^1 free amino group may be alkylated (methyl or allyl groups to give agonists and antagonists), but it must retain its basic character. The structural resemblance between morphine and the Tyr^1 group of opioid peptides is especially obvious.
3. In addition to the phenol and amine groups of Tyr^1, the next most important moiety in the enkephalin structure is the phenyl group of Phe^4. Removal of this group or changing its distance from Tyr^1 results in full or substantial loss in activity.
4. The enkephalins have several low-energy conformations, and different conformations likely are bound at different opioid receptor types and subtypes.
5. The replacement of the natural L-amino acids with unnatural D-amino acids can make the peptides resistant to the actions of several peptidases that generally rapidly degrade the natural endorphins. The use of a D-Ala in place of Gly^2 has been

especially useful for protecting the peptides from the action of nonselective aminopeptidases. The placement of bulky groups into the structure (e.g., the addition of N-Me to Phe^4) also will slow the action of peptidases. When evaluating new peptides for opioid activity, it often is difficult to tell if changes are caused by metabolic stability or receptor affinity.

6. Conversion of the terminal carboxyl group into an alcohol or an amide will protect the compound from carboxy peptidases.
7. Any introduction of unnatural D- or L-amino acids or bulky groups into the enkephalin structure will affect its conformational stability. The resultant peptides will have an increase or decrease in affinity for each of the opioid receptor types. The right combination of increases and/or decreases in receptor affinity will result in selectivity for a receptor type.
8. Structural changes that highly restrict the conformational mobility of the peptides (e.g., substitution of proline for Gly^2 or cyclization of the peptide) have been especially useful for the discovery of receptor-selective opioid peptides.

For examples of the above SARs, see the structures of the peptides given in Figures 24.4, 24.5, and 24.6.

Enkephalin Peptides

The effect of lengthening the amino acid chain of the enkephalin peptides deserves special consideration. As previously noted, the endogenous opioids found in mammals most often have Leu- or Met-enkephalin at their amino terminus end. Lengthening the carboxyl terminus can give the peptide greater affinity or selectivity for an opioid receptor type. This effect can be illustrated by the dynorphins, for which incorporation of the basic amino acids (especially Arg^7) into the C-terminus chain results in a marked increase in affinity for κ receptors. The message-address analogy has been used to describe this effect. The first four amino acids [Tyr-Gly-Gly-Phe] are essential for peptide ligands to bind to and to activate all opioid receptor types. The N-terminus amino acids can then be referred to as carrying the "message" to the receptors. Adding additional amino acids to the C-terminus can "address" the message to a specific receptor type. The additional peptide chain may be affecting the address (selectivity) by providing new and favorable binding interactions to one of the receptor types. Alternatively, the additional peptide could be inducing a conformational change in the message portion of the peptide that favors interaction with one of the receptor types.

METABOLISM OF THE OPIOIDS

Knowledge of the metabolism of the opioid drugs is essential to the understanding of the uses of these agents.

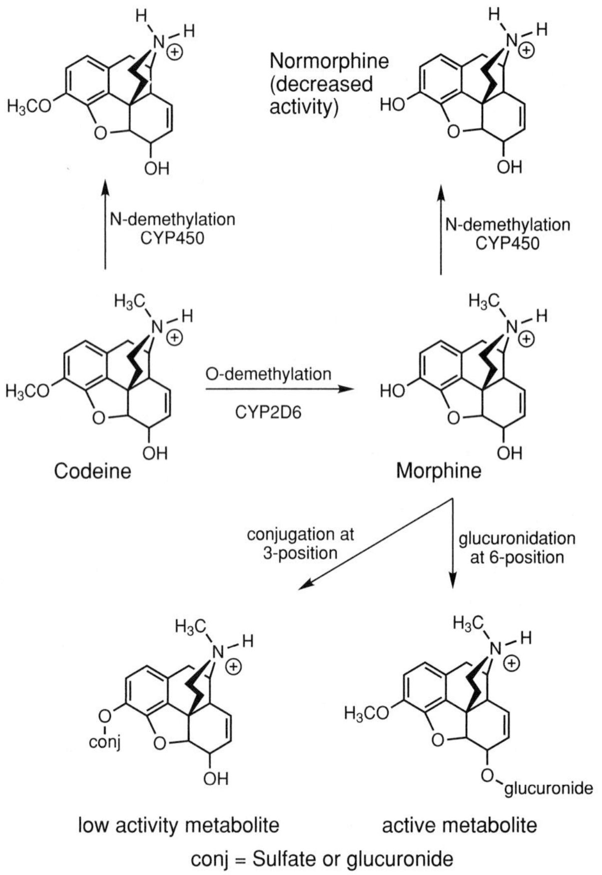

Fig. 24.10. Metabolism of morphine and codeine.

The poor oral versus parenteral dose ratio (~6:1) of morphine is caused by extensive first-pass metabolic conjugation of morphine at the phenolic (3-OH) position (Fig. 24.10). The metabolism occurs predominantly in the liver and requires the action of sulfotransferase or glucuronyltransferase enzymes. The conjugates have low activity and poor distribution properties. The 3-glucuronide does undergo enterohepatic cycling, which explains the need for high initial oral doses of morphine, followed by lower maintenance doses. Glucuronidation of morphine at the 6-OH position results in the formation of an active metabolite. Morphine is also N-demethylated to give normorphine, a compound that has decreased opioid activity and decreased bioavailability to the CNS. Normorphine undergoes N- and O-conjugations and excretion. Geriatric patients metabolize morphine at a slower rate than normal adult patients; thus, they are likely to show greater sensitivity to the drug and require lower doses.

In human subjects, approximately 10% of an oral dose of codeine is O-demethylated by CYP2D6 to produce morphine. The morphine produced as a metabolite of codeine is essential for the analgesic effect. A significant portion of the American population (8–10%) lacks CYP2D6, and these individuals do not experience analgesia

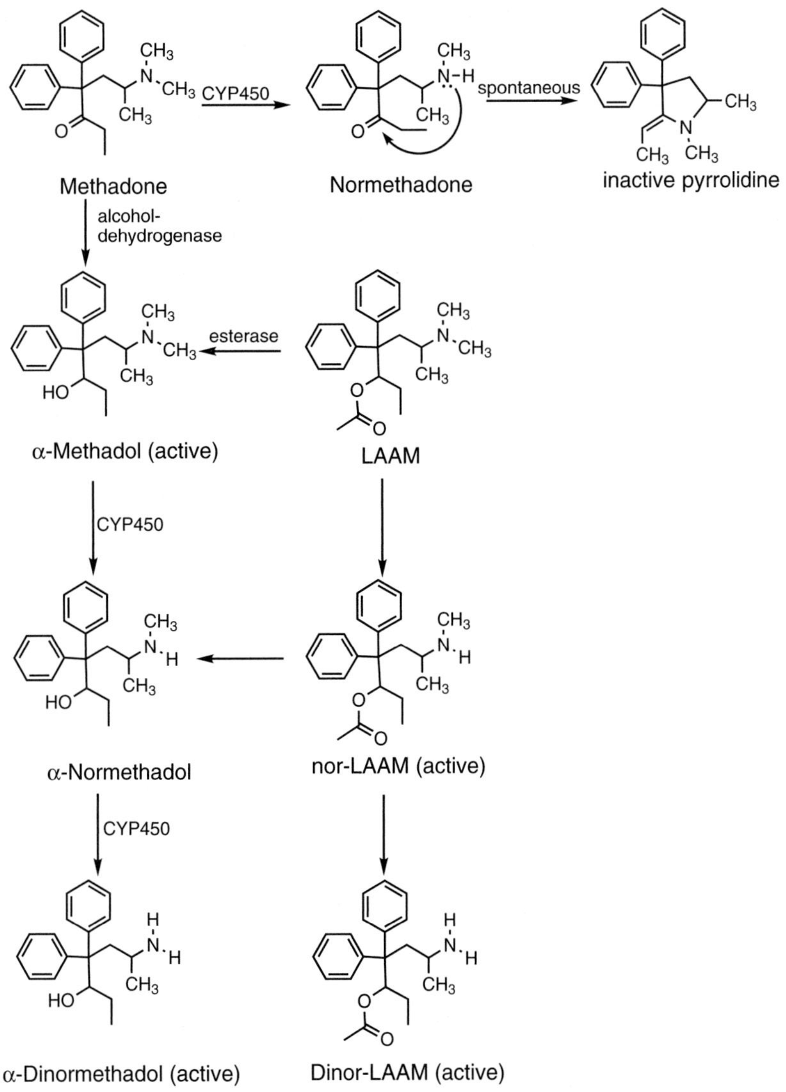

Methadone → (CYP450) → Normethadone → (spontaneous) → inactive pyrrolidine

Methadone → (alcohol-dehydrogenase) → α-Methadol (active)

LAAM → (esterase) → α-Methadol (active)

α-Methadol (active) → (CYP450) → α-Normethadol

LAAM → nor-LAAM (active) → α-Normethadol

α-Normethadol → (CYP450) → α-Dinormethadol (active)

nor-LAAM (active) → Dinor-LAAM (active)

Fig. 24.11. Metabolism of methadone and levomethadyl (LAAM).

when dosed with codeine (82). The antitussive activity of codeine is produced by the unmetabolized drug at nonopioid receptors and is not affected by the lack of CYP2D6. The bioactivation of codeine (versus the bioinactivation of morphine) results in an oral:parenteral dose ratio for codeine of 1.5:1; however, codeine is seldom given parenterally because of its strong effect to release histamine from mast cells.

Other rigid-structured opioid analogues undergo routes of metabolism similar to that of morphine. The amount of first-pass 3-O-conjugation varies from compound to compound; thus, the relative oral:parenteral dosages of the agents will vary. In general, compounds that are more potent and lipophilic than morphine (e.g., levorphanol) tend to have better oral activity. Compounds with N-alkyl groups larger than methyl get N-dealkylated as a major route of inactivation.

The short duration of action of meperidine is the result of rapid metabolism. Plasma esterases cleave the ester bond to leave the inactive zwitterionic 4-carboxylate derivative. Meperidine also undergoes N-demethylation to give normeperidine. Normeperidine has little analgesic activity, but it contributes significantly to the toxicity of meperidine.

The metabolism of methadone, as outlined in Figure 24.11, is important to its action. The major route of inactivation results from N-demethylation and cyclization of the secondary amine into an inactive pyrrole derivative. If the keto group is reduced by alcohol dehydrogenase to give methadol, the demethylation product can no longer cyclize to the pyrrole derivatives. Methadol is less active than methadone as an analgesic, but the N-demethylation products of methadol, normethadol and dinormethadol, are active analgesics with increased half-lives compared to that of methadone. The buildup of these metabolites is responsible for the long duration of action and the mild, prolonged withdrawal symptoms associated with methadone.

Levo-α-acetylmethadol (LAAM, levomethadyl acetate) is longer acting than methadone. Its slow onset of action after oral dose (and the isolation of at least three active metabolites) suggests that LAAM itself is a pro-drug. The relative contributions of LAAM and its active metabolites to the analgesic and addition maintenance properties in humans have not been determined. It is clear that a 75- to 100-mg oral dose of this agent will suppress withdrawal symptoms in opioid addicts for 3 to 4 days.

μ OPIOID RECEPTOR MODELS

A number of models have been proposed to represent the bonding interactions of agonists at μ opioid receptors. These models are "reflections" of complementary bonding interactions of μ agonists to the receptor as revealed from SAR studies. Beckett and Casy (83) published the first such receptor drawing in 1954. They studied the configurations and conformations of the μ agonists known at that time and proposed that all opioids could bind to the template (receptor model) shown in Figure 24.12. The model presumed that nonrigid opioids (e.g., meperidine and methadone) took a shape like that of morphine when binding to the receptor. It soon became apparent that the most stable conformations of meperidine and methadone were not able to be superimposed on the structure of morphine. New compounds that could not assume the shape of morphine also were being discovered, and it became apparent that the Beckett and Casy model could not explain the activity of all μ agonists.

In the mid-1960s, Portoghese (84) attempted to correlate the structures and analgesic activities of rigid and nonrigid opioids that contained the same series of N-substituents. He argued that if all opioids bound the receptor in the same conformation, then a substituent at a like position on any of the compounds should fall on the same surface area of the receptor. One would expect the same structural modification on any opioid structure to give the same type and degree of bonding interaction and, thus, the same contribution to analgesic activity. Portoghese found that parallel changes of the N-substituent on rigid (morphine, morphinan, or benzomorphan) analgesic parent structures gave parallel changes in activity. This finding supported the notion that rigid-structured opioid compounds bound to the receptor for analgesia in the same manner. When the same test was applied to nonrigid (meperidine-like) opioid structures, however, varying the N-substituent did not produce an activity change that paralleled that seen for the rigid-structured series. Apparently, the N-substituents in the rigid and nonrigid opioid series were falling on different surfaces of a receptor and, thus, making different contributions to analgesic activity. Portoghese concluded that the rigid and nonrigid series of compounds either were binding to different receptors or were interacting with the same receptor by different binding modes. He introduced the bimodal receptor binding model (Fig. 24.13) as one possible explanation of the results. Later, it was discovered that the activity of the rigid opioid compounds (Series 1) was enhanced by a 3-OH substituent on the aromatic ring, whereas a like substituent in some nonrigid opioids (Series 2) caused a loss of activity. Again, like substituents produced nonparallel changes in activity, indicating that the aromatic rings in the two series were not binding to the same receptor site. To provide an explanation for these results, the bimodal binding model was modified to incorporate the structure of the enkephalin (Fig. 24.14) (85). The rigid-structured opioids that benefit from the inclusion of a phenolic

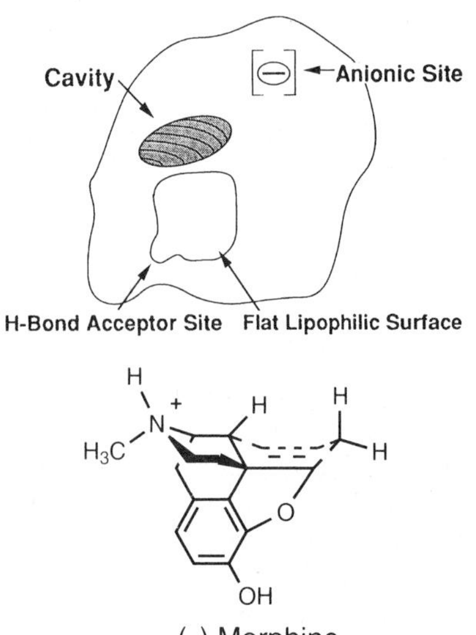

Fig. 24.12. A representation of the original model for the opioid receptor as proposed by Beckett and Casy (83). The morphine structure would have to rotate 180° about a vertical axis before it could bind to the receptor site. The model is only good for μ-selective agents.

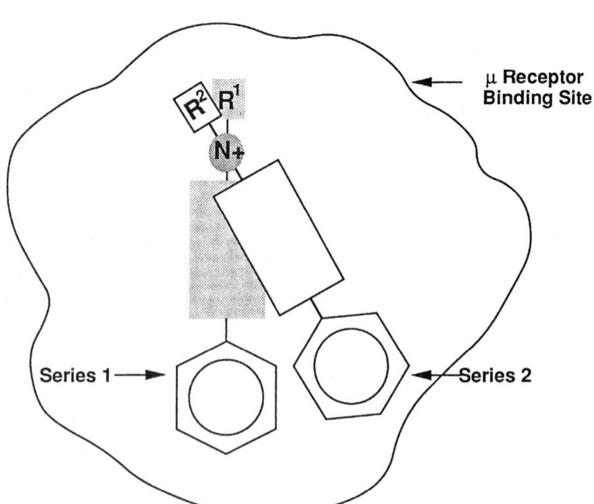

Fig. 24.13. A representation of the bimodal binding model of the μ opioid receptor as proposed by Portoghese (84). Different opioid series bind to different surface areas of the same receptor protein.

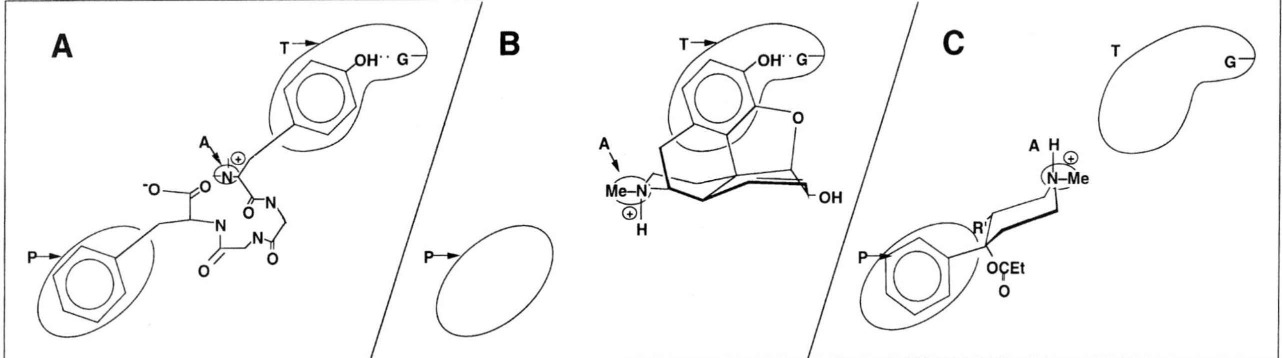

Fig. 24.14. A representation of the enkephalin binding site of μ opioid receptors (85). (A) An enkephalin bound to the receptor. (B) Morphine binding the receptor by utilizing the T-subsite (i.e., the tyrosine-binding site). (C) A meperidine-type opioid binding the receptor by utilizing the P-subsite (i.e., the phenylalanine-binding site).

hydroxyl group were proposed to bind the μ receptor in a manner equivalent to the tyrosine (Tyr[1] or T-subsite) of enkephalin. The nonrigid-structure opioids, which lose activity on introduction of a phenolic hydroxyl group into their structure, were proposed to interact with the receptor in a manner equivalent to the phenylalanine (Phe[4] or P-subsite) of enkephalin. The free amino group of Tyr[1] occupies the anionic binding site of the receptor that is the common binding point of both opioid series. This model closely resembles original bimodal binding proposal.

Models that attempt to explain the ability of Na^+ to decrease the binding affinity of agonists, but not antagonists, for the opioid receptor have been made (86). Sodium ions also protect the receptor from alkylation by nonselective alkylating agents.

The Beckett and Casy model was extended to explain the increased potency of the oripavine analogues, such as etorphine (Fig. 24.15) (76). The affinity of the oripavines for the μ opioid receptor can be much greater than that seen for morphine. It is likely that the increased receptor affinity comes from auxiliary drug–receptor bonding interactions similar to those depicted in the receptor model.

Martin (87) has proposed a receptor model for κ opioid receptors. Martin's model considers just the binding of rigid morphine-related opioid structures. The relationship of how rigid morphine-related agents interact with the κ receptor compared to the arylacetamide κ agonist derivatives has not been well studied.

Models for the δ opioid receptors have not been proposed.

SPECIFIC DRUGS

μ Agonists

Structures of specific drugs and compounds are given in Table 24.3.

(−)-Morphine Sulfate

Morphine sulfate is the analgesic used most often for severe, acute, and chronic pain. Morphine is a μ agonist and is a Schedule II drug. It is available in intramuscular, subcutaneous, oral, rectal, epidural, and intrathecal dosage forms. The epidural and intrathecal preparations are formulated without a preservative. Morphine is three- to six times more potent when given intramuscularly than when given orally. The difference in activity results from extensive first-pass 3-O-glucuronidation of morphine—an inactive metabolite. The half-life of intramuscularly dosed (10 mg) morphine is approximately 3 hours. The dose of morphine, by any dosage route, must be reduced in patients with renal failure and in geriatric and pediatric patients. The enhanced effects of morphine in renal failure is believed to be caused by a buildup of the active 6-glucuronide metabolite, which depends on renal function for elimination.

The analgesic effect of orally dosed morphine can equal that obtained by parenteral administration, if proper doses are given. When given orally, the initial

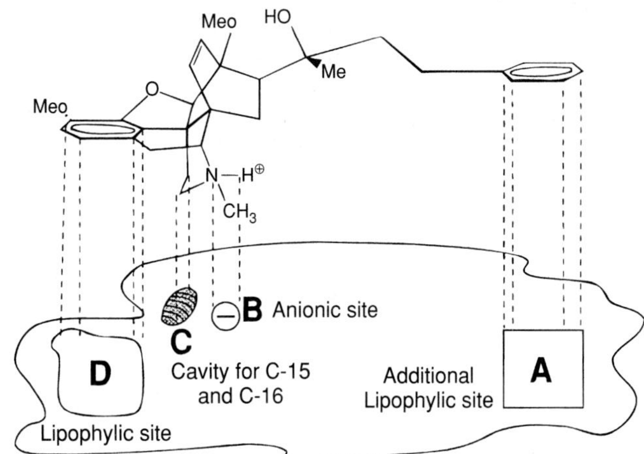

Fig. 24.15. A representation of the binding of an oripavine-type analgesic to the μ opioid receptor (76). The hydroxyl and phenyl groups in the side chain are believed to form additional bonding interactions with the receptor compared to the Beckett and Casy receptor model.

Table 24.3. Marketed Drugs that are Derivatives of Morphine

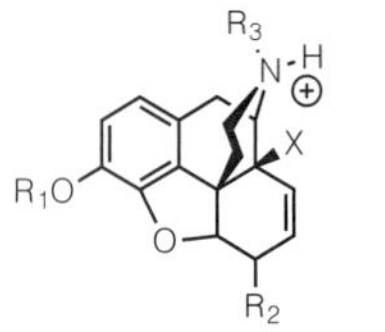

Generic name	R_1	R_2	R_3	X	Other
(-)-Morphine	H	OH	$-CH_3$	H	None
(-)-Codeine	CH_3	OH	$-CH_3$	H	None
(-)-Hydromorphone	H	Keto	$-CH_3$	H	No 7,8-double bond
(-)-Oxymorphone	H	Keto	$-CH_3$	OH	No 7,8-double bond
(-)-Hydrocodone	CH_3	Keto	$-CH_3$	H	No 7,8-double bond
(-)-Oxycodone	CH_3	Keto	$-CH_3$	OH	No 7,8-double bond
(-)-Nalbuphine	H	OH	$-CH_2-cBu$	OH	No 7,8-double bond
(-)-Naloxone	H	Keto	$-CH_2-CH=CH_2$	OH	No 7,8-double bond
(-)-Naltrexone	H	Keto	$-CH_2-cPr$	OH	No 7,8-double bond

dose of morphine is usually 60 mg, followed by maintenance doses of 20 to 30 mg every 4 hours. Addiction to clinically used morphine by the oral route generally is not a problem.

Overdoses of morphine, as well as all μ agonists in this section, can be effectively reversed with naloxone.

(−)-Codeine Phosphate

Codeine is used extensively to treat moderate to mild pain. Codeine is a weak μ agonist, but approximately 10% of an oral dose (30–60 mg) is metabolized to morphine (see the section on metabolism in this chapter), which contributes significantly to its analgesic effect. The plasma half-life of codeine after oral dose is 3.5 hours. The dose of codeine needed to produce analgesia after parenteral dose causes releases of histamine sufficient to produce hypotension, pruritus, and other allergic responses. Thus, administration of codeine by parenteral route is not recommended.

(−)-Hydromorphone Hydrochloride (Dilaudid)

Hydromorphone is a potent μ agonist (eight times greater than morphine) that is used to treat severe pain. It is available in intramuscular, intravenous, subcutaneous, oral, and rectal dosage forms. Like all strong μ agonists, hydromorphone is addicting and is a Schedule II drug. Hydromorphone has an oral:parenteral potency ratio of 5:1. The plasma half-lives after parenteral and oral dosage are 2.5 and 4 hours, respectively.

(−)-Oxymorphone Hydrochloride (Numorphan)

Oxymorphone is a potent μ agonist (10 times greater than morphine) that is used to treat severe pain. It is used by intramuscular, subcutaneous, intravenous, and rectal routes of administration. The intramuscular dose of oxymorphone (1 mg) has a half-life of 3 to 4 hours. It is a Schedule II drug. Oxymorphone, because of its 14-hydroxy group, has low antitussive activity.

(−)-Levorphanol Bitartrate (Levo-Dromoran)

Levorphanol is a potent μ agonist (approximately sixfold greater than morphine), and its uses, side effects, and physical dependence liability are like those of oxymorphone or hydromorphone. Levorphanol is available in oral, subcutaneous, and intravenous dosage forms. The oral dose of levorphanol is approximately twice the parenteral dose. This drug is unique among the μ agonists in that its analgesic duration of action is 4 to 6 hours, whereas its clearance half-life is 11.4 hours. Thus, effective analgesic doses of this agent can lead to a buildup of the drug in the body and result in excessive sedation.

(−)-Hydrocodone Bitartrate (Lortab, Vicodin in Combinations with Acetaminophen)

Hydrocodone is a Schedule III drug that is used to treat moderate pain. It is used mostly by the oral route (5-mg tablets and solutions) in combination with acetaminophen. The compound has good oral bioavailability and is metabolized in a manner similar to codeine.

(−)-Oxycodone Hydrochloride (Roxicodone, Oxycontin Sustained Release; and Percocet, Percodan, Tylox; in Combinations)

Oxycodone is about equipotent with morphine, but because of the 3-OCH group, it has a much lower oral:parenteral dose ratio. Thus, oxycodone is used orally to treat severe to moderate pain. It is a Schedule II drug as a single agent and when combined in strong analgesic mixtures. Oxycodone has a plasma half-life of approximately 4 hours and requires dosing every 4 to 6 hours. Metabolism of this agent is comparable to that of codeine.

Meperidine Hydrochloride (Demerol)

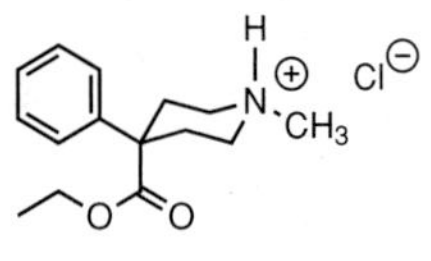

Meperidine is a μ agonist with approximately one-tenth the potency of morphine after intramuscular dose. Meperidine produces the analgesia, respiratory depression, and euphoria caused by other μ opioid agonists, but it causes less constipation and does not inhibit cough. When given orally, meperidine has 40 to 60% bioavailability because of significant first-pass metabolism. Because of the limited bioavailability, it is one-third as potent after an oral dose compared to a parenteral dose.

Meperidine has received extensive use in obstetrics because of its rapid onset and short duration of action. When it is given intravenously in small (25-mg) doses during delivery, the respiratory depression in the newborn child is minimized. Meperidine is used as an analgesic in a variety of nonobstetric anesthetic procedures. Meperidine is extensively metabolized in the liver, with only 5% of the drug being excreted unchanged. Prolonged dosage of meperidine may cause an accumulation of the metabolite normeperidine (see the section on metabolism in this chapter). Normeperidine has only weak analgesic activity, but it causes CNS excitation and can initiate grand mal seizures. It is recommended that meperidine be discontinued in any patient who exhibits signs of CNS excitation.

Meperidine has a strong adverse reaction when given to patients receiving a monoamine oxidase inhibitor. This drug interaction has been seen recently in patients with Parkinson's disease taking the monoamine oxidase–selective inhibitor selegiline (Eldepryl).

The elimination half-life of meperidine is 3 to 4 hours, and it can double in patients with liver disease. Acidification of the urine will cause enhanced clearance of meperidine, but there is a lesser effect on the clearance of the toxic metabolite normeperidine.

(±)Tramadol HCl (Ultram)

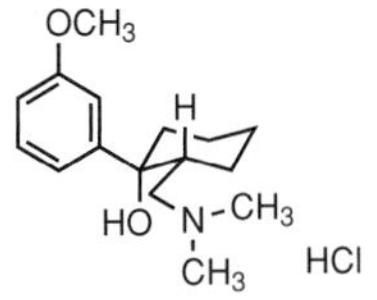

OCH_3 H HO N-CH_3 CH_3 HCl

The analgesic activity of tramadol is attributed to a synergistic effect caused by the opioid activity of the (+)-isomer and the neurotransmitter reuptake blocking effect of the (−)-isomer. The (+)-isomer possesses weak μ opioid agonist activity equivalent to approximately 1/3,800 that of morphine. The O-desmethyl metabolite (CYP2D6) of (±)-tramadol has improved μ opioid activity equivalent to 1/35 that of morphine. Affinity for both δ and κ receptors is improved. Despite its higher opioid potency, the contribution of O-desmethlytramedol to the overall analgesic effect has been questioned but not well studied. Individuals who lack CYP2D6 or are taking a CYP2D6 inhibitor have a reduced effect to tramadol (88). The fact that naloxone causes a decrease in the analgesic potency of tramadol argues strongly for an opioid component to the analgesic activity. (−)-Tramadol possesses only 1/20 the opioid activity of its (+)-isomer, but it has good activities for inhibition of norepinephrine (K_i = 0.78 μM) and serotonin (K_i = 0.99 μM) reuptake. Tramadol's neurotransmitter reuptake activity is approximately 1/20 that of imipramine, a tricyclic antidepressant agent that is used widely in pain management. Although none of the individual pharmacological activities of tramadol is impressive, they interact to give a synergistic analgesic effect that is clinically useful.

Tramadol has been used in Europe since the 1980s and was introduced to the U.S. market in 1995. The drug is nonaddicting and, thus, is not a scheduled agent. In addition, tramadol does not cause respiratory depression or constipation.

(±)-Methadone Hydrochloride (Dolophine Hydrochloride)

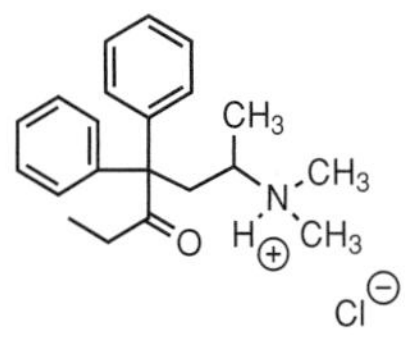

CH_3 N CH_3 O H⊕ CH_3 Cl⊖

Methadone is a synthetic agent with about the same μ opioid potency as morphine. The drug is used as a racemic mixture in the United States, but nearly all of the activity is caused by the *R*-(−)-isomer. Methadone's usefulness is a result of its greater oral potency and longer duration compared to most other μ agonists. When given orally, a 20-mg dose given every 8 to 12 hours can provide effective analgesia. Methadone is an excellent analgesic for use in patients with cancer, and it often is used in hospice programs. Oral doses of 40 mg are commonly used for 24-hour suppression of withdrawal symptoms (addiction maintenance) in opioid addicts. When given parenterally in doses of 2.5 to 10 mg, methadone (Schedule II drug) has all the effects of morphine and other μ agonists.

The metabolism of methadone is extremely important in determining its long duration of action (see the section on metabolism in this chapter). The elimination of methadone is dependent on liver function and urinary pH. The typical half-life is 19 hours. When urinary pH is raised from normal values of 5.2 to 7.8, the half-life becomes 42 hours. At the higher pH, a lower percentage of methadone exists in the ionized form, and there is more renal reabsorption of the drug. The metabolism of methadone by liver enzymes is extensive, and there are at least two active metabolites. CYP3A4 is the major enzyme catalyzing methadone metabolism. Enzyme inducers (e.g., phenytoin and rifampin) can lead to the initiation of opioid withdrawal symptoms in patients using methadone for maintenance of addiction. Toxic concentrations of methadone can accumulate in patients with liver disease, in geriatric patients with a decreased oxidative metabolism capacity, or in patients taking an inhibitor of CYP3A4 (e.g., nifedipine, diazepam, and fluvoxamine).

Methadone is a good drug for maintenance of addiction, but it is not ideal. Methadone requires once-a-day dosing, usually at a clinic, to suppress withdrawal symptoms. Once-a-day dosing is expensive and, sometimes, logistically difficult to achieve. Levomethadyl acetate is available and is used in some treatment programs to overcome the problems of methadone. Levomethadyl acetate is more potent than methadone, and it has a longer duration of action. A single oral dose of this agent can suppress abstinence withdrawal for up to 3 days. Both methadone and levomethadyl are associated with rare induction of cardiac arrhythmias through increases in the QT interval.

Propoxyphene Hydrochloride or Napsylate (Darvon, Dolene, Darvon-N & Generics)

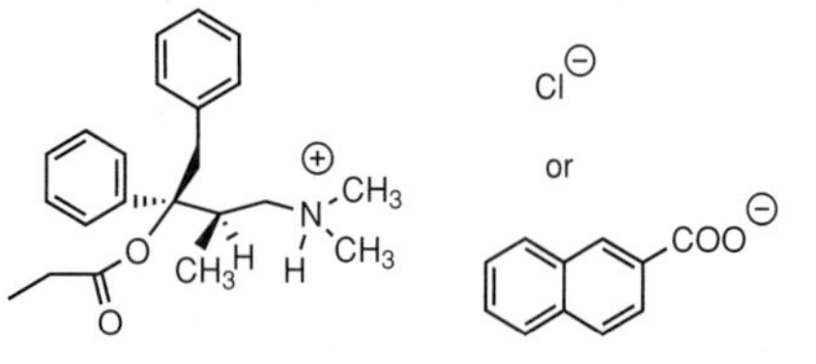

$Cl^{\ominus}$ or $COO^{\ominus}$

Propoxyphene is a weak μ agonist that is used as a single agent and in mixtures with nonsteroidal anti-inflammatory agents to treat mild or moderate pain. The active (+)-isomer has (2*S*,3*R*) absolute configuration. Propoxyphene is only available in oral dosage forms. Propoxyphene has approximately one-twelfth the potency of morphine, and most studies show it to be equally or less effective than aspirin as an analgesic. Doses of propoxyphene that approach the analgesic efficacy of morphine are toxic. Propoxyphene's popularity results from the fact that physicians prescribe it for its lower abuse potential (Schedule IV) compared to that of codeine.

Fentanyl Citrate (Sublimaze; Also in Combination with Droperidol)

The structure of fentanyl and related compounds are given in Table 24.4. Fentanyl is a μ agonist with approximately 80 times greater potency than morphine. Fentanyl has been used in combination with nitrous oxide for "balanced" anesthesia and in combination with droperidol for "neurolepalgesia." The advantages of fentanyl over morphine for anesthetic procedures are its shorter duration of action (1–2 hours) and the fact that it does not cause histamine release on intravenous injection.

A fentanyl patch is available for the treatment of severe chronic pain. This dosage form delivers fentanyl transdermally and provides effective analgesia for periods of up to 72 hours. In 1999, fentanyl also became available in a lollipop dose form for absorption from the oral cavity.

Fentanyl's short duration of action after parenteral dose is caused by redistribution rather than by metabolism or excretion. Repeated doses of fentanyl can result in accumulation and toxicities. Elderly patients usually are more sensitive to fentanyl and require lower doses.

Opioids have a wide spectrum of P-glycoprotein (P-gp) activity, acting as both substrates and inhibitors, which might contribute to their varying CNS-related effects. Although fentanyl, sufentanil, and alfentanil did not behave as P-gp substrates, they inhibited the in vitro P-gp–mediated efflux of drugs known to be P-gp transported, such as digoxin, increasing their blood levels and the potential for important drug interactions by inhibition of P-gp efflux transporter.

Table 24.4. Analogues Related to Fentanyl [4-(phenylpropionamido) piperidines]

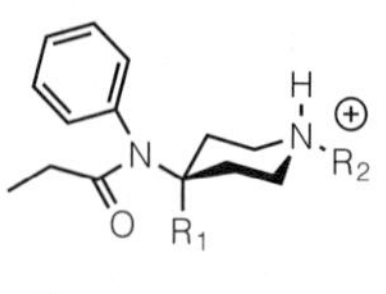

Generic name	Trade name	R_1	R_2
Fentanyl	Sublimaze Duragesic	H	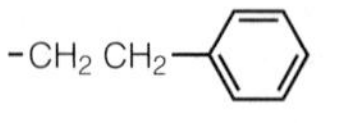 $-CH_2CH_2-$phenyl
Sufentanil	Sufenta	$-CH_2OCH_3$	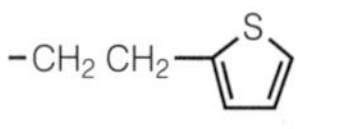 $-CH_2CH_2-$2-thienyl
Alfentanil	Alfenta	$-CH_2OCH_3$	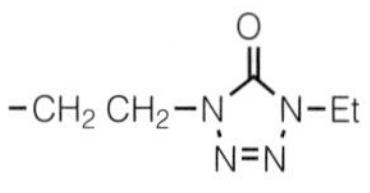 $-CH_2CH_2-$N(tetrazol-5-one)N–Et
Remifentanil	Ultiva	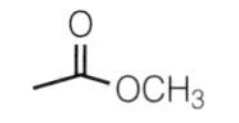 $-C(=O)OCH_3$	$-H_2C-CH_2-C(=O)-OCH_3$

Sufentanil Citrate (Sufenta)

Addition of the 4-methoxymethyl group and bioisosteric replacement of the phenyl with a 2-thiophenyl on the fentanyl structure results in a 10-fold increase in μ opioid activity (Table 24.4). The resultant compound, sufentanil, is 600 to 800 times more potent than morphine. Despite its greater sedative and analgesic potency, sufentanil produces less respiratory depression at effective anesthetic doses. Sufentanil is available in an intravenous dosage form, and it is used for anesthetic procedures. It has a faster onset and shorter duration of action than fentanyl. The short duration is caused by redistribution from brain tissues after intravenous dosage.

Alftentanil Hydrochloride (Alfenta)

Substitution of tetrazol-5-one for the thiophene ring in sufentanil results in a decrease in potency (~25 times that of morphine) and a decrease in the pK_a of the resultant compound, alfentanil (Table 24.4). The lower pK_a of alfentanil results in a lower percentage of the drug existing in the ionized form at physiological pH. Being more un-ionized, alfentanil penetrates the blood-brain barrier faster than other fentanyl derivatives and has a faster onset and shorter duration of action. Alfentanil is 99% metabolized in the liver and has a half-life of only 1.3 hours. Alfentanil is available as an intravenous dosage form for use in ultrashort anesthetic procedures.

Remifentanil HCl (Ultiva)

Remifentanil is much like alfentanil in its pharmacodynamic effects. It is a selective μ opioid agonist with 15 to 20 times greater potency than alfentanil (Table 24.4). Remifentanil has an onset of action of 1 to 3 minutes when given intravenously. Its unique property is its rapid offset of action, which is independent of the duration of administration of the compound. Thus, it is very useful for titration of antinociceptive effect, followed by a rapid and predictable recovery time of 3 to 5 minutes. The short duration of action is a result of the ester group, which has been rationally designed into the substituent on the piperidine nitrogen. This ester group is rapidly hydrolyzed to the inactive carboxylic acid by serum and tissue esterases, making the drug's duration of action essentially independent of the liver or renal function of the patient. Remifentanil is used extensively for analgesia associated with general anesthesia procedures. It often is used in combination with injectable general anesthetic agents, such as midazolam or propofol.

Mixed Agonist/Antagonists

(−)-Buprenorphine Hydrochloride (Buprenex)

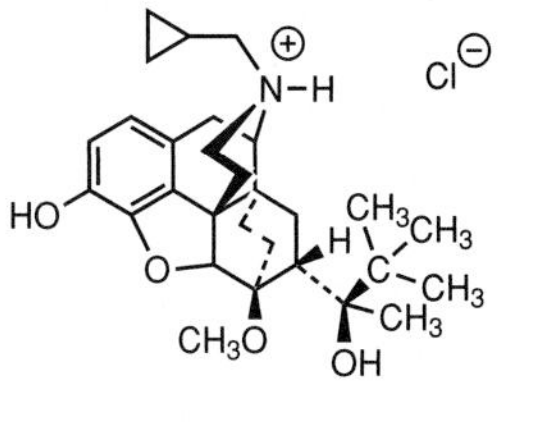

Buprenorphine is 20 to 50 times more potent than morphine in producing an ED50 analgesic effect in animal studies; however, it cannot produce an ED100 (compared to morphine) in these tests. Thus, buprenorphine is a potent partial agonist at μ opioid receptors. It also is a partial agonist at κ receptors but more of an antagonist at δ receptors. Buprenorphine, at 0.4 mg intramuscular dose, will produce the same degree of analgesia as 10 mg of morphine. Because of its partial agonist properties, it has a maximal analgesic action but also produces less severe respiratory depression. It is incapable of producing tolerance and addiction comparable to full μ agonists. In fact, buprenorphine's partial agonist action, very high affinity for opioid receptors, and high lipophilicity combine to give buprenorphine a tolerance, addiction, and withdrawal profile that is unique among the opioids. When given by itself to opioid-naive patients, little tolerance or addictive potential (Schedule 5) is observed. A mild withdrawal can occur some 2 weeks after the last dose of buprenorphine. Buprenorphine will precipitate withdrawal symptoms in highly addicted individuals, but it will suppress symptoms in individuals who are undergoing withdrawal from opioids. It blocks the effect of high doses of heroin. Because of these properties, buprenorphine has been approved for office-based use in treating opioid dependence (64). It also has been reported to suppress cocaine use and addiction.

Buprenorphine undergoes extensive first-pass 3-O-glucuronidation, which negates its usefulness after oral dose. It is available in parenteral and sublingual dosage forms. The typical dose is 0.3 to 0.6 mg three times per day by intramuscular injection for analgesia or 8 mg/day as a sublingual tablet for opioid-dependence maintenance. The duration of analgesic effect is 4 to 6 hours. After parenteral dose, approximately 70% of the drug is excreted in the feces, and the remainder appears as N-dealkylated and conjugated metabolites in the urine.

Naloxone is not an effective antagonist to buprenorphine because of the latter's high binding affinity to opioid receptors.

(−)-Butorphanol Tartrate (Stadol)

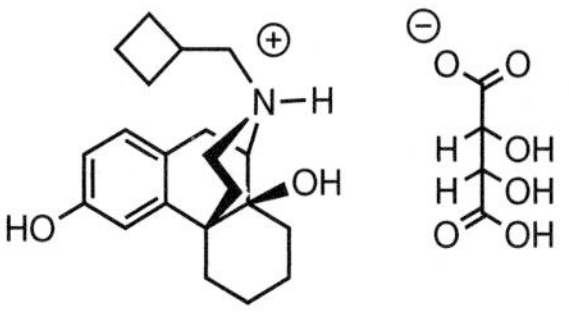

Butorphanol is a strong agonist at κ opioid receptors, and through this interaction, it is five times more potent than morphine as an analgesic. The κ agonists have a lower ceiling analgesic effect than full μ agonists; thus, they are not as effective in treating severe pain. Butorphanol is an antagonist at μ opioid receptors with approximately one-sixth the potency of naloxone. If given to a person addicted to a μ agonist, butorphanol will induce an immediate onset of abstinence syndrome.

Butorphanol has a different spectrum of side effects than μ opioid analgesics. Respiratory depression occurs. There is a lower ceiling on this effect, however, and it is not generally lethal, as is the case with high doses of μ agonists. Major side effects after normal analgesic doses are sedation, nausea, sweating, and dysphoric (hallucinogenic) effects at higher doses. Butorphanol causes an increase in pulmonary arterial pressure and pulmonary vascular resistance. There is an overall increased workload on the heart, and it should not be used in patients with congestive heart failure or to treat pain from acute myocardial infarction. Butorphanol has low abuse potential and is not a scheduled drug.

Because of first-pass metabolism, butorphanol is not used in an oral dose form. Given parenterally, it has a plasma half-life and duration of analgesic effectiveness of 3 to 4 hours. The outpatient use of butorphanol has been greatly increased by the introduction of a metered inhalant dosage form of the drug. The major metabolite of butorphanol is the inactive *trans*-3-hydroxycyclobutyl product, which is excreted primarily in the urine.

Nalbuphine Hydrochloride (Nubain)

Nalbuphine (Table 24.3) is an antagonist at μ receptors and an agonist at κ receptors. As an antagonist, it has approximately one-fourth the potency of naloxone, and it produces withdrawal when given to addicts. On a weight basis, the analgesic potency of nalbuphine approaches that of morphine. An intramuscular injection of 10 mg will give about the same degree and duration of analgesia as an equivalent dose of morphine.

Side effects of nalbuphine are like those of other κ agonists. Dysphoria is not as common as with pentazocine. Sedation is the most common side effect. Nalbuphine does not have the adverse cardiovascular properties found with pentazocine and butorphanol. Nalbuphine has low abuse potential and is not listed under the Controlled Substances Act.

Nalbuphine is only available for parenteral dosage. Its elimination half-life is 2 to 3 hours. Metabolism of nalbuphine is by conjugation of the 3-OH group, and greater than 90% of the drug is excreted as conjugates in the feces.

(−)-Pentazocine Hydrochloride and Lactate (Talwin Nx and Talwin)

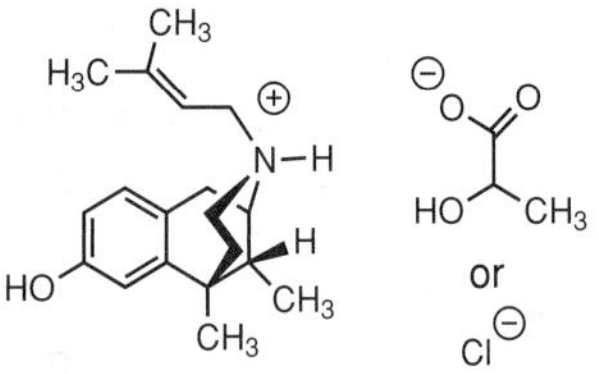

Pentazocine is a weak antagonist (one-thirtieth the potency of naloxone) at μ receptors and an agonist at κ receptors. Pentazocine is one-sixth as potent as an analgesic compared to morphine after parenteral doses. Pentazocine also is dosed orally and has an oral:parenteral dose ratio of approximately 2:1. It is used to treat moderate pain. The μ antagonist properties of pentazocine are sufficient to induce abstinence signs in opioid addicts.

The side effects of pentazocine are like other κ agonists. It has a greater tendency to produce dysphoric episodes, and it causes an increase in blood pressure and heart rate similar to butorphanol. Pentazocine is a Schedule IV drug. The major abuse of pentazocine has been its injection along with the antihistaminic drug tripelennamine (the "T's and blues"). Inclusion of the antihistaminic drug reportedly causes an increase in the euphoric, while decreasing the dysphoric, effects of the pentazocine. The manufacturers of pentazocine have attempted to thwart this use by including naloxone in the oral dose formulation of pentazocine. When taken orally, as intended, the naloxone has no bioavailability, and the pentazocine is able to act as normal. When the tablet is dissolved and injected, the naloxone will effectively block the opioid actions of the pentazocine.

The elimination half-life of pentazocine is approximately 4 hours after parenteral dosage and 3 hours after oral dosage. Bioavailability after oral dose is only 20 to 50% because of first-pass metabolism. Pentazocine is metabolized extensively in the liver and is excreted via the urinary tract. The major metabolites are 3-O-conjugates and hydroxylation of the terminal methyl groups of the N-substituent. All metabolites are inactive.

Dezocine (Dulgan)

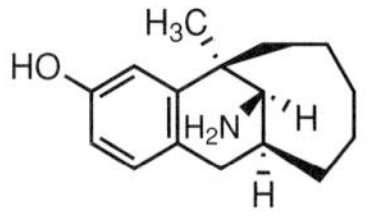

Dezocine is classified as a mixed agonist/antagonist. The SAR of dezocine is unique among the opioids. It is a primary amine, whereas all other nonpeptide opioids are tertiary amines. Its exact receptor selectivity profile has not been reported; however, its pharmacology is most similar to that of buprenorphine. It seems to be a partial agonist at μ receptors, to have little effect at κ receptors, and to exert some agonist effect at δ receptors. On a weight basis, it is about equipotent with morphine, and like morphine, it is useful for the treatment of moderate to severe pain. It is available for intramuscular and intravenous dose. The drug is indicated for postoperative and cancer-induced pain.

Dezocine has a half-life of 2.6 to 2.8 hours in healthy patients and 4.2 hours in patients with liver cirrhosis. The onset of action of dezocine is faster (30 minutes) than equivalent analgesic doses of morphine, and its duration of action is longer (4–6 hours). Dezocine is extensively metabolized by glucuronidation of the phenolic hydroxyl group and by N-oxidation. Metabolites are inactive and excreted mostly via the renal tract.

Dezocine causes respiratory depression, but like buprenorphine, there is a ceiling to this effect. Presumably, there also is a ceiling to the analgesic effect of dezocine, but this point is not well documented. Dezocine has lower affinity for μ receptors than buprenorphine, allowing its respiratory depressant effect to be readily reversed by naloxone.

The major side effects of dezocine are dizziness, vomiting, euphoria, dysphoria, nervousness, headache, pruritus, and sweating. Normal volunteers and recovered addicts report the subjective effects of single doses of dezocine to be like morphine. Because of the partial agonist mechanism of dezocine, one would not expect it to have a high abuse potential.

Opioids Used as Antidiarrheal Agents

Structure modification of 4-phenylpiperidines has led to the discovery of opioid analogues that are used extensively as antidiarrheal agents. Opioid agonists that act on μ and δ receptors have a strong inhibitory action on the peristaltic reflex on the intestine. This action occurs because endogenous opioid tracts innervate the intestinal wall, where they synapse onto cholinergic neurons. When opioids are released onto cholinergic neurons, they inhibit the release of acetylcholine and, thus, inhibit peristalsis. Any μ agonist used in medicine causes constipation as a side effect. Most μ agonists are not used as antidiarrheal agents because of their potential for abuse and addiction.

Opium tincture and camphorated opium tincture (Paregoric) have long been used as effective antidiarrheal agents. The bad taste of these liquid preparations and their abuse potential (Schedule II and III, respectively) serve to limit their use and to favor newer agents. Codeine sulfate or phosphate salt, as a single agent, is sometimes used for the short-term treatment of mild diarrhea.

Synthetic agents that are structural combinations of meperidine and methadone are used extensively as antidiarrheal agents. Structures and uses of these agents are given below.

Diphenoxylate HCl with Atropine Sulfate (Lomotil)

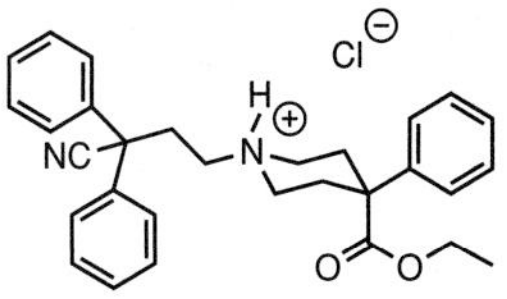

Diphenoxylate HCl (2.5 mg) and atropine (0.025 mg) are combined in tablets or 5 mL liquid and are used effectively as symptomatic treatment for diarrhea. The typical dose is two tablets or 10 mL every 3 to 4 hours. The combination with atropine enhances the block of acetylcholine-stimulated peristalsis, and the adverse effects of atropine helps to limit the abuse of the opioid. The combination is Schedule V under the Controlled Substances Act. Diphenoxylate itself has low μ opioid agonist activity. After oral dosing it is metabolized rapidly by ester hydrolysis to the zwitterionic free carboxylate (difenoxin), which is five times more potent. The zwitterionic properties of difenoxin probably limits its penetration into the CNS and explains the low abuse potential of this agent. High doses of diphenoxylate (40–60 mg) will cause euphoria and addiction.

Difenoxin HCl with Atropine Sulfate (Motofen)

Difenoxin, the active metabolite of diphenoxylate (as described above), also is used as an antidiarrheal agent. Tablets contain 1 mg of difenoxin and 0.025 mg of atropine sulfate. Dosage, uses, and effectiveness are similar to those of diphenoxylate.

Loperamide HCL (Imodium)

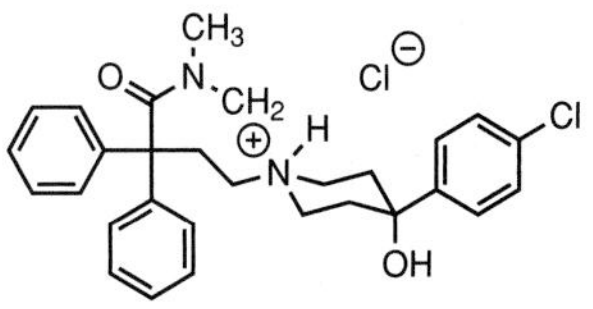

Loperamide is a safe and effective opioid-derived antidiarrheal agent, and it is not listed under the Controlled Substances Act. This medication is now available as a nonprescription item in the United States. It is used extensively for traveler's diarrhea. It exerts its antidiarrheal effects through interaction with μ-opiate receptors in the intestine to reduce peristalsis. Loperamide is marketed as capsules (2 mg) and liquid (1 mg/5 mL) preparations. The recommended dose is 4 mg initially and an additional 2 mg following each diarrheal stool. The dose should not exceed 16 mg/day. It is too lipophilic to dissolve in water for an intravenous dosage form, a property that limits its abuse potential. The compound is highly lipophilic and undergoes slow dissolution, thus limiting the bioavailability of the agent to approximately 40% of the dose. Its low oral bioavailability also can be attributed to first-pass metabolism by both CYP2C8 and CYP3A4 to its primary N-demethyl metabolite. Peak plasma levels are reached in approximately 5 hours, with an elimination half-life of approximately 11 hours. Approximately 1% of the dose is excreted into the urine unchanged. Loperamide also is a potent inhibitor of intestinal CYP3A4, increasing the intestinal absorption of other CYP3A4 substrates. The clinically significant drug interactions of loperamide with coadministered CYP3A4 and CYP2C8 substrates or inhibitors would be limited, however, because of its two metabolic pathways.

The efflux transporter P-gp is a major determinant of the pharmacokinetics and pharmacodynamics of loperamide, a potent opiate. The main reason that loperamide does not produce opioid CNS effects at usual doses in patients is a combination of slow dissolution, first-pass metabolism, and P-gp–mediated efflux, which prevents brain absorption, perhaps contributing to its low addiction potential. Loperamide produced no respiratory depression when administered alone, but when administered with a P-gp inhibitor, respiratory depression occurred, which could not be explained by increased plasma loperamide concentrations. This effect demonstrates the potential for important drug interactions by inhibition of P-gp efflux transporter. The lack of respiratory depression produced by loperamide, which allows it to be safely used therapeutically, can be reversed by a drug causing P-gp inhibition, resulting in serious toxic and abuse potential.

Enkephalinase Inhibitors as Antidiarrheal Agents

Although not available in the United States, inhibitors of enkephalinase, the major enzyme for the inactivation of endogenous opioid peptides, are available in Europe and much of the world for the treatment of diarrhea. Acetorphan (racecadotril), a pro-drug of thiorphan, is a good example of a clinically useful enkephalinase inhibitor used to treat diarrhea. The free thio group of thiorphan binds tightly to the zinc ion in the active site of the enzyme and inhibits its proteolytic action. Orally dosed acetorphan causes its antidiarrheal effect by inhibition of intestinal secretions and has a complementary effect when used in combination with loperamide, which exerts its effects by decreasing gastrointestinal transit time.

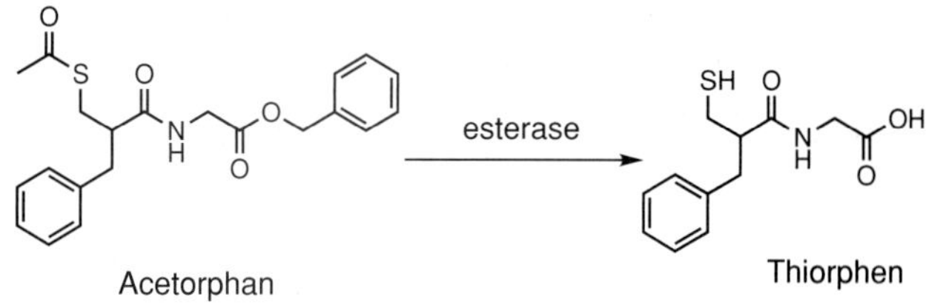

Acetorphan —esterase→ Thiorphen

Opioid Agents Used as Cough Suppressants (Antitussives)

Many of the rigid-structured opioids have cough suppressant activity. This action is not a true opioid effect in that it is not always antagonized by opioid antagonists, the (+)-isomers are equally effective with the analgesic (−)-isomers as cough suppressants, and the SARs for opioid analgesia and cough suppression do not parallel each other. The 3-methoxy derivatives of morphine (codeine and hydrocodone) are nearly as effective antitussive agents as free phenolic agents. The better oral activity and decreased abuse potential of the methoxy derivatives make them preferred as antitussive agents. Incorporation of the 14α-hydroxyl into the structure (oxycodone) greatly decreases antitussive activity. If no cough suppression is desired in a patient being treated for pain, meperidine is the preferred agent.

Codeine is used extensively as a cough suppressant. It is available as a single agent or as mixtures in a variety of tablet and liquid cough suppressant formulations. As a simple agent, codeine is Schedule II, and in mixtures, it is Schedule V under the Controlled Substances Act. When used properly as a cough suppressant, codeine has little abuse potential; however, cough formulas of codeine often are abused.

Hydrocodone bitartrate is approximately threefold more effective on a weight basis as an oral antitussive medication compared to codeine. Hydrocodone also has greater analgesic activity and abuse potential than codeine. Hydrocodone is only available as a Schedule III prescription agent in combination formulations for cough suppression.

Dextromethorphan HBr is the (+)-isomer of the 3-methoxy form of the synthetic opioid levorphanol. It lacks the analgesic, respiratory depressant, and abuse potential of μ opioid agonists but retains the centrally acting antitussive action. Dextromethorphan is not an opioid and is not listed in the Controlled Substances Act. Its effectiveness as an antitussive is less than that of codeine. Dextromethorphan is available in a number of nonprescription cough formulations.

CASE STUDY

Victoria F. Roche and S. William Zito

SJ is a 75-year-old native Hawaiian woman with debilitating degenerative arthritis of the spine. She has been stabilized on 50 μg/hour transdermal patches of fentanyl for 2 years, and these patches have allowed her to resume normal activities of daily living, including playing bridge with friends, visiting grandchildren, walking, and gardening. Her quality of life was good until last month, when she began having significant bouts of breakthrough pain that compromised both her abilities and her spirit. She sought help from her physician to achieve better pain control, and he prescribed compound 1, administered intranasally. SJ has just presented the prescription at your pharmacy.

On checking SJ's patient profile, you find that she is a poor CYP2C9 metabolizer who is on low-dose, delayed-release sodium valproate for the treatment of complex partial seizure disorder. Her seizures are being well-controlled on this medication. You evaluate the physician's therapeutic recommendation against the other analgesics you have available in your pharmacy and prepare to make a therapeutic decision on SJ's behalf.

1. Identify the therapeutic problem(s) in which the pharmacist's intervention may benefit the patient.
2. Identify and prioritize the patient-specific factors that must be considered to achieve the desired therapeutic outcomes.
3. Conduct a thorough and mechanistically oriented structure-activity analysis of all therapeutic alternatives provided in the case.
4. Evaluate the SAR findings against the patient-specific factors and desired therapeutic outcomes, and make a therapeutic decision.
5. Counsel your patient.

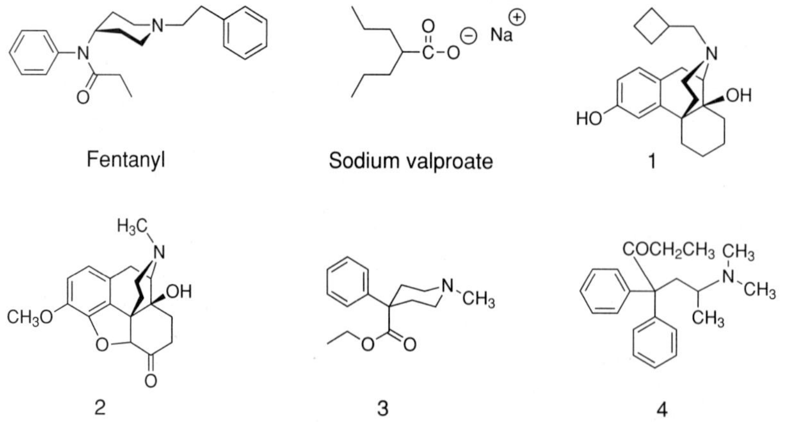

Fentanyl

Sodium valproate

1

2

3

4

References

1. Hughes J, Smith TW, Kosterlitz HW, et al. Identification of two related pentapeptides from the brain with potent opiate agonist activity. Nature 1975;258: 577–579.
2. Terenius L. Stereospecific interaction between narcotic analgesics and synaptic plasma membrane fraction of rat cerebral cortex. Acta Pharmacol Toxicol 1973;32:317–320.
3. Pert CB, Snyder SH. Opiate receptor: demonstration in nervous tissue. Science 1973;70:2243–2247.
4. Simon EJ, Hiller JM, Edelman I. Stereospecific binding of the potent narcotic analgesic [^{3}H]etorphine to rat brain homogenate. Proc Natl Acad Sci U S A 1973;70:1947–1949.
5. Goldstein A, Lowney LI, Pal BK. Stereospecific and nonspecific interactions of the morphine congener levorphanol in subcellular fractions of mouse brain. Proc Natl Acad Sci U S A 1971;68:1742–1747.
6. Li CH, Lemaire S, Yamashiro D, et al. The synthesis and opiate activity of β-endorphin. Biochem Biophys Res Commun 1976;71:19–25.
7. Goldstein A, Tachibana S, Lowney LI, et al. Procaine pituitary dynorphin: complete amino acid sequence of the biologically active heptadecapeptide. Proc Natl Acad Sci U S A 1979;76: 6666–6670.
8. Zadina JE, Hackler L, Ge LJ, et al. A potent and selective endogenous agonist for the μ-opiate receptor. Nature 1997;386:499–502.
9. Goldstein A, Barrett RW, James IF, et al. Morphine and other opiates from beef brain and adrenal. Proc Natl Acad Sci U S A 1985;82:5203–5207.
10. Akil H, Watson SJ, Young E, et al. Endogenous opioids: biology and function. Annu Rev Neurosci 1984;7:233–255.
11. Brantl V, Teshemacher H. A material with opioid activity in bovine milk and milk products. Naunyn Schmiedebergs Arch Pharmacol 1979;306:301–304.
12. Montecucchi PC, de Castiglioni R, Piani S, et al. Amino acid composition and sequence of dermorphin, a novel opiate-like peptide from the skin of *Phyllomedusa sauvagei.* Int J Pept Protein Res 1981;17:275–283.
13. Gilbert PE, Martin WR. The effects of morphine and nalorphine-like drugs in the nondependent, morphine-dependent, and cyclazocine-dependent chronic spinal dog. J Pharmacol Exp Ther 1976;198:66–82.
14. Lord JAH, Waterfield AA, Hughes J, et al. Endogenous opioid peptides: multiple agonists and receptors. Nature 1977;267:495–499.
15. Satoh M, Minami M. Molecular pharmacology of the opioid receptors. Pharmacol Ther 1995;68:343–364.
16. Dhawan BN, Cesselin R, Raghbir R, et al. International Union of Pharmacology. XII. Classification of opioid receptors. Pharmacol Rev 1996;48:567–592.
17. Pan L, Xu J, Yu R, et al. Identification and characterization of six new alternatively spliced variants of the human mu opioid receptor gene, *Oprm.* Neuroscience 2005;133;209–220.
18. Henderson G, McKnight AT. The orphan opioid receptor and its endogenous ligand—nociceptin/orphanin FQ. Trends Pharmacol Sci 1997;18:293–300.
19. Meunier JC, Mollereau C, Toll L, et al. Isolation and structure of the endogenous agonist of opioid receptor-like ORL1 receptor. Nature 1995;377:532–535.
20. Reinscheid RK, Nothacker HP, Bourson A, et al. Orphanin FQ: a neuropeptide that activates an opioid-like G protein–coupled receptor. Science 1995;270:792–794.
21. Inoue M, Kobayashi M, Kozaki S, et al. Nociceptin/orphanin FQ-induced nociceptive responses through substance P release from peripheral nerve endings in mice. Proc Natl Acad Sci U S A 1998;95:10949–10953.
22. Zeilhofer HU, Calo G. Nociceptin/orphanin FQ and its receptor-potential targets for pain therapy? J Pharmacol Exp Ther 2003;306:423–429.
23. Leslie FM. Methods used for the study of opioid receptors. Pharmacol Rev 1987;39:197–249.
24. Childers SR. Opioid receptor-coupled second messengers systems. Life Sci 1991;48:1991–2003.
25. Connor M, Christie MD. Opioid receptor signaling mechanisms. Clin Exp Pharmacol Physiol 1999;26:493–499.
26. Handa BK, Land AC, Lord JA, et al. Analogues of β-LPH61–64 possessing selective agonist activity at μ-opiate receptors. Eur J Pharmacol 1981;70: 531–540.
27. Negri L, Erspamer GF, Severini C, et al. Dermorphin-related peptides from the skin of *Phyllomedusa bicolor* and their amidated analogues activate two μ opioid receptor subtypes that modulate antinociception and catalepsy in the rat. Proc Natl Acad Sci U S A 1992;89:7203–7207.
28. Kieffer BL. Opioids: first lessons from knockout mice. Trends Pharmacol Sci 1999;20:19–25.
29. Schmidhammer H, Burkhard WP, Eggstein-Aeppi L, et al. Synthesis and biological evaluation of 14-alkoxymorphinans. 2. (−)-N-(cyclopropylmethyl)-4,14-dimethoxymorphinan-6-one, a selective μ opioid receptor antagonist. J Med Chem 1989;32:418–421.
30. Pelton JT, Kazmierski W, Gulya K, et al. Design and synthesis of conformationally constrained somatostatin analogues with high potency and specificity for μ opioid receptors. J Med Chem 1986;29:2370–2375.
31. Paul D, Pasternak GW. Differential blockade by naloxonazine of two mu opiate actions: analgesia and inhibition of gastrointestinal transit. Eur J Pharmacol 1988;149:403–404.
32. Szmuszkovicz J, Von Voigtlander PF. Benzeneacetamide amines: structurally novel non-μ opioids. J Med Chem 1982;25:1125–1126.
33. Clark CR, Halfpenny PR, Hill RG, et al. Highly selective κ opioid analgesics. Synthesis and structure–activity relationships of novel N-[(2-aminocyclohexyl)aryl]acetamide and N-[(2-aminocyclohexyl)aryloxy]acetamide derivatives. J Med Chem 1988;31:831–836.
34. Hunter JC, Leighton GE, Meecham KG, et al. CI-977, a novel and selective agonist for the κ-opioid receptor. Br J Pharmacol 1990;101:183–189.
35. Barber A, Bartoszyk GD, Bender HM, et al. A pharmacological profile of the novel, peripherally-selective κ-opioid receptor agonist, EMD 61753. Br J Pharmacol 1994;113:843–851.
36. Rothman RB, Bykov V, de Costa BR, et al. Evidence for four opioid κ binding sites in guinea pig brain. Prog Clin Biol Res 1990;328:9–12.
37. Choi H, Murray TF, DeLander GE, et al. N-terminal alkylated derivatives of [D-Pro10]dynorphin A-(1–11) are highly selective for κ-opioid receptors. J Med Chem 1992;35:4638–4639.
38. Lung FDT, Meyer JP, Li G, et al. Highly κ receptor–selective dynorphin A analogues with modifications in position 3 of dynorphin A(1–11)-NH_2. J Med Chem 1995;38:585–586.
39. Portoghese PS, Lipkowski AW, Takemori AE. Bimorphinans as highly selective, potent κ opioid receptor antagonists. J Med Chem 1987;30:238–239.
40. James IF, Goldstein A. Site-directed alkylation of multiple opioid receptors. I. Binding selectivity. Mol Pharmacol. 1984;25:337–342.
41. Gacel G, Fournie-Zaluski M-C, Roques BP. D-Tyr–Ser-Gly–Phe–Leu–Thr, a highly preferential ligand for δ-opiate receptors. FEBS Lett 1980;118:245–247.
42. Mosberg HI, Hurst R, Hruby VJ, et al. Bis-penicillamine enkephalins possess highly improved specificity toward δ opioid receptors. Proc Natl Acad Sci U S A 1983;80:5871–5874.
43. Portoghese PS, Larson DL, Sultana M, et al. Opioid agonist and antagonist activities of morphindoles related to naltrindole. J Med Chem 1992;35: 4325–4329.
44. Bilsky EJ, Calderon SN, Wang T, et al. SNC 80, a selective, nonpeptidic, and systemically active opioid δ agonist. J Pharmacol Exp Ther 1995;273:359–366.
45. Jiang Q, Takemori AE, Sultana M, et al. Differential antagonism of opioid δ antinociception by [D-Ala^2,Leu^5,Cys^6]- enkephalin and naltrindole 5′-isothiocyanate: evidence for δ receptor subtypes. J Pharmacol Exp Ther 1991;257:1069–1075.
46. Portoghese PS, Sultana M, Takemori AE. Naltrindole, a highly selective and potent nonpeptide δ opioid receptor antagonist. Eur J Pharmacol 1988;146: 185–186.
47. Takemori AE, Sultana M, Nagase H, et al. Agonist and antagonist activities of ligands derived from naltrexone and oxymorphone. Life Sci 1992;149:1–5.
48. Schiller PW, Nguyen TM, Weltrowska G, et al. Differential stereochemical requirements of μ vs. δ opioid receptors for ligand binding and signal transduction: development of a class of potent and highly δ-selective peptide antagonists. Proc Natl Acad Sci U S A 1992;89:11871–11875.
49. Schiller PW, Weltrowska G, Nguyen TM, et al. TIPP[ψ]: a highly potent and stable pseudopeptide δ opioid receptor antagonist with extraordinary delta selectivity. J Med Chem 1993;36:3182–3187.
50. Portoghese PS, Larson DL, Jiang JB, et al. Synthesis and pharmacologic characterization of an alkylating analogue (chlornaltrexamine) of naltrexone with ultralong-lasting narcotic antagonist properties. J Med Chem 1979;22: 168–173.
51. Portoghese PS, Larson DL, Sayre LM, et al. A novel opioid receptor site directed alkylating agent with irreversible narcotic antagonistic and reversible agonistic activities. J Med Chem 1980;23:233–234.
52. Burke TR Jr, Bajwa BS, Jacobson AE, et al. Probes for narcotic receptor mediated phenomena. 7. Synthesis and pharmacological properties of irreversible ligands specific for μ or δ opiate receptors. J Med Chem 1984;27: 1570–1574.
53. Burke TR Jr, Jacobson AE, Rice KC, et al. Probes for narcotic receptor mediated phenomena. 12. *cis*-(+)-3-Methylfentanyl isothiocyanate, a potent site-directed acylating agent for δ opioid receptors. Synthesis, absolute configuration, and receptor enantioselectivity. J Med Chem 1986;29:1087–1093.
54. de Costa BR, Band L, Rothman RB, et al. Synthesis of an affinity ligand ('UPHIT') for in vivo acylation of the κ-opioid receptor. FEBS Lett 1989;249:178–182.
55. Chang AC, Takemori AE, Ojala WH, et al. κ Opioid receptor selective affinity labels: electrophilic benzeneacetamides as κ-selective opioid antagonists. J Med Chem 1994;37:4490–4498.
56. Goldstein A. Some thoughts about endogenous opioids and addiction. Drug Alcohol Depend 1983;11:11–14.
57. Nestler EJ, Aghajanian GK. Molecular and cellular basis of addiction. Science 1997;278:58–63.
58. Hyytia P. Involvement of μ-opioid receptors in alcohol drinking by alcohol-preferring AA rats. Pharmacol Biochem Behav 1993;45:697–701.
59. Kenny PJ, Markou A. Nicotine self-administration acutely activates brain reward systems and induces a long-lasting increase in reward sensitivity. Neuropsychopharmacology 2006;31:1203–1211.
60. Sharma SK, Klee WA, Nirenberg M. Dual regulation of adenylate cyclase accounts for narcotic dependence and tolerance. Proc Natl Acad Sci U S A 1975;72:3092–3096.
61. Comparison of a single dose combination of methadone and morphine with morphine alone for treating postoperative pain. Available at: http://www.clinicaltrials.gov/ct/gui/show/NCT00142519?order=1. Accessed May 30, 2007.

62. Marsch LA. The efficacy of methadone maintenance interventions in reducing illicit opiate use, HIV risk behavior, and criminality: a meta-analysis. Addiction 1998;93:515–532.
63. Rawson RA, Hasson AL, Huber AM, et al. A 3-year progress report on the implementation of LAAM in the United States. Addiction 1998;93:533–540.
64. Fiellin DA, O'Connor PG. Office-based treatment of opioid-dependent patients. N Engl J Med 2002;347:817-823.
65. Gonzalez JP, Brogden RN. Naltrexone. A review of its pharmacodynamic and pharmacokinetic properties and therapeutic efficacy in the management of opioid dependence. Drugs 1988;35:192–213.
66. Volpicelli JR, Alterman AI, Hayashida M, et al. Naltrexone in the treatment of alcohol dependence. Arch Gen Psychiatry 1992;49:876–880.
67. Walsh SL, Sullivan JT, Preston KL, et al. Effects of naltrexone on response to intravenous cocaine, hydromorphone, and their combination in humans. J Pharmacol Exp Ther 1996;279:524–538.
68. Compton PA, Ling W, Charuvastra VC, et al. Buprenorphine as a pharmacotherapy for cocaine abuse: a review of the evidence. J Addict Dis 1995;14: 97–114.
69. Horan PJ, Mattia A, Bilsky EJ, et al. Antinociceptive profile of biphalin, a dimeric enkephalin analogue. J Pharmacol Exp Ther 1993;265:1446–1454.
70. Miyamoto Y, Portoghese PS, Takemori AE. Involvement of δ_2 opioid receptors in acute dependence on morphine in mice. J Pharmacol Exp Ther 1993;265: 1325–1327.
71. Dewey SL, Morgan AE, Ashby CR Jr, et al. A novel strategy for the treatment of cocaine addiction. Synapse 1998;30:119–129.
72. Kreek MJ. Opiate and cocaine addictions: challenge for pharmacotherapies. Pharmacol Biochem Behav 1997;57:551–569.
73. Iigima I, Minamikawa J, Jacobson AE, et al. Studies in the (+)-morphine series. 4. A markedly improved synthesis of (+)-morphine. J Org Chem 1978; 43:1462–1463.
74. Casy AF, Parfitt RT. Opioid Analgesics: Chemistry and Receptors. New York: Plenum Press, 1986.
75. Rees DC, Hunter JC. Opioid receptors. In Emment JC, ed. Comprehensive Medicinal Chemistry: The Rational Design, Mechanistic Study, and Therapeutic Application of Chemical Compounds, vol 3, Membranes and Receptors. Oxford, UK: Pergamon Press, 1990:805–846.
76. Lewis JW, Bently KW, Cowan A. Narcotic analgesics and antagonists. Annu Rev Pharmacol 1971;11:241–270.
77. Grewe R. Synthetic drugs with morphine action. Angew Chem 1947;A59: 194–199.
78. Eisleb O, Schaumann O. Dolantin, a new antispasmodic and analgesic. Dtsch Med Wschr 1939;65: 967–968.
79. Calderon SN, Coop A. SNC 80 and related δ opioid agonists. Curr Pharm Des 2004;10:733–742.
80. Broom DC, Nitsche JF, Pinter JE, et al. Comparison of receptor mechanisms and efficacy requirements for δ-agonist–induced convulsive activity and antinociception in mice. J Pharmacol Exp Ther 2002;303:723–729.
81. Janecka A, Fichna J, Janecki T. Opioid receptors and their ligands. Curr Top Med Chem 2004;4:1–17.
82. Lotsch J, Skarke C, Liefhold J, et al. Genetic predictors of the clinical response to opioid analgesics: clinical utility and future perspectives. Clin Pharmacokinet 2004;43:983–1013.
83. Beckett AH, Casy AF. Synthetic analgesics: stereochemical considerations. J Pharm Pharmacol 1954;6:986–1001.
84. Portoghese PS. A new concept on the mode of interaction of narcotic analgesics with receptors. J Med Chem 1965;8:609–616.
85. Portoghese PS, Alreja BD, Larson DL. Allylprodine analogues as receptor probes. Evidence that phenolic and nonphenolic ligands interact with different subsites on identical opioid receptors. J Med Chem 1981;24:782–787.
86. Feinberg AP, Creese I, Snyder SH. The opiate receptor: a model explaining structure–activity relationships of opiate agonists and antagonists. Proc Natl Acad Sci U S A 1976:73:4215–4219.
87. Martin WR. Pharmacology of opioids. Pharmacol Rev 1984;35:283–318.
88. Laugesen S, Enggaard TP, Pedersen RS, et al. Paroxetine, a cytochrome P450 2D6 inhibitor, diminishes the stereoselective O-demethylation and reduces the hypoalgesic effect of tramadol. Clin Pharmacol Ther 2005;77:312-323.

Suggested Readings

Aldrich JV, Virgil-Cruz SC. Narcotic analgesics. In: Abraham D, ed. Burger's Medicinal Chemistry and Drug discovery, 6th Ed. New York: John Wiley, 2003: 329–481.

Bloom FE. The endorphins: a growing family of pharmacologically pertinent peptides. Annu Rev Pharmacol Toxicol 1983;23:151–170.

Buschmann T, Christoph T, Friderichs E, et al. Analgesics: From Chemistry and Pharmacology to Clinical Application. Weinheim, Germany: Wiley-VCH, 2002.

Cami J, Farre M. Drug addiction. N Engl J Med 2003;349:975–986.

Childers SR. Opioid receptors: pinning down the opiate targets. Curr Biol 1997; 7:R695–R697.

Collier HOJ, Hughes J, Rance MJ, et al., eds. Opioids: Past, Present, and Future. London: Taylor and Francis, 1984.

Eisenstein TK, Hilburger ME. Opioid modulation of immune responses: effects on phagocyte and lymphoid cell populations. J Neuroimmunol 1998;83: 36–44.

Evans CJ. Secrets of the opium poppy revealed. Neuropharmacology 2004;47: 293–299.

Fowler CJ, Fraser GL. μ-, δ-, and κ-opioid receptors and their subtypes. A critical review with emphasis on radioligand binding experiments. Neurochem Intl 1994;24:836–846.

Fries DS. Analgesic agonists and CNS receptors. In: Cannon JG, ed. CNS drug–receptor interactions. Greenwich, CT: JAI Press, 1991:1–21.

Gutstein HB, Akil H. Opioid analgesics. In: Burton L, Lazo J, Parker K, eds. Goodman and Gilman's The Pharmacological Basis of therapeutics, 11th Ed. New York: McGraw-Hill, 2006:547–590.

Höllt VR. Opioid peptide processing and receptor selectivity. Annu Rev Pharmacol Toxicol 1986:26:59–77.

Hruby VJ, Gehrig CA. Recent developments in the design of receptor specific opioid peptides. Med Res Rev 1989;9:343–401.

Jordan B, Devi LA. Molecular mechanisms of opioid receptor signal transduction. Br J Anaesth 1998;81:12–19.

Koob GF, Nestler EJ. The neurobiology of drug addiction. J Neuropsychiatry Clin Neurosci 1997;9:482–497.

Lentz R, Evans SM, Walters DE, et al. Opiates. Orlando, FL: Academic Press, 1986.

Olson GA, Olson RD, Kastin AJ. Endogenous opiates: 1996. Peptides 1997;18: 1651–1688.

Ossipov MH, King LJ, Vanderah TW, et al. Antinociceptive and nociceptive actions of opioids. J Neurobiol 2004;61:126–148.

Reisine T, Bell GI. Molecular biology of opioid receptors. Trends Neurosci 1993;16:506–510.

Ulett GA, Han S, Han JS. Electroacupuncture: mechanisms and clinical application. Biol Psychiatry 1998;44:129–138.

Vallejo R, de Leon-Casasola O, Benyamin R. Opioid therapy and immunosuppression: a review. Am J Ther 2004;11:354–365.

Varga EV, Navratilova E, Stropova, et al. Agonist-specific regulation of δ-opioid receptor. Life Sci 2004;76:599–612.

Von Zastrow M. A cell biologist's perspective on physiological adaptation to opiate drugs. Neuropharmacology 2004;47:286–292.

Waldhoer M, Bartlett SE, Whistler JL. Opioid receptors. Annu Rev Biochem 2004;73:953–990.

Williams M, Kowaluk EA, Arneric SP. Emerging molecular approaches to pain therapy. J Med Chem 1999:42:1481–1500.

Zeilhofer HU, Calo G. Nociceptin/orphanin FQ and its receptor—potential targets for pain therapy. J Pharmacol Exp Ther 2003;306:423–429.

Zimmerman DM, Leander JD. Selective opioid receptor agonists and antagonists: research tools and potential therapeutic agents. J Med Chem 1990;33:895–902.

25. *Drugs Used to Treat Neuromuscular Disorders: Antiparkinsonian and Spasmolytic Agents*

RAYMOND G. BOOTH

DRUGS COVERED IN THIS CHAPTER:

AMANTADINE	LEVODOPA	SELEGILINE
BACLOFEN	MEMANTINE	TIZANIDINE
BROMOCRIPTINE	PERGOLIDE	TOLCAPONE
DANTROLENE	PRAMIPEXOLE	
DIAZEPAM	RASAGILINE	
ENTACOPONE	ROPINIROLE	

OVERVIEW OF NEUROMUSCULAR DISORDERS

Neuromuscular disorders covered in this chapter include the neurodegenerative movement disorder, Parkinson's disease, and various spasticity disorders. Parkinson's disease is characterized by debilitating tremor, rigidity, and bradykinesia. The neuropathology (but not the etiology) of Parkinson's disease, with resulting dopamine neurotransmitter deficit, has been well defined for decades; however, pharmacotherapy of the disorder remains far from satisfactory. The development of prophylactic and, perhaps, curative pharmacotherapy of Parkinson's disease requires advances in our understanding of the causes and pathogenesis of the disease, and this chapter reviews some current research in these areas in addition to available drugs.

Spasticity disorders covered here generally are characterized by an increase in tonic stretch reflexes and flexor muscle spasms together with muscle weakness. Muscle spasticity may accompany a number of different disorders but mostly is associated with cerebral palsy, multiple sclerosis, spinal cord injury, and stroke. These disorders do not share a similar pathophysiology with neurodegenerative diseases, such as parkinsonism. Accordingly, drugs used to treat spastic neuromuscular disorders have mechanisms of action that differ from those used to treat Parkinson's disease. Nevertheless, most drugs described in this chapter to treat neurodegenerative or spastic neuromuscular disorders have in common the ability to reduce muscle tone by virtue of their action on the central nervous system (CNS).

PARKINSON'S DISEASE

Clinical Features and Neuropathology

Parkinson's disease, first described by James Parkinson in 1817, affects approximately 0.3% of the general population and 1 to 2% of individuals who are 65 years or older. The average onset age is approximately 60 years, and the disorder presents clinically as a classic triad of signs: resting tremor, rigidity, and bradykinesia. Dementia also is a common feature of Parkinson's disease and occurs 6.6-fold more frequently in elderly patients with the disease than in elderly patients without the disease. Along with this morbidity, mortality is two- to five-fold higher among patients with Parkinson's disease than in age-matched controls, greatly reducing life expectancy among affected individuals (1).

Neuropathologically, Parkinson's disease is a slowly progressive, neurodegenerative disorder of the extrapyramidal dopaminergic nigrostriatal pathway (Fig. 25.1). The disease is characterized by the destruction of dopaminergic cells in the pars compacta region of the substantia nigra in the midbrain, leading to a deficiency of dopamine in the nerve terminals of the striatum in the forebrain (2). Degenerative changes in the pigmented nuclei of the noradrenergic locus ceruleus region also are typical, as is the appearance of intraneuronal inclusions called Lewy bodies. Neurochemically, the striatal dopamine deficiency accounts for the major motor symptoms of the disease, but loss of noradrenergic nerve terminals with concomitant reductions in norepinephrine may account for several of the nonmotor features seen in Parkinson's disease, including fatigue and abnormalities of blood pressure regulation. The mainstay of pharmacological treatment (3), developed in the mid-1960s, continues to be replacement therapy with the α-amino acid L-dihydroxyphenylalanine (L-dopa), the biochemical precursor to the catecholamine neurotransmitters dopamine and norepinephrine (Fig. 25.2).

Pathophysiology

Parkinson's disease primarily affects the part of the brain known as the basal ganglia, which consists of five interconnected, subcortical nuclei that span the telencephalon

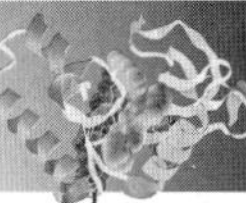

CLINICAL SIGNIFICANCE

The identification and description of Parkinson's disease in the early 1800s started us down a road to understanding and discovery that would be revolutionized almost 140 years later. This revolution centered on elucidating the nigrostriatal pathway and its important role in facilitating motor function and movement. Through better characterization of the structure and function of this anatomy and an understanding of the interrelationship of GABAergic, glutamatergic, dopaminergic, and cholinergic pathways, progress has been—and continues to be—made in relation to pharmacotherapy. In addition, understanding the contributions of genetics and environment to the development of diseases affecting motor function may ultimately lead to preventative therapies and, perhaps, cures. While reading this chapter, pay particular attention to the chemistry of agents that are used to treat movement disorders and how they affect the neuropharmacology of critical pathways. Applying this same knowledge to other agents with opposing pharmacology will help to reveal their potential to cause movement disorders. Ultimately, better clinical application will occur through a thorough comprehension of neuropharmacology as it relates to motor function and movement as well as the chemical nature and pharmacology of agents that affect it.

David Hayes, Pharm.D.
Clinical Assistant Professor
Department of Clinical Sciences and Administration
University of Houston College of Pharmacy

(forebrain), diencephalon, and mesencephalon (midbrain). These nuclei include the striatum (caudate and putamen), globus pallidus, subthalamic nucleus, substantia nigra pars compacta, and substantia nigra pars reticulata. The neuroanatomical connections of the basal ganglia, cerebral cortex, and motor neurons of the spinal cord are complex, and current understanding is incomplete. However, recent models of basal ganglia function (Fig. 25.3) have helped to understand pharmacological management of Parkinson's disease (4).

In normal striatum, dopamine, which is released from nerve terminals of dopaminergic cells originating in the substantia nigra, modulates the activity of inhibitory

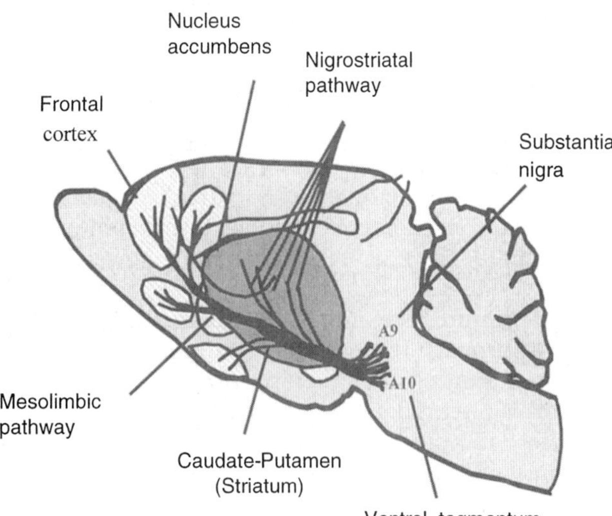

Fig. 25.1. Some dopaminergic pathways in the brain. The nigrostriated pathway (A9 cell bodies in substantia nigra; nerve terminals in striatum) is degenerated in Parkinson's disease.

γ-aminobutyric acid (GABA) neurons. In turn, striatal GABAergic neurons, through a series of complex "direct" and "indirect" neuronal pathways, modulate neuronal outflow to the thalamus, which provides excitatory (glutamatergic) input to the motor cortex. In the direct pathway are two sequential inhibitory GABAergic links that provide input directly to the thalamus. The first set of striatal GABAergic neurons in the direct pathway contains a predominance of excitatory dopamine D_1-type receptors. Thus, the net effect of dopamine D_1-mediated stimulation of striatal GABA neurons in the direct pathway is increased excitatory outflow from the thalamus to the motor cortex (Fig. 25.3). The indirect pathway uses two sequential GABAergic links, like the direct pathway, that are followed by an excitatory glutamatergic link and another inhibitory GABAergic input to the thalamus. The first set of striatal GABAergic neurons in the indirect pathway contains a predominance of inhibitory D_2-type receptors; thus, the net effect of dopamine D_2-mediated modulation of striatal GABAergic neurons in the indirect pathway is to reduce excitatory outflow from the thalamus to the motor cortex (Fig. 25.3). In the normal condition, the direct pathway is dominant, but in Parkinson's disease, the reduced levels of striatal dopamine negates this preference, and the indirect pathway becomes more apparent, with a net effect of decreased excitatory input to the motor cortex (Fig. 25.3).

Etiology

Although the neuropathology is well defined, the cause of Parkinson's disease is unknown. The development of effective pharmacotherapeutic and prophylactic therapy will require advances in our understanding of the etiology of the disease. Currently, there are several, sometimes convergent theories regarding the cause of

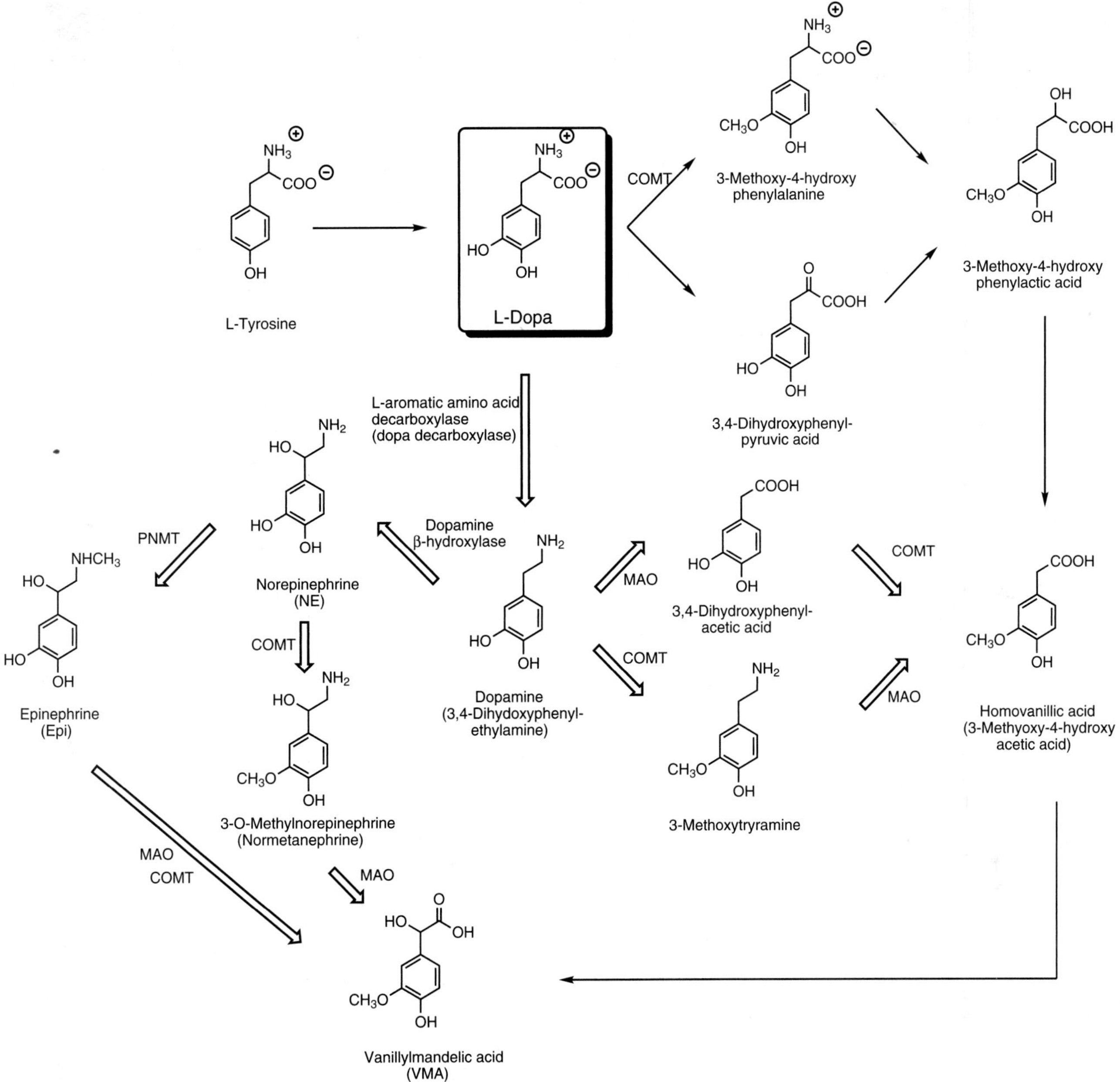

Fig. 25.2. Important pathways in the biosynthesis and metabolism of levodopa. Major pathways are shown by heavy arrows. COMT, catechol-O-methyltransferase; MAO, monoamine oxidase, PNMT, phenylethanolamine N-methyltransferase.

Parkinson's disease: "proteolytic stress," which recently has been characterized in connection with rare Parkinson's disease genetic mutations as well as environmental and/or endogenous neurotoxicants, mitochondrial dysfunction, and oxidative metabolism—any and all of which may lead to "oxidative stress." This section describes these and some alternative proposals regarding the etiology of Parkinson's disease.

Several neurodegenerative disorders (including the movement disorder Huntington's disease) are genetically determined; thus, researchers have investigated a possible genetic influence in Parkinson's disease. Epidemiological studies have found that apart from age, a family history of Parkinson's disease is the strongest predictor of an increased risk of the disorder (5,6); however, the role of shared environmental exposure in families must be considered. One familial form of the disease is characterized by mutations in the α-synuclein gene, originally reported in a single large Italian family, three smaller Greek families, and a German family (7,8). α-Synuclein is a highly conserved, abundant, 140-amino-acid protein that is expressed mainly in presynaptic nerve terminals in the brain; however, its function is unclear (9). Aggregation of α-synuclein protein leads to pathological inclusions (synucleinopathy)

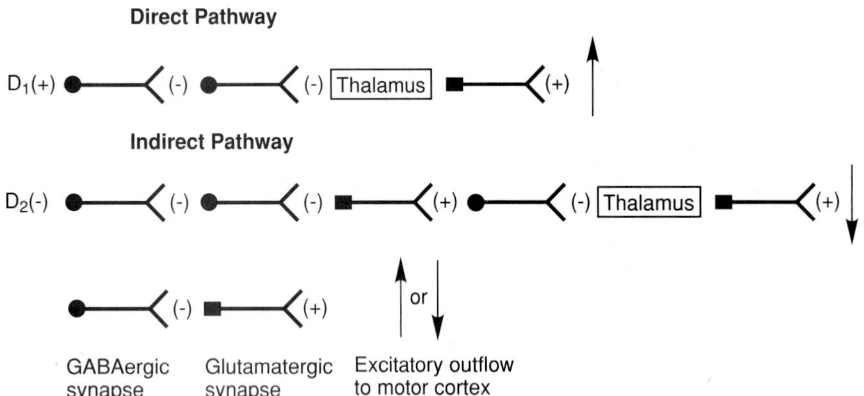

Fig. 25.3. Striatal dopaminergic stimulation of the direct and indirect pathways modulates the thalamus excitatory outflow to the motor cortex.

that characterize many neurodegenerative disorders, including Parkinson's disease (10).

Mutations in four other genes, parkin, DJ-1, PINK1, and LRRK2 codes for dardarin protein, are unequivocally associated with the development of familial Parkinson's disease (11), and a number of other mutations also are implicated. It is proposed that such mutations may lead to excessive production of damaged proteins and/or dysfunction of protein clearance mechanisms in the brain (12). In normal physiological conditions, damaged proteins usually are degraded and cleared by the ubiquitin–proteasome system (UPS). Increased production of damaged proteins and/or decreased UPS-mediated degradation and clearance of proteins may lead to protein aggregation and proteolytic stress. Proteolytic stress affects a variety of cellular structures and processes, and it can lead to cell death (13,14). In cases of familial Parkinson's disease associated with LRRK2/dardarin mutations, protein accumulation and Lewy body formation have been documented in postmortem analysis (15), but such data currently are unavailable for the parkin (a UPS enzyme), DJ-1, and PINK-1 mutations. Meanwhile, several studies have failed to detect mutations in the α-synuclein gene in a large sampling of families (16,17), and studies using both identical and heterozygous twins, which provide a rigorous genetic analysis, have failed to reveal a genetic component of Parkinson's disease (18). Thus, although compelling evidence exists for apparently rare cases of genetically linked Parkinson's disease, primarily involving early onset of the disorder, the majority of cases are not associated with known genetic mutations and are considered to be sporadic (19). It should be noted, however, that synucleinopathy has been detected in sporadic cases of Parkinson's disease (20), suggesting that hypotheses involving protein aggregation may be relevant to the etiology of the more common forms of the disease. Moreover, although Parkinson's disease associated with genetic mutation is rare (<10% of cases), the study of these cases has facilitated understanding of the molecular pathways that lead to neurodegeneration, especially involving dopaminergic neurons.

In contrast to Parkinson's disease forms that are associated with genetic mutations, little evidence suggests that the disorder is autoimmune-related (21). Likewise, although a form of parkinsonism associated with influenza virus–induced encephalitis did occur in a 1918 epidemic, recent studies indicate no evidence for a communicable infectious etiology (22). Strong evidence, however, suggests that some cases of Parkinson's disease may be caused by environmental toxicants. For instance, manganese miners in South America have a high risk of developing the disease (23), and in the major agricultural region of the Quebec province of Canada, a remarkably high correlation between the incidence of Parkinson's disease and the sale of pesticides is documented (24). An interesting link to the environment and/or endogenous milieu is that the incidence of Parkinson's disease is lower in cigarette smokers than in nonsmokers (25). It has been proposed that something in cigarette smoke may protect against a toxicant (environmental or endogenous) relevant to parkinsonian neuropathology. For example, the carbon monoxide in cigarette smoke may detoxify free radicals from environmental or endogenous sources. It also has been suggested that compounds in cigarette smoke, or the metabolites of these compounds, may inhibit monoamine oxidase (MAO)-B activity (26), the main enzyme responsible for metabolism of monoamine neurotransmitters, such as dopamine.

In fact, dopamine itself has been implicated in the disease process through production of chemically reactive oxidation products, suggesting that endogenously formed substances may be etiologic factors in Parkinson's disease (27). For example, the MAO-catalyzed oxidation of the monoamine neurotransmitters (dopamine, norepinephrine, and serotonin) generates hydrogen peroxide (see Equation 1 in Fig. 25.4), which can undergo a redox reaction with superoxide in the Haber-Weiss reaction (28) to form the extremely cytotoxic hydroxy radical (see Equation 2 in Fig. 25.4). Moreover, the auto-oxidation of dopamine to the corresponding electrophilic semiquinone and quinone (Fig. 25.4) species has received attention, because these oxidation

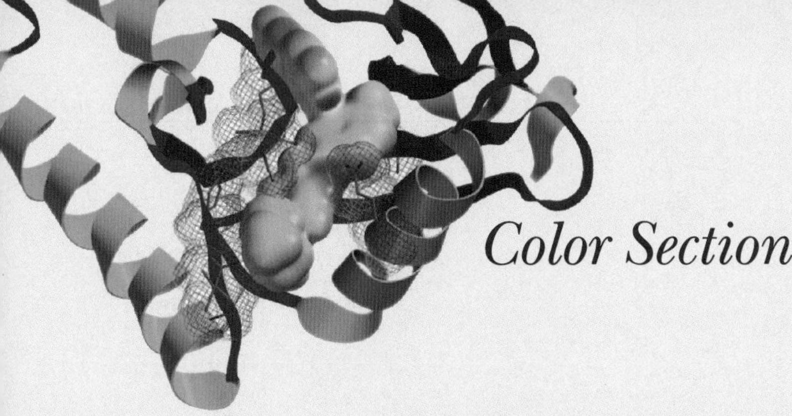

Color Section

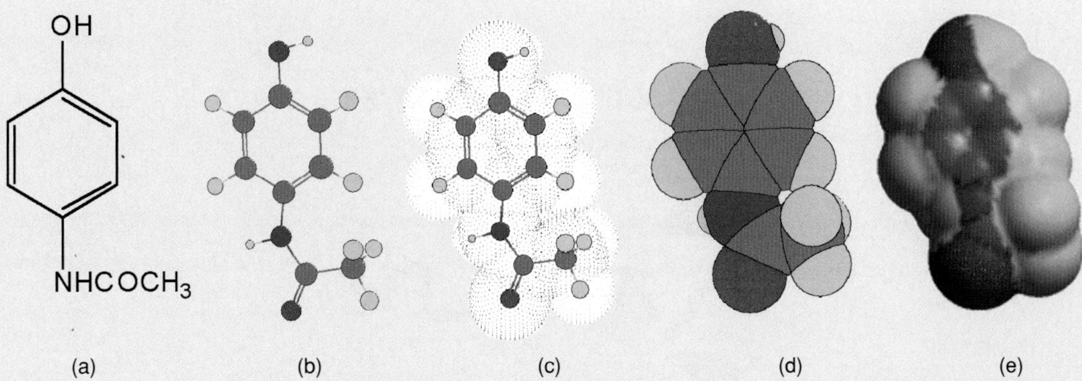

Fig. 3.1. Visualization of a drug molecule N-(4-hydroxy-phenyl)-acetamide (Tylenol or acetaminophen) computerized with different levels of graphic representations. (A) Molecular structure of the drug Tylenol. (B) Ball-stick model showing atomic positions and types. (C) Ball-stick model with van der Waals dot surfaces. (D) Space-filled model showing van der Walls radii of the oxygen, nitrogen, and carbon atoms. (E) Solvent accessible surface model (solid) (solvent radius, 1.4Å).

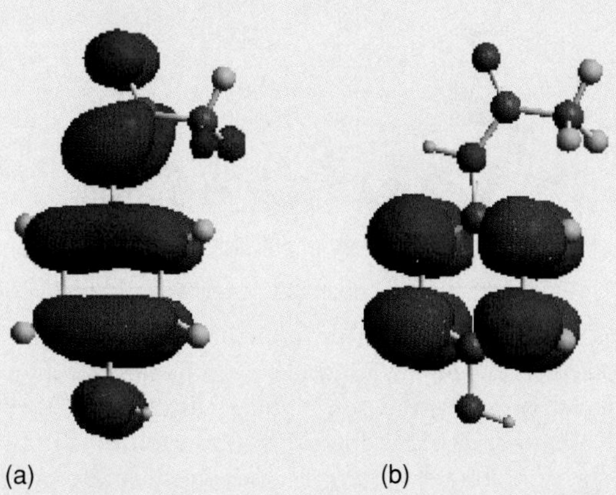

Fig. 3.3. Graphic visualization of molecular orbital surface HOMO/LUMO calculation for the drug molecule acetaminophen.

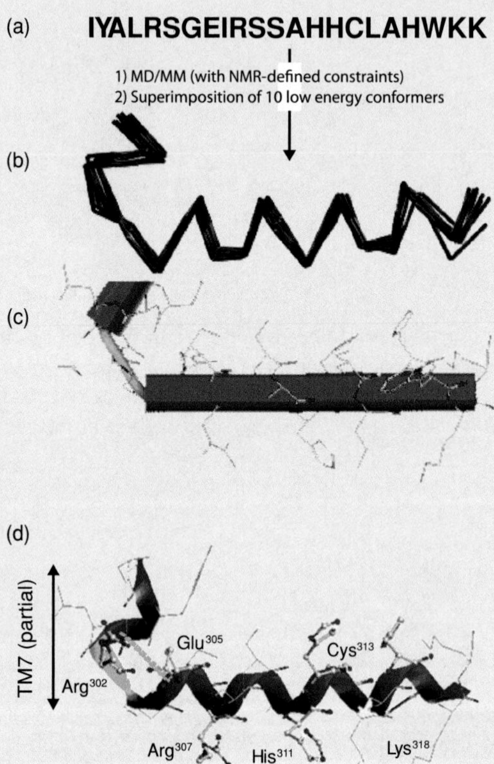

Fig. 3.7. Nuclear magnetic resonance NOE-constrained molecular dynamics/molecular mechanics structure calculation of (A) the polypeptides CB_2I298-K319; (B) the amino acid backbone superimposition of 10 low-energy conformers; (C) the cylinder representation with a turn at the fifth residue, arginine; (d) and the ribbon display of the two helical segments, showing a curve side chain of Arg302 forming a salt bridge (green line) with Glu305..

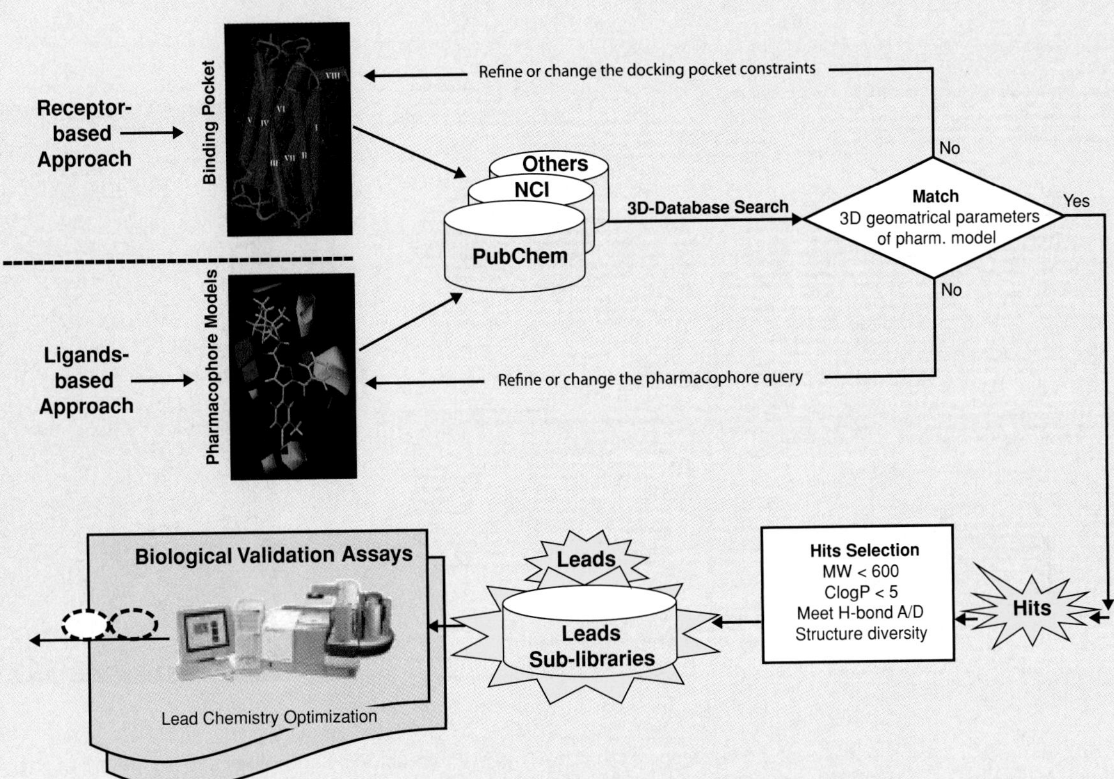

Fig. 3.8. A workflow of in silico virtual screening process: receptor-based and ligand-based approaches.

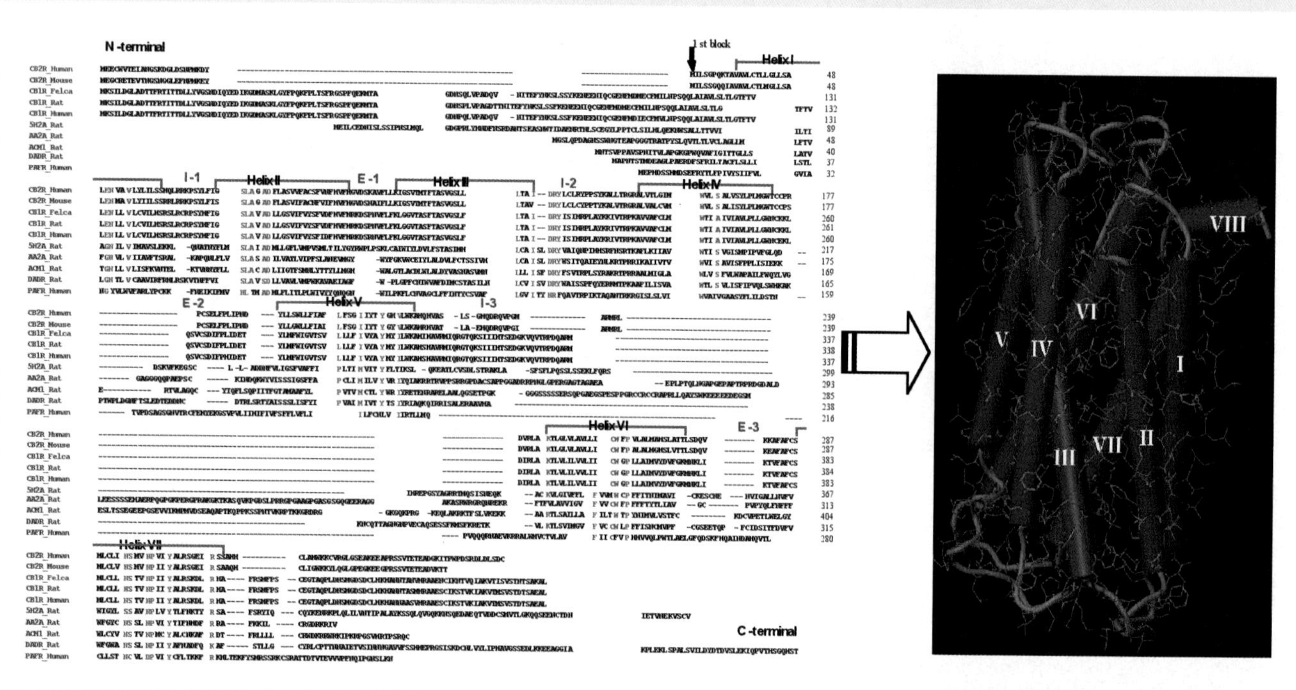

Fig. 3.9. Three-dimensional G protein–coupled CB_2 receptor structure (right) constructed by homology and multiple sequence alignment method (left), including the seven transmembrane helices (cylinders, I–VII) and loop regions (ribbons). (From Xie XQ, Chen JZ, Billings EM. 3D structural model of the G protein-coupled cannabinoid CB2 receptor. Proteins: Structure, Function, and Genetics 2003;53:307–319; with permission.)

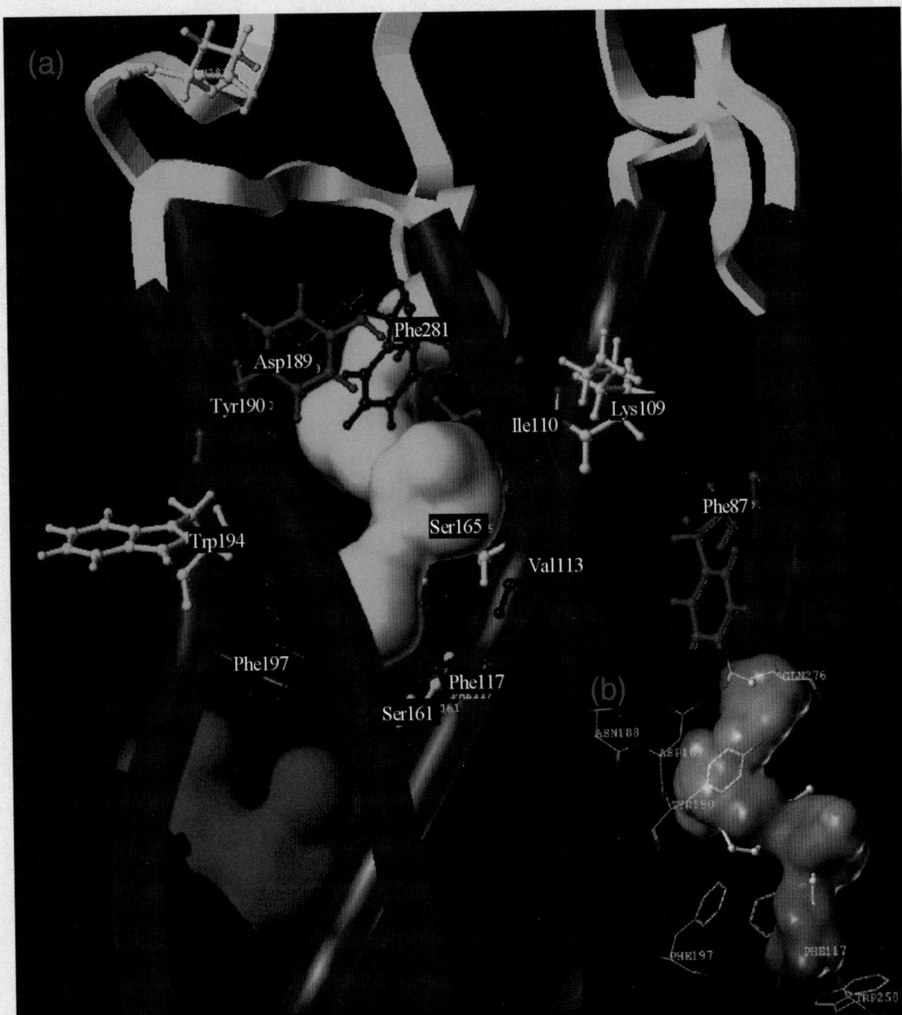

Fig. 3.10. MOLCAD-predicted CB_2-binding pocket surrounded by active amino acid residues, showing an amphipathic contour, hydrophilic center (blue), and hydrophobic cleft (brown). The site-directed mutagenesis–detected binding residues are color-coded in terms of their distance to the pocket (magenta > yellow > green > blue) as the interaction weakens.

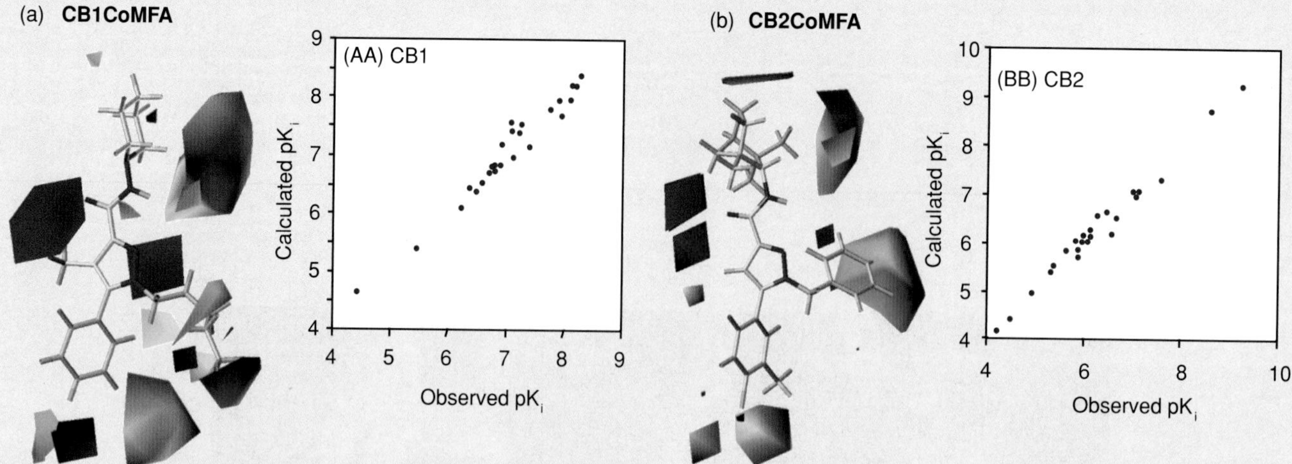

Fig. 3.11. CoMFA contour maps for arylpyrazole antagonists of cannabinoid receptor subtypes CB_1 (A) and CB_2 (B). Sterically favored areas (contribution level, 80%) are shown in green. Sterically unfavored areas (contribution level, 20%) are shown in yellow, and positive-potential favored areas (contribution level, 80%) are shown in blue. Positive-potential unfavored areas (contribution level, 20%) are shown in red. Plots of the corresponding CoMFA-calculated and experimental values of binding affinity (given as pK_i) of arylpyrazole compounds at CB_1 (AA) and CB2 (BB) receptor, respectively are shown as well. (Adapted with permission from Chen J, Han X, Lan R, et al. 3D-QSAR studies of arylpyrazole antagonists of cannabinoid receptor subtypes CB1 and CB2. A combined NMR and CoMFA approach. J Med Chem 2006;49:625–636; with permission.)

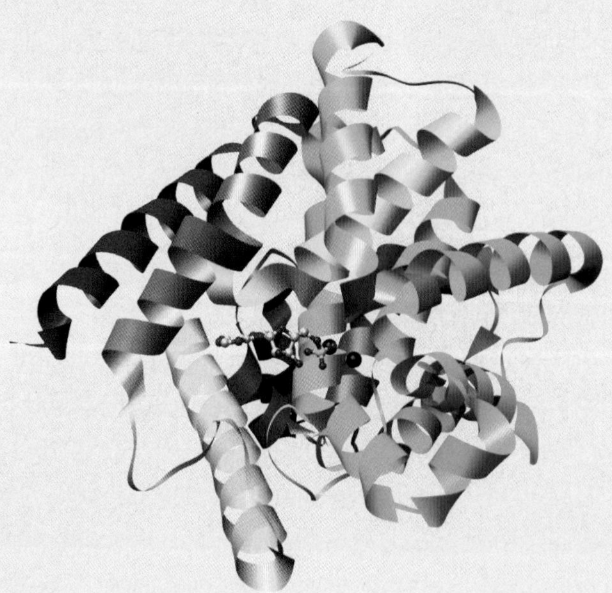

Fig. 17.4. Ribbon diagram of monomeric PDE4D2 (PDB 1PTW). 5′-AMP is shown as balls-and-sticks, whereas two divalent metal icons are shown as solid spheres. (From Manallack DT, Hughes RA, Thompson PE. The next generation of phosphodiesterase inhibitors: structural clues to ligand and substrate selectivity of phosphodiesterases. J Med Chem 2005;48:3449–6342; with permission.)

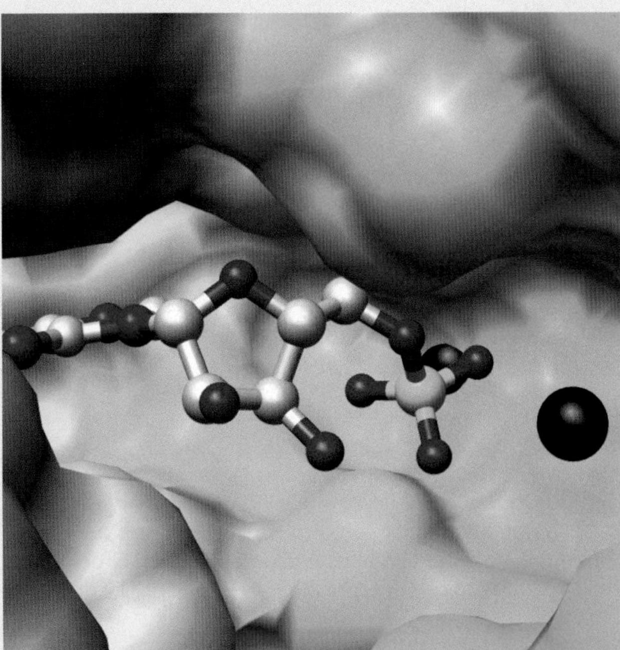

Fig. 17.5. Surface representation showing 5′-AMP in the nucleotide binding pocket of PDE4D2 (PDB 1PTW). 5′-AMP is shown as balls-and-sticks, while two divalent zinc icons are shown as solid spheres. (From Manallack DT, Hughes RA, Thompson PE. The next generation of phosphodiesterase inhibitors: structural clues to ligand and substrate selectivity of phosphodiesterases. J Med Chem 2005;48:3449–6342; with permission.)

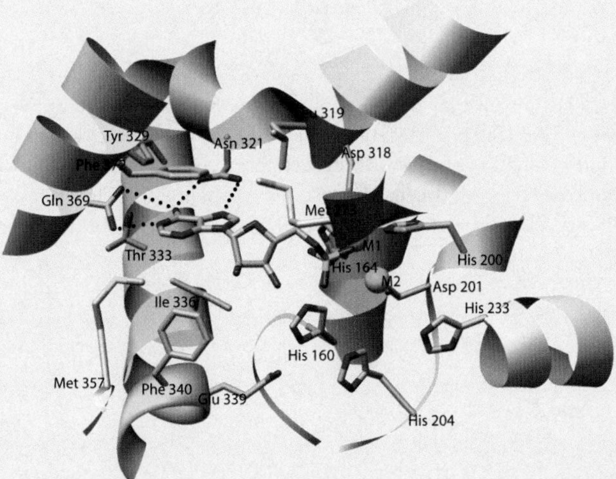

Fig. 17.7. Ribbon diagram of the active site of PDE4D2. The AMP phosphate group binds two divalent zinc icons and forms hydrogen bonds with His-160, Asp-201, and Asp-318. The adenine group of AMP adopts an anticonformation and orients toward the hydrophobic pocket made up of residues Tyr-159 (not shown), Leu-319, Asn-321, Thr-333, Ile-336, Gln-369, and Phe-372. It forms three hydrogen bonds with Gln-369 and Asn-321 and buttresses against Phe-372. The ribose of AMP has a C3′-endo puckering configuration and makes van der Waals contacts with residues His-160, Met-273, Asp-318, Leu-319, Ile-336, Phe-340, and Phe-372. (From Manallack DT, Hughes RA, Thompson PE. The next generation of phosphodiesterase inhibitors: structural clues to ligand and substrate selectivity of phosphodiesterases. J Med Chem 2005;48:3449–6342; with permission.)

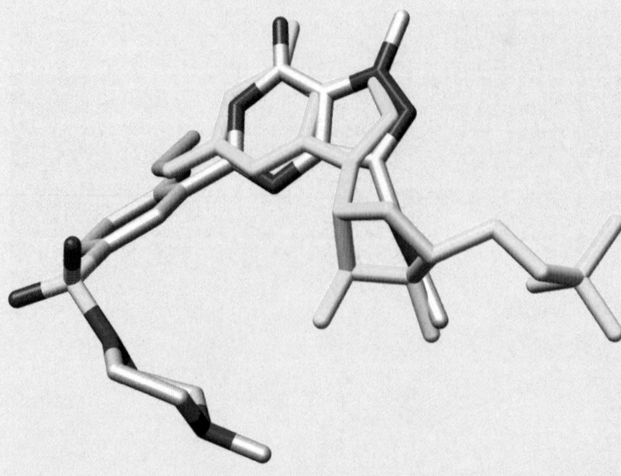

Fig. 17.9. Overlay of sildenafil with 5′-GMP in the active site of PDE5. (From Matot I, Gozal Y. Pulmonary responses to selective phosphodiesterase-5 and phosphodiesterase-3 inhibitors. Chest 2004;125:644–651; with permission.)

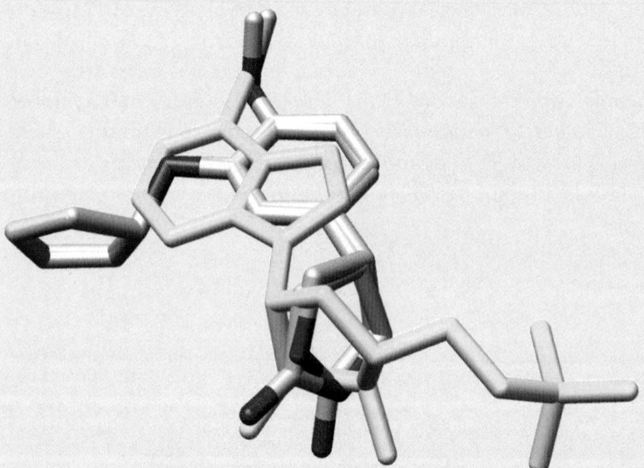

Fig. 17.11. Overlay of (R,S)-rolipram with 5′-AMP in the active site of PDE4D. (From Maurice DH, Palmer D, Tilley DG, et al. Cyclic nucleotide phosphodiesterase activity, expression, and targeting in cells of the cardiovascular system. Mol Pharmacol 2003;64:533–546; with permission.)

Equation 1:

$$RCH_2CH_2NH_2 + O_2 + H_2O \longrightarrow RCH_2CHO + NH_3 + H_2O_2$$

Equation 2:

$$H_2O_2 + O_2^{\cdot} \longrightarrow O_2 + {}^{-}OH + {}^{\cdot}OH$$

Dopamine Semi-quinone Quinone

Fig. 25.4. Formation of cytotoxic chemical species.

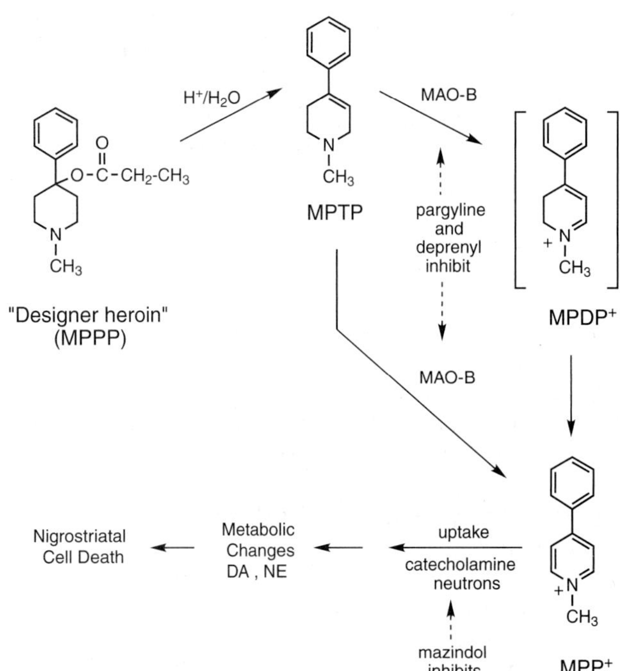

Fig. 25.5. Chemical conversion of MPPP and probable mechanism of MPTP neurotoxicity.

products also are cytotoxic (29). Manganese ion can catalyze oxidation of dopamine, and the resulting semiquinone and quinone species have been implicated in manganese neurotoxicity (30). The auto-oxidation of dopamine also leads to the formation of the polymeric black pigment neuromelanin (29). The physiologic role of neuromelanin is poorly understood. The pigment is increasingly deposited in catecholaminergic neurons with advancing age, however, and it has been suggested that its accumulation in nigral neuronal cells eventually causes cell death (2).

It has been postulated that Parkinson's disease might be the consequence of normal aging superimposed on a lesion in the substantia nigra that occurred earlier in life (31). Dopamine neurons degenerate with advancing age, and in normal adults, dopamine levels in striatum decline by approximately 13% per decade (32). Parkinsonian symptoms usually become apparent when striatal dopamine levels decline by approximately 80% (33). Conceivably, the symptoms of parkinsonism could be produced by two processes, a specific disease-related insult combined with pathological changes resulting from normal aging. This two-pronged pathophysiology may explain why Parkinson's disease is a progressive disorder of late onset. The discovery of the potent and selective dopaminergic neurotoxicant N-methyl-4-phenyl-1, 2,3,6-tetrahydropyridine (MPTP) has greatly aided scientists conducting studies to determine the etiology of Parkinson's disease.

Parkinsonism Caused by MPTP

The cyclic tertiary amine MPTP (Fig. 25.5) induces a form of parkinsonism in humans and monkeys similar in neuropathology and motor abnormalities to idiopathic Parkinson's disease (34–36). The role of MPTP in parkinsonian disorders was revealed by a serendipitous series of events. In 1977, a 23-year-old college student suddenly developed parkinsonian symptoms, with severe rigidity, bradykinesia, and mutism. The abrupt and early onset of symptoms was so atypical that the patient initially was thought to have catatonic schizophrenia. The subsequent diagnosis of parkinsonism was substantiated by a therapeutic response to L-dopa, whereupon the patient was referred to the National Institute of Mental Health in Bethesda, Maryland. The patient admitted having synthesized and used several illicit drugs, after which the psychiatrist who had elicited the patient's history visited his home and collected glassware that had been used for chemical syntheses. Chemical analysis revealed several pyridines, including MPTP, formed as by-products in synthesizing the reverse ester of the narcotic analgesic meperidine known as N-methyl-4-propionoxy-4-phenylpiperidine (MPPP), "designer heroin," or "synthetic heroin." This substance also is an analogue of another narcotic analgesic, α-prodine (Fig. 25.6). It was initially unclear, however, whether MPTP or other constituents of the injected mixture accounted for the neurotoxicity.

After the patient returned home, he continued to abuse drugs and died of an overdose; autopsy revealed degeneration of the substantia nigra—the hallmark

"Designer heroin" (MPPP) α-Prodine (Nisentil) Meperidine (Demerol)

Fig. 25.6. Phenylpiperidine synthetic analgesics.

neuropathological feature of Parkinson's disease. Subsequently, other patients were identified with virtually identical parkinsonian symptoms who had also been receiving intravenous injections of MPPP preparations containing varying amounts of MPTP. In several patients, MPTP was the principal or sole constituent injected, providing the first definitive evidence that MPTP is a parkinsonism-producing neurotoxicant. Both the clinical and neuropathological features of MPTP-induced parkinsonism resemble idiopathic Parkinson's disease more closely than any previous animal or human disorder elicited by toxins, metals, viruses, or other means. Accordingly, understanding the molecular pathophysiology of MPTP neurotoxicity has shed light on the neurodegenerative mechanisms in idiopathic parkinsonism.

Mechanisms of Neuronal Cell Death in MPTP-Induced Parkisonism

Consideration of the chemical structure of MPTP would suggest that the compound is relatively chemically inert, because no highly reactive functional group is present. Almost immediately, it was recognized that MPTP might undergo some type of metabolic activation to a more reactive metabolite. Researchers soon discovered that brain MAO-B catalyzes the two-electron oxidation of MPTP at the allylic α-carbon to give the unstable intermediate product 1-methyl-4-phenyl-2,3-dihydropyridinium ($MPDP^+$), which subsequently undergoes a further two-electron oxidation to the stable 1-methyl-4-phenylpyridinium species (MPP^+) via auto-oxidation, disproportionation, and enzyme-catalyzed mechanisms (Fig. 25.5) (37–39). Inhibitors of MAO-B subsequently were shown to prevent MPTP-induced parkinsonism in primates (40), and it currently is accepted that MPP is the major metabolite of MPTP responsible for the destruction of dopamine neurons, although a role for the unstable dihydropyridinium species $MPDP^+$ has not been ruled out.

The relationship of MAO and MPTP has neurobiological relevance beyond MPTP neurotoxicity. Monoamine oxidase catalyzes the α-carbon oxidation of the monoamine neurotransmitters (e.g., dopamine, norepinephrine, and serotonin) (Fig. 25.2). Oxidation of a heterocyclic tertiary amine (i.e., MPTP) by MAO is unprecedented and suggests a novel physiologic role for this enzyme. For example, MAO could be important in regulating the oxidation state of pyridine systems, such as those involving nucleic acids and NADH (41), which may be involved in the neurotoxicity of MPTP (vide infra). Interestingly, biochemical and epidemiologic evidence suggests that cigarette smokers have depressed MAO-B activity (42) and a lower incidence of Parkinson's disease (43). Nicotine is not a particularly potent inhibitor of MAO, and in fact, nicotine increases the neurotoxicity of MPTP (44). Other components of cigarette smoke, however, do inhibit MAO, and cigarette smoke protects against MPTP-induced depletion of striatal dopamine in mice (45).

Although extensive metabolic, biochemical, and toxicological investigations have established that the nigrostriatal neurodegenerative properties of MPTP are mediated by the MAO-B derived metabolite, MPP^+, this bioactivation reaction must proceed outside of the target nigrostriatal dopamine neurons, because they apparently do not contain MAO-B (46). It is thought that MPTP is oxidized to MPDP in MAO-B–rich glial cells near striatal nerve terminals and nigral cell bodies; the conjugate base MPDP presumably diffuses out of glial cells and is subsequently oxidized to the MPP^+ metabolite. The MPP^+ is sequestered into striatal dopaminergic nerve terminals via the dopamine neurotransporter, which accepts MPP^+ as a substrate (Fig. 25.5) (47). Intraneuronally, MPP^+ is concentrated into mitochondria, where it selectively inhibits complex I of the electron-transport chain, inhibiting NADH oxidation and, eventually, depleting the nigrostriatal neuronal cell of adenosine triphosphate (48,49). Thus, the current hypothesis regarding the mechanism of nigrostriatal cell death induced by MPTP (via MPP^+) is energy failure at the level of the mitochondrial respiratory chain (50,51).

Several sequential factors may account for the selective damage of nigrostriatal dopamine neurons by MPTP (Fig. 25.5). First, MPTP binds selectively to MAO-B, which is highly concentrated in glial cells in human substantia nigra and corpus striatum. Then, the MPP^+ produced from MPTP is selectively accumulated by dopamine neurotransporters into nigral dopamine cells and striatal dopamine nerve terminals. Finally, within nigral cell bodies, MPP^+ binds to neuromelanin and may be gradually released in a depot-like fashion, maintaining a toxic intracellular concentration of MPP^+ that inhibits mitochondrial respiration.

The serendipitous discovery and subsequent scientific investigation of the mechanism of parkinsonism produced by MPTP refocused study of the etiology and pathogenesis of idiopathic Parkinson's disease. For example, evidence suggests that a defect of mitochondrial respiratory chain function may occur in idiopathic Parkinson's disease (52,53). Specifically, it has been documented that there is a 30 to 40% reduction in mitochondrial complex I activity in the substantia nigra of patients with Parkinson's disease (52,53). In general, mitochondrial dysfunction and disorders of oxidative metabolism (oxidative stress), which can include a genetic component (11), now are considered to be critical components of most theories of nigral cell degeneration in Parkinson's disease. Discovery of the selective ability of MPTP to induce nigral cell death has stimulated broad interest in identifying potential environmental or endogenous compounds that may be causative agents in Parkinson's disease.

Pharmacotherapy of Parkinson's Disease

So far, clinical studies to evaluate the effectiveness of coadministration of an MAO-B inhibitor plus the antioxidant vitamin E to slow the progression of neurodegeneration in Parkinson's disease have not yielded encouraging results (54–56). Thus, currently available pharmacotherapy continues to be symptomatic, involving replacement of the dopamine deficiency in striatum by one or more of the following means: 1) augmentation of the synthesis of brain dopamine, 2) stimulation of dopamine release from presynaptic sites, 3) direct stimulation of dopamine receptors, 4) decreasing reuptake of dopamine at presynaptic sites, or 5) decreasing dopamine catabolism.

Levodopa Therapy

About 40 years after its introduction, levodopa remains the most effective pharmacotherapy in Parkinson's disease (57). Despite controversy regarding long-term efficacy, side effects, and even potential neurotoxicity, most patients derive a substantial benefit from levodopa over the entire course of their illness. Moreover, levodopa increases life expectancy among patients with Parkinson's disease, and survival is significantly reduced if the initiation of levodopa therapy is delayed (58).

The seminal report by Cotzias et al. (59) in 1967, describing dramatic symptomatic improvement of parkinsonian patients given high oral doses of racemic dopa, was followed by more clinical trials that confirmed the efficacy and safety of the levo isomer. The effectiveness of levodopa requires penetration of the drug into the CNS and its subsequent enzymatic decarboxylation to dopamine. Dopamine does not cross the blood-brain barrier, because it exists primarily in its protonated form under physiologic conditions ($pK_a = 10.6\ [NH_2]$) (60). When administered orally, levodopa is absorbed rapidly from the GI tract and also transported into the CNS by the amino acid transporter system.

Biosynthesis and Metabolism. Levodopa is an intermediary metabolite in the biosynthesis of catecholamines, formed from L-tyrosine in a rate-limiting hydroxylation step by tyrosine hydroxylase (Fig. 25.2). Levodopa subsequently is decarboxylated by the cytoplasmic enzyme L-aromatic amino acid decarboxylase (dopa decarboxylase) to form dopamine. The effects observed following systemic administration of levodopa have been attributed to its catabolites, dopamine, norepinephrine, and epinephrine, acting at various sites in the periphery and in the brain. The principal metabolic pathways for levodopa are shown in Figure 25.2. A small amount is methylated to 3-O-methyldopa, which accumulates in the CNS because of its long half-life. Most levodopa, however, is decarboxylated to dopamine, small amounts of which are metabolized to norepinephrine and epinephrine. The activity of dopa decarboxylase, however, is greater in the liver, heart, lungs, and kidneys than in the brain (61). Therefore, ingested levodopa is converted to dopamine in the periphery in preference to the brain. It is thought that in humans, levodopa thus enters the brain only when administered in doses high enough to overcome losses caused by peripheral metabolism (3–6 g daily). Inhibition of peripheral decarboxylase activity, by coadministration of a peripheral decarboxylase inhibitor such as carbidopa, can markedly increase the proportion of levodopa that crosses the blood-brain barrier (Fig. 25.7).

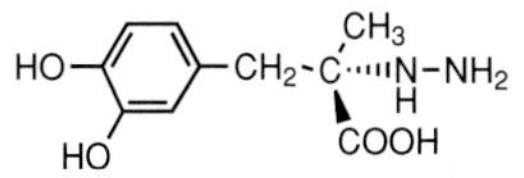

HO, HO, CH_3, CH_2-C, N-NH_2, H, COOH

S(-)-Carbidopa

The greater amount of dopamine that is formed in the brain after orally administered levodopa/carbidopa presumably provides symptomatic relief of parkinsonian symptoms, such as rigidity and bradykinesia. Parkinsonian patients not previously treated with levodopa usually are started on a combination therapy with Sinemet, which is available in a fixed ratio of 1 part carbidopa and 10 parts levodopa. Once formed from levodopa, metabolism of dopamine then proceeds relatively rapidly to the principal excretion products 3,4-dihydroxyphenylacetic acid and 3-methoxy-4-hydroxyphenylacetic acid (homovanillic acid) (Fig. 25.2).

Pyridoxine (a coenzyme for dopa decarboxylase) can reverse the therapeutic effects of levodopa by increasing decarboxylase activity, which results in more levodopa being converted to dopamine in the periphery and, consequently, less being available for penetration into the CNS. When peripheral dopa decarboxylation is blocked with carbidopa, however, the pyridoxine effect on peripheral levodopa metabolism is negligible (Fig. 25.7).

Side Effects. One of the most common side effects of levodopa therapy is gastric upset with nausea and vomiting. This appears to be the result of direct gastrointestinal irritation as well as stimulation by dopamine of the chemoreceptor trigger zone in the area postrema of the brainstem that activates the emetic center of the medulla. The blood-brain barrier is poorly developed in the area postrema, and the chemoreceptor trigger zone is accessible to emetic substances in the circulation. One of the advantages of combining levodopa with a peripheral decarboxylase inhibitor, such as carbidopa, is that a 75 to 80% reduction of the dosage of levodopa is permitted; thus, some side effects may be avoided or lessened in severity. Administration of carbidopa with levodopa results in a significant decrease in the incidence and severity of nausea and vomiting associated with levodopa alone. Other side effects of levodopa involve activation of peripheral adrenergic and dopaminergic receptors by dopamine (Fig. 25.7). For example, dopamine stimulation of peripheral α-adrenergic receptors causes vasoconstriction, and stimulation of β-adrenergic receptors enhances heart rate. Either of these may lead to increased blood pressure, and stimulation of peripheral dopamine receptors causes renal and mesenteric vasodilation. These cardiovascular side effects of levodopa (via dopamine) also can be diminished by coadministration of carbidopa to allow a lower dose of levodopa.

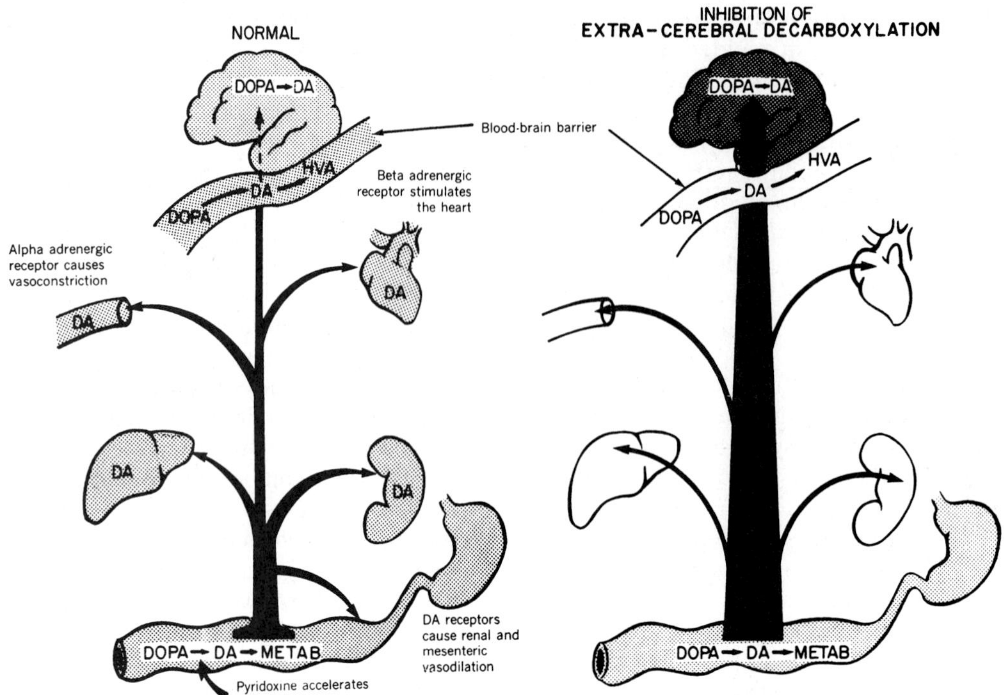

Fig. 25.7. Diagrammatic representation of the peripheral decarboxylation of levodopa to form dopamine (DA) and the mode of action of extracerebral decarboxylase on levodopa metabolism and distribution in vivo. The concurrent administration of levodopa and a decarboxylase inhibitor decreases the amount of levodopa required to elicit a therapeutic response in parkinsonism. HVA, homovanillic acid.

After approximately 5 years of levodopa therapy, 50% of patients develop motor fluctuations; the proportion of patients affected increases to 70% after 15 years of therapy (62). Motor complications include "off" periods of immobility or greater severity of other parkinsonian symptoms and various abnormal involuntary movements. This phenomenon may be caused by progression of the disease, with resulting striatal nerve terminal degeneration and decreased synthesis and storage of dopamine generated from endogenous or exogenous levodopa. In addition to these presynaptic changes, changes in postsynpatic D_1-type and D_2-type receptor systems in the striatum also may occur.

Psychiatric disturbances, such as visual hallucinations, mania, hypersexuality, and paranoid psychosis, also are complications of levodopa therapy. It generally is believed that these psychiatric disturbances result from dopamine (produced from levodopa) stimulation of dopamine receptors outside the motor striatum (i.e., in the mesolimbic dopaminergic system).

MAO-B Inhibitors

C_6H_5–CH_2–C(CH_3)(H)–N(CH_3)–$CH_2C{\equiv}CH$

(*R*)-(-)Selegiline (Eldepryl)

HN–CH_2–$C{\equiv}CH$ (on indan)

(*R*)-(+)Rasagiline (Agilect)

Selegiline and rasagiline. Selegiline and rasagiline are propargylamine-type selective inhibitors of MAO-B, which inactivates dopamine in the brain. The MAO-B inhibitors extend the duration of response to levodopa by reducing metabolism of dopamine; thus, the dose of levodopa can be reduced without loss of therapeutic benefit (3). It has been proposed that MAO-B inhibitors may prevent formation of neurotoxic oxidation products of dopamine and slow neurodegeneration in Parkinson's disease; however, data from recent clinical studies do not support this attractive "neuroprotective" hypothesis (54,55). Nevertheless, MAO-B inhibitors have a beneficial effect on motor fluctuations because of their levodopa-sparing effect (56).

Selegiline and rasagiline undergo extensive hepatic metabolism. Selegiline is N-dealkylated via CYP2B6 and CYP2C19 to (–)-methamphetamine and, subsequently, to (–)-amphetamine, which has vasoactive activity similar to (+)-amphetamine (63). The amphetamine metabolites of selegiline may contribute to its other pharmacological property of dopamine and norepinephrine reuptake inhibition, thus potentiating the pharmacological effects of levodopa (50). The amphetamine metabolites of selegiline have been associated with cardiovascular (orthostatic hypotension) and psychiatric (hallucinations) side effects. Rasagiline is N-dealkylated primarily by CYP1A2 to (*R*)-1-aminoindan, which does not have vasoactive activity (63).

Catechol-O-Methyltransferase Inhibitors

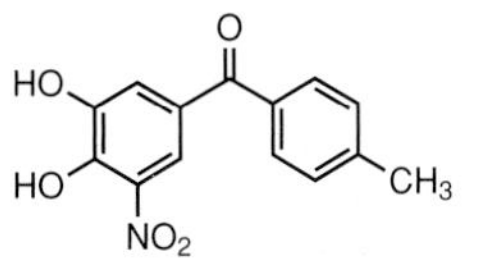

Tolcapone (Tasmar)

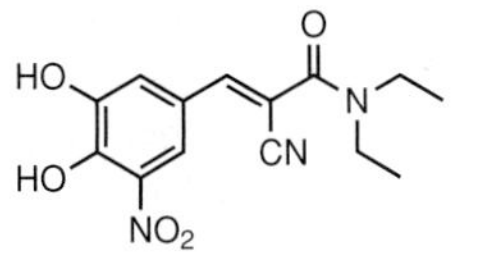

Entacapone (Comtun)

TOLCAPONE AND ENTACOPONE. Tolcapone and entacopone are reversible inhibitors of catechol-O-methyltransferase (COMT), which normally transfers a methyl group from the metabolic intermediate S-adenosyl-L-methionine to the 3-phenolic moiety of dopamine, resulting in inactivation of the neurotransmitter (Fig. 25.2). Therefore, because tolcapone and entacopone block the activity of COMT, they prolong the activity of dopamine. Because COMT also inactivates levodopa, COMT inhibitors prolong the action of levodopa. (Fig. 25.2).

Examination of the chemical structures of tolcapone and entacapone reveal obvious similarities, and the molecular mechanisms by which these drugs interact with human COMT are proposed to be similar (64). Although the mechanisms of action and pharmacotherapeutic effects are similar for tolcapone and entacapone, they differ with respect to pharmacokinetic properties and adverse effects. Tolcapone has a relatively longer duration of action (8–12 hours) and acts both in the brain and periphery, whereas entacapone has a shorter duration of action (2 hours) and acts mostly in the periphery to inhibit COMT. Some common adverse effects of these agents are predictable and attributable to increased brain dopamine (e.g., nausea, vivid dreams, confusion, and hallucinations). A potentially fatal adverse effect, however, occurs only with tolcapone—after marketing, three fatal cases of fulminant hepatic failure were observed, leading to its restriction to only those patients who have not responded to other therapies and who have appropriate monitoring for hepatic toxicity. The unforeseen hepatotoxicity associated with tolcapone has left entacapone as the only COMT inhibitor in wide clinical use (65). The mechanism by which liver damage is induced exclusively by tolcapone is believed to involve uncoupling of mitochondria oxidative phosphorylation, significantly reducing cellular generation of adenosine triphosphate (66,67). Additionally, it recently was shown that tolcapone (but not entacapone) induces cytotoxic pro-oxidant radical formation in hepatocytes (68). Finally, both COMT inhibitors may cause severe diarrhea and produce increased dyskinesias that may require a reduction in the dose of levodopa (69).

Dopamine Release Agents and Dopamine Reuptake Inhibitor Agents

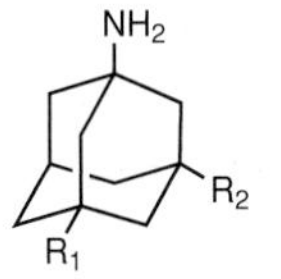

Amantadine (Symmetrel): R_1, R_2 = H
Memantine (Namenda): R_1, R_2, = CH_3

AMANTADINE AND MEMANTINE. Amantadine demonstrates clinically significant antiparkinsonian effects during the initial stages of the disease. Relief of symptoms generally is attributed to its activity to promote dopamine release from intraneuronal storage sites and to prevent dopamine reuptake (70). Both amantadine and its dimethyl derivative memantine (approved for Alzheimer's disease) are glutamic acid (N-methyl-D-aspartate [NMDA]) receptor antagonists that may be neuroprotective by preventing excessive influx of calcium into neuronal cells that may lead to excitotoxicity (70).

Amantadine is a primary amine, with a pK_a of 10.8, and most of the drug is in the protonated form at physiologic pH. Nevertheless, the drug may enter the brain because of its cage-like structure that not only increases its lipophilicity but also precludes its catabolism by oxidative enzymes; metabolism studies have shown that amantadine is excreted in the urine unchanged.

Dopamine Receptor Agonists

MECHANISM OF ACTION. The nigrostriatal neurodegeneration that proceeds over the course of Parkinson's disease limits the number of striatal nerve terminals that are available to decarboxylate levodopa to dopamine. Drugs that act directly to stimulate dopamine receptors, however, do not require functioning dopaminergic nerve terminals and can be useful in the management of late-stage disease problems during levodopa therapy. Dopamine receptor agonists currently available are nonselective and without balanced activity at D_1-type and D_2-type receptors–clinically used agents are full or partial agonists primarily at D_2-type receptors. Use of dopamine agonist monotherapy (i.e., without levodopa) has been suggested as initial therapy for Parkinson's disease based on the hypothesis that oxidative metabolites of dopamine (formed from exogenous and endogenous levodopa) may be neurotoxic. At present, however, no substantial evidence supports an indirect neuroprotective effect of dopamine receptor agonists. Meanwhile, dopamine receptor agonists have a longer duration of action (8–24 hours) compared to levodopa (6–8 hours) and may be less likely than levodopa to induce on/off effects and dyskinesias. In fact, the dopamine receptor agonists pramipexole and ropinirole (Fig. 25.8) do produce reduced motor fluctuations compared to levodopa; however, they also produce increased incidence of other adverse effects (71,72), such as nausea and vomiting (presumably from activation of the chemoreceptor trigger zone), sedation, and hallucinations and other psychiatric disturbances that are particularly troublesome for elderly patients. Thus, the dopamine agonists usually are given in combination with a reduced dose of levodopa/carbidopa, but monotherapy may be used for younger patients better able to tolerate side effects (3).

BROMOCRIPTINE. Bromocriptine (Fig. 25.8) is an ergot peptide derivative that is a partial agonist at D_1-type and a full agonist at D_2-type postsynaptic dopamine receptors

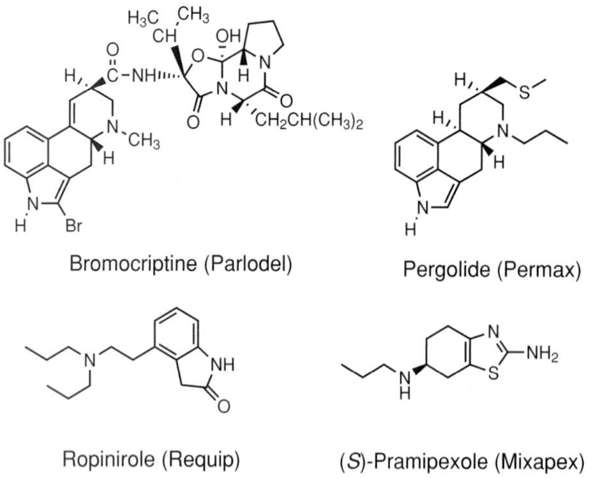

Bromocriptine (Parlodel)

Pergolide (Permax)

Ropinirole (Requip)

(*S*)-Pramipexole (Mixapex)

Fig. 25.8. Structures of the dopamine agonists bromocriptine, pergolide, ropinirole, and pramipexole.

(73), usually given in combination with levodopa therapy. It was the first direct dopamine receptor agonist used in treatment of Parkinson's disease after its development as an inhibitor of prolactin release (via activation of anterior pituitary D_2 receptors). At low doses (typically 1–5 mg/day), bromocriptine is an effective prolactin inhibitor, and at higher doses (typically 10–20 mg/day), the antiparkinsonism and mood-elevating effects of bromocriptine become apparent. Bromocriptine is absorbed after oral administration, but approximately 90% of a dose undergoes extensive first-pass hepatic metabolism, with the remainder hydrolyzed in the liver to inactive metabolites that are eliminated mostly in the bile. The half-life is relatively short (~3 hours).

PERGOLIDE. Pergolide (Fig. 25.8) is a nonpeptide ergot derivative with higher potency and efficacy as a D_1 agonist and equivalent D_2 agonist activity when compared to bromocriptine (73). For Parkinson's disease, as well as for inhibition of lactation, pergolide is more potent than bromocriptine and may be effective in patients who have become tolerant to bromocriptine. After oral administration, pergolide undergoes hepatic metabolism to 10 metabolites, some of which are pharmacologically active. Elimination of the drug is primarily renal, with a half-life is approximately 27 hours.

ROPINIROLE AND PRAMIPEXOLE. Ropinirole and pramipexole (Fig. 25.8) are nonergot compounds that are full agonists selective for dopamine D_2 and D_3 receptors, in contrast to ergot derivatives that also have activity at D_1-type and other nondopaminergic neurotransmitter receptors. Both ropinirole and pramipexole are indicated for treatment of early Parkinson's disease, either as monotherapy and as combination therapy with levodopa. A slower decline of dopaminergic neuronal function is noted for pramipexole monotherapy compared to initial treatment with levodopa (74). Ropinirole also is approved to treat restless leg syndrome, and although the mechanism is not clear, neuropharmacological studies suggest that dopaminergic neurotransmission is involved. Ropinrole is orally active and metabolized principally via CYP1A2 to form hydroxylated and N-dealkylated inactive products, with an elimination half-life of approximately 6 hours. Pramipexole is orally absorbed and primarily eliminated via the kidneys unchanged, with an elimination half-life of approximately 8–12 hours.

STRUCTURE–ACTIVITY RELATIONSHIPS OF DOPAMINE RECEPTOR AGONISTS. As described in Chapter 22, molecular cloning technology has been used to identify five genes that code for dopamine receptor proteins: two D_1-type receptors (D_1 and D_5), and three D_2-type receptors (D_2, D_3, and D_4). Whereas antipsychotic drug design (see Chapter 22) is directed toward discovery of molecules that act as antagonists at, especially, dopamine D_2-type receptors (albeit, an important role for the D_1 family has not been ruled out), the dopamine deficiency that characterizes Parkinson's disease naturally directs research toward discovery of ligands that act as agonists at dopamine receptors. Currently, however, no validated three-dimensional orientation of the amino acid residues at the ligand binding site has been reported for D_1-type or D_2-type receptors. Thus, development of selective agonists and antagonists for dopamine receptors still is guided by quantitative structure–activity relationships based on probe molecules.

The side chain of dopamine possesses unlimited flexibility and unrestricted rotation about the β-carbon–phenyl bond; thus, little information can be obtained concerning the conformational requirements for activation of dopamine receptors using the endogenous ligand. Accordingly, various compounds in which the catechol ring and the amino-ethyl moiety of dopamine are held in rigid conformation have been synthesized to probe the molecular determinants for binding and activation of dopamine receptors. One such compound is the aporphine alkaloid apomorphine (Fig. 25.9), which is obtained by the acid-catalyzed rearrangement of morphine. Apomorphine directly stimulates central dopamine receptors to produce effects similar to those of dopamine, including emetic and antiparkinson actions, which provide its pharmacotherapeutic usefulness.

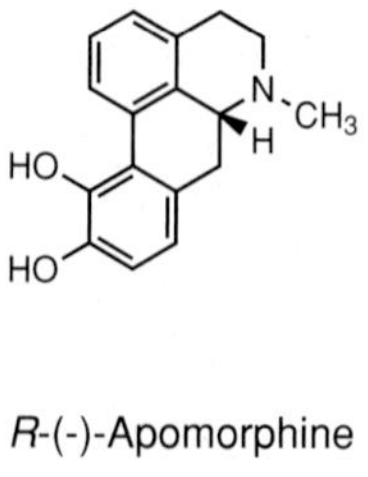

R-(-)-Apomorphine

Although the pK_a of apomorphine is approximately nine (mostly protonated at physiologic pH), the molecule

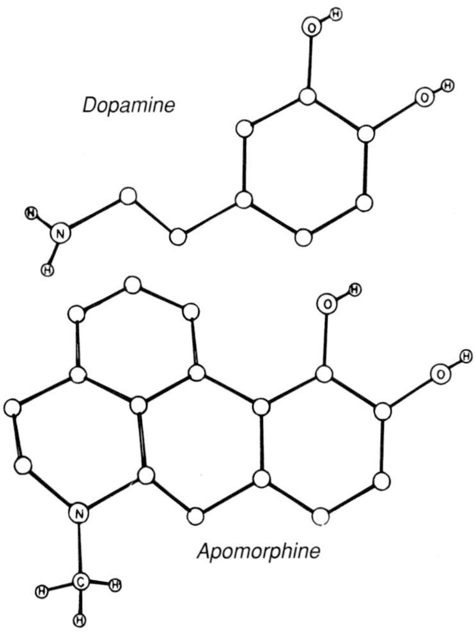

Dopamine

Apomorphine

Fig. 25.9. Model of apomorphine molecule as determined by the x-ray crystal data of Giesecke (77) showing the structural relationship to dopamine in the *trans* α-rotameric conformation.

apparently is lipophilic enough to pass across the blood-brain barrier, whereas dopamine ($pK_a = 10.6$) cannot. In the brain, (*R*)-(−)-apomorphine is a potent D_1 and D_2 agonist and produces an antiparkinsonian effect equivalent to that of levodopa. Interestingly, *S*-(+)-apomorphine is a postsynaptic D_2-type antagonist and a presynaptic D_2-type autoreceptor agonist that decreases dopamine synthesis (theoretically, such neurobiochemical activity would be desirable in an antipsychotic drug) (75). Unfortunately, apomorphine is difficult to administer because of first-pass enterohepatic metabolism and potent emetic effects. Apomorphine can be administered by subcutaneous injection and is approved to treat late-stage Parkinson's disease (76).

To help characterize the structure and function of dopamine receptors at the molecular level, the x-ray crystal structure of apomorphine (77) was compared to a structural model of dopamine (Fig. 25.9). It is obvious that apomorphine contains molecular features in common with the structure of dopamine in the *trans* α-rotamer conformation (Figs. 25.9 and 25.10). Isoapomorphine, which embeds the structure of dopamine in the *trans* β-rotameric conformation (Fig. 25.10), is less active than apomorphine as a dopamine agonist. The 1,2-dihydroxyaporphine analogue, which mimics the *cis* α-rotamer conformation of dopamine, is inactive (78). In other studies, the semirigid aminotetralin 2-amino-6,7-dihydroxy-1,2,3,4-tetrahydronaphthalene (A-6,7-DTN), which has a *trans* β-rotamer conformation between the benzene ring and the amino side chain (Fig. 25.10), was found to be a more potent dopamine agonist than 2-amino-5,6-dihydroxy-1,2,3,4-tetrahydronaphthalene (A-5,6-DTN), which has a *trans* α-rotamer conformation (Fig. 20.10) (79). Thus, results of experiments using these rigid dopamine-mimetic compounds suggest that the preferred conformation of dopamine is the extended *trans* conformation (α- or β-rotamer). Results from other experimental and molecular modeling/computational chemistry studies indicate that ligand activity at D_1 vs. D_2 receptors is critically dependent on the position of a ligand protonated nitrogen moiety that can form a high-affinity ionic bond with an anionic aspartic acid residue in the third transmembrane α-helix of the receptor (80).

Adjunct Therapy—Anticholinergic and Antihistamine Drugs

Cholinergic interneurons in the striatum exert mainly excitatory effects on GABAergic output from the striatum. Historically, it had been observed that drugs which increase cholinergic neurotransmission (e.g., the cholinesterase inhibitor physostigmine and the cholinergic agonist carbachol) aggravate parkinsonism in humans. Accordingly, before the discovery of levodopa, drug therapy for parkinsonism depended primarily on the limited efficacy of the natural belladonna alkaloids (e.g., atropine), which are cholinergic muscarinic receptor antagonists. With newer synthetic alkaloids (Table 25.1), attempts were made to increase central anticholinergic effects as well as to reduce undesirable peripheral effects, such as dry mouth, blurred vision, constipation, urinary retention, and tachycardia. Unfortunately, the CNS side effects of these agents also are very troublesome and include delusions, hallucinations, somnolence, ataxia, and dysarthria. In general, anticholinergic drugs rarely produce more than 20% improvement, and despite continued use, the symptoms of the disease continue to progress. The most important present usage of the anticholinergic agents is as adjunct therapy with L-dopa. The antihistamines, particularly those with central anticholinergic effects, generally are better tolerated in the elderly and may produce slightly greater relief from tremor, but this therapy is rarely used today.

SPASTICITY DISORDERS

Clinical Evaluation

Spasticity is characterized by skeletal muscle spasms and an increase in tonic stretch reflexes, sometimes with accompanying muscle weakness. Spasticity often is associated with cerebral palsy, multiple sclerosis, spinal cord injury, or stroke. The mechanisms that underlie clinical spasticity appear to involve damage to descending pathways in the spinal cord that results in hyperexcitability of α motor neurons. In addition to lack of accurate experimental models, a limiting factor in characterizing the pathophysiology of spasticity and effectiveness of antispasmodic drugs continues to be lack of quantitative methodology for assessment of the spasmodic condition

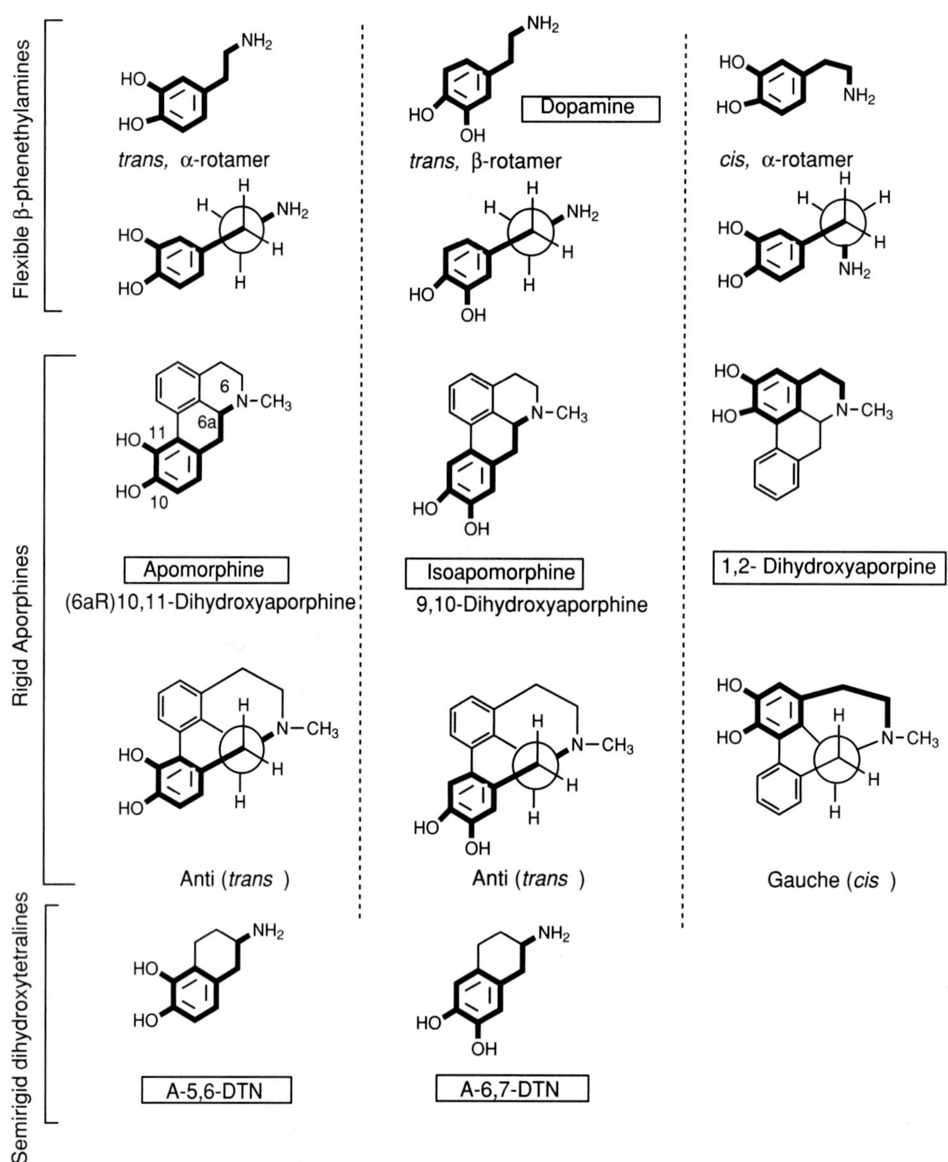

Fig. 25.10. Conformations of dopamine in the *trans* α-rotameric, *trans* β-rotameric, and *cis* α-rotameric forms and structural relationships to the rigid dopamine analogues apomorphine, isoapomorphine, and 1,2-dihydroxyaporphine. Also shown are the corresponding semirigid analogue s of dopamine, the dihydroxytetralins, A-5,6-DTN and A-6,7-DTN.

(87,88). Simple tests of muscle tone or reflex latency have not been fruitful; however, global clinical assessments, such as the number of painful spasms per day, have been more useful. Even the combined subjective impressions of improvement by the patient, family, and physician, however, may not establish that a particular drug is efficacious. Furthermore, spasm frequently coexists with pain and spasmolytic drug efficacy may be related to both skeletal muscle relaxation and analgesia. A straightforward strategy to establish whether a spasmolytic drug produces any benefit is gradual withdrawal of the drug (89). The diversity of neurological disorders that culminate in spasticity and the subjectivity of many of the measurements make it difficult to establish efficacy of any one of the spasmolytic drugs (90). In summary, clinical evidence for efficacy of oral antispasmodic agents is scarce and weak.

Spasmolytic Drugs

Skeletal Muscle Relaxants

Background. The drugs used for spasmolytic conditions are diverse in their chemical structures and their sites and mechanisms of action. The first drug recognized to exhibit spasmolytic activity was antodyne or 3-phenoxy-1,2-propanediol. In guinea pigs and rabbits,

Table 25.1. Drugs Used for Parkinsonism

Class and Generic Name	Trade Name	Chemical Structure	Initial Single Oral Dose
Synthetic anticholinergic agents			
Benztropine mesylate	Cogentin		0.5-1.0 mg
Trihexyphenidyl hydrochloride	Artane Pipanol (x = 2) Tremin	$(CH_2)_x$ N-CH_2CH_2C-OH $Cl^{\ominus}$	1.0-2.0 mg
Procyclidine hydrochloride	Kemadrin (x=1)		2.0-5.0 mg
Biperiden hydrochloride	Akineton	N-CH_2CH_2C-OH $Cl^{\ominus}$	1.0-2.0 mg
Antihistamine			
Diphenhydramine hydrochloride	Benadryl	CHO-CH_2CH_2-N CH_3 CH_3 $Cl^{\ominus}$	25.0 mg
Phenothiazine (Antihistamine)			
Ethopropazine hydrochloride	Parsidol	N-CH_2C-N C_2H_5 C_2H_5 CH_3 $Cl^{\ominus}$	50.0 mg

antodyne produced prolonged paralysis without impairing consciousness. Antodyne was introduced into clinical medicine in 1910 as an analgesic and antipyretic. The duration of its skeletal muscle relaxant effect, however, was too short-lived to be clinically useful. In 1943, structure–activity relationship studies of a series of simple glyceryl ethers related to antodyne led to the development and introduction of mephenesin (Table 25.2) in 1946 (91). Pharmacological studies revealed that mephenesin selectivity depressed polysynaptic, while sparing monosynaptic, spinal cord reflexes. The relative safety and selective action of mephenesin on the spinal cord led to its use as the first widely prescribed centrally acting skeletal muscle relaxant. Accordingly, mephenesin is the prototype of the interneuronal blocking type of muscle relaxant, albeit mephenesin itself no longer is used. In general, the pharmacology of the mephenesin-like muscle relaxants is remarkably similar to that of sedative-hypnotics. Indeed, the only apparent difference is that the spasmolytics have greater selectivity for modulating effects mediated by the spinal cord, thus producing less sedation than general sedative-hypnotics. Both classes produce a reversible, nonspecific depression of the CNS, and sedation, dizziness, and muscle weakness are common side effects.

Table 25.2 shows several compounds with mephenesin-like pharmacological profiles that have been developed and marketed as antispasmodic muscle relaxants. Chlorphenesin carbamate and methocarbamol are carbamate analogues of mephenesin that are designed to be longer lasting. Their duration of action, however, has not been reported. The alcohol carbon of methocarbamol is chiral, and the *R*-(+)-enantiomer was found to have greater muscle relaxant activity in mice (92). The drug, however, is prescribed as the racemate. Meprobamate is the principal metabolite of carisoprodol; thus, the pharmacology of the two overlap. In clinical studies, carisoprodol has modest efficacy for treatment of low-back pain associated with sprain or strain. Carisoprodol and meprobamate have sedative and anxiolytic effects similar to benzodiazepines, such as diazepam, and carry a similar liability for abuse and dependency (88). Metaxalone, on the other hand, is not associated with abuse, and although no data from high-quality clinical trials are available, it generally is reported to achieve muscle

Clinical Applications: Radiopharmaceuticals in Diagnosis of Parkinson's Disease

Even for an experienced neurologist, a diagnosis of Parkinson's disease can be difficult to confirm, especially during the early stages of this disease. Disease progression is highly variable. The degree of disability can fluctuate dramatically, and no two people have exactly the same symptoms. In addition, a number of conditions mimic Parkinson's disease, but these conditions cannot be treated effectively with antiparkinsonism drugs.

Imaging techniques are increasingly applied to neuropharmacological studies of brain function. Positron-emission tomography (PET) and single-photon emission computed tomography (SPECT) are sensitive methods that can be used in such studies. Although spatial resolution remains somewhat greater with PET, several advantages are offered by SPECT technology. Positron-emitting nuclides have such short half-lives (^{11}C, 20 min; ^{18}F, 109 min) that they usually require an on-site cyclotron for their production, whereas SPECT nuclides have longer half-lives (^{123}I, 13 hr) so that they can be supplied commercially. Quantitative assessment of nigrostriatal presynaptic dopaminergic nerve terminal function also has been a useful diagnostic tool for the early diagnosis of Parkinson's disease (81). Previously, 6-[^{18}F]fluoro-L-dopa ([^{18}F]-DOPA) has been used in PET to assess dopamine nerve terminal function in human brain. Meanwhile, it has been known for some time that cocaine and its radiolabeled derivatives bind to the dopamine neurotransporter located on presynaptic dopaminergic nerve terminals. Researchers have investigated whether it might be possible to depict these dopamine neurotransporter proteins using radiolabeled analogues of cocaine (82). Although radiolabeled cocaine analogues have been shown to bind to the neurotransporter, rapid hydrolysis of its benzoyl ester function limits its use in SPECT imaging. By removal of the ester group and directly linking the phenyl ring to the heterocyclic ring system, more stable tropane molecules are obtained that can be radiolabeled for imaging purposes.

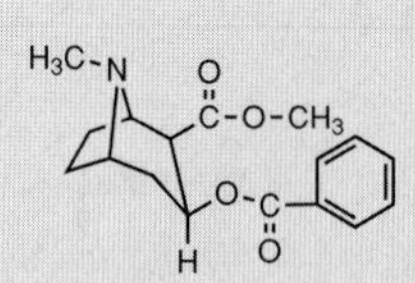

Cocaine

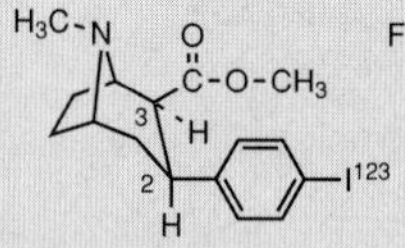

[^{123}I]-β-CIT (DopaScan®)

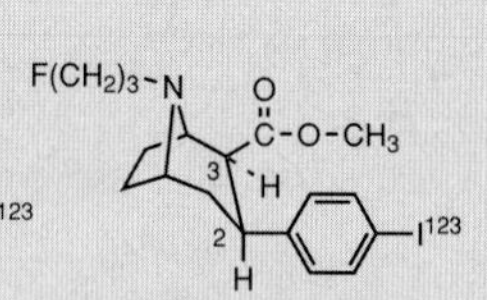

[^{123}I]-FP-CIT (DAT Scan®)

The first radiopharmaceutical to emerge from this research, [^{123}I]2-β-carbomethoxy-3β-(4-iodophenyl)tropane, is known as [^{123}I]β-CIT or RTI-55 (83,84). The radioactive iodine atom in the para position of the phenyl ring provides for the imaging properties of [^{123}I]β-CIT. A limiting factor with [^{123}I]β-CIT, however, is that it must be administered 8 hours before imaging to achieve peak uptake to dopamine nerve terminal regions. In an effort to improve the pharmacokinetic profile of [^{123}I]β-CIT, Neumeyer et al. (85) developed the N-3-fluoropropyl analogue of β-CIT, known as [^{123}I]FP-CIT. This dopamine nerve terminal imaging agent rapidly reaches its target sites (dopamine reuptake proteins) so that patients can be imaged 1 to 2 hours after injection of [^{123}I]FP-CIT. Moreover, researchers developed a radioligand suitable for PET imaging by replacement of the fluorine atom with [^{18}F] and replacement of the [^{123}I] atom with iodine in [^{123}I]FP-CIT (86). In Europe, [^{123}I]FP-CIT is approved for clinical use, and both [^{123}I]β-CIT and [^{123}I]FP-CIT are used as research tools to assess dopamine nerve terminal function in neurodegenerative and neuropsychiatric disorders.

relaxation without excessive sedation. Chloroxazone is another agent marketed as a skeletal muscle relaxant, but with unclear efficacy in spasmodic conditions. A considerable drawback to empirical use of chloroxazone is that idiosyncratic hepatotoxicity and several sensitivity reactions (urticaria, erythema, and pruritus) have been reported (88). Orphenadrine is an ethanolamine ether that is related both chemically and pharmacologically to diphenhydramine-type histamine H_1 antagonists. Although its efficacy is not clearly established, any muscle relaxant effects of orphenadrine may be caused by CNS anticholinergic activity, because this drug shows significant muscarinic receptor antagonism. Orphenadrine also is an NMDA receptor antagonist; however, it is unclear if this activity may lead to antispasmodic effects. The antimuscarinic activity of orphenadrine certainly leads to unpleasant peripheral side effects, such as dry mouth, blurred vision, and urinary retention. Cyclobenzaprine is another agent with prominent antimuscarinic activity that is used as a skeletal muscle relaxant, although its efficacy is modest. It is proposed that the muscle relaxant effects of cyclobenzaprine may result from antagonism of serotonin 5-HT_2 receptors in descending neurons of the spinal cord (93), but anticholinergic mechanisms cannot be ruled out. Although the presence of a double bond in the cycloheptyl ring of cyclobenzaprine is the only structural difference from the tricyclic antidepressant amitriptyline, cyclobenzaprine is not an efficacious antidepressant. Cyclobenzaprine has a long plasma half-life (1–3 days) and accumulation on multiple dosing contributes to its high incidence of sedation.

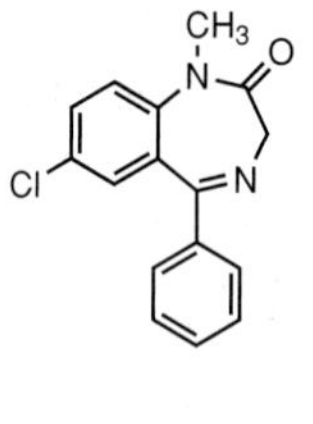

Diazepam (Valium)

DIAZEPAM. The second group of antispastic drugs to be developed were the benzodiazepines, typified by diazepam. Diazepam exerts its skeletal muscle relaxant effect by binding as an agonist at the benzodiazepine

Table 25.2. Skeletal Muscle Relaxants

Class and Generic Name	Trade Name	Chemical Structure	Initial Single Oral Dose
Glycerol monoethers and derivatives			
Mephenesin		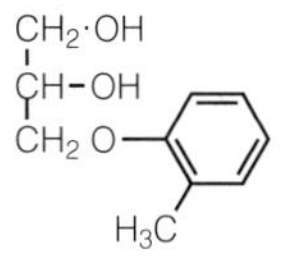 $CH_2 \cdot OH$ / CH–OH / CH_2 O–(2-methylphenyl)	1-2 g (oral)
Chlorphenesin carbamate	Maolate (R_1 = H, R_2 = Cl)	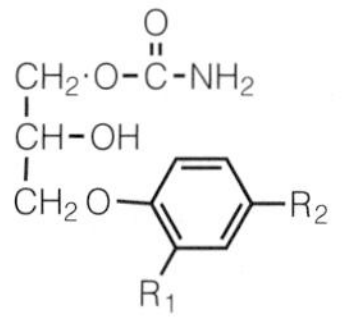 $CH_2 \cdot O-C(=O)-NH_2$ / CH–OH / CH_2 O–(phenyl with R_1, R_2)	800 mg (oral)
Methocarbamol	Robaxin ($R_1 = OCH_3$, R_2= H)		1-2 g (oral) 500 mg IM 1-3 g daily (IV)
Subtituted alkanediols and derivatives			
Meprobamate	Equanil Miltown (R = H)	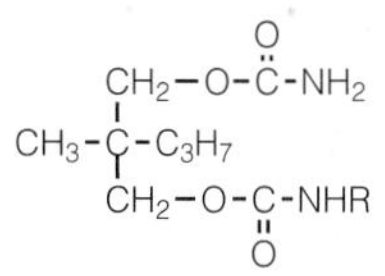 $CH_2-O-C(=O)-NH_2$ / $CH_3-C-C_3H_7$ / $CH_2-O-C(=O)-NHR$	400 mg
Carisoprodol	Rela Soma (R =$CH(CH_3)_2$)		250-350 mg
Metaxalone	Skelaxin	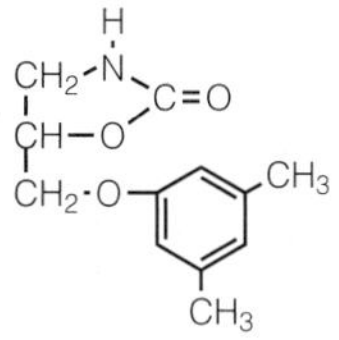 CH_2–NH–C(=O)–O–CH / $CH_2 \cdot O$–(3,5-dimethylphenyl)	800 mg
Benzazole			
Chlorzoxazone	Paraflex	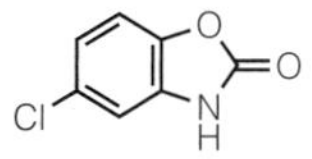 (5-chloro-benzoxazolone; Cl, O, =O, NH)	250-750 mg
Miscellaneous			
Orphenadrine citrate	Norflex	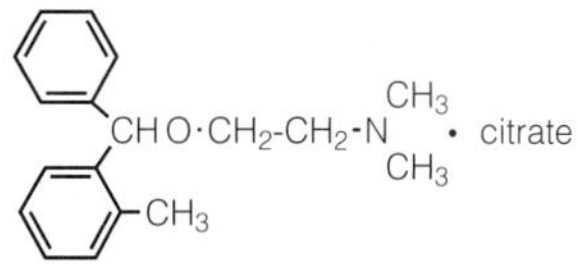 (phenyl)(2-methylphenyl)CH O·CH_2-CH_2·N(CH_3)$_2$ • citrate	100 mg (oral) 60 mg IM or IV
Cyclobenzaprine	Flexaril	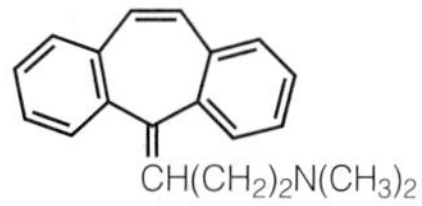 (dibenzocycloheptene)=$CH(CH_2)_2N(CH_3)_2$	10 mg

receptor of the $GABA_A$ receptor complex, which enhances GABA potency to increase chloride conductance (see Chapter 22). The muscle relaxant properties of classical benzodiazepines, such as diazepam, appear to be mediated mainly by the $GABA_A$ α_2 and α_3 subunits (94,95). The result is neuronal hyperpolarization, probably at both supraspinal and spinal sites for spasmolytic activity. Its actions are sufficient to relieve spasticity in patients with lesions affecting the spinal cord and in some patients with cerebral palsy (96). Few high-quality clinical trials have evaluated diazepam as a muscle relaxant, but these few suggest that diazepam is no more efficacious than, for example, carisoprodol, cyclobenzaprine, or tizanidine (i.e., efficacy is marginal) (87,88). Moreover, diazepam produces drowsiness and fatigue in most patients at doses required to significantly reduce muscle tone.

BACLOFEN. Baclofen (β-*p*-chlorophenyl-GABA) is a $GABA_B$ receptor agonist and is one of the most commonly used antispastic agents.

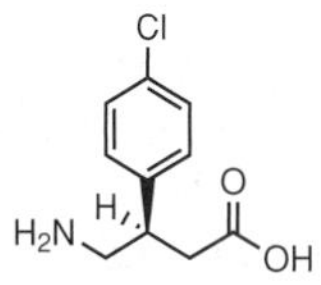

Cl, H_2N, H, O, OH

Baclofen
Racemic mixture (Lioresal)

The (*R*)-(−)-enantiomer is the active isomer at $GABA_B$ receptors, but the racemate (Lioresal) is approved for use as a spasmolytic agent. The molecular mechanisms of $GABA_B$ receptors in muscle spasticity are not understood any better than other putative receptor-based mechanisms discussed above. It is proposed that baclofen inhibits spinal cord monosynaptic and polysynaptic reflexes via $GABA_B$ receptor-mediated opening of neuronal potassium channels that leads to hyperpolarization of primary afferent fiber terminals. Baclofen also may reduce the release of excitatory neurotransmitters and substance P in the brain and/or spinal cord via $GABA_B$-mediated neuronal hyperpolarization (90,96). Adverse effects of oral baclofen include sedation, excessive weakness, vertigo, and psychological disturbances. It is used for the treatment of spasticity in paraplegia and quadriplegia, patients with multiple sclerosis, and traumatic lesion to the spinal cord (96). Baclofen is completely absorbed after oral administration, undergoes minimal hepatic metabolism, and is excreted mainly as the parent compound in urine and feces, with a half-life of approximately 3 to 4 hours. Intrathecal administration via an implanted infusion pump is used to control severe spasticity and pain that is not responsive to medication given by oral or other parenteral routes.

DANTROLENE. Dantrolene is a hydantoin derivative that acts peripherally to reduce spasticity and is indicated for use in spinal cord injury, stroke, cerebral palsy, and multiple sclerosis (97).

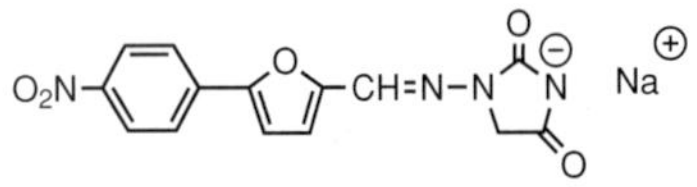

Dantrolene sodium (Dantrium)

The site of action of dantrolene is believed to be at the sarcoplasmic reticulum in skeletal muscle cells. Dantrolene binds to a calcium channel protein (ryanodine receptor) on the sarcoplasmic reticulum to close the channel and inhibit the release of calcium; the alkaloid ryanodine activates the same receptor to open the channel. Dantrolene is believed to act directly on the contractile mechanism of skeletal muscle to decrease the force of contraction in the absence of any demonstrated effects on neural pathways, on the neuromuscular junction, or on the excitable properties of the muscle fiber membranes (97). Cardiac muscle and smooth muscle are minimally affected by dantrolene, likely because calcium release from sarcoplasmic reticulum of these muscle cell types occurs via a mechanism that differs from skeletal muscle. The muscle relaxant effect of dantrolene on skeletal muscle, however, is not specific, and generalized muscle weakness occurs as a major adverse side effect. Like other hydantoins, dantrolene is a weak base (pK_a = 7.5) that can cross the blood-brain barrier; thus, CNS depressant side effects (e.g., sedation) are common. Dantrolene sodium salt is slowly absorbed from the gastrointestinal tract. The mean half-life of the drug in adults is approximately 9 hours after a 100-mg dose. It is slowly metabolized by the liver to give the 5-hydroxy and acetamido (nitro reduction and acetylation) metabolites, as well as unchanged drug, excreted in the urine. Interestingly, dantrolene also is valuable in alleviating the signs of malignant hyperthermia. This rare, genetically determined condition, which can be triggered by a variety of stimuli, including inhalation anesthetics and neuromuscular blocking drugs, involves an impaired ability of the sarcoplasmic reticulum to sequester calcium. For treating malignant hyperthermia, dantrolene is administered intravenously.

TIZANIDINE. Tizanidine is a centrally acting adrenergic α_2 receptor agonist used to treat chronic muscle spasticity conditions, such as multiple sclerosis.

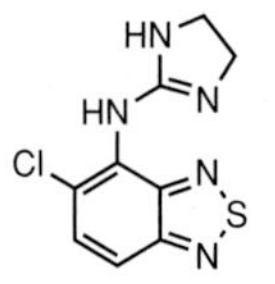

Tizanidine (Zanaflex)

Postulated mechanisms include α_2 receptor-mediated decreased release of norepinephrine and serotonin from spinal interneurons (98). Tizanidine is structurally related to the α_2 agonist clonidine that is used to treat hypertension; however, the blood pressure–lowering potency of tizanidine is approximately 10 to 20% that of clonidine. Nevertheless, patients may experience hypotension with tizanidine, together with muscle weakness, that may result in dizziness and falls in mobile patients. Tizanidine is rapidly and almost completely absorbed from the gastrointestinal tract; however, the estimated bioavailability is only 10 to 15% because of extensive first-pass metabolism, mainly by CYP1A2 (99), which results in oxidative degradation of the imidazoline ring and hydroxylation of the aromatic system (100). Elevated liver enzyme values are not frequent with tizanidine use. Hepatic injury and death because of liver failure have been reported, however, and this complication should be considered in view of its marginal antispasmodic efficacy (87,88). Other frequently reported side effects of tizanidine are drowsiness and dry mouth. Clonidine also has been used to treat spasticity; however, even less high-quality clinical study data are available for this agent.

ACKNOWLEDGEMENTS

The author wishes to express his gratitude to Drs. John L. Neumeyer and Ross J. Baldessarini for guidance in preparing this chapter.

CASE STUDY

Victoria F. Roche and S. William Zito

ST is a 68-year-old female who traded in her stressful job as an academic administrator at a major academic health center for the relaxed life of Northern California. Heading to "wine country" with her cats, retirement funds, and a few family heirlooms, she purposefully sought a new life, making new friends and doing the things she loves most. She's been very politically and culturally active in her community, and she thoroughly enjoys her job as the social events planner at a small, family-owned winery that is just now beginning to gain regional notoriety. Attendance at her nightly "wine and cheese" gatherings has increased dramatically over the past year, giving ST a chance to network with clients and to showcase the high quality of her employer's "vino."

Life seemed perfect until a diagnosis of Parkinson's disease was established three months ago. ST's symptoms are characteristic of this dopamine deficiency disorder and include rigidity, difficulty speaking, and slowed movements. She is still able to function at work but is obviously worried about what the future holds. She began levodopa therapy immediately (400 mg b.i.d.) but is struggling to cope with drug-induced nausea and vomiting severe enough to limit her usually passionate involvement with a local Parkinson's research advocacy group. In addition, although previously normotensive, she has experienced an increase in blood pressure that is now being treated with a thiazide diuretic.

You meet up with ST at a wine-tasting event at the vineyard, and in a private moment, she asks for your professional advice and counsel. Consider the structure of the compounds drawn below, and decide which might benefit this patient.

1. Identify the therapeutic problem(s) in which the pharmacist's intervention may benefit the patient.
2. Identify and prioritize the patient-specific factors that must be considered to achieve the desired therapeutic outcomes.
3. Conduct a thorough and mechanistically oriented structure-activity relationship analysis of all structures provided in the case.
4. Evaluate the structure–activity relationship findings against the patient-specific factors and desired therapeutic outcomes, and make a therapeutic decision.
5. Counsel your patient

HO, HO, CH_2–C–COOH, NH_2, H

Levodopa

H, N, NH_2

1

HO–C–CH_2 CH_2 N⊕, H_3C, ⊖ Cl

2

H, N⊕⊖ Cl, NH, O

3

N, CH_3

4

HO, HO, CH_2–C–COOH, NH_2, CH_3

5

References

1. Lang AE, Lozano AM. Parkinson's disease. Part 1. N Engl J Med 1998; 339:1044–1053.
2. Forno LS. Neuropathology of Parkinson's disease. J Neuropathol Exp Neurol 1996;55:259–272.
3. Lang AE, Lozano AM. Parkinson's disease. Part 2. N Engl J Med 1998; 339:1130–1143.
4. Parent A, Cicchetti F. The current model of basal ganglia organization under scrutiny. Mov Disord 1998; 13:199–202.
5. Semchuk KM, Love EJ, Lee RG. Parkinson's disease: a test of the multifactorial etiologic hypothesis. Neurology 1993;43:1173–1180.
6. Gwinn-Hardy K. Genetics of parkinsonism. Mov Disord 2002;17:645–656.
7. Polymeropoulos MH, Lavedan C, Leroy E, et al. Mutation in the α-synuclein gene identified in families with Parkinson's disease. Science 1997;276: 2045–2047.
8. Kruger R, Kuhn W, Muller T, et al. Ala30Pro mutation in the gene encoding α-synuclein in Parkinson's disease. Nat Genet 1998;18:106–108.
9. Goedert M. Familial Parkinson's disease. The awakening of α-synuclein. Nature 1997;388:232–233.
10. Norris EH, Giasson BI, Lee VM. α-Synuclein: normal function and role in neurodegenerative diseases. Curr Top Dev Biol 2004;60:17-54.
11. Jain S, Wood NW, Healy DG. Molecular genetic pathways in Parkinson's disease: a review. Clin Sci (Lond) 2005;109:355–364.
12. McNaught KS, Olanow CW. Protein aggregation in the pathogenesis of familial and sporadic Parkinson's disease. Neurobiol Aging 2006;27:530–545.
13. Ciechanover A, Brundin P. The ubiquitin–proteasome system in neurodegenerative diseases. Sometimes the chicken, sometimes the egg. Neuron 2003;40: 427–446.
14. Goldberg AL. Protein degradation and protection against misfolded or damaged proteins. Nature 2003;426:895–899.
15. Biskup S, Mueller JC, Sharma M, et al. Common variants of LRRK2 are not associated with sporadic Parkinson's disease. Ann Neurol 2005;58: 905–908.
16. Gasser T, Muller-Myhsok B, Wszolek ZK, et al. Genetic complexity and Parkinson's disease. Science 1997;277:388–389.
17. Scott WK, Staijich JM, Yamaoka LH, et al. Genetic complexity and Parkinson's disease. Deane Laboratory Parkinson Disease Research Group. Science 1997;277:387–388.
18. Ward CD, Duvoisin RC, Ince SE, et al. Parkinson's disease in 65 pairs of twins and in a set of quadruplets. Neurology 1983;33:815–824.
19. Gasser T. Genetics of Parkinson's disease. Curr Opin Neurol 2005;18: 363–369.
20. Baba M, Nakajo S, Tu PH, et al. Aggregation of α-synuclein in Lewy bodies of sporadic Parkinson's disease and dementia with Lewy bodies. Am J Pathol 1998;152:879–884.
21. Duvoisin RC. The cause of Parkinson's disease. In: Marsden CD, Fahn S, eds. Movement Disorders. London: Butterworth Scientific, 1982:8–24.

22. Gajdusek DC, Salazar AM. Amyotrophic lateral sclerosis and parkinsonian syndromes in high incidence among the Auyu and Jakai people of West New Guinea. Neurology 1982; 32:107–126.
23. Cotzias GC. Manganese in health and disease. Physiol Rev 1958; 38:503–532.
24. Barbeau A, Roy M, Cloutier T, et al. Environmental risk and genetic factors in the etiology of Parkinson's disease. In: Yahr M, Bergmann K, eds. Advances in Neurology, vol 45. New York: Raven Press, 1986:299–306.
25. Kessler II, Diamond EL. Epidemiologic studies of Parkinson's disease. I. Smoking and Parkinson's disease: a survey and explanatory hypothesis. Am J Epidemiol 1971;94:16–25.
26. Yu PH, Boulton AA. Irreversible inhibition of monoamine oxidase by some components of cigarette smoke. Life Sci 1987;41:675–682.
27. Langston JW, Irwin I, Ricaurte GA. Neurotoxins, parkinsonism, and Parkinson's disease. Pharmacology and Therapeutics 1987;32:19–49.
28. Haber F, Weiss J. The catalysis of hydrogen peroxide. Naturwissenschaften 1932;20:948–950.
29. Graham DG, Tiffany SM, Bell WR Jr, et al. Autoxidation versus covalent binding of quinones as the mechanism of toxicity of dopamine, 6-hydroxydopamine, and related compounds toward C1300 neuroblastoma cells in vitro. Mol Pharmacol 1978;14:644–653.
30. Graham DG. Catecholamine toxicity: a proposal for the molecular pathogenesis of manganese neurotoxicity and Parkinson's disease. Neurotoxicology 1984;5:83–95.
31. Calne DB, Langston JW, Martin WR, et al. Positron-emission tomography after MPTP: observations relating to the cause of Parkinson's disease. Nature 1985;317:246–248.
32. Carlsson A, Winblad B. Influence of age and time interval between death and autopsy on dopamine and 3-methoxytyramine levels in human basal ganglia. J Neural Transm 1976;38:271–276.
33. Riederer P, Woketich S. Time course of nigrostriatal degeneration in Parkinson's disease. A detailed study of influential factors in human brain amine analysis. J Neural Transm 1976;38:277–301.
34. Davis GC, Williams AC, Markey SP, et al. Chronic parkinsonism secondary to intravenous injection of meperidine analogues. Psychiatr Res 1979;1: 249–254.
35. Langston JW, Ballard P, Tetrud JW, et al. Chronic parkinsonism in humans due to a product of meperidine-analog synthesis. Science 1983;219:979–980.
36. Burns RS, Chiueh CC, Markey SP, et al. A primate model of parkinsonism: selective destruction of dopaminergic neurons in the pars compacta of the substantia nigra by N-methyl-4-phenyl-1,2,3,6-tetrahydropyridine. Proc Natl Acad Sci U S A 1983;80:4546–4550.
37. Chiba K, Trevor A, Castagnoli N Jr. Metabolism of the neurotoxic tertiary amine, MPTP, by brain monoamine oxidase. Biochem Biophys Res Commun 1984;120:574–578.
38. Salach JI, Singer TP, Castagnoli N Jr, et al. Oxidation of the neurotoxic amine 1-methyl-4-phenyl-1,2,3,6-tetrahydropyridine (MPTP) by monoamine oxidases A and B and suicide inactivation of the enzymes by MPTP. Biochem Biophys Res Commun 1984;125:831–835.
39. Peterson LA, Caldera PS, Trevor A, et al. Studies on the 1-methyl-4-phenyl-2,3-dihydropyridinium species 2,3-$MPDP^+$, the monoamine oxidase catalyzed oxidation product of the nigrostriatal toxin 1-methyl-4-phenyl-1,2,3,6-tetrahydropyridine (MPTP). J Med Chem 1985;28:1432–1436.
40. Langston JW, Irwin I, Langston EB, et al. Pargyline prevents MPTP-induced parkinsonism in primates. Science 1984; 225:1480–1482.
41. Snyder SH, D'Amato RJ. MPTP: a neurotoxin relevant to the pathophysiology of Parkinson's disease. The 1985 George C. Cotzias Lecture. Neurology 1986;36:250–258.
42. Yong VW, Perry TL. Monoamine oxidase B, smoking, and Parkinson's disease. J Neurol Sci 1986;72:265–272.
43. Nefzger MD, Quadfasel FA, Karl VC. A retrospective study of smoking in Parkinson's disease. Am J Epidemiol 1968;88:149–158.
44. Behmand RA, Harik SI. Nicotine enhances 1-methyl-4-phenyl-1,2,36-tetrahydropyridine neurotoxicity. J Neurochem 1992;58:776–779.
45. Shahi GS, Das PN, Moochhala SM. 1-Methyl-4-phenyl-1,2,36-tetrahydropyridine-induced neurotoxicity: partial protection against striato-nigral dopamine depletion in C57BL/6J mice by cigarette smoke exposure and by β-naphthoflavone-pretreatment. Neurosci Lett 1991;127:247–250.
46. Berry MD, Juorio AV, Paterson IA. The functional role of monoamine oxidases A and B in the mammalian central nervous system. Prog Neurobiol 1994;42:375–391.
47. Javitch JA, D'Amato RJ, Strittmatter SM, et al. Parkinsonism-inducing neurotoxin, N-methyl-4-phenyl-1,2,3,6-tetrahydropyridine: uptake of the metaboliteN-methyl-4-phenylpyridine by dopamine neurons explains selective toxicity. Proc Natl Acad Sci U S A 1985;82:2173–2177.
48. Vyas I, Heikkila RE, Nicklas WJ. Studies on the neurotoxicity of 1-methyl-4-phenyl-1,2,3,6-tetrahydropyridine: inhibition of NAD-linked substrate oxidation by its metabolite, 1-methyl-4-phenylpyridinium. J Neurochem 1986;46: 1501–1507.
49. Ramsay RR, McKeown KA, Johnson EA, et al. Inhibition of NADH oxidation by pyridine derivatives. Biochem Biophys Res Commun 1987;146:53–60.
50. Castagnoli N Jr, Rimoldi JM, Bloomquist J, et al. Potential metabolic bioactivation pathways involving cyclic tertiary amines and aza-arenes. Chem Res Toxicol 1997;10:924–940.
51. Watanabe H, Muramatsu Y, Kurosaki R et al. Protective effects of neuronal nitric oxide synthase inhibitor in mouse brain against MPTP neurotoxicity: an immunohistological study. Eur Neuropsychopharmacol 2004;14: 93–104.
52. Schapira AH, Mann VM, Cooper JM, et al. Mitochondrial function in Parkinson's disease. The Royal Kings and Queens Parkinson's Disease Research Group. Ann Neurol 1992;32:S116–S124.
53. Mann VM, Cooper JM, Krige D, et al. Brain, skeletal muscle, and platelet homogenate mitochondrial function in Parkinson's disease. Br Res 1992;115:33–42.
54. The Parkinson's Disease Study Group. Impact of tocopherol and deprenyl in DATATOP subjects not requiring levodopa. Ann Neurol 1996;39:29–36.
55. The Parkinson's Disease Study Group. Impact of tocopherol and deprenyl in DATATOP subjects requiring levodopa. Ann Neurol 1996 39:37–45.
56. Macleod AD, Counsell CE, Ives N, et al. Monoamine oxidase B inhibitors for early Parkinson's disease. Cochrane Database Syst Rev 2005;3:CD004898, www.cochrane.org/reviews/en/ab004898.html. Accessed April 2007.
57. Olanow CW, Agid Y, Mizuno Y, et al. Levodopa in the treatment of Parkinson's disease: current controversies. Mov Disord 2004;19:997–1005.
58. Rajput AH, Uitti RJ, Offord KO. Timely levodopa administration prolongs survival in Parkinson's disease. Parkinsonism and Related Disorders 1997;3: 159–165.
59. Cotzias GC, Van Woert MH, Schiffer LM. Aromatic amino acids and modification of parkinsonism. N Engl J Med 1967;276:374–379.
60. Nagatssu T. In: Biochemistry of Catecholamines. Baltimore: University Park Press, 1973:289–651.
61. Vogel WH. Determination and physiological disposition of p-methoxyphenylethylamine in the rat. Biochem Pharmacol 1970;19:2663–2665.
62. Miyawaki E, Lyons K, Pahwa R. Motor complications of chronic levodopa therapy in Parkinson's disease. Clin Neuropharmacol 1997;20:523–530.
63. Glezer S, Finberg JP. Pharmacological comparison between the actions of methamphetamine and 1-aminoindan stereoisomers on sympathetic nervous function in rat vas deferens. Eur J Pharmacol 2003;472:173–177.
64. Lautala P, Ulmanen I, Taskinen J. Molecular mechanisms controlling the rate and specificity of catechol O-methylation by human soluble catechol O-methyltransferase. Mol Pharmacol 2001;59:393–402.
65. Gordin A, Kaakkola S, Teravainen H. Clinical advantages of COMT inhibition with entacapone—a review. J Neural Transm 2004;111:1343–1363.
66. Korlipara LV, Cooper JM, Schapira AH. Differences in toxicity of the catechol-O-methyl transferase inhibitors, tolcapone and entacapone, to cultured human neuroblastoma cells. Neuropharmacology 2004;46:562–569.
67. Haasio K, Nissinen E, Sopanen L, et al. Different toxicological profile of two COMT inhibitors in vivo: the role of uncoupling effects. J Neural Transm 2002;109:1391–1401.
68. Tafazoli S, Spehar DD, O'Brien PJ. Oxidative stress mediated idiosyncratic drug toxicity. Drug Metab Rev 2005;37:311–332.
69. Kurth MC, Adler CH, St. Hilaire MS, et al. Tolcapone improves motor function and reduces levodopa requirement in patients with Parkinson's disease experiencing motor fluctuations: a multicenter, double-blind, randomized, placebo-controlled trial. Neurology 1997;48:81–87.
70. Geldenhuys WJ, Malan SF, Bloomquist JR, et al. Pharmacology and structure–activity relationships of bioactive polycyclic cage compounds: a focus on pentacycloundecane derivatives. Med Res Rev 2005;25:21-48.
71. Parkinson Study Group. Pramipexole vs. levodopa as initial treatment for Parkinson's disease: a randomized, controlled trial. JAMA 2000;284: 1931–1938.
72. Rascol O, Brooks DJ, Korczyn AD, et al. A five-year study of the incidence of dyskinesia in patients with early Parkinson's disease who were treated with ropinirole or levodopa. 056 Study Group. N Engl J Med 2000;342: 1484–1491.
73. Perachon S, Schwartz JC, Sokoloff P. Functional potencies of new antiparkinsonian drugs at recombinant human dopamine D_1, D_2, and D_3 receptors. Eur J Pharmacol 1999;366:293–300.
74. Parkinson Study Group. Dopamine transporter brain imaging to assess the effects of pramipexole vs levodopa on Parkinson's disease progression. JAMA 2002;287:1653–1661.
75. Booth RG, Baldessarini RJ, Kula NS, et al. Presynaptic inhibition of dopamine synthesis in rat striatal tissue by enantiomeric mono- and dihydroxyaporphines. Mol Pharmacol 1990;38:92–101.
76. Neumeyer JL, Baldessarini RJ. Apomorphine: new uses for an old drug. Pharmaceutical News 1997;4:12–16.
77. Giesecke J. The absolute configuration of apomorphine. Acta Cryst 1977;B33:302–303.
78. Neumeyer JL, McCarthy M, Battista S, et al. Aporphines. 9. The synthesis and pharmacological evaluations of (±)-9,10-dihyroxyaporphine, ([±]-isoapomorphine), (±)-, (−)-, and (+)-1,2-dihydroxyaporphine, and (+)-1,2,9,10-tetrahydroxyaprophine. J Med Chem 1973;16:1228–1233.
79. Westerink BHC, Dijkstra D, et al. Dopaminergic pro-drugs: brain concentrations and neurochemical effects of 5,6- and 6,7-ADTN after administration as dibenzoyl esters. Eur J Pharmacol 1980;61:7–15.
80. Wilcox RE, Tseng T, Brusniak MY, et al. CoMFA-based prediction of agonist affinities at recombinant D_1 vs D_2 dopamine receptors. J Med Chem 1998;41:4385–4399.

81. Garnett ES, Firnau G, Chan PKH, et al. [^{18}F]Fluoro-dopa, and analogue of dopa, and its use in direct external measurements of storage, degradation, and turnover of intracerebral dopamine. Proc Natl Acad Sci USA 1978;75: 464–467.
82. Volkow N, Fowler J, Wang G, et al. Decreased dopamine transporters with age in healthy human subjects. Ann Neurol 1994;36:237–239.
83. Neumeyer JL, Wang S, Milius R, et al. [^{123}I]-2β-carbomethoxy-3β-(4-iodophenyl)tropane: high-affinity SPECT radiotracer of monoamine reuptake sites in brain. J Med Chem 1991;34: 3144–3146.
84. Innis R, Seibyl J, Scanley B, et al. Single-photon emission computed tomographic imaging demonstrates loss of striatal dopamine transporters in Parkinson disease. Proc Natl Acad Sci U S A 1993;90:11965–11969.
85. Neumeyer JL, Wang S, Gao Y, et al. N-(w-fluoroalkyl analogues of (1R)-2β-carbomethoxy-3β-(4-iodophenyl) tropane (β-CIT): radiotracers for PET and SPECT imaging of dopamine transporters. J Med Chem 1994;37: 1558–1561.
86. Ishikawa T, Dhawan V, Kazumata K, et al. Comparative nigrostriatal dopaminergic imaging with [^{123}I]β-CIT-FP/SPECT and [^{18}F]F-DOPA/PET. J Nucl Med 1996;37:1760–1765.
87. Montane E, Vallano A, Laporte JR. Oral antispastic drugs in nonprogressive neurologic diseases: a systematic review. Neurology 2004;63:1357–1363.
88. Beebe FA, Barkin RL, Barkin S. A clinical and pharmacologic review of skeletal muscle relaxants for musculoskeletal conditions. Am J Ther 2005;12: 151–171.
89. Young RR, Delwaide PJ. Drug therapy: spasticity (first of two parts). N Engl J Med 1981;304:28–33.
90. Gracies JM, Nance P, Elovic E, et al. Traditional pharmacological treatments for spasticity. Part II: general and regional treatments. Muscle Nerve Suppl 1997;6:S92–S120.
91. Berger FM, Bradley W. The pharmacological properties of an alpha, beta-dihydroxy-gama-(2-methylphenoxy)-propane (Myanesisn). Br J Pharmacol Chemother 1946;1:265–272.
92. Souri E, Sharifzadeh M, Farsam H, et al. Muscle relaxant activity of methocarbamol enantiomers in mice. J Pharm Pharmacol 1999;51: 853–855.
93. Kobayashi H, Hasegawa Y, Ono H. Cyclobenzaprine, a centrally acting muscle relaxant, acts on descending serotonergic systems. Eur J Pharmacol 1996;5:29–35.
94. Crestani F, Low K, Keist R, et al. Molecular targets for the myelorelaxant action of diazepam. Mol Pharmacol 2001;59:442–445.
95. Basile AS, Lippa AS, Skolnick P. Anxioselective anxiolytics: can less be more? Eur J Pharmacol 2004;500:441–451.
96. Young RR, Delwaide PJ. Drug therapy: spasticity (second of two parts). N Engl J Med 1981;304:96–99.
97. Zafonte R, Lombard L, Elovic E. Antispasticity medications: uses and limitations of enteral therapy. Am J Phys Med Rehabil 2004;83:S50–S58.
98. Coward DM. Tizanidine: neuropharmacology and mechanism of action. Neurology 1994;44:S6–S10.
99. Granfors TM, Backman JT, Laitila J, et al. Tizanidine is mainly metabolized by cytochrome P450 1A2 in vitro. Br J Clin Pharmacol 2004;**57**:349–353.
100. Koch P, Hirst DR, von Wartburg BR. Biological fate of sirdalud in animals and man. Xenobiotica 1989;19:1255–1265.

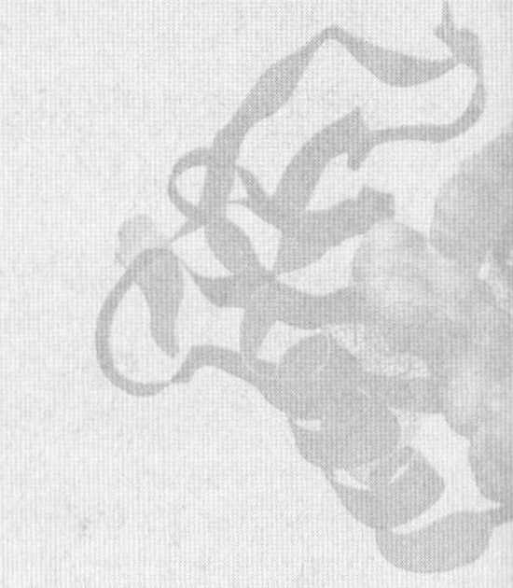

26. *Cardiac Agents: Cardiac Glycosides, Antianginal, and Antiarrhythmic Drugs*

AHMED S. MEHANNA

DRUGS COVERED IN THIS CHAPTER:

CARDIAC GLYCOSIDES POSITIVE INOTROPIC DRUGS
- Digoxin
- Digitalis products
- Digitoxin BP
- Lanatoside C BP
- Ouabain BP (G-Strophanthin)
- Deslanatoside C BP

NONGLYCOSIDIC POSITIVE INOTROPIC DRUGS
- Inamrinone
- Dobutamine
- Milrinone

ANTIANGINAL NITRATES AND NITRITES
- Amyl nitrite (isoamyl nitrite)
- Nitroglycerin
- Isosorbide dinitrate
- Erythrityl tetranitrate
- Pentaerythritol tetranitrate
- Nesiritide citrate

NITRIC OXIDE DONOR
- Molsidomine

CALCIUM CHANNEL BLOCKERS
- Verapamil
- Diltiazem
- Nifedipine
- Nicardipine
- Amlodipine
- Felodipine
- Nitredipine
- Bepridil

MODULATORS OF MYOCARDIAL METABOLISM
- Ranotazine

ANTIARRHYTHMIC AGENTS
- Class IA
  - Quinidine
  - Procainamide
  - Disopyramide
- Class IB
  - Lidocaine
  - Phenytoin
  - Tocainide
  - Mexiletine
- Class IC
  - Flecainide
  - Encainide
  - Propafenone
  - Moricizine
- Class II
  - Propranolol
- Class III
  - Sotalol
  - Ibutilide
  - Dofetilide
  - Bretylium
  - Amiodarone
- Class IV
  - Verapamil
  - Diltiazem
  - Bepridil

Those drugs with BP (British Pharmacopeia) designation are available only in Canada and countries other than the United States.

Heart diseases are grouped into three major disorders: cardiac failure or contractile dysfunction, ischemic heart disease (with angina as its primary symptom), and cardiac arrhythmia.

DRUGS FOR THE TREATMENT OF HEART FAILURE

Congestive Heart Failure

Cardiac failure can be described as inability of the heart to pump blood effectively at a rate that meets the needs of metabolizing tissues. This is the direct result of a reduced contractility of the cardiac muscles, especially those of the ventricles, which causes a decrease in cardiac output, increasing the blood volume of the heart (hence the term "congested"). As a result, the systemic blood pressure and the renal blood flow are both reduced, which often lead to the development of edema in the lower extremities and the lung (pulmonary edema) as well as renal failure. A group of drugs known as the cardiac glycosides were found to reverse most of these symptoms and complications.

Drugs for the Treatment of Congestive Heart Failure

CARDIAC GLYCOSIDES: POSITIVE IONOTROPIC DRUGS. The cardiac glycosides are an important class of naturally occurring drugs, the actions of which include both beneficial and toxic effects on the heart. Their desirable cardiotonic action is of particular benefit in the treatment of congestive heart failure (CHF) and associated edema, and their preparations have been used as medicinal agents as well as poisons since 1500 BC. This dual application serves to highlight the toxic potential for this class of life-saving drugs. Despite the extended use and obvious therapeutic benefits of the cardiac glycosides, it was not until the famous monograph by William Withering in 1785, "An Account of the Foxglove and Some of its Medical Uses," that cardiac glycoside therapy started to become more standardized and rational (1–3). The therapeutic use of purified cardiac glycoside preparations has occurred only over the last century. Today, the cardiac glycosides represent one of the most important drug classes available to the physician for the treatment of treat CHF.

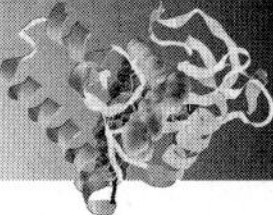

CLINICAL SIGNIFICANCE

Cardiovascular disease is by far the leading cause of death in industrialized nations. Although improved treatments have lowered this death rate, an additional result is a growing number of patients who are surviving with diseased hearts and who require intensive drug therapy regimens.

The cardiac glycosides and, most recently, digoxin have been used for centuries, but only within the last decade has their role been clarified by modern clinical trials. Still, many questions remain, including the precise mechanism(s) of action beyond the positive inotropic effect, the ideal dose and serum concentration, and the best methods to avoid toxicity and drug interactions. In particular, understanding how the structure of digoxin affects its pharmacokinetics allows the clinician to anticipate problems when it is used with potentially interacting drugs or in patients with organ dysfunction.

In many clinical situations, antiarrhythmic drugs have given way to implantable defibrillators for potentially life-threatening arrhythmias, but they are still commonly used both as adjunct therapy and in other arrhythmias, such as atrial fibrillation. The sheer number of antiarrhythmic agents with diverse mechanisms of action and the possibility of serious or even lethal adverse effects makes understanding how the structure of these drugs contributes to their efficacy and toxicity a high priority for pharmacists.

Jeffrey T. Sherer, Pharm.D., MPH, BCPS, CGP
Clinical Assistant Professor
University of Houston College of Pharmacy

Chemistry of the cardiac glycosides. Cardiac glycosides and other similar glycosides are composed of two portions: the sugar moiety, and the nonsugar (the aglycone) moiety.

Aglycones. The aglycone portion of the cardiac glycosides is a steroid nucleus with a unique set of fused rings, which makes these agents easily distinguished from the other steroids. Rings A-B and C-D are *cis* fused, whereas rings B-C have a *trans* configuration. Such ring fusion gives the aglycone nucleus of cardiac glycosides the characteristic "U-shape," as shown in Figure 26.1. The steroid nucleus also carries, in most cases, two angular methyl groups at C-10 and C-13. Hydroxyl groups are located at C-3, the site of the sugar attachment, and at C-14. The C-14 hydroxyl is normally unsubstituted; however, additional hydroxyl groups may be found at C-12 and C-16, the presence or absence of which distinguishes the important genins: digitoxigenin, digoxigenin, and gitoxigenin (Fig. 26.2). These additional hydroxyl groups have significant impact on the partitioning and pharmacokinetics for each glycoside, as discussed later.

The lactone ring at C-17 is another major structural feature of the cardiac aglycones. The size and degree of unsaturation of the lactone ring varies with the source of the glycoside. In most cases, the cardiac glycosides of plant origin, the cardenolides, possess a 5-membered, α,β-unsaturated lactone ring, whereas those derived from animal origin, the bufadienolides, possess a 6-membered lactone ring with two conjugated double bonds (generally referred to as α-pyrone) (Fig. 26.1).

Sugars. The hydroxyl group at C-3 of the aglycone portion usually is conjugated to a monosaccharide or a polysaccharide with β-1,4-glucosidic linkages. The number and identity of sugars vary from one glycoside to another, as

R'	Class
	Cardenolide (digitoxigenin shown)
	Bufadienolide (bufalin shown)

Fig. 26.1. Cardenolide and bufadienolide aglycones.

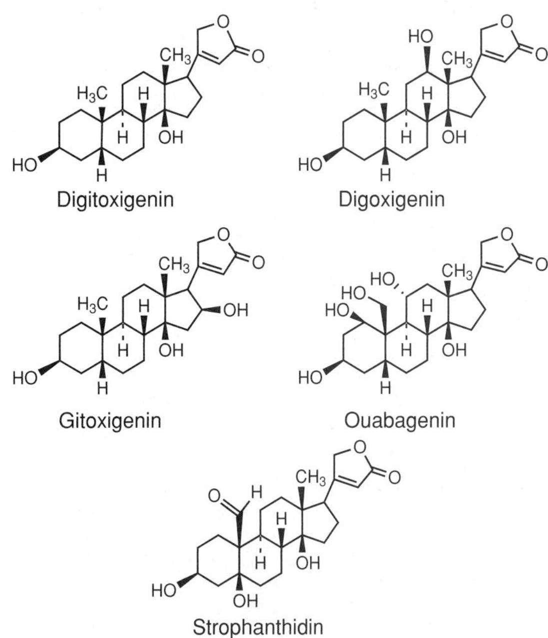

Fig. 26.2. Major cardenolide aglycones.

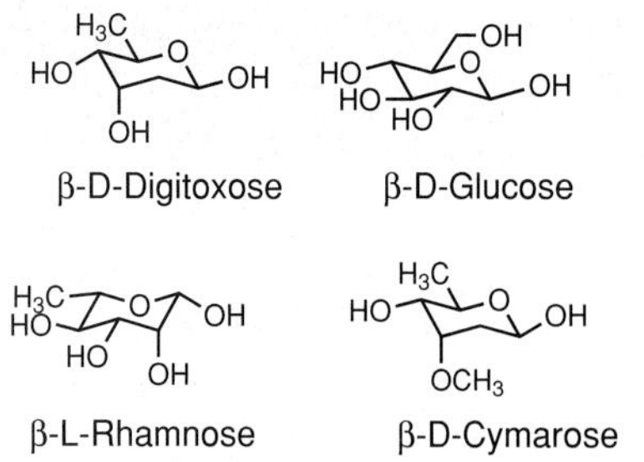

β-D-Digitoxose β-D-Glucose

β-L-Rhamnose β-D-Cymarose

Fig. 26.3. Selected sugars found in naturally occurring cardiac glycosides.

detailed subsequently. The most commonly found sugars in the cardiac glycosides are D-glucose, D-digitoxose, L-rhamnose, and D-cymarose (Fig. 26.3). These sugars predominately exist in the cardiac glycosides in the β-conformation. In some cases, the sugars exist in the acetylated form. The presence of an O-acetyl group on a sugar greatly affects the lipophilic character and pharmacokinetics of the entire glycoside, as discussed subsequently.

Sources and common names of cardiac glycosides. The cardiac glycosides occur mainly in plants and, in rare cases, in animals, such as poisonous toads. *Digitalis purpurea* or the foxglove plant, *Digitalis lanata, Strophanthus gratus,* and *Strophanthus kombe* are the major plant sources of the cardiac glycosides. Based on the nature and number of sugar molecules and the number of hydroxyl groups on the aglycone moiety, each combination of sugars and aglycones assumes different generic names. The site of the glycosides concentration in the plant, the types of glycosides, and the names of the structural components of these glycosides are summarized in Table 26.1.

Digitalis lanata. Lanatoside A is composed of the aglycone digitoxigenin (genin indicates no sugar) connected to three digitoxose sugar molecules, the third of which carries a 3-acetyl group, and a terminal glucose molecule. In other words, the structure sequence is glucose$_4$-3-acetyldigitoxose$_3$-digitoxose$_2$-digitoxose$_1$-digitoxigenin.

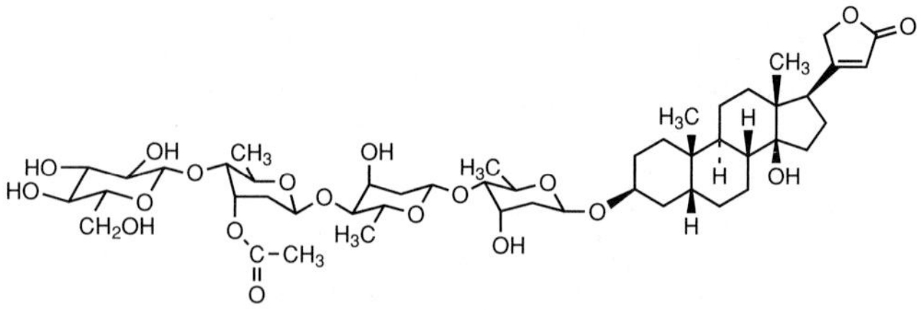

Lanatoside A

Lanatoside B has the identical sugar portion to lanatoside A, except that the aglycone has extra hydroxyl group at C-16 and is given the name gitoxigenin. The structural sequence is glucose$_4$-3-acetyldigitoxose$_3$-digitoxose$_2$-digitoxose$_1$-gitoxigenin.

Lanatoside C also has the same sugars found in both lanatosides A and B; however, the aglycone has the nucleus of lanatoside A plus an additional hydroxyl group at C-12. This cardenolide is named digoxigenin. The structural sequence is glucose$_4$-3-acetyldigitoxose$_3$-digitoxose$_2$-digitoxose$_1$-digoxigenin.

Partial hydrolysis of the glucose molecule and the acetate group from lanatoside A and C produces, respectively, two new and most important cardiac glycosides, digitoxin and digoxin, with the following sequences: digitoxin, (digitoxose)$_3$-digitoxigenin; and digoxin, (digitoxose)$_3$-digoxigenin.

Digitalis purpurea. Purpurea glycosides A and B have structures identical to those of lanatosides A and B, but with no acetyl group on the third digitoxose. Therefore, the purpurea glycosides A and B sometimes are called desacetyl digilanides A and B. Their sequences are as follows: purpurea glycoside A, glucose-(digitoxose)$_3$-digitoxigenin; and purpurea glycoside B, glucose-(digitoxose)$_3$-gitoxigenin. There is no purpurea glycoside C.

Table 26.1. Selected Natural Cardiac Glycosides and Their Sources

Source	Glycoside	Aglycone	Sugar[a]
Digitalis lanata (leaf)	Lanatoside A (digilanide A)	Digitoxigenin	Glucose-3-acetyldigitoxose-digitoxose-digitoxose
	Lanatoside B (digilanide B)	Gitoxigenin	
	Lanatoside C (digilanide C)	Digoxigenin	
Digitalis purpurea (leaf)	Purpurea glycoside A (desacetyl digilanide A)	Digitoxigenin	Glucose-digitoxose-digitoxose-digitoxose
	Purpurea glycoside B (desacetyl digilanide B)	Gitoxigenin	
Strophanthus gratus (seed)	G-Strophanthin	Oubagenin	Rhamnose
Strophanthus kombe (seed)	k-Strophanthoside	Strophanthidin	Glucose-glucose-cymarose

[a]Conjugated with the C-3 hydroxyl of the aglycone via the sugar to the far right. All sugars are conjugated via β-1,4-glucosidic bond.

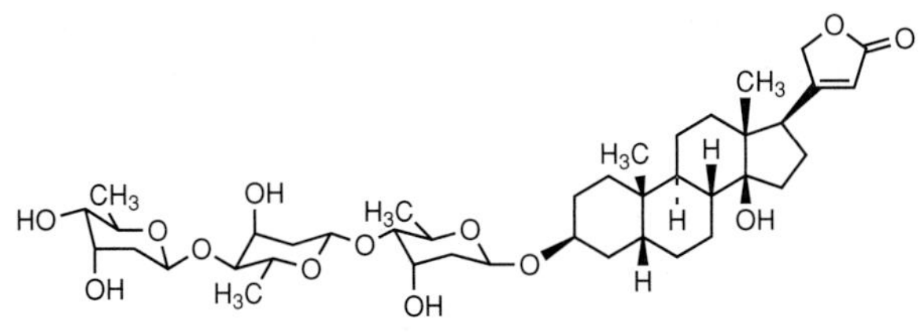

Digitoxin

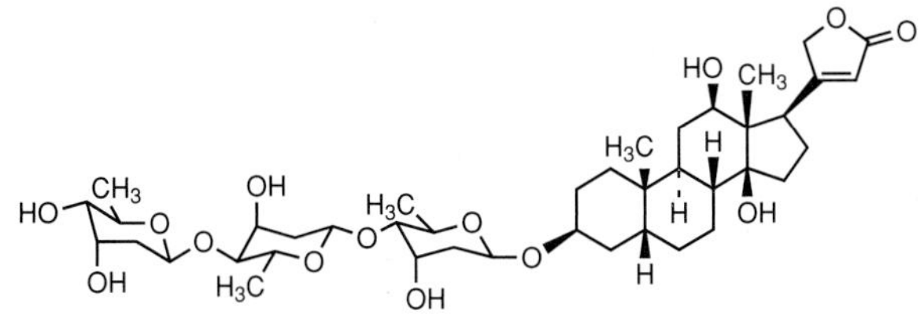

Digoxin

Strophanthus gratus and Strophanthus kombe. The glycosides extracted from the plants *Strophanthus gratus* and *Strophanthus kombe* are called g-strophanthin (or ouabain) and k-strophanthoside, respectively. The corresponding aglycone for ouabain is ouabagenin, and that for k-strophanthoside is strophanthidin. Ouabagenin has a polyhydroxylated steroidal nucleus, and strophanthidin has an additional hydroxyl group at C-5 with an angular aldehyde group at C-10, replacing the traditional methyl group at that position (Fig. 26.2). Ouabagenin is conjugated only to a single molecule of L-rhamnose, whereas strophanthidin is conjugated to a molecule of cymarose, which is further linked to two molecules of glucose.

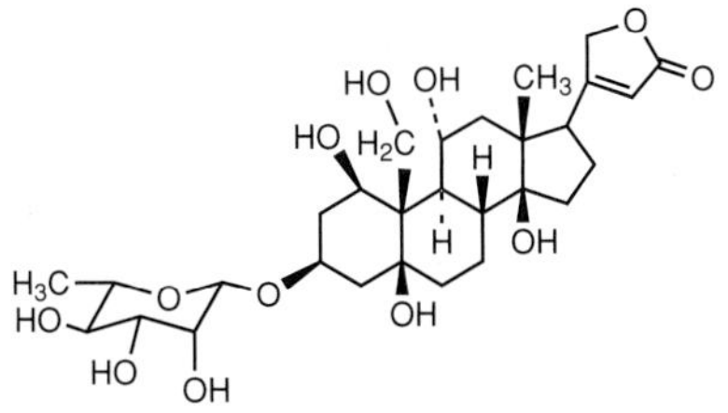

Ouabain

The medicinally used preparations are mainly obtained from *Digitalis purpurea* and *Digitalis lanata* plants. These glycosides generally are referred to as digitalis glycosides, cardiac glycosides, or simply, cardenolides. *Strophanthus* glycosides (e.g., ouabain) are no longer used therapeutically but were previously administered only intravenously because of poor oral absorption. Cardiac glycosides from animal sources (generally referred to as bufadienolides) are rare and of far less medicinal importance because of their high toxicity. Pharmaceutical preparations of whole plants and partially hydrolyzed glycosides of *Digitalis lanata* and *Digitalis purpurea* have been widely used clinically. Advancements in isolation and purification techniques, however, have made it possible to obtain highly purified digoxin preparations.

Pharmacology. Cardiac glycosides affect the heart in a dual fashion, both directly (on the cardiac muscle and the specialized conduction system of sinoatrial [SA] node, atrioventricular [AV] node, and His-Purkinje system) and indirectly (on the cardiovascular system mediated by the autonomic nervous reflexes). The combined direct and indirect effects of the cardiac glycosides lead to changes in the electrophysiological properties of the heart, including alteration of the contractility; heart rate; excitability; conductivity; refractory period; and automaticity of the atrium, ventricle, Purkinje fibers, AV node, and SA node. The heart response to the cardiac glycosides is a dose-dependent process and varies considerably between the normal hear and the heart with CHF. The effects observed after the administration of low doses (therapeutic doses) differ considerably from those observed at high doses (cardiotoxic doses). The pharmacological effects discussed consequently relate mainly to therapeutic doses administered to patients with CHF. The effects of cardiac glycosides on the properties of the heart muscle and different sites of the conduction system are summarized in Table 26.2. The increased force and rate of myocardial contraction (positive inotropic effect) and the prolongation of the refractory period of the AV node are the effects most relevant to the CHF problem. Both of these effects result from the direct action of the cardiac glycosides on the heart. The indirect effects are manifested as increased vagal nerve activity, which probably results from the glycoside-induced sensitization of the baroreceptors of the carotid sinus to changes in the arterial pressure; in other words, any given increase in the arterial blood pressure results in an increase in the vagal activity (parasympathetic) coupled with a greater decrease in the sympathetic activity. The vagal effect with uncompensated sympathetic response results in decreased heart rate and decreased peripheral vascular resistance (afterload). Therefore, cardiac glycosides reverse most of the symptoms associated with CHF as a result of increased sympathetic system activity, including increased heart rate, vascular resistance, and afterload. The administration of cardiac glycosides to a patient with CHF increases cardiac muscle contraction, reduces heart rate, and decreases both edema and the heart size.

Table 26.2. Effects of Cardiac Glycosides on the Heart

		Purkinje	AV	SA	
	Atrium	Ventricle	Fiber	Node	Node
Contractility	↑	↑	—	—	—
Excitability	0	Variable	↑	—	—
Conductivity	↑	↑	↓	↓	—
Refractory period	↓	↓	↑	↑	—
Automaticity	—	—	↑	—	↓

AV, atrioventricular; SA, sinoatrial; ↑ increased action; ↓ decreased action; 0, no action; —, no data available.

Biochemical mechanism of action. The mechanism whereby cardiac glycosides cause a positive inotropic effect and electrophysiological changes is still not completely known despite years of active investigation. Several mechanisms have been proposed, but the most widely accepted mechanism involves the ability of cardiac glycosides to inhibit the membrane-bound Na^+/K^+–adenosine triphosphatase (Na^+/K^+-ATPase) pump responsible for sodium/potassium exchange. To understand better the correlation between the pump and the mechanism of action of cardiac glycosides on the heart muscle contraction, one has to consider the sequence of events associated with cardiac action potential that ultimately leads to muscular contraction. The process of membrane depolarization/repolarization is controlled mainly by the movement of the three ions, Na^+, K^+, Ca^{2+}, in and out of the cell.

At the resting state (no contraction), the concentration of sodium is high outside the cell. On membrane depolarization, Na^+ fluxes in, leading to an immediate elevation of the action potential. Elevated intracellular sodium triggers the influx of Ca^{2+}, which occurs slowly and is represented by the plateau region of the cardiac action potential. The influx of calcium results in efflux of potassium out of the myocardium. The Na^+/K^+ exchange occurs at a later stage of the action potential to restore the membrane potential to its normal level (for further detail, see the discussion of antiarrhythmic agents and their classification at the end of this chapter). The Na^+/K^+ exchange requires energy and is catalyzed by the enzyme Na^+/K^+-ATPase. Cardiac glycosides are proposed to inhibit this enzyme, with a net result of reduced sodium exchange with potassium (i.e., increased intracellular sodium), which in turn results in increased intracellular calcium. Elevated intracellular calcium concentration triggers a series of intracellular biochemical events that ultimately result in an increase in the force of the myocardial contraction, or a positive inotropic effect. (The events that lead to muscle contraction are covered in further detail in the discussion of the mechanism of action of the calcium channel blockers later in this chapter.)

This mechanism of the cardiac glycosides via inhibiting the Na^+/K^+-ATPase pump is in agreement with the fact that the action of the cardiac glycosides is enhanced by low extracellular potassium and inhibited by high extracellular potassium. The cardiac glycosides–induced changes in the electrophysiology of the heart also can be explained based on the inhibition of Na^+/K^+-ATPase. It has been suggested that the intracellular loss of potassium because of inhibition of the pump causes a decrease in the cellular transmembrane potential approaching zero. This decrease in the membrane potential is sufficient to explain the increased excitability and other electrophysiological effects observed following cardiac glycosides administration.

Structural requirements for intrinsic activity. Many hypotheses have been put forth to explain the cardiac glycoside structure–activity relationships (SARs). Some of the difficulty in arriving at a universally acceptable SAR model has been attributed to the early method of testing cardiac glycoside preparations and the lack of a well-characterized cardiac glycoside "receptors." Until the early 1970s, nearly all the cardiac glycosides were evaluated based on their cardiac toxicity rather than on the more therapeutically relevant criteria. This was partly because of the belief that the cardiac toxicity was, in fact, an extension of the desired cardiotonic action. Thus, comparisons of cardiac glycoside preparations were based on the amount of drug required to cause cardiac arrest in test animals, usually anesthetized cats. More recently, most SAR studies have relied, at least initially, on results obtained with isolated cardiac tissue or whole-heart preparations. In these models, inotropic activity, contractility, and so forth can be directly assessed. In addition, the recognition of cardiac Na^+/K^+-ATPase as the probable receptor for the cardiac glycosides has made the inhibition of this enzyme system an important criterion for the cardiac glycosides activity.

Much of the interest in the effects of structural modification on cardiotonic activity results from the desire to develop agents with less toxic potential. Early studies based primarily on cardiac toxicity testing data suggested the importance of the steroid "backbone" shape, the 14-β-hydroxyl and the 17-unsaturated lactone for activity. More recent studies have been directed toward characterizing the interaction of the cardiac glycosides with Na^+/K^+-ATPase, the putative cardiac glycoside receptor. Using this enzyme model with enzyme inhibition as the biological end point, a number of hypotheses for cardiac glycoside receptor–binding interactions have been put forth. Many of these suggested that the 17-lactone plays an important role in receptor binding. Using synthetic analogues, it was found that unsaturation in the lactone ring was important, with the saturated lactone analogue showing diminished activity (4,5). Further investigations of synthetic compounds in which the lactone was replaced with open-chain structures of varying electronic and steric resemblance to the lactone showed that, in fact, the α,β-unsaturated lactone ring at C-17 was not an absolute requirement and that several α,β-unsaturated open-chain groups could be replaced with little or no loss in activity (4,5). For example, analogs possessing an α,β-unsaturated nitrile at the 17-β position had high activity. In light of this, most current theories point toward a key interaction of the carbonyl oxygen (or nitrile nitrogen) with the cardiac glycoside binding site on Na^+/K^+-ATPase (6,7). Some controversy, however, exists regarding this point. The importance of the "rest" of the cardiac glycoside molecule must not be ignored. Despite the apparently dominant role of the 17-lactone, it is the steroid (A-B-C-D) ring system that provides the lead structure for cardiac glycoside activity. Lactones alone, when not attached to the steroid ring system, show no Na^+/K^+-ATPase inhibitory activity. Some important steroid structural features have become apparent.

The C-D *cis* ring juncture appears to be critical for activity in compounds possessing the unsaturated butyrolactone in the normal 17-β position. This apparent requirement may be a reflection of changes in the spatial orientation of the 17-substituent (7). Moreover, the 14-β-OH is now believed to be dispensable, and the contribution to activity previously attributed to this group is thought to be related to the need to retain the sp^3 and *cis* character of the C-D ring juncture. The earlier interpretation arose from the fact that 14-deoxy analogues often had unsaturation in the D ring in place of the 14-β-OH. This double bond markedly influenced the position of the C-17 substituent, thereby complicating interpretation of 14-β-OH group importance. Finally, the A-B *cis* ring juncture also appears not to be mandatory for cardiac glycosides activity. This feature, however, is characteristic of all clinically useful cardiac glycosides, and conversion to an A-B trans ring system generally leads to a marked drop in activity unless compensating modifications are made elsewhere in the molecule.

Pharmaceutical preparations. The cardiac glycoside preparations that have been used range from powdered digitalis leaf to purified individual glycosides, including gitalin, lanatoside C, its partially hydrolyzed product deslanatoside C (desacetyl lanatoside C), digoxin, and ouabain (Table 26.3). Currently, digoxin is the only cardiac glycoside commercially available for therapeutic use in the United States. To arrive at an effective plasma concentration, a large initial dose (i.e., digitalizing or loading dose) often is given. The purpose of this large initial dose is to achieve a therapeutic blood and tissue level in the shortest possible time. Depending on the condition of the patient and the desired therapeutic goal, the loading dose may be much less than, or almost equal to, the dose that is likely to cause toxicity. Once the desired effect is obtained, the amount of drug lost from the body per day is replaced with a maintenance dose.

Absorption, metabolism, and excretion. The therapeutic effects of all cardiac glycosides on the heart are qualitatively similar; however, the glycosides largely differ in their pharmacokinetic properties. The latter are greatly influenced by the lipophilic character of each glycoside.

Table 26.3. Cardiac Glycosides and Their Dosage Forms

Name[a]	Dosage Forms
Digoxin USP and BP	Tablets, elixir, pediatric
Digitalis powder (Leaf) BP	Tablets, capsules
Digitoxin BP	Tablets, injection
Lanatoside C BP	Tablets
Ouabain BP	Injection (G-Strophanthin)
Deslanatoside C BP	Injection (desacetyllanatoside C)

[a]Those cardiac glycosides with *only* the BP (British Pharmacopeia) designation are available only in Canada and other countries except the United States.

Table 26.4. Effect of Glycoside Structure on Partition Coefficient

Glycoside	Partition Coefficient ($CHCl_3$/16% aq.MeOH)
Lanatoside C (glucose-3-acetyldigitoxose–digitoxose$_2$–digoxigenin)	16.2
Digoxin (digitoxose$_3$-digoxigenin)	81.5
Digitoxin (digitoxose$_3$-digitoxigenin)	96.5
Acetyldigoxin (3-acetyldigitoxose-digitoxose$_2$-digoxigenin)	98.0
G-Strophanthin (rhamnose-ouabagenin)	very low

In general, cardiac glycosides with more lipophilic character are absorbed faster and exhibit longer duration of action as a result of a slower urinary excretion rate. The lipophilicity of a cardiac glycoside is measured by its partitioning between chloroform and water mixed with methanol: The higher the concentration of the cardiac glycoside in the chloroform phase, the higher its partition coefficient, and the more lipophilic it is. The partition coefficients for five cardiac glycosides are listed in Table 26.4. It is evident from a comparison of the coefficients that their lipophilicity is markedly influenced by the number of sugar molecules and the number of hydroxyl groups on the aglycone part of a given glycoside. Lanatoside C, with a partition coefficient of 16.2, is far less lipophilic than that of acetyldigoxin (partition coefficient, 98), which structurally differs only in lacking the terminal glucose molecule. Likewise, a comparison of digitoxin and digoxin structures reveals that they only differ by an extra hydroxyl in digoxin at C-12. This seemingly minor difference in their partition coefficients from 96.5 to 81.5 for digitoxin and digoxin, respectively, results in significant differences in their pharmacokinetic behavior (Table 26.5). Table 26.4 also illustrates that the

Table 26.5. Comparison of the Pharmacokinetic Properties for Digoxin and Digitoxin

	Digoxin	Digitoxin
Gastrointestinal absorption	70–85%	95–100%
Average half life	1–2 days	5–7 days
Protein binding	25–30%	90–95%
Enterohepatic cycling	5%	25%
Excretion	Kidneys; largely unchanged	Liver metabolism
Therapeutic plasma level	0.5–2.5 ng/ml	20–35 ng/ml
Digitalizing dose (mg)	Oral: 0.75–1.5 IV: 0.5–1.0	Oral: 0.8–1.2 IV: 0.8–1.2
Maintenance dose (oral mg)	0.125–0.5	0.05–0.2

presence of the 3-O-acetyl group on acetyldigoxin enhances its lipophilic character more than that of desacetyl analogue, digoxin (partition coefficients of 98 and 81.5, respectively). The glycoside G-strophanthin (ouabain) possesses a very low lipophilic character because of the presence of five free hydroxyl groups on the steroid nucleus of the aglycone ouabagenin.

Digoxin is the most frequently used cardiac glycoside. The absorption of digoxin from the gastrointestinal tract is a passive process that depends on its lipid solubility, dissolution, and membrane permeability of the drug. The oral bioavailability of digoxin following oral administration exhibits interindividual variability, ranging from 70 to 85% of an administered dose. This interindividual variability has been attributed to intestinal P-gp efflux and P-gp–dependent renal elimination. Although digoxin is not extensively metabolized, it is transported from intestinal enterocytes along its epithelium into the intestinal lumen (effluxed) by P-glycoprotein (P-gp), which is also expressed in the kidney and liver. Alterations in P-gp transport may be the basis for several digoxin–drug interactions. For this reason, it is important to establish carefully the effective dose of digoxin for each patient to avoid digitalis toxicity.

Once the cardiac glycosides are absorbed, they bind to plasma proteins; digoxin has only 30% binding. The half-life of digoxin in patients with normal renal function is 1.5 to 2.0 days. Biliary excretion of digoxin is minimal. Digoxin is eliminated primarily unchanged by renal tubule excretion.

Contributing to the discontinuance of digitoxin as a therapeutic agent was a half-life range between 5 and 7 days because of its enterohepatic circulation. Approximately 25% of an absorbed dose of digitoxin is excreted in the bile unchanged, to be reabsorbed via enterohepatic circulation. Digitoxin, however, is extensively metabolized by the liver to a variety of metabolites, including $(\text{digitoxose})_2$-digitoxigenin, $(\text{digitoxose})_1$-digitoxigenin, and $(\text{digitoxose})_1$-digitoxigenin. Trace amounts of digoxin have been discovered in the urine. The pharmacokinetic data for digoxin and digitoxin is summarized in Table 26.5.

Drug interactions. Digoxin–drug interactions are common causes of digitalis toxicity. Recently, the clinical significance of the P-gp–dependent renal tubular secretion of digoxin associated with the well-documented digoxin–quinidine interaction has been reported (8). The discovery that digoxin is actively secreted into the urine by the renal tubular cell via the P-gp efflux pump has led to the conclusion that the digoxin–quinidine interaction can be attributed to inhibition of renal tubular secretion of digoxin by quinidine (a P-gp substrate). Quinidine competitively binds to P-gp in the renal tubule reducing the renal secretion of digoxin by as much as 60%, raising digoxin's plasma concentration to toxic levels. Other drugs that are substrates for renal P-gp also are likely to be associated with digoxin–drug interactions. Another documented digoxin–drug interaction associated with increased digoxin blood levels and toxicity is with verapamil. Unlike quinidine, verapamil inhibits intestinal P-gp efflux of digoxin, thereby blocking the intestinal secretion of digoxin into the lumen of the intestine and raising digoxin blood levels to toxic levels. On the other hand, the rifampin–digoxin interaction involves the rifampin induction of intestinal P-gp expression, thereby increasing the P-gp–mediated secretion of digoxin. This results in the lowering of digoxin blood levels to subtherapeutic concentrations. The P-gp transporters and their substrates, inhibitors, or inducers (see Table 10.16 for list) appear to play an important role in controlling the digoxin area under the curve (AUC) values through the renal tubular and intestinal secretion of digoxin and, subsequently, to digoxin–drug interactions and digitalis toxicity. Concurrent use of the cardiac glycosides with antiarrhythmics, sympathomimetics, β-adrenergic blockers, and calcium channel blockers that are substrates for P-gp may alter control of arrhythmias.

The absorption of digoxin after oral administration also can be significantly altered by other drugs concurrently present in the gastrointestinal tract. For example, laxatives may interfere with the absorption of digoxin because of increased intestinal motility. The presence of the drug cholestyramine, an agent used to treat hyperlipoproteinemia, decreases the absorption of digoxin by binding to and retaining digoxin in the gastrointestinal tract. Antacids, especially magnesium trisilicate, and antidiarrheal adsorbent suspensions also may inhibit the absorption of the digoxin. Potassium-depleting diuretics, such as thiazides, may increase the possibility of digitalis toxicity because of the additive hypokalemia. Several other drugs that are known to bind to plasma proteins, such as thyroid hormones, have the potential to displace digoxin from its plasma-binding sites, thereby increasing its free drug concentration to a toxic level.

Therapeutic uses. Although the primary clinical use for digoxin is in the treatment of CHF, this agent also is used in cases of atrial flutter or fibrillation and paroxysmal atrial tachycardia.

Toxicity. All cardiac glycosides preparations have the potential to cause toxicity. Because the minimal toxic dose of the glycosides is only two- to threefold the therapeutic dose, intoxication is quite common. In mild to moderate toxicity, the common symptoms are anorexia, nausea and vomiting, muscular weakness, bradycardia, and ventricular premature contractions. The nausea is a result of excitation of the chemoreceptor trigger zone in the medulla. In severe toxicity, the common symptoms are blurred vision, disorientation, diarrhea, ventricular tachycardia, and AV block, which may progress into ventricular fibrillation. It generally is accepted that the toxicity of the cardiac glycosides results from inhibition of the Na^+/K^+-ATPase pump, which results in increased intracellular levels of Ca^{2+}. Hypokalemia (decreased potassium), which can be induced by coadministration of thiazide diuretics, of glucocorticoids, or by other means, can be an important factor in initiating a toxic response. It has been shown that low levels of extracellular K^+ partially inhibit the Na^+/K^+-ATPase pump. In a patient stabilized on a cardiac glycoside, the Na^+/K^+-ATPase pump already is partially inhibited, and the hypokalemia only further inhibits the pump, causing an intracellular buildup of sodium, which leads to an increase in intracellular calcium levels. The high levels of calcium are responsible for the observed cardiac arrhythmias characteristic of the cardiac glycosides toxicity.

A common procedure used in treating cardiac glycoside toxicity is to administer potassium salts to increase extracellular potassium level, which stimulates the Na^+/K^+-ATPase pump, resulting in decreased intracellular sodium levels and, thus, decreased intracellular calcium. In treating any cardiac glycoside–induced toxicity, it is important to discontinue administration of the drug in addition to administering a potassium salt. Other drugs that may be useful in treating the tachyarrhythmias present during toxicity are lidocaine, phenytoin, and propranolol. Specific antibodies directed toward digoxin (Dig-Bind) have been used experimentally and proven to be very effective.

Nonglycosidic Positive Inotropic Agents

Nonglycosidic positive inotropic drugs can be divided into two main classes: those that act via stimulating the synthesis of cyclic adenosine monophosphate (cAMP), such as adrenergic and dopaminergic agonists; and those that inhibit the hydrolysis of cAMP, such as phosphodiesterase 3 (PDE3) inhibitors.

PHOSPHODIESTERASE 3 INHIBITORS. The mechanism of cardiac contraction involves a G-protein signal transduction pathway, which regulates intracellular calcium concentrations. Activation of the G_s-protein involves the formation of intracellular cAMP, which thereby increases intracellular calcium, stimulating cardiac muscle contraction (see Chapter 4). Relaxation occurs when the released cAMP is hydrolyzed by cytosolic cAMP-dependent PDE3, one of the phosphodiesterase isofoms. Therefore, inhibition of PDE3 increases intracellular cAMP, promoting cardiac muscle contraction but vasodilation of vascular smooth muscle. (See Chapter 17 for more information about phosphodiesterases.)

The overall cardiostimulatory and vasodilatory actions of PDE3 inhibitors make them suitable for the treatment of heart failure, because vascular smooth muscle relaxation reduces ventricular wall stress and the oxygen demands placed on the failing heart. The cardiostimulatory effects of the PDE3 inhibitors increases inotropy, which further enhances stroke volume and ejection fraction. Clinical trials have shown that long-term therapy with PDE3 inhibitors increases mortality in heart failure patients. Therefore, these PDE3 inhibitors are not used for the long-term, chronic therapy of CHF. They are very useful, however, in treating acute, decompensated heart failure or temporary bouts of decompensated chronic failure. They are not used as a monotherapy. Instead, they are used in conjunction with other treatment modalities, such as diuretics, angiotensin-converting enzyme inhibitors, β-blockers, or cardiac glycosides. The PDE3 inhibitors contract cardiac muscle and are used for treating heart failure, whereas the phosphodiesterase 5 (PDE5) inhibitors are vasodilators and are used for treating male erectile dysfunction. Note that the generic names for PDE3 inhibitors end in "one," and those for the PDE5 inhibitors end in "fil."

Side effects and contraindications. The most common and severe side effect of PDE3 inhibitors is ventricular arrhythmias, some of which may be life-threatening. Other side effects included headaches and hypotension, which are not uncommon for drugs that increase cAMP in cardiac and vascular tissues, with other examples being β-agonists.

Milrinone (Primacor®) and imamrinone (Inocor®). Although the digitalis glycosides may be the principal therapeutic agents for the treatment of CHF, they are not the only positive inotropic agents available. Among the "nonglycoside" inotropic agents are the bipyridines, inamrinone and milrinone, which are selective PDE3 inhibitors (Fig. 26.4). Inamrinone and milrinone are positive inotrope and vasodilators indicated for the short-term intravenous management of CHF in patients who have not responded adequately to digitalis, diuretics, and/or vasodilators (9,10). Milrinone is the drug of choice from among the currently available PDE3 inhibitors because of its greater selectivity for PDE3, shorter half-life (30–60 min), and fewer side effects. Imamrinone is associated with thrombocytopenia in 10% of patients. Inamrinone was introduced in 1978, and it produces both positive inotropic and concentration-dependent vasodilatory effects. Despite similar positive inotropic action to the cardiac glycosides, the inotropic action involves inhibition of PDE3, as previously described. Inamrinone was approved for the short-term intravenous administration in patients with severe heart failure refractory to other measures. Although inamrinone is orally active, several adverse side effects have dampened enthusiasm for long-term oral inamrinone therapy. These effects include gastrointestinal disturbances, thrombocytopenia, and impairment of the liver function. For intravenous infusion, inamrinone lactate and milrinone lactate injection solutions may be

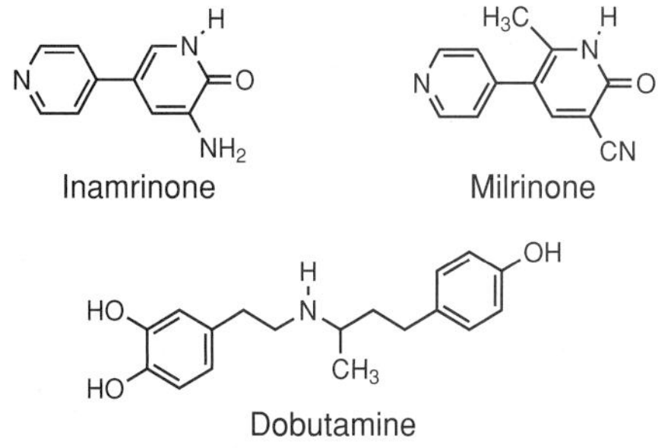

Inamrinone

Milrinone

Dobutamine

Fig. 26.4. Miscellaneous inotropic agents.

diluted in sodium chloride injection. Inamrinone lactate for injection is preserved with sodium metabisulfite and needs protection from light. It should not be diluted with solutions containing dextrose because a chemical reaction occurs in 24 hours. For milrinone, an immediate chemical interaction with furosemide with the formation of a precipitate is observed when furosemide is injected into an infusion of milrinone. Patients sensitive to bisulfites may also be sensitive to inamrinone lactate injection, which contains sodium metabisulfite.

The pharmacokinetics for inamrinone shows a half-life in healthy volunteers of approximately 3 to 4 hours, whereas in patients with CHF, the plasma half-life increases approximately 50% (5–8 hours). For infants younger than 4 weeks, the half-life life is 12.7 to 22.2 hours, and infants older than 4 weeks, the half-life is 3.8 to 6.8 hours. Time to peak effect is less than 10 minutes, with its duration of action ranging from 30 minutes to 2 hours depending on the dosage. Approximately 63% of imamrinone is eliminated via the urine as unchanged drug, and 18% is eliminated in the feces. Elderly patients are more likely to have age-related impairment of renal function, which may require adjustment of dosage in patients receiving inamrinone.

The limited success of inamrinone led to the development of structurally related newer agents, such as milrinone, with a mechanism of action similar to inamrinone. Milrinone, however, is an order of magnitude more potent than inamrinone. Furthermore, preliminary reports show it to be better tolerated, with no apparent thrombocytopenia or gastrointestinal disturbances. Milrinone is excreted largely unchanged in the urine, and accordingly, patients with impaired renal function require reduced dosages.

The pharmacokinetics for milrinone following intravenous injections to patients with CHF showed an elimination half-life of 2 to 3 hours. Its primary route of excretion is via the urine as unchanged milrinone (83%) and its O-glucuronide metabolite (12%). In patients with renal function impairment, elimination of unchanged milrinone is reduced, suggesting that a dosage adjustment may be necessary.

β-Adrenergic Receptor Agonists. Another promising area for the development of new positive inotropic agents is that of β-adrenergic receptor agonists (11) (see Chapter 13). The myocardium has mostly β_1-adrenergic receptors, and stimulation of these receptors by a variety of β-adrenergic agonists produces a potent positive inotropic response involving the G-protein signal transduction process increasing intracellular cAMP levels that lead to a cascade of events that ultimately produce an increase in intracellular Ca^{2+}, thereby increasing myocardial contractility (discussed in Chapters 4 and 13). Although many drugs possess β-adrenergic agonist activity, most have side effects that make them inappropriate for the treatment of CHF. For example, the well-known catecholamines, norepinephrine and epinephrine, are potent nonselective adrenergic receptor agonists. Because the actions of these agents are not limited to the myocardial β_1-receptors, however, they produce undesirable positive chronotropic effects, exacerbate arrhythmias, and result in vasoconstriction. These effects limit their utility in the treatment of CHF.

Dobutamine (Dobutrex). Among the most promising β_1 adrenergic agonists are those derived from dopamine, the endogenous precursor to norepinephrine. Dopamine itself is a potent stimulator of the β_1-receptors, but it results in many of the undesirable side effects described in Chapter 13. The new analogs of dopamine that have been developed retain the potent inotropic effect but possess fewer effects on heart rate, vascular tone, and arrhythmias. Dobutamine is a prime representative of this group of agents. Dobutamine is a potent β_1-adrenergic agonist on the myocardium (as well as α_1-agonist and -antagonist activities; see Chapter 13 for details concerning its mechanism of action) with beneficial effects, the composite of a variety of actions on the heart and the peripheral vasculature. Dobutamine is active only by the intravenous route because of its rapid first-pass metabolism via COMT (catechal-O-methyl transferase). Therefore, its use is limited to critical care situations. Nonetheless, its parenteral success has led to the search and development of orally active drugs. One of the major limitations associated with β_1-agonists is the phenomenon of myocardial β-receptor desensitization. This lowered responsiveness (desensitization) of the receptors appears to be due to a decrease in the number of β_1-receptors and partial uncoupling of the receptors from adenylate cyclase.

DRUGS FOR THE TREATMENT OF ANGINA

Angina Pectoris

Angina pectoris is the chronic disease affecting the coronary arteries, which supply oxygenated blood from the left ventricle to all heart tissues, including the ventricles themselves. When the lumen of the coronary artery becomes restricted, it becomes less efficient in supplying blood and oxygen to the heart, and the heart is said to be "ischemic" (oxygen deficient). Angina is the primary symptom of ischemic heart disease and is characterized by a sudden, severe pain originating in the chest, often radiating to the left shoulder and down the left arm. Angina is further subclassified into typical or variant angina based on the precipitating factors and the electrophysiological changes observed during the attack. Typical angina usually is the result of an advanced state of atherosclerosis and is provoked by food, exercise, and emotional factors. It is characterized by low ST segment of the electrocardiogram. Variant or acute angina results from sudden spasm in the coronary artery unrelated to atherosclerotic narrowing of the coronary circulation and can occur at rest. It is characterized by an increase in the ST segment of the electrocardiogram.

Antianginal Drugs

Therapy of angina is directed mainly toward alleviating and preventing anginal attacks by altering the oxygen supply/oxygen demand ratio to the cardiac muscle or dilating the coronary vessels. Three classes of drugs are found to be very efficient in this regard, although via different mechanisms. These include organic nitrates, calcium channel blockers, and β-adrenergic blockers.

Organic Nitrates

Organic nitrates have dominated the treatment of acute angina over the last 100 years. Although the recent introduction of the calcium channel blockers and the β-blockers as antianginal agents has expanded the physician therapeutic arsenal, organic nitrates are still the class of choice in the treatment of acute anginal episodes.

OVERVIEW. Organic nitrates are esters of simple organic alcohols or polyols with nitric acid. This class was developed after the antianginal effect of amyl nitrite (ester of isoamyl alcohol with nitrous acid) was first observed in 1857. Five members of this class are in clinical use today: amyl nitrite (amyl nitrite inhalant USP), nitroglycerin, isosorbide dinitrate, erythrityl tetranitrate, and pentaerythritol tetranitrate (Fig. 26.5). Two additional organic nitrates, tenitramine and propatylnitrate, are currently available in Europe (Fig. 26.5). This class usually is referred to as organic nitrates, because all of these agents, except amyl nitrite, are nitrate esters. It should be noted that the generic names do not always precisely describe the chemical nature of the drug but, rather, are used for simplicity. For example, the drug nitroglycerin is not really a nitro compound, because a nitro compound means a nitro group attached to a carbon atom (i.e., NO_2-C); the correct chemical name of nitroglycerin is glyceryltrinitrate. Another example is amyl nitrite, the structure of which indicates that it is an ester of isoamyl alcohol with nitrous acid; the correct chemical name of this drug is isoamyl nitrite.

The chemical nature of these molecules as esters constitutes some problems in formulating these agents for clinical use. The small lipophilic ester character makes them volatile. Volatility is an important concern in drug formulation because of the potential loss of the active principle from the dosage form. In addition, moisture should be avoided during storage to minimize the hydrolysis of the ester bond, which can lead to a decrease in the therapeutic effectiveness. Lastly, because these agents are nitrate esters, they possess explosive properties, especially in the pure concentrated form. Dilution in a variety of vehicles and excipients eliminates this potential hazard. The lipophilic nature of these esters, however, makes these agents very efficient in emergency treatment of anginal episodes as a result of their rapid absorption through biomembranes.

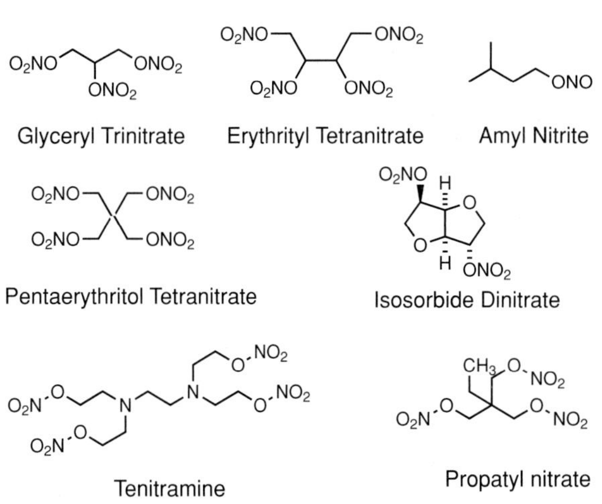

Glyceryl Trinitrate — Erythrityl Tetranitrate — Amyl Nitrite — Pentaerythritol Tetranitrate — Isosorbide Dinitrate — Tenitramine — Propatyl nitrate

Fig. 26.5. Organic nitrates and nitrites.

PHARMACOLOGICAL ACTIONS. The oxygen requirements of the myocardial tissues are related to the workload (oxygen demand) of the heart, which is, in part, a function of the heart rate, the systolic pressure, and the peripheral resistance of the blood flow (oxygen supply). Myocardial ischemia occurs when the oxygen supply is insufficient to meet the myocardial oxygen demand. This can occur, as explained previously, because of atherosclerotic narrowing of the coronary circulation (typical) or vasospasm of the coronary artery (variant). The nitrates have been shown to be effective in treating angina resulting from either cause. The vasodilating effect of organic nitrates on the veins leads to pooling of the blood in the veins and decreased venous return to the heart (decreased preload), whereas vasodilation of the coronary arterioles decreases the resistance of the peripheral tissues (decreased afterload). The decrease in both preload and afterload results in a generalized decrease in the myocardial workload, which translates into a reduced oxygen demand by the myocardium. Organic nitrates restore the balance between oxygen supply by venous dilation and oxygen demand by decreasing the myocardial workload.

BIOCHEMICAL MECHANISM OF ACTION. The organic nitrates (Fig. 26.5) are pharmacological sources of nitric oxide (NO) for the body. In the cardiovascular system, NO is naturally produced by vascular endothelial cells. This endothelial-derived NO has several important functions, including relaxation of vascular smooth muscle, inhibiting platelet aggregation (antithrombotic), and inhibiting leukocyte-endothelial interactions (anti-inflammatory). These actions involve NO-stimulated formation of cyclic guanosine monophosphate (cGMP) (see Chapter 29). Nitrodilators are drugs that mimic the actions of endogenous NO by releasing NO or forming NO within tissues. Free tissue sulfhydryl groups play a key role in the venodilation effect of nitroglycerin, which is supported by experimental evidence showing that prior administration of N-acetylcysteine, which should increase the availability of free sulfhydryl groups, resulted in an increase in the venodilating effect of organic nitrates. Similarly, pretreatment with reagents that react with free sulfhydryl groups, such as ethacrynic acid, blocked glyceryl trinitrate venodilation in vitro (13). A more complex mechanism for nitrate venodilation, however, was proposed by Ignarro et al. (14). They suggested that the nitrates act indirectly, by stimulating the enzyme guanylate (also known as guanylyl) cyclase and, thereby, producing elevated levels of cGMP, which in turn leads to venodilation. The initial stimulation of soluble guanylate cyclase is believed to be mediated by a nitrate-derived nitrosothiol metabolite produced intracellularly. In support of this mechanism is the observation that a variety of synthetic nitrosothiols were found to increase markedly soluble guanylate cyclase activity and to produce venodilation in vitro (15–19). Such a mechanism is consistent with the requirement for free sulfhydryl groups described previously. A unifying mechanism suggests that the organic nitrates through the formation of NO via a nitrosothiol-intermediate activate soluble guanylate cyclase, increasing intracellular cGMP concentrations, which in turn blocks the Ca^{2+}-catalyzed vascular contractions (Fig. 29-3) (20–23). Depletion of sulfhydryl groups during this metabolic process may be a major factor in the development of nitrate tolerance, along with compensatory physiologic mechanisms. Data also exist suggesting that organic nitrates increase intraplatelet cGMP concentrations, thereby inhibiting platelet aggregation. These pharmacological actions of organic nitrates appear to preferentially occur within portions of blood vessels containing damaged endothelium, thus making them extremely useful in the pharmacotherapy of acute ischemic events.

Pharmaceutical preparations and dosage forms. Organic nitrates are administered by inhalation; by infusion; as sublingual, chewable, and sustained-release tablets; as capsules; as transdermal disks; and as ointments.

Absorption, metabolism, and therapeutic effects. Organic nitrates are used for both treatment and prevention of painful anginal attacks. The therapeutic approaches to achieve these two goals, however, are distinctly different. For the treatment of acute anginal attacks (i.e., attacks that have already begun), a rapid-acting preparation is required. In contrast, preventative therapy requires a long-acting preparation with more emphasis on duration and less emphasis on onset. The onset of organic nitrate action is influenced not only by the specific agent chosen but also by the route of administration. Sublingual administration is used predominantly for a rapid onset of action. The duration of nitrate action is strongly influenced by rate of metabolism. All of the organic nitrates are subject to rapid first-pass metabolism not only by the action of glutathione-nitrate reductase in the liver, but also in extrahepatic tissues, such as the blood vessel walls themselves (24,25). In addition, rapid uptake into the vessel walls plays a significant role in the rapid disappearance of organic nitrates from the bloodstream. Sublingual, transdermal, and buccal administration routes have been used in an attempt to avoid at least some of the hepatic metabolism.

Acute angina most frequently is treated with sublingual glyceryl trinitrate. This sublingual preparation is rapidly absorbed from the sublingual, lingual, and buccal mucosa and usually provides relief within 2 minutes. The duration of action also is short (~30 minutes). Other treatments include amyl nitrite by inhalation and sublingual isosorbide dinitrate. Amyl nitrite is by far the fastest-acting preparation, with an onset of action in approximately 15 to 30 seconds, but the duration of action is only approximately 1 minute. Isosorbide dinitrate, although usually used as a long-acting agent, may be used to treat acute angina. Sublingually administered isosorbide dinitrate has a somewhat slower onset than glyceryl trinitrate (~3 minutes), but its action may last for 4 to 6 hours. Although the onset appears to be almost as rapid as that of glyceryl trinitrate, waiting an additional minute for relief may be deemed unacceptable by some patients.

To prevent recurring angina, long-acting organic nitrate preparations are used. Several agents fall into this category, such as orally administered isosorbide dinitrate, pentaerythritol tetranitrate, and erythrityl tetranitrate. In addition, a number of long-acting glyceryl trinitrate preparations are available. These include oral sustained-release forms, glyceryl trinitrate ointment, transdermal patches, and buccal tablets. Of these therapeutic options, isosorbide dinitrate and glyceryl trinitrate preparations are by far the most frequently used. At first, the whole concept of prophylactic nitrate use was met with skepticism by many physicians, both because early studies indicated that oral nitrates were almost completely broken down by first-pass metabolism (24,25) and because blood levels of the parent drug appeared to be virtually nil. These findings, in conjunction with several clinical studies showing equivocal efficacy, led Needleman et al. (25) to conclude, "There is no rational basis for the use of 'long-acting' nitrates (administered orally) in the prophylactic therapy of angina pectoris." More recent studies, however, suggest that oral prophylactic nitrates may be effective if appropriate doses are used (26). Moreover, some metabolites of long-acting nitrates are active as venodilators, albeit less potent than the parent drug. An example of this is isosorbide dinitrate, which is metabolized primarily in the liver by glutathione-nitrate reductase, which also participates in the metabolism of other organic nitrates, catalyzing the denitration of the parent drug to yield two metabolites, 2- and 5-isosorbide mononitrate (27). Of these, the 5-isomer is still a potent vasodilator, and its plasma half-life of approximately 4.5 hours is much longer than that of isosorbide dinitrate itself. The extended half-life, because of the metabolite's resistance to further metabolism, indicates that it may be contributing to the prolonged duration of action associated with use of isosorbide dinitrate (27).

Adverse effects. Most patients tolerate the nitrates fairly well. Headache and postural hypotension are the most common side effects of organic nitrates. Dizziness, nausea, vomiting, rapid pulse, and restlessness are among the additional side effects reported. These symptoms may be controlled by administering low doses initially and then gradually increasing the dose. Fortunately, tolerance to nitrate-induced headache develops after a few days of therapy. Because postural hypotension may occur in some individuals, advise the patient to sit down when taking a rapid-acting nitrate preparation for the first time. An effective dose of nitrate usually produces a fall in upright systolic pressure of 10 mm Hg and a reflex rise in heart rate of 10 beats per minute.

Another concern associated with prophylactic nitrate use is the development of tolerance (26,28). Tolerance, usually in the form of shortened duration of action, is commonly observed with chronic nitrate use. The clinical importance of this tolerance is, however, a matter of controversy. Because tolerance to nitrates has not been reported to lead to a total loss of activity, some physicians feel that it is not clinically relevant. In addition, an adjustment in dosage can compensate for the reduced response (26). It also has been reported that intermittent use of long-acting and sustained-release preparations may limit the extent of tolerance development.

Drug interactions. The most significant interactions of organic nitrates are with those agents that cause hypotension, such as other vasodilators, alcohol, and tricyclic antidepressants, in which the potential for orthostatic hypotension may arise. On the other hand, concurrent administration with sympathomimetic amines, such as ephedrine and norepinephrine, may lead to a decrease in the antianginal efficacy of the organic nitrates.

Nitric oxide donor. Molsidomine (Corvaton) is an oral NO donor known as a sydnone imine, a mesionic compound that is soluble in both water and organic solvents. Molsidomine is enzymatically metabolized by liver esterases to its active metabolite, linsodimine, which is spontaneously converted in the blood into its nitroso metabolite SIN-1A (Fig. 26.6). Molecular oxygen is required to release NO from SIN-1A. The beneficial effects of molsidomine in treatment of angina were recognized before the role of endogenous NO for causing vasodilation was identified. A possible explanation may revolve around activation of K^+ channels. Molsidomine has a slower onset and longer duration of action than conventional nitrates because of the relatively slow rate of conversion to linsodimine, which has a rapid onset and short duration of action. Nitric oxide acts as a cellular messenger, leading to activation of soluble guanylate cyclase to release cGMP (see Chapter 29) and vasodilation. Because the metabolites of molsidomine generate NO without the need for enzymes or cofactors, other than the presence of oxygen, tolerance to prolonged exposure does not occur. This mechanism differs from organic nitrates in which cysteine or thiol donors are required for conversion into NO. It is believed that cysteine depletion is the major factor in the development of nitrate tolerance.

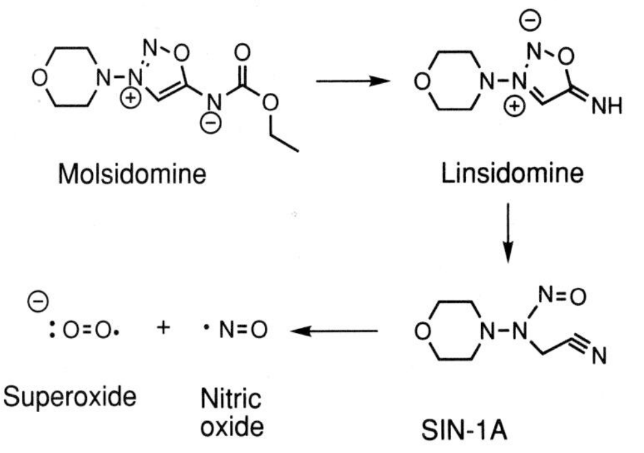

Fig. 26.6. Molsidomine metabolism to nitric oxide.

Molsidomine and lindosimine are therapeutic alternatives to traditional organic nitrates in treatment of stable angina, coronary vasospasm, and heart failure. Unlike organic nitrates, however, molsidomine and lindosimine have significant antiplatelet activity at therapeutic doses. The cogeneration of superoxide during the release of NO is a major concern limiting its therapeutic potential in the treatment of angina. Its short duration of action necessitates an increased dose frequency, which might be inconvenient in a clinical setting. The light sensitivity of molsidomine necessitates careful protection of infusion bags and tubing during administration.

Calcium Channel Blockers

The second major therapeutic approach to the treatment of angina is the use of calcium channel blockers (29.30) (see also the corresponding subsection in Chapter 28). In the 1906s, it was recognized that inhibition of calcium ion (Ca^{2+}) influx into myocardial cells may be advantageous in preventing angina. Currently, three classes of calcium channel blockers are approved for use in the prophylactic treatment of angina: the dihydropyridines nifedipine, nicardipine, and amlodipine; the benzothiazepine derivative diltiazem; as well as the aralkyl amine derivative verapamil and the diaminopropanol ether bepridil (Fig. 26.7). The last-mentioned are reserved for treatment failures in that serious arrhythmias may occur.

Chemistry

The structural dissimilarity of these agents is apparent and serves to emphasize the fact that each is distinctly different from the others in its profile of effects. Although nifedipine and similar drugs belong to the dihydropyridine family, diltiazem belongs to the benzo[*b*-1,5]thiazepine family. Verapamil is structurally characterized by a central basic nitrogen to which alkyl and aralkyl groups are attached. It is noteworthy that diltiazem and verapamil are both chiral, possessing asymmetric centers. In each case, the dextro-rotatory (i.e., the (+)-enantiomer) is approximately one order of magnitude more potent as a calcium channel blocker than the levo-rotatory (i.e., (−)-enantiomer).

Pharmacological Effects

Calcium ions are known to play a critical role in many physiologic functions. Physiologic calcium is found in a

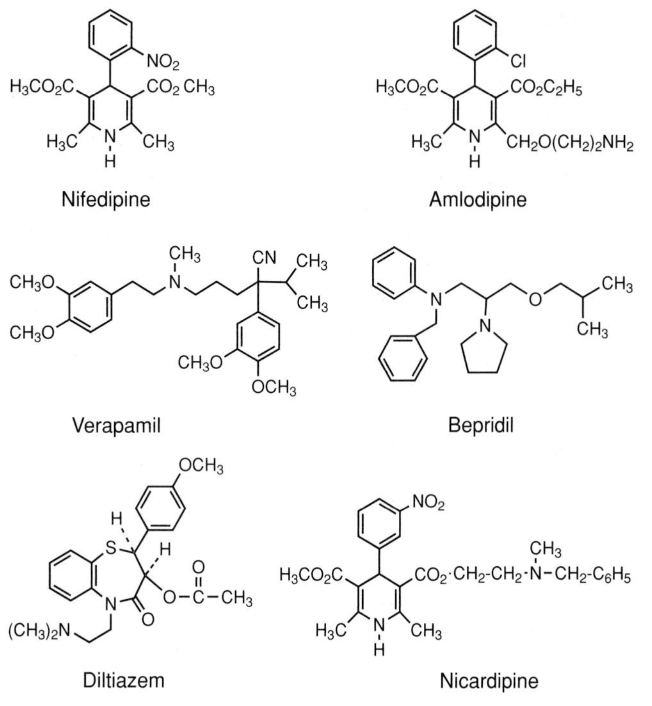

Fig. 26.7. Calcium channel blockers.

variety of locations, both intracellular and extracellular. Because calcium plays such a ubiquitous role in normal physiology, the overall therapeutic effect of the calcium channel blockers often is the composite of numerous pharmacological actions in a variety of tissues. The most important of these tissues associated with angina are the myocardium and the arterial vascular bed. Because of the dependency of myocardial contraction on calcium, these drugs have a negative inotropic effect on the heart. Vascular smooth muscle also depends on calcium influx for contraction. Although the underlying mechanism is somewhat different, inhibition of calcium channel influx into the vascular smooth muscles by the calcium channel blockers leads to arteriolar vasodilation. The venous beds appear to be less affected by the calcium channel blockers. The negative inotropic effect and arterial vasodilation result in decreased heart workload and afterload, respectively. The preload is not affected because of a lesser sensitivity of the venous bed to the calcium channel blockers.

Mechanism of Action

The depolarization and contraction of the myocardial cells are mediated, in part, by calcium influx. As previously explained, the overall process consists of two distinct, inward ion currents: First, sodium ions flow rapidly into the cell through the "fast channels," and subsequently, calcium enters more slowly through the "slow channels." The calcium ions trigger contraction indirectly by binding and inhibiting troponin, a natural suppressor of the contractile process. Once the inhibitory effect of troponin is removed, actin and myosin can interact to produce the contractile response. The calcium channel blockers produce a negative inotropic effect by interrupting the contractile response. In vascular smooth muscles, calcium causes constriction by binding to a specific intracellular protein calmodulin to form a complex that initiates the process of vascular constriction. The calcium channel blockers inhibit vascular smooth muscle contraction by depriving the cell from the calcium ions.

The effects of the three classes of calcium channel blockers on the myocardium and the arteries vary from one class to the other. Although verapamil and diltiazem affect both the heart and the arteriolar bed, the dihydropyridines have much less effect on the cardiac tissues and higher specificity for the arteriolar vascular bed. Therefore, both verapamil and diltiazem are used clinically in the management of angina, hypertension, and cardiac arrhythmia, whereas the dihydropyridines are used more frequently as antianginal and antihypertensive agents. Because nicardipine has a less negative inotropic effect than nifedipine, it may be preferred over nifedipine for patients with angina pectoris or hypertension who also have CHF dysfunction.

The recognition of the pivotal role of calcium flux on biological functions led to the reexamination of several therapeutic agents already in clinical use to see if their effects also were mediated through calcium-dependent mechanisms. Interestingly, many drugs were found to influence calcium movement and availability. In many cases, however, this effect was not found to contribute significantly to the desirable pharmacological activity, with other mechanisms playing more dominant roles.

Pharmaceutical Preparations

Calcium channel blockers are administered as oral tablets and capsules as regular or sustained-release forms. Verapamil and diltiazem also are administered by injection.

Absorption, Metabolism, and Excretion

The calcium channel blockers are rapidly and completely absorbed after oral administration (see Table 28.11 for summary of pharmacokinetic parameters). Prehepatic first-pass metabolism by CYP3A4 enzymes occurs with some orally administered calcium channel blockers, especially verapamil, with its low bioavailability of 20 to 35%. The bioavailability of diltiazem is 40 to 67%, of nicardipine 35%, of nifedipine 45 to 70%, and of amlodipine 64 to 90%. Verapamil is metabolized by CYP3A4 N-demethylation to its principal metabolite, norverapamil, which retains approximately 20% of the activity of verapamil, and by O-demethylation (CYP2D6) into inactive metabolites. Diltiazem is metabolized by enzyme hydrolysis to its primary metabolite, desacetyl derivative, which retains approximately 25 to 50% of the activity of diltiazem. The oral bioavailability of diltiazem and verapamil may be increased with chronic use and increasing dose (i.e., bioavailability is nonlinear). Diltiazem undergoes

N-demethylation by CYP3A4 and O-demethylation by CYP2D6. The N-demethylated metabolism pathway results in mechanism-based inhibition of CYP3A4. The major metabolite, detected following oral and continuous intravenous administration but not following rapid intravenous administration, is desacetyl diltiazem, which has one-quarter to one-half the arteriolar vasodilation activity of the parent compound. Its elimination half-life ranges from 5 to 8 hours, depending on the dosage. Its onset of action following oral administration is 30 to 60 minutes; 2 to 4% is excreted unchanged. For extended-release capsules, the onset of action is 2 to 3 hours. CYP3A4 inhibition by diltiazem and substrate for CYP2D6 provide a rational basis for pharmacokinetically significant interactions when they are coadministered with drugs that are cleared primarily by CYP3A4 or CYP2D6 mediated pathways. Considerable variability for verapamil may be observed in the elimination half-life of 1.5 to 7 hours. In addition, the plasma half-life may not always accurately predict the duration of action because of the presence of active metabolites. Less than 5% of an orally administered dose of verapamil is excreted unchanged into the urine. Its protein binding is approximately 90%.

A well-documented drug interaction between digoxin and verapamil that increases the AUCs for digoxin has been attributed to verapamil blocking the intestinal P-gp efflux of digoxin (previously described under digoxin–drug interactions). The fact that verapamil is a substrate for P-gp transport of drugs may be a potential source of other drug interactions. The oral coadministration of verapamil with CYP3A4 inhibitors (see Table 10.10 for a list of inhibitors) has resulted in at least a 100 to 200 times increase in the blood AUCs for verapamil and, thereby, a toxic dose.

The dihydropyridines are metabolized largely to a variety of inactive metabolites. Their binding to plasma proteins is high, ranging from 70 to 98% depending on the individual agent: For verapamil, protein binding is 90%; for diltiazem, 70 to 80%; for nifedipine, 92–98%; for nicardipine, greater than 90%; and for amlodipine, greater than 90%. Less than 4% of the dihydropyridine dose is excreted unchanged into the urine. The duration of action of the calcium channel blockers ranges from 4 to 8 hours (verapamil, 4 hours; diltiazem, 6–8 hours; nifedipine, 4–8 hours; and nicardipine, 6–8 hours). Amlodipine has a 24-hour duration of action. Thus, it is the only calcium channel blocker that can be given once daily as a nonsustained-release product.

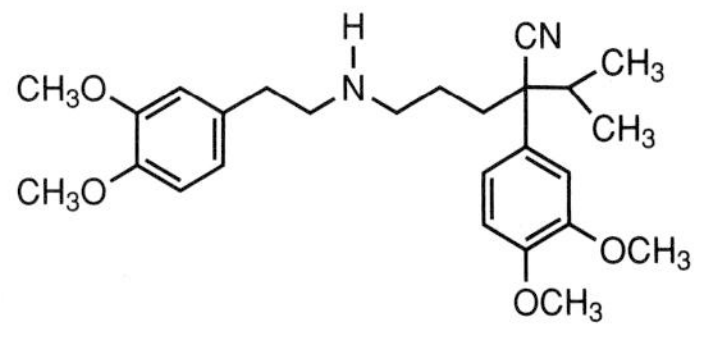

Norverapamil

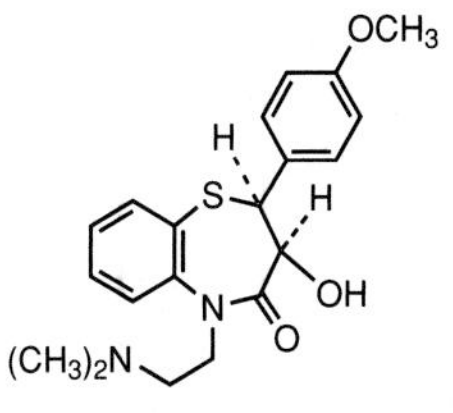

Desacetyldiltiazem

Adverse Effects

The most common side effects of the calcium channel blockers include dizziness, hypotension, headache, and peripheral and pulmonary edema. These symptoms are related mainly to the excessive vasodilation, especially with the dihydropyridines. Verapamil was reported to cause constipation to some patients.

Drug Interactions

Clinically significant drug interactions between calcium channel blockers and coadministration of CYP3A4 inhibitors, such as 6 to 8 oz. of grapefruit juice, HIV protease inhibitors, and erythromycin, have resulted in a 100- to 200-fold increase in the AUC for some calcium channel blockers (31). On the other hand, the coadministration of CYP3A4 inducers, such as rifampin or phenobarbital, result in an approximately 50% decrease in the AUC of calcium channel blockers. With other vasodilators, antihypertensive drugs, and alcohol, excessive hypotension may arise because of an additive effect. The high-protein-binding nature of these drugs precipitates a potential for mutual plasma displacement with other drugs known to possess the same property, such as oral anticoagulants, digitalis glycosides, oral hypoglycemic agents, sulfa drugs, and salicylates. Dose adjustment may be necessary in some cases.

Therapeutic Uses

Calcium channel blockers are clinically used as antianginal, antiarrhythmic, and antihypertensive agents (see corresponding subsection in Chapter 28).

β-Adrenergic Blocking Agents

The use of β-adrenergic blockers as antianginal agents is limited to the treatment of exertion-induced angina. Propranolol is the prototype drug in this class, but several newer agents have been approved for clinical use in the United States (see Chapter 13). Although these agents may be used alone, they often are used in combination therapy with nitrates, calcium channel blockers, or both. In several instances, combination therapy was found to provide more improvement than with either agent alone. This, however, is not always the case.

Modulators of Myocardial Metabolism

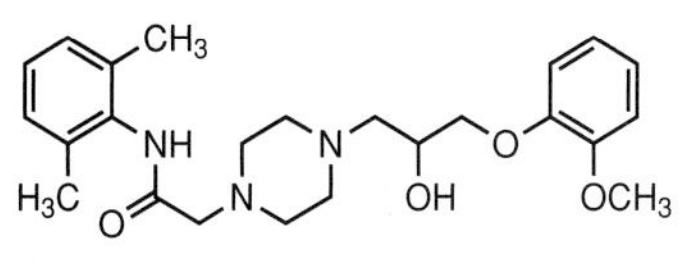

Ranolazine

Ranolazine (Ranexa) is a novel metabolic modulator approved for the treatment of chronic angina in combination with amlodipine, β-adrenoceptor antagonists, or nitrates in patients who have not achieved an adequate response with other antianginals. Although the exact mechanism of its antianginal and anti-ischemic effect is unknown, its antianginal and anti-ischemic action is not dependent on heart rate or blood pressure reduction, and it does not increase myocardial workload. Numerous studies suggest that ranolazine modulates myocardial metabolism by shifting myocardial energy metabolism from free fatty acids to glucose by inhibition of fatty acid oxidation, increasing glucose oxidation and, thus, generating more adenosine triphosphate (ATP) per molecule of oxygen consumed. Ranolazine mainly affects the late sodium current across the membrane with the potential to reduce the cardiac ischemic burden without significantly changing blood pressure and heart rate.

The oral bioavailability of ranolazine from extended-release tablets is 76%, and plasma concentration is not effected by food. Metabolism is mainly by CYP3A4 and, to a lesser degree, by CYP2D6, with less than 5% being excreted unchanged in the urine and feces. After a single oral dose of ranolazine solution, approximately 75% of the dose is excreted in the urine and approximately 25% in feces. Its elimination half-life for extended-release tablets is 7 to 9 hours. Ranolazine is an inhibitor of P-gp transporter. Ranolazine plasma concentrations are increased by CYP3A4 inhibitors. The CYP2D6 inhibition has a negligible effect on ranolazine exposure.

Miscellaneous Coronary Vasodilators

Another approach to the treatment of myocardial insufficiency is the use of the coronary vasodilators dipyridamole and papaverine. Dipyridamole, a PDE3 inhibitor, (Fig. 26.8) causes a long-acting and selective coronary vasodilation by increasing coronary blood flow via selective dilation of the coronary arteries. The state of the coronary arteries may determine the effect of dipyridamole on coronary blood flow and metabolic responses. Blood flow increased by 80% in unobstructed coronary vessels, whereas in stenotic coronary arteries, flow increased by approximately 40%. In patients with single-vessel coronary artery disease, intravenous dipyridamole increases flow to the ischemic area, probably by increasing collateral blood flow. Dipyridamole increases intracellular concentrations of the coronary vasodilator adenosine and cAMP and inhibits adenosine metabolism and uptake by vascular endothelial cells. The increased concentration of adenosine in vascular smooth muscle stimulates adenylate cyclase activity, leading to increased cAMP synthesis and, consequently, to relaxation of vascular smooth muscle (vasodilation). The effect of dipyridamole may not result only from its effect on adensoine but also from its ability to increase prostacyclin (vasodilator and platelet inhibitor) production by increasing cAMP concentration. Dipyridamole also increases intracellular cAMP by inhibiting PDE3, decreasing cAMP breakdown. Adenosine is a natural vasodilatory substance released by the myocardium during hypoxic episodes. Some structural similarity of adenosine to dipyridamole is apparent and substantiates this mechanism. Dipyridamole generally is used prophylactically, but its efficacy in reducing the incidence and severity of anginal attacks is not universally accepted.

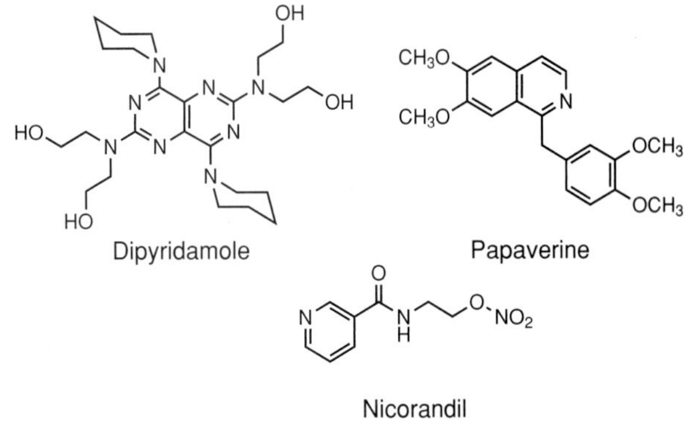

Dipyridamole

Papaverine

Nicorandil

Fig. 26.8. Miscellaneous coronary vasodilators.

Papaverine (Fig. 26.8) is a benzoisoquinoline vasodilator that produces generalized, nonspecific arteriolar dilatation and smooth muscle relaxation. Its oral bioavailability ranges from 30 to 50%, suggesting first-pass metabolism. Increased levels of intracellular cAMP secondary to inhibition of phosphodiesterase may contribute to its vasodilatation and relaxation effects without involving nerve supply. Large doses of papaverine can cause hypotension and tachycardia. Other studies suggest that it also depresses cardiac conduction and prolongs the refractory period.

The natriuretic polypeptide nesiritide (Natrecor) is manufactured in the United States using recombinant DNA technology for intravenous use to treat cases of angina and CHF. Nesiritide has the same amino acid sequence of the natural, 32-amino-acid natriuretic peptide that normally is released during cardiac ischemia and acts as vasodilator. Nesitride acts as a coronary vasodilator by binding to the soluble guanylate cyclase receptors in vascular smooth muscles, leading to increased intracellular concentrations of the vasodilator cGMP.

Nicorandil (Dancor, Ikorel) is a nicotinamide-nitrate ester (Fig. 26.8) used for the treatment of angina pectoris and CHF and has a dual mechanism of action. Structurally, it is a hybrid between organic nitrates and potassium channel activators. Although nicorandil contains a nitrate moiety, its pharmacological properties differ from organic nitrates. The nicotinamide moiety is responsible for the effect on K^+-ATP channels, which produces vascular smooth muscle relaxation by increasing potassium flux through ATP-sensitive sarcolemmal potassium channels. This leads to hyperpolarization of the cell membrane and subsequent decreases in levels of cytoplasmic calcium (calcium channel blockade) and dilation of arterial resistance vessels. Other agents in this class are minoxidil and diazoxide. The nitrate group explains its NO-like vasodilation on large coronary arteries, whereas its potassium channel–opening action is responsible for the dilatation of coronary resistance vessels, enabling it to decrease both preload and afterload and to increase coronary blood flow.

Nicorandil induces nitrate-like activation of soluble guanylate cyclase, increasing intracellular levels of cGMP with resultant dilation of venous capacitance vessels. Increases in cGMP are less than those observed with conventional nitrates, although the degree of vasodilation produced appears to be similar. Its oral bioavailability ranges from 75 to 80%. Food reduces the rate, but not the extent, of absorption. Nicorandil is extensively metabolized via denitration to inactive N-(2-hydroxyethyl)-nicotinamide, which undergoes further side-chain degradation to nicotinuric acid and, subsequently, nicotinamide and nicotinamide metabolites (e.g., nicotinic acid and N-methylnicotinamide). The nicotinamide derived from nicorandil merges into the endogenous pool of nicotinamide adenine dinucleoside coenzymes. Its elimination half-life is approximately 1 hour. Approximately 30% of nicorandil is excreted into the urine as metabolites, with less than 1% excreted unchanged.

DRUGS FOR THE TREATMENT OF CARDIAC ARRHYTHMIA

Arrhythmia

Arrhythmia is an alteration in the normal sequence of electrical impulse rhythm that leads to contraction of the myocardium. It is manifested as an abnormality in the rate, the site from which the impulses originate, or in the conduction through the myocardium. The rhythm of the heart normally is determined by a pacemaker site called the SA node, which consists of specialized cells that undergo spontaneous generation of action potentials at a rate of 100 to 110 action potentials ("beats") per minute. This intrinsic rhythm is strongly influenced by the vagus nerve, overcoming the sympathetic system at rest. This "vagal tone" brings the resting heart rate down to a normal sinus rhythm of 60 to 100 beats per minute. Sinus rates below this range are termed "sinus bradycardia," and sinus rates above this range are termed "sinus tachycardia." The sinus rhythm normally controls both atrial and ventricular rhythm. Action potentials generated by the SA node spread throughout the atria, depolarizing this tissue and causing atrial contraction. The impulse then travels into the ventricles via the AV node. Specialized conduction pathways within the ventricle rapidly conduct the wave of depolarization throughout the ventricles to elicit ventricular contraction. Therefore, normal cardiac rhythm is controlled by the pacemaker activity of the SA node. Abnormal or irregular cardiac rhythms (heartbeats) may occur when the SA node fails to function normally, when other pacemaker sites (e.g., ectopic pacemakers) trigger depolarization, or when a dysfunction occurs along the normal conduction pathways.

Causes of Arrhythmias

Many factors influence the normal rhythm of electrical activity in the heart. Arrhythmias may occur either because pacemaker cells fail to function properly or because of a blockage in transmission through the AV node. Underlying diseases, such as atherosclerosis, hyperthyroidism, or lung disease, also may be initiating factors. Some of the more common arrhythmias are those termed "ectopic," which occur when electrical signals spontaneously arise in regions other than the pacemaker and then compete with the normal impulses. Myocardial ischemia, excessive myocardial catecholamine release, stretching of the myocardium, and cardiac glycoside toxicity have all been shown to stimulate ectopic foci. A second mechanism for the generation of arrhythmias is from a phenomenon called reentry. This occurs when the electrical impulse does not die out after firing but, rather, continues to circulate and reexcite resting heart cells into depolarizing. The result of this reexcitation may be a single, premature beat or runs of ventricular tachycardia. Reentrant rhythms are common in the presence of coronary atherosclerosis.

Drugs for the Treatment of Antiarrhythmias and Their Classification

It is widely accepted that most currently available antiarrhythmic drugs may be classified into four categories, which are grouped on the basis of their effects on the cardiac action potential and, consequently, on the electrophysiological properties of the heart. To understand the basis of classification and the pharmacology of these agents, an understanding of normal cardiac electrophysiology is necessary.

Normal Physiologic Action

Normal cardiac contractions largely are a function of the action of a single atrial pacemaker, a fast and generally uniform conduction in predictable pathways, and a normal duration of the action potential and refractory period. Figure 26.9 depicts a normal cardiac action potential from a Purkinje fiber. The resting cell has a membrane potential of approximately −90 mV, with the

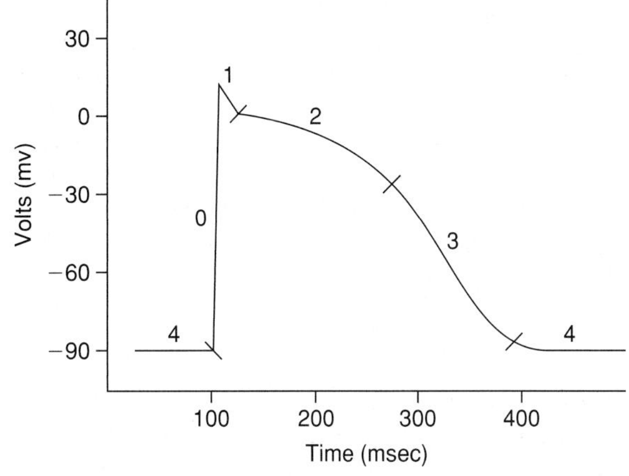

Fig. 26.9. Cardiac action potential recorded from a Purkinje fiber.

inside of the cell being electronegative relative to the outside of the cell. This is termed the "transmembrane resting potential." On excitation, the transmembrane potential reverses, and the inside of the membrane rapidly becomes positive with respect to the outside. On recovery from excitation, the resting potential is restored. These changes have been divided into five phases: Phase 0 represents depolarization and reversal of the transmembrane potential, phases 1–3 represent different stages of repolarization, and phase 4 represents the resting potential. During phase 0, which also is referred to as rapid depolarization, the permeability of the membrane for sodium ions increases, and sodium rapidly enters the cell, causing it to become depolarized. Phase 1 results from the ionic shift, which creates an electrochemical and concentration gradient that reduces the rate of sodium influx but favors the influx of chloride and efflux of potassium. Phase 2, the plateau phase, results from the slow inward movement of calcium, which is triggered by the rapid inward movement of sodium in phase 0. During this time, there also is an efflux of potassium that balances the influx of calcium, thus resulting in little or no change in membrane potential. Phase 3 is initiated by a slowing of the calcium influx coupled with a continued efflux of potassium. This continued efflux of potassium from the cell restores the membrane potential to normal resting potential levels. During phase 4, the Na^+, K^+-ATPase pump restores the ions to their proper local concentrations. The action potential is a coordinated sequence of ion movements in which sodium initially enters the cell, followed by a calcium influx, and finally, a potassium efflux returns the cell to its resting state. Several antiarrhythmic agents exert their effects by altering these ion fluxes.

Classification of Antiarrhythmic Drugs

CLASS IA ANTIARRHYTHMIC DRUGS. Class IA drugs generally are local anesthetics acting on nerve and myocardial membranes to slow conduction by blocking fast Na^+ channels, inhibiting phase 0 of the action potential (Fig. 26.9). Myocardial membranes show the greatest sensitivity. Class IA drugs decrease the maximal rate of depolarization without changing the resting potential. They also increase the threshold of excitability, increase the effective refractory period, decrease conduction velocity, and decrease spontaneous diastolic depolarization in pacemaker cells. The decrease in diastolic depolarization tends to suppress ectopic foci activity. Prolongation of the refractory period tends to abolish reentry arrhythmias. Table 26.6 summarizes these effects. Quinidine is considered to be the prototype drug for class IA.

Quinidine. Quinidine (Fig. 26.10) is widely used for acute and chronic treatment of ventricular and supraventricular arrhythmias, especially supraventricular tachycardia. It is a member of a family of alkaloids found in Cinchona bark (*Cinchona officinalis* L.) and is the diastereomer of quinine. Despite their structural similarity, quinidine and quinine differ markedly in their effects on the cardiac muscles, with the effects of quinidine being much more pronounced. Structurally, quinidine is composed of a quinoline ring and the bicyclic quinuclidine ring system, with a hydroxymethylene bridge connecting these two components. Examination of quinidine reveals two basic nitrogens, with the quinuclidine nitrogen (pK_a = 11) being the stronger of the two. Because of the basic character of quinidine, it is always used as water-soluble salt forms. These salts include quinidine sulfate, gluconate, and polygalacturonate. Good absorption (~95%) is observed with each of these forms after oral administration. In special situations, quinidine may be administered intravenously as the gluconate salt. The use of intravenous quinidine, however, is rare. The gluconate salt is particularly suited for parenteral use because of its high water solubility and lower irritant potential.

Quinidine's bioavailability appears to depend on a combination of metabolism and P-gp efflux. The bioavailabilities of quinidine sulfate and gluconate are 80 to 85% and 70 to 75%, respectively. Once absorbed, quinidine is subject to hepatic first-pass metabolism and is approximately 85% plasma protein bound, with an elimination half-life of approximately 6 hours. Quinidine is metabolized mainly in the liver, and renal excretion of unchanged drug also is significant (~10–50%). The metabolites are hydroxylated derivatives at either the quinoline ring through first-pass O-demethylation or at the quinuclidine ring through oxidation of the vinyl group. These metabolites possess only about one-third the activity of quinidine. Their contribution to overall therapeutic effect of quinidine is unclear. Recently, the clinical significance of the well-documented digoxin–quinidine interaction was described previously under digoxin–drug interactions. Apparently, quinidine (a P-gp substrate) inhibits the renal tubular secretion of digoxin via the P-gp efflux pump, resulting in increased plasma concentration for digoxin.

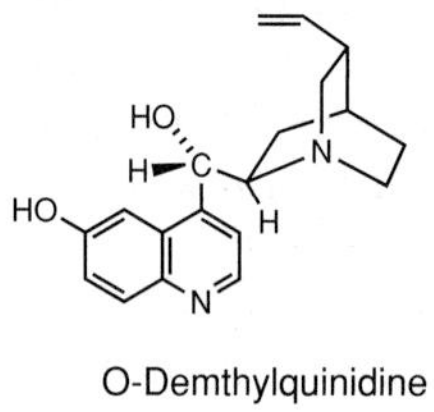

O-Demthylquinidine

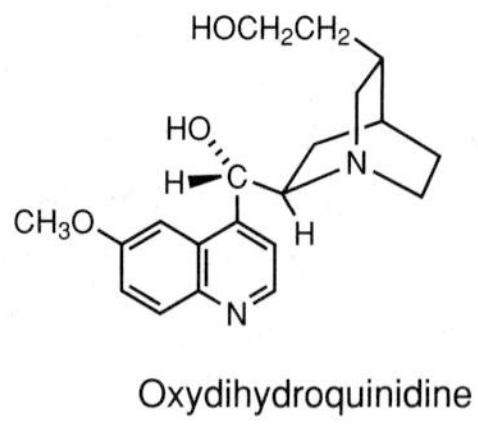

Oxydihydroquinidine

In addition, a common contaminant in quinidine preparations, dihydroquinidine, which is derived from reduction of the quinuclidine vinyl group at C-3 to an ethyl group, also may contribute to its activity (32). Although similar to quinidine in pharmacodynamic and pharmacokinetic behavior, this contaminant is both more potent as an antiarrhythmic and more toxic. Thus, levels of this contaminant may contribute to variability between commercial preparations. The most frequent adverse effects associated with quinidine therapy are gas-

Table 26.6. Summary of the Cardiac Physiological Effects of the Antiarrhythmic Drugs

Classification	Mechanism of Action	Primary Sites of Action	Drug Examples
Class IA	-Na^+ channel blockade -intermediate rate of dissociation from sodium channels -slows phase 0 depolarization -prolongs action potential duration -slows conduction	Atrial and ventricular tissue	Quinidine Procainamide Disopyramide
Class IB	-Na^+ channel blockade -rapid rate of dissociation from sodium channels -shorten phase 3 repolarization -shortens action potential duration	Ventricular tissue	Lidocaine Mexiletine Phenytoin Tocainide
Class 1C	- Na^+ channel blockade -slow rate of dissociation from sodium channels -markedly slows phase 0 depolarization -slows conduction	Ventricular tissue	Flecainide Encainide Propafenone Moricizine
Class II	- blocks sympathetic stimulation of β_1 adrenergic receptors -slow phase 4 depolarization -slows firing of SA node and conduction through AV node prolonging repolarization	SA node AV node	Propranolol Sotalol β_1 blockers
Class III	- K^+ channel blockade (block delayed rectifier current) -prolong phase 3 repolarization -prolongs duration of action potential which prolongs refractory period	Atrial and ventricular tissue	Amiodarone Sotalol Bretylium Ibutilide
Class IV	-Ca^{+2} channel blockade -slow phase 4 depolarization -slows firing of SA node and conduction through AV node prolonging repolarization of AV node	SA node AV node	Verapamil Diltiazim

trointestinal disturbances, such as nausea, diarrhea, and vomiting.

Procainamide. Procainamide (Fig. 26.10) is effective in the treatment of several types of cardiac arrhythmias. Its actions are similar to those of quinidine, yet procainamide may be effective in patients who are unresponsive to quinidine. The initial development of procainamide was stimulated by the observation that the local anesthetic procaine (the ester bio-isostere of procainamide), when administered intravenously, produced significant though short-lived antiarrhythmic effects.

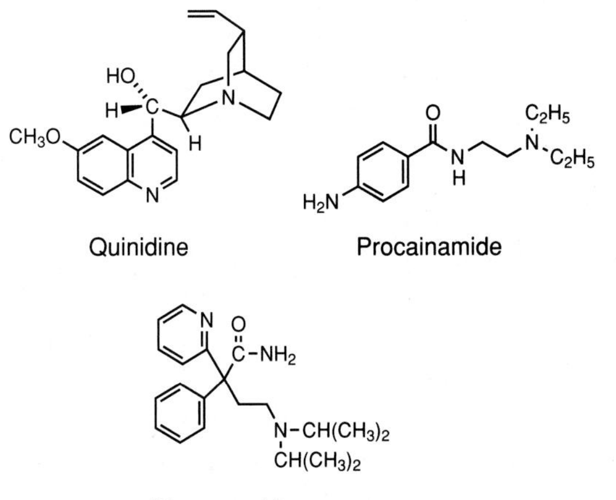

Quinidine

Procainamide

Disopyramide

Fig. 26.10. Class IA antiarrhythmics.

Unfortunately, considerable central nervous system toxicity, in addition to the short duration, limited the usefulness of this agent. Moreover, procaine is not active orally because of its short duration of action caused by both chemical and plasma esterase hydrolysis. A logical modification of this molecule was the isosteric replacement of the ester with an amide group. This produced orally active procainamide, which is more resistant to both enzymatic and chemical hydrolysis. Peak plasma levels of procainamide are observed within 45 to 90 minutes after oral administration, and approximately 70 to 80% of the dose is bioavailable. Approximately half of this dose is excreted unchanged, and the remaining half undergoes acetylation metabolism in the liver. Metabolites of procainamide include p-aminobenzoic acid and N-acetylprocainamide. Interestingly, the acetylated metabolite is also active as an antiarrhythmic. Its formation accounts for up to one-third of the administered dose and is catalyzed by the liver enzyme N-acetyl transferase. Because acetylation is strongly influenced by an individual's genetic background, marked variability in the amounts of this active metabolite may be observed from patient to patient. Renal excretion dominates, with approximately 90% of a dose excreted as unchanged drug and metabolites. The elimination half-life is approximately 3.5 hours. A substantial percentage (60–70%) of patients on procainamide show elevated levels of antinuclear antibodies after a few months. Of these patients, between 20 and 30% develop a drug-induced lupus syndrome if therapy is continued. These adverse effects, which are attributed to the aromatic amino group, are observed more frequently and more rapidly in "slow acetylators." Usually, the symptoms associated with procainamide-induced lupus syndrome subside fairly rapidly after the drug is discontinued. These problems, however, have discouraged long-term procainamide therapy.

Disopyramide. Disopyramide phosphate is used orally for the treatment of certain ventricular and atrial arrhythmias. Despite its structural dissimilarity to procainamide (Fig. 26.10), its cardiac effects are very similar. Disopyramide is rapidly and completely absorbed from the gastrointestinal tract. Peak plasma level is usually reached within 1 to 3 hours, and a plasma half-life of 5 to 7 hours is common. Approximately half of an oral dose is excreted unchanged in the urine. The remaining drug undergoes hepatic metabolism, principally to the corresponding N-dealkylated form. This metabolite retains approximately half the antiarrhythmic activity of disopyramide and also is subject to renal excretion. Adverse effects of disopyramide frequently are observed. These effects are primarily anticholinergic in nature and include dry mouth, blurred vision, constipation, and urinary retention.

CLASS IB ANTIARRHYTHMIC DRUGS

Lidocaine. Lidocaine, similar to procaine, is an effective, clinically used local anesthetic (Fig. 26.11) (see Chapter 16). Its cardiac effects, however, are distinctly different from those of procainamide or quinidine. Lidocaine normally is reserved for the treatment of ventricular arrhythmias and, in fact, usually is the drug of choice for emergency treatment of ventricular arrhythmias. Its utility in these situations results from the rapid onset of antiarrhythmic effects on intravenous infusion. In addition, these effects cease soon after the infusion is terminated. Thus, lidocaine therapy may be rapidly modified in response to changes in the patient's status. Lidocaine is effective as an antiarrhythmic only when given parenterally, and the intravenous route is the most common. Antiarrhythmic activity is not observed after oral administration because of the rapid and efficient first-pass metabolism by the liver. Parenterally administered lidocaine is approximately 60 to 70% plasma protein bound.

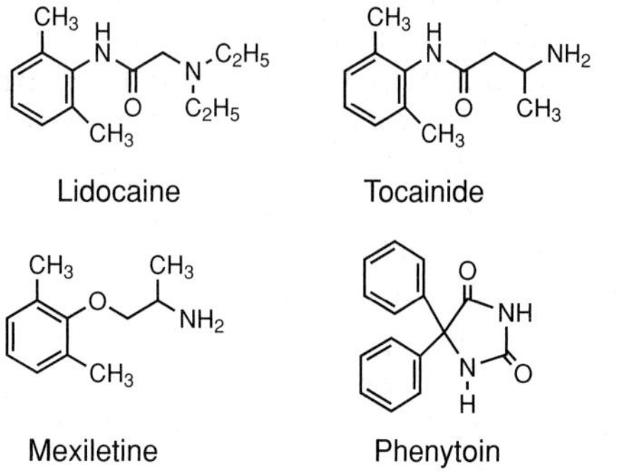

Lidocaine Tocainide Mexiletine Phenytoin

Fig. 26.11. Class IB antiarrhythmics.

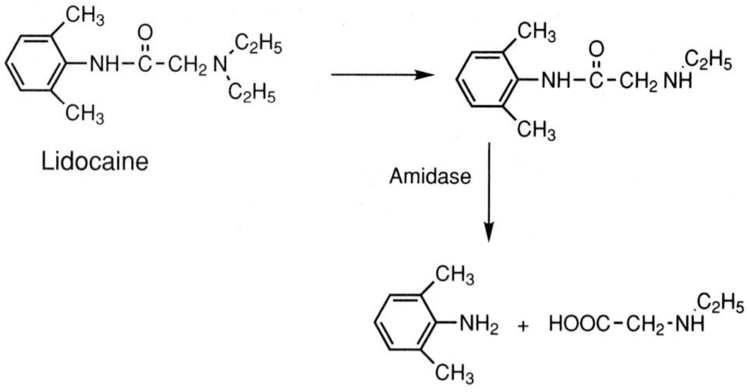

Lidocaine Amidase

Fig. 26.12. Metabolism of lidocaine.

Hepatic metabolism is rapid (plasma half-life, ~15–30 minutes) and primarily involves N-deethylation to yield monoethylglycinexylide, followed by amidase-catalyzed hydrolysis into N-ethylglycine and 2,6-dimethylaniline (2,6-xylidine) (Fig. 26.12).

Monoethylglycinexylide has good antiarrhythmic activity. It is not clinically useful, however, because it undergoes rapid enzymatic hydrolysis. The adverse effects of lidocaine include emetic and convulsant properties that predominantly involve the central nervous system and heart. The central nervous system effects may begin with dizziness and paresthesia and, in severe cases, ultimately lead to epileptic seizures.

Tocainide. Tocainide (Tonocard) (Fig. 26.11) is an α-methyl analogue structurally related to monoethylglycinexylide, the active metabolite of lidocaine, which possesses very similar electrophysiologic effects to lidocaine. In contrast to lidocaine, tocainide is orally active, and its oral absorption is excellent. Like lidocaine, it usually is reserved for the treatment of ventricular arrhythmias. The α-methyl group is believed to slow the rate of metabolism and, thereby, to contribute to oral activity. The plasma half-life of tocainide is approximately 12 hours, and nearly 50% of the drug may be excreted unchanged in the urine. Adverse effects associated with tocainide are like those observed with lidocaine—specifically, gastrointestinal disturbances and central nervous system effects.

Mexiletine. Mexiletine (Mexitil) (Fig. 26.11) is similar to both lidocaine and tocainide in its effects and therapeutic application. It is used principally to treat and prevent ventricular arrhythmias. Like tocainide, mexilitine has very good oral activity and absorption properties. Clearance depends on metabolism and renal excretion. A relatively long plasma half-life of approximately 12 to 16 hours is common. Adverse effects are similar to those experienced with tocainide and lidocaine.

Phenytoin. For 50 years, phenytoin (Fig. 26.11) has seen clinical use in the treatment of epileptic seizures (see Chapter 20). During this time, it was noticed that phenytoin also produced supposedly adverse cardiac effects. On closer examination, these adverse effects actually were found to be beneficial in the treatment of certain arrhythmias. Currently, phenytoin is used in the treatment of atrial and ventricular arrhythmias resulting from digitalis toxicity. It is not, however, officially approved for this use.

Phenytoin may be administered either orally or intravenously and is absorbed slowly after oral administration, with peak plasma levels achieved after 3 to 12 hours. It is extensively plasma protein bound (~90%), and the elimination half-life is between 15 and 30 hours. These large ranges reflect the considerable variability observed from patient to patient. Parenteral administration of phenytoin is usually limited to the intravenous route. Phenytoin for injection is dissolved in a highly alkaline vehicle (pH 12). This alkaline vehicle is required because phenytoin is weakly acidic and has very poor solubility in its un-ionized form. Reportedly, however, its phosphate ester fosphenytoin has water solubility advantages over phenytoin for injection. Intramuscular phenytoin generally is avoided, because it results in tissue necrosis at the site of injection and erratic absorption because of high alkalinity. In addition, intermittent intravenous infusion is required to reduce the incidence of severe phlebitis.

Phenytoin metabolism is relatively slow and predominantly involves aromatic hydroxylation to p-hydroxylated inactive metabolites (see Chapter 20). Phenytoin also induces its own metabolism and is subject to large interindividual variability. The major metabolite, 5-p-hydroxyphenyl-5-phenylhydantoin, accounts for approximately 75% of a dose. This metabolite is excreted through the kidney as the β-glucuronide conjugate. Phenytoin clearance is strongly influenced by its metabolism; therefore, agents that affect phenytoin metabolism may cause intoxication. In addition, because phenytoin is highly plasma protein bound, agents that displace phenytoin also may cause toxicity.

CLASS IC ANTIARRHYTHMIC DRUGS

Flecainide. Flecainide (Tamborcor) exhibits properties distinctly different from those of Class IA or IB antiarrhythmic drugs. Flecainide is a fluorinated benzamide derivative (Fig. 26.13), available as the acetate salt. Flecainide has been approved by the U.S. Food and Drug Administration (FDA) for the treatment of ventricular arrhythmias. Clinical studies suggest that this agent may be more effective than either quinidine or disopyramide in suppressing premature ventricular contractions. Oral flecainide is well absorbed, and the plasma half-life is approximately 14 hours. About half of an oral dose is metabolized in the liver, and one-third is excreted unchanged in the urine. As with other antiarrhythmics, flecainide may produce adverse effects. The most severe is flecainide's occasional tendency to aggravate existing arrhythmias or to induce new ones. Although fewer than 10% of patients experience this effect, it may be life-threatening. Accordingly, it may be desirable to start therapy in the hospital. Other less serious side effects include blurred vision, headache, nausea, and abdominal pain.

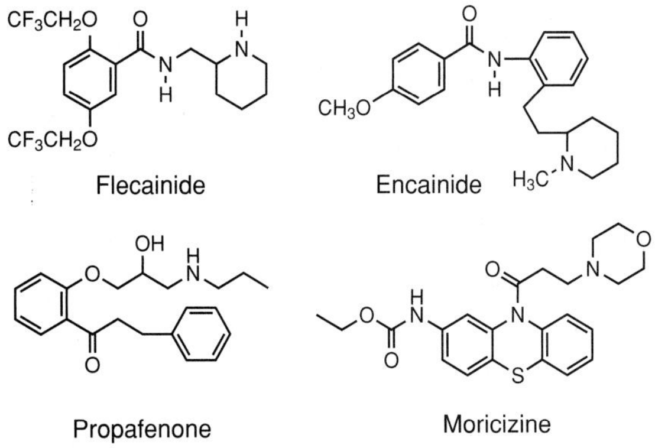

CF_3CH_2O CF_3CH_2O Flecainide

CH_3O H_3C Encainide

Propafenone

Moricizine

Fig, 26.13. Class IC antiarrhythmics.

Encainide. Encainide (Enkaid) (Fig. 26.13) represents another benzamide derivative, with similar pharmacological properties to flecainide but with less negative inotropic effect.

Propafenone. Propafenone (Rythmol) (Fig. 26.13) is a Class I, local anesthetic–type antiarrhythmic agent. Propafenone is structurally related to other Class IC antiarrhythmic drugs and also to β-adrenergic receptor blockers. It is used primarily for ventricular and supraventricular arrhythmias. The drug is administered orally and intravenously; however, the parenteral dosage forms are not commercially available in the United States. After oral administration, the drug is rapidly and almost completely absorbed from the gastrointestinal tract. Propafenone metabolism involves hepatic CYP2D6 enzymes. Its rate of metabolism is genetically determined by an individual's ability to metabolize the so-called phenotype compounds (fast or slow metabolizers) (see Chapter 10).

Moricizine. Moricizine (Ethmozine) (Fig. 26.13) is a phenothiazine analogue that processes the same electrophysiological effects on the heart as those of Class IC antiarrhythmics. Despite its short half-life after oral administration, its antiarrhythmic effects can persist for many hours, suggesting that some of its metabolites may be active.

CLASS II ANTIARRHYTHMIC DRUGS. Class II antiarrhythmic drugs (Fig. 26.14) are β-adrenergic receptor blocking agents, which block the role of the sympathetic nervous system in the genesis of certain cardiac arrhythmias. Their dominant electrophysiological effect is to depress adrenergically enhanced calcium influx through β-receptor blockade. Drugs in this class decrease neurologically induced automaticity at normal therapeutic doses. At higher doses, these drugs also may exhibit anesthetic properties, which cause decreased excitability, decreased conduction velocity, and a prolonged effective refractory period. In normal therapeutic situations, the β-blocking effects are more important than any local anesthetic effects that these

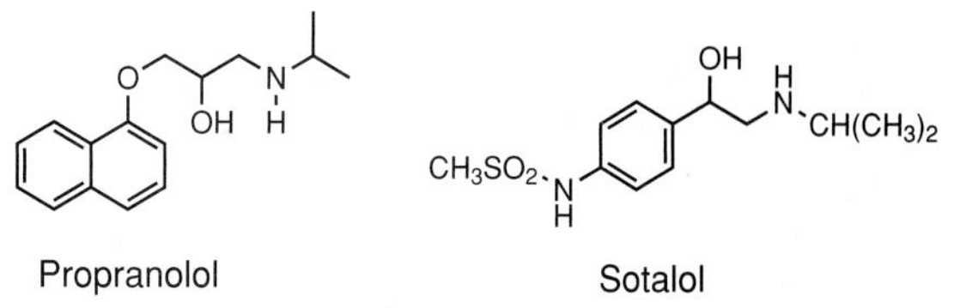

Fig. 26.14. Class II inhibitors of depolarization.

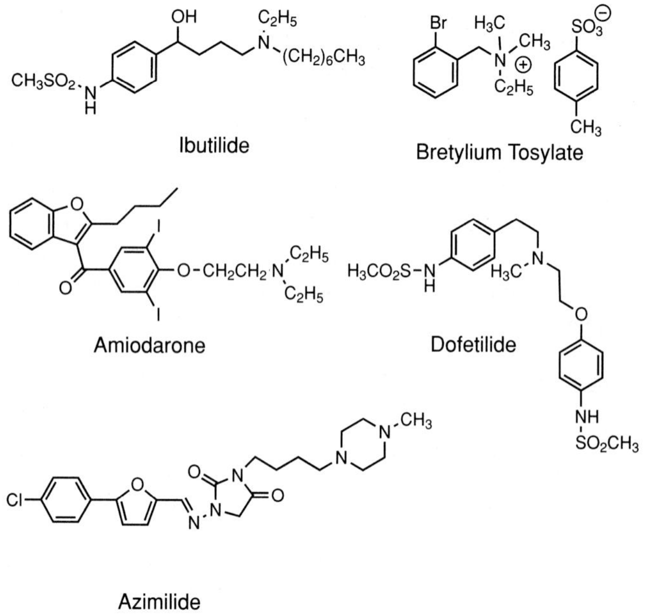

Fig. 26.15. Class III antiarrhythmic agents.

drugs may have. Propranolol is the prototype β-adrenergic blocker drug for class II (see Chapter 13).

Propranolol. (+)-Propranolol, a nonselective β-adrenergic blocker, is the prototype for Class II antiarrhythmics. Its pharmacology and pharmacokinetics are discussed in detail in Chapters 13 and 29. Its use as an antiarrhythmic usually is for the treatment of supraventricular arrhythmias, including atrial flutter, paroxysmal supraventricular tachycardia, and atrial fibrillation. Propranolol also is reported to be effective in the treatment of digitalis-induced ventricular arrhythmias. Moreover, beneficial results may be obtained when propranolol is used in combination with other agents. For example, in certain cases, quinidine and propranolol together have proved to be more successful in alleviating atrial fibrillation than either agent has alone. Few serious adverse effects are associated with propranolol therapy.

Sotalol. (±)-Sotalol (Betapace, Sotacor), a nonselective β-adrenergic blocker, is a methanesulfonanilide antiarrhythmic agent. As an antiarrhythmic, it is dually classified as Class II and Class III because of the similarity of its cardiac effects to both classes. Sotalol is used orally to suppress and prevent the recurrence of life-threatening ventricular arrhythmia.

CLASS III INHIBITORS OF REPOLARIZATION. Class III drugs cause a homogeneous prolongation of the duration of the action potential. This results in a prolongation of the effective refractory period. It is believed that most of Class III antiarrhythmic agents act through Phase 3 of the action potential by blocking potassium channels. Figure 26.15 illustrates the chemical structures of members of Class III. Bretylium is the prototype drug for this class.

Bretylium tosylate. Bretylium tosylate is a quaternary ammonium salt derivative (Fig. 26.15) originally developed for use as an antihypertensive. Its antiarrhythmic use is limited to emergency, life-threatening situations in which other agents, such as lidocaine and procainamide, have failed. Generally, bretylium is used only in intensive care units and may be administered either intravenously or intramuscularly. The plasma elimination half-life usually is approximately 10 hours, and it is eliminated largely unchanged in the urine. The major adverse effect associated with bretylium tosylate is hypotension, including orthostatic hypotension, which may be very severe.

Amiodarone. Initially developed as an antianginal (coronary vasodilator), amiodarone (Fig. 26.15) has antiarrhythmic effects that are somewhat similar to those of bretylium. It is approved by the U.S. FDA for the treatment of life-threatening ventricular arrhythmias that are refractory to other drugs. Its cardiac effects are not well characterized, but clinical studies indicate that it is primarily a Class III agent but also acts as a Class I, II, and IV antiarrythmic. It has a unique mechanism of action that involves alteration of the lipid membrane in which ion channels and receptors are located. Its severe toxicity, however, makes it the drug of last choice. As with bretylium tosylate, use of this agent should be initiated in a hospital setting.

Ibutilide. Ibutilide (Corvert) is another methanesulfonanilide derivative (Fig. 26.15), but unlike sotalol, it lacks any β-adrenergic blocking activity. Like sotalol, it exhibits electrophysiologic effects characteristic of Class III. Ibutilide is used only by intravenous infusion as its fumarate salt.

Dofetilide. Dofetilide (Tikosyn) is a bis-methanesulfonanilide derivative that is essentially the non-β-blocking moiety of the sotalol molecule (Fig. 26.15). It exhibits only Class III electrophysiological effects, but like ibutilide, it lacks any β-adrenergic blocking activity. Dofetlide is used orally to suppress atrial fibrillation and flutter. It is more potent and selective than other Class III methanesulfonanilides, including sotalol. Dofetilide is well absorbed from the gastrointestinal tract, with a bioavailability of 96 to 100%. The bioavailability of oral dofetilide is not affected by food or antacids. Protein binding is 60 to 70%. Dofetilide is metabolized by the hepatic CYP3A4 enzyme system via N-dealkylation and N-oxidation to inactive or minimally active metabolites. Of the approximately 80% of a dose excreted in urine, approximately 80% is excreted unchanged, with the other 20% as metabolites.

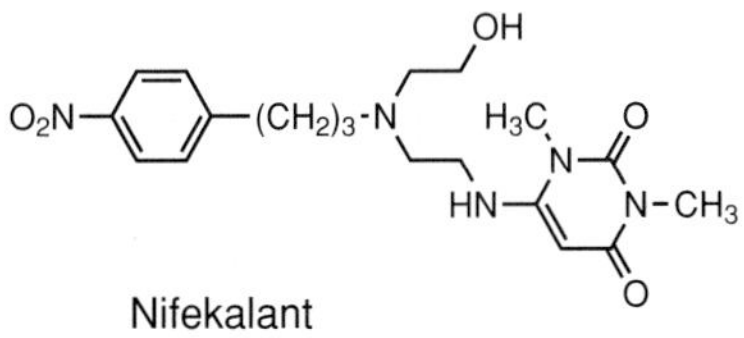

Fig. 26.16. Antiarrhythmic drugs in Phase III clinical trials.

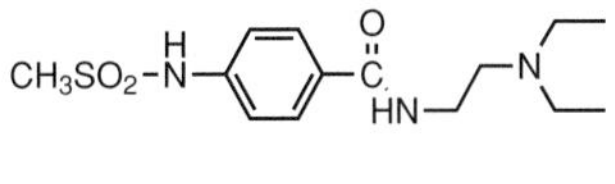

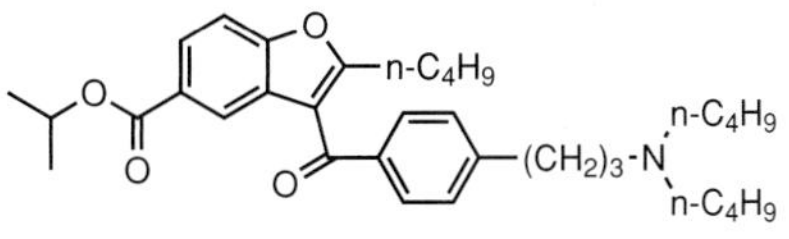

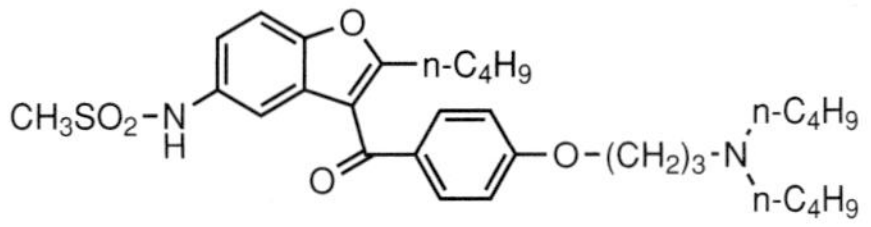

Azimilide. Azimilde is another Class III antiarrhythmic agent structurally unrelated to any of the above agents (Fig. 26.15). Azimilide is not available in the United States; it is only available in Europe. Following oral administration, the drug is completely absorbed, with no effect of food. Protein binding is 94%. It is metabolized in the liver to an active carboxylate metabolite, but its concentration in plasma is less than 5% of the parent compound. Thus, it is considered to be therapeutically inactive. Renal excretion is approximately 10%. Its elimination half-life is 3 to 4 days.

CLASS IV CALCIUM CHANNEL BLOCKERS. Class IV calcium channel antiarrhythmic drugs (Fig. 26.7) comprise a group of agents that selectively block the slow inward current carried by calcium (i.e., calcium channel blockers). The slow inward current in cardiac cells has been shown to be of importance for the normal action potential in SA node cells. It also has been suggested that this inward current is involved in the genesis of certain types of cardiac arrhythmias. Administration of a Class IV drug causes a prolongation of the refractory period in the AV node and the atria, a decrease in AV conduction, and a decrease in spontaneous diastolic depolarization. These effects block conduction of premature impulses at the AV node and, thus, are very effective in treating supraventricular arrhythmias. Verapamil and diltazem are prototype drugs for this class (Fig. 26.7), but dihydropyridine drugs are less effective in cardiac tissues. Refer to the section on calcium channel blocker under antianginal drugs for pharmacokinetic information.

ANTIARRHYTHMIC DRUGS IN PHASE III CLINICAL TRIALS

Antiarrhythmic drugs in Phase III clinical trials are shown in Figure 26.16. Nifekalant is a pyrimidinone Class III agent. Sematilide is a Class III agent that is a benzamide derivative of ibutilide, and SSR-149744c and dronedarone are noniodinated analogues of amiodarone, reportedly with fewer adverse effects than amiodarone.

CASE STUDY

Victoria F. Roche and S. William Zito

BZ shows up at the hospital where you work. He is a 30-year-old computer jock who works for one of the high-tech Internet companies. He has no history of any health-related problems, but today, he reports that he has been coming in from playing basketball on the company grounds feeling dizzy and thinking he is going to faint. At first, he thought it was the result of too much exertion in the heat of the summer; however, these symptoms have continued even when he is not strenuously exercising. In the emergency department, BZ is still experiencing these symptoms, and on questioning, he says he can feel his heart beating, is anxious, and is visibly out of breath when speaking. A physical examination reveals a pulse of 220 beats per minute, with normal temperature and lung sounds. An electrocardiogram reveals a regular narrow QRS complex at 200 to 220 beats per minutes. He is diagnosed with paroxysmal supraventricular tachycardia (PSVT) and treated with intravenous adenosine after vagal maneuvers fail (blowing on his thumb, "bearing down" as if he were forcing a bowel movement, or splashing his face with ice water) to restore him to normal sinus rhythm. BZ is admitted to the hospital for observation. Overnight and into the next day, BZ continues to have mild PSVTs; therefore, the cardiologist decides that prophylactic therapy is necessary. Evaluate structures 1 to 4 for possible use in this case.

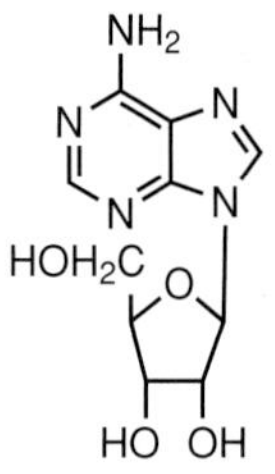

Adenosine 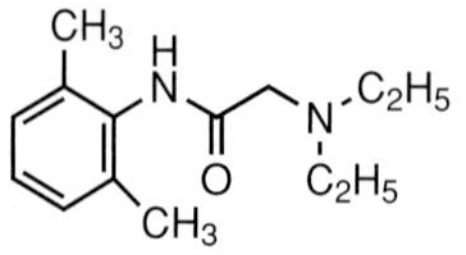 1 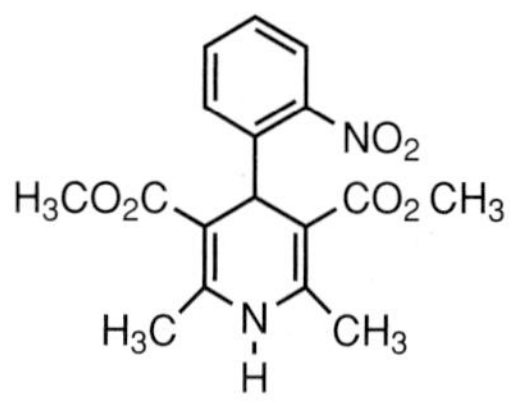 2

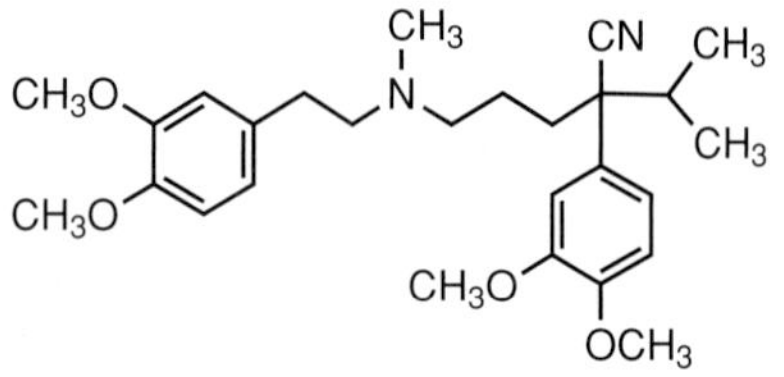

3 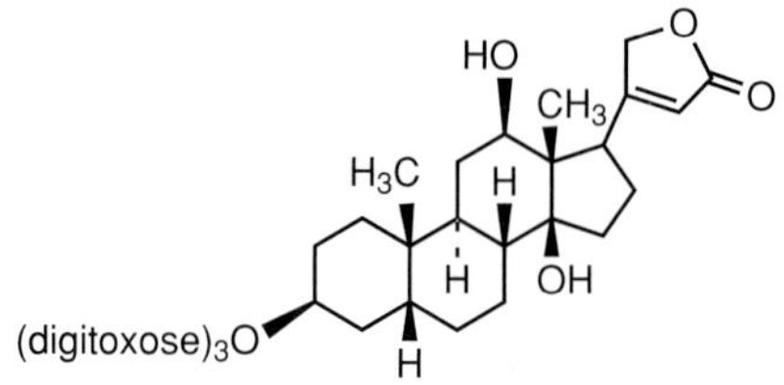 4

1. Identify the therapeutic problem(s) in which the pharmacist's intervention may benefit the patient.
2. Identify and prioritize the patient-specific factors that must be considered to achieve the desired therapeutic outcomes.
3. Conduct a thorough and mechanistically oriented structure-activity analysis of all therapeutic alternatives provided in the case.
4. Evaluate the SAR findings against the patient-specific factors and desired therapeutic outcomes, and make a therapeutic decision.
5. Counsel your patient.

References

1. Smith TW, Antman EM, Friedman PL, et al. Digitalis glycosides: mechanisms and manifestations of toxicity. Part II. Prog Cardiovasc Dis 1984;26:495–540.
2. Smith TW, Antman EM, Friedman PL, et al. Digitalis glycosides: mechanisms and manifestations of toxicity. Part III. Prog Cardiovasc Dis 1984; 27:21–56.
3. Rietbrock N, Woodcock BG. Two-hundred years of foxglove therapy: *Digitalis purpurea* 1785–1985. Trends Pharmacol Sci 1985;6:267–269.
4. Thomas R, Bontagy J, Gelbart A. Synthesis and biological activity of semisynthetic digitalis analogues. J Pharm Sci 1974;63:1649–1683.
5. Thomas R. Cardiac drugs. In: Wolff ME, ed. Burger's Medicinal Chemistry, 4th Ed., Part III. New York: John Wiley and Sons, 1981, pp 47–102.
6. Repke K. New developments in cardiac glycoside structure–activity relationships. Trends Pharmacol Sci 1985;6:275–278.
7. Fullerton DS, Griffin JF, Rohrer DC, et al. Using computer graphics to study cardiac glycoside–receptor interactions. Trends Pharmacol Sci 1985;6: 279–282.
8. Koren G, Woodland C, Ito S. Toxic digoxin–drug interactions: the major role of renal P-glycoprotein. Vet Human Toxicol 1998;40:45–46.
9. Colucci WS, Wright RF, Braunwald E. New positive inotropic agents in the treatment of congestive heart failure. 1. Mechanisms of action and recent clinical developments. N Engl J Med 1986;314:290–299.
10. Colucci WS, Wright RF, Braunwald E. New positive inotropic agents in the treatment of congestive heart failure. 2. Mechanisms of action and recent clinical developments. N Engl J Med 1986;314:349–358.
11. Westfall T, Westfall DP, Adrenergic Agonists and Antagonists. In: Goodman & Gilman's The Pharmacological Basis of Therapeutics, Brunton L, Lazo T, Barker K, 11th ed. New York, McGraw-Hill, 2006, pp 237–296.
12. Needleman P, Johnson EM Jr. Mechanism of tolerance development to organic nitrates. J Pharmacol Exp Ther 1973;184:709–715.
13. Needleman P, Jakschik B, Johnson EM Jr. Sulfhydryl requirement for relaxation of vascular smooth muscle. J Pharmacol Exp Ther 1973;187:324–331.
14. Ignarro LJ, Lippton H, Edwards JC, et al. Mechanism of vascular smooth muscle relaxation by organic nitrates, nitrites, nitroprusside and nitric oxide: evidence for the involvement of S-nitrosothiols as active intermediates. J Pharmacol Exp Ther 1981;218:739–749.
15. Ignarro LJ, Barry BK, Gruetter DY, et al. Guanylate cyclase activation of nitroprusside and nitroguanidine is related to formation of S-nitrosothol intermediates. Biochem Biophys Res Commun 1980;94:93–100.
16. Ignarro LJ, Barry BK, Gruetter DY, et al. Selective alterations in responsiveness of guanylate cyclase to activation by nitroso compounds during enzyme purification. Biochim Biophys Acta 1981;673:394–407.
17. Ignarro LJ, Edwards JC, Gruetter DY, et al. Possible involvement of S-nitosothiols in the activation of guanylate cyclase by nitroso compounds. FEBS Lett 1980; 110:275–278.
18. Ignarro LJ, Gruetter CA. Requirement of thiols for activation of coronary arterial guanylate cyclase by glyceral trinitrate and sodium nitrite: possible involvement of S-nitrosothiols. Biochim Biophys Acta 1980;631: 221–231.
19. Ignarro LJ, Kadowitz PJ, Baricos WH. Evidence that regulation of hepatic guanylate cyclase activity involves interactions between catalytic site -SH groups and both substrate and activator. Arch Biochem Biophys 1981;208: 75–86.
20. Moncada S, Plamer RM, Higgs EA. Nitric oxide: physiology, pathophysiology, and pharmacology. Pharmacol Rev 1991;43:109–142.
21. Snyder SH, Bredt DS. Nitric oxide as a neuronal messenger. Trends Pharmacol Sci 1991;12:125–128.
22. McCall T, Vallance P. Nitric oxide takes centre-stage with newly defined roles. Trend Pharmacol Sci 1992;13:1–6.
23. Feldman PL, Criffen OW, et al. Surprising life of nitric oxide. Chem Eng News 1993;71(51):26–38.
24. Fung HL, Sutton SC, Kamiya A. Blood vessel uptake and metabolism of organic nitrates in the rat. J Pharmacol Exp Ther 1984;228:334–341.
25. Needleman P, Lang S, Johnson EM Jr. Organic nitrates: relationship between biotransformation and rational angina pectoris therapy. J Pharmacol Exp Ther 1972;181:489–497.
26. Abrams J. Pharmacology of nitroglycerin and long-acting nitrates. Am J Cardiol 1985;56:12A–18A.
27. Fung HL. Pharmacokinetics of nitroglycerin and long-acting nitrate esters. Am J Med 1983;72(Suppl):13–19.
28. Corwin S, Reiffel JA. Nitrate therapy for angina pectoris. Current concepts about mechanism of action and evaluation of currently available preparations. Arch Intern Med 1985;145:538–543.
29. Rahwan RG, Witiak DT, Muir WW. Newer antiarrhythmics. Annu Rep Med Chem 1981;16:257–268.
30. Yedinak KC. Use of calcium channel antagonists for cardiovascular disease. Am Pharm 1993;33:49–65.
31. Michalets EL. Update: clinically significant cytochrome P-450 drug interactions. Pharmacotherapy 1998;18: 84–112.

32. Conn HL Jr, Luchi RJ. Some cellular and metabolic considerations relating to the action of quinidine as a prototype antiarrhythmic agent. Am J Med 1964;37:685–699.

Suggested Readings

Fozzard HA, Sheets MF. Cellular mechanism of action of cardiac glycosides. J Am Coll Cardiol 1985;5:10A–15A.

Hansten PD, ed. Drug Interactions: Clinical Significance of Drug–Drug Interactions, 5th Ed. Philadelphia: Lea and Febiger, 1985.

Kaplan HR. Advances in antiarrhythmic drug therapy: changing concepts.' Federation Proc 1986;45:2184–2213.

Katz AM. Effects of digitalis on cell biochemistry: sodium pump inhibition. J Am Coll Cardiol 1985;5:16A–21A.

Kowey PR. Pharmacological effects of antiarrhythmic drugs. Arch Intern Med 1998;158:325–332.

Mangini RJ, ed. Drug Interaction Facts. St. Louis: JB. Lippincott, 1983.

Michel T. Drugs used for the treatment of myocardial ischemia. In: Goodman and Gilman's The Pharmacological Basis of Therapeutics, 11th Ed. New York: McGraw-Hill, New York, 2006, pp 823–844.

Rocco T, Fong JG, Treatment of congestive heart failure. In: Goodman & Gilman's The Pharmacological Basis of Therapeutics, Brunton L, Lazo T, Barker K, 11th ed. New York: McGraw-Hill, 2006, pp 869–898.

Thomas RE. Cardiac drugs. In: Wolff ME, ed. Burger's Medicinal Chemistry and Drug Discovery, 5th Ed., Part IIA, vol 2. New York: John Wiley and Sons, 1996. pp 153–261.

27. *Diuretics*

GARY O. RANKIN

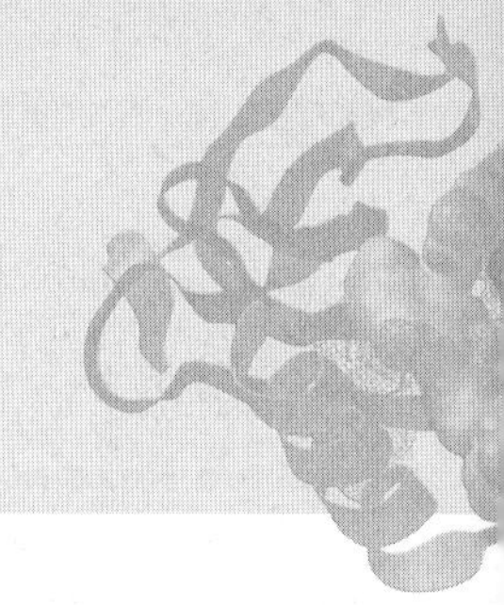

DRUGS COVERED IN THIS CHAPTER:

OSMOTIC DIURETICS
- Isosorbide
- Mannitol

CARBONIC ANHYDRASE INHIBITORS
- Acetazolamide

THIAZIDE DIURETICS
- Chlorothiazide
- Benzthiazide
- Hydrochlorothiazide
- Trichloromethiazide
- Methyclothiazide
- Polythiazide
- Hydroflumethiazide
- Bendroflumethiazide

THIAZIDE-LIKE DIURETICS
- Metolazone
- Quinethazone
- Chlorthalidone
- Indapamide

LOOP DIURETICS
- Furosemide
- Ethacrynic acid
- Bumetanide
- Torsemide

POTASSIUM-SPARING DIURETICS
- Amiloride
- Triameterene

ALDOSTERONE ANTAGONISTS (MINERALOCORTICOID RECEPTOR ANTAGONISTS)
- Spironolactone
- Canrenone
- Eplerenone

INTRODUCTION

Diuretics are chemicals that increase the rate of urine formation (1). By increasing the urine flow rate, diuretic usage leads to increased excretion of electrolytes (especially sodium and chloride ions) and water from the body without affecting protein, vitamin, glucose, or amino acid reabsorption. These pharmacological properties have led to the use of diuretics in the treatment of edematous conditions resulting from a variety of causes (e.g., congestive heart failure, nephrotic syndrome, and chronic liver disease) and in the management of hypertension. Diuretic drugs also are useful as the sole agent or as adjunct therapy in the treatment of a wide range of clinical conditions, including hypercalcemia, diabetes insipidus, acute mountain sickness, primary hyperaldosteronism, and glaucoma.

The primary target organ for diuretics is the kidney, where these drugs interfere with the reabsorption of sodium and other ions from the lumina of the nephrons, which are the functional units of the kidney. The amount of ions and accompanying water that are excreted as urine following administration of a diuretic, however, is determined by many factors, including the chemical structure of the diuretic, the site or sites of action of the agent, the salt intake of the patient, and the amount of extracellular fluid present. In addition to the direct effect of diuretics to impair solute and water reabsorption from the nephron, diuretics also can trigger compensatory physiological events that have an impact on either the magnitude or the duration of the diuretic response. Thus, it is important to be aware of the normal mechanisms of urine formation and renal control mechanisms to understand clearly the ability of chemicals to induce a diuresis.

NORMAL PHYSIOLOGY OF URINE FORMATION

Two important functions of the kidney are 1) to maintain a homeostatic balance of electrolytes and water and 2) to excrete water-soluble end products of metabolism. The kidney accomplishes these functions through the formation of urine by the nephrons (Fig. 27.1). Each kidney contains approximately 1 million nephrons and is capable of forming urine independently. The nephrons are composed of a specialized capillary bed called the glomerulus and a long tubule divided anatomically and functionally into the proximal tubule, loop of Henle, and distal tubule. Each component of the nephron contributes to the normal functions of the kidney in a unique manner; thus, all are targets for different classes of diuretic agents.

Urine formation begins with the filtration of blood at the glomerulus. Approximately 1,200 mL of blood per minute flows through both kidneys and reaches the nephron by way of afferent arterioles. Approximately 20% of the blood entering the glomerulus is filtered into Bowman's capsule to form the glomerular filtrate. The glomerular filtrate is composed of blood components with a molecular weight less than that of albumin (~69,000 daltons) and not bound to plasma proteins. The glomerular filtration rate (GFR) averages 125 mL/min in humans but can vary widely even in normal functional states.

The glomerular filtrate leaves the Bowman's capsule and enters the proximal convoluted tubule (S1, S2 segments, Fig 27.1), where the majority (50–60%) of filtered sodium is reabsorbed osmotically. Sodium reabsorption is coupled electrogenetically with the reabsorption of

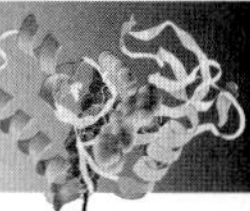

CLINICAL SIGNIFICANCE

It is important for the clinician to understand the medicinal chemistry of the diuretics to appropriately use them in individual patients. This diverse group of medications is classified in many ways: mechanism of action, site of action, chemical class, and effect on urine contents. Knowledge of structure-activity relationships helps to predict indications, possible off-label uses, magnitude of diuresis, potency, and side effect profile.

Consequently, diuretics have a variety of uses. Thiazide diuretics may be used either alone or in combination with other pharmacotherapy for the treatment of hypertension. Loop diuretics can provide immediate diuresis and are used for heart failure and in lieu of thiazides in patients with compromised renal function. In addition to more traditional uses, certain potassium-sparing diuretics provide added benefit to other pharmacotherapy in patients with primary hyperaldosteronism, heart failure, or post-acute myocardial infarction. Carbonic anhydrase inhibitors have limited use for diuresis; however, they may be used to reduce intraocular pressure and treat acute mountain sickness.

A thorough understanding of the medicinal chemistry, mechanisms of action, and pharmacokinetics helps the clinician to use available diuretics appropriately. As new medications are developed, the clinician will rely on these basic concepts to continue tailoring therapy to the individual patient with the goals to maximize outcomes, improve quality of life, and minimize adverse events.

Kimberly Birtcher, Pharm.D.
Clinical Assistant Professor
Department of Clinical Sciences and Administration
University of Houston College of Pharmacy

glucose, phosphate, and amino acids and nonelectrogenetically with bicarbonate reabsorption. Glucose and amino acids are completely reabsorbed in this portion of the nephron, whereas phosphate reabsorption is between 80 and 90% complete. The early proximal convoluted tubule also is the primary site of bicarbonate reabsorption (80–90%), a process that is mainly sodium dependent and coupled to hydrogen ion secretion. The reabsorption of sodium and bicarbonate is facilitated by the enzyme carbonic anhydrase, which is present in proximal tubular cells and catalyzes the formation of carbonic acid from water and carbon dioxide. The carbonic acid provides the hydrogen ion, which drives the reabsorption of sodium bicarbonate. Chloride ions are reabsorbed passively in the proximal tubule, where they follow actively transported sodium ions into tubular cells.

Fig. 27.1. The nephron. BC, Bowman's capsule; G, glomerulus; PCT, proximal convoluted tubule; PST, proximal straight tubule; DLH, descending limb of the Loop of Henle; TALH, thick ascending limb of the loop of Henle; DCT, distal convoluted tubule; CD, collecting duct.

The reabsorption of electrolytes and water also occurs isosmotically in the proximal straight tubule or pars recta (S3 segment, Fig. 27.1). By the end of the straight segment, between 65 and 70% of water and sodium, chloride, and calcium ions; 80 to 90% of bicarbonate and phosphate; and essentially 100% of glucose, amino acids, vitamins, and protein have been reabsorbed from the glomerular filtrate. The proximal tubule also is the site for active secretion of weakly acidic and weakly basic organic compounds. Thus, many of the diuretics can enter luminal fluid not only by filtration at the glomerulus but also by active secretion.

The descending limb of the loop of Henle is impermeable to ions, but water can freely move from the luminal fluid into the surrounding medullary interstitium, where the higher osmolality draws water into the interstitial space and concentrates luminal fluid. Luminal fluid continues to concentrate as it descends to the deepest portion of the loop of Henle, where the fluid becomes the most concentrated. The hypertonic luminal fluid next enters the water-impermeable, thick ascending limb of the loop of Henle. In this segment of the nephron, approximately 20 to 25% of the filtered sodium and chloride ions are reabsorbed via a cotransport system ($Na^+/K^+/2Cl^-$) on the luminal membrane. Reabsorption of sodium and chloride in the medullary portion of the thick ascending limb is important for maintaining the medullary interstitial concentration gradient. Reabsorption of sodium chloride in the cortical component of the thick ascending limb of the loop of Henle and the early distal convoluted tubule contributes to urinary dilution, and as a result, these two nephron sections sometimes are called the cortical diluting segment of the nephron.

Luminal fluid leaving the early distal tubule next passes through the late distal tubule and cortical collecting tubule (collecting duct), where sodium is reabsorbed in exchange for hydrogen and potassium ions. This process is partially controlled by mineralocorticoids (e.g., aldosterone) and accounts for the reabsorption of between 2 and 3% of filtered sodium ions. Although the reabsorption of sodium ions from these segments of the nephron is not large, this sodium/potassium/hydrogen ion exchange system determines the final acidity and potassium content of urine. Several factors, however, can influence the activity of this exchange system, including the amount of sodium ions delivered to these segments, the status of the acid-base balance in the body, and the levels of circulating aldosterone.

The urine formed during this process represents only approximately 1 to 2% of the original glomerular filtrate, with more than 98% of electrolytes and water filtered at the glomerulus being reabsorbed during passage through the nephron. Thus, a change in urine output of only 1 to 2% could double urine volume. Urine leaves the kidney through the ureters and travels to the bladder, where it is stored until urination removes the it from the body.

NORMAL REGULATION OF URINE FORMATION

The body contains several control mechanisms that regulate the volume and contents of urine. These systems are activated by changes in solute or water content of the body, by changes in systemic or renal blood pressure, and by a variety of other stimuli. Activation of one or more of these systems by diuretic drugs can modify the effectiveness of these drugs to produce their therapeutic response and may require additional therapeutic measures to ensure a maximal response.

The kidney has the ability to respond to changes in the GFR through the action of specialized distal tubular epithelial cells called the macula densa. These cells are in close contact with the glomerular apparatus of the same nephron and detect changes in the rate of urine flow and luminal sodium chloride concentration. An increase in the urine flow rate at this site (as can occur with the use of some diuretics) activates the macula densa cells to communicate with the granular cells and vascular segments of the juxtaglomerular apparatus. Stimulation of the juxtaglomerular apparatus causes renin to be released, which leads to the formation of angiotensin II and subsequent renal vasoconstriction. Renal vasoconstriction leads to a decrease in GFR and, possibly, a decrease in the effectiveness of the diuretic. Renin release also can be stimulated by factors other than diuretics, including decreased renal perfusion pressure, increased sympathetic tone, and decreased blood volume.

Another important regulatory mechanism for urine formation is antidiuretic hormone (ADH), also known as vasopressin, which is released from the posterior pituitary in response to reduced blood pressure and elevated plasma osmolality. In the kidney, ADH acts on the collecting tubule to increase water permeability and reabsorption. As a result, the urine becomes more concentrated, and water is conserved in the presence of ADH.

DISEASE STATES

The diuretic drugs are used primarily to treat two medically important conditions, edema and hypertension. Both conditions are common, although some patients exhibit refractory disease states that require additional modification of the drug regimen to include alternative diuretics or addition of nondiuretic drugs. Edema (excessive extracellular fluid) normally results from disease to the heart, kidney, or liver. Decreased cardiac function (e.g., congestive heart disease) can result in decreased perfusion of all organs (e.g., kidney) and limbs and an accumulation of edema fluid in the extremities, particularly around the ankles and in the hands. Left-sided heart failure can lead to the development of acute pulmonary edema, which is a medical emergency. Right-sided heart failure shifts extracellular fluid volume from the arterial circulation to the venous circulation, which leads to general edema formation.

Kidney dysfunction can lead to edema formation as a result of decreased formation of urine and the subsequent imbalance of water and electrolyte (e.g., sodium ion) homeostasis. Retention of salt and water results in an expansion of the extracellular fluid volume and, thus, edema formation. Thus, when salt intake exceeds salt excretion, edema can form. Edema formation also is associated with deceased protein levels in blood, as seen in nephrotic syndrome and liver disease. Cirrhosis of the liver leads to increased lymph in the space of Disse. Eventually, the increased lymph volume results in movement of fluid into the peritoneal cavity and ascites develops.

Hypertension develops from many causes and will be discussed in more detail elsewhere (see Chapter 29). In general, hypertension occurs when blood pressure is sustained at greater than 140/90 mm Hg. At this blood pressure level, patients are at increased risk for developing cardiovascular disease. One key element in controlling blood pressure is sodium ion, and early antihypertensive effects of diuretics are related to increased salt and water excretion. Additionally, however, diuretics have long-term effects resulting in decreased vascular resistance that contribute to blood pressure control. Although effects on vascular calcium-activated potassium channels have been proposed as contributing to the chronic antihypertensive effects of thiazide diuretics, the exact mechanisms of long term effects remain to be determined.

Diuretics also are useful in treating a number of other conditions including increased cranial (trauma or surgery) or intraocular (glaucoma) pressure (i.e., osmotic diuretics), diabetes insipidus (i.e., thiazides), hypercalcemia (i.e., loop diuretics), acute mountain sickness (i.e., carbonic anhydrase inhibitors), primary hyperaldosteronism (i.e., aldosterone antagonists), and osteoporosis (i.e., thiazides).

GENERAL THERAPEUTIC APPROACHES

Diuretic drugs may be administered acutely or chronically to treat edematous states. When immediate action to reduce edema (e.g., acute pulmonary edema) is needed, intravenous administration of a loop diuretic often is the approach of choice. Thiazide or loop diuretics normally are administered orally to treat nonemergency edematous states. The magnitude of the diuretic response is directly proportional to the amount of edema fluid that is present. As the volume of edema decreases, so does the magnitude of the diuretic response with each dose. If concern exists about diuretic-induced hypokalemia developing, then a potassium supplement or potassium-sparing diuretic may be added to the drug regimen. The development of hypokalemia is particularly important for patients with congestive heart failure who also are taking cardiac glycosides, such as digitalis. Digitalis has a narrow therapeutic index, and developing hypokalemia can potentiate digitalis-induced cardiac effects with potentially fatal results.

Diuretic drugs (thiazide and loop diuretics) are administered orally to help control blood pressure in the treatment of hypertension. Diuretics often are the first drugs used to treat hypertension, and they also may be added to other drug therapies used to control blood pressure with beneficial effects.

DIURETIC DRUG CLASSES

History

Compounds that increase the urine flow rate have been known for centuries. One of the earliest substances known to induce diuresis is water, an inhibitor of ADH release. Calomel (mercurous chloride) was used as early as the 16th century as a diuretic, but because of poor absorption from the gastrointestinal tract and toxicity, calomel was replaced clinically by the organomercurials (e.g., chlormerodrin). The organomercurials represented the first group of highly efficacious diuretics available for clinical use. The need to administer these drugs parenterally, the possibility of tolerance, and their potential toxicity, however, soon led to the search for newer, less toxic diuretics. Today, the organomercurials are no longer used as diuretics, but their discovery began the search for many of the diuretics used today. Other compounds previously used as diuretics include the acid-forming salts (ammonium chloride) and methylxanthines (theophylline).

Structure Classification

The diuretics currently in use today (Table 27.1) are classified by their chemical class (thiazides), mechanism of action (carbonic anhydrase inhibitors and osmotics), site of action (loop diuretics), or effects on urine contents (potassium-sparing diuretics). These drugs vary widely in their efficacy (i.e., their ability to increase the rate of urine formation) and their site of action within the nephron. Efficacy often is measured as the ability of the diuretic to increase the excretion of sodium ions filtered at the glomerulus (i.e., the filtered load of sodium) and should not be confused with potency, which is the amount of the diuretic required to produce a specific diuretic response.

Efficacy is determined, in part, by the site of action of the diuretic. Drugs (e.g., carbonic anhydrase inhibitors) that act primarily on the proximal convoluted tubule to induce diuresis are weak diuretics because of the ability of the nephron to reabsorb a significant portion of the luminal contents in latter portions of the nephron. Likewise, drugs (potassium-sparing diuretics) that act at the more distal segments of the nephron are weak diuretics,

Table 27.1. Diuretics: Sites and Mechanisms of Action

Class of Diuretic	Site of Action	Mechanism of Action
Osmotics	Proximal tubule	Osmotic effects decrease sodium and water reabsorption
	Loop of Henle	Increases medullary blood flow to decrease medullary hypertonicity and reduce sodium and water reabsorption
	Collecting tubule	Sodium and water reabsorption decreases because of reduced medullary hypertonicity and elevated urinary flow rate
Carbonic anhydrase inhibitors	Proximal convoluted tubule	Inhibition of renal carbonic anhydrase decreases sodium bicarbonate reabsorption
Thiazides and thiazide-like	Cortical portion of the thick ascending limb of loop of Henle and distal tubule	Inhibition of Na^+/Cl^- symporter
Loop or high-ceiling	Thick ascending limb of the loop of Henle	Inhibition of the luminal $Na^+/K^+/2Cl^-$ transport system
Potassium-sparing	Distal tubule and collecting duct	Inhibition of sodium and water reabsorption by: Competitive inhibition of aldosterone (spironolactone) Blockade of sodium channel at the luminal membrane (triamterene and amiloride)

because most of the glomerular filtrate has already been reabsorbed in the proximal tubule and ascending limb of the loop of Henle before reaching the distal tubule. Thus, the most efficacious diuretics discovered so far, the high-ceiling or loop diuretics, interfere with sodium chloride reabsorption at the ascending limb of the loop of Henle, which is situated after the proximal tubule but before the distal portions of the nephron and collecting tubule.

Osmotic Diuretics

Mechanism of Action

Osmotic diuretics are low-molecular-weight compounds that are freely filtered through the Bowman's capsule into the renal tubules, are nonreabsorbable solutes, and are not extensively metabolized except for glycerin and urea (see Table 27.2) for their pharmacokinetic properties). Once in the renal tubule, osmotic diuretics have a limited reabsorption because of their high water solubility. When administered as a hypertonic (hyperosmolar) solution, these agents increase intraluminal osmotic pressure, causing water to pass from the body into the tubule. Since the osmotic agent and associated water are not reabsorbed from the nephron, a diuretic effect is observed. Osmotic diuretics increase the volume of urine and the excretion of water and almost all of the electrolytes.

Polyols, such as mannitol, sorbitol, and isosorbide, provide this effect. Sugars, such as glucose and sucrose, also can have a diuretic effect by this mechanism. Although not a polyol, urea has a similar osmotic effect and has been used in the past as an osmotic diuretic.

Mannitol

Sorbitol

Isosorbide

Therapeutic Applications

Osmotic diuretics are not frequently used in medicine today except in the prophylaxis of acute renal failure, in which these drugs inhibit water reabsorption and main-

Table 27.2. Pharmacokinetic Properties of the Nonthiazide Diuretics

Drug	Trade Name	Relative Potency	Oral Absorption (%)	Peak Plasma	Duration of Effect	Half-life	Route of Elimination
Osmotic diuretics							
Glycerin			>80	1–1.5 h	4–6 h	0.5–0.75 h	>90% metabolism
Isosorbide			>80	NA	NA	5–9.5 h	Urine unchanged
Mannitol			<20	1–3 h IV	3–8 h	1.5 h	Urine unchanged
Urea			<10	1–2 h IV	3–10 h	NA	Metabolized
Loop diuretics: high-ceiling diuretics							
Furosemide	Lasix	1	11–90[a]	4–5 h	6–8 h	0.5–4 h (>3 h)[b]	80% urine unchanged (20% metabolized)
Bumetanide	Bumex	40	80–100	<2 h	5–6 h	0.3–1.5 h (>3 h)[b]	50% urine unchanged 45% metabolized
Ethacrynic acid	Edecrin	0.7	>90	2 h	6–8 h	0.5–1 h	30–50% urine unchanged 30% mercapturate
Torsemide	Demadex	3	80–100%	NA	NA	0.8–4 h	30% urine 70% metabolized
Inhibitor of carbonic anhydrase							
Acetazolamide	Diamox		>90	1–3 h	NA	<6 h	Urine unchanged
Potassium-sparing diuretics (inhibitors of renal epithelial Na^+ channels)							
Amiloride	Midamor	1	~50[a]	3–4 h	10–24 h	6–9 h normal (21 h)[b]	50% urine unchanged
Triameterene	Dyrenium	0.1	>70	2–4 h	>24 h	2–3 h	Metabolized to active metabolites
Aldosterone antagonists; potassium-sparing diuretics (mineralocorticoid receptor antagonists)							
Spironolactone	Aldactone		>90[c]	1–2 h	2–3 d	1–3 h	Active metabolite
Canrenone (7α-thiospironolactone) active metabolite			NA		13–24 h	3–4 h	Urine

[a]Food affects bioavailability.
[b]In patients with renal insufficiency.
[c]Formulation affects bioavailability.
Data from McEvoy GK, ed. AHFS 2000 Drug Information. Bethesda, MD: American Society of Health-System Pharmacists, 2000.
NA, no data available.

tain urine flow. They also may be helpful in maintaining urine flow in cases where urinary output is diminished because of severe bleeding or traumatic surgical experiences. The osmotic diuretics also have been used to acutely reduce increased intracranial or intraocular pressure. They are not considered to be primary diuretic agents in treating ordinary edemas, because osmotic diuretics can expand extracellular fluid volume.

Adverse Effects

Osmotic diuretics induce few adverse effects, but expansion of the extracellular fluid volume can occur, as noted above. Alteration of blood sodium levels can be seen, and these drugs should not be used in anuric or unresponsive patients. If cranial bleeding is present, mannitol or urea should not be used.

Specific Drugs

MANNITOL. Mannitol is the agent most commonly used as an osmotic diuretic. Sorbitol also can be used for similar reasons. These compounds can be prepared by the electrolytic reduction of glucose or sucrose.

Mannitol is administered intravenously in solutions of 5 to 50% at a rate of administration that is adjusted to maintain the urinary output at 30 to 50 ml/hour. Mannitol is filtered at the glomerulus and is poorly reabsorbed by the kidney tubule. The osmotic effect of mannitol in the tubule inhibits the reabsorption of water, and the rate of urine flow can be maintained. It also is used to reduce intracranial pressure by reducing cerebral intravascular volume.

ISOSORBIDE. Isosorbide is basically a bicyclic form of sorbitol that is used orally to cause a reduction in intraocular pressure in glaucoma cases. Although a diuretic effect is noted, its ophthalmologic properties are its primary value.

Carbonic Anhydrase Inhibitors

Mechanism of Action

In 1937, it was proposed that the normal acidification of urine was caused by secretion of hydrogen ions by the tubular cells of the kidney. These ions were provided by the action of the enzyme carbonic anhydrase, which catalyzes the formation of carbonic acid (H_2CO_3) from carbon dioxide and water.

$$CO_2 + H_2O \longrightarrow H_2CO_3 \longrightarrow H^{\oplus} + HCO_3^{\ominus}$$

It also was observed that sulfanilamide rendered the urine of dogs alkaline because of the inhibition of carbonic anhydrase. This inhibition of carbonic anhydrase resulted in a lesser exchange of hydrogen ions for sodium ions in the kidney tubule. Sodium ions, along with bicarbonate ions, and associated water molecules were then excreted, and a diuretic effect was noted. The large doses required and the side effects of sulfanilamide prompted a search for more effective carbonic anhydrase inhibitors as diuretic drugs.

It was soon learned that the sulfonamide portion of an active diuretic molecule could not be monosubstituted or disubstituted. It was reasoned that a more acidic sulfonamide would bind more tightly to the carbonic anhydrase enzyme. Synthesis of more acidic sulfonamides produced compounds more than 2,500-fold more active than sulfanilamide. Acetazolamide was introduced in 1953 as an orally effective diuretic drug. Before that time, the organic mercurials, which commonly required intramuscular injection, were the principal diuretics available.

Carbonic anhydrase inhibitors induce diuresis by inhibiting the formation of carbonic acid within proximal (proximal convoluted tubule; S2) and distal tubular cells to limit the number of hydrogen ions available to promote sodium reabsorption. For a diuretic response to be observed, more than 99% of the carbonic anhydrase must be inhibited. Although carbonic anhydrase activity in the proximal tubule regulates the reabsorption of approximately 20 to 25% of the filtered load of sodium, the carbonic anhydrase inhibitors are not highly efficacious diuretics. An increased excretion of only 2 to 5% of the filtered load of sodium is seen with carbonic anhydrase inhibitors because of increased reabsorption of sodium ions by the ascending limb of the loop of Henle and more distal nephron segments.

Therapeutic Applications

With prolonged use of the carbonic anhydrase inhibitor diuretics, the urine becomes more alkaline, and the blood becomes more acidic. When acidosis occurs, the carbonic anhydrase inhibitors lose their effectiveness as diuretics. They remain ineffective until normal acid-base balance in the body has been regained. For this reason, this class of compounds is limited in its diuretic use. Today, they are most commonly used in the treatment of glaucoma, in which they reduce the rate of aqueous humor formation and, subsequently, reduce the intraocular pressure. These compounds also have found some limited use in the treatment of absence seizures, to alkalinize the urine, to treat familial periodic paralysis, to reduce metabolic alkalosis, and prophylactically, to reduce acute mountain sickness.

Specific Drugs

ACETAZOLAMIDE. Acetazolamide was the first of the carbonic anhydrase inhibitors to be introduced as an orally effective diuretic, with a diuretic effect that lasts approximately 8 to 12 hours (see Table 27.2 for its pharmacokinetic properties). As mentioned earlier, its diuretic action is limited because of the systemic acidosis it produces. Acetazolamide reduces the rate of aqueous humor formation and is used primarily for reducing intraocular pressure in the treatment of glaucoma. The dose is 250 mg to 1 g per day.

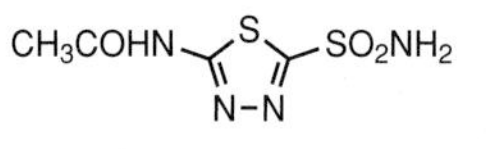

Acetazolamide

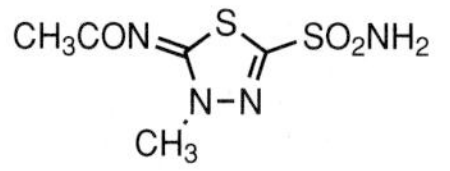

Methazolamide

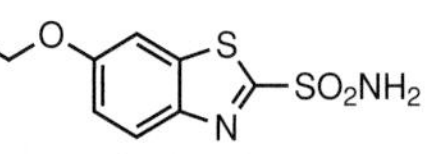

Ethoxzolamide

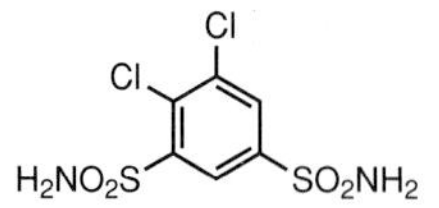

Dichlorphenamide

Glaucoma

The following carbonic anhydrase inhibitors are used orally in the treatment of glaucoma.

METHAZOLAMIDE. Methazolamide is a derivative of acetazolamide in which one of the active hydrogens has been replaced by a methyl group. This decreases the polarity and permits a greater penetration into the ocular fluid, where it acts as a carbonic anhydrase inhibitor, reducing intraocular pressure. Its dose for glaucoma is 50 to 100 mg two to three times a day.

ETHOXZOLAMIDE AND DICHLORPHENAMIDE. Ethoxzolamide is another carbonic anhydrase inhibitor with properties and uses resembling those of acetazolamide. Dichlorphenamide is a disulfonamide derivative that shares the same pharmacological properties and clinical uses as the previously discussed compounds. The dose of dichlorphenamide is 25 to 100 mg one to three times a day.

Benzothiadiazine or Thiazide Diuretics

Further study of the benzene disulfonamide derivatives was undertaken to find more efficacious carbonic anhydrase inhibitors. These studies provided some compounds with a high degree of diuretic activity. Chloro and amino substitution gave compounds with increased activity, but these compounds were weak carbonic anhydrase inhibitors. When the amino group was acylated, an unexpected ring closure took place. These compounds possessed a diuretic activity independent of the carbonic anhydrase inhibitory activity, and a new series of diuretics called the benzothiadiazines was discovered.

Mechanism of Action

The mechanism of action of the benzothiadiazine diuretics is primarily related to their ability to inhibit the Na^+/Cl^- symporter located in the distal convoluted tubule. These diuretics are actively secreted in the proximal tubule and are carried to the loop of Henle and to the distal tubule. The major site of action of these compounds is in the distal tubule, where these drugs compete for the chloride binding site of the Na^+/Cl^- symporter and inhibit the reabsorption of sodium and chloride ions. For this reason, they are referred to as saluretics. They also inhibit the reabsorption of potassium and bicarbonate ions, but to a lesser degree.

Structure–Activity Relationship

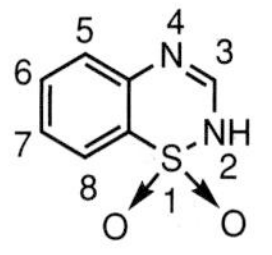

The thiazide diuretics are weakly acidic (see Appendix A for their pK_a values), with a benzothiadiazine 1,1-dioxide nucleus. The structure for the thiazide diuretics, relative activities, and pharmacokinetic properties for the thiazides are shown in Table 27.3. Chlorothiazide is the simplest member of this series, having a pK_a of 6.7 and 9.5. The hydrogen atom at the 2-N is the most acidic because of the electron-withdrawing effects of the neighboring sulfone group. The sulfonamide group that is substituted at C-7 provides an additional point of acidity in the molecule but is less acidic than the 2-N proton. These acidic protons make possible the formation of a water-soluble sodium salt that can be used for intravenous administration of the diuretics.

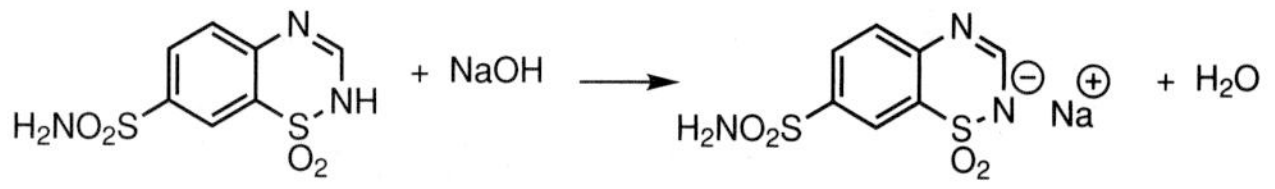

An electron-withdrawing group is necessary at position 6 for diuretic activity. Little diuretic activity is seen with a hydrogen atom at position 6, whereas compounds with a chloro or trifluoromethyl substitution are highly active. The trifluoromethyl-substituted diuretics are more lipid-soluble and have a longer duration of action than their chloro-substituted analogues. When electron-releasing groups, such as methyl or methoxyl, are placed at position 6, the diuretic activity is markedly reduced.

Replacement or removal of the sulfonamide group at position 7 yields compounds with little or no diuretic activity. Saturation of the double bond to give a 3,4-dihydro derivative produces a diuretic that is 10-fold more active than the unsaturated derivative. Substitution with a lipophilic group at position 3 gives a marked increase in the diuretic potency. Haloalkyl, aralkyl, or thioether substitution increases the lipid solubility of the molecule and yields compounds with a longer duration of action. Alkyl substitution on the 2-N position also decreases the polarity and increases the duration of diuretic action. Although these compounds do have carbonic anhydrase activity, there is no correlation of this activity with their saluretic activity (excretion of sodium and chloride ions).

Therapeutic Applications

The thiazide diuretics are administered once a day or in divided daily doses. Some have a duration of action that permits administration of a dose every other day. Some of these compounds are rapidly absorbed orally and can show their diuretic effect in an hour (Table 27.3). These compounds are not extensively metabolized and are primarily

Table 27.3. Pharmacological and Pharmacokinetic Properties for the Thiazide Diuretics

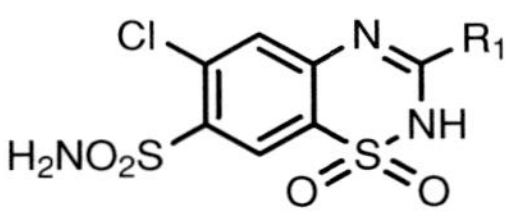

Structure I 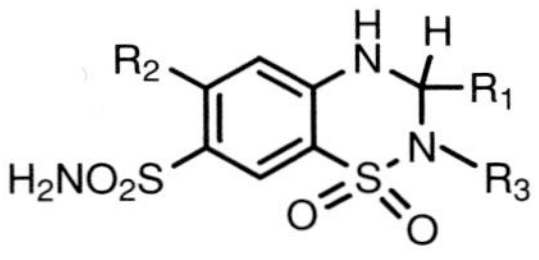   Structure II

Generic Name	Trade Name	Structure	Relative Potency[a]	Carbonic Anhydrase Inhibition[b]	Bioavail-ability	Peak Plasma (hours)	Half-life (hours)	Duration (hours)	Route of Elimination
Chlorothiazide	Diuril	Structure I: R_1 = H	0.8	2×10^{-6}	<25%	4	1–2 e: 13	6–12	U
Benzthiazide	Exna	Structure I: R_1 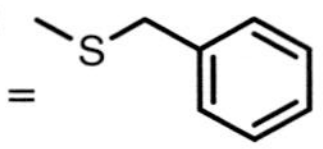 =	1.3	~10^{-7}	NA	NA	NA	12–18	NA
Hydrochlorothiazide	HydroDiuril Esidrix Oretic	Structure II: R_1 = H R_2 = Cl; R_3 = H	1.4	2×10^{-5}	>80%	4	6–15	6–12	U
Trichloromethiazide	Diurese Metahydrin Naqua	Structure II: R_1 = $CHCl_2$ R_2 = Cl; R_3 = H	1.7	6×10^{-5}	Var	6	NA	24	U
Methyclothiazide	Enduron Aquatensen	Structure II: R_1 = CH_2Cl R_2 = Cl; R_3 = CH_3	1.8	—	Var.	6	NA	>24	U
Polythiazide	Renese	Structure II: R_1 = $-CH_2$-S-CH_2-CF_3 R_2 = Cl; R_3 = CH_3	2.0	5×10^{-7}	var	6	NA	24–48	U 30% M
Hydroflumethiazide	Saluron Diucardin	Structure II: R_1 = H R_2 = CF_3; R_3 = H	1.3	2×10^{-4}	Inc	3–4	17 active metab.	18–24	U active metab.
Bendroflumethiazide	Naturetin	Structure II: R_1 = benzyl R_2 = CF_3; R_3 = H	1.8	3×10^{-4}	>90%	4	8.5	6–12	U

[a]The numerical values refer to potency ratios (in humans) with the natriuretic response to that of a standard dose of meralluride, which is given a value of one.
[b]50% inhibition of carbonic anhydrase in vitro.
Data from AHFS 2000 Drug Information. Bethesda, MD: American Society of Health-System Pharmacists, 2000; and USPDI Vol. I Drug Information for the Health Care Professional, 20th Ed. Rockville, MD: U.S. Pharmacopeial Convention. 2000.
U, urine unchanged; M, metabolized; NA, data not available; Var, variables absorption; Inc, incomplete absorption.

excreted unchanged in the urine. Thiazide diuretics are used to treat edemas caused by cardiac decompensation as well as in hepatic or renal disease. They also commonly are used in the treatment of hypertension. Their effect may be attributed to a reduction in blood volume and a direct relaxation of vascular smooth muscle.

Adverse Effects

Thiazide diuretics may induce a number of adverse effects, including hypersensitivity reactions, gastric irritation, nausea, and electrolyte imbalances, such as hyponatremia, hypokalemia, hypomagnesemia, hypochloremic alkalosis, hypercalcemia, and hyperuricemia. Individuals who exhibit hypersensitivity reactions to one thiazide are likely to have a hypersensitivity reaction to other thiazides and sulfamoyl-containing diuretics (e.g., thiazide-like and some high-ceiling diuretics). Potassium and magnesium supplements may be administered to treat hypokalemia or hypomagnesemia, but their use is not always indicated. These supplements usually are administered as potassium chloride, potassium gluconate, potassium citrate, magnesium oxide, or magnesium lactate. The salts are administered as solutions, tablets, or timed-release tablets. Generally, approximately 20 mEq of potassium is given daily. In cases of hypokalemia, 40 to 100 mEq/day may be administered. Potassium-sparing diuretics (e.g., triamterene or amiloride) also may be used to prevent hypokalemia. Combination preparation of hydrochlorothiazide or a potassium-sparing diuretic are available (e.g., Diazide and Moduretic).

Long-term use of thiazide diuretics also may result in decreased glucose tolerance and increased blood lipid (low-density lipoprotein cholesterol, total cholesterol, and total triglyceride) content.

Quinazolinone Derivatives—Quinethazone and Metolazone

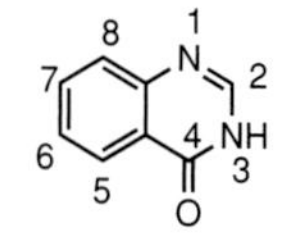

quinazolin-4-one

Overview

The quinazolin-4-one molecule has been structurally modified in a manner similar to the modification of the thiazide diuretics. Quinethazone and metolazone (pK_a = 9.7) are examples of this class (Table 27.4). The structural difference between the quinazolinone diuretics is the replacement of the 4-sulfone group ($-SO_2-$), with a 4-keto group ($-CO-$).

Because of their similar structures, it is not surprising that the quinazolinones have a diuretic effect similar to that of the thiazides.

Mechanism of Action and Therapeutic Applications

The pharmacokinetic properties for the quinazolinone diuretics are listed in Table 27.4. They have a long duration of action, usually as a result of protein binding. Although chlorothiazide has a duration of action of 6 to 12

Table 27.4. Pharmacokinetic Properties for the Thiazide-Like Diuretics

Generic name	Trade name	Structure	Bioavailability	Peak Plasma	$t_{1/2}$	Duration	Route of Elimination
Metolazone	Zaroxylon Mykrox #	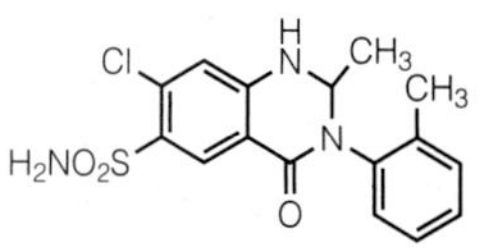	<65%a >90%	8–12h	14	12–24h	U: 70–95% EHC: 10–30%
Quinethazone	Hydromox	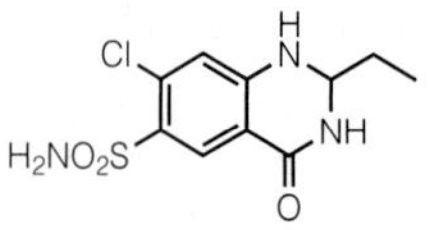	NA	6 h	6–15	18–24h	U
Chlorthalidone	Hygroton Thalitone #	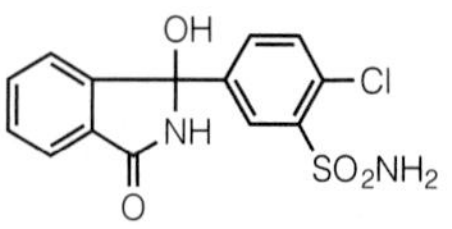	inc/var. >90%	4 h 2 h	35–50* e: 54	48–72 h	U: 30–60%
Indapamide	Lozol	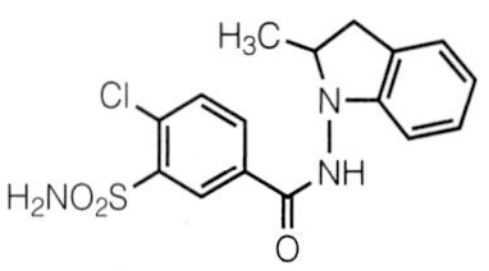	>90%	2–3h	14–18	8wks	M: 60–70% EHC: 20–30%

Data from AHFS 2000 Drug Information. Bethesda, MD: American Society of Health-System Pharmacists; 2000 and USPDI Vol. I Drug Info. for the Hlth Care Prof. 20th ed. Rockville, MD; United States Pharmacopeial Convention. 2000.

*Strongly bound to red blood cells. # = not interchangable with similar drug. U = urine unchanged; M = metabolized. NA = data not available. var. = variable absorption. inc. = incomplete absorption.

hours, quinethazone a duration of 18 to 24 hours, and metolazone a duration of 12 to 24 hours. Metolazone has a bioavailability of 65% (Zaroxolyn) and a prolonged onset to reach peak plasma concentrations of action ranging from 8 to 12 hours. When reformulated as for Mykrox™, however, metolazone is almost completely absorbed, with peak plasma concentrations reached in 2 to 4 hours. Thus, other versions of metolazone cannot be interchanged with Mykrox. Approximately 50 to 70% of metolazone is bound to carbonic anhydrase in the erythrocytes. Metolazone also has an increased potency, and the mode of action for both compounds is similar to that of the thiazide derivatives. In contrast to thiazide diuretics, metolazone may be effective as a diuretic when the GFR falls below 40 mL/min. The dose of quinethazone is 50 to 100 mg daily and that of metolazone 2.5 to 20 mg given as a single oral dose. Side effects are similar to adverse effects induced by the thiazide diuretics.

Phthalimidine Derivatives—Chlorthalidone

Overview

Chlorthalidone (pK_a = 9.4) is an example of a diuretic in this class of compounds that bears a structural analogy to the quinazolinones (Table 27.4). This compound may be named as a 1-oxo-isoindoline or a phthalimidine. Although the molecule exists primarily in the phthalimidine form, the ring may be opened to form a benzophenone derivative.

The benzophenone form illustrates the relationship to the quinazolinone series of diuretics. It may be regarded as an open ring variation.

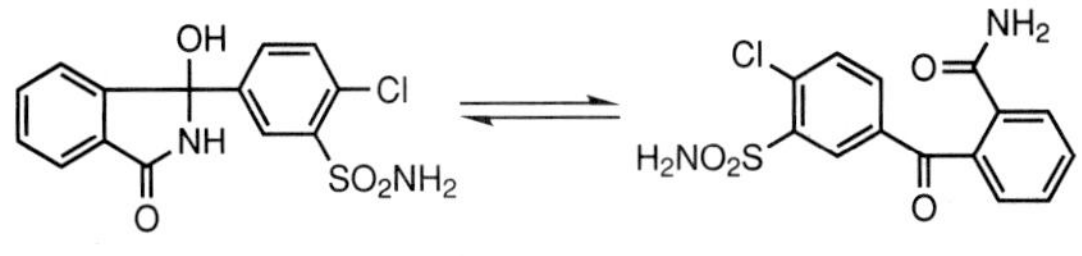

OH NH O Cl SO_2NH_2 ⇌ Cl NH_2 O H_2NO_2S O

Therapeutic Application

Chlorthalidone has a long duration of action (48–72 hours) (see Table 27.3 for its other pharmacokinetic properties). Although quinethazone and metolazone are administered daily, chlorthalidone may be administered in doses of 25 to 100 mg three times a week. When chlorthalidone is formulated with the excipient povidone, the product, Thalitone, has greater bioavailability (>90%) and reaches peak plasma concentrations in a shorter time compared with its other products. Similar to the quinazolinones, it also is extensively bound to carbonic anhydrase in the erythrocytes. Chlorthalidone-induced effects on urine content and side effects are similar to those induced by thiazide diuretics.

Indolines—Indapamide

Mechanism of Action

The prototypic indoline diuretic is indapamide, which was reported as a diuretic in 1984. Indapamide contains a polar chlorobenzamide moiety and a nonpolar lipophilic methylindoline group. In contrast to the thiazides, indapamide does not contain a thiazide ring, and only one sulfonamide group is present within the molecular structure (pK_a = 8.8). It is rapidly and completely absorbed from the gastrointestinal tract and reaches its peak plasma level in 2 to 3 hours, with a duration of action of up to 8 weeks. This prolonged duration of action is associated with its extensive binding to carbonic anhydrase in the erythrocytes. It exhibits biphasic kinetics, with a half-life of 14 to 18 hours and an elimination half-life of 24 hours. Indapamide is extensively metabolized, with 60 to 70% of the oral dose being eliminated in the urine as glucuronide and sulfate metabolites and less than 10% being excreted unchanged. The remaining 20 to 30% is eliminated via extrahepatic cycling.

Therapeutic Application

Uses of indapamide include the treatment of essential hypertension and edema resulting from congestive heart failure. Like metolazone, indapamide is an effective diuretic drug when GFR falls below 40 mL/min. The duration of action is approximately 24 hours, with the normal oral adult dosage starting at 2.5 mg given each morning. The dose may be increased to 5.0 mg/day, but doses beyond this level do not appear to provide additional results. Effects on urine content and side effects are similar to effects induced by thiazide diuretics.

High-Ceiling or Loop Diuretics

Mechanism of Action

This class of drugs is characterized more by its pharmacological similarities than by its chemical similarities. These diuretics produce a peak diuresis much greater than that observed with the other commonly used diuretics, hence the name high-ceiling diuretics. Their main site of action is believed to be on the thick ascending limb of the loop of Henle, where they inhibit the luminal $Na^+/K^+/2Cl^-$ symporter. These diuretics are commonly referred to as loop diuretics. Additional effects on the proximal and distal tubules also are possible. High-ceiling diuretics are characterized by a quick onset and short duration of activity. Their diuretic effect appears in approximately 30 minutes and lasts for approximately 6 hours. The pharmacokinetic properties for the loop diuretics are listed in Table 27.2.

Specific Drugs

FUROSEMIDE

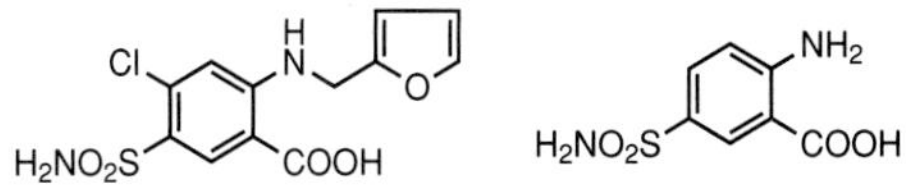

Cl H N O H_2NO_2S COOH

Furosemide

NH_2 H_2NO_2S COOH

5-Sulfamoyl-anthranilic acid

Structure–Activity Relationships. Furosemide is an example of a high-ceiling diuretic and may be regarded as a derivative of anthranilic acid or o-aminobenzoic acid.

Research on 5-sulfamoylanthranilic acids at the Hoechst Laboratories in Germany showed them to be effective diuretics. The most active of a series of variously substituted derivatives was furosemide.

The chlorine and sulfonamide substitutions are features also seen in previously discussed diuretics. Because the molecule possesses a free carboxyl group, furosemide is a stronger acid than the thiazide diuretics ($pK_a = 3.9$). This drug is excreted primarily unchanged. A small amount of metabolism, however, can take place on the furan ring, which is substituted on the aromatic amino group (see Table 27.2 for its other pharmacokinetic properties).

Therapeutic Applications. Furosemide has a saluretic effect 8- to 10-fold that of the thiazide diuretics; however, it has a shorter duration of action (~6–8 hours). Furosemide causes a marked excretion of sodium, chloride, potassium, calcium, magnesium, and bicarbonate ions, with as much as 25% of the filtered load of sodium excreted in response to initial treatment. It is effective for the treatment of edemas connected with cardiac, hepatic, and renal sites. Because it lowers the blood pressure similar to the thiazide derivatives, one of its uses is in the treatment of hypertension.

Furosemide is orally effective but may be used parenterally when a more prompt diuretic effect is desired, such as in the treatment of acute pulmonary edema. The dosage of furosemide, 20–80 mg/day, may be given in divided doses because of the short duration of action of the drug and carefully increased up to a maximum of 600 mg/day.

Adverse Effects. Clinical toxicity of furosemide and other loop diuretics primarily involves abnormalities of fluid and electrolyte balance. As with the thiazide diuretics, hypokalemia is an important adverse effect that can be prevented or treated with potassium supplements or coadministration of potassium-sparing diuretics. Increased calcium ion excretion can be a problem for postmenopausal osteopenic women, and furosemide generally should not be used in these individuals. Hyperuricemia, glucose intolerance, increased serum lipid levels, ototoxicity, and gastrointestinal side effects might be observed as well. Hypersensitivity reactions also are possible with furosemide (a sulfonamide-based drug), and cross-reactivity with other sulfonamide containing drugs is possible.

BUMETANIDE

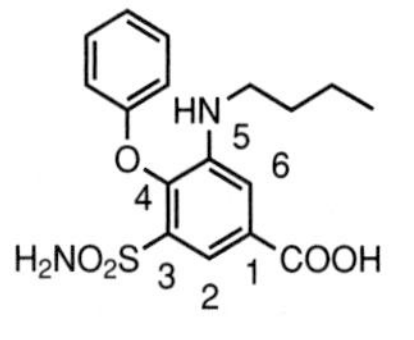

HN 5 6 O 4 H_2NO_2S 3 2 1 COOH

Bumetanide

Therapeutic Applications. A diuretic structurally related to furosemide is bumetanide. This compound also functions as a high-ceiling diuretic in the ascending limb of the loop of Henle. It has a duration of action of approximately 4 hours. The uses of this compound are similar to those described for furosemide. The dose of bumetanide is 0.5 to 2 mg/day given as a single dose. Adverse effects are similar to those induced by furosemide.

Structure–Activity Relationships. For bumetanide, a phenoxy group has replaced the customary chloro or trifluoromethyl substitutions seen in other diuretic molecules. The phenoxy group is an electron-withdrawing group similar to the chloro or trifluoromethyl substitutions. The amine group customarily seen at position 6 has been moved to position 5. These minor variations from furosemide produced a compound with a mode of action similar to that of furosemide, but with a marked increase in diuretic potency. The short duration of activity is similar, but the compound is approximately 50-fold more potent. Replacement of the phenoxy group at position 4 with a C_6H_5NH- or C_6H_5S- group also gives compounds with a favorable activity. When the butyl group on the C-5 amine is replaced with a furanylmethyl group, such as in furosemide; however, the results are not favorable.

TORSEMIDE

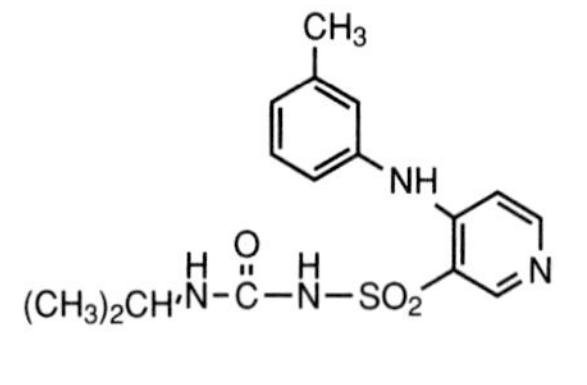

CH_3 NH H O H $(CH_3)_2CH$-N-C-N-SO_2 N

Torsemide

Further modification of furosemide-like structures has led to the development of torsemide. Instead of the sulfonamide group found in furosemide and bumetanide, torsemide contains a sulfonylurea moiety. Similar to other high-ceiling diuretics, torsemide inhibits the luminal $Na^+/K^+/2Cl^-$ symporter in the ascending limb of the loop of Henle to promote the excretion of sodium, potassium, chloride, calcium, and magnesium ions and water. An additional effect on the peritubular side at chloride channels may enhance the luminal effects of torsemide. In contrast to furosemide and bumetanide, however, torsemide does not act at the proximal tubule and, therefore, does not increase phosphate or bicarbonate excretion. Peak diuresis is observed 1 to 2 hours following oral or intravenous administration, with a duration of action of approximately 6 hours. Torsemide is indicated for the treatment of edema resulting from congestive heart failure and for the treatment of hypertension. In patients with cirrhosis and ascites, Torsemide should be used with caution. Adverse effects are similar to those induced by furosemide.

ETHACRYNIC ACID

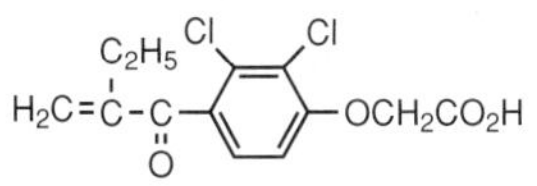

Ethacrynic acid

Mechanism of Action. Another major class of high-ceiling diuretics is the phenoxyacetic acid derivatives, of which ethacrynic acid is the prototypical agent. These compounds were developed at about the same time as furosemide but were designed to act mechanistically similar to the organomercurials (i.e., via inhibition of sulfhydryl-containing enzymes involved in solute reabsorption). The mechanism of action of ethacrynic acid appears to be more complex than the simple addition of sulfhydryl groups of the enzyme to the drug molecule. When the double bond of ethacrynic acid is reduced, the resultant compound is still active, although the diuretic activity is diminished. The sulfhydryl groups of the enzyme would not be expected to add to the drug molecule in the absence of the α,β-unsaturated ketone. The pharmacokinetic properties for ethacrynic acid are listed in Table 27.2.

In 1984, a new series of diuretics was reported (2,3). The following substance is representative of this series:

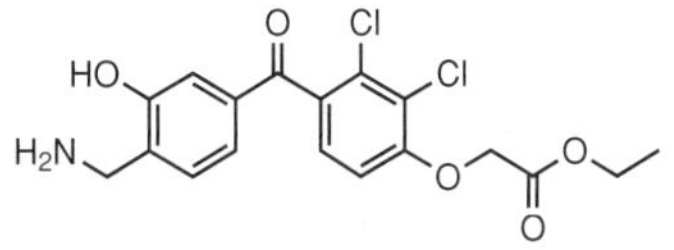

These compounds are potent high-ceiling diuretics that resemble ethacrynic acid in their mechanism of action. The ethyl ester group represents a pro-drug that can be easily hydrolyzed to the free carboxyl group. As in ethacrynic acid, a 2,3-dichloro substitution is necessary. In addition, a para-hydroxyl group and an unsubstituted aminomethyl group on the benzene ring are highly beneficial. The carbonyl group can be replaced with an ether or sulfide group. These compounds have no ability to add the sulfhydryl groups of the kidney enzymes. The complete mechanism of action of these compounds remains in doubt.

Similar to the other high-ceiling diuretics, ethacrynic acid inhibits the $Na^+/K^+/2Cl^-$ symporter in the ascending limb of the loop of Henle to promote a marked diuresis. Sodium, chloride, potassium, and calcium excretion are increased following oral or intravenous administration of ethacrynic acid. Oral administration of ethacrynic acid results in diuresis within 1 hour and a duration of action of 6 to 8 hours. Toxicity induced by ethacrynic acid is similar to that induced by furosemide and bumetanide. Ethacrynic acid is not widely used, however, because it induces a greater incidence of ototoxicity and more serious gastrointestinal effects than those of furosemide or bumetanide.

Structure–Activity Relationship. Optimal diuretic activity was obtained when an oxyacetic acid group was positioned para to an α,β-unsaturated carbonyl (or other sulfhydryl-reactive group) and chloro or methyl groups were placed at the 2- or 3-position of the phenyl ring. In addition, hydrogen atoms on the terminal alkene carbon also provided maximum reactivity. Thus, a molecule with a weakly acidic group to direct the drug to the kidney and an alkylating moiety to react with sulfhydryl groups and lipophilic groups seemed to provide the best combination for a diuretic in this class. These features led to the development of ethacrynic acid as the prototypic agent in this class.

NEW DRUGS

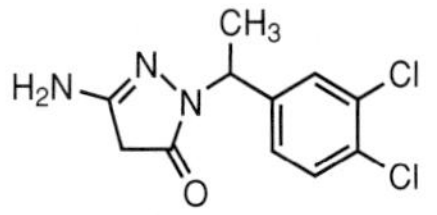

Muzolimine

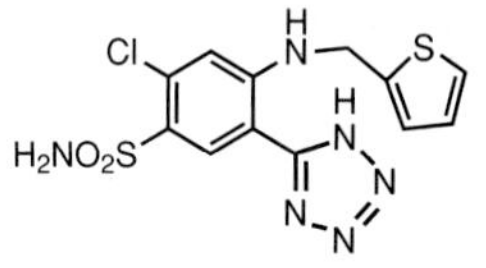

Azosemide

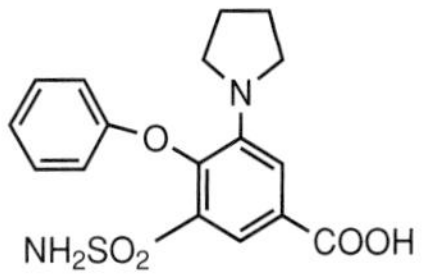

Piretanide

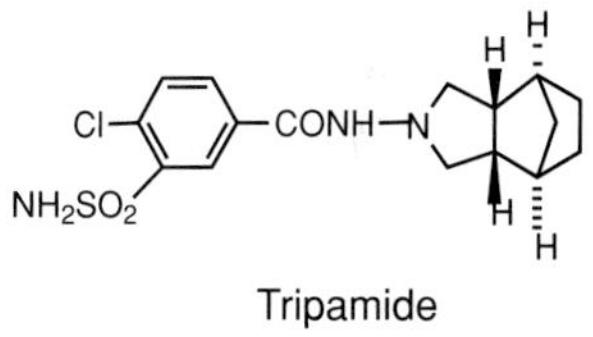

Tripamide

Four additional high-ceiling diuretics are azosemide, muzolimine, piretanide, and tripamide. Azosemide has low oral bioavailability (~10–15%) because of high first-pass metabolism in the liver, whereas piretanide has comparable pharmacokinetics to bumetanide.

As can be seen by these varied structures, the high-ceiling diuretics are characterized more by their pharmacological similarities than by their chemical similarities.

Potassium-Sparing Diuretics (Mineralocorticoid Receptor Antagonists)—Antihormone Diuretics

Mechanism of Action

The adrenal cortex secretes a potent mineralocorticoid called aldosterone, which promotes salt and water retention and potassium and hydrogen ion excretion.

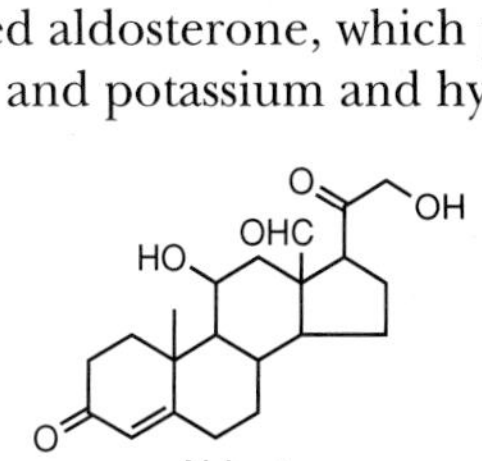

Aldosterone (aldol from)

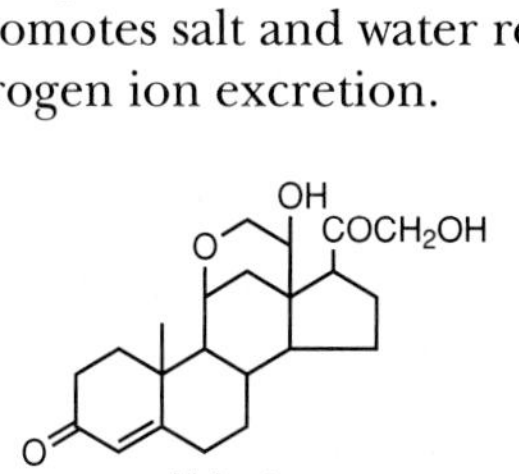

Aldosterone (hemiacetal from)

Other mineralocorticoids have an effect on the electrolytic balance of the body, but aldosterone is the most potent. Its ability to cause increased reabsorption of sodium and chloride ion and increased potassium ion excretion is approximately 3,000-fold that of hydrocortisone. A substance that antagonizes the effects of aldosterone could conceivably be a good diuretic drug. Spironolactone is such an antagonist.

Specific Drugs

SPIRONOLACTONE. Spironolactone is a competitive antagonist to the mineralocorticoids, such as aldosterone. The mineralocorticoid receptor is an intracellular protein that can bind aldosterone. Spironolactone binds to the receptor and competitively inhibits aldosterone binding to the receptor. The inability of aldosterone to bind to its receptor prevents reabsorption of sodium and chloride ions and the associated water. The most important site of these receptors is in the late distal convoluted tubule and collecting system (collecting duct).

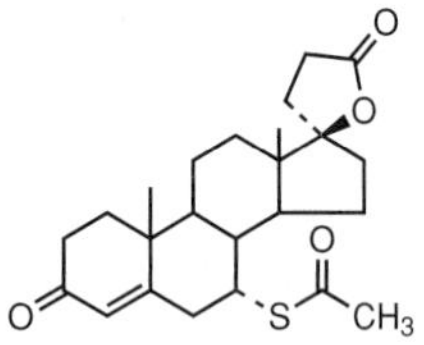

Spironolactone

Metabolism. On oral administration, approximately 90% of the dose of spironolactone is absorbed and is significantly metabolized during its first passage through the liver to its major active metabolite, canrenone (see Table 27.2 for their pharmacokinetic properties), which is interconvertible with its canrenoate anion. Canrenone is an antagonist to aldosterone.

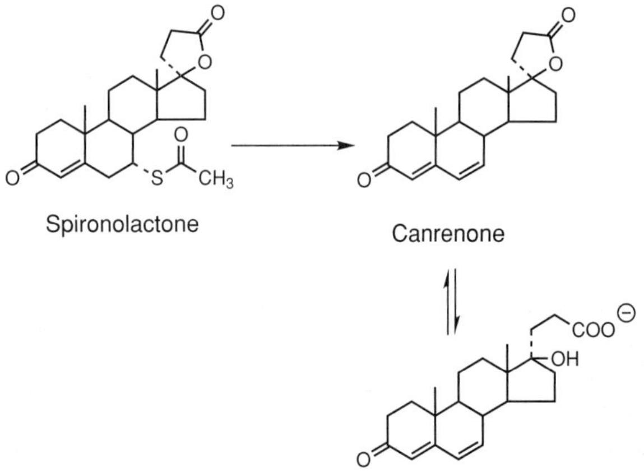

Spironolactone

Canrenone

Canrenoic acid anion

The canrenoate anion is not active per se but acts as an aldosterone antagonist because of its conversion to canrenone, which exists in the lactone form. Canrenone has been suggested to be the active form of spironolactone as an aldosterone antagonist. The formation of canrenone, however, cannot fully account for the total activity of spironolactone. Both canrenone and potassium canrenoate are used as diuretics in other countries, but they are not yet available in the United States.

Therapeutic Applications. Spironolactone is useful in treating edema resulting from primary hyperaldosteronism and refractory edema associated with secondary hyperaldosteronism. Spironolactone is considered to be the drug of choice for treating edema resulting from cirrhosis of the liver. The dose of spironolactone is 100 mg/day given in single or divided doses. Another use of spironolactone is coadministration with a potassium-depleting diuretic (e.g., a thiazide or loop diuretic) to prevent or treat diuretic-induced hypokalemia. Spironolactone can be administered in a fixed-dose combination with hydrochlorothiazide for this purpose, but optimal individualization of the dose of each drug is recommended.

Adverse Effects. The primary concern with the use of spironolactone is the development of hyperkalemia, which can be fatal. Spironolactone may cause hypersensitivity reactions, gastrointestinal disturbances, peptic ulcer, gynecomastia, decreased libido, and impotence. It also has been implicated in tumor production during chronic toxicity studies in rats, but human risk has not been documented.

EPLERENONE

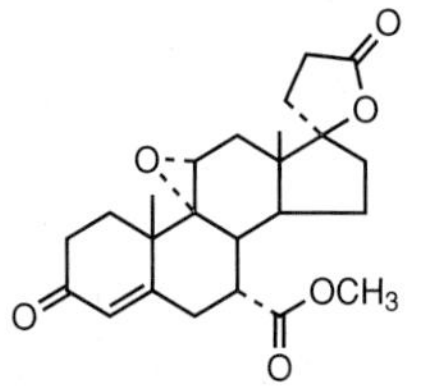

Eplerenone

A newer drug, eplerenone, has a structure similar to that of spironolactone and a similar mechanism of action. It was initially approved for use in the treatment of hypertension but it can now be used in the treatment of patients with left ventricular systolic dysfunction and congestive heart failure after myocardial infarction. It has a half-life of approximately 5 hours and undergoes hepatic metabolism to inactive metabolites as its main route of elimination. Clinical experience with eplerenone is currently limited.

Pteridines—Triamterene

Pteridines have a marked potential for influencing biological processes. Early screening of pteridine derivatives revealed that 2,4-diamino-6,7-dimethylpteridine was a fairly potent diuretic. Further structural modification led to the development of triamterene.

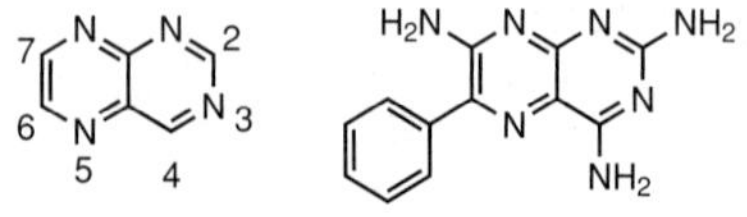

Pteridine

Triamterene

MECHANISM OF ACTION. Triamterene interferes with the process of cationic exchange by blocking luminal sodium channels in the late distal convoluted tubule and collecting duct. Sodium channel inhibitors block the reabsorption of sodium ion and inhibit the secretion of potassium ion. Aldosterone is not antagonized by triamterene. The net result is increased sodium and chloride ion excretion in the urine and almost no potassium excretion. Triamterene is more than 70% absorbed on oral administration (see Table 27.2 for its other pharmacokinetic properties). The diuretic effect occurs rapidly (~30 minutes) and reaches a peak plasma concentration in 2 to 4 hours, with a duration of action of more than 24 hours. Triamterene is extensively metabolized, and some of the metabolites are active as diuretics. Both the drug and its metabolites are excreted in the urine.

STRUCTURE–ACTIVITY RELATIONSHIPS. Modifications of the triamterene structure are not usually beneficial in terms of diuretic activity. Activity is retained if an amine group is replaced with a lower alkylamine group. Introduction of a para-methyl group on the phenyl ring decreases the activity by approximately half. Introduction of a para-hydroxyl group on the phenyl ring yields a compound that is essentially inactive as a diuretic.

THERAPEUTIC APPLICATIONS. Triamterene is useful in combination with a thiazide or loop diuretic in the treatment of edema or hypertension. Liddle's syndrome also may be treated with a sodium channel blocking drug, such as triamterene. Triamterene is administered initially in doses of 100 mg twice a day. A maintenance dose for each patient should be individually determined. This dose may vary from 100 mg a day to as low as 100 mg every other day.

ADVERSE EFFECTS. The most serious side effect associated with the use of triamterene is hyperkalemia. For this reason, potassium supplements are contraindicated, and serum potassium levels should be checked regularly. Triamterene also is used in combination with hydrochlorothiazide. Here, the hypokalemic effect of the hydrochlorothiazide counters the hyperkalemic effect of the triamterene. Other side effects that are seen with the use of triamterene are nausea, vomiting, and headache.

Aminopyrazines—Amiloride

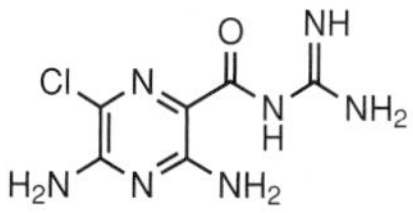

Cl, N, O, NH, N H, NH_2, H_2N, N, NH_2

Amiloride

Amiloride, another potassium-sparing diuretic, is an aminopyrazine structurally related to triamterene as an open-chain analogue. Similar to triamterene, it interferes with the process of cationic exchange in the distal convoluted tubule by blocking luminal sodium channels. It blocks the reabsorption of sodium ion and the secretion of potassium ion. It has no effect on the action of aldosterone. Oral amiloride is approximately 50% absorbed (see Table 27.2 for its other pharmacokinetic properties), with a duration of action of 10 to 12 hours, which is slightly longer than that for triamterene. Although triamterene is extensively metabolized, approximately 50% of amiloride is excreted unchanged. Renal impairment can increase its elimination half-life. Like triamterene, amiloride combined with a thiazide or loop diuretic is used to treat edema or hypertension. Aerosolized amiloride has shown some benefit in improving mucociliary clearance in patients with cystic fibrosis. As with triamterene, the most serious side effect associated with amiloride is hyperkalemia, and it also has the other side effects associated with triamterene. The dose of amiloride is 5 to 10 mg per day. Amiloride also is combined with hydrochlorothiazide in a fixed-dose combination.

Therapeutic Application of Diuretics

BD is a 67-year-old man who was admitted with a complaint of shortness of breath that has increased over the last few months. He also indicated that he has recently gained more than 12 pounds without changing his eating or exercise habits and that he often has trouble breathing when climbing stairs at home. Physical examination reveals signs and symptoms consistent with both right-sided (systemic edema, hepatomegaly, neck vein distension) and left-sided (weakness, fatigue, rales, cyanosis) heart failure. A diagnosis of congestive heart failure (CHF) is established, and a decision is made to limit sodium intake (low sodium diet) and to initiate oral therapy with digitalis to improve heart function. A diuretic also will be added to help remove edema fluid and decrease the workload on the heart. What diuretics would be appropriate to use in this patient?

ANSWER:

Selection of a diuretic would be based on the drug's ability to mobilize edema fluid and to help reduce the workload on the heart. Thiazide and loop (high-ceiling) diuretics are effective in mobilizing edema fluid and could be used in this patient. Osmotic diuretics are not effective at mobilizing edema fluid and will expand extracellular fluid, which would worsen the workload on the heart. Carbonic anhydrase inhibitors are weak diuretics and would not provide adequate diuresis to effectively reduce the workload on the heart. Potassium-sparing diuretics also are less effective than thiazides or loop diuretics in mobilizing edema fluid and would not be a diuretic of first choice in this patient.

Choosing between a thiazide or a loop diuretic depends on many factors, including the amount of edema present, severity of symptoms, and the patient's renal function. Loop diuretics (e.g., furosemide and torsemide) are more efficacious than thiazides and can remove edema fluid faster than thiazides can, thus providing quicker relief. Loop diuretics also have direct effects on the pulmonary venous system to help improve pulmonary symptoms related to the failing heart. Additionally, however, loop diuretics can cause more dramatic imbalances in extracellular volume and electrolyte levels than thiazides can, and loop diuretics can alter these levels sooner than with thiazide use. Thus, loop diuretics should be employed when moderate to severe CHF is present, but thiazides may be preferred when mild CHF is present.

Continued

Because this patient has moderate to severe symptoms, furosemide is chosen as the diuretic to use in this patient.

If BD had been seen when his CHF was mild but his renal function was already impaired (glomerular filtration rate [GFR], 25 mL/min), how would these circumstances affect your selection of a diuretic?

ANSWER:

Although a thiazide diuretic normally would be the diuretic of choice in treating mild CHF, a thiazide generally is less effective in patients with renal insufficiency. Thiazides can reach their site of action (the luminal sodium ion–chloride ion transporter of the distal convoluted tubule) following filtration at the glomerulus. The amount of drug filtered at the glomerulus depends on the extent of plasma protein binding for that drug. In addition, because thiazides are weakly acidic drugs ($pK_a \sim 7.0$–9.0), they are substrates for active secretion by the organic anion transport system of the proximal tubular cells. With the exception of metolazone and indapamide, however, most thiazides are ineffective as diuretics when the GFR is 30 to 40 mL/min (normal GFR, 125 mL/min).

Loop diuretics reach their site of action (luminal sodium ion–potassium ion–2 chloride ion transporter of the ascending limb of the loop of Henle) primarily via active secretion by the organic anion transport system of proximal tubular cells. As stronger organic acids than thiazide diuretics (e.g., pK_a of furosemide = 4.7), loop diuretics are good substrates for secretion. Extensive plasma protein binding by these drugs limits their access to the lumina of nephrons via filtration. Thus, a marked reduction in GFR does not limit access of loop diuretics to tubular lumina or markedly alter the therapeutic efficacy of these drugs. As a result, a loop diuretic would still be a preferred choice for treating BD if his CHF had been mild but his renal function reduced.

Following 6 weeks on his low-salt diet and drug therapy, BD's condition seems to be greatly improved. His serum potassium levels, however, have decreased from 4.2 to 3.1 mEq/L (normal value, 3.8–5.6 mEq/L). What caused his serum potassium levels to decrease over time? Why is this change a concern? What can be done to remedy this problem?

ANSWER:

One of the major side effects of using a loop diuretic is excessive excretion of electrolytes, including potassium ions. Loss of potassium can eventually lead to hypokalemia (low blood potassium), and hypokalemia alone can lead to the development of cardiac arrhythmias. Potassium loss, however, also potentiates the actions of digitalis (cardiac sodium–potassium–adenosine triphosphatase inhibition) and can lead to digitalis-induced cardiac arrhythmias as well. Hypokalemia can be treated/prevented by the use of potassium supplements or the use of a potassium-sparing diuretic (e.g., triamterene and amiloride). Because potassium-sparing diuretics are weakly basic drugs, they do not alter the active secretion of loop diuretics.

CASE STUDY

Victoria F. Roche and S. William Zito

You often eat lunch with your favorite grandma, who is 85 years old and generally in good health except for infrequent bouts of gout. During the last few years when you meet with her, you have noticed that she has been gaining weight around her middle and that her legs and ankle seem to be puffy. During your most recent lunch date, grandma shares with you a problem she has been having at night. It doesn't happen every night, but every now and then she wakes gasping for air, which requires her to get out of bed and open the window to get relief. She has taken to propping herself up using two or three pillows to get back to sleep. The next day, you accompany grandma to the family doctor, who based on physical examination and a chest radiograph makes a diagnosis of mild (New York Heart Association [NYHA] Functional Classification of Class II) congestive heart failure (CHF). A recommendation is made to limit sodium intake, institute a regimen of exercise and initiate diuretic therapy to remove pulmonary and pedal edema fluid, and decrease the workload on grandma's heart. The doctor knows you are a pharmacy student who likes medicinal chemistry and asks you to make an appropriate choice from structures 1 to 4.

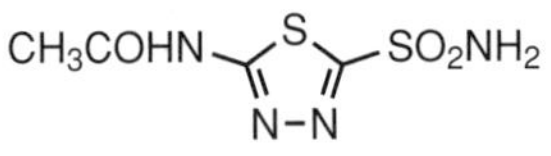

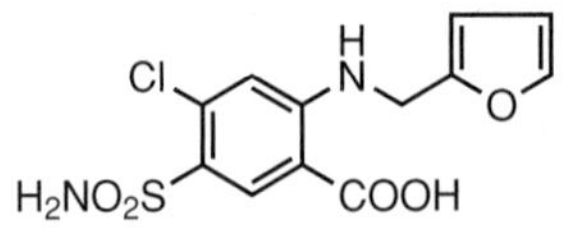

1. Identify the therapeutic problem(s) in which the pharmacist's intervention may benefit the patient.
2. Identify and prioritize the patient-specific factors that must be considered to achieve the desired therapeutic outcomes.

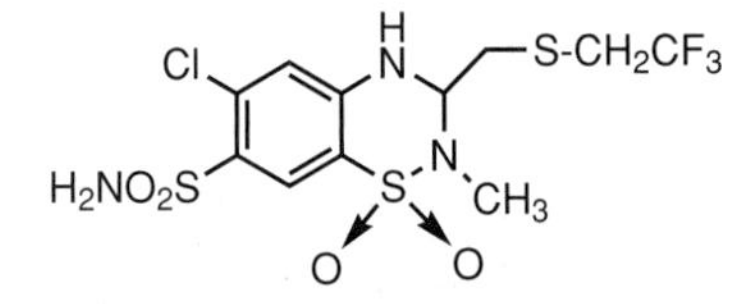

CH_3COHN S SO_2NH_2 N–N

1

Cl H N $S\text{-}CH_2CF_3$ H_2NO_2S S N CH_3 O O

2

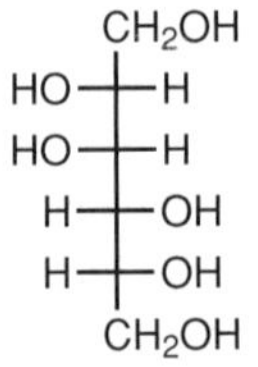

CH_2OH HO H HO H H OH H OH CH_2OH

3

Cl H N O H_2NO_2S COOH

4

3. Conduct a thorough and mechanistically oriented structure–activity analysis of all therapeutic alternatives provided in the case.
4. Evaluate the structure–activity relationship findings against the patient-specific factors and desired therapeutic outcomes, and make a therapeutic decision.
5. Counsel your patient.

References

1. Jackson EK. Diuretics. In: Brunton L, Lazo JS, Parker KL, eds. Goodman and Gilman's The Pharmacological Basis of Therapeutics, 11th Ed. New York, McGraw-Hill, 2006, pp 757–769.
2. Lee CM, Plattner JJ, Ours CW, et. al. [(Aminomethyl)aryloxy]acetic acid esters. A new class of high-ceiling diuretics. 1. Effects of nitrogen and aromatic nuclear substitution. J Med Chem 1984;27:1579–1587.
3. Plattner JJ, Fung AK, Smital JR, et al. [(Aminomethyl)aryloxy]acetic acid esters. A new class of high-ceiling diuretics. 2. Modifications of the oxyacetic side chain. J Med Chem 1984;27:1587–1596.

Suggested Readings

Acara MA. Renal pharmacology—diuretics. In: Smith CM, Reynard AM, eds. Textbook of Pharmacology. Philadelphia, WB Saunders, 1992, pp 554–588.

Friedman PA, Berndt, WO. Diuretic drugs. In: Craig CR, Stizel RE, eds. Modern Pharmacology with Clinical Applications, 6th Ed. Philadelphia: Lippincott Williams & Wilkins, 2004; pp 239–255.

Brenner BM, Rector FC Jr, eds. The Kidney, 4th Ed. Philadelphia, WB Saunders, 1991.

Breyer J, Jacobson HR. Molecular mechanisms of diuretic agents. Annu Rev Med 1990;41:265–275.

Kalantarinia K, Okusa MD. Diuretics: Drugs that increase the excretion of water and electrolytes. In: Minneman KP, Wecker L, eds. Brody's Human Pharmacology; Molecular to Clinical, 4th Ed. Philadelphia: Elsevier Mosby, 2005; pp 163–182.

Jackson EK. Diuretics. In: Brunton L, Lazo JS, Parker KL, eds. Goodman and Gilman's The Pharmacological Basis of Therapeutics, 11th Ed. New York: McGraw-Hill, 2006; pp 737–769.

28. *Angiotensin-Converting Enzyme Inhibitors, Antagonists and Calcium Blockers*

MARC HARROLD

DRUGS COVERED IN THIS CHAPTER:

ANTIOTENSIN II INHIBITORS	ANGIOTENSIN II BLOCKERS	CALCIUM CHANNEL BLOCKERS
• Captopril	• Candesartan	• Amlodipine
• Enalapril	• Eprosartan	• Bepridil
• Fosinopril	• Irbesartan	• Diltiazem
• Lisinopril	• Losartan	• Felodipine
• Quinapril	• Telmisartan	• Nifedipine
• Ramipril	• Olmesartan	• Nisoldipine
	• Valsartan	• Verapamil
		• Ziconotide

THE RENIN-ANGIOTENSIN PATHWAY

The renin-angiotensin system is a complex, highly regulated pathway that is integral in the regulation of blood volume, electrolyte balance, and arterial blood pressure. It consists of two main enzymes, renin and angiotensin-converting enzyme (ACE), the primary purpose of which is to release angiotensin II from its endogenous precursor, angiotensinogen (Fig. 28.1). Angiotensin II is a potent vasoconstrictor that affects peripheral resistance, renal function, and cardiovascular structure (1).

History and Overview of Pathway

Historically, the renin-angiotensin system dates back to 1898, when Tiegerstedt and Bergman demonstrated the existence of a pressor substance in crude kidney extracts. A little over 40 years later, two independent research groups discovered that this pressor substance, which had previously been named renin, actually was an enzyme and that the true pressor substance was a peptide formed by the catalytic action of renin. This peptide pressor substance initially was assigned two different names, angiotonin and hypertensin; however, these names eventually were combined to produce the current designation, angiotensin. In the 1950s, it was discovered that angiotensin exists as both an inactive decapeptide, angiotensin I, and an active octapeptide, angiotensin II, and that the conversion of angiotensin I to angiotensin II is catalyzed by an enzyme distinct from renin (3).

Angiotensinogen is an α_2-globulin with a molecular weight of 58,000 to 61,000 daltons. It contains 452 amino acids, is abundant in the plasma, and is continually synthesized and secreted by the liver. A number of hormones, including glucocorticoids, thyroid hormone, and angiotensin II, stimulate its synthesis. The most important portion of this compound is the N-terminus, specifi-

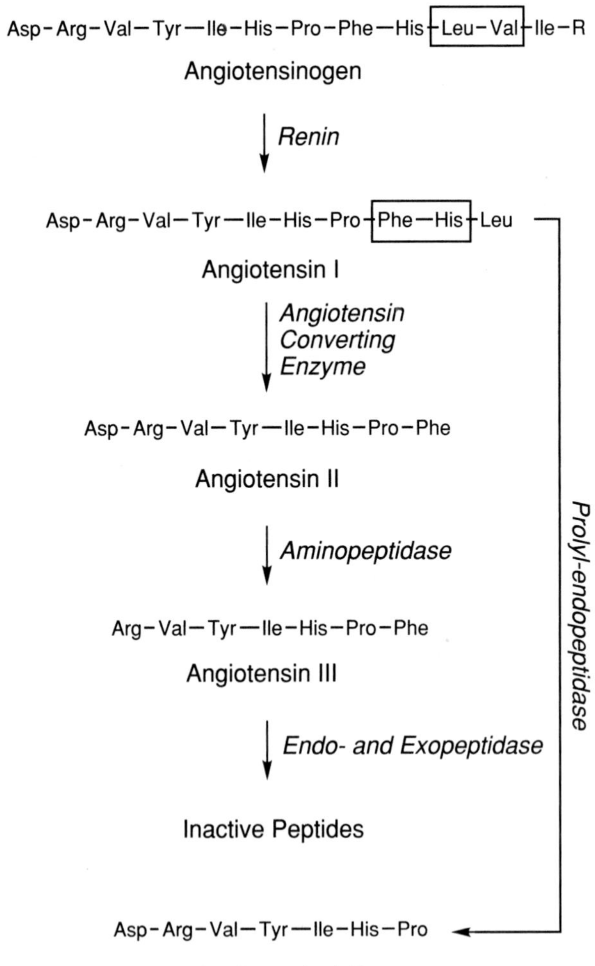

Fig. 28.1. Schematic representation of the renin-angiotensin pathway. The labile peptide bonds of angiotensinogen and angiotensin I are highlighted.

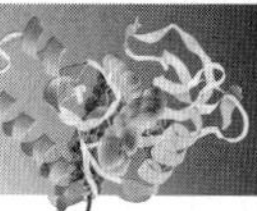

CLINICAL SIGNIFICANCE

The treatment of hypertension and congestive heart failure (CHF) has improved significantly with the introduction of angiotensin-converting enzyme (ACE) inhibitors, angiotensin receptor blockers, and calcium channel blockers. The SARs and structural modifications of these agents have produced major therapeutic advances. These drugs have become cornerstones of therapy today. For example, more than 25 years ago, captopril was the first ACE inhibitor to be developed. Subsequent molecular modifications led to the development of newer agents, such as lisinopril. Although lisinopril exerts comparable ACE inhibition, it possesses a superior pharmacokinetic profile. Instead of having to administer captopril three times daily, lisinopril can be administered once daily.

Medication compliance is notoriously poor in cardiovascular patients. Administering an ACE inhibitor such as lisinopril once daily results in greatly enhanced medication compliance. The therapeutic outcomes of patients with hypertension and CHF have improved immensely as a result. Similar molecular enhancements have been made with angiotensin receptor blockers and calcium channel blockers.

The application of basic science in modifying the chemical structure of these agents has ultimately resulted in patients living longer and suffering fewer cardiovascular events, such as myocardial infarction or worsening CHF. Importantly, their day-to-day quality of life is preserved as well.

Thomas L. Rihn, Pharm.D.
Senior Vice President and Chief Clinical Officer
University Pharmacotherapy Associates
Associate Professor of Clinical Pharmacy
Duquesne University
School of Pharmacy

cally the Leu_{10}-Val_{11} bond. This bond is cleaved by renin and produces the decapeptide angiotensin I. The Phe_8-His_9 peptide bond of angiotensin I is then cleaved by ACE to produce the octapeptide angiotensin II. Aminopeptidase can further convert angiotensin II to the active heptapeptide angiotensin III by removing the N-terminal arginine residue. Further actions of carboxypeptidases, aminopeptidases, and endopeptidases result in the formation of inactive peptide fragments. An additional compound can be formed by the action of a prolyl-endopeptidase on angiotensin I. Cleavage of the Pro_7-Phe_8 bond of angiotensin I produces a heptapeptide known as angiotensin 1-7. The actions of all of these compounds are discussed below.

Actions and Properties of Renin-Angiotensin Pathway Components

Renin is an aspartyl protease that determines the rate of angiotensin II production. It is a much more specific enzyme than ACE. Its primary function is to cleave the leucine-valine bond at residues 10 and 11 of angiotensinogen. The stimulation of renin release is controlled very closely by hemodynamic, neurogenic, and humoral signals (Fig. 28.2). Hemodynamic signals involve the renal juxtaglomerular cells. These cells are sensitive to the hemodynamic stretch of the afferent glomerular arteriole. An increase in the stretch implies a raised blood pressure and results in a reduced release of renin, whereas a decrease in the stretch increases renin secretion. Additionally, these cells also are sensitive to NaCl flux across the adjacent macula densa. Increases in NaCl flux across the macula densa inhibit renin release, but decreases in the flux stimulate release. Further, neurogenic enhancement of renin release occurs via activation of β_1 receptors. Finally, a variety of hormonal signals influence the release of renin. Somatostatin, atrial natriuretic factor, and angiotensin II inhibit renin release, whereas vasoactive intestinal peptide, parathyroid hormone, and glucagon stimulate renin release (4).

In contrast, ACE, also known as kininase II, is a zinc protease that is under minimal physiological control. It is not a rate-limiting step in the generation of angiotensin II and is a relatively nonspecific dipeptidyl carboxypeptidase that requires only a tripeptide sequence as a

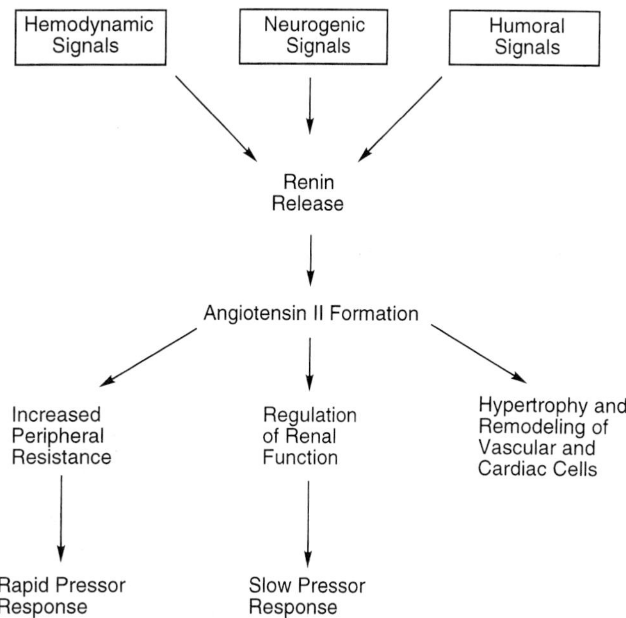

Fig. 28.2. Summary of the factors involved in renin release and the effects medicated by angiotensin II.

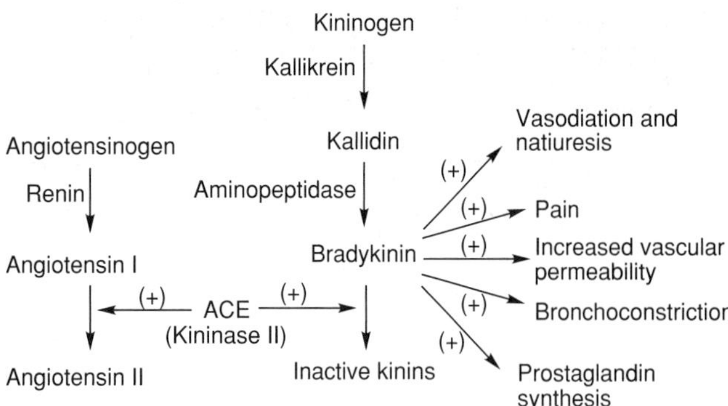

Fig. 28.3. Schematic representation of the bradykinin pathway and its relationship to ACE and the renin-angiotensin pathway.

substrate. The only structural feature required by ACE is that the penultimate amino acid in the peptide substrate cannot be proline. For this reason, angiotensin II, which contains a proline in the penultimate position, is not further metabolized by ACE. The lack of specificity and control exhibited by ACE results in its involvement in the bradykinin pathway (Fig. 28.3). Bradykinin is a nonapeptide that acts locally to produce pain, cause vasodilation, increase vascular permeability, stimulate prostaglandin synthesis, and cause bronchoconstriction. Similar to angiotensin II, bradykinin is produced by proteolytic cleavage of a precursor peptide. Cleavage of kininogens by the protease kallikrein produces a decapeptide known as either kallidin or lysyl-bradykinin. Subsequent cleavage of the N-terminal lysine by aminopeptidase produces bradykinin. The degradation of bradykinin to inactive peptides occurs through the actions of ACE. Thus, ACE not only produces a potent vasoconstrictor but also inactivates a potent vasodilator (1,4,5).

Angiotensin II is the dominant peptide produced by the renin-angiotensin pathway (Fig. 28.2). It is a potent vasoconstrictor that increases total peripheral resistance through a variety of mechanisms: direct vasoconstriction, enhancement of both catecholamine release and neurotransmission within the peripheral nervous system, and increased sympathetic discharge. The result of all these actions is a rapid pressor response. Additionally, angiotensin II causes a slow pressor response, resulting in a long term stabilization of arterial blood pressure. This long-term effect is accomplished by the regulation of renal function. Angiotensin II directly increases sodium reabsorption in the proximal tubule. It also alters renal hemodynamics and causes the release of aldosterone from the adrenal cortex. Finally, angiotensin II causes the hypertrophy and remodeling of both vascular and cardiac cells through a variety of hemodynamic and nonhemodynamic effects (1).

Although secondary peptides, angiotensin III and angiotensin 1-7, also are thought to contribute to the overall effects of the renin-angiotensin pathway, angiotensin III is equipotent with angiotensin II in stimulating aldosterone secretion; however, it is only 10 to 25% as potent in increasing blood pressure. In contrast, angiotensin 1-7 does not cause either aldosterone secretion or vasoconstriction, but it does have potent effects that are distinct from those of angiotensin II. Similar to angiotensin II, angiotensin 1-7 causes neuronal excitation and vasopressin release. Additionally, it enhances the production of prostaglandins via a receptor-mediated process that does not involve an increase in intracellular calcium levels. It has been proposed to be important in the modulation of cell-to-cell interactions in cardiovascular and neural tissues (6).

ROLE OF THE RENIN-ANGIOTENSIN PATHWAY IN CARDIOVASCULAR DISORDERS

Because the renin-angiotensin pathway is central to the maintenance of blood volume, arterial blood pressure, and electrolyte balance, abnormalities in this pathway (e.g., excessive release of renin and overproduction of angiotensin II) can contribute to a variety of cardiovascular disorders. Specifically, overactivity of this pathway can result in hypertension or heart failure via the mechanisms previously described. Abnormally high levels of angiotensin II can contribute to hypertension through both rapid and slow pressor responses. Additionally, high levels of angiotensin II can cause cellular hypertrophy and increase both afterload and wall tension. All of these events can cause or exacerbate heart failure.

High blood pressure is a relatively common disorder, affecting more than 50 million Americans. It is more prevalent in males than in females and in blacks than in Caucasians. Onset usually begins during the third, fourth, and fifth decades of life, and the incidence of the disorder increases with age. Hypertension is classified as either primary or secondary. Primary hypertension, also known as essential hypertension, is the most prevalent form of the disorder and is defined as high blood pressure of an unknown etiology. Most cases of primary hypertension are thought to result from a variety of underlying pathophysiological mechanisms and not from a single, specific cause. Additionally, genetic factors appear to be important in the development of primary hypertension. Secondary hypertension is associated with a specific disorder (e.g., chronic renal disease, pheochromocytoma, and Cushing's syndrome), is present in approximately 5% of individuals with high blood pressure and, in some instances, is potentially curable. Secondary hypertension is much more common in children than in adults (7).

Heart failure (previously designated as congestive heart failure) affects approximately 5 million Americans and is the most common hospital discharge diagnosis in patients older than 65 years. The overall 5-year survival rate is approximately 50% for all patients, with women having an overall lower mortality rate than men. The disease results from conditions in which the heart is unable to supply blood at a rate sufficient to meet the demands of the body. Similar to hypertension, this pathophysiological state can occur via a variety of mechanisms. Any pathophysiological event that causes either systolic or diastolic dysfunction will result in heart failure. Systolic dysfunction, or decreased contractility, can be caused by dilated cardiomyopathies, ventricular hypertrophy, or a reduction in muscle mass. Diastolic dysfunction, or restriction in ventricular filling, can be caused by increased ventricular stiffness, mitral or tricuspid valve stenosis, or pericardial disease. Both ventricular hypertrophy and myocardial ischemia can contribute to increased ventricular stiffness. Angiotensin II causes and/or exacerbates heart failure by increasing systemic vascular resistance, promoting sodium retention, stimulating aldosterone release, and stimulating ventricular hypertrophy and remodeling (8).

OVERVIEW OF DRUG THERAPY AFFECTING THE RENIN-ANGIOTENSIN PATHWAY

Because angiotensin II produces the majority of the effects attributed to the renin-angiotensin pathway, compounds that can block either the synthesis of angiotensin II or the binding of angiotensin II to its receptor should attenuate the actions of this pathway. Indeed, enzyme inhibitors of both renin and ACE, as well as receptor antagonists of angiotensin II, have all been shown to produce beneficial effects in decreasing the actions of angiotensin II. Inhibitors of ACE were the

Development of Orally Active Renin Inhibitors

Renin is a very specific enzyme. The octapeptide, His-Pro-Phe-His-Leu-Leu-Val-Tyr, is the smallest substrate recognized by the enzyme and is similar to the eight-amino-acid sequence, His_6-Pro_7-Phe_8-His_9-Leu_{10}-Val_{11}-Ile_{12}-His_{13}, which is found in angiotensinogen. Using this octapeptide, Boger (9) replaced the labile Leu-Leu bond with the stable dipeptide mimic statine and replaced the two C-terminal residues (Val–Tyr) with similar hydrophobic amino acids (Leu-Phe).

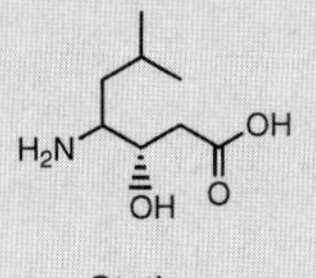

Statine

The resulting compound, N-isovaleryl-His-Pro-Phe-His-Sta-Leu-Phe-NH_2 (SCRIP), showed effective, although short-lived, inhibition of renin when given intravenously (IV). Infusion experiments with SCRIP were the first to demonstrate that a small molecule renin inhibitor could maintain a lowered blood pressure for an extended period of time. Susceptibility to proteolytic cleavage, however, limited the therapeutic utility of SCRIP and other analogous peptides.

Structure–activity studies with SCRIP revealed that the N-terminal His-Pro-Phe sequence could be replaced with an acylated phenylalanine or tyrosine without any significant loss in inhibitor activity. Additional changes to SCRIP resulted in the clinical drug candidate enalkiren, also known as A-64662 (Fig. 28.4). The histidine residue (His_6), which is present in angiotensinogen and all previous inhibitors, was thought to be essential for enzyme recognition and was left unchanged. The acylated tyrosine protects the compound from aminopeptidase enzymes and also contributes to enzyme active-site recognition. The remainder of the molecule is a stable dipeptide isostere. The cyclohexylmethylene and iso-butyl side chains are lipophilic and approximate the lipophilic side chains present in Leu_{10} and Val_{11} of angiotensinogen. Additionally, the use of a C-terminal alcohol instead of a C-terminal carboxylate protects enalkiren from carboxypeptidase enzymes (10,11).

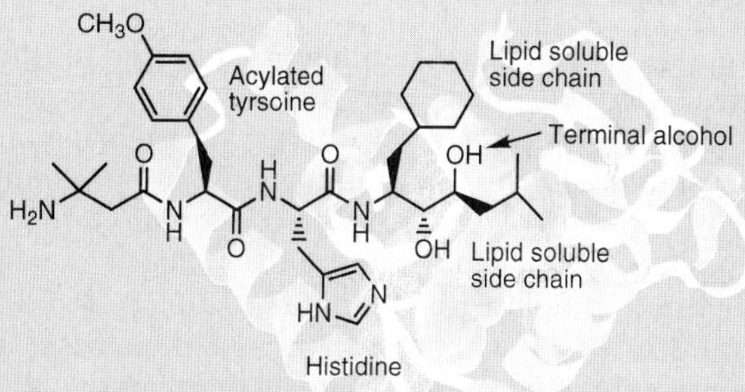

Enalkiren (A-64662)

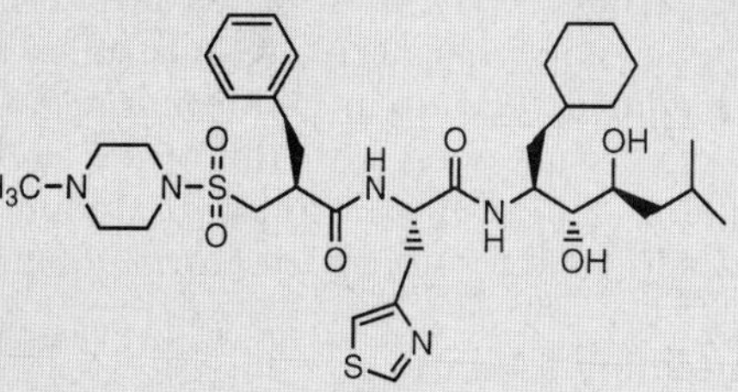

Zankiren (A-72517)

Fig. 28.4. Structures of enalkiren and zankiren.

Enalkiren has been extensively studied in preclinical and clinical trials and has been shown to be efficacious if given IV. It lacks significant bioavailability, however, mainly because of a lack of lipid solubility. A more lipophilic analogue, zankiren (A-72517) (Fig. 28.4), has demonstrated increased oral bioavailability and efficacy. Preclinical and clinical trials with orally administered zankiren showed good bioavailability and significant reduction in blood pressure (11,12). Zankiren has since been withdrawn from clinical trials for undisclosed reasons; however, the FDA recently approved Aliskiren (Tektournan), the first, non-peptidic orally active renin inhibitor. It is approved for the treatment of hypertension and will be available for use in 2007. See Drug update: http://thepoint./www.com/foyebe.

first class of compounds to be marketed. This occurred in 1981 with the approval by the U.S. Food and Drug Administration of captopril. Fourteen years later, losartan was approved as the first angiotensin II receptor blocker (previous referred to as an angiotensin II receptor antagonist). The development, structure–activity relationship (SAR), physicochemical properties, interactions, and indications of these classes of drugs are discussed below.

Attempts to develop orally active, bioavailable renin inhibitors actually predate the development of ACE inhibitors. Research in this area continues today; however, one of the main attractions of renin inhibitors, specificity, has proven to be a significant hurdle to the clinical development (9) of these agents.

ANGIOTENSIN-CONVERTING ENZYME INHIBITORS

Currently, there are 11 ACE inhibitors approved for therapeutic use in the United States. These compounds can be subclassified into three groups based on their chemical composition: sulfhydryl-containing inhibitors (exemplified by captopril), dicarboxylate-containing inhibitors (exemplified by enalapril), and phosphonate-containing inhibitors (exemplified by fosinopril). Captopril and fosinopril are the lone representatives of their respective chemical subclassifications, whereas the majority of the inhibitors contain the dicarboxylate functionality. All of these compounds effectively block the conversion of angiotensin I to angiotensin II and have similar therapeutic and physiological effects. The compounds differ primarily in their potency and pharmacokinetic profiles (1). Additionally, the sulfhydryl group in captopril is responsible for certain effects not seen with the other agents. Detailed descriptions of the rationale for the development of captopril, enalapril, and fosinopril are provided below.

Sulfhydryl-Containing Inhibitors: Development of Captopril

In 1965, Ferreira et al. (13) reported that the venom of the South American pit viper (*Bothrops jararaca*) contained factors that potentiated the action of bradykinin. These factors, originally designated as bradykinin-potentiating factors (BPFs), were isolated and found to be a family of peptides containing 5 to 13 amino acid residues. Their actions in potentiating bradykinin were subsequently linked to their ability to inhibit the enzymatic degradation of bradykinin. Soon thereafter, Bakhle et al. (14) reported that these same peptides also inhibited the enzymatic conversion of angiotensin I to angiotensin II. This latter enzyme, ACE, is now known to be identical with the former bradykininase enzyme (kininase II). Even at the time of these initial discoveries, however, BPFs were seen as lead compounds for the development of new antihypertensive agents, because they possessed dual activities—inhibition of the degradation of bradykinin, a potent vasodilator, and inhibition of the biosynthesis of angiotensin II, a potent vasoconstrictor (15).

A nonapeptide, SQ 20,881 (teprotide), isolated from the original BPFs had the greatest in vivo potency in inhibiting ACE and was shown to consistently lower blood pressure in patients with essential hypertension. It also exerted beneficial effects in patients with heart failure; however, because of its peptide nature and lack of oral activity, teprotide had limited activity in the therapeutic treatment of these diseases (15,16).

SQ 20,881

Cushman, Ondetti, and coworkers (17–19) used SQ 20,881 and other peptide analogues to provide an enhanced understanding of the enzymatic properties of ACE. Using knowledge of substrate-binding specificities and the fact that ACE has properties similar to those of pancreatic carboxypeptidases, these researchers developed a hypothetical model of the enzyme active site. Carboxypeptidase A, like ACE, is a zinc-containing exopeptidase. The binding of a substrate to carboxypeptidase A involves three major interactions (Fig. 28.5A).

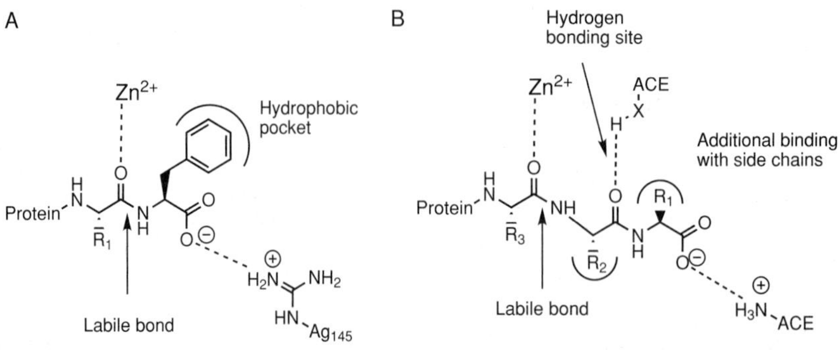

Fig. 28.5. A model of substrate binding to carboxypeptidase A (A) and ACE (B).

First, the negatively charged carboxylate terminus of the amino acid substrate binds to the positively charged Arg-145 on the enzyme. Second, a hydrophobic pocket in the enzyme provides specificity for a C-terminal aromatic or nonpolar residue. Third, the zinc atom is located close to the labile peptide bond and serves to stabilize the negatively charged tetrahedral intermediate, which results when a molecule of water attacks the carbonyl bond between the C-terminal and penultimate amino acid residues (20). Similarly, the binding of substrates to ACE was proposed to involve three or four major interactions (Fig. 28.5B). First, the negatively charged carboxylate terminus of angiotensin I and other substrates was assumed to occur via an ionic bond with a positively charged amine on ACE. Second, the role of the zinc atom in the mechanism of ACE hydrolysis was assumed to be similar to that of carboxypeptidase A. Because ACE cleaves dipeptides instead of single amino acids, the position of the zinc atom was assumed to be located two amino acids away from the cationic center for it to be adjacent to the labile peptide bond. Third, the side-chains R_1 and R_2 could contribute to the overall binding affinity; however, ACE, unlike carboxypeptidase A, does not show specificity for C-terminal hydrophobic amino acids and was not expected to have a hydrophobic binding pocket. Finally, the terminal peptide bond is nonlabile and was assumed to provide hydrogen bonding between the substrate and ACE.

The development of captopril and other orally active ACE inhibitors began with the observation that D-2-benzylsuccinic acid was an extremely potent inhibitor of carboxypeptidase A (17–19). The binding of this compound to carboxypeptidase A (Fig. 28.6A) is very similar to that seen for substrates with the exception that the zinc ion binds to a carboxylate group instead of the labile peptide bond. Byers and Wolfenden (21) proposed that this compound is a by-product analogue that contains structural features of both products of peptide hydrolysis. Most of the structural features of the compound are identical to the terminal amino acid of the substrate (Fig. 28.5A), whereas the additional carboxylate group is able to mimic the carboxylate group that would be produced

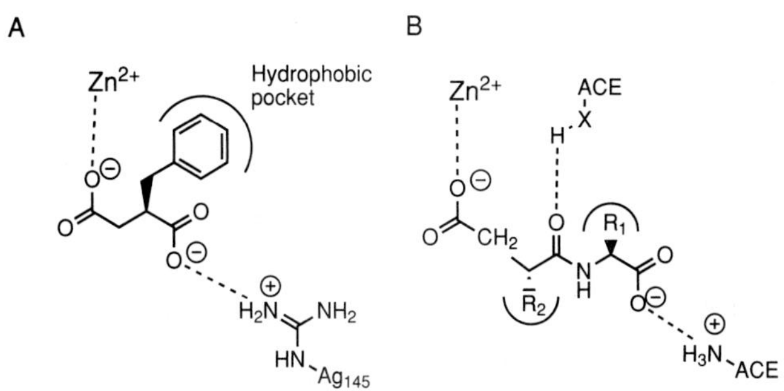

Fig. 28.6. Inhibitor binding models of (A) D-2-benzylsuccinic acid to carboxypeptidase A and (B) succinic acid derivatives to ACE.

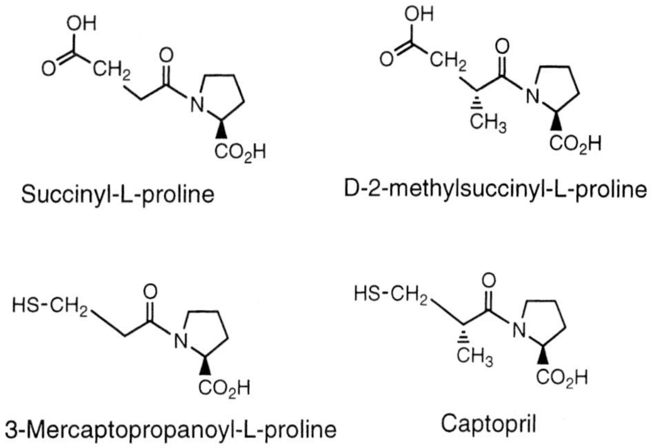

Succinyl-L-proline

D-2-methylsuccinyl-L-proline

3-Mercaptopropanoyl-L-proline

Captopril

Fig. 28.7. Compounds prepared in the development of captopril.

during peptide hydrolysis (21). Applying this concept to the hypothetical model of ACE described above resulted in the synthesis and evaluation of a series of succinic acid derivatives (Fig. 28.6B). Because proline was present as the C-terminal amino acid in SQ 20,881 as well as in other potent, inhibitory snake venom peptides, it was included in the structure of newly designed inhibitors. The first inhibitor to be synthesized and tested was succinyl-L-proline (Fig. 28.7). This compound proved to be somewhat disappointing. Although it provided reasonable specificity for ACE, it was only approximately 1/500 as potent as SQ 20,881.

Substitution of other amino acids in place of proline produced compounds that were even less potent; hence, all subsequent SAR studies were conducted using analogues of L-proline (Fig. 28.7). The addition of a methyl group to the 2 position of succinyl-L-proline to mimic the amino acid side chain, R_2, of the substrate enhanced activity but only marginally. D-2-Methylsuccinyl-L-proline had effects similar to SQ 20,881 but was still only 1/300 as potent. The D-isomer, rather than the L-isomer normally seen for amino acids, was necessary because of the isosteric replacement of an NH_2 with a CH_2 present in succinyl-L-proline. A comparison of the R_2 group of the substrate (Fig. 28.5B) with the methyl group of D-2-methylsuccinyl-L-proline, illustrates that this methyl group occupies the same binding site as the side chain of an L-amino group.

One of the most important alterations to succinyl-L-proline was the replacement of the succinyl carboxylate with other groups having enhanced affinity for the zinc atom bound to ACE. Replacement of this carboxylate with a sulfhydryl group produced 3-mercaptopropanoyl-L-proline. This compound has an IC_{50} value of 200 nM and is greater than 1000-fold more potent than succinyl-L-proline (Fig. 28.7). Additionally, it is 10- to 20-fold more potent than SQ 20,881 in inhibiting contractile and vasopressor responses to angiotensin I. Addition of a 2-D-methyl group further enhanced activity. The resulting compound, captopril (Fig. 28.7), is a competitive inhibitor of ACE with a K_i value of 1.7 nM and was the first ACE inhibitor to be marketed.

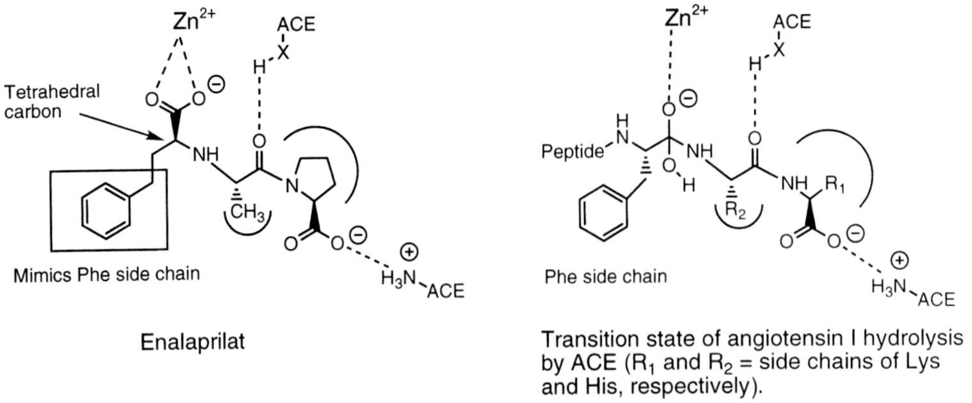

Fig. 28.8. A comparison of enalaprilat and the transition state of angiotensin I hydrolysis by ACE.

The sulfhydryl group of captopril proved to be responsible not only for the excellent inhibitory activity of the compound but also for the two most common side effects, skin rashes and taste disturbances (e.g., metallic taste and loss of taste). These side effects usually subsided on dosage reduction or discontinuation of captopril. They were attributed to the presence of the sulfhydryl group, because similar effects had been observed with penicillamine, a sulfhydryl containing agent used to treat Wilson's disease and rheumatoid arthritis (22,23).

Dicarboxylate-Containing Inhibitors

Development of Enalapril

Researchers at Merck (24) sought to develop compounds that lacked the sulfhydryl group of captopril yet maintained some ability to chelate zinc. Compounds having the general structure shown below were designed to meet this objective.

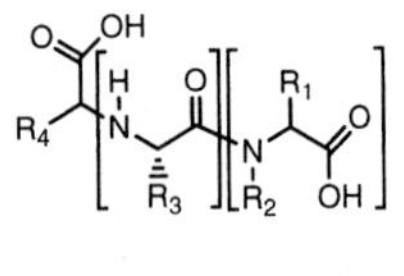

These compounds are tripeptide substrate analogues in which the C-terminal (A) and penultimate (B) amino acids are retained but the third amino acid is isosterically replaced by a substituted N-carboxymethyl group (C). Similar to the results seen in the development of captopril, C-terminal proline analogues provided optimum activity. The use of a methyl group at R_3 (i.e., B = Ala) and a phenylethyl group at R_4 resulted in enalaprilat (Fig. 28.8). In comparing the activity of captopril and enalaprilat, it was found that enalaprilat, with a K_i of 0.2 nM, was approximately 10-fold more potent than captopril. Studies investigating the binding of enalaprilat revealed that its ability to chelate the enzyme-bound zinc atom was significantly less than that of captopril. The enhanced binding was proposed to be caused by the ability to mimic the transition state of angiotensin I hydrolysis. As shown in Figure 28.8, enalaprilat possess a tetrahedral carbon in place of the labile peptide bond. The secondary amine, the carboxylic acid, and phenylethyl groups all contribute to the overall binding of the compound to ACE. The secondary amine is located at the same position as the labile amide nitrogen, the ionized carboxylic acid can form an ionic bond with the zinc atom, and the phenylethyl group mimics the hydrophobic side chain of the Phe amino acid, which is present in angiotensin I.

Despite excellent IV activity, enalaprilat has very poor oral bioavailability. Esterification of enalaprilat produced enalapril (Fig. 28.9), a compound with superior oral bioavailability. The combination of structural features in enalaprilat, especially the two carboxylate groups and the secondary amine, are responsible for its overall low lipophilicity and poor oral bioavailability. Zwitterion formation also has been suggested to contribute to the low oral activity (25), and a comparison of the pK_a values for the secondary amine of enalaprilat and enalapril supports this explanation. Ionization of the adjacent carboxylate in enalaprilat greatly enhances the basicity of the secondary amine such that the pK_a of the amine in this compound is 8.02, whereas in enalapril, it is only 5.49. Thus, in the small intestine, the amine in enalaprilat will be primarily ionized and form a zwitterion with the adjacent carboxylate, but the amine in enalapril will be primarily un-ionized (26).

Intravenous administration of either enalapril or enalaprilat produced similar effects on angiotensin II pro-

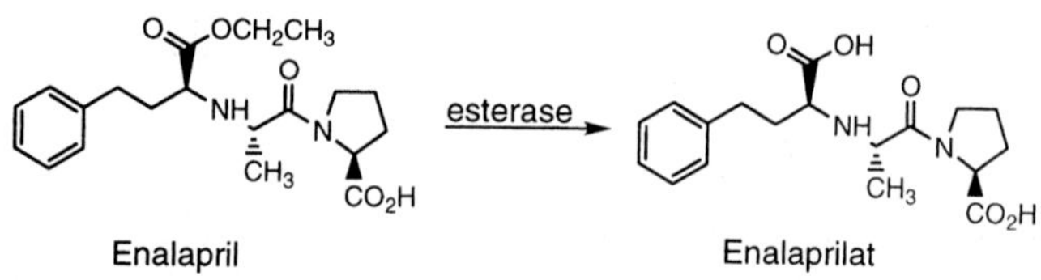

Fig. 28.9. Bioactivation of enalapril.

duction despite the fact that enalapril showed a 1,000-fold decrease in in vitro activity. Subsequent studies showed that enalapril undergoes bioactivation and, thus, is a pro-drug of enalaprilat. Because human plasma was reported to lack enalapril esterolytic activity, bioactivation by hepatic esterases (Fig. 28.9) has been suggested as the most probable mechanism for enalaprilat formation (27,28).

Additional Dicarboxylate Inhibitors

Eight other dicarboxylate inhibitors (Table 28.1) have been approved for various therapeutic indications; however, spirapril has never been marketed. Lisinopril is chemically unique in two respects. First, it contains the basic amino acid lysine (R_1 = $CH_2CH_2CH_2CH_2NH_2$) instead of the standard nonpolar alanine (R = CH_3)

Table 28.1. Additional Dicarboxylate-containing Angiotensin Converting Enzyme Inhibitors

General structure: R_3, OR_2, O, N, H, O, RING, R_1

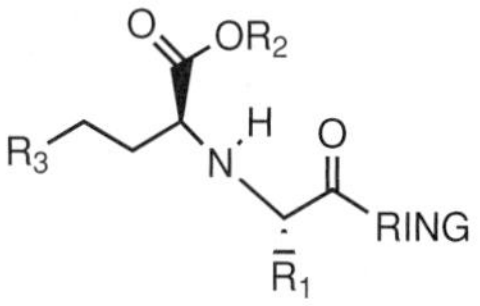

Benazepril: OC_2H_5, O, HN, N, O, CH_2COOH

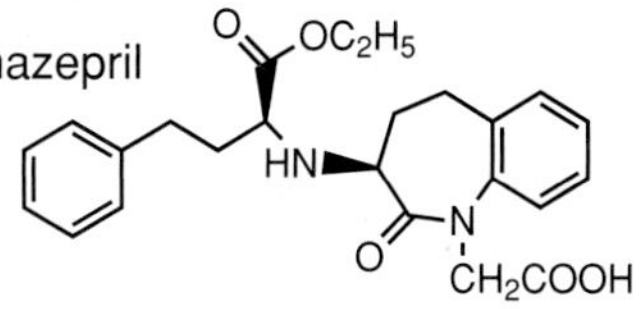

Compounds	Ring	R_1	R_2	R_3
Lisinopril	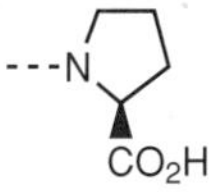 ---N, CO_2H	$(CH_2)_4NH_2$	H	
Moexipril	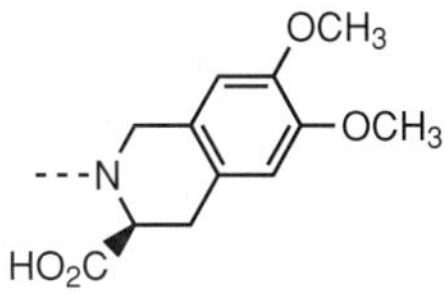 ---N, HO_2C, OCH_3, OCH_3	CH_3	CH_2CH_3	
Perindopril	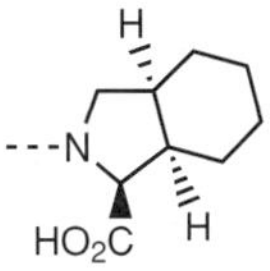 ---N, HO_2C, H, H	CH_3	CH_2CH_3	CH_3
Quinapril	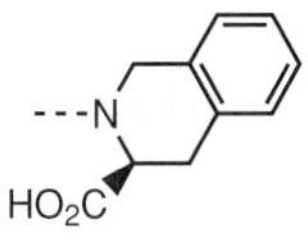 ---N, HO_2C	CH_3	CH_2CH_3	
Ramipril	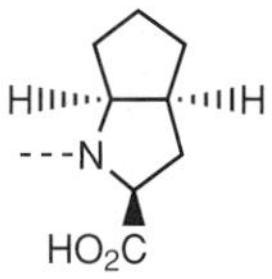 H, H, ---N, HO_2C	CH_3	CH_2CH_3	
Spirapril	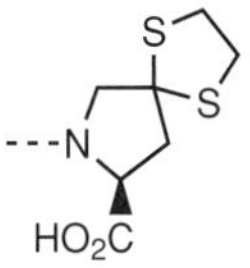 ---N, HO_2C, S, S	CH_3	CH_2CH_3	
Trandolapril	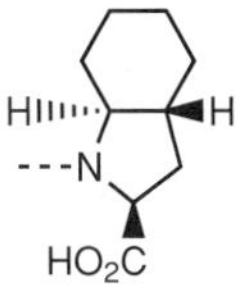 H, H, ---N, HO_2C	CH_3	CH_2CH_3	

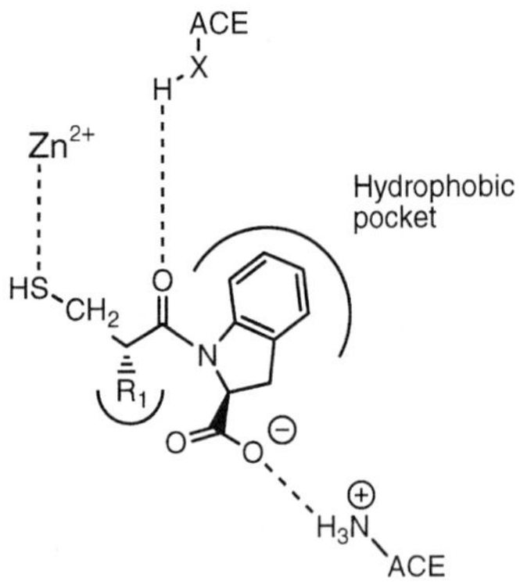

Fig. 28.10. A modified model of ACE inhibitor binding.

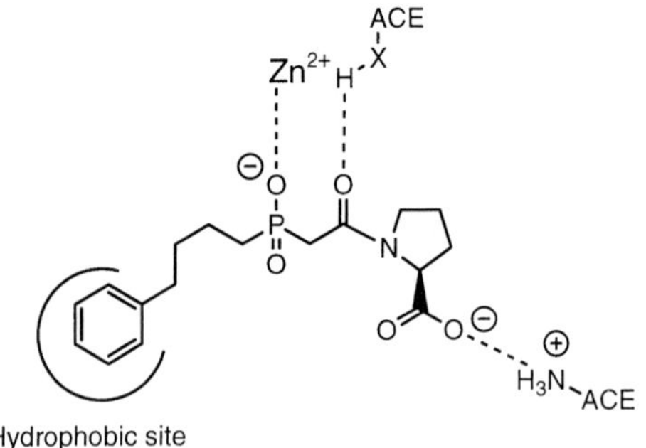

Fig. 28.11. The binding of phosphinate analogues to ACE.

residue. Second, it does not require bioactivation, because neither of the carboxylic acid groups are esterified (i.e., $R_2 = H$). Lisinopril was developed at the same time as enalapril. Despite the addition of another ionizable group, the oral absorption of lisinopril was found to be superior to that of enalaprilat but less than that of enalapril. In vitro studies of enalaprilat and lisinopril showed lisinopril to be slightly more potent than enalaprilat (27,28). Lisinopril, along with captopril, currently are the only two ACE inhibitors that are not pro-drugs.

The major structural difference among the remaining ACE inhibitors is in the ring of the C-terminal amino acid. Lisinopril, like enalapril and captopril, contains the pyrrolidine ring of proline, whereas all the other compounds contain larger bicyclic or spiro ring systems. Studies of indoline analogues of captopril indicated that a hydrophobic pocket similar to that seen in carboxypeptidase A also was present in ACE. This led to a modification (Fig. 28.10) of Ondetti and Cushman's original model and the development of inhibitors that contained larger hydrophobic ring systems (29). Although this modified model was proposed for captopril analogues, it is readily adaptable to include enalaprilat analogues. In general, the varied ring systems seen in benazepril, moexipril, perindopril, quinapril, ramipril, spirapril, and trandolapril provide enhanced binding and potency. They also lead to differences in absorption, plasma protein binding, elimination, onset of action, duration of action, and dosing among the drugs. These differences are discussed in more detail in *Pharmacokinetic Properties* below.

Phosphonate-containing Inhibitors: the Development of Fosinopril

The search for ACE inhibitors that lacked the sulfhydryl group also lead to the investigation of phosphorous-containing compounds (30). The phosphinic acid shown in Figure 28.11 is capable of binding to ACE in a manner similar to enalapril. The interaction of the zinc atom with the phosphinic acid is similar to that seen with sulfhydryl and carboxylate groups. Additionally, this compound is capable of forming the ionic, hydrogen, and hydrophobic bonds similar to those seen with enalapril and other dicarboxylate analogues. A feature unique to this compound is the ability of the phosphinic acid to more truly mimic the ionized, tetrahedral intermediate of peptide hydrolysis. Unlike enalapril and other dicarboxylate analogues, however, the spacing of this tetrahedral species is shorter, being only two atoms removed from the proline nitrogen. Additionally, the spacing between the proline nitrogen and the hydrophobic phenyl ring is one atom longer than that seen in the dicarboxylates.

Structural modification to investigate more hydrophobic, C-terminal ring systems, similar to that described above for the dicarboxylate compounds, lead to a 4-cyclohexylproline analogue of the original phosphinic acid. This compound, fosinoprilat (Fig. 28.12), was more potent than captopril but less potent than enalaprilat. The above-mentioned differences in the spacing of the phosphinic acid and phenyl groups may be responsible for this latter difference in potency. Similar to the dicarboxylates, fosinoprilat was too hydrophilic and exhibited poor oral activity. The pro-drug fosinopril contains an (acyloxy)alkyl group that allows better lipid solubility and improved bioavailability (30). Bioactivation via esterase activity in the intestinal wall and liver produces fosinopril (Fig. 28.12).

Mechanism of Action

The ACE inhibitors attenuate the effects of the renin-angiotensin system by inhibiting the conversion of angiotensin I to angiotensin II (Fig. 28.1). They also inhibit the conversion of [des-Asp^1]angiotensin I to angiotensin III; however, this action has only a minor role in the overall cardiovascular effects of these drugs. They are selective in that they do not directly interfere with any other components of the renin-angiotensin system; however, they do cause other effects that are unrelated to the decrease in angiotensin II concentration. Inhibitors of ACE increase bradykinin levels that, in turn, stimulate prostaglandin biosynthesis (Fig. 28.3). Both of these compounds have been proposed to contribute to the overall action of ACE inhibitors. Additionally, decreased angiotensin II levels increase the release of renin and the production of angiotensin I. Because ACE is inhibited,

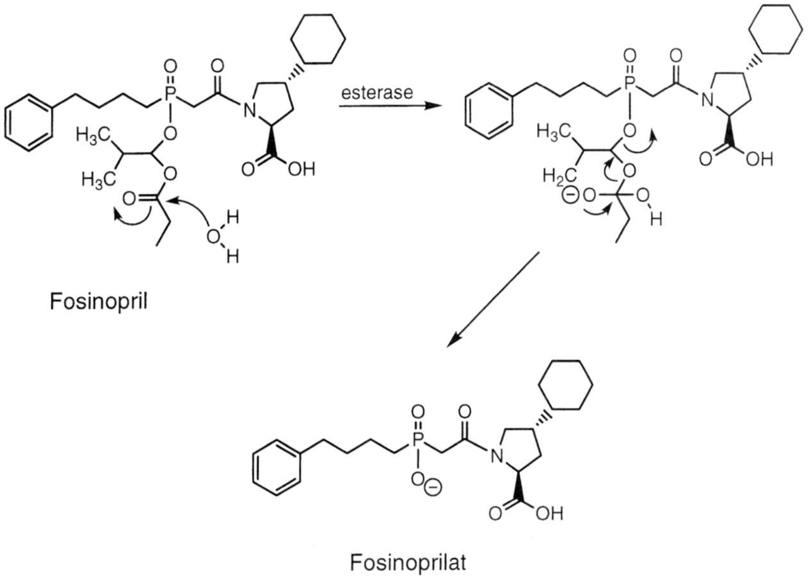

Fosinopril

esterase

Fosinoprilat

Fig. 28.12. Bioactivation of fosinopril.

angiotensin I is shunted toward the production of angiotensin 1-7 and other peptides. The contribution of these peptides to the overall effect of ACE inhibitors is unknown (1).

Structure–Activity Relationships

The structural characteristics for ACE inhibitory activity are given in Table 28.2. Angiotensin-converting enzyme is a stereoselective drug target. Because currently approved ACE inhibitors act as either di- or tripeptide substrate analogues, they must contain a stereochemistry that is consistent with the L-amino acids present in the natural substrates. This was established very early in the development of ACE inhibitors when compounds with carboxyl-terminal D-amino acids were discovered to be very poor inhibitors (31). Later work by Patchett et al. (24) reinforced this idea. They reported a 100- to 1,000-fold loss in inhibitor activity whenever the configuration of either the carboxylate or the R_1 substituent (Table 28.1) was altered. The *S,S,S*-configuration seen in enalapril and other dicarboxylate inhibitors meets the above-stated criteria and provides for optimum enzyme inhibition.

Physicochemical Properties

Captopril and fosinopril are acidic drugs, but all other ACE inhibitors are amphoteric. The carboxylic acid attached to the N-ring is a common structural feature in all ACE inhibitors. It has a pK_a in the range of 2.5 to 3.5 and will be ionized primarily at physiological pH. As discussed above

Table 28.2. Structure activity relationship of ACE inhibitors.

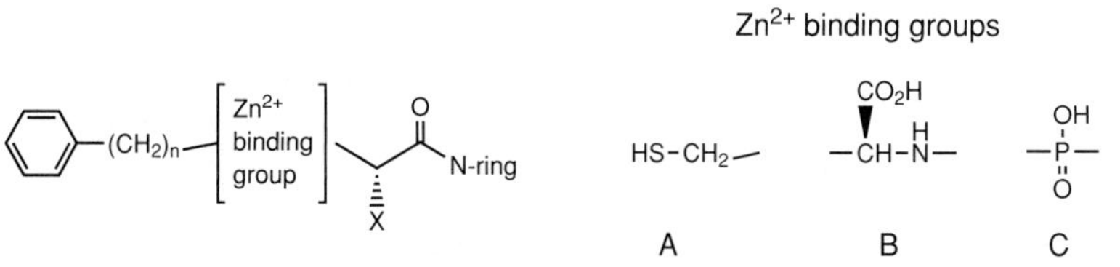

Zn^{2+} binding groups

$(CH_2)_n$ [Zn^{2+} binding group] N-ring X

HS-CH_2— (A) —CH-NH— with CO_2H (B) —P(OH)(=O)— (C)

a. The N-ring must contain a carboxylic acid to mimic the C-terminal carboxylate of ACE substrates.
b. Large hydrophobic heterocyclic rings (i.e., the N-ring) increase potency and alter pharmacokinetic parameters.
c. The zinc binding groups can be either sulfhydryl (A), a carboxylic acid (B), or a phosphinic acid (C).
d. The sulfhydryl group shows superior binding to zinc (the side chain mimicking Phe in carboxylate and phosphinic acid compounds compensates for the lack of a sulfhydryl group).
e. Sulfhydryl-containing compounds produce high incidence of skin rash and taste disturbances.
f. Sulfhydryl-containing compounds can form dimers and disulfides which may shorten duration of action.
g. Compounds which bind to zinc through either a carboxylate or phosphinate mimic the peptide hydrolysis transition state.
h. Esterification of the carboxylate or phosphinate produces an orally bioavailable prodrug.
i. X is usually methyl to mimic the side chain of alanine. Within the dicarboxylate series, when X equals n-butylamine (lysine side chain) this produces a compound which does not require prodrug for oral activity.
j. Optimum activity occurs when stereochemistry of inhibitor is consistent with L-amino acid stereochemisty present in normal substrates.

Table 28.3. Pharmacokinetic Parameters of ACE Inhibitors

Drug	Calculated Log P	Oral Bioavailability (%)	Effect of Food on Absorption	Active Metabolite	Protein Binding (%)	Onset of Action (hours)	Duration of Action (hours)	Major Route(s) of Elimination
Benazepril	5.504	37	Slows absorption	Benazeprilat	>95	1	24	Renal (primary) Biliary (secondary)
Captopril	0.272	60–75	Reduced	NA	25–30	0.25–0.50	6–12	Renal
Enalapril	2.426	60	None	Enalaprilat	50–60	1	24	Renal/Fecal
Enalaprilat	1.545	NA	NA	NA	—	0.25	6	Renal
Fosinopril	6.092	36	Slows absorption	Fosinoprilat	95	1	24	Renal (50%) Hepatic (50%)
Lisinopril	1.188	25–30	None	NA	25	1	24	Renal
Moexipril	4.055	13	Reduced	Moexiprilat	50	1	24	Fecal (primary) Renal (secondary)
Perindopril	3.363	65–95	Reduced	Perindoprilat	60–80	1	24	Renal
Quinapril	4.318	60	Reduced	Quinaprilat	97	1	24	Renal
Ramipril	3.409	50–60	Slows absorption	Ramiprilat	73	1–2	24	Renal (60%) Fecal (40%)
Spirapril	3.162	50	—	Spiraprilat	—	1	24	Renal (50%) Hepatic (50%)
Trandolapril	3.973	70	Slows absorption	Trandolaprilat	80	0.5–1.0	24	Fecal (primary) Renal (secondary)

NA, not applicable, —, data not available.

with enalapril, the pK_a and ionization of the secondary amine in the dicarboxylate series depends on whether the adjacent functional group is in the pro-drug or active form. In the pro-drug form, the amine is adjacent to an ester, is less basic, and is primarily un-ionized at physiological pH. Following bioactivation, the amine is adjacent to an ionized carboxylic acid that enhances both the basicity and ionization of the amine. Similarly, the basic nitrogen enhances the acidity of the adjacent carboxylic acid such that it usually has a lower pK_a than the carboxylic acid attached to the N-ring. As an example, the pK_a values of enalapril are 3.39 and 2.30. These values correspond to the carboxylic acid on the N-ring and the carboxylic acid adjacent to the amine, respectively. The analogous values for these functional groups in lisinopril are 3.3 and 1.7 (26).

The calculated log P values (26) along with other pharmacokinetic parameters for the ACE inhibitors are shown in Table 28.3. With three notable exceptions, captopril, enalaprilat, and lisinopril, all of the compounds possess good lipid solubility. Compounds that contain hydrophobic bicyclic ring systems are more lipid soluble than those that contain proline. A comparison of the log P values of benazepril, fosinopril, moexipril, perindopril, quinapril, ramipril, spiropril, and trandolapril to those for captopril and enalapril illustrates this fact. As previously discussed, enalaprilat is much more hydrophilic than its ester pro-drug and is currently the only ACE inhibitor marked for IV administration. In terms of solubility, lisinopril probably is the most interesting compound in that it is the most hydrophilic inhibitor, yet unlike enalaprilat, it is orally active. One possible explanation for this phenomenon is that in the duodenum, lisinopril will exist as a di-zwitterion in which the ionized groups can internally bind to one another. In this manner, lisinopril may be able to pass through the lipid bilayer with an overall net neutral charge.

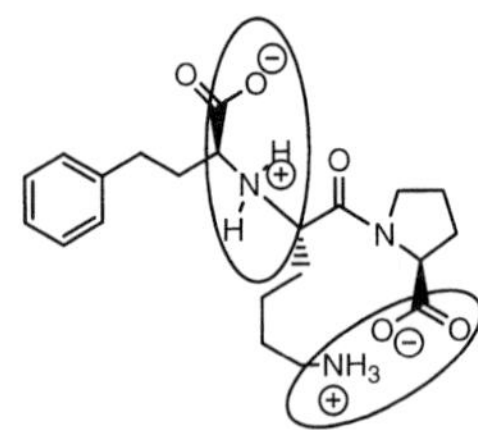

Metabolism

Lisinopril and enalaprilat are excreted unchanged, whereas all other ACE inhibitors undergo some degree of metabolic transformation (1,32–34). As previously discussed and illustrated (Figs. 28.9 and 28.12), all dicarboxylate and phosphonate pro-drugs must undergo bioactivation via hepatic esterases. Additionally, based on their structural features, specific compounds can undergo metabolic inactivation via various pathways (Fig. 28.13). Because of its sulfhydryl group, captopril is subject to oxidative dimerization or conjugation. Approximately 40 to 50% of a dose of captopril is excreted unchanged, whereas the remainder is excreted as either a disulfide dimer or a captopril-cysteine disulfide. Glucuronide conjugation has been reported for benazepril, fosinopril, quinapril, and ramipril. This conjugation can occur either with the parent pro-drug or with the activated drug. Benazepril, with the N-substituted glycine, is especially susceptible to this reaction because of a difference in steric hindrance. For all ACE inhibitors, except

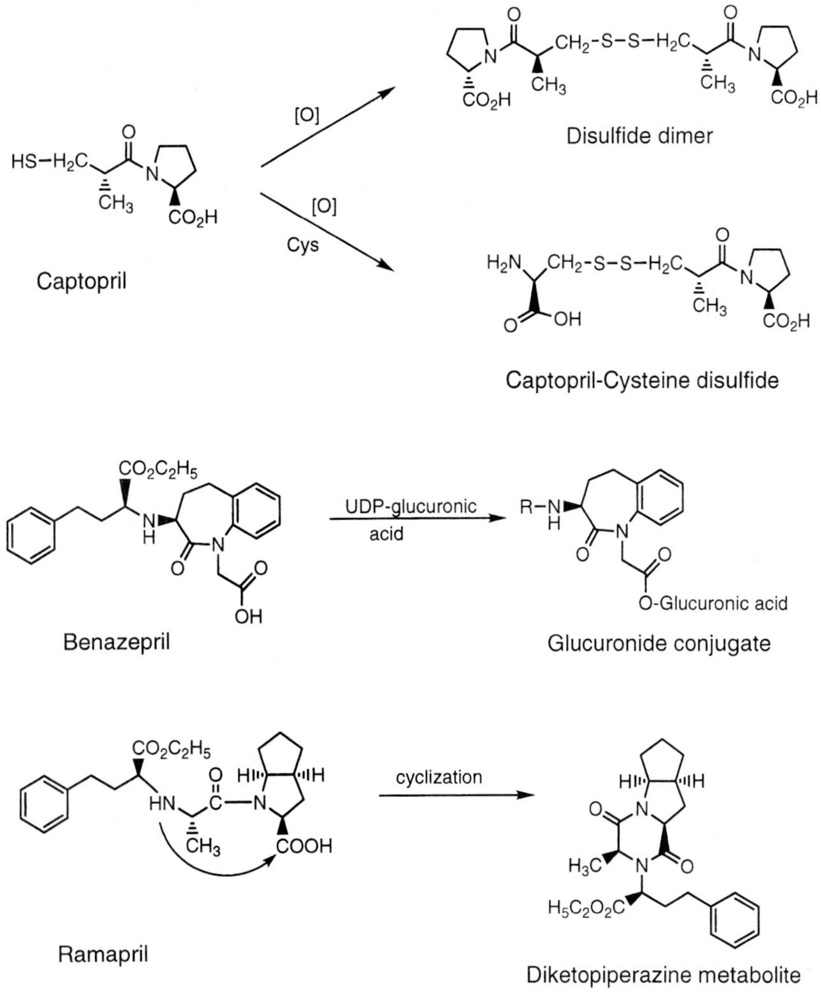

Captopril → [O] → Disulfide dimer

Captopril → [O], Cys → Captopril-Cysteine disulfide

Benazepril → UDP-glucuronic acid → Glucuronide conjugate

Ramapril → cyclization → Diketopiperazine metabolite

Fig. 28.13. Metabolic routes of ACE inhibitors.

benazepril, the carbon atom directly adjacent to the carboxylic acid is part of a ring system and provides some steric hindrance to conjugation. The unsubstituted methylene group (i.e., $-CH_2-$) of benazepril provides less steric hindrance and, thus, facilitates conjugation. Moexipril, perindopril, and ramipril can undergo cyclization to produce diketopiperazines. This cyclization can occur with either the parent or active forms of the drugs.

A comparative study of the metabolism and biliary excretion of lisinopril, enalapril, perindopril, and ramipril revealed that whereas neither lisinopril nor enalapril underwent any appreciable metabolism beyond bioactivation of enalapril to enalaprilat, both perindopril and ramipril were extensively metabolized beyond the initial bioactivation. It was proposed that these differences in hepatic metabolism could be explained, in part, by the larger, more hydrophobic rings present on perindopril and ramipril (35).

Pharmacokinetic Parameters

The pharmacokinetic parameters and dosing information for ACE inhibitors are summarized in Tables 28.3 and 28.4, respectively (1,32–34). The oral bioavailability of this class of drugs ranges from 13 to 95%. Differences in both lipid solubility and first-pass metabolism are most likely responsible for this wide variation. Both parameters should be considered when comparing any two or more compounds. With the exceptions of enalapril and lisinopril, the concurrent administration of food adversely affects the oral absorption of ACE inhibitors. Product literature specifically instructs that captopril should be taken 1 hour before meals and that moexipril should be taken in the fasting state. Although not specifically stated, similar instructions also should benefit patients taking an ACE inhibitor whose absorption is affected by food.

The extent of protein binding also exhibits wide variability among the different compounds. The data suggests that this variation has some correlation with the calculated log P values for the compounds (Table 28.3). Three of the more lipophilic compounds—fosinopril, quinapril, and benazepril—exhibit protein binding of greater than 90%, whereas three of the least lipophilic compounds—lisinopril, enalapril, and captopril—

exhibit much lower protein binding. The lack of a protein binding value for spirapril prevents a more definitive statement on this correlation.

Renal elimination is the primary route of elimination for most ACE inhibitors. With the exceptions of fosinopril and spirapril, altered renal function significantly diminishes the plasma clearance of ACE inhibitors, including those that are eliminated primarily by the feces. Therefore, the dosage of most ACE inhibitors should be reduced in patients with renal impairment (1). Studies of fosinopril in patients with heart failure demonstrated that it is eliminated by both renal and hepatic pathways and does not require a dosage reduction in patients with renal dysfunction (36). Spirapril also exhibits similar properties; however, it is not currently available for use. It should be noted that the literature data for routes of elimination are not always consistent. The designation of renal elimination is quite clear, but it is difficult to correlate what some sources call renal/hepatic elimination with what others call renal/fecal elimination. Additionally, it is uncertain whether the designation of fecal elimination also includes unabsorbed drug. As a result, there is some variability for major routes of elimination listed in Table 28.3.

With one exception, all ACE inhibitors have a similar onset of action, duration of action, and dosing interval. Captopril has a more rapid onset of action; however, it also has a shorter duration and requires a more frequent dosing interval than any of the other compounds. When oral dosing is inappropriate, enalaprilat can be used IV. The normal dose administered to hypertensive patients is 0.625 to 1.25 mg every 6 hours. The dose usually is administered over 5 minutes and may be titrated up to 5 mg IV every 6 hours.

Chemical/Pharmacological Classes Used to Treat Hypertension

Diuretics (see Chapter 27), ACE inhibitors, angiotensin II blockers, calcium channel blockers (see Chapter 28), central α_2-agonists, peripheral α_1-antagonists, β-blockers, ganglionic blockers, and vasodilators (see Chapter 29).

Therapeutic Applications

The ACE inhibitors have been approved for the treatment of hypertension, heart failure, left ventricular dysfunction (either post–myocardial infarction [MI] or asymptomatic), improved survival post-MI, diabetic nephropathy, and reduction of the risk of MI, stroke, and death from cardiovascular causes. Although all ACE inhibitors possess the same physiological actions and, thus, should produce similar therapeutic effects, the approved indications differ among the currently available agents (Table 28.4).

Table 28.4. Dosing Information for Orally Available ACE Inhibitors

Generic Name	Trade Name(s)	Approved Indications	Dosing Range (Treatment of Hypertension)	Maximum Daily Dose	Dose Reduction with Renal Dysfunction	Available Tablet Strengths (mg)
Benazepril	Lotensin	Hypertension	10–40 mg q.d. or b.i.d.	80 mg	Yes	5, 10, 20, 40
Captopril	Capoten	Hypertension, heart failure, left ventricular dysfunction (post-MI), diabetic nephropathy	25–150 mg b.i.d. or t.i.d.	450 mg	Yes	12.5, 25, 50, 100
Enalapril	Vasotec	Hypertension, heart failure, left ventricular dysfunction (asymptomatic)	2.5–40 mg q.d. or b.i.d.	40 mg	Yes	2.5, 5, 10, 20
Fosinopril	Monopril	Hypertension, heart failure	10–40 mg q.d.	80 mg	No	10, 20, 40
Lisinopril	Prinivil, Zestril	Hypertension, heart failure, Improve survival post-MI	10–40 mg q.d.	40 mg	Yes	2.5, 5, 10, 20, 30, 40
Moexipril	Univasc	Hypertension	7.5–30 mg q.d. or b.i.d.	30 mg	Yes	7.5, 15
Perindopril	Aceon	Hypertension	4–8 mg q.d. or b.i.d.	16 mg	Yes	2, 4, 8
Quinapril	Accupril	Hypertension, heart failure	10–80 mg q.d. or b.i.d.	80 mg	Yes	5, 10, 20, 40
Ramipril	Altace	Hypertension, heart failure, reduce risk of MI, stroke, and death from cardiovascular causes	2.5–20 mg q.d. or b.i.d.	20 mg	Yes	1.25, 2.5, 5, 10
Trandolapril	Mavik	Hypertension, heart failure, left ventricular dysfunction (post-MI)	1–4 mg q.d.	8 mg	Yes	1, 2, 4

MI, myocardial infarction.

Combination Products That Include an ACE Inhibitor

ACE Inhibitor/Diuretic: benazepril/hydrochlorothiazide, captopril/hydrochlorothiazide, enalapril/hydrochlorothiazide, fosinopril/hydrochlorothiazide, lisinopril/hydrochlorothiazide, moexipril/hydrochlorothiazide, and quinapril/hydrochlorothiazide

ACE Inhibitor/Calcium Channel Blocker: benazepril/amlodipine, enalapril/felodipine, trandolapril/verapamil

Unlabeled Uses

Hypertensive crises, renovascular hypertension, neonatal and childhood hypertension, stroke prevention, migraine prophylaxis, nondiabetic nephropathy, chronic kidney disease, diagnosis of scleroderma renal crisis, and Bartter's syndrome (32,33)

Inhibitors of ACE have been designated as first-line agents for the treatment of hypertension (37) and are effective for a variety of cardiovascular disorders. They can be used either individually or with other classes of compounds. They are especially useful in treating patients with hypertension who also suffer from heart failure, left ventricular dysfunction, or diabetes. Arterial and venous dilation seen with ACE inhibitors not only lowers blood pressure but also has favorable effects on both preload and afterload in patients with heart failure. Additionally, the ability of ACE inhibitors to cause regression of left ventricular hypertrophy has been demonstrated to reduce the incidence of further heart disease in patients with hypertension. The use of ACE inhibitors in patients with MI is similarly based on the ability of ACE inhibitors to decrease mortality by preventing postinfarction left ventricular hypertrophy and heart failure. Current recommendations to give ACE inhibitors to all patients with impaired left ventricular

Peptide Mimetics: Design of Agonists/Antagonists

Peptide mimetics have been defined as molecules that mimic the action of peptides, have no peptide bonds (i.e., no amide bonds between amino acids), and a molecular weight of less than 700 Daltons. In comparison with peptide drugs, peptide mimetics have numerous pharmaceutical advantages. Foremost among these are increased bioavailability and increased duration of action. The majority of known peptide mimetics have been discovered by random screening techniques; however, this process is costly, labor intensive, and unpredictable.

A more logical and rational approach is de novo peptide mimetic design (40), and an example of this approach is illustrated in Figure 28.14. In this example, the overall process is divided into three steps (A–C). Initially, the amino acids that comprise the pharmacophore of the peptide must be identified. Thus, a knowledge of the SARs for the peptide under consideration is essential. In Figure 28.14A, the side chains present on amino acid residues 1, 3, and 5 of a hypothetical heptapeptide are assumed to comprise the pharmacophore, and the remainder of the peptide is assumed to provide the proper structural support for these key groups. In the second step of this de novo design process, the proper spatial arrangement of the pharmacophoric groups must be elucidated. Nuclear magnetic resonance spectroscopy, x-ray diffraction studies, and molecular modeling programs that allow energy-minimization procedures and molecular dynamics simulation can be used to construct a model of the biologically active conformation. Returning to the example, the side chains representing the pharmacophore are assumed to be located on the inside of the peptide, whereas the remaining residues are assumed to be located on the outside of the peptide (Fig. 28.14B). In the final step of the process, the pharmacophoric groups must be mounted on a nonpeptide template in such a manner that they retain the proper spatial arrangement found in the original peptide. This is shown in Figure 28.14C, where side chains 1, 3, and 5 of the original peptide are connected to a rigid template (represented by the polygon). A variety of aromatic ring systems (e.g., benzene, biphenyl, phenanthrene, and benzodiazepine) can be used to provide the rigid template, and appropriately placed alkyl groups can be used to enhance spacing and increase flexibility. Additionally, isosteres of the original pharmacophoric groups may be used to circumvent specific synthetic problems (41).

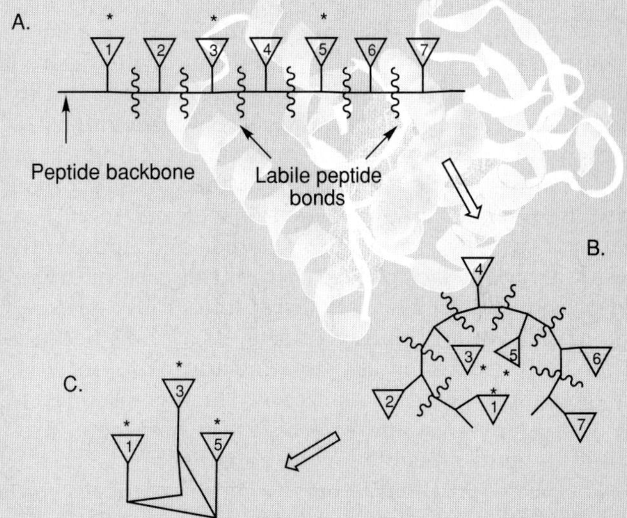

Fig. 28.14. A general process for the rational design of peptide mimetics: (A) identification of crucial pharmacophoric groups, (B) determination of the spatial arrangement of these groups, and (C) use of a template to mount the key functional groups in their proper conformation. Groups highlighted with an asterisk comprise the pharmacophore of the heptapeptide. (From Harrold MW. Preparing students for future therapies: the development of novel agents to control the renin-angiotensin system. Am J Pharm Educ 1997;61:173–178; with permission.)

systolic impairment regardless of the presence of observable symptoms also are based on the ability of these inhibitors to block the vascular and cardiac hypertrophy and remodeling caused by angiotensin II. Inhibitors of ACE also have been reported to slow the progression of diabetic nephropathy and, thus, are preferred agents in the treatment of hypertension in a patients with diabetes. It also has been suggested that ACE inhibitors be used in patients with diabetic nephropathy regardless of the presence or absence or hypertension (1,7,8,33).

Adverse Effects and Drug Interactions

The most prevalent or significant side effects of ACE inhibitors are listed below while drug interactions for ACE inhibitors are listed in Table 28.5 (1,32,33). Some adverse effects can be attributed to specific functional groups within individual agents, whereas others can be directly related to the mechanism of action of this class of compounds. The higher incidence of maculopapular rashes and taste disturbances observed for captopril have been linked to the presence of the sulfhydryl group in this compound. All ACE inhibitors can cause hypotension, hyperkalemia, and a dry cough. Hypotension results from an extension of the desired physiological effect, whereas hyperkalemia results from a decrease in aldosterone secretion secondary to a decrease in angiotensin II production. Cough is by far the most prevalent and bothersome side effect seen with the use of ACE inhibitors. It is seen in 5 to 20% of patients, usually is not dose related, and apparently results from the lack of selectivity of this class of drugs. As previously discussed, ACE inhibitors also prevent the breakdown of bradykinin (Fig. 28.3), and because bradykinin stimulates prostaglandin synthesis, prostaglandin levels also increase. The increased levels of both bradykinin and prostaglandin have been proposed to be responsible for the cough (38).

The use of ACE inhibitors during pregnancy is contraindicated. This class of compounds is not teratogenic during the first trimester, but administration during the second and third trimester is associated with an increased incidence of fetal morbidity and mortality. Inhibitors of ACE can be used in women of childbearing age; however, they should be discontinued as soon as pregnancy is confirmed.

Adverse Effects of ACE Inhibitors

Hypotension, hyperkalemia, cough, rash, taste disturbances, headache, dizziness, fatigue, nausea, vomiting, diarrhea, acute renal failure, neutropenia, proteinuria, and angioedema

Table 28.5. Drug Interactions for ACE Inhibitors

Drug	ACE Inhibitor	Result of Interaction
Allopurinol	Captopril	Increased risk of hypersensitivity
Antacids	All	Decreased bioavailability of ACE inhibitor (more likely with captopril and fosinopril)
Capsaicin	All	Exacerbation of cough
Digoxin	All	Either increased or decreased plasma digoxin levels
Diuretics	All	Potential excessive reduction in blood pressure; the effects of loop diuretics may be reduced.
Iron Salts	Captopril	Reduction of captopril levels unless administration is separated by at least 2 hours
K^+ preparations or K^+-sparing diuretics	All	Elevated serum potassium levels
Lithium	All	Increased serum lithium levels
NSAIDs	All	Decreased hypotensive effects
Phenothiazides	All	Increased pharmacological effects of ACE inhibitor
Probenecid	Captopril	Decreased clearance and increased blood levels of captopril
Rifampin	Enalapril	Decreased pharmacological effects of enalapril
Tetracycline	Quinapril	Decreased absorption of tetracycline (may result from high magnesium content of quinapril tablets)

NSAIDs, nonsteroidal anti-inflammatory agents.

ANGIOTENSIN II RECEPTOR BLOCKERS

From an historical perspective, the angiotensin II receptor was the initial target for developing compounds that could inhibit the renin-angiotensin pathway. Efforts to develop angiotensin II receptor antagonists began in the early 1970s and focused on peptide-based analogues of the natural agonist. The prototypical compound that resulted from these studies was saralasin, an octapeptide in which the Asp_1 and Phe_8 residues of angiotensin II were replaced with Sar (sarcosine, N-methylglycine) and Ile, respectively. Saralasin as well as other peptide analogues demonstrated the ability to reduce blood pressure; however, these compounds lacked oral bioavailability and expressed unwanted partial agonist activity. More recent efforts have used peptide mimetics to circumvent these inherent problems with peptide-based antagonists. The culmination of these efforts was the 1995 approval of losartan, a nonpeptide angiotensin II receptor blocker (ARB) (1,39).

Development of Losartan

The development of losartan can be traced back to two 1982 patent publications (42), which described the antihypertensive effects of a series of imidazole-5-acetic acid analogues. These compounds are exemplified by S-8308

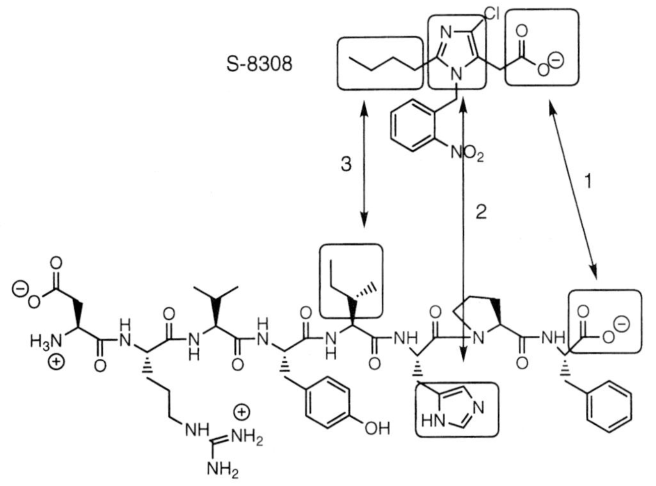

Fig. 28.15. Structural comparison of S-8308, an imidazole-5-acetic acid analogue, with angiotensin II. (Adapted from Timmermans PB, Wong PC, Chiu AT, et al. Angiotensin II receptors and angiotensin II receptor antagonists. Pharmacol Rev 1993;45: 205–213; with permission.)

(Fig. 28.15) and were later found to block the angiotensin II receptor specifically. Although these compounds were relatively weak antagonists, they did not possess the unwanted agonist activity previously seen in peptide analogues. A computerized molecular modeling overlap of angiotensin II with the structure of S-8308 revealed three common structural features: The ionized carboxylate of S-8308 correlated with the C-terminal carboxylate of angiotensin II, the imidazole ring of S-8308 correlated with the imidazole side chain of the His_6 residue, and the n-butyl group of S-8308 correlated with the hydrocarbon side chain of the Ile_5 residue (Fig. 28.15). The benzyl group of S-8308 was proposed to lie in the direction of the N-terminus of angiotensin II; however, it was not believed to have any significant receptor interactions.

From S-8308, a number of molecular modifications were carried out in an attempt to improve receptor binding and lipid solubility, with the latter being important to assure adequate oral absorption. These changes resulted in the preparation of losartan, a compound with high receptor affinity (IC_{50}, 0.019 M) and oral activity (Fig. 28.16).

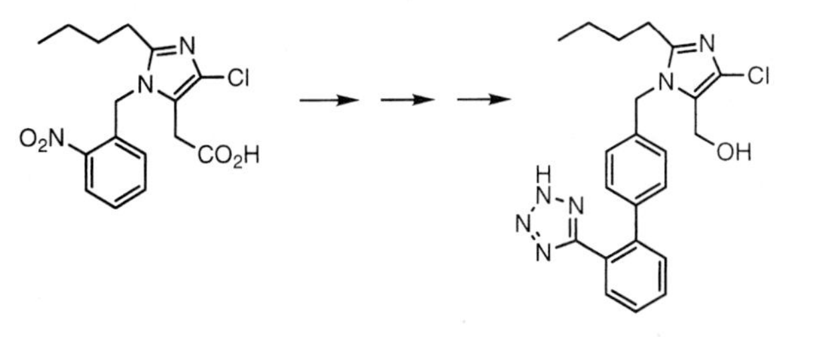

S-8308 (IC_{50} = 15 μM) Losartan (IC_{50} = 0.019μM)

Fig. 28.16. The development of losartan from S-8308.

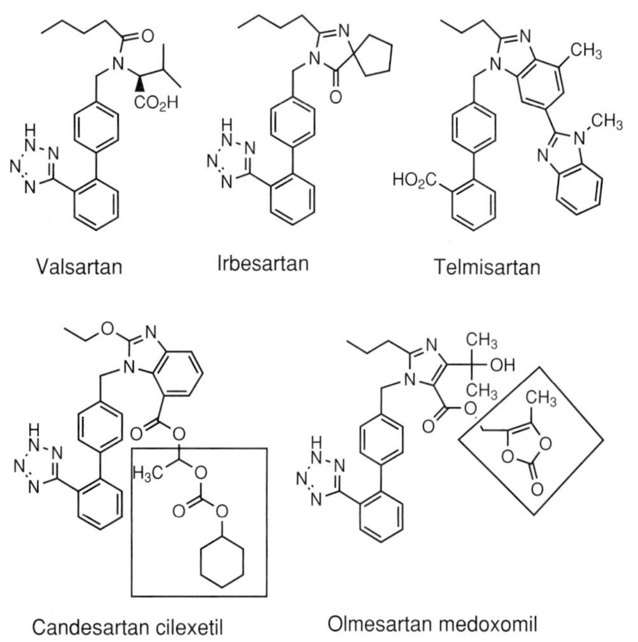

Valsartan Irbesartan Telmisartan

Candesartan cilexetil Olmesartan medoxomil

Fig. 28.17. Structures of losartan analogues. The highlighted portions of candesartan cilexitil and olmesartan medoxomil are hydrolyzed via esterases to produce their respective active, carboxylate metabolites.

Additional Angiotensin II Receptor Blockers

Valsartan, irbesartan, telmisartan, candesartan, and olmesartan are biphenyl analogues of losartan (Fig. 28.17). These compounds possess structural features that are similar to those seen in losartan. Valsartan, named for the valine portion of the compound, is the first nonimidazole-containing ARB and is slightly more potent (IC_{50}, 0.0089 μM) than losartan. The amide carbonyl of valsartan is isosteric with the imidazole nitrogen of losartan and can serve as a hydrogen bond acceptor similar to the imidazole nitrogen. Irbesartan is a spirocompound that lacks the primary alcohol of losartan but that has a 10-fold greater binding affinity (IC_{50}, 0.0013 μM) for the angiotensin II receptor. Hydrogen bonding, or ion–dipole binding, of the carbonyl group can mimic the interaction of the primary alcohol of losartan, whereas the spirocyclopentane can provide enhanced hydrophobic binding. Both candesartan cilexitil and telmisartan contain benzimidazole rings that provide some enhanced hydrophobic binding, similar to that seen with the spirocyclopentane ring of irbesartan. Both candesartan cilexitil and olmesartan medoxomil are pro-drugs that are rapidly and completely hydrolyzed during absorption from the gastrointestinal tract to their active carboxylic acid metabolites, candesartan and olmesartan, respectively. These carboxylic acids lie in exactly the same locations as the hydroxyl group of losartan, the carboxylic acid of valsartan, and the ketone of irbesartan and can participate in both ionic and dipole interactions.

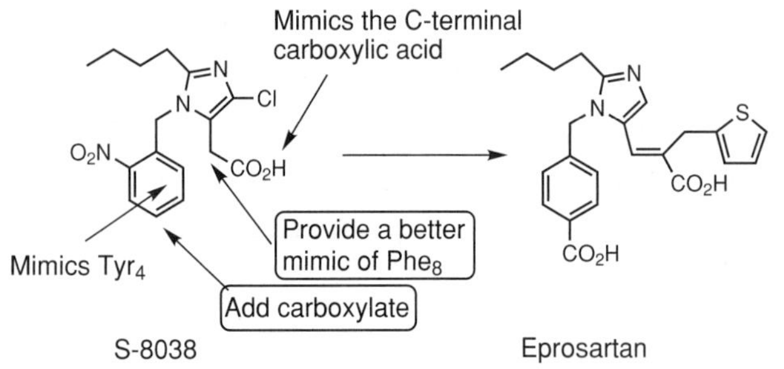

Fig. 28.18. The development of eprosartan from S-8308. The Phe_8 residue of angiotensin II contains the C-terminal carboxylic acid.

Eprosartan was developed using a different hypothesis than that for losartan (Fig. 28.18). Similar to the rationale for losartan, the carboxylic acid of S-8308 was thought to mimic the Phe_8 (i.e., C-terminal) carboxylate of angiotensin II. The benzyl group of S-8308 was proposed to be an important structural feature that mimicked the aromatic side chain of Tyr_4 present in the agonist. Thus, the major structural change was not an extension of the N-benzyl group but, rather, an enhancement of the compound's ability to mimic the C-terminal end of angiotensin II. This was accomplished by substituting the 5-acetic acid group with an α-thienylacrylic acid. In addition, a para-carboxylate (a functional group investigated during the development of losartan) also was added. The thienyl ring isosterically mimics the Phe_8 phenyl ring of angiotensin II and, along with the para-carboxylate, is responsible for the excellent potency ($IC_{50} = 0.0015$ μM) of this compound (39).

Mechanism of Action

The angiotensin II receptor exists in at least two subtypes, type 1 (AT_1) and type 2 (AT_2). The AT_1 receptors are located in brain, neuronal, vascular, renal, hepatic, adrenal, and myocardial tissues and mediate the cardiovascular, renal, and central nervous system (CNS) effects of angiotensin II. All currently available ARBs are 10,000-fold more selective for the AT_1 receptor subtype and act as competitive antagonists at this site. In terms of relative affinity for the AT_1 receptor, candesartan and olmesartan have the greatest affinity; irbesartan and eprosartan have a somewhat lower affinity; and telmisartan, valsartan, and losartan have the lowest affinity. All ARBs prevent and reverse all of the known effects of angiotensin II, including rapid and slow pressor responses, stimulatory effects on the peripheral sympathetic nervous system, CNS effects, release of catecholamines, secretion of aldosterone, direct and indirect renal effects, and all growth-promoting effects. The function of the AT_2 receptors is not as well characterized; however, they have been proposed to mediate a variety of growth, development, and differentiation processes. Some concern has arisen that unopposed stimulation of the AT_2 receptor in conjunction with AT_1 receptor antagonism may cause long-term adverse effects. As a result, compounds that exhibit balanced antagonism at both receptor subtypes are currently being sought (1,43).

Structure–Activity Relationships

All commercially available ARBs are analogues of the following general structure:

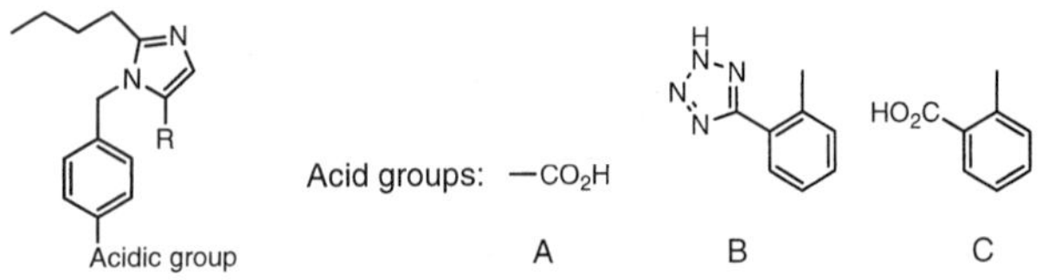

1. The "acidic group" is thought to mimic either the Tyr_4 phenol or the Asp_1 carboxylate of angiotensin II. Groups capable of such a role include the carboxylic acid (A), a phenyl tetrazole (B), or a phenyl carboxylate (C).
2. In the biphenyl series, the tetrazole and carboxylate groups must be in the ortho position for optimal activity (the tetrazole group is superior in terms of metabolic stability, lipophilicity, and oral bioavailability).
3. The n-butyl group of the model compound provides hydrophobic binding and, most likely, mimics the side chain of Ile_5 of angiotensin II. As seen with candesartan, telmisartan, and olmesartan, this n-butyl group can be replaced with either an ethyl ether or an n-propyl group.
4. The imidazole ring or an isosteric equivalent is required to mimic the His_6 side chain of angiotensin II.
5. Substitution can vary at the "R" position. A variety of R groups, including a carboxylic acid, a hydroxymethyl group, a ketone, or a benzimidazole ring, are present in currently available ARBs and are thought to interact with the AT_1 receptor through either ionic, ion–dipole, or dipole–dipole bonds.

Physicochemical Properties

All ARBs are acidic drugs. The tetrazole ring found in losartan, valsartan, irbesartan, candesartan, and olmesartan has a pK_a of approximately 6 and will be at least 90% ionized at physiological pH. The carboxylic acids found on valsartan, candesartan, olmesartan, telmisartan, and eprosartan have pK_a values in the range 3–4 and also will be primarily ionized. Currently, available agents have adequate, but not excellent, lipid solubility. As previously mentioned, the tetrazole group is more lipophilic than a carboxylic. Additionally, the four nitrogen atoms present in the tetrazole ring can create a greater charge distribution than that available for a carboxylic acid. These properties have been proposed to be responsible for the enhanced binding and bioavailability of the tetrazole-containing compounds (44). Similar to ACE inhibitors,

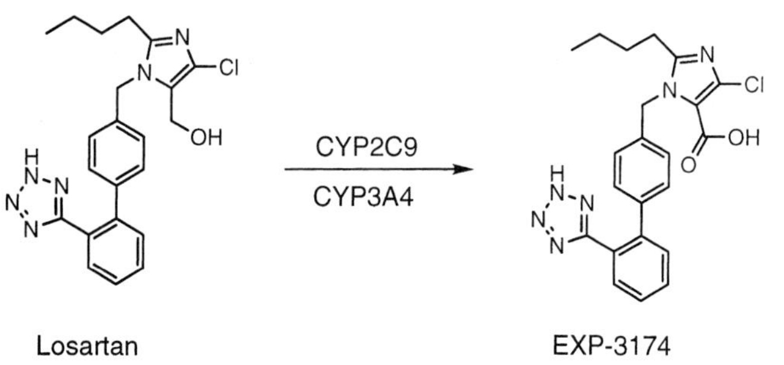

Losartan → (CYP2C9, CYP3A4) → EXP-3174

Fig. 28.19. The metabolic conversion of losartan to EXP-3174 by cytochrome P450 isozymes.

the stereochemistry of valsartan is consistent with the L-amino acids in the natural agonist.

Metabolism

Approximately 14% of a dose of losartan is oxidized by the isozymes CYP2C9 and CYP3A4 to produce EXP-3174, a noncompetitive AT_1 receptor antagonist that is 10- to 40-fold more potent than losartan (Fig. 28.19). The overall cardiovascular effects seen with losartan result from the combined actions of the parent drug and the active metabolite; thus, losartan should not be considered to be a pro-drug (1). As previously mentioned, candesartan cilexetil and olmesartan medoxomil are rapidly and completely hydrolyzed to candesartan and olmesartan, respectively, in the intestinal wall.

None of the other compounds are converted to active metabolites. All of these compounds are primarily (80%) excreted unchanged. Approximately 20% of valsartan is metabolized to inactive compounds via mechanisms that do not appear to involve the CYP450 system. The primary circulating metabolites for irbesartan, telmisartan and eprosartan, are inactive glucuronide conjugates. A small amount of irbesartan is oxidized by CYP2CP; however, irbesartan does not substantially induce or inhibit the CYP450 enzymes normally involved in drug metabolism (1,32–34).

Pharmacokinetic Parameters

The pharmacokinetic parameters and dosing information for angiotensin receptor antagonists are summarized in Tables 28.6 and 28.7, respectively (32–34). With the exception of irbesartan (60–80%) and, possibly, telmisartan (42–58%), all of the compounds have low, but adequate, oral bioavailability (15–33%). Given the fact that most of the compounds are excreted unchanged, the most probable reasons for the low bioavailability are poor lipid solubility and incomplete absorption. Effects of food on the absorption of losartan, eprosartan, valsartan, and eprosartan is to reduce absorption; however, these effects have been deemed to be clinically insignificant; thus, the compounds can be taken either with or without food. All of the compounds have similar onsets, are highly protein bound, have elimination half-lives that allow once- or twice-daily dosing, and with the exception of olmesartan, are primarily eliminated via the fecal route. Candesartan and telmisartan appear to require a slightly longer time to reach peak plasma concentrations. As with ACE inhibitors, literature designation of fecal elimination is unclear regarding whether it includes unabsorbed drug.

Candesartan cilexetil, losartan, and olmesartan differ from the other compounds in several respects. They are the only compounds with active metabolites, and they have the highest renal elimination of all of the agents. Product labeling indicates that renal impairment does not require a dosage reduction for losartan, but area under the curve values are increased by 50% in patients with a creatinine clearance of less than 30 mL/min and are doubled in hemodialysis patients. These increases are not seen for the other agents. Losartan and telmisartan are the only two agents that require initial dose reductions in patients with hepatic impairment. Because of significantly increased plasma concentration, patients with

Table 28.6. Pharmacokinetic Parameters of Angiotensin II Receptor Blockers

Drug	Oral Bioavailability (%)	Active Metabolite	Protein Binding (%)	Time to Peak Plasma Concentration (hours)	Elimination Half-Life (hours)	Major Route(s) of Elimination
Candesartan Cilexetil	15	Candesartan	99	3–4	9	Fecal (67%) Renal (33%)
Eprosartan	15	None	98	1–2	5–9	Fecal (90%) Renal (10%)
Irbesartan	60–80	None	90	1.5–2.0	11–15	Fecal (80%) Renal (20%)
Losartan	33	EXP-3174	98.7 (losartan) 99.8 (EXP-3174)	1 (losartan) 3–4 (EXP-3174)	1.5–2.0 (losartan) 6–9 (EXP-3174)	Fecal (60%) Renal (35%)
Olmesartan Medoxomil	26	Olmesartan	99	1.5–3.0	10–15	Fecal (35–50%) Renal (50–65%)
Telmisartan	42–58	None	100	5	24	Fecal (97%)
Valsartan	25	None	95	2–4	6	Fecal (83%) Renal (13%)

Table 28.7. Dosing Information for Angiotensin II Receptor Blockers

Generic Name	Trade Name(s)	Approved Indications	Dosing Range (Treatment of Hypertension)	Maximum Daily Dose	Initial Dose Reduction with Hepatic Dysfunction	Dose Reduction with Renal Dysfunction	Available Tablet Strengths (mg)
Candesartan Cilexetil	Atacand	Hypertension, heart failure	8–32 mg q.d.	32 mg	No	Only with severe impairment	4, 8, 16, 32
Eprosartan	Teveten	Hypertension	400–800 mg q.d. or b.i.d.	900 mg	No	Decrease maximum daily dose to 600 mg	400, 600
Irbesartan	Avapro	Hypertension, nephropathy in type II diabetics	150–300 mg q.d.	300 mg	No	No	75, 150, 300
Losartan	Cozaar	Hypertension, nephropathy in type II diabetics, hypertension with left ventricular hypertrophy	25–100 mg q.d. or b.i.d.	100 mg	Yes	Adults, no Children, yes	25, 50, 100
Olmesartan Medoxomil	Benicar	Hypertension	20–40 mg q.d.	40 mg	No	No	5, 20, 40
Telmisartan	Micardis	Hypertension	40–80 mg q.d.	80 mg	Yes (avoid)	No	20, 40, 80
Valsartan	Diovan	Hypertension, heart failure	80–320 q.d.	320 mg	No	No	40, 80, 160, 320

impaired hepatic function or biliary obstructive disorders should avoid the use of telmisartan.

Therapeutic Applications

All ARBs are currently approved for the treatment of hypertension and, along with ACE inhibitors, diuretics, β-blockers, and calcium channel blockers, have been designated as first-line agents either alone or in combination with other antihypertensive agents (37). All ARBs are available as single agents and as combination products with hydrochlorthiazide. Additionally, irbesartan and losartan have been approved for the treatment of nephropathy in type II diabetes, losartan for the treatment of hypertension with left ventricular hypertrophy, and candesartan and valsartan for the treatment of heart failure. Based on their ability to attenuate the renin-angiotensin system, one should expect a gradual increase in the number of uses and approved indications for this class of agents.

Adverse Effects

The most prevalent side effects of ARBs are listed above and discussed below. (1,32–34). Overall, this class of agents is well tolerated, with CNS effects being the most commonly reported complaint. Similar to ACE inhibitors, some of the adverse effects are directly related to attenuation of the renin-angiotensin pathway. Notably absent are the dry cough and angioedema seen with ACE inhibitors. Because ARBs are specific in their actions, this class of drugs does not affect the levels of bradykinin or prostaglandins and, thus, does not cause these bothersome side effects. Like ACE inhibitors, the use of ARBs during pregnancy is contraindicated, especially during the second and third trimesters. The use of ARBs should be discontinued as soon as pregnancy is confirmed unless the benefits outweigh the potential risks.

Adverse Effects of Angiotensin II Receptor Antagonists

Headache, dizziness, fatigue, hypotension, hyperkalemia, dyspepsia, diarrhea, abdominal pain, upper respiratory tract infection, myalgia, back pain, pharyngitis, and rhinitis

Drug Interactions

Coadministration of ARBs with potassium salts, potassium-sparing diuretics, or drospirenone may cause hyperkalemia. Nonsteroidal anti-inflammatory drugs may alter the response to ARBs and other antihypertensive agents (including ACE inhibitors and calcium channel blockers) because of inhibition of vasodilatory prostaglandins. Studies have shown that indomethacin, naproxen, and piroxicam have a greater propensity for causing this interaction. Telmisartan has been reported to increase digoxin levels and to slightly decrease warfarin levels; however, the reduced warfarin levels were not sufficient to alter the international normalized ratio. Rifampin, because of its ability to induce CYP3A4, can decrease the plasma levels of losartan and its active metabolite, EXP-3174. The clinical significance of drug interactions between ARBs and compounds that can inhibit either CYP3A4 or CYP2C9 has yet to be established.

ROLE OF CALCIUM AND CALCIUM CHANNELS IN VASCULAR SMOOTH MUSCLE CONTRACTION

Calcium is a key component of the excitation-contraction coupling process that occurs within the cardiovascular system. It acts as a cellular messenger to link internal or external excitation with cellular response. Increased cytosolic concentrations of Ca^{2+} result in the binding of Ca^{2+} to a regulatory protein, either troponin C in cardiac and skeletal muscle or calmodulin in vascular smooth muscle. This initial binding of Ca^{2+} uncovers myosin binding sites on the actin molecule, and subsequent interactions between actin and myosin result in muscle contraction. All of these events are reversed once the cytosolic concentration of Ca^{2+} decreases. In this situation, Ca^{2+} binding to troponin C or calmodulin is diminished or removed, myosin binding sites are concealed, actin and myosin can no longer interact, and muscle contraction ceases (45,46).

Mechanisms of Calcium Movement and Storage

The regulation of cytosolic calcium levels occurs via specific influx, efflux, and sequestering mechanisms (Fig. 28.20). The influx of calcium can occur through receptor-operated channels (site 1), the Na^+/Ca^{2+} exchange process (site 2), "leak" pathways (site 3), and potential-dependent channels (site 4). Influx via either receptor-operated or voltage-dependent channels has been proposed to be the major entry pathway for Ca^{2+}. Receptor-operated channels have been defined as those associated with cellular membrane receptors and activated by specific agonist–receptor interactions. In contrast, potential-dependent channels, also known as voltage-dependent or voltage-gated calcium channels, have been defined as those activated by membrane depolarization. The Na^+/Ca^{2+} exchange process can promote either influx or efflux, because the direction of Ca^{2+} movement depends on the relative intracellular and extracellular ratios of Na^+ and Ca^{2+}. The "leak" pathways, which include unstimulated Ca^{2+} entry as well as entry during the fast inward Na^+ phase of an action potential, play only a minor role in calcium influx.

Efflux can occur through either an ATP-driven membrane pump (site 5) or via the Na^+/Ca^{2+} exchange process previously mentioned (site 2). In addition to these influx and efflux mechanisms, the sarcoplasmic reticulum (site 6) and the mitochondria (site 7) function as internal storage/release sites. These storage sites work in concert with the influx and efflux processes to assure that cytosolic calcium levels are appropriate for cellular needs. Although influx and release processes are essential for excitation–contraction coupling, efflux and sequestering processes are equally important for terminating the contractile process and for protecting the cell from the deleterious effects of Ca^{2+} overload (47,48).

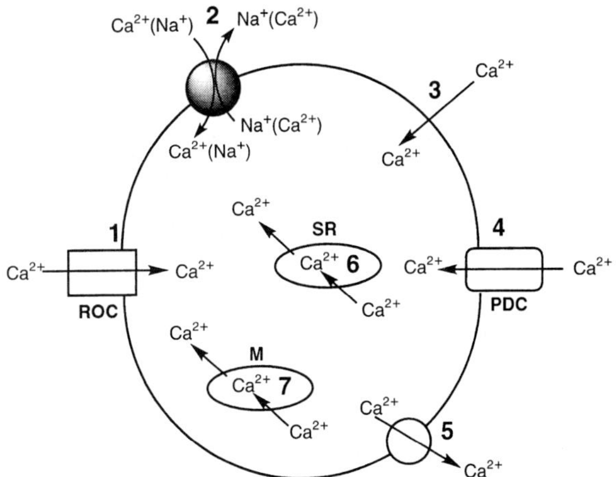

Fig. 28.20. Cellular mechanisms for the influx, efflux, and sequestering of Ca^{2+}. ROC, receptor-operated Ca^{2+} channels; PDC, potential-dependent Ca^{2+} channels; SR, sarcoplasmic reticulum; M, mitochondria.

Potential-Dependent Calcium Channels

The pharmacological class of agents known as calcium channel blockers produces their effects through interaction with potential-dependent channels. To date, six functional subclasses, or types, of potential-dependent Ca^{2+} channels have been identified: T, L, N, P, Q, and R. These types differ in location and function and can be divided into two major groups: low-voltage activated (LVA) channels, and high-voltage activated (HVA) channels. Of the six types, only the T (transient, tiny) channel can be rapidly activated and inactivated with small changes in the cell membrane potential. It is thus designated as an LVA channel. All of the other types of channels require a larger depolarization and are thus designated as HVA channels. The L (long-lasting, large) channel is the site of action for currently available calcium channel blockers and, therefore, has been extensively studied. It is located in skeletal, cardiac, and smooth muscle and, thus, is highly involved in organ and vessel contraction within the cardiovascular system. The N channel is found in neuronal tissue and exhibits kinetics and inhibitory sensitivity distinct from both L and T channels. The functions, sensitivities, and properties of the other three types of channels are not as well known. The P channel has been named for its presence in the Purkinje cells, whereas the Q and R channels have been characterized by their abilities to bind to certain polypeptide toxins (49–51).

The L channel is a pentameric complex consisting of α_1, α_2, β, γ, and δ polypeptides (see Fig. II.12). The α_1 subunit is a transmembrane-spanning protein that consists of four domains and that functions as the pore-forming subunit. The α_1 subunit also contains binding sites for all the currently available calcium channel blockers. The other four subunits surround the α_1 portion of the channel and contribute to the overall hydrophobicity of the pentamer. This hydrophobicity is important in that it allows the channel to be embedded in the cell membrane. Additionally, the α_2, δ, and β subunits modulate the α_1 subunit. Other types of potential-dependent channels are similar to the L channel. They all have a central α_1 subunit; however, molecular cloning studies have revealed that there are at least six α_1 genes: α_{1S}, α_{1A}, α_{1B}, α_{1C}, α_{1D}, and α_{1E}. Three of these genes, α_{1S}, α_{1C}, and α_{1D}, have been associated with L channels. The L channels found in skeletal muscle result from the α_{1S} gene; those in the heart, aorta, lung, and fibroblast result from the α_{1C} gene; and those in endocrine tissue result from the α_{1D} gene. Both α_{1C} and α_{1D} are used for L channels in the brain. Thus, there are some differences among the L channels located in different organs and tissues. Additionally, differences in α_1 genes as well as differences among the other subunits are responsible for the variations seen among the other five types of potential-dependent channels. As an example, the N channel lacks the γ subunit and contains an α_1 subunit derived from the α_{1B} gene (49,51).

CARDIOVASCULAR DISORDERS ASSOCIATED WITH POTENTIAL-DEPENDENT CALCIUM CHANNELS

As described above, the movement of calcium underlies the basic excitation–contraction coupling process. Thus, vascular tone and contraction primarily are determined by the availability of calcium from extracellular or intracellular sources. Potential-dependent Ca^{2+} channels are important in regulating the influx of Ca^{2+}; therefore, inhibition of Ca^{2+} flow through these channels results in both vasodilation and decreased cellular response to contractile stimuli. Arterial smooth muscle is more sensitive to this action than venous smooth muscle. Additionally, coronary and cerebral arterial vessels are more sensitive than other arterial beds (48,51). As a result of these actions, calcium channel blockers are useful in the treatment of hypertension and ischemic heart disease. A brief overview of hypertension is provided in the renin-angiotensin section of this chapter.

The term "ischemic heart disease," encompasses a variety of syndromes. These include angina pectoris, silent myocardial ischemia, acute coronary insufficiency, and MI. The overall incidence of ischemic heart disease is higher in men than in women and increases with age. Myocardial infarction is the primary initial event in men, whereas angina is the most common initial presentation in women. The average annual incidence rate (i.e., number of new cases/population) of angina pectoris is 1.5% and depends on the patient's age, gender, and risk-factor profile. A 1998 estimate from the American Heart Association places the prevalence of angina at approximately 6.4 million (52).

Angina pectoris is a clinical manifestation that results from coronary atherosclerotic heart disease. It is characterized by a severe constricting pain in the chest that often radiates to the left shoulder, the left arm, or the back. Clinically, angina pectoris can be classified as either exertional, variant, or unstable. Exertional angina, otherwise known as stable angina or exercise-induced angina, is the most common form and results from an imbalance between myocardial oxygen supply and demand. Variant angina, otherwise known as Prinzmetal's angina, results from the vasospasm of large, surface coronary vessels or branches. Unstable angina is the most difficult to treat and may occur as a result of advanced atherosclerosis and coronary vasospasm (53).

Excitation–contraction coupling in the heart is different from that in vascular smooth muscle in that a portion of the inward current is carried by Na^+ through the fast channel. In the sinoatrial and atrioventricular (AV) nodes, however, depolarization depends primarily on the movement of Ca^{2+} through the slow channel. Attenuation of this Ca^{2+} movement produces a negative inotropic effect and decreased conduction through the AV node. This latter effect is especially useful in treating paroxysmal supraventricular tachycardia (PSVT), an arrhythmia primarily caused by AV nodal reentry and AV reentry (51).

CALCIUM CHANNEL BLOCKERS

Historical Overview

Identification of compounds that could block the inward movement of Ca^{2+} through slow cardiac channels occurred in the early 1960s. Verapamil and other phenylalkylamines were shown to possess negative inotropic and chronotropic effects that were distinct from other coronary vasodilators. Further investigations revealed that these agents mimicked the cardiac effects of Ca^{2+} withdrawal: they reduced contractile force without affecting the action potential. The effects of these compounds could be reversed by the addition of Ca^{2+}, thus suggesting that the negative inotropic effect was linked to an inhibition of excitation–contraction coupling. Subsequently, derivatives of verapamil, as well as other chemical classes of compounds, were shown to competitively block Ca^{2+} movement through the slow channel and, thus, alter the cardiac action potential. Therefore, calcium channel blockers also are known as slow channel blockers, calcium entry blockers, and calcium antagonists (47,51).

Chemical Classifications

Overview

Currently, nine calcium channel blockers are available for therapeutic use. These compounds have diverse chemical structures and can be grouped into one of four chem-

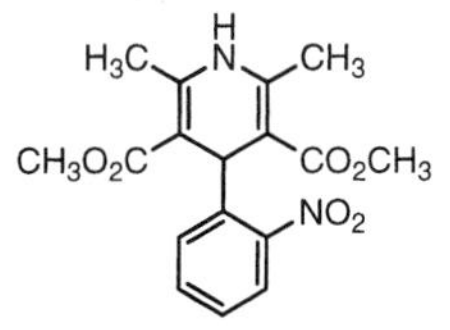

Nifedipine
(a 1,4-dihydropyridine)

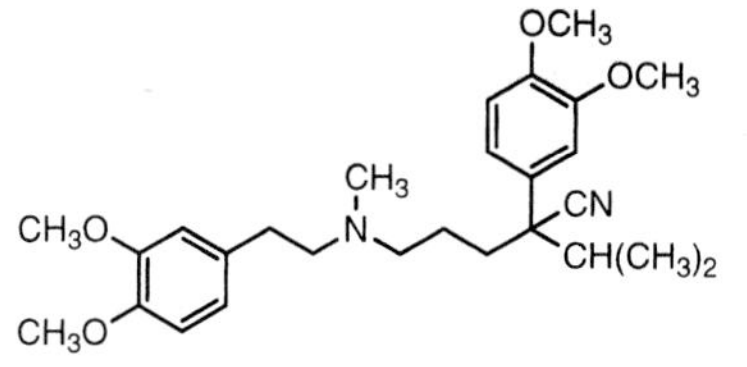

Verapamil
(a phenylalkylamine)

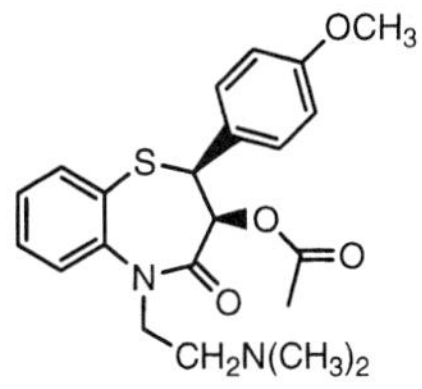

Diltiazem
(a benzothiazepine)

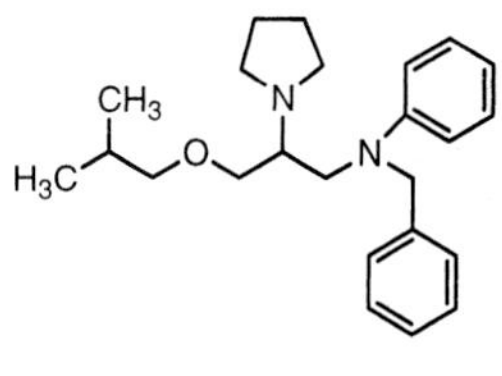

Bepridil
(a diaminopropanol ether)

Fig. 28.21. Chemical classes of calcium channel blockers.

ical classifications (Fig. 28.21), each of which produces a distinct pharmacological profile: 1,4-dihydropyridines (1,4-DHPs; e.g., nifedipine), phenylalkylamines (e.g., verapamil), benzothiazepines (e.g., diltiazem), and diaminopropanol ethers (e.g., bepridil). The majority of calcium channel blockers are 1,4-DHPs, and a detailed description of the SAR for this chemical class is provided below. In contrast, verapamil, diltiazem, and bepridil are the lone representatives of their respective chemical classes and, thus, are discussed as individual agents. Verapamil and diltiazem are discussed along with the 1,4-DHPs. Bepridil is a nonselective agent that is no longer available in the United States.

1,4-Dihydropyridines

History and Development. The chemistry of dihydropyridines can be traced back to an 1882 paper in

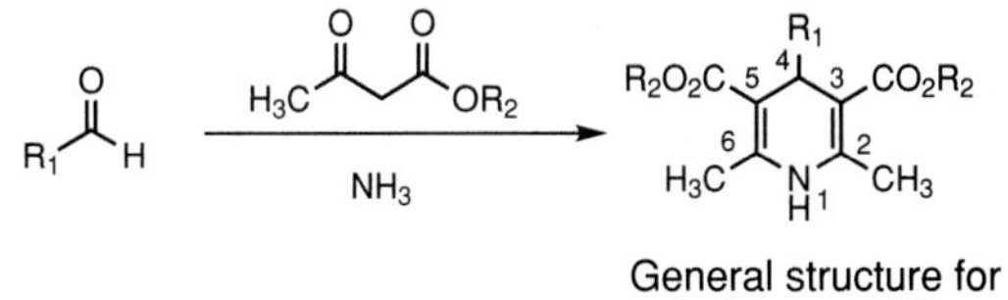

> Bepridil is unique among all the calcium channel blockers in that its actions are not based solely on its ability to block potential-dependent L-type (i.e., slow) Ca^{2+} channels (32,51). Unlike other calcium channel blockers, bepridil also blocks fast Na^{+} channels as well as receptor-operated calcium channels. These additional actions are responsible for bepridil's ability to inhibit cardiac conduction, to slow AV nodal conduction, to increase the refractory period, to slow the heart rate, and to prolong the QT interval.
>
> Bepridil was indicated for the oral treatment of chronic stable angina pectoris; however, its manufacturer voluntarily removed it from the U.S. market, primarily because of its ability to cause torsades de pointes. It also should be noted that bepridil was never highly prescribed, most likely because of the significant number of cardiovascular warnings and contraindications associated with its use.

NH_3

General structure for 1,4-dihydropyridines

Fig. 28.22. Synthesis of 1,4-DHPs using the Hantzsch reaction.

which Hantzsch described their utility as intermediates in the synthesis of substituted pyridines. Fifty years later, interest in this chemical class of compounds increased when it was discovered that a 1,4-DHP ring was responsible for the "hydrogen-transfer" properties of the coenzyme NADH. Numerous biochemical studies followed this discovery; however, it was not until the early 1970s that the pharmacological properties of 1,4-DHPs were fully investigated. Loev and coworkers at Smith, Klein & French laboratories investigated the activities of "Hantzsch-type" compounds. As shown in Figure 28.22, the Hantzsch reaction produced a symmetrical compound in which both the esters (i.e., CO_2R_2) and the C_2 and C_6 substituents (i.e., CH_3) are identical with each other. Structural requirements necessary for activity were identified by sequentially modifying the C_4 substituent (i.e., the R_1 group), the C_3- and C_5-esters (i.e., the R_2 groups), the C_2- and C_6-alkyl groups, and the N_1-H substituent (54–57).

Structure–Activity Relationships. The SARs for 1,4-DHP derivatives (see *General Structure* in Table 28.8) indicates that the following structural features are important for activity:

Table 28.8. Structure of the Dihydropyridine Ca^{2+} Channel Blockers

General structure:

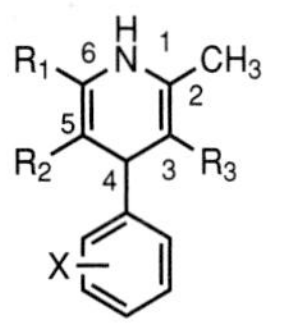

Isradipine:

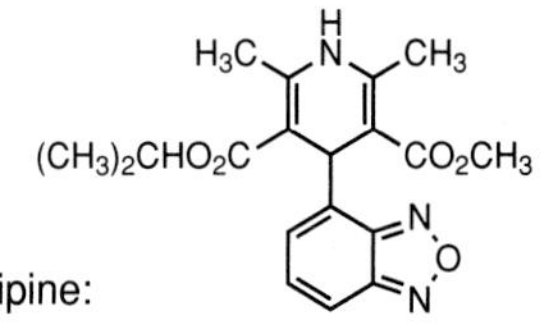

Compounds	R_1	R_2	R_3	X
Amlodipine	$CH_2O(CH_2)_2NH_2$	$CO_2CH_2CH_3$	CO_2CH_3	2-Cl
Felodipine	CH_3	$CO_2CH_2CH_3$	CO_2CH_3	2,3-Cl_2
Nicardipine	CH_3	$CO_2(CH_2)_2$-N(CH_3)-CH_2-C_6H_5	CO_2CH_3	3-NO_2
Nifedipine	CH_3	CO_2CH_3	CO_2CH_3	2-NO_2
Nimodipine	CH_3	$CO_2CH_2CH_2OCH_3$	$CO_2CH(CH_3)CH_3$	3-NO_2
Nisoldipine	CH_3	$CO_2CH_2CH(CH_3)_2$	CO_2CH_3	2-NO_2

1. A substituted phenyl ring at the C_4 position optimizes activity (heteroaromatic rings, such as pyridine, produce similar therapeutic effects but are not used because of observed animal toxicity), and C_4 substitution with a small nonplanar alkyl or cycloalkyl group decreases activity.
2. Phenyl ring substitution (X) is important for size and position rather than for electronic nature. Compounds with ortho or meta substitutions possess optimal activity, whereas those that are unsubstituted or that contain a para-substitution show a significant decrease in activity. Despite the fact that all commercially available 1,4-DHPs have electron-withdrawing ortho and/or meta substituents, this is not an absolute requirement. Compounds with electron-donating groups at these same positions also have demonstrated good activity. The importance of the ortho and meta substituents is to provide sufficient bulk to "lock" the conformation of the 1,4-DHP such that the C_4 aromatic ring is perpendicular to the 1,4-DHP ring (Fig. 28.23). This perpendicular conformation has been proposed to be essential for the activity of the 1,4-DHPs.
3. The 1,4-DHP ring is essential for activity. Substitution at the N_1 position or the use of oxidized (piperidine) or reduced (pyridine) ring systems greatly decreases or abolishes activity.
4. Ester groups at the C_3 and C_5 positions optimize activity. Other electron-withdrawing groups show decreased antagonist activity and may even show agonist activity. For example, the replacement of the C_3 ester of isradipine with a NO_2 group produces a calcium channel activator, or agonist (Fig. 28.24). Thus, the term "calcium channel modulators" is a more appropriate classification for the 1,4-DHPs.
5. When the esters at C_3 and C_5 are nonidentical, the C_4 carbon becomes chiral, and stereoselectivity between the enantiomers is observed. Additionally, evidence suggests that the C_3 and C_5 positions of the dihydropyridine ring are not equivalent positions. Crystal structures of nifedipine, a symmetrical 1,4-DHP, have shown that the C_3 carbonyl is synplanar to the C_2-C_3 bond but that the C_5 carbonyl is antiperiplanar to the C_5-C_6 bond (Fig. 28.25). Asymmetrical compounds have shown enhanced selectivity for specific blood vessels and are being preferentially developed. Nifedipine, the first 1,4-DHP to be marketed, is the only symmetrical compound in this chemical class.
6. With the exception of amlodipine, all 1,4-DHPs have C_2 and C_6 methyl groups. The enhanced potency of amlodipine (vs. nifedipine) suggests that the 1,4-DHP receptor can tolerate larger substituents at this position and that enhanced activity can be obtained by altering these groups.

Mechanism of Action

Despite the name, calcium channel blockers do not simply "plug the hole" and physically block the Ca^{2+} channel. Instead, they exert their effects by binding to specific receptor sites located within the central α_1 subunit of L-type, potential-dependent channels. Three

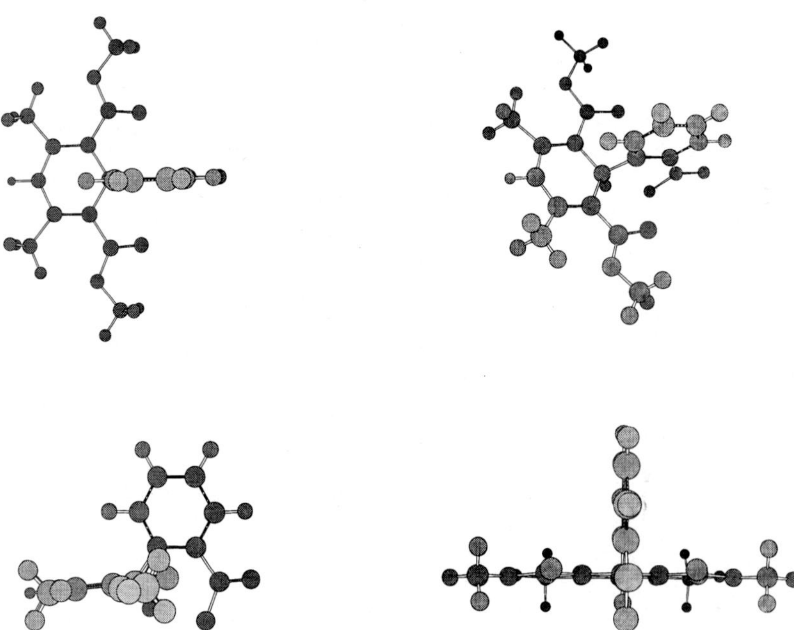

Fig. 28.23. Molecular models of nifedipine. The ortho-nitro group of nifedipine provides steric bulk and ensures that the required perpendicular nature of the phenyl and dihyropyridine rings is maintained.

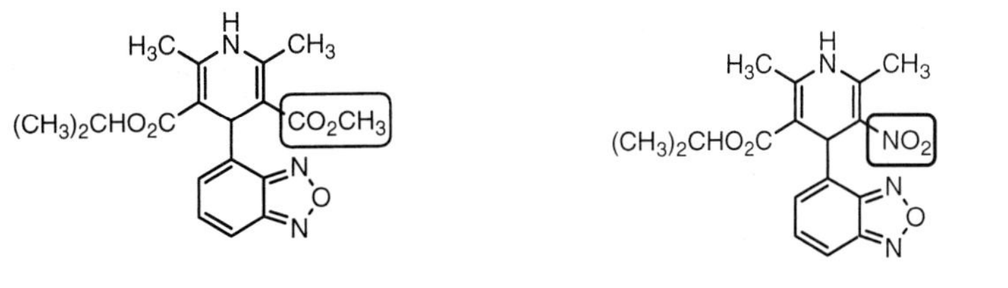

Isradipine
(Calcium channel blocker)

PN 202.791
(Calcium channel activator)

Fig. 28.24. Structures of isradipine and its analogous 3-nitro derivative.

distinct, but allosterically interacting, receptors have been identified for verapamil, diltiazem, and the 1,4-DHPs. As shown in Table 28.9, the binding of verapamil to its receptor inhibits the binding of both diltiazem and the 1,4-DHPs to their respective receptors. Likewise, the binding of either diltiazem or the 1,4-DHPs inhibits the binding of verapamil. In contrast, diltiazem and the 1,4-DHPs mutually enhance the binding of each other (54).

Potential-dependent channels can exist in one of three conformations: a resting state, which can be stimulated by membrane depolarization; an open state, which allows the Ca^{2+} to enter; and an inactive state, which is refractory to further depolarization. Calcium channel blockers have been shown to be more effective when membrane depolarization is either longer, more intense, or more frequent. This use-dependency suggests that these compounds preferentially interact with their receptors when the Ca^{2+} channel is in either the open or inactive state. This state dependence is not identical for all classes of Ca^{2+} blockers and, in combination with the different binding sites, allosteric interactions, acidity, and solubility, may be responsible for the pharmacological

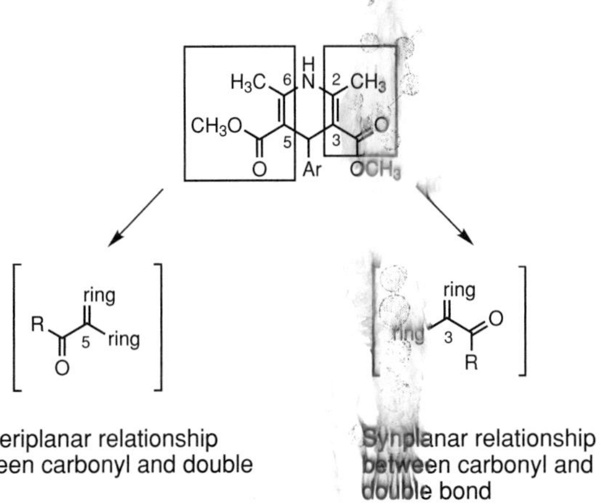

Fig. 28.25. Conformation of the C_3 and C_5 esters of nifedipine (Ar = 2-nitrophenyl). The C_3 carbonyl is synplanar to the C_2-C_3 bond, and the C_5 carbonyl antiperiplanar to the C_5-C_6 bond.

Ziconotide: An N-Type Calcium Channel Blocker

Ziconotide is a synthetic analogue of a naturally occurring conopeptide found in the piscivorous marine snail (*Conus magus*). It is structurally, mechanistically, and therapeutically different from the other calcium channel blockers discussed in this chapter. Structurally, it is a polybasic peptide containing 25 amino acids and three disulfide bridges.

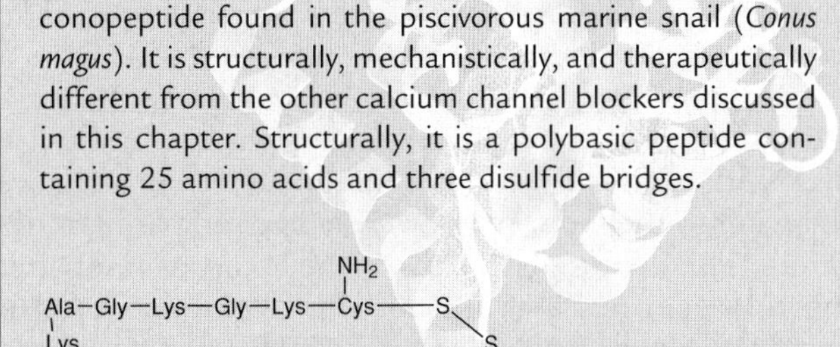

It selectively binds to N-type potential-dependent calcium channels located on the primary nociceptive (A-d and C) afferent nerves in the superficial layers (Rexed laminae I and II) of the dorsal horn in the spinal cord. Analgesic effects result from a blockade of neurotransmitter release and a disruption of normal nociceptive signal transmission. Ziconotide is indicated for the management of severe chronic pain in patients who are intolerant of or refractory to other systemic analgesics, adjunct therapies, or intrathecal morphine. Because of its peptide structure, ziconotide is not effective orally. It is administered by continuous intrathecal infusion. The initial recommended dose is 2.4 μg/day (0.1 μg/hour) and can be titrated up to a maximum daily dose of 19.2 mg (0.8 μg/hour). Ziconotide has a half-life of approximately 4.5 hours. It is metabolized by endopeptidases and exopeptidases in numerous organs and tissues. Common adverse effects of ziconotide include dizziness, nausea, confusion, headache, somnolence, nystagmus, asthenia, and pain. The most serious adverse effects appear to be the development of severe psychiatric symptoms and neurological impairment. As a result, ziconotide should not be used in patients with a preexisting history of psychosis. Frequent monitoring for evidence of cognitive impairment, hallucinations, or changes in mood or consciousness is essential. These effects are potentially additive with those of other CNS-depressant drugs (32,33,58).

Table 28.9. Actions of Calcium Channel Blockers and Interactions Among Their Receptor Sites

		Allosteric Effect on the Binding of		
Calcium Channel Blocker	Effect on Ca^{2+} Channel	Verapamil	Diltiazem	1,4-DHPs
Verapamil	Antagonist; blocks channel	NA	Inhibits	Inhibits
Diltiazem	Antagonist; blocks channel	Inhibits	NA	Enhances
1,4-Dihydropyridines	Antagonist/agonist; can either block or open channel	Inhibits	Enhances	MA

NA, not applicable.

differences among verapamil, diltiazem, and the 1,4-DHPs. A summary of these differences is listed in Table 28.10. The 1,4-DHPs, as exemplified by nifedipine, are primarily vasodilators, whereas verapamil and diltiazem have both vasodilator and cardiodepressant actions. The increased heart rate seen with nifedipine results from a reflex mechanism that tries to overcome the vasodilation and subsequent drop in blood pressure caused by the 1,4-DHPs. In contrast, the compensatory mechanism does not occur to the same extent with either verapamil or diltiazem. This is caused, in part, by the ability of verapamil and diltiazem to block AV nodal conductance and, in part, by the increased ability of 1,4-DHPs to activate the baroreceptor reflex. Ultimately, these pharmacological differences are reflected in the clinical use of these agents (48,53,54).

Physicochemical Properties

A comparison of the acid-base properties of verapamil, diltiazem, and the 1,4-DHPs reveals that whereas all of the compounds are basic, the 1,4-DHPs are considerably less basic than verapamil and diltiazem. Verapamil and diltiazem both contain tertiary amines with pK_a values of 8.9 and 7.7, respectively (26). In contrast, the nitrogen of the 1,4-DHPs is part of a conjugated carbamate. Its electrons are involved in resonance delocalization and are much less available for protonation. Thus, at physiological pH, verapamil and diltiazem are primarily ionized, whereas 1,4-DHPs are primarily un-ionized. There are two exceptions to this. Amlodipine and nicardipine contain basic amine groups as part of the side chains connected to the 1,4-DHP ring. Although the 1,4-DHP ring of these compounds is un-ionized, the side-chain amines will be primarily ionized at physiological pH. Because ionic attraction often is the initial interaction between a drug and its receptor, the differences in basicity between the 1,4-DHP ring and the tertiary amines of verapamil and diltiazem are consistent with the previously noted fact that the binding site for the 1,4-DHPs is distinct from those for verapamil and diltiazem.

The calculated log P values for the calcium channel blockers are listed in Table 28.11 (26). As evidenced by the data, all of these compounds possess good lipid solubility and, hence, excellent oral absorption (not shown in Table 28.11). Within the 1,4–DHP class, enhanced lipid solubility occurs in compounds that contain either larger ester groups or disubstituted phenyl rings. A comparison of the log P values of nifedipine and nisoldipine illustrates this fact. It should be noted that the calculated log P values listed in Table 28.11 are for the un-ionized compounds. These values significantly decrease for the ionized forms of amlodipine, nicardipine, verapamil, and diltiazem such that the latter three agents possess sufficient water solubility to be used both orally and parenterally.

Table 28.10. Comparison of the Cardiovascular Effects of Verapamil, Diltiazem, and Nifedipine

Cardiovascular Effect	Verapamil	Diltiazem	Nifedipine (a 1,4-DHP)
Peripheral vasodilation	oo	o	ooo
Blood pressure	•	•	•
Heart rate	Variable	•	oo
Coronary vascular resistance	•	•	•
Coronary blood flow	oo	oo	ooo
Atrioventricular node conduction	••	•	NE
Contractility	•	NE/•	NE/o

The number of circles represents the magnitude of response: o, = increase; •, decrease; NE = no effect.
Adapted from Swamy VC, Triggle DJ. Calcium channel blockers. In: Craig CR, Stitzel RE, eds. Modern Pharmacology with Clinical Applications, 5th Ed. Boston: Little, Brown, 1997:229–234 and Triggle DJ. Drugs acting on ion channels and membranes. In: Hansch C, Sammes PG, Taylor JB, eds. Comprehensive Medicinal Chemistry, vol 3. Oxford, UK: Pergamon Press, 1990:1047–1099; with permission.

Table 28.11. Pharmacokinetic Parameters of Calcium Channel Blockers

Drug	Calculated Log P	Oral Bioavailability (%)	Effect of Food on Absorption	Active Metabolite	Protein Binding (%)	T_{max} (hours)	Elimination Half-life (hours)	Major Route(s) of Elimination
1,4-Dihydropyridines								
Amlodipine	2.76	64–90	None	None	93	6–12	35–50	Renal (60%) Fecal (20–25%)
Felodipine	4.69	10–20	Increase	None	>99	2.5–5.0	11–16	Renal (70%) Fecal (10%)
Isradipine	3.19	15–24	Reduced rate, same extent	None	95	7–18 (CR)	8	Renal (60–65%) Fecal (25–30%)
Nicardipine	4.27	35	Reduced	None	>95	0.5–2.0 (IR) 1–4 (SR)	2–4	Renal (60%) Fecal (35%)
Nifedipine	2.40	45–70 86% (SR)	None	None	92–98	0.5 (IR) 6 (SR)	2–5 (IR) 7 (SR)	Renal (60–80%) Biliary/fecal (15%)
Nimodipine	3.14	13	Reduced	None	>95	1	8–9	Renal
Nisoldipine	3.86	5	High-fat meal increases immediate release but lowers overall amount	Hydroxylated analogue	>99	6–12	7–12	Renal (70–75%) Fecal (6–12%)
Phenalkylamines								
Verapamil	3.53	20–35	Reduced (SR form only)	Norverapamil	90	1–2 (IR) 7–11 (SR) 0.1–0.2 (IV)	3–7 (IR) 12 (SR)	Renal (70%) Fecal (16%)
Benzothiazepines								
Diltiazem	3.55	40–60	None	Deacetyl-diltiazem	70–80	2–4 (IR) 6–14 (SR)	3.0–4.5 (IR) 4.0–9.5 (SR) 3.4 (IV)	Renal (35%) Fecal (60–65%)

T_{max} time to maximum blood conentration; IR, immediate-release product; CR, controlled-release product; SR, sustained-release product; IV, intravenous administration.

All calcium channel blockers, with the exception of nifedipine, contain at least one chiral center; however, they are all marketed as their racemic mixtures. As previously noted, 1,4-DHPs with asymmetrically substituted esters exhibit stereoselectivity between the enantiomers. Additionally, the S-(−)-enantiomers of verapamil and other phenylalkylamines are more potent than the R-(+)-enantiomers. Very few SAR studies are available for diltiazem; however, the *cis* arrangement of the acetyl ester and the substituted phenyl ring is required for activity (54).

Metabolism

All calcium channel blockers undergo extensive first-pass metabolism in the liver and are substrates for the CYP3A4 isozyme (32,34). Additionally, several of these compounds can inhibit CYP3A4. All 1,4-DHPs are oxidatively metabolized to a variety of inactive compounds. In many cases, the dihydropyridine ring is initially oxidized to an inactive pyridine analogue (Fig. 28.26). These initial metabolites are then further transformed by hydrolysis, conjugation, and additional oxidation pathways. Nisoldipine also is subject to these processes; however, hydroxylation of its isobutyl ester produces a metabolite that retains 10% of the activity of the parent compound. In addition to the drug–drug interactions listed below (see Table 28.13), an interesting drug–food interaction occurs with the 1,4-DHPs and grapefruit juice (59). Coadministration of 1,4-DHPs with grapefruit juice produces an increase systemic concentration of the 1,4-DHPs. The mechanism of this interaction appears to result from inhibition of intestinal CYP450 by flavanoids and furanocoumarins specifically found in grapefruit juice (see Chapter 10). It has been proposed that limiting daily intake to either an 8-oz. glass of grapefruit juice or half of a fresh grapefruit would likely avoid significant drug interactions with most CYP3A4-metabolized drugs (60).

Verapamil is primarily metabolized to the N-demethylated compound, norverapamil, which retains approximately 20% of the pharmacological activity of verapamil and can reach or exceed the steady-state plasma levels of verapamil. Interestingly, the more active *S*-(−)-isomer undergoes more extensive first-pass hepatic metabolism than does the less active *R*-(+)-isomer. This is important to note, because when given IV, verapamil prolongs the PR interval to a greater extent than when it is given orally (61). This is because the preferential metabolism of the more active enantiomer does not occur with parenteral

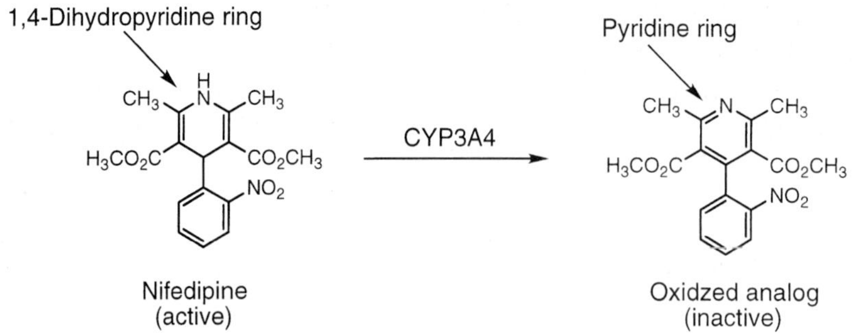

1,4-Dihydropyridine ring — Pyridine ring

Nifedipine (active) —CYP3A4→ Oxidzed analog (inactive)

Fig. 28.26. Oxidation of the 1,4-dihydropyridine ring of nifedipine.

administration. Diltiazem is primarily hydrolyzed to deacetyldiltiazem. This metabolite retains 25 to 50% of the coronary vasodilatory effects of diltiazem and is present in the plasma at levels of 10 to 45% of the parent compound.

Pharmacokinetic Parameters

The pharmacokinetic parameters and oral dosing information for calcium channel blockers are summarized in Tables 28.11 and 28.12, respectively (32–34). Some doses (specifically, those for diltiazem and verapamil) may vary for either specific indications (i.e., hypertension versus angina) or different brand names, and the reader should consult the product literature for additional information. The primary differences among the compounds are onset of action, half-life, and oral bioavailability. All calcium channel blockers have excellent oral absorption; however, because they also are subject to rapid first-pass metabolism in the liver, the actual oral bioavailability of these compounds varies considerably depending on the extent of metabolism. All compounds are highly plasma protein bound and primarily eliminated as inactive metabolites in the urine. Because of extensive hepatic transformation, calcium channel blockers should be used cautiously in patients with hepatic disease. Recommendations for these patients include dosage reductions,

Table 28.12. Oral Dosing Information for Calcium Channel Blockers

Generic Name	Brand Name(s)	Approved Indications	Normal Dosing Range	Maximum Daily Dose	Precautions with Hepatic Dysfunction	Available Tablet or Capsule Strengths (mg)
1,4-Dihydropyridines						
Amlodipine	Norvasc	Angina (V, CS), hypertension	5–10 mg q.d.	10 mg	Reduce dosage	2.5, 5, 10
Felodipine	Plendil	Hypertension	2.5–10.0 mg q.d.	10 mg	Reduce dosage	2.5, 5, 10
Isradipine	DynaCirc CR	Hypertension	5–20 mg q.d.	20 mg	Titrate dosage	5, 10
Nicardipine	Cardene, Cardene IV	Angina (CS), hypertension	20–40 mg t.i.d. (SR: 30–60 mg b.i.d.) (IV: 5–15 mg/hour)	120 mg	Titrate dosage	20, 30 (SR: 30, 45, 60) (IV: 2.5 mg/mL)
Nifedipine	Procardia, Adalat	Angina (V, CS), hypertension	10–20 mg t.i.d. (SR: 30–60 mg q.d.)	180 mg (SR: 90 mg)	Reduce dosage	10, 20 (SR: 30, 60, 90)
Nimodipine	Nimotop	Subarachnoid hemorrhage	60 mg every 4 hours for 21 days	360 mg	Reduce dosage	30
Nisoldipine	Sular	Hypertension	20–40 mg q.d.	60 mg	Closely monitor blood pressure	10, 20, 30, 40
Phenylalkylamines						
Verapamil	Calan, Covera, Isoptin, Verelan	Angina (V, CS, U), hypertension, atrial fibrillation/ flutter, PSVT	80–120 mg t.i.d. or q.i.d. (SR: 240–480 mg q.d. or b.i.d.)	480 mg (540 mg for Covera HS only)	Reduce dosage	40, 80, 120 (SR: 100, 120, 180, 200, 240, 300, 360) (IV: 2.5 mg/mL)
Benzothiazepines						
Diltiazem	Cardizem, Dilacor	Angina (V, CS), hypertension, atrial fibrillation/ flutter, PSVT	30–120 mg t.i.d. or q.i.d. (SR: 120–480 mg q.d.)	540 mg	Reduce dosage	30, 60, 90, 120 (SR: 60, 90, 120,180, 240, 300, 360, 420) (IV: 5 mg/mL)

Types of angina: V, vasospastic; CS, chronic stable; U, unstable; CR, controlled release; SR, sustained release; IV, intravenous; PSVT, paroxysmal supraventricular tachycardia.

Chemical/Pharmacological Classes Used to Treat Angina Pectoris

Organic nitrates, β-blockers (see Chapter 26), and calcium channel blockers

Unlabeled Uses

Migraine headache, Raynaud's syndrome, pulmonary hypertension, preterm labor, and hypertrophic cardiomyopathy

careful titrations, and close therapeutic monitoring. Diltiazem and verapamil also require dosage adjustments in patients with renal dysfunction, because renal impairment can significantly increase the concentrations of the active metabolites of these compounds. Dosage adjustments usually are not required for the other seven compounds, because six of them produce inactive metabolites and nisoldipine produces active metabolites with significantly lower activity.

Felodipine and nisoldipine are only available as sustained-release (or extended-release) formulations. Nifedipine, isradipine, nicardipine, verapamil, and diltiazem are available as both immediate-release and sustained-release formulations. The latter three compounds also are available as parenteral preparations. Unlike regular tablets and capsules, sustained-release (or extended-release) formulations cannot be chewed or crushed, because this may lead to an immediate, rather than a sustained, release of the compound. This effect not only will decrease the duration of the dose but also could produce an overdose and subsequent toxicities in the patient. Parenteral preparations of nicardipine and verapamil are incompatible with IV solutions containing sodium bicarbonate. In each case, sodium bicarbonate increases the pH of the solution, resulting in the precipitation of the calcium channel blocker. Although this interaction is not listed for diltiazem, it is reasonable to assume that a similar interaction may occur. Additionally, nicardipine is incompatible with lactated Ringer's solution, and verapamil will precipitate in solutions having a pH greater than or equal to six (32,33).

Therapeutic Applications

As illustrated in Table 28.12, calcium channel blockers have been approved for the treatment of hypertension, angina pectoris, subarachnoid hemorrhage, and specific types of arrhythmias (32,33). All calcium channel blockers cause vasodilation and decrease peripheral resistance. With the exceptions of nimodipine, all are approved to treat hypertension. Recent studies have indicated that immediate-release formulations of short-acting calcium channel blockers, especially nifedipine, can cause an abrupt vasodilation that can result in MI. As a result, only the sustained-release formulations of nifedipine and diltiazem should be used in the treatment of essential hypertension (62). Five of the nine agents are approved for the treatment of angina pectoris. Verapamil is the most versatile agent in that it is indicated for all three types of angina: vasospastic, chronic stable, and unstable. Amlodipine, nifedipine, and diltiazem are indicated for both vasospastic and chronic stable angina, whereas nicardipine is indicated only for chronic stable angina. Nimodipine is unique in that it has a greater effect on cerebral arteries than on other arteries. As a result, nimodipine is indicated for the improvement of neurological deficits because of spasm following subarachnoid hemorrhage from ruptured congenital intracranial aneurysms in patients otherwise in good neurological condition after the episode. Verapamil and diltiazem are pharmacologically different from the 1,4-DHPs in that they block sinus and AV nodal conduction. As a result, IV formulations of verapamil and diltiazem are indicated for the treatment of atrial fibrillation, atrial flutter, and PSVT. Verapamil also can be used orally, either alone (for prophylaxis of repetitive PSVT) or in combination with digoxin (for atrial flutter or atrial fibrillation).

Adverse Effects and Drug Interactions

The most prevalent or significant side effects of calcium channel blockers are listed below (32,33,48,51,53). Drug interactions for calcium channel blockers are listed in Table 28.13. In most instances, these side effects do not cause long-term complications, and they often resolve with time or dosage adjustments. Many of these effects are simply extensions of the pharmacological effects of this class of compounds. Excessive vasodilation results in edema, flushing, hypotension, nasal congestion, headache, and dizziness. Additionally, the palpitations, chest pain, and tachycardia seen with 1,4-DHPs are a result of sympathetic responses to the vasodilatory effects of this chemical class. The use of a β-blocker in combination with a 1,4-DHP can minimize these compensatory effects and can be very useful in treating hypertension. Verapamil and diltiazem can cause bradycardia and AV block because of their ability to depress AV nodal conduction. Because of risks associated with additive cardiodepressive effects, they should not be used in combination with β-blockers.

Adverse Effects of Calcium Channel Blockers

Edema, flushing, hypotension, nasal congestion, palpitations, chest pain, tachycardia, headache, fatigue, dizziness, rash, nausea, abdominal pain, constipation, diarrhea, vomiting, shortness of breath, weakness, bradycardia, and AV block

Table 28.13. Drug Interactions for Calcium Channel Blockers

Drug	Calcium Blocker(s)	Result of Interaction
Alpha$_1$-Blockers (Prazosin, Terazosin)	Verapamil	Increased prazosin and terazosin levels
Amiodarone	Diltiazem, Verapamil	Increased bradycardia and cardiotoxicity; decreased cardiac output
Aspirin	Verapamil	Increased incidence of bruising
Azole Antifungals	Felodipine, Isradipine, Nifedipine, Nisoldipine	Increased serum concentrations of the calcium channel blockers
Barbiturates	Felodipine, nifedipine, Verapamil	Decreased pharmacological effects of the calcium channel blockers
β-Blockers	All	Coadministration may cause additive or synergistic effects; increased cardiodepressant effects (more extensive with verapamil and diltiazem); inhibition of β-Blocker metabolism by diltiazem, isradipine, nicardipine, nifedipine, and verapamil
Buspirone	Diltiazem, Verapamil	Increase buspirone levels
Carbamazepine, Oxcarbazepine	Felodipine, Diltiazem, Verapamil	Carbamazepine and oxcarbazepine decrease felodipine levels; verapamil and diltiazem increase carbamazepine levels
Cimetidine	All	Increased 1,4-DHP levels
Cyclosporine	Felodipine Nicardipine, Nifedipine, Diltiazem, Verapamil	Increased cyclosporine levels when used with all of these except for nifedipine; cyclosporine increases felodipine and nifedipine levels
CYP3A4 Inhibitors	All	Potentially can increase the plasma levels of calcium channel blockers
Digoxin	Nifedipine, Diltiazem, Verapamil	Increased digoxin levels
Disopyramide, Flecainide	Verapamil	Additive cardiodepressant effects
Dofetilide	Verapamil	Increased dofetilide levels
Doxorubicin	Verapamil	Increased doxorubicin levels
Erythromycin, Clarithromycin	All	Increased 1,4-DHP levels and increased toxicity
Fentanyl	All	Severe hypotension and/or bradycardia
General Anesthetics	All	Potentiation of the cardiac effects and vascular dilation associated with anesthetics
HMG CoA Reductase Inhibitors	Diltiazem, verapamil	Increase levels of HMG CoA reductase inhibitor
Imipramine	Diltiazem, verapamil	Increased imipramine levels
Lithium	Diltiazem, Verapamil	Decreased lithium levels with verapamil; neurotoxicity with diltiazem
Lovastatin	Isradipine	Decreased effects of lovastatin
Melatonin	All	Decreased therapeutic effects of calcium channel blockers
Methylprednisolone	Diltiazem, Verapamil	Increased methylprednisolone levels
Midazolam, Triazolam	Diltiazem, Verapamil	Increased effects of these benzodiazepines
Moricizine	Diltiazem	Increased moricizine levels; decreased diltiazem levels
Phenobarbital	All	Decreased bioavailability of calcium channel blocker
Phenytoin	All	Decreased effectiveness of calcium channel blocker due to induction of metabolism
Quinidine	Diltiazem, Nifedipine, Nisoldipine, Verapamil	Variable responses: Quinidine decreases AUC of nisoldipine, but increases actions of nifedipine; Diltiazem and verapamil increase the effects of quinidine; while nifedipine decreases quinidine levels and actions
Rifampin	Diltiazem, Isradipine, Nicardipine, Nifedipine, Verapamil	Decreased levels of calcium channel blocker
Sirolimus, Tacrolimus	Diltiazem, Nifedipine, Verapamil	Increased sirolimus and tacrolimus levels
St. John's Wort	Nifedipine	Decreased nifedipine levels (St. John's wart most likely increases the metabolism of all calcium channel blockers)
Theophylline	Diltiazem, Verapamil	Increased theophylline levels and toxicity
Valproic acid	Nimodipine	Increased nimodipine levels
Vecuronium	Verapamil	Increased vecuronium levels
Vincristine	Nifedipine	Increased vincristine levels

CASE STUDY

Victoria F. Roche and S. William Zito

BB is a 58-year-old divorced woman who owns her own travel agency. She has a family history of alcoholism, and that, coupled with the social nature and constant pressures of her job, led BB to become an alcoholic. Five years ago, BB was diagnosed with diabetes, and since then, she has joined Alcoholics Anonymous and been successful in controlling her drinking. Her diabetes is under control with glyburide (5 mg daily with breakfast). Lately, however, she has experienced a loss of energy and difficulty breathing on her daily walk uptown to her office. In addition, BB often wakes during the night frightened by a sense that she has stopped breathing and finds it necessary to prop herself up with a couple of pillows to get a good night's sleep. On physical examination, her physician notices a tender abdomen with slight hepatomegaly and pedal edema, and an echocardiogram reveals cardiomegaly. A diagnosis of mild congestive heart failure was made, and BB was prescribed captopril (25 mg t.i.d.) and advised to control salt intake and to continue her normal exercise routine. On a follow-up visit to her physician, BB's symptoms have moderated, but she complains of an irritating cough and rash, that her medication makes everything taste like rust, and that her lips feel like they have silicon implants. BB's physician wants to change her medication, and you have the following choices available. What do you think?

1. Identify the therapeutic problem(s) in which the pharmacist's intervention may benefit the patient.
2. Identify and prioritize the patient-specific factors that must be considered to achieve the desired therapeutic outcomes.
3. Conduct a thorough and mechanistically oriented structure-activity analysis of all therapeutic alternatives provided in the case.
4. Evaluate the SAR findings against the patient-specific factors and desired therapeutic outcomes, and make a therapeutic decision.
5. Counsel your patient.

HS–H_2C O N CH$_3$ CO_2H

Captopril

O OH NH O N CO_2H NH_2

1

O OCH_2CH_3 O NH N CH_3 CO_2H

2

H_3C N CH_3 OH N CH_3 CH_3 O O O O O H N N N N

3

H_3C N Cl N OH H N N N N

4

References

1. Jackson EK. Renin and angiotensin. In: Brunton L, Lazo J, Parker K, et al., eds. Goodman & Gilman's The Pharmacological Basis of Therapeutics, 11th Ed. New York: McGraw-Hill, 2006:789–821.
2. Vaczek D. Top 200 prescription drugs of 2004. Pharmacy Times 2005; 71:41–46.
3. Skeggs L. Historical overview of the renin-angiotensin system. In: Doyle AE, Bearn AG, eds. Hypertension and the Angiotensin System: Therapeutic Approaches. New York: Raven Press, 1984:31–45.
4. Vallotton MB. The renin-angiotensin system. Trends Pharmacol Sci 1987; 8:69–74.
5. Brown NJ, Roberts LJ. Histamine, bradykinin, and their antagonists. In: Hardman JG, Limbird LE, Gilman AG, eds. The Pharmacological Basis of Therapeutics, 10th Ed. New York: McGraw-Hill, 2001:645–667.
6. Ferrario CM, Brosnihan KB, Diz DI, et al. Angiotensin-(1-7): a new hormone of the angiotensin system. Hyperten 1991;18(5 Suppl):III 126–133.
7. Saseen JJ, Carter BL. Hypertension. In: Dipiro JT, Talbert RL, Yee GC, et al., eds. Pharmacotherapy: A Pathophysiologic Approach, 6th Ed. New York: McGraw-Hill, 2005:185–217.
8. Parker RB, Patterson JH, Johnson JA. Heart failure. In: Dipiro JT, Talbert RL, Yee GC, et al., eds. Pharmacotherapy: A Pathophysiologic Approach, 6th Ed. New York: McGraw-Hill, 2005:219–260.

9. Boger J. Clinical goal in sight for small molecule renin inhibitors. Trends Pharmacol Sci 1987;8:370–372.
10. Petrillo EW Jr, Trippodo NC, DeForrest JM. Antihypertensive agents. Annu Rep Med Chem 1990;25:51–60.
11. Kleinert HD, Rosenberg SH, Baker WR, et al. Discovery of a peptide-based renin inhibitor with oral bioavailability and efficacy. Science 1992;257:1940–1943.
12. Buchholz RA, Lefker BA, Ravi Kiron MA. Hypertension therapy: what next? Annu Rep Med Chem 1993;28:69–78.
13. Ferreira SH, Bartelt DC, Lewis LJ. Isolation of bradykinin-potentiating peptides from *Bothrops jararaca* venom. Biochemistry 1970;9:2583–2593.
14. Bakhle YS. Conversion of angiotensin I to angiotensin II by cell-free extracts of dog lung. Nature 1968;220:919–921.
15. Garrison JC, Peach MJ. Renin and angiotensin. In: Gilman AG, Rall TW, Nies AS, et al., eds. The Pharmacological Basis of Therapeutics, 8th Ed. New York: Pergamon Press, 1990:749–763.
16. Silverman RB. The Organic Chemistry of Drug Design and Drug Action. San Diego: Academic Press, 1992:162–170.
17. Ondetti MA, Rubin B, Cushman DW. Design of specific inhibitors of angiotensin-converting enzyme: new class of orally active antihypertensive agents. Science 1977;196:441–444.
18. Cushman DW, Cheung HS, Sabo EF, et al. Design of potent competitive inhibitors of angiotensin-converting enzyme. Carboxyalkanoyl and mercaptoalkanoyl amino acids. Biochemistry 1977;16:5484–5491.
19. Ondetti MA, Cushman DW. Enzymes of the renin-angiotensin system and their inhibitors. Annu Rev Biochem 1982;51:283–308.
20. Stryer L. Biochemistry, 4th Ed. New York: Freeman and Company, 1995:218–222.
21. Byers LD, Wolfenden R. Binding of the by-product analogue benzylsuccinic acid by carboxypeptidase A. Biochemistry 1973;12:2070–2078.
22. Klaassen CD. Heavy metals and heavy-metal antagonists. In: Hardman JG, Limbird LE, Gilman AG, eds. The Pharmacological Basis of Therapeutics, 10th Ed. New York: McGraw-Hill, 2001:1851–1875.
23. Atkinson AB, Robertson JIS. Captopril in the treatment of clinical hypertension and cardiac failure. Lancet 1979;ii:836–839.
24. Patchett AA, Harris E, Tristram EW, et al. A new class of angiotensin-converting enzyme inhibitors. Nature 1980;288:280–283.
25. Gringauz A. Introduction to Medicinal Chemistry. New York: Wiley, 1997: 450–461.
26. SciFindeer. Calculated using Advanced Chemistry Development (ACD/Lab) Software V8.14 for Solaris (1994–2005 ACD/Lab) (V8.19 used for Perindolpril).
27. Gross DM, Sweet, CS, Ulm EH, et al. Effect of N-[(S)-1-carboxy-3-phenylpropyl]-L-Ala-L-Pro and its ethyl ester (MK-421) on angiotensin converting enzyme in vitro and angiotensin I pressor responses in vivo. J Pharmacol Exp Ther 1981;216:552–557.
28. Ulm EH, Hichens M, Gomez HJ, et al. Enalapril maleate and a lysine analogue (MK-521): disposition in man. Br J Clin Pharmacol 1982;14:357–362.
29. Kim DH, Guinosso CJ, Buzby GC Jr, et al. (Mercaptopropanoyl)indoline-2-carboxylic acids and related compounds as potent angiotensin-converting enzyme inhibitors and antihypertensive agents. J Med Chem 1983;26:394–403.
30. Krapcho J, Turk C, Cushman DW, et al. Angiotensin-converting enzyme inhibitors. Mercaptan, carboxyalkyl dipeptide, and phosphinic acid inhibitors incorporating 4-substituted prolines. J Med Chem 1988;31:1148–1160.
31. Oparil S, Koerner T, Tregear GW, et al. Substrate requirements for angiotensin I conversion in vivo and in vitro. Circ Res 1973;32:415–423.
32. Clinical Pharmacology Online. Gold Standard Multimedia, 2005. Available at: http://www.cp.gsm.com. Accessed October 15, 2005.
33. Drug Facts and Comparisons. St. Louis, MO: Wolters Kluwer Health, 2005.
34. Micromedex Online. The Thompson Corporation, 2005. Available at: http://www.micromedex.com. Accessed October 15, 2005.
35. Drummer OH, Nicolaci J, Iakovidis D. Biliary excretion and conjugation of diacid angiotensin-converting enzyme inhibitors. J Pharmacol Exp Ther 1990; 252:1202–1206.
36. Kostis JB, Garland WT, Delaney C, et al. Fosinopril: pharmacokinetic and pharmacodynamics in congestive heart failure. Clin Pharmacol Ther 1995;58:660–665.
37. Chobanian AV, Bakris GI, Black HR, et al., and the National High Blood Pressure Education Program Coordinating Committee. The Seventh Report of the Joint National Committee on Prevention, Detection, Evaluation, and Treatment of High Blood Pressure. JAMA 2003;289:2560–2572.
38. Lacourciere Y, Brunner H, Irwin R, et al. Effects of modulators of the renin-angiotensin-aldosterone system on cough. Losartan Cough Study Group. J Hypertens 1994;12:1387–1393.
39. Timmermans PB, Wong PC, Chiu AT, et al. Angiotensin II receptors and angiotensin II receptor antagonists. Pharmacol Rev 1993;45:205–213.
40. Moore GJ. Designing peptide mimetics. Trends Pharmacol Sci 1994;15:124–129.
41. Harrold MW. Preparing students for future therapies: the development of novel agents to control the renin-angiotensin system. Am J Pharm Educ 1997;61:173–178.
42. Furakawa Y, Kishimoto S, Nishikawa K. Hypotensive imidazole derivatives and hypotensive imidazole-5-acetic acid derivatives. U.S. Patents 4,340,598 and 4,355,040. Osaka, Japan, 1982.
43. Bauer JH, Reams GP. The angiotensin II type 1 receptor antagonists: a new class of antihypertensive drugs. Arch Intern Med 1995;155:1361–1368.
44. Carini DJ, Duncia JV, Aldrich PE, et al. Nonpeptide angiotensin II receptor antagonists: the discovery of a series of N-(biphenylylmethyl)imidazoles as potent, orally active antihypertensives. J Med Chem 1991;35:2525–2547.
45. Cutler SJ, Cocolas GH. Cardiovascular agents. In: Block JH, Beale, JM, eds. Wilson and Gisvold's Textbook of Organic Medicinal and Pharmaceutical Chemistry, 11th Ed. Philadelphia: Lippincott Williams & Wilkins, 2004:627–632.
46. Silverthorn DU. Human Physiology: An Integrated Approach. Upper Saddle River, NJ: Prentice Hall, 1998:325–361.
47. Janis RA, Triggle DJ. New developments in Ca^{2+} channel antagonists. J Med Chem 1983;26:775–785.
48. Swamy VC, Triggle DJ. Calcium channel blockers. In: Craig CR, Stitzel RE, eds. Modern Pharmacology with Clinical Applications, 5th Ed. Boston: Little, Brown, 1997:229–234.
49. Varadi G, Mori Y, Mikala G, et al. Molecular determinants of Ca^{2+} channel function and drug action. Trends Pharmacol Sci 1995;16:43–49.
50. Gilmore J, Dell C, Bowman D, et al. Neuronal calcium channels. Annu Rep Med Chem 1995;30:51–60.
51. Michel T. Treatment of myocardial ischemia. In: Brunton L, Lazo J, Parker K, et al., eds. Goodman and Gilman's The Pharmacological Basis of Therapeutics, 11th Ed. New York: McGraw-Hill, 2006:823–844.
52. Talbert RL. Ischemic heart disease. In: Dipiro JT, Talbert RL, Yee GC, et al., eds. Pharmacotherapy: A Pathophysiologic Approach, 6th Ed. New York: McGraw-Hill, 2005:261–290.
53. Vaghy PL. Calcium antagonists. In: Brody TM, Larner J, Minneman KP, et al., eds. Human Pharmacology: Molecular to Clinical, 2nd Ed. St. Louis: Mosby, 1994:203–213.
54. Triggle DJ. Drugs acting on ion channels and membranes. In: Hansch C, Sammes PG, Taylor JB, eds. Comprehensive Medicinal Chemistry, vol 3. Oxford, UK: Pergamon Press, 1990:1047–1099.
55. Loev B, Ehrreich SJ, Tedeschi RE. Dihydropyridines with potent hypotensive activity prepared by the Hantzsch reaction. J Pharm Pharmacol 1972;24:917–918.
56. Loev B, Goodman MM, Snader KM, et al. "Hantzsch-type" dihydropyridine hypotensive agents. J Med Chem 1974;17:956–965.
57. Triggle AM, Shefter E, Triggle DJ. Crystal structures of calcium channel antagonists: 2,6-dimethyl-3,5-dicarbomethoxy-4-[2-nitro, 3-cyano-, 4-(dimethylamino)-, and 2,3,4,5,6-pentafluorophenyl]-1,4-dihydropyridine. J Med Chem 1980;23:1442–1445.
58. Product information for Prialt. Available at: http://www.prialt.com. Accessed November 1, 2005.
59. Bailey DG, Arnold JMO, Spence JD. Grapefruit juice and drugs: how significant is the interaction? Clin Pharmacokinet 1994;26:91–98.
60. Drug interactions with grapefruit juice. The Medical Letter 2004;46:2–4.
61. Roden DM. Antiarrhythmic drugs. In: Brunton L, Lazo J, Parker K, et al., eds. Goodman & Gilman's The Pharmacological Basis of Therapeutics, 11th Ed. New York: McGraw-Hill, 2006:899–932.
62. Safety of calcium-channel blockers. The Medical Letter 1997;39:13–14.

29. *Central and Peripheral Sympatholytics and Vasodilators*

DAVID A. WILLIAMS

DRUGS COVERED IN THIS CHAPTER:

β-NONSELECTIVE BLOCKERS
- Carteolol
- Nadolol
- Penbutolol
- Pindolol
- Propranolol
- Timolol

β_1-SELECTIVE BLOCKERS
- Acebutolol
- Atenolol
- Betaxolol
- Bisoprolol
- Esmolol
- Metoprolol

α_1-BLOCKERS
- Prazosin
- Doxazosin
- Temazosin

MIXED α/B-BLOCKERS
- Carvedilol
- Labetalol

CENTRALLY ACTING SYMPATHOLYTICS
- Methyldopa
- Clonidine
- Moxonidine
- Rilmenidine
- Guanabenz
- Guanfacine
- Metyrosine

ADRENERGIC NEURON BLOCKING AGENTS
- Reserpine
- Guanethidine
- Guanadrel

VASODILATORS
- Hydralazine
- Minoxidil
- Diazoxide

PHOSPHODIESTERASE INHIBITORS
- Inamrinone
- Milrinone
- Sildenafil

NITRODILATOR
- Sodium nitroprusside

GANGLIONIC BLOCKERS
- Mecamylamine
- Trimethaphan

ENDOTHELIAL ANTAGONISTS
- Bosentan

PROSTANOIDS
- Epoprostenol
- Treprostinil
- Beraprost
- Iloprost

CARDIOVASCULAR HYPERTENSION

Hypertension is the most common cardiovascular disease and is the major risk factor for coronary artery disease, heart failure, stroke, and renal failure. Approximately 50 million Americans have a systolic or diastolic blood pressure above 140/90 mm Hg. The onset of hypertension is defined as having a blood pressure of 140/90 mm Hg or greater and most commonly appears during the fourth, fifth, and sixth decades of life (1).

The importance of controlling blood pressure is well documented (1), although the rates of awareness, treatment, and control of hypertension have not risen as expected in the National Health and Nutrition Examination Survey (2). This survey showed that 68% of Americans are aware that they have high blood pressure but that only 53% are receiving treatment and only 27% have their blood pressure under control. Since 1976, there had been a significant improvement in the rates of awareness, treatment, and control of hypertension, but since 1990, whatever progress had been achieved has now reached a plateau (2). Although the age-adjusted death rates from stroke and coronary heart disease during this period have fallen by 59 and 53%, respectively, these rates of decline also appear to have reached a plateau (2). These troubling trends should awaken clinicians to be more aggressive in the treatment of patients with hypertension.

When the decision to initiate hypertensive therapy is made, physicians often are presented with the dilemma of which of more than 80 antihypertensive products, representing more than 8 different drug classes, to use for their patients (Table 29.1) (1,3). Those factors that can affect the outcomes from the treatment of hypertension include potential adverse effects, clinically significant drug–drug interactions (especially when so many different drug classes are involved), patient compliance, affordability (especially for the elderly and those on fixed incomes), risk/benefit ratios, and dosing frequency must be considered (3). Having considered these factors, the health care provider (clinician or pharmacist) arrives at an appropriate choice of antihypertensive drug (3). Once the patient is stabilized on a antihypertensive medication, some of these issues need to be reevaluated. Patients should be continually asked about side effects, because many of the antihypertensive drugs possess side effects that the patient may not tolerate (1). This problem and the cost of drug therapy can affect compliance to drug therapy especially for the elderly and those on fixed incomes (4).

Drug therapy in the management of hypertension must be individualized and adjusted based on coexisting risk factors, including the degree of blood pressure elevation, severity of the disease (e.g., presence of target organ damage), presence of underlying cardiovascular or other risk factors, response to therapy (single or multiple

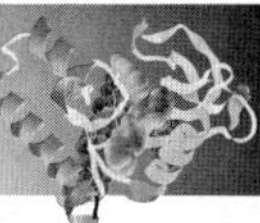

CLINICAL SIGNIFICANCE

Understanding the pathophysiology of hypertension and the medicinal chemistry of the treatment options allows the clinician to tailor pharmacotherapy to each individual patient. The patient with hypertension may start on a single oral agent but, eventually, will need a combination of medications from different drug classes, especially if the patient has diabetes, heart failure, or renal disease. A through understanding of the basic chemical properties of the drugs and their respective mechanism of action will be invaluable to making appropriate clinical decisions. The therapy for patients with hypertension must be "fine-tuned" as the clinical presentation of the hypertension changes or the patient's ability to metabolize and eliminate the medications changes. The therapeutic benefits can be maximized, and the side effects or other toxicities can be minimized. The ultimate goal for these patients would be to maximize the quality of life by controlling blood pressure and preventing long-term complications.

The astute clinician understands the differences between the medications in the individual medication classes. All β-blockers are not considered to be equally safe and effective in treating patients with peripheral arterial disease, reactive airway disease, heart failure, or a cocaine overdose. Not all calcium channel blockers and β-blockers may be safely combined for angina treatment, and only certain antihypertensive agents may be used safely during pregnancy.

The study of medicinal chemistry gives us hope for future treatment options for hypertension. Knowledge of structure-activity relationships and mechanisms of action foster the development of new medications and administration techniques. Clinicians will have to stay up to date with the new developments in the etiology of the disease state, the molecular bases of the drugs' actions, and the pharmacokinetic properties of the drugs to provide the best therapeutic outcomes for patients.

Kimberly Birtcher, Pharm.D.
Clinical Assistant Professor
University of Houston College of Pharmacy

drugs), and tolerance to drug-induced adverse effects (1,3). Antihypertensive therapy generally is reserved for patients who fail to respond to nondrug therapies along with lifestyle modifications, such as diet including sodium restriction and adequate potassium intake, regular aerobic physical activity, moderation of alcohol consumption, and weight reduction (3).

It is not surprising that compliance with antihypertensive therapy may be as low as 40% when one considers that the patient, if he or she has other chronic diseases, may be taking as many as 10 different drugs and up to 40 tablets or capsules per day (4). To achieve better compliance requires educating the patient and simplification of the drug regimen by reducing the number of drugs being taken.

Table 29.1. Classification of Antihypertensive Activity According to Mechanism of Action

I. Diuretics (Chapter 24)
II. Sympatholytic drugs
  1. Centrally acting drugs (methyldopa, clonidine, guanabenz, guanfacine) (Chapter 29)
  2. Ganglionic blocker drugs (Chapter 29)
  3. Adrenergic neuron blocking drugs (Chapter 29)
  4. β-Adrenergic blocking drugs (Chapters 12 and 29)
  5. α-Adrenergic blocking drugs (Chapters 12 and 29)
  6. Mixed α/β-adrenergic blocking drugs (Chapters 12 and 29)
III. Vasodilator (Chapter 29)
  Arterial (hydralazine, minoxidil, diazoxide)
  Arterial and venous (sodium nitroprusside)
IV. Calcium channel blockers (Chapter 27)
V. Angiotensin-converting enzyme inhibitors (Chapter 23)
VI. Angiotensin receptor antagonists (Chapter 27)

Hypertension in pregnancy presents a formidable therapeutic challenge and requires comprehensive management with close monitoring for both maternal and fetal welfare (5). Mechanisms involved with pregnancy-related hypertension include an hyperadrenergic state, plasma volume reduction, reduction in uteroplacental perfusion, hormonal control of vascular reactivity, and prostacyclin deficiency may result from or activate the mechanisms that elevate blood pressure. Effective blood pressure control for pregnancy-related hypertension often can be achieved with methyldopa (recommended), β-blockers, or mixed α/β-blockers (combinations of β-blockers with α-blockers). The vasodilating agent hydralazine is used to treat hypertensive emergencies associated with eclampsia (1,6). The presence or development of proteinuria (preeclampsia) in a hypertensive pregnant woman implies a major increase in risk to the fetus and warrants immediate admission to a hospital for specialist management (5).

Combination Antihypertensive Therapy

It is well-documented that monotherapy adequately controls hypertension only in approximately 50% of patients (7,8). Therefore, a large percentage of patients will require at least two drugs to control their blood pressure and symptoms of hypertension. By combining different antihypertensive drug classes in low doses, their different mechanisms of action result in synergistic blood pressure lowering as well as in minimizing the adverse effects and improving compliance issues (1,8). For example, the addition of a low-dose thiazide diuretic dramatically increases the response rates to methyldopa, angiotensin-

Table 29.2. Risk Factors for Cardiovascular Disease

Correctable	Noncorrectable
Cigarette smoking	Age > 60 years
Hypertension	Sex (men and postmenopausal women)
Elevated cholesterol	Family history of cardiovascular disease or stroke (women <65 years, men <55 years)
Reduced HDL cholesterol	
Diabetes mellitus	
Obesity	Target oral damage

HDL, high-density lipoprotein.

converting enzyme (ACE) inhibitors, and β-blockers without producing the undesirable side effects. In the latest guidelines for treatment of hypertension, the Joint National Committee for Prevention, Detection, Evaluation, and Treatment of High Blood Pressure (JNC VI), clinicians are encouraged to use either diuretics or mixed α/β blockers or β_1-blockers for initial monotherapy in patients with uncomplicated hypertension, because both of these drug classes have been shown to decrease morbidity and mortality in long-term clinical trials (2). In the presence of other cardiovascular diseases, however, the other antihypertensive classes that could be used as first-line agents include ACE inhibitors, calcium-channel blockers, α_1-blockers, or mixed α/β-blockers. In patients with risk factors for heart disease or with clinical manifestations of cardiovascular disease (Table 29.2), treatment should be more aggressive, with the goal of reducing blood pressure to less than 140/90 mm Hg (1). These recommendations reflect the current awareness of the importance of addressing other cardiovascular conditions aside from just lowering the blood pressure.

Arterial pressure is the product of cardiac output and peripheral vascular resistance and, therefore, can be lowered by decreasing or inhibiting either or both of these physiologic responses with the drug classes represented in Table 29.1 and summarized in Figure 29.1. This chapter will discuss those antihypertensives that are classified as either sympatholytics (i.e., having a central or peripheral mechanism of action) or vasodilators. These classes of drugs are less commonly used today because of the higher incidence of side effects associated with inhibition of the sympathetic nervous system (sympathoinhibition) or vasodilation. In many instances, they have been replaced because of availability of newer and more effective antihypertensive drugs with fewer side effects, such as ACE inhibitors.

Overview of Vascular Tone (1)

Before beginning the discussion of the sympatholytics and vasodilators, it is important to review the nature of vascular tone. The term "vascular tone" refers to the degree of constriction experienced by a blood vessel relative to its maximally dilated state. All resistance (arteries) and capacitance (venous) vessels under basal conditions exhibit some degree of smooth muscle contraction, which determines the diameter and, hence, the tone of the vessel.

Basal vascular tone varies among organs. Those organs having a large vasodilatory capacity (e.g., myocardium, skeletal muscle, skin, and splanchnic circulation) have high vascular tone, whereas organs having relatively low vasodilatory capacity (e.g., cerebral and renal circulations) have low vascular tone. Vascular tone is determined by

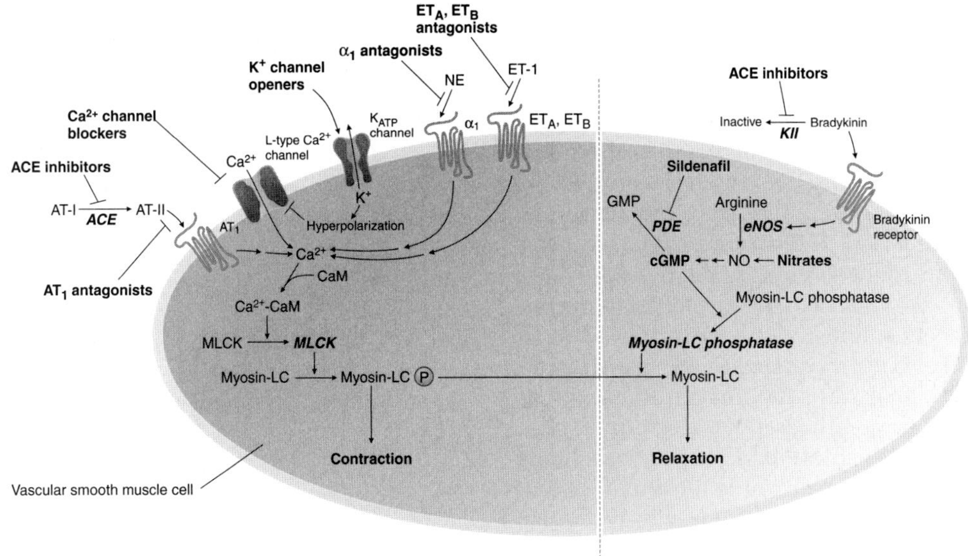

Fig. 29.1. Calcium second messenger mechanism of vascular smooth muscle contraction and relaxation and sites of action of the peripheral and centrally acting sympatholytics and vasodilators. (From Yeh DC, Michel T. Pharmacology of Vascular Tone. In: Golan DE, Tashjian A, Armstrong E, et al., eds. Principles of Pharmacology: The Pathophysiologic Basis of Drug Therapy. Baltimore: Lippincott Williams & Wilkins, 2004; 317–330; with permission.)

many different competing vasoconstrictor and vasodilator influences acting on the blood vessel. Influences such as sympathetic nerves and circulating angiotensin II regulate arterial blood pressure by increasing vascular tone (i.e., cause vasoconstriction). On the other hand, mechanisms for local blood flow regulation within an organ include endothelial factors (e.g., nitric oxide [NO] and endothelin) or local hormones/chemical substances (e.g., prostanoids, thromboxanes, histamine, and bradykinin) that can either increase or decrease tone. The mechanisms by which the above influences either constrict or relax blood vessels involve a variety of signal transduction mechanisms that, ultimately, influence the interaction between actin and myosin in the smooth muscle.

Overview of the Regulation of Vascular Smooth Muscle Contraction and Relaxation (1)

The contractile characteristics and the mechanisms that cause contraction of vascular smooth muscle (VSM) are very different from those of cardiac muscle. The VSM undergoes slow, sustained, tonic contractions, whereas cardiac muscle contractions are rapid and of relatively short duration (a few hundred milliseconds). Whereas VSM contains actin and myosin, it does not have the regulatory protein troponin, as is found in the heart. Furthermore, the arrangement of actin and myosin in VSM is not organized into distinct bands, it is in cardiac muscle. This is not to imply that the contractile proteins of VSM are disorganized and not well-developed. Actually, they are highly organized and well-suited for their role in maintaining tonic contractions and reducing lumen diameter.

Contraction of the VSM can be initiated by mechanical, electrical, and chemical stimuli. Passive stretching of VSM can cause contraction that originates from the smooth muscle itself and, therefore, is termed a "myogenic response." Electrical depolarization of the VSM cell membrane also elicits contraction, most likely by opening voltage-dependent calcium channels (L-type calcium channels) and causing an influx (increase) in the intracellular concentration of calcium. Finally, a number of chemical stimuli, such as norepinephrine, angiotensin II, vasopressin, endothelin-1, and thromboxane A_2, can cause contraction. Each of these substances bind to specific receptors on the VSM cell (or to receptors on the endothelium adjacent to the VSM), which then leads to VSM contraction. The mechanism of contraction involves different signal transduction pathways, all of which converge to increase intracellular calcium.

The mechanism by which an increase in intracellular calcium stimulates VSM contraction is illustrated in the left panel of Figure 29.1 An increase in free intracellular calcium results from either increased flux of calcium into the cell through calcium channels or by release of calcium from intracellular stores, such as the sarcoplasmic reticulum. The free calcium binds to a special calcium binding protein called calmodulin. Calcium–calmodulin activates myosin light-chain kinase (MLCK), an enzyme that is capable of phosphorylating myosin light chains in the presence of adenosine triphosphate (ATP). Myosin light-chain phosphorylation leads to actin–myosin cross-bridge formation between the myosin heads and the actin filaments and, hence, VSM contraction. Dephosphorylation of myosin light-chain phosphorylation by myosin light-chain phosphorylase yields myosin light chain which results in relaxation. The concentration of intracellular calcium depends on the balance between the calcium that enters the cells, the calcium that is released by intracellular storage sites (e.g., sarcoplasmic reticulum), and the removal of calcium either back into storage sites or out of the cell. Calcium is resequestered by the sarcoplasmic reticulum by an ATP-dependent calcium pump. Calcium is removed from the cell to the external environment either by an ATP-dependent calcium pump or by the sodium-calcium exchanger.

The activation of the calcium second messenger system by hormones, neurotransmitters, local mediators, and sensory stimuli is very important in regulating VSM contraction. Several signal transduction mechanisms modulate intracellular calcium concentration and, therefore, the state of vascular tone. These calcium second messenger systems are the phosphatidylinositol (PIP_2)/G_q protein–coupled pathway, the cyclic adenosine monophosphate (cAMP)/G_s protein–coupled pathway, and the NO/cyclic guanosine monophosphate (cGMP) pathway.

The PIP_2 pathway in VSM is similar to that found in the heart (Fig. 29.2). The VSM membrane is lined with spe-

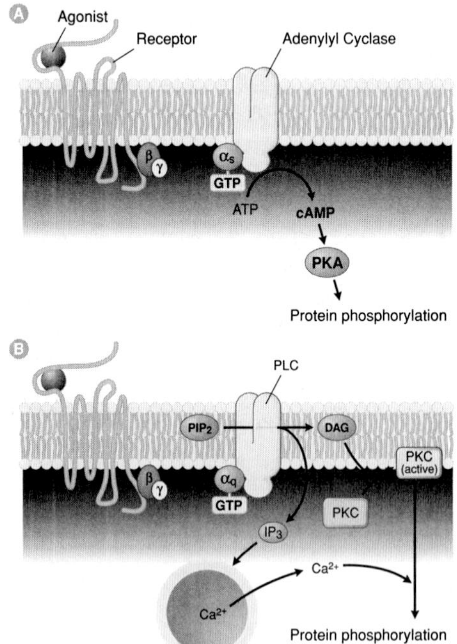

Fig. 29.2. The mechanism of activation of the cyclic adenosine monophosphate (cAMP)/G_s protein-coupled pathway and the phospholipase C/phosphatidylinositol (PIP_2) pathway in vascular smooth muscle. (From Yeh DC, Michel T. Pharmacology of Vascular Tone. In: Golan DE, Tashjian A, Armstrong E, et al., eds. Principles of Pharmacology: The Pathophysiologic Basis of Drug Therapy. Baltimore: Lippincott Williams & Wilkins, 2004; 317–330; with permission.)

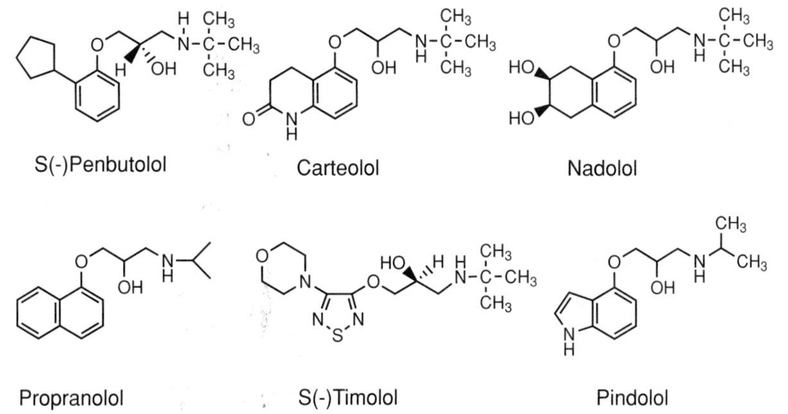

S(-)Penbutolol Carteolol Nadolol

Propranolol S(-)Timolol Pindolol

Fig. 29.3. Nonselective β-adrenergic blockers.

cific receptors for norepinephrine (α_1-adrenoceptors), angiotensin II (AT-II), or endothelin-1 (ET_A receptors) that stimulate G_q protein, activating phospholipase C and resulting in the formation of inositol triphosphate (IP_3) from PIP_2 in the membrane. Then, IP_3 stimulates the sarcoplasmic reticulum to release calcium, which in turn activates the phosphorylation of myosin light chain, causing contraction. The formation of diacylglycerol activates protein kinase C, which also contributes to VSM contraction via protein phosphorylation.

The cAMP/G_s protein–coupled pathway stimulates adenylate (also known as adenylyl) cyclase, which catalyzes the formation of cAMP (Fig. 29.2). In VSM, unlike the heart, an increase in intracellular cAMP concentrations stimulated by a β_2-adrenoceptor agonist, such as epinephrine or isoproterenol, binding to the β-receptor inhibits myosin light-chain phosphorylation, causing VSM relaxation. Therefore, drugs that increase cAMP (e.g., β_2-adrenoceptor agonists, PDE3 phosphodiesterase inhibitors) cause vasodilation. On the other hand, stimulation of G_i protein inhibits adenylyl cyclase.

A third mechanism that is also very important in regulating VSM tone is the NO/cGMP Pathway (Fig. 29.1, right). The formation of NO in the endothelium activates guanylate (also known as guanylyl) cyclase, which causes increased formation of cGMP and vasodilation. The precise mechanisms by which cGMP relaxes VSM is unclear; however, cGMP can activate a cGMP-dependent protein kinase, inhibit calcium entry into the VSM, activate K^+ channels, and decrease IP_3.

Drug Therapy of Hypertension

Peripherally Acting Sympatholytics

β-ADRENERGIC RECEPTOR BLOCKERS. β-blockers are drugs that bind to β-adrenoceptors and, thereby, block the binding of norepinephrine and epinephrine to these receptors, causing inhibition of normal sympathetic effects. Therefore, β-blockers are sympatholytic drugs. Some β-blockers, when they bind to the β-adrenoceptor, partially activate the receptor while preventing norepinephrine from binding to the receptor. These partial agonists therefore provide some "background" of sympathetic activity while preventing normal and enhanced sympathetic activity. These particular β-blockers (partial agonists) are said to possess intrinsic sympathomimetic activity (ISA). Some β-blockers also possess what is referred to as membrane-stabilizing activity. This effect is similar to the membrane-stabilizing activity of sodium channel blockers that represent Class I antiarrhythmics.

The first generation of β-blockers were nonselective, meaning that they blocked both β_1- and β_2-adrenoceptors (Fig. 29.3). Second-generation β-blockers are more cardioselective, because they are relatively selective for β_1-adrenoceptors (Fig. 29.4). Note that this relative selectivity can be lost at higher drug doses. Finally, the third-generation β-blockers are drugs that also possess vasodilator actions through blockade of vascular α-adrenoceptors (mixed α_1/β_1-adrenergic blockers) (see Fig. 29.7). Their structure–activity relationship, pharmacokinetics, and metabolism are discussed in Chapter 13 and also presented in Table 29.3. In addition to uncomplicated hypertension, they also may be used as monotherapy in the treatment of angina, arrhythmias, mitral valve prolapse, myocardial infarction, migraine headaches, performance anxiety, excessive sympathetic tone, or "thyroid storm" in hyperthyroidism (6).

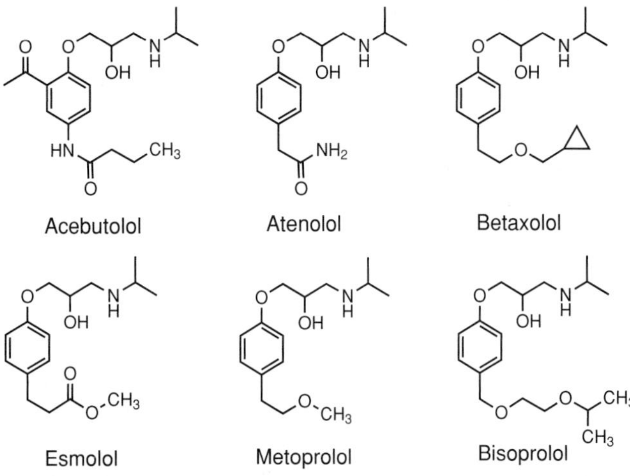

Acebutolol Atenolol Betaxolol

Esmolol Metoprolol Bisoprolol

Fig. 29.4. β_1-selective adrenergic blockers.

Table 29.3. Pharmacologic/Pharmacokinetic Properties of Antihypertensive β-Adrenergic Blocking Agents

Drug	Adrenergic Receptor Blocking Activity	Membrane Stabilizing Activity	Intrinsic Sympatho-mimetic activity	Lipid Solubility	Extent of Absorption (%)	Absolute Oral Bioavailability (%)	Half-life (hours)	Protein Binding (%)	Metabolism/Excretion
Acebutolol (Sectral)	β_1[a]	+	+	Low	90	20–60	3–4	26	Hepatic; renal excretion 30–40%, nonrenal excretion 50–60% (bile)
Atenolol (Tenormin)	β_1[α]	0	0	Low	50	50–60	6–9	5–16	~50 excreted unchanged in feces
Betaxolol (Kerlone)	β_1[α]	%	0	Low	~100	89	14–22	50	Hepatic; > 80% recovered in urine, 15% unchanged
Bisoprolol (Zebeta)	β_1[α]	0	0	Low	≥0	80	9–12	30	~50% excreted unchanged in urine, remainder as inactive metabolites; <2% excreted in feces
Esmolol (Brevibloc)	β_1[α]	0	0	Low	NA	NA	0.15	55	Rapid metabolism by esterases in cytosol of red blood cells
Metoprolol (Lopressor)	β_1[α]	0[b]	0	Moderate	95	40–50	3–7	12	Hepatic; renal excretion, <5% unchanged
Metoprolol, LA						77			
Carteolol (Cartrol)	β	0	++	Low	80	85	6	23–30	50–70% excreted unchanged in urine
Nadolol (Corgard)	β_1 β_2	0	0	Low	30	30–50	20–24	30	Urine, unchanged
Penbutolol (Levatol)	β_1 β_2	0	+	High	~100	>90	5	80–98	Hepatic (conjugation, oxidation); renal excretion of metabolites (17% as conjugate)
Pindolol (Visken)	β_1 β_2	+	+++	Moderate	95	>90	3–4[c]	40	Urinary excretion of metabolites (60–65%) and unchanged drug (35–40%)
Propranolol (Inderal)	β_1 β_2	++	0	High	90	30	3–5	90	Hepatic; <1% excreted unchanged in urine
Propranolol, LA						9–18	8–11		
Timolol (Blocadren)	β_1 β_2	0	0	Low to moderate	90	75	4	10	Hepatic; urinary excretion of metabolites and unchanged drug
Labetalol[d] (Normodyne)	β_1 β_2 α_1	0	0	Moderate	100	30–40	5.5–8.0	50	55–60% excreted in urine as conjugates or unchanged drug
Carvedilol (Coreg)	β_1 β_2 α_1	0	0	Moderate to high	>90	25–35	7–10	98	

[a]Inhibits β_2-receptors (bronchial and vascular) at higher doses.
[b]Detectable only at doses much greater than required for β-blockade.
[c]In elderly hypertensive patients with normal renal function; half-life variable, 7–15 hours.
[d]Not labetalol monograph.
Adapted from Drug Facts and Comparison 2000; with permission.
NA, not applicable (available as intravenous only); 0, none; +, low; ++, moderate; +++, high.

Mechanism of Action. The VSM are lined with β_2-adrenoceptors that normally are activated by norepinephrine released from sympathetic adrenergic nerves or by circulating epinephrine. These receptors, like those in the heart, are coupled to a G_s protein, which stimulates the formation of cAMP. Although increased cAMP enhances cardiac contraction, with VSM an increase in cAMP leads to smooth muscle relaxation (Fig. 29.2). Therefore, increases in intracellular cAMP caused by β_2-agonists inhibits MLCK, thereby producing less contractile force (i.e., promoting relaxation). Inhibition of cardiac β_1- and β_2-adrenoceptors reduce the contractility of the myocardium (negative inotropic), decreasing heart rate (negative chronotropic), blocking sympathetic outflow from the central nervous system (CNS), and suppressing renin release (9). The antianginal and antiarrhythmic effects of the β-blockers are discussed in Chapter 26.

Therapeutic Applications (1,6,10). β-Blockers decrease arterial blood pressure by reducing cardiac output. Many forms of hypertension are associated with an increase in blood volume and cardiac output. Therefore, reducing cardiac output by β-blockade can be an effective treatment for hypertension, especially when used in conjunction with a diuretic. Hypertension in some patients is caused by emotional stress, which causes enhanced sympathetic activity. β-Blockers are very effective in these patients and are especially useful in treating hypertension caused by a pheochromocytoma, which results in elevated circulating catecholamines. β-Blockers have an additional benefit as a treatment for hypertension in that they inhibit the release of renin by the kidneys (the release of which is partly regulated by a β_1-adrenoceptors in the kidney). Decreasing circulating plasma renin leads to a decrease in angiotensin II and aldosterone, which enhances renal loss of sodium and water and further diminishes arterial pressure. Acute treatment with a β-blocker is not very effective in reducing arterial pressure because of a compensatory increase in systemic vascular resistance. This may occur because of baroreceptor reflexes working in conjunction with the removal of β_2 vasodilatory influences that normally offset, to a small degree, α-adrenergic–mediated vascular tone. Chronic treatment with β-blockers lowers arterial pressure more than acute treatment, possibly because of reduced renin release and effects of β-blockade on central and peripheral nervous systems.

The selection of oral β-blockers as monotherapy for uncomplicated hypertension is based on several factors, including their cardioselectivity and preexisting conditions, ISA, lipophilicity, metabolism, and adverse effects (exception is esmolol) (Table 29.3). Esmolol is a very short-acting cardioselective β_1-blocker administered by infusion because of its rapid hydrolysis by plasma esterases to a rapidly excreted zwitterionic metabolite (plasma half-life, 9 minutes). Following the discontinuation of esmolol infusion, blood pressure returns to preexisting conditions in approximately 30 minutes. Oral β-blockers are recommended as initial therapy for uncomplicated hypertension or in the stepped-care approach to antihypertensive drug therapy (as step 1). The elderly hypertensive patient (age, >65 years) may not tolerate or respond to these drugs because of their mechanism of lowering cardiac output and increasing systemic vascular resistance (11).

Adverse Effects. Common adverse effects for the β-blockers include decreased exercise tolerance, cold extremities, depression, sleep disturbance, and impotence, although these side effects may be less severe with the β_1-selective blockers, such as metoprolol, atenolol, or bisoprolol (12). The use of lipid-soluble β-blockers, such as propranolol (Table 29.3), has been associated with more CNS side effects, such as dizziness, confusion, or depression (1,6). These side effects can be avoided, however, with the use of hydrophilic drugs, such as nadolol or atenolol. The use of β_1-selective drugs also helps to minimize adverse effects associated with β_2-blockade, including suppression of insulin release and increasing the chances for bronchospasms (asthma) (1,6). It is important to emphasize that none of the β-blockers, including the cardioselective ones, is cardiospecific. At high doses, these cardioselective agents can still adversely affect asthma, peripheral vascular disease, and diabetes (1,6). Nonselective β-blockers are contraindicated in patients with bronchospastic disease (asthma), and β_1-selective blockers should be used with caution in these patients. β-Blockers with ISA, such as acebutolol, pindolol, carteolol, or penbutolol (Table 29.3), partially stimulate the β-receptor while also blocking it (13). The proposed advantages of β-blockers with ISA over those without ISA include less cardiodepression and resting bradycardia as well as neutral effects on lipid and glucose metabolism. Neither cardioselectivity nor ISA, however, influences the efficacy of β-blockers in lowering blood pressure (6).

α_1-ADRENERGIC BLOCKERS. The structures for the available α_1-receptor blockers are shown in Figure 29.5. These include prazosin, doxazosin, and temazosin, the structure–activity relationships of which were previously discussed in Chapter 13, along with their pharmacokinetics and metabolism.

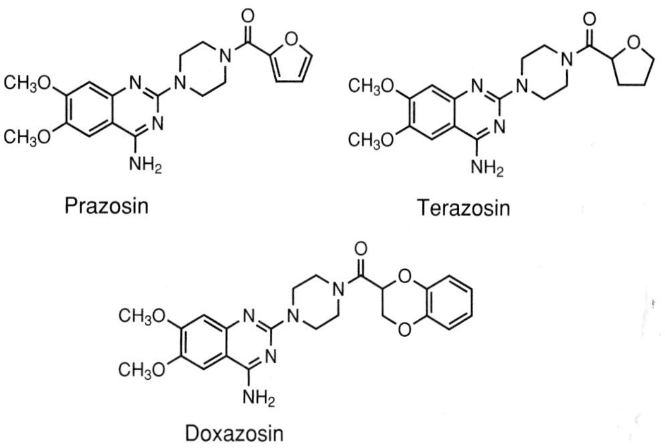

Prazosin

Terazosin

Doxazosin

Fig. 29.5. α_1-Selective adrenergic blockers.

Mechanism of Action. These drugs block the effect of sympathetic nerves on blood vessels by selectively binding to α_1-adrenoceptors located on the VSM (Fig. 29.1), stimulating G_q protein, and activates smooth muscle contraction through the IP_3 signal transduction pathway. Most of these drugs act as competitive antagonists by competing with the binding of norepinephrine to α_1-adrenergic receptors on VSM. Some α-blockers are noncompetitive (e.g., phenoxybenzamine) (see Chapter 12), which greatly prolongs their action. Prejunctional α_2-adrenoceptors located on the sympathetic nerve terminals serve as a negative feedback mechanism for norepinephrine release.

α-Blockers dilate both arteries and veins, because both vessel types are innervated by sympathetic adrenergic nerves. The vasodilator effect is more pronounced, however, in the arterial resistance vessels. Because most blood vessels have some degree of sympathetic tone under basal conditions, these drugs are effective dilators. They are even more effective under conditions of elevated sympathetic activity (e.g., during stress) or during pathologic increases in circulating catecholamines caused by an adrenal gland tumor (pheochromocytoma) (9). α_2-Adrenoceptors also are abundant in the smooth muscle of the bladder neck and prostate and, when inhibited, cause relaxation of the bladder muscle increasing urinary flow rates and the relief.

Therapeutic Applications (6,14). α_1-Blockers are effective agents for the initial management of hypertension and are especially advantageous for older men who also suffer from symptomatic benign prostatic hyperplasia. In the stepped-care approach to antihypertensive drug therapy, α_1-blockers are suggested as a step 1 drug. They have been shown to be as effective as other major classes of antihypertensives in lowering blood pressure in equivalent doses. α_1-Blockers possess a characteristic "first-dose" effect, which means that orthostatic hypotension frequently occurs with the first few doses of the drug. This side effect can be minimized by slowly increasing the dose and by administering the first few doses at bedtime.

Side Effects and Contraindications. The most common side effects are related directly to α_1-adrenoceptor blockade. These side effects include dizziness, orthostatic hypotension (because of loss of reflex vasoconstriction on standing), nasal congestion (because of dilation of nasal mucosal arterioles), headache, and reflex tachycardia (especially with nonselective α-blockers). Fluid retention also is a problem that can be rectified by use of a diuretic in conjunction with the α_1-blocker. α-Blockers have not been shown to be beneficial in heart failure or angina and should not be used in these conditions.

MIXED α/β-BLOCKERS. The two available mixed α/β-receptor blockers are carvedilol (15) and labetalol (16) (pK_a = 9.3) (Fig. 29.6), and their structure–activity relationships were previously discussed in Chapter 13 along with their pharmacokinetics and metabolism (Table 29.3).

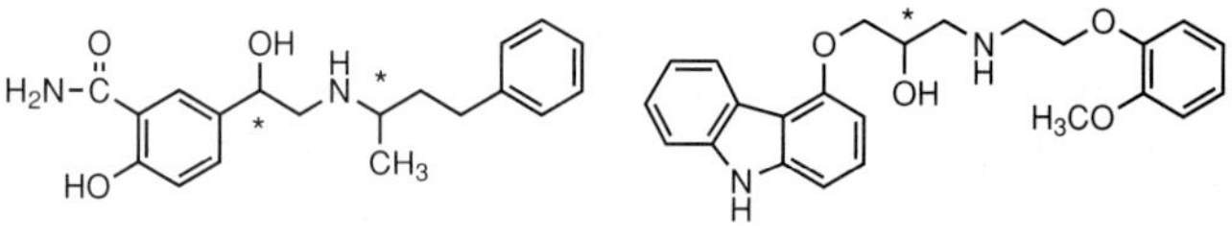

Labetalol Carvedilol

Fig. 29.6. Mixed α/β-selective adrenergic blockers.

The α-methyl substituent attached to the N-arylalkyl group appears to be responsible for the α-adrenergic blocking effect. Carvedilol is administered as its racemate. Its *S*-(−)-enantiomer is both an α- and nonselective β-blocker, whereas its *R*-(+)-enantiomer is an α_1-blocker. Labetalol possesses two chiral centers and, therefore, is administered as a mixture of four stereoisomers, of which $R(CH_3),R(OH)$ is the active β-blocker diastereomer with minimal α_1-blocking activity and the $S(CH_3),R(OH)$ diastereomer is predominantly an α_1-blocker. The *R,R* diastereomer is also known as dilevalol. The $S(CH_3),S(OH)$ and $R(CH_3),S(OH)$ diastereomers are both inactive. The comparative potency for labetalol reflects the fact that 25% of the diastereomeric mixture is the active *R,R*-diastereomer.

Mechanism of Action. The mixed α/β-receptor blocking properties in the same molecule confer some advantages in the lowering of blood pressure. Vasodilation via α_1-blockade lowers peripheral vascular resistance to maintain cardiac output, thus preventing bradycardia more effectively when compared to β-blockers (17). β-Blockade helps to avoid the reflex tachycardia sometimes observed with the other vasodilators listed below.

Therapeutic Applications. Monotherapy with these mixed-acting antihypertensive drugs reduces blood pressure as effectively as other major antihypertensives and their combinations (15–17). In the stepped-care approach to antihypertensive drug therapy, mixed α/β-blockers are recommended for initial management of mild to moderate hypertension (step 1). Both drugs effectively lower blood pressure in essential and renal hypertension. Carvedilol also is effective in ischemic heart disease.

Adverse Effects. Any adverse effects usually are related to β_1- or α_1-blockade. The β-effects usually are less bothersome, because the α_1-blockade reduces the effects of β-blockade.

Centrally Acting Sympatholytics

The sympathetic adrenergic nervous system plays a major role in the regulation of arterial pressure. Activation of these nerves to the heart increases the heart rate (positive chronotropy), contractility (positive inotropy), and velocity of electrical impulse conduction (positive dromotropy). Within the medulla are located preganglionic sympathetic excitatory neurons, which travel from the spinal cord to the ganglia. They have significant basal activity, which generates a level of sympathetic tone to the heart and vasculature even under basal conditions. The sympathetic neurons within the medulla receive input from other neurons within the medulla and together, these neuronal systems regulate sympathetic (and parasympathetic) outflow to the heart and vasculature. Sympatholytic drugs can block this sympathetic adrenergic system are three different levels. First, peripheral sympatholytic drugs, such as α-adrenoceptor and β-adrenoceptor antagonists, block the influence of norepinephrine at the effector organ (heart or blood vessel). Second, there are ganglionic blockers that block impulse transmission at the sympathetic ganglia. Third, there are drugs that block sympathetic activity within the brain, centrally acting sympatholytic drugs. Centrally acting sympatholytics block sympathetic activity by binding to and activating α_2-adrenoceptors, which reduces sympathetic outflow to the heart, thereby decreasing cardiac output by decreasing heart rate and contractility. Reduced sympathetic output to the vasculature decreases sympathetic vascular tone, which causes vasodilation and reduced systemic vascular resistance, which in turn decreases arterial pressure.

SPECIFIC DRUG

Methyldopa and Methyldopate Ester Hydrochloride

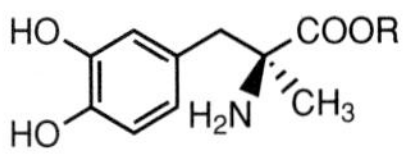

L-Methyldopa R = H
Methyldopate ethyl ester hydrochloride R = C_2H_5

Physicochemical Properties. Methyldopa is structurally and chemically related to L-DOPA and the catecholamines. To increase its water solubility for parenteral administration, the zwitterion methyldopa is esterified and converted to its hydrochloride salt, methyldopate ethyl ester hydrochloride (referred to as methyldopate). Methyldopate ester hydrochloride is used to prepare parenteral solutions of methyldopa, having a pH in the range of 3.5 to 6.0. Methyldopa is unstable in the presence of oxidizing agents (i.e., air), alkaline pH, and light. Being related to the catecholamines, which are subject to air oxidation, metabisulfite/sulfite may be added to dosage formulations to prevent oxidation. Some patients, especially those with asthma, may exhibit sulfite-related hypersensitivity reactions. Methyldopate hydrochloride injection has been reported to be physically incompatible with drugs that are poorly soluble in an acidic medium (e.g., sodium salts of barbiturates and sulfonamides) and with drugs that are acid labile. Incompatibility depends on several factors (e.g., concentrations of the drugs, specific diluents used, resulting pH, and temperature).

Mechanism of Action. As discussed in Chapter 12, the central mechanism for the antihypertensive activity of the prodrug methyldopa is not caused by its inhibition of norepinephrine biosynthesis but, rather, by its metabolism in the CNS to α-methylnorepinephrine, an α_2-adrenergic agonist (9). Other more powerful inhibitors of aromatic L-amino acid decarboxylase (e.g., carbidopa) have proven to be clinically useful, but not as antihypertensives. Rather, these agents are used to inhibit the metabolism of exogenous L-DOPA administered in the treatment of Parkinson's disease (see Chapter 24).

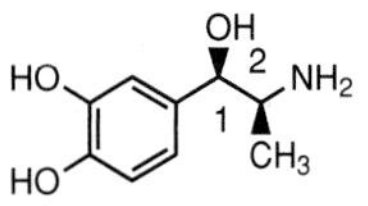

α–Methylnorepinephrine
direct acting stereoisomer

The mechanism of the central hypotensive action for methyldopa is attributed to its transport into the CNS via an aromatic amino acid transport mechanism, where it is decarboxylated and hydroxylated into α-methylnorepinephrine (9). This active metabolite of methyldopa decreases total peripheral resistance, with little change in cardiac output and heart rate, through its stimulation of central inhibitory α_2-adrenoceptors. A reduction of plasma renin activity also may contribute to the hypotensive action of methyldopa. Postural hypotension and sodium and water retention also are effects related to a reduction in blood pressure. If a diuretic is not administered concurrently with methyldopa, tolerance to the antihypertensive effect of the methyldopa during prolonged therapy can result.

Pharmacokinetics (18). The oral bioavailability of methyldopa ranges from 20 to 50% and varies among individuals. Optimum blood pressure response occurs in 12 to 24 hours in most patients. After withdrawal of the drug, blood pressure returns to pretreatment levels within 24 to 48 hours. Methyldopa and its metabolites are weakly bound to plasma proteins. Although 95% of a dose of methyldopa is eliminated in hypertensive patients with normal renal function, with a plasma half-life of approximately 2 hours, in patients with impaired renal function the half-life is doubled to approximately 3 to 4 hours, with about 50% of it excreted. Orally administered methyldopa undergoes presystemic first-pass metabolism in the gastrointestinal (GI) tract to its 3-O-monosulfate metabolite. Sulfate conjugation occurs to a greater extent when the drug is given orally than when it is given intravenously (IV). Its rate of sulfate conjugation is decreased in patients with renal insufficiency. Methyldopa is excreted in urine as its mono-O-sulfate conjugate. Any peripherally decarboxylated α-methylnorepinephrine is metabolized by catecho-o-methyltransferase (COMT) and monoamine oxidase (MAO).

Methyldopate is slowly hydrolyzed in the body to form methyldopa. The hypotensive effect of IV methyldopate begins in 4 to 6 hours and lasts 10 to 16 hours.

Therapeutic Applications (1,6). Methyldopa is used in the management of moderate to severe hypertension and is considered to be a step 2 drug reserved for patients who fail to respond to therapy with step 1 drugs. Methyldopa also is coadministered with diuretics and other classes of antihypertensive drugs, permitting a reduction in the dosage of each drug and minimizing adverse effects while maintaining blood pressure control. Methyldopa has been used in the management of hypertension during pregnancy without apparent substantial adverse effects on the fetus and also for the management of pregnancy-induced hypertension (i.e., preeclampsia) (5).

Intravenous methyldopate may be used for the management of hypertension when parenteral hypotensive therapy is necessary. Because of its slow onset of action, however, other agents, such as sodium nitroprusside, are preferred when a parenteral hypotensive agent is employed for hypertensive emergencies.

Adverse Effects (6). The most common adverse effect for methyldopa is drowsiness, which occurs within the first 48 to 72 hours of therapy and may disappear with continued administration of the drug. Sedation commonly recurs when its dosage is increased. A decrease in mental acuity, including impaired ability to concentrate, lapses of memory, and difficulty in performing simple calculations, may occur and usually necessitates withdrawal of the drug. Patients should be warned that methyldopa may impair their ability to perform activities requiring mental alertness or physical coordination (e.g., operating machinery or driving a motor vehicle). Nightmares, mental depression, orthostatic hypotension, and symptoms of cerebrovascular insufficiency may occur during methyldopa therapy and is an indication for dosage reduction. Orthostatic hypotension may be less pronounced with methyldopa than with guanethidine but may be more severe than with reserpine, clonidine, hydralazine, propranolol, or thiazide diuretics. Nasal congestion commonly occurs in patients receiving methyldopa. Positive direct antiglobulin (Coombs') test results have been reported in approximately 10 to 20% of patients receiving methyldopa, usually after 6 to 12 months of therapy. This phenomenon is dose related. Methyldopa should be used with caution in patients with a history of previous liver disease or dysfunction, and it should be stopped if unexplained drug-induced fever and jaundice occurs. These effects commonly occur within 3 weeks after initiation of treatment.

Dosage forms of methyldopa and methyldopate may contain sulfites, which can cause allergic-type reactions, including anaphylaxis and life-threatening or less severe asthmatic episodes. These allergic reactions are observed more frequently in asthmatic than in nonasthmatic individuals. Methyldopa is contraindicated in patients receiving MAO inhibitors.

α_2-ADRENERGIC AGONISTS. The mechanism of action, therapeutic applications, and adverse effects common to the α_2-adrenergic agonists clonidine, guanabenz, and guanfacine (Fig. 29.7) will be discussed together, but any significant differences between these specific agents will be included in the discussions of the individual drugs.

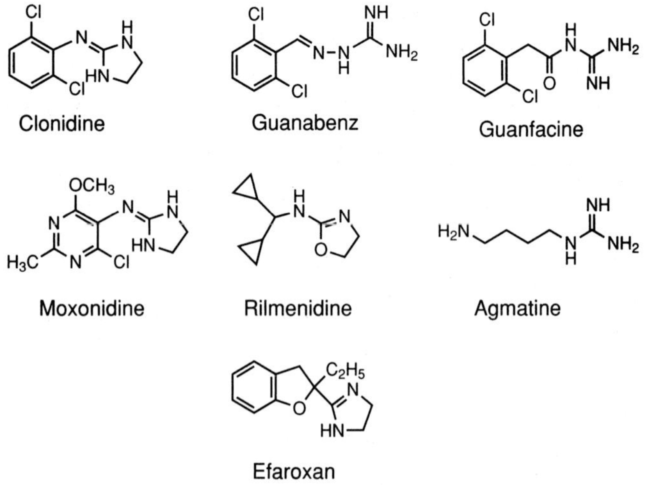

Clonidine Guanabenz Guanfacine
Moxonidine Rilmenidine Agmatine
Efaroxan

Fig. 29.7. Centrally acting sympatholytics.

Mechanism of Action. The overall mechanism of action for the centrally active sympatholytics, clonidine, guanabenz, and guanfacine, appears to be stimulation of α_2-adrenoceptors and specific binding to nonadrenergic imidazoline binding sites (I_1-IBS) in the CNS (mainly in the medulla oblongata), causing inhibition of sympathetic output (sympathoinhibition) (19,20). This effect results in reduced peripheral and renovascular resistance and leads to a decrease in systolic and diastolic blood pressure. Through the use of imidazoline and α_2-adrenergic antagonists, specific I_1-IBS have recently been characterized in CNS control of blood pressure (21). Specific I_1-IBS are G protein-coupled receptors, with agmatine being the endogenous ligand for IBS. Specific I_1-IBS are pharmacologically distinct from α_2-receptors, because they are not activated by catecholamines but characterized by their high affinity for 2-iminoimidazolines (or 2-aminoimidazolines) and low affinity for guanidines (21). Thus, the central hypotensive action for clonidine, other 2-aminoimidazolines, and structurally related compounds need both the I_1-IBS and α_2-adrenoceptors to produce their central sympatholytic response (20). As a result of this discovery, a new generation of centrally acting antihypertensive agents selective for the I_1-IBS receptor has been developed, moxonidine (a pyrimidinyl aminoimidazoline) and rilmenidine (an alkylaminooxazoline) (Fig. 29.7). Rilmenidine and moxonidine are both highly selective for the I_1-IBS while having low affinity for α_2-adrenoceptors, and both control blood pressure effectively without the adverse effects associated with binding to α_2-receptors (e.g., sedation, bradycardia, and mental depression) (20). Clonidine appears to be more selective for α_2-adrenoceptors than for I_1-IBS. Another antihypertensive is efaroxan which exhibits good affinity for I_1-IBS but is an antagonist at α_2-receptors.

Pharmacokinetics. The effective oral dose range for rilmenidine is 1 to 3 mg, with a dose-dependent duration of action of 10 to 20 hours. Moxonidine is administered once a day at a dose range of 0.2 to 0.4 mg. The oral bioavailability of moxonidine in humans is greater than 90%, with approximately 40 to 50% of the oral dose excreted unmetabolized in the urine (22,23). The principal route of metabolism for moxonidine is oxidation of the 2-methyl group in the pyrimidine ring to 2-hydroxymethyl and 2-carboxylic acid derivative as well as the formation of corresponding glucuronides. Following an oral dose of monoxidine, peak hypotensive effects occur within 2 hours, with an elimination half-life of greater than 8 hours (23,24). Rilmenidine is readily absorbed from the GI tract, with an oral bioavailability greater than 95%. It is poorly metabolized and is excreted unchanged in the urine, with an elimination half-life of 8 hours (25,26).

Following IV or oral administration of these drugs in normotensive patients, an initial hypertensive response to the drug occurs that is caused by activation of the peripheral α_2-adrenoceptors and the resulting vasoconstriction. This response is not observed, however, in patients with hypertension.

Therapeutic Applications (1,6). The selection of these drugs for monotherapy or in the stepped-care approach is based on several factors, including their similar mechanism of action, preexisting conditions, pharmacokinetics, distribution, and metabolism. The α_2-adrenergic antagonists show a similarity in adverse effects.

Clonidine, guanabenz, and guanfacine are used in the management of mild to moderate hypertension (1,6). They have been used as monotherapy or to achieve lower dosages in combination with other classes of antihypertensive agents. In the stepped-care approach to antihypertensive drug therapy, centrally acting sympatholytics generally are step 2 drugs and reserved for patients who fail to respond to therapy with a step 1 drug (e.g., diuretics, β-adrenergic blocking agents, ACE inhibitors, and α_1-blockers). Clonidine, guanabenz, and guanfacine have been used in conjunction with diuretics and other hypotensive agents, permitting a reduction in the dosage of each drug, minimizing adverse effects while maintaining blood pressure control. Geriatric patients, however, may not tolerate the adverse cognitive effects of these sympatholytics. All three drugs reduce blood pressure to essentially the same extent in both supine and standing patients; thus, orthostatic effects are mild and infrequently encountered. Exercise does not appear to affect the blood pressure response to guanabenz and guanfacine in patients with hypertension. Plasma renin activity may be unchanged or reduced during long-term therapy with these drugs.

Adverse Effects (6). Overall, the frequency of adverse effects produced by clonidine, guanabenz, and guanfacine are similar and appear to be dose related. Drowsiness, tiredness, dizziness, weakness, bradycardia, headache, and dry mouth are common adverse effects for patients receiving clonidine, guanabenz, and guanfacine. The sedative effect for these centrally acting sympatholytics may result from their central α_2-agonist activity. The dry mouth induced by these drugs may result from a combination of central and peripheral α_2-adrenoceptor mechanisms, and the decreased salivation may involve inhibition of cholinergic transmission via stimulation of peripheral α_2-adrenoceptors. Orthostatic hypotension does not appear to be a significant problem with these drugs, because there appears to be little difference between supine and standing systolic and diastolic blood pressures in most patients. Other adverse effects include urinary frequency and sexual dysfunction (e.g., decreased libido and impotence), nasal congestion, tinnitus, blurred vision, and dry eyes. These symptoms most often occur within the first few weeks of therapy and tend to diminish with continued therapy, or they may be relieved by a reduction in dosage. Although adverse effects of the drug generally are not severe, discontinuance of therapy has been necessary in some patients because of intolerable sedation or dry mouth. Sodium and fluid retention may be avoided or relieved by administration of a diuretic.

Drug Interactions (6). The hypotensive actions for clonidine, guanabenz, and guanfacine may be additive with, or may potentiate the action of, other CNS depressants, such as opiates or other analgesics, barbiturates or other sedatives, anesthetics, or alcohol. Coadministration of opiate analgesics with clonidine also may potentiate the hypotensive effects of clonidine. Tricyclic antidepressants (i.e., imipramine and desipramine) have reportedly inhibited the hypotensive effect of clonidine, guanabenz, and guanfacine, and the increase in blood pressure usually occurs during the second week of tricyclic antidepressant therapy. Dosage should be increased to adequately control hypertension if necessary. Sudden withdrawal of clonidine, guanabenz, and guanfacine may result in an excess of circulating catecholamines; therefore, caution should be exercised in concomitant use of drugs that affect the metabolism or tissue uptake of these amines (MAO inhibitors or tricyclic antidepressants, respectively). Because clonidine, guanabenz, and guanfacine may produce bradycardia, the possibility of additive effects should be considered if these drugs are given concomitantly with other drugs, such as hypotensive drugs or cardiac glycosides.

Specific Drugs

Clonidine. Clonidine is an aryl-2-aminoimidazoline that is more selective for α_2-adrenoceptors than for I_1-IBS (Fig. 29.7) in producing its hypotensive effect. It is available as oral tablets, injection, or a transdermal system.

Mechanism of Action. In addition to its central stimulation of I_1-IBS and α_2-adrenoceptors (20,21), clonidine (as well as other α_2-adrenergic agonists), when administered epidurally, produces analgesia by stimulation of spinal α_2-adrenoceptors, inhibiting sympathetically mediated pain pathways that are activated by nociceptive stimuli, thus preventing transmission of pain signals to the brain (9). Activation of α_2-adrenoceptors also apparently stimulates acetylcholine release and inhibits the release of substance

P, an inflammatory neuropeptide. Analgesia resulting from clonidine therapy is not antagonized by opiate antagonists.

Pharmacokinetics. Clonidine has an oral bioavailability of more than 90%, with a pK_a of 8.3 and a log P(exp) of 1.56 (6). It also is absorbed when applied topically to the eye. Clonidine is well absorbed percutaneously following topical application of a transdermal system to the arm or chest (27–29). Following application of a clonidine transdermal patch, therapeutic plasma concentrations are attained within 2 to 3 days. Studies have indicated that release of clonidine from the patch averages from 50 to 70% after 7 days of wear. Plasma clonidine concentrations attained with the transdermal systems generally are similar to twice-daily oral dosing regimens of the drug. Percutaneous absorption of the drug from the upper arm or chest is similar, but less drug is absorbed from the thigh (29). Replacement of the transdermal system at a different site at weekly intervals continuously maintains therapeutic plasma clonidine concentrations. Following discontinuance of transdermal therapy, therapeutic plasma drug concentrations persist for approximately 8 hours and then decline slowly over several days; over this time period, blood pressure returns gradually to pretreatment levels.

Blood pressure begins to decrease within 30 to 60 minutes after an oral dose of clonidine, with the maximum decrease in approximately 2 to 4 hours (6). The hypotensive effect lasts up to 8 hours. Following epidural administration of a single bolus dose of clonidine, it is rapidly absorbed into the systemic circulation and into cerebrospinal fluid (CSF), with maximal analgesia within 30 to 60 minutes. Although the CSF is not the presumed site of action of clonidine-mediated analgesia, the drug appears to diffuse rapidly from the CSF to the dorsal horn. After oral administration, clonidine appears to be well distributed throughout the body, with the lowest concentration in the brain. Clonidine is approximately 20 to 40% bound to plasma proteins, and it crosses the placenta. The plasma half-life of clonidine is 6 to 20 hours in patients with normal renal function and 18 to 41 hours in patients with impaired renal function. Clonidine is metabolized in the liver to its inactive major metabolite, 4-hydroxyclonidine, and its glucuronide and sulfate conjugates (10–20%) (Fig. 29.8). In humans, 40 to 60% of an oral or IV dose of clonidine is excreted in urine as unchanged drug within 24 hours. Approximately 85% of a single dose is excreted within 72 hours, with 20% of the dose excreted in feces, probably via enterohepatic circulation.

Therapeutic Applications (6). Clonidine is administered twice a day for the management of mild to moderate hypertension (6). Transdermal clonidine also has been successfully substituted for oral clonidine in some patients with mild to moderate hypertension whose compliance with a daily dosing regimen may be a problem (28).

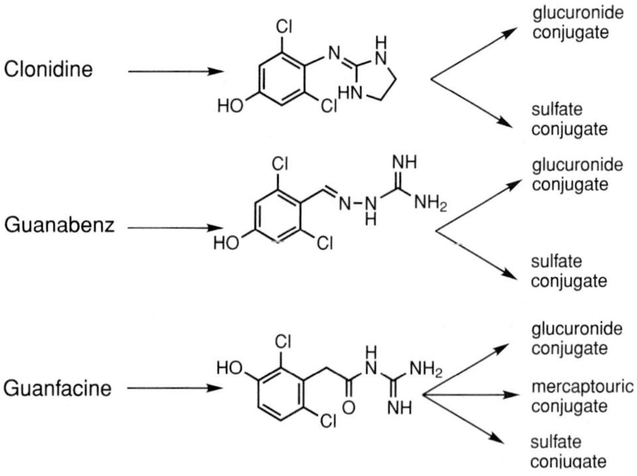

Fig. 29.8. Metabolites formed from clonidine, guanabenz, and guanfacine.

When administered by epidural infusion, clonidine is used as adjunct therapy in combination with opiates for the management of severe cancer pain not relieved by opiate analgesics alone. Other nonhypertensive uses for clonidine include the prophylaxis of migraine headaches, the treatment of severe dysmenorrhea, menopausal flushing, rapid detoxification in the management of opiate withdrawal in opiate-dependent individuals, in conjunction with benzodiazepines for the management of alcohol withdrawal, and for the treatment of tremors associated with the adverse effects of methylphenidate in patients with attention-deficit disorder. Clonidine has been used to reduce intraocular pressure in the treatment of open-angle and secondary glaucoma.

Adverse Effects (6). Adverse effects occurring with transdermal clonidine generally appear to be similar to those occurring with oral therapy (28,29). They have been mild and have tended to diminish with continued treatment. Hypotension has occurred in patients receiving clonidine by epidural infusion as adjunct therapy with epidural morphine for the treatment of cancer pain. With the transdermal system, localized skin reactions, such as erythema and pruritus, have occurred in some patients.

Within 2 to 3 hours following the abrupt withdrawal of oral clonidine therapy, a rapid increase in systolic and diastolic blood pressures occurs, and blood pressures may exceed pretreatment levels. Associated with the clonidine withdrawal syndrome, the symptoms observed include nervousness, agitation, restlessness, anxiety, insomnia, headache, sweating, palpitation, increased heart rate, tremor, and increased salivation. The exact mechanism of the withdrawal syndrome following discontinuance of α_2-adrenergic agonists has not been determined but may involve increased concentrations of circulating catecholamines, increased sensitivity of adrenoceptors, enhanced renin-angiotensin system activity, decreased vagal function, failure of autoregulation of cerebral blood flow, and failure of central α_2-adrenoceptor mechanisms to regulate sympathetic outflow from the CNS (6). The clonidine withdrawal syndrome is more pronounced after abrupt cessation of long-term therapy and with administration of high oral dosages (>1.2 mg daily). Withdrawal symptoms have been reported following discontinuance of transdermal therapy or when absorption of the drug is impaired because of dermatologic changes (e.g., contact dermatitis) under the transdermal system. Epidural clonidine may prolong the duration of the pharmacologic effects, including both sensory and motor blockade, of epidural local anesthetics.

Guanabenz Acetate. Guanabenz, a centrally active hypotensive agent, is pharmacologically related to clonidine but differs structurally from clonidine by the presence of an aminoguanidine side chain rather than an aminoimidazoline ring (Fig. 29.7). At pH 7.4, guanabenz (pK_a = 8.1) is predominately (80%) in the nonionized, lipid-soluble base form. Guanabenz can be given as a single daily dose administered at bedtime to minimize adverse effects.

Pharmacokinetics (30). The oral bioavailability of guanabenz is 70 to 80%. Following an oral dose, the hypotensive effect of guanabenz begins within 1 hour, peaks within 2 to 7 hours, and is diminished within 6 to 8 hours. It has an elimination half-life averaging 4 to 14 hours. The blood pressure response can persist for at least 12 hours. Following IV dosing, guanabenz is distributed into the CNS, with brain concentrations 3 to 70 times higher than concurrent plasma concentrations. Guanabenz is approximately 90% bound to plasma proteins. In patients with hepatic or renal impairment, its elimination half-life may be prolonged.

Guanabenz is metabolized principally by hydroxylation to its inactive metabolite, 4-hydroxyguanabenz, which is eliminated in the urine as its glucuronide (major) and sulfate conjugates (Fig. 29.8). Guanabenz and its inactive metabolites are excreted principally in urine, with approximately 70 to 80% of its oral dose excreted in urine within 24 hours and approximately 10–30% in feces via enterohepatic cycling. Approximately 40% of an oral dose of guanabenz is excreted in urine as 4-hydroxyguanabenz and its glucuronide, and less than 5% is excreted unchanged. The remainder is excreted as unidentified metabolites and their conjugates.

Therapeutic Applications (6,30). Overall, the therapeutic applications for guanabenz are similar to those of clonidine and other α_2-adrenergic agonists. One advantage for guanabenz is its once-a-day dosing schedule. Guanabenz has been used in diabetic patients with hypertension without adverse effect on the control of or therapy for diabetes, and it has been effective in hypertensive patients with chronic obstructive pulmonary disease, including asthma, chronic bronchitis, or emphysema. Guanabenz has been used alone or in combination with naltrexone in the management of opiate withdrawal in patients physically dependent on opiates and undergoing detoxification. Guanabenz also has been used as an analgesic in a limited number of patients with chronic pain.

Adverse Effects (6,30). Overall, the frequency of adverse effects produced by guanabenz is similar to that produced by clonidine and the other α_2-adrenergic agonists, but the incidence is lower. As with the other centrally active sympatholytics (e.g., clonidine), abrupt withdrawal of guanabenz may result in rebound hypertension, but the withdrawal syndrome symptoms appear to be less severe.

Guanfacine Hydrochloride. Guanfacine, a phenylacetyl guanidine derivative (pK_a = 7) (Fig. 29.7), is a centrally acting sympatholytic that is more selective for α_2-adrenoceptors than is clonidine. Its mechanism of action is similar to clonidine and is an effective alternative to that of the other centrally acting antihypertensive drugs. Although guanfacine is 5- to 20-fold less potent than clonidine on a weight basis, comparable blood pressure–lowering effects have been achieved when the two drugs were given in equipotent dosages. Its relatively long elimination half-life permits a once-a-day dosing schedule. Guanfacine activates peripheral α_2-adrenoceptors, because a transient increase in blood pressure is observed in normotensive, but not in hypertensive, patients.

Pharmacokinetics (31–33). The pharmacokinetic properties for guanfacine differ from those of clonidine, guanabenz, and α-methyldopa. At pH 7.4, guanfacine is predominately (67%) in the nonionized, lipid-soluble base form, which accounts for its high oral bioavailability (>80%). Following an oral dose, peak plasma concentrations occur in 1 to 4 hours, with a relatively long elimination half-life of 14 to 23 hours. The maximum blood pressure response occurs in 8 to 12 hours after oral administration and is maintained up to 36 hours following its discontinuation. Following IV dosing, guanfacine achieves the highest concentrations in liver and kidney, with low concentrations in the brain. Guanfacine is 64% bound to plasma proteins. In patients with hepatic or renal impairment, its elimination half-life may be prolonged.

Guanfacine is metabolized principally by hepatic hydroxylation to its inactive metabolite, 3-hydroxyguanfacine (20%), which is eliminated in the urine as its glucuronide (30%), sulfate (8%), or mercapturic acid conjugate (10%), and 24 to 37% is excreted as unchanged guanfacine (Fig. 29.8). Its nearly complete bioavailability suggests no evidence of any first-pass effect. Guanfacine and its inactive metabolites are excreted principally in urine, with approximately 80% of its oral dose excreted in urine within 48 hours.

Therapeutic Applications (6,32). Overall, the therapeutic applications for guanfacine are similar to those of the other centrally acting α_2-adrenergic agonists and methyldopa. It has been effective as monotherapy in the treatment of patients with mild to moderate hypertension. One advantage for guanfacine is its once-a-day dosing schedule. The use of diuretics to prevent accumulation of fluid may allow a reduction in the dosage for guanfacine.

Adverse Effects (6,32). Overall, although the frequency of troublesome adverse effects produced by guanfacine is similar to that produced by clonidine and the other centrally acting sympatholytics, their incidence and severity are lower with guanfacine. Unlike clonidine, abrupt discontinuation of guanfacine rarely results in rebound hypertension. When a withdrawal syndrome has occurred, its onset was slower and its symptoms less severe than the syndrome observed with clonidine.

Metyrosine

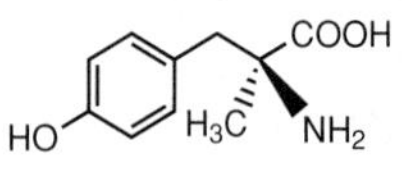

Metyrosine

Hypothetically, inhibitors of any of the three enzymes involved in the conversion of L-tyrosine to norepinephrine (see Fig. 13.1) could be used as drugs to moderate adrenergic transmission. Inhibitors of the rate-limiting enzyme tyrosine hydroxylase would be the most logical choice. One inhibitor of tyrosine hydroxylase, metyrosine or α-methyl-L-tyrosine, a competitive inhibitor of tyrosine hydroxylase, is in limited clinical use to help control hypertensive episodes caused by excess catecholamine biosynthesis. The drug also can control other symptoms of catecholamine overproduction in patients with the rare adrenal tumor pheochromocytoma. Although metyrosine is useful in treating hypertension associated with pheochromocytoma, it is not useful for treating essential hypertension. The drug metyrosine is the S-enantiomer of α-methyltyrosine. The R-enantiomer, R-α-methyltyrosine, does not bind to the active site of tyrosine hydroxylase and, thus, has no useful pharmacologic activity.

Adrenergic Neuron Blocking Agents

Bretylium, guanethidine, and guanadrel are three drugs with similar mechanisms of action involving norepinephrine storage granules. These drugs are transported into the adrenergic neurons by uptake-1, where they bind to the storage vesicles and prevent release of neurotransmitter in response to a neuronal impulse. Reserpine, guanethidine, and guanadrel are orally active antihypertensives that actually replace norepinephrine in the storage vesicles, resulting in a slow release in the amount of norepinephrine that is present. At usual doses, guanethidine and guanadrel act as "false neurotransmitters" in that they are released into the synapse but do not effectively stimulate the receptors. At higher acute doses, their principal mechanism is a poorly understood inhibition of neurotransmitter release. Bretylium is a quaternary ammonium salt and must be given IV, because it has poor oral absorption. Initially, it can cause a release of norepinephrine and a transient rise in blood pressure, but its clinical utility is limited to cardiac arrhythmias and so will not be discussed in this chapter (see Chapter 26).

RESERPINE

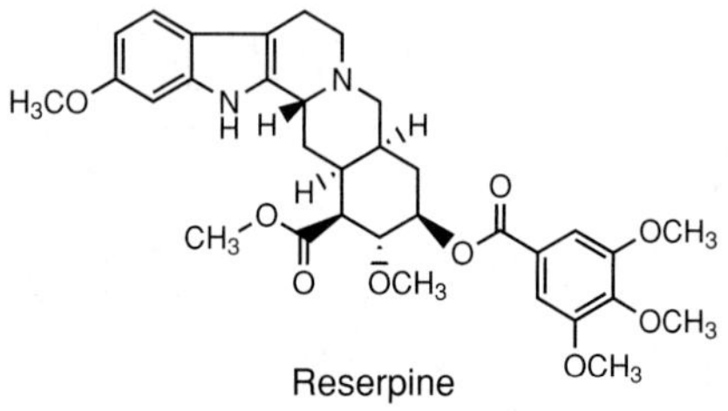

Reserpine

An old and historically important drug that affects the storage and release of norepinephrine is reserpine. Reserpine is one of several indole alkaloids isolated from the roots of *Rauwolfia serpentina*; these roots were used in India for centuries both as a remedy for snake bites and as a sedative. The antihypertensive effects of the root extracts were first reported in India in 1918 and in the West in 1949. Shortly thereafter, reserpine was isolated and identified as the principal active agent. Reserpine was the first effective antihypertensive drug introduced into Western medicine, but it has largely been replaced in clinical use by agents with fewer side effects.

Mechanism of Action (9). Reserpine acts to replace and deplete the adrenergic neurons of their stores of norepinephrine by inhibiting the active transport Mg-ATPase responsible for sequestering norepinephrine and dopamine within the storage vesicles. The norepinephrine and dopamine that are not sequestered in vesicles are destroyed by MAO. As a result, the storage vesicles contain little neurotransmitter, adrenergic transmission is dramatically inhibited, and sympathetic tone is decreased, leading to vasodilation. Reserpine has the same effect on epinephrine storage in the adrenal medulla. Reserpine readily enters the CNS, where it also depletes the stores of norepinephrine and serotonin. The CNS neurotransmitter depletion led to the use of reserpine in treating certain mental illnesses.

Pharmacokinetics (6,9). Limited information is available regarding the pharmacokinetics of reserpine. Peak blood concentrations for reserpine occur within 2 hours following oral administration, and the full effects for reserpine usually are delayed for at least 2 to 3 weeks. Both CNS and cardiovascular effects may persist for several days to several weeks after chronic oral therapy is discontinued. Reserpine appears to be widely distributed in body tissues, especially adipose tissue; crosses the blood-brain barrier and the placenta; and is distributed into milk. The elimination of reserpine appears to be biphasic, with a plasma half-life averaging 4.5 hours during the first phase and approximately 11.3 days during the second phase. Reserpine is metabolized to unidentified inactive compounds. Unchanged reserpine and its metabolites are excreted slowly in urine and feces, with an average of 60% reserpine recovered in feces within 96 hours after oral administration of 0.25 mg of radiolabeled reserpine.

Therapeutic Application (6). Reserpine has been used in the management of mild to moderate hypertension, but because of very significant CNS adverse effects and its cumulative action in the adrenergic neurons, reserpine is rarely used. Reserpine and related *Rauwolfia* alkaloids have been used in the symptomatic treatment of agitated psychotic states, such as schizophrenic disorders, although other antipsychotic agents generally have replaced reserpine and the alkaloids.

Adverse Effects (6). The common adverse CNS effects for reserpine include drowsiness, fatigue, or lethargy. Mental depression is one of the most serious potential adverse effects for reserpine, which may be severe enough to require hospitalization or result in suicide attempts. Reserpine-induced depression may persist for several months after the drug is discontinued.

GUANETHIDINE MONOSULFATE. Guanethidine contains two basic nitrogen atoms with pK_a values of 9.0 and 12.0 and, therefore, can form guanethidine monosulfate ($C_{10}H_{22}N_4 \cdot H_2SO_4$) or guanethidine sulfate [$(C_{10}H_{22}N_4)_2 \cdot H_2SO_4$] salts. Caution should be exercised when interchanging between these sulfate forms, because the potency of guanethidine may be expressed in terms of guanethidine sulfate or guanethidine monosulfate, a significant difference in molecular weight.

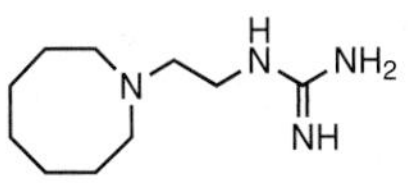

Guanethidine

Mechanism of Action. Guanethidine is an adrenergic neuronal blocking agent that produces a selective block of peripheral sympathetic pathways by replacing and depleting norepinephrine stores from adrenergic nerve endings, but not from the adrenal medulla (6,9). It prevents the release of norepinephrine from adrenergic nerve endings in response to sympathetic nerve stimulation. The chronic administration of guanethidine results in an increased sensitivity of these effector cells to catecholamines. Following the oral administration of usual doses of guanethidine, depletion of the catecholamine stores from adrenergic nerve endings occurs at a very slow rate, producing a more gradual and prolonged fall in systolic blood pressure than in diastolic pressure. Associated with the decrease in blood pressure is an increase in sodium and water retention and expansion of plasma volume (edema). If a diuretic is not administered concurrently with guanethidine, tolerance to the antihypertensive effect of the guanethidine during prolonged therapy can result.

Pharmacokinetics (6). Guanethidine is incompletely absorbed from the GI tract and is metabolized in the liver to several metabolites, including guanethidine N-oxide (from flavin mononucleotide). These metabolites of guanethidine are excreted in the urine and have less than 10% of its hypotensive activity. The amount of drug that reaches the systemic circulation after oral administration is highly variable from patient to patient and may range from 3 to 50% of a dose. Guanethidine accumulates in the neurons with an elimination half-life of 5 days.

Therapeutic Applications (6). Guanethidine is used in the management of moderate to severe hypertension and in the management of renal hypertension. In the stepped-care approach to antihypertensive drug therapy, guanethidine has been suggested as a step 2 or step 3 drug and generally is reserved for patients who fail to respond adequately to an antihypertensive regimen that includes a diuretic and other step 1 drugs, such as β-blockers, ACE inhibitors, or calcium-channel blocking agents. Its coadministration with other hypotensive agents permits a reduction in the dosage of each drug and a minimization of adverse effects while maintaining blood pressure control. It has been administered as ophthalmic drops in the treatment of chronic open-angle glaucoma and for endocrine ophthalmopathy, ophthalmoplegia, lid lag, and lid retraction.

Adverse Effects (6). Adverse effects of guanethidine frequently are dose related, including dizziness, weakness, lassitude, and syncope resulting from postural or postexercise hypotension. A hot environment (i.e., a hot bath) may aggravate postural hypotension. Patients should be warned about possible orthostatic hypotension and about the effect of rapid postural changes on blood pressure (e.g., arising in the morning) that may cause fainting, especially during the initial period of dosage adjustment. Sodium retention (edema) usually is controlled by the coadministration of a diuretic.

Drug Interactions (6). Diuretics and other hypotensive drugs can potentiate the hypotensive effects of guanethidine. Reportedly, MAO inhibitors antagonize the hypotensive effect of guanethidine. Oral sympathomimetic, nasal decongestants, and other vasopressor agents should be used cautiously in patients receiving guanethidine, because guanethidine may potentiate their pressor effects. The mydriatic response to ophthalmic administration of phenylephrine is markedly increased in patients receiving guanethidine either ophthalmically or orally.

Tricyclic antidepressants and some phenothiazines block the uptake of guanethidine into adrenergic neurons and, thus, prevent the hypotensive activity of guanethidine. Orthostatic hypotension may be increased by concomitant administration of alcohol with guanethidine, and patients receiving guanethidine should be cautioned to limit alcohol intake.

GUANADREL SULFATE. Guanadrel sulfate is a adrenergic neuronal blocking agent that is structurally and pharmacologically related to guanethidine: Both are guanidine derivatives. Guanadrel differs structurally from guanethidine by the presence of a dioxaspirodecyl ring system linked to guanidine by a methyl group rather than a hexahydroazocinyl ring linked by an ethyl group.

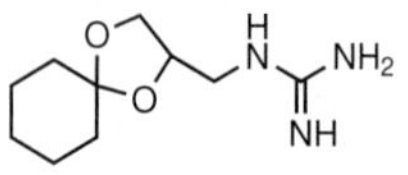

Guanadrel

Mechanism of Action. Guanadrel, like guanethidine, produces a selective block of efferent, peripheral sympathetic pathways by replacing and depleting norepinephrine stores from adrenergic nerve endings, thus preventing the release of norepinephrine from adrenergic nerve endings in response to sympathetic nerve stimulation (9,34). Unlike guanethidine, it does not release norepinephrine from the adrenal medulla and reportedly depletes norepinephrine stores in the GI tract to a lesser extent than guanethidine does. Guanadrel decreases systolic blood pressure more than diastolic blood pressure.

Pharmacokinetics (34). Guanadrel, unlike guanethidine, is rapidly and almost completely absorbed following oral administration. Following oral administration, its peak plasma concentrations usually are achieved in approximately 2 hours, and its hypotensive effect usually has an onset of 0.5 to 2.0 hours, with peak activity at 4 to 6 hours and a duration of action of 4 to 14 hours. Approximately 20% of guanadrel is bound to plasma proteins, and little, if any, of the drug crosses the blood-brain barrier or distributes into the eye. Guanadrel has a plasma half-life of approximately 2 hours and an elimination half-life of approximately 10 to 12 hours in patients with normal renal function. Approximately 40 to 50% of guanadrel is metabolized in the liver to 2,3-dihydroxypropylguanidine and several unidentified metabolites, which are excreted principally in the urine (Fig. 29.9). Unlike guanethidine, approximately 85% of an oral dose of the drug is excreted in the urine within 24 hours, with 40 to 50% of the dose excreted in the urine unchanged. In patients with impaired renal function, the half-life of guanadrel is prolonged, and apparent total body clearance and renal clearances are decreased.

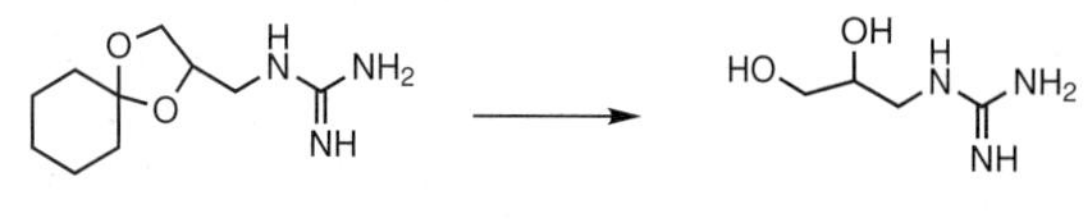

Guanadrel

Fig. 29.9. Metabolism of guanadrel.

Therapeutic Application (6,34). Guanadrel is used in the management of hypertension, and its efficacy is similar to that of guanethidine. Guanadrel generally is considered to be a step 2 drug and is reserved for patients who fail to respond to therapy with a step 1 drug or for cases requiring more prompt or aggressive therapy. Postural and postexercise hypotension is common in patients receiving guanadrel, and it also is likely that heat-induced vasodilation will augment its hypotensive effect. There is a possibility that geriatric patients may not tolerate the postural hypotensive effects of guanadrel. Being a peripheral adrenergic neuron blocking drug, guanadrel shares the toxic potentials of guanethidine, and the usual precautions of this drug should be observed.

Adverse Effects (6). Overall, the frequency of adverse effects produced by guanadrel is similar or less than those produced by guanethidine and by methyldopa. In patients with impaired renal function, the elimination half-life of unmetabolized guanadrel is prolonged and its clearance decreased, thus increasing the incidence of adverse effects if the usual dosage is maintained in these patients.

Drug Interactions. Being a peripheral adrenergic neuron blocking drug, guanadrel shares the same potential for drug interactions as guanethidine, and the usual precautions of this drug should be observed.

Vasodilators

Vasodilator drugs relax the smooth muscle in blood vessels, which causes the vessels to dilate. Dilation of arterial vessels leads to a reduction in systemic vascular resistance, which leads to a fall in arterial blood pressure. Dilation of venous vessels decreases venous blood pressure.

Arterial dilator drugs commonly are used to treat systemic and pulmonary hypertension, heart failure, and angina. They reduce arterial pressure by decreasing systemic vascular resistance, thereby reducing the afterload on the left ventricle and enhancing stroke volume and cardiac output. They also decrease the oxygen demand of the heart and, thereby, improve the oxygen supply/demand ratio. The primary functions of venous dilators in treating cardiovascular hypertension include reduction in venous pressure, thus reducing preload on the heart and decreasing cardiac output and capillary fluid filtration and edema formation (a decrease in capillary hydrostatic pressure). Therefore, venous dilators sometimes are used in the treatment of heart failure along with other drugs, because they help to reduce pulmonary and/or systemic edema that results from heart failure.

There are three potential drawbacks in the use of vasodilators: First, vasodilators can lead to a baroreceptor-mediated reflex stimulation of the heart (increased heart rate and inotropy) from systemic vasodilation and arterial pressure reduction. Second, they can impair the normal baroreceptor-mediated reflex vasoconstriction when a person stands up, which can lead to orthostatic hypotension and syncope on standing. Third, they can lead to renal retention of sodium and water, increasing blood volume and cardiac output.

Vasodilator drugs are classified either based on their site of action (arterial vs. venous) or, more commonly, by their primary mechanism of action.

DIRECT-ACTING VASODILATORS

Hydralazine Hydrochloride

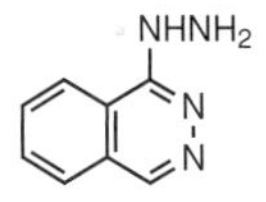

Hydralazine

Mechanism of Action. The only drug in this group, hydralazine, does not fit neatly into the other mechanistic classes, in part because its mechanism of action is not entirely clear. It appears to have multiple, direct effects on the VSM. Hydralazine, a phthalazine-substituted hydrazine antihypertensive drug with a pK_a of 7.3, is highly specific for arterial vessels, producing its vasodilation by a couple of different mechanisms. First, it causes smooth muscle hyperpolarization, quite likely through the opening of K^+ channels. Activation therefore increases the efflux of potassium ions from the cells, causing hyperpolarization of VSM cells and, thus, prolonging the opening of the potassium channel and sustaining a greater vasodilation on arterioles than on veins (9). It also may inhibit the second messenger, IP_3-induced release of calcium from the smooth muscle sarcoplasmic reticulum (the PIP_2 signal transduction pathway) (Fig. 29.2). Finally, hydralazine stimulates the formation of NO by the vascular endothelium, leading to cGMP-mediated vasodilation (Fig. 29.1). The arterial vasodilator action of hydralazine reduces systemic vascular resistance and arterial pressure. Diastolic blood pressure usually is decreased more than systolic pressure is. The hydralazine-induced decrease in blood pressure and peripheral resistance causes a reflex response, which is accompanied by increased heart rate, cardiac output, stroke volume, and an increase in plasma renin activity. It has no direct effect on the heart (6). This reflex response could offset the hypotensive effect of arteriolar dilation, limiting its antihypertensive effectiveness. Hydralazine also causes sodium and water retention and expansion of plasma volume, which could develop tolerance to its antihypertensive effect during prolonged therapy. Thus, coadministration of a diuretic improves the therapeutic outcome.

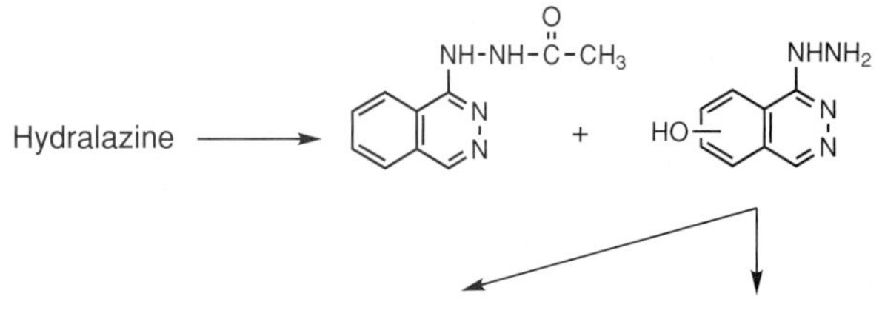

Hydralazine → N-acetyl (NH-NH-C(=O)-CH₃) phthalazine + HO-hydroxylated hydralazine (NHNH₂) → N-glucuronide conjugate, O-glucuronide conjugate

Fig. 29.10. Metabolism of hydralazine.

Pharmacokinetics (6,9). Hydralazine is well absorbed from the GI tract and is metabolized in the GI mucosa (prehepatic systemic metabolism) and in the liver by acetylation, hydroxylation, and conjugation with glucuronic acid (Fig. 29.10; see Table 8.17). Little of the hydralazine dose is excreted unchanged in urine but mainly as metabolites, which are without significant therapeutic activity. A small amount of hydralazine is reportedly converted to a hydrazone, most likely with vitamin B_6 (pyridoxine), which may be responsible for some its neurotoxic effects. Following the oral administration of hydralazine, its antihypertensive effect begins in 20 to 30 minutes and lasts 2 to 4 hours. The plasma half-life of hydralazine generally is 2 to 4 hours but, in some patients, may be up to 8 hours (i.e., slow acetylators). In slow acetylator patients or those with impaired renal function, the plasma concentrations for hydralazine are increased and, possibly, prolonged. Approximately 85% of hydralazine in the blood is bound to plasma proteins following administration of usual doses.

First-pass acetylation in the GI mucosa and liver is related to genetic acetylator phenotype (8). Acetylation phenotype is an important determinant of the plasma concentrations of hydralazine when the same dose of hydralazine is administered orally. Slow acetylators have an autosomal recessive trait that results in a relative deficiency of the hepatic enzyme N-acetyl transferase, thus prolonging the elimination half-life of hydralazine (see Chapter 10). This population of hypertensive patients will require an adjustment in dose to reduce the increased overactive response. Approximately 50% of African Americans and Caucasians, and the majority of American Indians, Eskimos, and Orientals are rapid acetylators of hydralazine. This population of patients will have subtherapeutic plasma concentrations of hydralazine because of its rapid metabolism to inactive metabolites and shorter elimination times. Patients with hydralazine-induced systemic lupus erythematosus frequently are slow acetylators.

Therapeutic Applications (6). Hydralazine is used in the management of moderate to severe hypertension. In the stepped-care approach to antihypertensive drug therapy, hydralazine has been suggested as a step 2 or step 3 drug and generally is reserved for patients who fail to respond adequately to an antihypertensive regimen that includes a diuretic and other hypotensive drugs, such as β-blockers, ACE inhibitors, or calcium-channel blockers. Hydralazine is recommended for use in conjunction with a diuretic and another hypotensive drugs, such as β-adrenergic blockers, and has been effectively used in conjunction with cardiac glycosides, diuretics, and other vasodilators for the short-term treatment of severe congestive heart failure. Patients who engage in potentially hazardous activities, such as operating machinery or driving motor vehicles, should be warned about possible faintness, dizziness, or weakness. Hydralazine should be used with caution in patients with cerebrovascular accidents or with severe renal damage.

Parenteral hydralazine may be used for the management of severe hypertension when the drug cannot be given orally or when blood pressure must be lowered immediately. Other agents (e.g., sodium nitroprusside) are preferred for the management of severe hypertension or hypersensitive emergencies when a parenteral hypotensive agent is employed.

Drug interactions. The coadministration of diuretics and other hypotensive drugs may have a synergistic effect, resulting in a marked decrease in blood pressure.

POTASSIUM CHANNEL OPENERS

Specific drugs

Minoxidil. Although several potassium channel openers have been used in research for many years, only one, minoxidil, is approved for use in humans for treating hypertension. Minoxidil is the N-oxide of a piperidinopyrimidine hypotensive agent, with a pK_a of 4.6, and is not an active hypotensive drug until it is metabolized by hepatic sulfotransferase to minoxidil N-O-sulfate (9).

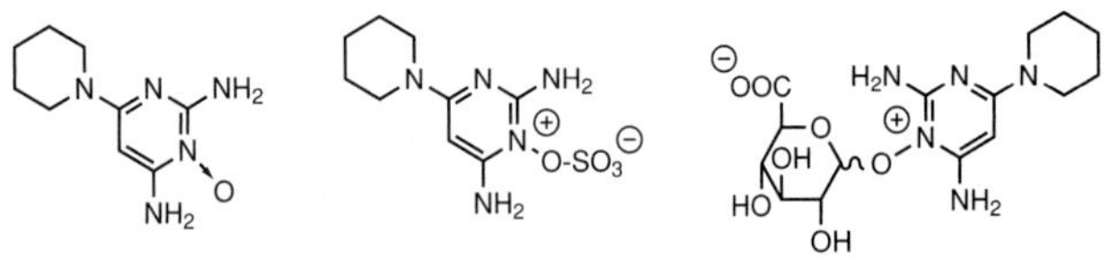

Minoxidil Minoxidil N-O-sulfate Minoxidil N-O-glucuronide

Mechanism of Action. Potassium channel openers are drugs that activate (i.e., open) ATP-sensitive K^+ channels in the VSM (Fig. 29.1). By opening these potassium channels, there is increased efflux of potassium ions from the cells, causing hyperpolarization of VSM, which closes the voltage-gated calcium channels and, thereby, decreases intracellular calcium. With less calcium available to combine with calmodulin, there is less activation of MLCK and phosphorylation of myosin light chains. This leads to relaxation and vasodilation. Because small arteries and arterioles normally have a high degree of smooth muscle tone, these drugs are particularly effective in dilating these resistance vessels, decreasing systemic vascular resistance, and lowering arterial pressure. The fall in arterial pressure leads to reflex cardiac stimulation (baroreceptor-mediated tachycardia).

Minoxidil, as its active metabolite minoxidil O-sulfate, prolongs the opening of the potassium channel, sustaining greater vasodilation on arterioles than on veins. The drug decreases blood pressure in both the supine and standing positions, and there is no orthostatic hypotension. Associated with the decrease in peripheral resistance and blood pressure is a reflex response that is accompanied by increased heart rate, cardiac output, and stroke volume, which can be attenuated by the coadministration of a β-blocker (6). Along with this decrease in peripheral resistance is increased plasma renin activity and sodium and water retention, which can result in expansion of fluid volume, edema, and congestive heart failure. The sodium- and water-retaining effects of minoxidil can be reversed by coadministration of a diuretic. When minoxidil is used in conjunction with a β-adrenergic blocker, pulmonary artery pressure remains essentially unchanged.

Pharmacokinetics (35). Minoxidil is absorbed from the GI tract and is metabolized to its active sulfate metabolite. Plasma concentrations for minoxidil sulfate peak within 1 hour and then decline rapidly. Following an oral dose of minoxidil, its hypotensive effect begins in 30 minutes, is maximal in 2 to 8 hours, and persists for approximately 2 to 5 days. The delayed onset of the hypotensive effect for minoxidil is attributed to its metabolism to its active metabolite. The drug is not bound to plasma proteins. The major metabolite for minoxidil is its N-O-glucuronide, which unlike the sulfate metabolite is inactive as a hypotensive agent. Approximately 10 to 20% of an oral dose of minoxidil is metabolized to its active metabolite, minoxidil O-sulfate, and approximately 20% of minoxidil is excreted unchanged.

Therapeutic Applications

HYPERTENSION (6,35). Being effective arterial dilators, potassium-channel openers are used in the treatment of hypertension. These drugs are not first-line therapy for hypertension because of their side effects; therefore, they are relegated to treating refractory, severe hypertension. They generally are used in conjunction with a β-blocker and a diuretic to attenuate the reflex tachycardia and retention of sodium and fluid, respectively.

Minoxidil is used in the management of severe hypertension and is considered to be a step 3 drug. It generally is reserved for resistant cases of hypertension that have not been managed with maximal therapeutic dosages of a diuretic and two other hypotensive drugs or for patients who have failed to respond adequately to step 3 therapy that includes hydralazine. To minimize sodium retention and increased plasma volume, minoxidil must be used in conjunction with a diuretic. A β-adrenergic blocker (e.g., propranolol) must be given before minoxidil therapy is begun and should be continued during minoxidil therapy to minimize minoxidil-induced tachycardia and increased myocardial workload.

ANDROGENETIC ALOPECIA (6,36). Minoxidil is used topically to stimulate regrowth of hair in patients with androgenic alopecia (male pattern alopecia, hereditary alopecia, or common male baldness) or alopecia areata. Commercially available topical minoxidil preparations should be used rather than the extemporaneous topical formulations from tablets to reduce the potential of minoxidil being absorbed systemically.

Drug Interactions. When minoxidil is administered with diuretics or other hypotensive drugs, the hypotensive effect of minoxidil increases, and concurrent use may cause profound orthostatic hypotensive effects.

Diazoxide

Metabolism

Diazoxide

Diazoxide is a nondiuretic hypotensive and hyperglycemic agent that is structurally related to the thiazide diuretics. Being a sulfonamide with a pK_a of 8.5, it can be solubilized in alkaline solutions (pH of injection is 11.6). Solutions or oral suspension of diazoxide are unstable to light and will darken when exposed to light. Such dosage forms should be protected from light, heat, and freezing. Darkened solutions may be subpotent and should not be used.

Mechanism of Action. Diazoxide reduces peripheral vascular resistance and blood pressure by a direct vasodilating effect on the VSM with a mechanism similar to that described for minoxidil by activating (opening) the ATP-modulated potassium channel (36). Thus, diazoxide prolongs the opening of the potassium channel, sustaining greater vasodilation on arterioles than on veins (9). The greatest hypotensive effect is observed in patients with malignant hypertension. Although oral or slow IV administration of diazoxide can produce a sustained fall in blood pressure, rapid IV administration is required for maximum hypotensive effects, especially in patients with malignant hypertension (6). Diazoxide-induced decreases in blood pressure and peripheral vascular resistance are accompanied by a reflex response, resulting in an increased heart rate, cardiac output, and left ventricular ejection rate. In contrast to the thiazide diuretics, diazoxide causes sodium and water retention and decreased urinary output, which can result in expansion of plasma and extracellular fluid volume, edema, and congestive heart failure, especially during prolonged administration.

Diazoxide increases blood glucose concentration (diazoxide-induced hyperglycemia) by several different mechanisms: by inhibiting pancreatic insulin secretion, by stimulating release of catecholamines, or by increasing hepatic release of glucose (6,9). The precise mechanism of inhibition of insulin release has not been elucidated but, possibly, may result from an effect of diazoxide on cell-membrane potassium channels and calcium flux.

Pharmacokinetics (6). Following rapid IV administration, diazoxide produces a prompt reduction in blood pressure, with maximum hypotensive effects occurring within 5 minutes. The duration of its hypotensive effect varies from 3 to 12 hours, but ranges from 30 minutes to 72 hours have been observed. The elimination half-life of diazoxide following a single oral or IV dose has been reported to range from 21 to 45 hours in adults with normal renal function. In patients with renal impairment, the half-life is prolonged. Approximately 90% of the diazoxide in the blood is bound to plasma proteins. Approximately 20 to 50% of diazoxide is eliminated unchanged in the urine, along with its major metabolites, resulting from the oxidation of the 3-methyl group to its 3-hydroxymethyl- and 3-carboxyl-metabolites.

Therapeutic Applications

SEVERE HYPERTENSION (6). Intravenous diazoxide has been used in hypertensive crises for emergency lowering of blood pressure when a prompt and urgent decrease in diastolic pressure is required in adults with severe nonmalignant and malignant hypertension and in children with acute severe hypertension. Generally, however, other IV hypotensive agents are preferred for the management of hypertensive crises. Diazoxide is intended for short-term use in hospitalized patients only. Although diazoxide also has been administered orally for the management of hypertension, its hyperglycemic and sodium-retaining effects make it unsuitable for chronic therapy.

HYPOGLYCEMIA (6). Diazoxide is administered orally in the management of hypoglycemia caused by hyperinsulinism associated with inoperable islet cell adenoma or carcinoma or extrapancreatic malignancy in adults.

PHOSPHODIESTERASE INHIBITORS

Mechanism of Action of cAMP-Dependent Phosphodiesterase Inhibitors (PDE3). The PDE3 is one of the isoforms of phosphodiesterase found in the heart and VSM. The mechanism by which cAMP and cGMP relaxes VSM has been described previously in the section on VSM contraction and relaxation (Fig. 29.1) (see also Chapter 17). The cAMP released is broken down by a cAMP-dependent phosphodiesterase (PDE3). Therefore, inhibition of PDE3 increases intracellular cAMP, which further inhibits MLCK, thereby producing less contractile force (i.e., promoting relaxation). The overall cardiac and vascular effects of cAMP-dependent phosphodiesterase inhibitors cause cardiac stimulation, increasing cardiac output and reducing systemic vascular resistance, thereby lowering arterial pressure. Because cardiac output increases and systemic vascular resistance decreases, the change in arterial pressure depends on the relative effects of the phosphodiesterase inhibitor on the heart versus the VSM. At normal therapeutic doses, PDE3 inhibitors, such as milrinone, have a greater effect on VSM than cardiac muscle so that arterial pressure is lowered in the presence of augmented cardiac output. Because of the dual cardiac and vascular effects of these compounds, they sometimes are referred to as inodilators.

Mechanism of Action of cGMP-Dependent Phosphodiesterase Inhibitors (PDE5). A second isoenzyme form of phosphodiesterase found in VSM is PDE5, a cGMP-dependent phosphodiesterase, which also is found in the corpus cavernosum of the penis (erectile dysfunction). This enzyme is responsible for breaking down cGMP that forms in response to increased NO (Fig. 29.1). Increased cGMP leads to smooth muscle relaxation primarily by reducing calcium entry into the cell. Inhibitors of cGMP-dependent phosphodiesterase increases intracellular cGMP, thereby enhancing VSM relaxation and vasodilation.

Therapeutic Indications. The cardiostimulatory and vasodilatory actions of PDE3 inhibitors make them suitable for the treatment of heart failure, because VSM relaxation reduces ventricular wall stress and the oxygen demands placed on the failing heart. The cardiostimulatory effects of the PDE3 increase inotropy, which further enhances stroke volume and ejection fraction. A baroreceptor reflex, which occurs in response to hypotension, may contribute to the tachycardia. Clinical trials have shown that long-term therapy with PDE3 inhibitors increases mortality in patients with heart failure; therefore, these drugs are not used for long-term, chronic therapy. They are very useful, however, in treating acute, decompensated heart failure or temporary bouts of decompensated chronic failure. They are not used as a monotherapy. Instead, they are used in conjunction with other treatment modalities, such as diuretics, ACE inhibitors, β-blockers, or digitalis. The somewhat selective vasodilatory actions of PDE5 inhibitors have made these compounds very useful in the treatment of male erectile dysfunction and as a combination therapy for pulmonary hypertension. The PDE3 inhibitors are used for treating heart failure, whereas the PDE5 inhibitors are used for treating male erectile dysfunction. Note that the generic names for PDE3 inhibitors end in "one" and those for the PDE5 inhibitors end in "fil".

Specific Drugs

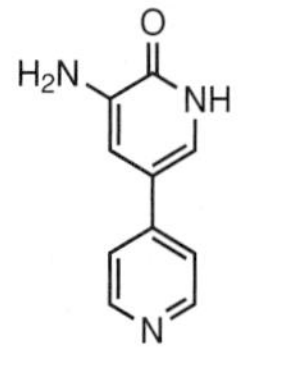

Inamrinone

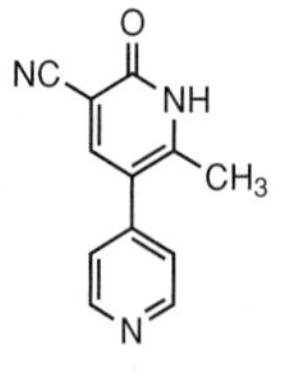

Milrinone

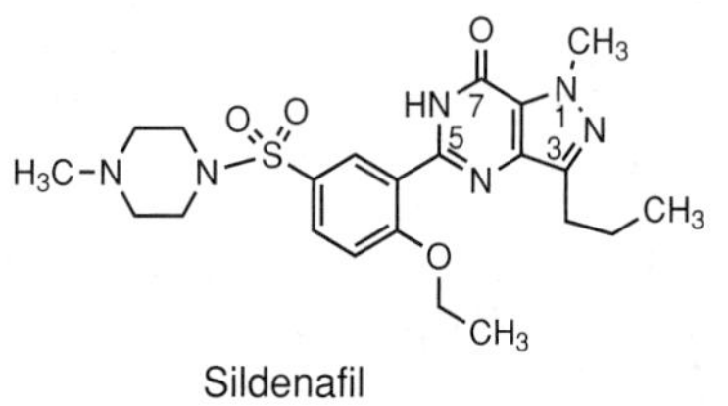

Sildenafil

Milrinone (Primacor as Lactate Salt) and Inamrinone (Inocor as Lactate Salt). Inamrinone and milrinone are positive inotropes and vasodilators indicated for the short-term IV management of congestive heart failure in patients who have not responded adequately to digitalis, diuretics, and/or vasodilators.

For IV infusion, inamrinone lactate and milrinone lactate injection solutions may be diluted in sodium chloride solution for injection. Inamrinone lactate for injection is preserved with sodium metabisulfite and needs protection from light. It should not be diluted with solutions containing dextrose, because a chemical interaction occurs over 24 hours. For milrinone, an immediate chemical interaction with furosemide with the formation of a precipitate is observed when furosemide is injected into an infusion of milrinone. Patients who are sensitive to bisulfites also may be sensitive to inamrinone lactate injection, which contains sodium metabisulfite.

The pharmacokinetics for inamrinone shows protein binding from 10 to 49%. Its half-life in healthy volunteers is approximately 3.6 hours, whereas in patients with congestive heart failure, the plasma half-life increases to approximately 5.0 to 8.3 hours. For infants younger than 4 weeks, the half-life is 12.7 to 22.2 hours, and for infants older than 4 weeks, the half-life is 3.8 to 6.8 hours. Time to peak effect is less than 10 minute. Its duration of action is dose related, ranging from 30 minutes at low dose to 2 hours at the higher dosages. Approximately 63% of the administered dose is eliminated via the urine as unchanged drug, and 18% is eliminated in the feces. Elderly patients are more likely to have age-related renal function impairment, which may require adjustment of dosage in patients receiving inamrinone.

The pharmacokinetics for milrinone following IV injections to patients with congestive heart failure showed a volume of distribution of 0.38 to 0.45 L/kg, a mean terminal elimination half-life of 2.3 hours, and a clearance of 0.13 L/kg/hour. These pharmacokinetic parameters were not dose-dependent, and the area under the plasma concentration versus time curve following injections was significantly dose-dependent. Milrinone is approximately 70% bound to human plasma protein. The primary route of excretion for orally administered milrinone is via the urine, with unchanged milrinone (83%) and its O-glucuronide metabolite (12%) being present. Elimination in normal subjects via the urine is rapid, with approximately 60% recovered within the first 2 hours following dosing and approximately 90% within the first 8 hours following dosing. In patients with renal function impairment, elimination of unchanged milrinone is reduced, suggesting that a dosage adjustment may be necessary.

The selective PDE5 inhibitor most commonly used is sildenafil (Viagra). Studies in vitro have shown that sildenafil is selective for PDE5. Its effect is more potent on PDE5 than on other known phosphodiesterases (10 times for PDE6, >80 times for PDE1, and >700 times for PDE2, PDE3, PDE4, PDE7, PDE8, PDE9, PDE10, and PDE11). The approximately 4,000 times selectivity for PDE5 versus PDE3 is important, because PDE3 is involved in control of cardiac contractility. Sildenafil is only approximately 10 times as potent for PDE5 compared to PDE6, an enzyme found in the retina that is involved in the phototransduction pathway of the retina. This lower selectivity is thought to be the basis for abnormalities related to color vision observed with higher doses or plasma levels. (For a complete discussion of the pharmacokinetics including drug metabolism, see Chapter 45.)

Side Effects and Contraindications. The most common and severe side effect for PDE3 inhibitors is ventricular arrhythmias, some of which may be life-threatening. Other side effects include headaches and hypotension, which are not uncommon for drugs that increase cAMP in cardiac and vascular tissues (e.g., β-agonists).

In addition to human corpus cavernosum smooth muscle, PDE5 also is found in lower concentrations in other tissues, including platelets, vascular and visceral smooth muscle, and skeletal muscle. The inhibition of PDE5 in these tissues by sildenafil may be the basis for the enhanced platelet antiaggregatory activity of NO observed in vitro, an inhibition of platelet thrombus formation in vivo, and peripheral arterial-venous dilatation in vivo. The most common side effects for PDE5 inhibitors include headache and cutaneous flushing, both of which are related to vascular dilation caused by increased vascular cGMP. Clinical evidence suggests that nitrodilators may interact adversely with PDE5 inhibitors. The reason for this adverse reaction is that nitrodilators stimulate cGMP production, whereas PDE5 inhibitors inhibit cGMP degradation. When combined, these two drug classes greatly potentiate cGMP levels, which can lead to hypotension and impaired coronary perfusion.

NITRODILATORS

Mechanism of Action. Nitric oxide, a molecule produced by many cells in the body, has several important actions. NO is a highly reactive gas that participates in many chemical reactions. It is one of the nitrogen oxides ("NOx") in automobile exhaust and plays a major role in the formation of photochemical smog, but NO also has many physiological functions. It is synthesized within cells by an enzyme NO synthase (NOS). There are three isoenzymes, neuronal NOS (nNOS or NOS-1), inducible NOS (iNOS or NOS-2) found in macrophages, and endothelial NOS (eNOS or NOS-3) found in the endothelial cells that line the lumen of blood vessels. Whereas the levels of nNOS and eNOS are relatively steady, expression of iNOS genes awaits an appropriate stimulus. All types of NOS produce NO from arginine with the aid of molecular oxygen and NADPH. Because NO diffuses freely across cell membranes, there are many other molecules with which it can interact, and NO is quickly consumed close to where it is synthesized. Thus, NO affects only cells adjacent to its point of synthesis. NO relaxes the smooth muscle in the walls of the arterioles. At each systole, the endothelial cells that line the blood vessels release a puff of NO, which diffuses into the underlying smooth muscle cells, causing them to relax and, thus, to permit the surge of blood to pass through easily. The signaling functions of NO begin with its binding to protein receptors on or in the cell, triggering the formation of cGMP from soluble guanylyl cyclase (Fig. 29.1). Mice in which the genes for the NOS found in endothelial cells (eNOS) has been "knocked out" suffer from hypertension. Nitroglycerin, which often is prescribed to reduce the pain of angina, does so by generating NO, which relaxes venous walls and arterioles improving the oxygen supply/decreased ratio (see Chapter 24). Nitric oxide also inhibits the aggregation of platelets and, thus, keeps inappropriate clotting from interfering with blood flow. Other actions on smooth muscle include penile erection and peristalsis aided by the relaxing effect of NO on the smooth muscle in intestinal walls; NO also inhibits the contractility of the smooth muscle wall of the uterus, but at birth, the production of NO decreases, allowing contractions to occur. Nitroglycerin has helped some women who were at risk of giving birth prematurely to carry their baby to full term. The NO from iNOS inhibits inflammation in blood vessels by blocking the release of mediators of inflammation from the endothelial cells, macrophages, and T lymphocytes. The NO from iNOS has been shown to S-nitrosylate COX-2, increasing its activity, and drugs that prevent this interaction could work synergistically with the nonsteroidal anti-inflammatory drugs inhibiting COX-2. Nitric oxide affects hormonal secretion from several endocrine glands. Hemoglobin transports NO at the same time that it carries oxygen, and when it unloads oxygen in the tissues, it also unloads NO. Fireflies use NO to turn on their flashers.

Since the dawn of recorded human history, nitrates have been used to preserve meat from bacterial spoilage. Harmless bacteria in our throat convert nitrates in our food into nitrites. When the nitrites reach the stomach, the acidic gastric juice (pH ~1.4) generates NO from these nitrites, killing almost all the bacteria that have been swallowed in our food.

In the cardiovascular system, NO is produced primarily by vascular endothelial cells. This endothelial-derived NO has several important functions, including relaxing VSM (vasodilation), inhibiting platelet aggregation (antithrombotic), and inhibiting leukocyte–endothelial interactions (anti-inflammatory). These actions involve NO-stimulated formation of cGMP (Fig. 29.1). Nitrodilators are drugs that mimic the actions of endogenous NO by releasing NO or forming NO within tissues. These drugs act directly on the VSM to cause relaxation and, therefore, serve as endothelial-independent vasodilators.

Sodium Nitroprusside (Sodium Nitroferricyanide; Nitropress; Nipride)

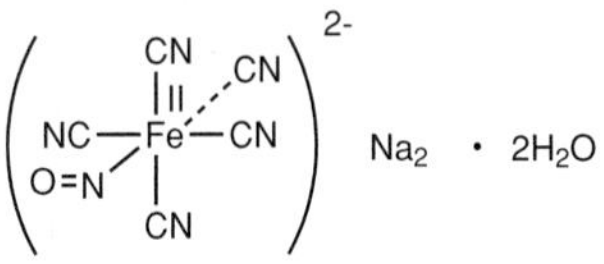

Sodium nitroprusside

There are two basic types of nitrodilators: those that release NO spontaneously (e.g., sodium nitroprusside), and those that require an enzyme activation to form NO (organic nitrates). Sodium nitroprusside is a direct-acting vasodilator on VSM, producing its vasodilation by the release of NO. Since 1929, it has been known as a rapidly acting hypotensive agent when administered as an infusion. It is chemically and structurally unrelated to other available hypotensive agents. As a reminder in preparing extemporaneous infusions, the potency of sodium nitroprusside is expressed in terms of the dihydrated drug. When reconstituted with 5% dextrose injection, sodium nitroprusside solutions are reddish-brown in color, with a pH of 3.5 to 6.0. Its crystals and solutions are sensitive and unstable to light and should be protected from extremes of light and heat. The exposure of sodium nitroprusside solutions to light causes deterioration, which may be evidenced by a change from a reddish-brown to a green to a blue color, indicating a rearrangement of the nitroso to the inactive isonitro form. Sodium nitroprusside solutions in glass bottles undergo approximately 20% degradation within 4 hours when exposed to fluorescent light and even more rapid degradation in plastic bags. Sodium nitroprusside solutions should be protected from light by wrapping the container with aluminum foil or other opaque material. When adequately protected from light, reconstituted solutions are stable for 24 hours. Trace metals, such as iron and copper, can catalyze the degradation of nitroprusside solutions, releasing cyanide. Any change in color for the nitroprusside solutions is an indication of degradation, and the solution should be discarded. No other drug or preservative should be added to stabilize sodium nitroprusside infusions.

Mechanism of Action. Sodium nitroprusside is not an active hypotensive drug until metabolized to its active metabolite, NO, the mechanism of action of which has been previously described (Fig. 29.1). Studies with sodium nitroprusside suggest that it releases NO by its interaction with glutathione or with sulfhydryl groups in the erythrocytes and tissues to form a S-nitrosothiol intermediate, which spontaneously produces NO, which in turn freely diffuses into the VSM, thereby increasing intracellular cGMP concentration (6,9). NO also activates K^+ channels, which leads to hyperpolarization and relaxation.

The hypotensive effect of sodium nitroprusside is augmented by concomitant use of other hypotensive agents and is not blocked by adrenergic blocking agents. It has no direct effect on the myocardium, but it may exert a direct coronary vasodilator effect on VSM. When sodium nitroprusside is administered to hypertensive patients, a slight increase in heart rate commonly occurs, and cardiac output usually is decreased slightly. Moderate doses of sodium nitroprusside in patients with hypertension produce renal vasodilation without an appreciable increase in renal blood flow or decrease in glomerular filtration (6).

Intravenous infusion of sodium nitroprusside produces an almost immediate reduction in blood pressure. Blood pressure begins to rise immediately when the infusion is slowed or stopped and returns to pretreatment levels within 1 to 10 minutes.

Pharmacokinetics. Sodium nitroprusside undergoes a redox reaction that releases cyanide (6,9). The cyanide that is produced is rapidly converted into thiocyanate in the liver by the enzyme thiosulfate sulfotransferase (rhodanase) and is excreted in the urine (6,9). The rate-limiting step in the conversion of cyanide to thiocyanate is the availability of sulfur donors, especially thiosulfate. Toxic symptoms of thiocyanate begin to appear at plasma thiocyanate concentrations of 50 to 100 mg/mL. The elimination half-life of thiocyanate is 2.7 to 7.0 days when renal function is normal but longer in patients with impaired renal function.

Therapeutic Applications (6). Intravenous sodium nitroprusside is used as an infusion for hypertensive crises and emergencies. The drug is consistently effective in the management of hypertensive emergencies, irrespective of etiology, and may be useful even when other drugs have failed. It may be used in the management of acute congestive heart failure.

Adverse Effects (6). The most clinically important adverse effects of sodium nitroprusside are profound hypotension and the accumulation of cyanide and thiocyanate. Thiocyanate may accumulate in the blood of patients receiving sodium nitroprusside therapy, especially in those with impaired renal function. Thiocyanate is mildly neurotoxic at serum concentrations of 60 μg/mL and may be life-threatening at concentrations of 200 μg/mL. Other adverse effects of thiocyanate includes inhibition of both the uptake and binding of iodine producing symptoms of hypothyroidism.

Sodium nitroprusside can bind to vitamin B_{12} interfering with its distribution and metabolism, and it should be used with caution in patients having low plasma vitamin B_{12} concentrations. Excess cyanide also can bind to hemoglobin, producing methemoglobinemia.

Ganglionic Blockers

Mechanism of Action. Ganglionic blockers block impulse transmission at the sympathetic ganglia. Neurotransmission within the sympathetic and parasympathetic ganglia involves the release of acetylcholine from preganglionic efferent nerves, which binds to nicotinic receptors on the postganglionic efferent nerves. Ganglionic blockers inhibit autonomic activity by interfering with neurotransmission within autonomic ganglia. This reduces sympathetic outflow to the heart, thereby decreasing cardiac output by decreasing heart rate and contractility. Reduced sympathetic output to the vasculature decreases sympathetic vascular tone, which causes vasodilation and reduced systemic vascular resistance, which decreases arterial pressure. Parasympathetic outflow also is reduced by ganglionic blockers.

Therapeutic Indications. Ganglionic blockers are not commonly used in the treatment of chronic hypertension largely because of their side effects and because numerous more effective and safer antihypertensive drugs can be used. They are, however, occasionally used for hypertensive emergencies.

The ganglionic blockers available for clinical use include trimethaphan camsylate and mecamylamine.

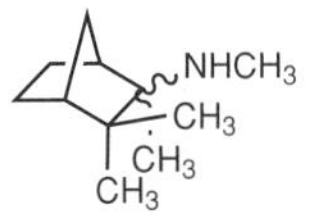

± Mecamylamine 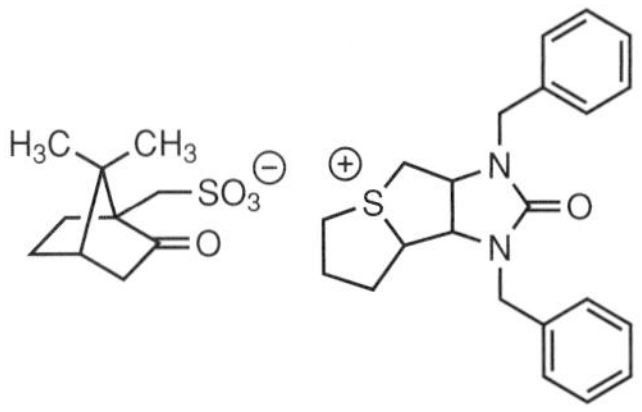   Trimethaphan camsylate

They are competitive antagonists at nicotinic acetylcholine receptors. Trimethaphan is a quaternary sulfonium ion and cannot cross lipid cell membranes, whereas mecamylamine is a secondary amine. Therefore, trimethaphan is a short-acting peripheral direct vasodilator that must be given as an IV infusion, whereas mecamylamine can be given orally. Mecamylamine rapidly disappears from the blood with a plasma half-life of 1 hour, and crosses the blood-brain barrier into the CNS. Trimethaphan is rapidly excreted in unchanged form by the kidney. Mecamylamine is excreted by the kidney much more slowly. Trimethaphan is the drug of choice for managing acute aortic dissection and for hypertensive emergencies. Both drugs are of limited use, because of the availability of more specific acting vasodilators. Mecamylamine has been used for labeling CNS nicotinic receptors and crosses into the CNS, where it can block neuronal nicotinic acetylcholine receptors. Mecamylamine has been studied for use with nicotine for smoking cessation.

Side Effects and Contraindications. Side effects of trimethaphan include prolonged neuromuscular blockade and potentiation of neuromuscular blocking agents. It can produce excessive hypotension and impotence (because of its sympatholytic effect) as well as constipation, urinary retention, and dry mouth (because of its parasympatholytic effect).

PULMONARY ARTERIAL HYPERTENSION

Pulmonary hypertension, which was once a rare life-threatening disease, reportedly affects about 160,000 people today. Pulmonary arterial hypertension (PAH) is defined as a group of diseases characterized by a progressive increase of pulmonary vascular resistance, leading to right ventricular failure. It includes a variety of pulmonary hypertensive diseases with different etiologies but similar clinical presentation (36). Primary pulmonary hypertension can occur, without any apparent cause (idiopathic), or can be inherited. Pulmonary arterial hypertension is a disease of the small pulmonary arteries, characterized by progressive narrowing of the pulmonary vascular bed. Vasoconstriction and scarring (or fibrosis) cause the pulmonary wall to become stiffer and thicker, contributing to an increased pulmonary vascular resistance. This extra stress causes the heart to enlarge and become less flexible. Less blood flows from the heart, through the lungs, and into the body, resulting in additional symptoms. One direct effect of these abnormally elevated pressures is blood leakage from the pulmonary vessels. A blood-producing cough often is an indicator of leakage from the pulmonary vessels. The pulmonary arterial walls produce a substance called endothelin, which causes these blood vessels to constrict. The reasons for this overproduction are unknown. In some cases, the cause is genetically programmed or the person is predisposed genetically to primary pulmonary hypertension after being exposed to a certain drug (e.g. the diet drugs Fen-Phen [fenfluramine/phentermine], Redux [dexfenfluramine], or Pondimin [fenfluramine]).

Often, primary pulmonary hypertension is not diagnosed in a timely manner, because its early symptoms can be confused with those of many other conditions (Table 29.4). To establish a diagnosis of pulmonary hypertension, a series of tests are performed that show how well a person's heart and lungs are working. These tests may include assessment of daily living tasks, such as a 6-minute walk test, a computed tomography scan to rule out a pulmonary embolism or lung disease, a pulmonary function test to rule out obstructive lung disease, a formal sleep study to rule out sleep apnea, and laboratory tests to rule out hepatitis, collagen disease, HIV, or other conditions.

Rationale for Pharmacologic Treatment

If PAH has an identifiable cause, then measures can be taken to correct the underlying problem. If the diagnosis

Table 29.4. Symptoms of Primary Pulmonary Hypertension

Breathlessness or shortness of breath
Feeling tired all the time
Dizziness, especially when climbing stairs or standing up
Fainting (often the symptom that brings people to their doctors)
Swollen ankles and legs
Chest pain, especially during physical activity

is primary PAH, then pharmacologic intervention is required to reduce the pressure. This is done using vasodilator drugs to decrease pulmonary vascular resistance and, thereby, to lower the pressure. Adjunct therapy may include diuretics to reduce blood volume, which will reduce central venous pressure and right ventricular stroke volume, as well as to reduce some of the signs and symptoms of edema and shortness of breath associated with PAH. Anticoagulants are administered to prevent the formation of pulmonary thrombi. Patients with cardiovascular hypertension generally are treated with antihypertensive drugs that reduce blood volume (which reduces central venous pressure and cardiac output), reduce systemic vascular resistance, or reduce cardiac output by depressing heart rate and stroke volume.

Drugs Used to Treat Pulmonary Hypertension

Classes of drugs used in the treatment of PAH include thiazide diuretics, loop diuretics, vasodilators, calcium channel blockers, prostaglandins, endothelin receptor antagonists, NO, and PDE5 inhibitors (38). During the last decade, substantial improvements in the therapeutic options for PAH have emerged that target the mechanisms involved in the pathogenesis of this devastating disease. Intravenous epoprostenol was the first drug to improve symptoms and survival of patients with PAH (40). Novel prostanoids, including subcutaneous treprostinil and inhaled iloprost, have beneficial effects in many patients, although their long-term efficacy is less well known. Among the newer treatments for PAH, endothelin receptor antagonists and PDE5 inhibitors have reshaped clinical practice. The endothelin receptor antagonist bosentan has been approved, and most guidelines recommend this drug as first-line treatment for patients with PAH and New York Heart Association (NYHA) functional class III heart failure (i.e., patients with marked limitation of activity; they are comfortable only at rest). Novel endothelin receptor antagonists, such as sitaxsentan sodium and ambrisentan, are currently being investigated. The combination of the PDE5 inhibitor sildenafil and iloprost, prostacyclin analogue, are being intensively studied in patients with pulmonary hypertension. Targeting a single pathway cannot be expected to be uniformly successful, because PAH is a complex disorder. Thus, combining substances with different modes of action is expected to improve symptoms, hemodynamics, and survival in PAH patients, although combination therapy has yet to undergo the scrutiny of large randomized clinical trials.

Specific Drugs

Phosphodiesterase Inhibitors

SILDENAFIL (REVATIO). Sildenafil has recently been approved for treatment of PAH through its inhibition of cGMP and smooth muscle relaxation of the pulmonary vasculature. The reader is referred to the previous discussion of phosphodiesterase inhibitors under the topic of vasodilators.

Endothelin Receptor Antagonists

MECHANISM OF ACTION. Endothelin-1 (ET-1) is a 21-amino-acid peptide that is produced by the vascular endothelium. It is a very potent vasoconstrictor that binds to VSM endothelin receptors ET_A and ET_B(Fig. 29.1). The ET-1 receptors are linked to the G_q protein and IP_3 signal transduction pathway (Fig. 29.11). Therefore, ET-1 causes sarcoplasmic reticulum release of calcium, increasing the VSM contractility. Vascular endothelial cells secrete the majority of ET-1. The endothelins bind to two receptor subtypes: ET_A, and ET_B. In vascular tissue, ET_A is located predominantly on smooth muscle cells, whereas ET_B is found on both endothelial and smooth muscle cells. Activation of ET_A by ET-1 leads to potent vasoconstriction from an increase in cytosolic calcium levels via influx of extracellular calcium and release from intracellular stores (Fig. 29.1). The actions of ET_B are more complicated. Like ET_A, ET-1 activation of ET_B on VSM cells leads to vasoconstriction. Furthermore, some studies suggest that in the pulmonary hypertensive state, blockade of both ET_A and ET_B is necessary to achieve maximal vasodilation. Activation of ET-B by

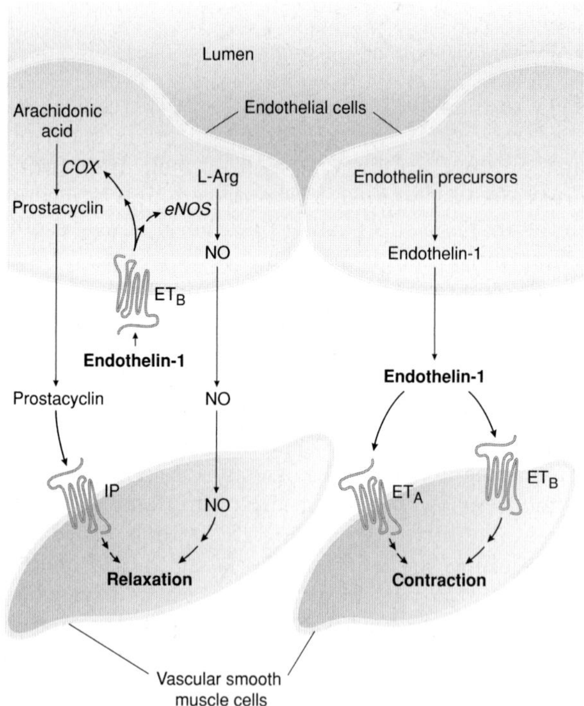

Fig. 29.11. The effects of endothelin-1, prostacyclin and nitric oxide on the contraction and relaxation (vasodilation) of vascular smooth muscle cells. (From Yeh DC, Michel T. Pharmacology of Vascular Tone. In: Golan DE, Tashjian AH, Armstrong E, et al., Principles of Pharmacology: The Pathophysiologic Basis of Drug Therapy. Baltimore: Lippincott Williams & Wilkins, 2004; with permission)

ET-1 stimulates cyclooxygenase (COX) which catalyzes the formation of prostacyclin from arachidonic acid. Prostacyclin then binds to and activates the isoprostanoid receptor (IP) on VSM. ET-1 also activates ET-B which stimulates endothelial nitric oxide synthease (eNOS) to produce NO from L-arginine. Both prostacyclin and NO are potent vasodilators of VSM (relaxation). Additionally, ET-1 binds to the ET_B receptors on the endothelium of pulmonary smooth muscle and stimulate the formation of NO, which produces vasodilation in the absence of smooth muscle ET_A and ET_B receptor activation. This receptor distribution helps to explain the phenomenon that ET-1 administration causes transient vasodilation (initial endothelial ET_B activation) and hypotension, followed by prolonged vasoconstriction (smooth muscle ET_A and ET_B activation) and hypertension.

Therapeutic indications. Because of its powerful vasoconstrictor properties and its effects on intracellular calcium, ET-1 has been implicated in the pathogenesis of hypertension, coronary vasospasm, and heart failure. A number of studies suggest a role for ET-1 in pulmonary hypertension as well as in systemic hypertension. Additionally, ET-1 has been shown to be released by the failing myocardium, where it can contribute to cardiac calcium overload and hypertrophy.

Endothelin receptor antagonists, by blocking the vasoconstrictor and cardiotonic effects of ET-1, produce vasodilation and cardiac inhibition. Endothelin receptor antagonists have been shown to decrease mortality and to improve hemodynamics in experimental models of heart failure.

At present, the only approved indication for endothelin antagonists is pulmonary hypertension.

Specific drugs

Bosentan (Tracleer)

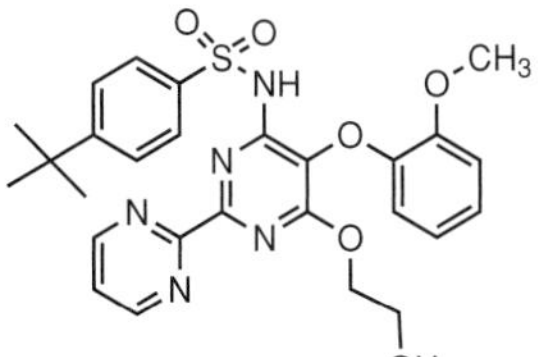

Bosentan

Bosentan is an orally administered, nonselective ET-1 receptor antagonist blocking ET_A and ET_B receptors and is approved for the treatment of patients with PAH. Following oral administration, bosentan attains peak plasma concentrations in approximately 3 hours, with an absolute bioavailability of approximately 50%. Food has no clinically relevant effect on its absorption recommended doses. Bosentan is approximately 98% bound to albumin, with a volume of distribution of 30 L. Its terminal half-life after oral administration is 5.4 hours and is unchanged at steady state. Steady-state concentrations are achieved within 3 to 5 days after multiple-dose administration. Bosentan is mainly eliminated from the body by hepatic metabolism and subsequent biliary excretion of the metabolites. Three metabolites have been identified, formed by CYP2C9 and CYP3A4 (Fig. 29.12). The pharmacokinetics of bosentan are dose-proportional up to 500 mg/day (multiple doses). The pharmacokinetics of bosentan in pediatric patients with PAH are comparable to those in healthy subjects, whereas adult patients with PAH show a twofold increase in clearance. Severe renal impairment and mild hepatic impairment do not have a clinically relevant influence on its pharmacokinetics. Bosentan generally should be avoided in patients with moderate or severe hepatic impairment and/or elevated liver aminotransferases. Inhibitors of CYP3A4 increase the plasma concentration of bosentan as well as cause an increase in the clearance of drugs metabolized by CYP3A4 and CYP2C9 because of induction of these metabolizing enzymes. The possibility of reduced efficacy of CYP2C9 and CYP3A4 substrates coadministered with bosentan is increased. No clinically relevant interaction was detected for P-glycoprotein. Bosentan can increase plasma levels of ET-1. Adverse effects include hypotension, headache, flushing, increased liver aminotransferases, leg edema, and anemia. Bosentan may cause birth defects and, therefore, is contraindicated in pregnancy. It also can cause liver injury.

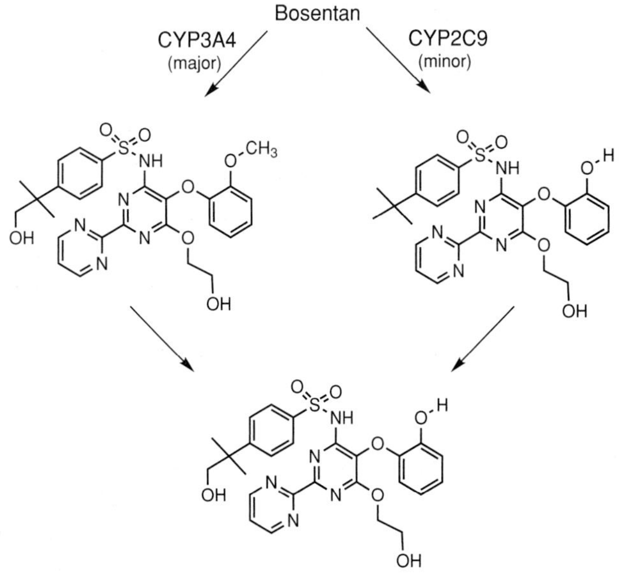

Bosentan
CYP3A4 (major)
CYP2C9 (minor)

Fig. 29.12. Metabolism of bosentan.

Prostanoids (39)

Epoprostenol (Flolan). Prostacyclin and its analogs (prostanoids) (Fig. 29.13) are potent vasodilators and possess antithrombotic and antiproliferative properties. Prostacyclin is derived from the endothelium of VSM, and its synthesis is reduced in patients with PAH. Its physiological antagonist, thromboxane A_2, is increased, however, causing vasoconstriction. Prostacyclin produces its vasodilation via activation of the PIP_2 signal transduction pathway, increasing concentrations of cAMP (Fig. 29.11). Epoprostenol is the sodium salt of prostacyclin and is administered as an implanted, continuous IV infusion because of its very short duration of action (2–3 minutes). It must be reconstituted with a special glycine buffer diluent, giving a reconstituted solution with pH 10 to 11 that is stable for 15 minutes at 4°C and for less than 10 minutes at 37°C. Its injection solution is unstable at a lower pH because of acid-catalyzed hydrolysis of the vinylether structure to 6-oxo-$PGF_{1\alpha}$ (Fig. 29.13). It is short acting because of rapid metabolism at the 15-hydroxy group to the inactive 15-oxo metabolite.

Treprostinil (Remodulin). Treprostinil (Fig. 29.13) is a synthetic, stable form of prostacyclin for the treatment for advanced pulmonary hypertension with NYHA class III or IV symptoms as well as for late-stage peripheral vascular disease (PVD). Its sodium salt injectable form is administered either as a continuous subcutaneous infusion directly into the skin or, if the subcutaneous infusion is not tolerated, as a continuous IV infusion without an implanted catheter. Treprostinil is rapidly absorbed from the subcutaneous site of infusion, with an almost 100% bioavailability and a mean half-life of 85 minutes (34 minutes for the IV infusion). The IV solution must be diluted with normal saline or sterile water before starting the infusion. Unlike epoprostenol, treprostinil is stable at room temperature for up to 5 years, with vasodilation action lasting from 4 to 6 hours, compared with the short, 2- to 3-minute action for epoprostenol. Because of its long life in the body, it can be administered under the skin with a microinfusion subcutaneous infusion pump rather than into the bloodstream and, thus, without hospitalization, as contrasted with the central IV infusion of epoprostenol.

Side effects include jaw pain, headaches, nausea, diarrhea, flushing, and localized pain at the delivery site under the skin. This pain has been reported as slight to severe irritation. Patients using the drug seem to experience improvement in their condition, including decreased fatigue, decreased shortness of breath, and decreased pulmonary artery pressures, as well as overall improvement in quality of life.

Beraprost. Beraprost is an oral formulation of a prostacyclin analog for the treatment of early stage pulmonary hypertension as well as early stage PVD. Beraprost is a chemically stable, oral form of prostacyclin that is readily absorbed from GI tract. Like natural prostacyclin, beraprost dilates blood vessels, prevents platelet aggregation, and prevents proliferation of smooth muscle cells surrounding blood vessels. It may be an important treatment for early stage PVD and for early stage pulmonary hypertension. Intermittent oral doses of beraprost, however, do not seem to provide the consistent blood levels

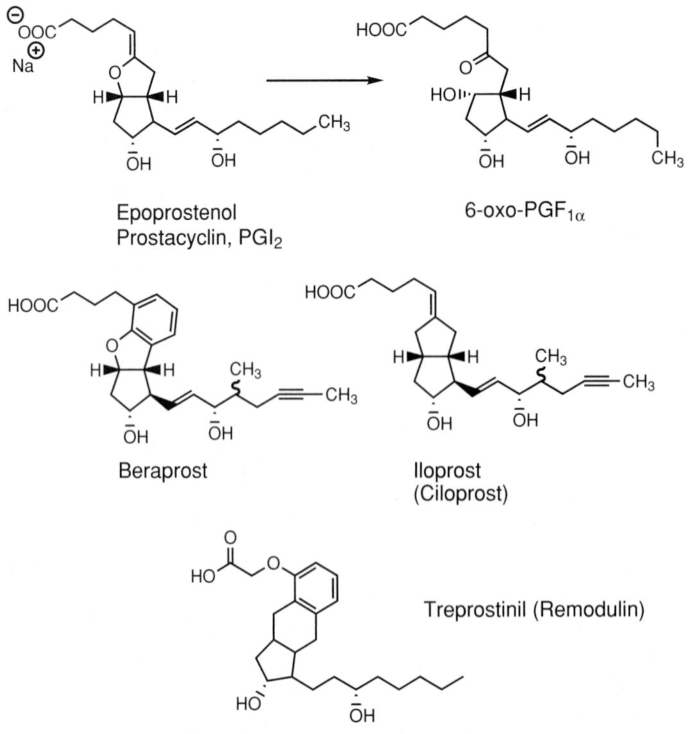

Fig. 29.13. Prostacyclin analogs.

necessary to treat the advanced stages of pulmonary hypertension. Beraprost has proven to be safe and effective for the treatment of PVD in the clinical studies conducted, and it has been approved for the treatment of PVD in Japan since 1994. It may soon be available for use in patients with pulmonary hypertension in the United States. Adverse effects include headache, flushing, jaw pain, and diarrhea.

Iloprost (Ventavis). Iloprost is administered as an inhalation solution of a prostacyclin analog for the treatment of NYHA class III and class IV PAH. The drug also can be administered as an IV infusion. It is stable at room temperature and to light, with a body half-life of 30 minutes. Iloprost has approximately 10 times greater potency than prostacyclin as a vasodilator of the pulmonary blood vessels; this greater potency of inhaled iloprost results from coating of the drug on the alveoli of the lungs. It relieves pulmonary vascular resistance. Patients inhale six to eight puffs every 2 to 3 hours. Each puff lasts approximately 15 minutes. This therapy is used mainly in Europe and is not available in United States. Studies have reported minor side effects, such as coughing, headaches, and jaw pain.

CASE STUDY

Victoria F. Roche and S. William Zito

KG is a 73-year-old, single, retired bank executive living in Paris who is in the early stages of Alzheimer's disease. Four months ago, she began therapy with tacrine HCl (Cognex currently 20 mg q.i.d.), which seems to be halting the advance of dementia. She experienced some dyspepsia from the tacrine which is being treated with omeprazole (Prilosec), as well as mild bradycardia which is not currently interfering with her function. Although she no longer smokes cigarettes, KG does have mild emphysema from her years as a pack-a-day smoker. Most recently, she has experienced urinary incontinence. "Accidents" have been few, but she now wears protective undergarments. Her only other medication is calcium atorvastatin (Lipitor, 10 mg q.d.) for elevated plasma low-density lipoprotein and total cholesterol. KG invested wisely as a young woman, owns a chalet on the outskirts of the city, and is able to afford quality in-home assistance. An attentive niece who studies art at the Sorbonne lives with her.

KG has been borderline hypertensive for several years and elected to keep things under control with diet and a walking regimen. She did well restricting her fat and overall calorie consumption, but she found it very difficult to effectively monitor her sodium intake. Her blood pressure is now elevated to the point that antihypertensive therapy is no longer optional. Consider the sympatholytic choices shown below, and prepare to make a therapeutic recommendation (en Francais).

1. Identify the therapeutic problem(s) in which the pharmacist's intervention may benefit the patient.
2. Identify and prioritize the patient-specific factors that must be considered to achieve the desired therapeutic outcomes.
3. Conduct a thorough and mechanistically oriented structure–activity analysis of all therapeutic alternatives provided in the case.
4. Evaluate the structure–activity relationship findings against the patient-specific factors and desired therapeutic outcomes, and make a therapeutic decision.
5. Counsel your patient

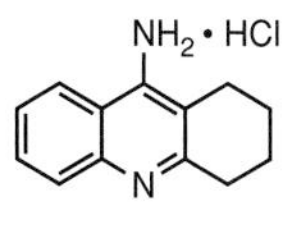

Tacrine

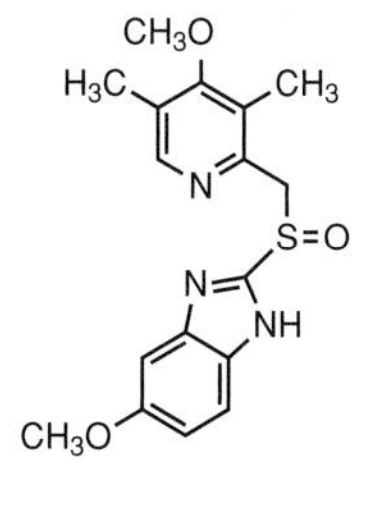

Omeprazole

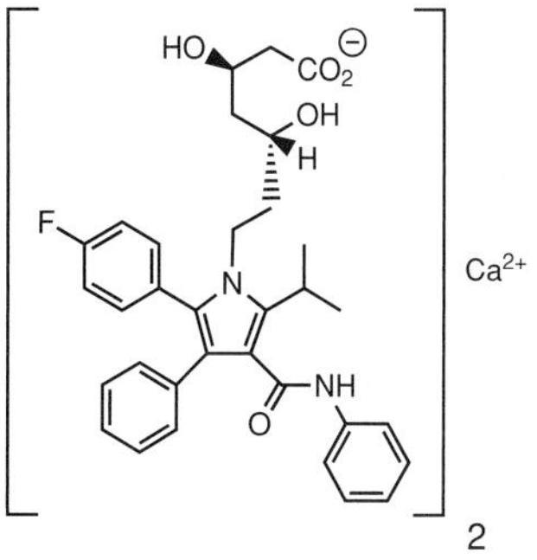

Atorvastatin

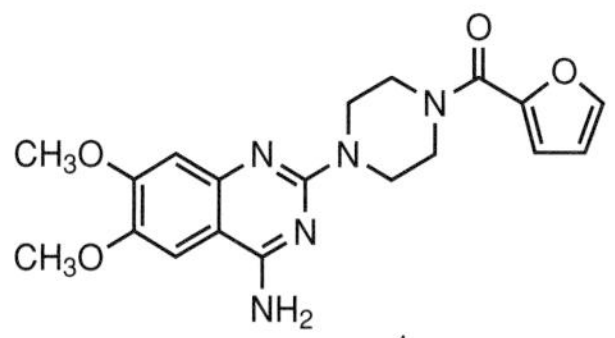

1

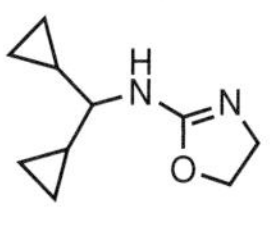

2

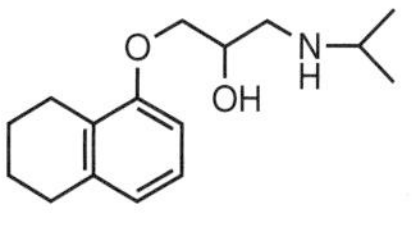

3

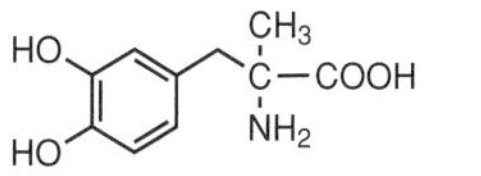

4

References

1. Yeh D, Michel T. Pharmacology of vascular tone. In: Goan DE, Tashjian A, Armstrong E, et al., eds. Principles of Pharmacology: The Pathophysiologic Basis of Drug Therapy. Baltimore: Lippincott Williams &Wilkins, 2004, pp. 317–330.
2. Weibert RT. Hypertension. In: Herfindal ET, Gourley DR, eds. Textbook of Therapeutics: Drug and Disease Management, 7th Ed. Baltimore: Lippincott Williams & Wilkins, 2000:795–824.
3. The Sixth Report of the Joint National Committee on Prevention, Detection, Evaluation, and Treatment of High Blood Pressure (JNC VI). Arch Intern Med. 1997;157:2413–2446.
4. Brown MJ. Haydock S. Pathoetiology, epidemiology, and diagnosis of hypertension. Drugs 2000;59(Suppl. 2):1–12.
5. Sibai B. Treatment of hypertension in pregnant women. N Engl J Med 1996;335:257–265.
6. McEvoy GK, ed. AHFS 2000 Drug Information. Bethesda, MD: American Society of Health-System Pharmacists, 2000:1658–1726.
7. Kaplan NM. Combination therapy for systemic hypertension. Am J Cardiol 1995;76:595–597.
8. Abernethy DR. Pharmacological properties of combination therapies for hypertension. Am J Hypertens 1997;10:13S–16S.
9. Hoffman B. Therapy of hypertension. In: Brunton LL, Lazo JS, Parker KL, eds. Goodman and Gilman's The Pharmacologic Basis of Therapeutics, 11th Ed. New York: McGraw-Hill, 2006:845–869.
10. Robertson JIS. State-of-the-art review: β-blockade and the treatment of hypertension. Drugs 1983;25(Suppl. 2):5–11.
11. Freis ED, Papademetriou V. Current drug treatment and treatment patterns with antihypertensive drugs. Drugs 1996;52:1–16.
12. Husserl FE, Messerli FH. Adverse effects of antihypertensive drugs. Drugs 1981;22:188–210.
13. Goldberg M, Fenster PE. Clinical significance of intrinsic sympathomimetic activity of beta blockers. Drug Therapy 1991:35–43.
14. Cauffield JS, Gums JG, Curry RW. Alpha blockers: A reassessment of their role in therapy. Am Fam Physician 1996;54:263–270.
15. Dunn CJ, Lea AP, Wagstaff AJ. Carvedilol. A reappraisal of its pharmacologica properties and therapeutic use in cardiovascular disorders. Drugs 1997;54: 161–185.
16. Goa KL, Benfield P, Sorkin EM. Labetalol: A reappraisal of its pharmacology, pharmacokinetics, and therapeutic use in hypertension and ischemic heart disease. Drugs 1989;37:583–627.
17. Van Zwieten PA. An overview of the pharmacodynamic properties and therapeutic potential of combined α- and β-adrenoreceptor antagonists. Drugs 1993;45:509–517.
18. Skerjanec A, Campbell NRC, Robertson S, et al. Pharmacokinetics and presystemic gut metabolism of methyldopa in healthy human subjects. J Clin Pharmacol 1995;35:275–280.
19. Bousquet P, Feldman J. Drugs acting on imidazoline receptors. A review of their pharmacology, their use in blood pressure control, and their potential interest in cardioprotection. Drugs 1999;58:799–812.
20. Piletz JE, Regunathan S, Ernsberger P. Agmatine and imidazolines: their novel receptors and enzymes. Ann N Y Acad Sci 2003;1009–1043.
21. Dardonville C, Rozas I.. Imidazoline binding sites and their ligands: an overview of the different chemical structures. Med Res Rev 2004;24:639–661
22. Ziegler D, Haxhiu MA, Kaan EC, et al. Pharmacology of moxonidine, an I_1–imidazoline receptor agonist. J Cardiovascular Pharmacol 1996;27(Suppl. 3):S26–S37.
23. Theodor R, Weimann HJ, Weber W, et al. Absolute bioavailability of moxonidine. Eur J Drug Metab Pharmacokinet 1991;16:153–159.
24. Chrisp P, Faulds D. Moxonidine: a review of its pharmacology, and therapeutic use in essential hypertension. Drugs 1992;44:993–1012.
25. Genissel P, Bromet N, Fourtillan JB, et al. Pharmacokinetics of rilmenidine in healthy subjects. Am J Cardiol 1988;61:47D–53D.
26. Genissel P, Bromet N. Pharmacokinetics of rilmenidine. Am J Med 1989;87:8S–23S.
27. Langley MS, Heel RC. Transdermal clonidine. A preliminary review of its pharmacodynamic properties and therapeutic efficacy. Drugs 1988;35:123–142.
28. Fujimura A, Ebihara A, Ohashi K-I, et al. Comparison of the pharmacokinetics, pharmacodynamics, and safety of oral (Catapres) and transdermal (M-5041T) clonidine in healthy subjects. J Clin Pharmacol 1994;34:260–265.
29. Ebihara A, Fujimura A, Ohashi K-I, et al. Influence of application site of a new transdermal clonidine, M-5041T, on its pharmacokinetics and pharmacodynamics in healthy subjects. J Clin Pharmacol 1993;33:1188–1191.
30. Holmes B, Brogden RN, Heel RC, et al. Guanabenz. A review of its pharmacodynamic properties and therapeutic efficacy in hypertension. Drugs 1983;26:212–229.
31. Sorkin EM, Heel RC. Guanfacine: a review of its pharmacodynamic and pharmacokinetic properties, and therapeutic efficacy in the treatment of hypertension. Drugs 1986;31:301–336.
32. Cornish LA. Guanfacine hydrochloride. A centrally acting antihypertensive agent. Clinical Pharmacy 1988;7:187–197.
33. Carchman SH, Crowe JT Jr, Wright GJ. The bioavailability and pharmacokinetics of guanfacine after oral and intravenous administration to healthy volunteers. J Clin Pharmacol 1987;27:762–767.
34. Finnerty FA Jr, Brogden RN. Guanadrel. A review of its pharmacodynamic and pharmacokinetic properties and therapeutic use in hypertension. Drugs 1985;30:22–31.
35. Campese VM. Minoxidil: a review of its pharmacological properties and therapeutic use. Drugs 1981;22:257–278.
36. Clissold SP, Heel RC. Topical minoxidil: a preliminary review of its pharmacodynamic properties and therapeutic efficacy in alopecia areata and alopecia androgenetica. Drugs 1987;33:107–122.
37. Duty S, Weston AH. Potassium channel openers. Pharmacological effects and future uses. Drugs 1990;40:785–791.
38. Golpon HA, Welte T, Hoeper MM. Pulmonary arterial hypertension: pathobiology, diagnosis, and treatment. Minerva Med 2005;96:303–314.
39. Hoeper MM. Drug treatment of pulmonary arterial hypertension: current and future agents. Drugs 2005;65:1337–1354.
40. Olschewski H, Rose F, Schermuly R, et al. Prostacyclin and its analogues in the treatment of pulmonary hypertension. Pharmacol Ther 2004;102:139–153.
41. Velliquette R-A, Kossover R, Previs S-F, et al. Lipid-lowering actions of imidazoline antihypertensive agents in metabolic syndrome X. Naunyn Schmiedebergs Arch Pharmacol 2006;372:300–312.

30. *Antihyperlipoproteinemics and Inhibitors of Cholesterol Biosynthesis*

MARC HARROLD

DRUGS COVERED IN THIS CHAPTER:

- Atorvastatin
- Cholestyramine
- Clofibric acid
- Colesevelam
- Colestipol
- Ezetimibe
- Fenofibric acid
- Fluvastatin
- Gemfibrozil
- Lovastatin
- Mevastatin
- Nicotinic acid/Niacin
- Pravastatin
- Rosuvastatin
- Simvastatin

THE CHEMISTRY AND BIOCHEMISTRY OF PLASMA LIPIDS

The major lipids found in the bloodstream are cholesterol, cholesterol esters, triglycerides, and phospholipids. An excess plasma concentration of one or more of these compounds is known as hyperlipidemia. Because all lipids require the presence of soluble lipoproteins to be transported in the blood, hyperlipidemia ultimately results in an increased concentration of these transport molecules, a condition known as hyperlipoproteinemia. Hyperlipoproteinemia has been strongly associated with atherosclerotic lesions and coronary heart disease (CHD) (1,2). Before discussing lipoproteins, their role in cardiovascular disease, and agents to decrease their concentrations, it is essential to examine the biochemistry of cholesterol, triglycerides, and phospholipids.

Synthesis and Degradation of Cholesterol

Cholesterol is a C_{27} steroid that serves as an important component of all cell membranes and as the precursor for androgens, estrogens, progesterone, and adrenocorticoids (Fig. 30.1). It is synthesized from acetyl coenzyme A (CoA), as shown in Figure 30.2 (4). The first stage of the biosynthesis is the formation of isopentenyl pyrophosphate from three acetyl CoA molecules. The conversion of 3-hydroxy-3-methylglutaryl (HMG)–CoA to mevalonic acid is especially important, because it is a primary control site for cholesterol biosynthesis. This reaction is catalyzed by HMG-CoA reductase and reduces the thioester of HMG-CoA to a primary hydroxyl group. The second stage involves the coupling of six isopentenyl pyrophosphate molecules to form squalene. Initially, three isopentenyl pyrophosphate molecules are condensed to form farnesyl pyrophosphate, a C_{15} intermediate. Two farnesyl pyrophosphate molecules are then combined using a similar type of reaction. The next stage involves the cyclization of squalene to lanosterol. This process involves an initial epoxidation of squalene, followed by a subsequent cyclization requiring a concerted flow of four pairs of electrons and the migration of two methyl groups. The final stage

Squalene Synthase: A Potential Drug Target

Inhibitors of squalene synthase, the enzyme responsible for catalyzing the two-step conversion of two molecules of farnesyl pyrophosphate to squalene, are currently being investigated as antihyperlipidemic agents. Squalene synthase catalyzes the first committed step in sterol biosynthesis and offers some potential advantages over 3-hydroxy-3-methylglutaryl–coenzyme A (HMG-CoA) reductase as a drug target. The latter group of compounds inhibits cholesterol synthesis at an early stage of the pathway and, thus, lacks specificity. Mevalonic acid, the immediate product of HMG-CoA reductase, is a common intermediate in the biosynthesis of other isoprenoids, such as ubiquinone (an electron carrier in oxidative phosphorylation), dolichol (a compound involved in oligosaccharide synthesis), and farnesylated proteins (the farnesyl portion targets the protein to cell membrane as opposed to the cytosol). Inhibitors of squalene synthase target an enzyme involved in a later stage of cholesterol biosynthesis and could potentially accomplish the same desired outcomes as currently available agents without interfering with the biosynthesis of other essential, nonsteroidal compounds. One class of compounds currently under investigation are the squalestatins. These compounds were originally isolated as fermentation products produced by a species of *Phoma*. Squalestatin 1 is a potent inhibitor of squalene synthetase and has been shown to produce a marked decrease in serum cholesterol. Additional analogues as well as other structural classes continue to be investigated and, ultimately, may produce alternatives to currently available therapy (5,6).

Squalestatin 1

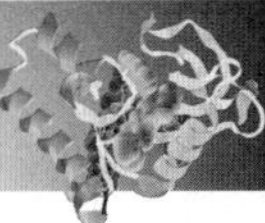

CLINICAL SIGNIFICANCE

The development and availability of cholesterol and triglyceride-lowering agents has evolved significantly over the past 10 to 15 years. The structure–activity relationships and structural modifications of bile acid sequestrants, fibrates, and 3-hydroxy-3-methylglutaryl–coenzyme A reductase inhibitors form the basis for this evolution and the therapeutic advances that have resulted.

The most widely used cholesterol-lowering agents in cardiovascular medicine today are the "statins" (vastatins). Lovastatin was the first statin to be used clinically on a large scale. Structural modifications of the early statin molecules have produced superior agents in terms of their pharmacokinetic profile, potency, drug interactions, and perhaps, selective adverse effects. This has resulted in the widespread clinical use of superior agents, such as atorvastatin. Such agents have been demonstrated in randomized clinical trials to exert a potent effect in lowering low-density lipoprotein (LDL) cholesterol as well as an important anti-inflammatory action.

The net effect of applying basic science in modifying the chemical structure of cholesterol-lowering drugs is that patient outcomes such as death, myocardial infarction, and other cardiovascular events have been vastly improved. This is clearly a situation in which the application of basic science has produced a profound effect on tens of millions of patients.

Thomas L. Rihn, Pharm.D.
Senior Vice President and Chief Clinical Officer
University Pharmacotherapy Associates
Associate Professor of Clinical Pharmacy
Duquesne University
School of Pharmacy

involves the conversion of lanosterol to cholesterol. This process removes three methyl groups from lanosterol, reduces the side-chain double bond, moves the other double bond within the ring structure, and requires approximately 20 steps.

Cholesterol is enzymatically transformed by two different pathways. As illustrated in Figure 30.1, cholesterol can be oxidatively cleaved by the enzyme desmolase (side chain–cleaving enzyme). The resulting compound, pregnenolone, serves as the common intermediate in the biosynthesis of all other endogenous steroids. As illustrated in Figure 30.3, cholesterol also can be converted to bile acids and bile salts. This pathway represents the most important mechanism for cholesterol catabolism. The enzyme 7α-hydroxylase catalyzes the initial, rate-limiting step in this metabolic pathway and, thus, is the key control enzyme for this pathway. Cholic acid and its derivatives are primarily (99%) conjugated with either glycine (75%) or taurine (24%). Bile salts, such as glycocholate, are surface-active agents that act as anionic detergents.

The bile salts are synthesized in the liver, stored in the gallbladder, and released into the small intestine, where they emulsify dietary lipids and fat-soluble vitamins. This solubilization promotes the absorption of these dietary compounds through the intestinal mucosa. Bile salts are predominantly reabsorbed through the enterohepatic circulation and returned to the liver, where they exert a negative feedback control on 7α-hydroxylase and, thus, regulate any subsequent conversion of cholesterol (4,7).

The terms "bile acid" and "bile salt" refer to the un-ionized and ionized forms, respectively, of these compounds. For illustrative purposes only, Figure 30.3 shows cholic acid as a un-ionized bile acid and glycocholate as an ionized bile salt (as the sodium salt). At physiologic and intestinal pH values, both compounds would exist almost exclusively in their ionized forms.

Overview of Triglycerides and Phospholipids

Triglycerides (or, more appropriately, triacylglycerols) are highly concentrated stores of metabolic energy. They are formed from glycerol 3-phosphate and acylated CoA (Fig. 30.4) and accumulate primarily in the cytosol of adipose cells. When required for energy production, triglycerides are hydrolyzed by lipase enzymes to liberate free fatty acids that are then subjected to β-oxidation, the citric acid cycle, and oxidative phosphorylation.

Phospholipids, or phosphoglycerides, are amphipathic compounds that are used to make cell membranes, generate second messengers, and store fatty acids for use in the generation of prostaglandins. They can be synthesized from phosphatidate, an intermediate in triglyceride synthesis. Two common phospholipids, phosphatidyl choline and phosphatidyl inositol, are shown below (4).

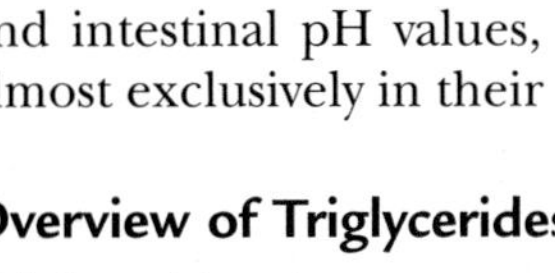

Phosphatidyl choline

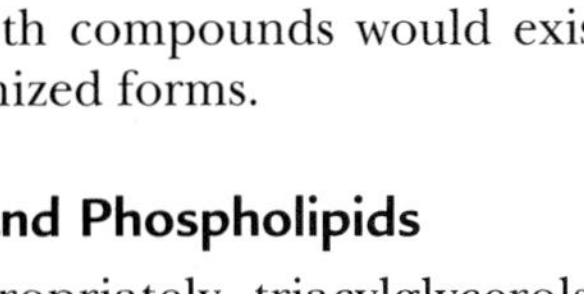

Phosphatidyl inositol

Lipoproteins and Transport of Cholesterol and Triglycerides

Cholesterol, triglycerides, and phospholipids are freely soluble in organic solvents, such as isopropanol, chloroform, and diethyl ether, but are relatively insoluble in

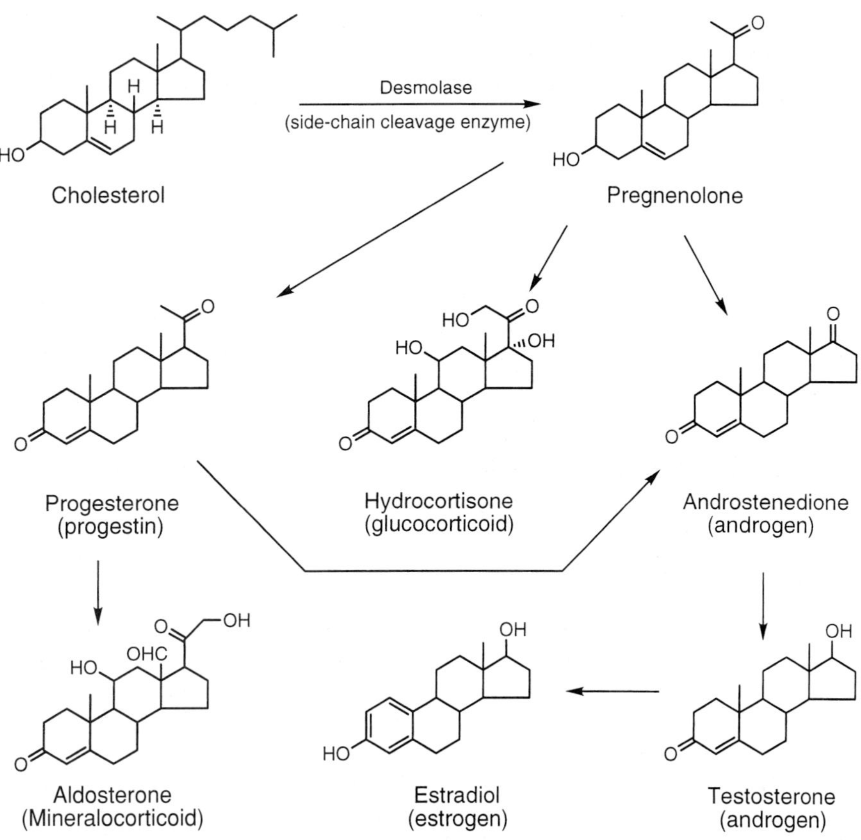

Fig. 30.1. Cholesterol's role as a key intermediate in the biosynthesis of endogenous steroids.

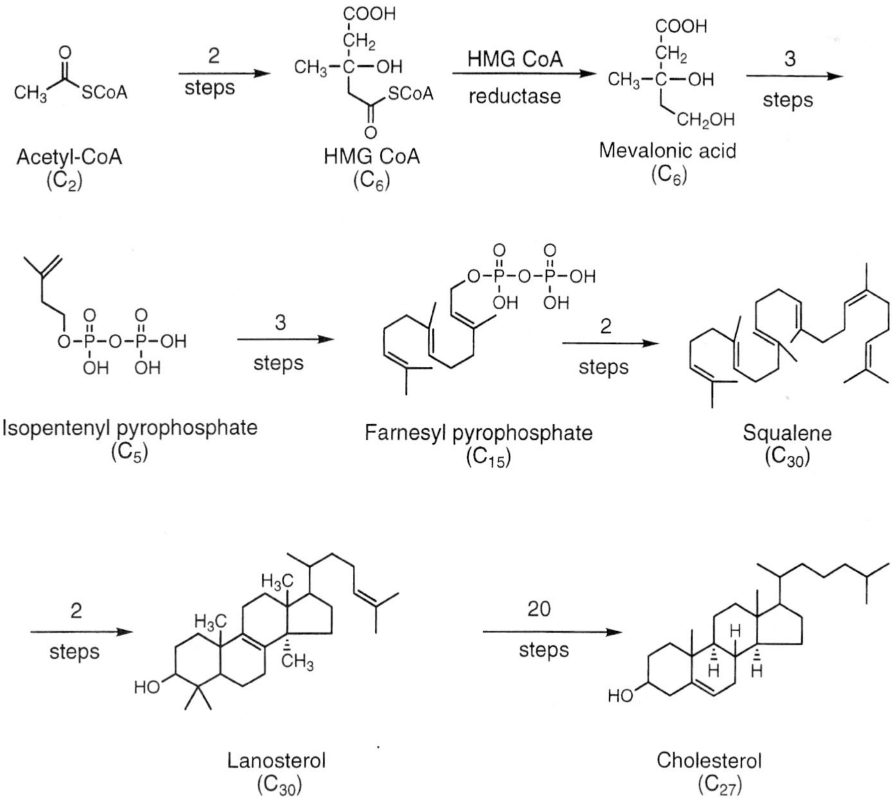

Acetyl-CoA (C_2)
2 steps
HMG CoA (C_6)
HMG CoA reductase
Mevalonic acid (C_6)
3 steps
Isopentenyl pyrophosphate (C_5)
3 steps
Farnesyl pyrophosphate (C_{15})
2 steps
Squalene (C_{30})
2 steps
Lanosterol (C_{30})
20 steps
Cholesterol (C_{27})

Fig. 30.2. The biosynthesis of cholesterol.

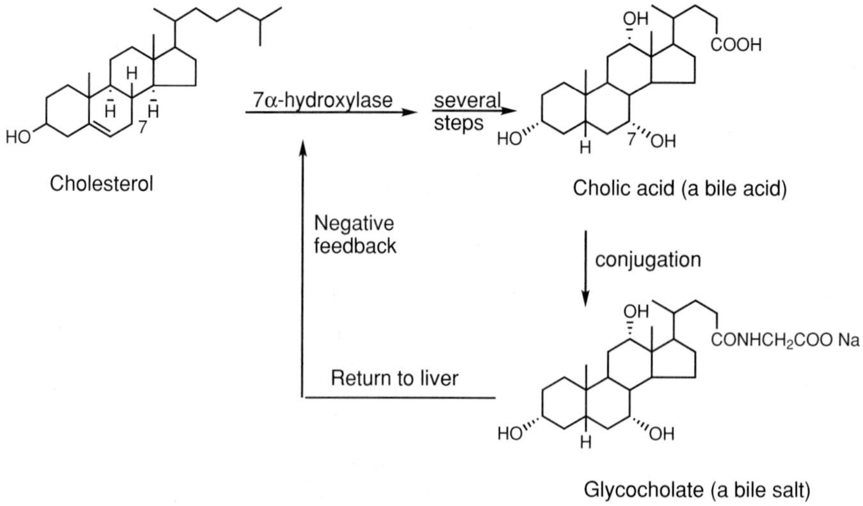

Fig. 30.3. The conversion of cholesterol to bile acids and bile salts.

aqueous, physiologic fluids. To be transported within the blood, these lipids are solubilized through association with macromolecular aggregates known as lipoproteins. Each lipoprotein is associated with additional proteins, known as apolipoproteins, on their outer surface. These apolipoproteins provide structural support and stability, bind to cellular receptors, and act as cofactors for enzymes involved in lipoprotein metabolism. The compositions and primary functions of the six major lipoproteins are listed in Table 30.1 (7,8).

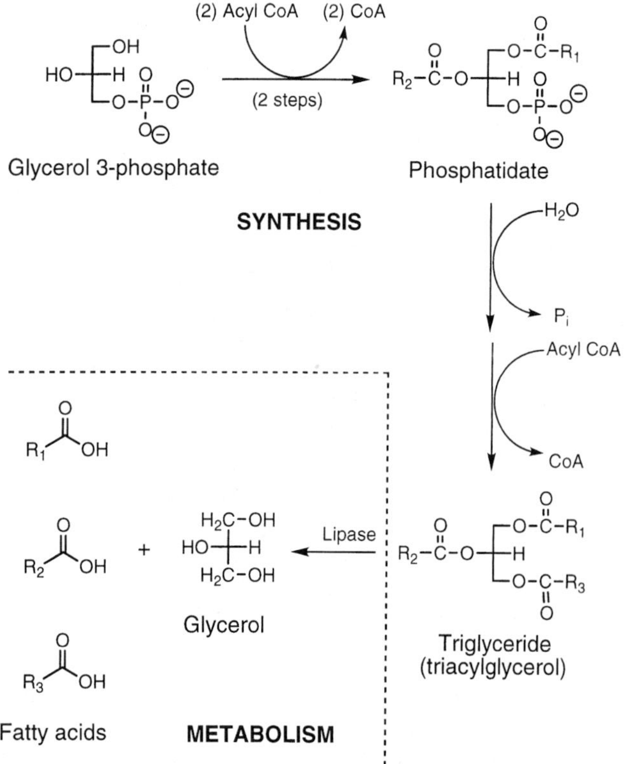

Fig. 30.4. The biosynthesis and metabolism of triglycerides.

Lipoprotein nomenclature is based on mode of separation. When preparative ultracentrifugation is used, lipoproteins are separated according to their density and identified as very-low-density lipoproteins (VLDLs), intermediate-density lipoproteins (IDLs), low-density lipoproteins (LDLs), and high-density lipoproteins (HDLs). When electrophoresis is employed in the separation, lipoproteins are designated as pre-β, β, and α. The IDLs are mainly found in the pre-β fraction as a second electrophoretic band and are currently believed to be an intermediate lipoprotein in the catabolism of VLDL to LDL. Chylomicron remnants and IDLs may show similar electrophoretic and ultracentrifugation separation characteristics. In general, VLDL, LDL, and HDL correspond to pre-β, β, and α lipoprotein, respectively.

The interrelationship among the lipoproteins is shown in Figure 30.5 (7,8). As illustrated, the pathway can be divided into both exogenous (dietary intake) and endogenous (synthetic) components. The exogenous pathway begins following the ingestion of a fat-containing meal or snack. Dietary lipids are absorbed in the form of cholesterol and fatty acids. The fatty acids are then reesterified within the intestinal mucosal cells and, along with the cholesterol, are incorporated into chylomicrons, the largest lipoprotein. During circulation, chylomicrons are degraded into remnants by the action of lipoprotein lipase, a plasma membrane enzyme located on capillary endothelial cells in adipose and muscle tissue. The interaction of chylomicrons with lipoprotein lipase requires apolipoprotein (apo) C-II, and the absence of either the enzyme or the apolipoprotein can lead to hypertriglyceridemia and pancreatitis. The liberated free acids are then available for either storage or energy generation by these tissues. The remnants are predominantly cleared from the plasma by liver parenchymal cells via recognition of the apoE portion of the carrier.

Table 30.1. Classification and Characteristics of Major Plasma Lipoproteins

Classification	Composition	Major Apolipoproteins	Primary Function(s)
Chylomicrons	Triglycerides 80–95%, free cholesterol 1–3%, cholesterol esters 2–4%, phospholipids 3–9%, apoproteins 1–2%	apoA-I, apoA-IV, apoB-48, apoC-I, apoC-II, apoC-III	Transport dietary triglycerides to adipose tissue and muscle for hydrolysis by lipoprotein lipase.
Chylomicron remnants	Primarily composed of dietary cholesterol esters.	apoB-48, apoE	Transport dietary cholesterol to liver for receptor-mediated endocytosis.
VLDL	Triglycerides 50–65%, free cholesterol 4–8%, cholesterol esters 16–22%, phospholipids 15–20%, apoproteins 6–10%	apoB-100, apoE, apoC-I, apoC-II, apoC-III	Transport endogenous triglycerides to adipose tissue and muscle for hydrolysis by lipoprotein lipase.
IDL	Intermediate between VLDL and LDL	apoB-100, apoE, apoC-II, apoC-III	Transport endogenous cholesterol for either conversion to LDL or receptor-mediated endocytosis by the liver.
LDL	Triglycerides 4–8%, free cholesterol 6–8%, cholesterol esters 45–50%, phospholipids 18–24%, apoproteins 18–22%	apoB-100	Transport endogenous cholesterol for receptor-mediated endocytosis by either the liver or extrahepatic tissues.
HDL	Triglycerides 2–7%, free cholesterol 3–5%, cholesterol esters 15–20%, phospholipids 26–32%, apoproteins 45–55%	apoA-I, apoA-II, apoE, apoC-I, apoC-II, apoC-III	Removal of cholesterol from extrahepatic tissues via transfer of cholesterol esters to IDL and LDL

apo, apolipoprotein; VLDL, very-low-density lipoprotein; IDL, intermediate-density lipoprotein; LDL, low-density lipoprotein; HDL, high-density lipoprotein.

The endogenous pathway begins in the liver with the formation of VLDL. Similar to chylomicrons, triglycerides are present in a higher concentration than either cholesterol or cholesterol esters; however, the concentration difference between these lipids is much less than that seen in chylomicrons. The metabolism of VLDL also is similar to chylomicrons in that lipoprotein lipase reduces the triglyceride content of VLDL and increases the availability of free fatty acids to the muscle and adipose tissue. The resulting lipoprotein, IDL, either can be further metabolized to LDL or can be transported to the liver for receptor-mediated endocytosis. This latter effect involves an interaction of the LDL receptor with the apolipoproteins, apoB-100 and apoE, on IDL. The amount of IDL delivered to the liver is approximately the same as that converted to LDL. The half-life of IDL is relatively short as compared to that of LDL and, thus, accounts for only a small portion of total plasma cholesterol. In contrast, LDL accounts for approximately two-thirds of total plasma cholesterol and serves as the primary source of cholesterol for both hepatic and extrahepatic cells. As with IDL, the uptake of LDL by these cells is mediated by a receptor interaction with the apoB-100 on LDL. The number of LDL receptors on the cell surface mediates regulation of cellular LDL uptake. Cells requiring increased amounts of cholesterol will increase the biosynthesis of LDL receptors. Conversely, it has been demonstrated that increased hepatic concentrations of cholesterol will inhibit both HMG-CoA reductase as well as the production of LDL receptors. As previously discussed, hepatic cholesterol can be converted to bile acids and bile salts and reenter the endogenous pathway through the bile and enterohepatic circulation.

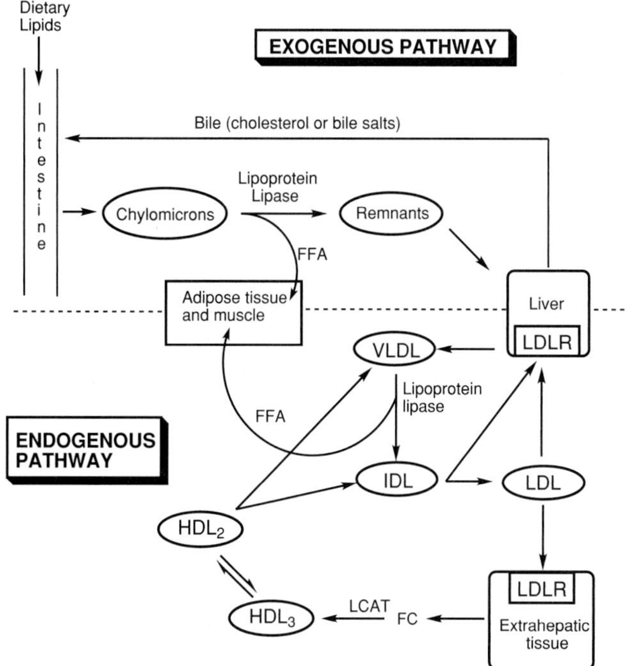

Fig. 30.5. Endogenous and exogenous pathways for lipid transport and metabolism. FFA, free fatty acids; LDLR, low-density lipoprotein receptor; FC, free unesterified cholesterol; LCAT, lecithin-cholesterol acyltransferase.

Synthesized in the liver and intestine, HDL initially exists as a dense, phospholipid disk composed primarily of apoA-I. The primary function of HDL is to act as a scavenger to remove cholesterol from extrahepatic cells and to facilitate its transport back to the liver. Nascent HDL accepts free, unesterified cholesterol. A plasma enzyme, lecithin-cholesterol acyltransferase, then esterifies the cholesterol. This process allows the resulting cholesterol esters to move from the surface to the core and results in the production of spherical HDL_3 particles. As cholesterol content is added, HDL_3 is converted to HDL_2, which is larger and less dense than HDL_3. The ultimate return of cholesterol from HDL_2 to the liver is known as reverse cholesterol transport and is accomplished via an intermediate transfer of cholesterol esters from HDL_2 to either VLDL or IDL. This process regenerates spherical HDL_3 molecules that can recirculate and acquire excess cholesterol from other tissues. In this manner, HDL serves to prevent the accumulation of cholesterol in arterial cell walls and other tissue and may serve as the basis for its cardioprotective properties (7,8).

Classification of Hyperlipoproteinemias

Hyperlipoproteinemia can be divided into primary and secondary disorders. Primary disorders are the result of genetic deficiencies or mutations, whereas secondary disorders are the result of other conditions or diseases. Secondary hyperlipoproteinemia has been associated with diabetes mellitus, hypothyroidism, renal disease, liver disease, alcoholism, and certain drugs (1,7,8).

In 1967, Fredrickson et al. (9) classified primary hyperlipoproteinemias into six phenotypes (I, IIa, IIb, III, IV, and V) based on which lipoproteins and lipids were elevated. Current literature and practice, however, appear to favor the more descriptive classifications and subclassifications listed in Table 30.2 Primary disorders are currently classified as those that primarily cause hypercholesterolemia, those that primarily cause hypertriglyceridemia, and those that cause a mixed elevation of both cholesterol and triglycerides. Subclassifications are based on the specific biochemical defect responsible for the disorder. Classifications developed by Fredrickson have been included in Table 30.2 under the heading *Previous Classification* for comparative and reference purposes.

As shown in Table 30.2, some disorders are well characterized, whereas others are not (1,7,8). Familial hypercholesterolemia is caused by a deficiency of LDL receptors. This results in a decreased uptake of IDL and LDL by hepatic and extrahepatic tissues and an elevation in plasma LDL levels. The homozygous form of this disorder is rare but results in extremely high LDL levels and early morbidity and mortality because of the total lack of LDL receptors. A related disorder, familial defective apoB-100, also results in elevated LDL levels but is caused by a genetic mutation rather than a deficiency. Alteration of apoB-100 decreases the affinity of LDL for the LDL receptor and thus hinders normal uptake and metabolism. Elevations in chylomicron levels can result from a deficiency of either lipoprotein lipase or apoC-II. These deficiencies cause decreased or impaired triglyceride hydrolysis and result in a massive accumulation of chylomicrons in the plasma. Dysbetalipoproteinemia results from the presence of an altered form of apoE and is the only mixed hyperlipoproteinemia with a known cause. Proper catabolism of chylomicron and VLDL remnants requires apoE. The presence of a binding-defective form of apoE, known as $apoE_2$, results in elevated levels of VLDL and IDL triglyceride and cholesterol levels.

DISEASES AND DISORDERS CAUSED BY HYPERLIPIDEMIAS

Coronary heart disease, which includes acute myocardial infarction, ischemic heart disease, and angina pectoris, is the leading cause of mortality in the United States. In 2002, more than 494,382 deaths were caused by CHD. Additionally, mortality from CHD often occurs rapidly, either in an emergency room or before hospitalization. The highest mortality is seen in patients older than 65 years; however, the vast majority of deaths in patients younger than 65 years occur during an initial attack. Risk factors associated with CHD include hypertension, cigarette smoking, elevated plasma cholesterol levels, physical inactivity, diabetes, and obesity (10).

Atherosclerosis, which is named from the Greek terms for "gruel" (*athere*) and "hardening" (*sclerosis*), is the underlying cause of CHD. It is a gradual process in which

Table 30.2. Characteristics of the Major Primary Hyperlipoproteinemias

Current Classification	Biochemical Defect	Elevated Lipoproteins	Previous Classification
Hypercholesterolemias			
Familial hypercholesterolemia	Deficiency of LDL receptors	LDL	IIa
Familial defective apoB-100	Mutant apoB-100	LDL	IIa
Polygenic hypercholesterolemia	Unknown	LDL	IIa
Hypertriglyceridemias			
Familial hypertriglyceridemia	Unknown	VLDL	IV
Familial lipoprotein lipase deficiency	Deficiency of lipoprotein lipase	Chylomicrons, VLDL	I (chylomicron elevation only), V
Familial apoC-II deficiency	Deficiency of apoC-II	Chylomicrons, VLDL	I (chylomicron elevation only), V
Mixed hypercholesterolemia and hypertriglyceridemia			
Familial combined hyperlipidemia	Unknown	VLDL, LDL	IIb
Dysbetalipoproteinemia	Presence of $apoE_2$ isoforms	VLDL, IDL	III

LDL, low-density lipoprotein; apo, apolipoprotein; VLDL, very-low-density lipoprotein; IDL, intermediate-density lipoprotein.

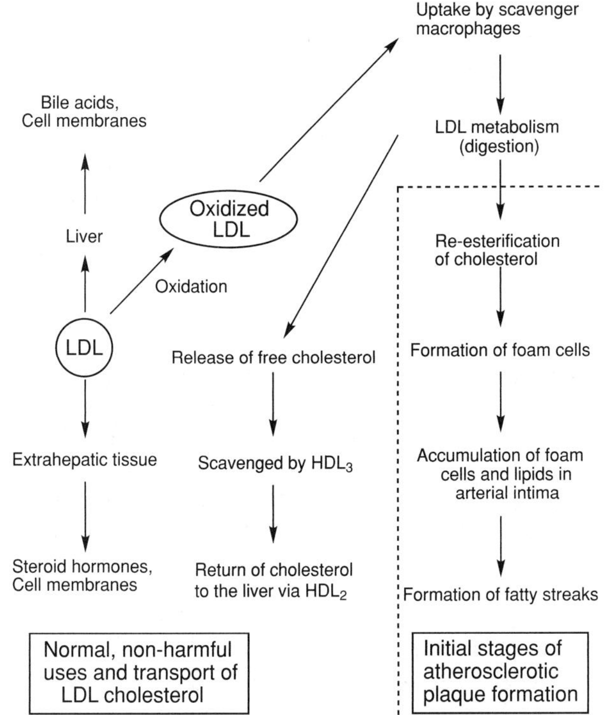

Fig. 30.6. The role of LDL cholesterol in the development of atherosclerotic plaques. The mechanism by which HDL provides a cardioprotective action also is shown.

an initial accumulation of lipids in the arterial intima leads to thickening of the arterial wall, plaque formation, thrombosis, and occlusion (11–13). The involvement of LDL cholesterol in this process is shown in Figure 30.6. Within the extracellular space of the intima, LDL is more susceptible to oxidative metabolism, because it is no longer protected by plasma antioxidants. This metabolism alters the properties of LDL such that it is readily scavenged by macrophages. Unlike normal LDL, the uptake of oxidized LDL is not regulated; thus, macrophage cells can readily become engorged with oxidized LDL. Subsequent metabolism produces free cholesterol, which either can be released into the plasma or reesterified by the enzyme acyl CoA–cholesterol acyltransferase (ACAT). Cholesterol released into plasma can be scavenged by HDL_3 and returned to the liver, thus preventing any accumulation or damage. In this manner, HDL acts as a cardioprotective agent, because high concentrations of reesterified cholesterol can morphologically change macrophages into foam cells. Accumulation of lipid-engorged foam cells in the arterial intima results in the formation of fatty streaks, the initial lesion of atherosclerosis. Later, the deposition of lipoproteins, cholesterol, and phospholipids causes the formation of softer, larger plaques. Associated with this lipid deposition is the proliferation of arterial smooth muscle cells into the intima and the laying down of collagen, elastin, and glycosaminoglycans, leading to fibrous plaques. Ultimately, the surface of the plaque deteriorates, and an atheromatous ulcer is formed with a fibrous matrix, accumulation of necrotic tissue, and appearance of cholesterol and cholesterol ester crystals. A complicated lesion also shows calcification and hemorrhage with the formation of organized mural thrombi. Thrombosis results from changes in the arterial walls and in the blood-clotting mechanism.

Obviously, individuals with higher cholesterol and LDL levels are more susceptible to these detrimental effects than those with normal cholesterol and LDL levels. Total plasma cholesterol levels less than 200 mg/dL are considered desirable. Levels above 240 mg/dL are considered high, and levels between 200 and 239 mg/dL are considered borderline. For LDL, plasma levels of less than 100 mg/dL are considered optimal, plasma levels equal to or greater than 160 are considered high, plasma levels between 130 and 159 mg/dL are considered borderline, and plasma levels between 100 and 129 are considered above optimal. Current guidelines (8,13) also recommend an LDL level below 70 mg/dL as a goal for very high-risk patients (i.e., those with multiple risk factors and known cardiovascular disease).

Elevated plasma triglyceride levels can contribute to atherosclerosis and CHD in mixed hyperlipoproteinemias, whereas pure hypertriglyceridemias are primarily associated with pancreatitis and show little to no relationship to CHD (7,8).

ACAT: A Potential Drug Target

Inhibitors of acyl CoA-cholesterol acyltransferase (ACAT) are currently being investigated as cholesterol-lowering or antiatherosclerotic agents. In addition to its role in foam cell formation, ACAT also is required for esterification of cholesterol in intestinal mucosal cells and for synthesis of cholesterol esters in hepatic VLDL formation. Thus, ACAT inhibitors have the potential of providing three beneficial effects in patients with hypercholesterolemia: decreased cholesterol absorption, decreased hepatic VLDL synthesis, and decreased foam cell formation. Initial successes at inhibiting ACAT were dampened by the discovery of accompanying adrenal toxicity. Subsequent structural modifications have lead to the development of potent, orally active ACAT inhibitors (e.g., CI1011), which lack this toxicity and have given new hope that inhibitors of this enzyme may provide an alternative treatment of atherosclerotic disorders (12,14).

CI1011

OVERVIEW OF DRUG THERAPY AFFECTING LIPOPROTEIN METABOLISM

Bile acid sequestrants, HMG-CoA reductase inhibitors (HMGRIs), ezetimibe, fibrates, and niacin are all used in the treatment of hyperlipoproteinemia. In general, successful use of these compounds depends on proper identification and classification of the hyperlipoproteinemia affecting the patient. With the possible exceptions of niacin, atorvastatin, and rosuvastatin, currently available compounds do not have equal efficacy in reducing both hypercholesterolemia and hypertriglyceridemia and, thus, are used primarily for their ability to decrease either cholesterol or triglyceride levels. Bile acid sequestrants, inhibitors of HMG-CoA reductase, and ezetimibe are effective in decreasing plasma cholesterol and LDL levels. The fibrates also have some actions on plasma cholesterol; however, their main effect is to stimulate lipoprotein lipase and to increase the clearance of triglycerides. Niacin, through its ability to decrease VLDL formation, has been shown to decrease the plasma levels of both triglycerides and cholesterol. All of these compounds are discussed below. References for these sections have been limited to current reviews and texts, selected papers, and product literature, both traditional and electronic. Readers requiring additional references for any of these compounds should consult either the previous edition of this text or the references contained within the cited reviews and texts.

BILE ACID SEQUESTRANTS

Historical Overview

Cholestyramine was originally developed in the 1960s to treat pruritus secondary to elevated plasma concentrations of bile acids in patients with cholestasis. Its ability to bind (i.e., to hold or to sequester) bile acids and to increase their fecal elimination was subsequently shown to produce beneficial effects in lowering serum cholesterol levels. In 1973, cholestyramine was approved for the treatment of hypercholesterolemia in patients who do not respond to dietary modifications. Colestipol and colesevelam, which retain the key structural features required to bind bile acids, were approved in 1977 and 2000, respectively (7,15).

Cholestyramine, colestipol, and colesevelam are chemically classified as anion-exchange resins. This term arises from their ability to selectively bind and exchange negatively charged atoms or molecules with one another. The selectivity comes from the fact that these positively charged resins do not bind equally to all anions. For example, the chloride ion of cholestyramine can be displaced by, or exchanged with, other anions (e.g., bile acids) that have a greater affinity for the positively charged functional groups on the resin.

Mechanism of Action

Cholestyramine, colestipol, and colesevelam lower plasma LDL levels by indirectly increasing the rate at which LDL is cleared from the bloodstream. Under normal circumstances, approximately 97% of bile acids are reabsorbed into the enterohepatic circulation. As previously discussed, these compounds are returned to the liver where they regulate their own production. Bile acid sequestrants are not orally absorbed but, rather, act locally within the gastrointestinal tract to interrupt this process. They bind the two major bile acids, glycocholic acid and taurocholic acid, and greatly increase their fecal excretion. As a result, decreased concentrations of these compounds are returned to the liver. This removes the feedback inhibition of 7α-hydroxylase and increases the hepatic conversion of cholesterol to bile acids (Fig. 30.3). The decrease in hepatic cholesterol concentrations leads to several compensatory effects: increased expression of LDL receptors, increased hepatic uptake of plasma LDL, induction of HMG-CoA reductase, and increased biosynthesis of cholesterol. The latter two effects are insufficient to counteract the increases in cholesterol clearance and catabolism; however, concurrent use of an HMGRI can provide an additive effect in lowering LDL cholesterol. Bile acid sequestrants do not alter the removal of plasma LDL by nonreceptor-mediated mechanisms and, thus, are ineffective in treating homozygous familial hypercholesterolemia (7,15–17).

The decreased return of bile acids to the liver also will produce an increase in triglyceride synthesis and a transient rise in VLDL levels. Subsequent compensatory mechanisms will increase VLDL removal, most likely through the increased LDL receptors, and return VLDL levels to predrug levels. For those patients with preexisting hypertriglyceridemia, the compensatory mechanisms are inadequate, and a persistent rise in VLDL levels occurs (7).

Structure–Activity Relationships

Cholestyramine (Fig. 30.7) is a copolymer consisting primarily of polystyrene, with a small amount of divinylbenzene as the cross-linking agent. In addition, it contains approximately 4 mEq of fixed quaternary ammonium groups per gram of dry resin. These positively charged groups function as binding sites for anions. Virtually all of these sites are accessible to bile acids. Increasing the amount of divinylbenzene from 2 to 4 to 8% increases the cross-linkage and reduces the porosity of the resin. This prevents binding of bile acids to interior sites and decreases the efficacy of the compound.

Colestipol (Fig. 30.7) is a copolymer of tetraethylenepentamine and epichlorhydrin and is commercially marked as its hydrochloride salt. The key functional groups on colestipol are the basic secondary and tertiary amines. Although the total nitrogen content of colestipol is greater than that of cholestyramine, the functional anion-exchange capacity of the resin depends on intestinal pH and may be less than cholestyramine. Recent in vitro studies indicate that cholestyramine has a higher adsorption capacity than colestipol for bile salts (18). Quaternization of colestipol with methyl iodide increases the capacity in vitro for glycocholate (19).

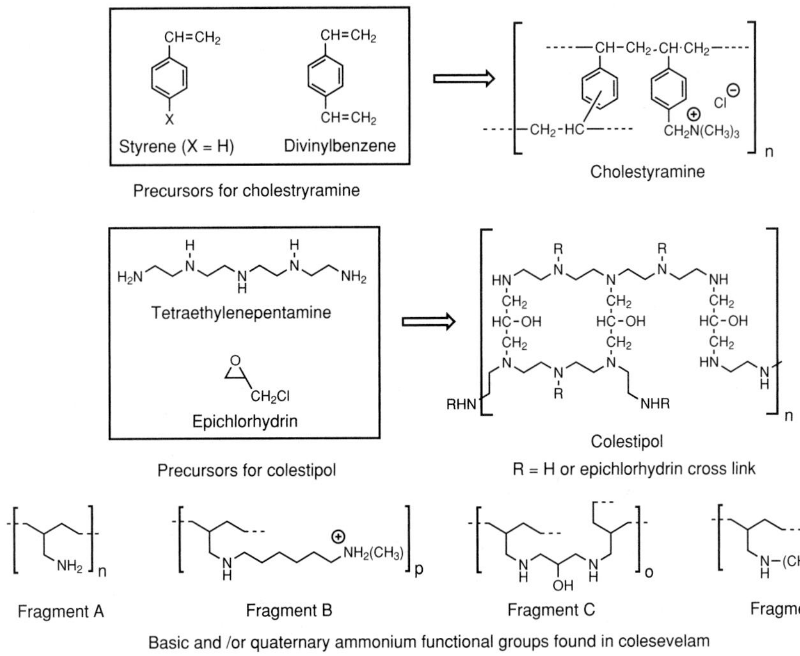

CH=CH2
CH=CH2
X
CH=CH2
Styrene (X = H)
Divinylbenzene
Precursors for cholestryramine
CH-CH2-CH-CH2
Cl⊖
CH2-HC
CH2N(CH3)3
n
Cholestyramine
H2N NH2
Tetraethylenepentamine
CH2Cl
Epichlorhydrin
Precursors for colestipol
HC-OH
RHN
NHR
Colestipol
R = H or epichlorhydrin cross link
Fragment A
Fragment B
Fragment C
Fragment D
Basic and /or quaternary ammonium functional groups found in colesevelam

Fig. 30.7. Structures of cholestyramine, colestipol, and precursors for these polymeric resins. Also included are the basic and quaternary functional groups found on colesevelam. Note that cholestyramine will contain a fraction of unsubsituted aromatic rings (i.e., those that are neither cross-linked nor contain a quaternary ammonium group).

Colesevelam is a more diverse polymer; however, its initial formation is similar to colestipol. In the case of colesevelam, poly(allyamine) is initially cross-linked with epichlorhydrin and then alkylated with 1-bromodecane and (6-bromohexyl)-trimethylammonium bromide. The resulting polymer contains four basic and/or quaternary functional groups, as shown in Figure 30.7. Fragment A is a primary amine, fragment B is a pair of secondary amines, fragment C is an alkylated amine attached to a quaternary ammonium group, and fragment D is a decylated amine. The overall polymer is a hydrophilic gel and is insoluble in water (7).

Physicochemical Properties

All bile acid sequestrants are large, hygroscopic, water-insoluble resins. The molecular weight of cholestyramine is reported to be greater than 1,000,000 daltons; however, no specific molecular weight has been assigned to either colestipol or colesevelam. Cholestyramine contains a large number of quaternary ammonium groups and, thus, has multiple permanent positive charges. Colestipol contains a large number of secondary and tertiary amines, whereas colesevelam contains quaternary ammonium groups as well as primary and secondary amines. Normal pK_a values for the amines range from 9.0 to 10.5; thus, all of these groups should be primarily ionized at intestinal pH.

Pharmacokinetic Parameters, Metabolism, and Dosing

Cholestyramine, colestipol, and colesevelam are not orally absorbed and are not metabolized by gastrointestinal enzymes. They are excreted in the feces as an insoluble complex with bile acids. Their onset of action occurs within 24 to 48 hours; however, it may take up to 1 month to achieve peak response (7,15,20).

Cholestyramine is available as a powder that is mixed with water, juice, or other noncarbonated beverages to create a slurry to drink. Patients should experiment with various liquids to find the most palatable combination; however, patient acceptance and compliance with this dosage formulation can limit its use. Each packet or scoop of cholestyramine is equivalent to 4 g of cholestyramine. The recommended daily dose for the treatment of hypercholesterolemia is 8 to 16 grams (two to four packets or scoops) per day divided into two doses and taken with meals. The maximum daily dose for hypercholesterolemia is 24 g. Colestipol is available as either granules or 1-g tablets. The granules should be taken in a manner similar to that described for the cholestyramine powder. The starting dose for the granules is 5 g once or twice daily. This dose can be increased in 5 g increments every 1 to 2 months until therapeutic goals or a maximum of 30 g/day have been reached. The starting dose for the tablets is 2 g once or twice daily. This dose can then be increased in 2 g segments up to a maximum daily dose of 16 g. Patients must be advised that colestipol tablets should not to be chewed, crushed, or cut and should be taken with plenty of water (15,21). Colesevelam is available as 625-mg tablets and should be taken with a meal. The starting dose is three tablets (1.875 g) twice a day or six tablets (3.75 g) once a day. The dose may be increased to a maximum of seven tablets per (4.375 g) per day.

Unlabeled Uses

Diarrhea, digitalis toxicity, and pseudomembranous colitis

Therapeutic Applications

Bile acid sequestrants are indicated for the treatment of hypercholesterolemia in patients who do not adequately respond to dietary modifications. They may be used either alone or in combination with HMGRIs or niacin. These combinations often can achieve a 50% reduction in plasma LDL levels. Cholestyramine, but neither colestipol nor colesevelam, also is approved for the relief of pruritus associated with partial biliary obstruction. Bile acid sequestrants should not be used to treat hypertriglyceridemias or mixed hyperlipoproteinemias in which hypertriglyceridemia is the primary concern. These compounds also are contraindicated in patients with cholelithiasis or complete biliary obstruction because of the impaired secretion of bile acids caused by these conditions. Finally, cholestyramine and colestipol are contraindicated in patients with primary biliary cirrhosis, because this can further raise serum cholesterol (7,15,21).

Adverse Effects

Because bile acid sequestrants are not orally absorbed, they produce minimal systemic side effects and, thus, are one of the safest drugs to use for hypercholesterolemia. Constipation is by far the most frequent patient complaint. Increasing dietary fiber or using bulk-producing laxatives, such as psyllium, often can minimize this adverse effect. Other gastrointestinal symptoms, such as bloating and abdominal discomfort, usually disappear with continued use; however, the possibility of fecal impaction requires that extreme caution be used in patients with preexisting constipation. All three of these compounds release chloride ions as part of their exchange mechanism and can cause hyperchloremic acidosis. This is not a common occurrence, but it may limit the use of bile acid sequestrants in patients with renal disease. Hypoprothrombinemia and bleeding are caused by the ability of bile acid sequestrants to bind with and impair the absorption of dietary vitamin K. These effects also are rare, but they may limit the use of these agents in patients with preexisting clotting disorder and in those being concurrently treated with anticoagulants (2,7,15,21).

Drug Interactions

Because of their mechanism of action, bile acid sequestrants can potentially bind with and decrease the oral absorption of almost any other drug. Because these anion-exchange resins contain numerous positive charges, they are much more likely to bind to acidic compounds than to basic compounds or nonelectrolytes. This is not an absolute, however, because cholestyramine and colestipol have been reported to decrease the oral absorption of propranolol (a base) and the lipid-soluble vitamins, A, D, E, and K (nonelectrolytes). As a result, the current recommendation is that all other oral medication should be administered at least 1 hour before or 4 hours after cholestyramine and colestipol. Interestingly, this drug interaction has been used in a beneficial manner to treat digitalis overdose and toxicity.

Adverse Effects of Bile Acid Sequestrants

Bloating, abdominal discomfort, constipation, bowel obstruction, steatorrhea, anorexia, cholelithiasis, pancreatitis, hyperchloremic acidosis, hypoprothrombinemia, and bleeding.

Colesevelam appears to be less likely to interfere with the absorption of concurrently administered drugs. No significant decreases in absorption were seen when colesevelam was coadministered with either digoxin, lovastatin, warfarin, metoprolol, quinidine, or valproic acid. Because of potential interactions, especially for drugs with a low therapeutic index, the administration of drugs that have not been directly studied in combination with colesevelam should be spaced accordingly, as described above for cholestryamine and colestipol (7,15).

HMG-CoA REDUCTASE INHIBITORS

Currently, six HMGRIs are approved for therapeutic use in the United States. Chemically, they can be divided into two groups, natural products and synthetic agents. All of these compounds effectively block the conversion of HMG-CoA to mevalonic acid and have similar effects on plasma cholesterol levels. The compounds differ somewhat in their indications, potencies, and pharmacokinetic profiles. They often are referred to as statins or, more recently, vastatins. Because of the potential confusion of the terms "statin" and "statine" (i.e., a stable dipeptide mimic [see Chapter 28]), it is suggested here that classifying an HMGRI as a vastatin is preferable to classifying it as a statin.

Historical Overview and Development

The development and use of HMGRIs began in 1976 with the discovery of mevastatin. Originally named compactin, this fungal metabolite was isolated from two different species of *Penicillium* and demonstrated potent, competitive inhibition of HMG-CoA reductase. Its affinity for the enzyme was shown to be 10,000-fold greater than that of the substrate HMG-CoA (22). Several years later, a structurally similar compound was isolated from *Monascus ruber* and *Aspergillus terreus*. This compound was originally known as mevinolin, was later renamed lovastatin, and was more than twofold more potent than mevastatin (Fig. 30.8). Structurally, it differed from mevastatin only by the presence of a methyl group at

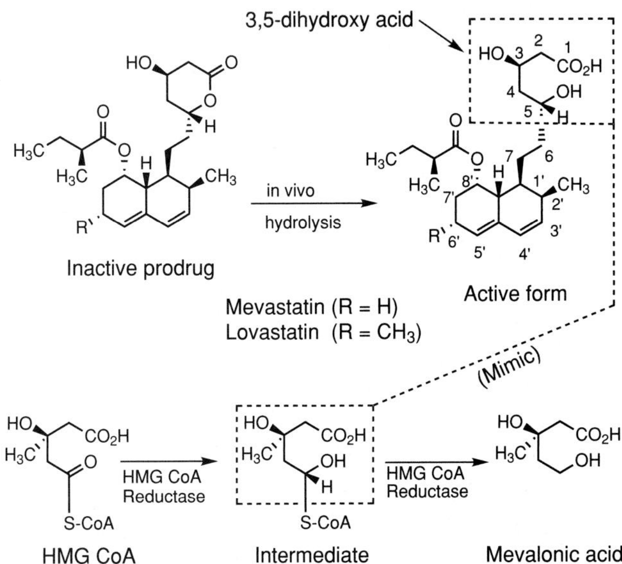

Fig. 30.8. Mechanism of action of mevastatin and lovastatin. Hydrolysis of these pro-drugs produces a 3,5-dihydroxy acid that mimics the tetrahedral intermediate produced by HMG-CoA reductase.

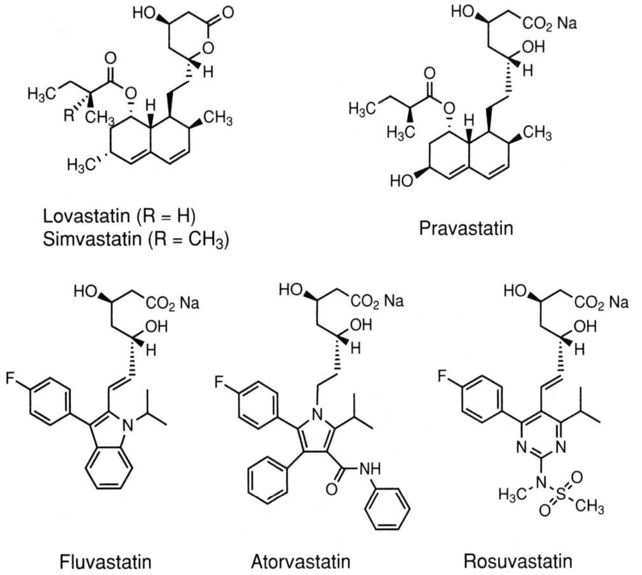

the 6′ position of the bicyclic ring. As illustrated in Figure 30.8, mevastatin and lovastatin can bind very tightly with HMG-CoA reductase, because their hydrolyzed lactones mimic the tetrahedral intermediate produced by the reductase enzyme (7). Studies published in 1985 confirmed this theory and also established that the bicyclic portions of these compounds bind to the CoA site of the enzyme (23). Clinical trials of mevastatin were halted after reports of altered intestinal morphology in dogs (24); however, lovastatin received approval by the U.S. Food and Drug Administration (FDA) in 1987, representing the first HMGRI to be available in the U.S. for therapeutic use.

Structure–Activity Relationship

Mevastatin and lovastatin served as lead compounds in the development of additional HMGRIs. Initial research published by Merck Pharmaceuticals examined alterations of the lactone and bicyclic rings as well as the ethylene bridge between them. The results demonstrated that the activity of HMGRIs is sensitive to the stereochemistry of the lactone ring, the ability of the lactone ring to be hydrolyzed, and the length of bridge connecting the two ring systems. Additionally, it was found that the bicyclic ring could be replaced with other lipophilic rings and that the size and shape of these other ring systems were important to the overall activity of the compounds (25).

Minor modifications of the bicyclic ring and side-chain ester of lovastatin produced simvastatin and pravastatin (Fig. 30.9). Pravastatin, a ring-opened dihydroxy acid with a 6α-hydroxyl group, is much more hydrophilic than either lovastatin or simvastatin. Proposed advantages of this enhanced hydrophilicity are minimal penetration into the lipophilic membranes of peripheral cells, better selectivity for hepatic tissues, and a reduction in the incidence of side effects seen with lovastatin and simvastatin. (26,27).

Lovastatin (R = H)
Simvastatin (R = CH_3)

Pravastatin

Fluvastatin

Atorvastatin

Rosuvastatin

Fig. 30.9. Commercially available HMG-CoA reductase inhibitors.

The replacement of the bicyclic ring with various substituted, aromatic ring systems led to the development of fluvastatin, atorvastatin, and rosuvastatin (Fig. 30.9). The initial rationale centered on a desire to simplify the structures of mevastatin and lovastatin. The 2,4-dichlorophenyl analogue (compound A) was one of the first compounds to demonstrate that this type of substitution was possible; however, compound A was considerably less potent than mevastatin. Subsequent research investigated a variety of aromatic substitutions and heterocyclic ring systems to optimize HMGRI activity. The substituted pyrrole (compound B) retained 30% of the activity of mevastatin (28) and was a key intermediate in the development of atorvastatin. The 4-fluorophenyl and isopropyl substitutions found in compound B also are seen in the indole and pyrimidine ring systems of fluvastatin and rosuvastatin, respectively, and most likely represent the optimum substitutions at their respective positions. The design of all three of these compounds included the ring-opened dihydroxyacid functionality first seen in pravastatin.

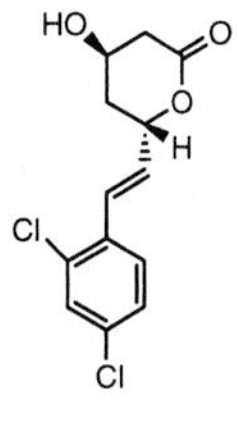

Compound A

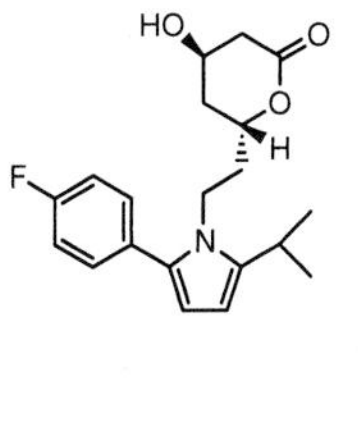

Compound B

Table 30.3. Structure-activity Relationship of HIMG CoA Reductase Inhibitors

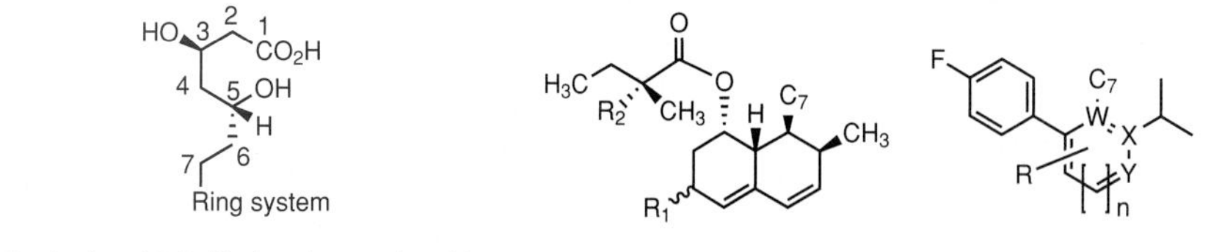

7-substituted-3,5-dihydroxyheptanoic acid	Ring A	Ring B

Common for all HMGRIs:

1. The 3,5-dihydroxycarboxylate is essential for inhibitory activity. Compounds containing a lactone are prodrugs requiring in vivo hydrolysis.
2. The absolute stereochemistry of the 3- and 5-hydroxyl groups must be the same as that found in mevastatin and lovastatin.
3. Altering the two carbon distance between C5 and the ring system diminishes or fails to improve activity.
4. A double bond between C6 and C7 can either increase or decrease activity. The ethyl group provides optimal activity for compounds containing ring A and some heterocyclic rings (e.g., pyrrole ring of atorvastatin). The ethenyl group is optimal for compounds with other ring systems, including the indole and pyrimidine rings seen in fluvastatin and rosuvastatin, respectively.

Ring A subclass:

-The decalin ring is essential for anchoring the compound to the enzyme active site. Replacement with a cyclohexane ring resulted in a 10,000 fold decrease in activity
-Stereochemistry of the ester side chain is not important for activity; however, conversion of this ester to an ether results in a decrease in activity.
-Methyl substitution at the R2 position increases activity (*i.e.,* simvastatin is more potent than lovastatin).
-β-Hydroxyl group substitution at the R1 position enhances hydrophilicity and may provide some cellular specificity.

Ring B subclass:

-Substituents W, X, and Y can be either carbon or nitrogen, n is equal to either zero or one (i.e., five or six member heterocyclic).
-The para-fluorophenyl cannot be coplanar with the central aromatic ring. (Structural restraints to cause coplanarity have resulted in a loss of activity).
-R substitution with aryl groups, hydrocarbon chains, amides, or sulfonamides enhances lipophilicity and inhibitory activity.

All HMGRIs can be chemically classified as 7-substituted-3,5-dihydroxyheptanoic acids, the general structure of which is shown in Table 30.3. Additionally, these compounds can be subclassified based on their lower ring. Compounds structurally related to the natural products mevastatin and lovastatin have structural features common to ring A, whereas those that are completely synthetic have structural features common to ring B (25,27–35).

Mechanism of Action

Inhibitors of HMG-CoA reductase lower plasma cholesterol levels by three related mechanisms: inhibition of cholesterol biosynthesis, enhancement of receptor-mediated LDL uptake, and reduction of VLDL precursors (15,21). As previously discussed, HMG-CoA reductase is the rate-limiting step in cholesterol biosynthesis. Inhibition of this enzyme causes an initial decrease in hepatic cholesterol. Compensatory mechanisms result in an enhanced expression of both HMG-CoA reductase and LDL receptors. The net result of all these effects is a slight to modest decrease in cholesterol synthesis, a significant increase in receptor-mediated LDL uptake, and an overall lowering of plasma LDL levels. Evidence to support the theory that enhanced LDL receptor expression is the primary mechanism for lowering LDL levels comes from the fact that most statins do not lower LDL levels in patients who are unable to produce LDL receptors (i.e., homozygous familial hypercholesterolemia). The increased number of LDL receptors also may increase the direct removal of VLDL and IDL. Because these lipoproteins are precursors to LDL, this action may contribute to the overall lowering of plasma LDL cholesterol. Finally, all HMGRIs can produce a modest (8–12%) increase in HDL (15).

Atorvastatin, rosuvastatin, and simvastatin appear to have some effects beyond those seen with the other HMGRIs. These compounds have been shown to decrease plasma LDL levels in patients with homozygous familial hypercholesterolemia, an effect that is proposed to result from their ability to produce a more significant decrease in the hepatic production of LDL cholesterol. Additionally, atorvastatin and rosuvastatin can produce a significant lowering in plasma triglycerides. In the case of atorvastatin, this effect has been attributed to its ability to produce an enhanced removal of triglyceride-rich VLDL (15,36,37).

Physicochemical Properties

In their active forms, all HMGRIs contain a carboxylic acid. This functional group is required for inhibitory activity, has a pK_a in the range of 2.5 to 3.5, and will be primarily ionized at physiologic pH. Lovastatin and simvastatin are neutral, lactone pro-drugs and should be classified as nonelectrolytes. Pravastatin, fluvastatin, and atorvastatin can be classified as acidic drugs. The nitrogen atoms in the indole and pyrrole rings of fluvastatin and atorvastatin, respectively, are aromatic nitrogens that are not ionizable. This is because the lone pair electrons of these atoms are involved in maintaining the aromaticity of their respective rings and are not available to bind protons. Rosuvastatin is technically an amphoteric compound; however, its pyrimidine ring is weakly basic and most likely will not be ionized at physiologic pH.

The calculated log P values for the HMGRIs are shown in Table 30.4. Although some variation exists among the values for lovastatin, pravastatin, and simvastatin, the general trends are the same regardless of what program was used to calculate the values. Atorvastatin, fluvastatin, and the pro-drugs lovastatin and simvastatin have a much higher lipid solubility than either pravastatin and rosuvastatin. Hydrolysis of the lactone ring for the two pro-drugs

Table 30.4. Pharmacokinetic Parameters of HMG-CoA Reductase Inhibitors

Drug	Calculated Log P[a]	Oral Bioavailability (%)	Active Metabolite(s)	Protein Binding (%)	Time to Peak Conc. (hours)	Elimination Half-Life (hours)	Major Route(s) of Elimination
Atorvastatin	4.13	12–14	ortho- and para-hydroxylated	98	1–2	14–19	Biliary/fecal (>90%) Renal (<2%)
Fluvastatin	3.62	20–30	None	98	0.5–1.0	1	Biliary/fecal (95%) Renal (5%)
Lovastatin	4.07 (4.04)[b]	5	3,5-Dihydroxy acid	>95	2	3–4	Fecal (83%) Renal (10%)
Pravastatin	1.44 (0.5)[b]	17	None	43–55	1.0–1.5	2–3	Fecal (70%) Renal (20%)
Rosuvastatin	0.42	20	N-desmethyl	88	3–5	19–20	Fecal (90%) Renal (10%)
Simvastatin	4.42 (4.2)[b]	5	3,5-Dihydroxy acid	95	4	3	Fecal (60%) Renal (13%)

[a]A commercial program was used for calculated values (45).
[b]Calculated using the CLOG program (38).

produces a 3,5-dihydroxycarboxylate with significantly improves water solubility.

The HMG-CoA reductase enzyme is stereoselective. The 3R,5R stereochemistry seen in the active forms of mevastatin and lovastatin (Fig. 30.8) is required for inhibitory activity and is present in all other HMGRIs. Stereochemistry of the substituents on the bicyclic rings of lovastatin, simvastatin, and pravastatin is less crucial to activity, as indicated in the summary of the structure–activity relationships (SARs).

Metabolism

As previously mentioned, lovastatin and simvastatin are inactive pro-drugs that must undergo in vivo hydrolysis to produce their effects (Fig. 30.8). The active forms of these two compounds as well as most HMGRIs undergo extensive first-pass metabolism (15,20,36,37). The CYP3A4 isozyme is responsible for the oxidative metabolism of atorvastatin, lovastatin, and simvastatin. In the case of atorvastatin, the ortho- and para-hydroxylated metabolites are equiactive with the parent compound and contribute significantly to the overall activity of the drug (Table 30.4). Rosuvastatin is metabolized to a limited extent by CYP2C9 to form an N-desmethyl metabolite that can contribute to activity, but is sevenfold less potent. In contrast, the activity of lovastatin and simvastatin resides primarily in the initial hydrolysis product (i.e., further oxidation decreases activity). Fluvastatin is metabolized by the CYP2C9 and CYP3A4 isozymes to active hydroxylated metabolites; however, these metabolites do not circulate systemically and do not contribute to the overall activity. Pravastatin also undergoes oxidative metabolism, but the resulting compounds retain only minimal activity and are not significant. Neither pravastatin nor rosuvastatin is metabolized by CYP3A4; therefore, these drugs are potentially advantageous for patients who must take concurrent medication that alters the activity of this isozyme.

Pharmacokinetic Parameters

The pharmacokinetic parameters and dosing information for HMGRIs are summarized in Tables 30.4 and 30.5 respectively (2,7,15,20,21,36,38,39). With a few exceptions, all of these compounds have similar onsets of action, durations of action, dosing intervals, and plasma protein binding. Despite the ability to attain a peak

Table 30.5. Dosing Information for HMG-CoA Reductase Inhibitors

Generic Name	Brand Name(s)	Dosing Range	Maximum Daily Dose	Dose Reduction with Renal Dysfunction	Tablet Strengths (mg)
Atorvastatin	Lipitor	10–80 mg q.d.	80 mg	No	10, 20, 40,80
Fluvastatin	Lescol Lescol XR	20–80 mg q.d. or b.i.d.	80 mg	Caution in severe impairment	20, 40, 80 (XR)
Lovastatin	Mevacor Altoprev (XR)	20–80 mg q.d. or b.i.d.	80 mg (60 mg if XR) (20 mg with fibrate)	Yes	10, 20, 40, 60 (XR)
Pravastatin	Pravachol	10–40 mg q.d.	80 mg	Yes	10, 20, 40, 80
Resuvastatin	Crestor	5–40 mg q.d.	40 mg (10 mg with fibrate)	Only with severe impairment	5, 10, 20, 40
Simvastatin	Zocor	5–40 mg q.d.	80 mg (10 mg with fibrate)	Only with severe impairment	5, 10, 20, 40, 80

plasma concentration in 1 to 4 hours, HMGRIs require approximately 2 weeks to demonstrate an initial lowering of plasma cholesterol. Peak reductions of plasma cholesterol occur after 4 to 6 weeks of therapy for most compounds. Studies with atorvastatin, however, indicate that it may only need 2 weeks to produce its peak reduction. Atorvastatin and rosuvastatin also are unique in that they have much longer durations of action than the other compounds. With the exception of pravastatin, which is one of the more hydrophilic compounds in this class, most HMGRIs bind extensively to plasma proteins.

Because of first-pass metabolism, the oral bioavailability of this class of drugs generally is low and does not reflect the actual absorption of the individual drugs. For example, 60 to 80% of a dose of simvastatin is orally absorbed, but only 5% is actually available to produce an effect. The same is true with fluvastatin, pravastatin, and lovastatin, which have oral absorptions of 90%, 34%, and 35%, respectively, but much lower bioavailabilities (Table 30.4). With the exception of lovastatin, the concurrent administration of food does not affect the overall therapeutic effects of HMGRIs. Lovastatin should always be administered with food to maximize oral bioavailability. Failure to do this results in a 33% decrease in plasma concentrations. In general, HMGRIs should be administered in the evening or at bedtime to counteract the peak cholesterol synthesis, which occurs in the early morning hours. Exceptions to this are atorvastatin and rosuvastatin, which because of their long half-lives are equally effective regardless of when they are administered.

The primary route of elimination of these compounds is through the feces. Because of extensive hepatic transformation and the ability to elevate hepatic enzymes, HMGRIs are contraindicated in patients with active hepatic disease or unexplained persistent elevations in serum aminotransferase concentrations. Dosage reductions in patients with renal dysfunction depend on the individual agent. Atorvastatin, which has minimal renal excretion, requires no dosage reduction and may be the best agent for patients with renal disorders. Fluvastatin, rosuvastatin, and simvastatin require dosage reductions only in cases of severe renal impairment and are better choices than lovastatin and pravastatin, which require dosage reductions in mild or moderate impairment.

Therapeutic Applications

All HMGRIs are approved for the treatment of primary hypercholesterolemia and familial combined hyperlipidemia (Fredrickson's type IIa and IIb) (Table 30.2) in patients who have not responded to diet, exercise, and other nonpharmacological methods (Table 30.6) (15,21). They may be used either alone or in combination with bile acid sequestrants, ezetimibe, or niacin. As previously mentioned, they should be administered at least 1 hour before or 4 to 6 hours after bile acid sequestrants when this combination is desired. Fluvastatin, lovastatin, pravastatin, and simvastatin have been specifically indicated to reduce the mortality of CHD and stroke. By reducing plasma LDL levels, these compounds slow the progression of atherosclerosis and reduce the risk of myocardial infarction and other ramifications of vascular occlusion. Atorvastatin, rosuvastatin, and simvastatin have been shown to be effective in homozygous familial hyperlipidemia and are indicated for this use. Additionally, atorvastatin, pravastatin, and simvastatin are indicated for primary dysbetalipoproteinemia (Fredrickson's type III) (Table 30.2). Finally, atorvastatin, pravastatin, rosuvastatin, and simvastatin are indicated for the treatment of hypertriglyceridemia.

Table 30.6. Approved Therapeutics Conditions for HMG CoA Reductase Inhibitors

Therapeutics Condition	Atorvastatin	Fluvastatin	Lovastatin	Pravastatin	Rosuvastatin	Simvastatin
Primary hypercholesterolemia	√	√	√	√	√	√
Primary dysbetalipoproteinemia	√			√		√
Mixed dyslipidemia	√	√	√	√	√	√
Hypertriglyceridemia	√			√	√	√
Homozygous familial hyperlipidemia	√				√	√
Primary prevention of cardiovascular events			√	√		√
Secondary prevention of cardiovascular events		√	√	√		√

Inhibitors of HMG-CoA reductase are contraindicated in pregnancy. Fetal development requires cholesterol as a precursor for the synthesis of steroids and cell membranes; thus, inhibition of its synthesis may cause fetal harm. Additionally, HMGRIs are excreted in breast milk and should not be used by nursing mothers.

Adverse Effects

The most prevalent or significant side effects of HMGRIs are listed below (7,15,21). In general, this class of drugs is well tolerated. Gastrointestinal disturbances are the most common complaint; however, these and other adverse reactions tend to be mild and transient. Elevations in hepatic transaminase levels can occur with all HMGRIs. These increases usually occur shortly after the initiation of therapy and resolve after the discontinuation of med-

Combination Products That Include an HMGRI

- HMGRI and antithrombotic
  - Pravastatin/aspirin (Pravigard PAC)
- HMGRI and calcium channel blocker
  - Atrovastatin/amlodipine (Caduet)
- HMGRI and additional antihypercholesterolemic agent
  - Lovastatin/niacin (Advicor)
  - Simvastatin/ezetimibe (Vytorin)

Potential Nonlipid-Lowering Uses of HMGRIs

Cellular metabolites derived from mevalonic acid are required for cell proliferation. Cholesterol is an essential component of cell membranes, farnesyl pyrophosphate is required to covalently bind to intracellular proteins and modify their function, ubiquinone is required for mitochondrial electron transport, and dolichol phosphates are required for glycoprotein synthesis.

Farnesyl pyrophosphate (Fig. 30.2) is an intermediate in the biosynthesis of cholesterol, ubiquinone, and dolichol phosphates. Based on their site of action, HMGRIs will decrease the availability of all four of these compounds and, thus, decrease cell proliferation. Potential applications of this antiproliferative effect include the prevention of restenosis following angioplasty, prevention of glomerular injury in renal disease, treatment of malignant disease, and prevention of organ transplantation rejection (40).

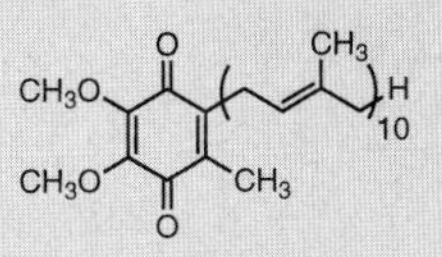

Ubiquinone

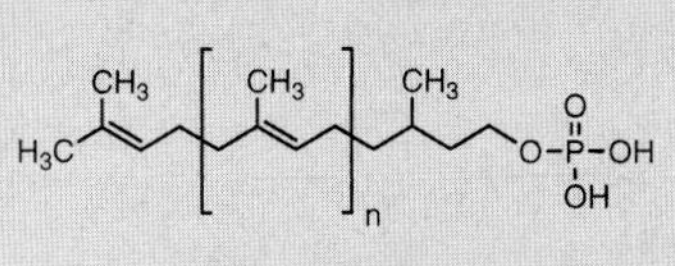

Dolichol phosphate (n = 15-19)

ication. In a small percentage of patients, these levels can increase to more than threefold the upper limit of normal. Therefore, liver function tests should be done at the initiation of therapy, at 6 and 12 weeks after the initiation of therapy, and at periodic intervals (e.g., every 6 months) thereafter. Similar testing should be done with dosage increases. Approximately 5 to 10% of patients will experience mild increases in creatine phosphokinase levels; however, less than 1% will develop symptoms of myalgia and myopathy (e.g., fever, muscle aches or cramps, and unusual tiredness or weakness). Tests for creatine phosphokinase levels should be performed in patients reporting muscle complaints. Rhabdomyolysis (i.e., massive muscle necrosis with secondary acute renal failure) has occurred, but this is rare. The risk of this very serious adverse effect increases when an HMGRI is taken with certain other medications, such as cyclosporine, erythromycin, niacin, or fibrates (Table 30.7). Specific dosage reductions have been suggested for the combination use of fibrates with lovastatin, rosuvastatin, or simvastatin. Despite reports that some HMGRIs present more of a risk of rhabdomyolysis than others, a U.S. FDA advisory statement in 2005 suggests that the risk is similar for all members of this drug class (15).

Adverse Effects of HMGRIs

Constipation, flatulence, dyspepsia, abdominal pain, diarrhea, nausea, vomiting, headache, rhinitis, sinusitis, elevated hepatic enzymes, arthralgia, myalgia, myopathy, muscle cramps, rhabdomyolysis, and chest pain

Drug Interactions

Drug interactions for HMGRIs are listed in Table 30.7

EZETIMIBE, A CHOLESTEROL ABSORPTION INHIBITOR

Historical Overview

The discovery of ezetimibe and its mechanism of action began with a desire to develop novel ACAT inhibitors, a potential target for hypercholesterolemia described earlier in this chapter (41). Compound C was one of the initial azetidinones tested for the ability to inhibit ACAT and to lower plasma cholesterol. Interestingly, this compound's ability to decrease plasma cholesterol exceeded its ability to inhibit ACAT. Further SAR studies resulted in the development of compound D and confirmed that the cholesterol-lowering activity of this class of compounds was independent of its ability to inhibit ACAT. Using compound D as a lead, as well as in vivo data suggesting that metabolic transformations produced the active compound ultimately responsible for the cholesterol lowering effect, structural modifications were made that, eventually, led to the development of ezetimibe. The most important changes involved the introduction of hydroxyl groups to help localize the compound in the intestine and the introduction of *p*-fluoro groups to block undesirable metabolism.

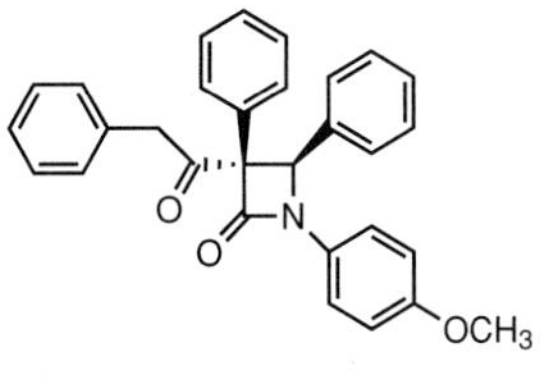

Compound C

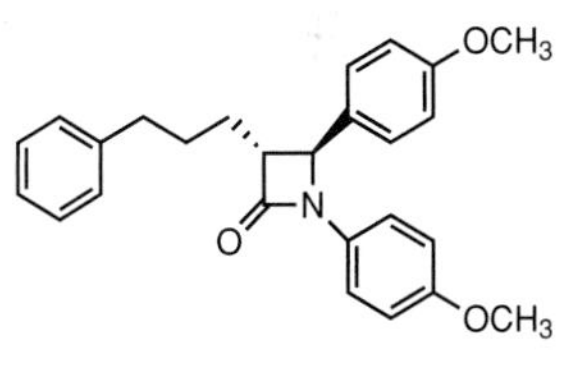

Compound D

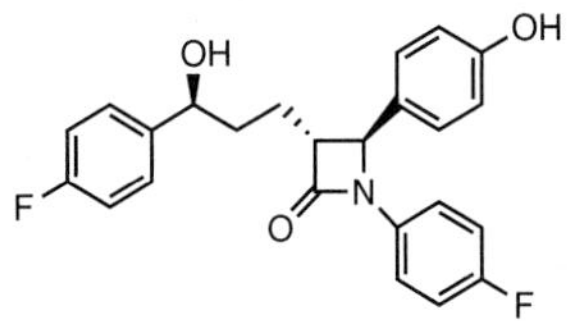

Ezetimibe

Mechanism of Action

Ezetimibe lowers plasma cholesterol levels by inhibiting the absorption of cholesterol at the brush border of the small intestine (15). Specifically, it has been proposed to bind to a specific transport protein located in the wall of the small intestine, resulting in a reduction of cholesterol transport and absorption (42). Ezetimibe appears to be selective in its actions in that it does not interfere with the absorption of triglycerides, lipid-soluble vitamins or other nutrients. The decreased absorption of cholesterol

Table 30.7. Drug Interactions for HMG-CoA Reductase Inhibitors (HMGRIs)

Drug	HMGRIs	Result of Interaction
Amiodarone	Lovastatin, Simvastatin	Increased risk of myopathy
Antacids	Atorvastatin, Rosuvastatin	Decreased levels of atorvastatin rosuvastatin; no change in plasma LDL reduction; administer rosuvastatin at least 2 hours after antacid
Azole antifungal agents	All	Increased risk of severe myopathy or rhabdomyolysis; increased plasma levels of atorvastatin, lovastatin, and simvastatin because of inhibition of CYP3A4; additive decreases in concentrations or activity of endogenous steroid hormones
Bile acid sequestrants	All	Decreased bioavailability of HMGRI if administration is not adequately spaced
Cimetidine	Fluvastatin	Increase in plasma fluvastatin levels
Cyclosporine	All	Increased risk of severe myopathy or rhabdomyolysis
Danazol	Lavastatin	Increased risk of severe myopathy or rhabdomyolysis
Digoxin	Atorvastatin, Fluvastatin, Simvastatin	Slight elevation in plasma concentrations of digoxin
Diltiazem	Atorvastatin, Lovastatin, Simvastatin	Increased risk of severe myopathy
Erythromcyin Clarithromycin	All	Increased risk of severe myopathy or rhabdomyolysis; increased plasma levels of atorvastatin, lovastatin, and simvastatin because of inhibition of CYP3A4
Ethanol	Fluvastatin, Lovastatin	Increased risk of hepatotoxicity
Fibrates	All	Increased risk of severe myopathy or rhabdomyolysis
Grapefruit juice (>1 quart/day)	Atorvastatin, Lovastatin, Simvastatin	Elevated plasma levels of the HMGRIs and increased risk of myopathy
HIV protease inhibitors	Atorvastatin, Lovastatin, Simvastatin	Elevated plasma levels of the HMGRIs and increased risk of myopathy
Isradipine	Lovastatin	Increased clearance of lovastatin and its metabolites
Niacin	All	Increased risk of severe myopathy or rhabdomyolysis
Omeprazole	Fluvastatin	Increase in plasma fluvastatin levels
Oral contraceptives	Atorvastatin, Rosuvastatin	Increased plasma concentrations of norethindrone and ethinyl estradiol
Phenytoin	Fluvastatin	Increased plasma concentrations of both compounds because of CYP2C9 interaction
Ranitidine	Fluvastatin	Increase in plasma fluvastatin levels
Rifampin	Fluvastatin	Increased plasma clearance of fluvastatin
Ritonavir, Squinavir	Pravastatin	Decreased plasma levels of pravastatin
Spironolactone	All	Additive decreases in concentrations or activity of endogenous steroid hormones
St. John's wort	Lovastatin, Simvastatin	Decreased HMGRI plasma levels
Warfarin	Fluvastatin, Lovastatin, Rosuvastatin, Simvastatin	Anticoagulant effect of warfarin may be increased

eventually leads to enhanced receptor-mediated LDL uptake similar to that seen with bile acid sequestrants and HMGRIs. When used as monotherapy, the decreased absorption of cholesterol causes a compensatory increase in cholesterol biosynthesis. This is similar to that described for bile acid sequestrants and is insufficient to override the overall LDL lowering effects of ezetimibe.

Physicochemical Properties

Ezetimbie is a crystalline powder that is practically insoluble in water but is freely soluble in ethanol and other organic solvents. Its calculated log P value is 3.50 (38). The phenol present in ezetimibe allows this compound to be classified as an acidic compound; however, the phenol has a pK_a of 9.72 and is predominantly un-ionized at physiologic pH.

Metabolism

Following oral administration, ezetimibe is rapidly and extensively metabolized in the intestinal wall and the liver to its active metabolite, a corresponding phenol glucuronide. This glucuronide is reexcreted in the bile back to its active site. A small amount (<5%) of ezetimibe undergoes oxidation to covert the benzylic hydroxyl group to a ketone; however, ezetimibe does not appear to exert any significant effect on the activity of CYP450 enzymes (15,20,42).

Pharmacokinetic Parameters

Ezetimibe is administered orally; however, its absolute bioavailability cannot be determined because of its aqueous insolubility and the lack of an injectable formulation. Based on area under the curve values, the oral absorption ranges from 35 to 60%. Mean peak concentrations of the active glucuronidated metabolite are reached within 1 to 2 hours. Both ezetimibe and its glucuronide conjugate are extensively bound (>90%) to plasma proteins. The relative plasma concentrations of ezetimibe and its glucuronide conjugate range from 10 to 20% and from 80 to 90%, respectively. Both compounds have a long half-life of approximately 22 hours. The coadministration of food with ezetimibe has no effect on the extent of absorption.

Table 30.8. Drug Interactions for Ezetimibe

Drug	Result of Interaction
Antacid	Aluminum and magnesium-containing antacids decrease the C_{max} of ezetimibe
Bile Acid Sequestrants	Decreased bioavailability of ezetimibe if administration is not adequately spaced
Cyclosporine	Increased ezetimibe concentration.
Fibrates	Increased ezetimibe concentration and possible increased risk of cholelithiasis. Concomitant use is not recommended.

The normal dose of ezetimibe is 10 mg once daily. Dosage reduction for patients with renal impairment, intermittent hemodialysis, or mild hepatic impairment is not necessary. Because of insufficient data, the use of ezetimibe is not recommended in patients with moderate to severe hepatic impairment (15,20,21).

Therapeutic Applications

Ezetimibe is indicated as monotherapy or in combination with an HMGRI for the reduction of elevated total cholesterol, LDL cholesterol, and apoB in patients with primary (heterozygous familial and nonfamilial) hypercholesterolemia. When used as monotherapy, ezetimibe reduces LDL cholesterol by approximately 18%. When used in combination therapy with an HMGRI, LDL levels are reduced by 25 to 65% depending on the dose of the HMGRI inhibitor. Ezetimibe also is indicated for homozygous familial hypercholesterolemia in combination with either atorvastatin or simvastatin and for homozygous familial sitosterolemia. All indications are for patients who have not responded to diet, exercise, and other nonpharmacological methods.

Adverse Effects of Ezetimibe

Abdominal pain, diarrhea, arthralgia, back pain, cough, pharyngitis, sinusitis, fatigue, and viral infection

Adverse Effects

Ezetimibe generally is well tolerated. The most common adverse effects are listed above. Whenever ezetimibe is used in combination with an HMGRI, the incidence of myopathy or rhabdomyolysis does not increase above that seen with HMGRI monotherapy (15,21).

Drug interactions for ezetimibe are listed in Table 30.8.

FIBRATES

Historical Overview and Development

The use of this class of drugs to treat hyperlipoproteinemias can be traced back to 1962 and, thus, predates the use of bile acid sequestrants and HMGRIs. A random screening test on a series of aryloxyisobutyric acids demonstrated that these compounds could lower both plasma cholesterol and total lipid levels (43). The compound that produced the best balance between activity and toxicity was ethyl *p*-chlorophenoxyisobutyrate (Fig. 30.10). Later renamed clofibrate, this compound was subsequently shown to be a pro-drug for *p*-chlorophenoxyisobutyric acid (clofibric acid). It was approved for therapeutic use in 1967, and for a time, it was a very popular and widely prescribed drug. Results from a 1978 World Health Organization trial changed the acceptance of clofibrate and dramatically decreased its use. These trials indicated that despite a 9% lowering of cholesterol, patients taking clofibrate showed no reduction of

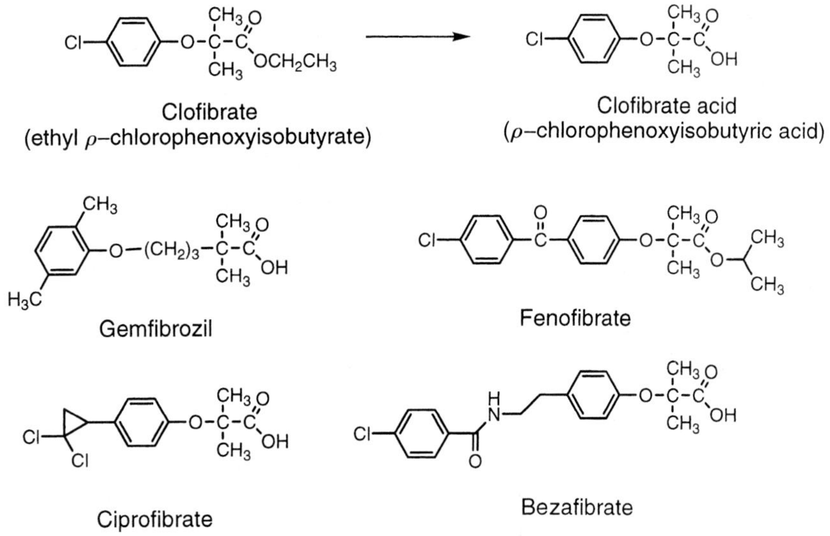

Clofibrate (ethyl *p*-chlorophenoxyisobutyrate)

Clofibrate acid (*p*-chlorophenoxyisobutyric acid)

Gemfibrozil

Fenofibrate

Ciprofibrate

Bezafibrate

Fig. 30.10. Bioactivation of clofibrate and chemical structures of other fibrates.

cardiovascular events and actually had an increase in overall mortality (7). Although clofibrate is no longer available in the United States, it has served as the prototype for the design of safer and more effective fibrates. Structural modifications, focused primarily on ring substitutions and the addition of spacer groups, have produced a number of active compounds (Fig. 30.10). Gemfibrozil and fenofibrate became available for therapy in 1981 and 1998, respectively. Fenofibrate was actually approved in 1993; however, its marketing was voluntarily delayed until a more bioavailable, micronized formulation of the drug was available (44). Both of these compounds are safer and more effective than clofibrate in lowering plasma triglyceride levels and increasing plasma HDL levels. Additional compounds, such as ciprofibrate and bezafibrate, are not currently available in the United States but have been used in other countries.

Mechanism of Action

Overall, fibrates decrease plasma triglyceride levels much more dramatically than they decrease plasma cholesterol levels. They significantly decrease VLDL levels, cause a moderate increase in HDL levels, and have variable effects on LDL concentrations. As an example of this latter point, gemfibrozil will raise LDL levels in patients with hypertriglyceridemia but lower LDL levels in patients with normal triglyceride levels. The exact mechanisms for these actions have not been fully elucidated; however, studies have shown that this class of compounds can produce a variety of beneficial effects on lipoprotein metabolism. Many of these effects have been proposed to be mediated through the activation of peroxisome proliferator-activated receptors (PPARs) and an alteration of gene expression. Specifically, fibrates bind to PPARα (7,15,27,44).

Decreases in plasma VLDL primarily result from the ability of these compounds to stimulate the activity of lipoprotein lipase, the enzyme responsible for removing triglycerides from plasma VLDL (Fig. 30.5). Additionally, fibrates can lower VLDL levels through PPARα-mediated stimulation of fatty acid oxidation, inhibition of triglyceride synthesis, and reduced expression of apoC-III. This latter effect enhances the action of lipoprotein lipase, because apoC-III normally serves as an inhibitor of this enzyme. Favorable effects on HDL levels appear to be related to increased transcription of apoA-I and apoA-II as well as a decreased activity of cholesteryl ester transfer protein.

All fibrates accelerate the turnover and removal of cholesterol from the liver. This increases the biliary secretion of cholesterol, enhances its fecal excretion, and may cause cholelithiasis (i.e., gallstone formation).

Structure–Activity Relationships

Fibrates can be chemically classified as analogues of phenoxyisobutyric acid. Literature references to the SARs for this class of drugs are sparse; however, all compounds are analogues of the following general structure.

[Aromatic ring]-O-[Spacer group]—C(CH_3)(CH_3)—C(=O)OH

The isobutyric acid group is essential for activity. Fenofibrate, which contains an ester, is a pro-drug and requires in vivo hydrolysis. Substitution at the para position of the aromatic ring with a chloro group or a chlorine containing isopropyl ring produces compounds with significantly longer half-lives. Although most compounds contain a phenoxyisobutyric acid, the addition of an n-propyl spacer, as seen in gemfibrozil, results in an active drug.

Physicochemical Properties

Similar to HMGRIs, the active forms of all fibrates contain a carboxylic acid. The pK_a of this functional group on clofibric acid is reported to be 3.5 (45) and, thus, will be primarily ionized at physiologic pH. Although not reported, the pK_a and ionization values of gemfibrozil and fenofibric acid can reasonably be assumed to be similar. Both clofibrate and fenofibrate are neutral, ester pro-drugs and should be classified as nonelectrolytes. Gemfibrozil can be classified as an acidic drug. The calculated log P values for fenofibrate and gemfibrozil are shown in Table 30.9 (45). Both compounds are highly lipid soluble despite the fact that gemfibrozil contains a water-soluble carboxylic acid. This can be partially explained by examining the π values for the substituents on fenofibrate and gemfibrozil (46). The 2,5-dimethyl ring in gemfibrozil is predicted to be much more hydrophobic than the 4-chloro ring of fenofibrate. Additionally, the propyl bridge seen in gemfibrozil, but not in fenofibrate, significantly adds to its hydrophobicity. The isopropyl ester as well as the additional aromatic ring account for the enhanced lipid solubility of fenofibrate. All currently available fibrates are achiral molecules and not subject to stereochemical concerns.

Table 30.9. Pharmacokinetic Parameters of Fibrates

Drug	Calculated Log P	Oral Bioavailability (%)	Active Metabolite	Protein Binding (%)	Time to Peak Conc (hrs)	Elimination Half-Life (hrs)	Major Route(s) of Elimination
Fenofibrate	5.24	60-90	Fenofibric acid	99	4-8	20-22	Renal (60-90%) Fecal (5-25%)
Gemfibrozil	3.9	> 90	none	99	1-2	1.5	Renal (70%) Fecal (6%)

Table 30.10. Dosage Information for Fibrates

Generic Name	Brand Name	Dosing Range	Maximum Daily Dose	Dose Reduction with Renal Dysfunction	Tablet/Capsule Strengths (mg)
Fenofibrate	TriCor	48-145 mg q.d. 54-160 mg q.d. 67-200 mg q.d.	145mg 160 mg 200 mg	Only with severe impairment	48, 145 54, 160 (generic) 67, 134, 200 (generic)
Gemfibrozil	Lopid	600 mg b.i.d.	1200 mg	Yes	600

Metabolism

The pro-drug fenofibrate undergoes rapid hydrolysis to produce fenofibric acid. This active metabolite can then be further metabolized by oxidative or conjugative pathways. Gemfibrozil is slightly different in that it does not require initial bioactivation; however, similar to fenofibric acid, it can be oxidized or conjugated. Oxidation of the aromatic methyl groups produces inactive hydroxymethyl and carboxylic acid analogues. As a drug class, fibrates and their oxidized analogues are primarily excreted as glucuronide conjugates in the urine. Oxidization requires the CYP3A4 isozyme; however, because of the ability of these compounds to be conjugated and eliminated either with or without oxidation, drug interactions with other compounds affecting the CYP3A4 system are less important here than with other drug classes.

Pharmacokinetic Parameters

The pharmacokinetic parameters and dosing information for the fibrates are summarized in Tables 30.9 and 30.10, respectively (7,15,20,21,45). The pro-drug, fenofibrate, requires a longer time to reach peak concentrations compared with gemfibrozil. Because of differences in aromatic substitution, fenofibrate also has a much longer half-life than gemfibrozil. As previously mentioned, the 2,5-dimethyl substitution in gemfibrozil is much more susceptible to oxidative metabolism than the para-chloro group present in fenofibrate. Similar to HMGRIs, changes in lipid levels are not seen immediately, and up to 2 months may be required to reach maximal clinical effects and to determine the overall clinical efficacy.

Fibrates have excellent bioavailability and are extensively bound to plasma proteins. Because food can significantly enhance their oral absorption, these compounds should be taken either with or just before meals. Fenofibrate was available in Europe and elsewhere as standard tablet and capsule formulations for many years before its approval and marketing in the United States, where it was introduced only after the development of a micronized formulation that allowed better oral absorption, a lower daily dose, and once-daily administration. A 67-mg dose of micronized fenofibrate is bioequivalent to a 100-mg dose of nonmicronized drug. Since that time, two additional tablet formulations have been developed. Abbott Laboratories currently markets TriCor as 48- and 145-mg tablets. The 48-mg formulation is equivalent to previous 54- and 67-mg formulations, and the 145-mg tablet is equivalent to previous 160- and 200-mg formulations. As noted in Table 30.10, fenofibrate is currently available in all of these strengths.

Renal elimination is the primary route through which these compounds are excreted from the body. Patients with mild renal dysfunction often can be managed with minor dosage adjustments, whereas those with severe impairment or renal failure may have to discontinue its use.

Therapeutic Applications

Fibrates are approved to treat hypertriglyceridemia and familial combined hyperlipidemia (Fredrickson's type IIa, IIb, IV, and V) (Table 30.2) in patients who are at risk of pancreatitis and have not responded to dietary adjustments or in patients who are at risk of CHD and have not responded to weight loss, dietary adjustments, and other pharmacological treatment. They can be used either alone or in combination with niacin, bile acid sequestrants, or HMGRIs. If used with bile acid sequestrants, fibrates must be taken either 1 hour before or 4 to 6 hours after the sequestrant. As discussed previously and reemphasized below, caution should be used if fibrates are combined with HMGRIs. Fibrates are not effective in the treatment of hypertriglyceridemia associated solely to elevated chylomicron levels (Fredrickson's type I).

Adverse Effects

The most prevalent or significant side effects caused by the fibrates are listed below (7,15,21). Despite the potential to cause serious side effects, fibrates usually are well tolerated. Gastrointestinal complaints are the most common but do not usually cause discontinuation of therapy. In general, gemfibrozil and fenofibrate appear to be less problematic than the original compound, clofibrate. In fact, many of the concerns regarding fibrate therapy are based on the effects of clofibrate and the results of a 1978 clinical trial in which patients taking clofibrate had a significantly higher morbidity and mortality from causes other than CHD. These causes included malignancy, gallbladder disease, pancreatitis, and postcholecystectomy

Unlabeled Uses

Polymetabolic syndrome X (fenofibrate)

Adverse Effects

Abdominal pain, dyspepsia, nausea, vomiting, diarrhea, constipation, cholestasis, jaundice, cholelithiasis, pancreatitis, headache, dizziness, drowsiness, blurred vision, mental depression, impotence, decreased libido, myopathy, myositis, rhabdomyolysis, anemia, leukopenia, eosinophilia, pruritus, and rash

complications. Studies with gemfibrozil and fenofibrate have not shown similar increases; however, because all fibrates have similar pharmacological actions, cautions and contraindications generally are applied to the entire drug class. As an example, even though gemfibrozil and fenofibrate have not demonstrated a significant increase in gallbladder disease, as seen with clofibrate, all three of these compounds are contraindicated in patients with preexisting gallbladder disease or cholelithiasis. Similar to HMGRIs, fibrates can cause myopathy, myositis, and rhabdomyolysis. Although rare, the risk of these serious effects increases when these two classes of agents are used together. Fibrates also cause increases in plasma aspartate transaminase (AST), alanine transaminase (ALT), and creatine phosphokinase levels.

Drug interactions for fibrates are listed in Table 30.11.

NICOTINIC ACID

Historical Overview

The history of nicotinic acid (niacin) began in 1867, when it was first synthesized by oxidation of nicotine. The name niacin was derived later from the words *ni*cotinic *ac*id and vitam*in* in an effort to avoid confusing nicotinic acid and nicotinamide with nicotine. Although the terms "niacin" and "nicotinic acid" are today used interchangeably, only the more chemically descriptive term, "nicotinic acid," will be used in the following discussions.

Nicotine Nicotinic acid Nicotinamide

Discovery of the biochemical and pharmacological actions of nicotinic acid began in the early 1900s, when brewer's yeast was demonstrated to prevent pellagra in humans. The subsequent isolation of nicotinic acid from brewer's yeast established its role as an essential dietary requirement. In the 1930s, its amide metabolite, nicotinamide, was isolated from liver extracts and found to be a required structural feature of nicotinamide adenine dinucleotide phosphate ($NADP^+$), a cofactor involved in electron transport and intermediary metabolism (47). In 1955, Altschul et al. (48) observed that high doses of nicotinic acid lowered cholesterol levels in humans, an activity unrelated to its properties as a vitamin. Subsequent studies have shown that nicotinic acid also lowers serum triglyceride levels and is effective against a variety of hyperlipoproteinemias. None of these antihyperlipidemic effects are seen with nicotinamide.

Mechanism of Action

Nicotinic acid exerts a variety of effects on lipoprotein metabolism (7,16,49). One of its most important actions is the inhibition of lipolysis in adipose tissue. This initial inhibition, like those of previously discussed antihyperlipidemic agents, produces a sequence of events that ultimately result in the lowering of plasma triglycerides and cholesterol. Impaired lipolysis decreases the mobilization of free fatty acids, thus reducing their plasma levels and their delivery to the liver. In turn, this decreases hepatic triglyceride synthesis and results in a decreased production of VLDL. Enhanced clearance of VLDL through stimulation of lipoprotein lipase also has been proposed to contribute to the reduction of plasma VLDL levels. Because LDL is derived from VLDL (Fig. 30.5), the decreased production of VLDL ultimately leads to a decrease in LDL levels. The sequential nature of this process has been clinically demonstrated. The reduction in triglyceride levels occurs within several hours after

Table 30.11. Drug Interactions for Fibrates

Drug	Fibrate	Result of Interaction
Antidiabetic agents	All	Increased hypoglycemic effect through increased sensitivity and decreased glucagon secretion
Bexarotene	Gemfibrozil	Increased bexarotene plasma concentrations
Bile acid sequestrants	All	Decreased bioavailability of fibrate if administration is not adequately spaced
Cyclosporine	Fenofibrate	Increased potential for nephrotoxicity
Ezetimibe	All	Increased ezetimibe concentration and possible increased risk of cholelithiasis; concomitant use is not recommended
HMG-CoA reductase inhibitors	All	Increased risk of severe myopathy or rhabdomyolysis
Oral anticoagulants	All	Increased hypoprothrombinemic effect
Repaglinide	Gemfibrozil	Increased repaglinide plasma concentrations
Ursodiol	All	Increased hepatic cholesterol secretion which may increase the possibility of gallstone formation and counteract the effectiveness of ursodiol

initiation of nicotinic acid therapy, whereas the reduction in cholesterol does not occur until after several days of therapy. Nicotinic acid also increases HDL levels because of a reduction in the clearance of apoA-I, an essential component of HDL. Unlike bile acid sequestrants and HMGRIs, nicotinic acid does not have any effects on cholesterol catabolism or biosynthesis.

Physicochemical Properties

Nicotinic acid (niacin) is a stable, nonhygroscopic, white, crystalline powder. Its carboxylic acid has a pK_a of 4.76 and, thus, is predominantly ionized at physiologic pH. The pyridine nitrogen is a very weak base (pK_a = 2.0) and, therefore, primarily exists in the un-ionized form. Nicotinic acid is freely soluble in alkaline solutions and has a measured log P of −0.20 at pH 6.0 (45).

Metabolism

Nicotinic acid is a B-complex vitamin that is converted to nicotinamide, NAD^+, and $NADP^+$. The latter two compounds are coenzymes and are required for oxidation/reduction reactions in a variety of biochemical pathways. Additionally, nicotinic acid is metabolized to a number of inactive compounds, including nicotinuric acid and N-methylated derivatives. Normal biochemical regulation and feedback prevent large doses of nicotinic acid from producing excess quantities of NAD^+ and $NADP^+$. Thus, small doses of nicotinic acid, such as those used for dietary supplementation, will be primarily excreted as metabolites, whereas large doses, such as those used for the treatment of hyperlipoproteinemia, will be primarily excreted unchanged by the kidney (15).

Pharmacokinetic Parameters

Nicotinic acid is readily absorbed. Peripheral vasodilation is seen within 20 minutes, and peak plasma concentrations occur within 45 minutes. The half-life of the compound is approximately one hour, thus necessitating frequent dosing or an extended-release formulation. Extended release tablets produce peripheral vasodilation within 1 hour, reach peak plasma concentrations within 4 to 5 hours, and have a duration of 8 to 10 hours.

Dosing of nicotinic acid should be titrated to minimize adverse effects. An initial dose of 50 to 100 mg t.i.d. often is used with immediate-release tablets. The dose then is gradually increased by 50 to 100 mg every 3 to 14 days, up to a maximum of 6 g/day, as tolerated. Therapeutic monitoring to assess efficacy and prevent toxicity is essential until a stable and effective dose is reached. Similar dosing escalations are available for extended-release products, with doses normally starting at 500 mg once daily at bedtime. (7,15,21).

Therapeutic Applications

Nicotinic acid is approved for the treatment of hypercholesterolemia, hypertriglyceridemia, and familial combined hyperlipidemia (Fredrickson's type IIa, IIb, IV, and V) (Table 30.2) in patients who have not responded to diet, exercise, and other nonpharmacological methods. It also is approved for nutritional supplementation, the prevention of pellagra, and as adjunct therapy for peripheral vascular disease and circulatory disorders. It is contraindicated in patients with hepatic disease and peptic ulcer disease. Additionally, because of its ability to elevate glucose and uric acid levels, especially when taken in large doses, nicotinic acid should be used with caution in patients who have or are predisposed to diabetes mellitus and gout (15,20,21).

Table 30.12. Drug Interactions for Nicotinic Acid

Drug	Result of Interaction
Adrenergic blocking agents	Enhanced vasodilation and postural hypotension
Bile acid sequestrants	Decreased bioavailability of nicotinic acid if administration is not adequately spaced
Ethanol	Potential enhanced hepatotoxicity and excessive peripheral or cutaneous vasodilation
HMG-CoA reductase inhibitors	Increased risk of myopathy and rhabdomyolysis
Vasodilating agents (calcium channel blockers, epoprostenol, nitrates)	Enhanced cutaneous vasodilation

Adverse Effects

The most common (and, often, dose-limiting) side effects of nicotinic acid treatment are cutaneous vasodilation (flushing and pruritus) and gastrointestinal intolerance, which may occur in 20 to 50% of treated patients. Flushing and pruritus are prostaglandin-mediated effects and may be prevented by taking aspirin or indomethacin before nicotinic acid. Gastrointestinal side effects, such as flatulence, nausea, vomiting, and diarrhea, can be minimized if nicotinic acid is taken either with or immediately after meals. As previously mentioned, all of these effects can be minimized by slowly titrating the dose of nicotinic acid. Hepatic dysfunction is one of the more serious complications of high dose nicotinic acid. Plasma AST, ALT, lactate dehydrogenase, and alkaline phosphatase levels often are elevated but usually return to normal when therapy is either adjusted or discontinued (7,15,21).

Drug interactions for nicotinic acid are listed in Table 30.12.

Adverse Effects of Niacin

Flushing, pruritus, headache, nausea, vomiting, diarrhea, flatulence, hepatic dysfunction, jaundice, hyperglycemia, hyperuricemia, blurred vision, and tachycardia

CASE STUDY

Victoria F. Roche and S. William Zito

MK is a 38-year-old female with a history of congenital cardiomyopathy that resulted in aortic value replacement surgery 3 years ago. MK opted for a mechanical valve and is now on chronic coumadin anticoagulant therapy and doing well. She is a fibromyalgia patient and manages her pain with oxycodone, 5 mg as needed (not to exceed every 4 hours). She manages the constipation that has accompanied her regular use of opioids with Senna (two tablets at bedtime and two in the morning). Feeling somewhat helpless about her health situation, she has begun tai-chi and yoga and to meditate regularly, and she has joined her husband in his vegetarian lifestyle (he's the sous-chef at the world-famous "Meatless in Seattle" restaurant). While difficult at first, she now religiously restricts her intake of fats and cholesterol-rich foods. She has been taking St. John's wort (purchased at the local Health & Nutrition outlet) for a mild, self-diagnosed depression that she hopes is temporary. After trying unsuccessfully for several years to conceive a child, MK and her husband are actively exploring adoption.

At her annual medical checkup, it was noted that MK's total serum cholesterol and LDL levels were mildly elevated, although her triglycerides and HDL levels were hovering around normal. Given her cardiovascular history, the physician wishes to implement therapy to bring her blood lipids down to National Cholesterol Education Program (NCEP)-recommended levels.

1. Identify the therapeutic problem(s) in which the pharmacist's intervention may benefit the patient.
2. Identify and prioritize the patient-specific factors that must be considered to achieve the desired therapeutic outcomes.
3. Conduct a thorough and mechanistically oriented structure–activity analysis of all therapeutic alternatives provided in this case.
4. Evaluate the SAR findings against the patient-specific factors and desired therapeutic outcomes, and make a therapeutic decision.
5. Counsel your patient

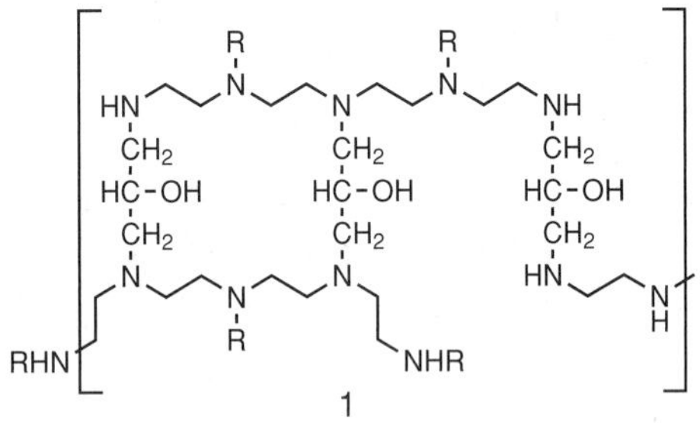

1 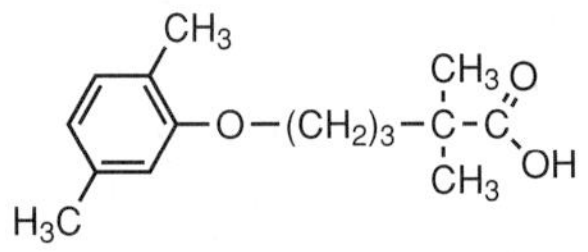 2 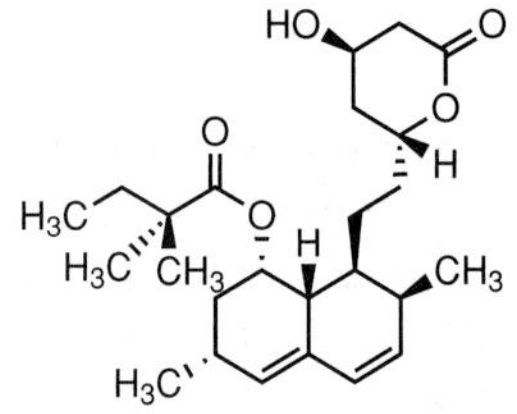 3

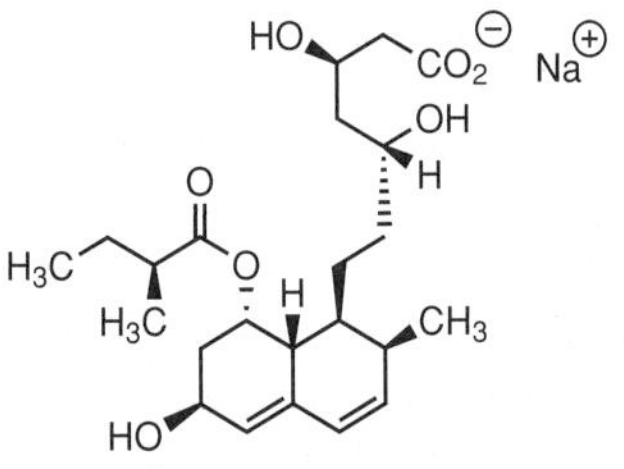

4 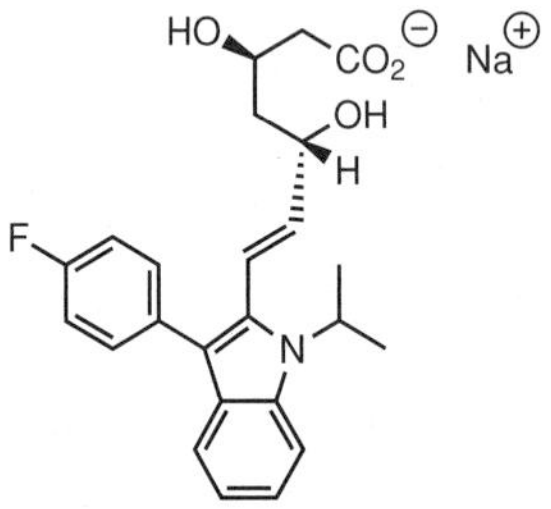 5 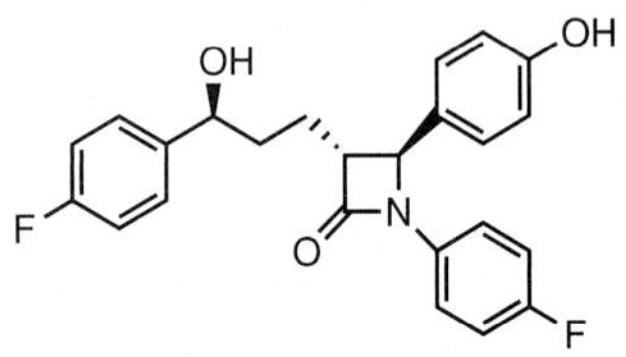 6

References

1. Ginsberg HN, Goldberg IJ. Disorders of lipoprotein metabolism. In: Fauci AS, Braunwald E, Isselbacher KJ, et al., eds. Harrison's Principles of Internal Medicine, 14th Ed. New York: McGraw-Hill, 1998:2138–2149.
2. Drugs for lipids. The Medical Letter 2005;3:15–22.
3. Vaczek D. Top 200 prescription drugs of 2004. Pharmacy Times 2005;71:41–46.
4. Berg JM, Tymoczko JL, Stryer L. Biochemistry, 5th Ed. New York: Freeman and Company, 2002:715–743.
5. Bamford MJ, Chan C, Craven AP, et al. The squalestatins: synthesis and biological activity of some C_3–modified analogues; replacement of a carboxylic acid or methyl ester with an isoelectronic heterocyclic functionality. J Med Chem 1995;38:3502–3513.
6. Chan C, Andreotti D, Cox B, et al. The squalestatins: decarboxy and 4-deoxy analogues as potent squalene synthase inhibitors. J Med Chem 1996;39:207–216.
7. Mahley RW, Bersot, TP. Drug therapy for hypercholesterolemia. In: Hardman JG, Limbird LE, Gilman AG, eds. The Pharmacological Basis of Therapeutics, 10th Ed. New York: McGraw-Hill, 2001:971–1002.
8. Talbert RL. Hyperlipidemia. In: Dipiro JT, Talbert RL, Yee GC, et al., eds. Pharmacotherapy: A Pathophysiologic Approach, 6th ed. New York: McGraw-Hill, 2005:429–452.
9. Fredrickson DS, Levy RI, Lees RS. Fat transport in lipoproteins—an integrated approach to mechanisms and disorders. N Engl J Med 1967;276:34–42.
10. American Heart Association. Heart and stroke statistics—2005 update. Available at: http://www.americanheart.org/presenter.jhtml?identifier=1200026. Accessed July 29, 2005.
11. Libby P. Atherosclerosis. In: Fauci AS, Braunwald E, Isselbacher KJ, et al., eds. Harrison's Principles of Internal Medicine, 14th Ed. New York: McGraw Hill, 1998:1345–1352.
12. Sliskovic DR, White AD. Therapeutic potential of ACAT inhibitors as lipid lowering and antiatherosclerotic agents. Trends Pharmacol Sci 1991;12:194–199.
13. Grundy SM, Cleeman JI, Bairey CN, et al. Implications of recent clinical trials for the National Cholesterol Education Program Adult Panel III guidelines. Circulation 2004;110:227–239.
14. Roth B. ACAT inhibitors: evolution from cholesterol-absorption inhibitors to antiatherosclerotic agents. Drug Discov Today 1998;3:19–25.

15. Clinical Pharmacology Online. Gold Standard Multimedia, 2005. Available at: http://www.cp.gsm.com. Accessed October 25, 2005.
16. Cendella RJ. Cholesterol and hypocholesterolemic drugs. In: Craig CR, Stitzel RE, eds. Modern Pharmacology with Clinical Applications, 5th Ed. Boston: Little, Brown and Co., 1997:279–289.
17. Brown MS, Goldstein JL. A receptor-mediated pathway for cholesterol homeostasis. Science 1986;232:34–47.
18. Zhu XX, Brown GR, St-Pierre LE. Polymeric sorbents for bile acids. I: Comparison between cholestyramine and colestipol. J Pharm Sci 1992;81:65–69.
19. Clas SD. Quaternized colestipol, an improved bile salt adsorbent: in vitro studies. J Pharm Sci 1991;80:128–131.
20. Micromedex Online. The Thompson Corporation, 2005. Available at http://www.micromedex.com. Accessed October 25,2005.
21. Drug Facts and Comparisons. St. Louis, MO: Wolters Kluwer Health, 2005:533–549.
22. Heathcock CH, Hadley CR, Rosen T, et al. Total synthesis and biological evaluation of structural analogues of compactin and dihydromevinolin. J Med Chem 1987;30:1858–1873.
23. Adams JL, Metcalf BW. Therapeutic consequences of the inhibition of sterol metabolism. In: Hansch C, Sammes PG, Taylor JB, eds. Comprehensive Medicinal Chemistry, vol 2. Oxford: Permagon Press, 1990;333–363.
24. Cutler SJ, Cocolas GH. Cardiovascular agents. In: Block JH, Beale, JM, eds. Wilson and Gisvold's Textbook of Organic Medicinal and Pharmaceutical Chemistry, 11th Ed. Philadelphia: Lippincott Williams & Wilkins, 2004: 657–663.
25. Stokker GE, Hoffman WF, Alberts AW, et al. 3-Hydroxy-3-methylglutaryl–coenzyme A reductase inhibitors. 1. Structural modification of 5-substituted 3,5-dihydroxypentanoic acids and their lactone derivatives. J Med Chem 1985;28:347–358.
26. Sliskovic DR, Blankley CJ, Krause BR, et al. Inhibitors of cholesterol biosynthesis. 6. trans-5-[2-(-N-heteroaryl-3,5-disubstituted-pyrazol-4-yl)ethyl/ethenyl]tetrahydro-4-hydroxy-2H-pyran-2-ones. J Med Chem 1992;35:2095–2103.
27. Bone EA, Davidson AH, Lewis CN, et al. Synthesis and biological evaluation of dihydroeptastatin, a novel inhibitor of 3-hydroxy-3-methylglutaryl–coenzyme A reductase. J Med Chem 1992;35:3388–3393.
28. Roth BD, Ortwine DF, Hoefle ML, et al. Inhibitors of cholesterol biosynthesis. 1. trans-6-(2-Pyrrol-1-ylethyl)-4-hydroxypyran-2-ones, a novel series of HMG-CoA reductase inhibitors. 1. Effects of structural modifications at the 2-and 5-positions of the pyrrole nucleus. J Med Chem 1990;33:21–31.
29. Hoffman WF, Alberts AW, Cragoe EJ Jr, et al. 3-Hydroxy-3-methylglutaryl–coenzyme A reductase inhibitors. 2. Structural modification of 7-(substituted aryl)-3,5-dihydroxy-6-heptenoic acids and their lactone derivatives. J Med Chem 1986;29:159–169.
30. Stokker GE, Alberts AW, Anderson PS, et al. 3-Hydroxy-3-methylglutaryl-coenzyme A reductase inhibitors. 3. 7-(3,5-Disubstituted [1,1′-biphenyl]-2-yl)-3,5-dihydroxy-6-heptenoic acids and their lactone derivatives. J Med Chem 1986;29:170–181.
31. Heathcock CH, Davis BR, Hadley CR. Synthesis and biological evaluation of a monocyclic, fully functional analogue of compactin. J Med Chem 1989;32:197–202.
32. Lee TJ, Holtz WJ, Smith RL, et al. 3-Hydroxy-3-methylglutaryl–coenzyme A reductase inhibitors. 8. Side chain ether analogues of lovastatin. J Med Chem 1991;34:2474–2477.
33. Hoffman WF, Alberts AW, Anderson PS, et al. 3-Hydroxy-3-methylglutaryl-coenzyme A reductase inhibitors. 4. Side chain ester derivatives of mevinolin. J Med Chem 1986;29:849–852.
34. Stokker GE, Alberts AW, Gilfillan JL, et al. 3-Hydroxy-3-methylglutaryl–coenzyme A reductase inhibitors. 5. 6-(Fluoren-9-yl)- and 6-(fluoren-9-ylidenyl)-3,5-dihydroxyhexanoic acids and their lactone derivatives. J Med Chem 1986;29:852–855.
35. Procopiou PA, Draper CD, Hutson JL, et al. Inhibitors of cholesterol biosynthesis. 2. 3,5-Dihydroxy-7-(N-pyrrolyl)-6-heptenoates, a novel series of HMG-CoA reductase inhibitors. J Med Chem 1993;36:3658–3662.
36. Atorvastatin—a new lipid-lowering drug. The Medical Letter 1997;39:29–31.
37. Rosuvastatin—a new lipid-lowering drug. The Medical Letter 2003;45:81–83.
38. Craig PN. Drug compendium. In: Hansch C, Sammes PG, Taylor JB, eds. Comprehensive Medicinal Chemistry, vol 6. Oxford: Permagon Press, 1990: 237–991.
39. Zocor (simvastatin) product literature. Merck, 1999.
40. Wheeler DC. Are there potential nonlipid-lowering uses of statins? Drugs 1998;56:517–522.
41. Clader JW. The discovery of ezetimibe: a view from outside the receptor. J Med Chem 2004;47:1–9.
42. Kosoglou T, Statkevich P, Johnson-Levonas AO, et al. Ezetimibe: a review of its metabolism, pharmacokinetics, and drug interactions. Clin Pharmacokinet 2005;44:467–494.
43. Thorp JM, Waring WS. Modification and distribution of lipids by ethyl chlorophenoxyisobutyrate. Nature 1962;194:948–949.
44. Hussar DA. New drugs of 1998. J Am Pharm Assoc 1999;39:170–172.
45. Values calculated by author using ACD/ChemSketch, Version 8.17, 2005. Obtained from Advanced Chemistry Development, Inc. Available at: http://www.acdlabs.com.
46. Hansch C, Leo A. Substituent constants for correlation analysis in chemistry and biology. New York: Wiley, 1979:49–54.
47. Garrett RH, Grisham CM. Biochemistry. Fort Worth, TX: Saunders College Publishing, 1995:468–473.
48. Altschul R, Hoffer A, Stephen JD. Influence of nicotinic acid on serum cholesterol in man. Arch Biochem 1955;54:558–559.
49. Drood JM, Zimetbaum PJ, Frishman WH. Nicotinic acid for the treatment of hyperlipoproteinemia. J Clin Pharmacol 1991;31:641–650.

31. *Antithrombotics, Thrombolytics, Coagulants, and Plasma Extenders*

MATTHIAS C. LU AND THOMAS L. LEMKE

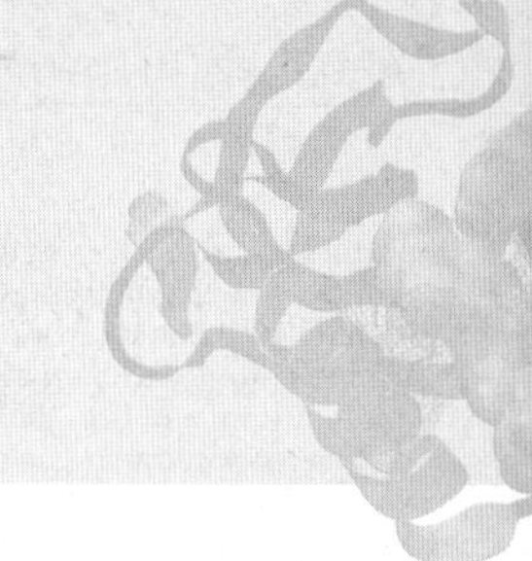

DRUGS COVERED IN THIS CHAPTER:

WARFARIN

HEPARINS

- High molecular weight heparin
- Low molecular weight haparin
  - Ardeparin
  - Dalteparin
  - Enoxaparin
- Fondaparinux

DIRECT THROMBIN INHIBITORS

- Argatroban
- Bivalirudin
- Desirudin
- Lepirudin
- Melagatran
- Ximelagatran

ANTIPLATELET DRUGS

- Abciximab
- Aspirin
- Cilostazol
- Clopidogrel
- Dipyridamole
- Eptifibatide
- Indobufen
- Sulfinpyrazone
- Ticlopidine
- Tirofiban
- Triflusal

THROMBOLYTIC DRUGS

- Alteplase
- Prourokinase
- Reteplase
- Streptokinase
- Tenecteplase
- Urokinase

COAGULANTS

- Protamine
- Vitamin K

ANTIFIBRINOLYTIC AGENTS

- Aprotinin

INTRODUCTION

Venous thromboembolism (VTE) is a complicating condition responsible for high morbidity and mortality in North America and Europe. This disease commonly is linked to advanced age but has both hereditary and acquired risk factors, such as surgery, any form of trauma, and childbirth, associated with it. It encompasses the conditions of deep vein thrombosis (DVT) and pulmonary embolism. In excess of 60,000 deaths annually are attributed to pulmonary embolism. Preventative therapy consists of the use of two different classes of antithrombotic agents, namely anticoagulants and antiplatelet drugs (1,2).

Heparin was discovered serendipitously in 1916 by a young coal miner turned medical student, Jay McLean, while working in the research laboratory of Professor W.H. Howell (3). Its beneficial effects were not realized until the early 1970s, when Kakkar et al. (4) established in a prospective, double-blind trial that low doses of heparin can prevent DVT after major surgery. In 1933, Dr. K.P. Link discovered that hydroxycoumarins are contained in sweet clover after finding cattle hemorrhaging to death (3). This discovery lead to the development of orally active anticoagulants for prophylaxis in VTE and other thrombotic disorders. Optimal therapy with warfarin and other coumarin derivatives are not easy, however, because of their narrow therapeutic indexes. The need to carefully assess the benefit and risks for anticoagulation with frequent drug monitoring and dose adjustment also is troublesome (5). Thus, further development of novel antithrombotic agents with greater specificity on the coagulation cascade, with more predictable pharmacodynamic and pharmacokinetic profiles, and with fewer or no laboratory monitoring requirements is still needed for optimal treatment of thrombotic disorders (6,7).

Thrombolytics, on the other hand, are drugs needed to dissolve the newly formed thrombi in conditions such as DVT, acute pulmonary embolism, or myocardial infarction. Because of their lack of specificity, however, these agents actually may cause internal bleeding and, thus, are contraindicated with the use of many other therapeutic agents.

A variety of pathological and toxicological conditions can result in excessive bleeding from inadequate coagulation. Depending on the etiology and severity of the hemorrhagic episode, select coagulants that induce blood coagulation are therapeutically used to prevent excessive bleeding in these conditions.

Plasma extenders and blood substitutes are used to maintain blood volume and blood circulation for resuscitation of severely anemic patients in emergency conditions. Although notable progress has been made in the development of oxygen-carrying blood substitutes that will someday bring effective replacements for whole blood into clinical practice, most still concentrate only on reproducing the function of hemoglobin, the molecule that carries oxygen through the body, and do not attempt to replicate the blood's other functions.

DISEASE STATES REQUIRING ANTITHROMBOTIC THERAPY

A number of serious medical conditions are thrombotic in nature. In fact, in Western society, thrombotic conditions are the major cause of morbidity and mortality, and

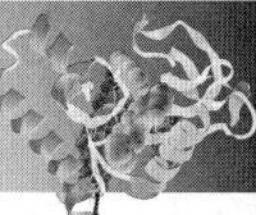

CLINICAL SIGNIFICANCE

Thrombotic disorders are among the most common causes of morbidity and mortality in the United States. More than 2 million people die each year from arterial or venous thrombosis or the consequences thereof. Antithrombotic and thrombolytic agents are the most commonly used pharmacological therapies to prevent and treat the whole spectrum of thrombotic disorders. The management of patients with thrombotic disorders involves multidisciplinary specialties, such as medicine, pharmacy, and nursing. Approaching clinical thrombosis in a multidisciplinary manner has the ultimate goal of rendering the best possible care to our patients. Regardless of the discipline involved, mastering the basic chemical and pharmacological principles of the major drug classes used in the prevention and treatment of thrombotic disorders is the first and most critical step to implementing a successful treatment approach.

Understanding the intricacies and the determinants of the coagulation cascade, along with the primary and secondary hemostatic and fibrinolytic pathways, allows us to clinically select and apply the best pharmacological agents targeted at these pathways. Furthermore, mastering the chemical and pharmacological properties of the various antithrombotic therapies is a necessary tool for clinicians involved in caring for patients with thrombosis. Often, selection of the safest and most effective therapeutic agent in certain specific patient circumstances will depend on our ability to differentiate among the characteristics of various options available. For example, in a patient with an allergic reaction to heparin (because of a suspected pork allergy), a good alternate anticoagulant for treatment of an acute thrombotic event is a synthetic agent, such as fondaparinux. In a patient with a deficiency of antithrombin (formerly known as antithrombin III), none of the heparin products or indirect factor Xa inhibitor products would work, because all of these have a mechanism of action dependent on Antithrombin. Alternate agents, such as direct inhibitors of thrombin, would need to be considered. In patients taking chronic warfarin therapy, dosing adjustments are made in increments of 5 to 20% of the patient's total weekly dose, because warfarin does not follow linear kinetics. Are there situations when using a combination of various antithrombotic agents would be appropriate? In certain indications, such as acute coronary syndromes, a combination of aspirin and clopidogrel is used, because these two agents have a complementary mechanism of action. The examples given above show just a few scenarios of how some of the basic concepts presented in this chapter are applied in clinical practice and how they eventually will aid clinicians to apply this knowledge toward providing specific and tailored treatment plans for their patients.

Edith A. Nutescu, Pharm.D.
Clinical Associate Professor
Director, Antithrombosis Center
College of Pharmacy
University of Illinois at Chicago

it is speculated that these disorders will be the leading cause of death worldwide within 20 years (1,8). As would be expected from the gravity of thrombotic disorders, many of the conditions involve the major vasculature, heart, brain and lungs.

In the heart, a thrombotic condition may be involved in the disease state of acute myocardial infarction, valvular heart disease, unstable angina, and atrial fibrillation as well as surgical procedures, such as percutaneous transluminal coronary angioplasty and prosthetic heart valve replacement. Thrombotic conditions involving the vasculature include VTE, primary and secondary prevention of arterial thromboembolism, and peripheral vascular disease. The most significant such condition involving the lungs is pulmonary embolism and, in the brain, cerebrovascular accidents. Anticoagulation therapy is indicated for all of these conditions.

Venous Thromboembolism and Pulmonary Embolism

Venous thromboembolism occurs when red bloods cells, fibrin, and to a lesser extent, platelets and leukocytes coagulate to form a thrombus within an intact cardiovascular system (9). A patient undergoing orthopaedic surgery incurs the greatest risk for VTE (10). Pulmonary embolism occurs when a segment of a thrombus within the deep venous system detaches itself from the blood vessel, travels to the lungs, and lodges within the pulmonary arteries. Both of these conditions, if not properly detected and treated, can have serious consequences, such as sudden death or recurrent VTE and postthrombotic syndrome characterized by persistent pain, swelling, and skin discoloration or necrosis and ulceration of the affected limb (6,7).

Atrial Fibrillation

Atrial fibrillation is the most common cardiac arrhythmia, being found in more than 2 million Americans. It is characterized as a storm of electrical energy that travels in spinning wavelets throughout the atria, causing the upper chambers to quiver or fibrillate. It also is one of the leading risk factors for ischemic stroke for those individuals older than 50 years (11–13). Atrial fibrillation is more prevalent in men than in women, and the median age of patients with atrial fibrillation is approximately 72 years. Anticoagulation with warfarin and lifestyle modification are the most effective treatment modalities for patients with atrial fibrillation.

Pathophysiology of Thrombogenesis

Arterial thrombosis usually is initiated by the exposure of the thrombogenic material as a result of spontaneous or mechanical rupture of an atherosclerotic plaque (6,14). Arterial thrombi usually form in medium-sized vessels as a result of surface lesions on endothelial cells roughened by atherosclerosis. In most cases, circulating platelets adhere to the areas of abnormal vascular endothelium. More platelets then aggregate with those stuck to the vascular wall, forming a clot known as an occlusive thrombus (14). The formation of the occlusive thrombus at the site of the lesion is the major cause of complications of stroke and myocardial infarction. Venous thrombosis results from either an excessive activation of the coagulation cascade (hypercoagulability) or from some disease process or venous pooling (stasis) of the blood. Venous thrombus is initiated in the same fashion as the arterial thrombus formation, except that the bulk of the clot is formed of long fibrin tails that enmesh red blood cells. Venous thrombosis also can occur from vascular trauma caused by damage to the vessel wall, especially after major orthopedic surgery (9). Hypercoagulability, venous stasis, and vascular injury are known as Virchow's triad. As a general rule, arterial thrombi cause serious conditions through localized occlusive ischemia, whereas venous thrombi fragment give rise to pleural embolic complications.

Biochemical Mechanism of Blood Coagulation: The Coagulation Cascade

The formation of a blood clot is the result of an intricate and elegant cascade of biochemical events (Fig. 31.1).

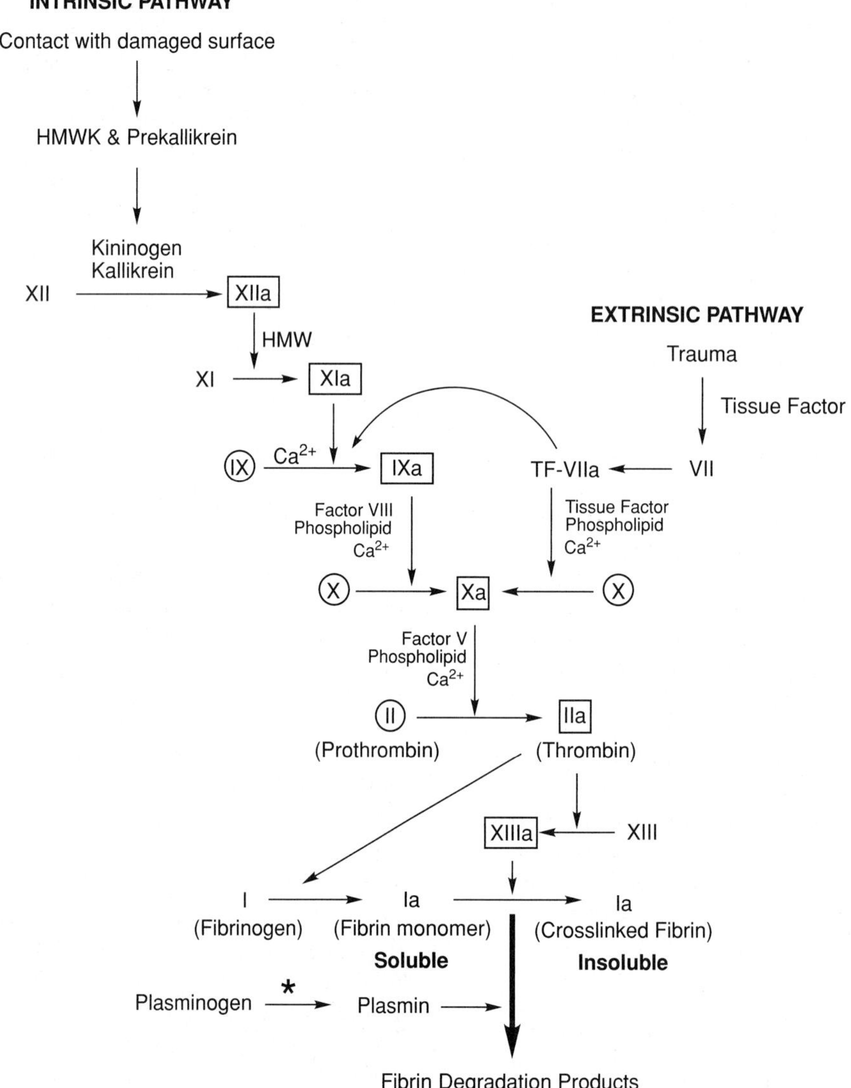

Fig. 31.1. The coagulation cascade. Circled factors are those inhibited by warfarin-like drugs; boxed factors are those affected by heparin. The star indicates the site of action of thrombolytic drugs, such as streptokinase and urokinase.

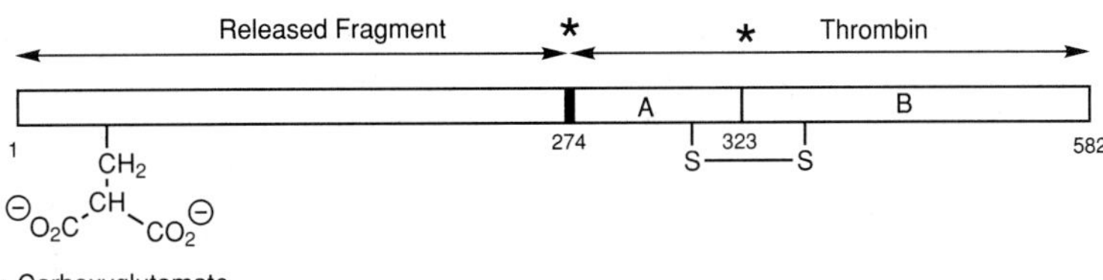

Fig. 31.2. Structure of prothrombin. Thrombin is liberated through the cleavage of the Arg 274–Thr 275 and Arg 323–Ile 324 peptide bonds (indicated by the stars). The γ-carboxyglutamate residues are in the released N-terminal portion of prothrombin and are not part of thrombin. The A and B chains of thrombin are joined by a disulfide bond.

The coagulation in arteries or veins is triggered by tissue factor (TF), a small-molecular-weight glycoprotein that initiates the extrinsic clotting cascade. The TF glycoprotein is expressed on the surface of macrophages, and TF is a major initiating factor of arterial thrombogenesis. Tissue factor binds and activates factor VII to form TF/VIIa complex, which in turn activates factor IX and factor X from either the intrinsic or extrinsic pathways shown in Figure 31.1.

Initiation of the intrinsic pathway involves the sequential activation of factors XII, XI, and IX. (The activated form of a coagulation factor is indicated by a lowercase "a.") In the presence of calcium, factor IXa binds to an activated factor VIII on the surface of activated platelets to form an intrinsic Xase complex, which initiates the activation of factor X to Xa. In addition, initiation of the extrinsic pathway involves activation of factor VII by TF to form TF/VIIa, which, like factor IXa, also catalyzes the conversion of factor X to Xa. The underlying purpose of the intrinsic pathway is maintenance of homeostasis, whereas the extrinsic pathway is activated by trauma. The intrinsic and extrinsic pathways come together with the conversion of factor X to its activated form, factor Xa. The coagulation cascade is unique in that the product of a given reaction (i.e., activated form of a specific factor) catalyzes the activation of the next factor in the cascade. The final steps in the coagulation cascade involve the conversion of prothrombin (factor II) to thrombin (factor IIa) by prothrombinase complex, consisting of factor Xa and activated factor V (Fig. 31.2). In turn, thrombin catalyzes the conversion of fibrinogen to soluble fibrin, which then becomes insoluble fibrin through the action of factor XIIIa. In its activated state, factor XIIIa actually is a transamidase enzyme. This enzyme catalyzes the formation of isopeptide bonds between lysine and glutamine side chains of distinct fibrin molecules, resulting in cross-linked (insoluble) fibrin aggregates (Fig. 31.3) (15).

Strategies for Regulating Coagulation

Coagulation can be regulated at several levels (6). These include TF pathway inhibitor (TFPI), antithrombin, and the protein C pathways. Because the design of many new anticoagulant drugs are aimed at enhancing endogenous anticoagulant or fibrinolytic mechanisms, a brief review of these pathways is warranted here.

Tissue factor pathway inhibitor is now recognized as a major physiological inhibitor of TF-initiated coagulation (16). Its main role is to modulate factor VIIa/TF catalytic activity by a two-step process. First, TFPI binds and inactivates factor Xa by forming a TFPI/factor Xa complex. Then, the inactivated factor Xa/TFPI complex binds factor VIIa within the TF/VIIa complex to modulate its catalytic activity. Additionally, TFPI potentiates the effect of heparins (i.e., TFPI is released from the vascular endothelium after injection of either unfractionated heparin or low-molecular-weight heparins [LMWHs]), which may then provide high concentrations of TFPI at sites of tissue damage and ongoing thrombosis (17). The propagation of coagulation occurs when TFPI concentrations are low (6).

Antithrombin is a potent inhibitor of thrombin, factors IXa and Xa. It also has inhibitory actions on other activated clotting factors, including the TF/VIIa complex. In the absence of heparin, however, the action of antithrombin is slow. The action of antithrombin is enhanced 1,000-fold in the presence of heparin. It should be pointed out that even though heparin is not normally found in the blood, the vascular endothelium is rich in heparin sulfate, which contains the antithrombin-binding pentasaccharide sequence of the heparin. Drugs such as fondaparinux and idraparinux block the propagation of coagulation by inactivating factor Xa and, thereby, inhibiting the thrombin formation (6). Direct

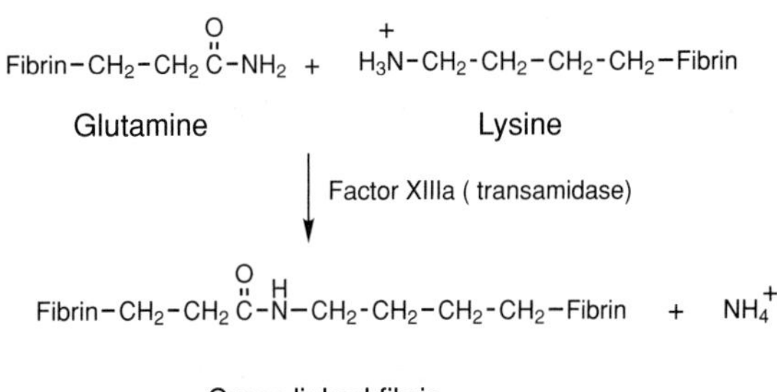

Fig. 31.3. Cross-linking of soluble fibrin monomers (factor Ia) through the activity of factor XIIIa, a transamidase enzyme.

thrombin inhibitors, such as hirudin and argatroban, work by inhibiting both the clot-bound and free thrombin and, thus, preventing fibrin formation, the final step in the coagulation cascade (6).

In the protein C pathway, thrombin also is inhibited by binding to thrombomodulin, a thrombin receptor found in the endothelium. On binding to thrombomodulin, thrombin changes conformation, converting it from a procoagulant into a potent activator of protein C, a vitamin K–dependent protein, which degrades and inactivates factors Va and VIIa, thereby attenuating thrombogenesis (18).

GENERAL APPROACHES TO ANTICOAGULANT THERAPY

Overview

Because current clinically available antithrombotic drugs target only a few specific areas within the coagulation cascade, the selection of an appropriate anticoagulant for a given patient should be based on the patient's medical and drug history, age and location of the clot, underlying diagnosis of the disease state, and ultimate goal of the therapeutic intervention. If dissolving of an existing clot is needed, activation of plasminogen with the thrombolytic agents, which degrades insoluble fibrin, is the typical approach. If the therapeutic goal is prevention of thrombus formation or extension, however, inhibition of factor activation higher in the cascade with heparin and other oral anticoagulants is the most appropriate.

An ideal anticoagulant should have reproducible pharmacodynamic and pharmacokinetic properties such that no coagulation monitoring is necessary. It also should have a wide therapeutic window, a rapid onset and offset of action, and minimal adverse effects, particularly with minimal interactions with food and other drugs.

Laboratory Assessment and Monitoring

Anticoagulant drug dosing represents a fine balance between reducing the morbidity and mortality associated with the thrombotic condition and minimizing the risk of serious hemorrhage from excessive therapeutic anticoagulation. Because of the potentially life-threatening consequences of either inadequate or excessive anticoagulation, patients receiving antithrombotic medications, such as warfarin and unfractionated heparin, often are closely monitored with specific clinical laboratory assays. A baseline assessment of the patient's coagulation features is performed before the initiation of anticoagulant therapy. This allows detection of congenital coagulation factor deficiencies, thrombocytopenia, hepatorenal insufficiency, and vascular abnormalities, which could prove to be catastrophic if anticoagulant therapy was instituted empirically.

For monitoring oral anticoagulant therapy (i.e., vitamin K antagonists), the prothrombin time (PT) is measured (19,20). This test is used to assess the activity of the vitamin K–dependent clotting factors (II, VII, IX and X). The PT is particularly sensitive to factor VII, which is not of great clinical significance in itself but serves as a rough estimate for the ability of the liver to synthesize proteins or the extent of vitamin K depletion from warfarin therapy. The PT assay measures the time that it takes for a clot to form in citrated plasma after the addition of tissue thromboplastin and calcium. In normal (i.e., warfarin-free) plasma, this clot formation takes 10 to 13 seconds (19,20). Because of variances in commercially available thromboplastins, most clinical laboratories now report PT results in terms of international normalized ratios (INRs). Patients on warfarin therapy are optimally maintained with an INR of 2.0 to 3.0. In cases of patients who have had mechanical prosthetic heart valves placed, an INR of 2.5 to 3.5 often is recommended. At the initiation of warfarin therapy, daily PT's are performed. As the drug dosage is adjusted appropriately based on these results, the length of time between PT assessments can be extended to weekly. Finally, after warfarin therapy has been optimized and the patient's PT results have stabilized within an acceptable range, monthly or bimonthly PT checks are reasonable.

Heparin directly deactivates clotting factors II and X. Therapy with this drug is monitored based on the activated partial thromboplastin time (aPTT) assay (19,20). This assay monitors factors II and X as well as several others. Deficiencies of clotting factors that affect the aPTT result can be of little clinical significance (e.g., prekallikrein and factor XII), of potential clinical significance (e.g., factor XI), or of great clinical significance (e.g., factors VIII and IX and the hemophilic factors). In the aPTT assay, a surface activator, such as elegiac acid, kaolin, or silica, is used to activate the intrinsic pathway. When this activator comes in contact with citrated plasma in the presence of calcium and phospholipid, clot formation begins. As with the PT, the time taken for this clot to form is measured. In normal (nonheparinized) plasma, the average aPTT result is 25 to 45 seconds. A therapeutic aPTT in a patient receiving heparin typically is 70 to 140 seconds. In vivo, the platelet membrane rather than the phospholipid is the source of several clotting factors and the site of many of the coagulation reactions in the intrinsic pathway. The phospholipid used in the aPTT assay does not completely substitute for the in vivo actions of the platelets. Although this phospholipid does potentiate the intrinsic pathway, it does so without activating factor VII. This "partial activation" of the intrinsic pathway is the genesis of the name of the assay (aPTT).

Several other laboratory assays are used to assess function at various points within the clotting cascade. Quantitative levels of fibrinogen and fibrin degradation products are used to assess the extent of the effects of conditions, such as acute inflammation, disseminated intravascular coagulation (DIC), and severe liver disease. The specific clotting factors in which a given patient may be deficient also can be determined using various mixing studies (19,20). These assessments are far more specialized and performed much less frequently than the PT and aPTT.

ORAL ANTICOAGULANTS

There are two different chemical classes of orally active anticoagulants, namely coumarin derivatives and 1,3-

indandiones. It has been known since 1921 that cattle eating spoiled sweet clover hay often would die from uncontrollable bleeding after suffering a very minor injury. This discovery and other subsequent findings eventually led to the isolation of bishydroxycoumarin (i.e., dicoumarol) in 1934 by Link and Campbell and its use in humans in 1954 as the first orally active anticoagulant drug (21).

Coumarin Derivatives

Warfarin and other vitamin K antagonists have been the mainstay of oral anticoagulant therapy for more than 50 years. Although their effectiveness in the prophylaxis of thrombotic disorders has been established through many well-designed clinical trials, their usages in clinical practice are challenging because of their narrow therapeutic index, potential for drug–drug/food interactions, and patient variability that requires close assessment and drug monitoring (20).

Mechanism of Action

Vitamin K antagonists, such as warfarin, produce their effect on blood coagulation by interfering with the cyclic interconversion of vitamin K and vitamin K 2,3-epoxide (Fig. 31.4) (22). Vitamin K is an essential cofactor necessary for the posttranslational carboxylation of the glutamic acid residues on the N-terminal portions of the specific clotting factors (II, VII, IX, and X) and anticoagulant proteins, such as protein C (22). This γ-glutamyl carboxylation results in a new amino acid, γ-carboxyglutamate, which through chelation of calcium ions causes the proteins to undergo a conformational change. This change in tertiary structure allows the four vitamin K–dependent clotting factors to become activated and bind to the negatively charged phospholipid membranes during clotting cascade activation.

The specific enzyme that carboxylates vitamin K–dependent coagulation factors requires a reduced form of vitamin K (vitamin K hydroquinone [KH_2]), molecular oxygen, and carbon dioxide as cofactors. In the process of this reaction, KH_2 is oxidized to vitamin K 2,3-epoxide. The return of the epoxide to the active KH_2 form is the result of a two-step reduction. First, the epoxide is reduced to vitamin K quinone by vitamin K 2,3-epoxide reductase in the presence of NADH. This quinone intermediate is then further reduced back to KH_2 by vitamin K quinone reductase. The warfarin-like anticoagulants (i.e., vitamin K antagonists) exert their anticoagulant activity through the inhibition of vitamin K 2,3-epoxide reductase and, possibly, through inhibition of vitamin K quinone reductase, which in turn inhibits activation of the four affected coagulation factors. Unlike heparin, and as a direct result of their mechanism of action, the vitamin K antagonists only inhibit blood coagulation in vivo.

Structure–Activity Relationship of Coumarin Derivatives

All of the coumarin derivatives (Fig. 31.5) are water-insoluble lactones. Structure–activity relationship requirements typically are based on substitution of the lactone ring, specifically in positions 3 and 4. Although coumarin is a neutral compound, the clinically available derivatives are weakly acidic because of the presence of a 4-hydroxy substitution. The acidity of the proton on the 4-hydroxy group allows formation of water-soluble sodium salts for commercial preparations. Furthermore, warfarin (and, possibly,

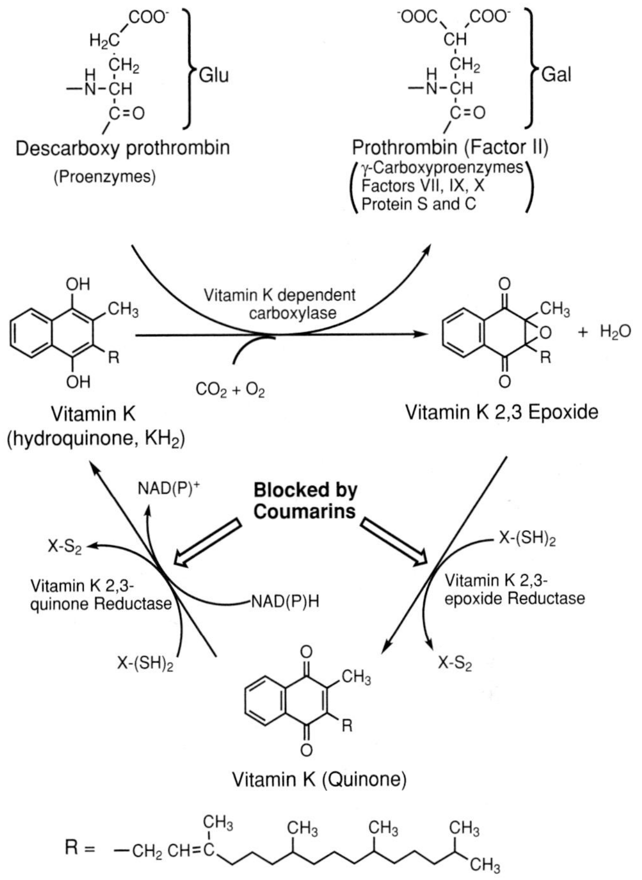

Fig. 31.4. Redox cycling of vitamin K in the activation of blood clotting, which involves conversion of glutamate residues to γ-carboxyglutamates.

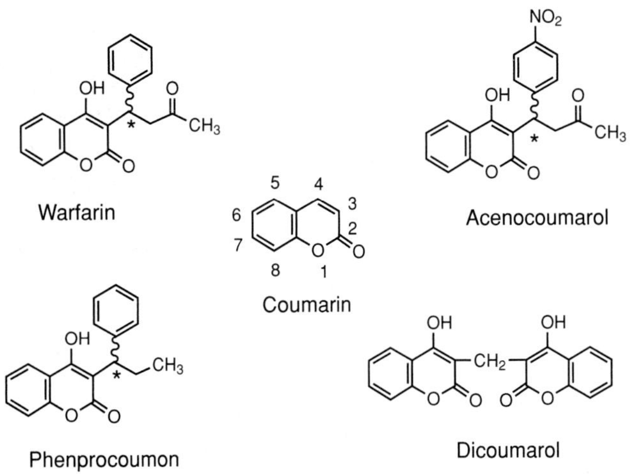

Fig. 31.5. Chemical structures of coumarin and coumarin-derived drugs.

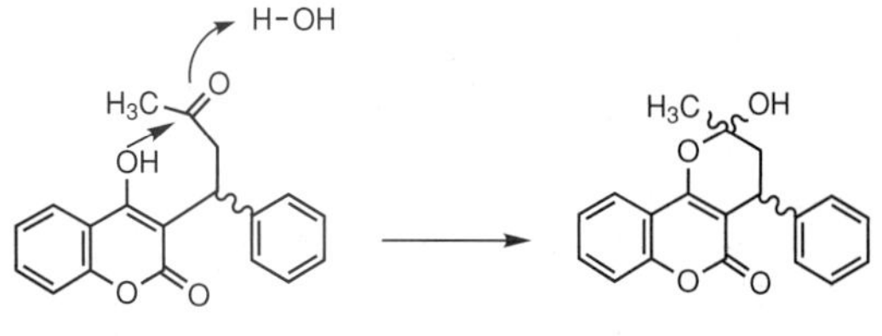

Fig. 31.6. Formation of a cyclic hemiketal of warfarin.

acenocoumarol) also can exist in solution as two diastereomeric cyclic hemiketal conformers in addition to its open-chain conformer (Fig. 31.6). Because it has been suggested that vitamin K forms an active hemiketal in vivo, the cyclic hemiacetals of the vitamin K antagonists, such as warfarin, also may be the active conformers in vivo (23).

Pharmacokinetics

The substituents at position 3 greatly affect the pharmacokinetic and toxicological properties of warfarin and its derivatives (Table 31.1) (24). Dicoumarol is not completely absorbed in the gastrointestinal tract, often is associated with gastrointestinal discomfort, and is very rarely used clinically. Today, the only coumarin used in the United States is warfarin, but phenprocoumon and acenocomumarol are used in Europe.

Warfarin

Warfarin sodium is rapidly and completely absorbed (~100% bioavailability) following oral, intramuscular, intravenous, or rectal administration. Peak plasma concentrations occur at approximately 3 hours. Its anticoagulant effect is not immediately present, however, following initiation of therapy. Instead, a delay in onset of anticoagulation occurs while the clotting factors with normal activity are cleared and those that have not been carboxylated because of the actions of warfarin reach physiologically significant levels. On average, this delay is approximately 5 hours for factor V turnover and 2 to 3 days for factor II (thrombin). Consequently, because of the rapid decline in protein C levels, the anticoagulated state frequently is preceded by a period of hypercoagulability (25).

Warfarin also is highly protein bound (95–99%) and, as a result, has numerous interactions with other drugs. The free drug (i.e., that not bound to plasma proteins) is the active constituent. Therefore, any other substance that displaces bound drug from protein binding sites increases the levels of free drug and, as a result, can cause warfarin toxicity, which usually is manifested by hemorrhage. The volume of distribution (V_d) is quite small (0.1–0.2 L/kg), and the plasma half-life is quite long, both of which presumably result from the high degree of plasma protein binding (20,26).

"Superwarfarin" Rodenticides

Brodifacoum is a member of the second-generation anticoagulant rodenticides known as "superwarfarins" (27). This compound and others like it (e.g., bromadiolone and difenacoum) were developed to combat rodent resistance to warfarin (27).

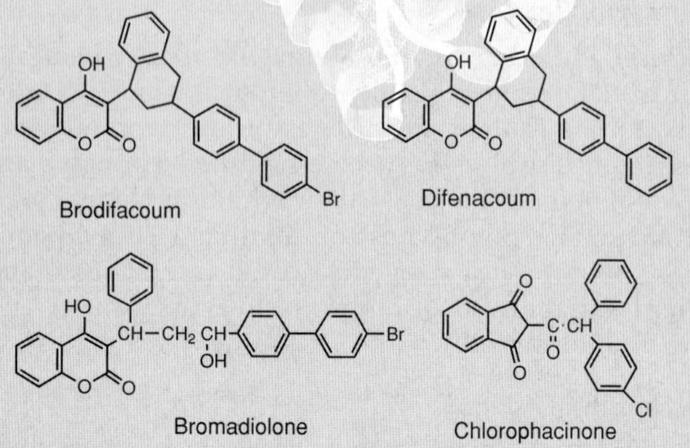

Human ingestion of brodifacoum typically is accidental in children but usually is intentional in adults (i.e., to commit suicide) (28). In cases when large quantities are ingested, severe and potentially fatal hemorrhaging can result. Brodifacoum is readily available over-the-counter in hardware stores and supermarkets, and it is marketed under numerous trade names in North America, Europe, Australia, and New Zealand. Brodifacoum, like warfarin, is thought to exhibit its anticoagulant effects through inhibition of vitamin K epoxide reductase. Despite the similarity in mechanism of action between brodifacoum and warfarin, brodifacoum is at least fivefold more potent as an anticoagulant rodenticide (27,29). The half-life of brodifacoum in humans is approximately 24.2 days, which is roughly ninefold longer than that of warfarin (27,30,31). Brodifacoum also has a volume of distribution roughly six times that of warfarin (30). For these reasons, vitamin K therapy may be needed for weeks to months after ingestion of a superwarfarin rodenticide (32).

Table 31.1. Pharmacokinetic Properties of the Coumarins and Anisindione

Drug	Trade Name	Onset (hours)	Duration (days)	Half-life (days)	Time to Peak Plasma Concentration (hours)
Warfarin	Coumadin	1.5–3.0	2–5	0.62–2.5	4
Dicoumerol		1–5	2–10	1–4	1–9
Phenprocoumon	Marcumar[a]		7–14	5–6	
Acenocoumarol	Sinthrom[a]		2	0.3–1.0	1–3
Anisindione	Miradon	~6	1–3	3–5	2–3

[a]Not available in the United States but available in Europe.

The clinically used preparation of warfarin is racemic, but the enantiomers are not equipotent. In fact, (*S*)-warfarin is at least fourfold more potent as an anticoagulant than the (*R*)-warfarin. The difference in the activities and metabolism of the enantiomers is the key to understanding several stereoselective drug interactions. Similar stereochemical properties are noted for the other asymmetric coumarins (Fig. 31.5). In the case of acenocoumarol, the (*R*)-isomer is responsible for the majority of its activity.

Warfarin and other coumarin derivatives undergo extensive hepatic oxidative metabolism catalyzed by CYP2C9 isozyme to give 6- and 7-hydroxywarfarins as the major inactive metabolites. Warfarin also undergoes, to a lesser extent, reductive metabolism of the ketone on the C-3 side chain to a pair of pharmacologically active, diastereomeric 2-hydroxywarfarins (Fig. 31.7). Almost no unchanged drug is excreted in the urine. As expected, those individuals with compromised hepatic function are at greater risk for warfarin toxicity secondary to diminished clearance. Many of the drug–drug interactions are associated with enhanced or inhibited metabolism of warfarin via CYP2C9 induction or inhibition. Many additional drugs and conditions have profound effects on warfarin therapy. A partial list of these factors is shown in Table 31.2 (24).

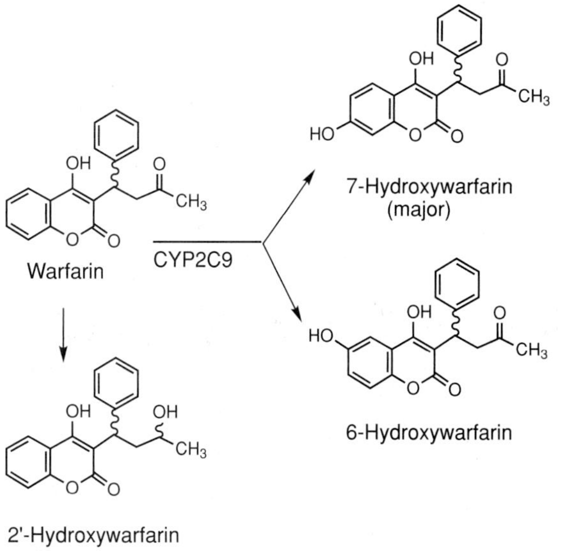

Warfarin → CYP2C9 → 7-Hydroxywarfarin (major); 6-Hydroxywarfarin

Warfarin → 2'-Hydroxywarfarin

Fig. 31.7. Metabolism of warfarin.

Table 31.2. Factors Affecting Warfarin Therapy

Potentiate Anticoagulation		Antagonize Anticoagulation	Drug Enhanced by Oral Anticoagulation
Drugs:		**Drugs:**	
Acetaminophen	Miconazole	Alcohol (chronic abuse)	Phenytoin
Alcohol/ethanol (acute intoxication)	Nalidixic acid	Aminoglycosides	
Allopurinol	Naproxen	Antacid	
Amiodarone	Omeprazole	Antihistamines	
Anabolic & androgenic steroids	Oral hypoglycemics	Barbiturates	
Aspirin	Pentoxiphylline	Carbamazepine	
Bromelains	Phenylbutazone	Chlordiazepoxide	
Cephalosporins	Phenytoin	Cholestyramine	
Chenodiol	Piroxicam	Colestipol	
Chloral hydrate	Propafenone	Corticosteroids	
Cimetidine	Propranolol	Dextrothyroxine	
Clofibrate	Quinidine, quinine	Griseofluvin	
Clofibrate	Sulfamethoxazole–trimethoprim	Haloperidol	
Clorpropamide	Sulfonylureas	Meprobamate	
Cotrimoxazole	Sulfinpyrazone	Nafcillin	
Dextran	Sulindac	Oral contraceptives	
Diazoxide	Tamoxifen	Penicillins (large doses)	
Diflunisal	Thyroxine	Phenytoin	
Disulfiram	Ticlopidine	Primadone	
Erythromycin	Tolmetin	Rifampin	
Ethacrynic acid	Tricyclic antidepressants	Sucralfate	
Fenoprofen		Trazodone	
Fluconazole		Vitamin K (large doses)	
Glucagon	**Other Factors:**		
Heparin	Fever	**Other Factors:**	
Ibuprofen	Stress	High–Vitamin K	
Indomethacin	Congestive heart failure	diet: spinach,	
Inhalation anesthetics	Radioactive compounds	cheddar cheese	
Isoniazid	Diarrhea	cabbage	
Ketoconazole	Cancer	Edema	
Lovastatin	X-rays	Hypothyroidism	
Mefenamic acid	Hyperthyroidism	Nephrotic	
Metronidazole	Hepatic dysfunction	syndrome	

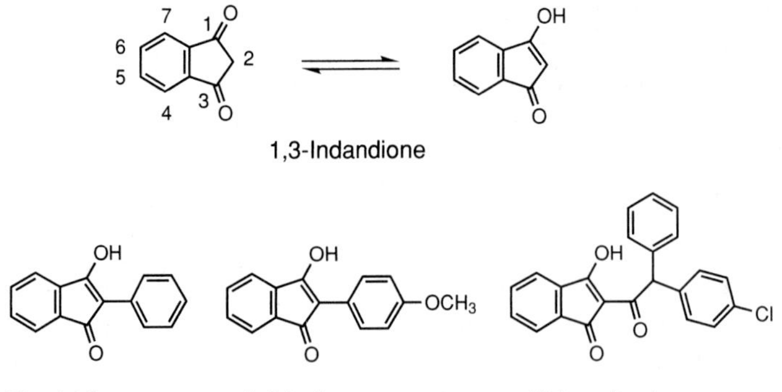

1,3-Indandione

Phenindione Anisindione Chlorophacinone

Fig. 31.8. Chemical structures of 1,3-indandione and 1,3-indandione-derived drugs.

Indandiones

Indane-1,3-dione derivatives (Fig. 31.8), such as phenindione and anisindione, are orally active anticoagulants having a similar mechanism of action to the coumarins but are rarely used clinically today because of their significant renal and hepatic toxicities. Furthermore, because of the structural similarity, patients who are allergic to warfarin will experience cross-sensitivity with anisindione and other indandione anticoagulants (33). Although anisindione reportedly has fewer significant side effects, most clinicians still prefer warfarin for oral anticoagulation. The pharmacokinetic properties also are similar to those of the coumarins (Table 31.1). Most of the newer indandione drugs, such as chlorophacinone, are marketed as potent rodenticides.

HEPARIN-BASED ANTICOAGULANTS

Chemistry

The heparin anticoagulants are represented by a variety of structures, including the natural heparan sulfate that lines the vascular endothelium, unfractionated heparin, LWMHs, and most recently, the synthetic pentasaccharide fondaparinux. Heparin is composed of a heterogeneous mixture of straight-chain, sulfated, and negatively charged mucopolysaccharides of a molecular weight range of 5 to 30 kDa, isolated from bovine lung or porcine intestinal mucosa. Heparin, also known as heparinic acid, is an acidic molecule similar to chondroitin and hyaluronic acid. The polysaccharide polymer chains are composed of two alternating sugar units, N-acetyl-D-glucosamine and uronic acid (either D-glucuronic or L-iduronic), linked by α, 1 → 4 bonds (Fig. 31.9) (34).

These chains are called glycosaminoglycans and typically are composed of 200 to 300 monosaccharide units. In mast cells, approximately 10 to 15 of these chains are bound to a core protein to yield a proteoglycan (i.e., a protein/sugar conglomerate molecule) with a molecular weight of 750 to 1,000 kDa. Before the molecule is capable of binding to antithrombin, the proteoglycan must undergo a series of structural modifications (34). These modifications include O-sulfation and N-sulfation of the D-glucosamine residues at carbons 6 and 2, respectively; O-sulfation of the D-glucuronic acid at carbon 2; epimerization of the D-glucuronic acid at carbon 5 to form L-iduronic acid; O-sulfation at carbon 2 of the L-iduronic acid; and N-deacetylation of the glucosamine and O-sulfation of the glucosamine at position 3. None of these reactions goes to completion, so the resulting polysaccharide chains are structurally quite diverse (35,36). The heparin proteoglycan then undergoes degradation by an endo-β-glucuronidase in mast cell granules to release the active 5- to 30-kDa polysaccharide chains.

Under physiological pH conditions, heparin exists primarily as polysulfate anions and, therefore, usually is administered as a salt. In clinical use, standard heparin most often is the sodium salt, but calcium heparin also is effective. Lithium heparin is used in blood sample collection tubes to prevent clotting of the blood samples both in vitro but not in vivo. The use of heparin salts also is important to maintain aqueous solubility, which is necessary for injection. Heparin can be administered intravenously or subcutaneously but not orally, because the polysaccharide

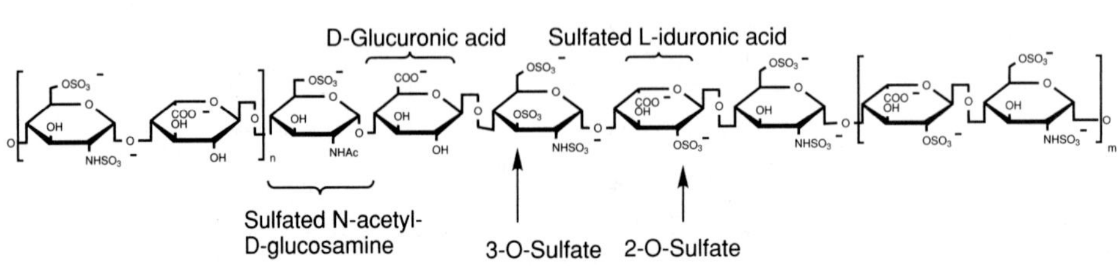

Fig. 31.9. Chemical structure of heparin polymer.

chains are broken down by gastric acid. Intramuscular injection of heparin is associated with a high risk of hematoma formation and is not recommended.

Mechanism of Action

Heparin (unfractionated heparin) was the first parenteral anticoagulant to show efficacy in the treatment of VTE and has been in use since 1937. Heparin acts at multiple sites in the coagulation cascade (34). Anticoagulation occurs when heparin binds, via a distinct pentasaccharide sequence in its molecule, to the circulating antithrombin III (a serine protease inhibitor) and potentates the antithrombin III–mediated inhibition of thrombin (factor IIa) and factor Xa, two of the key proteases in the blood coagulation cascade (Fig. 31.10) (37). The binding between heparin and antithrombin III consists of ionic bonding between sulfate and carboxylate anions in the pentasaccharide chain of heparin and arginine and lysine cations in the antithrombin III (38). Antithrombin III works by forming a stable 1:1 complex with both thrombin and factor Xa. Although the rates of these reactions (with IIa and Xa) are slow in the absence of heparin, binding is accelerated 1,000-fold when heparin is added (39). The reason for this enhancement is that when heparin binds to the antithrombin III, it induces a conformational change, resulting in increased accessibility of its active site and more rapid interaction with its protease substrates (i.e., thrombin and factor Xa). It should be noted that the ability of heparin to expose the active sites of antithrombin III is related to the large molecular size of heparin. With smaller molecules, such as LMWH and fondaparinux, the binding of antithrombin to thrombin is diminished, and the drugs become more selective (see discussions of LMWH and fondaparinux). Interestingly, the role of heparin in this process is only catalytic in nature (i.e., it is not consumed, inactivated, or degraded

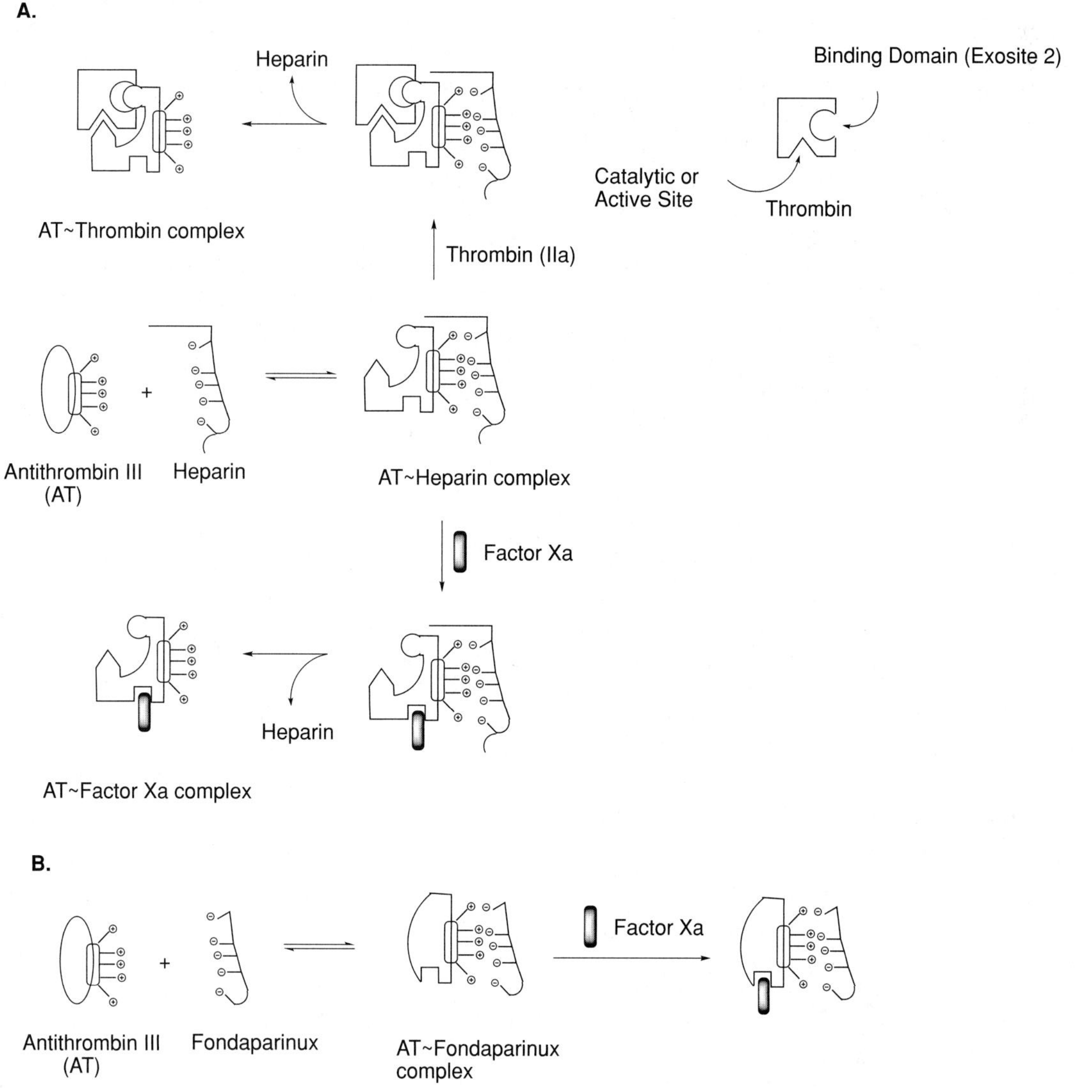

Fig. 31.10. Schematic representation of catalytic role of the heparin drugs in promoting (**A**) antithrombin–factor Xa and antithrombin–thrombin complexes and (**B**) antithrombin–fondaparinux complex.

by the reaction). In fact, once the complex of antithrombin and protease is formed, the heparin is released, with no loss of activity, to catalyze formation of more antithrombin/protease complexes (Fig. 31.10) (37). Additional effects of heparin on the coagulation of blood are a result of heparin's effects on plasminogen activator inhibitor, protein C inhibitor, and TFPI (17,18).

Pharmacokinetics

The pharmacokinetic profiles of heparin and LMWHs are quite different. Whereas heparin is only 30% absorbed following subcutaneous injection, 90% of LMWH is systemically absorbed (40). The binding affinity of heparin to various protein receptors, such as those on plasma proteins, endothelial cells, platelets, platelet factor 4 (PF4), and macrophages, is very high and is related to the high negative-charged density of heparin. This high nonspecific binding decreases bioavailability and patient variability. Additionally, heparin's nonspecific binding may account for heparin's narrow therapeutic window and heparin-induced thrombocytopenia (HIT), a major limitation of heparin. These same affinities are quite low, however, in the case of LMWHs. These parameters explain several of the benefits of the LMWH's. The favorable absorption kinetics and low protein binding affinity of the LMWHs results in a greater bioavailability compared with heparin. The lowered affinity of LMWHs for PF4 seems to correlate with a reduced incidence of HIT. Heparin is subject to fast zero-order metabolism in the liver, followed by slower first-order clearance from the kidneys (41,42). The LMWHs are renally cleared and follow first-order kinetics. This makes the clearance of LMWHs more predictable as well as resulting in a prolonged half-life. Finally, the incidence of heparin-mediated osteoporosis is significantly diminished with use of LMWHs as opposed to heparin.

Metabolism

Independent of molecular weight, the metabolic fate of the heparins is essentially the same. The distribution of the compounds is limited primarily to the circulation, but heparins also are taken up by the reticuloendothelial system (26). Once this uptake occurs, rapid depolymerization of the polysaccharide chains ensues, resulting in products that are inactive as anticoagulants. Desulfation also occurs in mononuclear phagocytes, which also produces inactive metabolites. These metabolites, as well as some of the parent compound, are then excreted in the urine (26). Because of the depolymerization of heparin in the liver and ultimate renal elimination of both metabolites and parent drug, half-life is prolonged in patients with hepatic or renal dysfunction. Another heparin-like medication is danaparoid sodium (43). The drug is composed of 84% heparan sulfate, 12% dermatan sulfate, and 4% chondroitin sulfate. The average molecular weight is 5.5 kDa, and like the LMWHs, danaparoid is dosed in terms of antifactor Xa activity. Danaparoid is completely bioavailable intravenously or subcutaneously and attains maximal antifactor Xa activity 2 to 5 hours after administration. The elimination half-life is approximately 24 hours, and clearance is through the kidneys. Coagulation assays (e.g., PT and aPTT) are not routinely monitored in patients receiving danaparoid therapy, because the drug has a very limited effect on factor II (thrombin) activity.

Specific Heparin Drugs

High-Molecular-Weight Heparin (Unfractionated Heparin)

Standard heparin is unfractionated and contains mucopolysaccharides ranging in molecular weight from 5 to 30 kDa (mean, ~15 kDa) and is referred to as high-molecular-weight heparin (Table 31.2). This group of compounds has a very high affinity for antithrombin III and causes significant in vivo anticoagulant effects. Because heparin is a heterogeneous mixture of polysaccharides with different affinities for the target receptor, dosing based on milligrams of drug is inappropriate (i.e., there frequently is a limited correlation between the concentration of heparin given and the anticoagulant effect produced). Therefore, heparin is dosed in terms of standardized activity units that must be established by bioassay. One USP unit for heparin is the quantity of heparin required to prevent 1.0 mL of citrated sheep blood from clotting for 1 hour after the addition of 0.2 mL of 1% calcium chloride (19). Commercially available heparin sodium USP must contain at least 120 USP units per milligram. Heparin therapy typically is monitored by the aPTT. A therapeutic aPTT is represented by a clotting time in the assay that is 1.5- to 2.5-fold the normal mean aPTT (19). Monitoring therapy with laboratory testing is critical.

Low-Molecular-Weight Heparins

In the past two decades, an increased interest has surfaced in a group of compounds known as LMWHs (41). The LMWHs typically are in the 4- to 6-kDa molecular weight range and are isolated as fractions from heparin using gel filtration chromatography or differential precipitation with ethanol (39). The LMWHs have more favorable pharmacokinetic and pharmacodynamic profiles relative to standard heparins (Table 31.3) (44). The mechanism of action of LMWHs is similar to conventional heparin, but the binding of LMWHs is more selective (i.e., LMWHs have more targeted activity against activated factor Xa and less against activated factor IIa [thrombin]) (Fig. 31.10). The reason for this difference is that even though LMWHs still possess the exact same specific pentasaccharide sequence as that of heparin needed for binding and potentiating the antithrombin III–mediated inhibition of activated factor Xa, most of the LMWH/antithrombin III complex is of insufficient length to bind and inhibit factor Xa and thrombin at the same time (44). Thus, although all LMWHs inactivate factor Xa, only 25 to 50% of these molecules also inactivate thrombin (41). This factor selectivity typically is defined as a higher factor Xa:thrombin (anti-Xa:anti-IIa) activity ratio. In fact, although standard (unfractionated) heparin has an anti-Xa:anti-IIa ratio of 1:1, the same ratio in the LMWHs varies from 2:1 to 4:1 (Table 31.3) (41).

Table 31.3. Properties of Heparin Derivatives

Drug	Trade Name	Dosing	Molecular Weight (daltons)	Binding Ratio
Unfractionated heparin				
Heparin	Calciparine, Calcilean	b.i.d., t.i.d.	5–30	1:1
Low-molecular-weight heparins				
Dalteparin	Fragmin	q.d.	3–8	2.2:1
Enoxaparin	Lovenox	q.d., b.i.d.	3.5–5.5	2.7–3.9:1
Tinzaparin	Innohep	q.d.	5.5–7.5	2.8:1
Pentasaccharide fondaparinux	Arixtra	q.d.	1.728	Xa only

Three LWMHs are commercially available in the United States. The LWMHs are shown in Table 31.3. The three drugs differ slightly in their medical indications for use as well as in their molecular weight ranges. All three compounds are indicated for perioperative thromboembolism prevention for specific abdominal and orthopaedic surgeries. Enoxaparin and dalteparin are approved for use, in combination with aspirin, for the prophylaxis of ischemic complications of unstable angina and non-Q-wave myocardial infarction (45). Enoxaparin also is used in therapy for DVT with or without concomitant pulmonary embolism (45). Because of the increased homogeneity of enoxaparin compared to heparin, dosing of this drug is based on drug weight rather than on USP unitage. A typical dosing scheme for enoxaparin is the administration of 1 mg/kg once or twice daily. In the cases of dalteparin and ardeparin, dosage is based on antifactor Xa units (a-Xa U). Dalteparin is given as a once-daily subcutaneous injection at a dose of 2,500 to 5,000 a-Xa U. Typical dosing for tinzaparin is 175 a–Xa U/kg once daily. The LMWHs have a limited anticoagulant effect on in vitro clotting assays, such as the aPTT. In contrast to the heparin, coagulation parameters, such as aPTT, usually are not monitored in patients receiving LMWHs, nor is monitoring these assays really necessary, because the LMWHs have a highly predictable dose–response relationship (41,44).

Newer Heparin Developments

Many recent studies involving heparin have been directed toward either increasing oral bioavailability or decreasing unwanted side effects (35,46). The poor bioavailability of heparin results from its high molecular weight and high anionic charge density. These properties combined with the instability of the polysaccharides to gastric acid make penetration of biological membranes, such as the gut wall, extremely difficult for heparin. Various approaches to increase heparin absorption following oral administration have been investigated (47). Formulations of heparin including the use of amine salts in enteric-coated tablets (48), salts from organic bases such as lipophilic amines (49), oil-water emulsions (50,51), liposomes (52), and microsphere encapsulation (53,54) have been examined. Combinations of heparin with assorted calcium binding substances and non-α-amino acids (N-acylated aminoalkanoic acids) for simultaneous oral administration also have been studied (47). None of these formulations has yet been approved for clinical use. Attempts to use structural modifications to heparin to attenuate undesirable side effects also have been investigated (46). Heparin-induced thrombocytopenia is caused by the interaction of heparin with PF4. The PF4 binding domain appears to be distinct from the thrombin binding domain. Therefore, it should be possible to use shorter oligosaccharides that bind specifically to the thrombin inhibitory sites without binding to PF4 (46). These observations were used to develop and synthetically produce a series of oligosaccharides with good thrombin binding profiles that have limited interaction with PF4. This preliminary work is quite promising, but these compounds are not yet clinically available.

Fondaparinux

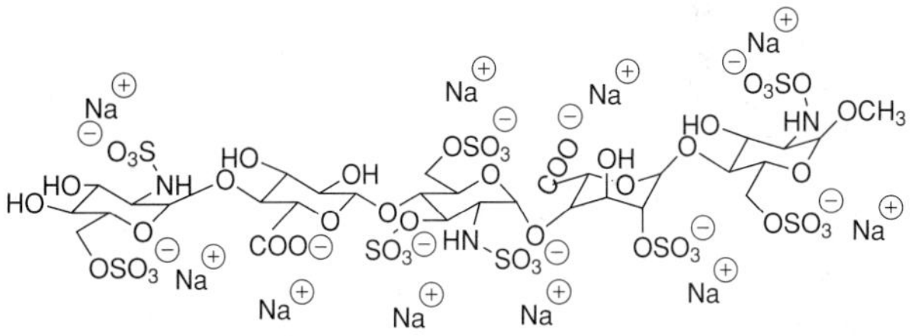

Fondaparinux is a prototype of a novel class of anticoagulants with significant advantages compared to their structurally related heparin (55). Based on the active site of the heparins, fondaparinux is a synthetic, highly sulfonated pentasaccharide. The immediate advantage of fondaparinux is that as a synthetic drug, its composition will not change, which results in improved pharmacokinetics and a more selective anticoagulant action.

Mechanism of Action. The development of fondaparinux, a synthetically derived pentasaccharide that binds specifically to and activates antithrombin III, is a further refinement on the mechanism of action of heparin (56). Fondaparinus and a related analogue, idraparinux, are specific, indirect inhibitors of activated factor Xa via their activation of antithrombin (Fig. 31.10). Fondaparinux has strategically located sulfonates that bind to antithrombin. Fondaparinux is structurally related to the antithrombotic binding site of heparin (57,58). Unlike heparin or LMWHs, however, these inhibitors have no effect on thrombin, because they lack the longer saccharide chains required for binding to thrombin. The highly sulfated heparins exhibit nonselective binding to a number of additional proteins, resulting in decreased bioavailability and significant variation in activity.

Therapeutic Application. Fondaparinux is the first selective factor Xa inhibitor that is approved for the prophylaxis of DVT, which may occur in patients undergoing hip fracture surgery or hip or knee replacement surgery

Idraparinux is a polymethylated derivative of fondaparinux that may soon be marketed. Like fondaparinux, this drug is an indirect inhibitor of factor Xa, which binds to antithrombin with high affinity (62). The drug has a plasma half-life of 80 hours and can be administered once a week. Idraparinux is administered subcutaneously, is 100% bioavailable, and does not bind to other plasma proteins.

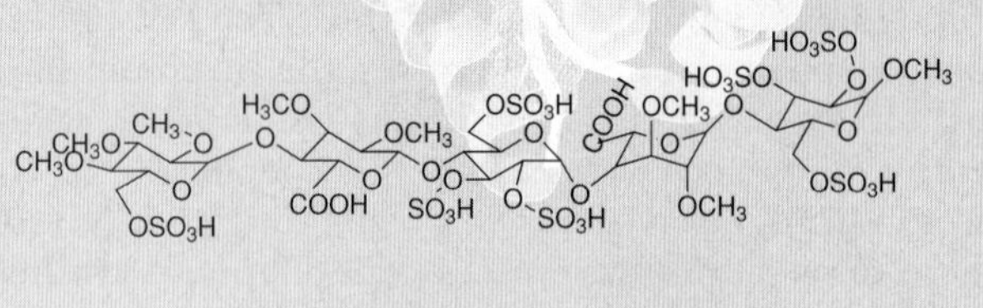

Idraparinux

(59). The most common side effect is major and minor bleeding, and the patient must be carefully monitored. The drug is not to be used when spinal anesthesia or spinal puncture is employed because of the potential for developing a blood clot in the spine. Fondaparinux has not been reported to cause thrombocytopenia, a condition seen with heparin (56,59,60). It is 100% bioavailable, with little or no protein binding.

Pharmacokinetics. Fondaparinux is administered via subcutaneous injection with a single daily dose and shows complete absorption. The drug is highly bound to antithrombin III (~94%), with no significant binding to other plasma proteins. Because of the predictable anticoagulant effect, the drug does not require routine coagulation monitoring (61). The drug is not metabolized and is excreted in the urine unchanged within 72 hours in patients with normal renal function. Fondaparinux has an elimination half-life of 17 hours. Presently, no clinically significant drug interactions have been reported.

DIRECT THROMBIN INHIBITORS

In the last 10 years, with a better understanding of the molecular mechanisms of blood coagulation, the availability of molecular modeling and recombinant technologies, and the structure-based drug design strategies, many new anticoagulants that target almost every step in the coagulation pathway have been developed (6,63). Among these, five direct thrombin inhibitors (DTIs; hirudin, bibalirudin, lepirudin, argatroban, and ximelagatran) have been approved for clinical use in recent years (Table 31.4). Many other anticoagulants that act on the endogenous anticoagulation mechanisms, such as activated protein C pathway, TFPI, as well as additional orally active DTIs, currently are undergoing clinical trials (63,64).

Discovery and Design of Direct Thrombin Inhibitors

Hirudin, the lead compound for the design of DTIs, is a small protein (65 amino acids) that was originally isolated from the salivary glands of the medicinal leech, *Hirudo medicinalis* (65). This protein has potent and specific inhibitory effects on thrombin through the formation of a 1:1 complex with the clotting factor. The anticoagulant activity of hirudin seems to be contained within its highly anionic C-terminus. Several clinical studies have compared hirudin and a small peptidomimetic analogue, hirulog, with heparin in the treatment of several thrombotic disorders. In many cases, hirudin seems to be more efficacious and the responses to it more predictable. Furthermore, some of the studies also indicate a lower incidence of bleeding complications with hirudin compared with heparin. Hirudin is now produced by recombinant technology, and many hirulogs continue to be screened (66,67). Significant progress in the design and development of direct thrombin inhibition has been achieved. The recent emergence of orally active DTIs may simplify the prevention and treatment of various thrombotic disorders (68–70).

Mechanism of Action

The DTIs bind and inactivate both free thrombin and thrombin bound to fibrin. Unlike heparin, DTIs, such as lepirudin, bivalirudin, argatroban, and ximelagatran, bind directly and reversibly to the active site of thrombin. Unlike the heparins, these inhibitors do not require an activated antithrombin III as a cofactor for their anticoagulant activity. Furthermore, contrary to the heparins,

Table 31.4. Direct Thrombin Inhibitors (DTIs)

Drug	Trade Name	Route of Administration	Site of Binding	Reversibility	Half-life (minutes)	Route of Excretion	Protein Binding
Hirudin		IV	CS, exosite-1	Irreversible			
Lepirudin	Refludan	IV	CS, exosite-1	Irreversible	80		
Desiruden	Iprivask	SC	CS, exosite-1	Irreversible	120–180	Kidney	0
Bivalirudin	Angiomax	IV	CS, exosite-1	Reversible	25	Kidney	0
Argatroban	Novastan	IV	CS	Reversible	39–51	Hepatobiliary	54%
Melagatran		SC, IV	CS	Reversible	150	Kidney	<15%
Ximelagatran	Exanta[a]	PO	CS	Reversible	180–228	Kidney	

CS, catalytic site; IV, intravenous, PO, oral; SC, subcutaneous.
[a]AstraZeneca announced the withdrawal of Exanta from the market on February. 14, 2006.

these agents inhibit only the activity of thrombin, whereas heparin indirectly inhibits factors IIa (thrombin), IXa, Xa, XIa, and XIIa (64). There are three different domains where DTIs bind to and block the action of thrombin: the active site (or catalytic site, CS) as well as two additional exosites. Exosite-1 acts as a dock for substrates such as fibrin and, thereby, orients the appropriate peptide bonds in the active site for its biotransformation. Exosite-2 is the heparin binding domain. Bivalent DTIs, such as lepirudin and bivalirudin, block thrombin at the active site and exosite-1, whereas argatroban, melagatran, and dabigatran are univalent DTIs and, thus, bind only to the active site of the thrombin.

Specific Drugs

Recombinant Hirudin Derivatives: Lepirudin and Desirudin

Lepirudin and desirudin have been approved for the treatment of HIT and of HIT with thrombotic syndrome (71). Both lepirudin and desirudin are recombinant hirudin derivatives that consists of a 65-amino-acid protein (72,73). Lepirudin is related to the recombinant product desirudin differing in the two N-terminal amino acids. The N-terminal amino acids in lepirudin are leucine-1 and threonine-2, whereas in desirudin, the N-terminal amino acids are valine-1 and valine-2. Additionally, desirudin lacks a sulfated tyrosine at amino acid 63. The antithrombin activity of the two drugs is slightly different.

Lepirudin and desirudin are both bivalent DTI that bind to both the active site and the exosite-1 of thrombin. The result of this binding is that they create a nearly irreversible inhibition of thrombin. Lepirudin and desirudin inhibit both free thrombin and thrombin bound to fibrin (74).

Lepirudin is administered via intravenous bolus injection, followed by continuous infusion, whereas desirudin is administered subcutaneously twice daily (Table 31.4) (73,75). The drugs are cleared via the kidneys. Lepirudin is nearly totally degraded before excretion (~90%), whereas desirudin is excreted 50% unchanged. Lepirudin has immunogenic properties, and a significant number of patients develop antihirudin antibodies. In addition, hemorrhages may occur in patients treated with lepirudin. The drug half-life is approximately 1.3 hours (76).

Bivalirudin

Bivalirudin, a 20-amino-acid peptide, has been approved for use in patients with unstable angina undergoing percutaneous coronary intervention (Fig. 31.11) (77).

Bivalirudin is a rapid-onset, short-acting DTI that binds to both the active site and the exosite-1 of thrombin. Unlike lepirudin, bivalirudin is a reversible inhibitor of both free thrombin and thrombin bound to fibrin. This reversibility is possible because the bound bivalirudin undergoes cleavage at the second N-terminal proline to release the portion of the drug bound to the active site. The carboxyl-terminal portion of bivalirudin dissociates from thrombin to regenerate thrombin (Fig. 31.11) (76). Bivalirudin does not bind to plasma protein.

Bivalirudin is administered via intravenous bolus injection, followed by continuous infusion (Table 31.4). The drug exhibits a rapid onset and a short duration of action. Bivalirudin is eliminated by renal excretion. It has been suggested that dosage adjustments be made in patients with severe renal impairment and in patients undergoing dialysis. Approximately 30% is eliminated unchanged along with proteolytic cleavage products. Because of the reversible nature of bivalirudin the drug exhibits less risk of bleeding than other antithrombotics, and there have been no reported cases of antibody formation to bivalirudin (78).

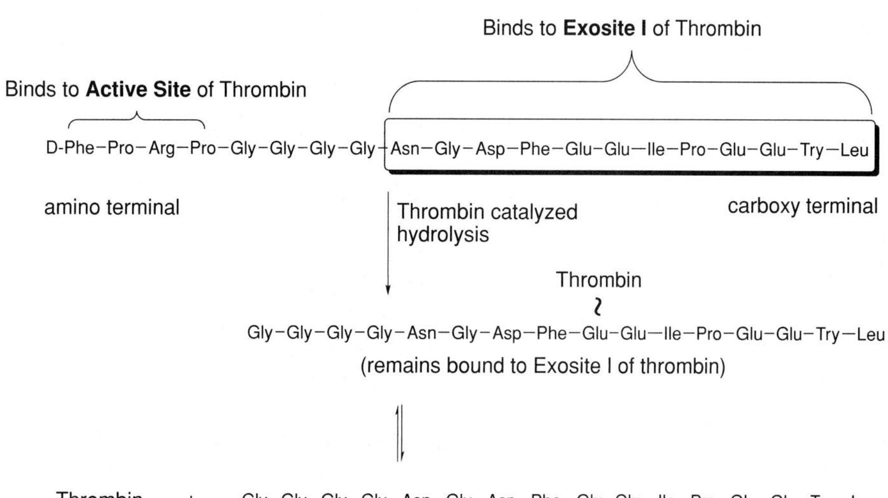

Fig. 31.11. Chemical structure of bivlirudin, binding sites to thrombin, and release from thrombin.

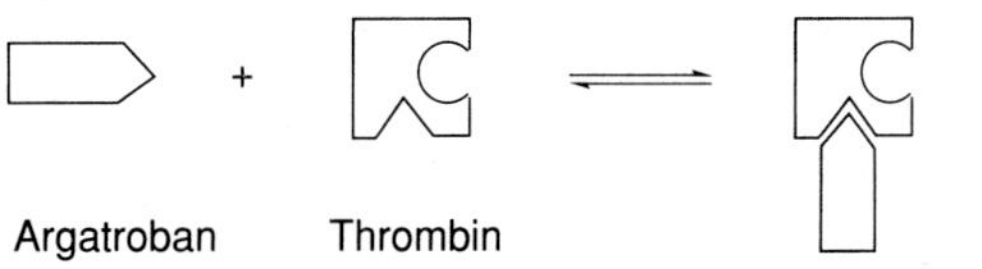

Argatroban Thrombin

Fig. 31.12. Schematic representation of mechanism of action of argatroban.

Argatroban

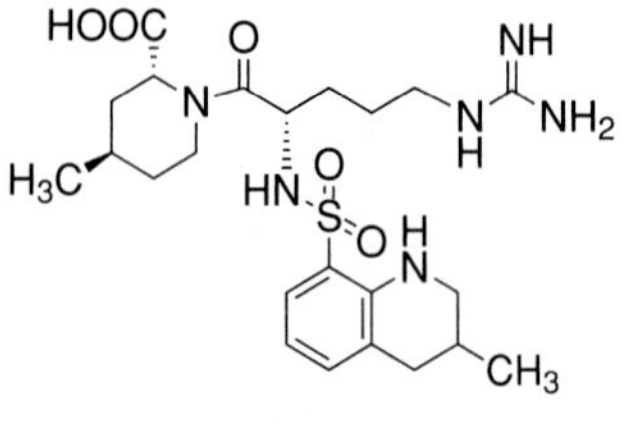

Argatroban

Argatroban has been approved for the prophylaxis and treatment of thrombosis in patients with HIT (79). Argatroban is a peptidomimetic that binds selectively to the catalytic site of thrombin as a univalent competitive DTI (Fig. 31.12). Argatroban is available as a mixture of 21-*R* and 21-*S* diastereomers (64:36), with the *S*-isomer approximately twice as potent as the *R*-isomer (80). The drug is a reversible inhibitor of both free thrombin as well as clot-bound thrombin.

PHARMACOKINETICS (TABLE 31.4). Argatroban is administered subcutaneously because of the low lipophilicity of the drug. The drug is bound to plasma protein and is metabolized via CYP3A4/5 to the aromatized metabolite and the two hydroxylated metabolites (Fig. 31.13). The M-1 metabolite retains 20 to 30% of the antithrombotic activity. Coadministration of argatroban with inhibitors of CYP3A4 does not appear to produce clinically significant effects. Argatroban is eliminated via biliary secretion into the feces (81).

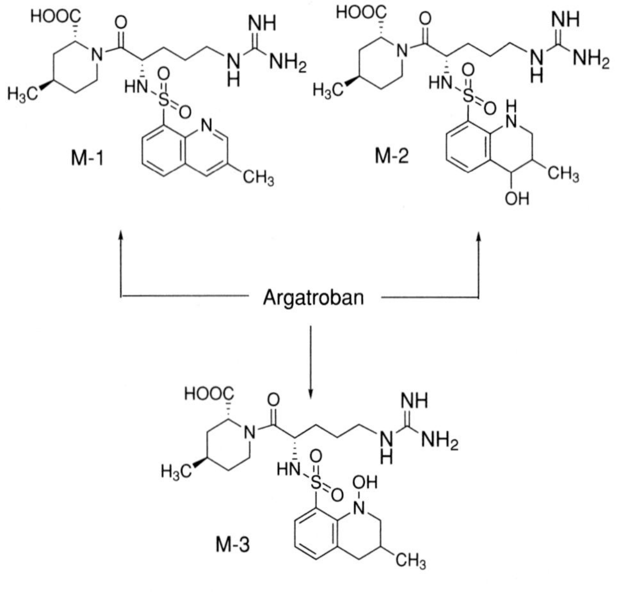

M-1 M-2 Argatroban M-3

Fig. 31.13. Metabolism of argatroban.

Ximelagatran was the first orally active DTI, approved in 2004 for the prevention of venous thromboembolism for patients undergoing total knee replacement surgery and in patients with atrial fibrillation (82,83). Ximelagatran is a pro-drug that, following metabolism, gives rise to the DTI melagatran. Melagatran inhibits both free thrombin and thrombin bound to fibrin by reversibly binding to a single site in thrombin; thus, it is referred to as a univalent DTI. This is in contrast to lepirudin and bivalirudin, which bind nearly irreversibly to two sites in thrombin. Melagatran also inhibits platelet activation and cleavage of protease-activated receptor-1 in a dose-dependent manner (84,85).

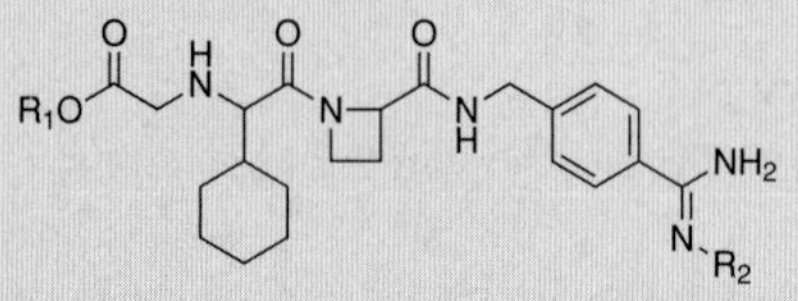

Ximelagatran ($R_1 = C_2H_5$, $R_2 = OH$)
Melagatran ($R_1 = H$, $R_2 = H$)

Ximelagatran was reported to be well tolerated, with a low incidence of adverse effects. It had been reported, however, that the drug caused liver toxicity, although studies have indicated that this is a rare event (86).

On February 14, 2006, AstraZeneca announced that the company had decided to withdraw melagatran/ximelagatran from the market and terminate its development because of a potential risk of severe liver injury when the drug was used beyond the approved 11 days. Previous studies had reported elevated liver transaminases in 7.9% of the patients and suggested monitoring with long-term use of the drug. This effect appeared after 1.5 to 4.0 months.

ANTIPLATELET DRUGS

Another site for regulating blood coagulation and subsequent thrombus formation is at the level of the platelets (87). Antiplatelet drugs work by inhibiting platelet activation via a number of different mechanisms (87,88). The major role of antiplatelet drugs is in the prevention of ischemic complications in patients with coronary diseases (89). These drugs also are effective in combination with moderate-intensity anticoagulants for patients with atrial fibrillation.

Pathophysiology of Arterial Thrombosis

The pivotal role of platelets in thrombus formation and potential sites for drug interventions is illustrated in Figure 31.14 (89). Normal endothelial cells in the vascular wall synthesize and release prostacyclin (PGI_2), which

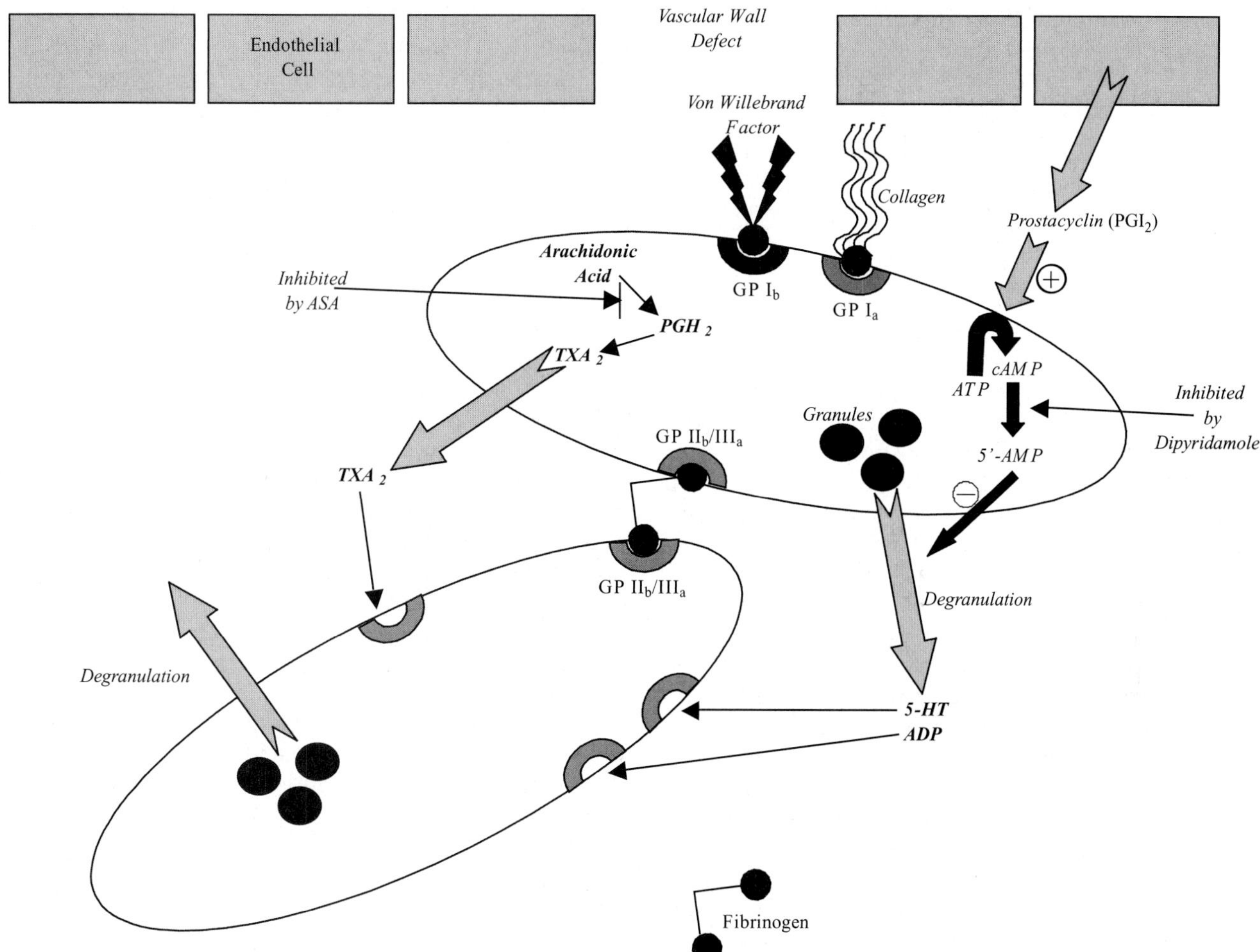

Fig. 31.14. Scheme describing platelet activation as it relates to blood clot formation. The thrombus is formed at the site of a damaged wall in the vasculature. Normal endothelial cells in vascular wall provide prostacyclin, which stimulates the conversion of adenosine triphosphate (ATP) to cyclic adenosine monophosphate (cAMP), preventing platelet aggregation. In injury, glycoprotein (GP) receptors bind substances such as von Willebrand factor and collagen, activating the platelet. The GPIIb/IIIa receptors cross-link platelets via fibrinogen binding. As the platelet degranulates, additional aggregating substances including thromboxane A_2 (TXA_2), serotonin (5-HT), and adenine diphosphate (ADP) are released. The substances bind to other platelets, activating them and resulting in a cascade effect. Also shown are the sites of inhibition of platelet aggregation.

stimulates the conversion of adenosine triphosphate (ATP) to cyclic adenosine monophosphate (cAMP), thus preventing platelet aggregation and degranulation. In the case of an injury to the vascular wall, glycoprotein (GP) receptors (i.e., GPI_a and GPI_b) bind substances such as von Willebrand factor (vWf) and collagen from the exposed subendothelial surface, thereby activating the platelets. The $GPII_b/III_a$ receptors (also known as the fibrinogen receptor or integrin αIIbβ3 receptor) then mediate the final step of platelet aggregation by binding to fibrinogen or vWf, thus cross-linking platelets to form aggregates (Fig. 31.14).

The adherent platelets degranulate and release additional aggregating substances, such as thromboxane A_2 (TXA_2), serotonin (5-HT), and adenosine diphosphate (ADP). These substances serve as secondary chemical messengers to recruit more platelets to the site of vascular injury and, thereby, amplify platelet aggregation. For example, thrombin production releases ADP, which is a potent inducer of platelet aggregation and stimulates prostaglandin synthesis from arachidonic acid in the platelet. The prostaglandins synthesized, PGI_2 and TXA_2, have opposite effects on thrombogenesis. The PGI_2 is synthesized in the walls of the vasculature and inhibits thrombus formation. Conversely, TXA_2, which is synthesized in the platelets, induces vasoconstriction and thrombogenesis. Serotonin, which also is released from the platelets, has similar and additive effects to those of TXA_2.

This rapid platelet aggregation and thrombus formation at the site of vascular injury is the main mechanism of hemostasis (stoppage of bleeding, a normal process of wound healing). When platelets are activated on the ruptured atherosclerotic plaques or in regions of restricted blood flow, however, it can lead to thromboembolic complications that contribute to common diseases, such as myocardial infarction or ischemic stroke.

Mechanism of Action of Antiplatelet Drugs

Most of the current available antiplatelet drugs, such as aspirin, dipyridamole, ticlopidine, and sulfinpyrazone, exert their actions by affecting only the secondary platelet aggregation pathways (87). For example, aspirin and sulfinpyrazone work by inhibiting the biosynthesis of TXA_2 in the platelets (see Fig. 36.4). Aspirin works by irreversibly and permanently inactivating cyclooxygenase (COX) through covalent acetylation of a serine residue in close proximity to the active site of the enzyme. A cumulative inactivation effect occurs on platelets with long-term therapy, because platelets do not synthesize new COX (i.e., platelets are unable to synthesize, via de novo pathway, COX-1, because they are anucleated cells). Therefore, the effects of aspirin last for the lifetime of the platelet (7–10 days). Sulfinpyrazone also is a potent but reversible COX inhibitor that does not affect PGI_2 synthesis in endothelial cells. Like nonsteroidal anti-inflammatory agents (NSAIDs), such as aspirin, this action inhibits the aggregation of platelets into thrombi. Dipyridamole interrupts platelet function through its effect of increasing cellular concentration of cAMP by inhibiting phosphodiesterase, an enzyme needed for degradation of cAMP. Dipyridamole also may stimulate PGI_2 release and inhibits TXA_2 formation. Ticlopidine and clopidogrel selectively inhibit ADP-induced platelet aggregation with no direct action on prostaglandin production. New and more selective antiplatelet drugs, such as integrin $\alpha IIb\beta 3$ receptor antagonists (GPIIa/IIIb blockers), thromboxane synthase inhibitor, and TXA_2 receptor antagonists, are currently being developed (88).

COX-1 Inhibitors

Because TXA_2 is a potent vasoconstrictor as well as a labile platelet aggregation inducer, inhibition of production of TXA_2 effectively blocks platelet aggregation. Aspirin and related analogues (Fig. 31.15) exhibit their effectiveness through such a blocking mechanism.

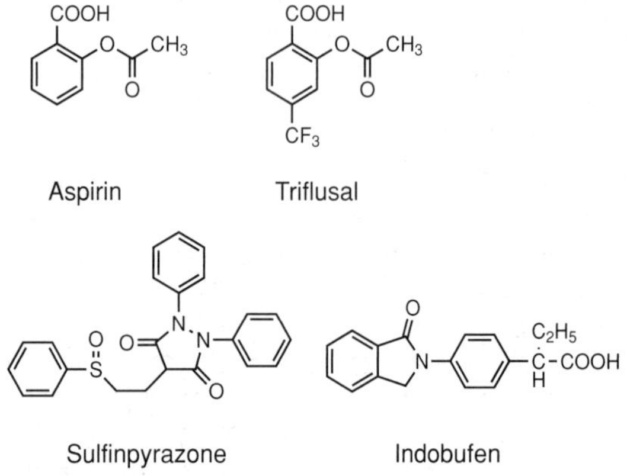

Aspirin Triflusal

Sulfinpyrazone Indobufen

Fig. 31.15. Cyclooxygenase (COX)-1 inhibitors.

Aspirin

Aspirin is a well-established antiplatelet drug in the treatment of atherothrombotic vascular disease (87–89). As stated earlier, aspirin works by its ability to acetylate and irreversibly deactivate platelet COX (COX-1), and its antithrombotic effect remains for the life span of the platelet (7–10 days). Aspirin also has been shown to have other antithrombotic effects that are unrelated to its action on COX-1 (87). These effects include the dose-dependent inhibition of platelet function, the enhancement of fibrinolysis, and the suppression of blood coagulation.

Aspirin is rapidly absorbed in the stomach and quickly degraded by plasma cholinesterases (half-life, 15–20 min). A once-daily dose of 160 mg of aspirin, which is much lower than dosages needed for its anti-inflammatory/analgesic actions, is sufficient to completely inactivate platelet COX-1 irreversibly (90). Higher doses of aspirin only contribute to its side effects, especially internal bleeding and upper gastrointestinal irritations.

In recent years, the term "aspirin resistance" has been used to denote those situations in which the use of aspirin is unable to protect a patient from thrombotic complications, to cause a prolongation of the bleeding time, or to produce an anticipated effect on one or more in vitro tests of platelet function (87,90,91). One possible explanation for aspirin-resistant TXA_2 biosynthesis is the transient expression of COX-2 in newly formed platelets (92). Many other clinical, pharmacodynamic, biological, and genetic factors, however, such as tobacco use, drug interaction, alternate pathways for platelet activation, and genetic polymorphism or mutations of the COX-1 gene, may be involved (93). Currently, many questions regarding the biochemical mechanism, diagnosis, prevalence, clinical relevance, and optimal therapeutic intervention for aspirin resistance remain unanswered (93).

Triflusal

Triflusal (2-acetoxy-4-trifluoromethyl benzoic acid) is an antiplatelet drug that despite its structural similarity to aspirin (Fig. 31.15) exhibits quite different pharmacological and pharmacokinetic properties (94). Unlike aspirin, 2-hydroxy-4-trifluoromethylbenzoic acid (HTB), the deacetylated metabolite of triflusal, retains significant antiplatelet activity. Triflusal is rapidly absorbed and metabolized. The area under the concentration–time curve for triflusal is 20.26 mg/L/hour after a 900-mg dose, whereas that for HTB is 42.27 mg/L/hour. Much of the pharmacokinetic data for triflusal activity is associated with HTB. The inhibition of COX, as measured by reduced production of thromboxane B_2, is 25% after 2 hours and 85% after 7 days with triflusal, whereas the effects of aspirin on thromboxane B_2 is more than 90% reduction after 2 hours and is maintained at this level after 7 days (95). It would appear that the presence of a 4-trifluoromethyl group also greatly enhances triflusal's ability to inhibit the activation of nuclear factor κB, which in turn regulates the expression of the mRNA of vascular cell adhesion molecule-1 (96) needed for platelet aggregation. In addition, triflusal increases nitric oxide synthesis in neutrophils, which results in an increased vasodilatory potential (97). Finally, an additional site of action for triflusal/HTB is the inhibition of cAMP phosphodiesterase, leading to increased levels of cAMP. Elevated cAMP levels decrease platelet aggregation through decreased mobilization of calcium. Aspirin and salicylic acid do not significantly increase cAMP levels.

Although recent trials comparing triflusal and aspirin for the prevention of vascular events in patients following a stroke revealed no significant differences between these two antiplatelet drugs, triflusal's use was associated with a significantly lower rate of hemorrhagic complications (94).

Sulfinpyrazone (Anturane)

Sulfinpyrazone is a structural derivative of the anti-inflammatory drug phenylbutazone. Unlike phenylbutazone, however, sulfinpyrazone does not have significant anti-inflammatory activity. It does have potent uricosuric effects and frequently is used in the treatment of gout. At least four metabolites of sulfinpyrazone have been identified, including the sulfide, sulfone, *p*-hydroxysulfide, and *p*-hydroxysulfinpyrazone derivatives (Fig. 31.16) (24). Only the parent sulfinpyrazone and its reduced sulfide metabolite, however, are active as COX inhibitors (98). Because these compounds are reversible inhibitors, the antithrombotic activity lasts only as long as blood levels of the drug and metabolite persist (half-life, 4–6 hours for parent sulfinpyrazone, 11–14 hours for the sulfide metabolite). Sulfinpyrazone is not yet approved in the United States for use in acute myocardial infarction or for transient ischemic attack prophylaxis.

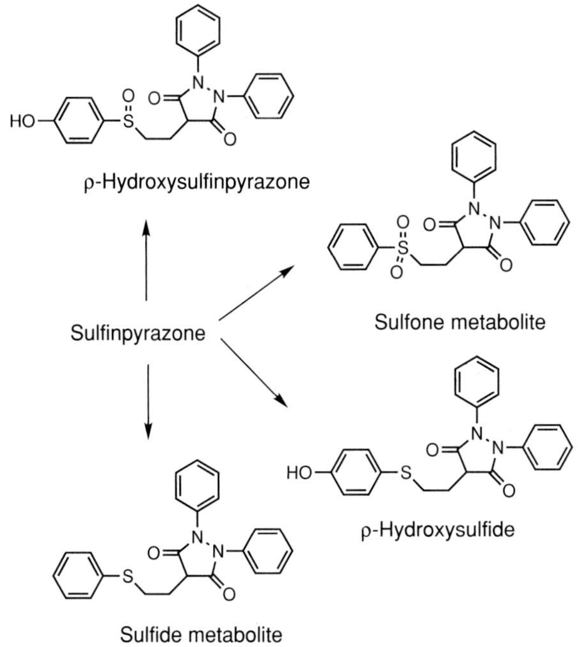

p-Hydroxysulfinpyrazone

Sulfinpyrazone

Sulfone metabolite

p-Hydroxysulfide

Sulfide metabolite

Fig. 31.16. Metabolism of sulfinpyrazone.

Indobufen

Many NSAIDs also inhibit TXA_2-dependent platelet function through a competitive, reversible inhibition of COX-1 (see Chapter 36 for their structures). At a conventional analgesic dosage, these drugs only inhibit COX-1 activity by 70 to 90%, which is inadequate for controlling platelet aggregation. Thus, unlike aspirin, most of the clinically available NSAIDs are not used clinically for their antithrombotic properties.

In contrast, indobufen (Fig. 31.15), a reversible but very potent inhibitor of platelet COX-1 activity, was shown to have comparable clinical efficacy to that of aspirin in prevention of DVT after myocardial infarction and in blocking exercise-induced increase in platelet aggregation (99). In the secondary prevention of thromboembolic events, 100 or 200 mg of indobufen twice daily is as effective as warfarin or aspirin in patients with or without atrial fibrillation (100). Currently, indobufen is only available for routine clinical use in Europe.

Phosphodiesterase Inhibitors

Phosphodiesterase-3 (PDE3) is an enzyme responsible for degradation of cAMP to AMP in platelets and blood vessels. Selective cAMP PDE3 inhibitors, such as dipyridamole and cilostazol (Fig. 31.17), inhibit the degradation of cAMP, thereby increasing cellular concentration of cAMP and leading to inhibition of platelet aggregation and vasodilation (see Chapter 17 for additional information) (101).

Dipyridamole (Aggrenox)

Dipyridamole is a pyrimidopyrimidine derivative with vasodilatory and antiplatelet properties (Fig. 31.17). Dipyridamole exerts its antiplatelet function by increasing cellular concentrations of cAMP via its inhibition of the degradating enzyme, cyclic nucleotide PDE3. It also blocks adenosine uptake, which acts at A_2 adenosine receptors to stimulate platelet adenyl cyclase. Less common uses for this drug include inhibition of embolization from prosthetic heart valves when used in combination with warfarin (the only currently recommended use) and reduction of thrombosis in patients with thrombotic disease when used in combination with aspirin. Alone, dipyridamole has little, if any, benefit in the treatment of thrombotic conditions (102).

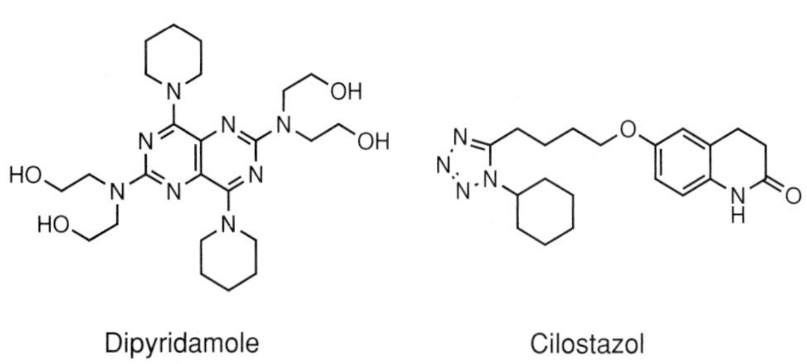

Dipyridamole

Cilostazol

Fig. 31.17. Chemical structures of phosphodiesterase inhibitors.

Cilostazol (Pletal)

Cilostazol, a quinolinone derivative, is a potent orally active antiplatelet drug approved for the treatment of intermittent claudication (a peripheral artery disease resulting from blockage of blood vessels in the limbs). Cilostazol exhibits greater selectivity than dipyridamole as an inhibitor of PDE3A (Fig. 31.18) (102). The drug does not affect the other PDEs (PDEs 1, 2, or 4). Cilostazol reversibly inhibit platelet aggregation induced by a number of stimuli, such as thrombin, ADP, collagen, or stress from exercise (103,104). Additionally, cilostazol inhibits adenosine uptake, leading to increased activity of adenosine at A_1 and A_2 receptors. Adenosine's action on A_2 receptors in platelets increase cAMP levels, which, as previously indicated, leads to decreased platelet aggregation (105).

Cilostazol is rapidly absorbed after oral administration, particularly with a high-fat meal, which greatly increases its bioavailability to approximately 90%. It is extensively metabolized in the liver by various cytochromes. The most important cytochromes appear to be CYP3A4 and, to lesser extent, by CYP2C19, with an elimination half-life of approximately 11 to 13 hours. Among the various metabolites produced (11 metabolites are known), the two major metabolites are 3,4-dehydrocilostazol and 4′-trans-hydroxycliostazol (Fig. 31.19). These two metabolites are pharmacologically active. Studies indicate that the concomitant administration of cilostazol with CYP3A inhibitors can greatly increase cilostazol blood concentrations, and a dose reduction may be required (106). Similar results are seen when CYP2C19 is inhibited, leading to decreased formation of 4-trans-hydroxycliostazol and significant increases in cilostazol and 3,4-dehydrocilostazol (107).

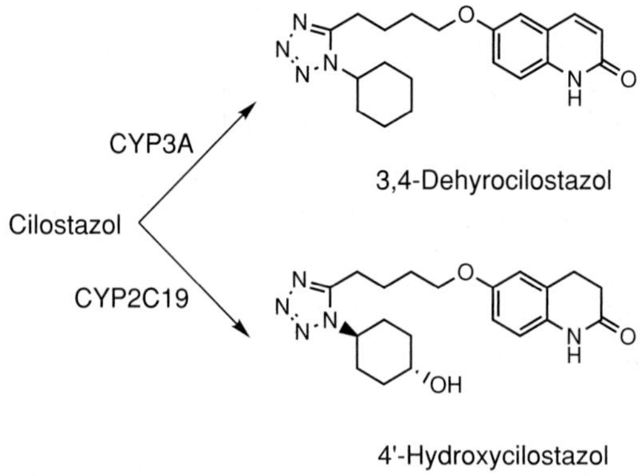

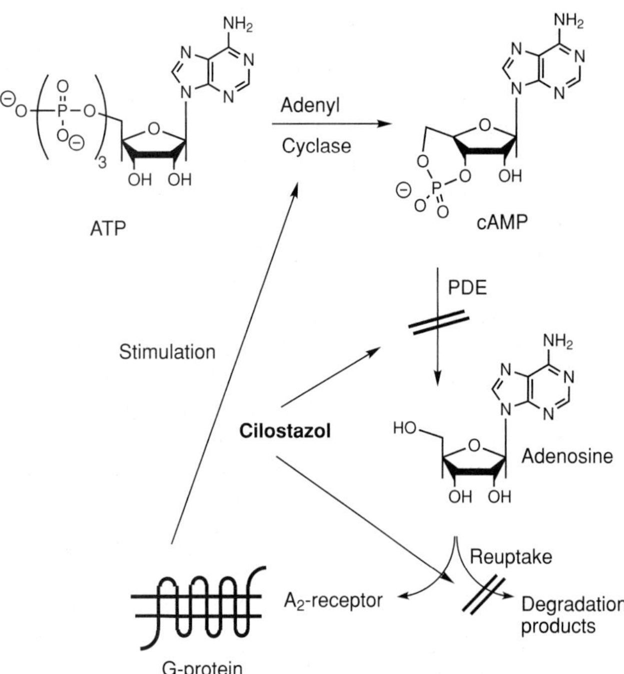

Fig. 31.18. Sites of action of cilostazol, blocking phosphodiesterase 3A (PDE) and adenosine uptake, leading to increased levels of cyclic adenosine monophosphate (cAMP) directly by inhibition of cAMP breakdown and indirectly through adenosine binding to adenosine 2 receptors (A_2-receptor), which through G-protein coupling stimulates adenyl cyclase.

Cilostazol — CYP3A → 3,4-Dehyrocilostazol; CYP2C19 → 4'-Hydroxycilostazol

Fig. 31.19. Metabolism of cilostazol.

Platelet P2Y Purinergic Receptor

The crucial role that ADP plays in platelet activation and aggregation has been extensively investigated (108). The molecular targets of ADP in the platelet are G protein–coupled P2Y purinergic receptors. There are three nucleotide receptors: $P2X_1$, a cation channel receptor activated by ATP, and purinergic receptors $P2Y_1$ and $P2Y_{12}$, both of which are activated by ADP. Initial binding of ADP to the $P2Y_1$ purinergic receptor (373-amino-acid protein) induces platelet shape changes, causes intracellular calcium mobilization, and initiates aggregation. Subsequent binding of ADP to the $P2Y_{12}$ purinergic receptors (342 amino acids) leads to sustained platelet aggregation by inhibiting adenylate cyclase and, thereby, decreasing cellular cAMP levels (109). The $P2Y_{12}$ receptor is coupled to the $G\alpha_{i2}$ G protein. The antithrombotic drugs ticlopidine and clopidogrel are irreversible antagonists of this $P2Y_{12}$ purinergic receptor (108). The clinical relevance of this $P2Y_{12}$ receptor as a new target for antiplatelet drug development of novel reversible antagonists has been extensively reviewed (109–111).

Ticlopidine (Ticlid) and Clopidogrel (Plavix)

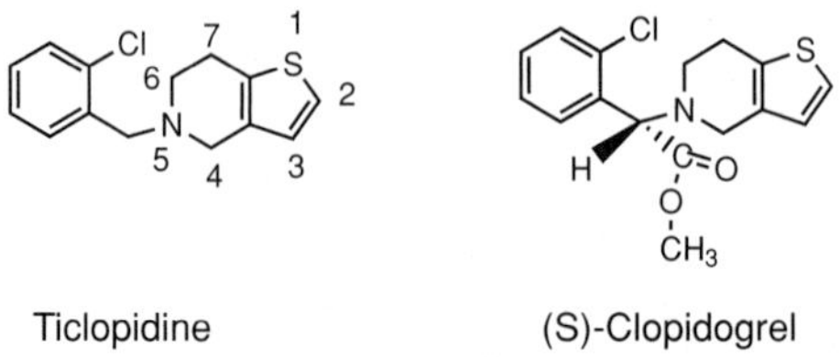

Ticlopidine (S)-Clopidogrel

Ticlopidine and clopidogrel are thienopyridines, which through inhibition of platelet aggregation prolong bleeding time and delay clot retraction. The thienopyridines are prescribed for reduction of myocardial infarction and stroke, for treatment of peripheral arterial disease, and in combination with aspirin for acute coronary syndromes. This latter utility appears to result from the fact that both aspirin and the thienopyridines block major amplification pathways, leading to platelet aggregation and, thus, producing enhanced effectiveness. Triclopidine has major safety concerns in that in a small population (1–2%), neutropenia occurs that is potentially fatal, may cause thrombotic thrombocytopenic purpura, and is largely replaced with clopidogrel. These same side effects are rare with clopidogrel. Additional side effects include diarrhea, nausea, vomiting, and skin rash (112).

The thienopyridine class exhibit selective inhibition of ADP-induced platelet aggregation. The action of ticlopidine and clopidogrel appear to be irreversible in that there is still antiplatelet activity for 7 to 10 days after discontinuation of the medications (despite the fact that the elimination half-life of ticlopidine is only 24–36 hours after a single dose) (24). Support of the theory of irreversible inhibition of $P2Y_{12}$ is provided by the observation that ticlopidine is not effective in blocking platelet aggregation in vitro when compared to the effect of the drug on the platelets of people taking ticlopidine. The thienopyridines both function as pro-drugs requiring cytochrome P450 activation. The thienopyridines are rapidly absorbed and extensively metabolized in the liver. The most significant metabolites of clopidogrel are shown in Figure 31.20. An inactive carboxylic acid represents the major circulating metabolite, which through oxidation by CYP3A4 gives rise to the 2-oxo derivative, which in turn is hydrolyzed to the thiol. The thiol is thought to bind irreversibly to $P2Y_{12}$ by forming a disulfide bridge to a cysteine in $P2Y_{12}$ (113–115). Specially, clopidogrel is thought to bind to Cys17 or Cys270 and, thus, block the binding of the agonist. In the case of ticlopidine, additional metabolites have been identified, dihydrothienopyridinium (M5) and thienodihydropyridinium metabolites (M6). These short-lived metabolites may be responsible for the toxic adverse reactions (116).

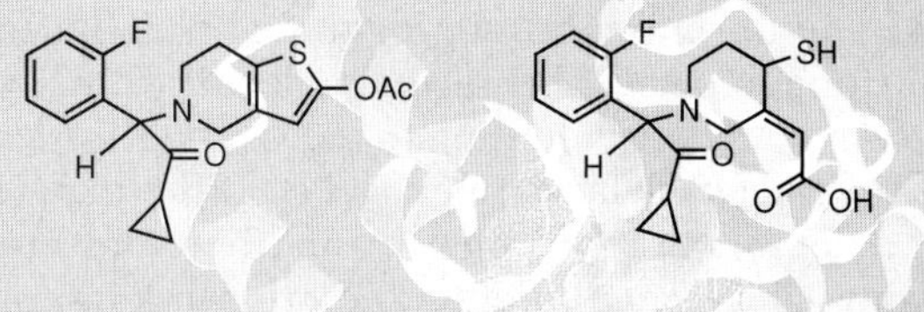

Prasugrel R-99224

In light of various limitations posed by clopidogrel, such as patient variability, resistance, and bleeding events, newer compounds continue to be developed. One such agent is parsugrel, which presently is in Phase II/III clinical studies. Prasugrel and its active metabolite R-99224 exhibit a more rapid onset, a higher potency, and a low rate of bleeding (117).

Glycoprotein II_b/III_a Receptor Antagonists

One of the newest groups of antithrombotic agents is the platelet receptor $GPII_b/III_a$ antagonists (87). This novel class of compounds has been shown to provide more comprehensive inhibition of platelet aggregation than the usual combination of aspirin and heparin. The final common pathway in platelet aggregation is the expression of functional $GPII_b/III_a$ (integrin αIIbβ3) receptors. These protein receptors are expressed regardless

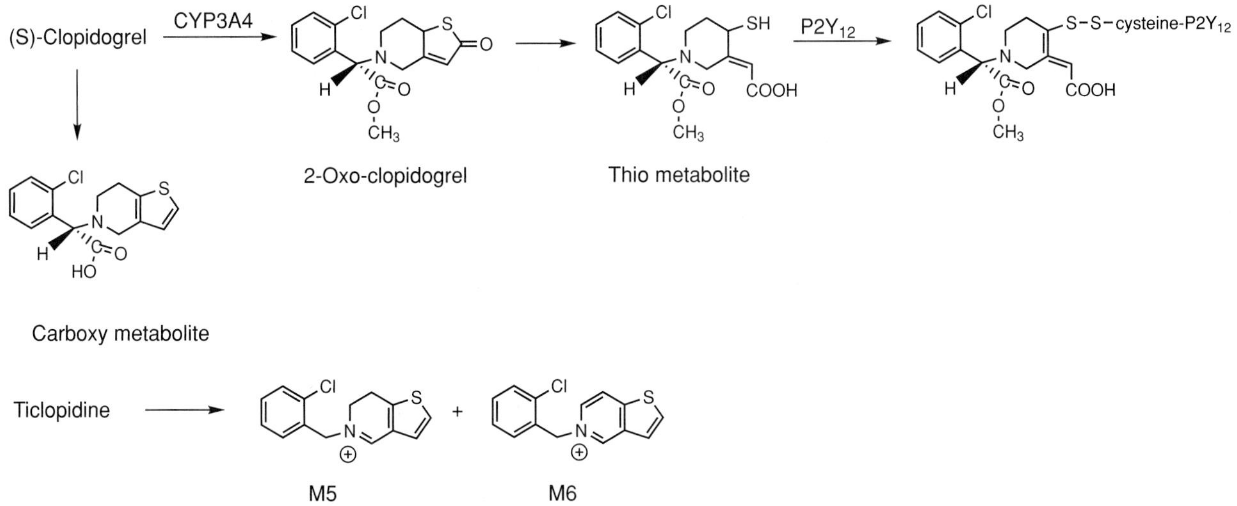

(S)-Clopidogrel → CYP3A4 → 2-Oxo-clopidogrel → Thio metabolite → $P2Y_{12}$ → S–S–cysteine-$P2Y_{12}$

Carboxy metabolite

Ticlopidine → M5 + M6

Fig. 31.20. Metabolism of clopidogrel and ticlopidine.

of the origin of the stimulus initiating the clotting cascade. The normal substrate for the $GPII_b/III_a$ receptor is fibrinogen. One fibrinogen molecule acts to cross-link two platelets via binding to the $GPII_b/III_a$ receptors on the platelet surfaces (Fig. 31.14). If the platelet surface receptors are occupied by another substrate that prevents fibrinogen binding and cross-linking, platelet aggregation will not occur. To this end, a number of novel compounds representing diverse structural groups have been prepared as $GPII_b/III_a$ receptor antagonists (Fig. 31.21) (118). Included in this list of antagonists are monoclonal antibodies against the natural $GPII_b/III_a$ receptor, naturally occurring peptides isolated from snake venom that contain the Arg-Gly-Asp (RGD) sequence, synthetic peptides containing either the RGD or Lys-Gly-Asp (KGD) sequences, and peptidomimetic and nonpeptide RGD mimetics that compete with fibrinogen and other ligands for occupancy of the receptor (87). The natural binding ligands, such as vWf and fibronectin, contain the natural RGD sequence.

The $GPII_b/III_a$ receptor antagonists are indicated in therapy for unstable angina, non-Q-wave myocardial infarction, and percutaneous coronary procedures. Like other antithrombotic agents, the main concern associated with $GPII_b/III_a$ receptor antagonists is bleeding. Additionally, these drugs have been suggested to possibly increase the risk of thrombocytopenia (87). Although a number of orally active $GPII_b/III_a$ receptor antagonists have been prepared and evaluated, their clinical efficacy in acute treatment of patients with unstable angina and in those undergoing angioplasty has not been fully established (118).

Abciximab

The initial antibodies against the $GPII_b/III_a$ receptor were murine in origin. Because of concerns about the antigenicity of a pure murine antibody, a chimeric human–mouse 7E3 Fab was developed (119). This chimera, marketed as abciximab, is the clinically available form of the antibody (120). For an adult patient, the usual dosing scheme is 0.25 mg/kg as an intravenous bolus given 10 to 60 minutes before percutaneous coronary intervention, followed by the continuous infusion of 0.125 μg/kg/minute for 12 hours to a maximum of 10 μg/kg. Elimination of abciximab is biphasic. The initial phase has a half-life of 10 minutes, whereas the half-life of the second phase is approximately 30 minutes and results from platelet binding. Platelet function returns to normal within 48 hours after infusion, even though abciximab is bound to circulating platelets for approximately 2 weeks (Table 31.5) (42).

Eptifibatide

Eptifibatide is a cyclic heptapeptide composed of six amino acids and one mercaptopropionyl residue. The cyclization is completed via a disulfide linkage between the cysteine and the mercaptopropionyl moieties. The lysine-glycine-aspartate component of eptifibatide is highly specific for the $GPII_b/III_a$ receptor, with low

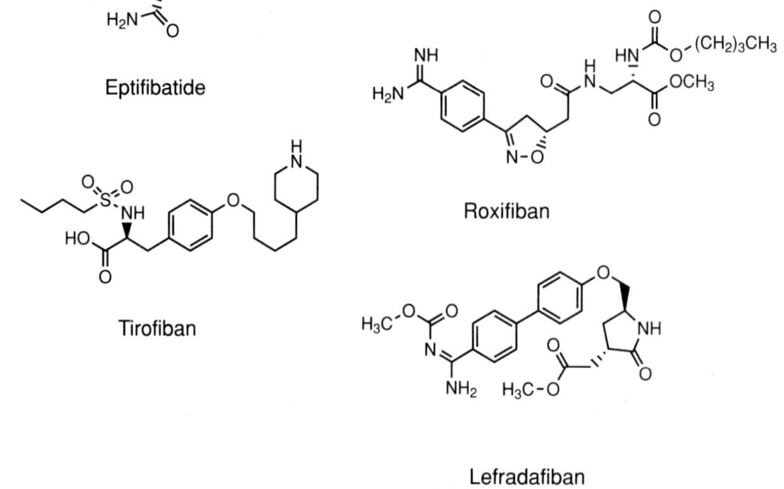

Eptifibatide

Lamifiban

Roxifiban

Tirofiban

Lefradafiban

Fig. 31.21. Structures of selected glycoprotein (GP) II_b/III_a receptor antagonists.

Table 31.5. Pharmacokinetic Properties of the Glycoprotein IIb/IIIa Receptor Antagonists

Drug	Trade Name	Molecular Weight (daltons)	Dissociation Constant (nmol/L)	Plasma Half-Life (hours)	Protein Binding (%)
Abciximab	ReoPro	47,615	5	72	
Eptifibatide	Integrelin	800	120	4	25
Tirofibin	Aggrastat	495	15	3–4	65

binding affinity, as indicated by the rapid dissociation constant (Table 31.5). Because of this, eptifibatide is a reversible, parenterally administered antagonist of platelet aggregation.

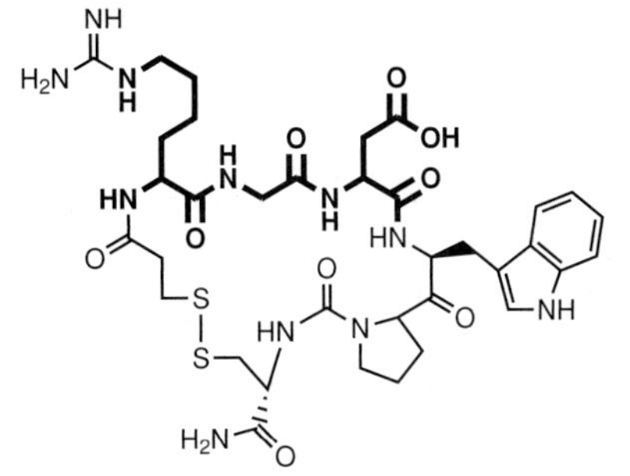

Eptifibatide (bolding indicates KGD portion of drug)

The drug is eliminated primarily via renal mechanisms as eptifibatide and deaminated eptifibatide. The clinical importance of eptifibatide and its benefits in comparison with other therapeutic agents used in the treatment of acute coronary syndromes and percutaneous coronary intervention have recently been reviewed by Curran and Keating (121).

Tirofiban

Tirofiban is a member of a new class of antithrombotic agents known as the "fibans" (Fig. 31.21). These compounds have a structural similarity to disintegrin, which was originally isolated from snake venoms. The location of the $-COO^-$ and NH_3^+ in the fibans is identical to the distance between the same functional groups of the RGD loop of disintegrin, and as a result, the fibans are able to effectively block the binding of fibrinogen to the GPIIb/IIIa receptor in an reversible manor. Tirofiban, like eptifibatide, has a rapid dissociation constant (Table 31.5). Tirofiban is a peptidomimetic (nonpeptide) that is parenterally administered and exhibits a reduced risk of bleeding because of its shorter biological half-life than abciximab. Additionally, it is less costly than other GPIIb/IIIa receptor antagonists. The remaining fibans shown in Figure 31.21 are in various stages of development. Lamifiban is administered parenterally, whereas roxifiban and lefradafiban are used orally.

New Developments in Antiplatelet Drugs

Several newer approaches to antiplatelet drug development have been recently discovered (122). These include inhibitions of the vWf/GPIb interaction, the platelet/collagen interaction, and the thrombin-induced platelet activation. Other approaches to platelet inhibition include the use of serotonin antagonists (because serotonin induces platelet aggregation), nitric oxide–donating antiplatelet agents, phosphodiesterase inhibitors, and inducers of adenyl cyclase.

Specific inhibitors of thromboxane synthase have been tested for their ability to block this enzyme without inhibiting the entrie acachidonic acid cascade (123). This allows an accumulation of prostaglandin G (PGG_2) and Prostaglandin H_2 (PGH_2) which can then be channeled into an increased production of prostacyclin (PGI_2) which also has antithrombotic activity.

THROMBOLYTIC DRUGS

Early application of reperfusion therapy with thrombolytic agents has significantly improved the outcomes of acute myocardial infarction and other conditions, such as pulmonary embolism, DVT, arterial thrombosis, acute thrombosis of retinal vessel, extensive coronary emboli, and peripheral vascular thromboembolism (124).

Although, the beneficial effect of the thrombolytic drugs, such as streptokinase and urokinase, for dissolving

Snake Venom–Induced Coagulopathy

The venom of snakes of the Crotalinae family, which includes rattlesnakes, produces a state of impaired coagulation. This can lead to both local and systemic hemorrhagic events. Venom consists of many components, including phospholipases and hemolysins, which cause cell lysis by disrupting platelet and red blood cell membranes. The venoms also contain procoagulant components that induce the formation of intravascular clots as well as hemorrhagins that destroy vascular integrity. Typically, both PT and aPTT are elevated with total fibrin levels being lowered and fibrin degradation products being increased. All of the findings are consistent with a consumptive coagulopathy. Because of the multiple mechanisms affecting coagulation, coagulopathies caused by snake venom are best managed using antivenin.

newly formed thrombus in patients with acute myocardial infarction were first reported in 1958, their full acceptance into clinical practice was not realized until the early 1980s as a result of several prospective, randomized, controlled trials. Today, with the approval of many second- and third-generation thrombolytic drugs, thrombolytic therapy has become a standard treatment for patients presenting with acute myocardial infarction or stroke (124,125).

Mechanism of Action

Normally, newly formed blood clots (fibrin) are dissolved by the actions of the fibrinolytic system. the purpose of which is the removal of unwanted clots without damaging the integrity of the vascular system. This system works via a relatively nonspecific protease enzyme called plasmin, the function of which is to digest fibrin (the very last step of the coagulation cascade) (Fig. 31.1). The lack of substrate specificity of plasmin is illustrated by the fact that it degrades fibrin clots as well as some plasma proteins and coagulation factors.

The fibrinolytically active plasmin is produced from the circulating inactive "proenzyme" plasminogen following the cleavage of a single peptide bond by a group of trypsin-like serine proteases known as the plasminogen activators. The principal activator, tissue-type plasminogen activator (tPA), is released from the vascular endothelium. Thrombolytic drugs, such as streptokinase and urokinase, act like a plasminogen activator that converts this proenzyme to the active plasmin. Endogenously, plasmin activity is regulated by two specific inactivators known as tPA inhibitors 1 and 2.

First-Generation Thrombolytic Agents

Streptokinase (Streptase)

Streptokinase is a drug of choice for thrombolytic therapy based on its cost-effectiveness consideration, and it is the only thrombolytic drug approved by the U.S. Food and Drug Administration (FDA) for peripheral vascular disease (126). The drug is approved for treatment of myocardial infarction but rarely is used for this condition today, having been replaced with the fibrin-specific agents discussed below (127).

Mechanism of action. Streptokinase is a protein purified from culture broths of group C β-hemolytic streptococci bacteria. Streptokinase contains a single polypeptide chain of 414-amino-acid residues with a molecular weight of 47 kDa (126). Streptokinase by itself has no intrinsic enzymatic activity. To be active, it must bind with plasminogen to form an activator complex (1:1 complex). This complex then acts to convert uncomplexed plasminogen to the active fibrinolytic enzyme, plasmin. The streptokinase/plasminogen complex not only degrades fibrin clots but also catalyzes the breakdown of fibrinogen and factors V and VII (124,126). As a result, streptokinase is considered to be a fibrin-nonspecific drug.

Pharmacokinetics. Unfortunately, the half-life of the activator complex is less than 30 minutes, which frequently is too short to completely lyse a thrombus. Anistreplase (APSAC; Eminase) is a 1:1 streptokinase/lysine-plasminogen complex that has been acylated with an anisoyl group at the active-site serine within the lysine-plasminogen. Anistreplase is inactive as such, but following complexation with fibrin, the anisoyl group is slowly cleaved, exposing the active site and, thus, leading to degradation of fibrin. The pro-drug nature of anistreplase exhibits an improved pharmacokinetic profile, with anistreplase acting as a semiselective lysis agent at the clot site. The inactivity of the circulating anistreplase also allows this drug to be given as a very rapid intravenous infusion (typically, 30 U over 3–5 minutes). Tissue reperfusion following anistreplase therapy compares favorably to streptokinase because of the extended half-life (90 minutes).

Side effects. Because it is a foreign protein, streptokinase is associated with significant hypersensitivity reactions. Most people have, at some point in their lives, had a streptococcal infection and, therefore, have developed circulating antistreptococcal antibodies. These antibodies frequently are active against streptokinase as well. The response of the streptokinase to these antibodies can vary widely, from inactivation of the fibrinolytic properties of the protein to rash, fever, and rarely, anaphylaxis. Significant allergic reactions to streptokinase occur in approximately 3% of patients.

Urokinase (Abbokinase)

Urokinase is an enzyme with the ability to directly degrade fibrin and fibrinogen. It is now isolated from cultures of human fetal kidney cells and is composed of two polypeptide chains with molecular weights of 32 and 54 kDa. This method of isolation is much more efficient than the original isolation of urokinase from human urine (128). Because of its source, the human body does not see urokinase as a foreign protein. Therefore, it lacks the antigenicity associated with streptokinase and frequently is used for patients with a known hypersensitivity to streptokinase (129). Plasmin cannot be used directly because of the presence of naturally occurring plasmin antagonists in plasma. No such inhibitors of urokinase exist in the plasma, however, allowing this enzyme to have clinical utility. Even so, urokinase is much more expensive (threefold the price of streptokinase) and has an even shorter half-life (15 minutes). Urokinase also has other fibrin-nonspecific actions similar to streptokinase.

Currently, urokinase is only approved for treatment of pulmonary embolism.

Second-Generation Thrombolytic Agents

Alteplase (Activase)

Alteplase (tPA) is a serine protease with a low affinity for free plasminogen but a very high affinity for the plasminogen bound to fibrin in a thrombus (fibrin-specific agent) (Fig. 31.22). Both streptokinase and urokinase lack this specificity (i.e., are nonspecific) and act on free plasminogen, inducing a generalized thrombolytic state. Alteplase also has a greater specificity for older clots compared with newer clots relative to streptokinase and urokinase. Alteplase was originally isolated from cultures of human melanoma cells but is now produced commercially using recombinant DNA technology. Alteplase is unmodified human tPA, whereas reteplase (see below) is human tPA that has had several specific amino acid sequences removed (130). At low doses, alteplase is quite selective for degrading fibrin without concomitant lysis of other proteins, such as fibrinogen. At the higher doses currently used therapeutically, however, alteplase activates free plasminogen to some extent and, therefore, can cause hemorrhage. Many of the therapeutic indications for the other thrombolytic agents also are indications for alteplase (i.e., myocardial infarction, massive pulmonary embolism, and acute ischemic stroke). The half-life of alteplase is very short (~5 minutes), necessitating its administration as a 15-mg intravenous bolus, followed by a 85-mg intravenous infusion over 90 minutes, or as 60 mg infused over the first hour, with the remaining 40 mg given at a rate of 20 mg/hour.

Prourokinase (scuPA, r-ProUK)

Prourokinase is a single-chain, urokinase-like plasminogen activator of 411 amino acids that displays clot-lysis activity yet does not interfere with hemostasis (131). It is nonimmunogenic and has a more favorable dose-related safety and efficacy profile than both urokinase and streptokinase. Thus, it is a potentially useful thrombolytic drug in the treatment of peripheral vascular occlusion (132).

Third-Generation Thrombolytic Agents

Many third-generation thrombolytic agents currently are under clinical trials. These agents are derived from

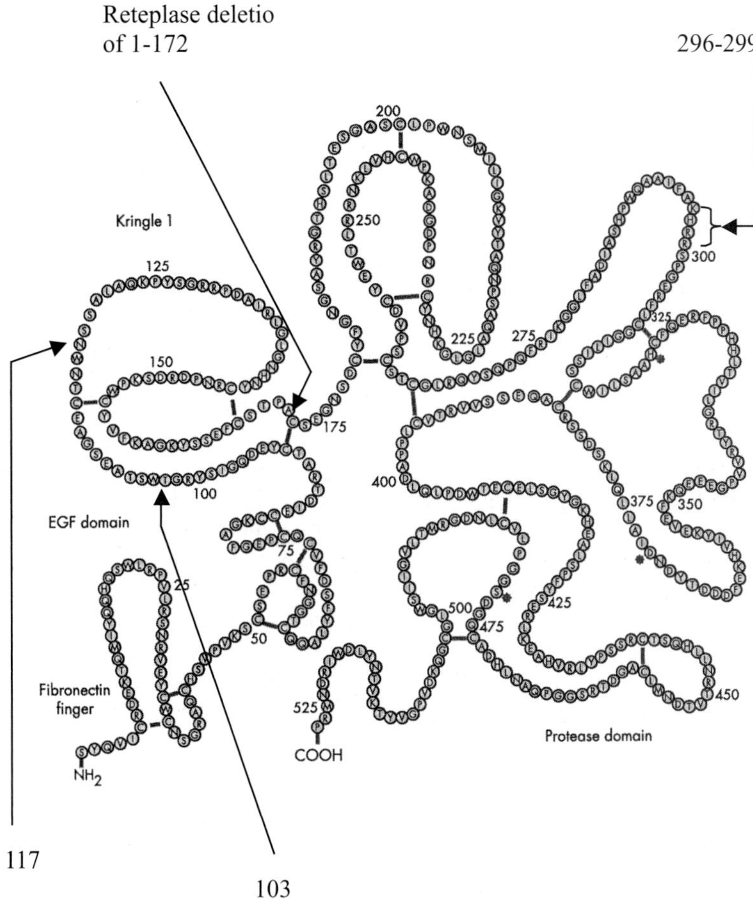

Fig. 31.22. Schematic diagram of alteplase, reteplase (removal of amino acids 1–172), and tenecteplase in which threonine (T) at position 103 is replaced with asparagines, asparagine (N) at position 117 is replaced with glutamine, and lysine (K)-histadine-arginine-asparagine at positions 296 to 299 are replaced with four alanines. (Adapted from Nordt TK. Bode C. Thrombolysis: Newer thrombolytic agents and their role in clinical medicine. Heart 2003;89: 1358–1362; with permission.)

structural modifications of the basic plasminogen activators (tPA or other tPA of animal origins) using technologies such as mutations, conjugation with monoclonal antibodies, or hybridization with another thrombolytic agent. Some of these agents are amediplase (hybrid of tPA and prourokinase), lanoteplase (mutant tPA), staphylokinase (from bacterial tPA) (125).

Reteplase (Retavase)

Reteplase is a recombinant deletion mutant of tPA lacking the finger, epidermal growth factor, kringle 1 domain, and carbohydrate side chain (Fig. 31.22) (133). As a highly fibrin-specific thrombolytic agent, reteplase is missing the first 172 amino acids that are present in alteplase and has 355 amino acids with a molecular weight of 39 kDa. Because of the removal of the finger kringle 1 domain, reteplase binding to fibrin is reduced from that of alteplase, and reteplase has reduced fibrin selectivity. In addition, the structural modification reduces hepatic elimination, leading to a longer half-life (reteplase, 14–18 minutes; alteplase, 3–4 minutes).

Administered as a double bolus of 10 U every 30 minutes, reteplase is approved for use in acute myocardial infarction.

Tenecteplase (TNKase)

Tenecteplase is composed of 527 amino acids with 17 disulfide bridges. It differs structurally from anteplase by three point mutations (Fig. 31.22). The mutations were bioengineered to occur at amino acid 103, where threonine (T) is replaced by asparagine; at amino acid 117, where asparagine (N) is replaced by glutamine; and at amino acids 296 to 299, where lysine (K)-histidine-arginine-arginine are replaced with four alanines. Thus, the name TNK is derived from the mutations. The replacement of these amino acids along with their attached carbohydrate side chains results in a prolonged half-life (~17 minutes) and allows a single bolus application (133). These point-mutation changes also change the binding of tenecteplase to plasminogen activator inhibitor-1 (PAI-1) by 80-fold, thus improving activity. A physiological enzyme, PAI-1 inhibits fibrinolysis. Finally, tenecteplase shows a 15-fold higher fibrin specificity. The drug is still eliminated via hepatic mechanisms.

TOXICITY OF ANTITHROMBOTICS AND THROMBOLYTICS

Antithrombotic Toxicity

Recall that warfarin exhibits its anticoagulation effects by preventing γ-carboxylation of specific glutamate residues necessary for vitamin K–dependent coagulation (Fig. 31.4). However, γ-carboxyglutamate proteins are not unique to coagulation factors. These types of proteins are synthesized in bone as well. As would be expected, warfarin also interferes with the carboxylation of these proteins, resulting in an inhibition of the effects of vitamin K on osteoblast development. It has been suggested that this is the mechanism responsible for bone abnormalities in neonates born to mothers who were treated with warfarin while pregnant (134). No evidence suggests that bone metabolism or development is affected by warfarin when the drug is administered to children or adults. Because of the mechanism of action of the warfarin-like drugs, the management of their toxicity is based largely on vitamin K therapy (see *Coagulants* below).

Unlike warfarin, heparin is safe for anticoagulant therapy during pregnancy (134). Although warfarin is known to cause serious fetal malformations when used in pregnancy, heparin does not cross the placental barrier and has shown no tendency to induce fetal damage. Furthermore, heparin does not increase fetal mortality or prematurity. To minimize the risk of postpartum hemorrhage, it is recommended that heparin therapy be withdrawn 24 hours before delivery.

Despite its safety in pregnancy, several potential problems are associated with heparin therapy. Because heparins (high-molecular-weight heparins and LMWHs) are isolated from animal sources, the chance of antigenic hypersensitivity exists but is rarely observed. Heparin competitively binds many other plasma proteins (i.e., vitronectin and PF4) in addition to the antithrombin, resulting in inactivation of the heparin as an anticoagulant (36). This may be the reason for heparin resistance and for a serious condition known as HIT. Typically, this condition occurs 7 to 14 days after initiation of heparin therapy, but it may occur earlier in some patients who have had previous exposures to heparin. In these cases, heparin-induced platelet aggregation occurs and may result in the production of antiplatelet antibodies. Development of this condition necessitates termination of heparin therapy and institution of antiplatelet drugs or oral anticoagulants. On withdrawal of heparin, the thrombocytopenia usually is reversible. Mild increases in liver function tests frequently are associated with heparin therapy. Long-term use of full therapeutic doses of heparin (>20,000 U/day for 3–6 months) has been associated with osteoporosis, and spontaneous vertebral fractures have been infrequently reported (36).

Hemorrhagic complications of heparin therapy are managed, in part, with the specific antagonist protamine sulfate (36). This agent is discussed in greater detail in the *Coagulants* section of this chapter.

The structural and mechanistic diversity of the antiplatelet drugs disallows a cohesive description of their toxicities. Hemorrhage is certainly a concern, but other, more drug-specific toxicities may be of greater immediate concern. It is suggested that toxicity information for antiplatelet medications be obtained from appropriate references for the specific agent in question and from the most recent reviews of antiplatelet agents (87).

Thrombolytic Toxicities

As discussed earlier, plasmin, because of its lack of specificity, not only digests fibrin but also degrades many other plasma proteins, including several coagulation factors and the anticoagulating factor, activated protein C. Thus, as expected, most thrombolytic drugs not only attack pathological clots but also exert their actions on any other site of compromised vascular integrity. The dissolution of necessary clots results in the principal side effect of thrombolytic therapy, hemorrhage. Its action on the activated protein C also may be responsible for their neurovascular toxicities (135).

Multiple studies have examined the incidence of life-threatening hemorrhage (i.e., intracranial hemorrhage) with the various thrombolytic medications. These studies indicate that the rate of significant hemorrhagic complication is essentially the same (0.1–0.7%) regardless of the specific therapeutic agent used. Supportive care is indicated in cases of thrombolytic toxicity. No specific antagonist exists to manage thrombolytic medication-induced hemorrhage, but antifibrinolytic drugs, such as aminocaproic acid and tranexamic acid, often are used. These compounds are described in detail in the *Coagulants* section of this chapter.

COAGULANTS

A variety of pathological and toxicological conditions can result in excessive bleeding from inadequate coagulation. Depending on the etiology and severity of the hemorrhagic episode, several possible blood coagulation inducers can be therapeutically employed.

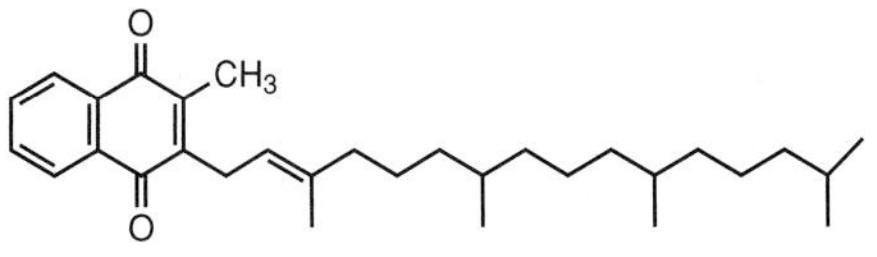

Vitamin K_1

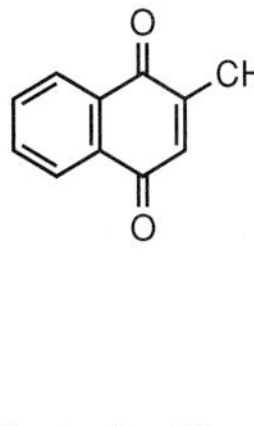

Vitamin K_3

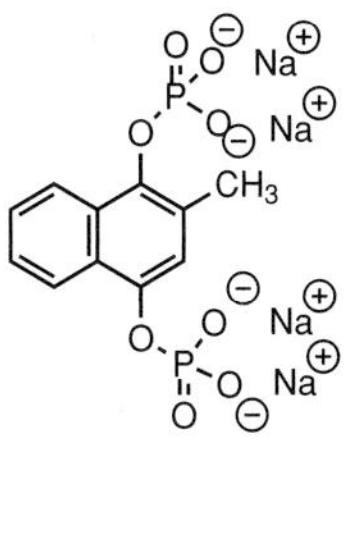

Vitamin K_4

Vitamin K

Because the orally active anticoagulants, such as warfarin and the indandiones, act through interruption of the normal actions of vitamin K, it stands to reason that vitamin K should be effective in the treatment of bleeding induced by these agents (122). Vitamin K_1 (phytonadione, Mephyton) is the form of vitamin K most often used therapeutically. Vitamin K_1 is safe for use in infants, pregnant women, and patients with glucose-6-phosphate deficiency. Furthermore, phytonadione, being more lipid soluble, has a faster onset than other vitamin K preparations and requires smaller doses than vitamin K_3 (menadione) or vitamin K_4 (menadiol sodium diphosphate). Both vitamins K_3 and K_4 may produce hyperbilirubinemia and kernicterus in neonates as well as hemolysis in neonates and glucose-6-phosphate–deficient patients. In fact, the only advantage of vitamins K_3 and K_4 over vitamin K_1 is that whereas absorption of vitamin K_1 requires the presence of bile, absorption of vitamins K_3 and K_4 does not, because they are absorbed via a passive process directly from the intestine (122). This may be a slight advantage for patients with cholestasis or severe pancreatic dysfunction. Only vitamin K_1, however, is appropriate therapy for bleeding associated with warfarin and superwarfarin anticoagulation. Vitamin K_2 is not used therapeutically.

Vitamin K_1 is effective at inducing coagulation when administered orally, subcutaneously, intramuscularly, or intravenously. Although the oral route is preferred, it is not always practical in a patient who is critically hemorrhaging. The other routes of administration, though used clinically, all have significant potential drawbacks. Larger doses (e.g., volume >5 mL) are not appropriate for subcutaneous administration, and intramuscular injection generally is avoided in patients who are at risk for significant hematoma formation (e.g., hemophiliacs). Intravenous dosing of vitamin K has been associated with severe anaphylactoid reactions (including death) presumably secondary to colloidal formulation.

The half-life of vitamin K_1 is quite short—only 1.7 hours via the intravenous route and 3–5 hours via the oral route. When given orally, vitamin K_1 is absorbed directly from the proximal small intestine in an energy-dependent and saturable process that requires the presence of bile salts. These kinetic features argue for administration in divided doses rather than larger, single daily doses. The typical starting point for adults with drug-induced hypoprothrombinemia is 2.5 to 10 mg of vitamin K_1 orally, repeating in 12 to 48 hours if needed. In cases of ingestion of long-acting superwarfarin rodenticides (e.g., brodifacoum), therapy may be 125 mg/day for weeks or months. Practically speaking, because vitamin K_1 is dispensed as 5-mg tablets, superwarfarin-poisoned patients may require 10 to 30 tablets every 6 hours.

Because of the short half-life of vitamin K_1, dosing must be repeated two to four times per day for the duration of treatment. Furthermore, regardless of the route of administration, coagulant effects are not evident for up to 24 hours. Because of this delay in onset, severe acute hemorrhage is better managed initially with intravenous infusion of fresh-frozen plasma, followed by vitamin K therapy.

Protamine

Mechanism of Action

Protamine sulfate has been approved in the United States as a specific antagonist to heparin since 1968 (134). Protamines are an arginine-rich, highly basic group of simple proteins derived from salmon sperm. The highly acidic heparin polysaccharides exhibit their anticoagulant activity through binding to antithrombin III. Because of the basicity of protamine, heparin has an increased affinity for protamine relative to antithrombin III. In fact, its binding affinity for protamine is so much greater than that of antithrombin III that protamine actually will induce dissociation of the heparin/ antithrombin III complex. If protamine is administered in the absence of heparin, it can have marked effects on coagulation. Protamine is not completely selective for heparin and, in vivo, also interacts with fibrinogen, platelets, and other plasma proteins causing anticoagulation. For this reason, use of the minimal amount of protamine necessary to antagonize heparin-associated bleeding should be employed (usually 1 mg of protamine intravenously for every 100 U of heparin remaining in the patient).

Side Effects

Anaphylaxis also has been associated with the use of protamine. Although development of protamine anaphylaxis is not limited to diabetics, those patients with diabetes that have used protamine-containing insulin (NPH or protamine zinc) do have a slightly increased risk of anaphylaxis. Some less common reactions to protamine include pulmonary vasoconstriction, hypotension, and thrombus formation.

Antifibrinolytic Agents

Mechanism of Action

Control of a variety of fibrinolytic states can be achieved using a number of synthetic antifibrinolytic agents, such as tranexamic acid (Cyklokapron) and ε-aminocaproic acid (Amicar), that completely inhibit plasminogen activation. Plasmin binds to fibrin through a lysine binding site to activate the final stages of fibrinolysis (Fig. 31.1). Aminocaproic acid, a lysine analogue, and tranexamic acid are antifibrinolytic agents with high affinity for the five lysine binding sites of plasminogen, thus effectively competing and preventing the binding of plasmin to fibrin.

$H_2N-CH_2-CH_2-CH_2-CH_2-CH_2-COOH$

Aminocaproic acid

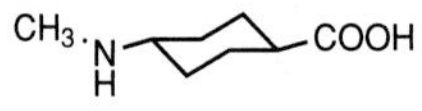

$CH_3 \cdot NH$–(cyclohexane)–COOH

Tranexamic acid

$H_2N-CH_2-CH_2-CH_2-CH_2-CH(NH_2)-COOH$

Lysine

Pharmacokinetics

Both ε-aminocaproic acid and tranexamic acid are readily absorbed when administered orally. They also can be given intravenously, although significant hypotension can result if the infusion is given too quickly. Elimination of the drugs is primarily renal, with little metabolism taking place. The half-lives of ε-aminocaproic acid and tranexamic acid are each approximately 2 hours.

Therapeutic Use

These drugs find clinical utility in settings such as prevention of rebleeding in intracranial hemorrhages, as adjunctive therapy in hemophilia, and of course, in treatment of bleeding associated with fibrinolytic therapy. In most bleeding conditions, however, ε-aminocaproic acid therapy has not been shown to be of definitive benefit. In recent trials, tranexamic acid was found to reduce red cell transfusion better than ε-aminocaproic acid or placebo in patients undergoing liver transplantation (136).

Side Effects

The major risk associated with ε-aminocaproic or tranexamic acid therapy is intravascular thrombosis as a direct result of the inhibition of plasminogen activator. Thrombi that form during therapy are not easily lysed and, therefore, can have additional ischemic consequences. Additional possible complications include hypotension, abdominal discomfort, and rarely, myopathy and muscle necrosis.

Aprotinin (Traysylol)

Operative procedures, such as heart valve replacement, frequently have effects on platelet function and endogenous coagulation factors (137). These effects may result in significant peri- or postoperative bleeding. Aprotinin is a serine protease inhibitor that blocks kallikrein and plasmin and provides some protection to platelets from mechanical injury. The inhibition of fibrinolysis results in profound antihemorrhagic effects (137). Side effects of aprotinin therapy usually are minor, but anaphylaxis has possibly been implicated in a small population ($<0.5\%$). For this reason, it is suggested that a small test dose be given before initiation of the therapeutic infusion.

Plasma Fractions

Spontaneous bleeding can result from dysfunction or deficiencies of specific coagulation factors. A list of coagulation factors and deficiency states is given in Table 31.6.

Spontaneous bleeding usually occurs when the activity of coagulation factors falls below 5% of normal. Typically, these deficiencies are the result of a chronic disease state, such as von Willebrand's disease or hemophilia. Management of an acute hemorrhagic event in a coagulation factor–deficient patient includes administration of the appropriate factors in concentrated form. The most

Table 31.6. Clotting Factors

Factor	Common Name	Deficiency State	Source	Half-Life of Infused Factor (days)	Target for Action of
I	Fibrinogen	Afibrinogenemia, defibrination syndrome	Liver	4	
II	Prothrombin	Prothrombin deficiency	Liver (requires vitamin K)	3	Heparin (IIa), warfarin (synthesis)
III	Tissue thromboplastin, thrombokinase, tissue factor		Liver (may require vitamin K)		
IV	Calcium (Ca^{2+})				
V	Proaccelerin, labile factor	Factor V deficiency	Liver	1	
VI	Deleted factor				
VII	Proconvertin, stable factor	Factor VII deficiency	Liver (requires vitamin K)	0.25	Heparin (VIIa); warfarin (synthesis)
VIII	Antihemophilic A factor (AHF), antihemophilic globulin (AHG)	Hemophilia A (classic) Von Willebrand's disease	Liver	0.5 Unknown	
IX	Antihemophilic B factor, plasma thromboplastin component (PTC), Christmas factor	Hemophilia B (Christmas disease)	Liver (requires vitamin K)	1	Heparin (IXa); warfarin (synthesis)
X	Stuart or Stuart-Prower factor	Stuart-Prower defect	Liver (requires vitamin K)	1.5	Heparin (IXa); warfarin (synthesis)
XI	Plasma thromboplastin antecedent (PTA)	PTA deficiency	Unknown	3	
XII	Hageman factor, contact factor	Hageman defect	Unknown	Unknown	
XIII	Fibrin-stabilizing factor, fibrinase	Fibrin-stabilizing factor deficiency	Unknown	6	
	Fletcher factor, prekallikrein factor		Liver		
	Fitzgerald factor, high-molecular-weight kininogen		Liver		
Antithrombin III		Antithrombin III deficiency		3	
Proteins C & S					Warfarin (synthesis)
Plasminogen					Thrombolytic enzymes, aminocaproic acid

common inherited clotting factor deficiencies involve factor VIII (classic hemophilia A) and factor IX (hemophilia B, or Christmas disease).

Two forms of factor VIII concentrate are clinically available, cryoprecipitate and lyophilized factor VIII concentrate. Cryoprecipitate is a factor VIII–rich plasma protein fraction (PPF) prepared from whole blood that also contains approximately 300 mg of fibrinogen per unit. Immediately before infusion, the required number of cryoprecipitate units are thawed in a sterile saline/citrate solution and pooled. The lyophilized factor VIII concentrates are prepared from large plasma pools and also are rich in fibrinogen. Lyophilized factor VIII concentrates are not useful in therapy for von Willebrand's disease, because during the extraction and lyophilization process, the polymeric structure of factor VIII in the von Willebrand protein that supports platelet adhesion is destroyed, rendering the preparation inactive. Because of the pooling of blood from multiple donors in the preparation of lyophilized factor VIII concentrates, it generally is held that cryoprecipitate, which is isolated from a single donor, is safer.

The major concern associated with the use of concentrated clotting factors is the risk of viral transmission (primarily HIV and hepatitis B). This fear has somewhat attenuated the use of concentrated plasma fractions, even in diseases such as hemophilia. Ultrapure factor VIII concentrates produced using recombinant DNA technology have been approved for use. Frequently, however, the expense of these recombinant agents is the reason why the more traditional plasma isolates are used—despite the possibility of viral transmission.

Lyophilized preparations of prothrombin, factor IX, and factor X also are available. The manufacturing process involves plasma extraction with solvents and detergents that renders the preparations virally inactive but still able to activate clotting factors. To prevent excessive thrombus formation in these situations, heparin often is added to the therapeutic regimen.

At times, a hemorrhagic event is possible but the patient does not require immediate coagulation therapy. For example, if a patient with mild hemophilia A needs to have a dental extraction performed, the potential for hemorrhage exists. In these cases, it is possible to increase the activity of the endogenous factor VIII through pretreatment with desmopressin acetate. This preoperative measure may alleviate the need for clotting factor replacement.

PLASMA EXTENDERS AND BLOOD SUBSTITUTES

Maintenance of circulation is secondary only to airway and breathing in the American Heart Association chain of survival (138). Circulation is governed by the three components of the Fick Principle: 1) on-loading of oxygen onto the erythrocytes (red blood cells), 2) delivery of oxygen-laden erythrocytes to the various cells and tissues, and 3) off-loading of the oxygen from the erythrocytes to the tissue cells (139). Interruption of any of these three components results in physiologic compromise. Inadequate blood volume (i.e., a loss of red blood cells) will disallow the transport of oxygen to tissues.

Severe anemia, such as that secondary to major hemorrhage, is a complicated condition to manage. Simply replacing lost blood with new blood may not always be practical—or even beneficial to the patient. Numerous approaches and theories exist that attempt to define the best method of emergently managing severe blood loss. Two basic types of fluid infusion are used for the resuscitation of severely anemic patients. These are sanguinous (blood-containing) infusions, in which fluids (e.g., whole blood and fractionated blood products) are used, and asanguinous (i.e., nonblood-containing) infusions, in which various crystalloids, colloids, blood substitutes, and plasma expanders are employed.

Sanguinous Resuscitation

It seems intuitive that resuscitation following severe blood loss would be best accomplished by replacing lost blood with fresh blood (i.e., sanguinous resuscitation); however, this is not always in the best interest of the resuscitation. Nonetheless, infusion of blood and blood products is recommended in certain hypovolemic circumstances. Generally, if hemodynamic instability exists in a hypovolemic adult following the infusion of 2 L of crystalloid (three successive 20 mL/kg body weight infusions in a child), addition of blood to the resuscitative regimen is recommended (140). The most significant advantage of sanguinous resuscitation is that infusion of red blood cells can replace both volume and oxygen-carrying capacity. Significant disadvantages of sanguinous resuscitation include limited supply, risk of transfusion reaction, expense, and possible transmission of bloodborne diseases.

At one time, a significant controversy existed regarding whether survivability was increased with the use of whole-blood transfusion or infusion of packed red blood cells (known as component therapy). Traditionally, this decision was based on cost and the fact that few hospitals actually stored whole blood. Fortunately, however, scientists reached the same decision as the fiscal experts (140). The three major conclusions drawn from the scientific community were as follows:

1. "Whole blood out" does not require "whole blood in." Banked whole blood stored at 4°C lacks functional platelets and also suffers a progressive deterioration in the activities of various clotting factors. There is little difference in these parameters between banked whole blood and packed red blood cells. Because trauma patients require red blood cells, clotting factors, and platelets to varying degrees, it makes more sense to use functional components to replace what is specifically needed at that time.
2. Whole blood is not infused more rapidly than packed red blood cells. In fact, infusion technology exists that allows replacement of packed red blood cells suspended in normal saline as fast as 1,600 mL/min.
3. The overall risk of antigenic hypersensitivity reactions is greatly increased when using whole blood as opposed to specific components. The standard of care at this time is judicious use of the individual components with crystalloid infusion to maintain volume while the defect resulting in the blood loss is repaired.

Asanguinous Resuscitation

Crystalloids are aqueous electrolyte-containing solutions without proteins or large molecules. Examples of crystalloids are normal saline (0.9% NaCl) and lactated Ringer's solution. Colloids are aqueous solutions that contain various proteins or other larger molecules as well as electrolytes. Protein-containing colloids include albumin and PPF. Nonproteinaceous colloids include the dextrans and hetastarch. A list detailing the compositions of several common crystalloids and colloids is given in Table 31.7.

Crystalloids

Crystalloids have several advantages, including being inexpensive and free of risk of transferring bloodborne pathogens or inducing anaphylaxis. Furthermore, they largely are compatible with drugs and undergo rapid

Table 31.7. Composition of Common Intravenous Fluids

Solution	Common/ Trade Name	Concentration Solute	Ionic Concentration g/dL	mEq/L	Indications	Contraindications
CRYSTALLOIDS						
0.9% Saline	Normal Saline	NaCl	0.90	Na^+ 154 Cl^- 154	Hypovolemia Heat-related emergencies Freshwater drowning Diabetic ketoacidosis	CHF
0.45% Saline	Half-Normal Saline	NaCl	0.45	Na^+ 77 Cl^- 77	Compromised cardiac function	Emergent rehydration
3% Saline	Hypertonic Saline	NaCl	3.0	Na^+ 513 Cl^- 513	Hypovolemia, hyponatremia, TCA OD*	Hypernatremia Hyperchloremia
5% Dextrose in water	D_5W	Glucose	5.0		Intravenous drug route Dilution of concentrated drugs for intravenous infusion	Volume replacement
Lactated Ringer's	Hartman's Solution	NaCl KCl $CaCl_2$ Na Lactate	0.86 0.03 0.02 0.31	Na^+ 130 K^+ 4 Ca^{2+}:3, Cl^-:109 Lactate 28	Hypovolemic shock Obstetric emergencies	CHF Renal failure Lactic Acidosis
COLLOIDS						
Plasma protein Fraction	Plasmanate	Albumin Globulin	4.4 0.6	Na^+ 130–160 Cl^- 130–160	Hypovolemic shock	Coagulopathy (relative)
Albumin		Albumin	5 25	Na^+ 130–160 Cl^- 130–160	Hypovolemic shock	Coagulopathy (relative)
Hetastarch	Hespan	Hydroxyethyl Starch	6 (in saline)	Na^+ 154 Cl^- 154	Hypovolemic shock	Factor VIII deficiency

*TCA OD, Tricyclic antidepressant overdose

renal clearance. The crystalloids, however, have a very short resident time in the intravascular space—only 30% remains in the vasculature within a few minutes following infusion. These fluids rapidly leak out of the vasculature into the interstitial space and can result in significant extravascular fluid accumulations ("third spacing"). Furthermore, crystalloids do not have any oxygen-carrying capacity.

Attempts at lengthening intravascular resident time of the solution and limit third spacing have resulted in the development of "hypertonic" crystalloid solutions. An example of a hypertonic solution is 3% NaCl ("hypertonic saline"). It has been suggested that the increased electrolyte concentration will result in an osmotic gradient pulling fluid from the interstitial and intracellular spaces into the vasculature. These fluid shifts therefore would require less total volume to be infused. As expected, the possibility of severe hypernatremia and hyperchloremia, among other electrolyte disturbances, exists.

Protein Colloids

Protein colloids contain larger molecules and have a longer intravascular residence time than crystalloids, but eventual fluid loss to the extravascular space does occur. Protein colloids, such as albumin and PPF, are prepared from pooled human blood and, therefore, carry with them a risk of transmission of viral infection or induction of anaphylaxis. The PPF is a 5% mixture (5 g of protein in 100 ml of 0.9% NaCl solution) of proteins that is osmotically equivalent to human plasma. The composition of the protein mixture is 83 to 90% albumin. Albumin typically is administered as either a 5 or 25% solution. By definition, albumin preparations must be composed of a protein mixture that is more than 90% albumin. Generally, PPF is favored over albumin for fluid resuscitation, because albumin appears to cause more interstitial edema.

Nonproteinaceous Colloids

Dextrans

Nonproteinaceous colloids also are used in fluid resuscitation. These compounds generally are complex mixtures of sugar polymers. Dextrans are glucose polymers produced by bacteria linked in an α-1,6 chain and having an α-1,3 or α-1,4 branch about every fifth residue. The specific positioning of the branching varies by the bacterium producing it. The molecular weights of these chains generally are 40 or 70 kDa (dextran-40 and dextran-70, respectively), and the compounds work via an osmotic gradient similar to the colloids and hypertonic crystalloid solutions. Dextran-70 is a 4% solution, whereas dextran-40 is a 10% preparation. Dextrans have a longer intravascular residence time

Dextran polymer

than albumin, which limits interstitial edema. As with the crystalloids and other colloids, the dextrans have no oxygen-carrying capacity. Furthermore, because they are bacterial products, the dextrans have the potential to be potent antigens and induce anaphylaxis. The incidence of serious antigenic response seems to increase if the dextran used has a significant fraction of components with a molecular weight of greater than 100 kDa. In these cases, administration of dextran-1 (molecular weight, 1 kDa) before the higher-molecular-weight dextrans minimizes formulation of the very large immunogenic complexes. This approach has been shown to decrease sensitivity responses to high-molecular-weight dextrans by as much as 15- to 20-fold. This is particularly important in a number of European countries, where dextran-150 (molecular weight, ~150 kDa) is routinely used.

Hetastarch. Hetastarch, another nonproteinaceous colloid, is a complex mixture of ethoxylated amylopectins ranging in molecular weight from 10 to 1,000 kDa (average molecular weight, ~450 kDa). When infused as a 6% solution, hetastarch approximates the activity of human albumin. The larger molecular weights, however, increase its intravascular residence time as well as its plasma expansion effects relative to albumin. Hetastarch is synthetically produced, so it is degraded more slowly and is less antigenic than other colloids. Despite these advantages, hetastarch is quite expensive and also has no oxygen-carrying capacity.

Plasma substitutes, such as dextrans and hetastarch, have some additional unusual disadvantages specific to the various classes. High-molecular-weight (70-kDa) dextran coats erythrocytes, making subsequent blood typing and cross-matching difficult. On the other hand, low-molecular-weight (40-kDa) dextran coats platelets, which can induce a bleeding disorder. Hetastarch has a dilutional effect on factor VIII and, therefore, should not be used to treat patients with factor VIII deficiency (e.g., hemophilia)–related hemorrhage.

Combination use of hypertonic crystalloids with nonproteinaceous colloids has been investigated. For example, 7.5% NaCl in 6% dextran-70 (hypertonic saline–dextrose) has been studied in a variety of animal models and in human trauma patients with some success. Particularly promising are animal studies of closed head injury, which suggest not only a hemodynamic benefit but also a sustained decrease in intracranial pressure. Studies in this system as well as in burn and trauma patients are ongoing.

Red-Cell Substitutes ("Synthetic Blood")

Concerns about the safety and adequacy of the blood supply and the increasing need to rigorously screened human blood because of HIV and hepatitis B and C virus have stimulated extensive search for "blood substitutes" (or, more accurately "red-cell substitutes") for resuscitation of trauma patients (140,141). Three different classes of materials have been evaluated clinically as potential blood substitutes (140). They are perfluorocarbon (PFC)-based emulsion, hemoglobin-based oxygen carriers (HBOCs), and liposome-enclosed hemoglobin. Thus far, only the PFCs and HBOCs have reached various phases of their clinical trials, whereas liposome-enclosed hemoglobin is still in the preclinical stage of development. Several excellent reviews have been published in recent years summarizing the clinical progress, efficacy, and toxicity of these agents (142–146).

Perfluorocarbon-Based Oxygen Carriers

Some of the common ingredients of the synthetic blood substitutes are shown in Fig. 31.23. The most significant benefit of PFCs is their ability to transport oxygen to the body tissues via the circulatory system and their in vivo metabolic stability (145). This ability results from the high solubility of gases, such as oxygen and carbon dioxide, in the PFC preparations. Red blood cells with fully functional hemoglobin have an oxygen solubility of 17 to 20 mL/dL. Red blood cells without hemoglobin can only dissolve approximately 0.3 mL/dL of oxygen. The oxygen solubility of PFC preparations is approximately 7 mL/dL.

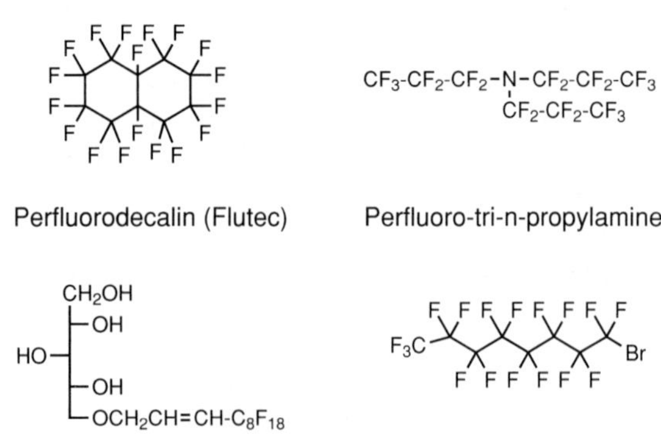

Fig. 31.23. Chemical structures of perfluorocarbon-based blood substitutes.

The PFCs are formulated as stable aqueous emulsions with dextrose, egg yolk phospholipids, and physiologic electrolytes. These emulsions are somewhat less viscous than whole blood at 37°C. The PFCs have a dose-dependent half-live of 8 to 24 hours. Normal doses are 10 mL/kg, but short-term doses of up to 30 mL/kg have been reported. The PFCs are not metabolized and are eliminated unchanged in expired respiratory gases. Because they are highly lipophilic, multiple doses can cause PFC accumulation in the liver and spleen. Therefore, it is recommended that these compounds not be administered more than once in a 6-month period.

During the early 1980s, PFC emulsions, such as Fluosol (a 20% emulsion of perfluorodecalin and perfluoro-tri-n-propylamine), were used as an oxygen carrier in the preoperative treatment of severely anemic patients, but often with significant toxicities, high incidence of hypertension, and potential to cause anaphylaxis reactions (143,147).

Another use for PFC emulsions is decreasing or preventing myocardial ischemia during percutaneous transluminal coronary angioplasty in high-risk patients. The emulsion is preoxygenated and injected transluminally through the coronary angioplasty balloon to deliver the oxygenated emulsion to areas distal to the point of balloon inflation. Less common but also investigated uses of PFC emulsions include therapy for carbon monoxide intoxication, oxygenation in cases of cerebral hypoxia, autoimmune hemolytic anemia, and nonavailability of compatible blood products. Newer PFCs, such as perflubron, that are less toxic have been used with some success in limited clinical trials during orthopaedic surgery (148).

Genetically Engineered and Chimeric Hemoglobin-Based Oxygen Carriers

Stroma-free hemoglobin appears to hold significant promise as a potential acellular oxygen transporter. These preparations have no effect on colloid osmotic pressure and are not effective as plasma expanders. A number of potential advantages exist with this technology. For example, stroma-free hemoglobin can be prepared from bovine or outdated human erythrocytes, no cross-match is necessary, it is lyophilized for convenient and space-efficient storage, and it is reconstituted in normal saline (149).

Two major problems that are currently being addressed are large-scale production of the material and the fact that stroma-free hemoglobin does not readily release oxygen to the tissues at normal oxygen tensions. Recombinant DNA technology has allowed the production of large amounts of hemoglobin through synthetic gene expression in *Escherichia coli* and *Saccharomyces cerevisiae.* New developments in hemoglobin polymerization also show promise (142,149).

Another approach to stroma-free hemoglobin technology is the development of chimeric hemoglobins. Human hemoglobin stripped from red blood cells is not functional. Diphosphoglycerate (DPG) is required for oxygen release from hemoglobin, and insufficient DPG is available outside the red cell to induce oxygen release (i.e., oxygen affinity for hemoglobin is too high in the absence of DPG). Tetrameric human hemoglobin decomposes into dimers when infused into the bloodstream. These dimers precipitate in the kidneys, potentially causing severe renal damage. In native red cell–bound hemoglobin, this decomposition is prevented by the high concentration of proteins inside the red blood cells. Interestingly, not all species require ATP and DPG to diminish oxygen affinity for hemoglobin. The crocodile is one such animal in which red blood cells do not contain DPG, and this phosphate has no effect on oxygen affinity to their hemoglobin. Crocodile hemoglobin cannot be used directly in humans, because certain features of human hemoglobin are necessary for recognition and signaling. Genetic engineering technology has allowed the creation of a chimeric hemoglobin that is part human and part crocodile and that is useful in humans (149). It has the advantage of providing hemoglobin oxygen-carrying capacity without transmitting human bloodborne diseases. One major disadvantage is that the chimeric hemoglobins are not endogenous proteins and, therefore, may be potent antigens. A great deal of investigation is still necessary before chimeric hemoglobins will see any clinical usage.

The most successful HBOCs clinically are polymerized hemoglobin solution (142). Among these, Hemolink, Hemopure, and PolyHeme are undergoing U.S. FDA–approved phase III clinical trials. Hemolink is a product consisting of human hemoglobin polymerized using an oxidized trisaccharide, O-raffinose, followed by a reduction. Hemopure and PolyHeme, on the other hand, are produced by using glutaraldehyde as the polymerizing agent and with either bovine hemoglobin (Hemopure) or human hemoglobin (PolyHeme) as the source of hemoglobins.

Newer HBOCs without the nitric oxide–scavenging properties of the first-generation HBOCs have been prepared and are being investigated as red-cell substitutes (150–153).

Liposome-Encapsulated Hemoglobin

The successful use of liposomes as drug-delivery vehicles has prompted the preparations of liposome-encapsulated hemoglobins as artificial red-cell substitutes (154). This represents a promising approach for the design of longer storage half-life red-cell substitutes, because it has no blood group antigens on its surface and, thus, could be stored for long period of times (154). The circulatory half-life of liposome-encapsulated hemoglobin is further improved with the design of cellular-based red-cell substitutes with an actin matrix underlying the lipid bilayer as a structure support (155).

CASE STUDY

Victoria F. Roche and S. William Zito

DF is a 24-year-old Hispanic man who appeared in the emergency department with a chief complaint of right leg swelling and pain. He reports that he received a severe trauma to his right calf 5 days ago from the crush of people at a protest rally in support of equal rights for immigrant farm workers. A review of DF's patient history reveals him to be a healthy male except for a previous HIT that resulted from low-dose heparin prophylaxis associated with a laparoscopic repair of an inguinal hernia several years ago. On examination, the physician observes the classic signs of DVT, including pain when asked to pull his foot up toward himself against resistance, tenderness, swelling, and warmth. The presence of DVT was confirmed by Doppler ultrasonography, and the physician wants to begin anticoagulation treatment and asks your opinion of the following choices

1. Identify the therapeutic problem(s) where the pharmacist's intervention may benefit the patient.
2. Identify and prioritize the patient-specific factors that must be considered to achieve the desired therapeutic outcomes.
3. Conduct a thorough and mechanistically oriented structure-activity analysis of all therapeutic alternatives provided in the case.
4. Evaluate the structure–activity relationship findings against the patient-specific factors and desired therapeutic outcomes, and make a therapeutic decision.
5. Counsel your patient.

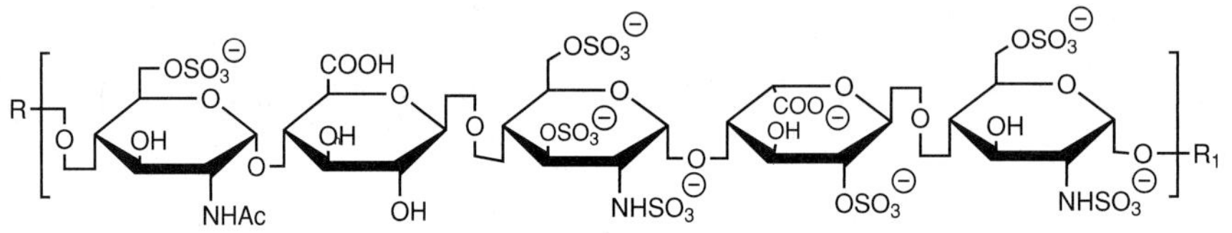

1

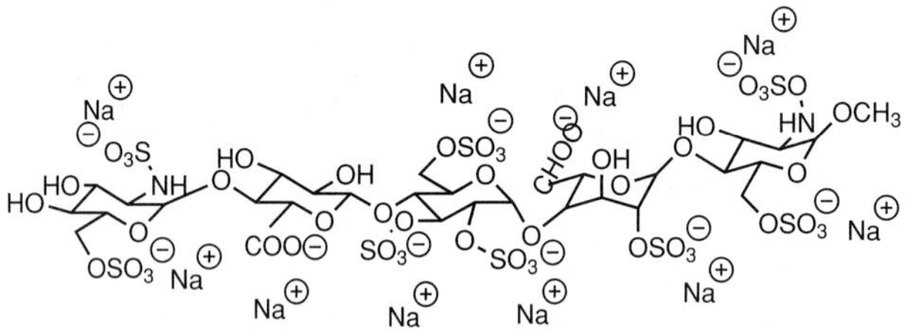

2

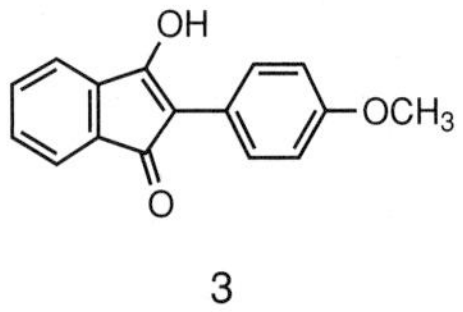

3

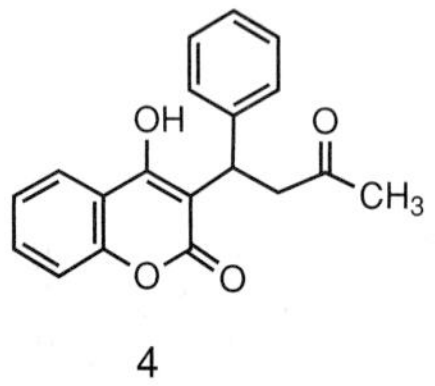

4

References

1. Ansell J, Bergqvist D. Current options in the prevention of thromboembolic disease. Drugs 2004;64(Suppl 1):1–5.
2. Hirsh J, Guyatt G, Albers GW, et al. Evidence-based guidelines: the Seventh ACCP Conference on Antithrombotic and Thrombolytic Therapy. Chest 2004;126:172S–173S.
3. Wright IS. The discovery and early development of anticoagulants: a historical perspective. Circulation 1959;19:73–134.
4. Kakkar VV, Corrigan TP, Spindler J, et al. Efficacy of low doses of heparin in prevention of deep vein thrombosis after major surgery. Lancet 1972; 300:101–106.
5. Blanchard E, Ansell J. Extended anticoagulation therapy for the primary and secondary prevention of venous thromboembolism. Drugs 2005;65:303–311.
6. Weitz JI, Hirsh J, Samama MM. New anticoagulant drugs: the Seventh ACCP Conference on Antithrombotic and Thrombolytic Therapy. Chest 2004; 126:265S–286S.
7. Nutescu E. Emerging options in the treatment of venous thromboembolism. Am J Health-Syst Pharm 2004;61(Suppl 7):12S–17S.
8. Fevig JM, Wexler RR. Anticoagulants: thrombin and factor Xa inhibitors. In: Doherty AM, ed. Ann Rep in Med Chem. San Diego: Academic Press, 1999; 34:81–100.
9. Kyrle PA, Eichinger S. Deep vein thrombosis. Lancet 2005;365:1163–1174.
10. Geerts WH, Pineo GF, Heit JA, et al. Prevention of venous thromboembolism: the Seventh ACCP Conference on Antithrombotic and Thrombolytic Therapy. Chest 2004;126:338S–400S.
11. Singer DE. Anticoagulation to prevent stroke in atrial fibrillation and its implications for managed care. Am J Cardiol 1998;81:35C–40C.
12. Nutescu EA, Helgason CM. Concomitant drug, dietary, and lifestyle issues in patients with atrial fibrillation receiving anticoagulation therapy for stroke prophylaxis. Curr Treatment Options Cardiovasc Med 2005;7:241–250.
13. Singer DE, Albers GW, Dalen JE, et al. Antithrombotic therapy in atrial fibrillation: the Seventh ACCP Conference on Antithrombotic and Thrombolytic Therapy. Chest 2004;126:429S–456S.
14. Khrenov AV, Anayeva NM, Griffin JH, et al. Coagulation pathways in atherothrombosis. Trends Cardiovasc Med 2002;12:317–324.
15. Stryer L. Biochemistry. 3rd Ed. New York: W.H. Freeman and Company, 1988.
16. Broze GJ Jr. Tissue factor pathway inhibitor. Thromb Haemost 1995;74: 90–93.
17. Sandset PM, Bendz B, Hansen JB. Physiological function of tissue factor pathway inhibitor and interaction with heparins. Haemostasis 2000;30: 48–56.
18. Esmon CT. The protein C pathway. Chest 2003;124:26S–32S.
19. Brookoff D. Hematologic evaluation. In: Flomenbaum N, Goldfrank L, Jacobson S, eds. Emergency Diagnostic Testing. 2nd Ed. St. Louis, MO: Mosby, 1995.

20. Ansell J, Hirsh J, Poller L, et al. The pharmacology and management of the vitamin K antagonists: the Seventh ACCP Conference on Antithrombotic and Thrombolytic Therapy. Chest 2004;126:204S–233S.
21. O'Reilly RA. Vitamin K and the oral anticoagulant drugs. Annu Rev Med 1976;27:245–261.
22. Hirsh J, Dalen JE, Anderson DR, et al. Oral anticoagulants: mechanism of action, clinical effectiveness, and optimal therapeutic range. Chest 2001; 119:8S–21S.
23. Valente EJ, Lingafelter EC, Porter WR, et al. Structure of warfarin in solution. J Med Chem 1977;20:1489–1493.
24. USPDI Drug Information for the Health Care Professional. 16th Ed. Rockville, MD: United States Pharmacopeial Convention, Inc., 1996:236–246.
25. Ansell J, Hirsh J, Dalen J, et al. Managing oral anticoagulant therapy. Chest 2001;119:22S–38S.
26. Baselt RC, ed. Disposition of Toxic Drugs and Chemicals in Man. 5th Ed. Foster City, CA: Chemical Toxicology Institute, 2000.
27. Hollinger BR, Pastoor TP. Case management and plasma half-life in a case of brodifacoum poisoning. Arch Intern Med 1993;153:1925–1928.
28. Palmer RB, Alakija P, Cde Baca JE, et al. Fatal brodifacoum rodenticide poisoning: autopsy and toxicologic findings. J Forensic Sci 1999;44:851–855.
29. Redfern R, Gill JE, Hadler MR. Laboratory evaluation of WBA8119 (brodifacoum) as a rodenticide for use against warfarin-resistant and non-resistant rats and mice. J Hygiene 1976;77:419–426.
30. Bachmann KA, Sullivan TJ. Dispositional and pharmacodynamic characteristics of brodifacoum in warfarin-sensitive rats. Pharmacol 1983;27:281–288.
31. Slattery J, Yacobi A, Levy G. Comparative pharmacokinetics of coumarin anticoagulants. XXV: Warfarin–ibuprofen interaction in rats. J Pharm Sci 1977;66:943–947.
32. Hoffman RS. Anticoagulants. In: Goldfrank LR, Flomenbaum NE, Lewin NA, et al., eds. Goldfrank's Toxicologic Emergencies. 6th Ed. Stamford, CT: Appleton & Lange, 1998 pp. 703–718.
33. Spyropoulos AC, Hayth KA, Jenkins P. Anticoagulation with anisindione in a patient with a warfarin-induced skin eruptions. Pharmacotherapy 2003;23: 533–536.
34. Linhardt RJ. Heparin: structure and activity. J Med Chem 2003;46: 2551–2554.
35. Codée JDC, Overkleeft HS, Van der Marel GA, et al. The synthesis of well-defined heparin and heparin sulfate fragments. Drug Discovery Today: Technologies 2004;1:317–326.
36. Hirsh J, Raschke R. Heparin and low-molecular weight heparin: the Seventh ACCP Conference on Antithrombotic and Thrombolytic Therapy. Chest 2004;126:188S–203S.
37. De Kort M, Buijsman RC, Van Boeckel CAA. Synthetic heparin derivatives as new anticoagulant drugs. Drug Discovery Today 2005;10:769–779.
38. Jin L, Abrahams JP, Skinner R, et al. The anticoagulant activity of antithrombin by heparin. Proc Natl Acad Sci U S A 1997;94:14683–14688.
39. Hambleton J. Drugs used in disorders of coagulation. In: Katzung BG, ed. Basic and Clinical Pharmacology. 9th Ed. New York: McGraw-Hill, 2004, 543–560.
40. Weitz JI. Low-molecular-weight heparins. N Engl J Med 1997;337:688–698.
41. Hovanessian HC. New generation anticoagulants: the low-molecular-weight heparins. Ann Emerg Med 1999;34:768–779.
42. Rosenberg RD. Biochemistry and pharmacology of low-molecular-weight heparin. Semin Hematol 1997;4(Suppl 4):2–8.
43. Physician's Desk Reference. 53rd Ed. Montvale, NJ: Medical Economics Company, 1999.
44. Kakkar AK. Low- and ultralow-molecular-weight heparins. Best Pract Res Clin Hematol 2004;17:77–87.
45. Siddiqui MAA, Wagstaff AJ. Enoxaparin—a review of its use as thromboprophylaxis in acutely ill, nonsurgical patients. Drugs 2005;65:1025–1036.
46. Petitou M, Herault J, Bernat A, et al. Synthesis of thrombin-inhibiting heparin mimetics without side effects. Nature 1999;398:417–422.
47. Leone-Bay A, Paton DR, Freeman J, et al. Synthesis and evaluation of compounds that facilitate the gastrointestinal absorption of heparin. J Med Chem 1998;41:1163–1171.
48. Zoppetti G, Caramazza I, Murakami Y, et al. Structural requirements for duodenal permeability of heparin–diamine complexes. Biochim Biophys Acta 1992;1156:92–98.
49. Andriuoli G, Caramazza I, Galimberti G, et al. Intraduodenal absorption in the rabbit of a novel heparin salt. Haemostasis 1992;22:113–116.
50. Engel RH, Riggi SJ. Intestinal absorption of heparin facilitated by sulfated or sulfonated surfactants. Proc Soc Exp Biol Med 1969;130:706–710.
51. Guarini S, Ferrari W. Olive oil–provoked, bile-dependent absorption of heparin from the gastrointestinal tract in rats. Pharm Res Commun 1986;17:685–694.
52. Ueno M, Nakasake T, Horikoshi I, et al. Oral administration of liposomally entrapped heparin to beagle dogs. Chem Pharm Bull 1982;30:2245–2247.
53. Steiner S, Rosen R. Delivery systems for pharmacological agents encapsulated with proteinoids. U.S. Patent 4,925,673 (1990).
54. Leone-Bay A, Leipold H, Agarwal R, et al. The evolution of an oral heparin dosing solution. Drugs Future 1997;22:885–891.
55. Nutescu EA. Evolving concepts in the treatment of venous thromboembolism: the role of factor Xa inhibitors. Pharmacotherapy 2004;24:82S–87S.
56. Bauer KA. Fondaparinux: a new synthetic and selective inhibitor of factor Xa. Best Pract Res Clin Hematol 2004;17:89–104.
57. Koopman MMW, Buller HR. Short- and long-acting synthetic pentasaccharides. J Intern Med 2003;254:335–342.
58. Petitou M, Duchaussoy P, Jaurand G, et al. Synthesis and pharmacological properties of a close analogue of an antithrombotic pentasaccharide (SR 90107A/ORG 31540). J Med Chem 1997;40:1600–1607.
59. Cheng JWM. Fondaparinux: a new antithrombotic agent. Clin Ther 2002;24:1757–1769.
60. Dager WE, Andersen J, Nutescu EA. Special considerations with fondaparinux therapy: heparin-induced thrombocytopenia and wound healing. Pharmacotherapy 2004;7:88S–94S.
61. Hawkins D. Limitation of traditional anticoagulants. Pharmacotherapy 2004;7:62S–65S.
62. Weitz JI, Bates SM. New anticoagulants. Journal of Thrombosis and Haemostasis 2005;3:1843–1853.
63. Hirsh J. New anticoagulants. Am Heart J 2001;142:3S–8S.
64. Nisio MD, Misswlsoep S, Buller HR. Direct thrombin inhibitors. N Engl J Med 2005;353:1028–1040.
65. Johnson PH. Hirudin: clinical potential of a thrombin inhibitor. Annu Rev Med 1994;45:165–177.
66. Krstenansky JL, Owen TJ, Yates MT, et al. Design, synthesis, and antithrombin activity for conformationally restricted analogues of peptide anticoagulants based on the C-terminal region of the leech peptide, hirudin. Biochim Biophys Acta 1988;957:53–59.
67. Maraganore JM, Bourdon P, Jablonski J, et al. Design and characterization of hirulogs: A novel class of bivalent peptide inhibitors of thrombin. Biochemistry 1990;29:7095–7101.
68. Nutescu EA, Wittkowsky AK. Direct thrombin inhibitors for anticoagulation. Am Pharmacother 2004;38:99–109.
69. Agnelli G. Clinical potential of oral direct thrombin inhibitors in the prevention and treatment of venous thromboembolism. Drugs 2004;64:47S–52S.
70. Haas S. Oral direct thrombin inhibition: an effective and novel approach for venous thromboembolism. Drugs 2004;64:7S–16S.
71. Eikelboom JW, French J. Management of patients with acute coronary syndromes. What is the clinical role of direct thrombin inhibitors? Drugs 2002;62:1839–1852.
72. Greinacher A, Lubenow N. Recombinant hirudin in clinical practice. Focus on lepirudin. Circulation 2001;103:1479–1484.
73. Matheson AJ, Goa KL. Desirudin: a review of its uses in the management of thrombotic disorders. Drugs 2000;60:679–700.
74. Hirsh J. Current anticoagulant therapy—unmet clinical needs. Thromb Res 2003;109:S1–S8.
75. Levy JH. Novel intravenous antithrombins. Am Heart J 2001;141:1043–1047.
76. Warkentin TE. Bivalent direct thrombin inhibitors: hirudin and bivalirudin. Best Pract Res Clin Hematol 2004;17:105–125.
77. Caron MF, McKendall GR. Bivalirudin in percutaneous coronary intervention. Am J Health-Sys Pharm 2003;60:1841–1849.
78. Chesebro JH. Direct thrombin inhibitor therapy in the cardiovascular patient. Am J Health-Sys Pharm 2003;60:S19–S26.
79. Lewis BE, Hursting MJ. Argatroban therapy in heparin-induced thrombocytopenia. In: Warkentin TE, Greinacher A, eds. Heparin-Induced Thrombocytopenia. 3rd Ed. New York: Marcel Dekker, 2004:437–474.
80. Nagashima H. Studies on the different modes of action of the anticoagulant protease inhibitors DX-9065a and argatroban. J Biol Chem 2002;277: 50439–50449.
81. Hauptmann J. Pharmacokinetics of an emerging new class of anticoagulant/antithrombotics drugs. Eur J Clin Pharmacol 2002;57:751–758.
82. Francis CW. Ximelagatran: a new oral anticoagulant. Best Pract Res Clin Hematol 2004;17:139–152.
83. Halperin JL. Ximelagatran: oral direct thrombin inhibition as anticoagulant therapy in atrial fibrillation. J Am Coll Cardiol 2005;45:1–9.
84. Nylander S, Mattsson C. Thrombin-induced platelet activation and its inhibition by anticoagulants with different modes of action. Blood Coagul Fibrinolysis 2003;14:159–167.
85. Sarich TC, Wolzt M, Eriksson UG, et al. Effects of ximelagatran, an oral direct thrombin inhibitor, r-hirudin and enoxaparin on thrombin generation and platelet activation in healthy male subjects. J Am Coll Cardiol 2003;41:557–564.
86. Eriksson UG, Bredberg U, Gislen K, et al. Pharmacokinetics and pharmacodynamics of ximelagatran, a novel oral direct thrombin inhibitor, in young healthy male subjects. Eur J Clin Pharmacol 2003;59:35–43.
87. Patrono C, Coller B, FitzGerald GA, et al. Platelet-active drugs: the relationships among dose, effectiveness, and side effects: the Seventh ACCP Conference on Antithrombotic and Thrombolytic Therapy. Chest 2004;126: 234S–264S.
88. Hankey GJ, Eikelboom JW. Antiplatelet drugs. Med J Aust 2003;178:568–574.
89. Patrono C. Aspirin as an antiplatelet drug. N Engl J Med 1994;330: 1287–1294.
90. Patrono C, Rodríguez LAG, Landolfi R, et al. Low-dose aspirin for the prevention of atherothrombosis. N Engl J Med 2005;353:2373–2383.
91. Sztriha LK, Sas K, Vecsei L. Aspirin resistance in stroke: 2004. J Neurol Sci 2005;229–230:163–169.

92. Rocca B, Secchiero P, Ciabattoni G, et al. Cyclooxygenase-2 expression is induced during human megakaryopoiesis and characterizes newly formed platelets. Proc Natl Acad Sci U S A 2002;99:7634–7639.
93. Mason PJ, Jacobs AK, Freedman JE. Aspirin resistance and atherothrombotic disease. J Am Coll Cardiol 2005;46:986–993.
94. Matías-Guiu J, Ferro JM, Alvarez-Sabin J, et al. Comparison of triflusal and aspirin for prevention of vascular events in patients after cerebral infarction. Stroke 2003;34:1–8.
95. McNeely W, Goa KL. Triflusal. Drugs 1998;55:823–833.
96. Bayón Y, Alonso A, Crespo MS. 4-Trifluoromethyl derivatives of salicylate, triflusal and its main metabolite 2-hydroxy-4-trifluoromethylbenzoic acid, are potent inhibitor of nuclear factor κB activation. Br J Pharmacol 1999;126: 1359–1466.
97. Sanzhez de Miguel L, Jimenez A, Monton M, et al. A 4-trifluoromethyl derivative of salicylate, triflusal, stimulates nitric oxide production by human neutrophils: role in platelet function. Eur J Clin Invest 2000;30:811–817.
98. Kuo BS, Ritschel WA. Correlation between inhibitory effect on platelet aggregation and disposition of sulfinpyrazone and its metabolites in rabbits. Part II: multiple-dose study. Biopharm Drug Dispos 1987;8:11–21.
99. Fornaro G, Rossi P, Mantica PG, et al. Indobufen in the prevention of thromboembolic complications in patients with heart disease—a randomized, placebo-controlled, double-blind study. Circulation 1993;87:162–164.
100. Bhana N, McClellan KJ. Indobufen: an updated review of its use in the management of atherothrombosis. Drugs Aging 2001;18:369–388.
101. Lee S-W, Park S-W, Hong M-K, et al. Triple versus dual antiplatelet therapy after coronary stenting. J Am Coll Cardiol 2005;46:1833–1837.
102. Diener H-C, Bogousslavsky J, Brass LM, et al. Aspirin and clopidogrel compared with clopidogrel alone after recent ischemic stroke or transient ischemic attack in high-risk patients (MATCH): randomized, double-blind, placebo-controlled trial. Lancet 2004;364:331–337.
103. Lee SW, Park SW, Hong MK, et al. Comparison of cilostazol versus ticlopidine therapy after successful coronary stenting. Am J Cardiol 2005;95:859–862.
104. Ahn JC, Song WH, Kwon JA, et al. Effects of cilostazol on platelet activation in coronary stenting patients who already treated with aspirin and clopidogrel. Korean J Intern Med 2004;19:230–236.
105. Schror K. The pharmacology of cilostazol. Diabetes Obes Metab 2002;4 (Suppl 2):S14–S19.
106. Suri A, Forbes WP, Bramer SL. Effects of CYP3A inhibition on the metabolism of cilostazol. Clin Pharmacokinet 1999;37(Suppl 2):61–68.
107. Suri A, Bramer SL. Effect of omeprazole on the metabolism of cilostazol. Clin Pharmacokinet 1999;37(Suppl 2):53–59.
108. Gachet C. The platelet P2 receptor as molecular targets for old and new antiplatelet drugs. Pharmacol Ther 2005;108:180–192.
109. Nguyen TA, Diodati JG, Pharand C. Resistance to clopidogrel: a review of the evidence. J Am Coll Cardiol 2005;45:1157–1164.
110. Conley PB, Delaney SM. Scientific and therapeutic insights into the role of the platelet P2Y12 receptor in thrombosis. Curr Opin Hematol 2003;10:333–338.
111. Dorsam RT, Kunapuli SP. Central role of the P2Y12 receptor in platelet activation. J Clin Invest 2004;113:340–345.
112. Dorsam RT, Murugappan S, Ding Z, et al. Clopidogrel: interactions with the P2Y12 receptor and clinical relevance. Hematology 2003;8:359–365.
113. Quinn MJ, Fitzgerald DJ. Triclopidine and clopidogrel. Circulation 1999; 100:1667–1672.
114. Savi P, Pereillo JM, Uzabiaga MF, et al. Identification and biological activity of the active metabolites of clopidogrel. Thromb Haemost 2000;84:891–896.
115. Ding Z, Kim S, Dorsam RT, et al. Inactivation of the human P2Y12 receptor by thiol reagents requires interaction with both extracellular cysteine residues, Cys17 and Cys270. Blood 2003;101:3908–3914.
116. Dalvie DK, O'Connell TN. Characterization of novel dihydrothienopyridinium and thienopyridinium metabolites of ticlopidine in vitro: role of peroxidases, cytochromes P450, and monoamine oxidases. Drug Metab Dispos 2004;32:49–57.
117. Wiviott SD, Antman EM, Winters KJ, et al. Randomized comparison of prasugrel (CS-747, LY640315), a novel thienopyridine P2Y12 antagonist, with clopidogrel in percutaneous coronary intervention: results of the joint utilization of medications to block platelets optimally (JUMBO)-TIMI 26 trial. Circulation 2005;111:3366–3373.
118. Mousa SA. Antiplatelet therapies: from aspirin to GPIIb/IIIa-receptor antagonists and beyond. Drug Discovery Today 1999;4:552–561.
119. Reverter JC, Beguin S, Kessels H, et al. Inhibition of platelet-mediated, tissue factor–induced thrombin generation by the mouse/human chimeric 7E3 antibody: potential implications for the effect of c7E3 Fab treatment on acute thrombosis and "clinical restenosis." J Clin Invest 1996;98:863–874.
120. Genetta TB, Mauro VF. ABCIXIMAB: a new antiaggregant used in angioplasty. Ann Pharmacother 1996;30:251–257.
121. Curran MP, Keating GM. Eptifibatide. Drugs 2005;65:2009–2035.
122. Gresele P, Agnelli G. Novel approaches to the treatment of thrombosis. Trends Pharmacol Sci 2002;23:25–32.
123. De la Cruz JP, Villalobos MA, Escalante R, et al. Effects of the selective inhibition of platelet thromboxane synthase on the platelet-subendothelium interaction. Br J Pharmacol 2002;137:1082–1088.
124. Khan IA, Gowda RM. Clinical perspective and therapeutics of thrombolysis. Int J Cardiol 2003;91:115–127.
125. Benchenane K, Lopez-Atalaya JP, Fernandez-Monreal M, et al. Equivocal roles of tissue-type plasminogen activator in stroke-induced injury. Trends Neurosci 2004;27:155–160.
126. Banerjee A, Chisti Y, Banerjee UC. Streptokinase—a clinically useful thrombolytic agent. Biotechnol Adv 2004;22:287–307.
127. Perler B. Thrombolytic therapies: the current state of affairs. J Endovasc Ther 2005;12:224–232.
128. Hansen AP, Petros AM, Meadows RP, et al. Solution structure of the amino terminal fragment of urokinase-type plasminogen activator. Biochemistry 1994;33:4847–4864.
129. Belkin M, Belkin B, Buckman CA, et al. Intra-arterial fibrinolytic therapy, efficacy of streptokinase vs urokinase. Arch Surg 1986;121:769–773.
130. Antman EM, Braunwald E. Coronary thrombosis. In: Braunwald E, Zipes DP, Libby P, Eds. Baunwald's Textbook of Cardiovascular Medicine. 6th Ed. Philadelphia, PA:WB Saunders. 2001:1145–1218.
131. Orsini G, Brandazza A, Sarmientos P, et al. Efficient renaturation and fibrinolytic properties of prourokinase and a deletion mutant expressed in *Escherichia coli* as inclusion bodies. Eur J Biochem 1991;195:691–697.
132. Ouriel K, Kandarpa K, Schuerr DM, et al. Prourokinase versus urokinase for recanalization of peripheral occlusions, safety and efficacy: the purpose trial. J Vasc Interv Radiol 1999;10:1083–1091.
133. Nordt TK, Bode C. Thrombolysis: newer thrombolytic agents and their role in clinical medicine. Heart 2003;89:1358–1362.
134. Bates SM, Greer IA, Hirsh J, et al. Use of antithrombotic agents during pregnancy: the Seventh ACCP Conference on Antithrombotic and Thrombolytic Therapy. Chest 2004;126:627S–644S.
135. Liu D, Cheng T, Guo H, et al. Tissue plasminogen activator neurovascular toxicity is controlled by activated protein C. Nat Med 2004;10:1379–1383.
136. Dalmau A, Sabate A, Acosta F, et al. Tranexamic acid reduces red cell transfusion better than epsilon-aminocaproic acid or placebo in liver transplantation. Anesth Analg 2000;91:29–34.
137. Greilich PE, Okada K, Latham P, et al. Aprotinin but not ε-aminocaproic acid decreases interleukin-10 after cardiac surgery with extracorporeal circulation–Randomized, double-blind, placebo-controlled study in patients receiving aprotinin and ε-aminocaproic acid. Circulation 2001;104 (Suppl I):265–269.
138. Cummins RO, ed. Textbook of Advanced Cardiac Life Support, 1997–1999 ed. Dallas, TX: American Heart Association, 1997.
139. McSwain NE, Frame S, Paturas, JL, eds. Shock and Fluid Resuscitation in Basic and Advanced Prehospital Trauma Life Support. 4th Ed. St. Louis, MO: Mosby, 1999.
140. Pollack C. Prehospital fluid resuscitation of the trauma patient. Emerg Med Clin North Am 1993;11:61–70.
141. Klein HG. The prospects for red-cell substitutes. N Engl J Med 2000;342: 1666–1668.
142. Stowell CP. Hemoglobin-based oxygen carriers. Curr Opin Hematol 2002; 9:537–543.
143. Moore EE. Blood substitutes: the future is now. J Am Coll Surg 2003; 196:1–17.
144. Schwarz KW, Dulchavsky SA, Silbergleit A. Blood substitutes: an update. Curr Surg 2002;59:378–382.
145. Bloomfield EL, Leone BJ. The safety of hemoglobin blood substitutes. Anesth Analg 2003;97:323–332.
146. Scott MG, Kucik DF, Goodnough LT, et al. Blood substitutes: evolution and future applications. Clin Chem 1997;43:1724–1731.
147. Tremper KK, Friedman AE, Levine EM, et al. The preoperative treatment of severely anemic patients with a perfluorochemical oxygen-transport fluid, Fluosol-DA. N Engl J Med 1982;307:277–283.
148. Spahn DR, van Brempt R, Theilmeier G, et al. Perflubron emulsion delays blood transfusions in orthopedic surgery. European Perflubron Emulsion Study Group. Anesthesiology 1999;91:195–208.
149. Komiyama N, Tame J, Nagai K. A hemoglobin-based blood substitute: transplanting a novel allosteric effect of crocodile hemoglobin. Biol Chem 1996;377:543–548.
150. Fizpatrik CM, Savage SA, Kerby JD, et al. Resuscitation with a blood substitute causes vasoconstriction without nitric oxide scavenging in a model of arterial hemorrhage. J Am Coll Surg 2004;199:693–710.
151. Olson JS, Foley EW, Rogge C, et al. No scavenging and the hypertensive effect of hemoglobin-based blood substitutes. Free Radic Biol Med 2004; 36:685–697.
152. Haney CR, Buehler PW, Galati A. Synthesis and characterization of a novel DTPA polymerized hemoglobin-based oxygen carrier. Biochem Biophys Acta 2005;1725:358–369.
153. Jia Y, Wood F, Menu P, et al. Oxygen binding and oxidation reactions of human hemoglobin conjugated to carboxylate dextran. Biochem Biophys Acta 2004;1672:164–173.
154. Sakai H, Tomiyama K, Sou K, et al. Poly(ethylene glycol)-conjugation and deoxygenation enable long-term preservation of hemoglobin-vesicles as oxygen carriers in a liquid state. Bioconjug Chem 2000;11:425–432.
155. Li S, Nickels J, Palmer AF. Liposome-encapsulated actin-hemoglobin (LEAcHb) artificial blood substitutes. Biomaterials 2005;26:3759–3769.

32. *Insulin and Drugs Used for the Treatment of Diabetes*

ROBIN M. ZAVOD, JOHN L. KRSTENANSKY, AND BRUCE L. CURRIE

DRUGS COVERED IN THIS CHAPTER:

ACARBOSE

AMYLIN

EXENATIDE

INSULIN
- Aspart
- Detemir
- Glulisine
- Glargine
- Lispro

LIRAGLUTIDE

METFORMIN

MIGLITOL

NATEGLINIDE

PIOGLITAZONE

PRAMLINTIDE

REPAGLINIDE

ROSIGLITAZONE

SULFONYLUREAS
- Acetohexamide
- Chlorpropamide
- Glimepiride
- Glipizide
- Glyburide
- Tolazamide
- Tolbutamide

TROGLITAZONE

VOGIBOSE

INTRODUCTION

History and Epidemiology

The term "diabetes mellitus" is derived from the Greek word for siphon (diabetes) and the Latin word for sweet (mellitus). The Greek physician Arateus, in the first century AD, described diabetes as "the melting down of flesh and limbs into urine" (1). The term "mellitus" was added 1,000 years later in medieval times when physicians noticed the sweet taste of urine from some of their patients. Diabetes is not a single disease but, rather, is a group of metabolic diseases characterized by hyperglycemia caused by inadequate insulin secretion with or without a simultaneous decrease in hormone action at its receptor (2). The World Health Organization estimates that 177 million people worldwide have diabetes. It is predicted that by 2010, there will be a 50% increase in this number, with the most significant increases in Africa, Asia, and South America (3). In the United States, it is estimated that 18.2 million people have diabetes. During the last 40 years, the prevalence of this disease has increased sixfold (4). Currently, diabetes is the fifth deadliest disease, killing 400,000 annually.

In 1869, Paul Langerhans determined that the pancreas is comprised of two cell types: acinar cells, which secrete digestive enzymes, and cells clustered in islets with a different biological function (5). Twenty years later, in Strasbourg, France, Mehring and Minkowski induced diabetes in a dog by removing its pancreas. In doing this type of experiment, they determined that the pancreas is the origin of diabetes mellitus (6). By 1909, the German scientist Georg Zuelzer had created the first pancreatic extract; unfortunately, the side effects were too extreme for the extract to be of therapeutic benefit. In 1921, in a laboratory provided by John J. R. MacLeod, Frederick G. Banting (orthopaedic surgeon), and Charles H. Best (medical student) isolated insulin from the pancreas and initially tested it in dogs (7). On January 11, 1922, their pancreatic extract was administered to a 14-year-old diabetic boy, Leonard Thompson, who was near death, and he quickly recovered. On May 31, 1922, a bovine pancreatic extract was developed by William Sansum, M.D., and chief chemist Norman Blatterwick and was injected into 51-year-old Charles Cowan, who recovered and lived to age 90 (8). In 1922, insulin could be readily isolated and purified in large quantities from both cattle and pigs in Great Britain, so the British Medical Research Council introduced insulin as a therapeutic agent. In 1923, Eli Lilly made insulin available in the United States and Canada, and the Nobel Prize for Medicine or Physiology was given to Banting and MacLeod, who shared it with Collip and Best (7). By 1924, large companies in both the United States and Britain were producing insulin and marketing it worldwide. In 1960, the primary amino acid sequence of insulin was identified, and by 1963, the complete synthesis of insulin was possible. Hodgkin and coworkers determined the three-dimensional structure of insulin in 1972 (5).

Type 1 Diabetes

Type 1 diabetes, which represents the diagnosis for 5 to 10% of the diabetic population, is caused by an absolute deficiency in insulin secretion. This overt absence of insulin production results from immune system–mediated destruction of the insulin-producing pancreatic β cells. Without insulin, the body's primary source of energy and the brain's only source of energy, glucose, is unable to

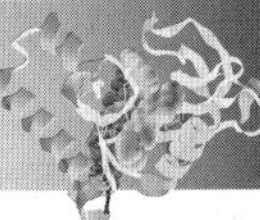

CLINICAL SIGNIFICANCE

Diabetes is a condition wherein the body no longer produces insulin (β-cell dysfunction) or uses insulin efficiently (insulin resistance). Insulin is a hormone that is needed to convert carbohydrates and other food into energy needed for life. The cause of diabetes remains unknown, although genetics and environmental factors, such as obesity and a sedentary lifestyle, appear to play important roles.

More than 20.8 million Americans, or 7% of the population, have diabetes. Unfortunately, an estimated 6.2 million people remain unaware that they have the disease. Diabetes is the leading cause of new-onset blindness, kidney failure, and nontraumatic amputations and has a major role in the development of heart disease, hypertension, sexual dysfunction, and dental disease.

Many oral diabetes medications are available with different mechanisms of action. Combination therapy, using medications from the different classes to address the deficiencies causing diabetes, is standard in diabetes care. Secretagogues, such as the sulfonylureas and the meglitinides, increase pancreatic insulin secretion and usually are used early in the disease process, when pancreatic β cells still produce insulin. Sulfonylureas typically can reduce a patient's hemoglobin A_{1c} by 2%, whereas meglitinides can cause a reduction of approximately 1%. Metformin blocks hepatic output of glucose, is used throughout the disease spectrum, and can reduce hemoglobin A_{1c} by 2%. Metformin is particularly advantageous in its ability to delay the onset of diabetes and to promote weight loss in patients. Thiazolidinediones (TZDs) enhance insulin sensitivity and may have a role early in preserving β-cell function in diabetes. The initial concern about the hepatotoxicity of TZDs has been relaxed, with few cases being reported with available agents. The efficacy typically seen with TZDs is an approximately 1.0 to 1.5% decrease in hemoglobin A_{1c}.

When the β cells of the pancreas cease to make insulin suddenly (type 1) or over time (type 2), exogenous insulin must be administered. The overall goal of insulin is to mimic physiological insulin secretion. This is achieved by using a combination of basal and bolus insulin. Types of basal insulin include neutral protamine Hagedorn, glargine, and detemir. Their role as basal insulin is to provide a constant, relatively peakless supply of insulin throughout the day, regardless of meals. Types of bolus insulin include aspart, glulisine, lispro, and regular. The role of bolus insulins is to provide insulin coverage for meals.

With the introduction of incretin mimetics, the first new class of diabetes agents in nearly 20 years is now available. Incretins improve glucose control but also have the potential to improve insulin resistance and to restore β-cell function.

One important aspect of treating a patient with diabetes is not to focus on blood sugar alone. The leading cause of death for patients with diabetes is heart disease; therefore, health care providers need to assess cholesterol, blood pressure, and other risk factors for heart disease.

Nathan A. Painter, Pharm.D.
Assistant Professor of Pharmacy Practice
School of Pharmacy
Loma Linda University

enter cells. This ultimately leads to the cells being energy starved as well as to elevated plasma blood glucose levels (hyperglycemia). Administration of exogenous insulin currently is the only method to effectively resolve this hormone deficiency.

Type 2 Diabetes

Type 2 diabetes, for which 800,000 new cases are diagnosed per year, is a more complex disease. If one parent has type 2 diabetes, the risk of developing it is 38%, whereas if both parents are affected then, the risk of developing diabetes before age 60 is 60% (3). Type 2 diabetes is characterized by end-organ insulin resistance and/or a relative deficiency in insulin secretion (9). Unlike the abrupt loss of β-cell function characteristic of type 1 diabetes, the pancreatic β cells in type 2 diabetes undergo progressive deterioration over a fairly long time. In many patients, insulin resistance causes an initial increase in plasma insulin levels as a result of a compensatory increase in insulin secretion. At this point, blood glucose levels likely appear normal and the patient is asymptomatic. As β-cell function falters and insulin resistance worsens, hyperglycemia results (2). For most patients with type 2 diabetes, resolution of their metabolic disease may occur with appropriate lifestyle changes, including a well balanced diet and regular exercise. For those type 2 patients who are unable to achieve normal blood glucose levels nonpharmacologically, several classes of oral agents are available that target various biochemical processes associated with insulin secretion and/or insulin receptor sensitivity.

Gestational Diabetes

Gestational diabetes (GDM) complicates approximately 4% of all pregnancies in the United States (135,000 cases annually) (9). It is classified as any degree of glucose intolerance that first occurs during pregnancy, typically during the third trimester. The risk factors associated with developing GDM include previous history of GDM, obesity, glycosuria, or a family history that includes diabetes (10). It is found more frequently in the following populations: African American, Hispanic American, Pacific Islander, and Native American (10). If GDM develops during pregnancy, then the woman has a 50% risk of developing type 2 diabetes in the future and a 50% risk of experiencing GDM in a subsequent pregnancy (10). Babies born to women with preexisting diabetes that is poorly controlled are two- to fourfold more likely

Table 32.1. Maturity-Onset Diabetes of the Young: Classifications and Genetic Loci (9,11)

Type	Genetic Loci	Biochemical Effect	Treatment
1	HNF-4α	Regulation of gene transcription in pancreatic β cells is abnormal. Defect in metabolic signaling of insulin secretion results.	Oral agent or insulin
2	Glucokinase	Defective enzyme produced. Enzyme is required in conversion of glucose to glucose-6-phosphate (the rate limiting step in glucose metabolism). Defect in β-cell sensitivity to glucose and hepatic storage of glucose as glycogen results.	Diet and exercise
3	HNF-1α	Regulation of gene transcription in pancreatic β cells is abnormal. Defect in metabolic signaling of insulin secretion results.	Oral agent or insulin
4	IPF-1	Transcriptional regulation of β-cell development/function is abnormal.	Oral agent or insulin
5	HNF-1β	Regulation of gene transcription in pancreatic β-cells is abnormal. Defect in metabolic signaling of insulin secretion results.	Insulin
6	NeuroD1	Transcriptional regulation of β-cell development/function is abnormal.	Insulin

to have a serious birth defect (e.g., eye defects, respiratory tract defects, cleft palate, anal atresia/stenosis, urinary tract defects, and positional defects of the foot) (10). Whether the mother has preexisting diabetes or develops GDM, she is at risk for delivering a large baby (≥10 pounds). It therefore is recommended that those women with preexisting diabetes maintain tight blood glucose control for 3 to 6 months before conception and that insulin therapy replace all oral hypoglycemic medications during the pregnancy.

Maturity-Onset Diabetes of the Young

Maturity-onset diabetes of the young may account for 1 to 5% of all cases of diabetes in the United States. It is not a single disease but, rather, represents several types of genetic disorders. To date, there have been abnormalities detected at six genetic loci (Table 32.1). It generally is characterized by impaired insulin secretion with minimal or no defects in insulin action. In this scenario, the onset of hyperglycemia is early (<25 years) (9,11).

Metabolic Syndrome

Metabolic syndrome, also known as Syndrome X or the insulin resistance syndrome, was defined by the World Health Organization in 1999 as the presence of diabetes, impaired fasting glycemia, impaired glucose tolerance or insulin resistance, and two or more of the following: obesity, dyslipidemia, hypertension, or microalbuminuria (Table 32.2) (12). Somewhat similar definitions are used by other organizations. The prevalence of this syndrome is highly age dependent (7% in ages 20–29, 44% in ages 60–69, and 42% in ages ≥70). Individuals with this syndrome are predicted to develop cardiovascular disease and diabetes.

Drug-Induced Diabetes

A number of drugs impair insulin secretion or insulin action at its receptor (Table 32.3) and, potentially, cause drug-induced diabetes. Generally speaking, impairment in insulin secretion may not be sufficient to cause a patient to develop diabetes; however, it may be enough for those who are already predisposed to develop the disease or already experiencing insulin resistance (9). In a limited number of cases, patients develop diabetes and their blood glucose levels remain uncontrolled despite treatment with insulin, oral agents, and diet modification (13). The greatest likelihood of developing drug-induced diabetes is associated with the glucocorticoids.

Prediabetes: Impaired Fasting Glucose and Impaired Glucose Tolerance

Impaired fasting glucose (IFG; fasting blood glucose, ≥100 mg/dL and <126 mg/dL) and impaired glucose tolerance (IGT; 2-hour values for oral glucose tolerance, ≥140 mg/dL and <200 mg/dL) are two additional metabolic states that must be mentioned. In addition to those diagnosed with diabetes, 16 million Americans experience IGT (4). Patients with either IFG or IGT could be classified as prediabetic, because the disease has not yet progressed far enough to cause hyperglycemia yet the blood glucose levels are too high to be considered normal (9). Approximately 7% of those patients who present with IFG or IGT progress to overt diabetes annually (3).

Table 32.2. Clinical Measures Associated with Metabolic Syndrome (12)

Condition	Measurement	Gender Differences
Obesity	BMI >30	Waist to hip ratio: Males: >0.9 Females: >0.85
Dyslipidemia	Triglycerides ≥1.7 mmol/L	HDL cholesterol Males: <0.9 mmol/L Females: <1.0 mmol/L
Hypertension	BP >140/90 mm Hg	
Microalbuminurea	Albumin excretion >20 μg/min	

BMI, body mass index; BP, blood pressure; HDL, high-density lipoprotein.

Table 32.3. Drugs that Impair Insulin Secretion or Insulin Action

Thyroid hormone	β-Adrenergic agonists
Nicotinic acid	Thiazides
Glucocorticoids	Dilantin
Atypical antipsychotic agents	α-Interferon

BIOCHEMISTRY AND PATHOGENESIS OF DIABETES

Glucose Metabolism

After consuming a meal, complex carbohydrates are broken down into simpler sugars in the gastrointestinal (GI) tract. Glucose can then be absorbed and serve as the primary source of energy for the body as well as the only source of energy for the brain. If too much glucose is absorbed, then hyperglycemia can result. Normally, the liver is able to prevent hyperglycemia by storing up to two-thirds of the glucose absorbed from the intestines and releasing it when the body requires additional energy (2). In addition to glucose being taken up and converted by glucokinase (hexokinase IV) to glucose-6-phosphate (G6P) and then, ultimately, to glycogen in the liver, it can be taken up or used by several other types of cells. In the presence of insulin, glucose is taken up into muscle (heart, skeletal, and smooth) cells and serves as a source of energy for those cells. Glucose can be taken up by pancreatic β cells via the glucose transporter 2 (GLUT2) and is then, in the rate-limiting step, phosphorylated by glucokinase to G6P (3). In this reaction, glucokinase effectively serves as a glucose sensor for the pancreatic β cells, because it controls the rate of entry of glucose into the glycolytic pathway and the subsequent metabolism of G6P to adenosine triphosphate (ATP) (11). Then, depending on the resulting ratio of adenosine diphosphate to ATP in the pancreatic islet cell, activation of the sulfonylurea receptor 1 (SUR1) protein occurs, followed by a cascade of biochemical events (3). These events include initial closure of potassium channels, which alters the membrane potential of the cell. Calcium channels then open, allowing calcium to flow into the pancreatic islet cell. This increase in intracellular calcium concentration triggers the movement and ultimate release of preformed insulin granules from the islet cells (3).

Role of Insulin and Insulin Receptors

Insulin plays a vital role in a number of biochemical processes, including more than 100 examples of gene regulation. In the liver and muscle tissues, insulin promotes the storage of excess glucose as glycogen. Insulin suppresses hepatic glucose production and the breakdown of fats into fatty acids and glycerol (2). Insulin facilitates absorption of amino acids into cells and their conversion into proteins. Insulin converts excess carbohydrates, which cannot be used as glycogen, into fats and then promotes the storage of fat in adipose tissue (2). When bound to cell surface receptors, insulin initiates a cascade of events that are integral to the transport of glucose into cells. The insulin receptor is a large, transmembrane glycoprotein composed of two α subunits and two β subunits linked by disulfide bonds (5). The α subunits, which possess the insulin binding domain, are located extracellularly. The β subunits are transmembrane proteins that also possess enzymatic activity. When insulin binds to and activates this receptor, intramolecular autophosphorylation of several β-subunit tyrosine residues occurs (2). This enhances the receptor's tyrosine kinase activity, which is responsible for phosphorylating insulin receptor substrates (IRS-1 to IRS-4). These phosphorylated proteins serve as intracellular signals for processes essential to cell survival and proliferation. This includes translocation of the glucose transporters to the cell surface and synthesis of glycogen, protein, mRNAs, and nuclear DNA (3).

Role of Glucose Transporters

Glucose transport into cells is regulated, in part, by glucose transporters. These integral membrane glycoproteins (~50,000 daltons) are comprised of 12 membrane-spanning α-helical domains (5). Several members of this family (GLUT1 to GLUT5) use a sodium-independent mechanism to facilitate glucose entry into the cell. When insulin binds to and activates its cell surface receptors, the intracellular vesicles, in which the GLUT1 and GLUT4 transporters normally reside, migrate toward the plasma membrane (5). This is an energy-dependent process. These vesicles fuse with the membrane, and the transporters orient themselves such that they become channels through which glucose can enter the cell. This process is reversible in that once insulin dissociates from the receptor, the intracellular vesicles re-form (via endocytosis), thereby moving the glucose transporters back into the intracellular pool. The rate-limiting step in glucose transport into muscle and adipose tissue is the initial translocation of intracellular vesicles toward the plasma membrane. Alteration of one or more steps in this sequence can lead to an insulin-resistant state. For example, a decrease in GLUT4 expression limits glucose entry into the cell (14).

Insulin Resistance

Insulin resistance often is a component of type 2 diabetes, IGT, and metabolic syndrome. It can be caused by obesity, physical inactivity, and aging, or it can be secondary to other disease states (e.g., Cushing's syndrome and pheochromocytoma) or medication usage (e.g., β-adrenergic blocking agents, glucocorticoids, oral contraceptives, and thiazide diuretics) (15). Clinically, insulin resistance presents itself as hyperglycemia because of a decrease in insulin-stimulated glucose transport into adipose tissue and skeletal muscle. There are many potential reasons for the development of resistance, including downregulation of GLUT4 expression (14), downregulation of GLUT4 translocation to the cell membrane, a decrease in the number of available insulin receptors, and/or a decrease in the affinity of insulin for its receptor (15). It also is possible that downstream insulin signaling may be blocked. This may be caused by dephosphorylation of the β-subunit tyrosine side chains by cellular protein–tyrosine phosphatases; phosphorylation of IRS-1, which reduces its ability to act as a substrate for the β-subunit tyrosine kinase; and/or degradation of the IRS proteins (3).

Hemoglobin A_{1c} and Glucose Control

Hemoglobin normally undergoes glycosylation of its amino terminal valine residue. The product of this glycosylation, hemoglobin A_{1c} (HbA_{1c}), is a valuable endogenous marker for glycemic control over the previous 4 to 12 weeks (16). This endogenous substance has a half-life equivalent to that of an erythrocyte. Measurement of an individual's HbA_{1c} is an assessment of the concentration of plasma glucose and the length of time that hemoglobin was exposed to those glucose concentrations. Clinical trials (e.g., Diabetes Control and Complications Trial [DCCT] and UK Prospective Diabetes Study) have clearly demonstrated that if a patient's HbA_{1c} is maintained below 7%, the development and progression of neuropathy, nephropathy, and retinopathy in type 1 or 2 patients can be significantly decreased (17).

Diabetic Complications

Uncontrolled or poorly controlled plasma glucose levels will result in the development and progression of microvascular and macrovascular diabetic complications that involve the eyes (retinopathy), kidneys (nephropathy), nerves (neuropathy), heart, and blood vessels (9).

Diabetes is the leading cause of new blindness in adults (10,000 cases in diabetic patients per year) and represents 15% of all blindness (2,4). Typically asymptomatic in its earliest, most treatable stages, diabetic eye disease (e.g., retinopathy, glaucoma, and cataracts) represents the most common microvascular diabetic complication. Diabetic retinopathy begins to develop as early as 7 years before the diagnosis of type 2 diabetes. It is caused by the accumulation of polyols, the formation of advanced glycation end products, oxidative stress, and the activation of protein kinase C. These products or processes have adverse effects on cellular metabolism, cell signaling, and growth factors (18).

Diabetes is the leading cause of end-stage renal disease and represents 35% of all end-stage renal disease (2,4). This complication is experienced by approximately 40% of all patients with diabetes and is correlated with increased cardiovascular mortality. Diabetic nephropathy, which is caused by both tubular and interstitial changes in kidney structure, is characterized by stage. Microalbuminuria or incipient nephropathy is defined as increased urinary albumin excretion (>30 mg/24 hours and ≤299 mg/24 hours), whereas macroalbuminuria or overt neuropathy is defined as urinary albumin excretion of more than 300 mg/24 hours (19). It is more prevalent in the African-American, Asian, and Native-American populations than in the Caucasian population. Even acute episodes of hyperglycemia can cause an increase in glomerular filtration rate or vascular damage resulting in glomerular dysfunction (12).

When plasma glucose levels remain high for an extended period of time, peripheral nerves are injured. Nerve damage, which can affect virtually every nerve fiber in the body, occurs in 60 to 70% of all diabetic patients (2). Peripheral neuropathy can lead to foot ulcerations, amputations, and Charcot joints (9). Cardiovascular autonomic neuropathy, a key cause of morbidity and mortality in the diabetic population, causes symptoms of orthostatic hypotension and decreased heart rate variability, contributes to exercise intolerance, and contributes to left ventricular dysfunction. Gastrointestinal autonomic neuropathy can result in gastroparesis, gastroesophageal reflux disease, delayed gastric emptying, and colon abnormalities. Genitourinary autonomic neuropathy can have adverse effects on both male and female sexual function and urinary continence. What most people associate with diabetic neuropathy actually is termed "sensorimotor neuropathy," which is characterized by pain, abnormal sensations and sensory loss (20). The pathology of diabetic neuropathy is similar to that described for retinopathy. A staggering statistic is that diabetic neuropathy can be linked to between 50 and 75% of all nontraumatic amputations (4).

There are macrovascular complications to consider as well, including ischemic heart disease, cerebrovascular disease, and peripheral vascular disease. These complications are the primary cause of morbidity in type 2 patients. Diabetic patients have a two- to fourfold greater risk than the nondiabetic population of dying from a myocardial infarction or stroke (17). Insulin resistance has been shown to stifle the action of nitric oxide and increase the levels of prothrombotic factors (e.g., fibrinogen). Without nitric oxide an increase in vascular smooth muscle cell proliferation, an increase in platelet adhesiveness (as well as vasoconstriction) is likely. Insulin resistance also can interfere with the fibrinolytic process via an increase in the synthesis of plasminogen activator inhibitor-1 (PAI-1) (15).

Abnormalities in lipid metabolism also contribute to the macrovascular complications. When the body is unable to use glucose as its source of energy, it relies on the metabolism of fats and proteins for energy. Lipolysis results in the release of fatty acids and glycerol from adipose tissue into circulation. The liver converts excess fatty acids into cholesterol and phospholipids. Along with triglycerides, these substances are organized by the liver into lipoproteins and released into the circulation. This results in the development of hypercholesterolemia and atherosclerosis. When the body increases fat utilization, there is a corresponding increase in the formation and release of keto acids into the circulation, which can result in metabolic ketoacidosis (diabetic ketoacidosis) (2).

Diagnosis of Diabetes

Some, but not all, diabetic patients display the classic signs and symptoms of hyperglycemia before diagnosis. This includes polydipsia (excessive thirst), polyuria (excessive urination), as well as weight loss and a lack of energy despite the consumption of large amounts of food. The diagnosis of any of the previously discussed metabolic disorders, including type 1 and 2 diabetes, requires the measurement of fasting plasma glucose levels and/or plasma glucose levels after an oral glucose challenge. The clinical criteria for the diagnosis of diabetes mellitus are found in Table 32.4. Different clinical criteria exists for the clinical values associated with the diagnosis of IFG and IGT, as previously presented (9). This also is true for GDM in pregnant women when the fasting plasma glucose is greater than 126 mg/dL or the casual plasma glucose is greater than 200 mg/dL. If a patient's plasma level exceeds these thresholds, then a glucose challenge test typically is ordered on a subsequent day. This test, which does not require that the patient be fasting, involves consumption of a 50-g oral glucose load by the patient, followed by evaluation of their plasma glucose after 1 hour. A value of greater than 140 mg/dL indicates that the patient should undergo a subsequent 3-hour, 100-g oral glucose load on another day (10). A 3-hour postload plasma glucose level of 140 mg/dL or greater indicates that a provisional diagnosis of GDM should be made (9).

Role of Hormones Other than Insulin

In addition to insulin, the pancreas produces glucagon from α cells, somatostatin from δ cells, and amylin from β cells. Each of these hormones has an influence on blood glucose concentrations.

Glucagon

Glucagon stimulates glycogenolysis and gluconeogenesis through a receptor-mediated action in the liver. Hyperglycemia in patients with diabetes can be associated with elevated levels of glucagon in the blood. Thus, there is interest in developing glucagon antagonists as an approach to glycemic control (21).

Table 32.4. Diagnosis Criteria for Diabetes Mellitus (9)

Clinical Values	Symptoms
Non-fasting plasma glucose level ≥200 mg/dL	Polydipsia, polyuria, unexplained weight loss
OR	
Fasting plasma glucose level ≥126 mg/dl	
OR	
2-hour postload glucose ≥200 mg/dL after consumption of a 75-g oral glucose load	

Somatostatin

Originally isolated from hypothalamic tissue, somatostatin is characterized as an inhibitor of growth hormone (GH) release. The structure was determined in 1971. Subsequent investigations led to the recognition that somatostatin also was released from the pancreas and has a role of inhibiting the secretion of both insulin and glucagon. A total of five somatostatin receptor subtypes have been characterized and cloned (sst1 to sst5). Subtype sst4 is associated with the inhibition of insulin release, and an sst4-selective inhibitor has been reported (22). The somatostatin analogue SOM230 has exhibited selectivity for sst1, sst2, sst3, and sst5 in rats and effectively decreased plasma GH and insulin-like growth factor-1 (IGF-1) levels by 75% without significant effects on insulin or glucagon (23). Another analogue, PTR3173, with selectivity for recombinant human somatostatin receptor (hsst2, hsst4, hsst5) was substantially more effective in inhibiting GH secretion compared to glucagon and insulin release in rats (24). Nocturnal GH release and subsequent elevation of IGF-1 is thought to contribute to insulin resistance. Somatostatin analogues that can selectively control GH or glucagon release could be developed and aid in glycemic control (25). Recent investigations of somatostatin receptors in the retina have led to the proposed use of somatostatin or analogues for the treatment of diabetic retinopathy (26).

Amylin

Amylin normally is cosecreted with insulin from secretory granules in pancreatic β cells in response to meals and works with insulin to provide postprandial glucose control. Native amylin is a single-chain peptide of 37 amino acids. Observed deficiencies of amylin in both type 1 and type 2 patients treated with insulin have led to research and drug development related to amylin (27).

Glucagon-like Peptide-1

Glucagon-like peptide-1 (GLP-1) is an incretin, a natural peptide hormone secreted in response to food intake. Incretins have multiple physiological effects to lower blood sugar, including the stimulation of insulin release and the inhibition of glucagon release following meals (28).

Adiponectin

Adiponectin is a cytokine produced by adipocytes and is termed an "adipokine." Adiponectin functions as an insulin sensitizer. Downregulation of adiponectin receptors and low levels of adiponectin have been associated with obesity-linked insulin resistance (29). Exercise and dietary changes have been shown to raise low levels of adiponectin in obese adolescents (30). Additionally, sarpogrelate hydrochloride, a 5-HT_{2A} antagonist, elevates low adiponectin levels and normalizes other factors associated with vascular changes seen in type 2 diabetes (31).

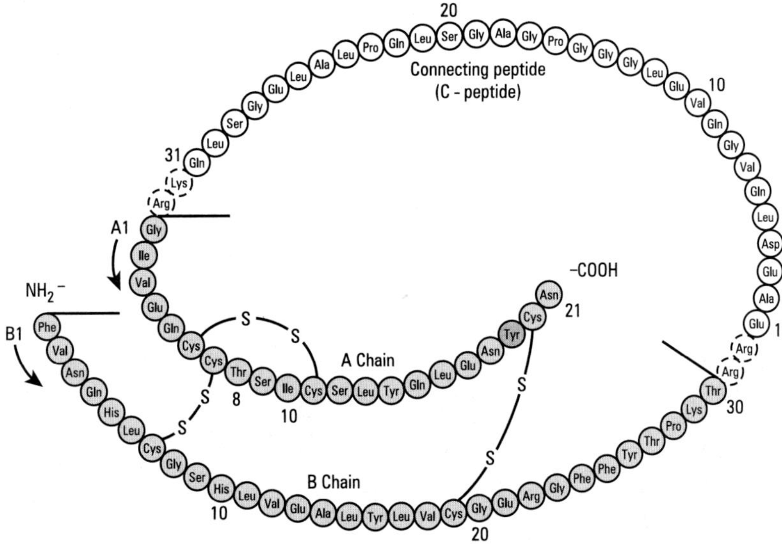

Fig. 32.1. Primary structure of proinsulin, showing cleavage sites to produce insulin.

INSULIN

Biosynthesis of Insulin

Insulin has a place in the biochemistry "hall of fame" in that it was the first protein for which the chemical structure and molecular weight were determined and was the first genetically engineered drug approved by the U.S. Food and Drug Administration (7). The active insulin hormone is composed of a 21-amino-acid A chain and a 30-amino-acid B chain that are linked by two disulfide bonds. Separately, each chain is biologically inactive. Insulin is initially synthesized as a 110-amino-acid preprohormone in the pancreatic β cells. The preprohormone then undergoes translocation through the membrane of the rough endoplasmic reticulum. During this process, the cleavage of 24-amino-acids from the N-terminus of the B chain occurs to produce proinsulin. Inside the rough endoplasmic reticulum, the protein folds, and the three critical disulfide bonds form. In the Golgi complex, proinsulin undergoes additional modification that is catalyzed by calcium-dependent endopeptidases (PC2 and PC3). In this process, four basic amino acids as well as the connecting C-peptide are removed via proteolysis (Fig. 32.1). The resulting insulin protein represents the active form of the hormone found in the plasma. In solution, insulin can exist as a monomer, dimer, or hexamer. In the pancreas, insulin is stored in its hexameric form. In this form, two zinc ions are coordinated per insulin hexamer. The half-life of insulin is 5 to 6 minutes, whereas the half life of proinsulin is approximately 17 minutes (5).

Secretion of Insulin

Secretion of insulin from the pancreas is very tightly regulated. When glucose enters the β cell (GLUT-2–facilitated transport), it is phosphorylated by glucokinase to G6P. The G6P is used to generate ATP, thereby changing the ratio of ATP to adenosine diphosphate (ADP) and prevents an ATP-sensitive potassium channel from functioning, which in turn leads to depolarization of the β cells. This prompts activation of a voltage-gated calcium channel and calcium flows into the β cells. The elevated intracellular calcium concentrations causes activation of phospholipases A_2 and C, and levels of inositol triphosphate rise (5). Inositol triphosphate, an intracellular second messenger, facilitates additional release of calcium into the cytosol. The intracellular concentrations of calcium are now sufficiently high to promote insulin secretion from the β cells. Several classes of pharmacological agents alter the regulation of insulin release. A list of these agents and their respective effect on insulin secretion can be found in Table 32.5.

Insulin interacts with its cell surface receptor via key amino acid residues located along the N- and C-termini of the A chain of insulin and along the carboxy terminus of the B chain of insulin (Table 32.6). The binding of insulin occurs to amino acid residues located within the N- and C-terminal regions of the α subunit of the receptor, which includes a cysteine-rich region (5). Binding and activation of the insulin receptor results in a cascade of biochemical events previously described.

Table 32.5. Agents that Alter Insulin Secretion (5)

Pharmacological Class	Effect on Insulin Secretion
α_2-Adrenergic receptor agonist	Inhibits insulin secretion
α_2-Adrenergic receptor antagonist	Promotes insulin secretion
β_2-Adrenergic receptors agonists	Promotes insulin secretion
β_2-Adrenergic receptors antagonists	Inhibits insulin secretion

Table 32.6 Amino Acid Interactions with Insulin Receptor

Chain	N-terminus	C-terminus
A	Gly A1, Glu A4, Gln A5	Tyr A19, Asn A21
B	Val B12	Tyr B16, Gly B23, Phe B24, Phe B25, Tyr B26

Metabolism of Insulin

Insulin degradation occurs primarily in the liver and kidney. Of that which is secreted from the pancreatic islet cells, 50% reaches the liver via the portal vein and undergoes disulfide bond cleavage catalyzed by glutathione insulin transhydrogenase (insulinase). This is followed by proteolytic degradation before entry into the general circulation. Insulin is filtered by the renal glomeruli and can then be reabsorbed or degraded by the tubules (5). At the tissue level, insulin degradation occurs to a limited extent at the cell surface.

Sources of Insulin

Four types of cells are found within the islet of Langerhans, and each cell type secretes its own polypeptide hormone (Table 32.7). The β cells produce a basal level of endogenous insulin at the rate of 0.25 to 1.5 IU/hour. Consumption of a meal causes a biphasic bolus secretion of insulin. There is an immediate release of insulin, followed by an additional release 30 to 45 minutes after eating. Within 2 to 4 hours of a meal, insulin secretion returns to basal levels (8). Under fasting conditions (e.g., overnight), the pancreas produces 40 μg (1 IU)/hour.

In the treatment of all patients with type 1 or some type 2 diabetes, exogenous insulin must be administered to achieve a euglycemic state. Initially, patients only had the option of administering either bovine- or porcine-based insulins. Insulins derived from these animals were considered to be viable alternatives to human insulin, because the amino acid sequence homology between species was superb (Table 32.8). As early as the 1950s, it became obvious that there were limitations to these sources of insulin, because 100% of these patients developed both high- and low-affinity insulin antibodies. As a result, immunologic insulin resistance (a syndrome in and of itself) was reported in those patients with elevated levels of insulin antibodies that bound tightly to insulin (32).

Table 32.7. Polypeptides Secreted by Cells in the Islet of Langerhans

Type of Cell	Hormone Secreted
α	Glucagon
β	Insulin and amylin
δ	Somatostatin
PP or F cell	Pancreatic polypeptide

Table 32.8. Insulin Sequence Homology Between Species

	Insulin Amino Acid Substitutions		
	A Chain		B Chain
Source	Position 8	Position 10	Position 30
Beef	Alanine	Valine	Alanine
Pork	Threonine	Isoleucine	Alanine
Human	Threonine	Isoleucine	Threonine

Once the complete synthesis of human insulin was accomplished (1963), human insulin could be synthesized via two possible routes. One method involved the synthesis of each chain separately, followed by linkage of the chains to produce the active hormone (7). The other, more favored route involved the use of fermentation to synthesize the peptide hormone, followed by isolation of the pure substance. In 1978, Genentech and City of Hope National Medical Center were able to produce human insulin by recombinant DNA methods (7). This involved the insertion of synthesized genes for each of the two chains into *Escherichia coli* and then the use of fermentation methods developed by Eli Lilly to generate commercial quantities of human insulin. Clinical trials started in 1980, and by 1982, Humulin (regular insulin) became the first genetically engineered drug approved by the U.S. Food and Drug Administration (7). Once this recombinant technology was established, it was rapidly applied to the production of a variety of insulin analogues.

Solution Structure of Insulin

The secondary and tertiary structure is substantially the same for all insulins despite differences in the primary structure from various species. The A chain has two α-helices and the B-chain an α-helix and a β-turn, with the B21 to B30 region as a β-strand. This conformation buries a number of hydrophobic A-chain residues in the interior of the peptide, which improves water solubility and stability. The presence of phenol and cresol that often are used as preservatives in insulin formulations results in substantial changes in the insulin conformation. Phenol, in the presence of zinc ions, causes the formation of a B1-B8 helix, which involves movement of more than 25 Å in the B1 residue (33).

Only the insulin monomer is able to interact with insulin receptors, and native insulin exists as a monomer at low, physiological concentrations (<0.1 μM). Insulin dimerizes at the higher concentrations (0.6 mM) found in pharmaceutical preparations, and at neutral pH in the presence of zinc ions, hexamers form (34). These zinc-associated hexamers also are the storage form of insulin in β cells. At concentrations greater than 0.2 mM, hexamers form even in the absence of zinc ions.

Changes in the insulin concentration can profoundly change absorption after subcutaneous administration

(35). Insulin given at a concentration of 40 IU/mL (previously used commercially) is absorbed quite rapidly, but insulin at 100 IU/mL (now used commercially) is absorbed significantly more slowly. This apparently reflects the decrease in monomer concentration, the only absorbable form, as the concentration of insulin increases.

Stability of Insulin

The importance of zinc ions for stabilizing insulin preparations has been known since the first reported crystallization of insulin in the presence of zinc ions in 1934 (36). Suspensions of zinc insulin were used at that time. Presently, all pharmaceutical preparations are either solutions of zinc insulin or suspensions of insoluble forms of zinc insulin. A longer-acting and more stable form of insulin is protamine zinc insulin, which is prepared by precipitating insulin in the presence of zinc ions and protamine, a basic protein. This precipitate is known to contain two zinc ions per insulin hexamer. A somewhat shorter-acting and more useful preparation is neutral protamine Hagedorn (NPH) insulin, which includes m-cresol as a preservative. This also is known as isophane insulin. Six m-cresol molecules occupy cavities in the hexamer involving the B1-B8 helix formed as a result of the presence of the m-cresol. Later, it was reported that when small additional amounts of zinc ions were added to hexameric two-zinc insulin in neutral acetate buffer, insulin could be made to crystallize in several forms with varying rates of dissolution in water. Thus, the rapidly soluble amorphous semilente insulin is a two-zinc insulin, and the crystalline, more slowly soluble ultralente insulin is a four-zinc form (37,38).

An additional form of insulin, partially unfolded insulin, can form a viscous or insoluble precipitates known as fibrils. Shielding of hydrophobic domains is the principal driving force for the aggregation. Further studies revealed that when the exposed hydrophobic domain (A2, A3, B11, and B15) interacts with the normally buried aliphatic residues (A13, B6, B14, and B18) in the hexameric structure, fibrils form (Fig. 32.1) (39). Fibrils also have been studied by electron microscopy, and packing considerations in the crystal lattice explain why fibril formation is accelerated when insulin is in the monomeric state (40). Insulin fibrils do not resuspend on shaking; thus, they are pharmaceutically inactive.

Insulin fibril formation is particularly important with the advent of infusion pumps to deliver insulin. In these devices, insulin is exposed to elevated temperatures, the presence of hydrophobic surfaces, and shear forces, all factors that increase insulin's tendency to aggregate. These problems can be overcome if the insulin is prepared with phosphate buffer or other additives. Another physical stability problem associated with insulin is adsorption to tubing and other surfaces. This normally occurs if the insulin concentration is less than 5 IU/mL (0.03 mM), and it can be prevented by adding albumin to the dosage form if a dilute insulin solution must be used (34).

There also are chemical instability issues associated with insulin. For 40 years, the only rapid-acting form of insulin was a solution of zinc insulin, with pH 2 to 3. If this insulin is stored at 4°C, deamidation of the asparagine at A21 occurs at a rate of 1 to 2% per month. The C-terminal Asn, under acidic conditions, undergoes cyclization to the anhydride, which in turn can react with water, leading to deamidation. The anhydride also can react with the N-terminal Phe of another chain to yield a cross-linked molecule. If stored at 25°C, the inactive deamidated derivative constitutes 90% of the total protein after 6 months (Fig. 32.2) (34).

If insulin is stored at neutral pH, a different reactions may occur. Deamidation occurs on the Asn at B3, and the products, the aspartate and isoaspartate-containing insulins, are equiactive with native insulin (Fig. 32.2). Deamidation is virtually undetectable in suspensions of bovine insulin zinc (37). More problematic transformations are possible, including chain cleavage between A8 Thr and A9 Ser and covalent cross-linking, either with a second insulin chain or with protamine, if present. These processes are relatively slow compared to the deamidations, but they have the potential of leading to products that may cause allergic reactions. Specific antibodies against insulin dimers have been found in 30% of diabetic patients receiving insulin (41).

Use of Insulin for Treatment of Diabetes

According to the DCCT and the UK Prospective Diabetes study, insulin and/or insulin analogues are the standard treatment for type 1, gestational, and some type 2 diabetes.

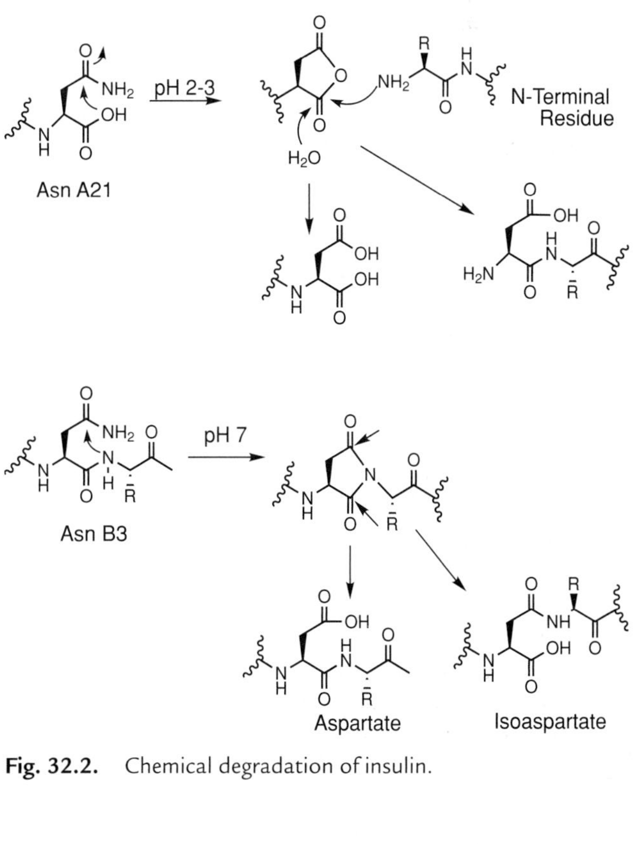

Fig. 32.2. Chemical degradation of insulin.

Table 32.9. Factors that Affect the Onset, Degree, and Duration of Insulin Activity (13)

Primary structure	Additions, deletions, insertions, modifications, and rearrangement of amino acid residues at the N- and/or C-terminus of the B chain
Insulin crystal type	soluble, amorphous, crystalline, microcrystalline
Concentration of zinc	
Presence of modifying protein	protamine
Site of injection	abdomen, upper arms, thighs, buttocks

Table 32.10. Insulin Analogues

Generic Name	Trade Name	Change in A Chain	Change in B Chain
Lispro	Humalog	None	B28 Pro → Lys; B29 Lys → Pro
Aspart	NovoLog	None	B28 Pro → Asp
Glulisine	Apidra	None	B3 Val → Lys; B29 Lys → Glu
Glargine	Lantus	A21 Asn → Gly	Add: B31 Arg and B32 Arg
Detemir	Levemir	None	Remove: B30 Thr Add: C14 fatty acid to B29 Lys

These drugs represented $9 billion in sales in 2006, with an anticipated $20 billion in sales by 2012. Although prescribing habits are different between and within countries, the most common factors that influence insulin selection generally include awareness and availability of insulin preparations as well as differences in eating habits and lifestyles (6). As with most medications that treat chronic conditions, the dosage and type of insulin and/or insulin analogue should be individualized and take into consideration the degree to which the patient adheres to recommended diet and exercise regimens. In the evaluation of which types of insulin to prescribe, a number of factors should be considered that affect the onset, degree, and duration of insulin activity. A list of these factors can be found in Table 32.9. These factors relate to the solubility and stability of insulin discussed above.

Insulin Overdose and Diabetic Coma

The most common and serious reaction to insulin therapy is hypoglycemia. It is important that patients with diabetes, especially those receiving insulin therapy, be able to recognize the signs and symptoms of hypoglycemia. Symptoms of hypoglycemia may be evident with a plasma glucose level at 60 to 80 mg/dL. Severe hypoglycemia can lead to convulsions and coma. Patients that vigorously attempt to achieve euglycemia to avoid various vascular complications risk increased frequency of hypoglycemic episodes (42). In the DCCT, the incidence of severe hypoglycemic reactions was threefold higher in the intensive insulin therapy group than in the conventional therapy group (43). It is now known that hypoglycemia kills neurons actively rather than by starvation from within. Thus, significant damage to regions of the brain can result from severe hypoglycemia (44). Because of these dangers, patients receiving insulin therapy should carry packets of sugar or candy to be used at the onset of the symptoms of hypoglycemia.

Insulin Analogues

Structure–activity relationship studies have been conducted over several years. These studies revealed that variations or removal of amino acid residues from the C-terminus of the insulin B chain did not drastically change the biological activity but could influence the rate of dimer formation or separation. If dimer formation can be inhibited, rapid-acting insulins may be obtained. Thus, the various insulin analogues that have been developed have substitutions in or additions to the C-terminus starting at residue B28. The resulting analogues have either a faster onset or a longer duration of action relative to native insulin. These analogues are all produced by recombinant DNA technology using a modified DNA template. Various analogues are summarized in Table 32.10.

Faster-Acting Analogues

As indicated in Table 32.10, both insulin lispro and insulin aspart B28 Pro is replaced with a linear amino acid. This change also results in a conformational change at the C-terminus and, therefore, the ability of the insulin to dimerize. Both of these analogues dissociate into monomers faster, and this produces a faster onset of action. Both insulin lispro and insulin aspart can be injected immediately before meals providing for more convenient timing and more accurate calculation of appropriate dosing. These analogues also can be used in combination with regular or NPH insulin (45).

Longer-Acting Analogues

The first long-acting analogue to be introduced to the market was insulin glargine. This analogue results from the replacement of A21 Asn by Gly and the addition of two Arg amino acids to the C-terminus of the B chain, as indicated in Table 32.10. The resulting analogue has an isoelectric point close to seven, which results in precipitation on subcutaneous injection. The analogue is slowly released from the resulting depot. Insulin glargine produces minimal peak effects and has a duration of action of 22 ± 4 hours. It has been demonstrated to be comparable or slightly better than NPH insulin at maintaining or reducing HbA_{1c} levels without nocturnal hypoglycemia (45).

Insulin detemir is a long-acting analogue that was recently introduced to the market. This analogue results from N-acylation of the B29 Lys with 14-carbon myristic acid (Table 32.10). The fatty acid side chain binds to plasma albumin to produce a depot and longer action. It is not as long-lasting as insulin glargine, and is injected twice daily by patients with type 1 and type 2 diabetes (45,46).

DRUG DEVELOPMENT RELATED TO OTHER HORMONES

Significant efforts are underway, in addition to those discussed earlier, to develop therapeutic approaches for the treatment of diabetes that are based on hormones other than insulin.

Glucagon Antagonists

Several nonpeptide glucagon antagonist are being investigated as potential agents for the treatment of diabetes (Fig. 32.3). Presently, several of these drugs are in early clinical trials, whereas other antagonists of potential interest have not yet entered the clinic (47,48). BAY-27-9955 is an especially interesting antiglucagonemic agents. The drug is being investigated in patients with poorly controlled type 2 diabetes.

Amylin Agonists

Native amylin is a single-chain peptide of 37 amino acids. As previously discussed, amylin is cosecreted with insulin from the β cells in response to meals. Amylin has various actions, including a slowing of gastric emptying and a lowering of blood glucose levels by decreasing glucagon release. It has been reported that amylin levels are abnormally low in patients with type 1 diabetes and are insufficient at mealtime in insulin-using patients with type 2 diabetes. Amylin appears to produce these effects by binding to specific receptors in the central nervous system. The administration of amylin in patients with type 1 diabetes is unsuitable because of a physicochemical property of amylin, which is that the peptide is insoluble and aggregates in solution. Recently, an analogue of amylin has been approved for use in type 1 and type 2 diabetes.

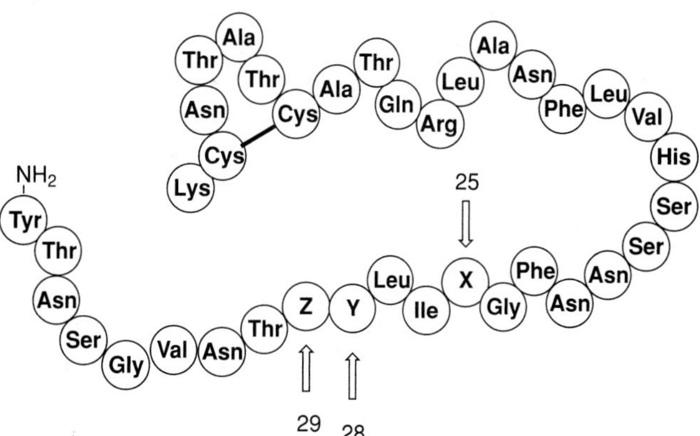

Amylin (human) X = Ala, Y = Z = Ser

Pramlintide (Symlin) X = Y = Z = Pro

NNC-92-1687

Skyrin

BAY 27-9955

Fig. 32.3. Glucagon receptor antagonists.

Pramlintide

Pramlintide is an analogue of amylin in which proline has replaced the normal amino acids at positions 25, 28, and 29, as indicated above. The result of these substitutions is an increase in water solubility and a reduced tendency for self-aggregation.

PHARMACOKINETICS. Pramlintide is administered via subcutaneous injection immediately before meals, reaches maximum circulating concentrations within 20 minutes, and has a half-life of 29 minutes. The drug is eliminated from the body primarily through the kidney. The plasma concentrations are similar to those seen with postprandial amylin. Because the drug is formulated at pH 4.0, it is potentially incompatible with insulin (pH 7.8) if administered within the same syringe, although one study of pramlintide combined with Novolin or Humulin did not show changes in the pharmacokinetics of either drugs (49,50).

MECHANISM OF ACTION. Amylin receptors have been identified in distinct areas of the brain, including the nucleus accumbens and the dorsal vagal complex. Stimulation of these receptors reduces food intake and depresses GI motility. It is assumed that pranlintide stimulates these receptors, leading to the reported benefits of the drug in patients with diabetes, although the exact mechanism is still poorly understood. Pranlintide causes a moderate reduction in HbA_{1c} and postprandial glucose levels when used in combination with insulin, which has benefits in normalizing fluctuations of circulating glucose levels.

SIDE EFFECTS. The major side effects reported for pramlintide consist of mild to moderate nausea, with severe nausea appearing in patients using large doses of the drug. The nausea may decrease on continued use of the drug. The rate of hypoglycemia appears to be quite low.

Glucagon-like Peptide-1 Agonists

Glucagon-like peptide-1 (GLP-1), a mammalian incretin hormone, consists of two peptides secreted by the endocrine L cells located in the small intestine. The two forms of GLP-1 differ by one amino acid, with 80% of the GLP-1 possessing 30 amino acids (the minor peptide contains 31 amino acids). The role of GLP-1 appears to be to prepare the body for a glucose surge following a sudden rise in plasma glucose. The early insulin response (first-phase insulin secretion) appears to be lost in patients with type 2 diabetes. The GLP-1 stimulates the first-phase release of insulin from the pancreatic β cells and, additionally, inhibits the release of glucagon, thus controlling the release of glucose from the liver. In addition, GLP-1 slows stomach empting, causing a feeling of fullness that reduces additional food intake; it does this by binding to GLP-1–specific receptors in the β cells of the pancreas. The release of GLP-1 is only associated with elevated glucose levels; thus, its release drops when glucose serum levels drop. The GLP-1 itself would appear to have drug potential if not for the fact that GLP-1 has a half-life of 90 seconds. The enzyme dipeptidyl peptidase IV (DPP-IV) metabolizes GLP-1 by removal of two amino acids from the N-terminus of GLP-1. The resulting peptide has a half-life of less than 2 minutes. The enzyme DPP-IV is found in intestinal capillaries and in the liver. Diabetic patients in which GLP-1 was continuously administered exhibited a significant drop in HbA_{1c} (1.3%), a steady weight loss, and an improvement in pancreatic β-cells function. Although continuous administration GLP-1 is not practical, this work did suggest two potential drug avenues: the development of GLP-1 mimics, and the other DPP-IV inhibitors (51–53).

Exenatide

H-His-Gly-Glu-Gly-Thr-Phe-Thr-Ser-Asp-Leu-Ser-Lys-Gln-Met-Glu
-Glu-Glu-Ala-Val-Arg-Leu-Phe-Ile-Glu-Trp-Leu-Lys-Asn-Gly-Gly-Pro
-Ser-Ser-Gly-Ala-Pro-Pro-Pro-Ser-NH_2

Exenatide (Byetta)

During the 1990s, it was discovered that saliva of Gila monsters contained a 39-amino-acid peptide, which had glucoregulatory activity. This peptide, exendin-4, has the ability to bind to the GLP-1 receptor and mimics the action of GLP-1. The synthetic version of exendin-4 is named exenatide. Exenatide shares 53% of the amino acid sequence with GLP-1 and also is a substrate for peptidase hydrolysis. Unlike GLP-1, however, exenatide has a half-life of 2 to 4 hours following subcutaneous injection. Exenatide is thought to exhibit its action via stimulation of GLP-1 receptors, resulting in the positive effects of improved insulin secretion, reduced glucagon release, reduced stomach emptying, as well as a reportedly slowing the loss of β cells and stimulating the differentiation and production of new β cells. The latter effect appearing to be different from that experienced by GLP-1 release. Exenatide is approved for use in certain patients with type 2 diabetes that is not adequately controlled on metformin and/or a sulfonylurea. The drug is administered via subcutaneous administration in combination with metformin or a sulfonylurea. It has not been approved for use in patients with type 1 diabetes. Some patients have experienced desired weight loss with long-term exenatide use (54). The most commonly reported adverse effects include nausea, vomiting, diarrhea, jittery feelings, headaches, and dizziness. The drug should not be administered prior to marks, but after meals.

Additional Experimental Agents Affecting GLP-1

Liraglutide. Liraglutide is a GLP-1 derivative in which a 16-carbon fatty acid has been attached to 26-amino-acid lysine. The fatty acid side chain promotes binding to albumin and limits degradation by DPP-IV, resulting in a prolonged duration of action (55). The drug requires once-daily injection and leads to prolonged release of the GLP-1 derivative. The released drug has been shown in animal models to reduce food intake and body weight and, like exenatide, to increase insulin secretion, decrease gastric empting, and reduce blood glucose levels. In addition, glucagon secretion is inhibited. In humans, the half-life of liraglutide has been shown to be extended to 10 hours, with a bioavailability of 55%.

Dipetidyl peptidase IV inhibitors. A serine protease, DPP-IV is the primary protease responsible for degrading GLP-1. This enzyme is found in both intestinal capillaries and the liver. The enzyme removes two amino acids from GLP-1, thus inactivating GLP-1. Unfortunately, DPP-IV is not selective for GLP-1 and its derivatives, but it has protease activity on a variety of substrates, including neuropeptides and enzymes involved in the immune system. A number of pharmaceutical companies have DPP-IV inhibitors in various stages of clinical investigation. Two such agents are saxagliptin (56) and vildagliptin (57). A new drug application has been submitted for vildagliptin with approval expected in 2007.

Saxagliptin

Vildagliptin (Galvus)

ORAL HYPOGLYCEMIC AGENTS

First- and Second-Generation Sulfonylureas

History

In the 1940s, 2-(*p*-aminobenzenesulfonamide)-5-isopropylthiadiazole was used to treat typhoid fever but caused a number of deaths through prolonged hypoglycemia. About this same time, it was found that carbutamide was significantly more active and safer as a hypoglycemic agent. It became the first sulfonylurea hypoglycemic agent to be marketed but, because of effects on bone marrow, ultimately was withdrawn from the market.

After the discovery of carbutamide, many sulfonylureas were examined, and a number are still marketed today. Until 1994 they were the only oral hypoglycemic agents available (58).

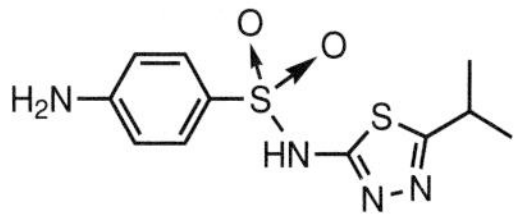

IPTD

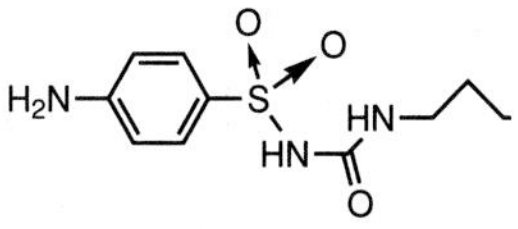

Carbutamide

Structure–Activity Relationships

The typical sulfonylurea is a mono substituted (usually para) aromatic sulfonylurea that has a bulky aliphatic substituent on the nonsulfonyl-attached nitrogen of the urea. Small alkyl groups, such as methyl or ethyl, are not active. In first-generation analogues, the aromatic substituent is a relatively simple atom or group of atoms (e.g., methyl, amino, acetyl, chloro, bromo, methylthio, or trifluoromethyl); however, the second-generation analogues have a larger *p*-(β-arylcarboxyamidoethyl) group that leads to significantly higher potency (Tables 32.11 and 32.12). Glimepiride typically is classified as a second-generation sulfonylurea, and it has a similar extended binding group like glyburide and glipizide; however, differences in its pharmacological profile may justify a separate classification.

Sulfonylureas are weak acids, with pK_a values of approximately 5.0 with proton dissociation from the sulfonyl-attached nitrogen of the urea. Serum protein binding is high (Table 32.12), so care must be taken when administering with other highly protein bound drugs.

Mechanism of Action

The principal action of the sulfonylureas is to stimulate the release of insulin from β cells. They act by affecting the ATP-sensitive potassium channel. This channel is a hetero-octameric complex of two subunits: a sulfonylurea receptor (SUR1), and an inwardly rectifying potassium channel (Kir6.2). On binding to SUR1, potassium efflux is blocked, leading to depolarization of the membrane. This depolarization opens voltage-dependent calcium channels, resulting in an influx of calcium. At higher intracellular calcium concentrations, calcium-sensitive proteins act to promote the release of stored insulin from the cells. There are two phases to the release of insulin: The first phase involves the insulin granules at the plasma membrane, and a second phase involves newly formed insulin granules that migrate to the membrane (59). These drugs are effective in patients with type 2 diabetes whose insulin-secreting capacity is intact but whose ability to produce adequate insulin in the presence of elevated glucose has been lost. Sulfonylureas can cause hypoglycemia, because these drugs can stimulate insulin secretion even when glucose levels are low.

All sulfonylureas exhibit both insulin-secreting and extrapancreatic activities. Glimepiride relies on extrapancreatic effects for a greater proportion of its

Table 32.11. First and Second Generation Sulfonylureas

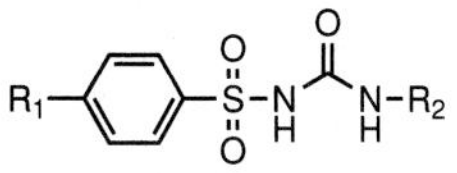

Generic name	Trade name	R_1	R_2
1st Generation:			
Tolbutamide	Orinase	CH_3-	$-CH_2CH_2CH_2CH_3$
Chlorpropamide	Diabinese	Cl–	$-CH_2CH_2CH_3$
Tolazamide	Tolinase	CH_3-	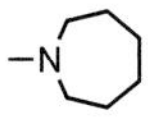 –N(azepane)
Acetohexamide	Dymelor	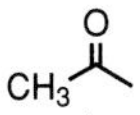 $CH_3C(O)-$	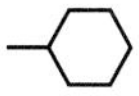 cyclohexyl
2nd Generation:			
Glyburide (Glibenclamide)	Diabeta Micronase Glynase PresTab	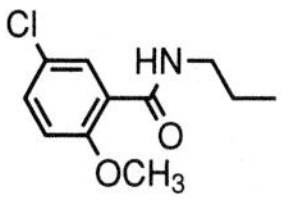 Cl, OCH_3-substituted benzamide–HN– (ethyl)	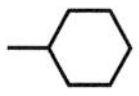 cyclohexyl
Glipizide	Glucotrol	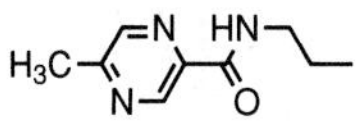 H_3C-pyrazine–C(O)–HN– (ethyl)	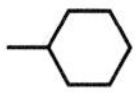 cyclohexyl
Glimepiride	Amaryl	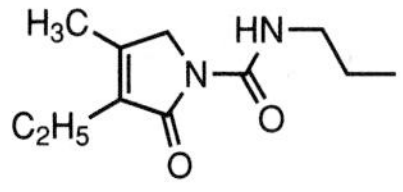 H_3C, C_2H_5-pyrrolinone–N–C(O)–HN– (ethyl)	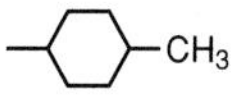 4-CH_3-cyclohexyl

Table 32.12. Pharmacokinetic Properties of the Sulfonylureas

Drug (Sulfonylureas)	Equivalent Dose (mg)	Serum Protein Binding (%)	$t_{1/2}$ (hour)	Duration (hour)	Renal Excretion (%)
Tolbutamide	1000	95–97	4.5–6.5	6–12	100
Chlorpropamide	250	88–96	36	up to 60	80–90
Tolazamide	250	94	7	12–14	85
Acetohexamide	500	65–88	6–8	12–18	60
Glyburide	5	99	1.5–3.0	up to 24	50
Glipizide	5	92–97	4	up to 24	68
Glimepiride	2	99	2–3	up to 24	40

hypoglycemic effect, and it is possibly because of this that it is considered less likely to produce unwanted hypoglycemia. Glimepiride binds well to not only SUR1 in β cells but also to SUR2A (as found in cardiac smooth muscle) and SUR2B (brain and smooth muscle). In contrast, tolbutamide is more selective for SUR1 (60).

Pharmacokinetics and Metabolism

Sulfonylureas are highly protein bound, primarily to albumin, which leads to a large volume of distribution (~0.2 L/kg) (Table 32.12). Food can delay the absorption of these drugs but does not typically affect bioavailability. Metabolism takes place in the liver, and the metabolites are renally excreted.

Chlorpropamide has a considerably longer half life than the other sulfonylureas, and as a result has a greater tendency for adverse effects. One explanation for the long half-life is that its metabolism (ω and ω-1 hydroxylation of the propyl group) is slow. A significant amount of the drug (~20%) is secreted unchanged.

In contrast, tolbutamide and tolazamide undergo a more rapid benzylic oxidation, leading to an inactive benzoic acid derivative (Fig. 32.4). An alternative hydroxylation of the aliphatic ring of tolazamide to an active metabolite results in a prolonged duration of action relative to tolbutamide.

The major metabolite of acetohexamide is reduction of the keto group, forming an alcohol. The hydroxy metabolite exhibits 2.5-fold the hypoglycemic activity of the parent molecule. An additional reported metabolite results from hydroxylation of the cyclohexyl group at the 4′-position, leading to inactivity.

Glipizide and glyburide are extensively metabolized (Fig. 32.5) to less active or inactive metabolites. Glipizide metabolites are excreted primarily in the urine, whereas glyburide's metabolites are excreted equally in the urine and bile.

Glimepiride is metabolized in the liver, primarily by CYP2C9, to the active metabolite M-1 (Fig. 32.6). It is then further metabolized to the inactive metabolite M-2.

Therapeutic Applications

Until the introduction of metformin and more recent antidiabetic treatments, sulfonylureas were the first line of pharmacological treatment. Both the first- and second-generation sulfonylureas appear to have the same clinical effectiveness, despite the large differences in potency. All produce a reliable glucose level reduction in patients with type 2 diabetes. These agents work best in patients whose type 2 diabetes is relatively mild (fasting serum glucose of <200 mg/dL or who can be controlled on ≤20 U of insulin daily). Frequency of administration varies among the compounds but is typically only once or twice daily.

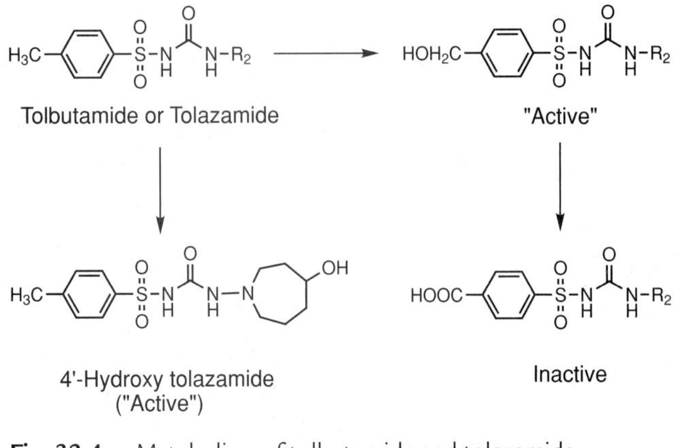

Tolbutamide or Tolazamide → "Active" → Inactive; 4′-Hydroxy tolazamide ("Active")

Fig. 32.4. Metabolism of tolbutamide and tolazamide.

Glyburide or Glipizide → trans-4′-metabolite + cis-3′metabolite

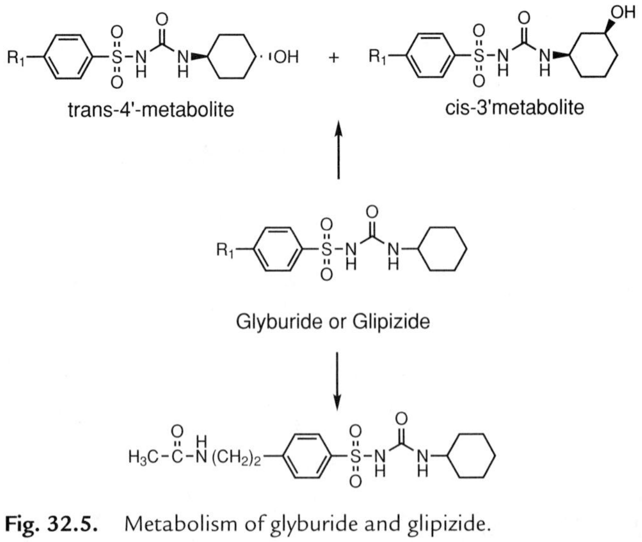

Fig. 32.5. Metabolism of glyburide and glipizide.

Meglitinides

Repaglinide

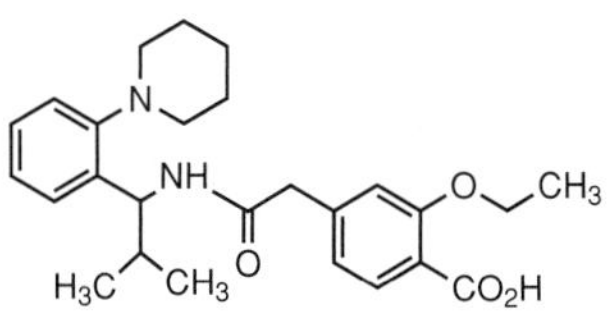

Repaglinide (Prandin)

Repaglinide is a nonsulfonylurea insulin secretagogue that was introduced in the United States in 1998 for type 2 diabetes. Like glimepiride described above, it binds well to SUR1, SUR2A, and SUR2B to block ATP-sensitive K^+ channels, resulting in insulin secretion from β cells in addition to having extrapancreatic effects (60). In an interesting conformational study, it was shown that repaglinide, several other active nonsulfonylurea hypoglycemics, as well as the sulfonylureas glyburide and glimepiride displayed a comparable "U"-shaped conformation, as indicated in molecular modeling studies. In this conformation, hydrophobic cycle groups were placed at the end of each branch, and a peptidic bond was at the bottom of the "U." Several inactive analogues of repaglinide and the poorly active drug meglitinide displayed a different conformation, with a greater distance between the hydrophobic cycle groups (61).

Repaglinide has a rapid onset and short duration of action compared to other hypoglycemic drugs. It is not associated with the prolonged hyperinsulinemia seen with the sulfonylureas, and possibly for this reason, it produces fewer side effects, including weight gain and potentially dangerous hypoglycemia. Repaglinide is at least fivefold more potent than glyburide on intravenous administration and nearly 10-fold more active on oral administration.

Nateglinide

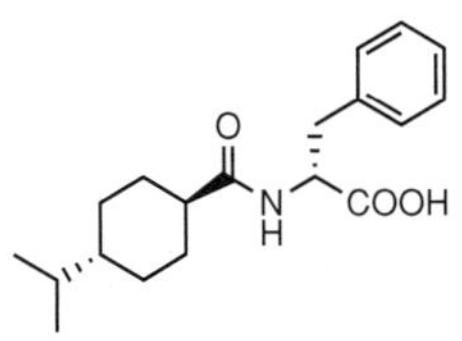

Nateglinide (Starlix)

Approved in the United States in late 2000, nateglinide is a rapidly absorbed insulin secretagogue that has a mechanism of action similar to that of repaglinide, with effects appearing within 20 minutes following oral dosing. Bioavailability is 73%, and it is 98% protein bound, primarily to albumin. Nateglinide is tissue selective, with low affinity for cardiac and skeletal muscle. It is metabolized in the liver, with 16% excreted in the urine unchanged. The major metabolites are hydroxyl derivatives (CYP2C9, 70%; CYP3A4, 30%) that are further conjugated to the glucuronide derivatives (Fig. 32.7). The drug has an elimination half-life of 1.5 hours.

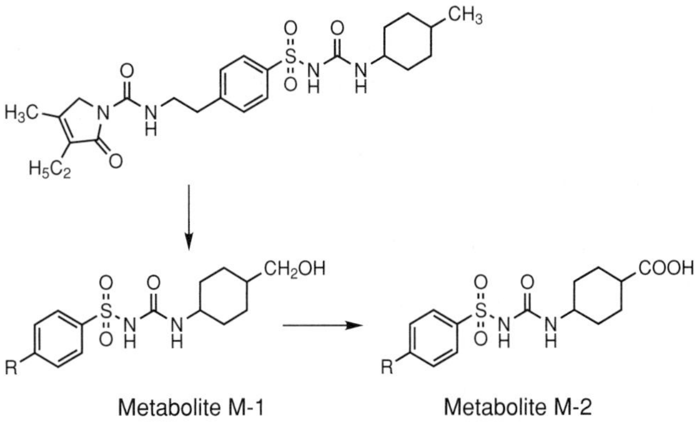

Metabolite M-1 Metabolite M-2

Fig. 32.6. Metabolism of glimepiride.

Like repaglinide, the insulin secretion produced by nateglinide is not as prolonged as that of the sulfonylureas and may result in less instances of hypoglycemia than other insulin-secreting agents. This also may be a result of the glucose-dependence of the insulin secretion caused by the drug. Low glucose levels lead to a diminished release of insulin.

Biguanides

Historically, goat's rue (*Galega officinalis*) had been used in Europe as a traditional remedy for diabetes (62). It was discovered that the active principle in this herb, galegine (isoamyleneguanidine), apparently also was the toxic principle in the plant, which caused the deaths of grazing animals. In 1918, guanidine itself was found to lower blood glucose levels in animals; however, it was too toxic for therapeutic use. In the 1950s, phenformin was found

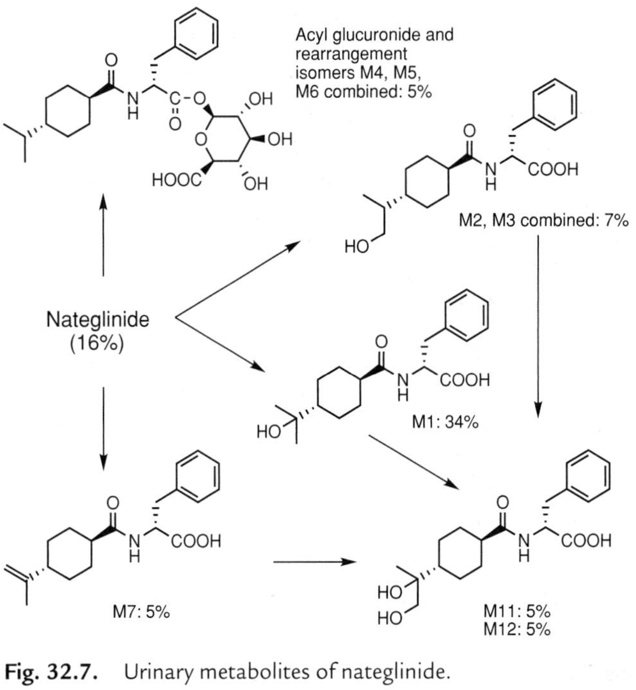

Acyl glucuronide and rearrangement isomers M4, M5, M6 combined: 5%

M2, M3 combined: 7%

Nateglinide (16%)

M1: 34%

M7: 5%

M11: 5%
M12: 5%

Fig. 32.7. Urinary metabolites of nateglinide.

to have antidiabetic properties and was used in the United States until 1977, when it was removed from the market because of patient deaths associated with lactic acidosis. Metformin was introduced in 1995 in the United States after a track record of safe and effective use for decades overseas, and it is currently in wide use.

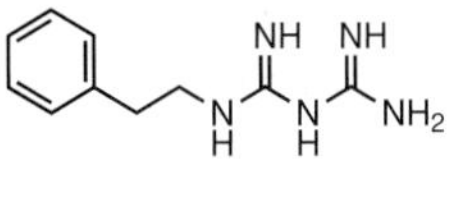

Phenformin

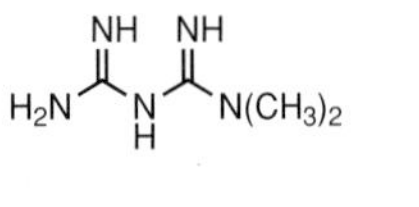

Metformin (Glucophage)

Mechanism of Action

Metformin and the other biguanides are described as insulin sensitizers. Their complete mechanism of action has not been fully elucidated. The biguanides act in the liver by decreasing excessive glucose production, most likely via reduced gluconeogenesis resulting from an increased sensitivity to insulin. They also improve glucose utilization by restoring tissue sensitivity to insulin (63). They appear to have their main action in the liver mitochondria via activation of adenosine 5′-monophosphate–activated protein kinase (AMPK) (64). Additional favorable effects resulting from metformin therapy, such as an improved lipid profile, have been reported. Metformin can lower free fatty acid concentrations by 10 to 30%. This antilipolytic effect may help to explain the reduction in gluconeogenesis through reduced levels of available substrate (65). When given as a monotherapy, metformin treatment does not lead to hypoglycemia, so it is better described as an antihyperglycemic agent rather than a hypoglycemic agent. The therapeutic effect of metformin requires the presence of insulin, and metformin does not stimulate the release of insulin or other factors, such as glucagon. In fact, the secretion of adiponectin, an insulin-sensitizing hormone, appears to be suppressed by metformin (66).

Pharmacokinetics and Metabolism

Metformin is quickly absorbed from the small intestine. Bioavailability is from 50 to 60%, and the drug is not protein bound. Peak plasma concentrations occur at approximately 2 hours. The drug is widely distributed in the body and accumulates in the wall of the small intestine. This depot of drug serves to maintain plasma concentrations. Metformin is excreted in the urine, via tubular excretion, as unmetabolized drug with a half-life of approximately 2 to 5 hours; therefore, renal impairment as well as hepatic disease are contraindications for the drug (63,65). One key drug–drug interaction of note is the competitive inhibition of renal excretion of metformin by cimetidine, which can lead to increased metformin blood levels (67).

Therapeutic Applications

Metformin is widely used as a monotherapy or in combination with a sulfonylurea in type 2 diabetes. For overweight and obese patients, it is the agent of choice. It is effective in patients of normal weight as well. Other benefits of metformin therapy are the potential for weight reduction and a 15 to 20% lowering of plasma triglycerides. Additional benefits of metformin therapy, particularly for patients with metabolic syndrome, are increased fibrinolysis and decreased plasminogen activator inhibitor-1 (PAI-1), an antithrombolytic protein (63). One study with overweight patients given metformin versus conventional treatment reported a statistically significant, 39% reduced risk of myocardial infarction (68).

Contraindications for metformin include renal insufficiency, liver disease, alcohol abuse, cardiac insufficiency, metabolic acidosis or any hypoxia-related condition. An additional consideration is that chronic metformin therapy can decrease oral absorption and subsequent serum concentrations of cyanocobalamin (vitamin B_{12}); nevertheless, this effect, which is seen in approximately one in four patients, does not appear to result in anemia.

Thiazolidinediones ("Glitazones")

The thiazolidinediones (Fig. 32.8), also known as "glitazones," sometimes are referred to as insulin enhancers. They are exemplified by ciglitazone, the first of the glitazones. Ciglitazone's antihyperglycemic effects were discovered serendipitously. The first drug in this class to be marketed was the drug troglitazone, which was introduced in the United States in 1997. Although clinical studies did indicate hepatic and cardiac toxicity, the toxicities were not considered to be severe, and it was felt that the drug could be used if liver function was closely monitored. In a 96-week study of patients with type 2 diabetes, little or no cardiac toxicity was noted (69). Unfortunately, rare cases of liver failure, liver transplants, and deaths were reported during postmarketing use, and the drug was voluntarily withdrawn in 2000 (70). More recently, two new glitazones have been approved and marketed. These include rosiglitazone and pioglitazone, both of which were introduced in 1999. Both drugs have been approved for monotherapy and combination therapy with metformin, sulfonylureas, or insulin. The

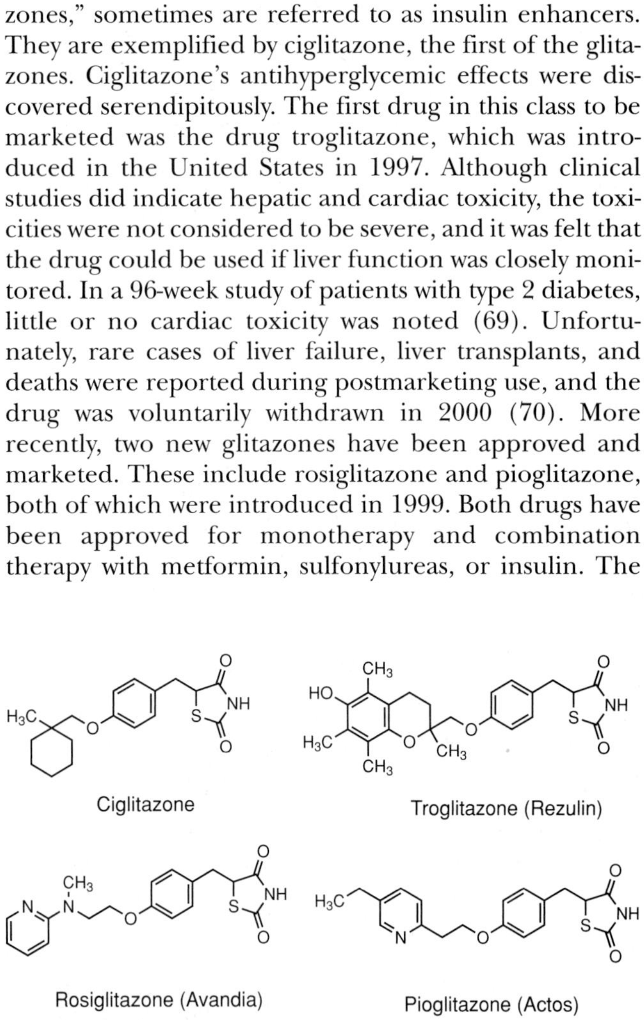

Ciglitazone

Troglitazone (Rezulin)

Rosiglitazone (Avandia)

Pioglitazone (Actos)

Fig. 32.8. Thiazolidinedione hypoglycemic agents ("glitazones").

glitazones lower blood glucose concentrations by improving sensitivity to insulin in target tissue, which includes adipose tissue, skeletal muscle, and liver. These agents are dependent on insulin for their activity.

Mechanism of Action

Like biguanides, thiazolidinediones are insulin sensitizers; however, they have a different mechanism of action from that of the biguanides. The thiazolidinediones stimulate peroxisome proliferator-activated receptor (PPAR)-γ stimulation. The PPARγ expression is highest in adipose tissue. In association with the retinoid X receptor, PPARγ binds to nuclear response elements, leading to the transcription of insulin-sensitive genes and, subsequently, a wide variety of actions including increases in: glucose uptake (adipose, muscle, liver), lipogenesis (adipose, liver), fatty acid uptake and preadipocyte differentiation (adipose), and glycolysis and glucose oxidation (muscle); in addition to decreases in gluconeogenesis, and glycogenolysis (liver).

Pharmacokinetics and Metabolism

The thiazolidinediones differ by the nature of the groups attached to the 2,4-thiazolidinedione nucleus (Fig. 32.8). These agents are extensively metabolized, with all metabolic changes occurring on or adjacent to the second aryl group. Considerable interest in the metabolism of troglitazone exists, because hepatic toxicity may be associated with a metabolite of troglitazone. Metabolic studies in rats, mice, dogs, monkeys, and humans report the presence of the four metabolites shown in Figure 32.9, with sulfate conjugation (M-1) being the primary metabolite in humans (71,72). The more interesting metabolite is the quinone product M-3, which is thought to arise through the action of CYP2C8 and CYP3A4. Quinone-type metabolites are considered to be reactive intermediates that may induce hepatic toxicity.

The metabolism of pioglitazone has been studied in rats and dogs and has led to the discovery of up to eight metabolic products. These products result from oxidation at either carbon adjacent to the pyridine ring and are found as various conjugates in the urine and bile (Fig. 32.10) (73,74). Metabolites M-1, M-2, and M-3 appear to contribute to the biological activity of pioglitazone.

The metabolism of rosiglitazone has been reported in humans, and in excess of 14 metabolites have been identified (75). The primary metabolites consist of sulfate and glucuronic acid conjugates of hydroxylation and N-demethylation products (Fig. 32.11). It is unlikely that these metabolites contribute to the biological activity of rosiglitazone.

Therapeutic Applications

The thiazolidinediones are beneficial in type 2 diabetes through a unique set of pharmacological effects. In a 6-month study of type 2 diabetes, a 600-mg daily dose of troglitazone lowered fasting serum glucose by 60 mg/dL, HbA_{1c} by 1.1%, insulin by 2.4 μU/mL, and triglycerides by 72 mg/dL versus placebo (76). The drugs appear to enhance insulin action, especially in liver, muscle, and fat tissue, where insulin-dependent glucose transport is essential.

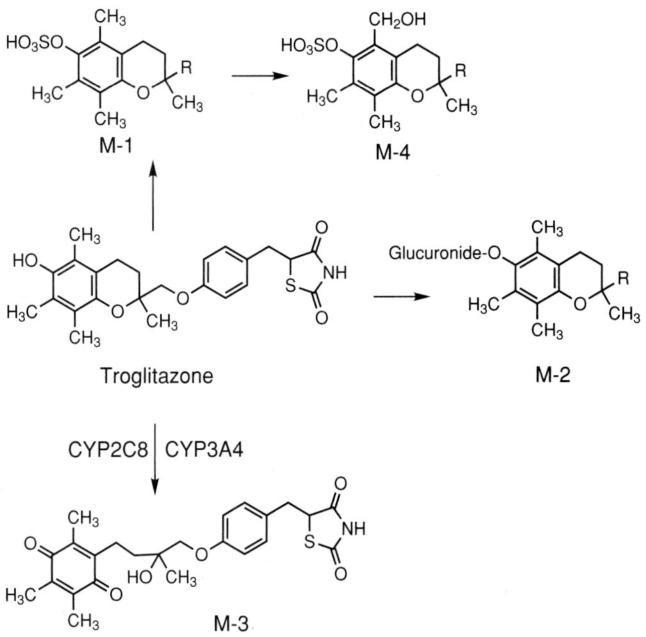

Fig. 32.9. Metabolic pathway of troglitazone.

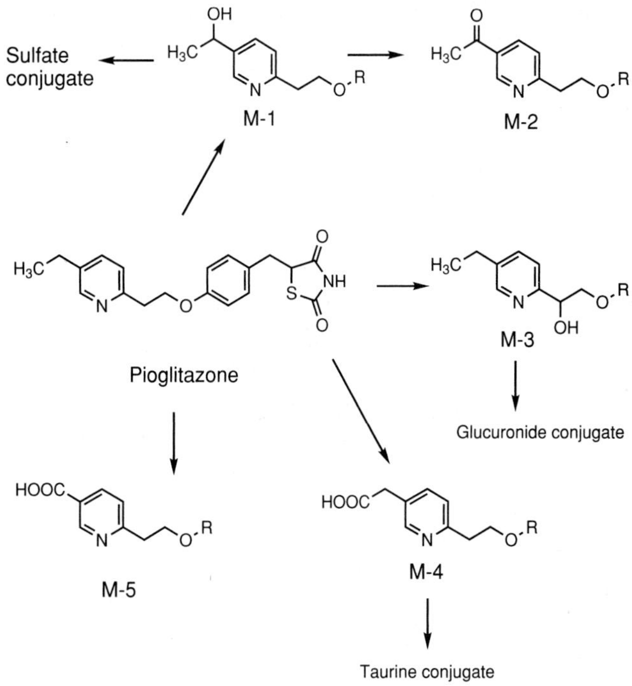

Fig. 32.10. Metabolic pathway of pioglitazone.

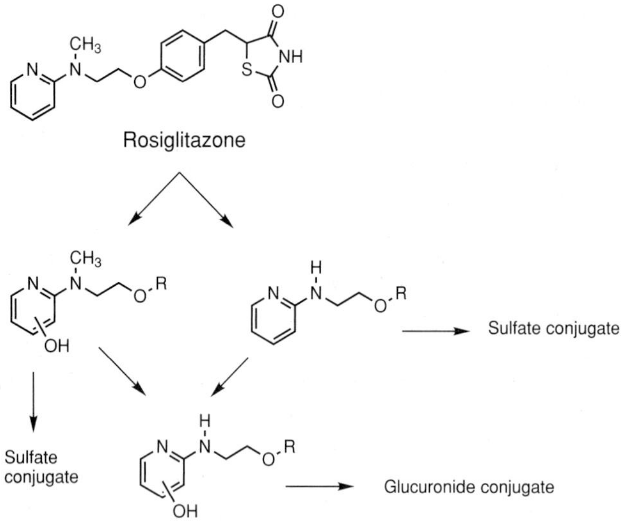

Rosiglitazone

Sulfate conjugate

Sulfate conjugate

Glucuronide conjugate

Fig. 32.11. Metabolic pathway of rosiglitazone.

Dual PPARα and PPARγ Coactivators

Because of the adipocyte differentiation effect of PPARγ activators (e.g., thiazolidinediones), weight gain can occur as an undesirable effect. In theory, a drug that activated both PPARα and PPARγ may be less prone to this side effect because of promotion of fatty acid oxidation. Activation of PPARα also is reported to reduce plasma triglyceride levels and to increase high-density lipoprotein levels; these are very desirable actions for the populations prone to type 2 diabetes. Two such agents that act on both of these targets are muraglitazar and tesaglitazar (Fig. 32.12). Others are in the clinic as well. Clinical trials demonstrated the expected benefits for muraglitazar, and it is intended as a monotherapy or in combination with metformin. Some concerns from the trials, however, are an increase, compared to placebo, in serious cardiovascular events, including death, myocardial infarction, transient ischemic attack, and congestive heart failure (77).

α-Glucosidase Inhibitors

Mechanism of Action

To be absorbed from the GI tract into the bloodstream, the complex carbohydrates that we ingest (i.e., starch) as

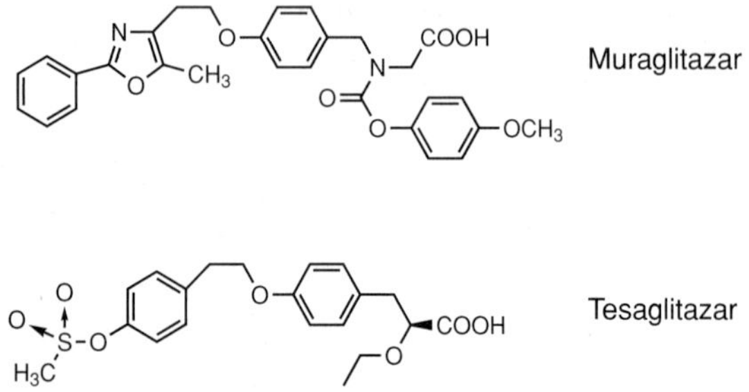

Muraglitazar

Tesaglitazar

Fig. 32.12. Dual PPARα and PPARγ activators.

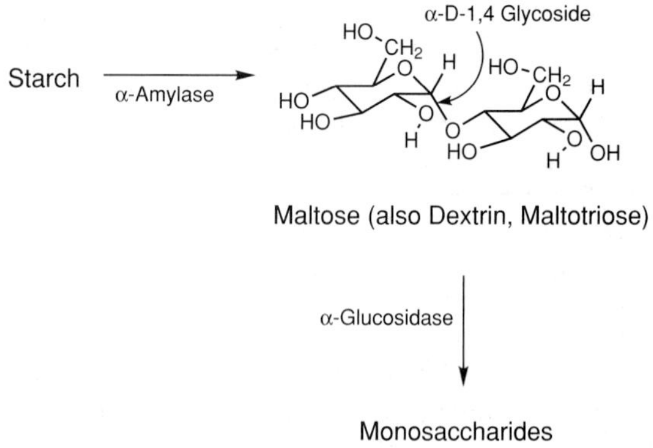

Starch → α-Amylase → Maltose (also Dextrin, Maltotriose)

α-D-1,4 Glycoside

α-Glucosidase

Monosaccharides

Fig. 32.13. Metabolism of complex carbohydrates.

part of our diet must first be hydrolyzed to monosaccharides (Fig. 32.13). The rationale for the α-glucosidase inhibitor class of drugs is that by preventing the hydrolysis of carbohydrates, their rate of absorption could be reduced. Starch normally is digested by salivary and pancreatic α-amylases to yield disaccharides (maltose), trisaccharides (maltotriose), and oligosaccharides (dextrin). The oligosaccharidases responsible for final hydrolysis of these materials are all located in the brush border of the small intestine and consist of two classes. The β-galactosidases hydrolyze β-disaccharides, such as lactose, whereas the α-glucosidases act on α-disaccharides, such as maltose, isomaltose, and sucrose (78).

Structure Activity Relationships

An extensive search for α-glucosidase inhibitors from microbial cultures led to the isolation of acarbose from an actinomycete (Fig. 32.14) (79). Extensive structure–activity investigations revealed that active α-glucosidase inhibitors have a common pharmacophore, comprising a substituted cyclohexane ring and a 4,6-dideoxy-4-amino-D-glucose unit known as carvosine. It appears that the

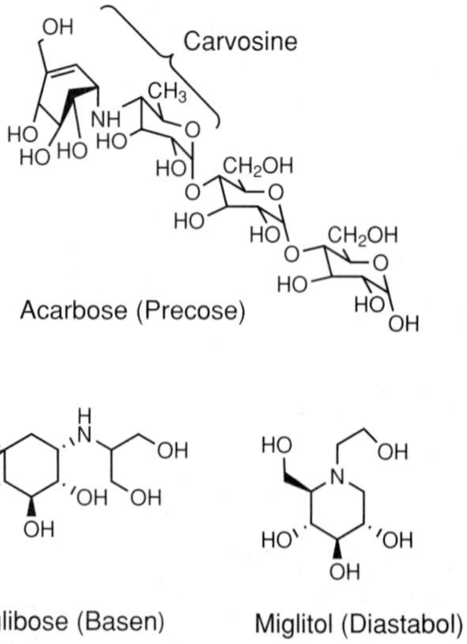

Carvosine

Acarbose (Precose)

Voglibose (Basen)

Miglitol (Diastabol)

Fig. 32.14. α-Glucosidase inhibitors.

secondary amino group of this core structure prevents an essential carboxyl group of the α-glucosidase from protonating the glycosidic oxygen bonds of the substrate (80).

More recently, screening programs of small molecules have yielded several other α-glucosidase inhibitors resembling simple amino sugars, such as miglitol and voglibose (Fig. 32.14).

Therapeutic Applications

Clinical studies on α-glucosidase inhibitors reveal that disaccharide hydrolysis is not blocked but, rather, is delayed. Because acarbose impacts end-stage hydrolysis of both starch and sucrose, however, it affects all primary dietary sources of glucose. Patients with type 2 diabetes have an insulin response that is slow as well as inadequate; therefore, slowing the rate of absorption of glucose following a meal should be helpful in preventing the large postprandial increases in serum glucose, which are associated with degenerative complications of diabetes. Treatment with acarbose in insulin-requiring patients with type 2 diabetes was associated with significantly decreased levels of HbA_{1c} (0.4%) and total daily insulin dose (8.3%) (81). Additionally, significant decreases in fasting glucose and in area under glucose–time curves following a meal. Overall, 45% of patients in the study showed a good clinical response to acarbose therapy. Acarbose is only minimally absorbed (0.5–1.7%) into the bloodstream; therefore, it is not associated with any significant systemic toxicity at normal doses. In the small intestine, amylases and bacteria degrade acarbose. Some of the by-products are systemically absorbed and eliminated in the urine. Because doses in excess of 100 mg three times daily are associated with increased serum transaminase levels indicative of liver damage, doses in excess of 100 mg are not recommended. Acarbose also is not recommended in patients with significant renal dysfunction or who suffer from inflammatory bowel disease, colonic ulceration, or partial intestinal obstruction. The drug does cause annoying flatulence and bloating in approximately 60% of the patients who use it, and it is suggested that this may be overcome by starting with a low dose of the drug and then titrating the dose upward. Acarbose (50–100 mg) is taken with the first bite of each meal.

The small molecule α-glucosidase inhibitor voglibose was marketed in Japan in 1994. It also slows the release of monosaccharides from polymeric materials and, thereby, lowers postprandial glucose levels. Additionally, the drug maintains low levels of glucose, triglycerides, and insulin in genetically obese rats, indicating possible effectiveness in conditions other than diabetes, such as obesity.

Miglitol, introduced in 1998, seems to produce therapeutic results similar to those of acarbose. It causes significant lowering of HbA_{1c} and of postprandial and fasting serum glucose. Unlike acarbose, however, miglitol is rapidly and completely absorbed into the bloodstream following oral administration. It is distributed primarily to the extracellular space, and it is rapidly cleared through the kidney without evidence of hepatic metabolism. It is not transferred into the central nervous system (82,83).

Rimonabant

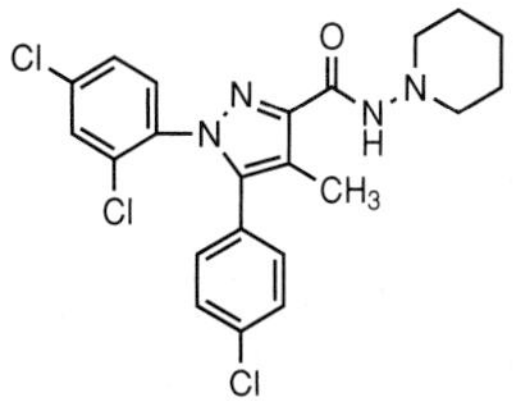

Rimonabant (Acomplia)

Obesity is a major factor leading to type 2 diabetes. As such, effective treatment of obesity may prevent or slow the onset of diabetes. Researchers at Sanofi-Aventis hypothesized that if cannabinoids stimulate appetite in a receptor-specific fashion (e.g., "the munchies"), then blocking central cannabinoid receptors might lead to decreased appetite. Rimonabant was discovered as part of a screening effort directed at the CB1 endocannabinoid receptor. It was found to be a selective and potent antagonist of the receptor. Both preclinical studies with animals and human trials with obese patients indicated that administration of rimonabant led to the decreased consumption of fats and sugar, resulting in weight loss. Additionally, a Phase III trial (the RIO-Diabetes trial) in patients with type 2 diabetes using oral antidiabetic medications demonstrated significant improvement in HbA_{1c}, high-density lipoprotein cholesterol, triglycerides, and systolic blood pressure, along with a reduction in waist circumference (84).

Approaches in Discovery and Development Phases

Considering the medical and economic importance of type 2 diabetes and the need for improvement over existing treatments, new agents for existing targets and the development of new therapeutic targets are being actively pursued in the laboratory and the clinic. Many promising targets are only in the early stages of preclinical development (e.g., small molecule insulin mimetics or glucagon antagonists, glucokinase activators, and β-cell potassium channel openers). Listed below are some selected new classes of therapeutics, some of which are in clinical trials or earlier in research.

Retinoid X Receptor Modulators

The retinoid X receptor (RXR) forms a functional heterodimer with PPARγ as well as other nuclear hormone receptors. The RXR modulators can activate the RXR-PPARγ complex, improving glucose tolerance in animal models; however, selectivity for this particular heterodimer is required to avoid undesirable side effects. Analogues acting by this mechanism are in earlier stages of development.

Protein Tyrosine Phosphatase 1B Inhibitors

It has been observed that mice lacking the protein tyrosine phosphatase 1B (PTP1B) gene generally are normal but have greater insulin sensitivity and gain less weight when given a high-fat diet. The enzyme dephosphorylates both the insulin receptor and the insulin receptor substrate-1, leading to decreased insulin sensitivity. Hence, PTP1B has been an active target for type 2 diabetes drug research. Creating a bioavailable inhibitor has proved to be challenging, however, and research is still ongoing. As an alternative approach, ISIS 113715, which is in Phase II clinical trials, is an antisense oligonucleotide designed to block transcription of PTP1B. The low doses from this trial reduced HbA_{1c} and plasma glucose without causing hypoglycemia.

CASE STUDY

Victoria F. Roche and S. William Zito

BA is an African American male and a former professional football player who at 68 years of age is obese, with a body weight 40% greater than his ideal weight. Along with his obesity, BA has hypertension, hyperlipidemia, and type 2 diabetes. His hypertension is under control with enalapril (10 mg q.d.), and his hyperlipidemia is controlled with atorvastatin (20 mg q.d.). His blood glucose, however, was uncontrollable by diet and glipizide (20 mg q.d.) or by various regimens of insulin (currently regular insulin and NPH insulin administered subcutaneously in the morning and at bedtime, respectively). Last week, BA had laboratory tests, and his results showed that he had developed mild diabetic nephropathy (creatinine clearance, 75 mL/min; urine albumin, 590 g/24 hours). His blood tests showed continued uncontrollable fasting plasma glucose (202 mg/dL; HbA_{1c}, 11%), and now his physician wants to add an oral antidiabetic drug to his insulin therapy. Evaluate structures 1 thought 4 for use in this case.

1. Identify the therapeutic problem(s) in which the pharmacist's intervention may benefit the patient.
2. The physician seeks your advice in selecting an oral antidiabetic agent (other than glipizide) to add to BA's insulin treatment. Identify and prioritize the patient-specific factors that must be considered to achieve the desired therapeutic outcomes.
3. Conduct a thorough and mechanistically oriented structure–activity analysis of all therapeutic alternatives provided in the case.
4. Evaluate the structure–activity relationship findings against the patient-specific factors and desired therapeutic outcomes, and make a therapeutic decision.
5. Counsel your patient.

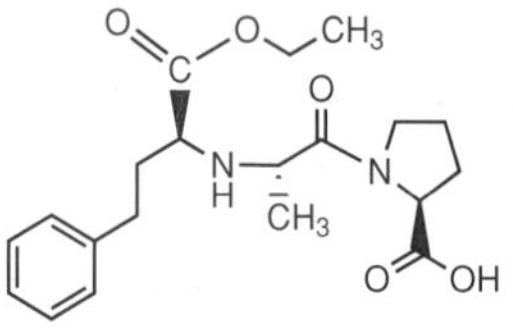

Enalapril

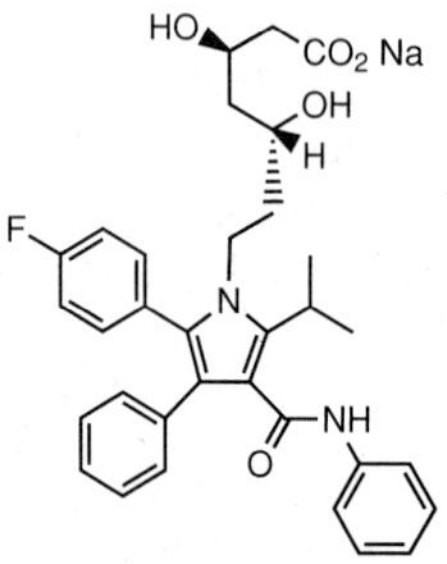

Atorvastatin

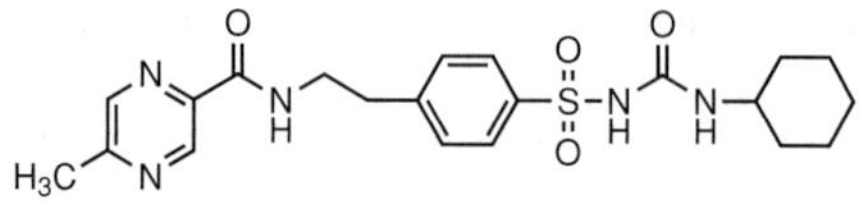

Glipizide

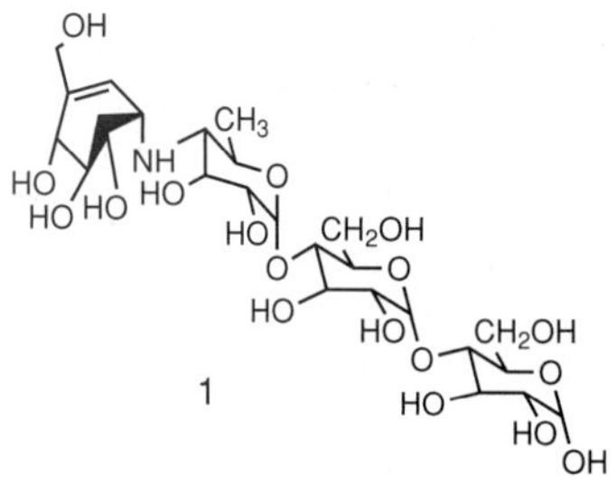

1

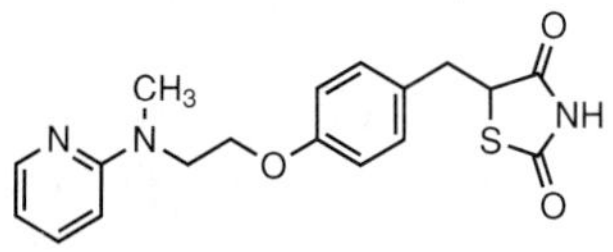

2

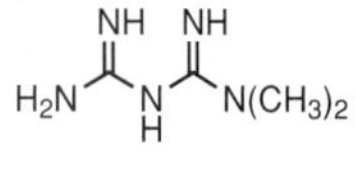

3

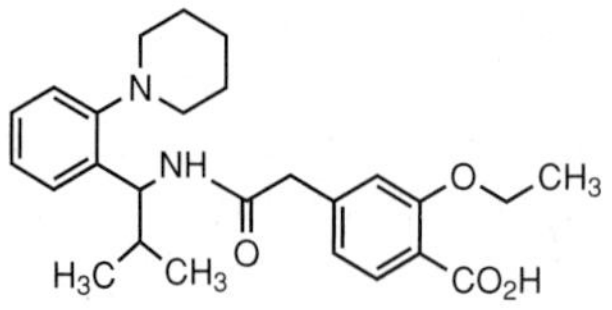

4

References

1. Pizzi RA. Defying diabetes: The discovery of insulin. Modern Drug Discovery 2000(July/Aug)3(6):77–80.
2. APhA Special Report. New approaches to insulin therapy for diabetes. American Pharmaceutical Association, Washington DC 2001.
3. Stumvoll M, Goldstein BJ, Van Haeften TW. Type 2 diabetes: principles of pathogenesis and therapy. Lancet 2005;365:1333–1346.
4. White JR, Campbell RK. Type 2 diabetes and insulin resistance: counseling patients in the pharmacy. US Pharmacist 2003(Apr)28(4):65–87.
5. Davis SN, Granner DK. Insulin, oral hypoglycemic agents, and the pharmacology of the endocrine pancreas. In: Jardman JG, Limbird LE, eds. Goodman & Gilman's The Pharmacological Basis of Therapeutics. 10th Ed. New York: McGraw-Hill Medical Publishing Division, 2001:1679–1714.
6. Owens DR, Zinman B, Bolli GB. Insulins today and beyond. Lancet 2001;358:739–746.
7. Thayer A. Insulin. Chem Engineering News 2005(June 20)83:74–75.
8. Peragallo-Dittko V. Current strategies in insulin replacement therapy. Diabetes Trends 2004(Sept, Suppl):17–23.
9. American Diabetes Association. Diagnosis and classification of diabetes mellitus. Diabetes Care 2004;27:S5–S10.
10. Saljoughian M. Gestational diabetes. US Pharmacist 2004(Sept)29(4):HS-3-7.
11. Fajans SS, Bell GI, Polonsky KS. Molecular mechanisms and clinical pathophysiology of maturity-onset diabetes of the young. N Engl J Med 2001;345: 971–980.
12. Sheehan JP. Fasting hyperglycemia: etiology, diagnosis, and treatment. Diabetes Technology & Therap 2004;6:525–533.
13. American Diabetes Association. Insulin administration. Diabetes Care 2004;27:S106–S109.
14. Yang Q, Graham TE, Mody N, et al. Serum retinol binding protein 4 contributes to insulin resistance in obesity and type 2 diabetes. Nature 2005;436: 356–362.
15. APhA Special Report. Managing insulin resistance. American Pharmaceutical Association, Washington DC 1999.
16. Brownlee M. The pathological implications of protein glycation. Clin Invest Med 1995;18:275–281.
17. New drug review. US Pharmacist 2004(Oct);29:86–87.
18. Fong DS, Aiello LP, Ferris FL, et al. Diabetic retinopathy. Diabetes Care 2004;27:2540–2553.
19. Gross JL, De Azevedo MJ, Silveiro SP, et al. Diabetic nephropathy: diagnosis, prevention, and treatment. Diabetes Care 2005;28:176–188.
20. Duby JJ, Campbell RK, Setter SM, et al. Diabetic neuropathy: an intensive review. Am J Health-Syst Pharm 2004;61:160–176.
21. Madsen P, Knudsen LB, Wiberg FC, et al. Discovery and structure–activity relationship of the first nonpeptide competitive human glucagon receptor antagonists. J Med Chem 1998;41:5150–5157.
22. Rossowski WJ, Coy DH. Potent inhibitory effects of a type four receptor-selective somatostatin analogue on rat insulin release. Biochem Biophys Res Commun 1993;197:366–371.
23. Bruns C, Lewis I, Briner U, et al. SOM230: a novel somatostatin peptidomimetic with broad somatotropin release inhibiting factor (SRIF) receptor binding and a unique antisecretory profile. Eur J Endocrinol 2002;146:707–716.
24. Afargan M, Tiensuu Janson E, Gelerman G, et al. Novel long-acting somatostatin analogue with endocrine selectivity: potent suppression of growth hormone but not of insulin. Endocrinology 2001;142:477–486.
25. Campbell PJ, Bolli GB, Gerich JE. Prevention of the dawn phenomenon (early morning hyperglycemia) in insulin-dependent diabetes mellitus by bedtime intranasal administration of a long-acting somatostatin analogue. Metabolism 1988;37:34–37.
26. Casini G, Catalani E, Dal Monte M, et al. Functional aspects of the somatostatinergic system in the retina and the potential therapeutic role of somatostatin in retinal disease. Histol Histopathol 2005;20:615–632.
27. Buse JB, Weyer C, Maggs DG. Amylin replacement with pramlintide in type 1 and type 2 diabetes: a physiological approach to overcome barriers with insulin therapy. Clin Diabetes 2002;20:137–144.
28. Kolterman O, Buse J, Fineman M, et al. Synthetic exendin-4 (exenatide) significantly reduces postprandial and fasting glucose in subjects with type 2 diabetes. J Clin Endocrinol Metab 2003;88:3082–3089.
29. Kadowaki T, Yamauchi T. Adiponectin and adiponectin receptors. Endocr Rev 2005;26:439–451.
30. Balagopal P, George D, Yarandi H, et al. Reversal of obesity-related hypoadiponectinemia by lifestyle intervention—a controlled randomized study in obese adolescents. J Clin Endocrinol Metab 2005;90:6192–6197.
31. Nomura S, Shouza A, Omoto S, et al. 5-HT_{2A} receptor antagonist increases circulating adiponectin in patients with type 2 diabetes. Blood Coagul Fibrinolysis 2005;16:423–428.
32. Heise T, et al. The effect of insulin antibodies on the metabolic action of inhaled and subcutaneous insulin. Diabetes Care 2005;28:2161–2169.
33. Wollmer A, Rannefeld B, Johansen BR, et al. Phenol promoted structural transformation of insulin in solution. Biol Chem Hoppe Seyler 1987;368: 903–911.
34. Brange J, Langkjaer J. Insulin structure and stability. In: Wang YL, Pearlman R, eds. Stability and Characterization of Protein and Peptide Drugs. New York: Plenum Press, 1993:315–350.
35. Polaschegg E. Effect of physicochemical variables of regular insulin formulations on their absorption from the subcutaneous tissue. Diabetes Res Clin Pract 1998;40:39–44.
36. Scott DA. Crystalline insulin. Biochem J 1934;28:1592–1602.
37. Constantino HR, Liauw S, Mitragotri S, et al., The pharmaceutical development of insulin: historical perspectives and future directions. In: Shahrokh Z, Sluzky V, Cleland JL, et al., Eds. Therapeutic protein and peptide formulation and delivery. American Chemical Society Symposium Series, Washington DC, American Chemical Society 1997;675:29–66.
38. Smith GD, Swenson DC, Dodson EJ, et al. Structural stability in 4-zinc human insulin hexamer. Proc Natl Acad Sci U S A 1984;81:7093–7097.
39. Brange J, Andersen L, Laursen ED, et al. Toward understanding insulin fibrillation. J Pharm Sci 1997;86:517–525.
40. Brange J, Whittingham J, Edwards D. Insulin structure and diabetes treatment. Current Science India 1997;72:470–476.
41. Maislos M, Mead PM, Gaynor DH, et al. The source of the circulating aggregate of insulin in type I diabetic patients is therapeutic insulin. J Clin Invest 1986;77:717–723.
42. Davis SN. Insulin, oral hypoglycemic agents, and the pharmacology of the endocrine pancreas. In: Brunton LL, Lazo JS, Parker KL, eds. Goodman & Gilman's The Pharmacological Basis of Therapeutics. 11th Ed. New York: McGraw-Hill, 2006:1613–1645.
43. DCCT Research Group. Retinopathy and nephropathy in patients with type 1 diabetes four years after a trial of intensive therapy. The Diabetes Control and Complications Trial/Epidemiology of Diabetes Interventions and Complications Research Group. N Engl J Med 2000;342:381–389.
44. Auer RN. Hypoglycemic brain damage. Metab Brain Dis 2004;19:169–175.
45. Hirsch IB. Insulin analogues. N Engl J Med 2005;352:174–183.
46. Chapman TM, Perry CM. Insulin detemir: a review of its use in the management of type 1 and 2 diabetes mellitus. Drugs 2004;64:2577–2595.
47. Parker JC, McPherson RK, Andrews KM, et al. Effects of skyrin, a receptor-selective glucagons antagonist, in rat and human hepatocytes. Diabetes 2000;49:2079–2086.
48. Sarabu R, Tilley J. Recent advances in therapeutic approaches to type 2 diabetes. Annu Rep Med Chem 2004;39:41–56.
49. Ryan GJ, Jobe LJ, Martin R. Pramlintide in the treatment of type 1 and type 2 diabetes mellitus. Clin Ther 2005;27:1500–1512.
50. Kruger DF, Gloster MA. Pramlintide for the treatment of insulin-requiring diabetes mellitus: rationale and review of clinical data. Drugs 2004;64: 1419–1432.
51. Dalton LW. Drugs for diabetes. Chem Engineering News 2004(Oct 25); 82:59–67.
52. Fehse F, Trautmann M, Holst JJ. et al. Exenatide augments first- and second-phase insulin secretion in response to intravenous glucose in subjects with type 2 diabetes. J Clin Endocrinol Metab 2005;90:5991–5997.
53. Keating GM. Exenatide. Drugs 2005;65:1681–1692.
54. Poon T, Nelson P, Shen L, et al. Exenatide improves glycemic control and reduces body weight in subjects with type 2 diabetes: a dose-ranging study. Diabetes Technol Ther 2005;7:467–477.
55. Nauck MA, Meier JJ. Glucagon-like peptide 1 and its derivatives in the treatment of diabetes. Regul Pept 2005;128:135–148.
56. Augeri DJ, Robl JA, Betebenner DA, et al. Discovery and preclinical profile of saxagliptin (BMS-477118): a highly potent, long-acting, orally active dipeptidyl peptidase IV inhibitor for the treatment of type 2 diabetes. J Med Chem 2005;48:5025–5037.
57. Ahren B, Pacini G, Foley JE, et al. Improved meal-related β-cell function and insulin sensitivity by the dipeptidyl peptidase-IV inhibitor vildagliptin in metformin-treated patients with type 2 diabetes over 1 year. Diabetes Care 2005;28:1936–1940.
58. Sheehan MT. Current therapeutic options in type 2 diabetes mellitus: a practical approach. Clin Med Res 2003;1:189–200.
59. Rorsman P, Renstrom E. Insulin granule dynamics in pancreatic beta cells. Diabetologica 2003;46:1029–1045.
60. Proks P, Reimann F, Green N, et al. Sulfonylurea stimulation of insulin secretion. Diabetes 2002;51:S368–S376.
61. Lins L, Brasseur R, Malaisse WJ. Conformational analysis of nonsulfonylurea hypoglycemic agents of the meglitinide family. Biochem Pharmacol 1995;50: 1879–1884.
62. Jellin JM, Gregory P, Batz F, et al. Goat's Rid. In: Pharmacist's Letter/Prescriber's Letter Natural Medicines Comprehensive Database. 3rd Ed. Stockton, CA Therapeutic Research Faculty; 2000:501.
63. Krentz AJ, Bailey CJ. Oral antidiabetic agents: current role in type 2 diabetes. Drugs 2005;65:385–411.
64. Zhou GC, Myers R, Chen YL, et al. Role of AMP-activated protein kinase in mechanism of metformin action. J Clin Invest 2001;108:1167–1174.
65. Zangeneh F, Kudva YC, Basu A. Insulin sensitizers. Mayo Clin Proc 2003;78:471–479.
66. Huypens P, Quartier E, Pipeleers D, et al. Metformin reduces adiponectin protein expression and the release in 3T3-L1 adipocytes involving activation of AMP activated protein kinase. Eur J Pharmacol 2005;518:90–95.
67. Somogyi A, Stockley C, Keal J, et al. Reduction of metformin renal tubular secretion by cimetidine in man. Br J Clin Pharmacol 1987;23: 545–551.

68. UK Prospective Diabetes Study Group. Effect of intensive blood-glucose control with metformin on complications in overweight patients with type 2 diabetes (IKPDS 34). Lancet 1998;352:854–865.
69. Driscoll J, Ghazzi M, Perez PE, et al. 96-Week follow up on cardiac safety in patients with type II diabetes treated with troglitazone. Diabetes 1997; 46(Suppl 1):149A.
70. Valiquett T, Huang S, Whitcomb R. Effects of troglitazone monotherapy in patients with NIDDM: a 6-month multicenter study. Diabetes 1997;46(Suppl 1):43A.
71. Kawai K, Kawasaki-Tokui Y, Odaka T, et al. Disposition and metabolism of the new oral antidiabetic drug troglitazone in rats, mice, and dogs. Arzneimittelforschung 1997;47:356–368.
72. Yamazaki H, Shibata A, Suzuki M, et al. Oxidation of troglitazone to a quinone-type metabolite catalyzed by cytochrome P-450 2C8 and P-450 3A4 in human liver microsomes. Drug Metab Dispos 1999;27:1260–1266.
73. Krieter PA, Colletti AE, Doss GA, et al. Disposition and metabolism of the hypoglycemic agent pioglitazone in rats. Drug Metab Dispos 1994;22:625–630.
74. Tanis SP, Parker TT, Colca JR, et al. Synthesis and biological activity of metabolites of the antidiabetic, antihyperglycemic agent pioglitazone. J Med Chem 1996;39:5053–5063.
75. Cox PJ, Ryan DA, Hollis FJ, et al. Absorption, disposition, and metabolism of rosiglitazone, a potent thiazolidinedione insulin sensitizer, in humans. Drug Metab Dispos 2000;28:772–780.
76. Substituting for troglitazone (Rezulin). Med Lett 2000;42:36.
77. Buse JB, Rubin CJ, Frederich R, et al. Muraglitazar, a dual (α/γ) PPAR activator: a randomized, double-blind, placebo-controlled, 24-week monotherapy trial in adult patients with type 2 diabetes. Clin Ther 2005;27:1181–1195.
78. Clissold SP, Edwards C. Acarbose. A preliminary review of its pharmacodynamic and pharmacokinetic properties, and therapeutic potential. Drugs 1988;35:214–243.
79. Schmidt DD, Frommer W, Junge B, et al. α-Glucosidase inhibitors. New complex oligosaccharides of microbial origin. Naturwissenschaften 1977;64: 535–536.
80. Heiker FR, Boeshagen H, Junge B, et al. Studies designed to localize the essential structural unit of glycoside-hydrolase inhibitors of the carbose type. In: Crutzfeld W, ed. Proceedings of the First International Symposium on Acarbose. Montreux: Excerpta Medica, 1981:137–141.
81. Coniff RF, Shapiro JA, Seaton TB, et al. A double-blind placebo-controlled trial evaluating the safety and efficacy of acarbose for the treatment of patients with insulin-requiring type II diabetes. Diabetes Care 1995;18:928–932.
82. Segal P, Feig PU, Schernthaner G, et al. The efficacy and safety of miglitol therapy compared with glibenclamide in patients with NIDDM inadequately controlled by diet alone. Diabetes Care 1997;20:687–691.
83. Ahr, HJ, Boberg M, Brendel E, et al. Pharmacokinetics of miglitol. Absorption, distribution, metabolism, and excretion following administration to rats, dogs, and man. Arzneimittelforschung 1997;47:734–745.
84. Boyd ST, Fremming BA. Rimonabant. A selective CB1 antagonist. Ann Pharmacother 2005;39:684–690.

33. *Adrenocorticoids*

DUANE D. MILLER, ROBERT W. BRUEGGEMEIER AND JAMES T. DALTON

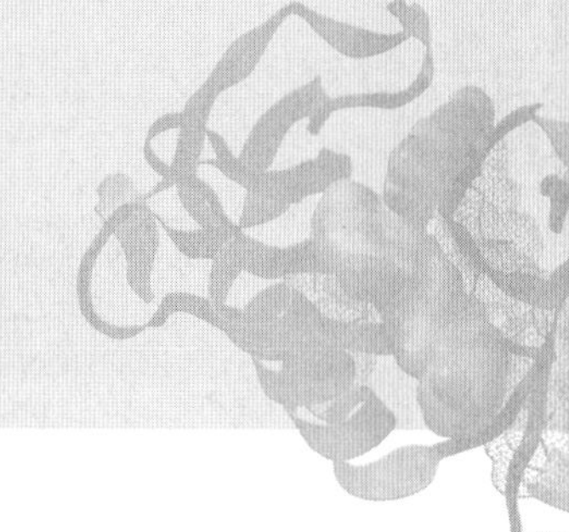

DRUGS COVERED IN THIS CHAPTER:

GLUCOCORTICOSTEROIDS
- Betamethasone
- Dexamethasone
- Fludrocortisone
- Hydrocortisone and derivatives
- Methylprednisolone
- Prednisone and prednisolone
- Triamcinolone

GLUCORTICOSTEROIDS USED TOPICALLY OR FOR INHALATION
- Beclomethasone dipropionate
- Budesonide
- Clobetasol propionate
- Flunisolide
- Fluocinolone acetonide
- Fluocinonide
- Fluorometholone
- Flurandrenolide
- Fluticasone propionate
- Halcinonide
- Halobetasol propionate
- Mometasone furoate
- Triamcinolone acetonide

MINERALOCORTICOSTEROIDS
- Aldosterone
- 11-Desoxycorticosterone

ADRENOCORTICOID ANTAGONISTS
- Aminoglutethimide
- Metyrapone
- Trilostane

INTRODUCTION

The adrenal glands are flattened, cap-like structures located above the kidneys. The inner core (medulla) of the gland secretes catecholamines, whereas the shell (cortex) of the gland synthesizes steroid hormones known as the adrenocorticoids. The adrenocorticoid steroids include the glucocorticoids, which regulate carbohydrate, lipid, and protein metabolism, and the mineralocorticoids, which influence salt balance and water retention. A third class of steroids produced by the adrenal glands is called the adrenal androgens, which have weak androgenic activity in men and women and can serve as precursors to the sex hormones, estrogens and androgens.

The adrenocorticoids (this chapter) and sex hormones (see Chapters 45 and 46) have much in common. All are steroids; consequently, the rules that define their structures, chemistry, and nomenclature are the same. The rings of these biochemically dynamic and physiologically active compounds have a similar stereochemical relationship. Changes in the geometry of the ring junctures generally result in inactive compounds regardless of the biological category of the steroid. Similar chemical groups are used to render some of these agents water soluble or active when taken orally or to modify their absorption.

In addition, the adrenocorticoids and the sex hormones, which include the estrogens, progestins, and androgens, are biosynthesized mainly from cholesterol (see Chapter 30), which in turn is synthesized from acetyl–coenzyme A. Cholesterol and steroid hormone catabolism take place primarily in the liver. Although the products found in the urine and feces depend on the hormone undergoing catabolism, many of the metabolic reactions are similar for these compounds. For example, reduction of double bonds at positions 4 and 5 or 5 and 6, epimerization of 3α-hydroxyl groups, reduction of 3-keto groups to the 3α-hydroxyl function, and oxidative removal of side chains are transformations common to these agents.

Despite the similarities in chemical structures and stereochemistry, each class of steroids demonstrates unique and distinctively different biological activities. Minor structural modifications to the steroid nucleus, such as changes in or insertion of functional groups at different positions, cause marked changes in physiologic activity. The first part of this chapter focuses on the similarities among the steroids and reviews steroid nomenclature, stereochemistry, and general mechanism of action. The second portion of the chapter focuses on the adrenocorticoids and discusses the biosynthesis, metabolism, medicinal chemistry, pharmacology, and pharmacokinetics of endogenous steroid hormones, synthetic agonists, and synthetic antagonists.

STEROID NOMENCLATURE AND STRUCTURE

Steroids consist of four fused rings (A, B, C, and D) (Fig. 33.1). Chemically, these hydrocarbons are cyclopentanoperhydrophenanthrenes; they contain a five-membered cyclopentane (D) ring plus the three rings of phenanthrene. A perhydrophenanthrene (rings A, B, and C) is the completely saturated derivative of phenanthrene. The polycyclic hydrocarbon known as 5α-cholestane will be used to illustrate the numbering system for a steroid (Fig. 33.1). The term "cholestane" refers to a steroid with 27 carbons that includes a side chain of eight carbons at position 17. Numbering begins

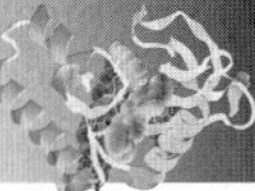

CLINICAL SIGNIFICANCE

Few groups of drugs can rival the adrenocorticoids, which are used for the widest variety of conditions. From asthma to rheumatologic diseases to dermatological disorders, the adrenocorticoids are commonly prescribed for their beneficial action, but unfortunately, they also exhibit toxicity. Only by understanding their complicated mechanisms of action can pharmacists help in maximizing the therapeutic benefits while minimizing the numerous adverse effects of these agents.

Pharmacists must be familiar with the numerous steroid products and dosage forms that are available as well as with the structure-activity relationships that determine their effects at different receptors. By understanding these factors, the likelihood that patients will derive significant benefits without untoward toxicities is significantly increased.

Finally, an appreciation concerning the role of endogenous mineralocorticoids in the pathophysiology of other diseases, such as heart failure and hypertension, is growing. An understanding of how the structure of endogenous and exogenous mineralocorticoids affects their physiologic properties provides insight regarding how drugs that antagonize this system may provide therapeutic benefits for these and other conditions.

Jeffrey T. Scherer, Pharm.D., MPH, BCPS, CGP
Clinical Assistant Professor
University of Houston College of Pharmacy

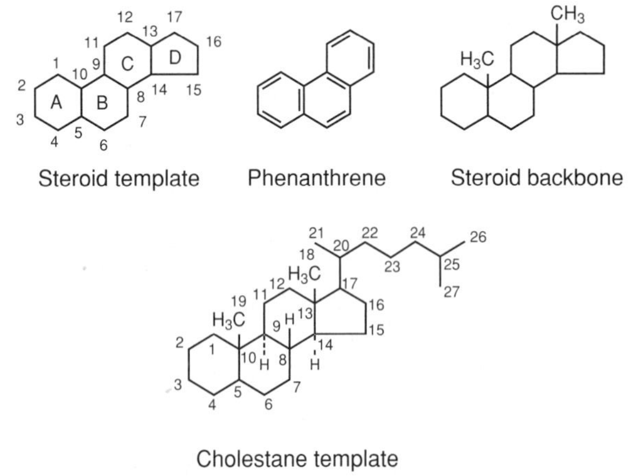

Steroid template Phenanthrene Steroid backbone

Cholestane template

Fig. 33.1. Basic steroid structure and numbering system.

in ring A at C1 and proceeds around rings A and B to C10, then into ring C beginning with C11, and snakes around rings C and D to C17. The angular methyl groups are numbered 18 (attached to C13) and 19 (attached to C10). The 17 side chain begins with C20, and the numbering finishes in sequential order. Using the planar representation for drawing the steroid structure (Fig. 33.2), the basic steroid structure becomes a plane with two surfaces: A top or β surface is pointing out toward the reader, and the bottom or α surface is pointing away from the reader. Hydrogens or functional groups on the β side of the molecule are denoted by solid lines; those on the α side are designated by dotted lines. The 5α notation is used to denote the configuration of the hydrogen atom at C5, which is opposite from the C19 angular methyl group, making the A/B ring juncture *trans*. The C19 angular methyl group is assigned the β side of the molecule. Similarly, the configuration of the 8β and 9α hydrogens, and the 14α hydrogen and C18 angular methyl group, denote *trans* fusion for rings B/C and C/D. The side chains at position 17 are always β unless indicated by dotted lines or in the nomenclature of the steroid (e.g., 17β or 17α).

Just as cyclohexane can be drawn in a chair conformation, the three-dimensional representation for 5α-cholestane is shown by the following conformational formula. Although cyclohexane may undergo a flip in conformation, steroids are rigid structures, because they generally have at least one *trans* fused ring system and these rings must be diequatorial to each other.

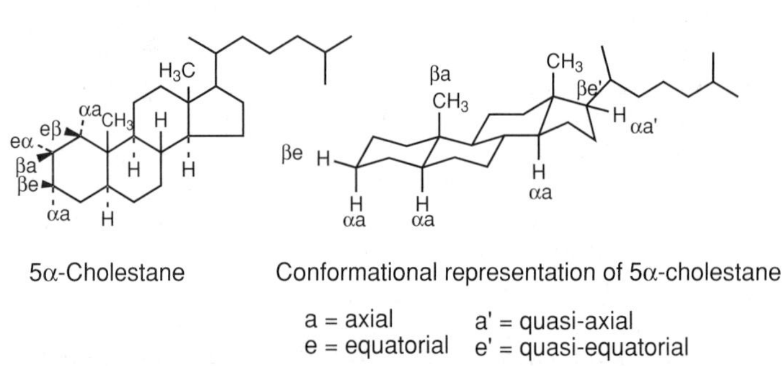

5α-Cholestane Conformational representation of 5α-cholestane

a = axial a' = quasi-axial
e = equatorial e' = quasi-equatorial

Fig. 33.2. Planar and conformational structures of 5α-cholestane.

β-cholestane.

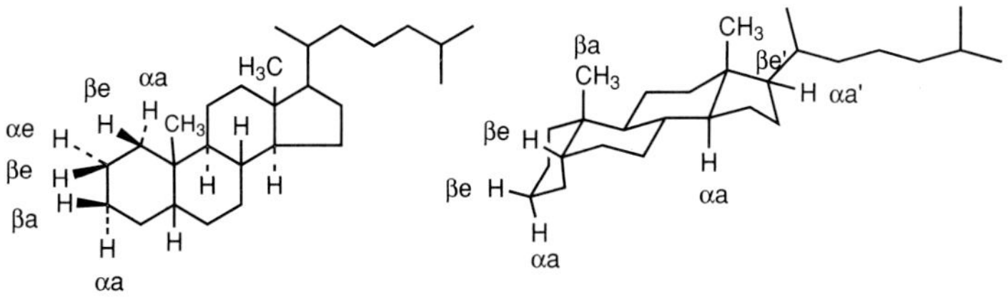

5β-Cholestane

Conformational representation of 5β-cholestane

a = axial a' = quasi-axial
e = equatorial e' = quasi-equatorial

Fig. 33.3. Planar and conformational structures of 5β-cholestane.

If one is aware that the angular methyl groups at positions 18 and 19 are β and have an axial orientation (i.e., perpendicular to the plane of the rings), the conformational orientation of the remaining bonds of a steroid can be easily assigned. For example, in 5α-cholestane, the C19 methyl group attached at position 10 is always β-axial; the two bonds at position 3 must be β-equatorial and α-axial, as indicated. The orientation of the remaining bonds on a steroid may be determined if one recalls that groups on a cyclohexane ring that are positioned on adjacent carbon atoms (vicinal, —C_1H—C_2H—) of the ring (i.e., 1,2 to each other) are *trans* if their relationship is 1,2-diaxial or 1,2-diequatorial and are *cis* if their relationship is 1,2-equatorial-axial.

Steroid chemists often refer to the series of carbon–carbon bonds shown with heavy lines as the backbone of the steroid (Fig. 33.1). The *cis* or *trans* relationship of the four rings may be expressed in terms of the backbone. The compound 5α-cholestane (Fig. 33.2) is said to have a *trans-anti-trans-anti-trans* backbone. In this structure, all the fused rings have *trans* (diequatorial) stereochemistry; in other words, the A/B fused ring, the B/C fused ring, and the C/D fused ring are *trans.* The term *anti* is used in backbone notation to define the orientation of rings that are connected to each other and have a *trans*-type relationship. For example, the bond equatorial to ring B, at position 9, which forms part of ring C, is *anti* to the bond equatorial to ring B, at position 10, which forms part of ring A. 5β-Cholestane (Fig. 33.3) has a *cis-anti-trans-anti-trans* backbone in which the A/B rings are fused *cis.* The term *syn* is used in a similar fashion as *anti* to define a *cis*-type relationship. No natural steroids exist with a *syn*-type geometry, although such compounds can be chemically synthesized. Thus, the conventional drawing of the steroid nucleus is the natural configuration and does not show the hydrogens at 8β, 9α, or 14β positions. If the carbon at position 5 is saturated, the hydrogen is always drawn as either 5α or 5β. Also, the conventional drawing of a steroid molecule has the C18 and C19 methyl groups shown only as solid lines (no CH_3 drawn).

The stereochemistry of the rings markedly affects the biological activity of a given class of steroids. Nearly all biologically active steroids have the cholestane-type backbone. In most of the important steroids discussed in this chapter, a double bond is present between positions 4 and 5 or 5 and 6; consequently, there is no *cis* or *trans* relationship between rings A and B. The symbol Δ often is used to designate a carbon–carbon double bond (C═C) in a steroid. If the C═C is between positions 4 and 5, the compound is referred to as a Δ^4-steroid. If the C═C is between positions 5 and 10, the compound is designated a $\Delta^{5(10)}$-steroid.

Cholesterol (cholest-5-en-3α-ol) is a Δ^5-steroid or, more specifically, a Δ^5-sterol, because it is an unsaturated alcohol. Biologically active compounds include members of the 5α-pregnane, 5α-androstane, and 5α-estrane steroid classes (Fig. 33.4). Pregnanes are steroids with 21 carbon atoms, androstanes 19 carbon atoms, and estranes 18 carbon atoms, with the C19 angular methyl group at C10 replaced by hydrogen. Numbering is the same as in 5α-cholestane.

The adrenocorticoids (adrenal cortex hormones) are pregnanes and are exemplified by cortisone, which is a 17α,21-dihydroxypregn-4-ene-3,11,20-trione. The acetate ester is named 17α,21-dihydroxypregn-4-ene-3,11,20-trione 21-acetate (cortisone acetate) (Fig. 33.4). Progesterone (pregn-4-ene-3,20-dione), a female sex hormone synthesized by the corpus luteum, also is a pregnane analogue. The male sex hormones (androgens) are based on the structure of 5α-androstane. Testosterone, an important and naturally occurring androgen, is named 17β-hydroxyandrost-4-en-3-one. Dehydroepiandrosterone (DHEA) is the major adrenal androgen and is named 3β-hydroxyandrost-5-en-17-one (Fig. 33.4). The estrogens, which are female sex hormones synthesized by the graafian follicle of the ovaries, are estrane analogues containing an aromatic A ring. Although the A ring does not contain isolated C═C groups, these analogues are named as if the bonds were in the positions shown in 17β-estradiol. Hence, 17β-estradiol, a typical member of this class of

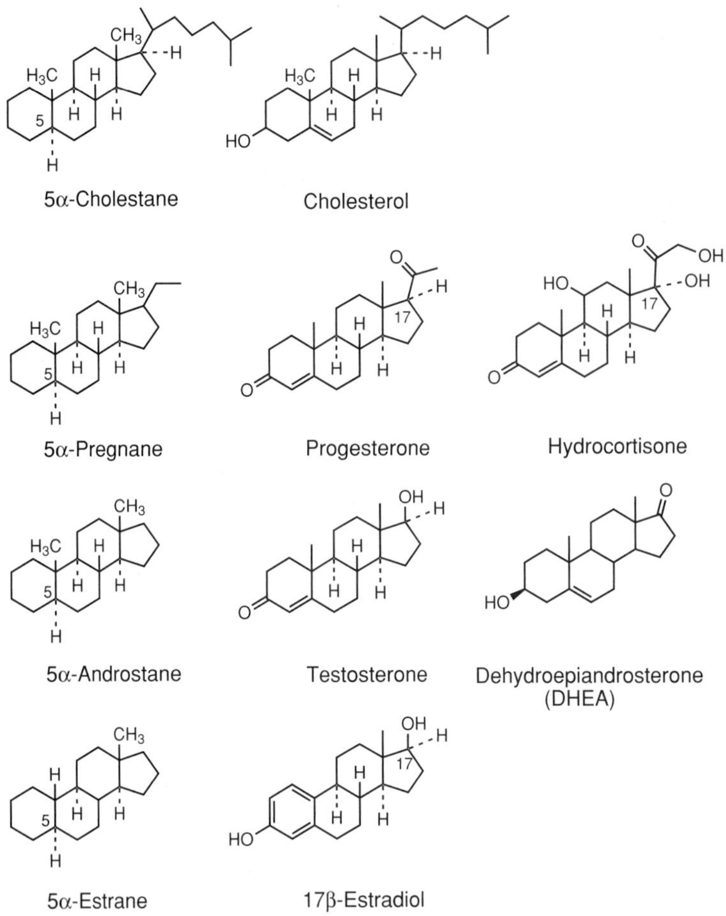

5α-Cholestane Cholesterol

5α-Pregnane Progesterone Hydrocortisone

5α-Androstane Testosterone Dehydroepiandrosterone (DHEA)

5α-Estrane 17β-Estradiol

Fig. 33.4. Steroid classes and corresponding natural hormones.

drugs, is named estra-1,3,5,(10)-triene-3,17β-diol. Other examples of steroid nomenclature are found throughout this chapter.

Aliphatic side chains at position 17 are always assumed to be β when cholestane or pregnane nomenclature is employed. Hence, the notation 17β need not be used when naming these compounds. If a pregnane has a 17α chain, however, this should be indicated in the nomenclature. Finally, the final "e" in the name for the parent steroid hydrocarbon is always dropped when it precedes a vowel, regardless of whether a number appears between the two parts of the word (e.g., note the nomenclature for cholesterol and testosterone versus that for cortisone). For a more extensive discussion of steroid nomenclature, consult the literature (1).

MECHANISM OF STEROID HORMONE ACTION

In addition to their structural similarities, adrenocorticoids, estrogens, progestins, and androgens share a common mode of action. They are present in the body only in extremely low concentrations (e.g., 0.1–1.0 nM), they exert potent physiologic effects on sensitive tissues, and they bind with high affinity to intracellular receptors. Extensive research activities directed at elucidation of the general mechanism of steroid hormone action have been performed for several decades, and many reviews have appeared (2–7).

The steroid hormones act on target cells to regulate gene expression and protein biosynthesis via the formation of steroid–receptor complexes, as outlined in Figure 33.5. The lipophilic steroid hormones are carried in the bloodstream, with the majority of the hormones reversibly bound to serum carrier proteins. The free steroids can diffuse through the cell membrane and enter cells. Those cells sensitive to the particular steroid hormone (referred to as target cells) contain steroid receptors capable of high-affinity binding with the steroid. These receptors are soluble intracellular proteins that can both bind steroid ligands with high affinity and act as transcriptional factors via interaction with specific DNA sites. Early studies suggested that the unoccupied steroid receptors were located solely in the cytosol of target cells (8). Recent investigations on estrogen, progestin, and androgen action, however, indicate that active, unoccupied receptors also are present in the nucleus of the cell (2,7,9). Before the binding of the

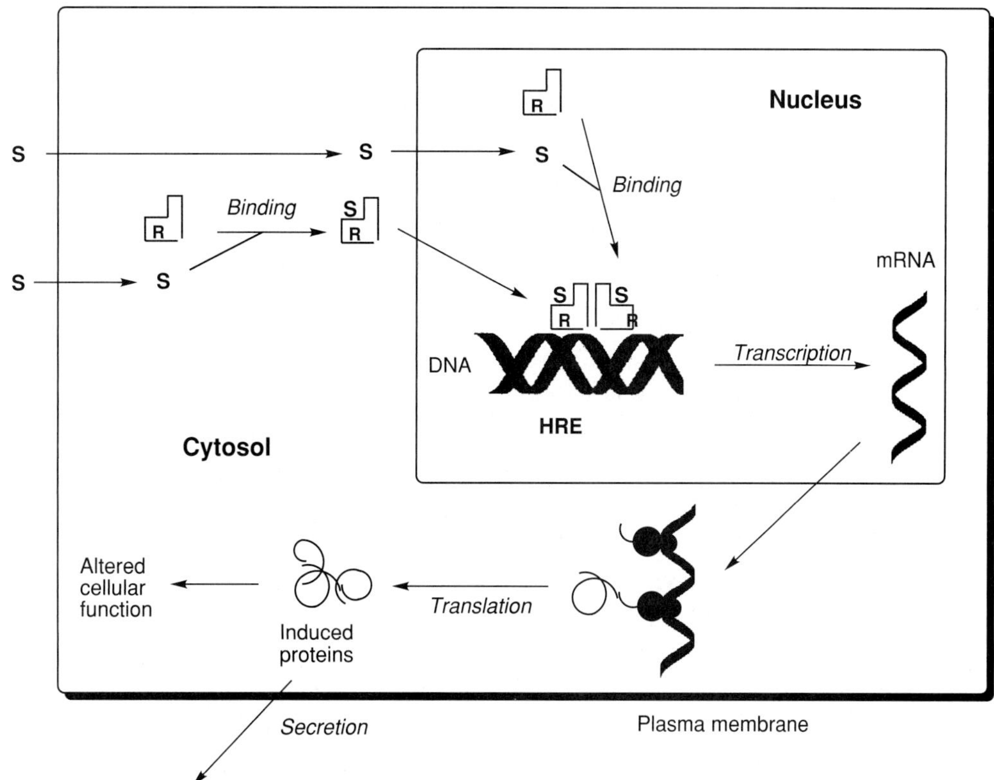

Fig. 33.5. Mechanism of steroid hormone action.

steroid, the steroid receptor is complexed with heat shock proteins. In the current model, the steroid enters the cell and binds to the steroid receptor in the cytoplasm or nucleus. This binding initiates a conformational change and dissociation of the heat shock protein, allowing steroid receptor dimerization and translocation to the nucleus. The receptor dimer interacts with particular regions of the cellular DNA, referred to as hormone-responsive elements (HRE), and with various coactivators and nuclear transcriptional factors. Binding of the nuclear steroid–receptor complex to DNA initiates transcription of the DNA sequence to produce mRNA. Finally, the elevated levels of mRNA lead to an increase in protein synthesis in the endoplasmic reticulum. These proteins include enzymes, receptors, and secreted factors that subsequently result in the steroid hormonal response regulating cell function, growth, and differentiation and playing central roles in normal physiological processes as well as in many important diseases.

The primary amino acid sequences of the various steroid hormone receptors have been deduced from cloned cDNA (3,5). The steroid receptor proteins are part of a larger family of nuclear receptor proteins that also include receptors for vitamin D, thyroid hormones, and retinoids. The overall structures of the receptors have strong similarities (Fig. 33.6). A high degree of homology (sequence similarities) in the steroid receptors is found in the DNA binding region that interacts with the HRE. The DNA binding region has critically placed cysteine amino acids that chelate zinc ions, forming finger-like projections, called zinc fingers, that bind to the DNA. Structure–function studies of cloned receptor proteins also identify regions of the molecules that are important for interactions with nuclear transcriptional factors, coactivator or corepressor proteins, activation of gene transcription, and protein-to-protein interactions. Recent evidence suggests that the protein–protein interactions with AP-1 and/or NFκB (other known transcriptional proteins) work to titrate out the effects of the steroid receptors on DNA. This may be critical for cross-talk between signaling pathways within the cell and may play an important role in feedback systems. Additional evidence suggests that steroid receptors may activate transcription in the absence of hormone, an effect that appears to depend on the phosphorylation of the receptor via cross-talk with membrane-bound adrenergic and/or growth factor receptors (10). The interactions necessary for formation of the steroid–receptor complexes and subsequent activation of gene transcription are complicated, involve multistage processes, and leave many unanswered questions.

The basic mechanism of steroid hormone action on target cells is similar for the various classes of agents. Differences in the actions of adrenocorticoids, estrogens, progestins, and androgens arise from the specificity of

Receptor Structures:

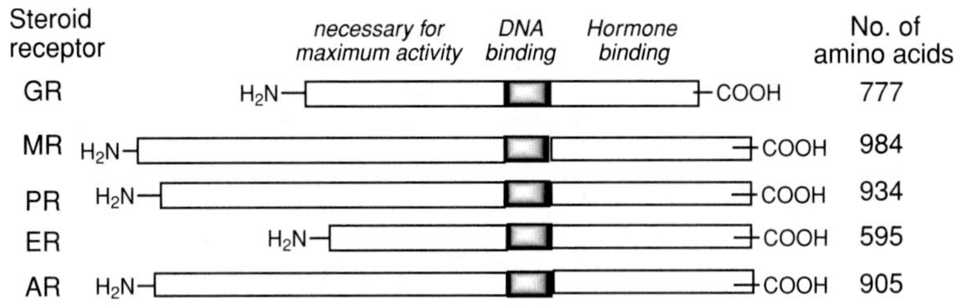

Steroid receptor		necessary for maximum activity	DNA binding	Hormone binding		No. of amino acids
GR	H_2N–		■		–COOH	777
MR	H_2N–		■		–COOH	984
PR	H_2N–		■		–COOH	934
ER	H_2N–		■		–COOH	595
AR	H_2N–		■		–COOH	905

Hormone responsive element (HRE):

	nucleotide sequence
GRE	G G T A C A n n n T G T T C T
MRE	G G T A C A n n n T G T T C T
PRE	G G T A C A n n n T G T T C T
ERE	G G T A C A n n n T G T T C T
ARE	A G G T C A n n n T G A C C T

Fig. 33.6. Structural features of steroid hormone receptors and hormone-responsive elements (HREs). Schematic comparison of the amino acid sequences of steroid receptors (GR, glucocorticoid; MR, mineralocorticoid; PR, progesterone; ER, estrogen; AR, androgen) with high homology in the DNA binding region. The HRE sequences also are compared (GRE, glucocorticoid; MRE, mineralocorticoid; PRE, progesterone; ERE, estrogen; ARE, androgen).

the particular receptor proteins, the particular genetic processes initiated, and the specific cellular proteins produced.

HISTORY AND DISEASE STATES

The importance of the adrenal glands was recognized long ago. Addison's disease, Cushing's disease, and Conn's syndrome are pathological conditions related to the adrenal cortex and the hormones produced by the gland.

Addison's disease was named after Thomas Addison. In 1855, Addison described a syndrome in which the physiologic significance of the adrenal cortex was emphasized (11). This disease is characterized by extreme weakness, anorexia, anemia, nausea and vomiting, low blood pressure, hyperpigmentation of the skin, and mental depression resulting from decreased secretion of steroid hormones by the adrenal cortex. Addison's disease is a rare affliction that affects roughly 1 in 100,000 people and is seen equally in both sexes and in all age groups.

Conditions of this type, generally referred to as hypoadrenalism, may result from several causes, including destruction of the cortex by tuberculosis or atrophy or decreased secretion of adrenocorticotropin (adrenocorticotropic hormone [ACTH]) because of diseases of the anterior pituitary (adenohypophysis). Cushing's disease, or hyperadrenalism, on the other hand, may result from adrenal cortex tumors or increased production of ACTH caused by pituitary carcinoma. Cushing's syndrome also is rare, occurring in only two to five people for every 1 million people each year. Approximately 10 percent of newly diagnosed cases are observed in children and teenagers.

Conn's syndrome is apparently caused by an inability of the adrenal cortex to carry out 17α-hydroxylation during the biosynthesis of the hormones from cholesterol. Consequently, the disease is characterized by a high secretory level of aldosterone, which lacks a 17α-hydroxyl functional group. In addition, hypernatremia, polyuria, alkalosis, and hypertension are observed (12).

The importance of the adrenocorticoids is most dramatically observed in adrenalectomized animals. There is an increase of urea in the blood, muscle weakness (asthenia), decreased liver glycogen, decreased resistance to insulin, lowered resistance to trauma (e.g., cold and mechanical or chemical shock), and electrolyte disturbances. Potassium ions are retained, and excretion of Na^+, Cl^-, and water is increased. Adrenalectomy in small animals causes death in a few days.

After Addison's observations in 1855, physiologists, pharmacologists, and chemists from many countries contributed to our understanding of adrenocorticoids. It was not until 1927, however, that Rogoff and Stewart found that extracts of adrenal glands, administered by intravenous (IV) injection, kept adrenalectomized dogs alive.

Since that discovery, similar experiments have been repeated many times. Originally, the biological activity of the extract was thought to result from a single compound. Later, 47 compounds were isolated from such extracts, and some were highly active. Among the biologically active corticoids isolated, hydrocortisone, corticosterone, aldosterone, cortisone, 11-desoxycorticosterone (17α-hydroxyprogesterone), 11-dehydrocorticosterone (11-desoxycortisol), and 17α-hydroxy-11-desoxycorticosterone were found to be most potent (13). The biosynthesis of these steroids is described below.

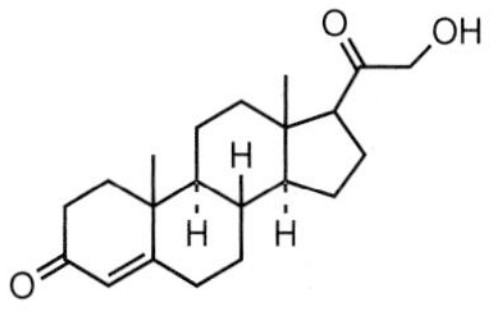

11-Desoxycorticosterone

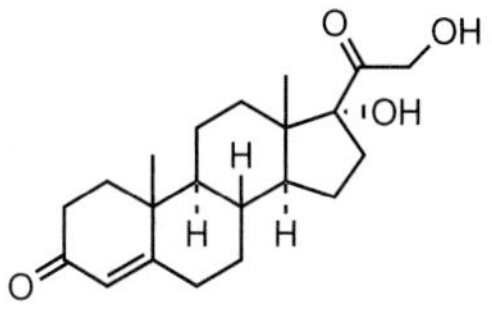

17α-Hydroxy-11-desoxycorticosterone

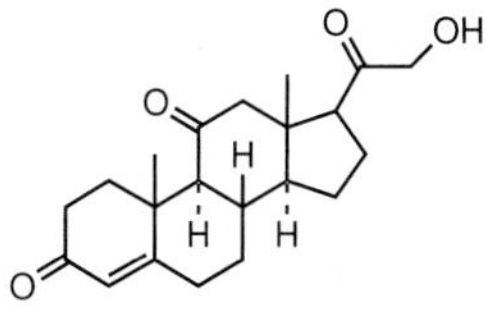

11-Dehydrocorticosterone

Cholesterol

O_2, NADPH

Cholest-5-ene-3β,22R-diol

O_2, NADPH

Cholest-5-ene-3β,20R,22R-triol

O_2, NADPH

Pregnenolone

\+

Isocaproic acid

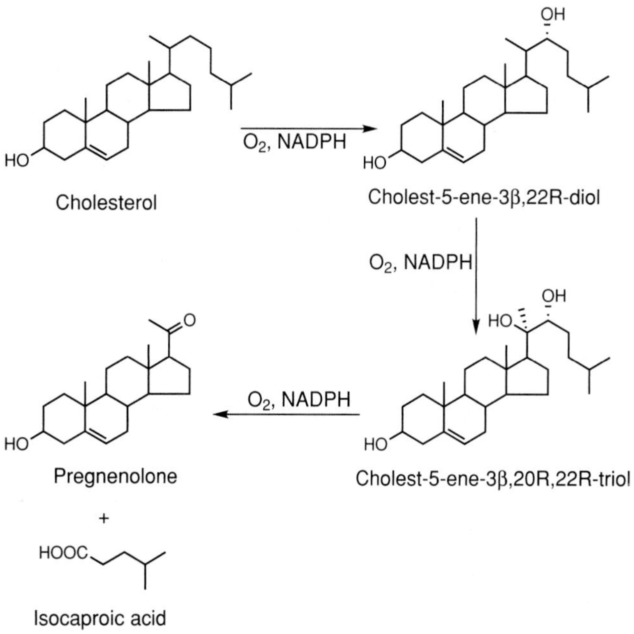

Fig. 33.7. Biosynthesis of pregnenolone from cholesterol.

BIOSYNTHESIS

Pregnenolone Formation

In the adrenal glands, cholesterol is converted by enzymatic cleavage of its side chain to pregnenolone (3β-hydroxypregn-5-en-20-one), which serves as the biosynthetic precursor of the adrenocorticoids (Fig. 33.7).This biotransformation is performed by a mitochondrial cytochrome P450 enzyme complex. This enzyme complex found in the mitochondrial membrane consists of three proteins: cytochrome P450 11A1 (CYP11A1; also known as $P450_{SCC}$), adrenodoxin, and adrenodoxin reductase (14). Defects in CYP11A1 lead to a lack of glucocorticoids, feminization, and hypertension. Three oxidation steps are involved in the conversion, and three moles of NADPH and molecular oxygen are consumed for each mole of cholesterol converted to pregnenolone. The first oxidation results in the formation of cholest-5-ene-3β,22R-diol (step a), followed by the second oxidation yielding cholest-5-ene-3β,20R,22R-triol (step b). The third oxidation step catalyzes the cleavage of the C20-C22 bond to release pregnenolone and isocaproic aldehyde (step c).

Pregnenolone serves as the common precursor in the formation of the adrenocorticoids and other steroid hormones. This C21 steroid is converted via enzymatic oxidations and isomerization of the double bond to a number of physiologically active C21 steroids, including the female sex hormone progesterone and the adrenocorticoids hydrocortisone (cortisol), corticosterone, and aldosterone. Oxidative cleavage of the two-carbon side chain of pregnenolone and subsequent enzymatic oxidations and isomerization lead to C19 steroids, including the androgens testosterone and dihydrotestosterone. The final group of steroids, the C18 female sex hormones, are derived from oxidative aromatization of the A ring of androgens to produce estrogens. More detailed information regarding these biosynthetic pathways are described in this and the following chapters under the particular class of steroid hormones.

Pregnenolone to Glucocorticoids and Mineralocorticoids

The biosynthesis of the glucocorticoids and mineralocorticoids are regulated by independent mechanisms. The glucocorticoids, such as cortisol, are biosynthesized and released under the influence of peptide hormones secreted by the hypothalamus and anterior pituitary (adenohypophysis) to activate the adrenal cortex (the hypothalamic-pituitary-adrenal [HPA] axis). Removal of the pituitary results in atrophy of the adrenal cortex and a marked decrease in the rate of glucocorticoid formation and secretion. On the other hand, the secretion of the mineralocorticoids, corticosterone and aldosterone, are under the influence of the octapeptide, angiotensin II. Angiotensin II is the active metabolite resulting from the renin-catalyzed proteolytic hydrolysis of plasma angiotensinogen to angiotensin I in the blood. In hypophysectomized animals, the rate of secretion of aldosterone is only slightly decreased or remains unchanged. Consequently, the electrolyte balance remains nearly normal.

The peptide hormone in the anterior pituitary that influences glucocorticoid biosynthesis is ACTH (corticotropin), whereas the peptide hormone in the hypothalamus is corticotropin-releasing factor (CRF). The production of both ACTH and CRF is regulated by the central nervous system and by a negative corticoid feedback mechanism. The CRF is released by the hypothalamus and is transported to the anterior pituitary, where it stimulates the release of ACTH into the bloodstream. Then, ACTH is transported to the adrenal glands, where it stimulates the biosynthesis and secretion of the glucocorticoids. The circulating levels of glucocorticoids act on the hypothalamus and anterior pituitary to regulate the release of both CRF and ACTH. As the levels of glucocorticoids rise, smaller amounts of CRF and ACTH are secreted, and a negative feedback is observed (HPA suppression). Stimuli, such as pain, noise, and emotional reactions, increase the secretion of CRF, ACTH, and consequently, the glucocorticoids. Once the stimulus is alleviated or removed, the negative feedback mechanism inhibits further production and helps to return the body to a normal hormonal balance (15,16).

Adrenocorticotropic hormone acts at the adrenal gland by binding to a receptor protein on the surface of the adrenal cortex cell to stimulate the biosynthesis and secretion of glucocorticoids. The only steroid stored in the adrenal gland is cholesterol, found in the form of cholesterol esters stored in lipid droplets. Adrenocorticotropic hormone stimulates the conversion of cholesterol esters to glucorticoids by initiating a series of biochemical events through its surface receptor. The ACTH receptor protein is coupled to a G protein and to adenylate cyclase. Binding of ACTH to its receptor leads to activation of adenylate cyclase via the G protein. The result is an increase in intracellular cyclic adenosine monophosphate (cAMP) levels. One of the processes influenced by elevated cAMP levels is the activation of cholesterol esterase, which cleaves cholesterol esters and liberates free cholesterol.

Free cholesterol is then converted within mitochondria to pregnenolone via the side-chain cleavage reaction described earlier (Fig. 33.7). Pregnenolone is converted to adrenocorticoids by a series of enzymatic oxidations and isomerization of the double bond (Fig. 33.8). The next several enzymatic steps in the biosynthesis of glucocorticoids occur in the endoplasmic reticulum of the adrenal cortex cell. Hydroxylation of pregnenolone at position 17 by the enzyme 17α-hydroxylase (CYP17) produces 17α-hydroxypregnenolone (step b). The 17α-hydroxyl group is important for adrenocorticoid hormone action. In one step, 17α-hydroxypregnenolone is oxidized to a 3-keto intermediate by the action of the enzyme 5-ene-3β-hydroxysteroid dehydrogenase (3β-HSD) and isomerized to 17α-hydroxyprogesterone by the enzyme 3-oxosteroid-4,5-isomerase (steps c and d). Another hydroxylation occurs by the action of 21-hydroxylase (CYP21) to give rise to 11-deoxycortisol, which contains the physiologically important ketol ($—COCH_2OH$) side chain at the 17β position (step e). A lack of CYP21 prevents cortisol biosynthesis, diverting excess 17α-hydroxypregnenolone and 17α-hydroxyprogesterone into overproduction of C19 androgens. The final step in the biosynthesis of hydrocortisone is catalyzed by the enzyme 11β-hydroxylase, a mitochondrial cytochrome P450 enzyme complex (CYP11B2). This last enzymatic step (step f) results in the formation of hydrocortisone (cortisol), the most potent endogenous glucocorticoid secreted by the adrenal cortex. Approximately 15 to 20 mg of hydrocortisone are biosynthesized daily. Several reviews (14,15,17–19) provide more detailed discussions about the enzymology and regulation of adrenal steroidogenesis.

The pathway for the formation of the potent mineralocorticoid molecule, aldosterone, is similar to that for hydrocortisone and uses several of the same enzymes (Fig. 33.8). The preferred pathway involves the conversion of pregnenolone to progesterone by 5-ene-3β-hydroxysteroid dehydrogenase and 3-oxosteroid-4, 5-isomerase (steps c and d). Hydroxylation at position 21 of progesterone by 21-hydroxylase results in 21-hydroxyprogesterone (11-deoxycorticosterone) (step e). Again, these first conversions occur in the endoplasmic reticulum of the cell, whereas the next enzymatic steps occur in the mitochondria. 11β-Hydroxylase (CYP11B2) catalyzes the conversion of 21-hydroxyprogesterone to corticosterone (step f), which exhibits mineralocorticoid activity. The final two oxidations involve hydroxylations at the C18 methyl group and are catalyzed by 18-hydroxylase (step g). These reactions produce first 18-hydroxycorticosterone (not shown) and then aldosterone, the most powerful endogenous mineralocorticoid secretion of the adrenal cortex. The aldehyde at C18 of aldosterone exists in equilibrium with its hemiacetal form.

METABOLISM

Hydrocortisone (hormonally active) and cortisone (the inactive metabolite of hydrocortisone) are biochemically interconvertible by the enzyme 11β-hydroxysteroid dehydrogenase (Fig. 33.9). Two isozymes of 11β-hydroxysteroid dehydrogenase are present, type 1 11β-hydroxysteroid dehydrogenase (11β-HSD1), referred to as the "liver" isozyme, and type 2 11β-hydroxysteroid dehydrogenase (11β-HSD2), referred to as the "kidney" isozyme (20–22). The 11β-HSD1 isozyme is a bidirectional enzyme, readily interconverts hydrocortisone and cortisone, and is found in many tissues in the body. This isozyme plays an important role in the regulation of hepatic gluconeogenesis in the liver and in fat production in adipose tissues. By contrast, the 11β-HSD2 isozyme is only unidirectional, catalyzing the 11β-dehydrogenation of hydrocortisone to give cortisone. The 11β-HSD2 is present in placenta and in kidney, specifically the distal convoluted tubules and cortical collecting ducts in the kidney. The 11β-HSD2 isozyme plays an important role in the rapid metabolism

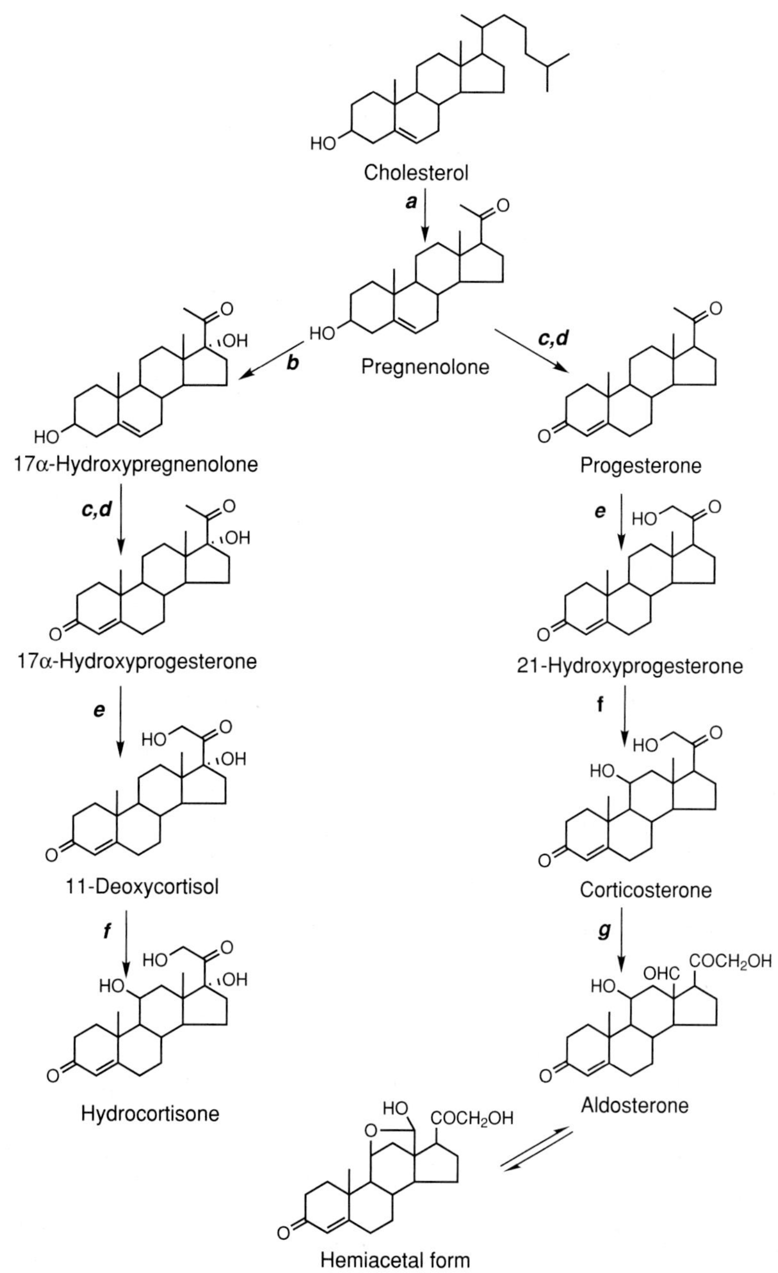

Fig. 33.8. Biosynthesis of the adrenocorticoids from cholesterol.

of hydrocortisone, thus preventing hydrocortisone from binding to the mineralocorticoid receptors present in the same kidney tissues. A deficiency of 11β-HSD2 is associated with the inherited genetic disease, apparent mineralocorticoid excess, which is characterized by hypertension, excessive salt retention, and hypokalemia caused by the elevated hydrocortisone levels in the kidney.

Hydrocortisone is metabolized by the liver following administration by any route, with a half-life of approximately 1.0 to 1.5 hours (23). Hydrocortisone is mainly excreted in the urine as inactive O-glucuronide conjugates and minor O-sulfate conjugates of urocortisol, 5β-dihydrocortisol, and urocortisone (Fig. 33.9). The tetrahydro metabolite urocortisol is the major metabolite formed and has the 5β-pregnane geometry and 3α-hydroxyl function. The 5β configuration is similar to the ring geometry for the nonhormonal bile acids. Several compounds of this type have been isolated (24,25). All of the biologically active adrenocorticoids contain a ketone at the 3-position and a double bond in the 4,5-position. The formation of 5β-metabolites from hydrocortisone is characterized by reduction of the 4,5-double bond to a 5β geometry for rings A and B (a *cis* configuration) by 5β-reductase or reduction of the 3-ketone by 3α-hydroxysteroid dehydrogenase (3α-hydroxyl configuration) or 3β-hydroxysteroid dehydrogenase (3β-hydroxyl configuration). These

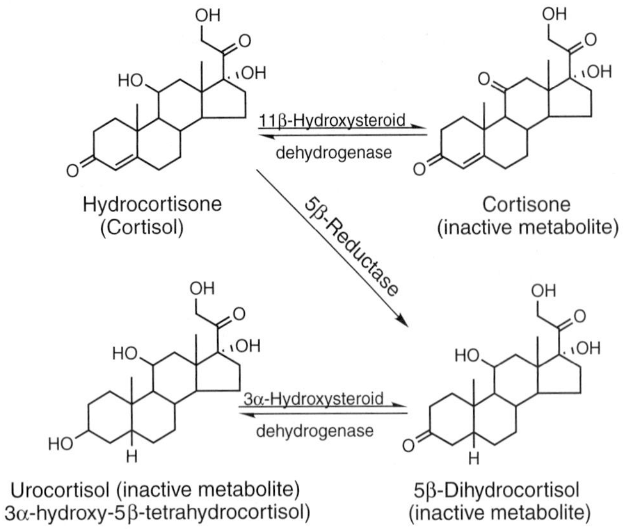

Fig. 33.9. Major routes of metabolism for hydrocortisone.

reactions represent the major pathways of metabolism for the glucocorticoids and their endogenous counterparts. Urocortisol and urocortisone are named after cortisol (hydrocortisone) and cortisone. Reversible oxidation of the 11β-hydroxyl group of many glucocorticoids (e.g., hydrocortisone, prednisolone, and methylprednisolone, but not dexamethasone and other 9α-fluorinated glucocorticoids) by 11β-hydroxysteroid dehydrogenase inactivates these drugs and limits their mineralocorticoid activity in the kidneys. Other routes of metabolism include 6β-hydroxylation (CYP3A4) and reduction of the 20-ketone (e.g., prednisolone) to form 20-hydroxyl analogues as well as oxidation of the 17-ketol side chain to 17β-carboxylic acids and loss of the 17-ketol side chain, resulting in 11β-hydroxy-17-keto-C19 steroids with the geometry of either 5α-androstane or 5β-androstane (15,17–19). In addition, some ring A aromatic adrenocorticoid metabolites that resemble the estrogens have been isolated (26). Biliary and fecal excretion contribute little to the elimination of the adrenocorticoids. The rate of formation of 6β-hydroxyhydrocortisone is a biomarker for determining the level of HPA suppression and adrenal insufficiency.

DEVELOPMENT OF ADRENOCORTICOID DRUGS

Systemic Corticosteroids

Overview

The route of administration depends on the disease being treated and the physicochemical, pharmacologic, and pharmacokinetic properties of the drug (Table 33.1). The clinically available adrenocorticoids may be administered by IV injection, oral tablets or solutions, topical formulations, intra-articular administration, and oral or nasal inhalation (Table 33.2). Only a handful of

Table 33.1. Pharmacological and Pharmacokinetic Properties for Some Adrenocorticoids

Adrenocorticoid	Oral Gluco-corticoid Dose[a] (mg)	Potency Relative to Hydrocortisone: Gluco-corticoid Activity[b]	Potency Relative to Hydrocortisone: Mineralo-corticoid Activity[c]	Protein Binding (%)[d]	Half-life (hours): Plasma	Half-life (hours): Biologic (tissue)	Duration of Action (days)
Short-acting							
Hydrocortisone	20	1	2+	>90	1.5–2.0	8–12	1.0–1.5
Cortisone	25	0.8	2+	>90	0.5	8–12	1.0–1.5
Intermediate-acting							
Prednisone	5	3.5	1+	>90	3.4–3.8	18–36	1.0–1.5
Prednisolone	5	4	1+	>90	2.1–3.5	18–36	1.0–1.5
Methylprednisolone	5	5	0[e]		>3.5	18–36	1.0–1.5
Triamcinolone	5	5	0[e]	>90	2–5	18–36	1.0–1.5
Long-acting							
Dexamethasone	0.75	20–30	0[e]	>90	3.0–4.5	36–54	2.8–3
Betamethasone	0.6	20–30	0[e]	>90	3–5	36–54	2.8–3
Fludrocortisone	Not employed	10	10	<90	3.5	18–36	1–2
Fluprednisolone	1.6	10	0[e]				
Aldosterone	Not employed	0.2	800				
11-Desoxycorticosterone	Not employed	0	40				
Corticosterone	IM	0.5	5				

[a]Based on the oral dose of an anti-inflammatory agent in rheumatoid arthritis.
[b]Anti-inflammatory, immunosuppressant, and metabolic effects.
[c]Sodium and water retention and potassium depletion effects.
[d]Hydrocortisone binds to transcortin (corticosteroid binding globulin [CBG]) and to albumin. Prednisone also binds to CBG, but betamethasone, dexamethasone, and tramincinolone do not.
[e]Although these glucocorticoids are considered not to have significant mineralocorticoid activity, hypokalemia and/or sodium and fluid retention may occur, depending on the dosage, duration of use, and patient predisposition.

Table 33.2. Adrenocorticoids, Their Trade Names, and Their Routes of Administration

Adrenocorticoid	Trade Name	PO	IV	IM	Inhaled/ Intranasal	Topical
Alclomethasone dipropionate	Alclovate					•
Amcinonide	Cyclocort					•
Beclomethasone dipropionate	Beclovent, Vanceril, Beconase				•	
Beclomethasone dipropionate monohydrate	Beconase AQ, Vancenase AQ				•	
Betamethasone	Celestone	•				
Betamethasone dipropionate	Diprosone, Maxivate					•
Betamethasone sodium phosphate	Celestone Phosphate			•		
Betamethasone valerate	BetaVal, Valisone,					•
Budesonide	Pulmicort, Rhinocort				•	
Clobetasol propionate	Temovate					•
Clocortolone pivalate	Cloderm					•
Cortisone acetate		•		•		
Desonide	Tridesolone					•
Dexamethasone	Decadron	•				•[a]
Dexamethasone acetate	Decadron-LA, Dalalone, Dexasone			•		
Dexamethasone sodium phosphate	Decadron Phosphate		•	•	•	
Desoximetasone	Topicort					•
Diflorasone diacetate	Maxiflor, Florone, Psorcon					•
Fludrocortisone acetate	Florinef	•				
Flumethasone pivalate	Flocort					•
Flunisolide	Aerobid, Nasalide, Nasarel				•	
Fluocinolone acetonide	Synalar, Flurosyn					•
Fluocinonide	Lidex, Fluonex					•
Fluoromethalone	FML, Fluor-Op					•[a]
Fluoromethalone acetate	Flarex					•[a]
Flurandenolide	Cordran					•
Fluticasone propionate	Cutivate, Flovent, Flonase				•	•
Halcinonide	Halog					•
Halobetasol propionate	Ultavate					•
Hydrocortisone	Hydrocortone	•				•[b]
Hydrocortisone acetate	Hydrocortone Acetate			•		•[c]
Hydrocortisone buteprate	Pandel					•
Hydrocortisone butyrate	Locoid					•
Hydrocortisone cypionate	Cortef	•				
Hydrocortisone sodium phosphate	Hydrocortone Phosphate		•	•		
Hydrocortisone sodium succinate	Solu-Cortef		•	•		
Hydrocortisone valerate						•
Methylprednisolone	Medrol	•				
Methylprednisolone acetate	Depo-Medrol, Depopred			•		•
Methylprednisolone sodium succinate	Solu-Medrol		•	•		
Mometasone furoate	Elocon					•
Mometasone furoate monohydrate	Nasonex				•	
Prednicarbate	Dermatop					•
Prednisolone	Deltacortef	•				
Prednisolone acetate	Predcor, Predalone, KeyPred	•		•		
Prednisolone acetate	Pred-Mild, Pred-Forte					•[a]
Prednisolone sodium phosphate	Pediapred, Inflamase, Hydeltrasol, AK-Pred	•		•		•[a]
Prednsiolone tebutate				•		
Prednisone	Deltasone, Meticorten, Orasone	•				•
Triamcinolone acetonide	Aristocort, Kenacort	•				
Triamcinolone acetonide	Kenalog, Triderm, Delta-Tritex, Flutex					•
Triamcinolone acetonide	Azmacort, Nasacort, Nasacort AQ				•	
Triamcinolone diacetate	Aristocort Forte, Triam Forte			•		
Triamcinolone hexacetonide	Aristospan			•		

PO, oral; IV, intravenous; IM, intramuscular.
[a]Ophthalmic formulations.
[b]Also in otic, ophthalmic, and rectal formulations (Cortenema).
[c]Also in intrarectal foam (Cortifoam).

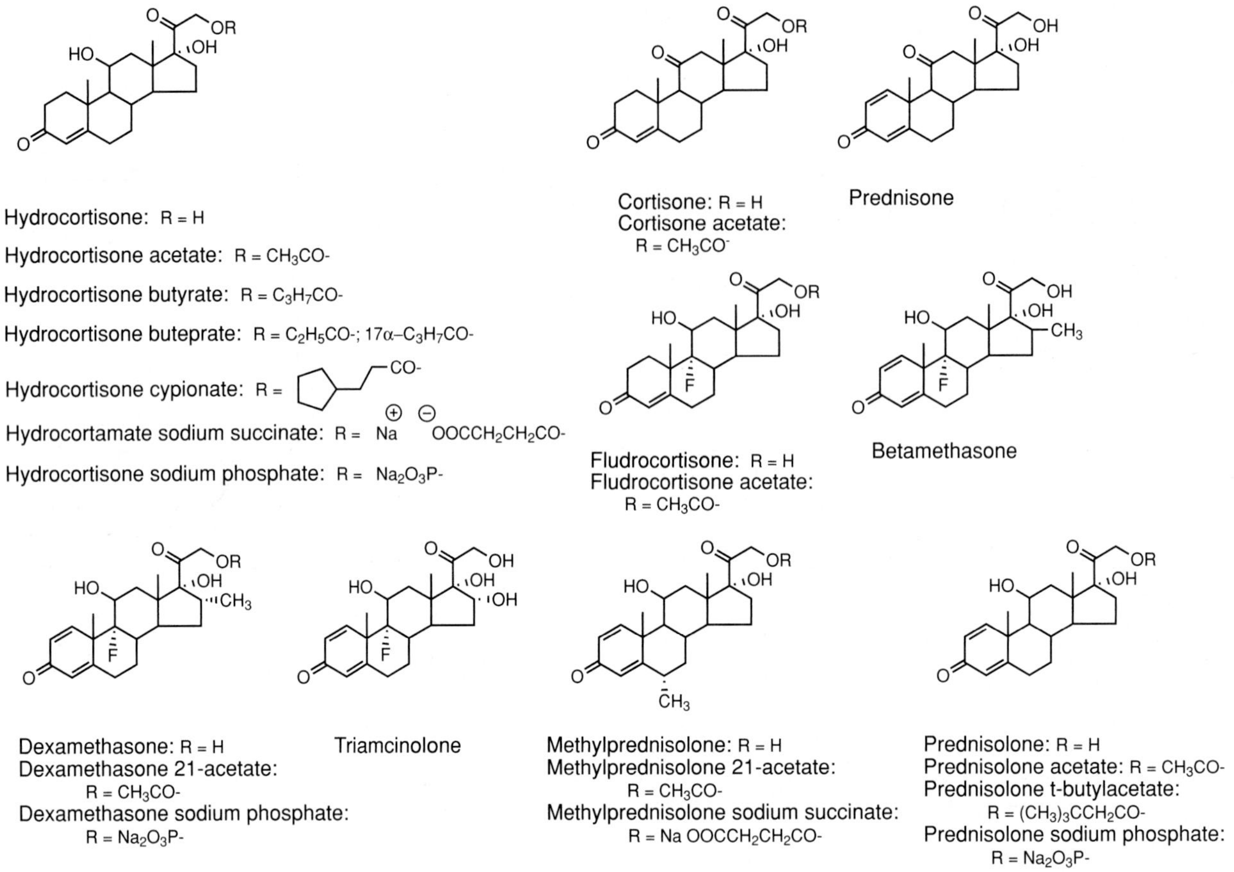

Hydrocortisone: R = H
Hydrocortisone acetate: R = CH_3CO-
Hydrocortisone butyrate: R = C_3H_7CO-
Hydrocortisone buteprate: R = C_2H_5CO-; 17α–C_3H_7CO-
Hydrocortisone cypionate: R = (cyclopentyl)–CH_2CH_2–CO-
Hydrocortamate sodium succinate: R = $Na^{\oplus}$ $^{\ominus}OOCCH_2CH_2CO$-
Hydrocortisone sodium phosphate: R = Na_2O_3P-

Cortisone: R = H
Cortisone acetate:
R = CH_3CO-

Prednisone

Fludrocortisone: R = H
Fludrocortisone acetate:
R = CH_3CO-

Betamethasone

Dexamethasone: R = H
Dexamethasone 21-acetate:
R = CH_3CO-
Dexamethasone sodium phosphate:
R = Na_2O_3P-

Triamcinolone

Methylprednisolone: R = H
Methylprednisolone 21-acetate:
R = CH_3CO-
Methylprednisolone sodium succinate:
R = Na $OOCCH_2CH_2CO$-

Prednisolone: R = H
Prednisolone acetate: R = CH_3CO-
Prednisolone t-butylacetate:
R = $(CH_3)_3CCH_2CO$-
Prednisolone sodium phosphate:
R = Na_2O_3P-

Fig. 33.10. Systemic corticosteroids.

corticosteroids are used clinically by the oral route, including hydrocortisone, prednisone, prednisolone, methylprednisolone, and dexamethasone (Fig. 33.10). These corticosteroids often are described as short-acting, intermediate-acting, or long-acting according to their biological half-life and duration of action (Table 33.2). They are well-absorbed, undergo little first-pass metabolism in the liver, and demonstrate oral bioavailabilities of 70 to 80%, except for triamcinolone (Table 33.3). The larger volume of distribution for methylprednisolone compared to prednisolone is thought to result from a combination of increased lipophilicity, decrease in metabolism, and better tissue penetration. Glucocorticoids vary in the extent to which they are bound to the plasma proteins, albumin, and corticosteroid-binding globulin (transcortin) (Table 33.3) (27).

Hydrocortisone is extensively bound to the plasma proteins, primarily to transcortin (corticosteroid-binding globulin), with only 5 to 10% of plasma hydrocortisone unbound. Prednisolone and methylprednisolone, but not the 9α-fluoro analogues betamethasone, dexamethasone, or triamcinolone, have a high affinity for transcortin and, thus, compete with hydrocortisone for this binding protein. The 9α-halo analogues bind primarily to albumin.

Table 33.3. Pharmacokinetics of Commonly Used Oral Adrenocorticoids

Adrenocorticoid	Bioavailability (%)	Half-Life (hours)	Protein Binding (%)	Volume Distribution (L/kg)	Log P (experimental)	Clearance (ml/min/70 kg)
Dexamethasone	78	3.0	90–95	0.2	1.83	260
Hydrocortisone	96	1.7	90	0.5	1.61	400
Methylprednisolone	90	2.3	90–95	1.5	1.76	430
Prednisone	80	3.6	~90	1.0	1.46	250
Prednisolone	82	2.8	90–95	0.7–1.5	1.62	60
Triamcinolone	23	2.6	~90	1.3	1.16	61

Only the unbound fraction of hydrocortisone and the synthetic corticosteroids are biologically active. Generally, the amount of transcortin in the plasma determines the distribution of glucocorticoids between free and bound forms, and free glucocorticoid concentrations determine the drug's half-life. Glucocorticoids cross the placenta and may be distributed into milk.

The degree of systemic side effects is dose-dependent, related to the half-life of the drug, frequency of administration, time of day when administered, and route of administration. In other words, the higher the plasma corticosteroid concentration and longer the half-life, the greater the systemic side effects will be (Table 33.3).

Regardless of the route of administration, all the synthetic adrenocorticoids are excreted from the body in a manner similar to the endogenous adrenocorticoids (i.e., they are metabolized in the liver and excreted into the urine primarily as glucuronide conjugates but also as sulfate conjugates) (28). In fact, hepatic oxidative metabolism rapidly converts many of the systemic and topical corticosteroids to inactive metabolites and, thus, serves to protect patients from the HPA-suppressive effects of these drugs on endogenous steroid production. The corticosteroids are metabolized in many tissues, including the liver, muscles, and red blood cells (15,18,29); however, the liver metabolizes them most rapidly. The fact that many of the endogenous corticosteroids are rapidly metabolized by the liver precludes their administration by the oral route. Catabolic products can be isolated from the urine and bile and can be formed in tissue preparations in vitro (30,31).

Specific Drugs

11-Desoxycorticosterone was the first naturally occurring corticoid to be synthesized. It was prepared, before its isolation from the adrenal cortex, by Steiger and Reichstein (32). As a result of his synthesis of 11-desoxycorticosterone and other early work with corticoids, Reichstein later shared the Nobel Prize with Kendall, another chemist who was instrumental in carrying out early steroid syntheses, and with Hench, a rheumatologist who in 1929 discovered that cortisone is effective in the treatment of rheumatoid arthritis. Kendall's basic research ultimately led to the synthesis of cortisone from naturally occurring bile acids (33).

CORTISONE, HYDROCORTISONE, AND THEIR DERIVATIVES. After the synthesis of 11-desoxycorticosterone in 1937, all the corticoids were synthesized and their structures confirmed. The first synthesis of cortisone from methyl 3α-hydroxy-11-ketobisnorcholanate was reported by Sarett (34) in 1946. Earlier work of Kendall and coworkers involving its preparation from the methyl ester of desoxycholic acid was used in his research (35). Later, several chemists, including Sarett (36), Kendall, and Tishler, found ways to improve the yields and to decrease the labor involved in the multistep conversion of bile acids to cortisone acetate. In 1949, Merck sold limited quantities of this glucocorticoid to physicians at $200 per gram for treating rheumatoid arthritis. Subsequent improvements in the methods of synthesis reduced the price to $10 per gram by 1951. In 1955, Upjohn used an efficient process involving the synthesis of cortisone acetate from progesterone, with the latter steroid being prepared from diosgenin. This further reduced the price to $3.50 per gram. In 2005, the cost was $8 per gram. Other pharmaceutical companies also began to sell cortisone synthesized from bile acids by a well-developed but lengthy procedure (33).

Cortisone is administered orally or by intramuscular (IM) injection as its 21-acetate (cortisone acetate). Cortisone acetate or hydrocortisone usually is the corticosteroid of choice for replacement therapy in patients with adrenocortical insufficiency, because these drugs have both glucocorticoid and mineralocorticoid properties. Following oral administration, cortisone acetate and hydrocortisone acetate are completely and rapidly deacetylated by first-pass metabolism (37). Much of the oral cortisone, however, is inactivated by oxidative metabolism (Fig. 33.9) before it can be converted to hydrocortisone in the liver. The pharmacokinetics for hydrocortisone acetate is indistinguishable from that of orally administered hydrocortisone. Oral hydrocortisone is completely absorbed, with a bioavailability of greater than 95% and a half-life of 1 to 2 hours (23). The metabolism of hydrocortisone (Fig. 33.9) has been previously described. Cortisone acetate is slowly absorbed from IM injection sites over a period of 24 to 48 hours and is reserved for patients who are unable to take the drug orally. The acetate ester derivative demonstrates increased stability and has a longer duration of action when administered by IM injection. Thus, smaller doses can be used. Similarly, hydrocortisone may be dispensed as its 21-acetate (hydrocortisone acetate), which is superior to cortisone acetate when injected intra-articularly. Systemic absorption of hydrocortisone acetate from intra-articular injection sites usually is complete within 24 to 48 hours. When administered intrarectally, hydrocortisone is poorly absorbed (38,39).

Other ester derivatives that are available include hydrocortisone cypionate [21-(3-cyclopentylpropionate) ester], hydrocortisone butyrate (17α-butyrate ester), hydrocortisone buteprate (17α-butyrate, 21-propionate esters), hydrocortisone valerate (17α-valerate ester), hydrocortisone sodium succinate (21-sodium succinate ester), and hydrocortisone sodium phosphate (the 21-sodium phosphate ester) (Fig. 33.10). The water-insoluble hydrocortisone cypionate is used orally in doses expressed in terms of hydrocortisone for slower absorption from the gastrointestinal (GI) tract. The extremely water-soluble 21-sodium succinate and 21-sodium phosphate esters are used for IV or IM injection in the management of emergency conditions that can be treated with anti-inflammatory steroids. The phosphate ester is completely and rapidly metabolized by phosphatases, with a half-life of less than 5 minutes (38). Peak hydrocortisone levels are reached in approximately 10 minutes. The sodium succinate ester is slowly and incompletely hydrolyzed, and peak hydrocortisone levels are attained in 30 to 45 minutes (38). Hydrocortisone butyrate, hydrocortisone buteprate, and hydrocortisone valerate are used topically.

After the introduction of cortisone (1948) and, later, hydrocortisone (1951) for the treatment of rheumatoid arthritis, many investigators began to search for superior agents having fewer side effects. When these drugs are used in doses necessary to suppress symptoms of rheumatoid arthritis, they also affect other metabolic processes. Side effects, such as excessive sodium retention and potassium excretion, negative nitrogen balance, increased gastric acidity, edema, and psychosis, are exaggerated manifestations of the normal metabolic functions of the hormones.

It was hoped that a compound with high glucocorticoid and low mineralocorticoid activity could be synthesized. Because it was recognized early that a carbonyl group at C3, a double bond between carbons 4 and 5, an oxygen (C=O or β-OH) at carbon 11, and a β-ketol side chain at position 17 are necessary for superior glucocorticoid activity, investigators began to synthesize analogues containing these functions. Additional groups were inserted into other positions of the basic steroid structure, with the expectation that these new substituents might modify the glucocorticoid and mineralocorticoid activities of the parent drugs.

The first potent analogues discovered, however, did not result from a concentrated effort to find a better drug but, rather, from basic chemical research concerned with the preparation of hydrocortisone from 11-epicortisol (11α-hydrocortisone).

11-Epicortisol

Fludrocortisone. A 9α-bromo analogue was prepared that had one-third the glucocorticoid activity of cortisone acetate (40). Other halogens were introduced into the 9α-position, and it was soon observed that glucocorticoid activity is inversely proportional to the size of the halogen at carbon 9. The 9α-fluoro analogue (fludrocortisone) is approximately 11 times as potent as cortisone acetate (Fig. 33.10). Fludrocortisone is orally administered as its 21-acetate derivative. When tested clinically in patients with rheumatoid arthritis, it was found to be effective at approximately one-tenth the dose of cortisone acetate. Although glucocorticoid activity is increased 11 times by insertion of the 9α-fluoro substituent, mineralocorticoid activity is increased 300 to 800 times (27). Because of its intense sodium-retaining activity, fludrocortisone is contraindicated in all conditions except those that require a high degree of mineralocorticoid activity, because it leads to edema. Fludrocortisone acetate is used orally for mineralocorticoid replacement therapy in patients with adrenocortical insufficiency, such as Addison's disease. This drug, introduced in 1954, helped to provide the impetus for the synthesis and biological evaluation of newer halogenated analogues.

Prednisone, prednisolone, and its derivatives. One year after the introduction of fludrocortisone, the Δ-corticoids were brought forth into clinical medicine. Investigators at Schering observed that the 1-dehydro derivatives of cortisone and hydrocortisone—namely, prednisone and prednisolone—are more potent antirheumatic and anti-allergenic agents than the parent compounds and produced fewer undesirable side effects. These compounds are known as Δ^1-corticoids, because they contain an additional double bond between positions 1 and 2 (Fig. 33.10).

The Δ^1-corticoids, which can be prepared by microbial dehydrogenation of cortisone or hydrocortisone with *Corynebacterium simplex* (41) and by several synthetic methods (33), represent the first chemical innovation leading to the creation of a modified compound that could be prescribed for rheumatoid arthritis. One high-yield route involves oxidation of 5α- or 5β-pregnane precursors that have appropriate oxygen substitutions with selenium dioxide (42).

Both prednisone and prednisolone were found to have adrenocortical activity (measured by eosinopenic response, liver glycogen decomposition, and thymus involution in adrenalectomized mice). In these tests, prednisone and prednisolone were found to be three- or fourfold more potent than cortisone and hydrocortisone. Antiphlogistic strengths in human subjects were similarly augmented, but their electrolyte activities were not proportionately increased.

The increased potency reflects the effect in the change in geometry of ring A caused by the introduction of C1=C2 function on glucocorticoid receptor (GR) affinity and altered pharmacokinetics (primarily metabolism). Although the remaining portions of the steroid are essentially unchanged (except for less easily visualized molecular perturbations), the conformation of ring A changes from a chair, as in 5α-pregnan-3-one, to a half-chair (pregn-4-en-3-one) and to a flattened boat (pregna-1,4-dien-3-one) on introduction of unsaturation (Fig. 33.11). The order of GR affinity is dexamethasone (10×) > triamcinolone (5×) > methylprednisolone (4×) > prednisolone (2×) > hydrocortisone (1×) (43).

When orally administered, prednisone and prednisolone are almost completely absorbed, with a bioavailability of greater than 80% (Table 33.3) (44,45). As with

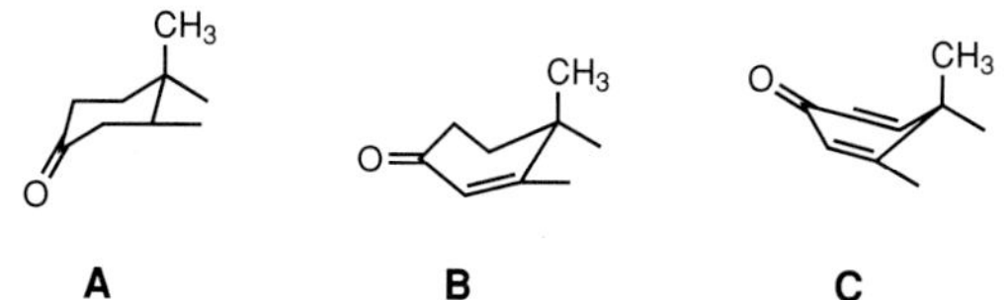

Fig. 33.11. Ring A conformations for 5α-pregnan-3-one (A), for pregn-4-en-3-one (B), and for pregna-1,4-dion-3-one (C).

the relationship between cortisone and hydrocortisone, prednisone and prednisolone are interconvertible by 11β-hydroxysteroid dehydrogenase in the liver. For practical purposes, prednisone and prednisolone are equally potent and may be used interchangeably. When prednisone or prednisolone is used in the treatment of rheumatoid arthritis, smaller doses are required than with hydrocortisone. The usual dose is 5 mg two to four times a day. Prednisolone is metabolized into a number of hydrophilic and less active metabolites, as shown in Figure 33.12, except there is no reduction of ring A as with hydrocortisone. The major metabolites (6β- and 16β-hydroxy) are primarily excreted as glucuronide conjugates in the urine. Prednisolone acetate is available in suspension and ointment forms for use externally. As with hydrocortisone, several other 21-esters of prednisolone are available. Prednisolone tert-butylacetate (3,3-dimethylbutyrate) is used in suspension form and by injection for the same reasons the 21-ester derivatives of hydrocortisone are employed. The butylacetate ester, which is suitable only for use by injection, has a long duration of action because of low water solubility and a slow rate of hydrolysis. The drug is administered in doses of 4 to 20 mg.

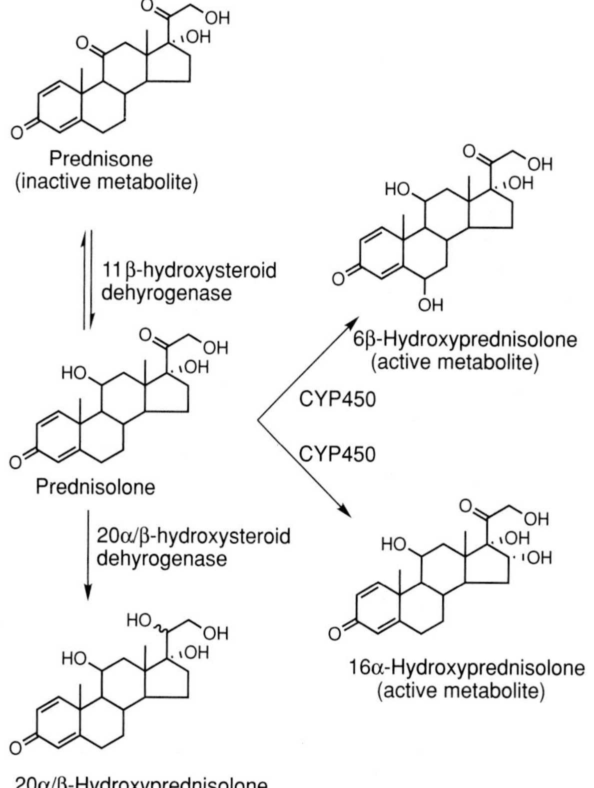

Fig. 33.12. Major routes of metabolism for prednisolone.

Prednisolone sodium phosphate is the water-soluble sodium salt of the 21-phosphate ester, with a half-life of less than 5 minutes because of rapid hydrolysis by phosphatases (44,46). Peak plasma levels for prednisolone are attained in approximately 10 minutes following its administration by injection (usual dose of 20 mg IV or IM). Topically, one or two drops of a 0.5% solution may be used four to six times daily for its anti-inflammatory action in the eye.

When doses of equivalent antirheumatic potency are given to patients not treated with steroids, the Δ^1-corticoids promote the same pattern of initial improvement as hydrocortisone. Statistical results of the improvement status during the first few months of therapy have been similar with prednisolone, prednisone, and hydrocortisone. The results of longer-term therapy have been significantly better with the modified compounds. Studies indicate that the Δ^1-corticoids may be used continuously in patients with rheumatoid arthritis without undue GI hazard. Although the Δ^1-corticoids are considered not to have significant mineralocorticoid activity, hypokalemia as well as sodium and fluid retention may occur, depending on the dosage and duration of use.

METHYLPREDNISOLONE. Between 1953 and 1962, many derivatives of the Δ^1-corticoids and the halogen-containing analogues (especially fluorinated compounds) were synthesized, and some became useful clinical agents. Studies with methylcorticoids revealed 2α-methyl derivatives to be inactive, whereas the 2α-methyl-9α-fluoro analogues had potent mineralocorticoid activity. Methyprednisolone (6α-methyl-11β,17,21-trihydroxypregna-1,4-diene-3,20-dione) was synthesized in 1956 and introduced into clinical medicine (Fig. 33.10). Methylprednisolone is extensively metabolized, with approximately 10% recovered unchanged in urine (47). The metabolic pathways include reduction of C20 ketone, oxidation of 17β-ketol group to C21-COOH and C20-COOH, and 6β-hydroxylation (CYP3A4). These compounds potentiated glucocorticoid activity with negligible salt retention for short-term therapy (Table 33.2) (48).

In human subjects, the metabolic effects did not differ appreciably from those of prednisolone. Its activities with respect to nitrogen excretion, ACTH suppression, and reduction of circulating eosinophils were similar to those of prednisolone. The sodium retention and potassium loss were slightly less than with prednisolone (49).

Methylprednisolone is administered IV as its water-soluble sodium salt of the 21-succinate ester. The succinate ester is slowly and incompletely hydrolyzed. Peak plasma levels for methylprednisolone is attained in approximately 30 to 60 minutes following its IV administration, and approximately 15% of its IV dose is recovered unchanged in urine (45,46). CYP3A4 inhibitors such as the antifungals, ketoconazole, and itraconazole can potentiate the effects of prednisolone.

Triamcinolone. A natural extension of corticoid research involved examination of compounds containing both a 9α-fluoro group and a double bond between positions 1 and 2. Triamcinolone (9-fluoro-11β, 16α, 17, 21-tetrahydroxypregna-1,4-diene-3,20-dione), introduced in 1958, combines the structural features of a Δ^1-corticoid and a 9α-fluoro corticoid (Fig. 33.10). As mentioned previously, the 9α-fluoro group increases the anti-inflammatory potency, but it also markedly increases the mineralocorticoid potency. This is undesirable if the drug is to be used internally for the treatment of rheumatoid arthritis. By inserting a 16α-hydroxy group into the molecule, one can decrease the mineralocorticoid activity.

The original interest in 16α-hydroxycorticosteroids stemmed from their isolation from the urine of a boy with an adrenal tumor. The desire of chemists to synthesize these corticoids, and the hope that such analogues might have potent biological activity furthered their development (50–52). Therefore, inserting a 16α-hydroxy group into 9α-fluoroprednisolone resulted in triamcinolone with glucocorticoid activity equivalent to prednisolone but decreased mineralocorticoid activity. In fact, 16α-hydroxy analogues of natural corticoids retain glucocorticoid activity and have a considerably reduced mineralocorticoid activity. The lower-than-expected oral anti-inflammatory potency for triamcinolone (Table 33.2) has been attributed to its low oral bioavailability (Table 33.3), in part because of increased hydrophilicity from the 16α-hydroxy group and first-pass metabolism, primarily to its 6β-hydroxy metabolite. These glucocorticoids actually may cause sodium excretion rather than sodium retention. Triamcinolone diacetate (17,21-diacetate) and its hexacetonide [16α, 17α-methylenedioxy-21-(3,3-dimethylbutyrate)] esters are administered IM or intra-articularly for a prolonged release of triamcinolone. Triamcinolone diacetate has a duration of action depending on its route of administration from 1 to 8 weeks, and triamcinolone hexacetonide has a duration of action of 3 to 4 weeks (53,54).

On a weight-for-weight basis, the antirheumatic potency of triamcinolone is greater than that of prednisolone (~20%) and approximately the same as that of methylprednisolone. Initial improvement following administration of triamcinolone is similar to that noted with other compounds. Reports in the literature, however, indicate that the percentage of patients maintained satisfactorily for long periods has been distinctly smaller than that with prednisolone.

Even though triamcinolone has an apparently decreased tendency to cause salt and water retention and edema and may induce sodium and water diuresis, it causes other unwanted side effects, including anorexia, weight loss, muscle weakness, leg cramps, nausea, dizziness, and a general toxic feeling (55). Intramuscular triamcinolone is reportedly effective and safe in the treatment of dermatoses, and in combination with folic acid antagonists, it is effective in the treatment of psoriasis (56,57).

Dexamethasone. Research with 16-methyl substituted corticoids was initiated in part because investigators hoped to stabilize the 17β-ketol side chain to metabolism in vivo and improve bioavailability (Fig. 33.10). These studies led to the development of dexamethasone (9-fluoro-16α-methyl-11β,17,21-trihydroxypregna-1,4-diene-3,20-dione), which was introduced for clinical trial. A 16α-methyl group does decrease the reactivity of the 20-keto group to carbonyl reagents and increases the stability of the drug in human plasma in vitro (58,59). Unlike 16α-hydroxylation, a methyl group increases the anti-inflammatory activity by increasing lipophilicity and, consequently, receptor affinity. Like the 16α-hydroxyl group, the methyl group appears to reduce markedly the salt-retaining properties of the corticosteroids (Table 33.2) (60–62). The activity of dexamethasone, as measured by glycogen deposition, is 20 times greater than that of hydrocortisone. It has five times the anti-inflammatory activity of prednisolone. Clinical data indicate that this compound has seven times the antirheumatic potency of prednisolone. It is roughly 30 times more potent than hydrocortisone. Its pharmacokinetics are presented in Table 33.3. Routes of metabolism for dexamethasone are similar to those for prednisolone, with its primary 6β-hydroxy metabolite being recovered in urine (63). Dexamethasone sodium phosphate is the water-soluble sodium salt of the 21-phosphate ester, with an IV half-life of less than 10 minutes because of rapid hydrolysis by plasma phosphatases (64). Peak plasma levels for dexamethasone usually are attained in approximately 10 to 20 minutes following its IV administered dose. A similar reaction occurs when the phosphate ester is applied topically or by inhalation.

In practical management, 0.75 mg of dexamethasone promotes a therapeutic response equivalent to that from 4 mg of triamcinolone or methylprednisolone, 5 mg of prednisolone, and 20 mg of hydrocortisone. Clinical investigations with small groups of patients indicate that this compound could control patients who did not respond well to prednisolone. Over long periods, the improved status of some patients deteriorated.

In summarizing the biological properties of this drug, it seems clear that with doses of corresponding antirheumatic strength, this steroid has approximately the same tendency as prednisolone to produce facial mooning, acne, and nervous excitation. Peripheral edema is uncommon (7%) and mild. The more common and most objectionable side effects are excessive appetite and weight gain, abdominal bloating, and distention. The frequency and severity of these symptoms vary with the dose (1 mg maximum for females, and 1.5 mg maximum for males). The longer biological half-life for dexamethasone significantly increases the potential for glucocorticoid-induced adrenal insufficiency (see *Adverse Effects*).

The striking increase in potency does not confer a general therapeutic index on dexamethasone that is higher than that of prednisolone. Again, this drug probably is best employed as a special-purpose corticoid. It may be useful when other steroids are no longer effective or when increased appetite and weight gain are desirable (64–69). Its efficacy may be increased when it is used in combination with cyproheptadine as an antiallergenic, antipyretic, and anti-inflammatory agent (60).

Betamethasone. Shortly after the introduction of dexamethasone, betamethasone, which differs from dexamethasone only in configuration of the 16-methyl group (Fig. 33.10), was made available for the treatment of rheumatic diseases and dermatologic disorders. This analogue, which contains a 16β-methyl group, has received sufficient clinical trial examination to indicate that it is as effective as dexamethasone or, perhaps, even slightly more active. Although this drug has been reported to be less toxic than other steroids, some clinical investigators suggest that it is best used for short-term therapy. Toxic side effects, such as increased appetite, weight gain, and facial mooning, occur with prolonged use. Generally, a 0.5-mg tablet of betamethasone is equivalent to a 5.0-mg tablet of prednisolone, and except for isolated instances, this drug is apparently on a par with dexamethasone (70).

Selective glucocorticoid receptor modulators. The long-term use of glucocorticoids is associated with severe adverse effects (see *Adverse Effects*), including osteoporosis, hyperglycemia, muscle wasting, hypertension, and impaired wound healing. Improved glucocorticoids that demonstrate potent anti-inflammatory activity without these serious side effects would provide a significant therapeutic advance and are the focus of intense research efforts by the pharmaceutical industry. The molecular mechanism of the GR makes it a particularly suitable target for this effort. The majority of unwanted side effects of the glucocorticoids arise from the interaction of the GR with DNA (i.e., GR-mediated transcription), whereas the anti-inflammatory effects are mediated via protein–protein interactions between the GR and pro-inflammatory transcription factors (i.e., AP-1 and NFκB) that results in repression of the inflammatory response. A variety of selective GR modulators with the ability to repress inflammation but with lesser ability to elicit GR-mediated transcription have been reported (71–73). Early investigations indicate that a variety of different nonsteroidal pharmacophores (e.g., spirocyclic dihydropyridines, triphenylmethanes, and benzoindazoles) bind with high affinity and selectivity to the GR. Importantly, some of these analogues demonstrate preferential ability to repress pro-inflammatory genes and a lesser ability to induce GR-mediated transcription. Although these nonsteroidal ligands have yet to be evaluated in clinical studies, these drugs may someday prove to be the first members of an improved class of anti-inflammatory drugs.

Discontinued oral glucocorticoids. Paramethasone acetate (6α-fluoro-16α-methyl-11β-17,21-trihydroxypregna-1,4-diene-3,20-dione 21-acetate), synthesized in 1960, retains the 16α-methyl group, but the 9α-fluoro substituent has been moved to the 6α position. It was thought that this manipulation would reduce the electrolyte loss associated with dexamethasone. Reports in the literature indicate that paramethasone causes a slight loss of sodium and chloride with little or no loss of potassium (with doses as large as 15 mg). An analysis of continuous therapy over 9 months, however, showed that the therapeutic efficacy of paramethasone did not differ greatly from that of fluprednisolone (74).

Fluprednisolone (6α-fluoro-11β,17,21-trihydroxypregna-1,4-diene-3,20-dione) is the 16-desmethyl analogue of paramethasone. Its activity is similar to that of paramethasone, and it has approximately 2.5 times the antirheumatic potency of prednisolone. With doses of 2 to 7 mg, evidence of salt and water retention has not been noted. The therapeutic index, however, probably is the same or only a little greater than that for prednisolone. Because no new adverse reactions have been noted during the administration of this drug on a short-term basis, it seems that a 6α-fluoro group does not deleteriously affect the activity of prednisolone (49,75).

Topical Glucocorticoids

Topically applied glucocorticoids are also capable of being systemically absorbed, although to a much smaller extent. The extent of absorption of topical adrenocorticoids is determined by several factors, including the type of cream or ointment, the condition of the skin to which it is being applied, and the use of occlusive dressings. Previous studies with halobetasol propionate showed that approximately 6% of the drug was systemically absorbed after topical application. Although this is a small fraction of the dose, the very high potency of halobetasol propionate contributed to its ability to cause mild adrenal suppression in some patients. The relative potency of the topical glucocorticoids is commonly determined using topical vasoconstriction assays and is dependent on the intrinsic activity of the drug, its concentration in the formulation, and the vehicle in which it is applied (Table 33.4).

Once absorbed through the skin, topical corticosteroids are handled through metabolic pathways similar to the systemically administered corticosteroids. They are metabolized, primarily in the liver, and are then excreted into the urine or in the bile (76). The fact that circulating

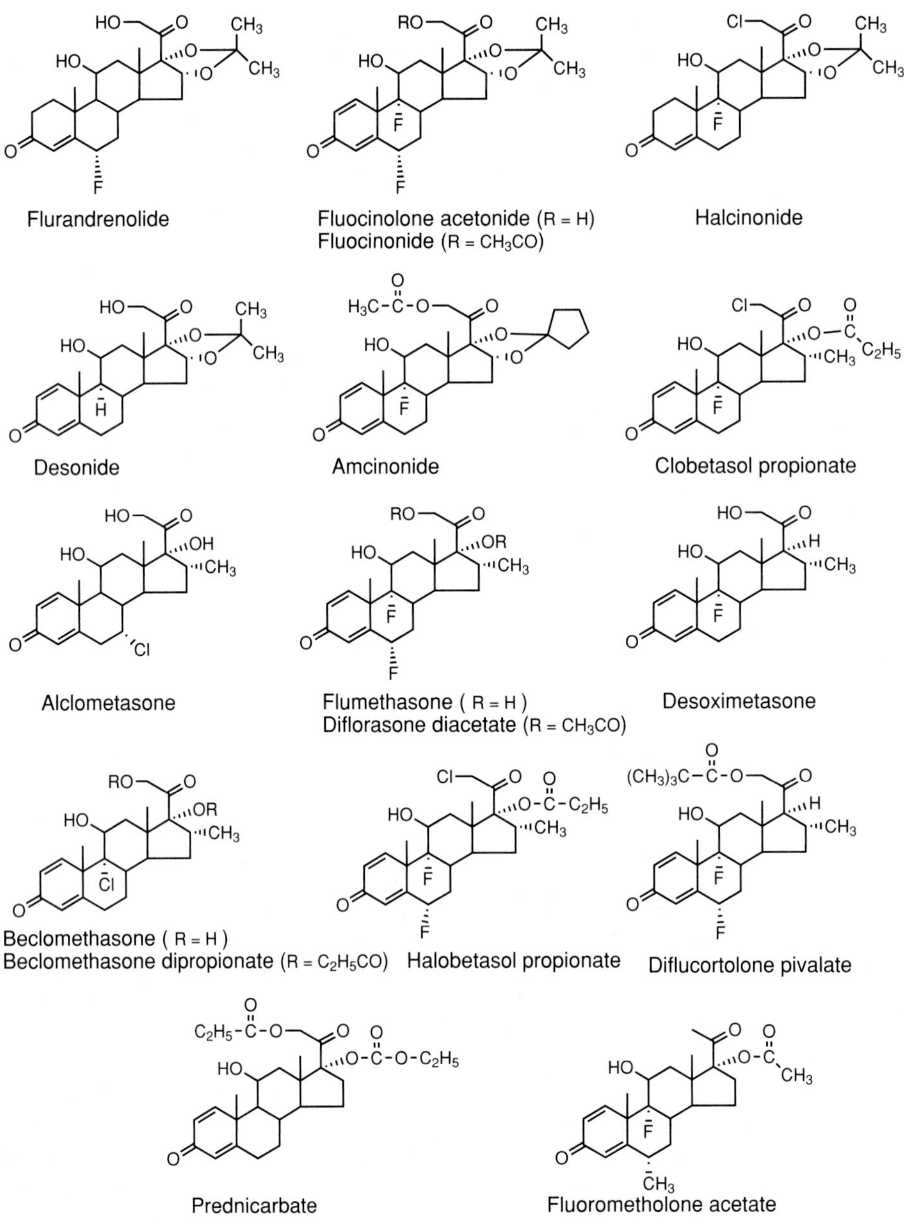

Fig. 33.13. Topical corticosteroids.

levels of the topical glucocorticoids often are well below the level of detection does not reduce the risk for potential adverse effects from systemic exposure of topical corticosteroids. The structures for the glucocorticoids applied topically are shown in Figure 33.13 and their relative potencies in Table 33.4. Topical dermatological products with a low potency ranking have a modest anti-inflammatory effect and are safest for chronic application. Those products with a medium potency ranking are used in moderate inflammatory dermatoses of limited duration. High potency preparations are used in more severe inflammatory dermatoses, but only for a short duration of treatment. Very high potency products are used primarily as an alternative to systemic corticosteroid therapy when local areas are involved and for only a short duration of therapy and on small surface areas.

Triamcinolone to be used topically is generally dispensed as its more potent and lipophilic acetonide, a 16α,17α-methylenedioxy cyclic ketal or isopropylidene derivative (Fig. 33.14) (see *Inhaled and Intranasal Glucocorticoids*). It is effective in the treatment of psoriasis and other corticoid-sensitive dermatologic conditions. Topically, triamcinolone acetonide is a more potent derivative of triamcinolone and is approximately eight times more active than prednisolone. The side effects of the drug, however, have occurred with sufficient frequency

Table 33.4. Potency Ranking for Topical Corticosteroids

I. Very high potency
- Augmented Betamethasone dipropionate
- Clobetasol propionate
- Diflorasone diacetate
- Halobetasol propionate

II. High potency
- Amcinonide
- Augmented betamethasone dipropionate
- Betamethasone dipropionate
- Betamethasone valerate
- Desoximetasone
- Diflorasone diacetate
- Fluocinolone acetonide
- Fluocinonide
- Halcinonide
- Triamcinolone acetonide

III. Medium potency
- Betamethasone benzoate
- Betamethasone dipropionate
- Betamethasone valerate
- Clocortolone pivalate
- Desoximetasone
- Fluocinolone acetonide
- Flurandrenolide
- Fluticasone propionate
- Hydrocortisone butyrate
- Hydrocortisone valerate
- Mometasone furoate
- Triamcinolone acetonide

IV. Low potency
- Alclometasone dipropionate
- Desonide
- Dexamethasone
- Dexamethasone sodium phosphate
- Fluocinolone acetonide
- Hydrocortisone
- Hydrocortisone acetate
- Prednicarbate

The relative potency is based on the drug concentration, type of vehicle used, and the vasoconstrictor assay as a measure of topical anti-inflammatory activity.

Triamcinolone acetonide

Flunisolide

Fluticasone propionate

Budesonide

Mometasone furoate

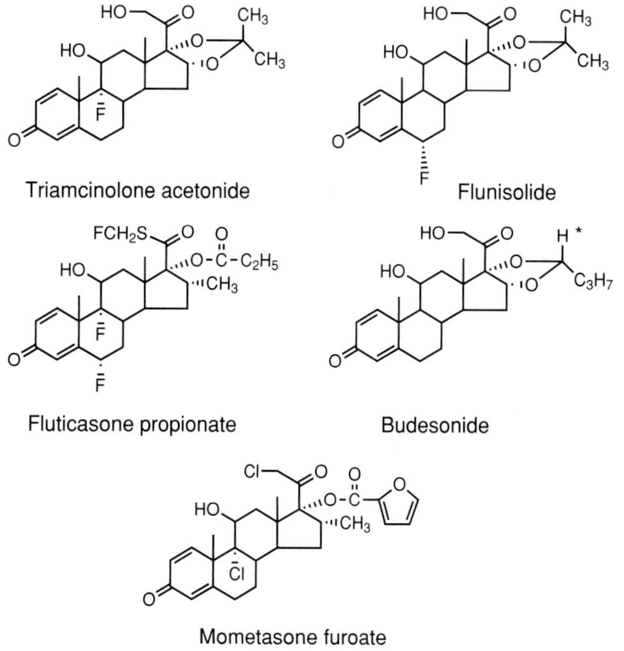

Fig. 33.14. Inhaled and intranasal corticosteroids.

to discourage its routine use for rheumatoid patients requiring steroid therapy. The drug may be employed advantageously as a special-purpose steroid for instances in which salt and water retention (from other corticoids, hypertension, or cardiac compensation) or excessive appetite and weight gain are problems in management.

Newer synthetic glucocorticoids have incorporated chlorine atoms onto the steroid molecule as fluorine substitutes. Beclomethasone, a 9α-chloro analogue of betamethasone, is a potent glucocorticoid with approximately half the potency of its fluoro analogue. It is used topically as its dipropionate derivative in inhalation aerosol therapy for asthma and rhinitis (see *Inhaled and Intranasal Glucocorticoids*) but not for treatment of steroid-responsive dermatoses (77). The topical anti-inflammatory potency for beclomethasone dipropionate (BDP) is approximately 5,000 times greater than hydrocortisone, 500 times greater than betamethasone or dexamethasone, and approximately five times greater than fluocinolone acetonide or triamcinolone acetonide, as measured by vasoconstrictor assay. Another potent topical glucocorticoid that contains a 7α-chloro group is alclometasone (78).

Additional mono- and difluorinated analogues for topical application include fluorometholone (6α-methyl-9α-fluoro; ophthalmic use), flurandrenolide (6α-fluoro-16α,17α-acetonide), fluocinolone acetonide (a 6α, 9α-difluoro-16α,17α-acetonide), and fluocinonide (21-acetate ester of fluocinolone acetonide) (Fig. 33.13). These compounds are classified as high to medium potency anti-inflammatory agents depending on the concentration and vehicle used (Table 33.4). The acetonide (ketal) derivatives at the 16,17-position enhance lipophilicity to provide potent topical anti-inflammatory agents (Table 33.4).

Psoriasis is one of the few inflammatory dermatoses that has not responded to routine topical steroid therapy, but these more potent steroids appear to work if a special occlusive dressing is used. In this technique, a thin layer of cream or ointment containing flurandrenolide is applied to the individual patch of psoriasis. The area is then covered with plastic food wrap or a similar pliable plastic film.

Clinical investigations generally show (0.05%) flurandrenolide to be more effective than 1% hydrocortisone acetate and to have approximately the same activity as 0.1% triamcinolone acetonide. Some investigators believe that its greater activity results from an increased biological half-life. In other words, these analogues are not metabolized as readily. Fluocinolone acetonide has about the same anti-inflammatory activity as fluorometholone.

Clobetasol propionate, halcinonide, halobetasol propionate, and mometasone furoate are examples of 21-chlorocorticoids, in which the 21-chloro group replaces the 21-hydroxyl group (79–82) (Figs. 33.13 and 33.14). Clobetasol propionate, the 21-chloro analogue of betamethasone 17-propionate, is approximately eight times more active as topical anti-inflammatory agent than betamethasone 17α-valerate, the standard of comparison for topical vasoconstrictor/anti-inflammatory activity. Mometasone furoate, a 9α,21-dichloro derivative (see *Inhaled and Intranasal Glucocorticoids*), also is approximately eight times more active than betamethasone 17α-valerate as a topical anti-inflammatory agent. Thus, substitution of a chlorine (or a fluorine) atom for the 21-hydroxyl group on the glucocorticoids greatly enhances topical anti-inflammatory activity (80). Clobetasol propionate and halobetasol propionate are classified as very high potency topical corticosteroid preparations (Table 33.4). The HPA suppression has occurred following the topical application of 2 g of the 0.05% clobetasol propionate ointment or cream (1 mg of clobetasol propionate total) daily. Because of its high potency and potential for causing adverse systemic effects during topical therapy, the usual dosage for very high potency topical steroids should not be exceeded. Fluticasone propionate is similar to the 21-chloro steroids, except that it has a 17α-fluoromethylcarbothioate group instead of the 17-ketol group derivative (see *Inhaled and Intranasal Glucocorticoids*) (Fig. 33.14). Although mometasone furoate and fluticasone propionate are very lipophilic and have the highest binding affinity for the GR (see *Inhaled and Intranasal Glucocorticoids*) when compared to triamcinolone acetonide and dexamethasone, their topical potency is listed as medium, in part because of their insolubility and poor dissolution into inflamed tissue.

Several nonfluorinated analogues of triamcinolone acetonide with the potency-enhancing cyclic ketal moiety are marketed, suggesting that halogens are not always necessary for topical activity. These nonfluorinated cyclic ketals include desonide and amcinonide (Fig. 33.13). Amcinonide's potency is greatly enhanced by the more lipophilic cyclopentanone ketal and 21-acetate. A recent addition to the nonhalogenated prednisolone derivatives is prednicarbate, a 17,21-diester (17α-ethylcarbonate-21-propionate) derivative of prednisolone (Fig. 33.13), which is used for the local treatment of corticoid-sensitive skin diseases (83). Any prednicarbate that is absorbed systemically is readily metabolized by hydrolysis of the 21-ester to its primary and pharmacologically active metabolite, prednisolone-17-ethylcarbonate. This metabolite has a half-life of approximately 1 to 2 hours and is further metabolized by the liver to prednisolone. In vitro binding studies with the GR suggest that the ethyl carbonate metabolite has a receptor binding affinity comparable to that of dexamethasone. The low systemic bioavailability for prednicarbate after dermal application has been attributed to its metabolism to less active prednisolone, which may be a factor for the low systemic side effects of prednicarbate.

Inhaled and Intranasal Glucocorticoids

Overview

It generally is accepted that the anti-inflammatory effect of glucocorticosteroids cannot be separated from their adverse effects at the receptor level. Therefore, pulmonary and nasal pharmacokinetics become important determinants for the potential of an inhaled or nasally applied corticosteroid to cause systemic effects, because the lung and nasal tissue provide an enormous surface area from which drug absorption can occur into the systemic circulation (84,85). The main areas of concern with regard to drug-induced systemic effects include HPA-axis suppression, change in bone mineral density and growth retardation in children, cataracts, and glaucoma. The degree of systemic side effects is dose-dependent, related to the half-life of the drug, the frequency of administration, the time of day when administered, and the route of administration; in other words, the higher the plasma corticosteroid concentration and longer the half-life, the greater the systemic side effects will be (86). Thus, the search is to develop inhaled/intranasal corticosteroids with the following desirable pharmacokinetic qualities: They would exhibit fast systemic clearance following GI absorption (high degree of first-pass intestinal/hepatic metabolism), short half-life, lack of active metabolites, and high affinity for the corticosteroid receptor. These qualities determine the proportion of the drug that reaches the target cells as well as the fraction of the dose that reaches the systemic circulation to produce side effects.

Modification of the pharmacokinetics through structural alterations has provided several new steroids with a better GR affinity and therapeutic index and a lower bioavailability than the older drugs (Fig. 33.14). The new inhaled/intranasal glucocorticosteroids like mometasone furoate, budesonide and fluticasone propionate are more lipophilic than those used in oral and systemic therapy and have greater affinity for the GR than does dexamethasone as a consequence of their greater lipophilicity (43). Several of the topical corticosteroids, such as mometasone furoate, BDP, triamcinolone acetonide, and flunisolide, were reintroduced as inhalation and intranasal dosage forms for treatment of respiratory diseases (e.g., asthma or rhinitis). Inhaled budesonide and flunisolide are readily absorbed from the airway mucosa into the blood and are rapidly biotransformed in the liver into inactive metabolites. Mometasone furoate and fluticasone propionate are very potent anti-inflammatory steroids with an oral bioavailability of less than 1%. Obviously, the risk of systemic side effects for these newer corticosteroids is greatly reduced when compared with

Table 33.5. Pharmacokinetics of Inhaled and Intranasal Corticosteroids

Parameters	Beclomethasone Dipropionate	Budesonide	Flunisolide[a]	Triamcinolone Acetonide	Fluticasone Propionate	Mometasone Furoate[a]
Receptor binding affinity[b]	0.4 13.5[c]	9.4 22R, 11.2 22S, 4.2	1.8	3.6	18 25–27	
Relative lipophilicity[d]	79,432 25,120 BMP	3,980	2,512	2,515	31,622	50,120[e]
Pulmonary bioavailability	~20%[f]	~39%	40%	25%[g]	~30% (aerosol)	<1% (aerosol)
Nasal bioavailability	~20%[f]	<20%	50%	25%[g]	13–16% (powder)	Not detectable (powder)
Oral bioavailability (systemic)	15–20%	~10%, oral	6–10%	23%	<2%	<1%
Protein binding	87% (transcortin & albumin)	85–90% (albumin)	Moderate (transcortin & albumin)	68%[g] (albumin)	91% (albumin)	90%
Half-life	30 min IV 10 min inhaled 6.5 hr BMP IV 2–7 hr BMP inhaled	2–3 hr IV	1–2 hr IV	1–2 hr IV 1–7 hr nasal 3.1 hr solution	~7.8 hr IV ~14 hr inhaled	4–6 h IV Aerosol (not detectable) Inhaled (not detectable)
Metabolism	Lung and liver esterase, liver (CYP3A4) first pass	Liver (CYP3A) first pass	Liver first pass	Liver first pass	Liver (CYP3A4) first pass	Liver
Onset of action	3–7 d	2–3 d	3–7 d	4–7 d	2–3d	7 hr
Excretion	Feces, urine 12–15%	~60% urine ~30% feces	~50% renal ~40% feces	~40% urine ~60% feces	80–90% feces <5% urine	50–90% feces 6–10% urine

BMP, beclomethasone IV, intravenous.
Data from McEvoy GK ed. AHFS 2001 Drug Information. Bethesda, MD: American Society of Health-System Pharmacists, 2001.
[a]Nasarel and Nasalide are not bioequivalent. Total absorption of Nasarel was 25% less, and the peak plasma concentration was 30% lower, than that of Nasalide. The clinical significance of this is likely to be small, however, because clinical efficacy is dependent on local effects on the nasal mucosa.
[b]Binding affinity to human glucocorticoid receptors in vitro relative to dexamethasone. Data from Kelly HW. Establishing a therapeutic index for the inhaled corticosteroids. Part 1: Pharmacokinetic pharmacodynamic comparison of the inhaled corticosteroids. J Allergy Clin Immunol 1998;102:S36–S51.
[c]Beclomethasone diproprionate is converted in the liver to the more active beclomethasone monopropionate.
[d]Measured from reverse-phase high-performance liquid chromatographic technique. Log k′ data from Brattsand R. Eur Respir Rev 1997;7:356–361 were converted to antilogs. k′ values: water = 1, hydrocortisone = 794, prednisolone = 316, dexamethasone = 400.
[e]Calculated log P for mometasone furoate = 4.7.
[f]Estimated for inhaled beclomethasone aerosol.
[g]Data from oral inhalation administration.

the older glucocorticosteroids (e.g., dexamethasone). Beclomethasone dipropionate was discovered to be a prodrug, and this discovery led to the reexamination of other 17α-monoesters as the active form of the corticosteroid esters. The absorption of budesonide, fluticasone propionate, and BDP into the airway tissue was 25 to 130 times greater than that for dexamethasone and hydrocortisone (86). The GR affinity and the pharmacokinetic properties for the inhaled and intranasal corticosteroids are listed in Table 33.5.

It is generally recognized that when administered by oral inhalation, 10 to 30% of a dose of the corticosteroid is deposited in the respiratory tract depending on type of inhaler (metered dose inhaler or dry powder inhaler [DPI]) and spacer used (87,88). The remainder of the dose is deposited primarily in the mouth and throat to be swallowed into the GI tract, where the drug may be absorbed, metabolized, and eliminated unchanged in the feces. Thus, systemic bioavailability of the inhaled/intranasal steroids is determined by the fraction of the dose absorbed from the lungs/nasal mucosa and the GI tract into systemic circulation and the degree of first-pass metabolism. Although these corticosteroids are very lipid soluble, they display variable degrees of absorption from respiratory and GI tissues, in part because of dissolution problems. When systemically absorbed, they are capable of suppressing the HPA and adrenal function with high and chronic dosing regimens (88,89). Although as much as 40% of the dose for the high-potency adrenocorticoids flunisolide, mometasone furoate, or fluticasone propionate is absorbed into airway and nasal tissues during oral inhalation, the remainder of the drug is swallowed to undergo extensive first-pass metabolism in the liver to essentially inactive metabolites, with no apparent suppression effects on adrenal function with long-term therapy.

Lipophilicity can positively or negatively alter the pharmacokinetic and pharmacodynamic actions of the inhaled/intranasal steroids (90). The lipophilic substituents attached to the corticosteroid nucleus may improve receptor affinity (Table 33.5), or they can affect pharmacokinetic properties, such as absorption, protein and tissue binding, distribution, and excretion. The inhaled/intranasal corticosteroids are inhaled as microcrystals and need sufficient water solubility to be dissolved in the nasal or lung epithelial tissue for local anti-inflammatory activity to occur. Lipophilicity, however, can delay their rate of dissolution into these tissues, which may be advantageous by prolonging their retention within these tissues, affecting their onset and duration of action, or a disadvantage by facilitating their transport away from these tissues via mucociliary clearance before full dissolution can occur. The systemic steroids prednisolone and hydrocortisone are less effective as inhaled/intranasal steroids because of their higher water solubility and lower lipophilicity. For inhaled/intranasal steroids, there is a sharp drop in water solubility when the lipophilicity is log $P \geq 4.5$ ($P = 30{,}000$), which is the case for fluticasone propionate, mometasone furoate, and BDP. High lipophilicity correlates well with low oral bioavailability (Table 33.5).

The use of dexamethasone sodium phosphate inhalation aerosol is not recommended because of the potential for extensive systemic absorption and the long metabolic half-life for dexamethasone after absorption, resulting in an increased risk of adverse effects with usual inhalation doses (27). Following the oral inhalation of dexamethasone sodium phosphate, a cumulative dose of 1,200 μg/day will result in the systemic absorption of 400 to 600 μg of dexamethasone, which is sufficient to cause HPA suppression. Dexamethasone sodium phosphate nasal aerosol delivers 100 μg per metered spray. The total daily adult nasal dose is 1,200 μg.

Specific Drugs

Triamcinolone Acetonide. Triamcinolone acetonide frequently is used by inhalation for the treatment of lung diseases (e.g., asthma). After inhalation, triamcinolone acetonide can become systemically available when the inhaled formulation is swallowed and absorbed unchanged from the GI tract, causing undesirable systemic effects (91–93). Triamcinolone acetonide that is swallowed is metabolized to 6β-hydroxytriamcinolone acetonide, 21-carboxytriamcinolone acetonide, and 21-carboxy-6β-hydroxytriamcinolone acetonide, all of which are more hydrophilic than their parent drug. Only approximately 1% of the dose was recovered from the urine as triamcinolone acetonide (94). Triamcinolone is not a major metabolite of triamcinolone acetonide in humans, suggesting that acetonide is resistant to hydrolytic cleavage. Triamcinolone acetonide is approximately eight times more potent than prednisolone.

Triamcinolone acetonide inhalation aerosol for pulmonary delivery is a microcrystalline suspension in a chlorofluorocarbon propellant that delivers 200 μg per metered spray, which is equivalent to 100 μg delivered at the mouthpiece. The total daily adult nasal dose for triamcinolone acetonide is 1.6 mg. Triamcinolone acetonide nasal aerosol is a microcrystalline suspension in a chlorofluorocarbon propellant that delivers 55 μg per metered spray. The total daily dose for triamcinolone acetonide is 440 μg.

Beclomethasone 17,21-Dipropionate. Beclomethasone dipropionate is used primarily as an inhalation aerosol therapy for asthma and rhinitis (77). A breakthrough in the discovery of new inhalation corticosteroids with reduced risks from systemic absorption was that the 17α-monopropionate ester of beclomethasone (17-BMP) was more active than BDP and 21-monopropionate (21-BMP) esters (95). Thus, BDP is a pro-drug that is rapidly metabolized by esterases in the lung and other tissues to its more active metabolite, 17-BMP, which has 30 times greater affinity for the GR than BDP and approximately 14 times dexamethasone (Table 33.5) (43).

Whether orally administered or swallowed from inhalation, BDP undergoes rapid first-pass metabolism of the unhindered 21-ester via enzymatic hydrolysis in the liver or GI tract primarily to 17-BMP but more slowly to 21-BMP and to beclomethasone and other unidentified metabolites and polar conjugates (96,97). The terminal half-life for 17-BMP is 6.5 hours. The portion of the inhaled dose of BDP that enters the lung is rapidly metabolized to 17-BMP in the respiratory tract before reaching systemic circulation, where it can be further metabolized by the liver. Following oral administration, BDP and its metabolites are excreted mainly in feces via biliary elimination, and 12 to 15% of a 4-mg dose of BDP is excreted in urine as free and conjugated metabolites. The usual therapeutic dose (<1,200 μg/day) for BDP oral inhalation does not produce systemic glucocorticoid effects, probably because the drug is rapidly metabolized to less active metabolites. At doses greater than 1,200 μg/ day, HPA suppression has been observed (27).

The BDP monohydrate nasal suspension is available as an aqueous microcrystalline suspension of BDP, which delivers 42 μg per metered spray. The BDP nasal aerosol or inhalation aerosol consists of microcrystalline suspension of BDP in chlorofluorocarbon propellant, both of which delivers 42, 50, or 84 μg per metered spray. The total daily adult dose for BDP is 600 μg from the nasal spray or nasal inhaler and 336 to 1,000 μg for the aerosol inhaler. Doses exceeding 2,000 μg/day need to be monitored for HPA suppression.

Flunisolide. When administered intranasally or by inhalation, flunisolide (Fig. 33.14) is rapidly absorbed from nasal or lung tissue (Table 33.5) (94). This corticosteroid is efficiently metabolized by the liver to inactive metabolites with no apparent effects on adrenal function with long-term therapy. Flunisolide that is swallowed undergoes extensive first-pass metabolism in the liver, and that which is absorbed directly from the nasopharyngeal mucosa or lung bypasses this initial metabolism (98). It is not known if the drug undergoes metabolism in the GI tract. Flunisolide is rapidly hydroxylated by CYP3A4 at the 6β position, followed by elimination of the 6α-fluoro group to its more polar 6β-hydroxy metabolite, which attains plasma concentrations that usually are greater than those for flunisolide (94,98).

Following IV administration of flunisolide, the 6β-hydroxy metabolite has 1/100 the potency of flunisolide and a plasma half-life of 3.9 to 4.6 hours. Flunisolide and its 6β-hydroxy metabolite are conjugated in the liver to inactive glucuronides and sulfates. After intranasal administrations of 100 μg, the plasma levels for flunisolide were undetectable within 4 hours. The duration of its systemic effects is short because of its short half-life.

Flunisolide nasal solution is available in an aqueous solubilized form, which delivers 25 μg per spray. The total daily adult dose for flunisolide from the nasal spray is 200 to 400 μg. Flunisolide inhalation aerosol for pulmonary delivery is a microcrystalline suspension in a chlorofluorocarbon propellant that delivers 250 μg per metered spray. The total daily adult inhalation dose for flunisolide is 1,000 μg. Doses exceeding 2,000 μg/day need to be monitored for HPA suppression.

Budesonide. Budesonide is a highly potent, nonhalogenated glucocorticoid intended for the local treatment of lung disease and rhinitis. It was designed to have a high ratio between local and systemic effects. Budesonide is composed of a 1:1 mixture of epimers of the 16,17-butylacetal, creating a chiral center (Fig. 33.14) (99). The 22R-epimer binds to the GR with higher affinity than does the 22S-epimer (Table 33.5) (43). The butyl acetal chain provided the highest potency for the homologous acetal chains. Its rate of topical uptake into epithelial tissue is more than 100 times faster than that for hydrocortisone and dexamethasone. Approximately 85% of the IV administered dose of budesonide undergoes extensive first-pass hepatic metabolism by CYP3A4 to its primary metabolites, 6β-hydroxybudesonide and 16α-hydroxyprednisolone, which have approximately 1/100 the potency of budesonide (100,101). This is an important inactivation step in limiting budesonide's systemic effect on adrenal suppression. Budesonide was metabolized three- to sixfold more rapidly than triamcinolone acetonide. The pharmacokinetics of budesonide after inhalation, oral, and IV administration displayed a mean plasma half-life of 2.8 hours and a systemic bioavailability of approximately 10% after oral administration (Table 33.5) (101). Pulmonary bioavailability is less than 40% after inhalation (70–75% after correction for the amounts of budesonide deposited in the inhalation device and oral cavity). No oxidative metabolism was observed in the lung. When given by inhalation, 32% of the dose is excreted in the urine as metabolites, 15% in the feces, and 41% of the dose remained in the mouthpiece of the inhaler. Following intranasal administration, very little of intranasal budesonide is absorbed from the nasal mucosa. Much of the intranasal dose (~60%) was swallowed, however, and remained in the GI tract to be excreted unchanged in the feces, whereas that fraction of the intranasal dose that was absorbed was extensively metabolized.

Inhaled budesonide, in spite of its lower lipophilicity, exhibits greater retention within the airways than other inhaled corticosteroids do (100,101). This unusual behavior for inhaled budesonide has been attributed to the subsequent formation of intracellular fatty acid esters of the 21-hydroxy group of budesonide in the airway and lung tissue (102,103). Following inhalation, approximately 70 to 80% of budesonide was reversibly esterified by free fatty acids in the airway tissue. These inactive esters behave like an intracellular depot drug by slowly regenerating free budesonide. Thus, this reversible esterification prolongs the local anti-inflammatory action of budesonide in the airways and may contribute to the high efficacy and safety of budesonide in the treatment of mild asthma when inhaled once daily.

The systemic availability of budesonide in children was estimated to be 6.1% of the nominal dose, and the terminal half-life was 2.3 hours (104,105). Approximately 6% of the nominal dose reached the systemic circulation of young children after inhalation of nebulized budesonide. This is approximately half the systemic availability found in healthy adults using the same nebulizer.

Budesonide nasal aerosol is supplied as a micronized suspension using a chlorofluorocarbon propellant, which delivers 32 μg from the nasal adapter supplied per metered spray. The total daily adult dose for budesonide is 256 μg. Budesonide powder for pulmonary inhalation uses micronized dry powder in a turboinhaler (DPI) that delivers 200 μg per metered sprayed. The total daily adult dose for budesonide from the DPI is 200 to 800 μg. Full benefit is attained in approximately 1 to 2 weeks.

Mometasone furoate. The development of mometasone furoate resulted from reexamination of the effect of 17α-ester functionalities on topical anti-inflammatory potency relative to the potent 17-benzoate ester of betamethasone. The structure–activity relationship study involved substitution of the 17-benzoate ester with heteroaromatic furoic, thienoic, and pyrrolic esters (81,106). Of the numerous 17α-heteroaryl esters studied, the 2-furoate ester displayed the greatest increase in potency. Therefore, combining the 17α-(2-furoate) ester with the potency-enhancing effect of the 21-chloro group, the resultant glucocorticoid (mometasone furoate) (Fig. 33.14) was 5 to 10 times more potent than the betamethasone benzoate ester, with a more rapid onset of action. Mometasone furoate was originally marketed as a topically applied corticosteroid, but because of its low systemic bioavailability, it was found to be more useful in the treatment of allergic disorders and lung diseases (107). It has the greatest binding affinity for the GR (Table 33.5), followed by fluticasone propionate, budesonide, triamcinolone acetonide, and dexamethasone (43). Mometasone furoate has strong local anti-inflammatory activity equivalent to that of fluticasone propionate. It has a quick onset of action relative to the other inhaled/intranasal steroids with the least systemic availability and, consequently, the fewest systemic side effects.

Following IV suspension or inhalation administration, mometasone furoate was detected in the plasma for up to 8 hours, with a half-life of 4 to 6 hours (Table 33.5) and an oral bioavailability of less than 1%. It is extensively metabolized with less than 10% of the administered dose recovered in the urine unchanged (108). Among the polar metabolites (~80%) and their conjugates (42%) that were recovered were 6β-hydroxymometasone furoate and its 21-hydroxy metabolite. In contrast, following intranasal administration, its plasma concentrations were below the limit of quantification, and the systemic bioavailability by this route was estimated to be less than 1%. The majority of the intranasal dose for mometasone furoate is deposited in the nasal mucosa and swallowed without absorption in the GI tract until eliminated in the feces (approximately 50–90% of the intranasal dose is recovered in the feces). That portion of the intranasal dose that was absorbed was extensively metabolized. These results indicate that inhaled mometasone furoate has negligible systemic bioavailability and is extensively metabolized, with reduced risk for causing systemic adrenal suppression effects.

Mometasone furoate nasal suspension is supplied as an aqueous suspension with an atomizing pump that dispenses 50 μg per metered spray. The total daily dose for mometasone furoate is 200 μg.

ANDROSTANE 17β-CARBOXYLATES AND 17β-CARBOTHIOATES

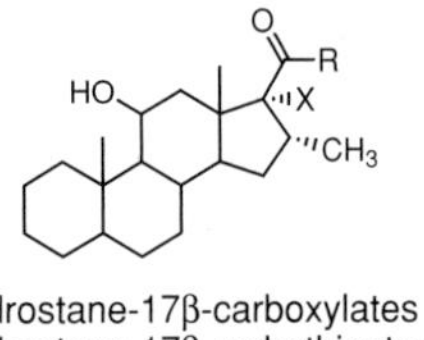

Androstane-17β-carboxylates (R = OCH_2F)
Androstane-17β-carbothioates (R = SCH_2F)
(X = acetate or propionate)

The androstane 17β-hydroxyl-17β-carboxylates and 17β-carbothioates were designed to be metabolically susceptible to hydrolysis and to have a low systemic bioavailability to minimize systemic glucocorticoid-induced adrenal suppression. The androstane 17α-hydroxyl-17β-carboxylates lacked the 17-ketol group found in most of the systemic corticosteroids. When these 17β-carboxylates were esterified to their 17α/β-diesters, however, they proved to be extremely potent anti-inflammatory corticosteroids, whereas the parent carboxylic acids were inactive (109). Thus, enzymatic hydrolysis of the 17-carboxylate ester function by intestinal or liver esterases would lead to formation of inactive metabolites. The greatest anti-inflammatory activity was observed with 17α-acetoxy and 17α-propionoxy groups and simple alkyl carboxylate esters, although the fluoromethyl esters showed the highest activity. Superseding the androstane 17β-carboxylates were the corresponding 17β-carbothioates (thioesters) derived from flumethasone. The 17β-fluoromethylcarbothioate when combined with the 17α-propionoxy group yielded fluticasone (Fig. 33.14) (110). The androstane 17β-carbothioates proved not only to be very potent anti-inflammatory agents but also to exhibit weak HPA suppression in the rat. Both the androstane 17β-carboxylates and the androstane 17β-carbothioates are very lipophilic and exhibit minimal oral bioavailability and very low systemic activity after inhalation because of intestinal and hepatic enzymatic hydrolysis to inactive metabolites, which have 1/2,000 the activity of the parent molecule (111).

Fluticasone Propionate. Fluticasone propionate, a trifluorinated glucocorticoid based on the androstane 17β-carbothioate nucleus (Fig. 33.14), was designed to be metabolically susceptible to hydrolysis and to have a low systemic bioavailability to minimize the systemic effects on plasma hydrocortisone levels. Its susceptibility to metabolic hydrolysis is doubly enhanced by the combination of a thioester and the high electronegativity of the fluorine group. Fluticasone propionate is approximately 0.5 times as lipophilic than BDP, eight times more lipophilic than budesonide, and 13 times more lipophilic than triamcinolone acetonide (Table 33.5) (90). It also displays high in vitro selectivity for the GR and a relative receptor affinity 1.5 times that of 17-BMP and mometasone furoate, three times that of budesonide, 18 times that of dexamethasone, and 20 times that of flunisolide and triamcinolone acetonide (43). The rate of association for fluticasone dipropionate with the receptor is faster, and the rate of dissociation is slower, than the other corticosteroids. The half-life of the fluticasone propionate active steroid–receptor complex is greater than 10 hours, compared with approximately 5 hours for budesonide, 7.5 hours for 17-BMP, and 4 hours for triamcinolone acetonide (43).

Following topical application to the nasal mucosa or after inhalation, fluticasone propionate produces potent anti-inflammatory effects, with an onset of action of approximately 2 to 3 days. The topical anti-inflammatory potency for fluticasone propionate is approximately equal to that for mometasone furoate, 13-fold greater than that for triamcinolone acetonide, ninefold greater than that for fluocinolone acetonide, threefold greater than that for betamethasone 17-valerate, and twofold greater than that for BDP (111). Because of its low systemic bioavailability when administered intranasally or by inhalation and nondetectability in plasma, most pharmacokinetic data for fluticasone propionate are based on IV or oral administration (Table 33.5). Its rate of topical uptake into epithelial tissue is more than 100-fold faster than that for hydrocortisone and dexamethasone but is similar to BDP and budesonide.

As a consequence of its high lipophilicity (Table 33.5), fluticasone propionate is very insoluble and, therefore, is poorly absorbed from the respiratory (10–13%) and GI tract following nasal inhalation of the drug (112–114). The majority of the intranasal dose for fluticasone propionate is deposited in the nasal mucosa and swallowed into the GI tract until eliminated in the feces (~80–90% of the intranasal dose is recovered metabolized and unchanged in the feces). After administration of an IV suspension, fluticasone propionate displayed a systemic bioavailability of less than 2% and underwent extensive hydrolysis and CYP3A4 first-pass metabolism in the liver, with an elimination half-life of approximately 3 hours. Its primary hydrolysis product is 17β-carboxylate metabolite, which has 1/2,000 the affinity for the GR, can be recovered from the urine along with other unidentified hydroxy metabolites and their conjugates. Following oral administration of 1 to 40 mg, fluticasone propionate is poorly absorbed from the GI tract because of hydrolysis and its insolubility, with an oral bioavailability of less than 1%. Less than 5% of the oral dose is excreted unchanged in the urine. Fluticasone propionate was not detected in plasma for up to 6 hours after IV or oral administration (113). Approximately 80 to 90% of the oral dose is excreted unchanged in the feces, of which approximately 3 to 40% is the hydrolyzed 17β-carboxylate metabolite. Pulmonary bioavailability ranges between 16 and 30% depending on the inhalation device used, with an elimination half-life of approximately 14 hours, increasing its potential for drug accumulation with repeated dosing (114). The long elimination half-life for fluticasone propionate results, in part, from its very high lipophilicity and very poor water solubility and, consequently, slow dissolution into lung tissue. Some suppression of overnight hydrocortisone levels has been reported with inhaled fluticasone propionate at higher dosages (indicative of HPA-axis suppression) (115).

Fluticasone propionate nasal suspension and inhalation aerosol are both available as micronized suspensions in a chlorofluorocarbon propellant that delivers 50 μg per metered spray. The total daily adult dose for fluticasone propionate is 200 μg for the nasal suspension and 880 μg for the inhalation aerosol.

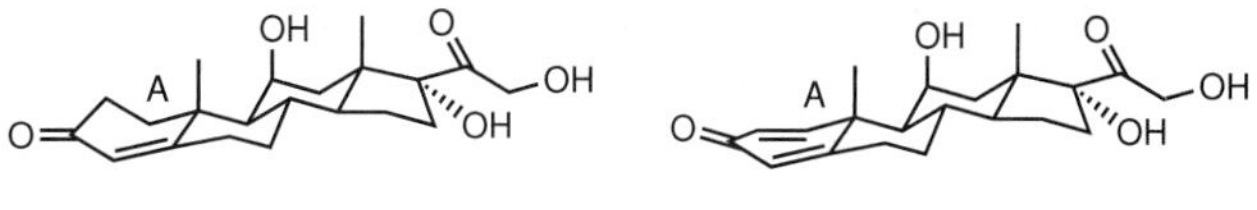

Hydrocortisone Prednisolone

Fig. 33.15. Conformations of hydrocortisone and prednisolone.

SUMMARY OF STRUCTURE–ACTIVITY RELATIONSHIPS

The structure in Figure 33.15 depicts the ring conformation and the absolute configuration of hydrocortisone and prednisolone. The all-*trans* (B/C and C/D) backbone that is necessary for activity is very evident.

As previously pointed out, the adrenocorticoids generally are classified as either glucocorticoids, which affect intermediary metabolism and are associated with inhibition of the inflammatory process, or mineralocorticoids. In fact, most naturally occurring and semisynthetic analogues exhibit both of these actions. The 17β-ketol (—$COCH_2OH$) side chain and the Δ^4-3-ketone functions are found in clinically used adrenocorticoids, and these groups do contribute to the potency of the agents. Modifications of these groups may result in derivatives that retain biological activity. For example, replacement of the 21-OH group with fluorine increases glucocorticoid and sodium-retaining activities, whereas substitution with chlorine or bromine abolishes activity. Some compounds that do not contain the Δ^4-3-ketone system have appreciable activity. It has been suggested that this group makes only a minor contribution to the specificity of action by these drugs or to the steroid–receptor association constant (116).

Based on structure–activity studies, the C and D rings, involving positions 11, 12, 13, 16, 17, 18, 20, and 21, are more important for receptor binding than the A and B rings. Generally, insertion of bulky substituents on the β-side of the molecule abolishes glycogenic activity, whereas insertion on the α-side does not. It has been suggested that association of these steroids with receptors involves β-surfaces of rings C and D and the 17β-ketol side chain (116). It is possible, however, that association with the α-surface of rings A, C, and D, as well as with the ketol side chain, is essential for sodium-retaining activity. Many functional groups, such as 17α-OH, 17α-CH_3, 16α-CH_3, 16β-CH_3, 16α-CH_3O, and 16α-OH substituents, abolish or reverse this activity in 11-desoxycorticosterone and 11-oxygenated steroids. Discussions of exceptions of these generalities are found in the literature (116).

Although some steroids cause sodium retention, many have glucocorticoid and either sodium-retaining or sodium-excreting action. Difficulties in correlating the structures of adrenocorticoids with biological action are compounded because of differences in assay methods, species variation, and mode of drug administration. For

Table 33.6. Biological Potencies of Modified Adrenocorticoids in the Rat and Humans*

		Potency Relative to Hydrocortisone (Cortisol)			
		Rat		Humans	
Adrenocorticoid	Thymus Involution	Liver Glycogen Deposition	Eosinopenic Potency	Hyperglycemic Potency	Antirheumatic Potency
Corticosterone	—	0.8	0.06	0.06	<0.1
Prednisone	—	3	—	4	4
Prednisolone	2	3.9	4	4	4
Methylprednisolone	10	11	5	5	5
Triamcinolone	4	47	5	5	5
Paramethasone	—	150	12	12	11
Dexamethasone	56	265	28	28	29
Fludrocortisone acetate	6	9	8	8	10
Fluprednisolone	6	81	9	9	10
Triamcinolone acetonide	33	242	3	3	3
Flurandrenoione	4	—	1	—	2
Fluorometholone	25	115	10	10	—
Fluocinolone	19	112	5	6	9

*Data from Ringler I. Steroidal activity in experimental animals and man. In: Dorfman RI, ed. Methods of Hormone Research, vol 3. Part A. New York: Academic Press, 1964.

example, whereas liver glycogen and anti-inflammatory assays in the rat correlate well, some drugs show high anti-inflammatory action in the rat but little or no antirheumatic activity in humans. The 9α-F analogue, fludrocortisone acetate, is more active than the 9α-Cl analogue in terms of sodium retention in the dog; the reverse is true in the rat. Although 16α-methylation and 16β-methylation enhance glucocorticoid activity, anti-inflammatory action is increased disproportionately to glycogenic action in both series.

In humans, eosinopenic and hyperglycemic potencies are essentially the same. There is a close correlation in efficacy ratios derived from these tests and antirheumatic potency (Table 33.6). Because the eosinopenic–hyperglycemic activity and antirheumatic potency show excellent agreement, it has been suggested that these assays afford advantages in the preliminary estimation of anti-inflammatory potency (27).

Structure–activity studies of glucocorticoids have been carried out mainly in animals and are not necessarily applicable to clinical efficacy in man. Relative activity and dose correlations for the clinically useful drugs are found in Table 33.2.

Several other compounds have been studied in animals and used to derive structure–activity relationships. For example, insertion of a double bond between positions 1 and 2 in hydrocortisone increases glucocorticoid activity. The Δ^1-corticoids have a much longer half-life in the blood than hydrocortisone. Ring A is much more slowly metabolized, but it is oxidatively metabolized at other positions, especially the 6β position and the 17β-ketol (Fig. 33.12). If, however, a double bond is inserted between positions 9 and 11 (no oxygen function at 11), a decrease in glucocorticoid activity is observed. Except for cortisone, which results in an analogue with decreased glucocorticoid activity when a double bond is inserted between position 6 and 7, such modification of other glucocorticoids generally produces no change in activity (16).

Insertion of α-CH_3 groups at positions 2 (in 11β-OH analogues), 6, and 16 increases glucocorticoid activity in animals. Again, insertion of a 2α-CH_3 group into the glucocorticoid almost completely prevents reduction of the Δ^4-3-ketone system in vivo and in vitro. Substitutions at positions 4α, 7α, 9α, 11α, and 21 decrease activity.

Although some analogues, such as 16α,17α-isopropylidinedioxy-6α-methylpregna-1,4-diene-3,20-dione and the 1,2-dihydro derivative, are 11-desoxysteroids and biologically active, the 11β-OH group of hydrocortisone does seem to be involved in the drug–receptor interaction (116). Cortisone, which contains an 11-keto function, is reduced in vivo to hydrocortisone. The drug 2α-methylhydrocortisone exhibits high glucocorticoid activity, probably because of steric hindrance to reduction (i.e., C=O → C-β-OH) by the methyl group, thus rendering the analogue inactive (40,117,118). Insertion of α-OH groups into most other positions (1, 6, 7, 9, 14, and 16) or reduction of the 20-ketone, however, decreases glucocorticoid activity, in part because of increased hydrophilicity.

The 9α-F group increases glucocorticoid activity and nearly prevents metabolic oxidation of the 11β-OH group to a ketone. Redox metabolism of Δ^4-steroids is mainly restricted to the Δ^4-3-ketone, 6 and 16 positions, and 17β-ketol side chains, whereas for Δ^4-steroids it is only the 6 and 16 positions and 17β-ketol side chains. The 9α-F group may increase activity by an inductive effect, which increases the acidic dissociation constant of the 11β-OH group and, thereby, increases the ability of the drug to hydrogen bonding to GRs.

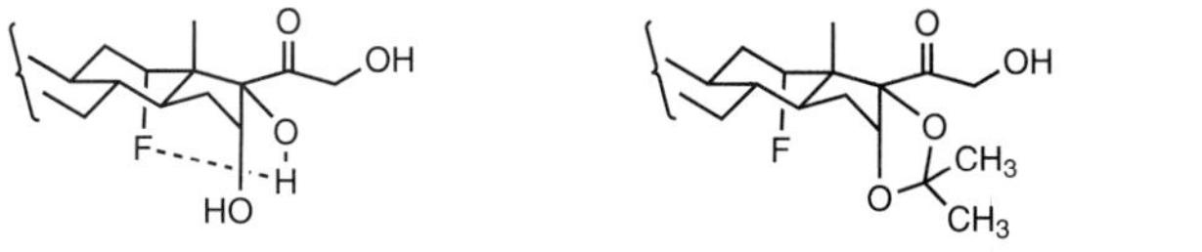

16α, 17α-Dihydroxy steroid 16α, 17α-Isopropylidenedioxy steroid

Fig. 33.16. Hydrogen bonding between 17α-hydroxyl and 12α-fluoro groups.

A 6α-F group also increases glucocorticoid activity, but it has less effect than the 9α-F function on sodium retention. Insertion of 2α-, 11α- (no OH group at 11), or 21-F groups decreases glucocorticoid activity. Of particular interest is a 12α-F group. When this function is inserted into corticosterone, which has no 17α-OH group, it potentiates activity to the same extent as a 9α-F group. Insertion of a 12α-F group into a 16α,17α-dihydroxy steroid, however, renders the compound inactive. A 9α-F group potentiates activity in such analogues.

It has been proposed that hydrogen bonding between the 12α-F and 17α-OH groups renders the analogue inactive (Fig. 33.16). Conversion to the 16α,17α-isopropylidinedioxy (acetonide) derivative, which cannot hydrogen bond, restores biological activity (119).

The mineralocorticoid activity of adrenocorticoids is another action of major significance. Many toxic side effects, making it necessary to withdraw steroid therapy in rheumatoid patients, are a result of this action. Highly active, naturally occurring mineralocorticoids have no OH function in positions 11 and 17. In fact, OH groups in any position reduce the sodium-retaining activity of the adrenocorticoid.

Generally, 9α-F, 9α-Cl, and 9α-Br substitution causes increased retention of urinary sodium with an order of activity in which F > Cl > Br, but species differences do exist. For these reasons, such compounds are not used internally in the treatment of diseases such as rheumatoid arthritis. Insertion of a 16α-OH group into the molecule affects the sodium retention activity so markedly that it not only negates the effect of the 9α-F atom but also causes sodium excretion.

A double bond between positions 1 and 2 (Δ^1-corticoids) also reduces the sodium retention activity of the parent drug. This functional group, however, contributes to the parent drug only approximately one-fifth the sodium-excreting tendency of a 16α-OH group (120).

The 12α-F, 2α-CH_3, and 9α-Cl substitutions contribute equally to sodium retention. A 21-OH group, found in all these drugs, contributes to this action to the same degree. Because 21-OH groups also contribute to glucocorticoid activity, it is easy to understand why it is difficult to develop compounds with only one major action.

A 2α-CH_3 group is approximately threefold, and a 21-F substituent twofold, as effective as unsaturation between positions 1 and 2 in reducing sodium retention. Other substituents reported to inhibit sodium retention include 16α-CH_3, 16β-CH_3, 16α-CH_3O, and 6α-Cl functions. A 17α-OH group, which is present in naturally occurring and semisynthetic analogues, reduces sodium retention to about the same extent as does unsaturation between positions 1 and 2.

Conversion of the 17α-hydroxy to either a 17α-ester or an ether, as with 16α,17α-isopropylidinedioxy (acetonide), greatly enhances the anti-inflammatory potency and GR affinity (Table 33.5). As evidenced with BDP, however, esterifying the 21-hydroxy group reduces activity and receptor affinity. On the other hand, 21-halogens or 21-halomethylene groups greatly increase topical anti-inflammatory activity with no change or a decrease in mineralocorticoid activity. Perhaps a hydrogen bonding group at position 21 enhances or retains mineralocorticoid receptor affinity.

ADRENOCORTICOID ANTAGONISTS

Antagonists of adrenocorticoids include agents that compete for binding to steroid receptors (antiglucocorticoids or antimineralocorticoids) and inhibitors of adrenosteroid biosynthesis. The action of adrenal steroids can be blocked by antagonists that compete with the endogenous steroids for binding sites on their respective cytosolic receptor proteins. The antagonist–receptor complexes are unable to stimulate the production of new mRNA and protein in the target tissues and, thus, are unable to elicit the biological responses of the hormone agonist. Spironolactone (Fig. 33.17) and related analogues bind to the mineralocorticoid receptor in the kidney and result in the diuretic response of increased Na^+ excretion and K^+ retention. The 3-keto-4-ene A ring is essential for this antagonistic activity, and the opening of the lactone ring dramatically reduces activity. The 7α-substituent increases both intrinsic activity and oral activity (121,122). Progesterone also has shown antimineralocorticoid activity at 10^{-4} molar concentrations.

Receptor antagonists of glucocorticoids have been described that are derivatives of 19-nortestosterone (123). Mifepristone, also referred to as RU-486 (Fig. 33.17), was originally developed as an antiprogestin and also exhibits very effective antagonism of glucocorticoids.

Several inhibitors of adrenocorticoid biosynthesis have been described, with the majority of nonsteroidal agents inhibiting one or more of the cytochrome P450 enzyme complexes involved in adrenosteroid biosynthesis (Fig. 33.17). Metyrapone reduces cortisol biosynthesis by primarily inhibiting mitochondrial 11β-hydroxylase (124, 125). It also inhibits, to a lesser degree, 18-hydroxylase and side-chain cleavage. This agent is used to test pituitary–adrenal function and the ability of the pituitary to secrete ACTH (125). Aminoglutethimide inhibits side-chain cleavage (125) and has been used as a medical adrenalectomy. Several azole antifungal drugs inhibit adrenocorticoid biosynthesis. Ketoconazole is one example of a potent inhibitor of fungal sterol biosynthesis at low con-

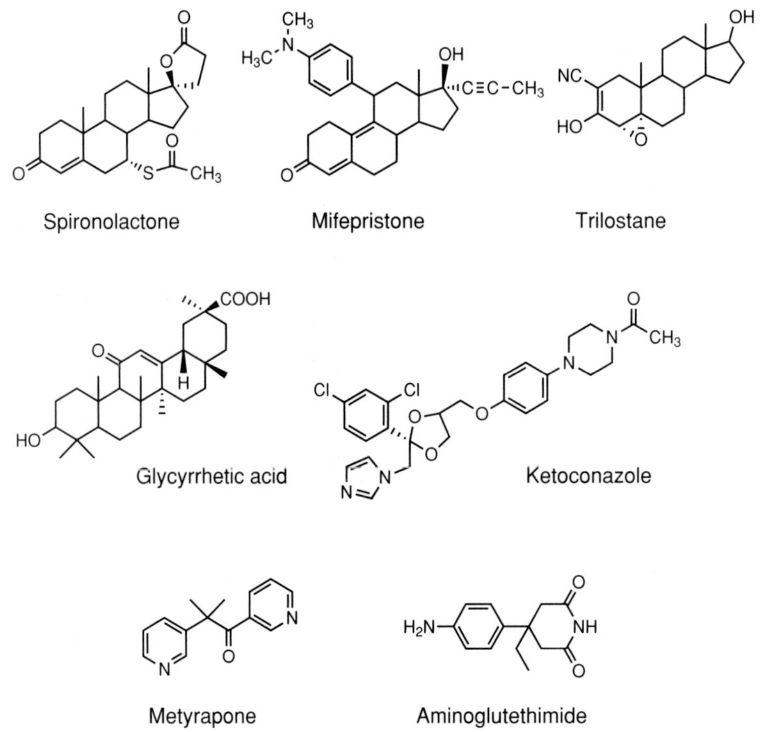

Fig. 33.17. Antagonists of adrenocorticoids.

centrations; however, at higher doses, ketoconazole inhibits CYP3A4 in adrenosteroid biosynthesis (126). Trilostane (4α,5α-epoxy-17β-hydroxy-3-oxoandrostan-2α-carbonitrile) is a steroidal inhibitor of 3β-hydroxysteroid dehydrogenase (127) and has been used in the treatment of Cushing's syndrome.

Inhibition of the two 11β-hydroxysteroid dehydrogenase isozymes has been described. Excessive ingestion of licorice, an extract of the roots of *Glycyrrhiza glabra*, produces undesirable mineralocorticoid-like intoxication (hypertension, excessive salt retention, and hypokalemia). The active components of licorice, glycyrrhetic acid (Fig. 33.17) and carbenoxolone, inhibit both 11β-HSD isozymes (128), with the undesirable side effects resulting from inhibition of 11β-HSD2 in the kidney. Bile acids, such as chenodeoxycholic acid and lithocholic acid, have recently shown selective inhibition of 11β-HSD1 (129,130), and nonsteroidal arylsulfoamidothiazoles also recently have been reported as 11β-HSD1 inhibitors (131). Such enzyme inhibitors may be useful in the treatment on metabolic syndromes to reduce elevated glucose concentrations and as possible antidiabetic agents.

MECHANISMS OF ADRENOCORTICOID ACTION

Molecular Interaction

Glucocorticoid action is mediated through the glucocorticoid receptor, which is found primarily in the cytosol of the cell when not bound to glucocorticoids. The GR is stabilized in the cytosol by complexation with phosphorylated proteins, including a 90-kDa protein referred to as a heat shock protein 90 (132). The steroid molecule binds to the GR, resulting in a conformational change of the receptor to dissociate the other proteins and initiate translocation of the steroid–receptor complex into the nucleus. The steroid–nuclear GR complex interacts with particular HRE regions of the cellular DNA, referred to as glucocorticoid-responsive elements and initiates transcription of the DNA sequence to produce mRNA. Finally, the elevated levels of mRNA lead to increased protein synthesis in the endoplasmic reticulum. These proteins then mediate glucocorticoid effects on carbohydrate, lipid, and protein metabolism. An alternative isoform of the GR has been identified. This isoform of the receptor does not bind known glucocorticoids, and its function remains to be determined (133,134). Some of the specific proteins induced by glucocorticoids have been identified and are discussed later. Mineralocorticoid effects are observed in several tissues, and specific mineralocorticoid receptors have been characterized that mediate mineralocorticoid functions (135).

Physiologic Effects

Glucocorticoids

Corticosteroids influence all tissues of the body and produce numerous and varying effects in cells (16).

These steroids regulate carbohydrate, lipid, and protein biosynthesis and metabolism (glucocorticoid effects), and they influence water and electrolyte balance (mineralocorticoid effects). Cortisol is the most potent glucocorticoid secreted by the adrenal gland, and aldosterone is the most potent endogenous mineralocorticoid. Both naturally occurring glucocorticoids and related, semisynthetic analogues can be evaluated in terms of their ability to sustain life, to stimulate an increase in blood glucose concentrations and a deposition of liver glycogen, to decrease circulating eosinophils (136), and to cause thymus involution in adrenalectomized animals (137,138). In addition, corticosteroids can affect immune system functions, inflammatory responses, and cell growth.

The primary physiologic function of glucocorticoids is to maintain blood glucose levels and, thus, ensure glucose-dependent processes critical to life, particularly brain functions. Cortisol and related steroids accomplish this by stimulating the formation of glucose, by diminishing glucose use by peripheral tissues, and by promoting glycogen synthesis in the liver to increase carbohydrate stores for later release of glucose. For glucose formation, glucocorticoids mobilize amino acids and promote amino acid metabolism and gluconeogenesis. These steroids, acting via the GR mechanism, induce the production of a variety of enzymes important for glucose formation. The synthesis of tyrosine aminotransferase increases within 30 minutes of glucocorticoid exposure (139–141). This enzyme promotes the transfer of amino groups from tyrosine to α-ketoglutarate to form glutamate and hydroxyphenylpyruvate. Another amino acid–metabolizing enzyme induced rapidly by glucocorticoids is tryptophan oxidase (142). This enzyme oxidizes tryptophan to formylkynurenine, which is subsequently converted to alanine. Alanine transaminase also is induced by glucocorticoids (143). Alanine and, to a lesser extent, glutamate are important for gluconeogenesis in the liver (144).

Several other enzymes important in gluconeogenesis and glycogen formation are elevated for several hours following glucocorticoid administration; these include glycogen synthetase, pyruvate kinase, phosphoenol pyruvate carboxykinase, and glucose-6-phosphate kinase (16,145,146). The delayed increases in these enzymes suggest that their biosyntheses are not regulated directly by glucocorticoids. In peripheral tissues, glucocorticoid-induced inhibition of phosphofructokinase is observed (146). This enzyme catalyzes the formation of D-fructose-1,6-diphosphate from D-fructose-6-phosphate during glycolysis. Inhibition of this enzyme decreases glucose utilization by peripheral tissues and results in maintaining blood glucose levels. Reviews of the multiple effects of glucocorticoids on carbohydrate metabolism have been published (16,146).

Additional effects of glucocorticoids in the body are preventing or minimizing inflammatory reactions and suppressing immune responses. These steroids interfere with both early events in inflammation (e.g., release of mediators, edema, and cellular infiltration) and later stages (e.g., capillary infiltration and collagen formation). Only a few of the mechanisms involved in glucocorticoid suppression of inflammation are known. Cortisol will induce the production of lipocortin and related proteins by increasing gene expression through the GR mechanism (147,148). Lipocortin inhibits the activity of phospholipase A_2, which liberates arachidonic acid and leads to the biosynthesis of eicosanoids (e.g., prostaglandins and leukotrienes) (149). Lipocortin also mediates the decreased production and release of platelet-activating factor (150), and glucocorticoids can suppress the expression of interleukin (IL)-1, tumor necrosis factor, and inducible nitric oxide synthase (151–153). These eicosanoids and peptide factors are important as mediators in the inflammatory response. Some of these factors also play important roles in cellular infiltration and capillary permeability in the inflamed region. Suppression of the immune responses are mediated by inhibition of the synthesis and release of important mediators as well. In macrophages, glucocorticoids inhibit IL-1 synthesis and, thus, interfere with proliferation of B lymphocytes, which are important for antibody production (154). Additionally, IL-1 is important for activation of resting T lymphocytes, which are important for cell-mediated immunity. The activated T cells produce IL-2, the biosynthesis of which also is reduced by glucocorticoids (154).

Mineralocorticoids

The primary physiologic function of mineralocorticoids is to maintain electrolyte balances in the body by enhancing Na^+ reabsorption and increasing K^+ and H^+ secretion in the kidney. Similar effects on cation transport are observed in a variety of secretory tissues, including the salivary glands, sweat glands, and mucosal tissues of the GI tract and the bladder. Aldosterone is the most potent endogenous mineralocorticoid. Deoxycorticosterone is approximately 20-fold less potent than aldosterone. Cortisol exhibits weak mineralocorticoid activity in vivo because of rapid metabolism of cortisol by 11β-hydroxysteroid dehydrogenase. The mechanism of action of aldosterone involves binding of the steroid to the mineralocorticoid receptor and initiation of gene transcription, mRNA biosynthesis, and protein production. A protein referred to as aldosterone-induced protein is produced through this mechanism and is thought to aid in Na^+ retention. One possible mode of action of aldosterone-induced protein is to act as a permease to increase the permeability of the cell membrane to Na^+ (155). This results in an accelerated rate of Na^+ influx and elevated activity of Na^+, K^+-ATPase to pump Na^+ into extracellular space (156).

PHARMACOLOGICAL EFFECTS AND CLINICAL APPLICATIONS

In addition to their natural hormonal actions, the adrenocorticoids have many clinical uses. Glucocorticoids and mineralocorticoids may be used for the treatment of adrenal insufficiency (hypoadrenalism), which results from failure of the adrenal glands to synthesize adequate amounts of the hormones. Adrenocorticoids also are used to maintain patients who have had partial or complete removal of their adrenal glands or adenohypophysis (adrenalectomy and hypophysectomy, respectively). Glucocorticoids can cross the placenta and can be distributed into milk.

Two major uses of glucocorticoids are in the treatment of rheumatoid diseases and allergic manifestations. Their use in the treatment of severe asthma is well documented, as is the utility of glucocorticoids in sepsis and acute respiratory distress syndrome (157,158). They are effective in the treatment of rheumatoid arthritis, acute rheumatic fever, bursitis, spontaneous hypoglycemia in children, gout, rheumatoid carditis, sprue, allergy (including contact dermatitis), and other conditions. The treatment of chronic rheumatic diseases and allergic conditions with glucocorticoids is symptomatic and continuous. Symptoms return after withdrawal of the drug.

In addition, these drugs are moderately effective in the treatment of ulcerative colitis, dermatomyositis, periarteritis nodosa, idiopathic pulmonary fibrosis, idiopathic thrombocytopenic purpura, regional ileitis, acquired hemolytic anemia, nephrosis, cirrhotic ascites, neurodermatitis, and temporal arteritis. The newer analogues with medium to high potency rankings (Table 33.4), such as diflorasone diacetate, desoximetasone, flurandrenolide, and fluocinonide (Fig. 33.12), are effective topically in the treatment of psoriasis. Glucocorticoids may be combined with antibiotics to treat pneumonia, peritonitis, typhoid fever, and meningococcemia.

When dosages with equivalent antirheumatic potency are given to patients not treated with steroids, the Δ^1-corticoids (prednisone and prednisolone) promote the same pattern of initial improvement as hydrocortisone. Statistical results of improvement during the first few months of therapy have been similar with prednisone, prednisolone, and hydrocortisone. The results of longer-term therapy have been significantly better with the modified compounds.

Satisfactory rheumatic control, lost after prolonged cortisone or hydrocortisone therapy, may be regained in an appreciable number of patients by changing to prednisone, prednisolone, or other modified drugs. Of patients whose conditions deteriorate below adequate levels during hydrocortisone administration, nearly half reach their previous level of improvement after Δ^1-corticoids (in doses slightly larger in terms of antirheumatic strength) are used. With further prolongation of steroid therapy, improvement again wanes in some patients, but in other patients, such management is successful for longer than 2 years. In some instances, the improvement is attributed to increased effectiveness of the drug because of correction of salt and water retention; in other instances, there is no adequate explanation.

When these drugs are administered in doses that have similar antirheumatic strengths, the general incidence of adverse reactions with prednisone and prednisolone is about the same as that with hydrocortisone. The compounds differ, however, in their tendencies to induce individual side effects. The incidence and degree of salt and water retention and blood pressure elevation are less with the Δ^1-corticoids. Conversely, these analogues are more likely to promote digestive complaints, peptic ulcer, vasomotor symptoms, and cutaneous ecchymosis.

Although these analogues have unwanted side effects, most clinical investigators prefer the Δ^1-corticoids to cortisone and hydrocortisone for rheumatoid patients who require steroid therapy. The reasons are that these drugs have less tendency to cause salt and water retention and potassium loss and that they restore improvement in a significant percentage of patients whose therapeutic control has been lost during cortisone and hydrocortisone therapy.

It seems desirable to administer prednisone and prednisolone in conjunction with nonabsorbable antacids. This affords improvement of long-term therapy. It appears that the therapeutic indices of these two analogues, especially when used in conjunction with nonabsorbable antacids, are higher than those for the naturally occurring glucocorticoids.

Most important, glucocorticoids should not be withdrawn abruptly in cases of acute infections or severe stress, such as surgery or trauma. Myasthenia gravis, peptic ulcer, diabetes mellitus, hyperthyroidism, hypertension, psychological disturbances, pregnancy (first trimester), and infections may be aggravated by glucocorticoid administration. Hormone therapy is contraindicated in these conditions and should be used only with the utmost precaution.

Semisynthetic analogues exhibiting high mineralocorticoid activity are not employed in the treatment of rheumatic disorders because of toxic side effects resulting from a disturbance of electrolyte and water balance. Some newer synthetic steroids (Table 33.2) are relatively free of sodium-retaining activity. They may show other toxic manifestations, however, and eventually need to be withdrawn.

Glucocorticoids sometimes are used in the treatment of scleroderma, discoid lupus, acute nephritis, osteoarthritis, acute hepatitis, hepatic coma, Hodgkin's disease, multiple myeloma, lymphoid tumors, acute leukemia, metastatic carcinoma of the breast, and chronic lymphatic leukemia. Glucocorticoids may be more or less effective in these diseases depending on the clinical condition.

Some modified compounds have been recommended for use when other analogues are no longer effective or when it is desirable to promote increased appetite and weight gain. Triamcinolone may be used advantageously when salt and water retention (from other glucocorticoids, hypertension, or cardiac compensation) or excessive appetite and weight gain are problems in management.

One factor must not be overlooked when applying potent anti-inflammatory agents with high mineralocorticoid activity to the skin. Consideration must be given to percutaneous absorption. Sodium retention and edema occur in patients with dermatitis who apply as much as 75 mg of fludrocortisone acetate (i.e., 30 mL of a 0.25% lotion) to the skin in 24 hours. The relative rate of percutaneous absorption, administered as a cream in rats, was triamcinolone acetate ≥ hydrocortisone > dexamethasone, but dexamethasone was deposited in skin longer than the other two drugs. Hydrocortisone disappeared most rapidly (159).

Topical Applications

Topical dermatological products with a low potency ranking have a modest anti-inflammatory effect and are safest for chronic application (Table 33.4). These products also are the safest products for use on the face with occlusion and in infants and young children. Those products with a medium potency ranking are used in moderate inflammatory dermatoses, such as chronic hand eczema and atopic eczema, and may be used on the face and intertriginous areas for a limited duration. High-potency preparations are used in more severe inflammatory dermatoses, such as severe eczema and psoriasis. They may be used for a limited duration and for longer periods in areas with thickened skin because of chronic conditions. High-potency preparations also may be used on the face and intertriginous areas, but only for a short treatment duration. Very-high-potency products are used primarily as an alternative to systemic corticosteroid therapy when local areas are involved. Examples of conditions for which very-high-potency products frequently are used include thick, chronic lesions caused by psoriasis, lichen simplex chronicus, and discoid lupus erythematosus. They may be used for only a short duration of therapy and on small surface areas. Occlusive dressings should not be used with these products. It has been suggested that patients using a lotion or ointment containing these drugs be instructed to apply them sparingly and to spread them lightly over the affected areas. The extent and frequency of applications should be carefully considered. A lotion vehicle is more effective when treating a dermatitis, but a greater degree of percutaneous absorption occurs than when ointments are used.

Intranasal and Inhaled Applications

The pulmonary and nasal bioavailability are important determinants for the potential of an inhaled or nasally applied corticosteroid to cause systemic effects, because the lung and nasal tissue provide an enormous surface area from which drug absorption can occur into the systemic circulation. The main areas of concern with regard to systemic effects include HPA-axis suppression, change in bone mineral density and growth retardation in children, cataracts, and glaucoma. The degree of systemic side effects is dose-dependent, related to the half-life of the drug, frequency administration, time of day when administered, and route of administration; in other words, the higher the plasma corticosteroid concentration and longer the half-life, the greater the systemic side effects will be (Table 33.5) (27). The amount of an inhaled or nasal corticosteroid reaching the systemic circulation is the sum of the drug concentration available following absorption from the lungs/nasal mucosa and from the GI tract. The fraction deposited in the mouth will be swallowed, and the systemic availability will be determined by its absorption from the GI tract and the degree of first-pass metabolism.

Delivery devices can produce clinically significant differences in activity by altering the dose deposited in the lung (10–25%) and, for orally absorbed drugs, the amount deposited in the oropharynx and swallowed (75–90%). Clinical studies have shown the following relative potency differences: mometasone furoate > fluticasone propionate > budesonide = BDP > triamcinolone acetonide = flunisolide. Potency differences can be overcome by giving larger doses of the less potent drug, which increases risks from systemic effects. Adrenal suppression may be associated with high doses of inhaled corticosteroids (>1.5 mg/day, or >0.75 mg/day for fluticasone propionate), although there is a considerable degree of interindividual susceptibility.

All currently used inhaled corticosteroids are rapidly cleared from the body but show varying levels of oral bioavailability, with fluticasone propionate having the lowest (Table 33.5). Following inhalation, there also is considerable variability in the rate of absorption from the lung, and pulmonary residence times are greatest for fluticasone propionate and triamcinolone acetonide and shortest for budesonide and flunisolide. Adrenal suppression has not been observed when intranasal fluticasone propionate was administered in dosages of 200 to 4,000 μg daily for up to 12 months.

Adverse Effects

Although short-term administration of corticosteroids are unlikely to produce harmful effects, these drugs, when used for longer than brief periods, can produce a variety of devastating effects, including glucocorticoid-induced adrenocortical insufficiency, glucocorticoid-

Table 33.7. Effect of an Oral Single Dose on the Duration of HPA Suppression

Adrenocorticoid	Duration of Suppression (days)
Hydrocortisone (250 mg)	1.25–1.5
Cortisone (250 mg)	1.25–1.5
Methylprednisolone (40 mg)	1.25–1.5
Prednisone (50 mg)	1.25–1.5
Prednisolone (50 mg)	1.25–1.5
Triamcinolone (40 mg)	2.25
Dexamethasone (5 mg)	2.75
Betamethasone (6 mg)	3.25

induced osteoporosis, and generalized protein depletion (16,27). The duration of anti-inflammatory activity of glucocorticoids approximately equals the duration of HPA-axis suppression. The duration of HPA-axis suppression after a single oral dose of glucocorticoids in one study is shown in Table 33.7. When given for prolonged periods, glucocorticoids suppress the HPA axis, thereby decreasing secretion of endogenous corticosteroids and adrenal atrophy. Glucocorticoids inhibit ACTH production by the adenohypophysis, and in turn, this reduces endogenous glucocorticoid production. With time, atrophy of the adrenal glands takes place. The degree and duration of adrenocortical insufficiency produced by the synthetic glucocorticoids is highly variable among patients and depends on the dose, frequency and time of administration, and duration of glucocorticoid therapy. This effect may be minimized by use of alternate-day therapy.

Patients who develop drug-induced adrenocortical insufficiency may require higher corticosteroid dosage when they are subjected to stress (e.g., infection, surgery, or trauma). In addition, acute adrenal insufficiency (even death) may occur if the drugs are withdrawn abruptly or if patients are transferred from systemic glucocorticoid therapy to oral inhalation therapy. Therefore, the drugs should be withdrawn very gradually following long-term therapy with pharmacological dosages. Adrenal suppression may persist up to 12 months in patients who receive large dosages for prolonged periods. Until recovery occurs, patients may show signs and symptoms of adrenal insufficiency when they are subjected to stress, and replacement therapy may be required. Because mineralocorticoid secretion may be impaired, sodium chloride or a mineralocorticoid also should be administered.

Although side effects and toxicities vary with the drug and, sometimes, with the patient, facial mooning, flushing, sweating, acne, thinning of the scalp hair, abdominal distention, and weight gain are observed with most glucocorticoids. Protein depletion (with osteoporosis and spontaneous fractures), myopathy (with weakness of muscles of the thighs, pelvis, and lower back), and aseptic necrosis of the hip and humerus are other side effects. These drugs may cause psychological disturbances, headache, vertigo, and peptic ulcer, and they may suppress growth in children.

Patients with well-controlled diabetes must be closely monitored and their insulin dosage increased if glycosuria or hyperglycemia ensues either during or following glucocorticoid administration. Patients should also be watched for signs of adrenocorticoid insufficiency after discontinuation of glucocorticoid therapy. Individuals with a history of tuberculosis should receive prophylactic doses of antituberculosis drugs.

Osteoporosis is one of the most serious adverse effects of long-term glucocorticoid therapy. Moderate-to high-dose glucocorticoid therapy is associated with loss of bone and an increased risk of fracture that is most rapid during the initial 6 months of therapy. These adverse effects of glucocorticoids appear to be both dose- and duration-dependent, with oral prednisone dosages of 7.5 mg or more daily for 6 months or longer often resulting in clinically important bone loss and increased fracture risk. Bone loss has even been associated with oral inhalation of glucocorticoids and is of great concern in children. Most patients receiving long-term glucocorticoid therapy will develop some degree of bone loss, and more than 25% will develop osteoporotic fractures. Vertebral fractures have been reported in 11% of patients with asthma who are receiving systemic glucocorticoids for at least 1 year, and glucocorticoid-treated patients with rheumatoid arthritis are at increased risk of fractures of the hip, rib, spine, leg, ankle, and foot. Muscle wasting or weakness and atrophy of the protein matrix of the bone resulting in osteoporosis are manifestations of protein catabolism, which may occur during prolonged therapy with glucocorticoids. These adverse effects may be especially serious in debilitated patients, in geriatric populations, and in postmenopausal women who are especially prone to osteoporosis.

To minimize the risk of glucocorticoid-induced bone loss (osteoporosis) and those with low mineral bone density, the smallest possible effective dosage and duration should be used. Topical and inhaled preparations should be used whenever possible. The immunosuppressive effects of glucocorticoids increase the susceptibility to and mask the symptoms of infections and may result in activation of latent infection or exacerbation of intercurrent infections. The most common adverse effect of oral inhalation therapy with glucocorticoids is fungal infections of the mouth, pharynx, and occasionally, the larynx. The mineralocorticoid effects are less frequent with synthetic glucocorticoids (except fludrocortisone) than with hydrocortisone or cortisone but may occur, especially when synthetic glucocorticoids are given in high dosage for prolonged periods.

CASE STUDY

Victoria F. Roche and S. William Zito

VS is a 42-year-old woman who presents at the ambulatory care clinic where you work with complaints of nausea, loss of appetite, and feeling tired all the time. She and her husband are vacationing in Maine, but she has not felt well enough to hike or accompany her husband on fishing excursions for the past 5 days. She has an apparent tan even though she has not been out of the house for several days. She denies fever, night sweats, visual disturbances, or changes in her menstrual cycle. She does admit to several months of nausea, anorexia, and a 15-lb weight loss. Examination and laboratory tests reveal a low blood pressure (97/73 mm Hg) with orthostatic hypotension, hyponatremia (127 mEq/L), low morning hydrocortisone (1.4 μg/dL), and elevated levels of ACTH (2,096 pg/mL), all of which confirm a diagnosis of Addison's disease. The physician feels that the symptoms are not severe enough to require parenteral cortisol and fluid replacement and, therefore, wants to begin oral adrenocorticoid therapy and asks your opinion of the following choices.

1. Identify the therapeutic problem(s) in which the pharmacist's intervention may benefit the patient.
2. Identify and prioritize the patient-specific factors that must be considered to achieve the desired therapeutic outcomes.
3. Conduct a thorough and mechanistically oriented structure-activity analysis of all therapeutic alternatives provided in the case.
4. Evaluate the structure-activity relationship findings against the patient-specific factors and desired therapeutic outcomes, and make a therapeutic decision.
5. Counsel your patient.

References

1. IUPAC-IUB Joint Commission on Biochemical Nomenclature (JCBN). The nomenclature of steroids. Recommendations 1989. Eur J Biochem 1989; 186:429–458. [Published erratum appears in Eur J Biochem 1993;213:2.]
2. Gustafsson JA, Carlstedt-Duke J, Poellinger L, et al. Biochemistry, molecular biology, and physiology of the glucocorticoid receptor. Endocr Rev 1987; 8:185–234.
3. Evans RM. The steroid and thyroid hormone receptor superfamily. Science 1988;240:889–895.
4. Ringold G, University of California Los Angeles. Steroid Hormone Action: Proceedings of a UCLA Symposium, Held in Park City, Utah, January 17–23, 1987. New York: Liss, 1988.
5. Beato M. Gene regulation by steroid hormones. Cell 1989;56:335–344.
6. O'Malley B. The steroid receptor superfamily: more excitement predicted for the future. Mol Endocrinol 1990;4:363–369.
7. Carson-Jurica MA, Schrader WT, O'Malley BW. Steroid receptor family: structure and functions. Endocr Rev 1990;11:201–220.
8. Jensen EV, Jacobson HI. Basic guide to the mechanism of estrogen action. Recent Prog Horm Res 1962;18:387–414.
9. Gorski J, Welshons WV, Sakai D, et al. Evolution of a model of estrogen action. Recent Prog Horm Res 1986;42:297–329.
10. Eickelberg O, Roth M, Lorx R, et al. Ligand-independent activation of the glucocorticoid receptor by β_2-adrenergic receptor agonists in primary human lung fibroblasts and vascular smooth muscle cells. J Biol Chem 1999;274:1005–1010.
11. Addison T. On the Constitutional and Local Effects of Disease of the Suprarenal Capsules by Thomas Addison. Special Ed. Birmingham, AL: Classics of Medicine Library, 1980.
12. Murison PJ. Hyperfunctioning adrenocortical diseases. Med Clin North Am 1967;51:883–901.
13. Shoppee CW. Chemistry of the steroids. 2nd Ed. London: Butterworths, 1964.
14. Simpson ER. Cholesterol side-chain cleavage, cytochrome P450, and the control of steroidogenesis. Mol Cell Endocrinol 1979;13(3):213–227.
15. Simpson ER, Waterman MR. Regulation of the synthesis of steroidogenic enzymes in adrenal cortical cells by ACTH. Annu Rev Physiol 1988;50: 427–440.
16. Schimmer BP, Parker KL. Adrenocorticotropic hormones. In: Hardman JG, Limbird LE, Molinoff PB, et al., editors. Goodman & Gilman's The Pharmacological Basis of Therapeutics. New York: McGraw-Hill, 2001:1459–1485.
17. Kremers P. Progesterone and pregnenolone 17α-hydroxylase: substrate specificity and selective inhibition by 17α-hydroxylated products. J Steroid Biochem 1976; 7:571–575.
18. Makin HLJ. Biochemistry of Steroid Hormones. 2nd Ed. Boston: Blackwell Scientific, 1984.
19. Miller WL. Molecular biology of steroid hormone synthesis. Endocr Rev 1988;9:295–318.
20. White PC, Mune T, Agarwal AK. 11β-Hydroxysteroid dehydrogenase and the syndrome of apparent mineralocorticoid excess. Endocr Rev 1997;18:135–156.
21. Penning TM. Molecular endocrinology of hydroxysteroid dehydrogenases. Endocr Rev 1997;18:281–305.

22. Tomlinson JW, Walker EA, Bujalska IJ, et al. 11β-Hydroxysteroid dehydrogenase type 1: a tissue-specific regulator of glucocorticoid response. Endocr Rev 2004;25:831–866.
23. Derendorf H, Mollmann H, Barth J, et al. Pharmacokinetics and oral bioavailability of hydrocortisone. J Clin Pharmacol 1991;31:473–476.
24. Romanoff LP, Morris CW, Welch PW, et al. The metabolism of cortisol-4-C14 in young and elderly men. I. Welch Secretion rate of cortisol and daily excretion of tetrahydrocortisol, allotetrahydrocortisol, tetrahydrocortisone, and cortolone (20α and 20β). J Clin Endocrinol Metab 1961;21:1413–1425.
25. Fukushima DK, Leeds NS, Bradlow HL, et al. The characterization of four new metabolites of adrenocortical hormones. J Biol Chem 1955;212:449–460.
26. Chang E, Dao TL. Adrenal estrogens. II. Further characterizations of isolated urinary 11β-hydroxyesterone and 11β-hydroxyestradiol. Biochim Biophys Acta 1962;57:609–612.
27. AHFS Drug Information 2006. Bethesda, MD: American Society of Health-System Pharmacists, 2006.
28. Gray CH, Green MA, Holness NJ, et al. Urinary metabolic products of prednisone and prednisolone. J Endocrinol 1956;14:146–154.
29. Robbins ED, Burton SD, Byers SO, et al. Hydrocortisone metabolism in the perfused isolated rat liver. J Clin Endocrinol Metab 1957;17:111–115.
30. Stevens W, Berliner DL, Dougherty TF. Conjugation of steroid by liver, kidney, and intestine of mice. Endocrinology 1961;68:875–877.
31. Glick JH. The isolation of two corticosteroids from cattle bile. Endocrinology 1957;60:368–375.
32. Steiger M, Reichstein T. Desoxy-cortico-steron (21-Oxy-progesteron) aus Δ^5-3-Oxy-ätio-cholensäure. Helv Chim Acta 1937;20:1164–1179.
33. Fieser LF, Fieser M. Steroids. New York: Reinhold, 1959.
34. Sarett LH. Partial synthesis of pregnene-4-triol-17(b),20(b),21-dione-3,11 and pregnene-4-diol-17(b),21-trione-3,11,20 monoacetate. J Biol Chem 1946; 162:601–631.
35. McKenzie BF, Marttox VR, Engel LL, et al. Steroids derived from bile acids. VI. An improved synthesis of methyl 3,9-epoxy-Δ^{11}-cholenate from desoxycholic acid. J Biol Chem 1948;173:271–281.
36. Sarett LH. Preparation of pregnane-17α,21-diol-3,11,20-trione acetate. Journal of the American Chemical Society 1949;71:2443–2444.
37. Heazelwood VJ, Galligan JP, Cannell GR, et al. Plasma cortisol delivery from oral cortisol and cortisone acetate: relative bioavailability. Br J Clin Pharmacol 1984;17:55–59.
38. Lima JJ, Jusko WJ. Bioavailability of hydrocortisone retention enemas in relation to absorption kinetics. Clin Pharmacol Ther 1980;28:262–269.
39. Mollmann H, Barth J, Mollmann C, et al. Pharmacokinetics and rectal bioavailability of hydrocortisone acetate. J Pharm Sci 1991;80:835–836.
40. Bush IE, Mahesh VB. Metabolism of 11-oxygenated steroids. 2. 2-Methyl steroids. Biochem J 1959;71:718–742.
41. Nobile A, Charney W, Perlman PL, et al. Microbiological transformation of steroids. I. Δ-1,4-diene-3-ketosteroids. Journal of the American Chemical Society 1955;77:4184.
42. Meystre C, Frey H, Voser W, et al. Gewinnung von 1,4-Bisdehydro-3-oxo-steroiden. Über Steroide, 139. Mitteilung. Helv Chim Acta 1956;39:734–742.
43. Smith CL, Kreutner W. In vitro glucocorticoid receptor binding and transcriptional activation by topically active glucocorticoids. Arzneimittelforschung 1998;48:956–960.
44. Barth J, Damoiseaux M, Mollmann H, et al. Pharmacokinetics and pharmacodynamics of prednisolone after intravenous and oral administration. Int J Clin Pharmacol Ther Toxicol 1992;30:317–324.
45. Rohatagi S, Barth J, Mollmann H, et al. Pharmacokinetics of methylprednisolone and prednisolone after single and multiple oral administration. J Clin Pharmacol 1997;37:916–925.
46. Mollmann H, Rohdewald P, Barth J, et al. Pharmacokinetics and dose linearity testing of methylprednisolone phosphate. Biopharm Drug Dispos 1989; 10:453–464.
47. Vree TB, Verwey-van Wissen CP, Lagerwerf AJ, et al. Isolation and identification of the C6-hydroxy and C20-hydroxy metabolites and glucuronide conjugate of methylprednisolone by preparative high-performance liquid chromatography from urine of patients receiving high-dose pulse therapy. J Chromatogr B Biomed Sci Appl 1999;726:157–168.
48. Spero GB, Thompsin JL, Lincoln FH, et al. Adrenal hormones related compounds. V. Fluorinated 6-methyl steroids. Journal of the American Chemical Society 1957;79:1515–1516.
49. Boland EW. Clinical comparison of the newer anti-inflammatory corticosteroids. Ann Rheumatic Dis 1962;21:176–187.
50. Hirschmann H, Hirschmann FB, Farrel GL. Partial synthesis of 16α,21-diacetoxyprogesterone. Journal of the American Chemical Society 1953;75: 4862–4863.
51. Allen WS, Bernstein S. Steroidal cyclic ketals. XII. The preparation of Δ^{16}-steroids. Journal of American Chemistry Society 1955;77:1028–1032.
52. Allen WS, Bernstein S. Steroidal cyclic ketals. XX. 16-hydroxylated steroids. III. the preparation of 16α-hydroxyhydrocortisone and related compounds. Journal of American Chemistry Society 1956;78:1909–1913.
53. Hochhaus G, Portner M, Barth J, et al. Oral bioavailability of triamcinolone tablets and a triamcinolone diacetate suspension. Pharm Res 1990;7:558–560.
54. Portner M, Mollmann H, Barth J, et al. [Pharmacokinetics of triamcinolone following oral administration]. Arzneimittelforschung 1988;38:1838–1840.
55. Boland EW. The treatment of rheumatoid arthritis with adrenocorticosteroids and their synthetic analogues: an appraisal of certain developments of the past decade. Ann N Y Acad Sci 1959;82:887–901.
56. Weiner AL. Intramuscular triamcinolone diacetate therapy of dermatoses: preliminary report. Antibiot Chemother 1962;12:360–366.
57. Dobes WL. The use of folic acid antagonists and steroids in treatment of psoriasis. South Med J 1963;56:187–192.
58. Arth GE, Johnson DBR, Fried J, et al. 16-Methylated steroids. I. 16α-Methylated analogues of Johnson cortisone, a new group of anti-inflammatory steroids. Journal of American Chemistry Society 1958;80:3160–3161.
59. Oliveto EP, Rausser R, Nussbaum AL, et al. 16-Alkylated corticoids. I. 16α-Methylprednisone and 16β-methylprednisone. Journal of American Chemistry Society 1958;80:4431.
60. Sperber PA. Cyproheptadine-dexamethasone combination in the treatment. Current Therapeutic Research 1962;4:70–73.
61. Silber RH. The biology of anti-inflammatory steroids. Ann N Y Acad Sci 1959;82:821–833.
62. Tolksdorf S. Laboratory evaluation of anti-inflammatory steroids. Ann N Y Acad Sci 1959;82:829–835.
63. Rohdewald P, Mollmann H, Barth J, et al. Pharmacokinetics of dexamethasone and its phosphate ester. Biopharm Drug Dispos 1987;8:205–212.
64. Nierman MM. Management of steroid-responsive dermatologic disorders with betamethasone. Clin Med 1962;69:1311–1320.
65. Cohen A, Coldman J. Use of a new corticosteroid in rheumatoid arthritis. Pennsylvania Medical Journal 1962;65:347–350.
66. Cohen AI. Treatment of allergy with oral betamethasone in 141 patients. Antibiot Chemother 1962;12:91–96.
67. Glyn JH, Fox DB. Preliminary clinical assessment of β-methasone. BMJ 1961;1:876–877.
68. Glyn JH, Fox DB. Betamethasone. BMJ 1961;2:650–651.
69. Wilkinson DS. Betamethasone. BMJ 1961;1:1319–1320.
70. Irwin GW, Priebe FH, Ridolfo AS. Metabolic effects of paramethasone acetate. Metabolism 1961;10:852–858.
71. Buijsman RC, Hermkens PH, van Rijn RD, et al. Nonsteroidal steroid receptor modulators. Curr Med Chem 2005;12:1017–1075.
72. Einstein M, Greenlee M, Rouen G, et al. Selective glucocorticoid receptor nonsteroidal ligands completely antagonize the dexamethasone mediated induction of enzymes involved in gluconeogenesis and glutamine metabolism. J Steroid Biochem Mol Biol 2004;92:345–356.
73. Miner JN, Hong MH, Negro-Vilar A. New and improved glucocorticoid receptor ligands. Expert Opin Investig Drugs 2005;14:1527–1545.
74. Stritzler C, Frank L, Rein R. Paramethasone, a new corticosteroid, in selected dermatoses. Arch Dermatol 1962;85:505–509.
75. Feinberg SM, Feinberg AR, Fisherman EW. Fluprednisolone, a new tropical corticosteroid in treating allergies. The Journal of New Drugs 1961;1:268–270.
76. Andersson P, Lihne M, Thalen A, et al. Effect of structural alterations on the biotransformation rate of glucocorticosteroids in rat and human liver. Xenobiotica 1987;17:35–44.
77. Brogden RN, Heel RC, Speight TM, et al. Beclomethasone dipropionate. A reappraisal of its pharmacodynamic properties and therapeutic efficacy after a decade of use in asthma and rhinitis. Drugs 1984;28:99–126.
78. Green MJ, Berkenkopf J, Fernandez X, et al. Synthesis and structure–activity relationships in a novel series of topically active corticosteroids. J Steroid Biochem 1979;11:61–66.
79. Asche H, Botta L, Rettig H, et al. Influence of formulation factors on the availability of drugs from topical preparations. Pharm Acta Helv 1985;60(8): 232–237.
80. Bodor N, Harget AJ, Phillips EW. Structure–activity relationships in the anti-inflammatory steroids: a pattern-recognition approach. J Med Chem 1983; 26:318–333.
81. Popper TL, Gentles MJ, Kung TT, et al. Structure–activity relationships of a series of novel topical corticosteroids. J Steroid Biochem 1987;27:837–843.
82. Shapiro EL, Gentles MJ, Tiberi RL, et al. 17-Heteroaroyl esters of corticosteroids. 2. 11β-Hydroxy series. J Med Chem 1987;30:1581–1588.
83. Barth J, Lehr KH, Derendorf H, et al. Studies on the pharmacokinetics and metabolism of prednicarbate after cutaneous and oral administration. Skin Pharmacol 1993;6:179–186.
84. Kelly HW. Comparison of inhaled corticosteroids. Ann Pharmacother 1998;32:220–232.
85. Derendorf H. Pharmacokinetic and pharmacodynamic properties of inhaled corticosteroids in relation to efficacy and safety. Respir Med 1997;91(Suppl A):22–33.
86. Derendorf H, Hochhaus G, Meibohm B, et al. Pharmacokinetics and pharmacodynamics of inhaled corticosteroids. J Allergy Clin Immunol 1998; 101:S440–S446.
87. Wales D, Makker H, Kane J, et al. Systemic bioavailability and potency of high-dose inhaled corticosteroids: a comparison of four inhaler devices and three drugs in healthy adult volunteers. Chest 1999;115:1278–1284.
88. Shaw RJ. Inhaled corticosteroids for adult asthma: impact of formulation and delivery device on relative pharmacokinetics, efficacy, and safety. Respir Med 1999;93:149–160.
89. Lipworth BJ. Systemic adverse effects of inhaled corticosteroid therapy: a systematic review and meta-analysis. Arch Intern Med 1999;159:941–955.

90. Greiff L, Andersson M, Svensson C, et al. Effects of orally inhaled budesonide in seasonal allergic rhinitis. Eur Respir J 1998;11:1268–1273.
91. Rohatagi S, Hochhaus G, Mollmann H, et al. Pharmacokinetic and pharmacodynamic evaluation of triamcinolone acetonide after intravenous, oral, and inhaled administration. J Clin Pharmacol 1995;35:1187–1193.
92. Argenti D, Shah B, Heald D. A pharmacokinetic study to evaluate the absolute bioavailability of triamcinolone acetonide following inhalation administration. J Clin Pharmacol 1999;39:695–702.
93. Derendorf H, Hochhaus G, Rohatagi S, et al. Pharmacokinetics of triamcinolone acetonide after intravenous, oral, and inhaled administration. J Clin Pharmacol 1995;35:302–305.
94. Mollmann H, Derendorf H, Barth J, et al. Pharmacokinetic/pharmacodynamic evaluation of systemic effects of flunisolide after inhalation. J Clin Pharmacol 1997;37:893–903.
95. Seale JP, Harrison LI. Effect of changing the fine particle mass of inhaled beclomethasone dipropionate on intrapulmonary deposition and pharmacokinetics. Respir Med 1998;92(Suppl A):9–15.
96. Lipworth BJ, Jackson CM. Pharmacokinetics of chlorofluorocarbon and hydrofluoroalkane metered-dose inhaler formulations of beclomethasone dipropionate. Br J Clin Pharmacol 1999;48:866–868.
97. Harrison LI, Soria I, Cline AC, et al. Pharmacokinetic differences between chlorofluorocarbon and chlorofluorocarbon-free metered dose inhalers of beclomethasone dipropionate in adult asthmatics. J Pharm Pharmacol 1999;51:1235–1240.
98. Dickens GR, Wermeling DP, Matheny CJ, et al. Pharmacokinetics of flunisolide administered via metered dose inhaler with and without a spacer device and following oral administration. Ann Allergy Asthma Immunol 2000;84:528–532.
99. Thalen BA, Axelsson BI, Andersson PH, et al. 6α-Fluoro- and 6α,9α-difluoro-11β,21-dihydroxy-16α,17α-propylmethylenedioxypregn-4-ene-3,20-dione: synthesis and evaluation of activity and kinetics of their C-22 epimers. Steroids 1998;63:37–43.
100. Ryrfeldt A, Andersson P, Edsbacker S, et al. Pharmacokinetics and metabolism of budesonide, a selective glucocorticoid. Eur J Respir Dis Suppl 1982; 122:86–95.
101. Szefler SJ. Pharmacodynamics and pharmacokinetics of budesonide: a new nebulized corticosteroid. J Allergy Clin Immunol 1999;104:175–183.
102. Miller-Larsson A, Mattsson H, Hjertberg E, et al. Reversible fatty acid conjugation of budesonide. Novel mechanism for prolonged retention of topically applied steroid in airway tissue. Drug Metab Dispos 1998;26:623–630.
103. Miller-Larsson A, Jansson P, Runstrom A, et al. Prolonged airway activity and improved selectivity of budesonide possibly due to esterification. Am J Respir Crit Care Med 2000;162:1455–1461.
104. Pedersen S, Steffensen G, Ekman I, et al. Pharmacokinetics of budesonide in children with asthma. Eur J Clin Pharmacol 1987;31:579–582.
105. Agertoft L, Andersen A, Weibull E, et al. Systemic availability and pharmacokinetics of nebulized budesonide in preschool children. Arch Dis Child 1999;80:241–247.
106. Shapiro EL, Gentles MJ, Tiberi RL, et al. Synthesis and structure–activity studies of corticosteroid 17-heterocyclic aromatic esters. 1. 9α,11β-Dichloro series. J Med Chem 1987;30:1068–1073.
107. Onrust SV, Lamb HM. Mometasone furoate. A review of its intranasal use in allergic rhinitis. Drugs 1998;56:725–745.
108. Affrime MB, Cuss F, Padhi D, et al. Bioavailability and metabolism of mometasone furoate following administration by metered-dose and dry-powder inhalers in healthy human volunteers. J Clin Pharmacol 2000;40: 1227–1236.
109. Phillipps GH, Bailey EJ, Bain BM, et al. Synthesis and structure–activity relationships in a series of antiinflammatory corticosteroid analogues, halomethyl androstane-17β-carbothioates and -17β-carboselenoates. J Med Chem 1994; 37:3717–3729.
110. Harding SM. The human pharmacology of fluticasone propionate. Respir Med 1990;84(Suppl A):25–29.
111. Johnson M. Development of fluticasone propionate and comparison with other inhaled corticosteroids. J Allergy Clin Immunol 1998;101:S434–S439.
112. Mollmann H, Wagner M, Meibohm B, et al. Pharmacokinetic and pharmacodynamic evaluation of fluticasone propionate after inhaled administration. Eur J Clin Pharmacol 1998;53:459–467.
113. Mackie AE, Ventresca GP, Fuller RW, et al. Pharmacokinetics of intravenous fluticasone propionate in healthy subjects. Br J Clin Pharmacol 1996;41:539–542.
114. Thorsson L, Dahlstrom K, Edsbacker S, et al. Pharmacokinetics and systemic effects of inhaled fluticasone propionate in healthy subjects. Br J Clin Pharmacol 1997;43:155–161.
115. Rohatagi S, Bye A, Falcoz C, et al. Dynamic modeling of cortisol reduction after inhaled administration of fluticasone propionate. J Clin Pharmacol 1996;36:938–941.
116. Bush IE. Chemical and biological factors in the activity of adrenocortical steroids. Pharmacol Rev 1962;14:317–336.
117. Glenn EM, Stafford RO, Lyster SC, et al. Relation between biological activity of hydrocortisone analogues and their rates of inactivation by rat liver enzyme systems. Endocrinology 1957;61:128–142.
118. Dulin WE, Bowman BJ, Stafford RO. Effects of 2-methylation on glucocorticoid activity of various C-21 steroids. Proc Soc Exp Biol Med 1957;94:303–305.
119. Fried J, Borman A. Synthetic derivatives of cortical hormones. Vitam Horm 1958;16:303–374.
120. Funder JW, Feldman D, Highland E, et al. Molecular modifications of antialdosterone compounds: effects on affinity of spirolactones for renal aldosterone receptors. Biochem Pharmacol 1974;23:1493–1501.
121. Peterfalvi M, Torelli V, Fournex R, et al. Importance of the lactonic ring in the activity of steroidal antialdosterones. Biochem Pharmacol 1980;29:353–357.
122. Duval D, Durant S, Homo-Delarche F. Effect of antiglucocorticoids on dexamethasone-induced inhibition of uridine incorporation and cell lysis in isolated mouse thymocytes. J Steroid Biochem 1984;20:283–287.
123. Agarwal MK, Hainque B, Moustaid N, et al. Glucocorticoid antagonists. FEBS Lett 1987;217:221–226.
124. Napoli JL, Counsell RE. New inhibitors of steroid 11β-hydroxylase. Structure–activity relationship studies of metyrapone-like compounds. J Med Chem 1977;20:762–766.
125. Shaw MA, Nicholls PJ, Smith HJ. Aminoglutethimide and ketoconazole: historical perspectives and future prospects. J Steroid Biochem 1988;31:137–146.
126. Sonino N. The use of ketoconazole as an inhibitor of steroid production. N Engl J Med 1987;317:812–818.
127. Potts GO, Creange JE, Hardomg HR, et al. Trilostane, an orally active inhibitor of steroid biosynthesis. Steroids 1978;32:257–267.
128. Monder C, Stewart PM, Lakshmi V, et al. Licorice inhibits corticosteroid 11β-dehydrogenase of rat kidney and liver: in vivo and in vitro studies. Endocrinology 1989;125:1046–1053.
129. Diederich S, Grossmann C, Hanke B, et al. In the search for specific inhibitors of human 11β-hydroxysteroid-dehydrogenases (11β-HSDs): chenodeoxycholic acid selectively inhibits 11β-HSD-I. Eur J Endocrinol 2000; 142:200–207.
130. Buhler H, Perschel FH, Fitzner R, et al. Endogenous inhibitors of 11β-OHSD: existence and possible significance. Steroids 1994;59:131–135.
131. Barf T, Vallgarda J, Emond R, et al. Arylsulfonamidothiazoles as a new class of potential antidiabetic drugs. Discovery of potent and selective inhibitors of the 11β-hydroxysteroid dehydrogenase type 1. J Med Chem 2002;45:3813–3815.
132. Pratt WB. Transformation of glucocorticoid and progesterone receptors to the DNA- binding state. J Cell Biochem 1987;35:51–68.
133. de Castro M, Elliot S, Kino T, et al. The nonligand binding β-isoform of the human glucocorticoid receptor (hGRβ): tissue levels, mechanism of action, and potential physiologic role. Mol Med 1996;2:597–607.
134. Bamberger CM, Bamberger AM, de Castro M, et al. Glucocorticoid receptor β, a potential endogenous inhibitor of glucocorticoid action in humans. J Clin Invest 1995;95:2435–2441.
135. Marver D. Aldosterone action in target epithelia. Vitam Horm 1980;38:55–117.
136. Speirs RS, Meyer RK. A method of assaying adrenal cortical hormones based on a decrease in the circulating eosinophil cells of adrenalectomized mice. Endocrinology 1951;48:316–326.
137. Ringer I, Brownfield R. The thymolytic activities of 16α, 17α ketals of triamcinolone. Endocrinology 1960;66:900–902.
138. Dorfman RI, Dorfman AS. The relative thymolytic activities of corticoids using the ovariectomized-adrenalectomized mouse. Endocrinology 1961;69:283–291.
139. Sereni F, Kenny FT, Kretchmer N. Factors influencing the development of tyrosine-α-ketoglutarate transaminase activity in rat liver. J Biol Chem 1959;234:609–612.
140. Kupfer D. Alteration in the magnitude of induction of tyrosine transaminase by glycocorticoids. The effects of phenobarbital, o,p'-DDD and β-diethylaminoethyl diphenylpropylacetate (SKF 525A). Arch Biochem Biophys 1968;127:200–206.
141. Lee K, Kenney FT. Induction of alanine transaminase by adrenal steroids in cultured hepatoma cells. Biochem Biophys Res Commun 1970;40:469–476.
142. Feigelson P, Beato M, Colman P, et al. Studies on the hepatic glucocorticoid receptor and on the hormonal modulation of specific mRNA levels during enzyme induction. Recent Prog Horm Res 1975;31:213–242.
143. Kenney F, Lee KL, Reel JR, et al. Regulation of tyrosine α-ketoglutarate transaminase in rat liver. IX. Studies of the mechanisms of hormonal inductions in cultured hepatoma cells. J Biol Chem 1970;245:5806–5812.
144. Felig P, Pozefsky T, Marliss E, et al. Alanine: key role in gluconeogenesis. Science 1970;167:1003–1004.
145. Landau BR. Adrenal steroids and carbohydrate metabolism. Vitam Horm 1965;23:1–59.
146. McMahon M, Gerich J, Rizza R. Effects of glucocorticoids on carbohydrate metabolism. Diabetes Metab Rev 1988;4:17–30.
147. Goulding NJ, Godolphin JL, Sharland PR, et al. Anti-inflammatory lipocortin 1 production by peripheral blood leucocytes in response to hydrocortisone. Lancet 1990;335:1416–1418.
148. Peers SH, Smillie F, Elderfield AJ, et al. Glucocorticoid and nonglucocorticoid induction of lipocortins (annexins) 1 and 2 in rat peritoneal leucocytes in vivo. Br J Pharmacol 1993;108:66–72.
149. Solito E, Parente L. Modulation of phospholipase A_2 activity in human fibroblasts. Br J Pharmacol 1989;96:656–660.
150. Parente L, Flower RJ. Hydrocortisone and 'macrocortin' inhibit the zymosan-induced release of lyso-PAF from rat peritoneal leucocytes. Life Sci 1985;36:1225–1231.
151. Beutler B, Cerami A. Cachectin: more than a tumor necrosis factor. N Engl J Med 1987;316:379–385.

152. Radomski MW, Palmer RM, Moncada S. Glucocorticoids inhibit the expression of an inducible, but not the constitutive, nitric oxide synthase in vascular endothelial cells. Proc Natl Acad Sci U S A 1990;87:10043–10047.
153. Lew W, Oppenheim JJ, Matsushima K. Analysis of the suppression of IL-1α and IL-1β production in human peripheral blood mononuclear adherent cells by a glucocorticoid hormone. J Immunol 1988;140:1895–1902.
154. Goodwin JS, Atluru D, Sierakowski S, et al. Mechanism of action of glucocorticosteroids. Inhibition of T cell proliferation and interleukin 2 production by hydrocortisone is reversed by leukotriene B_4. J Clin Invest 1986; 77:1244–1250.
155. Sharp GW, Leaf A. Studies on the mode of action of aldosterone. Recent Prog Horm Res 1966;22:431–471.
156. Koeppen BM, Biagi BA, Giebisch GH. Intracellular microelectrode characterization of the rabbit cortical collecting duct. Am J Physiol 1983;244:35–47.
157. Meduri GU, Kanangat S. Glucocorticoid treatment of sepsis and acute respiratory distress syndrome: time for a critical reappraisal [editorial; comment]. Crit Care Med 1998;26:630–633.
158. Meduri GU, Headley AS, Golden E, et al. Effect of prolonged methylprednisolone therapy in unresolving acute respiratory distress syndrome: a randomized controlled trial [see comments]. JAMA 1998;280:159–165.
159. Suzuki M. [Percutaneous absorption and systemic distribution of corticosteroids.] Nippon Hifuka Gakkai Zasshi 1982;92:757–776.

Suggested Readings

Avery MA, Woolfrey JR. Anti-inflammatory Steroids. In: Abraham DJ, editor. Burger's Medicinal Chemistry & Drug Discovery, Sixth Edition, Volume 3. Hoboken NJ: John Wiley & Sons, 2003:747–853.

Brueggemeier RW, Li PK. Steroid chemistry and biochemistry. In: Abraham DJ, ed. Burger's Medicinal Chemistry and Drug Discovery. 6th Ed. Vol 3. Hoboken NJ: John Wiley & Sons, 2003:593–627.

Carson-Jurica MA, Schrader WT, O'Malley BW. Steroid receptor family: structure and functions. Endocr Rev 1990;11:201–220.

Miller WL. Molecular biology of steroid hormone synthesis. Endocr Rev 1988;9: 295–318.

Schimmer BP, Parker KL. Adrenocorticotropic hormones. Adrenocortical steroids and their synthetic analogues. In: Brunton II, Lazo JS, Parker KL, ed. Goodman & Gilman's The Pharmacological Basis of Therapeutics. 11th Ed. New York: McGraw-Hill, 2006:1587–1612.

Simpson ER, Waterman MR. Regulation of the synthesis of steroidogenic enzymes in adrenal cortical cells by ACTH. Annu Rev Physiol 1988;50:427–440.

Tomlinson JW, Walker EA, Bujalska IJ, et al. 11β-Hydroxysteroid dehydrogenase type 1: a tissue-specific regulator of glucocorticoid response. Endocr Rev 2004;25:831–866.

34. *Thyroid Function and Thyroid Drugs*

ALI R. BANIJAMALI

DRUGS COVERED IN THIS CHAPTER:

DRUG FOR TREATMENT OF HYPOTHYROIDISM
- Thyroid gland products
- Levothyroxine
- Liotyronine
- Liotrix

DRUGS FOR TREATMENT OF HYPERTHYROIDISM
- Iodide
- Perchlorate
- Radioiodine
- Methimazole
- Propylthiouracil

INTRODUCTION

The thyroid gland is a highly vascular, flat structure located at the upper portion of the trachea, just below the larynx. It is composed of two lateral lobes joined by an isthmus across the ventral surface of the trachea. The gland is the source of two fundamentally different types of hormones, thyroxine (T_4) and triiodothyronine (T_3). Both hormones are vital for normal growth and development and control essential functions, such as energy metabolism and protein synthesis.

The word thyroid, meaning shield-shaped, was introduced by Wharton in his description of the gland (1). Like many before him, he attributed a solely cosmetic function to it because of the more frequent presence of enlarged glands in women, giving the throat region a more beautiful roundness. Later, however, it was observed that some characteristic symptoms for diseases always were accompanied by an obvious change in the size of the thyroid. This change was correctly interpreted as evidence that this structure plays a major role in normal body function.

An important step in the understanding of thyroid function was taken by Baumann (2), who discovered that the thyroid gland was the only organ in mammals that had the capability to incorporate iodine into organic substances. That discovery was important in research concerning the phylogeny of the thyroid.

Major clues to the physiological roles of thyroid hormones were provided when normal and abnormal thyroid function were related to oxygen uptake (3) and when thyroid hormones were found to induce metamorphosis in tadpoles (4). The first discovery led to investigations regarding the role of thyroid hormone in metabolism and calorigenesis, and the second inspired research concerning specific receptors as points of initiation of thyroid hormone expression. A patient lacking thyroid hormones may be treated with synthetic hormones or natural preparations. Better agents to treat hyperthyroidism are still being sought. Presently available drugs, other compounds affecting thyroid function, and current approaches in the search for new drugs are presented in this chapter within the context of thyroid biochemistry and physiology.

NORMAL BIOCHEMISTRY AND PHYSIOLOGY

Thyroid Follicular Cells

All vertebrates have a thyroid gland consisting of functional units, the follicles. The morphological and functional characteristics of the follicles are essentially similar in all vertebrate groups.

The follicle is a spherical, cyst-like structure approximately 300 μm in diameter, and it consists of a luminal cavity surrounded by a one-cell-deep layer of cells called follicular or acinar cells. The center of the follicles is filled with a gelatinous colloid, the main component of which is a glycoprotein called thyroglobulin. The follicular cells contain an extensive network of rough endoplasmic reticulum, a well-developed Golgi apparatus, and lysosomes of various sizes (5). Thyroglobulin is synthesized in the rough endoplasmic reticulum of the follicular cells and transported by way of the Golgi complex to the apical membrane and then secreted into the follicle lumen.

The follicular cell contains two major assembly lines operating in opposite directions (6). One line moves in an apical direction and produces thyroglobulin that is delivered to the follicle lumen; the other line begins at the apical cell surface with endocytosis of thyroglobulin and ends by delivering hormones at the basolateral cell membrane. The follicular cell seems, therefore, to fulfill the functions of secretory and absorptive cells simultaneously. In addition to the functions associated with these two lines, the follicle has the specific ability to metabolize iodine, comprising the accumulation of iodide, iodination of tryosyl residues in thyroglobulin, and coupling of the iodinated tyrosyls to form thyroid hormones.

Parafollicular cells, also called light cells or C cells, are located individually or in clusters between follicular cells but do not border on the colloid. These cells produce

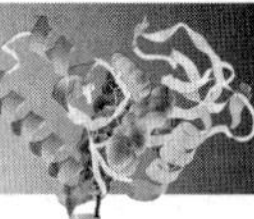

CLINICAL SIGNIFICANCE

Differences in the activity profiles of available treatments for thyroid disorders make patient-specific drug selection extremely important. The development of synthetic thyroid hormones has significantly improved treatment of hypothyroidism by decreasing the variations in thyroxine (T_4) and triiodothyronine (T_3) blood levels that often resulted from inconsistent bovine and porcine sources. Once-daily or once-weekly dosing, which has been associated with improved patient compliance, is another clinically significant benefit of synthetic T_4, resulting from its extended half-life. Knowledge of levothyroxine's pharmacokinetic profile also has prompted patient counseling efforts promoting premeal administration because of marked reduction in absorption when combined with meals.

The understanding of structure–activity relationships also enabled the development of synthetic T_3 (liothyronine), the metabolically more active form of thyroid hormone with a much shorter duration of action. This is especially useful for patients with thyroid carcinoma who are to undergo radioiodine imaging and possible treatment. Because of a half-life of only 24 hours, liothyronine substitution enables timelier radioiodine imaging and treatment, and as a result, patients experience less symptomatic hypothyroidism.

The study of medicinal chemistry has improved the treatment of thyroid disorders by reducing variability in plasma concentrations of T_3 and T_4 and by increasing the reliability of available monitoring methods. Accurate monitoring and therapy adjustments have resulted in fewer complications and increased quality of life among the millions of patients with thyroid disorders.

Dalia R. Mack, Pharm.D.
Assistant Clinical Specialist
Northeastern University
Department of Pharmacy Practice
Bouvé College of Health Sciences

thyrocalcitonin, a peptide hormone involved in calcium homeostasis. The extrafollicular space of the gland is occupied by blood vessels, capillaries, lymphatic vessels, and connective tissue.

Hormones of the Thyroid Gland

Thyroid hormones are iodinated amino acids derived from L-tyrosine. They are synthesized in the thyroid gland and stored as amino acid residues of thyroglobulin. The first known biologically active iodine-containing compound of the thyroid gland was isolated from thyroid extracts by Kendall (7) and named L-thyroxine (T_4). Later, its structure was established by Harington (8) as the 3,5,3′,5′-tetraiodo-L-thyronine (T_4) (Fig. 34.1), and its synthesis was accomplished by Harington and Bargar (9). Twenty-five years later, with the availability of chromatographic techniques and radioactive iodine, researchers discovered another major thyroid hormone, which was identified as 3,5,3′-triiodo-L-thyronine (T_3) (Fig. 34.1). This far more potent hormone is largely synthesized from T_4 by deiodinase enzymes outside the thyroid. The body is therefore able to use a dose of T_4 to produce its own T_3.

The thyroid hormones, T_4 and T_3, play numerous, profound roles in regulating metabolism, growth, and development and in maintaining homeostasis. Their reactions and products influence carbohydrate metabolism, protein synthesis and breakdown, and cardiovascular, renal, and brain function. It generally is believed that these actions result from effects of thyroid hormones on protein synthesis.

The thyroid gland also contains two quantitatively important iodinated amino acids, diiodo-L-tyrosine (DIT) and monoiodo-L-tyrosine (MIT). In addition, there are small amounts of other iodothyronines, such as 3,3′-diiodo-L-thyronine (T_2) and 3,3′,5′-triiodo-L-thyronine (reverse T_3 [rT_3]). None of the latter compounds possesses any significant hormonal activity. Chemically, MIT is 3-iodo-L-tyrosine, and DIT is 3,5-diiodo-L-tyrosine. The coupling of the two outer rings of DIT or of one outer ring of DIT with that of MIT (each with the net loss of

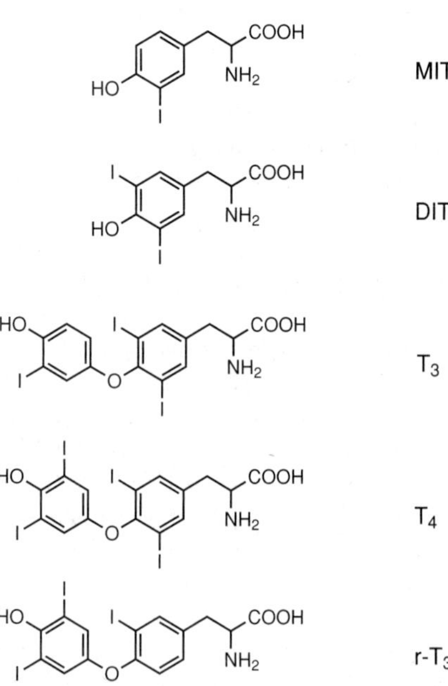

Fig. 34.1. Structure of the iodinated compounds of the thyroid gland.

alanine) leads to the formation of the two major thyroid hormones, T_4 and T_3, respectively.

Thyroglobulin is of special importance, because it serves as the matrix for the synthesis of T_4 and T_3 and as the storage form of the hormones and iodide. Thyroglobulin, a large glycoprotein with a molecular weight of 660,000 Da, accounts for about one-third of the weight of the thyroid gland. Thyroglobulin carries an average of 6 tyrosyl residues as monoiodo-L-tyrosine, 5 residues as diiodo-L-tyrosine, 0.3 residues as T_3, and 1 residue as T_4 (10). From these values, it can be estimated that a 20 g thyroid stores roughly 10 μmol (7.8 mg) of T_4 and 3 μmol (2.0 mg) of T_3 and that the normal human thyroid gland contains enough potential T_4 to maintain a euthyroid state for 2 months without new synthesis (11). The structures of the iodinated compounds of the thyroid gland are shown in Figure 34.1.

Biosynthesis of Thyroid Hormones

The synthesis of the thyroid hormones, T_3 and T_4, is regulated by thyrotropin (thyroid-stimulating hormone [TSH]), which stimulates the synthesis of thyroglobulin, thyroperoxidase (TPO), and hydrogen peroxide. The formation of the thyroid hormones depends on an exogenous supply of iodide. The thyroid gland is unique in that it is the only tissue of the body able to accumulate iodine in large quantities and incorporate it into hormones. Approximately 25% of the body's supply of iodide is located in the thyroid gland. The iodine atoms play a unique role in the conformational preferences for T_3 and T_4 because of their large steric bulkiness. The metabolism of iodine is so closely related to thyroid function that the two must be considered together. The formation of thyroid hormones involves the following complex sequence of events: 1) active uptake of iodide by the follicular cells, 2) oxidation of iodide and formation of iodotyrosyl residues of thyroglobulin, 3) formation of iodothyronines from iodotyrosines, 4) proteolysis of thyroglobulin and release of T_4 and T_3 into blood, and 5) conversion of T_4 to T_3. These processes are summarized in Figure 34.2 (12).

Active Uptake of Iodide by Follicular Cells

The first step in the synthesis of the thyroid hormones is the uptake of iodide from the blood by the thyroid gland. An adequate intake of iodide is essential for the synthesis of sufficient thyroid hormone. Dietary iodine is converted to iodide and almost completely absorbed from the gastrointestinal tract. Blood iodine is present in a steady state in which dietary iodide, iodide "leaked" from the thyroid gland, and reclaimed hormonal iodide provide the input. Thyroid gland iodide uptake, renal elimination, and a small biliary excretion providing the output. The thyroid gland regulates both the fraction of circulating iodide that it takes up and the amount of iodide that it leaks back into the circulation. A simplified scheme of iodide metabolism is shown in Figure 34.3.

The mechanism enabling the thyroid gland to concentrate blood iodide against a gradient into the follicular cell is the iodide pump (NIS, sodium/iodide symporter), which is regulated by TSH. The NIS, a Na^+-dependent active transporter, is located at the basolateral plasma membrane. The NIS-mediated I^- uptake is coupled to the inward translocation of Na^+. NIS expression is regulated by TSH at the posttranscriptional level. Decreased stores of thyroid iodine enhance iodide uptake; conversely, dietary iodide can reverse this process. The iodide pump maintains about a ratio of thyroid iodide to serum iodide (T:S ratio) of 20:1 under basal conditions but of more than 100:1 in hyperactive gland. The iodide pump also is found in the placenta and mammary tissue to enable the fetal thyroid and the natal thyroid glands to develop properly.

Iodide uptake may be blocked by several inorganic ions, such as thiocyanate and perchlorate. Because iodide uptake involves concurrent uptake of potassium, it also can be blocked by cardiac glycosides that inhibit potassium accumulation.

Oxidation of Iodide and Formation of Iodotyrosines

To serve as an iodinating agent, iodide must be oxidized to a higher oxidation state, a step that is hydrogen peroxide dependent and is catalyzed by TPO, a membrane-bound heme-enzyme that utilizes hydrogen peroxide as the oxidant. In addition to catalyzing the oxidation of iodide, TPO is essential for the incorporation of iodide into tyrosine residues in thyroglobulin (aromatic iodination) and coupling of the iodotyrosyl residues from DIT to form T_4 and T_3. The activity of TPO is increased by TSH from increased synthesis of TPO.

The second step in the synthesis of the thyroid hormones is a concerted reaction at the apical membrane in which the iodide in the follicle lumen is oxidized by TPO in the presence of hydrogen peroxide to an active iodine species that, in turn, iodinates selected tyrosyl residues of thyroglobulin. Consistent with the conditions necessary for aromatic halogenation, the iodination of the tyrosyl residues requires the iodinating species to be in a higher oxidation state compared with the iodide anion. The iodinating species is thought to be hypoiodate (OI^-) (12). The two-electron oxidation of iodide to its hypoiodate reactive species is accomplished by TPO. Although the diiodotyrosyl residues constitute the major products, some MIT peptides also are produced. TSH stimulates the generation of hydrogen peroxide and, thus, the process of iodination.

Hydrogen peroxide is an essential and limiting factor in the oxidation of iodide, aromatic iodination of tyrosyl residues, and the coupling reaction. The hydrogen peroxide–generating system is localized at the apical membrane, and its generation involves the oxidation of NADPH by an NADPH/FAD oxidase called thyroid oxidase. The reaction product of TPO with hydrogen peroxide is described as TPO-P, a π-cation radical, which generates hypoiodate. The generation of hydrogen peroxide is concentration controlled by iodide, which permits efficient hormone synthesis when iodide is scarce

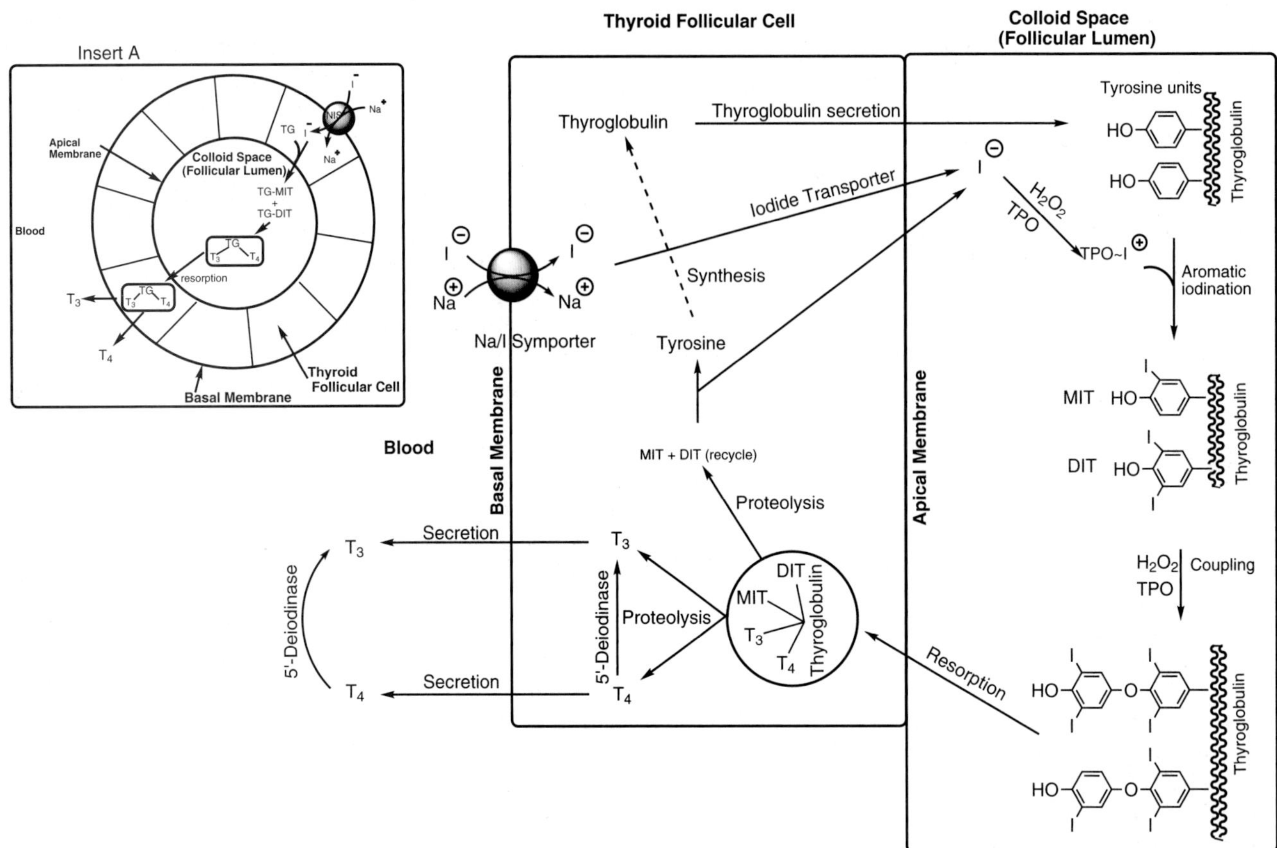

Fig. 34.2. Summary of the major pathways for the biosynthesis and secretion of the thyroid hormones. When thyrotropin (TSH) binds to the TSH receptor at the basal membrane of the follicular cell, the biosynthesis of thyroglobulin (TG) is stimulated, as is that of thyroperoxidase (TPO) and the production of hydrogen peroxide. Noniodinated TG is synthesized by the rough endoplasmic reticulum of the follicular cell and secreted through the apical membrane of the follicular cell into the follicular lumen. Iodide enters the follicular cell by the iodide pump (NIS, sodium iodide symporter) and is then transported into the follicular lumen. In the lumen, the iodide is oxidized by TPO-O (a π-cation radical intermediate formed from TPO and hydrogen peroxide) at the apical membrane to form hypoiodate anion (OI^-), followed by aromatic iodination of selected tyrosyl residues on TG to form diiodotyrosyl (DIT) and monoiodotyrosyl (MIT) residues. The tyrosyl ring of DIT couples with adjacent DIT and MIT residues with an ether linkage to form the outer ring of thyroxine (T_4) and of triiodothyronine (T_3), both of which remain attached to TG. Although shown as a sequential reaction, the iodination and coupling reactions occur simultaneously via TPO and hydrogen peroxide. Hydrogen peroxide is generated by a NADPH/FAD thyroid oxidase (THOX) at the apical membrane. Low plasma levels for T_4 cause the iodinated TG to be resorbed into the follicular cell, where complete proteolysis occurs by lysosomal protease to T_4, T_3, DIT, MIT, and noniodinated amino acids. Both T_4 and T_3 are secreted by the cell into the blood; T_4 is deiodinated to active T_3. Both DIT and MIT are recycled by a dehalogenase (or deiodinase) to free tyrosine and iodide, both of which are recycled back into iodinated thyroglobulin.

while avoiding excessive hormone synthesis when iodide is abundant. Deficient generation of hydrogen peroxide has been proposed as one explanation for goiter and decreased aromatic iodination in euthyroid patients. The in vitro addition of a hydrogen peroxide–generating system to thyroid homogenates or slices from these patients restored normal organification.

In the thyroid follicular cell, intracellular iodide taken up from blood is bound in organic form in a few minutes, so less than 1% of the total iodine of the gland is found as iodide. Therefore, inhibition of the iodide transport system requires blockade of organic binding. This can be achieved by the use of antithyroid drugs, of which n-propyl-6-thiouracil and 1-methyl-2-mercaptoimidazole (methimazole) are the most potent.

Coupling of Iodotyrosine Residues

Coupling is also catalyzed by TPO at the apical membrane, and although shown in Figure 34.2 as sequential steps, they occur simultaneously. This coupling reaction takes place at thyroglobulin and involves the coupling of the two outer rings from DIT residues to become T_4, whereas the coupling of the outer ring from MIT with DIT results in the formation of T_3. During the coupling

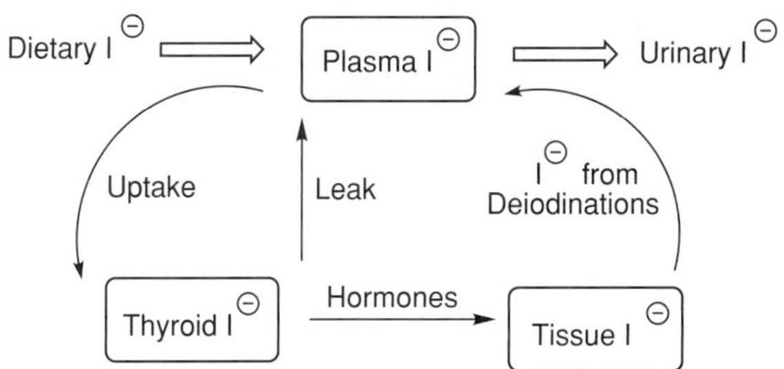

Fig. 34.3. Simplified scheme of iodide metabolism.

reaction as shown in Figure 34.2, a tyrosyl residue donates its iodinated phenyl group as a DIT radical to become the outer ring of the iodothyronine amino acid at an acceptor site, leaving dehydroalanine at the donor site. The location of the iodotyrosyl residues within thyroglobulin creates an optimal spatial alignment, facilitating the coupling reaction. These reactions are catalyzed by TPO and can be blocked by compounds such as thiourea, thiouracils, and sulfonamides.

Proteolysis of Thyroglobulin and Release of Iodothyronines

In response to demand for thyroid hormones, the release of thyroid hormones from thyroglobulin begins with the resorption of thyroglobulin via endocytosis into the follicular epithelial cells and its subsequent complete proteolysis by the lysosomal digestive enzymes of the follicular cells. Thyroglobulin proteolysis yields MIT, DIT, T_3, and T_4. Although MIT and DIT are formed, they do not leave the thyroid but, instead, are selectively deiodinated to tyrosine and recycled into new thyroglobulin. The iodide is recycled into hypoiodate for subsequent iodination, conserving the essential nutrients for the thyroid gland. Both T_3 and T_4 are secreted by the cell into the circulation. A defect in the recyclization of MIT and DIT can lead to hypothyroidism and goiter by increasing their elimination in the urine.

Conversion of Thyroxine to Triiodothyronine

Although T_4 is by far the major thyroid hormone secreted by the thyroid (~8 to 10 times the rate of T_3), it usually is considered to be a prohormone. Because T_4 has a longer half-life, much higher levels of T_4 than of T_3 are in the circulation. The enzymatic conversion of T_4 to T_3 is an obligate step in the physiological action of thyroid hormones in most extrathyroidal tissues. In the peripheral tissues, approximately 33% of the T_4 secreted undergoes 5′-deiodination to give T_3, and another 40% undergoes deiodination of the inner ring to yield the inactive material rT_3 (13). The deiodination of T_4 is a reductive process catalyzed by a group of enzymes named iodothyronine deiodinases, referred to as deiodinases and symbolized by D, found in a variety of cells. Approximately 80% of the T_3 is derived from circulating T_4.

Three types of deiodinases are currently known, and these are distinguished from each other primarily based on their location, substrate preference, and susceptibility to inhibitors. Type I deiodinase is found in liver and kidney and catalyzes both inner ring and outer ring deiodination (i.e., T_4 to T_3 and rT_3 to 3,3′-T_2). Type II deiodinase catalyzes mainly outer ring deiodination (i.e., T_4 to T_3 and T_3 to 3,3′-T_2) and is found in brain and the pituitary. Type III deiodinase is the principal source of rT_3 and is present in brain, skin, and placenta (14).

Transport of Thyroid Hormones in Blood

The iodothyronines secreted by the thyroid gland into thyroid vein blood are of limited solubility. They equilibrate rapidly, however, through noncovalent association with three major binding proteins: thyroid binding globulin (TBG), transthyretin (TTR; formerly called T_4 binding prealbumin), and albumin. Thyroid binding globulin is the primary serum binding protein because of its higher affinity for T_4. Under normal conditions, 75% of T_4 is bound to TBG, 10 to 15% to TTR, and 5 to 15% to albumin. When bound, T_4 is not physiologically active but does provide a storage pool of thyroid hormone, which can last 2 to 3 months (mean half-life of T_4, 6.7 days in adults). The plasma proteins involved in thyroid hormone transport and their approximate association constants (K_a) for T_3 and T_4 are shown in Table 34.1. This table indicates that TBG has a high affinity for T_4 ($K_a \sim 10^{10}$ M) and lower affinity for T_3. Additionally, TTR and albumin transport thyroid hormones in the blood; TTR has K_a values of approximately 10^7 and 10^6 M for T_4 and T_3, respectively. The equilibrium between the free hormone and that protein bound hormone determines the accessibility of the free thyroid hormone for the tissue receptors as well as to peripheral sites, where biotransformations take place. The lower binding affinity for T_3 to plasma proteins may be an important factor in the more rapid onset of action and the shorter biological half-life for T_3.

Thyroid hormones are taken into cells by facilitated diffusion or by active transport secondary to a sodium gradient (11). Once in the cell, thyroid hormones bind to cytosolic binding proteins and are not readily available for exchange with plasma hormones. Both T_3 and T_4 are not evenly distributed in body cells: A great part of T_4 is

Table 34.1. Plasma Proteins Involved in Thyroid Hormone Transport

		Binding of T_4		Binding of T_3	
Protein	Concentr. (mg/dL)	K_a	% Bound	K_a	% Bound
TBG	1.5	10^{10}	75	10^9	70
TTR	25	10^7	15	10^6	
Albumin	4,000	10^6	10	10^5	30

K_a, approximate association constant; TBG, tyroxine-binding globulin; TTR, transthyretin.

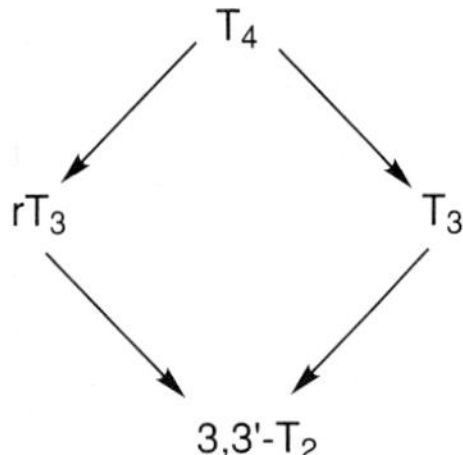

Fig. 34.4. Deiodination of thyroxine (T_4).

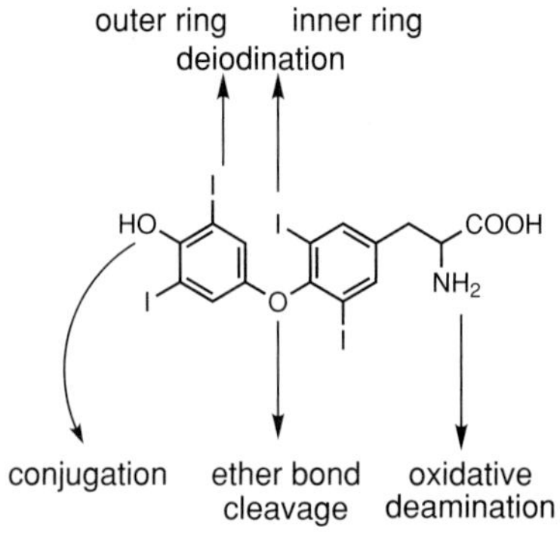

stored in liver and kidney, whereas most T_3 appears in muscle and brain (11).

Metabolism and Excretion

As discussed earlier, T_4 is considered to be a prohormone, and its peripheral metabolism occurs in two ways: outer ring deiodination by the enzyme 5′-D, which yields T_3, and inner ring deiodination by the enzyme 5-D, which yields rT_3, for which there is no known biological function (Fig. 34.4). In humans, deiodination is the most important metabolic pathway of the hormone, not only because of its dual role in the activation and inactivation of T_4 but also in quantitative terms.

Degradative metabolism of the thyroid hormones, apart from peripheral deiodination, occurs mainly in the liver, where both T_3 and T_4 are conjugated to form either glucuronide (mainly T_4) or sulfate (mainly T_3) with the phenolic hydroxyl group. The resulting iodothyronine conjugates are excreted via the bile into the intestine, where a portion is hydrolyzed by bacteria. The conjugates also undergo marginal enterohepatic circulation and are excreted unconjugated in feces.

T_4 is conjugated with sulfate in kidney and liver, and T_4-4′-O-sulfate, an excellent substrate for 5′-D (15), is believed to play a role in the regulation of T_4 metabolism.

Additional metabolism, involving side-chain degradation, proceeds by transamination, oxidative deamination, and decarboxylation to yield thyroacetic acid and thyroethanediol; cleavage of the diphenyl ether linkage has been detected as well, both in vitro and in vivo. The reactions through which thyroid hormone is metabolized are summarized in Figure 34.5.

Physiological Actions of Thyroid Hormones—Oxygen Consumption and Calorigenesis

The two most important actions of thyroid hormone are those related to oxygen consumption and those related to protein synthesis. Most effects of thyroid hormones can be related to the activation of genes following the binding of the hormone to high-affinity receptors of cell nuclei, but direct interactions of thyroid hormones with other cellular receptors cannot be excluded (16).

A respiratory component of the action of thyroid hormones was first observed almost a century ago. Respiratory

outer ring inner ring
deiodination
HO I I COOH NH2 O I I
conjugation ether bond cleavage oxidative deamination

Fig. 34.5. Metabolic pathways for thyroxine.

exchange was depressed in patients diagnosed as hypothyroid and increased in patients diagnosed as hyperthyroid (3). The increase in respiration that follows the administration of thyroid hormone reflects an increase in metabolic rate thyroid function has, indeed, long been assessed by measuring the basal or resting metabolic rate (BMR), a test in which the oxygen consumed, as measured in an individual at rest, is used to calculate total body energy production. The BMR of a hyperthyroid individual is above the normal range, or positive, and that of a hypothyroid individual below the normal range, or negative.

Thyroid hormones increase the oxygen consumption of most isolated tissues but not of isolated adult brain. This suggests that the behavioral changes seen in abnormal thyroid states (anxiety and nervousness in hyperthyroidism and impaired memory in hypothyroidism) in the adult are not directly linked to overall changes in brain oxygen consumption.

Because most of the energy produced by cellular respiration eventually appears as heat, an increase in cellular respiration necessarily leads to an increase in heat production (i.e., to a thermogenic or calorigenic effect). Thus, to the degree that thyroid hormones control BMR, they also control thermogenesis (17).

Clinically the inability to adjust to environmental temperature is symptomatic of departure from the euthyroid status. Patients with myxedema frequently have subnormal body temperature, have cold and dry skin, and tolerate cold poorly; the thyrotoxic patient, who compensates for excess heat production by sweating (warm, moist hands), does not easily tolerate a warm environment.

Thyroid hormones regulate the turnover of carbohydrates, lipids, and proteins. They promote glucose absorption, hepatic and renal gluconeogenesis, hepatic glycogenolysis, and glucose utilization in muscle and adipose tissue (18). They increase de novo cholesterol synthesis but increase low-density lipoprotein degradation and cholesterol disposal even more, leading to a net decrease in total and in low-density lipoprotein cholesterol plasma levels (19). Thyroid hormones are anabolic when present at normal concentrations; they then stimulate the expression of many key enzymes of metabolism.

Thyroid hormones at the levels present in hyperthyroidism are catabolic; they lead to the mobilization of tissue protein and, especially, of muscle tissue protein for gluconeogenetic processes (20). Thus, the depletion of liver glycogen, the increased breakdown of lipids, and the negative nitrogen balance observed in hyperthyroidism represent toxic effects. The metabolic processes of hypermetabolism are wasteful. In hyperthyroidism, a smaller-than-normal amount of liberated energy is available for useful work, and an excessive amount is wasted as heat.

Because of the role of mitochondria in cellular respiration and energy production, efforts to elucidate the mechanism of thyroid hormone action in metabolism and calorigenesis have focused on mitochondrial studies. Thyroid hormones in vitro are known to uncouple oxidative phosphorylation in isolated mitochondria, but these effects occur at unphysiological doses of T_4. In physiological concentrations, T_4 increases adenosine triphosphate (ATP) formation and the number and inner membrane surface area of mitochondria (21), but T_4 does not reduce the efficiency of oxidative phosphorylation. Furthermore, 2,4-dinitrophenol, a classic uncoupler of oxidative phosphorylation, can neither relieve hypothyroidism nor duplicate other physiological effects of thyroid hormones.

Because in most physiological circumstances oxygen consumption is controlled by energy metabolism, Ismail-Beigi and Edelman (22) proposed that the primary effect of thyroid hormones is to increase the amount of energy expended in translocating cations across cell membranes, probably as a response to an increased passive leak of sodium into, and potassium out of, cells. The extent to which this transport contributes to heat production and ATP utilization is uncertain. The stimulation of futile cycles by thyroid hormones (23) has been suggested to be an additional component of ATP disposal.

The effectiveness of β-blocking agents in treating the symptoms of thyrotoxicosis has led to investigations that have indicated thyroid hormones modulate adrenergic effects by increasing the number of β-adrenergic receptors (24) and, at least in cardiac tissue (25), by increasing the adrenergic receptors that are coupled with a membrane-bound adenylate cyclase (also known as adenyl cyclase) (26); both observations appear to be mutually consistent. The role of thyroid hormones in adaptive thermogenesis (17) could be affected by stimulating an increase in brown adipose tissue β-adrenergic receptors; catecholamines, which are known to activate the β receptor-linked adenylate cyclase in that tissue (23), would then start the lipolysis cascade resulting in heat production.

Differentiation and Protein Synthesis

Stimulation of amphibian metamorphosis by thyroid hormones has been known for a long time (4). Changes in amphibian morphogenesis, such as involution of the tail of *Xenopus* (toads) and metamorphosis of the axolotl (salamanders) and of *Rana* (frogs), have been repeatedly used as end points for the bioassay of thyroid analogues. In young mammals, thyroid hormone is necessary not only for general growth but also for proper differentiation of the central nervous system. The counterpart of amphibian metamorphosis in the developing mammalian brain is myelogenesis and the formation of axons and dendrites (27). Behavioral studies in neonate hypothyroid mammals show that impairment in learning capacity (27) paralleled impairment of proper anatomic development in the brain. A deficiency of thyroid hormone during the critical period when the developing human brain is sensitive to thyroid hormone results in an irreversible clinical entity termed cretinism, which is characterized by stunted growth and mental retardation.

A great deal of attention has been devoted to the events taking place in the roughly 48-hour interval between the administration of thyroid hormone and the manifestation of certain effects caused by that administration. After Tata (28) had observed that the anabolic effects observed in rats given T_4 could be blocked by inhibitors of protein synthesis, further investigations led Tata and Widnell (29) to the conclusion that thyroid hormones were activating protein synthesis at the ribosomal level. Subsequently, Dillmann et al. (30) showed that the T_3-induced formation of α-glycerophosphate dehydrogenase (E.C. 1.1.99.5) could be blocked by α-amanitin, an inhibitor of RNA polymerase II, inferring that thyroid hormones affected the transcription process. In 1972, when the partition of thyroid hormones between plasma and a number of tissues was investigated, Schadlow et al. (31) demonstrated that the uptake of T_3 by unfractionated pituitary tissue was inverse to the dose, suggesting that the pituitary was limited in its capacity to bind T_3. This finding prompted efforts to find the subcellular location of the binding sites and to search for the presence of specific binding sites in other tissues (32). The research revealed that the binding sites were located in cell nuclei and were also present in liver and kidney (32). Eventually, receptors were located in all mammalian tissues and also in tadpole erythrocytes (33). In cultured pituitary cells, the receptor was described as an acidic, nonhistone, 50,000-Da protein (34) with an equilibrium dissociation (K_d) constant of 2.9×10^{-11} for T_3 and of 2.6×10^{-10} for T_4, indicating that T_3 had a 10 times greater affinity than T_4 for the receptor. There were 6,000 nuclear binding sites in the pituitary, 4,000 in the liver, but only 16 in the testis, a tissue that is not responsive to thyroid hormone (35). The findings by Tata and Widnell (29) of the activation of one RNA polymerase were extended to all RNA polymerases, suggesting that thyroid hormones were involved in all phases of gene activation.

Receptors located on the plasma membrane, in the cytoplasm, and in mitochondria have been described as well (36). Plasma membrane receptors are believed to mediate the transport of hormone into the cell and, possibly, to mediate nonnuclear, immediate effects of thyroid hormone (36). The presence of a large number of low-affinity cytosol binding proteins has been known for some time (37), but these proteins have not been assigned a specific physiological role. The cytosolic binding proteins have been proposed as a large intracellular thyroid hormone reservoir, delaying the metabolic disposition of thyroid hormone.

Because thyroid hormones immediately increase oxygen uptake and ATP formation and, eventually, lead to an increase in the number, size, and inner membrane surface area of mitochondria as well as to the induction of many mitochondrial enzymes, many efforts to characterize mitochondrial thyroid hormone receptors have been made. Sterling et al. (38) have reported the presence of very high affinity receptors in mitochondria, but their work has not been duplicated. Additionally, many authors believe that most mitochondrial enzymes are synthesized on cytoplasmic ribosomes and then transferred into mitochondria (39).

Control of Thyroid Hormone Biosynthesis

The primary role of thyroid is to produce thyroid hormones. The primary regulator of thyroid, both its function and growth, is the pituitary hormone, thyrotropin (TSH). Thyrotropin is a glycoprotein with a molecular weight of approximately 28,000 daltons, which can dissociate into two equally large polypeptide chains: an α-chain, which is also present in other pituitary peptides, and a β-chain, which is present in TSH only. The TSH is produced by and released from the anterior pituitary gland, causing the thyroid hormone to initiate new thyroid hormone synthesis. Increases in iodide uptake, the iodination of thyroglobulin, and endocytosis of colloid are all observed in response to stimulation of TSH. The effects of TSH on the thyroid appear to be the consequence of binding to high-affinity receptors on the capillary membrane of follicular cells and activation of adenylate cyclase and protein kinase enzymes, found on the inner side of the membrane, with subsequent phosphorylation of cellular proteins. It is believed that most, if not all, effects of TSH are mediated through the cyclic adenosine monophosphate (cAMP) formed by adenylate cyclase and, possibly, also by cAMP-activated intracellular phosphokinases.

The amount of thyroid hormone circulating in body fluids and present in tissues remains fairly constant. Accounting for this constancy are the relatively long biological half-life of the thyroid hormones, the regulation of gland activity by the pituitary-hypothalamic system, and the availability of iodide. Thyroid hormone research points toward T_3 as the thyroid hormone; therefore, factors affecting peripheral T_3 formation by the 5′-D enzymes are highly relevant.

The relation of biological half-life to protein binding has already been alluded to. The T_4 is firmly bound to plasma proteins. Only 0.05% of T_4 is not protein bound, and T_4 has a biological half-life of 1 week, as compared to 1 day for the less firmly bound T_3.

The biosynthesis and secretion of TSH is, in turn, regulated by thyrotropin-releasing hormone (TRH) and the quantity of thyroid hormone in circulation through feedback control. The tripeptide pyroglutamylhistidylprolylamide, TRH is formed in the hypothalamus, reaches the thyrotrophs (i.e., the TSH-producing pituitary cells) by way of the hypophyseal portal system, and stimulates TSH release by binding to the TRH receptors of the thyrotrophs (40). The ability of thyroid hormones to prevent the release of TSH is referred to as feedback regulation. It is believed that T_3 prevents the TRH-stimulated release of TSH by stimulating the synthesis of a peptide that would compete with TRH for the TRH receptor sites on the thyrotroph (41). Inhibition of the transcription of the α and β subunits of TSH by thyroid hormone (42) also may contribute to the feedback effect.

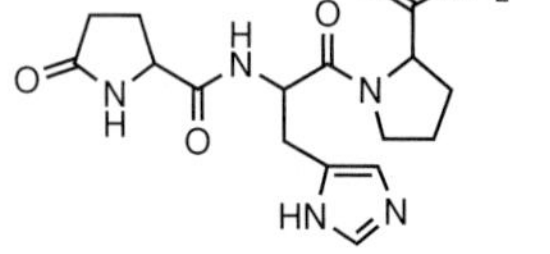

TRH

The amount of iodide available to the gland for hormone synthesis also is an important regulator of thyroid function. The efficiency of the thyroid pump mechanism and the rate of thyroglobulin and TPO synthesis are all TSH-dependent. In cases of iodide deficiency, the production of thyroid hormone is lowered, and TSH rises through the pituitary feedback mechanism described previously. The effect of the increased TSH is to produce more thyroid hormone by increasing efficiency of the iodide pump and increasing thyroglobulin and TPO synthesis. Thus, in iodide deficiency, there is an increased uptake of iodide (43) are larger MIT-to-DIT ratios, which leads to larger T_3-to-T_4 ratio. The T_3 is the more rapidly acting hormone, mitigating the effect of iodide deficiency. When iodide deficiency is severe, a persistent rise in TSH is observed. This then results in thyroid growth.

In the presence of an excess of circulating iodide, the absolute amount of iodide taken up remains approximately constant. There is a decrease in the fraction of the total iodide taken up and an increase in the amount of iodide leaked from the thyroid gland. In addition, there may be a decrease in organification (i.e., in the formation of iodinated thyroglobulin residues) and in the release of hormones from the gland. The decrease in organification that occurs at excessive physiological doses of iodide has been called the Wolff-Chaikoff block (44). This block may be caused by an interaction of iodide with NADPH (45), which depletes follicular NADPH and, in turn, depletes the H_2O_2 necessary for TPO activity. The decrease in hormone release occurs when iodide is given in pharmacological (mg) quantities; it may last for a few weeks.

The activity of deiodinases reflects thyroid status, general health, and food intake. In hypothyroidism, there is a decrease in hepatic 5′ D-I but an increase in 5′ D-II activity (46). There is a decrease in T_3 and an increase in rT_3 after hepatic disease (47), renal damage (48), chronic illness (49), and starvation (50), indicating a decrease in the activity of the quantitatively more important 5′ D-I. An increase in deiodinase activity has been observed after overfeeding subjects or after administering a high-carbohydrate or high-fat diet (51) to experimental animals. The mechanism of deiodinase control is presumably intricate, but the inhibiting effects of propranolol on 5′ D-I (52) and of prazosin on the 5′ D-II of BAT (53) infer the involvement of adrenergic components in the regulation. In addition, the rapid change in activity observed after asphyxia points toward a rapid, possibly cAMP-related control (54).

DISEASES INVOLVING THE THYROID GLAND

Hypothyroidism

Goiter

An enlarged, palpable thyroid gland is referred to as a goiter. When insufficient thyroid hormone is liberated from the thyroid gland, the breakdown of the thyroid-pituitary-hypothalamic feedback mechanism results in the release of excess TSH and in the formation of a thyroid hypertrophy referred to as a nontoxic goiter. The gland enlarges as it tries to take up more iodine, leading to goiter. Endemic goiters are those that occur in a significant segment of a given population. Goiters most frequently are caused by inadequate intake of dietary iodide in regions not reached by iodide-providing sea mists and, occasionally, by the prolonged intake of goitrogens derived from plant sources or aquifers. This condition can be prevented with iodine supplements, and many industrialized countries now iodize salt.

A characteristic sign of hypothyroidism is a decrease in metabolic rate, with a reduction in calorigenic effect and defective thermoregulation. The elevated serum cholesterol level seen in hypothyroidism is the result of a decrease in cholesterol degradation that exceeds the decrease in cholesterol biosynthesis; it reflects a general slowdown in catabolic processes. Shared symptoms of hypothyroidism and cognitive disorders include fatigue, mental dullness, lethargy, and inattention. Treatment of hypothyroidism includes supplementation of T_4 with the goal of returning TSH levels to normal.

Cretinism

Cretinism, the irreversible clinical entity characterized by defective physical and mental development, appears when thyroid hormone is not available during early childhood for normal bone formation and normal brain growth and differentiation.

Myxedema

Myxedema is used either as a specific term to describe the infiltration of the intercellular spaces of skin and muscle with mucopolysaccharide or as a general term, as in adult myxedema or pituitary myxedema, to denote hypothyroid status.

Hyperthyroidism

The increased metabolic rate of hyperthyroidism results in symptoms opposite to those seen in hypothyroidism. The increased oxygen demand in hyperthyroidism leads to an increased heart rate and increased cardiac output and, thereby, places strain on the heart. Exaggerated catabolic processes lead to decreased serum cholesterol and, possibly, to poor glucose tolerance and glucosuria as well, and the excessive calorigenic effect produced by catabolic processes causes anorexia and poor thermoregulation. Excessive hormone function is expressed by the word "toxic," as in toxic goiter, toxic adenoma, and thyrotoxicosis. Thyrotoxic crisis or thyroid storm is an emergency caused by a stress-triggered augmentation of the symptoms of thyrotoxicosis (55). Treatment models aim to decrease the overproduction of thyroid hormones using antithyroid medication or radioactive iodine ablation or surgery.

Graves' Disease

Graves' disease is the most frequently encountered form of hyperthyroidism and is caused by a generalized overactivity of the entire thyroid gland. Named after the physician who first described it, Graves' disease is an autoimmune condition in which the body's immune system tricks the thyroid into producing too much thyroid hormone. It is also called diffuse toxic goiter: "diffuse" because the entire thyroid gland is involved in the disease process; "toxic" because the patient appears hot and flushed, as if feverish due to an infection; and "goiter" because the thyroid gland enlarges in this condition. Signs of this disease may include goiter, a protrusion of the eyeballs called exophthalmos, and pretibial myxedema. Hyperthyroidism from Graves' disease is, in general, easily controlled and safely treated.

In the serum of most patients suffering from Graves' disease, an immunoglobulin (IgC) is present that, after a slow onset, elicits a long-lasting stimulation of the thyroid gland. Because the release of the long-acting thyroid stimulator is not controlled by thyroid hormone levels as is TSH, patients with long-acting thyroid stimulator have a hyperplastic, hypertrophied gland that produces and releases an excessive amount of hormone.

The indications are that the exophthalmos is caused by a substance produced by a distinct autoimmune system (56), possibly in response to a modified TSH of pituitary origin.

Hashimoto's Disease

Hashimoto's disease, named after the physician who first described it, is an autoimmune disorder in which plasma cells, lymphocytes, and fibrous tissue attack and destroy the thyroid gland. Pitt-Rivers and Tata (57) suggested that the sequence of events in Hashimoto's disease was initiated by injury to some thyroid structure, following which the normally sequestered thyroglobulin would be released and exposed to immunological mechanisms, thus setting into motion a progressive interaction between thyroglobulin and circulating autoantibodies. Hashimoto antibodies are present in adult-onset myxedema and in most persons with Graves' disease, but it is recognized that other antigenic factors are involved in these and other autoimmune diseases of the thyroid. Hypothyroidism resulting from Hashimoto's disease requires lifelong treatment with thyroid hormone replacement.

Generalized Resistance to Thyroid Hormone

Generalized resistance to thyroid hormone (GRTH) is a rare form of thyroid disorder and may be a heritable disorder characterized by reduced responsiveness of the pituitary and peripheral tissues to the action of thyroid hormones. Behavioral manifestations include hyperactivity, behavioral problems, and cognitive deficits. Physical traits representative of GRTH are small goiters, and GRTH is marked by genetic mutation of the thyroid receptor β gene on chromosome 3 (58).

Many have evaluated the association of GRTH to attention-deficit hyperactivity disorder and suggested that similar mechanistic pathways are shared between the two conditions (59,60). In GRTH, T_4 fails to block TSH production, leading to excess levels of T_3 and T_4 with either normal or elevated levels of TSH. In conditions of an improperly functioning thyroid, TH and TSH ratios are unregulated, producing symptoms that are characteristic of attention-deficit hyperactivity disorder.

Thyroid Cancer

Thyroid cancer is a disease in which malignant cells are found in the tissues of the thyroid gland. Four main types of cancer of the thyroid are differentiated based on how the cancer cells look under a microscope: papillary, follicular, medullary, and anaplastic. Follicular and papillary carcinomas have the highest incidence in young women but have low mortality; they represent a different disease than anaplastic types or undifferentiated carcinomas, both of which occur among the older patients and have high death rates. Each year in the United States, approximately 20,000 people are diagnosed with thyroid cancer, and it is more common in women than in men. A study published in Journal of National Cancer Institute (61) predicts that these numbers may rise as individuals who were exposed to radioactive iodine (^{131}I) from nuclear testing in the western states in the 1950s and 1960s reach middle age: A strong dose–response relationship was observed between radiation dose to the thyroid received in childhood and thyroid cancer risk. The risk of radiation-related thyroid cancer was threefold higher in iodine-deficient areas than elsewhere. Administration of potassium iodide as a dietary supplement appear to modify this risk. Treatment of thyroid cancer is straightforward and effective. Follow-up testing can be uncomfortable, however, because it requires a hypothyroid state. Follow-up takes two forms: serum thyroglobulin measurement, and a radioiodine whole-body scan, as described later.

THERAPEUTIC AGENTS

Thyroid Replacement Therapy

Hormone replacement appears to be the established therapy in the treatment of various forms of hypothyroidism, from the complete absence of thyroid function seen in myxedema to simple goiter and cretinism. Thyroid hormone drugs are natural or synthetic preparations containing T_4 sodium, T_3 sodium, or both. A large number of organic and some inorganic compounds stimulate or prevent thyroid hormone formation by interfering with iodide uptake into follicular cells, inhibiting TPO, preventing thyroid hormone binding to plasma proteins, or acting as effectors of thyroid deiodinases. Some of the agents described in this section are of therapeutic or diagnostic value, some illustrate potential side effects of drugs, and some are experimental compounds designed to achieve unmet therapeutic goals or to define structural parameters necessary for thyroid hormone actions.

Thyroid hormone preparations belong to two categories: natural hormone preparations derived from animal thyroid, and synthetic preparations.

Natural Thyroid Hormone Preparations

Natural preparations include desiccated thyroid and thyroglobulin. Desiccated thyroid and thyroglobulin are derived from thyroid glands of domesticated animals that are used for food by human. The hormones were released from the proteolytic activity of gut enzymes. Potency is based on total iodine content or bioassay and is somewhat variable with different preparations.

Desiccated thyroid preparations (Thyroid USP) are essentially acetone powders of bovine or porcine thyroid glands compressed into oral tablets. A diluent usually is present, because the preparations (especially those of porcine origin) commonly exceed the 0.17 to 0.23% iodine content required by the U.S. Pharmacopeia (USP). Because the iodine of desiccated thyroid is in the form of iodinated tyrosyl and thyronyl residues of the precipitated thyroglobulin, the preparation owes its efficacy to the hormones that eventually are liberated by intestinal proteases. In desiccated preparations, T_3 and T_4 may be present in a ratio of approximately the same as found in humans. Desiccated preparations are less expensive than synthetic hormones but have been shown to produce variable T_4/T_3 blood levels because of inconsistencies both between and within animal sources of the thyroid gland. Most comments regarding desiccated thyroid also apply to partially purified thyroglobulin, because the two preparations differ in their total and their relative amounts of T_4 and T_3.

Synthetic Thyroid Hormones

Synthetic, crystalline thyroid hormones are more uniformly absorbed than biological preparations and contain more precisely measured amounts of active ingredient in their dosage forms. Of present interest are T_4 (levothyroxine), T_3 (liothyronine), dT_4 (dextrothyroxine), and T_4-T_3 mixtures (Liotrix).

LEVOTHYROXINE. Because of its firmer binding to carrier proteins, synthetic crystalline L-T_4 sodium salt (levothyroxine sodium, Synthtoid, Euthyrox) has a slower onset of action than crystalline T_3 or a desiccated thyroid preparation. Its administration leads to a greater increase in serum T_4 but a lesser increase in serum T_3 than compared with Thyroid USP (62). The availability of 11 different tablet strengths, ranging from 25 to 300 μg, allows individual dosing.

LIOTHYRONINE. Crystalline T_3 (liothyronine sodium, Cytomel) has a rapid onset and short duration of action. It is the therapy of choice when it is desirable to have rapid onset or cessation of activity, such as in patients with heart disease.

LIOTRIX. A mixture of the sodium salts of T_4 and T_3 in a 4:1 ratio by weight is distributed as liotrix.

DEXTROTHYROXINE. Dextrothyroxine, the synthetic D-(+)-stereoisomer isomer of L-(−)-T_4, was introduced in hypocholesteremic-hypolipidemic therapy with the premise that it would be void of calorigenic effects. The possibility of trace contamination with and metabolic conversion to T_4 and congeners has restricted its use, however, especially in patients with coronary heart disease.

Thyroid Imaging A gents

Radioiodine

All isotopes of iodine are rapidly taken up in thyroid follicles. So far, only the isotopes ^{131}I and ^{125}I have been used consistently. The isotope ^{131}I, which decays to ^{131}Xe mainly with the emission of 0.6 meV β-particle and approximately 0.3 meV γ-rays, has a half-life of 8 days. The isotope ^{125}I, with a half-life of 60 days, decays to ^{125}Te by electron capture. The major component of its decay is a 27 keV x-rays, and the minor component is a 35.5 keV γ-ray.

The γ-radiation emitted by ^{131}I can be detected by a suitably placed scintillation crystal. This is the basis for the diagnostic use of this isotope in iodine uptake and in thyroid-scanning procedures.

The absorption of ^{131}I β-radiation, which leads to the highly localized destruction of the thyroid follicles in which the isotope is taken up, has promoted radioiodine as a therapeutic alternative to surgical removal of the gland. Advantages of radioiodine therapy over surgery include the simplicity of the procedure, its applicability to patients who are poor surgical risks, and the avoidance of surgical complications, such as hypoparathyroidism. The development of late hypothyroidism (63) and the fear of chromosomal damage are arguments against the use of radioiodine in patients under 20 years of age and during pregnancy.

A review of the use of ^{125}I in thyrotoxicosis has indicated that the potential advantages of the ^{125}I isotope, which are based on its lower penetrability and more localized action, have not been realized in practice (64).

Radioiodine whole-body scan and serum thyroglobulin measurement commonly are used as the follow-up testing in patients with thyroid cancer. Both follow-up tests have limitations and are uncomfortable, because they require a hypothyroid state. For thyroid cells to take up the labeled iodine, thyrotropin must be available, and for the pituitary to supply it, the body must be free of T_3 and T_4. This means that patients must completely stop taking medication for several weeks before the scan day. This results in a severe hypothyroidism, and approximately 25% of patients also produce antibodies against thyroglobulin, rendering the immunoassay useless. To make the follow-up tests easier, the U.S. Food and Drug Administration recently approved the use of Thyrogen (thyrotropin alfa for injection), a recombinant human thyrotropin produced in Chinese hamster ovary cells. Thyrogen has been shown to significantly enhance the sensitivity of thyroglobulin testing in patients maintained on thyroid hormone therapy, and it allows patients with thyroid cancer to avoid the debilitating effects of hypothyroidism when undergoing radioiodine imaging scans.

Perchlorate and Pertechnetate

The ability of large anions to be taken up into the thyroid by way of the iodide pump is linearly related to their molar volume (65). The affinity of iodide for the iodide pump was equal to that of thiocyanate but much smaller than that of the larger perchlorate and pertechnetate ions.

In contrast to iodide and SCN^-, TcO_4^- and ClO_4^- do not undergo intrathyroidal metabolism after they are trapped. This property has made TcO_4^- labeled with the short-lived technetium-99m a widely used radioisotope for thyroid trapping and for thyroid imaging.

Perchlorate, which competitively inhibits the uptake of iodide, has been used in both diagnosis and treatment of thyroid disease. In continental Europe, perchlorate has been used for surgical preparation and in the long-term treatment of thyrotoxicosis. In the United States, the use of perchlorate was drastically curtailed after aplastic anemia and severe renal damage were reported following its use.

Diagnostically, perchlorate is used to assess the intrathyroidal organification of iodine. When perchlorate is administered after a dose of radioactive iodine, perchlorate washes out or discharges intrathyroidal inorganic iodide but does not affect covalently bound organic iodide. When organification is inadequate, there is a sharp decrease in intrathyroidal radioactive iodine after perchlorate administration.

Antithyroid Drugs for the Treatment of Hyperthyroidism

Iodide

Inhibition of the release of thyroid hormone by iodide is the basis for its use in hyperthyroidism. Iodide decreases the vascularity of the enlarged thyroid gland and also lowers the elevated BMR. It also has been suggested that excess iodide might change the conformation of thyroglobulin, making the protein less susceptible to thyroidal proteolysis (66).

With the use of antithyroid drugs, the role of iodide in hyperthyroidism has been relegated to that of preparation for thyroid surgery. Iodide, as Lugol's solution

(Strong Iodine Solution USP) or as saturated potassium iodide solution, is administered for approximately 2 weeks to ensure decreased vascularity and firming of the gland. Iodism, a side effect of iodine administration, is apparently an allergic reaction characterized by dermatological and common cold-like symptoms (67).

Methimazole, Propylthiouracil, and Related Compounds

Thionamides are the most important class of antithyroid compounds in clinical practice used in nondestructive therapy of hyperthyroidism. These agents are potent inhibitors of TPO, which is responsible for the iodination of tyrosine residues of thyroglobulin and the coupling of iodotyrosine residues to form iodothyronines. These drugs have no effect on the iodide pump or on thyroid hormone release. The most clinically useful thionamides are thioureylenes, which are five- or six-membered heterocyclic derivatives of thiourea and include the thiouracil 6-n-propyl-2-thiouracil (PTU) and the thioimidazole 1-methyl-2-mercaptoimidazole (methimazole, Tapazole, MMI). The uptake of these drugs into the thyroid gland is stimulated by TSH and inhibited by iodide.

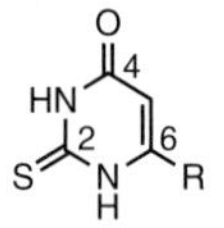

Thiouracil; R = H
Methylthiouracil; R = CH_3
Propylthiouracil (PTU); R = n-C_3H_7

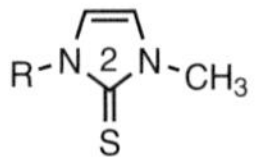

Methimazole(MMI, R = H)
Carbimazole (R = C_2H_5OCO)

Chemically, the grouping R-CS-N- as been referred to as thioamide, thionamide, thiocarbamide, or if R is N, as it is in thiouracil, PTU, and MMI, it is called a thioureylene. This structure may exist in either the thioketo or thioenol tautomeric forms.

Thioamide

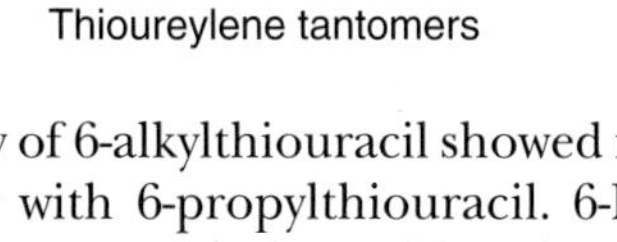

Thioketo Thioenol (SH form)

Thioureylene tantomers

The study of 6-alkylthiouracil showed maximal antithyroid activity with 6-propylthiouracil. 6-Methylthiouracil has less than one-tenth the activity of PTU.

The ability of PTU to inhibit the enzyme 5′-D-I (i.e., the peripheral deiodination of T_4 to T_3, in addition to its intrathyroidal inhibition of thyroid hormone formation) has made PTU the drug of choice in the emergency treatment of thyroid storm (68). Single doses of PTU in excess of 300 mg are capable of almost total blockage of peripheral T_3 production (69).

A number of studies have defined the structure–activity relationships (SARs) of the thiouracils and other related compounds as inhibitors of outer ring deiodinase (70). The C_2 thioketo/thioenol group and an unsubstituted N_1 position are essential for activity. The enolic hydroxyl group at C_4 in PTU and the presence of alkyl group at C_5 and C_6 enhance the inhibitory potency.

Methimazole has more TPO inhibitory activity and is longer-acting than PTU but, in contrast to PTU, is not able to inhibit the peripheral deiodination of T_4, presumably because of the presence of the methyl group at N_1 position. The suggested maintenance dosages listed in USP DI are 50 to 800 mg daily for PTU and 5 to 30 mg daily for MMI.

Efforts to improve the taste and decrease the rate of release of MMI led to the development of 1-carbethoxy-3-methylthioimidazole (carbimazole). Carbimazole, the pro-drug derivative of methimazole, gives rise to methimazole in vivo and is used in the same dosage.

The side effects of thioamides include diarrhea, vomiting, jaundice, skin rashes, and at times, sudden onset of agranulocytosis. There does not appear to be a great difference in toxicity among the compounds currently in use.

Both PTU and MMI are concentrated several-fold by the thyroid gland and inhibit the iodination and coupling reactions of TPO (12). Taurog (71) described the thioureylenes as potent inhibitors of thyroglobulin iodination. He suggested that a thioureylene, such as propylthiouracil (PTU-SH), would irreversibly inhibit TPO-catalyzed iodination of thyroglobulin when the thioureylene-to-iodide ratio was high and reversibly when the PTU-SH-to-iodide ratio was low. In the course of the iodination reaction, the thioureylene PTU-SH would be oxidized (72), possibly to a disulfide dimer, such as PTU-SS-PTU. Drug oxidation is the preferred reaction, and as long as sufficient drug is present, diverting hypoiodate (OI^-) from iodination to drug oxidation. Iodination of tyrosyl residues resumes once oxidation of the drug to disulfide products occurs by either hypoiodate or an enzyme-hypoiodate complex (EOI^-) is complete. Under these conditions, the thioureylenes act as competitive inhibitors by competing with tyrosyls for hypoiodate. Conversely, at high drug concentrations, the thioureylenes are only partially oxidized, and the partially oxidized intermediate can presumably inactivate TPO by covalent binding of an oxidized form of the drug to the prosthetic heme group of TPO to prevent formation of the hydrogen peroxide–TPO complex. As a result, iodination is irreversibly blocked. Data obtained from rats fed an iodide-deficient diet are consistent with this in vitro model in that intrathyroidal metabolism is radiolabeled PTU and MMI is decreased.

Thioureylene drugs also effectively inhibit the coupling of the DIT/MIT residues on thyroglobulin to yield the T_4 and T_3. This effect has been related to an alteration of the conformation of thyroglobulin brought on by the binding of the thioureylene to thyroglobulin (i.e., by the formation of a compound such as TPO-S-S-PTU) (73).

After the observation that PTU inhibited the peripheral deiodination of T_4 (68,74), attempts to relate deiodinase inhibitory activity to structural parameters were undertaken (74). These studies emphasized the need for tautomerization to a thiol form and for the presence of a polar hydrogen on the nitrogen adjacent to the sulfur-bearing carbon. A study of the relation of chemical structure to 5′-D-I inhibitory activity related to similar studies of structural requirements for TPO inhibition could prove fruitful in the design of improved antithyroid drugs.

Thyrotoxicosis

Because symptoms of thyrotoxicosis resemble those of adrenergic overstimulation, attempts to decrease such symptoms by adrenergic blockade have been undertaken. Reserpine and guanethidine, both of which are depletors of catecholamines, and propranolol, a β-blocking agent, have been used effectively to decrease the tachycardia, tremor, and anxiety of thyrotoxicosis. Because of its less serious side effects, propranolol has become the drug of choice in this adjunctive therapy. Reports of decreased T_3 plasma levels during propranolol treatment suggest that blocking of the peripheral deiodination of T_4 may contribute to the beneficial effects of propranolol. The use of propranolol as a preventive drug in acute thyrotoxicosis has been found to be beneficial by some investigators, but not by others.

Goitrogens and Drugs Affecting Thyroid Function

The presence of environmental goitrogens was suggested by the resistance of endemic goiters to iodine prophylaxis and iodide treatment in Italy and Colombia. In the past, endemic outbreaks of hypothyroidism have pointed toward calcium as a source of waterborne goitrogenicity, and it is presently believed that calcium is a weak goitrogen able to cause latent hypothyroidism to come to the surface.

Lithium salts have been used as safe adjuncts in the initial treatment of thyrotoxicosis (75). Lithium is concentrated by the thyroid gland (76), with a thyroid-to-serum ratio of more than 2:1, suggesting active transport. Lithium ion inhibits adenylate cyclase, which forms cAMP. Formed in response to TSH, cAMP is a stimulator of the processes involved in thyroid hormone release from the gland. Inhibition of hormone secretion by lithium has proved to be a useful adjunct in treatment of hyperthyroidism (77).

In view of the role of cysteine residues in the conformation of thyroglobulin, the mode of action of TPO, and the deiodination of T_4, the effect of sulfur-containing compounds on thyroid hormone formation is hardly surprising. Most naturally occurring sulfur compounds are derived from glucosinolates (formerly referred to as thioglucosides) (78), which are present in foods such as cabbage, turnip, mustard seed, salad greens, and radishes (most of these are from the genus *Brassica* or *Cruciferae*) as well as in the milk of cows grazing in areas containing Brassica weeds. Chemically, glucosinolates can give rise to many components, including thiocyanate (CNS^-), isothiocyanate (SCN^-), nitriles (RCN), and thiooxazolidones. Thiocyanate is a large anion that competes with iodide for uptake by the thyroid gland; its goitrogenic effect can be reversed by iodide intake. Goitrin, 5-R-vinyloxazolidine-2-thione, is a potent thyroid peroxidase inhibitor (79) that is claimed to be more effective than PTU in humans (80) and is held to be the cause of a mild goiter endemia in Finland. In rats, goitrin is actively taken up by the thyroid gland and appears to inhibit the coupling of thyroglobulin diiodotyrosyl residues (81). Many workers, however, believe that the goitrogenic effects of *Brassica* result from the additive effects of all goitrogenic components present.

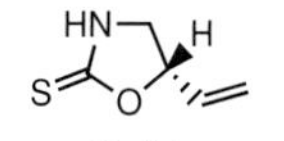

Goitrin

Other compounds affecting thyroid function include sulfonamides, anticoagulants, and oxygenated and iodinated aromatic compounds. The hypoglycemic agent carbutamide and the diuretic Diamox are examples of sulfonamides. Of the anticoagulants, heparin appears to interfere with the binding of T_4 to plasma transport proteins (82), but warfarin (Coumadin) and dicoumarol are competitive inhibitors of the substrate T_4 or rT_3 in the 5′-D reaction, with a dissociation constant (K_i) in the micromolar range (83). Other oxygenated compounds affecting the 5′-D include resorcinol, long known to be a goitrogen, and phloretin, a dihydrochalocone with an IC_{50} of 4 M.

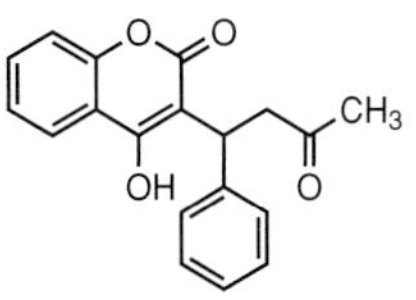

Warfarin

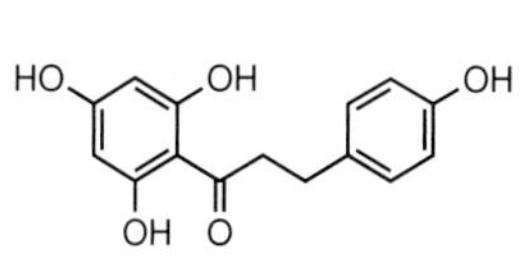

Phloretin

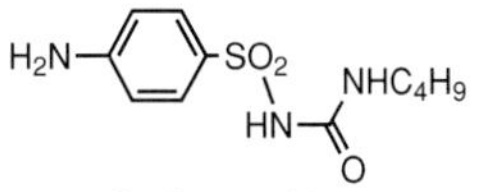

Carbutamide

The ability of oxidation products of 3,4-dihydroxycinnamic acid to prevent the binding of TSH to human thyroid membranes (84) suggests that other oxygenated phenols may interfere with thyroid hormone function in more than one way. Examples of iodinated drugs affecting thyroid function are the antiarrhythmic agent amiodarone and the radiocontrasting agents iopanoic acid and ipodoic acid. All of these compounds interfere with the peripheral deiodination of T_4 and are being tested as adjuncts in the treatment of hyperthyroidism.

The binding of thyroid hormones to plasma carrier proteins is affected by endogenous agents or by drugs that can change the concentration of these proteins or compete with thyroid hormones for binding sites. Examples of the first group are testosterone (and related anabolic agents) that are able to decrease and estrogens (and related contraceptive agents) that are able to increase the concentration of T_4 binding globulin. Salicylates, diphenylhydantoin, and heparin are members of the large group competing with thyroid hormones for binding sites. Alterations in the binding of T_3 and T_4 are of no large physiological consequence, because the steady-state concentrations of free hormone are rapidly restored by homeostatic mechanisms. Knowledge regarding the presence of agents affecting thyroid hormone binding, however, is important for the interpretation of diagnostic tests assessing the presence of free or total hormone in plasma.

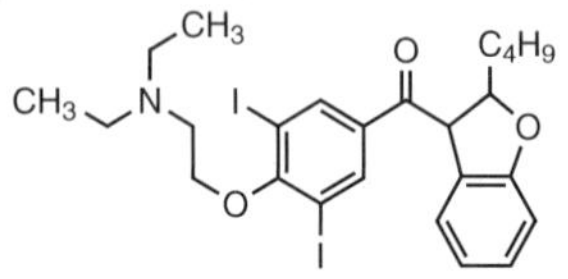

Amiodarone

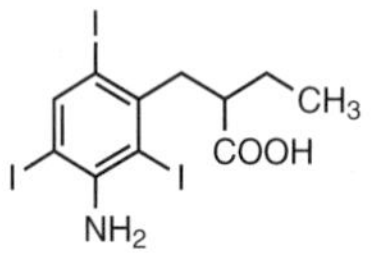

Iopanoic acid

THYROID HORMONE ANALOGUES

The search for thyroid hormone analogues was prompted by the desire to establish SARs for the hormone and by the need for a safe, specific antagonist able to block thyroid action without delay at a peripheral site. The reader will recall that TPO inhibitors, such as PTU, do not affect the extensive amount of hormone stored in thyroidal thyroglobulin.

Some early analogues designed as antagonists were butyl-3,5-diiodo-4-hydroxybenzoate (BHDB), which was designed as a deiodinase inhibitor and is, to a degree, effective as such, and 2′6′-diiodothyronine, which has a small antithyroid effect.

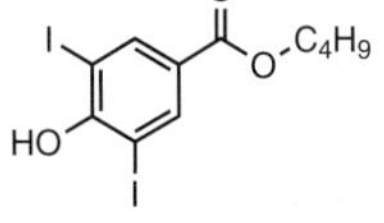

BHDB

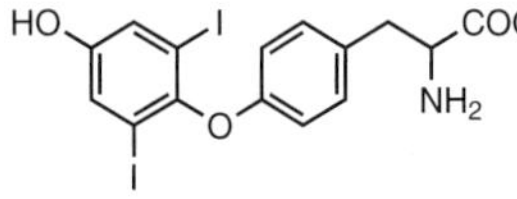

2′,6′-Diiodothyronine

When the activity of T_3 was discovered in 1955, and when none of the many analogues tabulated by Selenkow and Asper (85) demonstrated significant antithyroid activity, efforts were made to redefine the structural requirements for thyroid-like activity to provide a better rationale for the design of a peripheral thyroid antagonist. The biological assay methods used for the newer compounds included measurements of in vivo oxygen uptake, of hepatic lipogenic enzyme activity, of goiter formation, of the rate of amphibian metamorphosis, and more recently, of the binding to nuclear receptors.

The measurement of oxygen uptake provides a direct index of metabolic rate; this measurement can be done simply by placing experimental animals in a calibrated vessel maintained at constant temperature and connected to an oxygen analyzer (86). Repeatedly used as an index of thyromimetic activity have been the in vitro assay of oxygen uptake by suspended mitochondria and the spectrophotometric assays of rat liver mitochondrial α-glycerophosphate dehydrogenase (87) and of cytoplasmic malic enzyme (88).

In the "goiter" or "antigoiter" assay, goiter formation is induced by the administration of a TPO inhibitor, such as thiouracil. The inhibitor is blended with the food or added to the drinking water and given to experimental animals for 10 to 14 days. The increase in gland weight caused by the TPO inhibitor can be reversed by T_4 or by a test compound with thyromimetic activity. The effect of a given dose of thyromimetic agent compared with that of a given dose of T_4 yields the "antigoitrogenic effect" of the compound. Furthermore, when both a test compound and T_4 are given to an animal receiving a TPO inhibitor, the ability of the test compound to antagonize T_4, or the "antithyroid effect" of the test compound, can be assessed.

Discrepancies have been seen between the results obtained with amphibian metamorphosis and those obtained with other assays. These discrepancies have been attributed to the ability of test animals, such as tadpoles, to concentrate test compounds and, especially, lipophilic test compounds from the medium (89). The binding affinity of thyroid analogues to nuclear receptors correlates well with the effectiveness of these analogues in the antigoiter assay, provided that the metabolism of the analogues is taken into consideration (89).

Structure–Activity Relationships of Thyroid Analogues

The synthesis and biological evaluation of a wide variety of T_4 and T_3 analogues allowed a significant correlation of structural features with their relative importance in the production of hormonal responses. The key findings are summarized in Table 34.2. In general, only compounds with the appropriately substituted phenyl-X-phenyl nucleus (as depicted at the top of Table 34.2) have shown significant thyroid hormonal activities. Both single ring compounds such as DIT and a variety of its aliphatic and alicyclic ether derivatives showed no T_4-like activity in the rat antigoiter test (90), the method most often used in determining thyromimetic activity in vivo (91). The SARs

Table 34.2. Some Properties and Pharmacokinetics for Levothyroxine and Liothyronine[a]

Parameters	L-Thyroxine	Liothyronine
Trade name	Synthroid, Levothroid, Levoxyl	Cytomel
pK_a (phenolic)	6.7	8.4
Oral bioavailability (%)	50–80[b]	95
Peak response	Several weeks (hypothyroid)	2–3 days (hypothyroid)
Duration of action	Several weeks (hypothyroid)	Several days (hypothyroid)
Protein binding (%)	99% (weakly)	Weakly bound
Time to peak concentration (hours)	2–4	1–2
Volume of distribution (L/kg)	8.7–9.7	41–45
Elimination half-life (days)	6–7 euthyroid 9–10 hypothyroid 3–4 hyperthyroid	1 euthyroid 1–2 hypothyroid 1 hyperthyroid
Excretion (%)	50 urine 50 feces	urine

[a]Micromedex® Healthcare Series, Thompson Healthcare, Inc. Available at: http://www.thompsonhc.com. Accessed June 14, 2006.
[b]Food decreases bioavailability.

are discussed in terms of single structural variations of T_4 in the 1) alanine side chain, 2) 3- and 5-positions of the inner ring, 3) the bridging atom, 4) 3′- and 5′-positions of the outer ring, and 5) the 4′-phenolic hydroxyl group.

Aliphatic Side Chain

The naturally occurring hormones are biosynthesized from L-tyrosine and possess the L-alanine side chain. The L-isomers of T_4 and T_3 (compounds 1 and 3 in Table 34.2) are more active than the D-isomers (compounds 2 and 4) (Table 34.2). The carboxylate ion and the number of atoms connecting it to the ring are more important for activity than is the intact zwitterionic alanine side chain. In the carboxylate series, the activity is maximum with the two-carbon acetic acid side chain (compounds 7 and 8) but decreases with either the shorter formic acid (compounds 5 and 6) or the longer propionic and butyric acid analogues (compounds 9-12). The ethylamine side chain analogues of T_4 and T_3 (compounds 13 and 14) are less active than the corresponding carboxylic acid analogues. In addition, isomers of T_3 in which the alanine side chain is transposed with the 3-iodine or occupies the 2-position were inactive in the rat antigoiter test (92), indicating a critical location for the side chain in the 1-position of the inner ring.

Alanine-Bearing Ring

The phenyl ring bearing the alanine side chain, called the inner ring or α-ring, is substituted with iodine in the 3- and 5-positions in T_4 and T_3. As shown in Table 34.2, removal of both iodine atoms from the inner ring to form 3′,5′-T_2 (compound 15) or 3′-T_1 (compound 16) produces analogues devoid of T_4-like activity, primarily because of the loss of the perpendicular orientation of diphenyl ether conformation. Retention of activity observed on replacement of the 3- and 5-iodine atoms with bromine (compounds 17 and 18) implies that iodine does not play a unique role in thyroid hormone activity. Moreover, a broad range of hormone activity found with halogen free analogues (compounds 19 and 20) indicates that a halogen atom is not essential for activity. In contrast to T_3, 3′-isopropyl-3,6-dimethyl-L-thyronine (compound 20) has the capacity to cross the placental membrane and exerts thyromimetic effects in the fetus after administration to the mother. This could prove to be useful in treating fetal thyroid hormone deficiencies or in stimulating lung development (by stimulating lung to synthesize special phospholipids [surfactant], which ensure sufficient functioning of the infant's lungs at birth) immediately before premature birth (93). Substitution in the 3- and 5-positions by alkyl groups significantly larger and less symmetric than methyl groups, such as isopropyl and secondary butyl moieties, produces inactive analogues (compounds 21 and 22). These results show that 3,5-disubstitution by symmetric, lipophilic groups not exceeding the size of iodine is required for activity.

Bridging Atom

Several analogues have been synthesized in which the ether oxygen bridge has been removed or replaced by other atoms. The biphenyl analogue of T_4 (compound 23 in Table 34.2), formed by removal of the oxygen bridge, is inactive in the rat antigoiter test. The linear biphenyl structure is a drastic change from the normal diphenyl ether conformation found in the naturally occurring hormones. Replacement of the bridging oxygen atom by sulfur (compound 24) or by a methylene group (compound 25) produces highly active analogues. This provides evidence against the Niemann quinoid theory, which postulates that the ability of a compound to form a quinoid structure in the phenolic ring is essential for thyromimetic activity, and emphasizes the importance of the three-dimensional structure and receptor fit of the hormones. Attempts to prepare amino- and carbonyl-bridged analogues of T_3 and T_4 have been unsuccessful (94,95).

Phenolic Ring

The phenolic ring, also called the outer or β-ring, of the thyronine nucleus is required for hormonal activity. Variations in 3′- or 3′,5′-substituents on the phenolic ring have dramatic effects on biological activity and affinity for the nuclear receptor. The unsubstituted parent structure of this series L-T_2 (compound 26 in Table 34.2) possesses low activity. Substitution at the 3′-position by polar hydroxyl or nitro groups (compounds 27 and 28) causes a decrease in activity as a consequence of both lowered lipophilicity and intramolecular hydrogen bonding with the 4′-hydroxyl (96). Conversely, substitution by nonpolar halogen or alkyl groups results in an increase in activity in direct relation to the bulk and lipophilicity of the substituent—for example, F < Cl < Br < I (compounds 29-31) and CH_3 < CH_2CH_3 < $CH(CH_3)_2$ (compounds 32–34). Although 3′-isopropylthyronine (compound 34) is the most potent analogue

Table 34.3. Relative Rat Antigoiter Activity of Thyroxine Derivatives

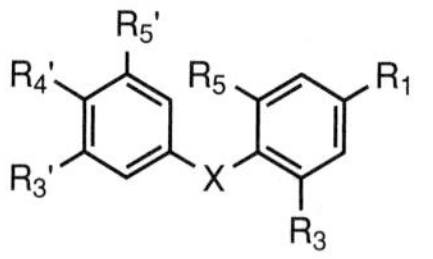

Compound	R_1	R_3	R_5	X	$R_{3'}$	$R_{5'}$	$R_{4'}$	Antigoiter Activity[a]
1. L-T_4	L-Ala	I	I	O	I	I	OH	100
2. D-T_4	D-Ala	I	I	O	I	I	OH	17
3. L-T_3	L-Ala	I	I	O	I	H	OH	550
4. D-T_3	D-Ala	I	I	O	I	H	OH	41
5.	COOH	I	I	O	I	I	OH	0.1
6.	COOH	I	I	O	I	H	OH	0.4
7.	CH_2COOH	I	I	O	I	I	OH	50
8.	CH_2COOH	I	I	O	I	H	OH	36
9.	$(CH_2)_2COOH$	I	I	O	I	I	OH	15
10.	$(CH_2)_2COOH$	I	I	O	I	H	OH	20
11.	$(CH_2)_3COOH$	I	I	O	I	I	OH	4
12.	$(CH_2)_3COOH$	I	I	O	I	H	OH	5
13.	$(CH_2)_2NH_2$	I	I	O	I	I	OH	0.6
14.	$(CH_2)_2NH_2$	I	I	O	I	H	OH	6
15.	L-Ala	H	H	O	I	I	OH	<0.01
16.	L-Ala	H	H	O	I	H	OH	<0.01
17.	DL-Ala	Br	Br	O	I	H	OH	93
18.	L-Ala	Br	Br	O	iPr	H	OH	166
19.	L-Ala	Me	Me	O	Me	H	OH	3
20.	L-Ala	Me	Me	O	iPr	H	OH	20
21.	DL-Ala	iPr	iPr	O	I	H	OH	0
22.	DL-Ala	sBu	sBU	O	I	H	OH	0
23.	DL-Ala	I	I	—	I	I	OH	0
24.	DL-Ala	I	I	S	I	H	OH	132
25.	DL-Ala	I	I	CH_2	I	H	OH	300
26.	L-Ala	I	I	O	H	H	OH	5
27.	L-Ala	I	I	O	OH	H	OH	1.5
28.	L-Ala	I	I	O	NO_2	H	OH	<1
29.	DL-Ala	I	I	O	F	H	OH	6
30.	L-Ala	I	I	O	Cl	H	OH	27
31.	DL-Ala	I	I	O	Br	H	OH	132
32.	L-Ala	I	I	O	Me	H	Oh	80
33.	L-Ala	I	I	O	Et	H	OH	517
34.	L-Ala	I	I	O	iPr	H	OH	786
35.	L-Ala	I	I	O	nPr	H	OH	200
36.	DL-Ala	I	I	O	Phe	H	OH	11
37.	DL-Ala	I	I	O	F	F	OH	2.3
38.	L-Ala	I	I	O	Cl	Cl	OH	21
39.	L-Ala	I	I	O	I	H	NH_2	<1.5
40.	DL-Ala	I	I	O	I	H	H	>150
41.	DL-Ala	I	I	O	CH_3	H	CH_3	0
42.	L-Ala	I	I	O	I	H	CH_3O	225

[a]See Ekins et al. (107) and Ahmad et al. (108). In vivo activity in rats relative to L-T_4 = 100% or DL-T_4 = 100% for goiter prevention.

known, being approximately 1.4 times as active as L-T_3, n-propylthyronine (compound 35) is only about one-fourth as active as isopropyl, apparently because of its less compact structure. As the series is further ascended, activity decreases with a further reduction for the more bulky 3′-phenyl substituent (compound 36). Substitution in both 3′- and 5′-positions by the same halogen produces less active hormones (compounds 37 and 38) than the corresponding 3′-monosubstituted analogues (compounds 29 and 30). The decrease in activity has been explained as resulting from the increase in phenolic hydroxyl ionization and the resulting increase in binding to TBG (the primary carrier of thyroid hormones in human plasma) (97). In general, a second substituent adjacent to the phenolic hydroxyl (5′-position) reduces activity in direct proportion to its size.

Phenolic Hydroxyl Group

A weakly ionized phenolic hydroxyl group at the 4′-position is essential for optimum hormonal activity. Replacement of the 4′-hydroxyl with an amino group (compound 39 in

Table 34.2) results in a substantial decrease in activity, presumably as a result of the weak hydrogen bonding ability of the latter group. The retention of activity observed with the 4′-unsubstituted compound (compound 40) provides direct evidence for metabolic 4′-hydroxylation as an activating step. Introduction of a 4′-substituent that cannot mimic the functional role of a phenolic group, such as a methyl group (compound 41), and that is not metabolically converted into a functional residue results in complete loss of hormonal activity. The thyromimetic activity of the 4′-methyl ether (compound 42) was ascribed to the ready metabolic cleavage to form an active 4′-hydroxyl analogue. The pK_a of 4′-phenolic hydroxyl group is 6.7 for T_4 (90% ionized at pH 7.4) and 8.5 for T_3 (~approximately 10% ionized). The greater acidity for T_4 is reflective of its stronger affinity for plasma proteins and, consequently, of its longer plasma half-life.

Conformational Properties of Thyroid Hormones and Analogues

The importance of the diphenyl ether conformation for biological activity was first proposed by Zenker and Jorgensen (98,99). Through molecular models, they showed that a perpendicular orientation of the planes of the aromatic rings of 3,5-diiodothyronines would be favored to minimize interactions between the bulky 3,5-iodines and the 2′,6′-hydrogens. In this orientation, the 3′- and 5′-positions of the ring are not conformationally equivalent, and the 3′-iodine of T_3 could be oriented either distal (away from) or 5′ proximal (closer) to the side chain–bearing ring (Fig. 34.6). Because the activity of compounds such as 3′,5′-dimethyl-3,5-diiodothyronine had demonstrated that alkyl groups could replace the 3′- and 5′-iodine substituents, model compounds bearing alkyl groups in the 3′-position and alkyl or iodine substituents in the 5′-position (in addition to the blocking 2′-methyl group) were synthesized for biological evaluation (99).

Biological evaluation of 2′,3′- and 2′,5′-substituted diiodothyronines (100) revealed that 3′-substitution was favorable for thyromimetic activity but that 5′-substitution was not. The structures of representative distal analogues, 2′,3′-dimethyl-3,5-DL-diiodothyronine (compound I) and O-(4′-hydroxy-1′-naphthyl)-3,5-DL-diiodotyrosine (compound II), and of the proximal analogues, 2′,5′-dimethyl-3,5-DL-diiodothyronine (compound III) and 2′-methyl-3,5,5′-DL-triiodothyronine (compound IV), are given in Figure 34.6. The effectiveness of these compounds in rat antigoiter assay (101) is presented in Table 34.4. These

Table 34.4. Effectiveness of Distal and Proximal Compounds Antigoiter Assay

Compound[a]	Dose (mg/kg/day)	% T_4 activity
I	0.025	50
II	0.013	>100
III	2.3	<1
IV	0.5	2

[a]See text for specific descriptions of compounds I–IV.

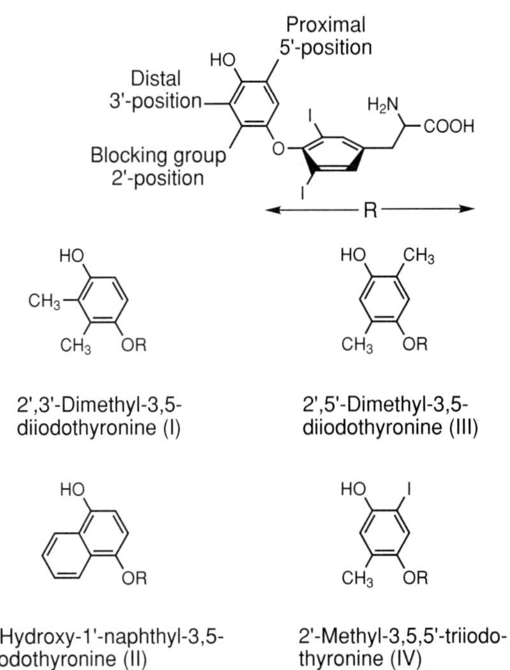

Fig. 34.6. Structures of representative distal and proximal compounds.

results clearly indicate that in 2′-blocked analogues, a distal 3′-substitution is favorable for thyromimetic activity, but a proximal 5′-substitution is not.

The perpendicular orientation of the rings of 3,5-diiodothyronines, which was postulated from molecular models, has been confirmed by x-ray crystallographic studies (102), molecular orbital calculations (103), and nuclear magnetic resonance studies (104,105).

In addition to being perpendicular to the inner ring, the outer phenolic ring can adopt conformations relative to the alanine side chain, which would be *cis* or *trans*. In other words, the cisoid and transoid conformations result from the methine group in the alanine side chain being either *cis* or *trans* to the phenolic ring (Fig. 34.7). Although the bioactive conformation of the alanine side chain in thyroid hormone analogues has not yet been defined, these conformations appear to be similar in energy, because both are found in thyroactive structures as determined by x-ray crystallography (106). The synthesis of conformationally fixed cyclic or unsaturated analogues may allow evaluation of the bioactivity of the two conformers.

Transthyretin Receptor Model

An additional tool in structural analysis and analogue design has been TTR (formerly called T_4 binding prealbumin), a plasma protein that binds as much as 27% of plasma T_3 (107). The amino acid sequence of the TTR T_3 binding site is known, and the protein has therefore served as a model, although admittedly an approximate model, for the T_3 receptor. The TTR model portrays the T_3 molecule as placed in an envelope near the axis of symmetry of the TTR dimer. In this envelope, hydrophobic

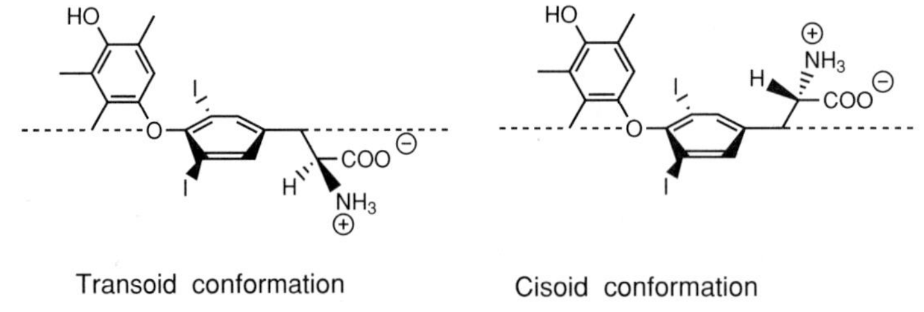

Transoid conformation Cisoid conformation

Fig. 34.7. Side-chain conformations of thyroid hormones: transoid (left), and cisoid (right).

residues, such as those of leucine, lysine, and alanine, are near pockets accommodating the 3,5,3′- and 5′-positions of T_3, whereas the hydrophilic groups of serine and threonine (hydrogen bonded to water), are between the 3′-substituent and the 4′-phenolic group. Taking this model into account, Ahmad et al. (108) suggested that 3′-acetyl-3,5-diiodothyronine might be a good analogue or a good inhibitor of T_3, because the carbonyl group of the 3′ acetyl substituent would form a strong hydrogen bond with the 4′ phenolic hydrogen, preventing thereby its bonding with the hydrated residue of the putative receptor.

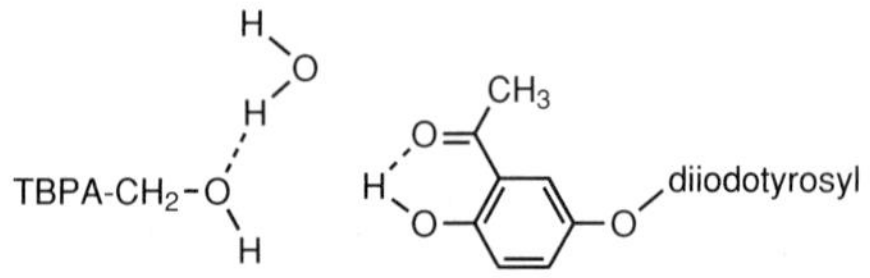

This compound, prepared by Benson et al. (109), was found to be indistinguishable from T_3 in oxygen uptake and glycerophosphate activity tests and to be half as active as T_3 in displacing labeled T_3 from rat liver nuclei in specific in vivo conditions.

Problems

What organs and functions of the body are regulated by thyroid hormones?

Thyroid hormones regulate the body's metabolism and organ function, affecting heart rate, cholesterol level, body weight, energy level, muscle strength, skin condition, menstrual regularity, memory and many other conditions.

List classes of drugs that interact (interfere) with thyroid hormones therapy.

- *Oral anticoagulants*—Thyroid hormones increase catabolism of vitamin K-dependent clotting factors.
- *Insulin or oral hypoglycemics*—Initiating thyroid replacement therapy causes increases in insulin or oral hypoglycemic requirements. The effects seen are poorly understood and depend on a variety of factors, such as endocrine status of the patient and type of thyroid preparations.
- *Cholestyramine*—Cholestyramine binds both T_4 and T_3 in the intestine, thus impairing absorption of these thyroid hormones.
- *Estrogen, oral contraceptives*—Estrogens tend to increase serum thyroxine-binding globulin (TBG), thus increasing thyroid requirements.
- Antidepressant drugs

Why is the use of thyroid hormones in therapy for obesity unjustified?

Drugs with thyroid hormone activity, either alone or together with other therapeutic agents, have been used for treatment of obesity. In euthyroid patients, doses within the range of daily hormonal requirements are ineffective for weight reduction. Larger doses may produce serious or even life-threatening manifestation of toxicity, particularly when given in association with sympathomimetic amines, such as those used for their anorectic effects.

What is the purpose of prescribing β-blockers along with thyroid drugs in treatment of hyperthyroidism?

β-Adrenergic blocking agents, such as atenolol, nadolol, metoprolol, or propranolol, block the action of circulating thyroid hormone on the body tissues, slowing heart rate and lessening nervousness. These drugs may be extremely helpful in reducing symptoms until one of the other forms of treatment have a chance to take effect. They are not used, however, in patients who have asthma or heart failure, which may be worsened with these drugs.

Patients with hypothyroidism and organic depression may need both levothyroxine and antidepressant drug therapy. In levothyroxine-treated patients with hypothyroidism who were treated with sertraline, there was an elevated serum thyrotropin concentration, indicative of a decrease in the efficacy of levothyroxine. What is the possible mechanism of interaction between the two drugs?

Sertraline may interfere by increasing the clearance of thyroxine.

REFERENCES

Harel Z, Biro FM, Tedford WL. Effect of long term treatment with sertraline (Zoloft) simulating hypothyroidism in an adolescent. J Adolesc Health 1995;16:232–234.

(*Continued*)

Problems (*Continued*)

McCowen K, Garber J, Spark R. Elevated serum thyrotropin in thyroxine-treated patients with hypothyroidism given sertraline. N Engl J Med 1997;337:1010–1011.

Shelton RC, Winn S, Ekhatore N, et al. The effects of antidepressants on the thyroid axis in depression. Biol Psychiatry 1993;33:120–126.

What are the tests for checking the thyroid function?

1. *Total serum T_4.* This includes both bound and free T_4 concentration.
2. *T_3 resin uptake (T_3RU).* The T_3 resin uptake test measures the amount of unsaturated binding sites on the thyroid hormone transport proteins. A proportion of the labeled T_3 will bind to available sites on the serum TBG; any excess will bind to the resin. Resin uptake is inversely proportional to the number of vacant binding sites and, therefore, inversely proportional to the total TBG.

   In thyrotoxicosis, fewer vacant binding sites are available on thyroxine binding globulin because of the high circulating levels of thyroid hormone. This means less radioactive T_3 will be able to bind to TBG and more will bind to the resin. Hence, resin uptake is higher in hyperthyroid patients than in normal patients. The converse is true in hypothyroid states. In high TBG states, such as pregnancy or estrogen therapy, the T_3RU will be low; however, the physiologically active free T_4 level will still be normal.
3. *Free thyroxine Index (FT_4I).* The FT_4I is a reflection of the amount of free T_4 in most situations. It is a calculated value and corrects for changes in TBG concentrations by using the following formula:

   $$FTI = (\text{total } T_4) \times (T_3 \text{ resin uptake}/T_3RU \text{ control})$$

   Mean normal T_3RU for the particular assay (normal range, 25–35%; mean normal, 30%). With extreme changes in TBG concentrations, acute medical illness, heparin therapy, or low protein states secondary to nephrotic syndrome, the FT_4I may not accurately reflect the amount of free T_4 concentrations.
4. *TSH test.* Measuring the serum TSH has become the screen test of choice for thyroid disease. Primary hypothyroidism produces elevated TSH levels, whereas patients with primary hyperthyroidism (i.e., Graves' disease) should have undetectable TSH values. This relationship is true only in individuals with an intact hypothalamic-pituitary-thyroid axis. Patients who present with a normal or detectable TSH level and elevated thyroid hormone concentrations require further evaluation to exclude central causes of hyperthyroidism.
5. *TRH test.* The administration of TRH causes a rise in TSH concentration in normal subjects (TSH, 2-30 mU/L). An exaggerated response occurs in primary hypothyroid subjects (TSH often is >30 mU/L, depending on the baseline TSH elevation.) Hyperthyroid patients have a mild or absent TSH response (TSH, <2 mU/L), because the suppressed TSH cannot be stimulated by exogenous TRH. The introduction of sensitive TSH assays that can detect low suppressed TSH levels, identifying patients with primary hyperthyroidism, has made the TRH stimulation test virtually obsolete.
6. *Iodine test.* Plasma iodine in the form of iodide is concentrated (trapped) in the thyroid cells by an energy-requiring active transport mechanism, where it is incorporated into T_3 and T_4 via organification. Therefore, iodine measures both trapping and organification by the thyroid gland.

What conditions are associated with decreased and increased levels of TBG?

TBG is synthesized by the liver under the influence of estrogen. An increase in TBG concentration in response to higher estrogen levels may result in higher measured total T_4 concentration. The amount of free T_4 concentration remains constant, however, and the patient remains clinically euthyroid.

Conditions associated with increased levels of TBG:

- *Estrogen effects*—pregnancy, oral contraceptives
- *Infectious hepatitis*
- *Biliary cirrhosis*
- *Genetic determination*

In contrast, factors that cause a decrease in TBG concentration or a lower affinity for T_4 binding to TBG may result in low measured total T_4 concentration without affecting free T_4 levels.

Conditions associated with decreased binding of T_4 by TBG:

- *Androgens and anabolic steroids*
- *Large doses of glucocorticoids*
- *Nephrotic syndrome*
- *Major systemic nonthyroidal illness*
- *Active acromegaly*
- *Chronic liver disease*
- *Drugs*—dilantin, tegretol
- *Genetic determination*

Considering that T_3 does not cross the placental membrane and, therefore, cannot be useful in treating fetal thyroid hormone deficiencies or in stimulating lung development immediately before premature birth, what would be your solution to overcome this problem?

(Refer to the *Structure-Activity Relationship of Thyroid Analogues* section)

3′-Isopropyl-3,6-dimethyl-L-thyronine has the capacity to cross the placental membrane and exerts thyromimetic effects in the fetus after administration to the mother.

List the major pathways for the metabolism of T_4.

1. Outer ring deiodination by the enzyme 5′-D, which yields T_3.
2. Inner ring deiodination by the enzyme 5-D, which yields rT_3.
3. Glucuronide conjugation through the phenolic hydroxy group, which yields T_4-4′-O-glucuronide.
4. Sulfate conjugation through the phenolic hydroxy group, which yields T_4-4′-O-sulfate.
5. Side-chain oxidative deamination and decarboxylation, which yields thyroacetic acid and thyroethanediol.

CASE STUDY

Victoria F. Roche and S. William Zito

GS is a 56-year-old women who, on her most recent visit to her physician, complains of always feeling cold. She says it is causing strife at home, because she always wants to turn up the thermostat and her husband wants to turn it down. In addition, she has been feeling tired for the last 6 months, and her skin has been dry and itchy. On further questioning, she reveals that she has been "grouchy" at work and finds it difficult to cope with the ordinary stresses of her job. Laboratory tests indicate elevated TSH (11 mIU/ml) and low levels of free T_4 (0.6 ng/dL). The physical and laboratory findings are consistent with a diagnosis of hypothyroidism. Her physician wants to treat the hypothyroidism with hormone replacement therapy. Evaluate the given structures for use in this case.

1. Identify the therapeutic problem(s) in which the pharmacist's intervention may benefit the patient.
2. Identify and prioritize the patient-specific factors that must be considered to achieve the desired therapeutic outcomes.
3. Conduct a thorough and mechanistically oriented SAR analysis of all therapeutic alternatives provided in the case.
4. Evaluate the SAR findings against the patient-specific factors and desired therapeutic outcomes, and make a therapeutic decision.
5. Counsel your patient.

1

2

3

References

1. Harington CR. Biochemical basis of thyroid function. Lancet 1935;I: 1199–1204,1261–1266.
2. Baumann E. Uber das normale Vorkommen von Jod in Tierkorper. Zeitschr f physiol Chem. 1896;21:319.
3. Magnus-Levy A. Uber den respiratorischen Gewechsel unter dem Einfluss der Thyroidea sowie unter verschiedenen pathologischen Zustanden. Berl Klin Wchnschr 1895;32:650.
4. Gudernatsch JF. Feeding experiments on tadpoles. Arch f Entwicklungs-mechanik der Organismen 1912;35:457.
5. Nadler NJ. Thyroid anatomical features. In: Greer MA, Solomon DH, eds. Handbook of Physiology, Sec 7, vol III. Washington, DC: American Physiological Society, 1974.
6. Ekholm R, Bjorkman U. Biochemistry of thyroid hormones. In: Martini L, ed. The Thyroid Gland. New York: Raven Press, 1990;83–125.
7. Kendall EC. JAMA 1915;64:2042.
8. Harington CR. Chemistry of thyroxine. II Constitution and synthesis of desiodothyroxine. Biochem J 1926;20:300–313.
9. Harington CR, Barger C. Chemistry of thyroxine. III. Constitution and synthesis of thyroxine. Biochem J 1927;21:169–183.
10. Sawin CT. The Hormones. Boston: Little, Brown, 1969:98.
11. de Groot LJ, Larsen PR, Retetoffs, et al. The Thyroid and Its Diseases. 5th Ed. New York: Wiley, 1984.
12. Taurog A. Hormone synthesis: thyroid iodine metabolism. In: Braverman L, Utiger R, eds. Werner and Ingbar's The Thyroid: A Fundamental and Clinical Text. 8th Ed. Philadelphia: Lippincott Williams & Wilkins, 2000:61–85.
13. Chopra IJ, Solomon DH, Chopra U, et al. Pathways of metabolism of thyroid hormones. Recent Prog Horm Res 1978;34:521—567.
14. Visser TJ, Docter R, Krenning EP, et al. Regulation of thyroid hormone bioactivity. Endocrinol Invest 1986;9(Suppl 4):17–26.
15. Visser TJ, Mol JA, Otten MH. Rapid deiodination of triiodothyronine sulfate by rat liver microsomal fraction. Endocrinology 1983;122:1547–1549.
16. Muller MJ, Seitz HJ. Pleiotypic action of thyroid hormones at the target cell level. Biochem Pharmacol 1984;33:1579–1584.
17. Himms-Hagen J. Cellular thermogenesis. Annu Rev Physiol 1976;38:315–351.
18. Muller MJ, Seitz HJ. Thyroid hormone action on intermediary metabolism. Part I: respiration, thermogenesis, and carbohydrate metabolism. Klin Wochenschr 1984;62:11–18.
19. Muller MJ, Seitz HJ. Thyroid hormone action on intermediary metabolism. Part II: lipid metabolism in hypo- and hyperthyroidism. Klin Wochenschr 1984;62:49–55.
20. Muller MJ, Seitz HJ. Thyroid hormone action on intermediary metabolism. Part III. Protein metabolism in hyper- and hypothyroidism. Klin Wochenschr 1984;62:97–102.
21. Sterling K. The mitochondrial route of thyroid hormone action. Bull N Y Acad Med 1977;53:260–266.
22. Ismail-Beigi F, Edelman IS. Mechanism of thyroid calorigenesis: role of active sodium transport. Proc Natl Acad Sci U S A 1970;67:1071–1078.
23. Sutherland EW, Robinson GA. The role of cyclic-3′,5′-AMP in responses to catecholamines and other hormones. Pharmacol Rev 1966;18:145–161.
24. Williams LT, Lefkowitz RJ, Watanabe AM, et al. Thyroid hormone regulation of β-adrenergic receptor number. J Biol Chem 1977;252:2787–2789.
25. Levey GS, Epstein SE. Myocardial adenyl cyclase: activation by thyroid hormones and evidence for two adenyl cyclase systems. J Clin Invest 1969;48: 1663–1669.
26. Stryer L. Biochemistry. 2nd Ed. San Francisco: Freeman, 1981:843.
27. Eayrs JT, Lishman WA. The mutation of behavior in hypothyroidism and salvation. Br J Anim Behav 1955;3:17–32.
28. Tata JR. Inhibition of the biological action of thyroid hormones by actinomycin D and puromycin. Nature 1963;197:1167–1168.
29. Tata JR, Widnell CC. Ribonucleic acid synthesis during the early action of thyroid hormones. Biochem J 1966;98:604–620.
30. Dillmann WH, Schwartz HL, Silva E, et al. α-Amanitin administration results in a temporary inhibition of hepatic enzyme induction by triiodothyronine: further evidence favoring a long-lived mediator of thyroid hormone action. Endocrinology 1977;100:1621–1627.
31. Schadlow AR, Surks MI, Schwartz HL, et al. Specific triiodothyronine binding sites in the anterior pituitary of the rat. Science 1972;176:1252–1254.
32. Oppenheimer JH, Koerner D, Schwartz HL, et al. Specific nuclear triiodothyronine binding sites in rat liver and kidney. J Clin Endocrinol Metab 1972;35:330–333.

33. Galton VA. Putative nuclear triiodothyronine receptors in tadpole erythrocytes: regulation of receptor number by thyroid hormone. Endocrinology 1984;114:735–742.
34. Samuels HH. Identification and characterization of thyroid hormone receptors using cell culture techniques. In: Oppenheimer JA, Samuels HH, eds. Molecular Basis of Thyroid Hormone Action. New York: Academic Press, 1983, pp. 35–65.
35. Oppenheimer JH, Samuels HH. The nuclear receptor-triiodothyronine complex: relationship to thyroid hormone distribution, metabolism and biological action. In: Oppenheimer JA, Samuels HH, eds. Molecular Basis of Thyroid Hormone Action. New York: Academic Press, 1983, pp. 1–34.
36. Barsano CP, DeGroot LJ. In: Oppenheimer JH, Samuels HH, eds. Molecular Basis of Thyroid Hormone Action. New York: Academic Press, 1983;139–177.
37. Robbins J, Rall JE. Proteins associated with the thyroid hormones. Physiol Rev 1960;40:415.
38. Sterling K, Milch PO, Brenner MA, et al. Thyroid hormone action: the mitochondrial pathway. Science 1977;197:996–999.
39. Schwartz HL, Oppenheimer JH. Physiologic and biochemical actions of thyroid hormone. Pharmacol Ther 1978;B3:349–376.
40. Barden N, Labrie F. J Receptor for thyrotropin-releasing hormone in plasma membranes of bovine anterior pituitary gland. Role of lipids. Biol Chem 1973;248:7601–7606.
41. Sterling K, Lazarus JH. The thyroid and its control. Annu Rev Physiol 1977;39:349–371.
42. Carr FE, Ridgeway EC, Chin WW. Regulation of the α and thyrotropin β-subunit messenger ribonucleic acids by thyroid hormones. Endocrinology 1985;116:873–878.
43. Greenspan FS, Forsham PH. Basic and Clinical Endocrinology. Los Altos: Lange Medical, 1983:141.
44. Wolff J, Chaikoff IL. Plasma inorganic iodide as homeostatic regulator of thyroid function. J Biol Chem 1948;174:555–564.
45. Virion A, Michot JL, Deme D, et al. NADPH oxidation catalyzed by the peroxidase/H_2O_2 system. Iodide-mediated oxidation of NADPH to iodinated NADP. Eur J Biochem 1985;148:239–248.
46. Leonard JL, Kaplan MM, Visser TJ, et al. Cerebral cortex responds rapidly to thyroid hormones. Science 1981;214:571–573.
47. McConnon J, Row VV, Volpe R. The influence of liver damage in man on the distribution and disposal rates of thyroxine and triiodothyronine. J Clin Endocrinol Metab 1972;34:144–153.
48. Lim VS, Fang VS, Katz AI, et al. Thyroid dysfunction in chronic renal failure. A study of the pituitary-thyroid axis and peripheral turnover kinetics of thyroxine and triiodothyronine. J Clin Invest 1977;60:522–534.
49. Carter JN, Eastmen CJ, Corcoran JM, et al. Inhibition of conversion of thyroxine to triiodothyronine in patients with severe chronic illness. Clin Endocrinol 1976;5:587–594.
50. Spaulding SW, Chopra IJ, Sherwin RS, et al. Effect of caloric restriction and dietary composition of serum T_3 and reverse T_3 in man. J Clin Endocrinol Metab 1976;42:197–200.
51. Chacon MA, Tildon JT. Mode of death and post-mortem time effects on 3,3′,5-triiodothyronine levels—relevance to elevated post-mortem T_3 levels in SIDS. Fed Proc 1984;43:866–868.
52. Heyma P, Larkins RG, Campbell DG. Inhibition by propranolol of 3,5,3′-triiodothyronine formation from thyroxine in isolated rat renal tubules: an effect independent of β-adrenergic blockade. Endocrinology 1980;106: 1437–1441.
53. Silva JE, Larsen PR. Adrenergic activation of triiodothyronime production in brown adipose tissue. Nuture 1983;305:712–713.
54. Zenker N, Chacon MA, Tildon JT. Mode of death effect on rat liver iodothyronine 5′-deiodinase activity: role of adenosine 3′,5′-monophosphate. Life Sci 1984;35:2213–2217.
55. Rosenberg IN. Thyroid storm. N Engl J Med 1970;283:1052–1053.
56. Mahaux JE, Chamla-Soumenkoff J, Delcourt R, et al. The effect of triiodothyronine on cervical lymphoid structures, thyroid activity, IgG and IgM immunoglobulin level, and exophthalmos in Graves' disease. Acta Endocrinol 1969;61:400–406.
57. Pitt-Rivers R, Tata JR, eds. The Chemistry of Thyroid Disease, Springfield, IL: Charles Thomas, 1960, p. 38.
58. Groenhout EG, Dorin RI. Generalized thyroid hormone resistance due to a deletion of the carboxy terminus of the C-erbAB receptor. Mol Cell Endocrinol 1994;99:81–88.
59. Weiss B, Landrian PJ. The developing brain and the environment: an introduction. Environ Health Prospect 2000;108(Suppl 3):373–374.
60. Hauser P, Zametkin AJ, Martinez P, et al. Attention-deficit hyperactivity disorder in people with generalized resistance to thyroid hormone. N Engl J Med 1993;328:997–1001.
61. Cardis E, Kesminiene A, Ivanov V, et al. Risk of thyroid cancer after exposure to ^{131}I in childhood. J Natl Cancer Inst 2005;97:724–732.
62. Jackson IM, Cobb WE. Why does anyone still use desiccated thyroid USP? Am J Med 1978;64:284–288.
63. Pittman JA Jr. In: Selenkow HA, Hoffman F, eds. Diagnosis and Treatment of Common Thyroid Disease. Amsterdam: Excerpta Medica, 1971:72–73.
64. Bremner WF, Spencer CA, Ratcliffe WA, et al. The assessment of ^{125}I treatment of thyrotoxicosis. Clin Endocrinol 1976;5:225–234.
65. Wolff J, Maurey JR. Thyroidal iodide transport. IV. The role of ion size. Biochem Biophys Acta 1963;69:58.
66. Lamas L, Ingbar SH. In: Robbins J, Braverman LE, eds. Thyroid Research. Amsterdam: Excerpta Medica, 1976:213.
67. Pittman JA Jr. Diagnosis and Treatment of Thyroid Disease. Philadelphia: FA Davis, 1963:48.
68. Morreale de Escobar G, Escobar del Rey R. Extrathyroid effects of some antithyroid drugs and their metabolic consequences. Rec Prog Horm Res 1967;23:87–137.
69. Cooper DS, Saxe VC, Meskell M, et al. Acute effects of propylthiouracil (PTU) on thyroidal iodide organification and peripheral iodothyronine deiodination: correlation with serum PTU levels measured by radioimmunoassay. J Clin Endocrinol Metab 1982;54:101–107.
70. Visser TJ, van Overmeeren E, Fekkes D, et al. Inhibition of iodothyronine 5′-deiodinase by thioureylenes: structur—activity relationship. FEBS Lett 1979;103:314–318.
71. Taurog A. The mechanism of action of the thioureylene antithyroid drugs. Endocrinology 1976;98:1031–1046.
72. Nakashima T, Taurog A, Riesco G. Mechanism of action of thioureylene antithyroid drugs: factors affecting intrathyroidal metabolism of propylthiouracil and methimazole in rats. Endocrinology 1978;103:2187–2197.
73. Papapetrou PD, Mothon S, Alexander WD. Binding of the 35-S of 35-S-propylthiouracil by follicular thyroglobulin in vivo and in vitro. Acta Endocrinol 1975;79:248–258.
74. Chopra IJ, Chua Teco GN, Eisenberg JB, et al. Structure–activity relationships of inhibition of hepatic monodeiodination of thyroxine to 3,5,3′-triiodothyronine by thiouracil and related compounds. Endocrinology 1982;110: 163–168.
75. Turner JG, Brownlie BE, Sadler WA, et al. An evaluation of lithium as an adjunct to carbimazole treatment in acute thyrotoxicosis. Acta Endocrinol 1976;83:86–92.
76. Berens SC, Wolff J, Murphy DL. Lithium concentration by the thyroid. Endocrinology 1970;87:1085–1087.
77. Temple R, Berman M, Robbins J, et al. The use of lithium in the treatment of thyrotoxicosis. J Clin Invest 1972;51:2746–2756.
78. Tookey HL, Van Ettén CH, Daxenbichler ME. Glucosinolates. In: Liener IE, ed. Toxic Constituents of Plant Foodstuffs. New York: Academic Press, 1980, pp. 103–142.
79. Langer P, Michajlovskij N. Effect of naturally occurring goitrogens on thyroid peroxidase and influence of some compounds on iodide formation during the estimation. Endocrinol Exp 1972;6:97–103.
80. Greer MA. Natural occurrence of goitrogenic agents. Rec Prog Hormone Res 1962;18:187–219.
81. Elfving S. Studies on the naturally occurring goitrogen 5-vinyl-2-thiooxazolidone. Metabolism and antithyroid effect in the rat. Ann Clin Res 1980; 12(Suppl 28):7–47.
82. Tabachnick M, Hao YL, Korcek L. Effect of oleate, diphenylhydantoin, and heparin on the binding of ^{125}I-thyroxine to purified thyroxine-binding globulin. J Clin Endocrinol Metab 1973;36:392–394.
83. Goswami A, Leonard JL, Rosenberg IN. Inhibition by coumadin anticoagulants of enzymatic outer ring monodeiodination of iodothyronine. Biochem Biophys Res Commun 1982;104:1231–1238.
84. Auf'mkolk M, Amir SM, Kubota K, et al. The active principles of plant extracts with antithyrotropic activity: oxidation products of derivatives of 3,4-dihydroxycinnamic acid. Endocrinology 1985;116:1677–1686.
85. Selenkow HA, Asper SP Jr. Biological activity of compounds struturally related to thyroxine. Physiol Rev 1955;35:426–474.
86. Zenker N, Goudonnet H, Truchot R. Effect of thyroid status and cold stress on tyrosine hydroxylase activity in adrenal gland and brown adipose tissue. Life Sci 1976;18:183–188.
87. Zenker N, Truchot R, Goudonnet H, et al. Isopropyldiiodothyronine and α-methylthyroxine: comparison of their in vitro and in vivo effects with those of thyroid hormones. Biochem Pharmacol 1976;25:1757–1762.
88. Tarentino AL, Richert DA, Westerfeld WW. The concurrent induction of hepatic α-glycerophosphate dehydrogenase and malate dehydrogenase by thyroid hormone. Biochim Biophys Acta 1966;124:295–309.
89. Jorgensen EC. Structure–activity relationships of thyroxine analogues. Pharmacol Ther 1976;B2:661–682.
90. Jorgensen EC, Lehman PA. Thyroxine analogues. IV. Synthesis of aliphatic and alicyclic ethers of 3,5-diiodo-DL-tyrosine. J Org Chem 1961;26:894.
91. Mussett MV, Pitt-Rivers R. The physiologic activity of thyroxine and triiodothyronine analogs. Metab Clin Exper 1957;6:18–25.
92. Jorgensen EC, Reid JAW. Thyroxine analogues. XI. Structural isomers of 3,5,3′-triiodo-DL-thyronine. J Med Chem 1964;7:701–705.
93. Gluckman PD, Ballard PL, Kaplan SL, et al. Prolactin in umbilical cord blood and the respiratory distress syndrome. Pediatr 1978;93:1011–1014.
94. Tripp SL, Block FB, Barile G. Synthesis of methylene- and carbonyl-bridged analogues of iodothyronine and iodothyroacetic acids. J Med Chem 1973;66:60–64.
95. Mukherjee R, Block P Jr. Thyroxine analogues: synthesis and nuclear magnetic resonance spectral studies of diphenylamines. J Chem Soc (C) 1971:1596–600.
96. Leeson PD, Ellis D, Emmett JC, et al. Thyroid hormone analogues. Synthesis of 3′-substituted 3,5-diiodo-L-thyronines and quantitative structure–activity

studies of in vitro and in vivo thyromimetic activities in rat liver and heart. J Med Chem 1988;31:37–54.
97. Jorgensen EC. Thyroid hormones and analogs II. Structure–activity relationships. In: Li CH, ed. Hormonal Proteins and Peptides, vol 6. New York: Academic Press, 1978:107–204.
98. Jorgensen EC. Thyroid hormones. In: Wolff ME, ed. Burger's Medicinal Chemistry, Part 3. 4th Ed. New York: Wiley, 1981:103–148.
99. Zenker N, Jorgensen EC. Thyroxine analogues. I. Synthesis of 3, 5-diiodi-4-(2′-alkylphenoxy)-DL-phenylalanine. J Am Chem Soc 1959;81: 4643–4647.
100. Jorgensen EC, Zenker N, Greenberg C. et al. Thyroxine analogues. III. Antigoitrogenic and calorigenic activity of some alkyl substituted analogues of thyroxine. J Biol Chem 1960;235:1732–1737.
101. Jorgensen EC, Lehman PA, Greenberg C, et al. Thyroxine analogues. VII. Antigoitrogenic, calorigenic, and hypocholesteremic activities of same aliphatic, alicyclic, and aromatic ethers of 3,5-diiodotyrosine in the rat. J Biol Chem 1962;237:3832–3838.
102. Cody V, Hazel J, Langs DA, et al. Molecular structure of thyroxine analogues. Crystal structure of 3,5,3′-triiodothyroacetic and 3,5,3′,5′-tetraoiodothyroacetic acid N-diethanolamine (1:1) complexes. J Med Chem 1977;20:1628-1631.
103. Kollman PA, Murray WJ, Nuss ME, et al. Molecular orbital studies of thyroid hormone analogues. J Am Chem Soc 1973;95:8518-8525.
104. Lehman PA, Jorgensen EC. Thyroxine analogues. XIII. NMR evidence for hindered rotation in diphenyl ethers. Tetrahedron 1965;21:363–380.
105. Duggan BM, Craik DJ. ^{1}H and ^{13}C NMR relaxation studies of molecular dynamics of the thyroid hormones thyroxine, 3,5,3′-triiodothyronine, and 3,5-diiodothyronine. J Med Chem 1996;39:4007-4016.
106. Cody V. Thyroid hormones: crystal structure, molecular conformation, binding, and structure-function relationships. Rec Prog Horm Res 1978;34:437-475.
107. Ekins R. Methods for the measurement of free thyroid hormones. In: Ekins R, Faglia G, Pennisi F, et al, eds. International Symposium on Free Thyroid Hormones. Amsterdam: Excerpta Medica, 1979:7–29.
108. Ahmad P. Fyfe CA, Mellors A. Parachors in drug design. Biochem Pharmacol 1975;24:1103-1110.
109. Benson MG, Ellis D, Emmett JC, et al. 3′-Acetyl-3,5-diiodo-L-thyronine: a novel highly active thyromimetic with low receptor affinity. Biochem Pharmacol 1984;33:3143-3149.

Suggested Readings

Gilbert ES, Tarone R, Bouville A, et al. Thyroid cancer rates and I-131 doses from Nevada atmospheric nuclear bomb tests. J Natl Cancer Inst 1998;90:1654–1660.
Ladenson PW, Braverman LE, Mazzaferri EL, et al. Comparison of administration of recombinant human thyrotropin with withdrawal of thyroid hormone for radioactive iodine scanning in patients with thyroid carcinoma. N Engl J Med 1997;337:888–896.
McCowen KC, Garber JR, Spark R. Elevated serum thyrotropin in thyroxine-treated patients with hypothyroidism given sertraline. N Engl J Med 1997;337:1010–1011.

35. *Calcium Homeostasis*

ROBIN M. ZAVOD

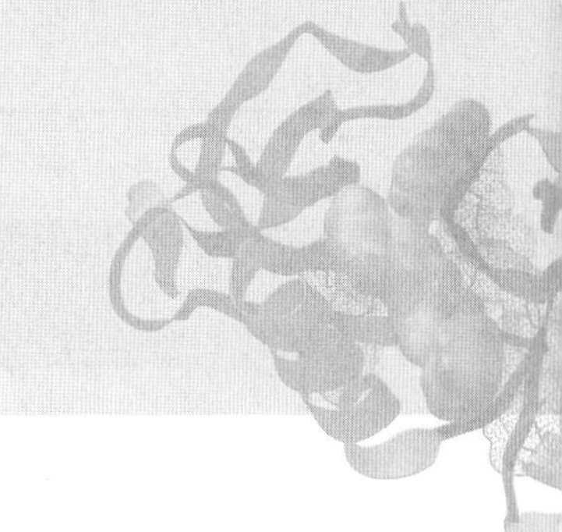

DRUGS COVERED IN THIS CHAPTER:

SELECTIVE ESTROGEN RECEPTOR MODULATORS
- Lasofoxifene
- Raloxifene

BISPHOSPHONATES
- Alendronate sodium
- Etidronate disodium
- Ibandronate sodium
- Pamidronate disodium
- Risedronate disodium
- Zoledronic acid

CALCITONIN

CINACALCET HYDROCHLORIDE

TERIPARATIDE

INORGANIC SALTS
- Calcium salts
- Gallium nitrate
- Sodium fluoride

INTRODUCTION

Three primary hormones—calcitonin, parathyroid hormone, and vitamin D—control the homeostatic regulation of calcium and its principle counterion, inorganic phosphate. Homeostatic control of these ions is essential not only for the moderation of longitudinal bone growth and bone remodeling but also for blood coagulation, neuromuscular excitability, plasma membrane structure and function, muscle contraction, glycogen and adenosine triphosphate (ATP) metabolism, neurotransmitter/hormone secretion, and enzyme catalysis (1). In an average 70-kg adult, approximately 1 kg of calcium is found, 99% of which is located in the bone. The principle calcium salt contained in the hydroxyapatite crystalline lattice of teeth and bones is $Ca_{10}(PO_4)_6(OH)_2$. Similarly, approximately 500 to 600 g of phosphate are present, 85% of which is found in the bone. The normal plasma concentration of calcium is approximately 4.5 to 5.7 mEq/L, 50% of which is protein bound. The remainder of the calcium is either complexed to corresponding counterions (46%) or exists in its ionized form (4%). It is only the ionized form of calcium that is tightly hormonally regulated (varies less than 5–10%) (1,2). Because serum calcium concentrations fluctuate, so do the plasma levels of the hormones associated with calcium homeostasis. Serum phosphorous levels vary with age, diet, and hormonal status. The most common form of phosphate in the blood (pH 7.4) is HPO_4^{2-}.

The bone is composed of two distinct tissue structures: cortical (compact) bone, and trabecular (cancellous) bone (3). Eighty percent of the skeleton is composed of cortical bone (e.g., long bones such as the humerus, radius, and ulna) (4,5), which is a relatively dense tissue (80–90% calcified) (4) that provides structure and support (3). Bone marrow cavities, flat bones, and the ends of long bones are all composed of trabecular bone, which is considerably more porous (5–20% calcified) (4,5). To maintain healthy, well-mineralized bone, a continuous process of bone resorption (loss of ionic calcium from bone) and formation occurs along the bone surface. Cortical bone is remodeled at the rate of 3% per year, whereas 25% of trabecular bone, which has considerably higher surface area, is remodeled annually (3). In terms of calcium turnover in bone, approximately 500 mg are removed and replaced on a daily basis.

Both inorganic and organic components are present in the bone. The highly crystalline inorganic component is hydroxyapatite, and the collagen matrix comprises the major portion (90%) of the organic component. The collagen matrix serves as the foundation for hydroxyapatite mineralization. Osteocalcin and osteonectin are minor organic constituents that promote binding of hydroxyapatite and calcium to the collagen matrix and regulate the rate of bone mineralization, respectively (5).

In general, peak bone mass occurs between 30 and 40 years of age (3,6) and is dependent on genetic factors as well as proper intake of calcium, maintenance of quality nutrition, and participation in weight-bearing exercise (6). Thereafter, peak bone mass progressively declines at the rate of 0.3 to 0.5% of cortical bone per year (3). After menopause, bone loss is accelerated (2% per year in the spine) (6) for a period of 5 to 10 years because of the loss of estrogen. This can result in up to a 30% decrease in bone mineral density.

HORMONAL REGULATION OF SERUM CALCIUM LEVELS

Arnaud (7) has developed a "butterfly model" that provides a diagrammatic view of the complex interrelationships among the three hormones (parathyroid, calcitonin, and vitamin D) that control calcium homeostasis (serum concentrations of ionic calcium) and their target organs (bone, kidney, and intestine) (Fig. 35.1). The right side (B loops) of the butterfly model describes the processes that increase the serum calcium concentration in response to hypocalcemia; the left side (A loops) depicts the events that occur in response to hypercalcemia.

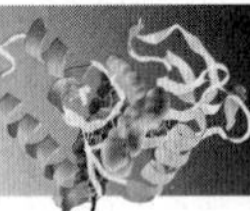

CLINICAL SIGNIFICANCE

As our knowledge about the development and risk factors associated with disruptions in calcium homeostasis has increased, so too have the modalities available to prevent and/or treat these disease processes. In general, disorders of calcium homeostasis involve the development of bone disease and/or alterations in serum calcium concentration. In the most basic sense, the development of bone disease is simply an inequity between bone breakdown and bone formation, which also may result in an altered serum calcium concentration. In addition to bone disease, disruptions in normal serum calcium concentrations may be related to an imbalance in calcium intake and renal calcium elimination. These disturbances can result from various factors, including increased activity of cells that cause bone breakdown, decreased activity of cells that form new bone, decreased absorption of calcium, or irregularities in levels of hormones that affect calcium absorption and influence cells involved in bone maintenance. Our understanding of these physiologic processes has led to the development of multiple classes of agents targeting the different mechanisms for evolution of these disease processes, including selective estrogen receptor modulators, bisphosphonates, and various calcium salts.

Application of the principles of medicinal chemistry has resulted in formulation of agents with additional routes of administration, increased potency, and decreased frequency of dosing. These advances have increased the utility of these agents and improved the quality of life for countless individuals affected by calcium homeostasis disorders. Understanding the development of individual disease processes involved in disorders of calcium homeostasis (e.g., osteoporosis, osteopetrosis, hyperparathyroidism, and Paget's disease) and the pharmacodynamic effects of individual compounds used to treat these disorders is paramount for the practitioner making therapeutic decisions. Incorporation of these factors into the therapeutic plan is necessary to target the valued pharmacodynamic effects of these agents while minimizing unwanted or harmful effects. An example would be the selection of raloxifene to treat osteoporosis in a patient with severe gastroesophageal reflux disease instead of an oral bisphosphonate, which could increase the likelihood of developing erosive esophagitis. Finally, it is also important for the clinician to recognize the capacity of certain entities used to treat calcium disorders to be allergenic or more prone to produce adverse effects so that selection of the best agent for an individual patient is facilitated.

Kathryn Neill, Pharm.D.
Assistant Professor
Critical Care Specialist
Department of Pharmacy Practice
College of Pharmacy
University of Arkansas for Medical Sciences

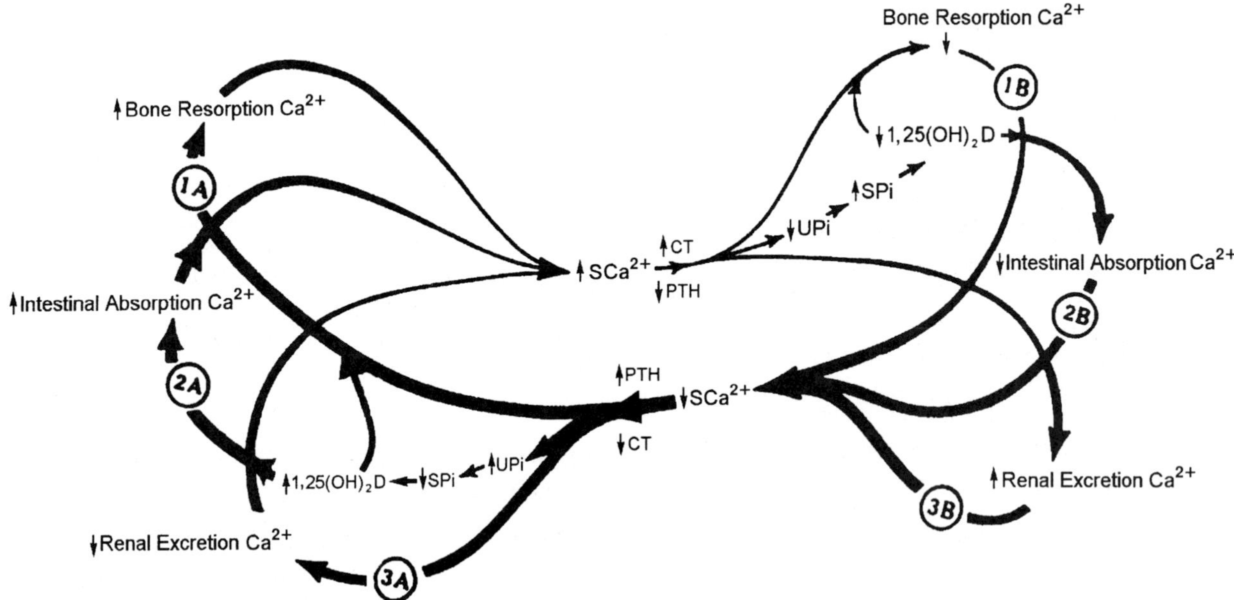

Fig. 35.1. The Arnaud's butterfly model for regulating calcium homeostasis consists of three overlapping loops that interlock and relate to one another through the serum concentrations of ionic calcium (SCa), parathyroid hormone (PTH), and calcitonin (CT). The right side (B loops, where B refers to the effects of CT) of the model describes the physiologic processes that increase the serum calcium concentration in response to hypocalcemia; the left side (A loops, where A refers to the effects of PTH) of the model depicts the events that decrease the serum calcium concentration in response to hypercalcemia. Loop 1 bone resorption; loop 2 intestinal absorption; loop 3 renal excretion; SPi, serium inorganic phosphate; UPi, urinary inorganic phosphate. (Adapted from Arnaud CD. Calcium homeostasis: regulatory elements and their integration. Fed Proc 1978; 37:2557-2560; with permission).

Calcitonin

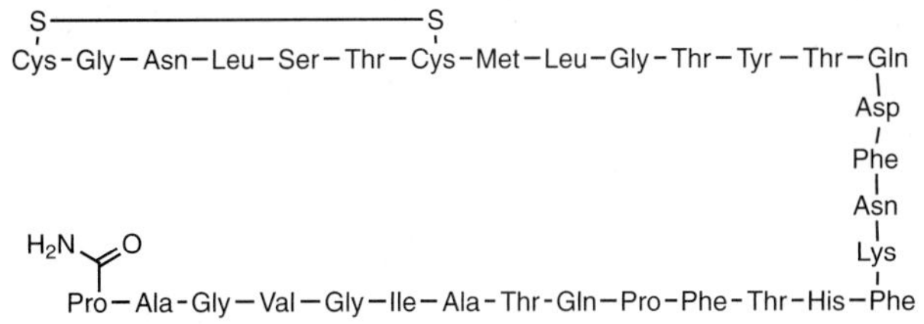

S————————S
Cys-Gly–Asn–Leu–Ser–Thr–Cys-Met–Leu–Gly-Thr–Tyr–Thr–Gln–Asp–Phe–Asn–Lys–Phe–His–Thr–Phe–Pro–Gln–Thr–Ala–Ile–Gly–Val–Gly–Ala–Pro($C(=O)NH_2$)

Human calcitonin

Human calcitonin is a 32-amino-acid peptide (molecular weight, 3,527 dalton) biosynthesized in the parafollicular "C" cells found within the thyroid gland. This hormone contains a critical disulfide bridge between residues 1 and 7, with the entire amino acid sequence required for biological activity. The carboxy terminal residue is a proline amide. "Pro-calcitonin," a precursor peptide, has been identified and proposed to facilitate intracellular transport and secretion. Calcitonin is secreted in response to elevated serum calcium concentrations (>9 mg/100 mL) and serves to oppose the hormonal effects of parathyroid hormone. In response to a hypercalcemic state (Fig. 35.1, B loops), increased calcitonin secretion drives serum calcium concentrations down via stimulation of urinary excretion of both calcium and phosphate (loop 3B), prevention of calcium resorption from the bone via inhibition of osteoclast activity (loop 1B), and inhibition of intestinal absorption of calcium (loop 2B). When serum calcium concentrations are low (hypocalcemia), the release of calcitonin is slowed, thereby activating loops 1A, 2A, and 3A.

Parathyroid Hormone

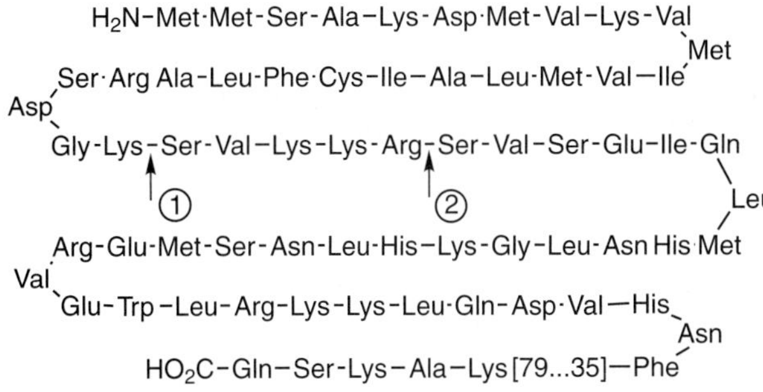

H_2N-Met-Met-Ser-Ala–Lys-Asp-Met-Val–Lys-Val-Met-Ile–Val-Met-Leu–Ala–Ile–Cys-Phe-Leu-Ala Arg-Ser-Asp-Gly-Lys-↑①-Ser-Val–Lys-Lys-Arg-↑②-Ser-Val-Ser-Glu-Ile-Gln-Leu-Met-His Asn-Leu-Gly-Lys–His–Leu-Asn-Ser-Met-Glu-Arg-Val-Glu-Trp–Leu–Arg-Lys-Lys-Leu-Gln-Asp-Val–His-Asn-Phe–Lys[79...35]–Ala–Lys–Ser–Gln–CO_2H

Human pre-proparathyroid hormone with site of cleavage leading to proparathyroid ① and site of cleavage leading to PTH ②.

Parathyroid hormone (PTH) is biosynthesized as a 115-amino-acid preprohormone in the rough endoplasmic reticulum of the parathyroid gland and is cleaved to the prohormone (90 amino acids) in the cisternal space of the reticulum. The active hormone is finally produced (84 amino acids; molecular weight, 9,500 dalton) in the Golgi complex and is stored in secretory granules in the parathyroid gland. This gland is exquisitely sensitive to serum calcium concentrations and is able to monitor these levels via calcium-sensing receptors (CaSR). These cell surface receptors help cells to react to micromolar changes in the concentration of ionized calcium in the serum (8). Binding of calcium to these receptors facilitates activation of phospholipase C and, ultimately, inhibition of PTH secretion. The relatively short-acting PTH is secreted from the parathyroid gland chief cells in response to a hypocalcemic state and serves to oppose the hormonal effects of calcitonin (1). Unlike calcitonin, the biological activity of PTH resides solely in residues 1 to 34 in the amino terminus. Parathyroid hormone decreases renal excretion of calcium (Fig. 35.1, loop 3A), indirectly stimulates intestinal absorption of calcium (Fig. 35.1, loop 2A), and in combination with active vitamin D, promotes bone resorption (Fig. 35.1, loop 1A) by a complex, unknown mechanism, thereby elevating serum calcium concentrations. In addition, the secretion of PTH stimulates the biosynthesis and release of the third hormone associated with calcium homeostasis, vitamin D. When serum calcium concentrations are high, the release of PTH is inhibited.

Vitamin D

Derived from cholesterol, vitamin D is biosynthesized from its prohormone cholecalciferol (D_3), the product of solar ultraviolet irradiation of 7-dehydrocholesterol in the skin (2). In 1966, it was first recognized that vitamin D must undergo activation *via* two oxidative metabolic steps (Fig. 35.2). The first oxidation to 25-hydroxycholecalciferol ($25(OH)D_3$: calcifediol; Calderol) occurs in the endoplasmic reticulum of the liver and is catalyzed by vitamin D 25-hydroxylase. This activation step is not

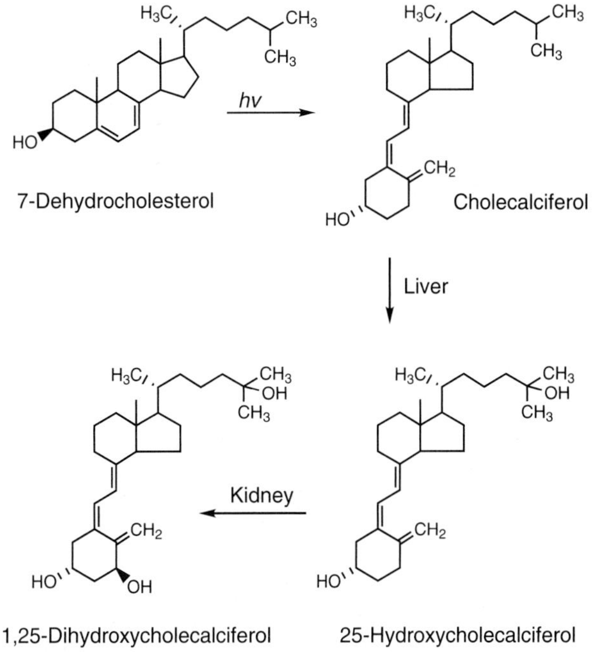

7-Dehydrocholesterol —hν→ Cholecalciferol —Liver→ 25-Hydroxycholecalciferol —Kidney→ 1,25-Dihydroxycholecalciferol

Fig. 35.2. Bioactivation of vitamin D.

regulated by plasma calcium concentrations. The major circulating form (10–80 μg/mL) is $25(OH)D_3$, which also is the primary storage form of vitamin D (2). In response to a hypocalcemic state and the secretion of PTH, a second oxidation step is activated in the mitochondria of the kidney, catalyzed by vitamin D 1α-hydroxylase (2,9). The product of this reaction, 1,25-dihydroxycholecalciferol ($1,25(OH)_2D_3$; 1,25-calcitriol; Rocaltrol, Calcijex) is the active form of vitamin D. Its concentration in the blood is 1/500 that of its monohydroxylated precursor. The biosynthesis of vitamin D is tightly regulated based on the serum concentrations of calcium, phosphate, PTH, and active vitamin D (2).

Sterol-specific cytoplasmic receptor proteins (vitamin D receptor) mediate the biological action of vitamin D (9). The active hormone is transported from the cytoplasm to the nucleus via the vitamin D receptor, and as a result of the interaction of the hormone with target genes, a variety of proteins are produced that stimulate the transport of calcium in each of the target tissues. Active vitamin D works in concert with PTH to enhance active intestinal absorption of calcium, to stimulate bone resorption, and to prohibit renal excretion of calcium (2,9). If serum calcium or 1,25-calcitriol concentrations are elevated, then vitamin D 24-hydroxylase (in renal mitochondria) is activated to oxidize $25(OH)D_3$ to inactive 24,25-dihydroxycholecalciferol and to further oxidize active vitamin D to the inactive 1,24,25-trihydroxylated derivative. Both the 1,24,25-trihydroxylated and the 24,25-dihydroxylated products have been found to suppress PTH secretion as well. Several factors have been identified in the regulation of the biosynthesis of vitamin D, including low phosphate concentrations (stimulatory) as well as pregnancy and lactation (stimulatory).

NORMAL PHYSIOLOGY

During growth periods in childhood and early adulthood, bone formation characteristically exceeds bone loss. In young adulthood, bone formation and bone resorption are nearly equal. After the age of 40 years, however, bone resorption is slightly greater than bone formation, and this results in a gradual decline in skeletal mass. Osteoblasts, osteoclasts, and osteocytes are the three types of cells that make up the bone remodeling unit (3) or bone metabolizing unit (4) and, therefore, are largely responsible for the bone remodeling process.

Osteoblasts, which are of mesenchymal origin and are formed in the bone marrow, stimulate bone formation (6). In the maturation process, osteoblasts undergo multiple cell divisions and, in so doing, express the gene products that are needed to form the bone matrix or osteoid (3) as well as those products responsible for mineralization of that tissue (6). Multiple endogenous substances are involved in osteoblast maturation, including many cytokines (interleukins and granulocyte-macrophage colony-stimulating-factor) (3) as well as hormones and growth factors (6). It is in the rough endoplasmic reticulum that the biosynthesis of the bone matrix protein occurs (4).

Osteoclasts are the large multinucleated cells of hemopoietic origin (6) that are responsible for carrying out the bone resorption or destroying process. Cytokines, PTH, and the active form of vitamin D activate these cells. Bone lining flat cells, derived from "retired" osteoclasts and osteoblasts, are located on the bone surface (3). The function of these flat cells is thought to serve to identify areas of the bone that have become weakened or misshapen and to send a signal to the bone remodeling unit to prepare the bone. Lining cells then digest the outer layer of the bone matrix in preparation for bone remodeling. The osteoclast membrane then comes into contact with the bone surface and forms an impermeable "sealing zone" of approximately 500 to 1,000 μm in size (2,6). The H^+ ATPase-rich osteoclast membrane that is in contact with the bone surface forms a ruffled border, the sealing zone becomes acidified, and ultimately, the bone minerals dissolve (6). Several types of lysosomal enzymes have been proposed to then digest the collagen matrix (3), thereby pitting the bone surface to a depth of 50 μm (4–6). Only calcitonin acts directly on the osteoclast to prevent bone resorption.

Yet another type of cell is found deep within the bone matrix, the osteocyte. The role of this type of cell has yet to be elucidated, but it has been proposed that it may be responsible for maintaining bone integrity (3) and for providing nutrition to the bone.

Parathyroid hormone stimulates bone resorption by several mechanisms: 1) Transformation of osteoprogenitor cells into osteoclasts is stimulated in the presence of PTH, 2) PTH promotes the deep osteocytes to mobilize calcium from perilacunar bone, and 3) surface osteocytes are stimulated by PTH to increase the flow of calcium out of the bone.

Quantification of bone mineral density (BMD) can be measured by noninvasive radiographic tests, such as single-photon (3) or dual-photon absorptiometry (spine, hip, and total body) (10), dual-energy x-ray absorptiometry (3,10,11) (spine, hip, total and body), peripheral dual-energy x-ray absorptiometry (wrist, heel, and finger), single energy x-ray absorptiometry (wrist or heel) (12), quantitative computed tomography (spine) and peripheral quantitative computed tomography (wrist) (10), and quantitative ultrasound (heel, shin bone, and knee cap) (12). Dual-energy x-ray absorptiometry is considered to be the gold standard for measuring bone density and has an accuracy that exceeds 95% (4). These techniques measure the attenuation of x-rays or gamma rays as they cross the spine, hip, or radius before they reach the detector (6). Other methods under development that measure BMD include ultrasound, traditional x-rays, and blood/urine tests (6). Traditional x-rays can identify the site of fracture, but they cannot measure BMD (3). Blood/urine tests can identify if the patient is suffering from a medical condition (3) that is contributing to the loss of BMD and can identify important biochemical markers that can assess the rate of

Table 35.1. Classification of Osteoporosis (14)

Etiology	Type I (postmenopausal) Increased Osteoclast Activity and Bone Resorption	Type II (senile) Decreased Osteoblast Activity and Bone Formation; Decreased GI Ca Absorption	Type III (secondary) Drug Therapies; Disease States
Typical age at diagnosis	50–75	>70	any age
Gender ratio	6:1 women/men	2:1 women/men	1:1 women/men
Typical fracture site	vertebrae, distal radius	femoral, neck, hip	vertebrae, hip, extremities
Bone morphology	decreased trabecular	decreased trabecular and normal cortical bone	decreased cortical bone
Rate of bone loss	2–3% per year	0.3–0.5% per year	variable

bone resorption and bone turnover. The measurement of serum calcium, phosphorous, and vitamin D levels also may provide insight regarding the cause of decreased BMD (3). Often, patients suffer from multiple vertebral compression fractures (3) without seeking treatment other than an over-the-counter analgesic, and the diagnosis of osteoporosis occurs only after the patient has already lost significant (as much as 30%) bone mass.

DISEASE STATES ASSOCIATED WITH ABNORMAL CALCIUM HOMEOSTASIS

Osteoporosis

Osteoporosis is a skeletal disease that is characterized by loss of bone mass as well as microarchitectural deterioration of the bone tissue. This disease is associated with increased bone fragility and susceptibility to fracture. It is a condition that is characterized not by inadequate bone formation but, rather, by a deficiency in the production of well-mineralized bone mass. Whereas no medical cause typically is evident in primary osteoporosis (3), secondary osteoporosis classically stems from medical illness or medication use. There are two types of primary adult osteoporosis, type I, or postmenopausal, and type II, or senile (Table 35.1). In type I osteoporosis, there is an accelerated rate of bone loss via enhanced resorption at the onset of menopause. In this form of the disease, the loss of trabecular bone is threefold greater than the loss of cortical bone. This disproportionate loss of bone mass is the primary cause of the vertebral crush fractures and the wrist and ankle fractures experienced by postmenopausal women. In type II osteoporosis, which is associated with aging, the degree of bone loss is similar in both trabecular and cortical bone (5) and is caused by decreased bone formation by the osteoblasts.

Drug- or disease-induced, or type III, osteoporosis (Table 35.2) accounts for up to 30% of the cases of vertebral fractures reported annually. It can be caused by a variety of factors, including long-term suppression of osteoblast function, an inhibition of calcium absorption from the gut, or excessive loss of calcium in the urine, as a result of estrogen deficiency, hyperparathyroidism (6,11), hyperthyroidism (6,11), hypogonadism (11,13), renal disease (6), depression, and treatment with glucocorticoids (13), thyroid hormone, anticonvulsants, methotrexate (13), cyclosporine (13), warfarin, lithium, or immunosuppressive therapy (6). Warfarin impairs the vitamin K–dependent biosynthesis of osteocalcin (13), it prevents the recycling of oxidized vitamin K to its active reduced form via inhibition of vitamin K epoxide reductase and vitamin K reductase. Long-term therapy with glucocorticoids has been shown to directly suppress osteoblast function and reduce calcium absorption from the gut (13). Vitamin D deficiency, as the cause of pseudohyperparathyroidism, is a common cause of osteoporosis in elder persons who are institutionalized and lack adequate sunlight exposure (2).

Osteoporosis is the cause of nearly 1.5 million fractures annually in the United States (3), including 250,000 hip fractures and 550,000 vertebral fractures. As it relates to the percentage of women older than 50 years who are at risk for developing osteoporosis because of low bone mass, the statistics are sobering: 52% of Caucasian and Asian women, 35% of African-American women, and 49% of Hispanic women. It has been predicted that one in every three women who live to the age of 90 years will experience a hip fracture (3,15). It has been estimated that 15 to 35% of hip fracture patients will require long-term nursing home care. A surprising 60% of hip fracture patients do not regain full function, and within 3 to 4

Table 35.2. Causes of Secondary (Type III) Osteoporosis (13,15)

Alcohol	Hypopituitarism
Algodystrophy	Mastocytosis
Anorexia nervosa	Mylenoma
Celiac disease	Organ transplant
Crohn's disease	Osteogenesis imperfecta
Diabetes mellitus	Primary biliary cirrhosis
Drug-induced (corticosteroids, heparin, warfarin)	Pregnancy
	Rheumatic diseases
Exercise induced amenorrhea	Thyrotoxicosis/thyroid replacement
Gastrectomy	Turner's syndrome
Hyperparathyroidism	Ulcerative colitis
Hypogonadism	

Table 35.3. Risk Factors for Osteoporosis (3)

Lifestyle Factors	Genetic Factors	Medical Disorders	Drugs
Smoking	White or Asian	Cushing's syndrome	Glucocorticoids
Sedentary lifestyle	Female	Hyperthyroidism	Thyroid hormone
Calcium intake	Family history	Congenital hypogonadism	Phenytoin
Milk intolerance	Small frame	Primary biliary cirrhosis	Carbamazepine
Excessive caffeine	Early menopause	Malabsorption syndromes	Heparin
Excessive alcohol		Gastrointestinal resection	Aluminum antacids
Nulliparity		Primary hyperparathyroidism	GnRH agonists
High protein intake		Anorexia nervosa	Furosemide
		Multiple myeloma	
		Depression	

GnRH, gonadotropin-releasing hormone.

months of hip fracture, as many as 25% die as a result of secondary complications (e.g., pneumonia or infection). Mortality also is increased 17% after both femoral and vertebral fractures. The risk factors associated with osteoporosis are presented in Table 35.3. Given these statistics, osteoporosis should be considered a significant health problem that only stands to worsen unless appropriate interventions are pursued.

Osteopetrosis

Osteopetrosis, also known as marble bone disease, describes a group of heritable disorders that are centered on a defect in osteoclast-mediated bone resorption. There are four autosomal recessive and one autosomal dominant forms of osteopetrosis (Table 35.4) (16). It generally is characterized by abnormally dense, brittle bone and increased skeletal mass. Unlike osteoporosis, this disorder results from decreased osteoclast activity, which has an effect on both the shape and structure of the bone. In very extreme cases, the medullary cavity, which houses bone marrow, fills with new bone, and production of hematopoietic cells is hampered. Like osteoporosis, this disease can be detected radiographically and appears as though there is a "bone within a bone." There is limited evidence that bisphosphonates can induce osteopetrosis via their inhibition of osteoclast activity (17).

Hypocalcemia

Hypocalcemia can be caused by PTH deficiency, vitamin D deficiency, various pharmacological agents, and miscellaneous disorders (Table 35.5) (18). A state of hypocalcemia will inhibit calcitonin release. This results in an elevation of PTH biosynthesis and release and indirectly causes an increase in the production of vitamin D. The left wing of Arnaud's butterfly model (Fig. 35.1) would be activated to increase serum calcium concentrations. In the absence of calcitonin, osteoclast activity is unregulated; therefore, bone resorption is accelerated. In acute cases of hypocalcemia, specifically in the case of hypocalcemic tetany, PTH is administered to correct the hormonal imbalance.

Hypercalcemia

A state of hypercalcemia (Table 35.6) will promote calcitonin biosynthesis and release. As a result, PTH biosynthesis and its secretion are inhibited, as is the production of vitamin D. The right wings of Arnaud's butterfly model (Fig. 35.1, B loops) would be activated to decrease serum calcium concentrations. In the presence of calcitonin,

Table 35.4. Human Osteopetrosis Genotypes

Gene Involved	Function of Gene	Clinical Symptoms	% Patients Affected
Autosomal Recessive Disorders			
CAII	Carbonic acid and proton production	Less severe: may improve with age, short stature, no hematologic failure	<5%
TCIRG1	Proton pump	Severe: apparent in infancy, visual impairment, hypocalcemia, death by 10 years of age	~60%
CLCN7	Chloride channel	Severe: apparent in infancy, similar to TCIRG1 symptoms Intermediate: apparent in infancy but less aggressive, osteomyelitis, fractures	~15%
gl/gl	Unknown	Extremely severe: death within months	<5%
Autosomal Dominant Disorder			
CLCN7	Chloride channel	Frequent fractures, osteomyelitis, some more severe (like recessive disorders)	

Table 35.5. Causes for Hypocalcemia

PTH Deficiency	Vitamin D Deficiency	Drugs	Miscellaneous
Hypoparathyroidism Pseudohypoparathyroidism	Nutritional deficiency Gastrointestinal malabsorption	Chemotherapeutic agents Diuretics • Furosemide	Osteoblastic metastases Phosphate infusion
Hypomagnesemia	Renal • Failure • Tubule disorders • Nephrotic syndrome Hepatobiliary disease (decreased synthesis) Pancreatic disease (malabsorption) Anticonvulsant therapy (malabsorption, abnormal metabolism)	Inhibitors of bone resorption • Calcitonin • Bisphosphonates • Estrogens Antiviral • Foscarnet Antifungal • Ketoconazole	Rapid infusion of citrate buffered plasma or blood or large amounts of albumin

osteoclast activity is inhibited, so bone resorption is slowed. In acute cases of hypercalcemia, calcitonin is administered to reestablish calcium homeostasis. Hypercalcemia also can be treated with sulfate salts, ethylenediaminetetraacetic acid, furosemide, ethacrynic acid, glucocorticoids, and plicamycin.

Hypoparathyroidism

Hypoparathyroidism is caused by decreased serum PTH concentrations. It is characterized by hypocalcemia, hyperphosphatemia, and reduced levels of circulating vitamin D. The right wings of Arnaud's butterfly model is predominant (Fig. 35.1), and serum calcium concentrations precipitously decrease. Administration of intravenous (IV) calcium gluconate and PTH serves to acutely correct plasma calcium levels. Chronic oral administration of active vitamin D as well as calcium supplements has been effective in maintaining appropriate serum calcium concentrations.

Pseudohypoparathyroidism

In this disease state, levels of PTH are normal or even elevated; however, serum calcium concentrations are low. End-organ insensitivity to PTH has been proposed to be the cause of the hypocalcemic state. Treatment of this condition with calcium and vitamin D has proven to be successful.

Hyperparathyroidism

Increased levels of PTH leads to moderately to severely elevated serum calcium concentrations (2) and, as a result, a significant loss of calcium from the bone. Deposits of calcium salts in soft tissue as well as formation of renal calculi also can result from this hormonal imbalance. Treatment of this condition with salmon calcitonin, loop diuretics, or other classical treatments for hypercalcemia has been favorable. The IV vitamin D analogue paricalcitol, which is used for both prevention and treatment of hyperparathyroidism secondary to chronic renal failure, has been shown to reduce parathyroid levels by an average of 30% after 6 weeks of treatment. Whereas paricalcitol is a fully active form of vitamin D, doxercalciferol requires activation by the liver. This analogue also is indicated for the treatment of secondary hyperparathyroidism. Doxercalciferol capsules should be administered three times weekly at the time of dialysis along with close monitoring of calcium and phosphate levels. Treatment of secondary hyperparathyroidism with vitamin D therapy is problematic, however, because it often leads to

Table 35.6. Calcium Homeostasis-Related Disorders

Type of Disorder	Treatment	Examples
Disorders leading to hypercalcemia	Fluids, low calcium diet, sulfate, loop diuretics, glucocorticoids, calcitonin, EDTA	Hyperparathyroidism Hypervitaminosis D Sarcoidosis Neoplasia Hyperthyroidism Immobilization Paget's disease of the bone Osteoporosis
Disorders of bone remodeling	Bisphosphonates, calcitonin, estrogen, calcitonin, calcium, fluoride, PTH + vitamin D	

EDTA, ethylenediaminetetra-acetic acid; PTH, parathyroid hormone.

hypercalcemia, hyperphosphatemia, or both because of increased intestinal absorption of both calcium and phosphorous (19). In patients with chronic renal failure, CaSR agonists are able to limit progression of hyperparathyroidism and growth of the parathyroid gland.

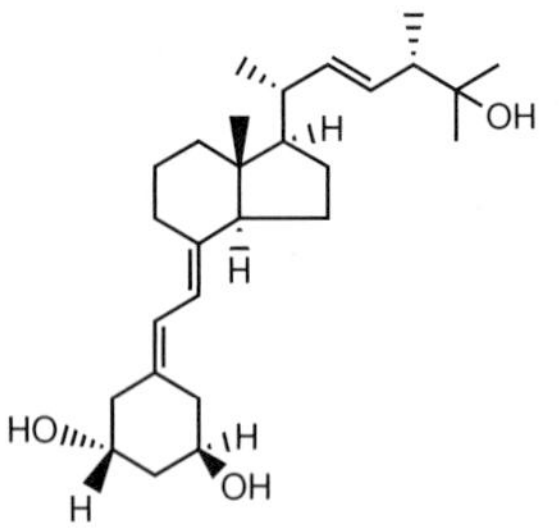

Paricalcitol (Zemplar)

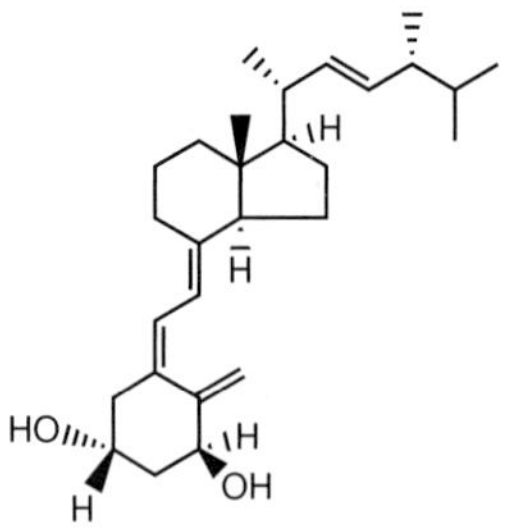

Doxercalciferol (Hectorol)

Rickets and Osteomalacia

During the Industrial Revolution, there was widespread incidence of rickets in both children and adults, because inadequate exposure to sunlight prevented the biosynthesis of active vitamin D in the skin. Both rickets and osteomalacia are metabolic bone diseases that are characterized by poor bone mineralization. Without adequate plasma levels of vitamin D and calcium, deposition of the calcium salts in the bone markedly decreases. Vitamin D supplementation (to improve intestinal absorption of calcium and mineralization of the bone) as well as oral calcium supplementation are required to treat these diseases once established. The incidence of rickets in the United States dropped dramatically through vitamin D–supplemented food programs. The increased use of milk substitutes (e.g., soy) and reduced exposure to sunlight has recently led to a rise in rickets. Rickets is still considered to be a worldwide health problem.

In addition to the classical environmental or nutritional cause of these diseases, both osteomalacia and rickets can have a pharmacological origin via chronic treatment with anticonvulsants (phenobarbital and phenytoin) or glucocorticoids. These agents interfere with intestinal absorption of calcium and, thereby, cause pseudohyperparathyroidism. As a result, an increase in bone turnover and a decrease in the formation of appropriately mineralized bone is observed. In these patients, treatment with vitamin D improves calcium absorption, ultimately enhancing mineralization of the bone.

Paget's Disease

Paget's disease (Table 35.6) is characterized by excessive bone resorption, followed by replacement of the normally mineralized bone with soft, poorly mineralized tissue (20). It has been determined that the osteoclasts have an abnormal structure, are hyperactive, and are present at elevated levels (20). Patients afflicted with this painful condition often suffer from multiple compression fractures. Administration of calcitonin and oral calcium and phosphate supplements had been the treatment of choice until the bisphosphonate risedronate was approved by the U.S. Food and Drug Administration (FDA). Daily administration of risedronate results in a decreased rate of bone turnover and a decrease in the levels of serum alkaline phosphatase and urinary hydroxyproline, two biochemical markers of bone turnover (4,20). A significant advantage to treatment with the bisphosphonates is long-term suppression of the disease (20). Calcium supplementation, which often is necessary in these patients, must be dosed separately from risedronate, because calcium- and aluminum- or magnesium-containing antacids interfere with absorption of the bisphosphonates.

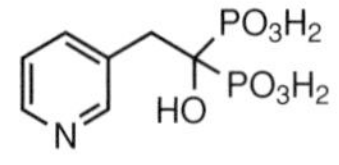

Risedronate

DRUG THERAPIES USED TO TREAT OSTEOPOROSIS

Agents used in the treatment and prevention of osteoporosis are categorized as antiresorptive agents, or bone-forming agents depending on the primary mechanism of action (21). For most effective therapies, bone mass increases for the first few years of treatment. Eventually, however, all the pits or lacunae will be filled in with new bone, and no additional increase in bone mass will occur. Antiresorptive agents have been shown to increase bone mass by as much as 8 to 9% at the lumbar spine and 3 to 6% in the femoral neck. Once a diagnosis of osteoporosis and the likely cause has been established, it is important to gather both patient fracture history and general medical history. This information is essential to select the appropriate treatment for a given patient (Table 35.7) (22).

Antiresorptive Agents

Estrogen Analogues—Estrogen Replacement Therapy

Mechanism of Action. The precise mechanism by which estrogen prevents bone resorption has not been elucidated; however, it has been proposed to be associated with inhibition of osteoclast activity. Limited evidence supports the presence of estrogen-specific receptors (present on osteoclasts) having a biochemical role in the regulation of

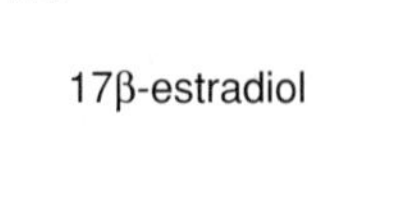

17β-estradiol

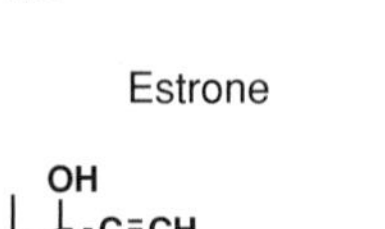

Estrone

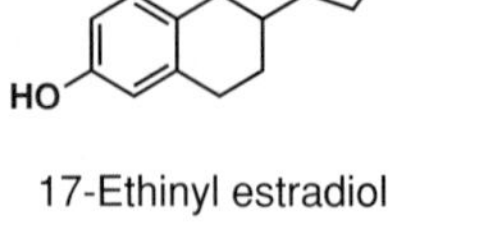

17-Ethinyl estradiol

Table 35.7. Osteoporosis Treatment Selection Criteria (22)

Patient Data	Aldendronate	Risedronate	Raloxifene	Calcitonin	Teriparatide
PM women: (+) osteoporosis/(+) fracture	√	√	√	√	√
PM women: (+) osteoporosis/(–) fracture	√				
Men: (+) osteoporosis	√				√
Corticosteroid induced osteoporosis	√		√		
(+) Esophageal or upper GI disorder	(–)	(–)	√	√	
(+) Vasomotor symptoms	√	√	(–)	√	
(+) Venous thromboembolic event	√	√	(–)	√	
(+) Vertebral compression fracture pain				√	

√ = Recommended; (–) = Not recommended

bone remodeling (14). Estrogen improves calcium absorption, promotes calcitonin biosynthesis, and increases the vitamin D receptors on osteoclasts. Although the primary mechanism of action remains unclear and its use is controversial at best, hormone replacement therapy is considered to be second-line therapy for the prevention of osteoporosis (23). Estrogen receptor therapy (ERT; e.g., 17β-estradiol, estrone sodium sulfate, or 17-ethinyl estradiol) (21) is classified as antiresorptive therapy in the prevention of osteoporosis. The pharmacokinetics of the estrogens is covered in detail in Chapter 46.

Therapeutic Effects. Fractures of the spine, wrist, and hips decrease by 50 to 70%, and spinal bone density increases by 5% (24), in those women treated with estrogen within 3 years of the onset of menopause and for 5 to 10 years thereafter (5,11,25). The minimum dose required and that which is considered to be standard therapy is 0.625 mg/day of conjugated estrogens (Premarin); however, a 0.3 mg/day dose of esterified estrogen (Estratab) has been shown to be adequate for the prevention of osteoporosis (5). Estrogen replacement therapy is available in several types of formulations, including transdermal patches (Climera, Estraderm, Menostar, or Vivelle).

Initiated at the onset of menopause, this therapy also has favorable effects on serum cholesterol levels (reduces low-density lipoprotein and elevates high-density lipoprotein levels). Women taking ERT have found relief from hot flashes, vaginal dryness, and urinary stress incontinence (21). It is recommended that the estrogen be combined with a progestin for those women with an intact uterus so as to decrease the risk of endometrial cancer (14). Hormone replacement therapy is not necessarily the treatment of choice for all women, because some are intolerant to this type of therapy or have a disease state in which ERT is contraindicated (e.g., breast cancer, liver disease, or active thromboembolic disease) (3).

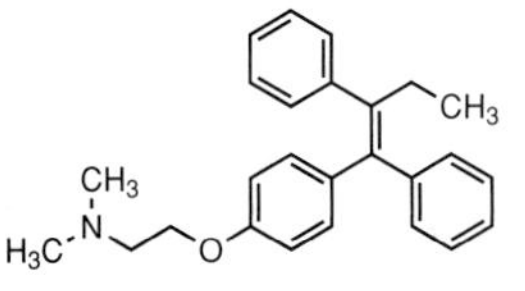

Selective Estrogen Receptor Modulators

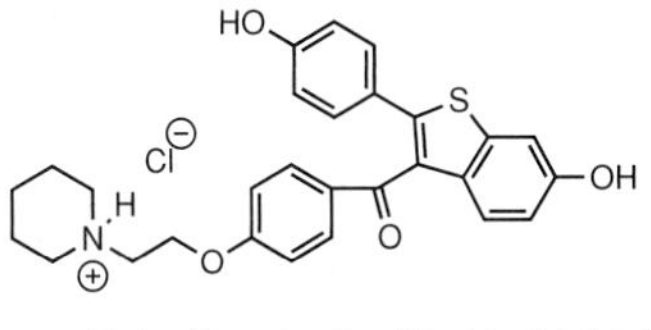

Raloxifene. Tamoxifen citrate, which is classified chemically as a triarylethylene, was developed as an antiestrogenic drug and as a selective estrogen receptor modulator (SERM). It is prescribed for the treatment of metastatic breast cancer. Raloxifene hydrochloride, a benzothiophene

Tamoxifen (Nolvadex)

Raloxifene hydrochloride (Evista)

> Tibolone is a synthetic steroid that has been shown to increase bone mineral density similar to alendronate. The U.S. FDA approval is pending; overseas, this agent is used for the treatment of menopausal symptoms as well as the prevention of osteoporosis. It is considered to be a viable alternative to conjugated equine estrogen plus micronized progesterone. With the 2.5-mg dose and calcium supplementation (800 mg/day), an increase in the lumbar spine and femoral neck bone density has been demonstrated. The ability of tibolone to prevent bone loss is proposed to be mediated through its estrogenic metabolites via the estrogen receptor (26). The most common reason for patient withdrawal from clinical trials was vaginal bleeding (also a common side effect when estrogen therapy is used). 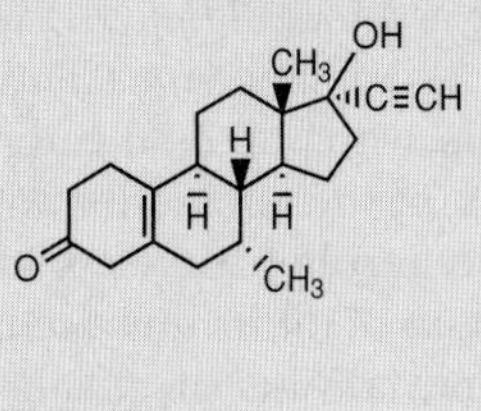
>
> Tibolone

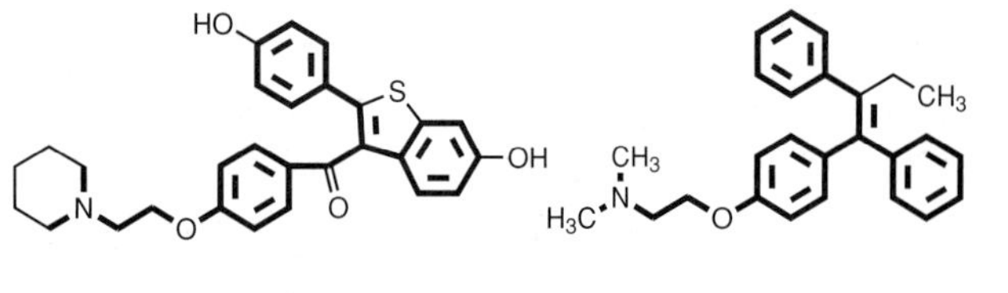

Raloxifene (Evista) Tamoxifen (Nolvadex)

Fig. 35.3. Structures of raloxifene and tamoxifen, highlighting the similarity between the two drugs.

derivative (24), also may be considered to be a semirigid analogue of tamoxifen (Fig. 35.3). The two drugs are similar in that they both possess agonist activity in certain tissues (e.g., bone and cardiovascular) and antagonist activity in others (e.g., breast and uterus) (6,21) (see Chapter 46). Raloxifene, the first SERM approved for the prevention of osteoporosis in postmenopausal women, acts as an estrogen agonist on receptors in osteoblasts and osteoclasts but as an antagonist at breast and uterine estrogen receptors. This selective action means that this agent does not increase the risk of endometrial or breast cancer, as is the case with long-term tamoxifen therapy. Because this agent does not have a stimulatory effect at its receptors on most tissues, it does not prevent the hot flashes and other symptoms of menopause as estrogen does (5).

Therapeutic Action. Clinical trials have shown that raloxifene, in combination with oral calcium supplementation, decreases the risk of vertebral fracture and promotes bone formation, albeit to a lesser extent than with estrogen. Raloxifene has been shown to have a beneficial effect on lipid profiles (11). Raloxifene should not be administered in combination with cholestyramine (decreased absorption), coumadin (prothrombin times and international normalized ratios must be monitored more closely), and those drugs that are highly protein bound, such as clofibrate, diazepam, ibuprofen, indomethacin, and naproxen.

Structure–Activity Relationship. From a structural perspective, the only pure antiestrogens are 7α-substituted estrogens (21). In the triarylethylene class of agents, the A ring phenol is critical for binding to the estrogen receptor, because it mimics the essential 3-phenolic group in estrogens (21). The orientation of the three aryl rings in a propeller type of arrangement also is important for tight receptor binding and biological activity (21).

Pharmacokinetics. Raloxifene is rapidly absorbed following oral administration, with an estimated 60% absorption, but it has a very low bioavailability (2%), associated with extensive phase II metabolism. The metabolites are excreted via the bile, with potential enterohepatic recycling that could account for the interaction with cholestyramine. Supportive of the enterohepatic recycling is the half-life of 28 hours. Metabolism of raloxifene occurs to a great extent in the intestine and consists of glucuronide conjugation catalyzed by uridine diphosphate glucuronosyltransferase

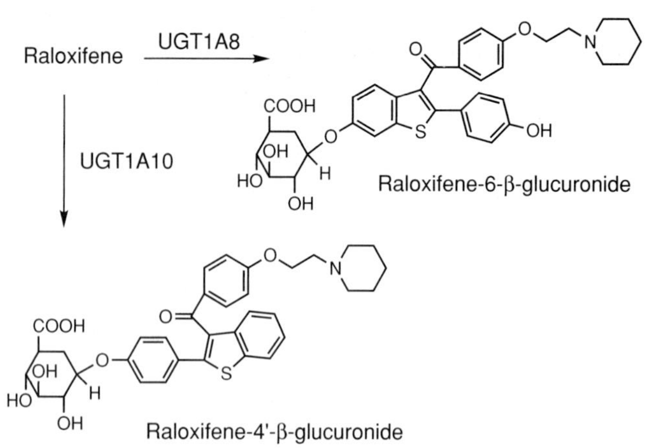

Raloxifene UGT1A8 UGT1A10

Raloxifene-6-β-glucuronide

Raloxifene-4'-β-glucuronide

Fig. 35.4. Metabolism of raloxifene.

(UGT) (27–29). The UGT1A family is responsible for intestinal human metabolism, as shown in Figure 35.4. Efflux by intestinal cells of the resulting glucuronide occurs via P-glycoprotein and multidrug resistance–related protein. The combination of rapid metabolism and efflux can account for the low bioavailability.

Lasofoxifene. Lasofoxifene is a very potent second-generation SERM currently in phase III clinical trials for the treatment and prevention of osteoporosis in postmenopausal women (Fig. 35.5). At low doses, this agent has been shown to prevent bone loss and decrease serum cholesterol (dose range, 0.01–20.0 mg/day). In early clinical trials, lasofoxifene improved BMD in the lumbar spine by 3% (after 12 months of therapy), which is twice the improvement observed with similar treatment using raloxifene. Improvement in hip BMD was similar for both agents. Interestingly, a more pronounced reduction

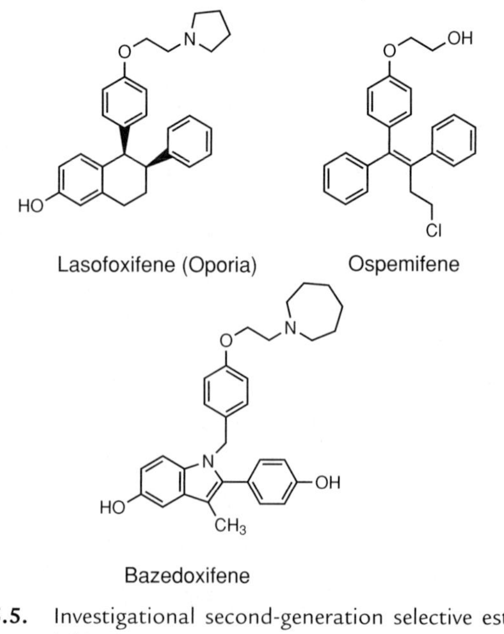

Lasofoxifene (Oporia) Ospemifene

Bazedoxifene

Fig. 35.5. Investigational second-generation selective estrogen receptor modulators.

in low-density lipoprotein cholesterol was observed with lasofoxifene treatment than with raloxifene treatment. As of September 2005, the U.S. FDA had rejected an New Drug Application (NDA) for lasofoxifene for undisclosed reasons.

Ospemifene is a SERM that is currently in Phase II/III clinical trials for the treatment of postmenopausal osteoporosis and urogenital atrophy (Fig. 35.5). It is a known metabolite of toremifene, a triphenylethylene derivative used to treat breast cancer. Ospemifene has been shown to have beneficial effects on the bone without significant estrogen-related side effects. The beneficial effect observed on bone stems from this agent's ability to increase osteoblast proliferation and, as a result, to enhance bone mineralization as well as bone formation. Unlike tamoxifen, ospemifene does not induce osteocyte apoptosis (30).

Bazedoxifene is an indole-based SERM that is under investigation for the treatment and prevention of postmenopausal osteoporosis (Fig. 35.5). It also is being evaluated in combination with Premarin (conjugated estrogens). Bazedoxifene displaces 17β-estradiol from estrogen receptors and has excellent binding affinity for the receptor itself. Unlike raloxifene, this agent does not cause hot flashes at the doses required to have a beneficial effect on bone. In addition, it does not cause uterine or mammary gland stimulation (31).

Bisphosphonates

Mechanism of Action. The bisphosphonates are synthetic in origin and are designed to mimic pyrophosphate, where the oxygen in P-O-P is replaced with a carbon atom to create a nonhydrolyzable backbone (24,25) (Fig. 35.6). Because pyrophosphate is a normal constituent of bone, these analogues selectively bind to the hydroxyapatite portion of the bone (25,32). The bisphosphonates (Fig. 35.7) effectively inhibit osteoclast

Pyrophosphate

Bisphosphonate
R_1 = hydroxy
R_2 = varies

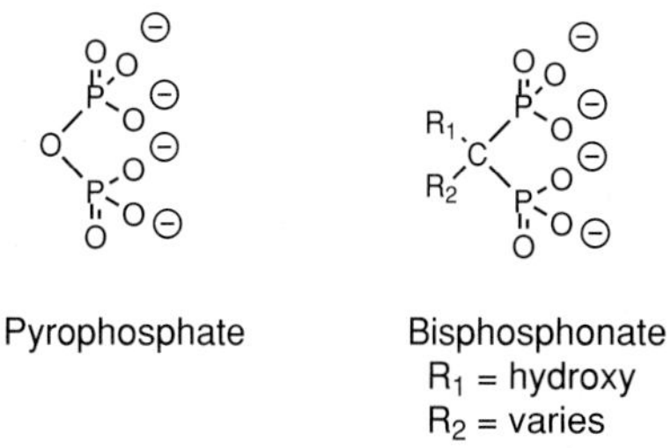

Fig. 35.6. Bisphosphonate structure-activity relationships.

proliferation, decrease osteoclast activity, reduce osteoclast life span, and as a result, decrease the number of sites along the bone surface where bone resorption occurs (25). By these three mechanisms, the bisphosphonates are able to limit bone turnover and allow the osteoblasts to form well-mineralized bone without opposition (3). The precise mechanisms of action of these antiresorptive agents has not been elucidated; it is equally uncertain whether all the bisphosphonates act by a similar mechanism (25). To date, cell surface receptors have not been identified, nor has a second messenger system been detected.

Structure–Activity Relationships. From a structural perspective, the bisphosphonates have been proposed to have specific molecular interactions with their biological target for drug action, even though precise structure–activity relationships (SARs) have not been elucidated. In fact, the exact molecular target is still under investigation. The central carbon of the geminal phosphonate has been substituted with a variety of functional groups to yield a large family of compounds with differing physicochemical and biological properties (25). The SAR studies (Fig. 35.6) have concluded that a hydroxyl substituent (R_1) maximizes the affinity of the agent for the hydroxyapatite

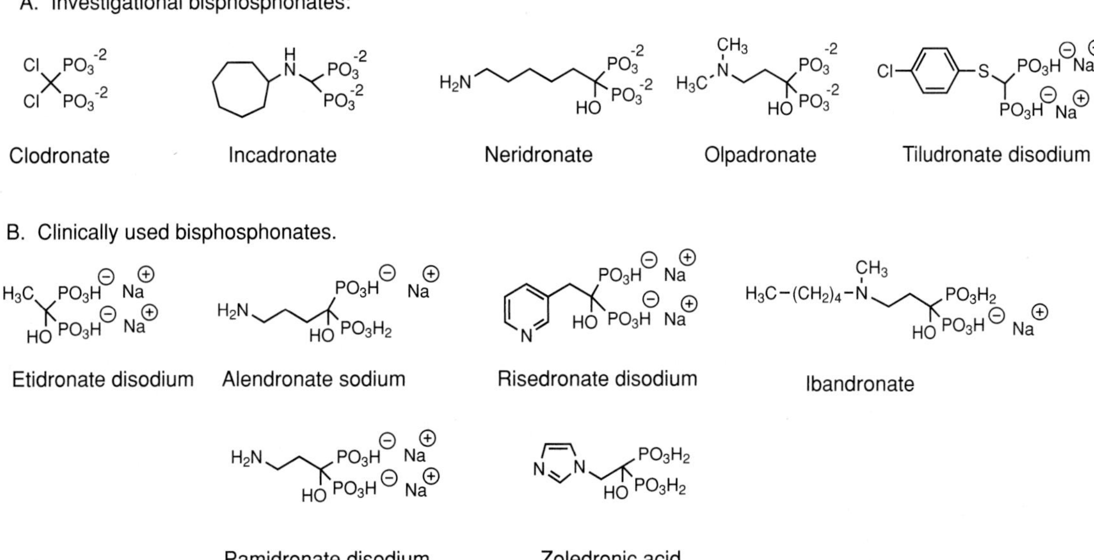

Fig. 35.7. Bisphosphonates, both investigational and clinically used.

as well as improves the antiresorptive character of the agent (21,33). The character of the R_2 substituent varies widely and clearly has a significant influence on the potency of this class of compounds (Fig. 35.7). The R_2 amino–substituted bisphosphonates (pamidronate, alendronate, and neridronate) are more potent than etidronate and clodronate (not available in the United States). The R_2 4-carbon amino linear chain for alendronate is more potent than the R_2 3-carbon derivative pamidronate and the R_2 6-carbon analogue neridronate (21). Alkylation of the amine functional group improving potency as is demonstrated by compounds with branched amine substituents at R_2 (e.g., olpadronate and ibandronate) and those that contain rings at R_2 (e.g., risedronate, incandronate, tiludronate, and zoledronate). The third-generation analogues contain a basic heterocyclic side chain at R_2 tethered to the central carbon by a variety of linkages (potency: $NH > CH_2 > S > O$) (21,33). Because structural variation of R_2 has a significant effect on potency, it can be surmised that R_2 interacts at an "active site" and participates in a specific molecular interaction. The bisphosphonate itself as well as the hydroxyl group at R_1 also should be included as critical SAR features (21).

Pharmacokinetics. To date, four generations of bisphosphonates have been developed for the treatment of osteoporosis (Fig. 35.7). Absorption of these agents from the gut is quite poor (1–5%) (11) because of their polar nature, and as a therapeutic class, they have limited cellular penetration. Up to 50% of the actual absorbed dose is taken up specifically by the bone within 4 to 6 hours, and the rest is exclusively excreted by the kidney (6,24). Uptake of these agents in the bone is concentrated in areas of the bone that are actively undergoing remodeling (32). Between the selective uptake and the rapid rate of clearance, the bisphosphonates enjoy a short circulating half-life and very limited drug exposure to nontarget tissues (25). Because the bisphosphonates are only released from the bone when the bone is resorbed, they have a tissue half-life of 1 to 10 years; however, these agents remain pharmacologically active only while they are exposed on bone resorption surfaces (32).

Specific Drugs

Etidronate Disodium (Didronel). Agents in the first generation (e.g., etidronate disodium and tiludronate) that were dosed continuously produced poorly mineralized bone (3), because there was no interval for appropriate bone mineralization to occur. Subsequent studies that used a cyclic dosing schedule (400 mg/day for 2 weeks, followed by 2.5 months of calcium supplementation only) showed improvement in bone mineralization (11,30). Etidronate has been approved for treatment of Paget's disease of the bone but not for treatment of osteoporosis (5). Tiludronate (6) is approximately 10-fold more potent than etidronate and, when given orally for 6 months (200, 400, or 800 mg/day), increases BMD by 2%. No further bone loss was detected in patients 6 months after cessation of therapy.

Alendronate Sodium (Fosamax). The second-generation agent alendronate sodium was the first bisphosphonate agent approved by the U.S. FDA for the prevention and treatment of osteoporosis and Paget's disease of the bone (32,34) and is 1,000-fold more potent than etidronate. This derivative, when dosed continuously (5–10 mg/day for osteoporosis and 40 mg/day for Paget's disease) and given with oral calcium supplements (500 mg/day), produced well-mineralized bone and significantly improved BMD (7% in the spine and 4% in the hip) within 18 months (6). In addition, the vertebral fracture rate was shown to decrease by 47%. A side effect associated with alendronate, chemical esophagitis (2,3,11,24), has been attributed to inadequate intake of water and lying down after taking the medication. Specific patient instructions were developed to limit the incidence of upper gastrointestinal problems and include: 1) taking the medication with 6 to 8 ounces of water on arising in the morning, 2) remaining in an upright position for at least 30 minutes after taking the medication, and 3) delaying drinking other liquids/eating for at least 30 minutes, if not 1 to 2 hours, to allow maximal absorption of the agent (3). To enhance absorption, calcium supplements and any aluminum- or magnesium-containing antacids should be dosed separately from the agents in this class. These agents are not recommended in patients with renal impairment (serum creatinine, <2.5 mg/dL), a history of esophageal disease, gastritis, or peptic ulcer (5).

Risedronate Disodium (Actonel). The third-generation agent risedronate disodium has been approved not only for the treatment of osteoporosis but also for the treatment of Paget's disease of the bone and glucocorticoid-induced osteoporosis. Risedronate is 1,000- to 5,000-fold more potent than etidronate. At the end of an 18-month study, 53% of those patients that took risedronate for 2 months remained in remission, as compared to 14% of the patients that took etidronate, an earlier-generation bisphosphonate, for 6 months. Oral administration of this agent suffers from the same problems as that of other bisphosphonate agents. Risedronate should not be given to patients with creatinine clearance of less than 30 mL/min.

A new formulation of alendronate, FOSAMAX PLUS D, was approved by the U.S. FDA in April 2005. This formulation includes 70 mg of alendronate and 2,800 IU of vitamin D_3 (i.e., a 7-day supply of both the bisphosphonate and vitamin D). This formulation should not be used in patients with severe kidney disease or low serum calcium levels and should not be the only therapy used to correct a vitamin D deficiency.

> Risedronate with calcium, which was approved by the U.S. FDA in August 2005, represents a novel type of packaging for this class of agents. It addresses the Surgeon General's Report on Bone Health and Osteoporosis, which states that treatments for osteoporosis need to be made simpler and more structured. Sold in units that contain a 1-month supply, each week of therapy includes a total of seven tablets, including one 35-mg tablet of risedronate and six 500-mg tablets of calcium carbonate.

Ibandronate Sodium (Boniva). Ibandronate sodium was approved in May 2003 for the treatment and prevention of osteoporosis in postmenopausal women. Its mechanism of action is identical to the other bisphosphonate agents. Administered daily (2.5 mg), ibandronate has been clinically shown to reduce the risk of vertebral fractures by 62% (35). If administered on an intermittent basis (20 mg), it reduces the risk of vertebral fractures by 50%. Ibandronate (2.5 mg daily), along with 500 mg of supplemental calcium, has been clinically shown to increase BMD in the hip (1.8%), femoral neck (2.0%), and lumbar spine (3.1%). The 150-mg formulation approved in March 2005 represents the first oral therapy for a chronic disease to be administered once monthly.

The oral bioavailability of this agent is extremely poor (0.6%) and is adversely affected by the presence of food, beverages other than water, and other medications, including calcium or vitamin D supplements and antacids. Because of the increased calcium content in mineral water, patients should not take this medication with this type of water. Drugs that inhibit gastric acid secretion (e.g., H_2 antagonists and proton-pump inhibitors) actually promote ibandronate absorption. Like the others in this therapeutic class, ibandronate is not metabolized, and that which is not bound to the bone (40–50% of the absorbed dose) is eliminated renally unchanged. It does not inhibit the cytochrome P450 (CYP450) isozymes. This agent does not require any dosage adjustment for patients with hepatic impairment or mild to moderate renal impairment (creatinine clearance, >30 mL/min). Ibandronate should not be prescribed for patients with severe renal impairment (creatinine clearance, <30 mL/min).

Osteonecrosis of the jaw has been reported in patients receiving IV bisphosphonate therapy. The majority of the patients who developed osteonecrosis of the jaw were undergoing chemotherapy, taking corticosteroids, and had undergone a dental procedure (e.g., tooth extraction). The U.S. FDA recommends that patients receive a thorough dental examination before initiation of IV bisphosphonate therapy and that they avoid invasive dental work during treatment.

The remaining two bisphosphonates, pamidronate and zoledronic acid, are approved for treatment of hypercalcemia of malignancy as well as other cancer conditions and will be discussed later in the chapter.

Calcitonin (Calcimar [IV, SC]; Miacalcin and Fertical [nasal spray])

Calcitonin (see earlier discussion in this chapter) has been approved for the treatment of postmenopausal osteoporosis, hypercalcemia of malignancy, and Paget's disease of the bone. Several sources are available (e.g., eel, human, salmon, and porcine). The calcitonin isolated from salmon is the preferred source, because it has greater receptor affinity and a longer half-life than the human hormone (3,7). Calcitonin is commercially available as synthetic calcitonin-salmon, which contains the same linear sequence of 32 amino acids, as occurs in natural calcitonin-salmon. Calcitonin-salmon differs structurally from human calcitonin at 16 of 32 amino acids (see Fig. 7.16 for primary structure differences between human and salmon calcitonin). The pharmacological activity of these calcitonins is the same, but calcitonin-salmon is approximately 50-fold more potent on a weight basis than human calcitonin with a longer duration of action. The duration of action for calcitonin salmon is 8 to 24 hours following intramuscular (IM) or subcutaneous (SC) administration and 0.5 to 12.0 hours following IV administration. The parenteral dose required for the treatment of osteoporosis is 100 IU/day (33). Initially only available by IM or SC injection, the peptide hormone calcitonin-salmon is available as a nasal spray (Miacalcin) and as a rectal suppository (6). A recombinant DNA form of calcitonin salmon was approved by the U.S. FDA in 2005 and is available as a nasal spray. The bioavailability of calcitonin-salmon nasal spray shows great variability (range, 0.3–30.6% of an IM dose). It is absorbed rapidly from the nasal mucosa, with peak plasma concentrations appearing 30 to 40 minutes after nasal administration, compared with 16 to 25 minutes following parental dosing. Calcitonin-salmon is readily metabolized in the kidney, with an elimination half-life calculated at 43 minutes. As a result, the intranasal dose required is 200 IU/day (3). Once the Miacalcin nasal pump has been activated, the bottle may be kept at room temperature until the medication is finished (2 weeks).

THERAPEUTIC APPLICATION. Calcitonin therapy requires the concomitant oral administration of elemental calcium (500 mg/day). Clinical studies have shown that the combination of intranasal calcitonin salmon (200 IU/day), oral calcium supplementation (>1,000 mg/day of elemental calcium), and vitamin D (400 IU/day) has decreased the rate of new fractures by more than 75% and has improved vertebral BMD by as much as 3% annually (3). Calcitonin prevents the abnormal bone turnover characteristic of Paget's disease of the bone and has antiresorptive activity. In the presence of calcitonin, the osteoclast brush borders disappear, and the osteoclasts move away from the bone surface undergoing remodeling (36). Side effects are significantly more pronounced when calcitonin-salmon is administered by injection and can include nausea, vomiting, anorexia, and flushing. Because calcitonin-salmon is protein in nature, the possibility of a systemic allergic reaction should be considered, and appropriate measures for treatment of hypersensitivity reaction should be readily available. Although calcitonin-salmon does not cross the placenta, it may pass into breast milk. Calcitonin-salmon is a possible alternative to ERT; however, only limited evidence suggests that it has efficacy in women who already have fractures. Resistance to calcitonin-salmon can result from the development of neutralizing antibodies (37).

In addition to its antiresorptive action via suppression of osteoclast activity, calcitonin-salmon exhibits a potent analgesic effect and has provided considerable relief to those patients suffering from the pain associated with Paget's disease and osteoporosis. This analgesic effect is a result of calcitonin-stimulated endogenous opioid release. The potency of this analgesic effect has been demonstrated to be 30- to 50-fold that of morphine in selected patients. Calcitonin is preferred over estrogen and the bisphosphonates when treatment of both osteoporosis and related bone pain is warranted.

Bone-Forming Agents

Teriparatide (Forteo)

In 2002, the U.S. FDA approved teriparatide for the treatment of postmenopausal osteoporosis in patients who have a high risk of fracture as well as to increase bone mass in men with primary or hypogonadal osteoporosis who have a high risk of fracture (38). Teriparatide is recombinant human PTH 1-34 (see p. 937), the biologically active portion of the endogenously produced preprohormone. Unlike the bisphosphonates, which are classified as bone restorative agents, teriparatide is the first approved bone-forming agent. Bone formation is possible because of the ability of this agent to increase the number of osteoblasts. Although teriparatide enhances the function of both osteoclasts and osteoblasts, the exposure incidence dictates its effect on the skeleton. If administered once daily or intermittently, teriparatide preferentially enhances osteoblastic function, and bone formation occurs. Continuous exposure to endogenous PTH may result in poor skeletal composition because of enhanced osteoclast-mediated bone resorption (36). After 18 months of treatment, lumbar BMD increased up to 12% in postmenopausal women. After 10 months of treatment, 53% of men had an increase of 5% or greater in spine BMD. The risk for developing new vertebral fractures was reduced by 65% after 21 months of treatment, and the number of nonvertebral fragility fractures was reduced by 53% (23).

Administered as a once-daily, 20-μg SC injection in the thigh or abdominal wall, teriparatide is a clear, colorless liquid that is available as a 750 μg/3 mL, prefilled, disposable pen that requires refrigeration. Concurrent calcium (1,000 mg) and vitamin D (400 IU) supplementation is recommended. Treatment for longer than 2 years is not recommended. Teriparatide is rapidly absorbed, demonstrates 95% bioavailability, and is quickly eliminated via both hepatic and extrahepatic routes. The half life is 1 hour when administered SC. Metabolic studies have not been performed on teriparatide; however, the entire PTH preprohormone has been shown to undergo enzyme-mediated transformations in the liver. Dizziness and leg cramps are the most commonly reported adverse side effects.

Temporary increases in serum calcium levels occur following administration of teriparatide. As a result, this agent is contraindicated in patients who are predisposed to hypercalcemia. Some evidence suggests that these elevations in serum calcium levels may cause a patient who is taking digitalis to experience digitalis toxicity (39). Teriparatide should not be prescribed to patients with Paget's disease, children, young adults, women who are pregnant or nursing, and those patients who have received skeletal radiation therapy (36). Because of an increased incidence of osteosarcoma (malignant bone tumors) observed in rats, teriparatide also carries a black box warning.

> An New Drug Application (NDA) for a full-length recombinant human parathyroid hormone (Preos) is currently under review by the U.S. FDA.

Inorganic Salts

Calcium salts. Appropriate intake of calcium during childhood, adolescence, and early adulthood increases peak BMD and may reduce the overall risk of developing osteoporosis. For those who are at low risk of developing osteoporosis and have adequate BMD, consumption of the recommended amounts of calcium (1,200–1,500 mg of elemental calcium per day for teenagers, 1,000 mg/day for premenopausal women and men, up to 1,500 mg/day for postmenopausal women not taking ERT, and 1,000 mg/day for postmenopausal women taking ERT) typically is sufficient to prevent bone loss (15). This often can be accomplished by eating a well-balanced diet. For those patients with established osteoporosis or areas of poorly mineralized bone, calcium supplementation alone is not sufficient to reverse the bone loss or to significantly improve mineralization of the bone (11).

The actual amount of elemental calcium that is present in the available calcium salts varies considerably; however, no one particular salt has been identified as an exceptional source of elemental calcium (Table 35.8). Absorption of calcium from the gastrointestinal tract (25–40%) improves under acidic conditions; therefore, those medications that change the acidic environment of the stomach (e.g., H_2 antagonists and proton-pump inhibitors) have an adverse effect on calcium absorption (3). Total daily doses of elemental calcium that exceed 500 mg should be spaced out over the day to improve absorption (5,15). The more water soluble and, therefore, more easily absorbed salts (e.g., citrate, lactate, and

Table 35.8. Percent of Elemental Calcium Content in Various Salts (3)

Salt	Calcium (%)	Elemental Calcium (mg/tablet)
Calcium carbonate	40	
Tums (500 mg chewable)		200 mg
Titrilac (1 g/5 mL suspension)		400 mg/5 mL
Alka-Mints (850 mg chewable)		340 mg
Os-Cal 500 (1,250 mg table)		500 mg
Viactive (1,250 mg chewable)		500 mg
Tricalcium phosphate	39	
Calcium chloride	27	
Tribasic calcium phosphate	23	
Posture (1,565.2 mg tablets)		600 mg
Calcium citrate	21	
Citrical (950 mg tablets)		200 mg
Citrical Liquitab (2,376 mg effervescent tabs)		500 mg
Calcium lactate	13	
Generics (325 mg tablets)		42 mg
Generics (650 mg tablets)		84 mg
Calcium gluconate	9	
Neo-Calglucon (1.8 g/5 mL syrup)		115 mg/5 mL

gluconate) are less dependent on the acidic environment for appropriate absorption and would be appropriate alternatives for patients who produce low levels of acid. Calcium carbonate is a poorly soluble form of calcium, but it is inexpensive and only requires the patient to take a few tablets per day with acidic food or beverages like citrus juice (15).

Sodium fluoride. Sodium fluoride (NaF) promotes the proliferation and activity of osteoblasts and is classified as a nonhormonal bone-forming agent. Because treatment with NaF induces bone formation, it is essential that this therapy be coupled with oral calcium supplementation (1,000 mg/day). Additionally, NaF exhibits moderate antiresorptive activity, because it inhibits osteoclastic activity when it is absorbed into the bone matrix. In the treatment of osteoporosis, the therapeutic window for this agent is fairly narrow: Doses less than 45 mg/day are subtherapeutic, and doses in excess of 75 mg/day impair bone mineralization. In addition, the bone that is formed in the presence of NaF is neither as well mineralized nor as strong as normal bone tissue. In fact, some studies have demonstrated that patients taking sodium fluoride have increased bone fragility despite the increase in bone mass and, as a result, have an increased nonvertebral fracture rate as compared to the placebo group (5,21,33). As a result, its use in the treatment of osteoporosis has not been approved and is considered to be somewhat controversial. Several studies have examined the benefits of continuous versus cyclic dosing of NaF in the treatment of osteoporosis. Intermittent dosing (25 mg b.i.d. for 12 months, followed by 2 months of calcium supplementation alone) of a slow-release formulation of sodium fluoride (SR-NaF; Neosten) with 400 mg of calcium citrate was shown to effectively improve bone mass (vertebra, 5% per year; femoral neck, 2% per year) as well as to decrease the number of vertebral fractures (40,41).

Miscellaneous Therapies

Various classes of drugs, such as thiazide diuretics, proton-pump inhibitors, androgens, PTH, statins, and human monoclonal antibody, have been shown to have beneficial effects in treatment of diseases associated with abnormal calcium homeostasis through various mechanisms.

The thiazide diuretics, which reduce urinary calcium excretion, also may reduce the rate of bone loss (33). This protective effect has been shown to vanish within 4 to 5 months after discontinuation of the thiazide.

Elevated concentrations of proton-pump inhibitors, such as omeprazole, have been shown to inhibit bone resorption via inhibition of H^+,K^+-ATPase, a potential energy pump located in the osteoclast ruffled border (30).

Androgens such as stanozolol (11), nandrolone (11), methandrostenolone, and the testosterone patch have been shown to increase bone mass by 5 to 10% and may be appropriate for men with a deficiency in testosterone.

An increase in trabecular bone mass by as much as 50% has been demonstrated in patients treated with low doses of PTH, but it comes at the expense of the cortical bone (1,11,25). Treatment with high doses of PTH is correlated with stimulation of bone resorption (20). Cyclical therapy with PTH and calcitonin has been shown to improve BMD in the spine without adverse effects in the cortical bone (11). When given in combination with estrogen, PTH promoted the formation of well-mineralized trabecular bone.

Strontium ranelate is an orally active agent that can be classified as both an antiresorptive agent and a bone-forming agent (42,43). It is able not only to stimulate replication of preosteoblastic cells to promote bone formation but also is able to decrease osteoclastic activity to prevent bone resorption. Biochemical markers for bone formation (e.g., bone-specific alkaline phosphatase), which normally decrease in the presence of antiresorptive therapy, are elevated in the presence of strontium ranelate (44). Lumbar spine BMD increased 11.4% in patients treated with this new agent.

The hydroxymethylglutaryl–coenzyme A (HMG-CoA) reductase inhibitors, otherwise known as the statins, have been found to increase bone formation via enhanced activity of the bone morphogenic protein 2 (*BMP-2*) gene. This gene increases osteoblast differentiation. In addition, by inhibiting HMG-CoA reductase, the statins not only prevent the biosynthesis of cholesterol but also prevent the formation of compounds associated with osteoclast activation (45). Unfortunately, clinical data from several large studies conflict, and further study is warranted before the statins can be considered as a viable treatment for osteoporosis (46).

AMG-162 (Amgen) is a fully human monoclonal antibody to the receptor activator of nuclear factor κB ligand (RANKL). Its receptor is located on the surface of osteoclasts and osteoclast precursors. When bound to its receptor, RANKL promotes the formation and activation of osteoclasts. To balance the effects of RANKL, the body produces osteopotegerin, which binds to RANKL and prevents it from binding to and activating its receptor, modulating the production and activation of osteoclasts (47). When an individual develops osteoporosis, this balance is "disrupted," and RANKL overwhelms osteopotegerin activity, causing significant bone loss. AMG-162 was designed to mimic the biochemical effects of osteopotegerin. Studies show that AMG-162 is more effective in improving BMD (4–7%) than weekly administration of alendronate (5%) (47). It is anticipated that this agent will be administered SC biannually. The most commonly reported adverse effect is dyspepsia.

There are a number of agents in the pipeline (Table 35.9), some with very novel mechanisms of action, including inhibitors of cathepsin B and protein tyrosine kinase Src, as well as antagonists at $\alpha_v\beta_3$ integrin receptors (48).

DRUG THERAPIES USED TO TREAT HYPERPARATHYROIDISM

Increased levels of PTH leads to moderately to severely elevated serum calcium concentrations (2) and alterations in phosphorous metabolism. To modulate the levels of PTH released from the parathyroid gland chief cells, regulation of CaSR sensitivity is required. An agonist at this receptor, a calcimimetic, serves to activate the receptor, whereas an antagonist at this receptor is classified as a calcilytic. There are two types of calcimimetic agents: those that activate the CaSR directly (type I), and those that require the presence of a cation, such as calcium or magnesium (type II) for activation (49). Type I calcimimetics are polycations (e.g., magnesium and neomycin). The first- and second-generation of type II calcimimetics are phenylalkylamine based. They have an indirect/allosteric action on CaSR mediated by a conformational alteration of these receptors.

Cinacalcet Hydrochloride (Sensipar)

Cinacalcet is the first type II calcimimetic agent approved that improves CaSR sensitivity to calcium (19,50). When calcium is bound to the CaSR, phospholipase C is activated, and the secretion of PTH is inhibited. In the presence of cinacalcet, not only is a drop in

Table 35.9. Experimental Agents for Treatment of Abnormal Calcium Homeostatis

Drug	Chemical Structure	Mechanism of Action	Stage of Clinical Trial
Precos (recombinant PTH)	34 amino acids	Treatment of osteoporosis	Phase III
SB-357114	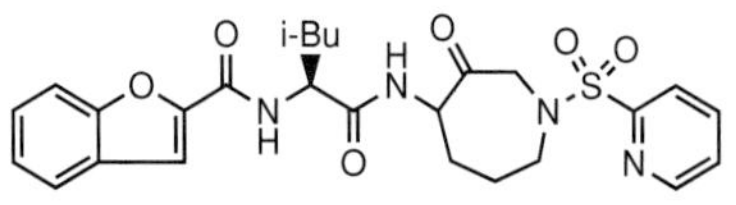 [structure]	Cathepsin K inhibitor	Phase I
Osteoprotegerin	—	Inhibitor of osteoclast differentiation and function	Phase II
Nitroflurbiprofen (HC–1026)	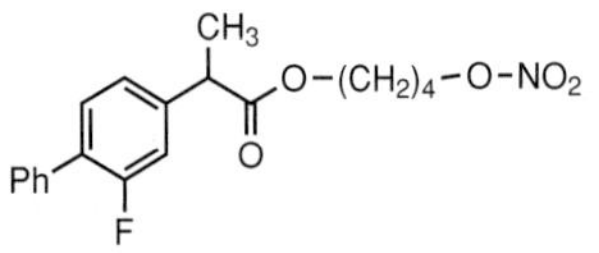 [structure: Ph, F, CH₃, O–(CH₂)₄–O–NO₂]	Nitrosylated nonsteroidal anti-inflammatory—decreases bone resorption	Phase II
CGP-77675 and	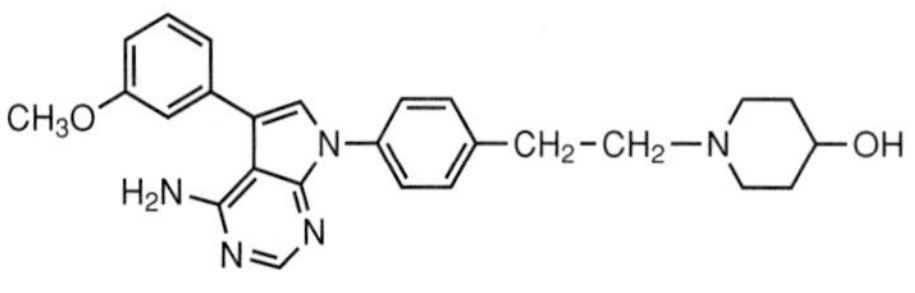 [structure: CH₃O, H₂N, N, –CH₂–CH₂–N, OH]	Protein tyrosine kinase Src inhibitor—decreases osteoclast mediated bone resorption	Preclinical
AP 23588	—		
SB-265123	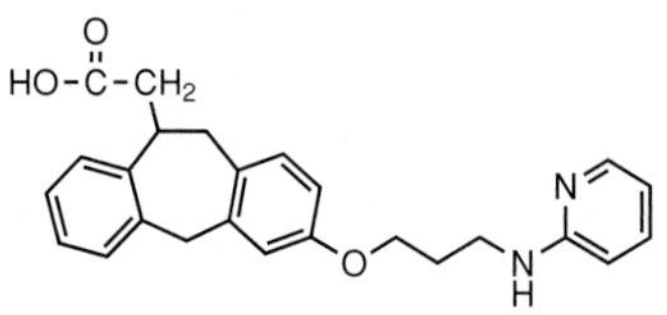 [structure: HO–C(=O)–CH₂]	$\alpha_v\beta_3$ Integrin receptor antagonist	Preclinical

PTH levels observed but also a decrease in serum calcium and phosphorous levels. This represents a significant therapeutic advantage over vitamin D–based treatments for secondary hyperparathyroidism (19). Cinacalcet hydrochloride is a second-generation calcimimetic approved for the treatment of secondary hyperparathyroidism in patients with chronic kidney disease on dialysis and for the treatment of hypercalcemia in patients with parathyroid cancer. It can be used alone, with vitamin D, and/or with a phosphate binder (51).

Cinacalcet hydrochloride (Sensipar)

DRUG THERAPIES USED TO TREAT HYPERCALCEMIA OF MALIGNANCY

Zoledronic Acid (Zometa)

Zoledronic acid, a bisphosphonate, was approved by the U.S. FDA in 2001 for the treatment of hypercalcemia of malignancy, a metabolic complication that can be life-threatening (Fig. 35.7). Hypercalcemia of malignancy can occur in up to 50% of patients diagnosed with advanced breast cancer, multiple myeloma, and nonsmall cell lung cancer. This condition arises when chemical moieties produced by the tumor cause overstimulation of osteoclasts. When there is an increase in bone degradation, there is a concomitant release of calcium into the plasma. When serum concentrations of calcium rapidly elevate, the kidneys are unable to handle the overload, and hypercalcemia results. This can lead to dehydration, nausea, vomiting, fatigue, and confusion. Zoledronic acid effectively decreases plasma calcium concentrations via inhibition of bone resorption (inhibition of osteoclastic activity and induction of osteoclast apoptosis). It also prevents the increase in osteoclastic activity caused by tumor-based stimulatory factors. Additionally zoledronic acid has been approved by the U.S. FDA for the treatment of multiple myeloma and bone metastases associated with solid tumor–based cancers (e.g., prostrate and lung). This agent is currently in late-stage clinical trials for the treatment and prevention of osteoporosis and, if approved, will be formulated as a 5-mg, once-yearly IV infusion.

The maximum recommended dose for the treatment of hypercalcemia of malignancy is 4 mg. A clinically significant deterioration in renal function occurs when single doses of this agent exceed 4 mg and the infusion duration is less than 15 minutes (52). It is recommended that patients be well hydrated before infusion. If serum calcium levels do not fall to normal levels, retreatment is appropriate, but retreatment is not recommended until 7 days have elapsed from the initial treatment. For the treatment of multiple myeloma and metastatic bone lesions, a 4-mg initial dose is recommended, followed by additional doses every 3 to 4 weeks for 9 to 15 months (prostate cancer, 15 months; breast cancer, 12 months; other solid tumors, 9 months).

Zoledronic acid is a white, crystalline powder that is available in vials for reconstitution for IV infusion over at least 15 minutes. It does not undergo metabolic transformation and does not inhibit CYP450 enzymes. Clearance of this agent is dependent on the patient's creatinine clearance, not on dose. Serum creatinine levels should be evaluated before every treatment. Zolendronic acid is contraindicated in patients with severe renal impairment.

Zolendronic acid should not be mixed with infusion solutions that contain calcium (e.g., lactated Ringer's) and should be administered via IV infusion in its own line. Because of the possibility of a serious deterioration in renal function, the manufacturer requires strict adherence to the infusion duration being no less than 15 minutes.

Pamidronate Disodium (Aredia)

Pamidronate, a second-generation bisphosphonate, is 100-fold more potent than etidronate (Fig. 35.7) (6). It has been approved for the treatment of hypercalcemia of malignancy, for Paget's disease, and for osteolytic bone metastases of breast cancer and osteolytic lesions of multiple myeloma. When used to treat bone metastases, pamidronate decreases osteoclast recruitment, decreases osteoclast activity and increases osteoclast apoptosis (53). Erosive esophagitis has been reported with the use of pamidronate sodium.

Gallium Nitrate (Ganite)

Gallium nitrate (Ganite) has been approved for the treatment of hypercalcemia of malignancy (33) in patients that do not respond to hydration. Its effectiveness stems from its ability to inhibit bone resorption despite the presence of tumor-derived factors that promote calcium loss from the bone. Administered by infusion over 24 hours, the typical dose is 200 mg/m^2/day for five consecutive days. A lower dose is recommended if the symptoms of hypercalcemia are mild (100 mg/m^2/day for 5 days). Steady state is achieved in 24 to 48 hours. Maintenance of patient hydration is essential during treatment. Gallium nitrate is not significantly metabolized and is largely excreted through the kidneys. It is contraindicated in patients with severe renal impairment. Renal function should be closely monitored in all patients receiving this agent.

CASE STUDY

Victoria F. Roche and S. William Zito

PA is a 62-year-old Caucasian female who presents to the emergency room with a complaint of persistent lower back pain for the past 2 weeks. She says that she "just woke up one morning with the back pain." While having her history taken, PA reveals that she was diagnosed with rheumatoid arthritis 6 years ago, which was 3 months after her second mastectomy for breast cancer. PA went through menopause 10 years ago, has not undergone hysterectomy, and has been on Synthroid (25 μg/daily) since she was surgically treated for hyperthyroidism at the age of 25. PA claims that her thyroid function was normal at her last visit to her endocrinologist. Currently, PA is being treated with the following drugs for her RA:

Sulfasalazine	(500-mg tablets, three tablets b.i.d.)
Oxycodone	(5-mg tablets; as needed for pain)
Methotrexate	(2.5-mg tablets, eight tablets weekly)
Prednisone	(10-mg tablets, one tablet daily for flare-ups)
Hydrochlorthiazide	(12.5-mg tablets; one tablet daily for ankle edema)

On further questioning, PA reports that flare-ups requiring her to go on prednisone have occurred at least twice a year since she was first diagnosed with rheumatoid arthritis. The emergency room physician ordered a dual-energy x-ray absorptiometry scan of the spine and requested a lateral spine image to be done at the same time. A diagnosis of osteoporosis was made based on the presence of vertebral fracture and a T value for bone mass density (BMD) of 2.0 standard deviations below the young adult mean. In addition to calcium carbonate (500 mg t.i.d.) and vitamin D (400 U q.d.), the physician wants to prescribe calcium antiresorptive therapy for PA, and you have the following drugs available from the hospital formulary. Make a recommendation.

OH, C≡CH, HO — 1

H_3C, $PO_3H^{\ominus}$ $Na^{\oplus}$, HO, $PO_3H^{\ominus}$ $Na^{\oplus}$ — 2

CH_3, H_3C-N, O, CH_3 — 3

$PO_3H^{\ominus}$ $Na^{\oplus}$, N, HO, $PO_3H^{\ominus}$ $Na^{\oplus}$ — 4

1. Identify the therapeutic problem(s) in which the pharmacist's intervention may benefit the patient.
2. Identify and prioritize the patient-specific factors that must be considered to achieve the desired therapeutic outcomes.
3. Conduct a thorough and mechanistically oriented structure–activity analysis of all therapeutic alternatives provided in the case.
4. Evaluate the SAR findings against the patient-specific factors and desired therapeutic outcomes, and make a therapeutic decision.
5. Counsel your patient.

References

1. Copp DH. Calcitonin: discovery, development, and clinical application. Clin Invest Med 1994;17:268–277.
2. Bouillon R, Carmeliet G, Boonen S. Aging and calcium metabolism. Bailliere's Clin Endocrinol Metab 1997;11:341–365.
3. Haines ST, Caceres B, Yancey L. Alternatives to estrogen replacement therapy for preventing osteoporosis. J Am Pharm Assoc 1996;36(12):707–715.
4. Christenson RH. Biochemical markers of bone metabolism: an overview. Clin Biochem 1997;30:573–593.
5. Miller DR, Hanel HJ. Prevention and treatment of osteoporosis. US Pharmacist 1999;24:81–90.
6. Rodan GA. Emerging therapies in osteoporosis. Ann Rpts Med Chem 1994;29:275–285.
7. Arnaud CD. Calcium homeostasis: regulatory elements and their integration. Fed Proc 1978;37:2557–2560.
8. Iqbal J, Zaidi M, Schneider AE. Cinacalcet hydrochloride. IDrugs 2003;6:587–592.
9. DeLuca HF, Zierold C. Mechanisms and functions of vitamin D. Nutr Rev 1998;56:S4–S10.
10. Schaefer B, Cone S. Increasing awareness of osteoporosis: a community pharmacy's experience. US Pharmacist 1998;23:72–85.
11. Francis RM. Management of established osteoporosis. Br J Clin Pharmacol 1998;45:95–99.
12. Saljoughian M. Postmenopausal osteoporosis. US Pharmacy 2003;28(9):18–35.
13. Reid DM, Harvie J. Secondary osteoporosis. Bailliere's Clin Endocrinol Metab 1997;11:83–99.
14. Hansen LB, Follin Vondracek S. Prevention and treatment of nonpostmenopausal osteoporosis. Am J Health-Syst Pharm 2004;61:2637–2656.
15. American Pharmaceutical Association. Special Report. Therapeutic Options for Osteoporosis. Washington, DC, 1993.
16. Tolar J, Teitelbaum SL, Orchard PJ. Osteopetrosis. N Engl J Med 2004;351:2839–2849.
17. Whyte MP, Wenkert D, Clements KL, et al. Bisphosphonate-induced osteoporosis. N Engl J Med 2003;349:457–463.
18. Pegoraro AA, Rutecki GM. Hypocalcemia. Available at: http://www.emedicine.com/med/topic1118.htm. Accessed June 13, 2005.
19. Block GA, Martin, KJ, De Franciso Al. Cinacalcet for secondary hyperparathyroidism in patients receiving hemodialysis. N Engl J Med 2004;350:1516–1525.
20. Reginster J-YL, LeCart M-P. Efficacy and safety of drugs for Paget's disease of bone. Bone 1995;17:485S–488S.
21. De Silva Jardine P, Thompson D. Antiosteoporosis agents. Ann Rpts Med Chem 1996;31:211–220.
22. Hisel TM, Phillips BB. Update on the treatment of osteoporosis. Formulary 2003;38:223–243.
23. Greenblatt D. Treatment of postmenopausal osteoporosis. Pharmacotherapy 2005;25:574–584.
24. Francis RM. Bisphosphonates in the treatment of osteoporosis in 1997: a review. Curr Ther Res 1997;58:656–678.
25. Yates AJ, Rodan GA. Alendronate and osteoporosis. Drug Discovery Today 1998;3:69–78.
26. Speroff L, Clarkson TB. Is tibolone a viable alternative to HT? Cont OB/GYN 2003;48(8):54–68.
27. Kemp DC, Fan PW, Stevens JC. Characterization of raloxifene glucuronidation in vitro: contribution of intestinal metabolism to presystemic clearance. Drug Metab Dispos 2002;30:694–700.
28. Jeong EJ, Lin H, Hu M. Disposition mechanisms of raloxifene in the human intestinal Caco-2 model. J Pharmacol Exp Ther 2004;310:376–386.
29. Jeong EJ, Liu Y, Lin H, et al. Species- and disposition model-dependent metabolism of raloxifene in gut and liver: role of UGT1A10. Drug Metab Dispos 2005;33:785–794.
30. Gennari L. Ospemifene. Curr Opin Investig Drugs 2004;5:448-455.
31. Gruber C, Gruber D. Bazedoxifene. Curr Opin Investig Drugs 2004;5: 1086–1093.
32. Diener KM. Bisphosphonates for controlling pain from metastatic bone disease. Am J Health-Syst Pharm 1996;53:1917–1927.
33. Caggiano TJ, Zask A, Bex F. Recent advances in bone metabolism and osteoporosis research. Ann Rpts Med Chem 1991;26.

34. Ashworth L. Focus on alendronate. Formulary 1996;31:23–30.
35. Riley TN, DeRuitter J. US Pharmacist 2003:95–104.
36. Reginster J. Calcitonin for prevention and treatment of osteoporosis. Am J Med 1993;95(Suppl 5A):44S–47S.
37. Gennari C, Agnusdei D, Camporeale A. Long-term treatment with calcitonin in osteoporosis. Horm Metab Res 1993;25:484–485.
38. Freeman TR. Teriparatide: a novel agent that builds new bone. J Am Pharm Assoc 2003;43:535–537.
39. LoBuono C. New osteoporosis drug is first to form bone. Drug Topics 2003:24.
40. American Pharmaceutical Association. New Product Bulletin. Miacalcin Nasal Spray. Washington, DC, 1996.
41. Pak CYC, Sakhaee K, Rubin C, et al. Update of fluoride in the treatment of osteoporosis. The Endocrinologist 1998;8:15–20.
42. Meunier PJ, et al. The effects of strontium ranelate on the risk of vertebral fracture in women with postmenopausal osteoporosis. N Engl J Med 2004;350:459–468.
43. Reginster J-Y, Lecart M-P, Deroisy R, et al. Strontium ranelate—a new paradigm in the treatment of osteoporosis. Expert Opin Investig Drugs 2004; 13:857–864.
44. Marie PJ. Strontium ranelate: a novel mode of action optimizing bone formation and resorption. Osteoporosis Int 2005;16(Suppl 1):S7–S10.
45. Gonyeau M. Statins and osteoporosis: a clinical review. Pharmacotherapy 2005;25:229–243.
46. Richard AA, Harrison TM. Efficacy of HMG-CoA reductase inhibitors in treating osteoporosis. Am J Health-Syst Pharm 2002;59:372–377.
47. Bekker PJ, et al. A single-dose placebo-controlled study of AMG 162, a fully human monoclonal antibody to RANKL in postmenopausal women. J Bone Miner Res 2004;19:1059–1066.
48. Biskobing DM. Novel therapies for osteoporosis. Expert Opin Investig Drugs 2003;12:611–621.
49. Joy MS, Kshirsagar A, Franceschini N. Calcimimetics and the treatment of primary and secondary hyperparathyroidism. Ann Pharmacother 2004;38:171–180.
50. Franceschini N, Joy MS, Kshirsagar A. Cinacalcet HCl: a calcimimetic agent for the treatment of primary and secondary hypoparathyroidism. Expert Opin Investig Drugs 2003;12:1413–1421.
51. Hussar DA. New drugs of 2004. J Am Pharm Assoc 2005;45:185–218.
52. Zometa prescribing information.
53. Van Poznak CH. The use of bisphosphonates in patients with breast cancer. Cancer Control 2002;9:480–489.

SECTION 4 Drugs Affecting the Immune System

36. *Nonsteroidal Anti-Inflammatory Drugs*

RONALD BORNE, MARK LEVI AND NORMAN WILSON

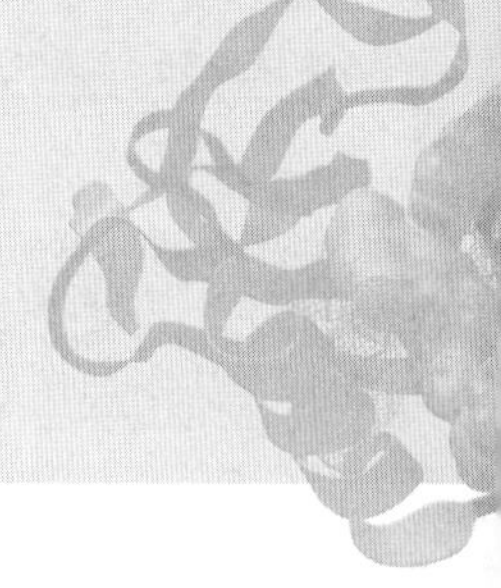

DRUGS COVERED IN THIS CHAPTER:

ANTIPYRETIC ANALGESICS
- Acetaminophen

ANTI-INFLAMATORY ANALGESICS
- Aspirin and other salicylates
- Diflunisal
- Indomethacin
- Diclofenac
- Etodolac
- Nabumetone
- Sulindac
- Tolmetin
- Ibuprofen
- Fenoprofen
- Flurbiprofen
- Ketoprofen
- Ketoraloc
- Naproxen
- Oxaprozin
- Suprofen
- Mefenamic acid
- Meclofenamic acid
- Piroxicam
- Meloxicam

COX-2 INHIBITORS
- Celecoxib
- Rofecoxib
- Valdecoxib
- Etoricoxib
- Lumiracoxib

DISEASE MODIFYING DRUGS FOR ARTHRITIS
- Gold salts
- Hydroxychloroquine
- Methotrexate
- Leflunomide
- Etanercept
- Infliximab
- Adalimumab
- Rituximab
- Anakinra
- Abatacept

DRUGS FOR THE TREATMENT OF GOUT
- Colchicine
- Probenecid
- Sulfinpyrazone
- Allopurinol

INTRODUCTION

The classification of drugs covered in this chapter as nonsteroidal anti-inflammatory drugs (NSAIDs) is somewhat misleading, because many of these entities possess antipyretic and analgetic properties in addition to anti-inflammatory properties, which are useful in the treatment of a number of rheumatic disorders. On the other hand, there are drugs that possess analgetic/antipyretic properties but are essentially devoid of anti-inflammatory activity. Additionally, drugs that possess uricosuric properties useful in the treatment of gout will be covered here. The prototype agent of this class is acetylsalicylic acid, aspirin, which has therapeutically useful analgetic, antipyretic, and anti-inflammatory actions; other drugs to be covered may possess only one or two of these properties. Steroids that are useful anti-inflammatory drugs are covered separately in Chapter 33.

Nonsteroidal anti-inflammatory drugs continue to be one of the more widely used groups of therapeutic drugs. The medicinal drugs covered in this chapter represent a major market in both prescription and nonprescription drugs. Other than caffeine or ethyl alcohol, aspirin may be the most widely used drug in the world (1). An estimated 70 to 100 million prescriptions are written annually for NSAIDs, with over-the-counter (OTC) use accounting for an additional use that may be up to sevenfold higher. Rheumatic diseases, which have been classified by the Arthritis Foundation (Table 36.1) (2), are inflammatory disorders affecting more individuals than any chronic illness. The Centers for Disease Control and Prevention estimates that more than 40 million Americans have some form of arthritis or chronic joint disorder. Approximately 7 million Americans suffer from arthritis in its most debilitating forms (3,4). Osteoarthritis is the most common form of arthritis in the United States, affecting about 12% of Americans between the ages of 25 and 74. Rheumatoid arthritis is thought to affect well over 2 million Americans (two to three times more females more than males), whereas juvenile arthritis affects 71,000 children under 16 years of age, 61,000 of whom are females. In addition, nonrheumatoid osteoporosis affects 24 million females (half of all women older than 45 years and 90% of all women older than 75 years) (3,4) and 16 million males. Because more than 80% of the U.S. population older than 55 years have joint abnormalities that are detectable radiographically (5), the use of NSAIDs will increase as Americans experience a greater life expectancy. It is not surprising, therefore, that the development of new NSAIDs continues at a steady pace—a pace slowed down by the recent controversies surrounding selective cyclooxygenase (COX)-2 inhibitors.

The diseases mentioned are considered to be host defense mechanisms. Inflammation is a normal and essential response to any noxious stimulus that threatens the host and may vary from a localized response to a generalized response (6). The resulting inflammation can be summarized as follows: 1) Initial injury causing release

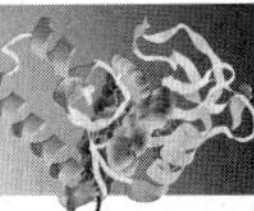

CLINICAL SIGNIFICANCE

The arachidonic acid pathway leading to the production of inflammatory mediators provides several targets for intervention on inflammation. The most widely used nonsteroidal anti-inflammatory drugs (NSAIDs) in practice today are drugs like aspirin, naproxen, ibuprofen, diclofenac, and others that inhibit the cyclooxygenase (COX) enzymes. Although specific NSAIDs have found their niches in particular disease states, the NSAIDs generally work by the same mechanism with little exception. Aspirin, a salicylate, is somewhat different from the other agents in that its property of irreversibly inhibiting platelet homeostasis works to its advantage and broadens its use in coronary artery disease prophylaxis, in which it has been shown to reduce mortality whereas the others have not. Other salicylate varieties lack the ability to irreversibly inhibit platelet function and, therefore, are not clinically useful this way.

Variations on the molecular structures have provided improved side effect profiles of agents used. For example, although phenacetin and acetaminophen are not anti-inflammatory agents, they are included in this chapter, because they are analgesics and antipyretics and illustrate the point that improvement in molecular structure from phenacetin to acetaminophen helped to reduce the hepatotoxicity and risk for drug-induced hemolytic anemia with which phenacetin was associated when it was on the market in the past.

Changes to the currently available NSAIDs are constantly being produced, hence the abundance of "me-too" drugs. With gastrointestinal (GI) bleeding and complications being the most feared consequence of taking these drugs, an emphasis on minimizing these risks has been one of the motivations to develop less offensive agents. Gastrointestinal side effects are believed to be related to indirect toxic effects (inhibiting COX enzymes) and direct toxic effects (local irritation to the GI mucosa). Molecular changes have been made to the various NSAIDs to produce more potent compounds, to reduce the direct irritant effects, and to create pro-drugs that lack the direct irritant effect altogether. Other changes have resulted in compounds with no more potency but with lower incidence of GI side effects, which still represents a therapeutic advantage.

As can be seen, a thorough understanding and appreciation of the chemical nature of the NSAIDs is directly linked to clinically significant end points and positive therapeutic outcomes.

Jill T. Johnson, Pharm.D., BCPS
Associate Professor
Department of Pharmacy Practice
College of Pharmacy
University of Arkansas for Medical Sciences

of inflammatory mediators (e.g., histamine, serotonin, leukokinins, SRS-A, lysosomal enzymes, lymphokinins, and prostaglandins); 2) vasodilation; 3) increased vascular permeability and exudation; 4) leukocyte migration, chemotaxis, and phagocytosis; and 5) proliferation of connective tissue cells. The most common sources of chemical mediators include neutrophils, basophils, mast cells, platelets, macrophages, and lymphocytes (6). The etiology of inflammatory and arthritic diseases has received a great deal of recent attention but remains, for the most part, unresolved, hindering the development of new agents that are curative in nature. Currently available drugs relieve the symptoms of the disease but are not curative.

Anti-inflammatory drugs may act by interfering with any one of several mechanisms, including immunological mechanisms such as antibody production or antigen–antibody complexation, activation of complement, cellular activities such as phagocytosis, interference with the formation and release of the chemical mediators of inflammation, or stabilization of lysosomal membranes. The role of complement in inflammation is of considerable interest (7–9). The complement system is one component of the host defense system that aids in the elimination of various microorganisms and antigens from blood and tissues. Although complement normally plays a functional role in the development of disease states, excessive complement activation, by promoting inflammation locally, is detrimental. Individuals with a deficiency of individual complement proteins, however, either acquired or hereditary, are more susceptible to infections caused by pyrogenic bacteria and diseases resulting from the generation of autoantibodies and immune complexes. Complement proteins are numbered C1 to C9, and their cleavage products are indicated by the suffixes a, b, and so on. The complement system consists of two activating pathways (an antibody-mediated classical pathway and a nonimmunologically activated alternate pathway), a single termination pathway, regulatory proteins, and complement receptors and involves approximately 30 membrane and plasma proteins (8). A major function of complement is to mark antigens and microorganisms with C3 fragments that direct them to cells containing C3 receptors, such as phagocytic cells (8). Complement has been implicated in numerous diseases, including allergic, hematologic, dermatologic, infectious, renal, hepatic inflammatory (rheumatoid arthritis and systemic lupus erythematosus), pulmonary, and others (e.g., multiple sclerosis and myasthenia gravis). Complement activation can induce the synthesis or release of inflammatory mediators, such as interleukin-1 (a potent proinflammatory cytokine) and prostaglandins (e.g., PGE_2). Leukotrienes (e.g., LTB_4) and thromboxanes also are released. Complement

Table 36.1. Classification of Rheumatic Diseases

A. Acute and chronic polyarthritis and other synovial diseases
   Rheumatoid arthritis
B. Infection-related rheumatic diseases
   Septic arthritis
   Osteomyelitis
   Lyme disease
   Rheumatic fever
C. Spondyloarthropathies
   Ankylosing spondylitis
   Reactive arthritis
   Psoriatic arthritis
   Enteropathic spondyloarthropathy (arthritis of inflammatory bowel disease)
D. Osteoarthritis and related degenerative related diseases
E. Crystal-induced arthropathies
   Gout (monosodium urate)
   Calcium pyrophosphate dehydrate, apatite, and other calcium crystals deposited in the joint
G. Metabolic bone disease
   Osteoporosis
H. Connective tissue disease
   Systemic lupus erythematosus
   Scleroderma/polymyositis
   Mixed connective tissue disease
I. Musculoskeletal diseases (regional pain syndromes)
   Neck, lower back and lumbar spine stenosis, shoulder, elbow, wrist and hand, hip, and knee
J. Inflammatory muscle (nonarticular) diseases
   Fibromyalgia
   Bursitis
   Tendinitis
K. Vasculitis
   Polymyalgia rheumatica
L. Sjogren's syndrome
M. Neoplasms
N. Drug-induced rheumatologic syndromes
   Systemic lupus erythematosus
   Glucocorticoid-induced arthritis
   Scleroderma (acrosclerosis)
   Vasculitis
   Statin-induced myositis

From Klippel JH, Wayand CM, Wortmann R, et al., eds. Primer on the Rheumatic Diseases. 12th Ed. Atlanta: Arthritis Foundation, 2001; with permission.

also aids the immigration of phagocytes associated with inflammation. Thus, inhibition of the complement system by controlling its activation or inhibiting those active fragments that are produced should be beneficial in reducing or eliminating tissue damage associated with inflammatory diseases.

Connective tissue diseases include the following states: rheumatoid arthritis, ankylosing spondylitis, systemic lupus erythematosus, polyarteritis nodosa, gout, rheumatic fever, and osteoarthritis, with the most common forms of which are rheumatoid arthritis, osteoporosis, and gout. Rheumatoid arthritis is a chronic, nonsuppurative inflammatory disease of unknown cause affecting primarily peripheral synovial joints. The onset is usually insidious, with immunological reactions playing a major role. The pathogenesis of rheumatoid arthritis has been summarized as follows (10): 1) An unknown initiation factor in the synovial joint causes the production of antigenic immunoglobulin (Ig) G, which stimulates the synthesis of the rheumatoid factors IgM and IgG, forming immune complexes; 2) IgG aggregates activate the complement system, leading to the generation of chemotactic factors (cytokines) that attract polymorphonuclear leukocytes into the articular cavity; 3) the polymorphonuclear leukocytes ingest immune complexes to become rheumatoid arthritis cells, which discharge hydrolases from lysosomal granules that, in turn, degrade extracellular tissue components, polysaccharides, and collagens in cartilage, thus provoking an inflammatory response in rheumatoid joints; and 4) all of which induce expression of cyclooxygenase. Clinical symptoms characteristically include symmetric swelling of at least three joints, accompanied by soft tissue swelling with tenderness, erythema, morning stiffness lasting at least an hour, and pain. The joints primarily involved are those of the extremities, and the patient often suffers a low-grade fever accompanied by malaise, anorexia, and fatigue. Serum protein irregularities and abnormal amounts of rheumatoid factors are common. It often is difficult to distinguish rheumatoid arthritis from other connective tissues disorders because of lack of definitive diagnostic features. Because bone erosions, uniform joint-space narrowing, and osteopenia (decreased bone density) develop within 6 months in about 40% of those with early rheumatoid arthritis, it is more effective to treat early rheumatoid arthritis with disease modifying drug therapy (DMARDs) before structural damage develops than attempting to correct the damage. Corticosteroids are used for controlling the symptoms, not disease modifying.

Osteoarthritis is a degenerative joint disease, and is the most common form of arthritis. It is characterized by degeneration of cartilage and hypertrophy of bone at the articular margin. Secondary inflammation of synovial tissue is common. The most common symptoms involve joint pain associated with movement, joints lose range-of-motion, minimal swelling of the involved joint, and, sometimes, bone enlargement. Weight-bearing joints and joints of the hands and fingers generally are involved. Treatment usually involves exercise and pain medication. Aspirin is considered first-choice therapy, with acetaminophen and NSAIDs being employed in patients who do not tolerate salicylates. Nutritional supplements such as glucosamine and hyaluronic acid have been shown to possibly slow progression of osteoarthritis.

Gout is a metabolic disease characterized by recurrent episodes of acute arthritis, usually monoarticular, and is associated with abnormal levels of uric acid in the body, particularly the presence of monosodium urate crystals in synovial fluid. Primary gout is a hereditary disease in which hyperuricemia is caused by an error in uric acid metabolism—either overproduction or an inability to excrete uric acid. Secondary gout refers to those cases in which hyperuricemia is caused by an acquired disease or disorder, such as chronic renal disease, lead poisoning, or myeloproliferative disorders. Gout generally occurs in mid-life and affects males significantly more than females (9:1). Treatment usually involves the use of uricosuric drugs, colchicine, NSAIDs, or corticosteroids.

The search for new and effective treatment modalities requires the availability of adequate screening tests. Although no model adequately reflects the events that occur in human arthritic conditions, several in vivo and in vitro assays are used. The most common in vivo animal assays measure the ability of anti-inflammatory drugs to inhibit edema induced in the rat paw by carrageenan (a mucopolysaccharide derived from a sea moss of the *Chondrus* species), to inhibit adjuvant arthritis in rats induced by *Mycobacterium butyricum* or *M. tuberculosis*, to inhibit granuloma formation usually induced by the implantation of a cotton pellet beneath the abdominal skin of rats, or to inhibit erythema of guinea pig skin as a result of exposure to ultraviolet radiation. In vitro techniques include the ability of NSAIDs to stabilize erythrocyte membranes or, more commonly, to inhibit the biosynthesis of prostaglandins, particularly in cultured human synoviocytes and chondrocytes, and monocyte culture fluid stimulated bovine synoviocytes and chondrocytes.

ROLE OF CHEMICAL MEDIATORS IN INFLAMMATION

As indicated previously, a number of chemical mediators have been postulated to play important roles in the inflammatory process. Before 1971, the proposal by Shen (11,12) that the NSAIDs exert their effects by interacting with a hypothetical anti-inflammatory receptor was widely accepted. The topography of the proposed receptor was based on known structure–activity relationships primarily within the series of indole acetic acid derivatives, of which indomethacin was the prototype. Most NSAIDs, whether they be salicylates, arylalkanoic acids, oxicams, or anthranilic acid derivatives, possess the common structural features of an acidic center, an aromatic or heteroaromatic ring, and an additional center of lipophilicity in the form of either an alkyl chain or an additional aromatic ring. The proposed receptor to which indomethacin was postulated to bind consisted of a cationic site to which the carboxylate anion would bind, a flat area to which the indole ring would bind through van der Waals forces, and an out-of-the-plane trough to which the benzene ring of the p-chlorobenzoyl group would bind through hydrophobic or charge-transfer interactions. Additional binding sites for the methoxy and carbonyl groups also were suggested. In 1971, Vane (13) published a classic paper in which he reported that indomethacin, aspirin, and salicylate, in this descending order of potency, inhibited the biosynthesis of prostaglandins from arachidonic acid using cell-free preparations of guinea pig lung, and he further suggested that the clinical actions of these drugs resulted from this inhibition. This theory has become the most widely accepted mechanism of action of NSAIDs. Gund and Shen (14) subsequently modified this hypothesis and proposed that the earlier anti-inflammatory receptor model actually described the active site of the key enzyme in prostaglandin biosynthesis (i.e., prostaglandin cyclooxygenase) (Fig. 36.1).

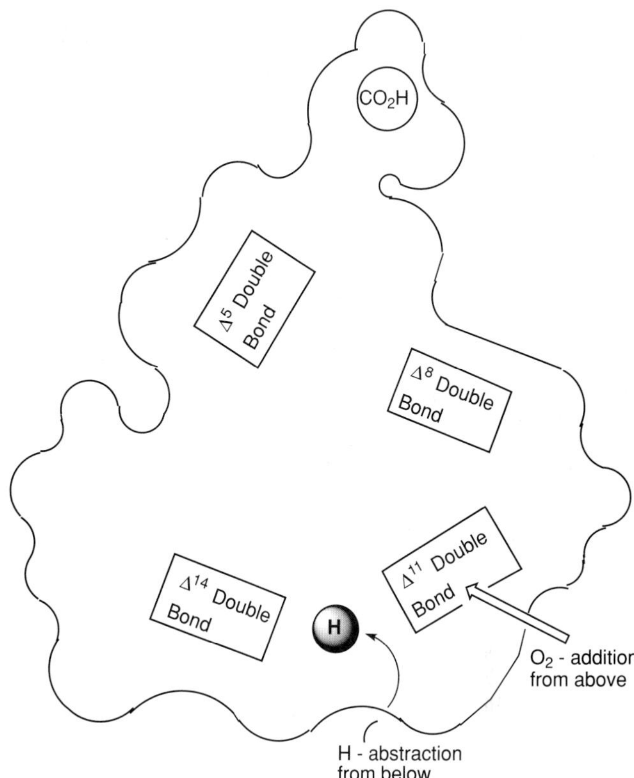

Fig. 36.1. Shen's proposed model of the fatty acid substrate binding site of prostaglandin synthetase. (Modified from Gund P, Shen TY. A model for the prostaglandin synthetase cyclooxygenation site and its inhibition by anti-inflammatory arylacetic acids. J Med Chem 1977;20:1146–1152; with permission.)

Prostaglandins, Thromboxanes, Prostacyclin, and Leukotrienes

Prostaglandins are naturally occurring, 20-carbon, cyclopentano–fatty acid derivatives produced in mammalian tissue from polyunsaturated fatty acids. They belong to the class of eicosanoids, a member of the group of autocoids derived from membrane phospholipids. The eicosanoids are derived from unsaturated fatty acids and include the following groups of compounds: prostaglandins, thromboxanes, prostacyclin, and leukotrienes. They have been found in essentially every compartment of the body. In 1931, Kurzrok and Lieb (15) reported that human seminal fluid possessed potent contractile and relaxant effects on uterine smooth muscle. Shortly thereafter, Goldblatt (16) in England and von Euler (17) in Sweden independently reported vasodepressor and smooth muscle–contracting properties in seminal fluid; von Euler identified the active constituent as a lipophilic acidic substance, which

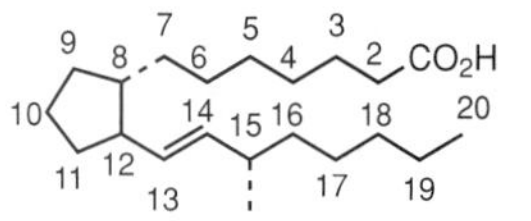

Fig. 36.2. General structure of the prostaglandins.

he termed "prostaglandin." These observations attracted little attention during World War II, but shortly thereafter, primarily through the efforts of Bergstrom and Samuelsson (18), it was realized that von Euler's prostaglandin was actually a mixture of a number of structurally related fatty acids. The first report of the structure of the prostaglandins in 1962 stimulated several studies relating to the chemical and biological properties of these potent substances.

The general structure of the prostaglandins is shown in Figure 36.2. All naturally occurring prostaglandins possess this substitution pattern, a 15α-hydroxy group and a *trans* double bond at C-13. Unless a double bond occurs at the C-8, C-12 positions, the two side chains (the carboxyl-bearing chain termed the α-chain and the hydroxyl-bearing chain termed the β-chain) are of the *trans* stereochemistry depicted. The prostaglandins are classified by the capital letters A, B, C. D, E, F, G, H, and I (e.g., PGA, PGB, and so on) depending on the nature and stereochemistry of oxygen substituents at the 9- and 11-positions. For example, members of the PGE series possess a keto function at C-9 and an α-hydroxyl group at C-11, whereas members of the PGF series possess α-hydroxyl groups at both of these positions. Members of the PGG and PGH series are cycloendoperoxide intermediates in the biosynthesis of prostaglandins, as depicted in Figure 36.3. The number of double bonds in the side chains connected to the cyclopentane ring is designated by subscripts 1, 2, or 3, indicative of the nature of the fatty acid precursor. The subscript 2 indicates an additional *cis* double bond at the C-5, C-6 positions, and the subscript 3 indicates a third double bond of *cis* stereochemistry at the C-17, C-18 positions.

Prostaglandins are derived biosynthetically from unsaturated fatty acid precursors. The number of double bonds contained in the naturally occurring prostaglandins reflects the nature of the biosynthetic precursors. Those containing one double bond are derived from 8,11,14-eicosatrienoic acid, those with two double bonds from arachidonic acid (5,8,11,14-eicosatetraenoic acid), and those with three double bonds from 5,8,11,14,17-eicosapentenoic acid. The most common of these fatty acids in humans is arachidonic acid; hence, prostaglandins of the 2 series play an important biological role. Arachidonic acid is derived from dietary linoleic acid or is ingested from the diet (19) and esterified to phospholipids (primarily phosphatidylethanolamine or phosphatidylcholine) in cell membranes. Various initiating factors interact with membrane receptors coupled to G proteins (guanine nucleotide–binding regulatory proteins) activating phospholipase A_2, which in turn

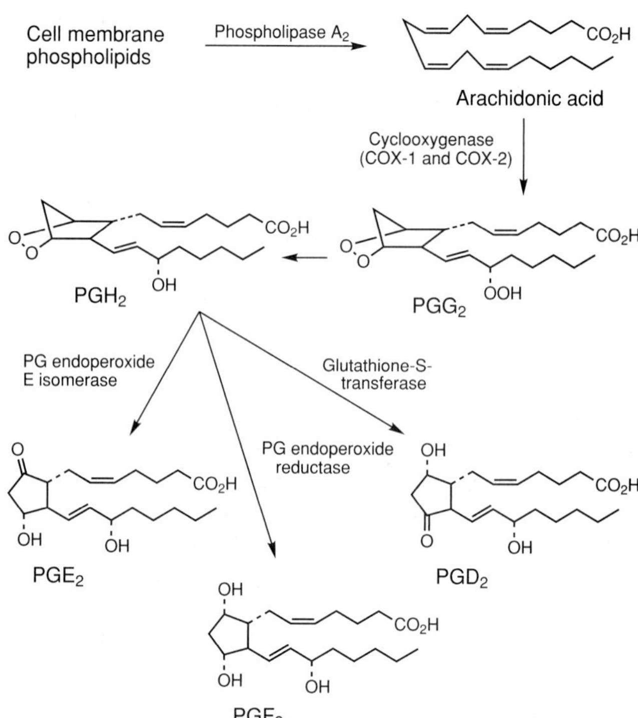

Fig. 36.3. Biosynthesis of prostaglandins from arachidonic acid.

hydrolyzes membrane phospholipids resulting in the release of arachidonic acid. Other phospholipases (e.g., phospholipase C) also are involved. Phospholipase C differs from phospholipase A_2 by inducing the formation of 1,2-diglycerides from phospholipids with the subsequent release of arachidonic acid by the actions of mono- and diglyceride lipases on the diglyceride (17). A polypeptide produced by leukocytes, interleukin-1, which mediates inflammation, increases phospholipase activity and, thus, prostaglandin biosynthesis. The steroidal anti-inflammatory drugs (corticosteroids) appear to act, in part, by inhibiting these phospholipases, particularly phospholipase A_2. The liberated arachidonic acid may then be acted on by two major enzyme systems: by arachidonic acid cyclooxygenase (prostaglandin endoperoxide synthetase, COX) to produce prostaglandins, thromboxanes, and prostacyclin, or by lipoxygenases to produce leukotrienes.

Interaction of arachidonic acid with cyclooxygenase (COX) in the presence of oxygen and heme produces, first, the cyclic endoperoxide, PGG_2, and then, through its peroxidase activity, PGH_2, both of which are chemically unstable and decompose rapidly (half-life, 5 minutes). The PGE_2 is formed by the action of PGE isomerase and PGD_2 by the actions of isomerases or glutathione-S-transferase on PGH_2, whereas $PGF_{2\alpha}$ is formed from PGH_2 via an endoperoxide reductase system (Fig. 36.3). It is the cyclooxygenase step at which the NSAIDs inhibit prostaglandin biosynthesis, preventing inflammation. Because PGG_2 and PGH_2 themselves may possess the ability to mediate the pain responses and produce vasoconstriction, and because PGG_2 may mediate the inflammatory response, cyclooxygenase inhibition would have a profound effect on the reduction of inflammation.

Three isoforms of COX have been identified: COX-1, COX-2, and COX-3. COX was first purified in 1976 and first cloned in 1988. Among the more significant advances of the past decade was the isolation of a second isoform of the COX enzyme, COX-2, the expression of which is inducible by cytokines and growth factors (20–24). A third distinct COX isoform, COX-3, has recently been reported in addition to two smaller COX-1–derived proteins (partial COX-1, or PCOX-1, proteins, termed PCOX-1α and PCOX-1β). It has been long known that acetaminophen possesses analgetic and antipyretic activity but little, if any, anti-inflammatory activity. Thus, the identification of this third isoform of the COX enzyme may be of importance, because COX-3 is selectively inhibited by analgetic/antipyretic drugs and is potently inhibited by some NSAIDs. Inhibition of COX-3 may represent a primary central mechanism by which acetaminophen decreases pain and fever (discussed later).

Both COX-1 and COX-2 are very similar in structure and almost identical in length, varying from 599 (human) to 602 (mice) amino acids for COX-1 and from 603 (mice) to 604 (human) for COX-2. Both isoforms possess molecular masses of 70 to 74 kDa and contain just over 600 amino acids, with an approximately 60% homology within the same species (25,26). Cyclooxygenase-2 contains an 18-amino-acid insert near the C-terminal end of the enzyme that is not present in COX-1, but all other residues that have been previously identified as being essential to the catalytic activity of COX-1 are present in COX-2. Both isoforms have been cloned from various species, including human, and are heme-containing membrane proteins that exist as dimers (25). The three-dimensional radiographic crystal structure of COX-2 derived from human or murine sources can be superimposed on that of COX-1. Residues that form the substrate binding channel, the catalytic sites, and those residues immediately adjacent are essentially identical with the exception of two minor differences. The isoleucine at positions 434 and 523 in COX-1 is exchanged for valine in COX-2. The smaller size of Val-523 in COX-2 allows inhibitor access to a side pocket off the main substrate channel, whereas the longer side chain of Ile in COX-1 sterically blocks inhibitor access. A major difference between COX-1 and COX-2 is that compared to COX-1, COX-2 lacks a sequence of 17 amino acids from the N-terminus but contains a sequence of 18 amino acids at the C-terminus. This causes a difference in the numbering systems of the two isoforms such that the serine residue acetylated by aspirin in COX-1 is numbered Ser-530, whereas in COX-2, the serine residue acetylated is Ser-516. Yet, the amino acid residues that are thought to be responsible for providing the catalytic role are the same, with both isoforms displaying similar ability to convert arachidonic acid to PGH_2. Cyclooxygenase-1 appears to be more specific than COX-2 for fatty acid substrates, because COX-2 accepts a wider range of fatty acid substrates than COX-1. Cyclooxygenase-1 primarily metabolizes arachidonic acid, and COX-2 metabolizes C-18 and C-20 fatty acid substrates. Selective inhibitors of COX-2 do not bind to Arg-120, which is used by the —COOH of arachidonic acid and the carboxylic acid selective or nonselective COX-1 inhibitors.

From a therapeutic viewpoint, the major difference between COX-1 and COX-2 lies in physiological function rather than in structure. Little COX-2 is present in resting cells, but its expression can be induced by cytokines in vascular smooth muscle, fibroblasts, and epithelial cells, leading to the suggestion that COX-1 functions to produce prostaglandins that are involved in normal cellular activity (protection of gastric mucosa, maintenance of kidney function) and COX-2 to produce prostglandins at inflammatory sites (27). Inducible COX-2 linked to inflammatory cell types and tissues is believed to be the target enzyme in the treatment of inflammatory disorders by NSAIDs. Until recently, most NSAIDs inhibited both COX-1 and COX-2, but with varying degrees of selectivity. Selective COX-2 inhibitors may eliminate side effects associated with NSAIDs because of COX-1 inhibition, such as gastric and renal effects.

Prostaglandins are rapidly metabolized and inactivated by various oxidative and reductive pathways. The initial step involves rapid oxidation of the 15α-OH to the corresponding ketone by the prostaglandin-specific enzyme, prostaglandin 15-OH dehydrogenase. This is followed by reduction of the C-13, C-14 double bond by prostaglandin Δ^{13}-reductase to the corresponding dihydro ketone, which for PGE_2 represents the major metabolite in plasma. Subsequently, enzymes normally involved in β- and ω-oxidation of fatty acids more slowly cleave the α-chain and oxidize the C-20 terminal methyl group to the carboxylic acid derivative, respectively. Hence, dicarboxylic acid derivatives containing only 16 carbon atoms are the major excreted metabolites of PGE_1 and PGE_2.

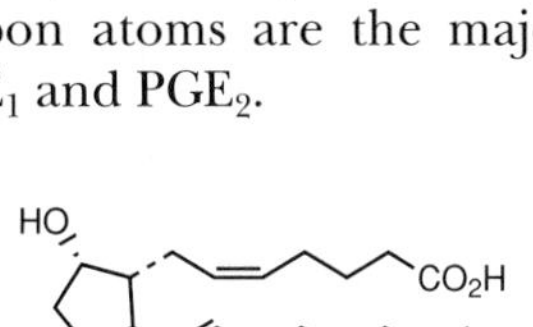

HO, CO_2H, HO, H_3C, OH

Carboprost

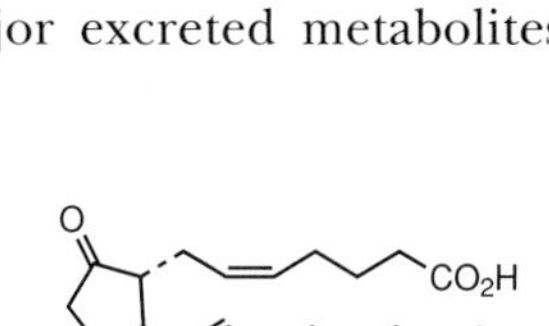

O, CO_2H, HO, H, OH

Dinoprostone

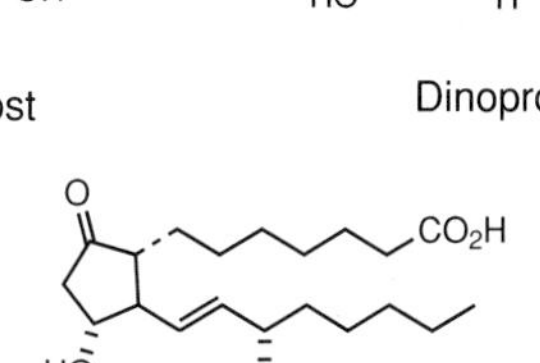

O, CO_2H, HO, OH

Alprostadil

The pharmacological actions of the various prostaglandins are quite diverse. When administered intravaginally, PGE_2 will stimulate the endometrium of the gravid uterus to contract in a manner similar to uterine contractions observed during labor. Thus, PGE_2 is therapeutically available as dinoprostone (Prostin E2) for use as an abortifacient at 12 to 20 weeks of gestation and for evacuation of uterine content in missed abortion or intrauterine fetal death up to 28 weeks of gestation. Additionally, PGE_2 is a potent stimulator of smooth muscle of the gastrointestinal (GI) tract and can elevate body temperature in addition to possessing potent vasodilating properties in most vascular tissue while possessing constrictor effects at certain sites. The PGEs in general cause pain when administered via the intradermal route. Many of these properties are shared by $PGF_{2\alpha}$ that also is therapeutically available as an abortifacient at 16 to 20 weeks of gestation and is available as dinoprost tromethamine (Prostin F2α). The synthetic 15-methyl derivative of $PGF_{2\alpha}$, carboprost, also is available as the tromethamine salt (Prostin 15/M) as an abortifacient at 13 to 20 of weeks gestation. However, $PGF_{2\alpha}$ differs from PGE_2 in that it does not significantly alter blood pressure in humans. The PGD_2 causes both vasodilation and vasoconstriction. The PGEs produce a relaxation of bronchial and tracheal smooth muscle, but the PGFs and PGD_2 cause contraction. The PGE_1 is available as alprostadil (Prostin VR Pediatric) to maintain patency of the ductus arteriosus in neonates until surgery can be performed to correct congenital heart defects.

The effects of prostaglandins on the GI tract deserve special mention. The PGEs and PGI_2 inhibit gastric secretion that may be induced by gastrin or histamine. Prostaglandins appear to play a major cytoprotective role in maintaining the integrity of gastric mucosa. The PGE_1 exerts a protective effect on gastroduodenal mucosa by stimulating secretion of an alkaline mucus and bicarbonate ion and by maintaining or increasing mucosal blood flow. Thus, inhibition of prostaglandin formation in joints produces favorable results, as indicated by a reduction in fever, pain, and swelling. Inhibition of prostaglandin biosynthesis in the GI tract is unfavorable, however, because it may cause disruption of mucosal integrity, resulting in peptic ulcer disease that, as will be discussed later, is commonly associated with the use of NSAIDs and aspirin.

Alternatively, nonprostanoids also can be formed from PGH_2, as illustrated in Figure 36.4. Thromboxane synthetase acts on PGH_2 to produce thromboxane A_2 (TXA_2), whereas prostacyclin synthetase converts PGH_2 to prostacyclin (PGI_2), both of which possess short biological half-lives. A potent vasoconstrictor and inducer of platelet aggregation, TXA_2 has a biological half-life of approximately 30 seconds, being rapidly nonenzymatically converted to the more stable, but inactive, TXB_2. Prostacyclin, a potent hypotensive and inhibitor of platelet aggregation, has a half-life of approximately 3 minutes and is nonenzymatically converted to 6-keto-$PGF_{1\alpha}$. Platelets contain primarily thromboxane synthetase, whereas endothelial cells contain primarily prostacyclin synthetase. Considerable research efforts are being expended in the development of stable prostacyclin analogues and thromboxane antagonists as

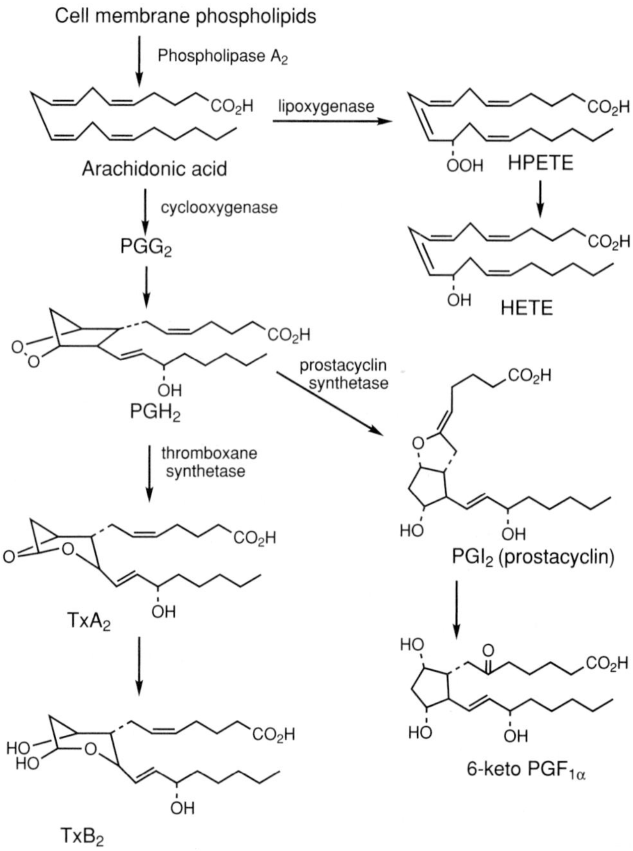

Fig. 36.4. Biosynthesis of thromboxanes, prostacyclin and leukotrienes.

cardiovascular drugs. The pharmacological effects of some prostaglandins, TXA_2, and prostacyclin are summarized in Table 36.2.

The existence of distinct prostaglandin receptors may explain the broad spectrum of action displayed by the prostaglandins. The nomenclature of these receptors is based on the affinity displayed by natural prostaglandins, prostacyclin, or thromboxanes at each receptor type. Thus, EP receptors are those receptors for which the PGEs have high affinity, FP receptors are those for PGFs, DP receptors are those for PGDs, IP receptors are those for PGI_2, and TP receptors are those for TXA_2. These receptors are coupled through G proteins to effector mechanisms that include stimulation of adenylate cyclase and, hence, increased cyclic adenosine monophosphate levels and phospholipase C that results in increased levels of inositol 1,4,5-triphosphate. Three distinct receptors for leukotrienes have been identified as well.

Lipoxygenases are a group of enzymes that oxidize polyunsaturated fatty acids possessing two *cis* double bonds separated by a methylene group to produce lipid hydroperoxides (19). Arachidonic acid is thus metabolized to a number of hydroperoxy-eicosatetraenoic acid

Table 36.2. Pharmacological Properties of Prostaglandins, Thromboxane, and Prostacyclin

	PGE_2	$PGF_{2\alpha}$	PGI_2	TxA_2
Uterus	Oxytocic	Oxytocic		
Bronchi	dilation	constriction		
Platelets			Inhibits aggregation	Aggregation
Blood vessels	Dilation	Constriction	Dilation	Constriction

derivatives (HPETEs). These enzymes differ in the position at which they peroxidize arachidonic acid and in their tissue specificity. For example, platelets possess only a 12-lipoxygenase, whereas leukocytes possess both a 12-lipoxygenase and a 5-lipoxygenase (28). The HPETE derivatives are not stable, being rapidly converted to a number of metabolites. Leukotrienes are products of the 5-lipoxygenase pathway and are divided into two major classes: hydroxylated eicosatetraenoic acids (LTs), represented by LTB_4, and peptidoleukotrienes (pLTs), such as LTC_4, LTD_4, and LTE_4. 5-Lipoxygenase will produce leukotrienes from 5-HPETE, as shown in Figure 36.5. LTA synthetase converts 5-HPETE to an unstable epoxide called LTA_4 that may be converted by LTA hydrolase to the leukotriene LTB_4 or by glutathione-S-transferase to LTC_4. Other cysteinyl leukotrienes (e.g., LTD_4, LTE_4, and LTF_4) can then be formed from LTC_4 by the removal of glutamic acid and glycine and then reconjugation with glutamic acid, respectively. Cysteinyl leukotrienes activate at least two receptors, designated as $CysLT_1$ and $CysLT_2$. A long-recognized mediator of inflammation, SRS-A (slow-reacting substance of anaphylaxis), is primarily a mixture of two leukotrienes, LTC_4 and LTD_4. The physiological roles of the various leukotrienes are becoming better understood. LTB_4 is a potent chemotactic agent for polymorphonuclear leukocytes, causes the accumulation of leukocytes at inflammation sites, and leads to the development of symptoms characteristic of inflammatory disorders. Both LTC_4 and LTD_4 are potent hypotensives and bronchoconstrictors. Because of the role played by LTs and pLTs in inflammatory conditions and asthma, it is not surprising that intensive research is being conducted in this area. The first cysteinyl leukotriene receptor antagonist, zafirlukast (Accolate) (Fig. 36.6), was approved in 1996 for the prophylaxis and chronic treatment of asthma and has been labeled "lukasts." It is a selective and competitive receptor antagonist of the cysteinyl leukotriene, LTD_4 and LTE_4. The cysteinyl leukotrienes, originally described as slow-reacting substances of anaphylaxis, produce airway edema, smooth muscle constriction, and altered cellular activity associated with the inflammatory process, all of which are associated with the pathophysiology of asthma. In humans, pretreatment with single oral doses of zafirlukast inhibited bronchoconstriction caused by sulfur dioxide and cold air and reduced the both early and late-phase reaction in patients with asthma caused by inhalation of various

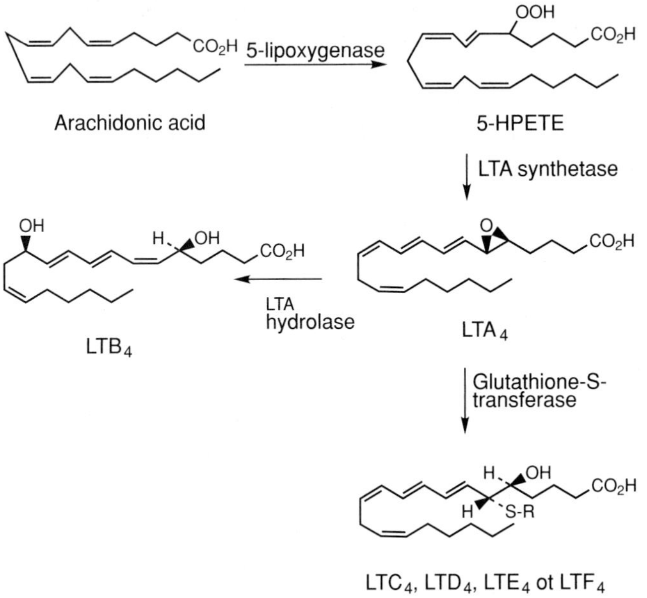

Arachidonic acid — 5-lipoxygenase → 5-HPETE — LTA synthetase → LTA_4 — LTA hydrolase → LTB_4; LTA_4 — Glutathione-S-transferase → LTC_4, LTD_4, LTE_4 ot LTF_4

Fig. 36.5. Biosynthesis of leukotrienes.

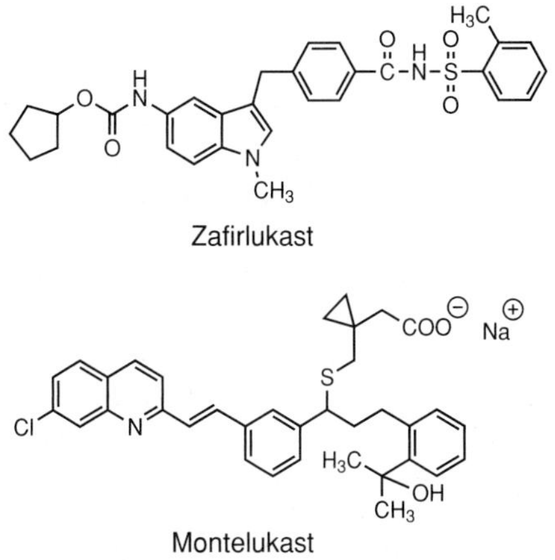

Zafirlukast

Montelukast

Fig. 36.6. Leukotriene antagonists.

antigens, such as grass, cat dander, and ragweed. Zafirlukast reduced the increase in bronchial hyperresponsiveness to inhaled histamine that followed inhaled allergen challenge. It is rapidly absorbed and food reduces bioavailability to approximately 40%. It is extensively metabolized via hydroxylation reactions mediated primarily by CYP2C9, and to a minor extent CYP3A4, to essentially inactive metabolites. Excretion is 90% fecal and 10% via urine. Its elimination half-life is approximately 10 hours. A second leukotriene antagonist, montelukast (Singulair) (Fig. 36.6), was approved shortly thereafter for prophylaxis and chronic treatment of asthma as an antagonist of LTD_4 at the $CysLT_1$ receptor. Its oral bioavailability ranges from 60 to 75% depending on the dosage form used. On oral administration, the time to peak concentration ranges from 2 to 4 h. Food can reduce its bioavailability, prolonging time to maximum plasma concentration. Protein binding is more than 99%. Montelukast is also extensively metabolized via hydroxylation reactions mediated by CYP2C9 and CYP3A4 to essentially inactive metabolites. Montelukast is excreted primarily in feces (86%), with an elimination half-life of 3 to 6 hours. The first inhibitor of leukotriene biosynthesis, zileuton (Zyflo), was approved shortly after zafirlukast for prophylaxis and chronic treatment of asthma. Zileuton is a specific inhibitor of 5-lipoxygenase and, thus, inhibits the formation of LTB_4, LTC_4, LTD_4, and LTE_4. The *R*- (+)- and *S*-(−)- enantiomers equally inhibit 5-lipoxygenase, and the drug is marketed as the racemic mixture. Zileuton is metabolized primarily to two diasteromeric glucuronide conjugates and the N-dehydroxylated metabolite.

Zileuton

THERAPEUTIC APPROACH TO ARTHRITIC DISORDERS

The goal of drug treatment in early rheumatoid arthritis is to induce remission or at least eliminate evidence of disease activity. Rheumatoid arthritis was traditionally treated with a stepwise approach starting with NSAIDs and progressing through more potent drugs such as glucocorticoids, DMARDs, and biologic response modifiers. The DMARDs were avoided early in the disease because of their potentially serious side effects and were usually reserved for people who showed signs of joint damage. Over time, however, this strategy was recognized as being faulty, because people treated early with DMARDs have better long-term outcomes, with greater preservation of function and less work disability.

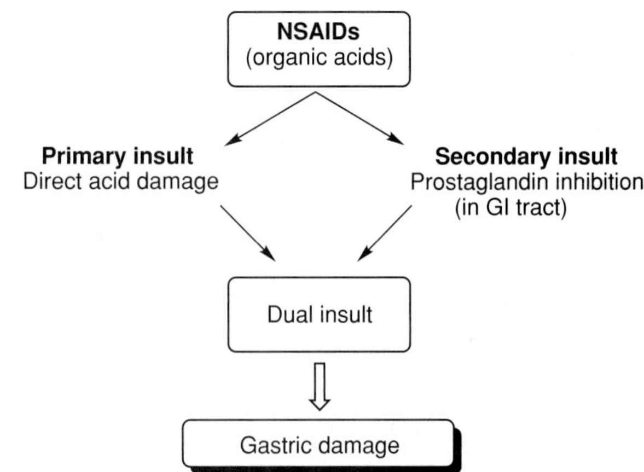

Fig. 36.7. NSAID-induced production of gastric damage by a dual-insult mechanism.

The current approach, therefore, is to treat rheumatoid arthritis aggressively with DMARDs and biologic response modifiers soon after diagnosis. Treating rheumatoid arthritis early with DMARDs, within 3–6 months after symptoms begin, controls inflammation better and is the best way to stop or slow progression of the disease and bring about remission and long term prevention of joint disease. Methotrexate is the cornerstone of DMARD therapy. Long-term treatment with methotrexate and biologic response modifiers may offer the best control of rheumatoid arthritis for the majority of people, which may eliminate the need for other NSAID medications.

A large number of NSAIDs are therapeutically available for the treatment of pain and inflammation associated with arthritic disorders, differing in efficacy but, perhaps more importantly, differing also in overall toxicity. As a group, NSAIDs can cause GI toxicity, such as dyspepsia, abdominal pain, heartburn, gastric erosion leading to wall perforation, peptic ulcer formation, bleeding, diarrhea, renal disorders (e.g., acute renal failure, tubular necrosis, and analgesic nephropathy), and other effects (e.g., tinnitus and headache). Gastric damage produced by NSAIDs generally involves a dual insult mechanism (Fig. 36.7). Most NSAIDs are acidic substances that produce a primary insult because of direct acid damage, an indirect contact effect, and a back diffusion of hydrogen ions. The secondary insult results from inhibition of prostaglandin biosynthesis in the GI tract, where prostaglandins exert a cytoprotective effect. The dual insult leads to gastric damage. A report from the Arthritis, Rheumatism, and Aging Medical Information System Post-Marketing Surveillance Program, before the introduction of COX-2–selective drugs, ranked the overall toxicity of NSAIDs in the following decreasing order: indomethacin > tolmetic > meclofenamate > ketoprofen > fenoprofen > salsalate > aspirin.

THERAPEUTIC CLASSIFICATIONS

Antipyretic Analgetics

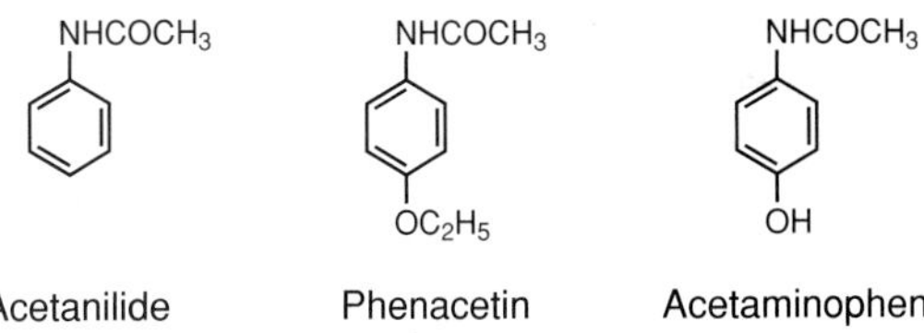

Mechanism of Action

Drugs included in this class possess analgetic and antipyretic actions but lack anti-inflammatory effects. Antipyretics interfere with those processes by which pyrogenic factors produce fever, but they do not appear to lower body temperature in afebrile subjects. It had been historically accepted that the antipyretics exert their actions within the central nervous system (CNS), primarily at the hypothalamic thermoregulatory center, but more recent evidence suggests that peripheral actions also may contribute. Endogenous leukocytic pyrogens may be released from cells that have been activated by various stimuli, and antipyretics may act by inhibiting the activation of these cells by an exogenous pyrogen or by inhibiting the release of endogenous leukocytic pyrogens from the cells once they have been activated by the exogenous pyrogen. Substantial evidence exists suggesting a central antipyretic mechanism, an antagonism that may result from either a direct competition of a pyrogen and the antipyretic agent at CNS receptors, or an inhibition of prostaglandins in the CNS (29). Despite the extensive use of acetaminophen, the mechanism of action has not been fully elucidated. Acetaminophen may inhibit pain impulses by exerting a depressant effect on peripheral receptors; an antagonistic effect on the actions of bradykinin may play a role. The antipyretic effects may not result from inhibition of release of endogenous pyrogen from leukocytes but, rather, from inhibiting the action of released endogenous pyrogen on hypothalamic thermoregulatory centers. The fact that acetaminophen is an effective antipyretic/analgetic but an ineffective anti-inflammatory agent may result from its greater inhibition of prostaglandin biosynthesis via inhibition of the COX-3 isoform in the CNS compared with that in the periphery.

Recent research in dogs has revealed a slice variant of COX-1 that was sensitive to inhibition by acetaminophen. This novel variant of the cyclooxygenase system was named COX-3, and it was hypothesized that inhibition of COX-3 could represent a primary CNS mechanism by which acetaminophen and phenacetin exerted their analgesic and antipyretic effects (30). The ability of selected analgesic/antipyretic drugs to inhibit COX-1, COX-2, and COX-3 is shown in Table 36.3 (30).

Further studies revealed that similar cyclooxygenase variants were present in rodents and humans, but these did not appear to be inhibited by acetaminophen (31,32). These cyclooxygenase variants are proposed to be COX-active, however, and to have a role in the biochemistry of these species (33,34). There is substantial nonhomology between the human, canine, and rodent COX-3 proteins.

The mode of action of acetaminophen therefore is still in question. Certainly, the analgetic and antipyretic properties parallel the decrease in PGE_2 levels in the CNS caused by acetaminophen. The COX-1–deleted, but not the COX-2–deleted, mice showed a decrease in these actions (35). Those authors suggest that in this species, it is COX-1, or a variant of it, that is affected by acetaminophen. Unlike other NSAIDs, such as ibuprofen or aspirin, acetaminophen does not have significant anti-inflammatory, antiplatelet, or gastric ulcerogenic activity. Other authors claim that the mechanism of action of acetaminophen is thought to involve inhibition of COX-2, and this fits with the therapeutic profile of the recently discovered, powerful, and selective COX-2 inhibitors (36). Acetaminophen is only effective, however, when COX-2 activity is at a low level. This view partially explains the lack of anti-inflammatory action, because COX-2 activity will be high in this situation (37).

Graham and Scott (37) also have put forward the interesting hypothesis that acetaminophen acts by depletion of the stores of glutathione, which is a known cofactor for PGE synthase. This would explain the decrease in PGE production and the concomitant analgetic effect. The depletion of glutathione is the main cause of acetaminophen toxicity. The highly reactive benzoquinoneimine, formed by CYP2E1 isoform, must be conjugated with glutathione before it can react with other crucial cell components. In overdose, failure of this molecular mechanism results in serious liver damage. The depletion of

Table 36.3. Binding Constants (IC_{50} mM) of Selected NSAIDs for the COX enzymes

Drug	COX-1	COX-2	COX-3
Acetaminophen	>1,000	>1,000	460
Phenacetin	>1,000	>1,000	102
Aspirin	10	>1,000	3.1
Diclofenac	0.035	0.041	0.008
Ibuprofen	2.4	5.7	0.24
Indomethacin	0.010	0.66	0.016

the body's supply of glutathione also should affect the biosynthesis of the inflammatory mediator leukotriene C4. At therapeutic acetaminophen levels, however, this does not seem to be significant.

A review paper discussing the dichotomies of the acetaminophen mechanism and COX-3 is available (38).

Historical Background

Acetanilide was introduced into therapy in 1886 under the name antifebrin as an antipyretic/analgetic agent but was subsequently found to be too toxic (methemoglobinemia and jaundice), particularly at high doses, to be useful. Phenacetin was introduced the following year and remained in use until the 1960s because of reports of nephrotoxicity. Phenacetin is longer acting than acetaminophen despite the fact that it is metabolized to acetaminophen but is a weaker antipyretic. Shortly thereafter, acetaminophen (paracetamol) was introduced in 1893 but remained unpopular for more than 50 years, until it was observed that it is a metabolite of both acetanilide and phenacetin. It remains the only useful agent of this group and is widely used as a nonprescription antipyretic/analgetic under a variety of trade names (Tylenol, Patrol, and Tempera). The analgetic activity of acetaminophen is comparable to that of aspirin, but acetaminophen lacks useful anti-inflammatory activity. Its advantages over aspirin as an analgetic, however, are that individuals who are hypersensitive to salicylates generally respond well to acetaminophen.

Structure–Activity Relationships

The structure–activity relationships of p-aminophenol derivatives have been widely studied. Based on the comparative toxicity of acetanilide and acetaminophen, aminophenols are less toxic than the corresponding aniline derivatives, although p-aminophenol itself is too toxic for therapeutic purposes. Etherification of the phenolic function with methyl or propyl groups produces derivatives with greater side effects than with ethyl groups. Substituents on the nitrogen atom that reduce basicity reduce activity unless that substituent is metabolically labile (e.g., acetyl). Amides derived from aromatic acids (e.g., N-phenylbenzamide) are less active or inactive.

ACETAMINOPHEN USP. Acetaminophen is weakly acidic (pK_a = 9.51) and synthesized by the acetylation of p-aminophenol. It is weakly bound to plasma proteins (18–25%). Acetaminophen is indicated for use as an antipyretic/analgetic, particularly in those individuals displaying an allergy or sensitivity to aspirin. It does not possess anti-inflammatory activity, but it will produce analgesia in a wide variety of arthritic and musculoskeletal disorders. It is available in various formulations, including suppositories, tablets, capsules, granules, and solutions. The usual adult dose is 325 to 650 mg every 4 to 6 hours. Doses of greater than 2.6 g/day are not recommended for long-term therapy because of potential hepatotoxicity issues. Acetaminophen, unlike aspirin, is stable in aqueous solution, making liquid formulations readily available, a particular advantage in pediatric cases.

Metabolism and Toxicity. The metabolism of acetanilide, acetaminophen, and phenacetin is illustrated in Figure 36.8 (39). As indicated earlier, both acetanilide and phenacetin are metabolized to acetaminophen. Additionally, both undergo hydrolysis to yield aniline derivatives that produce directly, or through their conversion to hydroxylamine derivatives, significant methemoglobinemia and hemolytic anemia, which resulted in their removal from the U.S. market. On the other hand, acetaminophen is undergoes rapid first-pass metabolism in the GI tract primarily by conjugation reactions, with the O-sulfate conjugate being the primary metabolite in children and the O-glucuronide being the primary metabolite in adults. A minor, but significant, product of both acetaminophen and phenacetin is the N-hydroxyamide produced by a CYP2E1 and CYP3A4. The CYP2E1 is the rate-limiting enzyme that initiates the cascade of events leading to acetaminophen hepatotoxicity; in the absence of this cytochrome P450 enzyme, toxicity will only be apparent at high concentrations. The N-hydroxyamide is then converted to a reactive toxic metabolite, an acetimidoquinone, which has been suggested (40) to produce the nephrotoxicity and hepatotoxicity associated with acetaminophen and phenacetin. Normally, this iminoquinone is detoxified by conjugation with hepatic glutathione. In cases of ingestion of large doses or overdoses of acetaminophen, however, hepatic stores of glutathione may be depleted by more than 70%, allowing the reactive quinone to interact with soft nucleophilic functional groups, primarily —SH groups, on hepatic proteins, resulting in the formation of covalent adducts that produce hepatic necrosis. Overdoses of acetaminophen can produce potentially fatal hepatic necrosis, renal tubular necrosis, and hypoglycemic coma. Various sulfhydryl-containing compounds were found to be useful as antidotes to acetaminophen overdoses. The most useful of these, N-acetylcysteine (Mucomyst, Acetadote), serves as a substitute for the depleted glutathione by enhancing hepatic glutathione stores and/or by enhancing disposition by nontoxic sulfate conjugation (41). N-Acetylcysteine also may inhibit the formation of the toxic iminoquinone metabolite (42). In cases of acetaminophen overdoses, N-acetylcysteine is administered as a 5% solution in water, soda, or juice or intravenously (IV) at 140 mg/kg followed by 17 maintenance doses of 70 mg/kg every 5 hours.

Drug Interactions. Hepatic necrosis develops at much lower doses of acetaminophen in some heavy drinkers than would be expected (39), perhaps because of the induction of the CYP2E1 system, depletion of glutathione stores, or aberrations in the primary sulfate and glucuronide conjugation pathways. At 4 g per day, acetaminophen has been reported to potentiate the response to oral anticoagulants, increasing prothrombin time (INR values) two to three times. Interactions with warfarin

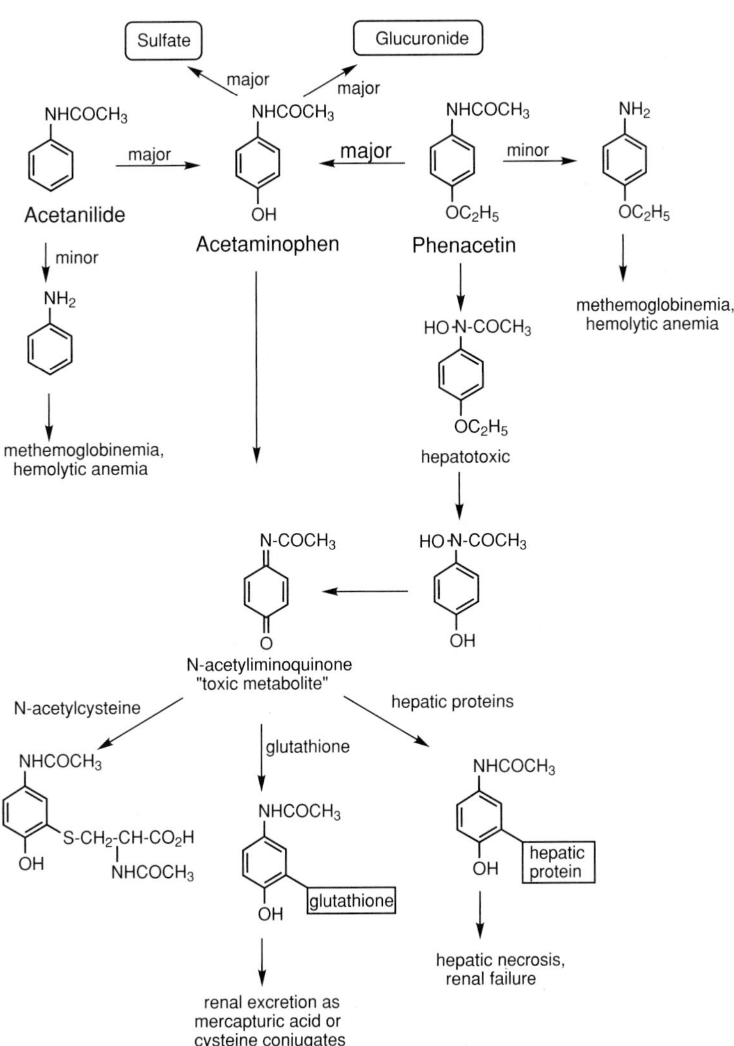

Fig. 36.8. Metabolism of acetaminophen.

(Coumadin), dicumarol, anisindione, and diphenadione have been suggested. The mechanism of these interactions has not been fully elucidated but may be associated with competition for plasma protein binding sites, because acetaminophen is a weak acid and is weakly bound, but may also interfere with the enzymes involved in vitamin K-dependent coagulation factor synthesis. The absorption of acetaminophen is enhanced by polysorbate and sorbitol and is reduced by anticholinergics and narcotic analgetics. Chemical incompatibilities also have been reported based on hydrolysis by strong acids or bases or by phenolic oxidation in the presence of oxidizing agents. Acetaminophen forms "sticky" mixtures with diphenhydramine HCl and discolors under humid conditions in the presence of caffeine or codeine phosphate.

Anti-Inflammatory Drugs

Salicylates

The use of salicylates dates back to the nineteenth century. Salicylic acid itself was first obtained in 1838 from salicin, a glycoside present in most willow and poplar bark. Interestingly, Hippocrates prescribed chewing willow bark for pain relief in the fifth century AD. In 1860, Kolbe synthesized salicylic acid from sodium phenoxide and carbon dioxide, a method that inexpensively produced large quantities. Derivatives of salicylic acid began to receive medical attention shortly thereafter. Sodium salicylate was employed as an antipyretic/antirheumatic agent in 1875, and the phenyl ester was used in 1886. Acetylsalicylic acid was prepared in 1853 but was not used medicinally until 1899. The term "aspirin" was given to acetylsalicylic acid by Dreser, the director of pharmacology at Frederich Bayer and Company in Germany, as a contraction of the letter "a" from acetyl and "spirin," an older name given to salicylic acid (spiric acid) that was derived from a natural source in spirea plants. Since then, numerous derivatives of salicylic acid have been synthesized and evaluated pharmacologically, yet only a relatively few derivatives have achieved therapeutic utility.

In addition to possessing antipyretic, analgetic, and anti-inflammatory properties, salicylates possess other actions that have been proven to be therapeutically beneficial. Because salicylates promote the excretion of uric acid, they are useful in the treatment of gouty arthritis. More recent attention has been given to the ability of salicylates to inhibit platelet aggregation, which may contribute to heart attacks and stroke. Aspirin appears to inhibit prostaglandin cyclooxygenase in platelet membranes, thus blocking formation of the potent platelet-aggregating factor TXA_2 in a manner that is irreversible. The Physicians Health Study concluded that in a group of 22,071 participants, there was a 44% reduction in the risk of myocardial infarction in the group taking a single 325-mg aspirin tablet taken every other day versus the placebo group (43). The role of aspirin in reducing cardiac mortality has been reviewed (44). Also, aspirin and other NSAIDs might be protective against colon cancer (45). Thus, the therapeutic utility of aspirin continues to increase. Unfortunately, a number of side effects are associated with the use of salicylates, most notably GI disturbances such as dyspepsia, gastroduodenal bleeding, gastric ulcerations, and gastritis.

Mechanism of Action. A number of possible mechanisms of action have been proposed for salicylates over the years. Among those that have been suggested are inhibition of the biosynthesis of histamine, antagonism of the actions of various kinins, inhibition of mucopolysaccharide biosynthesis, inhibition of lysosomal enzyme release, and inhibition of leukocyte accumulation. The most widely accepted mechanism of action currently is the ability of these drugs to inhibit the biosynthesis of prostaglandins at the cyclooxygenase stage discussed earlier. Aspirin is the only NSAID that covalently modifies cyclooxygenase by acetylating Ser-530 of COX-1 and Ser-516 of COX-2. Aspirin, however, is 10 to 100 times more potent against COX-1 than against COX-2 (46). Aspirin's actions on COX-1 prevent both endoperoxide and 15-peroxidation of arachidonic acid, but its action on COX-2 does not prevent formation of 15-OOH arachidonic acid (25).

Structure–Activity Relationships. Despite the vast effort that has been expended in the search to find a "better" aspirin—that is, one possessing fewer GI side effects but a greater potency and a longer duration of action yet is inexpensive and an antipyretic, analgetic, and anti-inflammatory agent that is overall superior to aspirin—none has yet to be discovered. The following structure–activity relationships have been established:

Salicylic acid

The active moiety appears to the salicylate anion. The side effects of aspirin, particularly the GI effects, appear to be associated with the carboxylic acid function. Reducing the acidity of this group (e.g., converting to an amide, salicylamide) maintains the analgetic actions of salicylic acid derivatives but eliminates the anti-inflammatory properties. Substitution on either the carboxyl or phenolic hydroxyl groups may affect potency and toxicity. Benzoic acid itself has only weak anti-inflammatory activity. Placing the phenolic hydroxyl group meta or para to the carboxyl group abolishes this activity. Substitution of halogen atoms on the aromatic ring enhances potency and toxicity. Substitution of aromatic rings at the 5-position of salicylic acid increases anti-inflammatory activity (e.g., diflunisal).

Absorption and Metabolism. Most salicylates are rapidly and effectively absorbed on oral administration with the rate of absorption and bioavailability being dependent on a number of factors, including the dosage formulation, gastric pH, food contents in the stomach, gastric emptying time, the presence of buffering agents or antacids, and particle size. Because salicylates are weak acids (acetylsalicylic acid $pK_a = 3.5$), absorption generally takes place primarily from the small intestine and, to a lesser extent, from the stomach by the process of passive diffusion of un-ionized molecules across the epithelial membranes of the GI tract. Thus, gastric pH is an important factor in the rate of absorption of salicylates. Any factor that increases gastric pH (e.g., buffering agents) will slow its rate of absorption, because more of the salicylate will be in the ionized form. The differences in the rates of absorption of aspirin, salicylate salts, and the numerous buffered preparations of salicylates actually are quite small, with absorption half-times in humans ranging from approximately 20 minutes for buffered preparations to 30 minutes for aspirin itself. The presence of food in the stomach also slows the rate of absorption. Formulation factors may contribute to the differences in absorption rates of the various brands of plain and buffered salicylate preparations. Tablet formulations consisting of small particles are absorbed faster than those of larger particle size. The bioavailability of salicylate from enteric-coated preparations may be inconsistent. Absorption of salicylate from rectal suppositories is slower and incomplete and is not recommended when high salicylate levels are required. Topical preparations of salicylic acid ester, e.g., methyl salicylate, are effective in that the rate of salicylate absorption from the skin is rapid. However, 3–5% solutions of salicylic acid are also applied topically as a keratolytic agent.

Salicylates are highly bound to plasma protein albumin, with binding being concentration dependent. At low therapeutic concentrations of 100 μg/mL, approximately 90% of aspirin is plasma protein bound, whereas at higher concentrations of approximately 400 μg/mL, only 76% binding is observed. Plasma protein binding is a major factor in the drug interactions observed for salicylates.

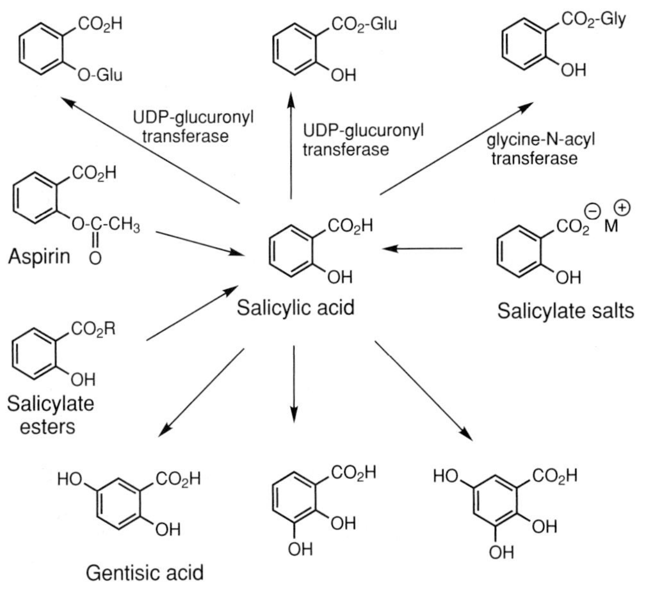

Fig. 36.9. Metabolism of salicylic acid derivatives. Glu, glucuronide conjugate; Gly, glycine conjugate.

The major metabolic routes of esters and salts of salicylic acid are illustrated in Figure 36.9. The initial route of metabolism of these derivatives is their conversion to salicylic acid, which may be excreted in the urine as the free acid (10%) or undergo conjugation with either glycine, to produce the major metabolite salicyluric acid (75%), or with glucuronic acid, to form the glucuronide ether and ester (15%). In addition, small amounts of metabolites resulting from microsomal aromatic hydroxylation are found. The major hydroxylation metabolite, gentisic acid, was once thought to be responsible for the anti-inflammatory actions of the salicylates, but its presence in trace quantities would rule out a major role for gentisic acid, or the other hydroxylation metabolites, in the pharmacological action of salicylates. The metabolism of pharmacokinetic properties of salicylates has been extensively reviewed (47).

Side effects. The most commonly observed side effects associated with the use of salicylates relate to disturbances of the GI tract. Nausea, vomiting, epigastric discomfort, intensification of symptoms of peptic ulcer disease (e.g., dyspepsia and heartburn), gastric ulcerations, erosive gastritis, and GI hemorrhage occur in individuals on high doses of aspirin. The incidence of these side effects is more rare at low doses, but a single dose of aspirin can cause GI distress in 5% of individuals. Gastric bleeding induced by salicylates generally is painless but can lead to fecal blood loss and may cause a persistent iron deficiency anemia. At dosages that generally are useful in anti-inflammatory therapy, aspirin may lead to a loss of 3 to 8 mL/day of blood. The mechanism by which salicylates cause gastric mucosal cell damage may be caused by a number of factors, including gastric acidity, ability of salicylates to damage the normal mucosal barrier that protects against the back diffusion of hydrogen ions, ability of salicylates to inhibit the formation of prostaglandins (particularly those of the PGE series, which normally inhibit gastric acid secretion), and inhibition of platelet aggregation (leading to an increased tendency toward bleeding). Thus, salicylate use before surgery or tooth extraction is contraindicated.

Reye's syndrome is an acute condition that may follow influenza and chickenpox infections in children from infancy to their late teens, with the majority of cases occurring between the ages of 4 and 12 years. It is characterized by symptoms including sudden vomiting, violent headaches, and unusual behavior in children who appear to be recovering from an often mild viral illness. Although a rare condition (60–120 cases per year, or an incidence of 0.15 per 100,000 population of those ≤18 years), it can be fatal, with a death rate of between 20 and 30%. Fortunately, the number of cases is declining, partly because of the observations that more than 90% of children with Reye's syndrome were on salicylate therapy during a recent viral illness. Based on these observations, the U.S. Food and Drug Administration (FDA) has proposed that aspirin and other salicylates be labeled with a warning against their use in children younger than 16 years with influenza, chickenpox, or other flu-like illness. Acetaminophen would appear to be the drug of choice in children with these conditions.

Salicylates account for approximately 25% of all accidental poisonings in the United States.

Drug interactions. Because of the widespread use of salicylates, it is not surprising that interactions with many other drugs used in therapeutic combinations have been observed. Several of these interactions are clinically significant. More data are available for aspirin than for any other specific salicylate product. As mentioned previously, acetylsalicylic acid is a weak acid that is highly bound to plasma proteins (50–80%), and it will compete for these plasma protein binding sites with other drugs that are highly bound to these sites. The interaction that results from the combination of salicylates with oral anticoagulants represents one of the most widely documented clinically significant drug interactions reported to date. The plasma concentration of free anticoagulant increases in the presence of salicylates, necessitating a possible decrease in the dosage of anticoagulant required to produce a beneficial therapeutic effect. The ability of salicylates to produce GI ulcerations and bleeding, coupled with the inhibition of the clotting mechanism, results in a clinically significant drug interaction. In addition, salicylates may inhibit the synthesis of prothrombin by antagonizing the actions of vitamin K. Additionally, NSAIDs can produce these interactions. The competition for plasma protein binding sites also can lead to an increase in free methotrexate levels (thus enhancing the toxicity of methotrexate), enhanced toxicity of long-acting sulfonamides, and a hypoglycemic effect (resulting from displacement of oral hypoglycemic drugs). In large doses, salicylates given concomitantly with uricosuric drugs, such as probenecid and sulfinpyrazone, may lead to a retention of uric acid and, thus, antagonize the uricosuric effect, despite the fact that salicylates when used alone increases urinary excretion of uric acid. The diuretic activity of aldosterone antagonists, such as spironolactone, may be antagonized by salicylates. Corticosteroids may decrease blood levels of salicylates because of their ability to increase the glomerular filtration rate. The incidence and severity of GI ulcerations may be increased if corticosteroids, salicylates, and NSAIDs are administered together. The GI bleeding induced by salicylates may be enhanced by the ingestion of ethanol. Numerous other interactions have been reported, but their clinical significance has not been fully established.

Salicylate hypersensitivity, particularly to aspirin, is relatively uncommon but must be recognized, because severe and potentially fatal reactions may occur. Signs of aspirin hypersensitivity appear soon after administration and include skin rashes, watery secretions, urticaria, vasomotor rhinitis, edema, bronchoconstriction, and anaphylaxis. Less than 1% of the U.S. population may experience aspirin hypersensitivity; this group consists primarily of middle-aged individuals. Females are more likely to experience aspirin intolerance or hypersensitivity. Aspirin-sensitive patients with asthma are especially at high risk. Mild salicylism may occur after repeated administration of large doses. Symptoms include dizziness, tinnitus, nausea, vomiting, diarrhea, and mental confusion. Doses of 10 to 30 g have been known to cause death in adults, but some individuals have ingested up to 130 g without fatality. More than 10,000 cases of serious salicylate toxicity occur in the United States each year.

AVAILABLE PREPARATIONS. The structures of the marketed preparations of salicylic acid are presented in Figure 36.10.

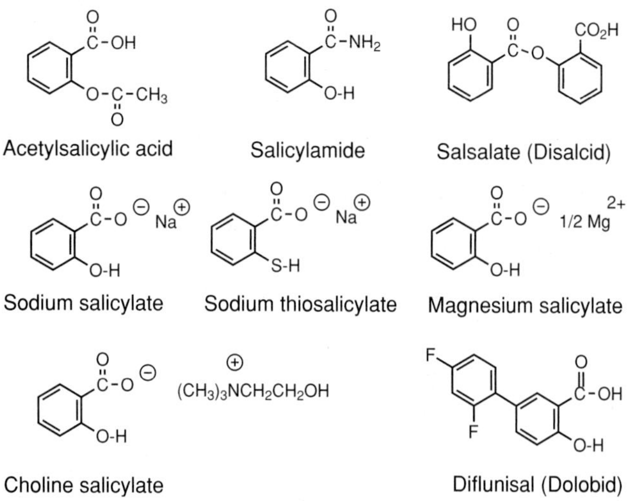

Acetylsalicylic acid | Salicylamide | Salsalate (Disalcid)

Sodium salicylate | Sodium thiosalicylate | Magnesium salicylate

Choline salicylate | Diflunisal (Dolobid)

Fig. 36.10. Structures of marketed derivatives of salicylic acid.

Aspirin USP. Acetylsalicylic acid, or aspirin, is a white powder that is stable in a dry environment but that is hydrolyzed to salicylic acid and acetic acid under humid or moist conditions. Hydrolysis also can occur when aspirin is combined with alkaline salts or with salts containing water of hydration. Stable aqueous solutions of aspirin are thus unobtainable despite the addition of modifying drugs that tend to decrease hydrolysis. Aspirin is rapidly absorbed largely intact from the stomach and upper small intestine on oral administration but is rapidly hydrolyzed by plasma esterases. Peak plasma levels usually are achieved within 2 hours after administration. Increasing the pH of the stomach by the addition of buffering agents may affect absorption, because the degree of ionization will be increased.

Aspirin is indicated for the relief of minor aches and mild to moderate pain (325–650 mg every 4 hours), for arthritis and related arthritic conditions (3.2–6.0 g/day), to reduce the risk of transient ischemic attacks (1.3 g/day), for myocardial infarction prophylaxis (300–325 mg/day), and as a platelet aggregation inhibitor (80–325 mg per day). It is available in a large number of dosage forms and strengths as tablets, suppositories, capsules, enteric-coated tablets, and buffered tablets.

Salicylamide. Salicylamide is less acidic (pK_a 8.2) than other salicylic acid derivatives. Although poorly soluble in water, stable solutions can be formed at pH 9 through ionization of the phenolic group. It is absorbed from the GI tract on oral administration and is rapidly metabolized to inactive metabolites by intestinal mucosa, but not by hydrolysis. Activity appears to reside in the intact molecule. Salicylamide is approximately 40 to 55% plasma protein bound, and it competes with other salicylates and acetaminophen for glucuronide conjugation, decreasing the extent of conjugation of these other drugs. Excretion occurs rapidly, primarily in the urine. The major advantages of salicylamide are its general lack of gastric irritation relative to aspirin, and its use in individuals who are hypersensitive to aspirin. Salicylamide enters the CNS more rapidly than other salicylates and will cause sedation and drowsiness when administered in large doses. Whereas salicylamide is reported to be as effective as aspirin as an analgetic/antipyretic and is effective in relieving pain associated with arthritic conditions, it does not appear to possess useful anti-inflammatory activity (48). Thus, indications for the treatment of arthritic disease states are unwarranted, and its use is restricted to the relief of minor aches and pain at a dosage of 325 to 650 mg three or four times per day. Its effects in humans are not reliable, however, and its use is not widely recommended.

Salicylate Salts. Several salts of salicylic acid, sodium salicylate USP, choline salicylate USP, and magnesium salicylate USP, and one salt of thiosalicylic acid, sodium thiosalicylate USP, are available. These salts are used primarily to decrease GI disturbances or because they form stable aqueous solutions. Sodium salicylate is half as potent, on a weight basis, as aspirin as an analgetic/

antipyretic, but it produces less GI irritation and equivalent blood levels and is useful in patients exhibiting hypersensitivity to aspirin. It generates salicylic acid in the GI tract, accounting for some GI irritation, and sodium bicarbonate sometimes is given concomitantly to reduce acidity. Sodium salicylate, unlike aspirin, does not affect platelet function, although prothrombin times are increased. It is available as tablets, enteric-coated tablets, and as a solution for injection.

Choline salicylate has a lower incidence of GI side effects compared with aspirin, and it has been shown to be particularly useful in treating juvenile rheumatoid arthritis, in which aspirin was ineffective. It is absorbed more rapidly than aspirin and produces higher salicylate plasma levels. It is available as a mint-flavored liquid.

Magnesium salicylate has a low incidence of GI side effects. Both sodium salicylate and magnesium salicylate should be used cautiously in individuals in whom excessive amounts of these electrolytes might be detrimental. The possibility of magnesium toxicity in individuals with renal insufficiency exists. It is available as tablets, but its safety in children under 12 years of age has not been fully determined.

Sodium thiosalicylate (Solate) is administered intramuscularly (IM) for the treatment of rheumatic fever, muscular pain, and acute gout.

Salsalate (Disalcid). Salsalate, or salicylsalicylic acid, (pK_a 3.5 [COOH], 9.8 [AR-OH]) is a dimer of salicylic acid. It is insoluble in gastric juice but is soluble in the small intestine, where it is partially hydrolyzed to two molecules of salicylic acid and absorbed. On a molar basis, it produces 15% less salicylic acid than aspirin. It does not cause GI blood loss and can be given to aspirin-sensitive patients. Salsalate is available as capsules and tablets.

Diflunisal (Dolobid). Diflunisal (pK_a 3.3) was introduced in the United States in 1982 and has gained considerable acceptance as an analgetic and as a treatment of rheumatoid arthritis and osteoarthritis. Diflunisal is metabolized primarily to ether and ester glucuronide conjugates. No metabolism involving changes in ring substituents has been reported. It is more potent than aspirin but produces fewer side effects and has a biological half-life three to four times greater than that of aspirin. It is rapidly and completely absorbed on oral administration, with peak plasma levels being achieved within 2 to 3 hours of administration. It is highly bound (99%) to plasma proteins after absorption. Its elimination half-life is 8 to 12 hours, and it is excreted into urine primarily as glucuronide conjugates. The most frequently reported side effects include disturbances of the GI system (e.g., nausea, dyspepsia, and diarrhea), dermatological reactions, and CNS effects (e.g., dizziness and headache).

Diflunisal is a moderately potent inhibitor of prostaglandin biosynthesis, but it differs from the manner in which aspirin inhibits the cyclooxygenase system in that the inhibition is competitive and reversible in nature. Diflunisal does not have an appreciable effect on platelet aggregation, however, and does not significantly produce gastric or intestinal bleeding.

Arylalkanoic Acids

$$\text{AR}-\underset{\text{}}{\overset{\text{R}}{\overset{|}{\text{CH}}}}-\overset{\text{O}}{\overset{\|}{\text{C}}}-\text{OH}$$

R = H, CH_3 or alkyl
AR = aryl or heteroaryl

The largest group of NSAIDs is represented by the class of arylalkanoic acids as typified by the general chemical structure, and several factors have caused this to be one of the most active areas of drug development in recent years. The impact that the introduction of phenylbutazone in the 1950s had on arthritis therapy was more than matched by the interest generated by the introduction of indomethacin in the mid-1960s. As a result of a study designed to investigate the anti-inflammatory activity of 350 indole acetic acid derivatives related structurally to serotonin and metabolites of serotonin, the Merck group led by Shen (49) reported the synthesis and antipyretic and anti-inflammatory activity of the most potent compound in the series, indomethacin. The observation that indomethacin possessed 1,085-fold the anti-inflammatory activity and 20-fold the antipyretic activity of phenylbutazone (and 10-fold the antipyretic activity of aminopyrine) generated considerable interest in the development of other aryl and heteroaryl acetic acid and propionic acid derivatives. The marketplace was ripe for new anti-inflammatory drugs and most pharmaceutical companies joined in the search for new arylalkanoic acids. The introduction of ibuprofen in the 1970s by Upjohn was quickly followed by the appearance of fenoprofen calcium, naproxen, and tolmetin. Sulindac, an analogue of indomethacin, was introduced in the late 1970s. The 1980s produced zomepirac, benoxaprofen, ketoprofen, flurbiprofen, suprofen, and diclofenac sodium. The 1990s produced ketorolac, etodolac, nabumetone, and most significantly, the development of selective COX-2 inhibitors, celecoxib, rofecoxib, and valicoxib, which reached the market during the period from 1997 to 2000. This rapid development has been accompanied by some setbacks, however. Zomepirac, introduced in 1980 as an analgetic, was withdrawn in 1983 because of severe anaphylactoid reactions, particularly in patients sensitive to aspirin. Benoxaprofen was withdrawn within 6 months of its introduction in 1982 because of several deaths caused by cholestatic jaundice in Europe and the United States. In addition, benoxaprofen produced photosensitivity reactions in patients when they were exposed to sunlight and onycholysis (loosening of the fingernails) in some patients. Suprofen, introduced as an analgetic in 1985, was removed from the market two years later because of flank pain and transient renal failure. In 1989, however, it was reintroduced for ophthalmic use. Numerous other arylalkanoic acids currently are being evaluated in various stages of clinical trials.

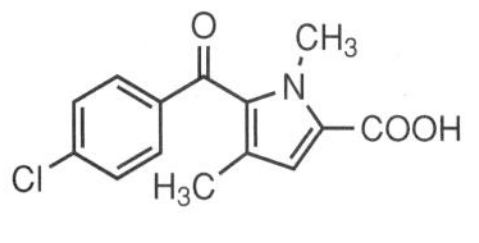

Zomepirac

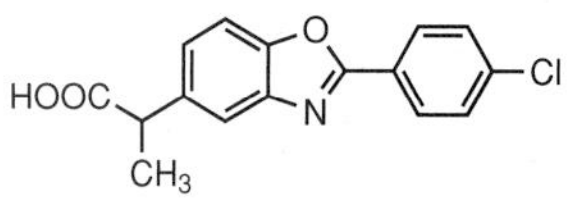

Benoxaprofen

As discussed earlier, most NSAIDs possess a number of biochemical and pharmacological actions. As was the case for the salicylates, the arylalkanoic acids share, to various extents, the property of inhibition of prostaglandin biosynthesis by inhibiting COX-1 and COX-2 with varying degrees of selectivity (Table 36.3).

General structure–activity relationships. Drugs of this class share a number of common structural features. These general structure–activity relationships will be discussed here as they pertain to the proposed mechanism of action. Specific structure–activity relationships for each drug or drug class will be presented separately, where appropriate.

All nonselective COX inhibitors possess a center of acidity, which can be represented by a carboxylic acid function, an enolic function, a hydroxamic acid function, a sulfonamide, or a tetrazole ring. The relationship of this acid center to the carboxylic acid function of arachidonic acid is obvious. The activity of ester and amide derivatives of carboxylic acids generally is attributed to the metabolic hydrolysis products. One nonacidic drug, nabumetone, has been recently introduced in the United States, but as will be discussed later, its activity is attributed to its bioactivation to an active acid metabolite. The center of acidity generally is located one carbon atom adjacent to a flat surface represented by an aromatic or heteroaromatic ring. The distance between these centers is crucial, because increasing this distance to two or three carbons generally diminishes activity. Derivatives of aryl or heteroaryl acetic or propionic acids are most common. This aromatic system appears to correlate with the double bonds at the 5- and 8-positions of arachidonic acid. Substitution of a methyl group on the carbon atom separating the acid center from the aromatic ring tends to increase anti-inflammatory activity. The resulting α-methyl acetic acid, or 2-substituted propionic acid, analogues have been given the class name "profens" by the U.S. Adopted Name Council. Groups larger than methyl decrease activity, but incorporation of this methyl group as part of an alicyclic ring system does not drastically affect activity. Introduction of a methyl group creates a center of chirality. Anti-inflammatory activity in those cases in which the enantiomers have been separated and evaluated, whether determined in vivo or in vitro by cyclooxygenase assays, is associated with the *S*-(+)-enantiomer. Interestingly, in those cases in which the propionic acid is administered as a racemic mixture, in vivo conversion of the *R*-enantiomer to the biologically active *S*-enantiomer is observed to varying degrees. A second area of lipophilicity that is noncoplanar with the aromatic or heteroaromatic ring generally enhances activity. This second lipophilic area may correspond to the area of the double bond in the 11-position of arachidonic acid. This lipophilic function may consist of an additional aromatic ring or alkyl groups either attached to or fused with the aromatic center.

R-COOH	Carboxylic acid; pKa 4-6
R-CONHOH	Hydroxamic acids; pKa (NH) 8-9
R-SO_2NH_2	Sulfonamide; pKa (NH) 9-10
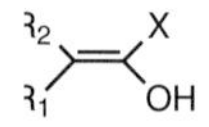 R_2, R_1, X, OH	Enolic (phenol); pKa (OH) 8-10
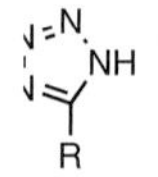 N, NH, R	Tetrazoles; pKa (NH) 4-6

General metabolism. Essentially all the arylalkanoic acid derivatives that are therapeutically available are extensively metabolized. Metabolism occurs primarily through hepatic microsomal enzyme systems and may lead to deactivation or bioactivation of the parent molecules. Metabolism of each drug will be treated separately.

Drug interactions. All the arylalkanoic acids are highly bound to plasma proteins and, thus, may displace other drugs from protein binding sites, resulting in an enhanced activity and toxicity of the displaced drugs. Interestingly, despite the high degree of plasma protein binding, indomethacin does not display this characteristic drug interaction. The most commonly observed interaction is that between the arylalkanoic acid and oral anticoagulants, particularly warfarin (Coumadin). Coadministration may prolong prothrombin time. Potential interactions with other acidic drugs, such as hydantoins, sulfonamides, and sulfonylureas, should be monitored. Concomitant administration of aspirin decreases plasma levels of arylalkanoic acids by as much as 20%. Probenecid, on the other hand, tends to increase these plasma levels. Interactions with drugs that may induce hepatic microsomal enzyme systems, such as phenobarbital, may enhance or diminish anti-inflammatory activity depending on whether the arylalkanoic acid is metabolically bioactivated or inactivated by this enzyme system. Certain diuretics, such as furosemide, inhibit the metabolism of prostaglandins by 15-hydroxyprostaglandin dehydrogenase, and the resulting increase in PGE_2 levels induce plasma renin activity. Because the arylalkanoic acids block the biosynthesis of prostaglandins, the effects of furosemide can be antagonized, in part, offering a potentially significant drug interaction.

Aryl- and heteroarylacetic acids. The structures of the aryl- and heteroarylacetic acid derivatives and the aryl- and heteroarylpropionic acids ("profens") available are presented in Figure 36.11.

Indomethacin. Aqueous solutions of indomethacin are not stable because of the ease of hydrolysis of the p-chlorobenzoyl group. The original synthesis of indomethacin by Shen et al. (49) involved the formation of 2-methyl-5-methoxyindole acetic acid and subsequent

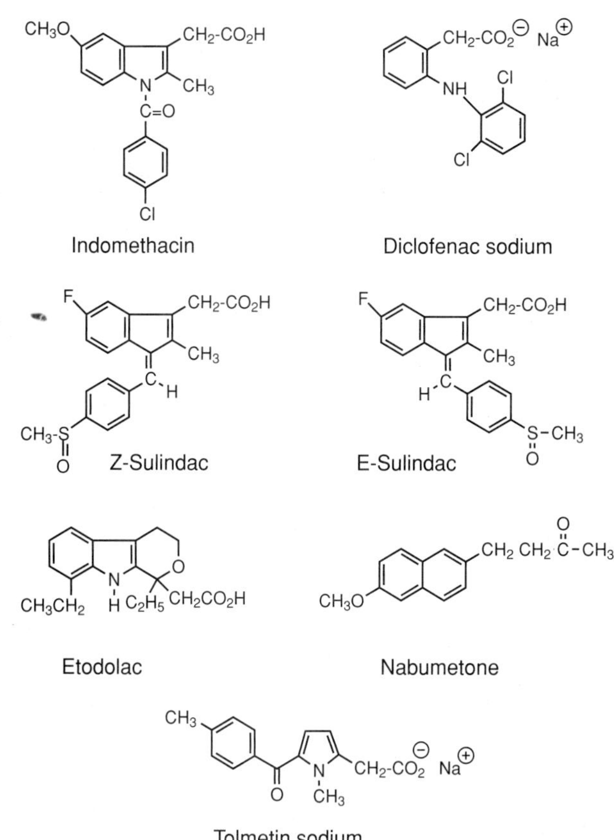

Fig. 36.11. Structures of aryl- and heteroarylacetic acid derivatives.

acylation after protection of the carboxyl group as the t-butyl ester. It was introduced in the United States in 1965. It is still one of the most potent NSAIDs in use. It also is a more potent antipyretic than either aspirin or acetaminophen, and it possesses approximately 10 times the analgetic potency of aspirin. The analgetic effect, however, is widely overshadowed by concern over the frequency of side effects.

Structure–Activity Relationships. Replacement of the carboxyl group with other acidic functionalities decreases activity. Anti-inflammatory activity generally increases as the acidity of the carboxyl group increases and decreases as the acidity is decreased. Amide analogues are inactive. Acylation of the indole nitrogen with aliphatic carboxylic acids or aralkylcarboxylic acids results in amide derivatives that are less active than those derived from benzoic acid. N-Benzoyl derivatives substituted in the para-position with fluoro, chloro, trifluoromethyl, or thiomethyl groups are the most active. The 5-position of the indole ring is most flexible with regard to the nature of substituents that enhance activity. Substituents such as methoxy, fluoro, dimethylamino, methyl, allyloxy, and acetyl are more active than the unsubstituted indole ring. The presence of an indole ring nitrogen is not essential for activity, because the corresponding 1-benzylidenylindene analogues (e.g., sulindac) are active. Alkyl groups, especially methyl, at the α-position are more active than aryl substituents. Substitution of a methyl group at the α-position of the acetic acid side chain (to give the corresponding propionic acid derivative) leads to equiactive analogues. The resulting chirality introduced in the molecules is important. Anti-inflammatory activity is displayed only by the *S*-(+)-enantiomer. The conformation of indomethacin appears to play a crucial role in its anti-inflammatory actions. The acetic acid side chain is flexible and can assume a large number of different conformations. The preferred and lower-energy conformation of the N-*p*-chlorobenzoyl group is one in which the chlorophenyl ring is oriented away from the 2-methyl group (or *cis* to the methoxyphenyl ring of the indole nucleus) and is noncoplanar with the indole ring because of steric hindrance produced by the 2-methyl group and the hydrogen atom at the 7-position. These conformations are represented as follows:

"*cis*-like" "*trans*-like"

Indomethacin

Absorption and Metabolism. Absorption of indomethacin occurs rapidly on oral administration, and peak plasma levels are obtained within 2 to 3 hours. Being an acidic substance ($pK_a = 4.5$), it is highly bound to plasma proteins (97%). Indomethacin is converted to inactive metabolites, approximately 50% of a single dose is 5-O-demethylated by CYP2C9 and 10% conjugated with glucuronic acid. Nonhepatic enzyme systems hydrolyze indomethacin to N-deacylated metabolites. The metabolism of indomethacin is illustrated in Figure 36.12.

The ability of indomethacin to potently inhibit prostaglandin biosynthesis may account for its anti-inflammatory, antipyretic, and analgetic actions. Pronounced side effects are frequently observed at antirheumatic doses. A large number of individuals taking indomethacin, especially those over the age of 70, experience undesirable effects of the GI tract (e.g., nausea, dyspepsia, diarrhea, and erosion of the stomach walls), the CNS (e.g., headache, dizziness, and vertigo), and the ears (tinnitus), and many patients must discontinue its use. As with other arylalkanoic acids, administration of indomethacin with food or milk decreases GI side effects.

Indomethacin is available for the short-term treatment of acute gouty arthritis, acute pain of ankylosing spondylitis, and osteoarthritis. An injectable form to be reconstituted also is available as the sodium trihydrate salt for IV use in premature infants with patent ductus arteriosus. Because of its ability to suppress uterine activity by inhibiting prostaglandin biosynthesis, indomethacin also has an unlabeled use to prevent premature labor.

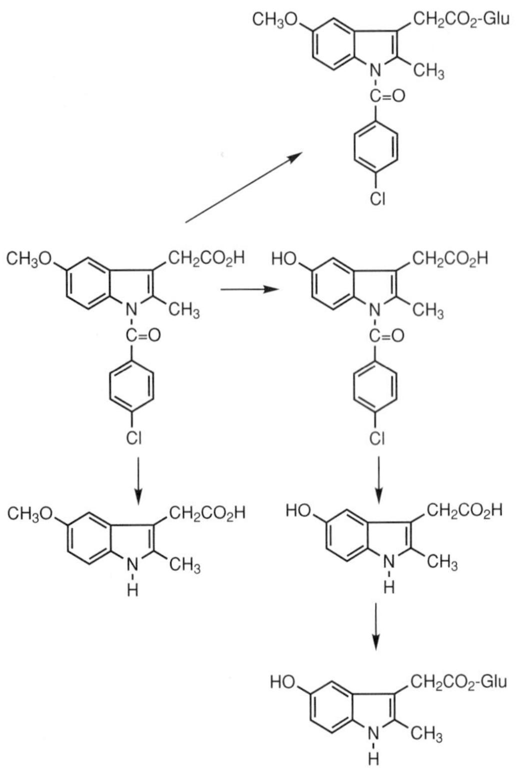

Fig. 36.12. Metabolism of indomethacin. Glu, glucuronide.

Sulindac. Sulindac was introduced in the United States in 1978 by Merck as a result of chemical studies designed to produce an analogue without the side effects commonly associated with the use of indomethacin, particularly GI irritation. It achieved wide popularity, and it remains one of the more widely used NSAIDs. Its synthesis also was reported by Shen et al. (50). Sulindac is a prodrug and is converted to a metabolite that appears to inhibit the cyclooxygenase system approximately eightfold as effectively as aspirin. In anti-inflammatory and antipyretic assays, it is only about half as potent as indomethacin but is equipotent in analgetic assays.

Structure–Activity Relationships. The use of classical bioisosteric changes in medicinal chemistry drug design was invoked in the design of sulindac. The isosteric replacement of the indole ring with the indene ring system resulted in a derivative with therapeutically useful anti-inflammatory activity and fewer CNS and GI side effects but with other undesirable effects, particularly poor water solubility and resultant crystalluria. The replacement of the N-p-chlorobenzoyl substituent with a benzylidiene function resulted in active derivatives. However, when the 5-methoxy group of the indene isostere was replaced with a fluorine atom, enhanced analgetic effects were observed. The decreased water solubility of the indene isostere was alleviated by replacing the chlorine atom of the phenyl substituent with a sulfinyl group. The importance of stereochemical features in the action of sulindac, introduced by the benzylidene double bond, is evidenced by the observation that the (Z)-isomer is a much more potent anti-inflammatory agent than the corresponding (E)-isomer (Fig. 36.10). This *cis*-relationship of the phenyl substituent to the aromatic ring bearing the fluoro substituent is similar to the proposed conformation of indomethacin, suggesting that both indomethacin and sulindac assume similar conformations at the active site of arachidonic acid cyclooxygenase.

Absorption and Metabolism. Sulindac is well absorbed on oral administration (90%), reaches peak plasma levels within 2 to 4 hours, and being acidic ($pK_a = 4.5$), is highly bound to serum proteins (93%). The metabolism of sulindac plays a major role in its actions, because all of the pharmacological activity is associated with its major metabolite. Sulindac is, in fact, a pro-drug, the sulfoxide function being reduced to the active sulfide metabolite. Sulindac is absorbed as the sulfoxide, which is not an inhibitor of prostaglandin biosynthesis in the GI tract. As discussed earlier, prostaglandins exert a protective effect in the GI tract, and inhibition of their synthesis here leads to many of the GI side effects noted for most NSAIDs. Once sulindac enters the circulatory system, it is reduced to the sulfide, which is an inhibitor of prostaglandin biosynthesis in the joints. Thus, sulindac produces less GI side effects, such as bleeding, ulcerations, and so on, than indomethacin and many other NSAIDs. In addition, the active metabolite has a plasma half-life approximately twice that of the parent compound (~16 hours versus 8 hours), which favorably affects the dosing schedule. In addition to the sulfide metabolite, sulindac is oxidized to the corresponding sulfone, which is inactive. A minor product results from hydroxylation of the benzylidene function and the methyl group at the 2-position. Glucuronides of several metabolites also are found. Sulindac as well as the sulfide and the sulfone metabolites are all highly protein-bound. Despite the fact that the sulfide metabolite is a major activation product and is found in high concentration in human plasma, it is not found in human urine, perhaps because of its high degree of protein binding. The major excretion product is the sulfone metabolite and its glucuronide conjugate. The complete metabolism of sulindac is illustrated in Figure 36.13.

Whereas the toxicity of sulindac is lower than that observed for indomethacin and other NSAIDs, the spectrum of adverse reactions is very similar. The most frequent side effects reported are associated with irritation of the GI tract (e.g., nausea, dyspepsia, and diarrhea), although these effects generally are mild. Effects on the CNS (e.g., dizziness and headache) are less common. Dermatological effects are less frequently encountered.

Sulindac is indicated for long-term use in the treatment of rheumatoid arthritis, osteoarthritis, ankylosing spondylitis, and acute gouty arthritis. The usual maximum dosage is 400 mg/day, with starting doses recommended at 150 mg twice a day. It is recommended that sulindac be administered with food.

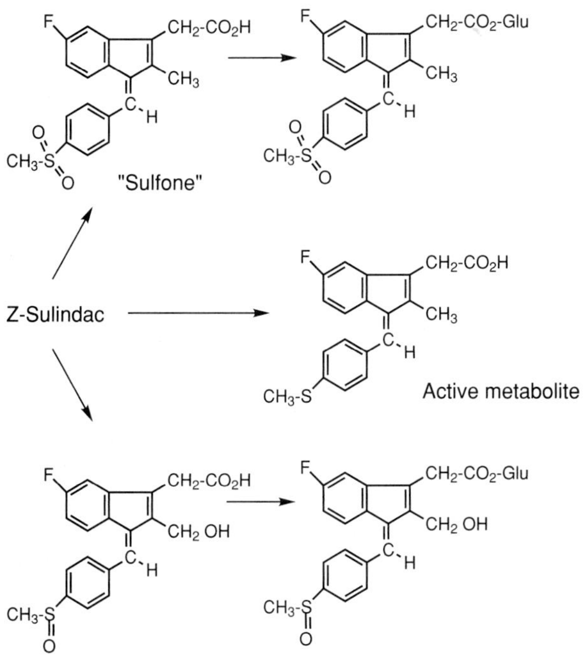

Fig. 36.13. Metabolism of sulindac. Glu, glucuronide.

Tolmetin Sodium. Tolmetin is synthesized straightforwardly from 1-methylpyrrole (51). It was introduced in the United States in 1976, and like other NSAIDs, inhibits prostaglandin biosynthesis. Tolmetin, however, also inhibits polymorph migration and decreases capillary permeability. Its anti-inflammatory activity, as measured in the carrageenan-induced rat paw edema and cotton pellet granuloma assays, is intermediate between those of phenylbutazone and indomethacin.

Structure–Activity Relationships. The relationship of tolmetin to indomethacin is clear, with each containing a noncoplanar *p*-chlorobenzoyl group and an acetic acid function. Tolmetin possesses a pyrrole ring instead of the indole ring in indomethacin. Replacement of the 5-*p*-toluoyl group with a *p*-chlorobenzoyl moiety produced little effect on activity, whereas introduction of a methyl group in the 4-position of the pyrrole ring produced interesting results. The 4-methyl-5-*p*-chlorobenzoyl analogue is approximately four times as potent as tolmetin. Substitution of the *p*-methyl group of tolmetin with a *p*-chloro group blocked oxidative metabolism, increasing duration of action to approximately 24 hours. McNeil marketed this compound in 1980 as zomepirac, an analgetic that was removed from the market in 1983 because of severe anaphylactic reactions, particularly in patients sensitive to aspirin. Unlike the previous structure–activity relationships discussed for arylalkanoic acids, the propionic acid analogue is slightly less potent than tolmetin.

Absorption and Metabolism. Tolmetin sodium is rapidly and almost completely absorbed on oral administration, with peak plasma levels being attained within the first hour of administration. It has a relatively short plasma half-life of approximately 1 hour because of extensive first-pass metabolism, involving hydroxylation of the *p*-methyl group to the primary alcohol, which is subsequently oxidized to the dicarboxylic acid shown below. This metabolite is inactive in standard in vivo anti-inflammatory assays. The free acid ($pK_a = 3.5$) is highly bound to plasma proteins (99%), and excretion of tolmetin and its metabolites occurs primarily in the urine.

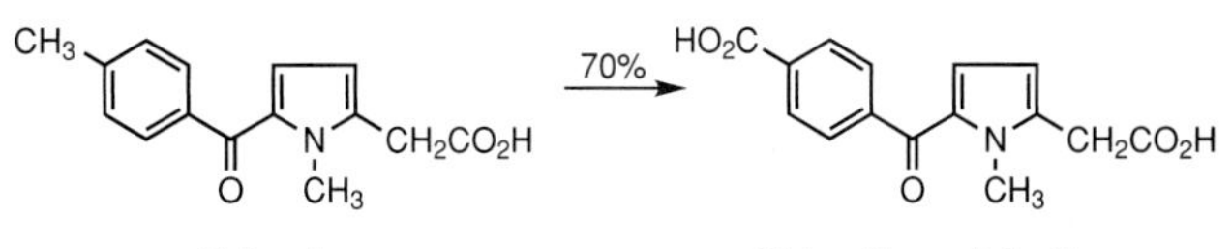

Tolmetin → (70%) → Tolmetin metabolite

Approximately 15 to 20% of an administered dose is excreted unchanged and 10% as the glucuronide conjugate of the parent drug. Conjugates of the dicarboxylic acid metabolite account for the majority of the remaining administered drug.

The most frequently adverse reactions are those involving the GI tract (e.g., abdominal pain, discomfort, and nausea) but appear to be less than those observed with aspirin. The CNS effects (e.g., dizziness and drowsiness) also are observed. Few cases of overdosage have been reported, but in such cases, recommended treatment includes elimination of the drug from the GI tract by emesis or gastric lavage and elimination of the acidic drug from the circulatory system by enhancing alkalinization of the urine with sodium bicarbonate.

Tolmetin sodium is indicated for the treatment of rheumatoid arthritis, juvenile rheumatoid arthritis, and osteoarthritis.

Diclofenac Sodium. Diclofenac is synthesized from N-phenyl-2,6-dichloroaniline (52). It is available in 120 different countries and, perhaps, is the most widely used NSAID in the world. It was introduced in the United States in 1989 but was first marketed in Japan in 1974. It ranks among the top prescription drugs in the United States. Diclofenac possesses structural characteristics of both arylalkanoic acid and the anthranilic acid classes of anti-inflammatory drugs, and it displays anti-inflammatory, analgetic, and antipyretic properties. In the carrageenan-induced rat paw edema assay, it is twice as potent as indomethacin and 450 times as potent as aspirin. As an analgetic, it is six times more potent than indomethacin and 40 times as potent as aspirin in the phenyl benzoquinone– induced writhing assay in mice. As an antipyretic, it is twice as potent as indomethacin and more than 350 times as potent as aspirin in the yeast-induced fever assay in rats. Diclofenac is unique among the NSAIDs in that it possesses three possible mechanisms of action: 1) inhibition of the arachidonic acid cyclooxygenase system (3 to 1,000 times more potent than other NSAIDs on a molar basis), resulting in a decreased production of prostaglandins and thromboxanes;

2) inhibition of the lipoxygenase pathway, resulting in decreased production of leukotrienes, particularly the pro-inflammatory LKB_4; and 3) inhibition of arachidonic acid release and stimulation of its reuptake, resulting in a reduction of arachidonic acid availability.

Structure–Activity Relationships. Structure–activity relationships in this series have not been extensively studied. It does appear that the function of the two *o*-chloro groups is to force the anilino-phenyl ring out of the plane of the phenylacetic acid portion, this twisting effect being important in the binding of NSAIDs to the active site of the COX, as previously discussed.

Absorption and Metabolism. Diclofenac is rapidly and completely (~100%) absorbed on oral administration, with peak plasma levels being reached within 1.5 to 2.5 hours. The free acid (pK_a = 4.0) is highly bound to serum proteins (99.5%), primarily albumin. Only 50 to 60% of an oral dose is bioavailable because of extensive hepatic metabolism. Four major metabolites resulting from aromatic hydroxylation have been identified. The major metabolite via CYP3A4 is the 4′-hydroxy derivative and accounts for 20 to 30% of the dose excreted, whereas the 5-hydroxy, 3′-hydroxy, and 4′,5-dihydroxy metabolites via CYP2C9 account for 10 to 20% of the excreted dose. The remaining drug is excreted in the form of sulfate conjugates. Although the major metabolite is much less active than the parent compound, it may exhibit significant biological activity, because it accounts for 30 to 40% of all of the metabolic products. The metabolism of diclofenac is illustrated in Figure 36.14.

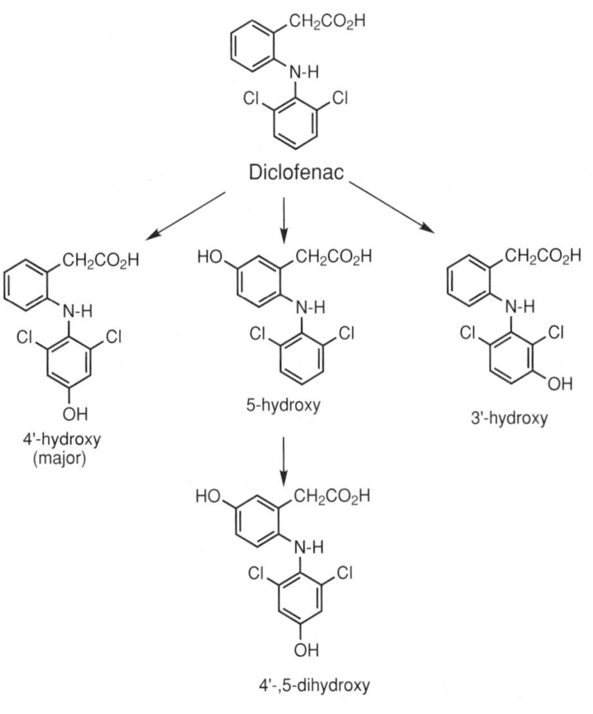

Fig. 36.14. Metabolism of diclofenac.

Diclofenac sodium is indicated for the treatment of rheumatoid arthritis, osteoarthritis, and ankylosing spondylitis.

Etodolac. Etodolac is promoted as the first of a new chemical class of anti-inflammatory drugs, the pyranocarboxylic acids. Although not strictly an arylacetic acid derivative (because there is a two-carbon atom separation between the carboxylic acid function and the heteroaromatic ring) (Fig. 36.10), it still possesses structural characteristics similar to those of the heteroarylacetic acids and is classified here. It was introduced in the United States in 1991 for acute and long-term use in the management of osteoarthritis and as an analgetic. It also possesses antipyretic activity. Etodolac is marketed as a racemic mixture, although only the *S*-(+)-enantiomer possesses anti-inflammatory activity in animal models. Etodolac also displays a high degree of enantioselectivity in its inhibitory effects on the arachidonic acid cyclooxygenase system. With regard to its anti-inflammatory actions, etodolac was approximately 50 times more active than aspirin, three times more potent than sulindac, and one-third as active as indomethacin. The ratio of the anti-inflammatory activity to the median effective dose (ED50) for gastric ulceration or erosion was more favorable for etodolac (median inhibitory dose [ID50]/ED50 = 10) than for aspirin, naproxen, sulindac, or indomethacin (ID50/ED50 = 4). At 2.5 to 3.5 times the effective anti-inflammatory dose, etodolac was reported to produce less GI bleeding than indomethacin, ibuprofen, or naproxen. The primary mechanism of action appears to be inhibition of the biosynthesis of prostaglandins at the cyclooxygenase step, with no inhibition of the lipoxygenase system. Etodolac, however, possesses a more favorable ratio of inhibition of prostaglandin biosynthesis in human rheumatoid synoviocytes and chondrocytes than by cultured human gastric mucosal cells compared to ibuprofen, indomethacin, naproxen, diclofenac, and piroxicam. Thus, although etodolac is no more potent an NSAID than many others, the lower incidence of GI side effects represents a potential therapeutic advantage.

Structure–Activity Relationships. During a search for newer, more effective antiarthritic drugs in the 1970s, the Ayerst group led by Humber investigated a series of pyranocarboxylic acids of the general structure shown below (53,54).

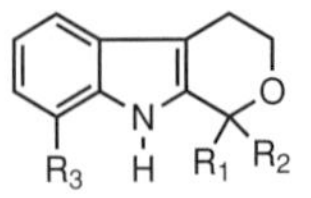

Structure–activity relationship studies indicated that alkyl groups at R_1 and an acetic acid function at R_2 enhanced anti-inflammatory activity. Lengthening the acid chain, or ester or amide derivatives, gave inactive compounds. The corresponding α-methylacetic acid derivatives also were inactive. Increasing the chain length of the R_1 substituent to ethyl or n-propyl gave derivatives that were 20 times more potent than methyl. A number of aromatic substituents in the aromatic ring were evaluated, and substituents at the 8-position were most beneficial. Among the most active were the 8-ethyl, 8-n-propyl, and 7-fluoro-8-methyl derivatives. Etodolac was found to possess the most favorable anti-inflammatory to gastric distress properties among these analogues.

Absorption and Metabolism. Etodolac is rapidly absorbed following oral administration, with maximum serum levels being achieved within 1 to 2 hours, and it is highly bound to plasma proteins (99%) with pK_a 4.7. The penetration of etodolac into synovial fluid is greater than or equal to that of tolmetin, piroxicam, or ibuprofen. Only diclofenac appears to provide greater penetration. Etodolac is metabolized to three hydroxylated metabolites and to glucuronide conjugates, none of which possesses important pharmacological activity. Metabolism appears to be the same in the elderly as in the general population, so no dosage adjustment appears necessary.

Etodolac is indicated for the management of the signs and symptoms of osteoarthritis and for the management of pain.

Nabumetone. Nabumetone is unique among the NSAIDs in that it represents a new class of nonacidic prodrugs, being rapidly metabolized after absorption to form a major active metabolite, 6-methoxynaphthalene-acetic acid. It was introduced in the United States in 1992 and is synthesized from 2-acetyl-6-methoxynaphthalene (55). Nabumetone, being nonacidic, does not produce a significant primary insult and is an ineffectual inhibitor of prostaglandin cyclooxygenase in gastric mucosa, thus producing minimum secondary insult. The result is that gastric side effects of nabumetone appear to be minimized. Once the parent drug enters the circulatory system, however, it is metabolized to an active metabolite, 6-methoxynaphthalene-2-acetic acid (6MNA), which is an effective inhibitor of cyclooxygenase in joints. Nabumetone thus represents a classic example of the prodrug approach in drug design.

In the carrageenan-induced rat paw assay, nabumetone is approximately 13 times more potent than aspirin, one-third as active as indomethacin, and half as active as diclofenac. It is only half as active as aspirin as an analgetic, as measured by the phenylquinone-induced writhing assay in mice. Despite its lower potency, the advantages of nabumetone may reside in its favorable gastric irritancy profile. The ratio of gastric irritancy dose in rats to anti-inflammatory activity in rats (ED50) for nabumetone is 21.25, whereas this ratio is 0.41 for aspirin, 0.55 for indomethacin, 0.72 for diclofenac, 3.00 for tolmetin, and 7.85 for zomepirac.

Structure–Activity Relationships. Introduction of methyl or ethyl groups on the butanone side chain greatly reduced anti-inflammatory activity. The ketone function can be converted to a dioxolane with retention of activity, whereas converting the ketone to an oxime reduced activity. Removal of the methoxy group at the 6-position reduced activity, but replacement of the methoxy with a methyl or chloro group gave active compounds. Replacement of the methoxy with hydroxyl, acetoxy, or N-methylcarbamoyl groups, or positional isomers of the methoxy group at the 2- or 4-positions, greatly reduced activity. The active metabolite, 6-MNA, is closely related structurally to naproxen, differing only by the lack of an α-methyl group. The ketone precursor, [4-(6-methoxy-2-naphthyl)pentan-2-one], that would be expected to produce naproxen as a metabolite was inactive in chronic models of inflammation.

Absorption and Metabolism. Nabumetone is absorbed primarily from the duodenum. Milk and food increase the rate of absorption and the bioavailability of the active metabolite. Plasma concentrations of unchanged drug are too low to be detected in most subjects after oral administration, so most pharmacokinetic studies have involved the disposition of the active metabolite. Pharmacokinetic properties are altered in elderly patients, with higher plasma levels of the active metabolite being noted. Nabumetone undergoes rapid and extensive metabolism in the liver, with a mean absolute bioavailability of the active metabolite of 38%. The metabolism of nabumetone is illustrated in Figure 36.15. The major,

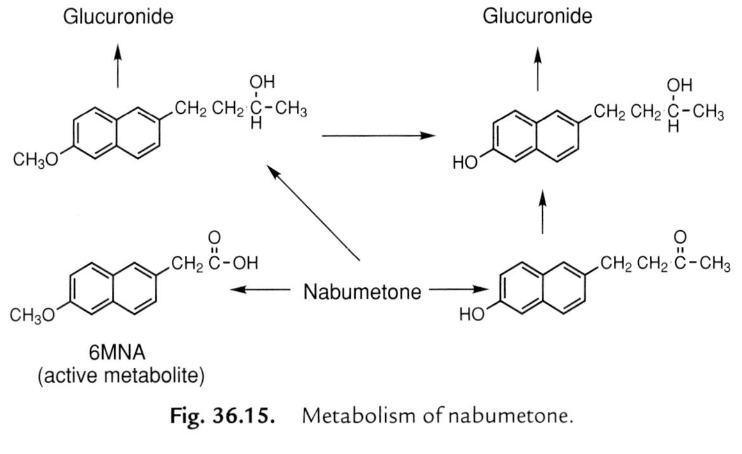

Fig. 36.15. Metabolism of nabumetone.

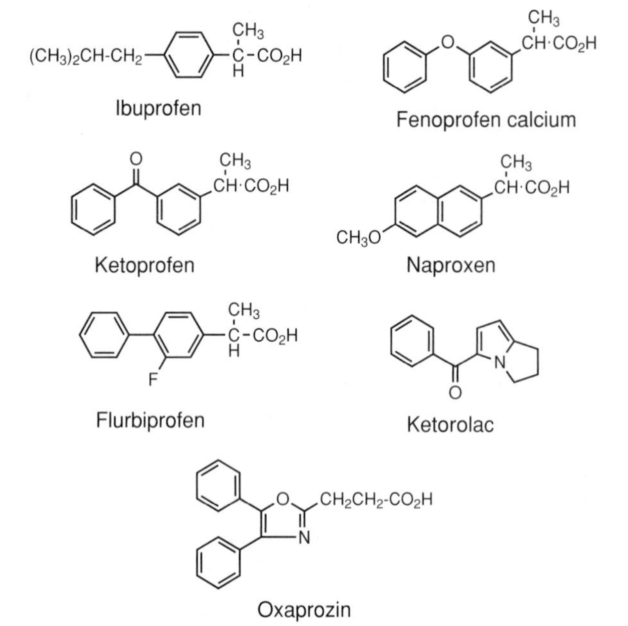

Ibuprofen

Fenoprofen calcium

Ketoprofen

Naproxen

Flurbiprofen

Ketorolac

Oxaprozin

Fig. 36.16. Structures of aryl- and heteroarylpropionic acid derivatives.

most active metabolite is 6MNA, but the initial alcohol metabolite, a minor product, and its esters also possess significant anti-inflammatory properties.

Nabumetone is indicated for the acute and chronic treatment of the signs and symptoms of osteoarthritis and rheumatoid arthritis. The recommended starting dosage is 1,000 mg as a single dose with or without food. More symptomatic relief of severe or persistent symptoms may be obtained at doses of 1,500 or 2,000 mg/day.

ARYL- AND HETEROARYLPROPIONIC ACIDS. Structures of aryl- and heteroarylpropionic acid derivatives are shown in Figure 36.16.

±-Ibuprofen. The synthesis of ibuprofen was originally reported in 1964 from p-isobutylacetophenone (56), but the drug was not marketed in the United States until 1974, despite the fact that it had been available for several years in Europe. It was the first NSAID approved since indomethacin, and was immediately accepted into therapy. Its success precipitated the introduction of many new drugs in the 1970s. This chemical class currently comprises the largest group of NSAIDs. Ibuprofen became the first prescription NSAID to become available as an OTC analgetic in almost 30 years and is available under a number of brand names. It is marketed as the racemic mixture, although biological activity resides almost exclusively in the *S*-(+)-isomer. Ibuprofen is more potent than aspirin but less potent than indomethacin in anti-inflammatory and prostaglandin biosynthesis inhibition assays, and it produces moderate degrees of gastric irritation.

Structure–Activity Relationships. The substitution of an α-methyl group on the alkanoic acid portion of acetic acid derivatives enhances anti-inflammatory actions and reduces many side effects. For example, the acetic acid analogue of ibuprofen, ibufenac (*p*-isobutylphenylacetic acid), is less potent and more hepatotoxic than ibuprofen. The stereochemistry associated with the chiral center in the arylpropionic acids, but lacking in the acetic acid derivatives, plays an important role in both the in vivo and in vitro activities of these drugs. As indicated earlier, although marketed as a racemic mixture, the (+)-enantiomer of ibuprofen possess greater activity in vitro than the (−)-isomer. The eudismic (*S*/*R*) ratio for the inhibition of bovine prostaglandin synthesis is approximately 160, but in vivo, the two enantiomers are equiactive (see next section on absorption and metabolism). The (+)-enantiomer of ibuprofen—and of most of the arylpropionic acids under investigation—has been shown to possess the (*S*)-absolute configuration.

Absorption and Metabolism. Ibuprofen is rapidly absorbed on oral administration, with peak plasma levels being generally attained within 2 hours and a duration of action of less than 6 hours. As with most of these acidic NSAIDs, ibuprofen (pK_a = 4.4) is extensively bound to plasma proteins (99%) and will interact with other acidic drugs that are protein bound. Metabolism occurs rapidly, and the drug is nearly completely excreted in the urine as unchanged drug and oxidative metabolites within 24 hours following administration (Fig. 36.17). Metabolism by CYP2C9 (90%) and CYP2C19 (10%) involves primarily ω-, and ω_1-, and ω_2-oxidation of the p-isobutyl side chain, followed by alcohol oxidation of the primary alcohol resulting from ω–oxidation to the corresponding carboxylic acid. All metabolites are inactive. When

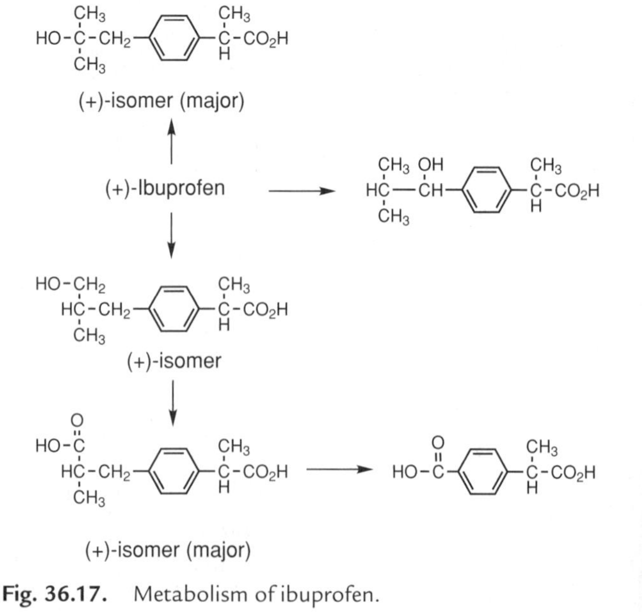

(+)-isomer (major)

(+)-Ibuprofen

(+)-isomer

(+)-isomer (major)

Fig. 36.17. Metabolism of ibuprofen.

ibuprofen is administered as the individual enantiomers, the major metabolite isolated is the *S*-(+)-enantiomer whatever the configuration of the starting enantiomer. Interestingly, the *R*-(−)-enantiomer is inverted to the *S*-(+)-enantiomer in vivo via an acetyl–coenzyme A intermediate, accounting for the observation that the two enantiomers are bioequivalent in vivo. This is a metabolic phenomenon that also has been observed for other arylpropionic acids, such as ketoprofen, benoxaprofen, fenoprofen, and naproxen (57).

Ibuprofen is indicated for the relief of the signs and symptoms of rheumatoid arthritis and osteoarthritis, the relief of mild to moderate pain, the reduction of fever, and the treatment of dysmenorrhea.

±-Fenoprofen Calcium. The calcium and sodium salts of fenoprofen possess similar bioavailability, distribution, and elimination characteristics. It is the calcium salt that is marketed, however, because it has the advantage of being less hygroscopic. Its original synthesis was reported in 1970 (58), and it was marketed in the United States in 1976. Fenoprofen is less potent in anti-inflammatory assays than ibuprofen, indomethacin, ketoprofen, or naproxen. As an inhibitor of prostaglandin biosynthesis, it is much less potent than indomethacin, more potent than aspirin, and about equipotent with ibuprofen. It also possesses analgetic and antipyretic activity. It possesses other pharmacological properties, such as inhibition of phagocytic and complement functions and stabilization of lysosomal membranes. Fenoprofen is marketed as a racemic mixture, because no differences have been observed in the in vivo anti-inflammatory or analgetic properties of the individual enantiomers. The ability of *R*-(−)-arylpropionic acids to undergo inversion to the *S*-(+)-enantiomers, however, may be involved. Like other NSAIDs, in vitro prostaglandin synthesis assays indicate that the *S*-(+)-enantiomer is more potent than the *R*-(−)-isomer.

Structure–Activity Relationships. Placing the phenoxy group in the ortho- or para-position of the arylpropionic acid ring markedly decreases activity. Replacement of the oxygen bridge between the two aromatic rings with a carbonyl group yields an analogue (ketoprofen) that also is marketed.

Absorption and Metabolism. Fenoprofen is readily absorbed (85%) on oral administration and is highly bound (99%) to plasma proteins. Peak plasma levels are attained within 2 hours of administration. The free acid has a pK_a of 4.5, which is within the range of the other arylalkanoic acids. Fenoprofen is rather extensively metabolized, primarily through glucuronide conjugation with the parent drug and the CYP2C9 4′-hydroxy metabolite.

Fenoprofen calcium is indicated for treatment of rheumatoid arthritis and osteoarthritis and for the relief of mild to moderate pain.

±-Ketoprofen. Ketoprofen (Fig. 36.10) was introduced in 1986 and was synthesized from 2-(p-amino- phenyl)propionic acid via a thiaxanthone intermediate (59). Ketoprofen, unlike many NSAIDs, inhibits the synthesis of leukotrienes and leukocyte migration into inflamed joints in addition to inhibiting the biosynthesis of prostaglandins. It stabilizes the lysosomal membrane during inflammation, resulting in decreased tissue destruction. Antibradykinin activity also has been observed. Bradykinin is released during inflammation and can activate peripheral pain receptors. In addition to anti-inflammatory activity, ketoprofen also possesses antipyretic and analgetic properties. Although it is less potent than indomethacin as an anti-inflammatory agent and an analgetic, its ability to produce gastric lesions is about the same (60).

Absorption and Metabolism. Ketoprofen is rapidly and nearly completely absorbed on oral administration, reaching peak plasma levels within 0.5 to 2 hours. It is highly plasma protein bound (99%) despite a lower acidity ($pK_a = 5.9$) than some other NSAIDs. Wide variation in plasma half-lives has been reported. It is metabolized by glucuronidation of the carboxylic acid, CYP3A4 and CYP2C9 hydroxylation of the benzoyl ring, and reduction of the keto function.

Ketoprofen is indicated for the long-term management of rheumatoid arthritis and osteoarthritis, for mild to moderate pain, and for primary dysmenorrhea.

Naproxen. Naproxen is synthesized from 2-methoxynaphthalene and the (+)-isomer obtained by resolution with cinchonidine (61). It was introduced in the United States in 1976 and, as a generic drug, has consistently been among the more popular NSAIDs. It is marketed as the *S*-(+)-enantiomer, but interestingly, the sodium salt of the (−)-isomer also is on the market as Anaprox. As an inhibitor of prostaglandin biosynthesis, it is 12 times more potent than aspirin, 10 times more potent than phenylbutazone, three to four times more potent than ibuprofen, and four times times more potent than fenoprofen, but it is approximately 300 times less potent than indomethacin. In vivo anti-inflammatory assays are consistent with this relative order of potency. In the carrageenan-induced rat paw edema assay, it is 11 times more potent than phenylbutazone and 55 times as potent as aspirin, but only 0.7 times as potent as indomethacin. In the phenylquinone writhing assay for analgesia, it is nine times as potent as phenylbutazone and seven times as potent as aspirin, but only 10% as potent as indomethacin. In the yeast-induced pyrexia assay for antipyretic activity, it is seven times as potent as phenylbutazone, 22 times as potent as aspirin, and 1.2 times as potent as indomethacin. The order of gastric ulcerogenic activity is sulindac < naproxen < aspirin, indomethacin, ketoprofen, and tolmetin.

Structure–Activity Relationships. In a series of substituted 2-naphthylacetic acids, substitution in the 6-position led to maximum anti-inflammatory activity. Small lipophilic groups, such as Cl, CH_3S, and CHF_2O, were active analogues, with CH_3O being the most potent. Larger groups were found to be less active. Derivatives of 2-naphthylpropionic acids are more potent than the corresponding acetic acid analogues. Replacing the carboxyl group with functional groups capable of being metabolized to the carboxyl function (e.g., —CO_2CH_3, —CHO, or —CH_2OH) led to a retention of activity. The S-(+)-isomer is the more potent enantiomer. Naproxen is the only arylalkanoic acid NSAID currently marketed as optically active isomers.

Absorption and Metabolism. Naproxen is almost completely absorbed following oral administration. Peak plasma levels are achieved within 2 to 4 hours following administration. Like most of the acidic NSAIDs (pK_a = 4.2), it is highly bound (99.6%) to plasma proteins. Approximately 70% of an administered dose is eliminated as either unchanged drug (60%) or as conjugates of unchanged drug (10%). The remainder is converted to the 6-O-desmethyl metabolite by both CYP3A4 and CYP1A2 and, further, to the glucuronide conjugate of the demethylated metabolite. The 6-O-desmethyl metabolite lacks anti-inflammatory activity. Like most of the arylalkanoic acids, the most common side effect associated with the use of naproxen is irritation to the GI tract. The most common other adverse reactions are associated with CNS disturbances (e.g., nausea and dizziness).

Naproxen is indicated for the treatment of rheumatoid arthritis, osteoarthritis, juvenile arthritis, ankylosing spondylitis, tendinitis, bursitis, acute gout, and primary dysmenorrhea and for the relief of mild to moderate pain.

±-Suprofen. Suprofen is a white, microcrystalline powder that is slightly soluble in water. It was originally synthesized from thiophene in 1974 (62) and was introduced in the United States in 1985 for the treatment of dysmenorrhea and as an analgetic for mild to moderate pain. Reports of severe flank pain and transient renal failure appeared, however, with the syndrome being noted abruptly within several hours after one or two doses of the drug; therefore, suprofen was removed from the U.S. market in 1987. Obviously, clinical trials are not always sufficient to determine a drug's safety, and postmarketing surveillance becomes most important. Suprofen was reintroduced in the United States in 1990 as a 1% ophthalmic solution for the prevention of surgically induced miosis during cataract extraction. Miosis complicates the removal of lens material and implantation of a posterior chamber intraocular lens that thus increases the risk of ocular trauma. The mechanism of action also involves inhibition of prostaglandin synthesis, because prostaglandins constrict the iris sphincter independent of a cholinergic mechanism. Additionally, prostaglandins also break down the blood-aqueous barrier, allowing the influx of plasma proteins into aqueous humor, resulting in an increase in intraocular pressure.

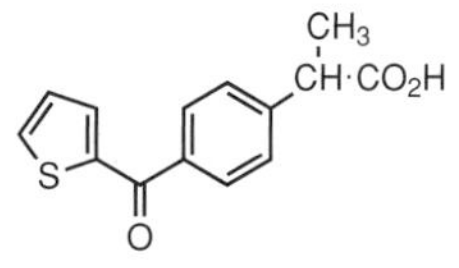

CH_3 CH·CO_2H S O

Suprofen

±-Flurbiprofen. Flurbiprofen (Fig. 36.10) synthesis was originally reported in 1974 (63). During a study of the pharmacological properties of a large number of substituted phenylalkanoic acids, including ibuprofen and ibufenac, the most potent were found to be substituted 2-(4-biphenyl)propionic acids. Further toxicological and pharmacological studies indicated that flurbiprofen possessed the most favorable therapeutic profile, so it was selected for further clinical development. It was not marketed until 1987, when it was introduced as the sodium salt as Ocufen, the first topical NSAID indicated for ophthalmic use in the United States. The indication for Ocufen is the same as that for Profenal—that is, to inhibit intraoperative miosis induced by prostaglandins in cataract surgery. Thus, flurbiprofen is an inhibitor of prostaglandin synthesis. The oral form was introduced in 1988 as Ansaid (another non-steroidal anti-inflammatory drug) and gained immediate acceptance. In acute inflammation assays in adrenalectomized rats, flurbiprofen was found to be 536-fold more potent than aspirin and 100-fold more potent than phenylbutazone. Orally, it was half as potent as methylprednisolone. As an antipyretic, it was 403 times as potent as aspirin in the yeast-induced fever assay in rats and was 26 times more potent than ibuprofen as an antinociceptive.

Absorption and Metabolism. Flurbiprofen is well absorbed after oral administration, with peak plasma levels being attained within 1.5 hours. Food alters the rate of absorption but not the extent of its bioavailability. It is extensively bound to plasma proteins (99%) and has a plasma half-life of 2 to 4 hours. Metabolism is extensive, with 60 to 70% of flurbiprofen and its metabolites being excreted as sulfate and glucuronide conjugates. Flurbiprofen shows some interesting metabolic patterns, with 40 to 47% as the 4′-hydroxy metabolite, 5% as the 3′,4′-dihydroxy metabolite, 20 to 30% as the 3′-hydroxy-4′-methoxy metabolite, and the remaining 20 to 25% of the drug being excreted unchanged. None of these metabolites demonstrates significant anti-inflammatory activity. The metabolism of flurbiprofen is presented in Figure 36.18.

Flurbiprofen is indicated as an oral formulation for the acute or long-term treatment of rheumatoid arthritis and osteoarthritis and as an ophthalmic solution for the inhibition of intraoperative miosis.

Ketorolac Tromethamine. Ketorolac (Fig. 36.10) represents a cyclized, heteroarylpropionic acid derivative, with the α-methyl group being fused to the pyrrole ring. It was introduced in 1990 and is indicated as a peripheral analgetic for

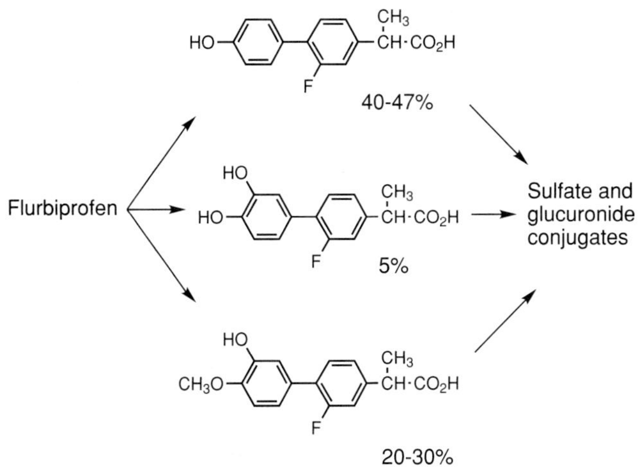

Flurbiprofen → HO–C₆H₄–C₆H₃(F)–CH(CH₃)–CO₂H 40-47% ; HO,HO–C₆H₃–C₆H₃(F)–CH(CH₃)–CO₂H 5% ; HO,CH₃O–C₆H₃–C₆H₃(F)–CH(CH₃)–CO₂H 20-30% → Sulfate and glucuronide conjugates

Fig. 36.18. Metabolism of flurbiprofen.

short-term use and for the relief of ocular itching caused by seasonal allergic conjunctivitis, although it exhibits anti-inflammatory and antipyretic activity as well. It was initially introduced only in an injectable form, but recently, an oral formulation has been made available. Its analgetic activity resembles that of the centrally acting analgetics, with 15 to 30 mg of ketorolac producing analgesia equivalent to a 12-mg dose of morphine, and it has become a widely accepted alternative to narcotic analgesia. Ketorolac inhibits prostaglandin synthesis. Although the analgetic effect is achieved within 10 minutes of injection, peak analgesia lags behind peak plasma levels by 45 to 90 minutes. The free acid has a pK_a of 3.5, and it is not surprising that it is highly plasma protein bound (>99%). Ketorolac is metabolized by CYP2C9 to its *p*-hydroxy derivative and to conjugates that are excreted primarily in the urine.

Oxaprozin. Oxaprozin (Fig. 36.10) was marketed in 1993 for acute and long-term use in the management of signs and symptoms of osteoarthritis and rheumatoid arthritis. Oxaprozin is synthesized by condensing benzoin with succinic anhydride and cyclizing the resulting benzoin hemisuccinate with ammonium acetate. Although not formally a propionic acid of the α-methylacetic acid type, it appears to be similar to the other propionic acid derivatives considered here. Oxaprozin is well absorbed (100%) following oral administration, but maximum plasma concentrations are not reached until 3 to 5 hours following ingestion. Oxaprozin is an anti-inflammatory agent possessing a rapid onset of action and a prolonged duration of action. In both the carrageenan raw paw edema assay and analgetic tests, it was equipotent with aspirin. Oxaprozin has been associated with the appearance of rash and/or mild photosensitivity. Some patients experience an increased incidence of rash on sun-exposed skin during clinical testing. Oxaprozin, aspirin, ibuprofen, indomethacin, naproxen, and sulindac have comparable efficacy in the treatment of rheumatoid arthritis, whereas oxaprozin, aspirin, naproxen, and piroxicam have comparable efficacy in osteoarthritis. It is highly bound to plasma proteins (99%), is highly lipophilic, and undergoes little first-pass metabolism. Metabolism is via hepatic microsomal oxidation and glucuronidation. Active phenolic metabolites are produced (<5%) but do not appear to contribute significantly to the overall pharmacological activity of oxaprozin.

Oxaprozin possesses a relatively long elimination half-life of 59 hours (range, 26–92 hours), enabling once-daily dosing. Administration with food appears to delay absorption but not bioavailability.

Several properties of the NSAIDs are summarized in Table 36.4.

N-Arylanthranilic Acids (Fenamic Acids)

The anthranilic acid class of NSAIDs is the result of the application of classical medicinal chemistry bio-isosteric drug design concepts, because these derivatives are nitrogen isosteres of salicylic acid. In the early 1960s, the Parke-Davis research group reported the development of a series of N-substituted anthranilic acids that have since been given the chemical class name of fenamic acids. The fact that this class of compounds possesses little advantage over the salicylates with respect to their anti-inflammatory and analgetic properties has diminished interest in their large-scale development relative to the arylalkanoic acids. Mefenamic acid was introduced in the United States in 1967 as an analgetic, and this remains the primary indication despite the fact that it possesses modest anti-inflammatory activity. Flufenamic acid has been available in Europe as an antirheumatic agent, but there are no apparent plans to introduce this drug in the United States. With regard to anti-inflammatory activity, mefenamic acid is approximately 1.5 times as potent as phenylbutazone and half as potent as flufenamic acid. Meclofenamic acid was introduced in the United States as its sodium salt in 1980, primarily as an antirheumatic agent and analgetic. The structures of these fenamic acids are shown in Figure 36.19.

The fenamic acids share a number of pharmacological properties with the other NSAIDs. Because these drugs are potent inhibitors of prostaglandin biosynthesis, it is tempting to speculate that this represents their primary mechanism of action. Scherrer, like Shen, had proposed a hypothetical receptor for NSAIDs and later modified (64) the receptor to represent the active site of arachidonic acid cyclooxygenase. Structurally, the fenamic acids fit the proposed active site of arachidonic acid cyclooxygenase proposed by Shen (12) (Fig. 36.1), because they possess an acidic function connected to an aromatic ring along with an additional lipophilic binding site—in this case, the N-aryl substituent. The greater anti-inflammatory activity of meclofenamic acid compared to that of mefenamic acid correlates well with its ability to inhibit prostaglandin synthesis. Scherrer (65) compared the in vivo anti-inflammatory activities, clinical

Table 36.4. Some Properties of the NSAIDs

Drug	Year Introduced	Anti-inflammatory Dose (mg)	Onset (Duration) of Action	Peak Plasma Levels (h)	Protein binding (%)	Biotransformation	Elimination Half-life (h)	pKa
Aspirin	1899	3200–6000	ND	2	90	Plasma hydrolysis and hepatic	< 30 min	3.5
Diclofenac (Voltaren)	1989	100–200	30 min (~8 h)	1.5–2.5	99	Hepatic; first-pass metabolism: 3A4	1–2	4.0
Diflunisal (Dolobid)	1982	500–1000	1 h (8–12 h)	2–3	99	Hepatic	8–12	3.3
Etodolac (Lodine)	1991	800–1200	30 min (4–6 h)	1–2	99	Hepatic : 2C9	6–7	4.7
Fenoprofen Ca (Nalfon)	1976	1200–2400	NR	2	99	Hepatic :2C9	3	4.5
Flurbiprofen (Ansaid)	1988	200–300	NR	1.5	99	Hepatic : 2C9	6 (2–12)	4.2
Ibuprofen (Motrin, Advil)	1974	1200–3200	30 min (4–6h)	2	99	Hepatic; first-pass metabolism: 2C9, 2C19	~2	4.4
Indomethacin (Indocin)	1965	75–150	2–4 h (2–3 d)	2–3	97	Hepatic : 2C9	5 (3–11)	4.5
Ketoprofen (Orudis)	1986	150–300	NR	0.5–2	99	Hepatic :2c9, 3A4	~2	5.9
Meclofenamate Na (Meclomen)	1980	200–400	1h (4–6h)	4.0	99	Hepatic :2C9	2–3	NR
Mefenamic acid (Ponstel)	1967	1000	NR	2–4	79	Hepatic: 2C9	2	4.2
Meloxicam (Mobic)	2000	7.5–15	NR	4–5	99	Hepatic 2C9	15–20	1.1 : 4.2
Nabumetone* (Relafen)	1992	1500–2000	NR	2.5 (1–8) 6-MNA	99**	Hepatic; first-pass metabolism to 6-MNA	6-MNA 23	Neutral
Naproxen (Naprosyn, Anaprox)	1976	500–1000	NR	2–4	99	Hepatic: 3A4, 1A2	13	4.2
Oxaprozin (Daypro)	1993	1200	NR	3–5	99	Hepatic: 2C9	25	4.3
Piroxicam (Feldene)	1982	20	2–4 h (24 h)	2	99	Hepatic: 2C9	50	1.8; 5.1
Sulindac* (Clinoril)	1978	400	NR	2–4	93	Hepatic; sulfide metabolite active	50	4.5
Tolmetin (Tolectin)	1976	1200	NR	<1	99	Hepatic	5	3.5

H= hours; m= min; NR=not reported.
* Pro-drug

anti-inflammatory doses in humans, and the in vitro inhibition of prostaglandin synthesis activities of mefenamic acid, meclofenamic acid, phenylbutazone, indomethacin, and aspirin and suggested an important role of prostaglandin synthesis inhibition in the production of therapeutic effects of the fenamic acids.

Side effects are those primarily associated with GI disturbances (e.g., dyspepsia, discomfort, and especially, diarrhea), some CNS effects (e.g., dizziness, headache, and drowsiness), skin rashes, and transient hepatic and renal abnormalities. Isolated cases of hemolytic anemia have been reported.

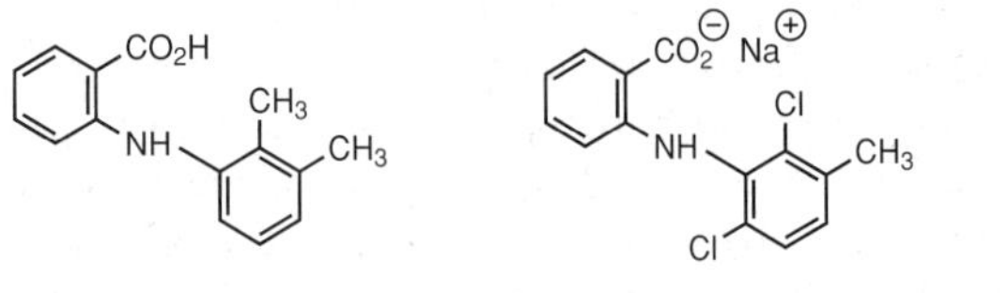

General structure–activity relationships. Substitution on the anthranilic acid ring generally reduces activity, whereas substitution of the N-aryl ring can lead to conflicting results. In the ultraviolet erythema assay for anti-inflammatory activity, the order of activity generally $3' > 2' \gg 4'$ for monosubstitution, with the $3'$-CF_3 derivative (flufenamic acid) being particularly potent.

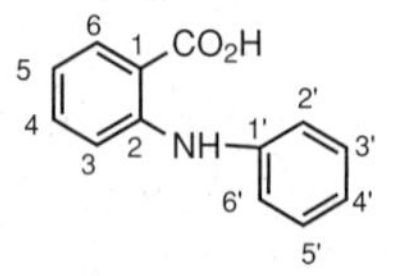

Mefenamic acid   Meclofenamate sodium

Fig. 36.19. Structures of N-arylanthranilic acids (fenamic acids).

The opposite order of activity was observed, however, in the rat paw edema assay, with the $2'$-Cl derivative being more potent than the 3′-Cl analogue. In disubstituted derivatives, in which the nature of the two substituents is the same, 2′,3′-disubstitution appears to be the most effective. A plausible explanation may be found in an examination of the proposed topography of the active sites of arachidonic acid cyclooxygenase using either the Shen or Sherrer models. Proposed binding sites include a hydrophobic trough to which a lipophilic group, noncoplanar with the ring bearing the carboxylic acid function, binds. Substituents on the N-aryl ring that force this ring to be noncoplanar with the anthranilic acid ring should enhance binding at this site and, thus, activity. This may account for the enhanced anti-inflammatory activity of meclofenamic acid, which has two ortho-substituents forcing this ring out of the plane of the anthranilic acid ring, over flufenamic acid (no ortho-substituents) and mefenamic acid (one ortho-substituent). Meclofenamic acid possesses 25 times greater anti-inflammatory activity than mefenamic acid. The NH-moiety of anthranilic acid appears to be essential for activity, because replacement of the NH function with O, CH_2, S, SO_2, N-CH_3, or N-$COCH_3$ functionalities significantly reduces activity. Finally, the position, rather than the nature, of the acidic function is critical for activity. Anthranilic acid derivatives are active, whereas the *m*- and *p*-aminobenzoic acid analogues are not. Replacement of the carboxylic acid function with the isosteric tetrazole moiety has little effect on activity.

Drug interactions. The pK_a values of the N-arylanthranilic acids (4.0–4.2) resemble those of the arylalkanoic acids; thus, it is not surprising that they are strongly bound to plasma proteins and that interactions with other highly protein bound drugs are very probable. The most common interactions reported are those of mefenamic acid and meclofenamic acid with oral anticoagulants. Concurrent administration of aspirin results in a reduction of plasma levels of meclofenamic acid.

Specific drugs

Mefenamic Acid. Mefenamic acid is synthesized from o-chlorobenzoic acid and 2,3-dimethylaniline under catalytic conditions (66). Mefenamic acid is the only fenamic acid derivative that produces analgesia centrally and peripherally. Mefenamic acid is indicated for the short-term relief of moderate pain and for primary dysmenorrhea.

Mefenamic acid is absorbed rapidly following oral administration, with peak plasma levels being attained within 2 to 4 hours. It is highly bound to plasma proteins (78.5%) and has a plasma half-life of 2 to 4 hours. Metabolism occurs through regioselective oxidation of the 3′-methyl group and glucuronidation of mefenamic acid and its metabolites. Urinary excretion accounts for approximately 50 to 55% of an administered dose, with unchanged drug accounting for 6%, the 3′-hydroxymethyl metabolite (primarily as the glucuronide) accounting for 25%, and the remaining 20% as the dicarboxylic acid (of which 30% is the glucuronide conjugate) (Fig. 36.20). These metabolites are essentially inactive.

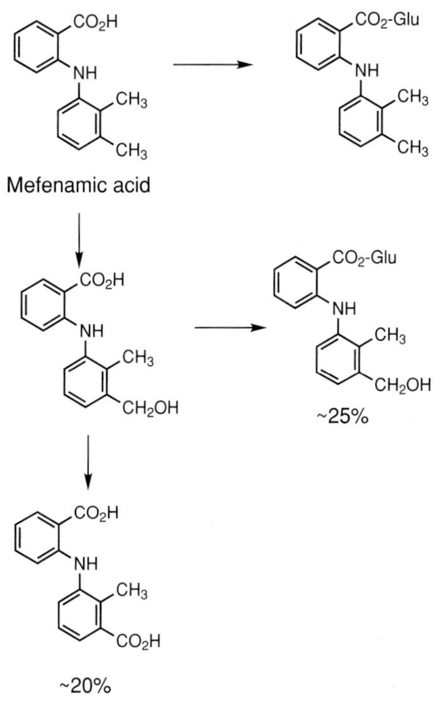

Fig. 36.20. Metabolism of mefenamic acid.

Meclofenamate Sodium. Meclofenamate sodium is rapidly and almost completely absorbed following oral administration, reaching peak plasma levels within 2 hours. It is highly bound to plasma proteins (99%) and has a plasma half-life of 2 to 4 hours. Metabolism involves oxidation of the methyl group, aromatic hydroxylation, monodehalogenation, and conjugation. Urinary excretion accounts for approximately 75% of the administered dose. The major metabolite is the product of 3′-methyl oxidation and has been shown to possess anti-inflammatory activity (Fig. 36.21).

Meclofenamate sodium is indicated for the relief of mild to moderate pain, the acute and chronic treatment of rheumatoid arthritis and osteoarthritis, the treatment of primary dysmenorrhea, and the treatment of idiopathic, heavy menstrual blood loss.

Oxicams

The enolic acid class of NSAIDs has been termed "oxicams" by the U.S. Adopted Name Council to describe the

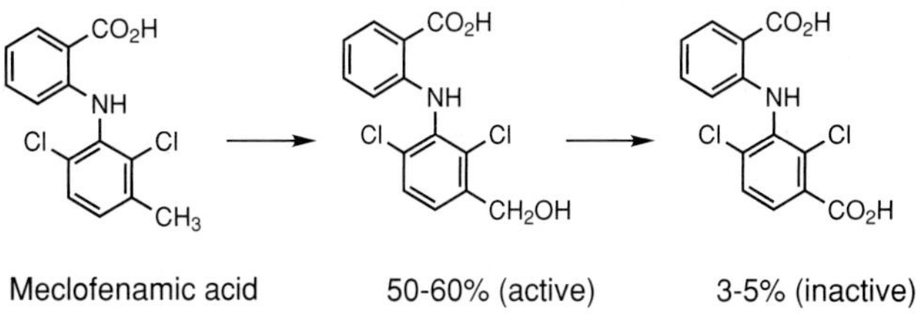

Fig. 36.21. Metabolism of meclofenamic acid.

series of 4-hydroxy-1,2-benzothiazine carboxamides that possess anti-inflammatory and analgetic properties. These structurally distinct substances resulted from extensive studies by the Pfizer group in an effort to produce noncarboxylic acid, potent, and well-tolerated anti-inflammatory drugs. Several series were prepared, including 2-aryl-1,3-indanediones, 2-arylbenzothiophen-3-(2H)-one 1,1-dioxides, dioxoquinoline-4-carboxamides, and 3-oxa-2H-1,2-benzothiazine-4-carboxamide 1,1-dioxides, and evaluated. These results, combined with the previously known activity of 1,3-dicarbonyl derivatives, such as phenylbutazone, led to the development of the oxicams. The first member of this class, piroxicam, was introduced in the United States in 1982 as Feldene and gained immediate acceptance.

Piroxicam is potent in standard in vivo assays, being 200 times more potent than aspirin and at least 10 times as potent as any other standard agent in the ultraviolet erythema assay, as potent as indomethacin and more potent than phenylbutazone or naproxen in the carrageenan-induced rat paw edema assay, and equipotent with indomethacin and 15 times more potent than phenylbutazone in the rat adjuvant arthritis assay. It is less potent than indomethacin, equipotent with aspirin, and more potent than fenoprofen, ibuprofen, naproxen, and phenylbutazone as an analgetic in the phenylquinone writhing assay. Piroxicam inhibits the migration of polymorphonuclear cells into inflammatory sites and inhibits the release of lysosomal enzymes from these cells. It also inhibits collagen-induced platelet aggregation. It is an effective inhibitor of arachidonic acid cyclooxygenase, being almost equipotent with indomethacin and more potent than ibuprofen, tolmetin, naproxen, fenoprofen, phenylbutazone, and aspirin in the inhibition of prostaglandin biosynthesis by methylcholanthrene-transformed mouse fibroblasts (MC-5) assay. A template for designing anti-inflammatory compounds based on CPK space-filling models of the peroxy radical precursor of PGG and inhibitors of cyclooxygenase was proposed (67), and the ability of oxicams, particularly piroxicam, to inhibit this enzyme was subsequently rationalized on the ability of oxicams to assume a conformation resembling that of the peroxy radical precursor (68).

Approximately 20% of individuals on piroxicam report adverse reactions. Not unexpectedly, the greatest incidence of side effects result from GI disturbances. The reported incidence of peptic ulcers, however, is less than 1%.

As will be discussed later, a new oxicam derivative, meloxicam, has been approved as a selective COX-2 inhibitor for the treatment of osteoarthritis.

General structure–activity relationships. Within the series of 4-hydroxy-1,2-benzothiazine carboxamides represented by the general structure shown below, optimum

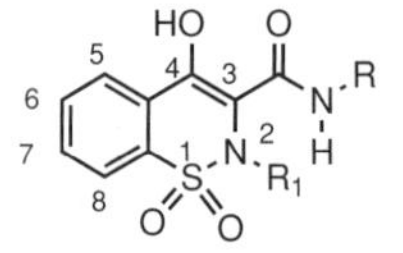

activity was observed when R_1 was a methyl substituent. The carboxamide substituent, R, generally is an aryl or heteroaryl substituent, because alkyl substituents are less active. Oxicams are acidic compounds, with pK_a values in the range of four to six. N-heterocyclic carboxamides generally are more acidic than the corresponding N-aryl carboxamides, and this enhanced acidity was attributed (69) to stabilization of the enolate anion by the pyridine nitrogen atom, as illustrated in tautomer A and additional stabilization by tautomer B:

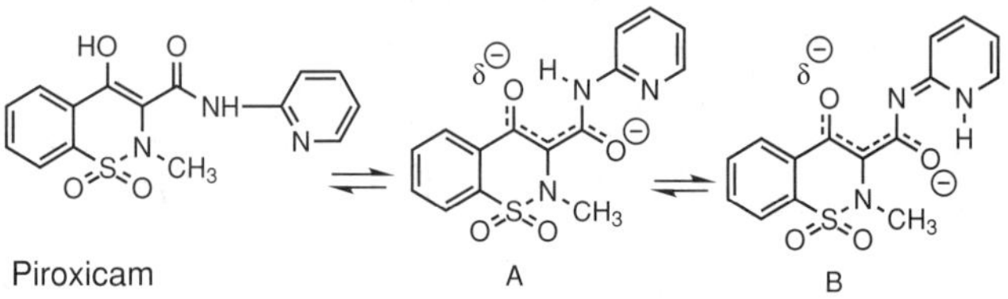

Piroxicam A B

This explains the observation that primary carboxamides are more potent than the corresponding secondary derivatives, because no N-H bond would be available to enhance the stabilization of the enolate anion. When the aryl group is *o*-substituted, variable results were obtained, whereas *m*-substituted derivatives generally are more potent than the corresponding *p*-isomers. In the aryl series, maximum activity is observed with a *m*-Cl substituent. No direct correlations were observed between acidity and activity, partition coefficient, and electronic or spatial properties in this series. Two major differences, however, are observed when R = heteroaryl rather than aryl: The pK_a values generally are two to four units lower, and anti-inflammatory activity increased as much as sevenfold. The greatest activity is associated with the 2-pyridyl (as in piroxicam), 2-thiazolyl, or 3-(5-methyl) isoxazolyl ring systems, with the latter derivative (isoxicam) having been withdrawn from the European market in 1985 following several reports of severe skin reactions. In addition to possessing activity equal to or greater than indomethacin in the carrageenan-induced rat paw edema assay, the heteroaryl carboxamides also possess longer plasma half-lives, providing an improvement in dosing scheduling regimens.

General metabolism. Although the metabolism of piroxicam varies quantitatively from species to species, qualitative similarities are found in the metabolic pathways of humans, rats, dogs, and rhesus monkeys. It is extensively metabolized in humans, with less than 5% of an administered dose being excreted unchanged. The major metabolites in humans result from CYP2C9 hydroxylation of the pyridine ring and subsequent glucuronidation; other metabolites are of lesser importance

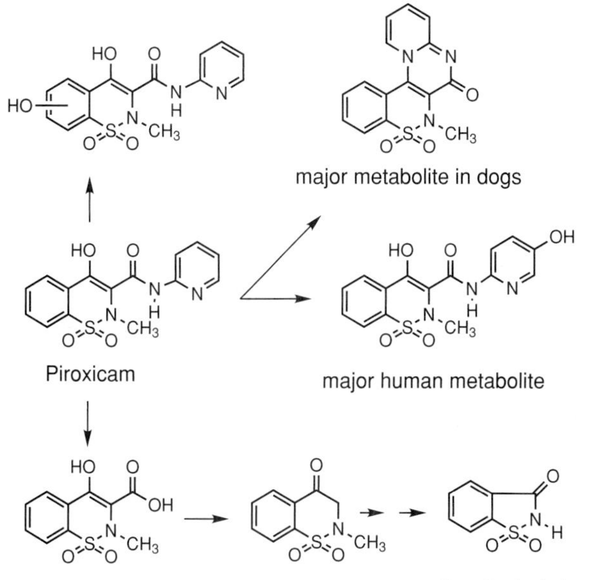

Fig. 36.22. Metabolism of piroxicam.

(Fig. 36.22). Aromatic hydroxylation at several positions of the aromatic benzothiazine ring also occurs; two hydroxylated metabolites have been extracted from rat urine. On the basis of NMR deuterium-exchange studies, hydroxylation at the 8-position was ruled out, indicating that hydroxylation occurs at two of the remaining positions. Other novel metabolic reactions occur. Cyclodehydration gave a tetracyclic metabolite (the major metabolite in dogs), whereas ring contraction following amide hydrolysis and decarboxylation eventually yields saccharin. All the known metabolites of piroxicam lack anti-inflammatory activity. For example, the major human metabolite is 1,000-fold less effective as an inhibitor of prostaglandin biosynthesis than piroxicam itself. Related oxicams undergo different routes of metabolism. For example, sudoxicam (the N-2-thiazolyl analogue) undergoes primarily hydroxylation of the thiazole ring, followed by ring-opening, whereas isoxicam undergoes primarily cleavage reactions of the benzothiazine ring.

DRUG INTERACTIONS. Few reports of therapeutically significant interactions of oxicams with other drugs have appeared. Concurrent administration of aspirin has been shown to reduce piroxicam plasma levels by approximately 20%, whereas the anticoagulant effect of acenocoumarin is potentiated, presumably as a result of plasma protein displacement.

Specific Drugs

Piroxicam. Prixoicam is synthesized by ring-expansion reactions of saccharin derivatives (70). Piroxicam is readily absorbed on oral administration, reaching peak plasma levels in approximately 2 hours. Peak plasma levels appear to be lower when given with food at low doses (30 mg), with no differences appearing with a 60-mg dose, but in general, food does not markedly affect bioavailability. Being acidic (pK_a = 6.3), it is highly bound to plasma proteins (99%). Piroxicam possesses an extended plasma half-life (38 hours), making single daily dosing possible. Piroxicam is indicated for long-term use in rheumatoid arthritis and osteoarthritis.

Meloxicam. In April 2000, the U.S. FDA approved meloxicam for the treatment of osteoarthritis. When meloxicam was initially introduced in the United Kingdom, it was promoted as a selective COX-2 inhibitor. Meloxicam, however, is less selective than celecoxib and much less selective than rofecoxib in in vitro studies (see *Selective COX-2 Inhibitors*). Meloxicam is readily absorbed when administered orally and is highly bound to plasma proteins. Meloxicam is extensively metabolized in the liver, primarily by CYP2C9 and, to a lesser extent, by CYP3A4. The advantages of meloxicam over celecoxib and rofecoxib in the treatment of osteoarthritis (or rheumatoid arthritis) are not readily apparent.

Meloxicam

Gastroenteropathy Induced By Nonselective COX NSAIDs

The effectiveness and popularity of the NSAIDs in the United States and Europe make this class one of the most commonly used classes of therapeutic entities. More than 75 million prescriptions are written annually for the NSAIDs, including aspirin. Unfortunately, until the introduction of the selective COX-2 inhibitors, almost all of the current drugs, which are nonselective COX-1 and COX-2 inhibitors, share the undesirable property of producing damaging effects to gastric and intestinal mucosa, resulting in erosion, ulcers, and GI bleeding, and these represent the major adverse reactions to the use of NSAIDs. As many as 20,000 deaths and 100,000 hospitalizations per year have been associated with GI complications resulting from the use of NSAIDs. Approximately 30 to 40% of patients taking NSAIDs report some type of gastric injury, and approximately 10% discontinue therapy because of these effects. These acute and chronic injuries to gastric mucosa result in a variety of lesions referred to as NSAID gastropathy, which differs from peptic ulcer disease by their localization more frequently in the stomach rather than in the duodenum. Additionally, NSAID-induced lesions occur more frequently in the elderly than typical peptic ulcers do. Normally, the stomach protects itself from the harmful effects of hydrochloric acid and pepsin by a number of protective mechanisms referred to as the gastric mucosal barrier, which consists of epithelial cells, the mucous and bicarbonate layer, and mucosal blood flow. Gastric mucosa actually is a gel consisting of polymers of glycoprotein, which limit the diffusion of hydrogen ions. These polymers reduce the rate at which hydrogen ions (produced in the lumen) and bicarbonate ion (secreted by the mucosa) mix; thus, a pH gradient is created across the mucus layer. Normally, gastric mucosal cells are rapidly repaired when they are damaged by factors such as food, ethanol, or acute ingestion of NSAIDs. Among the cytoprotective mechanisms is the ability of prostaglandins of the PGE series, particularly PGE_1, to increase the secretion of bicarbonate ion and mucus and to maintain mucosal blood flow. The prostaglandins also decrease acid secretion, permitting the gastric mucosal barrier to remain intact.

As mentioned earlier, Figure 36.7 illustrates the ability of aspirin and NSAIDs to induce gastric damage by a dual-insult mechanism. Aspirin and the NSAIDs are acidic substances that can damage the GI tract, even in the absence of hydrochloric acid, by changing the permeability of cell membranes, allowing a back diffusion of hydrogen ions. These weak acids remain un-ionized in the stomach, but the resulting lipophilic nature of these substances allows accumulation or concentration in gastric mucosal cells. Once inside these cells, however, the higher pH of the intracellular environment causes the acids to dissociate and become "trapped" within the cells. The permeability of the mucosal cell membrane is thus altered, and the accumulation of hydrogen ions causes mucosal cell damage. This gastric damage is a result, therefore, of the primary insult of acidic substances. As detailed earlier in this chapter, the primary mechanism of action of the NSAIDs is to inhibit the biosynthesis of prostaglandins at the cyclooxygenase step. The resulting nonselective inhibition of prostaglandin biosynthesis in the GI tract prevents the prostaglandins from exerting their protective mechanism on gastric mucosa; thus, the NSAIDs induce gastric damage through this secondary insult mechanism.

The use of PGE_1 to reduce NSAID-induced gastric damage is limited by the fact that it is ineffective orally and degrades rapidly on parenteral administration, primarily by oxidation of the 15-hydroxy group. To overcome these limitations, misoprostol was synthesized as a prostaglandin pro-drug analogue in which oral activity was achieved by administering the drug as the methyl ester, allowing the bioactive acid to be liberated after absorption. Oxidation of the 15-hydroxy group was overcome by moving the hydroxy group to the 16-position, thus "fooling" the enzyme prostaglandin 15-OH dehydrogenase. Oxidation was further limited by the introduction of a methyl group at the 16-position, producing a tertiary alcohol that is more difficult to oxidize than the secondary alcohol group of the prostaglandins. Misoprostol was introduced in 1989 as a mixture of stereoisomers at the 16-position as Cytotec for the prevention of NSAID-induced gastric ulcers (but not duodenal ulcers) in patients at high risk of complications from a gastric ulcer, particularly the elderly and patients with concomitant debilitating disease and in individuals with a history of gastric ulcers.

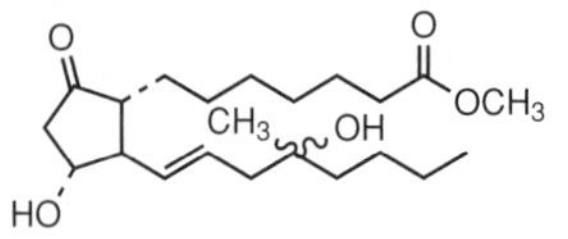

Misoprostol

Selective COX-2 Inhibitors

As previously discussed, the most notable achievement in the development of NSAIDs has been in the area of selective COX-2 inhibitors (coxibs). Classical NSAIDs share similar side effect profiles, particularly on the GI tract, many of which have been attributed to the inhibition of cyclooxygenase, the rate-limiting step in prostaglandin biosynthesis. With the discovery of two isoforms of cyclooxygenase, COX-1 and COX-2, and the realization that COX-1 is beneficial in maintaining normal processes in the GI tract by producing cytoprotective prostaglandins, stimulating bicarbonate secretion and mucus and producing an overall reduction in acid secretion, the search for drugs that selectively inhibit the COX-2 isoform has received much attention. The traditional NSAIDs inhibit COX-1, COX-2, and thromboxane synthetase to varying degrees of selectivity. Decreased gastric mucosal protection (resulting in an enhanced risk of ulceration) and stress-induced decreased renal perfusion result from nonselective inhibition of COX, whereas inhibition of thromboxane synthesis results in increased prostaglandin synthesis and a reduction in platelet aggregation and, thus, an increased bleeding tendency. Those NSAIDs with a greater selectivity for COX-1 generally cause greater GI bleeding and renal toxicity than those with greater selectivity for COX-2.

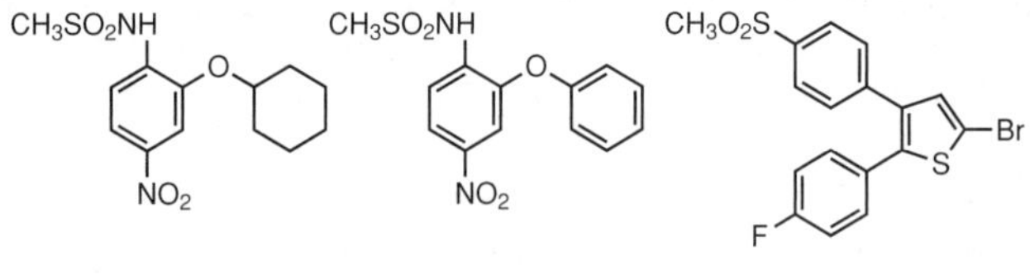

NS-398 Nimesulide DuP 697

These early studies led to extensive efforts by many laboratories to develop selective inhibitors of the COX-2 isoform with the goal of developing an "ideal" NSAID—that is, one that selectively inhibits COX-2, thus reducing the inflammatory response but not interfering with the GI-protective functions of COX-1. Two early lead compounds were developed, NS-398 and DuP 697, which have served as the basis of the development of two widely explored chemical classes. NS-398 and nimesulide are the prototypes of compounds known as "sulides,"

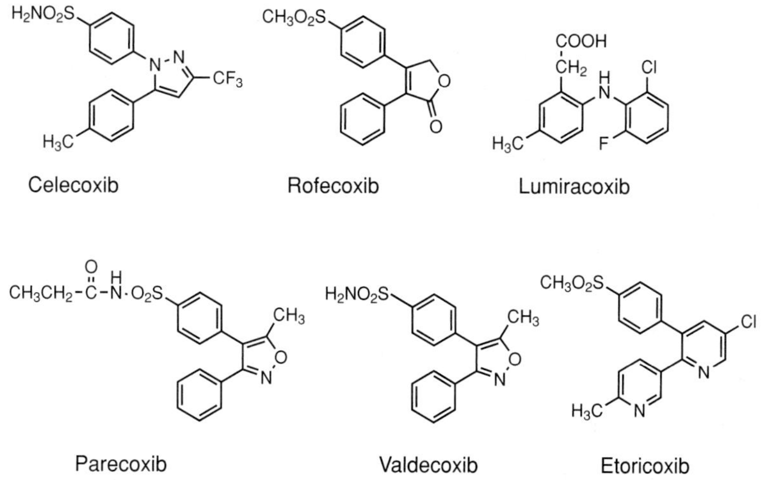

Celecoxib Rofecoxib Lumiracoxib

Parecoxib Valdecoxib Etoricoxib

Fig. 36.23. Structures of selective COX-2 inhibitors.

whereas DuP 697 is the prototype of a class of COX-2 inhibitors termed "coxibs." These efforts led to the introduction of three selective COX-2 inhibitors in the U.S. market (celecoxib, rofecoxib, and valdecoxib), whereas other selective inhibitors under investigation may have been halted (Fig. 36.23). An excellent review of the various chemical classes of selective COX-2 inhibitors has been published (71). Selective COX-2 inhibitors were designed to take advantage of the much larger NSAID binding site on COX-2 compared to the NSAID binding site on COX-1, resulting from the substitution of the smaller amino acid valine in COX-2 for isoleucine at position 523 in COX-1 (see earlier discussion). In COX-1, the larger isoleucine residue near the active site restricts access by larger, relatively rigid side-chain substituents, such as sulfamoyl or sulfonyl side chains usually seen in the selective COX-2 inhibitors.

A comparison of the selectivity of several NSAIDs and selective COX-2 inhibitors was recently presented (Fig. 36.24) (72). In another study regarding the pharmacological and biochemical profile of a new investigational selective COX-2 inhibitor, etoricoxib, the following comparison of COX-1/COX-2 selectivity for several selective and nonselective inhibitors in human whole blood assays was reported (Table 36.5) (73).

The U.S. FDA classifies only celecoxib, rofecoxib, and valdecoxib as selective COX-2 inhibitors. It classifies all other NSAIDs as nonselective.

Perhaps as interesting as the role that COX-2 selective inhibitors play in reducing the incidence of GI side effects among NSAIDs are the reports of other potential therapeutic uses for this new class of drugs, including potential use in the treatment of Alzheimer's disease and carcinomas of various types. The COX-2 appears to be induced in inflammatory plaques that are evident in the CNS in Alzheimer's disease. Several reports have appeared indicating that patients taking NSAIDs have a lower incidence and a decreased rate of progression of Alzheimer's disease. Epidemiological studies suggest a significant reduction in the risk for colon cancer in patients regularly taking aspirin. Additionally, NSAIDs have been reported to reduce the growth rate of polyps in the colon in humans as well as the incidence of tumors of the colon in animals. The expression of COX-2 appears to be significantly up-regulated in carcinoma of the colon. The effectiveness of NSAIDs in the prevention and treatment of other cancers, such as prostate cancer and mammary carcinoma, has been reported as well.

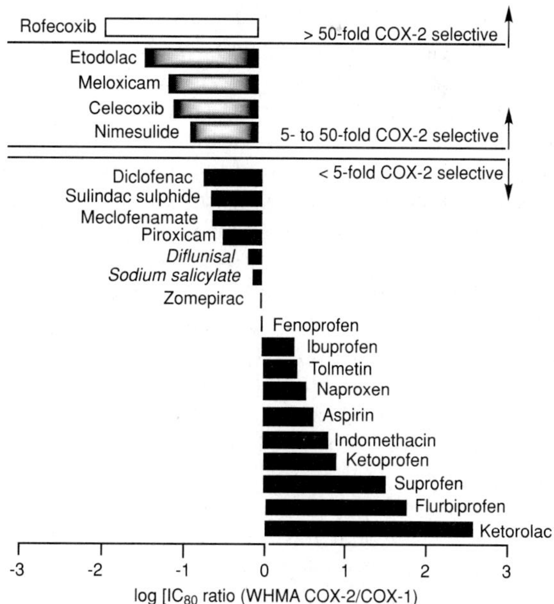

Fig. 36.24. Selectivity of COX-2 inhibitors and NSAIDs given as log inhibitory concentration (IC80) ratio. The "0" line indicates equipotency. (Adapted from Warner TD, Giuliano F, Vojnovic I, et al. Nonsteroid drug selectivities for cyclooxygenase-1 rather than cyclooxygenase-2 are associated with human gastrointestinal toxicity: a full in vitro analysis. Proc Natl Acad Sci U S A 1999; 96:7563–7568; with permission.)

Table 36.5. A Comparison of IC50 (μM) Binding Constants for Selective Versus Nonselective COX Inhibitors

Drug	COX-1	COX-2	COX-1/COX-2 Ratio
Etoricoxib	116	1.1	106
Rofecoxib	18.8	0.53	35
Valdecoxib	26.1	0.87	30
Celecoxib	6.7	0.87	7.6
Nimesulide	4.1	0.56	7.3
Diclofenac	0.15	0.05	3.0
Etodolac	9.0	3.7	2.4
Meloxicam	1.4	0.70	2.0
Indomethacin	0.19	0.44	0.4
Ibuprofen	4.8	24.3	0.2
6MNA	28.9	154	0.2
Piroxicam	0.76	9.0	0.08

6MNA, 6-methoxynaphthalene-2-acetic acid.

This effectiveness is more noticeable among COX-2 selective drugs.

Despite the promise of therapeutic effectiveness of the selective COX-2 inhibitors, the potential for severe cardiovascular effects prompted a critical review of these drugs. This concern was initiated through the revelation of long-term clinical trials of rofecoxib that indicated an increased risk of heart attack. One study completed in 2000, named VIGOR (74), showed an increased risk of myocardial infarction. A later retrospective analysis (75) of 1.4 million patients showed that daily rofecoxib doses of greater than 25 mg increased the risk of heart problems by 3.6-fold as compared with older NSAIDs. The coxibs were found (76) to suppress the formation of PGI_2, which may result in elevated blood pressure and accelerated atherogenesis as well as predisposing patients on coxib therapy to a heightened thrombotic response on the rupture of an atherosclerotic plaque (77). These effects may be related to the different consequences of inhibition of COX-1 and COX-2. Whereas COX-1 mediates the production of prostaglandins and the platelet aggregate stimulator TXA_2, COX-2 may mediate the production of the platelet aggregate inhibitor, prostacyclin. In an excellent review of the adverse cardiovascular effects of selective COX-2 inhibitors, it was suggested that the apparent consequence of selective inhibition of COX-2 is a significant reduction in the production of prostacyclins, whereas the production of TXA_2 by COX-1 is unaffected (78). Of practical interest is a report that resveratrol, an *m*-hydroxyquinone present in red wine that has been suggested to be one agent responsible for the cardioprotective effects observed with the consumption of red wine (i.e., the "French Paradox"), inhibits COX-1 with no apparent effect on COX-2 (79). Thus, the design of highly selective inhibitors of COX-2 would not be as desirable therapeutically as drugs that preferentially inhibit COX-2 but also inhibit COX-1 to a lesser extent.

In one of the most publicized drug withdrawals, Merck voluntarily withdrew rofecoxib from the U.S. market in September 2004, followed by Pfizer's withdrawal of valdecoxib in April 2005. Thus, the future of selective COX-2 inhibitors in the treatment of inflammatory disorders is very clouded.

SPECIFIC DRUGS

Celecoxib (Celebrex). Celecoxib is synthesized by condensing 4-methyl-acetophenone and ethyltrifluoroacetate with sodium methoxide and the resulting butanedione derivative cyclized with 4-hydrazinophenylsulfonamide (80). It was the first NSAID to be marketed as a selective COX-2 inhibitor. Celecoxib is well absorbed from the GI tract, with peak plasma concentrations generally being attained within 3 hours of administration. Peak plasma levels in geriatric patients may be increased, but dosage adjustments in elderly patients generally are not required unless the patient weighs less than 50 kg. Celecoxib is excreted in the urine and feces primarily as inactive metabolites, with less than 3% of an administered dose being excreted as unchanged drug. Metabolism occurs primarily in the liver by CYP2C9 and involves hydroxylation of the 4-methyl group to the primary alcohol, which is subsequently oxi-

> Celecoxib may cause an increased risk of serious cardiovascular thrombotic events, myocardial infarction, and stroke, which can be fatal. All NSAIDs may have a similar risk. This risk may increase with duration of use. Patients with cardiovascular disease or risk factors for cardiovascular disease may be at greater risk. The NSAIDs, including celecoxib, cause an increased risk of serious GI adverse events, including bleeding, ulceration, and perforation of the stomach or intestines, which can be fatal. These events can occur at any time during use and without warning symptoms. Elderly patients are at greater risk for serious GI events.

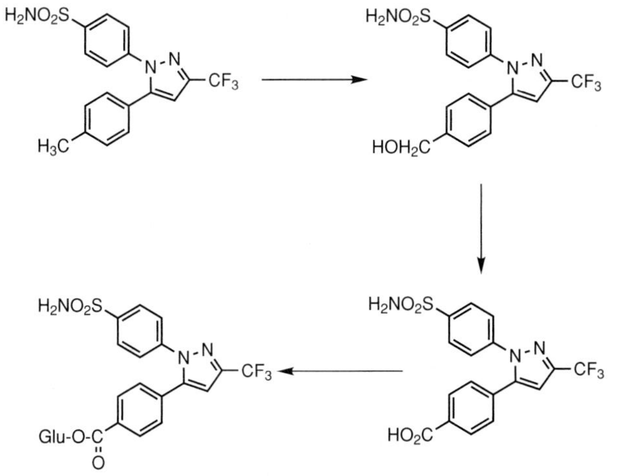

Fig. 36.25. Metabolism of celecoxib.

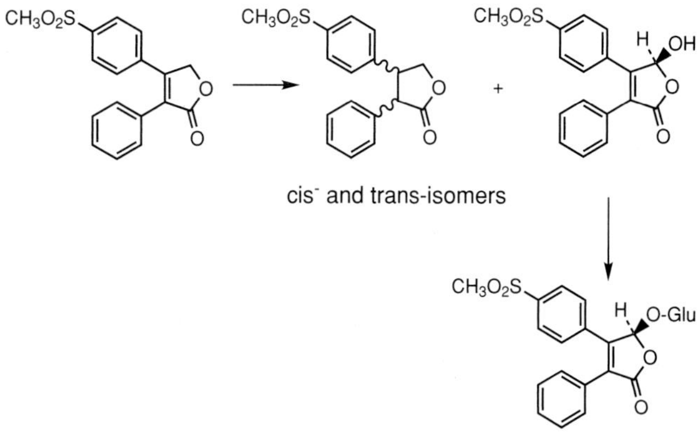

Fig. 36.26. Metabolism of refecoxib.

dized to its corresponding carboxylic acid, the major metabolite (73% of the administered dose) (Fig. 36.25). The carboxylic acid is conjugated, to a slight extent, with glucuronic acid to form the corresponding glucuronide. None of the isolated metabolites have been shown to exhibit pharmacological activity as inhibitors of either COX-1 or COX-2. Celecoxib also inhibits CYP2D6; thus, the potential of celecoxib to alter the pharmacokinetic profiles of other drugs inhibited by this isoenzyme exists. Celecoxib, however, does not appear to inhibit other CYP isoforms, such as CYP2C19 or CYP3A4. Other drug interactions related to the metabolic profile of celecoxib have been noted, particularly with other drugs that inhibit CYP2C. For example, coadministration of celecoxib with fluconazole can significantly increase plasma concentration of celecoxib, because fluconazole inhibits CYP2C9.

Celecoxib is currently indicated for the relief of signs and symptoms of osteoarthritis and rheumatoid arthritis and to reduce the number of adenomatous colorectal polyps in familial adenomatous polyposis as an adjunct to usual care. Celecoxib is at least as effective as naproxen in the symptomatic management of osteoarthritis and at least as effective as naproxen and diclofenac in the symptomatic treatment of rheumatoid arthritis, and it is less likely to cause adverse GI effects. Celecoxib appears to be effective in the management of pain associated with both of these arthritic conditions, but effectiveness in acute or chronic pain has not been fully demonstrated. Unlike aspirin, celecoxib does not exhibit antiplatelet activity. Concomitant administration of aspirin and celecoxib may increase the incidence of GI side effects. Another notable potential drug interaction with celecoxib is its ability, like other NSAIDs, to reduce the blood pressure response to angiotensin-converting enzyme inhibitors. A more detailed discussion of the chemical, pharmacological, pharmacokinetic, and clinical aspects of celecoxib is available (81).

Rofecoxib (Vioxx). Rofecoxib has been synthesized by a number of synthetic routes that have been summarized elsewhere (82). It was the second selective COX-2 inhibitor to be marketed. Rofecoxib is well absorbed from the GI tract on oral administration, with peak plasma levels generally being attained within 2 to 3 hours of dosing. Bioavailability averages 93% following administration of a single dose. The area under the plasma concentration–time curve is increased in patients older than 65 years compared to younger adults and is increased slightly in black and Hispanic patients compared with white patients, but the difference is not considered to be clinically significant.

Rofecoxib is excreted primarily in the urine (72%) as metabolites. Less than 1% is excreted in the urine as unchanged drug, whereas approximately 14% is excreted in the feces as unchanged drug. Although the metabolism of rofecoxib has not been fully determined, the microsomal cytochrome P450 system appears to play only a minor role—a major difference in the metabolic routes of rofecoxib and celecoxib. The major metabolic route appears to form reduction of the dihydrofuranone ring system by cystolic enzymes to the to *cis*- and *trans*-dihydro derivatives. Also isolated is the glucuronide of a hydroxy derivative that results from CYP2C9 oxidative metabolism. None of the isolated metabolites of rofecoxib possess pharmacological activity as COX-1 or COX-2 inhibitors. The metabolism of rofecoxib is presented in Figure 36.26.

> Rofecoxib (Vioxx) was voluntarily withdrawn from the United States and the worldwide market on September 30, 2004, because of safety concerns regarding an increased risk for cardiovascular events, including heart attack and stroke, in patients taking rofecoxib.

Rofecoxib was indicated for the relief of the signs and symptoms of osteoarthritis, for the management of acute pain in adults, and for the treatment of primary dysmenorrhea. Rofecoxib, diclofenac, and ibuprofen possess comparable efficacy in the treatment of osteoarthritis, but serious adverse effects on the GI tract are not observed with rofecoxib. In the treatment of pain, a single 50-mg dose of rofecoxib, a single 550-mg dose of naproxen sodium, and a single 400-mg dose of ibuprofen possess similar onsets of action. Rofecoxib, naproxen sodium, and ibuprofen displayed similar effectiveness in the treatment of postoperative dental pain. A 50-mg dose of rofecoxib was as effective as a 550-mg dose of naproxen sodium in the relief of primary dysmenorrhea in adults. Like celecoxib, rofecoxib does not affect platelet aggregation or bleeding and should not be used as a substitute for aspirin in the prevention of cardiovascular events. A more detailed discussion of the chemical, pharmacological, pharmacokinetic, and clinical aspects of rofecoxib is available (83).

Rofecoxib is approved for the relief of the signs and symptoms of osteoarthritis and the treatment of primary dysmenorrheal.

Valdecoxib (Bextra). Valdecoxib is freely soluble in alkaline aqueous solutions. At recommended doses, the mean oral bioavailability for valdecoxib is 83%, and the time to peak concentration is approximately 3 hours. Time to peak plasma concentration was delayed by 1 to 2 hours when administered with a high-fat meal. Protein binding is very high at 98%. Valdecoxib exhibits linear pharmacokinetics over the usual clinical dose range. Valdecoxib is extensively metabolized in humans. The primary metabolite for valdecoxib involved CYP2C9 hydroxylation of the 5-Me group, which was further metabolized to the inactive carboxylate, and N-hydroxylation at the sulfonamide moiety. Oxidative breakdown of the N-hydroxy sulfonamide function group led to the formation of the corresponding sulfinic acid and sulfonic acid metabolites. The O-and N-glucuronides were the major urinary metabolites. Only 3% of the administered dose was recovered in urine as unchanged valdecoxib. Its elimination half-life is 8 to 11 hours. Approximately 70% of a valdecoxib dose is eliminated in the urine as metabolites, and less than 5% is excreted in the feces and urine unchanged.

> Valdecoxib (Bextra) was voluntarily withdrawn from the U.S. market on April 7, 2005, because of safety concerns regarding increased risk of cardiovascular events and reports of serious and potentially life-threatening skin reactions, including deaths, in patients taking valdecoxib.

Valdecoxib is approved for the relief of the signs and symptoms of osteoarthritis and adult rheumatoid arthritis and for the treatment of primary dysmenorrhea. Valdecoxib is contraindicated for the treatment of post-operative pain immediately following coronary artery bypass graft surgery.

Precautions to consider for valdecoxib are that it may cause bronchoconstriction or anaphylaxis in aspirin-sensitive patients with asthma, who have experienced severe bronchospasm after taking aspirin or other NSAIDs.

Parecoxib (Parecoxib Sodium, Dynstat). As shown in Figure 36.23, parecoxib is a pro-drug of valdecoxib administered IM or IV for perioperative analgesic and anti-inflammatory use. As a pro-drug, it undergoes rapid in vivo hydrolysis to valdecoxib. It is the only parenterally administered coxib. Parecoxib at greater than 20 mg has analgesic activity superior to that of placebo and similar to that of parenteral 30 or 60 mg of ketorolac in patients with postoperative dental pain. A significant adverse effect is drug hypersensitivity. Parecoxib is currently marketed worldwide but has not been approved for use in the United States.

Etoricoxib (Arcoxia). Etoricoxib (Fig. 36.23) is a selective COX-2 inhibitor being developed for postsurgical treatment of dental pain (120 mg) and osteoarthritis. It has a methylsulfonyl group common to the other coxib inhibitors. Etoricoxib is rapidly absorbed, with an oral bioavailability of 80 to 100%, and reaches maximum plasma concentrations in 1 to 2 hours after dosing. Food decreases the rate of absorption but has no effect on the extent of absorption. It exhibits a long elimination half-life of approximately 22 hours, demonstrating linear plasma pharmacokinetics with no accumulation during multiple dosing. Etoricoxib is metabolized involving oxidation of its 6′-methyl group primarily by CYP3A4 but is not an inhibitor of CYP3A4. Other metabolites include 1′-N-oxide and glucuronides. Etoricoxib is primarily excreted as metabolites into the urine.

Lumiracoxib (Prexige). Lumiracoxib (Fig. 36.23) is a selective COX-2 inhibitor developed for the treatment of osteoarthritis, rheumatoid arthritis, and acute pain. It structurally differs from the other selective COX-2 inhibitors in being a phenylacetic acid with a carboxylic acid group (pK_a = 4.7). Lumiracoxib is rapidly absorbed, with an oral bioavailability of 74%, and reaches a maximum plasma concentration 2 hour after dosing. It is highly plasma protein bound and has a short elimination half-life of approximately 4 hours, demonstrating linear plasma pharmacokinetics with no accumulation during multiple dosing. Lumiracoxib is extensively metabolized involving oxidation of its 5-Me group and 4′-hydroxylation of the dihalogenated aromatic ring. The major in vitro oxidative pathways is catalyzed primarily by CYP2C9. Lumiracoxib and its metabolites are excreted via renal and fecal routes in approximately equal amounts. The COX-2 selectivity was confirmed by a lack of inhibition of arachidonic acid and collagen-induced platelet aggregation. As with other selective coxibs, lumiracoxib exhibits a reduced incidence of gastroduodenal erosions compared with that of naproxen. It was approved for use in the United Kingdom and the United States in 2007.

Disease-Modifying Antirheumatic Drugs

The drugs previously discussed as NSAIDs, both the nonselective COX and selective COX-2 inhibitors, have proven to be beneficial in the symptomatic treatment of arthritic disorders and to be a popular therapeutic regimen. Despite their effectiveness and popularity, however, it should be remembered that none of these drugs are effective in preventing or inhibiting the underlying pathogenic, chronic inflammatory processes. Recent interest has been generated by drugs that are effective in the treatment of arthritic disorders yet fail to demonstrate significant activity in the standard screening assays for antiarthritic drugs. Disease-modifying antirheumatic drugs (DMARDs) differ from the previously discussed drugs in that they are drugs that retard or halt the underlying progression, limiting the amount of joint damage that occurs in rheumatoid arthritis while lacking the anti-inflammatory and analgetic effects observed with NSAIDs. Although both NSAIDs and DMARDs improve symptoms of active rheumatoid arthritis, only DMARDs have been shown to alter the disease course and to improve radiographic outcomes. The DMARDs have an effect on rheumatoid arthritis that is different and more delayed in onset than either NSAIDs or corticosteroids. Once persistent disease activity (chronic synovitis) is established, a DMARD should be considered. The development of erosions or joint space narrowing on radiographs of the involved joints is a clear indication for DMARD therapy; however, one should not wait for radiographic changes to occur. They are much slower acting, taking as long as 3 months for measurable clinical benefits to be observed. Although these drugs also possess potentially dangerous adverse side effects, which in many cases limit their long-term use, DMARDs are effective in reducing joint destruction and the progression of early rheumatoid arthritis.

A 2004 study reported that taking DMARDs at early stages in the development of rheumatoid arthritis is especially important to slow the disease and to save the joints and other tissues from permanent damage. Typically, DMARDs are used with an NSAID or a corticosteroid. The NSAID or corticosteroid handles your immediate symptoms and limits inflammation, and the DMARD goes to work on the disease itself.

The DMARDS can be divided into two general categories: synthetic DMARDS, which can be taken orally, and biological DMARDS, which are given by IV infusion or subcutaneously, that target and inactivate cell proteins (cytokines) and T lymphocytes (T cells) from causing joint inflammation. The DMARD methotrexate, in combination with the biological DMARDs, may offer the best control of rheumatoid arthritis for the majority of people, eliminating the need for NSAID medications.

Synthetic Disease-Modifying Antirheumatic Drugs

The synthetic DMARDs include gold salts, hydroxychloroquine, and sulfasalazine. Less common synthetic DMARDs are penicillamine and minocycline. Synthetic immunosuppressants used for the treatment of inflammatory diseases include the antimetabolites methotrexate, leflunomide, and azathioprine.

Gold compounds

Historical Background. At the end of the 19th century, the chemotherapeutic applications of heavy metal derivatives were receiving considerable interest. Among those metals gaining the greatest attention were gold compounds (or gold salts). The first of these, gold cyanide, was effective in vitro against *Mycobacterium tuberculosis.* This discovery prompted others to extend the use of gold compounds in other disease states that are thought to be tubercular in origin. Early clinical observations had suggested similarities in the symptoms of tuberculosis and rheumatoid arthritis, and some thought rheumatoid arthritis to be an atypical form of tuberculosis. In 1927, aurothioglucose was found to relieve joint pain when used to treat bacterial endocarditis. The area of chrysotherapy had begun. Subsequent investigations led to an extensive study of gold compounds in Great Britain by the Empire Rheumatism Council, which reported in 1961 that sodium aurothiomalate was effective in slowing the development of progressive joint diseases. Both aurothioglucose and sodium aurothiomalate are orally ineffective and are administered by IM injection. In 1985, the first orally effective gold compound for arthritis, auranofin, was introduced in the United States. Several other gold compounds have been evaluated clinically but do not appear to offer advantages in terms of efficacy or toxicity.

Mechanism of Action. The biochemical and pharmacological properties shared by gold compounds are quite diverse. The mechanism by which they produce their antirheumatic actions has not been totally determined. The earlier observations that gold compounds were effective in preventing arthritis induced by hemolytic streptococci and by pleuropneumonia-like organisms led to the postulation that they acted through an antimicrobial mechanism. The inability of gold compounds to consistently inhibit mycoplasmal growth in vitro while inhibiting the arthritic process independent of microbial origins, however, suggested that they did not directly produce their effects by this mechanism. The involvement of immunological processes in the pathogenesis of arthritis suggested that a direct suppression of the immunologic response by gold compounds was involved. Available evidence, however, suggests that whereas enzymatic mediators released as a result of the immune response may be inhibited, no direct effect on either immediate or delayed cellular responses is evident to suggest any immunosuppressive mechanism. Suggestions have been made that protein denaturation and macroglobulin formation cause the proteins to become antigenic, thus initiating the immune response and producing biochemical changes in connective tissue, which ultimately leads to rheumatoid arthritis. The possibility that gold compounds inhibit the aggregation of macroglobulins and, in turn, inhibit the formation of immune complexes may account for their ability to slow connective tissue degradation. Interaction with collagen fibrils and, thus, reduction of collagen reactivity that alters the course of the arthritic process also have been postulated. Perhaps the most widely accepted mechanism of action is related to the ability of gold compounds to inhibit lysosomal enzymes, the release of which promotes the inflammatory response. The lysosomal enzymes glucuronidase, acid phosphatase, collagenase, and acid hydrolases are inhibited, presumably through a reversible interaction of gold with sulfhydryl groups on the enzymes. Gold thiomalate inhibits glucosamine-6-phosphate synthetase, a rate-limiting step in mucopolysaccharide biosynthesis and a property shared, to a lesser extent, by several NSAIDs. Gold sodium thiosulfate is a potent uncoupler of oxidative phosphorylation. Gold sodium thiomalate also is a fairly effective inhibitor of prostaglandin biosynthesis in vitro, but the relationship of this effect to the antiarthritic actions of gold compounds has not been clarified.

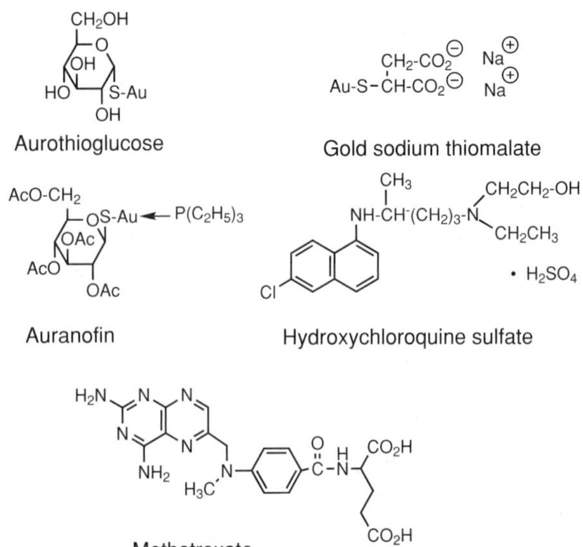

Fig. 36.27. Structures of disease-modifying antirheumatic drugs (DMARDs).

Side Effects. Toxic side effects have been associated with the use of gold compounds, with the incidence of reported adverse reactions in patients on chrysotherapy being as high as 55%. Serious toxicity occurs in 5 to 10% of reported cases. The most common adverse reactions include dermatitis (e.g., erythema, papular, vesicular, and exfoliative dermatitis), mouth lesions (e.g., stomatitis preceded by a metallic taste and gingivitis), pulmonary disorders (e.g., interstitial pneumonitis), nephritis (e.g., albuminuria and glomerulitis), and hematologic disorders (e.g., thrombocytopenic purpura, hypoplastic and/or aplastic anemia, and eosinophilia; blood dyscrasias are rare in incidence but can be severe). Less commonly reported reactions are GI disturbances (e.g., nausea, anorexia, and diarrhea), ocular toxicity (e.g., keratitis with inflammation and ulceration of the cornea and subepithelial deposition of gold in the cornea), and hepatitis. In those cases in which severe toxicity occurs, excretion of gold can be markedly enhanced by the administration of chelating agents, the two most common of which are dimercaprol (British Anti-Lewisite [BAL]) and penicillamine. Corticoids also suppress the symptoms of gold toxicity and the concomitant administration of dimercaprol, and corticosteroids have been recommended in cases of severe gold intoxication.

General Structure–Activity Relationships. Structure–activity relationships of gold compounds have not received a great amount of attention. Two important relationships, however, have been established: 1) Monovalent gold (aurous ion [Au^+]) is more effective than trivalent gold (auric ion [Au^{3+}]) or colloidal gold, and 2) only those compounds in which aurous ion is attached to a sulfur-containing ligand are active (Fig. 36.27). The nature of the ligands affects tissue distribution and excretion properties and, usually, are highly polar, water-soluble functions. Aurous ion has only a brief existence in solution and is rapidly converted to metallic gold or auric ion. Aqueous solutions decompose on standing at room temperature, posing a stability problem for the two injectable gold compounds therapeutically available (aurothioglucose and gold sodium thiomalate). Complexation of Au^+ with phosphine ligands stabilizes the reduced valence state and results in both nonionic complexes that are soluble in organic solvents and an enhancement of oral bioavailability. Other changes also occur. In the phosphine-Au-S compounds, gold has a coordination number of 2, and the molecules are nonconducting monomers in solution. The injectable gold compounds are monocoordinated. Whereas nongold phosphine compounds are ineffective in arthritic assays, the nature of the phosphine ligand in the gold coordination complexes appears to play a greater role in antiarthritic activity than the other groups bound to gold. Within a homologous series, the triethylphosphine gold derivatives provide greatest activity.

The structures of the three therapeutically available gold compounds in the United States are shown in Figure 36.27.

Absorption and Metabolism. Gold compounds generally are rapidly absorbed following IM injection, and the gold is widely distributed in body tissues, with the highest concentrations found in the reticuloendothelial system and in adrenal and renal cortices. Binding of gold from orally administered gold to red blood cells is higher than that of injectable gold. Gold accumulates in inflamed joints, where high levels persist for at least 20 days following injection. Although gold is excreted primarily in the urine, the bulk of injected gold is retained. Gold can be found in the urine months later.

Drug Interactions. The only significant drug interactions reported are the concurrent administration of drugs that also produce blood dyscrasias (most notably phenylbutazone and the antimalarial and immunosuppressive drugs).

Specific Drugs

Gold Sodium Thiomalate. Gold sodium thiomalate (actually a mixture of mono- and disodium salts of gold thiomalic acid) is very water soluble. It is available as a light-sensitive, aqueous solution of pH 5.8 to 6.5. The gold content is approximately 50%. It is administered IM, because it is not absorbed on oral administration and is highly bound (95%) to plasma proteins.

Gold sodium thiomalate is indicated in the treatment of active adult and juvenile rheumatoid arthritis as one part of a complete therapy program. It is recommended that injections be given to patients only when they are in a supine position. They must remain so for 10 minutes following injection.

Aurothioglucose. Aurothioglucose is highly water soluble, and its aqueous solutions decompose on long standing. It therefore is available as a suspension in sesame oil. Gold content is approximately 50%. Following IM injection, it is highly protein bound (95%), and peak plasma levels are achieved within 2 to 6 hours. Following a single 50-mg dose, the biological half-life ranges from 3 to 27 days, but following successive weekly doses, the half-life increases to 14 to 40 days after the third dose. The therapeutic effect does not correlate with serum plasma gold levels but appears to depend on total accumulated gold. Aurothioglucose is indicated for the adjunctive treatment of adult and juvenile rheumatoid arthritis.

Auranofin. Auranofin contains approximately 29% gold. The carbohydrate portion assumes a chair conformation, with all substituents occupying the equatorial position. It is the first orally effective gold compound used to treat rheumatoid arthritis. On a mg gold/kg basis, it is reported to be as effective in the rat adjuvant arthritis assay as the parenterally effective drugs. Daily oral doses produce a rapid increase in kidney and blood gold levels for the first 3 days of treatment, with a more gradual increase on subsequent administration. Plasma gold levels are lower than those attained with parenteral gold compounds. The major route of excretion is via the urine. Auranofin may produce fewer adverse reactions than parenteral gold compounds, but its therapeutic efficacy also may be less.

Auranofin is indicated in adults with active rheumatoid arthritis who have not responded sufficiently to one or more NSAIDs.

Aminoquinolines

BACKGROUND. The 4-aminoquinoline class of antimalarial drugs has been known to possess pharmacological actions that are beneficial in the treatment of rheumatoid arthritis. Two of these drugs, chloroquine and hydroxychloroquine (Fig. 36.27), have been used as antirheumatics since the early 1950s. The corneal and renal toxicity of chloroquine, however, has resulted in its discontinuance for this purpose, although it is still indicated as an antimalarial agent and an amebicide. Whereas hydroxychloroquine is less toxic, it also is less effective than chloroquine as an antirheumatic. The mechanism of action of these drugs as an antirheumatic remains unresolved. Interestingly, most of the data available relates to chloroquine rather than hydroxychloroquine but is assumed to be applicable to the latter. The spectrum of action of the 4-aminoquinolines differs from the NSAIDs in that chloroquine appears to be an antagonist of certain preformed prostaglandins. This effect, however, would indicate an acute, rather than a chronic, antirheumatic effect, whereas chloroquine has been shown to be similar to gold compounds in that it possesses a slow onset of action. Beneficial effects are noted only after 1 to 2 months of administration. Chloroquine inhibits chemotaxis of polymorphonuclear leukocytes in vitro but not in vivo. Its effects on collagen metabolism in connective tissue also are unclear. The most widely accepted mechanism of action of chloroquine and, presumably, of hydroxychloroquine is related to its ability to accumulate in lysosomes. Although evidence indicating stabilization of lysosomal membranes is not convincing, it may inhibit the activity of certain lysosomal enzymes, such as cartilage chondromucoprotease and cartilage cathepsin B. There does not appear to be a correlation of the antirheumatic effects of the 4-aminoquinolines with their antimalarial activity.

HYDROXYCHLOROQUINE SULFATE. Hydroxychloroquine sulfate is highly water soluble and exists in two different forms of different melting points. It is readily absorbed on oral administration, reaching peak plasma levels within 1 to 3 hours. It concentrates in organs such as the liver, spleen, kidneys, heart, lung, and brain, thereby prolonging elimination. Hydroxychloroquine is metabolized by N-dealkylation of the tertiary amines, followed by oxidative deamination of the resulting primary amine to the carboxylic acid derivative. In addition to possessing corneal and renal toxicity, hydroxychloroquine also may cause CNS, neuromuscular, GI, and hematological side effects. Hydroxychloroquine sulfate is indicated for the treatment of rheumatoid arthritis, lupus erythematosus, and malaria.

IMMUNOSUPPRESSANTS. The discovery of drugs that modify the immune response, whether as immunoregulatory, immunostimulatory, or immunosuppressive agents, has been the focus of much recent research activity. Several substances that suppress the immune system have been explored as antirheumatic drugs, because the etiology of rheumatoid arthritis may involve a destructive immune response (3,4). Thus, unlike drugs previously discussed, immunosuppressive drugs may act at the steps involved in the pathogenesis of the inflammatory disorders. As a group, however, these drugs are cytotoxic, as evidenced by the initial development of these drugs as anticancer agents. Among the more widely employed immunosuppressants are azathioprine, methotrexate, leflunomide, and cyclophosphamide. All of these drugs are quite toxic and, generally, are indicated for rheumatoid arthritis only in those patients with severe, active disease who have not responded to full-dose NSAID therapy and at least one DMARD and a corticosteroid. Interestingly, although aspirin and NSAIDs are effective in only one-third of children with juvenile arthritis, methotrexate, when given only once a week at low doses (<20 mg) to minimize side effects, is effective. Cyclosporine (Sandimmune) has been investigated in rheumatoid arthritis and appears to offer short-term benefits, although its toxic effects also limit its long-term use. Cyclosporine appears to inhibit the proliferation of T-helper/inducer lymphocytes, blocking the signaling pathway involved in the etiology of rheumatoid arthritis. The immunosupressants can have potentially serious side effects, such as increased susceptibility to infection.

Specific Drugs

Leflunomide. Leflunomide is a DMARD with anti-inflammatory and immunosuppressive activity used for the management of rheumatoid arthritis. It retards structural damage associated with arthritis in adults who have moderate to severe active rheumatoid arthritis. Leflunomide also is being investigated for use in patients with solid tumors and organ transplant recipients.

Leflunomide is a pro-drug that is rapidly and almost completely metabolized (half-life, <60 minutes) following oral administration to teriflunomide, the pharmacologically active α-cyanoenol metabolite (Fig. 36.28). The C_3-H of the isoxazole ring is essential for the ring opening to its active metabolite. The reaction is similar to CYP1A2-catalyzed dehydration of aldoximes. The exact mechanism of action of leflunomide in the management of rheumatoid arthritis has not been fully elucidated but appears to principally involve inhibition of B-lymphocyte (B-cell) proliferation, reducing antibody formation. Activated lymphocytes must proliferate and synthesize large quantities of cytokines, requiring increased de novo synthesis of uridine monophosphate (UMP) and other pyrimidine nucleotides for its cell life cycle. Therefore, any substance that reduces the intracellular concentration of pyrimidine nucleotides will affect the growth of these activated cells.

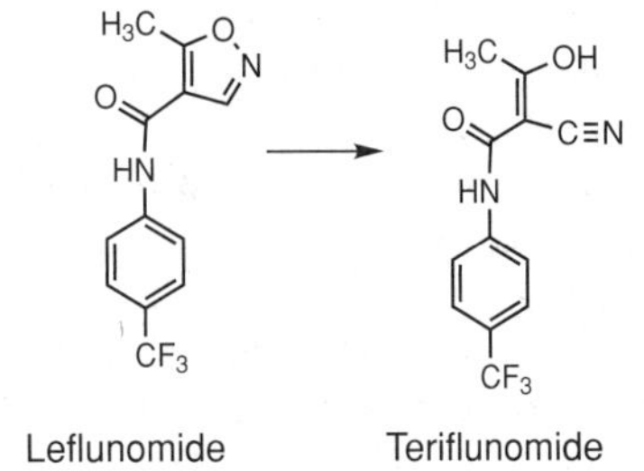

Leflunomide Teriflunomide

Fig. 36.28. Metabolism of leflunomide.

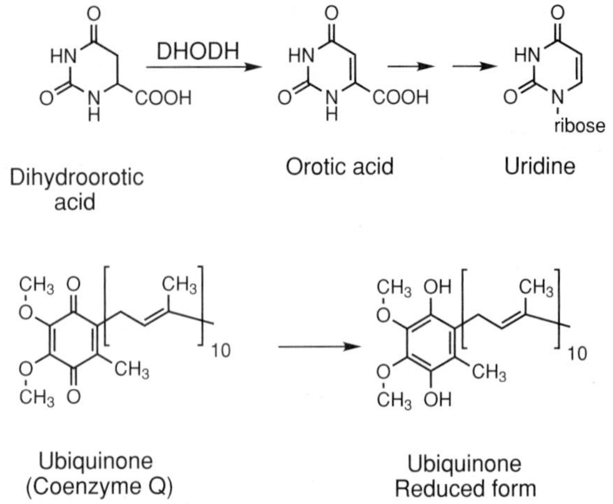

Dihydroorotic acid DHODH Orotic acid Uridine

Ubiquinone (Coenzyme Q) Ubiquinone Reduced form

Fig. 36.29. Dihydroorotate dehydrogenase (DHOH) pathway with cofactor, coenzyme Q.

Leflunomide is inactive, but teriflunomide inhibits pyrimidine de novo synthesis at low therapeutic doses by inhibiting dihydroorotate dehydrogenase (the rate-determining enzyme for the synthesis of UMP), decreasing DNA and RNA synthesis, and arresting the cell proliferation cycle and production of antibodies. The reduction of dihydroorotate to orotate occurs concurrently with the reduction of its cofactor, ubiquinone (coenzyme Q) (Fig. 36.29). The inhibition of dihydroorotate dehydrogenase by teriflunomide demonstrates noncompetitive and uncompetitive kinetics. Administration of leflunomide in patients with rheumatoid arthritis results in progressive removal of B cells and down-regulation of the immune process. Teriflunomide not only inhibits B-cell proliferation but also T-cell proliferation, blocking the synthesis of immunosuppressive cytokines. At high therapeutic doses, leflunomide inhibits protein tyrosine kinases.

Leflunomide is administered orally as a single daily dose without regard to meals. Therapy may be initiated with a loading dosage given for 3 days, followed by the usual maintenance dose. It undergoes primarily enterohepatic circulation, extending its duration of action. Cholestyramine can be used to enhance its elimination in cases of toxicity.

Methotrexate. Methotrexate (Fig. 36.27) is an antifolate drug approved for the treatment of severe active rheumatoid arthritis in adults who are intolerant to or have had an insufficient response to first-line therapy. Although the mechanism of action of methotrexate in rheumatoid arthritis is unknown, recent studies have shown that methotrexate reversibly inhibits dihydrofolate reductase, blocking the proliferation of B cells by interfering with DNA synthesis, repair, and replication. Oral absorption is dose-dependent, being well-absorbed at doses of 7.5–25 mg once a week. At this dose, oral bioavailability is approximately 60%, and food can delay absorption and reduce peak concentration. The volume of distribution is 0.4 to 0.8 L/kg. Protein binding is approximately 50%. It is metabolized to active metabolites, methotrexate polyglutamates and 7-hydroxymethotrexate. Some metabolism occurs by intestinal flora after oral administration. Methotrexate is actively transported into the urine (80–90% unchanged in the urine within 24 hours) via the folate transporter, an organic anion transporter. Its elimination half-life is 3 to 10 hours.

Life-threatening drug interactions are known to occur between methotrexate and NSAIDs, probenecid, and penicillin G. The NSAIDs (salicylate, ibuprofen, ketoprofen, piroxicam, and indomethacin), probenecid, and penicillin G dose dependently inhibited methotrexate elimination into urine by human organic anion transporters (hOAT1, hOAT3, and hOAT4). The inhibitory effects of these drugs on hOAT3 were comparable, with therapeutically relevant plasma concentrations of unbound drugs. Thus, patients with rheumatoid arthritis should not take NSAIDs while taking methotrexate.

Methotrexate therapy requires monitoring of liver enzymes and is contraindicated in those with hepatic disease and in women considering pregnancy.

Sulfasalazine (Azulfidine). Sulfasalazine is a pro-drug that is not active in its ingested form. It is broken down by colonic bacteria into 5-aminosalicylic acid (5-ASA; mesalamine) and sulfapyridine. Some controversy exists regarding which of these two products are responsible for the activity of azulfidine. 5-Aminosalicylic acid, however, is known to have a therapeutic benefit, although it is not clear whether sulfapyridine adds any further benefit. In the colon, the products created by the breakdown of sulfasalazine work as anti-inflammatory agents for treating colon inflammation. The beneficial effect of sulfasalazine is believed to result from a local effect on the bowel, although there also may be a beneficial systemic immune-suppressant effect. Sulfasalazine was approved in 1950.

Sulfasalazine → Metabolism → Sulfapyridine + 5-Aminosalicyclic acid

Following oral administration, sulfasalazine is poorly absorbed, with approximately 20% of the ingested sulfasalazine reaching the systemic circulation. The remainder of the ingested dose is metabolized by colonic bacteria into its components, sulfapyridine and mesalamine (5-ASA). Most of the sulfapyridine metabolized from sulfasalazine (60–80%) is absorbed in the colon following oral administration, and approximately 25% of the 5-ASA metabolized from sulfasalazine is absorbed in the colon. The apparent volume of distribution of sulfasalazine in eight healthy volunteers was 64 L/kg, and that of sulfapyridine was 0.4 to 1.2 L/kg. Protein binding is approximately 99% for sulfasalazine, approximately 50% for sulfapyridine, and approximately 43% for 5-ASA. The absorbed sulfapyridine is acetylated and hydroxylated in the liver, followed by conjugation with glucuronic acid and, for 5-ASA, acetylation in the intestinal mucosal wall and the liver. The elimination half-life is 5 to 10 hours for sulfasalazine and 6 to 14 hours for sulfapyridine, depending on acetylator status of the patient, and 0.6 to 1.4 hours for 5-ASA. Time to peak serum concentration is 1.5 to 6 hours for oral sulfasalazine and 9 to 24 hours for oral sulfapyridine; for enteric-coated tablets, time to peak serum concentration is 3 to 12 hours for sulfasalazine and 12 to 24 hours for sulfapyridine. Approximately 5% of sulfapyridine and approximately 67% of mesalamine are eliminated in the feces, and 75 to 91% of sulfasalazine and sulfapyridine metabolites are excreted in urine within 3 days, depending on the dosage form used. 5-Aminosalicyclic acid is excreted in urine mostly in acetylated form.

Sulfasalazine is used for the treatment of mild to moderate ulcerative colitis; as adjunct therapy in the treatment of severe ulcerative colitis, for the treatment of Crohn's disease, and for the treatment of rheumatoid arthritis or ankylosing spondylitis. Contraindications include hypersensitivity to sulfa drugs, salicylates, intestinal or urinary obstruction, and porphyria.

Biological Disease-Modifying Antirheumatic Drugs

CYTOKINE INHIBITORS

Tumor Necrosis Factor Blockers. T lymphocytes (T cells), a type of white blood cell, are important cells of the immune system. Patients with rheumatoid arthritis have increased numbers of T cells within the inflamed joints. These T cells are "activated"—that is, they multiply and release chemicals (cytokines) that promote the destruction of tissues surrounding the joints and cause the signs and symptoms of rheumatoid arthritis (84).

As discussed earlier in this chapter (see also Chapter 6 for a detailed discussion of cytokines), there is considerable expression of the cytokines, interleukin (IL)-1, IL-6, and tumor necrosis factor (TNF) α by the rheumatoid synovium. TNFα is a proinflammatory cytokine (cell protein) that plays a major role in the pathological inflammatory process of rheumatoid arthritis. TNF is an important mediator of local inflammation, and the release of TNFα from T-cells produces increased vascular permeability, release of nitric oxide with vasodilation, local activation of vascular endothelium, increased expression of adhesion molecules on endothelial blood vessels, and increased platelet activation and adhesion. As TNFα builds up in the joints, it leads to joint inflammation, which ultimately results in joint destruction. Because of its role in the progression of rheumatoid arthritis, methods for rendering TNFα inactive has become a key focus of therapies for rheumatoid arthritis (84). Patients with rheumatoid arthritis display elevated levels of the cytokines, TNFα, IL-1, and IL-6 in synovial fluid and tissue, and there appears to be a correlation between the amount of these products present and the severity of the disease. A significant advance in the treatment of arthritic diseases was the observation that therapy directed toward diminishing the effects of TNFα appeared to also improve the symptoms of ankylosing spondylitis and psoriatic arthritis.

Two different approaches have been developed to decrease TNF activity that has resulted in marketable drugs: administration of soluble TNF receptors (TNFRs; etanercept), and treatment with anti-TNFα antibodies (e.g., infliximab, adsalimumab). These compounds are designed to target and neutralize the effects of TNF, helping to reduce pain, morning stiffness, and tender or swollen joints, usually within 1 or 2 weeks after treatment begins. Evidence suggests that TNF blockers also may halt the progression of the disease. These medications work synergistically with methotrexate and therefore are often taken with methotrexate. The TNF blockers approved for treatment of rheumatoid arthritis are etanercept, infliximab, adalimumab, and rituximab. Potential side effects include injection site irritation (adalimumab and etanercept), worsening congestive heart failure (infliximab), blood disorders, lymphoma, demyelinating diseases, and increased risk of infection. These drugs should not be taken if an active infection is present. Effectiveness is lost if the drugs are discontinued.

Because TNF also is important for host defense against infections, the effects of long-term use on toxicity require further study. Substantial improvements in the course of the disease have been noted with both therapeutic approaches.

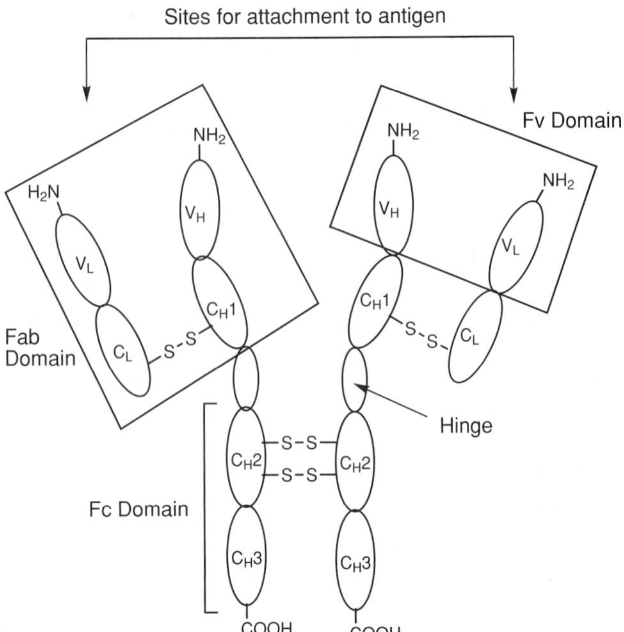

Fig. 36.30. Anti-tumor necrosis factor (TNF) agents. Etanercept is the extracellular portion of the human TNFR fused to the Fc domain of human immunoglobulin Ig G1. Infliximab is a partially humanized monoclonal antibody against TNFα. The Fv domains are derived from mouse antihuman sequences, whereas the Fc domain is composed of human IgG1 sequences. Adalimumab is fully humanized antibody to human TNFα (Fv and Fc derived from human sequences). Rituxan is a partially humanized monoclonal antibody against CD40. The Fv domains are derived from mouse antihuman sequences, and the Fc domain is composed of human IgG1 sequences.

Etanercept (Enbrel). Etanercept (Fig. 36.30) is produced by recombinant DNA technology in a Chinese hamster ovary mammalian cell line and is the first biotechnology-derived drug to be introduced for the reduction of the signs and symptoms of moderately to severely active rheumatoid arthritis in patients who have not adequately responded to one or more of the synthetic DMARDs. It is a dimeric soluble form of the p75 TNFR capable of binding to two TNF molecules in the circulation. It consists of the extracellular ligand binding portion of the 75-kDa human TNFR fused to the Fc portion of human IgG1 (Fig. 36.30). The Fc component of etanercept contains the C_H2 domain, the C_H3 domain, and the hinge region, but not the C_H1 domain of IgG1. It consists of 934 amino acids and has an apparent molecular weight of approximately 150 kDa. Two TNFRs have been identified, a 75-kDa protein and a 55-kDa protein, that occur as monomeric molecules on cell surfaces and soluble forms in the blood. The biological activity of TNF requires its binding to either of the two cell surface TNFRs. Etanercept can bind specifically to two molecules of TNFα in the circulation, preventing its interaction with cell surface TNFRs. It can be used as monotherapy or in combination with methotrexate. Some concern exists because of reports that etanercept may, in some cases, cause serious infections and may have contributed to the deaths of several patients using the drug. An excellent review of the properties and use of etanercept has recently appeared (6,85). Etanercept also binds TNFβ.

Etanercept is available as a powder for injection in single-use vials containing 25 mg of the drug. The reconstituted solution that is administered as a twice weekly subcutaneous injection should be clear and colorless.

Etanercept has been approved for reducing signs and symptoms, inhibiting the progression of structural damage, and improving physical function in patients with moderately to severely active rheumatoid arthritis; for reducing signs and symptoms in patients with active arthritis in patients with psoriatic arthritis; and for reducing signs and symptoms in patients with active ankylosing spondylitis.

Infliximab (Remicade). Infliximab is a chimeric ("humanized") IgG1κ monoclonal antibody to human TNFα (see Chapter 6 for detailed discussions for monoclonal antibodies). By combining the Fv domain of the mouse antibody responsible for recognizing TNFα with parts of the human Fc domain of IgG1 (IgG1κ), the fused protein looks more like normal human IgG1 molecule ("humanized"), so there is a better chance the fused protein will not be destroyed by the patient's own immune system. Infliximab has an approximate molecular weight of 149,100 daltons and binds specifically, with high affinity, to both the transmembrane and soluble forms of TNFα in the blood, thus neutralizing its biological activity (Fig. 36.30). It does not bind to TNFβ (lymphotoxin A), a related cytokine that uses the same receptors as TNFα. Infliximab is produced by a recombinant cell line cultured by continuous perfusion and is purified by a series of steps that includes measures to inactivate and remove viruses. Cells expressing transmembrane TNFα bound by infliximab can be lysed. The TNFα antibodies decrease synovitis and joint erosions in a murine model of collagen-induced arthritis and, when administered after disease onset, allows eroded joints to heal.

After treatment with infliximab, patients with rheumatoid arthritis or Crohn's disease exhibited reduced infiltration of inflammatory cells and TNFα production in inflamed tissues and decreased levels of serum IL-6 and C-reactive protein compared to baseline. In psoriatic arthritis, treatment with infliximab resulted in a reduction in the number of T cells and blood vessels in the synovium and psoriatic skin as well as a reduction of macrophages in the synovium. Single IV infusions showed a linear relationship between the dose administered and the maximum serum concentration. The volume of distribution at steady state was independent of dose and indicated that infliximab was distributed primarily within the vascular compartment. The terminal half-life of infliximab is 8.0 to 9.5 days. No systemic accumulation of infliximab occurred on continued repeated treatment at 4- or 8-week intervals.

Infliximab is supplied as a sterile, white, lyophilized powder formulated for IV infusion. Following reconstitution with Sterile Water for Injection, the solution should be used immediately after reconstitution, because the vials do not contain antibacterial preservatives. The reconstituted solution should be colorless to light yellow and opalescent.

Infliximab is indicated for the treatment of rheumatoid arthritis in combination with methotrexate and for Crohn's disease. Long-term use may be associated with the development of anti-infliximab antibodies, an effect that does not appear when it is used with methotrexate. Warnings associated with the use of infliximab include risks of autoimmunity, infections, and hypersensitivity reactions. An excellent review of the properties and use of infliximab has recently appeared (84). Infliximab is more specific than etanercept, because etanercept binds to both TNFα and TNFβ whereas infliximab is an antibody that binds only to TNFα. Infliximab possesses a longer half-life giving a dosing schedule of approximately every 6 to 8 weeks.

Infliximab, in combination with methotrexate, is indicated for reducing signs and symptoms, inhibiting the progression of structural damage, and improving physical function in patients with moderately to severely active rheumatoid arthritis; for reducing signs and symptoms and maintaining clinical remission in patients with moderately to severely active Crohn's disease who have had an inadequate response to conventional therapy; for reducing signs and symptoms in patients with active arthritis and in patients with psoriatic arthritis; and for reducing signs and symptoms in patients with active ankylosing spondylitis.

Adalimumab (Humira). Adalimumab is a recombinant human IgG1 monoclonal antibody targeted for human TNFα. Adalimumab is produced by recombinant DNA technology in a mammalian cell expression system using a protein-engineering strategy for creating a TNFα antibody with human-derived, heavy- and light-chain variable regions (Fab) and human IgG1κ constant regions. It consists of 1,330 amino acids and has a molecular weight of approximately 148 kDa (Fig. 36.30). Adalimumab, as an antibody, works by targeting and binding TNFα, thus neutralizing the effect of TNFα and, thereby, reducing the symptoms of rheumatoid arthritis and slowing the progression of structural joint damage caused by the disease. Adalimumab does not bind or inactivate TNFβ.

Adalimumab is supplied in single-use, prefilled, glass syringes as a sterile, preservative-free, colorless solution for subcutaneous administration. The pharmacokinetics of adalimumab were linear over the dose range of 0.5 to 10.0 mg/kg following a single IV dose. The mean elimination half-life was approximately 2 weeks.

Rituximab (Rituxan). Rituximab is a genetically engineered, fused mouse/human anti-CD40 monoclonal antibody that targets B lymphocytes by binding specifically to CD20 antigen, a protein found on the surface of B cells at certain stages in their life cycle. Rituximab is composed of two heavy chains of 451 amino acids and two light chains of 213 amino acids with an approximate molecular weight of 145 kDa (Fig. 36.30). Its binding affinity for the CD20 antigen is approximately 8.0 nM.. The mouse light- and heavy-chain Fab domains of rituximab, which binds to the CD20 antigen on B cells, is linked to the human Fc domains of IgG1κ. Once the rituximab molecule attaches to the B cells, it initiates B-cell lysis, inducing rapid and profound depletion of peripheral B cells, with patients showing near complete B-cell depletion within 2 weeks after receiving the first dose of rituximab. Because rituximab does not target B cells at the earliest stages of their development, however, these B-cell depletions usually are temporary. In clinical trials, the majority of patients showed peripheral B-cell depletion for at least 6 months, followed by subsequent gradual recovery. A small proportion of patients (4%) had prolonged peripheral B-cell depletion lasting more than 3 years after a single course of treatment.

Rituximab is a sterile, clear, colorless, preservative-free, liquid concentrate formulated for IV administration. It has changed the treatment of rheumatoid arthritis by showing that targeted B-cell therapy in combination with methotrexate can reduce signs and symptoms of rheumatoid arthritis in adult patients with moderately to severely active rheumatoid arthritis who have had an inadequate response to one or more TNF antagonist therapies. Although B cells once were considered to be one of the main contributing factors in the pathogenesis of rheumatoid arthritis, recent evidence has shown that T cells, dendritic cells, and macrophages also were involved. Rituximab has rekindled interest in B cells, highlighting their important role in perpetuating the inflammatory process and showing how they may interact with other cell types and contribute to joint inflammation.

For rheumatoid arthritis, rituximab is given as two 1,000-mg IV infusions separated by 2 weeks. Glucocorticoids also are recommended to reduce the incidence and severity of infusion reactions. Rituximab is given in combination with methotrexate. Its administration has been associated with hypersensitivity reactions (non-IgE-mediated reactions), which may respond to adjustments in the infusion rate and in medical management. People who have not found relief using TNF blockers might consider using rituximab. Side effects include flu-like signs and symptoms such as fever, chills, and nausea. Some people experience an "infusion-reaction complex," such as difficulty breathing and heart problems, that has resulted in fatalities.

Although originally approved for use in people with non-Hodgkin's lymphoma, rituximab was approved for rheumatoid arthritis in 2006.

Interleukin-1 Receptor Antagonist

Anakinra (Kineret). Anakinra is a recombinant, nonglycosylated form of the human IL-1 receptor antagonist (IL-1Rα) that neutralizes the inflammatory activity of IL-1 by competing with IL-1 for binding to its IL-1 type 1 receptor (IL-1R1). Interleukin-1 is a cytokine for which production is induced in response to inflammatory stimuli and which mediates various physiologic responses, including inflammatory and immunological responses that promotes inflammation. When IL-1 binds to IL-1R1, a signal is produced that increases the formation of nitric oxide, prostaglandin E_2 and collagenase in synovial cells, resulting in cartilage degradation as well as stimulation of bone resorption. Thus, IL-1Rα plays an important role for regulating synovial proinflammatory IL-1 activity by preventing IL-1 from binding to IL-1R1. Analysis of synovial fluid suggests that the rheumatoid synovium is characterized by an overexpression of IL-1. The resulting imbalance between IL-1 and IL-1Rα has been implicated in perpetuating the pro-inflammatory response and destructive tide of events in rheumatoid arthritis. If IL-1 is prevented from binding to IL-1R1, the inflammatory response decreases. The levels of the naturally occurring IL-lRα in synovium and synovial fluid from rheumatoid arthritis patients are insufficient to compete with the elevated amount of locally produced IL-1.

Therefore, anakinra neutralizes the proinflammatory activity of IL-1 by competitively inhibiting the binding of IL-1 to IL-1RI, similar to the endogenous antagonist, IL-1Rα. In vitro studies have shown that anakinra inhibits the induction of the inflammatory mediators, nitric oxide and prostaglandin E_2, and collagenase. Anakinra differs from native human IL-1Rα in that it has the addition of a single methionine residue at its amino terminus. Anakinra consists of 153 amino acids and has a molecular weight of 17.3 kDa. It is produced by recombinant DNA technology using an *Escherichia coli* bacterial expression system.

Anakinra is the first IL-1Rα to be approved for use in adults with moderate to severe active rheumatoid arthritis who have not responded adequately to conventional DMARD therapy. It may be used either alone or in combination with methotrexate. Anakinra is supplied in single-use, prefilled, glass syringes as sterile, clear, preservative-free solution that is administered daily as a self-administered subcutaneous injection under the skin. Some potential side effects include injection site reactions, decreased white blood cell counts, headache, and an increase in upper respiratory infections. There may be a slightly higher rate of respiratory infections in people who have asthma or chronic obstructive pulmonary disease. Persons with an active infection are advised not to use anakinra. Its elimination half-life after sc administration is 4 to 6 hours.

Costimulation Modulators. Two signals are required to activate a T-cell response to an antigen, called costimulation. Regulation of costimulatory molecules may be a mechanism whereby the immune system limits the extent of an immune response. If an unactivated antigen-presenting cell (APC; a cell that "presents" an antigen complex that is recognized by the T-cell receptor) presents an antigen to a T cell in the absence of an appropriate costimulatory signal, the T cell does not respond and becomes unreactive and nonresponsive to any further antigenic stimuli (Fig. 36.31). The T-cell costimulatory activation pathway is initiated, however, when an activated APC presents both an antigen and a costimulatory ligand, such as B7 (CD86) that interacts with CD28 on the surface of the T cell to form B7-CD28 complex, initiating T-cell proliferation and differentiation in response to the antigenic stimulus. This stimulus releases cytokines that bind to the T cell, further enhancing its activation. A counterbalance to CD28 is cytotoxic T-lymphocyte antigen-4 (CTLA-4), both of which are expressed on the surface of T cells. The CTLA-4, which is homologous with CD28, becomes expressed on T-cell activation, where it then competes with CD28 for binding to B7 ligands on the surface of APCs. The B7 ligands bind with much greater affinity to CTLA-4 than to CD28, preventing delivery of the costimulatory signal. This built-in limit prevents T-cell activation

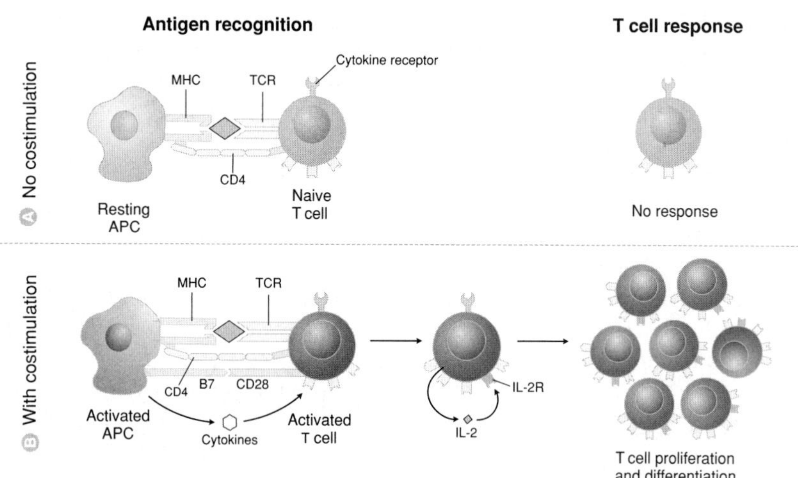

Fig. 36.31. Costimulation in the T-cell activation pathway.

from spiraling out of control. The CTLA-4 is not expressed constitutively, and its expression is up-regulated on T-cell activation. Eventually, however, CD28 is down-regulated.

Because the formation of a B7-CD28 complex between the APC and the T cell results in T-cell proliferation and the release of inflammatory cytokines, whereas the B7–CTLA-4 interaction inhibits the T-cell responses, the design of a pharmacological agent that prevents costimulation would preferentially inhibit only reactive T cells and be effective in treatment of rheumatoid arthritis. Thus, the discovery of abatacept.

Abatacept (Orencia). Abatacept, the first in a new class of immunosuppressant agents, known as costimulation modulators, acts by down-regulating T-cell activation for the treatment of rheumatoid arthritis (86). Abatacept is a novel chimeric CTLA-4–IgG1 fused protein created from the fusion of the extracellular domain of the mouse CTLA-4 with the modified heavy-chain constant region of human IgG1.

Abatacept, therefore, acts like an antibody that binds with great affinity to B7 ligands, preventing these ligands from interacting with CD28 on activated T cells. In patients with rheumatoid arthritis, blocking this response by abatacept prevents the generation of positive costimulation signals and stimulation of T-cell activation, suppressing the proliferation of reactive T-cells and the release of more cytokines that destroy tissue, causing the symptoms and signs of arthritis. The extracellular CTLA-4 portion of abatacept is responsible for the affinity of B7. Thus, abatacept slows the damage to bones and cartilage and relieves the symptoms and signs of arthritis.

People with moderate to severe active rheumatoid arthritis who have not been helped by TNF blockers might consider abatacept, which is administered IV monthly. Side effects may include headache, nausea, and mild infections, such as upper respiratory tract infections. Serious infections, such as pneumonia, can occur. There is some concern that blocking of the suppressive signal from B7 to CTLA-4 may have a negative effect on regulatory T cells and, thus, eventually, promote autoimmunity.

Herbs

At least a dozen different herbs are used to ease the symptoms of rheumatoid arthritis; most are considered to be anti-inflammatories. Herbs that have been tried include powdered ginger, borage seed oil, or devil's claw to reduce pain and swelling. Stinging nettles or turmeric also may lessen pain, stiffness, and inflammation. Because these herbs can interact with each other or with prescription comedications, lack of careful studies means that little is known about long-term effects and drug interactions.

Ayurvedic medicine also uses herbal compounds both internally and externally for symptom relief. Topical curcumin may relieve the inflammation of rheumatoid arthritis. When taken in capsule form, it can reduce morning stiffness and boost endurance. A combination of *Withania somnifera, Boswellia serrata,* and *Cucurma longa* also caused a significant drop in pain and disability for study participants with osteoarthritis.

Two herbs that have been used for centuries to treat headaches, fever, sore muscles, and rheumatism are white willow bark and meadowsweet, commonly described as "Nature's aspirin." White willow bark (*Salix alba*) contains salicin, a glycoside of salicylic acid. Once in the stomach, the salicin hydrolyzes into salicylic acid, which is the active principle for reducing pain and fever. White willow bark has been mentioned in ancient Egyptian, Assyrian, Greek, and Chinese manuscripts, and it was used to treat pain and fever by the ancient physicians Galen, Hippocrates, and Dioscorides. Native Americans used it for headaches, fever, sore muscles, rheumatism, and chills. In the mid-1700s, it was used to treat malaria. Salicin was isolated and identified in the early 1830s , but it was not conclusively shown to reduce the aches and soreness of rheumatism until 1874. White willow bark is recommended for headaches, backache, nerve pain, toothache, and injuries.

Meadowsweet (*Filipendula ulmaria*) is a common wild plant in Britain, Europe, and North America that also contains salicin, but it is not as potent as willow bark which has a higher salicin content. Its primary medicinal actions are antirheumatic, anti-inflammatory, carminative, antacid, antiemetic, astringent, and diuretic. The flower buds of meadowsweet are the source for salicin and methyl salicylate. Ingestion of the flower buds in a tea results in the breakdown of salicin to salicylic acid. Nicholas Culpeper, a seventeenth-century English pharmacist, mentioned the use of meadowsweet flower buds to help break fevers and promote sweating during a cold or flu.

DRUGS USED TO TREAT GOUT

Pathophysiology

Gout is an inflammatory disease characterized by elevated levels of uric acid (as urate ion) in the plasma and urine and may take two forms, acute and chronic. Acute gouty arthritis results from the accumulation of needle-like crystals of monosodium urate monohydrate within the joints, synovial fluid, and periarticular tissue and usually appears without warning. Initiating factors may be minor trauma, fatigue, emotional stress, infection, overindulgence in alcohol or food, or drugs, such as penicillin or insulin. Chronic gout symptoms develop as permanent erosive joint deformity appears. The increase in extracellular urate may result from increased uric acid biosynthesis, decreased urinary excretion of uric acid, or perhaps, a combination of both. The formation of uric acid from adenine and guanine is illustrated in Figure 36.32. Uric acid is formed by the oxidation of xanthine by the enzyme xanthine oxidase. Xanthine is a metabolic product of adenine (via hypoxanthine) and guanine formed by the enzymes adenine deaminase and guanine deaminase, respectively. Thus, uric acid is the excretory product of purine metabolism in humans as well as the scavenging of potential harmful oxygen free radicals in the body. In other mammals, uric acid is hydrolyzed to allantoin by the enzyme uricase, which is then subsequently hydrolyzed by allantoinase to allantoic acid. Hydrolysis of allantoic acid by allantoicase yields the final products, urea and glyoxylic acid.

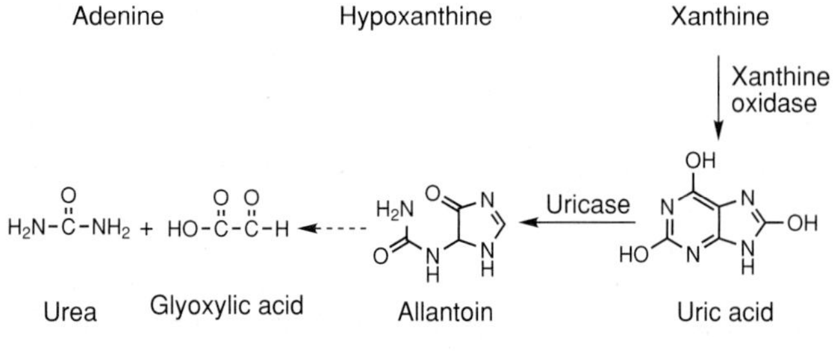

Normal pool levels of uric acid are approximately 1,000 to 1,200 mg in males and half that in females. In patients suffering from gout, these levels may be as high as two- or three times the normal levels. Uric acid is a weak acid with two pK_a values 5.7 and 10.3, with very low water solubility (~6 mg/100 mL). At physiological pH, it exists primarily as the monosodium salt, which is approximately 50 times more soluble in aqueous media than the free acid. Blood levels of urate are maintained by a careful balance between its formation and excretion. The kidney plays a dominant role in urate elimination, excreting about 70% of the daily urate production. The excretion of urate has been implicated in the development of hyperuricemia that leads to gout. In humans, the excretion of urate requires the urate anion transporter (URAT1) located in renal proximal tubule cells, which plays a central role in urate homeostasis. The URAT1 is targeted by uricosuric and antiuricosuric agents that affect urate excretion.

When levels of uric acid in the body increase, either as a result of decreased excretion or increased formation, the solubility limits of sodium urate are exceeded, and precipitation of the salt from the resulting supersaturated solution causes deposits of urate crystals to form. It is the formation of these urate crystals in joints and connective tissue that initiate attacks of gouty arthritis. The control of gout has been approached from the following therapeutic strategies: 1) control of acute attacks by drugs that reduce inflammation caused by the deposition of urate crystals (these drugs may possess only an anti-inflammatory component, such as colchicine, or both anti-inflammatory and analgetic actions, such as indomethacin, phenylbutazone and naproxen), 2) increasing the rate of uric acid excretion (by definition, these drugs are termed "uricosuric drugs" and include probenecid and sulfinpyrazone), and 3) inhibiting the biosynthesis of uric acid by inhibiting the enzyme xanthine oxidase by drugs such as allopurinol.

Fig. 36.32. Formation of uric acid, urea, and glyoxylic acid from purines.

Treatment of Acute Gout

The management of gout has been approached with the following therapeutic strategies: 1) control of acute attacks with drugs that reduce inflammation caused by the deposition of urate crystals, and 2) control of chronic gout by increasing the rate of uric acid excretion ("uricosuric drugs") and inhibiting the biosynthesis of uric acid by inhibiting the enzyme xanthine oxidase. Treatment of acute gout includes NSAIDs, such as indomethacin, colchicines, and glucocorticoids. The choice of an NSAID generally is based on the side effect profile.

Colchicine

Colchicine is a pale-yellow powder that is obtained from various species of *Colchicum*, primarily *Colchicum autum-*

nale L. Its total chemical synthesis has been achieved, but the primary source of colchicine currently remains alcohol extraction of the alkaloid from the corm and seed of *C. autumnale* L. It darkens on exposure to light and possesses moderate water solubility. Colchicine has a pK_a of 12.4. Its use in the treatment of gout dates back to the sixth century AD. Unlike those drugs that will be discussed next, colchicine does not alter serum levels of uric acid. It does, however, appear to retard the inflammation process initiated by the deposition of urate crystals. Acting on polymorphonuclear leukocytes and diminishing phagocytosis, it inhibits the production of lactic acid, causing an increase in the pH of synovial tissue and, thus, a decrease in urate deposition, because uric acid is more soluble at the higher pH. Additionally, colchicine inhibits the release of lysosomal enzymes during phagocytosis that also contributes to the reduction of inflammation. Because colchicine does not lower serum urate levels, it has been found to be beneficial to combine colchicine with a uricosuric agent, particularly probenecid. It is a potent drug, being effective at doses of approximately 1 mg, but doses as small as 7 mg have caused fatalities.

ABSORPTION AND METABOLISM. Colchicine is absorbed on oral administration, with peak plasma levels being attained within 0.5 to 2 hours after dosing. Plasma protein binding is only 31%. It concentrates primarily in the intestinal tract, liver, kidney, and spleen and is excreted primarily in the feces, with only 20% of an oral dose being excreted in the urine. It is retained in the body for considerable periods of time, being detected in the urine and leukocytes for 9 to 10 days following a single dose. Metabolism occurs primarily in the liver, with the major metabolite being the amine resulting from amide hydrolysis.

SIDE EFFECTS. Colchicine may produce bone marrow depression, with long-term therapy resulting in thrombocytopenia or aplastic anemia. At maximum dose levels, GI disturbances (e.g., nausea, diarrhea, and abdominal pain) may occur. Acute toxicity is characterized by GI distress, including severe diarrhea resulting in excessive fluid loss, respiratory depression, and kidney damage. Treatment normally involves measures that prevent shock as well as morphine and atropine to diminish abdominal pain. A number of drug interactions have been reported. In general, the actions of colchicine are potentiated by alkalinizing substances and are inhibited by acidifying drugs, consistent with its mechanism of action of increasing the pH of synovial fluid. Responses to CNS depressants and to sympathomimetic drugs appear to be enhanced. Clinical tests may be affected; most notably, elevated alkaline phosphatase and SGOT (serum glutamate oxaloacetate transaminase) values and decreased thrombocyte values may be obtained.

DOSING. Colchicine is indicated for the treatment of acute attacks of gout and is very effective. The usual dose is 1.0 to 1.2 mg, followed by 0.5 to 1.2 mg every 1 to 2 hours until either pain relief is observed or symptoms of GI distress are observed. When a rapid response is required, or if GI reactions warrant discontinuance of oral administration, IV administration (usually 2 mg initially) may be indicated. It is available as 0.5- or 0.6-mg tablets and as an injectable solution of 1 mg in 2-mL ampoules. It often is given in combination with probenecid, and combination products of the two are available in tablets containing 500 mg of probenecid and 0.5 mg of colchicine.

Treatment of Chronic Gout

Drugs That Increase Uric Acid Secretion

PROBENECID. Probenecid is insoluble in water and acidic solutions but is soluble in alkaline solutions buffered to pH 7.4. Probenecid initially was synthesized as a result of studies in the 1940s on sulfonamides that indicated the sulfonamides decreased the renal clearance of penicillin, extending the half-life of penicillin as supplies diminished. Probenecid thus was initially used—and is still indicated—for that purpose. Probenecid promotes the excretion of uric acid by inhibiting the urate anion exchange transporter (URAT1), decreasing the reabsorption of uric acid in the proximal tubules. The overall effect is to decrease plasma uric acid concentrations, thereby decreasing the rate and extent of urate crystal deposition in joints and synovial fluids. Within the series of N-dialkylsulfamyl benzoates from which probenecid is derived, renal clearance of these compounds is decreased as the length of the N-alkyl substituents is increased. Uricosuric activity increases with increasing size of the alkyl group in the series methyl, ethyl, and propyl.

Probenecid is essentially completely absorbed from the GI tract on oral administration, with peak plasma levels observed within 2 to 4 hours. Like most acidic compounds, probenecid (pK_a = 3.4) is extensively plasma protein bound (93–99%). The primary route of elimination of probenecid and its metabolites is the urine. It is extensively metabolized in humans, with only 5 to 10% being excreted as unchanged drug. The major metabolites detected result from glucuronide conjugation of the carboxylic acid, ω-oxidation of the n-propyl side chain and subsequent oxidation of the resulting alcohol to the carboxylic acid derivative, ω_1-oxidation of the n-propyl group, and N-dealkylation. Those metabolites possessing a free carboxylic acid function generally possess some uricosuric activity. Probenecid appears to be generally well tolerated, with few adverse reactions. The major side effect is GI distress (e.g., nausea, vomiting, and anorexia), but these occur in only 2% of patients at low doses. Other effects include headache, dizziness, urinary frequency, hypersensitivity reactions, sore gums, and anemia. Overdosages do not appear to present major difficulties; a case of a 49-year-old man who recovered from the ingestion of 47 g in a suicide attempt has been reported. Should overdosage occur, treatment consists of emesis or gastric lavage, short-acting barbiturates (if CNS excitation occurs), and epinephrine (for anaphylactic reactions). A number of drug interactions have been reported. Despite

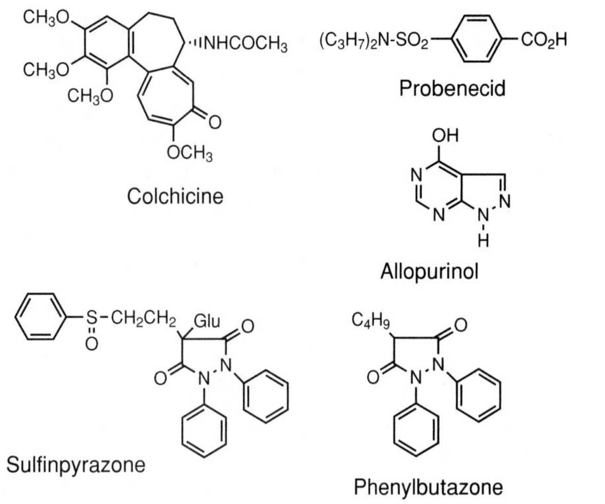

Colchicine

Probenecid

Allopurinol

Sulfinpyrazone

Phenylbutazone

Fig. 36.33. Structures of agents used to control gout.

the high degree of plasma protein binding, displacement interactions with other drugs bound to plasma proteins does not appear to occur to any significant extent. Salicylates counteract the uricosuric effects of probenecid. Because probenecid inhibits their renal excretion, increased plasma levels of the following drugs may be observed: aminosalicylic acid, methotrexate, sulfonamides, dapsone, sulfonylureas, naproxen, indomethacin, rifampin, and sulfinpyrazone. (The effects on penicillin plasma levels were discussed previously.)

Probenecid is indicated for the treatment of hyperuricemia associated with gout and gouty arthritis and for the elevation and prolongation of plasma levels of penicillins and cephalosporins. In gout, treatment should not begin until an acute attack has subsided. It is not recommended in individuals with known uric acid kidney stones or blood dyscrasias or for children under 2 years of age.

SULFINPYRAZONE. Sulfinpyrazone (Fig. 36.33) is soluble in alkaline solutions. Its synthesis is similar to that of phenylbutazone (87) (Fig. 36.33). It produces its uricosuric effect in a manner similar to that of probenecid. A dose of 35 mg produces a uricosuric effect equivalent to that produced by 100 mg of probenecid, whereas 400 mg/day of sulfinpyrazone produces an effect comparable to that obtained with doses of 1.5 to 2 g of probenecid. It also possesses, not surprisingly, some of the properties of phenylbutazone. It is an inhibitor of human platelet prostaglandin synthesis at the cyclooxygenase step, resulting in a decrease in platelet release and a reduction in platelet aggregation. This antiplatelet effect suggests a role for sulfinpyrazone in reducing the incidence of sudden death, which can occur in the first year following a myocardial infarction; however, it lacks the analgetic and anti-inflammatory effects of phenylbutazone.

Sulfinpyrazone is a strong acid (enolic OH $pK_a = 2.8$), a factor that is important in the production of the uricosuric effect, because within a series of pyrazolidinedione derivatives, the stronger the acid, the more potent the uricosuric effect. Polar substitution on the side chain also influences uricosuric activity, as discussed previously with regard to the pyrazolidinediones.

Oral administration results in rapid and essentially complete absorption, with peak plasma levels being attained within 1 to 2 hours of administration. It is highly bound (98–99%) to plasma proteins, and it is excreted in the urine primarily (50%) as unchanged drug.

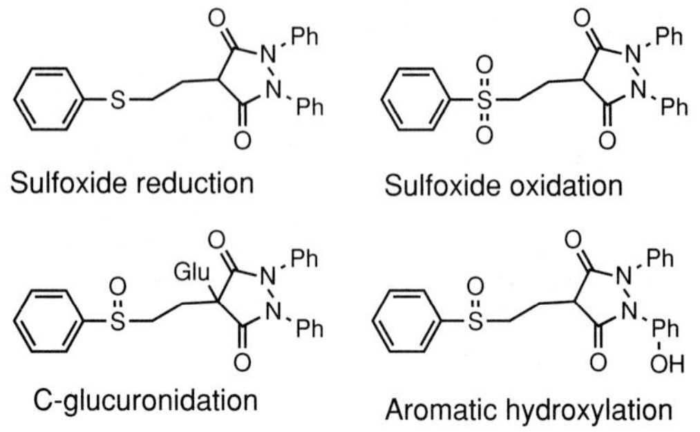

Sulfoxide reduction

Sulfoxide oxidation

C-glucuronidation

Aromatic hydroxylation

The metabolites produced result from sulfoxide reduction, sulfur and aromatic oxidation, and C-glucuronidation of the heterocyclic ring in a manner similar to that for phenylbutazone. The metabolite resulting from *p*-hydroxylation of the aromatic ring possesses uricosuric effects in humans. The sulfide metabolite, a major metabolic product, may contribute to the antiplatelet effects of sulfinpyrazone but not to the uricosuric effects. The most frequent adverse reactions are GI disturbances; however, the incidence is relatively low. It has been suggested that sulfinpyrazone is a much weaker inhibitor of prostaglandin synthesis in bovine stomach microsomes than either aspirin or indomethacin, a factor that may account for its gastric tolerance. Much rarer have been reports of blood dyscrasias and rash. Overdosage produces symptoms that are primarily GI in nature (e.g., nausea, diarrhea, and vomiting) but also may involve impaired respiration and convulsions. Treatment consists of emesis or gastric lavage and supportive care. Like probenecid, its uricosuric effects are antagonized by salicylates, and probenecid markedly inhibits the renal tubular secretion of sulfinpyrazone. It potentiates the actions of other drugs that are highly plasma protein bound, such as coumarin-type oral anticoagulants, antibacterial sulfonamides, and hypoglycemic sulfonylureas.

Sulfinpyrazone is indicated for the treatment of chronic and intermittent gouty arthritis.

Drugs That Decrease Uric Acid Formation

ALLOPURINOL

Mechanism of Action. The biosynthesis of uric acid from the immediate purine precursor xanthine that results from adenine, via the intermediate hypoxanthine, or from guanine is illustrated in Figure 36.32. The enzyme xanthine oxidase (a molybdenum hydroxylase enzyme) is involved in two steps, the conversion of hypoxanthine to xanthine, and the final step, the conversion of xanthine to uric acid. Allopurinol originally was designed as an antineoplastic antimetabolite to antagonize the actions of key purines inasmuch as it differs from normal purines only by the inversion of the nitrogen and carbon atoms at the 7- and 8-positions of the purine ring system but was found to have little or no effect on experimental tissues. It was subsequently found that allopurinol serves as a substrate for xanthine oxidase (15 to 20 times the affinity of xanthine) and reversibly inhibits that enzyme. Normally, uric acid is a major metabolic end product in humans. When allopurinol is administered, however, xanthine and hypoxanthine are elevated in the urine, and uric acid levels decrease. When the synthesis of uric acid is inhibited, plasma urate levels decrease, supersaturated solutions of urate are no longer present, and urate crystal deposits dissolve, eliminating the primary cause of gout. The increased plasma levels of hypoxanthine and xanthine pose no real problem, because they are more soluble than uric acid and are readily excreted.

Absorption and Metabolism. Allopurinol was synthesized in 1956 as part of a study of purine antagonists (88). It is well absorbed on oral administration, with peak plasma concentrations appearing within 1 hour. Decreases of uric acid can be observed within 24 to 48 hours. Excretion of allopurinol and its metabolite occurs primarily in the urine, with approximately 20% of a dose being excreted in the feces. Allopurinol is rapidly metabolized via oxidation and the formation of numerous ribonucleoside derivatives. The major oxidation metabolite, alloxanthine or oxypurinol, has a much longer half-life (18–30 hours versus 2–3 hours) than the parent drug and is an effective, although less potent, inhibitor of xanthine oxidase. The longer plasma half-life of alloxanthine results in an accumulation in the body during chronic administration, thus contributing significantly to the overall therapeutic effects of allopurinol. The major adverse effects are primarily dermatological in nature (e.g., skin rash and exfoliative lesions). Other effects, such as GI distress (e.g., nausea, vomiting, and diarrhea), hematopoietic effects (e.g., aplastic anemia, bone marrow depression, and transient leukopenia), neurological disorders (e.g., headache, neuritis, and dizziness), and ophthalmological effects (e.g., cataracts) are less commonly encountered. Allopurinol also may initiate attacks of acute gouty arthritis during the early stages of therapy and may require the concomitant administration of colchicine. Drug interactions include those drugs that normally also are metabolized by xanthine oxidase. For example, the oxidation of 6-mercaptopurine, a useful antineoplastic agent, is inhibiting, permitting a reduction in the therapeutic dose. Allopurinol also has an inhibitory effect on liver microsomal enzymes, thus prolonging the half-lives of drugs, such as oral anticoagulants, that normally are metabolized and inactivated by these enzymes, although this effect is quite variable. The incidence of ampicillin-related skin rashes increases with the concurrent administration of allopurinol.

Xanthine Oxidase

Allopurinol

Alloxanthine (oxypurinol)

Allopurinol is indicated for the treatment of primary and secondary gout, for malignancies such as leukemia and lymphoma, and for the treatment of patients with recurrent calcium oxalate calculi.

CASE STUDY

Victoria F. Roche and S. William Zito

PR is a 15-year-old female gymnast who has just been named to the U.S. Olympic Team after months of grueling and highly competitive trials. Her specialty events are the uneven parallel bars and the "horse," but she has performed well enough on all events to earn this coveted spot on the team. She is ecstatic but understandably nervous, because she is, by nature, a private person and the media spotlight has been intense since the announcement.

PR has consulted the team physician about dysmenorrhea that has become increasingly worse over the past 6 months. The cramping is now almost incapacitating for 2 to 3 days out of each period, and it has been interfering with her training. She knows just when the "big pain" will start, because PMS symptoms routinely begin 36 hours before the onset of bleeding. She has looked ahead, and if her cycles remain regular, she is due to have her period during the week of the summer Olympic games. From her medication history, the MD can see that PR takes OTC chlorpheniramine maleate (Chlortrimeton) fairly frequently for seasonal and pet-related allergies. Despite her young age, she has complained of a "nervous stomach," which has prompted her to try Prilosec OTC (omeprazole), especially before competitions when her emotions and GI distress are heightened. PR speaks of her very jam-packed schedule of school and training, and she asks for once-daily therapy to treat her menstruation-related pain if possible. As the pharmacist for the team, consider the following NSAID therapeutic choices, and prepare to make a recommendation.

1. Identify the therapeutic problem(s) in which the pharmacist's intervention may benefit the patient.
2. Identify and prioritize the patient-specific factors that must be considered to achieve the desired therapeutic outcomes.
3. Conduct a thorough and mechanistically oriented structure–activity analysis of all therapeutic alternatives provided in the case.
4. Evaluate the SAR findings against the patient-specific factors and desired therapeutic outcomes, and make a therapeutic decision.
5. Counsel your patient.

Chlorpheniramine maleate

Omeprazole

1 2 3 4

REFERENCES

1. Borne RF. Nonsteroidal anti-inflammatory agents, antipyretics, and uricosuric agents. In: Verderame M, ed. Handbook of Cardiovascular and Anti-Inflammatory Agents. Boca Raton, FL: CRC Press, 1986:27–104.
2. Klippel JH, Wegand CM, Wortmann R. Primer on the Rheumatic Diseases. 12th Ed. Atlanta: Arthritis Foundation, 2001.
3. Smith JB, Haynes MK. Rheumatoid arthritis—a molecular understanding. Ann Intern Med 2002;136:908–922.
4. Schwartz A. In a World of New Diseases, Arthritis Is Still the #1 Crippler. US Pharmacist 1990;15:8–12.
5. Bennett RW. Treatment strategies for osteo- and rheumatoid arthritis. US Pharmacist 1990;15:30–36.
6. Hamor GH. Nonsteroidal anti-inflammatory drugs. In: Foye WO, ed. Principles of Medicinal Chemistry. 3rd Ed. Philadelphia: Lea & Febiger, 1989:503–530.
7. Walport M. Complement. In: Roitt IM, Brostoff J, Male DK, eds. Immunology. 2nd Ed. St. Louis: CV Mosby, 1989 p 13.1–13.16.
8. Kinoshita T. Biology of complement: the overture. Immunol Today 1991;12:291–295.
9. Frank MM, Fries LF. The role of complement in inflammation and phagocytosis. Immunol Today 1991;12:322–326.
10. Shen TY. Nonsteroidal anti-inflammatory agents. In: Wolff M, ed. Burger's Medicinal Chemistry, Part III. 4th Ed. New York: John Wiley & Sons, 1981: 1205–1272.
11. Shen TY. Proc. Int. Symp. Milan, 1964. In: Grattini S, Dukes MNG, eds. Excerpta Medica, Amsterdam, 1965;13–20.
12. Shen TY. Anti-Inflammatory Agents. Top Med Chem 1967;1:29–38.
13. Vane JR Inhibition of prostaglandin synthesis as a mechanism of action for aspirin-like drugs. Nat New Biol 1971;231:232–235.
14. Gund P, Shen TY. A model for the prostaglandin synthetase cyclooxygenation site and its inhibition by anti-inflammatory arylacetic acids. J Med Chem 1977; 20:1146–1152.
15. Kurzrok R, Lieb C. Biochemical studies of human semen. II. The action of semen on the human uterus. Proc Soc Exp Biol N Y 1931;28:268–272.
16. Goldblatt MW. Properties of human seminal plasma. J Physiol (London) 1935;84:208–218.
17. von Euler US. The specific vasodilating and plain muscle-stimulating substances from accessory genital glands in man and certain animals (prostaglandin and vesiglandin). J Physiol (London) 1936;88:213–234.
18. Bergstrom S, Samuelsson B. The prostaglandins. Endeavour 1968;27: 109–113.
19. Smyth, EM, Burke A, Fitzgerald GA. Lipid-derived autacoids: Eicosanoids and platelet-activating factor. In: Brunton LL, Lazo JS, Parker KL, eds. Goodman and Gilman's The Pharmacological Basis of Therapeutics. 11th Ed. New York: Pergamon Press, 2006:653–670.
20. Hla T, Nielson K. Human cyclooxygenase-2 cDNA. Proc Natl Acad Sci U S A 1992;89:7384–7388.
21. Jones DA, Carlton DP, McIntyre TM, et al. Molecular cloning of human prostaglandin endoperoxide synthase type II and demonstration of expression in response to cytokines. J Biol Chem 1993;268:9049–9054.
22. Kennedy B, Chan C-C, Culp S, et al. Cloning expression of rat prostaglandin endoperoxide synthase (cyclooxygenase)-2 cDNA. Biochem Biophys Res Commun 1993;197:494–500.
23. Kujubu DA, Fletcher BS, Varnum C, et al. TIS10, a phorbol ester tumor promoter-inducible mRNA from Swiss 3T3 cells, encodes a novel prostaglandin synthase/cyclooxygenase homologue. J Biol Chem 1991;266: 12866–12872.
24. Xie W, Chipman JG, Robertson DL, et al. Expression of a mitogen-responsive gene encoding prostaglandin synthase is regulated by mRNA splicing. Proc Natl Acad Sci U S A 1991;88:2692–2696.
25. Chang HW, Jahng Y. Selective cyclooxygenase-2 inhibitors as anti-inflammatory agents. Korean J Med Chem 1998;8:48–79.
26. Vane JR, Bakhle YS, Botting YM. Cyclooxygenases 1 and 2. Annu Rev Pharmacol Toxicol 1998;38:97–120.
27. Botting JH. Nonsteroidal anti-inflammatory agents. Drugs Today 1999;35: 225–235.
28. Okazaki T, Sagawa N, Okita JR, et al. Diacylglycerol metabolism and arachidonic acid release in human fetal membranes and decidua vera. J Biol Chem 1981;256:7316–7321.
29. Clark WG. Mechanisms of antipyretic action. Gen Pharmacol 1979;10:71–77.
30. Chandrasekharan NV, Dai H, Roos KLT, et al. COX-3, a cyclooxygenase-1 variant inhibited by acetaminophen and other analgesic/antipyretic drugs: cloning, structure, and expression. Proc Natl Acad Sci U S A 2002;99: 13926–13931.
31. Hersh EV, Lally ET, Moore PA. Update on cyclooxygenase inhibitors: has a third COX isoform entered the fray? Curr Med Res Opin 2005;21: 1217–1226.
32. Qin N, Zhang SP, Reitz TL, et al. Cloning, expression, and functional characterization of human COX-1 splicing variants: evidence for intron-1 retention. J Pharmacol Exp Ther 2005;315:1298–1305.
33. Nurmi JT, Puolakkainen PA, Rautonen NE. Intro-1 retaining cyclooxygenase-1 splice variant is induced by osmotic stress in human intestinal epithelial cells. Prostaglandins Leukot Essent Fatty Acids 2005;73:343–350.
34. Snipes JA, Kis B, Shelness GS, et al. Cloning and characterization of cyclooxygenase-1b (putative cyclooxygenase-3) in rat. J Pharmacol Exp Ther 2005; 313:668–676.
35. Botting R. Ayoub SS. COX-3 and the mechanism of action of paracetamol/ acetaminophen. Prostaglandins Leukot Essent Fatty Acids 2005;72:85–87.
36. Kis B, Snipes JA, Simandle SA, et al. Acetaminophen-sensitive prostaglandin production in rat cerebral endothelial cells. Am J Physiol 2005;R897–R902.
37. Graham GG, Scott KF. Mechanism of action of paracetamol. Am J Ther 2005;12:46–55.
38. Kis B, Snipes JA, Busija DW. Acetaminophen and the cyclooxygenase puzzle: sorting out facts, fictions, and uncertainties. J Pharmacol Exp Ther 2005;315:1–7.
39. Kunkel DB. Emergency medicine. Geigy Pharmaceuticals, July 15, 1985.
40. Calder IC, Creek MJ, Williams PJ, et al. N-hydroxylation of p-acetophenetidide as a factor in nephrotoxicity. J Med Chem 1973;16:499–502.
41. Smilkstein MJ, Knapp GL, Kulig KW, et al. Efficacy of oral N-acetylcysteine in the treatment of acetaminophen overdose. Analysis of the national multicenter study (1976 to 1985). N Engl J Med 1988;319:1557–1562.

42. Buckpitt AR, Rollins DE, Mitchell JR. Varying effects of sulfhydryl nucleophiles on acetaminophen oxidation and sulfhydryl adduct formation. Biochem Pharmacol 1979;28:2941–2946.
43. Hennekens CH, Buting JE. Final report on the aspirin component of the ongoing physicians' health study. N Engl J Med 1989;321:129–135.
44. Gossel TA. Aspirin's role in reducing cardiac mortality. US Pharmacist 1988,13:34–38.
45. Thun MJ, Namboodiri MM, Heath CW. Unsuccessful emergency medical resuscitation—are continued efforts in the emergency department justified? N Engl J Med 1991;325:1393–1398.
46. Kalgutkar AS, Crews BC, Rowlinson SW, et al. Aspirin-like molecules that covalently inactivate cyclooxygenase-2. Science 1998;280:1268–1270.
47. Davison C. Salicylate metabolism in man. Ann N Y Acad Sci 1971;179: 249–268.
48. Paulus HE, Whitehouse MW. Some relevant clinical conditions and the available therapy. In: Rubin AA, ed. Search for New Drugs, vol 6. New York: Marcel Dekker, 1972:11–40.
49. Shen TY, Ellis RL, Windholz TB, et al. Nonsteroid anti-inflammatory agents. J Am Chem Soc. 1963;85:488–489.
50. Shen TY, Witzel BE, Jones H, et al. US Patent 3,654,349, 971. Chem Abstr 1971;74:141379v.
51. Carson JR, McKinstry DN, Wong S. 5-Benzoyl-1-methylpyrrol-2-acetic acids as anti-inflammatory agents. J Med Chem 1971;14:646–647.
52. Sallman A, Pfister R. German Patent 1,815,802. 1969. Chem Abstr 1970;72: 12385d.
53. Demerson CA, Humber LG, Dobson TA, et al. Chemistry and anti-inflammatory activities of prodolic acid and related 1,3,4,9-tetrahydropyrano[3,4,-b] indole-1-alkanoic acids. J Med Chem 1975;18:189–191.
54. Demerson CA, Humber LG, Phillip AH, et al. Etodolic acid and related compounds. Chemistry and anti-inflammatory actions of some potent di- and trisubstituted 1,3,4,9-tetrahydropyrano [3,4-b]indole-1-acetic acids. J Med Chem 1976;19:391–395.
55. Goudie AC, Gaster LM, Lake AW, et al. 4-(6-Methoxy-2-naphthyl)butan-2-one and related analogues, a novel structural class of anti-inflammatory compounds. J Med Chem 1978;21:1260–1264.
56. Nicholson JS, Adams SS. British Patent 971,700. Chem Abstr 1964;61: 14591d.
57. Hutt AJ, Caldwell J. The metabolic chiral inversion of 2-arylpropionic acids—a novel route with pharmacological consequences. J Pharm Pharmacol 1983;35:693–704.
58. Marshall WS. French Patent 2,015,728. 1970. Chem Abstr 1971;75:48707m.
59. Farge D, Messer MN, Moutonnier C. US Patent 3,641,127. 1972. Chem Abstr 1974;81:50040f.
60. Ueno K, Kubo S, Tagawa H, et al. 6,11-Dihydro-11-oxodibenz[be] oxepinacetic acids with potent anti-inflammatory activity J Med Chem 1976; 19:941–946.
61. Harrison IT, Lewis B, Nelson P, et al. Nonsteroidal anti-inflammatory agents. I. 6-Substituted 2-naphthylacetic acids. J Med Chem 1970;13:203–205.
62. Janssen PAJ, Van Deale GHP, Boey JM. German Patent 2,353,375. 1974. Chem Abstr 1973;79:104952j.
63. Adams SS, Bernard J, Nicholson JS, et al. US Patent 3,755,427. 1975. Chem Abstr 1974;81:49433e.
64. Scherrer RA. Introduction to the chemistry of anti-inflammatory and antiarthritic agents. In: Scherrer RA, Whitehouse MW, eds. Anti-Inflammatory Agents, vol 1. New York: Academic Press, 1974:35–55.
65. Scherrer RA. Aryl- and heteroarylcarboxylic acids. In: Scherrer RA, Whitehouse MW, eds. Anti-Inflammatory Agents, vol 1. New York: Academic Press, 1974:56–74.
66. Winder CV, Wax J, Scotti L, et al. Anti-inflammatory, antipyretic, and antinociceptive properties of N-(2,3-xylyl) anthranilic acid (mefenamic acid). J Pharmacol Exp Ther 1962;138:405–413.
67. Appleton RA, Brown K. Conformational requirements at the prostaglandin cyclooxygenase receptor site: a template for designing nonsteroidal anti-inflammatory drugs. Prostaglandins 1979;18:29–34.
68. Carty TJ, Stevens JS, Lombardino JG, et al. Piroxicam, a structurally novel anti-inflammatory compound. Mode of prostaglandin synthesis inhibition. Prostaglandins 1980;19:671–682.
69. Lombardino JG, Wiseman EH. Piroxicam and other anti-inflammatory oxicams. Med Res Rev 1982;2:127–152.
70. Lombardino JG, Wiseman EH, Chiaini J. Potent anti-inflammatory N-heterocyclic 3-carboxamides of 4-hydroxy-2-methyl-2H-1,2-benzothiazine 1,1-dioxide. J Med Chem 1973;16:493–496.
71. Prasit P, Riendeau D. Selective cyclooxygenase-2 inhibitors. Annu Rep Med Chem 1997;32:211–220.
72. Warner TD, Giuliano F, Vojnovic I, et al. Nonsteroid drug selectivities for cyclooxygenase-1 rather than cyclooxygenase-2 are associated with human gastrointestinal toxicity: a full in vitro analysis. Proc Natl Acad Sci U S A 1999;96:7563–7568.
73. Chan CC, Boyce S, Brideau C, et al. Rofecoxib [Vioxx, MK-0966; 4-(4′-methylsulfonylphenyl)-3-phenyl-2-(5H)-furanone]: a potent and orally active cyclooxygenase-2 inhibitor. Pharmacological and biochemical profiles. J Pharmacol Exp Ther 1999;290:551–560.
74. Bombardier C, Laine L, Reicin A, et al. Comparison of upper gastrointestinal toxicity of rofecoxib and naproxen in patients with rheumatoid arthritis. N Engl J Med 2000;343:1520–1528.
75. Aw T-J, Haas SJ, Liew D, et al. Meta-analysis of cyclooxygenase-2 inhibitors and their effects on blood pressure. Arch Intern Med 2005;165:1–7.
76. Fitzgerald GA. Coxibs and cardiovascular disease. N Engl J Med 2004;351:1709–1711.
77. Topol EJ. Failing the public health—rofecoxib, Merck, and the FDA. N Engl J Med 2004;351:1707–1709.
78. Dogne J-M, Supuran CT, Pratico D. Adverse cardiovascular effects of the coxibs. J Med Chem 2005;48:2251–2257.
79. Szewczuk LM, Penning TM. Mechanism-based inactivation of COX-1 by red wine m-hydroquinones. A structure–activity relationship study. J Nat Prod 2004;67:1777–1782.
80. Penning TD, Talley JJ, Bertenshaw SR, et al. Synthesis and biological evaluation of the 1,5-diarylpyrazole class of cyclooxygenase-2 inhibitors: identification of 4-[5-(4-methylphenyl)-3-(trifluoromethyl)-1H-pyrazol-1-yl] benzenesulfonamide (SC-58635, celecoxib). J Med Chem 1997;40:1347–1365.
81. McEvoy GK, ed. Non-steroidal Anti-inflammatory Agents. American Hospital Formulary Service Drug Information 2000:1872–1879.
82. Sorbera LA, Leeson PA, Castaner J. Rofecoxib. Drugs of the Future 1998;23:1287–1296.
83. McEvoy GK, ed. Non-steroidal Anti-inflammatory Agents. American Hospital Formulary Service Drug Information 2000:1879–1883.
84. Naguwa SM. Tumor necrosis factor inhibitor therapy for rheumatoid arthritis. N Y Acad Sci 2005;1051:709–715.
85. Jarvis B, Faulds D. Lamivudine. A review of its therapeutic potential in chronic hepatitis B. Drugs 1999;57:945–966.
86. Markham A, Lamb HM. Infliximab: a review of its use in the management of rheumatoid arthritis. Drugs 2000;59:1341–1359.
87. Bluestone JA, St. Clair EW, Turka LA. CTLA1g: bridging the basic immunology with clinical application. Imunity 2006;24:253–238.
88. Pfister R, Häflinger F. Über derivate und analoge de phenylbutazoins IV analoge mit schwefelhaltigen seitenkitten. Helv Chim Acta 1961;44:232–237.

37. *Antihistamines and Related Antiallergic and Antiulcer Agents*

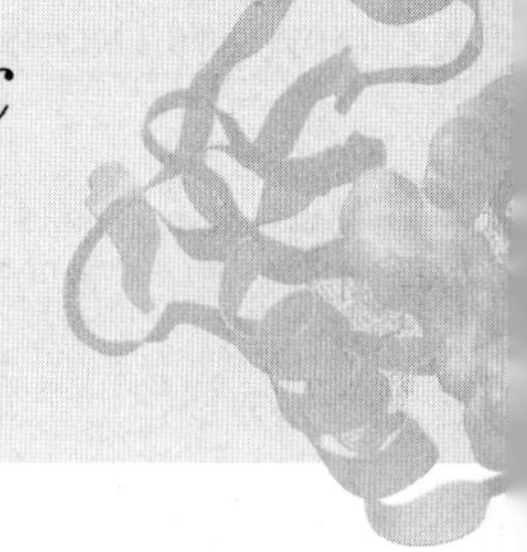

WENDEL L. NELSON

DRUGS COVERED IN THIS CHAPTER:

ANTIHISTAMINES

- Acrivastine
- Azelastine
- Carebastine
- Cetirizine
- Cromolyn
- Desloratadine
- Ebastine
- Emedastine
- Epinastine
- Fexofenadine
- Ketotifen
- Levocetirizine
- Levocobastine
- Lodoxamide
- Loratadine
- Mizolastine
- Nedocromil
- Olopatadine
- Pemirolast
- Terfenadine

ANTIULCER AGENTS

- Cimetidine
- Esomeprazole
- Famotidine
- Lansoprazole
- Metoclopromide
- Misoprostol
- Nizatidine
- Omeprazole
- Pantoprazole
- Rabeprazole
- Ranitidine
- Sucralfate

INTRODUCTION

Histamine [2-(imidazol-4-yl)ethylamine] was synthesized and its effects in model biological systems were studied before it was found physiologically. Its synthesis occurs in many tissues, including mast cells, parietal cells of the gastric mucosa, and neurons of the central nervous system (CNS) and the periphery. Early hypotheses about its physiological function were based on the observed, dramatic effects of histamine in guinea pigs. These effects include massive bronchial spasm and effects on smooth muscle and the vasculature that resemble anaphylactic shock. Marked species differences in the observed effects occur, however, and these dramatic effects are not observed in humans.

Histamine is located in many tissues, and on release, its effects are principally local ones, because it functions as an autocoid or paracrine (1). Its physiological function is complex and not completely understood. Histamine is one of the many mediators involved in allergic inflammatory responses, and it has an important role in regulating the secretion of gastric acid. These observations have led to development of many important drugs that antagonize its effects and are useful in treatment of allergic inflammatory disorders (H_1 antihistamines) and in the treatment of gastric hypersecretory disorders (H_2 antihistamines).

Besides its role in allergic inflammatory processes and gastric acid secretion, a physiological role at axons in several regions of the CNS has established its role in the regulation of sleeping and waking, in energy and endocrine homeostasis, and in cognition and memory. Histamine modulates the release of neurotransmitters via H_3 auto- and heteroreceptors located at histaminergic and nonhistaminergic neurons both centrally and peripherally. A novel H_4 receptor also been described where histamine facilitates the synthesis and release of other proinflammatory mediators and modulates the chemotactic responses, principally at mast cells and eosinophils.

CHEMISTRY

Histamine has pK_a values of 5.80 (imidazole) and 9.40 (aliphatic primary amine) (2). At physiological pH, it exists as an equilibrium mixture of tautomeric cations, with the monocation making up more than 96% of the total and the dication approximately 3%, with only a very small amount of the nonprotonated species. At lower pH values (e.g. the pH of acidic lipids), a much larger proportion of the dication exists. The two protonated species (mono- and dication) often are considered to be the biologically active forms. Penetration of membranes by histamine would be expected to occur via the nonprotonated species, and the unprotonated imidazole group would be expected to participate readily in proton-transfer processes physiologically. Several aromatic ring congeners of histamine with weakly and very weakly basic heteroaromatic rings (e.g., 4-chloroimidazole, 1,2,4-triazole, thiazole, and pyridine) exhibit histamine agonist activity (Table 37.1) (3), although they are less potent than histamine. These data suggest that the monocation (protonated aliphatic amine) is sufficient for agonist activity and that protonation of the heterocyclic ring is not an absolute requirement.

In aqueous solutions, the tautomeric equilibrium of the imidazole ring apparently favors the N^{τ}-H tautomer by approximately 4:1. The free base also prefers the N^{τ}-H tautomer. In the crystalline form of the monohydrochloride salt of histamine, however, where intermolecular crystal

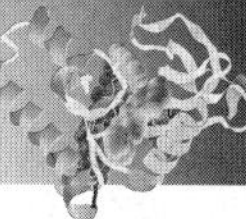

CLINICAL SIGNIFICANCE

The antihistamines and other agents presented in this chapter represent the extremes of many spectrums. Traditional antihistamines, like promethazine, have been marketed for more than 50 years; proton pump inhibitors have had new dosage forms approved as recently as 2005. Some of the agents are inexpensive, whereas others cost several dollars per dose. Indications for these medications range from minor allergic eye irritations to serious conditions, such as Zollinger-Ellison syndrome. The most important comparison to make between the drug classes and specific agents within each class is the chemical structure of the product. The differences and similarities of each structure define the function, potency, and side effect profile of the medication. Therefore, an understanding of the effect of chemical structure modifications is imperative to distinguish between the advantages and disadvantages of a treatment regimen.

This effort is well rewarded, because these products are commonly prescribed for medical treatments and many of these agents are available without a prescription. The accessibility of these drugs presents a significant opportunity for pharmacists to assist patients with proper product selections. To provide appropriate and pertinent therapeutic recommendations, the clinician must possess a thorough comprehension of the unique attributes for each medication, which can be determined by studying the chemical structure.

Heidi H. Bragg, R.Ph.
Clinical Assistant Professor
Department of Clinical Sciences and Administration
University of Houston
College of Pharmacy

pKa 9.40 pKa 5.80

pKa of histamine

Tautomers of histamine

packing forces are important, the N^{π}-H tautomer is preferred. Changes in tautomeric composition of analogues occur with changes in the 4-substituent (e.g., Me versus Cl), where the proportion of N^{τ}-H tautomer is decreased in the chlorine-substituted congener to 12%, compared with 70% for 4-methylhistamine, and decreased agonist potency is observed. An interpretation of these results is that tautomeric composition might be important in the agonist–receptor interaction (2).

Results of conformational studies performed on histamine and its congeners indicate both *trans* and gauche conformations exist in solution (Fig. 37.1) (2). The *trans* conformation of 4-methylhistamine, however, which is a selective H_2 agonist, cannot readily adopt the fully extended *trans* conformation because of interaction of the 4-methyl group with the aliphatic two-carbon chain. Because α- and β-methylhistamine exist predominantly as gauche conformers and both are very weak H_1 and H_2 agonists, it has been suggested that the *trans* conformation of histamine is preferred at both H_1 and H_2 receptors. A gauche conformation has been suggested for histamine at the H_3 receptor, because α-methylhistamine and some other more conformationally restricted analogues are potent H_3 agonists.

Addition of other alkyl substituents onto the histamine molecule generally produces compounds with decreased potency at H_1 and H_2 receptors. 2-Methylhistamine is a selective H_1 agonist (versus 4-methylhistamine, a selective H_2 agonist), but imidazole N-substitution (N^1 or N^3) with methyl groups results in nearly inactive agents. Similarly, aliphatic amine nitrogen substitution results in decreasing activity ($NH_2 > NHMe > NMe_2 > N^{+}Me_3$ [quaternary ammonium salt]) at both H_1 and H_2 receptors (2).

PHYSIOLOGICAL CHARACTERISTICS OF HISTAMINE

Synthesis and Metabolism of Histamine

Histamine is synthesized in the Golgi apparatus of mast cells and basophils by enzymatic decarboxylation of histidine.

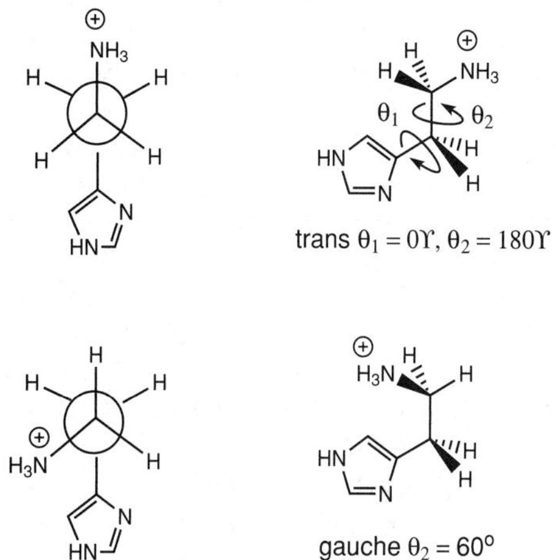

Fig. 37.1. Conformers of histamine.

Table 37.1. Histamine-Related Agonists[a]

	Relative H_1 activity vs. histamine	Relative H_2 activity vs. histamine	Relative H_3 activity vs. histamine
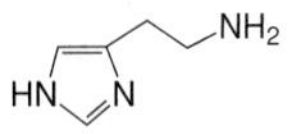	100	100	100
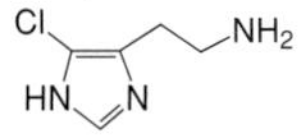	1.7	12	ND[b]
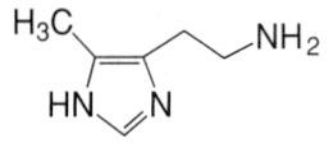	0.23	39	<0.008
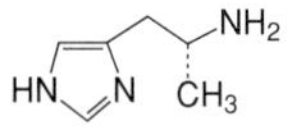	0.49	1.0	1550
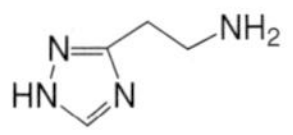	12.7	13.7	ND
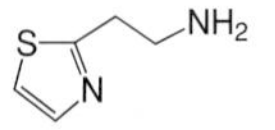	26	~0.3	<0.008
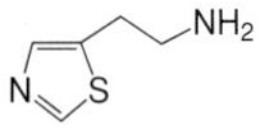	0.01	~0.1	ND
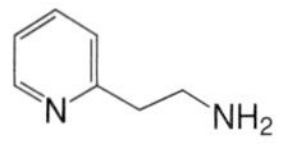	5.6	2.5	<0.06
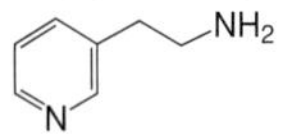	Inactive	Inactive	ND
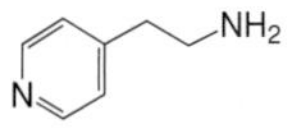	~0	~0.4	ND

ND = not determined.

[a]Activity expressed relative to histamine = 100, determined in vitro on guinea pig ileum (H_1),guinea pig atrium (H_2) and rat cerebral cortex (H_3)(3).

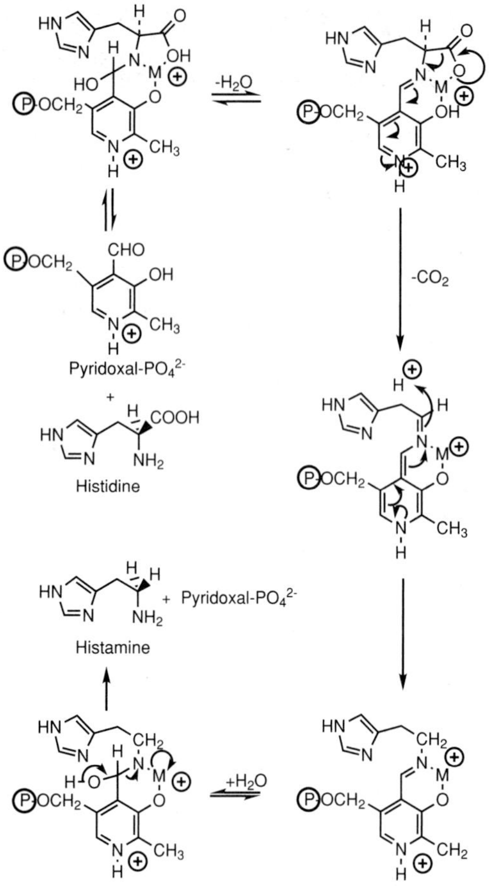

Fig. 37.2. Formation of histamine by decarboxylation of histidine.

This conversion is catalyzed by L-histidine decarboxylase, with pyridoxal phosphate serving as a cofactor for this process. The reaction mechanism for this decarboxylation probably involves the formation of an imine intermediate, followed by the loss of carbon dioxide, a mechanism demonstrated to occur for decarboxylation of many α-amino acids (Fig. 37.2). Pyridoxal phosphate provides an important catalytic function, and in the final step, the product is released by hydrolysis of the enzyme-bound Schiff base of histamine. Mechanism-based inhibitors of this process, such as α-fluoromethylhistidine, decrease the rate of synthesis of histamine and, thus, deplete cells of histamine. As such, α-fluoromethylhistidine is an important pharmacological tool (4). This approach, however, has not been successfully developed into agents for the treatment allergic inflammatory disorders, peptic ulcer, or motion sickness.

Once released, histamine is rapidly metabolized in vivo (based on products from radiolabeled histamine administered intradermally) to nearly inactive metabolites by two major pathways: N-methylation, and oxidation (Fig. 37.3). Methylation (S-adenosylmethionine), which is catalyzed by the intracellular enzyme N-methyltransferase, yields an inactive metabolite. A portion of the N-methylated metabolite is oxidized sequentially via monoamine oxidase and then via aldehyde oxidase to the corresponding N-methylimidazole acetic acid. Histamine also is oxidized to imidazole acetic acid by diamine oxidase (histaminase). A small amount of this acid intermediate is converted to the corresponding ribotide, an unusual metabolite (5).

Storage and Release of Histamine

In mast cells, histamine is stored in secretory granules as a complex with acidic residues of the proteoglycan heparin and in basophils in the blood as a complex with chondroitin sulfate (6,7). Mast cells are distributed in areas of skin and mucous membranes of the respiratory, gastrointestinal, and genitourinary tracts and in tissue adjacent to blood and lymph vessels. Although histamine is secreted at low levels from these mast cells and basophils, the primary mechanism of release is associated with cell activation by immunoglobulin (IgE)–mediated hypersensitivity processes (Fig. 37.4). Immediate hypersensitivity is initiated when allergen molecules cross-link to Fab components of adjacent IgE antibody molecules bound to high-affinity FcεRI receptors on the surface of these cells ($FcεRI^+$ cells). Dimerization of occupied IgE-Fc receptors results in several membrane and cytosolic events. These include release of preformed mediators

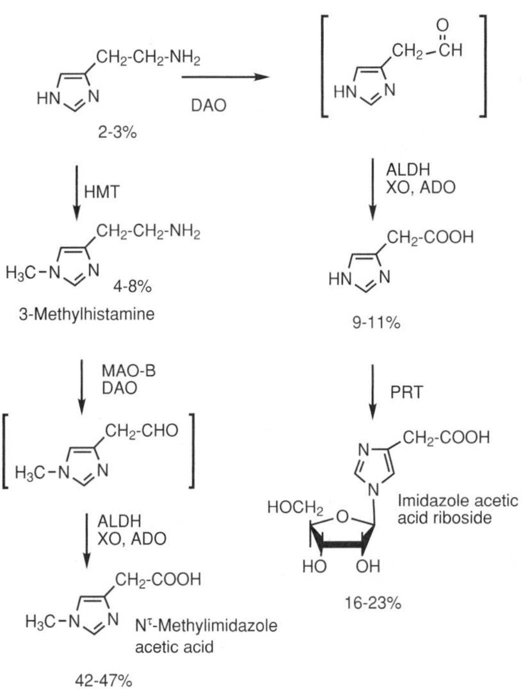

Fig. 37.3. Major metabolic pathways of histamine, from intradermal histamine as measured in the urine in 12 hours in human males (5). HMT, histamine N-methyltransferase; MAO-B, monoamine oxidase type B; DAO, diamineoxidase; ALDH, aldehyde dehydrogenase; ADO, aldehyde oxidase; XO, xanthine oxidase; PRT, phosphoribosyl transferase.

from secretory granules by exocytosis, synthesis and release of chemotactic mediators and neutral proteases (e.g., tryptase), synthesis and release of other lipid mediators (e.g., leukotrienes and prostaglandins), and stimulation of synthesis of cytokines and their subsequent release. Other cell activation stimuli for the release of histamine include concanavalin A, substance P, polyamines, opiates, and several lymphokines and cytokines. Different subpopulations of cells respond differently to these stimuli. With the exocytotic response, histamine rapidly dissociates from the partially solubilized granule matrix. In basophils, the release process may be slightly different, occurring without degranulation. Other cell types, including lymphocytes, platelets, neutrophils, monocytes, and some macrophages, secrete histamine-releasing factors. These cells also have distinct low-affinity receptors for IgE, which when occupied result in secretion of mediators that selectively recruit and activate secondary effector cells in the inflammatory process.

Mast cells play an important role in the early response to allergens, and they provide mediators that lead to initial and late stages of the process and, subsequently, to chronic inflammatory reactions (8–10). Early stages appear to be related to degranulation and the release of many mediators, including histamine, prostaglandin D_2 (PGD_2) and leukotriene C_4, platelet-activating factor, adenosine triphosphate (ATP), kinins, and some enzymes (e.g., tryptase and chymase). Thus, additional important mediators other than histamine have very significant roles. These mediators include platelet-activation factor, substance P, neurokinin A, and others. Besides processes of vasodilation and edema, activation of secondary inflammatory cells occurs, as do adherence of neutrophils and migration of eosinophils and T cells to postcapillary venule endothelial cells. This latter process is mediated by specific cell adhesion molecules. A further array of mediators and cellular responses follows. A series of interleukins are generated and secreted by subtypes of T cells. Stimulation of many NFκB-mediated gene transcription pathways occurs via H_1 receptor activation. Important cytokines are produced and liberated, including tumor necrosis factor α (TNF-α), interleukin-4 (IL-4), IL-5, IL-1, and IL-6, which are involved in chemokine secretion and regulation of cell maturation and proliferation processes, changes that occur in late-stage inflammatory processes. Thus, the inflammatory cascade is a complex and intricate one, and the effects of histamine are only a small part of the process. Inhibition of the production of many of the proinflammatory cytokines occurs in the presence of many of the H_1 antihistamines.

As a result of occupation of H_1 receptors by histamine, constriction of bronchial and gastrointestinal smooth muscle occurs. Spasm of the bronchi to inhaled histamine at one time was a test for airway reactivity. Intradermal injection of histamine produces vasodilation of arterioles as the first step in the "triple response" mediated via H_1 and H_2 receptors. A flare response follows this stimulation, resulting in release of substance P and other neuropeptides. Edema from exudation of plasma fluids follows because of contraction of endothelial cells of the postcapillary venules. The wheal and flare responses are mostly H_1 receptor mediated.

Histamine Receptors—Molecular and Mechanistic Aspects

Histamine receptors are found in various tissues. Among these are the H_1 receptors in smooth muscle of the bronchi, gut, and uterus. Contraction of the bronchi leads to restriction of air flow in the lungs. Histamine increases the permeability of capillary walls. Plasma constituents flow into extracellular spaces because of contraction of endothelial cells; this process leads to edema. At the level of the CNS, histamine secretion appears to be associated with wakefulness, because H_1 receptor antagonism centrally is associated with drowsiness. In the stomach, parietal cell stimulation increases production and secretion of acid, mediated through H_2 receptors. The H_2 receptors play a minor role in allergic inflammatory processes. The H_3 receptor is principally an autoreceptor in the CNS at histaminergic neurons, and it is a heteroreceptor on neurons that release other neurotransmitters, also in the brain. The H_4 receptor is expressed primarily on eosinophils and mast cells, where it is associated with chemotactic responses.

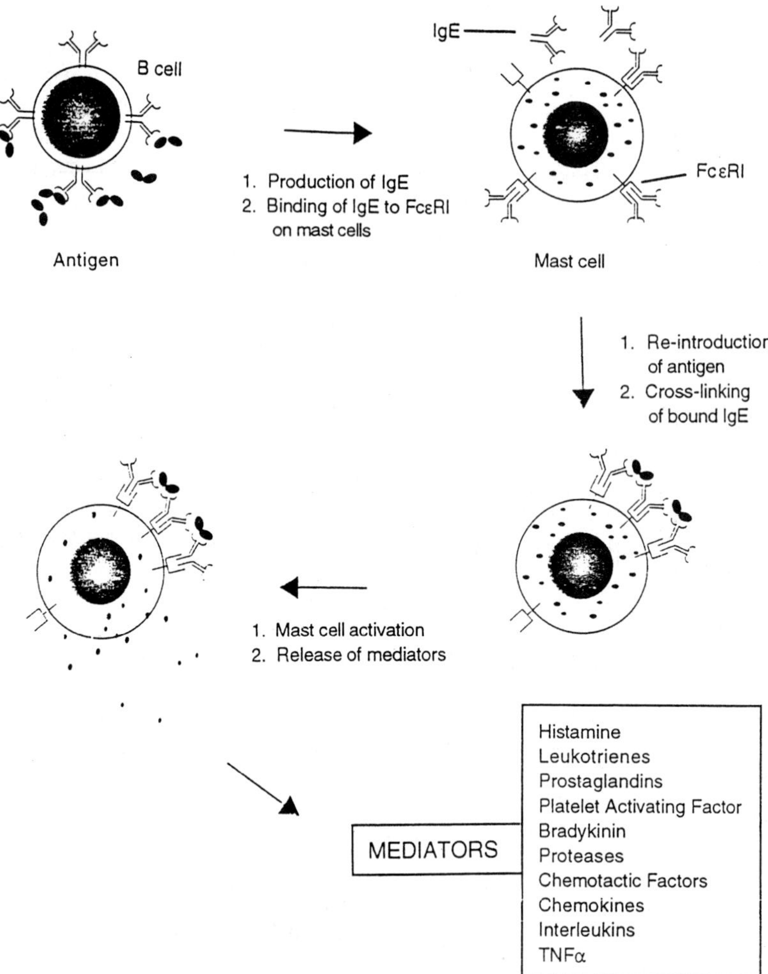

Fig. 37.4. Sequence of events in immediate hypersensitivity. Initial contact with an antigen leads to specific IgE synthesis by B cells. Secreted IgE binds to mast cells or basophils through high-affinity Fce receptors (FceRI). On subsequent exposure to the antigen, an immediate hypersensitivity reaction is triggered by cross-linking the IgE molecules.

All the histamine receptors appear to have constitutive receptor G-protein signaling activity independent of the presence of histamine (11). Most of the antihistamines studied are not antagonists, but some are inverse agonists. They reduce constitutive G-protein signaling activity. Occasionally, some antihistamines are neutral antagonists, i.e., they do not reduce the constitutive G protein–coupled activity of the receptor. A two-state model of inactive and active conformations of the receptor is consistent with this observation.

The human H_1 receptor gene encodes for a 487-amino-acid protein with the signature structural features of G protein–coupled receptors (seven transmembrane domains, N-terminal glycosylation sites, phosphorylation sites for protein kinases A and C, and a large intracellular loop with several serine and threonine residues) (11,12). It is coupled (via $G_{q/11}$ proteins) to phosphatidyl inositol turnover as the second-messenger system. The H_1 receptor shows 40% homology with the muscarinic M_1 receptor and the M_2 receptor. An aspartic acid in the third transmembrane domain is highly conserved in several species, and it is suggested to be a recognition site for the protonated aliphatic amine function of histamine at both H_1 and H_2 receptors. Based on mutation studies and homologous positions to α-adrenergic receptors, suggestions for sites of binding of the imidazole portion of histamine to amino acids threonine and/or asparagine in the fifth transmembrane have been made.

Signal transduction processes begin with $G_{q/11}$-coupled hydrolysis of phosphatidylinositide to inositol-1,4,5-triphosphate and 1,2-diacylglycerol, which occurs via activation of phospholipase C. Elevation of intracellular calcium ion from intracellular stores occurs. Voltage-gated calcium channels may be opened by activation of ion channels permeable to Na^+ and K^+ ions. Calcium channel antagonists block some effects of histamine on intestinal smooth muscle. In addition, the H_1 receptor can activate other signaling pathways, including phospholipase D and phospholipase A_2, and stimulate NFκB-mediated gene transcription.

The H_2 receptor is a 359-amino-acid protein in humans. It has some features similar to the H_1 protein (e.g., N-terminal glycosylation sites) and phosphorylation sites in the C-terminal. An aspartic acid residue in the third transmembrane loop appears to be critical to agonist and antagonist binding, and threonine/aspartate and tyrosine/aspartate couples in the fifth transmembrane domain appear to be important for interaction of the imidazole part of the histamine molecule. It is positively coupled via $G_{\alpha s}$ to activate adenylyl cyclase for synthesis of cyclic adenosine monophosphate (cAMP) as a second messenger. In some systems, it is coupled through G_q proteins to stimulate phospholipase C. It appears in some cells that other processes, such as breakdown of phosphoinositides, control of intracellular calcium ion levels, and phospholipase A_2 activity, can be regulated by other cAMP-independent pathways.

The highest density of H_3 receptors occurs in the brain, principally in the striatum, substantia nigra, and the cortex and to a much lesser extent at peripheral nerve terminals. It is a presynaptic auto- and heteroreceptor where activation leads to a decrease in neurotransmitter release. The most widely studied H_3 receptor is 445 amino acids, but many splice variants have been observed (13). It is activated via $G_{\alpha i/o}$ proteins (coupled negatively to adenylyl cyclase) to the activation of protein kinase A to modulate gene transcription. The H_3 receptors, via $G_{\alpha i/o}$ proteins, may activate phospholipase A_2, mitogen-activated protein kinase, and phosphatidyl inositol-3-kinase. The H_3 receptors have low sequence homology with H_1 and H_2 receptors (~20% each). Activation of histaminergic neurons centrally, which promotes arousal and attention and improves learning in animals, is a potential target for H_3 receptor antihistamines. Like the H_1 and H_2 antihistamines, the H_3 antihistamines function primarily as inverse agonists.

The H_4 receptors appear to be limited to cells of the hematopoietic system, with expression occurring primarily on eosinophils, basophils, dendritic cells, and T cells. Histamine stimulation results in a chemotactic response, cell migration. The presence of H_4 receptors on these cells suggests that this receptor plays a role in the inflammatory response. Evidence suggests that it may be regulated via inflammatory stimulation of TNF-α and IL-6. The H_4 receptor has 390 amino acids and is coupled to inhibition of adenylyl cyclase via $G_{\alpha i/o}$. It has highest homology with the H_3 receptor (~35–40%), with greater homology (58%) of the transmembrane segments. Thus, antihistamines could be useful agents to antagonize the inflammatory response. Agents studied to date also appear to be inverse agonists.

INHIBITORS OF HISTAMINE RELEASE

Mechanism of Action

The bronchodilatory activity of khellin, a chromone obtained from a plant source (*Ammi visnaga*) used by ancient Egyptians for spasmolytic activity, stimulated the search for related compounds with similar pharmacological properties (14). From a study of many bischromones, cromolyn sodium was developed and marketed (Fig. 37.5). Although it prevents bronchospasm, it does not reverse antigen-induced bronchiolar constriction. Thus, it and other agents like it that followed prevent the release of histamine and do not block the effects of histamine at its receptors.

The mechanism by which cromolyn and nedocromil inhibit degranulation of mast cells has been investigated (15). Both agents stimulate phosphorylation of moesin, a 78-kDa protein that is phosphorylated by isozymes of protein kinase C. It is suggested that phosphorylation results in conformational changes that exposes domains that promote association with actin and other proteins of the secretory granules. This association results in immobilization of the granules and inhibition of exocytosis. Cromolyn and nedocromil (vide infra) apparently inhibit function of cells other than mast cells; these effects may occur during later stages of inflammatory responses. Cromolyn does not have intrinsic antihistaminic or anti-inflammatory activity.

Mast cell stabilizers used in the treatment of asthma are additionally discussed in Chapter 44.

Therapeutic Applications of Specific Drugs

Cromolyn (Intal, Nasalcrom, Gastrocrom)

Cromolyn generally is used prophylactically for bronchial asthma (as an inhaled powder), for prevention of exercise-induced bronchospasm, and for seasonal and perennial allergic rhinitis (nasal solution). Topically, it also is used as eye drops for allergic conjunctivitis and keratitis. In

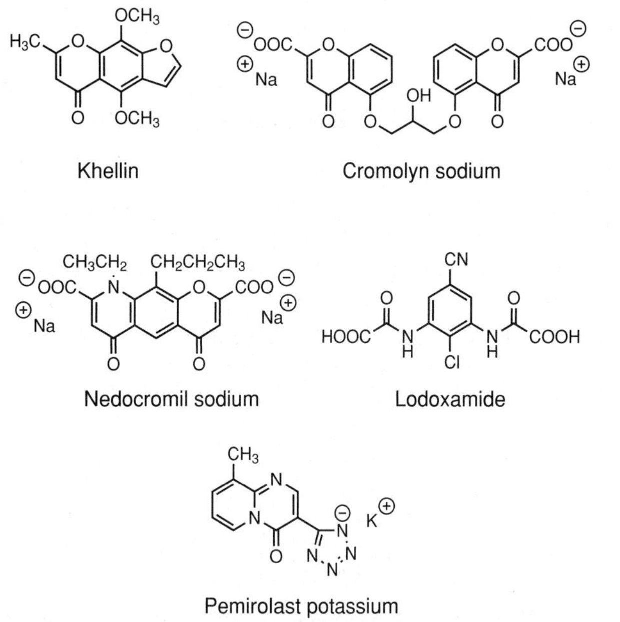

Khellin   Cromolyn sodium

Nedocromil sodium   Lodoxamide

Pemirolast potassium

Fig. 37.5. Mast cell degranulation inhibitors.

the management of asthmatic conditions, it is administered using a power-operated nebulizer. The bioavailability is very low with oral administration because of poor absorption. By inhalation, the powder is irritating to some patients. After inhalation, much less than 10% of the dose reaches the systemic circulation. An oral dosage form is used for mastocytosis.

Nedocromil (Alocril, Tilade)

Nedocromil is a chromone analogue also used by inhalation as an aerosol, primarily in the prophylaxis of asthma and reversible obstructive airway disease. It inhibits release of allergic mediators, and it is effective in a broad range of patients. An ophthalmic solution is available for the treatment of seasonal and perennial allergic conjunctivitis. Other structurally related compounds are not currently available in the United States but are available in other markets.

Lodoxamide (Alomide)

Lodoxamide, which shows some structural similarities to cromolyn and nedocromil, also is a mast cell stabilizer that inhibits the immediate hypersensitivity reaction, preventing increases in vascular permeability associated with antigen-IgE–mediated responses. Its precise mechanism of action is not completely understood. It is used topically in the eye, principally for conjunctivitis and keratitis associated with vernal allergens.

Pemirolast (Alamast)

Pemirolast, with an acidic tetrazole isosteric replacement for a carboxylic acid functionality, is used topically in the eye to prevent itching associated with allergic conjunctivitis. It is an inhibitor of the release of histamine and other inflammatory mediators, including leukotrienes. Significant use as a systemic agent has been reported, and it has been shown to be of value in preventing restenosis after percutaneous coronary angiopathy.

INHIBITORS OF RELEASED HISTAMINE

Historical Background

The first antihistamine was discovered by Forneau and Bovet (16), who observed that piperoxan protected guinea pigs against histamine-induced bronchospasm. The sensitivity of the guinea pig was initially thought to make it a good model for anaphylaxis. Piperoxan also has important effects related to antagonism of norepinephrine at α-adrenergic receptors.

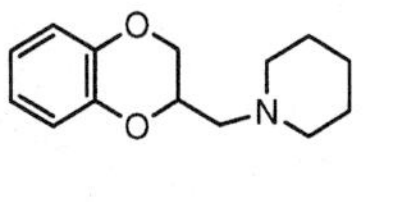

Piperoxan

Antihistamines, specifically H_1 antihistamines (17,18), are useful in the treatment of allergy and inflammatory disorders, in which many but not all effects are mediated via histamine. Compounds that had antagonistic effects in these assays did not antagonize the effects of histamine on the stomach (acid secretion) and heart (positive chronotropic and inotropic effects). These differences led to suggestion of the presence of H_1 and H_2 receptors and, ultimately, to the development of selective H_2 antihistamines to diminish the secretion of gastric acid. A third class of histamine receptors, H_3 receptors, appears primarily to consist of autoreceptors that control the synthesis and release of histamine presynaptically and of heteroreceptors that control the release of other transmitters, primarily in the CNS. The most recent class of histamine receptors, H_4 receptors, are expressed principally on eosinophils and mast cells, where they may play a role in the inflammatory response, especially during the late stages. Classical H_1 antihistamines do not bind to this histamine receptor, and H_4 receptors do not modulate degranulation of mast cells.

The first-generation H_1 antihistamines are useful and effective in the treatment of allergic responses (e.g., hay fever, rhinitis, urticaria, and food allergy). These agents also have effects at cholinergic, adrenergic, dopaminergic, and serotonergic receptors. Adverse central effects include sedation, drowsiness, decreased cognitive ability, and somnolence. Peripheral side effects associated with cholinergic blockade include blurred vision, dry mouth, urinary retention, and constipation. Other observed effects have included appetite stimulation, muscle spasm, anxiety, confusion, and occasionally, irritability, tremor, and tachycardia. Of all the side effects, CNS depression is the most common, and it can be so pronounced that some of these agents with short durations of action are used as over-the-counter (OTC) sleep aids. The separation of CNS depressant and anticholinergic effects from peripheral antihistaminic effects in later agents led to the second-generation antihistamines (vide infra).

Structural classes of H_1 antihistamines can be represented by a general structure of two aromatic groups linked through a short chain to a tertiary aliphatic amine (Fig. 37.6). The aromatic groups (Ar_1, Ar_2) usually are phenyl or substituted phenyl, thienyl, or pyridyl. These substituents are attached to the X group, which is a nitrogen atom in the ethylenediamines, a carbon attached to

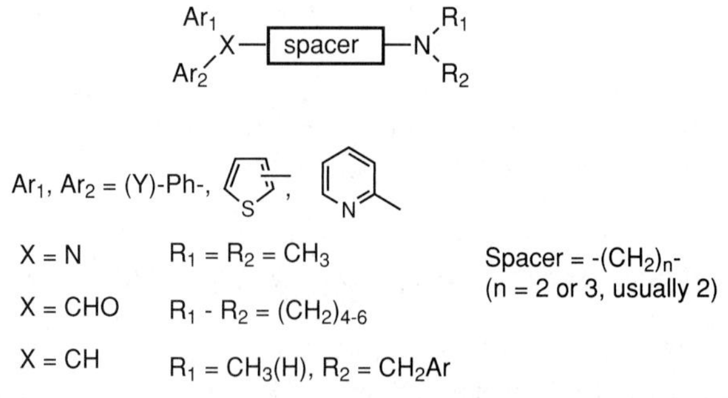

Ar_1, Ar_2 = (Y)-Ph-, [thienyl], [pyridyl]

X = N $R_1 = R_2 = CH_3$

X = CHO $R_1 - R_2 = (CH_2)_{4-6}$

X = CH $R_1 = CH_3(H)$, $R_2 = CH_2Ar$

Spacer = $-(CH_2)_n-$ (n = 2 or 3, usually 2)

Fig. 37.6. General structure of first-generation antihistamines.

an ether oxygen atom in the ethanolamine ether series, or only a carbon atom in the alkyl amines. The spacer usually is two or three carbons in length, and it may be in a ring, may be branched, and may be saturated or unsaturated. The R groups attached to the aliphatic amine usually are simple alkyl groups, generally methyl or, occasionally, aralkyl groups. One of the early thiophene-containing analogues was carcinogenic in rats. After thiophene versus benzene replacement in other series of compounds demonstrated some toxic effects, thiophene was relegated to one of the low-priority choices for isosteric replacement of a phenyl group.

Most H_1 antihistamines are inverse agonists rather than neutral antagonists. Like other histamine receptors, H_1 receptors have constitutive G protein–coupled activity in the absence of the agonist histamine that results in activation of second-messenger signaling pathways, such as phospholipase C activity and NFκB-mediated gene transcription (19). A model of active and inactive conformations of histamine receptors has been advanced to accommodate these biochemical findings. Inverse agonists bind to the inactive conformation of the receptor, shifting the equilibrium toward the inactive state. Neutral antagonists interact with both conformations of the receptor.

First-Generation H_1 Antihistamines

Ethylenediamines

The earliest series of H_1 antihistamines is the ethylenediamines. Two 2-carbon spacers may appear between the two nitrogen atoms in the piperazine series (vide infra). Examples of agents in the ethylenediamine class, of which phenbenzamine was the first of these agents, appear in Table 37.2. Compounds with several different but closely related aromatic rings are useful, such as phenyl, 2-pyridyl, halogen- and methoxy-substituted phenyl, or pyrimidyl. Thiazole-, furanyl-, and thiophene-ring congeners also were available in the past. The small alkyl substituents on basic nitrogen usually are methyl groups. A number of these agents are still used. With the exception of antazoline, all have the ethylenediamine spacer. In antazoline, the alkyl tertiary amine in phenbenzamine is replaced with an imidazoline group. Central nervous system effects, usually sedation, are very common among agents in this class.

Information regarding pharmacokinetic and metabolic disposition is limited, because this early group of compounds was not studied in depth. Only later, with second-generation H_1 antihistamines, and/or when issues of potential toxicity have arisen concerning some of the early compounds, has the metabolic disposition been examined more completely. Thus, the available information concerning the metabolism on these early antihistamines is sparse. From some of the ethylenediamines, expected products of N-demethylation and subsequent deamination have been reported. In addition, some produce quaternary N-glucuronides as urinary metabolites, a process that occurs, to some extent, in many relatively unhindered tertiary aliphatic amines among the antihistamines and also in other lipophilic aliphatic tertiary amine drug classes.

Table 37.2. Examples of Ethylenediamine Anthistamines

Drugs	X	Y	Ar
Phenbenzamine	CH	CH	phenyl
Tripelennamine (pyribenzamine)	N	CH	phenyl
Methapyrilene	N	CH	2-thienyl
Thonzylamine	N	N	CH_3O-phenyl
Related compound: Antazoline			

Ethanolamine Ethers

Structure Activity Relationships. The prototype of the aminoalkyl ethers is diphenhydramine, a benzhydryl ether which more than a half-century after its introduction remains still widely used for allergic conditions. Structural analogues with various ring substituents (Me, OMe, Cl, and Br) in one of the aromatic rings also have been developed, as have compounds with a 2-pyridyl group replacing one of the phenyl groups (Table 37.3).

Significant anticholinergic side effects are observed among members of the group (e.g., dry mouth, blurred vision, tachycardia, urinary retention, and constipation). It should be noted that diphenydramine is used in the treatment of parkinsonism because of its central anticholinergic properties. Other anticholinergic agents that are structurally related to the benzydryl ether antihistamines also are used in the treatment of parkinsonism (see Chapter 25). Sedative properties are very common as well. Sedation, accompanied by a short half-life and a wide margin of safety, allows some of these compounds to be used as OTC sleep aids. The 8-chlorotheophyllinate salt of diphenhydramine is marketed as dimenhydrinate for use in the treatment of motion sickness. The compound with the aryl groups *p*-Cl-Ph and 2-pyridyl is carbinoxamine, a potent antihistamine. Substitution of a methyl group at the carbon α to the ether function affords the related compound doxylamine, in which the aryl groups are phenyl and 2-pyridyl. Clemastine, a

Table 37.3. Ethanolamine Ether Antihistamines

Drugs	Trade Name	R_1	R_2	X
Diphenhydramine Dimenhydrinate	Benadryl Dramamine	H	H	CH
Bromodiphenhydramine		Br	H	CH
Chlorodiphenhydramine		Cl	H	CH
Carbinoxamine	Colistin	Cl	H	N
Doxylamine	Decapryn Unisom	H	CH_3	N

Related compounds:

Setastine (Loderix) Clemastine (Tavist)

Table 37.4. Antihistamine and Anticholinergic Activity of Enantiomers of Ring Substituted Ethanolamine Ethers (20)

		Antihistaminic Activity		Anticholinergic Activity	
$R_{2'}$	$R_{4'}$	pD_2	Ratio of Potency of (+)- to (−)- Isomer	pD_2	Ratio of Potency of (+)- to (−)- Isomer
$(CH_3)_3C$	H	(+) 8.76[a] (−) 6.87	78	(+) 6.14 (−) 5.89	1.9
H	CH_3	(+) 6.36 (−) 6.00	2.3	(+) 6.03 (−) 8.12[a]	0.008[b]

[a]Most potent enantiomer in each assay.
[b](−)-Enantiomer is ~125 times as potent as the (+)-enantiomer

homologue with an additional carbon atom between the oxygen and the basic nitrogen, which is incorporated into a ring, is a recent addition to the group, with less sedative properties. Other analogues are used elsewhere. For example, setastine, a compound with the alkyl amine substituent being incorporated into a 7-membered hexahydroazepine ring, is available in Europe.

Antihistaminic versus anticholinergic activity. Besides the structural analogues in Table 37.3 that possess increased selectivity for histamine H_1 receptors over muscarinic receptors, introduction of alkyl substituents at C-2' or C-4' of one aromatic ring results in significant changes in selectivity in tissue-based assays for antihistaminic versus anticholinergic activity. With increasing alkyl group size (Me, Et, iPr, and tBu) at C-2', large decreases in antihistaminic activity and increases in anticholinergic activity are observed (20). With larger alkyl groups, the possible spatial orientations of the two aromatic rings with regard to each other are limited because of increasing rotameric restrictions. Introduction of these alkyl substituents at C-4' decreases anticholinergic activity and yields small increases in antihistaminic activity. A chiral center is introduced with these changes, and differences in pharmacological properties of the enantiomers of each compound are observed. Two examples are shown in Table 37.4.

Stereochemical and structural effects. The observed differences in potency of enantiomers in tissue-based assays suggest significant stereoselective interactions of antagonists at the receptor level. Differences in affinity of 60- to 200-fold are noted between enantiomers in several analogues where the chiral center results because of differences in the two aromatic rings, such as Ph and 2-pyridyl, or Ph and *p*-Br-Ph (21). Enantiomers with the *S*-absolute configuration usually are more potent. Clemastine, a more complex homologue, is marketed as the *R,R*-enantiomer, which is the more potent of the *R,R*- and *S,S*-enantiomeric pair and more potent than either the *R,S*- and *S,R*-enantiomers of the other diastereomer (22). Consistent with results from related compounds, the chiral center at the benzhydryl carbon has a significant influence on potency, whereas the one in the pyrrolidine ring is of lesser importance (Table 37.5).

Very small changes in the arrangement of aromatic groups in the members of the ethanolamine ether series significantly alter the scope of their pharmacological properties. Previous work has shown that the two aromatic rings in diphenhydramine can be located slightly differently with respect to each other, as in phenyltoloxamine, a potent antihistamine. A retro arrangement of carbon and oxygen atoms, however, prepared in an

Table 37.5. Antihistamine Activity of Stereoisomers of Clemastine (22)

Drug	Diastereomers	pA_2	ED_{50}[a]
Clemastine	(R,R)	9.45	0.04 mg/kg
	(S,S)	7.99	5.0
	(R,S)	9.40	0.28
	(S,R)	8.57	11.0

[a]ED_{50} vs. lethal dose of histamine in guinea pigs (22).

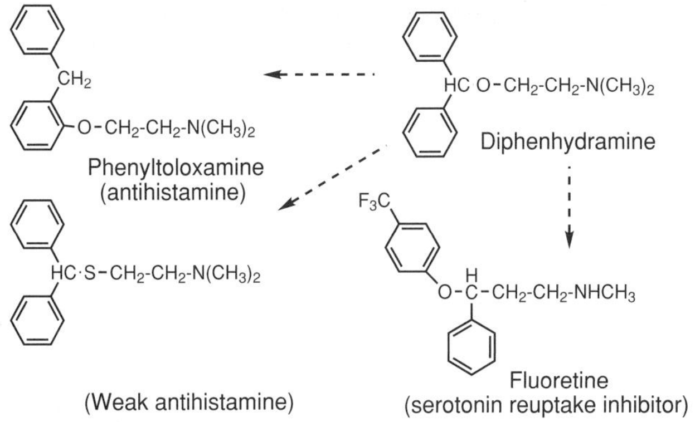

Phenyltoloxamine (antihistamine)

Diphenhydramine

(Weak antihistamine)

Fluoretine (serotonin reuptake inhibitor)

Fig. 37.7. Structural similarities among diphenhydramine-related structures.

attempt to investigate structural requirements for antihistamines, afforded significantly different pharmacological properties and, ultimately, led to a series of very important selective serotonin reuptake inhibitors, such as fluoxetine (Fig. 37.7). Unlike the bio-isosteric oxygen to nitrogen atom replacement, conversion of the oxygen atom to a sulfur atom in the diphenhydramine series results in a compound with greatly decreased antihistaminic activity (23).

Metabolism. Only limited information regarding the metabolic disposition of this group of compounds is available. As expected, N-demethylation (formation of the corresponding secondary amine) and subsequent deamination (formation of the carboxylic acid metabolite) is a major pathway for diphenydramine (Fig. 37.8) and some of its analogues. Although the early experiments are relatively incomplete, it appears that the N-demethylation products have shorter half-lives than the corresponding parent drugs, and they probably contribute very little to the observed antihistaminic properties. Minor metabolites that are conjugates of the carboxylic acid products of deamination or of ether cleavage products have been found in some animal species. Compounds with shorter half lives, like diphenhydramine, when used as antihistamines require repeated administration, but a very short half life is an advantage when the same drugs are used as sleep aids (17,18).

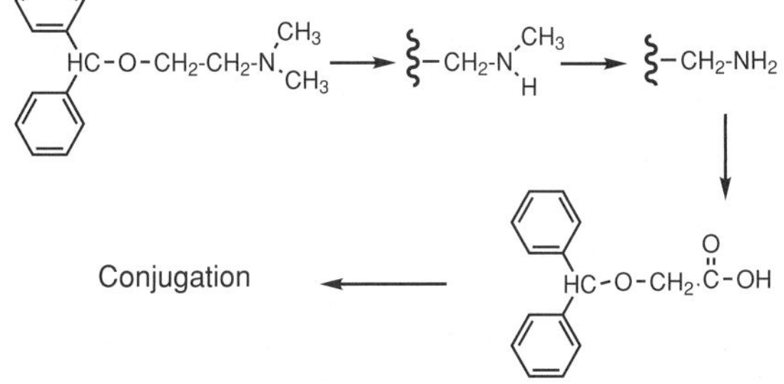

Conjugation

Fig. 37.8. Metabolism of diphenhydramine.

Alkyl Amines

A third class of analogues is one in which a carbon atom replaces the heteroatom spacer in the general structure. Examples are pheniramine, chlorpheniramine, brompheniramine, and the *E*-isomers of olefinic homologues (Fig. 37.9). The ring halogen–substituted compounds are widely used OTC antihistamines for mild seasonal allergies. These agents are characterized by a long duration of antihistaminic action and by a decreased incidence of central sedative side effects compared to the ethylenediamines and ethanolamine ether series. This structural change introduces a chiral carbon when the two aromatic rings are different (e.g., Ph and 2-pyridyl). These were the most extensively used antihistamines until the more selective second-generation antihistamines appeared.

Structural and Stereochemical Effects. *E*- and *Z*-isomers of the alkenes in this series show very large differences in potency in tissue-based assays. For example, *E*-pyrrobutamine is more potent than its *Z*-isomer by 165-fold, and *E*-triprolidine (Fig. 37.9) is more potent than its *Z*-isomer by approximately 1,000-fold (2). Dimethidene has many of the structural features of both of these two agents in a more complex, cyclized structure. The observed difference in potency between the *E*- and *Z*-isomers shows that the two aromatic rings probably have quite different binding environments at the receptor (24). These observations provide evidence suggesting that a 5- to 6-Å distance between the tertiary aliphatic amine and one of the aromatic rings is required at the site of receptor binding (Fig. 37.10) (25).

Differences in potency between the enantiomers of the conformationally mobile amino-alkanes also have been

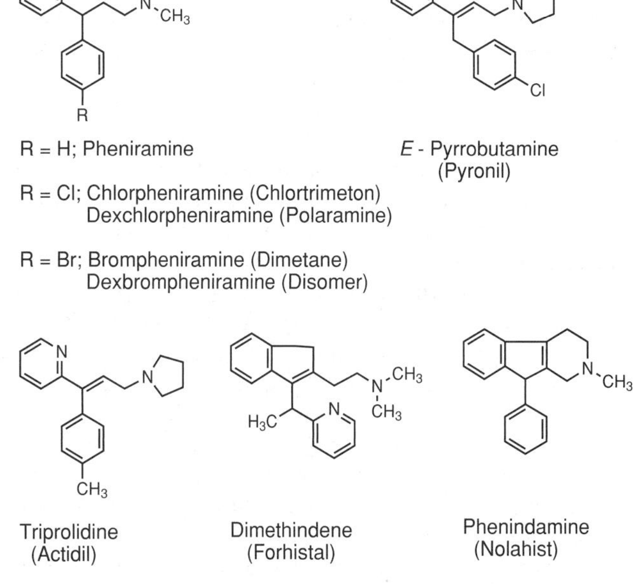

Fig. 37.9. Examples of alkane and alkene antihistamines.

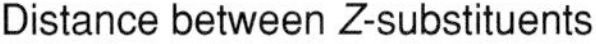

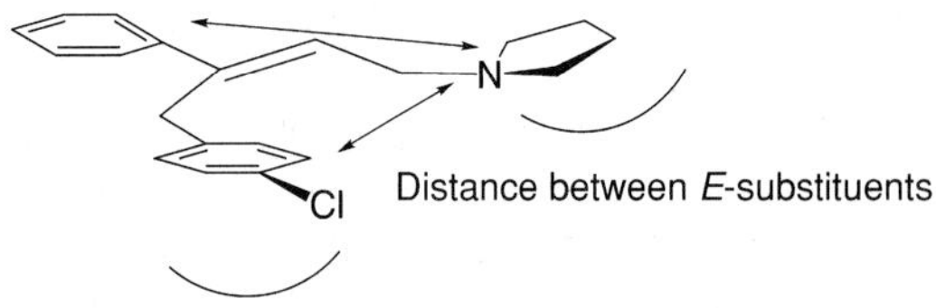

Fig. 37.10. Potential binding sites based on E/Z-configurations.

observed. The *S*-enantiomers have greater affinity for H_1 histamine receptors, occasionally by very large amounts, such as 200- to 1,000-fold in radioligand displacement assays and in tissue-based assays for *S*-(+)- versus *R*-(−)-chlorpheniramine, with the (+)-enantiomer being more potent (Ar=R-Ph, 2-pyridyl) (Fig. 37.9). Greater selectivity for H_1 receptors versus muscarinic and adrenergic receptors is observed as well. For members of the series, the chiral center of the more potent enantiomer correlates stereochemically with the more active enantiomer of the oxygen congener carbinoxamine (Table 37.3) (2,26). Single enantiomers of these agents are available (e.g., dexchlorpheniramine and dexbrompheniramine).

Half-life and Metabolism. The alkyl amines have significantly less CNS-depressant effects than benzhydryl ethers of ethanolamines. Additionally, these compounds have long half-lives and extended durations of action. These agents have decreased antiemetic effects and decreased anticholinergic properties compared to ethanolamine ethers. Many are available in OTC preparations for hay fever and other mild allergic conditions, sometimes in combination with adrenergic decongestants. Most are suitable for once-a-day dosing because of their long half-lives (up to 24 hours), although they are routinely administered more frequently.

Information concerning the metabolic disposition of some these agents has been reported. As expected, N-dealkylation is a major pathway, with the corresponding secondary and primary amines, as well as the parent drug, being found in the plasma.

Piperazines

Members of the piperazine class of agents are structurally related to both the ethylenediamines and the benzhydryl ethers of ethanolamines. Their structures include the 2-carbon separation between nitrogen atoms, which is incorporated into the piperazine ring (Table 37.6).

Diarylmethylene groups (benzhydryl substituents, as in diphenhydramine) are attached to one of the nitrogen atoms, and an alkyl or aralkyl substituent is attached to the other nitrogen. Early compounds, such as cyclizine, chlorcyclizine, meclizine, buclizine, and hydroxyzine, have been widely used as antihistamines and as agents for treatment of motion sickness, because they have useful central antiemetic effects.

These agents also have significant anticholinergic and antihistaminic properties. Anticholinergic side effects and drowsiness are common. The primary use of these compounds remains treatment of motion sickness and vertigo and suppression of nausea and vomiting. Although teratogenic effects of cyclizine and meclizine have been observed in rodents, large studies have not demonstrated adverse fetal effects in humans; however, these agents are used cautiously in pregnant women and children. Oxatomide is used in Europe principally in allergic rhinitis, urticaria, and in combination with albuterol in asthma. Drowsiness and sedation are noted. Hydroxyzine is used in treatment of pruritis, and at higher dosages, it is used in the management of anxiety and emotional stress. Its acid metabolite, cetirizine, which is formed from oxidation of the terminal primary alcohol to the corresponding carboxylic acid, usually is classified with the second-generation, nonsedating antihistamines. The amphoteric nature of cetirizine, having both the tertiary aliphatic amine and carboxylic acid functional groups, appears to be associated with decreased, but not absent, sedative side effects.

Table 37.6. Examples of Tricyclic Antihistamines

(General structure: benzhydryl-piperazine, N–R_2; R_1 on phenyl ring)

Drugs	Trade name	R_1	R_2
Cyclizine	Marezine	H	CH_3
Chlorcyclizine	Mantadil	Cl	CH_3
Meclizine	Antivert	Cl	H_2C–(phenyl)–CH_3
Buclizine	Bucladin-S	Cl	H_2C–(phenyl)–$C(CH_3)_3$
Oxatomide	Tinset	H	$CH_2CH_2CH_2$–N(benzimidazolone, C=O, NH)
Hydroxyzine	Atarax	Cl	$CH_2CH_2OCH_2CH_2OH$
Cetirizine	Zyrtec	Cl	$CH_2CH_2OCH_2COOH$

Tricyclic H_1 Antihistamines

The two aromatic groups noted in several of the classes of antihistamines can be connected to each other through additional atoms (e.g., heteroatoms like sulfur or oxygen) or through a short, 1- or 2-carbon chain. They have a general structure shown in Figure 37.11. The earliest potent tricyclic antihistamines (Table 37.7) were phenothiazines (Y=S, X=N). The phenothiazine antihistamines contain a 2- or 3-carbon, branched alkyl chain between the nonbasic phenothiazine nitrogen and the aliphatic amine. They differ from the antipsychotic phenothiazine derivatives in which the chain usually is three

X = C, CH, N, etc.
Y = CH_2, S, O, NH, CH_2O, CH_2CH_2, CH=CH, etc.
spacer = two or three carbons
R_1, R_2 = Me, or five membered ring

Fig. 37.11. General structure of tricyclic antihistamines.

carbons long, unbranched, and usually, without substituents in the aromatic ring. Besides useful antihistaminic effects, most have pronounced sedative effects and long durations of action. Other uses include the treatment of nausea and vomiting associated with anesthesia and for the treatment of motion sickness.

Conformational and Stereochemical Effects. In the active agents, the steric restrictions and decreased degrees of conformational freedom resulting from the connection of the two aromatic rings together suggests that certain spatial relationships between these two rings are acceptable in the drug–receptor interaction of H_1 antihistamines. These ring systems are not flat but, rather, are somewhat puckered, with the two aromatic rings not in the same plane. Usually, however, the conformations undergo rapid intraconversion. In some closely related systems, in which this intraconversion is very slow, conformational enantiomers (atropisomers) have been obtained and studied, including cyproheptadine, doxepine, and hydroxylated metabolites of loratadine (27,28). The enantiomers of 3-methoxycyproheptadine have significantly different pharmacological potency as

Table 37.7. Examples of Tricyclic Antihistamines.

Drugs	Trade name	Y	Z
Promethazine	Phenergan	S	
Pyrathiazine		S	
Trimeprazine	Temaril	S	
Methdilazine	Tacaryl	S	

Cyproheptadine (Periactin) Azatadine (Optimine)

antihistamines, antiserotonin, and anticholinergic agents (Fig. 37.12) (29). The (−)-isomer retained antihistaminic, antiserotonin, and appetite-stimulating effects similar to cyproheptadine, whereas the (+)-enantiomer had greater anticholinerigic potency. Differences of 9- to 60-fold have been observed in the reported assays.

Promethazine, an early agent in the series, has many useful pharmacological affects other than being an antihistamine. It has significant antiemetic and anticholinergic properties. It also has sedative-hypnotic properties and has been used to potentiate the effects of analgesic drugs. Subsequent analogues, such as trimeprazine and methdilazine, are used as antipruritic agents in the treatment of urticaria.

Compounds in which the sulfur atom is replaced with another bridge (e.g., two methylene groups) also are available. Some have a pyridine ring replacing one of the benzenoid systems. Cyproheptadine, with a 2-carbon spacer between the aromatic rings, also has anticholinergic, antiserotonergic, and appetite-stimulating properties, which are useful in treatment of anorexic nervosa and in cachexia. The pyridine analogue apparently lacks most of these qualities. Doxepine, an oxygen-containing congener of cyproheptadine, also has significant affinity for other receptors, and it has CNS-depressant qualities. It exists as a mixture of *Z*- and *E*-isomers (15:85) in its olefinic, nonpiperidine side chain. In tissue-based assays, the *Z*-isomer is more potent than the *E*-isomer by more than threefold (27). The most widely used among the group is loratadine, which is considered to be in the category of nonsedating, second-generation antihistamines (vide infra).

Metabolism. Information regarding the metabolic disposition and pharmacokinetic properties of agents in this group is limited, including incomplete identification of primary metabolic pathways, results of liver microsomal metabolic experiments, and only occasionally, pharmacokinetic information. In humans, products from the

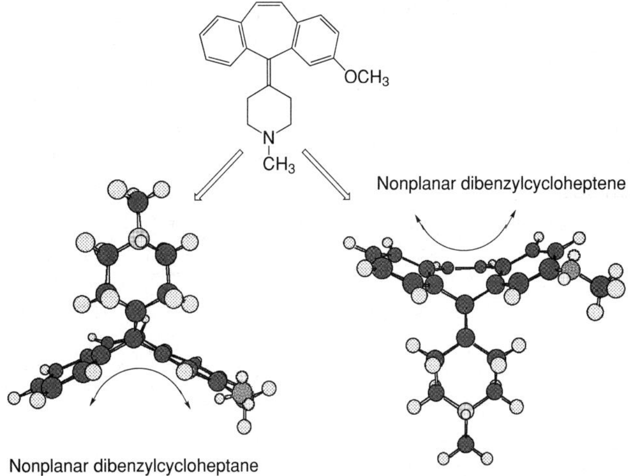

Fig. 37.12. Enantiomers (antropisomers) of 3-methoxycyproheptadine.

phenothiazines include products of N-demethylation, aromatic hydroxylation, and occasionally, sulfoxidation. From tricyclic analogues, metabolites resulting from N-demethylation, aromatic hydroxylation, and formation of N-quaternary glucuronides have been reported (30).

Second-Generation Nonsedating H_1 Antihistamines

Background

The second-generation antihistamines marketed over the last 20 to 25 years have improved H_1 selectivity, have little or no sedative qualities, and they may have antiallergic effects apart from antihistaminic activity (31). They vary widely in structure (Table 37.8) but less so in pharmacological properties, having effects principally in the periphery. Structural resemblance to the first-generation H_1 antagonists is not always obvious. because some of these agents were discovered while investigating new molecular structures for other pharmacological targets. These agents possess selective peripheral H_1 antihistaminic effects, and they usually have less anticholinergic activity. Furthermore, they also have decreased affinity for adrenergic and/or serotonergic receptors and limited CNS effects. The active agents apparently do not penetrate the blood-brain barrier significantly, perhaps because of their amphoteric nature (most are zwitterionic at physiological pH) and partitioning characteristics and/or because they are substrates for the drug efflux P-glycoprotein transporter or organic anion transporter proteins. A slow rate of dissociation from H_1 receptors also is reported for some of the agents. Several have antiallergic properties that are separate from their antihistaminic properties, which are not thoroughly understood. In most cases, the parent drug or its important metabolites have half-lives that are sufficiently long to account for the extended duration of action (32). Most are administered once daily.

Specific Drugs

FEXOFENADINE (ALLEGRA) AND TERFENADINE

Pharmacological Effects. This group of nonsedating antihistamines usually is thought to include fexofenadine and its parent terfenadine, astemizole, cetirizine, and loratadine and its metabolite desloratadine. Terfenadine was synthesized as an analogue of azacyclanol in a search for antipsychotic agents. The initial reports of its antihistaminic properties included the observation of similar effects of it acid metabolite fexofenadine (33). Whereas terfenadine is no longer available, it was once a very widely used nonsedating antihistamine. Extensive clinical experience resulted in the reports of dangerous cardiac arrhythmias occurring occasionally when certain other drugs were taken concomitantly. These cardiac arrhythmias included prolongation of the QT interval and torsades de pointes, a life-threatening ventricular arrhythmia. These cardiac effects are now known to be associated with blockade of the hERG (human ether-a-go-go) gene product, the α-subunit of an inward rectifying cardiac K^+ channel (34,35). These effects are associated only with the parent molecule. The side effects occur primarily at high concentrations of this lipophilic amine and, usually, in the presence of other CYP3A4 substrates, such as ketoconazole or macrolide antibiotics (e.g., triacetyloleandomycin). In the presence of competing CYP3A4 substrates and inhibitors,

Table 37.8. Second Generation Non-sedating Antihistamines

Terfenadine ($R = CH_3$)
Fexofenadine ($R = COOH$)

Astemizole

Desloratadine ($R = H$)
Loratadine ($R = COOCH_2CH_3$)

Cetirizine

Acrivastine

Ebastine ($R = CH_3$)
Carebastine ($R = COOH$)

Mizolastine

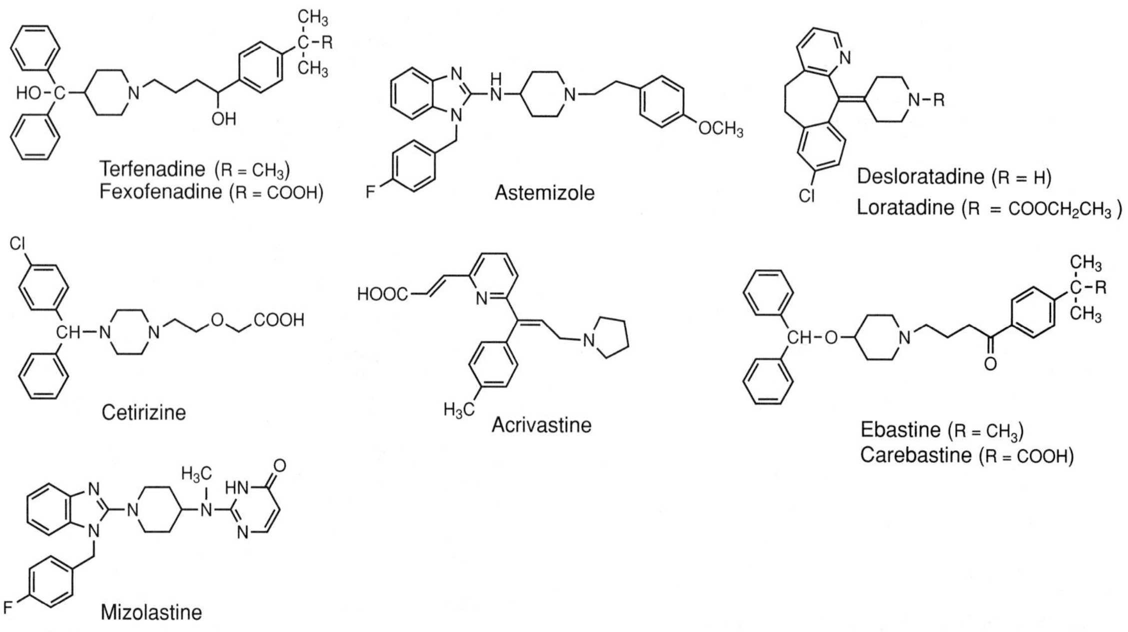

high plasma concentrations of the parent agent have resulted.

Metabolism. Fexofenadine, the carboxylic acid metabolite of terfenadine, is widely available (Fig. 37.13). It accounts for the antihistaminic properties of terfenadine, which is very rapidly metabolized via CYP3A4-catalyzed processes. Members of the organic anion transporter protein family and the drug efflux transporter P-glycoprotein are involved in the disposition of fexofenadine. Fexofenadine does not have the antiarrhythmic side effects of terfenadine.

Terfenadine and other lipophilic amines (e.g. astemizole, another second-generation antihistamine that is no longer marketed, grepafloxacin, thioridazine, sertrindole, and cisapride) are all aliphatic amines containing one or more aromatic groups (34). Each has been associated with life-threatening cardiac arrhythmias associated with binding to the hERG K^+ ion channel. The disposition of each depends significantly on CYP3A4 for its oxidative metabolism so that in the presence of inhibitors or competitive substrates, significantly elevated plasma levels are observed. Screening of potential drug candidates for interaction with this ion channel in radioligand displacement assays is done routinely to attempt to develop safe new drugs. Similarly, proof of safety of agents that are primarily CYP3A4 substrates is required. Studies regarding the effect of high-dose ketoconazole on the plasma levels of the drug in vivo usually are required.

LORATADINE (CLARITIN) AND DESLORATADINE (CLARINEX)

Pharmacological Effects. Loratadine (Table 37.8) is related to the first-generation tricyclic antihistamines and to antidepressants. It is nonsedating, and neither it nor its major metabolite, desloratadine (descarboethoxyloratadine), is associated with the potentially cardiotoxic effects reported for terfenadine and astemizole. On chronic dosing, the AUC (plasma concentration–time curve) for the metabolite is greater than that for the parent drug, and its half-life is longer. Desloratadine is a more potent H_1 antagonist and more potent inhibitor of histamine release. This metabolite, which probably accounts for the effects of loratadine, has been marketed. The hydroxylated metabolite of desloratadine, the 3′-hydroxylated product, may contribute to the pharmacological properties of desloratadine (36).

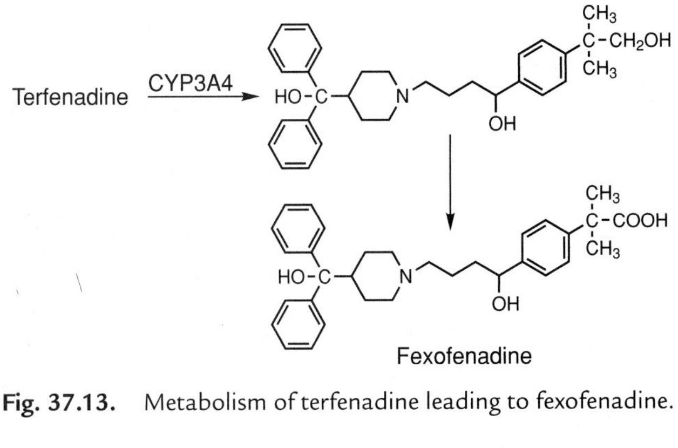

Terfenadine CYP3A4 → HO-C-…-N-…-OH (CH3-C-CH2OH-CH3) → HO-C-…-N-…-OH (CH3-C-COOH-CH3)
Fexofenadine

Fig. 37.13. Metabolism of terfenadine leading to fexofenadine.

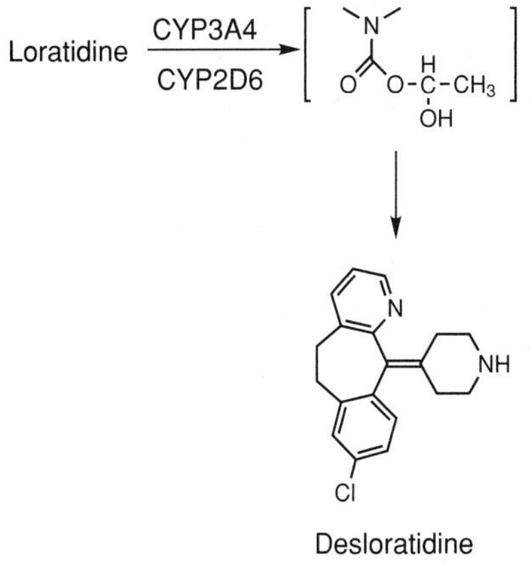

Loratadine CYP3A4 / CYP2D6 → [N; O, O-C(H)(OH)-CH3] → NH, N, Cl
Desloratadine

Fig. 37.14. Metabolism of loratadine.

Metabolism. The metabolic conversion of loratadine to descarboethoxyloratadine occurs via an oxidative process and not via direct hydrolysis (Fig. 37.14). Both CYP2D6 and CYP3A4 appear to be the CYP450 isozymes catalyzing this oxidative metabolic process (37). Apparently, the metabolite does not reach the CNS in significant concentrations. Among the nonsedating second-generation antihistamines, this metabolite appears to be the only nonzwitterionic species. The failure of zwitterionic molecules to reach CNS sites in significant concentrations can be rationalized readily, but a similar explanation is not apparent for loratadine or its metabolite. Competitive substrates for CYP3A4 do not produce a significant drug–drug interaction, because the parent molecule lacks effects on hERG K^+ channel in cardiac tissue.

CETIRIZINE (ZYRTEC) AND LEVOCETIRIZINE (XYSAL, XUSAL). Cetirizine, the acid metabolite from oxidation of the primary alcohol of the antihistamine hydroxyzine (Fig. 37.15 and Table 37.6), is a widely used antihistamine (38). It has a long duration of action and is highly selective for H_1 receptors. No cardiotoxicity has been reported, but some drowsiness occurs. The *R*-enantiomer of cetirizine, levocetirizine, is marketed in Europe. Levocetirizine has higher affinity than its *S*-enantiomer for the H_1 receptor (>30-fold) and is more slowly dissociated by more than 20-fold from the receptor (39). Thus, the antihistaminic

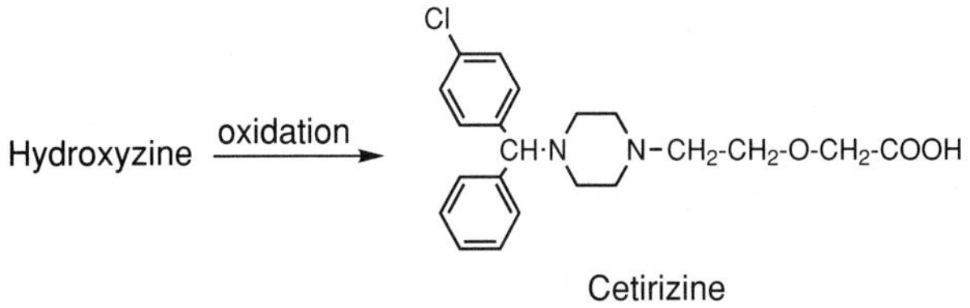

Hydroxyzine oxidation → Cl, CH·N N-CH2-CH2-O-CH2-COOH
Cetirizine

Fig. 37.15. Metabolism of hydroxyzine to cetirizine.

properties of cetirizine probably are accounted for by the *R*-enantiomer. Similar large differences in ratios of dissociation rates and K_i values for closely related enantiomers also are reported.

ACRIVASTINE (SEMPREX). Acrivastine, an acidic congener of triprolidine in which a carboxylic acid–substituted chain has been attached, also is a second-generation, nonsedating antihistamine. Penetration of the blood-brain barrier is limited, and it is less sedating than triprolidine. It is used principally in a combination with a decongestant.

EBASTINE (KESTINE) AND CAREBASTINE. Benzhydryl ethers of piperidinols also are useful antihistamines. Those with large N-substituents, like those in terfenadine and other nonsedating antihistamines, are most successful. Ebastine (Table 37.8), which is similar structurally to terfenadine, is a potent selective H_1 antihistamine as measured in radioligand displacement assays. In these assays, its acid metabolite has significantly higher affinity than the parent molecule. It is nonsedating and, apparently, free of anticholinergic effects (40). Like some other second-generation antihistamines, ebastine blocks release of PGD_2 and leukotriene C_4/D_4 in cellular assays. Pharmacokinetic data indicate that its acid metabolite carebastine is responsible for its antihistaminic properties, because the parent drug has a very short half-life and the active metabolite a much longer one (Fig. 37.16). In an animal model of torsades de pointes, ebastine, at a high dose, produced significant cardiac conduction abnormalities (e.g., prolongation of the QT interval), whereas the metabolite did not. At lower doses, these effects occurred only in the presence of competitive CYP3A4 substrates. Some in vitro data, however, suggest CYP450 isozymes other than CYP3A4 may be important in the initial hydroxylation. The pharmacologically active acid metabolite carebastine is metabolically analogous to fexofenadine (oxidation of a t-butyl group), the acid metabolite of terfenadine. Ebastine is marketed in several countries but not in the United States.

MIZOLASTINE (MIZOLLEN). Misolastine (Table 37.8) is a second-generation, nonsedating antihistamine that structurally resembles astemizole (41). It has an extended half-life of 7.3 to 17.1 hours and is highly bound to plasma protein (~95%). Metabolism occurs primarily through glucuronidation, and only small amounts of the compound are metabolized oxidatively. The AUC increases approximately twofold in the presence of ketoconazole, a CYP3A4 substrate and inhibitor. Only weak interaction with the hERG K^+ channel is reported, along with weak interactions with muscarinic receptors. Presently, it is only available in Europe.

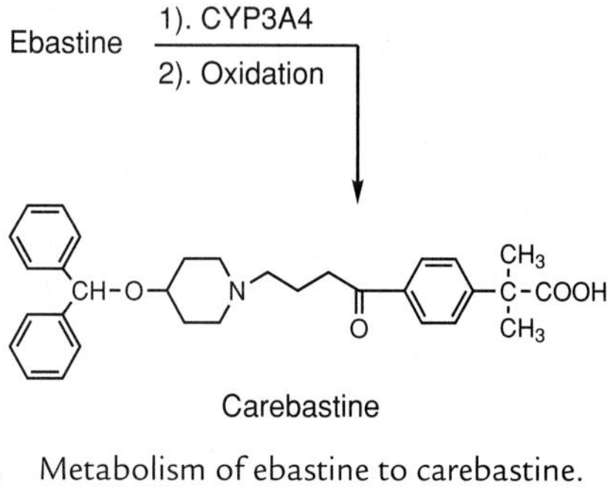

Ebastine → 1). CYP3A4 2). Oxidation → Carebastine

Fig. 37.16. Metabolism of ebastine to carebastine.

Topical H_1 Antihistamines

Therapeutic Applications

Topical application of H_1 antihistamines to the eye is made to relieve itching, congestion of the conjunctiva, and erythema (15,42). The density of mast cells in the conjunctiva is high, and the histamine concentrations in tear film are significant in the ocular allergic response. From eye drops, only small amounts of the antihistamine (1–5%) penetrate the cornea. More of the compound is absorbed via the conjunctiva and nasal mucosa, and still more ends up swallowed from tear duct and nasal drainage. Until recently, topical ocular antihistamines were limited to two classical agents: antazoline (Table 37.2), from the ethylenediamine series, and pheniramine (Fig. 37.9), from the alkylamine series. Both are used in combination with sympathomimetic vasoconstrictors.

A slow rate of receptor dissociation of H_1 antagonists is associated with long duration of action systemically, which occurs with the more recently available ocular antihistamines. Based on correlations of pK_a values and lipophilicity data, it appears that compounds with a log D (the sum of the partition coefficients of both the ionized and unionized species) near 1.0 ± 0.5 at pH 7.4 are most efficacious, and their water-soluble salts also show a low incidence of ocular irritation. Relationships between partitioning characteristics of these and other antihistamines indicate (at least moderate) receptor affinity and that a particular range of optimal lipophilicity for topical ocular antihistamines with minimal ocular irritation (43). Some of these compounds are currently available (Table 37.9) or are being evaluated as nasal sprays, and some also are occasionally used as systemic antihistamines.

Specific Drugs

OLOPATADINE (PATANOL). Olopatadine (Table 37.9) is structurally related to the tricyclic antihistamines. It has a long duration of action when applied topically, and it also appears to inhibit the release of inflammatory mediators (e.g., histamine, tryptase, and PGD_2) from mast cells. Its selectivity for H_1 receptors in tissue assays (over H_2 and H_3 receptors) is very high, and its selectivity for H_1 receptor blockade over α-adrenergic, dopaminergic, serotonergic, and muscarinic receptors also is very high. Olopatadine is reported to have a rapid onset of action and a long duration of action, consistent with high

Table 37.9. Topical Antihistamines

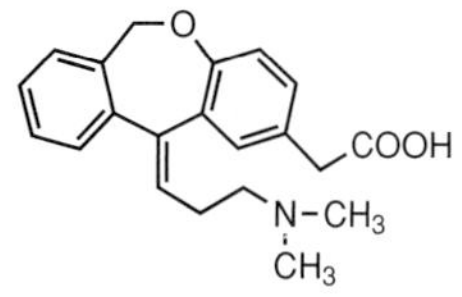

Olopatadine	Levocabastine
Emedastine	Azelastine
Ketotifen	Epinastine

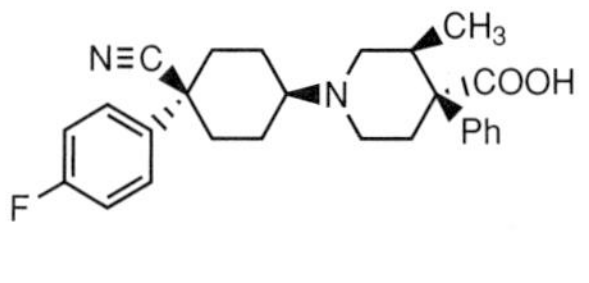

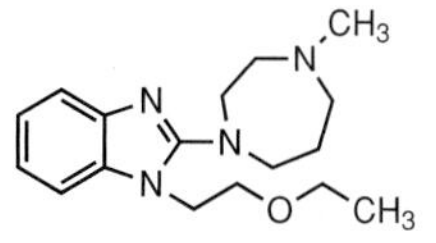

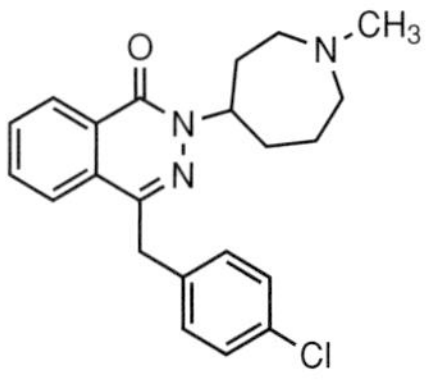

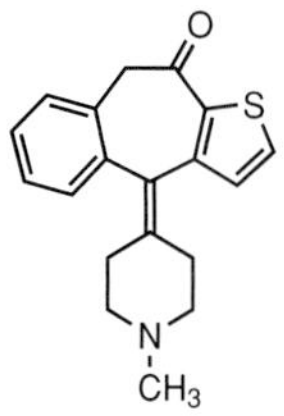

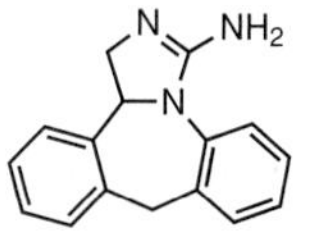

histamine receptor affinity and a slow rate of receptor dissociation. The presence of the carboxylic acid side chain apparently is responsible for the observed lack of muscarinic receptor affinity. This feature also may be responsible for limited penetration. Olapatadine also a mast cell stabilizer as well. The mechanism for this activity has not been delineated, but it has been shown to stabilize model cell membranes by interaction with phospholipid monolayers.

LEVOCOBASTINE (LIVOSTIN). Levocobastine is a potent, selective H_1 receptor antagonist used topically in eye drops for seasonal allergic conjunctivitis. A small amount of systemic absorption of the compound is reported. The agent also prevents release of transmitters from mast cells. A nasal spray used for allergic rhinitis is available outside the United States.

EMEDASTINE (EMADINE). Emedastine also is a newer antihistamine used topically in the eye for conjunctivitis. It has very high H_1 receptor selectivity characteristics, and it is structurally related to the benzimidazoles, such as astemizole. Inhibition of mast cell release of inflammatory mediators has been noted.

AZELASTINE (ASTELIN). Azelastine, although not a close structural analogue to the benzimidazoles, has some structural similarities to them. It is used as a nasal spray for allergic rhinitis and as eye drops for allergic conjunctivitis. Like olopatadine, azelastine also stabilizes mast cells, preventing degranulation and subsequent release of histamine, leukotrienes, and PGD_2. It is available in Europe for systemic use in the treatment of asthma and seasonal allergies. Besides antihistaminic effects, it also may block release of histamine and other inflammatory mediators from mast cells. When administered orally, the N-dealkylated metabolite appears to contribute significantly to its pharmacological effects.

KETOTIFEN (ZADITOR). Ketotifen is a potent, selective H_1 antihistamine that also prevents release of transmitters from mast cells. It is approved in the United States for topical use to prevent itching of the eye because of allergic conjunctivitis, It is used as a systemic antiallergy agent in several countries outside the United States for the treatment of seasonal allergic rhinitis, hay fever, and asthma. Being structurally analogous to the cyproheptadine-like antihistamines, differences in activity of the two enantiomers (atropisomers) has been noted, being approximately six- to seven-fold in ligand displacement and rodent-based assays (44). Ketotifen has been shown to stabilize mast cells and to inhibit degranulation of eosinophils. Like olopatadine, it has been shown to interact with model membranes, stabilizing them by interaction with phospholipids monolayers.

EPINASTINE (ELESTAT). Epinastine is a potent, long-acting H_1 antihistamine and an inhibitor of the release of histamine and other transmitters from mast cells. It has some affinity for H_2 receptors as well. It is used as an eye drop for allergic conjunctivitis. It does not penetrate into the CNS and is classified as a nonsedating antihistamine.

Antiulcer Agents

Background

The secretion of gastric acid occurs at the level of parietal cells of the oxyntic gland in the gastric mucosa (Fig. 37.17), producing 2 to 3 L of gastric juice per day, pH 1 in hydrochloric acid. Ultimately, this secretory process occurs via an H^+,K^+-ATPase that exchanges hydronium ion (H_3O^+) with uptake of a potassium ion. Several mediators regulate this secretion by way of receptor systems on the basolateral membrane. The H_2 histaminergic pathway is cAMP dependent. Gastrin and muscarinic receptors also regulate the secretion of gastric acid through calcium ion dependent pathways. In parietal cells, E-series prostaglandins work in opposition to the histaminergic pathway, inhibiting histamine-stimulated adenylyl cyclase activity. Other epithelial cells in the mucosal lining under the influence of prostaglandin-mediated pathways secrete bicarbonate and mucus, both of which are important in protecting the gastric lining from the effects of acid secretion. In many cases, hypersecretion of gastric acid appears to be associated with *Helicobacter pylori* infection, which may contribute to defects in mucosal protective defenses. Evidence suggests that some H_2 antihistamines, particularly cimetidine and ranitidine, have regulatory effects on T-cell lymphocyte proliferation by augmenting cytokine production and Ig

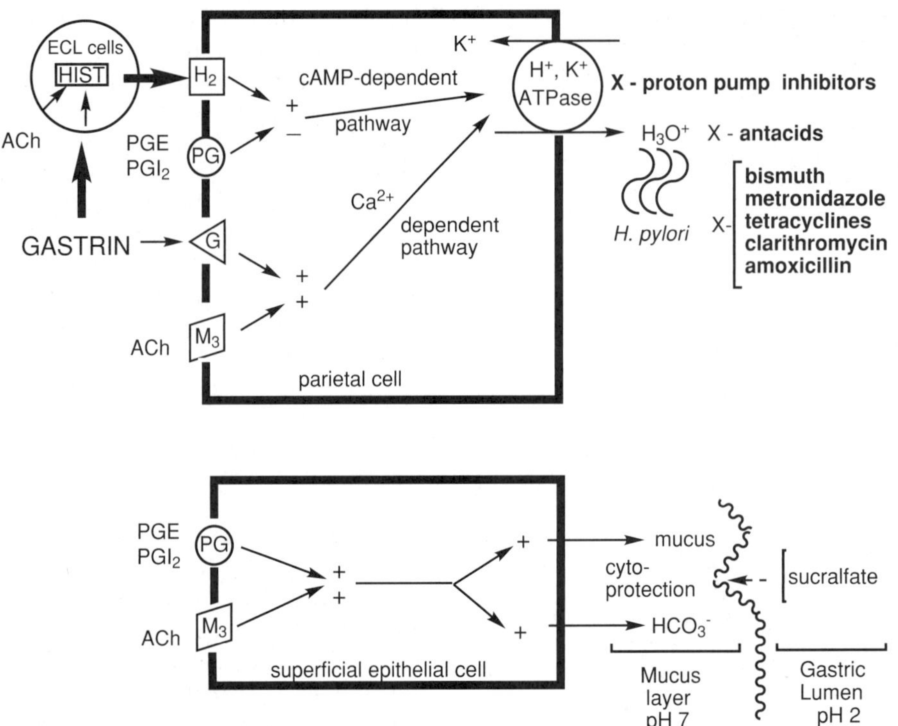

Fig. 37.17. Secretion of gastric acid and peptic ulcer disease. Histamine is secreted from and endochromaffin-like (ECL) cell, which is innervated by muscarinic receptors (M) via the enteric nervous system and by gastrin receptors (G). Agonist occupation of histamine H_2 receptors in parietal cells lead to gastric acid secretion. Other input at parietal cells includes the prostaglandins (PGs), gastrin, and muscarinic receptors. (Adapted from Hoogerwerf WA, Pasricha PJ. Pharmacotherapy of gastric acidity, peptic ulcers, and gastroesophageal reflux disease. In: Hardman JG, Limbird LE, Mollinoff PB, et al., eds. Goodman and Gilman's The Pharmacological Basis of Therapeutics. 11th Ed. New York: McGraw-Hill, 2005:968; with permission.)

production. These effects may not be associated with histamine receptors and may not be shared by nizatidine and famotidine.

Therapeutic Applications of H_2 Antihistamines

The H_2 antihistamines are used in the treatment of duodenal ulcers, gastric ulcers, gastroesophageal reflux disease (GERD), pathological hypersensitivity disorders, and upper gastrointestinal bleeding in critically ill patients and are sold OTC for acid indigestion (45). They also are included in multidrug treatment protocols for eradication of *H. pylori* in treatment of peptic ulcers and before surgery to prevent aspiration pneumonitis. Like H_1 antihistamines, H_2 antihistamines are inverse agonists that block the basal level of activity at this receptor. Combinations of H_1 and H_2 antihistamines are useful in idiopathic urticaria not responding to H_1 antihistamines alone and in itching and flushing of anaphylaxis, pruritis, and contact dermatitis.

STRUCTURAL REQUIREMENTS. The H_2 antihistamines specifically designed to decrease the secretion of gastric acid are based on an extensive investigative approach to drug design that began from the structures of partial agonist molecules very closely related to histamine (46). Ultimately, this work resulted in the development of cimetidine (Table 37.10), in which the imidazole ring like that of histamine is maintained. The imidazole ring is substituted with a C-4 methyl group, which in histamine agonists affords H_2 selectivity; a four-atom side chain, which includes one sulfur atom (the sulfur atom increases potency compared to carbon and oxygen congeners); and a terminal polar nonbasic unit, in this case an N-cyanoguanidine substituent. Guanidines substituted with electron-withdrawing groups have significantly decreased basicity compared to guanidine, and they are neutral (nonprotonated) at physiological pH. Thus, these are logical substituents to replace the terminal thiourea feature in unsuccessful earlier homologous candidates, metiamide and burimamide. The former agent was not marketed because of untoward effects, including agranulocytosis, and the latter agent lacked significant oral bioavailability. Subsequently, the nitromethylene unit was a replacement of the N-cyanoimino group in the substituted guanidine analogues, affording compounds of increased potency. Replacement for the imidazole ring with other heteroaromatic rings resulted in other useful analogues.

Table 37.10. H_2 Receptor Antihistamines

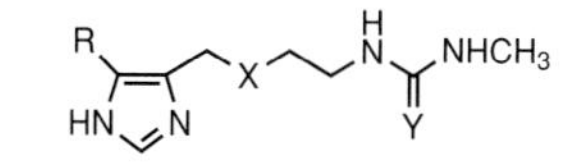

Drug	Trade name	R	X	Y
Burimamide		H	CH_2	S
Cimetidine	Tagamet	CH_3	S	N–C≡N
Metiamide		CH_3	S	S

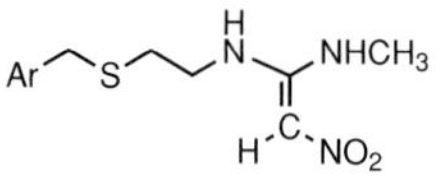

Drug	Trade name	Ar
Ranitidine	Zantac	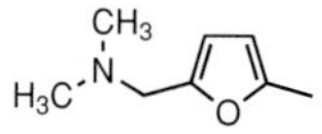
Nizatidine	Axid	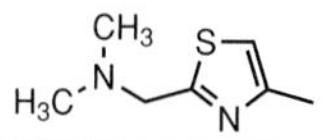

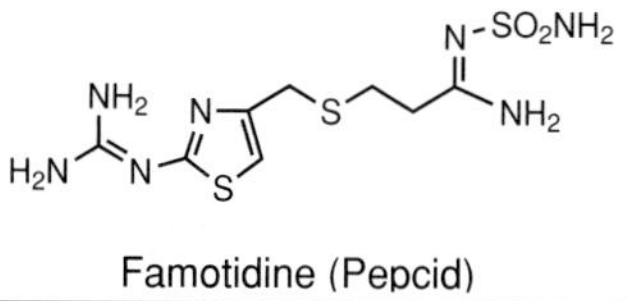

Famotidine (Pepcid)

METABOLISM. Cimetidine, ranitidine, and famotidine are subject to first-pass metabolism, and each has oral bioavailability of approximately 50%. The oral bioavailability of nizatidine is approximately 90%. All have half-lives of 1.5 to 4.0 hours, with that of nizatidine being the shortest. Significant amounts of each of these H_2 antihistamines are excreted unchanged, with small amounts of urinary products of sulfoxidation being a common metabolic feature. As expected, hydroxylation of the imidazole C-4 methyl group of cimetidine occurs. Ranitidine is excreted largely unchanged, but minor metabolic pathways include N-demethylation as well as N- and S-oxidation. The metabolites are not thought to contribute to the therapeutic properties of the parent drugs, with the exception of nizatidine, from which the N-desmethyl metabolite retains H_2 antihistamine activity (47).

SIDE EFFECTS AND DRUG INTERACTIONS. Cimetidine, the earliest of these agents, shows the greatest number of drug interactions (48). Among them are somnolence and confusion in elderly patients with decreased renal function. Gynecomastia, presumably related to increased prolactin secretion, has been reported. Cimetidine inhibits CYP450-dependent metabolic processes, affording increased concentration of several agents, the most important being those having narrow therapeutic concentration windows (e.g., phenytoin, theophylline, some benzodiazepines, warfarin, and quinidine). Inhibition of several CYP450 oxidative processes is associated with the presence of imidazole ring of cimetidine, which apparently replaces the histidine that serves as a ligand to the porphyrin iron in CYP450 enzymes. Other agents in this group contain heterocyclic rings other than imidazole and do not show this effect. Cimetidine is an inhibitor of renal tubular secretion of some drugs (e.g., procainamide). These tubular secretion effects also are less prevalent or even absent with other agents in this class. The other agents in the group are more potent than cimetidine, and significant differences are noted among them. Of these, ranitidine is the most widely used. The agents have OTC status and are widely available for gastric hyperacidity.

Proton Pump Inhibitors

Proton pump inhibitors are widely used in the treatment of duodenal and gastric ulcer, erosive esophagitis, GERD, GERD-related laryngitis, and hypersecretory conditions (e.g., Zollinger-Ellison syndrome) (49,50). The final step in acid secretion in parietal cells of the gastric mucosa is a process mediated by H^+,K^+-ATPase, the gastric proton pump, an enzyme with significant homology to Na^+,K^+-ATPase. This H^+,K^+-ATPase has some similarities to the H^+,K^+-ATPase in osteoclasts, which is involved in bone resorption. Gastric acid secretion can be inhibited in many ways. These include by antagonists at muscarinic, gastrin, or histamine H_2 receptors; by agonists at inhibitory receptors for prostaglandins and somatostatin; by proton pump inhibitors; or by carbonic anhydrase inhibitors.

MECHANISM OF ACTION. Omeprazole, lansoprazole, and related analogues (Table 37.11), produce inhibition of stimulated gastric acid secretion irrespective of the receptor stimulation process. Nearly all the compounds are close structural relatives, being weakly basic 2-pyridylmethylsulfinylbenzimidazoles. An analogue, tenatoprazole, which is an imidazopyridine isostere, is currently in clinical trials.

Table 37.11. H^+/K^+-ATPase Proton Pump Inhibitors

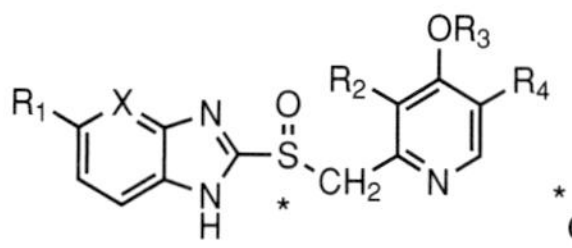

* chiral center

Drugs	Trade name	X	R_1	R_2	R_3	R_4
Omeprazole	Prilosec	CH	OCH_3	CH_3	CH_3	CH_3
Esomeprazole (S-enantiomer)	Nexium	CH	OCH_3	CH_3	CH_3	CH_3
Tenatoprazole		N	OCH_3	CH_3	CH_3	CH_3
Lansoprazole	Prevacid	CH	H	CH_3	CH_2CF_3	H
Rabeprazole	Aciphex	CH	H	CH_3	$(CH_2)_3OCH_3$	H
Pantoprazole	Protonix	CH	$OCHF_2$	OCH_3	CH_3	H

Only a few successful changes of the heterocyclic rings are possible (51). These agents have irreversible effects on the secretion of gastric acid, because the molecule rearranges in the strongly acidic environment of the parietal cell. Covalent binding of the rearranged inhibitor to the H^+,K^+-ATPase results in inactivation of the catalytic function of the proton pump. Evidence indicates that two molecules of the intermediate from omeprazole are bound to the active site; one of these sites has been identified as cysteine-813 (and, probably, cysteine-892 and/or -822) of the cysteine-rich H^+,K^+-ATPase (52). These cysteines are in different environments (e.g., exposed to the lumen or in the membrane), and different proton pump inhibitors bind differentially to them and other sulfhydryl groups. In the covalent binding, disulfide bonds are formed with the receptor. Analogous, but slightly different, results are reported for lansoprazole, pantoprazole, and rabeprazole (53). A chemical mechanism for the process is shown in Figure 37.18.

Because the initial rearrangement only occurs at a strongly acidic pH, acid-stable oral dosage forms are used that allow dissolution, release, and absorption of drug in the duodenum (e.g., enteric-coated granules in capsules or enteric-coated tablets). More recently, granular preparations of lansoprazole (enteric-coated granules) and omeprazole (with sodium bicarbonate) have become available. Intravenous dosage forms of lansoprazole, pantoprazole and esomeprazole are also available. The acid-catalyzed rearrangement of absorbed drug then occurs selectively in the acidic environment of the canaliculus, as it is secreted into the gastric lumen from the parietal cells. Some differences may occur in the sites of binding of the agents, and differences have been noted in recovery times, with rabeprazole have a shorter duration of action (54). Tenatoprazole has the longest plasma half-life and, in testing, appears to offer better control of nocturnal hyperacidity (55).

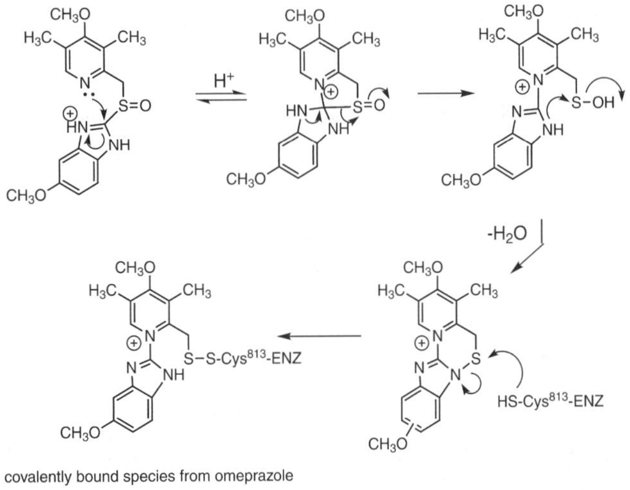

Fig. 37.18. Acid-catalyzed activation of omeprazole to reactive sulfonamide. At the parietal cell, H^+/K^+-ATPase, a cysteine residue, reacts to form disulfide-attached enzyme inhibitor.

CYP450 METABOLISM. Metabolism of omeprazole and other proton pump inhibitors occurs primarily in the liver (Fig. 37.19). The sulfone, hydroxylated, and O-demethylated metabolites have been reported as products. Omeprazole is a substrate primarily for CYP2C19 and may elevate concentrations of other substrates for this enzyme (e.g., diazepam) when given concurrently. The CYP3A4 contributes to a lesser extent. Further oxidation of the sulfone affords additional metabolites, which are excreted in the feces. Lansoprazole is metabolized by analogous routes (56). Fewer drug interactions with lansoprazole have been reported, although it also is a substrate for CYP2C19.

These sulfoxides have a chiral sulfur atom, and recent publications have been reported on the effects of stereochemistry on pharmacological and dispositional characteristics. The oxidative metabolism of omeprazole is catalyzed principally by CYP2C19 (primarily 5'-hydroxylation and, to a lesser extent, benzimidazole O-demethylation) (57). In human liver microsomes, the *R*-(+)-enantiomer is cleared more rapidly, and it is almost exclusively metabolized by CYP2C19. The clearance of the *S*-(−)-enantiomer is more dependent on oxidation by CYP2C19 than on CYP3A4-mediated metabolism, primarily sulfone formation. The marketed single enantiomer, esomeprazole, provides greater bioavailability in those who are CYP2C19 extensive metabolizers and less interindividual variation in those who are CYP2C19 poor metabolizers (~3% of Caucasians and up to 15–20% of Asians). Thus, the impact of variant alleles of CYP2C19 is less on the *S*-(−)-enantiomer than on the parent racemate. Higher blood levels and greater AUCs are observed, and increases in the time at a gastric pH greater than 4.0 are observed, which are correlated with healing rates.

Different proton pump inhibitors depend differently on CYP2C19 for oxidative metabolism, and the enantiomers show variation in dependence on CYP2C19 and other pathways (principally CYP3A4). Pantoprazole and lansoprazole show greater metabolism via CYP2C19, with the enantiomers being affected differently, than rabeprazole, which is metabolized only to a small extent by oxidative CYP450 enzymes.

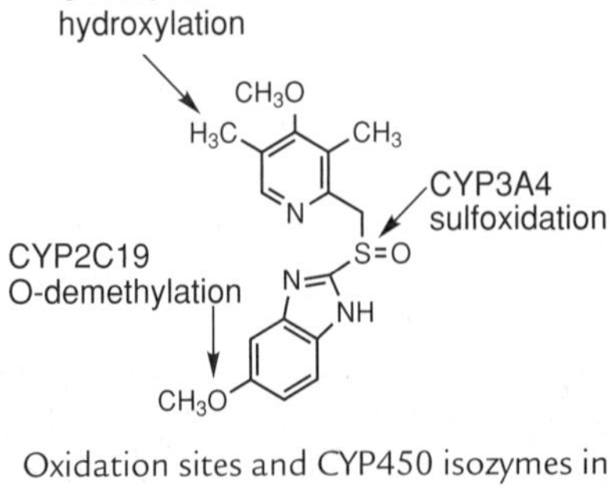

Fig. 37.19. Oxidation sites and CYP450 isozymes in the metabolism of omeprazole.

COMBINATION THERAPY IN *HELICOBACTER PYLORI* INFECTIONS. The majority of peptic ulcers are related to *H. pylori* infections and nonsteroidal anti-inflammatory drug (NSAID) therapy. *Helicobacter pylori* apparently penetrates the layer of gastric mucus by producing ammonia and carbon dioxide (urease-catalyzed hydrolysis of urea) to withstand the acidic environment of the stomach. More than 90% of patients with duodenal ulcer, excluding those with gastrinoma or taking NSAIDs, show the presence of *H. pylori*. Determination of *H. pylori* infection is routinely performed by measuring production of carbon dioxide (breath) or bicarbonate (blood) after oral administration of ^{13}C- or ^{14}C-labeled urea. Endoscopic examination and antigen-based serological tests may be used as confirmation (58). Eradication of *H. pylori* markedly decreases the incidence of ulcer recurrence. Several regimens of antibiotic therapy, widely used with proton pump inhibitors or less commonly with H_2-antagonists, are effective. Double- and triple-drug combinations, such as proton pump inhibitors with amoxicillin and clarithromycin or metronidazole, are used.

Competitive K^+ Inhibitors

Newer agents that block gastric acid secretion at the H^+,K^+-ATPase by binding as competitive inhibitors at the K^+ binding site are under development (Fig. 37.20) (45,49). An initial compound, SCH 28080, was hepatotoxic. Newer agents have included soraprazan and revaprazan. Each of them binds ionically to the proton pump at or near the K^+ binding site. Revaprazan has reached clinical trials. Studies to determine whether these or other related compounds can become useful drugs are ongoing.

Prokinetic Agents

Prokinetic drugs like metoclopramide, cisapride, and levosulpiride increase esophageal sphincter pressure and enhance peristalsis and gastric emptying, thus counteracting factors that lead to esophagitis (Fig. 37.21) (59). These agents appear to be 5-HT_4 partial agonists in the enteric nervous system, leading to release of acetylcholine. In addition, metoclopramide and levosulpiride are dopamine D_2 antagonists. Metoclopromide is used in GERD, in diabetic gastroparesis, and in nausea and vomiting of emetogenic cancer chemotherapy. Cisapride was removed from the U.S. prescription market because of metabolism-based interactions. In the presence of competing CYP3A4 substrates, high concentrations of the parent molecule lead to life-threatening cardiac arrhythmias via interaction with the hERG K^+ channel, similar to H_1 antihistamines terfenadine and astemizole. It is available only through an investigational limited-access program. Levosulpiride is available in Europe. Tegaserod (Zelnorm), also a selective 5-HT_4 partial agonist used in irritable bowel syndrome in women, has been used successfully in critically ill patients with gastroparesis.

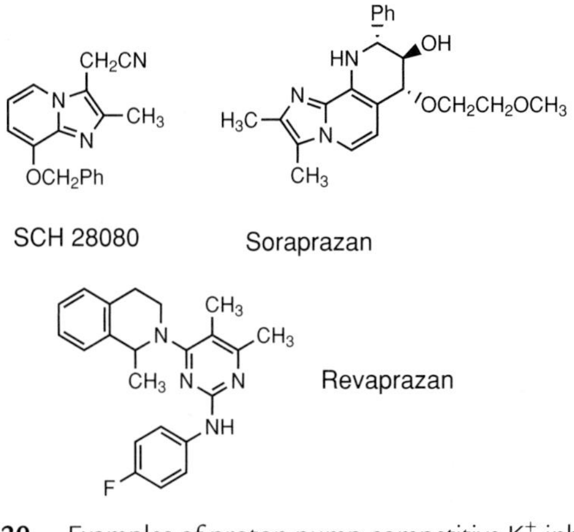

SCH 28080

Soraprazan

Revaprazan

Fig. 37.20. Examples of proton pump competitive K^+ inhibitors.

Metoclopramide

Levosulpiride

Cisapride

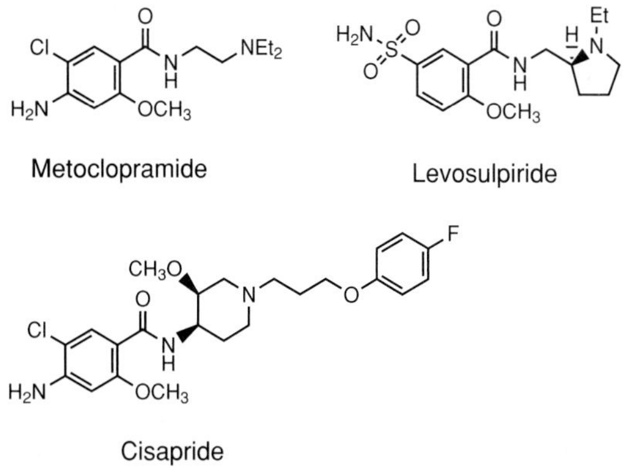

Fig. 37.21. Examples of prokinetic agents.

Prostaglandins

Prostaglandins have antisecretory effects on gastric acid (Fig. 37.17). Besides inhibiting adenylyl cyclase activity in parietal cells, which results in secretion of gastric acid, prostaglandins stimulate secretion of mucus and bicarbonate in adjacent superficial cells. Cytoprotective effects of endogenous E-series prostaglandins and of other, more stable synthetic congeners are observed. The only available oral prostaglandin in the United States is misoprostol. The orally administered carboxylic acid ester is hydrolyzed to the pharmacologically active carboxylic acid. It is a synthetic analogue of prostaglandin E_1, in which structural changes at C-13,14,15,16 are made to prevent rapid metabolic conversion to inactive products. The presence of the tertiary alcohol 1-carbon removed to C-16 obviates the usual conversion of the allylic secondary alcohol ($\Delta^{13,14}$-15-alcohol) of prostaglandins to the corresponding saturated ketones. A mixture of diastereomers of misoprostol is used; most of the activity arises from the 11*R*,16*S*-isomer (60). Misoprostol reduces basal levels of gastric acid secretion, but it has considerable smooth muscle contraction effects.

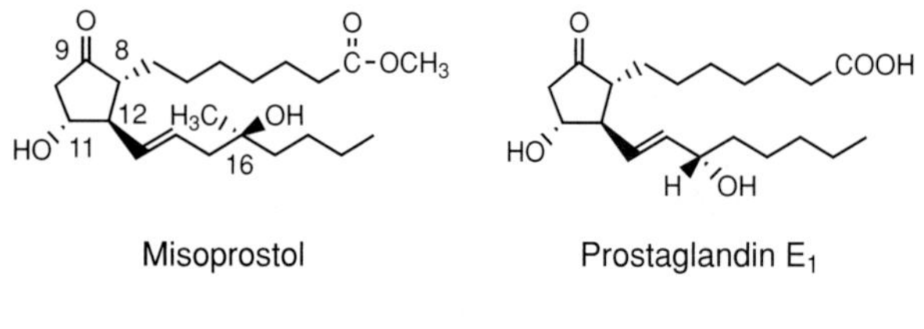

Misoprostol

Prostaglandin E_1

THERAPEUTIC APPLICATIONS AND SIDE EFFECTS. In the United States, misoprostol is administered with some current NSAIDs to reduce the risk of complications of gastric ulceration and bleeding. A primary mechanism of action by NSAIDs is derived from their inhibition of formation of prostaglandins from arachidonic acid. A prostaglandin may be added for the duration of NSAID therapy. A combination product of diclofenac (an NSAID) and misoprostol is available. Unlabelled uses of misoprostol include treatment of duodenal ulcers, for which it appears to be effective, and in the treatment of duodenal ulcers unresponsive to H_2 antagonists. In other countries, it has been used in the treatment of duodenal ulcers.

Significant side effects are those associated with its abortifacient properties and other smooth muscle contraction effects, e.g., diarrhea and abdominal pain. Misoprostol also is an effective cervical ripening agent (by vaginal application) for the induction of labor. Other unlabeled uses include the treatment of postpartum hemorrhage and, with mifepristone, termination of pregnancy.

Sucralfate and Insoluble Bismuth Preparations

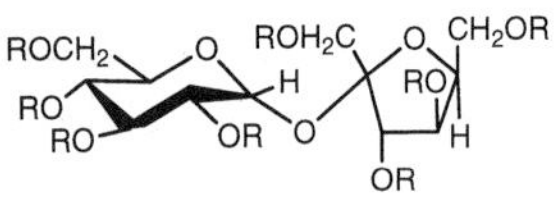

Sucralfate R = $SO_3[Al_2(OH)_5]$

Sucralfate is a complex of the sulfuric acid ester of sucrose and aluminum hydroxide. Secondary polymerization with aluminum hydroxide forms intermolecular bridges between molecules of sulfate esters with aluminum (61). Limited dissociation of the complex occurs in gastric acid, but these anionic sulfate esters form insoluble adherent complexes with the proteinaceous exudate at the abraded surface of a crater of the ulcerated area in the stomach. This physical complex protects the ulcer from the erosive action of pepsin and bile salts. Sucralfate also stimulates synthesis and release of prostaglandins, bicarbonate, and epidermal and fibroblast growth factors. Significant ulcer healing effects are noted in placebo-controlled trials. Only small amounts of sucralfate are absorbed systemically. In renal impairment, there is a risk of accumulation of absorbed aluminum from the drug. Sucralfate reduces absorption of other drugs, including H_2 antihistamines, quinolone antibiotics, phenytoin, and perhaps, warfarin (62).

Bismuth-containing preparations (e.g., those containing colloidal bismuth subcitrate) have effects similar to those of sucralfate, apparently because of their similar physical properties and coating effects. A combination of ranitidine–bismuth citrate is used with clarithromycin for eradication of *H. pylori* in the treatment and prevention of recurrence of duodenal ulcers. Combinations of bismuth subcitrate with other antibiotics and with H_2 antihistamines also are used. Bismuth subsalicylate is used in this way as well.

H3 RECEPTOR AGONISTS AND ANTAGONISTS

Physiological Role of H_3 Receptors

The H_3 receptor was identified as an autoreceptor that regulates the release of histamine. Histaminergic neurons are located primarily in the hippocampus, projecting to all major areas of the brain. These neurons are involved with the regulation of sleep and wakefulness and in feeding and memory (13). The H_3 receptor also is a heteroreceptor in the CNS, where it is involved in the regulation of synthesis and release of other neurotransmitters. In addition, H_3 heteroreceptors have been identified in peripheral tissues, including the airway and gastrointestinal tract.

H_3 Agonists and Antagonists

Several H_3 agonists and antagonists have been studied (Table 37.12). *R*-α-methylhistamine is a more potent agonist than histamine. The addition of methyl groups to the side chain or to the aliphatic amine nitrogen of histamine usually results in potent H_3 agonists, such as α,α-dimethylhistamine, *R*-α,*S*-β-dimethylhistamine, and N-methyl- and N-ethylhistamine, unlike the deleterious effect of these

Table 37.12. Examples of H_3 Agonists and Antagonists

H_3 Agonists

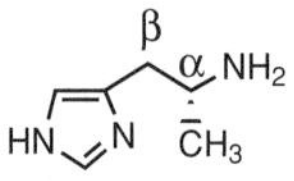

R-α-Methylhistamine; 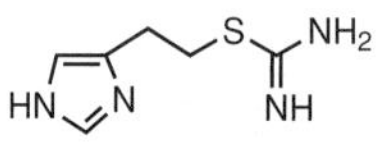 Imetit; 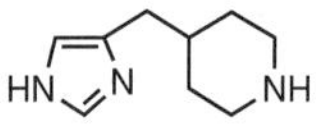 Immepip; 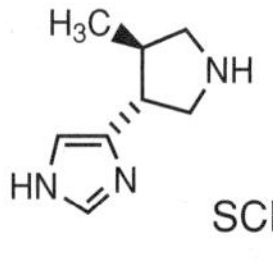 SCH 50971; 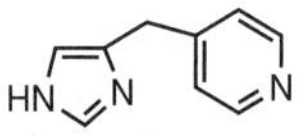 Immethridine

H_3 Antagonists

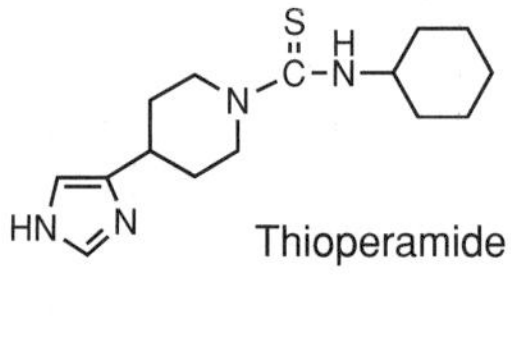

Thioperamide; 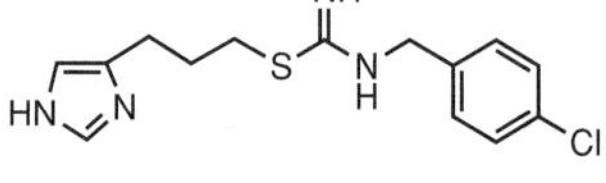 Clobenpropit; 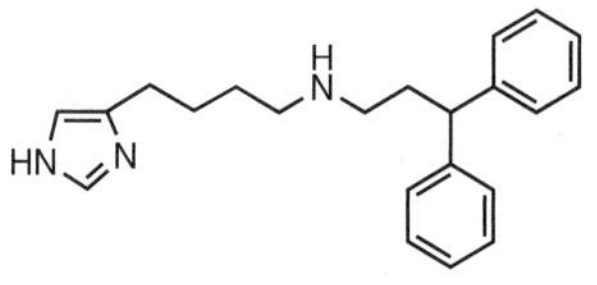 H_1/H_3-duel antagonist; 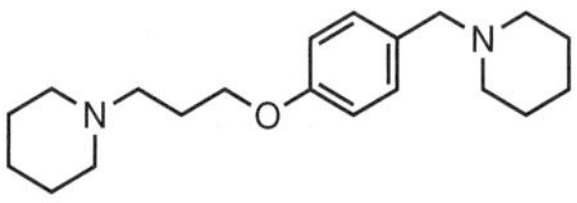 JNJ 5207852; 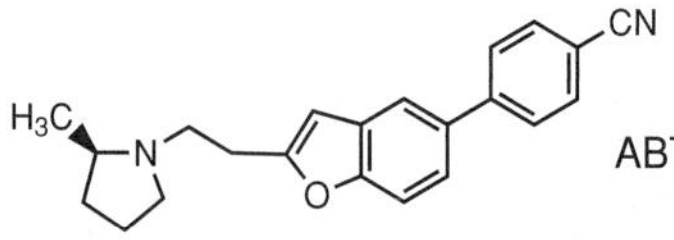 ABT-239

changes on H_1 and H_2 agonist activity. Other selective agonists are the isothiourea imetit, immepip and its N-methyl analogue (methimepip), both substituted piperidines, immethridine, a pyridine congener of immepip, and SCH 50971. All retain the imidazole ring of histamine.

Early H_3 antagonists, like thioperamide and clobenpropit analogues of immepip and imetit, respectively, are primarily pharmacological tools. Like the H_3 agonists, these agents retain the imidazole group but possess widely varying N-substituents. Some of the imidazole-containing agonist and antagonist analogues have affinity for other receptors (e.g., some α-adrenergic receptor subtypes), and they have the potential to interact with CYP450 enzymes as an iron–porphyrin ligand. Thus, nonimidazole-containing ligands have been sought.

Allergic rhinitis is one condition in which H_3 antihistamines may be useful. Thioperamide and clobenpropit are effective in animal models alone and in combination with H_1 antihistamines. Dual H_1/H_3 antihistamines are being studied, including a chlorpheniramine analogue that incorporates the imidazole alkylamine group of many H_3 antagonists (Table 37.12).

Centrally acting H_3 antagonists are under study by several drug companies. Agents are sought for a variety of disorders. These include treatment of depression, mild cognitive impairment, Alzheimer's disease, schizophrenia, narcolepsy, obesity, and attention-deficient hyperactivity disorder. Two examples are JNJ 5207852 (63), a compound that increases wakefulness, and ABT-239, a compound that is being evaluated for treatment of cognition related disorders (64).

H_4 RECEPTOR AGONISTS AND ANTAGONISTS

Physiological Role of H_4 Receptors

The H_4 receptor is expressed in mast cells, eosinophils, and other cells of hematopoietic lineage, including

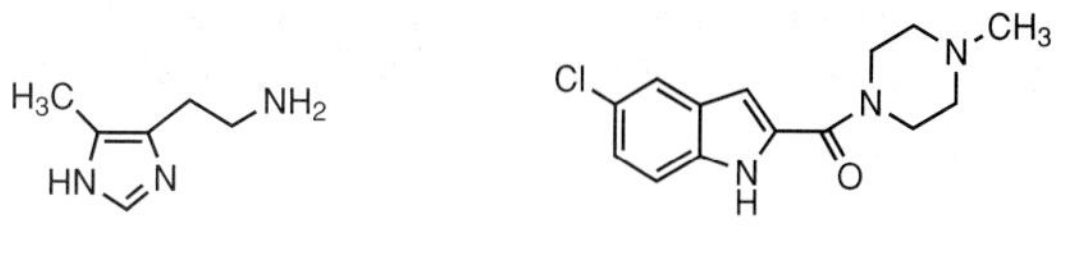

4-Methylhistamine

JNJ 7777120

Fig. 37.22. Other ligands at the H_4 receptor.

basophils and T cells. It is a relatively recent discovery; thus, much is not yet understood about its physiological role. It is thought to play a role in inflammatory responses, especially in the mediation of chemotactic responses. Its sequence homology is greatest with the H_3 receptor (35–40%) and is very low versus H_1 and H_2 receptors (65).

H_4 Agonists and Antagonists

Classical leukocyte chemoattractant effects that occur are blocked by thioperamide, an H_3/H_4 antihistamine. Other H_3 receptor ligands, such as *R*-α-methylhistamine and imetit, also are agonists at H_4 receptors, but they have lower affinity than at H_3 receptors (Table 37.12). Clobenpropit is a partial agonist at H_4 receptors, but it is an H_3 antihistamine (inverse agonist). Thioperamide is an inverse agonist at H_4 and H_3 receptors. 4-Methylhistamine (Fig. 37.22) has greater affinity (>100-fold) for H_4 receptors than other histamine receptor subtypes (66).

A selective H_4 antihistamine has recently been reported, JNJ 7777120 (Fig. 37.22). It blocks many mediated functions, including histamine-induced chemotaxis in mast cells and eosinophils (67). Conditions in which H_4 antagonists might be useful include autoimmune inflammatory and allergic disorders, including rheumatoid arthritis, asthma, and allergic rhinitis. Nasal stuffiness and blockage in allergic rhinitis, conditions that are poorly treated with H_1 and H_2 antihistamines, suggest the possible use of H_4 antihistamines in these conditions as well.

CASE STUDY

Victoria F. Roche and S. William Zito

BL is a 71-year-old financial advisor on vacation at the Gulf Coast with his wife of 47 years. It has been a therapeutic getaway, especially for Mrs. BL, who lost her central vision to exudative macular degeneration 18 months ago. While they hate to see their week of surf, sun, and relaxation come to an end, they are really looking forward to the drive to Albuquerque they will begin tomorrow for the wedding of their only granddaughter. On their last Gulf Shore night, they made reservations for a gala evening aboard the cruise ship *Chichibabin*, complete with dancing to the area's best Dixieland jazz band and a sumptuous buffet of Cajun foods. They had a ball, but unfortunately, BL experienced a severe allergic reaction to the crayfish he consumed (he ate two dozen) and had to be taken off the ship to the emergency room, where he received an injection of hydrocortisone. Although he can now breathe easier, he still has a red, itchy, and unsightly rash on the upper half of his body, including his arms, hands, and face. In addition to being uncomfortable, he is worried about how he will look for his granddaughter's big day.

Before heading out on their drive to Albuquerque, BL and his wife stop at a local pharmacy for some calamine lotion and an antihistamine to keep BL comfortable on the trip. He will be behind the wheel the whole way, because his wife can no longer see well enough to drive. As the pharmacist on duty that day, consider the antihistaminic structures below, and provide this couple with some much-needed pharmaceutical care.

1. Identify the therapeutic problem(s) in which the pharmacist's intervention may benefit the patient.
2. Identify and prioritize the patient-specific factors that must be considered to achieve the desired therapeutic outcomes.
3. Conduct a thorough and mechanistically oriented structure–activity analysis of all therapeutic alternatives provided in the case.
4. Evaluate the structure–activity relationship findings against the patient-specific factors and desired therapeutic outcomes, and make a therapeutic decision.
5. Counsel your patient.

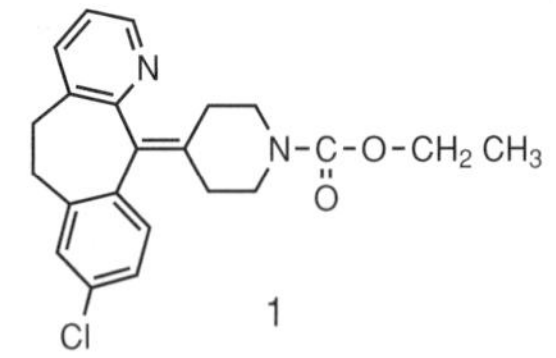

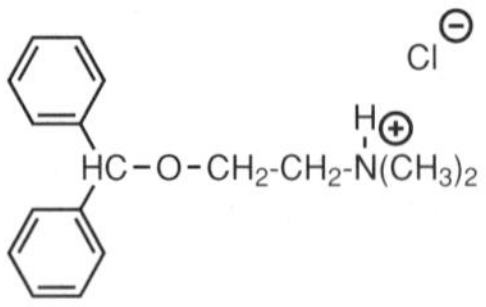

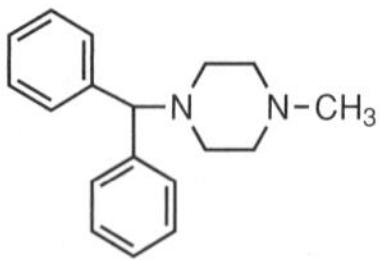

References

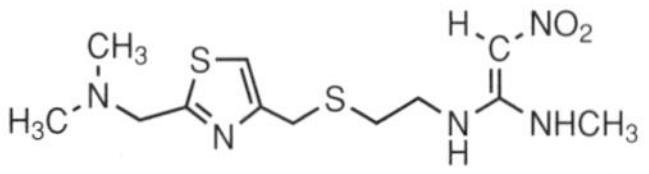

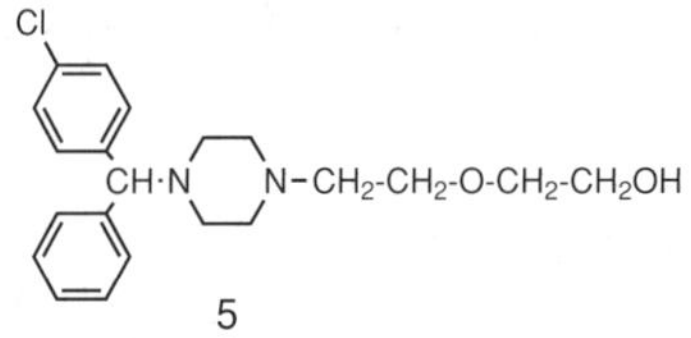

1. Babe KSJ, Serafin WE. Histamine, bradykinin, and their antagonists. In: Hardman JG, Limbird LE, Mollinoff PB, et al., editors. Goodman and Gilman's The Pharmacological Basis of Therapeutics. 9th Ed. New York: McGraw-Hill, 1995:581–600.
2. Cooper DG, Young RC, Durant GJ, et al. Histamine receptors. In: Emmett JC, ed. Comprehensive Medicinal Chemistry. The Rational design, Mechanistic Study, and Therapeutic Application of Chemical compounds, vol 3: Membranes and Receptors. Oxford: Pergamon Press; 1990:343–421.
3. Zhang M-Q, Leurs R, Timmerman H. Histamine H_1-receptor antagonists. In: Wolff ME, ed. Burger's Medicinal Chemistry and Drug Discovery. 5th Ed. New York: John Wiley & Sons, 1997:495–559.
4. Watanabe T, Yamatodani A, Maeyama K, et al. Pharmacology of α-fluoromethylhistidine, a specific inhibitor of histidine decarboxylase. Trends Pharmacol Sci 1990;11:363–367.
5. Schayer RC, Cooper JAD. Metabolism of ^{14}C-histamine in man. J Appl Physiol 1956;9:481–483.
6. Marone G, Genovese A, Granata F, et al. Pharmacological modulation of human mast cells and basophils. Clin Exp Allergy 2002;32:1682–1689.
7. Oliver JM, Kepley CL, Ortega E, et al. Immunologically mediated signaling in basophils and mast cells: finding therapeutic targets for allergic diseases in the human FcεR1 signaling pathway. Immunopharmacology 2000;48: 269–281.
8. Church MK, Shute JK, Jensen HM. Mast cell-derived mediators. In: Adkinson NF, Yunginer JW, Busse WW, et al., eds. Middleton's Allergy: Principles and Practice. 6th Ed. Philadelphia: Mosby; 2003:189–212.
9. Goetzl EJ. Lipid mediators of hypersensitivity and inflammation. In: Adkinson NF, Yunginer JW, Busse WW, et al., eds. Middleton's Allergy: Principles and Practice. 6th Ed. Philadelphia: Mosby, 2003:213–230.
10. Holgate ST, Robinson C, Church MK. Mediators of immediate hypersensitivity. In: Middleton E Jr, Reed CE, Ellis EF, Adkinson NF Jr, Yunginger JW, Busse WW, eds. Allergy: Principles and Practice. 4th Ed. St. Louis: Mosby, 1993:267–302.
11. Bakker RA, Timmerman H, Leurs R. Histamine receptors: specific ligands, receptor biochemistry, and signal transduction. In: Simons FER, ed. Histamine and H_1-antihistamines in allergic disease. 2nd Ed. New York: Marcel Dekker, 2002:27–64.
12. Leurs R, Smit MJ, Timmerman H. Molecular pharmacological aspects of histamine receptors. Pharmacol Ther 1995;66:413–463.
13. Leurs R, Bakker RA, Timmerman H, de Esch IJP. The histamine H_3 receptor: from gene cloning to H_3 receptor drugs. Nature Rev Drug Discovery 2005;4: 107–120.
14. Holgate ST. The chromones: cromolyn sodium and neodocromil sodium. In: Adkinson NF, Yunginer JW, Busse WW, et al., eds. Middleton's Allergy: Principles and Practice. 6th Ed. Philadelphia: Mosby; 2003:915–927.
15. Cook EB, Stahl JL, Barney NP, Graziano FM. Mechanisms of antihistamines and mast cell stabilizers in ocular allergic inflammation. Med Chem Revs Online 2004;1:333–347.
16. Forneau E, Bovet D. Recherches sur l'action sypmathicolytique d'un nouveau derive du dioxane. Arch Int Pharmacodyn 1933;46:178–191.
17. Simons FER. Advances in H_1-antihistamines. N Eng J Med 2004;351:2203–2217.
18. Simons FER. Antihistamines. In: Adkinson NF, Yunginer JW, Busse WW, et al., eds. Middleton's Allergy: Principles and Practice. 6th Ed. Philadelphia: Mosby; 2003:834–869.

19. Leurs R, Church MK, Taglialatela M. H_1-antihistamines: inverse agonism, anti-inflammatory actions, and cardiac effects. Clin Exp Allergy 2002;32:489–498.
20. Ariens EJ. Stereoselectivity of bioactive agents: general aspects. In: Ariens EJ, Soudijn W, Timmermans PBM, eds. Stereochemistry and Biological Activity. Oxford: Blackwell Scientific Publications, 1983:11–32.
21. Casy AF, Drake AF, Ganellin CR, et al. Stereochemical studies of chiral H_1 antagonists of histamine: the resolution, chiral analysis, and biological evaluation of four antipodal pairs. Chirality 1992;4:356–366.
22. Ebnoether A, Weber HP. Synthesis and absolute configuration of clemastine and its isomers. Helv Chim Acta 1976;59:2462–2468.
23. Timmerman H, Rekker RF, Harms AF, et al. Effect of alkyl substitution in drugs. XXII. Antihistaminic and anticholinergic activity of a series of thio ether analogues of substituted diphenhydramines. Arzneim-Forsch 1970;20: 1258–1259.
24. Towart R, Sautel M, Moret E, Costa E, Theraulaz M, Weitsch AF. Investigation of the antihistaminic action of dimethindene maleate (Fenistil) and its optical isomers. In: Timmerman H, van der Goot H, eds. Agents Actions Supplements. New Perspectives in Histamine Research. 1991;33:403–408.
25. Hanna PE, Ahmed AE. Conformationally restricted analogues of histamine H_1 receptor antagonists. *trans*- and *cis*-1,5-diphenyl-3-dimethylaminopyrrolidine. J Med Chem 1973;16:963–968.
26. Shafi'ee A, Hite G. The absolute configurations of the pheniramines, methyl phenidates, and pipradrols. J Med Chem 1969;12:266–270.
27. Otsuki I, Ishiko J, Sakai M, et al. Pharmacological activities of doxepin hydrochloride in relation to its geometrical isomers. Oyo Yakuri 1972;6: 973–984.
28. Piwinski JJ, Wong JK, Chan TM, et al. Hydroxylated metabolites of loratadine: an example of conformational diastereomers due to atropisomerism. J Org Chem 1990;55:3341–3350.
29. Remy DC, Rittle KE, Hunt CA, et al. (+)- And (−)-3-methoxycyproheptadine. A comparative evaluation of the antiserotonin, antihistaminic, anticholinergic, and orexigenic properties with cyproheptadine. J Med Chem 1977;20: 1681–1684.
30. Hawes EM. N^+-glucuronidation, a common pathway in human metabolism of drugs with a tertiary amine group. Drug Metab Dispos 1998;26:830–837.
31. Golightly LK, Greos LS. Second-generation antihistamines: actions and efficacy in the management of allergic disorders. Drugs 2005;65:341–384.
32. Molimard M, Diquet B, Strolin-Benedetti M. Comparison of pharmacokinetics and metabolism of desloratadine, fexofenadine, levocetirizine, and mizolastine in humans. Fundam Clin Pharmacol 2004;18:399–411.
33. Garteiz DA, Hook RH, Walker BJ, et al. Pharmacokinetics and biotransformation studies of terfenadine in man. Arzneim-Forsch 1982;32:1185–1190.
34. Pearlstein R, Vaz R, Rampe D. Understanding the structure-activity relationship of the human ether-a-go-go-related gene cardiac K^+ channel. A model for bad behavior. J Med Chem 2003;46:2017–2022.
35. Aronov AM. Predictive in silico modeling for hERG channel blockers. Drug Discovery Today 2005;10:149–155.
36. Gupta S, Banfield C, Kantesaria B, et al. Pharmacokinetic and safety profile of desloratadine and fexofenadine when coadministered with azithromycin: a randomized, placebo-controlled, parallel-group study. Clin Ther 2001;23: 451–466.
37. Yumibe N, Huie K, Chen KJ, et al. Identification of human liver cytochrome P450 enzymes that metabolize the nonsedating antihistamine loratadine. Formation of descarboethoxyloratadine by CYP3A4 and CYP2D6. Biochem Pharmacol 1996;51:165–72.
38. Curran MP, Scott LJ, Perry CM. Cetirizine: a review of its use in allergic disorders. Drugs 2004;64:523–561.
39. Gillard M, Van Der Perren C, Moguilevsky N, et al. Binding characteristics of cetirizine and levocetirizine to human H_1 histamine receptors: contribution of Lys191 and Thr194. Mol Pharmacol 2002;61:391–399.
40. van Cauwenberge P, De Belder T, Sys L. A review of the second-generation antihistamine ebastine for the treatment of allergic disorders. Expert Opin Pharmacother 2004;5:1807–1813.
41. Lebrun-Vignes B, Diquet B, Chosidow O. Clinical pharmacokinetics of mizolastine. Clin Pharmacokinet 2001;40:501–507.
42. Bielory L, Lien KW, Bigelsen S. Efficacy and tolerability of newer antihistamines in the treatment of allergic conjunctivitis. Drugs 2005;65:215–228.
43. Sharif NA, Hellberg MR, Yanni JM. Antihistamines, topical ocular. In: Wolff ME, ed. Burger's Medicinal Chemistry and Drug Discovery. 5th Ed. New York: John Wiley & Sons, 1997:255–279.
44. Polivka Z, Budesinsky M, Holubek J, et al. ^{4}H-Benzo[4,5-cyclohepta[1,2-b]thiophenes and 9,10-dihydro derivatives. Sulfonium analogues of pizotifen and ketotifen. Chirality of ketotifen. Synthesis of the 2-bromo derivative of ketotifen. Collect Czech Chem Commun 1989;54:2443–2469.
45. Roberts S, McDonald IM. Inhibitors of gastric acid secretion. In: Abraham DJ, ed. Burger's Medicinal Chemistry and Drug Discovery, vol 4. Autocoids, Diagnostics, and Drugs from New Biology. 6th Ed. Hoboken, NJ: Wiley-Interscience, 2003:85–127.
46. Ganellin CR. Discovery of cimetidine. In: Roberts SM, Price BJ, eds. Medicinal Chemistry, The Role of Organic Chemistry in Drug Research. London: Academic Press, 1985:93–118.
47. Price AH, Brogden RN. Nizatidine. A preliminary review of its pharmacodynamic and pharmacokinetic properties, and its therapeutic use in peptic ulcer disease. Drugs 1988;36:521–539.
48. Somogyi A, Muirhead M. Pharmacokinetic interactions of cimetidine. Clin Pharmacokinet 1987;12:321–366.
49. Vakil N. Review article: new pharmacological agents for the treatment of gastro-esophageal reflux disease. Aliment Pharmacol Ther 2004;19: 1041–1049.
50. Robinson M. Proton pump inhibitors: update on their role in acid-related gastrointestinal diseases. Int J Clin Pract 2005;59:709–715.
51. Lindberg P, Brandstrom A, Wallmark B, et al. Omeprazole: the first proton pump inhibitor. Med Res Rev 1990;10:1–54.
52. Shin JM, Cho YM, Sachs G. Chemistry of covalent inhibition of the gastric (H^+,K^+)-ATPase by proton pump inhibitors. J Am Chem Soc 2004;126: 7800–7811.
53. Besancon M, Simon A, Sachs G, Shin JM. Sites of reaction of the gastric H,K-ATPase with extracytoplasmic thiol reagents. J Biol Chem 1997;272: 22438–22446.
54. Horn J. Review article: relationship between the metabolism and efficacy of proton pump inhibitors—focus on rabeprazole. Aliment Pharmacol Ther 2004;20(Suppl 6):11–19.
55. Galmiche JP, des Varannes SB, Ducrotte P, et al. Tenatoprazole, a novel proton pump inhibitor with a prolonged plasma half-life: effects on intragastric pH and comparison with esomeprazole in healthy volunteers. Aliment Pharmacol Ther 2004;19:655–662.
56. Andersson T. Pharmacokinetics, metabolism, and interactions of acid pump inhibitors. Focus on omeprazole, lansoprazole, and pantoprazole. Clin Pharmacokinet 1996;31:9–28.
57. Andersson T. Single-isomer drugs: true therapeutic advances. Clin Pharmacokinet 2004;43:279–285.
58. Chisholm MA. Pharmacotherapy of duodenal and gastric ulcerations. Am J Pharm Ed 1998;62:196–203.
59. Corazza GR, Tonini M. Levosulpiride for dyspepsia and emesis: a review of its pharmacology, efficacy, and tolerability. Clin Drug Invest 2000;19:151–162.
60. Won-Kim S, Kachur JF, Gaginella TS. Stereospecific actions of misoprostol on rat colonic electrolyte transport. Prostaglandins 1993;46:221–231.
61. Nagashima R, Yoshida N. Sucralfate, a basic aluminum salt of sucrose sulfate. I. Behaviors in gastroduodenal pH. Arzneim-Forsch 1979;29:1668–1676.
62. Marks IN. Sucralfate: worldwide experience in recurrence therapy. J Clin Gastroenterol 1987;9(Suppl 1):18–22.
63. Barbier AJ, Berridge C, Dugovic C, et al. Acute wake-promoting actions of JNJ-5207852, a novel, diamine-based H_3 antagonist. Br J Pharmacol 2004;143: 649–661.
64. Fox GB, Esbenshade TA, Pan JB, et al. Pharmacological properties of ABT-239 [4-(2-{2-[(2R)-2-methylpyrrolidinyl]ethyl}-benzofuran-5-yl)benzonitrile]: II. Neurophysiological characterization and broad preclinical efficacy in cognition and schizophrenia of a potent and selective histamine H_3 receptor antagonist. J Pharmacol Exp Ther 2005;313:176–190.
65. Jablonowski JA, Carruthers NI, Thurmond RL. The histamine H_4 receptor and potential therapeutic uses for H_4 ligands. Mini-Revs Med Chem 2004;4:993–1000.
66. Lim HD, van Rijn RM, Ling P, et al. Evaluation of histamine H_1-, H_2-, and H_3-receptor ligands at the human histamine H_4 receptor: identification of 4-methylhistamine as the first potent and selective H_4 receptor agonist. J Pharmacol Exp Ther 2005;314:1310–1321.
67. Thurmond RL, Desai PJ, Dunford PJ, et al. A potent and selective histamine H_4 receptor antagonist with anti-inflammatory properties. J Pharmacol Exp Ther 2004;309:404–413.

38. *Antibiotics and Antimicrobial Agents*

LESTER A. MITSCHER, THOMAS L. LEMKE, AND ELMER J. GENTRY

DRUGS COVERED IN THIS CHAPTER:

ANTIBACTERIALS
- Methenamine
- Phosphomycin
- Quinolone class
- Sulfonamide class
- Trimethoprim

ANTIBIOTICS
- Penicillin class
  - Ampicillin
  - Amoxacillin
  - Bacampicillin
  - Benzylpenicillin
  - Carbenicillin and indanyl carbenicillin
  - Clavulanic acid
  - Methicillin
  - Mezlocillin and piperacillin
  - Nafcillin
  - Oxacillin, cloxacillin, and dicloxacillin
  - Phenoxymethyl penicillin
  - Piperacillin and tazobactam
  - Sulbactam
  - Ticarcillin
- Cephalosporin class
  - Cefaclor
  - Cefadroxil
  - Cefamandole nafate
  - Cefazolin
  - Cefdinir
  - Cefditoren pivoxil
  - Cefepime
  - Cefixime
  - Cefmetazole
  - Cefonicid
  - Cefoperazone
  - Cefotaxime
  - Cefotetan
  - Cefoxitin
  - Cefpodoxime proxetil
  - Cefprozil
  - Ceftazidime
  - Ceftibuten
  - Ceftizoxime
  - Ceftriaxone
  - Cefuroxime
  - Cephalexin
  - Cephapirin
  - Cephradine
  - Loracarbef
- Carbapenems
  - Ertapenem
  - Imipenem
  - Meropenem
- Monobactams
  - Aztreonam
- Aminoglycosides
  - Amikacin
  - Gentamicin
  - Kanamycin
  - Neomycin
  - Spectinomycin
  - Tobramycin
- Macrolides and ketolides
  - Azithromycin
  - Clarithromycin
  - Erythromycin estolate
  - Erythromycin ethylsuccinate
  - Erythromycin stearate
  - Telithromycin
  - Lincosamides
    - Clindamycin
    - Lincomycin
- Tetracyclines and glycylcyclines
  - Demeclocycline
  - Doxycycline
  - Oxytetracycline
  - Minocycline
  - Tetracycline
  - Tigecycline
- Bacitracin
- Chloramphenicol
- Daptomycin
- Linezolid
- Mupirocin
- Polymyxin B
- Quinupristin/dalfopristin
- Vancomycin

INTRODUCTION

Antibiotics are microbial metabolites or synthetic analogues inspired by them that, in small doses, inhibit the growth and survival of microorganisms without serious toxicity to the host. Selective toxicity is the key concept. Antibiotics are among the most frequently prescribed medications today, although microbial resistance resulting from evolutionary pressures and misuse threatens their continued efficacy. In many cases, the clinical utility of natural antibiotics has been enhanced through medicinal chemical manipulation of the original structure, leading to broader antimicrobial spectrum, greater potency, lesser toxicity, more convenient administration, and additional pharmacokinetic advantages. Through customary usage, the many synthetic substances that are unrelated to natural products but still inhibit or kill microorganisms are referred to as antimicrobial agents instead.

Because of a significant decrease in the pace of novel anti-infective discovery, increased regulatory constraints, and greater profits to be made by the use of medications for chronic conditions, there is presently a decreased research emphasis on antimicrobial agents. This coincides with a dramatic increase in microbial resistance to chemotherapy, that portends a bleak future in which humankind may once again face infectious diseases with few available countermeasures.

Our environment, body surfaces, and cavities support a rich and characteristic microbial flora. These cause us no significant illness or inconvenience as long as our neighbors or we do not indulge in behavior that exposes us to exceptional quantities or unusual strains of microbes or introduces bacteria into parts of the body where they are not normally resident. Protection against this happening is obtained primarily through public

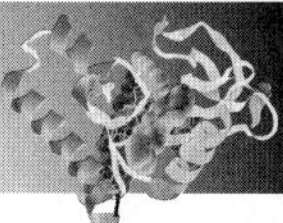

CLINICAL SIGNIFICANCE

The treatment of bacterial infections is one of the few disease states that all clinicians are guaranteed to be challenged with at some time in their career. Because bacteria are constantly changing, the selection of appropriate antimicrobial therapy is crucial in providing efficacious treatment of infections. It is of the utmost importance that clinicians understand the medicinal chemistry of antimicrobial agents to choose the most effective therapy for their patients. Antimicrobial resistance trends are constantly changing and vary from institution to institution, so a complete understanding of the structural relationship differences between antibiotics, even in the same class, is helpful in selecting the most appropriate therapy for an individual patient. In addition, side chains and subtle structural differences within antimicrobial classes can change the side-effect profiles of these agents. The informed clinician therefore can optimize their treatment choices from patient to patient while avoiding severe adverse effects.

The development of newer and more effective antimicrobial agents is essential in the fight against infectious diseases. Understanding the medicinal chemistry of the older and newer antimicrobial agents helps the clinician to comprehend their differences in antimicrobial spectrum and side-effect profile. Newer antibiotics are continuously being developed; however, many of them are from antimicrobial classes already established, with only small changes on the functional groups and/or side chains leading to dramatic differences in their antimicrobial spectrum. As stated previously, bacteria are constantly changing, as are antimicrobial susceptibility patterns. To optimize patient care, a clinician needs to stay informed about the effects of the medicinal chemistry differences as newer drugs come to market and antimicrobial resistance trends change.

Elizabeth Coyle, Pharm.D.
Clinical Assistant Professor
Department of Clinical Sciences & Administration
University of Houston College of Pharmacy

health measures, healthful habits, intact skin and mucosal barriers, and a properly functioning immune system. All parts of our bodies that are in contact with the environment support microbial life. It is estimated that 1 g of feces contains approximately 10^{13} microorganisms! All our internal fluids, organs, and body structures, however, are sterile under normal circumstances, and the presence of bacteria, fungi, viruses, or other organisms in these places is diagnostic evidence of infection. When mild microbial disease occurs, the otherwise healthy patient often will recover without requiring treatment. Here, an intact, functioning immune system is called on to kill invasive microorganisms. When this is insufficient to protect us, appropriate therapeutic intervention is indicated.

The chronicle of civilization before the discovery of bacteria and their role in infectious disease and, subsequently, the discovery of antibiotics and antimicrobial agents is punctuated by the outbreak of recurrent, devastating pandemics. An example is the successive waves of bubonic plague that dramatically decreased the population of Europe during the Middle Ages. Humankind was mystified as to the cause of infectious disease and what one might constructively do for prevention and cure. In warfare, infections often disabled or killed more individuals than the action of generals did. Our own family histories record the premature loss of loved ones, particularly small children, to one infection or another, and in the Third World, this pattern remains all too common today. This depressing picture was altered dramatically in the 20th century by the discovery and application of the powerful therapeutic agents described in this chapter. Fortunately, it no longer is common for persons to live short lives, and it now is rare for parents to bury their children. Public health measures, such as purification of water supplies, proper sewage disposal, routine preventive vaccination, pasteurization of milk, improved personal hygiene, and avoidance of unhealthy behavior (e.g., spitting in public places) also have greatly diminished our exposure to infection.

Considering that the first truly effective antimicrobial agents date from the mid-1930s (the sulfonamides) and the first antibiotics came into use in the 1940s (the penicillins), it is amazing that we have already grown complacent. Diseases that very recently seemed to be on their way to extinction, such as tuberculosis and gonorrhea, are once again becoming serious public health problems because of societal changes, persistent poverty, lack of education, ease of international travel, and the emergence of resistance by pathogens. It is disturbing to consider that previously unknown infectious diseases, such as acquired immunodeficiency syndrome (AIDS), Ebola virus infections, and Legionnaires' disease, are an increasing feature of modern life. Unfortunately, we can no longer confidently depend on the discovery of increasing numbers of novel antibiotics and antimicrobial agents to keep infectious diseases under control, but we must increasingly pay attention to neglected public health measures and concentrate on using antibiotics only when those measures fail.

HISTORY

Humankind has been subject to infection by microorganisms since before the dawn of recorded history. One presumes that humankind has been searching for suitable therapy for nearly as long. This was a desperately difficult enterprise given the acute nature of most infections and the nearly total lack of understanding about their origins that was prevalent until the last century. One can find indications in old medical writings of folkloric use of plant and animal preparations, soybean curd, moldy bread and cheese, counterinfection with other microbes, the slow development of public health measures, and an understanding of the desirability of personal cleanliness, but these factors were erratically and inefficiently applied and, when they were applied, often failed. Until the discovery of bacteria 300 years ago and the subsequent understanding of their role in infection about 150 years ago, there was no hope for rational therapy.

In Germany during the 19th century, Robert Koch showed that specific microorganisms could always be isolated from the excreta and tissues of people with particular infectious diseases and that these same microorganisms usually were absent in healthy individuals. They could then be grown on culture media and be administered to healthy individuals to reproduce in those healthy individuals all the classic symptoms of the same disease. Finally, the identical microorganism could then be isolated from this deliberately infected person. Following these rules, at long last, a chain of evidence connecting cause and effect was forged between certain microorganisms and specific infectious diseases. This work laid the foundation for rational prevention of and therapy for infectious diseases.

In 1877, Louis Pasteur reported that when what he termed "common bacteria" were introduced into a pure culture of anthrax bacilli, the bacilli died, and that an injection of deadly anthrax bacilli into a laboratory animal was harmless if "common bacteria" were injected along with it. This did not always work, but it did lead to the appreciation of antibiosis, wherein two or more microorganisms competed with one another for survival. Not until more than a half century later, however, did the underlying mechanisms begin to be appreciated and applied to achieve successful therapy.

The modern anti-infective era opened with the discovery of the sulfonamides in France and Germany in 1936 as an offshoot of Paul Ehrlich's earlier achievements in treating infections with organometallics and his theories of vital staining. The discovery of the utility of sulfanilamide was acknowledged by the awarding of a Nobel Prize in 1938. The well-known observation of a clear zone of inhibition (lysis) in a bacterial colony surrounding a colony of contaminating airborne *Penicillium* mold by Alexander Fleming in England in 1929, and the subsequent purification of penicillin from it in the late 1930s and early 1940s by Florey, Chain, Abraham, and Heatley, provided important additional impetus. With the first successful clinical trial of crude penicillin on February 12, 1941, and the requirements of wartime, an explosion of successful activity ensued that continues some 65 years later. In rapid succession, deliberate searches of the metabolic products of a wide variety of soil microbes led to the discovery of tyrothricin (1939), streptomycin (1943), chloramphenicol (1947), chlortetracycline (1948), neomycin (1949), and erythromycin (1952). These discoveries ushered in the age of the so-called "miracle drugs."

Microbes of soil origin remain to this day the most fruitful sources of antibiotics, although the specific means employed for their discovery are infinitely more sophisticated today than those employed 50 years ago. Initially, extracts of fermentations were screened simply for their ability to kill pathogenic microorganisms in vitro. Those that did were pushed along through ever more complex pharmacological and toxicological tests in attempts to discover clinically useful agents. Today, many thousands of such extracts of increasingly exotic microbes are tested each week, and the tests now include sophisticated assays for agents operating through particular biochemical mechanisms or possessing particular desirable properties.

Today, combinatorial chemical synthesis coupled with high-throughput screening make it possible to screen, in a short time, hundreds of thousands of compounds for antimicrobial activity. This is coupled with dramatic advances in all the relevant sciences. One would logically suppose that this would lead to the emergence of a large number of new antimicrobial agents. That this is yet to happen, however, is a measure of the complexity of the task. The impact of genomics and proteomics is predicted to have a favorable impact on this effort. The genome of *Haemophilus influenzae* was determined in 1995, and a decade later, more than 200 microbial genomes have been deciphered and are publicly available (http://www.ncbi.nlm.nih.gov/genomes/Complete.html). Of the 1,709 genes of *H. influenzae*, it is thought that 256 are potentially essential and, thus, are targets for antimicrobial drug development. These exciting new possibilities have yet to yield practical results, however, because of to the inherent complexity of the task.

In the year 2005, annual worldwide commerce in antibiotics was measured in multiple tons and was valued in excess of $10 billion. About half of this was associated with β-lactam antibiotics alone. Approximately 20% of the most frequently prescribed outpatient medications in the United States are anti-infective agents. Approximately 100 antibiotics have seen substantial clinical use, representing the most attractive of more than 20,000 known natural antibiotics and an order of magnitude more semisynthetic and totally synthetic antimicrobial agents. These agents have had a major impact on the practice of medicine and pharmacy and on the lives of persons still living, who remember well the perils and uncertainties of life before antibiotics became available.

This salubrious picture has an increasing dark side, however, because of the growing impact of bacterial resistance. Intrinsic resistance to antimicrobial agents (resistance present before exposure to antibiotics) was recognized from the beginning. Some bacteria are immune to treatment from the outset, because they do not take up the antibiotic or lack a susceptible target. Starting in the 1940s, however, and encountered with increasing frequency to this day, bacteria that previously were expected to respond were found to be resistant. Alarmingly, many became resistant during the course of chemotherapy, and others were simultaneously resistant to several different antibiotics. The latter were found to be capable of passing on this trait to other bacteria—even to those belonging to different genera. Similar findings are now encountered with fungi, viruses, and even tumors, indicating that this is a general biological phenomenon. The spread of this phenomenon is abetted by their short generation time (measured in fractions of an hour) and genetic versatility as well as by poor antibiotic prescription and utilization practices. Some authorities predict an impending return to the defenseless days of the preantibiotic era. For example, in the United Kingdom, resistance of the important Gram-positive pathogen *Staphylococcus aureus* has risen from approximately 2% in the 1990s to nearly 42% by the year 2000. Resistance to vancomycin in the United States among patients infected with *Enterococcus faecium* amounts to approximately 20 to 30%; such resistance was almost unknown a decade ago. Many other microbes and medicaments could be cited as well. An understanding of these phenomena and the devising of appropriate practical response measures are important contemporary priorities.

GENERAL THERAPEUTIC APPROACH

Drug Nomenclature

The names given to antimicrobials and antibiotics are as varied as their inventor's taste; however, some helpful unifying conventions are followed. For example, the penicillins are derived from fungi and have names ending in the suffix -cillin, as in ampicillin. The cephalosporins likewise are fungal products, although their names mostly begin with the prefix cef- (or, sometimes, following the English practice, ceph-). The synthetic fluoroquinolones mostly end in the suffix -floxacin. Although helpful in many respects, this nomenclature does result in many related substances possessing quite similar names. This can make remembering them a burden. Most of the remaining antibiotics are produced by fermentation of soil microorganisms belonging to various *Streptomyces* species. By convention, these have names ending in the suffix -mycin, as in streptomycin. Some prominent antibiotics are produced by fermentation of various soil microbes known as *Micromonospora* sp.; these antibiotics have names ending in -micin, as in gentamicin. The student has to take considerable care to avoid confusing them.

In earlier times, the terms "broad spectrum" and "narrow spectrum" had specific clinical meaning. The widespread emergence of microbes resistant to single agents and to multiple agents, however, has made these terms much less meaningful. Nonetheless, it still is valuable to remember that some antimicrobial families have the potential of inhibiting a wide range of bacterial genera belonging to both Gram-positive and Gram-negative cultures and so are called broad spectrum (e.g., the tetracyclines). Others inhibit only a few bacterial genera and are called narrow spectrum (e.g., the glycopeptides, typified by vancomycin, which are used almost exclusively for a few Gram-positive and anaerobic microorganisms).

The Importance of Pathogen Identification

Empiric-Based Therapy

Fundamental to appropriate antimicrobial therapy is an appreciation that individual species of bacteria are associated with particular infective diseases and that specific antibiotics are more likely to be useful than others for killing them. Sometimes, this can be used as the basis for successful empiric therapy. For example, first-course, community-acquired urinary tract infections in otherwise healthy individuals are most commonly caused by Gram-negative *Escherichia coli* of fecal origin. Even just knowing this much can give the physician several convenient choices for useful therapy. Likewise, skin infections, such as boils, are commonly the result of infection with Gram-positive *Staphylococcus aureus*. In most other cases, however, the cause of the disease is less obvious, and so, likewise, is the agent that might be useful against it. It is important to determine the specific disease that one is dealing with in these cases and what susceptibility patterns are exhibited by the causative microorganism. Knowing these factors

Gram Stain

Hans C.J. Gram, a Danish microbiologist, developed the Gram method for staining bacteria so that they were more readily visible under the microscope. The term has proven to be particularly useful in describing antibiotics as well, because antibiotics are conveniently classified by their activity against microorganisms depending on their reaction to this method. Gram-positive microorganisms are stained blue by contact with a methyl violet–iodine process. This is largely a consequence of their lack of an outer membrane and the nature of the thick cell wall surrounding them. Gram-negative microorganisms do not retain the methyl violet–iodine stain when washed with alcohol but, rather, are colored pink when subsequently treated with the red dye safranin. The lipopolysaccharides on their outer membrane apparently are responsible for the staining behavior of Gram-negative cells.

Because the Gram stain is dependent on the outer layers of bacterial cells and this also strongly influences the ability of antimicrobial agents to reach their cellular targets, knowing the Gram-staining behavior of infectious bacteria helps one to decide which antimicrobial might be effective in therapy.

Not all bacteria can be stained by the Gram procedure, however, and these often require special staining processes for visualization. Among the more prominent of these for our purposes are the mycobacteria (the causative agents of tuberculosis, for example). These very waxy cells are called acid-fast and are stained by carbol fuchsin instead.

enables the clinician to narrow the range of therapeutic choices. The only certainty, however, is that inability of a given antibiotic to kill or inhibit a given pathogen in vitro is a virtual guarantee that the drug will fail in vivo. Unfortunately, activity in vitro all too often also results in failure to cure in vivo, but here, at least, there is a significant possibility of success. Before the emergence of widespread bacterial resistance, identification of the causative microorganism often was sufficient for selecting a useful antibiotic. Today, however, this is only a useful first step, and much more detailed laboratory studies are needed to make a successful choice.

Experimentally Based Therapy

The modern clinical application of Koch's discoveries to the selection of an appropriate antibiotic involves sampling infectious material from a patient before instituting anti-infective chemotherapy, culturing the microorganism on suitable growth media, and identifying its genus and species. The bacterium in question is then grown in the presence of a variety of antibiotics to see which of them will inhibit its growth or survival and what concentrations will be needed to achieve this result. This is expressed in units of minimum inhibitory concentration (MIC). This term refers to that concentration that will inhibit 99% or more of the microbe in question, and it represents the minimum quantity that must reach the site of the infection to be useful. These concepts are illustrated in Figure 38.1.

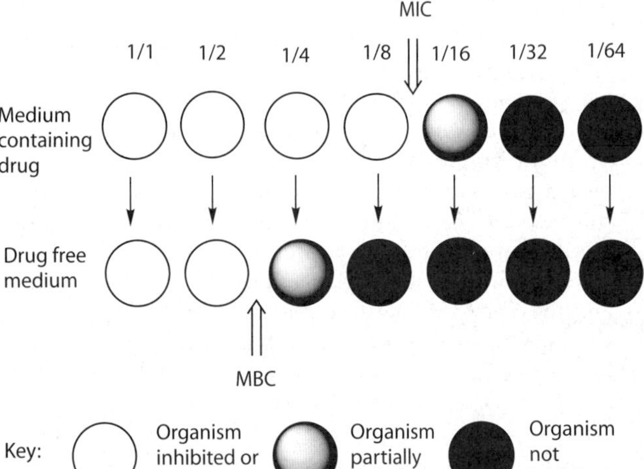

Fig. 38.1. In the top tubes (viewed from the top), a serially decreasing amount of antimicrobial agent is added to a suitable growth medium inoculated with a microorganism. Following incubation, microbial growth is detected by turbidity. The last concentration which produces no visible growth is scored as the minimum inhibitory concentration (MIC) (1/8). Next, a loopful is taken from each tube and placed in fresh medium not containing antibiotic (bottom row). In tubes where the organisms were killed by the drugs, there is no resumption of growth. Where the organisms were inhibited but not killed, removal of drug allows resumption growth. The last concentration that produces no visible growth under these conditions is scored as the minimum bactericidal concentration (MBC) (½).

To "cure" the infection, it usually is desirable to have several multiples of the MIC at the site of infection. This requires not only an understanding of the MIC but also an understanding of pharmacokinetic and pharmacodynamic considerations as well as the results of accumulated clinical experience. The choice of anti-infective agent is made from among those that are active. One of the most convenient experimental procedures is that of Kirby and Bauer. With their technique, sterile disks of filter paper impregnated with fixed doses of commercially available antibiotics are placed on the seeded Petri dish. The dish is then incubated at 37°C for 12 to 24 hours. If the antibiotic is active against the particular strain of bacterium isolated from the particular patient, a clear zone of inhibition will be seen around the disk. If a given antimicrobial agent is ineffective, the bacterium may even grow right up to the edge of the disk. The diameter of the inhibition zone is directly proportional to the degree of sensitivity of the bacterial strain and the concentration of the antibiotic in question. Currently, a given zone size in millimeters is dictated above which the bacterium is sensitive and below which it is resistant. When the zone size obtained is near this breakpoint (the breakpoint represents the maximum clinically achievable concentration of an anti-infective agent), the drug is regarded as being intermediate in sensitivity, and clinical failure can occur. This powerful methodology gives the clinician a choice of possible antibiotics to use in the particular patient and is illustrated in Figure 38.2. The widespread occurrence of resistance of individual strains of bacteria to given antibiotics reinforces the need to perform Kirby-Bauer susceptibility disk testing, but other laboratory methods can be employed for similar purposes. Of particular note are the E test strips, which utilize the

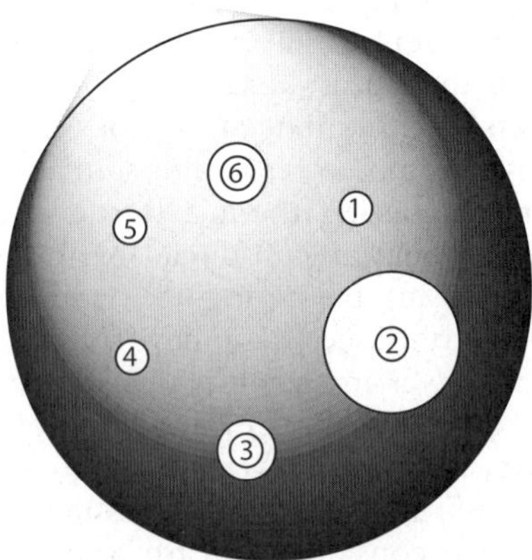

Fig. 38.2. Looking down on a Petri dish containing solidified nutrient agar to which had been added a suspension of a bacterial species. Next, six filter-paper disks containing six different antimicrobials was added followed by overnight incubation. The antimicrobials in disks 1, 4, and 5 were inactive. Of the active agents in disks 2, 3, and 6, antibiotic 2 was much more active, because the microorganism was not able to grow as near this impregnated disk.

same idea but employ a gradient of drug concentrations on a filter-paper strip.

This high level of scientific medicine requires significant expertise and equipment, so it is practiced mainly in urban medical centers. In office practice, the choice of medicinal agents is more commonly made empirically.

Bactericidal Versus Bacteriostatic

Almost all antibiotics have the capacity to be bactericidal in vitro; that is, they will kill bacteria if the concentration or dose is sufficiently high. In the laboratory, it is almost always possible to use such doses. Subsequent inoculation of fresh, antibiotic-free media with a culture that has been so treated will not produce growth of the culture, because the cells are dead. When such doses are achievable in live patients, such drugs are clinically bactericidal. At somewhat lower concentrations, bacterial multiplication is prevented even though the microorganism remains viable (bacteriostatic action).

The smallest concentration that will kill a bacterial colony is the minimum bactericidal concentration. The difference between a minimum bactericidal dose and a bacteriostatic dose is characteristic of given families of antibiotics. With gentamicin, for example, doubling or quadrupling the dose changes the effect on bacteria from bacteriostatic to bactericidal. Such bactericidal doses usually are achievable in the clinic. The difference between bactericidal and bacteriostatic doses with tetracycline is approximately 40-fold. It is not possible to achieve such doses safely in patients, so tetracycline is referred to as clinically bacteriostatic. If a bacteriostatic antibiotic is withdrawn prematurely from a patient, the microorganism can resume growth and the infection reestablish itself, because the culture is still alive. In this case, subsequent inoculation of fresh laboratory media not containing the antibiotic will result in colony development. Obviously, in immunocompromised patients who are unable to contribute natural body defenses to fight their own disease, having the drug kill the bacteria is essential for recovery. On the other hand, when a patient is immunocompetent or the infection is not severe, a bacteriostatic concentration will break the fulminating stage of the infection (when bacterial cell numbers are increasing at a logarithmic rate). With *Escherichia coli*, for example, the number of cells doubles every 2 hours. A bacteriostatic agent will interrupt this rapid growth and give the immune system a chance to deal with the disease. Cure usually follows if the numbers of live bacteria are not excessive at this time. Thus, whereas it is preferred that an antibiotic be bactericidal, bacteriostatic antibiotics are widely used and usually satisfactory. Obviously, however, patients should not skip doses or prematurely stop treatment.

Microbial Susceptibility

Resistance

Resistance is the failure of microorganisms to be killed or inhibited by antimicrobial treatment. Resistance can either be intrinsic (exist before exposure to drug) or acquired (develop subsequent to exposure to a drug). Resistance of bacteria to the toxic effects of antimicrobial agents and to antibiotics develops fairly easily both in the laboratory and in the clinic and is an ever-increasing public health hazard. Challenging a culture in the laboratory with sublethal quantities of an antibiotic kills the most intrinsically sensitive percentage of the strains in the colony. Those not killed or seriously inhibited continue to grow and have access to the remainder of the nutrients. A mutation to lower sensitivity also enables individual bacteria to survive against the selecting pressure of the antimicrobial agent. If the culture is treated several times in succession with sublethal doses in this manner, the concentration of antibiotic required to prevent growth becomes ever higher. When the origin of this form of resistance is explored, it almost always is found to result from an alteration in the biochemistry of the colony so that the molecular target of the antibiotic becomes less sensitive, or it can result from decreased uptake of antibiotic into the cells. This is genomically preserved and passes to the next generation by reproductive fission. The altered progeny may be weaker than the wild strain so that they die out if the antibiotic is not present to give them a competitive advantage. In some cases, additional compensatory mutations can occur that restore the vigor of the resistant organisms. Resistance of this type usually is expressed toward other antibiotics with the same mode of action and, therefore, is a familial characteristic—most tetracyclines, for example, show extensive cross-resistance with other agents in the tetracycline family. This is very enlightening with respect to discovery of the molecular mode of action, but it is not very relevant to the clinical situation.

In the clinic, resistance more commonly takes place by Resistance (R) factor mechanisms. In the more lurid examples, enzymes are elaborated that attack the antibiotic and inactivate it. Mutations leading to resistance occur by many mechanisms. They can result from point mutations, insertions, deletions, inversions, duplications, and transpositions of segments of genes or by acquisition of foreign DNA from plasmids, bacteriophages, and transposable genetic elements. The genetic material coding for this form of resistance very often is carried on extrachromosomic elements consisting of small, circular DNA molecules known as plasmids. A bacterial cell may have many plasmids or none. The plasmid may carry DNA for several different enzymes capable of destroying structurally dissimilar antibiotics. Such plasmid DNA may migrate within the cell from plasmid to plasmid or from plasmid to chromosome by a process known as transposition. Such plasmids may migrate from cell to cell by conjugation (passage through a sexual pilus), transduction (carriage by a virus vector), or transformation (excretion of DNA from cell A and its subsequent uptake by cell B). These mechanisms can convert an antibiotic-sensitive cell to an antibiotic-resistant cell. This can take place many times in a bacterium's already short generation time. The positive selecting pressure of inadequate levels of an antibiotic favors explosive spread of R-factor resistance. This provides a rationale for conservative but aggressive application of appropriate antimicrobial chemotherapy. Bacterial resistance generally is mediated through one of three mechanisms: 1) failure of the drug to penetrate into or stay in the cell, 2) destruction of the drug by defensive enzymes, or 3) alterations in the cellular target of the enzymes. It rarely is an all-or-nothing effect. In many cases, a resistant microorganism can still be controlled by achievable, though higher, doses than are required to control sensitive populations.

Persistence

Sensitive bacteria may not all be killed. Survivors are thought to have been resting (not metabolizing) during the drug treatment time and, therefore, to remain viable when tested subsequently. These bacteria are still sensitive to the drug even though they survived an otherwise toxic dose. Some bacteria also can aggregate in films. A poorly penetrating antibiotic may not reach the cells lying deep within such a film. Such cells, although intrinsically sensitive, may survive antibiotic treatment. Bacteria living in host cells or in cysts also are harder to reach by drugs and so are more difficult to control.

Postantibiotic Effect

Some antibiotics exert a significant toxicity to certain microorganisms that persists for a time after the drug is withdrawn and the concentration of drug in the blood falls below the MIC. A constant multiple of the MIC of a drug may not be essential for therapeutic success when a postantibiotic effect (PAE) is operating, because the microbe is still affected for a time after the drug is withdrawn. The PAE is defined by the time required for a 10-fold increase in viable bacterial colonies to occur after exposure to a single dose of the antimicrobial agent. The pharmacological basis for this effect is not clear. It is speculated that adherence to the intercellular target prevents some significant quantity of the antimicrobial agent from being washed away for a time. Others believe that there are other drug-related effects that injure the bacterium and that it is only slowly able to repair. Some as-yet-undiscovered cause might be at play. Under some conditions, a PAE can be detected for days in the chemotherapy of mycobacterial infections. The PAE has been observed for a variety of antibiotics, and its duration varies with the drug, the organism, the concentration of drug, and the duration of treatment. This phenomenon can be used to assist in patient compliance by decreasing the frequency and the length of chemotherapy; however, it also may lead to drug resistance and should be employed conservatively.

Biphasic ("Eagle") Effect

The biphasic effect is associated primarily with β-lactam antibiotics. It is a curious phenomenon in which low doses in vitro against certain bacteria (staphylococci and streptococci) produce lysis, whereas higher doses do not. This is believed to result from the differential sensitivity of the penicillin binding proteins (see below for an explanation of this term) in that higher doses of β-lactams inhibit the autolysins (this term also will be defined later). These are enzymes that also contribute to bacterial lysis.

Inoculum Effect

In a number of cases, microbial resistance is mediated by the production of bacterial enzymes that attack the antibiotic molecule, changing its structure to an inactive form. This can lead to a so-called inoculum effect, in which a susceptible antibiotic is apparently less potent when larger numbers of bacteria are present in the medium than when fewer cells are employed. The more bacteria that are present, the more antibiotic-destroying enzyme that is present, and the more antibiotic that is required to overcome this to achieve the desired response. An antibiotic that is not enzyme modified is comparatively free of inoculum effects.

Antimicrobial Dosing

Combination Therapy

The student may suppose that use of combinations of antibiotics would be superior to the use of individual antibiotics, because this would broaden the antimicrobial spectrum and make the accurate identification of the pathogen less critical. It has been found, however, by experiment that all too often, such combinations are antagonistic. A useful generalization, but one that is not always correct, is that one often may successfully combine two bactericidal antibiotics, particularly if their molecular mode of action is different. A common example is the use of a β-lactam antibiotic and an aminoglycoside for first-day empiric therapy of overwhelming sepsis of unknown etiology. Therapy must be instituted as soon after a specimen is obtained, or the patient may die. This often does not allow the microbiological laboratory sufficient time to identify the offending microorganism or to determine its antibiotic susceptibility. An emergency resort therefore is made to what is termed "shotgun therapy." Both of the antibiotic families applied in this example are bactericidal in readily achievable parenteral doses. As will be detailed later in this chapter, the β-lactams inhibit bacterial cell wall formation, and the aminoglycosides interfere with protein biosynthesis and membrane function. Their modes of action are supplementary. Because of toxicity considerations and the potential for untoward side effects, this empiric therapy is replaced by suitable specific monotherapy at the first opportunity after the sensitivity of the offending bacterium is experimentally established.

One also often may successfully combine two bacteriostatic antibiotics for special purposes, such as a macrolide and a sulfonamide. Occasionally, these are used in combination for the treatment of an upper respiratory tract infection caused by *Haemophilus influenzae,* because the combination of a protein biosynthesis inhibitor and an inhibitor of DNA biosynthesis gives fewer relapses than the use of either agent alone. The use of a bacteriostatic agent, such as tetracycline, in combination with a bactericidal agent, such as a β-lactam, usually is discouraged. The β-lactam antibiotics are much more effective when used against growing cultures, and a bacteriostatic agent interferes with bacterial growth, often giving an indifferent or antagonistic response when such agents are combined. Additional possible disadvantages of combination chemotherapy are higher cost, greater likelihood of side effects, and difficulties in demonstrating synergism in humans. The rising tide of antibiotic resistance is overcoming these reservations, however, and combination therapy is becoming more common.

Serum Protein Binding

The influence of serum protein binding on antibiotic effectiveness is fairly straightforward. It is considered in most instances that the percentage of antibiotic that is protein bound is not available at that moment for the treatment of infections and, therefore, must be subtracted from the total blood level to get the effective blood level. The tightness of the binding also is a consideration. Thus, a heavily and firmly serum protein-bound antibiotic would not generally be a good choice for the treatment of septicemias or infections in deep tissue, even though the microorganism involved is susceptible during in vitro tests. If the antibiotic is rapidly released from protein bondage, however, this factor decreases in importance, and the binding becomes a depot source. Distinguishing between these two types of protein binding is accomplished by comparing the percentages of binding to the excretion half-life. A highly bound but readily released antibiotic will have a comparatively short half-life and work well for systemic infections. Normally, an antibiotic that is not significantly protein bound will be rapidly excreted and have a short half-life. Thus, some protein binding of poorly water-soluble agents generally is regarded as being helpful. The student will recall that under most circumstances, the urine is a protein-free filtrate, so the proportion of an antibiotic that is firmly bound to serum proteins will be retained in the blood. Thus, a highly and firmly protein-bound antibiotic could be satisfactory for mild urinary tract infections.

Preferred Means of Dosing

Under ideal circumstances, it is desirable for an antibiotic to be available in both parenteral and oral forms. Whereas there is no question that the convenience of oral medication makes this ideal for outpatient and community use, very ill patients often require parenteral therapy. It would be consistent with today's practice of discharging patients "quicker and sicker" to send them home from the hospital with an efficacious oral version of the same antibiotic that led to the possibility of discharge in the first place. In that way, the patient would not have to come back to the hospital at intervals for drug administration, nor would one have to risk treatment failure by starting therapy with a new drug. For drugs with significant toxicities, the physician will prefer the injection form; the physician using this method is certain that the whole dose has been taken at the appropriate time. If the local pharmacist is adept at administration of parenteral medication, these considerations become less important. Employing directly observed therapy also avoids many aspects of noncompliance. For patients with highly contagious and dangerous infections, such as tuberculosis and HIV, directly observed therapy is increasingly the treatment mode of choice.

Initiation of Therapy

Because bacteria multiply rapidly—populations often double in 0.5 to 3.0 hours—it is important to institute antibiotic therapy as soon as possible. Thus, it often is desirable to initiate therapy with a double (loading) dose and then to follow this with smaller (maintenance) doses. To prevent relapse, the patient must be instructed not to skip doses and to take all of the medication provided, even though the presenting symptoms (e.g., diarrhea or fever) may resolve before the entire drug is taken. All too often, treatment failure and the emergence of resistance probably is caused by poor compliance or premature cessation of therapy by the patient.

Prophylactic Use of Antibiotics

Antibiotics often are used prophylactically, such as in preoperative bowel sanitization and orally for treatment of viral sore throats. These are not sound practices, because the patient is exposed to the possibility both of drug-associated side effects and a suprainfection by drug-resistant microorganisms. Moreover, the therapeutic gain from such practices often is marginal. As frustrating as this may be to the infectious diseases specialist, however, these are common medical practices and, hence, are difficult to stop.

Agricultural Use of Antibiotics

It is estimated that half of the antibiotics of commerce are used for agricultural purposes. Their use for treatment of infections of plants and animals is not to be discouraged so long as the drug residues from the treatment do not contaminate foods. In contamination, problems

> **Cost**
>
> Antibiotics often are expensive, but so are morbidity and mortality. Nonetheless, for many patients, cost is a significant consideration. The pharmacist is in an ideal position to guide both the physician and the patient on the question of possible alternative, equivalent treatments that might be more affordable. The most frequent comparisons are based on the cost of the usual dose of a given agent for a single course of therapy (usually the wholesale cost to the pharmacist for 10 days worth of drug).

such as penicillin allergy or subsequent infection higher up the food chain by drug-resistant microbes can occur. Several instances of death in humans have been recorded in the 1990s from such incidents. Animals grow demonstrably more rapidly to marketable size when antibiotics are added to their feed, even though the animals have no apparent infection. This is believed to result, in large part, from suppression of subclinical infections that, consequently, would divert protein biosynthesis from muscle and tissue growth into proteins needed to combat the infection. Under appropriate conditions, antibiotic feed supplementation is responsible, in part, for the comparative wholesomeness and cheapness of our food supplies. This practice has the potential, however, to contaminate the food that we consume or to provide reservoirs of drug-resistant enteric microorganisms. Occasionally, infections are traced to this cause, and resistance genes can originate in this manner and pass from strain to strain—and even to other species.

THERAPEUTIC CLASSES

Synthetic Antimicrobial Agents

Synthetic antimicrobial agents have not been modeled after any natural product, so they may not properly be termed "antibiotics." Some synthetics are extremely effective for treatment of infections and are widely used. Very few antibiotics are known to work in precisely the same way as these agents in killing bacteria. Also curious is the fact that those agents, for which the molecular mode of action is known, are at present nearly all effective against key enzymes needed for the biosynthesis or functioning of nucleic acids. Because they interrupt the biosynthesis or functions of nucleic acids rather than attack the finished products or substitute for them in nucleic acids, they are not genotoxic but are comparatively safe to use.

Sulfonamides

Introduction. The antibacterial properties of the sulfonamides were discovered in the mid-1930s following an incorrect hypothesis but after observing the results carefully and drawing correct conclusions. Prontosil rubrum, a red dye, was one of a series of dyes examined by Gerhard Domagk of Bayer of Germany in the belief that it might be taken up selectively by certain pathogenic bacteria and not by human cells, in a manner analogous to the way in which the Gram stain works, and, therefore, serve as a selective poison to kill these cells. The dye, indeed, proved to be active in vivo against streptococcal infections in mice. Curiously, it was not active in vitro. Trefouel and Bovet in France soon showed that the urine of prontosil rubrum–treated animals was bioactive in vitro. Fractionation led to identification of the active substance as *p*-aminobenzenesulfonic acid amide (sulfanilamide), a colorless cleavage product formed by reductive liver metabolism of the administered dye. Today, we would call prontosil rubrum a pro-drug. The discovery of the in vivo antibacterial properties of sulfanilamide ushered in the modern anti-infective era, and these investigators shared a Nobel Prize for medicine in 1938. For the first time in the long and weary chronicle of human struggle against infectious disease, physicians now had a comparatively safe and responsive oral drug to use. Considered along with the use of penicillin only 5 years later, the era of the so-called "wonder drugs" had dawned.

NH_2 SO_2NH_2 H_2N — Liver [H] → SO_2NH_2 H_2N

Prontosil Rubrum Sulfanilamide

Once mainstays of antimicrobial chemotherapy, the sulfonamides have decreased enormously in popularity and now are comparatively minor drugs. The relative cheapness of the sulfonamides is one of their most attractive features and accounts for much of their persistence in the market.

Mechanism of Action. The sulfonamides are bacteriostatic when administered to humans in achievable doses. They inhibit the enzyme dihydropteroate synthase, an important enzyme needed for the biosynthesis of folic acid derivatives and, ultimately, the thymidine required for DNA. They do this by competing at the active site with *p*-aminobenzoic acid (PABA), a normal structural component of folic acid derivatives. PABA is otherwise incorporated into the developing tetrahydrofolic acid molecule by enzyme-catalyzed condensation with 6-hydroxymethyl-7,8-dihydropterin-pyrophosphate to form 7,8-dihydropteroate and pyrophosphate. Thus, sulfonamides also may be classified as antimetabolites (Fig. 38.3). Indeed, the antimicrobial efficacy of sulfonamides can be reversed by adding significant quantities of PABA into the diet (in some multivitamin preparations and as metabolites of certain local anesthetics) or into the culture medium. Most susceptible bacteria are unable to take up preformed folic acid from their environment and convert it to a tetrahydrofolic acid but, instead, synthesize their own folates de novo. Folates are essential intermediates for the biosynthesis of thymidine, without which bacteria cannot multiply. This inhibition is strongly bacteriostatic and, ultimately, bactericidal. Humans are unable to synthesize folates from component parts, because we lack the necessary enzymes, including dihydropteroate synthase, and folic acid is supplied to us in our diet. Consequently, sulfonamides have no similarly lethal effect on human cell growth. The basis for the selective toxicity of sulfonamides thus is clear.

In a few strains of bacteria, however, the picture is somewhat more complex. Here, sulfonamides are attached to the dihydropteroate diphosphate in the place of the normal PABA. The resulting unnatural product, however, is not capable of undergoing the next necessary reaction (condensation with glutamic acid). This false metabolite

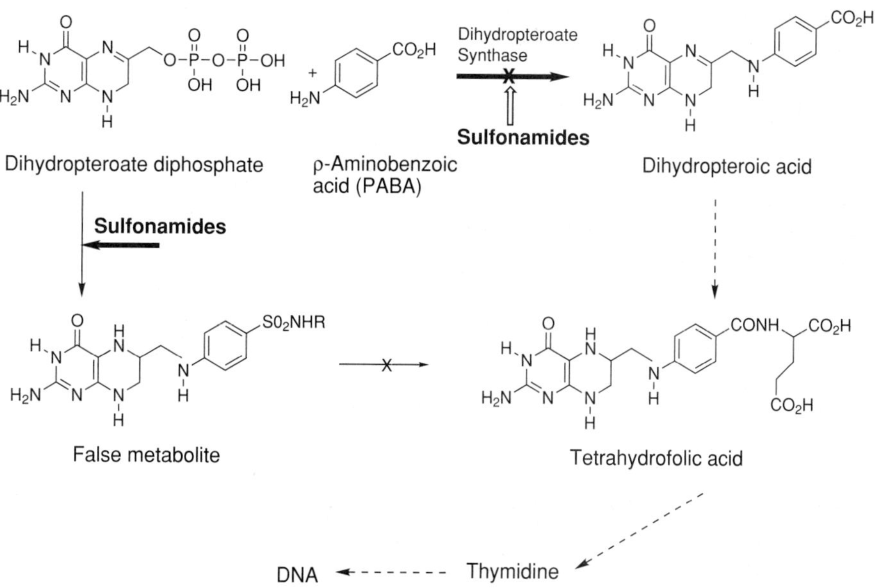

Fig. 38.3. Microbial biosynthetic pathway leading to tetrahydrofolic acid synthesis and major site of action (⟹) of sulfonamides as well as site of action seen in some bacteria (⟵) resulting in incorporation of sulfonamide as a false metabolite.

also is an enzyme inhibitor, and the net result is inability of the bacteria to multiply as soon as the preformed folic acid in their cells is used up and further nucleic acid biosynthesis becomes impossible. For these strains the result is the same, but the molecular basis of the effect is somewhat different (Fig. 38.3). Bacteria that are able to take up preformed folic acid into their cells are intrinsically resistant to sulfonamides.

STRUCTURE–ACTIVITY RELATIONSHIPS. The basis of the structural resemblance of sulfonamides to PABA that is so devastating to these bacteria is clear. The functional group that differs in the two molecules is the carboxyl of PABA and the sulfonamide moiety of sulfanilamide. The strongly electron-withdrawing character of the aromatic SO_2 group makes the nitrogen atom to which it is directly attached partially electropositive. This, in turn, increases the acidity of the hydrogen atoms attached to the nitrogen so that this functional group is slightly acidic (pK_a = 10.4). The pK_a of the carboxyl group of PABA is approximately 6.5. It was soon found, following a crash synthetic program, that replacement of one of the NH_2 hydrogens by an electron-withdrawing heteroaromatic ring was not only consistent with antimicrobial activity but also greatly acidified the remaining hydrogen and dramatically enhanced potency. With suitable groups in place, the pK_a is reduced to the same range as that of PABA itself. Not only did this markedly increase the antibacterial potency of the product, it also dramatically increased the water solubility under physiologic conditions. The pK_a of sulfisoxazole, one of the most popular of the sulfonamides in present use, is approximately 5.0. The poor water solubility of the earliest sulfonamides led to occasional crystallization in the urine (crystalluria) and resulted in kidney damage, because the molecules were un-ionized at urinary pH values. It is still recommended to drink increased quantities of water to avoid crystalluria when taking certain sulfonamides. This form of toxicity is now comparatively uncommon with the more important agents used today, however, because these agents form sodium salts that are at least partly ionized and, hence, reasonably water soluble at urinary pH values. They are poorly tolerated on injection, however, because these salts are corrosive to tissues.

Structural variation among the clinically useful sulfonamides is restricted primarily to installation of various heterocyclic aromatic substituents on the sulfonamide nitrogen.

NaOH → + HOH

Sulfisoxazole. pKa = 5 — Sodium Sulfisoxazole.

PHARMACOKINETICS. The orally administered sulfonamides are well absorbed from the gastrointestinal (GI) tract, distributed fairly widely, and excreted by the kidney. The drugs are bound to plasma protein (sulfisoxazole, 30–70% , sulfamethoxazole, 70%) and, as such, may displace other protein-bound drugs as well as bilirubin. The latter phenomenon disqualifies them for use in late term pregnancy as they can cause neonatal jaundice. Sulfonamides are partly deactivated by acetylation at N-4 and glucuronidation of the anilino nitrogen in the liver.

Plasmid-mediated resistance development is common, particularly among Gram-negative microorganisms and usually takes the form of decreased sensitivity of dihydropteroate synthase or increased production of PABA.

Therapeutic Applications. Of the thousands of sulfonamides that have been evaluated, sulfisoxazole acetyl in combination with erythromycin ethylsuccinate is currently the most popular. Sulfisoxazole acetyl is tasteless, which accounts for its use in pediatric preparations and is a pro-drug. The acetyl moiety is removed in the GI tract, giving rise to the active sulfisoxazole. Along with the surviving sulfonamides (Table 38.1), it has a comparatively broad antimicrobial spectrum in vitro, especially against Gram-negative organisms, but its clinical use generally is restricted because of the development of bacterial resistance. Susceptible organisms may include Enterobacteriaceae (*Escherichia coli, Klebsiella* sp., and *Proteus* sp.) and *Streptococcus pyogenes, Streptococcus pneumoniae,* and *Haemophilus* sp. Sulfamethoxazole, in combination with trimethoprim, is used for treatment of primary uncomplicated urinary tract infections and, occasionally, as a backup to other, normally more preferred agents in special situations.

The remaining sulfonamides are not used systemically. Sulfadiazine in the form of its silver salt is used topically for treatment of burns and is effective against a range of bacteria and fungus. Sulfacetamide is used ophthalmically for treatment of eye infections caused by susceptible organisms, and sulfasalazine is a pro-drug used in the treatment of ulcerative colitis and Crohn's disease.

Table 38.1. Clinically Relevent Sulfonamides

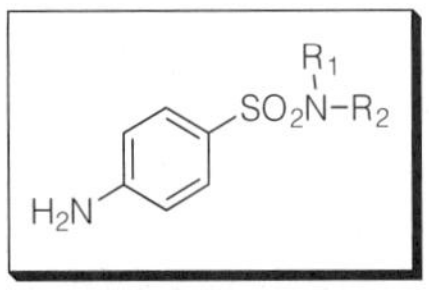

H_2N–C$_6$H$_4$–$SO_2N(R_1)$–R_2

Generic name	R_1	R_2	pKa
Sulfamethoxazole	H	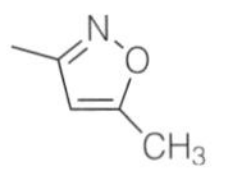 N, O, CH_3	5.6
Sulfadiazine	H	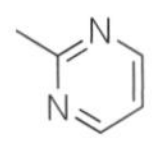 N, N	6.5
Silver Sulfadiazine	$Ag^{\oplus}$	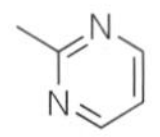 N, N	
Sulfisoxazole	H	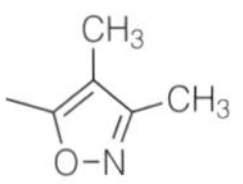 CH_3, CH_3, O–N	5.0
Acetyl Sulfisoxazole	$-C(=O)-CH_3$	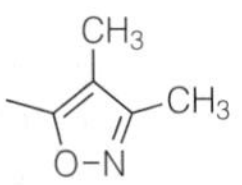 CH_3, CH_3, O–N	
Sulfacetamide	H	$COCH_3$	5.4

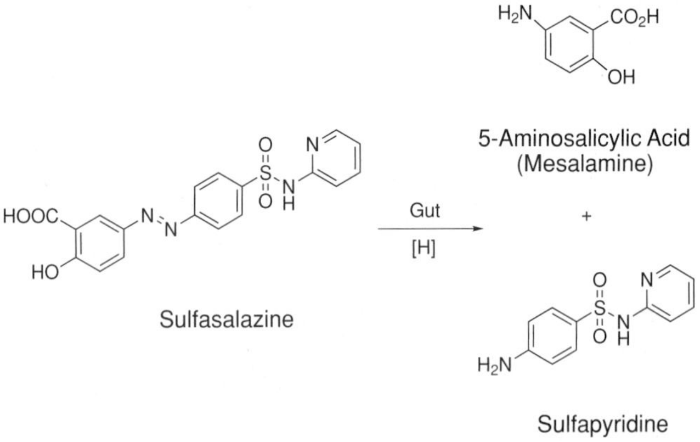

Sulfasalazine → (Gut, [H]) → 5-Aminosalicylic Acid (Mesalamine) + Sulfapyridine

Fig. 38.4. Activation of sulfasalazine to 5-aminosalicylic acid.

Adverse effects. Allergic reactions are the most common adverse effect and take the form of rash, photosensitivity, and drug fever. Less common problems are kidney and liver damage, hemolytic anemia, and other blood problems. The most serious adverse effect is the Stevens-Johnson syndrome characterized by sometimes-fatal erythema multiforme and ulceration of mucous membranes of the eye, mouth, and urethra. Fortunately, these effects are comparatively rare.

Sulfasalazine

Sulfasalazine stands out from the typical sulfonamide by the fact that although administered orally, the drug is not absorbed in the gut, so the majority of the dose is delivered to the distal bowel. In addition, the drug is a prodrug, which undergoes reductive metabolism by gut bacteria, converting the drug into sulfapyridine and 5-aminosalicyclic acid the active component (Fig. 38.4). The liberation of 5-aminosalicylic acid (mesalamine), an anti-inflammatory agent, is the purpose for administering this drug. This agent is used to treat ulcerative colitis and Crohn's disease. Direct administration of salicylates is otherwise irritating to the gastric mucosa.

Trimethoprim

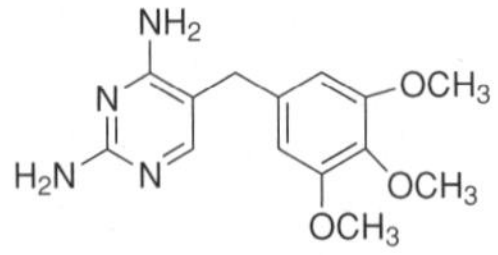

Trimethoprim (Proloprim, Trimpex)

Mechanism of action. A further step in the pathway leading from the pteroates to folic acid and on to DNA bases requires the enzyme dihydrofolate reductase. Exogenous folic acid must be reduced stepwise to dihydrofolic acid and then to tetrahydrofolic acid, an important cofactor essential for supplying a 1-carbon unit in thymidine biosynthesis and, ultimately, for DNA synthesis (Fig. 38.5). The same enzyme also must reduce endogenously produced dihydrofolate. Inhibition of this key

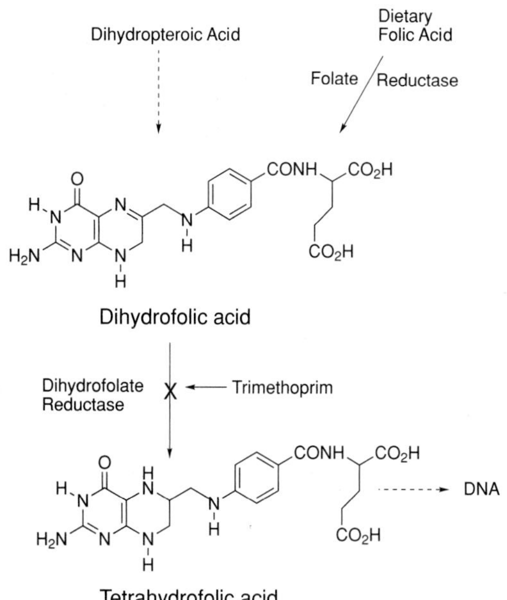

Fig. 38.5. Site of action of trimethoprim.

enzyme had been widely studied in attempts to find anticancer agents by starving rapidly dividing cancer cells of needed DNA precursors. The student will recall that methotrexate and its analogues came from such studies. Methotrexate is, however, much too toxic to be used as an antibiotic. Subsequently, however, trimethoprim was developed in 1969 by George Hitchings and Gertrude Elion (who shared a Nobel Prize for this and other contributions to chemotherapy in the 1980s). This inhibitor prevents tetrahydrofolic acid biosynthesis and results in bacteriostasis. Trimethoprim selectivity between bacterial and mammalian dihydrofolate reductases results from the subtle but significant architectural differences between these enzyme systems. Whereas the bacterial enzyme and the mammalian enzyme both efficiently catalyze the conversion of dihydrofolic acid to tetrahydrofolic acid, the bacterial enzyme is sensitive to inhibition by trimethoprim by up to 40,000-fold lower concentrations than the mouse enzyme is. This difference explains the useful selective toxicity of trimethoprim.

THERAPEUTIC APPLICATION. Trimethoprim frequently is used as a single agent clinically for the oral treatment of uncomplicated urinary tract infections caused by susceptible bacteria (predominantly community acquired *Escherichia coli* and other Gram-negative rods). It is, however, most commonly used in a 1:5 fixed concentration ratio with the sulfonamide sulfamethoxazole (Bactrim, Septra). This combination is not only synergistic in vitro but also is less likely to induce bacterial resistance than either agent alone. It is rationalized that microorganisms not completely inhibited by sulfamethoxazole at the pteroate condensation step will not likely be able to push the lessened amount of substrates that leak past a subsequent blockade of dihydrofolate reductase. Thus, these agents block sequentially at two different steps in the same essential pathway, and this combination is extremely difficult for a naive microorganism to survive. It also is comparatively uncommon that a microorganism will successfully mutate to resistance at both enzymes during the course of therapy. Of course, if the organism is already resistant to either drug at the outset of therapy, which happens more and more often, much of the advantage of the combination is lost.

Pairing these two particular antibacterial agents was based on pharmacokinetic factors and convenient availability. For such a combination to be useful in vivo, the two agents must arrive at the necessary tissue compartment where the infection is at the correct time and in the correct ratio. In this context, the optimum ratio of these two agents in vitro is 1:20. Of all the combinations tried, sulfamethoxazole came closest to being optimal for trimethoprim. Administration of a 1:5 combination of the two drugs orally produces the desired 1:20 ratio in the body once steady state is reached. Conveniently, sulfamethoxazole was already on the market, so it did not have to be approved specially by the U.S. Food and Drug Administration (FDA) for this purpose.

It is easier to demonstrate synergy in vitro than in vivo, and concerns about the toxic contribution of the sulfonamide (and, doubtless, commercial considerations as well) have led to a recent vogue for the use of trimethoprim alone. Trimethoprim has a broad spectrum in vitro, so it is potentially useful against many microorganisms. Combined with sulfamethoxazole, it is used for oral treatment of urinary tract infections, shigellosis, otitis media, traveler's diarrhea, methicillin-resistant *Staphylococcus aureus* (MRSA), *Legionella* infection, and bronchitis.

Among the opportunistic pathogens that afflict patients with AIDS is the pneumonia-causing fungus *Pneumocystis jiroveci* (previously classified as *Pneumocystis carinii*). Immunocompetent individuals rarely become infected with *P. jiroveci,* but it is a frequent pathogen in patients with AIDS and is nearly 100% fatal in such immunocompromised individuals. The combination of sulfamethoxazole–trimethoprim has proven to be useful and comparatively nontoxic for these patients. A form for injection is available for use in severe infections and is particularly useful in patients with AIDS. This treatment form leads to more frequent toxic reactions, however. The most frequent side effects of trimethoprim–sulfamethoxazole are rash, nausea, and vomiting. Blood dyscrasias are less common, as is pseudomembranous colitis (caused by nonantibiotic-sensitive opportunistic gut anaerobes, often *Clostridium difficile*). Many broad-spectrum antimicrobials can lead to such severe drug related diarrhea, and this side effect must be monitored carefully. Severe, nonresolving diarrhea can be fatal; therefore, it is a justification for withdrawing existing therapy in favor of antianaerobic antibiotic. Despite a significant effort, no structurally related analogue has emerged to compete with trimethoprim.

RESISTANCE. Bacterial resistance to trimethoprim is increasingly common. In pneumococcal infections, it can result from a single amino acid mutation (Ile-100 to Leu) in the dihydrofolate reductase enzyme. Overexpression of dihydrofolate reductase by *Staphylococcus aureus* has been reported in resistant strains as well.

Quinolones

INTRODUCTION

Nalidixic Acid   Cinoxacin

The quinolone antimicrobials comprise a group of synthetic substances possessing in common an N-1-alkylated 3-carboxypyrid-4-one ring fused to another aromatic ring, which itself carries other substituents. The first quinolone to be marketed (in 1965) was nalidixic acid. Nalidixic acid and cinoxacin are classified as first-generation quinolones based on their spectrum of activity and pharmacokinetic properties. While still available, they are considered to be minor urinary tract disinfectants that are effective primarily against certain susceptible Gram-negative bacteria. Thus, the quinolones were of little clinical significance until the discovery that the addition of a fluoro group to the 6-position of the basic nucleus greatly increased the biological activity. Brought to the market in 1986, norfloxacin, the first of the second-generation quinolones, has a broad spectrum and equivalent in potency to many of the fermentation derived antibiotics. Following its introduction, intense competition ensued, more than a thousand second-, third-, and fourth-generation analogues have now been made. Alatrofloxacin, ciprofloxacin, enoxacin, gatifloxacin, gemifloxacin, lomefloxacin, norfloxacin, ofloxacin, levofloxacin, moxifloxacin, sparfloxacin, and trovafloxacin are currently marketed in the United States (Fig. 38.6). Ciprofloxacin and levofloxacin dominate the worldwide fluoroquinolone market, accounting between them for over $3 billion in 2002.

It should be noted that the more recent quinolones also are referred to as the fluoroquinolones and that these agents are now an important class of antimicrobial agents.

MECHANISM OF ACTION. The quinolones are rapidly bactericidal, largely as a consequence of inhibition of DNA gyrase and topoisomerase IV, key bacterial enzymes that dictate the conformation of DNA. The *Escherichia coli* chromosome is a single, circular molecule of approximately 1 mm in length, whereas the cell is only 1 to 3 μm long. Thus, the DNA molecule must be dramatically compacted in a conformationally stable way so that it can fit. Using the energy generated by adenosine triphosphate (ATP) hydrolysis, the molecule is progressively wound about itself in a positive super coil. In the absence

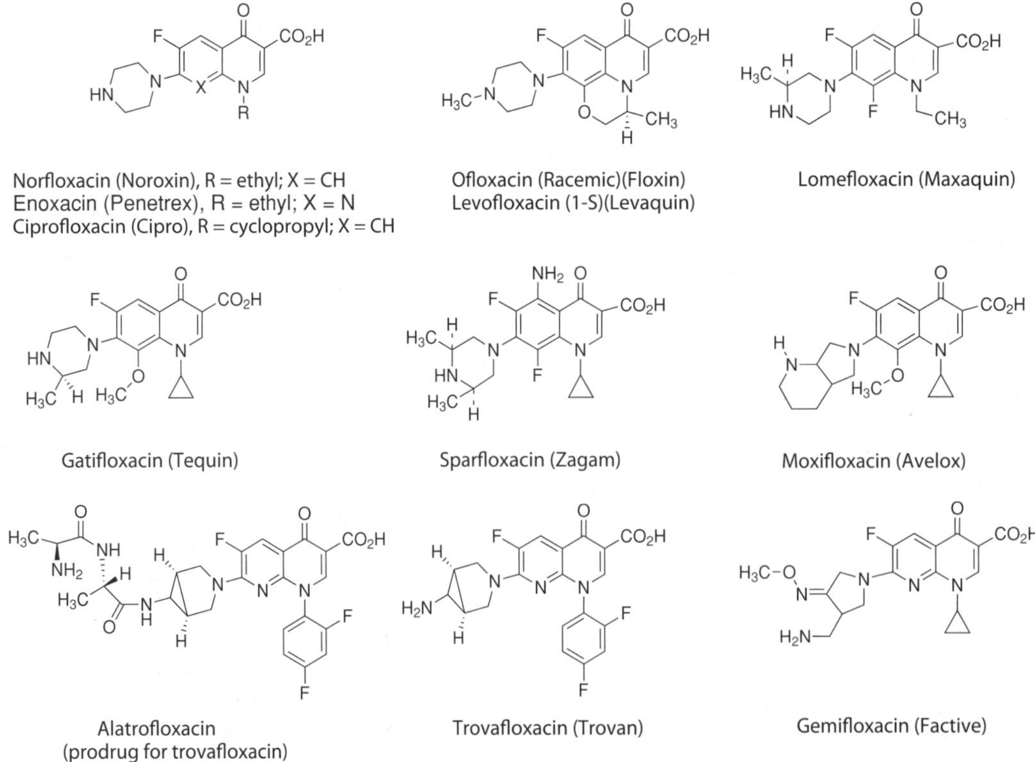

Fig. 38.6. Second-, third-, and fourth-generation quinolones.

of ATP, the process is reversed, relaxing the molecule. It also must be partially unwound so that the cell has access to the genetic information that it contains. This requires reversible conformational changes so that it can be stored properly, unwound, replicated, repaired, and transcribed on demand. These enzymes alter the conformation of DNA by catalyzing transient double-strand cuts staggered by four base pairs, passing the uncut portion of the molecule through the gap, and resealing the molecule back together. In this way, DNA gyrase alters the degree of DNA twisting by introducing negative DNA super coils, releasing tensional stress in the molecule. On the other hand, DNA topoisomerase IV decatenates (unties) enchained daughter DNA molecules produced through replication of circular DNA. Inhibition of DNA gyrase and topoisomerase IV makes a cell's DNA inaccessible and leads to cell death, particularly if the cell must deal with other toxic effects at the same time. These processes are shown schematically in Fig. 38.7. Different quinolones inhibit these essential enzymes to different extents. Topoisomerase IV seems to be more important to some Gram-positive organisms and DNA gyrase to some Gram-negative organisms.

The coumermycins, of which novobiocin (now archaic) was the most clinically relevant, bind to a different site in these topoisomerases (i.e., where the ATP binds). Resistance to the coumermycins develops rather easily, and they find little use today.

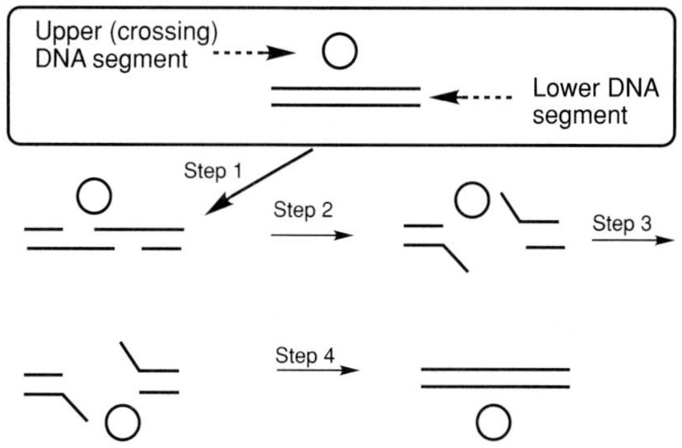

A. View from the top: Step 1. Stabilize positive node. Step 2. Break both strands of the back segment. Step 3. Pass unbroken segment through the break and reseal on the front side.

B. View from the side: Step 1. Staggered cuts in each strand. Step 2. Gate opens. Step 3. Transverse segment passed through the break. Step 4. Reseal cut segment.

Fig. 38.7. Schematic depicting supercoiling of circular DNA catalyzed by DNA gyrase.

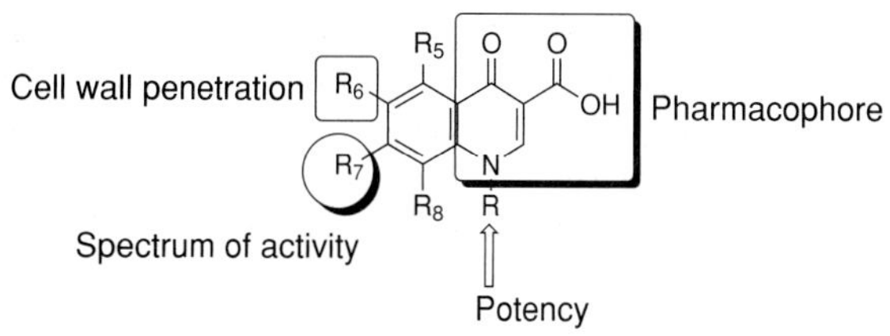

Fig. 38.8. Major structure–activity relationship features.

Humans shape their DNA with a topoisomerase II, an analogous enzyme that does not bind quinolones at normally achievable doses, so the quinolones of commerce do not kill host cells.

STRUCTURE–ACTIVITY RELATIONSHIP. The structural features of the quinolones strongly influence the antimicrobial and pharmacokinetic properties of this class of drugs. The essential pharmacophore for activity is the carboxy-4-pyridone nucleus (Fig. 38.8). Apparently, the carboxylic acid and the ketone are involved in binding to the DNA/DNA-gyrase enzyme system. Reduction of the 2,3-double bond or the 4-keto group inactivates the molecule, and substitution at C-2 interferes with enzyme– substrate complexation. Fluoro substitution at the C-6 position greatly improves antimicrobial activity by increasing the lipophilicity of the molecule, which in turn improves the drugs penetration through the bacterial cell wall. Additionally, C-6 fluoro increases the DNA gyrase inhibitory action. An additional fluoro group at C-8 further improves drug absorption and half-life but also may increase drug-induced photosensitivity. Heterocyclic substitution at C-7 improves the spectrum of activity especially against Gram-negative organisms. The piperazinyl (as in ciprofloxacin) and pyrrolidinyl (as in moxifloxacin) represent the most significant antimicrobial improvement. Unfortunately, the piperazinyl group at C-7 also increases binding to central nervous system (CNS) γ-aminobutyric acid (GABA) receptors, which accounts for CNS side effects. Alkyl substitution on the piperazine (lomefloxacin and ofloxacin) is reported to decrease binding to GABA, as does the addition of bulky groups at the N-1 position (sparfloxacin). The cyclopropyl substitution at N-1 appears to broaden activity of the quinolones to include activity against atypical bacteria, including *Mycoplasma, Chlamydia,* and *Legionella* species.

The introduction of a third ring to the nucleus of the quinolones gives rise to ofloxacin. Additionally, ofloxaxin has an asymmetric carbon at the C-3' position. The *S*-(−)-isomer (levofloxacin) is twice as active as ofloxacin and 8- to 128-fold more potent than the *R*-(+)-isomer resulting from increased binding to the DNA-gyrase.

Several of the quinolones produce mild to severe photosensitivity. A C-8 halogen appears to produce the highest incidence of photosensitivity via singlet oxygen and radical induction. Lomefloxacin has been reported to have the highest potential for producing phototoxicity. Substitution of a methoxy group at C-8 has been reported to reduce the photosensitivity (gatifloxacin).

Finally, a chemical incompatibility common to all the quinolones involves the ability of these drugs to chelate polyvalent metal ions (Ca^{2+}, Mg^{2+}, Zn^{2+}, Fe^{2+}, and Al^{3+}), resulting in decreased solubility and reduced drug absorption. Chelation occurs between the metal and the 3-carboxylic acid and 4-keto groups. Agents containing polyvalent metals should be administered at least 4 hours before or 2 hours after the quinolones.

PHARMACOKINETICS. The fluoroquinolones are well absorbed following oral administration, with excellent bioavailability. The maximum plasma concentration usually is reached within a few hours, and the drugs are moderately bound to plasma protein, leading to comparatively long half-lives (Table 38.2). Earlier quinolones were rapidly excreted into the urine, which limited their therapeutic application to urinary tract infections, whereas the newer drugs are distributed to alveolar macrophages, bronchial mucosa, epithelial lining fluid, and saliva, improving the use in various systemic infections. Several studies have suggested that the ratio of mean peak plasma concentration to MIC and the 24-hour area under the curve to MIC may correlate with therapeutic outcomes. If this proves to be true, it could greatly help the clinician in choosing the appropriate drug and dosing schedule.

THERAPEUTIC APPLICATIONS. The quinolones therapeutically fall into one of four classifications (Table 38.3). The specific drugs within each classification include nalidixic acid and cinoxin as first-generation agents, with utility limited to uncomplicated urinary tract infections. The second-generation quinolones include norfloxacin, lomefloxacin, enoxacin, ofloxacin, and ciprofloxacin. Whereas norfloxacin is used mainly for urinary tract infections (*Enterobacter* sp., *Enterococcus* sp., or *Pseudomonas aeruginosa*), ciprofloxacin also is used for prostatitis, upper respiratory tract infections, bone infections, septicemia, staphylococcal and pseudomonal endocarditis, meningitis, sexually transmitted diseases (gonorrhea and chlamydia), chronic ear infections, and purulent osteoarthritis. The third-generation quinolones, which include levofloxacin, sparfloxacin, gatifloxacin, and gemifloxacin, are used to treat infections caused by *Legionella* sp., *Chlamydia* sp., and *Mycoplasma* sp., as well as *Streptococcus pneumoniae.* These agents may find use in the treatment of acute bacterial exacerbation of chronic bronchitis and community-acquired pneumonia. Gemifloxacin has been approved for use against multidrug-resistant *S. pneumoniae.* Additional indications may include skin and skin structure infections and acute sinusitis caused by *S. pneumoniae, Haemophilus influenzae,* and *Moraxella catarrhalis.* The fourth-generation quinolines include trovafloxacin and moxifloxacin, which have a spectrum of activity that includes anaerobes, such as *Bacteroides fragilis.*

Table 38.2. Pharmacokinetic Properties for Selective Quinolones

Drug	Bioavailability (%)	Protein Binding (%)	Half-life (hours)
Ciprofloxacin	70	30	3.5
Enoxacin	90	40	3–6
Gatifloxacin	96	20	8.0
Gemifloxacin	71	60–70	8.0
Levofloxacin	99	31	6.9
Lomefloxacin	95	10	8
Moxifloxacin	86	47	12.1
Norfloxacin	30–40	10–15	3–4
Ofloxacin	98	32	9
Sparfloxacin	90	56	18.7
Trovafloxacin	88	73	11.0

Table 38.3. Therapeutic Classification of Quinolones

Generation	Characteristics
First generation	Poor serum and tissue concentration Not valuable for systemic infections Lack activity against *Pseudomonas aeruginosa*, Gram-positive organisms, and anaerobes
Second generation	Adequate serum and tissue concentration Good for systemic infections Active against Gram-negative organisms, including *P. aeruginosa*; weak activity against *Streptococcus pneumoniae*; no activity against anaerobes
Third generation	Once-daily dosing Active against *S. pneumoniae* and atypical bacteria; less active against *P. aeruginosa*
Fourth generation	Active against anaerobes and aerobic Gram-positive and Gram-negative organisms

RESISTANCE. Resistance to the quinolones is becoming more frequent and is associated with spontaneous mutations in two genes (*gyrA* and *gyrB*) that encode for the quinolone target protein, DNA gyrase. A single step mutation can lead to low-level resistance, whereas mutations in both genes lead to high-level resistance. This mechanism of resistance would be expected to produce cross-resistance within the class of quinolones. In addition, there are suggestions that resistance may be associated with an increase in drug efflux or a decrease in outer membrane permeability affecting drug influx. Such a mechanism of resistance would be expected to be more common in Gram-negative organisms with a more complex cell wall than in Gram-positive organisms with its cell envelope.

ADVERSE EFFECTS. The quinolone class is associated with more side effects than the β-lactam and macrolide classes but, nonetheless, see very widespread medicinal use.

Among the side effects associated with quinolones is a proconvulsant action, especially in epileptics, but this is mainly associated with the first-generation agents. Other CNS problems include hallucinations, insomnia, and visual disturbances. Some patients also experience diarrhea, vomiting, abdominal pain, and anorexia. These effects are most common with trovafloxacin. The quinolones are associated with erosion of the load-bearing joints of young animals. As a precaution, these drugs are not used casually in children younger than 18 years or in sexually active females of childbearing age. Ciprofloxacin is the fluoroquinolone of choice for children when use of a quinolone is required, because it has been extensively studied for this purpose. They also are potentially damaging in the first trimester of pregnancy because of a risk of severe metabolic acidosis and of hemolytic anemia. Coadministration with theophylline potentiates the action of the latter and should be monitored closely. Although it takes much higher concentrations of fluoroquinolones to inhibit human topoisomerase II than concentrations of either DNA gyrase or bacterial topoisomerase IV, some agents have a narrower margin of safety. With gemifloxacin, a mild to severe rash may develop.

Severe toxicities. Certain members of the fluoroquinolone family were marketed for a time but were subsequently severely limited in use or withdrawn because of the unacceptable toxicities experienced by some patients. These agents had been introduced with great hopes because of their breadth of spectrum and potency against resistant microorganisms. Temafloxacin, for example, was removed from the market because of hemolysis, renal failure, and thrombocytopenia (the hemolytic uremic syndrome). These effects only became apparent when large numbers of patients received the drug. Severe liver toxicity led to the removal from the market in Europe and restrictions on the use of trovafloxacin in the United States only for severe infections involving institutional care, where the patient can be closely monitored. Grepafloxacin was introduced to the market in late 1997 as a broad-spectrum fluoroqinolone and was withdrawn from the market in 1999 based on cardiovascular toxicity. Gatifloxacin, gemifloxacin, and moxifloxacin carry warnings about QT-interval prolongation but are still in use. Sparfloxacin also has been reported to produce cardio- and phototoxicity and should be used with great care. The drugs were reported to cause a prolonged QTc interval. Analogues with a C-8 chloro substituent, such as clinafloxacin and sitafloxacin, also were very potent but have largely fallen from favor because of excessive phototoxicity. All these drugs were well on the way to great popularity when these untoward events were detected. These phenomena were not apparently revealed during extensive previous animal and clinical studies. No consistent structural pattern is associated with these problems, with the exception that one would not use an N-1 2,4-difluorophenyl moiety except with great care.

Miscellaneous Agents

Nitroheteroaromatic compounds

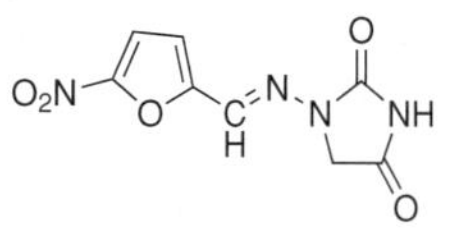

Nitrofurantoin (Furadantin, Macrodantin)

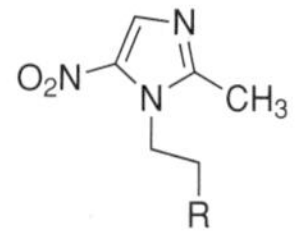

Metronidazole, R = OH (Flagyl)
Tinidazole R = $SO_2C_2H_5$(Fasigyn)

Nitrofurantoin, a widely used oral antibacterial nitrofuran, has been available since World War II. It is used for prophylaxis or treatment of acute urinary tract infections when kidney function is not impaired, and it inhibits kidney stone growth. Nausea and vomiting are common side effects. This is avoided, in part, by slowing the rate of absorption of the drug through use of wax-coated, large particles (Macrodantin). Nitrofurantoin inhibits DNA and RNA functions through mechanisms that are not well understood, although bioreductive activation is suspected to be an important component of this. Resistance is not commonly encountered. Rather severe side effects can be experienced when using this drug (e.g., acute pulmonary reactions, peripheral neuropathy, hemolytic anemia, liver toxicity, and fertility impairment), so caution is in order.

Metronidazole was initially introduced for the treatment of vaginal infections caused by amoeba. This nitroimidazole also is useful orally, however, for the treatment of trichomoniasis, giardiasis, and *Gardnerella vaginalis* infections. It has found increasing use of late in the parenteral treatment of anaerobic infections and in the treatment of pseudomembranous enterocolitis resulting from *Clostridium difficile*, an opportunistic pathogen that occasionally flourishes as a consequence of broad-spectrum antibiotic therapy. Infections with *C. difficile* can be life-threatening. The drug is believed to be metabolically activated by reduction of its nitro group to produce reactive oxygen species. Metronidazole also is a component of a multidrug cocktail used to treat *Helicobacter pylori* infections associated with gastric ulcers. Both drugs can cause disulfuram-like adverse reactions when alcohol is consumed. For many years, it had little competition from other therapies for its indications. Recently, tinidazole, another nitroimidazole, has been introduced in the United States as just such a competitor. It is too early to judge how competitive this agent will be, but it has a longer duration of action. Metronidazole use is associated with allergic rashes and CNS disturbances, including convulsions in some patients. It is carcinogenic in rodents. Thus, some caution is associated with its use.

Methenamine

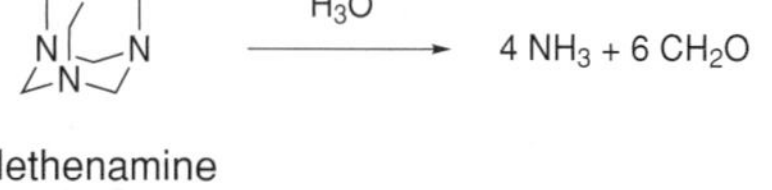

$$\xrightarrow{H_3O^{\oplus}} 4\ NH_3 + 6\ CH_2O$$

Methenamine
(Prosed, Urimax, Urised, Uroqid-Acid)

A venerable drug used for the disinfection of acidic urine, methenamine is a low-molecular-weight polymer of ammonia and formaldehyde that reverts to its components under mildly acidic conditions. Formaldehyde is the active antimicrobial component. Methenamine is used for recurrent urinary tract infections. The drug is available in various dosage forms as well as various salts, including the hippurate and mandelate.

Phosphomycin

H_3C PO_3H_2 O

Phosphomycin (Monurol)

Phosphomycin, introduced in 1972, inhibits enolpyruvial transferase, an enzyme catalyzing an early step in bacterial cell wall biosynthesis. Inhibition results in reduced synthesis of peptidoglycan, an important component in the bacterial cell wall. Phosphomycin is bactericidal against *Escherichia coli* and *Enterobacter faecalis* infections.

Antibiotics: Inhibitors of Bacterial Cell Wall Biosynthesis

Bacterial cell wall. Bacterial cells are enclosed within a complex and largely rigid cell wall. This differs dramatically from mammalian cells, which are surrounded by a flexible membrane, the chemical composition of which is dramatically different. This provides a number of potentially attractive targets for selective chemotherapy of bacterial infections. For one thing, enzymes that have no direct counterpart in mammalian cells construct the bacterial cell wall. Three of the main functions of the bacterial cell wall are 1) to provide a semipermeable barrier interfacing with the environment through which only desirable substances may pass, 2) to provide a sufficiently strong barrier so that the bacterial cell is protected from changes in the osmotic pressure of its environment, and 3) to prevent digestion by host enzymes. The initial units of the cell wall are constructed within the cell, but soon, the growing and increasingly complex structure must be extruded; final assembly takes place outside of the inner membrane. This circumstance makes the enzymes involved in the late steps more vulnerable to inhibition, because they are at or near the cell surface. Whereas individual bacterial species differ in specific details, the following generalized picture of the process is sufficiently accurate to illustrate the process.

Gram-Positive Bacteria. The cell wall of Gram-positive bacteria, although complex enough, is simpler than that of Gram-negative organisms. A schematic representation is shown in Figure 38.9. On the very outside of the cell is a set of characteristic carbohydrates and proteins that, together, make up the antigenic determinants that differ from species to species and that also cause adherence to particular target cells. There also may be a lipid-rich capsule surrounding the cell (not shown in Fig. 38.9). The next barrier that the wall presents is the peptidoglycan layer.

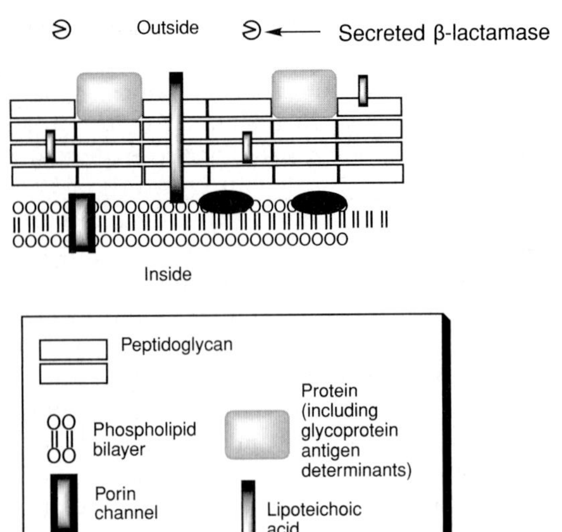

Fig. 38.9. Schematic of some features of the Gram-positive bacterial cell wall.

This is a spongy, gel-forming layer consisting of a series of alternating sugars (N-acetylglucosamine and N-acetylmuramic acid) linked (1,4)-β in a long chain (Fig. 38.10). To the lactic acid carboxyl moieties of the N-acetylmuramic acid units is attached, through an amide linkage, a series of amino acids, of which L-alanyl-D-glutamyl-L-lysyl-D-alanine is

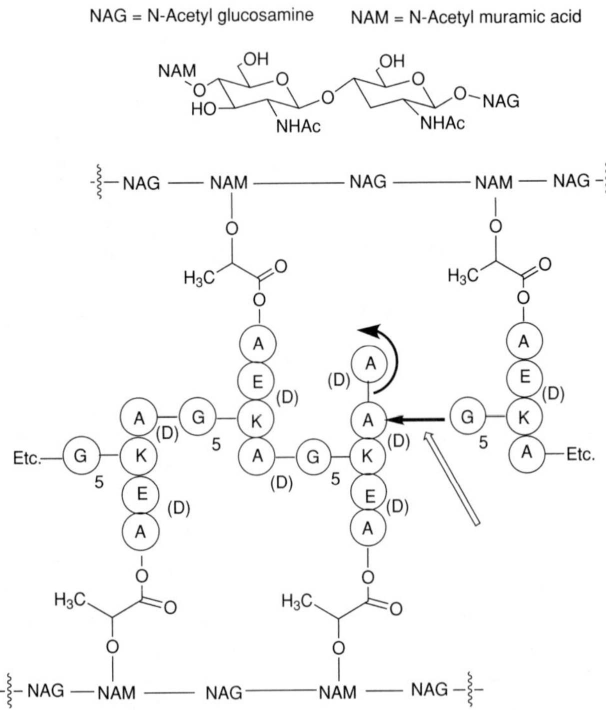

Fig. 38.10. Schematic of cell wall cross-linking. Pentaglycyl group replaces terminal D-alanine.

Table 38.4. Pencillins Binding Proteins (PBP) of E. coli

PBP	Function	Lethality?
1A	Cell elongation (peripheral wall extension)	Yes
1B	Cell elongation (peripheral wall extension)	Yes
2	Maintenance of rod shape	Yes
3	Septum formation	No
4	Limit the amount of cross linking of the peptidoglycan	No
5	Limit the amount of cross linking of the peptidoglycan	No
6	Limit the amount of cross linking of the peptidoglycan	No

V. Lorian, Ed., Antibiotics in Laboratory Medicine, Williams & Wilkins, Baltimore (1986).

typical of *Staphylococcus aureus*. One notes the D-stereochemistry of the glutamate and the terminal alanine. This feature is presumably important in protecting the peptidoglycan from hydrolysis by host peptidases, particularly in the GI tract. This unusual structural feature facilitates successful parasitism.

The early steps in the biosynthesis of the peptidoglycan unit result in formation of a complex polymeric sheet. This is then cross-linked to form a thickened wall. This bonds the terminal D-alanyl unit to the lysyl unit of an adjacent tetrapeptide strand through a pentaglycyl unit. This last step is an enzyme-catalyzed transamidation by which the terminal amino moiety on the last glycine unit of the A strand displaces the terminal D-Ala unit on the nearby B strand. The cell wall transamidase (one of the penicillin binding proteins [PBPs]) forms a transient, covalent bond during the synthesis phase with a particular serine hydroxyl on the enzyme. Completion of the catalytic cycle involves displacement of the enzyme by a glycine residue, which regenerates the enzyme. This process gives the wall additional rigidity, much as would be achieved by gluing the pages of a book together. This strong barrier protects against osmotic stress and accounts for the retention of characteristic morphological shape of Gram-positive bacteria (e.g., globes and rods). This step is highly sensitive to inhibition of β-lactam antibiotics. It also is the target of the glycopeptide antibiotics (e.g., vancomycin), as will be discussed later.

The peptidoglycan layer is traversed by complex glycophospholipids called teichoic and teichuronic acids. These are largely responsible for the acid mantle of Gram-positive bacteria. Beneath the peptidoglycan layer is the lipoidal cytoplasmic cell membrane in which a number of important protein molecules float in a lipid bilayer. Among these proteins are the β-lactam targets, known as the PBPs. These enzymes are important in cell wall formation and remodeling. In Gram-positive bacteria, the outer layers are relatively ineffective in keeping out antibiotics. It is the inner membrane and its protein components that provide the principal barrier to uptake of antibiotics. There are at least seven types of PBPs. Those of *Escherichia coli* are classified in Table 38.4. The functions of all of these are not entirely understood, but they are important in construction and repair of the cell wall. β-Lactam antibiotics bind to these proteins and kill bacteria by preventing the biosynthesis of a functional cell wall. Various β-lactam antibiotics display different patterns of binding to these proteins. The action of these proteins must alternate in a controlled and systematic way between their active and inert states so that bacterial cells can grow and multiply in an orderly manner. Selective interference by β-lactam antibiotics with the functioning of these proteins prevents normal growth and repair and creates serious problems for bacteria, particularly young cells needing to grow and mature cells needing to repair damage or to divide. The rapid bactericidal effect of penicillins on such cells can readily be imagined.

Gram-Negative Bacteria. With the Gram-negative bacteria, the cell wall is more complex and more lipoidal (Fig. 38.11). These cells usually contain an additional, outer lipid membrane that differs considerably from the inner membrane. The outer layer contains complex lipopolysaccharides that encode antigenic responses, cause septic shock, provide the serotype, and influence morphology. This exterior layer also contains a number of enzymes and exclusionary proteins. Important among these are the porins. These are transmembranal supermolecules made

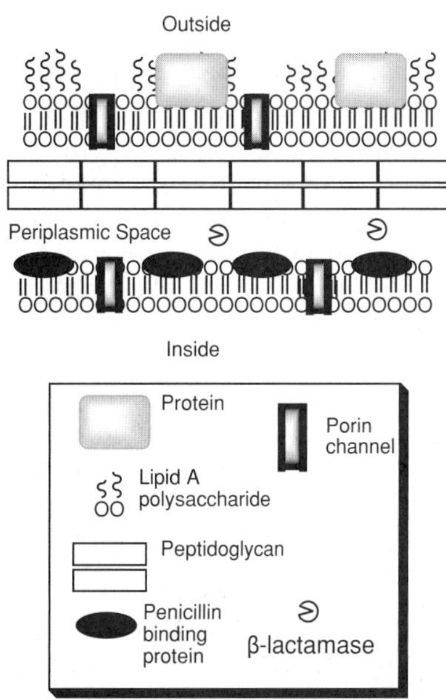

Fig. 38.11. Schematic of some features of the Gram-negative bacterial cell wall.

up of two or three monomeric proteins. The center of this array is a transmembranal pore of various dimensions. Some allow many kinds of small molecules to pass, and others contain specific receptors that allow only certain molecules to come in. The size, shape, and lipophilicity of drugs are important considerations controlling porin passage. Antibiotics have greater difficulty in penetrating into Gram-negative bacterial cells as a consequence. Next comes a periplasmic space containing a somewhat less impressive and thinner, as compared to the Gram-positive organisms, layer of peptidoglycan. Also present is a phospholipid-rich cytoplasmic membrane in which floats a series of characteristic proteins with various functions. The β-lactam targets (i.e., the PBPs) are found here.

Other inner membrane proteins are involved in transport, energy, and biosynthesis. In many such cells are proteins that actively pump out antibiotics and other substances at the expense of energy and that may require the simultaneous entrance of oppositely charged materials to maintain an electrostatic balance.

β-LACTAM ANTIBIOTICS

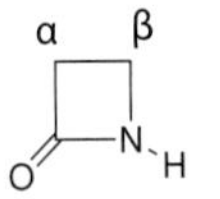

α β

N H

O

β -lactam
azetidinone

The name "lactam" is given to cyclic amides and is analogous to the name "lactone," which is given to cyclic esters. In an older nomenclature, the second carbon in an aliphatic carboxylic acid was designated α, the third β, and so on. Thus, a β-lactam is a cyclic amide with four atoms in its ring. The contemporary name for this ring system is azetidinone. This structural feature was very rare when it was found to be a feature of the structure of the penicillins, so the name "β-lactam" came to be a generic descriptor for the whole family. It is fortunate that this ring ultimately proved to be the main component of the pharmacophore, so the term possesses medicinal as well as chemical significance. The penicillin subclass of β-lactam antibiotics is characterized by the presence of a substituted 5-membered thiazoldine ring fused to the β-lactam ring. This fusion and the chirality of the β-lactam ring results in the molecule roughly possessing a "V"-shape. This drastically interferes with the planarity of the lactam bond and inhibits resonance of the lactam nitrogen with its carbonyl group. Consequently, the β-lactam ring is much more reactive and, therefore, more sensitive to nucleophilic attack when compared with normal planar amides.

History. The story of the discovery of the penicillins are widely known. In 1929, Alexander Fleming, a physician and a clinical microbiologist, was preserving a culture of a pathogen, and the plate became contaminated with an airborne fungus, *Penicillium notatum* (now named *Penicillium chrysogenum*), which not only grew on the plate but also produced a clear zone of inhibition around its colony. On returning from a vacation and finding this, he recognized the potential significance of this antibiotic effect, so he preserved the fungus and tried to identify its active constituent. The state of development of the art as well as his background and training were insufficient for the task at that time. It was not until a decade later that a group of English chemists, including Abraham, Chain, Florey, and Heatley, succeeded in purifying the unstable antibiotic. Finally, on February 12, 1941, following heroic efforts necessitated by wartime conditions, enough material was available for clinical examination and the demonstration that penicillin actually worked in humans. Much new technology had to be developed before large-scale use of penicillin could take place. The efforts of an international team solved, for example, the problems of large-scale sterile aerobic submerged fermentation, directed fermentation, strain improvement, and many other vexing problems. By 1943, penicillin was being produced in very large quantities for use by the armed forces. When peace came in 1945, production was in tons, and the drug was available very cheaply.

The earliest penicillins were produced by fungi from media constituents. The bicyclic heterocyclic nucleus of 6-aminopenicillanic acid (6-APA) was constructed by an involved process catalyzed by enzymes. The side chain was added essentially intact from media constituents. It was discovered that certain arylacetic acids, when added to the medium, were used to form the side chain amide moiety and that this was very important for stability and breadth of spectrum. It was later discovered that exclusion of such materials from the medium allowed the production of 6-APA without a side chain. Chemists could then add a much wider variety of side chains without being limited by the specific requirements of the enzymes. With this breakthrough, the penicillin field expanded to include orally active, broad-spectrum, and enzymatically stable penicillins. The cephalosporins were discovered as secondary metabolites of a different fungal species. Because it was stable to many activity-destroying β-lactamases, its core nucleus, 7-aminocephalosporanic acid, was substituted with a wide variety of unnatural side chains, and three generations of clinically useful analogues resulted. Later work produced the monobactams, carbapenems, and β-lactamase inhibitors. In the year 2005, about half of the money spent worldwide on antibiotics was for β-lactams. More than 100,000 of these compounds have been prepared by partial or total chemical synthesis, and a significant number of these remain on the market more than 60 years after their discovery.

Penicillins. The medicinal classifications, chemical structures, and generic names of the penicillins currently available are presented in Table 38.5.

Preparation of Penicillins. The original fermentation derived penicillins were produced by growth of the fungus

Table 38.5. Commercially Significant Pencillins and Related Molecules

Generic name	Trade name	R_1
Fermentation-Derived Penicillins		
6-Aminopenicillanic acid		H
Benzylpenicillin (Penicillin G)	Generic	C_6H_5-CH_2-
Phenoxymethylpenicillin (Penicillin V)	Generic	C_6H_5-OCH_2-
Semi-Synthetic Penicillinase-Resistant Parenteral Penicillins		
Methicillin		
Nafcillin	Nallpen, Unipen	
Semi-Synthetic Penicillinase-Resistant Oral Penicillins		
Oxacillin (X = Y = H)	Bactocill	
Cloxacillin (X = Cl, Y = H)	Cloxapen	
Dicloxacillin (X = Y = Cl)	Dycill, Pathocil	
Semi-Synthetic Penicillinase-Sensitive, Broad Spectrum, Parenteral Penicillins		
Carbenicillin (R_2 = H)	Geocillin	
Carbenicillin indanyl (R_2 = indanyl)		
Ticarcillin	Ticar	
Mezlocillin	Mezlin	
Piperacillin	Pipracil	
Semi-Synthetic Penicillinase-Sensitive, Broad-Spectrum, Oral Penicillins		
Ampicillin (X = H)	Principen, Omnipen	
Amoxicillin (X = OH)	Amoxil, Trimox, Wymox	

Penicillium chrysogenum on complex solid media, with the result that they were mixtures differing from one another in the identity of the side-chain moiety. When a sufficient supply of phenylacetic acid is present in liquid media, this is preferentially incorporated into the molecule to produce mainly benzylpenicillin (penicillin G in the old nomenclature). Use of phenoxyacetic acid instead leads to phenoxymethyl penicillin (penicillin V). More than two dozen different penicillins have been made in this way, but these two are the only ones that remain in clinical use. The bicyclic penicillin nucleus itself is prepared biosynthetically via a complex process from an acylated cysteinyl valyl peptide. The complete exclusion of side chain precursor acids from the medium produces the fundamental penicillin nucleus, 6-APA, but in poor yield. By itself, 6-APA has only very weak antibiotic activity, but when substituted on its primary amino group with a suitable amide side chain, its potency and antibacterial spectrum are profoundly enhanced. With this key precursor isolated, limitations caused by enzyme specificities in biosynthesis could be overcome by use of partial chemical synthesis. A more practical modern process for making 6-APA employs naturally occurring fungal enzymes that selectively hydrolyze away the side chain of natural penicillins without cleaving the β-lactam bond. These enzymes are found in certain Gram-negative bacteria but appear to be of negligible importance with respect to bacterial resistance to β-lactam antibiotics. More recently, ingeniously selective chemical processes have been devised for accomplishing removal of less interesting side chains from biosynthetic penicillins. The operational chemical freedom resulting from the convenient availability of 6-APA has led to partial synthesis of many thousands of analogues.

The sodium and potassium salts of penicillins are crystalline, hydroscopic, and water-soluble. They can be employed either orally or parentally. When dry, they are stable for long periods but hydrolyze rapidly when in solution. Their best stability is noted at pH values between 5.5 and 8.0 (especially at pH 6.0–7.2). The procaine and benzathine salts of benzylpenicillin, on the other hand, are water insoluble. Because they dissolve slowly, they are used for repository purposes following injection when long-term blood levels are required.

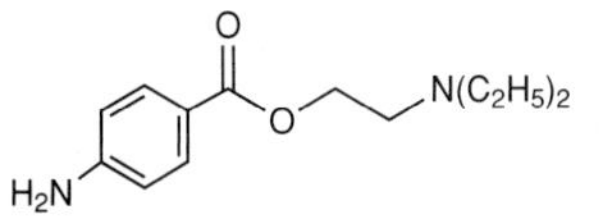

Procaine

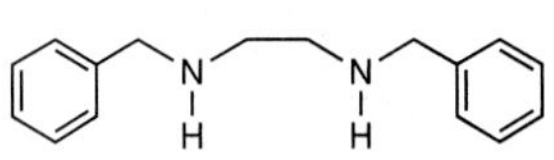

Benzathine

Nomenclature. The nomenclature of the penicillins, as with most antibiotics, is complex. The Chemical Abstracts system is definitive and unambiguous, but it is too complex for ordinary use (Fig. 38.12). For example, the chemical name for benzylpenicillin sodium is monosodium (2*S*,5*R*,6*R*)-3,3-dimethyl-7-oxo-6-(2-phenylacetamido)-4-thia-1-azabicyclo[3.2.0]heptane-2-carboxylate.

Confusingly, the U.S. Pharmacopeia uses a different system that results in the atoms being numbered differently. The simplest system has stood the test of time and involves taking the repeating radical, carbonyl-6-APA, and using the chemical trivial name for the radical that completes the structure. Thus, use of the names benzylpenicillin and phenoxymethylpenicillin makes practical sense. There are three asymmetric centers in the benzylpenicillin molecule, as indicated by the asterisk in Table 38.5. This absolute stereochemistry must be preserved for useful antibiotic activity.

Clinically Relevant Chemical Instabilities. The most unstable bond in the penicillin molecule is the highly strained and reactive β-lactam amide bond. This bond cleaves moderately slowly in water unless heated, but it breaks down much more rapidly in alkaline solutions to produce penicilloic acid, which readily decarboxylates to produce penilloic acid (Fig. 38.13). Penicilloic acid has a negligible tendency to re-close to the corresponding penicillin, so this reaction is essentially irreversible under physiologic conditions. Because the β-lactam ring is an essential portion of the pharmacophore, its hydrolysis deactivates the antibiotic. A fairly significant degree of hydrolysis also takes place in the liver. The bacterial enzyme, β-lactamase, catalyzes this reaction as well and is a principal cause of bacterial resistance in the clinic. Alcohols and amines bring about the same cleavage reaction, but the products are the corresponding esters and amides. These products are inactive. A reaction with a specific primary amino group of aminoglycoside antibiotics is of clinical relevance, because it inactivates penicillins and cephalosporins (discussed later). When proteins serve as the nucleophiles in this reaction, the antigenic conjugates that cause many penicillin allergies are produced. Small molecules that are not inherently antigenic but that react with proteins to produce antigens in this manner are called haptens. Commercially

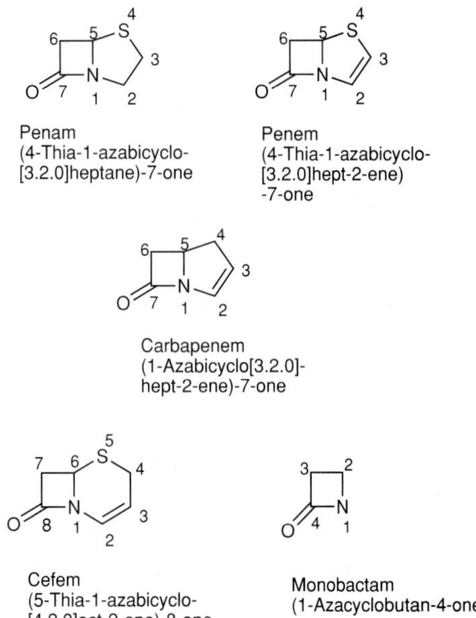

Fig. 38.12. Ring and numbering systems of clinically available β-lactam antibiotic types.

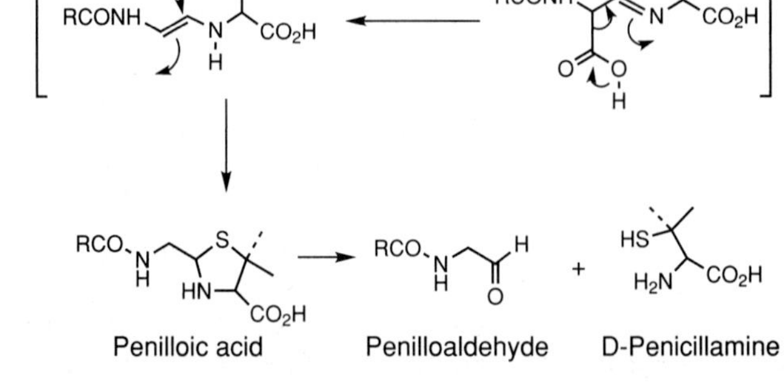

Penicillin → (OH⁻ or β-lactamase) → Penicilloic acid → Penilloic acid → Penilloaldehyde + D-Penicillamine

Fig. 38.13. Instability of β-lactams to nucleophiles.

available penicillin salts may be contaminated with small amounts of these antigenic penicilloyl proteins derived from reaction with proteins encountered in their fermentative production or by high-molecular-weight, self-condensation–derived polymers resulting when penicillins are concentrated and react with themselves. Both of these classes of impurities are antigenic and may sensitize some patients.

Solutions of penicillins for parenteral use should be refrigerated, used promptly, and not stored. In acidic solutions, thc hydrolysis of penicillins is complex. Hydrolysis of the β-lactam bond can be shown through kinetic analysis to involve participation of the side-chain amide oxygen, because the rate of this reaction differs widely depending on the nature of the R group. The main end products of the acidic degradation are penicillamine, penilloic acid, and penilloaldehyde (Fig. 38.14). The intermediate penicillenic acid is highly unstable and undergoes subsequent hydrolysis to the corresponding penicilloic acid. An alternate pathway involves sulfur ejection to a product that, in turn, fragments to liberate penicilloic acid as well. Penicilloic acid readily decarboxylates to penilloic acid. The latter hydrolyzes to produce penilloaldehyde and penicillamine (itself used clinically as a chelating agent). Several related fragmentations to a variety of other products take place. None of these products has antibacterial activity. At gastric pH (~2.0) and temperature of 37°C, benzylpenicillin has a half-life measured in minutes. The less water-soluble amine salts are more stable.

Structure–Activity Relationship. The chemical substituents attached to the penicillin nucleus can greatly influence

A penicillin

Penicilloic acid

Penilloic acid   Penilloaldehyde   D-Penicillamine

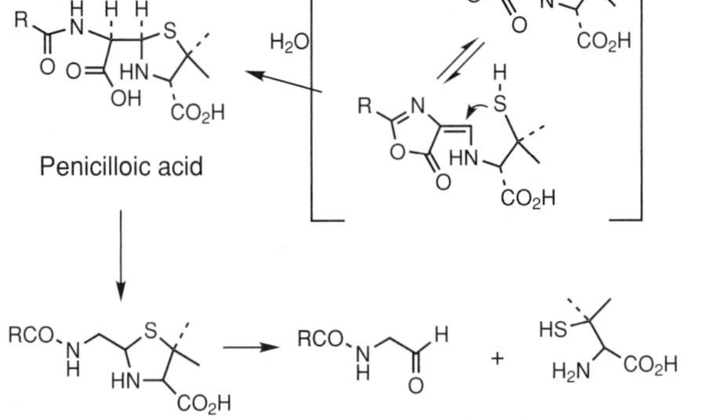

Fig. 38.14. Instability of penicillins in acid. Hydrolysis involves the C-6 side chain.

Table 38.6. Improved Acid Stability and Absorption of Substituted Penicillins

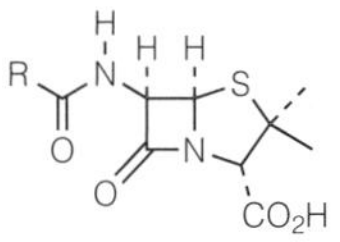

Drug	R	% Absorption intact drug
Benzylpenicillin	$C_6H_5-CH_2-$	15–30
Pen V	$C_6H_5-O-CH_2-$	60–73
Ampicillin	$C_6H_5-CH(NH_2)-$	30–50
Amoxicillin	$HO-C_6H_4-CH(NH_2)-$	75–90

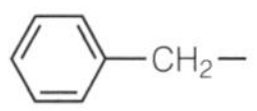

the stability of the penicillins as well as the spectrum of activity. It is important to recognize whether the structural changes affect drug stability on the shelf or in the GI tract (in vivo), improve stability toward bacterial metabolism, or enlarge the spectrum of activity.

The substitution of a side-chain R group on the primary amine with an electron-withdrawing group decreases the electron density on the side-chain carbonyl and protects these penicillins, in part, from acid degradation. This property has clinical implications, because these compounds survive passage through the stomach better and many can be given orally for systemic purposes. The survival of passage and degree of absorption under fasting conditions is shown in Table 38.6.

In addition, in vitro degradation reactions of penicillins can be retarded by keeping the pH of solutions between 6.0 and 6.8 and by refrigerating them. Metal ions, such as mercury, zinc, and copper, catalyze the degradation of penicillins, so they should be kept from contact with penicillin solutions. The lids of containers used today are routinely made of inert plastics, in part, to minimize such problems.

The more lipophilic the side chain of a penicillin, the more serum protein bound is the antibiotic (Table 38.7).

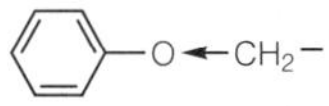

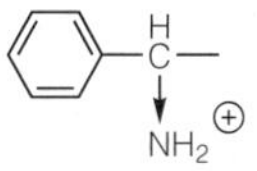

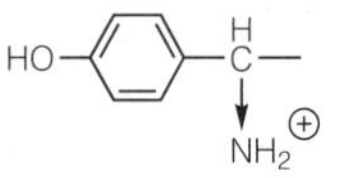

Table 38.7. Protein Binding of Penicillins

Penicillin	% Protein binding
Benzyl penicillin	45 - 68%
Phenoxymethyl penicillin	75 - 89%
Methicillin	35 - 80%
Ampicillin	25 - 30%
Amoxicillin	25 - 30%
Carbenicillin	~50%
Oxacillin	>90%
Cloxacillin	>90%

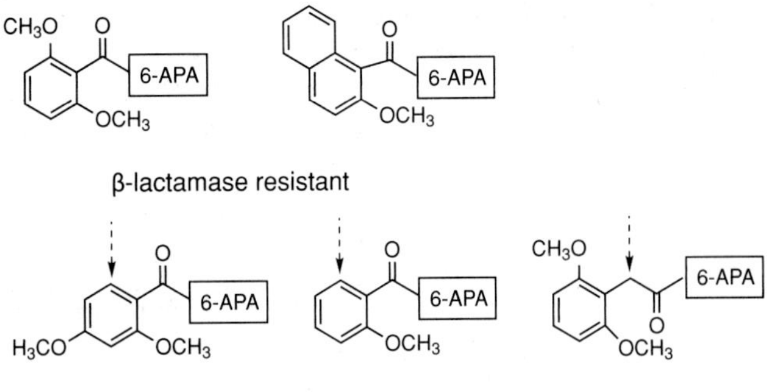

β-lactamase resistant

β-lactamase sensitive

Fig. 38.15. β-Lactamase resistant/sensitive structural features.

This has some advantages in terms of protection from degradation, but it does reduce measurably the effective bactericidal concentration of the drug in whole blood. Contrary to popular assumption, the degree of serum protein binding of the penicillins has comparatively little influence on their half-lives. The penicillins are actively excreted into the urine via an active transport system for negatively charged ions, and the rate of release from their bound form is sufficiently rapid that the controlling rate is the kidney secretion rate. The serum half-life of penicillin G is approximately 0.4 to 0.9 hours and that of phenoxymethyl penicillin approximately 0.5 hours. Both are excreted into the urine by tubular excretion. Probenicid, when present, competes effectively for excretion and, as a consequence, prolongs the half-life.

Stability of the penicillins toward β-lactamase is influenced by the bulk in the acyl group attached to the primary amine. β-Lactamases are much less tolerant to the presence of steric hindrance near the side-chain amide bond than are the penicillin binding proteins. When the aromatic ring is attached directly to the side-chain carbonyl and both ortho positions are substituted by methoxy groups, β-lactamase stability results (Fig. 38.15). Movement of one of the methoxy groups to the para position, or replacing one of them by a hydrogen, resulted in an analogue sensitive to β-lactamases. Putting in a methylene between the aromatic ring and 6-APA likewise produced a β-lactamase–sensitive agent (see Fig. 38.15). These findings provide strong support for the hypothesis that its resistance to enzyme degradation is based on differential steric hindrance. Prime examples of this effect are seen in the drugs methicillin, nafcillin, oxacillin, cloxicillin, and dicloxicillin (Table 38.5).

Mechanism of Action. The molecular mode of action of the β-lactam antibiotics is a selective and irreversible inhibition of the enzymes processing the developing peptidoglycan layer (Fig. 38.16). Just before cross-linking occurs, the peptide pendant from the lactate carboxyl of a muramic acid unit terminates in a D-alanyl-D-alanine unit. The terminal D-alanine unit is exchanged for a glycine unit on an adjacent strand in a reaction catalyzed by a cell wall transamidase. This enzyme is one of the penicillin biding proteins (carboxypeptidases, endopeptidases, and transpeptidases) that normally reside in the bacterial inner membrane and perform construction, repair, and housekeeping functions, maintaining cell wall integrity and playing a vital role in cell growth and division. They differ significantly from bacterium to bacterium, and this is used to rationalize different potency and morphologic outcomes following β-lactam attack on the different bacteria. The cell wall transamidase uses a serine hydroxyl group to attack the penultimate D-alanyl

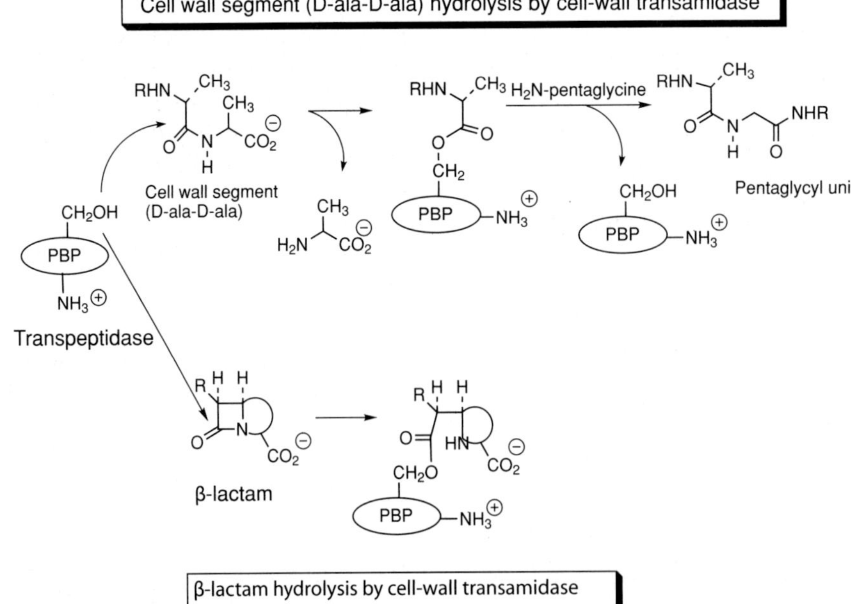

Fig. 38.16. Cell wall cross-linking and mechanism of action of β-lactams.

unit, forming a covalent ester bond, and the terminal D-alanine, which is released by this action, diffuses away. The enzyme–peptidoglycan ester bond is attacked by the free amino end of a pentaglycyl unit of an adjacent strand, regenerating the active site of transpeptidase for further catalytic action and producing a new amide bond, which connects two adjacent strands together.

The three-dimensional geometry of the active site of the enzyme perfectly accommodates to the shape and separation of the amino acids of its substrate. Because the substrate has unnatural stereochemistry at the critical residues, this enzyme is not expected to attack host peptides or even other bacterial peptides composed of natural amino acids.

The penicillins and the other β-lactam antibiotics have a structure that closely resembles that of acylated D-alanyl-D-alanine. The enzyme mistakenly accepts the penicillin as though it were its normal substrate. The highly strained β-lactam ring is much more reactive than a normal amide moiety, particularly when fused into the appropriate bicyclic system. The intermediate acyl–enzyme complex, however, is rather different structurally from the normal intermediate in that the hydrolysis does not break penicillin into two pieces, as it does with its normal substrate. In the penicillins, a heterocyclic residue is still covalently bonded and cannot diffuse away as the natural terminal D-alanine unit does. This presents a steric barrier to approach by the nearby pentaglycyl unit and, therefore, keeps the enzyme's active site from being regenerated and the cell wall precursors from being cross-linked. The resulting cell wall is structurally weak and is subject to osmotic stress. Cell lysis can result, and the cell rapidly dies, assisted by another class of bacterial enzymes, the autolysins. The result is a defective cell wall and an inactivated enzyme. The relief of strain that is obtained on enzymatic β-lactam bond cleavage is so pronounced that there is virtually no tendency for the reaction to reverse. Water also is an insufficiently effective nucleophile and cannot hydrolyze the complex either. Thus, the cell wall transamidase is stoichiometrically inactivated. The gaps in the cell wall produced by this covalent interruption are not filled in, because the enzyme is now inactivated. (More details of the putative drug–enzyme interaction will be discussed with the other classes of β-lactams.)

Binding of β-lactam antibiotics to PBP-1A and PBP-1B (transpeptidase) of *Escherichia coli* leads to cell lysis; to PBP-2 (transpeptidase) leads to oval cells deficient in rigidity and to inhibition of cell division; to PBP-3 (transpeptidase) leads to abnormally long, filamentous shapes by failure to produce a septum; and to PBP-4 through PBP-6 (carboxypeptidases) leads to no lethal effects. Approximately 8% of a dose of benzylpenicillin binds to PCP-1, 0.7% to PCP-2, 2% to PBP-3, 4% to PBP-4, 65% to PBP-5, and 21% to PBP-6. Thus, the majority of the penicillin dose bonds to PBPs for which the function remains obscure. Binding to PBP-1 is lethal. Other β-lactam antibiotics display different binding patterns. Amoxicillin and the cephalosporins bind more avidly to PBP-1, methicillin and cefotaxime to PBP-2, and mezlocillin and cefuroxime to PBP-3. All these drugs are lethal to susceptible bacteria.

Resistance. The first literature reports of a penicillinase were published in 1940 and 1944. This phenomenon was rare at the time and caused no particular alarm. Today, unfortunately, resistance to β-lactam antibiotics is increasingly common and is rather alarming. It can be intrinsic and involve decreased cellular uptake of drug, or it can involve lower binding affinity to the PBPs. This is particularly the case with MRSA, the PBP-2 of which has been mutated so that it no longer efficiently binds methicillin. Much more common, however, is the elaboration of a β-lactamase. β-Lactamases are enzymes (serine proteases) elaborated by microorganisms that catalyze hydrolysis of the β-lactam bond and inactivate β-lactam antibiotics to penicilloic acids before they can reach the PCPs (Fig. 38.17). In this, they somewhat resemble the cell wall transamidase from which they may have arisen. Hydrolytic regeneration of the active site is dramatically more facile with β-lactamases than is the case with cell wall transamidase so that the enzyme can turn over many times and a comparatively small amount of enzyme can destroy a large amount of drug. With Gram-positive bacteria, such as staphylococci, the β-lactamases usually are shed continuously into the medium and meet the drug outside the cell wall (Fig. 38.9). Thus, they are biosynthesized in significant quantities. With Gram-negative bacteria, a more conservative course is followed. Here, the β-lactamases are secreted into the periplasmic space between the inner and outer membrane, so although still distal to the PBPs, they do not readily escape into the medium and need not be resynthesized as often (Fig. 38.11). Numerous β-lactamases with various antibiotic substrate specificities are now known. Various classification systems are used for them, as illustrated in Tables 38.8 and 38.9. Elaboration of β-lactamases often is R factor–mediated and, in some cases, is even induced by the presence of β-lactam antibiotics. One now generally assumes that a *Staphylococcus aureus* strain will produce a

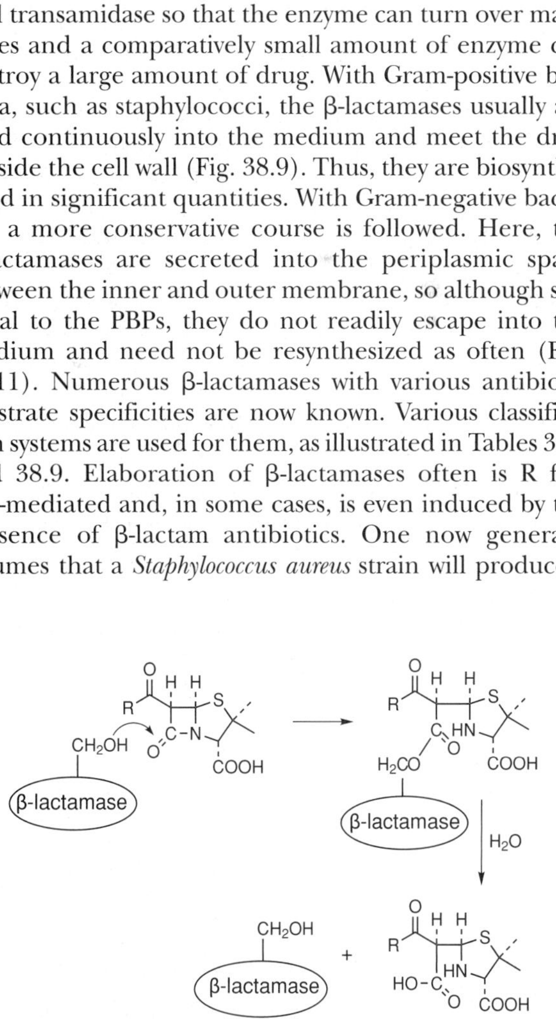

Fig. 38.17. β-Lactamase catalyzed hydrolysis of penicillins.

Table 38.8. β-lactamase Classifications According to Sykes and Matthew

Type	Substrate preferences	Gene location	Inducibility
Gram +/–	Penicillins mainly	r-Plasmid	Mostly
I	Cephalosponins mainly	Chromosome	Mainly
II	Penicillins mainly	Chromosome	Constituitive
III	Broad spectrum	r-Plasmid	Constituitive
IV	Broad spectrum	Chromosome	Constituitive
V	Methicillin, oxacillin, cloxacillin	r-Plasmid	Constituitive

Sykes RB, Matthew M. The beta-lactamases of gram-negative bacteria and their role in resistance to beta-lactam antibiotics. J Antimicrob Chemother 1976; 2: 115–117.

β-lactamase and that this will be less prevalent, but not uncommon, among *Haemophilus influenzae, Moraxella catarrhalis, Escherichia coli, and Klebsiella, Enterobacter, Serratia, Pseudomonas,* and *Bacteroides sp.* strains.

Allergenicity. Approximately 6 to 8% of the U.S. population is allergic to β-lactam antibiotics. Most commonly, this is expressed as a mild drug rash or itching and is of delayed onset. Occasionally, the reaction is immediate and profound. It may include cardiovascular collapse and shock and can even result in death. Sometimes, penicillin allergy can be anticipated by taking a medication history, and often, the patients who are likely to be allergic are those with a history of hypersensitivity to a wide variety of allergens (e.g., foods and pollens). A previous history of allergy to penicillins is a contraindicating factor to their use. Topical wheal-and-flare tests are available when there is doubt. When an allergic reaction develops, the drug must be discontinued, and, because cross-sensitivity is common, other β-lactam drugs should generally be avoided. Considering all therapeutic categories, penicillins, especially the ones most commonly employed (benzylpenicillin and ampicillin/amoxicillin), are probably the drugs most associated with allergy. Erythromycin and clindamycin are useful alternate choices for therapy in many cases of penicillin allergy.

In some cases, the patient may have become sensitized without knowing it because of previous passive exposure through contaminated foodstuffs or cross-contaminated medications. Penicillins are manufactured in facilities separate from those used to prepare other drugs to prevent cross-contamination and possible sensitization. Animals treated with penicillins are required to be drug-free for a significant time before products prepared from them can be consumed. The number of pharmacists who unknowingly override these protective measures by failing to cleanse their pill counters properly between prescriptions is unknown.

Because the origin of the allergy is a haptenic reaction with host proteins and the responsible bond in the drug is the β-lactam moiety, this side effect is caused by the pharmacophore of the drug and is unlikely to be overcome by molecular manipulation.

Table 38.9. β-Lactamase Classification According to Ambler[a] and Bush-Jacoby-Medeiros[b]

Class[a]	Characteristics
A	Penicillinases and TEM-type, broad-spectrum enzymes
B	Increased activity against cephalosporins
C	Chromosomal cephalosporinases of Gram-negative bacteria
D	Oxacillin-hydrolyzing enzymes
Group[b]	**Characteristics**
1	Cephalosporinases that are not inhibited by clavulanic acid
2	β-Lactamases inhibited by β-lactamase inhibitors
3	Metallo-β-lactamases that are poorly inhibited by all classical β-lactamase inhibitors
4	Penicillinases that are not inhibited by clavulanic acid

[a]Ambler RP. The structure of beta-lactamases. Phil Trans Royal Soc London B 1980;289:321–331.
[b]Bush K, Jacoby GA, Medeiros AA. A functional classification scheme for beta-lactamase and its correlation with molecular structure. Antimicrob Agents Chemother 1995;39:1211–1233.

Individual Penicillins. The penicillins usually are discussed under various groups based on spectrum of activity and sensitivity or resistance toward β-lactamase. One of the earliest and still most commonly used penicillin is benzylpenicillin.

Benzylpenicillin Group

BENZYLPENICILLIN (PENICILLIN G, TABLE 38.5). With the exception of *Neisseria gonorrhoeae* and *Haemophilus influenza* and a few bacteria encountered less frequently, the useful antimicrobial spectrum of benzylpenicillin is primarily against Gram-positive cocci. Because of its cheapness, efficacy, and lack of toxicity (except for acutely allergic patients), benzylpenicillin remains a remarkably useful agent for the treatment of diseases caused by susceptible microorganisms. As with most antibiotics, susceptibility tests must be performed, because many formerly highly sensitive microorganisms are now comparatively resistant. Infections of the upper and lower respiratory tract and of the genitourinary tract are the particular province of benzylpenicillin. Infections caused by group A β-hemolytic streptococci (pharyngitis, scarlet fever, cellulitis, pelvic infections, and septicemia) are commonly responsive. Group B hemolytic streptococci infections; especially of neonates (acute respiratory distress, pneumonia, meningitis, septic shock, and septicemia) usually respond. *Pneumococcal* pneumonia, *Haemophilus influenza* pneumonia of children, *Streptococcus pneumoniae*– and *Streptococcus pyogenes*–caused otitis media and sinusitis, meningococcal meningitis and brain abscess, meningococcal and pneumococcal septicemia, streptococcal endocarditis (often by *Streptococcus viridans*), pelvic inflammatory disease (often by *Neisseria gonorrhoeae* and *S. pyogenes*), uncomplicated gonorrhea (*N. gonorrhoeae*), meningitis (*Neisseria meningitidis*), syphilis (*Treponema pallidum*), Lyme disease (*Borrelia burgdorferi*), gas gangrene (*Clostridium perfringens*), and tetanus (*Clostridium tetani*) are among the diseases that commonly respond to benzylpenicillin therapy, either alone or sometimes with other drugs used in combination. Nonpenicillinase-producing *Staphylococcus aureus* and *Staphylococcus epidermidis* are quite sensitive but are all too rare today. Other, less common bacterial diseases also respond, such as those caused by *Bacillus anthracis* (anthrax) and *Corynebacterium diphtheriae* (diptheria).

Because of its cheapness, mild infections with susceptible microorganisms can be treated with comparatively large oral doses, although the most effective route of administration is parenteral, because fivefold the blood level can be regularly achieved in this manner. As previously indicated (see *Clinically relevant chemical instabilities* above), penicillin G is unstable under the acidic conditions of the stomach.

Very water-insoluble penicillin salts form with procaine and with N, N′-benzathine. These find therapeutic application for deep intramuscular (IM) injections. This produces lower but prolonged levels of penicillin as the drug slowly diffuses from the injection site.

The need to improve defects in benzylpenicillin stimulated an intense research effort that persists to this day. Overcoming such negative features as comparative instability (particularly to acid), comparatively poor oral absorption, allergenicity, sensitivity to β-lactamases, and relatively narrow antimicrobial spectrum have been objectives of this work. Only antigenicity has failed to respond significantly to this effort.

PHENOXYMETHYL PENICILLIN (PENICILLIN V, TABLE 38.5). Penicillin V is produced by fermentation in which the medium is enriched in phenoxyacetic acid. It also can be prepared by semisynthesis, and it is considerably more acid stable than benzylpenicillin, as indicated by oral absorption (Table 38.6). This is rationalized as being caused by the electronegative oxygen atom in the C-7 amide side chain inhibiting participation in β-lactam bond hydrolysis. In any case, penicillin V was the first of the so-called oral penicillins, giving higher and more prolonged blood levels than penicillin G itself. Its antimicrobial and clinical spectrum is roughly the same as that of benzylpenicillin, although it is somewhat less potent and is not, as a rule, used for acutely serious infections. Penicillin V has approximately the same sensitivity to β-lactamases and allergenicity as penicillin G.

Penicillinase-Resistant Parenteral Penicillins

METHICILLIN (TABLE 38.5). Although archaic today, methicillin was the first of the penicillinase-resistant agents to reach the clinic. It is unstable to gastric acid, having a half-life of 5 minutes at pH 2, so it must be administered via injection. As shown in Figure 38.15, increased bulk resulting from the addition of the dimethoxybenzoyl group to 6-APA leads to methicillin and a β-lactamase–resistant drug. Methicillin has a significantly narrower antimicrobial spectrum and less potency, so it was restricted to clinical use primarily for parenteral use in infections caused by β-lactamase—producing *Staphylococcus aureus* and a few other infections. Lately, an increasing number of infections have been found that are caused by MRSA. The mode of resistance in these cultures appears to be a reduced uptake and alteration in the PBPs. In particular, an altered PBP-2 is formed that has a very low affinity for β-lactams, including methicillin. Furthermore, methicillin is an efficient inducer of penicillinases, further counting against it. Consequently, this drug fell out of favor, and methicillin has now been supplanted by a number of agents.

NAFCILLIN (TABLE 38.3). Nafcillin has a fused benzene ring on one flank and an ethoxy moiety on the other of the side-chain amide linkage. Although slightly more acid stable than methicillin, it is virtually identical to it clinically.

OXACILLIN, CLOXACILLIN, AND DICLOXACILLIN. Using an isoxazolyl ring as a bio-isosteric replacement for the benzene ring and a methyl on one flank and a substituted benzene ring on the other in place of the methoxyls of methicillin produces the isoxazolyl penicillins. These are oxacillin, cloxacillin, and dicloxacillin (Table 38.5). Chemically, they differ from one another in the number of chlorine substituents on the benzene ring. Like methicillin, these generally are less potent than benzylpenicillin against Gram-positive microorganisms (generally staphylococci and streptococci) that do not produce a β-lactamase but retain their potency against those that do. An added bonus exists in that they are somewhat more acid stable. Thus, they may be taken orally, and they are more potent as well. Because they are highly serum protein bound (Table 38.7), they are not good choices for treatment of septicemia. Microorganisms resistant against methicillin generally also are resistant to the isoxazolyl group of penicillins.

Like nafcillin, the isoxazoyl group of penicillins is primarily used against *Staphylococcus aureus* in osteomyelitis, septicemia, endocarditis, and CNS infections.

Vancomycin (discussed later) is the current favorite for treatment of infections by MRSA with cotrimoxazole and rifampin often of value as well.

Penicillinase-Sensitive, Broad-Spectrum, Oral Penicillins

AMPICILLIN. The important first member of this group, ampicillin, is a benzylpenicillin analogue in which one of the hydrogen atoms of the side-chain methylene has been replaced with a primary amino group to produce an *R*-phenylglycine moiety (Table 38.5). In addition to significant acid stability, enhancing its successful oral use, the antimicrobial spectrum is shifted so that many common Gram-negative pathogens are sensitive to ampicillin. This is believed to result from greater penetration of ampicillin into Gram-negative bacteria. The acid stability generally is believed to be caused by the electron withdrawing character of the protonated primary amine group, reducing participation in hydrolysis of the β-lactam bond as well as to the comparative difficulty of bringing another positively charged species (H_3O^+) into the vicinity of the protonated amino group. The oral activity of ampicillin is abetted, in part, by active uptake assisted by the small intestine peptide carrier. Ampicillin has an apparent half-life of approximately 15 to 20 hours at pH 2.0 and 35°C. It unfortunately lacks stability toward β-lactamases, and resistance is an ever-increasing phenomenon. To assist in dealing with this, several additives for coadministration have been developed that inhibit the action of the β-lactamases (β-lactamase inhibitors).

In addition to the usual mode of penicillin allergenicity, concentrated preparations of ampicillin can self-condense to form high-molecular-weight aggregates through reaction of its primary amino group with the β-lactam bond of another molecule. These aggregates are thought to be antigenic and to be responsible for ampicillin allergenicity—a form of hypersensitivity that differs in some details from the usual penicillin allergenicity, which ampicillin also possesses. Ampicillin and amoxicillin are the penicillins most commonly associated with drug-induced rash. Avoiding use of old preparations is a somewhat effective means of dealing with this potential problem.

Ampicillin is essentially equivalent to benzylpenicillin for pneumococcal, streptococcal, and meningococcal infections, and many strains of Gram-negative *Salmonella, Shigella, Proteus mirabilis,* and *Escherichia coli,* as well as many strains of *Haemophilus influenzae* and *Neisseria gonorrhoeae,* respond well to oral treatment with ampicillin.

BACAMPICILLIN

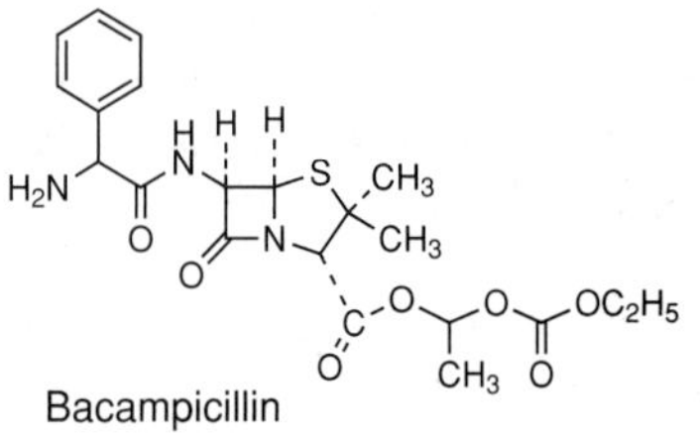

Bacampicillin

Although comparatively well absorbed (30–55%), the oral efficacy of ampicillin for systemic infections can be enhanced significantly through the preparation of pro-drugs. In contrast to ampicillin itself, which is amphoteric, bacampicillin is a weak base and is very well absorbed in the duodenum (80–98%). Enzymatic ester hydrolysis in the gut wall liberates carbon dioxide and ethanol, followed by spontaneous loss of acetaldehyde and production of ampicillin. The acetaldehyde is metabolized oxidatively by alcohol dehydrogenase to produce acetic acid, which joins the normal metabolic pool.

AMOXACILLIN (TABLE 38.5). Amoxicillin is a close analogue of ampicillin, in which a para-phenolic hydroxyl group has been introduced into the side-chain phenyl moiety. This adjusts the isoelectric point of the drug to a more acidic value, and this is believed to be partially responsible, along with the intestine peptide transporter, for the enhanced blood levels obtained with amoxicillin as compared to ampicillin itself (Table 38.6). Better oral absorption (74–92%) leads to less disturbance of the normal GI flora and, therefore, less drug-induced diarrhea. The antimicrobial spectrum and clinical uses of amoxicillin are approximately the same as those of ampicillin itself, and it is presently one of the most popular drugs in North America.

The addition of clavulanic acid (below) to amoxicillin (Augmentin) gives a combination in which the clavulanic acid serves to protect amoxicillin to a considerable extent against β-lactamases. This is now an extremely popular antimicrobial combination for outpatient use.

CLAVULANIC ACID

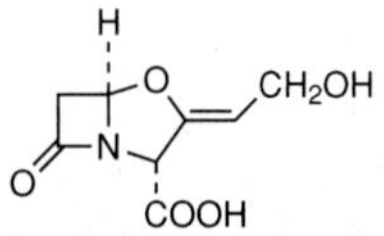

Clavulanic acid

Clavulanic acid is a mold product with only weak intrinsic antibacterial activity, but it is an excellent irreversible inhibitor of most β-lactamases. It is believed to acylate the active site serine by mimicking the normal substrate. Hydrolysis occurs with some β-lactamases, but in many cases, subsequent reactions occur that inhibit the enzyme irreversibly. This leads to its classification as a mechanism-based inhibitor (or so-called suicide substrate). The precise chemistry is not well understood (Fig. 38.18), but when clavulanic acid is added to ampicillin and amoxicillin preparations, the potency against β-lactamase–producing strains is markedly enhanced.

SULBACTAM

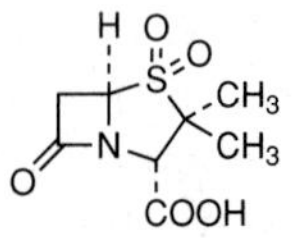

Sulbactam

Another β-lactamase–disabling agent is sulbactam. Sulbactam is prepared by partial chemical synthesis from penicillins. The oxidation of the sulfur atom to a sulfone greatly enhances the potency of sulbactam. The combination of sulbactam and ampicillin (Unasyn) is now clinically popular.

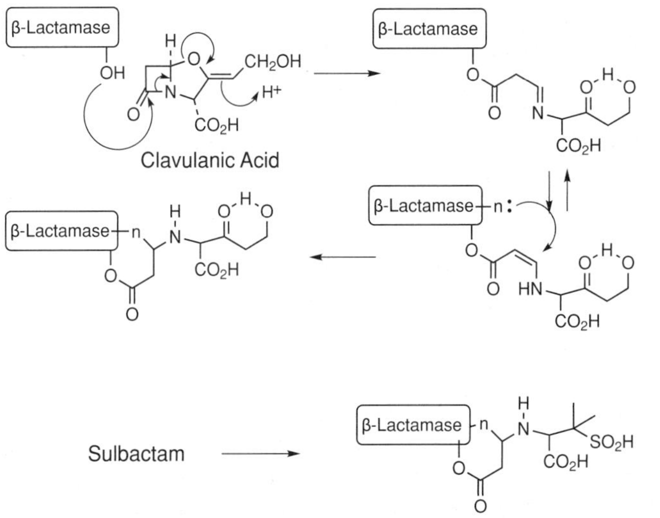

Fig. 38.18. Speculative mechanism for irreversible inactivation of β-lactamase by clavulanic acid and sulbactam.

If instead of a β-lactamase, ampicillin resistance is caused by a penetration barrier, clavulanic acid and sulbactam are not able to overcome this, because the underlying mechanism is different. Not all β-lactamases, however, are sensitive to the presence of clavulanic acid or to sulbactam.

Penicillinase-Sensitive, Broad-Spectrum, Parenteral Penicillins

MEZLOCILLIN AND PIPERACILLIN. Mezlocillin and piperacillin are ampicillin derivatives in which the D–side chain amino group has been converted by chemical processes to a variety of substituted urea analogues (Table 38.5). They are known as acylureidopenicillins. They preserve the useful anti-Gram-positive activity of ampicillin but have higher anti-Gram-negative potency. Even some strains of *Pseudomonas aeruginosa* are sensitive to these agents. It is speculated that the added side-chain moiety mimics a longer segment of the peptidoglycan chain than ampicillin does. It is recalled that this cell wall fragment usually is a tetrapeptide, so there certainly is room for an extension in this direction. This would give more possible attachment points to the penicillin biding proteins, and perhaps these features are responsible for their enhanced antibacterial properties. These agents are used parenterally with particular emphasis on Gram-negative bacteria, especially *Klebsiella pneumoniae* and the anaerobe *Bacteroides fragilis*. Resistance caused by β-lactamases is a prominent feature of their use, so disk testing and incorporation of additional agents (e.g., an aminoglycoside) for the treatment of severe infections is advisable.

PIPERACILLIN AND TAZOBACTAM COMBINATION (ZOSYN)

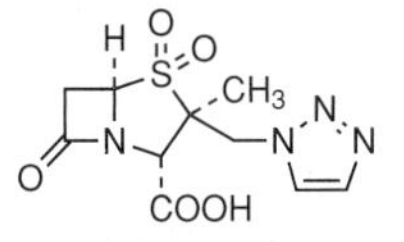

Tazobactam

Tazobactam often is coadministered with piperacillin because of tazobactam's ability to inhibit β-lactamases. Tazobactam, like other β-lactamase inhibitors, has little or no antibacterial activity. This effect is analogous to that of clavulanic acid and sulbactam (discussed above).

CARBENICILLIN AND INDANYL CARBENICILLIN. Carbenicillin is a benzylpenicillin analogue in which one of the methylene hydrogens of the side chain has been substituted with a carboxylic acid moiety (Table 38.5). The specific stereochemistry of this change is not very important, because both diastereoisomers are configurationally unstable and mutarotate with time to produce the same mixture of epimers. The introduction of the side-chain carboxyl produces enhanced anti-Gram-negative activity. In fact, carbenicillin is intrinsically one of the broadest spectrum penicillins. Carbenicillin is an order of magnitude less potent than the acylureidopenicillins. The drug is susceptible to β-lactamases and is acid unstable, so it must be given by injection.

Because it is a malonic acid hemiamide with a carbonyl (amide) moiety β to the carboxyl group, carbenicillin can decarboxylate readily to produce benzylpenicillin (Fig. 38.19). Although still an antibiotic, this degradation product has no activity against the organisms for which carbenicillin would be indicated, so this is still considered to be a degradation. In addition, the large doses of carbenicillin sodium that had to be employed (multigrams per day) resulted in ingestion of a significant amount of sodium ion, which could be a consideration with heart patients. Many of these problems were avoided by switching to the oral prodrug ester indanyl carbenicillin. This pro-drug is primarily used for oral treatment of urinary tract infections.

TICARCILLIN. Ticarcillin is a sulfur-based bio-isostere of carbenicillin that cannot decarboxylate as the carboxyl group of carbenicillin does (Table 38.5). This agent is somewhat more potent against pseudomonads compared with indanyl carbenicillin.

When potassium clavulanate is added to ticarcillin (Timentin), the combination has enhanced antipsedomonad activity because of its enhanced stability to lactamases.

Summary Statement. The penicillins ushered in the era of powerful antibiotics, and their use transformed the practice of antimicrobial chemotherapy. A significant percentage of the population alive today owe their

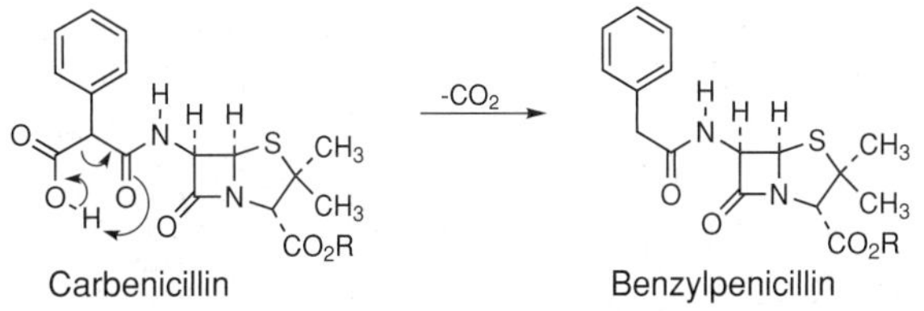

Carbenicillin → Benzylpenicillin ($-CO_2$)

Fig. 38.19. Decarboxylation of carbenicillin to benzylpenicillin.

longevity and relative freedom from morbidity to the use of these agents. The pace of discovery, however, has fallen off dramatically, and no new penicillin has been introduced into the market place for many years. The penicillins retain their important place in contemporary medicine, but research has turned elsewhere for novel agents.

Cephalosporins

History. In contrast to the discovery of the penicillins, in which the first agent had such outstanding biological antibiotic properties that it entered clinical use with comparatively little modification, the cephalosporins are remarkable for the level of persistence that was required before their initial discovery yielded economic returns. The original cephalosporin-producing fungus, *Cephalosporium acremonium,* was discovered in a sewage outfall off the Sardinian coast by Brotsu. In England, Abraham and Newton pursued it, because one of the constituents had the useful property of activity against penicillin-resistant cultures as a result of its stability to β-lactamases. Cephalosporin C, the component of special interest, is not potent enough to be a useful antibiotic, but removal, through chemical means, of the natural side chain produced 7-aminocephalosporanic acid (7-ACA), which, analogous to 6-APA, could be fitted with unnatural side chains (Fig. 38.20). Many of the compounds produced in this way are remarkably useful antibiotics. They differ from one another in antimicrobial spectrum, β-lactamase stability, absorption from the GI tract, metabolism, stability, and side effects (detailed below). Exploitation of sulfenic acid chemistry by Robert Morin, then at Eli Lilly and Company, resulted in the conversion of penicillins to cephalosporins, including 3-desacetoxy-7-ACA (7-ADCA). This process is practical because the penicillin fermentation is much more efficient than cephalosporin fermentation, making the transformation financially rewarding. Unfortunately, the chemistry involved is too complex to be covered in the space available here. Intensive investigation of the chemistry of 7-ACA and 7-ADCA has resulted in the subsequent preparation of many thousands of analogues from these two starting materials.

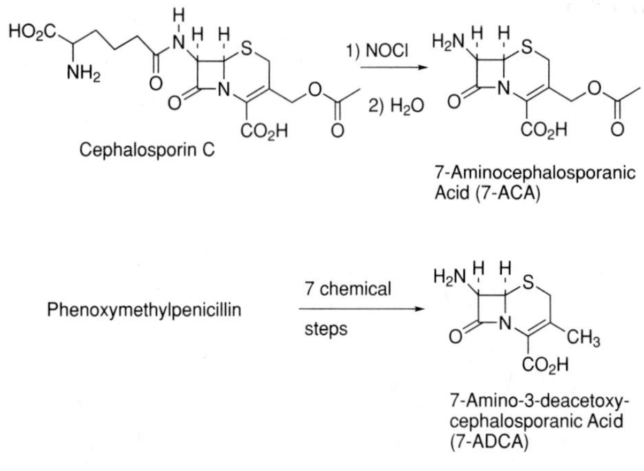

Cephalosporin C

1) NOCl

2) H_2O

7-Aminocephalosporanic Acid (7-ACA)

Phenoxymethylpenicillin

7 chemical steps

7-Amino-3-deacetoxy-cephalosporanic Acid (7-ADCA)

Fig. 38.20. Chemical preparation of 7-ACA and 7-ADCA.

Chemical Properties. The cephalosporins have their β-lactam ring annealed to a 6-membered dihydrothiazine ring in contrast to the penicillins, wherein the β-lactam ring is fused to a 5-membered thiazolidine ring. As a consequence of the bigger ring, the cephalosporins should be less strained and less reactive/potent. Much of the reactivity loss, however, is made up by possession of an olefinic linkage at C-2,3 and a methyleneacetoxy group at C-3. When the β-lactam ring is opened by hydrolysis, the acetoxy group can be ejected, carrying away the developing negative charge. This greatly reduces the energy required for the process. Thus, the facility with which the β-lactam bond of the cephalosporins is broken is modulated both by the nature of the C-7 substituent (analogous to the penicillins) as well as by the nature of the C-3 substituent and its ability to serve as a leaving group. Considerable support for this hypothesis comes from the finding that isomerization of the olefinic linkage to C-3,4 leads to great losses in antibiotic activity. In practice, most cephalosporins are comparatively unstable in aqueous solutions, and the pharmacist often is directed to keep injectable preparations frozen before use. Being carboxylic acids, they form water-soluble sodium salts, whereas the free acids are comparatively water insoluble. In many cases, when the free acids are supplied, the injectable forms contain sodium bicarbonate to facilitate solution.

Clinically Relevant Chemical Instabilities. The principal chemical instability of the cephalosporins is associated with β-lactam bond hydrolysis. The role of the C-7 and C-3 side chains in these reactions was discussed previously. Ejection of the C-3 substituent following β-lactam bond cleavage usually is drawn for convenience as though this is an unbroken (concerted) process. Evidence on this point being equivocal, ejection of the side chain may, at certain times and with specific cephalosporins, involve a discrete intermediate with the β-lactam bond broken, but with the C-3 substituent not yet eliminated, whereas other cephalosporins have nonejectable C-3 substituents. The methylthiotetrazole (MTT) group, found in a number of cephalosporins, is capable of elimination. When this happens, this moiety is believed to be responsible, in part, for clotting difficulties and acute alcohol intolerance in certain patients. The role of the C-7 side chain in all of these processes is clearly important, but active participation of the amide moiety in a manner analogous to the penicillins rarely is specifically invoked. The same considerations that modulate the chemical stability of cephalosporins also are involved in dictating β-lactamase sensitivity, potency, and allergenicity as well.

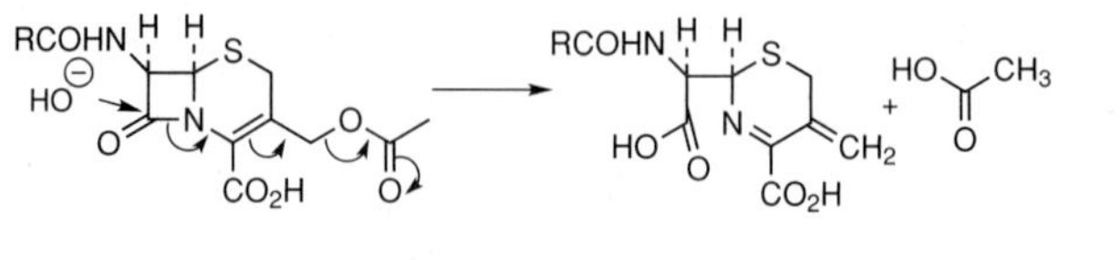

Metabolism. Those cephalosporins that have an acetyl group in the side chain are subject to enzymatic hydrolysis

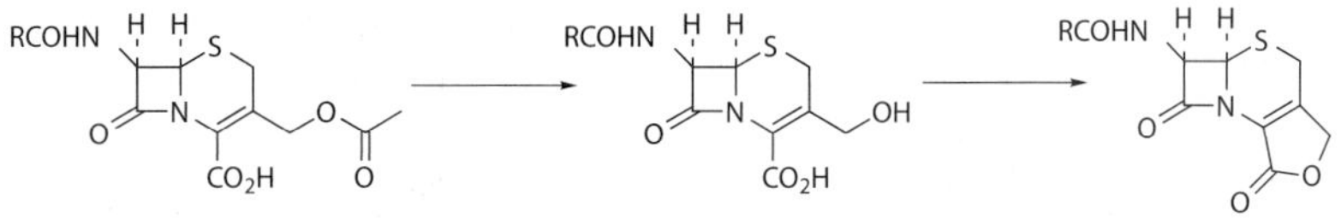

Fig. 38.21. Metabolism of C-3-acetyl-substituted cephalosporins.

in the body. The result is molecules with a hydroxymethyl moiety at C-3. A hydroxy moiety is a poor leaving group, so this change is considerably deactivating with respect to breakage of the β-lactam bond. In addition, the particular geometry of this part of the molecule leads to facile lactonization with the carboxyl group attached to C-2 (Fig. 38.21). In principle, this should result in formation of a different but reasonable leaving group; instead, the result is inactivation of the drugs involved. The penicillin biding proteins have an absolute requirement for a free carboxyl group to mimic that of the terminal carboxyl of the D-alanyl-D-alanine moiety in their normal substrate. Lactonization masks this docking functional group and, as a result, blocks affinity of the inhibitor for the enzyme.

Structure-Activity Relationship

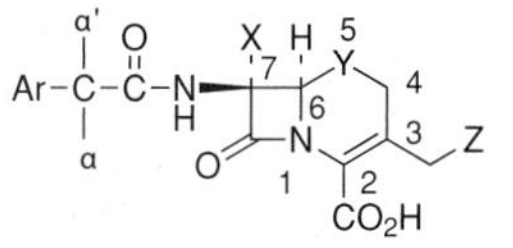

As with the penicillins, various molecular changes in the cephalosporin can improve in vitro stability, antibacterial activity, and stability toward β-lactamases. The addition of an amino and a hydrogen to the α and α′ position, respectively, results in a basic compound that is protonated under the acidic conditions of the stomach. The ammonium ion improves the stability of the β-lactam of the cephalosporin, leading to orally active drugs.

The 7β amino group is essential for antimicrobial activity (X = H), whereas replacement of the hydrogen at C-7 (X = H) with an alkoxy (X = OR) results in improvement of the antibacterial activity of the cephalosporin. Within specific cephalosporin derivatives, the addition of a 7α methoxy also improves the drugs stability toward β-lactamase. The derivatives where Y = S exhibit greater antibacterial activity than if Y = O, but the reverse is true when stability toward β-lactamase is considered. The 6α hydrogen is essential for biological activity. Finally, antibacterial activity is improved when Z is a 5-membered heterocycle versus a 6-membered heterocycle.

In a study examining the stability of cephalosporins toward β-lactamase, it was noted that the following changes improved β-lactamase resistance: 1) The L-isomer of an α amino α′ hydrogen derivative of a cephalosporin was 30- to 40-fold more stable than the D-isomer, 2) the addition of a methoxyoxime to the α and α′ positions increased stability nearly 100-fold, and 3) the Z-oxime was as much as 20,000-fold more stable than the E-oxime (Fig. 38.22). These changes have been incorporated into a number of marketed and experimental cephalosporins (Cefuroxime, Ceftizoxime, Ceftazidime, and Cefixime).

Mechanism of Action. The cephalosporins are believed to act in a manner analogous to that of the penicillins by binding to the penicillin biding proteins, followed by cell lysis (Fig. 38.16). The full details of the manner in which bacterial cells are killed are still obscure. Cephalosporins are bactericidal in clinical terms.

Resistance. Analogous to the penicillins, susceptible cephalosporins can be hydrolyzed by β-lactamases before they reach the penicillin biding proteins. Many β-lactamases are known. Some are more efficient at hydrolysis of penicillins, some at hydrolysis of cephalosporins and some are indiscriminate. Certain β-lactamases are constitutive (chromosomally encoded) in certain strains of Gram-negative bacteria (*Citrobacter, Enterobacter, Pseudomonas,* and *Serratia* sp.) and normally are repressed. These are induced (or derepressed) by certain β-lactam antibiotics (e.g., imipenem, cefotetam, and cefoxitin). As with the penicillins, specific examples will be seen below wherein resistance to β-lactamase hydrolysis is conveyed by strategic steric bulk near the side-chain amide linkage. Recently, an increasing number of metallo-β-lactamases have been discovered. The mechanism of these enzymes is dependent on divalent metal ions, commonly zinc. These are both chromosomally and plasmid derived and are as yet confined to the Gram-negative rods. Commonly, these enzymes attack some penicillins, cephalosporins, and carbapenems. Penetration barriers to the cephalosporins also are well known.

Allergenicity. Allergenicity is less commonly experienced and is less severe with cephalosporins than with penicillins. Cephalosporins frequently are administered to patients who have had a mild or delayed penicillin reaction. Cross-allergenicity is comparatively common, however, and cephalosporins should be administered with caution for patients who have a history of allergies. Patients who have had a rapid and severe reaction to penicillins should not be treated with cephalosporins.

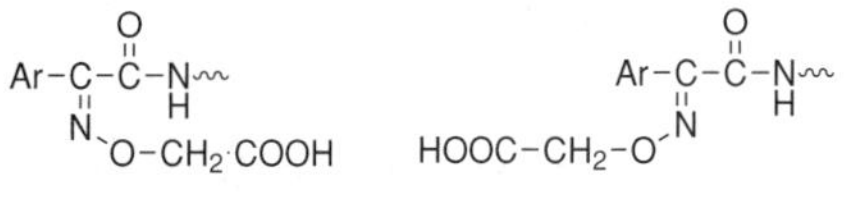

Z-oxime E-oxime

Fig. 38.22. Z- and E-oxime configuration.

Nomenclature and Classification. Most cephalosporins have generic names beginning with cef- or ceph-. This is convenient for classification, but it makes discriminating between individual members a true memory test. The cephalosporins are classified by a trivial nomenclature system loosely derived from the chronology of their introduction but more closely related to their antimicrobial spectrum. The first-generation cephalosporins primarily are active in vitro against Gram-positive cocci (penicillinase-positive and -negative *Staphylococcus aureus* and *S. epidermis*), group A β-hemolytic streptococci (*Streptococcus pyogenes*), group B streptococci (*Streptococcus agalactiae*), and *Streptococcus pneumoniae.* They are not effective against MRSA. They are not significantly active against Gram-negative bacteria, although some strains of *Escherichia coli, Klebsiella pneumoniae, Proteus mirabilis,* and *Shigella* sp. may be sensitive. The second-generation cephalosporins generally retain the anti-Gram-positive activity of the first-generation agents but include *Haemophilus influenzae* as well and add to this better anti-Gram-negative activity so that some strains of *Acinetobacter, Citrobacter, Enterobacter, Escherichia coli, Klebsiella, Neisseria, Proteus, Providencia,* and *Serratia* also are sensitive. Cefotetan, cefmetazole, and cefoxitin have some antianaerobic activity as well. The third-generation cephalosporins are less active against staphylococci than the first-generation agents but are much more active against Gram-negative bacteria than either the first- or the second-generation drugs. They frequently are particularly useful against nosocomial multidrug-resistant hospital-acquired strains. One also adds *Morganella* sp. and *Pseudomonas aeruginosa* to the list of species that often are sensitive. Unfortunately, the third-generation agents tend to be more expensive. The fourth-generation cephalosporins have an antibacterial spectrum like the third-generation drugs but add some enterobacteria that are resistant to the third-generation cephalosporins. They also are more active against some Gram-positive organisms.

Therapeutic Application. The incidence of cephalosporin resistance is such that it usually is preferable to do sensitivity disk testing before instituting therapy. Infections of the upper and lower respiratory tract, skin and related soft tissue, urinary tract, bones, and joints, as well as septicemias, endocarditis, intra-abdominal, and bile tract infections caused by susceptible Gram-positive organisms usually are responsive to cephalosporins. When a Gram-positive bacteria is involved, a first-generation agent is preferable. When the pathogen is Gram-negative and the infection is serious, parenteral use of a third-generation agent is recommended. For pelvic inflammatory disease, the number-one cause of sterility in sexually active young women, a combination with doxycycline is preferred. This infection often is mixed and frequently includes *Chlamydia trachomitis,* anaerobes, and penicillinase-producing *Neisseria gonorrhoeae.*

Adverse Effects. Aside from mild or severe allergic reaction, the most commonly experienced cephalosporin toxicities are mild and temporary nausea, vomiting, and diarrhea associated with disturbance of the normal flora. Rarely, a life-threatening pseudomembranous colitis diarrhea associated with the opportunistic and toxin-producing anaerobic pathogen, *Clostridium difficile,* can be experienced. Rare blood dyscrasias, which can even include aplastic anemia, also are seen. Certain structural types (details below) are associated with prolonged bleeding times and an antabuse-like acute alcohol intolerance.

First-generation Cephalosporins (Table 38.10)

Cephapirin. Cephapirin has a pyridylthiomethylene containing side chain at C-7. It is comparatively resistant to

Table 38.10. First Generation Cephalosporins

RCOHN, H, H, S, N, O, X, CO_2H

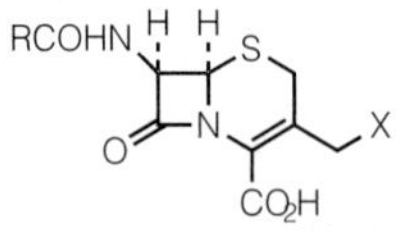

Generic names	Trade names	R	X	Salt
Parenteral Agents:				
Cephapirin	Cefadyl	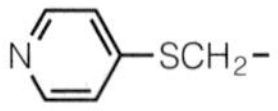 N, SCH_2–	OAc	Na
Cefazolin	Ancef, Kefzol, Zolicef	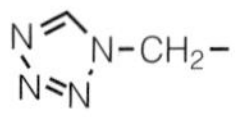 N, N, N, N–CH_2–	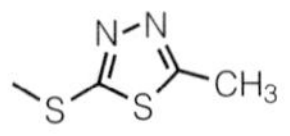 S, S, N–N, CH_3	Na
Oral Agents:				
Cephalexin	Keflex, Biocef Keftab	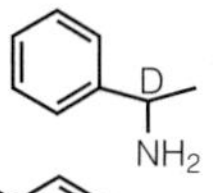 D, NH_2	H	HCl
Cefadroxil	Duricef	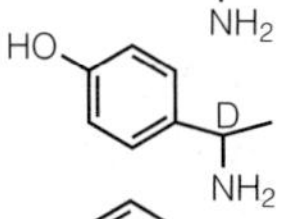 HO, D, NH_2	H	-
Oral and Parenteral Agent:				
Cephradine	Velosef	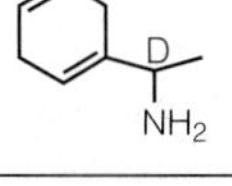 D, NH_2	H	-

staphylococcal β-lactamase, although it is sensitive to many other β-lactamases. Cephapirin also is sensitive to host deacetylation in the liver, kidneys, and plasma, which reduces potency by about half. Nonetheless, it finds significant use in the parenteral treatment of infections because of susceptible bacteria. It is a substitute for the nafcillin subgroup of penicillins. It is not orally active. It is comparatively painful on IM injection, and its doses must be reduced in the presence of renal impairment. Following injection, it is excreted primarily in the urine, partly by glomerular filtration and partly by tubular secretion.

Cefazolin. Cefazolin has the natural acetyl side chain at C-3 replaced by a thio-linked thiadiazole ring. Although this group is an activating leaving group, the moiety is not subject to the inactivating host hydrolysis reaction that characterizes cephapirin. At C-7, it possesses a tetrazoylmethylene unit. Cefazolin is less irritating on injection than its cohort in this generation of drugs and has a longer half-life than cephapirin. Its dosing should be reduced in the presence of renal impairment. It is comparatively unstable and should be protected from heat and light.

Cephalexin. Use of the ampicillin-type side chain conveys oral activity to cephalexin. Whereas it no longer has an activating side chain at C-3 and, as a consequence, is somewhat less potent, it does not undergo metabolic deactivation and, thus, maintains potency. It is rapidly and completely absorbed from the GI tract and has become quite popular. Somewhat puzzling is the fact that the use of the ampicillin side chain in the cephalosporins does not result in a comparable shift in antimicrobial spectrum. Cephalexin, like the other first-generation cephalosporins is active against many Gram-positive aerobic cocci but is limited against Gram-negative bacteria. It is a widely used drug, particularly against Gram-negative bacteria causing urinary tract infections, Gram-positive infections (*Staphylococcus aureus, Streptococcus pneumoniae* and *Streptococcus pyogenes*) of soft tissues, pharyngitis, and minor wounds.

Cefadroxil. Cefadroxil has an amoxicillin-like side chain at C-7 and is orally active. There are some indications that cefadroxil has some immunostimulant properties mediated through T-cell activation and that this is of material assistance to patients in fighting infections. The prolonged biological half-life of cefadroxil allows once-a-day dosage.

Cephradine. In cephradine, an interesting drug design device has been used. The aromatic ring in the ampicillin side chain has been partially hydrogenated by a Birch reduction such that the resulting molecule is still planar and π-electron excessive but has no conjugated olefinic linkages. It is comparatively acid stable and, therefore, is rapidly and nearly completely absorbed from the GI tract. Cephradine has the useful characteristic that it can be used both orally and IM so that parenteral therapy can be started in an institutional setting and then the patient can be sent home with the oral form, thus avoiding the risk of having to establish a different antibiotic. This is consistent with the present economics requiring sending patients home earlier than some physicians prefer. Unfortunately, however, for other reasons the IM and intravenous (IV) versions of cephradine are no longer available in the United States.

Second-Generation Cephalosporins (Table 38.11)

Cefamandole nafate. Cefamandole nafate has a formylated D-mandelic amide moiety at C-7. The formate ester is cleaved rapidly in the host to release the more active cefamandole. The esterification also apparently overcomes the instability of cefamandole when it is stored in dry form. This agent has increased activity against *Haemophilus influenzae* and some Gram-negative bacilli as compared with the first-generation cephalosporins. Loss of the 5-thio-l-methyl-l-H-tetrazole moiety (referred to sometimes by the acronym MTT) from C-3 is associated with prothrombin deficiency and bleeding problems as well as with an Antabuse-like acute alcohol intolerance. On the other hand, this grouping enhances potency and prevents metabolism by deacetylation. Like the other second-generation cephalosporins, cefamandole is more active against Gram-negative bacteria. The principle clinical use is for lower respiratory tract, skin and skin structures, and bone and joint infections as well as septicemia and urinary tract infections when the organisms are sensitive.

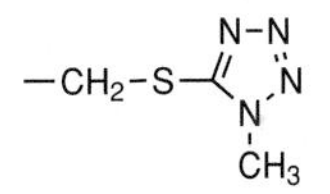

N–N
$-CH_2-S-$ (tetrazole ring) N
N
CH_3

MTT

Cefonicid. Cefonicid has an unesterified D-mandelic acid moiety at C-7 and a methylsulfothiotetrazole group at C-3. The latter is related to the MTT moiety mentioned above under cefamandole nafate; however, the clotting problems and Antabuse-like side effects associated with MTT have not been reported with cefonicid. The extra acid group in the C-3 side chain leads to this molecule being sold as an injectable disodium salt. Pain and discomfort at IM sites is experienced by some patients, as is a burning sensation and phlebitis. Cefonicid has a longer half-life than the other members of its group but achieves this at the price of somewhat lower potency against Gram-positive bacteria and aerobes. The drug is somewhat unstable, needs to be protected from light and heat, and may yellow or darken. If modest, however, this does not necessarily mean that the potency has decreased significantly, but overt precipitation does. Kirby-Bauer disk testing may overestimate the sensitivity of β-lactamase–producing bacteria to this agent, so some extra caution in interpretation of laboratory results is required.

Cefuroxime. Cefuroxime has a *Z*-oriented methoxyimino moiety as part of its C-7 side chain (Fig. 38.22). This conveys

Table 38.11. Second Generation Cephalosporins

Generic name	Trade name	R	X	Y	Z	Salt
Parenteral Agents						
Cefamandole nafate	Mandol	phenyl-CH(OCHO)- (D)	$-CH_2 \cdot S$-(1-methyltetrazol-5-yl) (MTT)	H	S	-
Cefonicid	Monocid	phenyl-CH(OH)- (D)	$-CH_2 \cdot S$-(1-(HO_3S-methyl)tetrazol-5-yl)	H	S	diNa
Cefuroxime	Ceftin Kefurox Zinacef	2-furyl-C(=$NOCH_3$)-	$-CH_2OCONH_2$	H	S	Na
Cefoxitin	Mefoxin	2-thienyl-CH_2-	$-CH_2OCONH_2$	OCH_3	S	Na
Cefotetan	Cefotan	(H_2NOC)(HO_2C)C=(1,3-dithietan-2-yl)-	MTT	OCH_3	S	diNa
Cefmetazole	Zefazone	$N{\equiv}C-CH_2-S-CH_2-$	MTT	OCH_3	S	Na
Oral Agents						
Cefaclor	Ceclor	phenyl-CH(NH_2)- (D)	Cl	H	S	-
Loracarbef	Lorabid	phenyl-CH(NH_2)- (D)	Cl	H	CH_2	-
Cefprozil	Cefzil	4-HO-phenyl-CH(NH_2)- (D)	$-CH=CH-CH_3$	H	S	-

considerable resistance to attack by many β-lactamases, but not by all. This is believed to result from the steric demands of this group. This hypothesis is supported by the finding that the *E*-analogue is attacked by β-lactamases. Resistance by *Pseudomonas aeruginosa*, on the other hand, is attributed to lack of penetration of the drug rather than to enzymatic hydrolysis. The carbamoyl moiety at C-3 is intermediate in metabolic stability between the classic acetyl moieties and the thiotetrazoles. Cefuroxime penetrates comparatively well into cerebral spinal fluid and is used in cases of *Haemophilus influenzae* meningitis.

In the form of its axetil ester (1-[acetyloxy]ethyl ester) pro-drug, cefuroxime axetil, a more lipophilic drug is produced that gives satisfactory blood levels on oral administration. The ester bond is cleaved metabolically, and the resulting intermediate form loses acetaldehyde spontaneously to produce cefuroxime itself. Conveniently for the patient, cefuroxime axetil is stable for approximately 24 hours when it is dissolved in apple juice. The axetil is the only antibiotic officially labeled for treatment of Lyme disease (although doxycycline often is the first choice even without a label indication for that purpose).

Cefuroxime axetil

Cefoxitin. Cefoxitin contains the same C-7 side chain as cephalothin and the same C-3 side chain as cefuroxime. The most novel chemical feature of cefoxitin is the possession of an α-oriented methoxyl group in place of the normal H-atom at C-7. This increased steric bulk conveys very significant stability against β-lactamases. The inspiration for these functional groups was provided by the discovery of the naturally occurring antibiotic cephamycin C derived from fermentation of *Streptomyces lactamdurans*. Cephamycin C itself has not seen clinical use but, rather, has provided the structural clue that led to useful agents such as cefoxitin. Agents that contain this 7α methoxy group are commonly referred to as cephamycins. Ingenious chemical transformations now enable synthetic introduction of such a methoxy group into cephalosporins lacking this feature.

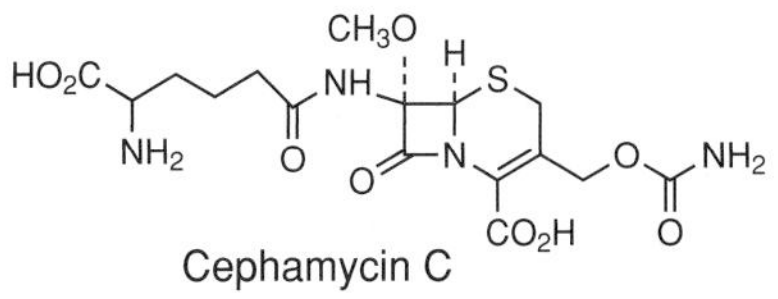

Cephamycin C

Cefoxitin has useful activity against gonorrhea and some anaerobic infections as compared with its second-generation relatives. On the negative side, cefoxitin has the capacity to induce certain broad-spectrum β-lactamases.

Cefotetan. Clearly, cefotetan also is inspired by cephamycin C but has a rather unusual sulfur-containing C-7 side-chain amide. Possession of two carboxyl groups leads to marketing it as a disodium salt. The C-3 MTT side chain suggests caution in monitoring prothrombin levels and bleeding times as well as in ingesting alcohol when using this agent. Like cefoxitin, cefotetan has better activity than the rest of this group against anaerobes. Cefotetan is comparatively stable, lasting for approximately 24 hours at room temperature when reconstituted. Slight yellowing and slight darkening produce materials that are still acceptable for therapy. Cefotetan is chemically incompatible with tetracycline, aminoglycosides, and with heparin, often forming precipitates with them. With respect to its molecular mode of action, it has a special affinity for PBP-3 of Gram-negative bacteria, consequently producing filamentous forms. It also binds well with PBP-1A and -1B, therefore leading to cell lysis and death. Whereas it is stable to a wide range of β-lactamases, it also is a potent inducer in some bacteria.

Cefaclor. Cefaclor differs from cephalexin primarily in the bio-isosteric replacement of methyl by chlorine at C-3 and is quite acid stable, allowing oral administration. It also is quite stable to metabolism. It is less active against Gram-negative bacteria compared with the other second-generation cephalosporins but is more active against Gram-negative bacteria compared with the first-generation drugs.

Loracarbef. Loracarbef is a synthetic C-5 "carba" analogue of cefaclor. The smaller methylene moiety (as compared to sulfur) would be expected to make loracarbef more reactive/potent, and this seems to be the case. It is more stable chemically, however, and this adds to its virtues. Diarrhea is the most common adverse effect with loracarbef and, along with certain other adverse effects, is seen more frequently with children, so this lessens enthusiasm for the drug in patients younger than 12 years.

Cefprozil. Cefprozil has an amoxicillin-like side chain at C-7, but at C-3, there is now a l-propenyl group conjugated with the double bond in the 6-membered ring. The double bond is present in its two geometric isomeric forms, both of which are antibacterially active. Fortunately, the predominant trans form (Table 38.11) is much more active against Gram-negative organisms. Cefprozil most closely resembles cefaclor in its properties but is a little more potent. It is approximately 90% bioavailable following oral administration, and peak levels are not significantly smaller when taken with food. The oral suspension of cefprozil is sweetened with aspartame, so phenylketonuric patients should be wary of this formulation.

Cefmetazole. Cefmetazole is a cephamycin with a nonaromatic side chain at C-7. In addition to a fairly characteristic second-generation cephalosporin antimicrobial spectrum, it possess fairly significant anti-antiaerobic activity. The ejection of its C-3 side chain leads to alcohol intolerance of the disulfuram type and prolonged clotting times.

Third-Generation Cephalosporins (Table 38.12)

Cefotaxime. Cefotaxime, like cefuroxime, has a *Z*-methoxyimino moiety at C-7 that conveys significant β-lactamase resistance. Microorganisms that produce chromosomally mediated β-lactamases usually are resistant following mutation to derepression of these enzymes. Cefoxitin, cefotetan, and imipenems are quite effective inducers of these enzymes. The enzymes that result either hydrolyze the drug in the usual way or bind tightly to them, preventing them from attaching to the PBPs. The clinical importance of this phenomenon is unclear.

The oxime moiety of cefotaxime is connected to an aminothiazole ring. Like other third-generation cephalosporins, it has excellent anti-Gram-negative activity and is useful institutionally. It has a metabolically vulnerable acetoxy group attached to C-3 and loses approximately 90% of its activity when this is hydrolyzed. This metabolic feature also complicates the pharmacokinetic data, because both active forms are present and have different properties. Cefotaxime should be protected from heat and light and may color slightly without significant loss of potency. Like other third-generation cephalosporins, cefotaxime has less activity against staphylococci but has greater activity against Gram-negative organisms.

Ceftizoxime. In ceftizoxime, the whole C-3 side chain has been omitted to prevent deactivation by hydrolysis. It rather resembles cefotaxime in its properties; however, not being subject to metabolism, its pharmacokinetic properties are much less complex.

Ceftriaxone. Ceftriaxone has the same C-7 side-chain moiety as cefotaxime and ceftizoxime, but the C-3 side chain consists of a metabolically stable and activating thiotriazinedione in place of the normal acetyl group. The C-3 side chain is sufficiently acidic that at normal pH, it forms an enolic sodium salt; thus, the commercial

Table 38.12. Third Generation Cephalosporins

(General structure: RCOHN, H H, S, O, N, X, COOH)

Generic name	Trade name	R	X	Salt
Parenteral Agents				
Cefotaxime	Claforan	N-OCH_3; H_2N, N, S	CH_2OAc	Na
Ceftizoxime	Cefizox	N-OCH_3; H_2N, N, S	H	Na
Ceftriaxone	Rocephin	N-OCH_3; H_2N, N, S	-CH_2S; CH_3, N, N, N, OH, O	diNa
Ceftazidime	Fortaz Ceptaz Tazidime Tazicef	CH_3, N-O-C-COOH, CH_3; H_2N, N, S	⊕ N (pyridinium)	H or Na
Cefoperazone	Cefobid	HO, D, NH; C_2H_5-N, N, O, O, O	—CH_2-S; N, N, N-N, H_3C	Na
Oral Agents				
Cefixime	Suprax	N-OCH_2CO_2H; H_2N, N, S	-HC=CH_2	-
Ceftibuten	Cedax	CH_2CO_2H; H_2N, N, S	H	-
Cefpodoxime proxetil (2-carboxyester= -O, O, O, CH_3, CH_3O, CH_3)	Vantin	N-OCH_3; H_2N, N, S	-CH_2OCH_3	-
Cefdinir	Omnicef	N-OH; H_2N, N, S	-HC=CH_2	-
Cefditoren pivoxil (2-carboxyester= -O, O, C$(CH_3)_3$, O)	Spectracef	N-OCH_3; H_2N, N, S	H, C=CH; S, N, CH_3	-

product is a disodium salt. It is useful for many severe infections and, notably, in the treatment of some meningitis infections caused by Gram-negative bacteria. It is quite stable to many β-lactamases but is sensitive to some inducible chromosomal β-lactamases.

Ceftazidime. In ceftazidime the oxime moiety is more complex, containing two methyl groups and a carboxylic acid. This assemblage conveys even more pronounced β-lactamase stability, greater anti–*Pseudomonas aeruginosa*, and increased activity against Gram-positive organisms. The C-3 side chain has been replaced by a charged pyridinium moiety. The latter considerably enhances water solubility and also highly activates the β-lactam bond toward cleavage. The drug must be protected against heat and light and may darken without significant loss of potency. It is not stable under some conditions. such as the presence of aminoglycosides and vancomycin. It also is attacked readily in sodium bicarbonate solutions. Resistance is mediated by chromosomally mediated β-lactamases and by lack of penetration into target bacteria. Otherwise, it has a very broad antibacterial spectrum.

Cefoperazone. Cefoperazone has a C-7 side chain reminiscent of piperacillin's and also possesses the C-3 side chain (MTT) that often is associated with the bleeding and alcohol intolerance problems among patients taking cephalosporins. Its useful activity against pseudomonads partly compensates for this, although it is not potent enough to be used as a single agent against this difficult pathogen. The C-7 side chain does not convey sufficient resistance to many β-lactamases, although the addition of clavulanic acid or sulbactam would presumably help.

There are comparatively few orally active third-generation agents. This group currently is represented by ceftibuten, cefixime, cefdinir, and cefpodoxime proxetil.

Cefixime. In cefixime, in addition to the β-lactamase–stabilizing *Z*-oximino acidic ether at C-7, the C-3 side chain is a vinyl group analogous to the propenyl group of cefprozil. This is believed to contribute strongly to the oral activity of the drug. Cefixime has anti-Gram-negative activity that is intermediate between that of the second- and third-generation agents described previously. It is poorly active against staphylococci, because it does not bind satisfactorily to PBP-2.

Ceftibuten. Ceftibuten has a *Z*-ethylidinecarboxyl group at C-7 instead of the *Z*-oximino ether linkages seen previously. This conveys enhanced β-lactamase stability and may contribute to oral activity as well. Ceftibuten has no C-3 side chain, so it is not measurably metabolized. It is highly (75–90%) absorbed on oral administration, but this is decreased significantly by food. Being lipophilic and acidic, it is significantly (65%) serum protein bound. Some isomerization of the geometry of the olefinic linkage appears to take place in vivo before excretion. It is mainly used for respiratory tract infections, otitis media, and pharyngitis as well as for urinary tract infections by susceptible microorganisms.

Cefpodoxime proxetil. Cefpodoxime proxetil is a pro-drug. It is cleaved enzymically to 2-propanol, carbon dioxide, acetaldehyde, and cefpodoxime in the gut wall. It has better anti–*Staphylococcus aureus* activity than cefixime and is used to treat pharyngitis, urinary tract infections, upper and lower respiratory tract infections, otitis media, skin and soft tissue infections, and gonorrhea.

Cefdinir. Cefdinir has an unsubstituted *Z*-oxime in its C-7 side chain, the consequence of which is attributed to its somewhat enhanced anti-Gram-positive activity—its main distinguishing feature. It has a vinyl moiety attached to C-3 that is associated with its oral activity. It has reasonable but not spectacular resistance to β-lactamases and is 20 to 25% absorbed on oral administration unless taken with fatty foods, which significantly diminishes blood levels.

Cefditoren Pivoxil. Cefditoren pivoxil is a new orally active pro-drug. Similar to cefpodoxime proxetil, the pivoxil ester is hydrolyzed following intestinal absorption to release the active drug, cefditoren, along with formaldehyde and pivalic acid. Cefditoren pivoxil should not be administered with drugs that reduce stomach acidity, because this may result in decreased absorption. The bioavailability of cefditoren pivoxil is increased if taken with food. Cefditoren pivoxil is indicated for mild to moderate infections in adults and adolescents with chronic bronchitis, pharyngitis/tonsillitis, and uncomplicated skin infections associated with Gram-negative bacteria. Effectiveness is reported against *Haemophilus influenzae* and *Moraxella catarrhalis* and includes β-lactamase–producing strains.

Fourth-Generation Cephalosporins

Cefepime

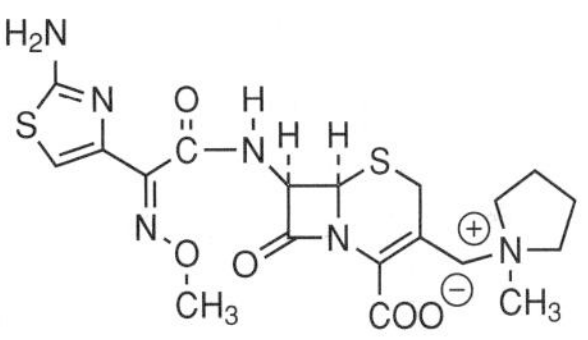

Cefepime (Maxipime)

Cefepime is a semisynthetic agent containing a *Z*-methoxyimine moiety and an aminothiazolyl group at C-7, broadening its spectrum and increasing its β-lactamase stability as well as increasing its antistaphylococcal activity. The quaternary N-methylpyrrolidine group at C-3 seems to help penetration into Gram-negative bacteria. The fourth-generation cephalosporins are characterized by enhanced antistaphylococcal activity and broader anti-Gram-negative activity than the third-generation group. Cefepime is used IM and IV against urinary tract infections, skin and skin structure infections, pneumonia, and intra-abdominal infections.

Summary Statement. With their broader spectrum, including many very dangerous bacteria, the cephalosporins have come to dominate β-lactam chemotherapy despite often lacking oral activity. Because the cephalosporin field is still being very actively pursued, the student can expect continual introduction of new agents into the foreseeable future.

Carbapenems. Thienamycin, the first of the carbapenems, was isolated from *Streptomyces cattleya.* Because of its extremely intense and broad-spectrum antimicrobial activity as well as its ability to inactivate β-lactamases, it combines in one molecule the functional features of the best of the β-lactam antibiotics as well as the β-lactamase inhibitors. It differs structurally in several important respects from the penicillins and cephalosporins. The sulfur atom is not part of the 5-membered ring but, rather, has been replaced by a methylene moiety at that position. Carbon is roughly half the molecular size of sulfur. Consequently, the carbapenem ring system is highly strained and very susceptible to reactions cleaving the β-lactam bond. The sulfur atom is now attached to C-3 as part of a functionalized side chain.

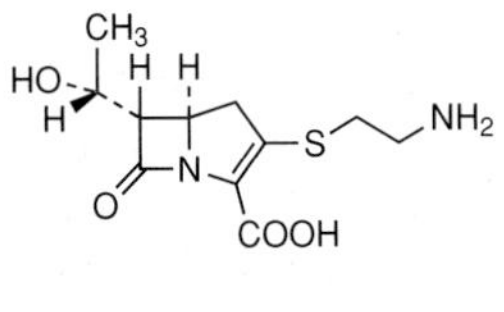

Thienamycin

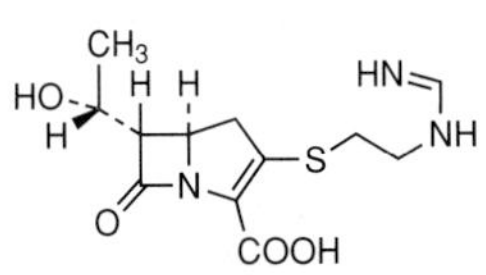

Imipenem

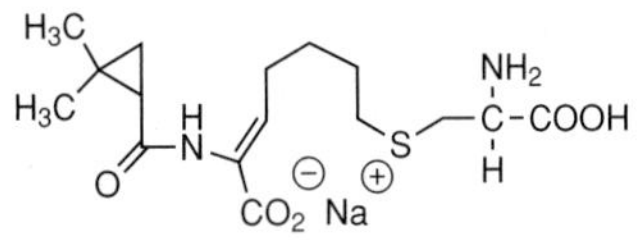

Cilastatin sodium

The endocyclic olefinic linkage also enhances the reactivity of the β-lactam ring. Both make thienamycin unstable, which caused great difficulties in the original isolation studies. The terminal amino group in the side chain attached to C-3 is nucleophilic and attacks the β-lactam bond of a nearby molecule through an intermolecular reaction destroying activity (Fig. 38.23). Ultimately, this problem was overcome by changing the amino group to a less nucleophilic N-formiminoyl moiety by a semisynthetic process to produce imipenem. At C-6, there is a 2-hydroxyethyl group attached with α-stereochemistry. Thus, the absolute stereochemistry of the molecule is 5*R*,6*S*,8*S*. With these striking differences from the penicillins and cephalosporins, it is not surprising that thienamycin analogues bind differently to the penicillin biding proteins (especially strongly to PBP-2), but it is gratifying that the result is very potent broad-spectrum activity.

Imipenem. Imipenem, as well as thienamycin, penetrates very well through porins and is very stable, even inhibitory, to many β-lactamases. Imipenem is not, however, orally active. When used to treat urinary tract infections, renal dehydropeptidase-1 hydrolyzes imipenem through hydrolysis of the β-lactam and deactivates it. An inhibitor for this enzyme, cilastatin, is coadministered with imipenem to protect it. Inhibition of human dehydropeptidase does not seem to have deleterious consequences to the patient, making this combination highly efficacious against urinary tract infections.

The combination of imipenem and cilastatin (Primaxin) is approximately 25% serum protein bound. On injection, it penetrates well into most tissues, but not cerebrospinal fluid, and is subsequently excreted in the urine. It is broader in its spectrum than any other antibiotic presently available in the United States. This very potent combination is especially useful for treatment of serious infections by aerobic Gram-negative bacilli, anaerobes, and *Staphylococcus aureus*. It is used clinically for severe infections of the gut in adults as well as of the genitourinary tract, bone, skin, and endocardia, with allergic reactions as its main risk factor; imipenem also has the unfortunate property of being a good β-lactamase inducer. Because of these features, imipenem–cilastatin is rarely a drug of first choice but, rather, is reserved for use in special circumstances.

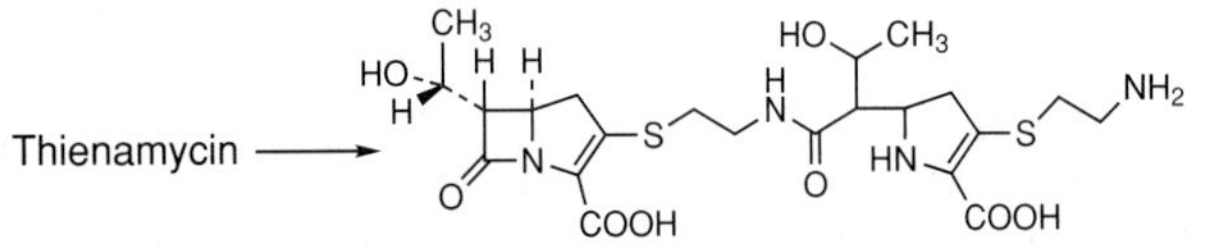

Thienamycin ⟶

Fig. 38.23. Intermolecular instability reaction of thienamycin.

Meropenem

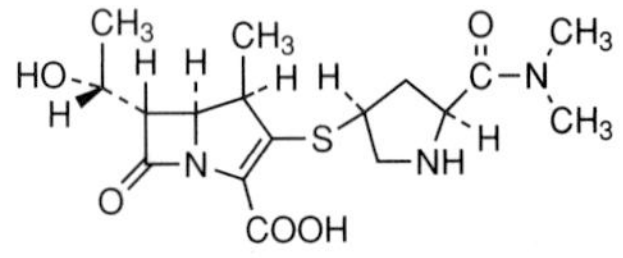

Meropenem (Merrem)

Meropenem is a synthetic carbapenem possessing a complex side chain at C-3. It also has a chiral methyl group at C-4. This methyl group conveys intrinsic resistance to hydrolysis by dehydropeptidase-1. As a consequence, it can be administered as a single agent for the treatment of severe bacterial infections.

Ertapenem

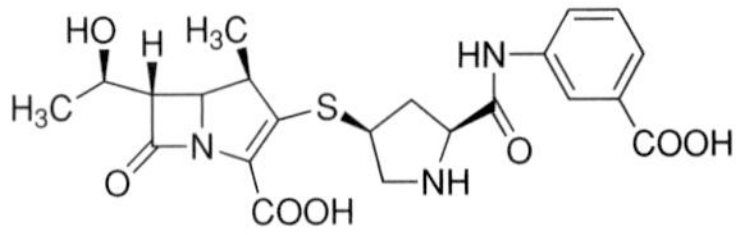

Ertapenem

Ertapenem is another synthetic carbapenem with a rather complex side chain at C-3. It is used once daily parenterally, with special application against anaerobes. As with meropenem, the 4-β-methyl group confers stability toward dehydropeptidase-1 It is not active against pseudomonads or acinetobacteria and, therefore, should not be substituted for imipenem or meropenem. It is relatively strongly bound to serum proteins, so it has a prolonged half-life, making it more convenient to use than the other carbapenems when its spectrum warrants this. Its reported indications include complicated intra-abdominal and complicated skin/skin structure infections caused by sensitive organisms (for intra-abdominal: *Escherichia coli, Clostridium clostridoforme, Bacteroides fragilis,* and *Peptostreptococcus* sp; for skin/skin structures: *Staphylococcus aureus* (methicillin-susceptible strains), *Streptococcus pyogenes, E. coli,* or *Peptostreptococcus* sp.). It can be administered once daily.

This class of antimicrobial agents is under intensive investigation, and several analogues were in various phases of preclinical investigation as of 2005.

Monobactams
Aztreonam

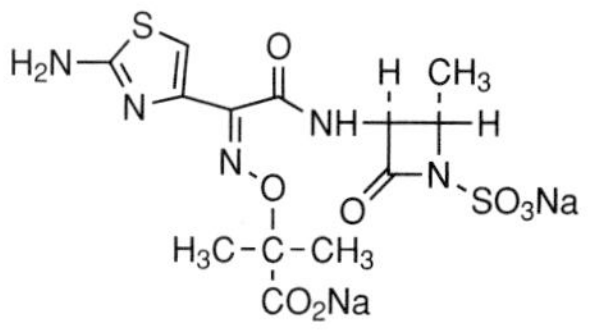

Aztreonam disodium (Azactam)

Fermentation of unusual microorganisms led to the discovery of a class of monocyclic β-lactam antibiotics, named monobactams. None of these natural molecules have proven to be important, but the group served as the inspiration for the synthesis of aztreonam. Aztreonam is a totally synthetic parenteral antibiotic, the antimicrobial spectrum of which is devoted almost exclusively to Gram-negative microorganisms, and it is capable of inactivating some β-lactamases. Its molecular mode of action is closely similar to that of the penicillins, cephalosporins, and carbapenems, the action being characterized by strong affinity for PBP-3, producing filamentous cells as a consequence. Whereas the principal side chain closely resembles that of ceftazidime, the sulfamic acid moiety attached to the β-lactam ring was unprecedented. Remembering the comparatively large size of sulfur atoms, this assembly may sufficiently spatially resemble the corresponding C-2 carboxyl group of the precedent β-lactam antibiotics to confuse the penicillin binding protons. The strongly electron-withdrawing character of the sulfamic acid group probably also makes the β-lactam bond more vulnerable to hydrolysis. In any case, the monobactams demonstrate that a fused ring is not essential for antibiotic activity. The α-oriented methyl group at C-2 is associated with the stability of aztreonam towards β-lactamases.

The protein binding is moderate (~50%), and the drug is nearly unchanged by metabolism. Aztreonam is given by injection and is primarily excreted in the urine. The primary clinical use of aztreonam is against severe infections caused by Gram-negative microorganisms, especially those acquired in the hospital. These are mainly urinary tract, upper respiratory tract, bone, cartilage, abdominal, obstetric and gynecologic infections, and septicemias. The drug is well tolerated, and adverse effects are infrequent. Interestingly, allergy would not be unexpected, but cross-allergenicity with penicillins and cephalosporins has not often been reported.

Antibiotics: Inhibitors of Protein Biosynthesis

BASIS FOR SELECTIVITY. Once the bacterial cell wall is traversed, complex cellular machinery deeper within the cell becomes available to antibiotics. Some of the most successful antibiotic families exert their lethal effects on bacteria by inhibiting ribosomally mediated protein biosynthesis. At first glimpse, this may seem to be anomalous, because eukaryotic organisms also construct their essential proteins on ribosomal organelles and the sequence of biochemical steps is closely analogous to that in prokaryotic microorganisms. At a molecular level, however, the apparent anomaly resolves itself, because the detailed architecture of prokaryotic ribosomes is rather different. In *Escherichia coli*, for example, the 70S ribosomal particle is composed not only of three RNA molecules but also of 55 different structural and functional proteins arranged in a nonsymmetrical manner. The small (30S) subunit has a 16S rRNA molecule and approximately 20 different proteins. The large subunit has a 23S and a 5S rRNA and more than 30 proteins. Quite recently, the x-ray crystal structure of the components of the bacterial ribosome has been determined. This is a landmark achievement given the size and complexity of this organelle. The available picture is still fuzzy but allows one to unravel the molecular details not only of how proteins are biosynthesized but also where important antibiotics bind when they interrupt this process. The functioning parts of the ribosome are the RNA molecules, and the proteins organize the whole and catalyze some portions of the biosynthetic cycle. The tRNA molecules bind roughly at the interface where the 50S and 30S subparticles come together. The codon–anticodon interaction with mRNA takes place in the 30S subunit, and the incoming amino acid and the growing peptide chain being made lies in the 50S subunit. Upsetting the view held for decades that the antibiotics bound to ribosomal proteins, it is now known that they bind to the rRNA instead. Aside from this important fact, most of the other key beliefs are still valid. Of key importance, the vital repeated movement of the tRNA bases mostly take place near interfaces between individual rRNA molecules, where this would be easiest. In agreement, it has been found that this region is comparatively disordered consistent with that movement (Fig. 38.24).

At normal doses, antibiotics do not bind to or interfere with the function of eukaryotic 80S ribosomal particles. The basis for the selective toxicity of these antibiotics is then apparent. Interference with bacterial protein biosynthesis prevents repair, cellular growth, and reproduction and can be clinically bacteriostatic or bactericidal.

AMINOGLYCOSIDES AND AMINOCYCLITOLS

Introduction. The aminoglycoside/aminocyclitol class of antibiotics contains a pharmacophoric 1,3-diaminoinositol moiety consisting of either streptamine, 2-deoxystreptamine, or spectinamine (Fig. 38.25). Several of the alcoholic functions of the 1,3-diaminoinositol are substituted through glycosidic bonds with characteristic amino sugars to form pseudo-oligosaccharides. The chemistry, spectrum, potency, toxicity, and pharmacokinetics of these agents are a function of the specific identity of the diaminoinositol unit and the arrangement and identity of the attachments. The various aminoglycoside antibiotics

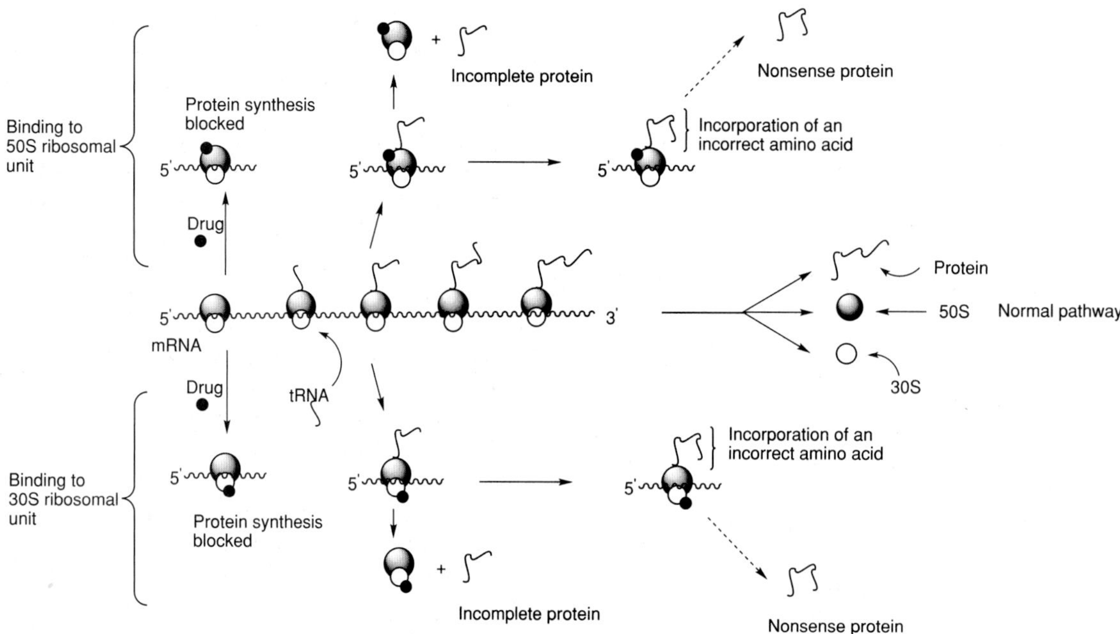

Fig. 38.24. General mechanism of action of drugs that block protein synthesis by binding to ribosomal units.

are freely water soluble at all achievable pH values, are basic and form acid addition salts, are not absorbed in significant amounts from the GI tract, and are excreted in active form in fairly high concentrations in the urine following injection. When the kidneys are not functioning efficiently, the concentrations injected must be reduced to prevent accumulation to toxic levels. When given orally, their action is primarily confined to the GI tract. They are more commonly given IM or by perfusion. Recently, tobramycin has been sprayed into the lungs to successfully treat *Pseudomonas aeruginosa* infections in patients with cystic fibrosis. This route of administration results in significantly reduced toxicity to the patient. These agents have intrinsically broad antimicrobial spectra, but their toxicity potential limits their clinical use to severe infections by Gram-negative bacteria. The aminoglycoside antibiotics are widely distributed (mainly in extracellular fluids) and have low levels of protein binding.

Mechanism of Action. The aminoglycosides are bactericidal because of a combination of toxic effects. At less than toxic doses, they bind to the 16S rRNA portion of the 30S ribosomal subparticle, impairing the proofreading function of the ribosome. A conformational change occurs in the peptidyl A site of the ribosome on aminoglycoside binding. This leads to mistranslation of RNA templates and the consequent selection of wrong amino acids and formation of so-called nonsense proteins (Fig. 38.24). The most relevant of these unnatural proteins are involved in upsetting bacterial membrane function. Their presence destroys the semipermeability of the membrane, and this damage cannot be repaired without de novo programmed protein biosynthesis. Among the substances that are admitted by the damaged membrane are large additional quantities of aminoglycoside. At these increased concentrations, protein biosynthesis ceases altogether. These combined effects are devastating to the target bacterial cells. Given their highly polar properties, the student may wonder how these agents can enter bacterial cells at all. Aminoglycosides apparently bind initially to external lipopolysaccharides and diffuse into the cells in small amounts. The uptake process is inhibited by Ca^{2+} and Mg^{2+} ions. These ions are, then, partially incompatible therapeutically. Passage through the cytoplasmic membrane is dependent on electron transport and energy generation. At high concentrations, eukaryotic protein biosynthesis also can be inhibited by aminoglycoside/aminocyclitol antibiotics.

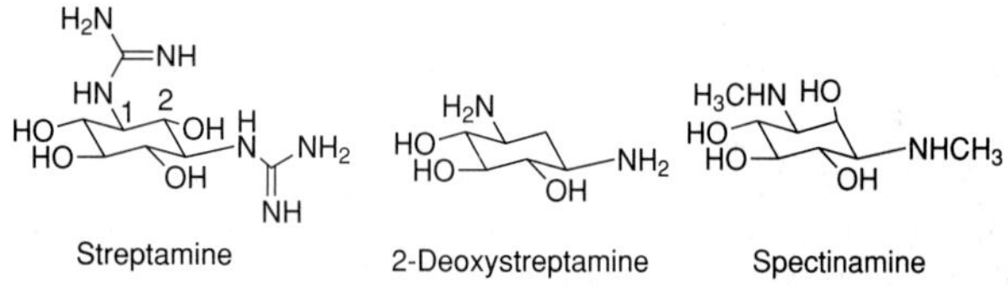

Streptamine 2-Deoxystreptamine Spectinamine

Fig. 38.25. 1,3-Diaminoinositol moieties in aminoglycosides.

Bacterial Resistance. Bacterial resistance to aminoglycoside antibiotics in the clinic is most commonly the result of bacterial elaboration of R factor–mediated enzymes that N-acetylate (aminoglycoside acetylase [AAC]), O-phosphorylate (aminoglycoside phosphorylase [APH]), and O-adenylate (aminoglycoside nucleotide transferase [ANT]) specific functional groups, preventing subsequent ribosomal binding (Fig. 38.26). In some cases, chemical deletion of the functional groups transformed by these enzymes leaves a molecule that is still antibiotic but is no longer a substrate; thus, agents with an intrinsically broader spectrum can be made semisynthetically in this way. In some other cases, novel functional groups can be attached to remote functionality that converts these antibiotics to poorer substrates for these R factor–mediated enzymes, and this expands their spectra (discussed later). Resistance also can involve point mutations of the ribosomal A site. These involve single-nucleotide residues at specific positions. The substituent at position 6′ of the aminoglycoside, the number of protonated amino groups, and the linkage between the sugar rings and the central deoxystreptamine moiety are particularly important in the interactions with the rRNA. Resistance caused by decreased aminoglycoside/aminocyclitol uptake into bacterial cells also is encountered.

Therapeutic Application. Intrinsically, aminoglycosides have broad antibiotic spectra against aerobic Gram-positive and Gram-negative bacteria but are reserved for use in serious infections caused by Gram-negative organisms because of serious toxicities that often are delayed in onset. They are active against Gram-negative aerobes, such as *Acinetobacter* sp., *Citrobacter* sp., *Enterobacter* sp., *Escherichia coli, Klebsiella* sp., *Proteus vulgaris, Providencia* sp., *Pseudomonas aeruginosa, Salmonella* sp., *Serratia marcescans, Shigella* sp., and Gram-positive aerobes (e.g., *Staphylococcus epidermidis).*

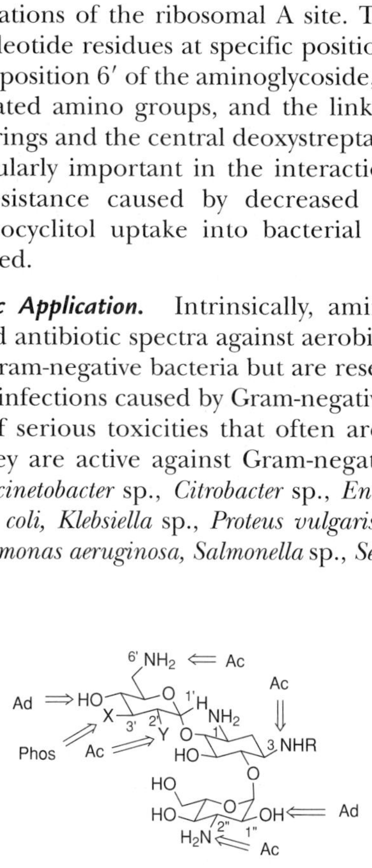

Tobramycin ($X=H$, $Y=NH_2$, $R=H$)

Kanamycin A ($X=OH$, $Y=OH$, $R=H$)

Amikacin ($X=Y=OH$, $R=COCHOHCH_2CH_2NH_2$)

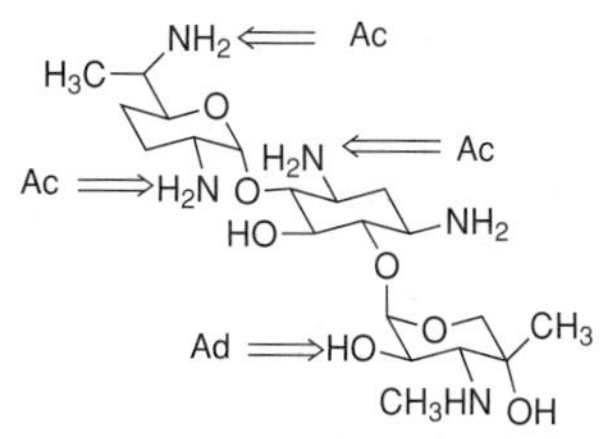

Gentamicin C-2

Fig. 38.26. Commercially important 2-desylstreptamine-containing aminoglycosides. Some points of inactivating attack by specific R factor–medicated enzymes are indicated by the following symbols. Ad ⇒ adenylation; Ac ⇒ acetylation; Phos ⇒ phosphorylation. APH(3′)-1, for example, is an acronym for an enzyme that phosphorylates aminoglycosides at the 3′-OH position.

Streptomycin and spectinomycin differ from the others in their useful antimicrobial spectra. Streptomycin is most commonly used for the treatment of tuberculosis and spectinomycin for treatment of gonorrhea. The other antibiotics of this class are inferior for these purposes.

These antibiotics have similar clinical spectra to those of the quinolones and are decreasing in popularity as quinolone use increases. Some aminoglycoside antibiotics in present clinical use are illustrated in Figure 38.26 along with some of their sites of enzymatic inactivation. There has not been a new aminoglycoside antibiotic introduced since the 1970s.

Adverse Effects. The toxicities associated with the aminoglycosides involve ototoxicity to functions mediated by the eighth cranial nerve, such as hearing loss and vertigo. Their use also can lead to kidney tubular necrosis, producing decreases in glomerular function. These toxic effects are related to blood levels and, apparently, are mediated by the special affinity of these aminoglycosides to kidney cells and to the sensory cells of the inner ear. The effects may have a delayed onset, making them all the more treacherous, because the patient can be injured significantly before symptoms appear. Less common is a curare-like neuromuscular blockade believed to be caused by competitive inhibition of calcium ion–dependent acetylcholine release at the neuromuscular junction. This effect can exaggerate the muscle weakness of patients with myasthenia gravis or Parkinson's disease. In current practice, all these toxic phenomena are well known; therefore, creatinine clearance should be determined and the dose adjusted downward accordingly so that these adverse effects are less common and less severe.

Specific Agents

Kanamycin (Kantrex). Kanamycin is a mixture of at least three components (A, B, and C, with A predominating) isolated from *Streptomyces kanamyceticus.* In addition to typical aminoglycoside antibiotic properties, kanamycin, along with gentamicin, neomycin, and paromomycin, is among the most chemically stable of the common antibiotics. Kanamycin can be heated without loss of activity for astonishing periods in acid or alkaline solutions and can even withstand autoclaving temperatures. Kanamycin, however, is unstable to R-factor enzymes, being O-phosphorylated on the C-3′hydroxyl by enzymes APH(3′)-I and APH(3′)-II and also is N-acetylated on the C-6′amino group, among others (Fig. 38.26). These transformation products are antibiotically inactive. Kanamycin is used parenterally against some Gram-negative bacteria, but *Pseudomonas aeruginosa* and anaerobes usually are resistant. Although it also can be used in combination with other agents against certain mycobacteria (*Mycobacterium kansasii, Mycobacterium marinum,* and *Mycobacterium intracellulare*), its popularity for this use is fading. Injections of kanamycin are painful enough to require use of a local anesthetic. Kanamycin occasionally is used in antitubercular admixtures.

Amikacin (Amikin). Amikacin is made semisynthetically from kanamycin A. Interestingly, the L-hydroxyaminobutyryl amide (HABA) moiety attached to N-3 inhibits adenylation and phosphorylation in the distant amino sugar ring (at C-2′ and C-3′), even though the HABA substituent is not where the enzymatic reaction takes place. This effect is attributed to decreased binding to the R factor–mediated enzymes. With this change, both potency and spectrum are strongly enhanced, and amikacin is used for the treatment of sensitive strains of *Mycobacterium tuberculosis, Yersinia tularensis,* and severe *Pseudomonas aeruginosa* infections resistant to other agents.

Tobramycin (Nebcin). Tobramycin is one component (factor 6) of a mixture produced by fermentation of *Streptomyces tenebrarius.* Lacking the C-3′ hydroxyl group, it is not a substrate for APH(3′)-1 and APH(3′)-II and so has an intrinsically broader spectrum than kanamycin. It is a substrate, however, for adenylation at C-2′ by ANT(2′) and acetylation at C-3 by AAC(3)-I and AAC(3)-II and at C-2′ by AAC(2′) (Fig. 38.26). It is widely used parenterally for difficult infections, especially those by gentamicin-resistant *Pseudomonas aeruginosa.* It is believed by some clinicians to be less toxic than gentamicin.

Gentamicin (Garamycin). Gentamicin is a mixture of several antibiotic components produced by fermentation of *Micromonospora purpurea* and other related soil microorganisms (hence its name is spelled with an "i" instead of a "y"). Gentamicins C-1, C-2, and C-1a are most prominent. Gentamicin is the most important of the aminoglycoside antibiotics still in use. Gentamicin was, for example, one of the first antibiotics to have significant activity against *Pseudomonas aeruginosa* infections. This water-loving, opportunistic pathogen frequently is encountered in burns, pneumonias, and urinary tract infections. It is highly virulent. As noted above, some of the functional groups that serve as targets for R factor–mediated enzymes are missing in the structure of gentamicins, so their antibacterial spectrum is enhanced. They are, however, inactivated through C-2′ adenylation by the enzyme ANT(2′) and acetylation at C-6′ by AAC(6′), at C-1 by AAC(1)-I and AAC(1)-II, and at C-2′ by AAC(2′). It often is combined with other anti-infective agents, and an interesting incompatibility has been uncovered. With certain β-lactam antibiotics, the two drugs react with each other so that N-acylation on C-1 of gentamicin by the β-lactam antibiotic takes place, thus inactivating both antibiotics (Fig. 38.27). The two agents should not, therefore, be mixed in the same solution and should be administered into different tissue compartments (usually one in each arm) to prevent this. This incompatibility is

Gentamicin C-2a (active) + β-lactam Antibiotic (active) → (inactive)

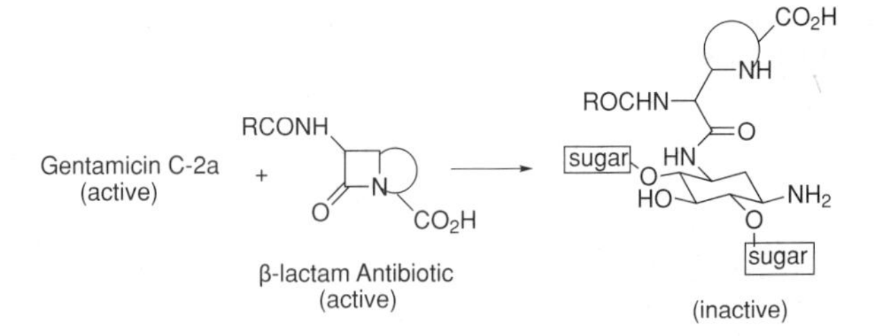

Fig. 38.27. A chemical drug–drug incompatibility between gentamicin C-2a and β-lactams.

likely to be associated with other aminoglycoside antibiotics as well.

Gentamicin is used for urinary tract infections, burns, some pneumonias, and bone and joint infections caused by susceptible Gram-negative bacteria. It often is used to prevent fouling of soft contact lenses. It also is used in polymer matrices in orthopaedic surgery to prevent sealed-in sepsis. It is given topically, sometimes in special dressings, to burn patients.

Spectinomycin (Trobicin)

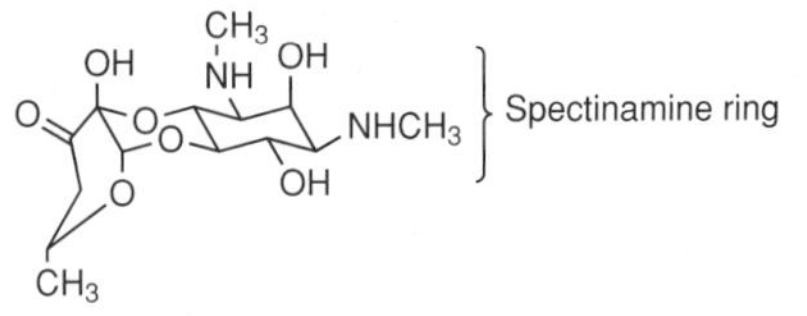

Spectinamine ring

Spectinomycin

An unusual aminoglycoside antibiotic, spectinomycin is produced by fermentation of *Streptomyces spectabilis* and differs substantially in its clinical properties from the others. The diaminoinositol unit (spectinamine) contains two mono-N-methyl groups, and the hydroxyl between them has a stereochemistry opposite to that in streptomycin. The glycosidically attached sugar also is unusual in that it contains three consecutive carbonyl groups, either overt or masked, and is fused by two adjacent linkages to spectinamine to produce an unusual, fused, three-ring structure. Spectinomycin is bacteriostatic as normally employed. It is used almost exclusively in a single bolus injection IM against *Neisseria gonorrhea,* especially penicillinase-producing strains, in cases of urogenital or oral gonorrhea and does not apparently produce any serious oto- or nephrotoxicity when used in this way. It is particularly useful for the treatment of patients allergic to penicillin and patients not likely to comply well with a medication scheme. It would likely be more widely used except that syphilis and chlamydia do not respond to it. It causes significant mistranslation following ribosomal binding but does not cause much inhibition of overall programmed protein biosynthesis. Resistance to spectinomycin by a kinase phosphorylating a hydroxyl group has been reported.

Streptomycin

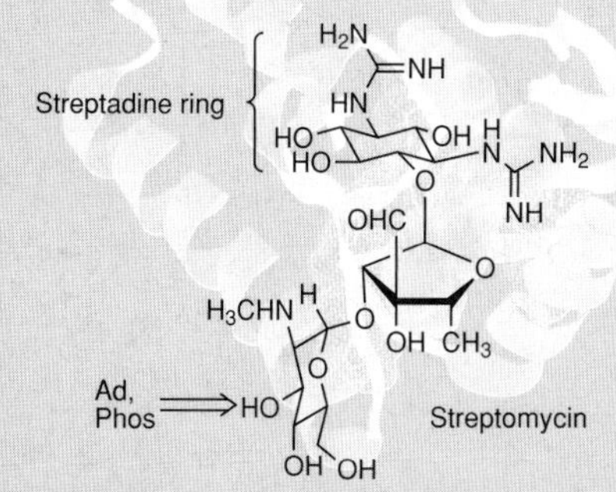

Streptadine ring

Ad, Phos

Streptomycin

Streptomycin is produced by fermentation of *Streptomyces griseus* and several related soil microorganisms. It was introduced in 1943 primarily for the treatment of tuberculosis (see Chapter 41). Control of this ancient scourge was greeted with such enthusiasm that Selmon Waksman, the discoverer of streptomycin, received a Nobel Prize in 1952. Streptomycin differs from the typical aminoglycosides with a modified pharmacophore in that the diaminoinositol unit is streptamine. Streptomycin also has an axial hydroxyl group at C-2 and two highly basic guanido groups at C-l and C-3 in place of the primary amine moieties of 2-deoxystreptamine. It is possible that the unusual pharmacophore of streptomycin accounts in large measure for its unusual antibacterial spectrum. Another molecular feature, the α-hydroxyaldehyde moiety, is a center of instability such that streptomycin cannot be sterilized by autoclaving, so streptomycin sulfate solutions that need sterilization are made by ultrafiltration. Streptomycin is rarely used today as a single agent.

Resistance to streptomycin takes the familiar course of N-acetylation, O-phosphorylation, and O-adenylation of specific functional groups.

Orally Used Aminoglycosides. Kanamycin and another archaic member of the aminoglycoside antibiotic group, paromomycin (Humatin) finds some oral use for the suppression of gut flora. Paromomycin is also used for the oral treatment of amoebic dysentery. Amoebas are persistent pathogens causing chronic diarrhea and are acquired most frequently by travelers who consume food supplies contaminated with human waste.

Neomycin

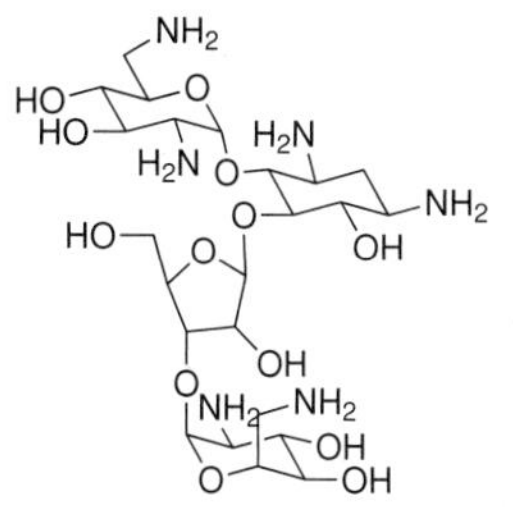

Neomycin B

Neomycin is a mixture of three compounds produced by fermentation of *Streptomyces fradiae,* with neomycin B predominating. It is most commonly used in preoperative bowel sanitation and the treatment of enteropathogenic *Escherichia coli* infections. It also is found in nonprescription ointments and is used topically for treatment of bacterial skin infections. When applied to intact skin, the drug is not absorbed, but when applied to large, denuded areas, systemic absorption occurs with the potential for toxic side effects. It also has seen some use in lowering serum cholesterol.

MACROLIDE ANTIBIOTICS

Introduction. The term "macrolide" is derived from the characteristic large lactone (cyclic ester) ring found in these antibiotics. The clinically important members of this antibiotic family (Fig. 38.28) have two or more characteristic sugars (usually cladinose and desosamine) attached to the 14-membered ring. One of these sugars usually carries a substituted amino group, so their overall chemical character is weakly basic ($pK_a \sim 8$). They are not very water-soluble as free bases. Salt formation with certain acids (glucoheptonic and lactobiononic acids in Fig. 38.28), however, increases water solubility, whereas other salts decrease solubility (laurylsulfate and stearic). Macrolide antibiotics with 16-membered rings are popular outside the United States, but one example, tylosin, finds extensive agricultural use in the United States. The 14-membered ring macrolides are biosynthesized from propionic acid units so that every second carbon of erythromycin, for example, bears a methyl group and the rest of the ring carbons, with one exception, are oxygen bearing. Two carbons bear so-called "extra" oxygen atoms introduced later in the biosynthesis (not present in a propionic acid unit), and two hydroxyls are glycosylated (Fig. 38.29).

Chemical Properties. The early macrolides of the erythromycin class are chemically unstable because of rapid acid-catalyzed internal cyclic ketal formation, leading to inactivity (Fig. 38.30). This reaction that occurs in the GI tract is clinically important. Most acid-susceptible macrolides are administered in coated tablets to minimize this effect. Semisynthetic analogues have been prepared that are structurally incapable of undergoing this reaction (clarithromycin, dirithromycin, and azithromycin) (Fig. 38.28) and have become very popular of late in the clinic.

Many macrolides have an unpleasant taste, which is partially overcome with water-insoluble dosage forms that also reduce acid instability and gut cramps. Enteric coatings are beneficial in reducing these adverse effects as well.

Mechanism of Action. The macrolides inhibit bacteria by interfering with programmed ribosomal protein biosynthesis by binding to the 23S rRNA in the polypeptide exit tunnel adjacent to the peptidyl transferase center in the 50S subparticle (Fig. 38.24). Binding appears to occur at two specific regions within the rRNA, which are referred to as domain V at adenine 2058 and 2059 and domain II

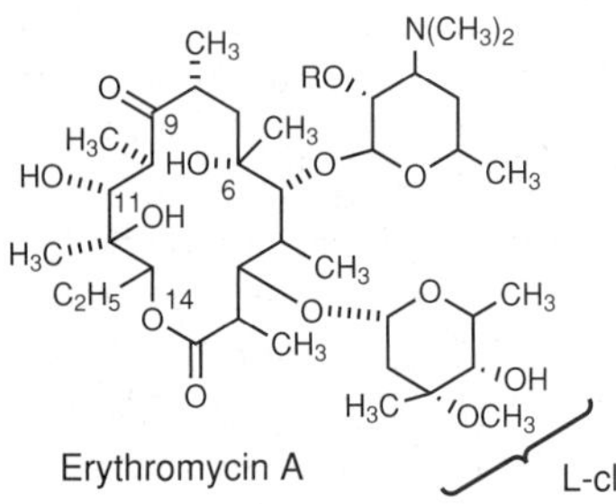

	R	Salt
Erythromycin base	H	—
Erythromycin hydrochloride	H	HCl
Erythromycin estolate	$COCH_2CH_3$	$CH_3(CH_2)_{11}OSO_3H$
Erythromycin ethylsuccinate	$CO(CH_2)CO_2C_2H_5$	—
Erythromycin lactobionate	H	Structure A
Erythromycin stearate	H	$CH_3(CH_2)_{16}CO_2H$

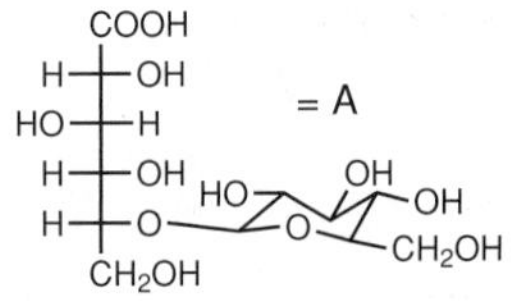

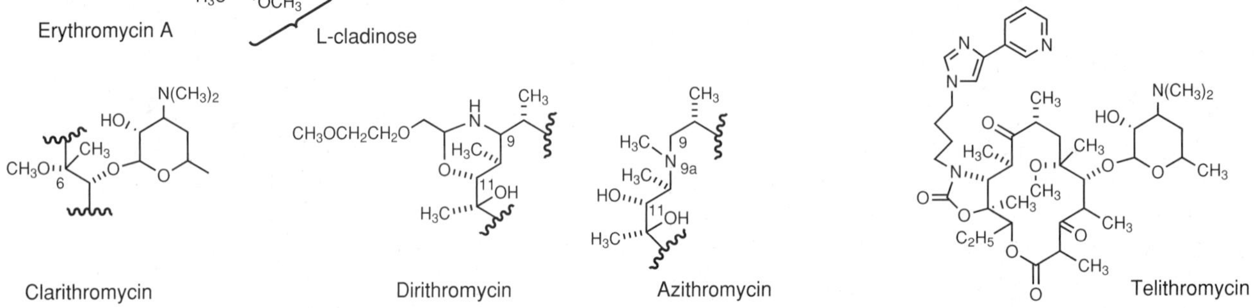

Erythromycin A — L-cladinose

Clarithromycin Dirithromycin Azithromycin Telithromycin

Fig. 38.28. Clinically important macrolide antibiotics.

at adenine 752. These sites are similar to those sites occupied by clindamycin, lincomycin, chloramphenicol, and streptogramin B antibiotics, leading to extensive cross-resistance. The ratio of binding is 1:1 between 23S and the macrolide. Binding of the macrolide to 23S rRNA prevents the growing peptide from becoming longer than a few residues, resulting in the dissociation of peptidyl tRNA molecules. The amino sugar moiety of the macrolides appears to be particularly important in the inhibition. Removal of the 3-L-cladinose results in reduced binding to domain V and an 100-fold decrease in biological activity. It also has been suggested that the L-cladinose is associated with GI distress resulting from the release of motilin

Resistance. Developed bacterial resistance is primarily caused by bacteria possessing R-factor enzymes that methylate a specific guanine residue on their own rRNA, making them somewhat less efficient protein biosynthesizers but comparatively poor binders of macrolides. The erythromycin-producing soil organism utilizes the same ribosomal methylation technique to protect itself against the toxic effects of its own metabolite. This leads to the speculation that the origin of some antibiotic resistance genes may lie in the producing organism itself and that this genetic material is acquired by bacteria from this source.

A second mechanism of resistance is associated with the mutation of adenine to guanine that occurs in domain V at adenine 2058. This change results in a 10,000-fold reduction of binding capacity of erythromycin and clarithromycin to the 23S rRNA. This mutation is much less likely to occur with the ketolide derivatives (telithromycin).

Some bacterial strains, however, appear to be resistant to macrolides because of the operation of an active efflux process in which the drug is expelled from the cell at the cost of energy. Intrinsic resistance of Gram-negative bacteria is primarily caused by lack of penetration, because the isolated ribosomes from these organisms often are susceptible.

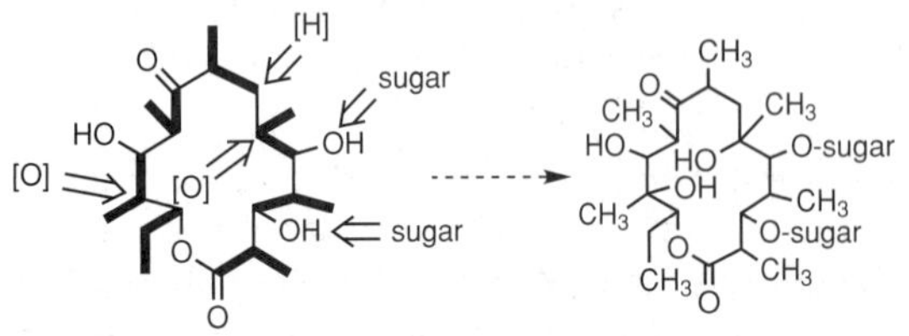

Fig. 38.29. Biosynthetic pathway to erythromycins from propionic acid units. [X] ⇒ refers to modifications to the basic ring skeleton.

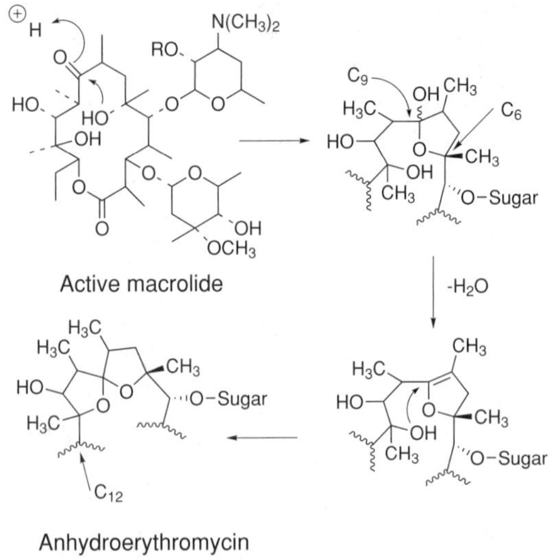

Active macrolide — $-H_2O$ — Anhydroerythromycin

Fig. 38.30. Acid-catalyzed intramolecular ketal formation with erythromycin.

Drug Interactions. Drug–drug interactions with macrolides are comparatively common and usually involve competition for oxidative liver metabolism by a member (CYP3A4) of the cytochrome P450 oxidase family. Such drugs as ergotamine, theophylline, carbamazepine, bromocryptine, warfarin, digoxin, oral contraceptives, carbamazepine, cyclosporine, astemizole, terfenadine, midazolam, triazolam, and methylprednisone can be involved. These interactions can have severely negative consequences for the patient. The result of this interaction is a longer half-life and enhanced potential toxicity by increasing the effective dose over time. The interaction with astemizole and terfenadine can lead to very serious cardiovascular effects. The main product of liver metabolism of erythromycin is the N-demethylated analogue.

Therapeutic Application. The macrolides are among the safest of the antibiotics in common use and often are used for the treatment of upper and lower respiratory tract and soft-tissue infections primarily caused by Gram-positive microorganisms like *Streptococcus pyogenes* and *Streptococcus pneumoniae,* Legionnaire's disease, prophylaxis of bacterial endocarditis by *Streptococcus viridans,* upper and lower respiratory tract infections and otitis media caused by *Haemophilus influenzae* (with a sulfonamide added), mycoplasmal pneumonia, and in combination with rifabutin in *Mycobacterium avium* complex infections in patients with AIDS, and it also finds some use for certain sexually transmitted diseases, such as gonorrhea and pelvic inflammatory disease, caused by mixed infections involving cell wall–free organisms, such as *Chlamydia trachomitis.* Clarithromycin also is used to treat gastric ulcers because of *Helicobacter pylori* infection as a component of multidrug cocktails. Thus, the macrolides have a comparatively narrow antimicrobial spectrum, reminiscent of the medium-spectrum penicillins, but the organisms involved include many of the more commonly encountered community-acquired diseases and the macrolides are remarkably free of serious toxicity to the host and, of course, do not cause β-lactam allergy. The utility of the macrolides against upper respiratory tract infections is aided by their particular affinity for these tissues. Tissue levels in the upper respiratory tract often are several multiples of that seen in the blood. The macrolides are primarily used orally for mild systemic infections of the respiratory tract, liver, kidneys, prostate, and milk gland even though absorption is somewhat irregular, especially when taken with food. Some derivatives are propropulsive through stimulation of gastrin production. The resulting hyperperistalsis causes uncomfortable GI cramps in some patients. They are bacteriostatic in the clinic in achievable concentrations.

Specific Agents

Erythromycin Esters and Salts

Estolate. One of the two most popular erythromycin pro-drugs, erythromycin estolate, is a C-2′-propionyl ester, N-laurylsulfate salt (Fig. 38.28). Administration of erythromycin estolate produces higher blood levels following metabolic regeneration of erythromycin. In a small number of cases, a severe, dose-related, cholestatic jaundice occurs in which the bile becomes granular in the bile duct, impeding flow so that the bile salts back up into the circulation. This seems to be partly allergic and partly dose related. If the drug causes hepatocyte damage, perhaps this releases antigenic proteins that promote further damage. When cholestatic jaundice occurs, the drug must be replaced by another, nonmacrolide antibiotic, such as one of the penicillins, one of the cephalosporins, or clindamycin. It is postulated that the propionyl ester group is transferred to a tissue component that is antigenic, although the evidence for this is not compelling.

Ethylsuccinate (EryPed, EES). Erythromycin ethyl succinate is a mixed double ester pro-drug in which one carboxyl of succinic acid esterifies the C-2′ hydroxyl of erythromycin and the other ethanol (Fig. 38.28). This pro-drug frequently is used in an oral suspension for pediatric use largely to mask the bitter taste of the drug. Film-coated tablets also are used to deal with this. Some cholestatic jaundice is associated with the use of EES.

Stearate. Erythromycin stearate is a very insoluble salt form of erythromycin. The water insolubility helps to mask the taste of the drug and enhances its stability in the stomach.

Lactobionate. Erythromycin lactobionate is a salt with enhanced water solubility that is used for injections.

Clarithromycin (Biaxin). Clarithromycin differs from erythromycin in that the C-6 hydroxy group has been converted semisynthetically to a methyl ether. The C-6 hydroxy group is involved in the process, initiated by protons, leading to internal cyclic ketal formation in erythromycin that results in drug inactivation (Fig. 38.30). This ketal, or one of the products of its subsequent degradation, also is associated with GI cramping. Conversion of the molecule to its more lipophilic methyl ether prevents internal ketal formation, which not only gives better blood levels through chemical stabilization but also results in less gastric upset. An extensive saturable first-pass liver metabolism of clarithromycin leads to formation of its C-14 hydroxy analogue, which has even greater antimicrobial potency, especially against *Haemophilus influenzae.* The enhanced lipophilicity of clarithromycin also allows lower and less frequent dosage for mild infections.

Azithromycin (Zithromax, Zmax). Azithromycin, called an "azalide," has been formed by semisynthetic conversion of erythromycin to a ring-expanded analogue in which an N-methyl group has been inserted between carbons 9 and 10, and the carbonyl moiety thus is absent (Fig. 38.28). Azithromycin has a 15-membered lactone ring.

This new functionality does not form a cyclic internal ketal. Not only is azithromycin more stable to acid degradation than erythromycin, it also has a considerably longer half-life, attributed to greater and longer tissue penetration, allowing once-a-day dosage. A popular treatment schedule with azithromycin is to take two tablets on the first day and then one tablet a day for the following 5 days and then to discontinue treatment. This is convenient for patients who comply poorly. The drug should be taken on an empty stomach. It does, however, give a metallic taste. Azithromycin tends to be broader spectrum than either erythromycin or clarithromycin. Both of these newer macrolides are quite similar in usage to erythromycin itself and are cross-resistant with it. Azithromycin has a significant postantibiotic effect against a number of pathogens. Azithromycin is commonly the first choice for treatment of infections that require a macrolide.

Ketolides. Research activity in the macrolide antibiotic class has been intense recently in attempts to reduce side effects and to broaden their antimicrobial spectra. The ketolides are a group of agents that are characterized by oxidation of the 3-position from an alcohol to a ketone. They are active against a significant number of erythromycin-resistant microorganisms. Recent investigation has been intense and a new agent has been introduced.

Telithromycin (Ketek). Telithromycin (Fig. 38.28) is orally effective in the treatment of community-acquired pneumonia, acute bacterial exacerbations of chronic bronchitis, and acute sinusitis. Its principal advantage appears to be activity against drug-resistant infections. Telithromycin possesses several structural modifications from the traditional erythromycin nucleus, including removal of the L-cladinose sugar at C-3. The L-cladinose is thought to be associated with the release of motilin and the resulting GI discomfort. Removal of L-cladinose and oxidation of the free hydroxy to a nonpolar ketone reduces biological activity through reduced binding to domain V, but this is offset by the addition of the chain at C-11/12, which greatly improves binding to domain II. Strong binding to domain V and II reduces bacterial resistance. The C-6 methoxy improves acid stability. Telithromycin was approved by the U.S. FDA following a mammoth (24,000 patient) clinical trial. The cost of this will no doubt inhibit further trials of replacement agents.

LINCOSAMIDES

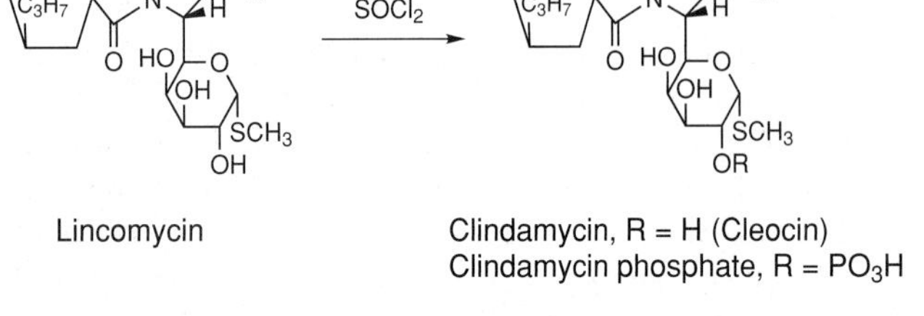

$SOCl_2$

Lincomycin

Clindamycin, R = H (Cleocin)
Clindamycin phosphate, R = PO_3H

Introduction. The lincosamides contain an unusual 8-carbon sugar, a thiomethyl amino-octoside (O-thio-lincosamide), linked by an amide bond to an n-propyl–substituted N-methylpyrrolidylcarboxylic acid (N-methyl-n-propyl-*trans*-hygric acid). Lincosamides are weakly basic and form clinically useful hydrochloric acid salts. They are chemically distinct from the macrolide antibiotics but possess many pharmacological similarities to them. The lincosamides bind to 50S ribosomal subparticles at a site partly overlapping with the macrolide site, are mutually cross-resistant with macrolides, and work through essentially the same molecular mechanism of action (Fig. 38.24). The lincoamides undergo extensive liver metabolism, resulting primarily in N-demethylation. The N-desmethyl analogue retains biological activity.

Specific Agents

Lincomycin (Lincocin). Lincomycin is a natural product isolated from fermentations of *Streptomyces lincolnensis* var. *lincolnensis.* It is active against Gram-positive organisms, including some anaerobes. It is indicated for the treatment of serious infections caused by sensitive strains of streptococci, pneumococci, and staphylococci. It generally is reserved for patients who are allergic to penicillin because of the increased risk of pseudomembranous colitis (described below). It also serves as the starting material for the synthesis of clindamycin (by a S_N-2 reaction that inverts the *R* stereochemistry of the C-7 hydroxyl to a C-7 *S*-chloride).

Clindamycin (Cleocin). The substitution of the chloride for the hydroxy group consequently make clindamycin more bioactive and lipophilic than lincomycin and, thus, is better absorbed following oral administration. It is significantly less painful than erythromycin when injected IM as a C-2 phosphate ester pro-drug and is approximately 90% absorbed when taken orally. It also is available as a palmitate ester hydrochloride salt that, interestingly, when reconstituted as instructed for use as an oral solution, has a pH between 2.5 to 5..0 Clindamycin has a clinical spectrum rather like the macrolides, although it distributes better into bones. Clindamycin works well for Gram-positive coccal infections, especially in patients who are allergic to β-lactams, and also has generally better activity against anaerobes. As with lincomycin, however, it is associated with GI complaints (nausea, vomiting, cramps, and drug-related diarrheas). The most severe of these is pseudomembranous colitis caused by release of two toxins by *Clostridium difficile,* an opportunistic anaerobe. Its overgrowth results from suppression of the normal flora, the presence of which otherwise preserves a healthier ecological balance. The popularity of clindamycin in the clinic has decreased even though pseudomembranous colitis is a comparatively rare side effect and also now is associated with several other broad-spectrum antibiotics. A less common side effect is exudative erythema multiform

(Stevens-Johnson syndrome). Clindamycin has excellent activity against *Propionobacterium acnes* when applied topically to comedones, and because it is white, it can be cosmetically tinted to match flesh tones better than the yellow tetracyclines. A very water-insoluble palmitate hydrochloride pro-drug of clindamycin also is available (lacks bitter taste).

TETRACYCLINES AND GLYCYLCYCLINES

Naphthacene

Tetracycline

(1,2,3,4,4a,5,5a,6,11,11a ,12,12a-dodecahydronaphthacene)

Introduction. The tetracycline family is widely, but not intensively, used in office practice. Of the agents in this family, minocycline and doxycycline are still frequently prescribed in the United States. This family of antibiotics is characterized by a highly functionalized, partially reduced naphthacene (four linearly fused, 6-membered rings) ring system, from which both the family name and the numbering system are derived. They possess a number of adverse effects, although most of them are annoying rather than dangerous. Because their antimicrobial spectrum is broad enough to include many of the pathogens encountered in a community setting, they were once very widely used. The advent of other choices and the high incidence of resistance that has developed has greatly decreased their medicinal prominence in recent years. Presently, they are recommended primarily for use against rickettsia, chlamydia, mycoplasma, anthrax, plague, and helicobacter organisms. A significant number of semisynthetic molecules derived from the antibacterial tetracyclines have shown potential activity in other therapeutic areas, such as antimetastasis, antitumor, anti-inflammatory, antiarthritic, antifungal, antineurotoxic, and antiperiodontal diseases, but discussion of these potential uses is beyond the scope of this chapter.

Chemical Properties. The tetracyclines are amphoteric substances with three pK_a values revealed by titration (2.8–3.4, 7.2–7.8, and 9.1–9.7) and have an isoelectric point at approximately pH 5. The basic function is the C-4-α-dimethylamino moiety. Commercially available tetracyclines (Table 38.13) generally are administered as comparatively water-soluble hydrochloride salts. The conjugated phenolic enone system extending from C-10 to C-12 is associated with the pK_a at approximately 7.5, whereas the conjugated trione system extending from C-1 to C-3 in ring A is nearly as acidic as acetic acid ($pK_a \sim 3$). These resonating systems can be drawn in a number of essentially equivalent ways with the double bonds in alternate positions. The formulae normally given are those settled on by popular convention.

Chelation. Chelation is an important feature of the chemical and clinical properties of the tetracyclines. The acidic functions of the tetracyclines are capable of forming salts through chelation with metal ions. The salts of polyvalent metal ions, such as Fe^{2+}, Ca^{2+}, Mg^{2+}, and Al^{3+}, are all quite insoluble at neutral pHs (Fig. 38.31). This insolubility not only is inconvenient for the preparation of solutions but also interferes with blood levels on oral administration. Consequently, the tetracyclines are incompatible with coadministered, multivalent ion–rich antacids and with hematinics, and concomitant consumption of daily products rich in calcium ion also is contraindicated. Further, the bones, of which the teeth are the most visible, are calcium-rich structures at nearly neutral pHs and so accumulate tetracyclines in proportion to the amount and duration

Table 38.13. Commercially Available Tetracyclines

Generic name	Trade name	X	R_1	R_2	R_3
Tetracycline	Achromycin Sumycin Tetralan	H	OH	CH_3	H
Demeclocycline	Declomycin	Cl	OH	H	H
Minocycline	Minocin	$N(CH_3)_2$	H	H	H
Oxytetracycline	Terramycin	H	OH	CH_3	OH
Doxycycline	Vibramycin Doryx	H	H	CH_3	OH

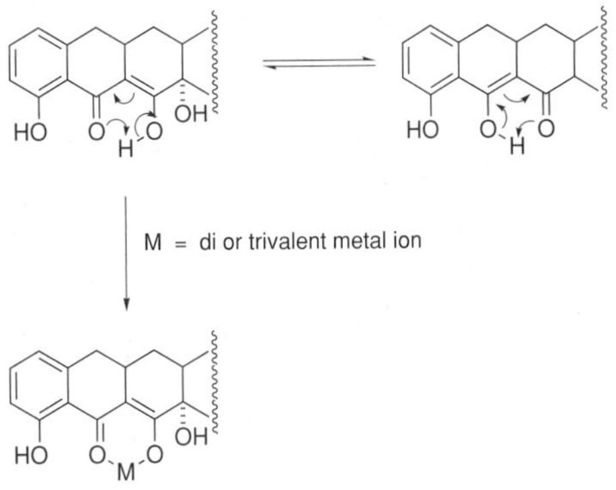

M = di or trivalent metal ion

Fig. 38.31. Metal chelation with the tetracyclines.

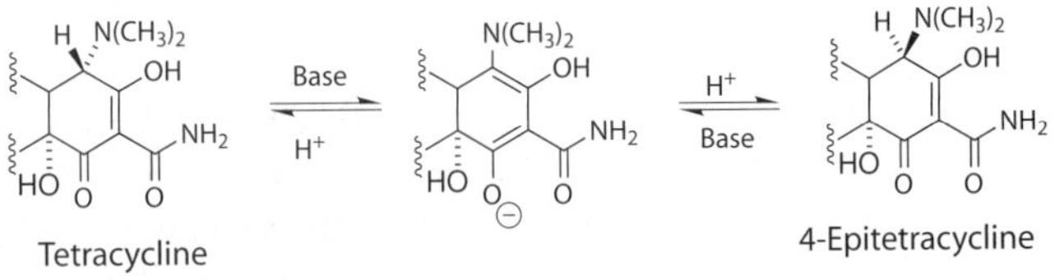

of therapy when bones and teeth are being formed. Because the tetracyclines are yellow, this leads to a progressive and, essentially, permanent discoloration in which, in advanced cases, the teeth are even brown. The intensification of discoloration with time is said to be a photochemical process. This is cosmetically unattractive but does not seem to be deleterious except in extreme cases, when so much antibiotic is taken up that the structure of bone is mechanically weakened. To avoid this, tetracyclines are not normally given to children once they are forming their permanent set of teeth (age, 6–12 years). In severe cases, the teeth can be treated with dilute HCl solution to dissolve away the colored antibiotic. This also significantly erodes the mineral matrix of the teeth, however, and must be repaired by plastic impregnation. People naturally prefer to avoid this heroic and expensive process. When concomitant oral therapy with tetracyclines and incompatible metal ions must be done, the ions should be given 1 hour before or 2 hours after the tetracyclines. Additionally, tetracyclines are painful on IM injection. This has been attributed, in part, to formation of insoluble calcium complexes. To deal with this, the injectable formulations contain ethylenediaminetetraacetic acid and are buffered at comparatively acidic pH levels where chelation is less pronounced and water solubility is higher.

Epimerization. The α-stereo orientation of the C-4 dimethylamino moiety of the tetracyclines is essential for their bioactivity. The presence of the tricarbonyl system of ring A allows enolization involving loss of the C-4 hydrogen (Fig. 38.32). Reprotonation can take place from either the top or bottom of the molecule. Reprotonation from the top of the enol regenerates tetracycline. Reprotonation from the bottom, however, produces inactive 4-epitetracycline. At equilibrium, the mixture consists of nearly equal amounts of the two diasteromers. Thus, old tetracycline preparations can lose approximately half their potency in this way. The epimerization process is most rapid at approximately pH 4 and is relatively slower in the solid-state.

Tetracycline 4-Epitetracycline

Fig. 38.32. Epimerization of tetracyclines.

Dehydration. Most of the natural tetracyclines have a tertiary benzylic hydroxyl group at C-6. This function has the ideal geometry for acid-catalyzed dehydration involving the C-5a α-oriented hydrogen (antiperiplanar *trans*). The resulting product is a naphthalene derivative, so there are energetic reasons for the reaction proceeding in that direction (Fig. 38.33). C-5a,6-anhydrotetracycline is much deeper in color than tetracycline and is biologically inactive.

Discolored old tetracyclines are suspect and should be discarded. Not only can inactive 4-epitetracyclines dehydrate to produce 4-epianhydrotetracyclines, anhydrotetracycline also can epimerize to produce the same product. This degradation product is toxic to the kidneys and produces a Fanconi-like syndrome that, in extreme cases, has been fatal. Commercial samples of tetracyclines are closely monitored for the presence of 4-epidehydrotetracycline, and injuries from this cause are now, fortunately, rare. Those tetracyclines, such as minocycline and doxycycline, which have no C-6-hydroxyl groups, cannot undergo dehydration and, therefore, are completely free of this toxicity.

Cleavage in Base. Another untoward degradation reaction involving a C-6-hydroxyl group is cleavage of the C-ring in alkaline solutions at or above pH 8.5 (Fig. 38.34). The lactonic product, an isotetracycline, is inactive. The clinical impact of this degradation under normal conditions is uncertain.

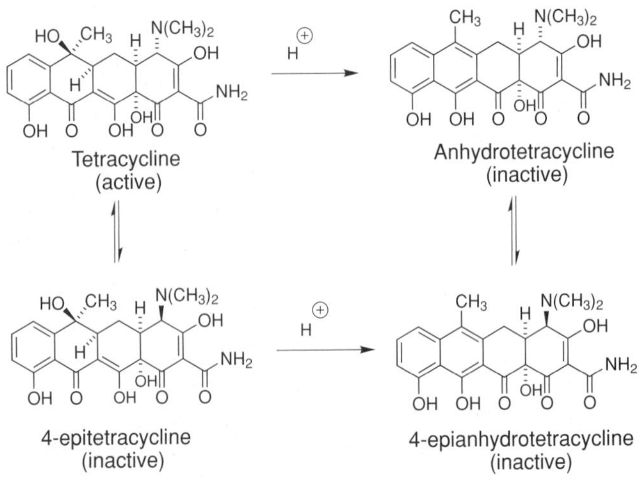

Tetracycline (active)

Anhydrotetracycline (inactive)

4-epitetracycline (inactive)

4-epianhydrotetracycline (inactive)

Fig. 38.33. Acid-catalyzed instability of tetracyclines.

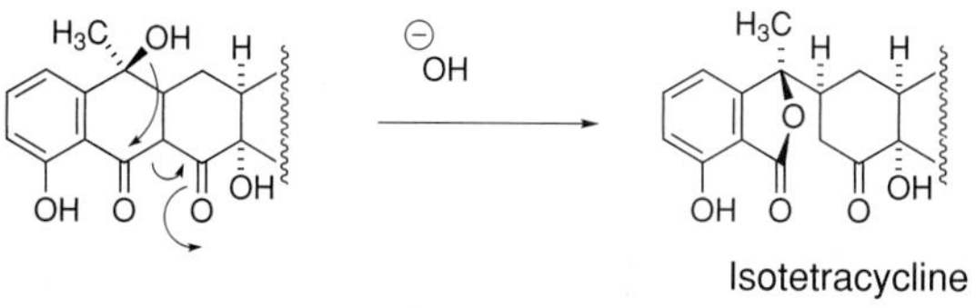

Fig. 38.34. Base-catalyzed instability of tetracyclines.

Phototoxicity. Certain tetracyclines, most notably those with a C-7-chlorine, absorb light in the visible region, leading to free radical generation and, potentially, cause severe erythema to sensitive patients on exposure to strong sunlight. Patients should be advised to be cautious about such exposure for at least their first few doses to avoid potentially severe sunburn. This effect is comparatively rare with most currently popular tetracyclines.

Mechanism of Action. The tetracyclines of clinical importance interfere with protein biosynthesis at the ribosomal level, leading to bacteriostasis. Tetracyclines bind to rRNA in the 30S subparticle with the possible cooperation of a 50S site by a process that remains imprecisely understood despite intensive study (Fig. 38.24). There is more than one binding site, but only one is believed to be critical for its action. The points of contact with the rRNA are those associated with antibiosis with the puzzling exception of the dimethylamino function. Studies have suggested that the tetracyclines bind to the 16S rRNA via the functional groups located at the 1- and 10- to 12a-positions (referred to as the southern face of the tetracycline) and at the 2- and 3-positions (referred to as the eastern face of the tetracycline) (Fig. 38.35). The dimethylamino function is known to be essential for activity but does not appear to bind in the x-ray pictures that are presently available. Once the tetracycline binds, it inhibits subsequent binding of aminoacyltransfer-RNA to the ribosomes, resulting in termination of peptide chain growth. Newer analogues of the tetracyclines suggest that substitution on the western and northern faces of the tetracycline are allowed as indicated by the newest glycylcyclines (see *Tigecycline* below).

The more lipophilic tetracyclines, typified by minocycline, also are capable of disrupting cytoplasmic membrane function, causing leakage of nucleotides and other essential cellular components from the cell, and have bactericidal properties. The more lipophilic tetracyclines enter bacterial cells partly by passive diffusion and the more water-soluble members partly through water-lined protein porin routes, perhaps assisted by the formation of highly lipophilic calcium and magnesium ion chelates. Deeper passage, however, through the inner cytoplasmic membrane is an energy-requiring active process, suggesting that the tetracyclines are mistaken by bacteria as food.

Resistance. Resistance to tetracyclines results in part from an unusual ribosomal protection process involving elaboration of bacterial proteins. These proteins associate with the ribosome, thus allowing protein

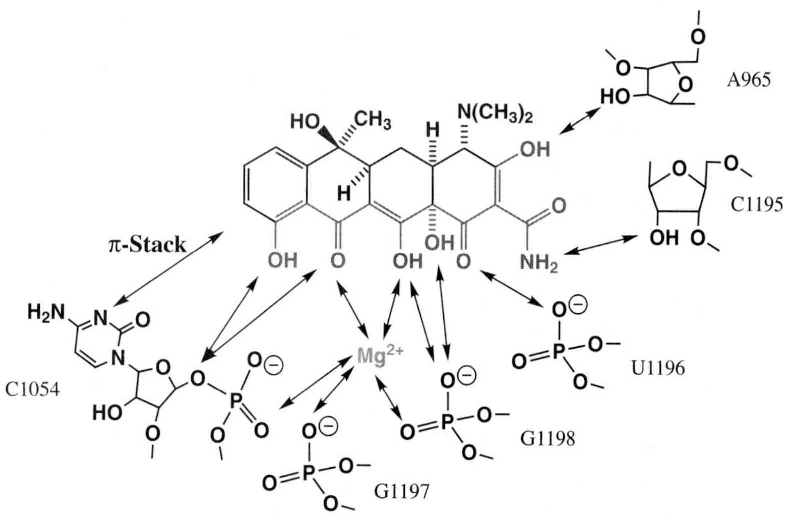

Fig. 38.35. Schematic representation of the primary binding site for a tetracycline and the sugar phosphate groups of 16S rRNA, which also involves a magnesium ion and the critical functional groups on the "southern" and "eastern" face of the tetracycline. (redrawn and modified from Brodersen et al. Cell, 2000;103: 1143–1154).

biosynthesis to proceed even in the presence of bound tetracycline, although exactly how this works is not well understood. Another important resistance mechanism involves R factor–mediated, energy-requiring, active efflux of tetracyclines from the bacterial cells. Some of the efflux proteins have activity that is limited to older tetracyclines, whereas others confer resistance to the entire family with the exception of glycylcyclines. Efflux resistance to glycylcylines, however, has been demonstrated in the laboratory, which suggests that it may occur clinically with extended use. Certain other microbes, such as *Mycoplasma* and *Neisseria* sp., seem to have modified membranes that either accumulate fewer tetracyclines or have porins through which tetracyclines have difficulty in passing. Because resistance is now widespread, these once extremely popular antibiotics are falling into comparative disuse.

Therapeutic Application. The tetracyclines possess very wide bacteriostatic antibacterial activity. Because of the resistance phenomenon and the comparative frequency of troublesome side effects, they are rarely the drugs of first choice today. Nonetheless, they are still popular for office use against susceptible microbes. The differences between the antimicrobial spectra of various tetracyclines are not large, although greater resistance to older agents may limit their use. They are used for low-dose oral and topical therapy for acne, first-course community-acquired urinary tract infections (largely caused by *Escherichia coli*), brucellosis, borreliosis, sexually transmitted diseases (especially chlamydia), rickettsial infections, mycoplasmal pneumonia, prophylaxis of malaria, prevention of traveler's diarrhea, cholera, *Enterobacter* infections, as part of *Helicobacter* cocktails, Lyme disease, Rocky Mountain spotted fever, anthrax, and for many other less common problems. The tetracyclines also are widely used for agricultural purposes.

Adverse Effects. In addition to the adverse effects mentioned earlier (tooth staining, phototoxicity, and potential kidney damage with outdated drug), the tetracyclines are associated with nausea, vomiting, diarrhea, and some CNS effects (dizziness and vertigo). Rapid administration or prolonged IV use can lead to thrombophlebitis. Therefore, tetracyclines generally are administered orally, because they are well absorbed. They also distinguish imperfectly between the bacterial 70S ribosomes and the mammalian 80S ribosomes, so in high doses or special situations (i.e., IV use during pregnancy), these drugs demonstrate a significant antianabolic effect. This may lead to severe liver and kidney damage; therefore, tetracyclines generally are not recommended in these situations. In cases of significant renal impairment, higher serum levels of tetracyclines can lead to azotemia. Additionally, inducers of cytochrome P450 metabolism (i.e., rifampin, barbiturates, and carbamazepine) increase metabolism of tetracyclines (especially doxycycline), so the dose of the tetracycline may require adjustment.

Specific Agents (Table 38.11)

Tetracycline. Tetracycline is produced by fermentation of *Streptomyces aureofaciens* and related species or by catalytic reduction of chlortetracycline. The blood levels achieved on oral administration often are irregular. Food and milk lower absorption by approximately 50%.

Demeclocycline. Demeclocycline lacks the C-6-methyl of tetracycline and is produced by a genetically altered strain of *Streptomyces aureofaciens*. Because it is a secondary alcohol, it is more chemically stable than tetracycline against dehydration. Food and milk co-consumption decrease absorption by half, although it is 60 to 80% absorbed by fasting adults. It is the tetracycline most highly associated with phototoxicity and has been shown to produce dose-dependent, reversible diabetes insipidus with extended use.

Oxytetracycline. It also is one of the classic tetracyclines. It is produced by fermentation of *Streptomyces rimosis* and other soil microorganisms. The most hydrophilic tetracycline on the market, it has largely now been replaced by its semisynthetic descendants. It is primarily used today for IM injections.

Minocycline. An important antibiotic produced by semisynthesis from demeclocycline is minocycline. It is much more lipophilic than its precursors, gives excellent blood levels following oral administration (90–100% available), and can be given once a day. Its absorption is lowered by approximately 20% when taken with food or milk. It is less dependent on active uptake mechanisms and has a somewhat broader antimicrobial spectrum. It also, apparently, is less painful on IM or IV injection, but it has vestibular toxicities (e.g., vertigo, ataxia, and nausea) not generally shared by other tetracyclines.

Doxycycline. It is produced by semisynthesis from other tetracycline molecules and is the most widely used of the tetracycline family. Doxycycline is well absorbed on oral administration (90–100% when fasting; reduced by 20% by co-consumption with food or milk), has a half-life permitting once-a-day dosing for mild infections, and is excreted partly in the feces and partly in the urine.

Once very widely used, tetracyclines have faded considerably in popularity because of widespread resistance and the introduction of newer broad-spectrum agents, such as amoxicillin with clavulanate. Research, however, continues, and novel analogues can be expected as indicated by the recent U.S. FDA approval of tigecycline, the first of a new class of tetracyclines referred to as the glycylcyclines.

Tigecycline

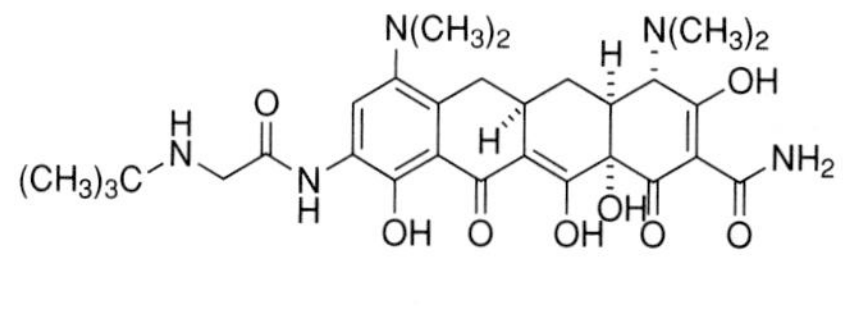

Tigecycline
(Tygacil)

The increased incidence of resistance to the tetracyclines led to a renewed research effort to find novel agents within this class. This effort led to the discovery of a new class of antibiotics, the glycylcyclines, that are closely related structurally to the tetracyclines but lack many of the clinical resistance issues. They are characterized by having an additional glycylamido substitution at the 9-position. As indicated earlier, substitution on the western face does not appear to interfere with binding of the drug to the rRNA. Tigecycline is the first of these agents to be marketed. Although it has limited indications (treatment of complicated skin/skin structure and complicated intra-abdominal infections), this agent is a broad-spectrum antibiotic based on the in vitro data. It is administered IV and, like the tetracyclines, can cause injection site pain and thrombophlebitis. It is expected to have other adverse effects similar to the tetracyclines.

SPECIAL PURPOSE ANTIBIOTICS. This group of antibiotics consists of a miscellaneous collection of structural types for which the toxicities or narrow ranges of applicability give them a more specialized place in antimicrobial chemotherapy than those covered to this point. They generally are reserved for special purposes.

Chloramphenicol (Chloromycetin)

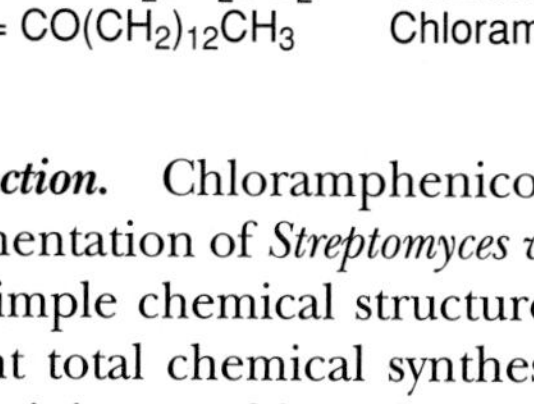

R = H Chloramphenicol (Chloromycetin)
R = $COCH_2CH_2CO_2H$ Chloramphenicol hemisuccinate
R = $CO(CH_2)_{12}CH_3$ Chloramphenicol palmitate

Introduction. Chloramphenicol was originally produced by fermentation of *Streptomyces venezuelae,* but its comparatively simple chemical structure soon resulted in several efficient total chemical syntheses. With two asymmetric centers, it is one of four diastereomers, only one of which (1*R*,2*R*) is significantly active. Because total synthesis produces a mixture of all four, the unwanted isomers must be removed before use. Chloramphenicol is a neutral substance that is only moderately soluble in water, because both nitrogen atoms are nonbasic under physiologic conditions (one is an amide and the other a nitro moiety). It was the first broad-spectrum oral antibiotic used in the United States (1947) and was once very popular. Severe potential blood dyscrasia has greatly decreased its use in North America. Although its cheapness and efficiency makes it still very popular in much of the rest of the world where it can often be purchased over-the-counter without a prescription.

Mechanism of action. Chloramphenicol is bacteriostatic by virtue of inhibition of protein biosynthesis in both bacterial and, to a lesser extent, host ribosomes. Chloramphenicol binds to the 50S subparticle in a region near where the macrolides and lincosamides bind (Fig. 38.24).

Resistance is mediated by several R-factor enzymes that catalyze acetylation of the secondary and, to some extent, the primary hydroxyl groups in the aliphatic side chain. These products no longer bind to the ribosomes and so are inactivated. *Escherichia coli* frequently is resistant because of chloramphenicol's lack of intercellular accumulation.

Metabolism. When given orally, it is rapidly and completely absorbed but has a fairly short half-life. It is mainly excreted in the urine in the form of its metabolites, which are a C-3 glucuronide, and, to a lesser extent, its deamidation product and the product of dehalogenation and reduction. These metabolites are all inactive. The aromatic nitro group also is reduced metabolically, and this product can undergo amide hydrolysis. The reduction of the nitro group, however, does not take place efficiently in humans but, rather, primarily occurs in the gut by the action of the normal flora. Chloramphenicol potentiates the activity of some other drugs by inducing liver metabolism. Such agents include anticoagulant coumarins, sulfonamides, oral hypoglycemics, and phenytoin.

Pro-Drug Forms. Two pro-drug forms of chloramphenicol are available (only the injectable form is available in the United States). The drug is intensively bitter, but this can be masked for use as a pediatric oral suspension by the C-3 palmitate, which is cleaved in the duodenum to liberate the drug. Chloramphenicol's poor water solubility is largely overcome by conversion to the C-3 hemisuccinoyl ester, which forms a water-soluble sodium salt. This is cleaved in the body by lung, liver, kidney, and blood esterases to produce active chloramphenicol. Because cleavage in muscles is slow, this pro-drug is used IV rather than IM.

Therapeutic Applications. Despite potentially serious limitations, chloramphenicol is an effective drug when used carefully. Its special value is in typhoid fever, *Haemophilus* infections (especially epiglottitis and meningitis, when given along with ampicillin), rickettsial infections, and in cases in which susceptible organisms have proven to be resistant to other therapies. Safer antibiotics should be used whenever possible. It is approximately 60% serum protein bound and diffuses well into tissues, especially into inflamed cerebrospinal fluid and, therefore, is of value for meningitis. It also penetrates well into lymph and mesenteric ganglions, rationalizing its particular value in typhoid fever.

Adverse Effects. Toxicities prevent chloramphenicol from being more widely used. Blood dyscrasias are seen in patients predisposed to them. The more serious form is a pancytopenia of the blood that is fatal in approximately 70% of cases and is believed to be caused by one of the reduction products of the aromatic nitro group. This side effect is known as aplastic anemia, and it has even occurred following use of the drug as an ophthalmic ointment. There seems to be a genetic predisposition toward this in a very small percentage of the population. This devastating side effect is estimated to occur once in every 25,000 to 40,000 courses of therapy. Less severe, but much more common, is a reversible inhibition of hematopoiesis seen in older patients or in those with renal insufficiency. If cell counts are taken, this can be controlled, because it is dose-related and marrow function will recover if the drug is withdrawn.

The so-called "gray" or "gray baby" syndrome, a form of cardiovascular collapse, is encountered when chloramphenicol is given to young infants (especially premature infants) if liver glucuronidation is underdeveloped, and successive doses will lead to rapid accumulation of the drug because of impaired excretion. A dose-related, profound anemia accompanied by an ashen-gray pallor is seen, as are vomiting, loss of appetite, and cyanosis. Deaths have resulted, often involving cardiovascular collapse.

Cyclic Peptides

Introduction. The usual physiologically significant peptides are linear. Several bacterial species, however, produce antibiotic mixtures of cyclic peptides, some with uncommon amino acids and some with common amino acids but with the D absolute stereochemistry. These cyclic substances often have a pendant fatty acid chain as well. One of the consequences of this unusual architecture is that these glycopeptide agents are not readily metabolized. These drugs usually are water soluble and are highly lethal to susceptible bacteria, because they attach themselves to the bacterial membranes and interfere with their semipermeability so that essential metabolites leak out and undesirable substances pass in. Unfortunately, they also are highly toxic in humans, so their use is reserved for serious situations in which there are few alternatives or to topical uses. Bacteria rarely are able to develop significant resistance to this group of antibiotics. They generally are unstable, so solutions should be protected from heat, light, and extremes of pH.

Vancomycin (Vancocin, Vancoled)

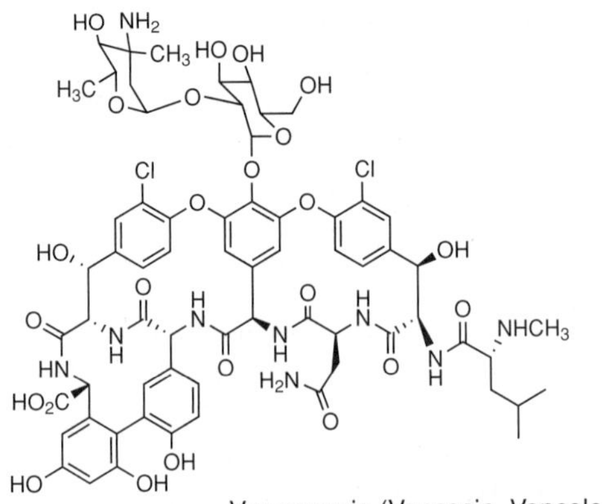

Vancomycin (Vancocin, Vancoled)

Vancomycin is produced by fermentation of *Amycolatopsis orientalis* (formerly *Nocardia orientalis*). It has been available for approximately 40 years, but its popularity has increased significantly with the emergence of MRSA in the early 1980s. Chemically, vancomycin has a glycosy lated hexapeptide chain that is rich in unusual amino acids, many of which contain aromatic rings cross-linked by aryl ether bonds into a rigid molecular framework.

Mechanism of Action. Vancomycin is a bacterial cell wall biosynthesis inhibitor. Evidence suggests that the active species is a homodimer of two vancomycin units. The binding site for its target is a peptide-lined cleft having high affinity for acetyl-D-alanyl-D-alanine and related peptides through five hydrogen bonds. It inhibits both transglycosylases (inhibiting the linking between muramic acid and acetyl glucosamine units) and transpeptidase (inhibiting peptide cross-linking) activities in cell wall biosynthesis (Fig. 38.10). Thus, vancomycin functions like a peptide receptor and interrupts bacterial cell wall biosynthesis at the same step as the β-lactams do, but by a different mechanism. By covering the substrate for cell wall transamidase, it prevents cross-linking resulting in osmotically defective cell walls.

Resistance. Only very recently, despite decades of intensive use, have some vancomycin-resistant bacteria emerged (vancomycin-resistant enterococcus [VRE] and vancomycin-resistant *Staphylococcus aureus*) [VRSA]. It is alleged that these resistant strains emerged as a consequence of the agricultural use of avoparcin, a structurally related antibiotic that has not found use for human infections in the United States but was used in Europe before its recent ban. The mechanism of resistance appears to be alteration of the target D-alanyl-D-alanine units on the peptidoglycan cell wall precursors to D-alanyl-D-lactate. This results in lowered affinity for vancomycin due to lack of a key hydrogen bonding interaction. It is greatly feared that this form of resistance will become common in the bacteria for which vancomycin is presently the last sure hope for successful chemotherapy. If so, such infection would become untreatable. These resistant strains are not yet common in clinically relevant strains, but most authorities believe that this is only a question of time. Vancomycin-intermediate *S. aureus*, also called glycoprotein-intermediate *S. aureus* (VISA), also has been reported. It appears to be resistant because of a thickened peptidoglycan layer.

Therapeutic Applications. Although a number of adverse effects can result from IV infusion (see below), vancomycin has negligible oral activity. It can be used orally for action in the GI tract, especially in cases of *Clostridium difficile* overgrowth. The useful spectrum is restricted to Gram-positive pathogens, with particular utility against multiply-resistant, coagulase-negative staphylococci and MRSA, which causes septicemias, endocarditis, skin and soft-tissue infections, and infections associated with venous catheters.

Adverse Effects. Vancomycin is highly associated with adverse infusion-related events. These are especially prevalent with higher doses and a rapid infusion rate. A rapid infusion rate has been shown to cause anaphylactoid reactions, including hypotension, wheezing, dyspnea, urticaria, and pruritus. A significant drug rash (the so-called red man syndrome) also can occur. These events are much less frequent with a slower infusion rate.

In addition to the danger of infusion-related events, higher doses of vancomycin can cause nephrotoxicity and auditory nerve damage. The risk of these effects is increased with elevated, prolonged concentrations, so vancomycin use should be monitored, especially in patients with decreased renal function. The ototoxicity may be transient or permanent and more commonly occurs in patients receiving high doses, patients with underlying hearing loss, and patients being treated concomitantly with other ototoxic agents (i.e., aminoglycosides).

Other Glycopeptides

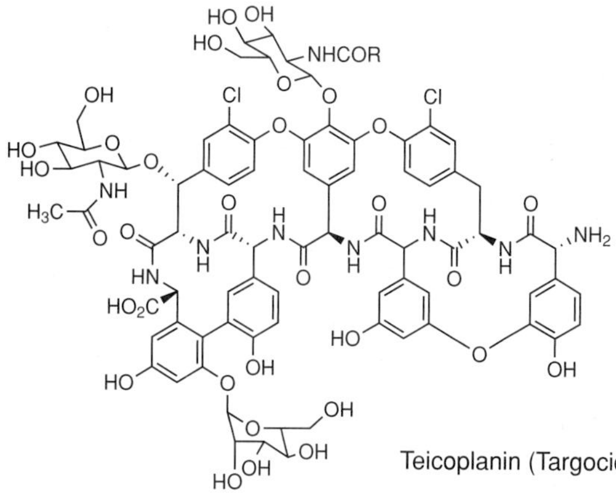

Teicoplanin (Targocid)

Teicoplanin is a mixture of five related fermentation products related to vancomycin. It is more lipid soluble and, therefore, distributes better into tissues and bacteria. It also is highly protein bound, so it can be used IM or IV once daily. It is markedly less irritating than vancomycin on injection; therefore, it appears to be better tolerated by patients and on IV administration. It is not presently available in the United States but is available in a number of other countries. The glycopeptide field is under intense investigation, and a number of agents are at various stages of preclinical evaluation.

Daptomycin (Cubicin)

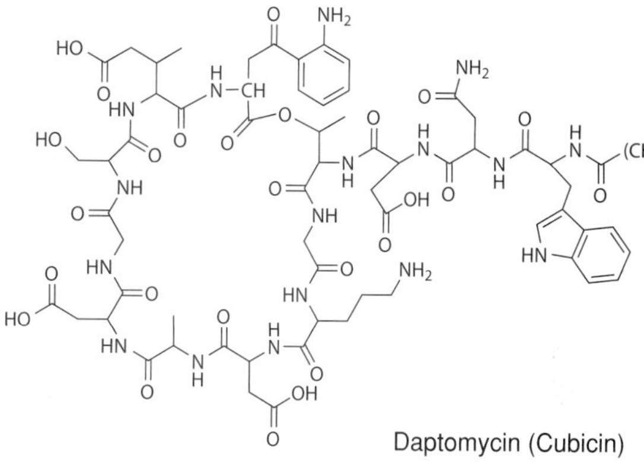

Daptomycin (Cubicin)

Daptomycin is a fermentation product having a cyclic lipopeptide structure. It is primarily active against Gram-positive infections, especially those involved in skin/skin structure infections. It is given IV but must be administered over a period of 30 minutes or more. It binds to cell membranes and causes depolarization, which interrupts protein, DNA, and RNA synthesis. Daptomycin is bactericidal. Although resistance can be achieved in vitro, resistance has been slow to emerge in the clinic. Patients should be monitored for muscle pain or weakness, because some incidence of elevated serum creatinine phosphokinase is associated with its use. A small number of clinical trial patients also developed conditions related to decreases in nerve conduction (e.g., paresthesias and Bell's palsy). Daptomycin is eliminated primarily by the kidney, so dose adjustment may be necessary in cases of renal insufficiency.

Streptogramins. The streptogramins are a group of natural occurring antibiotics isolated from *Streptomyces pristinasprialis.* The streptogramin antibiotics consist of A-type molecules and B-type molecules, which when combined have a synergistic activity. The mechanism of action of the two different types of molecules appear to be quite different.

Quinupristin/Dalfopristin. A drug combination of the streptogramins, quinupristin and dalfopristin was approved for IV use in the treatment of infections caused by vancomycin-resistant *Enterococcus faecium* bacteremia as well as skin/skin structure infections caused by MRSA and methicillin-sensitive *Streptococcus pyogenes.* Certain strains of *E. faecium* are resistant to essentially all

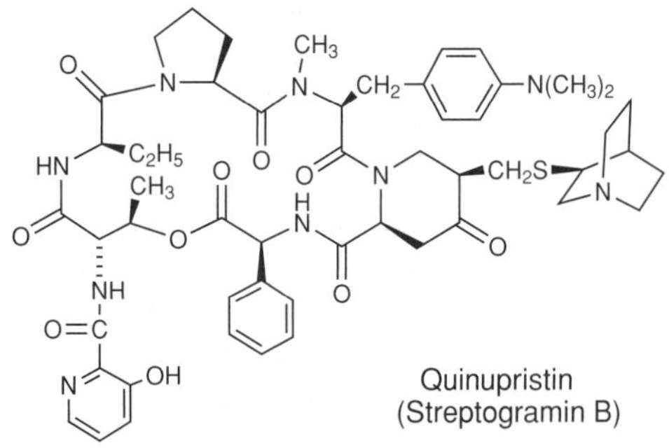

Quinupristin
(Streptogramin B)

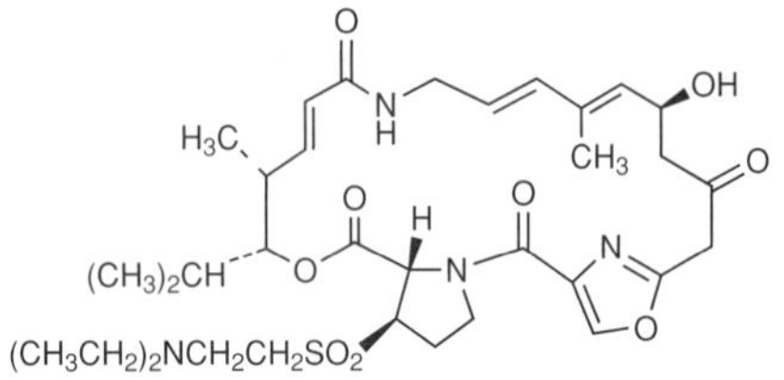

Dalfopristin
(Streptogramin A)

Synercid (30:70, quinupristin:dalfopristin)

other antibiotics, including vancomycin. The streptogramin type A compound dalfopristin binds to the 50S ribosomal subparticle, resulting in a conformational change in the substrate. It appears that dalfopristin binding creates a high-affinity binding site for quinupristin, accounting for the synergy. Its site of action appears to be similar to that of chloroamphenicol, with effects on both the 30S and 50S subparticles. Quinupristin, the type B streptogramin, binds to the 50S subparticle overlapping the sites occupied by the macrolides and lincosamides (MLS_B compounds) (Fig. 38.24). As a result, resistance to the later two classes of antibiotics confers resistance to quinupristin but not to dalfopristin. The two drugs are bacteriostatic when administered individually but act synergistically when combined (quinupristin:dalfopristin, 30:70 w/w) to produce a bactericidal effect. The combination is found to inhibit protein synthesis. Synercid is a strong inhibitor of the CYP3A4 isozyme, and a number of drug interactions are to be expected. Although the combination does not appear to prolong the QT_c interval, it inhibits the metabolism of a number of agents that have been shown to have this effect, so concomitant administration should be avoided. Synercid also can produce a number of other adverse effects, including infusion site reactions (e.g., pain, edema, and inflammation), arthralgia and myalgia, and hyperbilirubinemia.

Polymyxin B

Polymyxin B is produced by fermentation of *Bacillus polymyxa*. It is separated from a mixture of related cyclic peptides and is primarily active against Gram-negative microorganisms. It apparently binds to phosphate groups in bacterial cytoplasmic membranes and disrupts their integrity. It is used IM or IV as a sulfate salt to treat serious urinary tract infections, meningitis, and septicemia, primarily caused by *Pseudomonas aeruginosa*, but some other Gram-negative bacteria also will respond. Irrigation of the urinary bladder with solutions of polymyxin B sulfate is employed as well by some to reduce the incidence of infections subsequent to installation of indwelling catheters. Additionally, it is used ophthalmically to treat infections by *P. aeruginosa*. When given parenterally, the drug is neuro- and nephrotoxic and, therefore, is employed only after other drugs have failed.

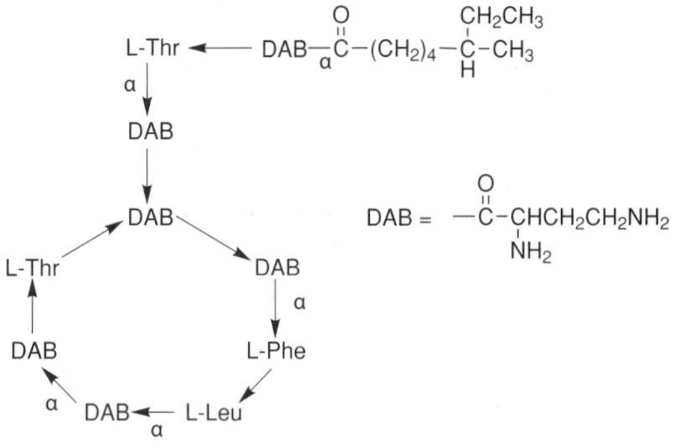

Bacitracin

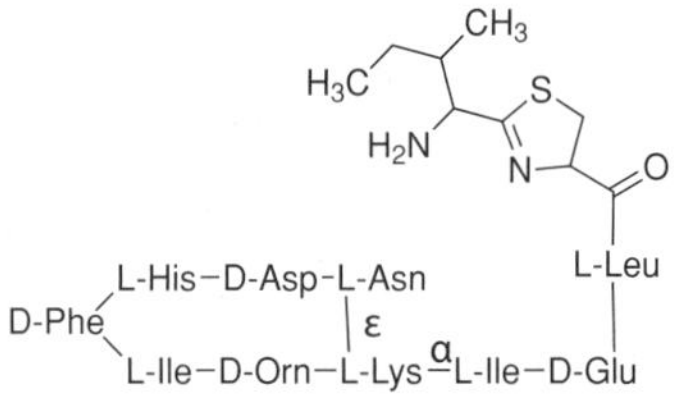

Bacitracin A

Bacitracin is a mixture of similar peptides produced by fermentation of the bacterium *Bacillus subtilis*. The A-type component predominates. Its mode of action is to inhibit both peptidoglycan biosynthesis at a late stage (probably at the dephosphorylation of the phospholipid carrier step) and disruptions of plasma membrane function. It is predominantly active against Gram-positive microorganisms, and parenteral use is limited to IM injection for infants with pneumonia and empyema caused by staphylococci resistant to other agents. It is rather neuro- and nephrotoxic and, therefore, is used in this manner with caution. Bacitracin also is widely employed topically to prevent infection in minor cuts, scrapes, and burns.

Linezolid

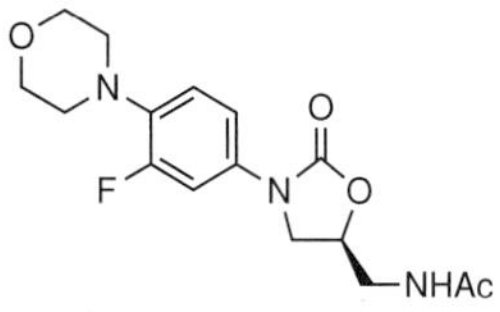

Linezolid (Zyvox)

Linezolid is the first member of the oxazolidinone class of agents and represents a new synthetic class of antibacterials. It is active primarily against Gram-positive aerobic organisms and is indicated for treatment of MRSA, nosocomial pneumonia, community-acquired pneumonia, complicated and uncomplicated skin/skin structure infections because of susceptible organisms, and vancomycin-resistant *Enterococcus faecium* infections. The mechanism of action is inhibition of protein synthesis, but at a stage different from that of other protein synthesis inhibitors. The oxazolidinones bind to the 23S rRNA of the 50S subparticle to prevent formation of a functional 70S initiation complex (Fig. 38.24). It is considered to be bacteriostatic against enterococci and staphylococci but bacteriocidal against streptococci. Resistance to oxazolidinones is encountered in the clinic because of a mutation in the 23S rRNA. This is believed to distort the linezolid binding site. Gram-negative microorganisms are intrinsically resistant to linezolid because of the presence of endogenous efflux pumps that keep it from accumulating in the cells. Linezolid is well absorbed orally and is generally well tolerated; however, some severe cases of reversible blood dyscrasias have been noted, resulting in a package insert warning that complete blood counts should be monitored weekly, especially in patients with poorly draining infections and who are receiving prolonged therapy with the drug. Some interference with monoamine oxidase action has been seen, so patients should be cautious about ingesting tyramine-rich foods. Coadministration with adrenergic and serotonergic agents also is unadvisable. Additionally, lactic acidosis has been reported in patients receiving linezolid. Significant oxidative metabolism of the morpholine ring occurs but is not caused by cytochrome P450, so it does not interfere with other drugs metabolized by this system. Significant activity is underway to prepare and evaluate other oxazolidinone analogues.

Mupirocin

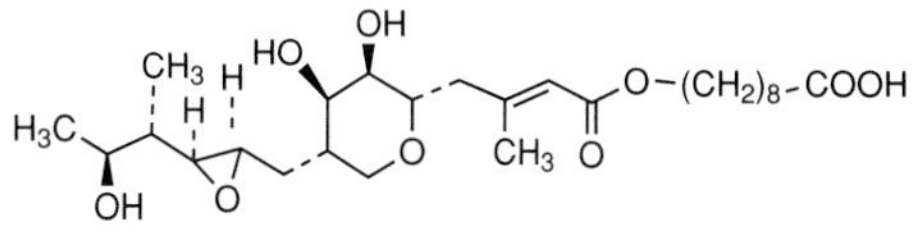

Mupirocin (Bactroban)

Mupirocin is a member of a group of lipid acids produced by fermentation of *Pseudomonas fluorescens.* It can only be used topically because of hydrolysis in vivo that inactivates the drug. It has an intrinsically broad spectrum, but its primary indication is topical use against staphylococcal and streptococcal skin infections. It is commonly used nasally in infection control programs to eradication nasal colonization by MRSA. Mupirocin binds to bacterial isoleucyl transfer-RNA synthase, preventing incorporation of isoleucine into bacterial proteins. Resistance is caused by alterations of the synthase target such that the enzyme still functions but does not bind mupirocin.

CASE STUDY

Victoria F. Roche and S. William Zito

MR is an 87-year-old, widowed woman living in a facility designed for healthy seniors capable of independent care. An unusually cold and harsh winter has curtailed the number of field trips and outings that could be planned, but the Activities Director has engaged the residents in many popular indoor events, such as line dancing, "chairobics" exercise sessions, board games, and musical entertainment. MR is a regular participant in these activities, because she gets lonely in her apartment and thoroughly enjoys the stimulation of interacting with her fellow residents (plus partaking of the refreshments served).

Recently, there has been an outbreak of community-acquired pneumonia in the facility, and unfortunately, MR has fallen victim. Although normally independent, she is somewhat frail and was sufficiently ill to require short-term hospitalization to identify appropriate therapy. The offending organism was confirmed to be *Streptococcus pneumoniae*, and the physician would like to maintain her on parenteral therapy for a few days before sending her home on oral medication. MR is concerned about out-of-pocket costs, because her late husband's insurance coverage, which she has been able to maintain, does not have a very extensive drug plan. MR's medical history includes a severe penicillin allergy and lactose intolerance, and her current medications include extended-release alprazolam (1 mg at bedtime for mild anxiety), simvastatin (Zocor, 20 mg q.d. in the evenings) for dyslipidemia, and low-dose micronized estradiol (0.5 mg q.d.), along with Viactive calcium chews (t.i.d.) to minimize bone loss. Her renal and hepatic function is suboptimal, as would be expected in someone of her advanced years. Consider the structures of the antibiotics drawn below, and prepare to make a therapeutic recommendation.

1. Identify the therapeutic problem(s) in which the pharmacist's intervention may benefit the patient.
2. Identify and prioritize the patient-specific factors that must be considered to achieve the desired therapeutic outcomes.
3. Conduct a thorough and mechanistically oriented structure–activity analysis of all therapeutic alternatives provided in the case.
4. Evaluate the SAR findings against the patient-specific factors and desired therapeutic outcomes, and make a therapeutic decision.
5. Counsel your patient.

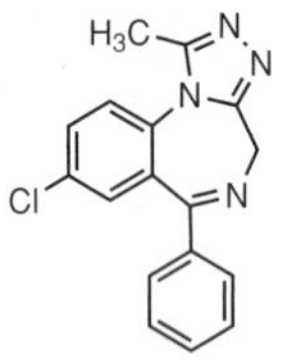

Alprazolam

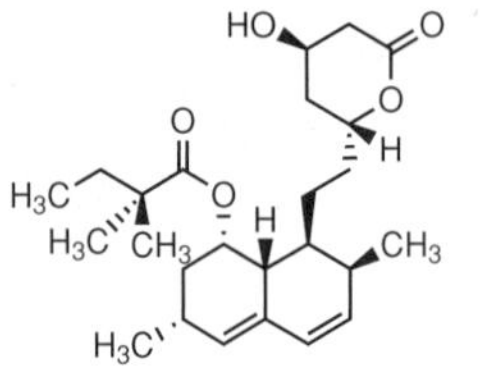

Simvastatin

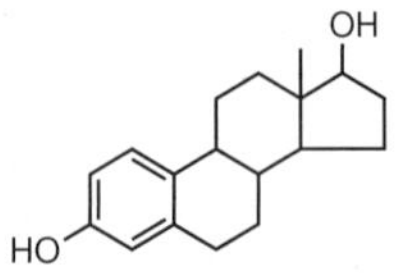

Estradiol

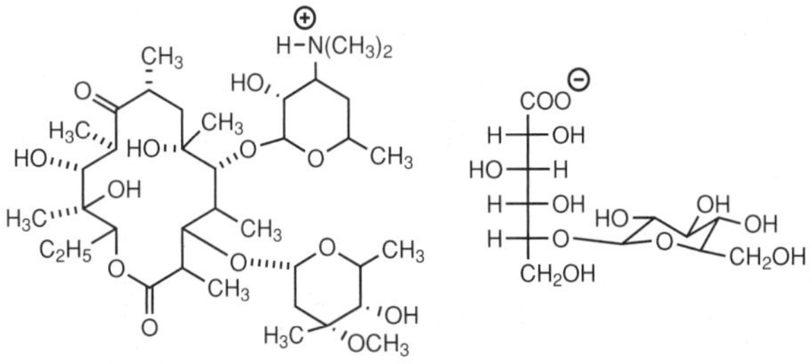

1

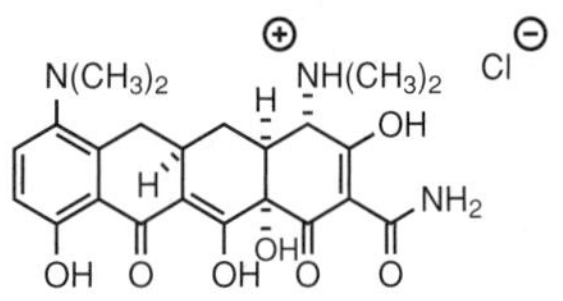

2

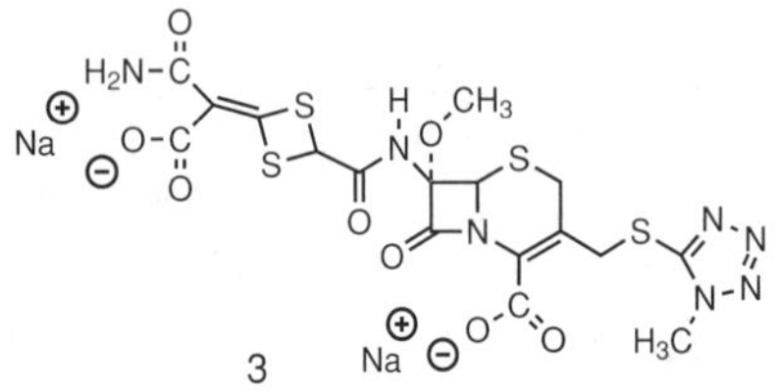

3

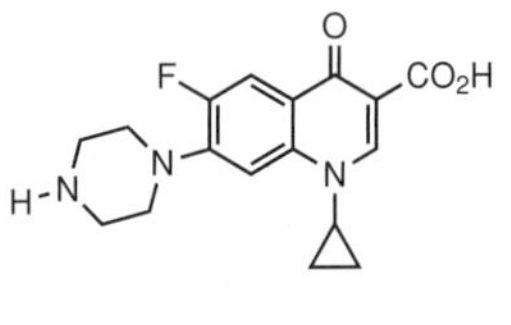

4

Suggested Readings

Albert A. Selective Toxicity. 6th Ed. New York: Chapman and Hall, 1979.

Association Franciaise las Enseignants de Chemie Therapeutique. Medicaments Antibiotiques. Paris: Tec & Doc Lavoisier, 1992:2

Bartmann K. Antitubercular drugs. In: Handbook of Experimental Pharmacology. New York: Springer-Verlag, 1988:84.

Burnet M, White DO. Natural History of Infectious Disease. 4th Ed. New York: Cambridge University Press, 1975.

Dax SL. Antibacterial Chemotherapeutic Agents. New York: Blackie Academic and Professional, 1997.

de Kruif P. Microbe Hunters. New York: Pocket Books, 1965 (Original Edition, New York: Harcourt, Brace, 1926).

Demain AL, Solomon NA, ed. Antibiotics Containing the β-Lactam Structure, Vols 1 and 2, Handbook of Experimental Pharmacology, Vol 67. New York: Springer-Verlag, 1983.

Drug Information. Bethesda, MD: American Society of Health-Systems Pharmacists, 2005.

Gale EF, Cundliffe E, Reynolds PE, et al., eds. The Molecular Basis of Antibiotic Action. New York: Wiley, 1981:2.

Garrett L. The Coming Plague. New York: Penguin, 1994.

Hitchings GH. Inhibition of folate metabolism in chemotherapy: the origins and uses of cotrimoxole. In: Hitchings GH, ed. Handbook of Experimental Pharmacology. New York: Springer, 1983:64.

Hlavka JJ, Boothe JH. The Tetracyclines. In: Handbook of Experimental Pharmacology. New York: Springer-Verlag, 1985:78.

Kuhlmann J, Dalhoff A, Zeiler H-J. Quinolone antibacterials. In: Handbook of Experimental Pharmacology. New York: Springer, 1998:127.

Kucers A, Bennet N McK. The Use of Antibiotics, 4th Ed. Philadelphia: Lippincott, 1987.

Levy SB. The Antibiotic Paradox. New York: Plenum Press, 1992.

Lukacs G, Ohno M, eds. Recent Progress in the Chemical Synthesis of Antibiotics. New York: Springer-Verlag, 1990.

Mandell GL, Douglas RG, Bennett JE. Principles and Practice of Infectious Disease, 3rd Ed. New York: Churchill Livingston, 1990.

The Medical Letter on Drugs and Therapeutics, Handbook of Antimicrobial Therapy. New Rochelle, NY: The Medical Letter, 1993.

Mitscher LA. The Chemistry of Tetracycline Antibiotics. New York: Decker, 1978.

Mitscher LA, Georg GI, Motohashi N. Antibiotic and antimicrobial drugs. In: DF Smith, ed. Handbook of Stereoisomers: Therapeutic Drugs. Boca Raton, FL: CRC Press, 1989:199–234.

Morin RB, Gorman M, eds. Chemistry and Biology of β-Lactam Antibiotics, Vols 1–3. New York: Academic Press, 1982.

Nagarajan R, ed. Glycopeptide Antibiotics. New York: Marcel Dekker, 1994.

Omura S, ed. Macrolide Antibiotics. New York: Academic Press, 1984.

Perlman D, ed. Structure–Activity Relationships among the Semisynthetic Antibiotics. New York: Academic Press, 1977.

Plempel M, Otten H. Walter/Heilmeyerís Antibiotika Fibel: Antibiotika und Chemotherapie, 5th Ed. Stuttgart: Georg Thieme Verlag, 1982.

Pratt WB. Fundamentals of Chemotherapy. New York: Oxford University Press, 1973.

Rosebury T. Microbes and Morals. New York: Balantine Books, 1976.
Ryan F. The Forgotten Plague: How the Battle Against Tuberculosis was Won—and Lost. Boston: Little, Brown and Co., 1993.
Sheehan JC. The Enchanted Ring: The Untold Story of Penicillin. Cambridge, MA: MIT Press, 1982.
Stewart GW. The Penicillin Group of Drugs. Amsterdam: Elsevier, 1965.
Sutcliffe J, Georgopapadakou NH, eds. Emerging Targets in Antibacterial and Antifungal Chemotherapy. New York: Chapman and Hall, 1992.
Umezawa H, Hooper IR, eds. Aminoglycoside antibiotics. In: Handbook of Experimental Pharmacology. New York: Springer-Verlag, 1982:62.
Verderame M. ed. Handbook of Chemotherapeutic Agents, Vols. 1 and 2. Boca Raton, FL: CRC Press, 1986:1–2.
Whelton A, Neu HC, eds. The Aminoglycosides. New York: Dekker, 1982.
Wolfson JS, Hooper DC, eds. Quinolone Antimicrobial Agents. 2nd Ed. Washington, DC: American Society for Microbiology, 1993.
Zinsser H. Rats, Lice, and History. Boston: Little, Brown and Co., 1950.

39. *Antiparasitic Agents*

THOMAS L. LEMKE

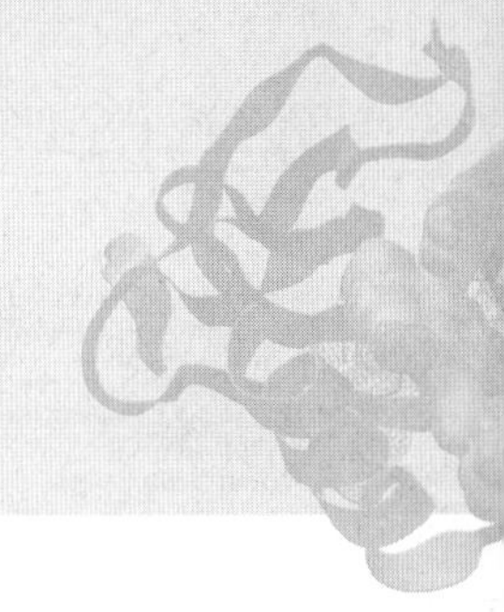

DRUGS COVERED IN THIS CHAPTER:

DRUG TREATMENT OF AMEBIASIS, GIARDIASIS, TRICHOMONIASIS
- Diloxanide furoate
- Metronidazole
- Nitazoxanide
- Tinidazole

TREATMENT OF PNEUMOCYSTIS
- Atovaquone
- Penamidine isethionate
- Sulfamethoxazole–trimethoprim
- Trimetrexate glucuronate

TREATMENT OF TRYPANOSOMIASIS
- Benznidazole
- Eflornithine
- Melarsoprol
- Niturtimox
- Pentamidine isethionate
- Suramin sodium

TREATMENT OF LEISHMANIASIS
- Sodium stibogluconate

ANTIMALARIALS
- Atovaquone–proguanil
- Chloroquine
- Halofantrine
- Mefloquine
- Pyrimethamine
- Quinine

ANTHELMINTICS
- Albendazole
- Diethylcarbamazine
- Ivermectin
- Mebendazole
- Oxamniquine
- Praziquantel
- Pyrantel pamoate
- Thiabendazole

SCABICIDES AND PEDICULOCIDES
- Crotamiton
- Lindane
- Permethrin
- Pyrethrin

GENERAL CONSIDERATIONS

An introduction to the topic of parasitic diseases usually emphasizes two points. First, parasitic infections affect huge numbers of individuals. It is estimated that well over 1 billion people are infected worldwide. Second, the majority of these parasitic infections are found in developing nations, in which the cost of health care is the dominant factor that determines whether the patient is (or is not) treated. The incidence of some parasitic diseases may exceed 80% of the population. The high cost of drug discovery and the low incidence of many of the parasitic infections in affluent Western countries have combined to reduce the incentive for both the study of the diseases and the development of effective therapy. This may be changing, however, because of global travel, improved communications, and growth of the developing countries, leading to an increased demand for more effective treatments.

The diseases associated with parasitic infections represent a large and diverse number of conditions, some common and some relatively unheard of by the general population. Included under the title of parasitic infections are the numerous types of protozoal infections: amebiasis, giardiasis, babesiosis, Chagas' disease, leishmaniasis, malaria, sleeping sickness, toxoplasmosis, trichomoniasis, and pneumocystosis (also considered to be a fungal infection). Helminth infections (worms) also are considered to be parasitic infections and may be caused by any of three classes of helminths: nematodes, cestodes, and trematodes. Insect infections, such as scabies, lice (pediculosis), and chiggers, also are considered to be parasitic infections.

PROTOZOAL DISEASES

Amebiasis

Amebiasis is a disease of the large intestine caused by *Entamoeba histolytica*. The disease occurs mainly in the tropics, but it also is seen in temperate climates. Amebiasis may be carried without significant symptoms or may lead to severe, life-threatening dysentery. The organism exists in one of two forms, the motile trophozoite form or the dormant cyst form. The trophozoite form is found in the intestine or wall of the colon and may be expelled from the body with the stools. The cyst form is encased by a chitinous wall that protects the organism from the environment, including chlorine used in water purification; thus, the organism may be transmitted through contaminated water and foods. It is the cyst form that is responsible for transmission of the disease. The cyst is spread by direct person-to-person contact and is commonly associated with living conditions in which poor personal hygiene, poor sanitation, poverty, and ignorance exist. The hosts may be rendered susceptible to infection by preexisting conditions, such as protein malnutrition, pregnancy, HIV infection, or high carbohydrate intake. Under these conditions, the organism is capable of invading body tissue. The protozoal invasion is not well understood. but it does appear to involve the processes indicated in Table 39.1. Symptoms may range from intermittent

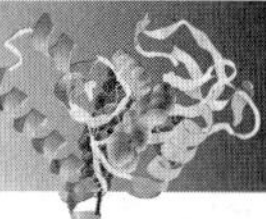

CLINICAL SIGNIFICANCE

Parasitic infections affect more than half the world's population and are responsible for significant health complications, especially in underdeveloped areas. Drug therapy for parasitic infections is quite challenging to practitioners for multiple reasons. Many practitioners lack experience with these agents and are unfamiliar with the toxicities and monitoring parameters associated with these drugs. Certain agents are available in only a limited number of countries, and opinions regarding safety and efficacy vary greatly among practitioners. Understanding the medicinal chemistry, pharmacodynamics, and pharmacokinetics of these agents is of utmost importance.

Despite efforts of vaccine development, drug therapy remains the most effective means to control parasitic infections. Limited introduction of new antiparasitic agents and drug shortages make the treatment of parasitic infestations challenging. Understanding which drugs work at different parts of the life cycle of the parasite also must be taken into consideration. Furthermore, the use of many antiparasitic agents are associated with toxicities, including precipitating severe inflammatory reactions, which may then be treated with anti-inflammatory agents and other supportive measures.

Laura Gerard, Pharm.D. BCPS
Clinical Assistant Professor
Department of Clinical Science & Administration
University of Houston College of Pharmacy.

diarrhea (foul-smelling loose/watery stools) to tenderness and enlargement of the liver (with the extraintestinal form) to acute amoebic dysentery. Many patients may experience no symptoms, and the organism remains in the bowels as a commensal organism.

Giardiasis

Giardiasis is a disease that shows considerable similarity to amebiasis. It is caused by *Giardia lamblia,* an organism that may be found in the duodenum and jejunum. The organism exists in a motile trophozoite form and an infectious cyst form. The cyst form can be deposited in water (lives up to 2 months), and the contaminated water may then be ingested by the human. The trophozoite, if expelled from the gastrointestinal (GI) tract, normally will not survive. *Giardia lamblia* is the single most common cause of waterborne diarrhea in the United States. Giardiasis is a common disease among campers who drink water from contaminated streams. It also may be spread between family members, children in day care centers, and dogs and their masters. The organism can attach to the mucosal wall via a ventral sucking disk, and similar to amebiasis, the patient may be asymptomatic or develop watery diarrhea, abdominal cramps, distention and flatulence, anorexia, nausea, and vomiting. Usually, the condition is self limiting in 1 to 4 weeks.

Trichomoniasis

Trichomoniasis is a protozoal infection caused by *Trichomonas vaginalis,* which exists only in a trophozoite form. The organs most commonly involved in the infection include the vagina, urethra, and prostate; thus, the disease is considered to be a venereal infection. The condition is transmitted by sexual contact, and it is estimated that trichomoniasis affects 180 million individuals worldwide. Infections in the male may be asymptomatic, whereas in the female, the symptoms may consist of vaginitis, profuse and foul-smelling discharge, burning and soreness on urination; and vulvar itching. Diagnosis is based on microscopic identification of the organism in fluids from the vagina, prostate, or urethra.

Pneumocystis

The organism responsible for pneumocystis (pneumocystosis) in humans is *Pneumocystis carinii.* It has the morphologic

Organisms that Commonly Cause Vaginitis

Vaginitis also may be caused by *Haemophilus vaginalis* (bacteria) or *Candida albicans* (fungus), which are treated differently from the protozoal infection.

Table 39.1. *Entamoeba Histolytidavasion* of Host

Intestinal form	a. Disintegration of cyst wall in small intestine
	b. Movement of trophozoites into the colon
	c. Adhesion of trophozoite to cells of the host which involves a change in composition and production of mucus
Extraintestinal form	d. Penetration of intestinal lining and entrance into portal circulation form
	e. Invasion of liver tissue

characteristics of a protozoan (i.e., lack of ergosterol in its cell membrane), but its rRNA and mitochondrial DNA pattern resembles that of fungi. Acute pneumocystis rarely strikes healthy individuals, although the organism is harbored in a wide variety of animals and most humans without any apparent adverse effect. *Pneumocystis carinii* becomes active only in those individuals who have a serious impairment of their immune systems. Thus, the organism is considered to be an opportunistic pathogen. More recently, this disease has appeared in patients with AIDS, 80% of whom ultimately contract *P. carinii* pneumonia (PCP), as one of the main causes of death. The disease also occurs in those receiving immunosuppressive drugs to prevent rejection following organ transplantation or for the treatment of malignant disease. Additionally, pneumocystis is seen in malnourished infants whose immunologic systems are impaired. The disease is thought to be transmitted via an airborne route. The disease is characterized by a severe pneumonia caused by rapid multiplication of the organisms, almost exclusively in lung tissue, with the organism lining the walls of the alveoli and gradually filling the alveolar spaces. Untreated, the acute form of the disease generally is fatal. Even patients who recover from pneumocystosis are at risk of recurrent episodes. Patients with AIDS experience a recurrence rate of approximately 50%.

Extrapulmonary pneumocystosis—that is, pneumocystosis outside of the lungs—also is known to exist and may be more common than presently recognized. This infection may be complicated by the presence of coinfectious organisms. Fortunately, drug therapy utilized for treatment of the pulmonary infection is beneficial for the extrapulmonary condition, although intravenous (IV) administration of the drugs may be necessary.

Tritryps

Three protozoan pathogens that belong to the family Trypanosomatidae, the order Kinetoplastida, and the genus *Trypanosoma* are *Leishmania major*, which is responsible for leishmaniasis; *Trypanosoma brucei*, which is responsible for African trypanosomiasis (African sleeping sickness); and *Trypanosoma cruzi*, which is responsible organism for Chagas' disease. Referred to as the "tritryps," these eukaryotic organisms share characteristic subcellular structures of a kinetoplast and glycosomes, are unicellular motile protozoa, are transmitted by various insect vectors, and infect mammalian hosts. The genomes of tritryps have recently been reported (1–3). Together, they infect hundreds of millions of people annually.

Trypanosomiasis (4)

There are two distinct forms of trypanosomiasis: Chagas' disease, and African sleeping sickness.

Chagas' disease. Chagas' disease, also known as American trypanosomiasis, is caused by the parasitic protozoa *Trypanosoma cruzi* and is found only in the Americas, primarily in Brazil but also in the southern United States. The protozoa lives in mammals and is spread by the bloodsucking insect known as the reduviid bug, assassin bug, or kissing bug. The insect becomes infected by drawing blood from an infected mammal and releasing the protozoa with discharged feces. The pathogen then enters the new host through breaks in the skin. Inflammatory lesions are seen at the site of entry. The disease also may be spread through transfusion with contaminated blood. Signs of initial infection may include malaise, fever, anorexia, and skin edema at the site where the protozoa entered the host. The disease ultimately may invade the heart, where after decades of infection with chronic Chagas' disease, the patient may experience an infection-associated heart attack. It is estimated that 5% of the Salvadorian and Nicaraguan immigrants to the United States may have chronic Chagas' disease.

African trypanosomiasis. African trypanosomiasis, or sleeping sickness, is caused by several subspecies of *Trypanosoma brucei* (*T. brucei rhodesiense* [east African sleeping sickness] and *T. brucei gambiense* [west African sleeping sickness]). In this case, the infected animal is bitten by the bloodsucking tsetse fly, which in turn transmits the protozoa via inoculation during a subsequent bite of a human. The protozoa, initially present in the gut of the vector. appears in the salivary gland for inoculation during the subsequent biting of a human. It is estimated that some 50 million people are at risk of African sleeping sickness, with 300,000 to 500,000 cases occurring in sub-Saharan Africa each year. The infection progresses through two stages. Stage I may present as fever and high temperatures lasting several days; hematologic and immunologic changes occur during this stage. Stage II occurs after the organism enters the central nervous system (CNS) and may involve symptoms suggesting the disease name—daytime somnolence, loss of spontaneity, halting speech, listless gaze, and extrapyramidal signs (e.g., tremors and choreiform movements). A breakdown of neurological function leading to coma and death may occur. Death may occur within weeks if untreated (*T. brucei rhodesiense*) or only after several years (*T. brucei gambiense*).

It should be noted that the sole source of energy for the trypanosomal organism is glycolysis, which in turn may account for the hypoglycemia seen in the host. In addition, the migration of the organism into the CNS may be associated with the organism's search for a rich source of available glucose.

Leishmaniasis

Leishmaniasis is a disease caused by a number of protozoa in the genus *Leishmania.* The protozoa may be harbored in diseased rodents, canines, and various other mammals and transmitted from the infected mammal to man by bites from female sandflies of the genus *Phlebotomus* and then appears in one of four major clinical syndromes: visceral leishmaniasis, cutaneous leishmaniasis, mucocutaneous leishmaniasis, or diffuse cutaneous leishmaniasis.

The sandfly, the vector involved in spreading the disease, breeds in warm, humid climates; thus, the disease is more common in the tropics. As many as 12 million individuals, worldwide are infected by this organism.

The visceral leishmaniasis, also known as kala azar (black fever), is caused by *Leishmania donovani.* This form of the disease is systemic and is characterized in patients by fever, typically nocturnal, diarrhea, cough, and enlarged liver and spleen. The skin of the patient may become darkened. Without treatment, death may occur in 20 months and is commonly associated with diarrhea, superinfections, or GI hemorrhage. Visceral leishmaniasis is most commonly found in India and Sudan.

Both cutaneous and monocutaneous leishmaniasis are characterized by single or multiple localized lesions. These slow-healing and, possibly, painful ulcers can lead to secondary bacterial infections. The Old World cutaneous leishmaniasis is caused by *Leishmania topica,* which is found most commonly in children and young adults in regions bordering the Mediterranean, the Middle East, Southern Russia, and India. *Leishmania major* is endemic to desert areas in Africa, the Middle East, and Russia, whereas *Leishmania aethiopica* is found in the Kenyan highlands and Ethiopia. The New World disease caused by *Leishmania peruviana, Leishmania braziliensis,* and *Leishmania panamensis* is found in South and Central America, whereas *Leishmania mexicana* may be endemic to south-central Texas. The incubation period for cutaneous leishmaniasis ranges from a few weeks to several months. The slow-healing lesions may be seen on the skin in various regions of the body depending on the specific strain of organism. Usually, these conditions exhibit spontaneous healing, but this also may occur over an extended period of time (1–2 years).

Malaria

Malaria is transmitted by the infected female *Anopheles* mosquito. The specific protozoan organisms causing malaria are from the genus *Plasmodium.* Only 4 of approximately 100 species cause malaria in humans. The remaining species affect birds, monkeys, livestock, rodents, and reptiles. The four species that affect humans are *Plasmodium falciparum, Plasmodium vivax, Plasmodium malariae,* and *Plasmodium ovale.* Concurrent infections by more than one of these species are seen in endemically affected regions of the world. Such multiple infections further complicate patient management and the choice of treatment regimens.

Malaria affects as many as 500 million humans globally and causes more than 2 million deaths annually. It is estimated that a third of these fatalities occur in children younger than 5 years. Although this disease is found primarily in the tropics and subtropics, it has been observed far beyond these boundaries.

Malaria has essentially been eradicated in most temperate-zone countries. However, more than 1,000 cases of malaria were documented recently in U.S. citizens returning from travel abroad. Today, malaria is found in most countries of Africa, Central and South America, and Southeast Asia. It is reported to be on the increase in Afghanistan, Bangladesh, Brazil, Burma, Cambodia, Colombia, China, Iran, India, Indonesia, Mexico, the Philippines, Thailand, and Vietnam. Infection from plasmodia can cause anemia, pulmonary edema, renal failure, jaundice, shock, cerebral malaria, and if not treated in a timely manner, even death.

Types of Malaria

Malarial infections are known according to the species of the parasite involved.

Plasmodium falciparum. Infection with *Plasmodium falciparum* has an incubation period (time from mosquito bite to clinical symptoms) of 1 to 3 weeks (average, 12 days). The *P. falciparum* life cycle in humans begins with the bite of an infected female mosquito. The parasites in the sporozoite stage enter the circulatory system, through which they can reach the liver in approximately 1 hour. These organisms grow and multiply 30,000- to 40,000-fold by asexual division within liver cells in 5 to 7 days. Then, as merozoites, they leave the liver to reenter the blood stream and invade the erythrocytes, or red blood cells (RBCs), where they continue to grow and multiply further for 1 to 3 days. Specific receptors on the surface of the erythrocytes serve as binding sites for the merozoite. These infected RBCs rupture, releasing merozoites in intervals of approximately 48 hours. Chemicals released by the ruptured cell in turn cause activation and release of additional substances associated with the patient's symptoms. The clinical symptoms include chills, fever, sweating, headaches, fatigue, anorexia, nausea, vomiting, and diarrhea. Some of the released merozoites are sequestered in vital organs (brain and heart), where they continue to grow. Recurrence of the clinical symptoms on alternate days leads to the terminology of tertian malaria. The *P. falciparum* parasite also can cause RBCs to clump and adhere to the wall of blood vessels. Such a phenomenon has been known to cause partial obstruction and, sometimes, restriction of the blood flow to vital organs like the brain, liver, and kidneys. Reinfection of RBCs can occur, allowing further multiplication and remanifestation of the malaria symptoms. Some merozoites develop into male and female sexual forms, called gametocytes, which can then be acquired by the female mosquito after biting the infected human. Gametocytes mature in the mosquito's stomach to form zygotes. Growth of the zygotes leads to the formation of oocysts (spherical structures located on the outside wall of the stomach). Sporozoites develop from the oocysts, are released into the body cavity of the mosquito, and migrate to the salivary gland of the insect, from which they can be transmitted to another human following a mosquito bite. The life cycle of the malaria parasites is shown in the Figure 39.1. The genome of the *P. falciparum* is now known and is expected to provide potential new

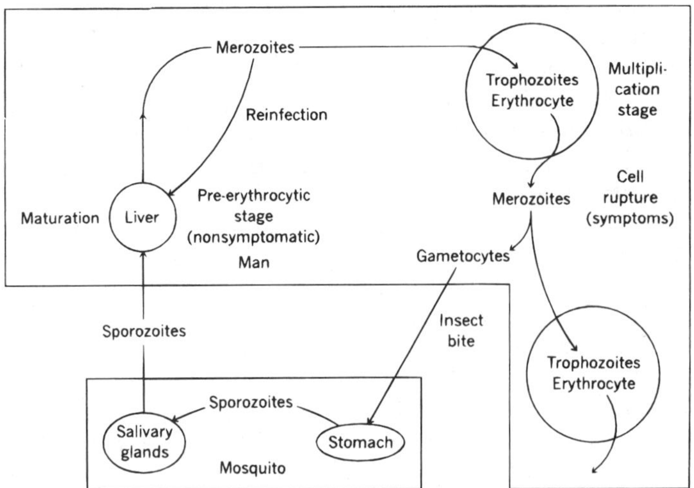

Fig. 39.1. Life cycle of malarial protozoa.

avenues for drug development. Genome information also is expected to give insight regarding the mechanisms of resistance and improve drug treatment.

Plasmodium vivax. *Plasmodium vivax* (benign tertian) is the most prevalent form of malaria. It has an incubation period of 1 to 4 weeks (average, 2 weeks). This form of malaria can cause spleen rupture and anemia. Relapses (renewed manifestations of erythrocytic infection) can occur. This results from the periodic release of dormant parasites (hypnozoites) from the liver cells. The erythrocytic forms generally are considered to be susceptible to treatment.

Plasmodium malariae. *Plasmodium malariae* is responsible for quartan malaria. It has an incubation period of 2 to 4 weeks (average, 3 weeks). The asexual cycle occurs every 72 hours. In addition to the usual symptoms, this form also causes nephritis. This is the mildest form of malaria and does not relapse. The RBC infection associated with *P. malariae* can last for many years. The *P. malariae* is quite unlikely to become resistant.

Plasmodium ovale. Infection with *Plasmodium ovale* has an incubation period of 9 to 18 days (average, 14 days). Relapses have been known to occur in individuals infected with this plasmodium. The relapse may be indicative of ovale tertian malaria and is associated with the ability of the organism to lie dormant in hepatic tissue for extended periods of time.

Types of Chemotherapy

Tissue schizonticides. These drugs eradicate the exoerythrocytic liver-tissue stages of the parasite, which prevents the parasite's entry into the blood. Drugs of this type are useful for prophylaxis. Some tissue schizonticides can act on the long-lived tissue form (hypnozoites of *P. vivax* and *P. ovale*) and, thus, can prevent relapses.

Blood schizonticides. These drugs destroy the erythrocytic stages of parasites and can cure cases of falciparum malaria or suppress relapses. This is the easiest phase to treat, because drug delivery into the blood stream can be accomplished rapidly.

Gametocytocides. Agents of this type kill the sexual forms of the plasmodia (gametocytes), which are transmittable to the *Anopheles* mosquito, thereby preventing transmission of the disease.

Sporontocides (sporozooiticides). These drugs act against sporozoites and are capable of killing these organisms as soon as they enter the bloodstream following a mosquito bite.

It should be noted that antimalarials may operate against more than one form of the organism and may be effective against one species of plasmodium but lack efficacy against others. In addition, antimalarial drugs may be classified according to their structural types.

GENERAL APPROACHES TO PROTOZOAL THERAPY

Amebiasis and Giardiasis

The most appropriate approach for treatment of this type of protozoal infection is through prevention. Because the infection usually occurs by consumption of contaminated drinking water and food, avoidance is the key to prevention. Drinking bottled water, or boiling or disinfecting the water, will reduce the risk. Improvement in personal hygiene and general sanitation also are beneficial.

Trypanosomiasis, Leishmaniasis, and Malaria

For these diseases that are spread by insect vectors, the use of insecticides, protective clothing, and insect repellents can greatly reduce the incidence of the disease. Unfortunately, many of these protozoal infections also can infect other hosts beside humans; thus, even the most successful insect irradiation methods cannot destroy all the reservoirs of the protozoa. The use of insect repellents and protective clothing may be useful for visitors to regions with endemic infections, but these procedures may prove to be ineffective for those living in the area. For such individuals, early detection and drug therapy is the method of treatment.

DRUG THERAPY FOR PROTOZOAL INFECTIONS

Treatment of Amebiasis, Giardiasis, and Trichomoniasis

Metronidazole (Flagyl, Metryl, Satric)

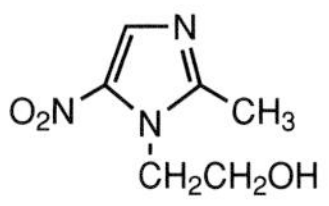

Metronidazole

Metronidazole was initially introduced for the treatment of vaginal infections caused by *Trichomonas vaginalis* but has since been shown to be effective for treatment of amebiasis, giardiasis, and anaerobic bacterial infections, including *Clostridium difficile.*

MECHANISM OF ACTION. Despite the availability of metronidazole since the late 1950s, the mechanism of action of the drug is still unknown. It generally is agreed that metronidazole is a pro-drug and that anaerobic organisms reduce the nitro group in metronidazole to a hydroxylamine, as shown in Figure 39.2, during which a reactive derivative or reactive species are produced that cause destructive effects on cell components (i.e., DNA, proteins, and membranes). Specifically, DoCampo (5) has reported that nitroaryl compounds (nitroimidazoles, metronidazole; nitrofurans, nifurtomox) are reduced to nitro radical anions, which in turn react with oxygen to regenerate the nitroaryl and the superoxide radical anion (Fig. 39.3). Further reduction of superoxide radical anion leads to hydrogen peroxide and homolytic cleavage of the latter leads to hydroxyl radical formation. Superoxide radical anion, hydrogen peroxide, and hydroxyl radicals are referred to as reactive oxygen species (ROS) and are the reactive substances that are implicated in damage to critical cellular components of the parasite.

METABOLISM. Liver metabolism of metronidazole leads to two major metabolites: hydroxylation of the 2-methyl

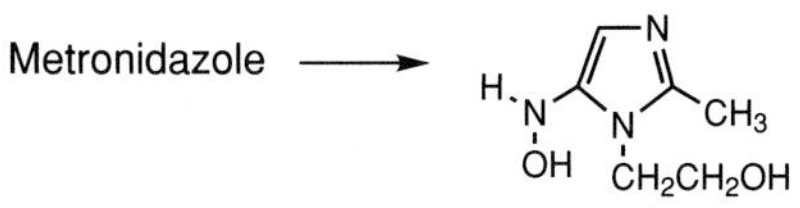

Metronidazole →

Fig. 39.2. Metabolic activation of metronidazole.

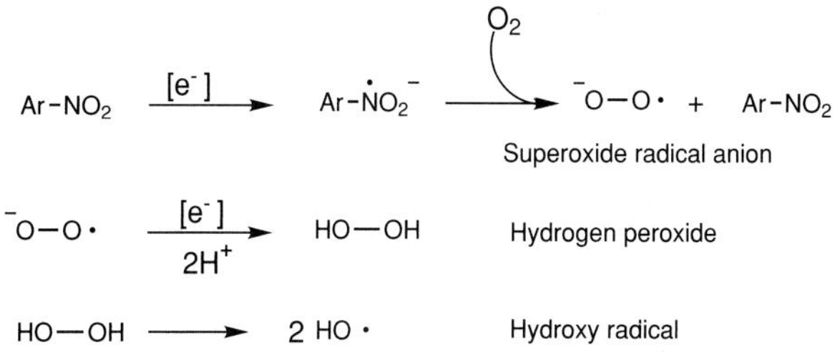

$$Ar\text{-}NO_2 \xrightarrow{[e^-]} Ar\text{-}\dot{N}O_2^- \xrightarrow{O_2} {}^-O\text{—}O\cdot + Ar\text{-}NO_2$$

Superoxide radical anion

$$^-O\text{—}O\cdot \xrightarrow[2H^+]{[e^-]} HO\text{—}OH$$ Hydrogen peroxide

$$HO\text{—}OH \longrightarrow 2\ HO\cdot$$ Hydroxy radical

Fig. 39.3. Formation of ROS from nitroaryl compounds.

group to 2-hydroxymethylmetronidazole (HM), and oxidation to metronidazole acetic acid (6). Both compounds possess biological activity. Additionally, HM is found in the urine as glucuronide and sulfate conjugates. In addition, a small amount of metronidazole is oxidized to acetamide, a known carcinogen in rats but not in humans, and to the oxalate derivative shown in Figure 39.4 (7).

PHARMACOKINETICS (6). Metronidazole is available in a variety of dosage forms, including IV, oral, rectal, and vaginal suppositories. The bioavailability of metronidazole is nearly 100% when administered orally but is significantly less when administered via the rectal route (67–82%) or the vaginal route (19–56%). The drug is not bound to plasma protein. Distribution of the drug is fairly uniform through out the body, including mother's milk.

THERAPEUTIC APPLICATION. Metronidazole is considered to be the drug of choice for treatment for the protozoal infections amebiasis (intestinal and extraintestinal), giardiasis, and trichomoniasis (8). It is the drug of choice for treatment of the Gram-positive bacilli *Clostridium difficile* and in combination is an alternative therapy for *Helicobacter pylori* infections (9). The common side effects exhibited with metronidazole include abdominal distress, a metallic taste, and a disulfiram-like effect if taken with alcohol. The drug is reported to be carcinogenic in mice, possibly related to the metabolite acetamide, and as a result should not be used during the first trimester of pregnancy.

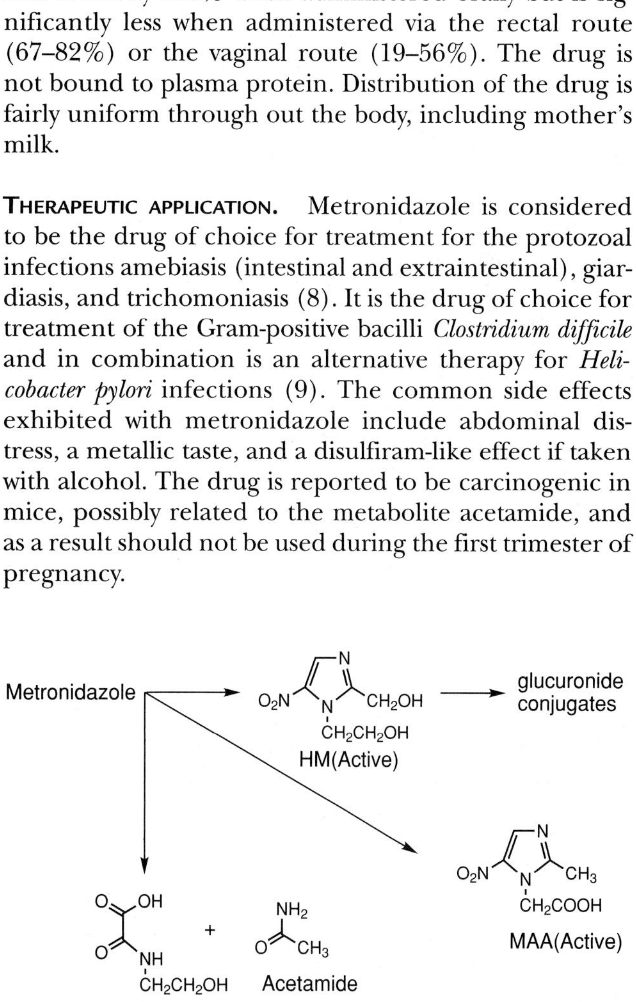

Metronidazole → HM(Active) → glucuronide conjugates

MAA(Active)

Acetamide

Fig. 39.4. Metabolism of metronidazole.

Tinidazole (Tindamax)

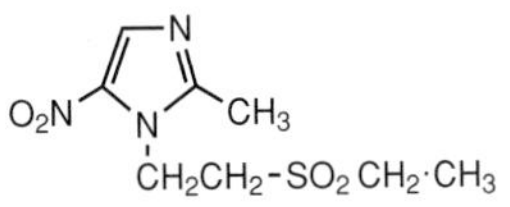

Tinidazole

Tinidazole has recently been approved by the U.S. Food and Drug Administration (FDA) for the treatment of amebiasis, giardiasis, and trichomoniasis. It also appears to be highly effective against *Helicobacter pylori* infections, although it is not approved for this use. The drug is rapidly and completely absorbed following oral administration and can be administered with food to reduce GI disturbance. Tinidazole has a mechanism of action that parallels that of metronidazole as well as a similar metabolic pathway leading to hydroxylation at the 2-methyl group catalyzed by CYP3A4. Basically, tinidazole appears to mimic the actions of metronidazole, although there are reports that it is effective against some protozoa which are resistant to metronidazole.

Nitazoxanide (Alinia)

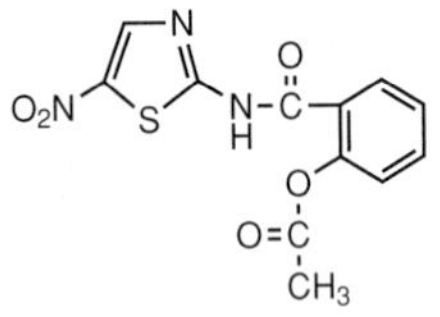

Nitazoxanide

Nitazoxanide (NTZ) has been approved as an orphan drug for the treatment of diarrhea in children (age, 1–11 years) and is associated with giardiasis, but it also is approved for diarrhea caused by crytosporidiosis in patients with AIDS. Crytosporidiosis is a protozoal infection caused by *Cryptosporidium parvum.* The condition is uncommon in healthy individuals but can be life-threatening in immunosuppressed patients and those with HIV infections.

Mechanism of Action (10). Nitazoxanide is a pro-drug that is metabolically converted into the deactylated drug tizoxanide (TIZ) (Fig. 39.5). The TIZ then undergoes a four-electron reduction of the 5-nitro group giving various short-lived intermediates, which may include the hydroxylamine derivative. It is these reduced products that represent the active form of NTZ. Whereas these intermediates would suggest that NTZ has the same mechanism of action as metronidazole, this does not appear to be the case. Nitazoxanide is thought to inhibit the enzyme pyruvate:ferredoxin oxidoreductase in *Trichomonas vaginalis, Entamoeba histolytica,* and *Clostridium perfingens.* The results of this inhibition is disruption of the bioenergetics of these organisms. Unlike metronidazole and tinidazole, which fragment DNA and are suspected mutagenic agents, NTZ and TIZ do not cause DNA fragmentation

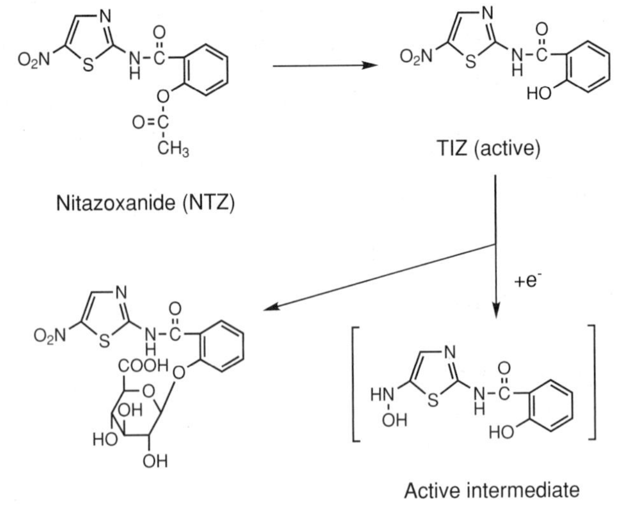

Nitazoxanide (NTZ)

TIZ (active)

Active intermediate

Fig. 39.5. Metabolic activation of nitazoxanide.

and are not considered to be mutagenic. This might be associated with the higher redox potential found for NTZ, a nitrothiazole, in comparison with very low redox potential found for the nitroimidazoles, such as metronidazole and tinidazole. Additional metabolites of TIZ also includes the glucuronide, which shows some biological activity, and small amounts of an aromatic hydroxylation product (Fig. 39.5).

Pharmacokinetics. Nitazoxanide is available as powder that is reconstituted and dispensed as an oral suspension. The drug is well absorbed from the GI tract and rapidly metabolized, with elimination products appearing in the urine and feces. The only identified products in the plasma are TIZ and its glucuronide (11). The product can be taken with food.

Therapeutic Application. Although NTZ has only been approved for treatment of diarrhea in children caused by *Giardia lamblia* and diarrhea caused by *Cryptosporidium parvum,* the drug may soon be approved for adults suffering from diarrhea caused *Giardia lamblia.* In addition, the drug has been shown to be effective against the protozoa *Entamoeba histolytica* and *Trichomonas vaginalis,* the bacteria *Helicobacter pylori* and *Clostridium perfringens,* and various helminths, including *Ascaris lumbricoides, Enterobius vermicularis, Ancylostoma doudenale,* and *Strongyloides stercoralis* (12).

Diloxanide Furoate

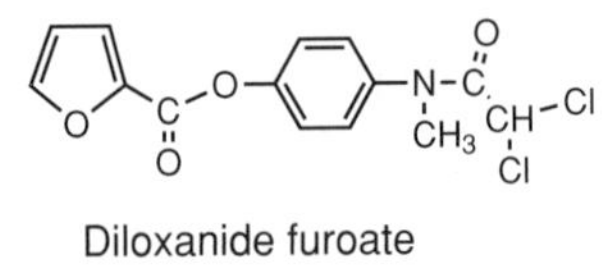

Diloxanide furoate

Diloxanide furoate (available from the Centers for Disease Control and Prevention [CDC]) is prescribed for the treatment of asymptomatic amebiasis but is ineffective as a single agent for the extraintestinal form of the disease. The drug is

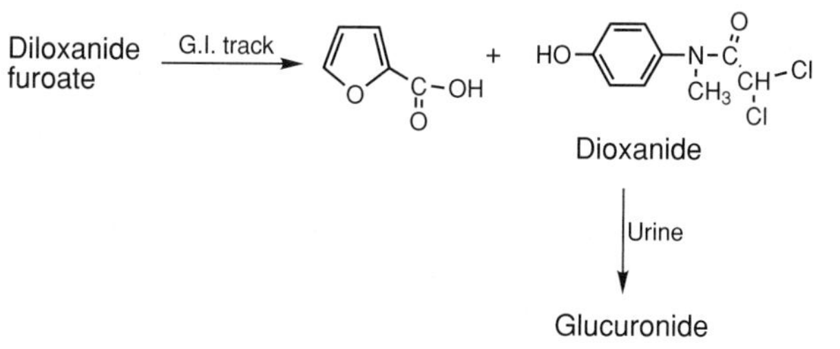

Diloxanide furoate → (G.I. track) furoic acid + Dioxanide → (Urine) Glucuronide

Fig. 39.6. Metabolism of diloxanide furoate.

administered orally and is hydrolyzed in the gut to give diloxanide, which is considered to be the active drug. Diloxanide is the only form identified in the bloodstream. The drug is found in the urine as the glucuronide (Fig. 39.6).

Treatment of Pneumocystis (13,14)

Sulfamethoxazole-Trimethoprim; Cotrimoxazole (Bactrim, Septra, Cotrim)

The combination of sulfamethoxazole and trimethoprim has proven to be the most successful method for treatment and prophylaxis of pneumocystis in patients with AIDS. This combination was first reported as being effective against PCP in 1975, and by 1980, it had become the preferred method of treatment, with a response rate of 65 to 94%. The combination is effective against both pneumocystic pneumonia and the extrapulmonary disease. *Pneumocystis carinii* appears to be especially susceptible to the sequential blocking action of cotrimazole, which inhibits both the incorporation of p-aminobenzoic acid (PABA) into folic acid as well as the reduction of dihydrofolic acid to tetrahydrofolic acid by dihydrofolate reductase (DHFR). (A detailed discussion of the mechanism of action and the structure–activity relationship of these drugs can be found in Chapter 38.) Depending on the severity of the infection, the combination is administered in doses of 20 mg/kg/day of trimethoprim and 100 mg/kg/day of sulfamethoxazole in four divided doses over a period of 14 to 21 days. The incidence of side effects of this combination are high and, generally, reflects the effects of the sulfa drug component. Side effects may be significant enough to terminate treatment.

Pentamidine Isethionate (Pentam 300, Nebupent)

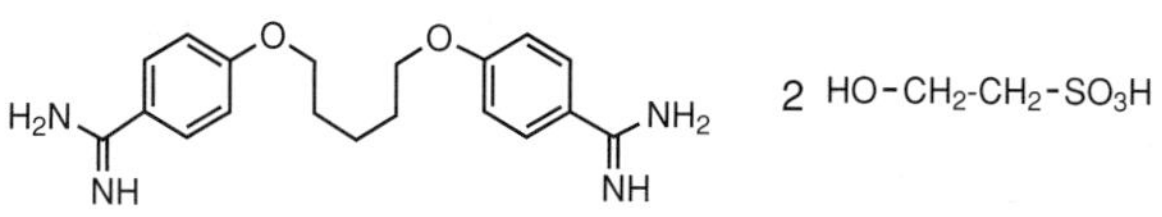

2 HO-CH_2-CH_2-SO_3H

Pentamidine isethionate

> **Orphan Drug Product**
>
> Dapsone plus trimethoprim also has been utilized for the treatment of pneumocystis, with effectiveness nearly equal to that of cotrimazole.

Pentamidine is available as the water-soluble isethionate salt, which is used both IV and as an aerosol. The drug can be used via the intramuscular route, but significant complications have been reported and. therefore, this route of administration is not recommended. The drug has fungicidal and antiprotozoal activity, but today, it is used primarily for treatment of PCP.

MECHANISM OF ACTION. The mechanism of action of pentamidine is not known with certainty, but strong evidence supports various mechanisms of action for pentamidine. Pentamidine selectively binds to the DNA in trypanosoma parasite (see below). Pentamidine has also been shown to inhibit topoisomerase in *Pneumocystis carinii,* which leads to double-strand cleavage of DNA in trypanosoma (12–14). It has been suggested that pentamidine's mechanism of action may be different in different organisms and, therefore, that the actions reported for trypanosoma may not carry over to pneumocystis.

PHARMACOKINETICS. Pentamidine must be administered IV and, after multiple injections daily or on alternate days, accumulates in body tissue. Plasma concentrations were measured up to 8 months following a single, 2-hour IV infusion. The accumulation aids in treatment as well as in prophylaxis. The drug shows poor penetration of the CNS.

THERAPEUTIC APPLICATION. Pentamidine is used as a second-line agent either by itself or in combination for the treatment and prophylaxis of PCP. For prophylaxis, the aerosol form of the drug is indicated and has minimum toxicity. The limitation of pentamidine—that is, the need for IV administration—may be associated with the potential for severe toxicity, which includes breathlessness, tachycardia, dizziness, headache, and vomiting. These symptoms may occur in as many as 50% of the patients. These effects are thought to be associated with a too rapid IV administration, resulting in the release of histamine.

Atovaquone (Mepron)

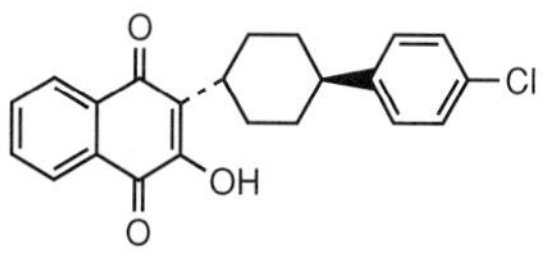

Atovaquone

Atovaquone, a chemical with structural similarity to the ubiquinone metabolites, was initially synthesized and investigated as an antimalarial, a use for which it has recently gained acceptance when used in combination therapy with other antimalarial agents. Today, its usefulness is primarily directed toward the treatment of PCP.

MECHANISM OF ACTION. Atovaquone is thought to produce its antiparasitic action by virtue of its ability to inhibit the mitochondrial respiratory chain. More specifically, atovaquone is a ubiquinone reductase inhibitor, inhibiting at the cytochrome bc_1 complex (15). This action leads to a collapse of the mitochondrial membrane potential. The compound shows stereospecific inhibition, with the *trans* isomer being more active than the *cis* isomer.

Pharmacokinetics. Atovaquone is poorly absorbed from the GI tract because of its poor water solubility and high fat solubility, but the absorption can be significantly increased if taken with a fat-rich meal. The drug is highly bound to plasma protein (94%) and does not enter the CNS in significant quantities. It is not significantly metabolized in humans and is exclusively eliminated in feces via the bile.

Therapeutic Applications. With as many as 70% of patients with AIDS developing pneumocystis and, of these, nearly 60% of the patients on cotrimoxazole developing serious side effects to this combination, atovaquone is an important alternative drug (16). Atovaquone also has been reported to be effective for the treatment of toxoplasmosis caused by *Toxoplasma gondii,* although it has not been approved for this use.

Trimetrexate Glucuronate (Neutrexin)

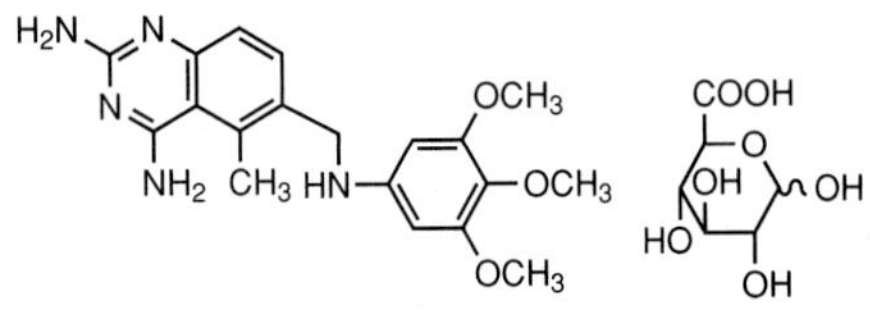

Trimetrexate glucuronate

Trimetrexate (TMQ) has been approved for the treatment of *Pneumocystis carinii* in patients with AIDS and also exhibits antiprotozoal activity against *Trypanosoma cruzi.* The drug is available as a single-ingredient medication, but it can be administered along with folinic acid in much the same way that methotrexate is administered with calcium leucovorin in cancer chemotherapy. Trimetrexate is a derivative of methotrexate.

Mechanism of Action. Trimetrexate is considered to be a nonclassical folate antagonist, whereas methotrexate, the structurally similar analogue of TMQ, is a classical folate antagonist. The difference between these two drugs is that methotrexate, with its polar glutamate side chain, is transported into the cell via a carrier-mediated transport system, whereas TMQ, without the glutamate moiety, is absorbed by the cell via a passive diffusion. Once in the cell, TMQ inhibits DHFR. Trimetrexate binds to *Pneumocystis carinii* DHFR 1,500 times more strongly than trimethoprim and somewhat more strongly than methotrexate. It also has been reported that TMQ readily enters the *P. carinii* cell because of the lipophilic nature of this drug (17). Methotrexate and leucovorin are not able to enter the cell, however, because the cell membrane of *P. carinii* does not possess the transporter protein (17).

Therapeutic Application. Trimetrexate, when combined with the cytoprotective agent leucovorin, is more effective and better tolerated than pentamidine in the treatment of PCP (18). Because the first- and second-line agents are successful in only 50 to 75% of these cases, and because adverse reactions severely limit the use of some of the older agents, TMQ may offer some advantages in treatment. Trimetrexate is administered by IV infusion over 60 to 90 minutes and should be combined with the cytoprotective drug leucovorin. The leucovorin protects against bone marrow suppression and against renal and hepatic dysfunction. Leucovorin administration should continue for 72 hours after the last dose of TMQ. Additionally, TMQ has been reported to be effective in the treatment of Chagas' disease.

Treatment of Trypanosomiasis (19)

Suramin Sodium (Available from the CDC)

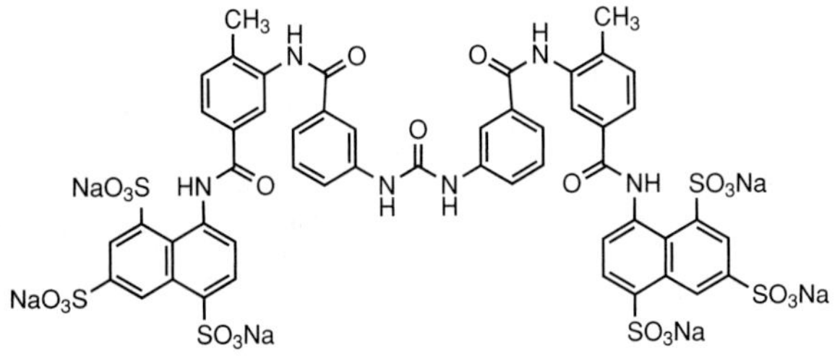

Suramin Sodium

Introduced into therapy for the treatment of early trypanosomiasis in the 1920s, suramin, a bis-hexasulfonatednaphthylurea, is still considered to be the drug of choice for treatment of non-CNS-associated African trypanosomiasis.

Mechanism of Action. The mechanism of action of suramin is unproven, but the drug is known to have a high affinity for binding to a number of critical enzymes in the pathogen. Among the enzymes to which suramin has been shown to bind are several dehydrogenases and kinases. As a result of binding, suramin has been shown to be an inhibitor of DHFR, a crucial enzyme in folate metabolism, and thymidine kinase. In addition, suramin is an inhibitor of glycolytic enzymes in *Trypanosoma brucei,* with binding constants much lower than those seen in mammalian cells. Inhibition of glycolysis would be expected to block energy sources of the pathogen, leading to lysis. Whether one or more of these inhibitor actions represent the toxic action of suramin on the pathogen remains unproven.

Pharmacokinetics. Suramin sodium is a water-soluble compound that is poorly absorbed via oral administration and must be administered IV in multiple injections.

Because of it highly ionic nature, suramin will not cross the blood-brain barrier and, therefore, is ineffective for the treatment of trypanosomal infections that reach the CNS. In addition, suramin is tightly bound to serum albumin. Despite this binding, the drug is preferentially absorbed by trypanosomes through a receptor-mediated endocytosis of serum protein. Because the drug remains in the bloodstream for an extended period of time, suramin has value as a prophylactic drug.

THERAPEUTIC APPLICATION. Seramin sodium is effective against east African trypanosomiasis, but it has limited value against west African trypanosomiasis. As indicated, because the drug will not enter the CNS, the drug is only useful for the treatment of early stages of the disease. The drug exhibits a wide variety of side effects, which can be severe in debilitated individuals, and include nausea, vomiting, and fatigue.

Pentamidine, Isethionate (Pentam 300, Nebupent)

First introduced as a therapy for trypanosomiasis in 1937, pentamidine is now used in a variety of protozoal and fungal infections and, as such, finds use in the treatment of trypanosomiasis, leishmaniasis, and pneumocystis (PCP). The drug is primarily used for treatment of PCP. When used for trypanosomiasis, pentamidine is only effective against *Trypanosoma brucei rhodesiense* (east African sleeping sickness) and, even then, only during the early stage of the disease,. because the drug does not readily cross the blood-brain barrier.

MECHANISM OF ACTION. As indicated above, several biochemical actions have been reported for pentamidine. The drug has been shown to bind to DNA through hydrogen-bonding of the amidine proton and AT-rich regions of DNA. More specifically, pentamidine binds to the N-3 of adenine, spans four to five base pairs, and binds to a second adenine to form interstrand cross-bonding (20). In addition to and, possibly, separate from this action, pentamidine appears to be a potent inhibitor of type II topoisomerase of mitochondria DNA (kinetoplast DNA) of the trypanosoma parasite (21). The mitochondrial DNA is a cyclic DNA. This inhibition leads to double-stand breaks in the DNA and linearization of the DNA. The relationship between binding to specific regions of the DNA and inhibition of topoisomerase is unclear.

In the case of *Trypanosoma brucei,* resistant strains are common. It is thought that resistance develops through an inability of the drug to reach the mitochondrial DNA (22). Transport into the mitochondria is a carrier-mediated process, with the absence of carrier in the resistant strains.

Eflornithine (Ornidyl)

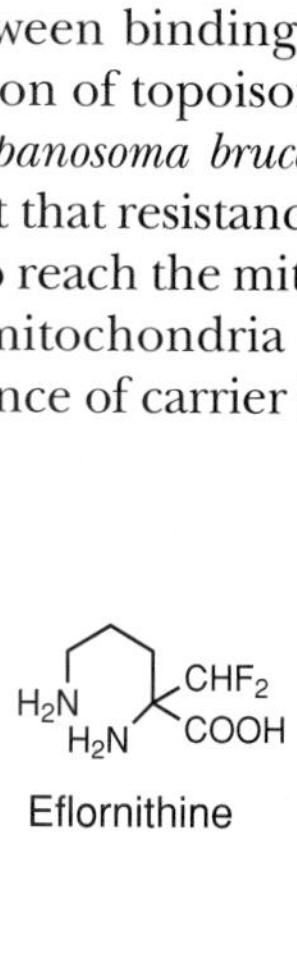

H_2N H_2N CHF_2 COOH

Eflornithine

Metcalf et al. (23) reported the synthesis of eflornithine (difluoromethyl ornithine [DFMO]) in 1978. Their interest arose from the desire to prepare ornithine decarboxylase (ODC) inhibitors as tools for studying the role of polyamines as regulators of growth processes. Ornithine decarboxylase catalyzes the conversion of ornithine to putrescine (1,4-diaminobutane), which in turn leads to the formation of the polyamines, spermine, and spermidine. It was not until 1980 that Bacchi et al. (24) demonstrated the potential of DFMO in the treatment of trypanosomiasis.

MECHANISM OF ACTION. Difluoromethyl ornithine is a suicide inhibitor of ODC, a pyridoxal phosphate–dependent enzyme, as shown in Figure 39.7. Evidence suggests that cysteine-360 in ODC is the site of eflornithine alkylation (25). Alkylation of ODC blocks the synthesis of putrescine, the rate-determining step in the synthesis of polyamines. Mammalian ODC also may be inhibited, but because the turnover of ODC is so rapid in mammals, eflornithine does not produce serious side effects.

PHARMACOKINETICS. Eflornithine may be administered either IV or orally. Administration IV requires large doses and frequent dosing, whereas poor oral absorption and rapid excretion because of the zwitterionic nature of the drug (an amino acid) has limited that route of administration. The drug does not bind to plasma protein and enters the CNS readily, most likely via an amino acid transport system. As a result, the drug can be used for both early and late stages of trypanosomiasis.

THERAPEUTIC APPLICATION. Eflornithine is indicated for the treatment of west African trypanosomiasis caused by

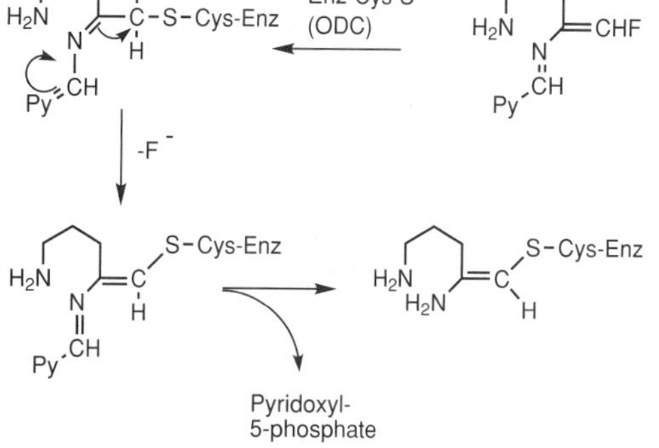

Eflornithine
Pyridoxyl-5-phosphate
$-CO_2$
$-F^-$
Enz-Cys-S$^-$ (ODC)
S-Cys-Enz
$-F^-$
Pyridoxyl-5-phosphate

Fig. 39.7. Inhibition of ornithine decarboxylase (Enz-Cys-SH) by eflornithine.

Trypanosoma brucei gambiense but has proven to be ineffective against east African trypanosomiasis. The cause of this ineffectiveness remains a mystery, although evidence suggests that in the resistant organism, endogenous ornithine plus increased activity of S-adenosylmethionine decarboxylase allows sufficient synthesis of spermidine and spermine to support cell division, thus bypassing the need for organism-synthesized ornithine (26). Side effects reported for eflornithine consist of anemia, diarrhea, and leukopenia.

Nifurtimox (Lampit)

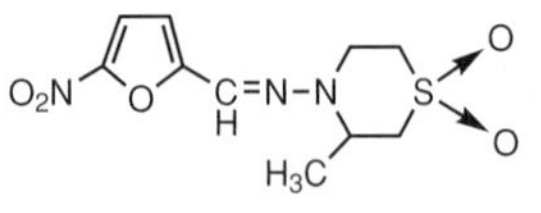

Nifurtoimox

Another of the nitroaryl compounds, nifurtimox has proven to be useful as a drug for the treatment of trypanosomiasis. It is one of two drugs approved for use in treatment of Chagas' disease.

MECHANISM OF ACTION. As discussed for metronidazole, nifurtimox is thought to undergo reduction followed by oxidation and, in the process, generate ROS, such as the superoxide radical anion, hydrogen peroxide, and hydroxyl radical (Fig. 39.3) (5). These species are potent oxidants, producing oxidative stress that may produce damage to DNA and lipids that may affect cellular membranes. In addition, Henderson et al. (27) have reported that nifurtimox inhibits trypanothione reductase, which results in the inhibition of trypanothione formation (93% inhibition). Trypanothione is a critical protective enzyme found uniquely in trypanosomal parasites.

THERAPEUTIC APPLICATION. Nifurtimox is the drug of choice for the treatment of acute Chagas' disease. The drug is not effective for the chronic stages of the disease. In the acute stage, the drug has an 80% cure rate. Side effects of the drug include hypersensitivity reactions, GI complications (nausea and vomiting), myalgia, and weakness.

Benznidazole (Rochagan)

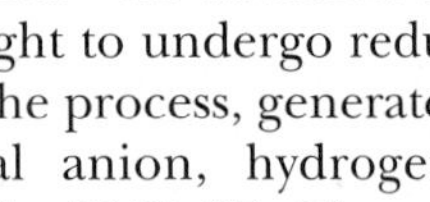

Benznidazole

Benznidazole is the second of the drugs approved for treatment of Chagas' disease. Like nifurtimox, it is effective against the circulating form of *Trypanosoma cruzi* during the acute phase of the disease, but also like nifurtimox, it is ineffective during the chronic stage of the disease.

MECHANISM OF ACTION. Studies suggest that benznidazole does not catalyze the formation of ROS and, therefore, has a mechanism of action different from that of nifurtimox. It has been proposed that benznidazole undergoes an one-electron transfer to the nitro group, which in turn dismutates to give back the nitroimidazole and a nitrosoimidazole (28). The latter product may then undergo an electrophilic addition to trypanothione, which leads to depletion of trypanothione, an essential enzyme system in the *Trypanosoma cruzi* (Fig. 39.8).

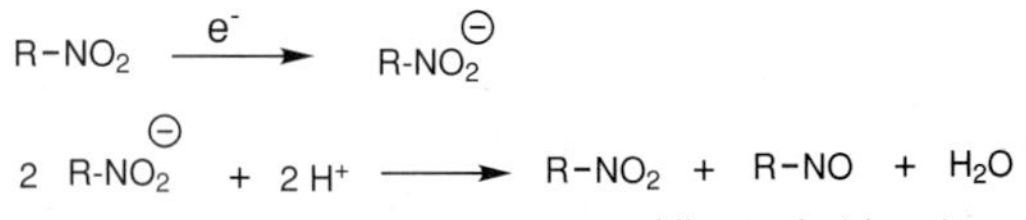

$$\text{R-NO}_2 \xrightarrow{e^-} \text{R-NO}_2^{\ominus}$$

$$2\ \text{R-NO}_2^{\ominus} + 2\,\text{H}^+ \longrightarrow \text{R-NO}_2 + \text{R-NO} + \text{H}_2\text{O}$$

Nitroso imidazole

Fig. 39.8. Proposed mechanism of action of benznidazole.

Benznidazole is not available in the United States but is available in South American countries. It is administered orally in a tablet form.

Melarsoprol (Available from the CDC)

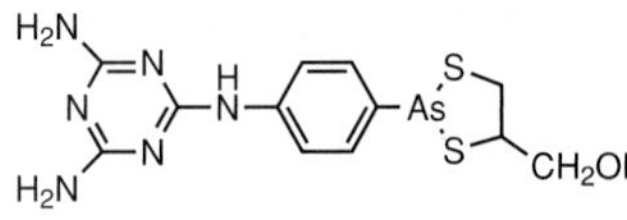

Melarsoprol

Knowingly or unknowingly, arsenic-containing drugs have been used for treatment of parasitic conditions for thousands of years. In the late 1800s and early 1900s, Paul Ehrlich introduced the use of trivalent arsenicals. Melarsoprol, an organoarsenical, came into use in the late 1940s, and it remains the first-choice drug in the treatment of trypanosomiasis. Until 1990, it also was the only treatment for late-stage sleeping sickness.

MECHANISM OF ACTION. It is known that trivalent arsenic reacts rapidly and reversibly with sulfhydryl-containing proteins, as shown in Figure 39.9. It generally is accepted that the enzyme with which melarsoprol reacts is an enzyme involved in glycolysis, and as a result, inhibition of pyruvate kinase occurs. It is argued, however, that the inhibition may not occur at pyruvate kinase but, rather, at a step before the pyruvate kinase. Blockage of glycolysis would be expected to lead to loss of motility and cell lysis. More recently, Fairlamb et al. (29) have proposed a mechanism of action that results in the inhibition of trypanothione reductase through the formation of a stable complex between melaroprol and trypanothione. Melarsoprol

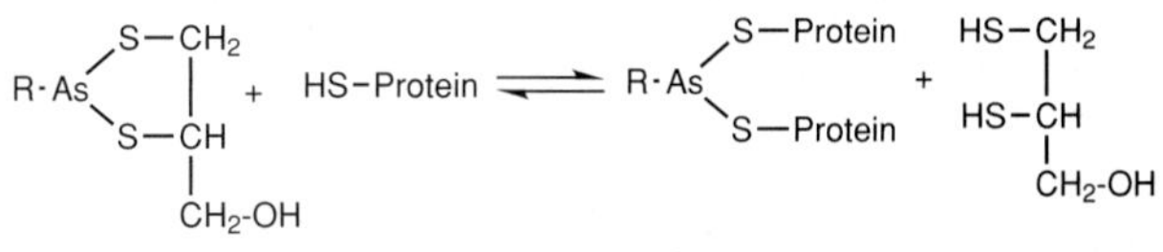

Fig. 39.9. Mechanism of action of trivalent arsenic compounds with trypanosome organism.

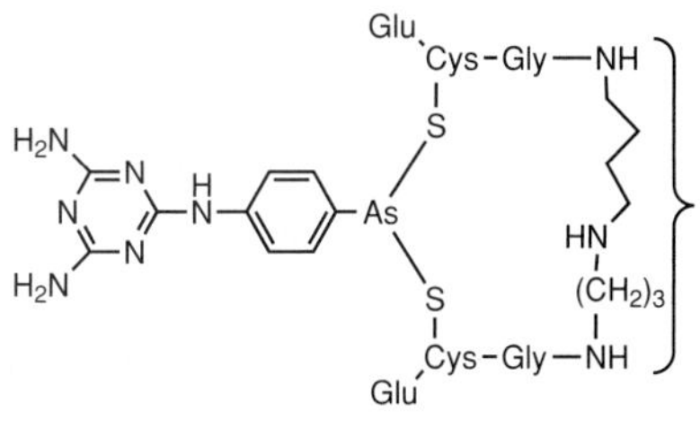

Fig. 39.10. Structure of melarsoprol trypanothione complex.

reacts with the cysteine sulfhydryl of trypanothione to form the stable adduct shown in Figure 39.10. Supportive of this mechanism is the synergistic action of melarsoprol with eflornithine (DMFO). Two drugs that produce sequential blockage of the synthesis of trypanothione.

PHARMACOKINETICS. Melarsoprol is administered IV in multiple doses and multiple sessions. Its major metabolite in humans is the lipophilic melarsen oxide, which can penetrate into the CNS. This metabolite apparently is responsible for the protein-binding characteristic for melarsoprol.

THERAPEUTIC APPLICATION. Melarsoprol is the drug of choice for the treatment of late-stage meningoencephalitic trypanosomiasis caused by the west and east African strains of the disease. Because the drug has the potential for serious nervous system toxicities (e.g., convulsions, acute cerebral edema, and coma), the drug usually is administered in a hospital setting with supervision. An additional problem with melarsoprol is the development of resistance by the parasite.

Treatment of Leishmaniasis

Sodium Stibogluconate (Pentostam, Available from the CDC)

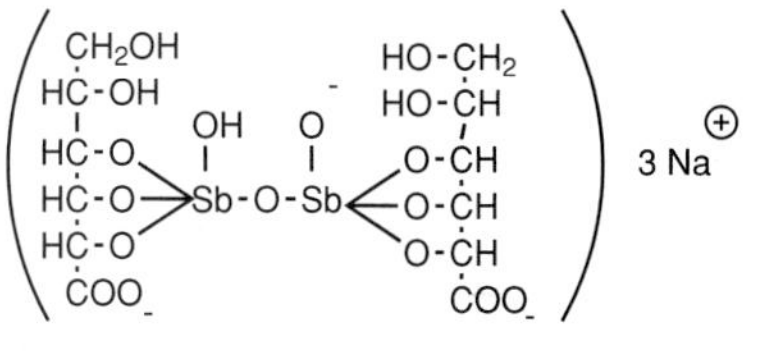

Sodium stibogluconate

Leishmaniasis was first described in the medical literature by Deishman and Donovan in 1903, and shortly after that, the use of antimony-based drugs were introduced as therapeutic agents to treat the condition (30). Although the structure of sodium stibogluconate is commonly drawn as shown, the actual compound probably is much more complex. The drug is a water-soluble preparation that is administered IM or IV. Pentavalent antimony compounds are thought to inhibit bioenergetic processes in the pathogen, with catabolism of glucose and inhibition of glycolytic enzymes being the primary sites of action (glucose catabolism is inhibited by 86–94%). This in turn results in inhibition of adenosine triphosphate (ATP)/guanosine triphosphate formation. Sodium sibogluconate is the drug of choice for the treatment of most forms of leishmaniasis (or meglumine antimonate, another pentavalent antimony agent). The recommended dose is 20 mg antimony/kg/day, not to exceed 850 mg antimony/day. A number of other drugs have been reported to be effective in the treatment of leishmaniasis, and these include pentamidine, amphotericin B, paromomycin, alkylphosphocholine analogues, rifampicin, and ketoconazole (31,32).

Treatment of Malaria

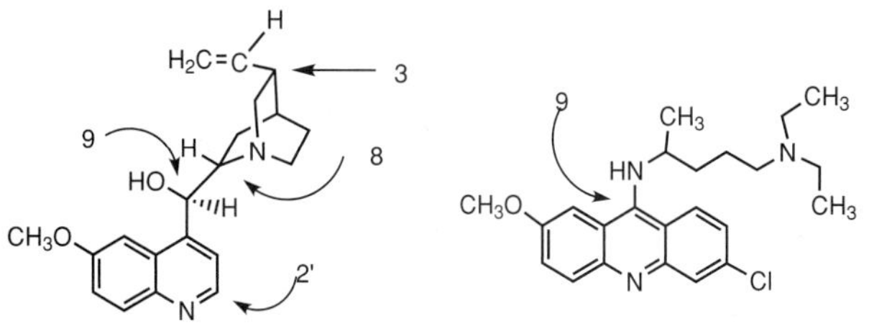

Quinine

Quinacrine

Quinine, was the first known antimalarial. It is a 4-quinolinemethanol derivative bearing a substituted quinuclidine ring. The use of quinine in Europe began in the seventeenth century, after the Incas of Peru informed the Spanish Jesuits about the antimalarial properties of the bark of an evergreen mountain tree they called quinquina (later called cinchona, after Dona Franciscoa Henriquez de Ribera [1576–1639], Countess of Chinchon and wife of the Peruvian Viceroy). The bark, when made into an aqueous solution, was capable of curing most forms of malaria. It was listed in the London Pharmacopeia of 1677. The alkaloid derived from it, quinine, was isolated in the mid-1820s. Quinine, a very bitter substance, has been used by millions of malaria sufferers. Recently, it has been employed successfully to treat chloroquine-resistant strains of *Plasmodium falciparum* and is considered to be the drug of choice for these resistant strains.

A second class of chemicals that played a role in the development of synthetic antimalarials were the 9-aminoacridines. 9-Aminoacridine itself was known to exhibit antibacterial activity, whereas a derivative of 9-aminoacridine synthesized in 1934, quinacrine, was found to possess weak antimalarial activity.

With the beginning of World War II and concern about an interruption in the supply of cinchona bark from the East Indies, a massive effort was begun to search for synthetic alternatives to quinine and to develop more effective antimalarial agents than quinacrine. With a basic understanding of the structure–activity relationship of quinine (see *Quinine*) and the chemical similarities seen with quinacrine, it is easy to visualize the relationship between these agents and the synthetic antimalarials. The 4-aminoquinolines, chloroquine and hydroxychloroquine, are structurally similar to the right half of quinacrine (Fig. 39.11). The 8-aminoquinolines, pamaquine and

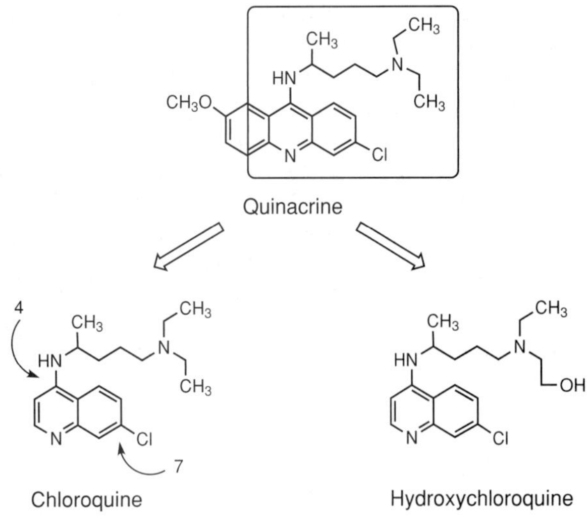

Fig. 39.11. Structural similarity between quinacrine and the 4-aminoquinolines.

primaquine, retain the methoxyquinoline nucleus of quinine and quinacrine (Fig. 39.12). The quinoline-4-methanols, mefloquine and halofantrine, show similarity to the 4-quinolinemethanol portion of quinine (Fig. 39.12).

4-Substituted Quinolines

Five compounds may be considered within this class of drugs: quinine, chloroquine and hydroxychloroquine,

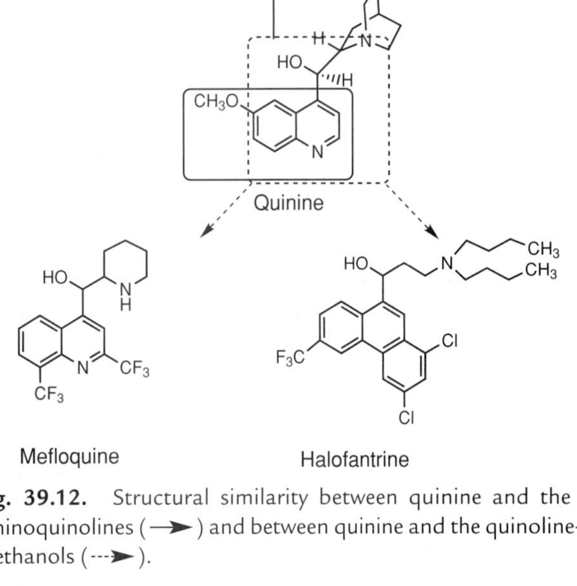

Fig. 39.12. Structural similarity between quinine and the 8-aminoquinolines (—➤) and between quinine and the quinoline-4-methanols (---➤).

mefloquine, and halofantrine (Figs. 39.11 and 39.12). These compounds not only share a structural similarity but also are thought to have similar mechanisms of action, are effective on the same stage of the parasite, and may share similar mechanisms of resistance.

Mechanism of action. The mechanism of action of chloroquine has been studied in depth, and the results of these studies have been assumed to be applicable to the other 4-substituted quinolines (33). Various mechanisms of actions have been offered to explain the action of this class of drugs, including the DNA intercalation mechanism, the weak base hypothesis, and the ferriprotoprophyrin hypothesis. The present understanding about the mechanism of action would appear to utilize various aspects of each of these previous mechanisms. It is known that hemoglobin is transported into the food vacuoles of the plasmodium, where digestion of the hemoglobin supplies the organism with a source of amino acids. One of the products of this digestion is free heme, a substance toxic to the plasmodium cells, which in the plasmodium vacuole is polymerized to hemozoin. It has been demonstrated that the quinolines bind to hemozoin through a drug–heme complex in which the aromatic quinoline ring π-bonds to the porphyrin nucleus (34). This drug–heme complex caps the growing hemozoin polymer, thus blocking further extension of the polymer. The result of this complexation is that newly formed, free toxic heme is now present, which leads to the death of the plasmodium. The accumulation of the 4-substituted quinolines in the acidic food vacuoles (pH 4.8–5.2) is based on the fact that these drugs are weak bases, as indicated by their pK_a values. The extracellular fluid of the parasite is at pH 7.4, and as a result, the weak base will move toward the more acidic pH of the vacuoles, reaching concentrations hundreds of times those in the plasma. Additionally, the binding of the quinoline to the heme draws additional quantities into the vacuole.

Mechanism of resistance. A limiting factor for most of the antimalarial drugs is the development of resistant strains of plasmodium. It should be noted that resistance differs from region to region, and in some cases, a resistant strain may develop to a particular drug without that drug ever having been introduced to the region (possible cross-resistance). The development of resistance is thought to be a spontaneous gene mutation. Several mechanisms of resistance appear to be operating. One of these mechanisms is based on the *Plasmodium falciparium* chloroquine-resistance transporter (*pfrcrt)* mechanism, which is sufficient and necessary to impart resistance (35). A gene encodes for a transmembrane transporter protein found in the membrane of the food vacuole. Multiple mutations within a specific region this gene result in reduced accumulation of chloroquine, resulting from the increased efflux of the drug. Additional transporter proteins also may be involved in resistance.

Rapid metabolism of the antimalarials by resistant strains of plasmodium also might be considered to play a significant role in the development of resistance. It has been shown that cytochrome P450 activity parallels increased resistance to specific drugs.

THERAPEUTIC APPLICATION. The 4-substituted quinolines are referred to as rapidly acting blood schizonticides, with activity against plasmodium in the erythrocytic stage. Chloroquine is the drug of choice, but unfortunately, the incidence of chloroquine-resistance infections are extremely common today. The spread of chloroquine resistance has reached almost all malarious areas of the world. In addition, multidrug-resistant and cross-resistant strains of plasmodium are now common. The drug of choice for the treatment of malaria caused by *Plasmodium falciparum, Plasmodium ovale, Plasmodium vivax,* and *Plasmodium malariae* in regions infected by chloroquine-resistant *P. falciparum* is quinine, in combination with traditional antibiotics, mefloquine, or various other combinations as alternative treatment agents (Table 39.2). Of interest is the observation that after years of nonuse of chloroquine, a reemergence of chloroquine-sensitive parasites has been found.

The 4-substituted quinolines, depending on the specific drug in question, also may be used for prophylaxis of malaria. Two types of prophylaxis are possible: causal prophylaxis, and suppressive prophylaxis. The former prevents the establishment of hepatic forms of the parasite, whereas the latter eradicates the erythrocytic parasites but has no effect on the hepatic forms. Several of the 4-substituted quinolines are effective suppressive prophylactics.

SPECIFIC 4-SUBSTITUTED QUINOLINES

Quinine. Quinine is the most prevalent alkaloid present in the bark extracts (~5%) of cinchona. Four stereochemical centers exist in the molecule (at C-3, C-4, C-8, and C-9) (Fig. 39-9). Quinine (absolute configuration of 3R:4S:8S:9R), quinidine (absolute configuration of 3R:4S:8R:9S), and their optical isomers all have antimalarial activity, whereas their C-9 epimers (i.e., the episeries having either 3R:4S:8R:9R or 3R:4S:8S:9S configurations) are inactive. Modification of the secondary alcohol at C-9, through oxidation, esterification, or similar processes, diminishes activity. The quinuclidine portion is not necessary for activity; however, an alkyl tertiary amine at C-9 is important.

Quinine is metabolized in the liver to the 2′-hydroxy derivative, followed by additional hydroxylation on the quinuclidine ring, with the 2,2′-dihydroxy derivative as the major metabolite. This metabolite has low activity and is rapidly excreted. The metabolizing enzyme of quinine is CYP3A4. With the increased use of quinine and its use in combination with other drugs, the potential for drug interactions based on the many known substrates for CYP3A4 (see Chapter 10) is of concern (36).

A quinine overdose causes tinnitus and visual disturbances; these side effects disappear on discontinuation of the drug. Quinine also can cause premature contractions during the late stages of pregnancy. Although quinine is suitable for parenteral administration, this route is considered to be hazardous because of its ability to cause hemolysis. Quinidine, the (+)-isomer of quinine, has been shown to be more effective in combating the disease, but it has undesirable cardiac side effects.

Table 39.2. Guidelines for Treatment of Malaria in the United States[a]

Clinical Diagnosis	Sensitivity	Drug Recommendation
Uncomplicated malaria *P. falciparum*	Chloroquine sensitive	Chloroquine phosphate
	Chloroquine resistant or unknown	A. Quinine sulfate + one of the following: Doxycycline Tetracycline Clindamycin B. Atovaquone–proquanil C. Mefloquine
Uncomplicated malaria *P. malariae*	Chloroquine sensitive	Chloroquine phosphate
Uncomplicated malaria *P. vivax* or *P. ovale*	Chloroquine sensitive	Chloroquine phosphate + Primaquine phosphate
Uncomplicated malaria *P. vivax*	Chloroquine resistant	A. Quinine sulfate + doxycycline, or Tetracycline + Primaquine phosphate B. Mefloquine + Primaquine phosphate
Severe malaria	Chloroquine sensitive/resistant	Quinidine gluconate + one of the following: Doxycycline Tetracycline Clindamycin

[a]Information taken from CDC Guideline for Treatment of Malaria in the United States. For more details, including infectious region and dosing, see http://www.cdc.gov/malaria/pdf/treatmenttable.pdf.

Chloroquine (Aralen). Chloroquine is the most effective of the hundreds of 4-aminoquinolines synthesized and tested during World War II as potential antimalarials. Structure–activity relationships demonstrated that the chloro at the 8-position increased activity, whereas alkylation at C-3 and C-8 diminished activity. The replacement of one of its N-ethyl groups with an hydroxyethyl produced hydroxychloroquine, a compound with reduced toxicity that is rarely used today except in cases of rheumatoid arthritis.

Chloroquine is commonly administered as the racemic mixture, because little is gained by using the individual isomers. The drug is well absorbed from the GI tract and distributed to many tissues, where it is tightly bound and slowly eliminated. The drug is metabolized by N-dealkylation by CYP2D6 and CYP3A4 isoforms. It has been reported that the level of metabolism correlates closely with the degree of resistance. The suggestion has been made to coadminister chloroquine with CYP2D6 and CYP3A4 inhibitors to potentate activity and reduce resistance. Although this may be possible, it is not commonly practiced.

Chloroquine is an excellent suppressive agent for treating acute attacks of malaria caused by *Plasmodium vivax* and *Plasmodium ovale.* The drug also is effective for cure and as a suppressive prophylactic for the treatment of *Plasmodium malariae* and susceptible *Plasmodium falciparum.*

Chloroquine generally is a safe drug, with toxicity occurring at high doses of medication if the drug is administered too rapidly via parenteral routes. With oral administration, the side effects primarily are GI effects, mild headache, visual disturbances, and urticaria.

Mefloquine (Lariam) (37). Mefloquine, which was synthesized with the intent of blocking the site of metabolism in quinine with the chemically stable CF_3 group, exists as four optical isomers of nearly equal activity. The drug is active against chloroquine-resistant strains of plasmodium, yet cross-resistance is not uncommon. Metabolism is cited as the possible mechanism of resistance. Mefloquine is slowly metabolized through CYP3A4 oxidation to its major inactive metabolite, carboxymefloquine (Fig. 39.13). Most of the parent drug is excreted unchanged into the urine. Its coadministration with CYP3A4 inhibitors (e.g., ketoconazole) has increased the area under the curve for mefloquine by inhibiting its metabolism to carboxymefloquine.

Mefloquine is only available in an oral dosage form, which is well absorbed. The presence of food in the GI tract affects the pharmacokinetic properties of the drug, usually enhancing absorption. The lipophilic nature of the drug accounts for the extensive tissue binding and low clearance of total drug, although the drug does not accumulate after prolonged administration. The drug has a high affinity for erythrocyte membranes.

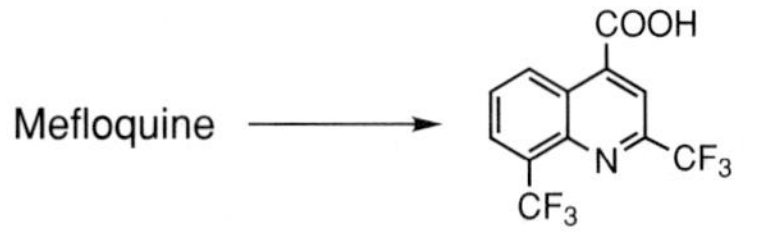

Mefloquine is an effective suppressive prophylactic agent against *Plasmodium falciparum* both in nonimmune populations (travelers coming into regions of malaria) and in resident populations. The drug also has high efficacy against falciparum malaria, with a low incidence of recrudescence. The drug is ineffective against sexual forms of the organism.

The incidence of side effects with mefloquine is considered to be high. The effects are classified as neuropsychiatric, GI, dermatologic, and cardiovascular. The neuropsychiatric effects may be serious (e.g., suicidal tendencies or seizures) or minor (e.g., dizziness, vertigo, ataxia, and headaches). Gastrointestinal side effects included nausea, vomiting, and diarrhea, whereas the dermatologic effects include rash, pruritus, and urticaria. Finally, cardiovascular side effects may include bradycardia, arrhythmias, and extrasystoles.

Mefloquine → COOH, N, CF_3, CF_3

Fig. 39.13. *Plasmodium falciparum* metabolism of mefloquine.

Halofantrine (Hafan). Halofantrine (38,39), a member of the 9-phenanthrenemethanol class (Fig. 39.12), originally came out of a synthesis program dating to World War II, but this particular agent was not fully developed until the 1960s. Halofantrine has one chiral center and has been separated into its enantiomers. There appears to be little difference between the enantiomers; thus, the drug is used as a racemic mixture.

Halofantrine is considered to be an alternative drug for treatment of both chloroquine-sensitive and chloroquine-resistant *Plasmodium falciparum* malaria, but its efficacy in mefloquine-resistant malaria may be questionable. The drug is metabolized via N-dealkylation to desbutylhalofantrine by CYP3A4 (Fig. 39.14). The metabolite appears to be several-fold more active than the administered drug.

At present, halofantrine is only available in a tablet form, which has significant implications as it relates to its

Additional Therapeutic Indications for Chloroquine

Chloroquine also is prescribed for treatment of rheumatoid arthritis, discoid lupus erythematosus, and photosensitivity diseases.

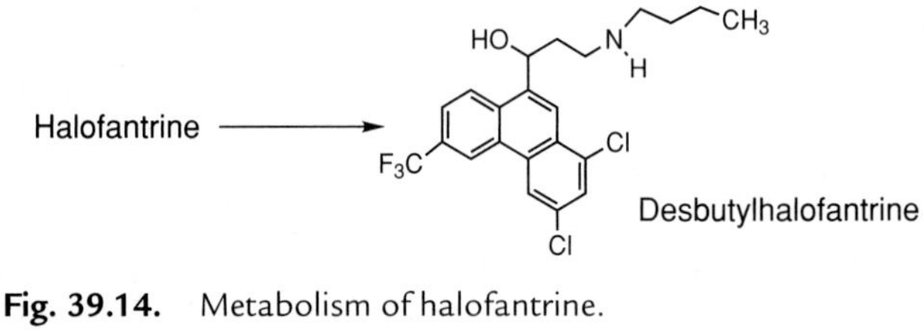

Halofantrine → HO, N, H, CH_3, F_3C, Cl, Cl — Desbutylhalofantrine

Fig. 39.14. Metabolism of halofantrine.

insolubility and drug absorption (bioavailability). Animal studies have shown that following oral administration, the drug is eliminated in feces, suggesting poor oral absorption. Its oral suspensions leads to as much as 30% lower plasma levels of the drug in comparison with the tablet. A micronized form of the drug has shown improved bioavailability. Its administration with or without food in the stomach also leads to considerable variation in plasma levels. A high lipid content in a meal taken 2 hours before dosing leads to a substantial increases in the rate and extent of absorption. Several cases of drug treatment failure appear to be related to poor absorption. Incomplete absorption and, as a result, low plasma levels, may play a role in the development of organism resistance. The elimination half-life of halofantrine and desbutylhalofantrine tend to be prolonged, which may be another factor in the development of resistance. Low levels of the drug may increase the likelihood of augmenting the emergence of halofantrine resistance.

Absorption problems with halofantrine cannot be solved by increasing the dosage of halofantrine because of significant toxicity problems. Toxicity, although minimal with short-term low doses, can be severe with high doses of halofantrine. Gastrointestinal side effects include nausea, vomiting, diarrhea, and abdominal pain. Cardiovascular toxicity include orthostatic hypotension and dose-dependent lengthening of QTc intervals.

8-AMINOQUINOLINES. Pamaquine, an 8-aminoquinoline, was first introduced for treatment of malaria in 1926 and has since been replaced with primaquine (Fig. 39.12). Primaquine is active against latent tissue forms of *Plasmodium vivax* and *Plasmodium ovale,* and it is active against the hepatic stages of *Plasmodium falciparum.* The drug is not active against erythrocytic stages of the parasite but does possess gametocidal activity against all strains of plasmodium.

Mechanism of Action. The mechanism of action of the 8-aminoquinolines is unknown, but primaquine can generate ROS via an autoxidation of the 8-amino group. The formation of a radical anion at the 8-amino group has been proposed by Augusto et al. (40). As a result, cell-destructive oxidants, such as hydrogen peroxide, superoxide, and hydroxyl radical, can be formed, as shown in Figure 39.3, leading to oxidative damage to critical cellular components.

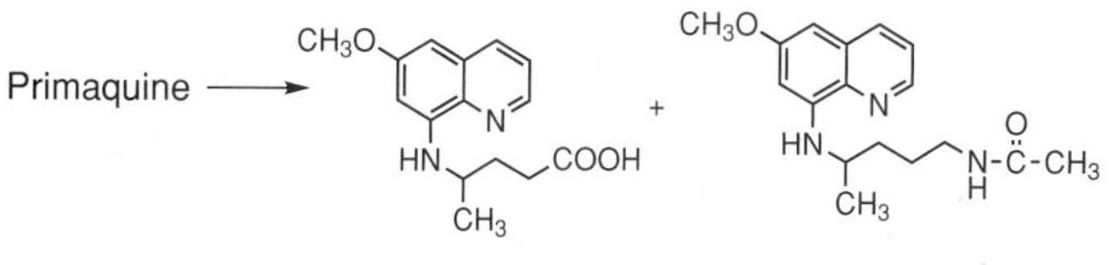

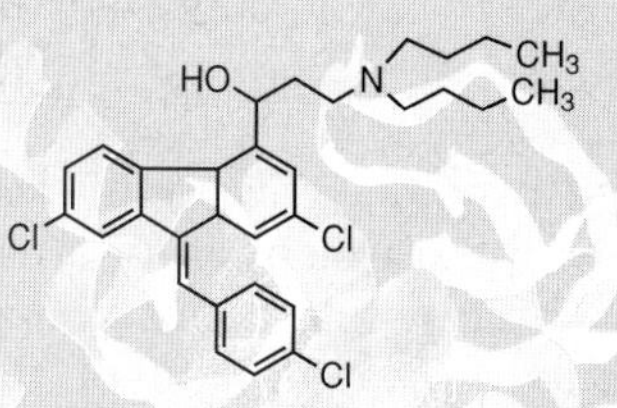

Lumefantrine (Riamet)

Lumefantrine is a derivative of halofantrine that has been reported to exhibit antimalarial activity when combined with artemether in the treatment of multidrug-resistant *Plasmodium falciparum.* No evidence of cardiotoxicity has been reported with this combination, which may offer promise for successful treatment of resistant organisms.

Primaquine → Carboxyprimaquine + N-Acetylprimaquine

Fig. 39.15. Metabolism of primaquine.

Metabolism. Primaquine is almost totally metabolized by CYP3A4 (99%), with the primary metabolite being carboxyprimaquine (Fig. 39.15) (41). Trace amounts of N-acetylprimaquine plus aromatic hydroxylation and conjugation metabolites also have been reported.

Therapeutic Application. Primaquine is classified as the drug of choice for the treatment of relapsing vivax and ovale forms of malaria and will produce a radical cure of the condition. It is recommended that the drug be combined with chloroquine to eradicate the erythrocytic stages of malaria. Primaquine is not given for long-term treatment because of potential toxicity and sensitization. The sensitivity appears most commonly in individuals who have glucose-6-phosphate dehydrogenase deficiency. In these cases, hemolytic anemia may develop.

PYRIMETHAMINE

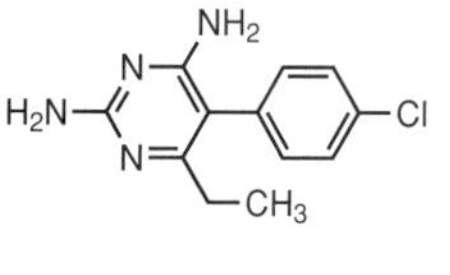

Pyrimethamine

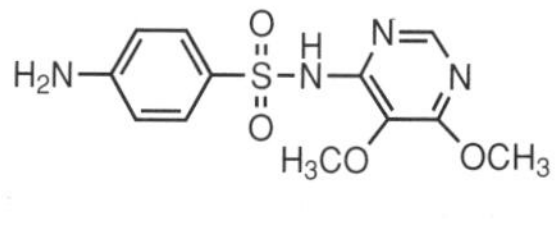

Sulfadoxine

Pyrimethamine (Daraprim) is a potent inhibitor of DHFR (42). The drug has been shown to have a significantly higher affinity for binding to the DHFR of plasmodium than to the host enzyme (>1,000 times in *Plasmodium berghei*) and, as a result, has been used to selectively treat plasmodium infections. The combination of pyrimethamine with a long-acting sulfonamide, sulfadoxine, which blocks dihydrofolate synthesis by blocking incorporation of PABA into the dihydrofolate, is called Fansidar, which produces sequential blockage of tetrahydrofolate synthesis similar to that reported for treatment of bacterial infections (see Chapter 38). *Plasmodium* enzymes catalyzing folic acid synthesis differ from those enzymes found in other organisms. A single bifunctional protein present in *Plasmodium* sp. catalyzes the phosphorylation of 6-hydroxymethyl-7,8-hydropterin (a pyrophosphokinase) and the incorporation of PABA into dihydropteroic acid. A second bifunctional enzyme catalyzes the reduction of dihydropteroic acid and thymidylic acid synthesis. As a result, the drug combination (Fansidar) appears to have improved drug-mediated disruption of folic acid in *Plasmodium* sp. (35,43). This combination has been used with quinine for the treatment and prevention of chloroquine-resistant malaria (*Plasmodium falciparum, Plasmodium ovale, Plasmodium vivax,* and *Plasmodium malaria*). The combination therapy (Fansidar) has the added advantage of being inexpensive, which is essential for successful therapy in developing countries. When used on its own, pyrimethamine is a blood schizonticide without effects on the tissue stage of the disease.

The mechanism of resistance to the folate inhibitor combination has been shown to be associated with point mutations in both DHFR and the dihydropteroate synthase enzymes (35).

ATOVAQUONE-PROGUANIL

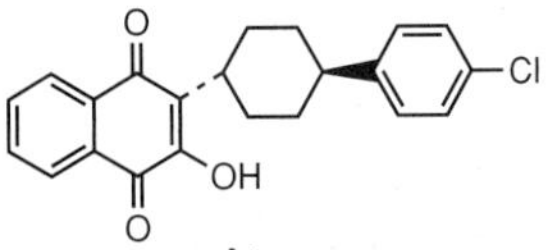

Atovaquone

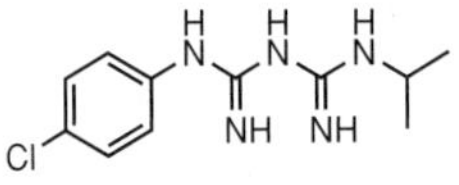

Proguanil

Atovaquone was originally developed as an antimalarial, but because of the high failure rate (~30%), it is not prescribed as a single chemical entity but, rather, is used to treat pneumocystis (see page 1092). More recently, however, atovaquone has been combined with proquanil as an effective prophylactic and therapeutic antimalarial (35). The two drug together (Malarone) exhibit synergy in which proguanil reduces the effective concentration of atovaquone needed to damage the mitochondrial membrane and atovaquone increases the effectiveness of proguanil but not its active metabolite (for the mechanism of action of atovaquone, see page 1091). Proguanil was developed decades earlier as a folic acid antagonist and functions as a pro-drug. The active form of proguanil is cycloguanil, which acts as a DHFR inhibitor (Fig. 39.16). Later, this discovery led to the development of pyrimethamine.

Resistance to atovaquone used as a monotherapy may have been associated with the pharmacokinetics of the drug. Atovaquone is quite lipophilic and has slow uptake, resulting in the pathogen experiencing low concentrations of the drug over an extended period of time, both of which encourage the development of resistance. A single-point mutation appears to be sufficient for resistance (44). To date, resistance to the combination has not been reported.

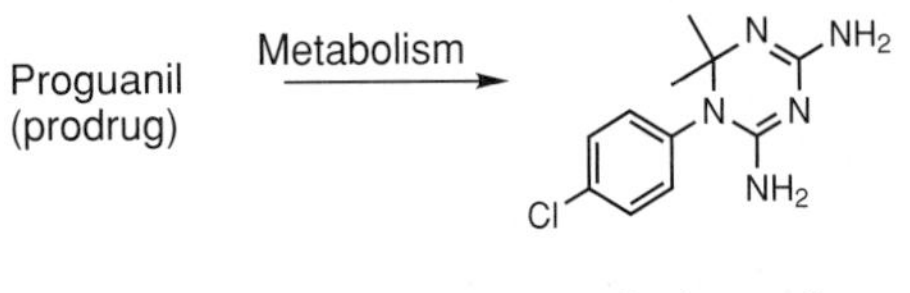

Proguanil (prodrug) → Metabolism → Cycloguanil

Fig. 39.16. Activation of proguanil leading to cycloguanil.

ARTEMISININS (45–48)

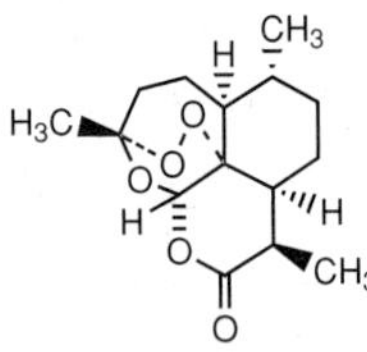

Artemisinin

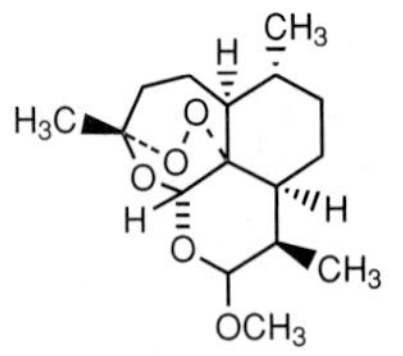

Artemether (Artenam)

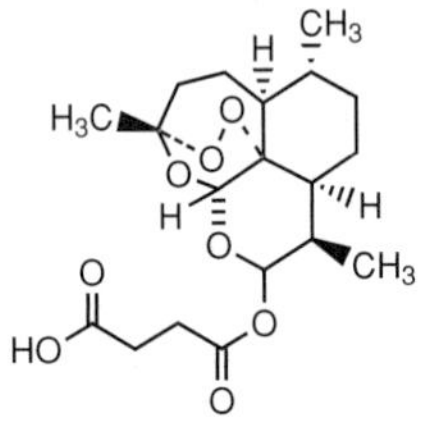

Artesunate

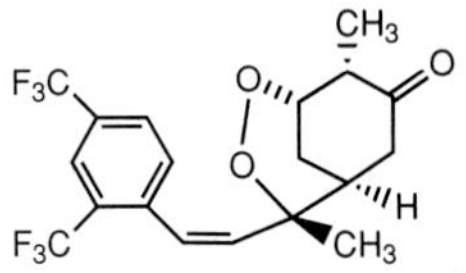

Arteflene

The most recent additions to the drug therapy for malaria are artemisinin and its derivatives. Isolated from *Artemisia annua* (qinghao, sweetworm wood), this material has been used by Chinese herbalists since 168 BC. Artemisinin and the synthetic and semisynthetic derivatives, artemether, arteflene, and artesunate, are active by virtue of the endoperoxide.

Mechanism of Action. The artemisinins appear to kill the parasite by a free radical mechanism—not by the generation of ROS but, rather, by virtue of a free radical associated with the endoperoxide, possibly involving a carbon radical. Evidence points toward activation of the endoperoxide via an iron-dependent mechanism. The resulting free radical selectively targets sarcoplasmic/endoplasmic reticulum Ca^{2+}-ATPase of the *Plasmodium falciparum* (PfATP6), altering calcium stores (49). The artemisinins actually may form covalent adducts to specific membrane-associated proteins after concentrating in infected erythrocytes.

THERAPEUTIC APPLICATION. The artemisinins are hydrophobic in nature with the exception of artesunate, which is available as a water-soluble hemisuccinate salt, and are partitioned into the membrane of the plasmodium. These compounds have gametocytocidal activity as well as activity against all asexual stages of the parasites. These agents are short acting, with relatively short half-lives. Little or no cross-resistance has been reported, with the drugs rapidly clearing the blood of parasites. The drugs have limited availability in the United States, but they are being utilized elsewhere as commercial or experimental agents, often in combination therapy. Combination therapy has the goal of reducing resistance with the hope for synergism and, when combined with longer-acting drugs, an improved therapy. Among the combinations reportedly used are artesunate–fosmidomycin, artemether–lumefantrine (Coartem), amodiaquine–artesunate, chloroquine–artemisinin, and artesunate–sulfadoxine–pyrimethamine (50). These combinations are referred to as artemisinin-based combination therapy (ACT). These ACTs have been reported to show cure rates of greater than 90%. The fixed-dose combination Coartem has been used in more than 10 million treatments, with significant increases being forecast.

HELMINTH INFECTIONS

Helminthiasis, or worm infestation, is one of the most prevalent diseases—and one of the most serious public health problems—in the world. Many worms are parasitic in humans and cause serious complications. Hundreds of millions (if not billions) of human infections by helminths exist worldwide, and with increased world travel and immigration from developing countries, one might expect to see this pattern of infection continue. It is estimated that one-fourth of the world population may be infected. It is interesting to note that helminths differ from many other parasites in that these organisms multiply outside of the definitive host and have the unique ability to evade host immune defenses for reasons that are not fully understood. As a result, helminth infections tend to be chronic, possibly lasting for the entire lifetime of the host (for a discussion of the uniqueness of helminth infections, see Maizels et al. in *Suggested Readings*). Helminths that infect human hosts are divided into two categories, or phyla: Platyhelminths (flatworms), and Aschelminths or nematodes (roundworms). The flatworms include the classes Cestode (tapeworms) and Trematode (flukes or schistosomes). The nematode class includes helminths common to the United States: roundworm, hookworm, pinworm, and whipworm. These worms are cylindrical in shape, with significant variations in size, proportion, and structure.

Nematode Infections

Ancylostomiasis or Hookworm Infection

The two most widespread types of hookworm in humans are the American hookworm (*Necator americanus*) and the "Old World" hookworm (*Ancylostoma doudenale*). The life cycles of both are similar. The larvae are found in the soil and are transmitted either by penetrating the skin or being ingested orally. The circulatory system transports the larvae via the respiratory tree to the digestive tract, where they mature and live for 9 to 15 years if left untreated. These worms feed on intestinal tissue and blood. Infestations cause pulmonary lesions, skin reactions, intestinal ulceration, and anemia. The worms are most prevalent in regions of the world with temperatures of 23 to 33°C, abundant rainfall, and well-drained, sandy soil.

Enterobiasis or Pinworm Infection (*Enterobius Vermicularis*)

These worms are widespread in temperate zones and are a common infestation of households and institutions. The pinworm lives in the lumen of the GI tract, attaching itself by the mouth to the mucosa of the cecum. Mature worms reach 10 mm in size. The female migrates to the rectum, usually at night, to deposit her eggs. This event is noted by the symptom of perianal pruritus. The eggs infect fingers and contaminate nightclothes and bed linen, where they remain infective for up to three weeks. Eggs resist drying and can be inhaled with household dust to continue the life cycle. Detection of the worm in the perianal region can be accomplished by means of a cellophane tape swabbed in the perianal region in the evening. The worms may be visible with the naked eye. The eggs can be collected in a similar manner but can only be seen under a microscope.

Ascariasis or Roundworm Infections (*Ascaris lumbricoides*)

These roundworms are common in developing countries, with the adult roundworm reaching 25 to 30 cm in length and lodging in the small intestine. Some infections are without symptoms, but abdominal discomfort and pain are common with heavy infestation. Roundworm eggs are released into the soil, where they incubate and remain viable for up to 6 years. When the egg is ingested, the larvae are released in the small intestine, penetrate the intestinal walls, and are carried via the blood to the lungs. The pulmonary phase of the disease lasts approximately 10 days, with the larvae passing through the bronchioles, bronchi, and trachea before being swallowed and returning to the small intestine. Some patients have reported adult worms exiting the esophagus through the oral cavity, and it is not unusual for live ascaris to be expelled with a bowel movement. Poor or lacking sanitary facilities expose the population to infestation through contaminated foods and beverages.

Trichuriasis or Whipworm Infections (*Trichuris trichiura*)

Infections by this parasite are caused by swallowing eggs from contaminated foods and beverages. The eggs are passed with the feces from an infected individual. These eggs may live in the soil for many years. The ingested eggs hatch in the small intestine, and the larvae embed in the intestinal wall. The worms then migrate to the large intestine, where they mature. Adult worms, which reach approximately 5 cm in length, thread their bodies into the epithelium of the colon. They feed on tissue fluids and blood. Infections from this worm cause symptoms of irritation and inflammation of the colonic mucosa, abdominal pain, diarrhea, and distention. Infections can last 5 or more years if not treated. Whipworm infections are commonly seen in individuals returning from visits to the subtropics and are more common in rural areas of the southeastern United States.

Trichinosis or Trichina Infection (*Trichinella spiralis*)

Trichinella spiralis produces an infection that may be both intestinal and systemic. The worm is found in muscle meat, where the organism exists as an encysted larvae. Traditionally, the worm has been associated with domestic pork that feeds on untreated garbage. More recently, outbreaks have occurred in individuals eating infected game, such as wild boar, bear, or walrus. Trichinosis infections are more likely to occur after consumption of homemade pork or wild-game sausages. After ingestion, the larvae are released from the cyst form and then migrate into the intestinal mucosa. After maturation and reproduction, the newly released larvae penetrate the mucosal lining and are distributed throughout the body, where they enter skeletal muscle. During the adult intestinal stage, diarrhea, abdominal pain, and nausea are the most common symptom, whereas the muscular form of the disease has symptoms that may include muscle pain and tenderness, edema, conjunctivitis, and weakness.

Filariasis

The term "filariasis" denotes infections with any of the Filarioidea, although it is commonly used to refer to lymphatic-dwelling filariae, such as *Wuchereria bancrofti, Brugia malayi,* and *Brugia timori.* Other filarial infections include *Loa loa* and *Onchocerca volvulus.* The latter two are known as the eyeworm and the river blindness worm, respectively. Elephantiasis is the most common disease associated with filariasis. These parasites vary in length from 6 cm for brugia to 50 cm for onchocerca. The incubation periods also vary from 2 months for brugia to 12 months for bancroftian filaria. It is estimated that 400 million persons are infected with human filarial parasites. Depending on the specific organism, various intermediate hosts are involved in spreading the infection. Mosquitoes are involved with the spread of *Wuchereria bancrofti, Brugia malayi,* and *Brugia timori,* whereas the female blackfly spreads river blindness. The larvae released by the female filaria are referred to as microfilariae and commonly may be found in the lymphatics.

Cestode and Trematode Infections

Cysticercosis or Tapeworm Infection

Helminths of this class that are of concern as potential parasites in humans include:

- **Beef tapeworm (*Taenia saginata*).** This worm is found worldwide and infects people who eat undercooked beef. The worm reaches a length of more than 5 m, and it contains approximately 100 segments/m. Each of these segments contains its own reproductive organs.
- **Pork tapeworm (*Taenia solium*).** Pork tapeworms sometimes are called bladder worms and occasionally are found in uncooked pork. The worm attaches itself to the intestinal wall of the human host. The adult worm reaches 5 m in length and, if untreated, survives in the host for many years.
- **Dwarf tapeworm (*Hymenolepis nana*).** This infection is transmitted directly from one human to another without an intermediate host. *Hymenolepis nana* reaches only 3 to 4 cm in length. It is found in temperate zones, and children are most frequently infected.
- **Fish tapeworm (*Diphyllobothrium latum*).** The fish tapeworm reaches a length of 10 m and contains approximately 400 segments/m. These tapeworms attach themselves to the intestinal wall and rob the host of nutrients. They especially absorb vitamin B_{12} and folic acid. Depletion of these critical nutrients, especially vitamin B_{12}, can lead to pernicious anemia. Tapeworm eggs are passed in the patient's feces, and contamination of food and drink may result in transmission of the infection.

Schistosomiasis or Blood Flukes

Three primary trematode species cause schistosomiasis in humans: *Schistosoma hematobium, Schistosoma mansoni,* and *Schistosoma japonicum.* Infections result from the penetration of normal skin by living (free-swimming) cercaria (the name given to the infectious stage of the parasite) with the aid of secreted enzymes. The cercaria develop to preadult forms in the lungs and skin. Then, these parasites travel in pairs via the bloodstream and invade various tissues. The adult worm reaches approximately 2 cm in length. The female deposits her eggs near the capillary beds, where granulomas form. Some of the eggs will move into the lumen of the intestines, bladder, or ureters and are released into the environmental surrounding, where the parasite will seek out the intermediate snail vector. Asexual reproduction occurs in the snail. After a period of time, the cercaria are again released from the snail to continue the cycle. The patients might experience headache, fatigue, fever, and GI disturbances during the early stages of the disease. Hepatic fibrosis and ascites occur during later stages. Untreated patients can harbor as many as 100 pairs of worms. Untreated worms can live 5 to 10 years within the host. It is estimated that as many as 200 million persons worldwide are infected with schistosomes. Depending on the species of schistosome, the disease is found in parts of South America, the Caribbean Islands, Africa, and the Middle East.

Drug Therapy for Helminth Infections (51)

Helminths represent a biologically diverse group of parasitic organisms differing in size, life cycle, site of infection (local and systemic), and susceptibility to chemotherapy. With such variation in infectious organisms, it is not surprising that the drugs used to control helminth infections also represent a varied group of chemical classes. As indicated in Table 39.3, the drugs may have fairly narrow spectra of activity (pyrantel pamoate) or a broad spectra of activity (benzimidazoles).

Benzimidazoles

The benzimidazoles (Table 39.4) are a broad-spectrum group of drugs discovered in the 1960s with activity against GI helminths. Several thousand benzimidazoles have been synthesized and screened for anthelmintic

Table 39.3. Therapeutic Application of Anthelmintics for Specific Helminth Infections

	M	A	DEC	IVM	PZQ	PP
Nematode Infections:						
Necator americanus	√	√				
Ancylostoma doudenale	√	√				√
Enterobius vermicularis	√			√		√
Ascaris lumbricoides	√	√		√		√
Trichuris trichiura	√	√		√		
Trichinella spiralis	√	√				
Wuchereria bancrofti			√	√		
Brugia malayi			√	√		
Brugia timori.			√			
Loa Loa		√	√	√		
Onchocerca volvulus		√	√	√		
Cestode Infections:						
Taenia saginata	√	√			√	
Taenia solium	√	√			√	
Hymenolepis nana	√				√	
Diphyllobothrium latum					√	
Trematode Infections:						
Schistosoma hematobium					√	
S. mansoni					√	
S. japonicum					√	

Benzimidazoles: M = Mebendazole, A = Albendazole; DEC = Diethylcarbamazine; IVM = Ivermectin; PZQ = Praziquantel; PP = Prantel pamoate.

activity, with albendazole, mebendazole, and thiabendazole representing the benzimidazole marketed today. The development and chemistry of this class of agents has been reviewed by Townsend and Wise (52).

Mechanism of Action. Two mechanisms have been proposed to account for the action of the benzimidazoles. Fumarate reductase is an important enzyme in helminths that appears to be involved in oxidation of NADH to NAD. The benzimidazoles are capable of inhibiting fumarate reductase (53). Inhibition of fumarate reductase ultimately uncouples oxidative phosphorylation, which is important in ATP production.

A second mechanism and, probably, the primary action of the benzimidazoles is associated with the ability of these drugs to bind to the protein tubulin and, thus, prevent tubulin polymerization to microtubules (54,55). Tubulin is a dimeric protein that is in dynamic equilibrium with the polymeric microtubules. Binding to the tubulin prevents the self-association of subunits and creates a "capping" of the microtubule at the associating end of the microtubule. The microtubulin continues to dissociate from the opposite end, with a net loss of microtubule length. What is interesting is the unique selectivity of the benzimidazoles. It has been shown that benzimidazole also can bind to mammalian tubulin, but when used as anthelmintics, these drugs are destructive to the helminth, with minimal toxicity to the host. It has been suggested that the selectivity is associated with differing pharmacokinetics between binding to the two different tubulin proteins.

Metabolism. The benzimidazoles have limited water solubility and, as a result, are poorly absorbed from the GI tract (a fatty meal will increase absorption). Poor absorption may be beneficial, because the drugs are used primarily to treat intestinal helminths. To the extent that the drugs are absorbed, they undergo rapid metabolism in the liver and are excreted in the bile (Fig. 39.17) (56,57). In most cases, the parent compound is rapidly and nearly completely metabolized with oxidative and hydrolytic processes predominating. The Phase I oxidative reaction commonly is a cytochrome P450–catalyzed reaction, which may then be followed by a Phase II conjugation.

Table 39.4. Benzimidazole Anthelmintics

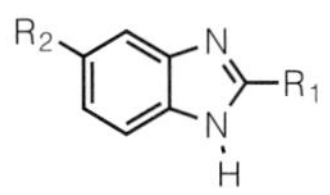

Drugs	Trade name	R_1	R_2
Thiabendazole	Mintezol	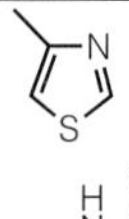 thiazolyl (N, S ring)	—H
Mebendazole	Vermox	$-NH-C(=O)-OCH_3$	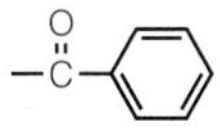 $-C(=O)-C_6H_5$
Albendazole	Zental	$-NH-C(=O)-OCH_3$	$-SCH_2CH_2CH_3$
Oxibendazole		$-NH-C(=O)-OCH_3$	$-OCH_2CH_2CH_3$
Parbendazole		$-NH-C(=O)-OCH_3$	$-CH_2CH_2CH_2CH_3$
Ciclobendazole		$-NH-C(=O)-OCH_3$	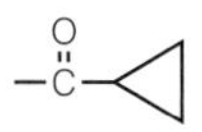 $-C(=O)-$cyclopropyl

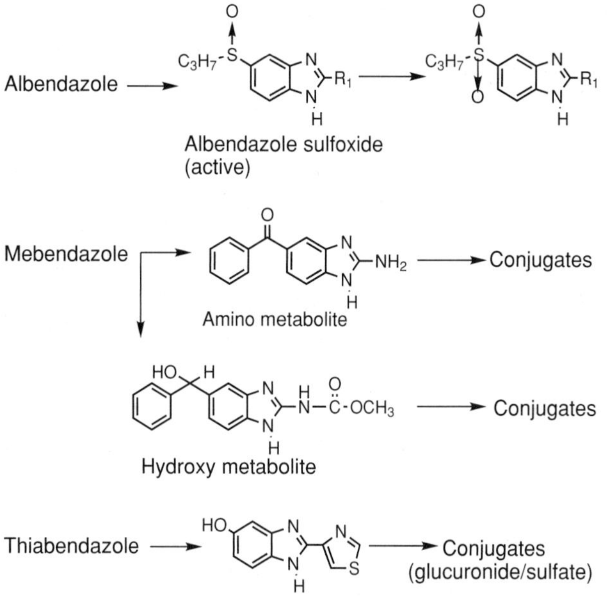

Albendazole → Albendazole sulfoxide (active) → sulfone

Mebendazole → Amino metabolite → Conjugates

Mebendazole → Hydroxy metabolite → Conjugates

Thiabendazole → hydroxy metabolite → Conjugates (glucuronide/sulfate)

Fig. 39.17. Metabolism of benzimidazoles.

Albendazole is unique in two ways. First, the presence of a thioether substituent at the five position increases the likelihood of sulfur oxidation. Second, the initial metabolite, albendazole sulfoxide, is a potent anthelmintic. This initial oxidation is catalyzed principally (70%) by CYP3A4 and CYP1A2 and(30%) by flavin-containing monooxygenase, giving rise to a compound that is bound to plasma protein. This intermediate has an expanded utility in that it has been shown to be active against the hydatid cyst found in echinococciasis, a tapeworm disease (58). Further oxidation by cytochrome P450 leads to the inactive sulfone. Additional metabolites of the sulfone have been reported that include carbamate hydrolysis to the amine and oxidation of the 5-propyl side chain. These reactions occur only to a minor extent.

Metabolism of mebendazole occurs primarily by reduction of the 5-carbonyl to a secondary alcohol, which greatly increases the water solubility of this compound. An additional Phase I metabolite resulting from carbamate hydrolysis has been reported as well. Both the secondary alcohol and the amine are readily conjugated (a Phase II metabolism). Evidence would suggest that the anthelmintic activity of mebendazole resides in the parent drug and none of the metabolites.

Thiabendazole is metabolized through aromatic hydroxylation at the five position catalyzed by CYP1A2. The resulting phenol is conjugated to 5-hydroxythiabendazole glucuronide and 5-hydroxythiabendazole sulfate, respectively. The initial metabolite, along with minor amount of N_1-methylthiabendazole (from a methylation Phase II reaction), have been reported to be teratogenic in mice and rats.

Therapeutic Application. As indicated in Table 39.3, mebendazole and albendazole have a wide spectrum of activity against intestinal nematodes. The drugs are useful and effective against mixed infections. The adverse reactions commonly are GI in nature (nausea, vomiting, and diarrhea). Both drugs have been reported to be teratogenic in rats and, therefore, should not be used during the first trimester of pregnancy. A third drug of this class is thiabendazole, which remains of some value in treatment of strongyloidiasis, as an alternate drug, and cutaneous larva migrans (creeping eruption), for which it is the drug of choice. Thiabendazole commonly is used in veterinary medicine. The drug is less commonly used because of associated toxicity. Thiabendazole has been reported to cause Stevens-Johnson syndrome and has the potential for hepatotoxicity and crystalluria.

Diethylcarbamazine (Hetrazan)

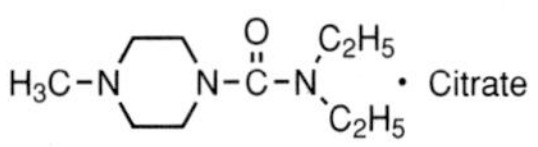

Diethylcarbamazine citrate

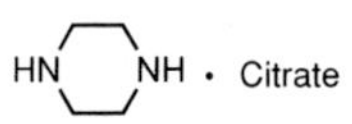

Piperazine citrate

Discovered in the 1940s, diethylcarbamazine (DEC) has proven to be especially effective as a filaricidal agent. The incidence of filariasis among American troops during World War II necessitated a search for drugs with an antifalarial spectrum of activity. The once-popular piperazine also was discovered during these initial screenings. Although chemically similar, the activity again helminths is quite different. Piperazine is active against nematodes, whereas DEC is active against falaria and microfalaria (59).

Mechanism of Action. Although studied extensively, the mechanism of action of DEC remains unknown. Diethylcarbamazine appears to be the active form of the drug, with a very rapid onset of action (within minutes), but of interest is the fact that the drug is inactive in vitro, suggesting that activation of a cellular component is essential to the filaricidal action. Three mechanisms have been suggested. The first is involvement of blood platelets triggered by the action of filarial excretory antigens. A complex reaction is thought to occur between the drug, the antigen, and platelets (60). Although these authors were unable to show a direct action of the drug on the microfalaria, a more recent study showed that DEC produced morphological damage to the microfalaria. The damage consisted of the loss of the cellular sheath, exposing antigenic determinants to immune defense mechanisms. Severe damage then occurred to microfalaria organelles, leading to death (61). The second is inhibition of microtubule polymerization and disruption of preformed microtubules (62). The third is interference with arachidonic acid metabolism (63). Diethylcarbamazine is known to have anti-inflammatory action, which appears to involve blockage at cyclooxygenase and leukotriene A_4 synthase (leukotriene synthesis). This action appears to alter vascular and cellular adhesiveness and cell activation. This latter action would suggest a possible relationship between the first and third mechanism.

Metabolism. The metabolism of DEC leads to the compounds shown in Figure 39.18 plus trace amounts of methylpiperazine and piperazine. Nearly all of the metabolites appear in the urine. As much as 10 to 20% of the drug is excreted unchanged. As indicated by the rapid action of the drug, it would appear that none of the metabolites are involved in the therapeutic action of DEC.

Therapeutic Application. Diethylcarbamazine citrate is freely soluble in water, is rapidly absorbed, and is effective against microfalariae. The drug does not appear to be effective against the adult worm. In general, the drug has mild adverse effects, but under some conditions, it

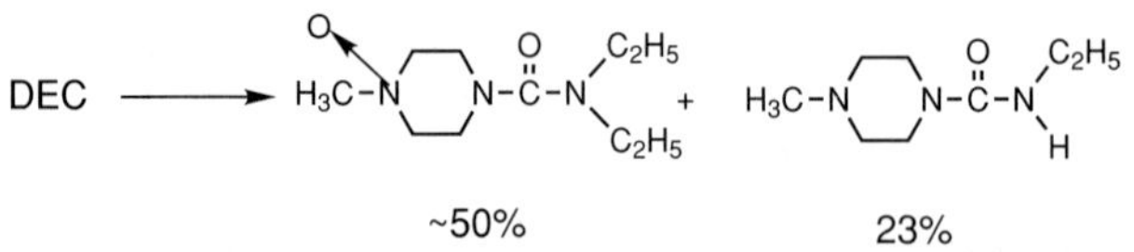

DEC → ~50% + 23%

Fig. 39.18. Metabolism of diethylcarbamazine (DEC).

may produce serve adverse reactions, including anaphylactic reactions, intense pruritus, and ocular complications (64). The severe anaphylactic reaction is known as the Mazzotti reaction, and it appears to be an immune response related to the presence of dead microfilariae. This reaction is more common in individuals who have a high-load microfilarial infection, and it may preclude the use of DEC in some patient populations (51).

Ivermectin (Mectizan)

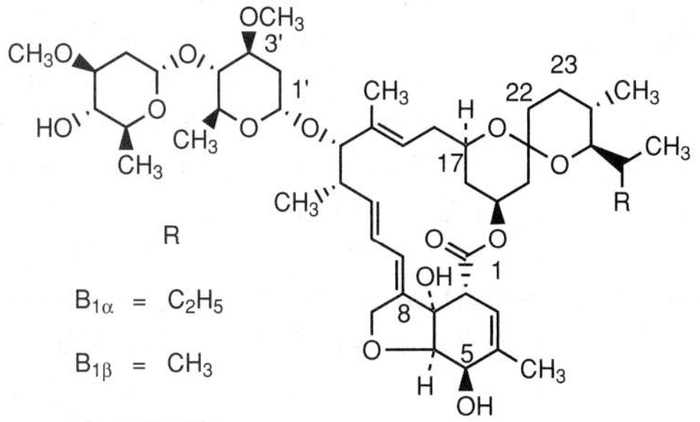

R

$B_{1\alpha}$ = C_2H_5

$B_{1\beta}$ = CH_3

Ivermectin

Extracted from the soil actinomycete *Streptomyces avermitilis,* the natural avermectins are 16-membered macrocyclic lactones that, on reduction of the $C_{22\text{-}23}$ double bond, give rise to ivermectin (IVM), which is an 80:20 mixture of dihydroavermectin $B_{1\alpha}$ and $B_{1\beta}$, respectively. The natural avermectins have minimal biological activity, but IVM has proven to be quite beneficial in the treatment of various nematode infections.

Mechanism of Action. Two mechanisms of action are thought to be involved in the action of IVM (51,65). The first is an indirect action in which motility of microfalaria is reduced, which in turn allows cytotoxic cells of the host to adhere to the parasite, resulting in elimination from the host. This action may occur by virtue of the ability of IVM to act either as a γ-aminobutyric acid (GABA) agonist or as an inducer of chloride ion influx, leading to hyperpolarization and muscle paralysis. The chloride ion influx appears to be the more plausible mechanism (66). Recently, it has been shown that IVM binds irreversibly to the glutamate-gated chloride channel of the nematode *Haemonchus contortus,* whereas the channel is in an open conformation. The binding then remains locked in the open conformation, allowing ions to cross the membrane, leading to the paralytic action of IVM (67). The result of this action is a rapid decrease in microfilarial concentrations.

A second action of IVM leads to the degeneration of microfilariae in utero. This action would result in fewer microfilariae being released from the female worms, and it occurs over a longer period of time. The presence of degenerated microfilariae in utero prevents further fertilization and production of microfilariae.

Metabolism. Ivermectin is rapidly absorbed, is bound to a great extent to plasma protein, and is excreted in the urine or feces either unchanged or as the 3′-O-demethyl-22,23-dihydroavermectin $B_{1\alpha}$ or as the dihydroavermectin $B_{1\alpha}$ monosaccharide. The absorption of IVM is significantly affected by the presence of alcohol. Administration of IVM as an alcoholic solution may result in as much as a 100% increase in absorption.

Therapeutic Application. Although IVM has activity against a variety of microfalaria, including *Wuchereria bancrofti, Brugia malayi, Loa loa,* and *Mansonella ozzardi,* as well as activity against *Strongyloides stercoralis,* the drug is used primarily in the treatment of onchocerciasis (African river blindness) caused by *Onchocerca volvulus.* It is estimated that 20 million people are affected by this condition and an additional 123 million are at risk of the infection. The drug is effective against both the eyeworm as well as skin infections of *O. volvulus.* Ivermectin has the distinct advantage over DEC in that IVM can be used as a single dose (150 μg/kg) once a year (although there is support for dosing every 6 months), has far less likelihood of causing the potentially fatal anaphylactic reaction (Mazzotti reaction), and can be used for mass treatment programs.

Praziquantel (Biltricide)

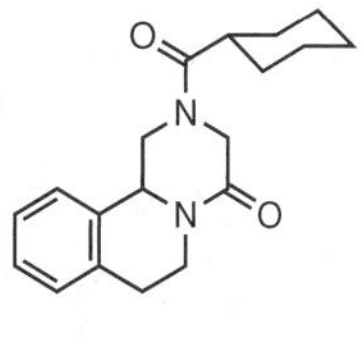

Praziquantel

Praziquantel (PZQ) is an isoquinoline derivative with most of the biological activity found in the levo enantiomer. The compound has no activity against nematodes, but it is highly effective against cestodes and trematodes.

Mechanism of Action. More than one mechanism of action may exist for PZQ, possibly depending on the type of parasite being treated. The mechanism of action appears to involve Ca^{2+} redistribution either directly or indirectly. In the case of helminths found in the lumen of the host (cestode infection), the drug leads to muscle contraction and paralysis, leading in turn to worm expulsion. Additionally, PZQ has been shown to inhibit phosphoinositide metabolism, which by an undetermined mechanism leads to the worm paralysis (68). With intravascular-dwelling schistosomes, PZQ leads to drug-induced damage of the tegument of the worm. As a result, antigens in the helminth are subject to attack by immune antibodies of the host (69,70). An antigen–antibody immunological reaction leads to the death of the parasite. Finally, PZQ affects glycogen content and energy metabolism (71,72).

Metabolism. Praziquantel is rapidly absorbed and undergoes hepatic first-pass metabolism. The metabolites are

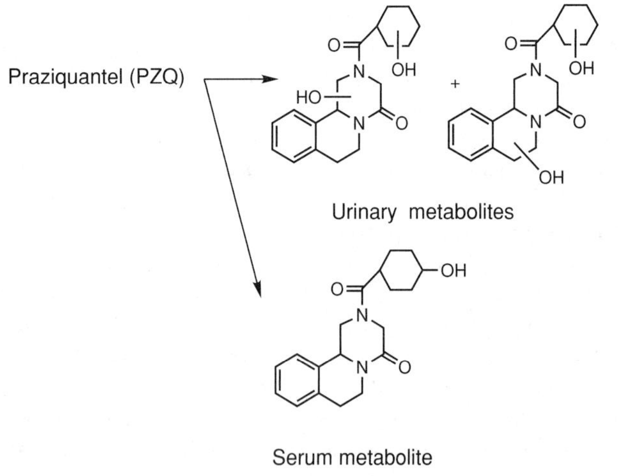

Praziquantel (PZQ)

Urinary metabolites

Serum metabolite

Fig. 39.19. Metabolism of praziquantel (PZQ).

either less active or inactive and consist of hydroxylated compounds. In the serum, the major metabolite appears to be the monohydroxylated 4-hydroxycyclohexylcarboxylate, whereas in the urine, 50 to 60% of the initial PZQ exists as dihydroxylated products (Fig. 39.19) (73). These hydroxylation reactions are catalyzed by CYP2B6 and CYP3A4. The metabolites would be expected to exist in the conjugated form in the urine.

Therapeutic Application. PZQ is the drug of choice for treatment of schistosomiasis and liver flukes (trematode and cestode infections). The drug is stage specific, with activity against the invasive stages, which includes the cercariae and young schistosomula and the mature worms, but not against the liver stages. Although an approved drug, PZQ is considered to be an investigational drug by the U.S. FDA in the treatment of schistosomiasis and liver flukes. The drug has a bitter taste and, therefore, should not be chewed. The side effects usually are not severe and consist of abdominal discomfort (pain and diarrhea). Mounting evidence suggests that resistance may become a significant problem.

Oxamniquine (Mansil, Vansil)

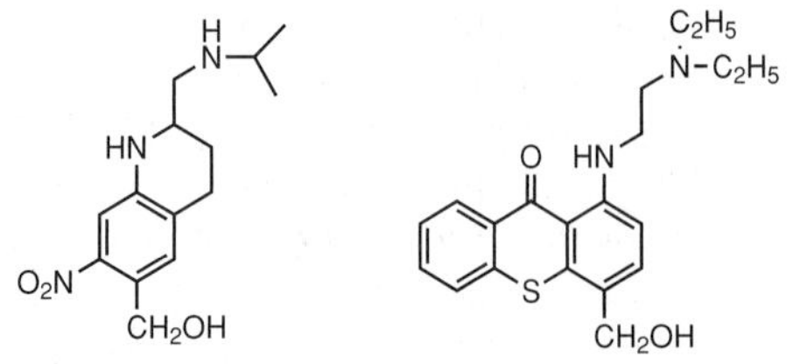

Oxamniquine Hycanthane

Oxamniquine was originally investigated in the 1960s and was found to have limited antiprotozoal activity, with activity against *Schistosoma mansoni* but no activity against the other two schistosomal organisms. In addition, the drug is stage specific, with activity against cercariae and very young schistosomula and adult worms. For reasons that remain unknown, the drug is more effective against adult male worms than against female worms. The drug has structural similarity to hycanthone, which is no longer used because of severe toxicity and teratogenic effects.

Mechanism of Action. Oxamniquine is activated via esterification to a biological ester that spontaneously dissociates to an electrophile, which alkylates the helminth DNA, leading to irreversible inhibition of nucleic acid metabolism (Fig. 39.20) (72). Resistant helminths do not esterify oxamniquine; therefore, activation does not occur. Other metabolic reactions consist of oxidative reactions, leading to inactivation (Fig. 39.20). The metabolites are excreted primarily in the urine.

Therapeutic Application. Oxamniquine is readily absorbed following oral administration and has a relatively short half-life. The drug has been highly effective against *Schistosoma mansoni* native to Brazil, where it is marketed under the trade name Mansil. It also is beneficial against West African *S. mansoni* and is supplied under the trade name Vansil. Side effects are minimal, with transient dizziness being reported. The major drawback is high cost. Encouraging outcomes have been reported with the combination of oxamniquine and PZQ.

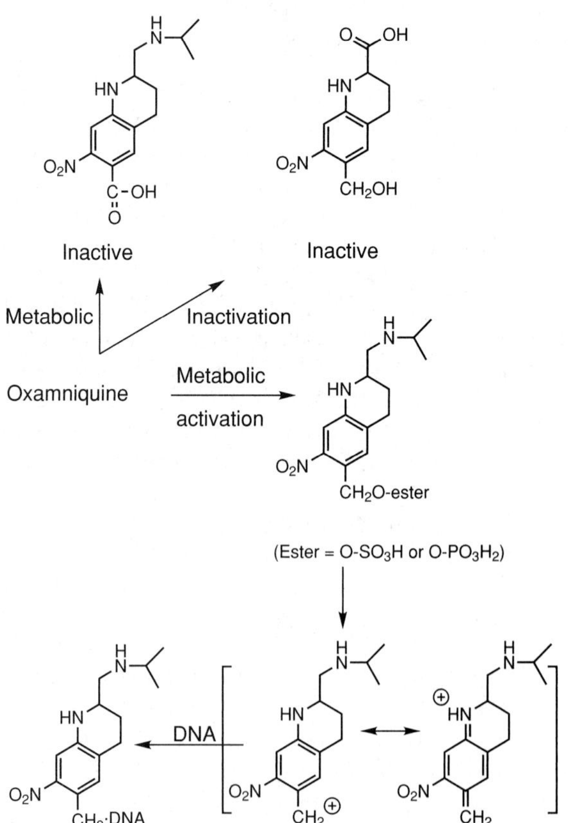

Fig. 39.20. Metabolism of oxamniquine accounting for the mechanism of action and inactivation.

Pyrantel Pamoate (Antiminth)

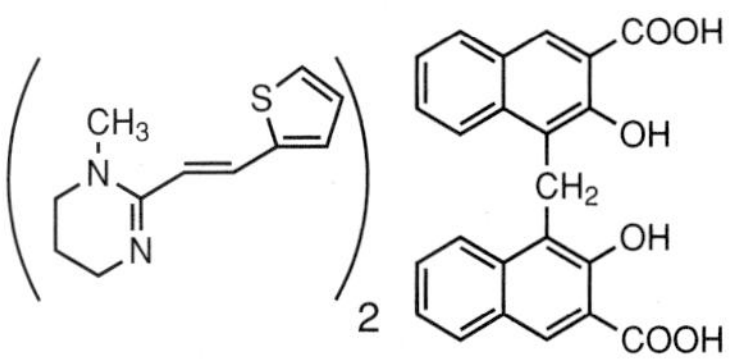

Pyrantel pamoate

Pyrantel was first reported for its anthelmintic activity in 1966 (74). Although it has activity against most intestinal roundworm infections, it has not been approved by the U.S. FDA for several of these infestations. It is considered to be the drug of choice in the treatment of pinworms. The drug is used as the pamoate salt, which is quite insoluble and, as a result, is not readily absorbed. This property improves the usefulness of the drug for treatment of intestinal helminths. In addition to its value in treating enterobiasis, the drug is effective for hookworm and roundworm (ascariasis) infections. Pyrantel acts as a depolarizing neuromuscular blocking agent that activates nicotinic receptors and inhibits cholinesterase, ultimately leading to worm paralysis.

ECTOPARASITIC INFECTIONS

Two parasitic organisms that cause common topical infections are *Sarcoptes scabiei,* which is responsible for scabies, and *Pediculus humanus,* which is responsible for lice infections.

Scabies

Scabies, commonly referred to as the "seven year itch," is a condition caused by *Sarcoptes scabiei,* or the itch mite. The condition commonly is spread by direct, person-to-person contact, although the organism is capable of living for 2 to 3 days in clothing, bedding, or house dust. Sharing of clothing is a common means whereby the condition spreads. The organism burrows into the epidermis, usually in the folds of the skin of the fingers, the elbows, female breast, penis, scrotum, and buttocks. The female parasite lays eggs in the skin, which then hatch and mature to adults. The itch mite can live for 30 to 60 days. The infections are most common in children, but they also may be found in adults in institutional settings. The primary symptom of severe itching may foster secondary infections at the site of scratching. Because of the potential for spread to other members of a family, it is common to treat all members of the family. This will prevent reinfection from a second family member after successful therapy of the first family member.

Lice

Pediculosis or lice is caused by any of the parasites *Pediculus humanus capitis,* the head louse; *Pediculus humanus corporis,* the body louse; or *Phthirius pubis,* the crab louse (found in the genital area). Lice are bloodsucking insects that live for 30 to 40 days on the body of the host. The organisms reproduce, and the female lays her eggs, the nits, which become attached to hair. The nits are white in color and hatch in 8 to 10 days. For the parasite to live, it must feed on blood, which it sucks through punctures in the skin. A hypersensitivity reaction occurs at these puncture sites, which then leads to pruritus, host scratching, and possible secondary infection. In addition to the scalp and skin, the eyebrows, eyelids, and beard may become sites of infection. The transfer of infection can occur through person-to-person contact and from infected clothing, on which the organism can survive for up to 1 week. The sharing of clothing is a common means for the spread of body lice. Head lice are quite common among children in grade school, whereas crab lice are common among individuals who are sexually active. Treatment of family members is recommended, and clothing and bed linen should be removed and washed in very hot water.

Drug Therapy for Scabies and Pediculosis

Lindane (Kwell)

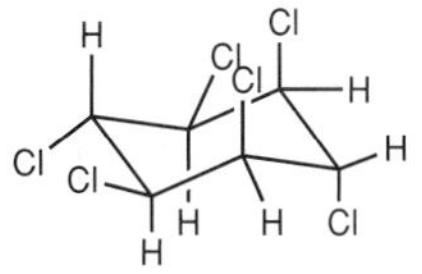

γ-Benzene hexachloride

Chlorination and reduction of benzene leads to a mixture of hexachlorocyclohexanes. The insecticidal activity resides primarily in the γ-isomer of hexachlorocyclohexane (γ-benzene hexachloride). The compound is thought to produce its insecticidal action by virtue of a CNS stimulatory action that occurs by blockage of GABA. The compound is readily absorbed through the chitinous exoskeleton of the parasite. Unfortunately, lindane also is readily absorbed through intact human skin, especially the scalp, and has the potential for systemic neurotoxicity in the host. Infants and children and, possibly, the elderly are most prone to the neurotoxic effects of the drug. Because the lindane is quite lipophilic and, is applied to the scalp as a shampoo, it may be absorbed where upon it can readily enter the CNS of the patient producing signs of neurotoxicity (convulsions, dizziness, clumsiness, and unsteadiness).

The drug is available in a lotion and a shampoo and is recommended for the treatment of both pediculosis and scabies. When using the lotion topically, it should be applied to dry skin, covering the entire surface and being left in place for 8 hours. The lindane then should be removed by washing thoroughly. If the shampoo is used for *Pediculosis capitis,* the hair should be cleaned of oil and dried before application of the lindane shampoo. The shampoo is then worked into the hair and scalp, being applied in such a way as to prevent other parts of the body from coming into contact with the drug. After approximately 4 minutes, the drug is removed by washing with water, and the hair is dried and then combed with a fine-toothed comb to remove nits.

Pyrethrum and Pyrethroids

The naturally occurring pyrethrums have been used as insecticides since the 1800s. These compounds are extracted from the flowering portion of the Chrysanthemum plant. The flowers produced in Kenya have, on average, 1.3% pyrethrins. These pyrethrum extracts are a major agricultural product for that country.

CHEMISTRY. The Chrysanthemum extract is a mixture of ester consisting of the acids chrysanthemic and pyrethric and the alcohols pyrethrolone and cinerolone (Fig. 39.21). The esters are prone to hydrolysis and oxidation and, as a result, should be stored in the cold and protected from light. Because of the high cost, limited availability, and rapid degradation, synthetic derivatives have been investigated. The result has been the preparation of pyrethroids, the synthetic derivatives of pyrethrins. The compound used therapeutically is permethrin, which exists as a 60:40 mixture of *trans:cis* isomers.

MECHANISM OF ACTION (75–78). The pyrethrins and pyrethroids (permethrin) are nerve membrane sodium channel toxins that do not affect potassium channels. The compounds bind to specific sodium channel proteins and slow the rate of inactivation of the sodium current elicited by membrane depolarization and, as a result, prolong the open time of the sodium channel. At low concentrations, the pyrethroids produce repetitive action potentials and neuron firing; at high concentrations, the nerve membrane is depolarized completely and excitation blocked.

The receptor interaction of the pyrethrums with the sodium channel complex is stereospecific and dependent on the stereochemistry of the carboxylic acid. In the case of the pyrethroids, the most active isomers are the 1R,3-*cis*- and 1R,3-*trans*-cyclopropanecarboxylates. The 1S-*cis*- and -*trans*-isomers are inactive and actually are antagonists to the action of the 1R-isomers.

METABOLISM. A property that enhances the usefulness of the pyrethrums and pyrethroids is that these compounds are highly toxic to the ectoparasites but relatively nontoxic to mammals if absorbed. The apparent lack of toxicity is associated with the rapid metabolism of these drugs through hydrolysis and or oxidation (Fig. 39.22) (79,80). The nature of the metabolism (i.e., hydrolysis versus oxidation) is dependent on the structure of the pyrethrins or pyrethroids. Oxidation of the *trans*-methyl of the isobutylene in the carboxyl moiety initially gives an alcohol, which then proceeds to the carboxylic acid, whereas epoxidation of the terminal alkene of the alcohol portion of pyrethrin I gives either the 1,2-diol or the 1,4-diol. No ester hydrolysis is reported. Permethrin is hydroxylated on the terminal aromatic ring at either the 4- or 2-position, is oxidized on the methyl group of the dimethylcyclopropane, and is hydrolyzed at the ester moiety. The rapid breakdown of these agents also accounts for their low persistence in the environment.

THERAPEUTIC APPLICATION

Pyrethrins (A-200, RID). Because of the high cost and rapid degradation of the pyrethrins, they usually are combined with piperonyl butoxide, a synergist (Fig. 39.21). Piperonyl butoxide has no insecticidal activity in it own right but is thought to inhibit the cytochrome P450 enzyme of the insect, thus preventing an oxidative inactivation of the pyrethrins by the parasite. The combination is used in a 10:1 ratio of piperonyl butoxide to pyrethrins. The mixture is used for treatment of *Pediculus humanus capitis*, *Pediculus humanus corporis*, and *Phthirius pubis*. Various dosage forms are available, including a gel, shampoo, and topical solution.

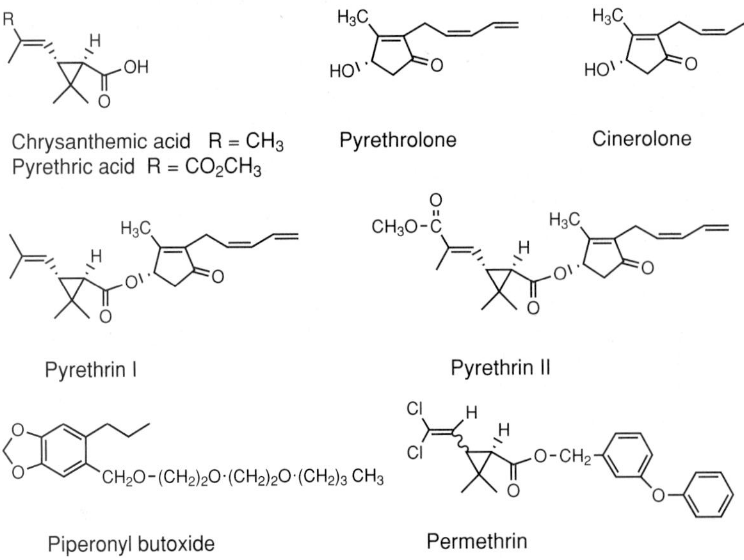

Fig. 39.21. Structures of pyrethrum and pyrethroid.

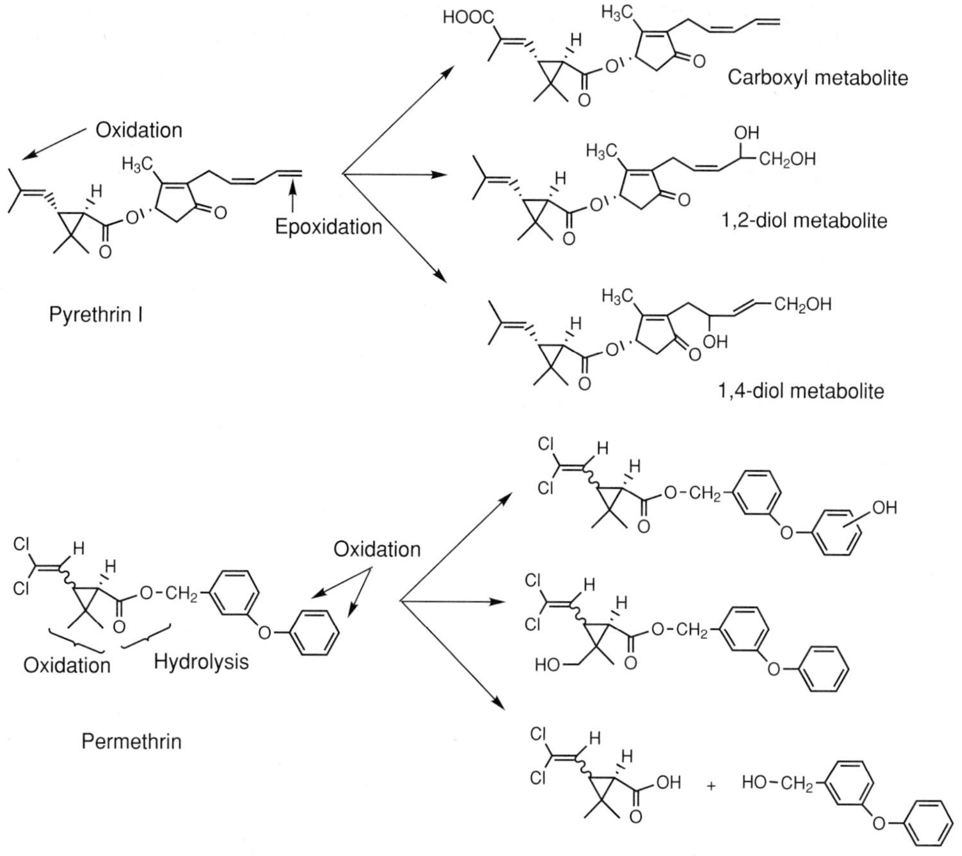

Fig. 39.22. Metabolism of pyrethrin I and permethrin.

Permethrin (Nix-1% lotion, Elimite-5% Cream). Permethrin, because of its increased stability and its availability synthetically, is not used with a synergist. The compound is used in a 1% lotion for the treatment of pediculosis capitis and in a 5% cream as a scabicide.

Crotamiton

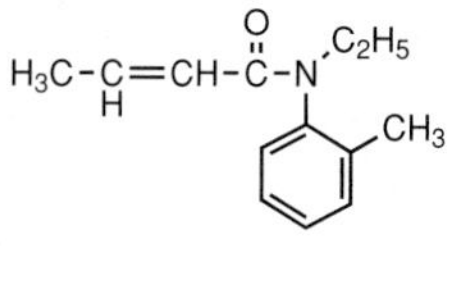

Crotamiton

Crotamiton is available as a 10% cream for the treatment of scabies, although it is less effective than pyrethrins or permethrin (81,82). Because crotamiton may need to be applied a second time for successful treatment of scabies but the pyrethrins or permethrin require a single application, poor patient compliance with crotamiton may reduce its effectiveness. The advantage of crotamiton over lindane comes from the fact that lindane has potential neurotoxicity if absorbed especially in infants and children, whereas crotamiton has less systemic neurotoxicity. The most common side effect reported for crotamiton is skin irritation.

CASE STUDY

Victoria F. Roche and S. William Zito

CQ is a strapping, 6-foot, 62-year-old, Caucasian male who presents to the emergency room with complaints of abdominal distention, flatulence, intermittent abdominal cramping, and diarrhea. In addition, he says he has not had his customary energy ever since he came back from a fishing trip to the Great Lakes. On further inquiry, CQ reveals that he is an avid fly fisherman and has had great success in catching a "trophy" salmon on light tackle. Although he generally practices conservation by releasing the fish he catches, he recalls that on one occasion, he kept a fish so that the cook at the resort he was staying at could teach him how to make his specialty of Scandinavian fish balls. To get the taste just right, CQ recalls that he had to taste the mixture before he cooked it. Hearing this, the physician suspects that CQ may have ingested a fish tapeworm, which was subsequently confirmed by finding operculate eggs (eggs with a lid) of the cestode, *Diphyllobothrium latum,* in the patient's feces on microscopic examination. You have the following antiparasitic agents in your hospital formulary. Which would be the best choice for this case?

1. Identify the therapeutic problem(s) in which the pharmacist's intervention may benefit the patient.
2. Identify and prioritize the patient-specific factors that must be considered to achieve the desired therapeutic outcomes.
3. Conduct a thorough and mechanistically oriented structure-activity analysis of all therapeutic alternatives provided in the case.
4. Evaluate the structure-activity relationship findings against the patient-specific factors and desired therapeutic outcomes, and make a therapeutic decision.
5. Counsel your patient.

O
N H O
N-C-O-CH3
N
H
1

C3H7-S N H O
N-C-O-CH3
N
H
2

O C2H5
H3C-N N-C-N
C2H5
3

O
N
N O
4

References

1. El-Sayed NM, Myler PJ, Blandin G, et al. Comparative genomics of trypanosomatid parasitic protozoa. Science 2005;309:404–409.
2. El-Sayed NM, Myler PJ, Bartholoneu DS, et al. The genome sequence of *Trypanosoma cruzi,* etiologic agent of Chagas' disease. Science 2005;309:409–415.
3. Berriamn M, Ghedin E, Hertz-Fowler C, et al. The genome of the African trypanosome *Trypanosoma brucei.* Science 2005;309:416–422.
4. Barrett MP, Burchmore RJB, Stich A, et al. The trypanosomiases. The Lancet 2003;362:1469–1480.
5. DoCampo R. Sensitivity of parasites to free radical damage by antiparasitic drugs. Chem Biol Interact 1990;73:1–27.
6. Lau AH, Lam NP, Piscitelli SC, et al. Clinical pharmacokinetics of metronidazole anti-infectives. Clin Pharmacokinet 1992;23:328–364.
7. Koch R, Beaulieu BB, Chrystal EJT, et al. Metronidazole metabolite in urine and its risk. Science 1981;211:399–400.
8. Drugs for parasitic infections. Med Lett 1998;40:1–12.
9. The choice of antibacterial drugs. Med Lett 1998;40:33–42.
10. Sisson G, Goodwin A, Raudonikiene A, et al. Enzyme associated with reductive activation and action of nitrazoxande, nitrofurans, and metronidazole in *Helicobacter pylori.* Antimicrob Agents Chemother 2002;46:2116–2123.
11. Stockis A, DeBruyn S, Gengler C, et al. Nitazoxanide pharmacokinetics and tolerability in man during 7 days dosing with 0.5 g and 1 g b.i.d. Int J Clin Pharmacol Ther 2002;40:221–227.
12. Nitazoxanide (Alinia)—a new antiprotozoal agent. Med Lett 2003;45:29–31.
13. Vohringer H-F, Arasteh K. Pharmacokinetic optimization in the treatment of *Pneumocystis carinii* pneumonia. Clin Pharmacokinet 1993;24:388–412.
14. Fishman JA. Treatment of infections due to *Pneumocystis carinii.* Antimicrob Agents Chemother 1998;42:1309–1314.
15. Fry M, Pudney M. Site of action of the antimalarial hydroxymaphthoquinoine, 2-[*trans*-4-(4′-chlorophenyl)cyclohexyl]-3-hydroxy-1,4-naphthoquinone (566C80). Biochem Pharmacol 1992;43:1545–1553.
16. Hughes WT, Gray VL, Gutteridge WE, et al. Efficacy of a hydroxynaphthoquinone, 566C80, in experimental *Pneumocystis carinii* pneumonitis. J Antimicrob Chemother 1990;34:225–228.
17. Allegra CJ, Kovacs JA, Drake JC, et al. Activity of antifolates against *Pneumocystis carinii* dihydrofolate reductase and indentification of a potent new agent. J Exp Med 1987;165:926–931.
18. Koda RT, Dube' MP, Li WY, et al. Pharmacokinetics of trimetrexate and dapsone in AIDS patients with *Pneumocystis carinii* pneumonia. J Clin Pharmacol 1999;39:268–274.
19. Wang CC. Molecular mechanisms and therapeutic approaches to the treatment of Africian trypanosomiasis. Annu Rev Pharmacol Toxicol 1995;35:93–127.
20. Edwards KJ, Jenkins T, Neidle S. Crystal structure of a pentamidine–oligonucleotide complex: implications for DNA-binding properties. Biochemistry 1992;31:7104–7109.
21. Shapiro T, Englund PT. Selective cleavage of kinetoplast DNA minicircles promoted by antitrypanosomal drugs. Proc Natl Acad Sci U S A 1990;87:950–954.
22. Dykstra CC, Tidwell RR. Inhibition of topoisomerase from *Pneumocystis carinii* by aromatic dicationic molecules. J Protozool 1991;38:78S–81S.
23. Metcalf BW, Bey P, Danzin C, et al. Catalytic irreversible inhibition of mammalian ornithine decarboxylase (E.C. 4.1.1.17) by substrate and product analogues. J Am Chem Soc 1978;100:2551–2553.
24. Bacchi CJ, Nathan HC, Hutner SH, et al. Polyamine metabolism: a potential therapeutic target in trypanosomes. Science 1980;210:332–334.
25. Poulin R, Lu L, Ackermann B, et al. Mechanism of the irreversible inactivation of mouse ornithine decarboxylase by α-difluoromethylornithine. J Biol Chem 1992;267:150–158.
26. Bacchi CJ, Garofalo J, Ciminelli M, et al. Resistance to DL-α-difluoromethylornithine by clinical isolates of *Trypanosoma brucei rhodeniense*: role of S-adenosylmethionine. Biochem Pharmacol 1993;46:471–481.
27. Henderson GB, Ulrich P, Fairlamb AH, et al. "Subversive" substrates for the enzyme trypanothione disulfide reductase. Alternative approach to chemotherapy of Chagas' disease. Proc Natl Acad Sci U S A 1988;85:5374–5378.

28. Maya JD, Bollo S, Nunez-Vergara LJ, et al. *Trypanosoma cruzi:* effect and mode of action of nitroimidazole and nitrofuran derivatives. Biochem Pharmacol 2003;65:999–1006.
29. Fairlamb AH, Henderson GB, Cerami A. Trypanothione is the primary target for arsenical drugs against African trypanosomes. Proc Natl Acad Sci U S A 1989;86:2607–2611.
30. Berman JD. Chemotherapy for leishmaniasis: biochemical mechanisms, clinical efficacy, and future strategies. Rev Infect Dis 1988;10:560–586.
31. Cook GC. Leishmaniasis: some recent developments in chemotherapy. J Antimicrob Chemother 1993;31:327–330.
32. Singh S, Sivakumar R. Challenges and new discoveries in the treatment of leishmaniasis. J Infect Chemother 2004;10:307–331.
33. Ward SA. Mechanisms of chloroquine resistance in malarial chemotherapy. Trends Pharmacol Sci 1988;9:241–246.
34. Sullivan DJ Jr, Gluzman IY, Russell DG, et al.. On the molecular mechanism of chloroquine's antimalarial action. Proc Natl Acad Sci U S A 1996;93: 11865–11869.
35. Arav-Boger R, Shapiro TA. Molecular mechanisms of resistance in antimalarial chemotherapy: the unmet challenge. Annu Rev Pharmacol Toxicol 2005;45: 565–585.
36. Zhao X-J, Ishizaki T. Metabolic interactions of selected antimalarial and nonantimalarial drugs with the major pathway (3-hydroxylation) of quinine in human liver microsomes. Br J Clin Pharmacol 1997;44:505–511.
37. Palmer KJ, Holliday SM, Brogden RN. Mefloquine: a review of its antimalarial activity, pharmacokinetic properties, and therapeutic efficacy. Drugs 1993; 45:430–475.
38. Bryson HM, Goa KL. Halofantrine: a review of its antimalarial activity, pharmacokinetic properties, and therapeutic potential. Drugs 1992;43:236–258.
39. Karbwang J, Bangchang KN. Clinical pharmacokinetics of halofantrine. Clin Pharmacokinet 1994;27:104–119.
40. Augusto O, Schrieber J, Mason RP. Direct ESR detection of a free radical intermediate drug in the peroxidase-catalyzed oxidation of the antimalarial drug primaquine. Biochem Pharmacol 1988;37:2791–2797.
41. Mihaly GW, Ward SA, Edwards G, et al. Pharmacokinetics of primaquine in man: identification of the carboxylic acid derivative as a major plasma metabolite. Br J Clin Pharmacol 1984;17:441–446.
42. Ferone R, Burchall JJ, Hitchings GH. *Plasmodium berghei* dihydrofolate reductase isolation, properties, and inhibition by antifolates. Mol Pharmacol 1969;5:49–59.
43. Triglia T, Cowman AF. Primary structure and expression of the dihydropteroate synthetase gene of *Plasmodium falciparum*. Proc Natl Acad Sci U S A 1994;91:7149–7153.
44. Olliaro P. Mode of action and mechanisms of resistance for antimalarial drugs. Pharmacol Ther 2001;89:207–219.
45. Cumming JN, Ploypradith P, Posner GH. Antimalarial activity of artemisinin (Qinghaosu) and related trioxanes: mechanism(s) of action. Adv Pharmacol 1997;37:253–297.
46. Meshnick SR, Taylor TE, Kamchonwongpaisan S. Artemisinin and the antimalarial endoperoxides: from herbal remedy to targeted chemotherapy. Microbiol Rev 1996;60:301–315.
47. Posner GH, Cumming JN, Woo S-H, et al. Orally active antimalarial 3-substituted trioxanes: new synthetic methodology and biological evaluation. J Med Chem 1998;41:940–951.
48. Cumming JN, Wang D, Shapiro TA, et al. Design, synthesis, derivatization, and structure–activity relationships of simplified, tetracyclic, 1,2,4-trioxane alcohol analogues of the antimalarial artemisinin. J Med Chem 1998;41:952–964.
49. Eckstein-Ludwig, Webb RJ, van Goethem DK, et al. Artemisinins target the SERCA of *Plasmodium falciparum*. Nature 2003;424:957–961.
50. Rosenthal PJ. Antimalarial drug discovery: old and new approaches. J Exp Biol 2003;206:3735–3744.
51. de Silva N, Guyatt H, Bundy D. Anthelmintics: a comparative review of their clinical pharmacology. Drugs 1997;53:769–786.
52. Townsend LB, Wise DS. The synthesis and chemistry of certain anthelmintic benzimidazoles. Parasitol Today 1990;6:107–112.
53. Prichard RK. Mode of action of the anthelmintic thiabendazole in *Haemonchus contortus*. Nature 1970;228:684–685.
54. Friedman PA, Platzer EG. Interaction of anthelmintic benzimidazoles and benzimidazole derivatives with bovine brain tubulin. Biochim Biophys Acta 1978;544:605–614.
55. Lacey E. Mode of action of benzimidazoles. Parasitol Today 1990;6:112–115.
56. Braithwaite PA, Roberts MS, Allan RJ, et al. Clinical pharmacokinetics of high-dose mebendazole in patients treated for hydatid disease. Eur J Clin Pharmacol 1982;22:161–169.
57. Gottschall DW, Theodorides EJ, Wang R. The metabolism of benzimidazole anthelmintics. Parasitol Today 1990;6:115–124.
58. Marriner SE, Morris DL, Dickson B, et al. Pharmacokinetics of albendazole in man. Eur J Clin Pharmacol 1986;30:705–708.
59. Hawking F. Diethylcarbamazine and new compounds for the treatment of filariasis. Adv Pharmacol Chemother 1979;16:129–194.
60. Cesbron J-Y, Capron A, Vargaftig BB, et al. Platelets mediate the action of diethylcarbamazine on microfilariae. Nature 1987;325:533–536.
61. Florencio MS, Peixoto CA. The effect of diethylcarbamazine on the ultrastructure of microfilariae of *Wuchereria bancrofti*. Parasitology 2003;126: 551–554.
62. Fujimaki Y, Ehara M, Kimura E, et al. Diethylcarbamazine, antifilarial drug, inhibits microtubule polymerization and disrupts preformed microtubules. Biochem Pharmacol 1990;39:851–856.
63. Maizels RM, Denham DA. Diethylcarbamazine (DEC): immunopharmacological interactions of an antifilarial drug. Parasitol 1992;105:S49–S60.
64. Mackenzie CD. Diethylcarbamazine: a review of its action in onchocerciasis, lymphatic filariasis, and inflammation. Trop Disease Bull 1985;82:R1–R37.
65. Goa KL, McTavish D, Clissold SP. Ivermectin: a review of its antifilarial activity, pharmacokinetic properties and clinical efficacy in onchocerciasis. Drugs 1991;42:640–658.
66. Ottesen EA, Campbell WC. Ivermectin in human medicine. J Antimicrob Chemother 1994;34:195–203.
67. Forrester SG, Beech RN, Prichard RK. Agonist enhancement of macrocyclic lactone activity at a glutamate-gated chloride channel subunit from *Haemonchus contortus*. Biochem Pharmacol 2004;67:1019–1024.
68. Wiest PM, Li Y, Olds GR, et al. Inhibition of phosphoinositide turnover by praziquantel in *Schistosoma mansoni*. J Parasitol 1992;78:753–755.
69. Xiao S-H, Catto BA, Webster LT Jr. Effects of praziquantel on different developmental stages of *Schistosoma mansoni* in vitro and in vivo. J Infect Dis 1985;151:1130–1137.
70. Fallon PG, Cooper RO, Probert AJ, et al. Immune-dependent chemotherapy of schistosomiasis. Parasitology 1992;105:S41–S48.
71. Utzinger J, Keiser J, Shuhua X, et al. Combination chemotherapy of schistosomiasis in laboratory studies and clinical trials. Antimicrob Agents Chemother 2003;47:1487–1495.
72. Cioli D, Pica-Mattoccia L, Archer S. Antischistosomal drugs: past, present . . . and future? Pharmacol Ther 1995;68:35–85.
73. Buhring KU, Diekmann HW, Muller H, et al. Metabolism of praziquantel in man. Eur J Drug Metab Pharmacokinet 1978;3:179–190.
74. Austin WC, Courtney WC, Danilewicz W, et al. Pyrantal tartrate, a new anthelmintic effective against infections of domestic animals. Nature 1966; 212:1273–1274.
75. Narahashi T. Nerve membrane ionic channels as the primary target of pyrethroids. Neurotoxicology 1985;6:3–22.
76. Vijverberg HPM, de Weille JR. The interaction of pyrethroids with voltage-dependent Na channels. Neurotoxicology 1985;6:23–34.
77. Grammon DW, Sanders G. Pyrethroid–receptor interactions: stereospecific binding and effects on sodium channels in mouse brain preparations. Neurotoxicology 1985;6:35–46.
78. Lombet A, Mourre C, Lazdunski M. Interaction of insecticides of the pyrethroid family with specific binding sites on the voltage-dependent sodium channel from mammalian brain. Brain Res 1988;459:44–53.
79. Soderund DM. Metabolic consideration in pyrethroid design. Xenobiotica 1992;22:1185–1194.
80. Ruzo LO, Casida JE. Metabolism and toxicology of pyrethroids with dihalovinyl substituents. Environ Health Perspect 1977;21:285–292.
81 Taplin D, Meinkin TL, Joaquin BA, et al. Comparison of critamiton 10% cream (Eurax) and permethrin 5% cream (Elimite) for the treatment of scabies in children. Pediatr Dermatol 1990;7:67–73.
82. Amer M, El-Ghariband I. Permethrin versus crotamiton and lindane in the treatment of scabies. Int J Dermatol 1992;31:357–358.

Suggested Readings

Freeman CD, Klutman EE, Lamp KC. Metronidazole: a therapeutic review and update. Drugs 1997;54:679–708.

Maizels RM, Bundy DAP, Selkirk ME, et al. Immunological modulation and evasion by helminth parasites in human populations Nature 1993;365: 797–805.

Wilson JD, Braunwald E, Isselbacher KJ, et al., eds. Harrison's Principles of Internal Medicine. 12th Ed. New York: McGraw-Hill, 1991:772.

40. *Antifungal Agents*

ROBERT K. GRIFFITH

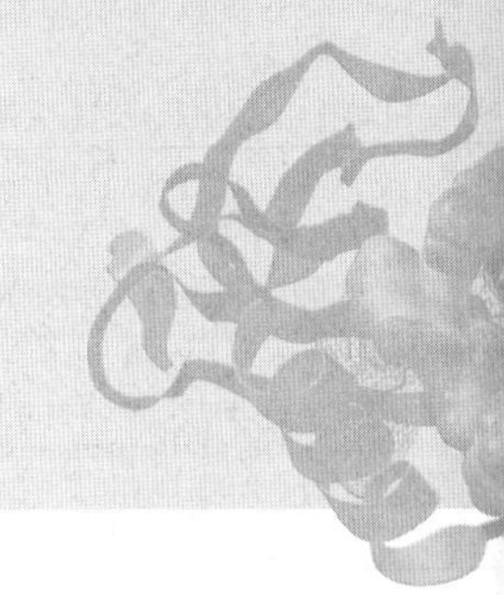

DRUGS COVERED IN THIS CHAPTER:

POLYENES
- Amphotericin B
- Natamycin
- Nystatin

AZOLES
- Fluconazole
- Itraconazole
- Ketoconazole
- Posaconazole
- Terconazole
- Voriconazole

ALLYL AMINES
- Butenafine
- Naftifine
- Terbinafine

ESCHINOCANDINS
- Anidulafingin
- Caspofungin
- Micafungin

CICLOPIROX

FLUCYTOSINE

GRISEOFULVIN

HALOGROGIN

TOLNAFTATE

UNDECYLENIC ACID

INTRODUCTION

Until recently, chemotherapy of fungal infections has lagged far behind chemotherapy of bacterial infections. This lack of progress has resulted, in part, because the most common fungal infections in humans have been relatively superficial infections of the skin and mucosal membranes and potentially lethal deep-seated infections have been quite rare. Because most humans with a normally functioning immune system are able to ward off invading fungal pathogens with little difficulty, the demand for improvements in antifungal therapy has been small. Immunocompromised patients, however, are very susceptible to invasive fungal infections. The onset of the AIDS epidemic, combined with the increased use of powerful immunosuppressive drugs for organ transplants and cancer chemotherapy, has resulted in a greatly increased incidence of life-threatening fungal infections and a corresponding increase in demand for new agents to treat these infections. The number of effective antifungal agents available is quite small compared to those available to treat bacterial infections, but research in this area is quite active. Several new agents have been introduced in the last few years.

FUNGAL DISEASES

The fungal kingdom includes yeasts, molds, rusts, and mushrooms. Most fungi are saprophytic, which means that they live on dead organic matter in the soil or on decaying leaves or wood. A few of these fungi can cause opportunistic infections if they are introduced into a human through wounds or by inhalation. Some of these infections can be fatal. There are relatively few obligate animal parasites (i.e., microorganisms that can only live on mammalian hosts) among the fungi, although *Candida albicans* is commonly found as part of the normal flora of the gastrointestinal tract and vagina. The obligatory parasites are limited to dermatophytes that have evolved to live on/in the keratin-containing hair and skin of mammals, where they cause diseases such as ringworm and athletes foot. (Ringworm is not caused by a parasitic worm but, rather, is named for the ring-like appearance of this fungal infection of the skin.) A detailed description of fungal infections is beyond the scope of this book, but comprehensive treatises are available (1).

Most fungal infections are caused primarily by various yeasts and molds. Yeasts, such as the opportunistic pathogen *Candida albicans* and the bakers' yeast *Saccharomyces cerevisiae*, typically grow as single oval cells and reproduce by budding. *Candida albicans* and some other pathogenic yeasts also can grow in multicellular chains called hyphae. Infection sites may contain both yeast and hyphal forms of the microorganism. Molds, such as *Trichophyton rubrum*, one of the causative agents of ringworm, grow in clusters of hyphae called a mycelium. All fungi produce spores, which may be transported by direct contact or through the air. Although most topical fungal infections are readily treated, the incidence of life threatening systemic fungal infections, including those caused by yeasts such as *Candida albicans* and molds such as *Aspergillus fumigans* are increasing, and mortality remains high (2).

Dermatophytes

Dermatophytes are fungi causing infections of skin, hair, and nails (3). The dermatophytes obtain nutrients from attacking the cross-linked structural protein keratin, which other fungi cannot use as a food source. Dermatophytic infections, known as tinea, are caused by various species of three genera (*Trichophyton, Microsporum,* and *Epidermophyton*) and are named for the site of infection rather than for the causative organism. Tinea capitis is a

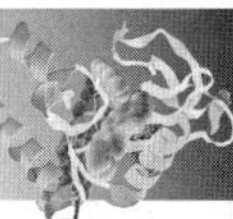

CLINICAL SIGNIFICANCE

Antifungal agents include diverse compounds with varied actions. A few key examples can highlight the importance of medicinal chemistry to clinical practice. Knowledge regarding the molecular structure of polyene antifungal agents, such as amphotericin B, is essential in understanding how they work. These agents are macrocyclic lactones with distinct hydrophilic and lipophilic regions. One of the putative mechanisms of polyene action involves the formation of pores in the fungal cell membrane. The lipophilic regions of the polyene molecules facilitate the binding to the cell membrane sterols. The hydrophilic portions of the molecule align to create a hydrophilic pore in the sterol-containing cell membrane. As a result, there is membrane depolarization and increased membrane permeability and, eventually, fungal cell death. The lipophilic regions of amphotericin B also contribute to its poor solubility in aqueous solutions. The traditional intravenous formulation of amphotericin B includes a dispersing agent, deoxycholate, which facilitates formation of the required micellular dispersion when administered in a 5% dextrose in water solution.

5-Flucytosine (5-FC) is an analogue of the natural pyrimidine cytosine that is converted to 5-fluorouracil (5-FU) in susceptible fungi. Formation of 5-FU is essential to the antimycotic effect of 5-FC; 5-FU acts as a pyrimidine antimetabolite and is phosphorylated to the cytotoxic agent 5-fluorodeoxyuridine monophosphate. All of these facts are commonly emphasized in a medicinal chemistry sequence, and readers probably are aware that 5-FU is a chemotherapeutic agent that causes myelosuppression as its major toxicity. Therefore, it should not be surprising that the same side effect can be seen in patients receiving 5-FC.

The newest antifungals, the echinocandins, are macromolecular structures with high molecular weights (>1,000 dalton), which a student can easily visualize by looking at the chemical structure. Their relatively low volume of distribution in the body can be partially explained by their size. Clinically, these agents have not achieved high concentrations in the central nervous system and the vitreous chamber of the eye, two compartments that are subject to fungal invasion.

Douglas Slain, Pharm.D. BCPS
Associate Professor
College of Pharmacy
West Virginia University

fungal infection of the hair and scalp. Tinea pedis refers to infections of the feet, including athlete's foot, tinea manuum to fungal infection of the hands, tinea cruris to infection of the groin (jock itch), and tinea unguium to infection of the fingernails. Athlete's foot in particular may be an infection involving several different fungi, including yeasts. Tinea unguium, also known as onychomycosis, whether of the fingernails or toenails, can be particularly difficult to treat, because the fungi invade the nail itself. Appropriate drug therapy prevents the fungus from spreading to the newly formed nail. Penetration of drugs into previously existing nail is problematic, however, and with some drug regimens, the infection is not cured until an entirely new, fungus-free nail has grown in. Because this can take months, patient compliance with a lengthy drug regimen can be a problem.

Yeasts

The most common cause of yeast infections is *Candida albicans,* which is part of the normal flora in a significant portion of the population where it resides in the oropharynx, gastrointestinal tract, vagina, and surrounding skin (4). It is the principal cause of vaginal yeast infections and oral yeast infections (thrush). These commonly occur in mucosal tissue when the normal population of flora has been disturbed by treatment of a bacterial infection with an antibiotic or when growth conditions are changed by hormonal fluctuations, such as occur in pregnancy. *Candida albicans* can cause infections of the skin and nails, although the latter are not common. In persons with healthy immune systems, *Candida* infections are limited to superficial infections of the skin and mucosa. In persons with impaired immune systems, however, *Candida albicans* also may cause deep-seated systemic infections, which can be fatal. Several other infections with *Candida* species occur, including *C. tropicalis, C. krusei, C. parapsilosis,* and *C. glabrata* (also known as *Torulopsis glabrata*). These organisms are becoming more common and often do not respond to antifungal therapy as readily as *Candida albicans.*

Cryptococcus neoformans is a yeast commonly found in bird droppings, particularly pigeon droppings (5). When dust contaminated with spores is inhaled by persons with a competent immune system, the organism causes a minor, self-limiting, lung infection. Such infections frequently are mistaken for a cold, and medical treatment is not sought. In immunocompromised persons, however, the organism can be carried by the circulatory system from the lungs to many other organs of the body, including the central nervous system (CNS). Infection of the CNS is uniformly fatal unless treated.

Although most yeast infections are caused by various species of *Candida* or *Cryptococcus,* other yeasts also can cause infections in humans, including *Malassezium furfur, Trichosporon beigelii,* and *Blastoschizomyces capitatus* (6). These infections are relatively rare, and they are difficult to treat.

Thermally Dimorphic Fungi (Endemic Mycoses)

Thermally dimorphic fungi are saprophytes that grow in one form at room temperature and in a different form in a human host at 37°C (7). The most common infectious agents are *Blastomyces dermatitidus, Paracoccidiodes brasiliensis, Coccidioides immitus,* and *Histoplasma capsulatum,* the causative agents of blastomycosis, paracoccidiomycosis, coccidiomycosis (valley fever), and histoplasmosis, respectively. All these organisms live in soil and cause disease through inhalation of contaminated dust. The resulting lung infections are often mild and self-limiting, but they may progress on to a serious lung infection. The circulatory system may transport the organisms to other tissues, where the resulting systemic infection may be fatal. *Blastomyces dermatitidus* is endemic to southcentral United States and *P. brasiliensis* to Central and South America, where it is the most common cause of fungal pulmonary infections. *Coccidioides immitus* is endemic to the dry areas of the southwestern United States and northern Mexico. It is particularly prevalent in the San Joaquin Valley of California, hence the name valley fever. *Histoplasma capsulatum* is endemic to the Mississippi and Ohio River valleys of the United States, where nearly 90% of the population tests positive for exposure to the organism.

Molds

Various *Aspergillus* species are found worldwide and are virtually ubiquitous in the environment. The most common organisms causing disease are *A. fumigatus, A. niger,* and *A. flavus.* Several other *Aspergillus* species are known to cause infection, and some, such as *A. nidulans,* are becoming more common. *Aspergillus* spp. very rarely cause disease in persons with normal immune systems but are very dangerous to persons with suppressed immune systems. Because *Aspergillus* spores are everywhere, inhalation is the most common route of inoculation, but infection through wounds, burns, and implanted devices (e.g., catheters) also is possible. Nosocomial (hospital-derived) aspergillosis is a major source of infection in persons with leukemia and in those receiving organ or bone marrow transplants. Aspergillosis of the lungs may be contained, but systemic aspergillosis has a high mortality rate.

Zygomycosis (mucormycosis) is a term used to describe infections caused by the genera *Rhizopus, Mucor,* and *Absidia* of the fungal order Mucorales (8). As with several other opportunistic fungal pathogens, these soil microorganisms generally are harmless to those with a competent immune system but can cause rapidly developing, fatal infections in an immunosuppressed patient. These organisms can infect the sinus cavity, from which they spread rapidly to the CNS. Blood vessels also may be attacked and ruptured. Zygomycoses spread rapidly and are often fatal.

BIOCHEMICAL TARGETS FOR ANTIFUNGAL CHEMOTHERAPY

Antifungal chemotherapy depends on biochemical differences between fungi and mammals (9,10). Unlike bacteria, which are prokaryotes, both fungi and mammals are eukaryotes, and the biochemical differences between them are not as great as one might expect. At the cellular level, the greatest difference between fungal cells and mammalian cells is that fungal cells have cell walls but that mammalian cells do not. Inhibitors of bacterial cell wall biosynthesis, such as penicillins and cephalosporins, have provided many powerful antibacterial agents with little toxicity to humans. The fungal cell wall therefore is a logical target for a similar class of drugs, which would be expected to be potent antifungals yet have little human toxicity. Only recently, however, have a few potent inhibitors of fungal cell wall biosynthesis become available for clinical use (11). Other targets for antifungal agents include inhibitors of DNA biosynthesis, disruption of mitotic spindles, and general interference with intermediary metabolism. The difference between fungal and mammalian cells that is most widely exploited, however, is that the cell membranes of fungi and mammals contain different sterols. Sterols are important structural components of fungal and mammalian cell membranes and are critical to the proper functioning of many cell membrane enzymes and ion-transport proteins. Mammalian cell membranes contain cholesterol as the sterol component, whereas fungi contain ergosterol (12).

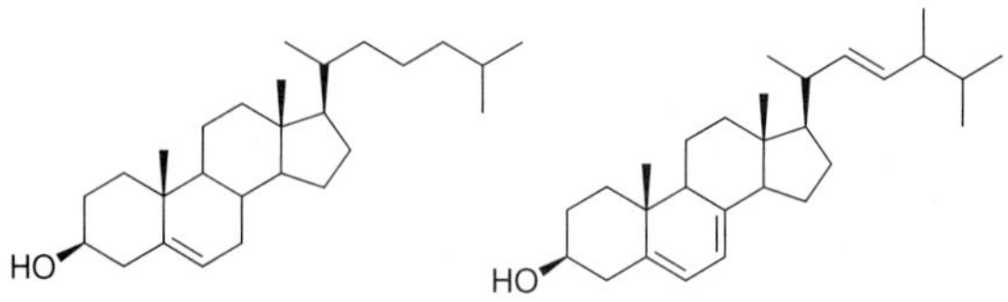

HO HO

Cholesterol Erogosterol

Although the two sterols are quite similar, the side chains are slightly different, and when three-dimensional models are constructed, the ring system of ergosterol is slightly flatter because of the additional double bonds in the B ring. Nevertheless, with only a few exceptions, this difference in sterol components provides the biochemical basis of selective toxicity for most of the currently available antifungal drugs.

Polyene Membrane Disruptors—Amphotericin B, Nystatin, and Congeners

Before the mid-1950s, effective antifungal therapy was limited to topical applications of undecylenic acid derivatives, mixtures of benzoic acid and salicylic acid, and a few other agents of modest efficacy. No reliable treatments existed for the few cases of deep-seated systemic fungal infections that did occur. The discovery of the polyene antifungal agents, however, provided a breakthrough into both a new class of antifungal agents and the first drug to be effective against deep-seated fungal infections. The polyenes are macrocyclic lactones with distinct hydrophilic and lipophilic regions. The hydrophilic region contains several alcohols, a carboxylic acid, and usually, a sugar. The lipophilic region contains, in part, a chromophore of four to seven conjugated double bonds. The number of conjugated double bonds correlates directly with antifungal activity in vitro and, inversely, with the degree of toxicity to mammalian cells. That is, not only are the compounds with seven conjugated double bonds, such as amphotericin B, approximately 10-fold more fungitoxic, they are the only ones that may be used systemically.

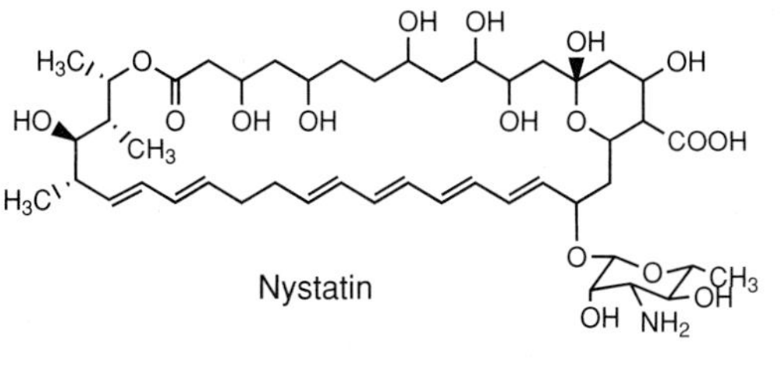

Nystatin

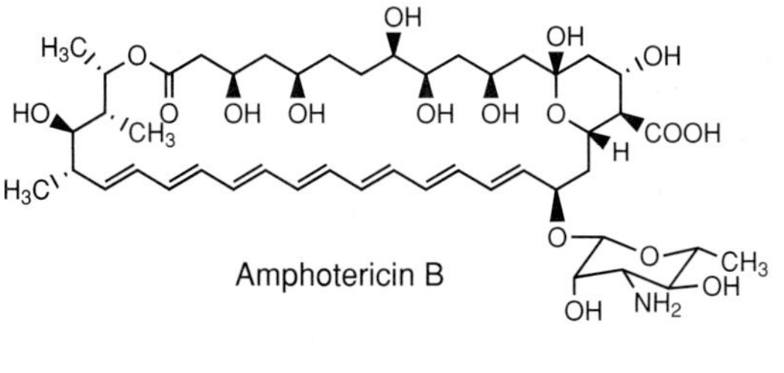

Amphotericin B

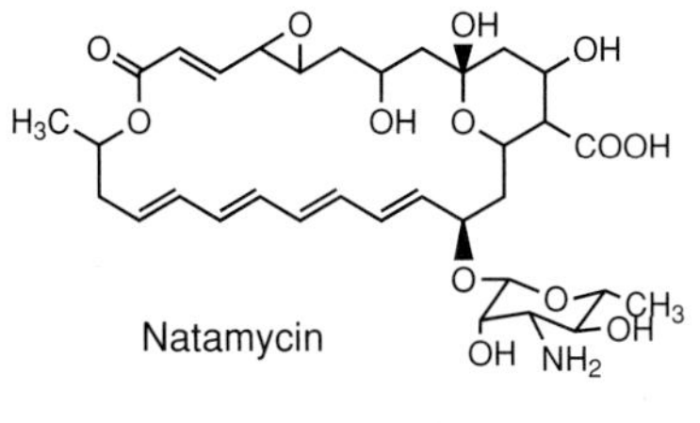

Natamycin

Mechanism of Action

The polyenes have an affinity for sterol-containing membranes, insert into the membranes, and disrupt membrane functions. The membranes of cells treated with polyenes become leaky, and eventually, the cells die because of the loss of essential cell constituents, such as ions and small organic molecules. Polyenes have a demonstrably higher affinity for membranes containing ergosterol over cholesterol-containing membranes. This is the basis for their greater toxicity to fungal cells. Some evidence suggests that the mechanism of insertion differs between the types of cells. Polyene molecules may insert individually into ergosterol-containing membranes but require prior formation of polyene micelles before inserting into cholesterol-containing membranes.

Specific Drugs

NYSTATIN. Nystatin, the first clinically useful polyene antifungal antibiotic, is a conjugated tetraene isolated from cultures of the bacterium *Streptomyces noursei* in 1951. Nystatin is an effective topical antifungal against a wide variety of organisms and is available in a variety of creams and ointments. Nystatin is too toxic to be used systemically, but because very little drug is absorbed following oral administration, it may be administered by mouth to treat fungal infections of the mouth and gastrointestinal tract (Table 40.1). Although nystatin itself was not a breakthrough in systemic antifungal therapy, the search for other polyenes led to the discovery of a polyene that can be used systemically.

AMPHOTERICIN B. Amphotericin B, which as a heptaene has low enough toxicity to mammalian cells to permit intravenous (IV) administration, was discovered in 1956. Amphotericin B is, nevertheless, a very toxic drug and must be used with caution. Adverse effects include fever, shaking chills, hypotension, and severe kidney toxicity. Despite its toxicity, amphotericin B is considered to be the drug of choice for many systemic, life-threatening fungal infections. The drug cannot cross the blood-brain barrier and must be administered intrathecally for treatment of fungal infections of the CNS. Closely related heptaenes are candicidin, hamycin, and trichomycin.

The nephrotoxicity of amphotericin B has been a serious drawback to the use of this drug since its introduction. Recently, however, the toxicity of the drug has been decreased substantially by changes in formulation (Table 40.2). The polyenes are only sparingly soluble in water, and amphotericin B has long been formulated as a complex with deoxycholic acid for IV administration. More recently developed formulations of amphotericin B, such as liposomal encapsulation and lipid complexes, have dramatically decreased the toxicity of the drug to humans, which permits higher plasma levels to be employed. The mechanisms by which the new formulations decrease the toxicity are not entirely clear, but altered distribution is clearly a factor. Because the blood vessels at the site of infection are more permeable than those of normal tissue, the large suspended particles of the lipid formulations can penetrate the site of infection more readily than they can penetrate healthy tissue. The result is selective delivery of drug to the site of infection. Some evidence also indicates that the newer formulations transfer amphotericin B to ergosterol-containing fungal cells more efficiently than to cholesterol-containing mammalian cells.

NATAMYCIN. Natamycin, a tetraene, is available in the United States as a 5% suspension applied topically for the treatment of fungal infections of the eye (Table 40.1).

Ergosterol Biosynthesis Inhibitors

A schematic of fungal ergosterol biosynthesis starting from squalene is shown in Figure 40.1. The biosynthetic pathway has been simplified to emphasize steps important to the action of currently employed antifungal drugs. The last nonsteroidal precursor to both ergosterol and cholesterol is the hydrocarbon squalene. Squalene is converted to squalene epoxide by the enzyme squalene epoxidase. Squalene epoxide is then cyclized to lanosterol, the first steroid in the biosynthetic pathway. The

Table 40.1. Topical Antifungals

Chemical Class	Generic Name	Trade Name	Dosage Form
Allylamine	Butenafine	Lotrimin Ultra	1% cream
		Mentax	
	Naftifine	Naftin	1% cream, gel
	Terbinafine	Lamisil	1% cream
		Lamisil DermGel	10 mg/g gel
	Tolnaftate (thiocarbamate)	Various	1% cream, solution
		Absorbine Athletes' Foot Cream	1% cream
		Genaspor	1% cream
		Tinactin	1% cream, solution, powder, spray powder, spray liquid
		Aftate	1% gel, spray powder, spray liquid
Imidizole	Clotrimazole	Cruex	1% cream
		Lotrimin AF	1% cream, lotion, solution
		Desenex	1% cream
	Econazole	Various	1% cream
		Spectazole	1% cream
	Sertaconazole	Ertaczo	2% cream
	Ketoconazole	Nizoral	2% cream, shampoo
	Miconazole	Micatin	2% cream, powder, spray powder, spray liquid
		Monistat-Derm	2% cream
		Maximum Strength Desenex	2% cream
		Fungoid Creme	2% cream
		Lotrimin AF	2% powder, spray powder
		Zeasorb AF	2% cream
		Prescription Strength Desenex	2% spray liquid
		Fungoid Tincture	2% solution
	Oxiconazole	Oxistat	1% cream, lotion
	Sulconazole	Exelderm	1% cream, solution
Triazole	Terconazole	Terazol	Topical 0.4–0.8% cream, suppository
Polyene	Nystatin	Mycostatin	100,000 U/g cream, ointment, powder
		Nilstat	100,000 U/g cream, ointment
		Nystex	100,000 U/g cream, ointment
	Natamycin	Alcon	5% ophthalmic suspension
Misc.	Ciclopirox	Loprox	0.77% cream, gel, suspension
			1% shampoo
		Penlac	8% nail lacquer
	Haloprogin	Halotex	1% cream, solution
	Undecylenic Acid	Protectol Medicated	15% powder
		Caldesene	10% powder
		Cruex	10% powder
		Cruex Aerosol	19% powder
		Desenex	25% powder
		Phicon F	8% cream
		Various	2–25% creams, powders, ointments

steps involved in converting the side chain of lanosterol to the side chain of ergosterol, and the steps in removal of the geminal dimethyl groups on position 4, are not shown, because none of these reactions is targeted by clinically employed antifungal agents.

A key step in conversion of lanosterol to both cholesterol and ergosterol is removal of the 14α-methyl group. This reaction is carried out by a cytochrome P450 (CYP450) enzyme, 14α-demethylase. The mechanism of this reaction involves three successive hydroxylations of the 14α-methyl group, converting it from a hydrocarbon through the alcohol, aldehyde, and carboxylic acid oxidation states (Fig. 40.2). The methyl group is eliminated as formic acid to afford a double bond between C-14 and C-15 of the D ring. This enzyme is the primary target of the azole antifungal agents discussed below.

Eventually, either before or after modification of the side chain, the Δ^{14} double bond is reduced by a Δ^{14}-reductase to form a *trans* ring juncture between the C and D rings. Several steps later, the double bond between C-8 and C-9 is isomerized to a Δ^7 double bond by the enzyme Δ^8,Δ^7-isomerase. Many of the steps are identical to those involved in mammalian cholesterol biosynthesis, and the basis for selective toxicity to fungal cells will be discussed under the specific agents.

Azoles—Imidazoles and Triazoles

Azole antifungal agents are the largest class of antimycotics available today, with more than 20 drugs on the market. Some are primarily used topically to treat superficial dermatophytic and yeast infections (Table 40.1), whereas others are administered orally for the treatment of systemic fungal infections (Table 40.2). The oral

Table 40.2. Systemic Antifungal Agents

Chemical Class	Generic Name	Trade Name	Dosage Form
Allylamine	Terbinafine	Lamisil	250-mg tablets
Imidazole	Ketoconazole	Various	200-mg tablets
		Nizoral	200-mg tablets
Triazole	Fluconazole	Diflucan	50-, 100-, 150-, and 200-mg tablets; 350-mg (10 mg/mL reconst.) powder for oral suspension; 100- and 200-mL (2 mg/mL) solution for injection
	Voriconazole	Vfend	50- and 200-mg tablets; 200-mg powder for injection; 45-g (40 mg/mL reconst.) powder for oral suspension
	Itraconazole	Various	100-mg capsules
		Sporanox	100-mg capsules; 10 mg/mL injection solution; 10 mg/mL oral solution
Echinocandins	Caspofungin	Cancidas	50- and 70-mg powder for injection
	Anidulafungin	Eraxis	50-mg powder for injection
	Micafungin	Mycamine	50-mg powder for injection
Polyene	Amphotericin B	Amphocin (desoxycholate)	50-mg powder for injection
		Fungizone (desoxycholate)	50-mg powder for injection
		Abelcet (lipid complex)	100 mg/20 mL suspension, single-use vials
		Amphotec (cholesteryl)	50 mg/20 mL and 100 mg/50 mL powder, single-use vials
		AmBisome (liposomal)	Powder, single-use vials
Misc.	Flucytosine	Ancobon	250- and 500-mg capsules
	Griseofulvin	Fulvicin, Grifulvin, Grisactin	250- and 500-mg microsize tablets; 125- to 330-mg ultramicrosize tablets

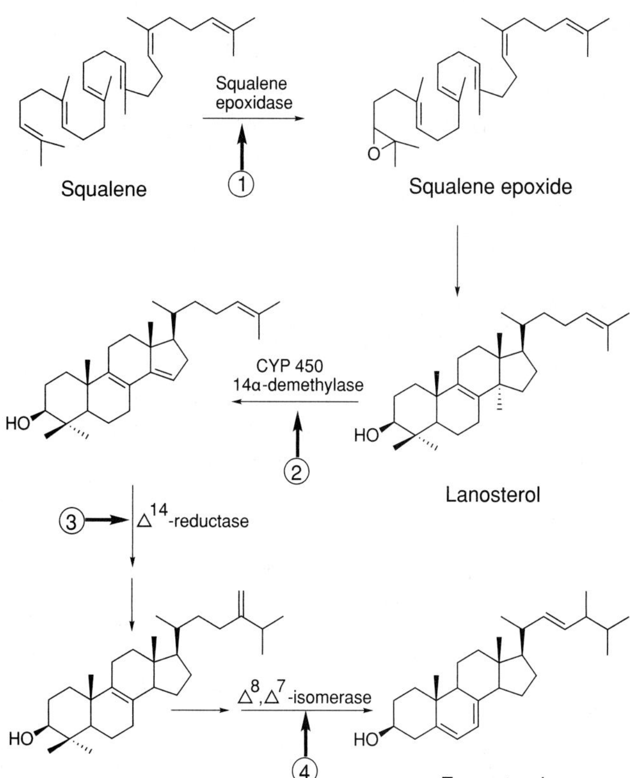

Fig. 40.1. Ergosterol biosynthesis from squalene, with key steps shown in the simplified figure. Enzymatic steps known to be the site of action of currently employed antifungal agents are indicated by a heavy black arrow and a number.

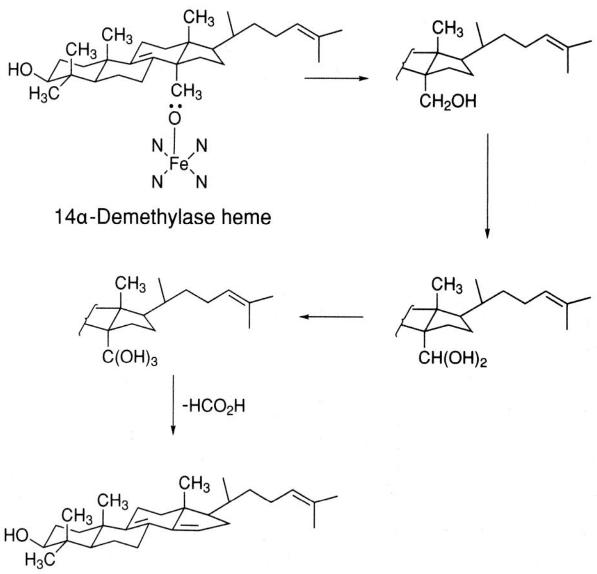

Fig. 40.2. Demethylation of the 14α-methyl group from lanosterol carried out by the cytochrome P450 enzyme sterol 14α-demethylase (CYP51). The mechanism involves three successive heme-catalyzed insertions of activated oxygen into the three carbon-hydrogen bonds of the 14α-methyl group, which raises the oxidation state of the methyl group to a carboxylic acid. The group is finally eliminated as formic acid to create a double bond between carbons 14 and 15.

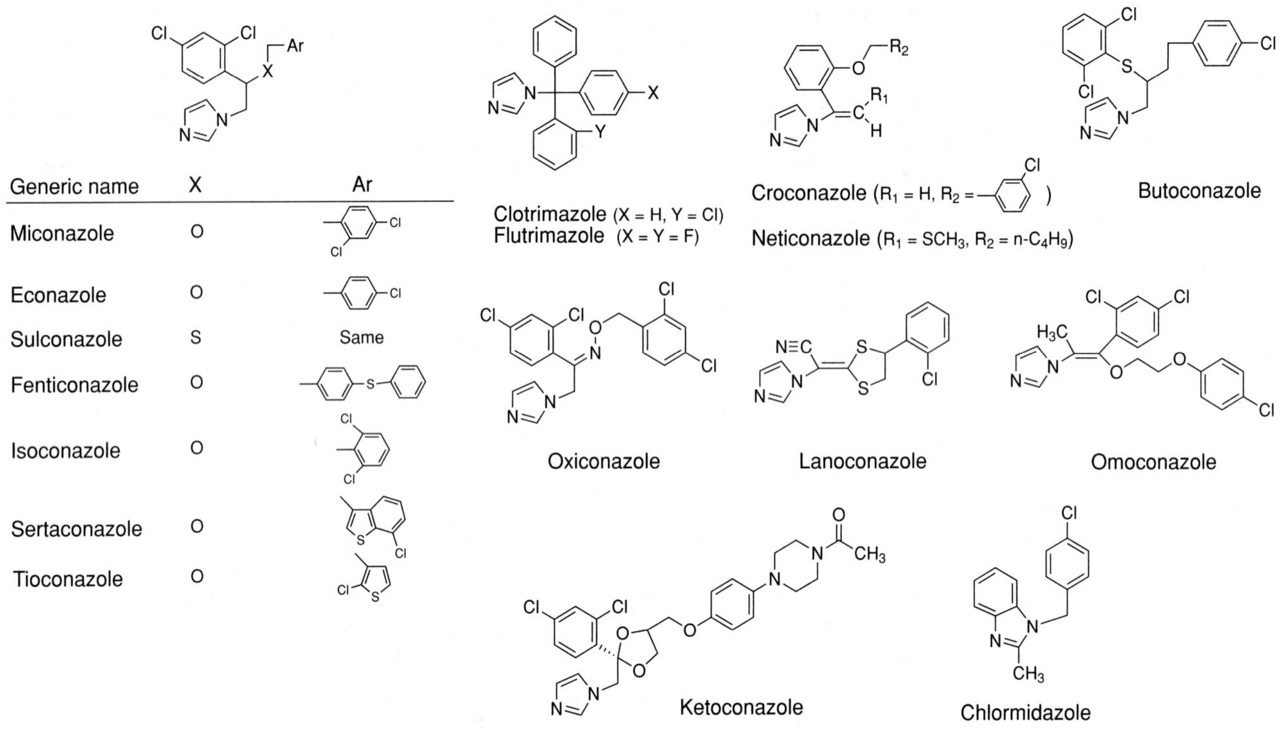

Generic name	X	Ar
Miconazole	O	
Econazole	O	
Sulconazole	S	Same
Fenticonazole	O	
Isoconazole	O	
Sertaconazole	O	
Tioconazole	O	

Clotrimazole (X = H, Y = Cl)
Flutrimazole (X = Y = F)

Croconazole (R_1 = H, R_2 =)
Neticonazole (R_1 = SCH_3, R_2 = n-C_4H_9)

Butoconazole

Oxiconazole

Lanoconazole

Omoconazole

Ketoconazole

Chlormidazole

Fig. 40.3. Imidazole antifungal agents.

bioavailability of some azoles, in contrast to amphotericin B, combined with their generally broad-spectrum of activity has led to their widespread use in treating a variety of serious infections. The characteristic chemical feature of azoles from which their name is derived is the presence of a five-membered aromatic ring containing either two or three nitrogen atoms. Imidazole rings have two nitrogens and triazoles three. In both cases, the azole ring is attached through N_1 to a side chain containing at least one aromatic ring. Imidazole-containing agents are shown in Figure 40.3 (for triazoles, see Fig. 40.6).

Mechanism of Action

All the azoles act by inhibiting ergosterol biosynthesis through inhibition of the 14α-demethylase discussed above under ergosterol biosynthesis (Fig. 40.1, Site 2). The basic N3 atom of the azole forms a bond with the heme iron of the CYP450 prosthetic group in the position normally occupied by the activated oxygen (Fig. 40.4). The remainder of the azole antifungal forms bonding interactions with the apoprotein in a manner that determines the relative selectivity of the drug for the fungal demethylase versus other CYP450 enzymes.

Inhibition of the 14α-demethylase results in accumulation in the fungal cell membrane of sterols still bearing a 14α-methyl group. These sterols do not have the exact shape and physical properties of the normal membrane sterol ergosterol. This results in permeability changes, leaky membranes, and malfunction of membrane-imbedded proteins. These effects taken together lead to fungal cell death. Because biosynthesis of the mammalian membrane sterol cholesterol also employs a CYP450 14α-demethylase, why do 14α-methyl sterols not accumulate in human cell membranes? The reason is in the relative strength of inhibition of the same enzyme from different species. For example, the median inhibitory concentration (IC_{50}) for ketoconazole against the enzyme from *Candida albicans* is approximately 10^{-9} M versus approximately 10^{-6} M for the human enzyme. This three orders of magnitude difference in strength of inhibition provides the therapeutic index with respect to this particular enzyme. As discussed below, however, many of the azoles are powerful inhibitors of other mammalian CYP450 enzymes.

The early azole antifungal drugs were all either extensively and rapidly degraded by first-pass metabolism or

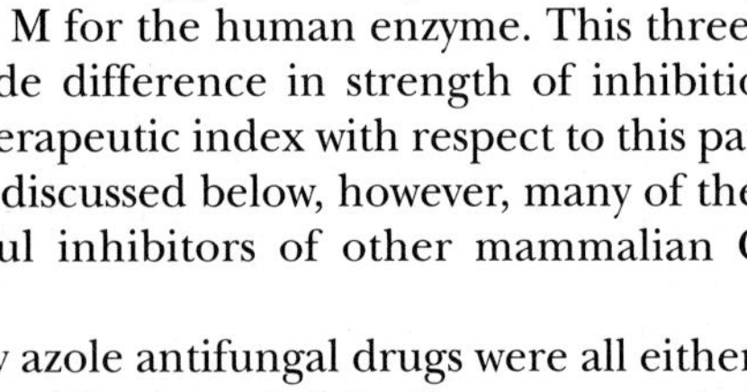

14α-Demethylase heme

Fig. 40.4. Mechanism of azole/CYP450 binding. The basic nitrogen of azole antifungal agents forms a bond to the heme iron of CYP450 enzymes, preventing the enzyme from oxidizing its normal substrates. Ketoconazole is representative of the azole antifungals.

too toxic for systemic use. As a result, only those drugs with reduced or slow first-pass metabolism (ketoconazole, fluconazole, itraconazole, voriconazole, and posaconazole) are used systemically. The other azoles (clotrimazole, tioconazole, terconazole, butoconazole, econazole, oxiconazole, sulconazole, miconazole, and ketoconazole) are available in a variety of creams and ointments for topical treatments of dermatophytic infections and intravaginal use for vaginal yeast infections. (Table 40.1).

SPECIFIC DRUGS

Ketoconazole. Ketoconazole (Fig. 40.3), an imidazole, was the first orally active antifungal azole to be discovered and, as a consequence, has been widely studied and employed for the treatment of systemic fungal infections, primarily candidiasis. Ketoconazole has little effect on *Aspergillus* or *Cryptococcus.* Ketoconazole is highly dependent on low stomach pH for absorption, and antacids or drugs that raise stomach pH will lower the bioavailability of ketoconazole. As with other azoles, it is extensively metabolized by microsomal enzymes (Fig. 40.5). All the metabolites are inactive. Evidence that CYP3A4 plays a significant role in metabolism of ketoconazole is that coadministration of CYP3A4 inducers, such as phenytoin, carbamazepine, and rifampin, can cause as much as a 50% reduction in levels of ketoconazole (13). Ketoconazole also is a powerful inhibitor of human CYP3A4 and, as a consequence, has many serious interactions with other drugs. For example, coadministration of ketoconazole with the hypnotic triazolam results in a 22-fold increase in triazolam's area under the curve (AUC) and a sevenfold increase in half-life. Interestingly, CYP3A4 also is present in the gut and may contribute substantially to the metabolism of many drugs, such as the immunosuppressant agent cyclosporine, thus the potential for drug–drug

Ketoconazole and Cyclosporine—A Clinical Useful Drug Interaction

Cyclosporine is an immunosuppressive agent used in transplant patients to help prevent organ rejection. Although effective, cyclosporine therapy is extremely expensive and the drug appears to be approximately 20% bioavailable following an oral dose. This low bioavailability results from the metabolism of cyclosporine by the CYP450 system to a number of metabolites. Early reports of coadministration of ketoconazole with cyclosporine described excessive adverse effects attributable to cyclosporine toxicity. From this and knowledge about the effects of ketoconazole on CYP450-mediated metabolism, investigators hypothesized that a much lower dose of cyclosporine could be given concomitantly with ketoconazole, producing blood levels of cyclosporine equivalent to those seen with the higher dose at a fraction of the cost. In fact, it appears that ketoconazole given concurrently with cyclosporine may allow up to an 80% reduction in cyclosporine dose.

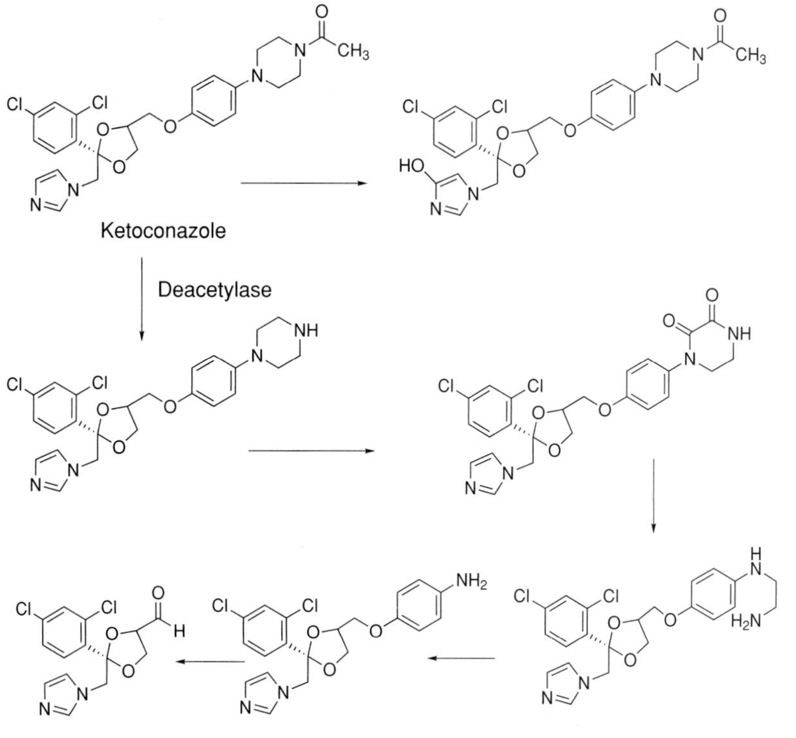

Ketoconazole

Deacetylase

Fig. 40.5. Extensive metabolism of ketoconazole involving hydrolysis of the N-acetyl by a deacetylase. The oxidation reactions are catalyzed by CYP3A4 and a flavin-linked mixed-function oxidase. All metabolites are inactive.

interaction (see box). Ketoconazole is a weak inhibitor of CYP2C9, which is the enzyme responsible for the metabolism of several narrow therapeutic index drugs, such as warfarin and phenytoin. As better systemic agents have become available, ketoconazole's clinical use has become limited to topical applications in a variety of dosage forms, including creams, lotions, suppositories, and shampoos.

Itraconazole. Itraconazole was, along with fluconazole, one of the first triazoles introduced into clinical use (Fig. 40.6) (14). Itraconazole's oral bioavailability is variable and is influenced by food and stomach pH, a strongly acidic pH being required for good absorption. Like ketoconazole, itraconazole is extensively metabolized by CYP3A4 following oral administration, and levels are markedly reduced by coadministration of the CYP3A4-inducers phenytoin, carbamazepine. and rifampin (13). Additionally, like ketoconazole, itraconazole has been demonstrated to be a strong inhibitor of CYP3A4 (15). This interaction has proven to be of clinical significance because the risk of developing rhabdomyolysis following lovastatin or simvastatin therapy with coadministration of itraconazole (16–18). Itraconazole therefore is likely to have serious interactions with any other drug metabolized by CYP3A4. Again like ketoconazole, itraconazole appears to have little or no effect on CYP2C9-mediated metabolism of warfarin and phenytoin.

Terconazole. Terconazole (Fig. 40.6) is a close analogue of ketoconazole and itraconazole. It is approved only for the treatment of vaginal candidiasis and is not used systemically (Table 40.1) (19,20).

Fluconazole. Fluconazole (Fig. 40.6), which was introduced at the same time as itraconazole, differs from ketoconazole and itraconazole in that it is equally bioavailable when given orally or IV. Two major advantages of fluconazole over other antifungal agents are that it can cross the blood-brain barrier and has efficacy against *Cryptococcus neoformans* (21). Fluconazole also differs in that it is only a weak inhibitor of CYP3A4 but a strong inhibitor of CYP2C9 (22). For instance, fluconazole doubles the AUC of (*S*)-warfarin (the active enantiomer) and greatly prolongs the prothrombin time in patients receiving warfarin anticoagulant therapy (23). Because warfarin has such a narrow therapeutic index and excessive anticoagulation can be extremely harmful, this interaction is considered to be of major clinical significance. Fluconazole also decreases the metabolism of the CYP2C9 substrate phenytoin, an antiepileptic agent that also has a narrow therapeutic index (24). Depending on the dose of fluconazole, coadministration with phenytoin can result in a 75 to 150% increase in the phenytoin AUC, and numerous case reports have documented substantial adverse effects following this regimen. Fluconazole also will inhibit CYP3A4, though not to the same degree as ketoconazole and itraconazole. Fluconazole exhibits a dose-dependent inhibition of triazolam metabolism (a CYP3A4 reaction) causing as much as a fourfold increase in triazolam AUC.

Voriconazole. Voriconazole (Fig. 40.6) is a fluconazole analogue that was developed to overcome some of the limitations of fluconazole (25) and does, indeed, have a broader spectrum of activity than fluconazole, having activity against *Aspergillus* and fluconazole-resistant strains of *Candida* and *Cryptococcus* (26). Voriconazole is orally absorbed and penetrates the blood-brain barrier. Unfortunately, voriconazole is extensively metabolized CYP450 enzymes (Fig. 40.7) and is an inhibitor of CYP2C19, CYP2C9, and CYP3A4, leading to many drug interactions (27,28). Voriconazole exhibits nonlinear, saturable kinetics, and because CYP2C19 exhibits genetic polymorphisms, plasma levels can be higher in poor metabolizers versus extensive metabolizers (29,30).

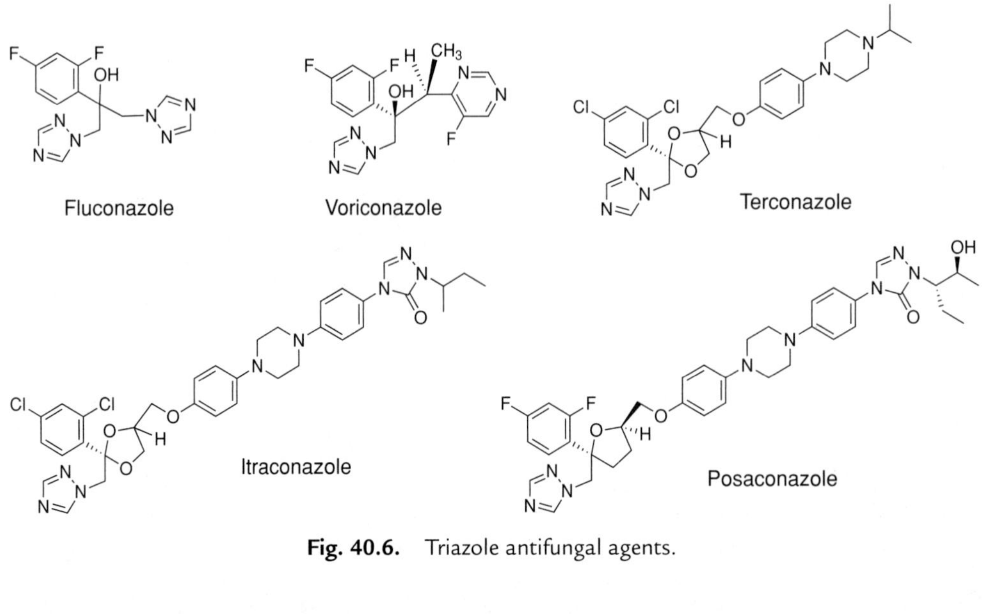

Fig. 40.6. Triazole antifungal agents.

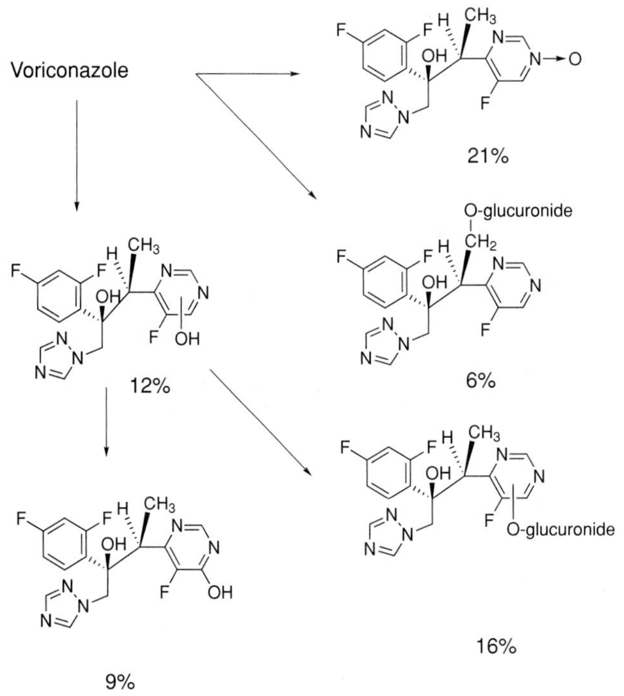

Fig. 40.7. Major metabolic products resulting from CYP450 metabolism of voriconazole.

Posaconazole. Posaconazole (Fig. 40.6), a recently introduced triazole, has a number of advantages over previous agents (31,32). Posaconazole has a wide spectrum of activity compared to other azoles, particularly against *Aspergillus* and other increasingly common nosocomial infections resistant to treatment by other antifungal drugs (32). Posaconazole is metabolized primarily by Phase II glucuronide conjugation and has little interaction with the oxidative CYP450 enzymes (33). Thus, posaconazole should have far fewer drug interactions than the other azole antifungal agents. Posaconazole is structurally similar to itraconazole and saperconazole, but it contains a tetrahydrofuran ring in place of the dioxolan ring of those agents, which may account for some of its unique properties.

Allyl Amines and Other Squalene Epoxidase Inhibitors

The group of agents generally known as allyl amines[34] strictly includes only naftifine and terbinafine, but because butenafine and tolnaftate function by the same mechanism of action, they are included in this class and are shown in Figure 40.8. One can, of course, consider the benzyl group of butenafine to be bio-isosteric with the allyl group of naftifine and terbinafine. Tolnaftate, a much older drug, is chemically a thiocarbamate but has the same mechanism of action as the allyl amines. These drugs have a more limited spectrum of activity than the azoles and are effective only against dermatophytes. Therefore, they are employed in the treatment of fungal infections of the skin and nails (35).

Mechanism of Action. All of the drugs in Figure 40.8 act through inhibition of the enzyme squalene epoxidase (Fig. 40.1, Site 1). Inhibition of this enzyme has two effects, both of which appear to be involved in the fungitoxic mechanism of this class (36). First, inhibition of squalene epoxidase results in a decrease in total sterol content of the fungal cell membrane. This decrease alters the physicochemical properties of the membrane, resulting in malfunctions of membrane-imbedded transport proteins involved in nutrient transport and pH balance. Second, inhibition of squalene epoxidase results in a buildup within the fungal cell of the hydrocarbon squalene, which is itself toxic when present in abnormally high amounts. Mammals also employ the enzyme squalene epoxidase in the biosynthesis of cholesterol, but a desirable therapeutic index arises from the fact that the fungal squalene epoxidase enzyme is far more sensitive to the drugs than the corresponding mammalian enzyme. Terbinafine has a K_i of 0.03 μM versus squalene epoxidase from *Candida albicans* but only 77 μM versus the same enzyme from rat liver—a 2,500-fold difference (37).

Specific Drugs

Naftifine. Naftifine (Fig. 40.8) was the first allyl amine to be discovered and marketed (34). It is subject to extensive first-pass metabolism to be orally active and, consequently, is only available in topical preparations (Table 40.1). The widest use of naftifine is against various tinea infections of the skin.

Terbinafine. Terbinafine (Fig. 40.8) is available in both topical and oral dosage forms (Tables 40.1 and 40.2) and is effective against a variety of dermatophytic

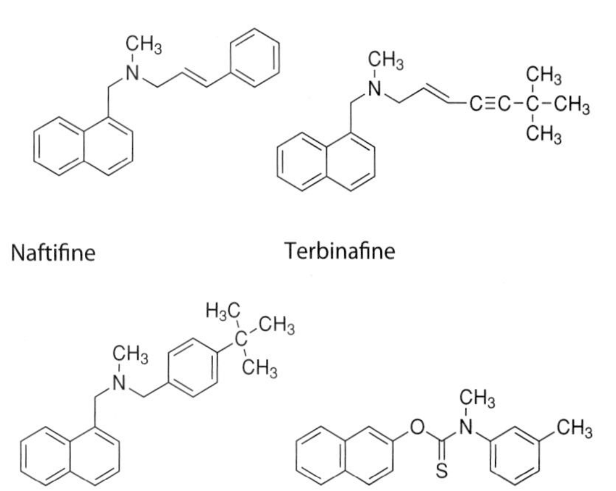

Fig. 40.8. The squalene epoxidase inhibitors, allyl amines. Naftifine was the first drug shown to act by inhibition of squalene epoxidase, as does the much older thinocarbamate, tolnaftate.

Azole Antifungals in Agriculture

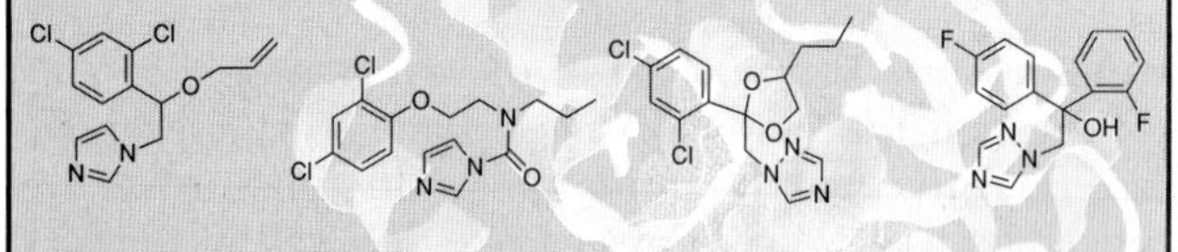

Imazalil Prochloraz Propiconazole Flutriafol

Every year, fungal infections of crops causes hundreds of millions of dollars worth of damage to a wide variety of food and other crops. Before the development of effective agricultural antifungals, crop diseases were the cause of several major famines. The infamous Irish Potato Famine of the nineteenth century was caused by a pathogenic fungus, *Phytophera infestans*. Tens of thousands of people starved to death, and thousands more emigrated to the United States to escape the famine. Today, both imidazole and triazole antifungal agents, such as imazalil and propiconazole, are among the most effective crop-protection agents known. More than 20 azole antifungals are used for crop protection, and a representative sample is shown. The mechanism of action of the agricultural antifungals is identical to that of the agents used for mammalian infections. In fact, they bear a remarkable resemblance to antifungal drugs employed in treating human disease.

infections when employed topically or systemically (38). A unique property of terbinafine is its effectiveness in the treatment of onychomycoses (nail infections) (39). Given orally, the highly lipophilic drug redistributes from the plasma into the nail bed and into the nail itself, where the infection resides (40), making terbinafine superior to other agents for treating this particular type of infection. Terbinafine is extensively metabolized by several CYP450 enzymes, including CYP1A2, CYP2C19, CYP2C9, CYP2C8, CYP3A4, and CYP2B6 (41). Because there are so many pathways for terbinafine metabolism, inhibition of any one has very little effect on overall clearance of the drug, although drugs that inhibit several CYP450 enzymes, such as cimetidine, can increase terbinafine plasma levels. Although not a substrate for the enzyme, terbinafine is a strong inhibitor of CYP2D6 and can have significant interactions with drugs that are metabolized by this enzyme, such as codeine and desipramine (22,42).

Butenafine and Tolnaftate. Butenafine and tolnaftate, like naftifine (Fig. 40.8), are only available in topical preparation for the treatment of dermatophytic infections (Table 40.1). Tolnaftate has been marketed in a variety of nonprescription drug preparations for decades. Butenafine, discovered more recently, has a somewhat wider spectrum of activity than tolnaftate. For example, butenafine is active against superficial *Candida albicans* infections, which are not affected by tolnaftate (43).

Agricultural Antifungal Morpholines

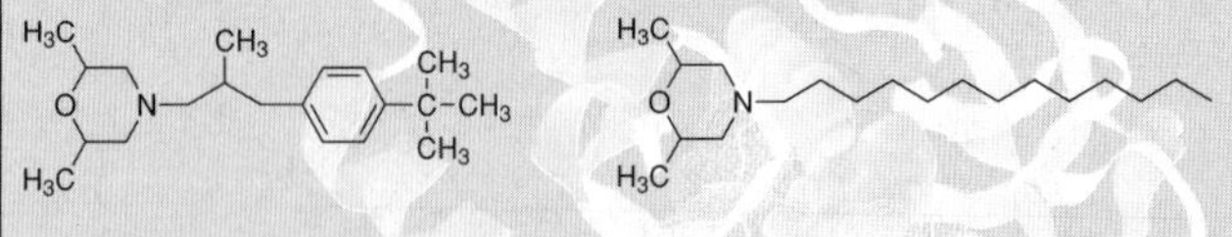

Fenpropimorph Tridemorph

Just as there are several classes of drugs to treat human fungal infections, there are several classes of "drugs" to treat fungal phytopathogens. The morpholines, fenpropimorph and tridemorph, are not used to treat human disease but have wide utility in protecting crops from phytopathogenic fungi.

Morpholines

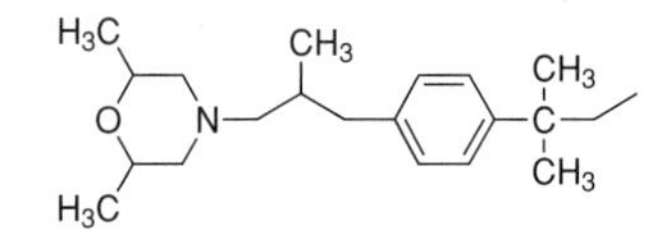

Amorolfine

Amorolfine is the only drug in this class that is employed clinically in the treatment of human fungal infections. Amorolfine is not currently available in the United States, but it is marketed in Europe and Asia for the topical treatment of dermatophytic infections (44).

Morpholine antifungals inhibit ergosterol biosynthesis by acting on the enzymes Δ^{14}-reductase and Δ^{8},Δ^{7}-isomerase (Fig. 40.1, Site 3 and 4) (45). Inhibition of these enzymes results in incorporation into fungal cell membranes of sterols retaining either a Δ^{14} double bond, a Δ^{8} double bond, or both. None of these will have the same overall shape and physicochemical properties as the preferred sterol, ergosterol. As with the antifungals already discussed, this results in membranes with altered properties and malfunctioning of membrane-embedded proteins.

Inhibitors of Cell Wall Biosynthesis—Echinocandins

The most notable difference between fungal and mammalian cells is that fungi have a cell wall and mammals do not. Drugs interfering with cell wall biosynthesis would be expected to be relatively nontoxic to mammals. Such drugs have been the foundation of antibacterial therapy since the discovery of penicillin and the development of dozens of effective penicillins and cephalosporins. Only recently, however, have a few drugs affecting fungal cell wall biosynthesis become available. Echinocandins, a group of cyclic peptides with long lipophilic side chains and sometimes called lipopeptides, have been under investigation for a number of years (Fig. 40.9) (46). Echinocandins interfere with cell wall biosynthesis through inhibition of the enzyme β-1,3-glucan synthase. β-Glucan is an important polymer component of many fungal cell walls, and reduction in the glucan content severely weakens the cell wall, leading to rupture of the fungal cell.

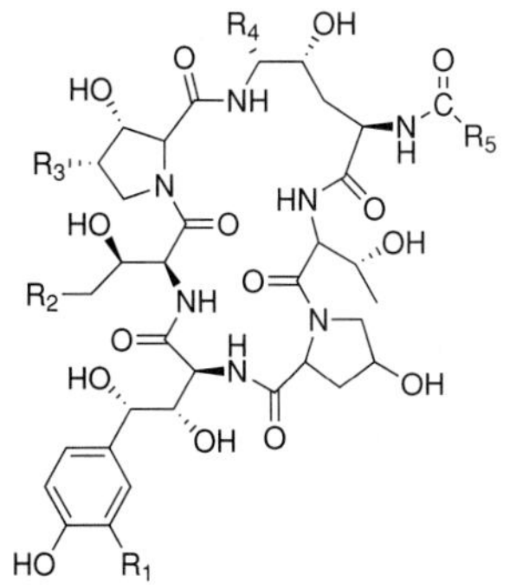

Drug	R_1	R_2	R_3	R_4	R_5
Caspofungin (Cancidas)	H	CH_2NH_2	H	$NHCH_2CH_2NH_2$	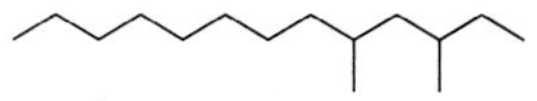
Anidulafungin (Eraxis)	H	H	CH_3	OH	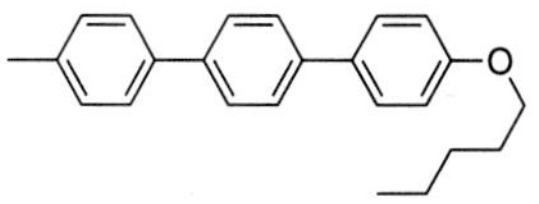
Micafungin (Mycamine)	OSO_3H	$CONH_2$	CH_3	OH	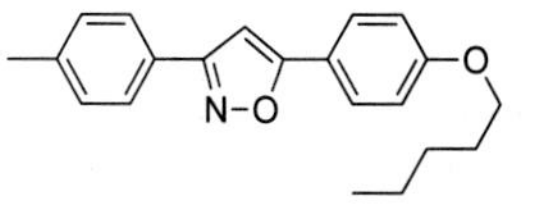

Fig. 40.9. Echinocandins.

Caspofungin, Anidulafungin, and Micafungin

Recently, three semisynthetic echinocandins have been approved for use in treating life-threatening systemic fungal infections (47). These are caspofungin, anidulafungin, and micafungin (Fig. 40.9). These drugs represent the first class of antifungal agents with a novel mechanism of action to be marketed in more than 30 years and are a very valuable contribution to therapy for systemic fugal infections. They are effective against a variety of *Candida* species that have proven to be resistant to other agents as well as effective against azole-resistant *Aspergillus*. Therefore, these drugs are truly life-saving for those afflicted with these previously resistant fungi. Unfortunately these echinocandins are not effective against *Cryptococcus neoformans*. None of these drugs is orally active, and all must be administered by IV infusion. Because of limited hepatic metabolism, drug–drug interactions are not a problem. Caspofungin is metabolized by hydrolysis in two portions of the hexapeptide ring (Fig. 40.10) (48), whereas anidulafungin does not appear to be actively metabolized but rather slowly degrades (49). Micafungin is metabolized by a sulfotransferase and by catechol-O-methyltransferase (COMT), but no significant drug interactions are known (50).

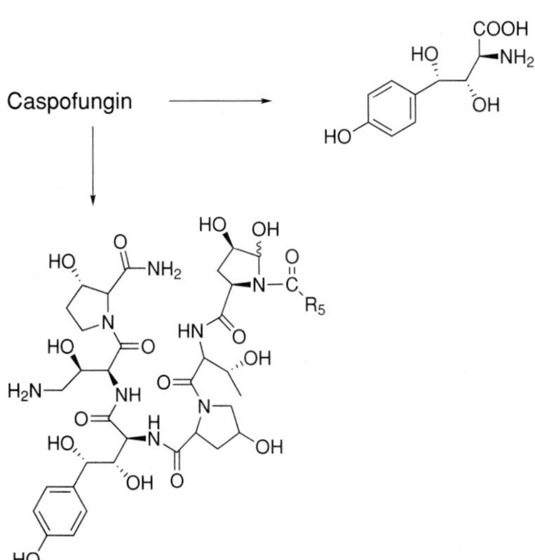

Fig. 40.10. Metabolic products formed from caspofungin.

Drugs Acting Through Other Mechanisms

Flucytosine

Flucytosine is a powerful antifungal agent used in the treatment of serious systemic fungal infections, such as *Cryptococcus neoformans* and *Candida* spp (Table 40.2). Flucytosine itself is not cytotoxic but, rather, is a pro-drug that is taken up by fungi and metabolized to 5-fluorouracil (5-FU) by fungal cytidine deaminase (Fig. 40.11) (51). Then, 5-FU is converted to 5-fluorodeoxyuridine, which as a thymidylate synthase inhibitor interferes with both protein and RNA biosynthesis. 5-Fluorouracil is cytotoxic and is employed in cancer chemotherapy (see Chapter 42). Human cells do not contain cytosine deaminase and, therefore, do not convert flucytosine to 5-FU. Some intestinal flora, however, do convert the drug to 5-FU, so human toxicity does result from this metabolism. Resistance rapidly develops to flucytosine when used alone, so it is almost always used in conjunction with amphotericin B. Use of flucytosine has declined since the discovery of fluconazole.

Griseofulvin

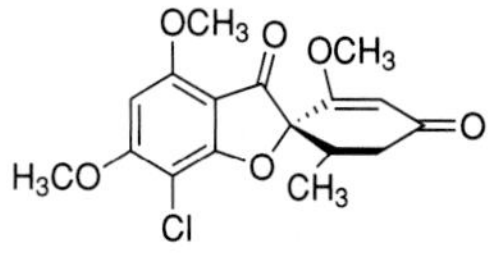

Griseofulvin

Griseofulvin is an antifungal antibiotic produced by an unusual strain of *Penicillium* (52). It is used orally to treat

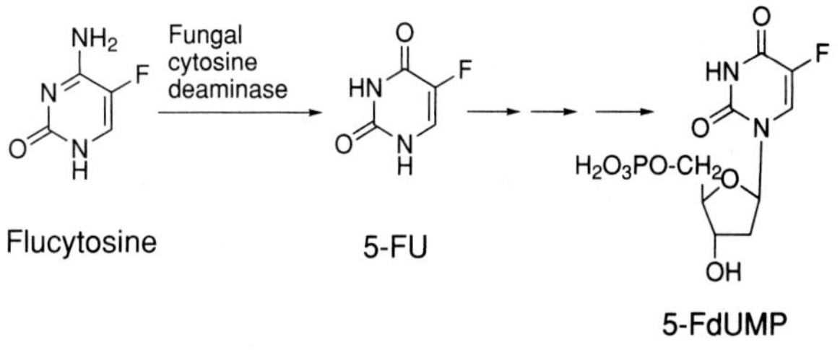

Fungal cytosine deaminase

Flucytosine 5-FU 5-FdUMP

Fig. 40.11. Flucytosine, a pro-drug, is converted by fungal cytosine deaminase to 5-fluorouracil (5-FU). This reaction does not occur in mammalian cells. A further transformation of 5-FU to the actual cytotoxic agent, 5-fluorodeoxyuridine monophosphate (5-FdUMP), also occurs.

superficial fungal infections, primarily fingernail and toenail infections, but it does not penetrate skin or nails if used topically (Table 40.2). When given orally, however, plasmaborne griseofulvin becomes incorporated into keratin precursor cells and, ultimately, into keratin, which cannot then support fungal growth. The infection is cured when the diseased tissue is replaced by new, uninfected tissue, which can take months. The mechanism of action of griseofulvin is through binding to the protein tubulin, which interferes with the function of the mitotic spindle and, thereby, inhibits cell division. Griseofulvin also may interfere directly with DNA replication. Griseofulvin is gradually being replaced by newer agents (53).

Haloprogin

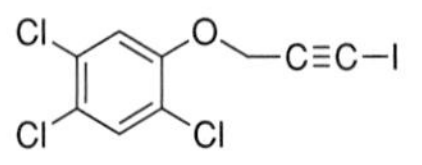

Cl, Cl, Cl, O, C≡C–I

Haloprogin

Haloprogin is an iodinated acetylene active against dermatophytes (54). Haloprogin is only used for topical applications (Table 40.1). The mechanism of haloprogin is not clear, but it appears to lead to nonspecific metabolic disruption. It has been demonstrated to interfere with DNA biosynthesis and cell respiration.

Ciclopirox

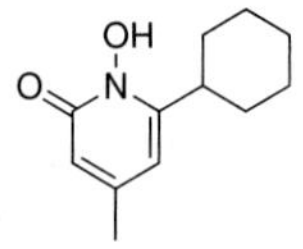

OH, O, N

Ciclopirox

Ciclopirox is a hydroxylated pyridinone that is employed for superficial dermatophytic infections, principally onychomycosis. Ciclopirox has a unique mechanism of action through chelation of polyvalent cations, such as Fe^{3+}, which causes inhibition of a number of metal-dependent enzymes within the fungal cell. Although ciclopirox has been available for more than 30 years, a new formulation of an 8% lacquer has been recently introduced for treating nail infections (55).

Undecylenic Acid

$H_2C{=}CH(CH_2)_8COOH$

Undecylenic acid

Undecylenic acid is widely employed, frequently as the zinc salt, in over-the-counter preparations for topical treatment of infections by dermatophytes (Table 40.1) (56). Undecylenic acid is fungistatic that acts through a nonspecific interaction with components in the fungal cell membrane.

CASE STUDY

Victoria F. Roche and S. William Zito

KK is a 42-year-old, Brazilian-born executive who works for Ronald Stump, an internationally famous investment mogul and entrepreneur who mentors (and generously rewards) go-getters like KK. KK's career potential seemed unlimited until he acquired AIDS from a previous partner who was unaware of his HIV-positive status at the time of their relationship. The last year has been tough for KK, who has always been athletic, adventurous, and seemingly indestructible, but he has fallen ill several times in the past 12 months with bacterial and viral infections, including a particularly nasty case of poststreptococcal nephritis. He is currently on antiviral therapy that includes indinavir sulfate (Crixivan, 800 mg every 8 hours) and zidovudine (Retrovir, 300 mg b.i.d.). Although he is still able to work and is managing fairly well, he is fearful about the anticipated final outcome of his disease and is employing spiritual and nontraditional strategies in an attempt to heal.

As part of this holistic approach to healing, KK flew to the Amazon and spent two nights alone on the edge of the jungle, seeking insight and peace through reflection and prayer. All he took in with him was his medication and a sufficient amount of food and water to last for 48 hours. He felt safe, however, because he was within a 20-minute walk of a tribal community and could sound an alarm that would alert people in case of danger or an emergency. He slept under the stars, pulling up ground vegetation into a "natural" bed each night. He felt emotionally restored after the experience—until it became known that he had inhaled dust contaminated with the soil fungus *P. brasiliensis* and a species of *Aspergillus* mold. He is now in the critical care wing of your hospital with a disseminated fungal infection. The therapeutic plan is to start him on an appropriate IV antifungal agent supplemented with oral therapy. Consider the structures of the antifungal agents drawn below, and identify suitable parenteral and oral antifungal drug products for KK.

1. Identify the therapeutic problem(s) in which the pharmacist's intervention may benefit the patient.
2. Identify and prioritize the patient-specific factors that must be considered to achieve the desired therapeutic outcomes.
3. Conduct a thorough and mechanistically oriented structure-activity analysis of all therapeutic alternatives provided in the case.
4. Evaluate the structure-activity relationship findings against the patient-specific factors and desired therapeutic outcomes, and make a therapeutic decision.
5. Counsel your patient.

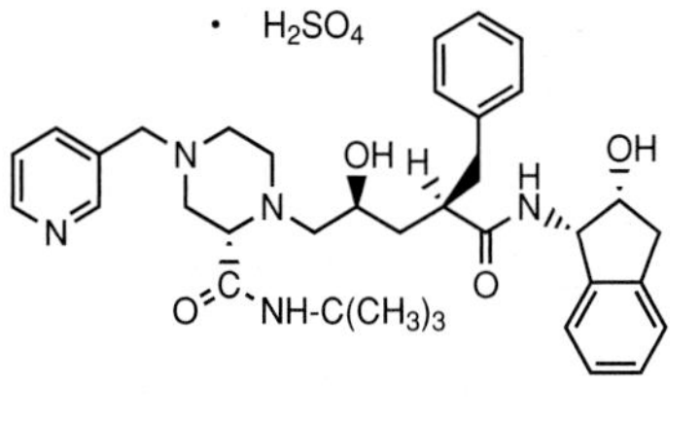

• H_2SO_4

Indinavir

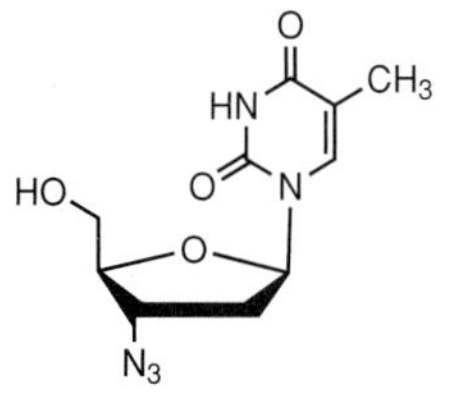

Zidovudine(AZT)

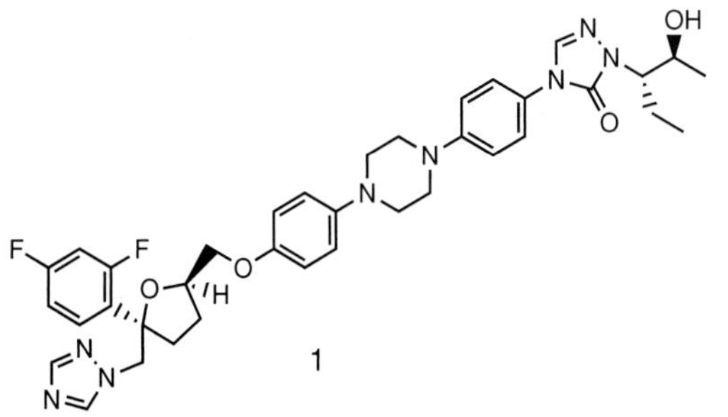

1

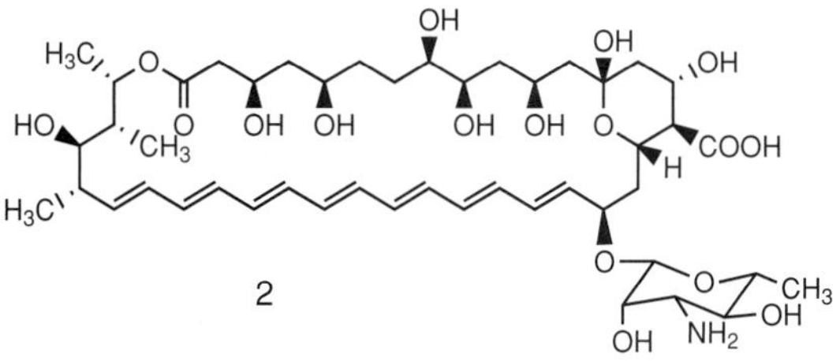

2

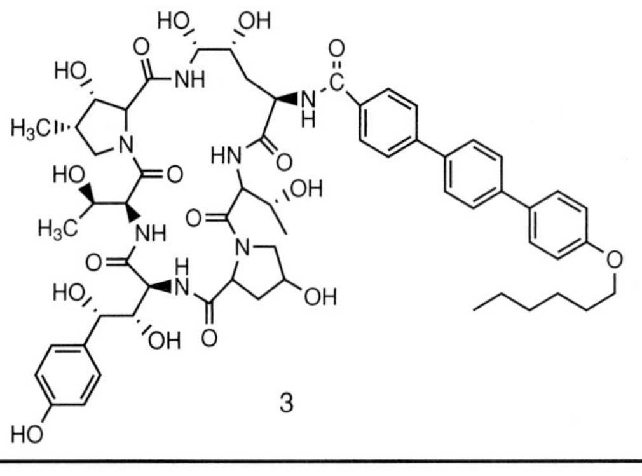

3

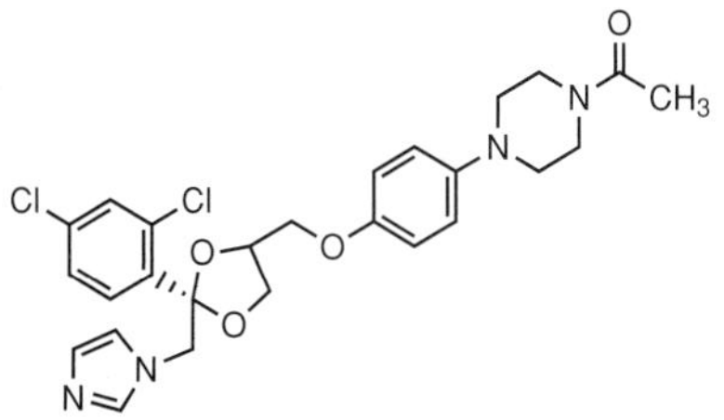

4

References

1. Anaissie EJ, McGinnis MR, Pfaller MA, eds. Clinical Mycology. New York: Churchill Livingstone, 2003.
2. Pfaller MA, Wenzel RP. The epidemiology of fungal infections. In: Anaissie EJ, McCinnis MR, Pfaller MA, eds. Clinical Mycology. New York: Churchill Livingstone, 2003:3–19.
3. Hiruma M, Yamaguchi H. Dermatophytes. In: Anaissie EJ, McCinnis MR, Pfaller MA, eds. Clinical Mycology. New York: Churchill Livingstone, 2003:370–379.
4. Digani MC, Solomkin JS, Anaissie EJ. Candida. In: Anaissie EJ, McCinnis MR, Pfaller MA, eds. Clinical Mycology. New York: Churchill Livingstone, 2003:195–241.
5. Viviani MA, Tortorano AM, Ajello L. Cryptococcus. In: Anaissie EJ, McCinnis MR, Pfaller MA, eds. Clinical Mycology. New York: Churchill Livingstone, 2003:240–259.
6. Maenza JR, Merz WG. Infections caused by non-*Candida*, non-*Cryptococcus* yeasts. In: Anaissie EJ, McCinnis MR, Pfaller MA, eds. Clinical Mycology. New York: Churchill Livingstone, 2003:260–272.
7. Perea S, Patterson TF. Endemic mycoses. In: Anaissie EJ, McCinnis MR, Pfaller MA, eds. Clinical Mycology. New York: Churchill Livingstone, 2003:352–369.
8. Dromer F, McGinnis MR. Zygomycosis. In: Anaissie EJ, McCinnis MR, Pfaller MA, eds. Clinical Mycology. New York: Churchill Livingstone, 2003:297–308.
9. Fernandes PB, ed. New Approaches for Antifungal Drugs. Boston: Birkhauser, 1992.
10. Koller W, ed. Target Sites of Fungicide Action. Boca Raton, FL: CRC Press, 1992.
11. Zaas AK, Alexander BD. Echinocandins: role in antifungal therapy, 2005. Expert Opin Pharmacother 2005;6:1657–1668.
12. Koller W. Antifungal agents with target sites in sterol functions and biosynthesis. In: Killer W, ed. Target Sites of Fungicide Action. Boca Raton, FL: CRC Press, 1992:119–206.
13. Tucker RM, Denning DW, Hanson LH, et al. Interaction of azoles with rifampin, phenytoin, and carbamazepine: in vitro and clinical observations. Clin Infect Dis 1992;14:165–174.
14. Warnock DW. Itraconazole and fluconazole: new drugs for deep fungal infection. J Antimicrob Chemother 1989;24:275–277.
15. Colburn DE, Giles FJ, Oladovich D, et al. In vitro evaluation of cytochrome P450–mediated drug interactions between cytarabine, idarubicin, itraconazole, and caspofungin. Hematology 2004;9:217–221.
16. Horn M. Coadministration of itraconazole with hypolipidemic agents may induce rhabdomyolysis in healthy individuals. Arch Dermatol 1996;132:1254.
17. Neuvonen PJ, Jalava KM. Itraconazole drastically increases plasma concentrations of lovastatin and lovastatin acid. Clin Pharmacol Ther 1996;60:54–61.
18. Vlahakos DV, Manginas A, Chilidou D, et al. Itraconazole-induced rhabdomyolysis and acute renal failure in a heart transplant recipient treated with simvastatin and cyclosporine. Transplantation 2002;73:1962–1964.
19. Van Cutsem J, Van Gerven F, Zaman R, et al. Terconazole—a new broad-spectrum antifungal. Chemotherapy 1983;29:322–331.
20. Doering PL, Santiago TM. Drugs for treatment of vulvovaginal candidiasis: comparative efficacy of agents and regimens. Drug Intelligence and Clinical Pharmacy 1990;24:1078–1083.
21. Bailey EM, Krakovsky DJ, Rybak MJ. The triazole antifungal agents: a review of itraconazole and fluconazole. Pharmacotherapy 1990;10:146–153.
22. Venkatakrishnan K, von Moltke LL, Greenblatt DJ. Effects of the antifungal agents on oxidative drug metabolism: clinical relevance. Clin Pharmacokinet 2000;38:111–180.
23. Kunze KL, Wienkers LC, Thummel KE, et al. Warfarin-fluconazole. I. Inhibition of the human cytochrome P450–dependent metabolism of warfarin by fluconazole: in vitro studies. Drug Metab Dispos 1996;24:414–421.
24. Niwa T, Shiraga T, Takagi A, Effect of antifungal drugs on cytochrome P450 (CYP) 2C9, CYP2C19, and CYP3A4 activities in human liver microsomes. Biol Pharm Bull 2005;28:1805–1808.
25. Sabo JA, Abdel-Rahman SM, Voriconazole: a new triazole antifungal. Ann Pharmacother 2000;34:1032–1043.
26. Herbrecht R, Denning DW, Patterson TF, et al. Voriconazole versus amphotericin B for primary therapy of invasive aspergillosis. N Engl J Med 2002;347:408–415.
27. Niwa T, Inoue-Yamamoto S, Shiraga T, et al. Effect of antifungal drugs on cytochrome P450 (CYP) 1A2, CYP2D6, and CYP2E1 activities in human liver microsomes. Biol Pharm Bull 2005;28:1813–1816.
28. Roffey SJ, Cole S, Comby P, et al. The disposition of vorixonazole in mouse, rat, guinea pig, dog, and human. Drug Metab Dispos 2003;31:731–741.
29. Cocchi S, Codeluppi M, Guaraldi G, et al. Invasive pulmonary and cerebral aspergillosis in a patient with Weil's disease. Scand J Infect Dis 2005;37: 396–398.
30. Ghannoum MA, Kuhn DM. Voriconazole—better chances for patients with invasive mycoses. Eur J Med Res 2002;7:242–256.
31. Barchiesi F, Schimizzi AM, Caselli F, et al. Activity of the new antifungal triazole, posaconazole, against *Cryptococcus neoformans*. J Antimicrob Chemother 2001;48:769–773.
32. Torres HA, Hachem RY, Chemaly RF, et al. Posaconazole: a broad-spectrum triazole antifungal. Lancet Infect Dis 2005;5:775–785.
33. Krieter P, Flannery B, Musick T, et al. Disposition of posaconazole following single-dose oral administration in healthy subjects. Antimicrob Agents Chemother 2004;48:3543–3551.
34. Petranyi G, Ryder NS, Stutz A. Allylamine derivatives: new class of synthetic antifungal agents inhibiting fungal squalene epoxidase. Science 1984;224: 1239–1241.
35. Gupta AK, Sauder DN, Shear NH. Antifungal agents: an overview. Part II. J Am Acad Dermatol, 1994;30:911–933.
36. Georgopapadakou NH, Bertasso A. Effects of squalene epoxidase inhibitors on *Candida albicans*. Antimicrob Agents Chemother 1992;36: 1779–1781.
37. Petranyi G, Stutz A, Ryde NS, et al. Experimental antimycotic activity of naftifine and terbinafine. In: Fromtling RA, ed. Recent Trends in the Discovery, Development, and Evaluation of Antifungal Agents. Barcelona: JR Prous Science, 1987:441–459.
38. Gupta AK, Ryder JE, Chow M, et al. Dermatophytosis: the management of fungal infections. Skinmed 2005;4:305–310.
39. Zaias N. Management of onychomycosis with oral terbinafine. J Am Acad Dermatol 1990;23:810–812.
40. Finlay AY. Pharmacokinetics of terbinafine in the nail. Br J Dermatol 1992;126 (Suppl 39):28–32.
41. Vickers AE, Sinclair JR, Zollinger M, et al. Multiple cytochrome P450s involved in the metabolism of terbinafine suggest a limited potential for drug–drug interactions. Drug Metab Dispos 1999;27:1029–3108.
42. Abdel-Rahman SM, Marcucci K, Boge T, et al. Potent inhibition of cytochrome P450 2D6–mediated dextromethorphan O-demethylation by terbinafine. Drug Metab Dispos 1999;27:770–775.
43. Odom RB. Update on topical therapy for superficial fungal infections: focus on butenafine. J Am Acad Dermatol 1997;36:S1–S2.
44. Zaug M, Bergstraesser M. Amorolfine in the treatment of onychomycoses and dermatomycoses (an overview). Clin Exp Dermatol 1992;17(Suppl 1):61–70.
45. Polak A. Preclinical data and mode of action of amorolfine. Dermatology 1992;184(Suppl 1):3–7.
46. Debono M, Gordee RS. Antibiotics that inhibit fungal cell wall development. Annu Rev Microbiol 1994;48:471–497.
47. Denning DW. Echinocandin antifungal drugs. Lancet 2003;362:1142–1151.
48. Balani SK, Xu X, Arison BH, et al. Metabolites of caspofungin acetate, a potent antifungal agent, in human plasma and urine. Drug Metab Dispos 2000;28:1274–1278.
49. Raasch RH. Anidulafungin: review of a new echinocandin antifungal agent. Expert Rev Anti-Infect Ther 2004;2:499–508.
50. Hebert MF, Smith HE, Marbury TC, et al. Pharmacokinetics of micafungin in healthy volunteers, volunteers with moderate liver disease, and volunteers with renal dysfunction. J Clin Pharmacol 2005;45:1145–1152.
51. Revankar SG, Graybill JR. Antifungal therapy. In: Anaissie EJ, McCinnis MR, Pfaller MA, eds. Clinical Mycology. New York: Churchill Livingstone, 2003:157–192.
52. Hunter PA, Darby GK, Russell NJ, eds. Fifty Years of Antimicrobials: Past Perspectives and Future Trends. Symposia of the Society for General Microbiology. Cambridge, UK: Cambridge University Press, 1995.
53. Cole GW, Stricklin G. A comparison of a new oral antifungal, terbinafine, with griseofulvin as therapy for tinea corporis. Arch Dermatol 1989;125: 1537–1539.
54. Rezabek GH, Friedman AD. Superficial fungal infections of the skin. Diagnosis and current treatment recommendations. Drugs 1992;43:674–682.
55. Gupta AK, Fleckman P, Baran R. Ciclopirox nail lacquer topical solution 8% in the treatment of toenail onychomycosis. J Am Acad Dermatol 2000;43 (Suppl 4):S70–S80.
56. Diehl KB. Topical antifungal agents: an update. Am Fam Physician 1996; 54:1687–1692.

41. *Antimycobacterial Agents*

THOMAS L. LEMKE

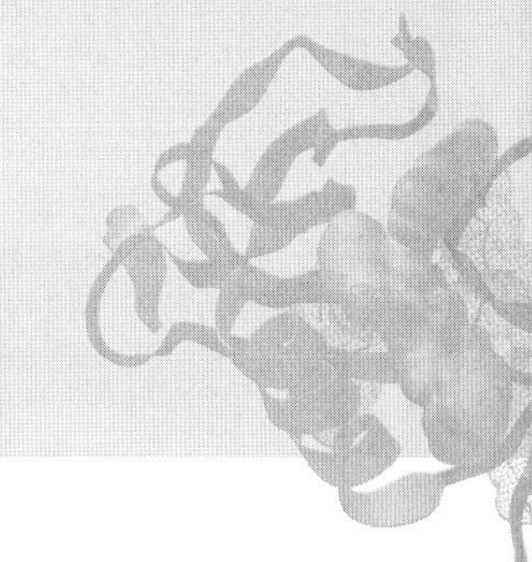

DRUGS COVERED IN THIS CHAPTER:

ANTIMYCOBACTERIAL AGENTS

ANTITUBERCULIN DRUGS

- Capreomycin
- Cycoserine
- Ethambutol
- Ethionamide
- Isoniazid
- Kanamycin
- Para aminobenzoic acid
- Pyrazinamide
- Rifampin
- Rifapentine
- Streptomycin

MAC THERAPY

- Azithromycin
- Clarithromycin

LEPROSTATIC DRUGS

- Clofazimine
- Dapsone
- Rifampin
- Thalidomide

GENERAL CONSIDERATIONS

Mycobacteria are a genus of acid-fast bacilli belonging to the Mycobacteriaceae, which include the organisms responsible for tuberculosis and leprosy as well as a number of other, less common diseases. Characteristic of mycobacteria is the fact that these organisms tend to be slow-growing, difficult to stain, and when they are stained with basic dye, can resist decolorization with acid alcohol. The staining characteristics relate to the abnormally high lipid content of the cell wall. In fact, the cell wall or cell envelope of the mycobacterium holds the secret to many of the characteristics of this genus of organisms. The cell envelope is unique in both structure and complexity. It has been suggested that the cell envelope is responsible for mycobacterium pathogenicity or virulence, multiple drug resistance, cell permeability, immunoreactivity and inhibition of antigen responsiveness, as well as disease persistence and recrudescence. In addition, several of the successful chemotherapeutic agents are know to inhibit the cell envelope synthesis as their mechanism of action. It is no wonder that significant effort has been put forth to define the chemical structure of the mycobacterium cell envelope.

A series of papers were presented and reported in 1991 dealing with the topic of the structure and functions of the cell envelope of mycobacterium (1). As illustrated in Figure 41.1, the mycobacterial cell envelope contains, on the interior surface, a plasma membrane similar to that found in most bacteria. A conventional peptidoglycan layer affording the organism rigidity appears next. This layer is composed of alternating N-acetyl-D-glucosamines (Glu) linked to N-glycoyl-D-muramic acids (Mur) through 1–4 linkages that, in turn, is attached to the peptido chain of D-alanine (A), D-glutamine (G), meso-diaminopimelic acid (DP), and L-alanine (A). A novel disaccharide phosphodiester linker made up of N-acetyl-D-glucosamine and rhamnose connects the muramic acid to a polygalactan and polyarabinose chain. The latter polysaccharides are referred to as the arabinogalactan (AG) portion of the cell envelope. The manner in which the arabinosyl and galactosyl resides are arranged is still under investigation. It is known that the arabinosyl chains terminate in mycolic acid residues. (The mycolates will be discussed in more detail later in this chapter.) Noncovalently bound to the mycolates are a number of free nonpolar and polar lipids (the phthiocerol lipids and the glycopeptidolipids, respectively). Finally, spanning from the interior, embedded in the plasma membrane, to the exterior is the lipoarabinomannan (LAM) polymer. As indicated, this unit is composed of polyarabinose, polymannan, and various lipids attached through a phosphatidylinositol moiety (2,3).

SPECIFIC DISEASES

Leprosy (Hansen's Disease)

Throughout the Bible, one finds reference to the condition of leprosy, such as that described in *Leviticus*: "[I]s there any flesh in the skin of which there is a burn by fire, and the quick flesh of the burn becomes a bright spot, reddish white or white, . . . and if the hair in the bright spot is turned white, and it appears deeper than the skin, it is leprosy broken out in the burn." Associated with the disease was a belief that individuals suffering from this disease were unclean. Today, leprosy (Hansen's disease) is recognized as a chronic granulomatous infection caused by *Mycobacterium leprae*. The disease may consist of lepromatous leprosy, tuberculoid leprosy, or a condition with characteristics between these two poles and referred to as borderline leprosy. The disease is more common in tropical countries but is not limited to warm climate regions. It is thought to afflict some 10 to 20 million individuals. Children appear to be the most susceptible population, but the signs and symptoms usually do not occur until much later in life. The incubation period usually is

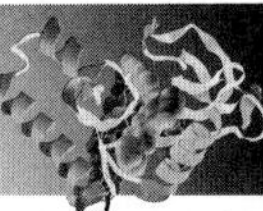

CLINICAL SIGNIFICANCE

Diseases caused by mycobacteria, such as tuberculosis and *Mycobacterium avium–intracellulare* complex, are of great concern to both health care workers and the public. Understanding the infectivity and pathophysiology of mycobacteria and the medicinal chemistry of the antimicrobials in the complex treatment of mycobacterial infections can help to facilitate a clinician's pharmacotherapy decisions. Mycobacteria are very-slow-growing organisms that grow both intracellularly and extracellularly. Because of their growth, the treatment of mycobacterial infections, especially tuberculosis, requires long-term treatment with a combination of agents to effectively eradicate the disease and prevent resistance. In addition, many of these agents are associated with significant side effects and drug interactions. A good understanding about the medicinal chemistry of the antimycobacterial agents helps the clinician to determine the most effective and safe combination for an individual patient.

The continuing interest in the study of the medicinal chemistry of antimycobacterial agents is prudent in the development of newer and safer agents. Researchers are continuously looking for agents that have more rapid antimycobacterial activity as well as lower resistance and fewer side effects. The discovery of such agents would have a significant effect on increasing the eradication of this worldwide epidemic. Shorter-course therapies would lead to an increase in patient compliance and possible decrease in mycobacterial resistance. As newer and more effective therapies are developed, clinicians will need to stay informed of these therapies, such as their pharmacokinetic and pharmacodynamic profiles, so that their patients can get the most optimal and effective treatment.

Elizabeth Coyle, Pharm.D.
Clinical Assistant Professor
Department of Clinical Sciences & Administration
University of Houston College of Pharmacy

three to five years. The disease is contagious, but the infectiousness is quite low. Person-to-person contact appears to be the means by which the disease is spread, with entrance into the body occurring through the skin or the mucosa of the upper respiratory tract. Skin and peripheral nerves are the regions most susceptible to attack.

The first signs of the disease consist of hypopigmented or hyperpigmented macules. Additionally, anesthetic or paresthetic patches may be experienced by the patient. Neural involvement in the extremities ultimately leads to muscle atrophy, resorption of small bones, and spontaneous amputation. When facial nerves are involved, corneal ulceration and blindness may occur. The identification of *M. leprae* in skin or blood samples is not always possible, but the detection of the antibody to the organism is an effective diagnostic test, especially for the lepromatous form of the disease.

Tuberculosis

Tuberculosis (TB) is a disease that has been known from the earliest of recorded history. It is characterized as a chronic bacterial infection caused by *Mycobacterium*

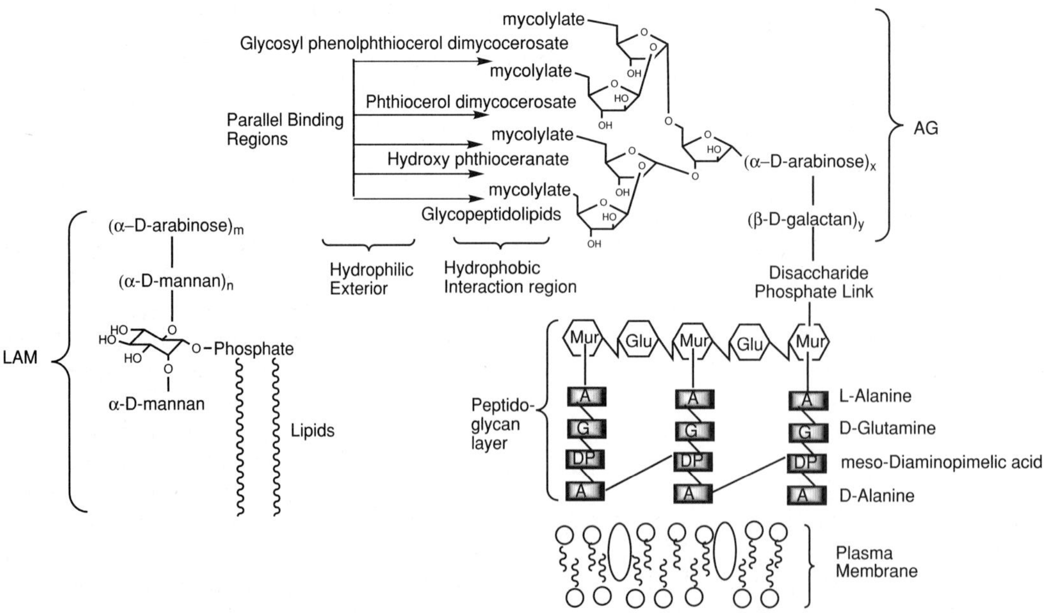

Fig. 41.1. Diagrammatic representation of the cell wall/cell envelope of mycobacterium.

tuberculosis, an acid-fast, aerobic bacillus with the previously discussed, unusual cell wall. The cell wall has a high lipid content, resulting in a high degree of hydrophobicity and resistance to alcohol, acids, alkali, and some disinfectants. After staining with a dye, the *M. tuberculosis* cell wall cannot subsequently be decolorized with acid wash, thus the characteristic of being an acid-fast bacillus. It is estimated that today, one-third to one-half of the world population is infected with *M. tuberculosis,* leading to approximately 6% of all deaths worldwide (~2 million deaths) (4,5). Tuberculosis is the leading worldwide cause of mortality resulting from an infectious bacterial agent. A steady decline in the reported cases of TB had been occurring in the United States from the 1950s until 1985. From 1985 until 1988, however, this decline leveled off, but beginning in 1989, an increase was noted. In 1991, the Centers for Disease Control and Prevention (CDC) reported 25,701 new cases of TB. Today, the press and professional publications announce the "epidemic" spread of TB. The resurgence has been linked to urban crowding, homelessness, immigration, drug abuse, the disappearance of preventive-medicine health clinics, crowded prisons, and the AIDS epidemic. "Most alarming is the emergence of multidrug-resistant TB" (MDR-TB) (6). Before 1984, only 10% of the organisms isolated from patients with TB were resistant to any drug. In 1984, 52% of the organisms were resistant to at least one drug, and 32% were resistant to more than one drug. MDR-TB may have a fatality rate as high as 50%. As a result of MDR-TB, isolates of *M. tuberculosis* should be tested for antimicrobial susceptibility. In fact, drug resistance is encountered in patients who have never been treated with any of the TB drugs.

Mycobacterium tuberculosis is transmitted primarily via the respiratory route. The organism appears in water droplets expelled during coughing, sneezing, or talking. Either in the droplet form or as the desiccated airborne bacilli, the organism enters the respiratory tract. The infectiousness of an individual will depend on the extent of the disease, the number of organisms in the sputum, and the amount of coughing. Usually, within 2 weeks of beginning therapy, the infected individual will no longer be infectious. TB is a disease that mainly affects the lungs (80–85% of the cases), but *M. tuberculosis* can spread through the bloodstream and the lymphatic system to the brain, bones, eyes, and skin (extrapulmonary TB). In pulmonary TB, the bacilli reach the alveoli and are ingested by pulmonary macrophages. Substances secreted by the macrophages stimulate surrounding fibroblasts to enclose the infection site, leading to formation of granulomas or tubercles. The infection, thus contained locally, may lie dormant, encapsulated in a fibrotic lesion, for years and then reappear later. Extrapulmonary TB is much more common in HIV-infected patients (40–75%).

Because of the effect of the AIDS virus on the immune system, all HIV-infected individuals should be screened for TB, and if infected, the patient should be treated for TB before an active infections develops. Patients with HIV infection and TB are 100-fold more likely of developing an active infection than noninfected patients. Individuals diagnosed with active TB should be counseled and tested for HIV, because the TB may have developed in conjunction with the weakened immune system seen in the patient with HIV infection.

Mycobacterium Avium–Intracellulare Complex

Mycobacterium avium and *Mycobacterium intracellulare* are atypical acid-fast bacilli that are ubiquitous in the environment and usually considered to be nonpathogenic in healthy individuals. Unfortunately, in immune-compromised individuals, these and possibly other, unidentified mycobacteria cause severe, life-threatening infections. Disseminated *Mycobacterium avium–intracellulare* complex (MAC) is the most common bacterial opportunistic infection seen in patients with AIDS and the third most common opportunistic infection behind candidal esophagitis and primary *Pneumocystis carinii* pneumonia reported in patients with AIDS. Between 1981 and 1987, and before the availability of effective antiretroviral medication, the incidence of MAC was reported as 5%. Today, approximately half of all patients with AIDS develop an infection caused by MAC. The lungs are the organs most commonly involved in patients without AIDS, but the infection may involve bone marrow, lymph nodes, liver, and blood in patients with AIDS. The CD4 T-lymphocyte count is used as a predictor for risk of disseminated MAC; a count of less than 50 cells/mm^3 in an HIV-infected person (adult or adolescent) is an indication of a potential infection and a recommendation for chemoprophylaxis. The MAC organisms grow within macrophages; therefore, the drug must be capable of penetration of the macrophage. Treatment of MAC, both prophylactically and for diagnosed infections, requires the use of multidrug therapy, and for disseminated MAC, this treatment is for the life of the patient.

GENERAL APPROACHES TO DRUG THERAPY

The mycobacteria have a number of characteristics in common, but it is important to recognize that the species vary widely in their susceptibility to the different drugs and that, in turn, this may relates to significant differences in the organisms. Some species, such as *M. tuberculosis,* are very slow-growing, with a doubling time of approximately 24 hours, whereas others, such as *Mycobacterium smegmatis,* doubles in 2 to 3 hours. The pathogenic mycobacterial organism can be divided into organism that are actively metabolizing and rapidly growing; semidormant bacilli, which exhibit spurts of metabolism bacilli in acid pH; and dormant or persisters. The latter characteristic is the most problematic and responsible for treatment failures. Most current TB drugs are those that are effective against actively metabolizing and rapidly growing bacilli. Thus, successful chemotherapy calls for drugs with bactericidal action against all stages of the organisms—but especially against the persisters. The use of combination therapy over an extended period of time is one answer to successful treatment.

DRUG THERAPY FOR TUBERCULOSIS

Drug therapy for the treatment of TB has been greatly hampered by the development of MDR-TB and the lack of new classes of drugs. In fact, no new drugs have been developed in the last 40 years. The only change in the treatment of TB has been the strategy of using direct observed treatment (DOT), with an emphasis on patient-centered care (7). Additionally, whereas the course of treatment has been reduced, through the use of drug combinations, to 6 months, patient compliance continues to be a serious problem, which in turn may be associated with the development of bacterial resistance.

First-Line Agents

Isoniazid (Isonicotinic Acid Hydrazide, Nydrazid, Laniazid)

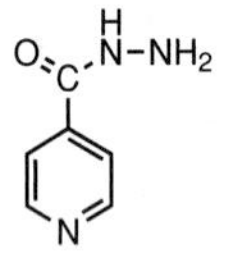

Isoniazid (INH) is a synthetic antibacterial agent with bactericidal action against *M. tuberculosis.* The drug was discovered in the 1950s as a beneficial agent effective against intracellular and extracellular bacilli, and it generally is considered to be the primary drug for treatment of *M. tuberculosis.* Its action is bactericidal against replicating organisms, but it appears to be only bacteriostatic at best against semidormant and dormant populations. After treatment with INH, *M. tuberculosis* loses its acid fastness, which may be interpreted as indicating that the drug interferes with cell wall development.

Mechanism of Action. Although extensively investigated, the mechanism of action of INH has remained unknown until recently. New investigations into mechanisms of bacterial resistance have shed light on the molecular mechanism of action of INH (8). It generally is recognized that INH is a pro-drug that is activated through an oxidation reaction catalyzed by an endogenous enzyme (9). This enzyme, katG, which exhibits catalase-peroxidase activity, converts INH to a reactive species capable of acylation of an enzyme system found exclusively in *M. tuberculosis.* Evidence in support of the activation of INH reveals that INH-resistant isolates have decreased catalase activity and that the loss of catalase activity is associated with the deletion of the catalase gene, *katG.* Furthermore, reintroduction of the gene into resistant organisms results in restored sensitivity of the organism to the drug. Reaction of INH with catalase-peroxidase results in formation of isonicotinaldehyde, isonicotinic acid, and isonicotinamide, which can be accounted for through the reactive intermediate isonicotinoyl radical or isonicotinic peroxide, as shown in Figure 41.2 (10). Evidence has been offered both for and against the reaction of catalase-peroxidase activated INH with a portion of the enzyme inhA, which is involved in the biosynthesis of the mycolic acids (Fig. 41.3) (11–13). The mycolic acids are important constituents of the mycobacterial cell wall in that they provide a permeability barrier to hydrophilic solutes. The enzyme inhA, produced under the control of the *inhA* gene, is an NADH-dependent, enoyl reductase protein thought to be involved in double-bond reduction during fatty acid elongation (Fig. 41.4). Isoniazid specifically inhibits long-chain fatty acid synthesis (>26 carbon atoms). It should be noted that the mycolic acids are α-branched lipids having a "short" arm of 20 to 24 carbons and a "long" arm of 50 to 60 carbons. It has been proposed that INH is activated to an electrophilic species that acylates the four position of the NADH (Fig. 41.5, on page 1132). The acylated NADH is no longer capable of catalyzing the reduction of unsaturated fatty acids, which are essential for the synthesis of the mycolic acids (14–16).

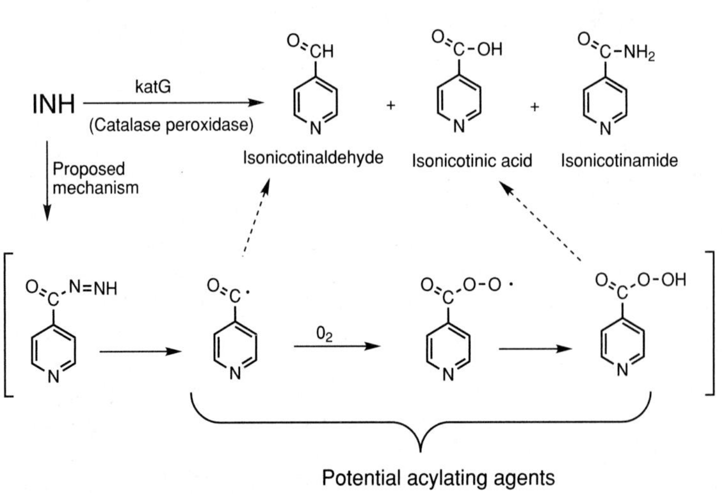

Fig. 41.2. Reaction products formed from catalase-peroxidase reaction with isoniazid (INH).

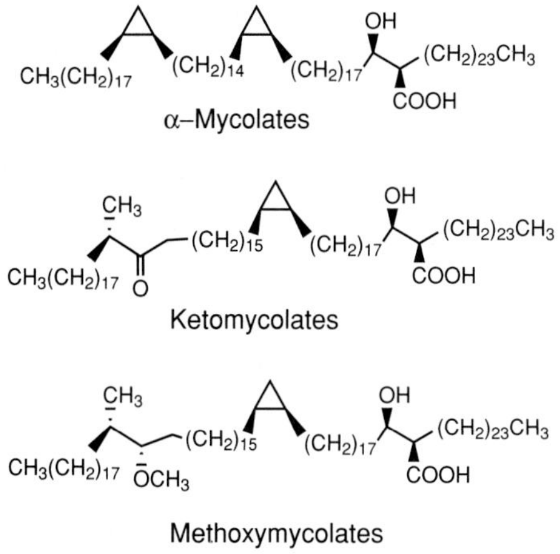

Fig. 41.3. Mycolic acids.

STRUCTURE–ACTIVITY RELATIONS. An extensive series of derivatives of nicotinaldehyde, isonicotinaldehyde, and substituted isonicotinic acid hydrazide have been prepared and investigated for their tuberculostatic activity. Isoniazid hydrazones were found to possess activity, but these compounds were shown to be unstable in the gastrointestinal (GI) tract, releasing the active isonicotinic acid hydrazide (i.e., INH). Thus, it would appear that their activity resulted from the INH and not from the derivatives (17,18). Substitution of the hydrazine portion of INH with alkyl and aralkyl substituents resulted in a series of active and inactive derivatives (19–22).

Substitution on the N-2 position resulted in active compounds (R1 and/or R2 = alkyl; R3 = H), whereas any substitution of the N-1 hydrogen with alkyl groups destroyed the activity (R1 and R2 = H; R3 = alkyl). None of these changes produced compounds with activity superior to that of INH.

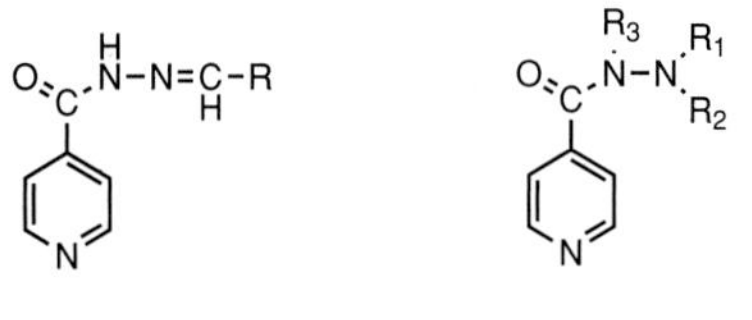

METABOLISM. Isoniazid is extensively metabolized to inactive metabolites (Fig. 41.6, on page 1132) (23,24). The major metabolite is N-acetylisoniazid. The enzyme responsible for acetylation, cytosolic N-acetyltransferase, is produced under genetic control in an inherited autosomal fashion. Individuals who possess high concentrations of the enzyme are referred to as rapid acetylators, whereas those with low concentrations are slow acetylators. This may result in a need to adjust the dosage for fast acetylators. The N-acetyltransferase is located primarily in the liver and small intestine. Other metabolites include isonicotinic acid, which is found in the urine as a glycine conjugate, and hydrazine. Isonicotinic acid also may result from hydrolysis of acetylisoniazid, but in this case, the second product of hydrolysis is acetylhydrazine. Acetylhydrazine is acetylated by N-acetyltransferase to the inactive diacetyl product. This reaction occurs more rapidly in rapid acetylators. The formation of acetylhydrazine is significant in that this compound has been associated with the hepatotoxicity, which may occur during INH therapy. Acetylhydrazine has been postulated to serve as a substrate for microsomal P450, resulting in the formation of a chemical that is capable of acetylating liver protein, in turn resulting in the liver necrosis (25). It has been suggested that a hydroxylamine intermediate is formed that results in an active acetylating agent (Fig. 41.7, on page 1132). The acetyl radical/cation acylates liver protein.

PHARMACOKINETICS. Isoniazid is readily absorbed following oral administration. Food and various antacids, especially aluminum-containing antacids, may interfere with or delay the absorption; therefore, it is recommended that the drug be taken on an empty stomach. The drug is well distributed to body tissues, including infected tissue. A long-standing concern about the use of INH during preventive therapy for latent TB has been the high incidence of hepatotoxicity. Recent studies have concluded that, excluding patients over 35 years of age, if relevant clinical monitoring is employed, the rate of hepatotoxicity is quite low (26). The risk of hepatotoxicity is associated with increasing age and appears to be higher in women than in men.

Rifamycin Antibiotics

The rifamycins are members of the ansamycin class of natural products produced by *Streptomyces mediterranei*. This chemical class is characterized as molecules with an

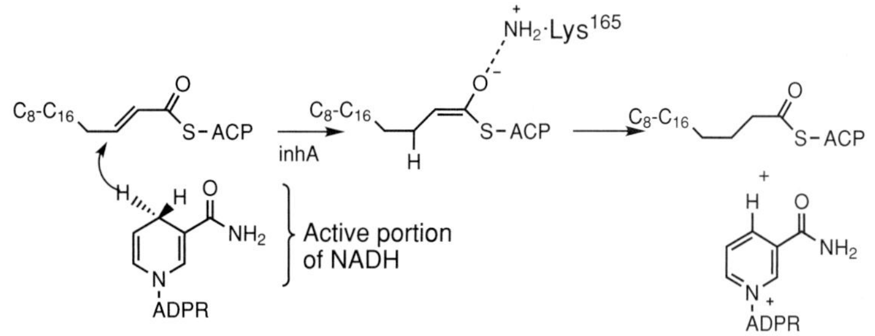

Fig. 41.4. Enoylthioester. ACP, acyl carrier (protein) reduction catalyzed by NADH and inhA.

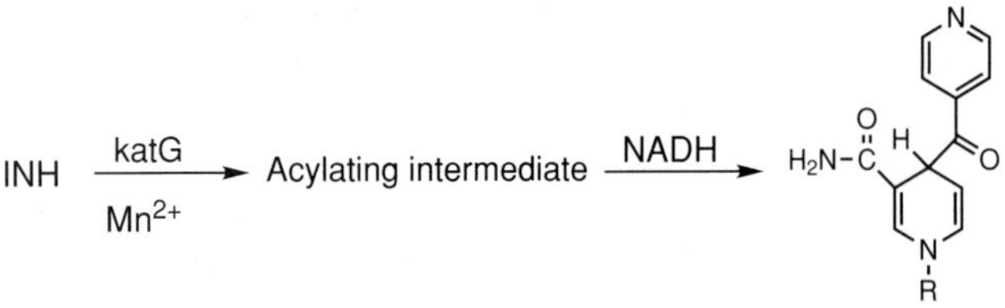

Fig. 41.5. Acylation of NADH and NADH-dependent enoylacyl protein (inhA).

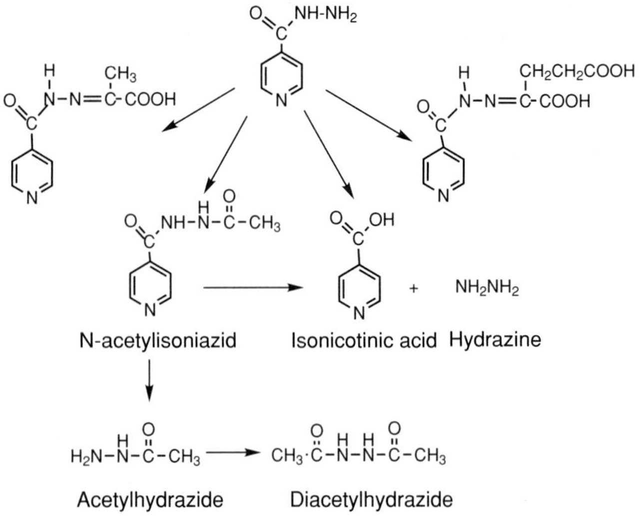

Fig. 41.6. Metabolism of isoniazid.

aliphatic chain forming a bridge between two nonadjacent positions of an aromatic moiety. While investigating the biological activity of the naturally occurring rifamycins (B, O, and S), a spontaneous reaction gave the biologically active rifamycin SV, which was later isolated from natural sources. Rifamycin SV was the original rifamycin antibiotic chosen for clinical development (27). Semisynthetic derivatives are prepared via conversion of the natural rifamycins to 3-formylrifamycin, which is derivatized with various hydrazines to give products such as rifampin (RIF) and rifapentine. Rifampin and rifapentine have significant benefit over previously investigated rifamycins in that they are orally active, are highly effective against a variety of both Gram-positive and Gram-negative organisms, and have high clinical efficacy in the treatment of TB. The rifamycin antibiotics are active against both growing and slow-metabolizing, nongrowing bacilli.

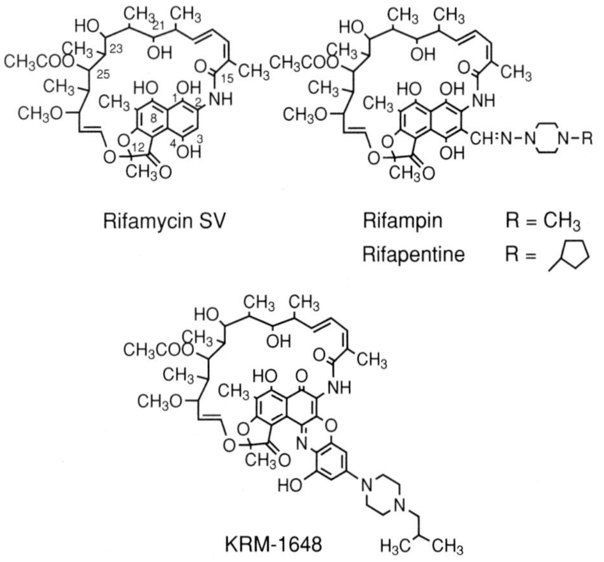

Mechanism of action. The rifamycins inhibit bacterial DNA-dependent RNA polymerase (DDRP) by binding to the β-subunit of the enzyme and are highly active against rapidly dividing intracellular and extracellular bacilli. Rifampin is active against DDRP from both Gram-positive and Gram-negative bacteria, but because of poor penetration of the cell wall of Gram-negative organisms by RIF, the drug has less value in infections caused by such organisms. Inhibition of DDRP leads to blocking the initiation of chain formation in RNA synthesis. It has been suggested that the naphthalene ring of the rifamycins π-π bonds to an aromatic amino acid ring in the DDRP protein (28). The DDRP is a metalloenzyme that contains two zinc atoms. It is further postulated that the oxygens at C-1 and C-8 of a rifamycin can chelate to a zinc atom, which increases the binding to DDRP, and finally, the oxygens at C-21 and C-23 form strong hydrogen bonds to the DDRP. The binding of the rifamycins to DDRP results in the inhibition of the RNA synthesis. Specifically, RIF has been shown to inhibit the elongation of full-length transcripts, but it has no effect on transcription initiation (8). Resistance develops when a mutation occurs in the gene responsible for the β-subunit of the RNA polymerase (*rpoB* gene), resulting in an inability of the antibiotic to readily bind to the RNA polymerase (29).

Structure–activity relationship. A large number of derivatives of the naturally occurring rifamycins have been prepared (30). From these compounds, the following generalizations can be made concerning the structure–activity relationship (SAR): 1) Free -OH groups are required at C-1, C-8, C-21, and C-23; 2) these groups appear to lie in a plane and to be important binding groups for attachment to DDRP, as previously indicated; 3) acetylation of C-21 and/or C-23 produces inactive compounds; 4) reduction of the double bonds in the macro ring results in a progressive decrease in activity; and 5) opening of the macro ring also gives inactive compounds. These latter two changes greatly affect the conformational structure of the rifamycins, which in turn

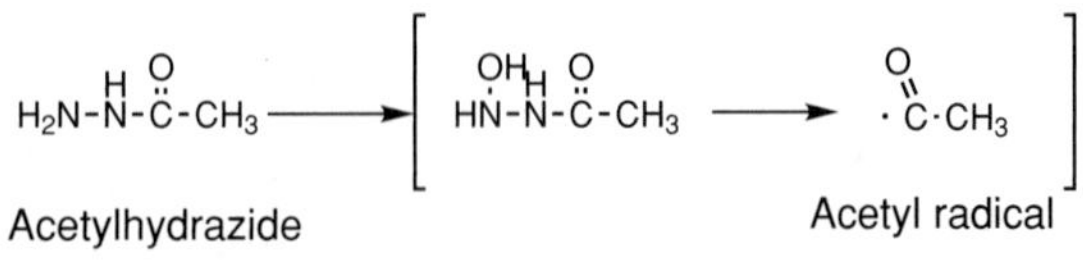

Fig. 41.7. Acylating metabolite of isoniazid.

decreases binding to DDRP. Substitution at C-3 or C-4 results in compounds with varying degrees of antibacterial activity. The substitution at these positions appears to affect transport across the bacterial cell wall. A compound incorporating such substitution is the benzoxazinorifamycin KRM-1648, which is proceeding through clinical investigation. In vitro studies have shown rapid tissue sterilization and encouraging results concerning combination therapy for TB and, possibly, MAC.

Metabolism. Rifampin and rifapentine are readily absorbed from the intestine, although food in the tract may affect absorption. Rifampin's absorption may be reduced by food in the intestine; therefore, the drug should be taken on an empty stomach (24). Intestinal absorption of rifapentine has been reported to be enhanced when taken after a meal (31). Neither drug appears to interfere with the absorption of other antituberculin agents, but there are conflicting reports on whether INH affects absorption of RIF. The major metabolism of RIF and rifapentine is deacetylation, which occurs at the C-25 acetate (Fig. 41.8). The resulting product, desacetylrifampin and desacetylrifapentine, are still active antibacterial agents. The majority of both desacetyl products are found in the feces, but desacetylrifampin glucuronide may be found in the urine as well. 3-Formylrifamycin SV has been reported as a second metabolite following both RIF and rifapentine administration. This product is thought to arise in the gut from an acid-catalyzed hydrolysis reaction. Formylrifamycin is reported to possess a broad spectrum of antibacterial activity (32).

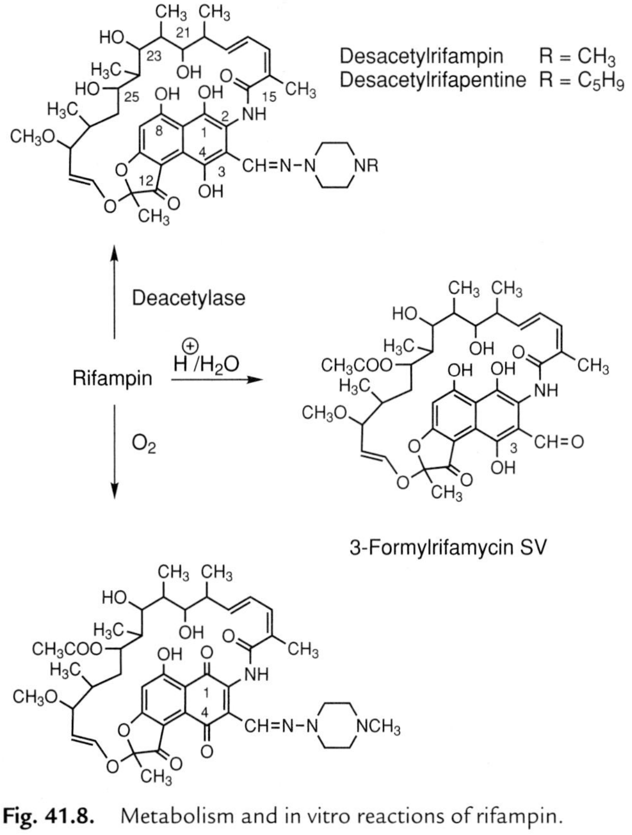

Fig. 41.8. Metabolism and in vitro reactions of rifampin.

Physicochemical properties. Rifampin and rifapentine are red-orange, crystalline compounds with zwitterionic properties. The presence of the phenolic groups results in acidic properties ($pK_a \sim 1.7$), whereas the piperazine moiety gives basic properties ($pK_a \sim 7.9$). These compounds are prone to acid hydrolysis, giving rise to 3-formylrifamycin SV, as indicated above. Rifampin and presumable rifapentine are prone to air oxidation of the *p*-phenolic groups in the naphthalene ring to give the *p*-quinone (C-1,4 quinone) (Fig. 41.8). Rifampin, rifapentine, and their metabolites are excreted in the urine, feces (biliary excretion), saliva, sweat, and tears. Because these agents have dye characteristics, one may note discoloration of the body fluids containing the drug. Notably, the tears may be discolored, and permanent staining of contact lenses may occur.

Therapeutic application

Rifampin (Rifadin, Rimactane). With the introduction of RIF in 1967, the duration of combination therapy for the treatment of TB was significantly reduced (from 18 to 9 months). Rifampin is nearly always used in combination with one or more other antituberculin agents. The drug is potentially hepatotoxic and may produce GI disturbances, rash, and thrombocytopenic purpura. Rifampin is known to induce hepatic microsomal enzymes (cytochrome P450) and may decrease the effectiveness of oral contraceptives, corticosteroids, warfarin, quinidine, methadone, zidovudine, clarithromycin, and the azole antifungal agents (see Chapter 10) (33).

Because of the decreased effectiveness of protease inhibitors and nonnucleoside reverse transcriptase inhibitors used in the treatment of HIV, the CDC has recommended avoidance of RIF in treatment of HIV-infected patients presently on these HIV therapies.

Rifapentine (Priftin). Rifapentine is the first new agent introduced for the treatment of pulmonary TB in the last 25 years. The drug's major advantage over RIF is the fact that when used in combination therapy, rifapentine can be administered twice weekly during the "intense" phase of therapy, followed by once-a-week administration during the "continuous" phase. In contrast, RIF normally is administered daily during the "intense" phase, followed by twice-a-week dosing during the "continuous" phase. Because relapse and the emergence of resistant strains of bacteria are associated with poor patient compliance, reduced dosing is expected to increase compliance. Initial clinical studies actually showed that the relapse rates in patients treated with rifapentine (10%) were higher than those in the patients treated with RIF (5%). It was found that poor compliance with the nonrifamycin antituberculin agents was responsible for the increased relapse (31).

Rifapentine is readily absorbed following oral administration and is highly bound to plasma protein (97.7% vs. 80% for RIF). Related to the higher plasma binding, refapentine has a longer mean elimination half-life (13.2 hours in healthy male volunteers) in comparison with the half-life reported for RIF (~2–5 hours). Greater than 70% of either drug is excreted in the feces. Rifapentine generally is considered to be more active than rifampin and can be used in patients with varying degrees of hepatic dysfunction without the need for dose adjustment (34). This drug, similar to what is seen with RIF, induces hepatic microsomal enzymes (cytochrome P450 3A4 and 2C8/9). Rifapentine has been reported to be teratogenic in rats and rabbits (31).

Pyrazinamide

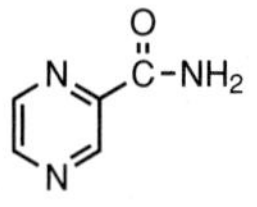

Pyrazinamide 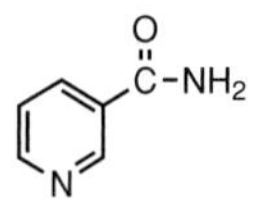 Nicotinamide

Pyrazinamide (pyrazinecarboxamide) was discovered while investigating analogues of nicotinamide. Pyrazinamide is a bio-isoster of nicotinamide and possesses bactericidal action against *Mycobacterium tuberculosis.* Pyrazinamide has become one of the more popular antituberculin agents despite the fact that resistance develops quickly. Combination therapy, however, has proven to be an effective means of reducing the rate of resistant strain development. The activity of pyrazinamide is pH dependent with good in vivo activity at pH 5.5, but the compound is nearly inactive at neutral pH.

Mechanism of Action. The mechanism of action of pyrazinamide is unknown, but recent findings suggest that pyrazinamide may be active either totally or in part as a pro-drug. Susceptible organisms produce pyrazinamidase, which is responsible for conversion of pyrazinamide to pyrazinoic acid intracellularly (8). Mutation in the pyrazinamidase gene (*pncA*) results in resistant strains of *M. tuberculosis* (36). Pyrazinoic acid has been shown to possess biological activity at a pH 5.4 or lower, in contract in vitro tests that show pyrazinoic acid is 8- to 16-fold less active than pyrazinamide (37). Pyrazinoic acid may lower the pH in the immediate surroundings of the *M. tuberculosis* to such an extent that the organism is unable to grow, but this physicochemical property appears to account for only some of the activity. The protonated pyrazinoic acid also can permeate the mycobacterial membrane to lower the pH of the cytoplasm. Recent evidence suggests that pyrazinoic acid decreases membrane potential in older, nonreplicating bacilli, thus decreasing membrane transport, and interferes with the energetics of the membrane (38).

Structure–Activity Relationship. Previous structural modification of pyrazinamide has proven to be ineffective in developing analogues with increased biological activity. Substitution on the pyrazine ring or use of alternate heterocyclic aromatic rings have given compounds with reduced activity (39). More recently, using quantitative SAR, a series of analogues have been prepared with improved biological activity. The requirements for successful analogues include 1) provision for hydrophilicity to allow sufficient plasma concentrations such that the drug can be delivered to the site of infection, 2) lipophilicity to allow penetration into the mycobacterial cell, and 3) susceptibility to hydrolysis such that the prodrug is unaffected by the "extracellular" enzymes but is readily hydrolyzed at the site of action. Two compounds have been found that meet these criteria: tert-butyl 5-chloropyrazinamide, and 2′-(2′-methyldecyl) 5-chloropyrazinamide (40).

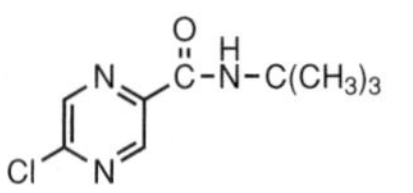

tert-butyl 5-chloropyrazinoate 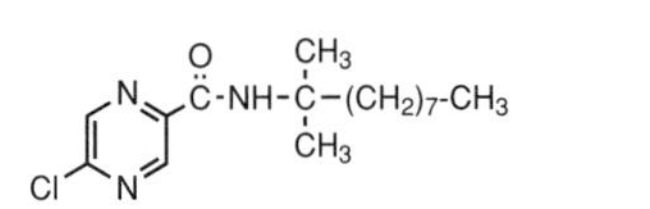 2'-(2'-methyldecyl) 5-chloropyrazinoate

Metabolism. Pyrazinamide is readily absorbed after oral administration, but little of the intact molecule is excreted unchanged (Fig. 41.9). The major metabolic route consists of hydrolysis by hepatic microsomal pyrazinamidase to pyrazinoic acid, which may then be oxidized by xanthine oxidase to 5-hydroxypyrazinoic acid. The latter compound may appear in the urine either free or as a conjugate with glycine (23).

Rifaximin (Xifaxan)

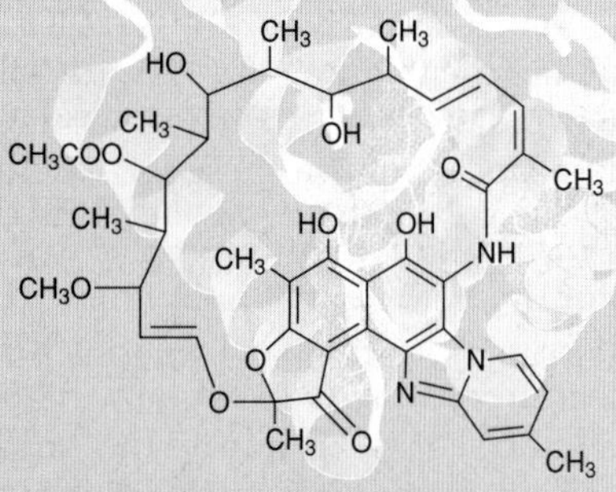

Rifaximin

Recently, the U.S. Food and Drug Administration (U.S. FDA) has approved the release of rifaximin, a rifamycin antibiotic, for the treatment of travelers' diarrhea (TD) caused by enterotoxigenic *Escherichia coli*. Although the drug is not intended for the treatment of TD, there are indications that the drug may be effective as a prophylactic agent. Rifaximin is administered orally, with less than 0.4% absorption; therefore, its actions are limited to the GI tract. Its mechanism of action is essentially the same as that of other reifamcyin antibiotics (35).

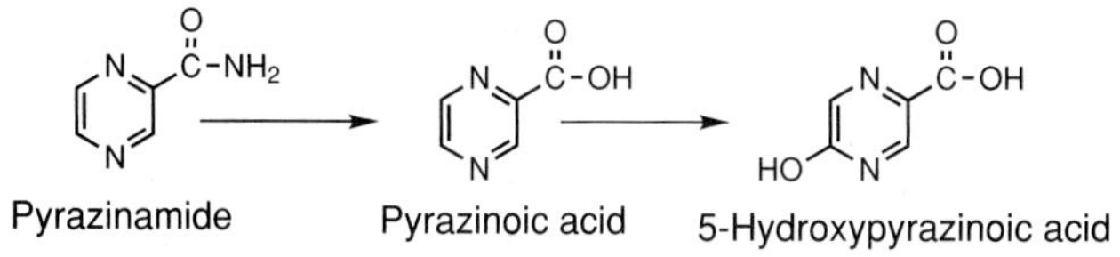

Pyrazinamide → Pyrazinoic acid → 5-Hydroxypyrazinoic acid

Fig. 41.9. Metabolism of pyrazinamide.

THERAPEUTIC APPLICATION. Pyrazinamide has gained acceptance as an essential component in combination therapy for the treatment of TB (component of Rifater with INH and RIF). The drug is especially beneficial in that it is active against semidormant intracellular tubercle bacilli that are not affected by other drugs (7,34). Evidence suggests that pyrazinamide is active against nonreplicating persister bacilli. The introduction of pyrazinamide combinations has reduced treatment regimens to 6 months from the previous 9-month therapy. The major serious side effect of pyrazinamide is the potential for hepatotoxicity. This effect is associated with dose and length of treatment. Pyrazinamide is not affected by the presence of food in the GI tract or by the use of aluminum-magnesium antacids (41).

Ethambutol (Myambutol)

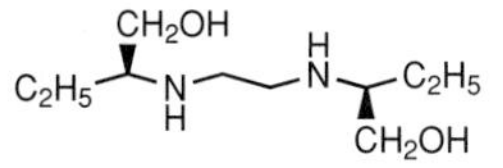

Ethambutol

Ethambutol (EMB), an ethylenediiminobutanol, is administered as its (+)-enantiomer, which is 200- to 500-fold more active than its (−)-enantiomer. The difference in activity between the two isomers suggests a specific receptor for its site of action. Ethambutol is a water-soluble, bacteriostatic agent that is readily absorbed (75–80%) following oral administration.

MECHANISM OF ACTION. The mechanism of action of EMB remains unknown, although mounting evidence suggests a specific site of action for EMB. It has been known for some time that EMB affects mycobacterial cell wall synthesis; however, the complicated nature of the mycobacterial cell wall has made pinpointing the site of action difficult. In addition to the peptidoglycan portion of the cell wall, the mycobacterium have a unique outer envelop consisting of arabinofuranose and galactose (AG), which is covalently attached to the peptidoglycan and an intercalated framework of lipoarabinomannan (LAM) (Fig. 41.1). The AG portion of the cell wall is highly branched and contains distinct segments of galactan and distinct segments of arabinan. At various locations within the arabinan segments (terminal and penultimate), the mycolic acids are attached to the C-5′ position of arabinan (42,43). Initially, Takayama et al. (44) reported that EMB inhibited the synthesis of the AG portion of the cell wall. More recently, it has been reported that EMB inhibits the enzymes arabinosyl transferase. One action of arabinosyl transferase is to catalyze the polymerization of D-arabinofuranose,

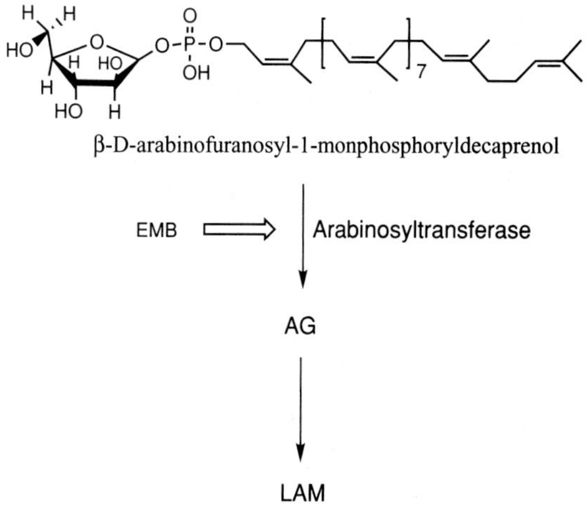

β-D-arabinofuranosyl-1-monphosphoryldecaprenol

EMB ⟹ Arabinosyltransferase

AG

LAM

Fig. 41.10. Site of action of ethambutol (EMB) in cell wall synthesis.

leading to AG (45,46). Ethambutol mimics arabinan, resulting in a buildup of the arabinan precursor β-D-arabinofuranosyl-1-monophosphoryldecaprenol and, as a result, a block of the synthesis of both AG and LAM (Fig. 41.10) (47). The mechanism of resistance to EMB involves a gene overexpression of arabinosyl transferase, which is controlled by the *embAB* gene (48).

This mechanism of action also accounts for the synergism seen between EMB and intracellular drugs, such as RIF. Damage to the cell wall created by EMB improves the cell penetration of the intracellular drugs, resulting in increased biological activity.

STRUCTURE–ACTIVITY RELATIONSHIP. An extensive number of analogues of EMB have been prepared, but none has proven to be superior to EMB itself. Extension of the ethylene diamine chain, replacement of either nitrogen, increasing the size of the nitrogen substituents, and moving the location of the alcohol groups are all changes that drastically reduce or destroy biological activity.

METABOLISM. The majority of the administered EMB is excreted unchanged (73%), with no more than 15% appearing in the urine as either Metabolite A or Metabolite B (Fig. 41.11). Both metabolites are devoid of biological activity.

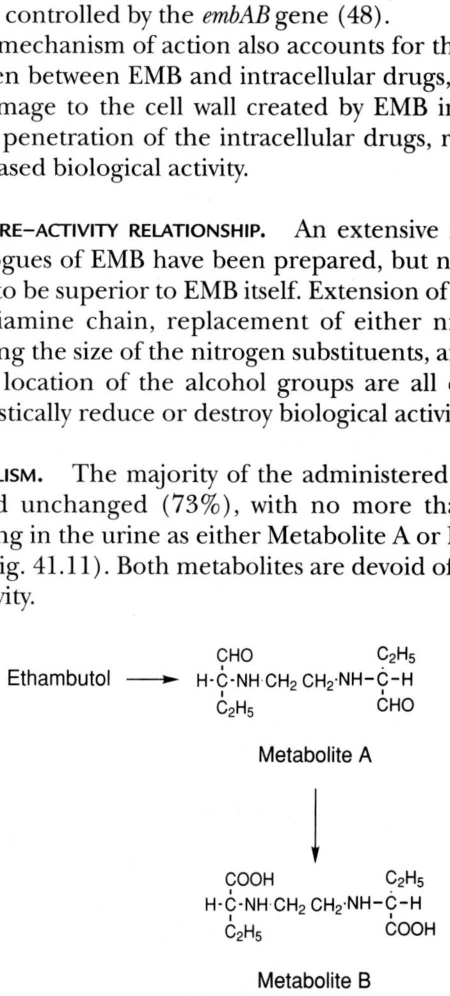

Ethambutol → Metabolite A → Metabolite B

Fig. 41.11. Metabolism of ethambutol.

Streptomycin

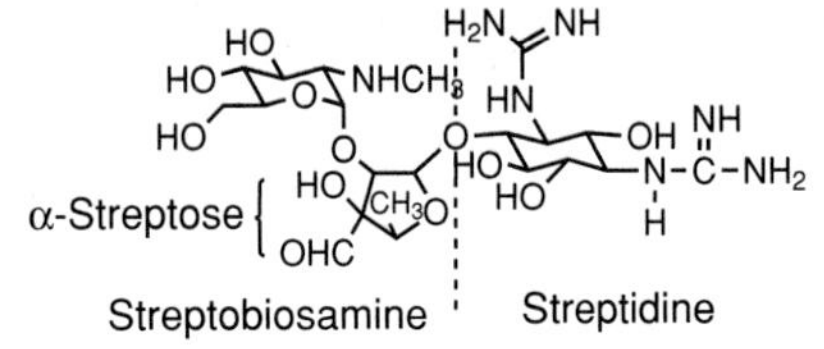

Streptobiosamine | Streptidine

α-Streptose

Streptomycin

Streptomycin (STM) was first isolated by Waksman and coworkers in 1944 and represented the first biologically active aminoglycoside. The material was isolated from a manure-containing soil sample and, ultimately, was shown to be produced by *Streptomyces griseus.* The structure was proposed and later confirmed by Kuehl et al. (49) in 1948. Streptomycin is water soluble, with basic properties. The compound usually is available as the trihydrochloride or sesquisulfate salt, both of which are quite soluble in water. The hydrophilic nature of STM results in very poor absorption from the GI tract. Orally administered STM is recovered intact from the feces, indicating that the lack of biological activity results from poor absorption and not chemical degradation.

MECHANISM OF ACTION. The mechanism of action of STM and the aminoglycosides in general has not been fully elucidated. It is known that the STM inhibits protein synthesis, but additional effects on misreading of an mRNA template and membrane damage may contribute to the bactericidal action of STM. Streptomycin is able to diffuse across the outer membrane of *Mycobacterium tuberculosis* and, ultimately, to penetrate the cytoplasmic membrane through an electron-dependent process. Through studies regarding the mechanism of drug resistance, it has been proposed that STM induces a misreading of the genetic code and, thus, inhibits translational initiation. In STM-resistant organisms, two changes have been discovered: First, S12 protein undergoes a change in which the lysine present at amino acids 43 and 88 in ribosomal protein S12 is replaced with arginine or threonine, and second, the pseudoknot conformation of 16S rRNA, which results from intramolecular base pairing between GCC bases in regions 524 to 526 of the rRNA to CGG bases in regions 505 to 507, is perturbed (50). It is thought that S12 protein stabilizes the pseudoknot, which is essential for 16S rRNA function. By some yet-to-be-defined mechanism, STM interferes with one or both of the normal actions of the 16S protein and 16S rRNA.

STRUCTURE–ACTIVITY RELATIONSHIP. All the aminoglycosides have very similar pharmacologic, pharmacodynamic, and toxic properties, but only STM and, to a lesser extent, kanamycin are used to treat TB. This is an indication for the narrow band of structurally allowed modifications giving rise to active analogues. Modification of the α-streptose portion of STM has been extensively studied. Reduction of the aldehyde to the alcohol results in a compound, dihydrostreptomycin, that has activity similar to STM but with a greater potential for producing delayed, severe deafness. Oxidation of the aldehyde to a carboxyl group or conversion to Schiff base derivatives (oxime, semicarbazone, or phenylhydrazone) results in inactive analogues. Oxidation of the methyl group in α-streptose to a methylene hydroxy gives an active analogue that has no advantage over STM. Modification of the aminomethyl group in the glucosamine portion of the molecule by demethylation or by replacement with larger alkyl groups reduces activity; removal or modification of either guanidine in the streptidine nucleus also decreases activity.

METABOLISM. No human metabolites of STM have been isolated in the urine of patients who have been administered the drug, with approximately 50 to 60% of the dose being recovered unchanged in the urine (24). Metabolism appears to be insignificant on a large scale, but it is implicated as a major mechanism of resistance. One problem with STM that was recognized early was the development of resistant strains of *Mycobacterium tuberculosis.* Combination drug therapy was partially successful in reducing this problem, but over time, resistance has greatly reduced the value of STM as a chemotherapeutic agent for treatment of TB. Various mechanisms may lead to the resistance seen in *M. tuberculosis.* Permeability barriers may result in STM not being transported through the cytoplasmic membrane, but the evidence appears to suggest that enzymatic inactivation of STM represents the major problem. The enzymes responsible for inactivation are adenyltransferase, which catalyzes adenylation of the C-3 hydroxyl group in the N-methylglucosamine moiety to give the O-3-adenylated metabolite, and phosphotransferase, which phosphorylates the same C-3 hydroxyl to give O-3-phosphorylate metabolite (Fig. 41.12). This latter reaction appears to be the most significant clinically. The result of these chemical modifications is that the metabolites produced will not bind to ribosomes.

Second-Line Agents

A number of drugs, including ethionamide, *p*-aminosalicylic acid, cycloserine, capreomycin, and kanamycin, are considered to be second-line agents (it should be noted that some authorities classify STM as a second-line agent). These agents are active antibacterial agents, but they usually are less well tolerated or have a higher incidence of adverse effects. These agents are utilized in cases of resistance, retreatment, or intolerance to the first-line drugs.

Ethionamide (Trecator-SC)

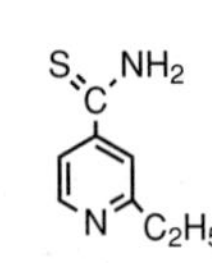

Ethionamide

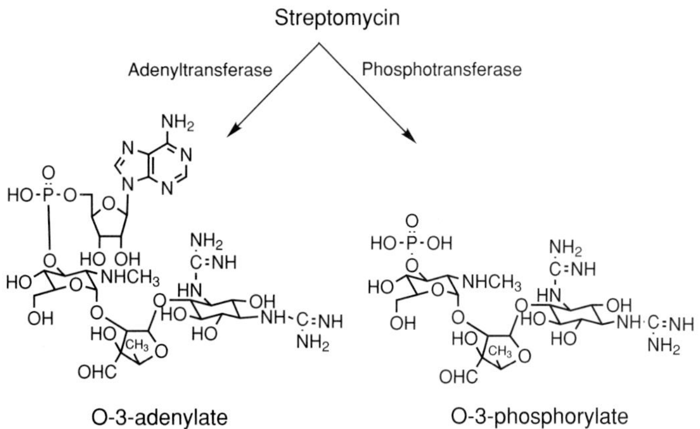

Fig. 41.12. Metabolism of streptomycin (STM) as a mechanism of resistance.

The synthesis of analogues of isonicotinamide resulted in the discovery of ethionamide and a homologue in which the ethyl group is replaced with a propyl (prothionamide). Both compounds have proven to be bactericidal against *Mycobacterium tuberculosis* and *Mycobacterium leprae.*

Mechanism of Action. Evidence has been presented suggesting that the mechanism of action of ethionamide is similar to that of INH (see *Mechanism of action* under *Isoniazid*) (11,15). Similar to INH, ethionamide is considered to be a pro-drug, which is converted via oxidation by catalase-peroxidase to an active acylating agent, ethionamide sulfoxide, which in turn inactivates the inhA enoyl reductase enzyme (Fig. 41.13). In the case of ethionamide, it has been proposed that the ethionamide sulfoxide acylates Cys-243 in inhA protein.

Metabolism. Ethionamide is orally active but is not well tolerated in a single large dose (>500 mg). The GI irritation can be reduced by administration with meals. Additional side effects may include central nervous system (CNS) effects, hepatitis, and hypersensitivities. Less than 1% of the drug is excreted in the free form, with the remainder of the drug appearing as one of six metabolites. Among the metabolites are ethionamide sulfoxide, 2-ethylisonicotinamide, and the N-methylated-6-oxodihydropyridines (Compounds A, B, and C in Fig. 41.14) (51).

p-aminosalicylic Acid

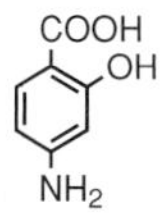

COOH, OH, NH_2

Para-aminosalicylic acid

Once a very popular component in TB therapy, *p*-aminosalicylic acid (PAS) is utilized as a second-line agent today. A combination of bacterial resistance and severe side effects has greatly reduced is value. As a bacteriostatic agent, PAS is used at a dose of up to 12 g/day, which causes considerable GI irritation. In addition, hypersensitivity reactions occur in 5 to 10% of the patients, with some of these reactions being life-threatening.

Mechanism of Action. *p*-aminosalicylic acid is thought to act as an antimetabolite interfering with the incorporation of p-aminobenzoic acid into folic acid. When coadministered with INH, PAS is found to reduce the acetylation of INH, itself being the substrate for acetylation, thus increasing the plasma levels of INH. This action may be especially valuable in patients who are rapid acetylators.

Metabolism. *p*-aminosalicylic acid is extensively metabolized by acetylation of the amino group and by conjugation

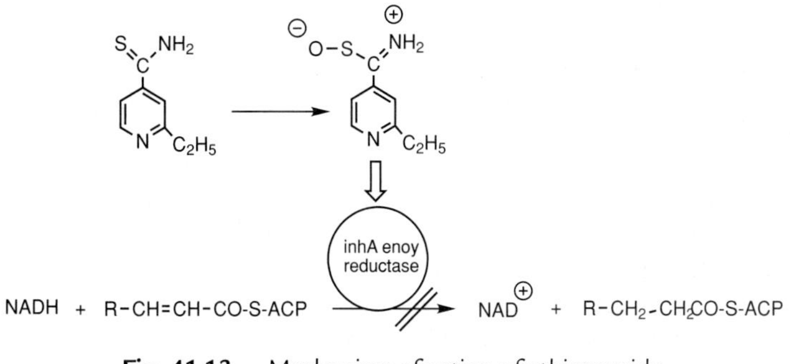

inhA enoy reductase

NADH + R-CH=CH-CO-S-ACP → $NAD^{\oplus}$ + R-CH_2-CH_2CO-S-ACP

Fig. 41.13. Mechanism of action of ethionamide.

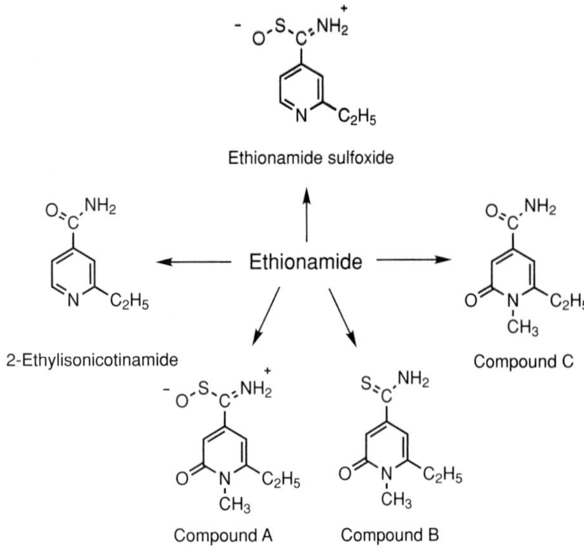

Fig. 41.14. Metabolism of ethionamide.

with glucuronic acid and glycine at the carboxyl group. It is used primarily in cases of resistance, retreatment, and intolerance of other agents and is available from the CDC.

Cycloserine (Seromycin)

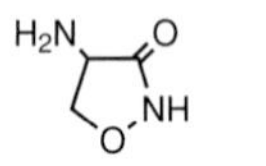

Cycloserine

Cycloserine is a natural product isolated from *Streptomyces orchidaceus* as the D-(+)-enantiomer.

Mechanism of Action. D-Cycloserine is considered to be the active form of the drug, having its action associated with the ability to inhibit two key enzymes, D-alanine racemase and D-alanine ligase. D-Alanine is an important component of the peptidoglycan portion of the mycobacterial cell wall. Mycobacterium are capable of utilizing natural occurring L-alanine and converting the L-alanine to D-alanine via the enzyme D-alanine racemase. The resulting D-alanine is coupled with itself to form a D-alanine–D-alanine complex under the influence of D-alanine ligase, and this complex is incorporated into the peptidoglycan of the mycobacterial cell wall (Fig. 41.15). D-Cycloserine is a rigid analogue of D-alanine; therefore, it competitively inhibits the binding of D-alanine to both of these enzymes and its incorporation into the peptidoglycan (Fig. 41.15) (52). Resistance is associated with an over expression of D-alanine racemase.

Side Effects. Cycloserine is readily absorbed after oral administration and is widely distributed, including the CNS. Unfortunately, D-cycloserine binds to neuronal N-methylasparate receptors and, in addition, affects synthesis and metabolism of γ-aminobutyric acid, leading to complex series of CNS effects. As a second-line agent, cycloserine should only be used when retreatment is necessary or when the organism is resistant to other drugs. Cycloserine should not be used as a single drug; it must be used in combination.

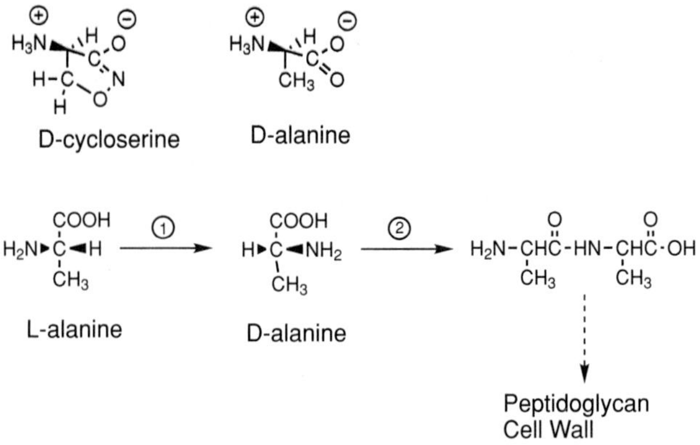

Fig. 41.15. Sites of action of D-cycloserine: 1, D-alanine racemase; 2, D-alanine ligase.

Capreomycin (Capastat)

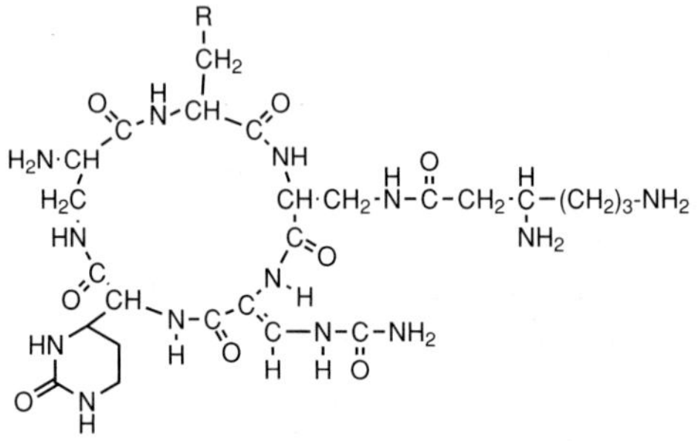

Capreomycin

Capreomycin is a mixture of four cyclic polypeptides, of which capreomycin Ia (R = OH) and Ib (R = H) make up 90% of the mixture. Capreomycin is produced by *Streptomyces capreolus* and is quite similar to the antibiotic viomycin. Little, if anything, is known about its mechanism of action, but if the chemical and pharmacological similarity to viomycin carries over to the mechanism of action, then one might expect something similar. Viomycin is a potent inhibitor of protein synthesis, particularly that which depends on mRNA at the 70S ribosome (53). Viomycin blocks chain elongation by binding to either or both the 50S or 30S ribosomal subunits. As a polypeptide, the drug must be administered parenterally, with the preferred route of administration being intramuscular. As a second-line bacteriostatic antituberculin drug, it is reserved for "resistant" infections and cases of treatment failure. The drug should not be given as a single agent; rather, it should be used in combination with EMB or INH. Reported toxicity of capreomycin includes renal and hepatic damage, hearing loss, and allergic reactions.

Kanamycin (Kanamycin A, R = OH; Kanamycin B, R = NH_2; Kantrex)

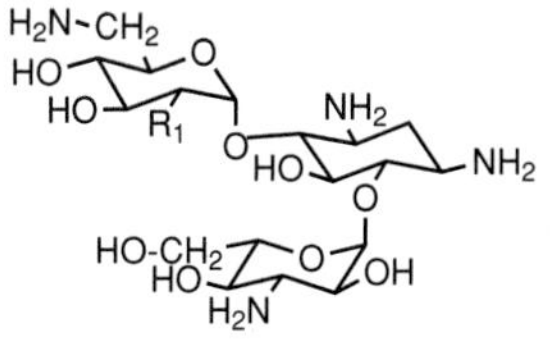

Kanamycin

A member of the aminoglycoside class, kanamycin is a second-line agent with very limited use in the treatment of *Mycobacterium tuberculosis.* The drug is only utilized to treat resistant organisms, and then should be used only in combination with other effective agents. The parenteral form of the drug is used, because as an aminoglycoside, the drug is poorly absorbed via the oral route. The narrow range of effectiveness and the severe toxicity, especially if the drug is administered over a long period of time, have limited is usefulness. (For additional information on kanamycin and aminoglycosides in general, see Chapter 38.)

Therapeutic Considerations for Treatment of Tuberculosis

Overview

Various stages of infectious organisms have been identified that may require special consideration for chemotherapy. The organism may be in a dormant stage, which usually is not affected by drugs. The continuously growing stage of the organism may find the bacteria either in an extracellular or an intracellular location. A stage of the organism, which is classified as the very slowly metabolizing bacteria, also exists in a relatively acidic environment. Finally, the organism may exhibit a stage in which it is dormant, followed by spurts of growth. As noted in the discussion of specific drugs, one stage or another may be more or less susceptible to a particular drug based on the above characteristics. It also is recognized that organisms from some geographic regions may show a low incidence of drug resistance. whereas those from other regions have a high incidence of drug resistance.

For patients with TB likely to be infected with organisms suspected of showing low rates of drug resistance, the American Thoracic Society currently recommends a minimum 26-week treatment period, consisting of an initial 2-month (8-week) phase, followed by a continuation phase of either 4 or 7 months. Four basic regimens are recommended for treatment of susceptible *Mycobacterium tuberculosis* infections in adults. During the initial phase, three of the four regimens use a combination of INH, RIF, pyrazinamide, and EMB, given either 7, 5, or 3 days per week. The fourth regimen utilizes INH, RIF, and EMB given 7 or 5 days per week (when drugs are administered DOT, the drugs can be given less often). The four-drug regimen is administered based on the assumption that a proportion of the organisms are resistant to INH. For treatment of children when visual acuity cannot be tested, EMB usually is not recommended. Several options for drug treatment exist for the continuation phase of treatment (54). In a majority of cases, the continuation phase will last 4 months. Here again, if DOT is utilized, the patient may only need to be treated two or three times weekly; without DOT, the treatment is daily. The drug combination of INH and RIF is used during the continuation phase. Typical daily doses are 300 mg of INH, 600 mg of RIF, 2 g of pyrazinamide, and 1 g of EMB. The addition of pyrazinamide to the drug regimen results in a reduction of treatment time from 9 to 6 months. Individuals on any of these regimen are considered to be noninfectious after the first 2 weeks. This same group of drugs is recommended for patients with both TB and AIDS. The "cardinal rules" for all TB regimens are: 1) get drug susceptibility information as soon as possible; 2) always begin therapy with at least three drugs; 3) at all costs, avoid a regimen employing only one effective drug; and 4) always add at least two drugs to a failing regimen (6,33,55). In addition, it is recommended that consideration be given to treating all patients with DOT.

The only proven treatment for prophylaxis of TB (patients with a positive skin test or a high risk factor) is INH used for 6 or 12 months. High risk factors are considered to be adults and children with HIV infection, close contacts of infectious cases, and those with fibrotic lesions on chest radiographs. Adverse effects when using INH over a long treatment period can be a serious problem. Isoniazid may cause severe liver damage, and the drug should be removed if serum aminotransferase activity increases to three to fivefold normal or the patient develops symptoms of hepatitis. Peripheral neuropathy may be seen with INH therapy. This condition may be prevented by coadministration of pyridoxine. Persons who are presumed to be infected with INH-resistant organisms should be treated with RIF rather than INH. Hepatitis, thrombocytopenia, and nephrotoxicity may be seen with RIF therapy. RIF is thought to potentiate the hepatitis caused by INH. Gastrointestinal upset and staining effects caused by RIF are of minor importance.

Fluoroquinolones

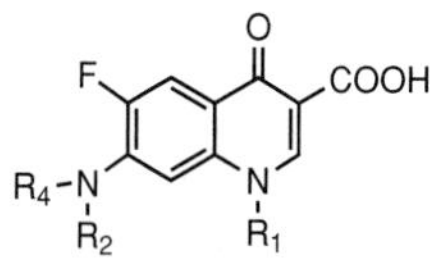

6-Fluoro- 4-quinolones

The fluoroquinolones are a broad-spectrum class of antibacterials that have been demonstrated to have activity against a wide range of Gram-negative as well as Gram-positive pathogens, including *Mycobacterium tuberculosis,*

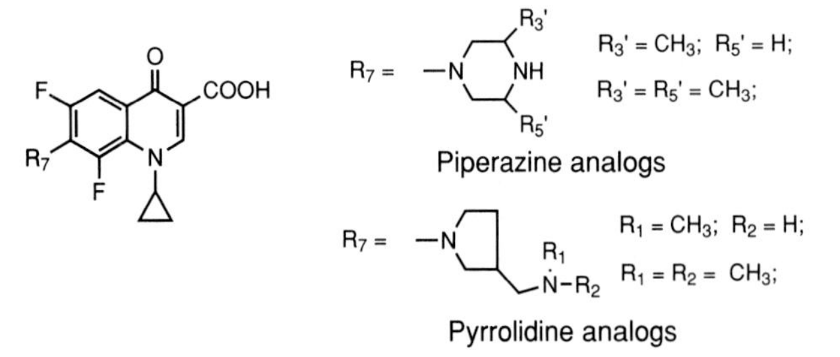

Fig. 41.16. 4-Quinolones demonstrating high activity against mycobacteria.

Mycobacterium kansasii, Mycobacterium xenopi, Mycobacterium fortuitum, MAC, and *Mycobacterium leprae.* The quinolones are attractive in that they are active at low concentrations, concentrate within macrophages, and have a low frequency of side effects.

MECHANISM OF ACTION. The mechanism of action of the fluoroquinolones is reported in detail in Chapter 38 and basically involves binding to DNA gyrase–DNA complex (GyrA and GyrB), inhibiting bacterial DNA replication and transcription. As a result, these drugs exhibit bactericidal activity.

STRUCTURE–ACTIVITY RELATIONSHIP. The structural requirements for activity against mycobacterium and, specifically, for activity against the MAC has been explored (56,57). It is known that nonfluorinated quinolones are inactive against mycobacteria. In addition, it has been reported that certain fragments or substructures within the quinolones improve activity toward the MAC (biophores), whereas other fragments deactivate the quinolones (biophobes). The important structural features acting as biophores include: 1) a cyclopropyl ring at the N-1 position, 2) fluorine atoms at positions C-6 and C-8, and 3) a C-7 heterocyclic substituent. Excessive lipophilicity at N-1 can decrease activity (i.e., 2,4-difluorobenzene). The C-7 substituents with greatest activity against mycobacteria include the substituted piperazines and pyrrolidines (Fig. 41.16). Two biophobes also have been reported and are shown in Fig. 41.17.

Several C-8 methoxy–substituted fluoroquinolones have been reported with superior activity over earlier quinolones (58,59). Moxifloxacin (BAY-12-8039) is reported to be active against *Mycobacterium tuberculosis* when combined with INH, and PD 161148 has been reported to have three to fourfold times the activity of ciprofloxacin as well as to demonstrate activity in GyrA-mutated resistant strains.

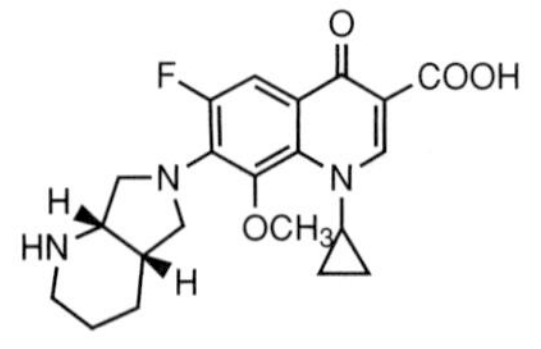

Moxifloxacin

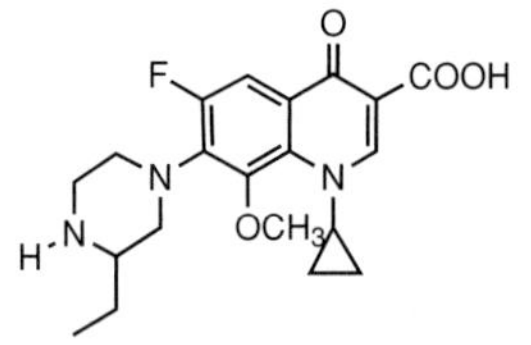

PD 161148

THERAPEUTIC APPLICATION. Fluoroquinolone therapy for TB is predominantly used in patients infected with multidrug-resistant organisms. Resistance to the quinolones has been reported and appears to be associated with mutations in the *gyrA* and *gyrB* genes, leading to single-amino-acid substitution in the DNA gyrase protein (8). As a result, use of the fluoroquinolones must be monitored in the treated patient population. The most active floroquinolones available for treatment of TB are ciprofloxacin (Cipro), sparfloxacin (Zagam), and ofloxacin (Floxin) (Fig. 41.18) (60).

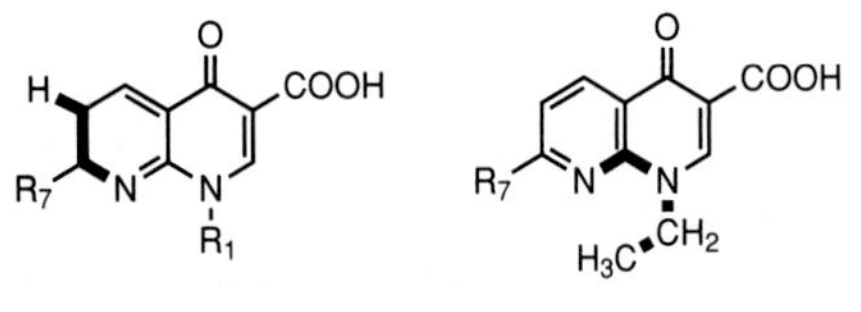

Fig. 41.17. Biophobes (bold) that inactivate 4-quinolones toward mycobacteria.

DRUG THERAPY FOR MAC

Drug therapy for the treatment of MAC is complicated. It underwent significant changes in the early 1990s, but little has changed during the last 10 years. Recommendations for treatment are presently based on small and, in some cases, incomplete studies; more changes can be expected in the future. For the most up-to-date information, the reader is referred to the CDC's homepage (http://www.cdc.gov). The 1997 guidelines for prophylaxis of MAC advise that all adults and adolescents with HIV infection and a CD4 lymphocyte count of less than 50 cells/mL receive clarithromycin, 500 mg b.i.d., or azithromycin, 1200 mg once a week. This recommendation is considered to be a standard of care (61–63). For treatment of MAC, it is recommended that a combination therapy be used that includes at least two drugs (either clarithromycin or azithromycin plus EMB for life). Other drugs that can be added to the combination consist of rifabutin, fluoroquinolones, and amikacin. It should be noted that INH and pyrazinamide are ineffective in the treatment of disseminated MAC.

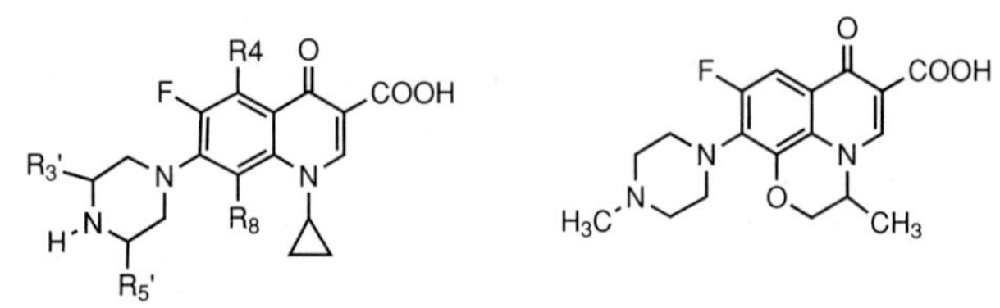

Ciprofloxacin: $R_4 = R_8 = R_3' = R_5' = H$
Sparfloxacin: $R_4 = NH_2$, $R_8 = F$; $R_3' = R_5' = CH_3$
Ofloxacin

Fig. 41.18. Fluoroquinolones active against *Mycobacterium tuberculosis.*

Macrolides

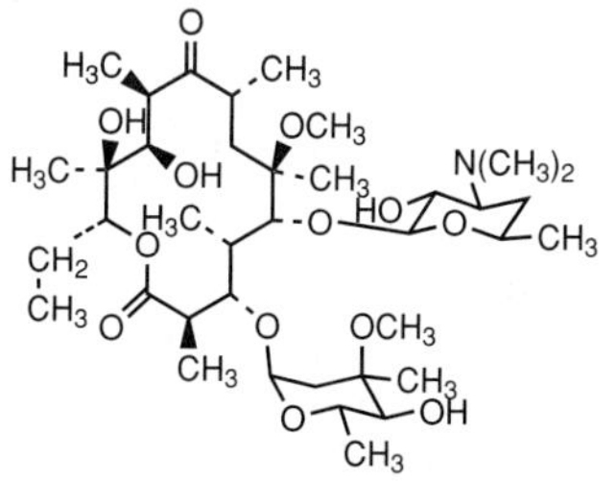

Clarithromycin

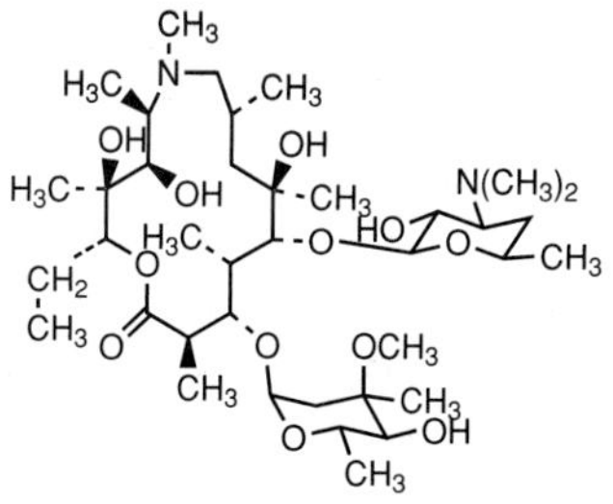

Azithromycin

Both clarithromycin or azithromycin are considered to be first-line agents for the prevention and treatment of MAC and have replaced rifabutin. Both macrolides are concentrated in macrophages (clarithromycin concentration is 17.3-fold higher in macrophage cells than in extracellular fluid) and appear to be equally effective, although clarithromycin has a lower MIC (minimum inhibitory concentration). Azithromycin has an intra-alveolar macrophage half-life of 195 hours, compared to a 4-hour half-life for clarithromycin. For prevention, the macrolides may be used as single agents, although there is a risk of resistant organisms forming and of a cross-resistance between clarithromycin and azithromycin. In one study, the combination of azithromycin and rifabutin proved to be more effective than either drug used alone. For the treatment of MAC, combination therapy is recommended.

Mechanism of Action

The macrolide antibiotics are bacteriostatic agents that inhibit protein synthesis by binding to the 50S ribosomal units. (For a more detailed discussion, see Chapter 38.)

Metabolism

Clarithromycin is metabolized in the liver to an active metabolite, 14-hydroxyclarithromycin, which is less active than the parent molecule. In addition, the drug is an inhibitor of CYP3A4, which could lead to increased concentrations of some drugs, such as rifabutin (see below). Azithromycin is primarily excreted unchanged in the gut, and at present, there is no evidence of CYP3A4 induction or inhibition.

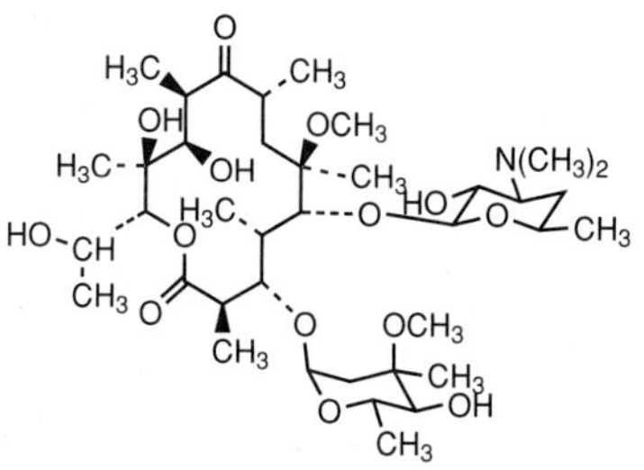

14-Hydroxyclarithromycin

Rifamycins

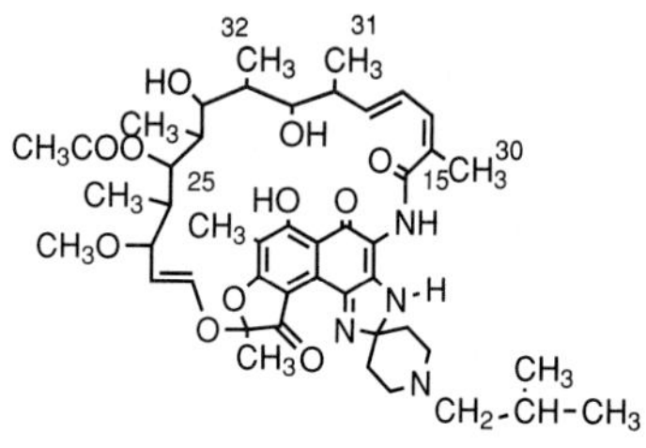

Rifabutin

Various rifamycin derivatives have been investigated or are under investigation for use in the prevention and treatment of MAC. Until recently (1997), rifabutin (Mycobutin) was considered to be the drug of choice for prophylaxis of MAC-infected patients. Studies since 1995, however, have suggested that the macrolides are more effective (survival rates), present fewer side effects, and cause less drug interactions than rifabutin. Early treatment of MAC bacteremia consists of multidrug regimens, usually involving four or five drugs. Drug interactions and, in some studies, exceptionally high drug doses have given confusing results. It generally is agreed that rifabutin should be used in treatment when macrolides have failed or can be combined with azithromycin for prophylaxis or treatment when clarithromycin is unsuccessful.

Drug Interactions

The most significant drug interaction identified with rifabutin is associated with the fact that the drugs in this class are inducers of CYP3A4 and the CYP2C family. As a result, certain drugs that are substrates for these isoforms will show reduced activity. Rifabutin has been shown to reduce the area under the curve and the maximum concentration of clarithromycin and most HIV protease inhibitors. This action could lead to inactivity or resistance to these agents. In addition, because the HIV protease inhibitors are inhibitors of CYP3A4, a combination of rifabutin plus an HIV protease inhibitor is expected to increase the rifabutin area under the curve and maximum concentration, thus increasing the risk of rifabutin side effects. The most serious side effect of rifabutin is uveitis (inflammation of the iris). Under these conditions, appropriate changes in dosing are required. If combination therapy is desirable for the treatment of MAC, the combination of azithromycin and rifabutin is recommended, because no significant change in mean serum drug concentration is reported to occur with either agent when used in combination.

Drug Metabolism

The hepatic metabolism of rifabutin is complex, with as many as 20 metabolites having been reported. The structure of most of the metabolites remains unknown, but several have been identified, including 25-desacetylrifabutin, 25-desacetylrifabutin-N-oxide, 31-hydroxyrifabutin,

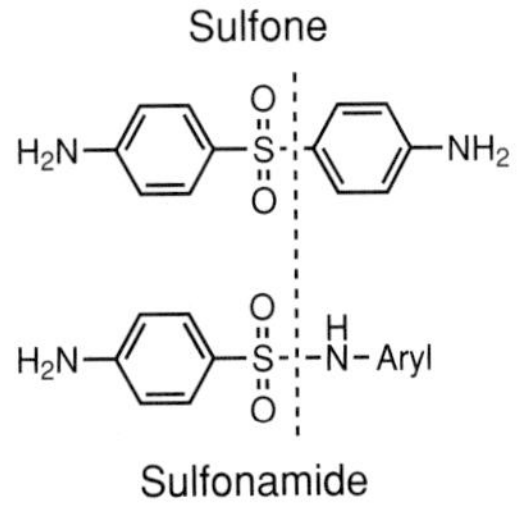

Sulfone

Sulfonamide

Fig. 41.19. Structural comparison of sulfones versus sulfonamide.

32-hydroxyrifabutin, and 32-hydroxy-25-desacetylrifabutin. The metabolites appear in the urine (50%) and in the feces (30%). Based on the activity of other rifamycins, it might be expected that one or more of the metabolites possess antimycobacterial activity.

Additional Drugs

Various other agents have been combined with the macrolides or RIF for the prophylaxis and treatment of MAC. As indicated above, the effectiveness of each component in multidrug treatment is not easily defined. The additional drugs utilized include EMB, ciprofloxacin, amikacin, and clofazimine. Ethambutol and ciprofloxacin appear to have good activity against MAC, but clofazimine has shown unfavorable results. The U.S. FDA has advised against the use of clofazimine during initial therapy for MAC (62).

LEPROSY

Sulfones

The diaryl sulfones represent the major class of agents used to treat leprosy. The initial discovery of the sulfones came about as a result of studies directed at exploring the SAR of sulfonamides (Fig. 41.19). A variety of additional chemical modifications have produced several other active agents, but none has proved to be more beneficial than the original lead, 4,4′-diaminodiphenylsulfone. Dapsone was first introduced into the treatment of leprosy in 1943.

> Dapsone has a variety of uses in addition to the treatment of leprosy. These include the treatment of dermatitis herpetiformis as well as an unlabeled use in the treatment of brown recluse spider bites, inflammatory bowel disorders, leishmaniasis, malaria prophylaxis, relapsing polychondritis, rheumatic and connective tissue disorders, and prophylaxis of *Pneumocystis carinii* pneumonia in HIV-infected patients and organ transplant patients. Recently, dapsone has been approved for the treatment of acne. Under the trade name of Aczone, the drug is available as a 5% gel. Glucose-6-phosphate dehydrogenase (G6PD) levels, blood hemoglobin, and reticulocyte counts should be followed in patients with G6PD deficiency anemia and predisposed to increased hemolytic effects.

Dapsone

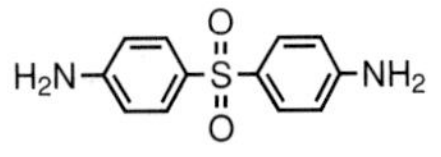

4,4′-Diaminodiphenylsulfone (Dapsone)

Dapsone, a diaminodiphenyl sulfone, is a nearly water-insoluble agent that is very weakly basic ($pK_a \sim 1.0$). The lack of solubility may account, in part, for the occurrence of GI irritation. Despite the lack of solubility, the drug is efficiently absorbed from the GI tract. Although dapsone is bound to plasma protein (~70%), it is distributed throughout the body.

Mechanism of Action

Dapsone, a bacteriostatic agent, is thought to act in a manner similar to that of the sulfonamides—namely, through competitive inhibition of *p*-aminobenzoic acid incorporation into folic acid (see *Sulfonamides* in Chapter 38). Bacteria synthesize folic acid, but host cells do not. As a result, coadministration of dapsone and *p*-aminobenzoic acid will inactivate dapsone. Both dapsone and clofazimine have significant anti-inflammatory actions, which may or may not play a role in the antimicrobial action. The anti-inflammatory action also may be a beneficial side effect, offsetting the complication of erythema nodosum leprosum seen in some patients. The anti-inflammatory action may come about by inhibition of myeloperoxidase-catalyzed reactions (64).

Structure–Activity Relationship

Several derivatives of dapsone have been prepared in an attempt to increase the activity. Isosteric replacement of one benzene ring resulted in the formation of thiazolsulfone. Although still active, it is less effective than dapsone. Substitution on the aromatic ring, to produce acetosulfone, reduced activity while increasing water solubility and decreasing GI irritation. A successful substitution consists of adding methanesulfinate to dapsone to give sulfoxone sodium. This water-soluble form of dapsone is hydrolyzed in vivo to produce dapsone. Sulfoxone sodium is used in individuals who are unable to tolerate dapsone because of GI irritation, but it must be used in a dose threefold that of dapsone because of inefficient metabolism to dapsone. The chemical modification of

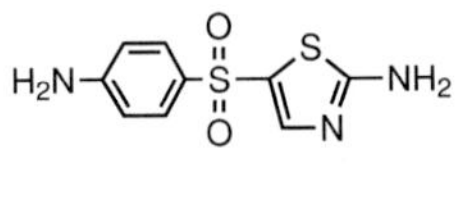

Thiazolsulfone

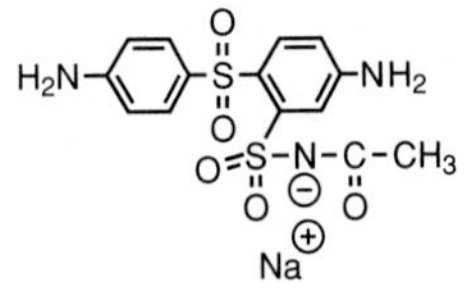

Acetosulfone

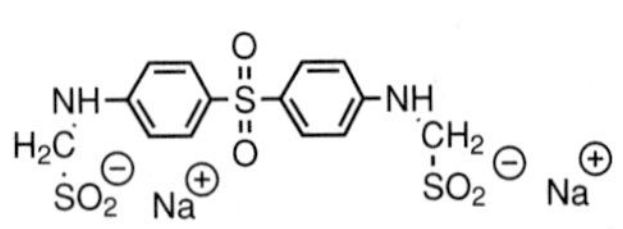

Sulfoxone sodium

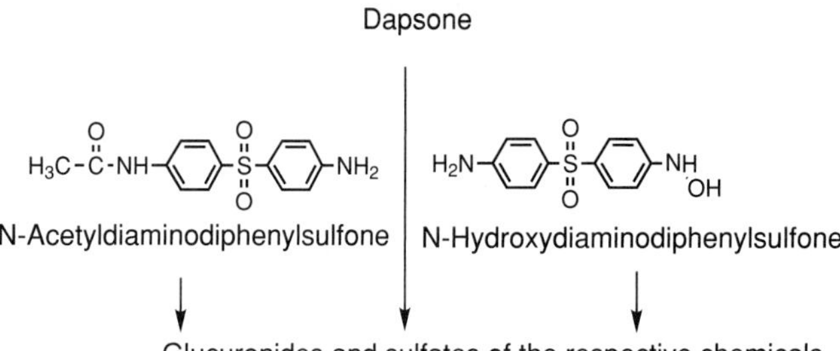

Fig. 41.20. Metabolites of dapsone.

dapsone derivatives continues to be pursued with the intent of finding newer agents useful for the treatment of resistant strains of *Mycobacterium leprae* (65).

Metabolism

The major metabolic product of dapsone results from N-acetylation in the liver by N-acetyltransferase. Dapsone also is N-hydroxylated to the hydroxylamine derivative. These metabolic reactions are catalyzed by CYP3A4 isoforms. Neither of these compounds possess significant leprostatic activity, although N-acetyldiaminodiphenylsulfone may be deacetylated back to dapsone. Products found in the urine consist of small amounts of dapsone, the metabolites N-acetyldiaminodiphenylsulfone and N-hydroxydiaminodiphenylsulfone, as well as glucuronide and sulfates of each of these substances (Fig. 41.20).

Although the acetylated metabolites of dapsone are inactive, there is growing concern over the adverse hematologic effects of the hydroxylated metabolite. The specific adverse effect reported for the N-hydroxydiaminodiphenylsulfone metabolite is methemoglobinemia (66).

Clofazimine (Lamprene)

Clofazimine

Although classified as a secondary drug for the treatment of leprosy and commonly used as a component of multidrug therapy, clofazimine appears to be increasing in use. Clofazimine was first used to treat advanced leprosy unresponsive to dapsone or STM in 1966. The chemical, a phenazine derivative, is a water-insoluble dye (dark-red crystals) that leads to pigmentation of the skin. In addition, discoloration (pink, red, or brownish-black) of the feces, eyelid lining, sputum, sweat, tears, and urine is seen.

Mechanism of Action

The mechanism of action remains unclear at the present time. The molecule possess direct antimycobacterial and immunosuppressive properties. It has been shown that clofazimine increases prostaglandin synthesis and the generation of antimicrobial reactive oxidants from neutrophils, which may play a role in the antileprosy effects. The host cell defense may be stimulated by clofazimine, resulting in the generation of oxidants, such as the superoxide anion, which in turn could have a lethal effect on the organism (67,68).

Structure-Activity Relationship

Several investigators have reported studies directed toward an understanding of the SAR of clofazimine (69–71). Substituents on the imino group at position 2, *p*-chloro substitution on the phenyls at C-3 and N-10, as well as substituents at position 7 have been investigated. The imino group at C-2 appears to be essential, with activity increased when the imino group is substituted with alkyl and cycloalkyl groups. Halogen substitution on the para position of the two phenyls at C-3 and N-10 enhance activity but are not essential to activity. The following order of activity has been reported: Br $>$ Cl $>$ CH_3 $>$ EtO $>$ H or F. In the analogues studied, the increased activity correlates well with pro-oxidative activities of the molecule (e.g., ability to generate superoxide anion) as well as increased lipophilicity.

Metabolism

Various metabolites of clofazimine have been identified, but these account for less than 1% of the administered dose. The lack of higher concentrations of the metabolites may, in part, result from the very slow elimination of clofazimine from the body, which has an estimated half-life of from 8.8 to 69 days. The lipophilic nature of clofazimine results in distribution and storage of the drug in fat tissue. There appears to be some discrepancy as to the structures of the metabolites (71,72). The most recent studies suggest the presence of two conjugates, with the possibility of intermediates (Fig. 41.21). Clofazimine is thought to undergo hydroxylic dehalogenation on the 3-chloroaniline, followed by sulfate conjugation and 4-hydroxylation, followed by glucuronic acid conjugation.

Rifampin (Rifadin, Rimactane)

Rifampin, an antituberculin drug, has already been discussed. Its actions against *Mycobacterium leprae* parallel those effects reported for *Mycobacterium tuberculosis.* Today, RIF is considered to be an effective antileprosy agent when used in combination with the sulfones.

Thalidomide(Thalomid)

Thalidomide

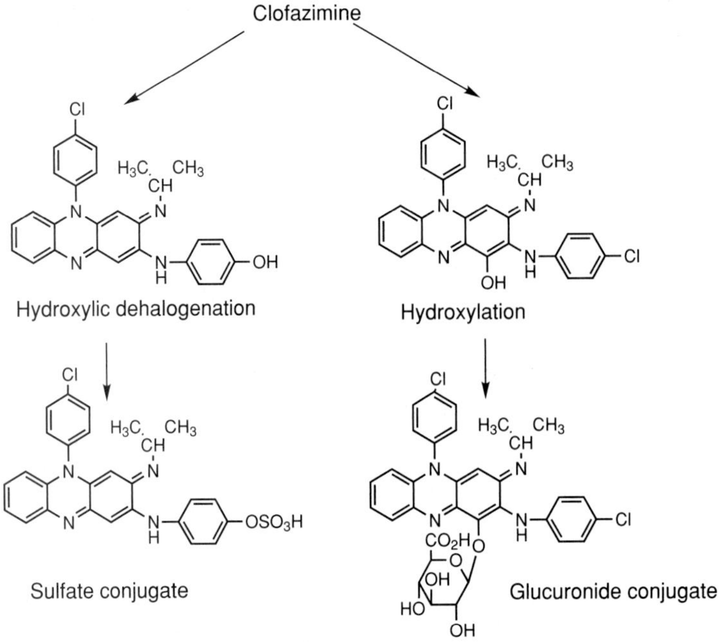

Clofazimine

Hydroxylic dehalogenation

Hydroxylation

Sulfate conjugate

Glucuronide conjugate

Fig. 41.21. Human metabolic products of clofazimine.

The development of painful, tender, inflamed, subcutaneous nodules that may last a week or two but may reappear and last for long periods is seen in a number of diseases. In the case of leprosy, the condition is referred to as erythema nodosum leprosum (ENL). The condition appears to by a hypersensitivity reaction, and although it may appear in nontreated patients, it commonly is seen as a complication of the chemotherapy of leprosy. In addition to painful nodules, the patient may experience fever, malaise, wasting, vasculitis, and peripheral neuritis. This condition has been successfully treated with thalidomide. Recently, thalidomide has been approved by the U.S. FDA for treatment of ENL and is considered to be the drug of choice (73,74). The mechanism whereby thalidomide produces relief is thought to be associated with the drug's ability to control inflammatory cytokines. Specifically, thalidomide inhibits the synthesis and release of tumor necrosis factor α, which is synthesized and released by blood mononuclear cells and appears in the serum during ENL; concentrations drop when the patient is treated with thalidomide. In addition to the treatment of ENL, thalidomide has been reported to exhibit beneficial effects in the treatment of aphthous ulcers in HIV-positive patients, Behcet's disease, chronic graft-versus-host disease, rash caused by systemic or cutaneous lupus erythematosus, pyoderma gangrenosum, and multiple myeloma.

Thalidomide is a very potent teratogenic agent, with a history of an estimated 10,000 deformed infants born to mothers who used the drug during pregnancy. It can be used safely in postmenopausal women, but strict controls are required for women of childbearing age. Additionally, although no evidence suggests that men can transmit the drug during sex, the use of condoms by male patients will be required.

Therapeutic Considerations

Since its introduction into the chemotherapy of leprosy in 1947, dapsone has proved to be the single most effective agent. This drug was used as a monotherapeutic agent despite the recognition that resistant strains were beginning to emerge. Since 1977, monotherapy with dapsone is no longer recognized as an acceptable method for the treatment of leprosy. Today, combination chemotherapy is the method of choice. The combination consists of RIF (600 mg monthly), dapsone (100 mg daily), and clofazimine (300 mg monthly, with 50 mg daily added for patients with multibacillary leprosy, which is defined as five or more skin lesions). Therapy is usually continued for at least 2 years or as long as skin smears are positive. The patient is kept under supervision for 5 years following completion of chemotherapy. A similar treatment regimen is recommended for treatment of paucibacillary leprosy (defined as five or fewer skin lesions) except that treatment is continued for 6 months and the patient kept under observation for an additional 2 years (75,76). It should be noted that the patient is noninfectious within 72 hours of starting treatment. Other combinations that have been reported include RIF plus ofloxacin and minocycline or ofloxicin plus minocycline. The new regimens allow a shortened treatment period and a reduced rate of relapse.

An important aspect of therapy for leprosy involves the treatment of peripheral nerve damage. This nerve damage can be treated with steroids, such as prednisolone. For severe cases, however, thalidomide is used.

CASE STUDY

Victoria F. Roche and S. William Zito

BB is a 73-year-old holy man living on the Apache reservation in western Arizona. Like too many of his heritage, he is diabetic, and the limited formulary at the reservation's health center provides him with tolbutamide to control his blood sugar levels. In the early 1990s, he was exposed to the hantavirus during the outbreak in the "Four Corners" region of the United States. Although he did suffer some hepatic damage as a result of his infection, he felt blessed to have escaped the usually fatal outcome of this disease. As a young man, he worked for a brief period in a reservation-based uranium mine, until an explosion caused him to lose all hearing in one ear. The accident, coupled with increasing years, has reduced the hearing in his other ear to approximately 60%. Fortunately, his vision is still good for a man of 73.

There has been a recent outbreak of tuberculosis on the reservation, and BB has presented to the IHS (Indian Health Service) facility where you are chief pharmacist with all the signs and symptoms of active, but early, disease. After determining that his metabolic acetylation rate is normal, although somewhat compromised by his liver dysfunction, you prepare to make a selection for combination therapy. Consider the structure of the four drug candidates drawn below.

1. Identify the therapeutic problem(s) in which the pharmacist's intervention may benefit the patient.
2. Identify and prioritize the patient-specific factors that must be considered to achieve the desired therapeutic outcomes.
3. Conduct a thorough and mechanistically oriented structure–activity analysis of all therapeutic alternatives provided in the case.
4. Evaluate the SAR findings against the patient-specific factors and desired therapeutic outcomes, and make a therapeutic decision.
5. Counsel your patient.

Tolbutamide

1

2

3

4

References

1. Rastogi N. Structure and functions of the cell envelope in relation to mycobacterial virulence, pathogenicity, and multiple drug resistance. 7th Form in microbiology. Res Microbiol 1991;142:419–481.
2. Minnikin DE. Chemical principles in the organization of lipid components in the mycobacterial cell envelope. Res Microbiol 1991;142:423–427.
3. McNeil MR, Brennan PJ. Structure, function and biogenesis of the cell envelope of mycobacteria in relation to bacterial physiology, pathogenesis, and drug resistance. Some thoughts and possibilities arising from recent structural information. Res Microbiol 1991;142:451–463.
4. Marwick C. Do worldwide outbreaks mean tuberculosis again becomes 'captain of all thes men of death'? JAMA 1992;267:1174–1175.
5. Daniel TM. Tuberculosis. In: Wilson JD, Braunwald E, Isselbacher KJ, et al., eds. Harrison's Principles of Internal Medicine. 12th Ed. New York, McGraw-Hill, 1991. 637–645.
6. Taylor HG. The tuberculosis epidemic and the pharmacist's role. Am Pharm 1992;32(7):41–44.
7. Zhang Y. The magic bullets and tuberculosis drug targets. Annu Rev Pharmacol Toxicol 2005;45:529–564.
8. Blanchard JS. Molecular mechanisms of drug resistance in *Mycobacterium tuberculosis*. Annu Rev Biochem 1996;65:215–239.
9. Zhang Y, Heym B, Allen B, et al. The catalase-peroxidase gene and isoniazid resistance of *Mycobacterium tuberculosis*. Nature 1992;358:591–593.
10. Johnsson K, Schultz PG. Mechanistic studies of the oxidation of isoniazid by the catalase-peroxidase from *Mycombacterium tuberculosis*. J Am Chem Soc 1994;116:7425–7426.
11. Banerjee A, Dubnau E, Quemard A, et al. *inhA*, a gene encoding a target for isonaizid and ethionamide in *Mycombacterium tuberculosis*. Science 1994;263: 227–230.
12. Mdluli K, Sherman DR, Hickey MJ, et al. Biochemical and genetic data suggest that inhA is not the primary target for activated isoniazid in *Mycobacterium tuberculosis*. J Infect Dis 1996;174:1085–1090.
13. Basso LA, Zheng R, Musser JM, et al. Mechanism of isoniazid resistance in *Mycobacterium tuberculosis*: enzymatic characterization of enoyl reductase mutants identified in isoniazid-resistant clinical isolates. J Infect Dis 1998;178:769–775.
14. Quemard A, Sacchettini JC, Dessen A, et al. Enzymatic characterization of the target for isoniazid in *Mycobacterium tuberculosis*. Biochemistry 1995;34: 8235–8241.
15. Johnsson K, King DS, Schultz PG. Studies on the mechanism of action of isoniazid and ethimamide in the chemotherapy of tuberculosis. J Am Chem Soc 1995;117:5009–5010.
16. Rozwarski DA, Grant GA, Barton DHR, et al. Modification of the NADH of the isoniazid target (Inha) from *Mycobacterium tuberculosis*. Science 1998;279:98–102.
17. Bavin EM, James B, Kay E, et al. Further observations on the antibacterial activity to *Mycobacterium tuberculosis* of a derivative of isoniazid, o-hydroxybenzal isonicotinylhydrazone (NUPASAL-213). J Pharm Pharmacol 1955;7:1032–1038.
18. Bavin EM, Drain DJ, Seiler M, et al. Some further studies on tuberculostatic compounds. J Pharm Pharmacol 1952:4:844–855.
19. Fox HH, Gibas JT. Synthetic tuberculostats. IV. Pyridine carboxylic acid hydrazides and benzoic acid hydrazides. J Org Chem 1952;17:1653–1660.
20. Fox HH, Gibas JT. Synthetic tuberculostats. VIII. Monoalkyl derivatives of isonicotinylhydrazine. J Org Chem 1953;18:994–1002.

21. Fox HH, Gibas JT. Synthetic tuberculostats. IX. Dialkyl derivatives of isonicotinylhydrazine. J Org Chem 1955;20:60–69.
22. Fox HH, Gibas JT. Synthetic tuberculostats. XI. Trialkyl and other derivatives of isonicotinylhydrazine. J Org Chem 1956;21:356–361.
23. Weber WW, Hein DW. Clinical pharmacokinetics of isoniazid. Clin Pharmacokinet 1979;4:401–422.
24. Holdiness MR. Clinical pharmacokinetics of the antituberculosis drugs. Clin Pharmacokinet 1984;9:511–544.
25. Timbrell JA, Mitchell JR, Snodgrass WR, et al. Isoniazid hepatotoxicity: the relationship between covalent binding and metabolism in vivo. J Pharmacol Exp Ther 1980;213:364–369.
26. Nolan CM, Goldberg SV, Buskin SE. Hepatotoxicity associated with isoniazid preventing therapy. JAMA 1999;281:1014–1018.
27. Lancini G. Ansamycins. In: Pape H, Rehm H-J, ed. Biotechnology: Microbial Products II, vol 4. Deerfield Beach, FL: VCH, 1986.
28. Arora SK. Correlation of structure and activity in ansamycins: structure, conformation, and interactions of antibiotic rifamycin S. J Med Chem 1985;28: 1099–1102.
29. Levin ME, Hatfull GF. *Mycobacterium smegmatis* RNA polymerase: DNA supercoiling, action of rifampicin, and mechanism of rifampicin resistance. Mol Microbiol 1993;8:277–285.
30. Lancini G, Zanchelli W. Structure–activity relationship in rifamycins. In: Perlman D, ed. Structure–Activity Relationship Among the Semisynthetic Antibiotics. New York: Academic Press, 1977.
31. Jarvis B, Lamb HM. Rifapentine. Drugs 1998;56:607–616.
32. Reith K, Keung A, Toren PC, et al. Disposition and metabolism of ^{14}C-rifapentine in healthy volunteers. Drug Met Dispos 1998;26:732–738.
33. Drugs for tuberculosis. The Medical Letter, 37, The Medical Letter, Inc., New Rochelle, NY, August 4, 1995; 67–70.
34. Keung ACF, Eller MG, Weir SJ. Pharmacokinetics of rifapentine in patients with varying degrees of hepatic dysfunction. J Clin Pharmacol 1998;38: 517–524.
35. Steffen R, Sack DA, Riopel L, et al. Therapy of travelers' diarrhea with rifaximin on various continents. Am J Gastroenterol 2003;98:1073–1078.
36. Scorpio A, Zhang Y. Mutations in *pncA*, a gene encoding pyrazinamidase/nicotinamidase, cause resistance to the antituberculous drug pyrazinamide in tubercle bacillus. Nat Med 1996;2:662–667.
37. Heifets LB, Flory MA, Lindholm-Levy PJ. Does pyrazinoic acid as an active moiety of pyrazinamide have specific activity against *Mycobacterium tuberculosis*? Antimicrob Agents Chemother 1989;33:1252–1254.
38. Zhang Y, Wade MM, Scorpio A, et al. Mode of action of pyrazinamide: disruption of mycobacterium tuberculosis membrane transport and energetics by pyrazinoic acid. Antimicrob Chemother 2003;790–795.
39. Kushner S, Dalalian H, Sanjurjo JL, et al. Experimental chemotherapy of tuberculosis. II. The synthesis of pyrazinamides and related compounds. J Am Chem Soc 1952;74:3617–3621.
40. Bergmann KE, Cynamon MH, Welch JT. Quantitiative structure–activity relationships for the in vitro antimycobacterial activity of pyrazinoic acid esters. J Med Chem 1996;39:3394–3400.
41. Peloquin CA, Bulpitt AE, Jaresko GS, et al. Pharmacokinetics of pyrazinamide under fasting conditions, with food, and with antacids. Pharmacotherapy 1998;18:1205–1211.
42. Daffe M, Brennan PJ, McNeil MR. Predominant structural features of the cell wall arabinogalactan of *Mycobacterium tuberculosis* as revealed through characterization of oligoglycosyl alditol fragments by gas chromatography/mass spectrometry and by ^{1}H and ^{13}C NMR analysis. J Biol Chem 1990;265: 6734–6743.
43. Wolucka BA, McNeil MR, de Hoffmann E, et al. Recognition of the lipid intermediate for arabinoglactan/arabinomannan structure of cell wall of mycobacterium: biosynthesis and its relation to the mode of action of ethambutol in mycobacteria. J Biol Chem 1994;269:23328–23335.
44. Takayama K, Kilburn JO. Inhibition of synthesis of arabinoglactan by ethambutol in *Mycobacterium smegmatis*. Antimicrob Agents Chemother 1989;33: 1493–1499.
45. Mikusova K, Slayden RAS, Besra GS, et al. Biogenesis of the mycobacterial cell wall and the site of action of ethambutol. Antimicrob Agents Chemo 1995;39:2484–2489.
46. Lee RE, Mikusova, Brennan PJ, et al. J Am Chem Soc 1995;117:11829–11832.
47. Khoo K-H, Douglas E, Azadi P, et al. Truncated structural variants of lopoarabinomannan in ethambutol drug-resistant strains of *Mycobacterium smegmatis*. J Biol Chem 1996;271:28628–28690.
48. Belanger AE, Besra GS, Ford ME, et al. The *embAB* genes of *Mycobacterium avium* encode an arabinosyl transferase involved in cell wall arabinan biosynthesis that is the target for the antimycobacterial drug ethambutol. Proc Natl Acad Sci U S A 1996;93:11919–11924.
49. Kuehl FA, Peck RL, Hoffhine CE Jr, et al. Streptomyces antibiotics. XVIII. Structure of streptomycin. J Am Chem Soc 1945;70:2325–2329.
50. Finken M, Kirschner P, Meier A, et al. Molecular basis of streptomycin resistance in *Mycobacterium tuberculosis*: alterations of the ribosomal protein S12 gene and point mutations within a functional 16S ribosomal RNA pseudoknot. Mol Microbiol 1993;9:1239–1246.
51. Bieder A, Brunel P, Mazeau L. Identification de Trois Nouveaux Metabolites de l'ethionamide: Chromatographie, Spectrophotometrie, Polarographie. Ann Pharmaceut Francais 1966;24:493–500.
52. Caceres NE, Harris NB, Wellehan JF, et al. Overexpression of the D-alanine racemase gene confers resistance to D-dycloserine in *Mycobacterium smegmatis*. J Bacteriol 1997;179:5046–5055.
53. Gale EF, Cundliffe E, Reynolds PE, et al. In: The Molecular Basis of Antibiotic Action. 2nd Ed. London: Wiley & Son, 1981.
54. American Thoracic Society, Centers for Disease Control and Prevention, Infectious Disease Society of America. Treatment of tuberculosis. Am J Respir Crit Care Med 2003;167:604–661.
55. Reinke CM, Albrant DH. An old scourge: tuberculosis in the 1990s. US Pharmacist Hospital Edition 1991;16(October): 37–72.
56. Jacobs MR. Activity of quinolones against mycobacteria. Drugs 1995;49(Suppl. 2):67–75.
57. Renau TE, Sanchez JP, Gage JW, et al. Structure–activity relationships of the quinolone antibacterials against mycobacteria: effect of structural changes at N-1 and C-7. J Med Chem 1996;39:729–735.
58. Miyazaki E, Miyazaki M, Chen JM, et al. Moxifloxacin (BAY-12-8039), a new 8-methoxyquinolone, is active in the mouse model of tuberculosis. Antimicrob Agents Chemother 1999;43:85–89.
59. Zhao BY, Pine R, Domagala J, et al. Fluoroquinolone action against clinical isolates of *Mycobacterium tuberculosis*: effects of a C-8 methoxy group on survival in liquid media and in human macrophages. Antimicrob Agents Chemo 1999;43:661–666.
60. Yew WW, Kwan SY, Ma WK, et al. In vitro activity of ofloxacin in *Mycobacterium tuberculosis* and its clinical efficacy in multiply resistant pulmonary tuberculosis. J Antimicrob Chemother 1990;26:227–236.
61. Amsdenn GW, Peloquin CA, Berning SE. The role of advanced generation macrolides in the prophylaxis and treatment of *Mycobacterium avium* complex (MAC) infections. Drugs 1997;54:69–80.
62. Wright J. Current strategies for the prevention and treatment of disseminated *Mycobacterium avium* complex infection in patients with AIDS. Pharmacotherapy 1998;18:738–747.
63. Faris MA, Raasch RH, Hopfer RL, et al. Treatment and prophylaxis of disseminated *Mycobacterium avium* complex in HIV-infected individuals. Ann Pharmacother 1998;32:561–573.
64. van Zyl JM, Basson K, Kriegler A, et al. Mechanisms by which clofazimine and dapsone inhibit the myeloperoxidase system. Biochem Pharmacol 1991;42: 599–608.
65. Dhople AM. In vitro and in vivo activity of K-130, a dihyrofolate reductase inhibitor, against *Mycobacterium leprae*. Arzneim-Forsch Drug Res 1999;49:267–271.
66. Ward KE, McCarthy MW. Dapsone-induced methemoglobinemia. Ann Pharmacother 1998;32:549–552.
67. Savage JE, O'Sullivan JF, Zeis BM, et al. Investigation of the structural properties of dihydrophenazines which contribute to their pro-oxidative interaction with human phagocytes. J Antimicrob Chemother 1989;23:691–700.
68. Franzblau SG, White KE, O'Sullivan JF. Structure–activity relationships of tetramethylpiperdine-substituted phenazines against *Mycobacterium leprae* in vitro. Antimicrob Agents Chemother 1989;33:2004–2005.
69. Arutla S, Arra GS, Prabhakar CM, et al. Pro- and antioxidant effects of some antileprotic drugs in vitro and their influence on super oxide dismutase activity. Arzneim-Forsch Drug Res 1998;48:1024–1027.
70. O'Sullivan JF, Conalty ML, Morrison NE. Clofazimine analogues active against a clofazimine-resistant organism. J Med Chem 1988;31:567–572.
71. Kapoor VK. Clofazimine. In: Florey K, ed. Analytical Profiles of Drug Substances , vol 18. San Diego: Academic Press, 1989.
72. Krishna DR, Mamidi RNVS, Hofmann U, et al. Characterization of clofazimine metabolites in humans by HPLC-electrospray mass spectrometry. Arzneim-Forsch Drug Res 1997;47:303–306.
73. Stirling D, Sherman M, Strauss S. Thalidomide: a surprising recovery. J Am Pharm Assoc 1997;37:306–313.
74. Thalidomide. The Medical Letter, 40, The Medical Letter, Inc., New Rochelle, NY, October 23, 1998; 103–104.
75. Lambert HP, O'Grady FW. Antibiotic and Chemotherapy. 6th Ed. Edinburgh: Churchill Livingstone, 1992.
76. Lockwood DNJ, Kumar B. Treatment of leprosy. BMJ 2004;1447–1448.

42. *Cancer and Chemotherapy*

VICTORIA F. ROCHE

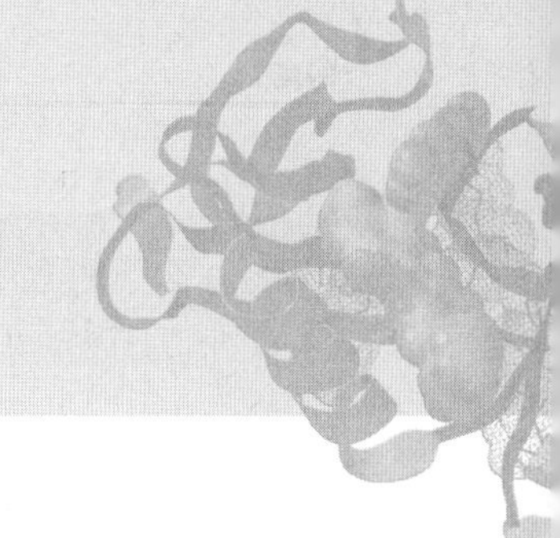

DRUGS COVERED IN THIS CHAPTER:

DNA ALKYLATING AGENTS
- Chlorambucil
- Cyclophosphamide
- Estramustine
- Ifosfamide
- Mechlorethamine
- Melphalan
- Thiotepa

NITROSOUREAS
- Carmustine
- Lomustine
- Streptozocin

PROCARBAZINE AND TRIAZENES
- Dacarbazine
- Procarbazine
- Temozolomide

MISCELLANEOUS ALKYLATING AGENTS
- Altretamine
- Busulfan

ORGANOPLATINUM COMPLEXES
- Carboplatin
- Cisplatin
- Oxaliplatin
- Satraplatin

ANTIBIOTICS
- Bleomycin
- Dactinomycin
- Daunorubicin
- Doxorubicin
- Epirubicin
- Idarubicin
- Mitoxantrone
- Mitomycin
- Valrubicin

ANTIMETABOLITES
- DNA polymerase inhibitors
  - Cladribine
  - Clofarabine
  - Cytarabine
  - Fludarabine
  - Gemcitabine
- Pyrimidine antagonists
  - Capecitabine
  - Floxuridine
  - Fluorouracil
  - Methotrexate
  - Pemetrexed
- Purine antagonists
  - Mercaptopurine
  - Thioguanine
- Miscellaneous antimetabolites
  - Hydroxyurea
  - Pentostatin

MITOSIS INHIBITORS
- Docetaxel
- Etoposide
- Irinotecan
- Paclitaxel
- Teniposide
- Topotecan
- Vinblastine
- Vincristine
- Vinorelbine

MISCELLANEOUS ANTICANCER AGENT
- Azacitidine

INTRODUCTION

Overview

Healthy cells are under strict biochemical control for growth and differentiation. Cells divide and proliferate under the influence of various growth stimulators and are subject to arrested growth (senescence) and programmed cell death (apoptosis). In cancer, these regulatory processes have gone awry, and cells grow and divide uncontrollably, consuming energy and losing both structure and function because of an inability to adequately differentiate. To add insult to injury, rampant cell division is accompanied by disabled cell-death processes, leading first to cellular immortality and, eventually, to genetic instability. The causes of cancer are many and varied (e.g., chemical, environmental, viral, and mutagenic), but all ultimately lead to an aberration in the expression of proto-oncogenes, the products of which control normal cell life. When these genes mutate to become oncogenes in a sequential, multistep process, cancer results. Oncogenes (e.g., *myc* and *ras*) can either overexpress or underexpress regulatory biochemicals, resulting in preferential and accelerated cellular growth. Concomitantly, tumor suppressor genes (e.g., anti-oncogenes like *p53, p21,* p^{INK4A}, and *retinoblastoma*) can be inhibited (1).

Initially, tumors grow exponentially, taking a consistent amount of time for every doubling of the tumor cell population size. In fact, the majority of a cancer cell's lifetime is spent before the tumor presents clinically. Initially, growth is very rapid (doubling time measured in days), but doubling time can slow to weeks or months as the tumor ages (2) because of increasingly poor vascularization and the resulting decrease in access to blood and essential nutrients.

Selected Definitions

Oncogenes and Tumor Suppressor Genes

Oncogenes are regulators of cellular communication with the outside environment. They are derived through the mutation of proto-oncogenes, which are normal and ubiquitous genes involved in the regulation of homeostatic cellular functions. Mutations in proto-oncogenes can occur as spontaneous point mutations, inherited germline mutations, chromosomal rearrangements or through augmentation of gene expression. Regardless of the mutational mechanism, when the mutated oncogenes are

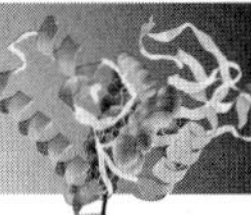

CLINICAL SIGNIFICANCE

Chemotherapy has significantly changed the treatment of cancer since the first agents were studied in the 1940s. Understanding the chemical mechanism of action for traditional chemotherapeutic agents, including whether the agent is cell-cycle specific or cell-cycle nonspecific, is important so that administration can be planned accordingly and coadministration of agents with similar toxicities can be avoided.

The disadvantage of traditional chemotherapeutic agents is the inability of the agent to recognize the difference between normal cells and cancer cells. So, although the agents may shrink or eliminate the tumor, the treatment is accompanied by many unwanted side effects. There are numerous examples in which a chemical understanding of the chemotherapeutic agent is needed. For example, hydration with chloride-containing fluid is necessary with cisplatin to keep cisplatin in its inactive form in the kidneys and to avoid renal toxicity. Another example can be found when using cyclophosphamide or ifosfamide. The dissociation of aldophosphamide produces the active compound phophoramide mustard, but it also produces acrolein, which can cause significant damage to the bladder. This bladder damage, or hemorrhagic cystitis, can be prevented with the use of mesna, which inactivates the effects of acrolein in the bladder. Understanding the chemical basis for the toxicities seen with chemotherapy is imperative in managing or preventing them in clinical practice.

Kelly Nystrom, Pharm.D., BCOP
Assistant Professor
Pharmacy Practice Department
School of Pharmacy and Health Professions
Creighton University

stimulated by exposure to chemical, environmental, or viral carcinogens, they produce proteins that are either wrongly expressed within their normal cell or expressed in inappropriate tissues. In either case, cellular proliferation leading to cancer results (1,3).

Tumor suppressor genes are intended to keep oncogenes in check by halting uncontrolled cellular growth. In direct opposition to oncogenes, which induce cancer when stimulated or amplified, tumor suppressor genes promote cancer when inactivated or attenuated. Two of the most prevalent tumor suppressor genes involved in the generation of cancer are *p53* and *retinoblastoma,* or *Rb.* When either of these two suppressor genes loses function, the negative control on cellular proliferation is lifted and cells gain immortality (an essential quality of a cancer cell). The loss or disruption of function of the *p53* tumor suppressor gene is found in approximately half of human cancers and is a harbinger of a poor prognosis.

Oncogenes and tumor suppressor genes that have been linked to specific types of cancer are identified in Table 42.1. Table 42.2 relates oncogenic markers of selected cancers to disease prognosis and treatment strategy.

Cell Cycle

When cells reproduce, they do so via a very specific game plan known as the cell cycle. Cell division (mitosis) kicks off the cycle, and after a period of 30 to 60 minutes, the cells go into either a resting phase (called G_0) or a presynthetic (gap) phase (called G_1), in which enzyme production occurs in preparation for de novo nucleic acid synthesis. Production of DNA then occurs in an S phase that can last up to 20 hours. The S phase is followed by a gap phase (G_2), in which RNA, critical proteins, and the mitotic spindle apparatus are generated for the next mitotic (M) phase (3,4).

This is important to our discussion, because some anticancer agents are specific for a certain phase of the cell cycle. For example, antimetabolite antineoplastics damage cells in the S phase, whereas mitosis inhibitors pack their greatest cell-killing punch in the M phase. The administration of cell-cycle phase–specific antineoplastics is carefully planned so that the drug encounters cancer cells at their most vulnerable moments. Other antineoplastic agents are toxic to cells regardless of cycle phase (e.g., DNA alkylating agents and most antineoplastic antibiotics). These cell-cycle phase–nonspecific agents can be administered at any time that is feasible for the provider and convenient for the patient.

In general, cancer cells undergoing rapid division are most vulnerable to the cytotoxic action of antineoplastic agents, and antineoplastic therapy holds its greatest

Table 42.1. Oncogenic Origin of Selected Cancers (1,3)

Cancer Type	Common Oncogenic or Tumor Suppressor Gene Origin
Chronic myelogenous leukemia	*bcr-abl* proto-oncogene translocation
Follicular lymphoma	*bcl-2* amplification, *myc* mutation
Sporadic thyroid cancer	*ret* mutation
Colorectal and gastric cancer	*APC* gene mutation
Familial breast and ovarian cancer	*BRCA1, BRCA2* mutation
Invasive ductal breast cancer	*HER-2* amplification
Familial melanoma	*p16^{INK4A}* mutation
Childhood neuroblastoma and small cell lung cancer	N-*myc* amplification
Leukemia, breast, colon, gastric, and lung cancer	*c-MYC* amplification
Renal cell cancer	Von Hippel-Lindaugene (VHL) dysfunction

Table 42.2. Oncogenic Markers and Therapeutic Strategies in Selected Cancers (1)

Cancer Type	Oncogenic Marker	Prognosis/Responsiveness to Chemotherapy	Approach
Breast cancer	HER-2 amplification	Poor	Aggressive chemotherapy, targeted therapy
Acute myelogenous leukemia	t(8;21) or inv(16) translocation	Good	Standard chemotherapy
Acute lymphocytic leukemia	*bcr-abl* rearrangement	Poor	Bone marrow transplantation

promise for positive outcomes if initiated when the tumor is small but growing aggressively. Conversely, slow-growing tumors with a high percentage of cells remaining in the G_0 phase (e.g., nonsmall cell lung cancer) often are nonresponsive to standard chemotherapy (4). If the tumor is not detected until it is quite large, therapy also can be compromised by inefficient or substandard drug delivery because of poor tumor vascularization.

Metastasis

Metastasis refers to the process by which malignant cells leave the parent tumor, migrate to distant sites, and invade new tissue. The primary metastatic "highways" utilized by meandering cancer cells are the blood and lymph fluids. Sloughed cells must find a biological environment with all of their essential growth factors in place before they can put down roots and evolve into a full-fledged metastatic tumor. Because many distinct and interdependent steps must be accomplished to establish metastatic disease, the process has been termed the "metastatic cascade" (5). Fortunately, there are many opportunities within the cascade for the body to mount a successful defense and destroy the potential invaders.

Cancer Staging

Clinicians need to have a common language through which to communicate about disease severity to make the best team-based decisions about the relative risks and benefits of treatment options. In the TNM cancer staging classification, the severity of solid tumor neoplastic growth is characterized by the size of the tumor mass (T_1–T_4), the extent of lymph node involvement (N_1–N_3), and whether distant metastasis has occurred (M_0 or M_1). The higher the subscripted number in each of these parameters, the more advanced and/or disseminated the disease. Taken together, the TNM characteristics of a tumor can be translated into a comprehensive staging scale ranging from I (localized) to IV (metastatic). The intermediate disease severity stages indicate local (Stage II) or regional (Stage III) tissue invasion (3). Staging is an essential prerequisite for the prediction of prognosis and the identification of the most appropriate treatment plan and optimal dosing regimen (2).

Response Criteria

In this era of patient-centered, team-based care, it is equally beneficial to quantify a patient's clinical response to therapy in a manner that is consistent and universally understood by all health care providers. Five discrete anticancer therapy response categories have been defined, with criteria established for each (3). Whereas "cure" is obviously the most noble goal, it is very difficult to achieve in most types of cancer. "Cure" for all cancers except breast and melanoma equates to no evidence of disease for a minimum of 5 years. More commonly, the response category viewed as the pinnacle is "complete response," in which the patient has no evidence of cancer for at least 1 month following the cessation of therapy but where relapses are still possible. A "partial response" is claimed when tumor size or disease severity has been cut at least in half and there is no evidence of new lesions at the primary site or elsewhere. If this level of clinical improvement is not reached, yet the patient has experienced significant attenuation of symptoms and/or enhancement of quality of life, the response is termed "clinical benefit." A less optimistic response category is "stable disease," in which tumor size or disease severity has changed by 25% or less in either direction. Most dire is "progression," a category that is characterized by tumor growth or worsening disease severity at the 25% or higher level.

Historical Background (6)

> "Those who have not been trained in chemistry or medicine, which after all is only applied chemistry, may not realize how difficult the problem of [cancer] treatment really is. It is almost, not quite, but almost as hard as finding some agent that will dissolve away the left ear, say, yet leave the right ear unharmed: so slight is the difference between the cancer cell and its normal ancestor."

Thus wrote noted cancer researcher and physician Dr. William H. Woglom in a monograph published by the American Association for the Advancement of Science in 1947 (7). Although somewhat predictive of what we now know to be true regarding the relationship between resident genes and oncogenes, Dr. Woglom's rather gloomy prognosis of our ability to meet cancer on its own ground and beat it was underpinned by centuries of unsuccessful attempts to treat neoplastic disease with toxic metals, including lead, arsenic, silver, zinc, antimony, mercury, and bismuth. The era of more promising chemotherapy was just on the horizon, however, even as Woglom penned his words of therapeutic woe.

Among the first nonmetallic therapeutic agents to show benefit in the treatment of cancer was cortisone and, later, prednisone. In the 1940s, these glucocorticoids were shown to induce tumor regression in a laboratory cancer model (murine lymphosarcoma) and in acute leukemia. In the same decade, the retrospective recognition that World War I soldiers exposed to sulfur mustard gas, used as an agent of war, suffered from damaged lymphoid tissue and bone marrow led to the development of the cytotoxic nitrogen mustards for the treatment of lymphoma. Chemists then used their scientific understanding of mustard reactivity to design agents that were either "superpotent" and nonselective (e.g., highly toxic) or of lower reactivity so as to provide oral activity and less systemic toxicity.

The discovery in 1940 that *p*-aminobenzenesulfonamide was effective against streptococcal infections ushered in the era of antimetabolite chemotherapy. The development of antifolate antineoplastics, which were shown to be effective in combating childhood leukemias, got its start in the late 1940s. In the mid- to late-1950s, on the heels of the success of antifolates, came the development of antimetabolites based on the structures of endogenous purine and pyrimidine bases. Perhaps the most exciting discovery in this regard was the recognition that a very simple analogue of the endogenous pyrimidine uracil (5-fluorouracil) was a potent inhibitor of deoxythymidine monophosphate biosynthesis and that inhibiting the production of this essential nucleotide produced positive results in patients suffering from colon, stomach, pancreatic, and breast cancers. Antimetabolites that target DNA polymerase (e.g., cytarabine) were conceptualized and synthesized in the late 1950s and subsequently shown to be effective in acute myeloblastic leukemia.

The antibiotic antineoplastics came into clinical utility when the highly toxic actinomycin (discovered in the 1940s) was found to be effective in the treatment of human testicular cancer and uterine choriocarcinoma. Other natural anticancer antibiotics, such as bleomycin, subsequently were found to be active against various hematological cancers and solid tumors (1960s), which led to the development of semisynthetic analogues with both high potency and wider margins of safety in more recent times. The antimitotic vinca alkaloids vincristine and vinblastine were shown to have activity against Hodgkin's disease and acute lymphoblastic leukemia around the same time that the antibiotic antineoplastics were being developed.

Cancer chemotherapy appears to have come full circle since the "metal-intense Renaissance," because some of the newest anticancer drugs to join the U.S. market are organometallic platinum complexes. The activity of cisplatin (the first such complex to be commercially available) against lymphosarcoma and solid tumors of the head, neck, and reproductive organs was first noted in the early 1970s. The fortuitous discovery of organoplatinum complexes in the treatment of cancer is attributed to Dr. Barnett Rosenberg, who was studying the impact of electromagnetic radiation on bacterial cell growth using platinum electrodes. He followed up on the astute observation that the bacteria exposed to the electrodes experienced profound changes in cellular structure, which ultimately were attributed to the in situ generation of cisplatin. Both Pt(II) and Pt(IV) analogues of cisplatin, which offer high potency coupled with lower resistance potential and fewer use-limiting side effects (e.g., oto-, nephro-, and hematotoxicity), are currently on the market and in clinical trials. In addition to organometallics, the efficacy of sex hormones and hormone antagonists in fighting hormone-dependent cancers (e.g., estrogen receptor–positive breast cancer or prostate cancer) and the advent of therapeutic biological response modifiers with direct antiproliferative effects (e.g., interferons) has added significantly to the therapeutic options available to providers and the cancer patients for whom they care.

Despite the wide range of antineoplastic agents currently available, it has been estimated that more than half of all patients with cancer ultimately succumb to their disease (8). Novel therapies based on an in-depth understanding of the molecular mechanisms involved in the complex cascade of events we call cancer are urgently needed. Fortunately, molecular targets for focused chemotherapeutic interventions are being discovered with increasing regularity, opening the door for the scientifically grounded development of new drugs. The critical role of computer-based technology in facilitating the ability of chemists to conceptualize and visualize molecular interactions between potential drugs and putative receptor targets that lead to rational drug design and development, as well as in analyzing and managing the overwhelming amounts of data that are generated from these studies, cannot be underestimated. Likewise, the availability of viable tumor cell lines has facilitated a disease-specific orientation to the hunt for more effective therapies. Currently, there are tumor cell lines for lung, colon, breast, and kidney cancers, as well as for melanoma and leukemia (8).

Several monoclonal antibodies targeted to tumor cell antigens or proteins critical to cellular proliferation (e.g., human epidermal growth factor, vascular endothelial growth factor, tyrosine kinase, and proteasomes) have found their way to the U.S. market. In addition, several new targets for anticancer drug development currently are being actively explored by biomedical scientists (1,3). For example, cancer cells overexpress the enzyme telomerase, which inhibits the natural destruction of chromosomal telomeres (DNA caps), leading to unwanted cellular immortality. Telomerase inhibitors would be expected to reestablish cellular senescence and to halt uncontrolled cell division by maintaining the integrity of the telomeres and are being pursued as a new biochemical approach to disease attenuation or control. Other potential antineoplastic drug targets being seriously investigated are aberrant genes or enzymes unique to specific tumors and P-glycoprotein, which is overexpressed in

Table 42.3. Estimated 2005 Incidence and Mortality of Common Cancers (3)

	Prostate/Breast		Lung		Colorectal	
	Men	Women	Men	Women	Men	Women
Incidence	232,090 (33%)	211,240 (32%)	93,010 (13%)	79,560 (12%)	71,820 (10%)	73,470 (11%)
Mortality	30,350 (10%)	40,410 (15%)	90,490 (31%)	73,020 (27%)	28,540 (10%)	27,750 (10%)

many cancers as a result of an amplified *mdr-1* gene and responsible for the rapid ejection of antineoplastic agents from target cells. Other multidrug resistance–associated proteins (the MRP family) involved in this devastating rebound of the cancer cell also are being investigated as potential sites of therapeutic intervention. The intense focus on resistance molecules such P-glycoprotein is warranted, because patients whose tumors express this efflux-promoting protein respond poorly to chemotherapy and have a poor prognosis (2).

In the future, it is hoped that clinicians will be able to generate a genetic expression profile for each patient with cancer to help them predict response to all possible therapies and to guide pharmacotherapy selection.

DISEASE STATE

Cancers generally can be classified as lymphatic, epithelial, nerve, or connective tissue related, and tumor nomenclature is based on tissue of origin as follows: carcinoma (epithelial origin), sarcoma (muscle or connective tissue origin), leukemia and lymphoma (lymphatic or hematologic origin), and glioma (neural origin). The risk of developing epithelial-derived cancers increases with age.

Incidence

Approximately 1.3 million cases of cancer are diagnosed each year in the United States, resulting in an estimated 570,280 annual deaths (3). The most commonly acquired cancers include those of the prostate, breast, lung, colon, and rectum. Lung cancer is the most fatal and is responsible for approximately 160,000 deaths each year. These prominent cancers (prostate/breast, lung, and colorectal) occur with very similar frequency in men and women, and little gender-related differences in mortality are noted (Table 42.3). Some geographical differences in incidence have been noted, with lung cancer being more prevalent in rural southern U.S. states, and breast and colon cancer more commonly diagnosed in the "northeast corridor" of the United States (9).

Signs and Symptoms

The clinical manifestations of cancer can vary widely depending on type and stage of neoplastic disease. The American Cancer Society has been promulgating its list of the major warning signs of cancer for decades (Table 42.4) (10,11). Patients are well-served by being familiar with these early warning signs, because cancer is most effectively treated when diagnosed before more life-threatening symptoms appear. One readily recognized symptom of cancer is persistent weight loss (especially in children), and severe, unrelenting pain is a hallmark symptom of cancer in the later stages. Solid tumors can become palpable or observable masses when the cancer is advanced.

Biochemical Bases and Causes of Cancer

Currently, it is understood that cancer is caused by mutations in "resident" or normal genes rather than by the introduction of foreign genes into otherwise healthy systems (1,3). The single-gene theory of cancer (where a single mutation could result in neoplastic disease) has been abandoned in favor of the multiple mutation prerequisite, and complex gene pathways, interactions, and communications are now the focus of study in the understanding of

Table 42.4. The American Cancer Society's Major Warning Signs of Cancer (10,11)

Cancer Warning Signs in Adults	Cancer Warning Signs in Children
Change in bowel or bladder habits	Continued, unexplained weight loss
A sore that does not heal	Frequent headaches, with vomiting
Unusual bleeding or discharge	Localized pain or persistent limping
Thickening or lump in breast or elsewhere	Any unusual mass or swelling
Indigestion or difficulty in swallowing	Sudden eye or vision changes
Obvious change in a wart or mole	Recurrent or unexplained fever
Nagging cough or hoarseness	Excessive bruising or bleeding
	Noticeable paleness or loss of energy

Table 42.5. RNA and DNA Viruses Associated with Cancer Development (12,13)

RNA Virus	Cancer
Human T-lymphotrophic virus	Adult T-cell leukemia (ATL)
Hepatitis C	Hepatocellular carcinoma (HCC)
DNA Virus	**Cancer**
Hepadnavirus	Hepatocellular carcinoma (HCC)
Papillomavirus	Skin cancer, cervical cancer
Epstein-Barr virus	Burkett's lymphoma, Hodgkin's disease, anaplastic nasopharyngeal carcinoma, gastric cancer
Herpesvirus	Karposi's sarcoma

Table 42.6. Some Environmental Precipitants of Cancer (9)

Environmental Cancer Precipitant	Cancer Type
Tobacco	Lung, oral, bladder, pancreatic, stomach, and renal cancer
Alcohol	Liver, rectal. and breast cancer
Tobacco plus alcohol	Oral cancers
Radon	Lung cancer
Halogenated compounds	Bladder cancer
Immunosuppressive agents	Lymphoma
Herbicides	Lymphoma
Ionizing or ultraviolet radiation	Leukemia, breast, thyroid, lung, and skin cancer

malignant processes and their treatments. Once determined, the "mutational profile" of malignant cells may very well predict such parameters as disease severity, most promising therapeutic interventions, and clinical outcome.

The development of cancer occurs in four discrete steps or phases. In the **initiation** phase, exposure to a precipitating carcinogen prompts irreversible mutation in a number of different genes. The **promotion** phase is a time during which mutated cells arising from altered genes grow preferentially compared to normal cells. This preferential growth can result from continued exposure to the original carcinogen or from promotion by environmental "accelerants." This stage is reversible, so cancer sometimes can be avoided with appropriate changes in diet and lifestyle. The **transformation** phase is the 5- to 20-year progression of a mutated cell to a cancer cell. Cellular proliferation, clonal colony development, tissue invasion and destruction, and metastasis defines the final **progression** phase of cancer development (3).

As previously mentioned, the genetic mutations leading to the diseases that we call cancer can be stimulated by a variety of chemical, environmental, and viral triggers. Both RNA retroviruses and DNA viruses have been implicated in human cancer causation (Table 42.5), although many more DNA than RNA viruses have oncogenic potential (12,13).

Individuals in certain occupations may be at enhanced risk for the development of some cancers because of unavoidable exposure to carcinogenic chemicals (9). Perhaps the best-known example of occupationally induced cancer involves exposure to asbestos, which has been conclusively linked with the development of lung, pleural, and peritoneal malignancies. Miners exposed to radon also are at a significantly enhanced risk for the development of lung cancer, as are individuals exposed through their work to soot, tars, hexavalent chromium, and nickel-containing compounds. The aromatic amines β-naphthylamine and 4-aminobiphenyl are known to induce bladder cancer, and exposure to the common organic solvent benzene has been linked to the development of leukemia.

Environmental carcinogens are all around us (Table 42.6). Fortunately, however, individuals can do many things to protect themselves from exposure or from negative consequences of limited exposure. The chemicals deposited in the lungs from inhaling cigarette smoke are the primary cause of lung cancer in the United States, but smokers who quit decrease their risk for this often-fatal cancer by 67% or more after 10 smoke-free years (9). Nonsmokers can protect themselves from the cancer-promoting effects of secondhand smoke by removing themselves from smoke-filled environments, although this is not always as simple as it sounds. Smoking combined with alcohol has a synergistic effect in promoting the development of oral cancer. In addition to quitting smoking, abstaining from alcohol or drinking in moderation is a choice that individuals can make in an effort to decrease their overall risk of developing cancer.

Other measures that patients can take to minimize the risk of cancer from environmental causes include protection from damaging ultraviolet rays through the use of high-SPF sunscreens and the consumption of foods that are low in fat but rich in carotenoids, vitamins A and C, folate, selenium, and/or fiber (9).

GENERAL THERAPEUTIC APPROACHES

Overview

Cancer treatment can be comprised of surgery, radiation, antineoplastic chemotherapy, and/or therapy with biological response modifiers, which stimulate the patient's own immunological defense mechanisms. Surgery and radiation (ionizing, thermal, or photodynamic) are favored for isolated or localized cancers; chemotherapy and biological response modifiers (with or without surgery and/or radiation) are reserved for disseminated or systemic cancers. Chemotherapy also can be used after surgery and/or radiation as an "insurance policy" against microscopic metastatic disease (adjuvant therapy) or before surgery to decrease the size of the mass to be removed (neoadjuvant therapy).

Unfortunately, cancer cells do not simply "lie down" in the face of chemotherapeutic intervention. Rather, these aggressive cells fight back in an attempt to retain their immortality. Some cancer cells acquire resistance to anticancer drugs by down-regulating enzymes essential for drug transport or for the activation of antineoplastic prodrugs or by up-regulating enzymes involved in inactivating biotransformation. As noted previously, other mechanisms of biochemical retaliation include down-regulation of target enzymes, altered drug uptake and efflux mechanisms (e.g., amplification of the gene that encodes for P-glycoprotein or the multidrug resistance–associated protein), inhibition of cellular repair proteins, and apoptosis inhibition (2–4).

Cancer Chemotherapy

The word "antineoplastic" means "against new growth." In general, the mechanism of cytotoxic action for all antineoplastic agents is interference with cellular synthesis or the function of RNA, DNA, and the proteins that sustain life. All antineoplastic agents are poisons, because they are designed to kill cells. An ideal antineoplastic, however, would be both tissue specific (i.e., would only target the diseased organ or physiological system) and cell specific (i.e., would only destroy malignant cells), leaving healthy cells and organ systems alone. Unfortunately, the ideal is not yet the reality, because currently available anticancer drugs are highly and, often, generally toxic, especially for cells with short half-lives. For example, nonspecific destruction of the rapidly dividing cells of the gastrointestinal (GI) tract leads to the severe nausea and vomiting associated with cancer chemotherapy, whereas alopecia and fatigue (as well as susceptibility to infection) are the result of the destruction of rapidly dividing cells in hair follicles and bone marrow, respectively. Factors such as the extent and severity of the disease, individual sensitivity to the antineoplastic mechanism employed by the drugs selected for use, and the kinetics controlling drug transport and cell-cycle specificity all impact the chance for chemotherapeutic success (2).

Because cancer chemotherapy often is given in several courses or "rounds," with an interval of several days or weeks in between to permit attenuation of side effects, three distinct aspects of drug dosing must be considered when determining the impact of antineoplastic therapy on overall patient welfare. First, the dose that ideally should be given per course has been identified for each commonly employed antineoplastic agent but can be altered significantly by individual patient health status (e.g., hepatic, renal, cardiovascular, hematopoietic, pulmonary, and/or other comorbidities), activity/performance status, genetic makeup, and the nature and anticipated severity of side effects. Each round of antineoplastic therapy kills a given percentage of cancer cells with each administration ("cell kill hypothesis"), and the percentage killed rises proportionally with the dose of drug. If chemotherapy can shrink the tumor to 10^4 or fewer cells, normal host defense systems usually are capable of eradicating them (2,3). Therefore, the dose of drug that comes as close as possible to the recommended dose is the goal. Expect significant interpatient variation in response to the same chemotherapeutic regimen secondary to individual genetics, level of debilitation, extent of tissue invasion, critical organ system function (including bone marrow), and past exposure to chemotherapeutic agents.

An ever-growing understanding of genetic polymorphism and its impact on the biosynthesis of target proteins and metabolizing enzymes is helping health care providers make wiser decisions about antineoplastic therapy and drug regimens. The length of the "drug-free" interval is the second important drug-dosing consideration, because a shorter interval (or higher dose intensity—the "one-two punch") is associated with a more aggressive inhibition of tumor growth. Often, however, patients cannot tolerate the debilitating side effects (e.g., myelosuppression) without a prolonged interval between rounds. The advent of genetically engineered biological response modifiers, such as granulocyte colony-stimulating factor, which boosts the ability of bone marrow to produce neutrophils, has had a positive impact on optimizing dosing intensity/density.

Finally, many chemotherapeutic agents produce serious chronic or delayed toxicities that may be irreversible, particularly in heart, lung, and kidneys, which demands that the total cumulative dose be taken into account when designing the regimen. The ultimate balancing act is to give the patient as much antineoplastic drug as normally is recommended in the time frame most likely to kill the greatest percentage of cancer cells without inducing intolerable or life-threatening toxicity in healthy organs and tissues. Armed with the knowledge of the biochemical and/or molecular basis of toxicity, the pharmacist is in an excellent position to employ appropriate pharmacotherapeutic agents to attenuate unavoidable side effects.

One approach for minimizing unwanted toxicity is to employ a chemotherapeutic regimen of several drugs that act by distinct mechanisms and/or precipitate different side effects. Attacking the tumor with different therapeutic "guns" should permit a lower dose of each to be used compared to single-agent therapy, and it should target a larger variety of the mutant cells that comprise the tumor. Minimizing side effect overlap provides a greater chance that the patient will be able to tolerate therapy and accommodate a shorter interval between courses (2,3).

As previously noted, it is essential that the oncology pharmacist be well versed in the pharmacotherapy-based management of severe pain, infection, and the nausea, vomiting, and fatigue associated with chemotherapy. The provision of contemporary and valid drug information to patients and families is essential, as is assistance in helping with the interpretation of information that patients and loved ones secure either through their health care providers or independently (e.g., from the Internet).

THERAPEUTIC CLASSES OF ANTICANCER DRUGS

DNA Cross-Linking Agents (Alkylators and Organic Metallics)

The primary target of DNA cross-linking agents is the actively dividing DNA molecule. The DNA cross-linkers are all extremely reactive electrophilic (δ^+) structures. When encountered, the nucleophilic groups on various DNA bases (particularly, but not exclusively, the N^7 of guanine) readily attack the electrophilic drug, resulting in irreversible alkylation or complexation of the DNA base.

Some DNA alkylating agents, such as the nitrogen mustards and nitrosoureas, are bifunctional, meaning that one molecule of the drug can bind two distinct DNA bases. Most commonly, the alkylated bases are on different DNA molecules, and interstrand DNA cross-linking through two guanine N^7 atoms results. The DNA alkylating antineoplastics are not cell-cycle specific, but they are more toxic to cells in the late G_1 or S phases of the cycle. This is the time when DNA is unwinding and exposing its nucleotides, enhancing the chance that vulnerable DNA functional groups will encounter the electrophilic antineoplastic drug and launch the nucleophilic attack that leads to its own destruction. The DNA alkylators have a great capacity for inducing both mutagenesis and carcinogenesis; in other words, they can promote cancer in addition to treating it.

Organometallic antineoplastics (platinum coordination complexes) also cross-link DNA, and many do so by binding to adjacent guanine nucleotides, called diguanosine dinucleotides, on a single strand of DNA. This leads to intrastrand DNA cross-linking. The anionic phosphate group on a second strand of DNA stabilizes the drug-DNA complex and makes the damage to DNA replication irreversible. Some organometallic agents also damage DNA through interstrand cross-linking.

Nitrogen Mustards and Aziridine-Mediated Alkylators

β α R α β
Cl-CH₂-CH₂-N-CH₂-CH₂-Cl

Bis-β-haloalkylamine

Nitrogen mustards are bis(β-haloalkyl)amines. The term "bis" means two, and the "halo" (short for "halogen") in the nomenclature is invariably chlorine. The two chlorine atoms dramatically decrease the basic strength of the amino nitrogen through a strong negative inductive effect. As a result, the un-ionized conjugate of these drugs predominates at physiological pH. This is intentional, because it is the unionized amine (with its lone pair of electrons) that allows the formation of the highly electrophilic aziridinium ion, which is the reactive DNA-destroying intermediate generated by all true mustards.

Mechanism of Action. The mechanism of action of the nitrogen mustards (14) is depicted in Figure 42.1. In step 1, the lone pair of electrons on the un-ionized amino group conducts an intramolecular nucleophilic attack at the β-carbon of the mustard, displacing chloride ion and forming the highly electrophilic aziridinium ion intermediate, a quaternary amine salt. The carbon atoms of this strained cyclic structure are highly electrophilic

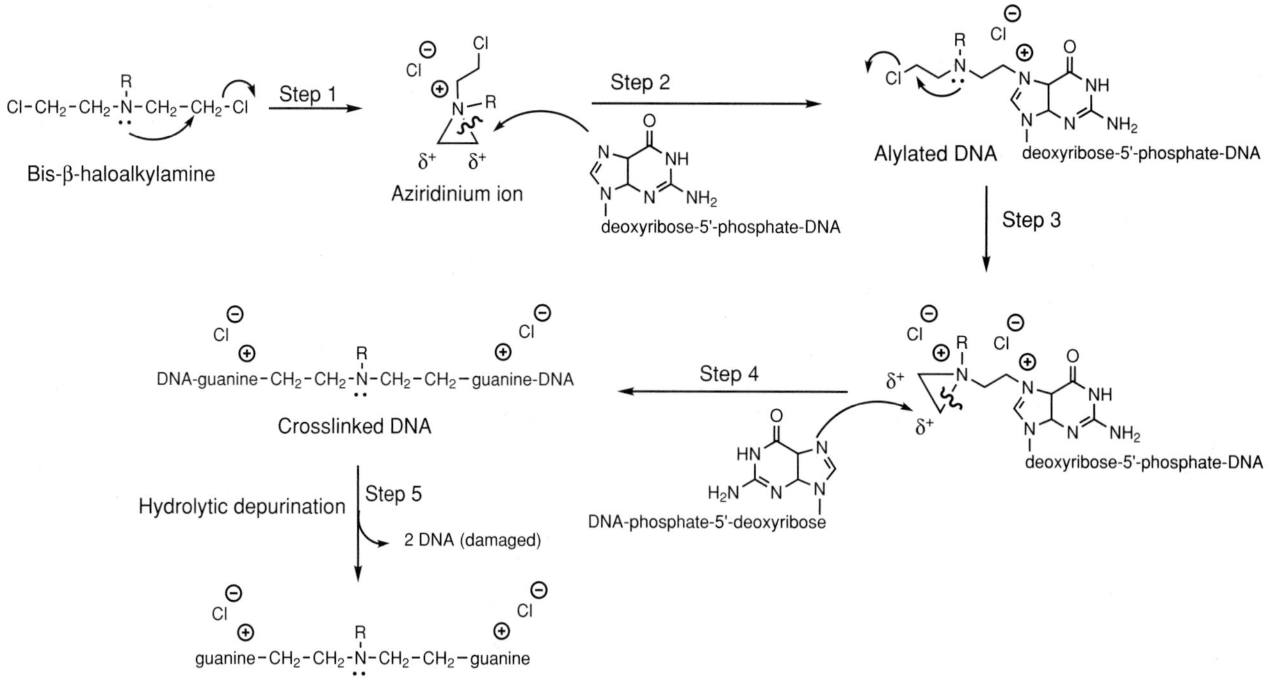

Fig. 42.1. DNA destruction through nitrogen mustard-mediated alkylation.

because of the strong negative inductive effect of the positively charged nitrogen atom.

In step 2, a DNA nucleophile conducts an intermolecular nucleophilic attack, which breaks the aziridine ring and alkylates DNA. Although guanine is the preferred nucleic acid base involved in the alkylation reaction, adenine also is known to react. Of critical importance is the fact that the lone pair of electrons on the mustard nitrogen is regenerated when the aziridine ring cleaves.

Steps 3 and 4 are simply repetitions of steps 1 and 2, respectively, involving the second arm of the mustard and a second molecule of DNA. Ultimately, two molecules of DNA will be cross-linked through the carbon atoms of what was once the nitrogen mustard. Finally, hydrolytic depurination (step 5) cleaves the bound guanine residues from the DNA strand. This is an attempt to liberate the DNA from the mustard's covalent "stranglehold," but the DNA released from this mustard trap is damaged and unable to replicate. Cell death is the inevitable result. If this is happening in a tumor cell, the therapeutic goal has been accomplished. If it is happening in a healthy cell, particularly one with a short half-life, then the patient may experience side effects that can be use-limiting.

STRUCTURE–ACTIVITY RELATIONSHIPS. The structure of nitrogen mustards differs only in the nature of the third group (R) attached to the amino nitrogen. This group, which can be either aliphatic or aromatic, is the prime determinant of chemical reactivity, oral bioavailability, and the nature and extent of side effects.

An aliphatic nitrogen substituent (e.g., CH_3) will push electrons to the amine through σ bonds. This electronic enrichment enhances the nucleophilic character of the lone pair of electrons and increases the speed at which the δ^+ β-carbon of the mustard will be attacked. Whether in a tumor cell or a healthy cell, the aziridinium ion, as soon as it forms, will react with unpaired DNA and/or other cell nucleophiles, such as electron-rich SH, OH, and NH groups of amino acids on enzymes or membrane-bound receptors. The body's water also can react with (and inactivate) the aziridinium ion. The intra- and intermolecular reactions designated as steps 1 through 4 in Figure 42.1 happen so rapidly that almost no chance exists for tissue or cell specificity, which means a greatly increased risk of serious side effects and use-limiting toxicity.

Conversely, an aromatic nitrogen substituent (e.g., phenyl) conjugated with the mustard nitrogen will stabilize the lone pair of electrons through resonance. Resonance delocalization significantly slows the rate of intramolecular nucleophilic attack, aziridinium ion formation, and DNA alkylation. Aromatic mustards have a reactivity sufficiently controlled to permit oral administration and attenuate the severity of side effects. The higher stability also provides the chance for enhanced tissue selectivity by giving the intact mustard time to reach malignant cells before generating the electrophilic aziridinium ion.

Nitrogen mustards can decompose in aqueous media through formation of the inactive dehalogenated diol

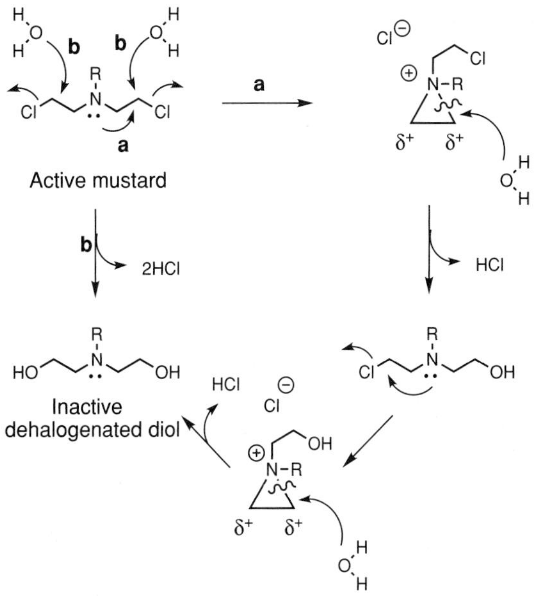

Fig. 42.2. Aqueous decomposition of nitrogen mustards.

shown in Figure 42.2. Both the mustard nitrogen (pathway a) and the oxygen of water (pathway b) can act as nucleophiles to advance this degradative process. The decomposition reactions can be inhibited if the nucleophilic character of these atoms is eliminated through protonation, so buffering solutions to a slightly acidic pH helps to enhance stability in aqueous solution.

SPECIFIC DRUGS

Mechlorethamine Hydrochloride. Mechlorethamine is the only aliphatic nitrogen mustard currently on the U.S. market (Fig. 42.3). Its use is limited by extremely high reactivity, which leads to rapid and nonspecific alkylation of cellular nucleophiles and excessive toxicity. It is a severe vesicant, and if accidental skin contact occurs, the drug must be inactivated with 2% sodium thiosulfate ($Na_2S_2O_3$) solution. This reagent reacts with the mustard to create an inactive, highly ionized, and water-soluble thiosulfate ester that can be washed away (Fig. 42.4). The affected tissue also should be treated with an ice compress for 6 to 12 hours.

Mechlorethamine is marketed in hydrochloride salt form to provide water solubility for intravenous (IV) or intracavitary administration. The strong electron-withdrawing effect of the two chlorine atoms reduces the pK_a of mechlorethamine to 6.1, which gives a ratio of unionized to ionized drug forms of approximately 20:1 at pH 7.4. This agent is too reactive for oral administration and too toxic to use alone. In addition to severe nausea and vomiting, myelosuppression (lymphocytopenia and granulocytopenia), and alopecia, it can cause myelogenous leukemia with extended use because of its mutagenic/carcinogenic effects on bone marrow stem cells. Mechlorethamine is still used in regimens for cancers of the blood (e.g., Hodgkin's disease, chronic myelocytic, or chronic lymphocytic leukemia); fortunately, however, safer and still highly potent antineoplastic agents are now available.

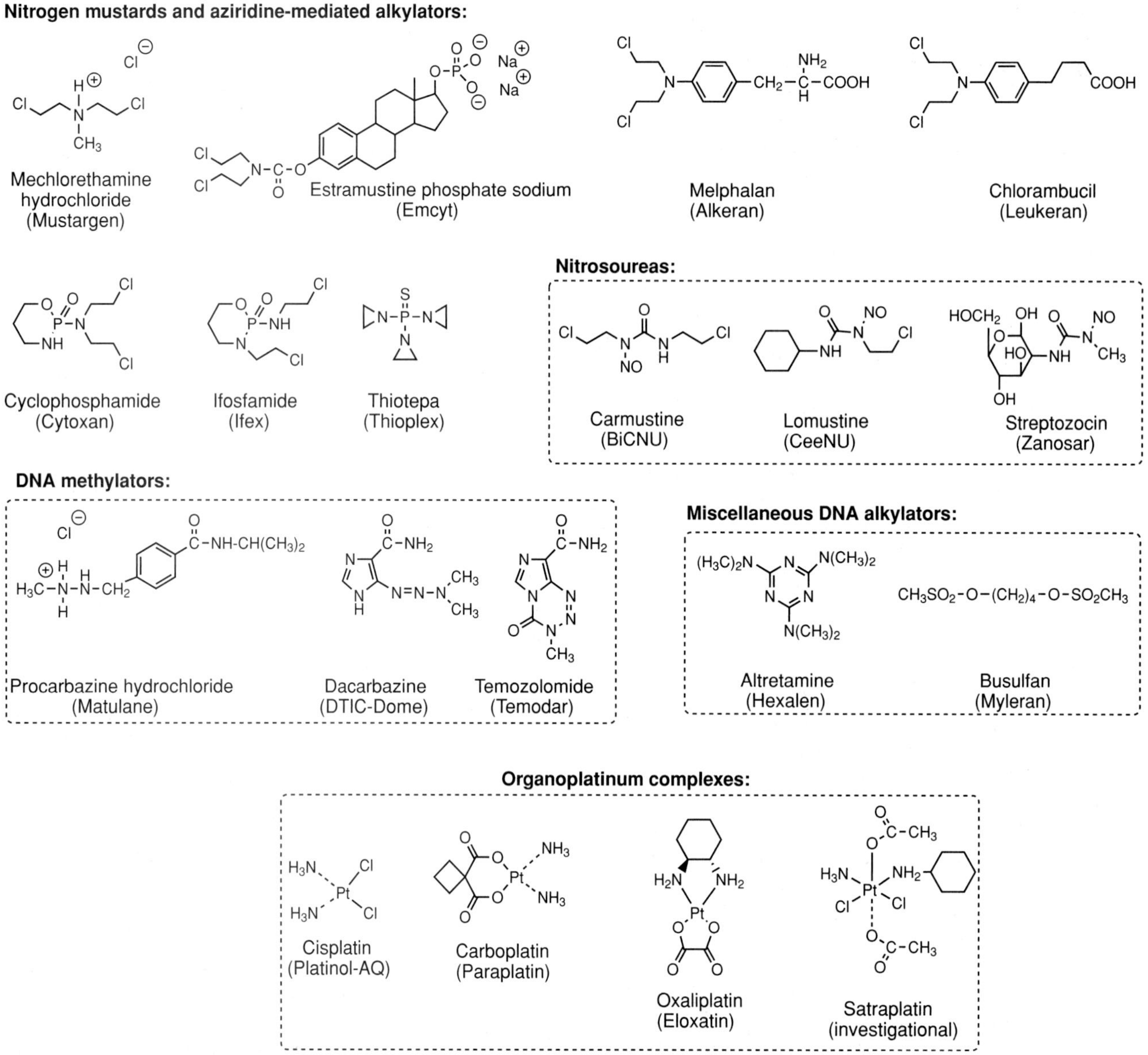

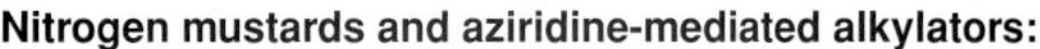

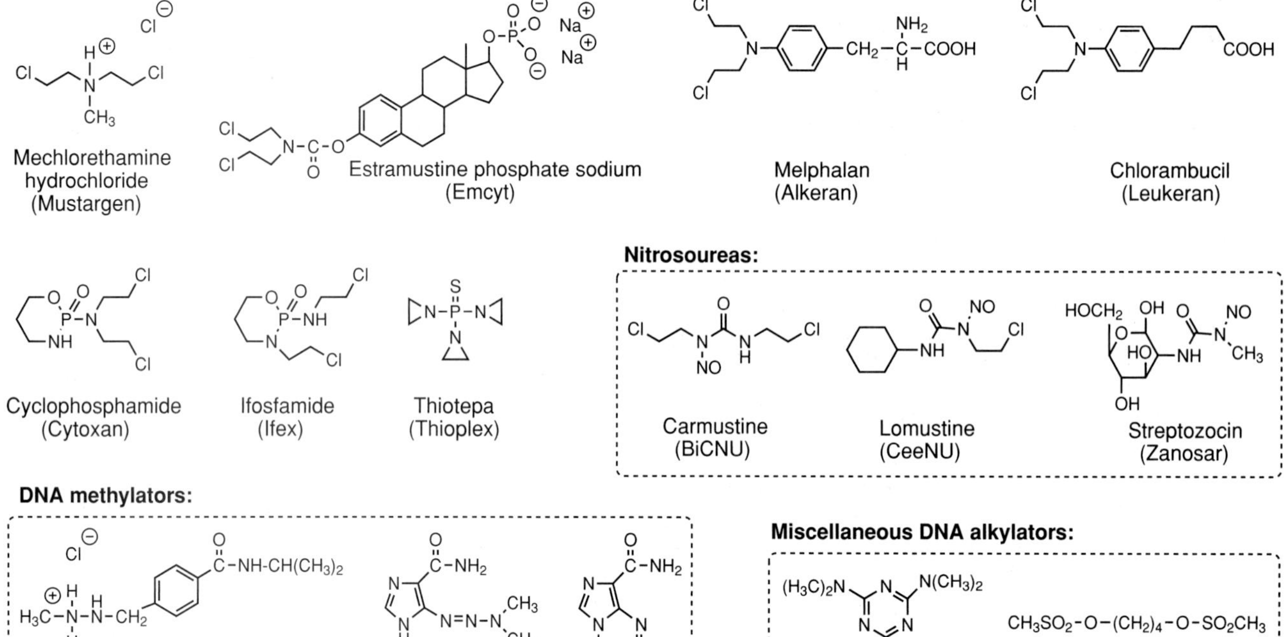

Fig. 42.3. DNA cross-linking agents.

Melphalan. This aromatic mustard, used primarily in the treatment of multiple myeloma, is able to stabilize the lone pair of electrons on the mustard nitrogen through resonance with the conjugated phenyl ring, slowing the formation of the reactive aziridinium ion. The L-isomer of the amino acid Phe was purposefully incorporated into this antineoplastic agent (Fig. 42.3), because naturally occurring L–amino acids are preferentially transported into cells by the action of specific amino acid carrier proteins. It was assumed that the L-Phe would act as a homing device and actively transport the toxic mustard inside the tumor cells, but some studies indicate that melphalan enters cells through facilitated diffusion rather than by active transport (15).

Because the lone pair of electrons of melphalan (and other aromatic mustards) is less reactive, there is a greater opportunity for distribution to cancer cells and a decreased incidence of severe side effects. There is a lower incidence of nausea and vomiting compared to mechlorethamine, but patients still experience myelosuppression, which can

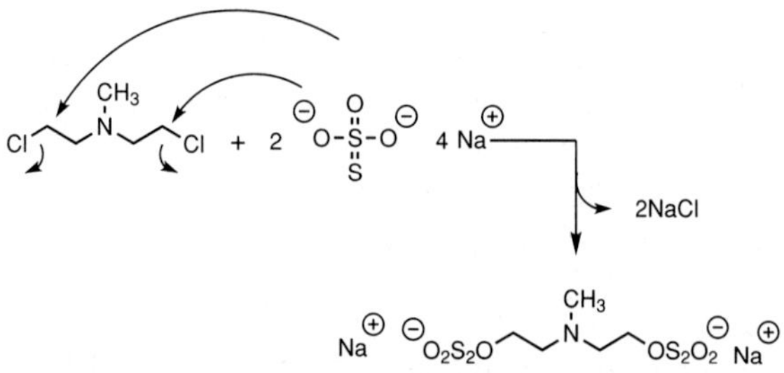

Fig. 42.4. Mechlorethamine inactivation by sodium thiosulfate.

be severe. This drug also is mutagenic and can induce leukemia.

Melphalan is orally active, but absorption can be erratic. Absorption is decreased with food, but dosing regimens do not demand an empty stomach. The drug can be formulated for IV administration, but the risk of serious side effects is higher. Melphalan distributes into body water, so toxicity can be pronounced in dehydrated patients or in those with renal dysfunction. Dehydration can be corrected, but dosage adjustments should be considered in patients with renal disease.

Chlorambucil. Like melphalan, chlorambucil (Fig. 42.3) has good oral bioavailability, which is decreased in the presence of food, and the potential to induce nonlymphocytic leukemia. This drug is active intact and also undergoes β-oxidation to provide an active phenylacetic acid mustard metabolite, which is responsible for some of the observed antineoplastic activity. It is used in the palliative treatment of chronic lymphocytic leukemia, malignant lymphoma, and Hodgkin's disease.

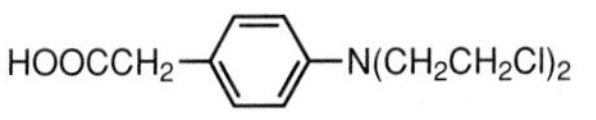

Phenylacetic acid mustard (an active chlorambucil metabolite)

Estramustine Phosphate Sodium. This resonance-stabilized, mustard-like antineoplastic agent utilizes an estradiol carrier (Fig. 42.3) to selectively deliver drug to steroid-dependent prostate tissue, and its use is limited to the palliative treatment of progressive prostate cancer. The essential 17β-OH group has been esterified with phosphoric acid, and the C_3-phenol has been carbamylated. The body still, however, transports the basic steroidal pharmacophore into cells. The ionized sodium phosphate ester of the active 17β-OH group makes the compound water soluble and able to distribute in the blood. The ester is readily cleaved during absorption to provide the active 17β-OH.

The nitrogen mustard moiety of estramustine is incorporated into a carbamate group made from the C_3-phenolic OH group of the estradiol structure. The resonance and negative induction capabilities of the carbamate extensively delocalize the lone pair of electrons on the mustard nitrogen. This stabilizes the lone pair in the same qualitative way that conjugation with the phenyl ring of melphalan and chlorambucil does, and it is very slow to attack the electrophilic β-carbon. Because the formation of the aziridinium ion is significantly delayed, DNA alkylation is controlled, and the drug can be given orally. Estramustine is considered to be a weak alkylating agent, and its primary mechanism of antineoplastic action actually is inhibition of cellular mitosis.

The carbamate group containing the mustard moiety can be cleaved in vivo to generate estradiol (Fig. 42.5). This is obviously not desired, because the chemically reactive mustard is being detached from the carrier molecule designed to take it to the prostatic tumor cell. The

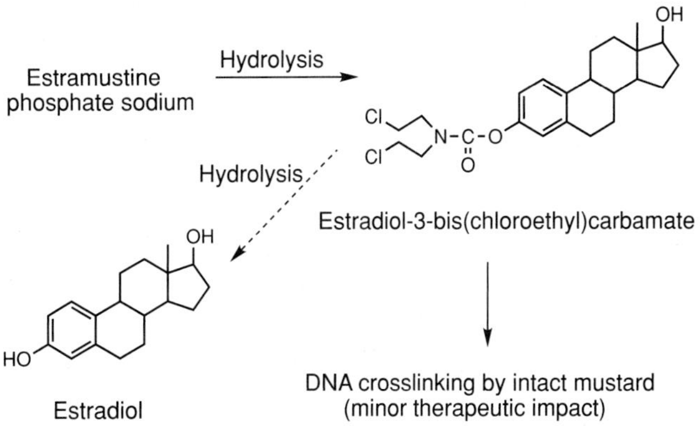

Fig. 42.5. Estramustine metabolism.

normal metabolites of estradiol (conjugates of estradiol and estriol) are found in the feces. The formation of active estrogens is why this drug is not used to treat estrogen-dependent tumors (e.g., estrogen-dependent breast cancer). The liberated estradiol also can increase blood pressure and induce blood clots, leading to myocardial infarction. Fortunately, the myocardial infarctions usually are nonfatal, but the drug should be used with extreme caution in men who are predisposed to clotting disorders or who have a history of cerebral vascular disease or coronary artery disease. Hepatotoxicity also is associated with estramustine use.

Cyclophosphamide. Cyclophosphamide (Fig. 42.3) is a prodrug, antineoplastic agent requiring activation by metabolic and nonmetabolic processes (Fig. 42.6). The initial metabolic step is mediated primarily by CYP2B6 (and, to a much lower extent, by CYP3A4) and involves hydroxylation of the oxazaphosphorine ring to generate a carbinolamine (16). This hydroxylation reaction must occur before the molecule will be transported into cells. CYP3A4 (but not CYP2B6) also catalyzes an inactivating N-dechloroethylation reaction, which yields highly nephrotoxic and neurotoxic chloroacetaldehyde (16). Chloroacetaldehyde toxicity is accompanied by glutathione depletion, indicating that, as expected, this electrophilic by-product alkylates Cys residues of critical cell proteins (17). Alkylation of Lys, adenosine, and cytidine residues also is possible.

The CYP-generated carbinolamine undergoes nonenzymatic hydrolysis to provide the aldophosphamide either in the bloodstream or inside the cell. If this hydrolysis occurs extracellularly, the aldophosphamide is still able to penetrate cell membranes to reach the intracellular space. Once inside the cell, acrolein (a highly reactive α,β-unsaturated aldehyde) splits off, generating phosphoramide mustard. With a pK_a of 4.75, the mustard will be persistently anionic at intracellular pH and trapped inside the cell.

The fate of phosphoramide mustard is varied. Most of it cyclizes to form the quaternary aziridinium ion, which alkylates DNA in the manner of all mustards. Some of it will decompose, losing phosphoric acid (H_3PO_4)

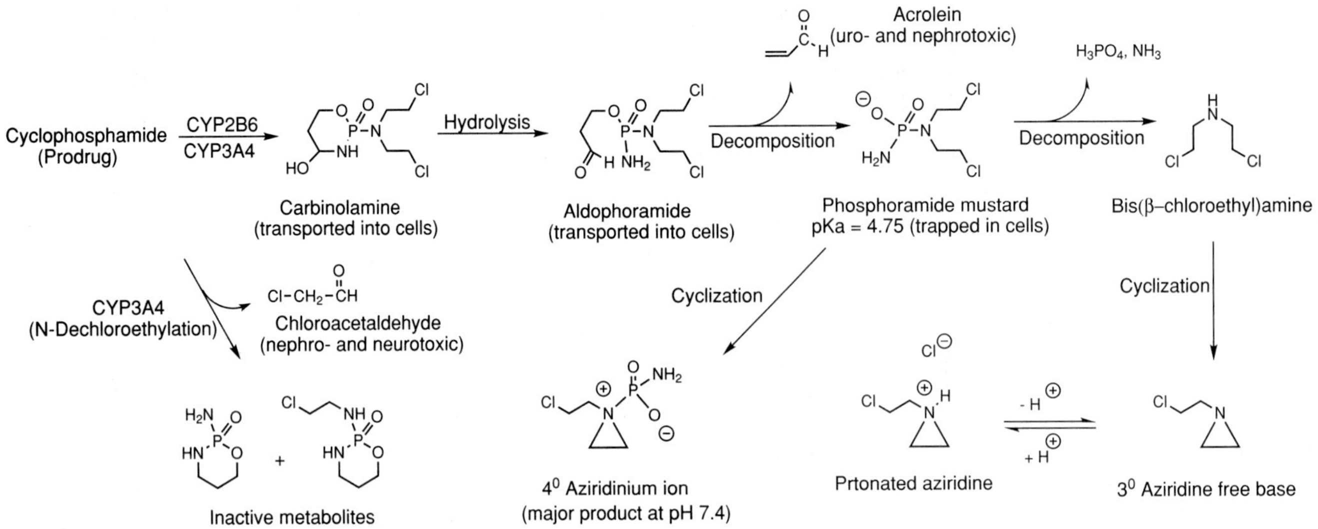

Fig. 42.6. Cyclophosphamide metabolism.

and ammonia (NH_3) and leaving the naked bis(β-chloroethyl)amine mustard. This secondary amine cyclizes in a manner similar to the tertiary phosphoramide mustard, forming a tertiary aziridine (rather than a quaternary aziridinium) species. The free tertiary aziridine can protonate at intracellular pH to provide the cationic aziridine species, which is in equilibrium with the free-base form. Some electrophilic character is lost, but the carbon atoms in both forms are still δ^+ enough to attract DNA nucleophiles, albeit less vigorously. The net result of this attack is DNA alkylation and cell death.

The need for metabolic activation in the liver means lowered GI toxicity and less nonspecific toxicity for cyclophosphamide compared with other DNA alkylating agents, but cyclophosphamide is not without its toxic effects. Acrolein, generated during the formation of phosphoramide mustard, is a very electrophilic and highly reactive species and causes extensive damage to cells of the kidney and bladder. Potentially fatal acute hemorrhagic cystitis is a significant risk of cyclophosphamide therapy.

Bladder damage from acrolein results from attack by Cys sulfhydryl groups at the δ^+ terminal carbon of the acrolein structure, resulting in renal cell alkylation and cell death. Physiological results can include severe hemorrhage, sclerosis, and on occasion, induction of bladder cancer. Acrolein also damages the nephron, particularly when used in high doses, in children, in patients with only one kidney, or when coadministered with other nephrotoxic agents (e.g., cisplatin). To minimize the risk of bladder toxicity from acrolein, fluids should be forced and the bladder irrigated. Mesna (Mesnex) also is available as adjuvant therapy in case of overt toxicity or as a prophylactic protectant. A sulfhydryl reagent, mesna competes with Cys residues for the alkylating arolein, as shown in Figure 42.7. Mesna concentrates in the bladder and will prevent damage to those cells. It does not concentrate to any appreciable extent in the nephron and, therefore, is not good protection against cyclophosphamide-induced nephrotoxicity.

As effective as mesna is for preventing acrolein-induced urotoxicity, it does little to spare the kidney and nerve cells from chloroacetaldehyde, the other toxic by-product of cyclophosphamide metabolism (18). Luckily, only approximately 10% of a standard dose of cyclophosphamide undergoes the dechloroethylation reaction, although this percentage can rise if higher doses are used (16).

Cyclophosphamide most commonly is used in combination with other antineoplastic agents to treat a wide range of neoplasms, including leukemias and malignant lymphomas, multiple myeloma, ovarian adenocarinoma, and breast cancer. The drug is metabolized in the liver

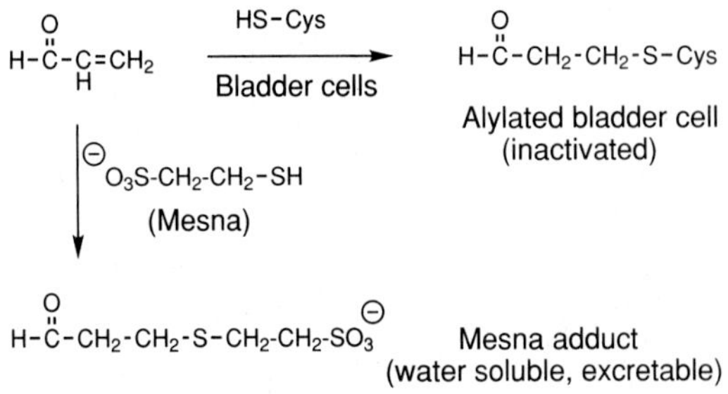

Fig. 42.7. Sulfhydryl alkylation by acrolein.

and is eliminated via the kidney, with approximately 15% of a given dose being excreted unchanged. Doses should be reduced in patients with levels of creatinine clearance less than 30 mL/min. Interestingly, hepatic dysfunction does not seem to alter metabolism of this drug, but caution should be exercised in patients with inhibited cytochrome P450 (CYP450) enzymes or with a combination of factors that could negatively impact drug activation/inactivation pathways.

Ifosfamide. This cyclophosphamide analogue has the two arms of the mustard on different nitrogen atoms (Fig. 42.3). Ifosfamide also requires metabolic activation (Fig. 42.8), but this time it is the CYP3A4 isoform that converts the majority of the dose to the carbinolamine, with CYP2B6 taking on a minor, supporting role (19). Because ifosfamide has a lower affinity for the hydroxylating CYP3A4 and CYP2B6 enzymes, presumably as a result of steric hindrance, bioactivation proceeds at a slower rate (20). Doses three- to fourfold higher than cyclophosphamide are required to achieve the same antineoplastic result.

Unlike cyclophosphamide, dechloroethylation is a significant metabolic pathway for ifosfamide, and approximately 45% of a standard dose will undergo this inactivating and toxicity-inducing biotransformation. CYP3A4 catalyzes approximately 70% of ifosfamide dechloroethylation, with CYP2B6 taking care of the remainder (16). The fact that this reaction can occur in the renal tubule, generating chloroacetaldehyde right in the nephron, contributes to its significantly higher nephrotoxicity (20). Ultimately, both chloroalkyl groups are lost before the compound is excreted.

It bears repeating that there is a significantly higher risk of bladder toxicity and nephrotoxicity with ifosfamide than with cyclophosphamide. This is because:

- Significantly more chloroacetaldehyde is generated through CYP3A4- and CYP2B6-mediated dechloroethylation. This biotransformation can take place in the nephron, which places the toxic by-product right where it will do the most damage.
- Ifosfamide is more water soluble than cyclophosphamide and will concentrate in the renal system. Between 20 and 50% of a dose is excreted unchanged in the urine.
- Acrolein also is formed when this alkylator generates the cytotoxic aziridiniun ion.
- Higher doses must be administered to achieve the same degree of antineoplastic action, so more molecules of acrolein and chloroacetaldehyde will be produced.

Because acrolein is formed, the same precautions against hemorrhagic cystitis that were previously outlined for cyclophosphamide must be taken: hydrate well, irrigate thoroughly, and administer with mesna. As previously stated, mesna will not prevent chloroacetaldehyde-induced toxicity.

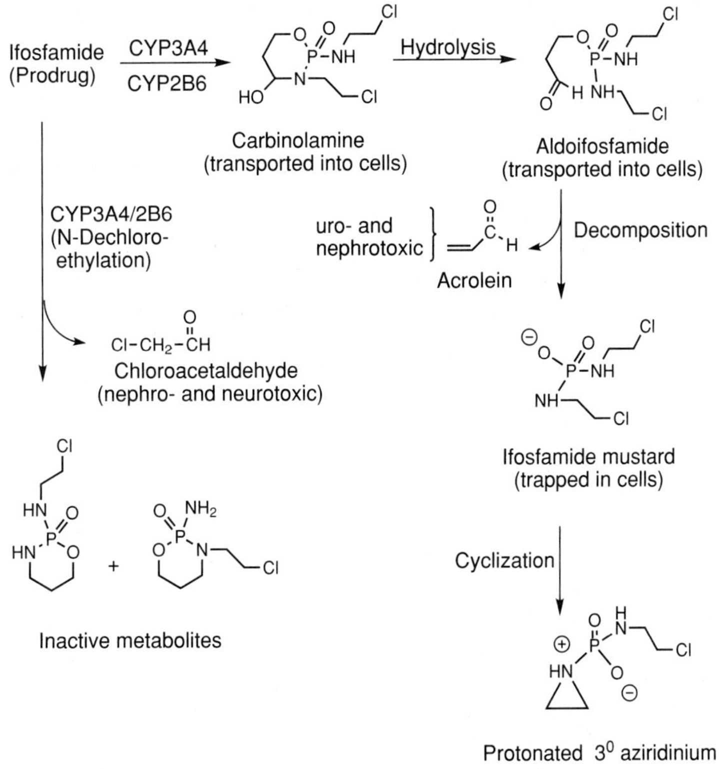

Fig. 42.8. Ifosfamide metabolism.

Ifosamide currently is used as "third-line" therapy against testicular cancer, although it also has shown activity in a number of solid tumors and hematologic cancers. Patients on ifosfamide (but not cyclophosphamide) commonly exhibit central nervous system (CNS) toxicity. In severe forms, CNS depression can progress to coma and death.

Thiotepa. Thiotepa (Fig. 42.3), a tertiary aziridine, is less reactive than quaternary aziridinium compounds and is classified as a weak alkylator. It is possible for the nitrogen atoms to be protonate before reacting with DNA (a positively charged aziridine is more reactive than the un-ionized aziridine), but the electron-withdrawing effect of the sulfur atom decreases the pK_a to approximately six, which keeps the percentage ionized at pH 7.4 relatively low. Thiotepa undergoes oxidative desulfuration, forming an active cytotoxic metabolite known as TEPA (triethylenephosphoramide). This antineoplastic agent is most commonly employed in the treatment of ovarian and breast cancers, as well as papillary carcinoma of the bladder.

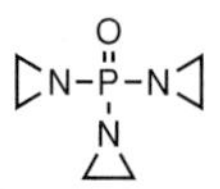

Triethylenephosphoramide
(an active thiotepa metabolite)

Thiotepa and the TEPA metabolite readily enter the CNS after systemic administration, leading to dizziness, blurred vision, and headaches. More critically, these agents also are severe myelosuppressants and can induce leukopenia, thrombocytopenia, and anemia. Patients treated with thiotepa are at high risk for infection and hemorrhage. Oral absorption is unreliable, so thiotepa is given IV or can be instilled intravesically in the treatment of bladder cancer. Even when administered locally in bladder cancer, high levels of this lipophilic drug reach the systemic circulation, resulting in bone marrow depression. Patients have died from myelosuppression after intravesically administered thiotepa. The drug also causes damage to the hepatic and renal systems. Dose and/or administration frequency should be increased slowly, even if the initial response to the drug is sluggish, or unacceptable toxicity may result.

Nitrosoureas

MECHANISM OF ACTION. The nitrosoureas are unstable structures that decompose readily in the aqueous environment of the cell. Nonenzymatic fragmentation is stimulated by the loss of proton from the urea moiety. Cyclization of the resultant anion to an unstable oxazolidine (pathway A) is followed by decomposition to vinyl diazotic acid and a substituted isocyanate, both of which release a gaseous fragment (nitrogen and carbon dioxide, respectively) to generate cytotoxic electrophiles (Fig. 42.9). Vinyl carbocation, acetaldehyde, and 2-chloroethylamine generated from the 2-chloroethylisocyanate moiety of carmustine are all capable of alkylating DNA in the standard manner (21). A second decomposition mechanism (pathway B) ultimately produces an electrophilic 2-chloroethylcarbocation capable of DNA alkylation at guanine-N^7 and O^6 as well as an isocyanate that can carbamylate amino acid residues (e.g., Lys).

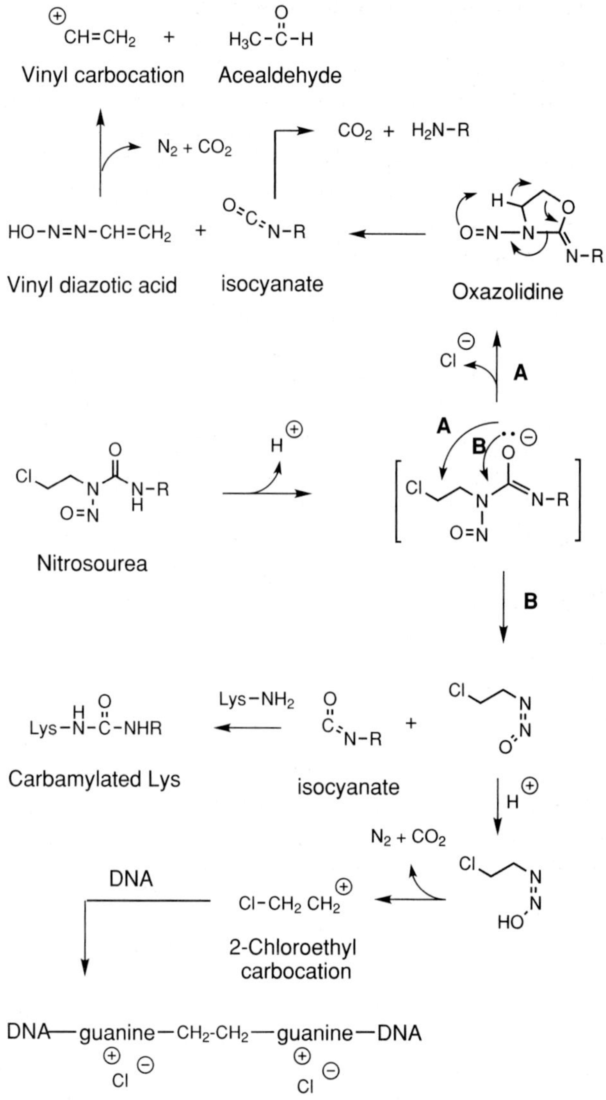

Fig. 42.9. Nitrosourea decomposition to active electrophiles.

SPECIFIC DRUGS

Carmustine and Lomustine. Carmustine and lomustine are both highly lipophilic chloroethylnitrosourea analogues marketed for use in brain tumors and Hodgkin's disease. Carmustine also has shown value in the treatment of non-Hodgkin's lymphoma and multiple myeloma, and it is given IV or incorporated into biodegradable wafers that are implanted directly into the CNS after tumor resection. The high lipophilicity of carmustine precludes a totally aqueous IV formulation, and the drug is administered in 10% ethanol. Although carmustine degrades within 15 minutes of IV administration, lomustine is stable enough for oral use and is marketed in capsule form. Carmustine also can decompose in vitro if exposed to temperatures around 90°F. Pure carmustine is a low-melting solid, but the decomposed product is an oil and, therefore, is readily detected. Vials of carmustine that appear oily should be discarded.

Both carmustine and lomustine can induce thrombocytopenia and leukopenia, leading to hemorrhage and massive infection. Acute (as well as potentially fatal delayed) pulmonary toxicity also is a risk. Pulmonary toxicity is dose-related, and individuals who received the drug in childhood or early adolescence are at higher risk for the delayed reaction. The grand mal seizures that are possible from the wafer formulation of carmustine appear to result from the wafer rather than from the nitrosourea.

Streptozocin. The glucopyranose moiety of streptozocin confers both islet cell specificity and high water solubility to this nitrosourea-based antineoplastic. As a result, it is used exclusively in metastatic islet cell carcinoma of the pancreas and is administered IV in D5W or normal saline. Lacking the 2-chloroethyl substituent of carmustine and lomustine, it is much less reactive as a DNA alkylating agent, and myelotoxicity is relatively rare but not unknown. Cumulative, dose-related renal toxicity can be severe or fatal, however, and 67% of patients receiving this drug will exhibit some kidney-related pathology. Good hydration is essential to successful therapy, and kidney function should be monitored weekly.

Procarbazine and Triazenes

MECHANISM OF ACTION. Procarbazine and the triazenes dacarbazine and temozolomide act by different mechanisms, but they all exert an antineoplastic effect through the O^6-methylation of guanine nucleotides. O^6-methylguanine pairs preferentially with thymine, and these "mispairs" prompt point mutations during subsequent DNA replication cycles and trigger cell destruction through the activation of the normal postreplication mismatch repair (MMR) system. Patients who are able to repair this damage through the action of O^6-alkylguanine-DNA-alkyltransferase, which transfers the offending CH_3 group to a Cys residue on the alkyltransferase protein, will exhibit resistance to these agents, whereas those who underexpress this protein should respond well (22). Because the alkyltransferase is irreversibly inactivated in the DNA rescue process, enzyme depletion (and subsequent loss of DNA repair capability) is a significant risk.

Procarbazine metabolism involves CYP1A and CYP2B enzymes (23), and DNA alkylation operates through a free radical mechanism (Fig. 42.10). The major degradation pathway involves benzylic oxidation of azoprocarbazine, producing methylhydrazine that generates a methyl radical through an unstable diazene intermediate (24,25) In addition to O^6, the reactive methyl radical formed can alkylate the C^8 and N^7 positions of guanine. In contrast, the triazenes methylate DNA guanine via diazomethane and/or methyl carbocation generated in situ. Although temozolomide is converted to the diazomethane precursor 3-methyl-(triazen-l-yl) imidazole-4-carboxamide (MTIC) through nonenzymatic mechanisms, the conversion of dacarbazine to MTIC depends on the action of CYP1A1 and CYP1A2 enzymes, with a smaller contribution by CYP2E1 (Fig. 42.11) (23,26). The O^6 and N^7 positions of guanine are the most vulnerable to triazene methylation.

SPECIFIC DRUGS

Procarbazine. This methyl radical generator is utilized predominantly in the treatment of Hodgkin's disease. It is administered as part of a multidrug regimen that also includes a nitrogen mustard (mechlorethamine), a mitosis inhibitor (vincristine), and prednisone. It is administered as capsules and is well absorbed after oral administration. Procarbazine is extensively metabolized in the liver, and 70% of an administered dose is excreted in the urine as N-isopropylterephthalamic acid (Fig. 42.10). In addition to

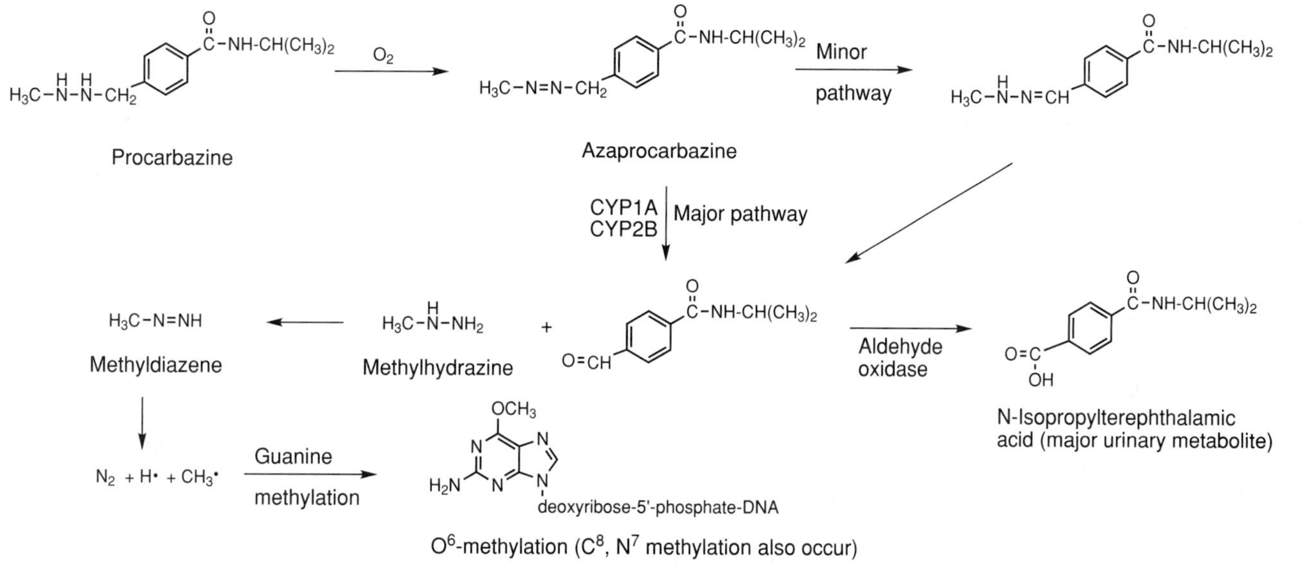

O^6-methylation (C^8, N^7 methylation also occur)

Fig. 42.10. Procarbazine metabolism and mechanism of action.

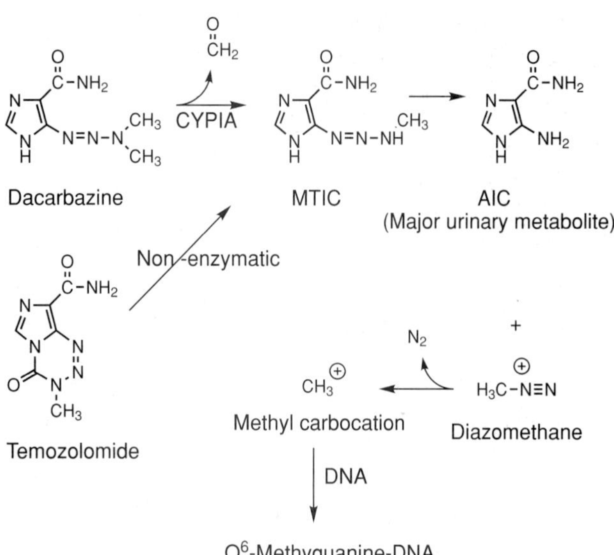

Fig. 42.11. Metabolic activation of triazenes.

methylating DNA guanine residues, it is proposed to inhibit the de novo synthesis of proteins and nucleic acids. Procarbazine inhibits monoamine oxidase, leading to several significant and potentially fatal drug–drug and drug–food interactions. Facial flushing and other disulfiram-like symptoms are noted when alcohol is concomitantly consumed, because the drug also inhibits enzymes involved in ethanol metabolism.

Dacarbazine. This DNA methylating agent is administered IV as a single agent in the treatment of malignant melanoma and in combination with other agents in the treatment of metastatic melanoma. Approximately 40% of the drug is excreted unchanged, but both the 5-aminoimidazole-4-carboxamide (AIC, formed through the action of CYP1A enzymes) and the carboxylic acid (AIC hydrolysis product) are major urinary metabolites (Fig. 42.11). Leukopenia and thrombocytopenia are the most common side effects and may be fatal. Patients also are at risk for hepatotoxicity, including hepatocellular necrosis.

Temozolomide. This imidazolotetrazine derivative is administered orally in capsule form for the treatment of glioblastoma multiforme or in patients with anaplastic astrocytoma who have not responded to procarbazine or the nitrosoureas. Oral absorption is rapid and complete. The CYP450 enzymes are not extensively involved in temozolomide metabolism, and less than 6% of the drug is excreted unchanged in the urine. Women clear the drug less effectively than men and have a higher incidence of severe neutropenia and thrombocytopenia in the initial therapy cycle. Food decreases temozolomide absorption, and myelosuppression is the most significant adverse effect.

Miscellaneous DNA Alkylating Agents

ALTRETAMINE. This unique structure (Fig. 42.3) is believed to damage tumor cells through the production of the weakly alkylating species formaldehyde, a product of CYP450-mediated N-demethylation. Administered orally, altretamine is extensively metabolized on first pass, producing primarily mono- and didemethylated metabolites. Additional demethylation reactions occur in tumor cells, releasing formaldehyde in situ before the drug is excreted in the urine. The carbinolamine (methylol) intermediates of CYP450-mediated metabolism also can generate electrophilic iminium species that are capable of reacting covalently with DNA guanine and cytosine residues as well as protein (Fig. 42.12). Iminium-mediated DNA cross-linking and DNA-protein interstrand cross-linking, mediated through both the iminium intermediate and formaldehyde, have been demonstrated (27,28), although the significance of DNA cross-linking on altretamine antitumor activity is uncertain. Resistance to altretamine has been shown to parallel resistance to formaldehyde-induced cytotoxicity (27). Its use currently is restricted to patients with ovarian cancer who have not responded to organoplatinum therapy. The toxicities induced by altretamine are GI, neurologic, and hematologic in nature.

BUSULFAN. Chemically, busulfan is classified as an alkyl sulfonate (Fig. 42.3). One or both of the methylsulfonate ester moieties can be displaced by the nucleophilic N^7 of guanine, leading to monoalkylated and cross-linked DNA, as shown in Figure 42.13. The extent of alkyl sulfonate–mediated DNA interstrand cross-linking has been shown to vary with the length of the alkyl chain between sulfonate esters, with the tetramethylene-containing busulfan showing less interstrand cross-linking capability than hexamethylene, methylene, or octamethylene analogues (29).

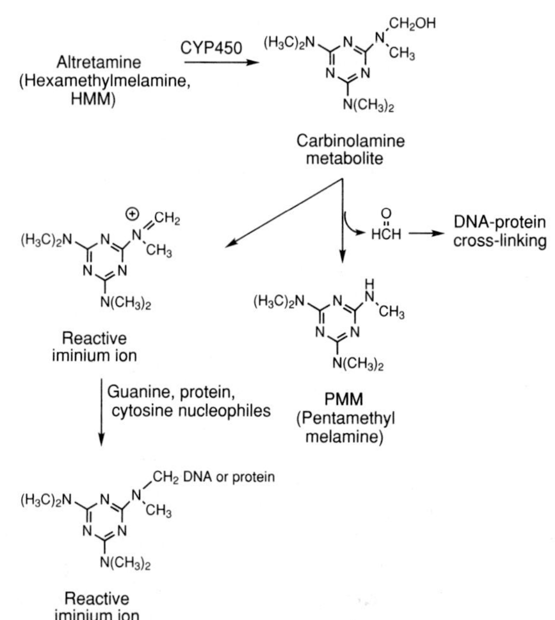

Fig. 42.12. Altretamine metabolism and mechanism of action.

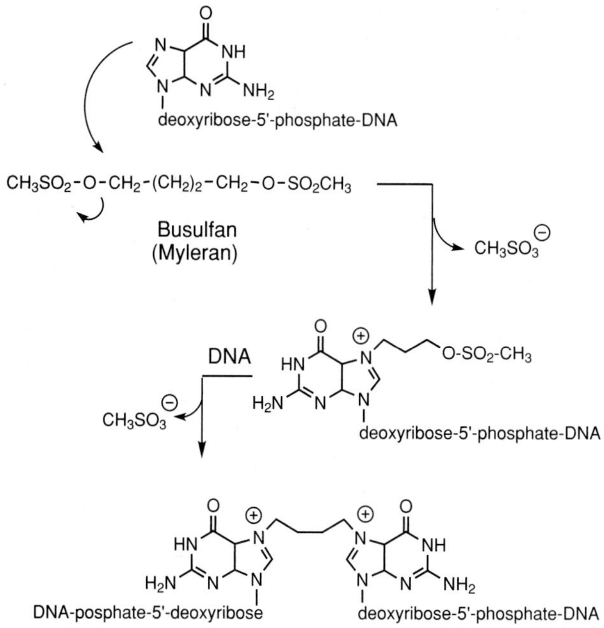

Fig. 42.13. Busulfan-mediated DNA alkylation.

Intrastrand cross-linking also occurs, preferentially at 5′-GA-3′ but also at 5′-GG-3′ sequences (30). Alkylation of Cys sulfhydryl groups is yet another mechanism of cytotoxicity. Busulfan is used in the treatment of chronic myelogenous leukemia and can be administered either orally or by IV infusion. Serious bone marrow hypoplasia and myelosuppression are possible with this agent, and recovery from busulfan-induced pancytopenia can take up to 2 years.

Organoplatinum Complexes

Mechanism of Action. Organoplatinum antineoplastic agents contain an electron-deficient metal atom that acts as a magnet for electron-rich DNA nucleophiles. Like nitrogen mustards, organoplatinum complexes are bifunctional and can accept electrons from two DNA nucleophiles. Intrastrand cross-links most frequently occur between adjacent guanine residues referred to as diguanosine dinucleotides (60–65%) or adjacent guanine and adenine residues (25–30%). Interstrand cross-linking, which occurs much less frequently (1–3%), usually involves guanine and adenine bases (31). All the currently marketed organoplatinum anticancer agents are Pt(II) complexes with square-planar geometry, although an octahedral Pt(IV) complex currently is undergoing clinical trials.

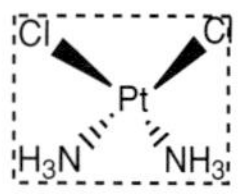

Cisplatin (square planar geometry)

Platinum is inherently electron deficient, but the net charge on the organometallic complex is zero because of the contribution of electrons by two of the four ligands bound to the parent structure. Most commonly, the electron-donating ligand is chloride. Before reacting with DNA, the electron-donating ligands most commonly are displaced through nucleophilic attack by cellular water. When the displaced ligands are chloride anions (e.g., in cisplatin), the chloride-poor environment of the tumor cell facilitates the process, driving the generation of the active, cytotoxic hydrated forms (Fig. 42.14). Because the original ligands leave the metal with their electrons, the hydrated organoplatinum molecule has a net positive charge (32).

The hydrated platinum analogues are readily attacked by DNA nucleophiles (e.g., the N^7 of adjacent guanine residues) because of the net positive charge that has

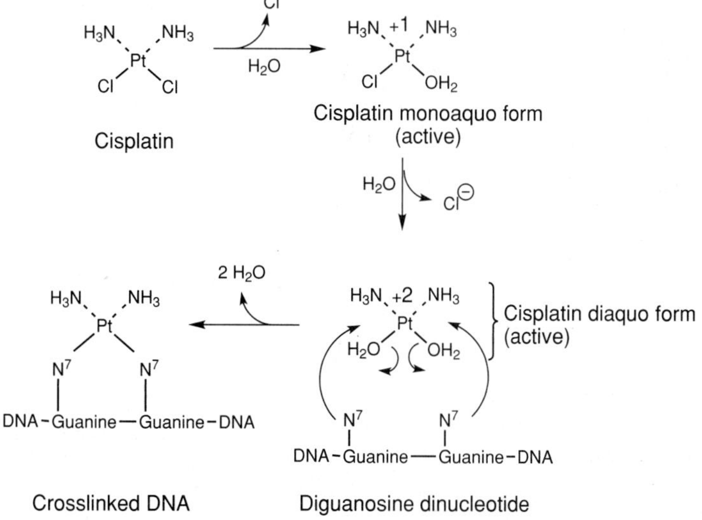

Fig. 42.14. Cisplatin activation and DNA cross-linking.

been regained on the Pt atom (Fig. 42.14). The DNA bases become coordinated with the platinum, and in the *cis* configuration, DNA repair mechanisms are unable to correct the damage. The net result is a major change in DNA conformation such that base pairs that normally engage in hydrogen-bond formation are not permitted to interact. The two ammine ligands of the complex are bound irreversibly to the Pt atom through very strong coordinate covalent bonds. They cannot be displaced by DNA nucleophiles, but they do stabilize the cross-linked DNA-platinum complex by forming strong ion–dipole bonds with the anionic phosphate residues on DNA.

SPECIFIC DRUGS

Cisplatin. The simplest of the organometallic antineoplastic agents, cisplatin is utilized IV in the treatment of metastatic testicular and ovarian cancer and advanced bladder cancer. It is rapidly hydrated, resulting in a short plasma half-life of less than 30 minutes. It is eliminated predominantly via the kidney, but approximately 10% of a given dose undergoes biliary excretion. It is highly nephrotoxic and can cause significant damage to the renal tubules, especially in patients with preexisting kidney disease or one kidney or who are concurrently receiving other nephrotoxic drugs (e.g., cyclophosphamide or ifosfamide). Dosages should be reduced in any of the above situations. Clearance decreases with chronic therapy, and toxicities can manifest at a late date.

To proactively protect patients against kidney damage, patients should be hydrated with chloride-containing solutions. Saline or mannitol diuretics can be administered to promote continuous excretion of the drug and its hydrated analogues. Sodium thiosulfate, which accumulates in the renal tubules, also has been used to neutralize active drug in the kidneys in an effort to avoid nephrotoxicity (Fig. 42.15). The reaction of sodium thiosulfate with cisplatin in the serum is much slower, because the drug does not concentrate there and what is there is very strongly bound to serum proteins. The very strong protein binding explains why dialysis, even when prolonged, cannot rescue patients from cisplatin toxicity. Myelosuppression and ototoxicity, including irreversible hearing loss, also can occur with cisplatin use. Cisplatin is a very severe emetogen, and vomiting almost always will occur unless antiemetic therapy is coadministered.

Cisplatin and the other organoplatinum anticancer agents react with aluminum and cannot be administered through aluminum-containing needles. The drug is photosensitive, is packaged in amber bottles, and must be protected from light.

Carboplatin. Carboplatin (Fig. 42.3), another square planar Pt(II) complex, forms the same cytotoxic hydrated intermediate as cisplatin but does so at a slower rate, making it a less potent chemotherapeutic agent. The ultimate damage done to cells as a result of carboplatin use, however, approaches that of cisplatin. The plasma half-life of carboplatin is 3 hours, and the drug is less extensively bound to serum proteins. Excretion is predominantly renal, and doses must be reduced in patients with kidney disease. Suppression of platelets and white blood cells is the most significant toxic reaction of carboplatin use. This drug induces fewer nonhematological toxicities (e.g., emesis, nephrotoxicity, and ototoxicity) compared to cisplatin, and it is approved for use only in the treatment of ovarian cancer. Unlabeled uses include combination therapy in lung, testicular, and head and neck cancers.

Oxaliplatin. This Pt(II) complex loses oxalic acid as oxalate anion ($^{-}$OOC-COO^{-}) in vivo to form the mono- and dihydrated diaminocyclohexane (DACH) platinum analogues shown in Figure 42.16. The *trans*-(*R*,*R*)-DACH structure serves as the carrier for the cytotoxic hydrated platinum and extends into the major groove of DNA when the DNA-Pt complex forms (33). Hydrophobic DNA intrusion is believed to contribute to the cytotoxicity of this organometallic agent. Oxaliplatin engages primarily in intrastrand cross-linking with diguanosine dinucleotides, adjacent A-G nucleotides, and guanines that are separated by one nucleotide (G-X-G). Interstrand cross-linking, although less common, also occurs.

The adduct formed between oxaliplatin and DNA diguanosine dinucleotides is conformationally distinct from the adduct formed with cisplatin. Specifically, whereas the cisplatin diguanosine dinucleotide adduct bends the DNA by 60 to 80° and presents a relatively wide minor groove, the oxaliplatin adduct produces a 31° bend with a comparatively narrow minor groove (34).

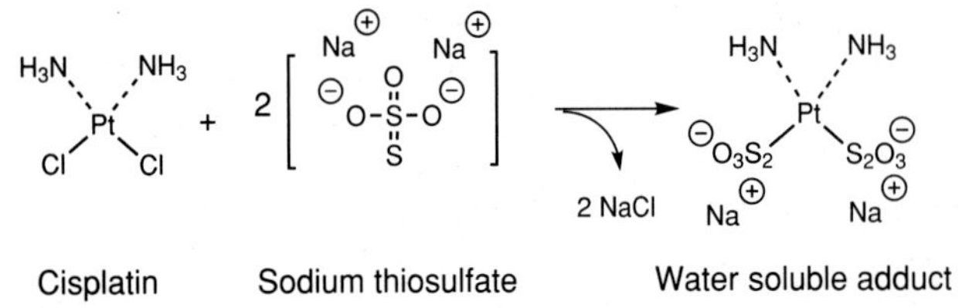

Cisplatin + 2 Sodium thiosulfate → Water soluble adduct + 2 NaCl

Fig. 42.15. Cisplatin inactivation by sodium thiosulfate.

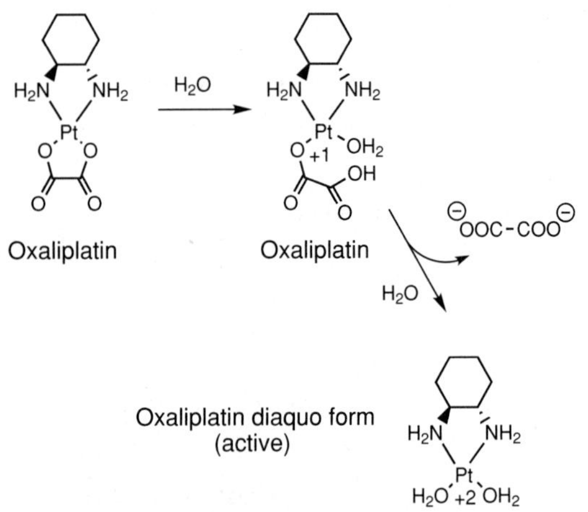

Oxaliplatin → (H_2O) Oxaliplatin → (H_2O, −$^{-}$OOC-COO^{-}) Oxaliplatin diaquo form (active)

Fig. 42.16. Activation of oxaliplatin.

This distinct oxaliplatin conformation is believed to result from the steric impact of the (*R,R*)-DACH carrier, which orients the hydrogen atoms on the ammine ligands such that the *cis*-NH_3 can form a hydrogen bond with a guanine-O^6, a bond that the inactive (*S,S*)-isomer is unable to form (35). The conformation of the oxaliplatin-DNA adduct is much less likely to be recognized by MMR proteins, and the effectiveness of oxaliplatin in MMR-deficient cells is believed to be responsible for the lack of resistance that has plagued cisplatin and carboplatin (36,37). Oxaliplatin often retains activity in patients who are no longer responding to the "first-generation" organometallics and also is significantly less mutagenic, nephrotoxic, hematotoxic, and ototoxic than cisplatin. Excretion is via the kidney.

Oxaliplatin decomposes in alkaline media and should not be coadministered with drugs that will increase the pH of the IV solution. Oxaliplatin is used in the treatment of metastatic colon or rectal cancer, either alone or in combination with 5-fluorouracil. Pulmonary fibrosis and peripheral sensory neuropathies that can be life-threatening are known to occur. It has been proposed that the latter adverse effect is caused by oxalate-based chelation of intracellular Ca^{2+}, which inhibits voltage-gated sodium channels in sensory nerve cells (38). This hypothesis is supported by the observation that infusions of calcium or magnesium salts can significantly attenuate oxaliplatin-induced neuropathy without compromising therapeutic efficacy (39). In the future, exploitation of genetic differences in the expression of various repair proteins, growth factors, and metabolizing enzymes may allow the tailoring of oxaliplatin therapy based on an individual's pharmacogenetic profile (37).

Satraplatin. This newest organometallic agent (Fig. 42.3) currently is in clinical trials as a second-line agent for the treatment of hormone-refractory prostate cancer (36). There is hope that it also will find value in ovarian cancer and small cell lung cancer. Satraplatin is a Pt(IV) complex. As with the Pt(II) complexes, the platinum has no net charge in the parent drug, because its original +4 charge has been "neutralized" by the donation of four electrons from the chloride and acetate ligands. Unlike the square-planar Pt(II) complexes currently on the market, it is active by the oral route. It is metabolized quickly in whole blood, producing up to six metabolites. The major metabolite is the desacetoxy analogue. As with other organoplatinum complexes, the diaquo form is active. At this early stage, the toxicity profile appears to be mild, with dose-related myelosuppression, particularly neutropenia and thrombocytopenia, being the major use-limiting side effect.

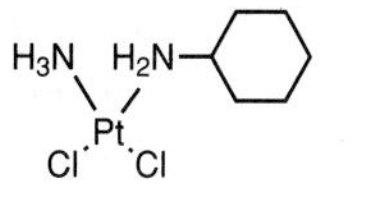

H_3N H_2N Pt Cl Cl

Desacetoxysatraplatin

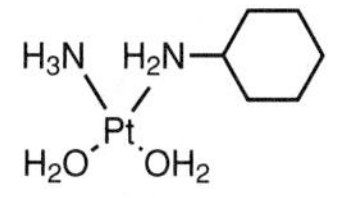

H_3N H_2N Pt H_2O OH_2

Diaquo satraplatin (active)

Antibiotics

The antibiotic antineoplastics (Fig. 42.17) are a broad category of natural or semisynthetic compounds that block DNA transcription by nicking and/or inducing point mutations in the DNA strand and/or by inhibiting enzymes critical to the DNA replication process. Antibiotic antineoplastics that interact directly with DNA first intercalate the double-stranded helix by inserting between the base pairs and forming strong noncovalent interactions with DNA bases. The highly stabilized complex deforms and uncoils the DNA, prohibiting proper replication. To bulldoze its way between the bonded DNA strands, a segment of the antibiotic must have the trigonal coplanar geometry guaranteed by aromaticity.

Many of the antineoplastic antibiotic compounds inhibit topoisomerase II, an enzyme responsible for maintaining proper DNA structure during replication and transcription to RNA. Topoisomerase II normally cleaves DNA during the replication phase but repairs its own damage after replication is complete. Topoisomerase II inhibitors act to stimulate the cleavage reaction but inhibit the DNA resealing activity of the enzyme, leaving the DNA irreversibly damaged and unable to replicate.

Yet another proposed mechanism of cytotoxic action is the generation of cytotoxic free radicals that cause single-strand breaks in DNA. One antibiotic (mitomycin) is capable of alkylating DNA, a mechanism more commonly associated with the nitrogen mustard antineoplastics but which is entirely predictable from the nucleophilic aziridine ring found within the structure of this anticancer agent.

Anthracyclines and Anthracenediones

Anthracycline antineoplastic antibiotics are very closely related to the tetracycline antibacterials. Structurally, they are glycosides and contain a sugar portion (L-daunosamine) and a nonsugar organic portion. The nonsugar portion of glycosides is generically referred to as an aglycone. In anthracyclines, the aglycone moiety is specifically called anthracyclinone or anthroquinone.

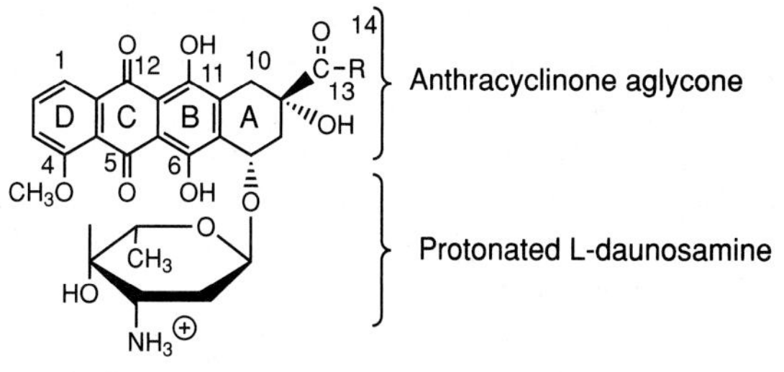

1 O 12 OH 11 10 O 14 C–R 13 D C B A OH 4 5 6 CH_3O O OH O O CH_3 HO $NH_3^{\oplus}$

Anthracyclinone aglycone

Protonated L-daunosamine

Mechanism of Action. As previously mentioned, DNA intercalation initiates the antineoplastic action of the anthracyclines. The anthracyclinone portion of the structure, particularly rings B, C, and D, is large and predominantly aromatic. This flat ring system slides between the two DNA strands, orienting itself in a perpendicular fashion relative to the long axis of DNA. Once intercalated, the anthracycline-DNA complex is stabilized through van

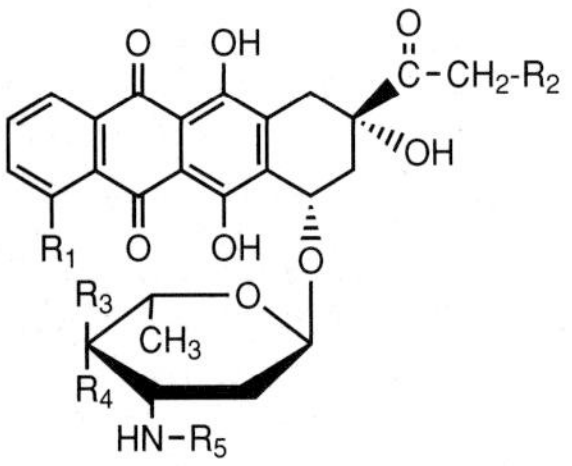

Drug Name	Trade Name	Salt	R_1	R_2	R_3	R_4	R_5
Doxorubicin	Adriamycin	HCl	CH_3O	OH	H	OH	H
Liposomal	Doxil	—					
Daunorubicin	Cerubidine	HCl	CH_3O	H	H	OH	H
Liposomal	DaunoXome	Citrate					
Idarubicin	Idamycin PFS	HCl	H	H	H	OH	H
Epirubicin	Ellence	HCl	CH_3O	OH	OH	H	H
Valrubicin	Valstar	—	CH_3O	$O\text{-}C(=O)\text{-}C_4H_9$	H	OH	$\text{—}C(=O)\text{-}CF_3$

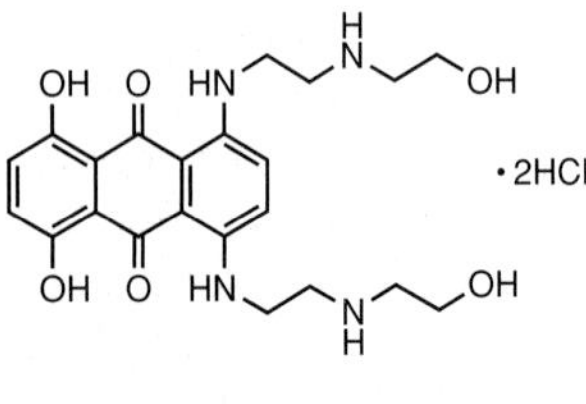

Mitoxantrone (Novantrone)

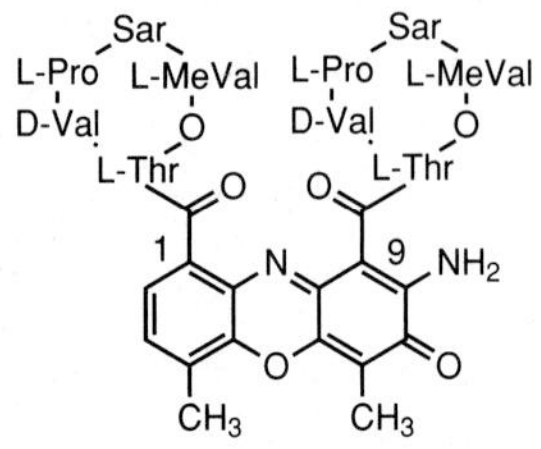

Dactinomycin (Cosmegen)

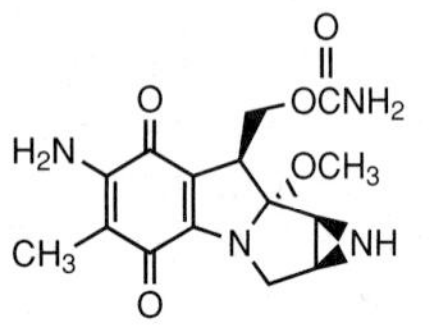

Mitomycin (Mutamycin)

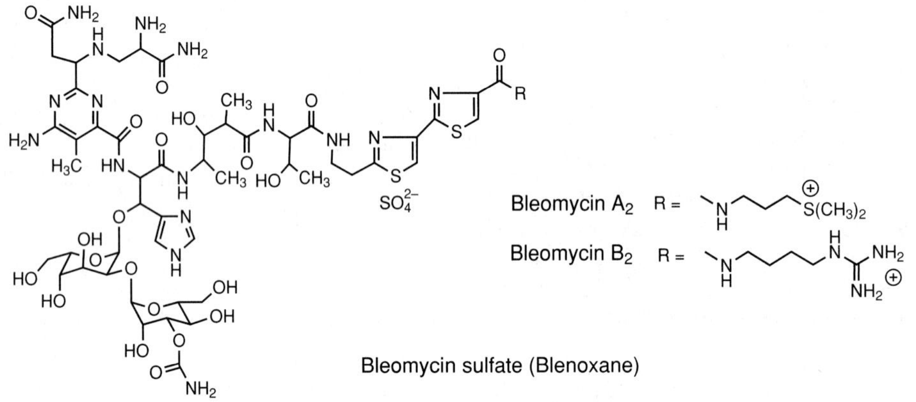

Bleomycin A_2 R =

Bleomycin B_2 R =

Bleomycin sulfate (Blenoxane)

Fig. 42.17. Anticancer antibiotics.

der Waals, hydrophobic, and hydrogen bonds. Binding is best in DNA regions that are rich in guanine and cytosine bases.

The protonated 3′-amino group on the daunosamine sugar has long been thought to stabilize the intercalated complex through interaction with an anionic DNA phosphate, but investigators recently have proposed that this substituent may link covalently to the C_2-NH_2 of guanine via a methylene bridging unit provided by formaldehyde (40). Regardless of the interaction, the daunosamine amino group is believed to play a crucial role in orchestrating the DNA sequence specificity of the intercalation process (41). The loss or epimerization of the 3′-amino moiety decreases, but does not destroy, DNA binding. In fact, the antitumor activity of these drugs is related more to the proper positioning and stabilization of the drug at its binding site than to the actual affinity of the drug for the DNA (41,42).

Even though DNA intercalation is required before the antineoplastic action of the anthracyclines can be realized, it alone does not kill the cell. Rather, the predominant cytotoxic effect is topoisomerase II inhibition. Anthracyclines bind to the DNA-enzyme complex in the area close to the DNA cleavage site. They stabilize a ternary cleavable complex that allows the DNA to be cut and covalently linked to topoisomerase Tyr residues but that does not permit the cleaved DNA to reseal. The aromatic portion of the anthracyclinone ring system and the daunosamine sugar bind to DNA, whereas the anthracyclinone A ring is believed to bind with the topoisomerase II enzyme (41). Removal of the 4-OCH_3 group found on all natural anthracycline anticancer products increases antitumor activity by facilitating the intercalation process and directing the binding of the dauosamine sugar in a way that stabilizes the ternary complex and promotes the cleavage (but not the resealing) of DNA (42). The daunosamine sugar is known to bind in the minor groove of DNA at the DNA-topoisomerase interface, but specific binding interactions between drug functional groups and topoisomerase residues have yet to be fully elucidated. Because a small number of anthracycline-induced DNA breaks can result in a high level of cell death, it has been hypothesized that the site of DNA cleavage, which contains an essential T-A dinucleotide, is particularly lethal to the cell (43).

Mechanism of Cardiotoxicity. A very important mechanism of use-limiting anthracycline cardiotoxicity involves the formation of cytotoxic free radicals. A free radical is a highly reactive species with an unpaired electron. Of particular importance to the antineoplastic action of these drugs is the formation of the superoxide radical anion ($\cdot O_2^-$) and the hydroxyl radical ($\cdot OH$), both of which are formed via reduction of the anthracyclinone quinone (ring C) to hydroquinone by NADPH/CYP450 reductase. The mechanism by which cytotoxic free radicals are generated is shown in Figure 42.18.

When NADPH/CYP450 reductase reduces the quinone ring to a hydroquinone, superoxide radical anions ($\cdot O_2^-$) are generated. Superoxide radical anions react to generate hydrogen peroxide (H_2O_2), a reaction that requires protons and is catalyzed by the enzyme superoxide dismutase in a Cu^{2+} mediated process. The fate of this hydrogen peroxide dictates the degree of cytotoxicity observed from the anthracycline.

In the presence of the enzyme catalase, hydrogen peroxide is rapidly converted to water and oxygen, which obviously are harmless chemicals as far as the body is concerned. In the presence of ferrous ion (Fe^{2+}), however, hydrogen peroxide is converted into the highly toxic hydroxyl radical through a process called the Fenton reaction. Hydroxyl radicals promote single-strand breaks in DNA, which is therapeutically desirable to treat the uncontrolled growth of cancer cells. Anthracycline anticancer agents also are known to interfere with normal ferritin-iron mobilization, resulting in iron accumulation (44). The anthracyclines chelate strongly with di- and trivalent cations, including intracellular Fe^{2+}, so the generation of cytotoxic hydroxyl radicals after the initial NADPH/CYP450 reductase reduction is essentially guaranteed. Hydroxide anion and ferric ion also are formed during the production of hydroxyl radicals.

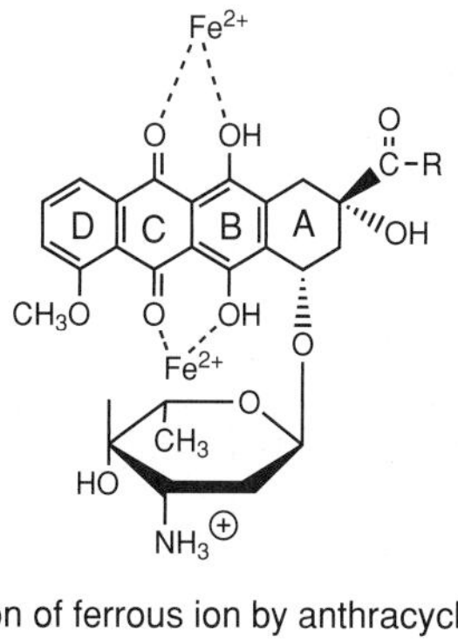

Chelation of ferrous ion by anthracyclines

The generation of hydroxyl radicals inside the tumor cell might augment the antineoplastic effect of the anthracyclines, but such generation is uncommon at standard antineoplastic doses (43). These cytotoxic radicals are generated within the heart, however, leading to acute and often severe cardiotoxicity. Cardiac tissue is particularly vulnerable to free radical damage by the anthracyclines because it does not contain the catalase enzyme (45). When hydrogen peroxide forms in the myocardium, it has no choice but to go down the Fenton pathway. Cardiac toxicity is the major use-limiting side effect of anthracycline use, but coadministration of dexrazoxane (an antioxidant and iron chelator) has been shown to lower its incidence (46). A role for nitric oxide metabolism, particularly nitric oxide synthase, in anthracycline-mediated cardiotoxicity recently has been proposed (47). In the future, nitric oxide metabolic enzymes may be key targets for drugs that, when coadministered with anthracyclines, could lower the risk of cardiotoxicity.

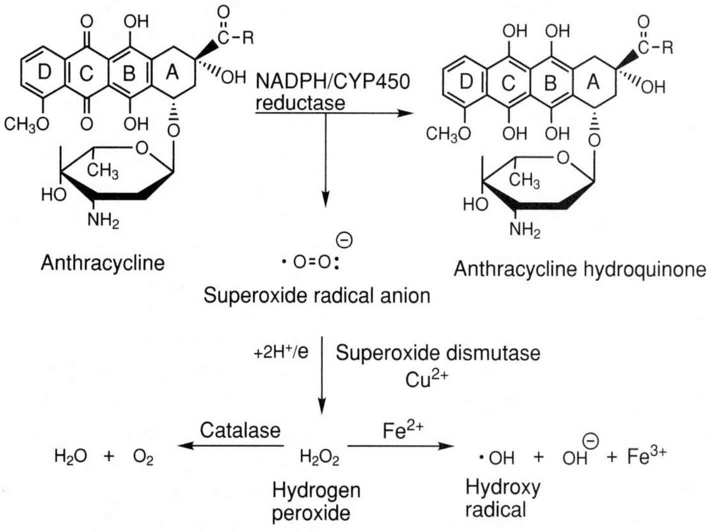

Fig. 42.18. Anthracycline-medicated free radical formation.

Although the rate of quinone metabolism influences the risk of acute anthracycline-induced cardiotoxicity, metabolism at C_{13} is believed to be responsible for the severe and chronic cardiotoxicity that some patients experience. The C_{13}-carbonyl is reduced to the active secondary alcohol via cytosolic aldoketoreductase enzymes (Fig. 42.19), and the larger the R group, the slower this reaction and the longer the duration of antineoplastic action. The C_{13}-substituents found on most marketed anthracyclines include CH_3 (daunorubicin and idarubicin) and CH_2OH (doxorubicin and epirubicin). Before excretion, anthracyclines are further metabolized to their aglycones, followed by O-dealkylation of the C_4 methoxy ether (if present) and conjugation with either glucuronic acid or sulfate.

The active secondary alcohol metabolites formed by aldoketoreductase induce a prolonged inhibition of calcium loading, opens a selective ion channel leading to increased cytosolic levels of Ca^{2+} in the sarcoplasmic reticulum, and inhibits Na^+,K^+–adenosine triphosphatase action in the sarcolemma. Collectively, these cellular events can induce a chronic cardiomyopathy that presents as severe congestive heart failure involving systolic and diastolic dysfunction (44). Chronic anthracycline-induced congestive heart failure can manifest without warning years after therapy, and it often is unresponsive to therapeutic intervention. Those at highest risk include the very young or very old, those with underlying cardiovascular disease, those receiving high cumulative doses, and those being treated with cyclophosphamide. Because toxicity is dose-dependent, patients with liver dysfunction who cannot adequately metabolize and clear the anthracycline also are at risk. Dosage adjustments in patients with liver disease must be made to avoid life-threatening toxicity.

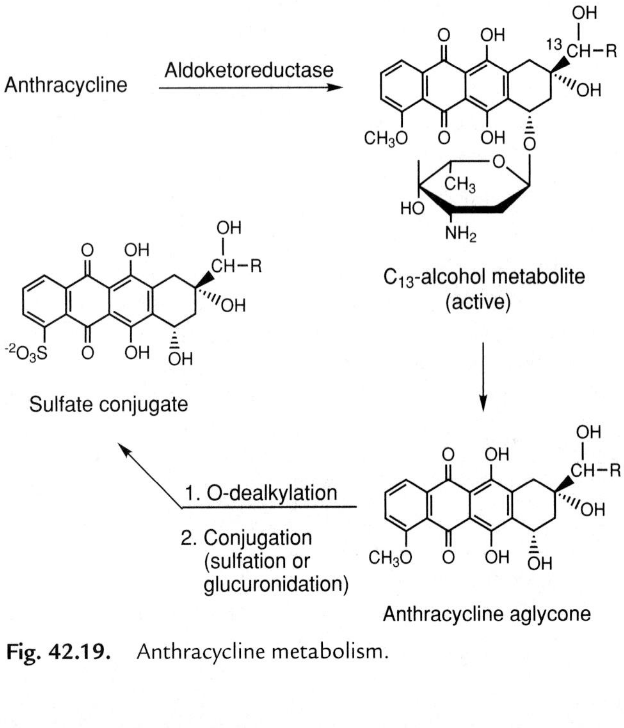

Anthracycline — Aldoketoreductase → C_{13}-alcohol metabolite (active) → Anthracycline aglycone → 1. O-dealkylation 2. Conjugation (sulfation or glucuronidation) → Sulfate conjugate

Fig. 42.19. Anthracycline metabolism.

ADDITIONAL SIDE EFFECTS. In addition to cardiac toxicity, all anthracycline antineoplastics can cause severe myelosuppression (especially leukocytopenia) as well as moderate to severe nausea and vomiting, mucositis leading to hemorrhage and potentially fatal infection, and alopecia. Side effects are dose-dependent. Most of the anthracyclines are orally inactive and must be given by IV injection. They are highly necrotic to skin and, if extravasation occurs, can cause such severe blistering and ulceration that skin excision, followed by plastic surgery, may be indicated. The anthracyclines contain photosensitive phenolic groups that must be protected from light and air. The highly conjugated structure imparts a reddish-orange color to these compounds (implied in the name "rubicin"), which is maintained when these compounds are excreted in the urine. Patients should be warned that the reddish urine they will experience is not hemorrhagic but, rather, simply the result of the conjugated chemistry of this class of drugs.

SPECIFIC DRUGS

Doxorubicin Hydrochloride. The C_{13} substituent of doxorubicin is hydroxymethyl (Fig. 42.17), which retards the action of cytosolic aldoketoreductase and slows the conversion to the equally active, but chronically cardiotoxic, doxorubicinol. This contributes to the longer duration of action compared to analogues that have CH_3 at this position (e.g., daunorubicin). Doxorubicin is highly lipophilic and concentrates in the liver, lymph nodes, muscle, bone marrow, fat, and skin. Elimination is triphasic, and the drug has a terminal half-life of 30 to 40 hours. The majority of an administered dose is excreted in the feces. Doxorubicin is utilized either alone or in combination therapy to treat a wide range of neoplastic disorders, including hematologic cancers and solid tumors in breast, ovary, stomach, bladder, and thyroid gland.

A liposomal formulation of doxorubicin (Fig. 42.17) is used in the treatment of AIDS-related Kaposi's sarcoma and organoplatinum-resistant ovarian cancer. Liposomes are taken up selectively into tumor cells, presumably because of their persistence in the bloodstream and enhanced permeability of tumor vascular membranes. In liposomal form, the drug is protected against enzymes that generate cardiotoxic free radicals, although this form of the drug can still induce potentially fatal congestive heart failure. Clinical experience with the liposomal formulation is limited, and few studies comparing the long-term toxicity with that of conventional doxorubicin therapy have been conducted. Therefore, all precautions outlined for the use of doxorubin also are employed when the liposomal formulation is used. The half-life of Doxil is extended to approximately 55 hours, and it is administered in doses ranging from 20 to 50 mg/m^2 every 3 to 4 weeks. The area under the curve of the liposomal formulation is approximately threefold that of the free drug formulation. It is cleared more slowly than conventional doxorubicin and generates very little of the doxorubicinol metabolite. Significant side effects have occurred when the liposomal formulation is erroneously dispensed, so pharmacists must be vigilant when interpreting therapeutic orders.

Epirubicin Hydrochloride. This stereoisomer of doxorubicin has the 4′-hydroxy group of the daunosamine sugar oriented in the β-position (Fig. 42.17). Epirubicin will be slowly reduced to the active C_{13} alcohol (epirubicinol), giving it a 30- to 38-hour half life, which is similar to that of doxorubicin. Unlike doxorubicinol, however, which was equally active with doxorubicin, epirubicinol has only one-tenth the activity of its parent drug and is not believed to contribute significantly to the therapeutic action of this agent. Cleavage of the epimerized sugar will occur before excretion, generating an aglycone that is indistinguishable from that generated by doxorubicin. Although excretion is primarily biliary, dosage reduction in severe renal impairment, as well as in hepatic dysfunction, is warranted.

Epirubicin is indicated for use in breast cancer, and the starting dose is 100 to 120 mg/m^2 (compared to a starting dose of 60–75 mg/m^2 for doxorubicin). The side effects and precautions are as outlined previously for doxorubicin, although there is a lower risk of serious myocardial toxicity or myelotoxicity.

Valrubicin. Chemically, valrubicin differs from its doxorubicin parent by the addition of a C_{14}-valerate ester and a 3′-trifluoroacetamide (Fig. 42.17). The carbon-rich valerate obviously is lipophilic, and acylation of the daunosamine amino group makes the 3′-substituent unionizable. Both of these structural changes promote a more rapid and extensive penetration into tumor cells.

Valrubicin currently has orphan drug status in the treatment of bacille Calmette-Guérin (BCG)–refractory bladder cancer (the total patient population is ~1,000 individuals) and is used with patients for whom surgical intervention would result in high morbidity or death. It is administered directly into the bladder through a catheter (intravesically). The lipophilic drug is water insoluble, but it dissolves in an aqueous vehicle that includes polyoxyethylene glycol and ethanol. The patient retains the drug in the bladder for 2 hours, then voids the solution in the normal fashion.

Valrubicin is active as administered, and despite the fact that hydrolysis of the ester and trifluoroacetamide can be envisioned, it is excreted essentially unchanged. Less than 1% of an administered dose is absorbed systemically, so there is essentially no exposure to metabolizing enzymes. The reduced C_{13}-alcoholic metabolite does not form to any appreciable extent during the 2-hour treatment period. Therapy is considered to be almost exclusively local, and there is little risk for cardiac toxicity, bone marrow suppression, drug–drug interactions, or other side effects. The most commonly reported adverse reactions are abdominal pain, urinary tract infection, hematuria, and dysuria. Systemic exposure to the drug and its metabolites would, of course, be greater in patients whose bladder wall integrity has been compromised by disease, and these patients should not receive valrubicin.

Daunorubicin Hydrochloride. The absence of the OH group at C_{14} in daunorubicin (Fig. 42.17) results in a faster conversion to the equally active and chronically cardiotoxic C_{13}-ol metabolite (daunorubicinol) compared to hydroxymethyl-substituted anthracyclines like doxorubicin. The 18.5-hour terminal half-life of daunorubicin is approximately half that of doxorubicin, and the terminal half-life of the active daunorubicinol metabolite is 26.7 hours. Excretion is approximately 40% biliary and 25% urinary. Daunorubicin is administered IV at a dose of 45 mg/m^2 for the treatment of lymphocytic and nonlymphocytic leukemia. The toxicity and side-effect profile of this anthracycline is similar to that of doxorubicin, and all previously identified precautions apply.

The citrate salt of daunorubicin is marketed as a liposomal formulation (Fig. 42.17), which promotes the use of this agent in solid tumors. Like Doxil (the liposomal formulation of doxorubicin), DaunoXome is indicated for use in AIDS-related Kaposi's sarcoma and is administered IV at a dose of 40 mg/m^2 every 2 weeks. The pharmacokinetic profiles of Doxil and DaunoXome are similar.

Idarubicin Hydrochloride. Idarubicin (Fig. 42.17) is the 4-desmethoxy analogue of daunorubicin. The loss of the C_4-ether flattens the D ring, facilitating intercalation between DNA base pairs. In turn, this orients the daunosamine sugar in the minor groove in a way that better stabilizes the ternary complex between drug, DNA, and topoisomerase (42).

The loss of the 4-methoxy moiety also makes this compound more lipophilic than either doxorubicin or daunorubicin. This results in a better penetration into tumor cells and an enhanced antineoplastic potency. Increased rates of remission have been noted with the use of idarubicin compared to other anthracyclines antineoplastic agents. Unlike its congeners, idarubicin shows significant oral bioavailability and is lipophilic enough to penetrate the blood-brain barrier. Currently, however, it is given only by the IV route and is not used in the treatment of brain cancer. Its primary indication is in acute myeloid leukemia, and it is administered in combination with other antileukemic drugs.

Idarubicin is reduced by aldoketoreductases to idarubicinol, which is as active as the parent drug. Because there is no aromatic methoxy group, there is no O-dealkylation to the C_4-phenol. The major metabolite is free, unconjugated idarubicinol. The half-lives of both idarubicin and idarubicinol are 22 and 45 hours, respectively. Idarubicin is administered IV at a dose of 10 to 12 mg/m^2/day for 3 to 4 days, and the idarubicinol metabolite can still be found in therapeutic concentrations in the blood 8 days after administration. Like other anthracyclines, excretion primarily is fecal, with a lesser dependence on renal elimination. Some authors have shown that idarubin is transported into cardiac tissue via a saturable transporter and that the coadministration of methylxanthines (e.g., caffeine) can increase both myocardial drug concentrations and the risk of idarubicin-induced cardiotoxicity (48).

Mitoxantrone Hydrochloride. Chemically, mitoxantrone is classified as an anthracenedione (Fig. 42.17). The sugar moiety is missing, but the cationic side-chain amino nitrogens could bind to the anionic phosphate residue of the DNA backbone in the same fashion that the cationic L-daunosamine amino group of the true anthracyclines has been presumed to do. This molecule has the structural features needed to intercalate DNA and inhibit topoisomerase II, but the enhanced stability of the quinone ring (possibly through an increased potential for intramolecular hydrogen bonding) makes the ring highly resistant to NADPH/CYP450 reductase. This limits the formation of the superoxide radicals that are required for the generation of the highly toxic hydroxyl radical. In addition, there is no active cardiotoxic metabolite to induce chronic toxicity by disrupting the flow of myocardial cations. The chance of cardiovascular toxicity from mitoxantrone is significantly decreased, although patients who have been previously treated with anthracycline antineoplastics may still be at risk. It is thought that any observed myocardial toxicity may be operating through mechanisms other than the generation of cytotoxic radicals.

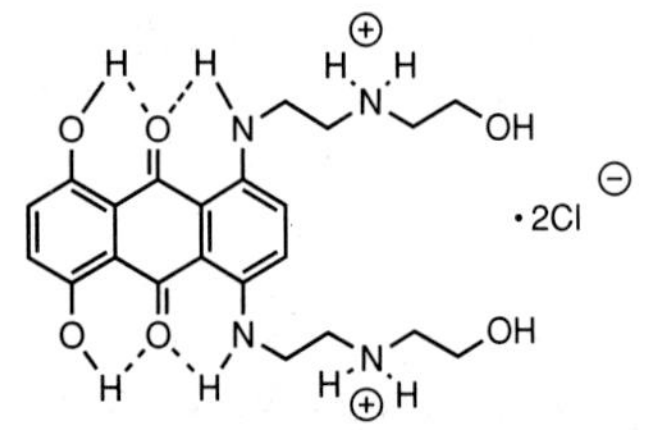

In addition, the risk of ulceration and necrosis on extravasation, as well as of nonmarrow-related toxicities such as nausea, vomiting, mucositis, and alopecia, is significantly less than observed with true anthracyclines. There is a significant risk of bone marrow suppression, however. The risk of myelosuppression increases with dose, but it can be observed even when low doses are used.

Mitoxantrone excretion primarily is biliary. Both the unchanged drug and inactive metabolites resulting from N-dealkylation, deamination, and oxidation of the resultant aldehyde to the carboxylic acid are observed. Both arms of the structure can be metabolized, leading to mono- or dicarboxylic acid metabolites (Fig. 42.20), which are excreted as the glucuronide conjugate. The conjugated metabolites are an intense, dark blue in color and will result in blue-green urine. The whites of the eyes and, in some cases, the skin also may take on a bluish cast.

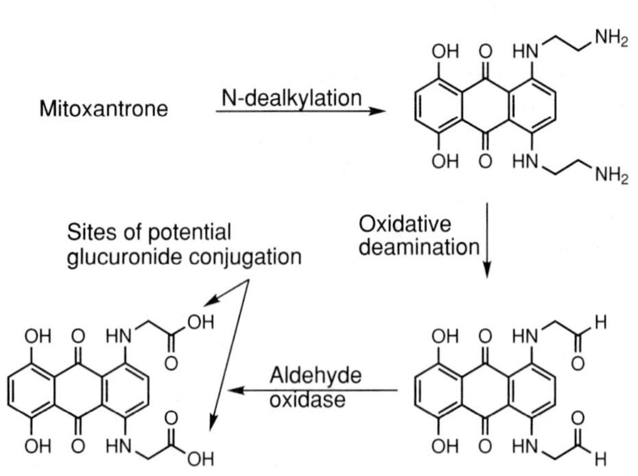

Mitoxantrone
N-dealkylation
Oxidative deamination
Aldehyde oxidase
Sites of potential glucuronide conjugation

Fig. 42.20. Mitoxantrone metabolism.

Mitoxantrone is used in combination with other agents during the initial treatment of acute nonlymphocytic leukemia and hormone-refractory prostate cancer. Recent studies have shown that mitoxantrone also decreases the rate of relapse and disease progression in patients with multiple sclerosis (49). Although too toxic for use in patients with primary progressive disease, it is available for the treatment of chronic progressive, progressive relapsing, or deteriorating relapsing-remitting multiple sclerosis.

Miscellaneous Antibiotics

DACTINOMYCIN. Dactinomycin (Fig. 42.17) has two pentapeptide lactones attached to an aromatic (and, therefore, flat) actinocin (or phenoxazinone) structure. It is capable of intercalating DNA and binds preferably between guanine and cytosine residues on a single DNA strand. This interaction results in DNA elongation and distortion, commonly referred to as a point mutation. When sliding between adjacent DNA base pairs, the actinocin orients itself perpendicular to the main DNA axis, allowing the pentapeptide lactone units to bind to residues in the minor groove of DNA through hydrophobic and hydrogen bonds. An affinity-enhancing bond between the threonine carbonyl oxygen and a protonated C_2-amino group of guanine also forms. Other hydrogen, hydrophobic, and van der Waals (π-stacking) interactions form between the lactone and DNA residues, particularly guanine and cytosine.

The binding of the actinocin and polypeptide lactone portions of dactinomycin to DNA is cooperative, meaning that the binding of one unit facilitates the binding of the other, most likely by promoting an optimal orientation. This significantly enhances drug-DNA affinity. The binding of dactinomycin to DNA, although noncovalent, is much stronger than that observed with the anthracyclines. Drug dissociation from DNA is slow, leading to a pseudoirreversible effect. As a result of very strong DNA binding interactions, topoisomerase II is inhibited, which results in nonrepairable double-strand breaks in DNA. Transcription and translation processes are blocked, resulting in a decrease in de novo RNA (especially mRNA) and protein synthesis.

The *p*-benzoquinoneimine segment of dactinomycin renders the molecule vulnerable to NADPH/CYP450 reductase. Free radicals can be generated, and additional single-strand DNA breaks can result. The loss of either aromatic methyl group results in a loss of activity. The reason for this profound impact on pharmacological action and therapeutic utility is unknown.

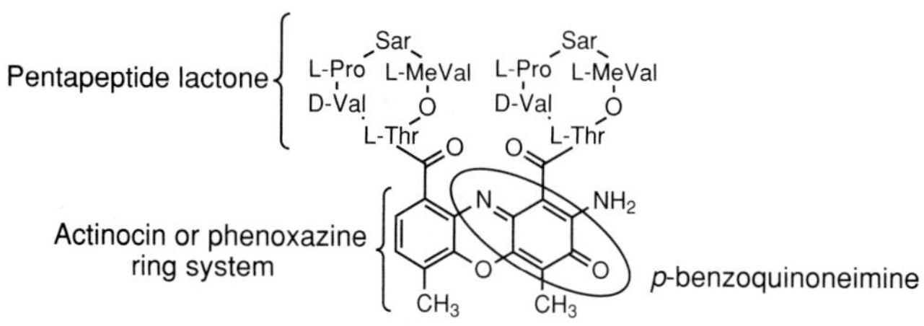

Pentapeptide lactone
Actinocin or phenoxazine ring system
p-benzoquinoneimine

Dactinomycin

Dactinomycin is used for the treatment of various solid tumors and muscle-related cancers. It induces severe side effects, and nausea and vomiting can be use-limiting. Myelosuppression also is common and, most often, is the dose-limiting toxic effect. The drug usually is given by the IV route, but toxicity can be limited if the tumor can be perfused with drug (assuming minimal distribution into the general circulation). Dactinomycin is a severe blistering agent, and extravasation can cause irreversible and profound tissue damage. The side effects of radiation therapy are significantly exaggerated by the concurrent use of dactinomycin. The drug's 36-hour half-life is the result of a very high affinity for DNA, a large volume of distribution, and minimal metabolic breakdown. Dactinomycin is photosensitive and must be protected from light.

Mitomycin. As shown in Figure 42.21, mitomycin is activated through a bioreductive process utilizing NADPH/CYP450 reductase and/or NAD(P)H quinone oxidoreductase 1 (NQ 01 reductase), an enzyme expressed in many neoplastic cells (50,51). Through these enzymes, the quinone ring of mitomycin is readily reduced to the hydroquinone, generating superoxide radicals in the process that ultimately will be converted to cytotoxic hydroxyl radicals through the Fenton reaction. As previously discussed, hydroxyl radicals induce single-strand breaks in DNA. Formation of the hydroquinone is followed by aromatization to the indole ring through the loss of methanol. Both the electrophilic aziridine ring and the δ^+ methylene group adjacent to the carbamate ester are vulnerable to attack by DNA nucleophiles, such as the 2-NH_2 group of guanine or the 4-NH_2 group of cytosine, resulting in cross-linked DNA and cell death.

Mitomycin is administered IV in the treatment of disseminated adenocarcinoma of the stomach or pancreas, and it has been used intravesically in superficial bladder cancer. Biotransformation pathways are saturable, and approximately 10% of an administered dose is eliminated unchanged via the kidneys. Myelosuppression is the major use-limiting side effect of this drug, which is slow to manifest but quite prolonged in duration. Severe skin necrosis can occur on extravasation, and potentially fatal pulmonary toxicities have been noted as well. Mitomycin can induce hemolytic uremia accompanied by irreversible renal dysfunction and thrombocytopenia, and the drug should not be administered to patients with serum creatinine levels greater than 1.7 mg/dL. Severe bronchospasm also has been noted in patients treated with vinca alkaloids who also are receiving (or who have previously received) mitomycin.

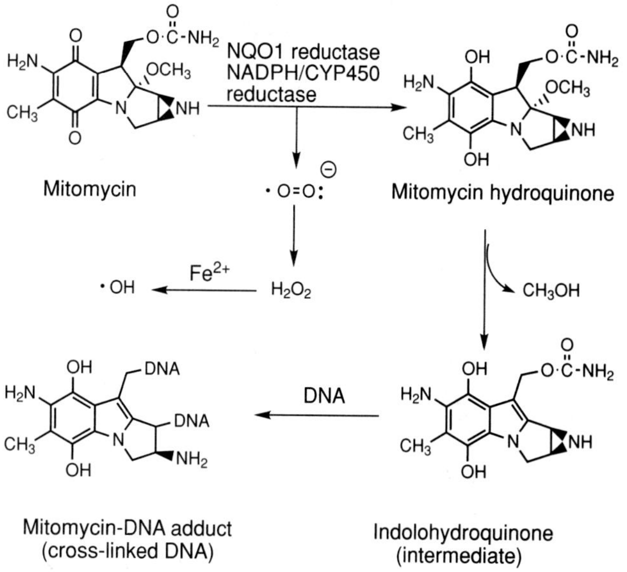

Mitomycin
NQO1 reductase NADPH/CYP450 reductase
Mitomycin hydroquinone
$\cdot O{=}O:^{\ominus}$
Fe^{2+}
$\cdot OH$
H_2O_2
CH_3OH
DNA
Mitomycin-DNA adduct (cross-linked DNA)
Indolohydroquinone (intermediate)

Fig. 42.21. Mitomycin metabolism.

Bleomycin sulfate. The commercially available bleomycin drug product is a mixture of naturally occurring glycopeptides, predominantly bleomycin A_2 (Fig. 42.17). The aromatic bithiazole ring system can intercalate DNA, but unlike most of the antibiotics discussed thus far, the molecule does not inhibit topoisomerase II. Rather, intercalation positions bleomycin for DNA destruction via cytotoxic free radicals. The disaccharide, polyamine, imidazole, and pyrimidine structures are very electron rich and readily chelate intracellular Fe^{2+}. Once chelated, Fe^{2+} is oxidized to Fe^{3+}, with a concomitant reduction of bound oxygen, and both superoxide and hydroxyl radicals are generated. The free radicals cleave deoxyribose and cause single-strand breaks in DNA, most commonly between guanine-cytosine or guanine-thymine residues. When the cyclic deoxyribose sugar breaks, it forms a highly electrophilic base propenal that inactivates essential cellular proteins by alkylating nucleophilic Cys residues (Fig. 42.22). Reduced glutathione is proposed to serve a protective role by acting as propenal scavenger and, until depleted, saves cellular proteins from alkylation (52).

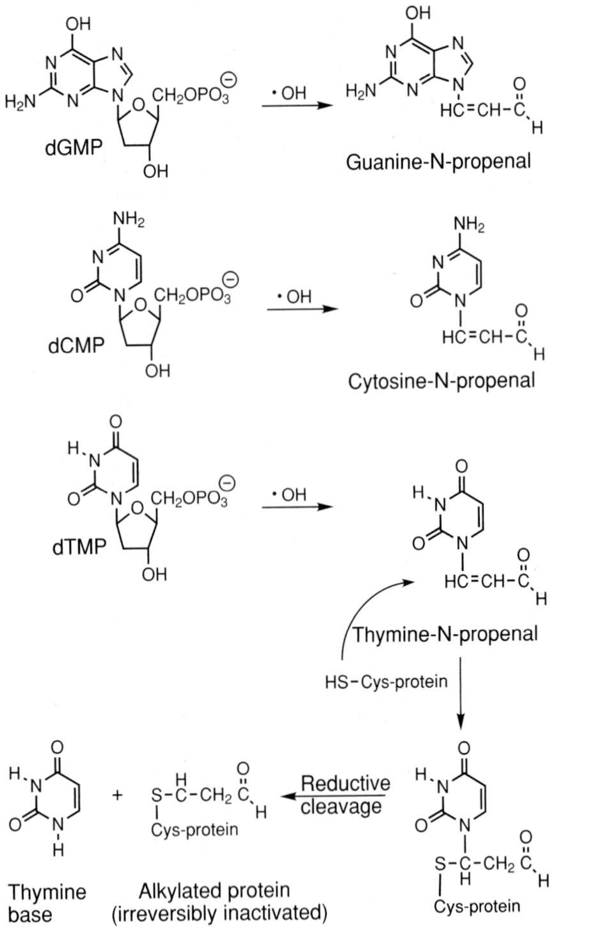

Fig. 42.22. Alkylation of Cys residues by hydroxyl radical-generated base propenals.

Bleomycin is a natural product isolated from *Streptomyces verticillus*. It normally is chelated with Cu^{2+}, which must be removed via catalytic reduction before marketing. This increases the cost of the drug, but it frees up the critical bleomycin functional groups for chelation with intracellular ferrous iron.

The action of bleomycin is terminated through the action of bleomycin hydrase, a cytosolic aminopeptidase that cleaves the terminal amide moiety to form the inactive carboxylate metabolite (Fig. 42.23). The metabolic replacement of the electron-withdrawing amide with an electron-donating carboxylate increases the pK_a of the α-amino group, which normally interacts with DNA in the un-ionized conjugate form. After hydrolysis, the ratio of ionized to un-ionized forms of this critical amine increases approximately 126-fold, destroying DNA affinity and leading to the loss of therapeutic action. Drug destruction via the bleomycin hydrase pathway is rapid, and tumors will be resistant to bleomycin if they contain high concentrations of the enzyme. Conversely, tumors that are poor in bleomycin hydrase (e.g., squamous cell carcinoma) respond well to this agent.

Bleomycin hydrase is found in all tissues except skin and lung. Approximately 10% of patients who are administered bleomycin will experience potentially fatal pulmonary fibrosis, which can occur during therapy or several months following termination of therapy, often without warning. Some studies have shown that the copper-complexing agent tetrathiomolybdate can reduce the risk of bleomycin-induced fibrosis by inhibiting the action of copper-dependent inflammatory cytokines (53). Erythema and hypertrophic modifications in skin also are common side effects that manifest after 2 to 3 weeks of bleomycin therapy.

Bleomycin is used IV in the palliative treatment of squamous cell head and neck cancers, testicular and other genital carcinomas, and Hodgkin's and non-Hodgkin's lymphoma. It is excreted via the kidneys, and serum concentrations of active drug are increased in patients with renal disease. The elimination half-life can rise from 2 to 4 hours to more than 20 hours in renal failure, resulting in significant toxicity, especially pulmonary toxicity. Dosage adjustments are warranted. Unlike many antineoplastic agents, bleomycin does not suppress the bone marrow, and it often is given in combination with compounds that do, so that the dose of all

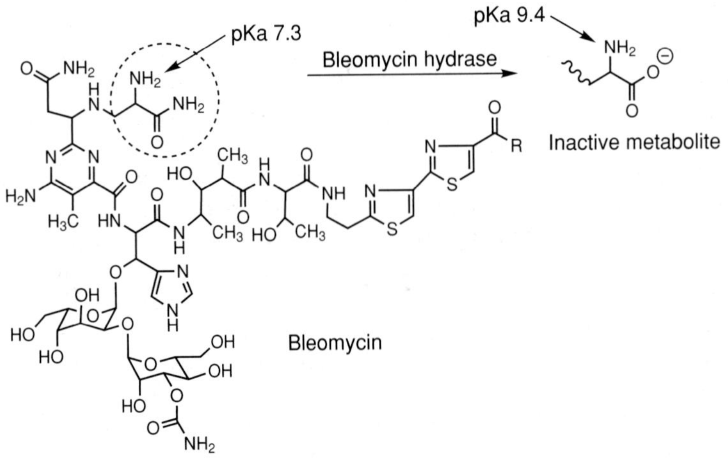

Fig. 42.23. Bleomycin hydrase mediated inactivation of bleomycin.

drugs can be optimized. Nausea and vomiting also are relatively mild, but approximately 1% of lymphoma patients who are treated with bleomycin will experience an immediate or delayed, severe idiosyncratic reaction that mimics anaphylaxis.

Antimetabolites

The antineoplastic agents discussed thus far have all damaged existing DNA and inhibited its ability to replicate. The antimetabolites, on the other hand, most commonly stop the de novo synthesis of DNA by inhibiting the formation of the nucleotides that make up these life-sustaining polymers. We will see that the rate-limiting enzymes of nucleotide biosynthesis often are the primary target for the antimetabolites, because inhibition of this key enzyme is the most efficient way to shut down any biochemical reaction sequence. Antimetabolites also are capable of inhibiting other enzymes required in the biosynthesis of DNA, and many can arrest chain elongation by promoting the incorporation of false nucleotides into the growing DNA strand.

The antimetabolites serve as false substrates for critical nucleotide biosynthesis enzymes. These enzyme inhibitors are structurally "dolled up" to look like a super attractive version of the normal (endogenous) substrate. Speaking anthropomorphically, through a form of chemical entrapment, they entice the enzymes to choose them over the endogenous substrate, and once they do, the antimetabolites bind them irreversibly. If the building block nucleotides cannot be synthesized, then DNA synthesis (and tumor growth) is stopped dead in its tracks. If tumor growth is arrested, then metastasis slows, and the patient has a fighting chance for remission and/or cure.

Antimetabolite antineoplastics are categorized by the class of nucleotide they inhibit. Purine antagonists inhibit the synthesis of the purine-based nucleotides adenylate monophosphate (AMP) and guanylate monophosphate (GMP), and the pyrimidine antagonists stop the production of the pyrimidine-based nucleotides, primarily deoxythymidine monophosphate (dTMP).

Pyrimidine Antagonists: dTMP Synthesis Inhibitors

dTMP BIOSYNTHESIS. Looked at simply, dTMP is produced via C_5-methylation of deoxyuridine monophosphate (dUMP). The rate-limiting enzyme of the dTMP synthetic pathway is the sulfhydryl-containing thymidylate synthase, with 5,10-methylenetetrahydrofolate (5,10-methylene-THF) serving as the methyl-donating cofactor. All dTMP synthesis inhibitors will inhibit thymidylate synthase either directly or indirectly, and this will result in a "thymineless death" in actively dividing cells. Without dTMP and its deoxythmidine triphosphate metabolite, DNA will fragment, and the cell will die.

To truly understand how an antimetabolite inhibits a biochemical pathway, we must first understand completely how the pathway normally functions. A quick look at the dTMP synthesis pathway (Fig. 42.24) will confirm that our "simple methylation reaction" is comprised of several important steps, each of which is analyzed in turn below.

The synthase enzyme is very large and contains a deep pocket for the binding of both substrate and cofactor.

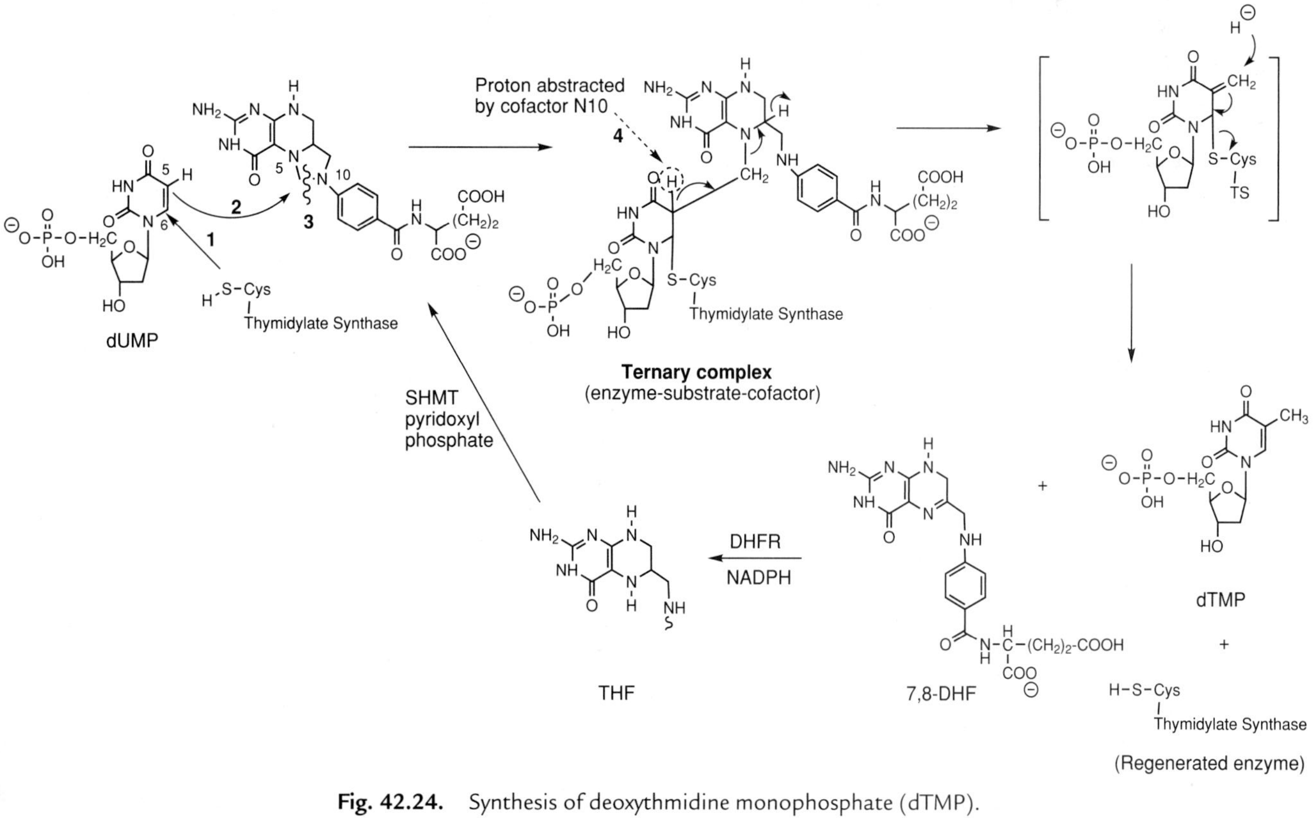

Fig. 42.24. Synthesis of deoxythmidine monophosphate (dTMP).

It may be illuminating to think of this binding pocket like a big cooking pot. Once the "ingredients" are added (substrate and cofactor), the process of making the product (dTMP) can begin. The active site binding motifs for both substrate and cofactor are highly conserved among all thymidylate synthase enzymes, regardless of source (54). Whereas early studies on substrate binding were conducted with bacteria-derived synthases, the human enzyme (hTS) has now been crystallized and some binding residues identified (55). With regard to substrate binding (hTS sequence numbers given where known):

- Four Arg residues at positions 50, 218, 175′, and 176′ form electrostatic bonds with the anionic 5′-phosphate of the substrate.
- Tyr (H-donor) and His (H-acceptor) residues form hydrogen bonds with the deoxyribose 3′-OH.
- The main-chain amide of aspartate (Asp^{218}) forms a hydrogen bond with the pyrimidine C_2 carbonyl oxygen.
- His^{196} forms a hydrogen bond with the pyrimidine C_4 carbonyl oxygen.
- An Asn residue (H-acceptor) forms a hydrogen bond with the pyrimidine C_3-NH.
- Cys^{195} forms a transient covalent bond with C_6 of the pyrimidine ring.

The glutamate tail of 5,10-methylene-THF binds to Lys and His residues of the synthase. Oxygen atoms of leucine (Leu^{221}) and phenylalanine (Phe^{225}) interact with the *p*-aminobenzoic acid component of the folate, whereas Asp^{218}, His, and Ile residues interact with additional cofactor functional groups (55,56). The binding of both substrate and cofactor promotes a conformational change in the synthase protein and causes the N-terminal portion of the synthase to change its location, which covers the opening of the binding "pot" like a big lid. The conformational change brings the folate cofactor "face to face" with the dUMP substrate, properly orienting all key functional groups for the reaction to come.

The C_6 position of the dUMP substrate is surrounded by electron-withdrawing nitrogen and oxygen atoms, leaving it highly electrophilic (δ^+) and ready to be attacked by the nucleophilic Cys^{195} of the synthase. The Cys sulfhydryl group launches an intermolecular nucleophilic attack, forming a new covalent bond between the sulfur and C_6 of the substrate (step 1). The bond that breaks in response to this attack is the 5,6-double bond of dUMP, which attacks the methylene group of the cofactor (step 2). With the release of the N_{10} nitrogen the cofactor imidazolidine ring breaks (step 3). Taken together, steps 1 to 3 generate a ternary complex of enzyme, substrate and cofactor (Fig. 42.24).

A series of reactions involving bond breaking and bond making are shown in Figure 42.24, leading to formation of dTMP, 7,8-dihydrofolate (7,8-DHF), and regenerated thymidylate synthase. The C_5-H abstraction by N_{10} of the cofactor (step 4) is essential for synthesis of dTMP. To complete the biochemical cycle, 7,8-DHF must be reduced to THF via dihydrofolate reductase (DHFR) utilizing NADPH. Finally, THF is converted to 5,10-methylene-THF through the action of serine hydroxymethyltransferase and vitamin B_6.

With the enzyme and cofactor both regenerated, and with plenty of dUMP stored in cellular pools, the cell is ready to synthesize another molecule of dTMP. This happens at a regular pace in healthy cells and at an uncontrolled rate in tumor cells.

DIRECT INHIBITORS OF THYMIDYLATE SYNTHASE (FIG. 42.25)

Fluorouracil. To bind to thymidylate synthase, this fluorinated pyrimidine prodrug must be converted to its deoxyribonucleotide form (Fig. 42.26). The active form of fluorouracil differs from the endogenous substrate only by the presence of the 5-fluoro group, which holds the key to the cell-killing action of this drug. The C_6 position of the false substrate is significantly more electrophilic than normal because of the strong electron-withdrawing effect of the C_5 fluorine. This greatly increases the rate of attack by Cys^{195}, resulting in a very fast formation of a fluorinated ternary complex (Fig. 42.27). The small size of the fluorine atom assures no steric hindrance to the formation of this false complex.

The next step in the pathway required the abstraction of the C_5-H (as proton) by N_{10} of the cofactor, but this is no longer possible. Not only is the C_5-fluorine bond stable to cleavage, the fluorine atom and N_{10} would repel one another because they are both electron rich. The false ternary complex cannot break down, no product is formed, no cofactor is released, and most importantly, the rate-limiting enzyme (thymidylate synthase) is not regenerated. Because dTMP can no longer be synthesized, the cell will die.

Fluorouracil is administered IV in the palliative treatment of colorectal, breast, stomach, and pancreatic cancers. Patients are treated for four consecutive days, followed by treatment on odd-numbered days up to a maximum of 12 days. Fluorouracil is rapidly cleared from the bloodstream, and although up to 20% of a dose is excreted unchanged in the urine, most undergoes hepatic catabolism via a series of enzymes that includes the polymorphic dihydropyrimidine dehydrogenase (Fig. 42.28). Patients who are genetically deficient in this enzyme will experience a more pronounced effect from this drug and are at significant risk for use-limiting toxicity (57). In general, women clear fluorouracil faster than men do. Dosage adjustments usually are not required in hepatic or renal dysfunction. Major toxicities are related to bone marrow depression, stomatitis/esophagopharyngitis, and potential GI ulceration. Nausea and vomiting are common. Solutions of fluorouracil are light sensitive, but discolored products that have been properly stored and protected from light are still safe to use.

Floxuridine. This deoxyribonucleoside prodrug (Fig. 42.26) is bioconverted via 2′-deoxyuridine kinase–mediated phosphorylation to the same active 5-fluoro-dUMP structure generated in the multistep biotransformation of

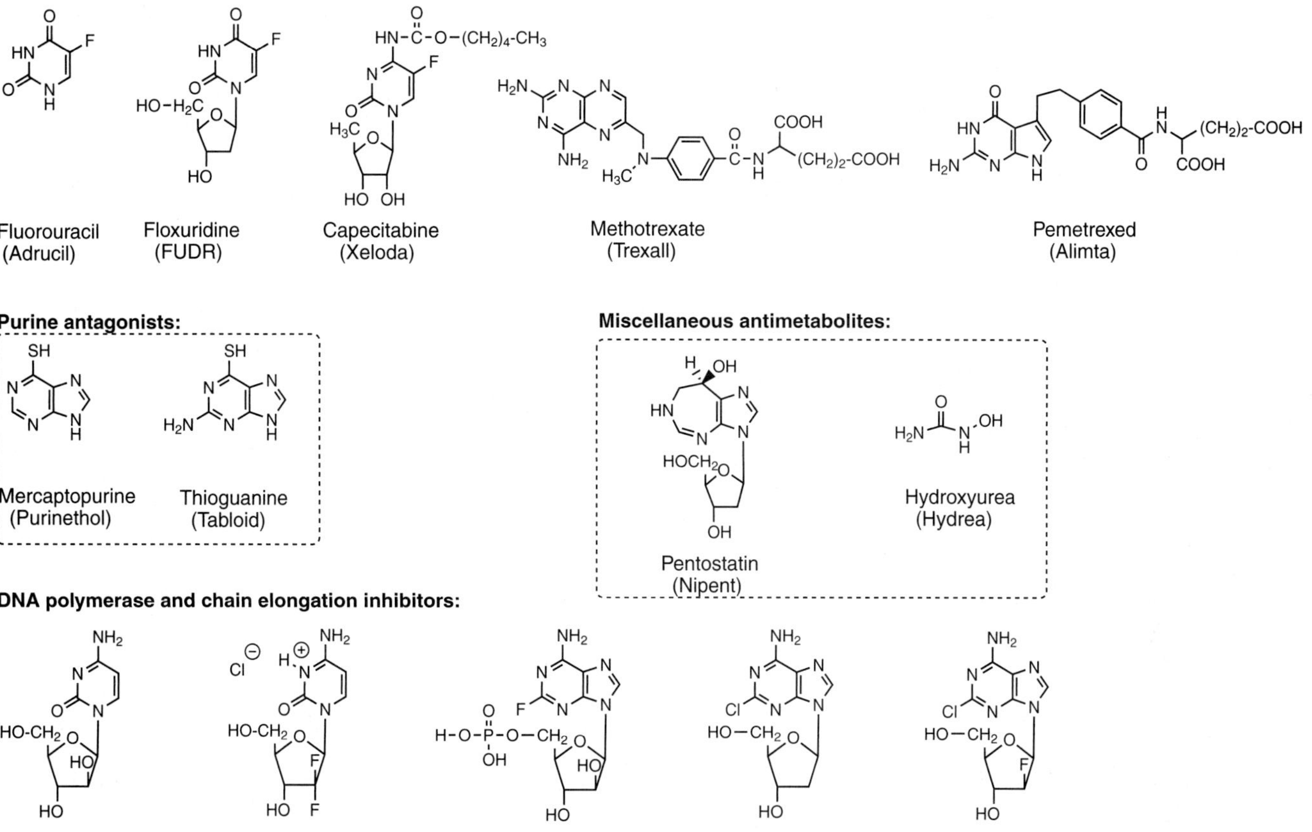

Fig. 42.25. Antimetabolites.

fluorouracil. It is given by intra-arterial infusion for the palliative treatment of GI adenocarcinoma that has metastasized to the liver and that cannot be managed surgically.

Capecitabine. Although capecitabine is a carbamylated analogue of cytidine (Fig. 42.29), the drug actually is another 5-fluoro-dUMP prodrug. Given orally, it is extensively metabolized to fluorouracil, which is then converted to the active fluorinated deoxyribonucleotide as previously described. Thymidine phosphorylase, an enzyme involved in this biotransformation, is much more active in tumors than in normal tissue, which improves the tumor-selective generation of fluorouracil. Levels of active drug in the tumor can be up to 3.5-fold higher than in surrounding tissue (58), leading to a lower incidence of side effects compared to fluorouracil therapy. Because capecitabine is biotransformed to fluorouracil, it follows the same catabolic and elimination pathways (Fig. 42.28) reported for 5-fluorouracil. Doses should be attenuated in moderate to severe renal impairment, and the caution relative to the augmented risk of toxicity in patients with dihydropyrimidine dehydrogenase deficiency applies.

Capecitabine is indicated for use as first-line therapy in patients with colorectal cancer. It also is used alone or in combination with docetaxel in patients with metastatic breast cancer who have experienced disease progression or recurrence after anthracycline therapy. Given b.i.d. in tablet form, the total daily dose is calculated based on patient body surface area and is taken 30 minutes after eating to avoid food-induced decreases in absorption. In addition to bone marrow suppression, nausea, and vomiting, the drug can induce severe diarrhea and a potentially disabling disorder termed "hand-and-foot syndrome" (palmar-plantar erythrodysethesia). Capecitabine inhibits CYP2C9 and, along with competition for serum protein binding sites, results in clinically significant drug–drug interactions with both warfarin and phenytoin. The interaction with warfarin can result in potentially fatal bleeding episodes, which can appear within days of combination therapy or be delayed up to 1 month after discontinuation of capecitabine therapy.

Indirect Inhibitors of Thymidylate Synthase

Methotrexate. Methotrexate (Fig. 42.25) is a folic acid antagonist structurally designed to compete successfully with 7,8-DHF for the DHFR enzyme. The direct inhibition of DHFR causes cellular levels of 7,8-DHF to build

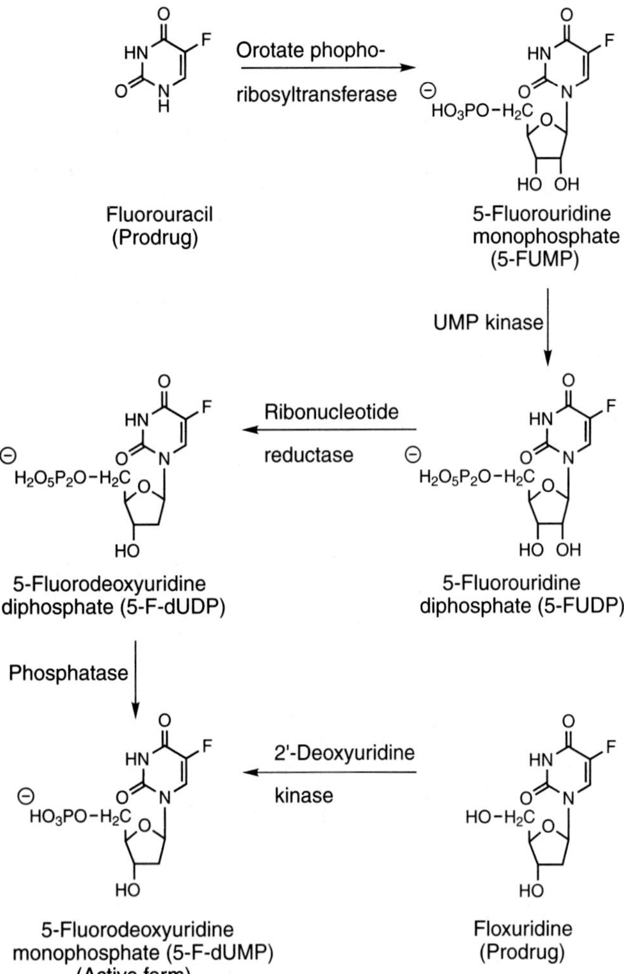

Fig. 42.26. Activation of fluorouracil and floxuridine.

up, which in turn results in feedback (indirect) inhibition of thymidylate synthase. Methotrexate also is effective in inhibiting glycine amide ribonucleotide (GAR) transformylase (see Fig. 42.31), a key enzyme in the synthesis of purine nucleotides. Take note of the structural differences between methotrexate and DHF, because these differences will be important to an understanding of the chemical mechanism of this anticancer agent.

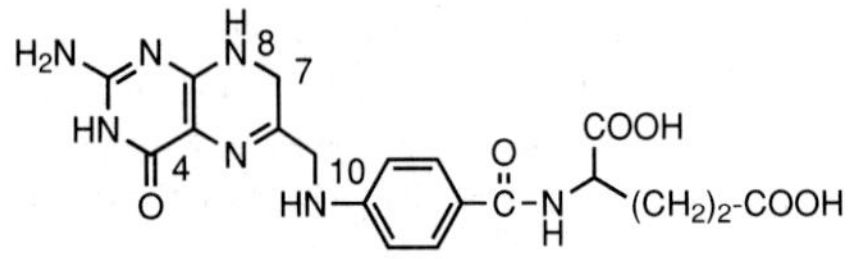

7,8-Dihydrofolate

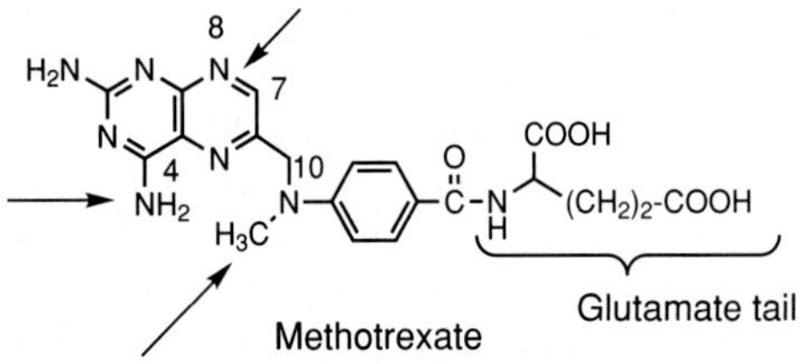

Methotrexate

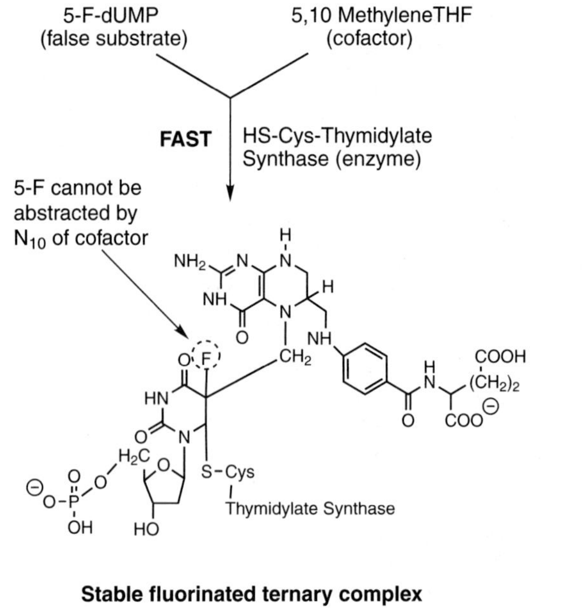

Glutamate tail

5-F-dUMP
(false substrate)

5,10 MethyleneTHF
(cofactor)

FAST

HS-Cys-Thymidylate
Synthase (enzyme)

5-F cannot be abstracted by N_{10} of cofactor

Thymidylate Synthase

Stable fluorinated ternary complex

Fig. 42.27. Mechanism of action of fluorouracil.

It has been proposed that the N_5 position of DHF is protonated by a Glu[30] of DHFR (59) and, in cationic form, binds to DHFR Asp[27] through an electrostatic bond (Fig. 42.30). N_5 is the strongest base in the DHF structure, in part because of attenuating the impact of the C_4 carbonyl on electron density around N_1. Additional affinity-enhancing interactions between enzyme and substrate also have been identified (60,61), and once bound, the substrate 5,6-double bond is positioned close to the NADPH cofactor so that the transfer of hydride can proceed.

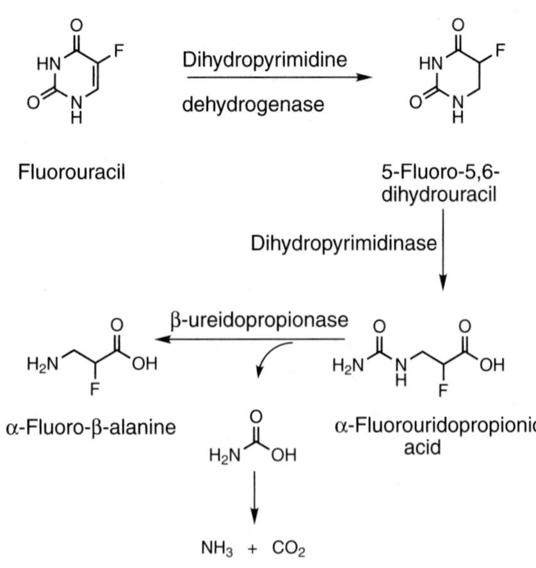

Fig. 42.28. Fluorouracil metabolism.

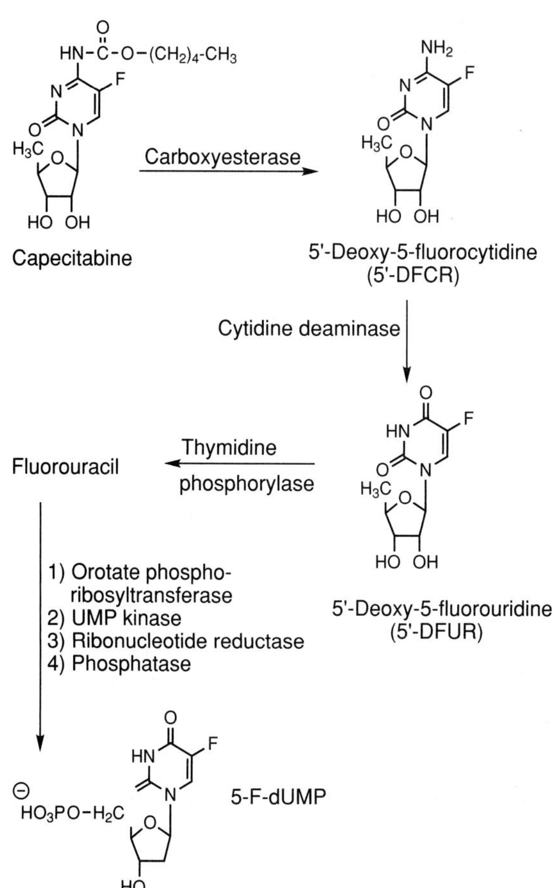

Fig. 42.29. Capecitabine activation.

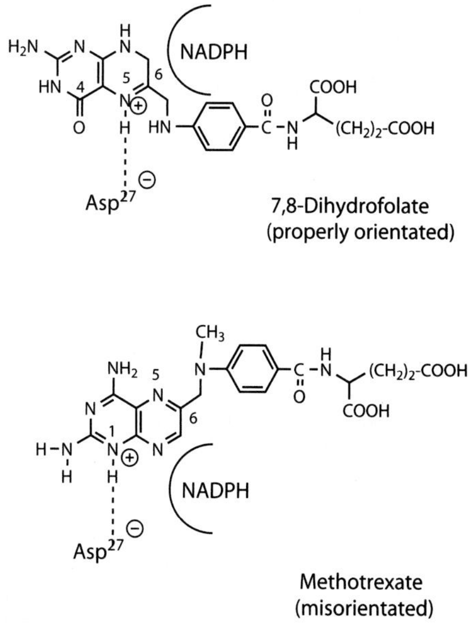

In contrast, the C_4 amino substituent of methotrexate enriches electron density at N_1 through π-electron donation, increasing its basic character between 10- and 1,000-fold and promoting protonation by Glu^{30} at the expense of N_5. Because N_1 and N_5 are across the pteridine ring from one another, the interaction of N_1 with the DHFR Asp^{27} will effectively stand the false substrate "on its head" relative to the orientation of 7,8-DHF (Fig. 42.30) (61,62). With the 5,6-double bond of methotrexate 180° away from the bound NADPH cofactor (61) and stabilized by the fully aromatic pteridine ring, the possibility for reduction is eliminated. The DHFR enzyme will be pseudoirreversibly bound to a molecule it cannot reduce, which ties up the DHFR enzyme and prevents the conversion of DHF to THF. In turn, this halts the synthesis of the 5,10-methylene-THF cofactor required for dTMP biosynthesis and causes feedback inhibition of the thymidylate synthase enzyme. The cell will die a "thymineless death."

Methotrexate can be given orally in the treatment of breast, head and neck, and various lung cancers as well as in non-Hodgkin's lymphoma. The sodium salt form also is marketed for IV, intramuscular, intra-arterial, or intrathecal injection. Oral absorption is dose-dependent and peaks at 80 mg/m^2 because of site saturation.

Fig. 42.30. Misorientation of methotrexate of dihydrofolate reductase (DHFR).

The monoglutamate tail of methotrexate permits active transport into cells, with carrier-mediated transport predominating at serum concentration levels lower than 100 μM. Once inside the cell, methotrexate undergoes a polyglutamation reaction that adds several anionic carboxylate groups to trap the drug at the site of action. Polyglutamation is more efficient in tumor cells than in healthy cells and, therefore, may promote selective toxicity of this drug. Cancer cells can become resistant to methotrexate over time which may involve impaired transport across tumor cell membranes, enhanced efflux from the tumor cell, and attenuated polyglutamation rates. The polyglutamated drug will be hydrolyzed back to the parent structure before renal elimination. Up to 90% of an administered dose of methotrexate is excreted unchanged in the urine within 24 hours.

Methotrexate toxicity can occur with high doses if "third space" fluids allow drug to accumulate in ascites and pleural effusions and/or when renal excretion is impaired by kidney disease. When used in high doses, methotrexate and its 7-hydroxymetabolite (which has a three- to fivefold lower water solubility) can precipitate in the renal tubule, causing damaging crystalluria. Methotrexate- induced lung disease is a particularly critical problem, because it can arise at any time and at any dose, and it can even be fatal. Methotrexate use also can precipitate severe GI side effects, including ulcerative stomatitis and hemorrhagic enteritis, leading to intestinal perforation. Potentially fatal skin reactions are a risk as well. As a Category X teratogen, this drug should not be given to women who are pregnant or planning to become pregnant.

If severe methotrexate toxicity occurs, reduced folate replacement therapy with 5-formyltetrahydrofolate (leucovorin) must be initiated as soon as possible. Leucovorin generates the folate cofactors needed by DHFR and GAR transformylase to ensure the continued synthesis of pyrimidine and purine nucleotides in healthy cells. "Leucovorin rescue" therapy often is given as prophylaxis after high-dose methotrexate therapy.

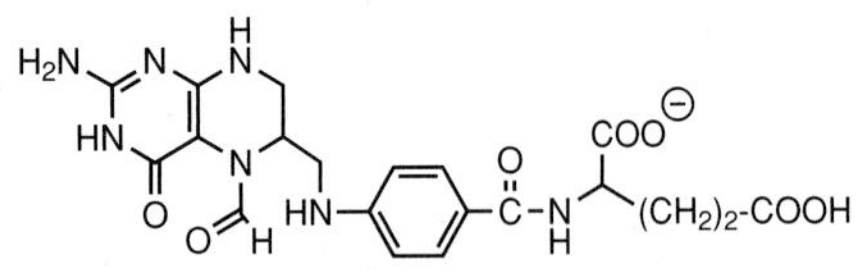

5-Formyltetrahydrofolate
(Leucovorin)

Pemetrexed. Pemetrexed (Fig. 42.25) is a novel multitarget antifolate used by the IV route for the treatment of advanced or metastatic nonsmall cell lung cancer and in combination with cisplatin in malignant pleural mesothelioma. Like methotrexate, it is actively transported into tumor cells through reduced folate carriers and, in polyglutamated form, inhibits the synthesis of pyrimidine and purine-based nucletotides by disrupting folate-dependent metabolic processes (63). In addition to DHFR, this pyrrolopyrimidine-based inhibitor binds tightly to thymidylate synthase and GAR transformylase (64,65). Patients on pemetrexed must take folate and vitamin B_{12} supplements to reduce the risk of bone marrow suppression (neutropenia, thrombocytopenia, and anemia) and GI side effects. Pretreatment with corticosteroids can reduce the risk of drug-induced skin rash. Pemetrexed has a half-life of 3.5 hours and is excreted primarily unchanged via the kidneys. Significant cross-resistance has been noted between pemetrexed and other pyrimidine and folate antagonists (63).

Purine Antagonists: Amidophosphoribosyl Transferase Inhibitors

AMP AND GMP BIOSYNTHESIS. The rate-limiting enzyme in the synthesis of purine nucleotides is amidophosphoribosyl transferase (also known as phosphoribosylpyrophosphate amido transferase), which is a major target for one of the two thiol-containing purine anticancer antimetabolites on the U.S. market.

The pathway outlining the normal synthesis of AMP and GMP is provided in Figure 42.31. It is important to recognize that the rate-limiting step is the first of the pathway; if that step is inhibited, no other step can proceed. Also, note that the rate-limiting transferase enzyme works on a phosphorylated ribose substrate. Because phosphorylated ribose is a component of every intermediate in the pathway, no enzyme in the sequence will function without its presence. Finally, note the reaction in the pathway catalyzed by GAR transformylase, which requires the methyl-donating 10-formyltetrahydrofolate. As previously mentioned, this step is inhibited by methotrexate.

THIOPURINE METABOLISM. The two currently marketed purine anticancer agents are both 6-thio analogues of the endogenous purine bases guanine and purine, also known as inosine (Fig. 42.25). They are prodrugs and must be converted to ribonucleotides by hypoxanthine guanine phosphoribosyl transferase (HGPRT) before they can exert their cytotoxic actions. Mercaptopurine, acting through a methylated ribonucleotide metabolite, inhibits the target amidophosphoribosyl transferase enzyme, leading to the true antimetabolic effect of lowered AMP and GMP biosynthesis (Fig. 42.32). A second mechanism of antineoplastic activity for mercaptopurine (and the predominant mechanism for thioguanine) involves the incorporation of di- and triphosphate deoxy- and ribonucleotides generated within the tumor cell into DNA and RNA, respectively (66). This illicit substitution further inhibits elongation of the strands and promotes apoptosis.

Thiopurines are metabolized by S-methylation via the polymorphic enzyme thiopurine methyl transferase (TPMT) with S-adenosylmethionine serving as cofactor. The methylated thiopurine bases cannot react with HGPRT and, therefore, cannot form the active false ribonucleotides. Drug manufacturers take this into account when establishing dosing regimens. The active false ribonucleotide 6-thioinosinic acid also is subject to extensive TPMT-catalyzed methylation. The S-methyl-6-thioinosinic acid metabolite is a potent inhibitor of the amidophosphoribosyl transferase enzyme and contributes to the cytotoxic action of the parent drug (Fig. 42.32). In contrast, little or no 6-methylthioguanylic acid is produced inside the cell (66,67).

Thiopurine methyl transferase is polymorphic in humans, and some individuals do not express this protein to any significant extent (68). Patients who are poor TPMT metabolizers (e.g., 10% of Caucasians, but also evident in other races) will not experience the activity-attenuating metabolic effect and will generate more active ribonucleotide per dose than patients with normal or excessive levels of the enzyme will. The TPMT genotype of patients should be assessed before initiating thiopurine therapy, because poor metabolizers are at a high risk of life-threatening myelosuppression from elevated levels of false ribonucleotides, even when standard doses are administered (67). In addition, the accumulation of mutagenic thiopurine-based ribonucleotides puts these patients at higher risk for secondary malignancies (66). Thiopurines can still be used in poor TPMT metabolizers, but the dose should be decreased significantly (e.g., 10- to 15-fold) and white blood cell counts monitored vigilantly.

Extensive TPMT metabolizers, who represent up to 90% of patients on thiopurine therapy, will form lower amounts of apoptotic 6-thiolated ribonucleotides. In the case of mercaptopurine, the molecules of ribonucleotide generated will be methylated very rapidly to the antimetabolic 6-methylthioinosinic acid, thus enhancing sensitivity to the drug (67). In contrast, extensive TPMT metabolizers show a decreased sensitivity to thioguanine,

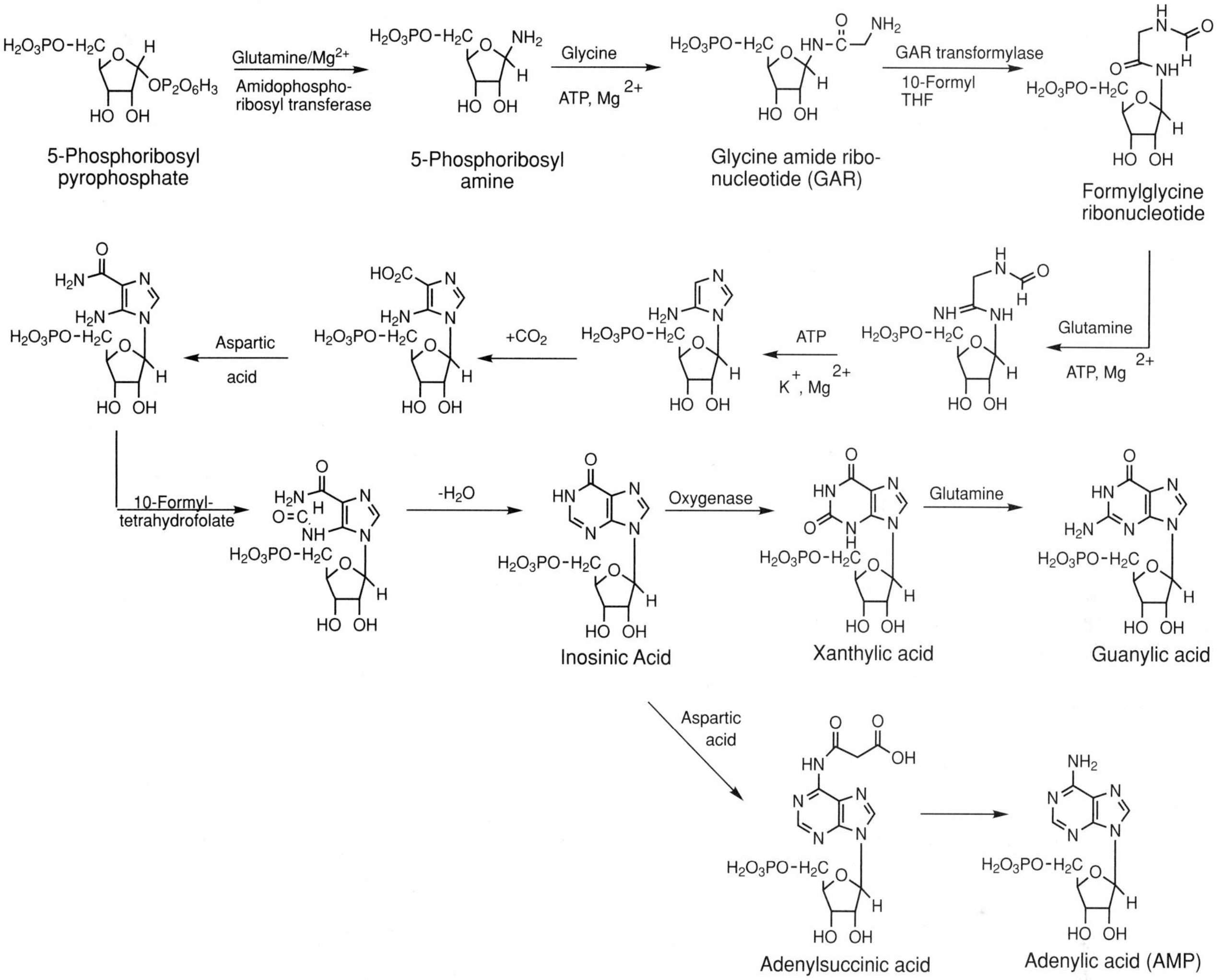

Fig. 42.31. Biosynthetic scheme for the synthesis of purines.

because there is no compensatory increase in the formation of methylated ribonucleotide to offset the decreased production of 6-thioguanylic acid (66).

Xanthine oxidase competes with TPMT for mercaptopurine (but not for thioguanine) and converts it to inactive 6-thiouric acid, which is excreted in the urine (Fig. 42.33) (68). 6-Thioinosinic acid also is subject to metabolism via the xanthine oxidase pathway, ultimately forming the same inactive metabolite. Allopurinol, which inhibits xanthine oxidase and increases levels of active 6-thioinosinic acid, can be coadministered with mercaptopurine to increase its duration of action and effective antineoplastic potency. The dose of mercaptopurine can be cut approximately in half when coadministered with allopurinol. Coadministration of allopurinol with thioguanine is not warranted, because the impact of xanthine oxidase on its metabolic degradation is minor.

SPECIFIC DRUGS

Mercaptopurine. Mercaptopurine (Fig. 42.32) is used in the treatment of acute lymphatic and myelogenous leukemias. It is available in an oral dosage form, but absorption can be erratic and is reduced by the presence of food. The drug is extensively metabolized on first pass and excreted by the kidneys. Bone marrow suppression is the major use-limiting toxicity, although the drug can be hepatotoxic in high doses. Dosage adjustments should be considered in the face of renal or hepatic impairment. Because the major mechanism of action of mercaptopurine is inhibition of de novo purine nucleotide biosynthesis rather than apoptosis secondary to the incorporation of false nucleotides into DNA, there is a lower risk for mutagenesis and secondary malignancy compared to thioguanine (66).

Thioguanine. Thiogunanine (Fig. 42.32) is administered orally in the treatment of nonlymphocytic leukemias. Like mercaptopurine, absorption is incomplete and variable, and the toxicity profiles are similar except where previously noted.

DNA Polymerase/DNA Chain Elongation Inhibitors

Five halogenated and/or ribose-modified DNA nucleoside analogues are marketed for the treatment of a wide

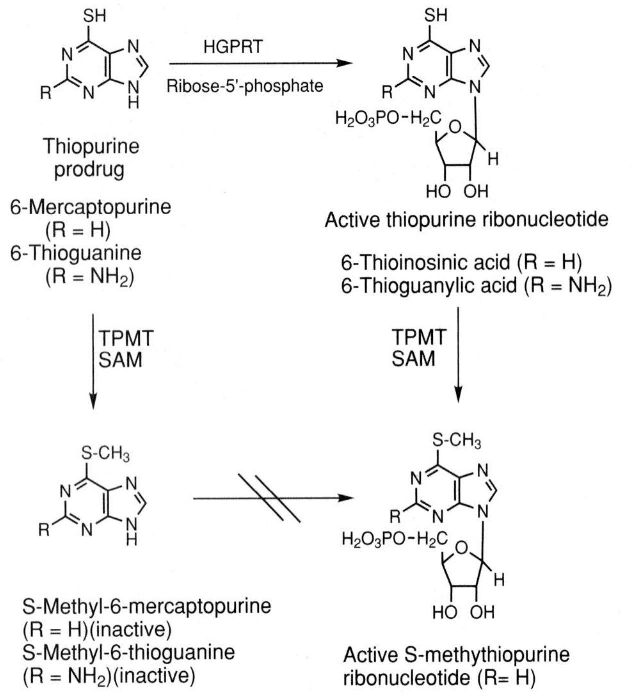

Fig. 42.32. Thiopurine metabolism leading to activation and inactivation.

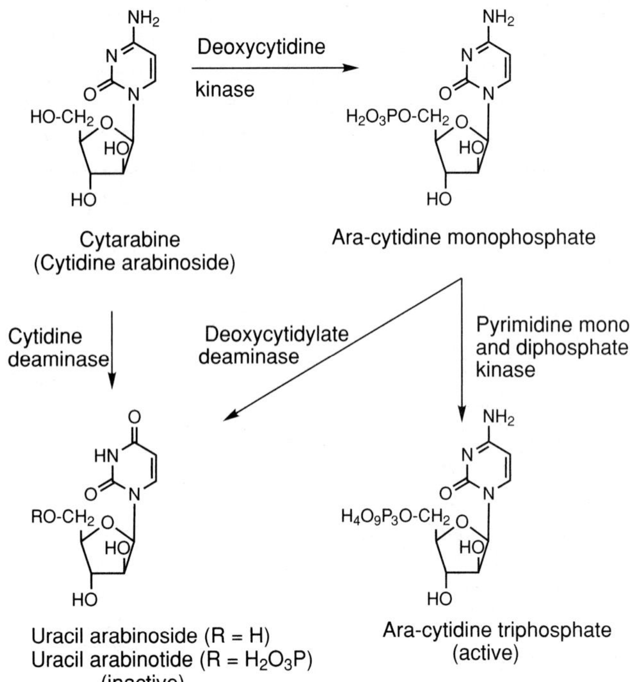

Fig. 42.34. Cytarabine metabolism.

variety of hematologic cancers and solid tumors (Fig. 42.25). These agents have complex and multifaceted mechanisms. All include inhibition of DNA polymerase and/or DNA chain elongation among their actions, however, and all must be converted to triphosphate nucleotides before activity is realized. As nucleosides, they are actively taken up into cells via a selective nucleoside transporter protein, so tumors deficient in this transporter system will be resistant to these anticancer agents. Once inside the cell, specific kinases conduct the essential phosphorylation reactions. In active triphosphate form, they can be mistakenly incorporated into the growing DNA chain, thus arresting further elongation, and/or inhibit enzymes essential for DNA synthesis.

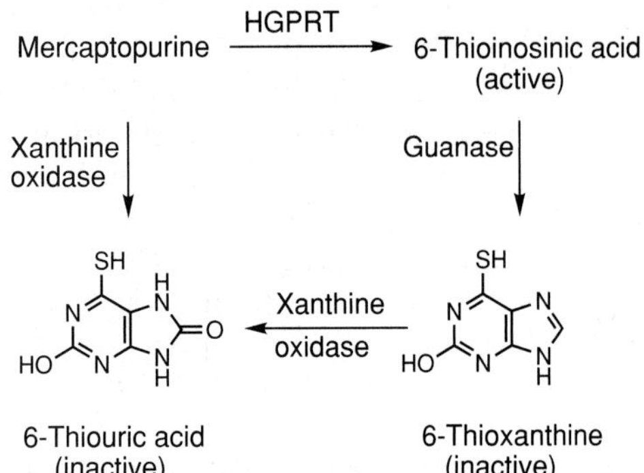

Fig. 42.33. Xanthine oxidase inactivation of mercaptopurine and 6-thioinosinic acid.

All drugs in this group are administered IV, are excreted via the kidneys, and induce myelosuppression as their major use-limiting side effect.

Cytarabine and Gemcitabine. Both of these cytidine-based anticancer agents (Fig. 42.25) undergo initial phosphorylation by deoxycytidine kinase to the monophosphate with subsequent phosphorylations catalyzed by pyrimidine monophosphate and diphosphate kinases. Cytaribine, an arabinoside, is catabolized by cytidine and deoxycytidylate (deoxycytidine monophosphate) deaminases to inactive uracil analogues (Fig. 42.34). The significantly longer half-life of gemcitabine (19 hours) compared to conventional cytarabine (3.6 hours) is caused by the inhibitory action of the difluorodeoxycytidine triphosphate metabolite on the potentially degradative deoxycytidine monophosphate deaminase enzyme (58). Gemcitabine elimination is gender-dependent, with women having the greater risk for toxicity because of lower renal clearance.

Gemcitabine is indicated in the treatment of breast, pancreatic, and nonsmall cell lung cancers. Cytarabine, which can be administered subcutaneously and intrathecally in addition to IV, is used in the treatment of various leukemias. A liposomal formulation of cytarabine is available for the treatment of lymphomatous meningitis.

Fludarabine, Cladribine, and Clofarabine. Like their pyrimidine counterparts, these 3-halogenated adenosine-based nucleosides undergo conversion to the active triphosphate nucleotides (Fig. 42.25) after active transport into tumor cells. All are initially phosphorylated by deoxycytidine kinase, and cells with high levels of this enzyme should respond well to these agents. The C_2-halogen renders the molecules relatively resistant to the degradative action of adenosine deaminase, and a significant fraction of the dose is eliminated unchanged via the kidneys. Fludarabine, an arabinoside, actually is marketed as the monophosphate nucleotide to enhance water solubility for IV administration, but this group is cleaved rapidly in the bloodstream, allowing the free nucleoside to take advantage of the nucleoside-specific transporting proteins.

Cladribine is indicated in the treatment of hairy cell leukemia, whereas fludarabine phosphate is utilized in chronic lymphocytic leukemia. In addition to myelosuppression, fludarabine phosphate can induce hemolytic anemia, and severe CNS toxicity has been noted with high doses.

Clofarabine is used in acute lymphoblastic leukemia patients of 21 years or less who have failed with at least two previous regimens. In addition to inhibiting DNA chain elongation, this drug also inhibits ribonucleotide reductase and facilitates the release of proapoptotic proteins from mitochondria. The rapid attenuation of leukemia cells after administration of this agent can result in a condition known as tumor lysis syndrome, and respiratory and cardiac toxicities can occur secondary to cytokine release. Toxicity can progress to potentially fatal capillary leak syndrome and organ failure, and patients should receive IV fluids for the entire 5-day course of therapy to minimize risk of serious adverse events.

Miscellaneous Antimetabolites

PENTOSTATIN. Pentostatin (Fig. 42.25) is a ring-expanded purine ribonucleoside that inhibits adenosine deaminase and is used in the treatment of hairy cell leukemia. The elevated levels of deoxyadenosine triphosphate that result from inhibition of this degradative enzyme inhibit the action of ribonucleotide reductase (the enzyme that converts ribose diphosphate to deoxyribose diphosphate), thus halting DNA synthesis within the tumor cell.

HYDROXYUREA. Hydroxyurea (Fig. 42.25) blocks the synthesis of DNA by trapping a tyrosyl free radical species at the catalytic site of ribonucleotide reductase, thereby inhibiting the enzyme that converts ribonucleotide diphosphates into their corresponding deoxyribonucleotides. It is used orally for the treatment of melanoma, metastatic or inoperable ovarian cancer, resistant chronic myelocytic leukemia, and as an adjunct to radiation in the treatment of squamous cell carcinoma and cancer of the head and neck. Hydroxyurea increases the effectiveness of radiation therapy through its selective toxicity to cells in the radiation-resistant S phase and by stalling the cell cycle in the G_1 stage, in which radiation therapy does the greatest damage. It addition, hydroxyurea thwarts the normal damage-repair mechanisms of surviving cells.

Hydroxyurea has excellent oral bioavailability (80–100%), and serum levels peak within 2 hours of consuming the capsules. If a positive response is noted within 6 weeks, toxicities generally are mild enough to permit long-term or indefinite therapy on either a daily or every-3-day basis. Leukopenia and, less commonly, thrombocytopenia and/or anemia are the most serious adverse effects. Excretion of the unchanged drug and the urea metabolite is via the kidneys. The carbon dioxide produced as a by-product of hydroxyurea metabolism is excreted in the expired air.

Mitosis Inhibitors

The mitotic process depends on the structural and functional viability of microtubules (polymeric heterodimers consisting of isotypes of α- and β- tubulin proteins). These distinct but nearly identical 50-kDa proteins lie adjacent to one another within the tubule and "roll up" to form an open, pipe-like cylinder akin to a hollow peppermint candy stick. A γ-tubulin protein is found at the organizational center of the microtubule. The nature of the tubulin isotypes found in the microtubule are conserved throughout specific tissues within a given species and will impact the cell's sensitivity to mitosis inhibitors.

During cell division, tubulin undergoes intense, sporadic, and alternating periods of structural growth and erosion known as "dynamic instability." The proteins alternatively polymerize and depolymerize through guanosine triphosphate– and Ca^{2+}-dependent processes. Polymerization involves the addition of tubulin dimers to either end of the tubule, although the faster-growing (+)-end is more commonly involved. Polymerization results in tubular elongation, whereas depolymerization results in the shortening of the structure. The frenetic alteration in structure, facilitated by microtubule-associated proteins (MAPs), ultimately allows the formation of the mitotic spindle and the attachment to chromosomes that is a prerequisite to cell division. Inhibiting the essential hyperdynamic changes in microtubular structure results in mitotic arrest and apoptosis. Two classes of mitosis inhibitors currently are marketed for the treatment of cancer, taxanes, and vinca alkaloids.

Taxanes

Anticancer taxanes initially were isolated from the bark of the Pacific yew (*Taxus brevifolia*) but are now produced semisynthetically from an inactive natural precursor found in the leaves of the European yew (*Taxus baccata*) a renewable resource. Taxanes bind to polymerized (elongated) β-tubulin at a specific receptor site located within the tubular lumen. At standard therapeutic doses (which should lead to intracellular concentrations of 1–20 μM), taxane-tubulin binding renders the microtubules resistant to depolymerization and prone to polymerization (69). This promotes the elongation phase of microtubule dynamic instability at the expense of the shortening phase, and it inhibits the disassembly of the tubule into the mitotic spindle. In turn, this interrupts the normal process of cell division. At these concentrations, extensive polymerization causes the formation of large and

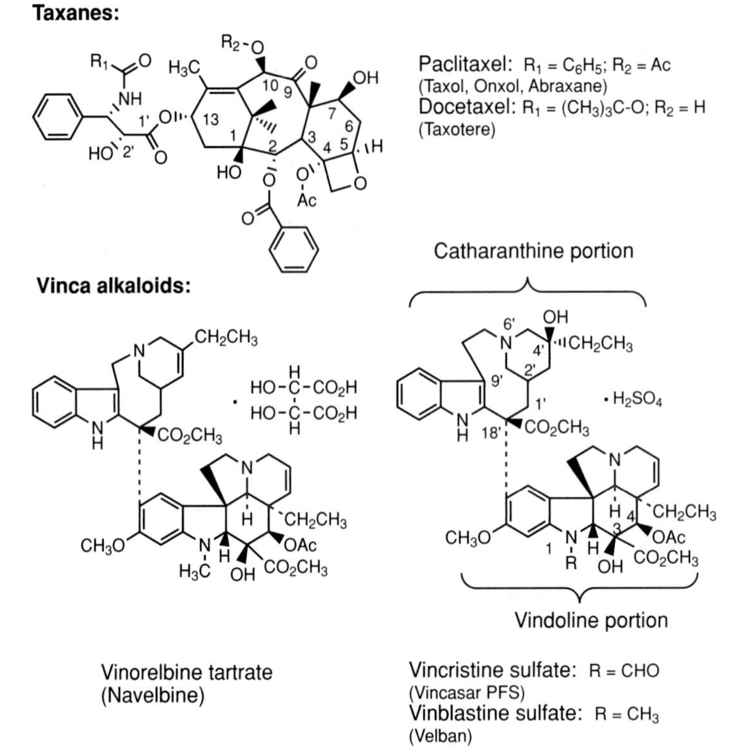

Taxanes:

Paclitaxel: $R_1 = C_6H_5$; $R_2 = Ac$
(Taxol, Onxol, Abraxane)
Docetaxel: $R_1 = (CH_3)_3C\text{-}O$; $R_2 = H$
(Taxotere)

Vinca alkaloids:

Catharanthine portion

Vindoline portion

Vinorelbine tartrate
(Navelbine)

Vincristine sulfate: R = CHO
(Vincasar PFS)
Vinblastine sulfate: $R = CH_3$
(Velban)

Fig. 42.35. Mitosis inhibitors.

dense aberrant structures, known as asters, that contain stabilized microtubule bundles.

Chemistry and Receptor Binding. Chemically, diterpenoid taxanes consist of a 15-membered tricyclic taxane ring system (tricyclo[9.3.1.0]pentadecane) fused to an oxetane (D) ring and contain an esterified β-phenylisoserine side chain at C_{13}. As shown in Figure 42.35, the two marketed taxane antineoplastics differ in substitution pattern at C_{10} (acetate ester or secondary alcohol) and C_{13} (benzamido or *t*-butoxycarboxamido). The taxane ring system often is conceptualized as having "northern" and "southern" halves. The "southern" segment is critical to receptor binding, whereas the "northern" section ensures the proper conformation of essential functional groups, including the C_{13}-isoserine side chain (with its $C_{1'}$-carbonyl, free $C_{2'}$-(R)-OH and $C_{3'}$-(S)-benzamido or *t*-butoxycarboxamido groups), the benzoyl and acetyl esters at C_2 and C_4, respectively, and the intact oxetane ring (70–72).

The key taxane-tubulin binding interactions are identified in Table 42.7, utilizing paclitaxel as ligand (70,73,74). Paclitaxel interacts at the β-tubulin binding site in a folded ("T" or "butterfly") conformation, that places C_2-benzoyl and the $C_{3'}$-benzamido groups in close proximity (70). Their independent intermolecular engagement with a critical β-tubulin His residue, however, which is perfectly positioned between them, keeps them from interacting with one another. The oxetane ring of taxanes, although capable of enhancing receptor affinity through hydrogen bonding (72,73), is believed to serve a more critical role in properly orienting the C_4-acetyl moiety for

Table 42.7. Paclitaxel–β-Tubulin Binding Interactions (70,73,74)

Paclitaxel Functional Group	β-Tubulin Binding Residues	Interaction
C_2-benzoyl phenyl	Leu^{217}, Leu^{219}, His^{229}, Leu^{230}	Hydrophobic
C_2-benzoyl carbonyl	Arg^{278}	Hydrogen bond
$C_{3'}$-benzamido-NH	Asp^{26}	Hydrogen bond
$C_{3'}$-benzamido carbonyl	His^{229}	Hydrogen bond
$C_{3'}$-phenyl	Ala^{233}, Ser^{236}, Phe^{272}	Hydrophobic
C_4-acetyl	Leu^{217}, Leu^{230}, Phe^{272}, Leu^{275}	Hydrophobic
C_7-OH	Thr^{276}, Ser^{277}, Arg^{278}	Hydrogen bond
C_{12}-CH_3	Leu^{217}, Leu^{230}, Phe^{272}, Leu^{275}	Hydrophobic
$C_{2'}$-OH	Arg^{369}, Gly^{370} (NH)	Hydrogen bond
$C_{1'}$-carbonyl	Gly^{370} (NH)	Hydrogen bond
Oxetane oxygen	Thr^{276} (NH)	Hydrogen bond

interaction within its hydrophobic binding pocket (71). The C_1-OH also promotes conformational stability through intramolecular interaction with the carbonyl oxygen of the C_2 benzoyl moiety (70). The areas of the paclitaxel structure where steric influences are most critical to receptor binding have been identified (72).

Taxane metabolism. The taxanes are metabolized to significantly less cytotoxic metabolites by CYP450 enzymes. In humans, CYP2C8 bioconverts paclitaxel to 6α-hydroxypaclitaxel, the major metabolite, which is 30-fold less active than the parent structure (75–77). CYP3A4 mediates the formation of additional minor *p*-hydroxylated metabolites of the benzamido and benzoyl at $C_{3'}$ and C_2 respectively (Fig. 42.36), and the 10-desacetyl metabolite has been documented in urine and plasma. Docetaxel is oxidized exclusively by CYP3A4/5, with CYP3A4 having a 10-fold higher affinity for the drug than CYP3A5. The major metabolite, known as hydroxydocetaxel, is the hydroxymethyl derivative of the 3′-*t*-butoxycarboxamide side chain (77). Hydroxydocetaxel is further oxidized and cyclized to isomeric oxazolidinediones before excretion. The elimination of taxanes is predominantly biliary.

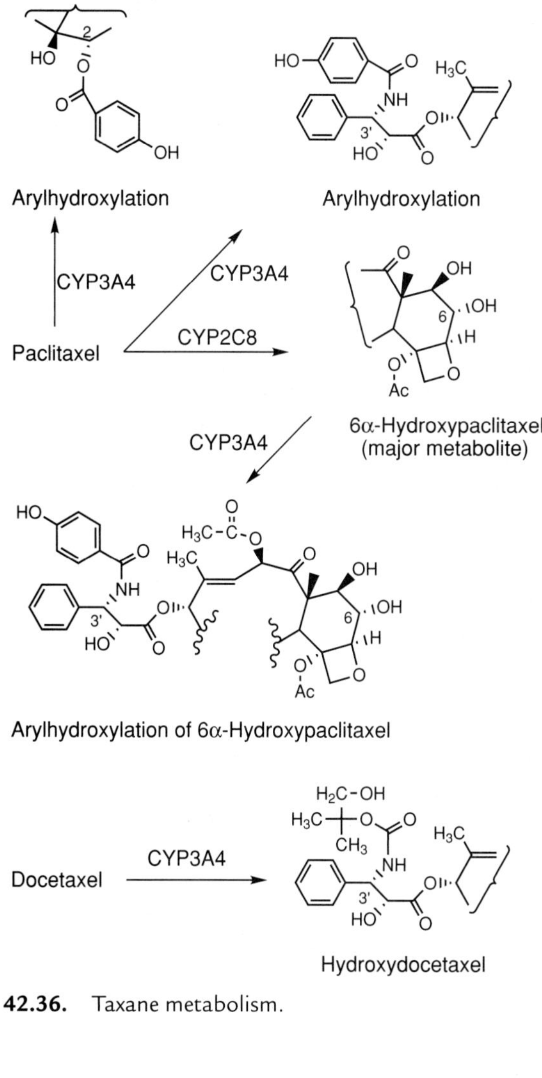

Fig. 42.36. Taxane metabolism.

The metabolic patterns of these closely related structures are distinct, and it has been hypothesized that the C_{13} side chain plays a major role in positioning the compounds in the catalytic site of CYP450 enzymes. Specifically, the 3′-phenyl ring of paclitaxel has been proposed to properly orient C_6 for hydroxylation through π-stacking interactions with CYP2C8 active site residues while decreasing affinity for CYP3A4 binding groups. The hydrophobic character of the 10-acetoxy group, found in paclitaxel, enhances CYP450-mediated hydroxylation two- to fivefold by facilitating substrate binding or augmenting catalytic capability. Both isoforms are impacted by the presence of this ester, often to the same extent (77).

Epothilones

Low water solubility is a significant drawback to the therapeutic utility of the taxanes. This is particularly true of paclitaxel, which has a more lipophilic acetate moiety at C_{10} compared to docetaxel's more polar hydroxyl group. Paclitaxel must be administered in a vehicle of 50% alcohol/50% polyoxyethylated caster oil, which can lead to an enhanced risk of hypersensitivity reactions (dyspnea, hypotension, angioedema, and uticaria) in patients not pretreated with H_1 and H_2 antagonists and dexamethasone (78). In addition, high P-glycoprotein–mediated cellular efflux of both taxane anticancer agents can result in drug resistance. To overcome these problems, epothilone B (Fig. 42.37), a 16-membered macrolide structurally unrelated to the taxanes but with functional groups properly positioned to mimic critical tubulin-binding groups, is being actively investigated for use in a variety of solid tumor and hematologic cancers. Epothilone B binds with very high affinity to the taxane binding site on polymerized β-tubulin, and it acts through the same cytotoxic

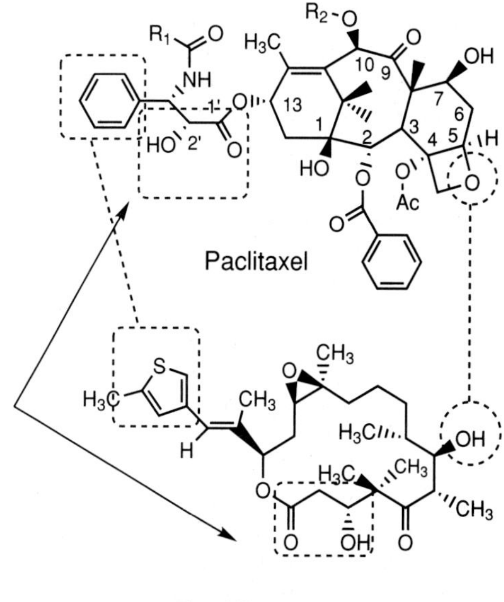

Fig. 42.37. Receptor binding-matched epothilone B and paclitaxel functional groups.

mechanism. In addition to enhanced water solubility and a lack of P-glycoprotein affinity, epothilone is more efficiently produced through fermentation with the myxobacterium *Sorangium cellulosum* and has a higher antineoplastic potency (74,79,80).

SPECIFIC DRUGS

Paclitaxel. Paclitaxel (Fig. 42.35), which is claimed to be "the best-selling anticancer drug in history" (70), is indicated for IV use in combination with cisplatin as first-line therapy for advanced ovarian and nonsmall cell lung cancer. It also is used alone or in combination with the fluorouracil prodrug capecitabine in anthracycline-resistant metastatic breast cancer. Paxclitaxel's ability to up-regulate thymidine phosphorylase, one of capecitabine's activating enzymes, is the rationale behind the combination therapy (81). Solution (Taxol, Onxol) and albumin-bound (Abraxane) formulations are available and cannot be used interchangeably. Abraxane also has been employed in various solid tumors of the GI and genitourinary tracts. Solution-based infusions generally are administered over 3 to 24 hours and can be passed through an in-line, 0.22-μm filter to reduce vehicle-related cloudiness. The albumin-bound form is given over 30 minutes and should be well-mixed (but not filtered) to ensure complete suspension of the protein–drug particles.

The major use-limiting adverse effect of paclitaxel is dose-dependent myelosuppression, particularly neutropenia, and first doses may need to be decreased in patients with hepatic dysfunction. Subsequent dose reductions, if any, should be tailored to individual response. The drug should not be given to patients who have baseline neutrophil counts below 1,500 cells/mm^3. The albumin-bound formulation also is associated with sensory neuropathy. As noted above, all patients receiving solution-based paclitaxel should be pretreated with antihistamines and a corticosteroid to minimize the risk of potentially fatal hypersensitivity reactions. Paclitaxel is a Category D teratogen and carries a high risk of fetal intrauterine mortality. Both male and female patients are advised not to attempt conception while on this drug. Due caution should be observed when coadministering paclitaxel with drugs that inhibit or compete for metabolizing enzymes, particularly CYP2C8 (e.g., 17α-ethinylestradiol and diazepam).

Docetaxel. The indications for docetaxel (Fig. 42.35) generally mirror those of paclitaxel, although docetaxel is not used in ovarian cancer. It has greater water solubility than paclitaxel because of presence of the free C_{10}-OH group, and it is formulated with polysorbate 80 rather than with polyoxyethylated castor oil. Hypersensitivity reactions are still possible, and all patients should receive corticosteroid premedication. In addition to neutropenia and teratogenicity, this taxane can induce significant fluid retention, and 2-kg weight gains are not uncommon. Although rare, onycholysis also has been reported. Drug–drug interactions have been noted when docetaxel is coadministered with drugs that inhibit or compete for CYP3A4 enzymes (e.g., "azole" antifungals, erythromycin, and cyclosporine) (82).

Vinca Alkaloids

Several alkaloids found naturally in *Catharanthus roseus* (periwinkle) have potent antimitotic activity. In opposition to the taxoids, vinca alkaloids halt cell division by inhibiting polymerization. They bind at the interface of two heterodimers within the inner tubular lumen at a single high-affinity site on the (+)-end of the tubules and attenuate the uptake of the guanosine triphosphate essential to tubule elongation (83). Simultaneous binding to α- and β-tubulin results in protein cross-linking, which promotes a stabilized protofilament structure (84). Inhibition of microtubule elongation occurs at "substoichiometric" concentrations, at which alkaloid occupation of only 1 to 2% of the total number of high-affinity sites can result in up to a 50% inhibition of microtubule assembly (85). At high concentrations, when alkaloid binding to high-affinity sites becomes stoichiometric and lower-affinity binding sites on the tubule wall also are occupied, microtubular depolymerization is stimulated, leading to the exposure of additional alkaloidal binding sites and resulting in dramatic changes in microtubular conformation. Spiral aggregates, protofilaments, and highly structured crystals form, and the mitotic spindle ultimately disintegrates (69,81). The loss of the directing mitotic spindle promotes chromosome "clumping" in unnatural shapes (balls and stars), leading to cell death (78). Other nonmitotic toxicities related to the microtubule-disrupting action of the vinca alkaloids include inhibition of axonal transport and secretory processes and disturbances in platelet structure and function (85).

CHEMISTRY. The specific chemical nature of the vinca binding site remains elusive because of difficulties encountered in binding assay development and implementation as well as in data analysis. It is known that the active site is close to residue 339 and residue 390 on α- and β-tubulin, respectively (86). Of the three marketed vinca alkaloids (vincristine, vinblastine, and vinorelbine), vincristine binds most tightly, whereas vinblastine has the lowest affinity (85). Because vinca alkaloids enter cells by simple passive diffusion, unbound vinorelbine and vinblastine (being more lipophilic than vincristine) may be more extensively taken up into tissues. Vincristine, however, is cleared more slowly from the system and has the longest terminal half-life of the three agents, resulting in a more prolonged tumor cell exposure (69,85). Like the taxanes, tumor resistance to vinca alkaloids is mediated through P-glycoprotein.

The vinca alkaloids are complex structures composed of two polycyclic segments known as catharanthine (or velbanamine) and vindoline (Fig. 42.35), both of which are essential for high-affinity tubulin binding. The three commercially available anticancer alkaloids differ in the length of the alkyl chain bridging positions 6′ and 9′ of the catharanthine moiety (methylene or ethylene), in the substituents at position 4′ (olefin or tertiary alcohol), and in the N_1 vindoline indole nitrogen (methyl or formyl). Although subtle, these structural changes lead to significant differences in clinical spectrum, potency, and toxicity. For example, vincristine's relative lack of bone marrow toxicity at standard therapeutic doses makes it popular in combination therapy with more myelosuppressive anticancer agents, whereas vinblastine's relative lack of neurotoxicity permits its coadministration with cisplatin. It is known that acetylation of either hydroxyl group destroys antineoplastic activity. Reduction of the vindoline olefinic linkage greatly attenuates action (78). The $C_{18'}$-methoxycarbonyl, as well as the stereochemistry at positions 18′ and 2′, also are believed to be critical to activity (87).

Vinca alkaloids undergo O_4-deacetylation to yield metabolites equally or more active than the parent drug. They also are subject to extensive CYP3A4-mediated metabolism before biliary excretion, although the structures of these metabolites are currently unknown (88–90).

Specific drugs

Vincristine. Vincristine (Fig. 42.35) is marketed as the sulfate salt and is given by the IV bolus or continuous infusion routes in the treatment of acute leukemia and various Hodgkin's and non-Hodgkin's lymphomas. Toxicity often is more pronounced by the latter route. Elimination is triphasic, with the first phase (5 minutes) representing rapid uptake into tissues and the last phase (85 hours) representing release back to the plasma from tubulin-containing cells. Because the drug is extensively metabolized in the liver, patients with hepatic dysfunction are at an increased risk for toxicity, and dosage reductions should be considered. The most significant dose-limiting adverse effect is neurotoxicity, which can manifest initially as numbness and painful paresthesias in the extremities and progress to muscular pain, severe weakness, and loss of coordination. Patients can experience constipation secondary to intestinal neurotoxicity, which may require treatment with cathartics. Myelosuppression is not particularly problematic, because it occurs at doses higher than those that can be tolerated. As previously noted, coadministration with mitomycin can induce acute or delayed pulmonary toxicity characterized by severe bronchospasm.

All vinca alkaloids are severe vesicants that can induce necrosis, cellulitis, and/or thrombophlebitis. Proper needle placement before administration should be assured to eliminate the risk of extravasation. Unlike the tissue damage caused by the vesicant action of nitrogen mustards and antibiotic antineoplastics, cold exacerbates tissue destruction. If extravasation occurs, apply heat for 1 hour fours time a day for 3 to 5 days, coupled with local hyaluronidase injections. Vinca alkaloids are all Category D teratogens and are fatal if administered by the intrathecal route.

Vinblastine. In addition to the hematologic indications that it shares with vincristine, vinblastine sulfate (Fig. 42.35) has found utility in the treatment of advanced testicular carcinoma (often in combination with bleomycin), advanced mycosis fungoides, Kaposi's sarcoma, and histiocytosis X. Leukopenia is the dose-limiting side effect, and dose reductions are warranted in patients with serum bilirubin levels greater than 3 mg/dL. The drug-related impact on erythrocyte and thrombocyte levels usually is insignificant. Like vincristine, it is administered as an IV bolus or infusion. The initial elimination half-life of 3.7 minutes is similar to vincristine, but the 24.8-hour terminal half-life is significantly shorter.

Vinorelbine. Vinorelbine tartrate (Fig. 42.35) is used alone or in combination with cisplatin for first-line treatment of nonsmall cell lung cancer. This semisynthetic alkaloid is unique in having oral bioavailability (85), but it currently is available only for IV injection. The initial phase elimination half-life is on par with that observed for vincristine and vinblastine, and the terminal phase half-life is between 28 and 44 hours. Although dose-limiting granulocytopenia is the major adverse effect, potentially fatal interstitial pulmonary changes have been noted, and patients with symptoms of respiratory distress should be promptly evaluated. As with all vinca alkaloids, elimination is primarily hepatobiliary, and dosage reduction should be considered in patients with liver dysfunction.

Estramustine. Because this anticancer agent contains a carbamylated nitrogen mustard moiety (Fig. 42.3), it is most commonly classified as a DNA alkylator; however, it is now known that its primary mechanism of antineoplastic action is inhibition of mitosis. Estramustine binds to MAP-4, prompting dissociation of this protein from the microtubule and promoting depolymerization and disassembly. It also can bind directly to α- and β-tubulin at a site distinct from the vinca alkaloid and taxane binding sites, although paclitaxel exerts a noncompetitive inhibition of estramustine binding to tubulin. A specific estramustine binding protein in prostate tissue is believed to facilitate its action in the treatment of metastatic carcinoma of the prostate. Estramustine has a low affinity for the β_{III} tubulin isotype, which often is overexpressed in estramustine-resistant prostatic neoplasms as one defense against this therapeutic intervention (81,91).

Topoisomerase Poisons

Epipodophyllotoxins

The epipodophyllotoxins (Fig. 42.38) are semisynthetic glycosidic derivatives of podophyllotoxin, the major component of the resinous podophyllin isolated from the dried roots of the American mandrake or mayapple plant (*Podophyllum peltatum*). Although these compounds are capable of binding to tubulin and inhibiting mitosis, their primary mechanism of antineoplastic action is poisoning topoisomerase II, a mechanism that they share

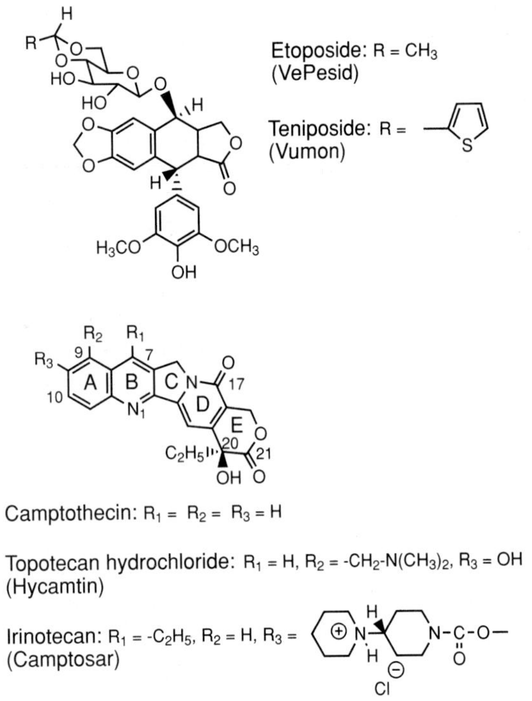

Etoposide: R = CH_3
(VePesid)

Teniposide: R = (thienyl)
(Vumon)

Camptothecin: R_1 = R_2 = R_3 = H

Topotecan hydrochloride: R_1 = H, R_2 = $-CH_2-N(CH_3)_2$, R_3 = OH
(Hycamtin)

Irinotecan: R_1 = $-C_2H_5$, R_2 = H, R_3 =
(Camptosar)

Fig. 42.38. Topoisomerase poisons.

with anthracyclines and dactinomycin (discussed with the antibiotic antineoplastics under *Antibiotics*). Topoisomerase IIα has two distinct DNA-independent binding sites for the epipodophyllotoxins, one within the catalytic domain and a second within the N-terminal ATP-binding domain (92). Once bound, the toxins stabilize the cleavable ternary drug-enzyme-DNA complex, stimulating DNA ligation but inhibiting resealing. The DNA-topoisomerase fragments accumulate in the cell, ultimately resulting in apoptosis. The RNA transcription processes also are disrupted by the interaction of epipodophyllotoxins with topoisomerase IIα (93).

Epipodophyllotoxins are cell-cycle specific and have their most devastating impact on cells in the S or early G_2 phase. For this reason, doses are divided and administered over several days. Resistance is multifaceted and involves down-regulation of topoisomerase IIα, attenuation of enzymatic activity levels, development of novel DNA repair mechanisms, and P-glycoprotein–mediated cellular efflux.

Chemistry. Structurally, the two marketed epipodophyllotoxins, etoposide and teniposide, differ only in the nature of one β-D-glucopyranosyl substituent (methyl or thienyl, respectively). Both are highly water insoluble, but teniposide's higher lipophilicity facilitates cellular uptake and results in a 10-fold enhancement of potency (93). The need for solubility enhancers, such as polysorbate 80 (Tween, etoposide) or polyoxyethylated castor oil (Cremophor EL, teniposide), in IV formulations puts patients at risk for hypersensitivity reactions that can manifest as hypotension and thrombophlebitis. Epinephrine, antihistamines, and corticosteroids often are coadministered to minimize risk. A water-soluble phosphate ester analogue of etoposide can be administered in standard aqueous vehicles, permitting higher doses than the oil-modified formulations would allow. The phosphate ester is rapidly cleaved to the free alcohol in the blood.

Metabolism. Epipodophyllotoxins are subject to metabolic transformation before renal and nonrenal elimination (Fig. 42.39). Etoposide is stable enough for oral administration, although a dose approximately twice that of the IV formulation must be administered. Teniposide is more extensively metabolized, presumably because of its enhanced ability to penetrate into hepatocytes, and no oral dosage form is marketed. Both drugs undergo lactone hydrolysis to generate the inactive hydroxy acid as the major metabolite, but the parent drugs also can be transformed by CYP3A4-catalyzed O-demethylation and Phase II glucuronide or sulfate conjugation. Phase II metabolism accounts for between 5 to 22% of the dose. Clinically significant interactions between epipodophyllotoxins and CYP3A4 inducers, such as phenytoin, phenobarbital, and St. John's wort, have been documented, and coadministration can enhance antineoplastic drug clearance by as much as

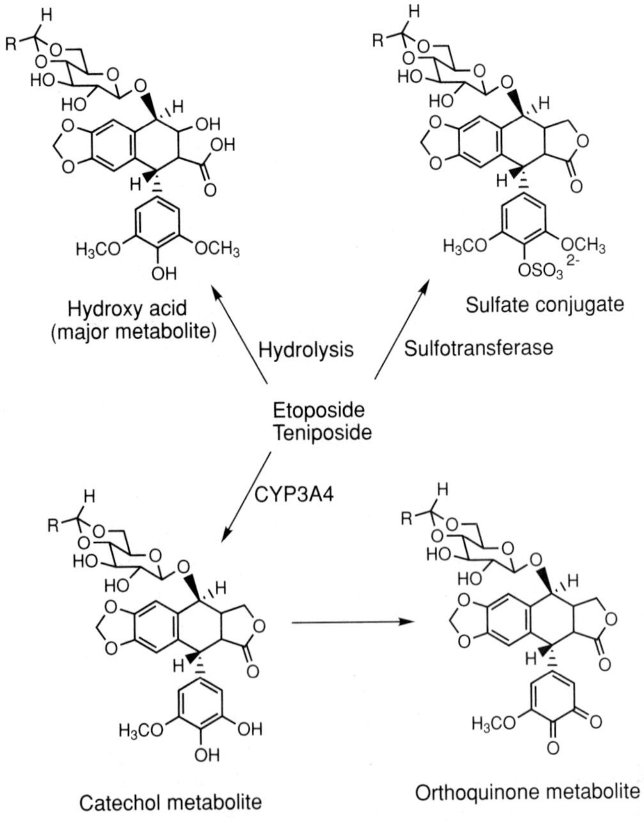

Hydroxy acid (major metabolite) — Hydrolysis
Sulfate conjugate — Sulfotransferase
Etoposide Teniposide
CYP3A4
Catechol metabolite
Orthoquinone metabolite

Fig. 42.39. Epipodophyllotoxin metabolism.

77%. Conversely, CYP3A4 inhibitors, such as cyclosporine or macrolide antibiotics, can decrease clearance, leading to unwanted toxicity.

The catechol metabolite can oxidize to a reactive orthoquinone, and both have been proposed to promote topoisomerase-mediated DNA cleavage, potentially enhancing the risk of the translocations that result in therapy-induced acute myeloid leukemia in children treated with these drugs. Epipodophyllotoxin-induced leukemia occurs in 2 to 12% of patients and is believed to result from translocation of the *MLL* gene at chromosome band 11q23. The mean latency period of 2 years is shorter than the 5- to 7-year latency for leukemia induced by DNA alkylators, and the drug-induced cancer often is resistant to standard treatment (including bone marrow transplantation) (94). Other serious adverse effects include dose-limiting mucositis and myelosuppression, particularly leukopenia. Alopecia is common, and nausea and vomiting, most noticeable with the oral dosage form, generally are mild.

SPECIFIC DRUGS

Etoposide. Etoposide (Fig. 42.38) is utilized in the treatment of small cell lung cancer and in combination with other agents in refractory testicular cancer. Both IV and oral formulations are available. Oral bioavailability is concentration dependent and runs approximately 50% for the 50-mg capsule. Little first-pass metabolism is noted with the gelatin capsule dosage form. The drug is more than 96% protein bound, undergoes biphasic elimination, and has a terminal half-life of 4 to 11 hours. Approximately 35 to 45% of a dose is eliminated via the kidneys, with less than 6% excreted in feces. The drug should be used with caution in patients with renal or liver disease. Specifically, doses should be decreased in patients with creatinine clearance of less than 50 mL/min or bilirubin levels of greater than 1.5 mg/dL, and the drug should not be used in patients with bilirubin levels of greater than 3.1 mg/dL. Organoplatinum anticancer agents (e.g., cisplatin) decrease etoposide clearance, especially in children. If used in combination, administration must be separated by at least 2 days.

Teniposide. Teniposide (Fig. 42.38) is used in combination with other agents for the treatment of refractory childhood acute lymphoblastic leukemia. Compared to etoposide, it is more tightly protein bound (>99%), more extensively metabolized, more slowly cleared (terminal half-life, 5–40 hours), and less dependent on renal elimination (10–21%). Exposure to heparin can cause teniposide to precipitate, so lines must be thoroughly flushed before and after teniposide administration. The drug also can spontaneously precipitate, particularly if solutions are overagitated, and patients receiving 24-hour infusions should be monitored for blockage of access catheters. Teniposide and etoposide are Category D teratogens and, if at all possible, should not be used in women of childbearing years.

Camptothecins

MECHANISM OF ACTION. Camptothecins are chiral, extensively conjugated, amine-containing pentacyclic lactones (Fig. 42.38). The biological target of camptothecins is topoisomerase I (rather than the topoisomerase II enzyme that serves as the receptor for the anthracyclines, dactinomycin and epipodophyllotoxins), but the mechanism of antineoplastic action is qualitatively similar (stabilization of a cleavable ternary DNA-enzyme complex that does not permit the resealing of nicked DNA). Although the fragmented DNA is capable of resealing in the absence of drug, when DNA replication forks encounter the fragmented DNA, a double-stranded DNA break occurs, killing the cell.

The binding of camptothecins occurs in such a way as to stabilize a covalent DNA-topoisomerase bond at the point of single-strand breakage (Tyr^{723} on the human enzyme). The binding pocket, located within the DNA strand, is revealed only after the normal DNA nicking has occurred, explaining why these poisons preferentially bind to the enzyme-DNA complex rather than to unoccupied DNA or enzyme. The flat camptothecin ring system intercalates DNA at the site of cleavage, mimicking a DNA base pair (95). The crystal structures of human ternary complexes involving the parent camptothecin alkaloid, camptothecin, and the semisynthetic analogue, topotecan (Fig. 42.38), have been solved, and important drug–protein interacting entities are noted in Table 42.8 (95,96). The bulky substituents at C_7, C_9, and C_{10} of the marketed compounds, which project into the major groove of DNA, do not hinder binding.

Camptothecins are most potent in cells undergoing active DNA replication and cell division (e.g., they are S-phase specific). Mechanisms of resistance are similar to those discussed for other drugs and include down-regulation or mutation of the target enzyme, down-regulation of enzymes needed for drug activation, and cellular efflux. Breast cancer resistance protein and multidrug resistance (MDR)-associated proteins, such as MAP-2 and MAP-3, rather than P-glycoprotein, appear to mediate resistance to these agents (78,93).

CHEMISTRY. The parent camptothecin alkaloid, isolated from bark of *Camptotheca acuminate*, has antitumor activity, but its limited water solubility necessitated delivery as

Table 42.8. Topotecan–Topoisomerase I Interactions (95,96)

Topotecan Functional Group	Topoisomerase I Residue
Pyridine N_1	Arg^{364}
C_{10}-OH	Enzyme associated water (H-bond)
C_{17}-pyridone carbonyl	Asn^{722}
C_{20}-OH	Asp^{533} (H-bond)
C_{21}-lactone carbonyl	Tyr^{723}-phosphate, Lys^{532}

the sodium salt of the significantly less active hydrolyzed lactone. Lactonization of the hydroxy acid in acidic urine was significant, and elevated levels of active intact alkaloid in the kidney accounted for the hemorrhagic cystitis induced by this compound. Currently marketed analogues have a basic side chain incorporated at either C_9 (tocotecan) or C_{10} (irinotecan), allowing the formation of water-soluble salts of the intact semisynthetic alkaloid. At pH 7.4, the active lactone exists in equilibrium with the hydroxy acid hydrolysis product, with the direction dictated by the extent of binding to serum albumin. The preferential protein binding of the lactone, which occurs with irinotecan, shifts the equilibrium to favor the production of the more active lactone, thus enhancing potency.

Specific Drugs

Irinotecan Hydrochloride. In combination with fluorouracil, this prodrug camptothecin (Fig. 42.38) analogue is considered to be first-line therapy in the treatment of metastatic colorectal cancer. It also has shown efficacy in small cell and nonsmall cell lung cancers when used in combination with cisplatin. Given IV, the drug is slowly bioactivated in the liver through hydrolysis of the C_{10}-carbamate ester. The catalyzing enzyme is a saturable carboxylesterase known as irinotecan-converting enzyme. Levels of active metabolite, known as SN-38 (Fig. 42.40), are 50- to 100-fold lower than the parent drug, but preferential protein binding of the lactone (95%) permits significant plasma levels of the optimally active SN-38 compared to the hydroxy acid metabolite. SN-38 has a terminal half-life of 11.5 hours (compared to 5.0–9.6 hours for the prodrug parent) and is glucuronidated at the C_{10} phenol before elimination. CYP3A4 also cleaves the terminal piperidine ring through oxidation at the α-carbons, followed by hydrolysis of the resultant amides, producing inactive metabolites. Excretion of the parent drug and metabolites is renal (14–37%) and, to a lesser extent, biliary.

Delayed diarrhea induced by irinotecan is dose-limiting and potentially fatal, and vigorous loperamide therapy should be instituted at the first sign of symptoms. Acute diarrhea is attributed to the drug's ability to inhibit acetylcholinesterase and can be addressed through anticholinergic pretreatment. Pretreatment also helps patients to avoid "cholinergic syndrome," a collection of annoying side effects that include flushing, sweating, blurred vision, lacrimation, and less commonly, bradycardia. Camptothecins also are myelosuppressive, and neutropenia can be severe, particularly in patients with elevated bilirubin levels. Extensive biotransformation also demands cautious use of irinotecan in patients with hepatic dysfunction. Prophylactic antiemetic therapy should be given at least 30 minutes before the administration of irinotecan to minimize the nausea and vomiting associated with this anticancer agent.

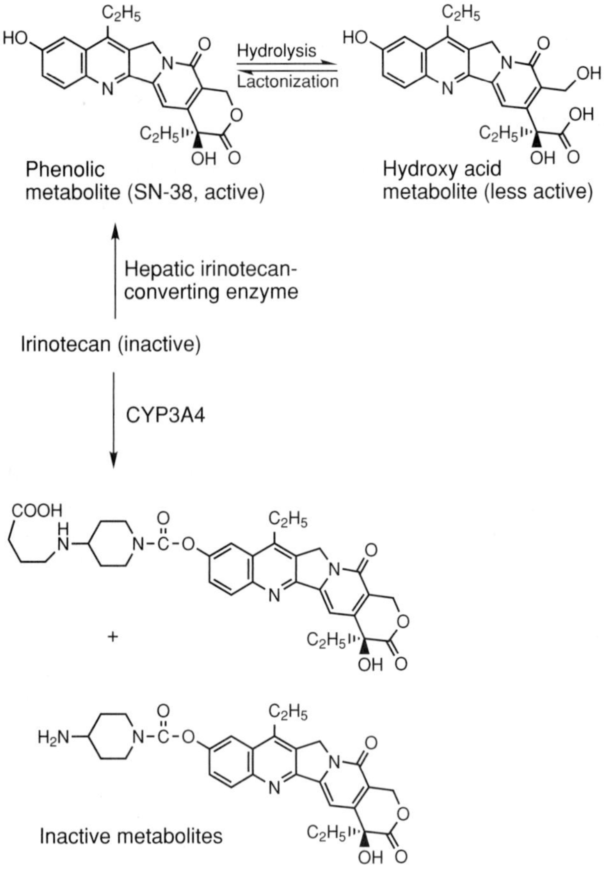

Fig. 42.40. Irinotecan metabolism.

Topotecan Hydrochloride. This active camptothecin analogue (Fig. 42.38) is used by the IV route in the treatment of ovarian and small cell lung cancer that has not responded to first-line therapy. Myelosuppression, particularly neutropenia, is use-limiting and has precluded combination therapy with other bone marrow-suppressing drugs. Thrombocytopenia and anemia occur in approximately one-third of treated patients. Schedules that call for daily (for 5 days) administration also can result in serious mucositis and diarrhea.

Topotecan elimination is biphasic, with a terminal half-life of 2.0 to 3.5 hours. Lactone hydrolysis is rapid, and binding to serum proteins is limited to between 25 and 40%. CYP3A4-mediated N-dealkylation to mono- and didealkylated metabolites occurs to a limited extent, and the O-glucuronides that form at multiple points along the metabolic path are excreted via the kidney (Fig. 42.41). Extensive renal clearance demands dosage adjustment in patients with kidney disease.

Because both topotecan and irinotecan are metabolized by CYP3A4, the potential for drug–drug interactions must be evaluated. Reduced clearance was noted when azole antifungal agents and cyclosporine were coadministered with irinotecan, and accelerated clearance

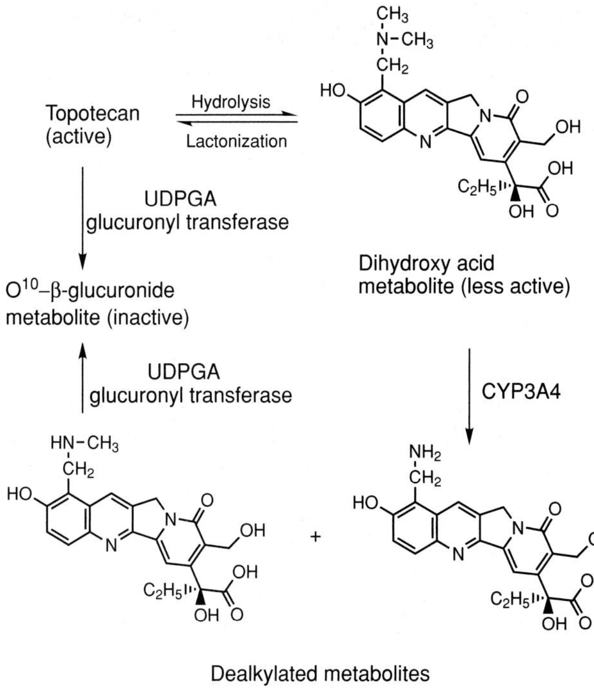

Topotecan (active) — Hydrolysis / Lactonization — Dihydroxy acid metabolite (less active)

UDPGA glucuronyl transferase

O^{10}–β-glucuronide metabolite (inactive)

UDPGA glucuronyl transferase

CYP3A4

Dealkylated metabolites

Fig. 42.41. Topotecan metabolism.

was observed when topotecan was coadministered with CYP3A4 inducers, such as phenobarbital and phenytoin.

Miscellaneous Anticancer Agents: DNA Demethylators

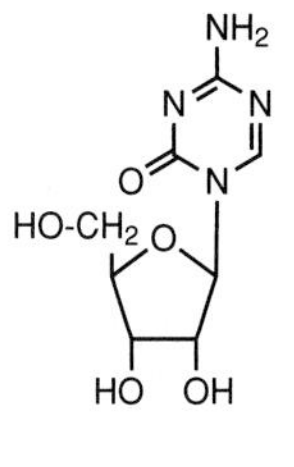

Azacitidine (Vidaza)

Azacitidine

In contrast to the DNA alkylating agents discussed earlier in this chapter, one nucleic acid–based chemotherapeutic agent, azacitidine, blocks abnormal cellular proliferation by dealkylating (specifically demethylating) DNA residues on genes responsible for differentiation and growth. The hypomethylation effect sometimes can restore normal gene function while selectively killing cells that have stopped responding to the body's cellular proliferation control processes. Azacitidine is given subcutaneously for the treatment of myelodysplastic syndrome, and serum levels generally are maximized within 30 minutes. The parent drug and its metabolites are excreted in the urine. Azacitidine is carcinogenic and teratogenic in rodents, and leukopenia, thrombocytopenia, and neutropenia are the most common reasons for drug discontinuation or dosage reduction.

Other Chemotherapeutic Approaches

Hormone Therapy

Glucocorticoids (e.g., prednisone and methylprednisolone) commonly are administered with anticancer agents to suppress lymphocytic activity and to enhance the chance of success in the treatment of leukemias and lymphomas. In addition, some tumors, such as estrogen-dependent breast cancer, endometrial cancer, and metastatic cancer of the prostate, depend on the presence of sex hormones for viability. In these neoplastic diseases, the use of steroid receptor antagonists, synthesis inhibitors, or gonadotropin secretion inhibitors, either alone or in combination with other antineoplastic drugs, is a common approach to chemotherapeutic care. Antiestrogens (e.g., tamoxifen), antiandrogens (e.g., flutamide), progestins (e.g., megestrol acetate), aromatase inhibitors (e.g., exemestane), and luteinizing hormone–releasing hormone agonists (e.g., leuprolide acetate) are all available for use in managing hormone-dependent tumors and often are employed after surgery, radiation therapy, and/or other chemotherapy. (Readers are referred to Chapters 45 and 46 for a more detailed discussion of the hormone agonists and antagonists currently used in the treatment of cancer.)

Enzyme Therapy

Exogenous asparagine is essential to the survival of malignant lymphocytic leukemia cells, because these cells lack asparagine synthetase enzymes. L-Asparaginase (also known as L-asparagine amidohydrolase) or its derivatives can be added to the chemotherapeutic regimen of patients with leukemia to deplete serum asparagine by hydrolysis to aspartate and ammonia. Being deprived of this avenue for asparagine acquisition, tumor cells die from an inability to synthesize essential proteins. Normal cells, which contain asparagine synthetase, are able to synthesize this essential nutrient and can withstand therapy.

Biological Response Modifiers

Several human or recombinant antiproliferative proteins are currently in use for the treatment of cancer. Interleukin-2, interferons, BCG vaccine, tyrosine kinase, epidermal growth factor, proteasome inhibitors, and several monoclonal antibodies directed against tumor cell antigens now augment the cancer chemotherapeutic arsenal. (Readers are directed to Chapter 5 for a more in-depth discussion of the peptides and proteins available for the treatment of neoplastic disease.)

CASE STUDY

Victoria F. Roche and S. William Zito

PR is a 37-year-old Portuguese man who survived Wilms' tumor during his childhood. Unfortunately, the chemotherapy used to treat his neoplasm induced a delayed and drug-resistant cardiomyopathy that ultimately resulted in a successful heart transplant when he was 25. Although he was managing fairly well, PR was recently dealt another health-related blow with a diagnosis of bladder cancer. The cancer was discovered last week and, although aggressive, appears to still be localized to the bladder. He is deemed not to be a candidate for surgery.

PR's current pharmacotherapy includes cyclosporine (an immunosuppressant that is metabolized predominantly by, and also inhibits, CYP3A4) and low-dose prednisone. In addition to the organoplatinum complex cisplatin, his oncologist wants to construct a chemotherapeutic regimen that combines an antimetabolite, a topoisomerase II inhibitor, and a mitosis inhibitor. Review the structure–activity relationships of the following five antineoplastic structures in preparation for your recommendation.

1. Identify the therapeutic problem(s) in which the pharmacist's intervention may benefit the patient.
2. Identify and prioritize the patient-specific factors that must be considered to achieve the desired therapeutic outcomes.
3. Conduct a thorough and mechanistically oriented structure–activity analysis of all therapeutic alternatives provided in the case.
4. Evaluate the structure–activity relationship findings against the patient-specific factors and desired therapeutic outcomes, and make a therapeutic decision.
5. Counsel your patient, and advise the physician.

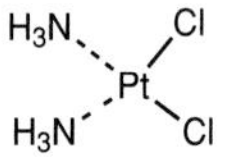

Cisplatin

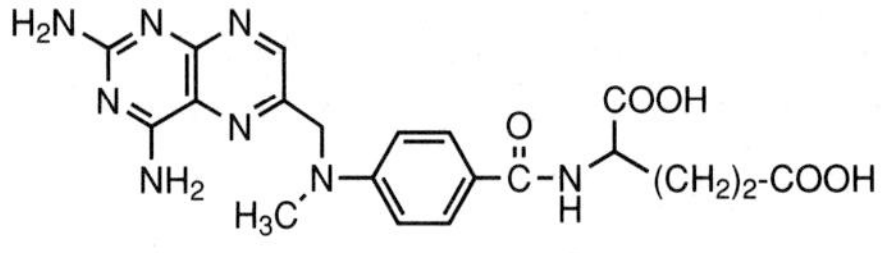

1

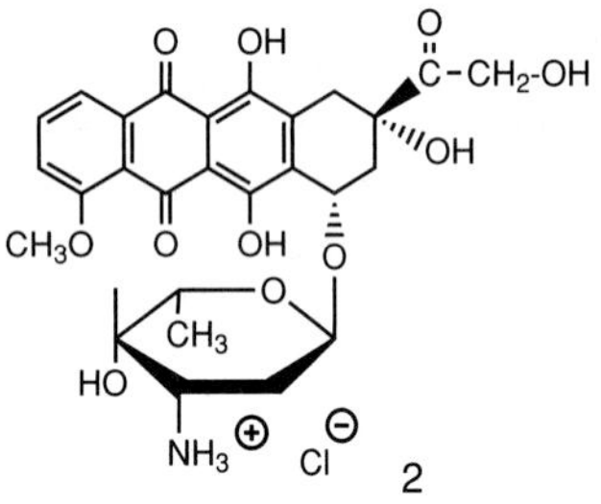

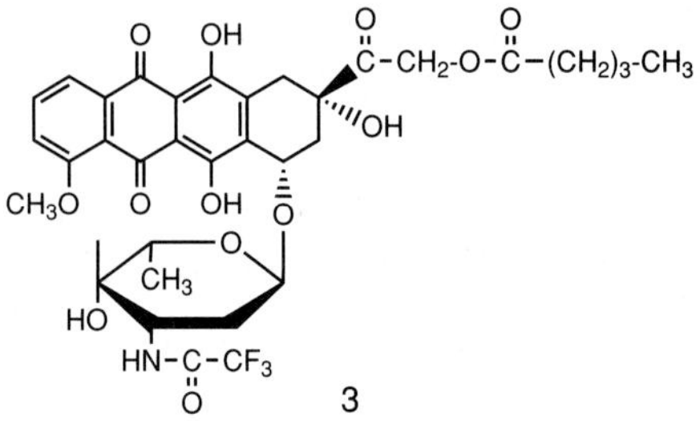

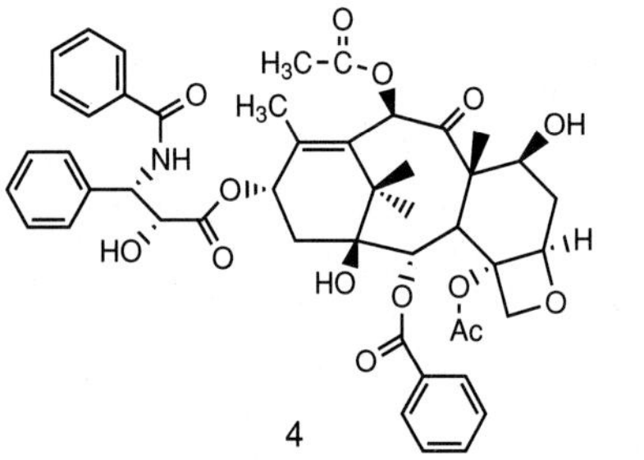

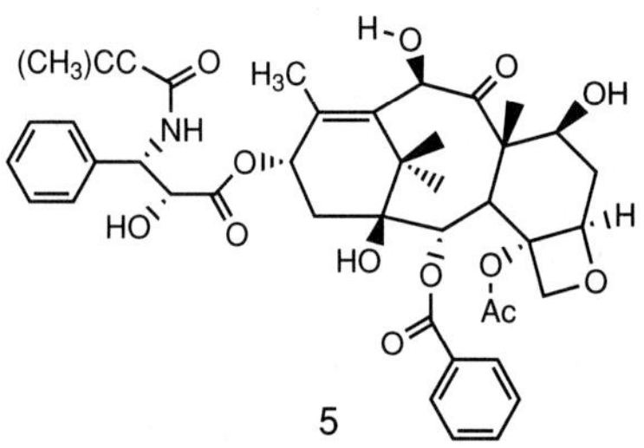

2

3

4

5

References

1. Liu ET. Oncogenes and suppressor genes: genetic control of cancer. In: Goldman L, Ausiello D, eds. Cecil Textbook of Medicine. 22nd Ed. Philadelphia: WB Saunders, 2004:1108–1116.
2. Bertino JR, Hait W. Principles of cancer therapy. In: Goldman L, Ausiello D, eds. Cecil Textbook of Medicine. 22nd Ed. Philadelphia: WB Saunders, 2004:1137–1150.
3. Balmer CM, Valley AW, Iannucci A. Cancer treatment and chemotherapy. In: DiPrio JT, Talbert RL, Yee GC, et al., eds. Pharmacotherapy: A Pathophysiologic Approach. 6th Ed. New York: McGraw-Hill, 2005:2279–2328.
4. Calabresi P, Chabner BA. Chemotherapy of neoplastic diseases. In: Hardman JG, Limbird LE, eds. Goodman & Gilman's The Pharmacological Basis of Therapeutics. 10th Ed. New York: McGraw-Hill, 2001:1386–1388.
5. Stetler-Stevenson WG. Invasion and metastases. In: DeVita VT Jr, Hellman S, Rosenberg SA, eds. Cancer: Principles and Practice of Oncology. 7th Ed. Baltimore: Lippincott Williams &Wilkins, 2005:117–118.
6. Burchenal JH. The historical development of cancer chemotherapy. Semin Oncol 1977;4:135–146.
7. Woglom WH. General review of cancer therapy. In: Moulton FR, ed. Approaches to Tumor Chemotherapy. Washington DC: Amer Assoc Advancement Sci, 1947:1.

8. Chu E. Pharmacology of cancer chemotherapy: drug development. In: DeVita VT Jr, Hellman S, Rosenberg SA, eds. Cancer: Principles and Practice of Oncology. 7th Ed. Baltimore: Lippincott Williams & Wilkins, 2005:307–317.
9. Blot WJ. Epidemiology of cancer. In: Goldman L, Ausiello D, eds. Cecil Textbook of Medicine. 22nd Ed. Philadelphia: WB Saunders, 2004: 1116–1120.
10. http://www.legacyofhope.org/warnsigns.html. Accessed 5/23/07.
11. http://www.healingdaily.com/conditions/7-warning-signs-of-cancer.htm. Accessed 5/23/07.
12. Buchschacher GL Jr, Wong-Staal F. Etiology of cancer: viruses: RNA viruses. In: DeVita VT Jr, Hellman S, Rosenberg SA, eds. Cancer: Principles and Practice of Oncology. 7th Ed. Baltimore: Lippincott Williams & Wilkins, 2005: 165–173.
13. Howley PM, Ganem D, Kieff E. Etiology of cancer: viruses: DNA viruses. In: DeVita VT Jr, Hellman S, Rosenberg SA, eds. Cancer: Principles and Practice of Oncology. 7th Ed. Baltimore: Lippincott Williams &Wilkins, 2005:173–184.
14. Ludeman SM. The chemistry of the metabolites of cyclophosphamide. Curr Pharm Des 1999;5:627–643.
15. Goldenberg GJ, Lee M, Lam HY, et al. Evidence for carrier-mediated transport of melphalan by L5178Y lymphoblasts in vitro. Cancer Res 1977:37:755–760.
16. Huang A, Roy P, Waxman DJ. Role of human liver microsomal CYP3A4 and CYP2B6 in catalyzing N-dechloroethylation of cyclophosphamide and ifosfamide. Biochem Pharmacol 2000;59:961–972.
17. Lind MJ, McGown AT, Hadfield JA, et al. The effect of ifosfamide and its metabolites on intracellular glutathione levels in vitro and in vivo. Biochem Pharmacol 1989;38:1835–1840.
18. Springate JE. Ifosfamide metabolite chloroacetaldehyde causes renal dysfunction in vivo. J Appl Toxicol 1997;17:75–79.
19. Roy P, Yu LJ, Crespi CL, et al. Development of a substrate-activity based approach to identify the major human liver P450 catalysts of cyclophosphamide and ifosfamide activation based on cDNA-expressed activities and liver microsomal P450 profiles. Drug Metab Dispos 1999;27:655–666.
20. Woodland D, Ito S, Granvil CP, et al. Evidence of renal metabolism of ifosfamide to nephrotoxic metabolites. Life Sci 2000;68:109–117.
21. Eisenbrand G, Muller, N, Denkel E, et al. DNA adducts and DNA damage by antineoplastic and carcinogenic N-nitrosocompounds. J Cancer Res Clin Oncol 1986;112:196–204.
22. Kyrtopoulos SA, Anderson LM, Chhabra SK, et al. DNA adducts and the mechanism of carcinogenesis and cytotoxicity of methylating agents of environmental and clinical significance. Cancer Detect Prev 1997;21:391–405.
23. Patterson LH, Murray GI. Tumor cytochrome P450 and drug activation. Curr Pharm Des 2002;8:1335–1347.
24. Moloney SJ, Wiebkin P, Cummings SW, et al. Metabolic activation of the terminal N-methyl group of N-isopropyl-α-(2-methylhydrazino)-p-toluamide hydrochloride (procarbazine). Carcinogenesis 1985;6:397–401.
25. Moloney SJ, Prough RA. Studies on the pathway of methane formation from procarbazine, a 2-methylbenzylhydrazine derivative, by rat liver microsomes. Arch Biochem Biophys 1983;221:577–584.
26. Yamagata S, Ohmori S, Suzuki N, et al. Metabolism of dacarbazine by rat liver microsomes: Contribution of CYP1A enzymes to dacarbazine N-demethylation. Drug Metab Dispos 1998;26:379–382.
27. Coley HM, Brooks N, Phillips DH, et al. The role of N-(hydroxymethyl) melamines as antitumor agents: mechanism of action studies. Biochem Pharmacol 1995;9:1203–1212.
28. Ames MM. Hexamethylmelamine: Pharmacology and mechanism of action. Cancer Treat Rev 1991;18(Suppl. A):3–14.
29. Ponti M, Souhami RL, Fox BW, et al. DNA interstrand cross-linking and sequence selectivity of dimethanesulfonates. Br J Cancer 1991;63:743–747.
30. Iwamoto T, Hiraku Y, Oikawa S, et al. DNA intrastrand cross-link at the 5′-GA-3′ sequence formed by busulfan and its role in the cytotoxic effect. Cancer Sci 2004;95:454–458.
31. Chaney SG, Campbell SL, Bassett E, et al. Recognition and processing of cisplatin- and oxaliplatin-DNA adducts. Crit Rev Oncol Hematol 2005;53:3–11.
32. Raymond E, Faivre S, Woynarowski JM, et al. Oxaliplatin: mechanism of action and antineoplastic activity. Semin Oncol 1998;25(Suppl. 5):4–12.
33. Mishima M, Samimi G, Kondo A, et al. The cellular pharmacology of oxaliplatin resistance. Eur J Cancer 2002;38:1405–1412.
34. Chaney SG, Campbell SL, Temple B, et al. Protein interactions with platinum-DNA adducts: from structure to function. J Inorg Biochem 2004;98: 1551–1559.
35. Barnes KR, Lippard SJ. Cisplatin and related anticancer drugs: recent advances and insights. Metal Ions in Biological Systems 2004;42:143–177.
36. McKeage MJ. New-generation platinum drugs in the treatment of cisplatin-resistant cancers. Expert Opin Invest Drugs 2005;14:1033–1046.
37. Kweekel DM, Gelderblom H, Guchelaar H-J. Pharmacology of oxaliplatin and the use of pharmacogenomics to individualize therapy. Cancer Treat Rev 2005;31:90–105.
38. Grolleau F, Gamelin L, Boisdron-Celle M, et al. A possible explanation for a neurotoxic effect of the anticancer agent oxaliplatin on neuronal voltage-gated sodium channels. J Neurophysiol 2001;85:2293–2297.
39. Gamelin L, Boisdron-Celle M, Delva R, et al. Prevention of oxaliplatin-related neurotoxicity by calcium and magnesium infusions: a retrospective study of 161 patients receiving oxaliplatin combined with 5-fluorouracil and leucovorin for advanced colorectal cancer. Clin Cancer Res 2004;10: 4055–4061.
40. Piestrzeniecwicz MK, Wilmanska D, Szemraj J, et al. Interactions of novel morpholine and hexamethylene derivatives of anthracycline antibiotics with DNA. Z Naturforsch 2004;59:739–748.
41. Binaschi M, Bigioni M, Cipollone A, et al. Anthracyclines: selected new developments. Curr Med Chem 2001;1:113–130.
42. Zunino F, Pratesi G, Perego P. Role of the sugar moiety in the pharmacological activity of anthracyclines: development of a novel series of disaccharide analogues. Biochem Pharmacol 2001;61:933–938.
43. Gerwirtz DA. A critical evaluation of the mechanisms of action proposed for the antitumor effects of the anthracycline antibiotics adriamycin and daunorubicin. Biochem Pharmacol 1999;57:727–741.
44. Kwok JC, Richardson DR. Examination of the mechanism(s) involved in doxorubicin-mediated iron accumulation in ferritin: studies using metabolic inhibitors, protein synthesis inhibitors and lysosomotropic agents. Mol Pharmacol 2004;65:181–195.
45. Lothstein L, Israel M, Sweatman TW. Anthracycline drug targeting: cytoplasmic versus nuclear—a fork in the road. Drug Res Updates 2001;4:169–177.
46. Swain SM, Vici P. The current and future role of dexrazoxane as a cardioprotectant in anthracycline treatment: expert panel review. J Cancer Res Clin Oncol 2004;130:1–7.
47. Fogli S, Nieri P, Breschi MC. The role of nitric oxide in anthracycline toxicity and prospects for pharmacologic prevention of cardiac damage. FASEB J 2004;18:664–675.
48. Kang W, Weiss M. Caffeine enhances the myocardial uptake of idarubicin but reverses its negative inotropic effect. Naunyn-Schmiedelbergs Arch Pharmacol 2003;367:151–155.
49. Correale J, Rush C, Amengual A, et al. Mitoxantrone as rescue therapy in worsening relapsing-remitting MS patients receiving IFN-β. J Neuroimmunol 2005;162:173–183.
50. Basu S, Brown JE, Flannigan GM, et al. The immunohistochemical analysis of NAD(P)H:quinone oxidoreductase and NADPH cytochrome P450 reductase in human superficial bladder tumors: relationship between tumor enzymology and clinical outcome following intravesical mitomycin C therapy. Int J Cancer 2004;109:703–709.
51. Zappa F, Ward T, Pedrinis E, et al. NAD(P)H:quinone oxidoreductase 1 expression in kidney podocytes. J Histochem Cytochem 2003;51:297–302.
52. Grollman AP, Takeshita M, Pillai KMR, et al. Origin and cytotoxic properties of base propenals derived from DNA. Cancer Res 1985;45:1127–1131.
53. Brewer GJ, Dick R, Ullenbruch MR, et al. Inhibition of key cytokines by tetrathiomolybdate in the bleomycin model of pulmonary fibrosis. J Inorg Biochem 2004;98:2160–2167.
54. Guliana S, Polkinghorne I, Smith GA, et al. Macropodid herpesvirus 1 encodes genes for both thymidylate synthase and ICP34.5. Virus-Genes 2002;24:207–213.
55. Schiffer CA, Clifton IJ, Davisson VJ, et al. Crystal structure of human thymidylate synthase: a structural mechanism for guiding substrates into the active site. Biochemistry 1995;34:16279–16287.
56. Kamb A, Finer-Moore J, Calvert AH, et al. Structural basis for recognition of polyglutamyl folates by thymidylate synthase. Biochemistry 1992;31: 9883–9890.
57. Lee A, Ezzeldin H, Fourie J, et al. Dihydropyrimidine dehydrogenase deficiency: impact of pharmacogenetics on 5-fluorouracil therapy. Clin Adv Hematol Oncol 2004;2:527–532.
58. Kummar S, Noronha V, Chu E. Antimetabolites. In: DeVita VT Jr, Hellman S, Rosenberg SA, eds. Cancer: Principles and Practice of Oncology. 7th Ed. Baltimore: Lippincott Williams &Wilkins, 2005:365–374.
59. Dummins PL, Gready JE. Energetically most likely substrate and active-site protonation sites and pathways in the catalytic mechanism of dihydrofolate reductase. J Am Chem Soc 2001;123:3418–3428.
60. Cody V, Luft JR, Ciszak E, et al. Crystal structure determination at 2.3 angstrom of recombinant human dihydrofolate reductase ternary complex with NADPH and methotrexate-γ-tetrazole. Anticancer Drug Des 1992;7: 483–491.
61. Cannon WR, Garrison BJ, Benkovic SJ. Consideration of the pH-dependent inhibition of dihydrofolate reductase by methotrexate. J Mol Biol 1997;271: 656–668.
62. Meiering EM, Li H, Delcamp TJ, et al. Contributions of tryptophan 24 and glutamate 30 to binding long-lived water molecules in the ternary complex of human dihydrofolate reductase with methotrexate and NADPH studies by site directed mutagenesis and nuclear magnetic resonance spectroscopy. J Mol Biol 1995;241:309–325.
63. Raymond E, Louvet, C, Tournigand C, et al. Premetrexed disodium combined with oxaliplatin, SN38, or 5-fluorouracil, based on the quantitation of drug interactions in human HT29 colon cancer cells. Int J Oncol 2002;21:361–367.
64. Mendelsohn LG, Shih C, Chen VJ, et al. Enzyme inhibition, polyglutamation, and the effect of LY231514 (MTA) on purine biosynthesis. Semin Oncol 1999;26(Suppl. 6):42–47.
65. Sayre PH, Finer-Moore JS, Fritz TA, et al. Multitargeted antifolates aimed at avoiding drug resistance form covalent closed inhibitory complexes with human and *Escherichia coli* thymidylate synthases. J Mol Biol 2001;313: 813–829.

66. Coulthard SA, Hogarth LA, Little M, et al. The effect of thiopurine methyltransferase expression on sensitivity to thiopurine drugs. Mol Pharmacol 2002;62:102–109.
67. Cara CJ, Pena AS, Sans M, et al. Reviewing the mechanism of action of thiopurine drugs: toward a new paradigm in clinical practice. Med Sci Mont 2004;10:247–254.
68. Coulthard S, Hogarth L. The thiopurines: an update. Invest New Drugs 2005; 23:523–532.
69. Rowinsky EK, Tolcher AW. Antimicrotubule agents. In: DeVita VT Jr, Hellman S, Rosenberg SA, eds. Cancer: Principles and Practice of Oncology. 7th Ed. Baltimore: Lippincott Williams &Wilkins, 2005:390–416.
70. Maccari L, Manetti F, Corelli F, et al. 3D QSAR studies for the β-tubulin binding site of microtubule-stabilizing anticancer agents (MSAAs). A pseudoreceptor model for taxanes based on the experimental structure of tubulin. Il Farmaco 2003;58:659–668.
71. Gueritte F. General and recent aspects of the chemistry and structure–activity relationships of taxoids. Curr Pharm Des 2001;7:1229–1249.
72. Islam MN, Song Y, Iskander MN. Investigation of structural requirements of anticancer activity at the paclitaxel/tubulin binding site using CoMFA and CoMSIA. J Mol Graph Model 2003;21:263–272.
73. Manetti F, Forli S, Maccari L, et al. 3D QSAR studies of the interaction between β-tubulin and microtubule stabilizing antimitotic agents (MSAA). A combined pharmacophore generation and pseudoreceptor modeling approach applied to taxanes and epothilones. Il Farmaco 2003;58:357–361
74. Manetti F, Maccari L, Corelli F, et al. 3D QSAR models of interactions between β-tubulin and microtubule stabilizing antimitotic agents (MSAA): A survey on taxanes and epothilones. Curr Topics Med Chem 2004;4:203–217.
75. Vaclavikova R, Soucek P, Svobodova L, et al. Different in vitro metabolism of paclitaxel and docetaxel in humans, rats, pigs, and minipigs. Drug Metab Dispos 2004;32:666–674.
76. Vaclavikova R, Horsky S, Simek P, et al. Paclitaxel metabolism in rat and human liver microsomes is inhibited by phenolic antioxidants. Naunyn-Schmiedelbergs Arch Pharmacol 2003;368:200–209.
77. Cresteil T, Monsarrat B, DuBois J, et al. Regioselective metabolism of taxoids by human CYP3A4 and 2C8: structure–activity relationship. Drug Metab Dispos 2002;39:438–445.
78. Chabner BA., Ryan DP, Paz-Ares L, et al. Antineoplastic agents. In: Hardman JG, Limbird LE, eds. Goodman & Gilman's The Pharmacological Basis of Therapeutics. 10th Ed. New York: McGraw-Hill, 2001:1389–1459.
79. Buey RM, Diaz JF, Andreu JM, et al. Interaction of epothilone analogues with the paclitaxel binding site: relationship between binding affinity, microtubule stabilization, and cytotoxicity. Chem Biol 2004;11:225–236.
80. Altmann K-H. Epothilong B and its analogues: a new family of anticancer agents. Mini Rev Med Chem 2003;3:149–158.
81. Hait WN, Rubin E, Goodin S. Tubulin-targeting agents. In: Giaconne G, Schilsky R, Sondel P, eds. Cancer Chemotherapy and Biological Response Modifiers, Annual 21. Amsterdam: Elsevier BV, 2003:41–67.
82. Engles FK, Ten-Tije AJ, Baker SD, et al. Effect of cytochrome P450 3A4 inhibition on the pharmacokinetics of docetaxel. Clin Pharmacol Ther 2004;75:448–454.
83. Pellegrini F, Budman DR. Review: tubulin function, actions of antitubulin drugs, and new drug development. Cancer Invest 2005;23:264–273.
84. Gigant B, Wang C, Ravelli RBG, et al. Structural basis for the regulation of tubulin by vinblastine. Nature 2005;435:519–522.
85. Beck WT, Cass CE, Houghton PJ. Microtubule-targeting anticancer drugs derived from plants and microbes: vinca alkaloids, taxanes, and epothiolones. In: Bast RC Jr, Kufe DW, Pollock RE, Weichselbaum RR, Holland JF, Frei E III, eds. Holland-Frei Cancer Medicine. 5th Ed. Hamilton, Ontario: BC Decker, 2000:680–698.
86. Islam MN, Iskander MN. Microtubulin binding sites as target for developing anticancer agents. Mini Rev Med Chem 2004;4:1077–1104.
87. Himes RH. Interactions of the Catharanthus (Vinca) alkaloids with tubulin and microtubules. Pharmacol Ther 1991;51:257–267.
88. Wu ML, Deng JF, Wu JC, et al. Severe bone marrow depression induced by the anticancer herb *Cantharanthus roseus.* J Toxicol Clin Toxicol 2005;43:667–671.
89. Beulz-Riche D, Grude P, Puozzo C, et al. Characterization of human cytochrome P450 isoenzymes involved in the metabolism of vinorelbine. Fundam Clin Pharmacol 2005;19:545–553.
90. Jakita J, Kuwabara T, Kobayashi H, et al. CYP3A4 is mainly responsible for the metabolism of a new vinca alkaloid, vinorelbine, in human liver microsomes. Drug Metab Dispos 2000;28:1121–1127.
91. Laing N, Dahllof B, Hartley-Asp B, et al. Interaction of estramustine with tubulin isotypes. Biochemistry 1997;36:871–878.
92. Vilain N, Tsai-Pflugfelder M, Benoit A, et al. Modulation of drug sensitivity in yeast cells by the ATP-binding domain of human DNA topoisomerase IIα. Nucleic Acids Res 2003;31:5714–5722.
93. Takimoto CH. Topoisomerase interactive agents. In: DeVita VT Jr, Hellman S, Rosenberg SA, eds. Cancer: Principles and Practice of Oncology. 7th Ed. Baltimore: Lippincott Williams &Wilkins, 2005:375–390.
94. Felix CA. Secondary leukemias induced by topoisomerase-targeted drugs. Biochim Biophys Acta 1998;1400:233–255.
95. Staker BL, Hjerrild K, Feese MD, et al. The mechanism of topoisomerase I poisoning by a camptothecin analogue. Proc Nat Acad Sci U S A 2002;99: 15387–15392.
96. Staker BL, Feese MD, Cushman M, et al. Structures of three classes of anticancer agents bound to the human topoisomerase I–DNA covalent complex. J Med Chem 2005;48:2336–2345.

43. *Antiviral Agents and Protease Inhibitors*

PATRICK M. WOSTER

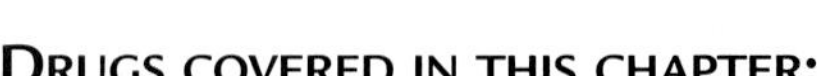

DRUGS COVERED IN THIS CHAPTER:

ACYCLOVIR
ADEFOVIR DIPIVOXIL
AMANTADINE
CIDOFOVIR
CYTARABINE
FAMCICLOVIR
FOMIVIRSEN
FOSCARNET
GANCICLOVIR
IDOXURIDINE
INTERFERON
RIBAVIRIN
RIMANTADINE
TRIFLUOROTHYMIDINE
VALACYCLOVIR
VIDARABINE
NEURAMINIDASE INHIBITORS
- Enfuvirtide
- Oseltamivir phosphate
- Zanamivir

ANTIRETROVIRAL AGENTS
- Nucleoside reverse transcriptase inhibitors
  - Abacavir
  - Didanosine
  - Emtricitabine
  - Lamivudine
  - Stavudine
  - Tenofovir disoproxil
  - Zalcitabine
  - Zidovudine
- Nonnucleoside reverse transcriptase inhibitors
  - Delavirdine
  - Efavirenz
  - Nevirapine
- Protease inhibitors
  - Amprenavir
  - Atazanavir
  - Fosamprenavir
  - Indinavir
  - Lopinavir/ritonavir
  - Nelfinavir
  - Ritonavir
  - Saquinavir
  Tipraqnavir

INTRODUCTION

Viruses are the smallest of the human infectious agents, ranging in size from approximately by 20 to 300 nm in diameter (1,2). They contain one kind of nucleic acid, either RNA or DNA, as their entire genome, which codes for a variety of enzymes and other proteins used in replication and transmission of the organism. It can be argued that a virus does not qualify as a true life form, because it is nothing more than a nucleic acid strand with associated proteins and cannot move under its own power. When it attaches itself to a host cell, however, it internalizes itself and forces the host to make additional copies of the virus, demonstrating a clear reproductive plan. During replication, it utilizes host cellular biochemicals and processes and, thus, in a sense, takes in "nutrients" to survive and multiply. In some cases, viruses respond to external conditions and escape the immune response by integrating into the host DNA, demonstrating the ability to respond to external stimuli. Although viruses are simple organisms, they are a significant causative agent for numerous human diseases and, as such, represent one of the major challenges in the area of drug discovery. Agents that are used clinically for a variety of viral diseases act by targeting processes that are specific to the virus, such as a unique viral enzyme, or a necessary process, such as transcription. To date, however, no drug has been discovered that is truly curative for viral infection. In addition, because viruses have the ability to undergo mutations, resistance to existing therapies can develop. The discovery of new antiviral agents is thus an important ongoing effort in medicinal chemistry.

VIRUS STRUCTURE AND CLASSIFICATION (1,2)

Numerous species of virus that infect bacteria, plants, and animals have been identified, and they exhibit a remarkable range of diversity. All viruses exist as obligate cellular parasites, and as such, they do not need to possess the complex biochemical machinery that is characteristic of higher organisms. They do, however, have a defined macromolecular structure that is designed to protect them from the environment and to facilitate their entry into cells. The basic subunit of a virus is its genome, which can be made up of either DNA or RNA. The nucleic acid portion of a virus can be single or double stranded and may be present in linear or circular form. Viral genomic DNA or RNA often is associated with basic nucleoproteins and may be surrounded by a symmetrical protein known as a capsid. The capsid is made up of repeating structural units known as protomers, which themselves are made up of nonidentical protein subunits. The combination of the nucleic acid core and the capsid is called the nucleocapsid, and in some cases, this comprises the entire virus. In other cases, the nucleocapsid structure is surrounded by a lipid-containing membrane that is derived during viral maturation, when the virus undergoes budding through the host cell membrane. The complete viral particle, with

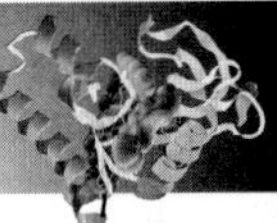

CLINICAL SIGNIFICANCE

Antiviral agents include diverse compounds with varied actions. A thorough clinical understanding about most of these compounds is dependent on a basic appreciation of biochemistry and medicinal chemistry. Viruses are mainly composed of either RNA or DNA nucleic acid strands. As such, one of the most ideal targets for treating viral pathogens has been the inhibition of viral replication. Successful viral replication is dependent on enzyme-mediated transcription of viral RNA or DNA. A significant number of antiviral agents, including HIV nucleoside reverse transcriptase inhibitors and a majority of antiherpes agents, are designed to be "false" substrates of viral transcription enzymes. It is through competitive inhibition that these agents are able to fulfill their intended effect. Their chemical structures are similar to naturally occurring substrate nucleoside purines (adenosine and guanosine) and pyrimidines (thymidine and cytidine). Their incorporation, however, will lead to termination of replication. These nucleoside antiviral agents typically require triphosphorylation to become active intracellularly. It is important to recognize that resistance to these antiviral medications can develop when genetic mutations alter the ability of viral enzymes to phosphorylate the drugs. Drugs like cidofovir and tenofovir are nucleotide analogues, which means they are already monophosphorylated. As a result, these agents can maintain activity against viruses that have developed resistance to other nucleoside agents through certain resistant mutations.

In clinical practice, HIV antiretroviral regimens usually require a pair of nucleoside reverse transcriptase inhibitors in the regimen. It is of paramount importance that combinations of "like" nucleosides analogues (i.e., two thymidines, two cytosines, etc.) are not used together, because they have displayed antagonism and reduced viral load suppression. Nonnucleoside reverse transcriptase inhibitors are not structurally related to nucleic purines and pyrimidines; therefore, they do not act as substrates of the target enzyme.

Protease inhibitors, which are the most potent antiretroviral agents currently available, were the end result of coordinated chemical design and structure-based computational analysis of the protease enzyme. With identification of the protease crystalline structure and identification of active binding sites, scientists were able to create compounds that would fit the protease enzyme with strong affinity and cause an inhibition of protease function. The clinical impact of these man-made drugs is regarded by many as being the greatest single advance in the treatment of HIV infection.

Douglas Slain, Pharm.D., BCPS
Associate Professor
College of Pharmacy
West Virginia University

or without an envelope, is called the virion. Viral architecture can be grouped into three types based on the arrangement of morphologic subunits, and each virus exhibits cubic (icosahedral) symmetry, helical symmetry, or a complex structure. Icosahedral virions are symmetrical structures that contain 20 surfaces, each of which is an equilateral triangle. A sufficient number of capsid structural units must be employed in the icosahedron to make a capsid large enough to encapsulate the viral genome. Morphologic units called capsomeres are seen on the surface of icosahedral viral particles. These structures are clusters of polypeptides, but they do not necessarily correspond to the chemically defined structural units. Some viruses arrange their structural subunits into a standard helical formation. In viruses with helical symmetry, protein subunits systematically bind to the viral nucleic acid, ultimately forming a nucleocapsid helix. The filamentous nucleocapsid is then coiled inside a lipid-containing envelope. Unlike icosahedral virions, the regular, periodic interaction between capsid protein and viral nucleic acid prevents the formation of "empty" helical particles. Finally, some viral particles, such as the large and complex poxviruses, do not exhibit cubic or helical symmetry but, instead, form more complicated structures that can be spherical, brick-shaped, or ovoid. A subset of complex viruses are called pleomorphic viruses, in that they assume multiple, complex morphologies.

Viral taxonomy is complex, and viruses are classified according to a number of factors, including morphology, properties of the genome (i.e., DNA versus RNA, single strand versus double strand, linear or circular, and sense or antisense), physicochemical properties, structure of associated proteins, replication strategy, and so on. Viruses are separated into major groups called families, with names that end in the suffix -viridae, and then into genera that end in -virus. Thus, poxviruses are in the family Poxviridae and in the genus *Poxvirus*. A comparison of the genetic and structural features of viral families with members that can infect humans appears in Table 43.1.

VIRAL REPLICATION, CELLULAR EFFECTS, AND PATHOGENESIS (2,3)

As mentioned above, all viruses exist as obligate intracellular parasites, and as such, they rely on the cellular machinery of the host for their growth, development, and replication. To synthesize the proteins needed for viral replication, the organism must be capable of producing usable mRNA in sufficient quantities to compete with host mRNA for protein synthesis. During viral replication, all of the macromolecules required by the virus are synthesized in a highly organized sequence. The replication cycle (Fig. 43.1) begins when the intact virion binds to a host cell through electrostatic adsorption to a specific "receptor"

Table 43.1. Characteristics of Virus Families Containing Members that Infect Humans

Family	Examples	Genome	Capsid Symmetry	Size (nm^{-1})	Envelope	Diseases
Parvoviridae	Parvovirus B19	ssDNA, sense or antisense	Icosa	18–26	No	Erythema infectiosum (fifth disease); polyarthralgia arthritis; aplastic crisis, anemia
Papillomaviridae	Human papilloma (wart)virus; polyoma virus; SV 40	dsDNA, circular DNA	Icosa	55	No	Warts; salivary gland infection; multifocal leukoencephalopathy; tumors
Adenoviridae	Multiple types (40 adenoviruses/ mastadenovirus)	dsDNA	Icosa	70–90	No	Infections of the eye and respiratory tract; tumors
Hepadnaviridae	Hepadnavirus, hepatitis B virus	dsDNA, circular, one ss region	Icosa	40–48	Yes	Hepatitis B; tumors
Herpesviridae	Herpes simplex I and II; varicella-zoster; herpes zoster; cytomegalovirus; Epstein-Barr virus	dsDNA	Icosa	150–200	Yes	Eye, skin, and genital infection; chickenpox; shingles; mononucleosis; tumors
Poxviridae	Variola; vaccinia	dsDNA	Comp	230–400	Complex	Smallpox; cowpox; chickenpox; tumors
Picornaviridae	Hepatitis A virus; poliovirus; enterovirus; rhinovirus, coxsackie virus A and B	ssRNA, sense	Icosa	28–30	No	Respiratory diseases; gastrointestinal diseases; polio; aseptic meningitis
Astroviridae	Astrovirus	ssRNA, sense	Icosa	28–30	No	Diarrhea in infants and immunocompromised patients
Caliciviridae	Norwalk virus	ssRNA, sense	Icosa	27–40	No	Epidemic gastroenteritis
Togaviridae	Rubella virus; alphavirus, arbovirus	ssRNA, sense	Icosa	50–70	Yes	Measles (rubella)
Flaviviridae	Hepatitis C virus; arbovirus; yellow fever virus; dengue virus; West Nile virus	ssRNA, sense	Comp	40–60	Yes	Hepatitis C; yellow fever; dengue fever; encephalitis; tumors
Coronaviridae	Coronavirus	ssRNA, sense	Comp	120–160	Yes	Colds; gastroenteritis in infants; SARS
Retroviridae	HIV-I and -II; lentavirus; human T-cell lymphotropic viruses	ssRNA as dimer	Comp	80–100	Yes	AIDS; AIDS-related complex; breast cancer; human T-cell leukemia; nasopharyngeal carcinoma
Arenaviridae	Arenavirus	ssRNA, antisense	Comp	50–300	Yes	Lassa fever; hemorrhagic fever; choriomeningitis
Orthomyxoviridae	Influenza virus A, B, and C	ss RNA, antisense	Hel	80–120	Yes	Influenza
Bunyaviridae	Hantavirus	ssRNA, antisense	Hel	80–120	Yes	Hemorrhagic fever
Rhabdoviridae	Rhabdovirus; rabies virus; encephalitis virus	ssRNA, antisense	Hel	75–180	Yes	Rabies; encephalitis
Paramyxoviridae	Syncytial virus; parainfluenza virus	ssRNA, antisense	Hel	150–300	Yes	Mumps; measles (rubeola)
Filoviridae	Marburg virus; Ebola virus	ssRNA, antisense	Hel	80–800	Yes	Marburg viral fever; Ebola hemorrhagic fever
Reoviridae	Rheovirus; rotavirus; orbivirus	dsRNA, in 10–12 pieces	Icosa	60–80	No	Mild respiratory and gastrointestinal infection; Colorado tick fever
Prion	Prion proteinaceous material	None	NA	NA	No	Bovine spongiform encephalopathy; Creutzfeldt-Jakob disease

ds, double-stranded; ss, single-stranded; Icos, icosahedral; Comp, complex; Hel, helical.

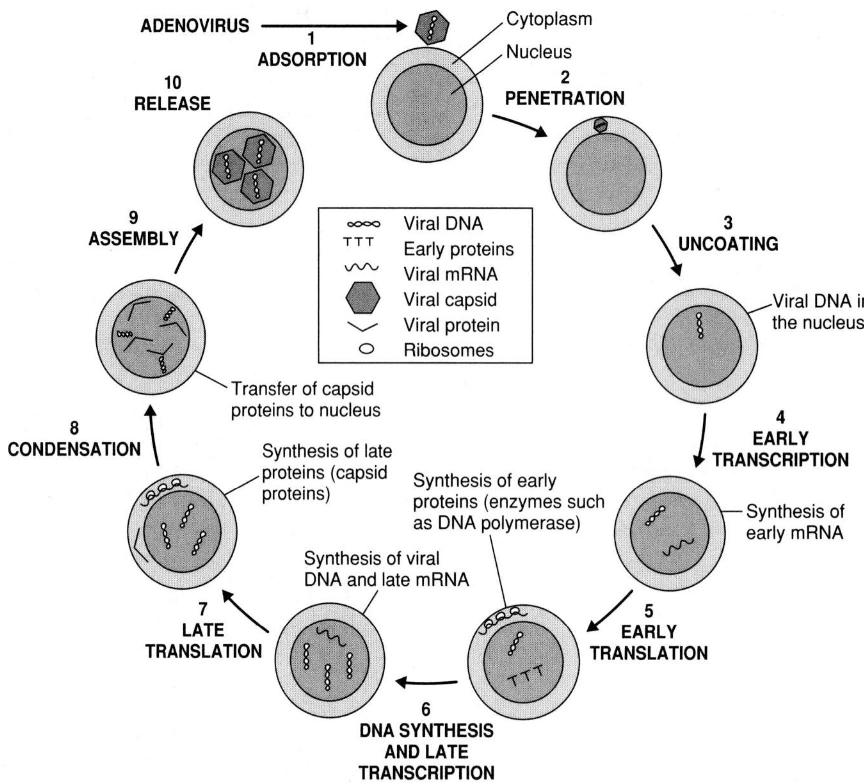

Fig. 43.1. Steps involved in the viral life cycle. (Adapted from Brooks GF, Butel JS, Morse SA, et al. Jawetz, Melnick, and Adelberg's Medical Microbiology. 23rd Ed. New York: McGraw-Hill, 2004; with permission. Copyright 2004 The McGraw-Hill Companies, Inc.)

site. This process is known as the attachment phase. Attachment is most likely a fortuitous event resulting from structural complementarity between the exterior structure of the virion and a normal cell surface structure on the host cell. For example, HIV binds to the CD4 receptor on cells of the immune system, rhinoviruses bind ICAM-1, and Epstein-Barr virus (EBV) recognizes the CD21 receptor on B cells. When attachment has been achieved, the virion enters the penetration phase, the process by which it gains entry into the host cell. Penetration may occur by receptor-mediated endocytosis, fusion of the viral envelope with the cell membrane, or in some cases, direct penetration of the membrane. Following penetration of the cell, viruses must be uncoated, resulting in either the naked nucleic acid or the nucleocapsid form, which usually contains polymerase enzymes. After they have been uncoated, viruses are no longer infectious.

Once the virus has penetrated the cell and uncoated, it enters a segment of its life cycle known as the eclipse period, the length of which varies with the type of virus. During this time, the virus utilizes host resources to replicate and produce necessary viral proteins. Cells that can support viral reproduction are called permissive. As a result, the infection is known as a productive infection, because it results in new viral particles. When new infectious viral particles are produced, host cellular metabolism may be completely directed toward the production of viral products, resulting in destruction of the cell. In other cases, host cell metabolism is not dramatically altered, and the infected cell can survive. During viral reproduction, up to 100,000 new virions can be produced, and the replication cycle can vary from a few hours to more than 3 days. Some cells types, called nonpermissive, are unable to support the reproduction of an infective virion, resulting in an abortive infection. Abortive infections also occur when the virus itself is defective. Either situation can lead to a latent infection, where the viral genome may persist in a surviving host cell. As will be described below, such an infection can lead to the transformation of a cell from normal to malignant.

DNA Virus

The strategies used by various viruses to replicate vary widely, but all are characterized by the need to transcribe mRNA that is suitable for translation of viral proteins. Several pathways lead to the required mRNA, after which the host enzymes and raw materials are used to make viral proteins. Early viral proteins used in replication are synthesized immediately after infection, whereas late proteins used to produce the complete virion structure are synthesized after viral nucleic acid synthesis. Most DNA viruses contain double-stranded DNA as their genome and, thus, can replicate using host cell machinery to produce mRNA directly. Papillomavirus, adenovirus, and herpesvirus are replicated in the host nucleus and, thus, use transcriptional enzymes of the host (i.e., DNA-dependent RNA polymerase) to synthesize mRNA. This mRNA is then translated to form proteins needed by the virus, including enzymes (e.g., DNA-dependent DNA polymerase) used to produce progeny DNA copies. These progeny DNA strands are infectious. By contrast, poxviruses replicate in the cytoplasm using a mechanism that is not well understood, wherein the genome initially is transcribed by a viral enzyme in the virion core. Parvoviruses contain a single-stranded DNA genome and must synthesize double-stranded DNA in the host nucleus before synthesis of mRNA and translation of proteins. This process may or may not require a helper virus, such as herpes simplex. The hepatitis B viral genome, comprised of double-stranded DNA, contains numerous gaps that must be repaired using a DNA polymerase packaged in the virion before transcription to form mRNA.

RNA Virus

Compared to DNA viruses, those viruses with RNA-based genomes have evolved a wide variety of reproductive strategies. The single-stranded RNA viruses may be divided into three groups that differ in the method by which the RNA genome is utilized. In all three groups, the RNA genome must serve two functions: to be translated to form protein, and to be replicated to form progeny RNA strands. The first group is comprised of viruses such as picornaviruses, flaviviruses, and togaviruses that have an RNA genome that can be used directly as mRNA. Viral RNA that can be used as mRNA is by convention termed (+) or sense-strand RNA. In most cases (e.g. picornaviruses), this sense-strand RNA binds to the host ribosome shortly after entering the cell, where it is read and used to produce a single polypeptide called the polyprotein. The polyprotein is then processed by autocatalysis and various proteolytic enzymes to produce the required viral proteins. In some cases (e.g. togaviruses), only a portion of the RNA genome is available to be translated by the host ribosome. Following the initial translation of the sense strand, it serves a second function—namely, to serve as a template for the synthesis of a (−) or antisense strand via an RNA-dependent RNA polymerase. This antisense strand then can be used to produce additional sense-strand RNAs that are infectious and also can serve as mRNA. These progeny sense-strand RNAs are then packaged into an intact virion before transmission to another host cell.

The second group of single-stranded RNA viruses, including orthomyxoviruses, bunyaviruses, arenaviruses, paramyxoviruses, filoviruses, and rhabdoviruses, all contain an antisense RNA genome that can be used only for transcription of new RNA. All antisense RNA viruses contain an RNA transcriptase as part of their virion, because the host cell does not have this type of RNA-dependent RNA polymerase. During the first round of genome expression, a series of short sense-strand RNAs are made, which are then translated to form the required viral enzymes for replication. Ultimately, these enzymes are used to produce a full-length sense RNA strand, which is then used to make multiple copies of the antisense viral genome. The progeny antisense DNA strands by themselves are not infectious, because they have not yet been packaged with the required RNA transcriptase. When the progeny antisense RNA has been synthesized, it is packaged into an intact virion, in which form it becomes infectious before transmission to another cell.

The third group of RNA viruses are the retroviruses, in which single-stranded RNA exists as a dimer of a sense and an antisense strand. The genomic RNA strands can be base-paired, although the structure of this complex is not well understood, or the strands can be hydrogen-bonded to other macromolecules in the virion. Retroviral genomic RNA serves a single function—namely, to act as a template for the formation of double-stranded viral DNA. Host cells do not contain an enzyme that can form DNA from viral RNA; thus, the virion of a retrovirus must contain a reverse transcriptase (RT) enzyme as well as various host tRNA molecules. Transcription of the genome begins when a complex of RT and tRNA binds to the viral genome. A complimentary DNA strand is then synthesized using one of the host tRNAs as a primer, and the original RNA strand is digested by RNAse H and viral ribonuclease packaged in the virion. A complimentary DNA strand is then synthesized, and the resulting double-stranded DNA is translocated to the nucleus, where viral enzymes incorporate genome-length viral DNA into the host genome. In some cases, the viral portion of the genome can remain dormant for long periods, or it may be immediately used to make progeny viral RNA, a process that is catalyzed by host RNA polymerase II. Transcription produces both shortened segments that are used to make polyproteins and full-length progeny RNA. The polyproteins are processed to form various viral proteins, whereas the full length RNA is packaged into an infectious virion.

Virus Protein

In addition to replication of the viral genome, a number of other structures associated with the complete virion also can be made. A number of viral proteins may be synthesized that have important functions in the structure, transmission, and survival of the virus. These proteins can protect the genetic material in the virus from destruction by nucleases, participate in the attachment process, and provide structure and symmetry to the virion. In addition, in certain cases where the virus requires an enzymatic process for which there is no host enzyme, a virion may include enzymes, such as RNA polymerases or a RT. Some viruses require a lipid envelope that contains transmembrane proteins specifically coded for by the virus and which envelopes the genetic material during viral budding. Viral envelopes contain glycoproteins that are involved in cell recognition during attachment to the host cell. These glycoproteins often reflect the composition of glycoproteins in the host cell. They are a determinant of the antigenic nature of viruses and, thus, facilitate recognition by the immune system of the host. Depending on their composition, however, they also can help the virus to elude neutralization by the immune system.

Cellular Egress

Viruses use one of two strategies for exiting infected cells. Nonenveloped viruses (e.g., picornaviruses and rheoviruses) complete their maturation by assembling into their corresponding virion within the cell nucleus or the cytoplasm. For example, picornaviruses assemble by clustering 60 copies of each of three viral proteins, called VP0, VP1, and VP3, into a structure called a procapsid. Viral RNA is then packaged into the procapsid, and proteolytic cleavage of VP0 produces two new viral proteins, called VP2 and VP4. The resulting conformational change produces a stable and symmetrical structure that shields the genome from degradation by host nucleases. In most cases, destruction of the host cell is required when the virion exits. Enveloped viruses (i.e., all antisense RNA viruses, togaviruses, flaviviruses, coronaviruses, hepadnaviruses, herpesviruses, and retroviruses) contain proteins that carry signal sequences and markers that cause them to be inserted into the inner and outer surfaces of the host cell cytoplasmic membrane. Viral proteins on the outer surface are glycosylated using host enzymes, then displace host cell surface proteins and collect into patches. Viral nucleocapsids that recognize proteins on the inner surface of the membrane, where they bind, are engulfed by the patch area of the membrane. The completed virion exits the cell by budding and release into the extracellular space. Viral egress can have a variety of effects on the host cell, ranging from destruction of the cell to minimal noncytolytic effects. Herpesviruses differ from other enveloped viruses in the manner in which they form their envelope. The nucleocapsid is formed in the nucleus, and final maturation of the virion occurs only on the inner surface of the host cell membrane, forming vesicles that are stored in between the inner and outer aspect of the cell membrane. Egress of the herpesvirus vesicle always occurs through destruction of the host cell.

Virus Pathogenesis

A complete discussion of viral pathogenesis is beyond the scope of this chapter. In general, however, the symptoms of a viral infection may be considered to arise from the response to viral replication and cell injury in the host. These responses range from asymptomatic or subclinical to severe clinical manifestations, and they may be either local or systemic. Understanding the biochemical events that produce viral diseases can aid in the design of effective and specific therapies. Not surprisingly, viral pathogenesis occurs in distinct steps: 1) viral entry into the host and primary viral replication, 2) viral spread, 3) cellular injury and host immune response, 4) viral clearance or establishment of persistent infection, 5) and viral shedding. Most viruses enter the host through the respiratory or gastrointestinal (GI) tract, but they also may penetrate the skin, urogenital tract, or conjunctiva. In a few cases, viral particles can enter through direct injection (e.g., HIV and hepatitis) or through insect bites (arboviruses). When a local infection occurs, the virus replicates near the site of entry, and the underlying tissue is not affected. Some viruses, however, are able to migrate to other sites, usually through the bloodstream or lymphatic system, to produce systemic infections. When infection occurs at a remote site, most viruses demonstrate tissue or organ preference (e.g. herpesvirus localizes in nerve ganglia, and the rabies virus migrates to the central nervous system [CNS]). Localization of a virus in a particular tissue can be the result of cell receptor specificity or can arise because a virus may be activated by proteolytic enzymes in a specific cell type.

Clinical disease develops through a complex series of events when virus-infected cells are destroyed or their function is impaired, and some symptoms, such as malaise and anorexia, can result from host responses, such as cytokine release. Disease-mediated damage may become chronic when cell types that do not regenerate (e.g., brain tissue) are involved. Ultimately, the host either succumbs to the infection; develops a chronic, latent, or subclinical infection; or completely recovers. In chronic infections, the virus can be continuously detected at low levels, and either mild or no clinical symptoms may present. By contrast, latent infections are those in which the virus persists for extended periods of time in an inactive form or a location not exposed to the immune response. Intermittent flare-ups of clinical disease can occur, during which time infectious virus can be detected. Subclinical infections are those that give no overt sign of their presence. Humoral and cell-mediated immunity, interferon and other cytokines, and other host defense factors, depending on the type of virus, are common mediators of recovery and begin to develop very soon after infection. Infiltration with mononuclear cells and lymphocytes is responsible for the inflammatory reaction in uncomplicated viral lesions. Virus-infected cells can be lysed by T lymphocytes through recognition of viral polypeptides on the cell surface, and humoral immunity protects the host against reinfection by the same virus. Neutralizing antibodies that are directed against capsid proteins can prevent viral infection by disrupting viral attachment or uncoating. Interestingly, viruses have evolved a variety of survival tactics that serve to suppress or evade the host immune response. Because viruses are obligate intracellular parasites, a method of transmission from one host to another is required for survival of the species. Thus, during an active infection, shedding of the infectious virion into the environment is a required step in the life cycle of the virus and ensures transmission of the virus to new hosts. Shedding usually occurs at the same site where the infection was initiated and can occur at various stages in the disease course.

VIRAL DISEASES

HIV (4,5)

The human immunodeficiency virus (HIV-1) was first identified in 1979 and was found to be the cause of acquired immune deficiency syndrome (AIDS) in 1981. Since that time, AIDS had become a serious worldwide epidemic that continues to expand. The Joint United Nations Program on HIV/AIDS estimated that by the end of 2005, a total of 40.3 million people worldwide were living with HIV/AIDS, the majority having been infected through heterosexual contact. It is estimated that in 2005, more than 3.1 million people died of AIDS, and 4.9 million new cases of HIV were diagnosed, including more than 700,000 children (6). The incidence of the disease varies by location, with sub-Saharan Africa having the highest incidence. Because it is sexually transmitted, a high percentage of infected individuals are young adult workers, and as such, the disease has a significant economic impact in some regions. In addition, infected mother-to-fetus transmission occurs between 13 and 40% of the time. Although a variety of drugs have been developed for treating patients with AIDS, none has proven to be successful in curing the disease. The basic difficulty experienced with this viral infection is the ability of virus to mutate, leading to rapid drug resistance.

The HIV-1 genome consists of two identical, 9.2-kb, single-stranded RNA molecules within the virion, each of which contains information for only nine genes. Following infection of the host cell, the persistent form of the HIV-1 genome is proviral double-stranded DNA. Mature HIV virions are spherical and consist of a lipid bilayer membrane surrounding a nucleocapsid that contains genomic RNA, a viral protease, RT, an integrase, and some other cellular factors. The HIV life cycle is depicted in Figure 43.2, and begins when the viral extracellular protein gp120 attaches to the CD4 receptor on T lymphocytes. Following attachment, the viral envelope and host cell membrane are fused, and the nucleocapsid is released into the cytoplasm. The nucleocapsid is uncoated, and the resulting RNA serves as a substrate for RT, producing a proviral double-stranded DNA that migrates to the nucleus and is incorporated into host DNA by integrase. This DNA is not expressed in resting T lymphocytes, but when the cell is activated, proviral DNA is transcribed by host RNA polymerase II. The viral RNA and proteins are transported to the cell membrane, where they assemble, form a viral bud, and are released from the lymphocyte membrane. This produces an immature virion, and processing of the viral surface proteins by HIV protease then affords the mature, infectious virus. Approximately 50% of HIV infections are asymptomatic, whereas the other 50% produce flu-like symptoms

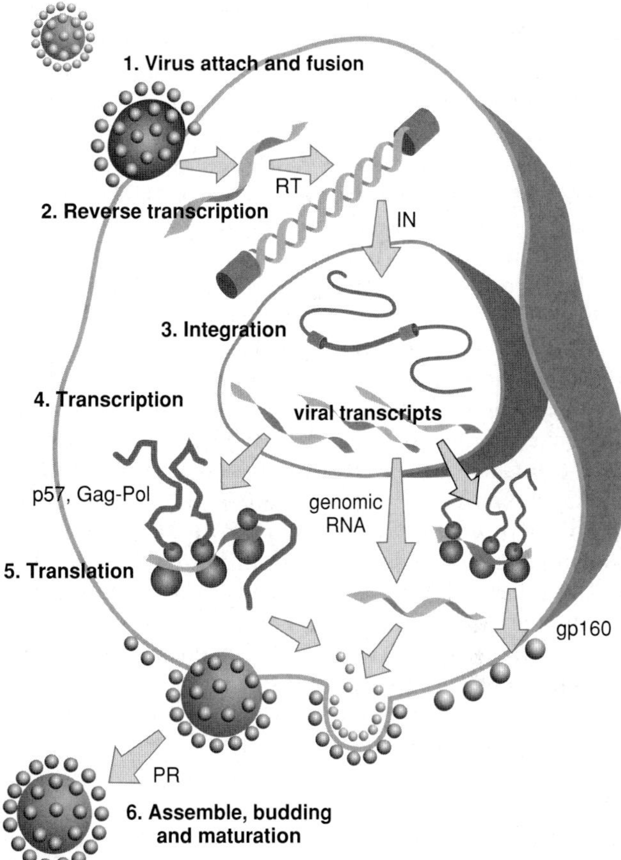

Fig. 43.2. Replicative cycle of HIV. (1) The virus gp120 protein binds to CD4 resulting in fusion of the viral envelope and the cellular membrane and the release of viral nucleocapsid into the cytoplasm. (2) The nucleocapsid is uncoated, and viral RNA is reverse transcribed by reverse transcriptase (RT). (3) The resulting double-stranded proviral DNA migrates into the cell nucleus and is integrated into the cellular DNA by integrase (IN). (4) Proviral DNA is transcribed by the cellular RNA polymerase II. (5) The mRNAs are translated by the cellular polysomes. (6) Viral proteins and genomic RNA are transported to the cellular membrane and assemble. Immature virions are released, and polypeptide precursors are processed by the viral protease (PR) to produce mature vital particles. (Adapted from Sierra S, Kupfer B, Kaiser R. Basics of the virology of HIV-1 and its replication. J Clin Virol 2005;34:233; with permission from Elsevier.)

within 4 weeks. During this initial phase, viral titers are very high but then decline as specific antibodies are formed. The latent period is mediated by factors that are not well understood and can last several years. During this time, viral replication continues, and the level of CD4-positive T lymphocytes steadily declines. Eventually, the patient's immune system becomes compromised, resulting in a variety of opportunistic infections. RT sometimes makes mistakes reading the viral RNA sequence, leading to mutations in the virus and changes in the structure of the surface proteins. Thus, vaccines, which induce the production of antibodies that recognize and bind to very specific viral surface molecules, are unlikely to be effective in HIV therapy. As will be discussed below, other viral processes, such as reverse transcription and proteolytic processing, are viable targets for small molecule therapy.

Kaposi's sarcoma is a common complication of AIDS and has been shown to arise from a complex interaction between HIV and the human herpesvirus (HHV)-8. This disease presents as a reddish or purple lesion on various areas of the skin and, in the advanced state, may involve the lungs or GI tract. HHV-8 does not work alone but, rather, in combination with a patient's altered response to cytokines and the HIV-1 transactivating protein Tat, which promotes the growth of endothelial cells. HHV-8 can then encode interleukin-6 viral proteins, which are specific cytokines that stimulate cell growth in the skin. HHV-8 further destroys the immune system by directing a cell to remove the major histocompatibility complex (MHC-1) proteins that protect it from invasion. These proteins are then transferred to the interior of the cell and are destroyed, leaving the cell unguarded and vulnerable to pathogens that normally would be cleared by the immune system. It recently has been discovered that xCT, the 12-transmembrane light chain of the human cystine/glutamate exchange transporter system, serves as a receptor for internalization of HHV-8 (7).

Herpesvirus (2)

The herpesvirus family contains several of the most important human pathogens and are responsible for causing a spectrum of common diseases. A common and significant feature of the herpesviruses is their ability to establish lifelong, persistent infections in their hosts and to undergo periodic reactivation. Herpesviruses possess a large number of genes, and some of the resulting proteins are targets for antiviral chemotherapy. The herpesviruses that commonly infect humans include herpes simplex virus (HSV)-1 and -2, varicella-zoster virus (VZV), cytomegalovirus (CMV), EBV, HHV-6 and -7, and Kaposi's sarcoma–associated HHV-8 (also known as KSHV). Herpesviruses are large viruses that have identical morphology and consist of a core of linear, double-stranded DNA surrounded by a protein coat that exhibits icosahedral symmetry and has 162 capsomeres. The genome is large and encodes at least 100 different proteins, including polypeptides involved in viral structure, the viral envelope, and enzymes involved in nucleic acid metabolism, DNA synthesis, and protein regulation. Oral cold sores and genital herpes infections are caused by HSV-1 and -2, respectively. These viruses can establish a latent infection in the ganglia of nerves that supply the site of the primary infection, and the latent disease is reactivated by a number of stress factors. It is estimated that virtually 100% of adult humans are infected with HSV-1, although many infections are subclinical and asymptomatic. The varicella virus is the cause of chickenpox, and the herpes zoster virus is responsible for shingles. Human CMV infection rarely causes disease in healthy people, but when infection occurs in adulthood, it may cause an infectious mononucleosis–like illness. Primary infection with the EBV is the cause of infectious mononucleosis, and this virus is thought to be a factor in the development of Burkitt's lymphoma and other malignancies. Human herpesvirus-6 is thought to cause roseola and mononucleosis, whereas HHV-7 probably is not involved in any human diseases. The role of HHV-8 in the pathogenesis of Kaposi's sarcoma has been discussed above.

Hepatitis (2)

Viral hepatitis is a systemic disease but primarily involves the liver. Hepatitis A virus (HAV) is responsible for infectious hepatitis, and hepatitis B virus (HBV) is associated with serum hepatitis. Hepatitis C virus (HCV) is a common cause of posttransfusion hepatitis. Another viral agent, hepatitis E virus (HEV), causes an enterically transmitted form of hepatitis. On occasion, disease can arise from hepatic infection with yellow fever virus, CMV, EBV, HSV, rubella virus, and the enteroviruses. Viral hepatitis usually involves acute inflammation of the liver, fever, nausea, vomiting, and jaundice, and all forms of hepatitis produce identical histopathologic lesions in the liver during acute disease. HAV is a member of the picornavirus family and carries a single-stranded RNA genome; only one strain of the virus exists. The onset of HAV hepatitis occurs within 24 hours, in contrast to the slower onset of clinical symptoms with HBV and HCV infection. Complete recovery occurs in most cases of hepatitis A, and chronic infection never occurs. HBV is classified as a hepadnavirus with a double-stranded, circular DNA genome. The outcome of HBV infection ranges from complete recovery to progression to chronic hepatitis and, rarely, death. HBV establishes chronic infections, especially in infants; 80 to 95% of infants and young children infected with HBV become chronic carriers and are at high risk of developing hepatocellular carcinoma. In adults, 65 to 80% of infections are asymptomatic, and 90 to 95% of all patients recover completely. HCV is a positive-stranded RNA flavivirus and exists in at least six major genotypes. Most cases of posttransfusion hepatitis are caused by HCV, and these infections usually are subclinical, with minor elevation of liver enzymes and a low incidence of jaundice. However, 70 to 90% of HCV-infected patients develop chronic hepatitis, and many are at risk of progressing to chronic active hepatitis and cirrhosis decades later. HEV is transmitted enterically and occurs in epidemic form in developing countries, where water supplies sometimes are contaminated with feces. The disease is more severe in adults than in children, who usually are asymptomatic.

Influenza (2)

Respiratory illnesses commonly known as colds and flu account for more than half of all acute illnesses in the United States each year. Influenza viruses belong to the orthomyxoviridae family and are a major source of morbidity and mortality caused by respiratory disease. Outbreaks of infection can occur in global epidemics that have resulted in millions of deaths worldwide. Genetic mutations often cause antigenic changes in the structure of viral surface glycoproteins, making influenza viruses extremely difficult to control. Three immunologic types of influenza viruses are known and are termed influenza A, B, and C. Antigenic changes are very common in influenza A, which is responsible for the majority of influenza epidemics. Influenza B undergoes more infrequent antigenic changes and is less often the cause of an influenza epidemic, whereas influenza C are antigenically stable and cause only mild illness in immunocompetent individuals. The viruses carry a single-stranded, negative-sense RNA genome that has eight segments in influenza A and B. Influenza C contains only seven segments of RNA and lack a neuraminidase gene (see below). The complete virion in each type contains nine different structural proteins. A nucleoprotein associates with viral RNA to form a ribonucleoprotein structure that makes up the viral nucleocapsid. Three other large proteins are bound to the viral ribonuclear protein and are responsible for RNA transcription and replication. A matrix protein also is included in the virion that forms a shell underneath the viral lipid envelope and comprises approximately 40% of all viral protein.

The influenza virion structure also includes a lipid envelope derived from the host cell. This envelope contains two viral surface glycoproteins called hemagglutinin and neuraminidase (NA). Mutations cause antigenic changes in the structure of these two surface glycoproteins; thus, they are the main determinants of antigenicity and host immunity. The ability of the virus to change the structure of hemagglutinin on the virus surface primarily is responsible for the continual evolution of new strains, sometimes leading to subsequent influenza epidemics. Neuraminidase is an enzyme that removes sialic acid from surface glycoproteins during viral maturation and is required to produce infectious particles and lower the viscosity of the mucin layer of the respiratory tract. Influenza virus spreads through airborne droplets or contact with contaminated hands or surfaces and has an incubation period that varies from 1 to 4 days. Transmission of the virus, however, begins to occur 24 hours before to the onset of symptoms. Interferon is detectable in respiratory secretions at the onset of symptoms, and the host response to interferon response contributes to recovery. Antibodies and other cell-mediated responses are seen 1 to 2 weeks after infection. It is well established that secondary infections from other viruses or bacteria can occur, and Reye's syndrome, an acute encephalopathy occurring in children and adolescents, is a rare complication of influenza B, influenza A, herpesvirus, and VZV infections. The chances of contracting Reye's syndrome are increased when salicylates are used in children suffering from influenza and related respiratory diseases.

Tumor Viruses (2,8–12)

Viruses are etiologic factors in the development of several types of human tumors, most notably cervical cancer and liver cancer. At least 15% of all human tumors worldwide have a viral cause. Tumor viruses can be found in both the RNA and DNA virus kingdoms (13). The list of human viruses presently known to be involved in tumor development includes four DNA viruses (EBV, certain papilloma viruses, HBV, and the Kaposi's sarcoma–associated HHV-8), and two RNA viruses (adult T-cell leukemia virus [HTLV-1] and HCV). Tumor viruses alter cellular behavior through the use of a small amount of genetic information, employing two general strategies. The tumor virus either introduces a new "transforming gene" into the cell (direct-acting), or the virus alters the expression of a preexisting cellular gene or genes (indirect-acting). In both cases, normal regulation of cellular growth processes is lost. Viruses alone cannot act as carcinogens, and other events are necessary to disable regulatory pathways and checkpoints to produce transformed, malignant cells. The processes used in the transformation of host cells by human tumor viruses are very diverse.

Cellular transformation may be defined as a stable, heritable change in the growth control of cells that results in tumor formation. Transformation from a normal to a neoplastic cell generally requires the retention of viral genes in the host cell. In the majority of cases, this is accomplished by the integration of certain viral genes into the host cell genome. Retroviruses incorporate their proviral DNA, formed through the action of RT, into host cell DNA. By contrast, DNA tumor viruses integrate a portion of the DNA of the viral genome into the host cell chromosome.

All RNA tumor viruses are members of the retrovirus family and belong to one of two classes (9,10,12). Class I RNA viruses are direct-transforming and carry an oncogene obtained through accidental incorporation from the host cell. No class I RNA viruses are known to produce tumors in humans. Class II or chronic RNA tumor viruses are weakly transforming and do not carry host cell–derived oncogenes. The two known cancer-causing retroviruses in humans act indirectly. They often act by inserting their proviral DNA into the immediate neighborhood of a host cellular oncogene. HTLV-1 acts in this manner, thus increasing the number of preneoplastic cells and facilitating secondary cellular changes leading to transformation.

DNA tumor virus strains exist among the papilloma-, polyoma-, adeno-, herpes-, hepadna-, and poxvirus groups (11). DNA tumor viruses encode viral oncoproteins that are important for viral replication but also affect cellular growth control pathways. For example, inactivation of the retinoblastoma gene (*Rb*) and the p53 pathway by viral transforming proteins is a common strategy used by papovaviruses and adenoviruses. As mentioned above, all DNA tumor viruses kill their host cell when the infectious virion is released to infect other cells. Thus, transformation and tumorigenicity are entirely dependent on a host cell interaction with the virus that does not involve viral spread to other cells, and cells transformed by DNA tumor viruses depend on the continued expression of the virally encoded oncogene.

Recent studies have revealed that the human tumor viruses EBV, HHV-8, human papillomavirus, HBV, HCV, and HTLV-1 express proteins that are targeted to the mitochondria (8). Because the mitochondria play a critical role in energy production, cell death, calcium homeostasis, and redox balance, these proteins have profound effects on host cell physiology. Further study of these proteins and their interactions with mitochondria will aid in the understanding the mechanisms of viral replication and tumorigenesis and could reveal important new targets for anti-tumor therapy.

Prion Diseases (14–16)

Although they are not viruses, the infective proteins known as prions have sufficient similarities to viruses to warrant their discussion in this chapter. Prions are small proteins that have been shown to cause a variety of transmissible spongiform encephalopathies, which are rare neurodegenerative disorders typified by symptoms in the CNS, such as spongiform changes, neuronal loss, glial activation, and accumulation of amyloid aggregates of an abnormally folded host protein. Human prion diseases include kuru, Creutzfeldt-Jakob disease (variant, sporadic, familial and iatrogenic), Gerstmann-Sträussler-Scheinker syndrome, and fatal familial insomnia. The disease in cattle known as bovine spongiform encephalopathy and the related disease scrapie exhibit similar pathologic features. Following exposure, prions accumulate in lymphoid tissue, such as the spleen, lymph nodes, tonsils, and Peyer's patches (specialized lymphoid follicles located in the submucosa of the small intestine). This accumulation of the infectious agent is necessary for invasion of the CNS. In humans, the incubation period of the disease can vary between 18 months and 40 years. Prions appear to be variant, improperly folded versions of a normal cellular protein called PrP^c, a 30- to 35-kDa protein with two sites for N-glycosylation that is anchored in the neuronal cell membrane. PrP^c protein contains three α-helices, a short β-pleated sheet region, and a long, unstructured portion that comprises half the molecule. The variant, infectious form of the protein is known as PrP^{sc} and is produced autocatalytically from PrP^c. Prion diseases are always fatal, with no known cases of remission or recovery. The host shows no inflammatory response or immune response and no production of interferon, and there is no effect on host B-cell or T-cell function. At present, there are no effective agents to treat prion diseases.

VIRAL CHEMOTHERAPY

General Approaches (17,18)

The principles involved in the design of antiviral agents are similar to those used in the design of all chemotherapeutic agents. Drugs in this category are targeted to some process in the virus that is not present in the host cell. The earliest examples of antiviral agents did not achieve this goal, and these drugs were toxic at therapeutic levels or had a limited spectrum of activity. A variety of factors make the design of effective antiviral agents difficult, including their ability to undergo antigenic changes, the latent period during which there are no symptoms, and their reliance on host enzymes and other processes. This problem is compounded by the facts that host immunity is not well understood and that symptoms of viral infection may not appear until replication is complete and the viral genome has been incorporated into infected cells. Nonetheless, the continuing identification of new targets for antiviral agents provides new avenues for the discovery of small molecule therapies. The following section includes information regarding currently marketed antiviral compounds that have been designed in eight general areas:

- Agents that disrupt virus attachment to host cell receptors, penetration, or uncoating
- Agents that inhibit virus-associated enzymes, such as DNA polymerases and others
- Agents that inhibit viral transcription
- Agents that inhibit viral translation
- Agents that interfere with viral regulatory proteins
- Agents that interfere with glycosylation, phosphorylation, sulfation, and so on.
- Agents that interfere with the assembly of viral proteins
- Agents that prohibit the release of viruses from cell surface membranes

The remainder of this chapter deals primarily with small molecule antiviral agents that have been approved by the U.S. Food and Drug Administration (FDA) and are clinically effective in the treatment of viral infection. Immunizing biological agents, such as vaccines as well as antineoplastic agents with antiviral activity, are not covered. Some compounds used primarily in the treatment of bacterial infections, such as rifampicin, bleomycin, adriamycin, and actinomycin, also inhibit viral replication. These antibiotics do not affect the transcription or translation of viral mRNA, however, and are only effective in high concentrations. Therefore, such antibiotics are not commonly used for viral infections. There is a continuing need for new antiviral agents, primarily because viral infections are not curable after the virus invades the host cell and begins to replicate. Vaccines are effective, but they are only able to prevent an infection, and only then in cases where specific virus strains are involved. For example, immunization against influenza, which is a yearly routine in many parts of the world, can only provide immunity against the specific strains that are represented in that preparation. New virulent strains may arise from nonhuman sources, such as the so-called swine flu or avian flu viruses, and currently available vaccines would have no effect against these new strains. With regard to small molecule antiviral agents, the ideal drug would have broad-spectrum antiviral activity, completely inhibit viral replication, maintain efficacy against mutant

Table 43.2. Antiviral Agents Interfering with Cellular Penetration and Early Replication

Generic Name	Trade Name	Spectrum of Activity	Dosage Form
Amantadine	Symmetrel	Influenza A	Capsule (100 mg), Syrup (50 mg/5 mL)
Rimantadine	Flumadine	Influenza A	Capsule (100 mg)
Interferon-α_{2a}	Roferon A, Alferon, Intron, Wellferon	Chronic hepatitis, CMV, HSV, papillomavirus, rhinovirus, and others	Injectable (3, 5, 10, 18, 25, and 50 million units/mL)
Interferon-α_{2b}	Interon A	Chronic hepatitis B and C, many other viruses	Injectable (3, 5, 10, 18, 25, and 50 million units/mL)
Interferon-γ	Actimmune		Injectable (100 μg/0.5 mL)
Zanamavir	Relenza	Influenza A and B	Inhaled powder (5 mg)
Oseltamivir	Tamiflu	Influenza A and B	Capsule (75 mg)
Enfurtizide	Fuzeon	HIV	Adult: 90 mg SQ b.i.d. Children (6–16 years): 2 mg/kg SQ b.i.d.

CMV, cytomegalovirus; HSV, herpes simplex virus, SQ, subcutaneous.

viral strains, and reach the target organ without interfering with normal cellular processes or the immune system of the host.

Agents Inhibiting Virus Attachment, Penetration, Uncoating, and Early Viral Replication (Table 43.2)

Amantadine

Amantadine

Mechanism of Action. Amantadine hydrochloride (1-adamantanamine hydrochloride) is a symmetric, tricyclic, primary amine that inhibits penetration of RNA viral particles into the host cell (19). It also inhibits the early stages of viral replication by blocking the uncoating of the viral genome and the transfer of nucleic acid into the host cell.

Clinical Application. Amantadine is clinically effective in preventing and treating all type A strains of influenza, particularly type A2 strains of Asian influenza virus, and to a lesser extent, German measles (rubella) or atoga virus. It also shows in vitro activity against influenza B, parainfluenza (paramyxovirus), respiratory syncytial virus (RSV), and some RNA viruses (murine, Rous, and Esh sarcoma viruses). Many prototype influenza A viruses of different human subtypes (H1N1; Fort Dix; H2N2, Asian type; and H3N2, Hong Kong type) also are inhibited by amantadine hydrochloride both in vitro and in animal model systems. If given within the first 48 hours of onset of symptoms, amantadine hydrochloride is effective in respiratory tract illness resulting from influenza A (but not influenza B), adenoviruses, and RSV.

Pharmacokinetics. Amantadine is well absorbed orally, and the usual dosage for oral administration is 100 mg twice daily. The drug has been approved as a capsule, tablet, and syrup for the treatment of keratoconjunctivitis caused by HSV infection. Amantadine hydrochloride oral solution should not be kept in a freezer but, rather, should be stored in a tight container at 15 to 30°C. Capsules and tablets should be protected from moisture and light. A 100 mg oral dose produces blood serum levels of 0.3 mg/mL within 1 to 8 hours. Maximum tissue concentration is reached in 48 hours when a 100 mg dose is given every 12 hours. In healthy adults receiving a 25, 100, or 150 mg dose of the drug twice daily, steady-state trough plasma concentrations were 110, 302, or 588 mg/mL, respectively. Usually, no neurotoxicity is observed if the plasma level of amantadine is no more than 1.00 mg/mL.

Amantadine crosses the blood-brain barrier and is distributed in saliva, nasal secretions, and breast milk (20). Approximately 90% of the drug is excreted unchanged by the kidney, primarily through glomerular filtration and tubular secretion, and there are no reports of metabolic products. Acidification of urine increases the rate of amantadine excretion. The half-life of the drug is 15 to 20 hours in patients with normal renal function.

Side Effects. Generally, the drug has low toxicity at therapeutic levels but may cause severe CNS symptoms, such as nervousness, confusion, headache, drowsiness, insomnia, depression, and hallucinations. The GI side effects include nausea, diarrhea, constipation, and anorexia. Convulsions and coma occur with high doses and in patients with cerebral arteriosclerosis and convulsive disorders. Chronic toxicity with amantadine is unexpected, because few side effects have been experienced when the drug has been used in long-term therapy for Parkinson's disease. Some serious reactions, however, include depression, orthostatic hypotension, psychosis, urinary retention, and congestive heart failure. Amantadine hydrochloride should be used with caution in patients who have a history of epilepsy, severe arteriosclerosis, liver diseases, and eczematoid dermatitis. Because amantadine does not appear to interfere with the immunogenicity of inactivated influenza A vaccine, patients may continue the use of amantadine for 1 week after influenza A vaccination. A virus that is resistant to amantadine has been obtained in cell culture and from animals, but these reports are not confirmed in humans.

Rimantadine

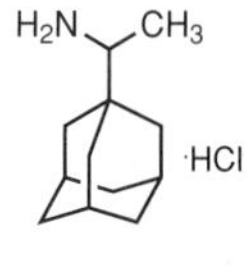

Rimantadine

Mechanism of Action. Rimantadine hydrochloride (α-methyl-1-adamantanemethylamine hydrochloride) is a synthetic adamatane derivative that is structurally and pharmacologically related to amantadine (21,22). It appears to be more effective than amantadine hydrochloride against influenza A, with fewer CNS side effects. Rimantadine hydrochloride is thought to interfere with virus uncoating by inhibiting the release of specific proteins. It may act by inhibiting RT or the synthesis of virus-specific RNA, but it does not inhibit virus adsorption or penetration. It appears to produce a virustatic effect early in the virus replication. It is used widely in Russia and Europe.

Clinical Application. Rimantadine hydrochloride has activity against most strains of influenza A, including H1N1, H2N2, and H3N2, but it has no activity against influenza B virus. It is used for prevention of infection caused by various human, animal, or avian strains of influenza A virus in adults and children. The side effects are nightmares, hallucinations, and vomiting. The most common side effects of rimantadine are associated with the CNS and the GI tract. Rimantadine is metabolized in the liver, and approximately 20% is excreted unchanged as hydroxylated compound.

Pharmacokinetics. The half-life of rimantadine in adults ranges from 24 to 36 hours. More than 90% of rimantadine doses were absorbed in 3 to 6 hours. Steady-state plasma concentrations are from 0.10 to 2.60 mg/mL at doses of 3 mg/kg/d in infants to doses of 100 mg twice daily in the elderly. Nasal fluid concentrations of rimantadine at steady state were 1.5-fold higher than plasma concentration.

Interferon (23,24)

Isaacs and Lindenmann discovered interferon in 1957. When they infected cells with viruses, interference with the cellular effects of viral infection were observed. Interferon was subsequently isolated and found to protect the cells from further infection. When interferon was administered to other cells or animals, it displayed biological properties such as inhibition of viral growth, cell multiplication, and immunomodulatory activities. These results led to the speculation that interferon may be a natural antiviral factor, possibly formed before antibody production, and may be involved in the normal mechanism of resistance displayed against viral infection. Some investigators relate interferon to the polypeptide hormones and suggest that interferon functions in cell-to-cell communication by transmitting specific messages. Recently, antitumor and anticancer properties of interferon have evoked worldwide interest in the possible use of this agent in therapy for viral diseases, cancer, and immunodeficiency disorders. Host cells synthesize interferons in response to various inducers.

Interferon Induction. Because viruses were found to induce the release of interferon, efforts were made to induce the production or release of interferon in humans by the administration of chemical "inducers" (25). Various small molecules (substituted propanediamine) and large polymers (double-stranded polynucleotides) were used to induce interferons. Statolon, a natural double-stranded RNA produced in *Penicillium stoloniferum* culture, and a double-stranded complex of polyriboinosinic acid and polyribocytidylic acid (poly I:C) have been used as nonviral inducers for releasing preformed interferons. A modification of poly I:C stabilized with poly-L-lysine and carboxymethylcellulose (poly ICLC) has been used experimentally in humans. Clinically, it has prevented coryza when used locally in the nose and conjunctival sacs. This substance is a better interferon inducer than poly I:C. Another interferon inducer is ampligen, a polynucleotide derivative of poly I:C with spaced uridines. It has anti-HIV activity in vitro and is an immunomodulator.

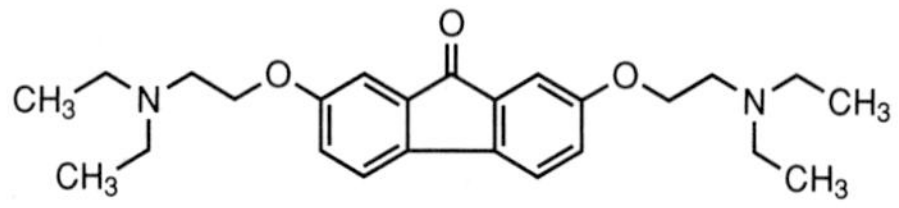

Tilorone

Other chemical inducers, such as pyran copolymers, tilorone, diethylaminoethyl dextran, and heparin, also have been used. Tilorone is an effective inducer of interferon in mice, but it is relatively ineffective in humans. Initial use of interferon and its inducers instilled intranasally after rhinovirus exposure was successful in the prevention of respiratory diseases. The clinical success of interferon and its inducers has not yet been established, although they may play a significant role in cell-mediated immunity to viral infections and cancer. Disadvantages of interferon use include unacceptable side effects, such as fever, headache, myalgias, leukopenia, nausea, vomiting, diarrhea, hypotension, alopecia, anorexia, and weight loss.

Interferon Structure. Interferon consists of a mixture of small proteins with molecular weights ranging from 20,000 to 160,000 daltons. They are glycoproteins that exhibit species-specific antiviral activity. Human interferons are classified into three types (26): α, β, and γ. The α-type is secreted by human leukocytes (white blood cells and non–T lymphocytes), and the β-type is secreted by human fibroblasts. Lymphoid cells (T lymphocytes), which either have been exposed to a presensitized antigen or have been stimulated to divide by mitogens, secrete interferon-α. Interferon-γ also is called "immune" interferon. Interferons are active in extremely low concentrations (for more details, see Chapter 6).

Clinical application. Interferon has been tested for use in chronic HBV infection, herpetic keratitis, herpes genitalis, herpes zoster, varicella-zoster, chronic hepatitis, influenza, and common cold infections. Other uses of interferon are in the treatment of cancers, such as breast cancer, lung carcinoma, and multiple myeloma. Interferon has had some success when used as a prophylactic agent for CMV infection in renal transplant recipients. The scarcity of interferon and the difficulty in purifying it have limited clinical trials. Supplies have been augmented by recombinant DNA technology, which allows cloning of the interferon gene (27), although the high cost still hinders clinical application. The U.S. FDA has approved recombinant interferon-α_{2a}, -α_{2b} and -γ for the treatment of hairy cell leukemia (a rare form of cancer), AIDS-related Kaposi's sarcoma, and genital warts (condyloma acuminatum). Subcutaneous injection of recombinant interferon-α_{2b} has been approved for the treatment of chronic hepatitis C. Some foreign countries have approved interferon-α for the treatment of cancers, such as multiple myeloma (cancer of plasma cells), malignant melanoma (skin cancer), and Kaposi's sarcoma (cancer associated with AIDS). Both interferon-β- and -γ as well as interleukin-2 may be commercial drugs of the future for the treatment of cancers and viral infections, including genital warts and the common cold.

Mechanism of action. Although interferons are mediators of immune response, different mechanisms for the antiviral action of interferon have been proposed. Interferon-α possesses broad-spectrum antiviral activity and acts on virus-infected cells by binding to specific cell surface receptors. It inhibits the transcription and translation of mRNA into viral nucleic acid and protein. Studies in cell-free systems have shown that the addition of adenosine triphosphate and double-stranded RNA to extracts of interferon-treated cells activates cellular RNA proteins and a cellular endonuclease. This activation causes the formation of translation inhibitory protein, which terminates production of viral enzyme, nucleic acid, and structural proteins (28). Interferon also may act by blocking synthesis of a cleaving enzyme required for viral release.

Pharmacokinetics. The pharmacokinetics of interferon is not well understood. Maximum levels in blood after intramuscular injection was obtained in 5 to 8 hours. Interferon does not penetrate well into cerebrospinal fluid (CSF). Oral administration of interferon does not indicate a detectable serum level, and as such, oral administration is clinically ineffective. After intramuscular or subcutaneous injection, drug concentration in plasma is dose related. Clinical use of interferon is limited to topical administration (nasal sprays) for prophylaxis and treatment of rhinovirus infections. Adverse reactions and toxicity include influenza-like syndrome of fever, chills, headache, myalgias, nausea, vomiting, diarrhea, bone marrow suppression, mental confusion, and behavioral changes. Intranasal administration produces mucosal friability, ulceration, and dryness.

Neuraminidase Inhibitors (29)

The role played by the surface glycoproteins hemagglutinin, an enzyme that is important for viral binding to host cell receptors via a terminal sialic acid residue, and neuraminidase (NA), an enzyme that is involved in various aspects of activation of influenza viruses, was discussed above. Freshly shed viral particles are coated with sialic acid residues. Neuraminidase is found in both influenza A and B viruses and is thought to be involved in catalytically cleaving glycosidic bonds between terminal sialic acid residues and adjacent sugars on hemagglutinin. The cleavage of sialic acid bonds facilitates the spread of viruses by enhancing adsorption to cell surface receptors and, thus, increases the infective level of the virus. In the absence of sialic acid cleavage from hemagglutinin, viral aggregation or inappropriate binding to hemagglutinin will occur, interfering with the spread of the infection. Neuraminidase also appears to play a role in preventing viral inactivation by respiratory mucus.

Mechanism of action. Because neuraminidase plays such an important role in the activation of newly formed viruses, it is not surprising that the development of neuraminidase inhibitors has become an important potential means of inhibiting the spread of viral infections. X-ray crystallography of neuraminidase has shown that whereas the amino acid sequence in the neuraminidase from various viruses is considerably different, the sialic acid binding site is quite similar for influenza A and B viruses. In addition, it is believed that the hydrolysis of sialic acid proceeds through a oxonium cation-stabilized carbonium ion, as shown in Figure 43.3. Mimicking the transition state with novel carboxylic derivatives of sialic acid has led to the development of transition state–based inhibitors (30). The first of these compounds, 2-deoxy-2,3-dehydro-N-acetylneuraminic acid (DANA) (Fig. 43.4), was found to be an active neuraminidase inhibitor but lacked specificity for viral neuraminidase. On determination of the crystal structure of neuraminidase, more sophisticated measurements of the binding site for sialic acid lead to the development of zanamivir and later oseltamivir.

Specific drugs

Zanamivir. Crystallographic studies of DANA (Fig. 43.4) bound to neuraminidase defined the receptor site to

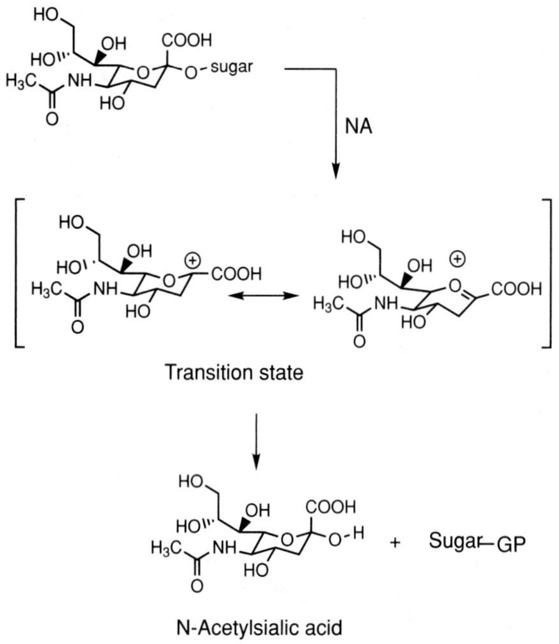

Fig. 43.3. Neuraminidase-catalyzed removal of a sialic acid residue from a glycoprotein chain. GP, glycoprotein; NA, neuraminidase.

which the sialic acid portion of the virus binds. These studies suggested that substitution of the 4-hydroxy with an amino group or the larger guanidino group should increase binding of the inhibitor to neuraminidase. The 4-amino derivative was found to bind to a glutamic acid (Glu^{119}) in the receptor through a salt bridge, whereas the guanidino was able to form both a salt bridge to Glu^{119} and a charge–charge interaction with Glu^{227}. The result of these substitutions was a dramatic increase in binding capacity to neuraminidase of the amino and guanidino derivatives, leading to effective competitive inhibition of the enzyme. The result has been the development of zanamivir (Fig. 43.4) as an effective agent against influenza A and B viruses.

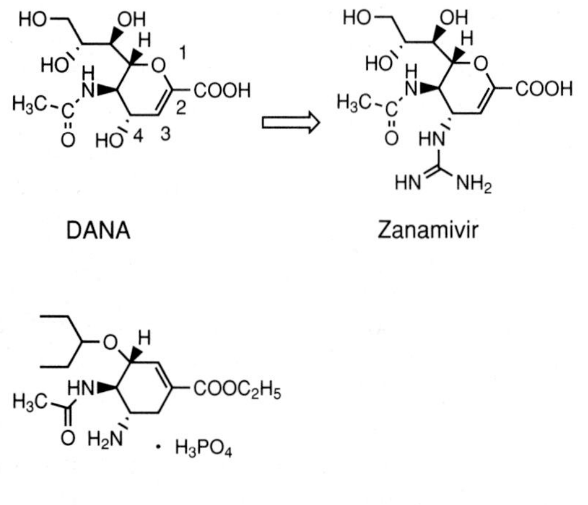

Fig. 43.4. Sialic acid derivatives 2-deoxy-2,3-dehydro-N-acetylneuraminic acid (DANA), zanamir, and oseltamivir phosphate, which act as inhibitors of neuraminidase.

Zanamirvir is effective when administered via the nasal, intraperitoneal, and intravenous (IV) routes, but it is inactive when given orally (Table 43.2). Animal studies have shown 68% recovery of the drug in the urine following intraperitoneal administration, 43% urinary recovery following nasal administration, and only 3% urinary recovery following oral administration. Human data gave results similar to those obtained in animal models. Human efficacy studies with nasal drops or sprays demonstrated that the drug was effective when administered before and after exposure to influenza A or B virus. When given before viral inoculation, the drug reduced viral shedding, infection, and symptoms. When administered beginning at either 26 or 32 hours after inoculation, there was a reduction in shedding, viral titer, and fever. Presently, the drug is available as a dry powder for oral inhalation by adults and adolescents who have been symptomatic for no more than 2 days. Zanamirvir is able to more rapidly resolve influenza symptoms and to improve recovery (from 7 days with placebo to 4 days with treatment). Additional studies have suggested the prophylactic benefit of zanamirvir when administered to family members after one member of the family developed flu-like symptoms. As a result, the manufacturer has submitted an application for the use of the drug for the prevention of influenza A and B infections.

Oseltamivir Phosphate. X-ray crystallographic studies further demonstrated that additional binding sites exist between neuraminidase and substrate involving the C-5 acetamido carbonyl and an arginine (Arg^{152}); the C-2 carboxyl and arginines at 118, 292, and 371; and the potential for hydrophobic binding to substituents at C-6 (with glutamic acid, alanine, arginine, and isoleucine). Structure–activity relationship studies showed that maximum binding occurred to neuraminidase when C-6 was substituted with the 3-pentyloxy side chain, such as the one found in oseltamivir. In addition, esterification with ethanol gave rise to a compound that is orally effective. Oseltamivir (Fig. 43.4) was approved as the first orally administered neuraminidase inhibitor used against influenza A and B viruses (Table 43.2). The drug is indicated for the treatment of uncomplicated acute illness caused by influenza infection. Recently, the drug has been approved for prevention of influenza A and B infections in adults, adolescents, and children 1 year of age and older. The drug is effective in treating influenza if administered within 2 days after onset of symptoms. The recommended dose is 75 mg twice daily for 5 days. The prophylactic dose is 75 mg taken once daily for 7 days in adults and teenagers, with lower doses for children 1 year or older (dosed based on body weight). Oseltamivir is readily absorbed from the GI tract following oral administration. It is a prodrug that is extensively metabolized in the liver, undergoing ester hydrolysis to the active carboxylic acid

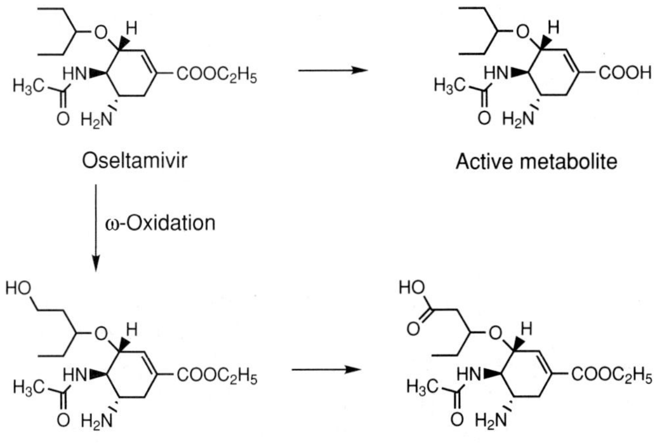

Oseltamivir

Active metabolite

ω-Oxidation

Fig. 43.5. Metabolism of oseltamivir by deethylation and ω-oxidation.

(Fig. 43.5). Two oxidative metabolites also have been isolated, with the major oxidation product being the ω-carboxylic acid (31). Side effects with oseltamivir are minor, consist of nausea and vomiting, and occur primarily in the first two days of therapy.

Enfuvirtide (32,33).

N-acetyl-Tyr-Thr-Ser-Leu-Ile-His-Ser-Leu-Ile-Glu-Glu-Ser-Gln-Asp-Gln-Gln-Glu-Lys-Asp-Glu-Gln-Glu-Leu-Leu-Glu-Leu-Asp-Lys-Try-Ala-Ser-Leu-Try-Asp-Try-Phe-NH_2

Enfuvirtide

Entry inhibitors, also known as fusion inhibitors, are a new class of drugs for the treatment of HIV infection, and enfuvirtide is the first compound of this family to be approved for clinical use. Enfuvirtide is an oligo peptide consisting of 36 amino acids. It is a synthetic peptide that mimics an HR2 fragment of gp41, blocking the formation of a six-helix bundle structure that is critical in the fusion of the HIV-1 virion to a CD4-positive T lymphocyte. Specifically, it binds to the tryptophan-rich region of the gp41 protein. Enfuvirtide is used in combination with other antiretrovirals and works against a variety of HIV-1 variants, but it is not active against HIV-2. Resistance to enfuvirtide can develop when the virus produces changes in a 10-amino-acid domain between residues 36 to 45 in the gp41 HIV surface glycoprotein.

The drug is administered twice daily as a subcutaneous injection and has a complex absorption pattern. Enfuvirtide is highly bound to plasma protein (~92%) and is prone to proteolytic metabolism. Adverse reactions are common at the site of injection (e.g., pain, erythema, and pruritus) and insomnia.

Agents Interfering with Viral Nucleic Acid Replication (Table 43.3)

Acyclovir and Valacyclovir

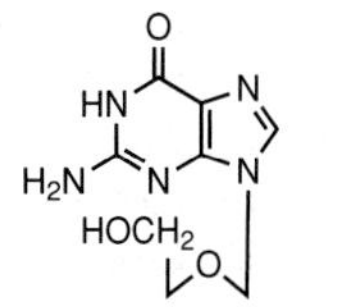

Acyclovir
(9-[(2-Hydroxyethoxy)methyl]guanine)

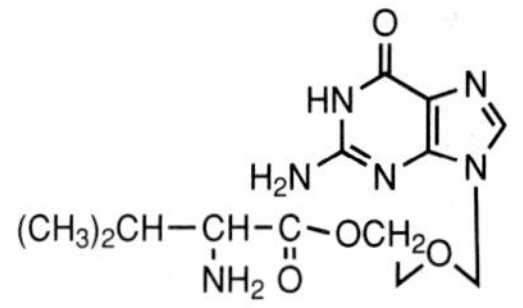

Valacyclovir

Mechanism of Action. Acyclovir is a synthetic analogue of deoxyguanosine in which the carbohydrate moiety is acyclic (34). Because of this difference in structure as compared to other antiviral compounds (idoxuridine, vidarabine, and

Table 43.3. Antiviral Agents Interfering with Viral Nucleic Acid Replication

Generic Name	Common Name	Trade Name	Spectrum of Activity	Dosage Form
Acyclovir	Acyclo-G	Zovirax	HSV-1, HSV-2, VZV, EBV	5% Ointment, injectable (5 mg/mL), capsule (200 mg), tablet (400 and 800 mg), suspension (200 mg/5 mL)
Valacyclovir		Valtrex	HSV-1, VZV, CMV	Tablet (500 mg)
Cidofovir	HPMPC	Vistide	CMV, HSV-1, HSV-2, VZV, CMV, EBV	Injectable (75 mg/mL)
Cytarabine	Ara-C	Cytosar	Herpes zoster	Injectable (10, 20, 50, and 100 mg/mL)
Famciclovir	FCV	Famvir	HSV, VZV, EBV, chronic HBV	Tablet (125, 250, and 500 mg)
Fomivirsen		Vitravene	CMV retinitis	Injectable (6.6 mg/mL)
Foscarnet	PFA	Foscavir	CMV retinitis, HSV	Injectable (24 mg/mL)
Ganciclovir	DHPG	Cytovene, Vitrasert	CMV retinitis	Injectable (50 mg/mL), capsule (250 and 500 mg), insert (4.5 mg/insert)
Idoxuridine	5-IUDR	Herplex	HSV keratitis	0.1% Solution, 0.5% ointment
Ribavirin		Virazole	RSV, influenza A and B, HIV-1, parainfluenza	Aerosol (20 mg/mL)
Trifluorothymidine	TFT, FT3	Viroptic	HSV-1	1% Solution
Vidarabine	Ara-A	Vira A	HSV-1, HSV-2	3% Ointment (monohydrate)
Adefovir dipivoxil		Hepsera	HBV	Tablet (10 mg)

CMV, cytomegalovirus; EBV, Epstein-Barr virus; HBV, hepatitis B virus; HSV, herpes simplex virus; VZV, varicella-zoster virus.

trifluridine), acyclovir possesses a unique mechanism of antiviral activity. The mode of action of acyclovir consists of three consecutive mechanisms (35). The first of these mechanisms involves conversion of the drug to active acyclovir monophosphate within cells by viral thymidine kinase (Fig. 43.6). This phosphorylation reaction occurs faster within cells infected by herpesvirus than in normal cells, because acyclovir is a poor substrate for the normal cell thymidine kinase. Acyclovir is further converted to di- and triphosphates by a normal cellular enzyme called guanosine monophosphate kinase. In the second mechanism, viral DNA polymerase is competitively inhibited by acyclovir triphosphate with a lower median inhibition concentration (IC50) than that for cellular DNA polymerase. Acyclovir triphosphate is incorporated into the viral DNA chain during DNA synthesis. Because acyclovir triphosphate lacks the 3′-hydroxyl group of a cyclic sugar, it terminates further elongation of the DNA chain. The third mechanism depends on preferential uptake of acyclovir by herpes-infected cells as compared to uninfected cells, resulting in a higher concentration of acyclovir triphosphate and leading to a high therapeutic index between herpes-infected cells compared to normal cells. Acyclovir is active against certain herpesvirus infections. These viruses induce virus-specific thymidine kinase and DNA polymerase, which are inhibited by acyclovir. Thus, acyclovir significantly reduces DNA synthesis in virus-infected cells without significantly disturbing the active replication of uninfected cells.

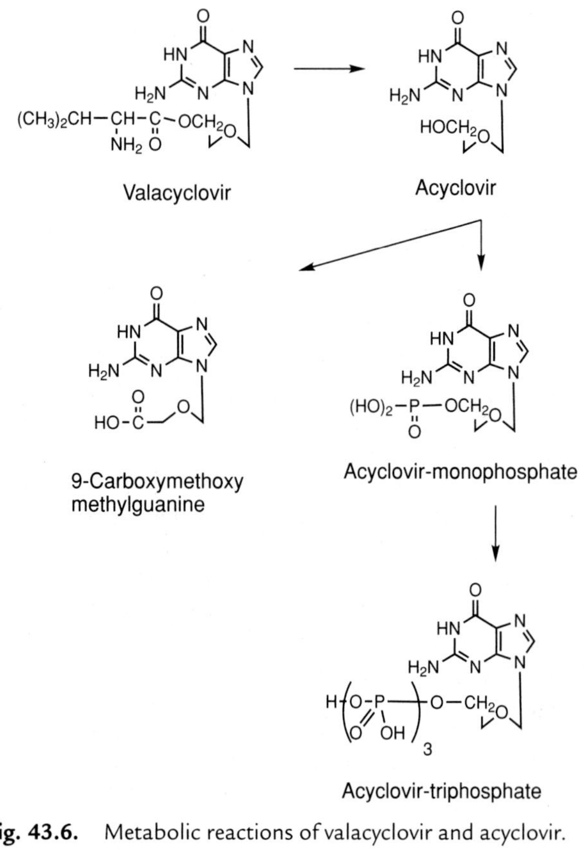

Valacyclovir

Acyclovir

9-Carboxymethoxy methylguanine

Acyclovir-monophosphate

Acyclovir-triphosphate

Fig. 43.6. Metabolic reactions of valacyclovir and acyclovir.

Clinical application. Acyclovir has potent activity against several DNA viruses including HSV-1, the common cause of labial herpes (cold sore), and HSV-2, the common cause of genital herpes (36). Varicella-zoster virus and some isolates of EBV are affected to a lesser extent by acyclovir. On the other hand, CMV is less sensitive to acyclovir, which has no activity against vaccinia virus, adenovirus, and parainfluenza infections. An ointment containing 5% acyclovir has been used in a regimen of five times a day for up to 14 days for the treatment of herpetic keratitis and of primary and recurrent infections of herpes genitalis. Mild pain, transient burning, stinging, pruritus, rash, and vulvitis have been noted. The U.S. FDA has approved topical and IV acyclovir preparations for initial herpes genitalis and HSV-1 and HSV-2 infections in immunocompromised patients (37). In these individuals, early use of acyclovir shortens the duration of viral shedding and lesion pain. Oral doses of 200 mg of acyclovir, taken five times a day for 5 to 10 days, have not proven to be successful because of the low bioavailability of current preparations. Oral doses of 800 mg of the drug given five times daily for 7 to 10 days have been approved by the U.S. FDA for the treatment of herpes zoster infection. This treatment shortens the duration of viral shedding in chickenpox and shingles. The IV injection of the drug (given 10 mg/kg three times a day for 10 to 12 days) has been approved for the treatment of herpes simplex encephalitis (38). Excessive and high doses of acyclovir have, however, caused viruses to develop resistance to the drug. This resistance results from reduction of virus-encoded thymidine kinase, which does not effectively activate the drug.

Pharmacokinetics. Pharmacokinetic studies show that IV dose administration of 2.5 mg/kg of acyclovir results in peak plasma concentrations of 3.4 to 6.8 mg/mL (39,40). The bioavailability of acyclovir is 15 to 30%, and it is metabolized to 9-carboxymethoxymethylguanine, which is inactive (Fig. 43.6). Plasma protein binding averages 15%, and approximately 70% of acyclovir is excreted unchanged in the urine by both glomerular filtration and tubular secretion. The half-life of the drug is approximately 3 hours in patients with normal renal function. In an individual with renal diseases, the half-life of the drug is prolonged. Therefore, acyclovir dosage adjustment is necessary for patients with renal impairment. Because of its low molecular weight and protein binding, acyclovir is easily dialyzed. Thus, a full dose of the drug should be given after hemodialysis. It should be infused slowly, over at least 30 minutes, to avoid acute transient and reversible renal failure. Acyclovir easily penetrates the lung, brain, muscle, spleen, uterus, vaginal mucosa, intestine, liver, and kidney. Acyclovir has relatively few side effects, except that IV injection causes reversible renal dysfunction and irritation, inflammation, and pain at the injection site. Infusion sites therefore should be inspected frequently and changed after every 72 hours. The drug is slightly toxic to bone marrow at higher doses. Less frequent side effects are nausea, vomiting, headache, skin rashes, hematuria, arthralgia, and insomnia.

Valacyclovir hydrochloride is an amino acid ester prodrug of acyclovir that exhibits antiviral activity only after metabolism first in the intestine walls or liver to acyclovir and then conversion to the triphosphate, as shown in Figure 43.6 (41). Structurally, it differs from acyclovir by the presence of the amino acid valine attached to the 5′-hydroxyl group of the nucleoside. Valacyclovir's benefit comes from an increased GI absorption, resulting in higher plasma concentrations of acyclovir, which normally is poorly absorbed from the GI tract. As with acyclovir, valacyclovir is active against HSV-1, VZV, and CMV (Table 43.3) because of its affinity for the viral form of the enzyme thymidine kinase. Oral valacyclovir is used for the treatment of acute, localized herpes zoster (shingles) in immunocompetent patients and may be given without meals. It also is used for the initial and recurrent episodes of genital herpes infections. The adverse effects are similar to acyclovir, which include nausea, headache, vomiting, constipation, and anorexia. The binding of valacyclovir to human plasma proteins ranges between 13.5 to 17.9%. The plasma elimination half-life of acyclovir is 2.5 to 3.3 hours. The bioavailability of valacyclovir hydrochloride is 54%, compared to approximately 20% for oral acyclovir, and it is as effective as acyclovir in decreasing the duration of pain associated with posttherapeutic neuralgia and episodes of genital lesion healing.

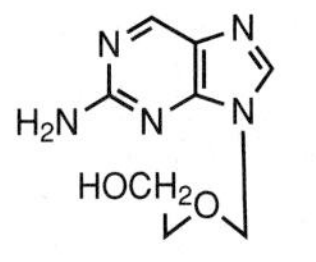

6-Deoxyacyclovir

The related analogue 6-deoxyacyclovir is a prodrug form of acyclovir that is activated through metabolism by xanthine oxidase. This drug, which has improved solubility characteristics compared to acyclovir, is used for the treatment of VZV infection.

Cidofovir

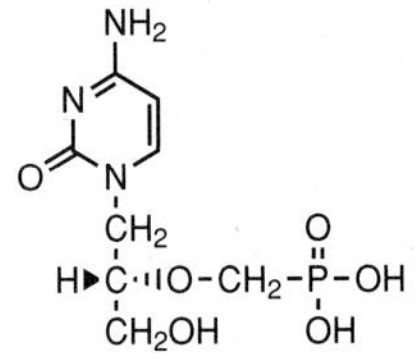

Cidofovir
1-[(*S*)-3-hydroxy-2-(phosphonomethoxy)propyl]cytosine

Mechanism of Action. Cidofovir is a synthetic acyclic pyrimidine nucleotide analogue of cytosine (42). It is a phosphorylated nucleotide that is additionally phosphorylated by host cell enzymes to its active intracellular metabolite, cidofovir diphosphate. This reaction occurs without initial virus-dependent phosphorylation by viral nucleoside kinases. It has antiviral effects by interfering with DNA synthesis and inhibiting viral replication.

Pharmacokinetics. Topical cidofovir (0.2%) is as effective as trifluridine (1%) in reducing HSV-1 shedding and healing time in rabbits with dendritic keratitis. Cidofovir is administered IV, topically, and by ocular implant (Table 43.3). Peak plasma concentration of 3.1 to 23.6 mg/mL is achieved with doses of 1.0 to 10.0 mg/kg, respectively. The terminal plasma half-life is 2.6 hours, and 90% of the drug is excreted in the urine. It has a variable bioavailability (2–26%).

Clinical Application. Cidofovir is active against herpesviruses, including HSV-1 and HSV-2, VZV, CMV, and EBV. It is effective against acyclovir-resistant strains of HSV and ganciclovir-resistant strains of CMV. Cidofovir is a long-acting drug for the treatment of CMV retinitis in patients with AIDS when given as an IV infusion or an intravitreal injection. It is not a curative drug, and its benefit over foscarnet or ganciclovir is yet to be determined. The major adverse effect is nephrotoxicity, which appears to result in renal tubular damage. Concomitant administration of cidofovir with probenecid is contraindicated because of increased risk of nephrotoxicity.

Cytarabine

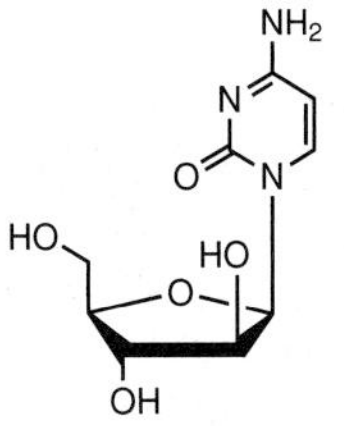

Cytarabine
1-β'-Arabinofuranosylcytosine (ara-C)

Mechanism of Action. Cytarabine is a pyrimidine nucleoside related to idoxuridine (43). It is used primarily as an anticancer rather than an antiviral agent. Cytarabine acts by blocking the utilization of deoxycytidine, thereby inhibiting the replication of viral DNA. The drug is first converted to mono-, di-, and triphosphates, which interfere with DNA synthesis by inhibiting both DNA polymerase and the reductase that promotes the conversion of cytidine diphosphate into its deoxy derivatives.

Clinical Application. Cytarabine is used to treat Burkitt's lymphoma and both myeloid and lymphatic leukemias. Its antiviral use is in the treatment of herpes zoster (shingles) infection (Table 43.3). It also is used to treat herpetic keratitis and viral infections resistant to idoxuridine. The drug generally is used topically, but it has been given by IV injection to individuals with serious herpesvirus infection (44). Cytarabine is deaminated rapidly in the body to an inactive compound, arabinosyluracil, which is excreted in

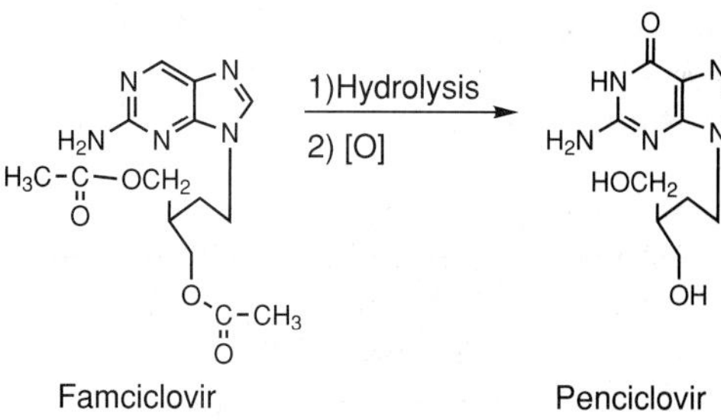

Famciclovir 1)Hydrolysis 2) [O] Penciclovir

Fig. 43.7. Metabolic activation of famciclovir.

the urine. The half-life of the drug in plasma is 3 to 5 hours. The toxic effects of cytarabine are chiefly on bone marrow, the GI tract, and the kidney. The drug is not given during the early months of pregnancy because of its teratogenic and carcinogenic effects in animals.

Famciclovir

Mechanism of Action. Famciclovir (Fig. 43-7) is a synthetic purine nucleoside analogue related to guanine (45,46). It is the diacetyl 6-deoxy ester of penciclovir, which is structurally related to ganciclovir. Its pharmacological and microbiological activities are similar to those of acyclovir. Famciclovir is a prodrug of penciclovir, which is formed in vivo by hydrolysis of the acetyl groups and oxidation at the 6-position by mixed function oxidases. Penciclovir and its metabolite penciclovir triphosphate possess antiviral activity resulting from inhibition of viral DNA polymerase.

Clinical Application. Famciclovir is active against recurrent HSV (genital herpes and cold sores), VZV, and EBV but is less active against CMV (Table 43.3). It is used in the treatment of recurrent localized herpes zoster and genital herpes in immunocompetent adults, and it also is promising for the treatment of chronic HBV reinfection after liver transplantation.

Pharmacokinetics. Famciclovir can be given with or without food. The most common adverse effects are headache and GI disturbances. Concomitant use of famciclovir with probenecid results in increased plasma concentrations of penciclovir. The recommended dose of famciclovir is 500 mg every 8 hours for 7 days. The absolute bioavailability of famciclovir is 77%, and the area under plasma concentration–time curve (AUC) is 86 μg/mL. Famciclovir with digoxin increased plasma concentration of digoxin to 19% as compared to digoxin given alone.

Fomivirsen

Fomivirsen sodium is used to treat CMV, which causes opportunistic retinitis in patients with AIDS. Such patients respond to fomivirsen but not to other treatment for CMV retinitis, which leads to blindness (47). Fomivirsen is the first antisense oligonucleotide agent that has been approved as an alternative medicine for patients with CMV retinitis for whom other agents did not work (see Chapter 8, Fomivirsen). It works by inhibiting the synthesis of proteins responsible for the regulation of viral gene expression that is involved in infection of CMV retinitis. Fomivirsen works only in the eye in which it is injected. It is not recommended if cidofovir is used within the last 2 to 4 weeks because of increased risk of eye inflammation. Fomivirsen is given in two induction doses, followed by monthly maintenance doses, each being 330 μg administered by intravitreal injection. It can cause increased pressure in the eye that requires treatment by an ophthalmologist. Fomivirsen also is used in the treatment of Crohn's disease and certain cancers. It causes eye inflammation, abnormal vision, cataract, eye pain, and retinal problems. In addition, it causes several other side effects, such as stomach pain, headache, fever, infection, rash, vomiting, and liver dysfunction.

Foscarnet

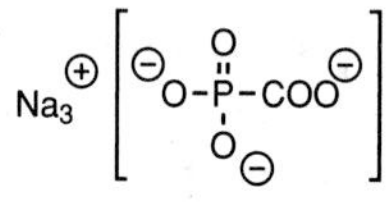

$Na_3^{\oplus}\left[{}^{\ominus}O-P(=O)(O^{\ominus})-COO^{\ominus}\right]$

Foscarnet sodium

Foscarnet sodium is a trisodium phosphoformate hexahydrate that inhibits DNA polymerase of herpesviruses, including CMV and retroviral RT (48). It is not phosphorylated into an active form by viral host cell enzymes. Therefore, it has the advantage of not requiring an activation step before attacking the target viral enzyme.

Clinical Application. Foscarnet sodium was approved by the U.S. FDA for the treatment of CMV retinitis in patients with AIDS. In combination with ganciclovir, the results have been promising, even in progressive disease with ganciclovir-resistant strains. Foscarnet sodium also is effective in the treatment of mucocutaneous diseases caused by acyclovir-resistant strains of HSV and VZV in patients with AIDS. Foscarnet sodium is administered IV at 60 mg/kg three times a day for initial therapy and at 90 to 120 mg/kg daily for maintenance therapy (Table 43.3). The plasma-half life is 3 to 6 hours. Foscarnet sodium penetrates into the CSF and the eye. The drug is neurotoxic, and common adverse effects include phlebitis, anemia, nausea, vomiting, and seizures. Foscarnet sodium carries the risk of severe hypocalcemia, especially with concurrent use of IV pentamidine. Foscarnet sodium used with zidovudine (ZDV) has an additive effect against CMV and acts synergistically against HIV.

Ganciclovir

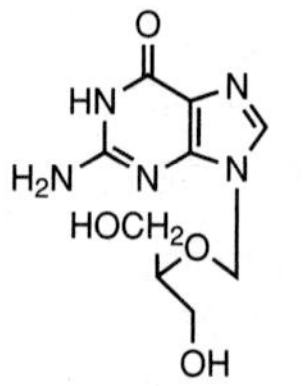

Ganciclovir (DHPG)

Mechanism of action. Ganciclovir sodium is an acyclic deoxyguanosine analogue of acyclovir (49). Ganciclovir inhibits DNA polymerase. Its active form is ganciclovir triphosphate, which is an inhibitor of viral rather than of cellular DNA polymerase. The phosphorylation of ganciclovir does not require a virus-specific thymidine kinase for its activity against CMV. The mechanism of action is similar to that of acyclovir; however, ganciclovir is more toxic than acyclovir to human cells.

Clinical significance. Ganciclovir has greater activity than acyclovir against CMV and EBV infection in immunocompromised patients. It also is active against HSV infection and in some mutants that are resistant to acyclovir. In patients with AIDS, ganciclovir stopped progressive hemorrhagic retinitis and symptomatic pneumonitis related to CMV infection. Ganciclovir is absorbed and phosphorylated by infection-induced kinases of HSV and VZV infections. Common side effects are leukopenia, neutropenia, and thrombocytopenia. Ganciclovir with ZDV causes severe hematologic toxicity. Ganciclovir is available only as an IV infusion, because its oral bioavailability is poor (Table 43.3). It is given in doses of 5 mg/kg twice daily for 14 to 21 days. When ganciclovir is given by IV administration, concentrations of the drug in the CSF and the brain vary from 25 to 70% of the plasma concentration. After minimal metabolism, ganciclovir is excreted in the urine. In adults with normal renal function, the serum half-life of the drug is approximately 3 hours. Ganciclovir has been approved by the U.S. FDA for the treatment of CMV retinitis in immunocompromised patients and in patients with AIDS.

Idoxuridine

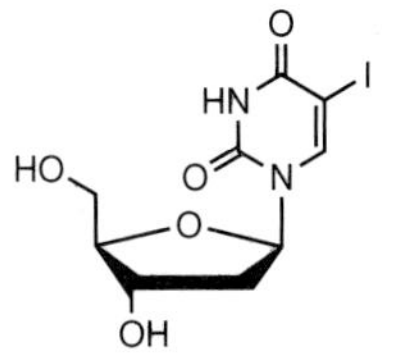

Idoxuridine

Mechanism of action. Idoxuridine is a nucleoside containing a halogenated pyrimidine and is an analogue of thymidine (49). It acts as an antiviral agent against DNA viruses by interfering with their replication based on the similarity of structure between thymidine and idoxuridine. Idoxuridine is first phosphorylated by the host cell virus-encoded enzyme thymidine kinase to an active triphosphate form. The phosphorylated drug inhibits cellular DNA polymerase to a lesser extent than HSV DNA polymerase, which is necessary for the synthesis of viral DNA. The triphosphate form of the drug is then incorporated during viral nucleic acid synthesis by a false pairing system that replaces thymidine. When transcription occurs, faulty viral proteins are formed, resulting in defective viral particles (51).

Clinical application. Idoxuridine is available as ophthalmic drops (0.1%) and ointment (0.5%) for the treatment of HSV keratoconjunctivitis, the leading cause of blindness in the United States (Table 43.3). Because of its poor solubility, the drug is ineffective in the treatment of labial or genital HSV or of cutaneous herpes zoster infection. Idoxuridine in dimethyl sulfoxide (DMSO), however, has been used in mucocutaneous HSV infection of the mouth and nose. Because DMSO facilitates drug absorption and also has some therapeutic effect, a 40% solution of idoxuridine in DMSO is more effective than idoxuridine used without this vehicle. Therefore, the U.S. FDA approved idoxuridine only for topical treatment of herpes simplex keratitis, and it is more effective in epithelial than in stromal infections. It is less effective for recurrent herpes keratitis, probably because of the development of drug-resistant virus strains.

Adverse reactions of idoxuridine include such local reactions as pain, pruritus, edema, burning, and hypersensitivity. Systemic administration of idoxuridine by IV injection may be given in an emergency, but this leads to bone marrow toxicities, such as leukopenia, thrombocytopenia, and anemia. It also may induce stomatitis, nausea, vomiting, abnormalities of liver functions, and alopecia. Idoxuridine has a plasma half-life of 30 minutes and is rapidly metabolized in the blood to idoxuracil and uracil.

Additional Hydrogenated Uridines

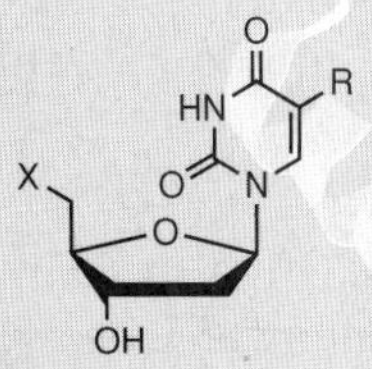

Fluorodeoxyuridine (R = F, X = OH)
Bromodeoxyuridine (R = Br, X = OH)
5'-aminoidoxuridine (R = I, X = NH_2)

Other halogenated uridine derivatives have been reported to exhibit antiviral activity. Fluorodeoxyuridine has in vitro antiviral activity but is not used in clinical practice. Bromodeoxyuridine is used in subacute sclerosing panencephalitis, a deadly, virus-induced CNS disease. This agent appears to interfere with DNA synthesis in the same way as idoxuridine. The 5′-amino analogue of idoxuridine (5-iodo-5′-amino-2′,5′-dideoxyuridine) is a better antiviral agent than idoxuridine, and it is less toxic. It is metabolized in herpesvirus-infected cells only by thymidine kinase to di- and triphosphoramidates. These metabolites inhibit HSV-specific late RNA transcription, causing reduction of less infective abnormal viral proteins. 5-Bromo-2′-deoxyuridine has an action similar to that of other iodinated compounds. None of these compounds are commercially available in the United States.

Ribavirin

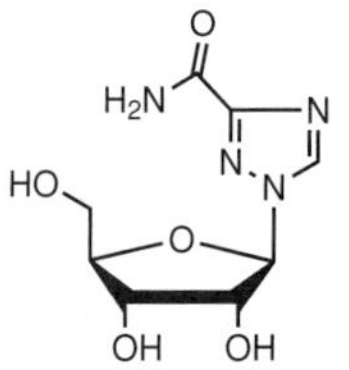

Ribavirin

Mechanism of Action. Ribavirin, a guanosine analogue, has broad-spectrum antiviral activity against both DNA and RNA viruses (52,53). It is phosphorylated by adenosine kinase to the triphosphate, resulting in the inhibition of viral specific RNA polymerase, disrupting messenger RNA and nucleic acid synthesis.

Clinical Application. Ribavirin is highly active against influenza A and B viruses and the parainfluenza group of viruses, genital herpes, herpes zoster, measles, and acute hepatitis types A, B, and C. Aerosolized ribavirin has been approved by the U.S. FDA for the treatment of lower respiratory tract infections (bronchiolitis and pneumonia) and serious RSV infections, but it can cause cardiopulmonary and immunologic disorders in children (Table 43.3). Ribavirin inhibits in vitro replication of HIV-1. Clinically, ribavirin has been shown to delay the onset of full-blown AIDS in patients with early symptoms of HIV infection. Some viruses are less susceptible, such as poliovirus, herpesviruses excluding varicella, vaccinia, mumps, reovirus, and rotavirus. A randomized, double-blind study of aerosolized ribavirin treatment of infants with RSV infections indicated significant improvement in the severity of infection, with a decrease in viral shedding (54).

Pharmacokinetics. Oral or IV forms of ribavirin are useful in the prevention and treatment of Lassa fever. The oral bioavailability is approximately 45%, and the serum half-life is 9 hours. Peak plasma level after 1 hour is 1 to 3 mg/mL. Intravenous administration of the drug has higher peak plasma levels. Aerosol preparation delivery of drug (0.8 mg/kg/hour) produced drug levels in respiratory secretions of 50 to 200 mg/mL (Table 43.3). The clinical benefits of this agent are yet to be confirmed. Its few side effects generally are limited to GI disturbances, such as nausea, vomiting, and diarrhea. The drug is contraindicated in patients with asthma because of deterioration of pulmonary function. Viral strains susceptible to ribavirin have not been found to develop drug resistance, as is the case with other antiviral agents, such as acyclovir, idoxuridine, and bromovinyldeoxyuridine.

Trifluorothymidine

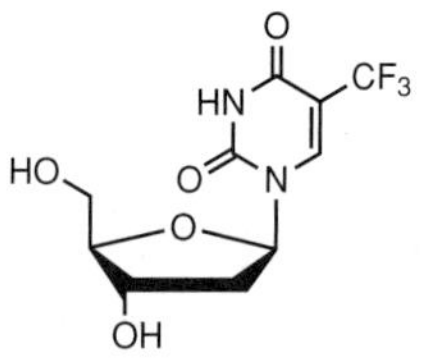

Trifluorothymidine (TFT, F3T)

Mechanism of Action. Trifluorothymidine is a fluorinated pyridine nucleoside structurally related to idoxuridine (55). It has been approved by the U.S. FDA and is a potent, specific inhibitor of replication of HSV-1 in vitro. Its mechanism of action is similar to that of idoxuridine. Like other antiherpes drugs, it is first phosphorylated by thymidine kinase to mono-, di-, and triphosphate forms, which are then incorporated into viral DNA in place of thymidine to stop the formation of late virus mRNA and subsequent synthesis of the virion proteins.

Clinical Application. Trifluorothymidine, because of its greater solubility in water, is active against HSV-1 and HSV-2. It also is useful in treating infections caused by human CMV and VZV infections (Table 43.3). The advantage of use of this agent over idoxuridine is its high topical efficacy in the cure of primary keratoconjunctivitis and recurrent epithelial keratitis. It also is useful for difficult cases of herpetic iritis and established stromal keratitis.

Pharmacokinetics. Trifluorothymidine is available as a 1% ophthalmic solution, which is effective in dendritic ulcers. Generally, a 1% eye solution of trifluorothymidine is well tolerated. Cross-hypersensitivity and cross-toxicity between trifluorothymidine, idoxuridine, and vidarabine are rare. The most frequent side effects are temporary burning, stinging, localized edema, and bone marrow toxicity. It is less toxic but more expensive than idoxuridine. Trifluorothymidine, when given IV, shows a plasma half-life of 18 minutes and is excreted in the urine either unchanged or as the inactive metabolite 5-carboxyuracil.

Vidarabine

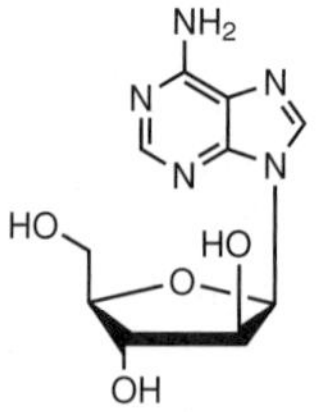

Vidarabine (ara-A)

MECHANISM OF ACTION. Vidarabine is an adenosine nucleoside obtained from cultures of *Streptomyces antibioticus* (56). Cellular enzymes convert vidarabine to mono-, di-, and triphosphate derivatives that interfere with viral nucleic acid replication, specifically inhibiting the early steps in DNA synthesis. This agent was used originally as an antineoplastic drug. Its antiviral effect is, in some cases, superior to that of idoxuridine or cytarabine.

CLINICAL APPLICATION. Vidarabine is used mainly in human HSV-1 and HSV-2 encephalitis, decreasing the mortality rate from 70 to 30%. Whitley et al. (57) reported that early vidarabine therapy is helpful in controlling complications of localized or disseminated herpes zoster in immunocompromised patients. Vidarabine also is useful in neonatal herpes labialis or genitalis, vaccinia virus, adenovirus, RNA viruses, papovavirus, CMV, and smallpox virus infections. Given the efficacy of vidarabine in certain viral infections, the U.S. FDA approved a 3% ointment for the treatment of herpes simplex keratoconjunctivitis and recurrent epithelial keratitis, and a 2% IV injection for the treatment of herpes simplex encephalitis and herpes zoster infections (Table 43.3). A topical ophthalmic preparation of vidarabine is useful in herpes simplex keratitis but shows little promise in herpes simplex labialis or genitalis. The monophosphate esters of vidarabine are more water-soluble and can be used in smaller volumes and even intramuscularly. These esters are under clinical investigation for the treatment of hepatitis B, systemic and cutaneous herpes simplex, and herpes zoster virus infections in immunocompromised patients.

PHARMACOKINETICS. Vidarabine is deaminated rapidly by adenosine deaminase, which is present in serum and red blood cells. The enzyme converts vidarabine to its principal metabolite, arabinosyl hypoxanthine (ara-HX), which has weak antiviral activity (Fig. 43.8) (58). The half-life of vidarabine is approximately 1 hour, whereas ara-HX has a half-life of 3.5 hours. The drug is detected mostly in the kidney, liver, and spleen, because 50% of it is recovered in the urine as ara-HX. Levels of vidarabine in CSF fluid are 50% of those in the plasma.

The most common side effects of vidarabine are GI disturbances, such as anorexia, nausea, vomiting, and diarrhea. The CNS side effects include tremors, dizziness, pain syndromes, and seizures. Bone marrow suppression is reported at higher doses. Because vidarabine is reported to be mutagenic, carcinogenic, and teratogenic in animal studies, its use in pregnant women is to be avoided. Allopurinol and theophylline may interfere with the metabolism of vidarabine at higher doses because of the xanthine oxidase metabolism of vidarabine. Therefore, this agent should be avoided or given with caution to patients receiving these medications concurrently. Also, adjustment of the dose is necessary in patients with renal insufficiency.

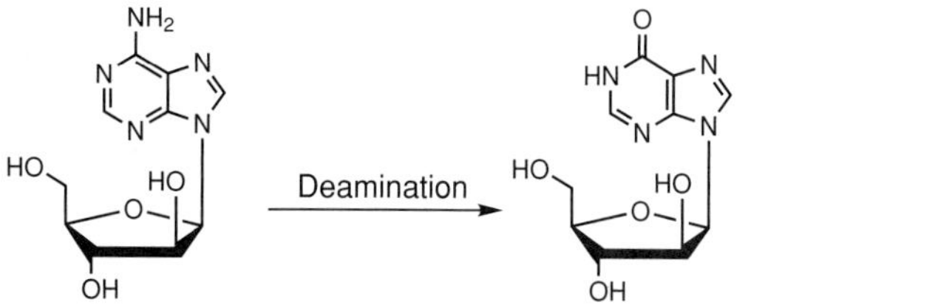

Vidarabine (ara-A) — Deamination → Arabinofuranosylhypoxanthine (ara-HX)

Fig. 43.8. Metabolism of vidarabine.

Adefovir Dipivoxil (59)

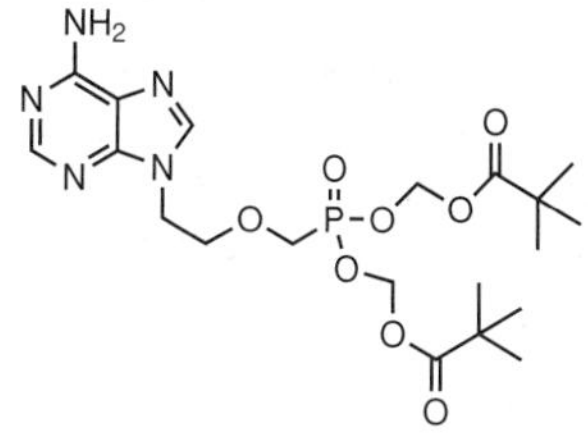

Adefovir dipivoxil

MECHANISM OF ACTION. Adefovir dipivoxil is an orally active prodrug indicated for the treatment of chronic hepatitis B. The drug is hydrolyzed by extracellular esterases to produce adefovir, which in turn is phosphorylated by adenylate kinase to adefovir diphosphate, which inhibits HBV DNA polymerase. Incorporation of adefovir into viral DNA also leads to DNA chain termination. As shown in Figure 43.9, adefovir dipivoxyl is activated in two steps involving an esterase that exposes a free phosphate group (adefovir), followed by addition of a second phosphate by adenylate kinase to form adefovir diphosphate, the active form of the drug.

PHARMACOKINETICS. Adefovir is poorly absorbed orally, but the bioavailability of adefovir dipivoxil reaches approximately 59%. The drug is absorbed to an equal extent with or without the presence of food. Adefovir is excreted renally unchanged.

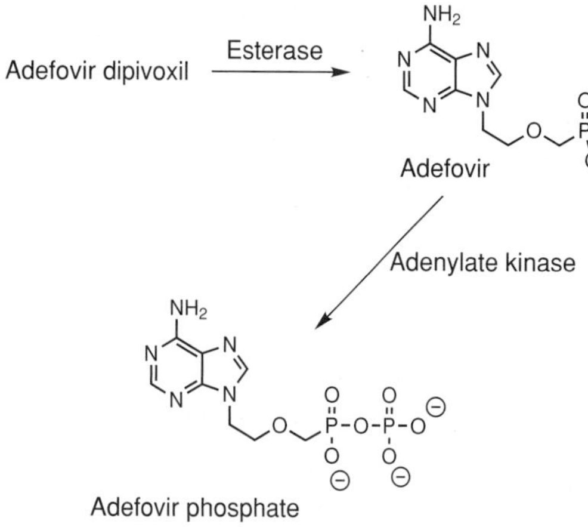

Adefovir dipivoxil — Esterase → Adefovir — Adenylate kinase → Adefovir phosphate

Fig. 43.9. Activation of the pro-drug adeflovir dipivoxyl by esterase and adenylate kinase.

Methisazone: An Agent Affecting Translation of Ribosomes

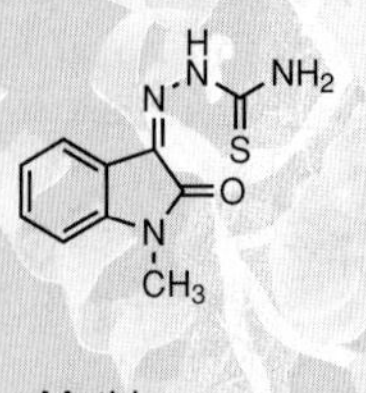

Methisazone

Historically, methisazone was one of the first antiviral compounds used in clinical practice. Methisazone (60) acts by interfering with the translation of mRNA message at the ribosome, preventing protein synthesis. Ultimately, it produced a defect in protein incorporation into the virus. Although viral DNA increases and host cells are damaged, an infectious virus is not produced. Methisazone displayed activity against poxviruses, including variola and vaccinia (61). Some RNA viruses, such as rhinoviruses, echoviruses, reoviruses, influenza, parainfluenza, and polioviruses, also were inhibited. Methisazone is not available in the United States and appears to have minimal usefulness today.

Clinical Application. Adefovir dipivoxil joins interferon and lamivudine in the treatment of chronic HBV. It can be used singly or in combination with lamivudine. Early clinical studies indicate benefit of the use of adefovir dipivoxil to treat lamivudine-resistant HBV with a low level of resistant virus developing to monotherapy with adefovir dipivoxil.

Antiretroviral (Anti-HIV) Agents Including Protease Inhibitors (62,63)

There can be no permanent cure of AIDS without the prevention or elimination of HIV infection, but patients with AIDS can prolong their life if the disease is diagnosed early and treatment is promptly initiated. Initial HIV treatment requires specific drugs that inhibit RT and HIV protease (i.e., protease inhibitors [PIs]). In advanced HIV infection, AIDS is complicated by other organisms that proliferate in immunocompromised hosts, known as opportunistic infections. Such patients are treated symptomatically with a variety of drugs depending on the opportunistic infections (64–66). Anti-HIV agents have side effects, but patients can be managed by a careful monitoring of the drugs. Opportunistic diseases include infections by parasites, bacteria, fungi, and viruses. Neoplasms, including Kaposi's sarcoma and Burkitt's lymphoma, also commonly occur.

Anti-HIV agents are classified according to the mode of action. The drugs inhibiting RT interfere with replication of HIV and stop synthesis of infective viral particles. They are further classified into nucleoside and nonnucleoside RT inhibitors. The drugs inhibiting HIV protease inactivate RT activity and block release of viral particles from the infected cells. The chemistry, pharmacokinetics, side effects, toxicity, and drug interactions of RT inhibitors and PIs are discussed below.

Nucleoside Reverse Transcriptase Inhibitors (67–69)

The synthesis of viral DNA under the direction of RT requires the availability of purines and pyrimidine nucleosides and nucleotides. Therefore, it is not surprising that a variety of chemical modifications of natural nucleosides have been investigated. Two such modifications have resulted in active drugs. Removal of the 3′-hydroxyl group of the deoxynucleosides has given rise to dideoxyadenosine (didanosine is the prodrug for this derivative) (70,71), dideoxycytodine (72–74), and didehydrodideoxythymidine (75). Replacement of the 3′-deoxy with an azido group has given 3′-azidothymidine (76–79) and 3′-azidouridine (no longer used as a drug) (80). All of these drugs have similar mechanisms of action in that their incorporation into the viral DNA will ultimately lead to chain-terminating blockade because of the lack of a 3′-hydroxyl needed for the DNA propagation.

Zidovudine

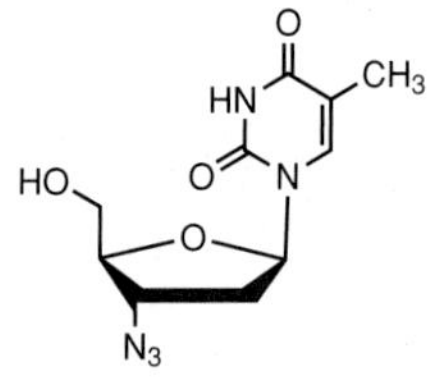

Zidovudine(AZT)

Mechanism of Action. Zidovudine (AZT, ZDV) is an analogue of thymidine in which the azido group is substituted at the 3-carbon atom of the dideoxyribose moiety. It is active against RNA tumor viruses (retroviruses) that are the causative agents of AIDS and T-cell leukemia. Retroviruses, by virtue of RT, direct the synthesis of a provirus (DNA copy of a viral RNA genome). Proviral DNA integrates into the normal cell DNA, leading to the HIV infection. Zidovudine is converted to 5′-mono-, di-, and triphosphates by the cellular thymidine kinase. These phosphates are then incorporated into proviral DNA, because RT uses ZDV-triphosphate as a substrate. This process prevents normal 5′,3′-phosphodiester bonding, resulting in termination of DNA chain elongation because of the presence of an azido group in ZDV. The multiplication of HIV is halted by selective inhibition of RT and, thus, viral DNA polymerase by ZDV-triphosphate at the required dose concentration. Zidovudine is a potent inhibitor of HIV-1, but it also inhibits HIV-2 and EBV.

Clinical Application. Zidovudine is used in AIDS and AIDS-related complex (ARC) to control opportunistic infections by raising absolute CD4 lymphocyte counts. It was first synthesized in 1964 (81), and its biological activity was reported in 1974 (82). In 1986, Yarchoan et al. (83) demonstrated application of ZDV in clinical trials of AIDS and related diseases. Zidovudine is recommended in the control of the disease in asymptomatic patients in whom absolute CD4 lymphocyte counts are less than $200/mm^3$. It prolongs the life of patients affected with

Pneumocystis carinii pneumonia and improves the condition of patients with advanced ARC by reducing the severity and frequency of opportunistic infections. Substantial benefits are obtained when the drug is given after the CD4 cell counts fall to less than 500/mm^3. Therefore, ZDV is used in early and advanced symptomatic treatment of patients with AIDS or ARC. Use with other RT inhibitors or in combination with PIs is more beneficial when resistance to ZDV occurs.

Human immunodeficiency virus attacks susceptible cells and interacts mainly with CD4 cell surface proteins of helper T cells. As discussed above, the viral glycoprotein gp120 forms a complex with CD4 receptor on host cells and enters the cells by endocytosis. The sequence of events is shown in Figure 43.2. Ultimately, the immune system of the host is altered, and symptoms of AIDS appear. Patients with AIDS have symptoms such as high fever, weight loss, lymphadenopathy, chronic diarrhea, myalgias, fatigue, and night sweats. Zidovudine is given in such conditions; however, the drug is toxic to the bone marrow and causes macrocytic anemia, neutropenia, and granulocytopenia. Other adverse reactions include headache, insomnia, nausea, vomiting, seizures, myalgias, and confusion.

Pharmacokinetics. Zidovudine is available in various dosage forms for oral or IV administration (Table 43.4). For asymptomatic adults, the initial recommended dosage is 1,200 mg daily (200 mg every 4 hours), which is reduced to 600 mg daily (100 mg every 4 hours) for patients with advanced disease. The maintenance dose is 600 mg daily in symptomatic patients. Zidovudine is sensitive to heat and light because of its azide group and should be stored in colored bottles at 15 to 25°C. It is well absorbed through the GI tract, and it concentrates in the body tissues and fluids, including the CSF. The bioavailability of the drug was found to be approximately 65%. Its half-life is approximately 1 hour. Intravenous doses of 2.5 mg/kg or oral doses of 5 mg/kg yielded peak plasma concentrations of 5 mmol/L. Plasma protein binding was approximately 30%. Most of the drug is converted to its inactive glucuronide metabolite and is excreted unchanged through urine. Additionally, ZDV crosses the blood-brain barrier. Pentamidine, dapsone, amphotericin B, flucytosine, and doxorubicin may increase the toxic effects of ZDV. Probencid prolongs the plasma half-life of the drug.

DIDANOSINE

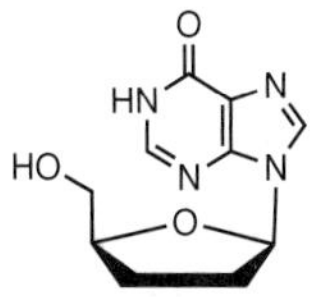

Didanosine(ddI)

Mechanism of Action. Didanosine (ddI) is a purine dideoxynucleoside, which is an analogue of inosine. Chemically, it is 2′,3′-dideoxyinosine, and it differs from inosine by having hydrogen atoms in place of the 2′- and 3′-hydroxyl groups on the ribose ring. Didanosine is a prodrug that is bioactivated by metabolism to dideoxyadenosine triphosphate, which is a competitive inhibitor of viral RT and is incorporated into the developing viral DNA in place of deoxyladenosine triphosphate. As such, this agent causes chain termination because of the absence of a 3′-hydroxyl group. Didanosine inhibits HIV RT and exerts a virustatic effect on the retroviruses. Combined with ZDV, antiretroviral activity of ddI is increased.

Pharmacokinetics. Didanosine has a plasma half-life of 1.5 hours and is given in a 200 mg dose twice daily. Oral bioavailability of the drug is approximately 25% at doses of 7 mg/kg or less. Didanosine significantly decreased p24 antigen levels and increased CD4 cell counts. Viral resistance to ddI occurred after treatment for 1 year. Didanosine is less toxic than ZDV. The CSF fluid/plasma

Table 43.4. HIV Reverse Transcriptase Inhibitors

Generic Name	Common Name	Trade Name	Dosage Form
		Nucleoside Reverse Transcriptase Inhibitors	
Zidovudine	AZT ZDV	Retrovir	Tablet (300 mg), Capsule (100 mg), syrup (50 mg/5 mL), injectable (10 mg/mL)
Didanosine	ddI	Videx	Tablet (25, 50, 100, 150, and 200 mg)
Dideoxyadenosine	ddA		Powder for oral solution (100, 167, and 250 mg)
Zalcitabine*	ddC	Hivid	Tablet (0.375 mg)
Stavudine	D4T	Zerit	Capsule (15, 20, 30, and 40 mg), powder for oral solution (1 mg/mL)
Lamivudine	3TC	Epivir	Tablet (150 mg), solution (10 mg/mL)
		Epivir HBV	Tablet (100 mg), solution (5 mg/mL)
Abacavir	ABC	Ziagen	Tablet (300 mg), solution (20 mg/mL)
Tenofovir disoproxil		Viread	Tablet (300 mg)
Emtricitabine		Emtriva	Caplet (200 mg)
		Nonnucleoside Reverse Transcriptase Inhibitors	
Nevirapine		Viramune	Tablet (200 mg)
Delavirdine	DLV	Rescriptor	Tablet (100 mg)
Efavirenz		Sustiva	Capsule (50, 100, and 200 mg)

*On December 31, 2006, Hoffmann-La Roche halted the sale and distribution of Hivid (zalcitabine) due to widespread availability of other more useful drugs to treat HIV infection.

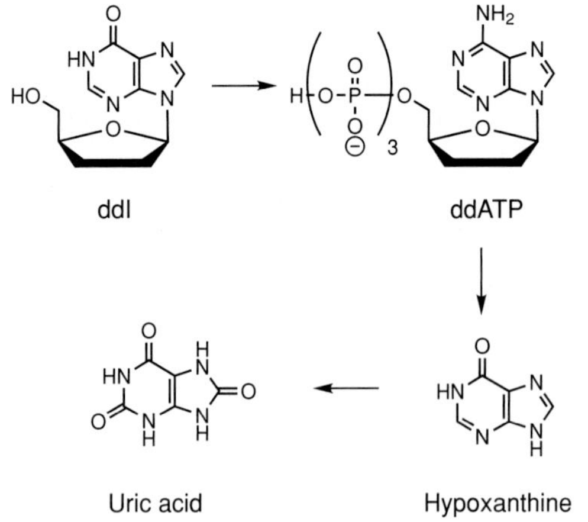

Fig. 43.10. Metabolism of didanosine.

ratio of ddI is 0.2. Didanosine is ultimately converted to hypoxanthine, xanthine, and uric acid through the usual metabolic pathway for purines (Fig. 43.10). The latter is a nontoxic metabolic product.

Didanosine is given in advanced HIV infection, ZDV intolerance, or significant clinical/immunologic deterioration. The major side effects of ddI are painful peripheral neuropathy and pancreatitis. Some of the minor side effects include abdominal pain, nausea, and vomiting. The use of products, such as pentamidine, sulfonamides, and cimetidine, should be avoided with ddI. The combination of ddI with ZDV is beneficial, however, because these drugs have different toxicity profile.

ZALCITABINE, LAMIVUDINE, AND EMTRICITABINE. These three synthetic pyrimidine nucleoside analogues are quite similar in structure and in mechanism of action (Fig. 43.11). The three compounds differ from 2′-deoxycytidine in that the 3′-hydroxymethylene group of 2′-deoxyriboribose moiety is replaced with either a methylene or a sulfur atom. Additionally, in the case of emtricitabine, the C_5 hydrogen is replaced with a fluoro atom. In all three cases, these drugs act as pro-drugs and must first be phosphorylated to the respective 5′-triphosphates derivatives, which are the active forms. The resulting triphosphates compete with the normal substrate (deoxycytidine-5′-triphosphate) for incorporation into the viral DNA by inhibiting HIV RT, which ultimately leads to termination of viral DNA elongation.

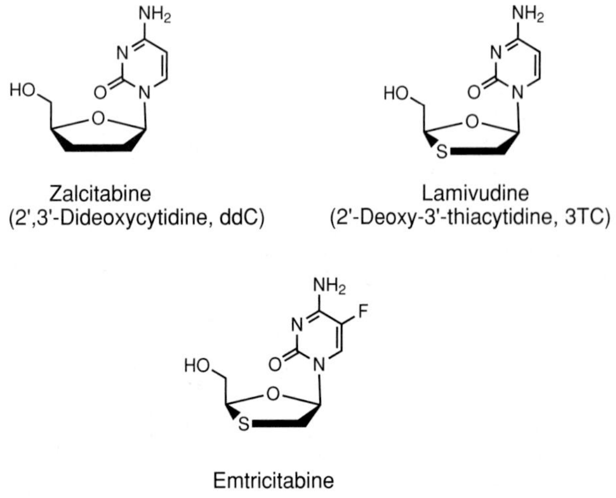

Fig. 43.11. Deoxycytidine analogues as nucleoside reverse transcriptase inhibitors.

Zalcitabine. Zalcitabine (ddC) (Table 43.4) was originally introduced as a useful alternate drug to ZDV when given in combination with ZDV when CD4 cell counts fall to less than 300 cells/mm^3. Monotherapy with ddC is more active than ZDV. Oral bioavailability is 87%, and plasma half-life is approximately 1 hour. It has various side effects, with peripheral neuropathy proving quite troublesome. In low doses (0.005 mg/kg every 4 hours), ddC produces sustained decrease in p24 antigen level and increase in CD4 cell counts. The CSF fluid/plasma ratio of ddC is 0.2.

Following oral administration, bioavailability of ddC is less than 80%, which is further reduced when taken with food. The mean maximum plasma concentration of the drug also is reduced from 25.2 to 15.5 ng/mL when the drug was taken with food. Dideoxyuridine is the major metabolite in urine and feces. The drug penetrates the blood-brain barrier. On December 31, 2006, Hoffmann-La Roche halted the sale and distribution of Hivid (zalcitabine) due to the widespread availability of other more useful drugs to treat HIV infection.

Lamivudine (84). Lamivudine (3TC) (Fig. 43.11) usually is given with other antiretroviral agents, such as ZDV or D4T. 3TC at a dose of 600 mg/day reduced HIV cells by 75%, and in combination with ZDV, the reduction in viral load was 94%. 3TC is rapidly absorbed through the GI tract. Its bioavailability is approximately 86% after oral administration of 2 mg/kg twice daily; peak serum 3TC concentration is approximately 2 mg/mL. 3TC binding to human plasma is approximately 36%. In vivo, it is converted to the *trans* sulfoxide metabolite, although a majority of the drug is eliminated unchanged in urine.

The U.S. FDA approved 3TC in combination with ZDV for the treatment of disease progression caused by HIV infection. The combinations of 3TC with ddI, ddC, or D4T also are used for advanced HIV infection. Such combinations have the ability to delay resistance to ZDV and restore ZDV sensitivity in patients with AIDS. Recently, oral therapy with lower doses of 3TC (Table 43.4) has been approved by the U.S. FDA for the treatment of chronic hepatitis B. Peripheral neuropathy and GI disturbances are the major side effects of 3TC. The minor side effects are nausea, vomiting, and diarrhea.

Emtricitabine (85). Emtricitabine (Fig. 43.11) is an orally active nucleoside RT inhibitor that is administered once daily. The (−)-enantiomer is the most active form of the drug, although the (+)-isomer also is active. The drug is not bound to plasma protein, and approximately 86% is excreted unchanged in the urine. The only metabolites identified consist of the 3′-sulfoxide and the 2′-O-glucuronide. Emtricitabine is reported to be more active than lamivudine, with a low level of resistance developing when used in combination therapy with efavirenz and didanosine.

STAVUDINE

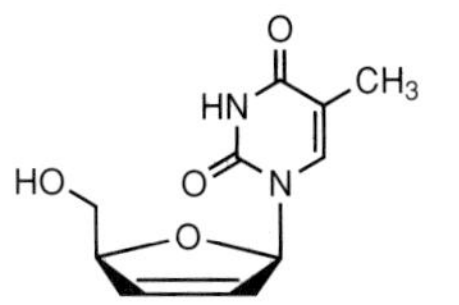

Stavudine
(2',3'-Dideoxy-2',3'-didehydrothymidine, D4T)

Stavudine (D4T) is a pyrimidine nucleoside analogue that has significant activity against HIV-1 after intracellular conversion of the drug to a D4T-triphosphate. It differs in structure from thymidine by the replacement of the 3′-hydroxyl group with a hydrogen atom and a double bond in the 2′,3′-positions on the deoxyribose ring. It decreases p24 antigen and raised CD4 cell counts. D4T is beneficial for patients where CD4 cell counts do not decrease to less than 300 cells/mm^3 with ZDV and ddI. It is more effective than ZDV or ddC in treating patients by delaying the progression of HIV infection. It is recommended for patients with advanced HIV infection.

Pharmacokinetics. D4T is rapidly absorbed, and absolute bioavailability in adults is 85% at an oral dose of 4 mg/kg (Table 43.4). A peak plasma concentration occurs in dose-dependent manner within 1 hour. It can be taken with food. The apparent volume distribution after oral dose is 66 L. The plasma half-life of D4T is approximately 1.5 hours, and the intracellular half-life of D4T-triphosphate is 3.5 hours. It is less toxic to bone marrow but causes peripheral neuropathic toxicity. The side effects include pain, tingling, and numbness in the hands and feet.

ABACAVIR.

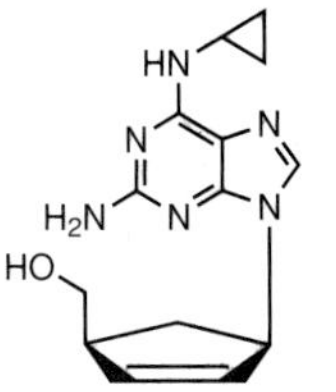

Abacavir (ABC)

Abacavir sulfate (ABC) was approved in 1998 as a nucleoside RT inhibitor to be used in combination with other drugs for the treatment of HIV and AIDS. The drug is extensively metabolized via stepwise phosphorylation to 5′-mono-, di-, and triphosphate. Abacavir is well absorbed (>75%) and penetrates the CNS. The drug can be taken without regard to meals. The drug does not show any clinically significant drug–drug interactions. Abacavir has been reported to produce life-threatening hypersensitivity reactions. The major use of abacavir appears to be in combination with other nucleoside RT inhibitors. A fixed-combination product has recently been approved by the U.S. FDA consisting of 300 mg of ABC, 150 mg of 3TC, and 300 mg of ZDV (Trizivar). The combination has been shown to be superior to other combinations in reducing viral load as well as to show improvement in CD4 cell count. The most common adverse effects reported with abacavir include headache, nausea, vomiting, malaise, and diarrhea.

TENOFOVIR DISOPROXIL (86)

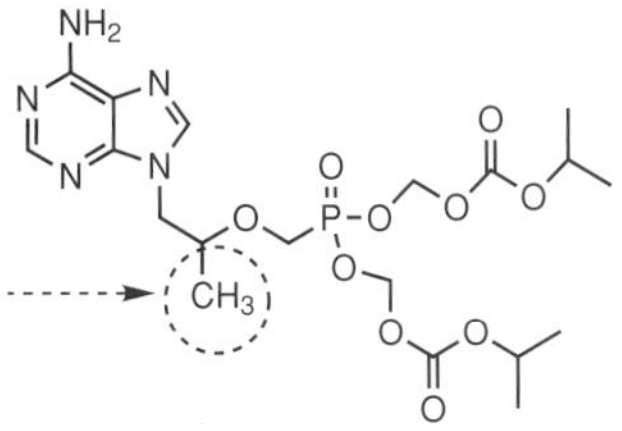

Tenofovir disoproxil

Tenofovir disoproxil is a prodrug in a manner similar to that of adefovir dipivoxil. In both cases, the phosphate esters are removed through the action of plasma esterase, leading in this case to tenofovir, which differs from adefovir by the presence of the indicated methyl group (Fig. 43.9). Tenofovir disoproxil exhibits good bioavailability (25%), which is improved in the presence of food (35%). The drug is approved for the treatment of HIV infections in adult patients. Tenofovir diphosphate is an HIV RT inhibitor. The active form of tenofovir is the tenofovir diphosphate, which competes with dATP for incorporation into viral DNA, and when incorporated, tenofovir diphosphate results in premature termination of DNA growth and inhibition of DNA polymerase. Tenofovir disoproxil is indicated for treatment-experienced patients with HIV-1. The drug also appears to be effective in treatment-naive patients, but initial approval is for treatment-experienced patients. The drug is administered as one tablet taken once daily (Table 43.4). It is recommended that the drug be combined with other RT inhibitors or HIV PIs, which results in additive or synergistic activity.

Nonnucleoside RT Inhibitors

The U.S. FDA recently approved several nonnucleosides that inhibit RT activity. They are used with nucleoside drugs to obtain synergistic activity in decreasing the viral load and increasing the CD4 cell count. These drugs are primarily designed and synthesized by protein structure–based drug design methodologies. Their use as monotherapy may be limited because of rapid onset of resistance and hypersensitivity reactions. Interaction of nonnucleoside drugs, however, with other PIs, such as saquinavir, indinavir, and ritonavir, is being investigated. Also, interaction of these drugs with clarithromycin, ketoconazole, rifabutin, and rifampin are currently being studied. Nonnucleosides that inhibit RT activity are discussed below.

NEVIRAPINE

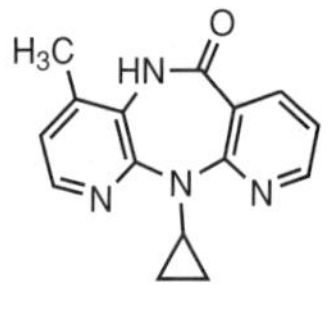

Nevirapine

Nevirapine and its analogues exhibit antiretroviral effect against azothymidine-resistant HIV strains (87). Nevirapine in combination with ZDV and ddI produced approximately 18% higher CD4 cell counts and a decrease in viral load compared with patients who took ZDV and ddI. Nevirapine is recommended with nucleosides for patients infected with HIV-1 who have experienced clinical or immunologic deterioration. The significant side effects of nevirapine are liver dysfunction and skin rashes.

Mechanism of Action. Nevirapine is a dipyridodiazepinone derivative that binds directly to RT. Thus, it blocks RNA- and DNA-dependent polymerase activities by causing a disruption of the enzyme's catalytic site. The activity of nevirapine does not compete with template or nucleoside triphosphate. The HIV-2 RT and human DNA polymerases are not inhibited by nevirapine. The 50% inhibitory concentration ranged within 10 to 100 nM against HIV-1.

Pharmacokinetics. Nevirapine is rapidly absorbed after oral administration, and its bioavailability is approximately 95%. Peak plasma nevirapine concentrations of 2 ± 0.4 mg/mL (7.5 mM) are obtained in 4 hours following a single 200 mg dose (Table 43.4). Following multiple doses, nevirapine concentrations appear to increase linearly in the dose range of 200 to 400 mg/day. Nevirapine is approximately 60% bound to plasma proteins in the plasma concentration range of 1 to 10 mg/mL. It readily crosses the placenta and is found in breast milk. Nevirapine is metabolized as glucuronide conjugates of hydroxylated metabolites, which are excreted in urine. In vivo, ketoconazole did not produce any significant inhibitory effect on nevirapine metabolism. The plasma concentrations of nevirapine were elevated or reduced in patients receiving cimetidine or rifabutin, respectively.

DELAVIRDINE

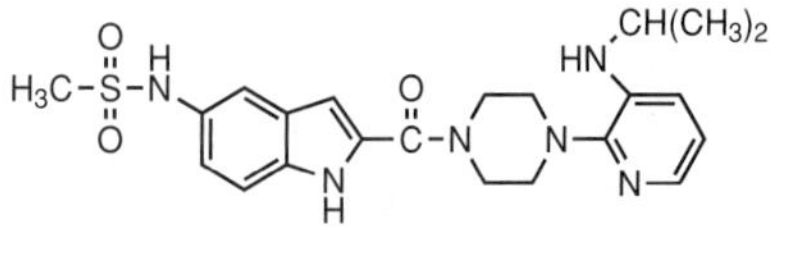

Delavirdine

Delavirdine, a bisheteroarylpiperazine derivative, is a potent nonnucleoside RT inhibitor of activity specific for HIV-1 (88). The U.S. FDA has approved this drug for use in combination with other anti-HIV agents (Table 43.4). In Phase I/II study trials, it demonstrated sustained improvements in CD4 cell counts, p24 antigen levels, and RNA viral load. Promising results were obtained when the drug was used in two- or three-drug combinations with nucleoside drugs. Combination of delavirdine with ddI, ddC, or ZDV demonstrated additive or synergistic effects. Delavirdine with ZDV, however, was more beneficial in early HIV infection. Combinations of nevirapine and delavirdine had an antagonistic effect on HIV-1 RT inhibition.

Mechanism of Action. Delavirdine directly inhibits RT and DNA-directed DNA polymerase activities of HIV-1 after the formation of the enzyme–substrate complexes, thereby causing chain-termination effects.

Pharmacokinetics. Delaviradine is rapidly absorbed by oral administration and peak plasma concentration was obtained in 1 hour. Administration of delaviridine at 400 mg three times daily resulted in peak plasma concentration of 45 mM. The single dose bioavailability of delaviridine tablets relative to oral solution was approximate 85%. The 50% inhibitory concentration for delavirdine against RT activity was 6.0 nM. Delaviridine is extensively bound to plasma protein (~98%). It is metabolized to its N-desisopropyl metabolite in liver, and the pharmacokinetics is nonlinear. Clarithromycin, rifabutin, or ergot alkaloid derivatives are predicted to increase plasma concentration of delaviridine. Skin rashes are the major side effect of delavirdine therapy. Cross-resistance between delavidine and PIs, such as indinavir, nelfinavir, ritonavir, and saquinavir, is unlikely because of action on different enzyme targets.

EFAVIRENZ

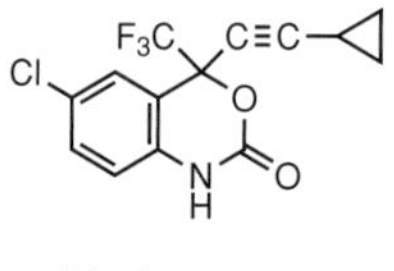

Efavirenz

Efavirenz is a nonnucleoside RT inhibitor that is a potent inhibitor of wild-type as well as resistant mutant HIV-1 (89). Inhibition of up to 95% is reported for efavirenz at concentrations of 1.5 mM. In combination with indinavir, a mean reduction in HIV RNA of 1.68 log and an increase in CD4 cell counts of 96 cells/mm^3 have been reported. Coadministration of efavirenz with indinavir reduced the indinavir concentration (AUC) by approximately 35%.

Efavirenz is administered once a day and can be used as a substitute for indinavir in combination therapy with standard drugs, such as ZDV and 3TC. Because it is given once a day, it cuts down the number of pills that a patient with AIDS must swallow. In the current cocktail therapy used for patients with AIDS, efavirenz is a good option to reduce the many side effects of cocktail therapy. It is administered to both adults and children and may be less expensive than indinavir.

The side effects of efavirenz include dizziness, insomnia, impaired concentration, abnormal dreams, and drowsiness. The most common adverse effect is a skin rash. Other side effects are diarrhea, headache, and dizziness. Efavirenz is recommended to be taken at bedtime with or without food. Patients on efavirenz should avoid driving or operating machinery and the intake of high fat meals. It should always be taken in combination with at least one other anti-HIV agent. Efavirenz is contraindicated with midazolam, triazolam, or ergot derivatives.

HIV Protease Inhibitors (Table 43.5) (90)

The HIV protease is an enzyme that is essential for viral growth and that mediates the posttranslational modification of core proteins into structural proteins. The structural proteins p7, p9, p17, and p24, which play important roles in infectivity of HIV, are products of a *pol* gene. The HIV genome contains various regions designated as genes, such as the *gag* and *gag-pol* genes, that are translated as polyproteins and form immature viral particles. These precursor protein molecules are cleaved by a viral *pol*-encoded aspartic proteinase to form the desired structural proteins of the mature viral particle. The HIV protease also activates RT and plays an important role in the release of infectious viral particles. Thus, an area of considerable interest has been the development of drugs that act as inhibitors of protease and *pol* gene. Such inhibitors act on HIV protease and prevent posttranslational processing and budding of immature viral particles from the infected cells. This group of drugs represents a major breakthrough in the treatment of HIV when used in combination with RT inhibitors, and their development is one of the most significant advances in medicinal chemistry.

MECHANISM OF ACTION. The HIV protease exists as a dimer in which each monomer contains one of two conserved aspartate residues at the active site. Drugs that inhibit HIV protease are designed as transition-state mimetics that align at the active site of HIV-1 protease, as defined by three-dimensional crystallographic analysis of the protein structure. A number of oligopeptide-like analogues have been synthesized that differentially inhibit viral and mammalian aspartic proteases, and the most useful of these are selective for the viral enzyme HIV-1 protease. Structurally, these agents are either peptidomimetic and nonpeptide compounds. Their effectiveness is related to their ability to inhibit the *gag-pol* gene, which processes p24, p55, and p160. Consequently, the infectivity of HIV-1 is diminished.

Although some compounds exhibit both in vitro and in vivo antiviral activities, optimization of their pharmacokinetic and pharmacodynamic properties has presented major problems. In view of the great demand for successful anti-AIDS drugs, the U.S. FDA has approved nine drugs as PIs under the accelerated approval process.

METABOLISM. The PIs have a high potential for drug interactions, stemming from the fact that they are substrates for and inhibitors of the CYP3A4 enzyme system. As a result, concurrent use of PIs with other drugs metabolized by CYP3A4 may be contraindicated, and in some cases, the drug interactions can be life-threatening. The most potent cytochrome P450 (CYP450) inhibitor in this class is ritonavir (used to advantage in combination with lopinavir); followed by indinavir, nelfinavir, and amprenavir as moderate inhibitors; and by saquinavir as the least potent inhibitor. Drug interactions have been reported with bepridil, dihydroergotamine, and a number of benzodiazepines. Marked increase in activity of amiodarone, lidocaine (systemic), quinidine, the tricyclic antidepressants, and warfarin might be expected. Other interactions have been reported to include rifampin, rifabutin phenobarbital, phenytoin, dexamethasone, or carbazepine. Because the PIs are themselves metabolized by CYP450, their action may be altered by other agents that induce or inhibit this system. In the case of rifabutin, which inhibits CYP3A4 in the gut, relative bioavailability of the PIs is increased, and the dose of the PIs may need to be decreased.

RESISTANCE. Resistance to the transition-state peptidomimetic PIs has already become problematic. Resistance is associated with point mutations among various amino acids within the peptide chain of the HIV protease. Single-amino-acid mutations reduce the activity of

Table 43.5. HIV Protease Inhibitors

Generic Name	Common Name	Trade Name	Dosage Form(mg/unit)
Saquinavir		Invirase	Capsule (200 mg)
		Fortovase	Capsule (200 mg)
Ritonavir	RTV	Norvir	Capsule (200 mg)
Indinavir	IDV	Crixivan	Capsule (200 and 400 mg)
Nelfinavir	NFV	Viracept	Tablet (250 mg), powder (50 mg/g)
Amprenavir	APV	Agenerase	Capsule (50 and 150 mg), solution (15 mg/mL)
Lopinavir/ritonavir	LPV/r	Kaletra	Capsule (133.3/33.3 mg), solution (80/20 mg/mL)
Atazanavir	ATZ	Reyataz	Capsule (150 and 200 mg)
Fosamprenavir	Fos-APV	Lexiva	Tablet (700 mg)
Tipranavir	TPV	Aptivus	Capsule (250 mg)

the PIs, but total resistance appears to require multiple mutations. The most susceptible mutations consist of Leu[33] to Ile, Val, or Phe; Val[82] to Ala, Phe, Leu, or Thr; Ile[84] to Val; and Leu[90] to Met. These changes are referred to a PI resistance–associated mutations. The presence of one or two such mutations leads to reduced susceptibility, whereas five or more mutations can lead to resistance.

SPECIFIC DRUGS

Saquinavir

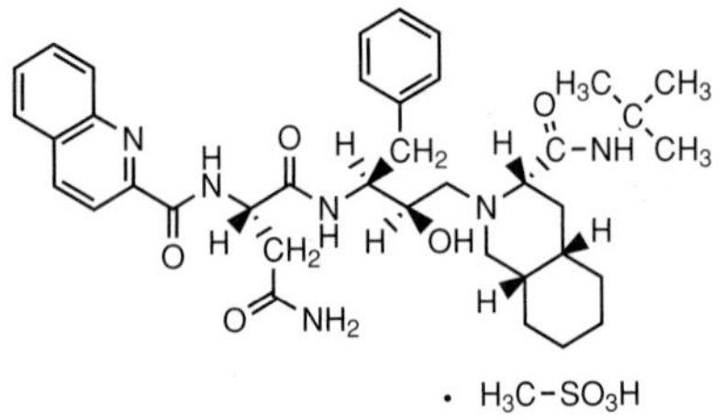

· H_3C-SO_3H

Saquinavir

Saquinavir

M-7

M-2, M-3

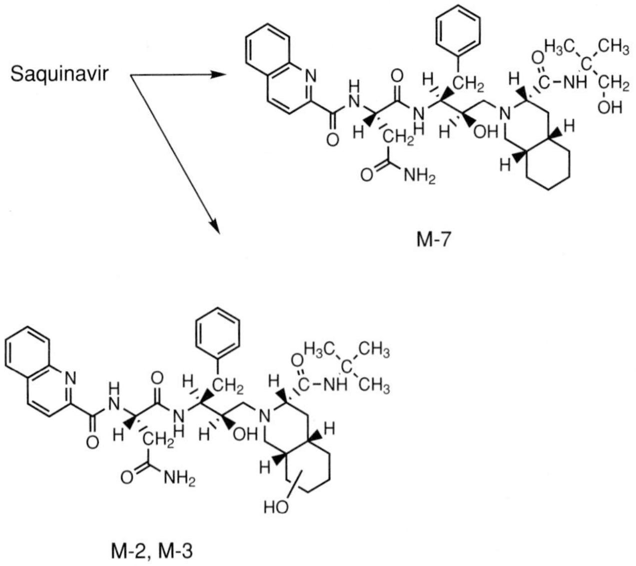

Fig. 43.12. Major metabolic products from saquinavir.

Saquinavir mesylate was the first PI approved by the U.S. FDA in December 1995 (91,92). It is a carboxamide derivative that is specifically designed to inhibit HIV protease, thus preventing posttranslational formation of viral proteins. It contains a hydroxyethylamine moiety rather than the Phe-Pro scissile bond present in the normal substrate for HIV protease.

Clinical Application. Saquinavir is used in the treatment of advanced HIV infection in selected patients. Saquinavir is used concomitantly with either ZDV in untreated patients or ddC in patients previously treated with prolonged ZDV therapy. Although combined therapy did not slow progression of disease, CD4 cell counts were increased in patients infected with HIV in the United States and European countries. Triple therapy with saquinavir, ZDV, and ddC has been more effective than double therapy with saquinavir plus ZDV or ddC. Thus, combination therapy slowed disease progression and mortality.

The IC50 concentration of saquinavir in both acutely and chronically infected cells was 1 to 30 nM. In combination with ZDV, ddC, or ddI, the activity of saquinavir was increased without increased cytotoxicity. The resistance of HIV isolates to saquinavir was observed as a result of substitution mutations in the HIV protease at amino acid positions 48 (glycine to valine) and 90 (leucine to methionine).

Pharmacokinetics. The bioavailability of saquinavir in a single, 600 mg dose following a high-fat meal was shown to be approximately 4%. Approximately 30% of a 600 mg dose of saquinavir reached the liver, where it showed first-pass metabolism. The poor bioavailability is associated with intestinal metabolism catalyzed by CYP3A4 and, possibly, CYP3A5. Additionally, P-glycoprotein found in intestinal epithelial cells acts as an efflux pump interfering with saquinavir absorption. The metabolites, mono- and dihydroxylated compounds (Fig. 43.12), are not active (93). Approximately 88 and 19% of a 600 mg oral dose was found in the feces and urine, respectively. The volume distribution following IV administration of a 12 mg dose of saquinavir was 700 L. The drug is 98% bound to plasma proteins, and a very low concentration of saquinavir was found in the CSF. As compared to multiple dosing, the steady-state AUC was 2.5-fold higher than that observed after a single dose of 600 mg in HIV-infected patients after a meal. Saquinavir has a plasma half-life of approximately 1.8 hours. Although the saquinavir hard-gel capsule used in combination with other antiretroviral drugs reduces the risk of disease progression or death, it has limited bioavailability. To overcome this limitation, the U.S. FDA has approved saquinavir soft-gel capsules. Saquinavir is well tolerated in combination with ZDV and/or ddC, and it has few side effects. Gastrointestinal disturbances, however, have been common adverse effects. Saquinavir also has a few mild side effects, such as headache, rhinitis, nausea, and diarrhea.

Ritonavir

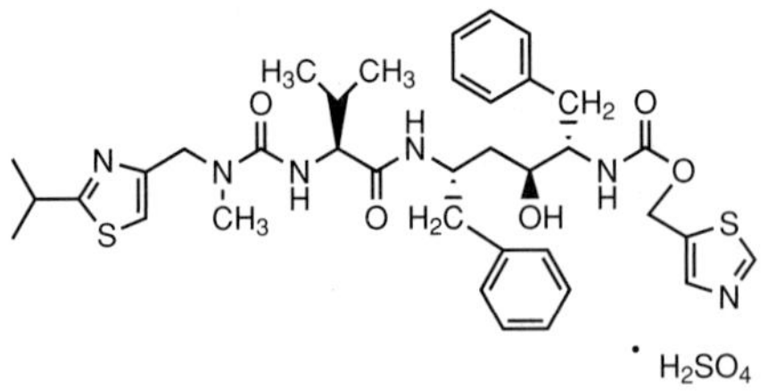

· H_2SO_4

Ritonavir

Ritonavir is another HIV PI and was approved by the U.S. FDA in March 1996 (94). Ritonavir is a peptidomimetic inhibitor of both the HIV-1 and HIV-2 proteases. A 50% reduction in viral replication was obtained at 3.8 to 153 nM of ritonavir.

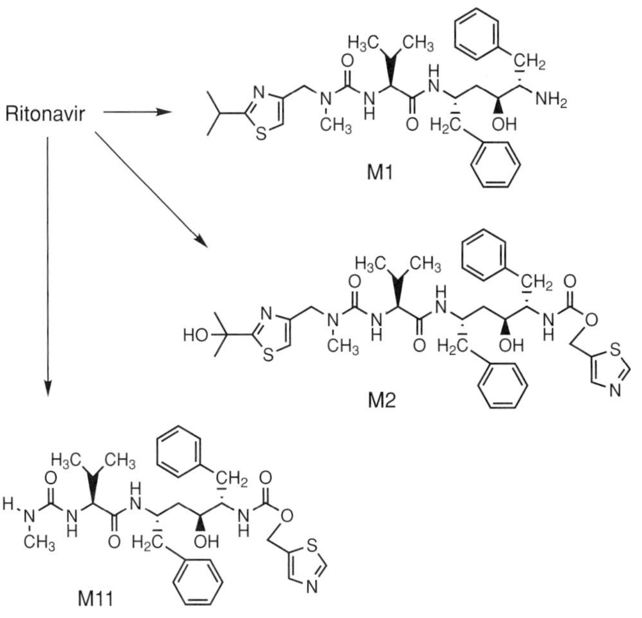

Fig. 43.13. Major metabolic products from CYP3A4 metabolism of ritonavir.

Pharmacokinetics. After a 600 mg dose of an oral solution, peak concentrations of ritonavir were obtained in approximately 2 or 4 hours under fasting or nonfasting conditions, respectively. Under nonfasting conditions, peak ritonavir concentrations decreased 23%, and the extent of absorption decreased 7% relative to fasting conditions. In two separate studies, the capsule and oral solution indicated AUC values of 129.5 ± 47.1 and 129.0 ± 39.3 mg/h/mL, respectively, when a 600 mg dose was given under nonfasting conditions. Five ritonavir metabolites have been isolated from human urine and feces, the most significant of which are shown in Figure 43.13 (95). The isopropylthiazole oxidation product was the major active metabolite (M2).

As with saquinavir, ritonavir is metabolized by CYP3A4 and is an inhibitor of the CYP450 system. Ritonavir is contraindicated with various compounds, such as astemizole, cisapride, clarithromycin, desipramine, ethinyl estradiol, rifabutin, several of the statins, sulfamethoxazole, and trimethoprim, because of increased concentrations of these drugs in the plasma as a result of inhibited oxidative metabolism as well as the fact that several of these drugs are CYP450 inducers. Ritonavir is the most potent PI in its ability to inhibit CYP450 and the efflux pump P-glycoprotein; as a result, the potential for severe drug interactions is quite great. Ritonavir alone or in combination with 3TC, ZDV, saquinavir, or ddC increased CD4 cell counts and decreased HIV RNA particle levels. Cross-resistance between ritonavir and RT inhibitors is unlikely because of the different mode of action and enzyme involved. Common adverse reactions, such as nausea, diarrhea, vomiting, anorexia, abdominal pain, and neurologic disturbances, have been reported with the use of ritonavir alone or in combination with other nucleoside analogues. Ritonavir is used for the treatment of advanced HIV infection, including opportunistic infections. In combination with nucleoside drugs, ritonavir has reduced the risk of mortality and clinical progression.

Because of the strong CYP450-inhibiting effects of ritonavir, the drug has found value when used in fixed-dosage combinations with other PIs to block their metabolism and act as a booster for these drugs (lopinavir/ritonavir and tipranavir/ritonavir). In these cases, ritonavir is used in a subtherapeutic dose but boosts the effectiveness of the coadministered drug. The utilization of ritonavir in a therapeutic dose for treating HIV infections appears to be decreasing, but its utilization as a booster drug is finding favor.

Indinavir

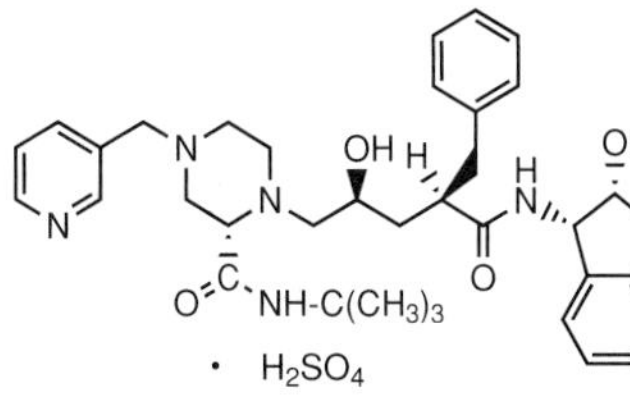

Indinavir

Indinavir sulfate, a pentanoic acid amide derivative, was approved by the U.S. FDA in March 1996 (96). The 95% inhibitory concentration against laboratory-adapted HIV variants, primary clinical isolates and clinically resistant virus to indinavir analogues, is 25 to 100 nM in drug combination studies with ZDV and ddI. In some patients, however, HIV has shown resistance to ritonavir. This resistance is caused by mutation of the virus that is correlated with the expression of amino acid substitutions in the viral protease. Cross-resistance to indinavir is observed with other PIs but not with the RT inhibitor. For this reason, indinavir is beneficial with ZDV and other nucleoside drugs.

Pharmacokinetics. Indinavir is rapidly absorbed in fasting patients, and plasma peak concentration is observed in approximately 1 hour. At a dose of 800 mg every 8 hours, peak plasma concentration is approximately 300 nM. The drug is approximately 60% bound to human plasma proteins. Indinavir is metabolized via oxidation and glucuronide conjugation (M1 in Fig. 43.14). At least seven metabolites have been identified, with the conjugate being the major metabolite (97). These metabolites were recovered in feces and urine, with approximately 20% of the drug excreted in the urine. The half-life of indinavir is approximately 1.8 hours.

Because of indinavir's metabolism, a number of drug interactions are possible. Indinavir interacts with rifabutin or ketoconazole, leading to increased or decreased indinavir concentration, respectively, in the blood plasma. Administration of drug combinations of indinavir with antiviral nucleoside analogues, cimetidine, quinidine, trimethoprim/sulfamethoxazole, fluconazole, or isoniazid resulted in an increased activity of indinavir. Indinavir is

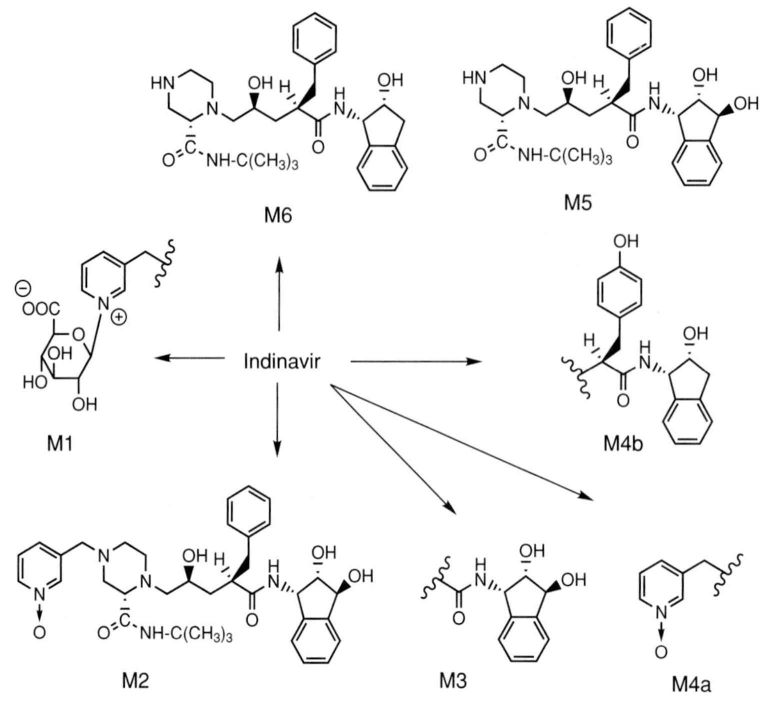

Fig. 43.14. Metabolic products formed from indinavir.

contraindicated in patients taking triazolam or midazolam, because the inhibition of metabolism of these drugs may result in prolonged sedation, nephrolithiasis, asymptomatic hyperbilirubinemia and GI problems (anorexia, constipation, dyspepsia, and gastritis). The usual oral dose for indinavir alone or in combination with other antiviral agents is one 800 mg capsule every 8 hours. The drug is well absorbed if given on an empty stomach or 1 hour before or 2 hours after a light meal with water. The dose is reduced to 600 mg every 8 hours if given concurrently with ketoconazole. Indinavir activity is increased when combined with RT inhibitors.

Nelfinavir

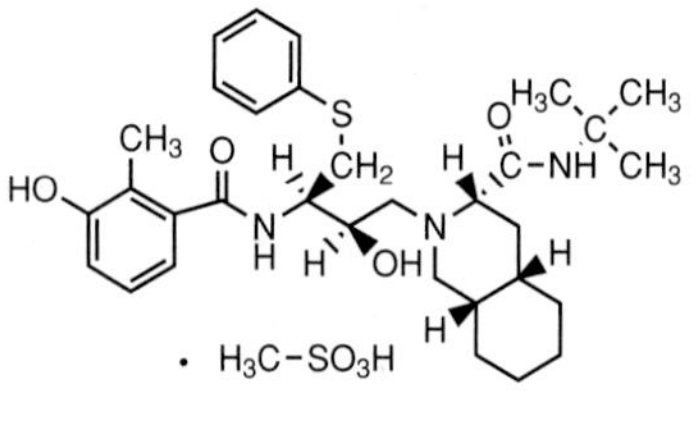

Nelfinavir

Nelfinavir mesylate is a peptidomimetic drug that is effective in HIV-1 and HIV-2 wild-type and ZDV-resistant strains, with median effective dose concentrations ranging from 9 to 60 nM (95% effective dose, 0.04 mg/mL) (98). After IV administration, the elimination half-life of nelfinavir was approximately 1 hour. In combination with D4T, nelfinavir reduced HIV viral load by approximately 98% after 4 weeks. It is well tolerated when used with azole antifungals (ketoconazole, fluconazole, or itraconazole) or macrolide antibiotics (erythromycin, clarithromycin, or azithromycin); however, it causes diarrhea and other side effects common to nonnucleoside drugs. Following oral administration, nelfinavir peak levels in plasma ranged from 0.34 mg/mL (10 mg/kg in the dog) to 1.7 mg/mL (50 mg/kg in the rat). In the dog, nelfinavir was slowly absorbed, and bioavailability was 47%. The drug appeared to be metabolized in the liver, and the major excretory route was in feces.

Amprenavir

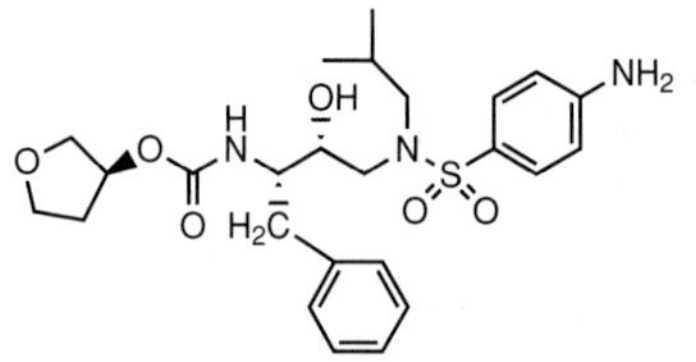

Amprenavir

Amprenavir is the fifth in a series of PIs to be approved for marketing in the United States. Although it is structurally unique from the previous agents, its pharmacological profile does not appear to differ significantly from those of the previously marketed agents. Early studies suggest that a different resistance profile may exist and that the drug may be effective against some resistant strains of HIV. Side effects appear to be more common than with other PIs and include nausea, vomiting, paresthesia, depression, and rash. Because amprenavir is a sulfonamide, there is some concern regarding cross-sensitivity with antibacterial sulfonamides. This has not been reported, but care should be taken if sensitivity to trimethoprim/sulfamethoxazole, used in *Pneumocystis carinii* pneumonia, is reported.

Amprenavir is rapidly absorbed following oral administration and may be taken with or without food. High-fat meals decrease the absorption of the drug and, therefore, should be avoided. The product is available in capsule and liquid form. The recommended adult and adolescent dose of 1,200 mg twice daily requires the patient to take eight capsules (150 mg each) twice daily. The liquid preparation is recommended for children between 4 and 12 years of age or for patients 13 to 16 years of age who weigh less than 50 kg. The dose is 22.5 mg/kg twice daily or 17 mg/kg three times a day. Because this preparation contains the excipient propylene glycol, it is not recommended for children less than 4 years of age and certain other individuals who are unable to metabolize this alcohol.

Lopinavir/Ritonavir

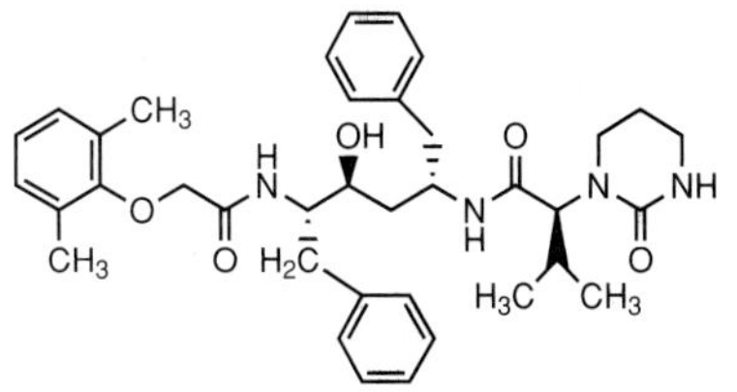

Lopinavir

Recently, the U.S. FDA has approved the release of lopinavir/ritonavir combination in patients who have not responded to other regimens for treatment of HIV. The product is available in a soft-gelatin capsule containing 133.3 mg of lopinavir and 33.3 mg of ritonavir as well as in oral solutions containing 80 mg/mL of lopinavir and 20 mg/mL of ritonavir. The small amount of ritonavir is not expected to have antiretroviral activity; rather, the ritonavir is meant to increase the plasma concentrations of lopinavir by inhibiting lopinavir's metabolism by CYP3A4 (ritonavir acts as a booster). These drugs, in combination with other antiretroviral agents, have been approved for use in adults as well as in patients between the ages of 6 months and 12 years. This is the first PI to be indicated for the very young.

Atazanavir (99)

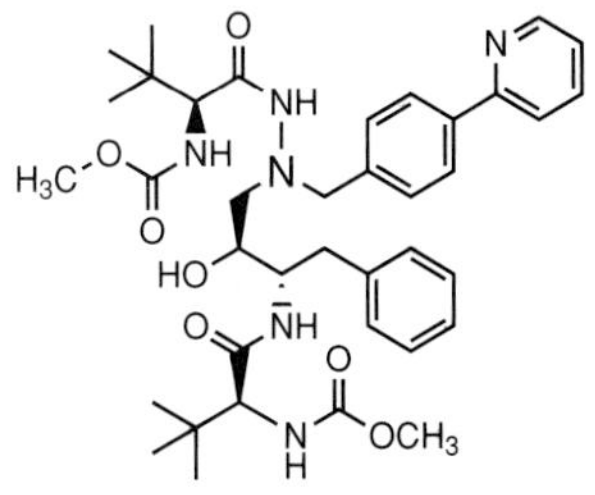

Atazanavir

Atazanavir is an antiretroviral agent approved for use in combination with other antiretroviral agents for the treatment of HIV infections. Atazanavir is a peptidomimetic transition-state inhibitor that targets HIV-1 protease and reduces the viral replication and, thus, the virulence of HIV-1. Similar to saquinavir, ritonavir, indinavir, nelfinavir, amprenavir, and lopinavir, the drug is used in combination with RT inhibitors to produce excellent efficacy in patients with AIDS.

Pharmacokinetics. Atazanavir is dosed orally once daily, thus reducing "pill burden," and it appears to have minimal impact on lipid parameters but does increase total bilirubin. The drug is well absorbed when administered orally with food (bioavailability, ~68%). The drug is highly bound to plasma protein (86%) and is metabolized by CYP3A isoenzyme. Atazanavir is a moderate inhibitor of CYP3A, and potential drug–drug interactions are possible with CYP3A inhibitors and inducers.

Fosamprenavir (100)

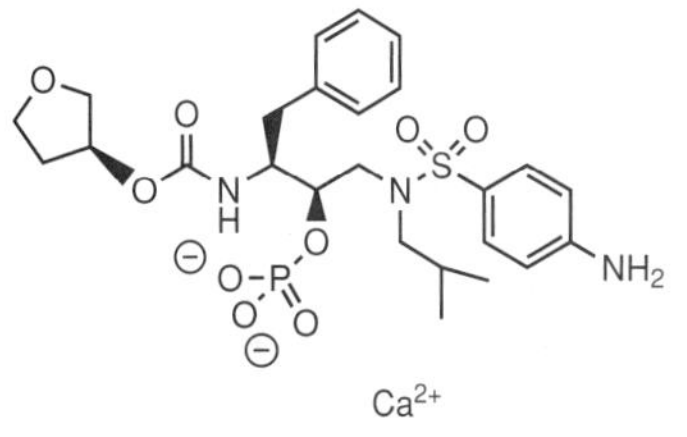

Fosamprenavir calcium

Fosamprenavir calcium has been approved for the treatment of HIV in adults when used in combination with other anti-HIV drugs. It is a prodrug that, on hydrolysis by serum phosphatases, gives rise to amprenavir, which is a peptidomimetic transition-state inhibitor that targets HIV-1 protease and reduces the viral replication and, thus, the infectiousness of HIV-1. It is commonly administered in combination with RT inhibitors to produce excellent efficacy in patients with AIDS. The drug is administered as two 700 mg tablets twice daily or, in combination with ritonavir, can be given as two 700 mg tables once daily or one 700 mg tablet twice daily. As a result, formaprenavir lowers the "pill burden" in patients with AIDS.

Tipranavir (101–104)

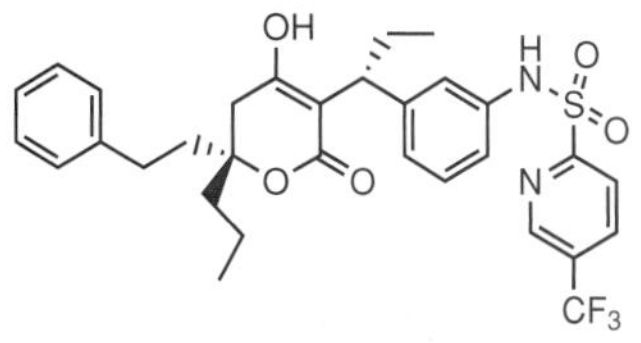

Tipranavir

Tipranavir was released as a nonpeptide PI in June 2005 for the treatment of HIV in adults. The drug was derived through a structure-based design and differs significantly from the design of the previously discussed transition-state peptidomimetics. Tipranavir appears to be bound to the same active site of HIV-1 protease as the peptidomimetics are, but because of its different chemical structure, cross-resistance is significantly less than that seen between the peptidomimetics. The drug suppresses viral replication in various strains of HIV-1 in vitro, and when combined with azothymidine or delaviridine, synergistic activity is noted in vitro. Tipranavir has an advantage over the other PIs in that it is not as strongly bound to plasma protein as the earlier PIs are, a property that reduces the 90% inhibition concentration.

Tipranavir is administered with a booster dose of ritonavir. The tipranavir/ritonavir must be taken with other anti-HIV drugs. Normal dosing consists of 500 mg of tipranavir and 200 mg of ritonavir twice daily. Whereas tipranavir is a substrate for CYP3A4, in the presence of ritonavir very little metabolism of tipranavir occurs, although the combination leads to induction of P-glycoprotein, which may increase the bioavailability of tipranavir. By itself, tipranavir exhibits increased absorption in the presence of food. Initially, tipranavir was available as the disodium salt, but it was demonstrated that the free acid, in the form of a self-emulsifying drug delivery system (soft-gel capsules), showed improved bioavailability.

Drug interactions occur between tipranavir and fluconazole and between tipranavir and clarithromycin, increasing the AUC over a 12 hour period for tipranavir by 56 and 59%, respectively. Care should be taken when administering tipranavir with CYP450 inhibitors and inducers, because clinically significant interactions are possible. Coadministration of tipranavir with antacids decreases the tripranavir AUC by up to 33%.

The most common side effects reported for tipranavir consist of diarrhea and nausea. These adverse events may be significant enough to lead to drug discontinuance.

Combination Drug Therapy (105,106)

Combination drug therapy for viral infections is another approach currently under investigation. The synergistic antiviral effects of rimantadine with ribavirin and tiazofurin against influenza B virus and of ganciclovir (DHPG) with foscarnet against HSV-1 and HSV-2 are noteworthy. The synergistic action of either trifluorothymidine or acyclovir with leukocyte interferon has been used in the topical treatment of human herpetic keratitis. During the past decade, research into combination antiretroviral therapy for patients with AIDS has made remarkable progress. The first approved drug for HIV-infected patients, ZDV, produced bone marrow toxicity. To overcome toxic effects, combinations of ZDV with foscarnet, ddC, or ddI have been used. Such combination therapy indicated improved efficacy and decreased side effects as compared to either drug when used alone. The combination of ZDV with interferon-α has been used to treat patients with AIDS-related Kaposi's sarcoma. This combination drug therapy delayed emergence of ZDV-resistant HIV strains.

A combination of granulocyte-macrophage colony-stimulating factor with ZDV and interferon-α has been successful in managing treatment-related cytopenia in HIV-infected patients. The advantages of combination therapy include therapeutic antiviral effect, decreased toxicity, and low incidence of drug-resistant infection. In recent years, emergence of drug resistance has been demonstrated in patients receiving single antiviral agent therapy. Resistance to amantadine, acyclovir, ribavirin, ganciclovir, ZDV and other antiviral agents is noteworthy.

Combined antiretroviral drug therapy serves different purposes. It prolongs the life of patients with AIDS; removes drug resistance, and/or reduces the toxicity of drugs. With these objectives, successful combinations of ZDV have been reported with ddC, ddI, 3TC, or D4T. Recently, combination of nucleosides drugs (ZDV, ddC, ddI, and 3TC) are used with PIs (saquinavir, indinavir, and ritonavir) for delaying HIV infection. Combined nucleoside drugs are known to delay progression of HIV infection.

Antiretroviral therapy includes nucleosides or nonnucleoside RT inhibitors and PIs. These drugs inhibit HIV replication at different stages of viral infection. Nucleoside and nonnucleoside drugs inhibit RT by preventing RNA formation or viral protein synthesis. Nonnucleoside drugs inhibit RT by inactivating the catalytic site of the enzyme. The PIs act after HIV provirus has integrated into the human genome. These drug inhibit protease, which is an enzyme responsible for cleaving viral precursor polypeptides into effective virions. Thus, PIs combined with RT inhibitors act by a synergistic mechanism to interrupt HIV replication.

Two-drug combinations, such as ZDV plus ddI or ddC, 3TC and ZDV, and D4T plus ddI, have been successful in raising CD4 cell counts and decreasing HIV RNA viral load. Triple-drug therapy consisting of ZDV, 3TC, and one PI (indinavir, ritonavir, or nelfinavir) has been more effective than double-drug therapy consisting of two nonnucleoside analogue combinations. Also, fewer opportunistic infections were noted when patients took the three-drug combination. Additionally, ZDV can be combined with immunomodulators to increase immunologic response in patients with AIDS. Zidovudine has been combined with interferon-α to obtain synergistic activity of the drug. An ideal approach of combined antiretroviral drug therapy would be drugs acting at different stages of HIV cell replication.

Investigational Antiviral Agents: Short Interfering RNA (107)

The field of directed RNA interference (RNAi) has rapidly developed into a highly promising approach for specifically interrupting gene function to alleviate disease pathology. RNAi is a mechanism for silencing gene expression that has been conserved through evolution in eukaryotes ranging from plants to humans. In this process, double-stranded duplexes of 21 to 25 nucleotides in length are created from a parent double-stranded RNA molecule. These short interfering RNAs (siRNAs) direct the cell to cleave target mRNAs that share sequence identity with the siRNAs. Many research groups are attempting to develop RNAi therapies that induce the degradation of target mRNA involved in inherited or acquired disorders. This technology is especially well-suited to treating viral infections, and numerous examples now illustrate that a wide range of viruses can be inhibited with RNAi, both in vitro and in vivo. Antiviral RNAi therapies can be tailored to the biochemical characteristics of each pathogen and can be made more specific through choice of delivery vehicle, route of administration, selection of gene targets, and regulation of RNAi induction. As has been mentioned above, successful antiviral therapeutics possess the ability to discriminate virus from host. Because viruses rely extensively on host cell machinery for many functions and activities involved in viral replication, however, they offer a very limited number of therapeutic targets. Because RNAi specifically targets a short stretch of viral nucleic acids rather than a viral protein, even a small viral genome can provide a large number of potential targets.

CASE STUDY

Victoria F. Roche and S. William Zito

You are an Oregon pharmacist mentoring the American Pharmacist Association Academy of Student Pharmacists chapter of a local pharmacy school in its service outreach program with an area shelter for abused women. This shelter serves about 50 women and their children, assisting the women with work placements when needed and providing day care services and transportation to area schools for the kids. All residents have breakfast together at 6:30 AM, and dinner is offered at 6:00 PM. with about three-quarters of the families partaking on any given evening. Various community groups make sure the pantry is well stocked, and one has provided supplies of aspirin and other over-the-counter products for as-needed use by the shelter's clients. The corporate headquarters of Sea Mist, a company that markets products made from locally grown cranberries, has selected this shelter as the primary beneficiary of its community service commitment, and it provides the residents with essentially limitless quantities of its products, including cranberry juice (enjoyed often by most of those living at the shelter).

A recent outbreak of influenza A has struck your community, and although only a few residents of the shelter have become ill, you and the MD who also donates her services to the facility realize that all the residents (including the children) are at risk. Because of a nationwide shortage of vaccine, vaccination of the residents is not possible, but together, you are trying to secure sufficient quantities of an orally active, antiviral agent to treat and/or protect these patients. The Sea Mist employees have volunteered to cover the cost of any medication not donated by the manufacturer. Taking advantage of a "teachable moment" in clinical practice, you ask your ASP students who are currently taking medicinal chemistry to identify the best agent of the four structural choices shown below to meet the needs of this diverse population.

1. Identify the therapeutic problem(s) in which the pharmacist's intervention may benefit the patient.
2. Identify and prioritize the patient-specific factors that must be considered to achieve the desired therapeutic outcomes.
3. Conduct a thorough and mechanistically oriented structure–activity analysis of all therapeutic alternatives provided in the case.
4. Evaluate the structure–activity relationship findings against the patient-specific factors and desired therapeutic outcomes, and make a therapeutic decision.
5. Counsel your patients.

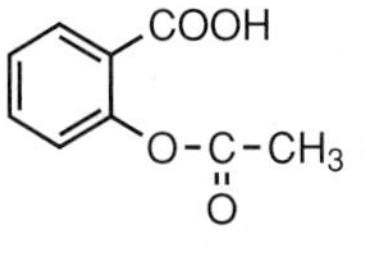

COOH
O–C–CH3
O

Aspirin

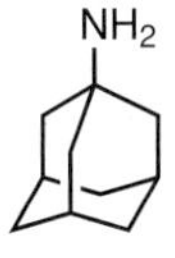

NH2

1

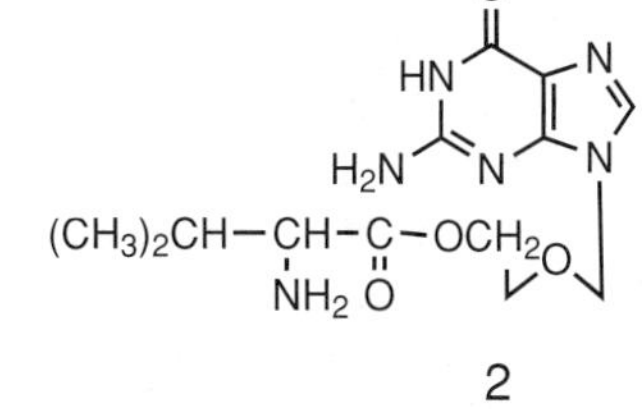

O
HN
N
H2N
N
N
(CH3)2CH–CH–C–OCH2
O
NH2 O

2

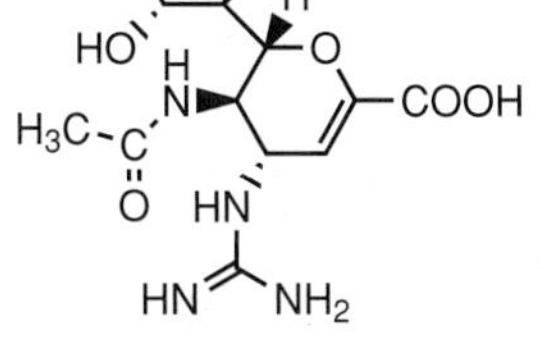

HO
OH
H
HO H
O
N
COOH
H3C–C
O HN
HN NH2

3

O H
HN
COOC2H5
H3C
O H2N

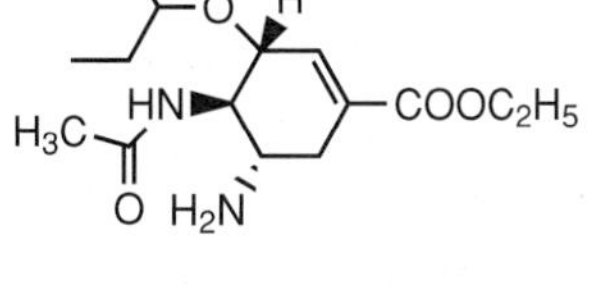

4

References

1. Baron S. Medical Microbiology 3rd Ed. New York: Churchill Livingstone, 1991:555–652.
2. Brooks GF; Butel JS; Morse SA, et al. Jawetz, Melnick, and Adelberg's Medical Microbiology. 23rd Ed. New York: McGraw-Hill, 2004.
3. Tyler KL, Fields BN. Fields Virology. 2nd Ed. New York: Raven Press, 1990:191–239.
4. Sierra S, Kupfer B, Kaiser R. Basics of the virology of HIV-1 and its replication. J Clin Virol 2005;34:233–244.
5. Gallo RC. History of the discoveries of the first human retroviruses: HTLV-1 and HTLV-2 Oncogene 2005. 24;5926–5930.
6. World Health Organization, Joint United Nations Programme on HIV/AIDS (UNAIDS). AIDS Epidemic Update 2005. Available at: http://www.who.int/hiv/epiupdates/en/index.html. Accessed April 12, 2006.
7. Kaleeba JAR, Berger EA. Kaposi's sarcoma–associated herpesvirus fusion-entry receptor: cystine transporter xCT. Science 2006;311:1921–1924.
8. D'Agostino DM. Bernardi P, ChiecoBianchi L, et al. Mitochondria as functional targets of protein coded by human tumor viruses. Adv Cancer Res. 2005;94:87–142.
9. Grassmann R, Aboud M, Jeang K-T. Molecular mechanisms of cellular transformation by HTLV-1 Tax. Oncogene 2005;24:5976–5985.
10. Mikkers H, Berns A. Retroviral insertional mutagenesis: tagging cancer pathways. Adv Cancer Res 2003;88:53–99.
11. O'Shea CC. DNA tumor viruses—the spies who lyse us. Curr Opin Genet Dev 2005;15:18–26.
12. Robinson HL. Retroviruses and cancer. Rev Infect Dis 1982;4:1015–1025.
13. Klein G. Perspectives in studies of human tumor viruses. Front Biosci 2002;7:268–274.
14. Mabbott NA, MacPherson GG. Prions and their lethal journey to the brain. Nat Rev Microbiol 2006;4:201–211.
15. Johnson RT. Prion diseases. Lancet Neurol 2005;4:635–642.
16. Weissmann C. Birth of a prion: spontaneous generation revisited. Cell 2005;122:165–168.
17. Mandell GL, Bennett SE, Dolin R, eds. Principles and Practice of Infectious Diseases. New York: Churchill Livingstone, 1995.
18. Mills J, Corey L, eds. Antiviral Chemotherapy: New Directions for Clinical Application and Research, vol. 3, Englewood Cliffs, NJ: Prentice Hall, 1993.
19. Burlington DB, Meiklejohn G, Mostow SR. Anti-influenza A virus activity of amantadine hydrochloride and rimantadine hydrochloride in ferret tracheal ciliated epithelium. Antimicrob Agents Chemother 1982;21:794–799.
20. Hayden FG. Combinations of antiviral agents for treatment of influenza virus infection. J Antimicrob Agents Chemother 1986;18(Suppl B):177–183.
21. Wingfield WL, Pollack D, Grunert RR. Therapeutic efficacy of an amantadine and rimantadine hydrochloride in naturally occurring influenza A2 respiratory illness in man. N Engl J Med 1969;28:579–584.
22. Wintermeyer SM, Nahata MC. Rimantadine: a clinical prospective. Ann Pharmacother 1995;29:299–310.
23. Francis ML, Meltzer MS, Gendelman HE. Interferons in the persistence, pathogenesis, and treatment of HIV infection. AIDS Res Hum Retroviruses 1992;8:199–207.
24. Hayden FG. Intra-nasal interferon for control of respiratory viril infections. In: Revel M, ed. Clinical Aspects of Interferons. Boston: Kluwer Academic Publishers, 1988.
25. Pollard RB. Interferons and interferon inducers: development of clinical usefulness and therapeutic promise. Drugs 1982;23:37–55.
26. Streuli M, Nagata S, Weismann C. At least three human type α interferons: structure of α2. Science 1980;209:1343–1347.
27. Taniguchi T, Guarente L, Roberts TM, et al. Expression of the human fibroblast interferon gene in *Escherichia coli*. Proc Nat. Acad Sci U S A 1980;77: 5230–5233.
28. Baglioni C, Maroney PA. Mechanisms of action of human interferons, induction of 2′,5′-oligo (A) polymerase. J Biol Chem 1980;255:8390–8393.
29. Calfee DP, Hayden FG. New approaches to influenza chemotherapy: neuraminidase inhibitors. Drugs 1998;56:537–553.
30. Kim CU, Lew W, Williams MA, et al. Influenza neuraminidase inhibitors possessing a novel hydrophobic interaction in the enzyme active site: design, synthesis, and structural analysis of carboxylic sialic acid analogues with potent anti-influenza activity. J Am Chem Soc 1997;119:681–690.
31. Sweeny DJ, Lynch G, Bidgood AM, et al. Metabolism of the influenza neuraminidase inhibitor pro-drug oseltamivir in the rat. Drug Met Dispos 2000;28:737–741.
32. Poveda E, Briz V, Soriano V. Enfuvirtide, the first fusion inhibitor to treat HIV infection. AIDS Rev 2005;7:139–147.
33 Lalezari JP, Henry K, O'Hearn M, et al. Enfuvirtide, an HIV-1 fusion inhibitor, for drug-resistant HIV infection in North and South America. N Engl J Med 2003;348:2175–2185.
34. Field HJ. A perspective on resistance to acyclovir in herpes simplex virus. Antimicrob Agents Chemother 1983;12(Suppl. B):129–135.
35. Elion GB, Furman PA, Fyfe JA, et al. Selectivity of action of an antiherpetic agent, 9-(2-hydroxyethoxymethyl) guanine. Proc Natl Acad Sci U S A 1977;74:5716–5720.
36. Whitley RJ, Alford CA. Antiviral agents: clinical status report. Hosp Pract 1981;16:109–121.
37. Mitchell CD, Bean B, Gentry SR, et al. Acyclovir therapy for mucocutaneous herpes simplex infections in immunocompromised patients. Lancet 1981;i:1389–1392.
38. Whitley RJ, Alford CA, Hirsch MS, et al. Vidarabine versus acyclovir therapy in herpes simplex encephalitis. N Engl J Med 1986;314:144–149.
39. Brigden D, Bye A, Fowle AS, et al. Human pharmacokinetics of acyclovir (an antiviral agent) following rapid intravenous injection. J Antimicrob Chemother 1981;7:399–404.
40. de Miranda P, Whitley RJ, Blum MR, et al. Acyclovir kinetics after intravenous infusion. Clin Pharmacol Ther 1979;26:718–728.
41. Perry CM, Faulds D. Valaciclovir, a review of its antiviral activity, pharmacokinetic properties and therapeutic efficacy in herpes virus infection. Drugs 1996;52:754–772.
42. Martinez CM, Lucks-Golger DB. Cidofovir use in acyclovir-resistant herpes infection. Ann Pharmacother 1997;31:1519–1521.
43. Ward RL, Stevens JG. Effect of cytosine arabinoside on viral-specific protein synthesis in cells infected with herpes simplex virus. J Virol 1975;15:71–80.
44. Nutter RL, Rapp F. The effect of cytosine arabinoside on virus production in various cells infected with herpes simplex virus types 1 and 2. Cancer Res 1973;33:166–170.
45. Schacker T, Hu HL, Koell DM, et al. Famciclovir for the suppression of symptomatic and asymptomatic herpes simplex virus reactivation in HIV-infected person. A double-blind, placebo-control trial. Ann Intern Med 1998;128: 21–28.
46. De Clerq E, Field HJ. Antiviral pro-drugs–the development of successful prodrug strategies for antiviral chemotherapy. Br J Pharmacol 2006;147:1–11.
47. Field AK. Viral targets for antisense oligonucleotides: a mini-review. Antiviral Res 1998;37:67–81.
48. Chrisp P, Clissold SP. Foscarnet: a review of its antiviral activity, pharmacokinetic properties, and therapeutic use in immunocompromised patients with cytomegalovirus retinitis. Drugs 1991;41:104–129.
49. Fletcher CV, Balfour HH. Evaluation of ganciclovir for cytomegalovirus disease. Drug Intel Clin Pharm 1989;23:5–11.
50. Whitley RJ. The past as prelude to the future: history, status, and future of antiviral drugs. Ann Pharmacother 1996;30:967–971.
51. Farah A, ed. Handbook of Experimental Biology, vol. 38/2. Berlin: Springer, 1975:272–347.
52. Sidwell RW, Huffman JH, Khare GP, et al. Broas-spectrum antiviral activity of virazole: 1-β-D-ribofuranosyl-1,2,4-triazole-3-carboxamide. Science 1972;177: 705–706.
53. Hall CB, McBride JT. Vapors, viruses, and views. Ribavirin and respiratory syncytial virus. Am J Dis Child 1986;140:331–332.
54. Fox CF, Robinson WS, eds. Virus Research. New York: Academic Press, 1973:415–436.
55. Power WJ, Benedict SA, Hillery M, et al. Randomized double-blind trial of bromovinyldeoxyuridine (BUVD) and trifluorothymidine (TFT) in dendritic corneal ulceration. Br J Ophthalmol 1991;75:649–651.
56. Whitley RJ, Soong SJ, Dolin R, et al. Adenine arabinoside therapy of biopsy-proved herpes simplex encephalitis. National Institute of Allergy and Infectious Diseases Collaborative Antiviral Study. N Engl J Med 1977;297: 289–294.
57. Whitley RJ, Soong SJ, Dolin R, et al. Early vidarabine therapy to control the complications of herpes zoster in immunocompromised patients. N Engl J Med 1982;307:971–975.
58. Chao DL, Kimblall AP. Determination of arabinosyladenine by adenosine deaminase and inhibition by arabinosyl-6-mercaptopurine. Cancer Res 1972;32:1721–1724.
59. Dando TM, Plosker GL. Adefovir dipivoxil: a review of its use in chronic hepatitis B. Drugs 2003;63:2215–2234.
60. Blair E, Darby G, eds. Antiviral Therapy. New York: BIOS Scientific Publishers, 1998.
61. do Valle LA, de Melo PR, de Gomes LF. Methisazone in prevention of variola minor among contacts. Lancet 1965;2:976–978.
62. Mohan P, Baba M, eds. Anti-AIDS drug development: challenges, strategies, and prospects. Chur, Switzerland: Harwood Academic, 1995.
63. Sethi ML. Current concepts in HIV/AIDS pharmacotherapy. The Consultant Pharmacists 1998;13:1224–1245.
64. Berger TG. Treatment of bacterial, fungal, and parasitic infections in the HIV-infected host. Semin Dermatol 1993;12:296–300.
65. Sattler FR, Feinberg J. New developments in the treatment of *Pneumocystis carinii* pneumonia. Chest 1992;101:451–457.
66. Goa KL, Barradell LB. Fluconazole. An update of its pharmacodynamic and pharmacokinetic properties and therapeutic use in major superficial and systemic mycosis in immunocompromised patients. Drugs 1995;50:658–690.
67. Mitsuya H, ed. Anti-HIV nucleosides: past, present, and future. New York: Chapman and Hall, 1997.
68. Whitley RJ. Antiviral Therapy. In: Gorbach SL, Barlett JG and Blacklow NR. eds. Infectious Diseases, Lippincott, Williams & Wilkins, Philiadelphia, 2003:299–316.
69. Barlett JG. Antiretroviral Therapy. In: Gorbach SL, Barlett JG, and Blacklow NR, eds. Infectious Diseases, Lippincott, Williams & Wilkins, Philiadelphia, 2003:1028–1037.

70. MacDonald L, Kazanjian P. Antiretroviral therapy in HIV-infection: an update. Formulary 1996;31:780–804.
71. Faulds D, Brogden RN. Didanosine. A review of its antiviral activity, pharmacokinetic properties and therapeutic potential in human immunodeficiency virus infection. Drugs 1992;44:94–116.
72. Beach JW. Chemotherapeutic agents for human immunodeficiency virus infection: mechanism of action, pharmacokinetics, metabolism, and adverse reactions. Clin Ther 1998;20:2–25.
73. Lipsky JJ. Zalcitabine and didanosine. Lancet 1993;341:30–32.
74. Shelton MH, O'Donnell AM, Morse GD. Zalcitabine. Ann Pharmacother 1993;27:480–489.
75. Neuzil KM. Pharmacologic therapy for HIV infection: a review. Am J Med Sci 1994;307:368–373.
76. Fischl MA, Richmann DD, Greico MH, et al. The efficacy of the azothymidine (AZT) in the treatment of patients with AIDS and AIDS-related complex: a double-blinded, placebo-controlled trial. N Engl J Med 1987;317: 185–191.
77. Fischl MA, Richmann DD, Hansen N, et al. The safety and efficacy of zidovudine (AZT) in the treatment of subjects with mildly symptomatic human immunodeficiency virus type 1 (HIV) infection: a double-blind, placebo-controlled trial. Ann Intern Med 1990;112:727–737.
78. Sethi ML. Zidovudine. In: Florey K, ed. Analytical Profiles of Drug Substances, vol 20. San Diego: Academic Press, 1991:729–765.
79. Nasr M, Littest C, McGowan J. Computer-assisted structure–activity correlations of dideoxynucleoside analogues as potential anti-HIV drugs. Antiviral Res 1990;14:125–148.
80. Hoth DF, Myers MW, Stein DS. Current status of HIV therapy I. Antiviral agents. Hosp Pract 1992;27:145–156.
81. Horowitz JP, Chua J, Noel M. Nucleosides V. The monomesylates of 1-(2′-deoxy-β-D-lyxofuranosyl) thymine. J Org Chem 1964;29:2076–2079.
82. Ostertag W, Roesler G, Krieg CJ, et al. Induction of endogenous virus and of thymidine kinase by bromodeoxyuridine in cell cultures transformed by Friend virus. Proc Natl Acad Sci U S A 1974;71:4980–4985.
83. Yarchoan R, Klecker RW, Weinhold KJ, et al. Administration of 3′-azido-3′-deoxythymidine, an inhibitor of HTLV-III/LAV replication to patients with AIDS or AIDS-related complex. Lancet 1986;i:575–580.
84. Perry CM, Faulds D. Lamivudine. A review of its antiviral activity, pharmacokinetic properties, and therapeutic efficacy in the management of HIV infection. Drugs 1997;53:657–680.
85. Bang LM, Scott LJ. Emtricitabine: an antiretroviral agent for HIV infection. Drugs 2003;63:2413–2424.
86. Barditch-Crovo P, Deeks SG, Collier A, et al. Phase I/II trial of the pharmacokinetics, safety, and antiretroviral activity of tenofovir disoproxil fumarate in human immunodeficiency virus-infected adults. Antimicrob Agents Chemother 2001;45:2733–2739.
87. Tan B, Ratner L. The use of new antiretroviral therapy in combination with chemotherapy. Curr Opin Oncol 1997;9:455–464.
88. Freimuth WW. Delaviridine mesylate, a potent nonnucleoside HIV-1 reverse transcriptase inhibitor. Adv Exp Med Biol 1996;394:279–289.
89. Graul A, Rabasseda X, Castaner J. Efavirenz. Drugs of the Future 1998;23: 133–141.
90. Deeks SG, Volberding PA. HIV-1 protease inhibitors. AIDS Clin Rev 1997–1998:145–185.
91. Hoetelmans RM, Meenhorst PL, Mulder JW, et al. Clinical pharmacology of HIV protease inhibitors: focus on saquanivir, indinavir, and ritonavir. Pharm World Sci 1997;19:159–175.
92. Perry CM, Noble S. Saquinavir soft-gel capsule formulation. Drugs 1998;56: 461–486.
93. Fitzsimmons ME, Collins JM. Selective biotransformation of the human immunodeficiency virus protease inhibitor saquinavir by human small-intestinal cytochrome P450 3A4. Drug Metab Dispos 1997;25:256–266.
94. Markowitz M, Saag M, Powderly WG, et al. A preliminary study of ritonavir, an inhibitor HIV-1 protease to treat HIV-1 infection. N Engl J Med 1995;333:1534–1539.
95. Kumar GN, Rodrigues AD, Buko AM, et al. Cytochrome P450–mediated metabolism of the HIV-1 protease inhibitor ritonavir (ABT-538) in human liver microsomes. J Pharmacol Exp Ther 1996;277:423–431.
96. Deeks SG, Smith M, Holodniy M, et al. HIV-1 protease inhibitor: a review for clinician. JAMA 1997;277:145–153.
97. Balani SK, Arison BH, Mathai L, et al. Metabolites of L-735,524, a potent HIV-1 protease inhibitor, in human urine. Drug Metab Dispos 1995;23:266–270.
98. Perry CM, Benfield P. Nelfinavir. Drugs 1997;54:81–88.
99. Colonno RJ, Thiry A, Limoli K, et al. Activities of atazanavir (BMS-232632) against a large panel of human immunodeficiency virus type 1 clinical isolates resistant to one or more approved protease inhibitors. Antimicrob Agents Chemother 2003;47:1324–1333.
100. Falcoz C, Jenkins JM, Bye C, et al. Pharmacokinetics of GW433908, a pro-drug of amprenavir in healthy male volunteers. J Clin Pharmacol 2002;42:887–898.
101. Thaisrivongs S, Skulnick HI, Turner SR. Structure-based design of HIV protease inhibitors: sulfonamide-containing 5,6-dihydro-4-hydroxy-2-pyrones as nonpeptidic inhibitors. J Med Chem 1996;39:4349–4353.
102. Poppe SM, Slade DE, Chong K-T, et al. Antiviral activity of the dihydropyrone PNU-140690, a new nonpeptidic human immunodeficiency virus protease inhibitor. Antimicrob Agents Chemother 1997;41:1058–1063.
103. Plosker GL, Figgitt DP. Tipranavir. Drugs 1997;63:1611–1618.
104. Katherine FC, Keam SJ. Tipranavir: a ritonavir-boosted protease inhibitor. Drugs 2005;65:1669–1677.
105. Fischl MA, Stanley K, Collier AC, et al. Combination and monotherapy with zidovudine and zalcitabine in patients with advanced HIV disease. The NIAID AIDS Clinical Trial Group. Ann Intern Med 1995;122:24–32.
106. Havlir DV, Lange JM. New antivirals and new combinations. AIDS 1998;12 (Suppl. A):S165–S174.
107. Leonard JN, Schaffer DV. Antiviral RNAi therapy: emerging approaches for hitting a moving target. Gene Ther 2006;13:532–540.

Suggested Readings

Bamford DH, Burnett RM, Stuart DI. Evolution of viral structure. Theoretical Population Biology 2002;61:461–470.
Brooks G F, Butel J S, Morse SA, et al. Jawetz, Melnick, and Adelberg's Medical Microbiology. 23rd Ed. New York: McGraw-Hill, 2004.
De Clercq E. Antivirals and antiviral strategies. Nat Rev Microbiol 2004;2:704–720.
De Clercq E. Antiviral drugs in current clinical use. J Clin Virol 2004;30:115–133.
De Clercq E. Recent highlights in the development of new antiviral drugs. Curr Opin Microbiol 2005;8:552–560.
De Clercq E. Antiviral drug discovery and development: where chemistry meets with biomedicine. Antiviral Res 2005;67:56–75.
De Clercq E, Field HJ. Antiviral pro-drugs–the development of successful prodrug strategies for antiviral chemotherapy. Br. J Pharmacol. 2006;147:1–11.
Fung SK, Lok AS. Drug insight: nucleoside and nucleotide analogue inhibitors for hepatitis B. Nat Clin Pract Gastroenterol Hepatol 2004;1:90–97.
Grassmann R, Aboud M, Jeang K-T. Molecular mechanisms of cellular transformation by HTLV-1 Tax. Oncogene 2005;24:5976–5985.
Mabbott NA, MacPherson GG. Prions and their lethal journey to the brain. Nat Rev Microbiol 2006;4:201–211.
Moscona A. Neuraminidase inhibitors for influenza. N Engl J Med 2005;353: 1363–1373.
O'Shea CC. DNA tumor viruses—the spies who lyse us. Curr Opin Genet Dev 2005;15:18–26.
Robinson HL. Retroviruses and cancer. Rev Infect Dis 1982;4:1015–1025.
Sierra S, Kupfer B, Kaiser R. Basics of the virology of HIV-1 and its replication. J Clin Virol 2005:34:233–244.

PART IV

DISEASE STATE MANAGEMENT

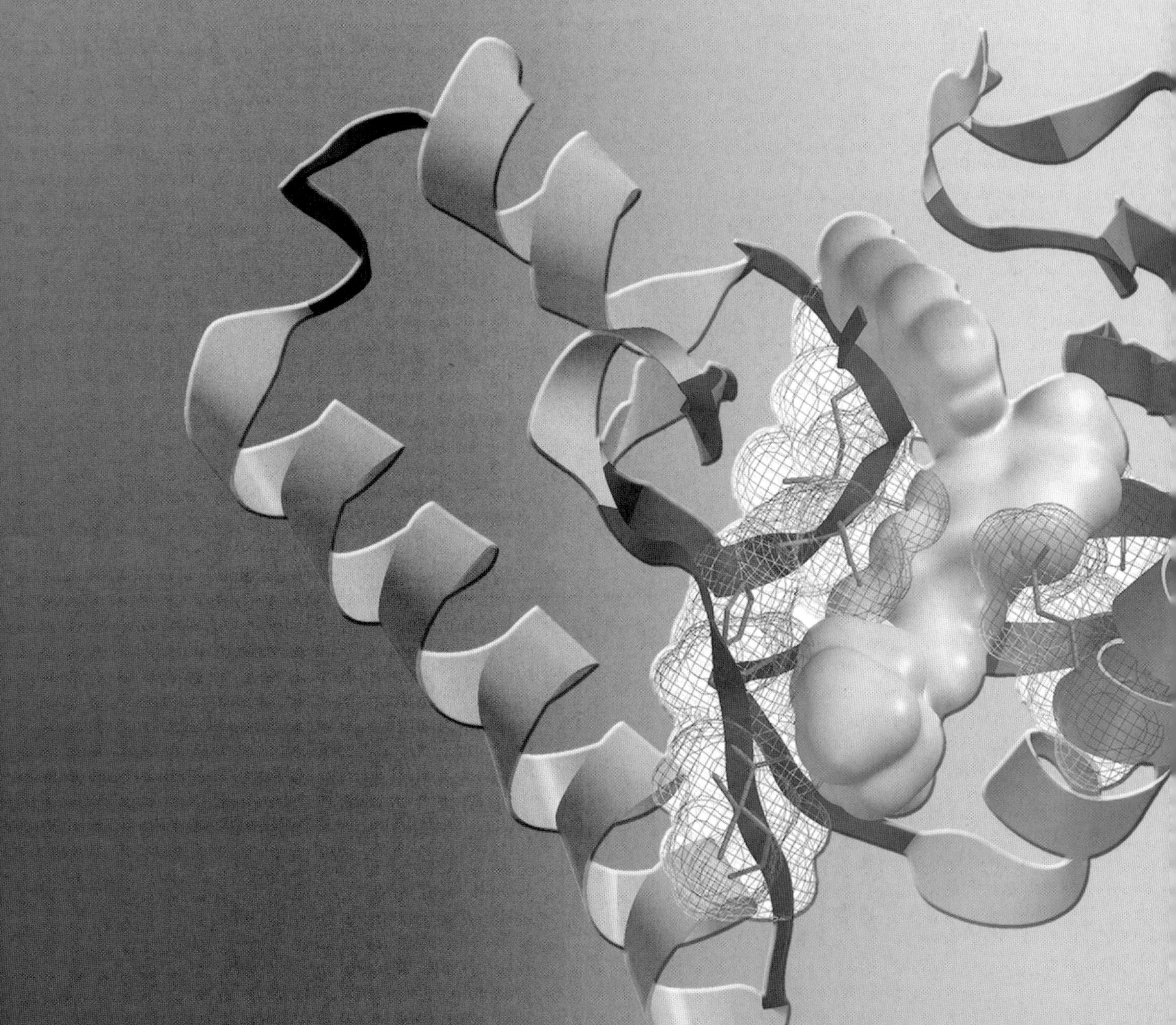

44. *Asthma and Chronic Obstructive Pulmonary Disease*

S. WILLIAM ZITO

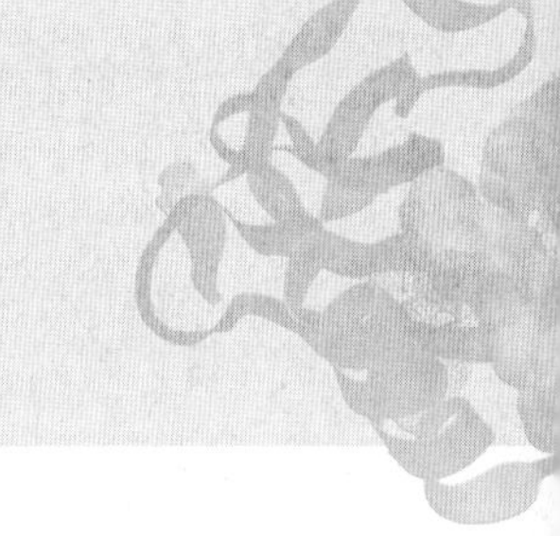

DRUGS COVERED IN THIS CHAPTER:

β_2-ADRENERGIC AGONISTS
- Albuterol
- Bitolterol mesylate
- Epinephrine (Adrenalin)
- Fenoterol hydrobromide
- Formoterol fumarate
- Isoetharine hydrochloride
- Metaproterenol sulfate
- Salmeterol xinafoate
- Terbutaline sulfate

ANTIMUSCARINICS
- Ipratropium hydrobromide
- Tiotropium bromide

METHYLXANTHINES
- Dyphylline
- Theophylline

ADRENOCORTICOIDS
- Beclomethasone dipropionate
- Budesonide
- Flunisolide
- Fluticasone propionate
- Hydrocortisone
- Methylprednisolone
- Mometasone furoate
- Prednisolone
- Triamcinolone acetonide

MAST CELL DEGRANULATION INHIBITORS
- Cromolyn sodium
- Nedocromil sodium

LEUKOTRIENE MODIFERS
- Montelukast
- Zafirlukast
- Zileutin

MONOCLONAL ANTI-IgE ANTIBODY
- Omalizumab

ASTHMA

Epidemiology

Asthma is a Greek word that is derived from the verb "aasein," meaning to pant or exhale with open mouth. The earliest use of the term as a medical condition dates back to Ancient Greece, in Hippocrates' *Corpus Hippocraticum* (1). The incidence of asthma is greatest in the developed world, and there has been an increase in asthma over the last two decades in the United States (2). According to 2002 U.S. population data gathered by the National Center for Health Statistics, the number of people who were ever diagnosed with asthma by a health professional (lifetime prevalence) is 30.8 million (111 per 1,000). Of that number, it is estimated that 20 million people are currently under treatment and that as many as 12 million had an asthma attack in the 12 months before the survey. Children aged 0 to 17 years have the highest rate of asthma (83 per 1,000), but the rate decreases significantly in adults, indicating that many children "outgrow" the disease. Race and gender seem to play a role in the prevalence of asthma. Puerto Ricans, blacks, and Native Americans have an asthma prevalence much higher than in Caucasians. The high Puerto Rican incidence is masked when they are included among all Hispanics. Boys have a higher incidence of asthma than girls; however, this reverses in adulthood, when females show a 30% higher prevalence compared to males. Asthma causes a significant loss of schooldays and workdays and results in nearly 2 million visits to the emergency department each year. If asthma is not controlled, it can result in death: almost 5,000 people died from asthma in 2002. Blacks had an asthma death rate more than 200% higher than that in Caucasians, and women had a death rate 40% higher than males. These data reinforce the influence of race and gender on the morbidity and mortality of asthma and point out the fact that asthma is a significant public health burden in the United States (3).

Etiology, Signs, and Symptoms

Asthma is a complex disorder involving biochemical, autonomic, immunologic, infectious, environmental, and psychological factors to varying degrees in different individuals. Patients with asthma demonstrate recurrent episodes of paroxysmal dyspnea, wheezing, and cough. Most asthmatic attacks are short-lived, with the patient being free from symptoms between exacerbations. Some patients may have persistent difficulty breathing that does not respond to any treatment and that is believed to be the result of airway remodeling (4). The National Institutes of Health (NIH) Expert Panel Report 2: Guidelines for the Diagnosis and Management of Asthma (EPR-2) simply defines asthma as a chronic inflammatory response of the airways (5).

The most common form of asthma is allergic asthma (atopic or extrinsic asthma), and it is associated with environmental allergens, such as plant pollens, house dust mites (*Dermatophagoides farinae*), domestic pet dander, molds, and foods. The less common form, intrinsic asthma, has no known allergic cause and usually occurs in adults older than 35 years. Intrinsic asthma may result from an autonomic dysfunction characterized by excess cholinergic and/or tachykinin activity, but this hypothesis has never been proven (6). Aside from environmental allergens, an asthmatic attack may be precipitated by

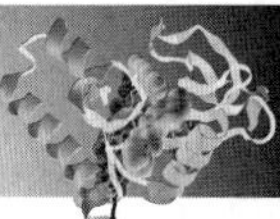

CLINICAL SIGNIFICANCE

The therapeutic approach to the management of asthma and chronic obstructive pulmonary disease (COPD) has changed dramatically over the past several decades. Treatment guidelines have evolved based on a better understanding of these disease states as well as on the development of newer and more efficacious treatment modalities through the application of structure-activity relationships (SARs) of chemical lead compounds. Although both disease states are characterized by pulmonary obstruction and chronic inflammation, the nature of such pulmonary abnormalities differ between the two conditions. Traditional therapy had focused on the symptomatic relief of airflow obstruction through the use of bronchodilators, such as adrenergic agonists and anticholinergics. Today, however, greater emphasis is placed on managing the underlying inflammation and minimizing disease progression.

The current therapeutic approach to managing these diseases includes the use of rapidly acting drugs to relieve acute symptoms as well as maintenance medications to minimize inflammation and control long-term symptoms. Short-acting adrenergic agonists are the agents most commonly used to manage acute exacerbations of these disease states. Although effective, older agents, such as epinephrine and isoproterenol, were limited in their pharmacokinetic profile as well as in their lack of pulmonary selectivity. Modifying the chemical structure of these compounds, however, has resulted in the development of agents with significant clinical advantages in terms of duration of action and adverse effect profiles. Similarly, the application of SAR principles to the development of anti-inflammatory agents, such as corticosteroids, leukotriene antagonists, and mast-cell stabilizers, has lead to the availability of superior long-term controlling agents in terms of potency, pharmacokinetic profile, and safety.

In treating patients with asthma and COPD clinicians should be mindful of the SARs of those agents being employed. The application of these principles should be used to determine the most appropriate drug therapy in light of patient-specific needs and desired therapeutic outcomes. Additionally, clinicians can look forward to the availability of newer and more clinically appropriate agents for the management of asthma and COPD as research in medicinal chemistry results in the development of increasingly selective drug entities and improved receptor targeting modalities.

Joseph V. Etzel, Pharm.D.
Assistant Dean of Student Affairs
Associate Clinical Professor of Pharmacy
College of Pharmacy & Allied Health Professions
St. John's University
Jamaica, New York

respiratory infection, exercise, polyps, drugs (e.g., aspirin and β-adrenergic antagonists), and environmental pollutants (e.g., sulfur dioxide, cigarette smoke, and occupational chemicals). In predisposed individuals, emotional stress and drugs or foods that contain tartrazine, sulfites, and preservatives also can precipitate an asthmatic onset (7).

Why has there been a marked increase in asthma in affluent industrialized countries? To answer this question, recent thought has focused on the "hygiene hypothesis," which implicates an imbalance of TH_1 and TH_2 lymphocytes as a major cause of the increased prevalence of asthma (8). The TH_1 lymphocytes are the type of CD4+ T lymphocyte associated with defense against bacterial infection, whereas the TH_2 type predominates in allergic inflammation. The hypothesis claims that because bacterial infections have significantly decreased in industrialized nations, there is an imbalance, in susceptible children, in favor of the TH_2-type lymphocytes, and this imbalance therefore favors allergic asthma (9).

Asthma frequently occurs in families, and studies have shown that this results, at least in part, from mutually shared genes (10,11). Asthma is a complex disorder and lacks a mendelian genetic pattern, so it is difficult to study. To date, however, genetic research indicates that what is inherited is the susceptibility to develop asthma. It is clear that genes alone are not responsible for the development of asthma, because environmental factors also play a major role. Numerous genes on various chromosomes have been linked to asthma. Table 44.1 shows several gene products that may influence the development of asthma (10–15). In reality, however, there is little correlation between gene expression and clinical symptoms. The one exception to this is the low-expression allele of macrophage migration inhibitory factor (MIF), which has been shown to have a strong association with patients that have mild asthma (16). Drug development of MIF inhibitors might lead to future treatments for asthma.

Table 44.1. Putative Asthma Associated Gene Products

Gene Products
β_2-Adrenergic receptor
Interleukin-4, -5, -9, and -13
Interleukin-4 receptor α (Il-4Rα)
β Chain of the high-affinity IgE receptor (FcεRIβ)
Tumor necrosis factor α (TNFα)
Major histochemical complex (MHC)
T-cell receptor α/δ complex
ADAM33 (a disintegrin and metalloproteinase)
Dipeptidyl peptidase 10
PHD finger protein 11
Prostanoid DP1 receptor
Macrophage migration inhibitory factor (MIF)

Pathogenesis of Asthma

For a long time, asthmatic symptoms were thought to be the result of airway smooth muscle abnormalities, resulting in episodic bronchoconstriction. Today, however, it is clear that the constriction of bronchial smooth muscle is only one of many effects of chronic airway inflammation. Evidence of inflammation appears very soon after the onset of symptoms; therefore, treatment algorithms for asthma now emphasize quick relief of the bronchoconstriction and the amelioration of the underlying inflammation (17).

Inflammation in asthma is characterized by mucous plugging, epithelial shedding, basement membrane thickening, inflammatory cell infiltration, and smooth muscle hypertrophy and hyperplasia (Fig. 44.1). An acute extrinsic asthmatic attack begins when mast cells become activated. Activation of mast cells occurs when an antigen cross-links with immunoglobulin (Ig) Es on their surface. This IgE complex triggers mast cell degranulation, leading to the rapid release of inflammatory mediators, such as histamine, prostaglandins, leukotrienes, and cytokines (including tumor necrosis factor α and interleukins). The initial attack generally resolves within an hour; however, a second phase begins 4 to 6 hours after exposure and can last up to 24 hours. This late phase is a result of recruitment of additional inflammatory cells, primarily eosinophils, by the release of cytokines from macrophages and TH_2-type lymphocytes in the lower lung (18).

Clinical Evaluation

Most patients with asthma are asymptomatic between acute exacerbations. The onset of symptoms can be sudden or gradual and frequently can occur during the night or early in the morning. Acute symptoms include shortness of breath, wheezing or whistling at the end of exhalation, cough, and chest tightness. Patients with chronic and poorly controlled asthma develop barrel chest and diminished diaphragm movement, both of which are evidence of chronic pulmonary hyperinflation.

Acute asthmatic attacks may be mild, moderate, or severe depending on the degree of airway obstruction. The determination of the degree of airflow obstruction is accomplished by pulmonary function testing. The most common pulmonary function test utilizes spirometry, which measures the rate at which the lung changes volume during forced breathing maneuvers. The most important spirometric measure is the forced vital capacity (FVC). This requires the patient to exhale as rapidly and as completely as possible after a maximal inhalation. Normal lungs generally can empty their volume in 6 seconds or less. When airflow is obstructed, however, the expiratory time may increase by as much as fivefold. In practice, the forced expiratory volume in the first second of expiration (FEV_1) is measured and compared to the FVC and then recorded as the ratio of FEV_1 to FVC (FEV_1/FVC) (Fig. 44.2) (measurement is done by means

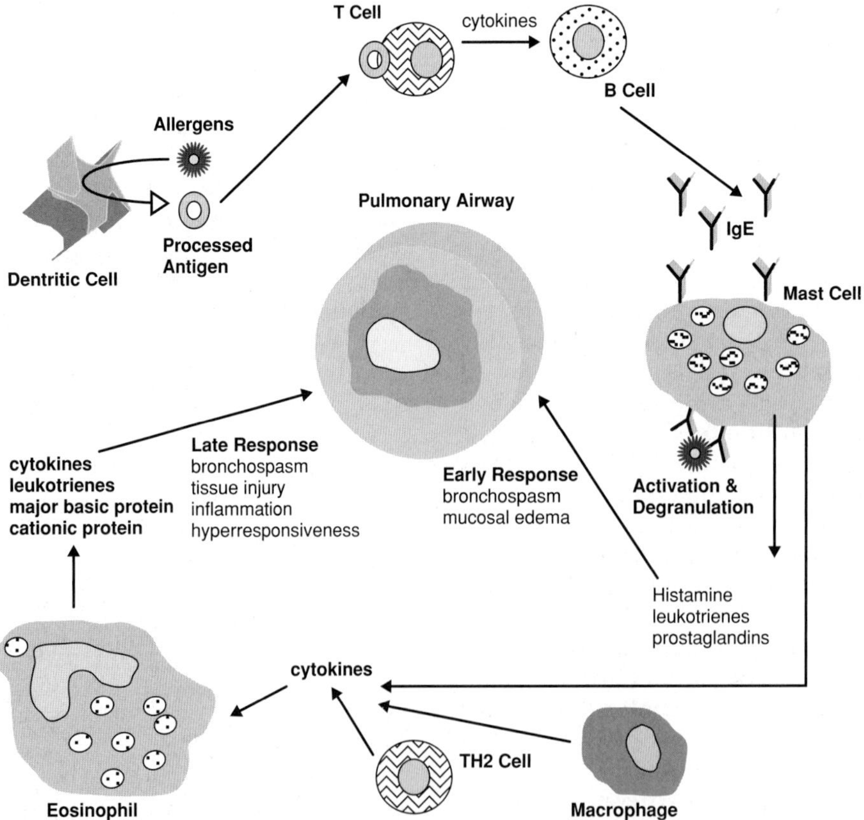

Fig. 44.1. Pictorial summary of asthma pathogenesis.

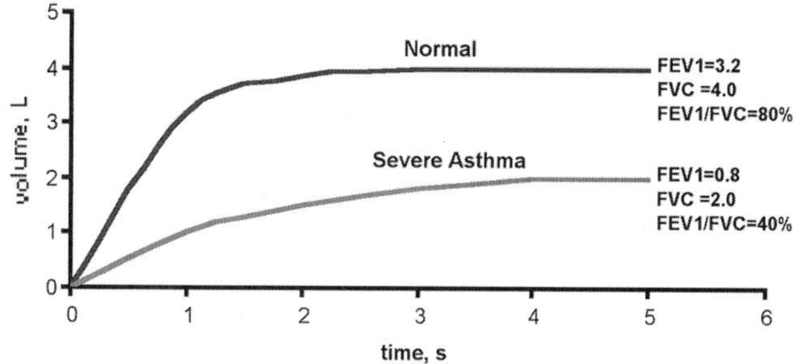

Fig. 44.2. Spirometric comparison of normal and severe asthma. FEV_1, forced expiratory volume in 1 second; FVC, forced vital capacity.

of a spirometer). Healthy persons normally can expel at least 75% of their FVC in the first second. Deceases in the FEV_1/FVC ratio indicate obstruction, and a decrease below 40% indicates severe asthma (17,18).

A more convenient way to measure airway obstruction is to determine the peak expiratory flow (PEF) rate. The PEF rate correlates well with the FEV_1; can be determined using inexpensive, handheld, peak flow meters; and is easily and simply measured at home. The PEF rate is the maximal rate of flow that is produced through forced expiration. Peak flow meters come with a chart that lists predicted PEF rates based on the patient's age, gender, and height. The patient or clinician can then compare the determined PEF rate with the predicted PEF rate and make an evaluation regarding the severity of an asthmatic attack. The PEF rate or the FEV_1, along with the frequency of daytime and nighttime symptoms, forms the basis for the classification of the severity of an asthmatic attack. Table 44.2 shows the severity classification of asthma established by the NIH Expert Panel Report 2: Guidelines for the Diagnosis and Management of Asthma (EPR-2) (5).

GENERAL THERAPEUTIC APPROACHES TO THE TREATMENT AND MANAGEMENT OF ASTHMA

Asthma symptoms are caused by bronchoconstriction and inflammation, and approaches to treatment are directed at both these physiological problems. Therefore, drugs that affect adrenergic/cholinergic bronchial smooth muscle tone and drugs that inhibit the inflammatory process are used to treat and control asthma symptoms. In the normal lung, bronchiole smooth muscle tone results from the balance between the bronchoconstrictive effects of the cholinergic system and the bronchodilating effects of the adrenergic system on the smooth muscles of the bronchioles. Pharmacological treatment of asthmatic bronchoconstriction consists of either increasing adrenergic tone with an adrenergic agonist or inhibiting cholinergic tone with an anticholinergic agent.

The inflammatory effects seen in asthma result from the release of physiologically active chemicals from a variety of inflammatory cells. Pharmacological treatment, therefore, uses anti-inflammatory drugs (corticosteroids), mast cell stabilizers, leukotriene modifiers, and IgE monoclonal antibodies. Figure 44.3 depicts the overall approach to the pharmacological treatment of asthma.

Therapeutic management of asthma requires the use of quickly acting drugs to relieve an acute attack as well as drugs that control symptoms over the long-term. The current approach to asthma management utilizes a stepwise approach (5). The quick-reliever medication is almost always an inhaled short-acting β_2-adrenergic agonist, whereas controller drugs are inhaled corticosteroids, long-acting β_2-agonists, leukotriene modifiers, cromolyn sodium, and/or methylxanthines. The dose, route of administration, and number of controller drugs depends on the severity of the patient's disease. Table 44.3 shows the stepwise approach to asthma management based on disease severity.

THERAPEUTIC CLASSES OF DRUGS USED TO TREAT ASTHMA AND CHRONIC OBSTRUCTIVE PULMONARY DISEASE

β_2-Adrenergic Agonists

Introduction

What structural features make a drug an adrenergic agonist? What features make it a selective β_2-agonist? The answers to these questions lie in the structural relationship

Table 44.2. Classification of Asthma Severity (5)

	Step 1 (Mild Intermittent)	Step 2 (Mild Persistent)	Step 3 (Moderate Persistent)	Step 4 (Severe Persistent)
Frequency of symptoms				
Days	≤2/week	3–6/week	Daily	Continual
Nights	≤2/month	3–4/month	≥5/month	Frequent
PEF or FEV_1	≥80%	≥80%	>60% <80%	≤60%
PEF or FEV_1 variability	<20%	20–30%	>30%	>30%

FEV_1, forced expiratory volume in 1 second; PEF, peak expiratory flow.

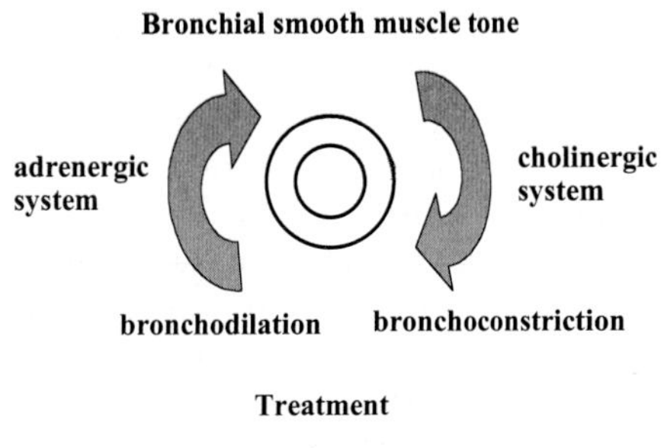

Treatment

Increase adrenergic tone by adding an adrenergic agonist
Decrease cholinergic tone by adding an anticholinergic

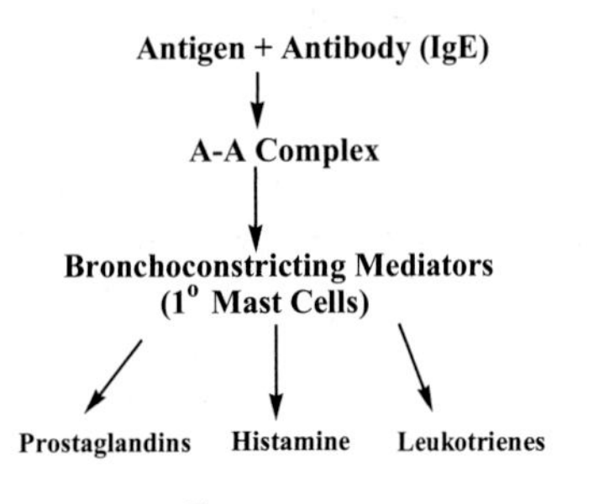

Treatment

Corticosteroids; Mast Cell Stabilizers; Leukotriene modifiers and monoclonal anti-IgE antibody

Fig. 44.3. Overview of pharmacological treatment for asthma.

Table 44.3. Stepwise Medication Management of Asthma

All Patients: Short-Acting Inhaled β_2-Agonist as Needed for Acute Episodes

Severity Classification	Long-Term Control
Mild Intermittent (Step 1)	No daily medication needed A course of systemic steroid may be necessary to treat a severe episode
Mild Persistent (Step 2)	Low-dose inhaled steroid Other treatment options: Cromolyn/nedocromil OR Leukotriene modifier OR Sustained-release theophylline
Moderate Persistent (Step 3)	Low- to medium-dose inhaled steroid PLUS an inhaled long-acting β_2-agonist Other treatment options: Medium-dose inhaled steroid PLUS cromolyn/nedocromil OR Medium-dose inhaled steroid PLUS leukotriene modifier OR Medium-dose inhaled steroid PLUS sustained-release theophylline
Severe Persistent (Step 4)	High-dose inhaled steroid PLUS a long-acting bronchodilator PLUS one or more of the following: Oral long-acting β_2-agonist Sustained-release theophylline Oral steroid Leukotriene modifier

of a drug to that of norepinephrine (NE), the physiological neurotransmitter of the sympathetic branch of the autonomic nervous system. Drugs that act on postsynaptic sympathetic receptors in the same way as NE are called sympathomimetics or, more commonly, adrenergic agonists. The related natural agonist epinephrine (EPI; adrenalin) is the predominant adrenergic hormone produced in the chromaffin cells of the adrenal medulla. Epinephrine interacts just like NE at all adrenergic receptors.

Chemistry and Biochemistry of Norepinephrine and Epinephrine

Chemically, NE is classified as a catecholamine. A catechol is a 1,2-dihydroxybenzene, and NE is a β-hydroxyethylaminodihydroxybenzene. Epinephrine is the N-methyl derivative of NE, and they both have acidic and basic functional groups. Physiologically, however, they behave as a base, being more than 90% protonated at pH 7.4 (pK_a = 9.6) and functioning as an ionized acid.

HO, HO, OH, NHR

Norepinephrine R = H
Epinephrine R = CH_3

Norepinephrine is biosynthesized in the neurons of both the central nervous system and the autonomic nervous system, whereas EPI is formed in the chromaffin cells of the adrenal medulla. Both NE and EPI are derived from L-tyrosine by a series of enzyme-catalyzed reactions (Fig. 44.4 depicts the overall pathway). L-Tyrosine hydroxylase hydroxylates the meta position of L-tyrosine, producing L-dihydroxyphenylalanine (L-DOPA) and is the rate-limiting step. The L-DOPA is then decarboxylated by L-aromatic amino acid decarboxylase to form dopamine, which is converted to NE by the action of dopamine β-hydroxylase. Dopamine β-hydroxylase occurs in storage vesicles of the nerve ending, and the NE formed is stored there until it is released into the synaptic cleft. In the chromaffin cells, the formed NE is converted to EPI by N-methylation catalyzed by phenylethanolamine N-methyltransferase.

Termination of Neurotransmission

Stimulated adrenergic neurons release NE into the synaptic cleft, which then binds reversibly with receptors to produce a characteristic adrenergic response. Termination of the adrenergic response occurs primarily by reuptake (uptake-1) into the presynaptic neuron; however, diffusion away from the receptors and extracellular metabolism also occurs to a limited extent. The NE that is taken back up into the presynaptic neuron is

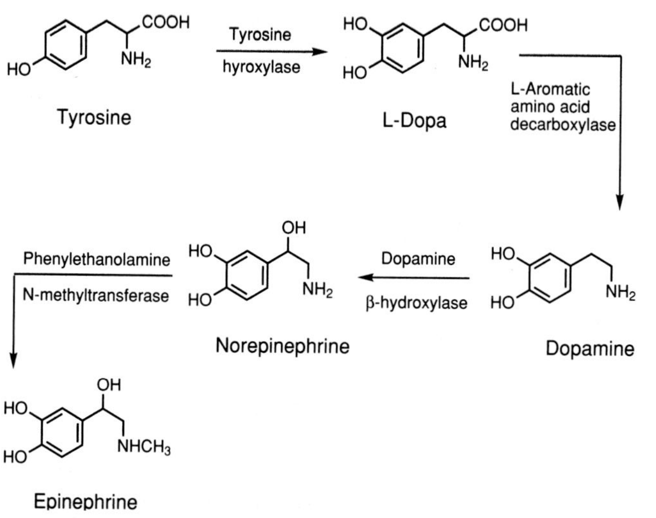

Tyrosine
Tyrosine hyroxylase
L-Dopa
L-Aromatic amino acid decarboxylase
Dopamine
Dopamine β-hydroxylase
Norepinephrine
Phenylethanolamine N-methyltransferase
Epinephrine

Fig. 44.4. The biosynthesis of norepinephrine and epinephrine from tyrosine.

either used again as a neurotransmitter or is metabolized by mitochondrial monoamine oxidase (MAO). The extraneuronal NE that diffuses away from the neurons is either metabolized by catechol O-methyl transferase (COMT) in situ or reaches the circulatory system and is metabolized by COMT and MAO in various tissues, most importantly the liver, gastrointestinal (GI) tract, and the lungs. Figure 44.5 depicts the possible metabolic pathways for both NE and EPI. It is important to note that agonists that are resistant to MAO and/or COMT have greater oral availability and longer duration of action.

Adrenergic Receptors

The adrenergic receptors have long been pharmacologically classified as α or β based on their interaction with NE, EPI, and the adrenergic prototype, isoproterenol (19).

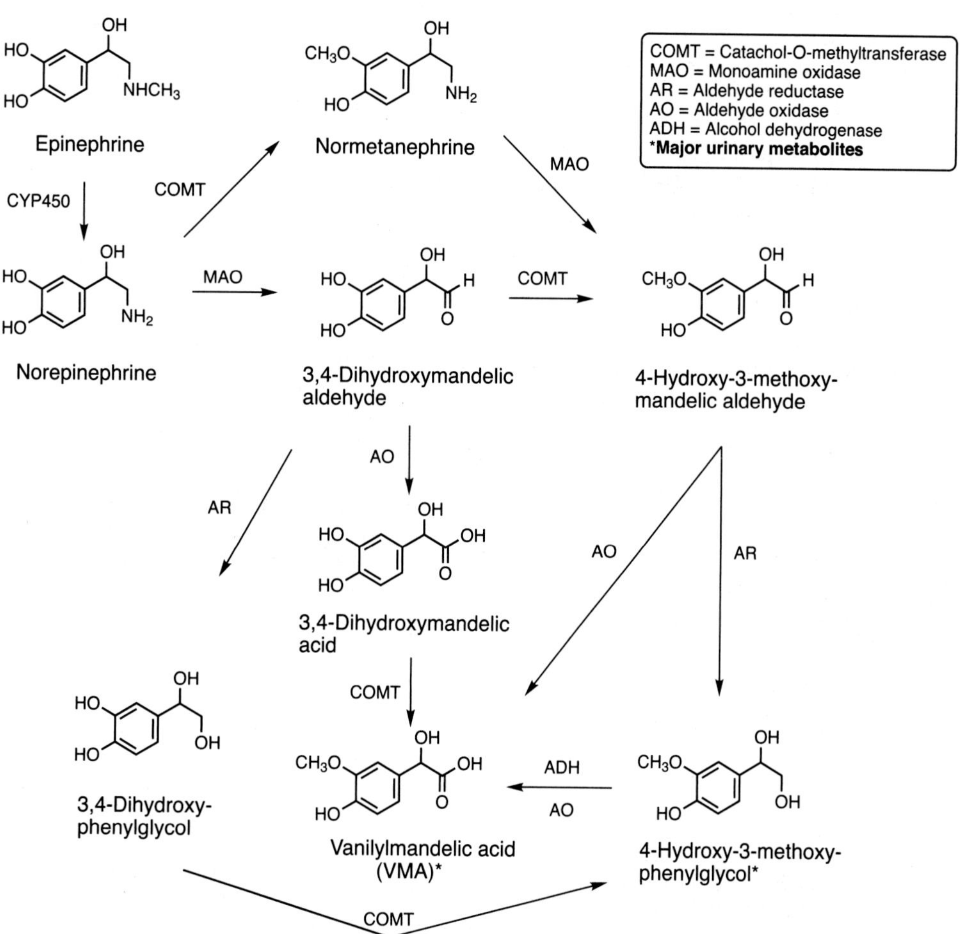

Fig. 44.5. Metabolic pathways for norepinephrine and epinephrine.

HO, HO, OH, NHR

Norepinephrine (NE)	R = H
Epinephrine (EPI)	R = CH_3
Isoproterenol (ISO)	R = $HC(CH_3)_2$

As mentioned above, NE and EPI are nonselective and interact with all adrenergic receptors, but isoproterenol selectively interacts only with the β-receptors. The adrenergic receptors have been further divided into three groups, α_1, α_2 and β, each of which has been further divided into three receptor subtypes based on their organ distribution and physiologic activities (20). Therefore, there are now a total of nine adrenergic receptor subtypes, but the most important in relation to the treatment of asthma and chronic obstructive pulmonary disease (COPD) are the β_1 and β_2 subtypes that are found primarily in the heart and the lung, respectively. As may be deduced from Table 44.4, adrenergic agonists that are selective for the β_2 subtype will cause bronchial dilation and might be expected to relieve the bronchospasm of an asthmatic attack. Nonselective β-agonists, however, will have stimulatory cardiac effects and, therefore, would have limited use in cardiac patients with asthma.

Adrenergic Receptor Structure and Agonist Interactions

The adrenergic receptors are a member of the guanine nucleotide binding regulatory protein–coupled receptor family more commonly referred to as G protein–coupled receptors. They affect biological activity by releasing secondary messenger molecules inside the cell after they bind an extracellular agonist. This process usually is referred to as signal transduction and is common to hormone and neurotransmitter receptors found in the muscarinic, serotonergic, dopaminergic, and adrenergic systems. All the G protein–coupled receptors are structurally similar, being comprised of seven transmembrane

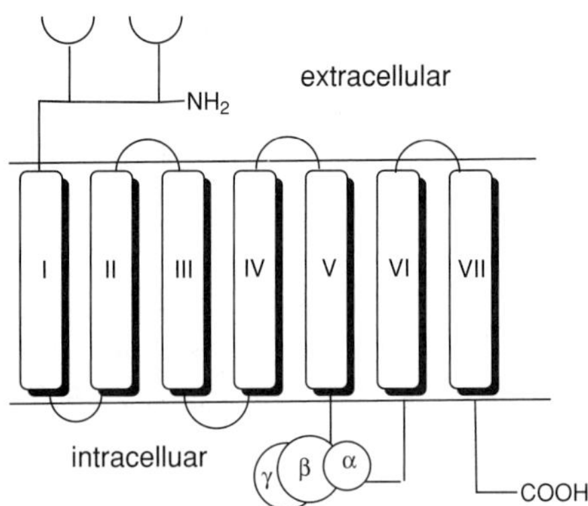

Fig. 44.6. Representation of the G protein–coupled receptor.

α-helix bundles. The helices are connected by short stretches of hydrophilic residues, which form multiple loops in the intracellular and extracellular domains. The G proteins generally are bound to the third intracellular loop and imbedded in the inner membrane (Fig. 44.6).

All the β-adrenergic receptors are coupled to adenylate cyclase via specific G stimulatory proteins (Gs). When agonist binds to the β-adrenergic receptors, the α-subunit migrates through the membrane and stimulates adenylate cyclase to form cyclic adenosine monophosphate (cAMP) from adenosine triphosphate. Once formed in the cell, cAMP activates protein kinase A, which catalyzes the phosphorylation of numerous proteins, thereby regulating their activity and leading to characteristic cellular responses. The intracellular enzyme phosphodiesterase (PDE) hydrolyzes cAMP to form AMP and terminates its action (Fig. 44.7).

A great deal of research has been done to identify the binding residues of the adrenergic receptors. Molecular modeling methods have been used to construct three-dimensional models for agonist complexes with the β-adrenergic receptors. The picture that has emerged is that NE binds ionically via its protonated amine to Asp-113 in helix 3 and hydrogen bonds to both hydroxyls of the catechol ring with Ser-204 and Ser-207 in helix 5. That binding limits configurational and rotational freedoms, which allows reinforcing van der Waals interactions between the aromatic ring with residues Phe-290 in helix 6 and Val-114 in helix 3. The N-alkyl substituents are believed to fit into a

Table 44.4. Physiological Response in Relationship to β-receptor Subtype and Organ Site

Receptor Subtype	Organ Location	Response
β_1	Heart	Increased rate and force Increased conduction velocity
β_2	Bronchiole smooth muscle	Dilation
	Intestine	Decreased motility
	Liver	Increased gluconeogenesis Increased glycogenolysis
	Uterus	Contraction
	Lungs	Bronchial dilation

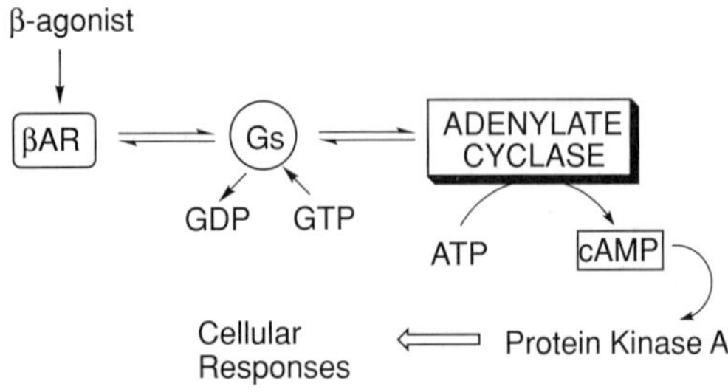

Fig. 44.7. β-Adrenergic receptor G protein coupling to adenylate cyclase.

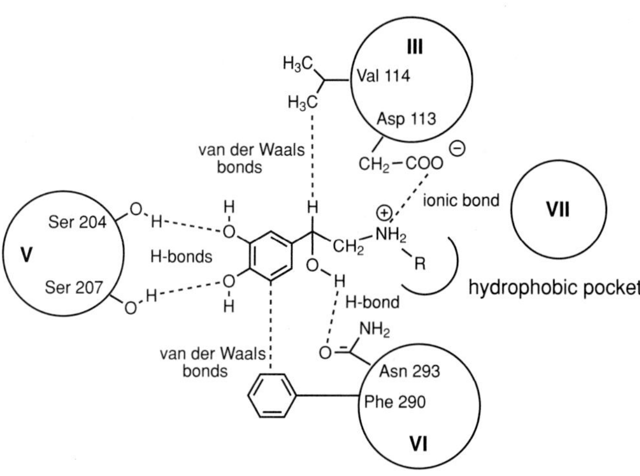

Fig. 44.8. Ligand binding to key residues in the adrenergic receptor.

pocket formed between aliphatic residues in helix 6 and helix 7. Stereochemistry also plays an important role in receptor binding. The β-carbon in NE/EPI is chiral and can be either *R* or *S* in configuration. Endogenous NE/EPI exists in the *R* configuration so that the β-hydroxyl oriented toward the receptor Asn-293. (Fig. 44.8) (21,22).

Adrenergic Agonist Structure–Activity Relationships

The fundamental pharmacophore for all adrenergic agonists is a substituted β-phenylethylamine (Table 44.5). The nature and number of substituents on the pharmacophore influences whether an analogue will be direct-acting or indirect-acting or have a mixture of direct and indirect action. In addition, the nature and number of substituents also influences the specificity for

Table 44.5. Relationship of Substituents to Adrenergic Agonist Mechanism of Action

Adrenergic agonist pharmacophore

Action	R_3	R_4	R_5
Direct[1]	OH	OH	OH
or	OH	OH	H
Indirect[2]	H	H	H
or	H	H	OH
Mixed[3]	H	OH	OH
or	OH	H	OH

[1] β-OH (R_3) necessary for direct action, optimal if in the R-configuration; *m*-OH (R_4) also necessary for direct action; *p*-OH (R_5) can be an H or OH, however catechol optimal.
[2] Without the catechol OH's (R_4 & R_5) or β-OH (R_3) there is little affinity for the β-receptor; *p*-OH doesn't contribute to β-receptor binding affinity.
[3] β-OH (R_3) or *m*-OH (R_4) contribute to direct action.

the β-receptor subtypes. Direct-acting adrenergic agonists bind the β-adrenergic receptors just like NE/EPI, producing a sympathetic response. Indirect-acting agonists cause their effect by a number of mechanisms. They can stimulate the release of NE from the presynaptic terminal, inhibit the reuptake of released NE, or inhibit the metabolic degradation of NE by neuronal MAO (i.e., MAO inhibitors). Mixed-acting agonists work as their name implies (i.e., they have both direct and indirect abilities). Table 44.5 shows the relationship between substituents and the mechanisms of action by adrenergic agonists.

Relationship of Structure to α- or β-Receptor Selectivity

The substituents on the amino group (R_1) determines α- or β-receptor selectivity. As was noted above, when the N-substituent was changed from hydrogen (NE) to methyl (EPI) to isopropyl, the receptor affinity went from nonselective for NE/EPI to β-selective for isopropyl. Therefore, one can say that the larger the bulk of the N-substituent, the greater the selectivity for the β-receptor. As a matter of fact, if R_1 is *t*-butyl or aralkyl, there is complete loss of α-receptor affinity, and the β-receptor affinity shows preference for the β_2-receptor. It must be said that receptor selectivity is dose related, and when the dose is high enough, all selectivity can be lost.

Substituents on the α-carbon (R_2) other than hydrogen will show an increased duration of action, because they make the compound resistant to metabolism by MAO. In addition, if the substituent is ethyl, there is a selectivity for the β_2-receptor, which is enhanced by a bulky N-substituent. Interestingly, α-methyl substitution shows a slight β-receptor enhancement and only for the *S*-configuration.

For an adrenergic agonist to demonstrate significant β_2-receptor selectivity, there needs to be in addition to the bulky N-substituent an appropriately substituted phenyl ring. The currently marketed adrenergic agonists contain a resorcinol ring, a salicyl alcohol moiety, or a m-formamide group (Fig. 44.9). In addition, these ring configurations are resistant to COMT metabolism and will increase the duration of action.

Specific Adrenergic Drugs Used to Treat Asthma

For a more detailed discussion of the chemistry of adrenergic agents, see Chapter 13.

Resorcinol   Salicyl alcohol   N-formamide

Fig. 44.9. Ring configurations that contribute to β_2-receptor selectivity.

Epinephrine (Adrenalin)

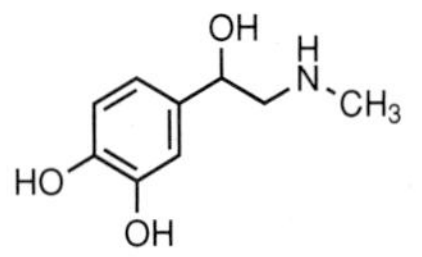

Epinephrine (Epi Pen)

The combination of the catechol nucleus, the β-hydroxyl group, and the N-methyl give EPI a direct action and a strong affinity for all adrenergic receptors. Epinephrine and all other catechols are chemically susceptible to oxygen and other oxidizing agents, especially in the presence of bases and light, quickly decomposing to inactive quinones. Therefore, all catechol drugs are stabilized with antioxidants and dispensed in air-tight amber containers.

Epinephrine is ultimately metabolized by COMT and MAO to 3-methoxy-4-hydroxy-mandelic acid (vanillylmandelic acid), which is excreted as the sulfate or glucuronide in the urine (Fig. 44.5). Only a very small amount is excreted unchanged.

Epinephrine usually is administered slowly by intravenous (IV) injection to relieve acute asthmatic attacks not controlled by other treatments. Intravenous injection produces an immediate response. Use of EPI with drugs that enhance cardiac arrhythmias (digitalis or quinidine) is not recommended. Tricyclic antidepressants and MAO inhibitors will potentiate the effects of EPI on the heart. Epinephrine should be used with caution in individuals suffering from hyperthyroidism, cardiovascular disease, hypertension, or diabetes. Adverse effects include palpitations, tachycardia, sweating, nausea and vomiting, respiratory difficulty, dizziness, tremor, apprehension, and anxiety.

Isoetharine Hydrochloride

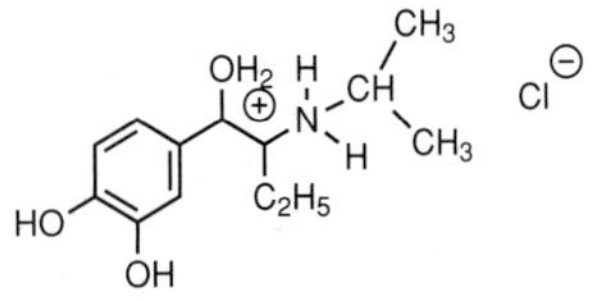

Isoetharine hydrochloride

The α-ethyl group confers β_2-selectivity, and the β-hydroxyl group and catechol nucleus makes this a direct-acting drug. It is susceptible to COMT metabolism; however, the α-ethyl group inhibits MAO. Therefore, one would expect some oral activity.

Isoetharine is dispensed as a solution only for inhalation administration to treat reversible bronchospasm of asthma. It has fallen into relative disuse, because with high doses, there is a significant incidence of cardiovascular (β_1-receptor) adverse effects and it has a low β_2-receptor potency compared to newer β_2-selective agonists. It has a 2- to 4-minute onset of action when inhaled and a duration of action of 3 hours. Isoetharine has adverse effects similar to those of EPI, including palpitations, tachycardia, nausea and vomiting, dizziness, tremor, and headache. Isoetharine may cause decreased levels of theophylline when coadministered. Cardiovascular effects are a concern when isoetharine is taken with other asthma drugs.

Metaproterenol Sulfate

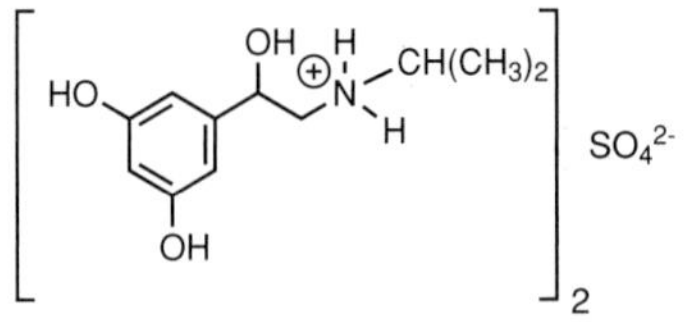

Metaproterenol sulfate
(Alupent, Metaprel)

Metaproterenol is a direct-acting resorcinol analogue of isoproterenol. The N-isopropyl is β-directing, and the combination with the resorcinol ring system enhances the selectivity for the β_2-receptors. It is the least potent of the β_2-selective agonists, however, most likely because of the poor β_2-selectivity of the isopropyl group. It has good oral bioavailability being resistant to COMT and only slowly metabolized by MAO. When administered orally, it has an onset of approximately 30 minutes with a 4-hour duration. Inhaled metaproterenol can have an onset as quick as 5 minutes; however, it can be as long as 30 minutes in susceptible individuals. Metaproterenol is available in tablet, syrup, and inhalation dosage forms and is recommended for bronchial asthma attacks and treatment of acute asthmatic attacks in children 6 years of age and older (5% solution for inhalation only). Metaproterenol has the same adverse effect profile as other adrenergic agonists, but with a decreased incidence of arrhythmias.

Terbutaline Sulfate

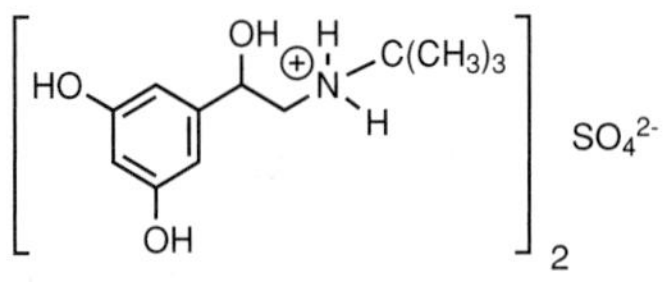

Terbutaline sulfate
(Brethine, Brethaire)

Terbutaline is the N-*t*-butyl analogue of metaproterenol and, as such, would be expected to have a more potent β_2-selectivity. When compared to metaproterenol, terbutaline has a threefold greater potency at the β_2-receptor. Like metaproterenol, it is resistant to COMT and slowly metabolized by MAO, therefore having good oral bioavailability with similar onset and duration. Terbutaline is available as tablets and solutions for injection and inhalation. Adverse effects are similar to other

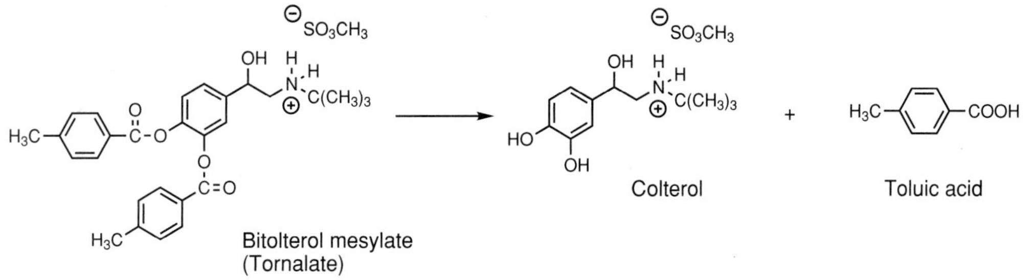

Bitolterol mesylate (Tornalate) → Colterol + Toluic acid

Fig. 44.10. Esterase hydrolysis of bitolterol.

direct-acting β_2-selective agonists, however, with a greater incidence of palpitations.

Bitolterol Mesylate

Bitolterol is a prodrug that releases colterol on activation by esterases in the lung (Fig. 44.10). Colterol is a direct-acting agonist, and the N-*t*-butyl group makes it β_2-selective with a binding potency equivalent to that of isoetharine and terbutaline. The ester form is lipophilic, which helps to keep it local in the lung and resistant to COMT, which tends to increase its duration of action. Onset begins 2 to 4 minutes after administration, and the effect can last as long as 8 hours. It has a adverse effect profile similar to that of other β_2-selective agonists, with less drowsiness and restlessness compared to other direct-acting agonists.

Albuterol

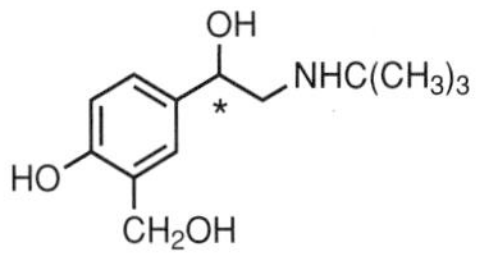

dl-Albuterol (Proventil, Ventolin)
Levalbuterol (Xopenex)

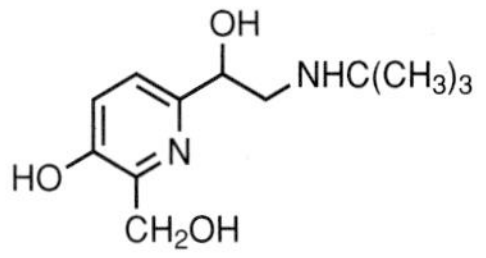

Pirbuterol (Maxair)

Albuterol has the N-*t*-butyl and a salicyl alcohol phenyl ring, which gives it optimal β_2-selectivity. It is resistant to COMT and slowly metabolized by MAO, giving it good oral bioavailability. Its onset by inhalation is within 5 minutes, with a duration of action between 4 and 8 hours. It currently is the drug of choice for relief of the acute bronchospasm of an asthmatic attack. Levalbuterol is the *R*-(−)-isomer of albuterol and is available only in solution to be administered via nebulizer. Because it is the active isomer, the dose is fourfold less than that of albuterol. Pirbuterol is the pyridine isostere of albuterol. It has pharmacokinetics similar to albuterol but is half as potent at the β_2-receptor. Pirbuterol is only available as an inhaler, whereas albuterol comes in tablet, syrup, solution, and aerosol formulations. Adverse effects of pirbuterol are nervousness, tremor, and headache, which is less than the profile for albuterol, which adds nausea, vomiting, dizziness, hypertension, insomnia, tachycardia, and palpitations.

Salmeterol Xinafoate

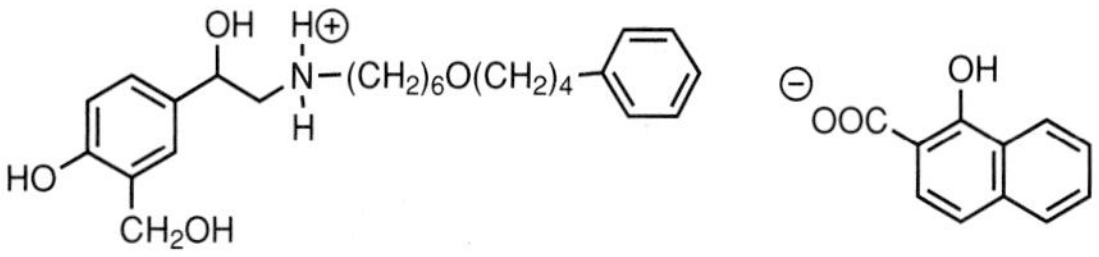

Salmeterol xinafoate
(Serevent diskus)

Salmeterol has an N-phenylbutoxyhexyl substituent in combination with a β-hydroxyl group and a salicyl phenyl ring for optimal direct-acting β_2-receptor selectivity and potency. Salmeterol has the greatest receptor affinity of all the adrenergic agonists. It is resistant to both MAO and COMT and that, together with its increased lipophilicity, gives salmeterol a long duration of action. It is postulated that the phenylbutoxyhexyl N-substituent binds outside of the receptor site and keeps the active pharmacophore moiety in position for prolonged stimulations. It is available only as a powder for inhalation, with a 20-minute onset of action, which lasts for 12 hours. It is used as a controller for the long-term treatment of asthma and is not recommended for quick relief of an acute attack. It also is available in combination with the steroid fluticasone proprionate (Advair Diskus). There was a small but significant increase in asthma-related deaths among patients receiving salmeterol during a large clinical trial. Subgroup analyses suggested that the risk may be greater in black patients compared with Caucasian patients (23).

Formoterol Fumarate

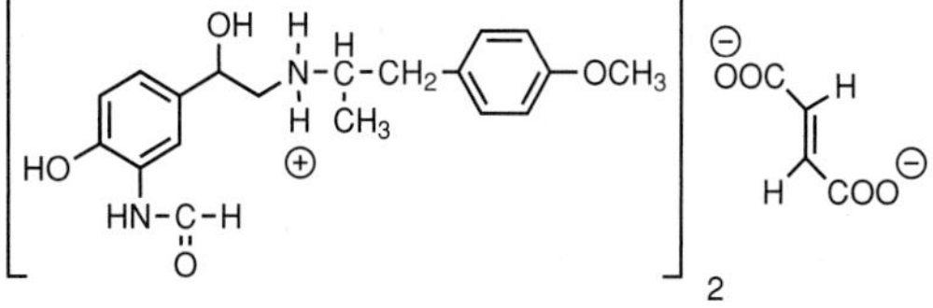

Formoterol fumarate
(Foradil aerosolizer)

Formoterol has a β-directing N-isopropyl-*p*-methoxyphenyl group and a unique *m*-formamide and *p*-hydroxyphenyl ring, which provides selectivity for β_2-receptors. It is resistant to MAO and COMT, making it a long-acting agonist. Formoterol has a more rapid onset as compared to salmeterol while maintaining the same long duration of action.

This is believed to result from formoterol's greater water solubility, allowing it to get to the receptor sites faster, whereas its moderate lipophilicity keeps it in the lungs longer. It is indicated for the long-term maintenance treatment of asthma and for patients with symptoms of nocturnal asthma who require regular treatment with inhaled, short-acting, β_2-agonists. It is not indicated for patients whose asthma can be managed by occasional use of inhaled, short-acting, β_2-agonists. Formoterol is available only as a powder in a capsule for administration via the aerosolizer. Patients should be cautioned not to take the capsules orally and to keep them in a safe place to avoid accidental oral administration.

Fenoterol Hydrobromide

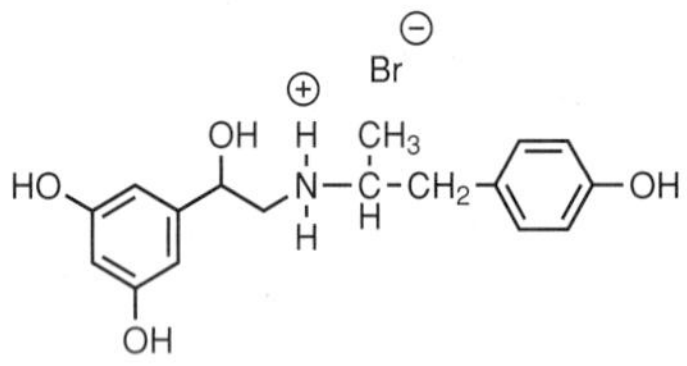

Fenoterol hydrobromide
(Berotec)

Fenoterol is an investigational drug in the United States that has been in use in Europe since 1970. It is the *p*-hydroxyphenyl derivative of metaproteronol, and the combination of the resorcinol ring and the bulky *p*-hydroxyphenyl isopropyl group on the nitrogen gives fenoterol significant β_2-receptor selectivity. It has approximately half the affinity for the β_2-receptor as compared to albuterol. The resorcinol ring is resistant to COMT metabolism, and the bulky nitrogen substituent greatly retards MOA metabolism as well giving fenoterol a reasonable oral bioavailability with pharmacokinetics similar to albuterol (i.e., rapid onset and a 4- to 6-hour duration of action after oral inhalation).

Antimuscarinics

Introduction

Acetylcholine is the endogenous neurotransmitter of the parasympathetic nervous system. The parasympathetic nerve fibers are found in both the autonomic and central nervous systems. These fibers are classified into those that are stimulated by muscarine and those that are stimulated by nicotine. Nicotine, an alkaloid from *Nicotiana tabacum*, stimulates preganglionic fibers in both the parasympathetic and sympathetic systems as well as the somatic motor fibers of the skeletal system. Muscarine, an alkaloid from the poisonous mushroom *Amanita muscaria*, stimulates postganglionic parasympathetic fibers with receptors found on autonomic effector cells. The central nervous system has fibers that contain both nicotinic and muscarinic receptors. In this chapter, we are most interested in the drugs that block the muscarinic fibers (antimuscarinics), because blocking them results in cardiovascular, mydriatic, antispasmodic, antisecretory, and bronchodilatory effects.

Biochemistry and Metabolism of Acetylcholine

Acetylcholine is the ester formed between acetylcoenzyme A and choline by the action of choline acetyltransferase in the presynaptic cholinergic neurons. Most of the choline used to biosynthesize acetylcholine comes via uptake from the synaptic space, where it is produced from the hydrolysis of acetylcholine by acetylcholinesterase, a serine hydroxylase. Additionally, some choline is biosynthesized in the presynaptic neurons from serine (Fig. 44.11). Once formed, acetylcholine is stored in vesicles from which it is released on stimulation.

The duration of action of acetylcholine is very short, because it is rapidly hydrolyzed by the acetylcholinesterase present in the synaptic space. This hydrolysis is a straightforward splitting of the acetylcholine into acetic acid and choline; however, the way this happens is very interesting and begins by the proper binding of acetylcholine in the catalytic pocket. Binding of the cationic N-end to tyrosine, glutamate, and tryptophan via a combination of π-cation and electrostatic forces places the acyl head of acetylcholine in the correct position for attack by the serine hydroxyl group (Fig. 44.12).

Once properly bound, the hydrolysis actually involves two hydrolytic steps. The first step is the hydrolysis of acetylcholine by nucleophilic attack at the carbonyl carbon by the serine hydroxyl group, which liberates choline and leaves the enzyme acetylated. A triad formed between glutamine, histidine, and the serine at the catalytic site activates the serine for the nucleophilic attack. The second step is the hydrolysis of the acetylated enzyme by water to regenerate the free enzyme. The water is activated by hydrogen-bonding to the histidine residue, which increases the nucleophilic character of

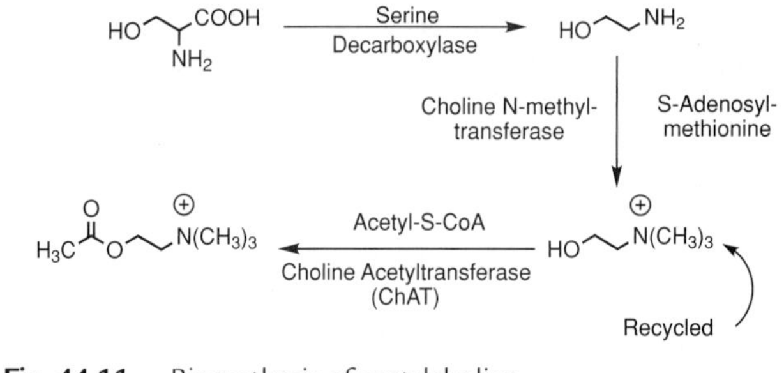

Serine Decarboxylase

Choline N-methyltransferase

S-Adenosylmethionine

Acetyl-S-CoA

Choline Acetyltransferase (ChAT)

Recycled

Fig. 44.11. Biosynthesis of acetylcholine.

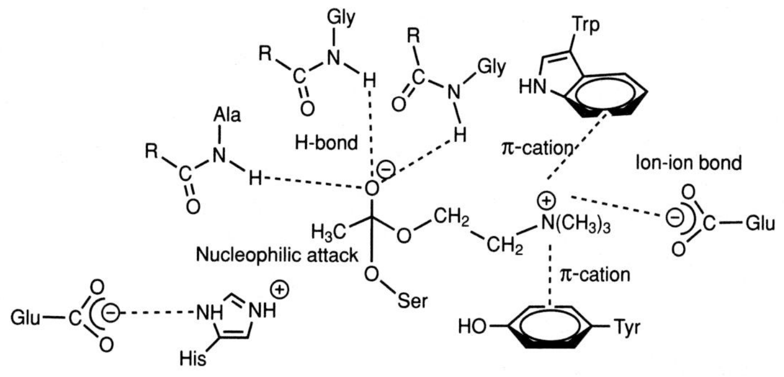

Fig. 44.12. Binding of acetylcholine in the catalytic site of acetylcholinesterase.

the oxygen of water. The activated water attacks the electrophilic carbonyl carbon of the acetyl group to generate acetate and regenerate the free hydroxyl group of serine (Fig. 44.13) (24).

Muscarinic Receptor Structure and Agonist/Antagonist Interactions

The muscarinic receptors are considered to be part of the superfamily of G protein–coupled receptors. They consist of seven transmembrane helices and are linked to their G protein through interaction with the second and third intracellular loops (25). There are five subtypes of receptor, designated M_{1-5}, and the odd-numbered receptors (M_1, M_3, and M_5) are coupled to the G_q/G_{11} class. This class of receptors activate intracellular phospholipase C to hydrolyze phosphatidylinositol 4,5-diphosphate to diacylglycerol and inositol triphosphate as intracellular messengers. The even-numbered receptors (M_2 and M_4) are coupled to the G_i/G_o class, which mediates the inhibition of adenylate cyclase (Fig. 44.14).

Table 44.6 lists the physiologic action of the M_3 receptors. Because the M_3 receptors cause bronchiole constriction, they counterbalance the bronchiole dilation of the β_2-adrenergic receptors in the lung, resulting in maintenance of bronchiole tone. This forms the basis for the therapeutic use of inhaled antimuscarinics, because they block cholinergic bronchiole constriction and allow

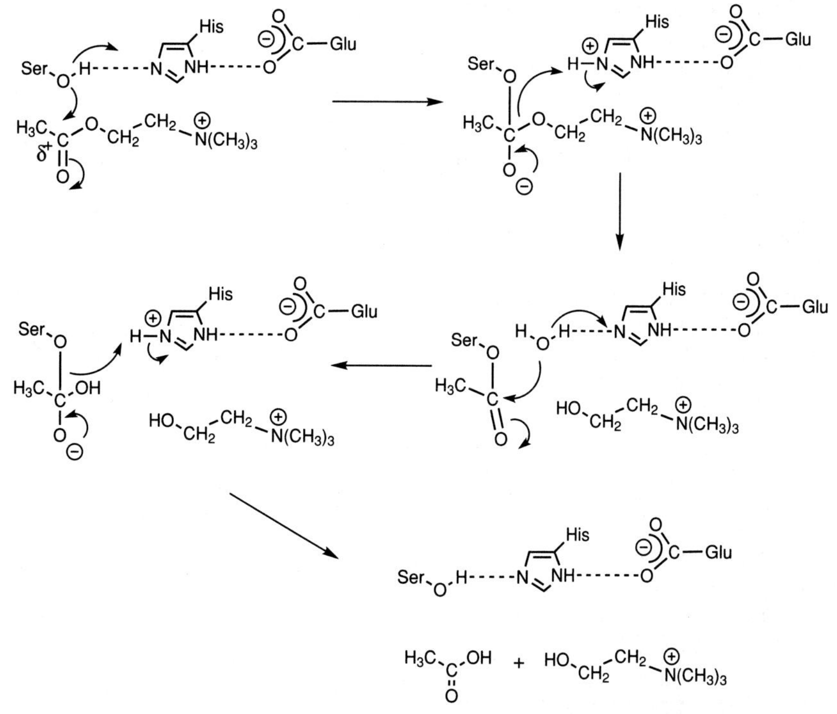

Fig. 44.13. The role of the triad formed between glutamine, histidine, and serine in the hydrolysis of acetylcholine by acetylcholinesterase.

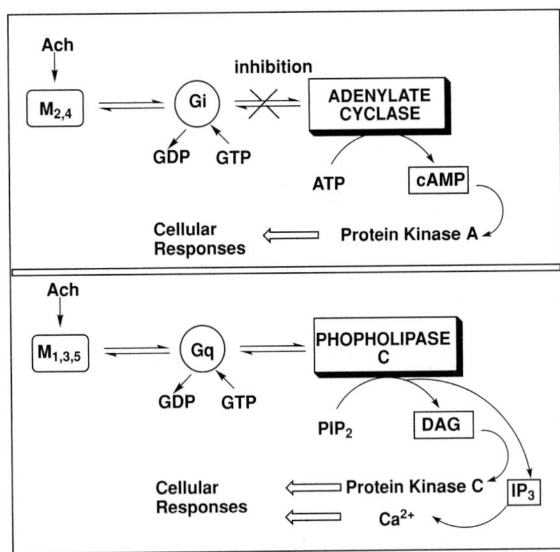

Fig. 44.14. Comparison of the role of G protein in odd- and even-numbered muscarinic receptors.

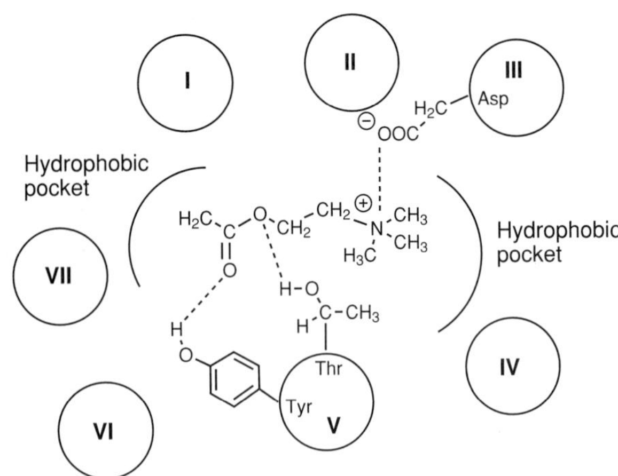

Fig. 44.15. Acetylcholine binding to residues in the muscarinic receptor.

adrenergic bronchiole dilation to help overcome the pulmonary constriction associated with an asthmatic attack.

Affinity labeling and mutagenic studies have established that acetylcholine binds to its receptor in a narrow region of the circular arrangement of the seven transmembrane helices approximately 10 to 15 angstroms away from the membrane surface. The cationic nitrogen of acetylcholine binds to the anionic carboxylate of an Asp located in helix 3 (26). As depicted in Figure 44.15, the ionic interaction is stabilized by hydrogen-bonding with a Tyr in helix 5 and a Thr in helix 5. It is postulated that muscarinic antagonists (see *Structure–Activity Relationships of Antimuscarinic Agents* below) bind to the Asp and contain hydrophobic substituents that bind to a hydrophobic pocket in the receptor, which does not allow the change in conformation needed to transfer the agonist signal to the coupled G protein (27).

Table 44.6. Physiological Action Associated with the M_3 Muscarinic Receptors

Organ	M_3-Receptor Effect
Eye	
Iris circular muscle	Contracts
Ciliary muscle	Contracts
Heart	
Sinoatrial node	Decelerates
Atrial contractility	Decelerates
Bronchiole smooth muscle	Contracts
Gastrointestinal tract	
Smooth muscle	Contracts
Secretions	Increases
Sphincters	Relaxes

From Katzung B. Introduction to autonomic pharmacology. In: Katzung B, ed. Basic and Clinical Pharmacology. 8th Ed. New York: Lange Medical Books/McGraw-Hill, 2001:75–191; with permission.

Structure–Activity Relationships of Antimuscarinic Agents

The structural pharmacophore for all antimuscarinic drugs is an acetylcholine analogue in which the acetyl methyl group is substituted with at least one phenyl ring. This pharmacophore generally is classified as an amino alcohol ester. The ester function can be replaced with different moieties to produce different classes of antimuscarinic drugs. When the ester function is replaced by an ether function, the amino alcohol ether class is produced. When the ester function is replaced by a saturated carbon, the amino alcohols are obtained when R_1 is a hydroxyl group, and the amino amides are obtained when R_1 is an amido group (Fig. 44.16).

The classic chemical prototype for the antimuscarinics is atropine, an alkaloid from *Atropa belladonna.* Buried within its structure is the amino alcohol ester pharmacophore, where R_1 is a hydroxymethyl group, R_2 is a hydrogen, and the nitrogen is part of a bicyclic ring system called tropine (Fig. 44.17).

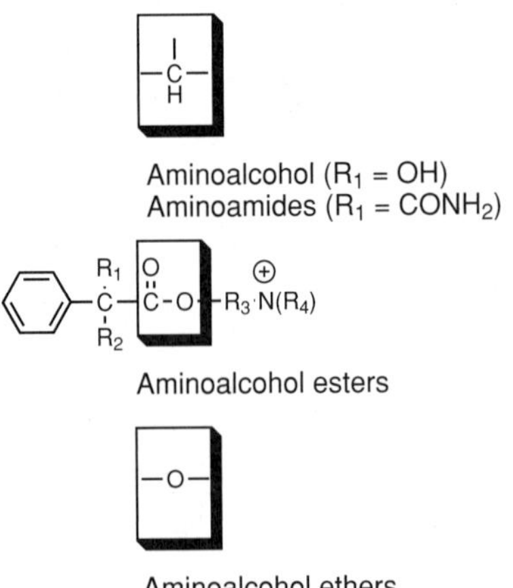

Fig. 44.16. The pharmacophore for all classes of antimuscarinic agents.

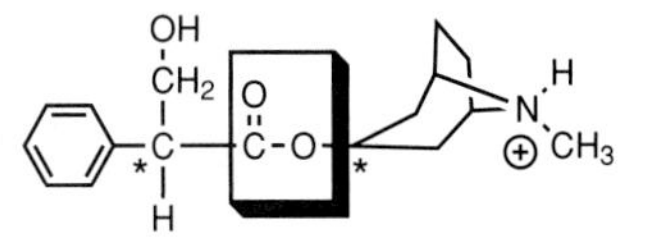

Fig. 44.17. Atropine is an example of the amino alcohol ester class of antimuscarinic agents.

Although atropine does not have a quaternary nitrogen, the nitrogen is protonated at physiologic pH; therefore, it can bind to the anionic Asp residue in the muscarinic receptor. The nitrogen is not absolutely necessary for activity and can be replaced with a carbon atom. This leads to a substantial lose of binding affinity, however, and there are no marketed drugs with this configuration. The nitrogen can be substituted with alkyl groups, and methyl is the optimal size. When the nitrogen is made quaternary, the molecule loses its oral availability but leads to compounds that can be administered effectively by inhalation. The asterisks in atropine (Fig. 49.17) refer to chiral carbons. When stereochemistry is present in the amino alcohol moiety (tropine), there is little difference between the activities of the *R*- and *S*-configurations. When stereochemistry is found in the acid moiety, however, the *R* configuration is approximately 100-fold more active than the *S*-isomer. This indicates the importance of the binding role for the phenyl ring in causing the uncoupling of the G protein, which leads to receptor inhibition (28).

Specific Antimuscarinic Drugs Used to Treat Asthma

For a more detailed discussion of the chemistry of cholinergic agents, see Chapter 12.

Ipratropium Hydrobromide

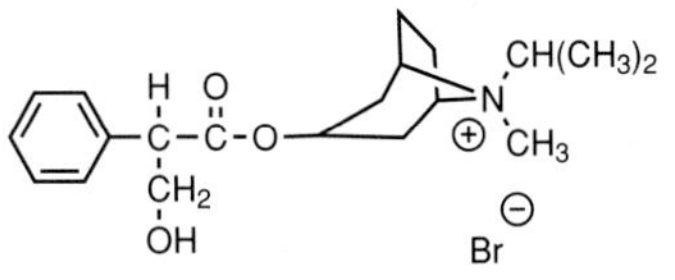

Ipratropium hydrobromide
(Atrovent)

Ipratropium is the N-isopropyl analogue of atropine. Its quaternary cationic nature makes it highly hydrophilic and poorly absorbed from the lungs after inhalation via solution or aerosol. Much of an inhaled dose is swallowed. There is no significant absorption, however, and the bronchodilation effect can be considered to be a local, site-specific effect. Ipratropium is indicated primarily for the relief of bronchospasms associated with COPD (chronic obstructive pulmonary disease) and has seen little application for the treatment of asthma. It also is administered by nasal spray for the relief of rhinorrhea associated with the common cold and perennial rhinitis. Inhaled ipratropium has a 15-minute onset of action and a rather short duration of action (<4 hours); therefore, it is dosed four times a day. Other drugs, including adrenergic agonists, methylxanthines, steroids, and cromolyn sodium, can be coadministered with ipratropium without adverse drug reactions. The little ipratropium that reaches the circulation is minimally protein bound and is partially metabolized to inactive esterase products. Most adverse effects from ipratropium are common to antimuscarinics and include blurred vision, dry mouth, tachycardia, urinary difficulty, and headache. Patients should be careful not to spray ipratropium into their eyes, because its dilation effects can precipitate or exacerbate narrow-angle glaucoma.

Tiotropium Bromide

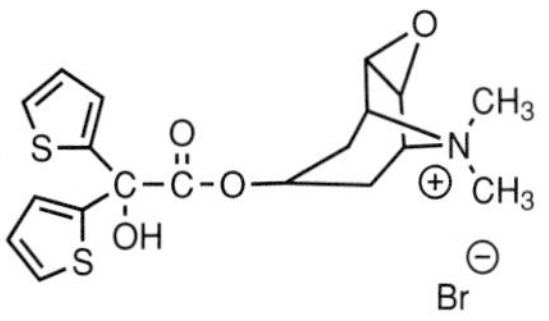

Tiotropium bromide
(Spiriva)

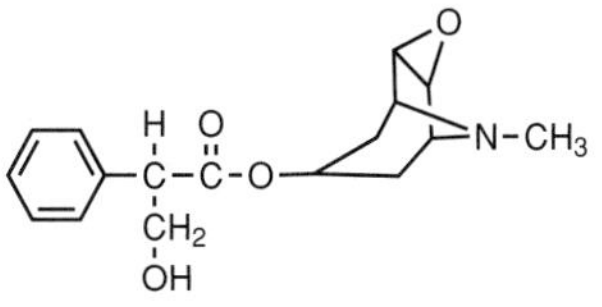

Scopolamine

Tiotropium is the dithienyl derivative of N-methyl scopolamine, a quaternary analogue of naturally occurring scopolamine in *Atropa belladonna*. It is indicated primarily for the relief of bronchospasms associated with COPD and can be considered to be a site-specific, local medication to the lung. Tiotropium is administered as a dry powder via inhalation using a HandiHaler, in which is placed the drug, contained in a green capsule. Patients should be cautioned not to be confused and take the medication orally. Systemic distribution following oral inhalation is minimal, essentially because of its hydrophilic character. If swallowed, only approximately 14% of the dose is eliminated in the urine, with the remainder being found in the feces. Inhaled tiotropium has a 30-minute onset of action but a much longer duration of action than ipratropium (24 versus <4 hours, respectively). Tiotropium is metabolized by both CYP3A4 and CYP2D6, followed by glutathione conjugation to a variety of metabolites. Only a very small amount is nonenzymatically hydrolyzed to inactive products. Tiotropium has an adverse reaction profile similar to that of ipratropium, with dry mouth being the most common adverse effect; however, blurred vision, tachycardia, urinary difficulty, headache precipitation, and exacerbation of narrow-angle glaucoma have been reported.

Methylxanthines

Introduction

The methylxanthines naturally occur in coffee (*Coffea arabica*), cacao (*Theobroma cacao*), and tea (*Camellia sinensis*) (29). The major methylxanthines are caffeine, theophylline, and theobromine, and they differ by the

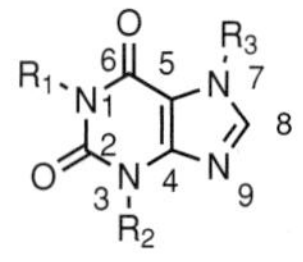

	R_1	R_2	R_3
Caffeine	CH_3	CH_3	CH_3
Theophylline	CH_3	CH_3	H
Theobromine	H	CH_3	CH_3

Fig. 44.18. Structural differences between the methylxanthines.

position and number of methyl groups on their xanthine ring system (Fig. 44.18).

The most common source of these xanthines is in the beverages coffee, tea, and cocoa, which are universally consumed mainly for their stimulant properties. A cup of coffee or tea contains between 60 and 85 mg of caffeine, and a cup of cocoa can have as much as 250 mg of theobromine. Caffeine frequently is added to cola drinks as well as to over-the-counter analgesics and stimulants. Theophylline is used for its bronchodilating effects in the treatment of asthma. Its importance has declined greatly since the development of the inhaled β_2-adrenergic agonists and inhaled steroids and because its narrow therapeutic window requires close patient monitoring and periodic blood level determination to avoid serious side effects.

Theophylline

In spite of a great deal of investigation, just how theophylline causes bronchodilation is not clearly understood. Inhibition of the enzyme PDE, which is responsible for the hydrolysis of cAMP and cyclic guanosine monophosphate (cGMP), generally is put forth as the mechanism of action; however, theophylline also is an adenosine antagonist and has been implicated in stimulation of the release of catecholamines. It has been clearly shown that theophylline does inhibit PDEs in vitro, and x-ray crystallographic studies have identified the binding residues that interact with the methylxanthines (Fig. 44.19).

Theophylline binds to a subpocket of the active site and appears to be sandwiched between a phenylalanine and a valine via hydrophobic bonds. Its binding affinity is reinforced by hydrogen-bonding between a tyrosine and N-7 and a glutamine and O-6 of the xanthine ring system. There are more than 11 families of PDEs, and studies have shown that theophylline binds in a similar manner to both the PDE4 and PDE5 family isoforms (30). (For a more detailed description of PDE subtypes and their inhibitors, see Chapter 17.)

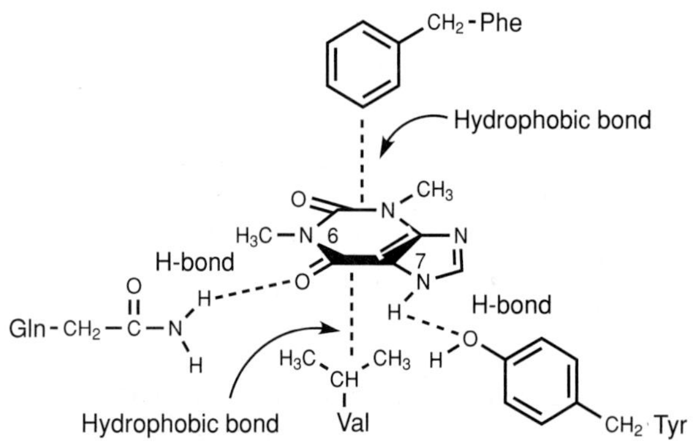

Fig. 44.19. Methylxanthine binding interactions in the catalytic pocket of phosphodiesterase.

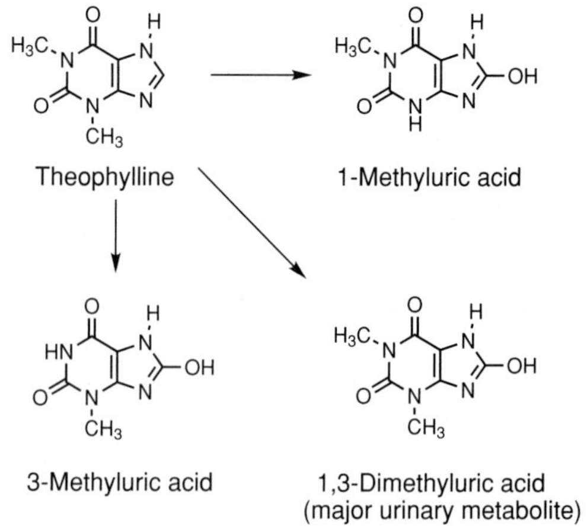

Fig. 44.20. Metabolism of theophylline.

Chemically, theophylline is 1,3-dimethylxanthine and contains both an acidic and a basic nitrogen (N-7 and N-9, respectively). Physiologically, it behaves as an acid (pK_a = 8.6), and its poor aqueous solubility can be enhanced by salt formation with organic bases. Theophylline is metabolized by a combination of C-8 oxidation and N-demethylation to yield methyluric acid metabolites (Fig. 44.20). The major urinary metabolite is 1,3-dimethyl uric acid, which is the product of the action of xanthine oxidase. Because none of the metabolites is uric acid itself, theophylline can be safely given to patients who suffer from gout.

Methylxanthine Drugs Used to Treat Asthma

Theophylline

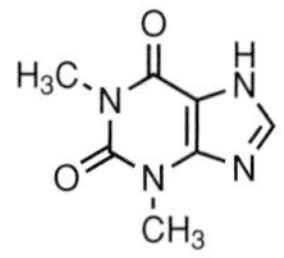

Theophylline
(Elixophylline, Bronkodyl,
various others)

The primary indication for theophylline is as a controller medication for the treatment of bronchospasm of asthma and COPD. In addition to bronchodilation effects, theophylline dilates pulmonary blood vessels, acts centrally to stimulate respiration, acts as a diuretic, increases gastric acid secretion, and inhibits uterine contractions. Dosing requires the determination of plasma levels with 10 to 20 μg/mL being associated with the least incidence of side effects. Overdose of theophylline can result in a quick onset of ventricular arrhythmias, convulsions, or even death without any previous warning. Many drugs increase the plasma concentration of theophylline, including quinolone and macrolide antibiotics, nonselective β-blockers, ephedrine, calcium channel blockers, cimetidine, and oral contraceptives. Theophylline is available in tablet, capsule, liquid, and parenteral dosage preparations. There also are combination products with guaifenesin and ephedrine available as tablet and liquid dosage forms. There are two products that are theophylline salts. Aminophylline is theophylline ethylenediamine, which contains 70% theophylline and is available in tablets, liquid, parenteral, and suppository dosage forms. Oxytriphylline is the choline salt of theophylline, and it contains 64% theophylline in tablets and liquid dosage forms. Care must be taken to correctly calculate the equivalent dose when switching a patient from theophylline to one of its salts.

Dyphylline (Dihydroxypropyl Theophylline)

Dyphylline

Dyphylline is the N-7 dihydroxypropyl derivative of theophylline and is not a theophylline salt. Dyphylline does not get metabolized to theophylline in vivo, and even though it contains 70% theophylline by molecular weight ratio, the equivalent amount to theophylline is not known. Dosing must be accomplished independently by monitoring dyphylline blood levels. Dyphylline has a diminished bronchodilator effect compared to theophylline, but it may have lower and less serious side effects. Dosage forms available are an elixir and tablets.

Adrenocorticoids Used to Treat Asthma and COPD

Introduction

Steroids are a large class of tetracyclic terpene compounds that are widely distributed in plants and animals. Many synthetic analogues have been made to take advantages of their various pharmacological activities. There are four major classes of steroids: the adrenocorticoids, the sex hormones, the bile acids, and the vitamins. The adrenocorticoids are formed in the adrenal cortex and are subdivided into the glucocorticoids and mineralocorticoids. The glucocorticoids are so named because they affect glucose homeostasis, but they also have significant anti-inflammatory activity. The mineralocorticoids affect sodium and water retention. The reproductive organs in both the male and female produce steroid hormones that are responsible for the differentiation of the sex characteristics and the development of muscle and hair. The bile acids are derived from cholesterol and are an essential aid to the action of lipase in the digestion of fats, and vitamin D and its derivatives are associated with calcium homeostasis. We will limit our discussion to the glucocorticoids, because their anti-inflammatory activity makes them useful for the treatment of asthma and COPD. Of note, because the major role of the glucocorticoids is to provide the body with levels of glucose that are compatible with life, they should be used with caution in patients with diabetes. Similarly, because the major role of the mineralocorticoids is to maintain blood volume and regulate electrolyte balance, their use in patients with hypertension should be monitored carefully. (For more detail regarding the adrenal corticosteroids, see Chapter 33.)

Steroid Nomenclature

The basic structure of a steroid is a tetracyclic cyclopentanoperhydrophenanthrene, referred to as the sterid nucleus, as depicted in Figure 44.21. The addition of methyl groups at C-10 and C-13 and of an ethyl group at C-17 to the sterid nucleus gives a 21-carbon base structure called pregnane. All glucocorticoids are substituted pregnanes. Rings A, B, and C are in the chair conformation, All ring junctions are *trans,* giving the glucocorticoids a rigid backbone with α and β faces. The glucocorticoids bind to their receptor via the β face. All glucocorticoids have at least one double bond in ring A and hydroxyl groups at C-11, C-17, and C-21 as well as 3- and 20-keto groups. For example, hydrocortisone is Δ^4-11β,17α,21-trihydroxy-3,20-pregnenedione. A more complete discussion of steroid nomenclature and stereochemistry has been published elsewhere (31).

Steroid Biosynthesis and Secretion

Steroids are biosynthesized from cholesterol. Cholesterol is obtained through our diet (~0.3 g/day), but the majority is biosynthesized from acetate in the liver (~1 g/day). The complete pathway can be seen in Figure 44.22. Of note is the central branching role played by pregnenolone, leading to both classes of the adrenocorticoids.

Cyclopentanoperhydrophenanthrene

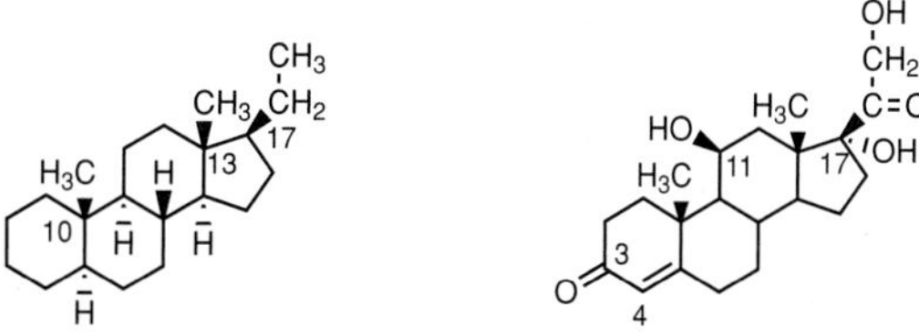

5α-Pregnane

Δ^4-11β,17λ,21-Trihydroxy-3,20-pregenedione (Hydrocortisone)

Fig. 44.21. Basic skeletons for steroid structures, numbering and nomenclature.

Once formed, the adrenocorticoids are secreted into the circulatory system, and circulating levels are maintained via a feedback mechanism (Fig. 44.23). When circulating levels are low, the hypothalamus secretes corticotrophin-releasing factor (CRF). In turn, CRF stimulates the anterior pituitary to secrete adrenocorticotrophic hormone, which stimulates the adrenal cortex to synthesize and secrete the adrenocorticoids (mainly hydrocortisone and aldosterone). When circulating levels of the adrenocorticoids are sufficiently high, they feedback-inhibit CRF secretion from the hypothalamus and adrenocorticotrophic hormone release from the anterior pituitary gland. It should be noted that chronic use of steroids inhibits the adrenal cortex from producing glucocorticoids. This is known as hypothalamus-pituitary-adrenal (HPA) suppression. If steroid therapy is stopped abruptly, the lack of endogenous glucocorticoids can be life-threatening. A slow and gradual withdrawal from exogenous steroid therapy is always warranted to allow the HPA axis to recover.

Steroid Pharmacological Action

The major pharmacological activities of the glucocorticoids are anti-inflammation, inhibition of cytokines, and inhibition of mast cell release of autocoids. The anti-inflammatory

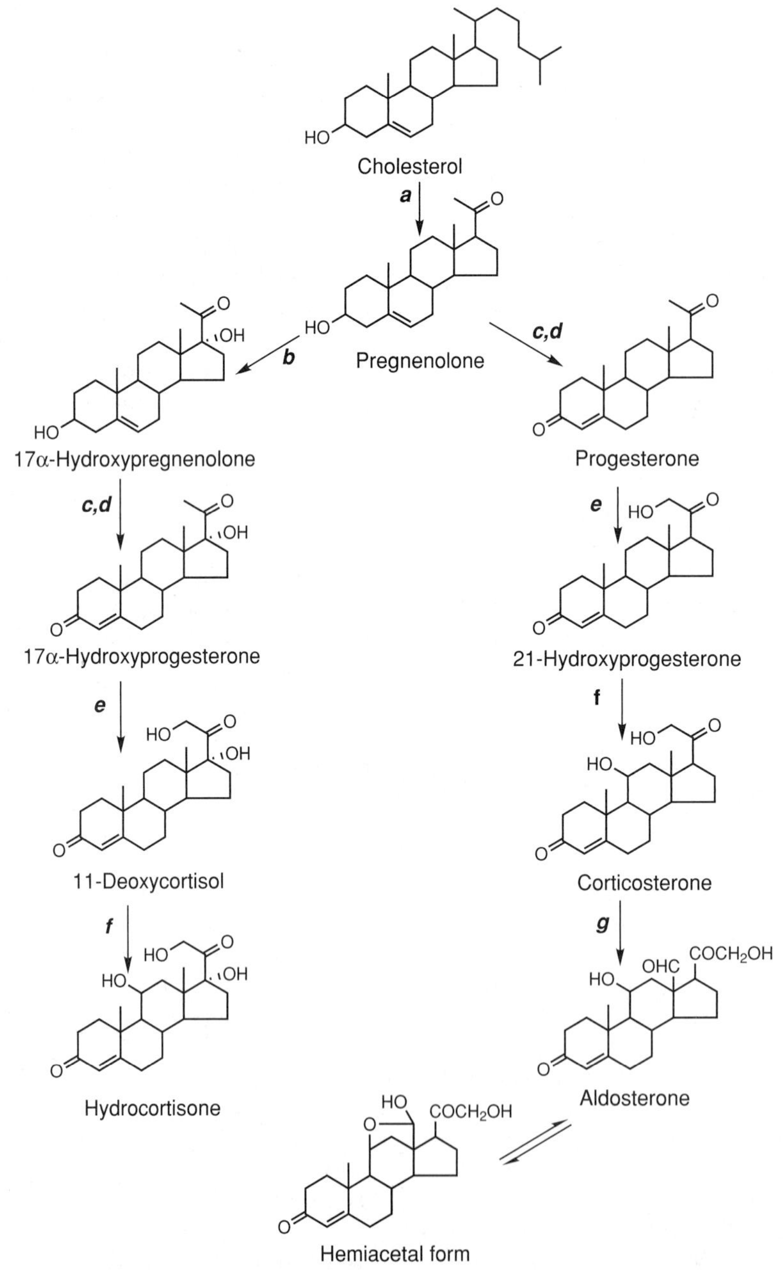

Fig. 44.22. Biosynthesis of the adrenocorticoids from cholesterol. The enzymes involved are (*a*) side chain cleavage, (*b*) 17α-hydroxylase, (*c*) 5-ene-3β-hydroxy-steroid dehydrogenase, (*d*) 3-oxosteroid-4,5-isomerase, (*e*) 21-hydroxylase, (*f*) 11β-hydroxylase, and (*g*) 18-hydroxylate.

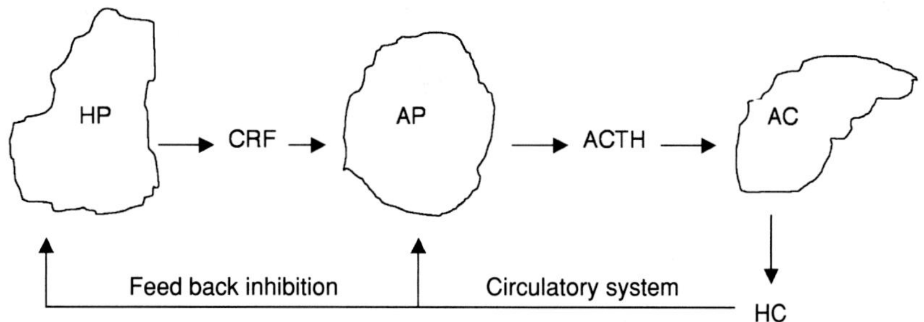

Fig. 44.23. Mechanism of adrenocorticoid secretion and control. HP=hypothalamus, CRF=corticotrophin releasing factor, AP=anterior pituitary, ACTH=adrenocorticotrophic hormone, AC=adrenal cortex, HC=hydrocortisone.

activity of the glucocorticoids is derived from their ability to affect protein synthesis. Specifically, they stimulate the synthesis of lipocortin, a protein that inhibits phospholipase A_2, which is an enzyme that catalyzes the breakdown of membranes to release arachidonic acid, the first step in the arachidonic acid cascade that results in the production of inflammatory prostaglandins and leukotrienes (Figs. 44.24 and 44.25). Therefore, inhibition of phospholipase A_2 ultimately results in the reduction of the inflammatory prostaglandins and leukotrienes.

Another way that glucocorticoids are anti-inflammatory involves their ability to inhibit interleukin-1, which stimulates the proliferation of T and B lymphocytes that are responsible for the production of the cytokines and antibodies that are important in the inflammatory and immune responses to antigens. Therefore, the glucocorticoids, by their ability to inhibit interleukin-1, cause a decrease in T and B lymphocytes, which makes them immunosuppressant, and must be used with caution in patients with infection. A third action of glucocorticoids is to inhibit the synthesis and release of histamine and other autocoids from mast cells. These pharmacological activities make the glucocorticoids especially useful for treating the

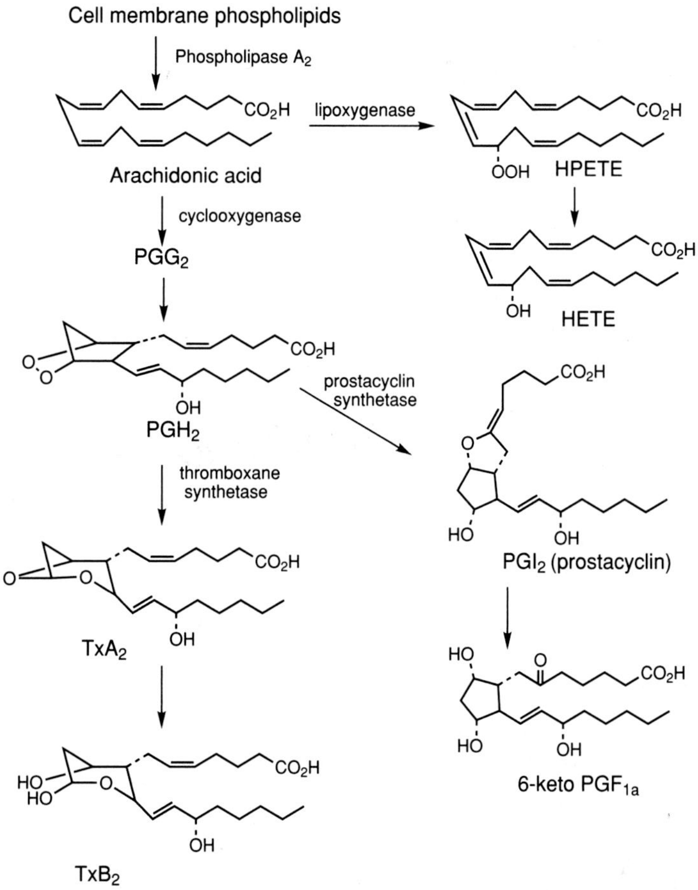

Cell membrane phospholipids
Phospholipase A_2
Arachidonic acid
lipoxygenase
HPETE
HETE
cyclooxygenase
PGG_2
PGH_2
prostacyclin synthetase
PGI_2 (prostacyclin)
6-keto PGF_{1a}
thromboxane synthetase
TxA_2
TxB_2

Fig. 44.24. Biosynthesis of thromboxanes, prostacyclin, and prostaglandins.

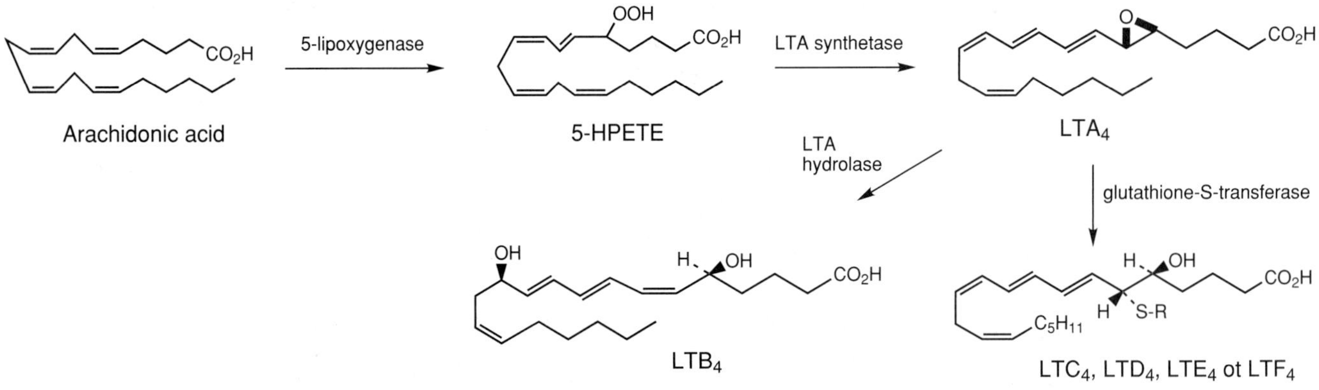

Arachidonic acid → 5-lipoxygenase → 5-HPETE → LTA synthetase → LTA_4

LTA_4 → LTA hydrolase → LTB_4

LTA_4 → glutathione-S-transferase → LTC_4, LTD_4, LTE_4 ot LTF_4

Fig. 44.25. Biosynthesis of leukotrienes.

inflammatory processes associated with asthma and COPD.

Steroid Mechanism of Action

How do glucocorticoids and other adrenocorticoids affect the levels of proteins and other biologically important compounds? The short answer is that they bind to their receptor in the cytoplasm and that the glucocorticoid–receptor complex travels into the nucleus, where it binds to DNA and affects gene transcription, which increases and, sometimes, decreases the production of important biologically active compounds. The detail of just how the glucocorticoids accomplish this is quite interesting and is depicted in Fig. 44.26.

Circulating glucocorticoids enter the target cell by simple diffusion, because they are relatively lipophilic. The glucocorticoid receptor occurs inside the cell in combination with a heat shock protein. The glucocorticoid receptor has three distinct regions: the amino terminal for maximum activity, a middle region for binding to DNA, and the carboxy terminal, where the glucocorticoids bind. When the glucocorticoid binds to its receptor, the heat shock protein is released, with a conformational change in the steroid–receptor complex and the glucocorticoid–receptor complex then translocates into the nucleus of the cell, where it binds to specific sequences of DNA called hormone-response elements (HREs), which are located in the promoter areas of hormone-responsive

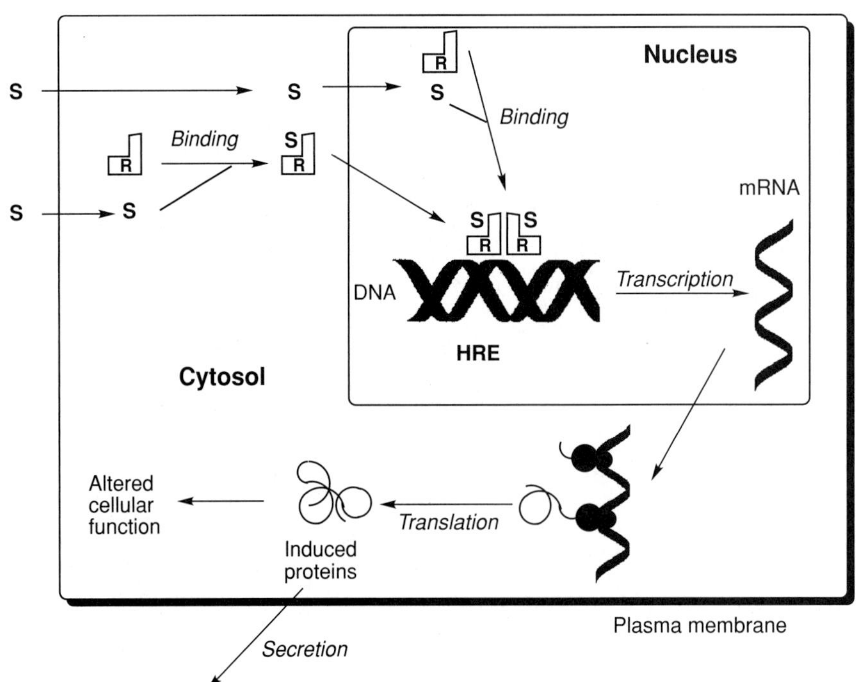

Fig. 44.26. Mechanism of steroid hormone action. (s = steroid; R = receptor).

genes. The DNA binding region of the glucocorticoid receptor contains eight cysteine amino acid residues that coordinate two zinc ions that form peptide loops called zinc fingers. When the zinc finger domains bind to the HRE of DNA, it dimerizes the glucocorticoid–receptor complex, placing each subunit in adjacent binding grooves. In most cases, binding causes gene transcription and protein synthesis; however, in some instances, binding will block transcription (32,33).

Steroid Receptor Structure and Glucocorticoid Binding

The glucocorticoid receptor is a member of the nuclear receptor superfamily, which includes the receptors for the steroid hormones, retinoids, peroxisomal activators, vitamin D, and thyroid hormones. The steroid receptor is a soluble protein found in the cytosol of the cell. The binding domain of all the steroid receptors consists of 11 α-helices and four β-strands. X-ray crystallographic structural analysis, however, has revealed a unique binding pocket for the glucocorticoid receptor, which makes it distinct from the estrogen receptor, androgen receptor, and mineralocorticoid receptor. When a glucocorticoid binds to the receptor, it is completely enclosed within a pocket formed by helices 3, 4, 5, 6, 7, and 10 and β-strands 1 and 2. The strong binding affinity for the glucocorticoids is a result of the hydrophobic and hydrophilic interactions with amino acid residues in the ligand binding domain. Nearly every atom of the glucocorticoid contacts one or more amino acid residues. The most significant contacts are the hydrogen-bonding between every hydrophilic group on the glucocorticoid structure (Fig. 44.27). The carbonyl group on ring A forms hydrogen bonds with both Arg-611 and the amide of Gln-570. The hydroxyls at C-11 and C-21 hydrogen bond with the side chain of Asn-564. The C-17 hydroxyl group hydrogen bonds with Gln-642, and the C-20 carbonyl group bonds with Thr-739. Glucocorticoid binding to the ligand binding domain releases the heat shock protein and stabilizes the receptor in an active form capable of dimerization subsequent to HRE site binding (34,35).

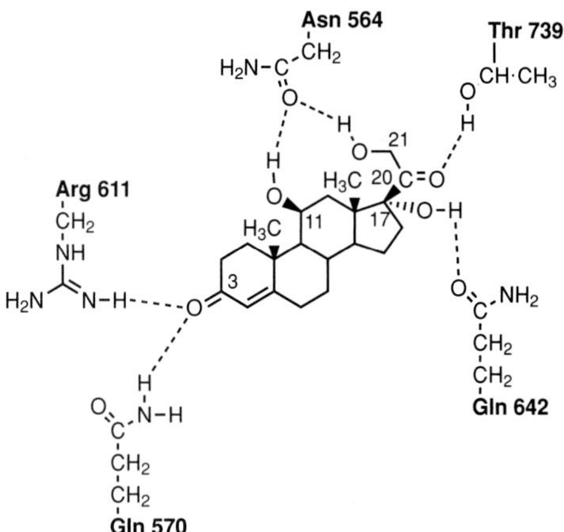

Fig. 44.27. Important glucocorticoid receptor–ligand binding residues.

Glucocorticoid Structure–Activity Relationships

There are essential structural features that are necessary for glucocorticoid activity. The natural glucocorticoids also interact with the mineralocorticoid receptor and, therefore, will have salt-retaining properties. A large number of synthetic analogues have been prepared to decrease the mineralocorticoid effects in favor of increasing the glucocorticoid (anti-inflammatory) effect of the steroids. In addition, many derivatives are prepared to enhance pharmacokinetic parameters, most notably the synthesis of lipophilic and hydrophilic esters.

Functional groups that are essential for both mineralocorticoid and glucocorticoid activity include the pregnane skeleton with an all-*trans* backbone, the ring A-en-one system (Δ^4-3-one ring A), and the 17β-ketol side chain (C-20-keto-C-21-hydroxy). The C-21 hydroxyl group must be free for both mineralocorticoid and glucocorticoid activity. An exception to this rule are the C-21 chloro and C-20 fluoromethyl thio ester ($-SCH_2F$) derivatives that retain anti-inflammatory activity when applied topically or by inhalation. Glucocorticoids that are used for their anti-inflammatory effects and that have both glucocorticoid and mineralocorticoid activity are hydrocortisone, cortisone, prednisone, and prednisolone.

Many derivatives of the fundamental glucocorticoid skeleton have been synthesized with the intention of enhancing anti-inflammatory activity and decreasing the salt-retaining properties of the glucocorticoids when administered in therapeutic doses. Figure 44.28 depicts those positions where substituents will affect anti-inflammatory and/or mineralocorticoid activity. The triangles indicate those positions where substitutions will increase the anti-inflammatory activity, and the open circles those positions where substituents will increase both anti-inflammatory and mineralocorticoid properties, the closed circle the position where substituents will decrease the mineralocorticoid activity, and the open box where specific substituents can either increase anti-inflammatory activity or decrease mineralocorticoid properties depending on the specific substituent. Therefore, the anti-inflammatory activity will be greatly increased by flattening ring A by adding a double bond at C-1 (Δ^1) and also by adding a hydroxyl group at C-11. A 17α-hydroxy increases both activities, as does 9α-fluoro or 9α-chloro. Mineralocorticoid activity is substantially eliminated by 16α- or 16β-methyl groups, a 16α-hydroxyl group, or a 16α,17α-acetonide. A C-6 α-methyl group only slightly enhances the anti-inflammatory activity, whereas a C-6α-fluoro has twice as much anti-inflammatory effect. Both substituents, in combination with a C-16 substituent, will greatly decrease the mineralocorticoid effects.

Therefore, synthetic compounds can be prepared with marked glucocorticoid activity that are devoid of any

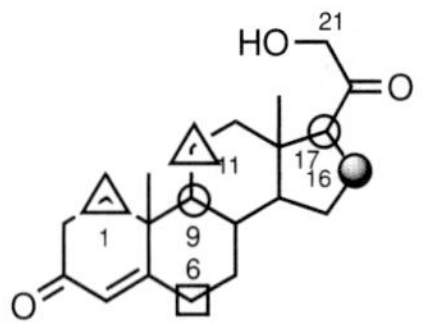

Both anti-inflammatory and mineralcorticoid activity increased (open circle)	Anti-inflammatory activity increased (triangle and square)	Mineralocorticoid activity decreased (closed circle and square)
17α-OH	1-dehydro	6α-CH_3
9α-F	6α-F	16α-& 16β-CH_3
9α-Cl	11β-OH	16α,17α-acetonide
21-OH		16α-OH

Fig. 44.28. Glucocorticoid structure-activity relationship.

significant mineralocorticoid activity. These include triamcinolone, methylprednisolone, fluticasone, beclomethasone, budesonide, and mometasone.

Glucocorticoid Metabolism

If one or more of the essential functional groups on the glucocorticoid skeleton are modified by metabolism, glucocorticoid activity will be lost. There are three major metabolic reactions that will eliminate the glucocorticoid activity. They are ring A reductions, C-17 oxidation, and C-11 keto-enol isomerization. Reduction of the ring A 3-keto to a 3α-hydroxy by 3α-hydroxysteroid dehydrogenase, and the reduction of the 4,5-double bond by 5β-reductase to produce the A/B *cis*-fused ring, gives rise to inactive metabolites (Fig. 44.29). Oxidation of the C-17 side chain to produce a 17-keto steroid requires both the C-17 hydroxyl group and a free C-21 hydroxyl group. Esterification of one or both will inhibit this metabolism and prolong the duration of action. The rapid in vivo equilibrium that exists between cortisone (11-keto) and hydrocortisone (11-β-hydroxy) is catalyzed by 11β-hydroxysteroid dehydrogenase, produces the keto form that is inactive but also the hydroxy form that is highly glucocorticoid enhancing and found on all glucocorticoids. Figure 44.29 summarizes the metabolism of hydrocortisone.

Synthetic Steroid Esters

The glucocorticoids are lipophilic in spite of having at least three hydroxyl groups. The hydroxyl groups can be esterified with an appropriate acid that will either enhance or decrease that lipophilicity. The C-21

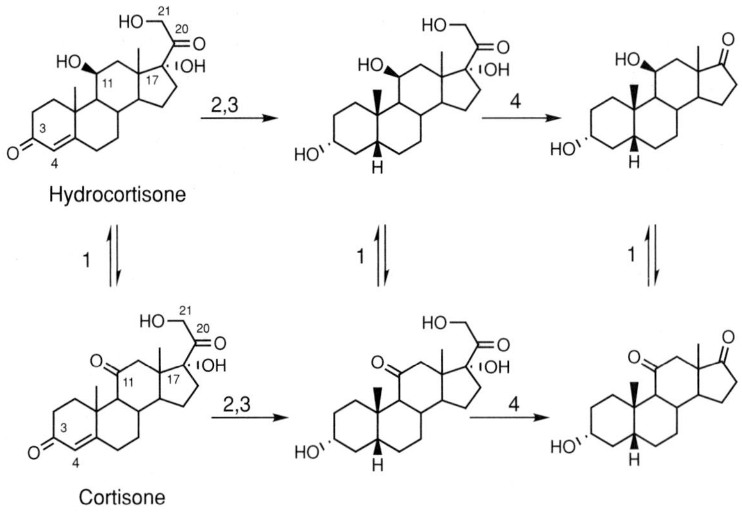

Metabolizing enzymes: 1 = 11β-hydroxysteroid dehydrogenase
2 = 3α-hydroxysteroid dehydrogenase
3 = 5β-reductase
4 = C-17 oxidase

Fig. 44.29. Metabolic pathways for hydrocortisone.

hydroxyl group is the most accessible and, therefore, is the easiest to esterify. The C-17 hydroxyl group also is easily esterified, but because it is slightly hindered by the C-17 side chain, it will react more slowly. The C-11 hydroxyl group is highly hindered by the C-10 and C-13 methyl groups and will not react with acids to form esters. In addition, esterification has an effect on both receptor affinity and glucocorticoid metabolism. Because the C-21 must be free to hydrogen bond to the Arg-564 in the glucocorticoid receptor, C-21 esters are prodrugs requiring hydrolysis to become active. Also, the C-17 hydroxyl group needs to be free to be metabolically oxidized; therefore, esterification of the C-17 hydroxyl group inhibits oxidation to the C-17 keto group, thus prolonging duration of action. Duration also is prolonged because of the fact that the lipophilic glucocorticoid esters do not concentrate in the urine (i.e., they undergo tubular reabsorption following glomerular filtration).

The lipophilicity of a glucocorticoid can be enhanced by esterification with lipophilic acids. Doing so results in a number of effects, including increasing the log P, which provides local activity with less systemic absorption and decreased side effects. The fact that C-21 lipophilic esters are prodrugs means that they have a longer duration of action. They also have a slower onset, because the lipophilic esters generally are bulky and retard hydrolytic enzymes.

These lipophilic prodrugs can be administered orally to treat a variety of conditions, by inhalation to treat asthma and COPD, and topically to treat various types of dermatitis. When administered orally, their longer duration of action means that they can be given less frequently, which often results in better compliance. Figure 44.30 shows the structures of the most common C-21 lipophilic esters found on commercially available glucocorticoids.

Diesters and ketals provide a further enhancement of log P (i.e., increased lipophilicity) and an increased duration of action, because they are slow to metabolize. It should be noted that diesters and hexacatonides (Fig. 44.31) are prodrugs, whereas plain ketals are not (i.e., they already have a free C-21 hydroxyl group). Diesters are formed at C-21 and at either the C-17 or, if present, the C-16 hydroxyl groups. The diesters are prodrugs; however, the esters at C-17 or C-16 are active intact. The most common diesters are either the diacetate or dipropionate.

A ketal is a cyclic derivative formed between hydroxyl groups on adjacent carbons and a carbonyl carbon of a ketone. The most common ketal found in glucocorticoids is called an acetonide and is the condensation product formed between the C-16 and C-17 hydroxyl groups and the carbonyl carbon of acetone (CH_3COCH_3) (Fig. 44.31). If the acetonide is found along with a C-21-*t*-butylacetate ester, it is named a hexacetonide; the "hex" refers to the total number of carbons found in the butylacetate group. The hexacetonides are prodrugs and must hydrolyze to become active. The buteprate (i.e., probutate) is a diester consisting of a propionate at C-21 and a butyrate at C-17 (Fig. 44.31). It also is a prodrug, and the C-21 ester must be hydrolyzed to yield the active form.

Esterification also can be used to increase the hydrophilicity of the glucocorticoids, making them water-soluble prodrugs. The synthetic approach here is to use either a dicarboxylic acid or phosphoric acid to condense with the C-21 hydoxyl group (Fig. 44.31). This

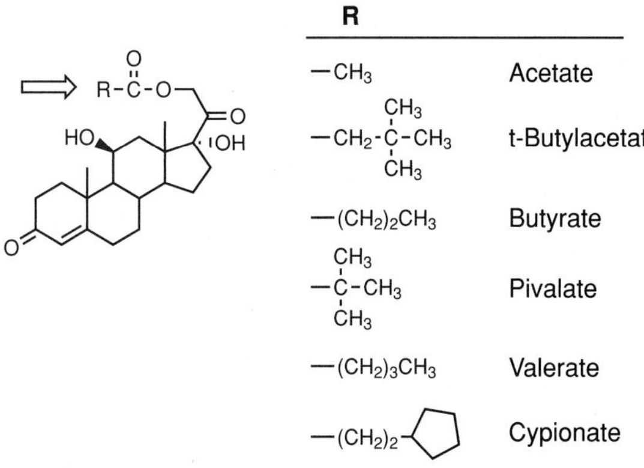

R	
$-CH_3$	Acetate
$-CH_2-C(CH_3)_2-CH_3$	t-Butylacetate
$-(CH_2)_2CH_3$	Butyrate
$-C(CH_3)_2-CH_3$	Pivalate
$-(CH_2)_3CH_3$	Valerate
$-(CH_2)_2$-cyclopentyl	Cypionate

Fig. 44.30. Common lipophilic esters of glucocorticoids.

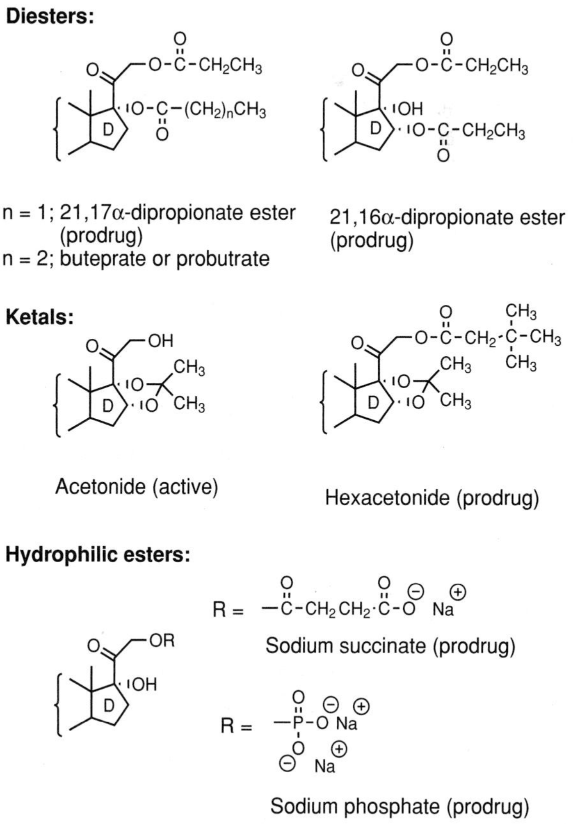

Diesters:

n = 1; 21,17α-dipropionate ester (prodrug)
n = 2; buteprate or probutrate

21,16α-dipropionate ester (prodrug)

Ketals:

Acetonide (active)

Hexacetonide (prodrug)

Hydrophilic esters:

R = $-C(=O)-CH_2CH_2-C(=O)-O^{\ominus}\ Na^{\oplus}$

Sodium succinate (prodrug)

R = $-P(=O)(O^{\ominus}Na^{\oplus})-O^{\ominus}\ Na^{\oplus}$

Sodium phosphate (prodrug)

Fig. 44.31. Examples of glucocorticoid lipophilic diesters and ketals and hydrophilic esters.

places an ionizable group (a carboxylate or phosphate) on the prodrug, yielding water-soluble esters. These derivatives are used to prepare aqueous injectable products that can be administered intramuscularly or IV.

Hydrophilic glucocorticoid prodrugs have a rapid onset, because they are readily hydrolyzed by plasma esterases. In contrast to the lipophilic prodrugs, their water solubility allows them to be easily excreted through the kidney, resulting in a shorter duration of action. Hydrophilic prodrugs have more systemic side effects because of their wide distribution that comes from their high solubility in the blood. Along with their ability to be injected IV, this property makes them useful in asthmatic emergencies (i.e., status asthmaticus) during which the patient is unable to take oral medication.

Table 44.7. Glucocorticoid Prodrug Derivatives

Drug	Trade Name	Site of Ester	Route of Administration
Hydrocortisone derivatives			
Hydrocortisone phosphate		C-21	IM, IV, SC
Sodium succinate	A-Hydrocort Sulucortef	C-21	IM, IV
Cypionate	Cortef	C-21	PO
Acetate	Cortaid	C-21	Topical
Butyrate	Locoid	C-21	Topical
Buteprate	Pandel	C-21	Topical
Valerate	Westcort	C-21	Topical
Prednisolone derivatives			
Phosphate	Hydeltrasol	C-21	IV, IM
Acetate	Key-Pred	C-21	Topical
Di-t-butylacetate (tebutate)	Prednisol TBA	C-17,21	Topical
Methylprednisolone derivatives			
Sodium succinate	Solu-medrol A-Methapred	C-21	IV, IM
Acetate	Depo-Medrol Depoject	C-21	IM

IM, intramuscular; IV, intravenous; PO, oral; SC, subcutaneous.

Glucocorticoid Drugs Used to Treat Asthma

Systemic Glucocorticoids

Hydrocortisone

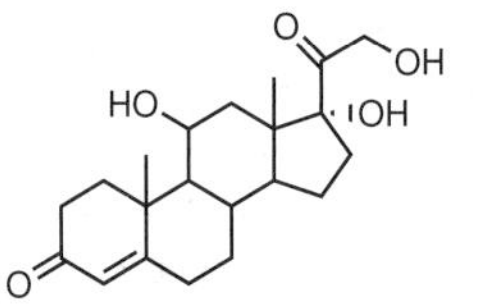

Hydrocortisone
(Cortisol)

Δ^4-11β,17α,21-trihydroxy-3,20-pregnenedione

Hydrocortisone is endogenous, and it has both glucocorticoid and mineralocorticoid activity. It is the fundamental structure by which the glucocorticoid and mineralocorticoid activities of all other corticosteroids are judged. Functional groups that are essential for both mineralocorticoid and glucocorticoid activity include the pregnane skeleton with an all-*trans* backbone, the ring A-en-one system (Δ^4-3-one ring A) and the 17β-ketol side chain (C-20-keto-C-21-hydroxy). The glucocorticoid activity is enhanced by the C-11 and C-17 hydroxyl groups. Hydrocortisone can be used to treat severe asthmatic attacks that do not respond to conventional treatment. It is available as various ester forms (Table 44.7).

Side Effects. Systemic administration of glucocorticoids can result in a large number of adverse effects on prolonged use. As already stated, there is the severe risk of HPA axis suppression, requiring the slow tapering off of the dose. In addition, glucocorticoids have cardiovascular effects (thromboembolism, hypertension, and arrhythmias), central nervous system effects (convulsions and steroid psychosis), dermatological effects (impaired wound healing and hair growth), endocrine effects (amenorrhea, postmenstrual bleeding, and suppression of growth in children), electrolyte disturbances (sodium and fluid retention, hypertension, and metabolic alkalosis), GI effects (pancreatitis, increased appetite, and peptic ulcer), musculoskeletal effects (muscle weakness, steroid myopathy, and osteoporosis), and ophthalmic effects (cataracts, increased intraocular pressure, and glaucoma).

Prednisolone

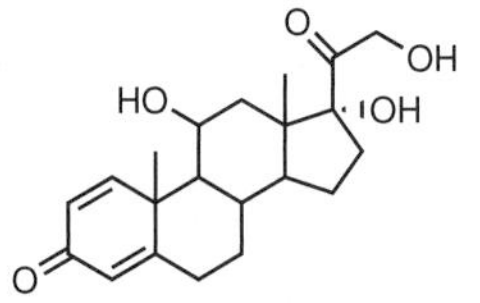

Prednisolone
(Delta-Cortef)

Δ^4-11β,17α,21-trihydroxy-pregnadiene-3,20-dione

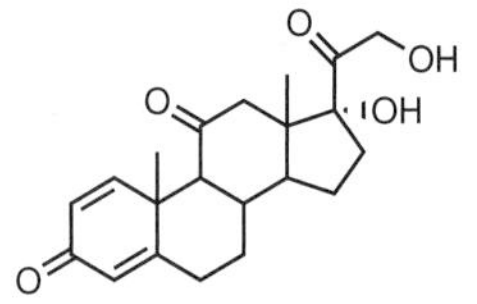

Prednisone
(Deltasone, Meticortin)

Δ^4-17α,21-dihydroxy-pregnadiene-3,11,20-trione

Prednisolone is hydrocortisone to which has been added a Δ^1 double bond. This places two double bonds in ring A, which flattens it and increases glucocorticoid action at the expense of mineralocorticoid activity. Prednisolone has fourfold the glucocorticoid activity of hydrocortisone while having approximately half its mineralocorticoid activity. In addition, prednisolone has an increased duration of action compared to hydrocortisone, because the extra double bond in ring A retards its metabolic reduction.

Prednisolone can be used to treat severe asthmatic attacks that do not respond to conventional treatment, and it is available as the free alcohol for oral administration. The C-21 sodium phosphate (Hydeltrasol) ester is available for parenteral use. Various ester prodrugs are available, as listed in Table 44.7. A prodrug of prednisolone is prednisone. It is the 11-keto analogue of prednisolone and must be converted in vivo to the active 11β-hydroxy compound, which is necessary to hydrogen bond to Asn-564 in the glucocorticoid receptor. Prednisone should not be used in patients with hepatic dysfunction, because their ability to reduce the 11-keto group with 11β-hydroxysteroid dehydrogenase to the active metabolite may be impaired.

METHYLPREDNISOLONE

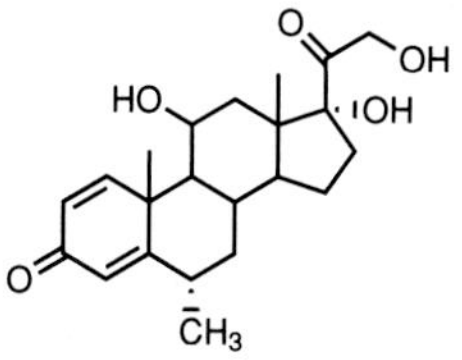

6-Methylprednisolone
(Medrol)

$\Delta^{1,4}$-6α-methyl-11α,17α,21-trihydroxy-pregnadiene-3,20-dione

Adding a 6α-methyl group to prednisolone increases the glucocorticoid activity and effectively abolishes mineralocorticoid action. It has fivefold the glucocorticoid activity of hydrocortisone (prednisolone has fourfold the glucocorticoid activity) and none of its mineralocorticoid properties. It is used almost exclusively as a systemic product and is available as the free alcohol for oral administration and as various esters (Table 44.7).

Glucocorticoids for Inhalation

BECLOMETHASONE DIPROPIONATE

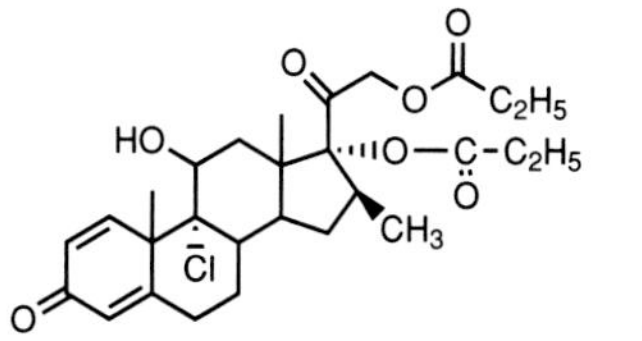

Beclomethasone dipropionate
(QVAR, Vanceril)

9α-Chloro-16β-methyl-11β,17α,21-trihydroxypregna-1,4-diene-3,20-dione 17,21-dipropionate

Beclomethasone dipropionate is a lipophilic prodrug that, when inhaled, shows a systemic bioavailability of approximately 20% of the administered dose. The 16β-methyl group decreases mineralocorticoid activity, and the 9α-chloro group increases both the glucocorticoid and mineralocorticoid activity, resulting in potent anti-inflammatory activity with little or no salt-retaining effects. The main adverse effects are headache, sinusitis, and pain. Beclomethasone dipropionate is metabolized to the more active 17α-monopropionate derivative during absorption from the lungs and then further metabolized to the free alcohol in the liver. The dipropionate also is metabolized to the inactive 21-monopropionate in the liver. Beclomethasone dipropionate and its metabolites are mainly excreted in the feces, with less than 10% excreted in the urine.

BUDESONIDE

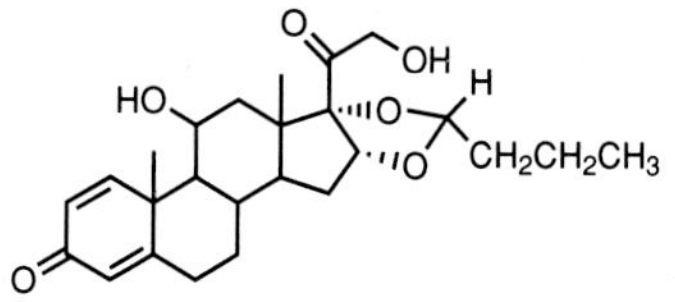

Budesonide
(Pulmacort tubuhaler, Respules)

16α,17–[(*R,S*-butylidenebis(oxy)]-11β,21-dihydroxypregna-1,4-diene-3,20-dione

Budesonide is an acetal formed between the 16α,17α-dihydroxyl groups and butanal. It is a nonhalogenated glucocorticoid with a 16,17-acetal that decreases the mineralocorticoid activity. In receptor affinity studies, the *R*-epimer was twofold more active than the *S*-epimer. Because the C-21 hydroxy is free, budesonide is not a prodrug and is active as administered. Only 34% of the metered dose of inhaled budesonide reaches the lung. Systemically absorbed budesonide is highly protein bound and metabolized to 16α-hydroxyprednisolone and 6β-hydroxybudesonide in the liver. Both metabolites have less than 1% of the glucocorticoid activity of the parent compound. Inhaled budesonide is excreted mainly as metabolites via both the feces (15%) and the urine (32%). Budesonide is available as a powder delivered through an aerosol or as a suspension for inhalation.

FLUNISOLIDE

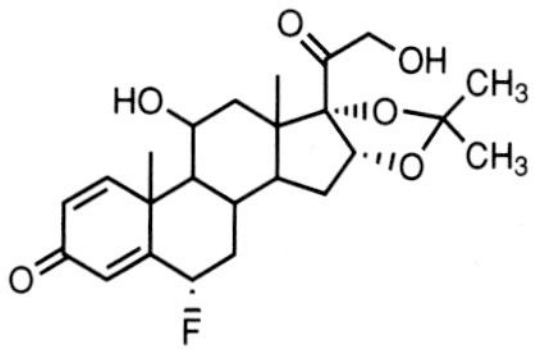

Flunisolide
(Aerobid)

6α–Fluoro-11β,21-dihydroxy-16α,17-[(1-methylethylidene)bis(oxy)]pregna-1,4-diene-3,20-dione

Flunisolide is an acetone ketal (acetonide) with a 6α-fluoro group and a free C-21 hydroxyl group. The acetonide decreases mineralocorticoid activity, and the 6α-fluoro group increases glucocorticoid activity. It is not a prodrug, because it has the free hydroxyl group at C-21. Flunisolide has approximately 20% of the receptor affinity as budesonide, and approximately 40% of the inhaled dose is systemically bioavailable. Flunisolide is quickly metabolized by CYP3A4 to the 6β-hydroxy metabolite, which has less than 1% of the activity of the parent compound. This, along with the rapid elimination of both flunisolide and its metabolite as glucuronides, greatly limits any systemic adverse effects. Flunisolide is available as a microcrystalline powder aerosol.

Fluticasone propionate

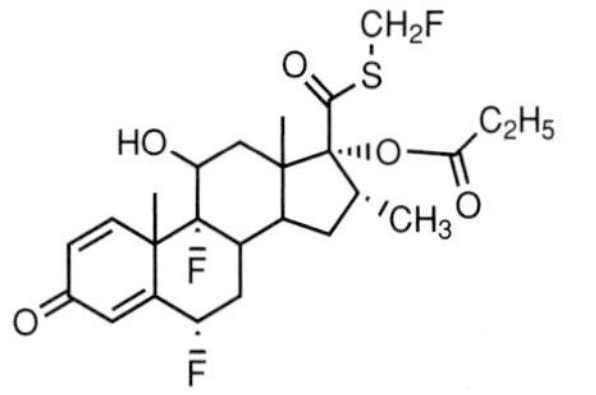

Fluticasone (Flovent, Flonase)

6α,9α-Difluoro-S-fluoromethyl-11β-hydroxy-16α-methyl-3-oxo-17α-propionyloxyandrosta-1, 4-diene-17α-carbothioate

Fluticasone propionate has a unique C-20 thioflouromethyl group, and that, in combination with the 17α-propionate ester, gives it 36-fold the glucocorticoid receptor affinity as compared to beclomethasone dipropionate and twofold the affinity as compared to budesonide. The 9α-flouro group increases both glucocorticoid and mineralocorticoid activities, and the 6α-flouro group enhances only the glucocorticoid action. Studies have determined that the effectiveness of inhaled fluticasone propionate results from a local rather than a systemic effect. Interestingly, less than 1% of the swallowed dose is bioavailable, in contrast to the fact that the majority of the inhaled dose is systemically available and highly protein bound. Fluticasone propionate is not a prodrug and is extensively metabolized by the liver. The only detectable metabolite is the 17β-carboxylic acid derived from CYP3A4 oxidation. This metabolite has 2,000-fold less affinity for the glucocorticoid receptor than the parent drug. Elimination is through both the feces and the urine, with the relative amounts determined by the route of administration. Fluticasone propionate is available in aerosol and powder inhalation formulations.

Mometasone furoate

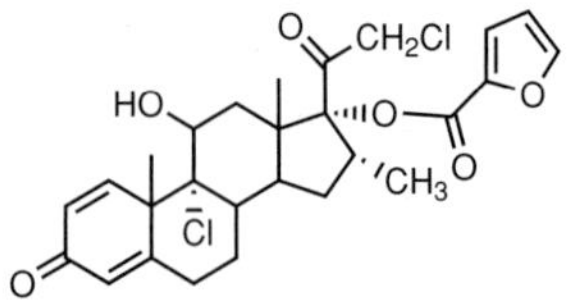

Mometasone furoate (Asmanex twisthaler)

9α,21-dichloro-17α–[(2-furanylcarbonyl)oxy]-11β-hydroxy-16α-methylpregna-1,4-diene-3,20-dione

Mometasone furoate is the most recent glucocorticoid to be developed and commercialized. It has a number of unique functional groups that confer enhanced glucocorticoid activity as well as pharmacokinetic advantages. The combination of the C-21 chloro and the furoic acid ester at C-17 results in the highest glucocorticoid receptor affinity of any topical corticosteroid. The 16α- methyl decreases the mineralocorticoid effects, and the 9α-chloro group increases both glucocorticoid and mineralocorticoid activities. Inhaled mometasone furoate acts locally as an anti-inflammatory treatment for asthma and has the least systemic bioavailability of all the inhaled glucocorticoids (<1%). It is extensively metabolized, with 6β-hydroxymometasone and 21-hydroxymometasone being found among the metabolites. Inhaled mometasone furoate in mainly excreted in the feces (~74%) as metabolites and only minimally excreted in the urine (~8%). It has a relatively long half-life in the lung and is administered once daily, usually in the evening.

Triamcinolone acetonide

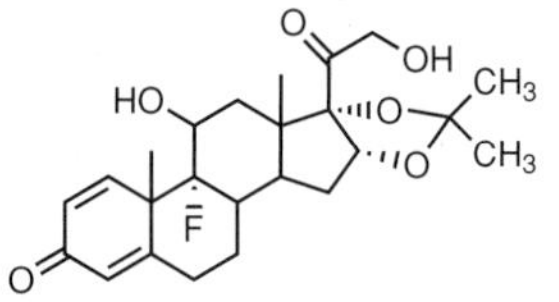

Triamcinolone acetonide (Azmacort)

9α–Fluoro-11β,17α,21-trihydroxypregna-1,4-diene-3,20-dione-16α,17-acetonide

Triamcinolone acetonide has the acetonide function, which greatly decreases its mineralocorticoid activity. The 9α-flouro group increases both the glucocorticoid and the mineralocorticoid activities. Triamcinolone acetonide has a receptor affinity that is 10-fold that of beclomethasone dipropionate but sixfold less that of mometasone furoate. After oral inhalation, as much of 25% of triamcinolone acetonide can be detected systemically; a good proportion of that is assumed to be from swallowing and absorbed from the GI tract unchanged. It is metabolized in the liver to a number of metabolites, including 6β-hydroxytriamcinolone acetonide and the C-21 carboxy-6β-hydroxytriamcinolone acetonide, both of which are readily excreted via the kidneys. The acetonide remains intact during metabolic reactions and, therefore, is highly resistant to hydrolytic cleavage. Triamcinolone acetonide is excreted mainly as metabolites in the urine (40%) and in the feces (60%), with less than 1% being excreted unchanged.

Mast Cell Degranulation Inhibitors

Introduction

The discovery that a Middle Eastern herb, *Ammi visnaga* (Khella, Bishop's weed), had mild bronchodilation effects led to the isolation of a benzopyrone (a chromone), khellin. Khellin had only weak bronchodilator effects, so synthetic analogues were prepared in an attempt to enhance the bronchodilation. All analogues

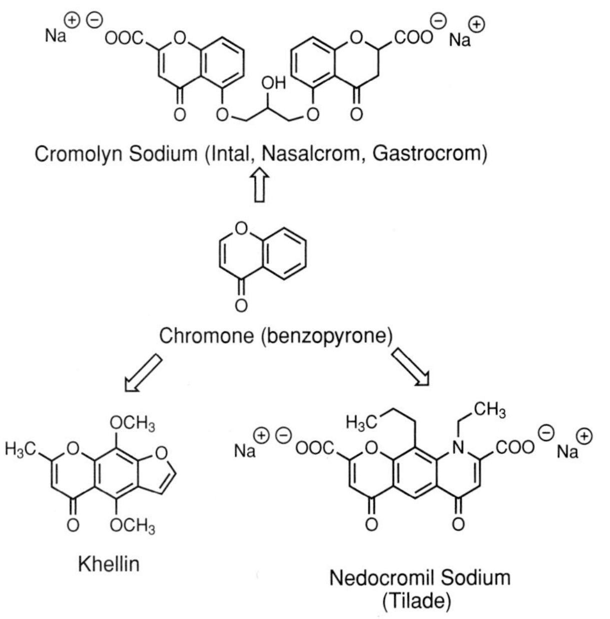

Cromolyn Sodium (Intal, Nasalcrom, Gastrocrom)

Chromone (benzopyrone)

Khellin

Nedocromil Sodium (Tilade)

Fig. 44.32. Structures of several chromone mast cell stabilizers.

were less active; however, it was noted by Dr. Roger Altounyans, who was experimenting on himself with these analogues, that one of them, if inhaled before an asthmatic attack, gave excellent protection against the attack's severity (36). The active compound was identified as a bischromone and named cromolyn sodium in the United States and sodium cromoglycate in Europe (Fig. 44.32).

This class of mast cell degranulation inhibitors prevents the release of histamine, leukotrienes, prostaglandins, and other inflammatory autocoids by interaction with the sensitized mast cell before antigenic challenge and does not inhibit the binding of IgE to the mast cell or the antigen to IgE. The exact mechanism of action is still not completely understood; however, it is clear that inhibition of the role of calcium in the degranulation process is involved. A number of membrane and cellular proteins that bind cromolyn sodium are known to regulate intracellular calcium levels and include basophilic membrane protein, nucleoside diphosphate kinase, calgranulins B and C, and annexins I through V (37,38). Mast cell degranulation inhibitors also are used topically in the eye to treat allergic reactions; in addition to cromolyn sodium, they include nedocromil sodium, lodoxamide tromethamine, and pemirolast potassium. (For additional details about this class of compounds, see Chapter 37.)

Mast Cell Stabilizers Used to Treat Asthma

Cromolyn sodium

Cromolyn sodium is a bischromone that contains the fundamental benzopyrone moiety of khellin (Fig. 44.32). The two chromone rings are necessary for activity and must be coplanar, with a linking chain of no longer than six carbons. If one changes the linking chain to positions 8 and 8′, coplanarity cannot be maintained, and the compound loses all activity. Cromolyn sodium is poorly absorbed from the lungs (~8%), insignificantly from the eye (~0.07%), and by approximately 1% from the GI tract. What little that finds its way into systemic circulation is eliminated intact in the urine and the bile. For the treatment of asthma, cromolyn sodium is available as a solution for both intranasal and inhalation administration. There also is an oral concentrate (100 mg/5 mL), which is administered as a 200-mg dose given four times a day.

Nedocromil Sodium

Nedocromil sodium was developed by changing the furan ring of khellin to a piperidinone ring (Fig. 44.32). In vitro, nedocromil sodium inhibits the release of inflammatory response mediators from a variety of cells, including neutrophils, mast cells, macrophages, and platelets. Inhaled nedocromil sodium is poorly absorbed into the systemic circulation, with approximately 3% of an inhaled dose excreted in the urine during the first 6 hours after administration. Only 2% of orally dosed nedocromil sodium is bioavailable, 89% of which is protein bound. When administered IV, nedocromil sodium is not metabolized and is excreted unchanged in the bile and the urine. Nedocromil sodium is available in aerosol canisters for oral inhalation via a mouthpiece.

Leukotriene Modifiers

Introduction

It has been known for more than 40 years that a substance called SRS-A (slow-reacting substance of anaphylaxis) produced a slowly developing, long-lasting contraction of isolated guinea pig ileum and that this same substance was associated with the pathophysiology of asthma. Subsequently, it was determined that SRS-A actually was a mixture of triene-containing lipids, designated as cysteine-leukotrienes: LTC_4, LTD_4, and LTE_4. Determination of the chemical structure of these biologically active compounds led to the development of biosynthesis inhibitors as well as receptor antagonists that are useful in the treatment of asthma (39).

Biosynthesis of leukotrienes

The leukotrienes occur in a variety of inflammatory cells that are abundant in asthma, including eosinophils, mast cells, and macrophages. They are derived from arachidonic acid via a branch of the common pathway to the prostacyclins and thromboxanes. Arachidonic acid itself is produced by the action of phospholipase A_2 on cell walls. Unlike the prostacyclins and thromboxanes, excess arachidonic acid does not activate the pathway. Instead, the first step in the conversion of arachidonic acid to produce the leukotrienes is controlled by an activating protein, 5-lipoxygenase–activating protein, which

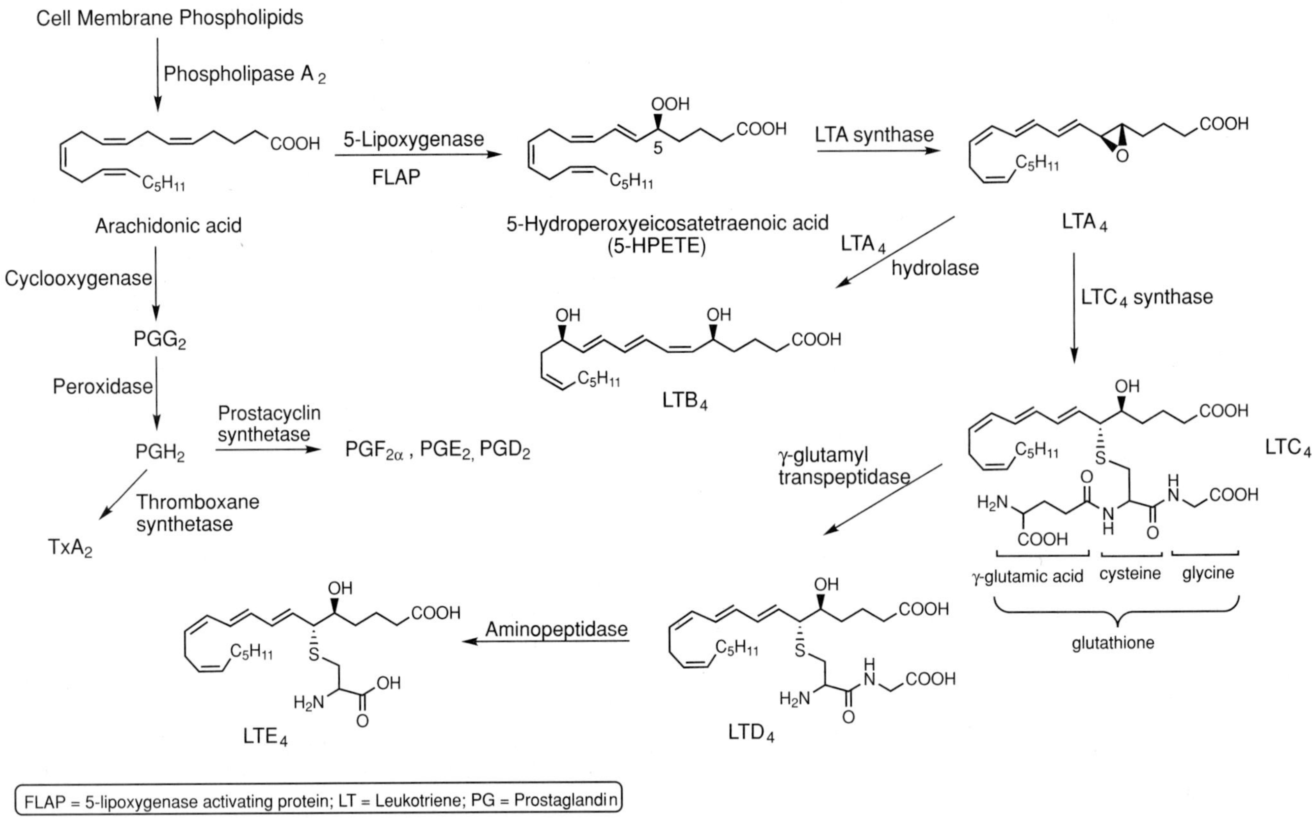

Cell Membrane Phospholipids
Phospholipase A 2
COOH 5-Lipoxygenase FLAP
OOH COOH LTA synthase
COOH
Arachidonic acid
5-Hydroperoxyeicosatetraenoic acid (5-HPETE)
LTA 4 hydrolase
LTA 4
LTC 4 synthase
Cyclooxygenase
PGG2
Peroxidase
PGH2
Prostacyclin synthetase
PGF2α, PGE2, PGD2
Thromboxane synthetase
TxA2
LTB 4
γ-glutamyl transpeptidase
LTC 4
γ-glutamic acid cysteine glycine
glutathione
Aminopeptidase
LTE 4
LTD 4

FLAP = 5-lipoxygenase activating protein; LT = Leukotriene; PG = Prostaglandin

Fig. 44.33. Biochemical pathways leading to the leukotrienes.

regulates the interaction of 5-lipoxygenase with its substrate. Figure 44.33 depicts the biosynthetic pathway and shows that 5-lipoxygenase oxidizes arachidonic acid to the unstable peroxide intermediate, 5-hydroperoxyeicosatetraenoic acid, which is quickly dehydrated to LTA_4, which in turn is further metabolized by LTA_4 hydrolase to LTB_4 and by LTA_4 synthase to the glutathione adduct, LTC_4. Cleavage of γ-glutamic acid by γ-glutamyl transpeptidase converts LTC_4 to LTD_4, which in turn is converted to LTE_4 by the removal of glycine under the action of dipeptidase. The three leukotrienes produced from LTA_4 have strong bronchoconstrictive activity: LTD_4 is the most potent bronchoconstrictor, with the fastest onset of action; however, LTB_4 has no bronchoconstrictive activity but is a potent neutrophil chemotactic agent.

Leukotriene Receptors

The cysteinyl leukotriene (cysLT) receptors are of the rhodopsin family of the G protein–coupled receptor family. As such, they consist of seven transmembrane-spanning helices that activate intracellular signaling pathways in response to their endogenous ligands (LTC_4, LTD_4, and LTE_4). Studies have identified two distinct cysLT receptors, and molecular biologists have cloned the human genes for both the $cysLT_1$ receptor and the $cysLT_2$ receptor (40). Pharmacology studies distinguished between the two cysLT receptors by evaluating their interaction with known antagonists, showing that the $cysLT_1$ receptor is competitively inhibited from binding LTD_4 whereas the $cysLT_2$ receptor was not. In addition, there is a slight difference in ligand-binding affinities between the two receptors. The $cysLT_1$ receptors have an affinity profile of $LTD_4 > LTC_4 = LTE_4$, whereas the $cysLT_2$ receptors show an affinity profile of $LTC_4 = LTD_4 > LTE_4$. Both receptor types occur in the lungs and spleen. The $cysLT_1$ receptor is found only in the placenta and small intestines, whereas the $cysLT_2$ receptor occurs only in the heart, lymph nodes, and brain. The incomplete overlap of tissue distribution along with their distinct ligand-binding properties suggests the $cysLT_1$ receptors and the $cysLT_2$ receptors might serve different functions in vivo (41), and because the $cysLT_1$ receptors are inhibited by selective antagonists, they have importance in the treatment of leukotriene related bronchoconstriction in asthma.

Leukotriene Modifier Drugs

Two approaches to the development of leukotriene modifiers have been taken. The first approach was to block their biosynthesis by looking for compounds that inhibit one or more of the enzymes involved in the biochemical pathway. The second approach was to identify antagonists with selective affinity for the $cysLT_1$ receptors.

Leukotriene Biosynthesis Inhibitors

The search for orally active 5-lipoxygenase inhibitors has resulted in only a few classes of compounds that are effective in animals and humans with the N-hydroxyureas, yielding a useful product (42). The 5-lipoxygenase inhibitors block the production of LTB_4 as well as LTC_4, LTD_4, and LTE_4, thereby decreasing both the bronchoconstrictive and chemotactic effects of the leukotrienes.

ZILEUTIN

Benzothienyl

N-hydroxyurea

Zileuton (Zyflo)

Zileutin is the first N-hydroxyurea 5-lipoxygenase inhibitor to be marketed. It is the ethylbenzothienyl derivative of N-hydroxyurea and occurs as the racemic mixture of *R*-(+)- and *S*-(−)-enantiomers, both of which are pharmacologically active. The N-hydroxyl group is essential for inhibitory activity, with the benzothienyl group contributing to its overall lipophilicity. Zileutin is rapidly absorbed orally and is 93% protein bound in the plasma. Metabolism occurs in the liver, with the inactive O-glucuronide being the major metabolite, along with less than 0.5% inactive N-dehydroxylated and unchanged zileutin. The glucuronidation is stereoselective, with the *S*-isomer being metabolized and eliminated more quickly (43). Greater than 90% of an oral dose is bioavailable, and 95% is excreted as metabolites in the urine, with a half-life of 2.5 hours, thus requiring four-times-a-day dosing. Zileutin increases the plasma levels of propranolol, theophylline, and warfarin, and dosing of these drugs should be reduced and the serum levels monitored carefully in patients taking both drugs. The most serious side effect of zileutin is elevation of liver enzymes; if symptoms of liver dysfunction (e.g., nausea, fatigue, pruritis, jaundice, or flu-like symptoms) occur, the drug should be discontinued.

LEUKOTRIENE RECEPTOR ANTAGONISTS. The search for leukotriene receptor antagonists began without the aid of ligand–receptor binding data and took the form of three approaches. These included the design of leukotriene structural analogues, quinoline analogues, and the random screening of compounds. The combination of these efforts led to a simple SAR: The lipophilic tetraene tail of LTD_4 can be mimicked by a variety of more stable aromatic rings, the thioether of the glycinyl-cysteinyl dipeptide can be replaced by an alkyl carboxylic acid, and the C_1 carboxylate of LTD_4 needs to be retained. Additional research focusing on the three-dimensional requirements for antagonist binding to the cysLT receptors further clarified that the pharmacophore needs to consist of an acidic or negative ionizable functional group, a hydrogen-bond acceptor function, and three hydrophobic regions (44). Based on this background, synthetic efforts resulted in the development of montelukast and zafirlukast as $cysLT_1$ receptor antagonists. Figure 44.34 demonstrates how both these antagonists fit the pharmacophore model.

MONTELUKAST

Montelukast (Singulair)

Montelukast was developed from other weakly antagonistic quinoline derivatives. A number of changes can be made to the structure without the loss of activity. These include changing the double bond between the two aromatic rings to an ether linkage, reducing the quinoline ring, changing the chlorine to a fluorine, and/or exchanging the sulfur for an amide group. Montelukast is a high-affinity, selective antagonist of the $cysLT_1$ receptor. It is rapidly absorbed orally, with a bioavailability of 64%. Montelukast is 99% bound to plasma proteins and is extensively metabolized in the

Hydrophobic region

Acidic region

Hydrogen-bond donor

Hydrophobic region

Montelukast

Hydrophobic region

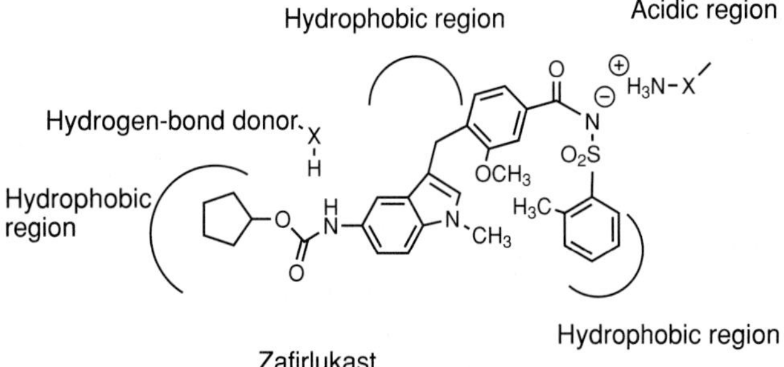

Fig. 44.34. Interaction of montelulast and zafirlukast with cysteinyl leukotriene (cysLT) receptor model.

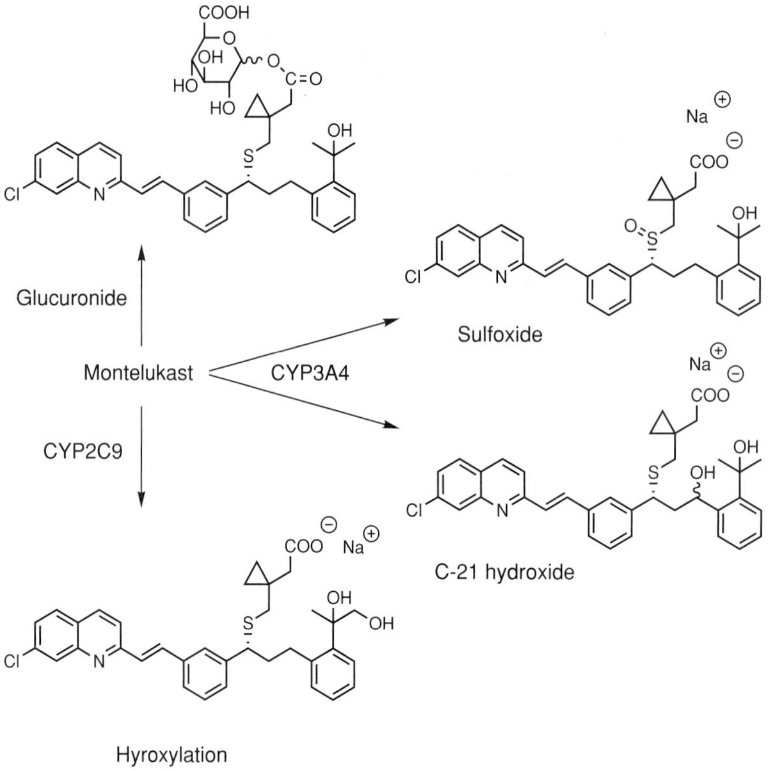

Fig. 44.35. Metabolism of montelukast.

liver by CYP3A4 and CYP2C9 to oxidated products. CYP3A4 oxidizes the sulfur and the C-21 benzylic carbon, whereas CYP2C9 is selectively responsible for the methyl hydroxylation. Figure 44.35 shows the primary metabolic pathway for montelukast in humans (45). More than 86% of an oral dose is eliminated as metabolites through the bile. Montelukast did not demonstrate any significant adverse effects greater than placebo in clinical trials; however, because it is metabolized by the cytochrome P450 (CYP450) enzymes, its plasma levels should be monitored when coadministered with CYP450-inducing drugs, such as phenobarbital, rifampin, and phenytoin. Montelukast is available in tablet, chewable tablet, and granules for administration mixed with food.

Zafirlukast

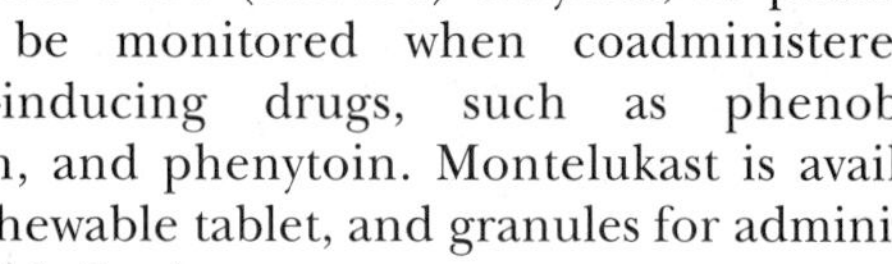

Zafirlukast (Accolate)

Zafirlukast is an indole derivative with a sulfonamide group that fulfills the need for an ionizable moiety on the pharmacophore. A large number of analogues have been prepared; however, they all resulted in a decrease in antagonist activity. Zafirlukast, like montelukast, is a selective antagonist for the $cysLT_1$ receptor and antagonizes the bronchoconstrictive effects of all leukotrienes (LTC_4, LTD_4, and LTE_4). Zafirlukast is well absorbed orally; however, food will decrease its absorption by as much as 40%. Zafirlukast is primarily metabolized in the liver by CYP2C9 and CYP3A4 to hydroxylated metabolites (46). Zafirlukast also has been shown to undergo carbamate hydrolysis, followed by N-acetylation. Additionally, zafirlukast in known to produce an idiosyncratic hepatotoxicity in susceptible patients. This is appears to result from the formation of an electrophilic α,β-unsaturated iminium intermediate evidenced by the formation of a glutathione adduct on the methylene carbon bridging the indole ring to the methoxybenzene moiety of the molecule (47).

Figure 44.36 summarizes the metabolism of zafirlukast. More than 90% if its metabolites are excreted in the feces, with the remaining found in the urine. Zafirlukast inhibits CYP3A4 and CYP2C9 in concentrations equivalent to clinical plasma levels and, therefore, should be used with caution in patients taking drugs metabolized by these enzymes. Specifically, coadministration with warfarin results in a significant increase in prothrombin time. Other drugs metabolized by CYP2C9 are phenytoin and carbamazepine. In addi-

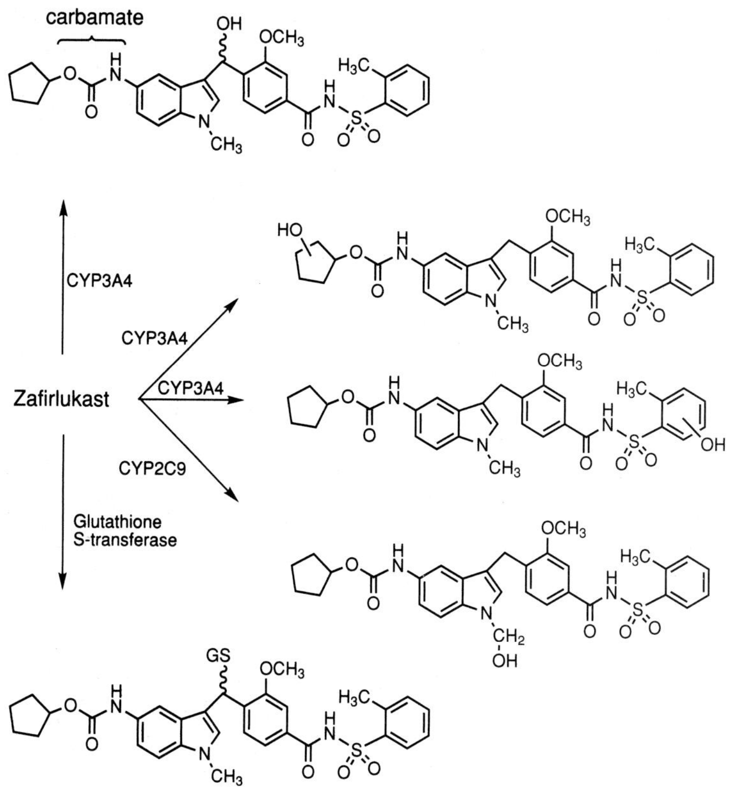

Fig. 44.36. Metabolism of zafirlukast to oxidative products and a glutathione adduct.

tion, CYP3A4-metabolized drugs are cyclosporine, cisapride, and the dihydropyridine class of calcium channel blockers. Of particular interest is the fact that aspirin increases the plasma levels of zafirlukast, and theophylline decreases the plasma levels of zafirlukast. Care should be taken when coadministering with erythromycin, because this decreases the bioavailability of zafirlukast. Zafirlukast is only available in tablet formulations.

Monoclonal Anti-IgE Antibody

Introduction

The pathophysiology of allergic asthma, as already discussed, involves the dendritic processing of the allergen, which ultimately results in the production of allergen-specific IgE by activated B lymphocytes. The IgE binds to high-affinity (FcεRI) receptors on mast cells. The site where IgE binds to the receptor is located on the Fc fragment area of the C-ε-3 region, hence the acronym FcεRI (Fig. 44.37A). Subsequent allergen exposure causes cross-linking of bound IgE molecules, which triggers degranulation of these cells, resulting in the release of asthma mediators. Monoclonal anti-IgE antibody development is designed to moderate the role of IgE in activating mast cells, thereby decreasing the severity of allergic asthmatic attacks, and may have beneficial effects in treating seasonal allergic rhinitis.

Omalizumab Development and Pharmacology

Omalizumab is a monoclonal antibody developed through somatic cell hybridization techniques and was identified as a murine anti-human IgE antibody, originally called MAE11 (48). It is designed to interact with the site that binds to FcεRI on mast cells. Additional amino acid sequences have been incorporated into the antibody so that a humanized product resulted that only differs by 5% nonhuman amino acid residues.

In vitro, omalizumab has been shown to complex with free IgE, forming trimers consisting of a 2:1 complex of IgE to omalizumab or a 1:2 complex of IgE to omalizumab. In addition, larger complexes also are formed, consisting of a 3:3 ratio of each (Fig. 44.37B). Omalizumab does not bind to IgE already bound to mast cells and, therefore, does not cause the degranulation that might be expected from such interaction. Thus, omalizumab effectively neutralizes free IgE and, aside from the obvious decrease of available IgE, also causes the down-regulation of FcεRI receptors on the mast cell surface, resulting in a decrease of IgE bound to the mast cell.

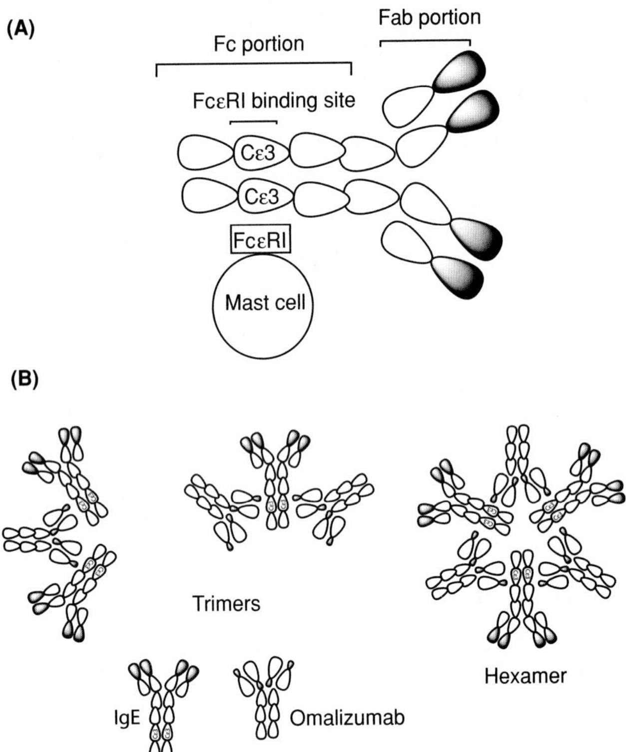

Fig. 44.37. (A) Graphic representation of IgE binding to the FCεRI on a mast cell. (B) Graphic representation of immune complexes formed between omalizumab. Hexamers predominate when components are in a 1:1 ratio, and the trimers predominate when one of the components is in excess.

Omalizumab (Xolaire)

The clinical role for omalizumab is in the treatment of allergic asthma. It is approved for the treatment of adults and adolescents 12 years of age and older whose symptoms are not controlled with inhaled glucocorticoids and who have a positive skin test for airborne allergens. The bioavailability after subcutaneous administration is 62%, with slow absorption resulting in peak serum levels in 7 to 8 days from a single dose. Steady-state plasma concentration is reached in 14 to 29 days with multiple dosing regimens. The elimination of omalizumab is not clearly understood; however, studies have determined that intact IgE is excreted via the bile and that omalizumab:IgE complexes are cleared faster than uncomplexed omalizumab and slower than free IgE. This means that over time, total IgE concentrations (free and complexed IgE) increase, because the complex is cleared more slowly. The metabolism of omalizumab is not known, and the clearance of the complex is similar to the liver elimination of another immunoglobulin, IgG. The reticuloendothelial system degrades IgG, and it is believed that the same process occurs for the omalizumab:IgE complex. Omalizumab is available as a lyophilized powder for injection in single-use, 5-mL vials.

CHRONIC OBSTRUCTIVE LUNG DISEASE

Definition and Epidemiology

Chromic obstructive lung disease is characterized by persistent breathing difficulty that is not completely reversible and is progressive over time. It usually is the result of an abnormal inflammatory response to airborne toxic chemicals. Thus, COPD is a general term and most commonly refers to chronic bronchitis and emphysema. Asthma is considered to be a disease entity unto itself and is not included in the definition of COPD. Both COPD and asthma are both considered to be inflammatory diseases; however, the nature of the inflammation is different. Asthma is associated with the release of inflammatory mediators from mast cells and eosinophils, whereas chronic bronchitis is primarily associated with neutrophils and emphysema with alveoli damage. In addition, asthma is more often than not allergenic, whereas chronic bronchitis and emphysema have no allergic component. Finally, it is uncommon for asthma to be associated with smoking, whereas there is a very high incidence of both chronic bronchitis and emphysema in smokers.

Patients with COPD display a variety of symptoms, ranging from chronic productive cough to severe dyspnea requiring hospitalization. Other chronic illnesses, including cardiac, endocrine, and renal disease, often occur along with COPD in many patients. In the United States, COPD is the fourth leading cause of death, being responsible for more than 100,000 deaths per year (49). It has been estimated that between 16 and 24 million people in the United States have COPD and that those with chronic bronchitis outnumber those with emphysema. Rates of COPD-related death among women have tripled over the last 30 years, and this is being attributed to their increase in smoking. Chronic obstructive pulmonary disease is recognized as a global health problem, and in 2001, the NIH and the World Health Organization developed the Global Initiative for Chronic Lung Disease (GOLD) guidelines, which present only evidence-based recommendations for the treatment of COPD (50,51).

Pathogenesis

The single most important risk factor for the development of COPD is smoking. It is estimated that 85% of COPD cases are attributable to cigarette smoking. Not all people who smoke, however, develop the disease, which means other factors are involved. It seems that genetics, environmental pollutants, and infection along with bronchial hyperreactivity all play an important role.

Cigarette smoke attracts inflammatory cells into the lungs and stimulates the release of the proteolytic enzyme elastase. Elastase breaks down elastin, which is a needed structural component of lung tissue. Normally, the lung is protected from elastase by an inhibitor, α_1-antitrypsin (ATT). Cigarette smoke, however, causes an abnormal amount of elastase to be produced that ATT cannot counter, leading to lung damage. Smokers with an inherited deficiency of ATT have a greatly increased risk of developing emphysema, especially at an early age. Patients with COPD show an accelerated decline in lung function (50–90 mL FEV_1/year) as compared to nonsmokers (20–30 mL/year) (see earlier discussion of FEV under *General Therapeutic Approaches to the Treatment and Management of Asthma*). Patients with COPD who stop smoking slow down the progression of the disease. Unfortunately, however, they do not improve, because the symptoms are an indication of irreparable lung tissue damage.

The role of other risk factors for developing COPD is not clear. Air pollution and occupational exposure to gases and particulates from the incomplete combustion of coal, diesel, and gasoline are related to the development of cough and sputum, but development of COPD seems to occur only in susceptible individuals. Passive cigarette smoke comes from the burning end of the cigarette and actually is higher in toxic substances compared with exhaled smoke. It has been established that respiratory infections as well as cough and sputum production are more common in children who live in households where one or both parents smoke. Chinese and Afro-Caribbean races have a reduced incidence of COPD, whereas COPD in American blacks is on the rise (49).

Permanent destructive enlargement of the airspaces distal to the terminal bronchioles without obvious fibrosis is the pathological characteristic of emphysema. On the other hand, chronic bronchitis is characterized by hypersecretion of mucus, most of which is produced by the trachea and first branches of the bronchi. The smaller bronchi and terminal bronchioles, however, are the site of the increased airway resistance in chronic bronchitis. In the early stages of chronic bronchitis, the mucus and inflammation contribute to "smoker's cough," with little effect on airway obstruction. As inflammation continues, cell wall edema and the production of large amounts of mucus contribute to airway narrowing and the difficulty in breathing associated with COPD. Even though bronchospasm may seem to be involved in COPD, there is little related pathogenesis. Chronic obstructive pulmonary disease is a disease of the small airways and their adjacent alveoli. In chronic bronchitis, there are structural changes in the small airways as a result of persistent inflammatory irritation, which leads to airway narrowing. Emphysema on the other hand is the result of loss of lung elastic recoil because of inflammation and alveolar wall destruction. Both diseases often occur together, with one predominate over the other. An important clinical manifestation between chronic bronchitis and emphysema is that there is significant hypoxia and carbon dioxide retention with chronic bronchitis, which does not happen with emphysema. Because of this, emphysema patients are referred to as "pink puffers," whereas patients with chronic bronchitis are called "blue bloaters" (52).

Pharmacotherapy

All the medications used to treat COPD have already been covered in the previous section on asthma. The GOLD guidelines base their treatment protocols on a classification of disease severity divided into five stages (50,51). Stages O and I are defined as "at risk" (O) and mild COPD (I). In stage O, the patient has normal lung function, with chronic cough and sputum production. Treatment at this stage is to counsel the patient to reduce risks and, especially, to stop smoking. In stage I, there is minor airway limitation, characterized as $FEV_1/FVC < 70\%$ but $FEV_1 \geq 80\%$ of the predicted value. Stage I treatment is to use a short-acting bronchodilator, usually as needed, but regular use is effective in patients with concurrent asthma. The most frequently used short-acting bronchodilator is the β_2-agonist albuterol, although pirbuterol and the anticholinergic ipratropium can be just as effective, but with a slightly longer onset of action. The patient also should take precautions to avoid bacterial or viral infections by receiving vaccinations against influenza and pneumococcal pneumonia.

Stage II COPD is a moderate disease condition in which the patient demonstrates shortness of breath on exertion and spirometry reveals $FEV_1/FVC < 70\%$ and FEV_1 between 50 and 80% of the predicted value. Stage II drug treatment requires the addition of a long-acting bronchodilator along with the short-acting bronchodilator. Salmeterol and formoterol are long-acting β_2-agonists, and tiotropium is the long-acting anticholinergic most often used. Alternatively, the addition of ipratropium along with the short-acting β_2-agonist also can be effective at this stage. Extended- release theophylline is an option for patients who do not receive adequate relief of symptoms or who cannot tolerate other bronchodilators.

Stage III is a severe form of COPD, with $FEV_1/FVC <$ 70% and FEV_1 between 30 and 50% of the predicted value. The patient experiences increasing dyspnea that affects his or her ability to perform routine tasks (i.e., climbing stairs). A course of oral glucocorticoids (i.e., prednisone) may be used to control a severe attack. The role of inhaled glucocorticoids is not clearly established, and no evidence suggests that an inhaled glucocorticoid has any advantage in patients who can maintain their FEV_1 with bronchodilators. As of this writing, no inhaled glucocorticoids are approved for the treatment of COPD; however, there is one combination formulation of fluticasone propionate and salmeterol dosage (250 μg/50 μg) approved for twice-daily administration.

Stage IV is the most severe form of COPD, with airflow restriction of $FEV_1/FVC < 70\%$ and $FEV_1 < 30\%$ of the predicted value along with chronic respiratory failure. At this stage, the patient is experiencing debilitating exacerbations that are not controlled by medication and requires daily oxygen for respiratory failure. Surgery also is an option, but it is not without serious risks. Surgical options include bullectomy (removal of large blebs in the lungs), lung transplant (uncommon), and lung volume reduction surgery (removal of lung sections affected by emphysema).

Patients with emphysema that is associated with ATT deficiencies can receive weekly IV infusions of to maintain acceptable antiprotease activity that can minimize their disease progression. The three approved ATT products are Aralast, Prolastin, and Zemaira. Because these protein products are derived from human plasma, there is the risk of transmission of viral infection and Creutzfeldt-Jakob disease.

New Drug Classes for Treatment of Asthma and COPD

Phosphodiesterase Inhibitors

Introduction. A number of important therapeutic agents owe their pharmacological action to their ability to inhibit the enzyme PDE. In the treatment of asthma, theophylline, at least in part, relaxes bronchospasm by relaxing bronchiole smooth muscles; amrinone and milrinone are ionotropic agents that relax vasculature, causing vasodilation; sildenafil and vardenafil relax smooth muscle of the vasculature in the penis; dipyramidole inhibits platelet aggregation; and the alkaloid papaverine relieves smooth and cardiac muscle spasms through its ability to inhibit PDE. These pharmacological effects are the result of inhibiting the ability of PDE to break down cAMP and cGMP and prolong their action as secondary messengers within a variety of cell types throughout the body. The PDE inhibitors also are implicated in an anti-inflammatory role by increasing cAMP and cGMP levels in cell types associated with the release of inflammatory chemicals from T and B cells, monocytes, neutrophils, and eosinophils. This last discovery is the impetus to develop new PDE inhibitors to treat asthma (eosinophils) and COPD (neutrophils).

New Phosphodiesterase Inhibitors

Progress in the development of PDE inhibitors to treat COPD and asthma awaited the basic pharmacological research that identified the specific PDE isoforms associated with inflammatory cells so that selective inhibitors could be designed and synthesized (53). (For additional discussion of PDE inhibitors and the structural characteristics of the PDE4 binding site, see Chapter 17.) As mentioned earlier, there are 11 families of PDEs, with PDE4 being associated with inflammatory processes. Specifically, three PDE4 subtypes (PDE4A, PDE4B, and PDE4D) are found in inflammatory cells (with PDE4B being predominant). Therefore, recent efforts in this area have been directed toward the development and synthesis of selective PDE4 inhibitors. Two PDE4 inhibitors are being investigated for their possible use in treating asthma and COPD. In the United States, cilomilast is being investigated for the treatment of COPD, and in Europe, roflumilast is being investigated for the treatment of both asthma and COPD.

Cilomilast

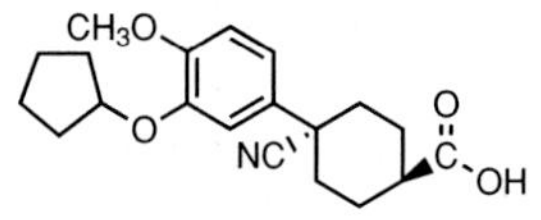

Cilomilast (Ariflo)

Cilomilast contains the dialkoxyphenyl ring characteristic of selective PDE4 inhibitors. The ether oxygens hydrogen bond to a glutamine in the binding pocket, and the cyclopentyl ring adds additional hydrophobic interactions. The oxygen atoms of the carboxyl group form hydrogen bonds with water that is coordinated with Mg^{2+} located in the distal end of the binding pocket. Orally administered cilomilast is 96% bioavailable. Food does not interfere with the overall absorption; however, food does slow down the rate. Cilomilast is 99% bound to albumin in the plasma and is metabolized in the liver by CYP2C8. The metabolism is extensive and results in oxidation, carboxyl group glucuronidation, and dealkylation of the cyclopentyl group, followed by glucuronidation or sulfation. A major difficulty with cilomilast is that in therapeutic doses, patients during clinical trials have experienced significant diarrhea and nausea. These effects appear to be tolerable and, theoretically, result from its inhibition of the PDE4D receptor subtype.

Roflumilast

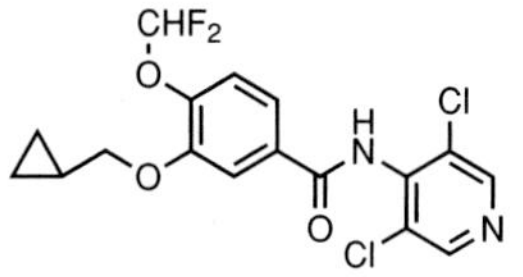

Roflumilast (Daxas)

The PDE4 receptor binding of roflumilast is similar to that of cilomilast. The dialkylphenyl oxygens hydrogen bonds to a glutamine deep inside the binding pocket. The diflouromethoxy group and the cyclopropyl group contribute hydrophobic bonds; however, the cyclopentyl group on cilomilast makes far more interactions compared with the cyclopropyl group. The water molecule coordinated to the Mg^{2+} hydrogen bonds to the dichloropyridyl group just like the carboxylic acid oxygens in cilomilast. These structural differences make roflumilast a more potent inhibitor than cilomilast toward PDE4B (54). Roflumilast is well absorbed on oral administration and has a half-life of 10 hours. Roflumilast is metabolized in the liver to its N-oxide derivative, which also is a PDE4 inhibitor, and it has a plasma half-life of 20 hours (see Chapter 17). Roflumilast is currently undergoing clinical trials in Europe for use in the treatment of both asthma and COPD.

CASE STUDY

Victoria F. Roche and S. William Zito

BJ is a Las Vegas blackjack dealer. He is a 38-year-old Caucasian man who has mild intermittent asthma treated with inhaled albuterol for occasional exacerbations. He works nights and sleeps during the day. He shows up at the emergency room early one morning complaining that he is not sleeping well lately. He says he wakes up about once a week gasping for breath. In addition, he has been having increased episodes of acute asthma during his job, which have caused him to use his inhaler at least once a night. He finds that his clients are disturbed by his wheezing and audible gurgling, and he fears he will lose his job unless something is done about it. On further inquiry, you determine that BJ is taking phenytoin (100 mg t.i.d.) to control the epilepsy he has had since he was an adolescent. The attending physician determines that BJ's asthma has progressed to the mild persistent stage and wants to prescribe an appropriate medication. Evaluate the following choices for use in this case.

1. Identify the therapeutic problem(s) in which the pharmacist's intervention may benefit the patient.
2. Identify and prioritize the patient-specific factors that must be considered to achieve the desired therapeutic outcomes.
3. Conduct a thorough and mechanistically oriented structure-activity analysis of all therapeutic alternatives provided in the case.
4. Evaluate the SAR findings against the patient specific factors and desired therapeutic outcomes and make a therapeutic decision.
5. Counsel your patient.

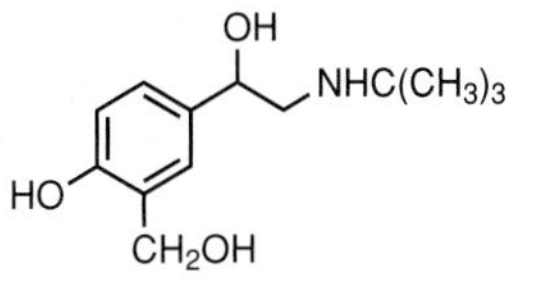

Albuterol

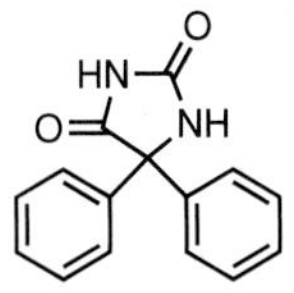

phenytoin

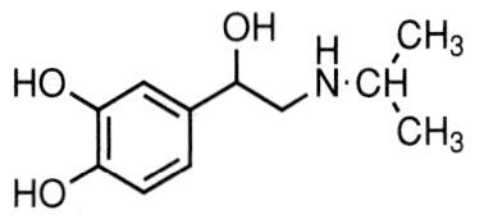

1

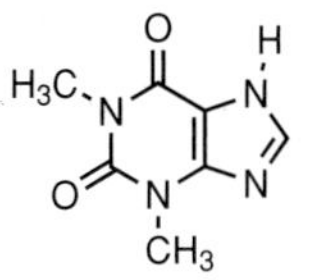

2

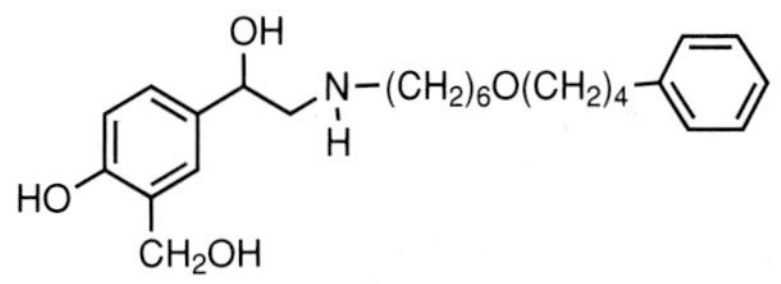

3

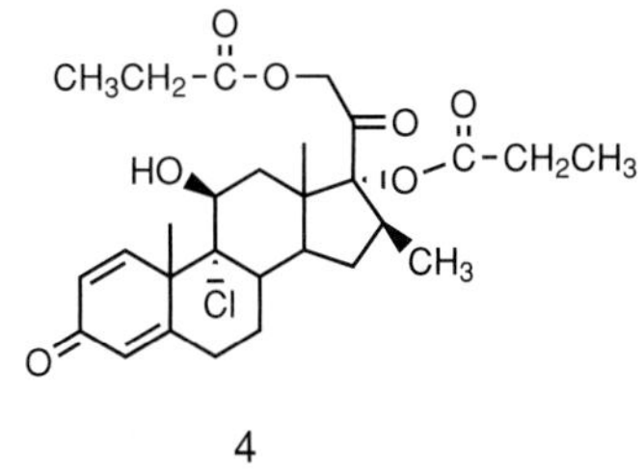

4

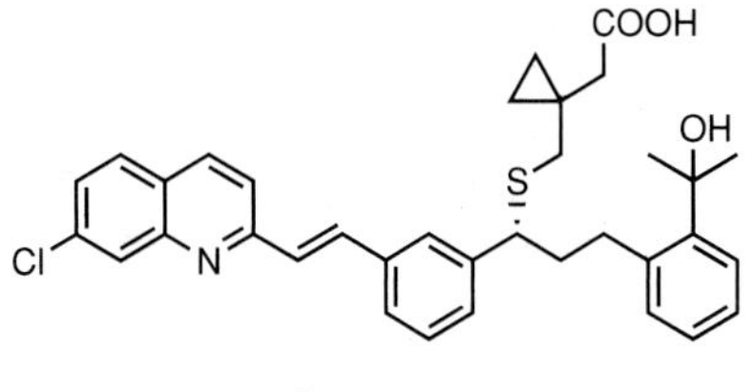

5

References

1. Marketos SG, Ballas CN. Bronchial asthma in the medical literature of Greek antiquity. J Asthma 1982;19:263–269.
2. Mannino DM, Homa DM, Akinbami LJ, et al. Surveillance for asthma—United States, 1908-1999. MMWR 2002;51:1–14.
3. Centers for Disease Control and Prevention, National Center for Health Statistics. Asthma prevalence, health care use, and mortality, 2002. Available at: http:/www. cdc.gov/nchs/products/pubs/pubd/hestats/asthma/asthma.htm. Accessed September 10, 2005.
4. Bethsda, MD. National Institutes of Health. National Asthma Education Program Expert Panel Report 2. Guidelines for the Diagnosis and Management of Asthma—Update on Selected Topics 2002. Bethsda, MD NIH publication 02-5075.
5. Bethsda, MD. National Institutes of Health. National Asthma Education Program Expert Panel Report 2: Guidelines for the Diagnosis and Management of Asthma, 1997. Bethsda, MD NIH publication 97-4051.
6. Elias JA, Lee CG, Zheng T, et al. New insights into the pathogenesis of asthma. J Clin Invest 2003;111:291–297.
7. Self TH. Asthma. In: Koda-Kimble MA, Young LY, Kradjan WA, et al., eds. Applied Therapeutics: The Clinical Use of Drugs. 8th Ed. Baltimore: Lippincott Williams & Wilkins, 2005:23-1–23-41.
8. Weiss ST. Eat dirt—the hygiene hypothesis and allergic diseases. N Engl J Med 2002;347:930–931.
9. Bach JF. The effect of infections on susceptibility to autoimmune and allergic diseases. N Eng J Med 2002;347:911–920.
10. Ober C. Perspectives on the past decade of asthma genetics. J Allergy Clin Immunol 2005;116:274–278.
11. Cookson W. The alliance of genes and environment in asthma and allergy. Nature 1999;402:5–11.
12. Sandford AJ, Pare PD. The genetics of asthma. The important questions. Am J Respir Crit Care Med 2000;161:202–206.
13. Tattersfield AE, Knox AJ, Britton JR, et al. Asthma. Lancet 2002;360:1313–1322.
14. Bochner BS, Busse WW. Allergy and asthma. J Allergy Clin Immunol 2005;115:953–959.
15. Lily CM. Diversity of asthma: evolving concepts of pathophysiology and lessons from genetics. J Allergy Clin Immunol 2005;115:S526–S531.
16. Mizue Y, Ghani S, Leng L, et al. Role of macrophage migration inhibitory factor in asthma. Proceedings of the National Academy of Science 2005;102:14410–14415.
17. Peters JI, Levine SM. Introduction to pulmonary function testing. In: DiPiro JT, Talbert RL, Yee GC, et al., eds. Pharmacotherapy: A Pathophysiologic Approach. 5th Ed. Stamford, CT: Appleton & Lange, 2002;23:467–473.

18. Welsh DA, Thomas DA. Obstructive lung disease. In: Ali J, Summer WR, Levitzky MG, eds. Pulmonary Pathophysiology. 2nd Ed. New York: Lange Medical Books/McGraw-Hill, 2005:85–91.
19. Ahlquist RP. A study of the adrenergic receptors. Am J Physiol 1948;153:586–600.
20. Philipp M, Hein L. Adrenergic receptor knockout mice: distinct functions of nine receptor subtypes. Pharmacol Ther 2004;101:65–74.
21. Bikker JK, Trumpp-Kallmeyer S, Humblet C. G protein–coupled receptors: models, mutagenesis, and drug design. J Med Chem 1998;41:2911–2927.
22. Furse KE, Lybrand TP. Three-dimensional models for β-adrenergic receptor complexes with agonists and antagonists. J Med Chem 2003;46:4450–4462.
23. Nelson HS, Weiss ST, Bleeker ER, et al. SMART Study Group. The Salmeterol Multicenter Asthma Research Trial: a comparison of usual pharmacotherapy for asthma or usual pharmacotherapy plus salmeterol. Chest 2006;129:15–26.
24. Kua J, Zhang, Y, Eslami AC, et al. Studying the roles of W86, E202, and Y337 on binding of acetylcholine to acetylcholinesterase using a combined molecular dynamics and multiple docking approach. Protein Sci 2003;12:2675–2684.
25. Kostenis E, Zeng FY, Wess J. Structure function analysis of muscarinic acetylcholine receptors. J Physiol 1998;92:265–268.
26. Katzung B. Introduction to autonomic pharmacology. In: Katzung B, ed. Basic and Clinical Pharmacology. 8th Ed. New York: Lange Medical Books/McGraw-Hill, 2001:75–191.
27. Wess J, Blin N, Mutschler E, et al. Muscarinic acetylcholine receptors: structural basis of ligand binding and G protein coupling. Life Sci 1995;56:915–922.
28. Lattin DL, Fifer EK. Drugs affecting cholinergic neurotransmission. In: Lemke TL, Williams DA, eds. Foyes Principles of Medicinal Chemistry. 5th Ed. Baltimore: Lippincott Williams & Wilkins, 2002:264–291.
29. Robbers JE, Speedie MK, Tyler VE. eds. Pharmacognosy and Pharmacobiotechnology. 1st Ed. Baltimore: Williams & Wilkins, 1996:182–185.
30. Huai Q, Liu Y, Francis SH, et al. Crystal structure of phosphodiesterases 4 and 5 in complex with inhibitor 3-isobutyl-1-methylxanthine suggest a conformation determinant of inhibitor selectivity. J Biol Chem 2004;279:13095–13101.
31. IUPAC-IUB Joint Commission on Biochemical Nomenclature (JCBN). The nomenclature of steroids. Recommendations 1989. Eur J Biochem 1989;186: 429–458 [published erratum in Eur J Biochem 1993;213:2].
32. Miller DD, Brueggemeier RW, Dalton JT. Adrenocorticoids. In: Lemke TL, Williams DA, eds. Foyes Principles of Medicinal Chemistry. 5th Ed. Baltimore: Lippincott Williams & Wilkins 2002:655–656.
33. Luis BF, Xu WX, Otwinowski Z, et al. Crystallographic analysis of the interaction of the glucocorticoid receptor with DNA. Nature 1991;352:497–505.
34. Bledsoe RK, Montana VG, Stanley TB, et al. Crystal structure of the glucocorticoid receptor ligand binding domain reveals a novel mode of receptor dimerization and coactivator recognition. Cell 2002;110:93–101.
35. Hammer S, Spika I, Sippl W, et al. Glucocorticoid receptor interactions with glucocorticoids: evaluation by molecular modeling and functional analysis of glucocorticoid receptor mutants. Steroids 2003;68:329–339.
36. Cohen S. The allergy archives: pioneers and milestones—Roger Altounyan and the discovery of cromolyn. J Allergy Clin Immunol April 2005;882–885.
37. Hemmerich S, Yarden Y, Pecht I. A cromoglycate binding protein from rat mast cells of a leukemia line is a nucleoside diphosphate kinase. Biochemistry 1992;31:4574–4579.
38. Oyama Y, Shishibori T, Yamashita K, et al. Two distinct antiallergic drugs, amlexanox and cromolyn, bind to the same kinds of calcium binding proteins, except calmodulin, in bovine lung extract. Biochem Biophys Res Commun 1997;240:341–347.
39. Samuelson SE, Dahlen JA, Lindgren CA, et al. Leukotrienes and lipoxins: structures, biosynthesis, and biological effects. Science 1987;237:1171–1176.
40. Capra V. Molecular and functional aspects of human cysteinyl leukotriene receptors. Pharmacol Res 2004;50:1–11.
41. Kanoak Y Boyce JA. Cysteinyl leukotrienes and the receptors: cellular distribution and function in immune and inflammatory responses. J Immunol 2004;173:1503–1510.
42. Brooks CD, Summers JB. Modulators of leukotriene biosynthesis and receptor activation. J Med Chem 1996;39:2629–2654.
43. Sweeny DJ, Nellans HN. Stereoselective glucuronidation of zileutin isomers by human hepatic microsomes. Drug Metab Dispos 1995;23:149–153.
44. Palomar A, Pascual J, Cabre F, et al. Derivation of pharmacophore and comfa models for leukotriene D_4 receptor antagonists of the quinolinyl(bridged) aryl series. J Med Chem 2000;43:392–400.
45. Chiba M, Xu X, Nishime JA, et al. Hepatic microsomal metabolism of montelukast, a potent leukotriene D_4 receptor antagonist, in humans. Drug Metab Dispos 1997;25:1022–1037.
46. Savidge RD, Bui KH, Birmingham BK, et al. Metabolism and excretion of zafirlukast in dogs, rats, and mice. Drug Metab Dispos 1998;26:1069–1076.
47. Kassahun K, Skordos K, McIntosh I, et al. Zafirlukast metabolism by cytochrome P450 3A4 produces an electrophilic α,β-unsaturated iminium species that results in the selective mechanism based inactivation of the enzyme. Chem Res Toxicol 2005;18:1427–1437.
48. Buhl R. Anti-IgE antibodies for the treatment of asthma. Curr Opin Pulm Med 2005;11:27–34.
49. Mannino DM, Homa DM, Akinbami LJ, et al. Chronic obstructive pulmonary disease surveillance: United States, 1971–2000. MMWR 2002;51:1–16.
50. Pauwels RA, Buist AS, Calverley PM, et al. Global strategy for the diagnosis, management, and prevention of chronic obstructive pulmonary disease. NHLBI/WHO Global Initiative for Chronic Obstructive Lung Disease (GOLD) Workshop summary. Am J Respir Crit Care Med 2001;63:1256–1276.
51. Workshop report: global strategy for diagnosis, management, and prevention of COPD—Updated 2005. Available at: http://www.goldcopd.org. Accessed on Feb 2005.
52. Konzem SL, Stratton MA. Chronic obstructive lung disease. In: DiPiro JT, Talbert RL, Yee GC, et al., eds. Pharmacotherapy: A Pathophysiologic Approach. 5th Ed. Stamford, CT: Appleton & Lange, 2002;27:511–529.
53. Lipworth BJ. Phosphodiesterase-4 inhibitors for asthma and chronic obstructive pulmonary disease. Lancet 2005;365:167–175.
54. Card GL, England BP, Suzuki Y, et al. Structural basis for the activity of drugs that inhibit phosphodiesterases. Structure (Cambridge) 2004;12:2233–2247.

45. *Men's Health*

DUANE D. MILLER, ROBERT W. BRUEGGEMEIER, AND JAMES T. DALTON

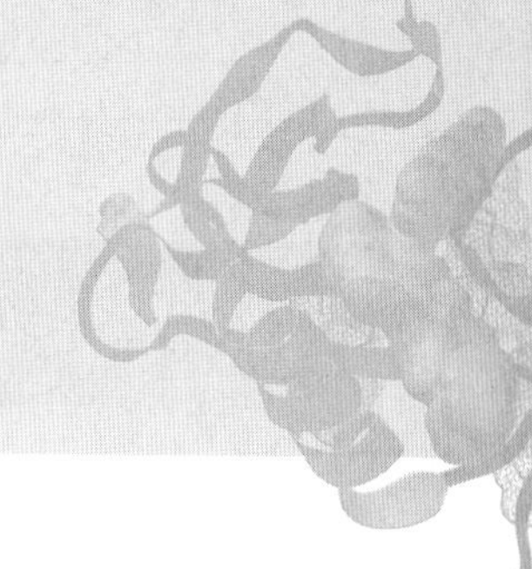

DRUGS COVERED IN THIS CHAPTER:

TESTOSTERONE PRODUCTS
- Oral testosterone
  - Methyltestosterone
  - Fluoxymesterone
- Testosterone esters
- Transdermal patches
- Transdermal gels
- Buccal

ANABOLIC AGENTS
- Nandrolone
- Oxandrolone
- Oxymetholone
- Stanozolol
- Testolactone

α_1-ADRENERGIC ANTAGONISTS
- Alfuzosin
- Doxazosin
- Tamsulosin
- Terazosin

ANTIANDROGENS
- Bicalutamide
- Flutamide
- Nilutamide

INHIBITORS OF ANDROGEN BIOSYNTHESIS
- 5α-Reductase inhibitors
  - Finasteride
  - Dutasteride
- 17α-Hydroxylase/17,20-lyase inhibitors
- Luteinizing hormone–releasing hormone agonists
  - Buserelin
  - Goserelin
  - Leuprolide

DRUGS FOR TREATMENT OF ERECTILE DYSFUNCTION
- Phosphodiesterase-5 inhibitors
  - Sildenafil
  - Vardenafil
  - Tadalafil
- OTHER DRUGS
  - Prostaglandin E_1
  - Papaverine
  - Phentolamine

INTRODUCTION

This chapter focuses on the physiology, pharmacology, metabolism, and structure–activity relationships for therapeutic and emerging classes of drugs that are used almost exclusively in men. Major differences in endocrine hormones and the anatomy and physiology of the reproductive system and genitourinary tract between males and females make men uniquely susceptible to a variety of disorders, including aging-related androgen insufficiency (hypogonadism and andropause), prostate and testicular cancer, benign prostatic hyperplasia (BPH), and erectile dysfunction (ED). The majority of these disorders and their treatments are associated with the male sex hormones (i.e., androgens), their pharmacological target (i.e., the androgen receptor [AR]), and the tissues that rely on the androgens.

Prostate problems are common in older men, particularly those aged 50 years and older. A man may have prostate problems for a number of reasons, including an infection of the prostate (prostatitis), a noncancerous enlargement of the prostate (BPH), or prostate cancer, the second most common cancer in men. Risk of prostate cancer increases with age; approximately 70 percent of all cases of the disease are diagnosed in men aged 65 years and older. Prostate problems often are discovered by men themselves. The signs of prostate problems include frequent urge to urinate, blood in the urine, painful or burning urination, difficulty urinating, or inability to urinate.

Aging-related androgen insufficiency (male hypogonadism) is a physiological condition characterized by the inability of the testes to produce sufficient testosterone to maintain sexual function, muscle strength, bone mineral density, and fertility (spermatogenesis). One in five men older than 50 years will exhibit symptoms of this condition. Symptoms of aging-related androgen insufficiency may include lethargy or decreased energy, decreased libido or interest in sex, ED (with loss of erections), muscle weakness and aches, inability to sleep, hot flashes, night sweats, depression, infertility, thinning of bones or bone loss, and cardiovascular disease. By the time that men are between the ages of 40 and 55 years, some may experience a phenomenon similar to the female menopause, called andropause. Whether andropause is more common than hypogonadism in the aging male is a matter for debate. The decline in testosterone occurs very gradually in men over several decades and may be accompanied by loss of bone mass (osteoporosis), loss of muscle mass and strength, and changes in fat distribution, cholesterol levels, spermatogenesis, sexual performance, quality of life, and impotence (i.e., ED). Studies show that a decline in testosterone actually can put men at risk for other health problems, such as heart disease and weak bones. Psychological stress, alcohol abuse, injuries or surgery, medications, obesity and infections, tobacco, and drugs, such as decongestants, antihypertensives, tranquilizers, statins, or antiseizure agents, can contribute to the onset of these conditions. There is no way of predicting who will experience the symptoms of androgen insufficiency that are of sufficient severity to seek medical help; neither is it predictable at what age the symptoms of aging-related androgen insufficiency will occur in a particular individual. Each man's symptoms also may be different. Because all this happens at a time of life when many men begin to question their values, accomplishments, and direction in life, it often is difficult to realize that the changes occurring are related to more than just external conditions.

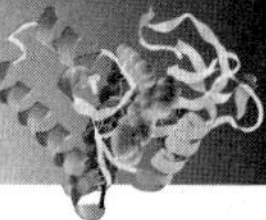

CLINICAL SIGNIFICANCE

Significant research is currently underway in the area of men's health. In less than a decade, we have gone from having minimally effective pharmacological agents for erectile dysfunction (ED) to having several options. The widespread use of these phosphodiesterase (PDE5) inhibitors is acknowledged by the fact that Viagra (sildenafil) was one of the Top 200 drugs dispensed in 2004.

There are advantages and disadvantages to each of these PDE5 inhibitors. Some can be taken with food and other cannot. Some have optimal durations of action, and others are much shorter. All, however, have been known to have adverse effects and drug interactions in common. Some of these adverse effects can be rather severe, and the drug interactions with nitrates can be fatal.

The development of newer, more effective, and less deleterious agents is essential for ED. Agents that are more selective for PDE5 and avoid other PDEs are critical to this endeavor. By studying the structure–activity relationships between the PDEs and the inhibitors, this can be achieved. Minor changes to the side chains or functional groups of the currently available PDE inhibitors can potentially eliminate the adverse effects and drug interactions that limit the use of these agents. As new agents become available, clinicians continually compare and contrast these new agents to the ones that are currently available in an effort to improve patient care. This is an ongoing, joint effort by chemists and clinicians alike to optimize patient care either indirectly or directly by continually making adjustments to either chemical structures or therapeutic treatment plans for the patient.

Catherine L. Hatfield, Pharm.D.
Clinical Assistant Professor
Department of Clinical Sciences and Administrations
University of Houston
College of Pharmacy

Now that men are living longer, there is heightened interest in aging-related androgen insufficiency, its risks for other health problems, and its treatment.

Testicular cancer is the most common form of cancer among males aged 15 to 44 years and is approximately four times more common in white men than in African–American men. After motor vehicle accidents and suicide, cancer is the leading cause of death in this age group, followed by homicide, heart disease, and HIV. Testicular cancer is known as "young man's cancer." Early detection is the key to survival. Testicular cancer is androgen-dependent, with a very fast onset. because the tumors can be very aggressive. When the cancer is confined to the testicles, there often is no pain, but by the time pain develops, it often is a sign that the cancer has already spread. Survival rates increase significantly if treatment has begun before the cancer has a chance to metastasize. Testicular cancer most often is discovered by men. Therefore, all men should conduct testicular self-examinations at least monthly and, preferably, every time they shower for any changes or lumps and to see a doctor immediately if any changes noted. The diagnosis is noninvasive and involves using ultrasound to look at the density, size, and shape of the testicles and other masses in the scrotum.

Men who experience any of these symptoms associated with the prostate, aging-related androgen insufficiency, and testicular cancer should see a doctor to find out the cause of the problem and to talk about possible treatment.

The discovery and clinical development of selective estrogen receptor modulators transformed the therapeutic use of estrogens (1). Similarly, nonsteroidal selective AR modulators (SARMs), with the ability to selectively stimulate or maintain muscle and bone mass or to reduce prostate mass in BPH without the androgenic effects of testosterone and 5α-dihydrotestosterone (DHT), now are leading a similar revolution in the therapeutic use of androgens. The discovery of SARMs not only provides a potentially significant therapeutic advance for androgen replacement therapy but also provides model compounds to further study the molecular mechanism of action of the AR (2). Results from in vitro and in vivo animal studies suggest that the therapeutic promise of SARMs as a treatment of muscle wasting, osteoporosis, hormonal male contraception, and BPH may be soon realized.

Testosterone and its metabolite, DHT, are the primary endogenous androgens and play crucial physiological roles in establishing and maintaining the male phenotype (3). Their actions are essential for the differentiation and growth of male reproductive organs, initiation and regulation of spermatogenesis, and control of male sexual behavior. In addition, androgens are important for the development of male characteristics in certain extragenital structures, such as muscle, bone, hair, larynx, skin, lipid tissue, and kidney (4). In females, the precise physiological roles of androgens are not completely understood, but the aging-related decline in circulating androgen levels has been linked to symptoms such as decreased libido and sexuality, lack of vigor, diminished well-being, and loss of bone mineral density in postmenopausal women (5–7).

THE SEX HORMONES

The sex steroid hormones are steroid molecules that are necessary for reproduction in females and males and that affect the development of secondary sex characteristics in both sexes. The sex steroids are comprised of three

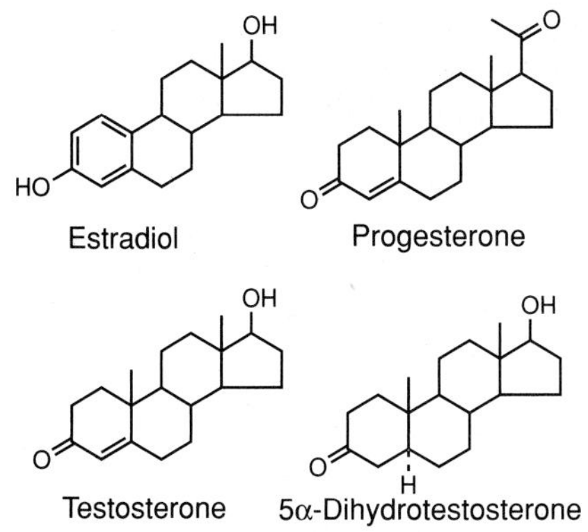

Fig. 45.1. The sex hormones.

classes: estrogens, progestins, and androgens (Fig. 45.1). The two principal classes of female sex steroid hormones are estrogens and progestins (for further discussion, see Chapter 46). Chemically, the naturally occurring estrogens are C-18 steroids and have in common a planar unsaturated A ring with a 3-phenolic group that aids in separation and purification from nonphenolic substances. The most potent endogenous estrogen is estradiol (Fig. 45.1). The naturally occurring progestins are C_{21} steroids and have in common a 3-keto-4-ene structure in the A ring and a ketone at the C-21 position. The most potent endogenous progestin is progesterone (Fig. 45.1). The principal class of the male sex steroid hormone is the androgens. The naturally occurring androgens are C-19 steroids and have in common oxygen atoms (as either hydroxyl or ketone groups) at both the C-3 and C-17 positions. The potent androgen found in the blood is testosterone (Fig. 45.1), with the more potent metabolite formed in certain androgen target tissues being DHT (Fig. 45.1). All three classes of endogenous steroids are present in both males and females. The production and circulating plasma levels of estrogens and progestins are higher in females, however, and the production and circulating plasma levels of androgens are higher in males.

DISCOVERY OF ANDROGENS

One of the early and unusual experiments with testicular extracts was carried out in 1889 by the French physiologist Brown-Séquard. He administered such an extract to himself and reported that he felt an increased vigor and capacity for work (8). In 1911, Pézard showed that extracts of testicular tissue increase comb growth in capons (9). Early attempts to isolate pure male hormones from the testes failed, because only small amounts are present in this tissue.

The earliest report of an isolated androgen was presented by Butenandt (10) in 1931. He isolated 15 mg of crystalline androsterone from 15,000 L of human male urine. A second crystalline compound, dehydroepiandrosterone, which has weak androgenic activity, was isolated by Butenandt and Dannenberg (11) in 1934. During the following year, testosterone was isolated from bull testes by David et al. (12). This hormone was shown to be 6 to 10 times as active as androsterone.

Shortly after testosterone was isolated, Butenandt and Hanisch (13) reported its synthesis. In that same year, extracts of urine from males were shown to cause nitrogen retention as well as the expected androgenic effects (14). Many steroids with androgenic activity have subsequently been synthesized. Steroid hormones may have many potent effects on various tissues, and slight chemical alterations of androgenic steroids may increase some of these effects without altering others.

Testosterone was the first androgen to be used clinically for its anabolic activity. New sources of the hormone were needed, however, because only 270 mg could be isolated from a ton of bull testes (15). Commercially, testosterone is prepared from various steroids, including sarsasapogenin, diosgenin, and certain androgens found in stallion urine. Because of its androgenic action, testosterone is limited in its use in humans as an anabolic steroid. Many steroids were synthesized in an attempt to separate the androgenic and the anabolic actions. Because testosterone had to be given parenterally, it also was desirable to find orally active agents.

In the United States, most of the androgens and anabolic steroid products are subject to control by the U.S. Federal Control Substances Act as amended by the Anabolic Steroid Control Act of 1990 as Schedule III drugs.

ANDROGEN PHYSIOLOGY

The overall physiological effects of endogenous androgens are contributed by testosterone and its active metabolites, DHT and estradiol. Testosterone and DHT execute their actions predominantly through the AR, which belongs to the nuclear receptor superfamily and functions as a ligand-dependent transcription factor. Circulating testosterone is essential for the differentiation and growth of male accessory reproductive organs (e.g., prostate and seminal vesicles), control of male sexual behavior, and the development and maintenance of male secondary characteristics that involve muscle, bone, larynx, and hair. Healthy young adult men produce approximately 3 to 10 mg of testosterone per day, with circulating plasma levels ranging from approximately 500 to 1,000 ng/dL in eugonadal (normal) men. Circulating testosterone participates in the feedback regulation of androgen production by the hypothalamus-pituitary-testis axis, as shown in Figure 45.2. Testosterone, luteinizing hormone (LH), and LH-releasing hormone (LHRH; a.k.a. gonadotropin-releasing hormone) constitute the elements of a negative feedback control mechanism, whereby testosterone controls its own release. Low circulating testosterone levels increase the hypothalamic secretion of LHRH, which leads to increased production of LH and, consequently, increased testosterone production by the Leydig cells. More than 95% of circulating testosterone is synthesized and secreted by the Leydig

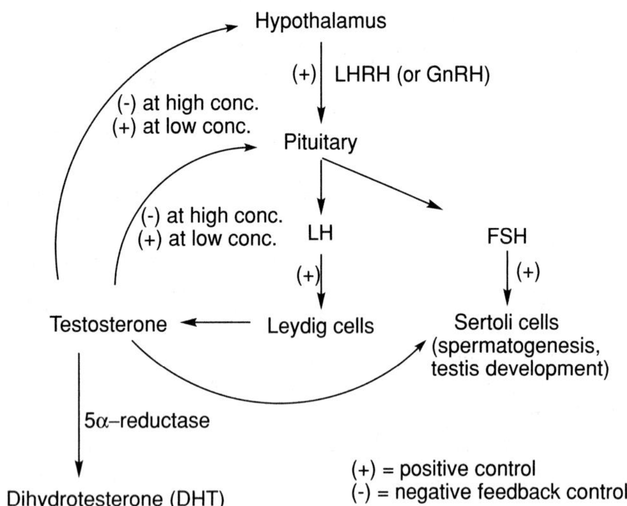

Fig. 45.2. Hypothalamus-pituitary-testicular axis. (+), positive control; (−), negative feedback control.

cells in the testes. High testosterone levels, on the other hand, inhibit LHRH release, thus suppressing both LH secretion and testosterone secretion. The LHRH is released from the hypothalamus in short, intermittent pulses every 2 hours and at greater magnitude in the morning, which in turn stimulates the pulsatile secretion of LH and follicle-stimulating hormone (FSH) from the pituitary. Follicle-stimulating hormone stimulates the Sertoli cells controlling spermatogenesis and development of the testis. Thus, testosterone secretion likewise is pulsatile and diurnal, with the highest concentration occurring at approximately 8:00 AM and the lowest at approximately 8:00 PM. In older men, especially those older than 60 years, the body does not produce enough testosterone that is needed to do all the intended work, and the testosterone levels remain relatively constant, without the morning pulses observed in young adult men. Average plasma testosterone concentrations in older men peak in the morning, with daily ranges of approximately 300 to 550 ng/dL by 70 years of age. The diurnal cycling is blunted as men age (16). In women, testosterone levels range from 15 to 100 ng/dL. Starting at approximately 40 years of age, testosterone levels drop by approximately 10 percent every decade. In the normal functioning of the male hormonal system, 97 to 98% of plasma testosterone is bound to sex hormone binding globulin, making it unavailable to the body's tissues. The remaining 2 to 3% is known as "bioavailable" or free testosterone. Furthermore, the receptor sites where testosterone must bind to be effective also can be occupied by estradiol, an estrogen also found in men that increases with age and body weight.

In the testis, FSH directly interacts with FSH receptors expressed in Sertoli cells and stimulates spermatogenesis, whereas LH indirectly stimulates spermatogenesis through testosterone synthesized by Leydig cells. Testosterone and its aromatized metabolite (estradiol) negatively regulate circulating levels of testosterone in the hypothalamus and pituitary. Activin and inhibin produced by Sertoli cells stimulate or inhibit, respectively, the secretion of FSH from the pituitary (17). High concentrations of intratesticular testosterone are essential for the initiation and maintenance of spermatogenesis, as evidenced by the infertility of hypogonadal men. Results from both animal models and humans, however, support the idea that both FSH and testosterone are required to achieve quantitative and qualitative spermatogenesis.

Androgens also are needed for the development of secondary sex characteristics. The male voice deepens because of thickening of the laryngeal mucosa and lengthening of the vocal cords. In both men and women, they play a role first in stimulating the growth of hair on the face, arms, legs, and pubic areas and later in the recession of the male hairline. The fructose content of human semen and both the size and the secretory capacity of the sebaceous glands also depend on the levels of testosterone.

Testosterone causes nitrogen retention by increasing the rate of protein synthesis and muscle mass while decreasing the rate of protein catabolism. The positive nitrogen balance therefore results from both decreased catabolism and increased anabolism of proteins that are used in male sex accessory apparatus and muscle. The actions of androgen in the reproductive tissues, including prostate, seminal vesicle, testis, and accessory structures, are known as the androgenic effects, whereas the nitrogen-retaining effects of androgen in muscle and bone are known as the anabolic effects. Although the precise mechanism of androgen action on muscle remains unknown, the common hypothesis is that androgens promote muscle protein synthesis. Evidence supports the idea that testosterone supplementation increases muscle protein synthesis in elderly men (18) and young hypogonadal men (19). Also, androgen-induced increases in muscle mass appear to arise from muscle fiber hypertrophy rather than hyperplasia (i.e., cellular enlargement rather than cellular proliferation) (20).

The thickness and linear growth of bones are stimulated and, later, limited by testosterone because of closure of the epiphyses. Androgens affect bone mineral density by changing overall osteoblast (bone-forming cell) activity and osteoclast (bone-resorbing cell) activity, resulting from changes in the total number of each cell type and individual cell functional capacity (21,22). Androgens seem to have the ability to decelerate the bone remodeling cycle and tilt the focal balance of that cycle toward bone formation. The loss of androgens is thought to increase the rate of bone remodeling by removing the restraining effects on osteoblastogenesis and osteoclastogenesis.

ANDROGEN BIOSYNTHESIS

The major pathways for the biosynthesis of the sex steroid hormones are summarized in Figure 45.3. Cholesterol is

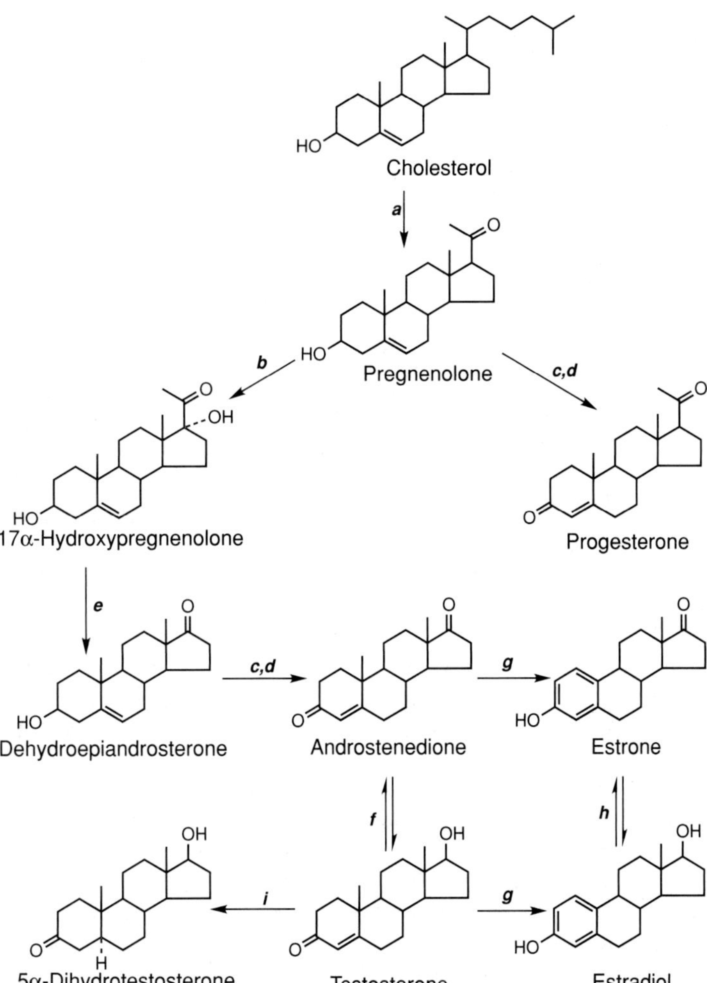

Fig. 45.3. Biosynthesis of androgens and other sex steroid hormones. The enzymes involved in this biosynthesis are (a) side-chain cleavage, (b) 17α-hydroxylase (c) 5-ene-3β-hydroxysteroid dehydrogenase, (d) 3-oxo-steroid-4,5-isomerase, (e) 17,20-lyase, (f) 17β-hydroxysteroid dehydrogenase, (g) aromatase, (h) estradiol dehydrogenase, and (i) 5α-reductase.

stored in endocrine tissues and is converted to androgen, estrogen, or progesterone when the tissue is stimulated by a gonadotropic hormone. Androgens (male sex hormones) primarily are synthesized from cholesterol in the testes, whereas estrogens are biosynthesized chiefly in the ovary in mature, premenopausal women. This is not surprising, because androgens are intermediates in the biosynthesis of estrogens. In the liver, androgens are formed from C-21 steroids. During pregnancy, the placenta is the main source of estrogen biosynthesis and pathways for production change (23,24). Small amounts of these hormones also are synthesized by the adrenal cortex, the hypothalamus, and the anterior pituitary in both sexes. The major source of estrogens in both postmenopausal women and men is adipose tissue (25).

Luteinizing hormone binds to its receptor on the surface of the Leydig cells to initiate testosterone biosynthesis. As in other endocrine cells, the binding of gonadotropin activates the G_S signal transduction pathway, increasing intracellular cyclic adenosine monophosphate (cAMP) levels via activation of adenylate cyclase. One of the processes influenced by elevated cAMP levels is the activation of cholesterol esterase, which cleaves cholesterol esters and liberates free cholesterol. The free cholesterol is then converted in mitochondria to pregnenolone via the side-chain cleavage reaction (Fig. 45.3). Pregnenolone is converted by 17α-hydroxylase to 17α-hydroxypregnenolone and then to dehydroepiandrosterone (DHEA; a C-19 steroid) via 17-20 lyase, which involves cleavage of the C-17 to C-20 carbon–carbon bond and loss of the 17β-acetyl side chain (26). The 17α-hydroxylase is found in the endoplasmic reticulum membrane and is comprised of the cytochrome $P450_{17\alpha}$ protein and the ubiquitous NADPH-cytochrome P450 reductase. Cytochrome $P450_{17\alpha}$ is expressed by the *CYP17* gene found on chromosome 10 in humans. Alternatively, progesterone can be formed from pregnenolone via the action of 5-ene-3β-hydroxysteroid dehydrogenase and

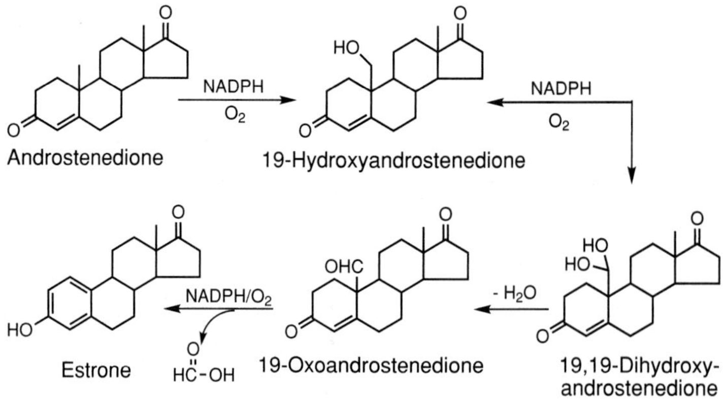

Androstenedione → (NADPH, O_2) → 19-Hydroxyandrostenedione → (NADPH, O_2) → 19,19-Dihydroxyandrostenedione → ($-H_2O$) → 19-Oxoandrostenedione → (NADPH/O_2, HCOOH) → Estrone

Fig. 45.4. Aromatase mechanism.

3-oxosteroid-4,5-isomerase. These same enzymes are responsible for the conversion of DHEA to the 17-ketosteroidal androgen, androstenedione.

Testosterone is formed by reduction of the 17-ketone of androstenedione by 17β-hydroxysteroid dehydrogenase (27,28). Testosterone and androstenedione are metabolically interconvertible. Loss of the C-19 angular methyl group and aromatization of the A ring of testosterone or androstenedione is catalyzed by the microsomal cytochrome P450 enzyme complex, called aromatase, and results in the C-18 steroids—namely, 17β-estradiol or estrone, respectively—as shown in Figure 45.4. 17β-Estradiol and estrone are metabolically interconvertible, catalyzed by estradiol dehydrogenase. Research interests in the aromatization reaction continue to expand from basic endocrinology and reproductive biology studies to aromatase inhibition for the treatment of estrogen-dependent cancers, as illustrated in several conferences and reviews (29–32). Androstenedione is the preferred substrate for aromatization, and three molecules of NADPH and three molecules of oxygen are necessary for conversion of one molecule of androgen to estrogen (33).

The most potent endogenous androgen is the 5α-reduced steroid, DHT, which is biosynthesized by two 5α-reductase isoforms, Type 1 and Type 2 (Fig. 45.1). Type 1 5α-reductase is expressed predominantly in sebaceous glands of the skin, scalp, and liver. Type 1 5α-reductase is responsible for approximately one-third of the circulating DHT. Type 2 5α-reductase is found primarily in prostate, seminal vesicles, epididymides, genital skin (scrotum), hair follicles, and liver, and it is responsible for two-thirds of the circulating DHT. Approximately 6 to 8% of testosterone is converted to DHT. 5α-Reductase has been found in both the microsomal fraction and the nuclear membrane of homogenized target tissues, and it catalyzes an irreversible reduction reaction, which requires NADPH as a cofactor, that provides the α-hydrogen at C-5 (34,35). Conversion to DHT amplifies the action of testosterone by three to five times because of the greater binding affinity of DHT as compared to testosterone for the ARs (36).

ANDROGEN METABOLISM

Testosterone can be metabolized in either its target tissues or the liver (37–39), as shown in Figure 45.5. In androgen target tissues, testosterone can be converted to physiologically active metabolites. In the prostate gland, skin, and liver (40), testosterone is reduced to DHT by 5α-reductase (Types 1 and 2) (41). On the other hand, a small amount of testosterone (0.3%) also can be converted to estradiol by aromatase through cleavage of the C-19 methyl group, and aromatization of ring A, which mainly occurs in adipose tissue. This process also occurs in the ovaries of women. In men, approximately 80% of the circulating estrogen arises from aromatization of testosterone in the adipose tissue (42), with the other 20% being secreted by the Leydig cells in the testes (43).

Both 5α-reduction and aromatization are irreversible processes. In addition to these pathways, testosterone also can be further inactivated in the liver through reduction and oxidation, followed by glucuronidation and renal excretion. It can be metabolized to androstenedione through oxidation of the 17β-OH group and to androstanedione with 5α-reduction of ring A. Androstanedione can be further converted to androsterone after 3-keto group reduction. Alternatively, androstenedione also can be converted to etiocholanolone through 5β- and 3-keto reduction. Similarly, DHT can be converted to androstanedione, androsterone, and androstanediol (44).

After the administration of radiolabeled testosterone, approximately 90% of the radioactivity is found in the urine, and 6% is recovered in the feces through enterohepatic circulation (45). Major urinary metabolites include androsterone and its 5α-diastereoisomer etiocholanolone, both of which are inactive metabolites. They are excreted mainly as glucuronide conjugates or, to a lesser extent, as sulfate conjugates (46). The reduction of testosterone to its *cis* A/B ring juncture (5β) conformation, etiocholanolone, explains its complete loss of activity, because the *cis* A/B ring no longer has affinity for the AR, as shown in Figure 45.6. Most of the other metabolites mentioned above undergo extensive glucuronidation of

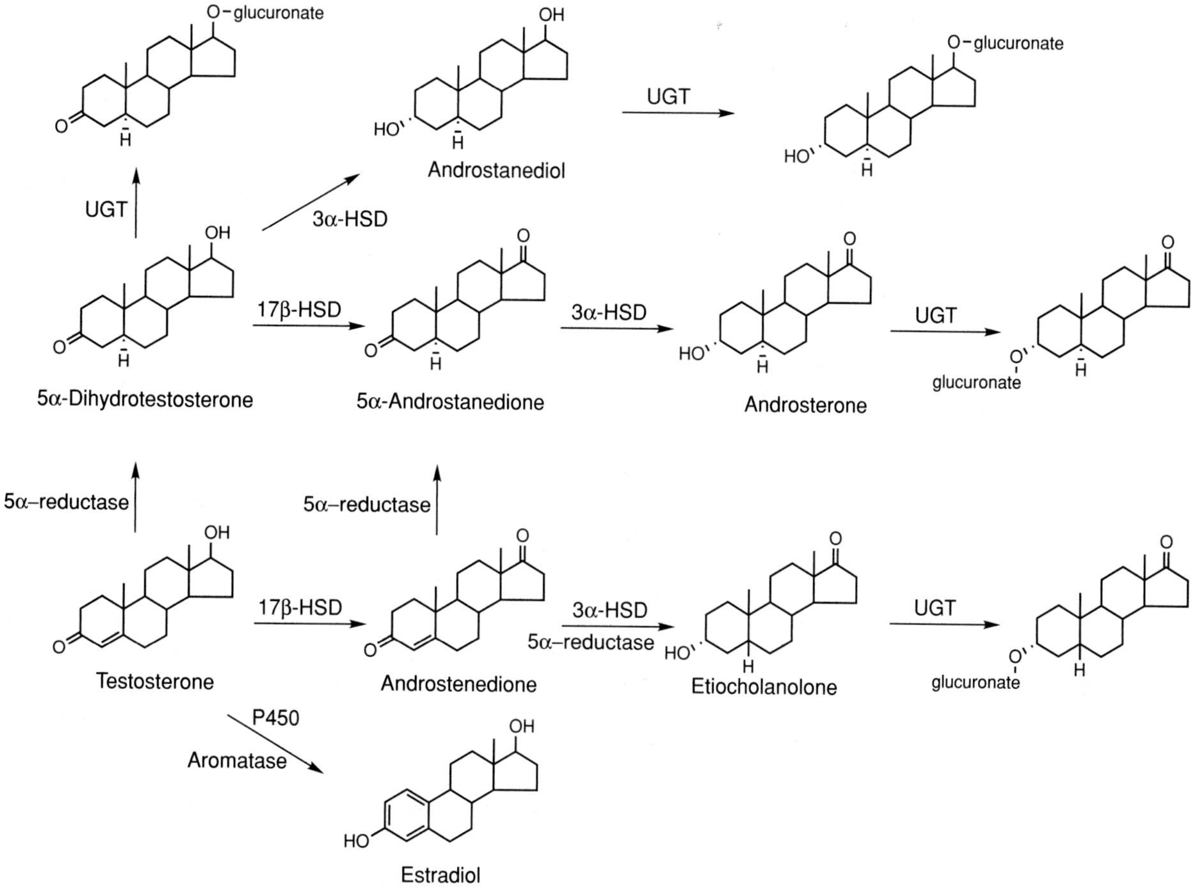

Fig. 45.5. Testosterone metabolism. G, glucuronide; HSD, hydroxy steroid dehydrogenase; UGT, uridine diphosphoglucuronosyltransferase.

the 3α- or 17β-OH groups as well, either in the target tissues or in the liver (46), and are further excreted in the urine. Therefore, following oral administration, the plasma testosterone half-life is less than 30 minutes because of extensive hepatic metabolism. Approximately 90% of an oral dose of testosterone undergoes first-pass metabolism before it reaches the systemic circulation. A number of minor metabolites of testosterone also have been isolated from urine and identified as 5α-androstanes and 5β-androstanes with a 3α-hydroxyl function. Most 17-ketosteroids isolated from the urine result from catabolism of the adrenocorticoids rather than from metabolism of androgens.

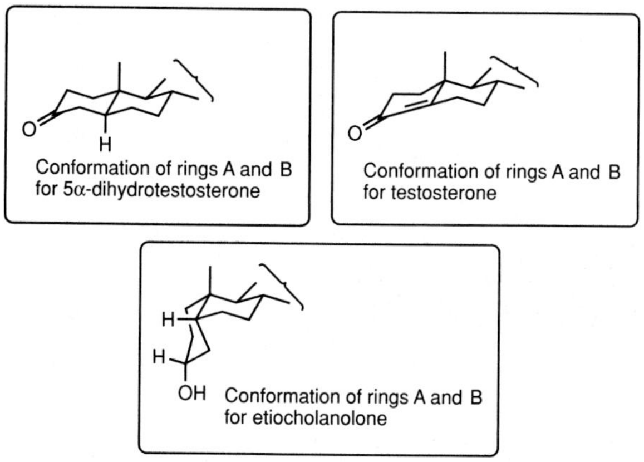

Fig. 45.6. Conformations of dihydrotestosterone (DHT), testosterone (T), and etiocholanolone A and B rings.

MECHANISMS OF ANDROGEN ACTION

Testosterone, DHT, and other androgens execute their actions predominantly through the AR. The AR is mainly expressed in androgen target tissues, such as the prostate, skeletal muscle, liver, and central nervous system, with the highest expression level being observed in the prostate, adrenal gland, and epididymis (47). Testosterone binds preferentially to the AR in muscle, bone, brain, and bone marrow, whereas DHT binds to the AR in genitalia, prostate, skin, and hair follicles. It is a member of the steroid and nuclear receptor superfamily, which is composed of more than 100 members and continues to grow. Among this large family of proteins, only five vertebrate steroid receptors (estrogen, progesterone, androgen, glucocorticoid, and mineralocorticoid receptors) are known. Like other steroid receptors, AR is a soluble protein that functions as an intracellular transcriptional factor. The

AR function is regulated by the binding of androgens, which initiates sequential conformational changes of the receptor that affect receptor–protein interaction and receptor–DNA interactions (48).

The AR gene is more than 90 kb long and codes for a protein of 919 amino acids that has three major functional domains, as illustrated in Figure 45.7. The N-terminal domain, which serves a modulatory function, is encoded by exon 1 (1,586 bp). The DNA binding domain (DBD) is encoded by exons 2 and 3 (152 and 117 bp, respectively). The ligand binding domain (LBD) is encoded by five exons, which vary from 131 to 288 bp in size. There also is a small hinge region between the DBD and LBD. Two transactivation functions have been identified. The N-terminal activation function (AF1) is not conserved in sequence and is ligand-independent (constitutively active), whereas the C-terminal activation function (AF2) is conserved in sequence and functions in a ligand-dependent manner (49). A nuclear localization signal spans the region between the DBD and the hinge region.

Similar to the other steroid receptors, unbound AR is mainly located in the cytoplasm and associated with a complex of heat shock proteins through interactions with LBD (50). On agonist binding (51), AR goes through a series of conformational changes: The heat shock proteins dissociate from AR, and the transformed AR undergoes dimerization, phosphorylation, and translocation to the nucleus, which is mediated by the nuclear localization signal, as shown in Figure 45.7. Translocated receptor then binds to androgen-response elements (AREs) in DNA, which are characterized by a six-nucleotide half-site consensus sequence 5′-TGTTCT-3′ spaced by three random nucleotides and are located in the promoter or enhancer region of AR gene targets. Recruitment of other transcription coregulators (including coactivators and corepressors) and transcriptional machinery further ensures the transactivation of AR-regulated gene expression. All these complicated processes are initiated by the ligand-induced conformational changes in the LBD.

Ligand-induced AR conformational changes provide the structural basis for the recruitment of cofactor proteins and transcriptional machinery, which also is required for the assembly of AR-mediated transcription complexes (52), as shown in Figure 45.8. The formation of an activation complex is known to involve AR, coactivators, and RNA polymerase II recruitment to both the enhancer and promoter, whereas the formation of a repression complex involves factors bound only at the promoter and not at the enhancer. Because the formation of a functional AF2 region provides a structural basis for ligand-induced protein–protein interaction, ligand-specific recruitment of coregulators might be crucial for the agonist or antagonist activity of AR ligands.

Binding of DNA also is required for AR-regulated gene expression, which is known as the classic genomic function of AR. The ARE half-site sequence can be arranged either as inverted repeats or as direct repeats (52,53), and AR recognizes and binds to the ARE site through two zinc fingers located in the DBD. Like other steroid receptors, ligand-bound AR forms homodimers and appears to form "head-to-head" dimers (54) even when it is bound to the direct repeats of ARE. Selective recognition of specific ARE sequences could be regulated by ligand binding (55) and/or the presence of other transcriptional factors, which bind to their own DNA binding sites as well (combinatorial regulation) (56).

Besides the genomic pathway, the nongenomic pathway of AR also has been reported in oocytes (57), skeletal muscle cells (58), osteoblasts (59,60), and prostate cancer cells (61,62). As compared to the genomic pathway, the nongenomic actions of steroid receptors are characterized by the rapidity of the action, which varies from seconds to an hour or so, and by interaction with plasma membrane–associated signaling pathways (63). Nevertheless, the structural basis for nongenomic action is direct interactions between AR and cytosolic proteins from different signaling pathways, which could be closely

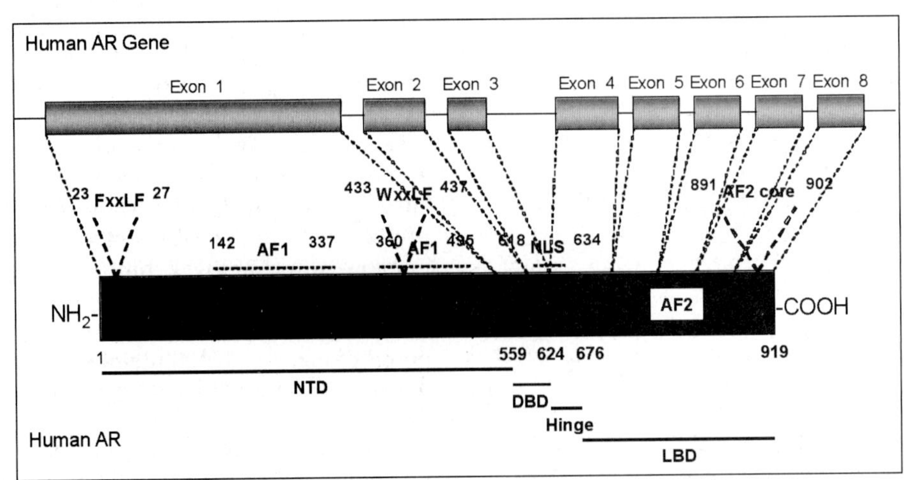

Fig. 45.7. Structural domains of the androgen receptor gene and protein.

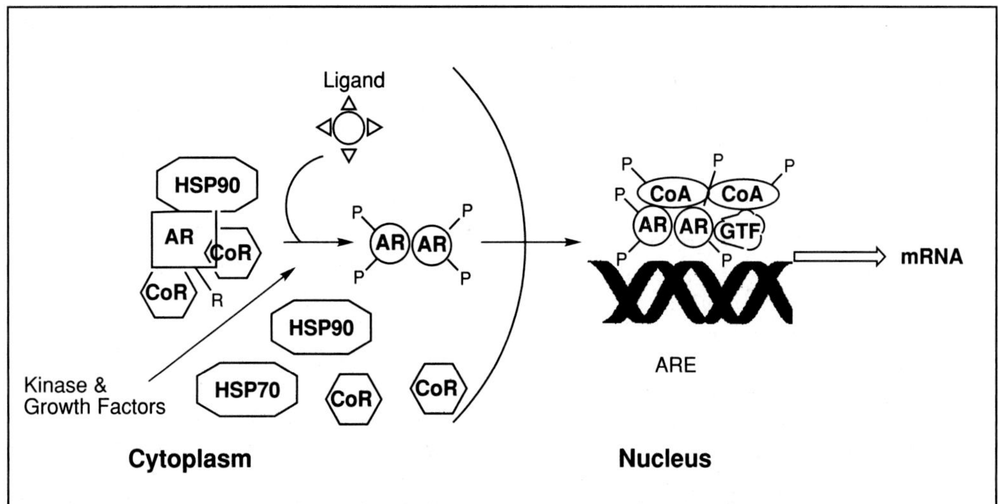

Fig. 45.8. Mechanism of androgen action. The androgen receptor (AR) is maintained in an inactive complex by heat shock protein (HSP) 70, HSP 90, and corepressors (CoR). On ligand binding, it homodimerizes and enters the nucleus. The receptor is basally phosphorylated (P) in the absence of hormone, and hormone binding increases the phosphorylation status of the receptor. The AR binds to the androgen-response element (ARE) on the promoter of androgen responsive genes, leading to the recruitment of coactivators (CoA) and general transcription factors (GTF), leading to gene transcription.

related to the ligand-induced conformational change of the LBD or, indirectly, the N-terminal domain. Functionally, the nongenomic action of androgen involves either rapid activation of kinase-signaling cascades or modulation of intracellular calcium levels, which could be related to stimulation of gap junction communication, neuronal plasticity, and aortic relaxation (64). Separation of the genomic and nongenomic functions of steroid receptors using specific ligands also was proposed as a new strategy to achieve tissue selectivity (63,65).

DRUGS USED IN THE TREATMENT OF AGING-RELATED ANDROGEN INSUFFICIENCIES

Male Hypogonadism

Male hypogonadism (testosterone deficiency) is the inability of the testes to produce sufficient testosterone to maintain sexual function, muscle strength, bone mineral density, and fertility (spermatogenesis). In men, there is a gradual decline of approximately 1% per year in the production of testosterone beginning around 40 years of age. For most men, testosterone levels naturally decline with advancing age but still remain within the physiological range throughout their lifetimes, causing no significant problems. Approximately 20% of men older than age 60 years and 30 to 40% of men older than 80 years have plasma testosterone levels indicative of hypogonadism (<325 ng/dL). Male hypogonadism is most commonly primary hypogonadism (testicular failure to produce testosterone for various reasons), secondary hypogonadism (hypothalamic-pituitary failure to stimulate testicles to produce testosterone), or a combination of both.

Testosterone and structurally related steroidal androgens have been used for decades to treat male hypogonadism, Klinefelter's syndrome (a chromosomal abnormality resulting in testicular dysfunction), anemia secondary to chronic renal failure, aplastic anemia, protein wasting diseases associated with cancer, burns, traumas, AIDS, short stature, breast cancer (as an antiestrogen), or hereditary angioedema (46). However, these agents have been demoted to the therapy of final resort because of serious hepatotoxicity and the recent development of more effective therapies (e.g., erythropoietin, aromatase inhibitors, and taxanes). Although severe hypogonadism is uncommon, aging-related androgen insufficiency is much more frequent. Low endogenous testosterone concentrations are associated with sarcopenia and frailty arising from decreased fat-free mass, lessened muscle strength, and reduced bone mineral density (osteoporosis). Low testosterone concentrations also are associated with decreased sexual libido and ED. More than 30 million men older than 40 years in the United States are estimated to suffer from ED. Although androgens are not essential for erection (66), transdermal and intramuscular (IM) testosterone replacement therapy often is employed in hypogonadal men with ED (67). Furthermore, selective phosphodiesterase (PDE5) inhibitors that increase penile blood flow are considered to be the treatment of choice for men with ED. Hormone replacement therapy with testosterone in aging men also improves body composition, bone and cartilage metabolism, and memory and cognition, and it even decreases cardiovascular risk (68).

Low testosterone concentrations frequently are seen in patients with ED, aging, type II diabetes, HIV/AIDS, osteoporosis, depression, obesity, alcohol abuse, anabolic steroid abuse, chronic inflammatory disease, cancer, and glucocorticoid use.

Andropause

Andropause was first described in the medical literature in the 1940s, but the ability to diagnose it is relatively new. The idea that men, as well as women, might be subject to sex hormone fluctuations in later life has been a topic of debate among endocrinologists and men's health professionals (69). Andropause affects men between the ages of 40 and 55 years, but unlike women, men do not have a clear-cut signpost, such as the cessation of menstruation to mark this transition. Men's "transition" may be much more gradual and expand over many decades, and men will very likely experience andropausal symptoms to include ED, loss of muscle mass, irritability, generalized fatigue, and even problems with memory and cognition. A decline in testosterone levels will occur in virtually all men, and there is no way of predicting who will experience andropausal symptoms of sufficient severity to seek medical help. It is estimated that 30% of men in their fifties, and up to 50% of men older than 65 years, will have testosterone levels low enough to cause noticeable symptoms. Once andropause is discovered, the process of replacing the missing testosterone is either by injection, locally applied hormone gel, transdermal patch, or implanted cartridge.

Testosterone Replacement Therapy

The acceptance of testosterone replacement therapy (TRT) has been hampered by the lack of orally active preparations with good efficacy and, particularly, a safe profile (70). Progress has been limited over the last three decades in developing synthetic molecules that could separate the desirable physiological functions normally regulated by endogenous androgens from the undesirable or dose-limiting side effects. The abuse of synthetic anabolic steroids by athletes and body builders has contributed to the general perception of certain undesirable side effects, such as aggressive behavior, liver toxicity, acne or impotency.

Current androgenic formulations for TRT largely are restricted to injectable formulations of testosterone esters, transdermal delivery formulations (scrotal or nonscrotal patches or gel), or buccal testosterone. Marketed injectable forms of testosterone esters (e.g., testosterone enanthate, propionate, or cypionate) produce undesirable fluctuations in testosterone blood levels, with supraphysiological concentrations early and subphysiological levels toward the end of the period before the next injection. These fluctuations provide an unsatisfactory benefits profile and, in some cases, undesired side effects. Skin patches provide a better blood level profile of testosterone, but skin irritation and daily application limit the usefulness and acceptability of this form of therapy. Oral preparations such as fluoxymesterone and 17α-methyltestosterone are not currently used because of concerns about liver toxicity linked to the 17α-alkyl group and because of somewhat lower efficacy (70). Thus, these oral androgens are considered to be obsolete and do not represent a viable form of therapy.

Benefits and Risks of Testosterone Replacement Therapy

Multiple large-scale and long-term clinical trials of TRT have been conducted in aging men to evaluate the risk–benefit ratio of TRT in aging men, but no agreement exists regarding the benefits and risks of TRT (Table 45.1) (for review, see (69,70). The potential benefits of TRT include increase in bone mineral density as well as improvement in muscle mass and strength, cognitive function, mood, and sexual function. The potential risks of TRT, however, including those in the cardiovascular system, blood (e.g., hematocrit and hemoglobin levels), and prostate, are routinely experienced. An

Table 45.1. Testosterone Replacement Therapy

Benefits	Risks
Improved sexual performance and desire	Stimulated growth of preexisting prostate cancer
More energy and improved quality of life	Greater chance for benign prostatic hyperplasia
More energy and sense of well-being	Increased hemoglobin levels to above the physiological range
Increased bone mineral density	Problems with voiding; symptoms includes poor urine flow and hesitancy before urinating
Improved muscle mass strength	Increased potential for liver damage from oral preparations
Improved (lower) low-density lipoprotein profile	Sleep apnea (stopping of breathing during sleep)
Decreased irritability and depression	Breast tenderness and swelling (gynecomastia)
Improved cognitive function	Testicular shrinkage (testicular atrophy)
Increased hemoglobin levels to the physiological range	Infertility (decreased spermatogenesis)
Thickened body hair and skin	Skin reaction from patches or gel
	Pain, soreness, or bruising from injection
	Increased fluid retention
	Increased skin problems (acne, oily skin)
	Increased body hair

emerging class of drugs known as SARMs may soon transform the therapeutic landscape of androgen use by selectively stimulating anabolic targets and avoiding steroid-related side effects. Because of the long-term effects of TRT in otherwise healthy men remain unclear, the Institute of Medicine recommends that TRT not be used to prevent or to relieve the physical or psychological effects of aging (71).

Clearly, TRT is beneficial for hypogonadal men with androgen insufficiency to restore sexual function and muscle strength, to prevent bone loss, and to protect against heart disease (atherosclerosis) (70). Increasing testosterone levels with TRT, however, may pose problems by stimulating the growth of the prostate. Long-term TRT could cause prostate gland enlargement, which might fuel the growth of prostate cancer that is already present and could cause breast enlargement in men (gynecomastia). This is especially worrisome, because prostate cancer is common in older men and many men may have prostate cancer that is undiagnosed.

In elderly men, testosterone effects on muscle mass and strength have not been consistent or impressive, possibly because of the low dosages used in clinical trials. The high correlation between the dose (and plasma concentration) and the anabolic actions of androgen in muscle suggests that androgen administration of higher doses in elderly men may significantly increase muscle mass and strength, but high doses might increase the adverse effects and the aromatization of testosterone to estrogen.

Types of Testosterone Replacement Therapy

Several types of TRT exist. Choosing a specific therapy depends on the patient's preference of a particular delivery system, the side effects, and the cost. Types include injection, transdermal, buccal mucosal, and oral (Table 45.2).

INJECTION. Because orally administered testosterone is ineffective in the treatment of male androgen insufficiency syndromes as a result of extensive presystemic first-pass metabolism, IM injections bypass the problems of first-pass metabolism. Intramuscular testosterone injections are depot esters that undergo differing rates of in vivo ester hydrolysis to release free testosterone over an extended period of time. Typically, the depot esters are administered IM into a large muscle once every 2 to 4 weeks depending on the depot ester used (Table 45.2). They are safe, effective, and the least expensive androgen preparations available. The major disadvantage with the IM route for the depot esters is that testosterone plasma concentrations exhibit a saw-toothed pattern, with supraphysiological levels within 2 to 4 days following the IM injection and subphysiological levels before the next injection. A more satisfactory physiological replacement therapy without the fluctuations in free testosterone plasma levels would be to IM administer a lower dose (i.e., 100 mg) on a weekly or biweekly schedule. Because IM injection of testosterone or its esters causes local irritation, the rate of absorption may be erratic.

Among the esters of testosterone available for IM administration include the 17β-propionate, 17β-enanthate, and the cypionate (17β-cyclopentylpropionate) (Fig. 45.9). Testosterone enanthate and cypionate are the depot esters commonly used with comparable pharmacokinetics. Testosterone enanthate (Delasteryl) is formed by esterification of the 17β-hydroxy group of testosterone with heptanoic acid and testosterone cypionate with cyclopentanepropionic acid. Sterile solutions of these esters are available in a suitable vegetable oil, such as cottonseed oil. Unlike oral testosterone, with a half-life of 10 to 100 minutes, IM testosterone administration avoids first-pass metabolism. Generally, the amount of sex hormone binding globulin in plasma determines the distribution of testosterone between free and bound forms, and free testosterone concentrations determine the drug's half-life. The bulky cypionate and enanthate esters of testosterone have a duration of action of up to 2 to 4 weeks, whereas the shorter propionate ester has a shorter duration of action of 1 to 2 weeks. Doses may be adjusted by aiming for midphysiological (400–600 ng/dL) testosterone values after 1 week or at the low end (300–400 ng/dL) just before the next injection is due.

TRANSDERMAL. Transdermal TRT systems are, perhaps, the most commonly used systems for delivering testosterone to bypass the rapid first-pass metabolism associated with oral testosterone. Clinical studies have shown that these formulations are effective forms of testosterone replacement, with peak response within 3 to 6 months. Discontinue use of the transdermal formulation if the desired response is not reached within this time period. Skin irritation is more common with the transdermal formulations, with more than 50% experiencing some form of skin irritation at some point during the treatment. Pretreatment with corticosteroid creams (not with the ointment) has been shown to reduce the severity and incidence of skin irritation without significantly affecting testosterone absorption from the formulation. With the transdermal formulations, testosterone levels were maintained within physiological values, and a beneficial effect was observed on general mood and sexual functioning. A plasma concentration in the midphysiological range (400–600 ng/dL) is the goal.

Matrix-Type Transdermal Systems. This type of patch (scrotal patch; Testoderm®) must be applied to dry, clean (shaven) scrotal skin, which is 5 to 30 times more permeable to testosterone than other skin sites, every 24 hours to produce an adequate testosterone plasma concentration. The matrix system is described as a "drug-in-adhesive film," in which the drug is located on the adhesive layer of the film; thus, it is thinner and less bulky than the reservoir system. The advantage of the matrix system is that it produces supraphysiological levels of DHT

Table 45.2. Testosterone Products and Properties[a]

Product	Trade Name	Onset of Peak Response	Duration of Action	Time to Peak Conc.	Time to Steady-State Conc.	Dose (mg)	Oral Frequency of Dosing	Bioavail-ability (%)	Elimination Half-life
Methyltestosterone	Android Testred Virilon Oreton Methyl	—	24 hours	2 h	—	10–50	Daily	70	3 hours
Fluoxymesterone	Halotestin Android-F	—	24 hours	—	—	5–40	Daily	80	9 hours
Testosterone undecanoate	Andriol	6 hours	10 hours	~6 hours	—	40–120	Daily	<10	3 hours
Testosterone propionate	Testex	6–24 hours	1–2 wks	3–36 hours	—	10–50	Two or three times per week	—	—
Testosterone cypionate	Andronate Depotestosterone Depotest	6–24 hours	2–4 weeks	24 hours	—	50–400	2–4 weeks	—	8 days
Testosterone enanthate	Andro-LA Andryl Delatesteryl Delatest Everone Testamone Testrin-PA	6–24 hours	2–4 weeks	24 hours	—	50–400	2–4 weeks	—	8 days
Trandermal patches	Androderm Testoderm TTS Testoderm	3–6 months	24 hours	2–4 hours	2–3 days	2–5	24 hours	—	10–100 minutes
Transdermal gels	AndroGel Testim	3–6 months	5 days	4 (2–6) hours	2–3 days	50–100	24 hours	—	10–100 minutes
Buccal muscosal	Striant	—	24 hours	5 (0.5–12) hours	2–3 days	30	Every 12 hours	—	6 hours

[a]Thonpson Healthcare, Inc. Micromedex Healthcare Series. Available at: http://www.Thompsonhc.com.

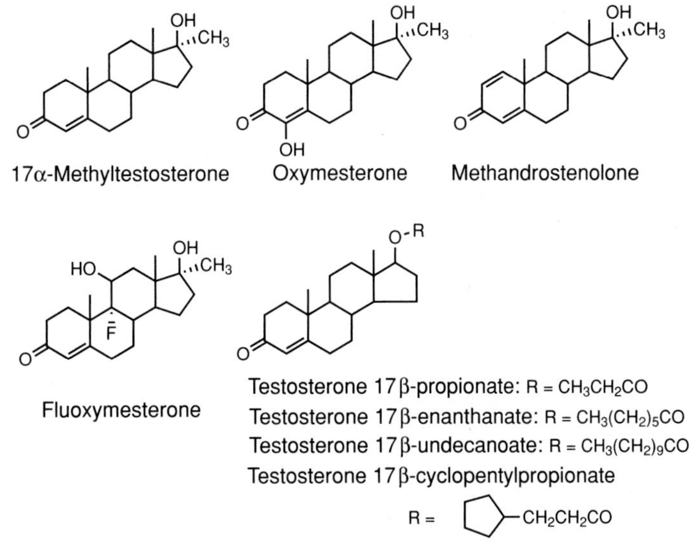

17α-Methyltestosterone Oxymesterone Methandrostenolone

Fluoxymesterone

Testosterone 17β-propionate: R = CH_3CH_2CO
Testosterone 17β-enanthanate: R = $CH_3(CH_2)_5CO$
Testosterone 17β-undecanoate: R = $CH_3(CH_2)_9CO$
Testosterone 17β-cyclopentylpropionate
R = cyclopentyl–CH_2CH_2CO

Fig. 45.9. Testosterone esters and synthetic testosterone derivatives.

because of the high 5α-reductase enzyme activity of the scrotal tissue. The patches have an occlusive backing that prevents sex partners from coming in contact with the active drug. A matrix transdermal system will not produce adequate plasma testosterone concentrations if applied to nonscrotal skin. Plasma testosterone concentrations are reached in approximately 2 to 4 hours. Although testosterone is absorbed throughout a 24-hour period, concentrations do not simulate the circadian rhythm of endogenous testosterone in normal (eugonadal) males. Within 24 hours after application of the matrix system, plasma testosterone concentration gradually falls to 60 to 80% of the peak plasma concentration, and when the system is removed, testosterone plasma concentration declines to baseline within 2 hours. Inadequate scrotal size and adherence problems are limitations. Skin irritation does occur in those with sensitive scrotal skins.

Reservoir-Type Transdermal Systems. The reservoir-type patch (nonscrotal patch; Androderm, Testoderm TTS) is not applied to scrotal skin but, rather, to the abdomen, back, thighs, or upper arms every 24 hours (see Table 45.4 for dosage strength). This type of patch is membrane-controlled for the drug to diffuse continuously over 24 hours from the reservoir into the skin. Thus, this type of patch is thicker than the matrix (scrotal) patch. The patches have an occlusive backing that prevents sex partners from coming in contact with the active drug. The site of the application is rotated at 7-day intervals between applications to lessen skin reactions at the same application site. The advantage of the reservoir transdermal system is that it achieves normal testosterone circadian rhythm as seen in younger men, peaking in the morning and decreasing throughout the rest of the day. The reservoir-type patch, when applied to nonscrotal skin, produced physiological DHT and estradiol plasma concentrations. Steady-state plasma concentrations of testosterone, which are approximately 10 times baseline values, are reached in about 6 hours (range, 4–10 hours depending on application patch location), which then fall to 60 to 80% of the peak plasma concentration within 24 hours after application of the transdermal system. Thus, physiological plasma testosterone concentrations are maintained over 24 hours with this type of patch. Drug accumulation does not occur with repeated applications. When the system is removed, testosterone plasma concentrations decline to baseline within 2 hours. A usual dose for the reservoir-type transdermal results in the systemic absorption of 2 to 10 mg daily in hypogonadal men.

Gel. Testosterone gel (AndroGel, Testim) is a 1% testosterone hydroalcoholic gel that provides continuous transdermal delivery of testosterone for 24 hours once the gel is rubbed into the skin on the lower abdomen, upper arm, or shoulder; do not apply to scrotal tissue (Table 45.2). Because there is a continuous release of testosterone over 24 hours, the normal circadian rhythm is not observed. As the gel dries, approximately 10% of the testosterone is absorbed through the skin. Gel application of TRT appears to cause fewer skin reactions than occur with the patches. Avoid showering or bathing for several hours after an application to ensure adequate absorption. A potential side effect of the gel is the possibility of transferring the medication to your partner; skin-to-skin contact should be avoided either until the gel is completely dry or by covering the area after an application. Following the application of 5 g of gel, which will deliver 50 mg of testosterone, the mean peak testosterone concentrations are reached in approximately 2 hours, which are about two to three times baseline values. For optimum results, the gel is best applied in the evening to allow maximum concentration to occur early in the morning hours. Doses of the gel may be adjusted by aiming for midphysiological (400–600 ng/dL) testosterone values after 1 week. When the gel treatment is discontinued, plasma testosterone levels remain in the physiological range for 24 to 48 hours, then return to their pretreatment levels within 5 days following the last application. An increase in plasma testosterone can be observed within 30 minutes of application. Plasma concentrations approximate the steady-state level by the end of the first 24 hours and are at steady state by the second or third day of dosing.

Buccal Mucosal. Striant is a gel-like substance that adheres to the gumline, which softens to deliver physiological amounts of testosterone to the systemic circulation, thereby producing circulating testosterone concentrations in hypogonadal males that approximate physiological levels seen in healthy young men (400–700 ng/dL). One buccal system (30 mg) is applied to the gum region twice daily, morning and evening, approximately 12 hours apart. Because there is a continuous release of testosterone over 24 hours, the normal circadian rhythm is not observed. Peak plasma testosterone concentrations are reached within 10 to 12 hours and are stable within a few days of the buccal preparation. The buccal preparation is difficult for patients to get used to, because the side effects may include gum irritation or pain, bitter taste, or headache. A study found that this form of TRT delivers a steadier dose of testosterone throughout the day without significant adverse effects, comparable to the gel.

ORAL. Orally administered testosterone is ineffective in the treatment of male androgen deficiency syndromes because of extensive presystemic first-pass metabolism, primarily to inactive 17-ketosteroid, etiocholanolone and androsterone, and androstanediol metabolites in the gastrointestinal mucosa during absorption and in the liver (Fig. 45.5). Oral administration results in supraphysiological elevations of testosterone and undesirable variability of plasma concentrations. The plasma half-life of testosterone is less than 30 minutes. Generally, the amount of sex hormone binding globulin in plasma determines the distribution of testosterone between free and bound forms, and free testosterone concentrations determine the drug's half-life. Approximately 90% of a dose of testosterone is metabolized, and its metabolites are excreted in the urine primarily as glucuronide conjugates, with approximately 6% of a dose being excreted in the feces as unmetabolized testosterone. Comparative dosage ranges for testosterone and its synthetic preparations are shown in Table 45.2. Taking testosterone orally (Android, Testred) is not recommended for long-term replacement. Oral testosterone may cause an unfavorable cholesterol profile and increase your risk of blood clots and heart and liver problems.

The androgenic activity of lipophilic long-chain ester testosterone 17β-undecanoate (Android Testocaps is not approved for use in the United States) (Fig. 45.9) has been attributed to formation of testosterone via systemic ester hydrolysis of lymphatically transported testosterone undecanoate (72). Its oral bioavailability was approximately 3%. Lymphatically transported testosterone undecanoate accounted for between 90 and 100% of the systemically available ester and that 83 and 85% of the systemically available testosterone resulted from systemic hydrolysis of lymphatically transported testosterone undecanoate. These data demonstrate that intestinal lymphatic transport of testosterone undecanoate produces increased systemic exposure of testosterone by avoiding the extensive first-pass hepatic metabolism responsible for the inactivation of testosterone after oral administration.

Testosterone also has been compressed into 75- or 200-mg testosterone pellets, which release 1 to 3 mg of testosterone/day. One to two pellets are implanted under the skin, typically in the buttocks or abdomen, through a special needle under local anesthesia. They usually are replaced every 3 to 4 months. Although the pellets have been used experimentally for approximately 15 years, the use of testosterone pellets is not approved by the U.S. Food and Drug Administration. Reportedly, the pellets offer the advantage of very consistent testosterone blood levels. Some users have reported problems with the pellets working their way out from under the skin.

Synthetic Derivatives of Testosterone

Some of the early studies with androgens included structural modifications of the naturally occurring hormones to avoid first-pass metabolism. Blocking the metabolism of the 17β-hydroxy group with substituents in the 17α-position resulted in androgens with an increased bioavailability and duration of action when given orally. The synthetic androgens include methyltestosterone and fluoxymesterone (Fig. 45.9). The long-term use of oral androgens has been related to liver cancer.

17α-METHYLTESTOSTERONE. The synthesis of 17α-methyltestosterone made available a compound that was orally active (73) in daily doses between 10 and 50 mg, which is equivalent to a 400 mg oral dose of testosterone. The presence of a 17α alkyl group reduces susceptibility to hepatic oxidative metabolism, thereby increasing oral bioavailability by slowing metabolism. Following oral administration, methyltestosterone is well absorbed from the gastrointestinal tract, with a half-life of approximately 3 hours. This drug has the androgenic and anabolic activities of testosterone. Although orally active, it is more effective when administered sublingually. The alkylated oral androgens should be viewed as potentially hepatotoxic and should not be used.

Fluoxymesterone. By substituting a 9α-fluoro group onto an analog of 17α-methyltestosterone, fluoxymesterone has 20 times the anabolic and 10 times the androgenic activity of 17α-methyltestosterone (Fig. 45.9) (73). It has a mean half-life of 9 hours, and less than 5% of the drug is excreted unchanged. An adverse effect of fluoxymesterone is sodium and water retention that could lead to edema.

Structure–Activity Relationships of Steroidal Androgens

For a substance to have androgenic activity, it must contain a steroid skeleton (74). Oxygen functional groups normally occurring at positions 3 and 17 are not essential, because the basic nucleus, 5α-androstane, has androgenic activity (Fig. 45.1). This appears to be the minimal structural requirement for hormonal activity. For derivatives of etiocholane, in which the hydrogen is in the 5β-position, thereby affording a *cis* A/B ring juncture, no active androgens and anabolic agents are known (74). Generally, both ring expansion (to form homo derivatives by inserting a methylene group into one of the rings in the steroid nucleus) or ring contraction (by removing a methylene group) significantly reduces or destroys the androgenic and anabolic activities.

Introduction of a 3-ketone function or a 3α-OH group enhances androgenic activity. A hydroxyl group in the 17α-position of androstane contributes no androgenic or anabolic activity; no known substituent can approach the effectiveness of a 17β-OH group. Evidence indicates that the longer-acting esters of the 17β-OH compounds are hydrolyzed in vivo to the free alcohol, which is the active species. It is thought that the 17β-oxygen atom is important for attachment to the receptor site and that 17α-alkyl groups are important for preventing metabolic changes at this position (73). Such 17α-substituents render the compounds orally active.

Increasing the length of the alkyl side chain at the 17α-position, however, resulted in decreased activity, and the incorporation of other substituents, such as the 17α-ethynyl group, produced compounds with useful progestational activity (progestins) (see Chapter 46), such as ethisterone. Attaching an isoxazole ring to ethisterone produced danazol (Danatrol, Danocrine), which exhibited potent antigonadotropic properties, weak androgen and anabolic properties, and no estrogen or progestin activity. As a gonadotropin inhibitor, danazol suppresses the surge of LH and FSH from the pituitary, thus suppressing ovarian steroidogenesis. For this reason, it is used in the treatment of endometriosis. Previous treatment of endometriosis had been surgical or medical, with progestins or a combination of estrogen and progestin. Danazol is metabolized by CYP3A4 to its inactive metabolite, 2-hydroxymethylethisterone.

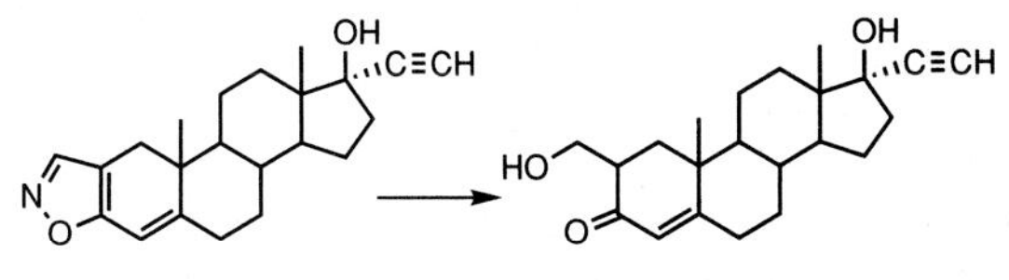

OH ..C≡CH N O Danazol → HO OH ..C≡CH O 2-Hydroxymethylethisterone (Danazol metabolite)

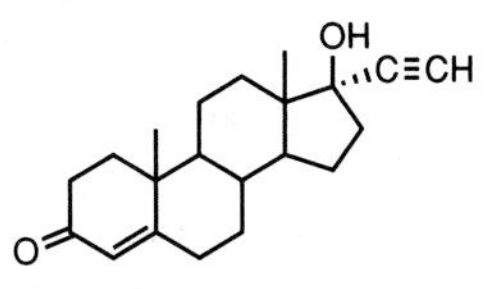

OH ..C≡CH O Ethisterone

Several modifications of 17α-methyltestosterone lead to potent, orally active anabolic agents. Two hydroxylated analogs include oxymesterone (Fig. 45.9) and oxymetholone (Fig. 45.10). These drugs have at least three times the anabolic and half the androgenic activity of testosterone (73).

Halogen substitution produces compounds with decreased activity except when inserted into positions 4 or 9 (e.g., fluoxymesterone). Replacement of a carbon atom in position 2 by oxygen has produced the only clinically successful heterocyclic steroid among a number of azasteroids and oxasteroids. Some of the 2-oxasteroids are potent anabolic agents.

Introduction of a sp^2 hybridized carbon atom into the A ring renders the ring more planar, and in turn, this may be responsible for greater anabolic activity. The 19-norsteroids are of interest, because these agents seem to produce a more favorable ratio of anabolic to androgenic activity. Vida (73) has extensively reviewed the replacement of various hydrogens on the androgen steroid skeleton by other functional groups. It appears that certain substitutions at positions 1, 2, 7, 17, and 18 may result in compounds with favorable activities that will be of clinical importance.

ADVERSE EFFECTS. Testosterone replacement therapy can have undesirable side effects depending on the type of delivery system used. The adverse effects from oral testosterone include stomach upset, headache, acne, increased hair growth on the face or body, jaundice (liver toxicity), anxiety, change in sex drive, sleeplessness, increased urination, depression, enlargement of breasts, and increased frequency and duration of erections (46). Breast enlargement can develop because testosterone can be converted to estradiol via aromatase. Other adverse effects include water retention, liver toxicity, cardiovascular disease, sleep apnea, and prostate enlargement. These risks are relatively uncommon when the dosage is closely monitored to maintain physiological plasma testosterone concentrations. Testosterone replacement therapy is contraindicated in men with carcinoma of the breast or with known or suspected carcinoma of the prostate. Therefore, pretreatment screening for any prostate dysfunction is mandatory before starting TRT.

Anabolic Agents

Because complete dissociation of anabolic and androgenic effects is not possible, many of the actions of anabolic

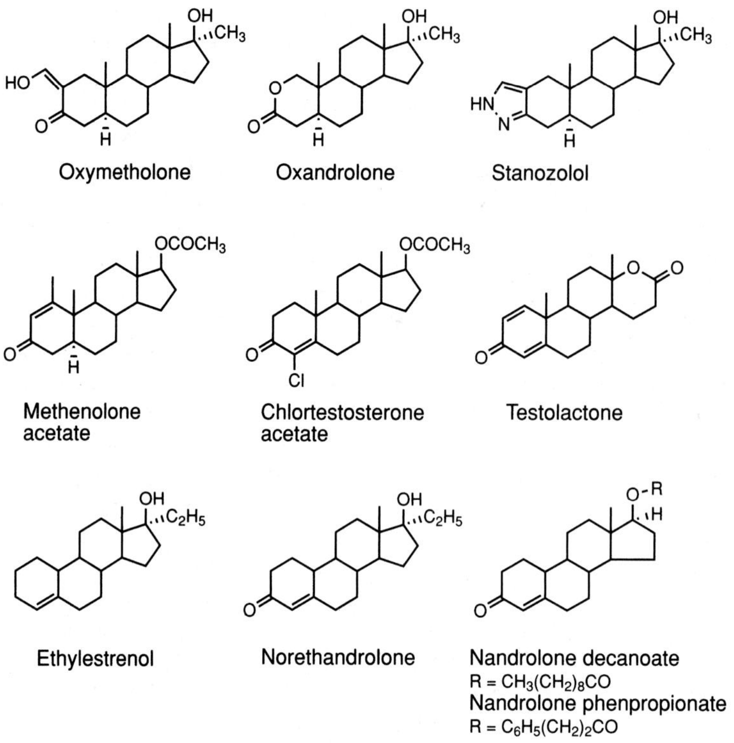

Oxymetholone

Oxandrolone

Stanozolol

Methenolone acetate

Chlortestosterone acetate

Testolactone

Ethylestrenol

Norethandrolone

Nandrolone decanoate
R = $CH_3(CH_2)_8CO$
Nandrolone phenpropionate
R = $C_6H_5(CH_2)_2CO$

Fig. 45.10. Anabolic steroids.

steroids are similar to those of androgens. Comparative dosage ranges for the anabolic steroids are shown in Table 45.2.

Selenium dioxide dehydrogenation of 17α-methyltestosterone yields the 1,4-diene analogue, methandrostenolone, as shown in Fig. 45.10, which has several-fold the anabolic activity of the starting material. It has low androgenic activity but, apparently, can produce mammogenic effects in men. These effects are thought to result from estrogenic metabolites.

The 17α-alkylated anabolic steroids in clinical use are oxandrolone (Anavar, Oxandrin), oxymetholone (Anadrol-50), stanozolol (Winstrol), nandrolone decanoate (Deca-Durabolin, Hybolin), and phenpropionate, as shown in Figure 45.10.

A 2-oxasteroid analogue of 17α-methyltestosterone is oxandrolone, which contains a lactone in the A ring (oxygen bio-isostere of ring A) and, therefore, is susceptible to in vivo hydrolysis. It has three times the anabolic activity of 17α-methyltestosterone but exhibits slight androgenic activity (75). A pyrazole heterocyclic compound used for its anabolic effects is stanozolol (75).

The anabolic steroid oxymetholone is used primarily to stimulate production of erythropoietin in the treatment of anemias resulting from bone marrow failure.

Testolactone (Teslac), a 18-oxasteroid, is a D-homo-oxoandrostandienedione analogue, with ring D being a 6-membered lactone ring. Although testolactone possesses some anabolic activity with weak androgenic effects, it is used primarily in the treatment of breast cancer as a noncompetitive irreversible inhibitor of aromatase to suppress the formation of estrogens that would stimulate the growth of breast tissue (46). It is primarily excreted in the urine unchanged, but it is metabolized in the liver by partial reduction of the 4-ene double bond in ring A to the 5β-metabolite (*cis* A/B ring juncture). Testolactone is available in both parenteral and oral forms.

Alkylation in the 1, 2, 7, and 18 positions of the androstane molecule generally increases anabolic activity (73). One of these derivatives, methenolone acetate, is an example of a potent anabolic agent that does not have an alkyl substituent at the 17α-position. A halogenated anabolic agent used in about the same dosage is chlortestosterone acetate.

Androgens, having no methyl group in position 10 of the steroid nucleus, are an important class of anabolic agents often referred to as the 19-norandrogens, as shown in Fig. 45.10. The removal of the 19-CH_3 group of the androgen results in reduction of its androgenic properties but retention of its anabolic, tissue-building properties. These steroids can be synthesized by the Birch reduction of the aromatic A ring of a 3-methoxy estrogen to a 2,5(10)-estradiene. Cleavage of the enol ether with HCl results in the 19-nortestosterone derivative. In animal assays, 19-nortestosterone has about the same anabolic activity as the propionate ester of testosterone, but its androgenic activity is much lower. Because 19-nortestosterone showed some separation of anabolic and androgenic activities, related analogues were synthesized and biologically investigated. Two of the more potent members of the series are norethandrolone and ethylestrenol, are shown in Figure 45.10. Norethandrolone has a better ratio of anabolic to androgenic activity than either 19-nortestosterone or 17α-methyl-19-nortestosterone does (46). Both androgenic and progestational side effects have been observed with this agent. Ethylestrenol is more potent than norethandrolone as an anabolic agent and is used in a dosage of 4 mg per day orally.

Nandrolone phenpropionate and nandrolone decanoate are esters of 19-nortestosterone, as shown in Figure 45.10, that when administered IM, slow in vivo hydrolysis of the ester occurs releasing free 19-nortestosterone over a prolonged period. Nandrolone decanoate is the longer-acting ester intended for deep IM injection, preferably into the gluteal muscle, in the treatment of anemia associated with renal insufficiency. Nandrolone phenpropionate has a shorter duration of action than the decanoate and is used in the treatment of metastatic breast cancer in women.

Abuse of Steroidal Anabolic Agents to Enhance Athletic Performance

Performance-enhancing substances are now a point of major interest for athletes, government, and news media. These substances are having a major impact on sports and the public in general. It appears that we are headed for much greater antidoping efforts in sports. A great deal of interest has recently been shown in "designer" anabolic steroids for their high-muscle-building effects, as shown in Fig. 45.11. Tetrahydrogestrinone and desoxymethyltestosterone (DMT), as shown in Figure 45.11, brought a great deal of interest to the performance-enhancing area, because their use was very difficult to detect (77,78). Tetrahydrogestrinone is thought to have been derived from gestrinone, a substance that has been used for the treatment of a variety of gynecological disorders. Tetrahydrogestrinone also is related to trenbolone, which has been used by body builders and by ranchers to build up cattle before marketing. Before tetrahydrogestrinone, both gestrinone and trenbolone had been on the banned anabolic steroid list of the International Olympic Committee. Tetrahydrogestrinone was very difficult to trace, however, because it was unstable under the normal conditions of testing for anabolic steroids. Once a suitable assay was developed, it was possible to go back and test samples of athletes around the world, and several were found to have taken tetrahydrogestrinone.

Nonsteroidal Androgens

Selective Androgen Receptor Modulators

In the past several years, the successful marketing and clinical application of selective estrogen receptor modulators (see Chapter 46) has raised the possibility of developing selective ligands for other members of the nuclear receptor superfamily. The concept of SARMs (2,78,79) also emerged—namely, a compound that is an antagonist or weak agonist in the prostate but agonist in the bone and muscle and is orally available with low hepatotoxicity. For an ideal SARM, the antagonist or weak agonist activity in the prostate will reduce concern for the potential to stimulate nascent or undetected prostate cancer; whereas the strong agonist activity in the muscle and bone can be used to treat muscle-wasting conditions, hypogonadism, and/or aging-related frailty. Currently, research on SARMs is in its early stages—namely, preclinical discovery and the early phase of clinical development. Phase II studies planned for the next 2 to 3 years, however, should reveal the true promise of this exciting new therapeutic class of drugs.

The SARM pharmacophores can be classified into four categories: N-arylpropionamide (81,82), bicyclic hydantoin (83), tricyclic quinolines (84), and tetrahydroquinoline (85) analogs, as shown in Figure 45.12. These nonsteroidal AR ligands are not substrates for aromatase or 5α-reductase but exhibit affinity as full AR agonists in anabolic organs (e.g., muscle and bone) or as partial AR agonists in androgenic tissues (e.g., prostate and seminal vesicles).

STRUCTURE–ACTIVITY RELATIONSHIPS FOR THE N-ARYLPROPIONAMIDES. The majority of published preclinical research has focused on a series of N-arylpropionamide analogues as AR agonists or partial agonists, utilizing the key structural elements of bicalutamide, an androgen antagonist (see below for a comparison of both structures) (2,81,82). A

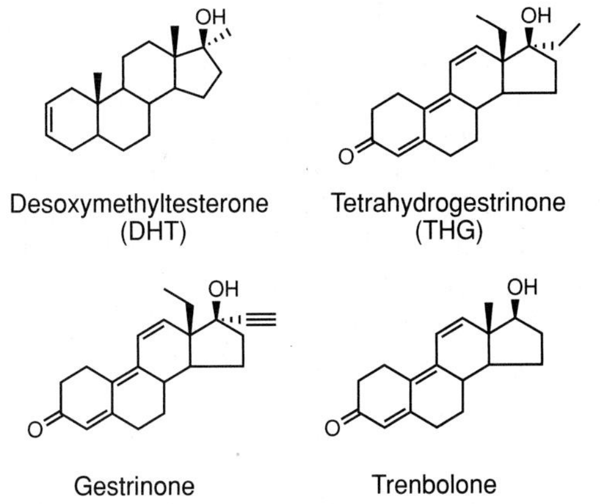

Desoxymethyltesterone (DHT)

Tetrahydrogestrinone (THG)

Gestrinone

Trenbolone

Fig. 45.11. Illegal anabolic agents.

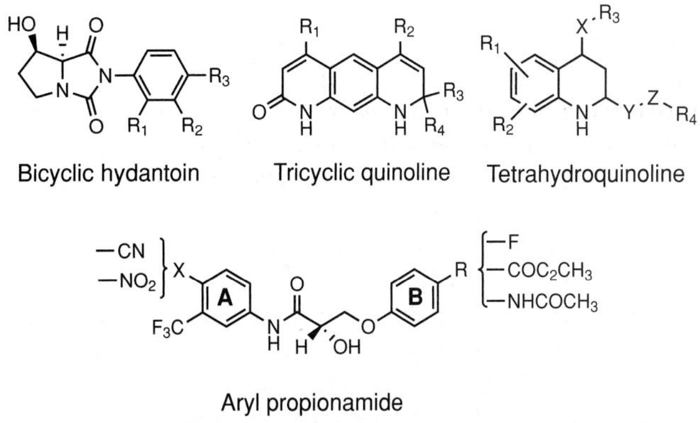

Bicyclic hydantoin

Tricyclic quinoline

Tetrahydroquinoline

Aryl propionamide

Fig. 45.12. Selective adrenergic receptor modulators.

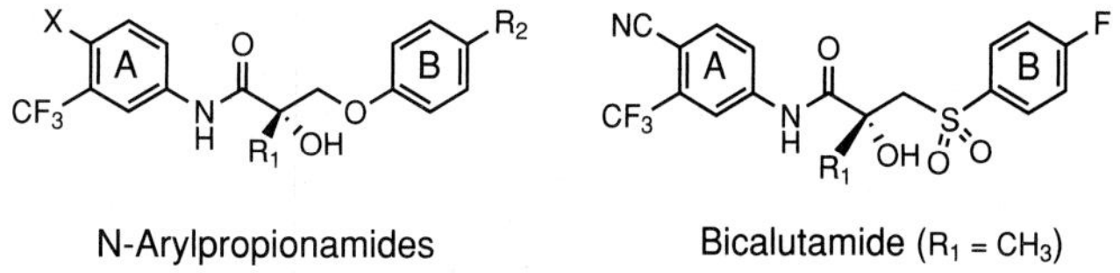

N-Arylpropionamides Bicalutamide (R_1 = CH_3)

SARM Comparison

series of chiral bicalutamide analogs, which bear electron-withdrawing groups (either a cyano or a nitro group at the 4-position and a trifluoromethyl group at the 3-position) in ring A, with a fluoro or acetylamino substituents at the para position in ring B (R_2) demonstrated high in vitro AR binding affinity and in vivo androgenicity and anabolic activity in rats (86,87). The *R*-isomer analogs which have a trifluoromethyl group instead of an Me group at the R2 position exhibited higher AR binding affinity and more potent activity than their corresponding *S*-isomers (88). The sulfide analogs (replacement of ether oxygen with sulfur) exhibited greater AR binding affinity, except that hepatic oxidation of the sulfur linkage led to rapid in vivo inactivation and reduced efficacy. Partial androgen agonist activity was observed when position 3 of ring A was substituted with a trifluoromethyl group (89). Replacing the aromatic ring A with a heterocyclic ring derivative failed to retain AR binding affinity, which probably arose from steric hinderance on binding with the AR; however, a heterocyclic B ring retained AR binding affinity. Small size electron-withdrawing moieties at R2, such as fluoro, chloro, nitro, or cyano groups, are optimum. Because aromatic nitro groups are associated with hepatotoxicity, the nitro group was replaced with a nonreducible electron-withdrawing group (i.e., a cyano group), which gave the most potent and efficacious N-arylpropionamide SARM with favorable pharmacokinetic properties. As evidenced from structure–activity relationship studies, minor differences in ligand structure can lead to either agonist or antagonist activity. Full or partial agonist binding to AR is influenced by stereoisomeric conformation as well as by steric and electronic effects of the substituents. Molecular modeling of N-arylpropionamide AR ligands was used in conjunction with pharmacology, pharmacodynamics, pharmacokinetics, and metabolism to examine and optimize structural properties.

Results from in vitro and in vivo animal studies suggest that the therapeutic promise of SARMs as treatment for muscle wasting, osteoporosis, hormonal male contraception, BPH, or other conditions associated with aging or androgen deficiency—without unwanted side effects associated with testosterone—may be soon realized (2,79). The AR specificity and lack of steroidal-related side effects clearly distinguish these drugs from their steroidal predecessors and open the door for expanded clinical use of androgens. As the molecular mechanisms of action of SARMs on target tissues become more fully understood, the discovery of novel SARMs and expansion into broader therapeutic applications will be more feasible. Currently, research concerning SARMs is in preclinical discovery and the early phase of clinical development with the expectations that SARMs with the beneficial pharmacological activity of androgens without the unwanted side effects will provide individual patients who have various androgen-dependent disorders with a significantly improved quality of life.

TREATMENT OF PROSTATIC DISEASES

Diseases of the prostate represent some of the greatest threats to men's health. Incidence rates for BPH escalate rapidly with age, from approximately 50% of men at age 50 years to approximately 90% at age 90 years in the United States. Drugs that inhibit the metabolism of testosterone to DHT (i.e., 5α-reductase inhibitors) (90) or block urethral constriction (α_1-adrenergic receptor antagonists) (91) are used as front-line treatment for urinary obstruction associated with BPH. Surgery also commonly is performed as treatment for early-stage prostate cancer (i.e., prostatectomy) and transurethral resection of the prostate, making these some of the most common surgeries performed on men.

Prostate cancer is the most common noncutaneous cancer and remains the second leading cause of death from cancer in American men (92). Androgen receptor antagonists (i.e., antiandrogens) and LHRH (or gonadotropin-releasing hormone) analogs are routinely used for medical management of patients with early stage prostate cancer, whereas patients with advanced prostate cancer are treated with anticancer chemotherapy.

Benign Prostatic Hyperplasia

Benign prostatic hyperplasia is the noncancerous proliferation of the prostate gland. The major problem associated with BPH is lower urinary tract symptoms. Approximately 80% of men will develop BPH within their lifetime. Although the cause of BPH is not well understood, it occurs mainly in older men, and it does not develop in men whose testes were removed before puberty. As men age, the amount of active testosterone in the blood decreases, leaving a higher proportion of estrogen. Animal studies have suggested that BPH may result from the increased concentration of estrogen or DHT within the gland, which promotes cell growth (93). Men who do not produce DHT do not develop BPH (94).

The symptoms of BPH stem from obstruction of the urethra by an enlarged prostate and the gradual loss of bladder function, which results in incomplete emptying of the bladder. The symptoms of BPH vary, but the most common symptoms involve changes or problems with urination. The typical symptoms of BPH are obstructive (e.g., poor urine stream, dribbling, and large residual urine volume) and irritative (e.g., hesitancy, increased frequency of urination, and nocturia), which can significantly compromise the quality of life for men. The enlarging prostate increases the adrenergic tone of the prostate in patients with BPH, which results in further tightening of the urethra. When partial obstruction is present, urinary retention also can be brought on by alcohol, cold temperatures, a long period of immobility, or the ingestion of over-the-counter cold or allergy medicines that contain a sympathomimetic decongestant drug or anticholinergics.

Severe BPH can cause serious problems over time, including urinary retention and strain on the bladder, which can lead to urinary tract infections, bladder or kidney damage, bladder stones, and incontinence.

Before and during adulthood, DHT plays a critical role in determining prostate size, and multiple lines of evidence suggest the importance of DHT in the development of BPH (95,96). For instance, BPH does not develop in males with certain type 2 5α-reductase mutations or in males with very low levels of androgen because of prepubertal castration or hypopituitarism-related hypogonadism. Moreover, clinical treatment of BPH either by chemical or surgical castration or by type 2 5α-reductase inhibitor (e.g., finasteride) induces apoptosis of epithelial cells, which in turn significantly decreases the volume of the prostate (96). Recently, the role of age-dependent changes in the intraprostatic hormonal environment in the development of BPH was evaluated (90). Despite the aging-related decrease in testosterone and intraprostatic DHT production, an increased estradiol/DHT ratio was observed in the aging human prostate, which can be relevant to the development of BPH. Furthermore, estradiol is capable of inducing precancerous lesions and prostate cancer in aging dogs (97). Therefore, TRT in older men raises concern regarding acceleration of BPH and/or prostate cancer.

Surgical procedures often are used to reduce a large prostate mass, but there are early pharmacological treatments of BPH with an α_1-adrenergic blocker, a 5α-reductase inhibitor, and phytotherapy.

The α_1-adrenergic antagonists treat the increased adrenergic tone of the sympathetic nervous system by relaxing the muscles at the neck of the bladder and in the prostate, thereby reducing the pressure on the urethra and increasing the flow of urine (91). They do not cure BPH but, rather, help to alleviate some of the symptoms. Approximately 60% of men find that symptoms improve significantly within the first 2 to 3 weeks of treatment with an α_1-antagonist. In addition to alfuzosin and tamsulosin, which are the first-line α_1-adrenergic antagonists, other α_1-antagonists include doxazosin and terazosin, which also have been used to treat high blood pressure. Tamsulosin and alfuzosin are uroseletive α_1-adrenergic antagonists developed specifically to treat BPH.

The 5α-reductase inhibitors work by suppressing the production of intraprostatic DHT, thereby reducing the size of the prostate (90). Finasteride and dutasteride are the most commonly used drugs for this purpose. Unlike α_1-antagonists, 5α-reductase inhibitors are able to reverse BPH to some extent and so may delay the need for surgery. Several months of treatment may be needed before the benefit is noticed.

α_1-Adrenergic Antagonists

Mechanism of action. α_1-Adrenoceptors are widely distributed in the human body and play important

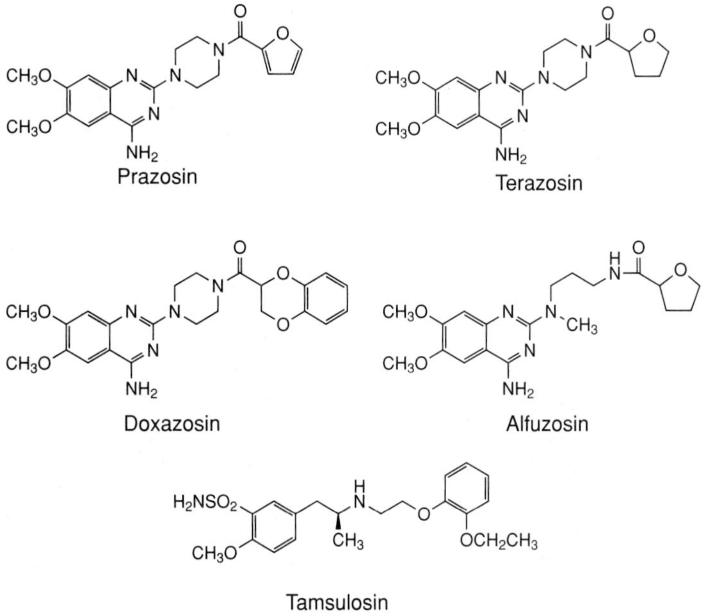

Prazosin

Terazosin

Doxazosin

Alfuzosin

Tamsulosin

Fig. 45.13. α_1-Adrenergic antagonists for treatment of benign prostatic hyperplasia.

physiological roles (see Chapter 13). Of the three α_1-adrenoceptor subtypes (α_{1A}, α_{1B}, and α_{1D}), α_{1A}-adrenoceptors are expressed in prostate and urethral tissue and mediate smooth muscle contraction. The fact that a single α_{1A}-adrenoceptor subtype is found in the prostatic and urethral smooth muscle cells led to the design of drugs with uroselectivity for this receptor subtype. Thus, alfuzosin (an aminoquinazoline) and tamsulosin (an N-substituted, catecholamine-related sulfonamide) were designed for the treatment of BPH, as shown in Figure 45.13 (96). Doxazosin and terazosin, along with prazosin, originally were used as antihypertensives but also were found to be effective for the treatment of BPH based on their common mechanism of action. A comparison of the affinities (K_i, nM) of the α_{1A}-adrenoceptor antagonists (Table 45.3) did not show substantial differences for the quinazoline α_{1A}-antagonists (alfuzosin, doxazosin, and terazosin) but some uroselectivity for tamsulosin (91). Although in vitro studies showed subtype uroselectivity, in vivo studies showed that those α_{1A}-adrenoceptor antagonists without adrenoceptor subtype selectivity, such as alfuzosin and doxazosin, showed uroselectivity (terazosin was not uroselective), whereas tamsulosin, which exhibited in vitro selectivity for the α_{1A}-adrenoceptor, did not show the expected in vivo uroselectivity (99). These differences between in vitro and in vivo studies suggest that these drugs modify urethral pressures in a manner that is not correlated with their selectivity for the cloned α_{1A}-adrenoceptor subtypes. It is apparent that the existing α_{1A}-adrenoceptor antagonists have different in vivo pharmacological profiles that are not yet predictable from their receptor based on the current state of knowledge regarding the α_{1A}-adrenoceptor classification (99).

Thus, tamsulosin and alfuzosin are first-line drugs for the treatment of BPH and have no utility in treating hypertension, because they have fewer cardiovascular effects than terazosin and doxazosin. Their clinical profiles are related to their pharmacokinetic differences (Table 45.3). Improvements in urine flow occur 4 to 8 hours after the first dose and in BPH symptoms after 1 week.

ADVERSE REACTIONS. In patients with BPH, the most common adverse effects for α_1-adrenergic antagonists are related to vasodilation, including dizziness, orthostatic hypotension, headache, and tachycardia, which occurred during the first 2 weeks of treatment (46). Therefore, a dose titration usually is required, especially in patients older than 60 years. These cardiovascular side effects are attributed to a nonselective blockade of α_1-adrenoceptors present in vascular smooth muscle in addition to the required blockade of α_1-adrenoceptors in prostate. No first-dose effect and fewer vasodilatory adverse events have been reported with the sustained-release formulations, which occur more frequently with the immediate-release formulation At higher doses, orthostatic hypotension occurs more frequently. The first-dose phenomenon of orthostatic hypotension and syncope has been reported occasionally in elderly patients and in those concurrently receiving calcium antagonists, diuretics, and β-blockers.

Quinazolines

Prazosin was the first selective quinazoline α_1-blocker to be discovered in the late 1960s as an antihypertensive. Alfuzosin, doxazosin, and terazosin are structurally similar (a 4-amino-6,7-dimethoxyquinazoline ring system) but differ in the attached side chain as a piperazine ring or open-chain analogue as shown in Figure 45.13. The other structural differences are the acyl groups attached to the second nitrogen of the piperazine or the aminopropyl chain. The differences in these groups afford

Table 45.3. Some Properties and Pharmacokinetics of the α-Adrenergic Antagonists

Drug	Alfuzosin	Doxazosin	Tamsulosin	Terazosin
Trade Name	Uroxatral	Cardura	Flomax	Hytrin
cLogP[a]	−1.0 ± 0.4	0.7 ± 0.4	2.2 ± 0.4	−1.0 ± 0.4
log D[a] (pH 7)	−1.3	−0.5	−0.5	−1.0
Oral Bioavailability (%)	65	65 (62–69)	<50 with food >90 fasted	90
Onset of Action (weeks)[b]	<2	1–2	1	2
Duration of Action (hours)	>48	18–36	>24	>18
Protein binding (%)	82–90	98	94	95
Time to Peak Conc. (hours)	1–2	2–5	4–5	1
Volume of Distribution (L/kg)	2.5–3.2	1.0–3.4	18	25–30
Elimination Half-life (hours)	3–10	18–22	9–13 14–15 elderly	9–12
Cytochrome Isoforms	3A4	3A4	3A4, 2D6	—
Excretion (%)	69 feces 24–30 urine (metabolites)	63–65 feces ~20 urine ~10 unchanged	21 feces 76 urine 10 unchanged	55–65 feces 30 urine 10–20 unchanged
K_i (nmol/L) for α_{1A}	2.4	2.7	0.5	2.5

[a]Chemical Abstracts, American Chemical Society, calculated using Advanced Chemistry Development (ACD/Labs) Software V8.14 for Solaris (1994–2006 ACD/Labs).
[b]Time for improvement in urine flow observed.

dramatic differences in some of the pharmacokinetic properties for these agents (see Table 45.5). Perhaps most significant are the long half-lives and durations of action for these drugs that permit once-a-day dosing and, generally, lead to increased patient compliance.

Alfuzosin is a first-line uroselective drug for the treatment of BPH, but with no utility in treating hypertension, because it has fewer cardiovascular effects than terazosin and doxazosin. Alfuzosin is hepatically metabolized by 7-O-demethylation and N-dealkylation, primarily by CYP3A4 to inactive metabolites. In patients with moderate or severe hepatic insufficiency, a reduction in clearance resulted in a three to four times increase in its plasma concentrations, which may require a reduction in dose.

Doxazosin is primarily metabolized by 7-O-demethylation, hydroxylation of the benzdioxan ring, and oxidation of the piperazine ring to inactive metabolites. In patients with renal insufficiency, the elimination half-life was not significantly different from healthy volunteers.

Terazosin is similarly metabolized via 7-O-demethylation and N-dealkylation to four metabolites: 6- and 7-O-demethyl terazosin, the piperazine derivative of terazosin, and the diamine metabolite of the piperazine compound.

Catecholamine-Sulfonamide

Tamsulosin exhibits uroselectivity and is a first-line drug for the treatment of BPH, with no utility for treating hypertension, because of its fewer cardiovascular effects. Tamulson is O-deethylated by CYP3A4 to phenolic metabolites that are conjugated to glucuronide or sulfate before renal excretion and by O-demethylation and 3′-hydroxylation to catechol metabolites that also are conjugated with glucuronide and sulfate.

5α-Reductase Inhibitors

The development of BPH requires a combination of intraprostatic DHT and the aging process. Although not elevated in BPH, levels of DHT in the prostate remain at a physiological levels with aging despite a decrease in plasma testosterone. Adult males with genetically inherited, type 2 5α-reductase deficiency also have decreased DHT levels. These 5α-reductase–deficient males have a small prostate gland throughout life and do not develop BPH. Except for the associated urogenital defects that are present at birth, no other clinical abnormalities related to 5α-reductase deficiency have been observed in these individuals.

MECHANISM OF ACTION. Inhibitors of DHT biosynthesis can result in a decrease in both circulating target-tissue DHT concentrations, thus blocking its androgenic action in these tissues. The critical enzyme targeted for DHT inhibition is 5α-reductase, which converts testosterone to DHT. The first agent to demonstrate 5α-reductase inhibition was a progestin analogue, medrogesterone (100) (Fig. 45.14). Two azasteroid-17-amide derivatives of medrogesterone have been developed as potent irreversible inhibitors of 5α-reductase and approved for the

Medrogesterone

Finasteride (R = $C(CH_3)_3$)

Dutasteride (R = 2,5-bis(CF_3)phenyl)

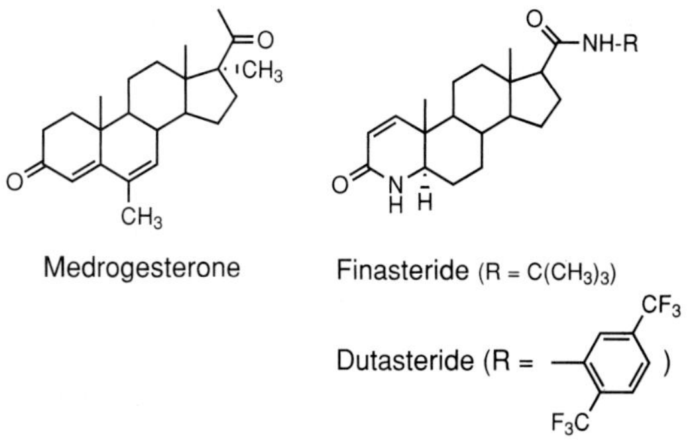

Fig. 45.14. 5α-Reductase inhibitors for the treatment of benign prostatic hyperplasia.

treatment of BPH: finasteride, a selective inhibitor of type 2 5α-reductase (101,102), and dutasteride, a nonselective inhibitor of type 1 and type 2 5α-reductase (103) (Fig. 45.14). Thus, the inhibition of type 2 5α-reductase suppresses the metabolism of testosterone to DHT, resulting in significant decreases in plasma and intraprostatic DHT concentrations (102–104).

Finasteride and dutasteride are both mechanism-based inhibitors of type 1 and type 2 5α-reductase isoenzymes that inactivate 5α-reductase by an apparent irreversible modification of 5α-reductase (105,106). The inhibition constants (median inhibitory concentrations [IC_{50s}]) in Table 45.5 suggest that finasteride is 30 times more selective for type 2 5α-reductase, whereas dutasteride appears to be approximately 10 times more potent as an inhibitor of type 2 5α-reductase than as a inhibitor of type 1 5α-reductase. The reduction of finasteride to dihydrofinasteride proceeds through an enzyme-bound, NADP-dihydrofinasteride adduct (see Chapter 5) (105). The mechanism- based inhibition explains the exceptional potency and specificity of finasteride and dutasteride in the treatment of BPH. This concept of mechanism-based inhibition may have application to the development of other inhibitors of pyridine nucleotide–linked enzymes.

DRUG INTERACTIONS. Because finasteride and dutasteride are metabolized primarily by CYP3A4, the CYP3A4 inhibitors, such as ritonavir, ketoconazole, verapamil, diltiazem, cimetidine, and ciprofloxacin, may increase the drugs' blood levels and, possibly, cause drug–drug interactions. Clinical drug interaction studies have shown no pharmacokinetic or pharmacodynamic interactions between dutasteride and tamsulosin or terazosin, warfarin, digoxin, and cholestyramine.

FINASTERIDE. The selective inhibition of the type 2 5α-reductase isozyme produces a rapid reduction in plasma DHT concentration, reaching 65% suppression within 24 hours of administering a 1-mg oral tablet (106). At steady state, finasteride suppresses DHT levels by approximately 70% in plasma and by as much as 85 to 90% in the prostate. The remaining DHT in the prostate likely is the result of type 1 5α-reductase. The mean circulating levels of testosterone and estradiol remained within their physiological concentration range. Long-term therapy with finasteride can reduce clinical significant end points of BPH, such as acute urinary retention or surgery. Finasteride is most effective in men with large prostates. Finasteride has no affinity for the AR and no androgenic, antiandrogenic, estrogenic, antiestrogenic, or progestational effects.

Pharmacokinetics. The mean oral bioavailability of finasteride is 65%, as shown in Table 45.4, and is not affected by food (99). Approximately 90% of circulating finasteride is bound to plasma proteins. Finasteride has been found to cross the blood-brain barrier, but levels in semen were undetectable (<0.2 ng/mL). Finasteride is extensively metabolized in the liver, primarily via CYP3A4 to two major metabolites: monohydroxylation of the t-butyl side chain, which is further metabolized via an aldehyde intermediate to the second metabolite, a monocarboxylic acid (Fig. 45.15). The metabolites show approximately 20% the inhibition of finasteride for 5α-reductase. The mean terminal half-life is approximately 5 to 6 hours in men between 18 and 60 years of age and 8 hours in men older than 70 years of age. Following an oral dose of finasteride, approximately 40% of the dose was excreted in the urine as metabolites and approximately 57% in the feces. Even though the elimination rate of finasteride is decreased in the elderly, no dosage adjustment is necessary. No dosage adjustment is necessary in patients with renal insufficiency. A decrease in the urinary excretion of metabolites was observed in patients with renal impairment, but this was compensated for by

Table 45.4. Some Properties and Pharmacokinetics of the 5α-Reductases

Drugs	Finasteride	Dutasteride
Trade Name	Proscar	Avodart
cLogP[a]	3.2 ± 0.4	5.6 ± 0.6
log D[a] (pH 7)	3.2	5.6
Oral Bioavailability (%)	65 (26–170)	60 (40–94)
Onset of Action (hours)	<24	—
Duration of Action (hours)	—	>5 weeks
Protein binding (%)	90	99
Time to Peak Conc. (hours)	—	2–3
Volume of Distribution (L/kg)	76 (44–96)	300–500
Elimination Half-life (hours)	5–6 (18–60 yr) >8 for 60+ yr	5 weeks
Cytochrome Isoforms	3A4	3A4
Active Metabolites	None	6-*p*-OH
Excretion (%)	57 feces and 40 urine as metabolites	40 feces metabolites 5 unmetabolized urine
IC50 (nmol/L)	313 Type 1 11 Type 2	3.9 Type 1 1.8 Type 2

[a]Chemical Abstracts, American Chemical Society, calculated using Advanced Chemistry Development (ACD/Labs) Software V8.14 for Solaris (1994–2006ACD/Labs).

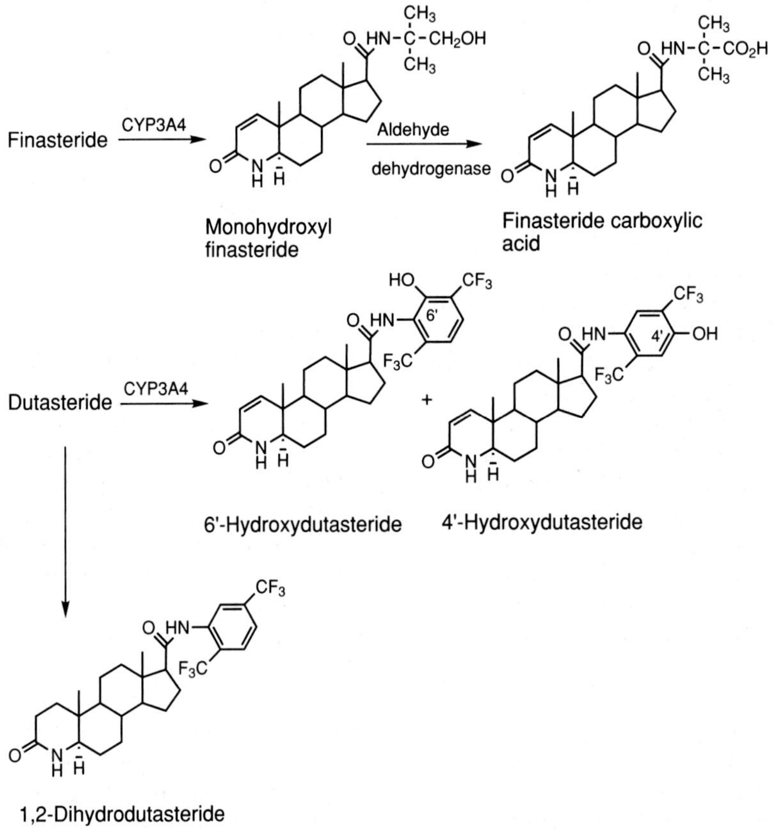

Fig. 45.15. Metabolites of finasteride and dutasteride.

an increase in fecal excretion of metabolites. Caution should be used during administration to patients with liver function abnormalities, because finasteride is metabolized extensively in the liver.

Dutasteride. Similar to finasteride, dutastèride is a competitive and mechanism-based inhibitor not only of type 2 but also of type 1 5α-reductase isoenzymes, with which stable enzyme-NADP adduct complexes are formed, inhibiting the conversion of testosterone to DHT (106). The suppression of both type 1 and type 2 isoforms results in greater and more consistent reduction of plasma DHT than that observed for finasteride (107–109). The more effective dual inhibition of type 1 and type 2 5α-reductase isoforms lowers circulating DHT to a greater extent than with finasteride and shows advantages in treating BPH and other disease states (e.g., prostate cancer) that are DHT-dependent.

The maximum effect of 0.5 mg daily doses of dutasteride on the suppression of DHT is dose-dependent and is observed within 1 to 2 weeks. After 2 weeks of 0.5 mg daily dosing, median plasma DHT concentrations were reduced by 90%, and after 1 year, the median decrease in plasma DHT was 94% (108,109). The median increase in plasma testosterone was 19% but remained within the physiological range. The drug also reduced serum prostatic specific antigen by approximately 50% at 6 months and total prostate volume by 25% at 2 years. Dutasteride produced improvements in quality of life and peak urinary flow rate and reduction of acute urinary retention without the need for surgery. The main side effects are ED, decreased libido, gynecomastia, and ejaculation disorders. Long-term use (>4 years), however, did not reveal increased onset of sexual side effects. In addition, the combination of dutasteride and tamsulosin is well-tolerated and has the added advantage of rapid symptomatic relief.

Pharmacokinetics. Following oral administration, peak plasma concentrations of dutasteride occurs in approximately 2 to 3 hours, with a bioavailability of approximately 60% (Table 45.4), and no meaningful reduction in absorption with occurs with food (107). Dutasteride is highly bound to plasma proteins 99%. The concentrations of dutasteride in semen averaged approximately 3 ng/mL, with no significant effects of on DHT plasma levels of sex partners. Dutasteride is extensively metabolized in humans by CYP3A4 to three major metabolites: 4′-hydroxydutasteride and 1,2-dihydrodutasteride, which are less potent than parent drug, and 6′-hydroxydutasteride, which is comparable to the parent drug as an inhibitor of both Type 1 and Type 2 5α-reductases. Dutasteride and its metabolites were excreted mainly (40%) in feces as dutasteride-related metabolites. The terminal elimination half-life of dutasteride is approximately 5 weeks. Because of its long half-life, plasma concentrations remain detectable for up to 4 to 6 months after discontinuation of treatment. No dose adjustment is necessary in elderly patients, even though its half-life increased with age from approximately 170 hours in men between 20 and 49 years to 300 hours in men older than 70 years (102). No adjustment in dosage is necessary for patients with renal impairment.

Phytotherapy

A number of plant extracts are popularly used to alleviate BPH, although formal evidence that they are effective is often scanty (110). Extracts of the saw palmetto berry (*Serenoa repens*) are widely used for the treatment of BPH, often as an alternative to pharmaceutical agents. In a national survey conducted in 2002, 1.1% of the adult male population in the United States, or approximately 2.5 million males, reported using saw palmetto. The herb is widely used in Europe, where half of the German urologists prefer prescribing plant-based extracts rather than synthetic drugs. The most common nonstandardized preparation used is either the hexane-extract (Permixon®) or the ethanol or carbon dioxide extraction of the dried ripe fruit from the American dwarf saw palmetto plant (*Serenoa repens*), which is rich in fatty acids and plant sterols. The plant sterols appear to be the primary active constituents. The U.S. Pharmacopeia states that the liposterolic extract product should contain 70 to 95% fatty acids and 0.2 to 0.5% sterols. Other substances in the extracts include polyprenic compounds and flavonoids. The usual therapeutic dose of the extracts is 320 mg daily.

Serenoa repens had been popular in the United States during the 19th century as a treatment for a variety of urogenital disorders and had been mentioned as a treatment for prostate problems as early as 1899. Research into the effects of *S. repens* in many European countries appeared to confirm a positive action on BPH. The mechanism of action for the saw palmetto is not clearly established, but the sterols may have, as one mechanism of action, the inhibition of 5α-reductase and a decrease in DHT production. Therapeutic results should be expected in 6 to 8 weeks, but clinical efficacy is observed with BPH for 6 months or longer. The liposterolic extract is largely devoid of the side effects noted for prescription BPH drugs.

Although most previous randomized trials of saw palmetto have reported small improvements in the symptoms of BPH or in urinary flow rates, these studies were limited by the small numbers of subjects enrolled, their short duration, failure to use standardized products, their failure to use standard outcome measures, and the lack of information from participants concerning how effectively the placebo was blinded. Using widely accepted outcome measures from the American Urological Association (AUA) and a matched placebo capsule, a randomized, 1-year, double-blind saw palmetto trial (funded by the National Institutes of Health National Institute on Complementary and Alternative Medicine) was performed to determine the efficacy of saw palmetto for the treatment of BPH (111) A total of 225 men aged

50 years and older with documented disease received 160 mg of a standardized saw palmetto extract twice a day or a matching-placebo capsule. Over the course of a year, the men made eight office visits and were evaluated for assessment of AUA standardized changes which induced maximal urine flow, postvoid residual urine volume, prostate size, and other health-related outcomes. In contrast to most previous studies, this study reported no significant benefit of saw palmetto on urinary symptoms in terms of objective measures of BPH over a 1-year period.

Despite the differences between these studies, the weight of evidence suggests that saw palmetto may induce mild to moderate improvements in urinary symptoms and flow measures.

Other Western herbs that have been investigated for the treatment of BPH include pumpkin seeds (*Cucurbita pepo*), nettle root (*Urtica dioica* or *Urtica urens*), bee pollen (particularly that from the rye plant), African potato (tubers of *Hypoxis rooperi*), and the African tree *Pygeum africanum*, also known as *Prunus africanum*. In most cases, but particularly with pumpkin seeds and African potato, the main active components are sterols, such as β-sitosterol, which also has been used for BPH. Triterpenoids in *Pygeum* sp. also have been proposed to be active components, potentially having the action of reducing prostate swelling. Among the Chinese herbs recommended for BPH, the iridoid glycosides may be the active components from plantago seed, catalpol from rehmannia, and morroniside from cornus (an ingredient in the rehmannia formulas). Iridoids have not been found in the Western herbal therapies for BPH and represent a potential new area for future investigation. Iridoids are the recognized active constituents of the Western herb chaste tree berry (*Vitex agnus costus*), which has been shown to reduce prolactin levels in women; elevated prolactin may be a risk factor for prostate enlargement in men. Triterpenoids found in vaccaria and alisma (an ingredient in rehmannia formulas) could contribute to their therapeutic effects in a manner similar to that suggested for pygeum.

Prostatic Cancer

Prostate cancer is the second leading cause of death in the United States and is the most commonly diagnosed cancer in American males (92). Prostate cancer is more common in African-American males, in whom it tends to be more aggressive and progressive, leading to advanced disease. The incidence of prostate cancer increases with age. Traditional treatments for prostate cancer include surgery (radical prostatectomy), radiotherapy, hormonal therapy, chemotherapy, cryosurgery (tissue is frozen to kill cancer cells), or watchful waiting.

Ever since Huggins and Hodges won the 1966 Nobel Prize for describing the relationship between testosterone and prostate cancer, androgen deprivation has become an important component in the treatment of prostate cancer by providing what amounts to chemical castration, reducing the need for testicular surgery. Testicular surgery (bilateral orchiectomy) to prevent testosterone production was once the standard treatment for advanced prostate cancer. Although this surgery is not a cure, it may delay the advance of the disease. Refinements in the therapy have occurred since this time, including androgen deprivation with antiandrogens, 5α-reductase inhibitor combinations, intravenous bisphosphonate infusions, and chemotherapy for advanced cases. If the cancer is no longer responding to hormonal treatment, chemotherapy may be tried for advanced disease.

Because prostate cancer typically grows slowly and causes no symptoms, the prostate-specific antigen (PSA) test is most often used as a screening test for prostate cancer, although it also may be used to evaluate and manage other prostate problems. Screening tests are able to detect prostate cancer at an early stage, but it is not clear whether this earlier detection and consequent earlier treatment leads to any change in the natural history and outcome of prostate cancer. The PSA screening test cannot tell the difference between prostate cancer and other prostate problems. The PSA is a protein made by the prostate tissue. Men with prostate cancer often have elevated PSA levels, because the cancer cells make excessive amounts of this protein.

Antiandrogens (Androgen Antagonists)

Treatment for advanced prostate cancer involves the use of hormone-blocking drugs called antiandrogens. The goal of antiandrogen therapy is to block the effects of testosterone and DHT on ARs. Antiandrogens, however, are not a cure for prostate cancer. Nonsteroidal antiandrogens (Fig. 45.16), such as flutamide, nilutamide, and bicalutamide, are referred to as pure antiandrogens, because they bind exclusively to AR and, thus, are devoid of antigonadotropic, antiestrogenic, and progestational effects (112). These agents have advantages over steroidal antiandrogens, such as megesterol acetate or cyproterone acetate (Fig. 45.17), in terms of specificity, selectivity, and pharmacokinetic properties.

Antiandrogens block the binding of DHT at the AR and, when administered with an androgen, blocks or diminishes the effectiveness of androgens in androgen-sensitive tissues. Such compounds have shown potential therapeutic use in the treatment of acne, virilization in women, and hyperplasia and neoplasia of the prostate (113). Several steroidal and nonsteroidal agents have demonstrated antiandrogenic activity. Cyproterone acetate suppresses gonadotropin release and binds with high affinity to the AR (114,115). Oxendolone also acts by competing for the receptor binding sites (116). A novel AR antagonist, WIN 49,596, has been described (117) which contains a fused pyrazole ring at carbons 2 and 3 of the steroid nucleus. A potent nonsteroidal antiandrogen, flutamide, has been shown to compete with DHT for the AR (118). Its hydroxylated metabolite is a more powerful antiandrogen in vivo, and it has a higher affinity for the receptor than the parent compound (119).

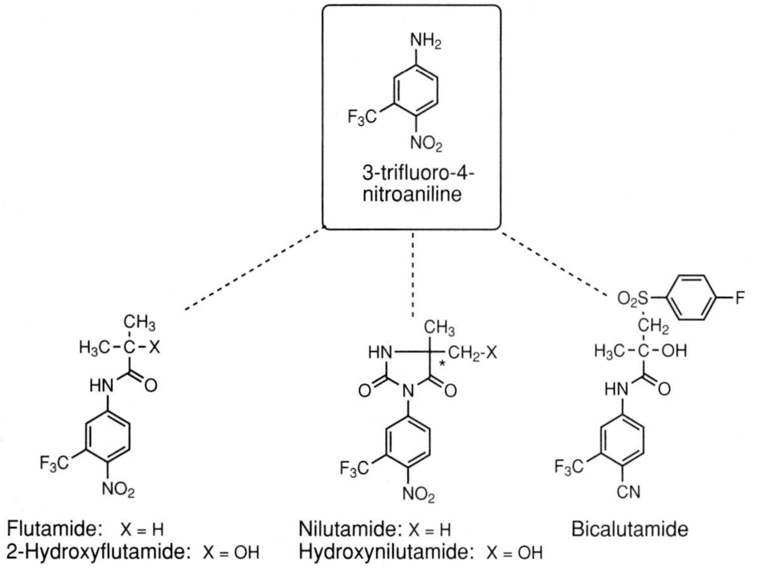

3-trifluoro-4-nitroaniline

Flutamide: X = H
2-Hydroxyflutamide: X = OH

Nilutamide: X = H
Hydroxynilutamide: X = OH

Bicalutamide

Fig. 45.16. Nonsteroidal antiandrogens.

Antiandrogens are particularly useful for the treatment of prostate cancer during its early stages. Often, however, prostate cancer advances to a "hormone-refractory" state, in which the disease progresses in the presence of continued androgen ablation or antiandrogen therapy, suggesting the development of androgen-independent prostate cancer cells or the ability of adrenal androgens to support tumor growth (as discussed above). Instances of antiandrogen withdrawal syndrome also have been reported after prolonged treatment with antiandrogens. Antiandrogen withdrawal syndrome is commonly observed clinically and is defined in terms of the tumor regression or symptomatic relief observed on cessation of antiandrogen therapy. The AR mutations that result in receptor promiscuity and the ability of these antiandrogens to exhibit agonist activity may account, at least in part, for this phenomenon. For example, hydroxyflutamide and bicalutamide act as AR agonists in AR mutants with an alanine residue at position 877 or leucine residue at position 741 (as opposed to threonine or tryptophan residues, respectively, that are present at these positions in the wild-type AR) (120,121).

The search for nonsteroidal antiandrogens lead to the development of the substituted toluidides, flutamide and bicalutamide, and nilutamide, a hydantoin that is structurally related to the toluidides (Fig. 45.16). These compounds are pure antiandrogens and compete with DHT for the human prostate AR. They are used in combination with other drugs in the treatment of metastatic prostate cancer. Although these compounds possess no intrinsic hormonal activity, their antiandrogenic mechanism of action is via competitive blockade of ARs for DHT in the hormone-sensitive tumor cells of the prostate (122). As a result of this antagonism, androgen-dependent DNA and protein synthesis is inhibited, causing arrest or regression of the prostatic tumor. Because these nonsteroidal antiandrogens are metabolized extensively in the liver, they should be used with caution in patients who have liver function abnormalities.

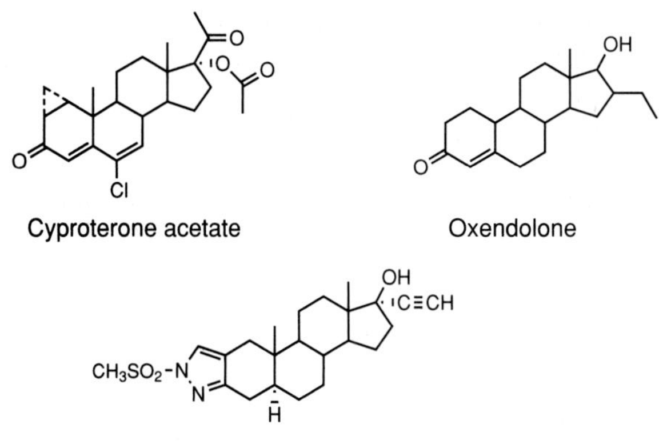

Fig. 45.17. Steroidal antiandrogens.

SPECIFIC DRUGS

Bicalutamide. Bicalutamide is a nonsteroidal pure antiandrogen given at a dosage of 150 mg once daily as monotherapy for the treatment of early (localized or locally advanced) nonmetastatic prostate cancer (123). It also can be used at a lower dosage in combination with a LHRH analogue or surgical castration for the treatment of advanced prostate cancer. Bicalutamide is a racemate and its antiandrogenic activity resides almost exclusively in the (*R*)-enantiomer, which has an approximately fourfold higher affinity for the prostate AR than hydroxyflutamide does. The (*S*)-enantiomer has no antiandrogenic activity. (*R*)-Bicalutamide is slowly absorbed, but absorption is unaffected by food (124). It has a long plasma elimination half-life of 1 week and accumulates approximately 10 times in plasma during daily administration

Table 45.5. Some Properties and Pharmacokinetics of the Antiandrogens

Drugs	Bicalutamide	Flutamide	Nilutamide
Trade Name	Casodex	Eulexin	Nilandron
cLogP[a]	4.9 ± 0.7	3.7 ± 0.4	3.3 ± 0.6
log D (pH 7)	4.9	3.7	3.3
Oral Bioavailability (%)	80–90	—	—
Onset of Action (weeks)[b]	8–12	2–4	1–2
Duration of Action	8 days	3 months to 2.5 years	1–3 months
Protein binding (%)	96	94–96	80–84
Time to Peak Conc. (hours)	31	2–3	1–4
Elimination Half-life (hours)	~6	8 (10 active metabolite) 10 elderly	40–60 60–120 met
Cytochrome Isoforms	3A4	1A2	Flavin monooxygenase, CYP2C
Active Metabolites	None	2-hydroxy	Yes
Excretion (%)	43 feces 34 urine/ glucunomide metabolites	<10 feces ~28 urine <10 unchanged	<10 feces 62 urine <2 unchanged

[a]Chemical Abstracts, American Chemical Society, calculated using Advanced Chemistry Development (ACD/Labs) Software V8.14 for Solaris (1994–2006 ACD/Labs).
[b]Time for significant improvement in prostate-specific antigen or other biomarkers.

(Table 45.5). (*S*)-Bicalutamide is much more rapidly absorbed and cleared from plasma. At steady state, the plasma levels of (*R*)-bicalutamide are 100 times higher than those of (*S*)-bicalutamide. Although mild to moderate hepatic impairment does not affect pharmacokinetics, evidence suggests slower elimination of (*R*)-bicalutamide in subjects with severe hepatic impairment (124). Bicalutamide metabolites are excreted almost equally in urine and feces, with little or no unchanged drug excreted in urine. Unmetabolized drug predominates in the plasma. Following oral administration, the racemate displays stereoselective oxidative metabolism of its (*R*)-enantiomer, with an elimination half-life of approximately 6 days. (*R*)-Bicalutamide is cleared almost exclusively by CYP3A4-mediated metabolism, but glucuronidation is the predominant metabolic route for (*S*)-bicalutamide. No evidence indicates CYP3A4 induction in humans.

Flutamide. Following oral administration, flutamide is completely absorbed from the gastrointestinal tract and undergoes extensive first-pass metabolism by CYP1A2 to its major metabolite, 2-hydroxyflutamide, and its hydrolysis product, 3-trifluoromethyl-4-nitroaniline (Fig. 45.16) (119). 2-Hydroxyflutamide is a more powerful antiandrogen in vivo, with higher affinity for the receptor than that of flutamide (123). 2-Hydroxyflutamide has an elimination half-life of approximately 8 hours. These studies show the principal role of CYP1A2 in the metabolism of flutamide to 2-hydroxyflutamide, with minor contribution from CYP3A4. 2-Hydroxyflutamide inhibits the metabolism of flutamide and both 2- and 4-hydroxylation of estradiol. Flutamide is a pure antagonist, whereas 2-hydroxyflutamide is a more potent AR antagonist but also can activate the androgenic receptor at higher concentrations (125). These findings raise the possibility that increased conversion of flutamide to 2-hydroxyflutamide or accumulation of 2-hydroxyflutamide in cells may contribute to the anomalous responses to flutamide that are observed in some advanced prostate cancers.

Nilutamide. Nilutamide is a hepatotoxic nitroaromatic antiandrogen used for the treatment of metastatic prostate carcinoma in men (114). It is a competitive antagonist of the AR. Nilutamide is a nitroaromatic hydantoin analog of flutamide, as shown in Figure 45.16, that is completely absorbed after oral administration, with a mean elimination half-life of approximately 50 hours (Table 45.5) (124). One of the methyl groups attached to the hydantoin ring is stereoselectively hydroxylated to a chiral metabolite, which subsequently is oxidized to its carboxylic acid metabolite. Less than 2% of nilutamide is excreted unchanged in the urine. In vitro, the nitro group of nilutamide was reduced to the amine and hydroxylamine moieties by nitric oxide (NO) synthases, a flavin monooxygenase (FMO) system (126). The therapeutic effects of nilutamide are overshadowed, however, by the occurrence of several adverse reactions mediated by toxic mechanisms, which are poorly investigated. The reduction of nilutamide is catalyzed by NO synthases via the formation of either or both a nitro anion free radical or its reduction to its hydroxylamino derivative could explain some of the toxic effects of this drug (127). Nitric oxide synthases also are involved in the formation of reactive NO and oxygen species and in the interactions with some xenobiotic compounds.

Inhibitors of Androgen Biosynthesis

The association between lifetime exposure to testosterone and DHT and the risk of developing prostate cancer suggests chemoprevention with specific inhibitors of key enzymes associated with androgen biosynthesis (127). Two key enzymes considered for inhibition are

5α-reductase, which inhibits the formation of DHT and 17α-hydroxylase/17,20-lyase, which inhibits testosterone biosynthesis (Fig. 45.3).

5α-REDUCTASE INHIBITORS. The 5α-reductase inhibitors have been discussed previously (see *Benign Prostatic Hyperplasia*). The results of the Prostate Cancer Prevention Trial (128) for finasteride showed a 25% relative risk reduction in prostate cancer in men aged 55 years or older, albeit at an increased risk of invasive tumors (129). The risk of invasive tumors may outweigh the benefit of these agents. The 5α-reductase inhibitors have not been proven to be effective as chemoprevention against clinically significant prostate cancer.

17α-HYDROXYLASE/17,20-LYASE INHIBITORS. A second enzyme system targeted for androgen inhibition is 17α-hydroxylase/17,20-lyase, which is the key enzyme that converts pregnenolone to DHA and, subsequently, to testosterone (Fig. 45.3). Because testosterone has androgenic activity, inhibition of its biosynthesis would be useful in treating androgen-dependent diseases, such as prostate cancer (130). Inhibitors of 17α-hydroxylase/17,20-lyase inhibitors could prevent androgen biosynthesis from both testes and adrenals and may provide effective treatment of patients with prostate cancer.

The antifungal agent ketoconazole (Fig. 45.18) is an effective inhibitor of 17α-hydroxylase (IC_{50}, 76 nM), which has demonstrated the promise of 17α-hydroxylase inhibitors for the treatment of metastatic prostate cancer patients (131). The nonsteroidal imidazole agent R 75251(Liarozole) (Fig. 45.18) (132), is under development as a potentially more selective inhibitor of 17α-hydroxylase/17,20-lyase. The steroidal compounds MDL 27302 (133) as well as abiraterone (CB7598) and Sa 40 (134) (Fig. 45.18), were designed as mechanism-based inhibitors of 17α-hydroxylase/17,20-lyase. For MDL 27302, inhibition is specific to the cyclopropylamino compound, because the isopropylamino- or the cyclobutylamino-analogs were not inhibitory. Enzymatic specificity of MDL 27,302 of 17α-hydroxylase/17,20-lyase was demonstrated by its failure to inhibit steroid 21-hydroxylase and the cholesterol side-chain cleavage enzyme (CYP450scc). Both the 17α-hydroxylase and 17/20-lyase activities of human testicular microsomes were inhibited by MDL 27,302. Abiraterone and Sa 40 are heterocyclic analogues of MDL 27,302 and potent irreversible inhibitors of 17α-hydroxylase (IC50s, 4 and 24 nM, respectively) (134). Inhibition studies show that the 16,17-double bond is necessary for irreversible binding of these 17-pyridyl and 17-pyrimidyl steroids to 17α-hydroxylase. Oxidation to an epoxide probably is not involved, however, because the epoxide was a weak inhibitor (IC50, 260 nM).

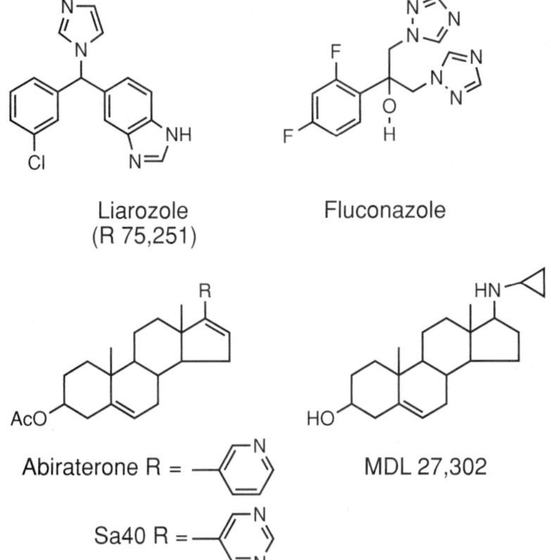

Fig. 45.18. 17-Hydroxylase/lyase inhibitors for prostate cancer.

LUTEINIZING HORMONE–RELEASING HORMONE AGONISTS. The goal of LHRH therapy for prostate cancer is to suppress the production of testosterone in the testis and/or block its effects at its tissue receptors. Androgen deprivation using LHRH agonists (Fig. 45.19), such as leuprolide acetate (Lupron Depot), goserelin (Zoladex), and buserelin (Suprefact), suppresses the secretion of LH and, consequently, testosterone synthesis to castration levels (i.e., chemical castration) (135). The LHRH agonists significantly suppress the synthesis of intraprostatic DHT from testosterone and the size of the prostate (see the hypothalamus-pituitary-testis axis in Fig. 45.2). This effect is not immediate, however, and occurs 2 to 4 weeks after initiation of therapy. LHRH therapy slows the spread of cancerous cells and helps to alleviate or ease the symptoms associated with advanced prostate cancer. However, LHRH agonists are not cures for prostate cancer. The most common side effects associated with LHRH therapy are hot flashes, but impotence and loss of libido may also occur. Long-term use of LHRH therapy is associated with osteoporosis, decreased cognitive abilities, fatigue, and vascular stiffness. Symptoms may worsen over the first few weeks of treatment. Periodic monitoring of PSA and plasma testosterone levels is recommended. Tumor flare reactions may occur transiently but can be prevented by antiandrogens or by short-term estrogens at low dose for several weeks.

H^{-5} oxoPro-His–Trp–Ser–Tyr–D-Leu—Leu-Arg—Pro-NH-C_2H_5

Leuprolide

H^{-5} oxoPro-His–Trp–Ser–Tyr-D-Ser(t-Bu)-Leu-Arg-Pro-NH-NH-C(=O)-NH_2

Goserelin

H^{-5} oxoPro-His–Trp–Ser–Tyr-D-Ser(t-Bu)-Leu-Arg-Pro-NHC_2H_5

Buserelin

[Note: H^{-5} oxoPro = pGlu (PyroGlu)]

Fig. 45.19. Luteinizing hormone-releasing hormone (LHRH) agonists used for the treatment of prostate cancer.

Chemotherapy

Chemotherapy usually is reserved for patients whose prostate cancer has spread outside of the prostate gland and are no longer responsive to hormonal therapy. Chemotherapeutic drugs that can be used for prostate cancer include a combination regimen of mitoxantrone/ corticosteroids or estramustane/docetaxel (Taxotere) (see Chapter 42).

Bone-Protecting Treatments

The most common site for the spread of prostate cancer is bone. Most symptoms of advanced prostate cancer are caused by the presence of disease in the bone. These symptoms can be mitigated with a drug called zoledronic acid (Zometa), a bisphosphonic acid administered by intravenous infusion that inhibits osteoclastic bone resorption, which can slow the spread of disease, reducing the development of bone pain and inhibiting bone fractures. Zoledronic acid is most commonly given to patients whose cancer is no longer responding to hormones, but it also may be given to prevent the bone thinning and weakening that results from hormonal treatments.

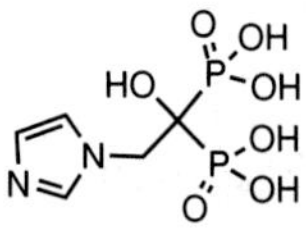

Zoledronic acid

Treatment of Prostatitis

Prostatitis is a broad term used to identify inflammation of the prostate gland associated with lower urinary tract symptoms in men (136). Prostatitis rarely occurs in males younger than 30 years; however, it is a common problem in older males, being described as acute bacterial prostatitis, chronic bacterial prostatitis, or nonbacterial prostatitis. Because antimicrobial drug penetration generally is poor into the prostate gland, with poor efficacy of the antimicrobial agents and long duration of treatment; a 30 to 40% failure rate occurs with common treatment modalities. Three major factors determine the diffusion and concentration of antimicrobial agents in prostatic fluid and tissue: the lipid solubility of the antimicrobial agent, its dissociation constant (pK_a), and the percentage plasma protein binding. The physiological pH of human prostatic fluid is 6.5 to 6.7, but it increases in chronic prostatitis, ranging from 7.0 to 8.3 (136). A greater concentration of antimicrobial agents in the prostatic fluid occurs in the presence of a pH gradient across the membrane separating plasma from prostatic fluid. Of the available antimicrobial agents, β-lactam drugs have a low pK_a and poor lipid solubility and, thus, penetrate poorly into prostatic fluid, except for some cephalosporins. Good to excellent penetration into prostatic fluid and tissue has been demonstrated with many antimicrobial agents, including tobramycin, tetracyclines, macrolides, fluoroquinolones, sulfonamides, and nitrofurantoin. The diagnosis and therapy of prostatitis remains a challenge. Because prostatitis usually requires prolonged therapy, patients must understand the importance of compliance, and physicians should screen for drug interactions that may decrease compliance and efficacy.

Acute bacterial prostatitis is the least common of the prostate infections and, usually, is accompanied by a urinary tract infection with positive cultures. The symptoms include sudden onset of fever, chills, and low back pain, as well as complaints of urinary obstruction (e.g., dysuria, nocturia, urgency, frequency, and burning) and urinary irritation (e.g., hesitancy, straining, dribbling, weak stream, and incomplete emptying). The most commonly prescribed antimicrobials for acute bacterial prostatitis are trimethoprim–sulfamethoxazole, doxycline, and the fluoroquinolones, ciprofloxacin, ofloxacin, and norfloxacin (see Chapter 38). The concentrations of these antimicrobial agents in the prostatic fluid are two to three times that in plasma, thus achieving adequate concentrations in prostatic tissues to eradicate the most common causative pathogens. The recommended duration of treatment for acute bacterial prostatitis is 4 to 6 weeks. A short-course therapy is not recommended because of the risk of relapse or progression to chronic bacterial prostatitis.

Chronic bacterial prostatitis occurs when acute bacterial prostatitis has been inadequately treated because of pathogen resistance, relapse, or short-course therapy or because of blocked drainage of secretions from the prostate. Most men with chronic prostatitis will have had a previous bout of acute prostatitis. The most common clinical feature of chronic prostatitis is recurrent urinary tract infections and the symptoms and complaints of acute bacterial prostatitis. Fluoroquinolones, trimethoprim–sulfamethoxazole, doxycycline, and nitrofurantoin are used in the management of chronic prostatitis. Chronic prostatitis warrants at least 10 to 12 weeks of therapy. Poor clinical outcomes, however, have been observed because of poor diffusion of antimicrobials into the prostate.

Nonbacterial prostatitis is the most common type of prostatitis. It occurs more frequently than bacterial prostatitis, with the same signs and symptoms as bacterial prostatitis except that prostatic fluid cultures are negative for presence of bacteria. Inflammation is evident on prostate gland examination. Treatment includes minocycline, doxycycline, or erythromycin. Treatment duration is approximately 2 to 4 weeks.

DRUGS USED FOR ERECTILE DYSFUNCTION

Phosphodiesterase Inhibitors

The currently available first- and second-generation oral PDE5 inhibitors, sildenafil, tadalafil, and vardenafil, have emerged as the first-line treatment for ED because of patient convenience, safety, and clinical efficacy and have markedly improved the quality of life in men with ED of various etiologies. As defined by the National Institutes of Health Consensus Development Panel on Impotence in

1993, ED is the inability to achieve or maintain an erection sufficient for satisfactory sexual performance. It is estimated that 10 to 30 million men in the United States, and more than 100 million men worldwide, experience some form of ED. This condition is strongly associated with age, and according to the community-based Massachusetts Male Aging Study, the prevalence of ED in men between 40 and 70 years of age is 52%. The general classification of ED includes psychogenic ED (e.g., depression, psychological stress, relationship problems, and performance anxiety), organic ED (e.g., diabetes, hypertension, spinal cord injuries, and some medications), and mixed psychogenic and organic ED.

Treatment options for men with ED have changed significantly over the past three decades and have progressed from psychosexual therapy and penile prostheses (1970s) through revascularization, vacuum constriction devices, and intracavernosal injection therapy (1980s) to transurethral and oral drug delivery (1990s). The introduction of the first PDE5 inhibitor, sildenafil citrate (Viagra), in 1998 has revolutionized the treatment of men with ED of a broad-spectrum of etiologies and acknowledged the need for pharmacological agents in the treatment of ED (137). With the recognition of the prevalence of ED by the public and the effectiveness of agents like Viagra, there was an increase effort in the search for new agents with fewer side effects that led to the development of the second-generation PDE5 inhibitors, vardenafil and tadalafil, which have since been introduced into the world market at differing potencies and pharmacokinetics.

Mechanism of Action

The physiological mechanism to achieve penile erection is mediated via an NO/cyclic guanosine monophosphate (cGMP) pathway. During sexual stimulation, parasympathetic neurons and vascular endothelial cells release NO, which activates soluble guanylate cyclase, thereby increasing the level of cGMP in the corpus cavernosum and relaxation (vasodilation) of vascular smooth muscle. Phosphodiesterase-5 is a cGMP-specific hydrolyzing enzyme (see Chapter 17) and is present at high concentrations in the smooth muscle of the penile corpus cavernosum (138,139). One of the more effective methods for elevating cGMP levels in this tissue is to use PDE5 inhibitors. Other PDE isoenzymes also found in the human cavernous smooth muscle include PDE3 (cGMP-inhibited PDE) and PDE4 (cAMP-specific PDE). Thus, inhibitors of PDE, especially PDE5, have been shown to be an effective means for treating ED by enhancing and maintaining erections during sexual stimulation through sustaining sufficient cellular levels of cGMP in both the corpus cavernosum and the blood vessels supplying it. The increased vasodilation of the corporeal sinusoids allows more blood flow into the penis, thereby enhancing an erection.

Structure–Activity Relationships

The chemical similarities and distinct differences between sildenafil, vardenafil, and tadalafil in regarding their selectivity for the inhibition of PDE5 and other PDE isoforms and their pharmacokinetic disparities largely affect the efficacy profile of these compounds. The obvious difference for the three drugs is the heterocyclic ring systems used to mimic the purine ring of cGMP. Although the heterocyclic ring systems and the N-substituent (ethyl versus methyl) attached to the piperazine side chain (Fig. 45.20) are the only two structural differences between sildenafil and vardenafil, these differences do not explain why vardenafil has a more than 20 times greater potency than sildenafil for inhibiting PDE5. A structure–activity relationship analysis for the difference in potency between sildenafil and vardenafil revealed that the methyl/ethyl group on the piperazine moiety plays very little role in the potency difference for inhibiting PDE5, whereas the differences in the heterocyclic ring systems play a critical role in higher potency for vardenafil (140).

A comparison of the in vitro inhibition values (IC_{50s}) reveals that vardenafil is approximately 10 times more selective as an inhibitor of PDE5 than sildenafil and tadalafil (Table 45.6) (140). Furthermore, vardenafil also was approximately four times more selective than sildenafil for the inhibition of PDE1 and PDE6, as shown by its IC_{50} selectivity ratios: a PDE5/PDE1 of 257 for valdenafil and 60 for sildenafil, and a PDE5/PDE6 of 16 for valdenafil

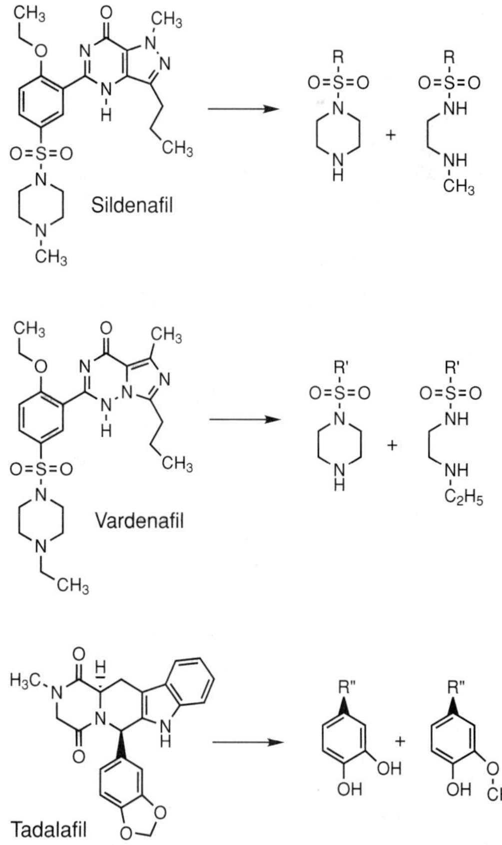

Fig. 45.20. Phosphodiesterase 5 inhibitors for erectile dysfunction and their primary metabolites.

Table 45.6. Some Properties and Pharmacokinetics of the Phosphodiesterase 5 Inhibitors

Drugs	Sildenafil	Vardenafil	Tadalafil
Trade Name	Viagra	Levitra	Tsailis
cLogP[a]	2.3 ± 0.7	3.0 ± 0.7	1.4 ± 0.8
log D (pH 7)	2.2	3.0	1.4
Oral Bioavailability (%)	38–40	15 (8–25)	~36
Onset of Action (hours)	<0.5	<1	0.5–1
Duration of Action (hours)	<4	<1	<36
Protein Binding (%)	96	94	94
Time to Peak Conc. (hours)	0.5–2	0.5–3	0.5–6
Volume of Distribution (L/kg)	105	208	63
Peak Plasma Conc. (nM/L)	1–2	0.03	0.84
Elimination Half-life (hours)	3–5	4–5	18
Cytochrome Isoforms	3A4 (major) 2C9 (minor)	3A4 (major) 2C9 (minor)	3A4 (primary)
Active Metabolites	N-desmethyl	N-desethyl	None
Excretion (%)	~80 feces/met ~13 urine/met	>90 feces/met <10 urine/met	~60 feces/met ~35 urine/met
PDE5 IC50 (nM)	3.9 (3–7)	0.16 (0.09–0.7)	1.8 (0.9–5)
PDE5/PDE6 IC50	7.4	16	85
PDE5/PDE1 IC50	60	257	—

[a]Chemical Abstracts, American Chemical Society, calculated using Advanced Chemistry Development (ACD/Labs) Software V8.14 for Solaris (1994–2006 ACD/Labs).
IC_{50}, median inhibitory concentration; PDE, phosphodiesterase.

and 7.4 for sildenafil (Table 45.6). The low PDE5/PDE6 selectivity ratio suggests that at therapeutic doses, sildenafil is only approximately 10 times as potent for PDE5 as for PDE6, which is a retinal enzyme found in the photoreceptors of the human retina. This lower PDE5/PDE6 selectivity ratio toward PDE6 for sildenafil indicates it is more likely to inhibit PDE6, which is presumed to be the cause for color vision abnormalities observed with high doses or plasma levels of sildenafil.

Pharmacokinetics

Sildenafil, vardenafil and tadalafil have only limited oral bioavailability because of extensive presystemic metabolism in the intestine and hepatic first-pass metabolism via CYP3A isoform family (Table 45.6) (141). The three drugs are rapidly absorbed after oral administration and reach peak plasma concentrations within 30 to 60 minutes. Rapid absorption and lipophilicity are considered to be a prerequisite for their rapid onset of efficacy and sexual satisfaction. Sildenafil and vardenafil are both rapidly absorbed, but with a significant difference in their mean bioavailability of approximately 15% for vadenafil and 40% for sildenafil. The administration of a high-fat meal had no significant effect on the rate and extent of absorption of tadalafil but did decrease the rate of absorption for sildenafil and vardenafil, which is consistent with their calculated lipophilicity (Table 45.6). It remains unclear whether food has any effect on their absorption and therapeutic efficacy. They are all highly protein bound, with free plasma concentration fractions of only 4 to 6%. Although the bioavailability for tadalafil has not been reported, pharmacokinetic studies and its long duration of action suggest that it is predominately metabolized by hepatic CYP3A4 to catechol metabolites, with minimal presystemic metabolism.

The major route of elimination for the three PDE5 inhibitors is hepatic metabolism, with renal excretion of unmetabolized drug accounting for 1% or less of the elimination pathways (141). CYP3A is the major drug-metabolizing enzymes for the three PDE5 inhibitors. CYP2C9, CYP2C19, and CYP2D6, however, also contribute to the metabolism of sildenafil, and CYP2C9 contributes to the metabolism of vardenafil. Both sildenafil and vardenafil have active metabolites that reach plasma concentrations high enough to contribute to the overall efficacy and safety profile of their parent-drug molecules. Grapefruit juice increases the bioavailability of sildenafil and vardenafil as well as delays their absorption. The pharmacokinetics of sildenafil and vardenafil may become less predictable in patients who also drink grapefruit juice. Although patients usually will not be endangered by concomitant use of grapefruit juice, it seems advisable to avoid this combination, which can cause systemic vasodilatation.

The larger differences in their volumes of distribution, together with the substantial differences in their systemic clearance, result in distinct differences in their elimination half-lives: 3 to 5 hours for sildenafil and vardenafil, compared with approximately 18 hours for tadalafil.

Hepatic CYP3A and CYP2C activity has been described as being age-dependent, with reduced activity being exhibited in elderly compared to young individuals. This decrease in metabolic activity is reflected by a corresponding increase in plasma concentrations of all three PDE5 inhibitors, warranting dose reductions for sildenafil and vardenafil in elderly patients. Similarly, ethnicity-dependent differences in the pharmacokinetics of all three PDE5 inhibitors may be expected based on known ethnic differences in CYP3A4/5 activity. Gender differences in pharmacokinetics have not been described for any of the three PDE5 inhibitors, which seems to be in agreement with the literature. Severe renal impairment resulted in an increase in plasma concentrations for all the drugs, and this warrants dose reductions for sildenafil and tadalafil in the affected patient population.

Drug Interactions

None of the three PDE5 inhibitors has been identified as CYP inhibitors, including CYP3A or CYP2C substrates. Because metabolism via CYP3A is the major elimination pathway for all three drugs (sildenafil, vardenafil, and tadalafil), all inducers and inhibitors of CYP3A activity have the potential to interfere with the elimination of these drugs. This interaction potential has been verified clinically for inducers of CYP3A activity only for rifampicin and tadalafil (141). The strong inhibitors of CYP3A4 (ritonavir, indinavir, saquinavir, erythromycin, and ketoconazole) increased the plasma levels for sildenafil, vardenafil, and tadalafil. Grapefruit juice, a selective inhibitor of CYP3A intestinal metabolism, also increased the plasma concentrations of sildenafil and vardenafil but not of tadalafil. Ritonavir, as an inhibitor of CYP3A4 and CYP2C9, increased the plasma levels for vardenafil by 50 to 300 times, most likely as a consequence of the simultaneous inhibition of both CYP3A4 and CYP2C9, the major metabolism pathways for vardenafil. The effect of ritonavir on sildenafil was much less pronounced (11 times), because other compensatory CYP-mediated metabolism pathways were still available. Ritonavir increased the plasma levels for tadalafil (CYP3A4) by approximately three times.

Adverse Effects

A number of side effects have been reported with these drugs, including nausea, cutaneous flushing, headache, and retinal effects, including a bluish haze and increased light sensitivity, and indigestion. It has been suggested that some of these side effects result from the inhibition of other PDEs, including the isoform PDE6 (141,142). The search is on for even more selective ED agents to see if additional side effects can be eliminated. If one is taking α-adrenergic blockers for high blood pressure, one should consult a physician before using the agents together (141). Other vasodilators associated with regulating the intracellular levels of cGMP, such as nitroglycerin, should not be used in combination with the PDE5 inhibitors.

Therapeutic Effects

The first line of treatment of ED is PDE5 inhibition, because the three drugs can be given orally. If the PDE5 inhibitors are not effective, then the cause may be low libido, and men should have their testosterone blood levels checked (in some instances, TRT may help to resolve ED). Other alternative drugs currently available for the treatment of ED include prostaglandin E_1, which is given by injection at the base of the penis or by suppository into the tip of the penis, as well as the α_1-adrenergic blocker and the nonselective PDE inhibitor papaverine. Apomorphine is a dopamine agonist that can be used for treating ED but, in humans, has the undesirable emetic side effect. Some selective dopamine D_4 agents are now being investigated for treatment of ED. Vacuum devices and penile implants are also available.

Specific Drugs for Erectile Dysfunction

SILDENAFIL. In 1998, sildenafil was the first selective PDE inhibitor to be approved and found to be effective in treating ED (137). Sildenafil has approximately one-tenth the selectivity for PDE5 as for PDE6, which is found in the photoreceptors of the human retina. In vitro metabolism studies for sildenafil have shown that the primary metabolite, N-desmethylsildenafil, and the minor metabolite, oxidative opening of the piperazine ring, are mediated by CYP3A4, CYP2C9, CYP2C19, and CYP2D6. The estimated relative contributions to clearance were 79% for CYP3A4, 20% for CYP2C9, and less than 2% for CYP2C19 and CYP2D6. These results demonstrate that CYP3A4 is the primary cytochrome mediating N-demethylation and that drugs inhibiting CYP3A4 likely impair sildenafil biotransformation and clearance. The pharmacokinetics of radiolabeled sildenafil were consistent with rapid absorption, first-pass metabolism, and primarily fecal elimination of N-demethylated metabolites. The absorption of sildenafil following oral administration was rapid (~92%), whereas the oral bioavailability was approximately 38% as a result of first-pass metabolism.

VARDENAFIL. Vardenafil was the second agent to be marketed and had the advantage that its onset time was not reduced by taking the medication on a full stomach (Table 45.6) (141,143). It is 30 times more potent as an inhibitor of PDE5 (mean IC_{50}, 3.9 nM) than sildenafil and 10 times more potent than tadalafil, with a greater selectivity (>1,000 times) for human PDE5 than for human PDE2, PDE3, and PDE4 and moderate selectivity (>80 times) for PDE1 (140,144) (Table 45.6). The PDE inhibitory selectivity and both the in vitro and in vivo potency of the new PDE5 inhibitor vardenafil. Vardenafil specifically inhibited the hydrolysis of cGMP by PDE5, with an IC50 of 0.7 nM (sildenafil 6..6 nM). The IC_{50} of vardenafil for PDE1 was 180 nM, for PDE6 11 nM, and for PDE2, PDE3 and PDE4 more than 1,000 nM.

TADALAFIL. Tadalafil was the last agent to be released and can be taken on a full stomach without slowing the onset (Table 45.6) (141). It has a much longer duration of action, lasting up to 48 hours, compared with sildenafil and vardenafil, which last for approximately 4 hours. The longer half-life of tadalafil results in a lengthened period of responsiveness as compared to sildenafil and vardenafil. This longer therapeutic window requires fewer time constraints for the effectiveness of tadalafil and has been interpreted as being advantageous through providing the option for more spontaneous sexual activity. Because of its long half-life, however, tadalafil, has been detected in plasma even 5 days after oral administration. This suggests the possibility of accumulation if taken regularly and in short intervals, which may result in an increased risk of side effects with the excessive use of this PDE5 inhibitor. The 3,4-methylenedioxy substitution on the phenyl ring was significant for increasing its potency as PDE5 inhibitor. Optimization of the chain on the piperazinedione ring resulted in no significant change in IC50s. Tadalafil is a highly potent PDE5 inhibitor (IC50, 5 nM), with high selectivity for PDE5 versus PDE1 through PDE4 (145). The PDE5/PDE6 selectivity ratio is 85.

Prostaglandin E_1. Prostaglandin E_1 (PGE1; Alprostadil) is approved for the intracavernosal (Caverject, Edex)or intraurethral suppository (Muse) treatment of ED. A three-drug combination of PGE1, papaverine, and phentolamine sometimes is used as an intracavernosal injection to achieve a synergistic action. Erectile dysfunction that is medication-induced or caused by endocrine problems, such as hypogonadism or hyper- or hypothyroidism, should be evaluated and appropriately treated before PGE1 treatment is considered. Prostaglandin E_1 is produced endogenously to relax vascular smooth muscle and cause vasodilation by activating the adenylate cyclase/cAMP pathway. Recent studies show that the cAMP is important in the PGE1 relaxation of penile erectile tissue and vasodilation of penile resistance arteries (146). Moreover, agents that stimulate the release of cAMP also cross-activate the NO/cGMP cascade.

When administered by intracavernosal injection or as an intraurethral suppository, PGE1 acts locally to relax the smooth muscle of the corpora cavernosa and the cavernosal arteries. Swelling, elongation, and rigidity of the penis result when arterial blood rapidly flows into the corpus cavernosum to expand the lacunar spaces. The entrapped blood reduces the venous blood outflow as sinusoids compress against the tunica albuginea. Adding papaverine and phentolamine to the PGE1 regimen synergistically increases arterial blood flow via separate mechanisms. Papaverine relaxes the sinusoid and the smooth muscle of the helicine arteries, whereas phentolamine relaxes arterial smooth muscle and blocks both of the α-adrenergic receptors that inhibit an erection. Prostaglandin E_1 is rapidly metabolized within the urethra, prostate, and corpus cavernosum to 7α-hydroxy-5,11-diketotetranorprosta-1,16-dioic acid and 5α,7α-dihydroxy-11-ketotetranorprostane-1,16-dioic acid (147). The major route of excretion of PGE1 metabolites is via the kidney. Its elimination half-life is 5 to 10 minutes. If any alprostadil is systemically absorbed, it is metabolized by a single pass through the lungs. The onset of action is within 10 minutes, and the time to peak effect is less than 20 minutes. The duration of action is 1 to 3 hours for the intracavernosal injection and 30 to 60 minutes for the intraurethral suppository.

Papaverine (Intracavernosal). Papaverine is used, sometimes in combination with phentolamine, by intracavernosal injection to facilitate erections in men with ED. In general, papaverine is most useful in patients with organic ED (neurogenic and, to a lesser extent, vascular). It is less useful in patients with ED resulting from endocrine problems (hypogonadism or hyper- or hypothyroidism) or medications. When administered by intracavernosal injection, papaverine, a weak and nonspecific PDE inhibitor, is thought to cause relaxation of the cavernous smooth muscles and vasodilation of the penile arteries by inhibition of PDE (148). These effects result in increased arterial blood flow into the corpus cavernosa and in swelling and elongation of the penis. Venous outflow also is reduced, possibly as a result of increased venous resistance. Adding phentolamine and PGE1 to the papaverine regimen synergistically increases arterial blood flow via their separate mechanisms. Papaverine is slowly released into the venous circulation with minimal systemic effects. The time to peak effect usually is within 10 minutes, and the duration of action is 1 to 6 hours with concurrent administration with phentolamine

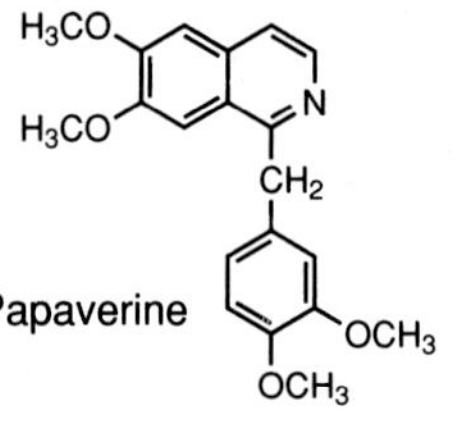

Papaverine

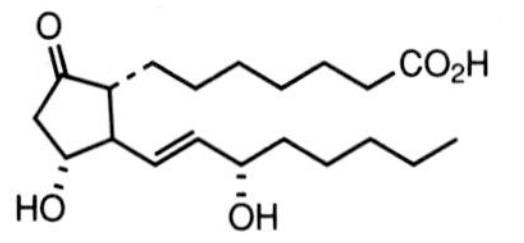

PGE_1

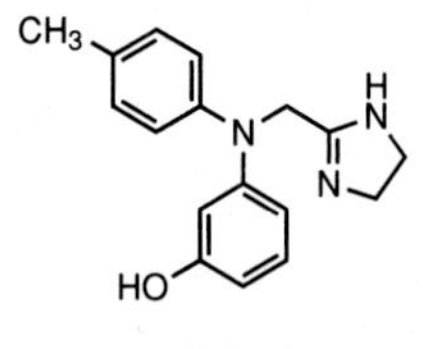

Phentolamine

Phentolamine (Intracavernosal; Rogitine). Phentolamine is used in combination with papaverine, by intracavernosal injection, to facilitate erections in men with impotence (see *Papaverine* above). Its mechanism of action is as an α-adrenergic antagonist (see Chapter 13) of both α_1- and α_2-receptors, causing vasodilation and reduction in peripheral resistance. When administered by intracavernosal injection, it is thought to cause relaxation of the cavernous smooth muscles and vasodilation of the penile arteries. This results in increased arterial blood flow into the corpus cavernosa as well as swelling and elongation of the penis. Venous outflow also is reduced, possibly as a result of increased venous resistance. Phentolamine is slowly released into venous circulation with minimal, if any, systemic effects. Time to peak effect is within 10 minutes, and duration of action when used with papaverine is 1 to 6 hours.

Testicular Cancer

Testicular cancer develops in the testicles and, according to the National Cancer Institute (NCI), accounts only for approximately 1% of all cancers in men. Compared with prostate cancer, testicular cancer is relatively rare. It is most common among males between 15 and 40 years of age and is approximately fourfold more common in white men than in black men.

Nearly all testicular tumors originate from germ cells, the specialized sperm-forming cells within the testicles. These tumors fall into one of two types, seminomas or nonseminomas (149). Seminomas account for approximately 40 percent of all testicular cancer and are made up of immature germ cells. Seminomas are slow-growing and tend to stay localized in the testicle for long periods. Nonseminomas arise from more mature, specialized germ cells and tend to be more aggressive than seminomas. According to the American Cancer Society, 60 to 70% of patients with nonseminomas have cancer that has spread to the lymph nodes. α-Fetoprotein is a tumor-associated marker in blood for testicular cancer. Its measurement can help to show how well the chemotherapeutic drugs are working. Because seminomas are slow-growing, they tend to stay localized and usually are diagnosed at stage 1 (confined to testicle) or stage 2 (spread to lymph nodes). Treatment might be a combination of testicle removal, radiation, or chemotherapy. Most nonseminomas are not diagnosed at stage 1. Advanced testicular cancer (stage 3, metastasized to other tissues) seminomas as well as stage 2 and stage 3 nonseminomas usually are treated with multidrug chemotherapy. The majority of cases are stage 1 when first identified; stage 3 cases are relatively rare.

Chemotherapy is the standard treatment, with or without radiation, when the cancer has spread to other parts of the body. The drugs approved to treat testicular cancer, including ifosfamide, etoposide, vinblastine, bleomycin, and cisplatin. Cisplatin usually is given in combination with bleomycin and etoposide or other chemotherapy drugs following surgery or radiation therapy. Testicular cancer has one of the highest cure rates of all cancers, essentially 100% at stage 1. Approximately 90% of men with advanced testicular cancer can be cured, according to the NCI. Because testicular cancer is curable when detected early, the NCI recommends regular monthly testicular self-examination after a hot shower, when the scrotum is looser, feeling for lumps or enlargement.

Male Osteoporosis

Osteoporosis is a common condition in men that usually develops after the age of 70 years and affects approximately 2 million men in the United States (150). Osteoporosis occurs less frequently in men because of greater skeletal bone mass during growth (i.e., greater bone size). Approximately 20 to 25% of all hip fractures occur in men, however, and the age-adjusted prevalence of vertebral deformities appears to be similar in men and in women. Currently, bisphosphonates (alendronate and risedronate) (see Chapter 35) are the therapy of choice for increasing bone mineral density to decrease the risk of fracture in the treatment of male osteoporosis, and a short course of parathyroid hormone (1-34; teriparatide) may be indicated for men with very low bone mineral density or for those in whom bisphosphonate therapy is unsuccessful. Antiandrogen therapy for the treatment of prostate cancer, hypogonadism, and diabetes are some of the risk factors for osteoporosis and fracture. Vitamin D and calcium have been shown to help improve bone mineral density. Testosterone replacement therapy is controversial except in men who clearly have hypogonadism and low levels of testosterone; in those men, treatment with testosterone appears to increase bone density.

CASE STUDY

Victoria F. Roche and S. William Zito

BD is a 84-year-old white man who is spry for his age and lives with his 72-year-old wife in a small house in the rural countryside of New York State. They have several cats, and BD is allergic to cat dander and takes Dytan (diphenhydramine tannate; 50 mg every 12 hours) to control his symptoms. He reports to the ambulatory care clinic that he has had a recent onset of urinary hesitancy, a weak stream, intermittent flow, and postmicturation dribble. In addition, he complains that he has to urinate more frequently, especially during the night. BD reports that when he has to get up to urinate at night, he feels dizzy and wobbly in his rush to get to the bathroom. On further questioning, BD states that he gets dizzy every time he rises quickly from a sitting position. After examination and elimination of other conditions that could cause his symptoms (urinary tract infections, bladder cancer, or bladder stones), a diagnosis of benign prostatic hyperplasia (BPH) is made, and the physician wants to treat BD with medication. Evaluate the following choices for use in this case:

1. Identify the therapeutic problem(s) in which the pharmacist's intervention may benefit the patient.
2. Identify and prioritize the patient-specific factors that must be considered to achieve the desired therapeutic outcomes.

3. Conduct a thorough and mechanistically oriented structure-activity analysis of all therapeutic alternatives provided in the case.
4. Evaluate the structure-activity relationship findings against the patient-specific factors and desired therapeutic outcomes, and make a therapeutic decision.
5. Counsel your patient.

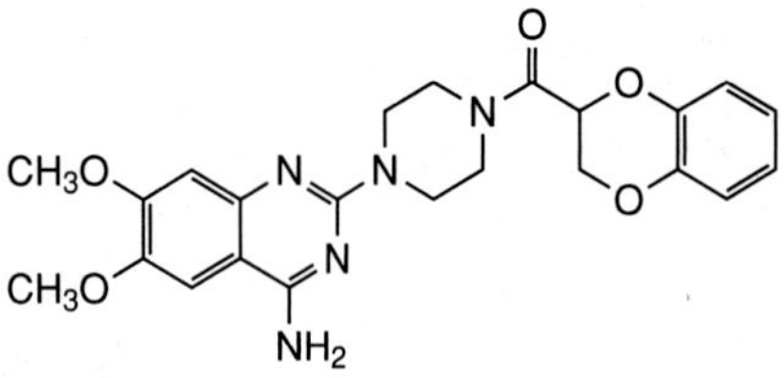

1

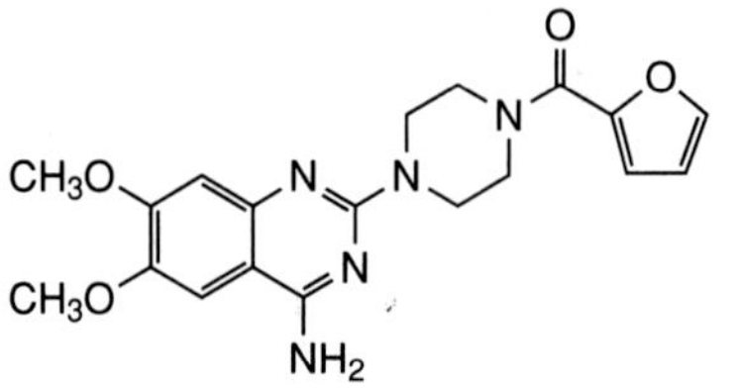

2

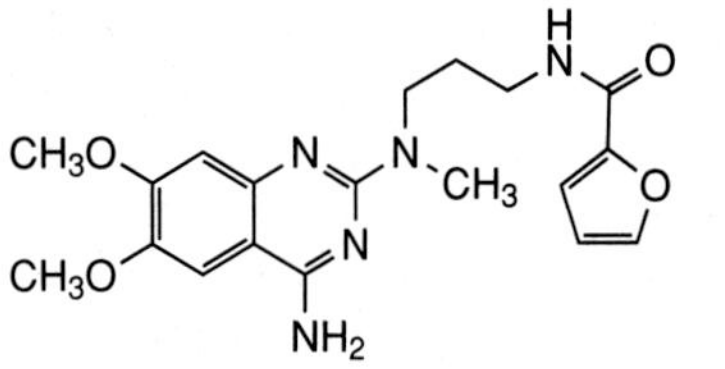

3

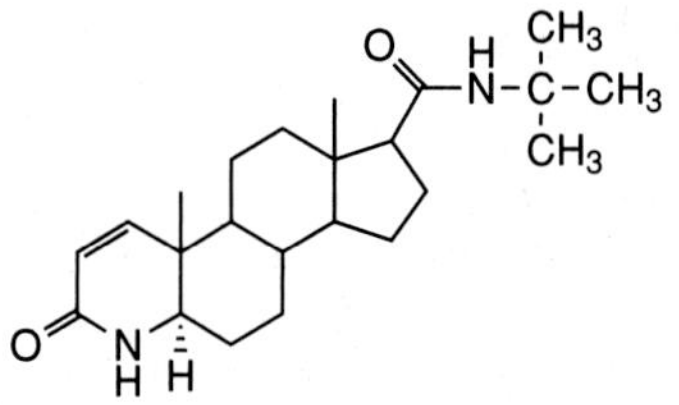

4

References

1. Jordan VC. Selective estrogen receptor modulators. In: Williams DA, Lemke T, eds. Foye's Principles of Medicinal Chemistry. Baltimore: Lippincott Williams & Wilkins, 2002;1059–1069.
2. Chen J, Kim J, Dalton JT. Discovery and therapeutic promise of selective androgen receptor modulators. Molecular Interventions 2005;5: 173–188.
3. Mooradian AD, Morley JE, Korenman SG. Biological actions of androgens. Endocr Rev 1987;8:1–28.
4. Takeda H, Chodak G, Mutchnik S, et al. Immunohistochemical localization of androgen receptors with mono- and polyclonal antibodies to androgen receptor. J Endocrinol 1990;126:17–25.
5. Davis S. Androgen replacement in women: a commentary. J Clin Endocrinol Metab 1999;84:1886–1891.
6. Davis SR. The therapeutic use of androgens in women. J Steroid Biochem Mol Biol 1999;69:177–184.
7. Davis SR, Burger HG. Clinical review 82: androgens and the postmenopausal woman. J Clin Endocrinol Metab 1996;81:2759–2763.
8. Brown-Sequard CE. Des effects produits chez Phomme par des injections sous cutanées d'un liquide retire des testicules frais de cobaye et de chien. CR Seanc Soc Biol 1889;1:420–430.
9. Pezard A. Sur la determination des caractéres sexuels secondaire chez les gallinacés. C R H Acad Sci 1911;153:1027–1034.
10. Butenandt A. Chemical investigation of the sex hormones. Angew Chem. 1931;44:905–908.
11. Butenandt AH, Dannenberg H. Androsterone, a crystalline male sex hormone. III. Isolation of a new physiologically inert sterol derivative from male urine, its relationship to dehydroandrosterone and androsterone. Z Physiol Chem 1934;229:192–208.
12. David K, Dingemanse E, Freud J, et al. Crystalline male hormone from testes (testosterone), more active than androsterone prepared from urine or cholesterol. Z Physiol Chem 1935:281–282.
13. Butenandt A, Hanisch G. Testosterone. Transformation of dehydroandrosterone into androstenediol and testosterone; a way to the preparation of testosterone from cholestrol. Chem Ber 1935;68B:1859–1862.
14. Kochakian CD, Murlin JR. Effect of male hormone on the protein and energy metabolism of castrate dogs. J Nutr 1935;10:437–459.
15. Kock FC. The chemistry and biology of the male sex hormones. Bull N Y Acad Med 1938;14:655–680.
16. Bremner WJ, Vitiello MV, Prinz N. Loss of circadian rhythmicity in blood testosterone levels with aging in normal men. J Clin Endocrinol Metab 1983;56:1278–1281.
17. Vale W, Wiater E, Gray P, et al. Activins and inhibins and their signaling. Ann N Y Acad Sci 2004;1038:142–147.
18. Ferrando AA, Sheffield-Moore M, Yeckel CW, et al. Testosterone administration to older men improves muscle function: molecular and physiological mechanisms. Am J Physiol Endocrinol Metab 2002;282:E601–E607.
19. Brodsky IG, Balagopal P, Nair KS. Effects of testosterone replacement on muscle mass and muscle protein synthesis in hypogonadal men—a clinical research center study. J Clin Endocrinol Metab 1996;81:3469–3475.
20. Bhasin S. Testosterone supplementation for aging-associated sarcopenia. J Gerontol A Biol Sci Med Sci 2003;58:1002–1008.
21. Manolagas SC, Kousteni S, Jilka RL. Sex steroids and bone. Recent Prog Horm Res 2002;57:385–409.
22. Wiren KM. Androgens and bone growth: it's location, location, location. Current Opinion Pharmacology 2005;5:626–632.
23. Fishman J, Brown JB, Hellman Leon, et al. Estrogen metabolism in normal and pregnant women. J Biol Chem 1962;237:1489–1494.
24. Gurpide E, Angers M, Vande Wiele RL, et al. Determination of secretory rates of estrogens in pregnant and nonpregnant women from the specific activities of urinary metabolites. J Clin Endocrinol Metab 1962;22:935–945.
25. Simpson ER, Merrill JC, Hollub AJ, et al. Regulation of estrogen biosynthesis by human adipose cells. Endocr Rev 1989;10:136–148.
26. Nakajin S, Hall PF. Microsomal cytochrome P-450 from neonatal pig testis. Purification and properties of a C-21 steroid side-chain cleavage system (17α-hydroxylase-C17,20-lyase). J Biol Chem 1981;256:3871–3876.
27. Baulieu EE, Wallace W, Lieberman S. The conversion in vitro of Δ^5-androstene-3β,17β-diol-17α-H3 to testosterone-17α-H3 by human adrenal and placental tissue. J Biol Chem 1963;238:1316–1319.
28. Rosner JM, Horita S, Forsham PH. Androstenediol, a probable intermediate in the in vitro conversion of dehydroepiandrosterone to testosterone by the rabbit testis. Endocrinology 1964;75:299–303.
29. Brodie A. Aromatase inhibitors: introduction and perspective. J Enzyme Inhib 1990;42:75–77.
30. Brueggemeier RW, Hackett JC, Diaz-Cruz ES. Aromatase inhibitors in the treatment of breast cancer. Endocr Rev 2005;26:331–345.
31. Miller WR, Anderson TJ, Evans DB, et al. An integrated view of aromatase and its inhibition. J Steroid Biochem Mol Biol 2003;86:413–421.
32. Osborne CK, Schiff R. Aromatase inhibitors: future directions. J Steroid Biochem Mol Biol 2005;95:183–187.
33. Thompson EA Jr, Siiteri PK. The involvement of human placental microsomal cytochrome P-450 in aromatization. J Biol Chem 1974;249:5373–5378.
34. Bruchovsky N, Wilson JD. The conversion of testosterone to 5-α-androstan-17-β-ol-3-one by rat prostate in vivo and in vitro. J Biol Chem 1968;243:2012–2021.

35. Ofner P. Effects and metabolism of hormones in normal and neoplastic prostate tissue. Vitam Horm 1968;26:237–291.
36. Liao S, Liang T, Fang S, et al. Steroid structure and androgenic activity. Specificities involved in the receptor binding and nuclear retention of various androgens. J Biol Chem 1973;248:6154–6162.
37. Brueggemeir R. Male sex hormones, analogues, and antagonists. In: Burger A, Abraham DJ, eds. Burger's Medicinal Chemistry and Drug Discovery. 6th Ed. Hoboken, NJ: Wiley, 2003.
38. Dorfman RI, Ungar F. Metabolism of Steroid Hormones. 2nd Ed. New York: New York, 1965:716.
39. Thigpen AE, Silver RI, Guileyardo JM, et al. Tissue distribution and ontogeny of steroid 5α-reductase isozyme expression. J Clin Invest 1993;92:903–910.
40. Russel DW, Berman DM, Bryant JT, et al. The molecular genetics of steroid 5α-reductases. Recent Prog Horm Res 1994;49:275–284.
41. Johansen KL. Testosterone metabolism and replacement therapy in patients with end-stage renal disease. Semin Dial 2004;17:202–208.
42. Vermeulen A, Kaufman JM, Goemaere S, et al. Estradiol in elderly men. Aging Male 2002;5(2):98–102.
43. Fotherby K, James F, Atkinson L, Dumasia M, et al. Studies in the aromatization of a synthetic progestin. J Endocrinol 1972;52(1):v–vi.
44. Belanger A, Pelletier G, Labrie F, et al. Inactivation of androgens by UDP-glucuronosyltransferase enzymes in humans. Trends Endocrinol Metab 2003;14:473–479.
45. Keller ET, Ershler WB, Chang C. The androgen receptor: a mediator of diverse responses. Front Biosci 1996;1:59–71.
46. Snyder PJ. Androgens. In: Bunton LL, Lazo JS, Parker KL, eds. Goodman & Gilman's The Pharmacological Basis of Therapeutics. 10th Ed. New York: McGraw-Hill, 2006, p. 1573–1586.
47. Gao W, Bohl CE, Dalton JT. Chemistry and structural biology of androgen receptor. Chem Rev 2005;105:3352–3370.
48. Chawnshang C. Androgens and androgen receptor: mechanisms, functions, and clinical applications. Boston: Kluwer Academic Publishers, 2002.
49. Freedman LP. Molecular Biology of Steroid and Nuclear Hormone Receptors. Progress in Gene expression. Boston: Birkhauser, 1998.
50. Pratt WB, Toft DO. Steroid receptor interactions with heat shock protein and immunophilin chaperones. Endocr Rev 1997;18:306–360.
51. Shang Y, Myers M, Brown M. Formation of the androgen receptor transcription complex. Mol Cell 2002;9:601–610.
52. Claessens F, Verrijdt G, Schoenmakers E, et al. Selective DNA binding by the androgen receptor as a mechanism for hormone-specific gene regulation. J Steroid Biochem Mol Biol 2001;76:23–30.
53. Haelens A, Verrijdt G, Callewaert L, et al. DNA recognition by the androgen receptor: evidence for an alternative DNA-dependent dimerization, and an active role of sequences flanking the response element on transactivation. Biochem J 2003;369(Pt 1):141–151.
54. Shaffer PL, Jivan Arif, Dollins DE, et al. Structural basis of androgen receptor binding to selective androgen response elements. Proc Natl Acad Sci U S A 2004;101:4758–4763.
55. Hsiao PW, Thin TH, Lin DL, et al. Differential regulation of testosterone vs. 5α-dihydrotestosterone by selective androgen response elements. Mol Cell Biochem 2000;206:169–175.
56. Remenyi A, Scholer HR, Wilmanns M. Combinatorial control of gene expression. Nat Struct Mol Biol 2004;11:812–815.
57. Lutz LB, Jamnongjit M, Yang WH, et al. Selective modulation of genomic and nongenomic androgen responses by androgen receptor ligands. Mol Endocrinol 2003;17:1106– 1116.
58. Estrada M, Espinosa A, Mueller M, et al. Testosterone stimulates intracellular calcium release and mitogen-activated protein kinases via a G protein–coupled receptor in skeletal muscle cells. Endocrinology 2003;144:3586–3597.
59. Kousteni S, Bellido T, Plotkin LI, et al. Nongenotropic, sex-nonspecific signaling through the estrogen or androgen receptors: dissociation from transcriptional activity. Cell 2001;104:719–730.
60. Zagar Y, Chaumaz G, Lieberherr M. Signaling cross-talk from Gβ4 subunit to Elk-1 in the rapid action of androgens. J Biol Chem 2004;279:2403–2413.
61. Kampa M, Papakonstanti EA, Hatzoglou A, et al. The human prostate cancer cell line LNCaP bears functional membrane testosterone receptors that increase PSA secretion and modify actin cytoskeleton. FASEB J 2002;16:1429–1431.
62. Unni E, Sun S, Nan B, et al. Changes in androgen receptor nongenotropic signaling correlate with transition of LNCaP cells to androgen independence. Cancer Res 2004;64:7156–7168.
63. Norman AW, Mizwicki MY, Norman DP. Steroid-hormone rapid actions, membrane receptors, and a conformational ensemble model. Nat Rev Drug Discov 2004;3:27–41.
64. Simoncini T, Genazzani AR. Nongenomic actions of sex steroid hormones. Eur J Endocrinol 2003;148:281–292.
65. Kousteni S, Chen J-R, Bellido T, et al. Reversal of bone loss in mice by nongenotropic signaling of sex steroids. Science 2002;298:843–846.
66. Bancroft J, Wu FC. Changes in erectile responsiveness during androgen replacement therapy. Arch Sex Behav 1983;12:59–66.
67. Arver S, Dobs AS, Meikle AW, et al. Improvement of sexual function in testosterone deficient men treated for 1 year with a permeation enhanced testosterone transdermal system. J Urol 1996;155:1604–1608.
68. Oettel M. Testosterone metabolism, dose–response relationships, and receptor polymorphisms: selected pharmacological/toxicological considerations on benefits versus risks of testosterone therapy in men. Aging Male 2003;6:230–256.
69. Hijazi RA, Cunningham GR. Andropause: is androgen replacement therapy indicated for the aging male? Annu Rev Med 2005;56:117–137.
70. Rhoben EL, Morgentaler A. Risks of testosterone replacement therapy and recommendations for monitoring. N Engl J Med 2004;350:482–492.
71. Testosterone and Aging: Clinical Research Directions. Institute of Medicine, November 2003.
72. Shackleford DM, Faassen WA, Houwing N, et al. Contribution of lymphatically transported testosterone undecanoate to the systemic exposure of testosterone after oral administration of two andriol formulations in conscious lymph duct–cannulated dogs. J Pharmacol Exp Ther 2003;306:925–933.
73. Vida JA. Androgens and Anabolic Agents: Chemistry and Pharmacology. New York: Academic Press, 1969.
74. Segaloff A, Gabbard RB. 5α-Androstane—an androgenic hydrocarbon. Endocrinology 1960;67:887–889.
75. Arnold A, Potts GO, Beyler AL. The ratio of anabolic to androgenic activity of (7,17) 17-dimethyltestosterone, oxymesterone, mestanolone, and rluoxymesterone. J Endocrinol 1963;28:87–92.
76. Clark AS, Harrold EV. Comparison of the effects of stanozolol, oxymetholone, and testosterone cypionate on the sexual behavior of castrated male rats. Behav Neurosci 1997;111:1368–1374.
77. Catlin DH, Sekera MH, Ahrens BD, et al. Tetrahydrogestrinone: discovery, synthesis, and detection in urine. Rapid Commun Mass Spectrom 2004;18: 1245–1249.
78. Jasuja R, Catlin DH, Miller A, et al. Tetrahydrogestrinone is an androgenic steroid that stimulates androgen receptor-mediated, myogenic differentiation in C3H10T1/2 multipotent mesenchymal cells and promotes muscle accretion in orchidectomized male rats. Endocrinology 2005;146:4472–4478.
79. Zhi L, Martinborough E. Selective androgen receptor modulators (SARMs). Annual Reports of Medicinal Chemistry 2001;36:169–180.
80. Negro-Vilar A. Selective androgen receptor modulators (SARMs): a novel approach to androgen therapy for the new millennium. J Clin Endocrinol Metab 1999;84:3459–3462.
81. Dalton JT, Mukherjee A, Zhu Z, et al. Discovery of nonsteroidal androgens. Biochem Biophys Res Commun 1998;244:1–4.
82. Tucker H, Crook JW, Chesterson GJ. Nonsteroidal antiandrogens. Synthesis and structure–activity relationships of 3-substituted derivatives of 2-hydroxypropionanilides. J Med Chem 1998;31:954–959.
83. Balog A, Salvati ME, Shan Weifang, et al. The synthesis and evaluation of [2.2.1]-bicycloazahydantoins as androgen receptor antagonists Bioorg Med Chem Lett 2004;14:6107–6111.
84. Higuchi RI, Edwards JP, Caferro TR, et al. 4-Alkyl- and 3,4-dialkyl-1,2,3,4-tetrahydro-8-pyridono[5,6-g]quinolines: Potent, nonsteroidal androgen receptor agonists. Bioorg Med Chem Lett 1999;9:1335–1340.
85. Zhi L, Tegley CM, Marschke KB, et al. Switching androgen receptor antagonists to agonists by modifying C-ring substituents on piperidino[3,2-g]quinolinone. Bioorg Med Chem Lett 1999;9:1009–1012.
86. Yin D, He Y, Perera MA, et al. Key structural features of nonsteroidal ligands for binding and activation of the androgen receptor. Mol Pharmacol 2003;63:211–223.
87. He Y, Yin D, Perera M, et al. Novel nonsteroidal ligands with high binding affinity and potent functional activity for the androgen receptor. Eur J Med Chem 2002;37:619–634.
88. Kirkovsky L, Mukherjee A, Yin D, et al. Chiral nonsteroidal affinity ligands for the androgen receptor. 1. Bicalutamide analogues bearing electrophilic groups in the B aromatic ring. J Med Chem 2000;43:581–590.
89. Bohl CE, Gao W, Miller DD, et al. Structural basis for antagonism and resistance of bicalutamide in prostate cancer. Proc Natl Acad Sci U S A 2005;102: 6201–6206.
90. Tarter TH, Vaughan ED Jr. Inhibitors of 5α-reductase in the treatment of benign prostatic hyperplasia. Curr Pharm Des 2006;12:775–783.
91. Martin DJ. Preclinical pharmacology of α1-adrenoceptor antagonists. Eur Urol 1999;36(Suppl. 1):35–41.
92. Greenlee RT, Hill-Harmon MB, Murray T, Thun M, et al. Cancer statistics, 2001. CA Cancer J Clin 2001;51:15–36 [erratum appears in CA Cancer J Clin 2001;51:144].
93. Shibata Y, Ito K, Suzuki K. Changes in the endocrine environment of the human prostate transition zone with aging: simultaneous quantitative analysis of prostatic sex steroids and comparison with human prostatic histological composition. Prostate 2000;42:45–55.
94. Lee M, Sharifi R. Benign prostatic hyperplasia: diagnosis and treatment guideline. Ann Pharmacother 1997;31:481–486.
95. Tan SY, Antonipillai I, Murphy BE. Inhibition of testosterone metabolism in the human prostate. J Clin Endocrinol Metab 1974;39:936–941.
96. Andriole G, Bruchovsky N, Chung LW, et al. Dihydrotestosterone and the prostate: the scientific rationale for 5α-reductase inhibitors in the treatment of benign prostatic hyperplasia. J Urol 2004;172:1399–1403.
97. Liang T, Cascieri MA, Cheung AH, et al. Species differences in prostatic steroid 5α-reductases of rat, dog, and human. Endocrinology 1985;117:571–579.

98. Amadesi S, Varani K, Spisani L, et al. Comparison of prazosin, terazosin, and tamsulosin: functional and binding studies in isolated prostatic and vascular human tissues. Prostate 2001;47:231–238.
99. Foglar R, Shibata K, Horie K, et al. Use of recombinant α_1-adrenoceptors to characterize subtype selectivity of drugs for the treatment of prostatic hypertrophy. Eur J Pharmacol 1995;288:201–207.
100. Peterson CM. Progestogens, progesterone antagonists, progesterone, and androgens: synthesis, classification, and uses. Clin Obstet Gynecol 1995;38: 813–820.
101. Rasmusson GH, Reynolds GF, Steinberg NG, et al. Azasteroids: structure–activity relationships for inhibition of 5α-reductase and of androgen receptor binding. J Med Chem 1986;29:2298.
102. McConnell JD, Wilson JD, George FW, et al. Finasteride, an inhibitor of 5α-reductase, suppresses prostatic dihydrotestosterone in men with benign prostatic hyperplasia. J Clin Endocrinol Metab 1992;74:505–508.
103. Djavan R, Milani S, Fong YK. Dutasteride : a novel dual inhibitor of 5α-reductase for benign prostatic hyperplasia. Expert Opin Pharmacother 2005;6:311–317.
104. Vermeulen A, Giagulli VA, De Schepper P, et al. Hormonal effects of an orally active 4-azasteroid inhibitor of 5α-reductase in humans. Prostate 1989;14:45–53.
105. Bull G, Garcia-Calvo, M, Andersson, S, et al. Mechanism-based inhibition of human steroid 5α-reductase by finasteride: enzyme-catalyzed formation of NADP-dihydrofinasteride, a potent bisubstrate analogue inhibitor. J Am Chem Soc 1996;118:2359–2365.
106. Darren SJ, Lee FW, Simpson ND, et al. Pharmacokinetic parameters and mechanisms of inhibition of rat type 1 and 2 steroid 5α-reductases: determinants for different in vivo activities of GI198745 and finasteride in the rat. Biochem Pharmacol 2001;62:933–942.
107. Frye SV. Discovery and clinical development of dutasteride, a potent dual 5α-reductase inhibitor. Curr Top Med Chem 2006;6:405–421.
108. Dolder CR. Dutasteride: a dual 5α-reductase inhibitor for the treatment of symptomatic benign prostatic hyperplasia. Ann Pharmacother 2006;40:658–665.
109. Roehrborn CG, Boyle P, Nickel JC, et al. Efficacy and safety of a dual inhibitor of 5α-reductase types 1 and 2 (dutasteride) in men with benign prostatic hyperplasia. Urology 2002;60:434–441.
110. Buck AC. Is there a scientific basis for the therapeutic effects of *Serenoa repens* in benign prostatic hyperplasia? Mechanisms of action. J Urol 2004;172: 1792–1799.
111. Bent S, Kane C, Shinohara K, et al. Saw palmetto for benign prostatic hyperplasia. N Engl J Med 2006;354:557–566.
112. Neumann F, Topert M. Pharmacology of antiandrogens. J Steroid Biochem 1986;25:885–895
113. Martini L, Motta M. Androgens and Antiandrogens. New York: Raven Press, 1977:77–89.
114. Neri RO. Antiandrogens. Adv Sex Horm Res 1976;2:233–262.
115. Yoshioka K, et al. Studies on antiandrogenic agents. Synthesis of 16β-ethyl-19-nortestosterone. Chem Pharm Bull (Tokyo) 1975;23:3203–3207.
116. Wakeling AE, et al. Receptor binding and biological activity of steroidal and nonsteroidal antiandrogens. J Steroid Biochem 1981;15:355–359.
117. Snyder BW, Winneker RC, Batzold FH. Endocrine profile of Win 49596 in the rat: a novel androgen receptor antagonist. J Steroid Biochem 1989;33: 1127–1132.
118. Liao S, Howell DK, Chang TN. Action of a nonsteroidal antiandrogen, flutamide, on the receptor binding and nuclear retention of 5α-dihydrotestosterone in rat ventral prostate. Endocrinology 1974;94:1205–1209.
119. Shet MS, Mcphaul M, Fisher CW, et al. Metabolism of the antiandrogenic drug (flutamide) by human CYP1A2. Drug Metab Dispos 1997;25: 1298–1303.
120. Suzuki H, Akakura K, Komiya A, et al. Codon 877 mutation in the androgen receptor gene in advanced prostate cancer: relation to antiandrogen withdrawal syndrome. Prostate 1996;29:153–158.
121. Hara T, Miyazaki J, Araki H, et al. Novel mutations of androgen receptor: a possible mechanism of bicalutamide withdrawal syndrome. Cancer Res 2003;63:149–153.
122. Fang S, Liao S. Antagonistic action of antiandrogens on the formation of a specific dihydrotestosterone-receptor protein complex in rat ventral prostate. Mol Pharmacol 1969;5:428–431.
123. Furr BJ, Tucker H. The preclinical development of bicalutamide: pharmacodynamics and mechanism of action. Urology 1996;47(Suppl. 1A):13–25.
124. Cockshott ID. Bicalutamide: clinical pharmacokinetics and metabolism. Clin Pharmacokinet 2004;43:855–878.
125. Marugo M, Bernasconi D, Miglietta L, et al. Effects of dihydrotestosterone and hydroxyflutamide on androgen receptors in cultured human breast cancer cells (EVSA-T). J Steroid Biochem Mol Biol 1992;42:547–554.
126. Ask K, Decologne N, Ginies C, et al. Metabolism of nilutamide in rat lung. Biochem Pharmacol 2006;71:377–385.
127. Ask K, Dijols S, Giroud C, et al. Reduction of nilutamide by NO synthases: implications for the adverse effects of this nitroaromatic antiandrogen drug. Chem Res Toxicol 2003;16:1547–1554.
128. National Cancer Institute. The prostate cancer prevention trial. Available at: http://www.cancer.gov/pcpt.
129. Thompson IM, Goodman PJ, Tangen CM, et al. The influence of finasteride on the development of prostate cancer. N Engl J Med 2003;349:215–224.
130. Van Wauwe J, Janssen PA. Is there a case for P-450 inhibitors in cancer treatment? J Med Chem 1989;32:2231–2239.
131. Barrie SE, Potter GA, Goddard PM, et al. Pharmacology of novel steroidal inhibitors of cytochrome P45017α (17β-hydroxylase/C17-20 lyase). J Steroid Biochem Mol Biol 1994;50:267–273.
132. Angelastro MR, Laughlin ME, Schatzman GL, et al. 17β-(Cyclopropylamino)-androst-5-en-3β-ol, a selective mechanism-based inhibitor of cytochrome P450(17α) (steroid 17α-hydroxylase/C17-20 lyase). Biochem Biophys Res Commun 1989;162:1571.
133. Haidar S, Ehmer PB, Barassin S, et al. Effects of novel 17α-hydroxylase/C17,20-lyase (P450 17, CYP 17) inhibitors on androgen biosynthesis in vitro and in vivo. J Steroid Biochem Mol Biol 2003;84:555–562.
134. Oottamasathien S, Crawford ED. Recent advances in hormonal therapy for advanced prostate cancer. Oncology 2003;17:1047–1052.
135. Stevermer JJ, Easley SK. Treatment of prostatitis. Am Fam Physician 2000;61:3015–3022.
136. Charalabopoulos K, Karachalios G, Baltogiannis D, et al. Penetration of antimicrobial agents into the prostate. Chemotherapy 2003;49:269–279.
137. Boolell M, Allen MJ, Ballard SA, et al. Sildenafil: an orally active type 5 cyclic GMP-specific phosphodiesterase inhibitor for the treatment of penile erectile dysfunction. Int J Impot Res 1996;8:47–52.
138. Setter SM, Iltz JL, Fincham JE, et al. Phosphodiesterase-5 inhibitors for erectile dysfunction. Ann Pharmacother 2005;39:1286–1295.
139. Pissarnitski D. Phosphodiesterase-5 (PDE5) inhibitors for the treatment of male erectile disorder: attaining selectivity versus PDE6. Med Res Rev 2006;26:369–395.
140. Saenz de Tejada I, Angulo J, Cuevas P, et al. The phosphodiesterase inhibitory selectivity and the in vitro and in vivo potency of the new PDE5 inhibitor vardenafil. Int J Impot Res 2001;13:282–290.
141. Gupta M, Kovar A, Meibohm B. The clinical pharmacokinetics of phosphodiesterase-5 inhibitors for erectile dysfunction. J Clin Pharmacol 2005;45: 987–1003.
142. Kloner RA. Cardiovascular effects of the three phosphodiesterase-5 inhibitors approved for the treatment of erectile dysfunction. Circulation 2004;110:3149–3155.
143. Porst H, Rosen R, Padma-Nathan H, et al. The efficacy and tolerability of vardenafil, a new, oral, selective phosphodiesterase type 5 inhibitor, in patients with erectile dysfunction: the first at-home clinical trial. Int J Impot Res 2001;13:192–199.
144. Corbin JD, Beasley A, Blount MA, et al. Vardenafil: structural basis for higher potency over sildenafil in inhibiting cGMP-specific phosphodiesterase-5 (PDE5). Neurochem Int 2004;45:859–863.
145. Kuan J, Brock G. Selective phosphodiesterase type 5 inhibition using tadalafil for the treatment of erectile dysfunction. Expert Opin Investig Drugs 2002;11:1605–1613.
146. Beckman TJ, Abu-Lebdeh HS, Mynderse LA. Evaluation and medical management of erectile dysfunction. Mayo Clin Proc 2006;81:385–390.
147. McDonald-Gibson WJ, McDonald-Gibson RG, Greaves MW. Prostaglandin E_1 metabolism by human plasma. Prostaglandins 1972;2:251–263.
148. Bechara A, Casabe A, Cheliz G, et al. Comparative study of papaverine plus phentolamine versus prostaglandin E_1 in erectile dysfunction. J Urol 1997; 157:2132–2134.
149. McGlynn KA, Devesa SS, Sigurdson AJ, et al. Trends in the incidence of testicular germ cell tumors in the United States. Cancer 2003;97:63–70.
150. Kamel HK. Male osteoporosis: new trends in diagnosis and therapy. Drugs Aging 2005;22:741–748.

Suggested Readings

Beato M. Gene regulation by steroid hormones. Cell 1989;56(3):335–344.

Bentley PJ. Endocrine Pharmacology. Cambridge, UK: Cambridge University Press, 1980.

Brueggemeier RW. Androgens, anabolics and antiandrogens. In: Verderame M, ed. Handbook of Hormones, Vitamins, and Radiopaques. Boca Raton, FL: CRC Press, 1986:1–49.

Brueggemeier RW, Male Sex Hormones, Analogs and Antagonists. In: Wolff ME, ed., Burger's Medicinal Chemistry, 5th ed., New York: Wiley Interscience, 1995:445–510

Evans RM. The steroid and thyroid hormone receptor superfamily. Science 1988;240(4854):889–895.

Magarian RA, et al. In: Verderame M, ed. Handbook of Hormones, Vitamins, and Radiopaques, Boca Raton, FL: CRC Press, 1986:51–92.

Makin HJL, ed. Biochemistry of Steroid Hormones. 2nd Ed. Oxford, UK: Blackwell Scientific Publications, 1984.

Proteau PL, Steroids and therapeutically related compounds. In: Block JH, Beale Jr JM eds,Wilson and Gisvold's Textbook of Organic Medicinal and Pharmaceutical Chemistry. Baltimore, 11th ed., Lippincott Williams & Wilkins, 2004:767–817.

Snyder PJ. Androgens. In: Brunton L, Lazo, J, Parker K, eds., Goodman & Gilman's The Pharmacological Basis of Therapeutics 11th ed., New York, McGraw-Hill, 2006:1573–1586

Witzman RF. Steroids: Keys to Life. New York, Van Nostrand-Reinhold, 1981.

Zeelen FJ. Medicinal Chemistry of Steroids. Amsterdam: Elsevier, 1990.

46. *Women's Health*

ROBIN M. ZAVOD

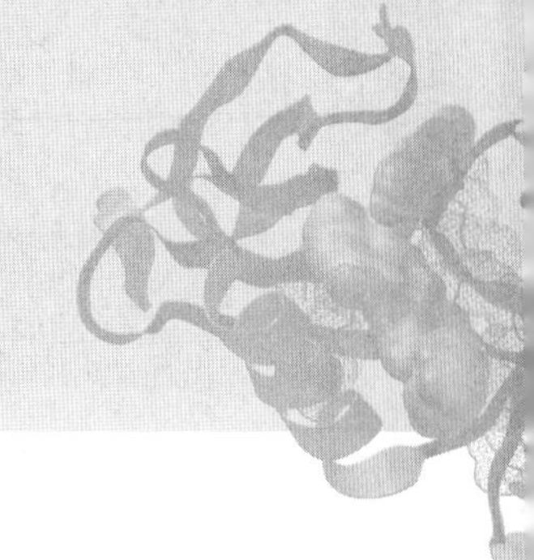

DRUGS COVERED IN THIS CHAPTER:

STEROIDAL ESTROGENS
- Conjugated Estrogens
- Estradiol
- Ethynyl estradiol
- Mestranol

PROGESTINS
- Desogestrel
- Dienogest
- Drospirenone
- Elcomdetrine
- Ethisterone
- Gestodene
- Medroxyprogesterone acetate
- Megestrol acetate
- Nomogestrel acetate
- Norethindrone
- Norgestimate
- Norgestrel/Levonorgestrel
- Trimegestone

Mifepristone

INFERTILITY DRUGS
- Clomiphene citrate
- Follicle Stimulating Hormone
- Gonadotropin Releasing Hormone
- Lutropin alfa

SELECTIVE ESTROGEN RECEPTOR MODULATORS
- Tamoxifen
- Toremifene

AROMATASE INHIBITORS
- Anastrozole
- Exemastane
- Letrozole

Fulvestrant

INTRODUCTION

The sex hormones are specific steroids necessary for reproduction as well as for the development of secondary sex characteristics in both sexes. The sex steroids are comprised of three classes—estrogens, progestins, and androgens. In this chapter, the two principal classes of female sex hormones, estrogens and progestins, will be discussed. The naturally occurring estrogens are C_{18} steroids and contain an aromatic A ring with a hydroxyl group at the 3 position. The most potent endogenous estrogen is estradiol. The naturally occurring progestins are C_{21} steroids and contain a 3-keto-4-ene structure in the A ring and a ketone at the C_{21} position. The most potent endogenous progestin is progesterone. The class of steroids that contains the male sex hormones is the androgen class. The naturally occurring androgens are C_{19} steroids and contain either a hydroxyl or ketone functional group at both the C_3 and C_{17} positions. The primary androgen found in the blood is testosterone, with the active metabolite 5α-dihydrotestosterone formed in certain target tissues. All three classes of endogenous steroids are present in both sexes, but the production and circulating plasma levels of estrogens and progestins are substantially higher in females.

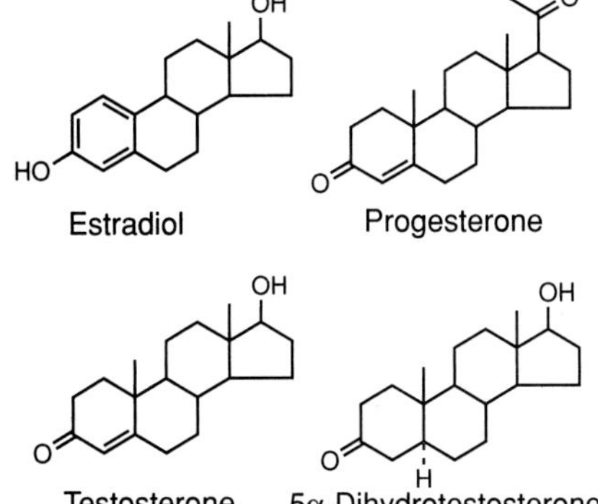

SEX HORMONES: REPRODUCTIVE CYCLE

The female reproductive cycle is controlled by an integrated system involving the hypothalamus, anterior pituitary gland, ovary, and reproductive tract (Fig. 46.1). The hypothalamus exerts its action on the pituitary gland via the hormone signal gonadotropin-releasing hormone (GnRH). This hormone is released by the hypothalamus in a pulsatile fashion and stimulates the release of the gonadotropins, follicle stimulating hormone (FSH) and luteinizing hormone (LH) from the anterior pituitary.

The two main gonadotropins, FSH and LH, regulate production of the sex hormones estrogen and progesterone. As the name implies, FSH promotes the initial development and growth of immature ovarian follicles, and as these follicles mature, they secrete estradiol. During the follicular phase, when estrogen levels are elevated, the endometrium undergoes proliferation as a direct result of estrogenic stimulation. As estradiol levels increase, the production of FSH decreases via feedback inhibition, and LH release is stimulated. The level of LH rises to a sharp peak (LH surge) at the midpoint of the menstrual cycle. This serves to cause the dominant follicle to rupture and release its egg (ovulation). The luteal phase follows ovulation and ends at menses. During this phase, the endometrium

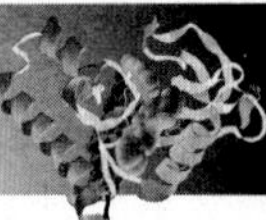

CLINICAL SIGNIFICANCE

Women's health issues encompass a variety of disease states and range from contraception to infertility, menopause, osteoporosis, and oncology. Pharmacological agents treating these disease states are numerous and wide-ranging with regards to their use. Recent developments of drugs dealing with women's health issues not only have focused on producing better oral contraceptives but also have expanded to designing drugs for the treatment of osteoporosis, infertility, and breast cancer.

With so many medications to choose from, the clinician must be knowledgeable about the drug's pharmacodynamic, pharmacokinetic, and medicinal chemistry properties to optimize therapy. For example, with so many oral contraceptives (OCs) on the market, the clinician must apply his or her knowledge about the drug to tailor the therapy. For patients with acne, OCs with low androgenic characteristics would be appropriate. Postpartum mothers who are breastfeeding and want to start on OCs will need to use a product containing progestin only. In addition to OCs, drugs used to treat infertility must be customized to fit the patient's clinical picture. A variety of medications are used to treat infertility, ranging from clomiphene citrate, an antiestrogen, to products containing follicle-stimulating hormone.

Advancement in the treatment of bone disorders and cancer in women have resulted from the increased knowledge of estrogen receptors and the development of selective estrogen receptor modulators (SERMs). Modifications in the structure–activity relationships of SERMs produce drugs with favorable side effect profiles that are effective for osteoporosis and breast cancer. Many ongoing research investigations continue to develop drugs for treating the assortment of health care issues facing women. An essential component in both the development and the clinical applications of these drugs is the utilization of knowledge regarding the drugs' medicinal chemistry properties.

Nancy Ordonez, Pharm.D.
Clinical Assistant Professor
University of Houston
College of Pharmacy

shows secretory activity, and cell proliferation declines. Once ovulation has occurred, LH induces luteinization of the tissue that remains from the ruptured follicle, which leads to formation of the corpus luteum. The corpus luteum is responsible for the biosynthesis and secretion of progesterone during the luteal phase of the menstrual cycle, when endometrial preparation for pregnancy occurs, as well as during the early weeks of a pregnancy.

If the egg remains unfertilized, the corpus luteum degrades, and the levels of progesterone and estrogen decline. This leads to sloughing off of the endometrial lining, known as menstruation. At this point in the menstrual cycle, estrogen and progesterone levels are low, and hormonal feedback to the hypothalamus ceases. Without the influence of these hormonal signals, the hypothalamus releases additional GnRH, and the cycle begins again. A single menstrual cycle starts with the onset of menses (day 1) and ends with the start of the next menstrual period. This interval varies from 20 to 35 days, with an average length of 28 days. The major events of the ovarian cycle are summarized in Figure 46.2.

If the egg is fertilized successfully, then the menstrual cycle is interrupted because of the release of gonadotropin synthesized in the placenta, human chorionic gonadotropin (hCG). The role of this glycoprotein is to maintain the corpus luteum. Fourteen days after egg fertilization, the level of urinary hCG reaches a concentration that can be detected by a home pregnancy test. Levels of this gonadotropin peak around the seventh week of pregnancy and then decrease to a level that is maintained throughout pregnancy.

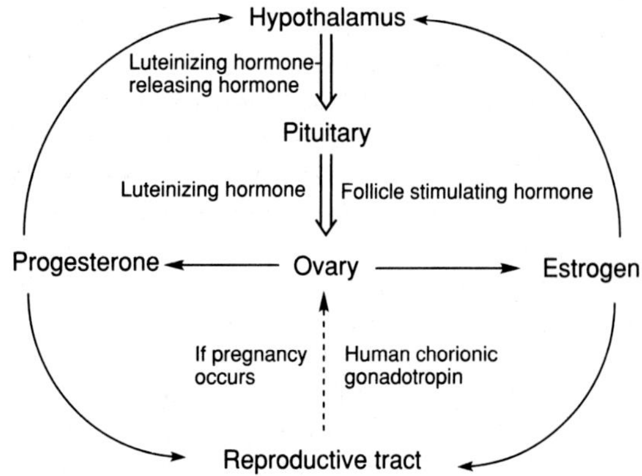

Fig. 46.1. Hypothalamic, ovarian, and reproductive tract interrelationships.

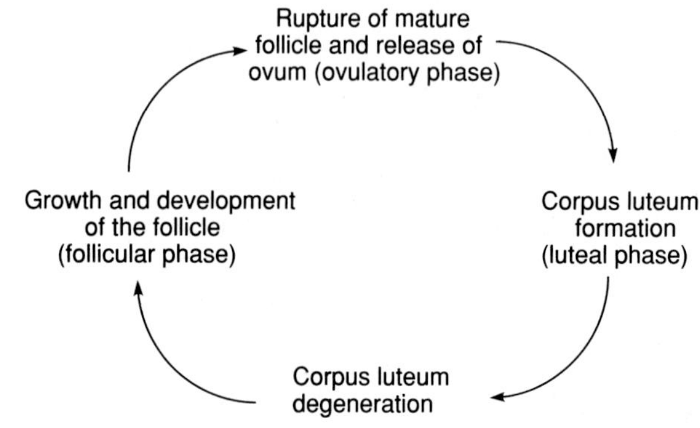

Fig. 46.2. Ovarian cycle.

Home Pregnancy Tests

With the increased availability of a variety of home diagnostic tests, the sale of home pregnancy, ovulation, and fertility tests alone was a $330 million dollar business in 2005. Home pregnancy tests have been utilized since 1976, with approximately 26 devices currently available in the United States. These tests claim that they can be utilized on the first day of a missed menstrual period (or, for certain devices, even earlier) with more than 99% diagnostic accuracy for pregnancy. Despite these claims, accurate results are obtained only a fraction of the time (Table 46.1) (1).

Home pregnancy tests are qualitative tests and simply detect the presence of the α and β subunits of hCG in a small sample of urine collected early in the day (Table 46.2) (2,3). Their detection limits range from 6.3 to 50 IU/L, and all are calibrated using regular hCG. A positive response indicates that the anti-hCG monoclonal or polyclonal antibodies found within the tests have successfully bound to a specific site along hCG. A second antibody linked to an enzyme that reacts with this anti-hCG complex causes a color change (3). What is not clear is if it is the regular hCG or the hyperglycosylated hCG (hCG) that is the source for the immunoreactivity observed during the weeks immediately following implantation. Compelling evidence suggests that hyperglycosylated hCG may be the principle source of hCG immunoreactivity, yet the detection limits for this glycoprotein are poorer than those reported for regular hCG. Only 6 of 15 home pregnancy tests evaluated were equally capable of detecting hyperglycosylated hCG and regular hCG (2).

False-positive results can stem from recent birth, miscarriage, or the use of menotropins or hCG injections in women experiencing infertility, in whom hCG levels may still be elevated (4). Although unlikely because of the use of monoclonal antibody technology, there also may be false-positive results from pharmacological sources, including methadone, promethazine, or chlorodiazepoxide (3). False-negative results generally are a consequence of errors in using the device or in handling the urine sample.

Table 46.1. Clinical Sensitivity Evaluation of Home Pregnancy Tests (1)

Name of Device	Confidence in Positive Results (%)	Clinical Sensitivity (%)
EPT	45	16
Clear Blue Easy Earliest Results	100	80
First Response Early Result	100	>95
Fact Plus Select	24	<16
Accu-Clear	22	<16

Table 46.2. Evaluation of Home Pregnancy Tests with Regular Human Chorionic Gonadotropin (hCG) and Hyperglycosylated hCG (H-hCG) Standards (2)

	Regular hCG (IU/L)				H-hCG (IU/L)				
Name of Device	6.3	13	25	50	6.3	13	25	50	hCG limit (IU/L)
EPT	−	−	+	++	−	+	+	++	40
Clear Blue Easy	+	+	++	++	−	−	+	+	50
First Response Early Result	−	+	+	++	−	−	+	++	~50
Fact Plus Select	−	−	+	+	−	−	+	+	100
Answer	−	−	+	++	−	−	±	+	100

(−), negative result observed; (±), exceptionally faint positive result observed; (+), clear positive result observed; (++), strongly positive result observed.

For the first 9 weeks of pregnancy, the corpus luteum produces an adequate level of estrogen and progesterone to maintain the pregnancy. After this period, the placenta assumes these responsibilities. Both estrogen and progesterone levels increase during pregnancy, finally reaching their maximal concentrations a few days before labor and delivery.

Over the course of a woman's lifetime, her hormonal status and ability to reproduce vary considerably. Sexual maturation and the onset of the reproductive period are correlated with the start of cyclic menstrual bleeding. This typically occurs between the ages of 8 and 17 years (average age, 11 years). Later in life, reproductive capacity begins to wane, and women gradually lose ovarian function, which causes intermittent maturation of follicles and, therefore, irregular production of the corpus luteum. This is referred to as perimenopause. Eventually, cessation of menses occurs, resulting in menopause and the loss of reproductive capacity. This typically occurs between the ages of 45 and 55 years. Throughout a woman's reproductive life cycle, various types of hormone therapy play key roles in regulating the hormone cycle. This chapter will focus primarily on hormonal therapies for the treatment and/or management of contraception, endometriosis, infertility, menopause, and breast cancer.

STEROID HORMONES

Estrogens

Three endogenous estrogens are present in women. Estradiol, the most potent of the three, represents 10 to 20% of the circulating estrogen. Estrone is 10-fold less potent than estradiol and accounts for 60 to 80% of the circulating estrogen. The remaining 10 to 20% is in the form of estriol, a very weak estrogen. Estrone was the first estrogen to be isolated in crystalline form from the urine of pregnant women. The two other C_{18} estrogen steroids, 17β-estradiol and estriol, were isolated and characterized later.

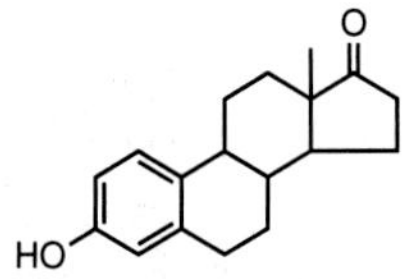

Estrone 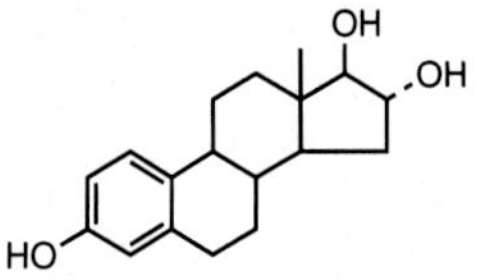 Estriol

Biosynthesis

Estrogens are biosynthesized in the maturing dominant follicle and in the corpus luteum in premenopausal women. During pregnancy, the placenta becomes the primary location of estrogen biosynthesis (5,6). Approximately 50% of estrone production occurs in the ovaries. The remaining estrone is biosynthesized from estradiol as well as from the conversion of estrone sulfate to estrone in the adrenal gland and the aromatization of androstenedione. In contrast to premenopausal women, in whom the natural estrone to estradiol ratio is 1:2, postmenopausal women have an estrone to estradiol ratio of 2:1, which reflects the loss of ovarian function.

In endocrine tissues, cholesterol is the steroid that is stored and converted to estrogen, progesterone, or androgen when the tissue is stimulated by a gonadotropic hormone. The major pathways for the biosynthesis of sex steroid hormones are summarized in Figure 46.3. In the ovary, FSH acts on the preovulatory follicle to stimulate the biosynthesis of estrogens. The thecal cells of the preovulatory follicle convert cholesterol into androgens, whereas the granulosa cells convert androgens to estrogens.

Cleavage of the side chain of cholesterol produces pregnenolone (step a in Fig. 46.3), which can then be transformed into progesterone or, via several biosynthetic

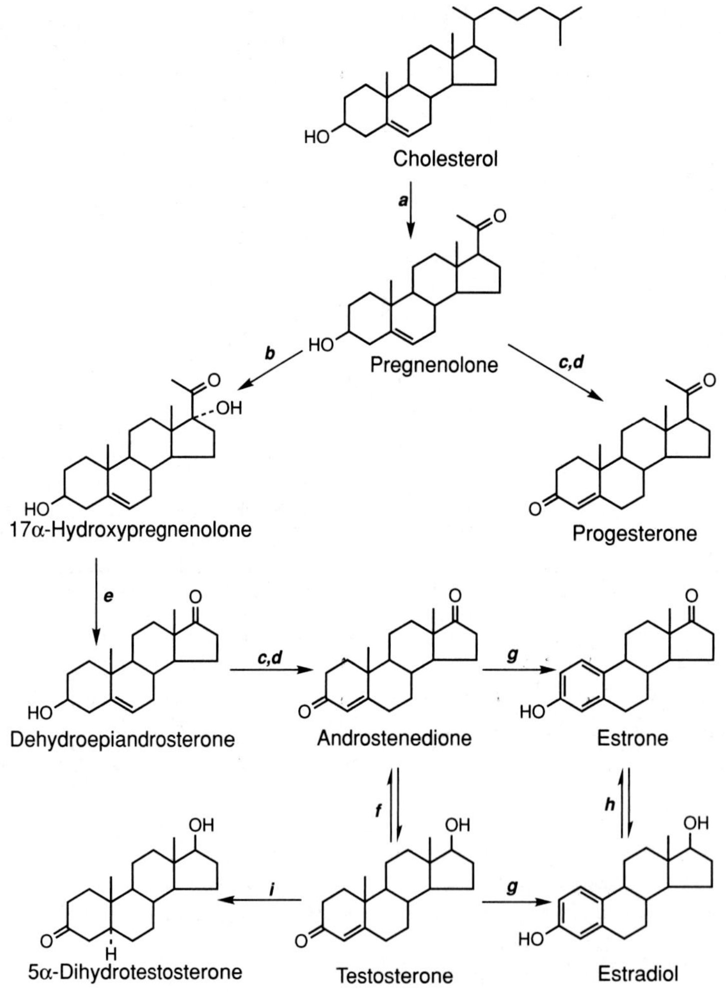

Cholesterol

Pregnenolone

17α-Hydroxypregnenolone

Progesterone

Dehydroepiandrosterone

Androstenedione

Estrone

5α-Dihydrotestosterone

Testosterone

Estradiol

Fig. 46.3. Biosynthesis of sex steroid hormones. The enzymes involved in this biosynthesis are (a) side-chain cleavage, (b) 17α-hydroxylase, (c) 5-ene-3β-hydroxysteroid dehydrogenase, (d) 3-oxosteroid-4,5-isomerase, (e) 17,20-lyase, (f) 17β-hydroxysteroid dehydrogenase, (g) aromatase, (h) estradiol dehydrogenase, and (i) 5α-reductase.

steps, to the aromatic A ring system found in estrogens (7). Pregnenolone is converted by 17α-hydroxylase to 17α-hydroxypregnenolone (step b), which then proceeds on to the intermediate dehydroepiandrosterone (DHEA) via 17,20-lyase reaction (step e) (8). DHEA is converted by 5-ene-3β-hydroxysteroid dehydrogenase and 3-oxosteroid-4,5-isomerase to the 17-ketosteroid, androstenedione (steps c and d), which is interconvertible with testosterone via 17β-hydroxysteroid dehydrogenase (step f). The final step in the biosynthesis is the conversion of the C_{19} androgens to the C_{18} estrogens via the loss of the C_{19} angular methyl group and aromatization of ring A to form 17β-estradiol or estrone (step g) catalyzed by aromatase. The interconversion of 17β-estradiol and estrone is catalyzed by estradiol dehydrogenase (step h), a member of the 17β-hydroxysteroid dehydrogenase family.

Metabolism

Metabolism of the estrogens to their water-soluble glucuronide and sulfate conjugates occurs mainly in the liver. Creation of a reservoir of estrogen occurs as a result of enterohepatic recycling, a process by which estrogens undergo desulfation followed by resulfation.

Approximately 50% of an exogenous dose of 17β-estradiol undergoes hepatic first-pass metabolism to metabolites that are readily excreted via the kidney, and the remaining 50% is found in bile fluid (9). Much of the material found in bile subsequently enters the intestine, where it is reabsorbed and returned to the liver. Only 10% of an administered dose is found in the feces (5). Both 17β-estradiol and estrone are converted by 16α-hydroxylase to yield estriol (Fig. 46.4A), which is found in the urine as the glucuronide conjugate.

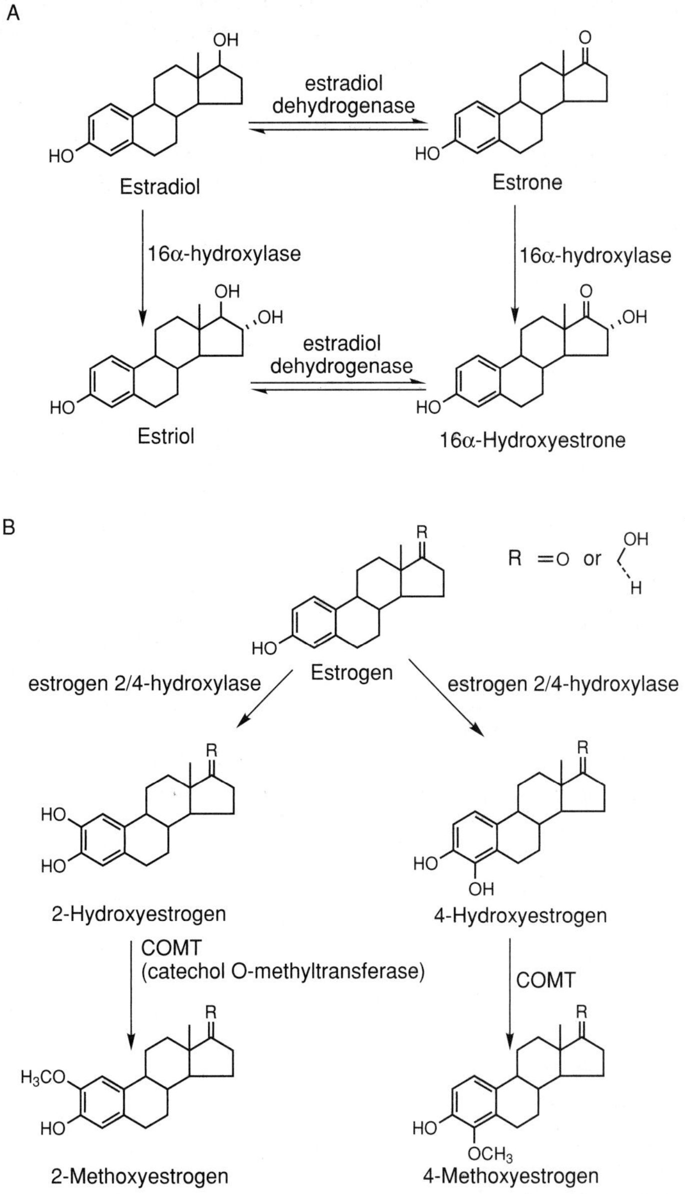

Fig. 46.4. Estrogen metabolism.

Table 46.3. Estrogenic Affinity for Binding Proteins and Metabolic Clearance Rate (11,12)

Estrogen	RBA to SHBG	% Bound to SHBG	% Bound to Albumin	Metabolic Clearance Rate (litter/day/m^2)
17β Estradiol	50	37	61	580
Estrone	12	16	80	1050
Estriol	0.3	1	91	1100
Estrone sulfate	0	0	99	80
Equilin sulfate	0			175

RBA, relative binding affinity (testosterone, 100%)
SHBG, Sex hormone binding glovulin

Estrogens are metabolized by estrogen 2/4-hydroxylase (CYP3A4) at positions ortho to the 3-phenolic group to form the 2-hydroxyestrogens and the 4-hydroxyestrogens (Fig. 46.4B). The resulting catechol estrogens bind to estrogen receptors (ERs) and produce weak to moderate estrogenic effects. These metabolites are unstable in vivo, however, and are rapidly converted to their 2-methoxy and 4-methoxyestrogen metabolites as well as to their glucuronide, sulfate, and glutathione conjugates. These metabolites are found in comparatively large amounts in the urine (9,10).

Estradiol is 37% bound to sex hormone binding globulin (SHBG) and 61% bound to albumin, leaving only 2% free in circulation (Table 46.3) (11,12). The affinity of estrone and of the sulfated esters of estrone and estradiol for SHBG is less than that that of estradiol; however, they are more tightly bound to albumin than estradiol is. These proteins are vital to the transport, distribution, and metabolic clearance rate of estrogens (13). In addition, estradiol is capable of inducing the synthesis of SHBG.

Mechanism of Estrogenic Action

Molecular interactions. Estradiol plays a key role in several physiological processes, including the development of secondary sex characteristics during puberty, stimulation of the mammary glands during pregnancy, and thermoregulatory capacity. Estradiol facilitates these processes via its biological target, the ER, of which there are two subtypes (ER-α and ER-β). The two receptors differ in size: ER-α is composed of 595 amino acids, and ER-β is composed of 485 amino acids. The expression and distribution of these subtypes is inconsistent between the various tissues and organs, which may explain the wide response that is observed (11). The predominant ER in the female reproductive tract and mammary glands is ER-α, whereas ER-β is found primarily in vascular endothelial cells, bone, and male prostate tissues. Expression of both ER-α and ER-β can be regulated hormonally via estradiol. Estradiol has similar affinities for both ER-α and ER-β (Table 46.4), which is not the case for certain nonsteroidal estrogenic compounds and antiestrogens (14).

Within each target cell are two receptor locations, one within the nucleus, where a genomic mechanism predominates, and a second within the cell membrane, where a nongenomic mechanism prevails. Unlike the nuclear receptors, the cell membrane receptors are coupled to G proteins that are linked to a cascade of intracellular signals. Nuclear ER-α and ER-β are virtually identical in their DNA binding sites but are only ~60% homologous in the C-terminal ligand binding domain (11,13).

When estradiol binds either ER-α or ER-β, the receptor protein is phosphorylated and undergoes a conformational change to produce either homo- or heterodimers (ER-α/ER-α, ER-β/ER-β, or ER-α/ER-β) (15). The dimeric ER complex then migrates from the cytosol to the cell nucleus, where it teams up with specific estrogen-response elements (ERE) found within an adaptor protein, typically a promoter, which aids in binding of the complex to estrogen activated genes (11,13). This complex also enlists a coactivator (CoA) complex to this promoter, which regulates DNA transcription (Fig. 46.5). Because the ER can interact with other nuclear receptors as well as with transcription factors, it is not easy to tease out all the factors that control estrogen-mediated biological responses.

Physiological effects. One of the principal actions of the estrogens is to promote the development of female secondary sex characteristics. These feminizing attributes include hair growth, skin softening, breast growth, and accumulation of fat in the thighs, hips, and buttocks. Estrogen also stimulates the growth and development of the female reproductive tract, including the uterine oviduct, cervix, and vagina.

Estrogens play a significant role in breast tissue as well. Considerable research has focused on understanding

Table 46.4. Relative Binding Affinities of Endogenous and Exogenous Estrogens (14)

Estrogen	ER-α Binding Affinity	ER-β Binding Affinity
17β-estradiol	100	100
Estrone	60	37
Estrone sulfate	<1	<1
Estriol	14	21
Coumestrol	94	185
Genistein	5	36
Tamoxifen	7	6
Clomiphene	25	12
Diethylstilbestrol	468	295

ER, estrogen receptor.

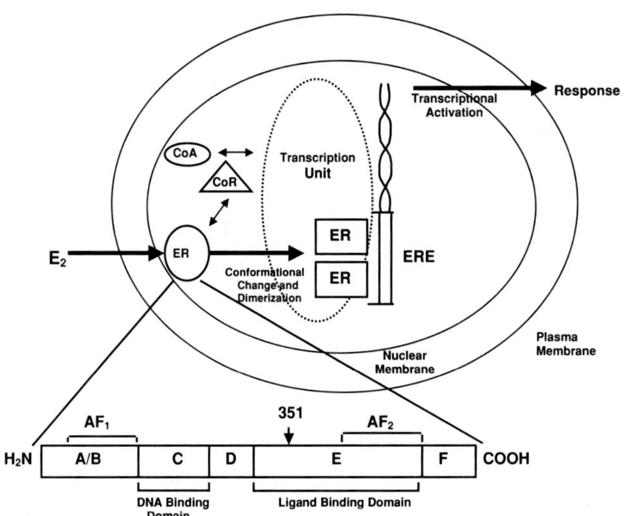

Fig. 46.5. A subcellular model of estradiol (E_2) action in a target tissue. The abbreviations used are as described in the text.

breast cancer and the factors that influence its growth. Estrogens serve as "fuel" for hormone-dependent mammary carcinoma and cause proliferation of breast cells. They also stimulate gene expression and, therefore, the production of several proteins, including those intracellular proteins important for breast cell function and growth as well as those proteins that influence tumor growth and metastasis. Some of these intracellular proteins include the enzymes needed for DNA synthesis, such as DNA polymerase, thymidine kinase, thymidylate synthetase, and dihydrofolate reductase (16,17).

Steroidal Estrogens

ESTRADIOL. Estradiol is the most potent endogenous estrogen, exhibiting high affinity for the ER and high potency when administered parenterally. When administered orally, estradiol is promptly conjugated in the intestine and oxidatively metabolized by the liver, resulting in its low oral bioavailability and therapeutic effectiveness.

ETHYNYL ESTRADIOL AND MESTRANOL. One method to increase the oral bioavailability of estradiol is to prevent metabolic oxidation of the estradiol C_{17} hydroxyl group to estrone. This is readily accomplished via alkylation of the C_{17} position with a chemically inert alkyne group (e.g., ethynyl estradiol [EE]) (Fig. 46.6). This synthetic analogue is several hundred-fold more potent than estradiol, with doses in the microgram rather than the milligram range (Table 46.5) (18). Following oral administration, EE is rapidly and almost completely absorbed, with an oral bioavailability of approximately 40% and an elimination half-life of 26 hours (Table 46.6). Ethynyl estradiol undergoes extensive first-pass metabolism to its 3-O-glucuronide and 3-O-sulfate metabolites and, via aromatic hydroxylation, to 2–hydroxyethynylestradiol and its O-methyl metabolites. Ethynyl estradiol undergoes extensive enterohepatic recycling. The bacteria in the GI tract hydrolyze the glucuronide and sulfate conjugates, thereby permitting reabsorption of EE. It is for this reason that a number of antibacterial agents have an adverse effect on oral contraceptive (OC) efficacy.

Another semisynthetic estrogen, mestranol, is the 3-O-methyl ether of EE (Fig. 46.6). Mestranol is a prodrug and, following oral administration, is rapidly metabolized to EE via hepatic O-demethylation. Mestranol and EE are used primarily in OC formulations (19).

ESTERS OF ESTRADIOL. To deliver estrogens with a longer duration of action, 17β-estradiol must be derivatized into an ester prodrug. In contrast to the ethynyl derivatives delivered orally, these estrogen analogues usually are administered intramuscularly. Slow hydrolysis of the ester releases free estradiol over a prolonged period of time. The therapeutically useful esters of estradiol include 17β-valerate and 17β-cyclopentylpropionate (cypionate) (Fig. 46.6). Estradiol cypionate is available as a sterile solution of the drug in oil (e.g., cottonseed oil), with a duration of action of 14 to 28 days. Estradiol valerate is available as a sterile solution in a vegetable oil (e.g., sesame oil or castor oil), with a duration of action of 14 to 21 days.

CONJUGATED ESTROGENS. Pregnant mares produce two unique estrogenic compounds, equilenin and equilin, that are excreted in the urine as sodium sulfate conjugates. These conjugated metabolites also are utilized as estrogen preparations (Fig. 46.7). Conjugated Estrogens USP is a mixture of the sodium salts of the sulfate esters of estradiol derived from equine urine or prepared synthetically from estrone and equilin. These preparations are composed of a mixture of sodium estrone sulfate (52.5–61.5%) and

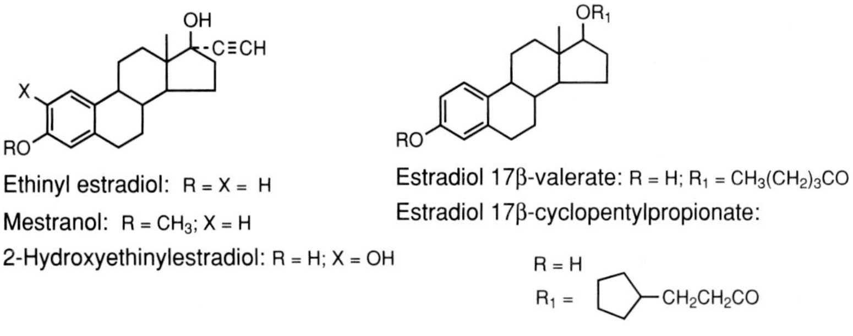

OH, C≡CH, X, RO

Ethinyl estradiol: R = X = H

Mestranol: $R = CH_3$; X = H

2-Hydroxyethinylestradiol: R = H; X = OH

OR_1, RO

Estradiol 17β-valerate: R = H; $R_1 = CH_3(CH_2)_3CO$

Estradiol 17β-cyclopentylpropionate:

R = H

R_1 = (cyclopentyl)$-CH_2CH_2CO$

Fig. 46.6. 17α-Ethynyl estrogens and estradiol esters.

Table 46.5. Potencies of Orally Administered Estrogens (12,13)

Type of Estrogen	FSH suppression	Serum SHBG suppression
Piperazine estrone sulfate	1.1	1
Micronized estradiol	1.3	1
Conjugated estrogens	1.4	3.2
Ethynyl estradiol	80–200	614

FSH, follicle-stimulating hormone; SHBG, sex hormone binding globulin.

sodium equilin sulfate (22.5–30.5%) as well as several lesser metabolites (e.g., 17α- and 17β-dihydroequilenin or 17α- and 17β-estradiol) as sodium sulfate conjugates. Esterified Estrogens USP is a blend of estrone sodium sulfate (75–85%) and sodium equilin sulfate (6–15%) (Fig. 46.7).

Synthetic Conjugated Estrogens A is a mixture of conjugated estrogens prepared synthetically from plant sources (i.e., soy and yams) containing a mixture of 9 of the 10 known conjugated estrogenic substances present in Conjugated Estrogens USP. Synthetic Conjugated Estrogens A is a

Table 46.6. Pharmacokinetic Properties for Some Estrogenic and Progestinal Agents[a]

Drug	Protein[b] binding	Oral Bioavailability	Biotransformation	Elimination half-life (hrs)	Time to peak conc. (hrs)	Peak serum conc.(ng/mL)	Elimination (%)
Estradiol	50–80%	Poor	Hepatic first pass metabolism	20 minutes		0.1–0.2	Renal: 90[d]
Ethynyl estradiol	98%	40%		26 (6–20)	1–2	33	
Progesterone							
Oral 200 mg micronized	>90%	<10%	Hepatic first pass metabolism	<5 minutes	2–4	24.3	Renal: 50–60[d]
IM 45 mg			Hepatic	10 weeks	28	39.1	Fecal: 10
IM 90 mg				19.6	9.2	53.8	
Vaginal gel 45 mg				34.8	6.8	14.9	
Medroxyprogesterone acetate: Oral 10 mg	>90%	High	Hepatic	30	2–4	19–35	Renal: 15–22[d]
IM 150 mg/mL every 3 months			No first-pass hepatic metabolism	50 days	3 weeks	1–7	Fecal: 45–80
Megestrol acetate							
Oral 160 mg	>90	ND	Hepatic	38 (13–104)	2–3	200	Renal: 66[d]
Oral 600 mg					2–3	753	Fecal: 20
Norgestrel	>90%	60%	Hepatic	20	24	ND	Renal: 45[d] Fecal: 32
Levonorgestrel 3/12/60 months implants 216 mg loading dose[d]	>90	60	No first-pass Hepatic metabolism	16 (8–30)	24	1.6 first week, then 0.26–0.4	Renal: 45[d] Fecal: 32
Desogestrel (Desogen) (as 3-keto-desgestrel)	>90	76	First pass to 3-ketodesogestrel active metabolite	12–58	1–2	2–6	Renal: 43[d] Fecal: 50
Norethindrone	>80	65	Hepatic first pass metabolism	8 (5–14)	0.5–4.0	5–10	Renal: 50[d] Fecal: 20–40
Norethindrone acetate	>80	65	Hepatic first pass metabolism	8 (5–14)	0.5–4.0	5–10	Renal: 50[d] Fecal: 20–40
Norgestimate as (desacetylnorgestimate)	>50–60 >90	60	First pass to desacetylnorgestimate	37	1–2	0.5–0.7	Renal: 47[d] Fecal: 37

[a]USP Drug Information 2000.
[b]Sex hormone binding globulin (SHBG) synthesis is stimulated by estrogens and inhibited by androgens; levels are twice as high in women as in men.
[c]Progesterone binds strongly to cortisol binding globulin (CBG; 17.7%) and SHBG (0.6%) and weakly to albumin (79.3%). Absorption is the rate-limiting step for the elimination half-life of Levonorgestrel: free, 1.1–1.7%; SHBG, 92–62%; and albumin, 37.56%; but suppresses SHBG by 33%. Norethindrone: free, 3.5%; SHBG, 35.5%; and albumin, 61%. Medroxyprogesterone does not bind SHBG. 3-Keto-desgestrel, 64%; albumin, 32%. Norgestimate >90% protein bound.
[d]A mean dose of 35 μg levonorgestrel is released daily.
ND, no data available.

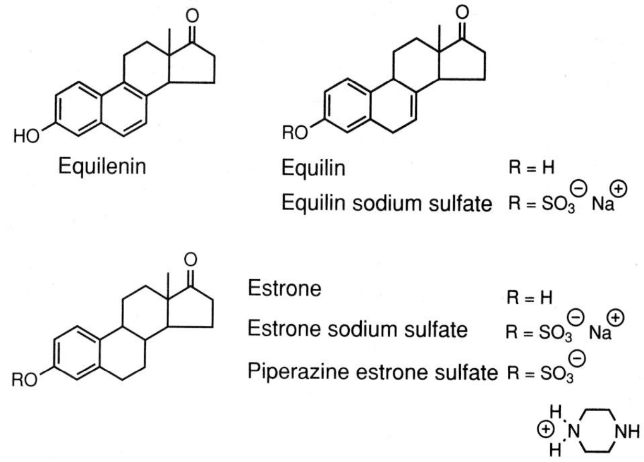

Fig. 46.7. Conjugated and esterified estrogens.

mixture of the sodium salts of estrogen sulfates, including estrone sulfate and sodium equilin sulfate.

Another sulfate conjugate that is orally effective is estropipate (piperazine estrone sulfate). This derivative has the same actions and utility as the conjugated, naturally occurring estrogens.

Nonsteroidal Estrogens

STILBENE DERIVATIVES. The steroid nucleus is not required for estrogenic action. Several derivatives of stilbene (diphenylethylene) that were used therapeutically demonstrate potent estrogenic activity. Diethylstilbestrol (DES), prepared in 1939, was one of these stilbenes (Fig. 46.8). A *trans* stilbene, DES has 10-fold the estrogenic potency of its *cis* isomer, largely because the *trans* isomer more closely resembles estradiol (20). Unfortunately, when DES was administered to relieve pregnancy-related symptoms, it was correlated with abnormal growth in the offspring.

Structure–Activity Relationships

As a result of numerous studies, there is an extensive body of knowledge regarding structure–activity relationships for estrogens (21–24). The aromatic A ring and the C_3 hydroxyl group are structural features essential for estrogenic activity. The 17β-hydroxyl, the distance between the C_3 and C_{17} hydroxyl groups, and the presence of planar hydrophobic scaffolding also are important structural contributors and help to optimize estrogenic activity. Ideally, the distance between the oxygen atoms of the C_3 and C_{17} hydroxyl groups should range from 10.3 to 12.1 Å.

Substitution of the estrogen steroid nucleus can significantly modify estrogenic activity. Functionality at the C_1 position greatly reduces activity, and only small groups can be accommodated at the 2 and 4 positions. Addition of hydroxyl groups at positions 6, 7, and 11 reduces activity. Removal of the oxygen function from position 3 or 17, or epimerization of the 17β-hydroxyl group of estradiol to the α-configuration, results in an estrogenic analogue that is less active (25). The equine estrogens contain one or two additional double bonds in the steroidal B ring (equilin and equilenin, respectively) (Fig. 46.7). The presence of this unsaturation substantially boosts the estrogenic potency of these estrogens. Substituents at the 11β position are tolerated; for example, 11β-methoxy or 11β-ethyl has significantly greater affinity for the ER as compared to estradiol.

Certain modifications at the 17α and 16 positions can lead to enhanced activity. For example, the 17α-ethynyl or 17α-vinyl groups provide the greatest activity, whereas highly polar substituents at this position are poorly tolerated. At the 16 position, moderate size and polarity are tolerated. Enlargement of the D ring (i.e., D-homoestradiol) greatly reduces estrogenic activity.

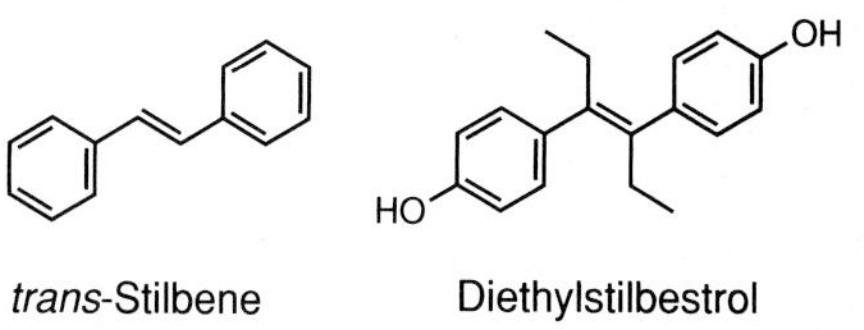

Fig. 46.8. Nonsteroidal estrogens.

Pharmacokinetics

The bioavailability observed varies with the route of estrogen administration. When administered subcutaneously, the order of bioavailability of the three naturally occurring steroids is estradiol > estrone > estriol. When administered orally, this order changes to estriol > estradiol > estrone (26). Although all three of these estrogens demonstrate at least minimal bioavailability when administered orally, chemical modifications have led to estrogen analogues with improved oral activity. For example, EE is a more effective oral estrogen because of its resistance to metabolism in the gastrointestinal tract and in the liver. Other types of highly active, orally bioavailable estrogen analogues include those with a labile ether (e.g., 3-(2-tetrahydropyranyl) and 17β-(2-tetrahydropyranyl) estradiol) (27). These drugs proved to be 12- and 15-fold as active, respectively, as estradiol.

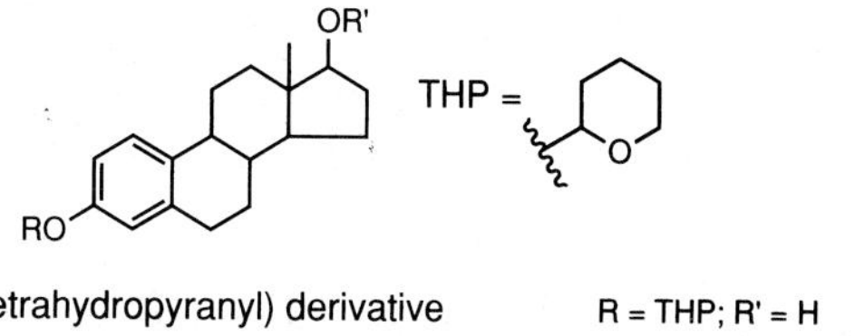

Estrogen Antagonists

Agents that antagonize the actions of estrogens are of particular interest for their contraceptive utility and for the treatment of estrogen-dependent breast cancer. There are three classes of agents that either interfere with estrogen activation of its receptor (e.g., impeded estrogens or triphenylethylene antiestrogens) or limit estrogen biosynthesis (e.g., inhibitors of aromatase).

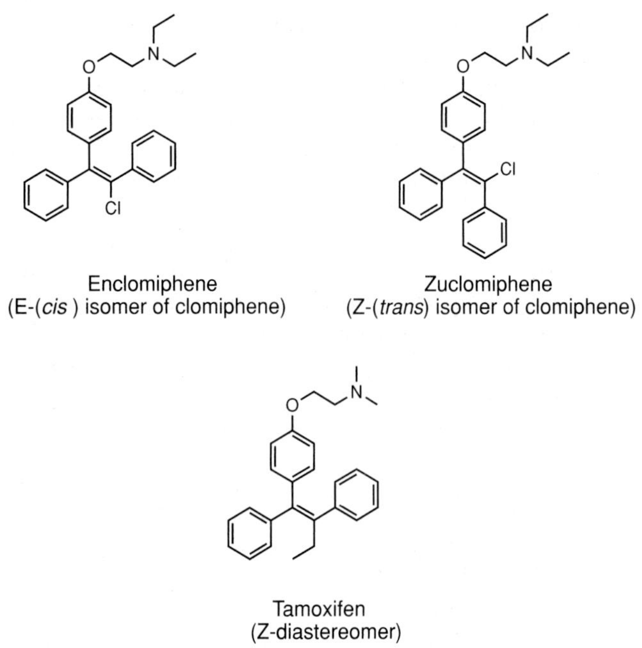

Enclomiphene
(E-(*cis*) isomer of clomiphene)

Zuclomiphene
(Z-(*trans*) isomer of clomiphene)

Tamoxifen
(Z-diastereomer)

Fig. 46.9. Antiestrogens—triphenylethylene analogues.

IMPEDED ESTROGENS. The impeded estrogens (e.g., estriol) interact with the ER in target tissues but dissociate from the receptor too rapidly to produce a significant estrogenic effect. If, however, the impeded estrogens are present in a high enough local concentration, they will compete with or impede estradiol access to its receptor site, thereby reducing the effect of estradiol on the cell (5,28).

ANTIESTROGENS—TRIPHENYLETHYLENE ANALOGUES. The triphenylethylene antiestrogens (Fig. 46.9) are structurally related to the stilbene family of estrogens and exhibit high affinity for the ER. They prevent translocation of the estrogen–receptor complex into the nucleus of target cells and interfere with the binding of the receptor–hormone complex to the acceptor site of the chromatin (29,30).

Advances in the molecular pharmacology of estrogen and ERs have led to the development of SERMs. These agents exhibit tissue-specific estrogen agonist or antagonist activity (31). The 3,4-dihydronaphthalene- and benzothiophene-containing SERMs are rigid analogues of the triphenylethylenes. The first SERM to be marketed for the treatment of osteoporosis was the benzothiophene raloxifene, an estrogen agonist at the bone (see Chapter 34). Discussion about the SERMs used in the treatment of breast cancer can be found later in this chapter.

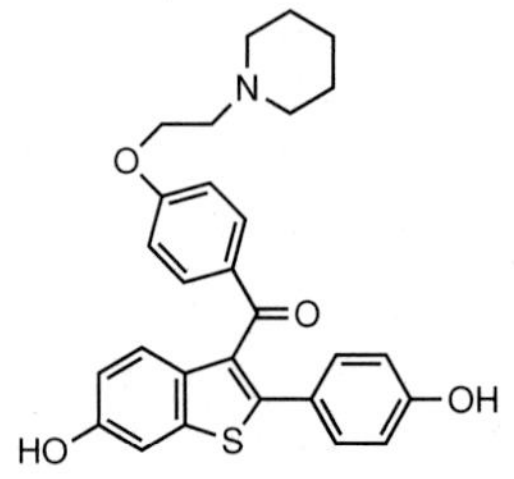

Raloxifene
(Evista)

AROMATASE INHIBITORS

Androstenedione Derivatives. Inhibitors of aromatase block the conversion of androgens to estrogens and, therefore, have the therapeutic potential to control reproductive functions and aid in the treatment of estrogen-dependent cancers, such as breast cancer. These steroidal agents compete with androstenedione for the active site of the aromatase enzyme. The structure–activity relationships for steroidal aromatase inhibitors indicate that the best agents are substrate analogues, with only small structural changes to the A ring and at C_{19} permitted (Fig. 46.10). Analogues

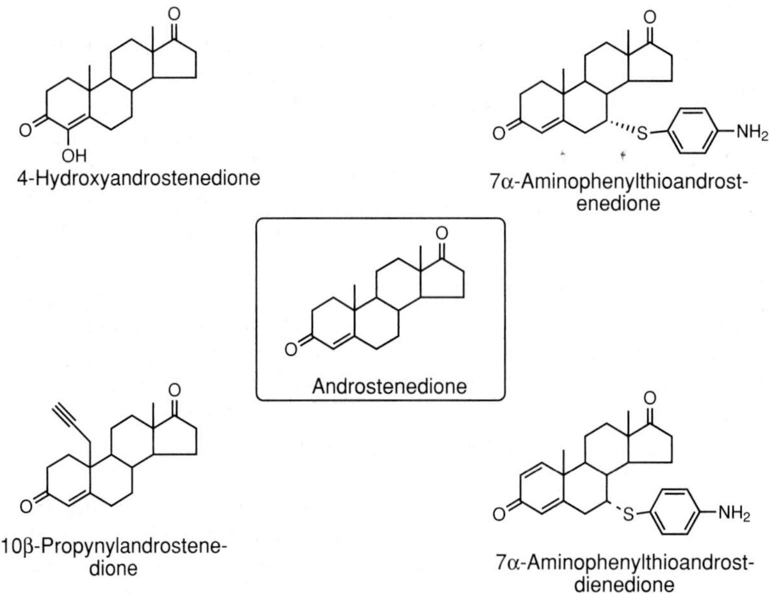

Fig. 46.10. Androstenedione aromatase inhibitors.

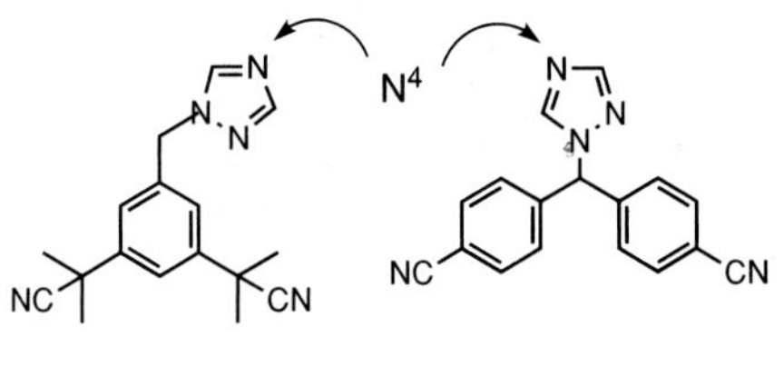

Anastrozole (Arimidex) Letrozole (Femara)

Fig. 46.11. Triazole aromatase inhibitors.

that contain aryl functionalities at the 7α position have enhanced affinity for the enzyme. In addition, 4-hydroxyandrostenedione, several androsta-1,4-diene-3,17-diones, and 10β-propynylestr-4-ene-3,17-dione act as enzyme-activated irreversible inhibitors (suicide substrates) in vitro. Additional information about the use of aromatase inhibitors in the treatment of breast cancer can be found later in this chapter.

Triazole Derivatives. Triazole based aromatase inhibitors were developed based on the aromatase inhibitor aminoglutethimide (32,33) and include anastrozole (34) and letrozole (35) (Fig. 46.11). The triazoles inhibit aromatase as a result of the N-4 nitrogen of the triazole ring interaction with the heme iron atom of this CYP19 enzyme complex. Anastrozole and letrozole are competitive inhibitors of aromatase and selectively inhibit the conversion of testosterone to estrogens in all tissues and, thereby, reduce serum concentrations of circulating estrone, estradiol, and estrone sulfate. Because estrogen acts as a growth factor for hormone-dependent breast cancer cells, reduction of serum and tumor concentrations of estrogen inhibits tumor growth and delays disease progression. Ovarian production of estrogen declines in postmenopausal women, so the conversion of androstenedione and testosterone to estrone and estradiol in peripheral tissues becomes the primary source of estrogen. The structure–activity relationships of these inhibitors have been reviewed elsewhere (36–38). Additional information about the triazole derivatives as it relates to the treatment of breast cancer can be found later in this chapter.

Clinical Applications

Estrogens are utilized in the treatment of a wide variety of menstrual-related disturbances, including the management of menopausal symptoms (e.g., vulvar and vaginal atrophy); female hypoestrogenism resulting from hypogonadism, castration, or primary ovarian failure; as well as amenorrhea, dysmenorrhea, and oligomenorrhea. They also are effective in the management of ovarian development failure, acne, and senile vaginitis. After childbirth, estrogens have been used to suppress lactation in those women who elect not to participate in breastfeeding. More detailed discussions about the clinical application of estrogens in the treatment of several disease states can be found later in this chapter.

Administration of estrogens may promote sodium retention and, as a result, cause retention of water and, possibly, edema. This effect, however, is less pronounced than that observed with the glucocorticoids. More detailed information regarding the pharmacology and toxicology of estrogens can be found in published reviews (5,21,39).

Progestins

Fraenkel (40) first observed in 1903 that removal of the corpus luteum shortly after conception resulted in pregnancy termination. In 1929, Corner and Allen (41) developed an assay method for progestogenic activity, and by 1934, the hormone progesterone had been isolated by several research groups (26).

Biosynthesis

Progesterone biosynthesis is initiated when LH, secreted from the anterior pituitary, binds to the target cell surface LH receptor. Activation of the LH receptor results in an increase of intracellular cyclic adenosine monophosphate (cAMP) levels via activation of a G protein and adenylate cyclase. In the presence of elevated concentrations of cAMP, cholesterol esterase activation occurs. This enzyme catalyzes the cleavage of cholesterol esters to free cholesterol, which is then converted in mitochondria to pregnenolone as described previously. The formation of progesterone from pregnenolone is catalyzed by 5-ene-3β-hydroxysteroid dehydrogenase and 3-oxosteroid-4,5-isomerase (steps c and d in Fig. 46.3).

Progesterone is secreted primarily from the ovaries (30 mg/day), particularly by the corpus luteum in reproductive-age women and by the placenta during pregnancy. Compared to the ovaries, the adrenal gland produces only a small fraction of progesterone (1 mg/day).

Metabolism

Progesterone is rapidly metabolized by the liver, regardless of the route of administration, and has a half-life of 5 to 10 minutes (Fig. 46.12). Progesterone is mainly excreted renally as the glucuronide and sulfate conjugates of 5β-pregnanediol. The glucuronide metabolite serves as an index of the corpus luteum activity, and a premature drop in its level may be a warning of possible miscarriage.

Other routes of metabolism include 6α-hydroxylation and reduction of the 20-ketone. These metabolites have no significant progestogenic activity. The formation of 5β-pregnanediol from progesterone is characterized by reduction of the 4,5-double bond to create a *cis* A/B ring juncture and reduction of the 3-ketone to a 3α-hydroxy group.

In the serum, progesterone is bound to either cortisol binding globulin or albumin, with only a small fraction being freely available. The metabolic clearance rate for progesterone is 2,100 to 2,500 L/day, for which protein binding has no role.

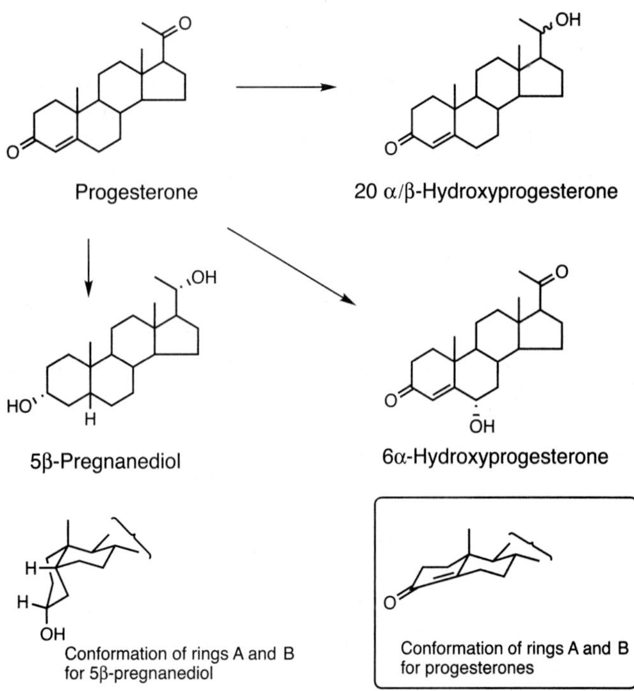

Fig. 46.12. Metabolism of progesterone.

Mechanism of Progestin Action—Molecular Interactions

The progesterone receptor is a ligand-activated transcription factor and a member of the nuclear receptor superfamily. All nuclear receptors have three conserved functional domains, including the DNA binding domain, the N-terminal domain, and the C-terminal ligand binding domain (42). Very little is known about the structure of the N-terminal domain. The DNA binding domain contains two asymmetric zinc fingers with four cysteine residues coordinated to each zinc atom. Between the zinc fingers is an α helix, which has specific interactions with the DNA. The ligand binding domain is composed of 12 α helices and four β sheets that ultimately form a hydrophobic cavity in which the receptor agonist binds (42). When progesterone binds to its receptor, a conformational change in the receptor occurs, transforming it into an active transcriptional factor. Phosphorylation of the receptor occurs at this point, but it is unclear what biochemical role that plays. The receptor then undergoes dimerization to form PR-A and PR-B, which are not structurally identical. These isoforms have similar activities as it relates to steroid hormone and DNA binding, but their functional activities are unique. The dimer interacts with specific nuclear DNA sequences (hormone-response elements) within progesterone-responsive genes. The receptor agonist–receptor dimer complex combines with coactivators that link the complex to gene transcription (43). The rate of gene transcription is then either increased or decreased. Once gene transcription is initiated, proteins are biosynthesized, and physiological effects are observed in target cells and organs.

Physiological Effects

The primary physiological site of action of progesterone is the uterus. It acts on both the endometrium (inner mucous lining) and the myometrium (muscle mass) of the uterus. The effect of progesterone on the endometrium, already primed by estrogens, is to induce the secretory phase of the menstrual cycle. During this phase, the endometrial glands grow and secrete large amounts of carbohydrates that can be utilized by the fertilized ovum as an energy source. The primary function of progesterone with respect to the myometrium is to stop spontaneous rhythmic contractions of the uterus.

Progesterone often is referred to as the "hormone of pregnancy." For the first trimester, the corpus luteum serves as the primary source of progesterone, at which point the developing placenta takes over as the major source of progesterone and estrogen. The high level of progesterone that is produced during pregnancy sends a signal to the hypothalamus via the negative feedback system to prevent release of the FSH and LH necessary for the development of new ova.

In general, the nonreproductive effects of progesterone are fairly insignificant. Progesterone is able to antagonize the actions of aldosterone, and as a result, there is an increase in sodium excretion. When sodium levels drop, aldosterone secretion is stimulated, and sodium is retained (44). It has been suggested that the temperature-raising effect of progesterone may be the result of a reduction in perspiration. This effect is not unique to progesterone, because other steroids in the pregnane and androstane series have a similar effect (45).

Ovarian biosynthesis and secretion of progesterone is controlled by the release of LH from the anterior pituitary during ovulation. The LH induces progesterone secretion from the corpus luteum during the second half of the menstrual cycle. If conception does not occur, the corpus luteum degenerates, and progesterone production decreases. As progesterone levels drop, endometrial sloughing occurs—otherwise known as menstruation.

Side Effects

Characteristic progestin-related side effects include nausea and vomiting, drowsiness, as well as breakthrough and irregular bleeding. With prolonged therapy, a greater incidence of these effects may occur, along with edema and weight gain, breast pain, decreased libido, and masculinization of the female fetus.

Structure–Activity Relationships

Progestin activity is restricted to those molecules with a steroid nucleus. The synthetic progestins generally can be divided into two classes of compounds: the androgens (19-norandrostane or estrane derivatives), and the 17α-hydroxyprogesterones (46–49). In the androgen series, a 17α-substituent, such as ethynyl, methyl, ethyl, and variations of these, provides oral bioavailability. Ethisterone (17β-hydroxy-17α-ethynylprogesterone) (see Fig. 46.14), the first androstane found to be effective, has only about one-third the activity of progesterone when delivered subcutaneously, but is 15-fold more active than progesterone when administered orally. Closely related to testosterone, this progestin has significant androgenic activity. Removal of the CH_3 group at position 19 leads to norethindrone (norethisterone) (Fig. 46.14), which has 5- to 10-fold more progestin activity. The activity of norethindrone is increased further by the addition of a chlorine substituent at position 21 (blocks metabolic hydroxylation) or by the addition of a methyl group at carbon 18 (norgestrel) (see Fig. 46.15). Ethynodiol acetate is an extremely potent oral progestin. It is more active when administered orally than parenterally and, when combined with an estrogen, is effective as an OC.

Progesterone

α-configuration

Further unsaturation of the B or C ring of 19-androstane derivatives usually enhances progestin activity. Introduction of a halogen or methyl substituent in the 6α or 7α positions generally increases hormonal activity. Acetylation of the 17β-OH of norethindrone increases the duration of action of the drug. Removal of the 3-keto function of norethindrone allows retention of potent progestin activity and no androgenic effects.

Activity of the 17α-hydroxyprogesterones is enhanced by unsaturation at C_6 and C_7 and by substitution of a methyl group or a halogen at C_6. This activity may be further increased by introducing a CH_3 group at C_{11}. These substitutions prevent metabolic reduction of the two carbonyl groups and metabolic oxidation at C_6. Substitution of a fluoro group at C_{21} prevents metabolic hydroxylation and enhances oral effectiveness.

Because glucocorticoid receptor activity is not desirable yet is innate to those derivatives that bind with high affinity to the progesterone receptor, structural alterations have been investigated to pare out this biological activity. Small B-ring substituents serve to decrease glucocorticoid action, as do substituents at the C_{17} position.

Synthetic Progestins

Early generations of the progestins were utilized primarily for contraceptive purposes, so antigonadotropic activity was considered to be desirable. Unfortunately, many of these agents were plagued by androgenic activity and the corresponding adverse effects (Table 46.7) (11). Development of newer progestins is now focused on analogues with improved progesterone receptor selectivity (Table 46.8) and little or no effect on the androgen, estrogen, or glucocorticoid receptors (43). From a structural perspective, these synthetic progestins contain either a pregnane or androstane steroid nucleus.

Androstane Pregnane

Not only can the progestins be classified structurally, they also can be organized by generation. The first-generation agents include 17-hydroxyprogesterone analogues (Fig. 46.13) as well as norethynodrel, norethindrone, and their derivatives (Fig. 46.14). Norgestrel and levonorgestrel are two of the predominant agents in the second-generation (Fig. 46.15). The levonorgestrel derivatives desogestrel, gestodene, and norgestimate compose the third generation (Fig. 46.16), and the new,

Table 46.7. Hormonal Activities of Representative Progestins (11)

Progestogen	Antiestrogenic	Androgenic	Antiandrogenic	Glucocorticoid	Antimineralo-corticoid
Progesterone	√√	0	√	√√	√√
Medroxyprogesterone acetate	√√	√	0	√√	0
Norethisterone (1)	√√	√√	0	0	0
Levonorgestrel (2)	√√	√√	0	0	0
Etonogestrel (3)	√√	√√	0	√	0
Norgestimate (3)	√√	√√	0	?	?
Drospirenone (4)	√√	0	√√	0	√√
Elcometrine (4)	√√	0	0	0	?
Nomegestrol acetate (4)	√√	0	√√	0	0
Trimegestone (4)	√√	0	√	0	√
Dienogest (4)	√√	0	√√	0	0

The number in parentheses indicates the generation of progestogen. √√, effective; √, weekly effective; 0, not effective;?, unknown.

Table 46.8. Steroid Receptor Binding Affinities (11,43)

Progestogen	Progesterone	Androgen	Glucocorticoid	Mineralo-corticoid
Progesterone	50	0	10	100
Medroxyprogesterone acetate (1)	115	5	29	160
Norethisterone (1)	75	15	0	0
Levonorgestrel (2)	150	45	1	75
Etonogestrel (3)	150	20	14	0
Norgestimate (3)	15	0	1	0
Gestodene (3)	90	85	27	290
Drospirenone (4)	35	65	6	230
Elcometrine (4)	136	0	38	?
Nomegestrol acetate (4)	125	42	6	0
Trimegestone (4)	330	1	9	120
Dienogest (4)	5	10	1	0

The number in parentheses indicates the generation of progestogen.

fourth-generation 19-norprogesterones include NES, nomegestrol acetate, and trimegestone (Fig. 46.17). In addition, there is one nonethynylated estrane, dienogest, and one spironolactone derivative, drospirenone, to round out the fourth generation (43). The antiandrogenic activity associated with several fourth-generation agents (e.g., trimegestone, drospirenone, and dienogest) makes this group of progestins unique (Table 46.7) (11). Trimegestone and elcometrine are the most potent progestins, with the third-generation levonorgestrel and etonogestrel (3-ketodesogestrel) being slightly less potent (Table 46.8).

Progesterone and Its Derivatives

Progesterone has a significant role in priming the uterine endometrium for implantation of a potential blastocyst. It also is involved in formation of the placenta postimplantation, the development of mammary glands, and by preventing contraction of the uterine musculature, pregnancy maintenance. Progesterone also has inhibitory roles, including ovulation prevention via an antigonadotropic effect and inhibition of the conversion of testosterone to dihydrotestosterone, an active metabolite, by virtue of its ability to be a substrate for 5α-reductase (43). Interestingly, progesterone reduces nuclear estradiol receptor levels and induces 17-hydroxysteroid dehydrogenase, the enzyme that catalyzes the conversion of estradiol to the less potent estrone (50).

There are some limitations as to how progesterone can be administered, because it has relatively low bioavailability when administered orally. The pharmacokinetics for progesterone and its derivatives are listed in Table 46.6. To achieve consistent therapeutic benefit, progesterone must be administered either by injection or intravaginally. Progesterone may need to be administered over a relatively long period of time to maintain a

Medroxyprogesterone acetate
Megestrol acetate
17α-Acetoxyprogesterone

Fig. 46.13. Progesterone and its derivatives.

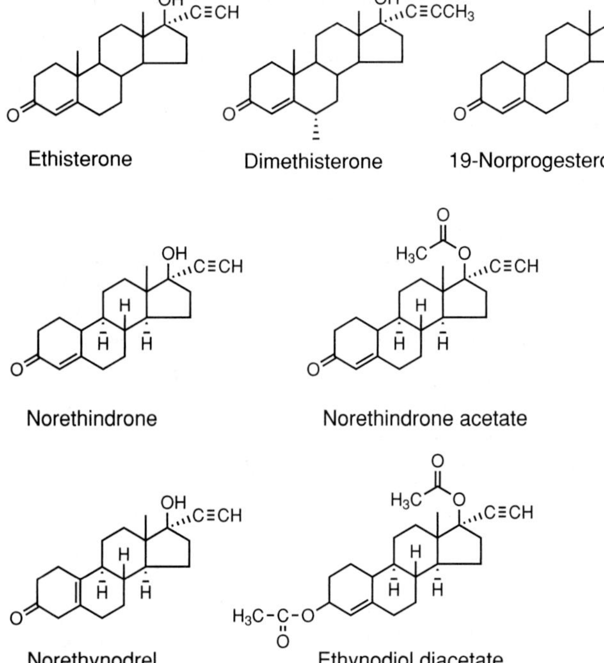

Fig. 46.14. Progestins and norethisterone/norethindrone-related, 19-nortestosterone androstanes.

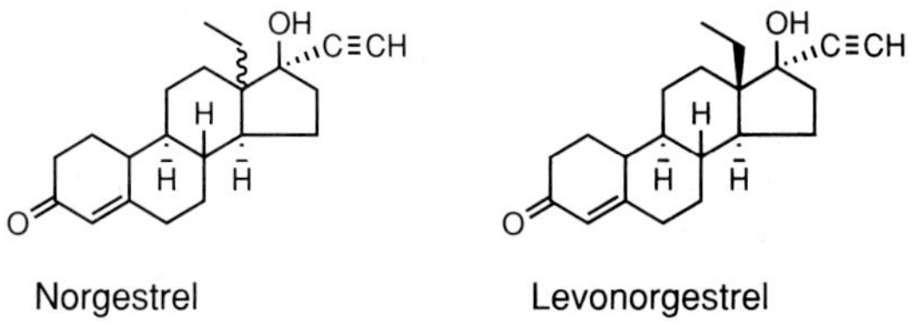

Fig. 46.15. Norgestrel and levonorgestrel.

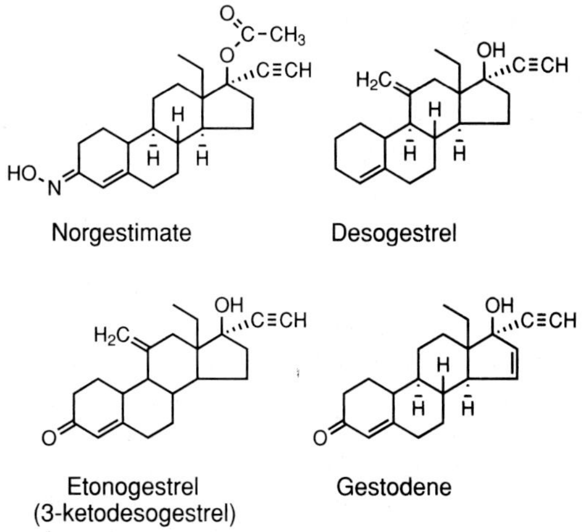

Fig. 46.16. Levonorgestrel-related, 19-nortesterone androstanes.

pregnancy, so it is important to note that neither of the two routes just mentioned is without significant adverse effects. As a result, development of orally active derivatives has been a significant priority.

MEDROXYPROGESTERONE ACETATE. The initial structural modifications made to progesterone led to only weakly active or inactive analogues. For example, 17α-acetoxyprogesterone had limited activity when administered orally (51). Further structural modification of 17α-acetoxyprogesterone was aimed at limiting metabolic hydroxylation at C_6. This was accomplished by the addition of a C_6 substituent, and the resulting analogue displayed improved biological activity (48).

Among the first of these substituted 17α-acetoxyprogesterone analogues to be utilized therapeutically was medroxyprogesterone acetate, a 6α-methyl progesterone analogue (Fig. 46.13) (52). This analogue is 25-fold more active than ethisterone. Following oral administration, medroxyprogesterone acetate is completely and rapidly deacetylated by first-pass metabolism to medroxyprogesterone. Medroxyprogesterone is extensively metabolized via pathways similar to those for progesterone, except for 6α-hydroxylation. Most medroxyprogesterone acetate metabolites are excreted in the urine, primarily as glucuronide conjugates. Plasma protein binding for medroxyprogesterone is approximately 86%, primarily to serum albumin, with no binding to SHBG.

MEGESTROL ACETATE (MEGACE). Progestin activity is further enhanced when a double bond is introduced between positions 6 and 7, as is found in megestrol acetate (Fig. 46.13). Megestrol is used primarily in the treatment of breast and endometrial carcinomas and in postmenopausal women with advanced hormone-dependent carcinoma. Less than 10% of an oral dose undergoes metabolism. Several major metabolites appear in the urine (e.g., 2-hydroxy and 6-hydroxymethyl megestrol and their glucuronide conjugates).

Synthetic Progestins

ETHISTERONE AND ITS ANALOGUES. Ethisterone (Fig. 46.14), a 17α-ethynyl derivative of testosterone, is one of the first synthetic progestins to be used therapeutically. In 1937, this agent was synthesized from male sex hormones (androstanes) in an attempt to find an orally active androgen (53). Ethisterone later proved to be an effective oral progestin and became useful in the treatment of menstrual dysfunctions (49). Several molecular modifications

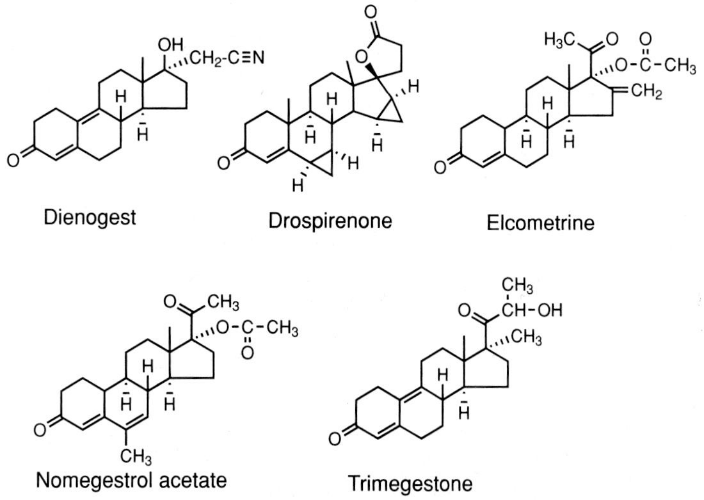

Fig. 46.17. 19-Norprogesterones (fourth-generation progestins).

of ethisterone have improved progestogenic action, including introduction of methyl groups in the $C_{6\alpha}$ and C_{21} positions (e.g., dimethisterone) (Fig. 46.14) (39).

A second breakthrough was made in 1944, when Ehrenstein (54) discovered that the C_{19} methyl group is not necessary for progestogenic activity. In fact, this work showed that loss of the C_{19} methyl results in analogues with activity equal to or greater than that of parenterally administered progesterone. In 1953, Djerassi et al. (55) synthesized 19-norprogesterone (Fig. 46.14). This drug differed from the natural hormone only in replacement of the C_{19} angular methyl group with a hydrogen atom. When administered parenterally, this analogue was eightfold more active than progesterone and, at the time, was the most potent progestin known.

NORETHINDRONE (NORETHISTERONE) AND NORETHYNODREL. Research on 19-norsteroids as potential progestins culminated in the synthesis of two potent, orally active progestins, norethindrone and norethynodrel (Fig. 46.14) (46). These two substances were among the first 19-norsteroids to be used clinically for progesterone-related disorders. When combined with estrogens, such as EE or mestranol, these agents were effective contraceptives. Because the progestogenic action of norethynodrel is approximately one-tenth that of norethindrone, it is no longer utilized in OC formulations. Although norethindrone is a weak androgen, it does not exhibit any glucocorticoid or antimineralocorticoid activity (Table 46.7).

Following oral administration, norethindrone acetate is completely and rapidly deacetylated by hepatic and intestinal first-pass metabolism to norethindrone, with an oral bioavailability of approximately 64%. Subsequent metabolism of norethindrone includes reduction of the Δ^4 double bond to both the 5α- and 5β-dihydronorethindrone products as well as reduction of the ketone. The pharmacokinetics for norethindrone acetate are indistinguishable from that of orally administered norethindrone. Roughly 36% of norethindrone is bound to SHBG, and 61% is bound to albumin (11).

Norethindrone acetate also can be administered transdermally along with estradiol when formulated as a patch. This combination of hormones can be utilized as part of either a continuous or a cyclic hormone replacement regimen.

NORGESTREL AND LEVONORGESTREL. Norgestrel is formulated as a racemic mixture despite the fact that only its levo isomer, levonorgestrel, is pharmacologically active (Fig. 46.15). Levonorgestrel exhibits some androgenic activity but no glucocorticoid or antimineralocorticoid action. Levonorgestrel can be administered orally, transdermally (combined with estradiol and formulated as a 7-day patch), and for prolonged, continuous use, via an intrauterine device (IUD). The oral bioavailability of levonorgestrel is approximately 95% (11). From a protein binding perspective, 48% of an oral dose is bound to SHBG, and 50% is bound to albumin. Levonorgestrel undergoes metabolic reduction of its ketone and is hydroxylated.

NORGESTIMATE AND DESOGESTREL. Norgestimate (Fig. 46.16) is considered to be a pro-progestin (prodrug), because it rapidly undergoes a two-step metabolic transformation to form two active products, norelgestromine (levonorgestrel 3-oxime) and levonorgestrel (Fig. 46.15). Deacetylation occurs in the intestine and liver, whereas conversion of the 3-oxime to the corresponding ketone occurs primarily in the liver. Unlike the other progestins mentioned, norgestimate and its metabolites are not bound to SHBG.

Norgestimate exhibits high selectivity for the progesterone receptor and low androgenic activity as a result of a large drug-induced increase in the production of SHBG. As a component of both mono- and triphasic OC formulations, this progestin exhibits fewer androgenic side effects, including less of a detrimental effect on the patient's lipid profile and lack of significant weight gain (56). Rates of breakthrough bleeding were lower with a triphasic regimen including norgestimate compared to a monophasic regimen containing norethindrone acetate. Norgestimate is metabolized to norelgestromin, the primary active metabolite and the active progestin found in the contraceptive patch (Ortho Evra).

Desogestrel also is a prodrug and is rapidly metabolized in the intestinal mucosa and on first pass through the liver to its active metabolite, etonogestrel (3-ketodesogestrel) (Fig. 46.16). Following oral administration, the relative bioavailability for desogestrel is approximately 84%. Desogestrel also exhibits high selectivity for the progesterone receptor and low androgenic activity, and it does not diminish the beneficial effects of estrogen on the lipid profile. The rates of breakthrough bleeding are low with the monophasic desogestrel/EE formulation, which has improved therapy discontinuation percentages. Unfortunately, there is conflicting evidence regarding the risk of venous thromboembolism with these preparations, with some studies suggesting a twofold increase in risk (56).

GESTODENE. Unlike the other members of the third generation of progestins, gestodene is not a prodrug (Fig. 46.16). It exhibits nearly 100% oral bioavailability and excellent receptor binding affinity for the progesterone receptor. Because the SHBG level is considered to be a surrogate marker for venous thromboembolism (VTE) risk, it is important to note that an increase in SHBG levels is evident both in monophasic combination OC preparations (200–300% increase) and in triphasic preparations (150% increase) that contain gestodene (57). Both the monophasic and triphasic preparations also cause an increase in triglyceride and total cholesterol levels, although the increase is smaller in magnitude than those associated with desogestrel and norgestimate. An increase in high-density lipoprotein (HDL) levels was not observed (58). The effectiveness of a gestodene/ethynyl estradiol combination transdermal patch is currently under investigation.

DIENOGEST, DROSPIRENONE, ELCOMDETRINE, NOMEGESTROL ACETATE, AND TRIMEGESTONE. Classified as a testosterone-like, norethindrone-related progestin, dienogest is structurally unique in that it contains an estrane skeleton, a C_{17} cyanomethyl group that replaces the C_{17} ethynyl group, and Δ^9 unsaturation (Fig. 46.17). An effective OC preparation results when dienogest is combined with EE. Similarly, correction of menopausal symptoms results when dienogest is combined with estradiol valerate. Limited evidence suggests that this combination has a positive impact on cognition, which is in direct opposition to the Women's Health Initiative (WHI) study data regarding the combination of medroxyprogesterone acetate and conjugated estrogens.

Derived from spironolactone, drospirenone (Fig. 46.17) is the only progestin with antimineralocorticoid activity. Its affinity for the mineralocorticoid receptor is fivefold greater than that of aldosterone. Drospirenone has progestogenic action, but only 10% that of levonorgestrel. Drospirenone also has antiandrogenic action, because it blocks testosterone from binding to androgenic receptors but does not exhibit estrogenic or glucocorticoid receptor activity.

This androstane-based progestin has several distinctive functional groups: two cyclopropyl groups, one that

Table 46.9. Components of a Representative Set of Oral Contraceptives (64)

Trade Name	Estrogen	Progestin
Monophasic combination oral contraceptives		
Alesse	EE (20 μg)	Levonorgestrel (0.1 mg)
Loestrin-21/Loestrin Fe 1/20	EE (20 μg)	Norethindrone acetate (1 mg)
Yasminelle[a]	EE (20 μg)	Drospirenone (3 mg)
Yasmin	EE (30 μg)	Drospirenone (3 mg)
YAZ	Estradiol (20 μg)	Drospirenone (3 mg)
Loestrin-21/Loestrin Fe 1.5/30	EE (30 μg)	Norethindrone acetate (1.5 mg)
Lo/Ovral	EE (30 μg)	Norgestrel (0.3 mg)
Desogen	EE (30 μg)	Desogestrel (0.15 mg)
Ortho-Cept	EE (30 μg)	Desogestrel (0.15 mg)
Levlen	EE (30 μg)	Levonorgestrel (0.15 mg)
Nordette	EE (30 μg)	Levonorgestrel (0.15 mg)
Seasonale	EE (30 μg)	Levonorgestrel (0.15 mg)
Seasonique	EE (30 μg) days 1–84 EE (10 μg) days 85–91	Levonorgestrel (0.15 mg) days 1–84 Levonorgestrel (0.15 mg) days 85–91
Ortho-Novum 1/35	EE (35 μg)	Norethindrone (1 mg)
Modicon	EE (35 μg)	Norethindrone (0.5 mg)
Ovcon-35 (chewable)	EE (35 μg)	Norethindrone (0.4 mg)
Ortho-Cyclen	EE (35 μg)	Norgestimate (0.25 mg)
Demulen	EE (35 μg)	Ethynodiol diacetate (1 mg)
Ovcon-50	EE (50 μg)	Norethindrone (1 mg)
Demulen 1/50	EE (50 μg)	Ethynodiol diacetate (1 mg)
Ovral	EE (50 μg)	Norgestrel (0.5 mg)
Ortho-Novum 1/35	Mestranol (50 μg)	Norethindrone (1 mg)
Biphasic combination oral contraceptives		
Mircette	EE (20 μg) days 1–21 EE (10 μg) days 24–28	Desogestrel (0.15 mg) Desogestrel (0.0 mg)
Ortho-Novum 10/11	EE (35 μg) EE (35 μg)	10 tablets Norethindrone (0.5 mg) 11 tablets Norethindrone (1 mg)
Triphasic combination oral contraceptives		
Estrostep 21 and Estrostep Fe	EE 20/30/35 μg	Norethindrone acetate (1 mg)
Cyclessa	EE (25 μg)	Desogestrel (0.1/0.125/0.15 mg)
Ortho TriCyclen Lo	EE (25 μg)	Norgestimate (0.18/0.215/0.25 mg)
Triphasil	EE (30/40/30 μg)	Levonorgestrel (0.05/0.075/0.125 mg)
Ortho TriCyclen	EE (35 μg)	Norgestimate (0.18/0.215/0.25 mg)
Ortho Novum 7/7/7	EE (35 μg)	Norethindrone (0.5/0.75/1 mg)
Progestin-only agents		
Ortho Micronor		Norethindrone (0.35 mg)
Ovrette		Norgestrel (0.075 mg)

[a]Not yet approved by the U.S. Food and Drug Administration.
EE, ethynyl estradiol.

includes C_6 and C_7 and the other C_{15} and C_{16}, and a C_{17} lactone. When combined with EE, drospirenone is effective in a monophasic OC (Table 46.9). Additionally, drospirenone plus estradiol (Angeliq) is used in the treatment of various menopausal symptoms. The unique antimineralocorticoid activity of drospirenone effectively negates the side effects related to angiotensinogen production (causing an increase in sodium and water retention) associated with EE. Remarkably, within the first several cycles, women actually lost weight when utilizing this combination of hormones (43). Regrettably, this benefit was lost, and statistically significant weight gain occurred as the number of cycles approached 13 (56).

Elcometrine (Fig. 46.17) is a member of the 19-norprogesterone class of progestins. When administered subcutaneously (implant), intravaginally (vaginal ring), or transdermally, elcometrine is an exceptionally potent progestin. It is 100-fold more potent when administered subcutaneously than when delivered orally. Its oral bioavailability is only 10%, with a half life of just 1 to 2 hours because of rapid metabolism (11). The C_{16} methylene functionality substantially increases its affinity for the progesterone receptor. Elcometrine does not bind to the androgenic receptor and, therefore, does not possess either androgenic or antiandrogenic activity (11). Unfortunately, like medroxyprogesterone acetate, elcometrine has affinity for the glucocorticoid receptor, although adverse effects were noted only at exceptionally high doses. Because of its antiestrogenic action, elcometrine also can be administered transdermally along with estradiol as a treatment for menopausal symptoms (43). From a protein binding perspective, elcometrine does not bind to SHBG but, rather, to albumin (11).

Nomogestrol acetate (Fig. 46.17) is structurally similar to megestrol acetate but lacks the angular C_{19} methyl group. It has substantially better selectivity for the progesterone receptor and higher potency than medroxyprogesterone acetate. Nomogestrol acetate has potent antigonadotropic action and, therefore, is an appropriate progestin to use in an OC preparation. It exhibits no glucocorticoid, antimineralocorticoid, or androgenic activity; however, it does demonstrate significant antiandrogenic action (11). Like NES, this progestin is bound primarily to albumin. Like desogestrel, it does not diminish the beneficial effects of estrogen on the lipid profile (11).

Trimegestone, the most potent of the 19-norprogesterones, contains an unusual C_{21} hydroxyl group (Fig. 46.17). It has very high affinity for the progesterone receptor but only weak affinity for the mineralocorticoid receptor. Trimegestone displays no glucocorticoid, androgenic, or antiandrogenic action. This progestin undergoes metabolic hydroxylation to produce metabolites with substantial progestogenic action. Either alone or in combination with estradiol, trimegestone has shown favorable results regarding bone loss and bone turnover (43). Given with estradiol, this hormone replacement therapy (HRT) combination is effective in the treatment of postmenopausal symptoms regardless of whether it is administered continuously or as part of cyclic therapy. Like desogestrel and nomogestrel acetate, this progestin does not diminish the beneficial effects of estrogen on the lipid profile (11).

Progestin Antagonists

MIFEPRISTONE. An antiprogestin is a substance that competes with progesterone for its receptor and, ultimately, prevents progesterone from binding to and activating its receptor. Because progesterone is integral to the continuation of an early pregnancy, it is expected that antiprogestins will interfere with pregnancy maintenance. In 1982, the first antiprogestin, mifepristone (RU 486), was reported (59). Mifepristone was shown to interrupt early stages of implantation and pregnancy in humans (60). Following oral administration, mifepristone is rapidly absorbed, with a peak plasma concentration in approximately 90 minutes, an oral bioavailability of approximately 70%, and a terminal elimination half-life of 18 hours. It is 98% protein bound, primarily to albumin and α_1-acid glycoprotein. Mifepristone is metabolized primarily via CYP3A4 pathways involving mono- and di-N-demethylation and terminal hydroxylation of the 17-propynyl chain. The fact that approximately 83% of the drug is recovered in the feces and 9% in the urine suggests a biliary route of elimination. Mifepristone also demonstrates antiglucocorticoid activity (61).

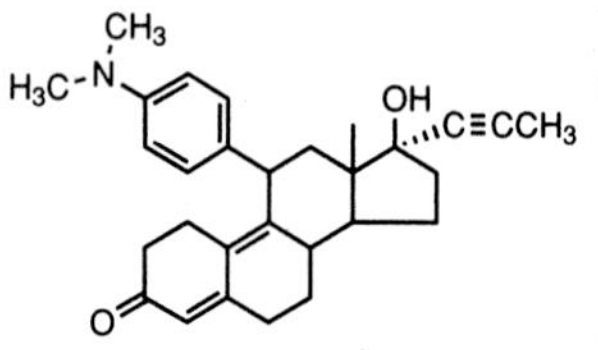

Mifepristone (Mifeprex)

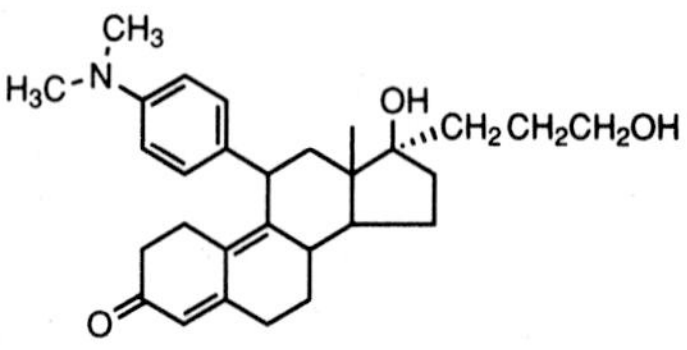

Onapristone

Additional antiprogestin analogues, such as onapristone (ZK 98,299), exhibit less antiglucocorticoid activity (62). These antiprogestins also have demonstrated therapeutic potential for the treatment of hormone-dependent breast cancer (63).

THERAPEUTIC APPLICATIONS

A woman's reproductive life cycle spans nearly four decades. During this time her hormonal status and ability to reproduce vary considerably. The need for hormonal intervention during this time period varies from person to person and, typically, requires highly individualized medication regimens. The remainder of this chapter will focus on hormonal and selected nonhormonal therapies for the treatment and/or management of contraception, endometriosis, infertility, menopause, and breast cancer.

Contraceptive Methods

Despite the availability of a wide variety of contraceptive methods and technologies, nearly half of all pregnancies in the United States are unplanned, and one-fourth are terminated. You might expect that cost, adverse effects, and inconvenience would be some of the hurdles to achieving contraceptive efficacy, but one of the greatest barriers is ineffective patient education (64). Despite ease of use, nearly 50% of those patients who have chosen an OC regimen discontinue their therapy within a year (65). If information regarding potential side effects, dosing requirements, and how the therapy is able to prevent pregnancy is provided in an accessible fashion, however, there may be many fewer patients who discontinue their contraceptive therapy (64,66,67).

Behavioral and Barrier Methods

Behavioral methods, such as natural family planning, fertility awareness, coitus interruptus, and lactation infertility, typically result in the highest pregnancy rates of all of the contraceptive methods. To be effective, these methods require disciplined effort on the part of the patient and her partner and somewhat detailed patient training. Barrier methods, such as male and female condoms, diaphragms, sponge (including nonoxynol-9 spermicide), and cervical caps, still require a very conscientious and often preplanned effort on the part of the patient as well as fairly detailed patient training. Unplanned pregnancy rates with these barrier methods are approximately 12 to 15%. Pharmacological contraception, including OCs, patches, vaginal rings, IUDs, and injectable medications, provides substantially lower pregnancy rates with diligent use, relatively limited patient effort, and patient education that is focused largely on adverse effects.

Combination Oral Contraceptives

Available since the early 1960s, most OC pills contain both an estrogen and a progestin component. The estrogen component, either EE or mestranol, suppresses FSH release and, therefore, prevents the formation of a dominant follicle during the follicular phase of the menstrual cycle. The dominant follicle is responsible for producing estradiol, which sends a negative feedback signal to the hypothalamus to prevent the secretion of additional gonadotropins and, therefore, prevent maturation of additional follicles. The estrogen component also is responsible for maintaining the stability of the endometrial lining (68). The progestin component, of which there are many available, suppresses the LH surge and, therefore, blocks ovulation.

In the more than 40 year evolution of OCs, the estrogen dose has dropped to one-sixth, and the progestin dose to one-tenth, of the original levels. This makes the newer OC agents substantially safer but also subject to adverse effects, such as irregular and breakthrough bleeding. In addition to these dosage changes, the progestin components have become progressively more selective in their binding to the progesterone receptor, thereby limiting the androgenic side effects that were characteristic of the older progestins (56).

OC agents are either monophasic or multiphasic in their hormone composition (Table 46.9). The multiphasic formulations more closely mimic the natural changes in both hormone concentrations that occur throughout the menstrual cycle. Most of the OC formulations are administered for 21 days, followed by 7 drug-free days to allow monthly withdrawal bleeding. Recently approved extended-cycle products, which allow the patient to experience only 7 drug-free days every 3 months, have efficacies similar to that of the standard 28 day regimen (Seasonale and Seasonique) (Table 46.9). Another nonstandard combination OC consists of estrogen plus progestin for 21 days, followed by 2 hormone-free days and then 5 days of EE (Mircette) (Table 46.9) (66). In Spring 2007 the FDA approved the first continuous regimen of low-dose EE and levonorgestrel (hybrel) that completely eliminates the menstrual cycle.

Two triphasic formulations that use a low dose of estradiol (25 μg) are currently under development. These formulations aim to minimize the side effect profile (e.g., breast tenderness, bloating, and nausea) and to maximize cycle control (e.g., minimal breakthrough bleeding). The formulation includes estradiol and a triphasic stair-step dose of either norgestimate or desogestrel.

A low-dose formulation was approved by the U.S. Food and Drug Administration (FDA) in early spring of 2006 (YAZ) (Table 46.9). This preparation is monophasic and is comprised of estradiol and drospirenone. The dosing regimen for this OC is comprised of 24 days of drug therapy, followed by 4 drug-free days to allow withdrawal bleeding. The 3-mg drospireneone component of this preparation is equivalent to 25 mg of spironolactone in terms of diuretic potential. Because of the diuretic action of drospirenone, the drug has the potential to cause hyperkalemia. Diminished fluid-related weight gain is an obvious advantage to this OC formulation, but caution is advised in patients with renal or adrenal insufficiency, with hepatic dysfunction, or who are receiving chronic pharmacotherapy that may increase serum potassium levels (e.g., angiotensin-converting enzyme inhibitors and potassium-sparing diuretics). This product joins a previous OC formulation that contains drospirenone (Yasmin) (Table 46.9). It should be noted that intracyclic bleeding (spotting) is more prevalent with EE doses of less than 30 μg, as is the case with these OCs. Studies have shown that the incidence of this adverse effect was greatest during the first cycle of OC use and diminished to very low incidence within three cycles (69).

Although the adverse effects of OC therapy include an increased risk of stroke, acute myocardial infarction, and venous thromboembolic disease, the incidence of cardiovascular disease in this patient population (age, <35 years) is already low (66). In women older than 35 years, the natural incidence of cardiovascular disease increases, so these adverse effects become more important to consider. From a metabolic perspective, the primary adverse effect of the estrogen component is an increase in hepatic production of proteins, including those that enhance venous and arterial thromboembolism (70). In addition, the progestin component has an adverse effect on the lipid profile, including an elevation of serum triglyceride and a decrease in HDL levels. Generally speaking, the estrogen component of a combination OC balances out this negative impact on a patient's lipid profile. Neoplastic effects are associated with OCs as well, such as an increased risk of cervical cancer and a decreased risk of colorectal, endometrial, and ovarian cancers that persists long after the discontinuation of therapy.

Progestin-Only Oral Contraceptives

A few contraceptive formulations only contain progestins (Table 46.9). Their contraceptive effects are accomplished via several mechanisms. From a hormonal perspective, progestins are able to suppress ovulation by preventing midmenstrual-cycle LH and FSH peaks via negative feedback inhibition. They also thicken cervical mucus to prevent entry of sperm into the endometrial cavity as well as transform the endometrium into an unsuitable environment for embryo implantation. Although the progestins suppress ovulation, they only do so 60% of the time, which generally is not sufficient for young women. The progestin-only OCs are an appropriate choice, however, for older women in whom fertility is diminished, for those patients with contraindications to exogenous estrogen (e.g., smoking or high blood pressure), or for a lactating patient who is already experiencing prolactin-induced ovulation suppression (64). Unlike the combination oral agents, timing of administration is critical, because the effect of the progestin on the cervical mucus lasts for only 27 hours. If there is more than a 3-hour delay in the time of administration from the previous day, that dose is considered to be "missed," and additional contraceptive methods are recommended.

The first progestin-only "mini-pills" contained either norethindrone or norgestrel. Their adverse effect profile is limited, because there is no estrogen component to increase the risk of venous thromboembolism or other cardiovascular related risks. Agents that induce metabolic enzymes (e.g., primidone, carbamazepine, topiramate, rifampin, ritonavir, and St. John's wort) may decrease the efficacy of the mini-pills by reducing the circulating levels of hormone (71). Antibiotics do not alter the enterohepatic recycling of progestins as they do with estrogens.

Transdermal Contraceptive Patch

Despite the ease of administration of the OCs, poor patient adherence rates have fueled the development of several long-acting contraceptive formulations. The contraceptive patch (Table 46.10), containing a combination of norelgestromin and EE, is applied to the upper arm, abdomen, or buttocks once per week on the same day of the week for 3 weeks, followed by a patch-free week to allow withdrawal bleeding. After several weeks of therapy (several patches applied), the mean and steady-state serum concentrations were in the range needed for contraceptive efficacy (72). Despite the absence of first-pass metabolism with this route of administration, the EE component undergoes hydroxylation and is conjugated to the corresponding glucuronide and sulfate derivatives. Contraceptive efficacy is compromised with coadministration of various metabolic enzyme inducers. If more than 48 hours elapse between patch removal and administration, it is recommended to start a new 4-week cycle with the newly administered patch, and an additional method of contraception should be used for one week (73). The patch provides equivalent efficacy to the OCs; however, it may not be as effective for women who weigh more than 90 kg (74). The adverse effects associated with the patch are headache, nausea, breast and abdominal pain, and application site irritation.

Contraceptive Vaginal Ring

The vaginal ring, another long-acting contraceptive, continually delivers a low dose of etonogestrel and EE directly into the vagina (Table 46.10). The ring is inserted into the vagina by the patient and remains in place for 3 weeks. Again, 1 drug-free week allows appropriate withdrawal bleeding. Unscheduled removal of the ring is allowed, but the ring must be reinserted within 3 hours to ensure continued therapeutic efficacy (67). This formulation has comparable efficacy with the OCs yet provides continuous hormone delivery, thereby minimizing the side effects caused by the pulsatile delivery associated with oral

Table 46.10. Contraceptive Methods Using Nonoral Routes of Administration

Trade Name	Estrogen	Progestin	Route of Administration
Ortho Evra	EE (0.75 mg)	Norelgestromin (6 mg)	Patch
NuvaRing	EE (15 μg)	Etonogestrel (120 μg)	Vaginal ring
Lunelle[a]	Estradiol cypionate (5 mg)	Medroxyprogesterone acetate (25 mg)	IM
Depo-Provera		Medroxyprogesterone acetate (150 mg/mL)	IM (400–1,000 mg weekly)
Norplant[a]		Levonorgestrel (36 mg/rod)	6 Subdermal rods (5 years)
Jadelle		Levonorgestrel	2 Subdermal rods (5 years)
Implanon		Etonogestrel	1 Subdermal rod (3 years)
Uniplant		Nomogestrel acetate	1 Subdermal rod
Nestorone		Elcometrine	1 Subdermal rod (2 years)
Mirena		Levonorgestrel (52 mg)	IUD (5 years)

[a]Not available in the United States.
EE, ethynyl estradiol; IM, intramuscular.

dosing regimens (67,75). This formulation is not without adverse effects, including decreased libido, nausea, vaginitis, and breast tenderness.

Contraceptive Injectables

An intramuscular formulation that contains an aqueous suspension of medroxyprogesterone acetate and estradiol cypionate is available but is not currently marketed in the United States (Table 46.10). The 28- to 33-day dosing interval provides excellent contraceptive effectiveness. There are several advantages to this contraceptive method, including scheduled withdrawal bleeding and a quick return to a fertile state on discontinuation of therapy. The adverse effects are similar to those seen with other combination OC formulations, including headache, weight gain, decreased libido, and breast tenderness (67).

Progestin-Only Injectables

The issue regarding timing of administration all but disappears when a progestin injection is administered every 3 months. In this formulation, medroxyprogesterone acetate is an aqueous microcrystalline suspension (Table 46.10). The mechanisms by which this progestin accomplishes contraceptive efficacy are the same as those discussed previously for other progestins. Despite the ease of use, the continuation rate after a year of injections is less than 30%, largely because of the adverse effects, including irregular and heavy bleeding, amenorrhea, and infertility that lasts for 9 to 21 months after the last injection (64). Improved patient education concerning the potential side effects may be a simple solution to discontinuation of therapy.

Several subdermal implants are available that provide contraceptive efficacy for 1 to 5 years depending on the formulation (Table 46.10). These implants consist of progestins contained within individual rods that are surgically implanted into the upper arm. As indicated in Table 46.10, varying durations of action can be expected depending on the number of rods implanted. Currently, Norplant is not available in the United States, and Implanon has only received "approval" status by the U.S. FDA. These formulation is subject to the same adverse effects as other progestin-only methods.

Intrauterine Devices

There are two forms of IUDs: one that releases the progestin levonorgestrel (Table 46.10), and one that is copper-coated. Both devices are T-shaped and must be inserted into the uterus by a physician. These devices mechanically irritate the endometrium and create an inflammatory environment that is toxic to sperm and ova and is not conducive to embryo implantation (64), The copper coating further enhances this inflammatory response. The copper-based IUD can be used continuously for 10 years, whereas the progestin-containing device is only approved for 5 years of use (76). Although generally well tolerated, ectopic pregnancy and infection (related to device insertion or to the device itself) are two serious potential complications. Discontinuation of use often is a result of breakthrough and/or heavy withdrawal bleeding.

Emergency Contraception

Emergency contraception is defined as any method that prevents pregnancy after intercourse. This type of therapy is available in either combination or single-agent formulations. The progestin only pills contain either levonorgestrel (Plan B) or norgestrel (Fig. 46.14). The two combination regimens include EE along with each of these progestins. Typically, these agents are administered as one dose within 72 hours of intercourse, with another dose taken 12 hours later. Nausea and vomiting are common side effects. If the patient is hormone adverse, then insertion of a copper IUD within 5 days of ovulation (the earliest estimated date) will prevent implantation (77).

Mifepristone (Mifeprex) is a 19-nortestosterone–based antiprogestogen that competes with the endogenous agonist for the progesterone receptor (see previous discussion). If administered within 5 days of unprotected intercourse, it also will prevent pregnancy. Despite the presence of the bulky 11β-diethylamino phenyl group, mifepristone has higher receptor affinity than progesterone itself. It is not completely understood how mifepristone inactivates the progesterone receptor. Of note is that mifepristone and progesterone do not interact similarly with the ligand binding domain, such that in the presence of mifepristone, the conformational change that occurs in this domain is unique from that produced by the natural agonist (42).

Endometriosis

Endometriosis, a condition present in 1 of 10 menstruating women, is characterized by implantation of endometrial tissue outside the uterus, typically within the pelvic region (78,79). During a normal menstrual cycle, hormonal signals cause the endometrial tissues to thicken in anticipation of embryo implantation. If a pregnancy does not occur, then these tissues are shed, resulting in a monthly period. When endometrial tissues implant outside the uterus, they respond identically to those within the uterus, such that when hormones fall in response to a nonpregnant state, these tissues are shed—yet have no natural exit. This tissue may form cysts, which in turn may form scar tissue and/or adhesions. Typically, the presence of one or more of these elicits significant pain and discomfort, especially during menstruation. Because the resulting scars and/or adhesions can cause infertility (78), treatment should be sought if the patient wishes to have children.

The cause of endometriosis is not completely understood. Sampson's hypothesis in 1927 suggests that menstrual fluids flow back (retrograde) through the fallopian tubes, where the endometrial cells can then implant and grow. Another theory proposes that the bloodstream is responsible for transporting the endometrial cells to regions outside the uterus. A third hypothesis is that endometriosis is a genetically acquired disease and that environmental factors trigger disease initiation (78,79). One of the hypotheses currently gaining some strength involves the immune system. Abnormal B- and T-cell function is evident in endometrial lesions, as are abnormal levels of cytokines, growth factors, and interleukins (80). Regardless of the cause, the growth of these endometrial lesions are controlled by both estrogen and progesterone (81), which means that hormonal intervention is likely to be effective in the treatment of this condition.

Pharmacological Management

Treatment of endometriosis largely depends on the severity of the symptoms experienced by the patient. Characteristics of the pain experienced by patients include dysmenorrhea, pelvic and lower abdominal pain, and dyspareunia (81). The American Association of Reproductive Medicine has a four-tiered system to describe the severity of the endometriotic disease, ranging from stage I (mild) to stage IV (severe) (80). Pharmacological management looks to achieve two primary goals: pain management, and prevention/delay of disease progression. Nonsteroidal anti-inflammatory drugs (e.g., ibuprofen), which inhibit prostaglandin biosynthesis, may be sufficient to ease menstrual pain, but this pain may not be adequately managed even at the maximum dose. Endometriotic pain is directly related to the fluctuating levels of endogenous hormones. Clear evidence indicates that endometriosis-related symptoms improve substantially during pregnancy and after menopause. Because OCs chemically produce a "pregnant" state, one might expect this type of hormone therapy to be a viable treatment option.

Combination oral contraceptives. There are a number of hormone-based pharmacological options for the treatment of endometriosis. If a woman wishes to achieve complete cessation of endometriosis-related pain, a 3- to 4-month regimen using a combination OC is recommended. This forces the body into a chemically "pregnant" state, such that hormone fluctuations and ovulation cease. As a result, menstrual flow decreases, and the size of the endometrial implants diminish. No evidence suggests that one OC combination is more efficacious than another (80). After 3 to 4 months of continuous OC therapy, 1 drug-free week is required to allow withdrawal bleeding to occur. If daily administration is difficult for the patient to manage, then selection of one of several delivery systems that allow less frequent dosing (e.g., transdermal patch or vaginal ring) is appropriate. Cyclic dosing is more appropriate if the patient does not experience symptoms continually throughout the menstrual cycle. Adverse effects include nausea, headache, and breakthrough bleeding.

Gonadotropin-releasing hormone agonists. The GnRH agonists leuprolide, goserelin, and nafarelin down-regulate the hypothalamic-pituitary GnRH receptors, thereby limiting the secretion of FSH and LH and causing suppression of ovarian function (78,80). This creates an estrogen-deficient environment that prevents menstruation and reduces the size of wayward endometrial implants. These agents have enjoyed success in the treatment of endometriosis (85–100% success with 6 months of therapy), but they come with a price. The GnRH agonists generate a state of artificial menopause, which can cause classical vasomotor symptoms (e.g., urogenital atrophy and insomnia). Bone mineral density suffers substantially after prolonged use, so the duration of this type of therapy is limited to 6 months (82). One way to extend the duration of therapy is to coadminister agents that address these side effects. Suggested "add-back" therapies include a progestin alone (e.g., norethindrone), a progestin and a bisphosphonate (e.g., etidronate), or a progestin and an estrogen (e.g., conjugated equine estrogen [CEE]). The amount of estrogen that is added back is enough to counteract the side effects of the GnRH agonists but insufficient to cause endometrial tissue growth (80). A serious limitation to multidrug therapy is the considerable cost associated with these agents as compared to the OCs or progestin injectables.

Androgenic agents. Danazol, a synthetic analogue of 17α-ethynyl testosterone, induces amenorrhea, anovulation and endometrial atrophy via suppression of the hypothalamic-pituitary-ovary (HPO) axis (78,80). This causes an estrogen-deficient state, but it also causes an increase in androgen production. Danazol generally is not well tolerated because of its androgenic and anabolic side effects, including acne, decreased breast size, facial hair, weight gain, and oily skin (78,79). This type of therapy is not a viable option for women with liver disease or hyperlipidemia. Because danazol is teratogenic, it is recommended that effective contraception be utilized during treatment (78,80).

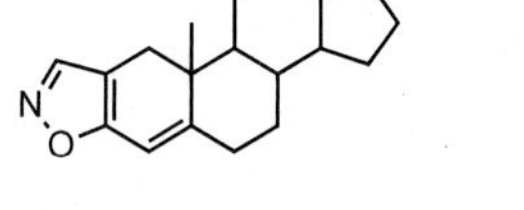

Danazol
(Danocrine)

Progestins. Medroxyprogesterone acetate (Fig. 46.13), administered by injection (Depo-Provera), orally, or delivered via IUD, effectively suppresses the HPO axis, induces anovulation, and reduces serum estrogen levels (83). This prevents menstruation and endometrial implant growth. As a result, endometriosis-related pain is minimized in approximately 90% of the patients. Drug therapy selection should reflect the fact that pharmacological therapy is likely to be required on a chronic basis. The progestins are fairly well tolerated and relatively inexpensive, but they are not without adverse effects, including nausea, breakthrough bleeding, weight gain, and mood swings, including depression.

Aromatase inhibitors. Normal endometrial tissues are devoid of aromatase activity. In patients with endometriosis, evidence suggests that high levels of aromatase are present in endometrial implants. Aromatase is the enzyme that catalyzes the conversion of androstenedione and testosterone to estrone and estradiol, respectively (Fig. 46.3). If an aromatase inhibitor, such as anastrozole (Fig. 46.11), is administered, then estrogen production will be decreased in the endometrial implants. A local state of estrogen deficiency will prevent growth of these implants (84). Unfortunately, one outcome of prolonged aromatase therapy is the development of osteoporosis. As a result, an OC typically is coadministered to provide baseline estrogen concentrations and limit the risk of osteoporosis.

Selective estrogen receptor modulators. To be effective in the treatment of endometriosis without therapy-limiting side effects, a SERM must behave as an estrogen antagonist at the endometrium and as an agonist at the bone. An investigational agent, TZE-5323, has antiestrogenic action by virtue of its ability to inhibit binding of estrogen to ER-α and ER-β and then limit subsequent transcriptional activation (85). This agent may prove to be beneficial in the treatment of endometriosis.

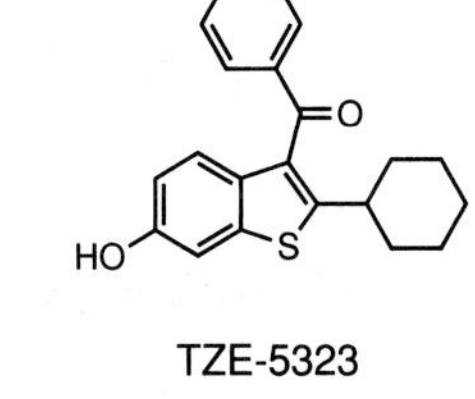

TZE-5323

Progesterone receptor modulators. Like the SERMs, the selective progesterone receptor modulators bind to the progesterone receptors and act as either an agonist or antagonist depending on the absence or presence of progesterone and the tissue that is being targeted. In the absence of progesterone, these agents demonstrate progestin activity. In the presence of progesterone, they exhibit antiprogestin activity in some target tissues, particularly the endometrium (81). Several investigational agents, including asoprisnil, have suppressed the growth of endometrial implants while estrogen concentrations remained at similar levels to those found during the follicular phase of the menstrual cycle (86). Asoprisnil undergoes metabolic O-dealkylation to an active metabolite.

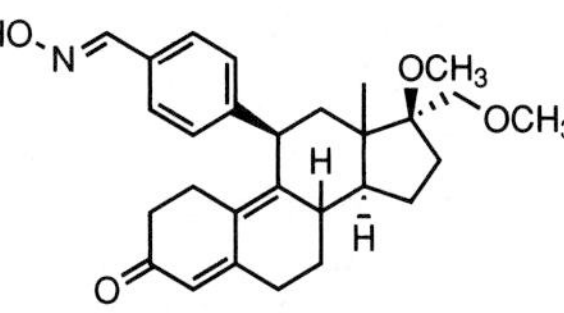

Asoprisnil

Surgical intervention. Laparoscopic surgical intervention to remove the endometrial implants is recommended for those patients who do not wish to utilize pharmacological methods because of their immediate interest in having children. It should be noted that as many as 20% of patients do not respond to surgical intervention. This results, in part, from a failure to identify and excise all the errant endometrial tissues (80). Adjunct therapy is not routinely utilized, because study data fail to consistently show efficacy (87).

Infertility

Infertility is not a disease state of the "individual" but, rather, often is considered to be a disease state of the "couple." Defined as the inability to conceive a pregnancy after 12 months of unprotected intercourse, infertility affects 10 to 13% of couples. Identification of the cause of infertility requires thorough medical histories as well as several diagnostic tests (Table 46.11) (88,89). The causes of infertility include ovulatory disorders as well as situations in which tubal factors, uterine factors, cervical factors, and/or immunologic and thrombophilic factors play a substantial role (Table 46.12) (90).

In 1994, nearly one-third of all first births were by women older than 35 years of age, an interesting statistic that highlights the recent trend to delay having children (88,91). With this delay comes an age-related reduction in fertility and the need to employ one or more pharmacological therapies to achieve a live birth. There have been more than 1 million babies born as a result of in vitro fertilization (IVF), with nearly one in three embryo-transfer cycles resulting in a live birth (92). Many infertility treatment options and protocols are available, most of which are highly individualized (Table 46.13) (89).

Intrauterine Insemination and In Vitro Fertilization

Intrauterine insemination (IUI) involves induction of ovulation, followed by transfer of motile sperm directly into the uterine cavity. This type of procedure is indicated if erectile dysfunction or male infertility (low motility, count, and/or poor morphology) has been identified, if the cervical environment is not conducive for effective sperm motility and/or sustenance, and if there are any physiological dysfunctions (93).

In vitro fertilization involves hyperstimulation of the ovaries to produce multiple mature follicles. Once the follicles reach 18 to 21 mm in diameter, hCG is administered, and within 34 to 36 hours, all the mature follicles are aspirated and their eggs removed from the ovaries. Depending on the couple, fertilization of the oocyte by the sperm may or may not require assistance. The resulting fertilized oocytes or embryos are then sustained and

Table 46.11. Infertility Medical Evaluation (88,89)

Male	Female
Fertility in other relationships	Previous pregnancies, fertility in other relationships; onset of menstrual cycle
Medication use	Medication use, including contraceptive use
Alcohol or recreational drug use, cigarette smoking	Alcohol or recreational drug use, cigarette smoking
Environmental exposure (e.g., sauna, hot tub), chemotherapy or radiation exposure	Environmental exposure (e.g., DES), chemotherapy or radiation exposure
Sexual dysfunction/frequency of intercourse	Frequency of intercourse
Semen analysis	Ovulation documentation
	Screening tests: pap smear, cervical cultures, mammogram, infectious disease screening
	Day 3 FSH levels (>10 mIU/mL = low rate of pregnancy)
	Thyroid panel, including TSH levels
	Fasting Prolactin levels
	Clomiphene citrate challenge test + FSH and estradiol levels (assess ovarian reserve)
	Hysterosalpingogram (assess tubal patency, shape of intrauterine cavity)
	Laparoscopy (assess endometriosis or if adhesions are present)
	Hysteroscopy (assess interuterine lesions or abnormalities)

DES, diethylstilbestrol; FSH, follicle-stimulating hormone; TSH, thyroid-stimulating hormone.

monitored for 3 to 5 days. Embryo characterization is performed daily to identify the most advanced embryos of good quality for subsequent transfer into the uterine cavity. Preimplantation genetic diagnosis can be performed with a single cell biopsied from each embryo that reaches the 6- to 8-cell stage by day 3. The genetic tests performed (only on 10 chromosomes) will help the physician and patient to identify those embryos with normal genetic makeup (including sex determination). Despite these advanced technologies and regardless of the age group the pregnancy rate does not exceed 50%, and the risk for multiple births is substantially higher than that observed in the general population.

Clomiphene Citrate (Clomid)

Clomiphene citrate is by far the most frequently prescribed agent to stimulate ovulation. It is administered orally as a mixture of two geometric isomers. The Z (*cis,*

Table 46.12. Infertility Classification and Causes (90)

Ovulatory Disorders	Characteristics	Therapeutic Regimen
WHO Class I		
Hypogonadotropic, hypogonadal anovulation	Low or low normal FSH, low estradiol due to decreased Gn-RH or pituitary not responding to Gn-RH	Weight gain, reduce exercise, pulsatile Gn-RH
WHO Class II		
Normogonadotropic, normoestrogenic anovulation	Normal gonadotropins and estrogens, FSH secretion during follicular stage is subnormal, includes women with PCOS	Weight loss, clomiphene with or without metformin, aromatase inhibitors
WHO Class III		
Hypergonadotropic, hypoestrogenic anovulation	Premature ovarian failure, ovarian resistance	
Hyperprolactinemic anovulation	Elevated levels of prolactin inhibits gonadotropin and therefore estrogen secretion	Dopamine agonists (bromocriptine)
Tubal Factor Infertility		Hysterosalpinogram, IVF, tubal reconstruction, laparoscopic surgery (endometriosis)
Uterine Factor Infertility		Leiomyoma, polyp removal
Cervical Factor Infertility		IUI, IVF
Immunologic and Thrombophilic Factor Infertility		Low dose aspirin and heparin, anticoagulation therapy
Unexplained Infertility		Clomiphene with or without IUI, gonadotropins with IUI, ART

ART, assisted reproduction technology; FSH, follicle-stimulating hormone; nGnRH, gonadotropin-releasing hormone; IUI, intrauterine insemination; IVF, invitro fertilization; PCOS, polycystic ovarian syndrome, WHO, World Health Organization.

Table 46.13. Representative Infertility Treatment Options (89)

Treatment Option	Patient characteristics	Pharmacological Therapy
Intrauterine insemination	Mild endometriosis Unexplained infertility Mild male factors	Clomiphene citrate (days 5–9), monitor LH levels
Ovulation induction	Ovulatory disorder PCOS Hyperprolactinemia Hypothalamic amenorrhea Premature ovarian failure	Progestin challenge test; gonadotropin therapy (hMG and/or FSH)
In vitro fertilization (with or without donor oocytes)	Tubal factor Severe endometriosis Unexplained infertility	Ovarian hyperstimulation, hCG
Therapeutic donor insemination	Women without partners Severe male factor	Sperm donor

FSH, follicle-stimulating hormone; hCG, human chorionic gonadotropin; hMG, human menopausal gonadotropin; LH, luteinizing hormone; PCOS, polycystic ovarian syndrome.

zuclomiphene)-diastereomer displays estrogenic activity, and the E (*trans*, enclomiphene)-diastereomer exhibits antiestrogenic activity (Fig. 46.9). Its ability to stimulate ovulation stems from its action at the hypothalamic ERs, where it serves to block these receptors and interfere with natural feedback inhibition. When an estrogen deficiency is perceived by the hypothalamus, it responds by secreting GnRH. This peptide hormone signals the pituitary to release the gonadotropins FSH and LH. Elevated FSH levels promote follicular development, which in turn causes the maturing follicles to secrete estradiol. Clomiphene is administered orally (50 or 100 mg) for 5 consecutive days, typically on days 5 to 9 of the menstrual cycle. Approximately 7 days after the last clomiphene tablet is taken, the hypothalamus finally is able to detect that estradiol levels are elevated, and it then signals the pituitary to secrete LH. This surge in LH causes the dominant follicle to rupture and release an egg, a process known as ovulation.

The clomiphene citrate challenge test is a diagnostic tool utilized to evaluate ovarian reserve in women older than 35 years of age. The protocol involves measurement of FSH and estradiol levels on day 3 of the cycle, followed by administration of 100 mg of clomiphene citrate on days 5 to 9 and measurement of FSH and estradiol on day 10 of the cycle. Elevated estrogen levels on day 3 are a good predictor of a poor pregnancy prognosis. Any FSH measurement that is high (>10 mIU/mL), even if other levels measured within the same cycle are within the normal range, is interpreted to mean a significantly limited reproductive potential because of poor ovarian reserve (88,91,94).

The adverse effects associated with clomiphene include thickening of the cervical mucus, which creates a substantial barrier for motile sperm. A postcoital test can be performed to determine if this, in fact, represents an insurmountable hurdle. If so, an IUI is warranted to bypass this cervical challenge. Another adverse effect is endometrial thinning, which is not conducive to embryo implantation; if this is the case, additional pharmacological therapies are recommended to thicken the endometrial lining. Other adverse effects include hot flashes and mood swings (95).

Women with low estrogen levels or hypothalamic disorders that result in irregular or absent ovulation are not candidates for clomiphene therapy. There is a 10% chance of having twins and a slightly higher risk of miscarriage in women stimulated with clomiphene (95). Clomiphene-based ovulatory stimulation should only be considered for a maximum of six cycles.

Clomiphene is readily absorbed from the GI tract following oral administration, with a half-life of approximately 5 days. It is metabolized in the liver, and its metabolites are excreted principally in the feces via enterohepatic recirculation.

Human Chorionic Gonadotropin (Pregnyl)

Human chorionic gonadotropin mimics LH both in structure and in function. It is produced by the placenta during pregnancy and is isolated from the urine of pregnant women. In the protocols for IUI or IVF, exogenous hCG must be administered to stimulate a scheduled ovulation. Between 36 and 72 hours after intramuscular administration, the dominant follicle ruptures and releases its egg. At that point, the scheduled IUI or IVF occurs. The hCG can be given in combination with clomiphene citrate to enhance ovulation (95). (For an in-depth discussion of hCG, see Chapter 7.)

Human Menopausal Gonadotropin (Reprondex)

Human menopausal gonadotropin (menotropins) is composed of equal parts FSH and LH and is derived from the urine of menopausal women. This type of therapy is utilized after clomiphene-based therapy has failed or if a patient does not produce sufficient levels of FSH or LH and experiences amenorrhea. These hormones directly stimulate the ovaries to develop multiple follicles per reproductive cycle (95).

Human menopausal gonadotropin has a substantial role in several IVF protocols. It typically is administered via injection (75 or 150 U) starting on day 2 or 3 of the menstrual cycle and is administered continuously (7–12 days) until shortly before the patient is ready to undergo follicle retrieval. The size and number of maturing follicles, as well as the patient's estrogen level, are closely monitored to maximize the number of follicles retrieved and to minimize the risk of ovarian hyperstimulation syndrome (OHSS) (95).

Adverse effects include injection site reactions and inflammation as well as the possibility of developing OHSS. Menopur, another formulation of menotropins that also contains equal parts FHS and LH, has been shown to cause fewer injection site reactions.

Follicle-Stimulating Hormone (Fertinex, Follistim, Gonal-F)

Two types of products are available that contain FSH. Fertinex contains FSH isolated from the urine of menopausal women and does not contain significant amounts of LH. Follistim and Gonal-F are products that contain only purified synthetic (recombinant) FSH. The recombinant products are more effective at stimulating the development of multiple follicles (92,93). All three agents are administered as a subcutaneous injection. Administration of exogenous FSH circumvents the influence of both the hypothalamus and the pituitary on the ovaries and causes direct stimulation of ovarian follicle growth. Women who fail to achieve pregnancy with clomiphene assistance or who are diagnosed with polycystic ovarian syndrome are candidates for this type of therapy (95). (For additional discussion of FSH, see Chapters 6 and 7).

Dopamine Agonists—Bromocriptine and Cabergoline

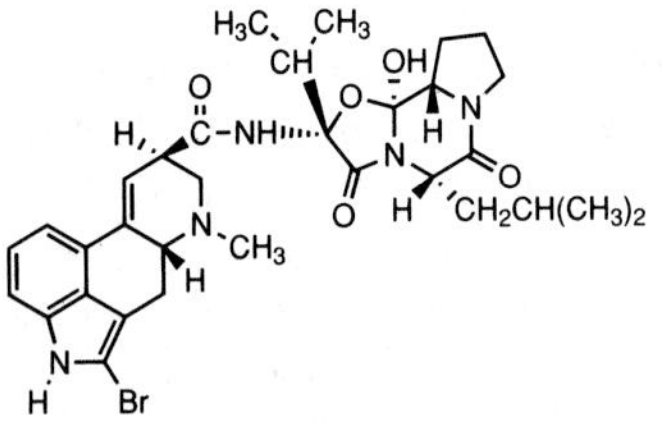

Bromocriptine (Pergonal, Parlodel)

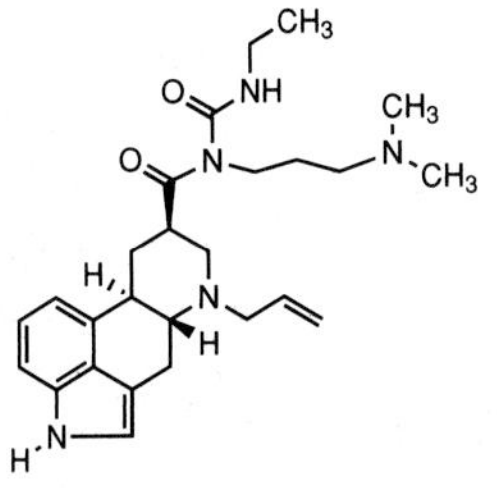

Cabergoline (Dostinex)

The hormone prolactin is responsible for stimulating the production of breast milk in mothers of newborns as well as for inducing lactation infertility. In this situation, FSH and LH secretion is inhibited; therefore, ovulation is prevented. In other populations of women, elevated levels of prolactin can result from the presence of an adenoma, a benign pituitary tumor, or because the pituitary cells that produce prolactin are hyperactive. This hyperactivity may have a pharmacological genesis (e.g., antipsychotics, tranquilizers, painkillers, and alcohol) or a pathophysiological origin (e.g., kidney or thyroid disease). Both bromocriptine and cabergoline suppress prolactin production. Bromocriptine is available as a tablet or capsule and is administered one to four times daily. It also is available as an intravaginal formulation. Cabergoline tablets are administered one to two times weekly. Once the prolactin levels drop to normal levels, the patient should experience improved fertility. If pregnancy is not achieved despite normal prolactin levels, then addition of clomiphene or gonadotropins is warranted (95).

Gonadotropin-Releasing Hormone

Gonadotropin-releasing hormone is secreted from the hypothalamus in a pulsatile fashion once roughly every 90 minutes. It is rapidly degraded by pituitary endopeptidases and has a circulatory half-life of 2 to 4 minutes. Degradation occurs primarily at the Gly^6 residue. Synthetic efforts to improve peptide stability have resulted in several successful GnRH agonists that contain hydrophobic D-amino acids replacing Gly^6 (96) (see Chapter 7).

When GnRH binds to and activates its pituitary cell surface receptor, it sends a signal for the pituitary to biosynthesize and secrete FSH and LH. This receptor is part of the family of G protein–coupled receptors and is composed of 7-transmembrane domains. Eventually, the receptor hormone complex is internalized, the ligand degraded, and the receptor partially recycled (96).

If a patient is unable to produce sufficient quantities of GnRH, then replacement therapy is available. To mimic normal secretion patterns, this hormone is delivered by infusion every 90 minutes via an external pump worn by the patient (95).

Gonadotropin-Releasing Hormone Agonists and Antagonists

Typically, GnRH agonists are administered continuously and not in normal physiological pulses. As a result of constant stimulation of the GnRH receptors, an initial hyperstimulation of the pituitary occurs, causing a surge in FSH and LH secretion, which is quickly followed by complete cessation of their release. Ultimately, this causes the production of estrogen and progesterone to stop, which prevents ovulation from occurring. In patients who do not have a regular ovulatory cycle, these medications are utilized to squelch all internal influence over ovulation. Once internal hormonal signaling has been silenced, human menopausal gonadotropin can be administered, permitting the physician exquisite control over the levels of pituitary hormones. With exogenous FSH and LH now present, follicle development is stimulated, and oocyte retrieval for IVF is possible. When used continuously, GnRH agonists stifle the natural LH surge associated with ovulation, so hCG must be administered 34 to 36 hours before oocyte retrieval to launch ovulation.

Several GnRH agonists are available, including leuprolide acetate (Lupron) and goserelin acetate (Zoladex), which are injectable agents, and nafarelin acetate (Synarel), which is administered via nasal spray. (Discussion about structure–activity relationships can be found in Chapter 7.)

Two GnRH antagonists, ganirelix acetate (Antagon) and cetrorelix (Cetrotide), are administered by intramuscular injection (95). The primary advantage of the GnRH antagonists over the agonists is that they interact with and effectively block the GnRH receptor without causing an initial surge of FSH and LH. The primary role of both the antagonists and agonists is to prevent a premature LH surge.

In an IVF cycle, the GnRH antagonist is not administered until the dominant follicle reaches 14 mm in diameter, which is nearly a week after gonadotropin therapy is initiated. The GnRH antagonists suffer from low solubility and the tendency to form gels in aqueous solutions (96). Ganirelix acetate has a short half-life and must be administered daily until hCG is administered, whereas cetrorelix has a longer half-life and can be administered once every 3 to 4 days (93). (Discussion about structure–activity relationships can be found in Chapter 7.)

Women whose ovulatory cycle has been managed by gonadotropin therapy have a 25% risk of multiple pregnancies. Some evidence suggests a lower pregnancy rate in patients utilizing protocols that include a GnRH antagonist (96,97). Adverse effects include injection site pain and inflammation, abdominal bloating, mood swings, and menopausal symptoms, including hot flashes and vaginal dryness. The likelihood of developing OHSS is fairly small in protocols that include GnRH agonists or antagonists. In these regimens, the physician has control over the hCG injection necessary to trigger ovulation and can delay—or even withhold—this injection if estrogen levels are too high, a factor that predisposes the patient to develop OHSS (95). It should be noted that GnRH down-regulation caused by these agents may have an adverse effect on oocyte quality, which has a negative impact on an IVF cycle (92).

As part of an assisted reproductive technology protocol, the use of both a GnRH agonist or antagonist and exogenous gonadotropins provides significant benefits, including enhanced stimulation of follicular development, improved oocyte quality, and LH surge suppression, all of which lead to fewer cycle cancellations and improved reproductive capability (92).

Lutropin alfa (Luveris)

Lutropin alfa is the first recombinant human form of LH approved by the U.S. FDA. This agent serves as LH replacement therapy for those women who are hypogonadotropic and hypogonadal with a substantial deficiency in LH (<1.2 IU/L). Lutropin alfa typically is utilized in combination with follitropin alfa to induce follicular growth and development. Both of these agents are administered subcutaneously.

The half-life of lutropin alfa is approximately 10 hours. Treatment should not exceed 14 days unless follicular development is clearly evident. Adverse effects include headache, breast and abdominal pain, and nausea. Lutropin alfa can contribute to the development of OHSS and should not be utilized in women primary ovarian failure or uncontrolled thyroid or adrenal dysfunction or who are pregnant.

Menopause

Physiologically, menopause is described as the loss of ovarian follicle function, followed by the cessation of menses. Before menopause, the body typically is engaged in a 2- to 4-year preamble, complete with the signs and symptoms of menopause (e.g., hot flashes and night sweats). This stage is termed perimenopause and is characterized by a gradual decline in the secretion of estrogen and progesterone. When the ovary no longer prepares follicles for ovulation and the resulting corpus luteum is not formed, a dramatic decrease in the production of estrogen and progesterone occurs, along with the resulting physiological changes, including bone loss, urogenital atrophy, and perhaps, incontinence, vasomotor symptoms, enhanced risk of cardiovascular disease, sexual dysfunction including decreased libido, as well as reduced skin elasticity (98). Many, if not most, of these changes have a negative effect on the quality of life for women during what is considered to be an exceptionally productive time in their lives. Identification of pharmacological and nonpharmacological methods to alleviate these symptoms is essential to improving quality of life during this turbulent hormonal phase at the end of a woman's reproductive lifetime.

History

As early as 1899, the Merck Manual listed several treatments for menopausal symptoms, including the drug Ovarin, which was composed of desiccated and pulverized cow ovaries flavored with vanilla. In 1932, this formulation was largely replaced by products that contained components isolated from the urine of pregnant women. By the late 1930s, these human-derived products were supplanted by Premarin, which contained components isolated from the urine of pregnant mares (99). Other formulations that take advantage of other routes of administration have been available for quite some time as well; for example, in 1928, the first estrogen patch was developed by Searle.

By the 1960s and 1970s, the first studies regarding serious adverse effects associated with estrogen therapy were reported, including severe hypertensive episodes and increased thromboembolic events. In 1978, the U.S. FDA mandated that a comprehensive warning be distributed with all estrogen products, including OCs. This document listed the approved indications and fully described the potential risks of using an estrogen-containing formulation. Despite these warnings, the use of estrogen-containing products actually increased as a result of the U.S. FDA notice that stated that these agents were effective for the prevention of osteoporosis (99).

Hormone Replacement Therapy

Until mid-2002, hormone replacement therapy (HRT) continued to be considered as first-line therapy for the pharmacological management of menopausal symptoms and for health preventive purposes in postmenopausal women. At that point, the results from the WHI study and, eventually, the WHI Memory Study (100) were released and clearly identified that although HRT (combination of 0.625 mg/day of CEE and 2.5 mg/day of medroxyprogesterone acetate) reduced the incidence of colorectal and endometrial cancers as well as hip fracture, it also increased the incidence of heart attacks, stroke, and breast cancer as well as increased global cognitive impairment (101). Ultimately, the U.S. FDA mandated that safety warnings appear on the package labels for both combination and estrogen-only products to warn women about these risks.

Medical management of menopause largely revolves around treatment of the symptoms caused by estrogen deficiency. Without regular maturation of ovarian eggs, follicles are not consistently formed and, therefore, do not consistently secrete the same levels of estrogen as found in premenopausal women. In postmenopausal women, the primary source of endogenous estrogen (albeit a fraction of that found in premenopausal women) comes from the transformation of androstenedione into estrone. Because the release of FSH and LH by the pituitary gland is governed by estrogen concentrations via negative feedback inhibition, it is no surprise that menopausal women have FSH levels 10- to 15-fold higher and LH levels four- to fivefold higher than those found in premenopausal women (50). In addition, low estrogen levels prevent launch of the normal LH surge that is key to follicular rupture, followed by formation of the corpus luteum. Because the corpus luteum is responsible for the secretion of progesterone, it is, again, no surprise that the levels of this hormone also are out of balance during menopause (102).

The vasomotor symptoms associated with menopause represent some of the most disturbing and, potentially, embarrassing menopause-related effects experienced by women. Since the early 1940s, estrogen replacement therapy with CEE (ERT) has been indicated for the treatment of these symptoms as well as for the treatment of urogenital atrophy and vaginal dryness. For those patients with an intact uterus, progesterone was administered along with the estrogen to prevent endometrial hyperplasia and endometrial cancer. This type of combination therapy is referred to as HRT. Nearly 90% of menopausal patients experience symptom relief after initiation of either ERT or HRT (Table 46.14) (103,104). Each patient requires individual dose titration to maximize menopausal symptom relief and to minimize side effects (e.g., breast tenderness, weight gain, and vaginal bleeding). Because of the WHI findings, HRT is considered as safe to administer if used short term and if dose reduction occurs after 2 to 3 years of treatment.

Despite the WHI findings, estrogen remains the gold standard in relief of menopausal symptoms. Recently, pharmaceutical manufacturers have concentrated on the development of alternate dosage forms that deliver the minimum dose of estrogen to minimize adverse effects, to maximize therapeutic benefit, and to maintain a more normal ratio of estrone to estradiol. These formulations include several different types of transdermal products, vaginal rings, and vaginal creams. The estrogens found in these products include estradiol, EE (synthetic), piperazine estrone sulfate, and conjugated estrogens. Unfortunately, these estrogens do not have identical potencies. Conjugated equine estrogens, esterified estrogens, and estrone sodium sulfate at 0.625 mg are equivalent to 1 mg of micronized estrogen, 0.75 μg of piperazine estrone sulfate, 5 to 10 μg of EE, or 0.50 μg of transdermal estrogen.

Although estradiol is the most potent endogenous estrogen, it has poor oral bioavailability. Oral administration of estrogen in a conjugated (e.g., estradiol valerate) or micronized (Estrace) form enhances absorption by the GI mucosa; however, when administered via this route, estradiol undergoes extensive hepatic metabolism (CYP3A4) to the corresponding ketone (estrone), which is much less potent. Only 10% of an oral dose of estradiol reaches the circulation (50). Estrone then undergoes sulfate conjugation to an inactive product. In effect, estrone sulfate represents a stable reservoir of circulating estradiol (12,13). Piperazine estrone sulfate (estropipate) also is quickly converted to estrone sulfate when administered orally. In premenopausal women, the physiological ratio of estradiol to estrone is 2:1, but after oral administration of estradiol, this ratio shifts substantially in favor of higher circulating estrone levels.

One mechanism to increase the oral bioavailability of estradiol is to prevent metabolic oxidation of the estradiol C_{17} hydroxyl group to the corresponding ketone. This is readily accomplished via alkylation of the C_{17} position with a chemically inert alkyne group (e.g., EE). This synthetic analogue is several hundred-fold more potent than estradiol, with doses in the microgram rather than the milligram range.

Conjugated equine estrogen, isolated from the urine of pregnant mares, currently is the most popular form of ERT. In addition to the ring-B saturated hormones already discussed (45% estrone sulfate), CEE also contains equilin estrogens that have an unsaturated B ring, including equilin sulfate (25%) and 17α-dihydroequilin (15%). Comparison between human and equine-derived estrogens yields nearly equivalent binding properties between equilin and estrone as well as similar metabolic fates (12).

Another method to keep the ratio of estrone to estradiol more equivalent is to utilize formulations that deliver estrogen via routes that are not subject to first-pass metabolism (e.g., transdermal, intravaginal, and intranasal). In addition, these routes permit ratios of estradiol to estrone similar to those found in premenopausal women (50). Transdermal formulations (Table 46.14) permits utilization

Table 46.14. Hormone Replacement Therapy for Treatment of Menopausal Vasomotor Symptoms (97,101,102)

Dosage Form	Trade Name	Estrogen	Progesterone
Tablets: estrogen only			
	Femtrace	Estradiol acetate	
	Premarin	Conjugated equine estrogens	
	Cenestin	Conjugated estrogens (plant derived)	
	Menest, Estratab	Esterified estrogen	
	Estrace	Micronized 17β-estradiol	
	Ortho-Est, Ogen	Estropipate	
	Enjuva[a]	Conjugated estrogens	
		$\Delta^{8,9}$-dehydroestrone sulfate	
Tablets: estrogen/progestin combination			
	Angeliq	Estradiol	Drospirenone
	Prempro	Conjugated estrogens	Medroxyprogesterone acetate (daily)
	Premphase	Conjugated estrogens	Medroxyprogesterone acetate (cyclic)
	FemHRT	Ethynyl estradiol	Norethindrone acetate
	Activella	Estradiol	Norethindrone acetate
	Ortho-Prefest	Estradiol	Norgestimate
Transdermal or percutaneous			
• Spray	Evamist[a]	Estradiol	
• Emulsion	Estrasorb	Estradiol	
• Gel	Estrogel	Estradiol	
• Patch (estrogen)	Climera	Estradiol	
	Estraderm	Estradiol	
	Vivelle	Estradiol	
	Vivelle dot	Estradiol	
	Ortho-Prefest		Norgestimate
• Patch (combo)	Menostar	Estradiol	Levonorgestrel
	Climera Pro	Estradiol	Norethindrone acetate
	Combipatch	Estradiol	Norethindrone acetate
Capsules			
	Prometrium		Micronized progesterone
Intravaginal delivery			
• Tablets	Vagifem	Estradiol	
• Cream	Estrace Vaginal	Estradiol	
	Premarin	Conjugated estrogens	
	Vaginal	Estropipate	
• Ring	Ogen Vaginal	Estradiol	
	Estring	Estradiol acetate	
• Gel (Controlled release)	Femring		Progesterone
	Crinone		

[a]Investigational agent.

of a lower drug dose and provides continuous systemic availability.

Intravaginal administration of micronized estradiol tablets (Table 46.14) represents another avenue for effective estradiol absorption without concern about first-pass metabolism (12). Unfortunately, vaginal creams containing estradiol only achieve 25% of the absorption expected for a similar oral dose. As a result, this formulation is best utilized for the treatment of urogenital atrophy. A sustained release depot formulation of estradiol is available in the form of a vaginal ring (Femring, Estring) (Table 46.14). This type of formulation elutes estradiol or estradiol acetate over a 90-day period, thereby limiting the effort required by the patient. Estring delivers 7.5 μg estradiol/day and is indicated for the treatment of urogenital atrophy. Available in two strengths, Femring releases the equivalent of 50 or 100 μg estradiol/day via estradiol acetate, which subsequently is hydrolyzed to estradiol after release. This ring is indicated for the treatment of several urogenital symptoms associated with postmenopausal atrophy as well as for the treatment of vasomotor symptoms as a result of delivery of sufficient systemic estrogen. Although easy to utilize, percutaneous preparations (topical emulsion, topical gel) (Table 46.14) suffer from inconsistent absorption. Estradiol also is formulated as an intranasal spray that is therapeutically equivalent to both oral and transdermal delivery.

In addition to those identified by the WHI study, the adverse effects of ERT include nausea, headache, breast tenderness, and heavy withdrawal bleeding. Transdermal delivery minimizes headache and nausea, and use of a low-dose oral regimen lessens breast tenderness (50).

Table 46.15. Combination Therapies for the Treatment of Menopausal Symptoms (50)

Type of Therapy	Effect of Therapy	Regimen
Oral continuous-cyclic (sequential)	Scheduled withdrawal bleeding	CEE (1-14) + [CEE + MPA] (15-28)
Transdermal continuous-cyclic (sequential)	Scheduled withdrawal bleeding	17β-Estradiol + norethindrone acetate
Oral continuous-combined	Prevents monthly bleeding; unpredictable breakthrough bleeding likely to occur for first 6–12 months	CEE + MPA, 17β-estradiol + norethindrone acetate, ethynyl estradiol + norethindrone acetate
Transdermal continuous-combined	Prevents monthly bleeding	17β-estradiol + norethindrone acetate
Continuous long cycle (cyclic withdrawal)	Reduced monthly bleeding	Estrogen administered daily, progestin given six times/year for 12–14 days
Intermittent-combined (Continuous pulse)	Prevents monthly bleeding	3 days of estrogen alone, followed by 3 days estrogen and progestin combo, repeat continuously

CEE, conjugated equine estrogen; MPA, medroxyprogesterone acetate.

Micronized progesterone (Table 46.14) in combination with oral CEE provides valuable therapeutic benefit in the treatment of menopausal symptoms without the risk of endometrial hyperplasia. Unless micronized, progesterone is poorly absorbed when administered orally (12). Intravaginal administration of a controlled-release progesterone gel (Table 46.14) results in excellent absorption and more consistent serum levels than orally administered micronized progesterone. Systemic absorption is limited when progesterone is delivered by this route. Intramuscular administration of a progesterone in oil formulation produces the highest serum concentrations but is least likely to be tolerated by patients. The adverse effects associated with the use of oral progestins include irritability, depression, weight gain, and headache. These can be minimized if other routes of administration are utilized (e.g., IUD).

To minimize patient effort and to maximize patient adherence, a number of estrogen/progesterone combination products are commercially available (Table 46.15). Four types of combination regimens are available (oral and transdermal), including both continuous and cyclic therapeutic options. Cyclic regimens require a minimum of 12 to 14 days of progestin administration to prevent endometrial hyperplasia.

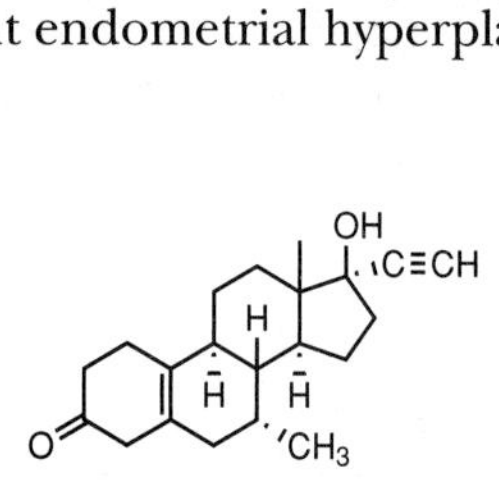

Tibolone

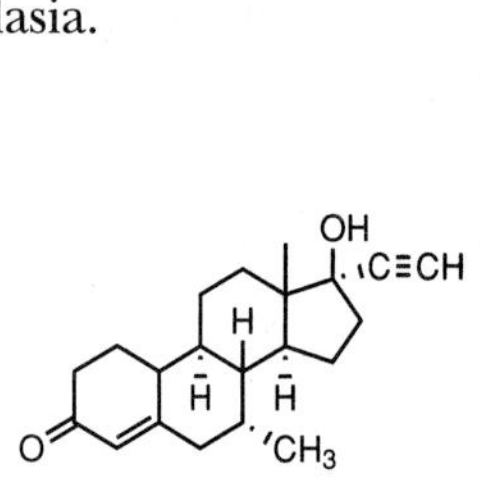

Δ^4 Isomer

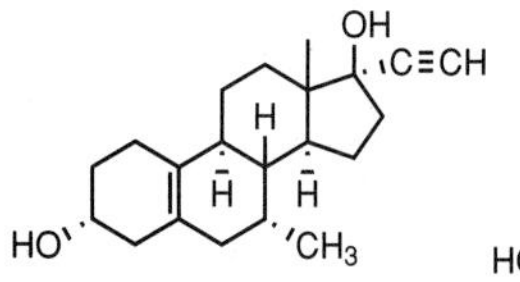

3α-Hydroxytibolone

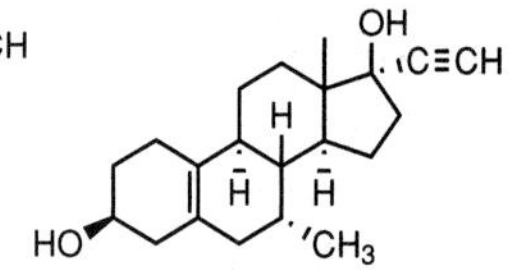

3β-Hydroxytibolone

Used in perimenopause, administration of a synthetic progestin supplements the waning progesterone produced in the luteal phase of the menstrual cycle. This helps to prevent endometrial hyperplasia and to ensure regular menses despite the irregularity of the menstrual cycle.

Tibolone is a synthetic 19-norpregnane with estrogenic, progestogenic, and androgenic action. With such varied activities, it is no surprise that tibolone is able to treat multiple psychological and physiological menopausal symptoms as well as to confer beneficial health preventive benefits. Administered as a prodrug, tibolone undergoes metabolism in the GI tract to active metabolites (Δ^4 unsaturated, 3α-OH, and 3β-OH derivatives). Although tibolone induces endometrial atrophy in menopausal and postmenopausal women and, therefore, does not cause withdrawal bleeding, it should not be used in perimenopausal women, because it can cause irregular bleeding.

With such concern and confusion surrounding the use of either ERT or HRT for the treatment of menopausal symptoms and postmenopausal health benefits, women have turned to other natural or nonhormonal pharmacological sources of relief (Table 46.16) (105,106). "Hormonal herbs," such as soy, black cohosh, and red clover,

Table 46.16. Nonhormone Replacement Remedies for Vasomotor Symptoms of Menopause (103,104)

Serotonin Based	Adrenergic Based	GABA Based	Herbals
Venlafaxine (SNRI)	Clonidine	Gabapentin	Soy
Paroxetine (SSRI)	Mirtazepine		Black cohosh
Fluoxetine (SSRI)			Garden sage
Citalopram (SSRI)			Dong quai
Sertraline (SSRI)			Kava
Mirtazepine			Valerian
			Red Clover
			Flaxseed

GABA, γ-aminobutyric acid; SNRI, serotonin and norepinephrine reuptake inhibitor; SSRI, selective serotonin uptake inhibitor.

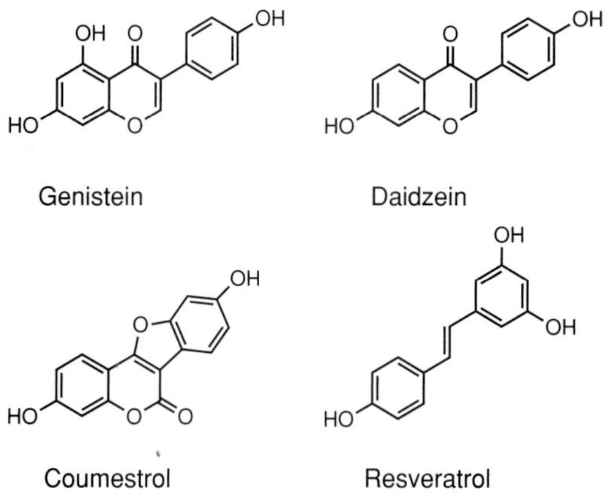

Fig. 46.18. Naturally occurring phytoestrogens.

are purported to contain some or all of the phytoestrogens genistein, daidzein, and coumestrol (Fig. 46.18), which possess at least weak estrogenic activity (Table 46.17) (105–107) but structurally are nonsteroidal. Other sources of nonsteroidal phytoestrogens, such as resveratrol from the skin of wine grapes (e.g., *Vitis vinifera*), currently are under investigation for their purported estrogenic effects (108). Small studies have indicated that the phytoestrogens may have additional beneficial effects on lipid profile and bone density (50). There is limited evidence that gabapentin and clonidine are effective in reducing the frequency of hot flashes, but their use is limited because of significant side effect profiles.

Several of the newer antidepressants, specifically those that modulate serotonergic neurotransmission, have become more prominent in the treatment of menopausal symptoms. Some even consider this as first-line treatment when hormone therapy is contraindicated. Venlafaxine, a dual serotonin and norepinephrine reuptake inhibitor, has been found to decrease the frequency and substantially reduce the intensity of vasomotor symptoms as well as to improve problems of fatigue and sleep difficulty in more than 50% of the participants in clinical trials (105,109). In comparison, fluoxetine and sertraline, which are selective serotonin reuptake inhibitors (SSRIs), only modestly improve the frequency and intensity of vasomotor symptoms. The effectiveness of paroxetine, another SSRI, mirrors that of venlafaxine. Interestingly, the SSRI citalopram not only is similarly effective as paroxetine but also is effective in those patients in whom vasomotor symptoms did not resolve with venlafaxine treatment. Mirtazepine is an α_2-receptor antagonist as well as a serotonergic (5-HT_2) antagonist. The role of serotonin in modulation of the thermoregulatory processes is only starting to become clear. New evidence indicates that activation of central 5-HT_2 receptors results in hyperthermia; therefore, administration of a 5-HT_2 receptor antagonist should alleviate the thermoregulatory dysfunction associated with estrogen deficiency (105). Interestingly, an endogenous estrogen deficiency causes a reduction in the expression of central 5-HT_2 receptors, which is reversible on administration of an exogenous source of estrogen. There are nonpharmacological avenues to consider when trying to limit the rise in body temperature, including avoidance of caffeine, alcohol, spicy foods, anxiety, and physical contact.

Hormone-Dependent Breast Cancer

Background and Introduction

In the United States, the lifetime risk of developing breast cancer is one in eight, with the greatest incidence in women older than 60 years of age (110). It is the second leading cause of death from cancer in women (lung cancer is number one). An evaluation of 51 studies that represented 52,000 women with breast cancer

Table 46.17. Herbal Products with Purported Utility in Postmenopausal Women (103–105)

Herb	Purported Use	Potential Problems
Soy (beans) *Glycine max*	Contains phytoestrogens—varied evidence for success in treatment of hot flashes	No concurrent treatment with tamoxifen
Black cohosh (root) *Actacea racemosa*	Contains phytoestrogens—purported use for hot flashes, additional studies needed	Possible liver issues
Sage (leaves, flowers) *Salvia officinalis*	Reduces night sweats and hot flashes	Kidney damage (large amounts)
Kava *Piper methysticum*	Reduces anxiety—no evidence for use in hot flashes	Liver damage
Red clover (leaf) *Trifolium pretense*	Contains phytoestrogens—not clinically significant reduction in hot flashes	Interaction with warfarin that can cause bleeding issues
Dong quai (root) *Angelica sinensis*	Not effective in treating hot flashes	Interaction with warfarin that can cause bleeding issues
Valerian (root) *Valeriana officinalis*	Treats hot flashes and insomnia	Morning drowsiness
Ginseng (root) *Panax ginseng*	May help with quality of life issues (mood, sleep) but does not help with hot flashes	
Flaxseed	No significant evidence that it helps hot flashes	Alters activity of antiplatelet and anticoagulant drugs

Menopause and Libido

Despite what you might gather from promotional ads on the television and radio, sexual dysfunction in women occurs much more frequently than in men. Regardless of age (18–59 years), the prevalence of a lack of interest in sex among U.S. women is approximately 30% (113). This loss of sexual desire, a general feeling of lethargy or loss of energy, and reduced muscle strength can be attributed largely to an androgen deficiency. Urogenital atrophy and a decrease in vaginal lubrication in postmenopausal women also are potential reasons for a woman to experience an arousal disorder. These symptoms are directly linked to an estrogen deficiency. Administration of an exogenous androgen, typically testosterone, eases some of these symptoms, but it is unclear if this is a result of androgen receptor activation or of conversion into estradiol. Testosterone can be administered via several routes, including intramuscularly, subcutaneously (implants), or transdermally (patches). Estrogen replacement therapy effectively manages vasomotor symptoms as well as urogenital atrophy and dryness and diminishes some of the psychological symptoms, but it has virtually no effect on the waning libido experienced by many menopausal women. A method to address both sets of symptoms is to administer an oral estrogen/androgen combination (Estratest [methyltestosterone + esterified estrogen]) daily (50). With this type of regimen, it is imperative that the testosterone dose only generates physiological serum testosterone levels so as to maximize therapeutic benefit and minimize undesirable side effects, including virilization and fluid retention (114).

Nonhormonal strategies also are available to treat female sexual arousal disorder. A transdermal formulation of alprostadil, used to treat male erectile dysfunction, has been shown to improve the arousal success rate. Applied 15 minutes before intercourse, this cream can cause local irritation, which is reversible on cleansing (115).

Menopause and Osteoporosis

Osteoporosis causes 1.5 million fractures annually, including hip and spine fractures that increase both morbidity and mortality. In women older than 50 years, one in six will experience a hip fracture, and only 40% of patients older than 55 years with a hip fracture actually recover their mobility (116). (A comprehensive review of pharmacological therapies available for the treatment and prevention of osteoporosis can be found in Chapter 35.)

The estrogen deficiency associated with menopause has a detrimental effect on bone composition and quality. Before 65 years of age, postmenopausal women lose 3 to 5% of their bone mass on an annual basis. After this point, bone loss occurs at a rate of 0.5 to 1.0% annually. This results, in part, from an increase in circulating cytokines (e.g., tumor necrosis factor α, interleukin-1, and interleukin- 6) when estrogen levels are low. These cytokines stimulate differentiation and proliferation of osteoclasts, the cells that normally degrade bone. The WHI study shows a positive correlation between HRT and a substantial decrease in fractures (24%). Currently, HRT (0.625 mg of CEE with 2.5 mg of medroxyprogesterone acetate) is recommended for the prevention, but not the treatment, of osteoporosis. This type of therapy should be initiated shortly after menopause and continued for at least 7 years (102). A lower dose of estrogen (0.3 mg) along with a progestin also may afford ample prevention. Despite the well-documented benefits of HRT in the prevention of osteoporosis, this should not be the primary therapeutic indication. In addition, no estrogen- or progestin-containing products have a U.S. FDA indication for the treatment of osteoporosis (99).

Studies that evaluate the benefit of combination OCs on bone mineral density have produced mixed results. Nearly one-third of these studies indicate no benefit, but the rest show a beneficial effect, including a 25% reduction of hip fractures in postmenopausal women (117). In those patients using a combination OC containing at least 50 μg of the estrogen component, this reduction in the risk of hip fracture improved to 44% (66). In general, the maximal benefits on bone mineral density are observed when the patients are older, have taken OCs for 5 or more years, and have used an OC preparation containing at least 50 μg of estradiol.

Climara Pro (transdermal patch with estradiol [0.045 mg/day] and levonorgestrel [0.015 mg/day]) is indicated for the treatment of the vasomotor symptoms related to menopause. Recently, it has been approved for the prevention of postmenopausal osteoporosis.

Tamoxifen and raloxifene are SERMs and represent effective nonsteroidal therapy for the treatment of breast cancer and bone loss, respectively. The SERMs are a unique drug class in that a single agent may act as a receptor agonist in select tissues but a receptor antagonist in other tissues. In theory, it might be possible to protect a woman from osteoporosis and to reduce her risk for endometrial, breast, and colorectal cancers without worsening menopausal vasomotor symptoms with one drug. To date, no SERM can meet all these goals simultaneously. Raloxifene, a second-generation SERM, is an estrogenic agonist at the bone and is very effective for preventing osteoporosis without negative endometrial consequences or increasing the risk of breast cancer (see Chapter 35) (50). It is classified as an antiresorptive agent and has been approved by the U.S. FDA for both the treatment and prevention of osteoporosis. It also has a beneficial role in reducing the risk of cardiovascular events in postmenopausal women because of its antiatherogenic effects (reduces low-density lipoprotein [LDL] levels) as well as in decreasing the risk of breast cancer (118). Unlike the bisphosphonates, which decrease both hip and vertebral fractures by 30 to 50%, raloxifene reduces only vertebral fracture by the same percentage. Raloxifene only has an effect on skeletal sites composed of cancellous bone. Unfortunately, raloxifene causes or worsens vasomotor symptoms in approximately 25% of patients, which represent a limitation to its use. In addition, raloxifene causes a threefold increase in the risk for venous thromboembolism, which makes it contraindicated in women with a history of thrombosis. Following oral administration, raloxifene undergoes rapid first-pass metabolism to form its glucuronide conjugates (see Fig. 35.4) and, thus, has an oral bioavailability (~2%).

Because raloxifene only reduces the risk of vertebral fracture, there is a need to identify agents that are effective at multiple skeletal sites with minimal side effects. The novel SERM HMR-3339 improves bone mineral density in adult ovariectomized rats at a variety of skeletal sites (e.g., lumbar spine, tibia, and femur), including those sites composed of cortical bone (118,119). An additional benefit afforded by HMR-3339 is a reduction in total cholesterol (10–15%) and LDL (10–24%). This antiatherogenic activity, coupled with promising reductions in fracture risk across multiple skeletal sites, makes HMR-3339 a very exciting drug candidate for the treatment of multiple postmenopausal conditions.

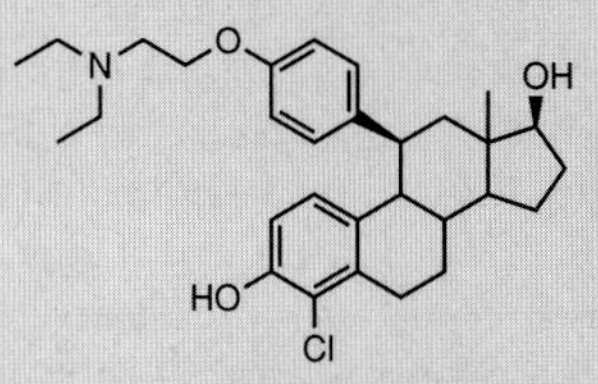

HMR-3339

Additional SERMs are presently undergoing clinical evaluation for treatment of osteoporosis and menopause-related vaginal atrophy (see Chapter 35).

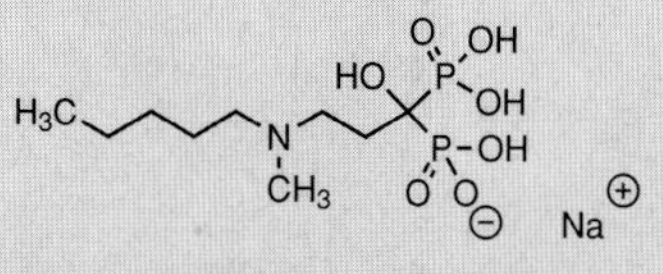

Ibandronate sodium

Ibandronate sodium (Boniva) is one example of the bisphosphonate class of antiresorptive agents and is effective in the treatment and prevention of postmenopausal osteoporosis (see Chapter 35) (120). It was first approved as a tablet (2.5 mg) to be administered daily and later approved as the first once-monthly formulation (150 mg) for the treatment and prevention of osteoporosis (120). In January 2006, the U.S. FDA approved an intravenous formulation of ibandronate sodium (3 mg) to be administered every three months for the treatment of osteoporosis. This type of formulation benefits those patients who have difficulty swallowing oral dosage forms or are unable to remain upright for 30 to 60 minutes. The injectable formulation generated a larger increase in lumbar spine bone mineral density compared to the oral formulations. Bone mineral density in the hip, femoral neck, and trochanter were improved as well. Adverse events associated with the injectable formulation included arthralgia, back and abdominal pain, and hypertension. There is a risk of renal toxicity that is inversely related to the rate of administration of this formulation. Caution is advised in patients who have renal impairment or who are receiving other pharmacological therapy that may negatively affect renal function (118).

showed a 15% increase in the risk of breast cancer in patients who had taken a combination of estrogen and progestin for less than 5 years. As treatment duration increased, this risk was amplified (111). In the HRT arm of the WHI study, the risk of breast cancer increased, yet in the ERT arm, there was no change in this risk (112). It should be noted that this increase in risk occurred 3 years after initiation of the study. To make matters worse, the breast cancers found in women of the HRT arm were likely to be more advanced than those found in women of the placebo arm of the study. Both arms of the WHI study were terminated prematurely, because the health risks incurred outweighed the benefits. No increased incidence of breast cancer was found in the ERT arm. The incidence of stroke did increase, however, and there was no benefit as it related to coronary heart disease (121).

According to the WHI study, there was no increased risk of endometrial cancer in patients taking HRT. If unopposed estrogen is administered to a patient with an intact uterus, then a significant increase in the risk of uterine cancer occurs within 2 years of treatment initiation (122). As the dose and duration of treatment increase, this risk grows.

Estrogen deficiency has been correlated with the development of colorectal cancer, the third most commonly diagnosed cancer. When estrogen levels are low, expression of the ER diminishes. Colorectal cells without ER expression are ripe to become cancerous. If estrogen levels are boosted by HRT, then ER expression should improve correspondingly, thereby reducing the number of colorectal cells primed to become malignant. The WHI study clearly shows a substantial decrease (37%) in the occurrence of colorectal cancer in patients treated with HRT.

Molecular Mechanism of Action of the SERMs

The precise mechanism of SERM action is not well understood, but clearly, the ER is a primary target, as a signal transduction pathway, to modulate drug action in different tissues. Different concentrations of ER are present in breast cancers, which can be explained by heterogeneity in the tumor cell population. The more cells in the tumor that contain ERs, the higher the overall ER content, and the more likely the tumor will respond to antiestrogen therapy. Approximately 60% of ER-positive (receptor-rich) tumors are responsive to any form of additive or ablative endocrine therapy, whereas only 10% of ER-negative (receptor-poor) tumors respond to endocrine therapy (123). The current standard of care is to determine the ER status of the tumor in all patients with breast cancer.

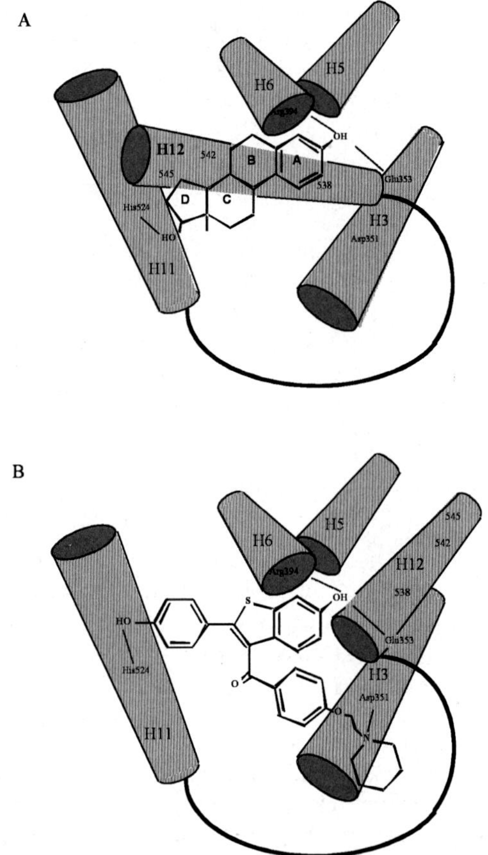

Fig. 46.19. Comparison of the binding of estradiol (A) and raloxifene (B) in the ligand binding domain of the human estrogen receptor (ER). The key event in estrogen action is the repositioning of helix 12 (H12) to seal the steroid into the hydrophilic pocket so that coactivators can bind at the key amino acids indicated on H12. This cannot happen in the raloxifene-ER complex.

The ER is divided into six regions (A–F, as shown in Fig. 46.5) (124). The DNA-binding domain (region C) is essential for the interaction of the ER with an estrogen-response element (125). The ligand-binding domain (region E) is the site of estradiol binding and the site of competitive binding by antiestrogens. The activating function (AF-1 and AF-2) regions are the areas of the ER that interact with coactivator molecules to form an effective transcription unit at an estrogen-responsive gene (126).

Crystallization of the ligand-binding domain (region E) of the ER with estradiol, DES, and raloxifene (127) as well as 4-hydroxytamoxifen (128) has provided an important insight regarding the conformational changes that occur with agonist or antagonist ER complexes. Figure 46.19 illustrates the crystal structure of the estradiol and raloxifene receptor complexes. The most important difference is the position of helix 12, which is essential for the correct binding of coactivators to form a transcription complex at an estrogen-responsive gene. Estradiol causes helix 12 to seal the ligand inside the hydrophobic pocket of the ligand-binding domain. It is hypothesized that this conformation allows coactivator binding. By contrast, raloxifene prevents helix 12 from sealing the hydrophobic pocket, and gene transcription is prevented (because coactivators cannot bind) (127). A similar model is proposed for the 4-hydroxytamoxifen ER complex, but it is clear from studies in vitro that the raloxifene– and 4-hydroxytamoxifen–receptor complexes have different efficacies (129).

The antiestrogenic and some of the estrogen-like actions of SERMs can be explained by the different conformations of the ER-α complexes attracting novel coactivators or corepressors (CoR) (Fig. 46.5) to modulate estrogen action at different sites. In this model, the receptor would be the same at each site, yet the coactivators and corepressors would be distributed differently at different targets (130).

Alternatively, ER-α could be modulated by different concentrations of ER-β at different sites. It has been suggested that ER-β could enhance estrogen-like gene activation through a protein–protein interaction at AP-1 (*fos* and *jun*) sites (131). At present, it is not entirely clear how SERM action is modulated at each target. Indeed, more than one mechanism may occur.

Selective Estrogen Receptor Modulators

Introduction. Lerner et al. (132) described the first nonsteroidal antiestrogen, ethamoxytriphetol (MER25) (Fig. 46.20). This compound is an antiestrogen, with no other hormonal or antihormonal action. Although MER25 behaved as a "morning after" pill in laboratory animals (133), clinical trials associated with other repro-

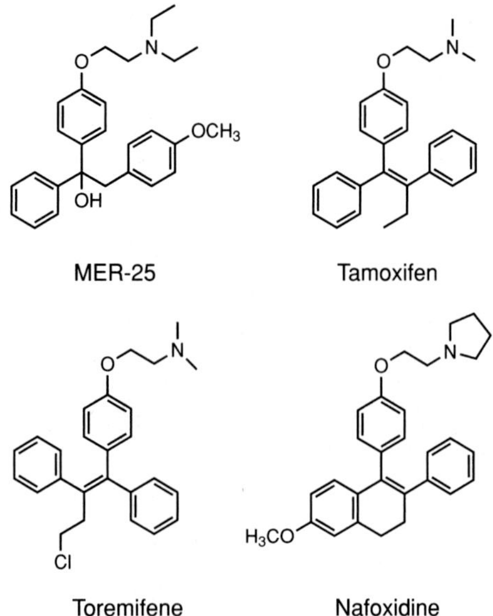

Fig. 46.20. Nonsteroidal antiestrogens.

ductive and gynecologic applications showed that the drug had low potency and that the dose required caused central nervous system toxicity (134). In the search for more potent antiestrogens, clomiphene also was identified as an effective postcoital contraceptive in laboratory animals (Fig. 46.9) (135). Clinical trials in humans, however, demonstrated that clomiphene induces ovulation (136) and does not prevent implantation. Tamoxifen, a related triphenylethylene (Fig. 46.9), also was discovered as part of a fertility-control program (137). This drug is administered as the Z-diastereomer and, in some countries, is used for ovulation induction (138). Interestingly tamoxifen, clomiphene, and a rigid analogue of tamoxifen, nafoxidine (Fig. 46.20), all inhibit the binding of [^{3}H]estradiol to ER; therefore, it was logical to test their efficacy as breast cancer treatments. Clomiphene and nafoxidine were not pursued after initial testing as a result of concerns about toxic side effects (139). Although a very low incidence of side effects is associated with tamoxifen, vasomotor symptoms often are evident and negatively affect patient quality of life (140–142). During the past 25 years, tamoxifen has become the endocrine treatment of choice for all stages of breast cancer and the first agent to reduce the incidence of breast cancer in high-risk pre- and postmenopausal women (143–145). Tamoxifen has now replaced endocrine ablative surgery in both pre- and postmenopausal patients with advanced breast cancer.

TAMOXIFEN (NOLVADEX). Tamoxifen (Fig. 46.20) is a SERM that is used as an antiestrogen in the treatment of estrogen-dependent breast cancer following primary treatment (chemotherapy and/or surgery). Therapy is limited to 5 years, because no additional benefit has been identified for treatment regimens of longer duration. Tamoxifen demonstrates only weak estrogenic effects at several sites, including the endometrium and bone, and on the lipid profile (142). Tamoxifen undergoes rapid N-demethylation to its major metabolite, N-demethyltamoxifen, by CYP3A4 and via CYP2D6 to its minor metabolite, 4-hydroxytamoxifen (Fig. 46.21). Evidence suggests that 4-hydroxytamoxifen is the active metabolite of tamoxifen (146,147), with a higher binding affinity than the parent drug for the ER (148). Circulating levels of the demethylated metabolite at steady state are up to twice the level of the parent drug, because the elimination half-life of N-demethyl tamoxifen is 14 days, compared with 7 days for tamoxifen (149). The aminoethyl ether side chain of the triphenylethylene antiestrogens is critical for the antiestrogenic activity of these agents.

Tamoxifen is rapidly absorbed from the GI tract with 100% bioavailability. It undergoes minimal first-pass metabolism and is highly protein bound, primarily to albumin. Tamoxifen's terminal elimination half-life is 5 to 7 days, which is indicative of enterohepatic recycling, elevated protein binding, and metabolic autoinhibition (142). For those patients receiving concurrent anticoagulation therapy, a dosage reduction of the anticoagulant may be warranted.

After 5 years of tamoxifen therapy, a significant number of patients experience a relapse, primarily because of tamoxifen resistance. What is observed clinically is that the weak estrogenic effects of tamoxifen begin to predominate and effectively "feed" the hormone-dependent tumor.

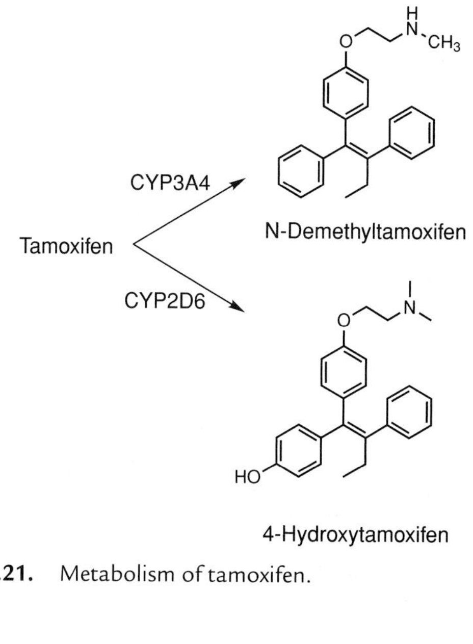

Tamoxifen → (CYP3A4) N-Demethyltamoxifen; Tamoxifen → (CYP2D6) 4-Hydroxytamoxifen

Fig. 46.21. Metabolism of tamoxifen.

TOREMIFENE (FARESTON). Toremifene is structurally and pharmacologically related to tamoxifen. It differs structurally from tamoxifen because of halogenation (chlorination) of the ethyl side chain, which reduces its antiestrogenic potency (Fig. 46.20). Toremifene demonstrates beneficial effects on the bone and cardiovascular system and increases HDL levels (142).

Toremifene is rapidly absorbed from the GI tract, with 100% bioavailability. It undergoes minimal first-pass metabolism and is highly protein bound, primarily to albumin. Toremifene, like tamoxifen, undergoes rapid N-demethylation, catalyzed by CYP3A4, to its active metabolite, N-demethyltoremifene. It also undergoes deamination-hydroxylation to ospemifene (Fig. 46.22) (142). Because toremifene is extensively metabolized in the liver, it should be used cautiously in patients with hepatic impairment. The terminal elimination half-life for toremifene is 5 to 6 days, which again is indicative of enterohepatic recycling and high protein binding (140).

Ospemifene is another SERM that is currently in Phase III clinical trials for the treatment of postmenopausal osteoporosis and urogenital atrophy (150). As a metabolite of toremifene, it also is under evaluation as an effective treatment for breast cancer. In addi-

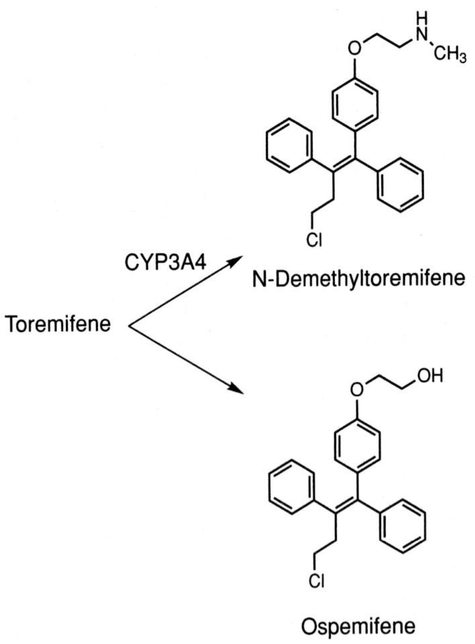

Toremifene → (CYP3A4) N-Demethyltoremifene; Toremifene → Ospemifene

Fig. 46.22. Metabolism of toremifene.

tion to its beneficial effects on the bone, ospemifene lowers LDL levels and improves the symptoms of vaginal dryness.

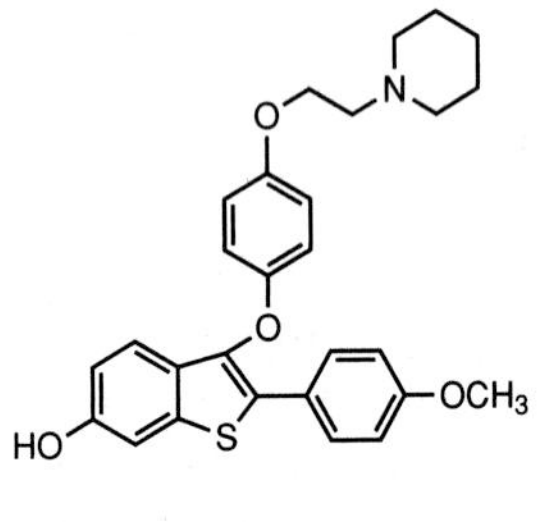

Arzoxifene

ARZOXIFENE. Arzoxifene is a third-generation SERM currently in Phase III clinical trials for the treatment of ER-positive recurrent/metastatic breast cancer. Similar to raloxifene, it is an ER antagonist in both breast and uterine tissues and an ER agonist on bone and the cardiovascular system (142,151). Arzoxifene is able to both preserve and build bone mineral density, which makes it a viable candidate for the treatment of osteoporosis. Ample evidence from early clinical trials indicates that arzoxifene also can be utilized as a chemopreventive agent against breast cancer (151,152). Adverse effects include hot flashes (major) and headache, nausea, vomiting, and constipation (minor) (142).

Pure Antiestrogens

Despite the fact that 30 to 40% of patients with advanced breast cancer respond to tamoxifen therapy, this response only lasts for 12 to 18 months. Tamoxifen resistance is caused, in part, by its intrinsic agonist activity at the ER. In addition, tamoxifen only inhibits the AF-2 activation pathway but does not play a role in AF-1 pathway inhibition. Pure antiestrogens do not possess any estrogenic activity in any species or target tissue and, therefore, offer an additional avenue of treatment when resistance to tamoxifen occurs. In addition, because they are devoid of estrogenic action, these agents cannot be classified as SERMs.

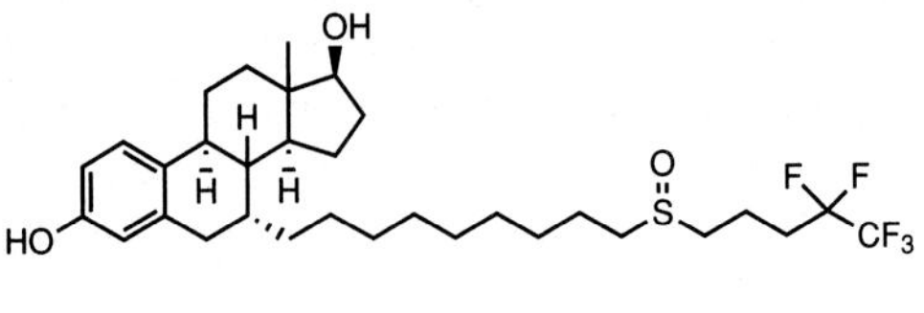

Fulvestrant

FULVESTRANT (FASLODEX). Fulvestrant is effective in preventing the growth of tamoxifen-resistant breast cancers (153) both in the laboratory (154,155) and in clinical trials. It is indicated following antiestrogen therapy for the treatment of ER-positive metastatic breast cancer that has continued to progress (156). Fulvestrant is an estradiol analogue with a hydrophobic side chain in the 7α position. Oral bioavailability is poor despite metabolic protection on the end of the hydrophobic side chain. The rationale for this stems from the fact that fulvestrant is virtually insoluble. As a result, it is administered by intramuscular injection once a month. Metabolism of fulvestrant to both active and less active metabolites is similar to that observed with the endogenous steroids (156). Side effects appear to be minimal and include several GI symptoms, headache, and hot flashes. There is no clinical evidence of uterine stimulation or laboratory evidence of stimulation of endometrial carcinoma models (157). Fulvestrant should not be administered to women who are pregnant, who are taking anticoagulants, or who have thrombocytopenia.

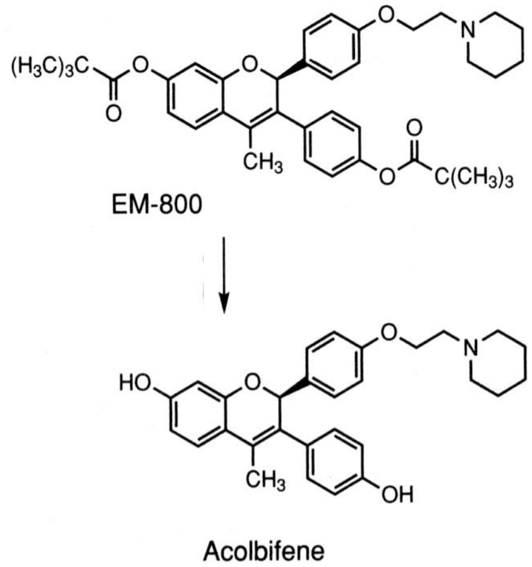

EM-800 → Acolbifene

ACOLBIFENE. The prodrug EM-800 is an orally active nonsteroidal antiestrogen and is a triphenylethylene rigid analogue. EM-800 undergoes ester hydrolysis to the active metabolite acolbifene (158). This fourth-generation antiestrogen is 200-fold more potent than tamoxifen in breast and uterine cancer cells and is effective in patients for whom tamoxifen therapy has failed. The mechanistic rationale for the effectiveness of acolbifene in tamoxifen-resistant tumors is based on the fact that it inhibits both the AF-1 and AF-2 activation pathways and does not possess any intrinsic estrogenic action. Acolbifene enjoys a 60% breast cancer cure rate (159). Structurally, acolbifene resembles raloxifene, with a benzopyran ring substituted for the benzothiophene ring. An additional benefit observed with acolbifene is its protective effect on bone loss. Adverse effects include nausea and vomiting.

Aromatase Inhibitors

Aromatase inhibitors are considered to be first-line therapy in postmenopausal women with metastatic, hormone receptor–positive breast cancer who do not tolerate tamoxifen. Aromatase is a viable target for drug action in the treatment of breast cancer, because it is the enzyme that catalyzes the conversion of androstenedione and testosterone to estrone and estradiol, respectively (Fig. 46.3, g and h). Inhibition of this enzyme limits estrogen production and effectively starves the hormone-dependent tumor. Studies do not clearly indicate that aromatase inhibitors are better first-line agents than tamoxifen and have not clearly identified a portion of this patient population that is more likely to benefit from this class of agents. It is recommended that postmenopausal women who have completed a 5-year regimen of tamoxifen for the treatment of early stage, hormone receptor–positive breast cancer consider extending their treatment with an aromatase inhibitor. It has not yet been definitively established what the optimum duration of treatment should be or whether an aromatase inhibitor should supplant or be sequenced after tamoxifen therapy. The aromatase inhibitors are associated with a lower risk of endometrial cancer and thromboembolic events but with higher rates of fractures and myalgia as compared to tamoxifen.

Letrazole (Femara). Letrazole (Fig. 46.11) is a nonsteroidal aromatase inhibitor that was approved for the treatment of postmenopausal women with hormone receptor–positive or hormone receptor–unknown, locally advanced or metastatic breast cancer. By binding to the heme group of aromatase, letrazole inhibits the aromatase and causes a reduction in plasma estrogen levels. Inhibition of aromatase by letrazole is competitive and highly specific, with no effect on enzymes that are responsible for the production of glucocorticosteroids and mineralocorticosteroids (160).

This agent is significantly more effective than tamoxifen in treating hormone-dependent cancer. Letrazole reduces the rate of tumor progression for 9.4 months, compared with 6 months for tamoxifen. Because tamoxifen therapy is limited to only 5 years, patients with breast cancer are left vulnerable to the return of their cancer. There is a 2 to 4% chance each year that the cancer might return. Taking letrazole after this 5-year period decreases the risk of the cancer returning by half. Letrazole also is used in patients who were treated for early forms of breast cancer to prevent disease from recurring. In clinical trials, it was shown that this type of preventive treatment cut the recurrence risk in half.

Letrazole is administered orally (2.5 mg daily) and is rapidly absorbed from the GI tract. Absorption is not affected by food. It is slowly metabolized (CYP3A4 and CYP2A6) to an inactive agent that is subsequently glucuronidated and eliminated renally. Letrazole strongly inhibits CYP2A6 and moderately inhibits CYP2C19. Its metabolism is induced by tamoxifen (142). Letrazole may increase the risk of osteoporosis and can cause hot flashes and night sweats. An increased incidence of hypercholesterolemia also has been documented.

Anastrozole (Arimidex). Anastrozole (Fig. 46.11) is a potent and highly selective, nonsteroidal aromatase inhibitor utilized in the treatment of advanced breast cancer that is hormone-responsive. It is considered to be second-line therapy (after tamoxifen) in the treatment of postmenopausal breast cancer. Anastrozole, a benzyltriazole derivative, competes with the natural substrate for binding to the active site of the aromatase. The mechanism of enzyme inhibition resides in the coordination of the triazole ring with the heme iron atom of the aromatase enzyme complex (161,162). This coordination ultimately prevents aromatization of androgens into estrogens and, therefore, deprives the tumor of estrogen. This effect is reversible. In the presence of anastrozole, estradiol levels are reduced to undetectable levels, with no adverse effects on levels of any other hormone, including cortisol and aldosterone.

Anastrozole is well absorbed orally, with biliary elimination as its primary route (85%) and an elimination half-life of approximately 50 hours (161). Approximately 60% of an oral dose is metabolized in the liver by N-dealkylation, hydroxylation, and glucuronidation to inactive triazole metabolites.

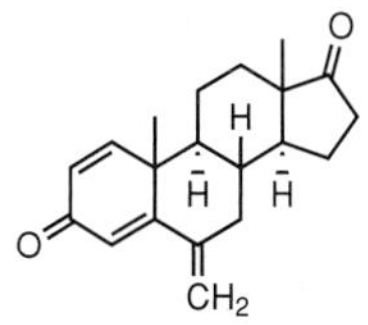

Exemestane

Exemastane (Aromasin). Exemastane is a steroid-based, irreversible aromatase inhibitor that is approved for the treatment of estrogen-dependent tumors and postmenopausal breast cancer. It also has been approved overseas as adjuvant therapy after 2 to 3 years of adjuvant tamoxifen treatment of ER-positive, invasive early breast cancer. The structure of exemastane is related to androstenedione. It is important to consider the woman's menstrual status when utilizing this agent, because the synthesis of ovarian aromatase is part of a negative feedback loop such that decreased levels of circulating estrogen will promote increased biosynthesis of aromatase. As a result, exemastane should not be administered to premenopausal women or those who are pregnant. Exemastane binds irreversibly to aromatase and, therefore, is classified as a suicide inhibitor. Because this agent has high binding affinity and specificity for aromatase, it is able to suppress the activity of this enzyme by 97.7% (anastrozole, 92–96%; letrozole, 98%) (163).

Exemastane is administered orally (25 mg daily); however, only 50% of a given dose is absorbed. Absorption is improved if the medication is taken following a high-fat meal. Approximately 90% of a dose is bound to plasma proteins. Exemastane undergoes extensive metabolism by CYP3A4, and dosage adjustments may be necessary if given concomitantly with a CYP3A4 inducer (163). Adverse reactions reported in patients with early breast cancer include hot flashes, arthralgia, and fatigue, whereas hot flashes and nausea were the primary adverse reactions noted in patients with advanced breast cancer.

Conclusions

Throughout a woman's reproductive life cycle there are a number of disease states or life circumstances that can be successfully managed with one or more hormone-related therapeutic strategies. Not only is it important to select an appropriate therapeutic regimen for each individual, it also is essential to determine which route of administration and, therefore, which formulation is the most therapeutically advantageous. A number of formulations are available for several single and multicomponent products, and maximizing patient compliance should be considered when recommending a particular product. There are no products devoid of adverse effects, so it is important that these be explained to the patient to minimize discontinuation of the recommended therapy.

The alarming results generated by the WHI studies have fueled the development of new estrogen-containing products designed to deliver lower doses of estrogen to minimize systemic exposure and decrease the risk of cardiovascular disease and development of cancer. In addition, a number of alternative therapies are under investigation for the treatment of menopausal symptoms. Agents that modulate serotonergic neurotransmission seem to be especially promising, because many of these therapies are already known commercial entities.

Pharmacological management of breast cancer continues to make progress with advanced characterization techniques and the use of aromatase inhibitors and SERMs. Future generations of SERMs will need to be completely devoid of estrogenic activity to prevent the development of resistance, as is occurring with tamoxifen.

CASE STUDY

Victoria F. Roche and S. William Zito

AF is a 55-year-old female forensic chemist who has always taken pride in her healthy lifestyle. She has exercised regularly all her life and enjoys sports such as tennis, bicycling, and strenuous hiking. More recently, she has been working out in a gym, running approximately 12 to 15 miles per week, and engaging in a strengthening routine using the gym's weight-training machines. The only medicines that she takes are multivitamins and atorvastatin (Lipitor, 10 mg q.d.) to keep her total cholesterol, triglyceride, and LDL levels low. AF's blood pressure is normal, and her cardiac function is good.

AF's medical history includes uterine cysts that developed during her early forties and, ultimately, resulted in hemorrhagic monthly bleeding. After being diagnosed as severely anemic, she underwent a partial hysterectomy (uterus only) when she was 44 years old. When she began to show signs and symptoms of menopause at age 48, her gynecologist put her on HRT to control regular and severe hot flashes and night sweats. She took her HRT religiously for 6 years, until information from the WHI indicated that she might be at risk for ovarian cancer. There is no history of cancer in AF's family, but she was concerned enough to halt HRT even though her hot flashes and night sweats returned with a vengeance. Her intake of calcium is moderate, with the consumption of one to two glasses of milk per day. She tries to avoid cheese because of a slow but steady gain in weight over the past 2 years.

On noting that AF had lost a quarter-inch in height since her last clinic visit, her gynecologist recommended a bone density determination. The results showed a thinning of the bone. That, along with the fact that her 83-year-old mother has significant osteoporosis, prompted a decision to initiate therapy. Consider the structures of the therapeutic agents drawn below, and prepare to make a recommendation to AF's gynecologist.

1. Identify the therapeutic problem(s) in which the pharmacist's intervention may benefit the patient.
2. Identify and prioritize the patient-specific factors that must be considered to achieve the desired therapeutic outcomes.
3. Conduct a thorough and mechanistically oriented structure–activity analysis of all therapeutic alternatives provided in the case.
4. Evaluate the structure–activity relationship findings against the patient-specific factors and desired therapeutic outcomes, and make a therapeutic decision.
5. Counsel your patient.

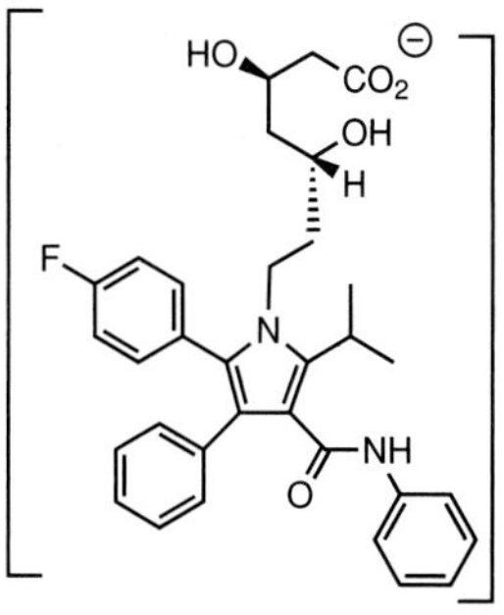

Atorvastatin Calcium 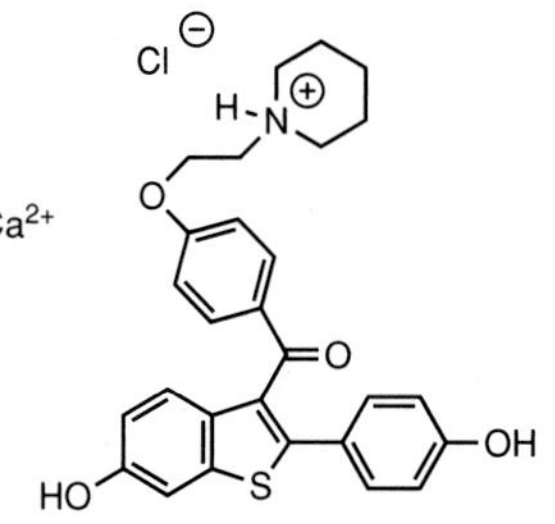 1 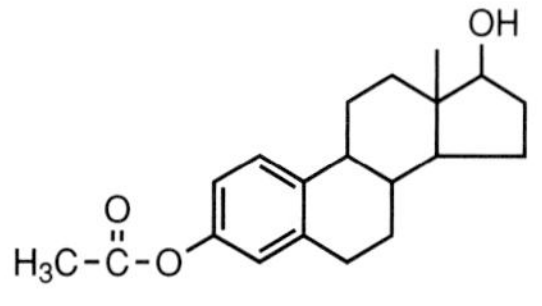 2 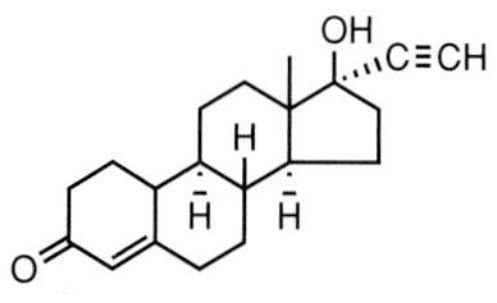 3

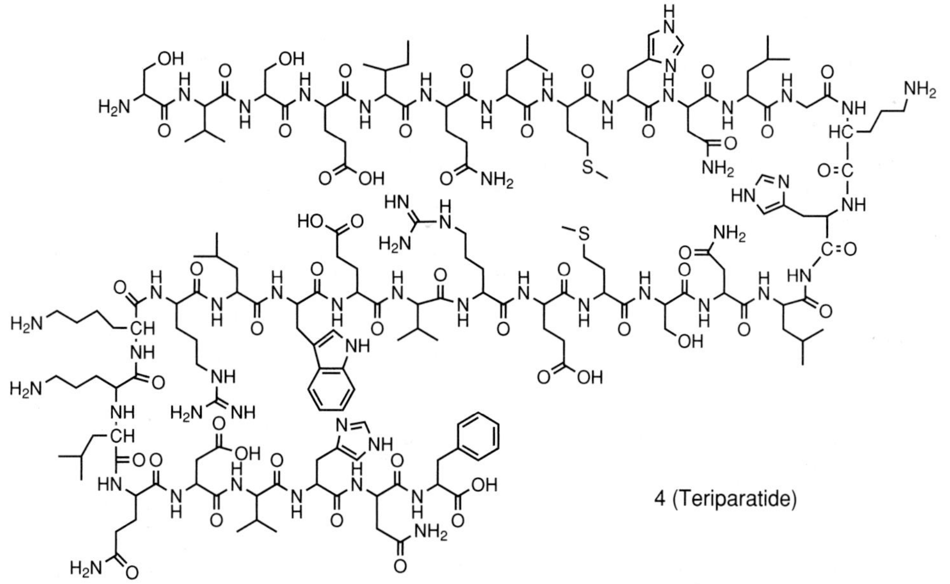

4 (Teriparatide)

References

1. Cole LA, Sutton-Riley JM, Khanlian SA, et al. Sensitivity of over-the-counter pregnancy tests: comparison of utility and marketing messages. J Am Pharm Assoc 2005;45:608–615.
2. Butler SA, Khanlian SA, Cole LA. Detection of early pregnancy forms of human chorionic gonadotropin by home pregnancy test devices. Clin Chem 2001;47:2131–2136.
3. Hulisz DT, Urbanski CM. Home pregnancy testing kits. US Pharmacist 2002;21:22–32.
4. Eichner SF, Timpe EM. Urinary-based ovulation and pregnancy: point-of-care testing. Ann Pharmacother 2004;38:325–331.
5. Williams C, Stancel GM. Estrogens and progestins. In: Hardman JG, Limbard LE, Moliwoff PB. eds. Goodman and Gilman's The Pharmacological Basis of Therapeutics. 9th Ed. New York: Pergamon Press, 1996:1411–1440.
6. Gurpide E, Anger H, Vande Wicke RL. et al. Determination of secretory rates of estrogens in pregnant and nonpregnant women from the specific activities of urinary metabolites. J Clin Endocrinol Metab 1962;22:935–945.
7. O'Malley BW, Means AR. Receptors for Reproductive Hormones. New York: Plenum Press, 1974.
8. Najakin S, Hall PF. Microsomal cytochrome P-450 from neonatal pig testis. Purification and properties of a C_{21} steroid side-chain cleavage system (17α-hydroxylase-C17,20 lyase). J Biol Chem 1981;256:3871–3876.
9. Brown JB. Determination and significance of the natural estrogens. Adv Clin Chem 1960;3:157–233.
10. Diczfalusy E, Lauritzen C. Oestrogen bein Menschen. Berlin: Springer, 1961.
11. Kuhl H. Pharmacology of estrogens and progestins: influence of different routes of administration. Climacteric 2005;8(Suppl. 1):3–63.
12. Grow DR. Metabolism of endogenous and exogenous reproductive hormones. Obstet Gynecol Clin North Am 2002;29:425–436.
13. Ansbacher R. The pharmacokinetics and efficacy of different estrogens are not equivalent. Am J Obstet Gynecol 2001;184:255–263.
14. Kuiper GGJM, Carlsson B, Grandien K.. et al. Comparison of the ligand binding specificity and transcript tissue distribution of estrogen receptors α and β. Endocrinology 1997;138:863–870.
15. Ray S, Rastogi R, Kumar A. Current status of estrogen receptors. Prog Drug Res 2002;59:201–232.
16. Aitken SC, Lippman ME. Hormonal regulation of de novo pyrimidine synthesis and utilization in human breast cancer cells in tissue culture. Cancer Res 1983;43:4684–4690.
17. Aitken SC, Lippman ME. Effect of estrogens and antiestrogens on growth-regulatory enzymes in human breast cancer cells in tissue culture. Cancer Res 1985;45:1611–1620.
18. Inhoffen HH, Hohlweg W. Neue per os-wirksame weibliche Keimdrüsenhormon-Derivate: 17-Aethynyl-oestradiol und Pregnen-in-on-3-ol-17. Naturwissenschaften 1938;26:96–100.
19. Colton LB, Nysted CN, Riegel B, et al. 17-Alkyl-19-nortestosterones. J Am Chem Soc 1957;79: 1123–1127.
20. Solmssen UV. Synthetic estrogens and the relation between their structure and their activity. Chem Rev 1945;37:481–598.
21. Bentley PJ. Endocrine Pharmacology. Cambridge, UK: Cambridge University Press, 1980.
22. Anstead GM, Carlson KE, Katzenellenbogen JA. The estradiol pharmacophore: ligand structure–estrogen receptor binding affinity relationships and a model for the receptor binding site. Steroids 1997;62:268–303.
23. Brzozowski AM, Pike ACW, Dauter Z et al. The crystallization of the ligand-binding domain (LBD) of the estrogen receptor (ER) with 17β-estradiol and raloxifene. Nature 1997;389:753–758.
24. Shiau AK, Barstad D, Loria PM, et al. The structural basis of estrogen receptor/coactivator recognition and the antagonism of this interaction by tamoxifen. Cell 1998;95:927–937.
25. Baran JS. Synthesis of 11β-hydroxyestrone and related 16- and 17-hydroxyestratrienes. J Med Chem 1967;10:1188–1190.
26. Fieser LF, Fieser M. Steroids. New York, Reinhold, 1959:421.
27. Cross AD, Denot E, Carpio H, et al. Steroids CCLXX. Biologically-active labile ethers. II. A new group of potent orally active estrogens. Steroids 1965;4:423–432.
28. Funder JW, Feldman D, Highheel E, et al. Molecular modifications of antialdosterone compounds: effects on affinity of spirolactones for renal aldosterone receptors. Biochem Pharmacol 1974;23:1493–1501.

29. Katzenellenbogen BS, Ferguson ER. Antiestrogen action in the uterus: biological ineffectiveness of nuclear bound estradiol after antiestrogen. Endocrinology 1975;97:1–12.
30. Clark JH, Peck EJ Jr, Anderson JN, et al. Estrogen receptors and antagonism of steroid hormone action. Nature 1974;251:446–448.
31. Jordan VC. Selective estrogen receptor modulators. In: Williams DA, Lemke T, eds. Foye's Principles of Medicinal Chemistry. 5th Ed. Baltimore: Lippincott Williams & Wilkins, 2002:1059–1069.
32. Salhanick HA. Basic studies on aminoglutethimide. Cancer Res 1982;42 (Suppl. 8):3315S–3321S.
33. Bhatnagar AS, Hausler A, Schieweck K, et al. Novel aromatase inhibitors. J Steroid Biochem Mol Biol 1990;37:363–367.
34. Buzdar AU, Jonat W, Howell A, et al. ARIMIDEX: a potent and selective aromatase inhibitor for the treatment of advanced breast cancer. J Steroid Biochem Mol Biol 1997;61:145–150.
35. Bhatnagar AS, Hausler A, Schieweck K, et al. Highly selective inhibition of estrogen biosynthesis by CGS 20267, a new nonsteroidal aromatase inhibitor. J Steroid Biochem Mol Biol 1990;37:1021–1027.
36. Brueggemeier RW. Biochemical and molecular aspects of aromatase. J Enzyme Inhib 1990;4:101–111.
37. Johnston JO, Metcalf BW. In: Sunkara P, ed. Novel Approaches to Cancer Chemotherapy. New York: Academic Press, 1984:307–358.
38. Banting L, Nicholls PJ, Shaw MA, et al. Recent developments in aromatase inhibition as a potential treatment for estrogen-dependent breast cancer. Prog Med Chem 1989;26:253–298.
39. Rucnitz PC. Female sex hormones and analogs. In: Wolff ME, ed. Burger's Medicinal Chemistry, vol 4. 5th Ed. New York: Wiley, 1997:553–588.
40. Fraenkel L. Arch Gynaek 1903;68:438.
41. Corner GW, Allen WM. Physiology of the corpus luteum. Am J Physiol 1929;88:326–339.
42. Leonhardt SA, Edwards DP. Mechanism of action of progesterone antagonists. Exp Biol Med 2002;227:969–980.
43. Sitruk-Ware R. New progestogens: a review of their effects in perimenopausal and postmenopausal women. Drugs Aging 2004;21:865–883.
44. Fotherby K. The biochemistry of progesterone. Vitam Horm 1964;22: 153–204.
45. Rothchild I. In: Salhanick HA, et al., eds. Metabolic Effects of Gonadal Hormones and Contraceptive Steroids. New York: Plenum Press, 1969:668.
46. Jaffe RB, et al. In: Lednicer D, ed. Contraception: The Chemical Control of Fertility. New York: Marcel Dekker, 1969.
47. Heftmann E. Steroid Biochemistry. New York: Academic Press, 1970:140.
48. Klopper A. Developments in steroidal hormonal contraception. Br Med Bull 1970;26:39–44.
49. Klimstra PD. Progestational agents. Am J Pharm Ed 1970;34:630–647.
50. Kalantaridou SN, Davis SR, Calis KA. Hormone therapy in women. In: DiPiro JT, et al., eds. Pharmacotherapy: A Pathophysiologic Approach. 6th Ed. New York: McGraw-Hill, 2005.
51. Davis ME, Wied GL. 17α-Hydroxyprogesterone caproate: a new substance with prolonged progestational activity: a comparison with chemically pure progesterone. J Clin Endocrinol Metab 1955;15:923–930.
52. Babcock JC, et al. 6α-Methyl-17α-Hydroxyprogesterone 17-acylates: a new class of potent progestins. J Am Chem Soc 1958;80:2904–2905.
53. Ruzicka L, Hofmann K. Sexual hormone XXIV. Über die Anlagerung von Acetylen an die 17-ständige Ketogruppe bei trans-Androsteron und Δ^5-trans-Dehydro-androsteron. Helv Chim Acta 1937;20:1280–1282.
54. Ehrenstein M. Investigations on steroids. VIII. Lower homologues of hormones of the pregnane series: 10-nor-11-desoxycorticosterone acetate and 10-norprogesterone. J Org Chem 1944;9:435–456.
55. Djerassi C, et al. Steroids. XLVIII. 19-Norprogesterone, a potent progestational hormone. J Am Chem Soc 1953;75:4440–4442.
56. Kaunitz AM. Enhancing oral contraceptive success: the potential for new formulations. Am J Obstet Gynecol 2004;190:S23–S29.
57. Sitruk-Ware R. Pharmacological profile of progestins. Maturitas 2004;47: 277–283.
58. Teichmann A. Metabolic profile of six oral contraceptives containing norgestimate, gestodene, and desogestrel. Int J Fertil Menopausal Stud 1995;40(Suppl. 2):98–104.
59. Philibert D, Deraedt R, et al. 64th Annual Meeting of the Endocrine Society, San Francisco, June 1982, Abstract No. 668.
60. Baulieu EE. Contragestion and other clinical applications of RU 486, an antiprogesterone at the receptor. Science 1989;245:1351–1357.
61. Agarwal MK, et al. Glucocorticoid antagonists. FEBS Lett 1987;217:221–226.
62. Elger W, et al. Studies on the mechanisms of action of progesterone antagonists. J Steroid Biochem Mol Biol 1986;25:835–845.
63. Horwitz KB. The molecular biology of RU486. Is there a role for antiprogestins in the treatment of breast cancer? Endocr Rev 1992;13:146–163.
64. Himmerick KA. Enhancing contraception: a comprehensive review. JAAPA 2005;7(18):26–33.
65. Mishell DR Jr. State of the art in hormonal contraception: an overview. Am J Obstet Gynecol 2004;190:S1–S4.
66. Edwards LA. An update on oral contraceptive options. Formulary 2004;39: 104–121.
67. Forinash AB, Evans SL. New hormonal contraceptives: a comprehensive review of the literature. Pharmacotherapy 2003;23:1573–1591.
68. Dickerson LM, Bucci KK. Contraception. In: DiPiro JT, et al., eds. Pharmacotherapy: A Pathophysiologic Approach. 6th Ed. New York: McGraw-Hill, 2005.
69. Cibula D, Weidenhammer HG, et al. Efficacy and safety of a low-dose 21-day combined oral contraceptive containing ethynyl estradiol 20 μg and drospirenone 3 mg. Clin Drug Invest 2006;26:143–150.
70. Mishell Dr Jr. The pharmacologic and metabolic effects of oral contraceptives. Int J Fertil 1989;34(Suppl.):21–26.
71. Erkkola R, Landren B-M. Role of progestins in contraception. Acta Obstet Gynecol Scand 2005;84:207–216.
72. Goa KL, Warner GT, Easthope SE. Transdermal ethynyl estradiol/norelgestromin: a review of its use in hormonal contraception. Treat Endocrinol 2003;2:191–206.
73. Hitchens K. Birth control now comes in a patch for women. Drug Topics 2002;19.
74. Zieman M, Guillebaud J, et al. Contraceptive efficacy and cycle control with the Ortho Evra/Evra transdermal system: the analysis of pooled data. Fertil Steril 2002;77(2 Suppl. 2):S13–S18.
75. Bjarnadottir RI, Tuppurainen M, Killick SR. Comparison of cycle control with a combined contraceptive vaginal ring and oral levonorgestrel/ethynyl estradiol. Am J Obstet Gynecol 2002;186:389–395.
76. Sivin I, Stern J. Health during prolonged use of levonorgestrel 20 micrograms/d and the copper TCu 380Ag intrauterine contraceptive devices: a multicenter study. International Committee for Contraception Research (ICCR). Fertil Steril 1994;61:70–77.
77. Glasier A. Emergency postcoital contraception. N Engl J Med 1997;337: 1058–1064.
78. Crosignani P, Olive D, et al. Advances in the management of endometriosis: an update for clinicians. Hum Reprod Update 2006;12:179–189.
79. Saljoughian M. Understanding endometriosis and its treatment. US Pharmacist 2005;HS5–HS8.
80. Sturpe DA, Patel AD. Endometriosis. In: DiPiro JT, et al., eds. Pharmacotherapy: A Pathophysiologic Approach. 6th Ed. New York: McGraw-Hill, 2005.
81. Garcia-Velasco JA, Quea G. Medical treatment of endometriosis. Minerva Ginecol 2005;57:249–255.
82. Valle RF, Sciarra JJ. Endometriosis: treatment strategies. Ann N Y Acad Sci 2003;997:229–239.
83. Luciano AA, Turksoy RN, Carleo J. Evaluation of oral medroxyprogesterone acetate in the treatment of endometriosis. Obstet Gynecol 1988;72:323–327.
84. Bulun SE, Fang Z, et al. Aromatase and endometriosis. Semin Reprod Med 2004;22:45–50.
85. Saito T, Yoshizawa M, et al. Effects of the novel orally active antiestrogen TZE-5323 on experimental endometriosis. Arzneimittelforschung/Drug Res 2003;53:507–514.
86. DeManno D, Elger W, et al. Asoprisnil (J867): a selective progesterone receptor modulator for gynecological therapy. Steroids 2003;68:1019–1032.
87. Olive DL, Pritts EA. The treatment of endometriosis: a review of the evidence. Ann N Y Acad Sci 2002;955:360–372 [discussion 389–393, 396–406].
88. Pal L, Santoro N. Age-related decline in fertility. Endocrinol Metab Clin North Am 2003;32:669–688.
89. Gharib S, Chapin MD, et al. Infertility: A Guide to Evaluation, Treatment and Counseling. Boston: Brigham and Women's Hospital Mary Horrigan Connors Center for Women's Health, 1–10.
90. Kuohung W, Barbieri RL. Overview of treatment of female infertility. Available at: http://uptodateonline.com/utd/content/topic.do?topicKey=gen_gyne/25217&type=A&selectedTitle=3~70. Accessed April 13, 2006.
91. Corson SL. Achieving and maintaining pregnancy after 40. Int J Fertil 1998;43:249–256.
92. Arslan M, Bocca S, et al. Controlled ovarian hyperstimulation protocols for in vitro fertilization: two decades of experience after the birth of Elizabeth Carr. Fertil Steril 2005;84:555–569.
93. Hugues J-N. Ovarian stimulation for assisted reproductive technologies. Available at: http://www.who.int/reproductive-health/infertility/14.pdf. Accessed June 6, 2006.
94. Scott RT, Leonardi MR. A prospective evaluation of clomiphene citrate challenge test screening of the general infertility population. Obstet Gynecol 1993;82:539–544.
95. Ovulation Drugs: A Guide for Patients. American Society for Reproductive Medicine, 2000:1–19.
96. Schultze-Mosgau A, Griesinger G, et al. New developments in the use of peptide gonadotropin-releasing hormone antagonists versus agonists. Expert Opin Investig Drugs 2005;14:1085–1097.
97. Al Inany H, Aboulghar M. GnRH antagonist in assisted reproduction: a Cochrane review. Hum Reprod 2002;17:874–885.
98. Utian WH. Psychosocial and socioeconomic burden of vasomotor symptoms in menopause: a comprehensive review. Health and Quality of Life Outcomes 2005;3:47–56.

99. Stefanick ML. Estrogens and progestins: background and history, trends in use, and guidelines and regimens approved by the U.S. Food and Drug Administration. Am J Med 2005;118:64S–73S.
100. Shumaker SA, Legault C, et al. Estrogen plus the incidence of dementia and mild cognitive impairment in postmenopausal women: The Women's Health Initiative Memory Study: a randomized, controlled study. JAMA 2003;2662.
101. Shumaker SA, Legault C, et al. Conjugated equine estrogens and incidence of probable dementia and mild cognitive impairment in postmenopausal women: Women's Health Initiative Memory Study. JAMA 2004;291:2947–2958, 2959–2968, 3005–3007.
102. Smoot LC. Hormone replacement therapy: where do we stand now? Drug Topics 2004;84–93.
103. Estrogen Monograph: Facts and Comparisons, Version 4.0. Available at: **XXX**. Accessed June 5, 2006.
104. Estrogens and Progestins Combined Monograph: Facts and Comparisons, Version 4.1. Available at: XXX. Accessed June 5, 2006.
105. Perez DG, Loprinzi CL. Newer antidepressants and other nonhormonal agents for the treatment of hot flashes. Compr Ther 2005;31:224–236.
106. Bhatti WH, Gaich CL, Menke GL. Natural hormone replacement therapy. US Pharmacist 2004;41–54.
107. National Institutes of Health State-of-the-Science. Conference statement: management of menopause-related symptoms. Ann Intern Med 2005;142: 1003–1013.
108. Gehm BD, McAndrews JM, et al. Resveratrol, a polyphenolic compound found in grapes and wine, is an agonist for the estrogen receptor. Proc Natl Acad Sci US A 1997;94:14138–14143.
109. Sulli M, See S, Kanmaz T. Nonhormonal therapy for hot flashes. US Pharmacist 2003;28(9):41–54.
110. Swanson GM. Breast cancer risk estimation: a translational statistic for communication to the public. J Natl Cancer Inst 1993;85:848–849.
111. Collaborative Group on Hormonal Factors in Breast Cancer. Breast cancer and hormone replacement therapy: collaborative reanalysis of data from epidemiological studies of 52,705 women with breast cancer and 108,411 women without breast cancer. Lancet 1997;350:1047–1059.
112. Stefanick ML, Anderson GL, Margolis KL, et al. Effects of conjugated equine estrogens on breast cancer and mammography screening in postmenopausal women with hysterectomy. JAMA 2006;295:1647–1657.
113. Warnock JK. Female hypoactive sexual desire disorder: epidemiology, diagnosis, and treatment. CNS Drugs 2002;16:745–753.
114. Arlt W. Androgen therapy in women. Eur J Endocrinol 2006;154:1–11.
115. Palkhivala A. Alprostadil cream may be effective against female sexual arousal disorder. ASRM 2005 Annual Meeting: Abstract O-322. Presented October 19, 2005.
116. Greenblatt D. Treatment of postmenopausal osteoporosis. Pharmacotherapy 2005;25:574–584.
117. Michaelsson K, Baron JA, Farahmand BY, et al. Oral contraceptive use and risk of hip fracture: a case-control study. Lancet 1999;353:1481–1484.
118. Vogelvang TE, Mijatovic V, Kenemans P, et al. HMR 3339, a novel selective estrogen receptor modulator, reduces total cholesterol, low-density lipoprotein cholesterol, and homocysteine in healthy postmenopausal women. Fertil Steril 2004;82:1540–1549.
119. Ammann P, Bourrin S, Brunner F, et al. A new selective estrogen receptor modulator HMR-3339 fully corrects bone alterations induced by ovariectomy in adult rats. Bone 2004;35:153–161.
120. Bisphosphonate Monograph, Facts and Comparisons 4.0, http://online.factsandcomparisons.com/MonoDisp.aspx?monoID=fandc-hcp10318&book=DFC Accessed 4/28/06.
121. Women's Health Initiative Steering Committee. Effect of conjugated equine estrogen in postmenopausal women with hysterectomy. JAMA 2004;291: 1701–1712.
122. Casper RF. Estrogen with interrupted progestin HRT: a review of experimental and clinical studies. Maturitas 2000;34:97–108.
123. McGuire WL, Carbone PP, Volliner EP. Estrogen Receptors in Human Breast Cancer. New York: Raven Press, 1975.
124. Kumar V, Green S, et al. Functional domains of the human estrogen receptor. Cell 1987;51:941–951.
125. Green S, Chambon P. Estradiol induction of a glucocorticoid-responsive gene by a chimeric receptor. Nature 1987;325:75–78.
126. Kraus WL, McInerney EM, Katzenellenbogen BS. Ligand-dependent, transcriptionally productive association of the amino- and carboxyl-terminal regions of a steroid hormone nuclear receptor. Proc Natl Acad Sci U S A 1995;92:12314–12318.
127. Brzozowski AM, Pike AC, et al. Molecular basis of agonism and antagonism in the estrogen receptor. Nature 1997;389:753–758.
128. Shiau AK, Barstad D, et al. The structural basis of estrogen receptor/coactivator recognition and the antagonism of this interaction by tamoxifen. Cell 1998;95:927–937.
129. Jordan VC. Antiestrogenic action of raloxifene and tamoxifen: today and tomorrow. J Natl Cancer Inst 1998;90:967–971.
130. Wijayaratne AL, Nagel SC, et al. Comparative analyses of mechanistic differences among antiestrogens. Endocrinology 1999;140:5828–5840.
131. Paech K, Webb P, et al. Differential ligand activation of estrogen receptors ER-α and ER-β at AP1 sites. Science 1997;277:1508–1510.
132. Lerner LJ, Holthaus JF, Thompson CR. A nonsteroidal estrogen antagonist 1-(p-2-diethylaminoethoxyphenyl)-1-phenyl-2-p-methoxyphenylethanol. Endocrinology 1958;63:295–318.
133. Segal JS, Nelson WO. An orally active compound with antifertility effects in rats. Proc Soc Exp Biol Med 1958;98:431–436.
134. Lerner LJ. The first nonsteroidal antiestrogen–MER 25. In: Nonsteroidal Antiestrogens: Molecular Pharmacology and Antitumor Activity. Sydney, Australia: Sydney Academic Press; 1981:1–6.
135. Holtkamp DE, Greslin SC, et al. Gonadotropin inhibiting and antifecundity effects of chloramiphene. Proc Soc Exp Biol Med 1960;105:197–201.
136. Greenblatt R, Roy S, Mahesh V. The induction of ovulation. Am J Obstet Gynecol 1962;84:900–912.
137. Harper MJ, Walpole AL. A new derivative of triphenylethylene: effect on implantation and mode of action in rats. J Reprod Fertil 1967;13:101–119.
138. Furr BJ, Jordan VC. The pharmacology and clinical uses of tamoxifen. Pharmacol Ther 1984;25:127–205.
139. Legha SS, Carter SK. Antiestrogens in the treatment of breast cancer. Cancer Treat Rev 1976;3:205–216.
140. Cole MP, Jones CT, Todd ID. A new antiestrogenic agent in late breast cancer. An early clinical appraisal of ICI46474. Br J Cancer 1971;25:270–275.
141. Ward HW. Antiestrogen therapy for breast cancer: a trial of tamoxifen at two dose levels. Br Med J 1973;1:13–14.
142. Morella KC, Wurz GT, DeGregorio MW. Pharmacokinetics of selective estrogen receptor modulators. Clin Pharmacokinet 2003;42:361–372.
143. Lerner LJ, Jordan VC. Development of antiestrogens and their use in breast cancer: Eighth Cain Memorial Award Lecture. Cancer Res 1990;50: 4177–4189.
144. Osborne CK. Tamoxifen in the treatment of breast cancer. N Engl J Med 1998;339:1609–1618.
145. Fisher B, Costantino JP, et al. Tamoxifen for prevention of breast cancer: report of the National Surgical Adjuvant Breast and Bowel Project P-1 Study. J Natl Cancer Inst 1998;90:1371–1388.
146. Jordan VC, et al. A monohydroxylated metabolite of tamoxifen with potent antiestrogenic activity. J Endocrinol 1977;75:305–316.
147. Jordan VC, Murphy CS. Endocrine pharmacology of antiestrogens as antitumor agents. Endocr Rev 1990;11:578–610.
148. Jordan VC, Collins MM, et al. A monohydroxylated metabolite of tamoxifen with potent antiestrogenic activity. J Endocrinol 1977;75:305–316.
149. Jordan VC. Biochemical pharmacology of antiestrogen action. Pharmacol Rev 1984;36:245–276.
150. Gennari L. Ospemifene hormos. Current Opin Invest Drugs 2004;5: 448–455.
151. Fabian CJ, Kimler BF, et al. Breast cancer chemoprevention Phase I evaluation of biomarker modulation by arzoxifene, a third-generation selective estrogen receptor modulator. Clin Cancer Res 2004;10:5403–5417.
152. Suh N, Glasebrook AL, et al. Arzoxifene, a new selective estrogen receptor modulator for chemoprevention of experimental breast cancer. Cancer Res 2001;61:8412–8415.
153. Howell A, DeFriend DJ, et al. Pharmacokinetics, pharmacological, and antitumor effects of the specific antiestrogen ICI 182780 in women with advanced breast cancer. Br J Cancer 1996;74:300–308.
154. Wakeling AE, Dukes M, Bowler J. A potent specific pure antiestrogen with clinical potential. Cancer Res 1991;51:3867–3873.
155. Osborne CK, Coronado-Heinsohn EB, et al. Comparison of the effects of a pure steroidal antiestrogen with those of tamoxifen in a model of human breast cancer. J Natl Cancer Inst 1995;87:746–750.
156. Faslodex (fulvestrant injection), Prescribing Information. AstraZeneca Pharmaceuticals, 2004.
157. O'Regan RM, Cisneros A, et al. Effects of the antiestrogens tamoxifen, toremifene, and ICI 182,780 on endometrial cancer growth. J Natl Cancer Inst 1998;90:1552–1558.
158. Simard J, Sanchez R, et al. Blockade of the stimulatory effect of estrogens, OH-tamoxifen, OH-toremifene, droloxifene, and raloxifene on alkaline phosphatase activity by the antiestrogen EM-800 in human endometrial adenocarcinoma Ishikawa cells. Cancer Res 1997;57:3494–3497.
159. Labrie F, Champagne P, et al. Activity and safety of the antiestrogen EM-800, the orally active precursor of acolbifene, in tamoxifen-resistant breast cancer. J Clin Oncol 2004;22:864–871.
160. Femara (letrazole tablets), Prescribing Information. Novartis, 2001.
161. Higa GM, Al-Khouri N. Anastrozole: a selective aromatase inhibitor for the treatment of breast cancer. Am J Health-Syst Pharm 1998;55:445–452.
162. Higa GM. Altering the estrogenic milieu of breast cancer with a focus on the new aromatase inhibitors. Pharmacotherapy 2000;20:280–291.
163. Higa GM. Exemestane: treatment of breast cancer with selective inactivation of aromatase. Am J Health-Syst Pharm 2002;59:2194–2201.

APPENDIX A. *pK_a Values for Some Drugs and Miscellaneous Organic Acids and Bases*

DAVID A. WILLIAMS

Table A.1. pK_a Values for Some Drugs and Miscellaneous Organic Acids and Bases

Drugs	pK_a Values HA	pK_a Values HB^+	Reference
Acebutolol		9.2	1
Acenocoumarol	4.7		1
Acetaminophen	9.7		1
Acetanilide		0.5	1
Acetazolamide	7.4, 9.1		3
Acetohydroxamic acid	9.4		1
α-Acetylmethadol		8.6	1
Acetysalicylic acid	3.5		1
Acyclovir	9.3	2.3	1
Adriamycin		8.2	1
Ajamaline		8.2	1
Albuterol	10.3	9.3	9
Alclofenac	4.3		1
Alfentanil		6.5	1
Allobarbital	7.8		1
Allopurinol	9.4		1,4
Alphaprodine		8.7	1
Alprenolol		9.7	1,5
Altretamine		10.3	1
Amantadine		9.0	1
Amidinocillin	3.4	8.9	1
Amiloride		8.7	1
Aminoacrine		10.0	1
p-Aminobenzoic acid	4.9	2.5	1
Aminocaproic acid	4.4	10.8	1
Aminohippuric acid	3.8		1
Aminopterin	5.5		1
Aminopyrine		5.0	1
p-Aminosalicylic acid	3.6	1.8	1
Aminothiadiazole		3.2	1
Amiodarone		6.6	1
Amitriptyline		9.4	15
Amobarbital	7.8		1
Amoxapine		7.6	1,4
Amoxicillin	2.4	9.6	12
Amphetamine		10.0	1
Amphotericin B	5.5	10.0	11
Ampicillin	2.5	7.2	16
Anileridine		3.7, 7.5	1
Antazoline		2.5, 10.1	1
Antipyrine		1.5	1
Apomorphine	8.9	7.0	1
Aprobarbital	8.0		1
Ascorbic acid	4.2, 11.6		1
Atenolol		9.6	6
Atropine		9.8	1
Azatadine		9.3	1
Azathioprine	8.0		9
Azlocillin	2.8		1
Aztrenam	0.7, 2.9	3.9	1
Bacampicillin		6.8	1
Baclofen	5.4	9.5	1
Barbital	7.9		1
Bendroflumethiazide	8.5		5

(Continued)

Table A.1. ***Continued***

Drugs	pK_a Values		Reference
	HA	HB^+	
Benzocaine		2.5	1
Benzphetamine		6.6	1
Benzquinamide		5.9	1
Benztropine		10.0	1
Betahistine		3.5, 9.8	1
Betaprodine		8.7	1
Bethanidine		10.6	1
Bromazepam	11.0	2.9	1
Bromocriptine[a]		9.8	1
Bromodiphenhydramine		4.9	7
Brompheniramine		3.6, 9.8	1
Brucine		8.2, 2.5	1
Bufuralol		8.9	1
Bumetanide	5.2, 10.0		1
Bunolol		9.3	1
Bupivacaine		8.1	1
Bupropion		7.0	8
Burimamide		7.5	1
Butabarbital	7.9		1
Butacaine		9.0	1
Butaclamol		7.2	1
Butamben		5.4	1
Butorphanol		8.6	1
Butylated hydroxytoluene	7.5		1
Butylparaben	8.5		3
Caffeine	>14.0	0.6	1
Camptothecin		10.8	1
Captopril	3.7, 9.8		4
Carbachol		4.8	1
Carbenicillin	2.7		1
Carbenoxolone	6.7, 7.1		1
Carbinoxamine		8.1	1
Carisoprodol		4.2	4
Carpindolol		8.8	1
Cefaclor	1.5	7.2	8
Cefamandole	2.7		9
Cefazolin	2.1		1
Cefoperazone	2.6		4
Cefotaxime	3.4		4
Cefoxitin	2.2		10
Ceftazidime	1.8, 2.7	4.1	11
Ceftizoxime	2.7	2.1	4
Ceftriaxone	3.2, 4.1	3.2	1
Cefuroxime			4
Cephacetrile			3
Cephalexin[b]	3.2		1
L-Cephaloglycin	4.6	7.1	1
Cephaloridine	3.4		1
Cephalothin	2.5		1
Cephapirin			4
Cephradine			4
Chenodiol	4.3		1,4
Chloral hydrate	10.0		16
Chlorambucil	5.8		4
Chlorcyclizine		2.1, 8.2	1
Chlordiazepoxide		4.8	1
Chlorhexidine		10.8	1
Chlorocresol	9.6		1
Chloroquin		8.1, 9.9	1
8-Chlorotheophylline	8.2		1
Chlorothiazide	6.8, 9.5		1
Chlorpheniramine		9.0	1
Chlorphentermine		9.6	1

Drugs	pK$_a$ Values		Reference
	HA	HB$^+$	
Chlorpromazine		9.3	1
Chlorpropamide	4.9		1
Chlorprothixene		8.8, 7.6	16
Chlortetracycline[c]	3.3, 7.4	9.3	1
Chlorthalidone	9.4	1	
Chlorzoxazone	8.3		1
Cimetidine		6.8	1
Cinchonine		4.3, 8.4	1
Ciprofloxacin	6.0	8.8	1
Clindamycin		7.5	9
Clofibrate	3.5		1
Clonazepam	10.5	1.5	1
Clonidine		8.3	1
Clopenthixol		6.7, 7.6	1
Clotrimazole		4.7	10
Cloxacillin	2.8		1
Clozapine		8.0	1
Cocaine		8.7	1
Codeine		8.2	1
Colchicine		1.9	1
Cromolyn	1.1, 1.9		1
Cyanocobalamin		3.4	9
Cyclacillin	2.7	7.5	4
Cyclazocine		9.4	1
Cyclizine		8.0, 2.5	1
Cyclobarbital	8.6		1
Cyclobenzapine		8.5	1
Cyclopentamine		11.5	1
Cyclopentolate		7.9	1
Cycloserine		4.5, 7.4	1
Cyclothiazide[c]	9.1, 10.5		1
Cyproheptadine		8.9	4
Cytarabine		4.3	1
Dacarbazine		4.4	1
Dantrolene	7.5		1
Dapsone		1.3, 2.5	1
Daunorubicin		8.4	1,4
Debrisoquin		11.9	1
Dehydrocholic acid	5.12		1
Demeclocycline	3.3, 7.2	9.4	1
Demoxepam		4.5, 10.6	1
Deserpidine[d]		6.7	1
Desipramine		10.4	1
Dextroamphetamine		9.9	1
Dextrobrompheniramine		9.3	1
Dextrochlorpheniramine		9.2	1
Dextrofenfluramine		9.1	1
Dextroindoprofen	4.6		1
Dextromethorphan		8.3	1
Dextromoramide		7.0	1
Diacetylmorphine (heroin)		7.8	1
Diatrizoic acid	3.4		1
Diazepam		3.4	1
Diazoxide	8.5		1
Dibenzepin		8.3	8
Dibucaine		8.9	1
Dichlorphenamide	7.4, 8.6		1
Diclofenac	4.5		1
Dicloxacillin	2.8		1
Dicoumarol	4.4, 8.0		1
Dicyclomine		9.0	1
Diethazine		9.1	1
Diethylcarbamazepine		7.7	1
Diflunisal	3.0		1
Dihydroergocriptine		6.9	1

(Continued)

Table A.1. ***Continued***

Drugs	pK$_a$ Values HA	HB$^+$	Reference
Dihydroergocristine		6.9	1
Dihydroergotamine		6.9	1
Dihydrostreptomycin		7.8	1
Dilevolol		9.5	1
Diltiazem		7.7	1
Dimethadione	6.1		1
Dimethisoquin		6.3	1
Dinoprost[e]	4.9		1
Dinoprostone	4.6		1
Diperodon		8.4	11
Diphenhydramine		9.1	1
Diphenoxylate		7.1	1
Diphenylpyraline		8.9	1
Dipipanone		8.5	1
Dipyridamole		6.4	1
Disopyramide	10.2	8.4	1
Dobutamine		9.5	1,4
Dopamine	10.6	8.9	1
Doxepin		9.0	1
Doxorubicin		8.2, 10.2	1
Doxycycline	3.4, 7.7	9.5	1
Doxylamine		4.4, 9.2	1
Droperidol		7.6	1
Emetine		8.2, 7.4	1
Enalapril	3.0	5.5	1
Enalaprilat	2.3, 3.4	8.0	1
Ephedrine		9.6	1
Epinephrine	8.9	10.0	1
Ergometrine		7.3	1
Ergonovine		6.8	1
Ergotamine		6.4	1
Erythromycin		8.8	1
Estrone[f]	10.8		13
Ethacrynic acid	3.50		1
Ethambutol		6.3, 9.5	1
Ethoheptazine		8.5	1
Ethopropazine		9.6	1
Ethosuximide	9.5		1
Ethoxazolamide	8.1		1
Ethyl biscoumacetate	7.5		1
Ethylmorphine		8.2	1
Ethylnorepinephrine		8.4	1
Etidocaine		7.9	1
Etileprine	9.0	10.2	1
Etomidate		4.2	1
Eugenol	9.8		1
Fenclofenac	4.5		1
Fenfluramine		9.1	1
Fenoterol	10.0	8.6	1
Fenprofen	4.5		1
Fentanyl		8.4	14
Floxuridine	7.4		1
Flubiprofen	4.3		1
Flucloxacillin	2.7		1
Flucytosine	10.7	2.9	1
Flufenamic acid	3.9		10
Flumizole	10.7		1
Flunitrazepam		1.8	1
Fluorouracil	8.0, 13.0		1
Flupenthixol		7.8	1
Fluphenazine enanthate		3.5, 8.2	1
Fluphenazine		3.9, 8.1	1
Flupromazine		9.2	1
Flurazepam	8.2	1.9	1

Drugs	pK$_a$ Values HA	HB$^+$	Reference
Furosemide	3.9		1
Fusidic acid	5.4		1
Gentamicin[b]		8.2	1
Glibenclamide	5.3		9
Glipizide	5.9		1
Glutethimide	9.2		1
Glyburide	5.3		1
Glycyclamine		5.5	1
Guanethidine		8.3, 11.9	1
Guanoxan		12.3	1
Haloperidol		8.3	1
Hexetidine		8.3	12
Hexobarbital	8.2		1
Hexylcaine		9.1	1
Hexylresorcinol	9.5		1
Hippuric acid	3.6		1
Histamine		5.9, 9.8	1
Homatropine		9.7	1
Hycanthone		3.4	1
Hydralazine		0.5, 7.1	1
Hydrochlorothiazide	7.0, 9.2		1
Hydrocodone		8.9	1
Hydrocortisone sodium succinate	5.1		1
Hydroflumethiazide	8.9, 10.7		1
Hydromorphone		8.2	1
Hydroquinone	10.0, 12.0		1
Hydroxyamphetamine		9.3	1
Hydroxyzine		2.0, 7.1	1
Hyoscyamine		9.7	1
Ibuprofen	5.2		1
Idoxuridine	8.3		1
Imipramine		9.5	1
Indapamide	8.8		5
Indomethacin	4.5		1
Indoprofen	5.8		1
Indoramin		7.7	1
Iocetamic acid[g]	4.1 or 4.3		4
Iodipamide	3.5		1
Iodoquinol	8.0		1
Iopanoic acid	4.8		4
Iprindole	8.2		1
Ipronidazole		2.7	1
Isocarboxazid		10.4	1
Isoniazid		2.0, 3.5, 10.8	1
Isoproterenol	10.1, 12.1	8.6	1
Isoxsuprine	9.8	8.0	1
Kanamycin		7.2	1
Ketamine		7.5	1,11
Ketobemidone		8.7	1
Ketoconazole		2.9, 6.5	1,4
Ketoprofen[h]	4.8		1,9
Labetalol	8.7	7.4	1
Leucovorin	3.1, 8.1, 10.4		1
Levallorphan tartrate	4.5	6.9	1
Levobunolol		9.2	1
Levodopa	2.3, 9.7, 13.4	8.7	1
Levomethorphan		8.3	1
Levomoramide		7.0	1
Levonordefrin	9.8	8.6	1
Levopropoxyphene		6.3	1
Levorphanol		9.2	1
Levothyroxine	2.2, 6.7	10.1	1
Lidocaine		7.8	1
Lincomycin		7.5	1

(Continued)

Table A.1. ***Continued***

Drugs	pK$_a$ Values HA	HB$^+$	Reference
Liothyronine	8.4		1
Lisinopril	1.7, 3.3, 11.1	7.0	1
Loperamide		8.6	1
Lorazepam	11.5	1.3	1
Loxapine		6.6	1
Lysergide		7.5	1
Maprotiline		10.2	4
Mazindol		8.6	1
Mecamylamine		11.2	1
Mechlorethamine		6.4	1
Meclizine		3.1, 6.2	1
Meclofenamic acid	4.0		4
Medazepam		6.2	1
Mefenamic acid	4.2		1
Mepazine		9.3	1
Meperidine		8.7	1
Mephentermine		10.4	1
Mephobarbital	7.7		1
Mepindolol		8.9	1
Mepivacaine		7.7	1
Mercaptomerin	3.7, 5.1		1
Mercaptopurine	7.8	11.0	1
Mesalamine	2.7	5.8	1
Mesna	9.1		1
Metaproterenol	11.8	8.8	1
Metaraminol		8.6	1
Methacycline	3.5, 7.6	9.5	1
Methadone		8.3	1
Methamphetamine		10.0	1
Methapyrilene		3.7, 8.9	1
Methaqualone		2.5	1
Metharbital	8.2		1
Methazolamide	7.3		1
Methdilazine		7.5	1
Methenamine		4.8	4
Methicillin	3.0		1
Methohexital	8.3		1
Methotrexate	3.8, 4.8	5.6	1
Methotrimeprazine		9.2	1
Methoxamine		9.2	1
Methoxyphenamine		10.1	1
Methyclothiazide	9.4		1
Methyl nicotinate		3.1	1
Methyl paraben	8.4		1
Methyl salicylate	9.9		1
Methyldopa	2.3, 10.4, 12.6	9.2	1
Methylergonovine		6.6	1
Methylphenidate		8.8	1
Methylthiouracil	8.2		1
Methyprylon	12.0		1
Methysergide		6.62	1
Metoclopramide		0.6, 9.3	1
Metolazone	9.7		1
Metopon		8.1	1
Metoprolol		9.7	1
Metronidazole		2.6	4
Metyrosine	2.7, 10.1		1
Mexiletine		9.1	1
Mezlocillin	2.7		1
Miconazole		6.7	1
Midazolam		6.2	1
Minocycline	2.8, 5.0, 7.8	9.5	1
Minoxidil		4.6	4

Drugs	pK$_a$ Values HA	HB$^+$	Reference
Mitomycin		10.9	1
Molindone		6.9	1
Morphine	9.9	8.0	1
Moxalactam	2.5, 7.7, 10.2		4
Nabilone[b]	13.5		9
Nadolol		9.4	5
Nafcillin	2.7		1
Nalbuphine	10.0	8.7	4
Nalidixic acid	6.0		1
Nalorphine		7.8	1
Naloxone		7.9	1
Naphazoline		10.9	1
Naproxen	4.2		1
Natamycin	4.6	8.4	8
Neostigmine		12.0	1
Niacin	2.0	4.8	1
Nicotinamide		0.5, 3.4	1
Nicotine		3.1, 8.0	1
Nikethamide		3.5	1
Nitrazepam	10.8	3.2	1
Nitrofurantoin	7.1		1
Norcodeine		5.7	1
Nordefrin	9.8	8.5	1
Norepinephrine	9.8, 12.0	8.6	1,2
Norfenephrine		8.7	1
Normorphine		9.8	1
Nortriptyline		9.7	1
Noscapine		6.2	1
Novobiocin	4.3, 9.1		1
Nystatin[i]	8.9	5.1	11
Octopamine	9.5	8.9	1
Orphenadrine		8.4	1
Oxacillin	2.7		1
Oxazepam	11.6	1.8	
Oxprenolol		9.5	5
Oxybutynin		7.0	4
Oxycodone		8.9	1
Oxymorphone	9.3	8.5	1
Oxyphenbutazone	4.7		1
Oxypurinol	7.7		1
Oxytetracycline[c]	3.3, 7.3	9.1	1
Pamaquine		1.3, 3.5, 10.0	1
Papaverine		6.4	1
Pargyline		6.9	1
Pemoline		10.5	1,2
Penbutolol[c]		9.3	1
Penicillamine	1.8, 10.5	7.9	1
Penicillin G	2.8		1
Penicillin V	2.7		1
Pentamidine		11.4	4
Pentazocine	10.0	8.5	2,9
Pentobarbital	8.1		1
Pentoxiphylline		0.3	1
Perphenazine		3.7, 7.8	1
Phenacetin		2.2	1
Phenazocine		8.5	1
Phencyclidine		8.5	2
Phendimetrazine		7.6	1
Phenethicillin	2.8		1
Phenformin		2.7, 11.8	1
Phenindamine		8.3	1
Phenindione	4.1		1
Pheniramine		4.2, 9.3	1
Phenmetrazine		8.5	1
Phenobarbital	7.4		1

(Continued)

Table A.1. ***Continued***

Drugs	pK$_a$ Values HA	HB$^+$	Reference
Phenolphthalein	9.7		1
Phenolsulfonphthalein	8.1		1
Phenothiazine		2.5	1
Phenoxybenzamine		4.4	4
Phenoxypropazine		6.9	1
Phentermine		10.1	1
Phentolamine		7.7	1
Phenylbutazone	4.5		1
Phenylephrine	10.1	8.8	1
Phenylpropanolamine		9.4	1
Phenyltoloxamine		9.1	1
Phenyramidol		5.9	1
Phenytoin	8.3		1
Physostigmine		2.0, 8.2	1
Pilocarpine		1.6, 7.1	1
Pimozide		7.3, 8.6	1
Pindolol		8.8	1
Piperazine		5.6, 9.8	1
Pipradrol		9.7	1
Pirbuterol		3.0, 7.0, 10.3	1
Piroxicam	4.6		1
Pivampicillin		7.0	1
Polymyxin		8.9	1
Polythiazide	9.8		1
Practolol		9.5	1
Pralidoxime		7.9	1
Pramoxine		6.2	1
Prazepam		2.9	1
Prazosin		6.5	1
Prenalterol	10.0	9.5	1
Prilocaine		7.9	1
Probenecid	3.4		1
Procainamide		9.2	1
Procaine		8.8	1
Procarbazine		6.8	1
Prochlorperazine		3.7, 8.1	1
Promazine		9.4	1
Promethazine		9.1	1
Proparacaine		3.2	11
Propiomazine		9.1	1
Propoxycaine		8.6	1
Propoxyphene		6.3	1
Propranolol		9.5	1
Propylhexedrine		10.4	1
Propylthiouracil	7.8		1
Pseudoephedrine		9.5	1
Pyrathiazine		8.9	1
Pyrazinamide		0.5	1
Pyridoxine	8.96	5.0	1
Pyrilamine		4.0, 8.9	1
Pyrimethamine		7.3	1
Pyrrobutamine		8.8	1
Quinacrine		8.2, 10.2	1
Quinethazone	9.3, 10.7		1
Quinidine		4.2, 7.9	1
Quinine		4.2, 8.5	1
Ranitidine		2.3, 8.2	4
Rescinnamine		6.4	4
Reserpine		6.6	1
Rifampin	1.7	7.9	1
Rimoterol	10.3	8.7	1
Ritodrine		9.0	1
Rolitetracycline	7.4		1

Drugs	pK$_a$ Values		Reference
	HA	HB$^+$	
Rotoxamine		8.1	1
Saccharin	1.6		1
Salicylamide	8.2		3
Salicylic acid	3.0, 13.4		1
Salsalate	3.5, 9.8		1,2
Scopolamine		7.6	1
Secobarbital	7.9, 12.6		1
Serotonin	9.8	4.9, 9.1	1
Sotalol	8.5	9.8	1
Sparteine		4.8, 12.0	1
Spiperone		8.3, 9.1	1
Streptozocin		1.3	4
Strychnine		2.3, 8.0	1
Succinylsulfathiazole	4.5		1
Sufentanil		8.0	4
Sulfacetamide	5.4	1.8	1
Sulfadiazine	6.5	2.0	1
Sulfadimethoxine	6.7	2.0	1
Sulfaguanidine	12.1	2.8	1
Sulfamerazine	7.1	2.3	1
Sulfamethazine	7.4	2.4	1
Sulfamethizole	5.5	2.0	1
Sulfamethoxazole	5.6		1
Sulfaphenazole	6.5	1.9	1
Sulfapyridine	8.43	2.6	1
Sulfasalazine	2.4, 9.7, 11.8		1
Sulfathiazole	7.1	2.4	1
Sulfinpyrazone	2.8		1
Sulfisoxazole	5.0		1
Sulindac	4.5		1
Sulpiride		9.1	1
Sulthiame	10.0		1
p-Synephrine	10.2	9.3	1
Talbutal	7.8		1
Tamoxifen		8.9	4
Temazepam		1.6	1
Terbutaline	10.1, 11.2	8.8	1
Tetracaine		8.4	1
Tetracycline	3.3, 7.7	9.7	1
Tetrahydrocannabinol (THC)	10.6		2
Tetrahydrozoline		10.5	1
Thenyldiamine		3.9, 8.9	1
Theobromine	10.1	0.1	1
Theophylline	8.6	3.5	1
Thiazbendazole		4.7	4
Thiamine		4.8, 9.0	1
Thiamylal	7.5		1
Thioguanine	8.2		3
Thiopental	7.5		1
Thiopropazate		3.2, 7.2	1
Thioridazine		9.5	1
Thiothixene		7.7, 7.9	1
Thiouracil	7.5		1
Thonzylamine		2.2, 9.0	1
L-Thyroxine	2.2, 6.7	10.1	1
Ticarcillin	2.6, 3.4		1
Ticrynafen	2.7		1
Timolol		8.8	1
Timoprazole		3.1, 8.8	1
Tiotidine		6.8	1
Tiprofenic acid	30.0		1
Tobramycin		6.7, 8.3, 9.9	2
Tocainide		7.5	1
Tolamolol		7.9	5
Tolazamide	3.1	5.7	1

(Continued)

Table A.1. ***Continued***

Drugs	pKa Values HA	HB^+	Reference
Tolazoline		10.3	1
Tolbutamide	5.4		1
Tolmetin	3.5		1
Tramzoline		10.7	1
Tranylcypromine		8.2	1
Trazodone		6.7	1
Triamterene		6.2	1
Trichlormethiazide	8.6		1
Trifluperazine		3.9, 8.1	1,3
Triflupromazine		9.2	1
Trimeprazine		9.0	1
Trimethobenzamide		8.3	1
Trimethoprim		6.6	3
Trimipramine		8.0	4
Tripelennamine		4.2, 8.7	1
Triprolidine		6.5	1
Troleandomycin		6.6	1
Tromethamine		8.1	1
Tropicamide		5.3	1
Tuaminoheptane		10.5	1
Tubocurarine		8.1, 9.1	1
Tyramine	10.9	9.3	1
Valproic acid	4.8		1,3
Verapamil		8.9	1
Vidarabine		3.5, 12.5	1
Viloxazine		8.1	1
Vinbarbital	8.0		1
Vinblastine		5.4, 7.4	1
Vincristine[j]		5.0, 7.4	1
Vindesine		6.0, 7.7	1
Warfarin	5.1		1
Xylometazoline		10.2	1
Zimeldine		3.8, 8.74	1
Miscellaneous organic acids and bases			
Acetic acid	4.8		
Allylamine		10.7	
6-Aminopenicillanic acid	2.3	4.9	
Ammonia		9.3	
Aniline		4.6	
Benzoic acid	4.2		
Benzyl alcohol	18.0		
Benzylamine		9.3	
Butyric acid	4.8		
Carbonic acid	6.4, 10.4		
Citric acid	3.1, 4.8, 5.4		
Diethanolamine		8.9	
Diethylamine		11.0	
Dimethylamine		10.7	
p-Dimethylaminobenzoic acid		5.1	
Ethanol	15.6		
Ethanolamine		9.5	
Ethylamine		10.7	
Ethylenediamine		7.2, 10.0	
Fumaric acid	3.0, 4.4		
Gluconic acid	3.6		
Glucuronic acid	3.2		
Guanidine		13.6	
Imidazole		7.0	
Isopropylamine		10.6	
Lactic acid	3.9		
Maleic acid	1.9		

Drugs	pK$_a$ Values HA	HB$^+$	Reference
Mandelic acid	3.4		
Monochloroacetic acid	2.9		
N-propylamine		10.6	
Nitromethane	11.0		
Phenol	9.9		
Phthalic acid	2.9		
Resorcinol	9.2, 11.3		
Sorbic acid	4.8		
Succinimide	9.6		
Tartaric acid	3.0, 4.4		
p-Toluidine		5.3	
Trichloroacetic acid	0.9		
Triethanolamine		7.8	
Triethylamine		10.7	
Tropic acid	4.1		
Tropine		10.4	
Uric acid	5.4		

[a]Determined in methyl cellosolve/water (8:2 w/w mixture).
[b]Determined in 66% dimethylformamide.
[c]Determined in 25 to 30% ethanol.
[d]Determined in 40% methanol.
[e]Prostaglandin $F_{2\alpha}$.
[f]Spectrophotometric determination.
[g]The pK$_a$ values of the four optical isomers are 4.1 for two isomers and 4.25 for two isomers.
[h]Determined in methanol/water (3:1 mixture).
[i]Determined in dimethylformamide/water (1:1 mixture).
[j]Determined in 33% dimethylformamide.

General References

Albert A, Serjeant EP. The Determination of Ionization Constants of Acids and Bases: A Laboratory Manual. 3rd Ed. New York, Chapman and Hall, 1984.

Florey, K. ed. Analytical Profiles of Drugs Substances. New York: Academic Press, 1978.

Hansch C, Sammes PG, Taylor JB, eds. Comprehensive Medicinal Chemistry, vol 6. Pergamon Press: Oxford, 1990.

O'Neil A, Heckelman PE, Koch C.B, et al. The Merck Index. 14th Ed. Rahway, NJ: Merck and Co, 2006.

Perrin DD, Dempsey B, Serjeant EP. pKa Prediction for Organic Acids and Bases. New York: Chapman and Hall, 1981.

Serjeant EP, Dempsey B. Ionization Constants of Organic Acids in Aqueous Solution. IUPAC Chemical Data Series No. 23. Oxford, UK: Pergamon Press, 1979.

Sinko P. Martin's Physical Pharmacy and Pharmaceutical Sciences. 5th Ed. Baltimore: Lippincott Williams & Wilkins, 2005.

APPENDIX B. *pH Values for Tissue Fluids*

DAVID A. WILLIAMS

Table B.1. pH Values for Tissue Fluids

Fluid	pH
Aqueous humor	7.2
Blood, arterial	7.4
Blood, venous	7.4
Blood, maternal umbilical	7.3
Cerebrospinal fluid	7.4
Colon[a]	
Fasting	5–8
Fed	5–8
Duodenum[a]	
Fasting	4.4–6.6
Fed	5.2–6.2
Feces[b]	7.1 (4.6–8.8)
Ileum[a]	
Fasting	6.8–8.6
Fed	6.8–8.0
Intestine, microsurface	5.3
Lacrimal fluid (tears)	7.4
Milk, breast	7.0
Muscle, skeletal[c]	6.0
Nasal secretions	6.0
Prostatic fluid	6.5
Saliva	6.4
Semen	7.2
Stomach[a]	
Fasting	1.4–2.1
Fed	3–7
Sweat	5.4
Urine	5.8 (5.5–7.0)
Vaginal secretions, premenopause	4.5
Vaginal secretions, postmenopause	7.0

[a]Dressman JB, Amidon GL, Reppas C, et al. Dissolution testing as a prognostic tool for oral drug absorption. Pharm Res 1998;15:11–22.
[b]Value for normal, soft, formed stools. Hard stools tend to be more alkaline, whereas watery, unformed stools are acidic.
[c]Studies conducted intracellularly on the rat.

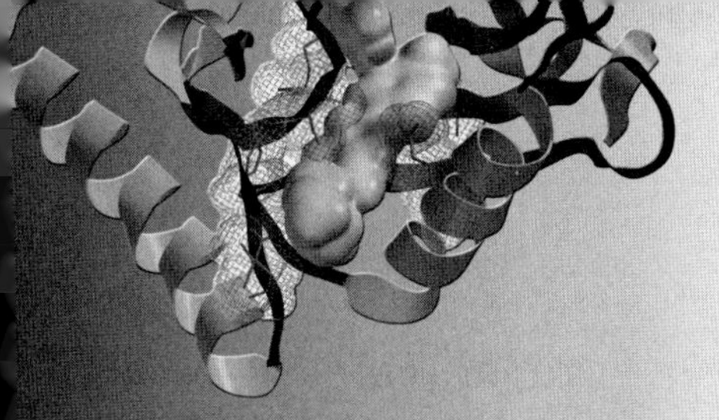

Drug Index

Page numbers followed by "f" indicate illustrations and chemical structures; those followed by "t" indicate to tables. Drugs are listed under the generic name.

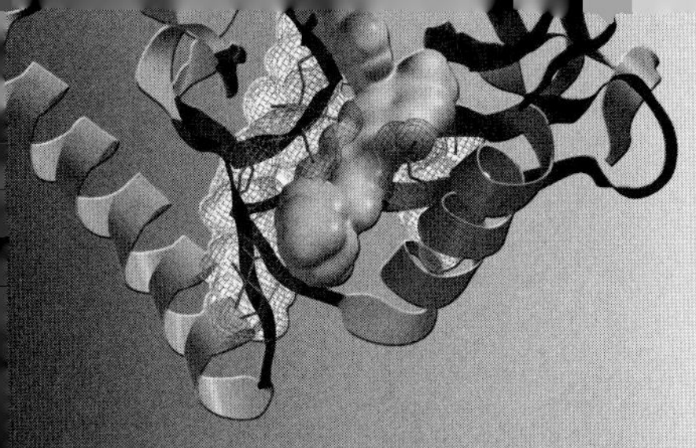

SUBJECT INDEX

Page numbers followed by "f" indicate illustrations and chemical structures; those followed by "t" indicate to tables. Drugs are listed under the generic name.

U

V

W

X

Y

Z